THE
5-MINUTE
VETERINARY
CONSULT
CANINE AND FELINE
THIRD EDITION

THE
5-MINUTE
VETERINARY
CONSULT

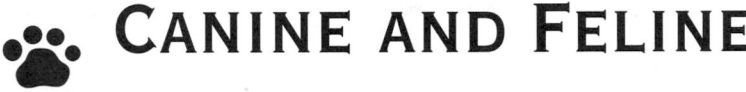

CANINE AND FELINE

THIRD EDITION

Larry Patrick Tilley, DVM
Diplomate, American College of Veterinary
Internal Medicine (Internal Medicine)
President, VetMed Consultants
Chief Medical Officer, Dr. Tilley & Associates
Sante Fe, New Mexico

Francis W. K. Smith, Jr., DVM
Diplomate, American College of Veterinary
Internal Medicine (Internal Medicine & Cardiology)
Vice-President, VetMed Consultants
Lexington, Massachusetts
Clinical Assistant Professor, Department of Medicine
Tufts University, School of Veterinary Medicine
North Grafton, Massachusetts

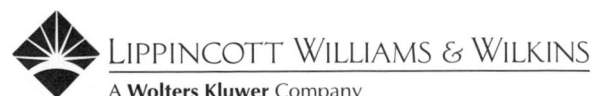

LIPPINCOTT WILLIAMS & WILKINS
A **Wolters Kluwer** Company

Philadelphia · Baltimore · New York · London
Buenos Aires · Hong Kong · Sydney · Tokyo

Executive Editor: David B. Troy
Managing Editor: Matthew J. Hauber
Senior Project Editor: Karen M. Ruppert
Marketing Manager: Samantha S. Smith
Designer: Doug Smock
Compositor: Maryland Composition
Printer: Quebecor

351 West Camden Street
Baltimore, MD 21201

530 Walnut St.
Philadelphia, PA 19106

The publisher is not responsible (as a matter of product liability, negligence, or otherwise) for any injury resulting from any material contained herein. This publication contains information relating to general principles of medical care that should not be construed as specific instructions for individual patients. Manufacturers' product information and package inserts should be reviewed for current information, including contraindications, dosages, and precautions.

Printed in the United States of America

First Edition, 1997
Second Edition, 2000

Library of Congress Cataloging-in-Publication Data

Tilley, Lawrence P.
    The 5-minute veterinary consult: canine feline / Larry Patrick Tilley, Francis W.K. Smith, Jr.—
3rd ed.
      p. cm.
    Includes index.
    ISBN 0-7817-4038-X
    1. Dogs—Diseases—Handbooks, manuals, etc.   2. Cats—Diseases—Handbooks,
manuals, etc.   I. Title: Five minute veterinary consult.   II. Smith, Francis W.K.   III. Title.

SF991 .T55 2003
636.7'0896—dc21   2003054602

The publishers have made every effort to trace the copyright holders for borrowed material. If they have inadvertently overlooked any, they will be pleased to make the necessary arrangements at the first opportunity.

To purchase additional copies of this book, call our customer service department at **(800) 638-3030** or fax orders to **(301) 824-7390**. International customers should call **(301) 714-2324**.

Visit Lippincott Williams & Wilkins on the Internet: http://www.LWW.com. Lippincott Williams & Wilkins customer service representatives are available from 8:30 am to 6:00 pm, EST.

04 05 06 07 08
2 3 4 5 6 7 8 9 10

To my wife, Jeri, and my son, Kyle, in honor of that secret correspondence within our hearts; to family and animals who represent the purity of life.

Larry Patrick Tilley

To my wife, May, my son, Ben, and my daughter, Jade, I cherish our time together and your constant love and support. To my father, Frank, thanks for being my perfect role model.

Francis W.K. Smith Jr.

PREFACE

Keeping abreast of advances in veterinary internal medicine is extremely difficult, especially for the busy general practitioner. To keep current with all the veterinary journals while practicing medicine is impossible. The veterinarian in practice can be overwhelmed by all of the findings and conclusions of thousands of studies conducted by veterinary specialists. *The 5-Minute Veterinary Consult* is designed to provide the busy veterinary practitioner and student of veterinary medicine with concise practical reviews of almost all the diseases and clinical problems in dogs and cats. Our goal in creating this textbook was also to provide up-to-date information in an easy-to-use format. Emphasis is placed on diagnosis and treatment of problems and diseases likely to be seen by veterinarians.

Our fondest dream was realized when the first two editions of this book were chosen as a comprehensive reference source for canine and feline medicine by veterinary students, practicing veterinarians, and board-certified specialists. The format has proven easy to use and very popular with busy practitioners. The scope of the book and the number of consulting editors and authors have been expanded. For the third edition, we have added a behaviorist to our team of consulting editors and greatly expanded the number of behavior topics. We have also increased the number of authors from outside North America, to provide the best advice in the world. The number of topics has been increased, and every topic has been updated to provide you with the most current information possible in a textbook. The Appendix has also been expanded to include more useful tables, and the Drug Formulary has been updated and expanded.

Several good veterinary internal medicine textbooks are available. The uniqueness and value of *The 5-Minute Veterinary Consult* as a quick reference is the consistency of presentation, the breadth of coverage, the contribution of large numbers of experts, and the timely preparation of the manuscript. The format of every topic is identical, making it easy to find information. An extensive list of topic headings ensures complete coverage of each topic.

For the third edition, we have eliminated the division of topics into different sections (i.e., Presenting Problems, Diagnostics—Lab Tests, Diagnostics—ECG, and Diseases), as some topics did not lend themselves to this classification and the system led to confusion when trying to find certain topics. As a result of this change, we changed the names of the laboratory test topics to reflect the clinical syndrome rather than the test name (e.g., Calcium, Hypercalcemia is now Hypercalcemia). Some topic names have also been changed to be consistent with the SNOMED (Systemized Nomenclature of Human and Veterinary Medicine) terminology.

As the title implies, one objective of this book is to make information quickly available. To this end, we have organized topics alphabetically. Most topics can be found without using the index. A table of contents broken out by organ system and a detailed index are provided. Large volumes of useful information are summarized in charts in the Appendix. Also included in the Appendix are an extensive and detailed Drug Formulary, toxicology tables, endocrine testing protocols, normal laboratory values, and conversion tables.

We are delighted and privileged to have had the assistance of numerous experts in veterinary internal medicine from around the world. For the third edition, we expanded the number of consulting editors and contributors. More than 300 veterinary specialists contributed to this text, allowing each chapter to be written by an expert on the subject. In addition to providing outstanding information, this large pool of experts allowed us to publish this major text in a timely manner.

Many large textbooks take several years to write, making some of the information outdated by the time the book is published. We are indebted to the many contributors and consulting editors, whose hard work allowed us to write, edit, and publish this work in 2 years, with most chapters completed within a year of publication. Our goal is to revise the text every 2 years, so that the contents will always be current.

We have also produced CD-ROM and PDA applications to accompany this textbook. These media combine text and graphics in an interactive format. Now veterinarians can quickly access information about necessary clinical skills and new developments in diagnosis and treatment on their computers or PDAs. Our *5-Minute Veterinary Consult* CD-ROM offers fast, affordable access to much of the accumulated wisdom in veterinary medicine by use of a simple search-and-retrieval process. This interactive computer technology brings to the clinic examination room and doctor's office an easy-to-use "dynamic textbook" that will markedly improve the quality of continuing education and clinical practice. The PDA application allows for timely updates to be released between editions of the book.

The third edition of this textbook constitutes an important, up-to-date medical reference source for your practice and clinical education. We strived to make it complete yet practical and easy to use. Our dreams are realized if this text helps you to quickly locate and use the "momentarily important" information that is essential to the practice of high-quality veterinary medicine. We would appreciate your input so that we can make future editions even more useful. If you would like to see any changes in content or format, additions, or deletions, please let us know. Send comments to the following:

Drs. Larry Tilley and Frank Smith
c/o Lippincott Williams & Wilkins
351 West Camden Street
Baltimore, MD 21201

ACKNOWLEDGMENTS

The completion of this textbook provides a welcome opportunity to recognize in writing the many individuals who have helped along the way. The editors gratefully acknowledge the consulting editors and the contributors who, by their expertise, have so unmistakably enhanced the quality of this textbook.

We would also like to acknowledge and thank our families for their support of this project and the sacrifices they made to allow us the time to complete the book.

In addition to thanking veterinarians who have referred patients to us, we would like to express our gratitude to each of the veterinary students, interns, and residents whom we have had the privilege of teaching. Their curiosity and intellectual stimulation have enabled us to grow and have prompted us to undertake the task of writing this book.

Finally, a special thank you goes to Matt Hauber and to all the rest of the staff at Lippincott Williams & Wilkins and everyone in the production and editing departments. The marketing and sales departments also must be acknowledged for generating such an interest in this book. They are all meticulous workers and kind people who have made the final stages of preparing this book both inspiring and fun. An important life goal of ours has been fulfilled: to provide expertise in small animal internal medicine worldwide and to teach the principles contained in this textbook to veterinarians and students everywhere.

CONSULTING EDITORS

LARRY G. ADAMS, DVM, PhD
Diplomate, ACVIM (Internal Medicine)
Purdue University School of
Veterinary Medicine
West Lafayette, Indiana
Subject: Nephrology/Urology

STEPHEN C. BARR, BVSc, MVS, PhD
Diplomate, ACVIM (Internal Medicine)
New York State College of
Veterinary Medicine
Cornell University
Ithaca, New York
Subject: Infectious Disease

SHARON A. CENTER, DVM
Diplomate, ACVIM (Internal Medicine)
New York State College of
Veterinary Medicine
Cornell University
Ithaca, New York
Subject: Hepatology

DEBORAH SUSAN GRECO, DVM, PhD
Diplomate, ACVIM (Internal Medicine)
Animal Medical Center
New York, New York
Subject: Endocrinology & Metabolism

KAREN HELTON RHODES, DVM
Diplomate, ACVD
Dermatology Consultations
Goshen, New York
Subject: Dermatology

DEBRA F. HORWITZ, DVM
Diplomate, ACVB
Adjunct Clinical Assistant Professor
University of Missouri, Veterinary
Medical Teaching Hospital
Veterinary Behavior Consultations
St. Louis, Missouri
Subject: Behavior

ALBERT E. JERGENS, DVM, PhD
Diplomate, ACVIM (Internal Medicine)
College of Veterinary Medicine
Iowa State University
Ames, Iowa
Subject: Gastroenterology

LYNELLE R. JOHNSON, DVM, MS
Diplomate, ACVIM (Internal Medicine)
University of California—Davis
Davis, California
Subject: Respiratory

STEPHEN A. KRUTH
Diplomate, ACVIM (Internal Medicine)
University of Guelph Ontario
Veterinary College
Guelph, Ontario
Subject: Hematology/Immunology

HEIDI B. LOBPRISE, DVM
Diplomate, AVDC
Veterinary Specialty Team
Pfizer Animal Health
McKinney, Texas
Subject: Dentistry

SARA K. LYLE, DVM, MS
Diplomate, ACT
Louisiana State University,
School of Veterinary Medicine
Baton Rouge, Louisiana
Subject: Theriogenology

PAUL E. MILLER, DVM
Diplomate, ACVO
School of Veterinary Medicine
University of Wisconsin—Madison
Madison, Wisconsin
Subject: Ophthalmology

WALLACE B. MORRISON, DVM, MS
Diplomate, ACVIM (Internal Medicine)
Purdue University School of
Veterinary Medicine
West Lafayette, Indiana
Subject: Oncology

CARL A. OSBORNE, DVM, PhD
Diplomate, ACVIM (Internal Medicine)
College of Veterinary Medicine
University of Minnesota
St. Paul, Minnesota
Subject: Nephrology/Urology

GARY D. OSWEILER, DVM, PhD
Diplomate, ABVT
Iowa State University
Ames, Iowa
Subject: Toxicology

MARK PAPICH DVM, MS
Diplomate, ACVCP
College of Veterinary Medicine
North Carolina State University
Raleigh, North Carolina
Subject: Drug Formulary

JOANE M. PARENT, DVM, MVSc
Diplomate, ACVIM (Neurology)
Ontario Veterinary College
University of Guelph
Guelph, Ontario
Subject: Neurology

PETER K. SHIRES, BVSc, MS
Diplomate, ACVS
Virginia-Maryland Regional College of
Veterinary Medicine
Blacksburg, Virginia
Subject: Musculoskeletal

FRANCIS W.K. SMITH, JR., DVM
Diplomate, ACVIM
(Internal Medicine & Cardiology)
VetMed Consultants
Lexington, Massachusetts
Subject: Cardiology

LARRY P. TILLEY, DVM
Diplomate, ACVIM (Internal Medicine)
VetMed Consultants
Sante Fe, New Mexico
Subject: Cardiology

Contributors

JONATHAN A. ABBOTT, DVM
Diplomate, ACVIM (Cardiology)
Associate Professor
Department of Small Animal
Clinical Sciences
Virginia-Maryland Regional College of
Veterinary Medicine Virginia Tech
Blacksburg, Virginia

GEORGE ABRAMS, DVM
Diplomate, ACVO
Ophthalmology
Postdoctoral Fellow
Department of Surgical Sciences
School of Veterinary Medicine
University of Wisconsin-Madison
Madison, Wisconsin

ANTHONY ABRAMS-OGG, DVM, DVSc
Diplomate, ACVIM (Internal Medicine)
Associate Professor
Clinical Studies
Ontario Veterinary College
University of Guelph
Guelph, Ontario
Canada

LARRY G. ADAMS, DVM, PHD
Diplomate, ACVIM (Internal Medicine)
Associate Professor of Small Animal
Internal Medicine
Department of Veterinary
Clinical Sciences
Purdue University
School of Veterinary Medicine
West Lafayette, Indiana

RENEE AL-SARRAF, DVM
Diplomate, ACVIM (Oncology)
Animal Emergency and Referral Center
West Caldwell, New Jersey

JAMES MUDIE GEORGE ANTHONY,
DVM, FAVD
Diplomate, AVDC, EVDC
Pacific Dental Service for Animals
Vancouver, British Columbia, Canada

MAX J. G. APPEL, DVM, PhD
Professor Emeritus
James A. Baker Institute for Animal Health
College of Veterinary Medicine
Cornell University
Ithaca, New York

LOUIS F. ARCHBALD, DVM, PhD
Diplomate, ACT
Professor
Department of Large Animal
Clinical Sciences
College of Veterinary Medicine
University of Florida
Gainesville, Florida

JULIE ARMSTRONG, DVM, MVSC
Diplomate, ACVIM (Internal Medicine)
Staff Veterinarian
Department of Small Animal Medicine
Ontario Veterinary College
University of Guelph
Guelph, Ontario
Canada

RODNEY S. BAGLEY, DVM
Diplomate, ACVIM
(Neurology and Internal Medicine)
Associate Professor
Department of Clinical Sciences
College of Veterinary Medicine
Washington State University
Pullman, Washington

E. MURL BAILEY, DVM, MS, PhD
Diplomate, ABVT
Professor
Department of Veterinary Physiology
and Pharmacology
College of Veterinary Medicine
Texas A & M University
College Station, Texas

MELISSA J. BAIN, DVM
Diplomate, ACVB
Lecturer
Veterinary Medical Teaching Hospital
School of Veterinary Medicine
University of California—Davis
Davis, California

LARRY BAKER, DVM
Fellow, Academy of Veterinary Dentistry
Northgate Veterinary Dentistry
Decatur, Illinois

CHERYL BALKMAN, DVM
Clinical Instructor
Department of Clinical Sciences
Cornell University
Ithaca, New York

STEPHEN C. BARR, BVSC, MVS, PhD
Diplomate ACVIM (Internal Medicine)
Associate Professor of Medicine
Department of Clinical Sciences
New York State College of Veterinary
Medicine Cornell University
Ithaca, New York

MARGARET C. BARR, DVM, PhD
Assistant Member
Vaccine Research Institute of
San Diego
San Diego, California

JOSEPH W. BARTGES, DVM, PhD
Diplomate, ACVIM
(Internal Medicine) and ACVN
Associate Professor of Medicine &
Nutrition, Clinical Internist and Nutritionist
Department of Small Animal
Clinical Sciences
University of Tennessee
Knoxville, Tennessee

BRIAN S. BEALE, DVM
Diplomate, ACVS
Gulf Coast Veterinary Surgery
Houston, Texas

ANDREW W. BEARDOW, BVM&S, MRCVS
Diplomate, ACVIM (Cardiology)
Vice-President, Cardiopet, Inc.
Little Falls, New Jersey

ELLEN N. BEHREND
Diplomate, ACVIM (Internal Medicine)
College of Veterinary Medicine
Auburn University
Auburn, Alabama

JAMIE R. BELLAH, DVM
Diplomate, ACVS
Adjunct Professor, University of Florida
Staff Surgeon
Affiliated Veterinary Specialists—
Orange Park
Orange Park, Florida

JAN BELLOWS, DVM
Diplomate, ABVP
Diplomate, AVDC
Hometown Animal Hospital
Westin, Florida

NICOLE BENNETT, DVM
Small Animal Internal Medicine Resident
Department of Clinical Sciences
College of Veterinary Medicine
Colorado State University
Fort Collins, Colorado

ELLISON BENTLEY, DVM
Diplomate, ACVO
Assistant Professor
Department of Surgical Sciences
School of Veterinary Medicine
University of Wisconsin-Madison
Madison, Wisconsin

MARC G. BERCOVITCH, DVM
Diplomate, ACVIM
(Internal Medicine)
Veterinary Referral Clinic
Cleveland, Ohio

LAURIE BERGMAN, VMD
Resident
Behavior Service
University of California, Davis
School of Veterinary Medicine
Davis, California

CHRISTINE BERTHELIN-BAKER, DVM,
Diplomate ACVIM (Neurology),
Diplomate, ECVN
Clinical Veterinary Neurologist
Neuropathology Unit
Weybridge, Addleston,
United Kingdom

ADAM BIRKENHEUER, DVM
Department of Clinical Sciences
Vector Borne Disease Laboratory
College of Veterinary Medicine
North Carolina State University
Raleigh, North Carolina

BONNIE BLOOM, DVM
Veterinary Dental Resident
Dallas Dental Service Animal Clinic
Dallas, Texas

JOHN D. BONAGURA, DVM, MS
Diplomate ACVIM
(Cardiology, Internal Medicine)
Professor
Department of Veterinary
Clinical Sciences
OSU Veterinary Hospital
Columbus, Ohio

MARIBETH J. BOSSBALY, VMD
Diplomate, ACVIM (Cardiology)
Cardiologist, Heartsound Consultants
Langhorne, Pennsylvania

DWIGHT BOWMAN
Department of Microbiology
College of Veterinary Medicine
Cornell University
Ithaca, New York

RANDI BRANNAN, DVM
Fellow, Academy of Veterinary
Dentistry
Portland, Oregon

JANICE MCINTOSH BRIGHT, BSN, MS, DVM
Diplomate ACVIM
(Cardiology & Internal Medicine)
Associate Professor of Cardiology
Department of Clinical Sciences
Colorado State University
College of Veterinary Medicine and
Biological Sciences
Fort Collins, Colorado

MARJORY BROOKS, DVM
Comparative Coagulation
Section Co-Director
Dept of Population Medicine &
Diagnostic Science
Animal Health Diagnostic Laboratory
Cornell University
Ithaca, New York

SCOTT A. BROWN, VMD, PhD
Diplomate, ACVIM (Internal Medicine)
Professor
Dept of Physiology & Pharmacology
Dept of Small Animal Medicine
College of Veterinary Medicine
Veterinary Medicine Teaching Hospital
University of Georgia
Athens, Georgia

DONALD J. BROWN, BS, MSE, DVM, PhD
Diplomate, ACVIM (Cardiology)
Assistant Professor
Department of Clinical Sciences
School of Veterinary Medicine
Tufts University
North Grafton, Massachusetts

JÖRG BÜCHELER, DVM, PhD, FTA
Diplomate, ACVIM (Internal Medicine)
Diplomate, ECVIM
Veterinary Specialist Consulting
Knoxville, Tennessee

SUSAN E. BUNCH, DVM, PhD
Diplomate, ACVIM (Internal Medicine)
Professor of Medicine
Department of Clinical Sciences
North Carolina State University
College of Veterinary Medicine
Raleigh, North Carolina

COLIN F. BURROWS, BVetMed, PhD, MRCVS
Diplomate, ACVIM (Internal Medicine)
Professor and Chair / Chief of Staff
Department of Small Animal Clinical
Sciences / Veterinary Medical
Teaching Hospital
University of Florida
College of Veterinary Medicine
Gainesville, Florida

NAOMI L. BURTNICK, MT (ASCP)
Owner and Ultrasonographer
New Mexico Veterinary Specialty
Referral Center
Santa Fe, New Mexico

CLAY ARNOLD CALVERT, DVM
Diplomate, ACVIM (Internal Medicine)
Professor
Department of Small Animal Medicine
College of Veterinary Medicine
University of Georgia
Athens, Georgia

KAREN CAMPBELL, DVM, MS
Diplomate, ACVIM
(Internal Medicine) and Diplomate, ACVD
Professor and Section Head,
Specialty Medicine
Department of Veterinary
Clinical Medicine
University of Illinois
College of Veterinary Medicine
Urbana, Illinois

LELAND CARMICHAEL, DVM, PhD
Diplomate, ACVM
John M. Olin Professor of
Virology, Emeritus
Department of Clinical Sciences
College of Veterinary Medicine
Cornell University
Ithaca, New York

LARRY G. CARPENTER, DVM, MS
Diplomate, ACVS
Surgeon
Department of Defense Military
Working Dog Center
Veterinary Services
Lackland Air Force Base
San Antonio, Texas

JANET K. CARRERAS, VMD
Diplomate ACVIM (Oncology)
Oncologist
Gulf Coast Veterinary Oncology
Gulf Coast Veterinary Specialists
Houston, TX

THOMAS L. CARSON, DVM, MS, PhD
Diplomate, ABVT
Veterinary Diagnostic Laboratory
Iowa State University
College of Veterinary Medicine
Ames, Iowa

SHARON A. CENTER, DVM
Diplomate, ACVIM (Internal Medicine)
Professor of Medicine
Department of Veterinary
Cornell University
New York State College of Veterinary
Medicine Clinical Sciences
Ithaca, New York

ERIN S. CHAMPAGNE, DVM
Diplomate, ACVO
Ophthalmologist
Sheridan Animal Hospital
Buffalo, New York

DENNIS J. CHEW, DVM
Diplomate ACVIM (Internal Medicine)
College of Veterinary Medicine
The Ohio State University
Columbus, Ohio

GEORGINA CHILD, BVSc
Diplomate, ACVIM (Neurology)
Veterinary Specialist (Neurology)
Veterinary Specialist Centre
North Ryde, New South Wales,
Australia

MARY M. CHRISTOPHER, DVM, PhD
Diplomate, ACVP (Clinical Pathology)
Department of Pathology,
Microbiology and Immunology
University of California—Davis
School of Veterinary Medicine
Davis, California

RUTHANNE CHUN, DVM
  Diplomate, ACVIM (Oncology)
  Assistant Professor
  Department of Clinical Sciences
  School of Veterinary Medicine /
  Veterinary Medical Teaching Hospital
  Kansas State University
  Manhattan, Kansas

EDWARD G. CLARK
  University of Saskatchewan
  Saskatoon, Saskatchewan
  Canada

SUSAN M. COCHRANE, DVM, DVSC
  Diplomate, ACVIM (Neurology)
  Staff Neurologist
  Veterinary Emergency Clinic/
  Referral Centre
  Toronto, Ontario

ELLEN C. CODNER, BS, DVM, MS
  Diplomate, ACVIM (Internal Medicine)
  Diplomate, ACVD
  Animal Dermatology Specialists
  San Ramon, California

STEPHEN COLES, BVSc (Melbourne),
MACVSc
  Diplomate, AVDC
  Dootor
  Melbourne, Victoria, Australia

CARMEN M.H. COLITZ, DVM, PhD
  Diplomate, ACVO
  Ophthalmology
  Department of Veterinary
  Clinical Sciences
  The Ohio State University
  College of Veterinary Medicine
  Columbus, Ohio

LESLIE L. COOPER
  School of Veterinary Medicine
  University of California–Davis
  Davis, California

ANGELYN CORNETTA, DVM
  Diplomate, ACVIM (Internal Medicine)
  Intern Director
  VCA South Shore Animal Hospital
  South Weymouth, Massachusetts

LARRY D. COWGILL, DVM, PhD
  Diplomate, ACVIM (Internal Medicine)
  Professor, Department of Medicine
  and Epidemiology
  Director, Companion Animal
  Hemodialysis Unit of the
  Veterinary Medical Teaching Hospital
  School of Veterinary Medicine,
  University of California—Davis
  Davis, California

JOHN CRANDALL
  Resident
  College of Veterinary Medicine
  Iowa State University
  Ames, Iowa

MITCHELL A. CRYSTAL, DVM
  Diplomate, ACVIM (Internal Medicine)
  Chief of Medicine
  North Florida Veterinary Specialists, P.A.
  Jacksonville/Orange Park, Florida

PAUL A. CUDDON, BVSc
  Diplomate, ACVIM (Neurology)
  Associate Professor
  Department of Clinical Sciences
  Vet Specialists of N. Colorado
  Loveland, Colorado

ELIZABETH A. CURRY-GALVIN, DVM
  Assistant Director, Scientific Activities
  American Veterinary Medical Association
  Schaumburg, Illinois

GEORGE H. D'ANDREA, BS, DVM, MS
  Diplomate, ACVP
  Diagnostic Specialist
  Department of Pathology/Toxicology
  CSR—Veterinary Diagnostic Laboratory
  Auburn, Alabama

TANIA N. DAVEY, BSC, BVMS, MACVSc
  Associate Clinician
  West Chermside Veterinary Clinic and
  Specialist Referral Service
  Brisbane, Australia

AUTUMN P. DAVIDSON
  Diplomate, ACVIM (Internal Medicine)
  Associate Clinical Professor /
  Director Veterinary Clinic
  University of California—Davis /
  Guide Dogs for the Blind, Inc.
  Davis, California / San Rafael, California

THOMAS KEVIN DAY, DVM, MS
  Diplomate, ACVA
  Diplomate, ACVECC
  Emergency & Critical Care Veterinarian
  Louisville Veterinary Specialty and
  Emergency Services
  Louisville, Kentucky

HELIO S. AUTRAN DE MORAIS, DVM,
MS, PhD
  Diplomate, ACVIM
  (Internal Medicine and Cardiology)
  Department of Medical Sciences
  University of Wisconsin-Madison School
  of Veterinary Medicine
  Madison, Wisconsin

TERESA C. DEFRANCESCO, DVM
  Diplomate, ACVIM (Cardiology)
  Clinical Assistant Professor
  Department of Clinical Sciences
  North Carolina State University
  College of Veterinary Medicine
  Raleigh, North Carolina

SAGI DENENBERG, DVM
  Doncaster, Animal Clinic
  Thornhill, Ontario, Canada

ROBERT C. DENOVO, DVM, MS
  Diplomate, ACVIM (Internal Medicine)
  Associate Professor of Medicine
  Department of Small Animal
  Clinical Science
  College of Veterinary Medicine
  University of Tennessee
  Knoxville, Tennessee

NISHI DHUPA, BVM, MRCVS
  Diplomate, ACVIM (Internal Medicine)
  Diplomate, ACVECC
  Director
  Emergency / Critical Care
  Cornell University Hospital for Animals
  Ithaca, New York

SHARON M. DIAL, DVM, PhD
  Director
  Animal Diagnostic Laboratory
  Tucson, Arizona

STEPHEN DiBARTOLO, DVM
  Diplomate, ACVIM (Internal Medicine)
  Professor Veterinary Clinical Sciences
  College of Veterinary Medicine
  Ohio State University
  Columbus, Ohio

KELLY J. DIEHL, DVM, MS
  Diplomate, ACVIM (Internal Medicine)
  Staff Internist Medicine
  Section Veterinary Referral
  Center of Colorado
  Englewood, Colorado

BRADFORD C. DIXON, DVM, MS
  Diplomate ACVS
  Staff Surgeon Southwest
  Veterinary Surgical Service
  Phoenix, Arizona

SUE DOWNING, DVM
  Diplomate, ACVIM (Oncology)
  Associate Veterinarian
  Department of Oncology
  Veterinary Cancer Referral Group
  Los Angeles, California

DAVID DUCLOS, DVM
  Diplomate, ACVD
  Owner
  Animal Skin and Allergy Clinic
  Lynnwood, Washington

DAVID F. EDWARDS, DVM
  Diplomate, ACVIM (Internal Medicine)
  Diplomate, ACVP (Clinical Pathology)
  Professor
  Department of Pathology
  University of Tennessee
  College of Veterinary Medicine
  Knoxville, Tennessee

ERICK L. EGGER, DVM
  Diplomate ACVS
  Affiliate Faculty, Veterinary
  Orthopedic Consultant
  Clinical Sciences
  Colorado State University
  Fort Collins, Colorado

BRUCE E. EILTS, DVM, MS
  Diplomate, ACT
  Professor of Theriogenology
  Department of Veterinary
  Clinical Sciences
  Louisana State University
  School of Veterinary Medicine
  Baton Rouge, Lousiana

MARC STEPHEN ELIE, DVM
    Diplomate, ACVIM (Internal Medicine)
    Staff Internist
    Department of Internal Medicine
    Michigan Veterinary Specialists
    Southfield, Michigan

ROBYN ELMSLIE, DVM
    Diplomate, ACVIM (Oncology)
    Oncologist
    Veterinary Cancer Specialists
    Englewood, Colorado

RICHARD FAYRER-HOSKEN, BVSc, PhD,
MRCVS
    Diplomate, ACT
    Professor
    Department of Large Animal Medicine
    University of Georgia
    College of Veterinary Medicine
    Athens, Georgia

BRETT M. FEDER, BS, DVM
    Diplomate, ACVIM (Internal Medicine)
    Director South Carolina
    Veterinary Internal Medicine
    Columbia, South Carolina

LINDA S. FINEMAN, DVM
    Diplomate, ACVIM (Oncology)
    Staff Oncologist
    Pacific Veterinary Specialists
    Capitola, California

SCOTT D. FITZGERALD, DVM, PhD
    Diplomate, ACVP
    Associate Professor
    Department of Pathology and
    Diagnostic Investigation
    College of Veterinary Medicine
    Michigan State University
    East Lansing, Michigan

CAROL S. FOIL, DVM, MS
    Diplomate, ACVD
    Professor of Dermatology
    Department of Veterinary
    Clinical Sciences
    Louisiana State University
    School of Veterinary Medicine
    Baton Rouge, Louisiana

S. DRU FORRESTER, DVM, MS
    Diplomate, ACVIM (Internal Medicine)
    College of Veterinary Medicine
    Western University of Health Sciences
    Pomona, California

THERESA W. FOSSUM, DVM, PhD
    Diplomate, ACVS
    Tom & Joan Read Chair, Internal
    Veterinary Surgery / Professor of Surgery
    Department of Small Animal
    Medicine and Surgery
    College of Veterinary Medicine
    Texas A & M University
    College Station, Texas

KIMBERLY PAIGE FREEMAN, DVM
    Gulf Coast Veterinary Oncology
    Gulf Coast Veterinary Specialists
    Houston, TX

JONI L. FRESHMAN, DVM, MS
    Diplomate, ACVIM (Internal Medicine)
    Director
    Canine Consultants
    Colorado Springs, Colorado

TAM GARLAND, DVM, PhD
    Diplomate, ABVT
    Texas A&M University
    College of Veterinary Medicine
    College Station, Texas

LAURA D. GARRETT, DVM
    Diplomate, ACVIM (Oncology)
    Assistant Professor, Oncology
    Department of Clinical Sciences
    Kansas State University
    Manhattan, Kansas

BRIAN C. GILGER, DVM, MS
    Diplomate, ACVO
    Associate Professor
    Department of Clinical Sciences
    North Carolina State University
    College of Veterinary Medicine
    Raleigh, North Carolina

JOHN G. GORDON, DVM
    Diplomate, ACVD
    Private Practice
    MedVet Associates, Inc.
    Columbus, Ohio

CECILIA GORREL, BSc, MA, Vet MB, DDS,
MRCVS
    Diplomate, EVCD, Hon FAVD
    Lecturer / Sole Trader
    Department of Dentistry and Oral Surgery
    VMTH University of California—Davis /
    Cedar Veterinary Group
    Davis, California / Dorset, UK

SHARON FOOSHEE GRACE, MS, DVM
    Diplomate, ACVIM
    (Internal Medicine) & ABVP
    Assistant Clinical Professor
    Department of Small Animal
    Internal Medicine
    Mississippi State University
    Mississippi State, Mississippi

JOANNE C. GRAHAM, DVM, MS
    Diplomate, ACVIM (Oncology)
    Veterinary Oncologist
    Arboretum View Veterinary Specialists
    Downers Grove, Illinois

W. DUNBAR GRAM, DVM
    Diplomate, ACVD
    Animal Allergy and Dermatology
    Virginia Beach, Virginia

GREGORY F. GRAUER, DVM, MS
    Diplomate, ACVIM (Internal Medicine)
    Professor and Head
    Department of Clinical Sciences
    College of Veterinary Medicine
    Kansas State University
    Manhattan, Kansas

THOMAS K. GRAVES, DVM, PhD
    Diplomate, ACVIM (Internal Medicine)
    Assistant Professor of Internal Medicine
    College of Veterinary Medicine
    University of Illinois
    Urbana, Illinois

DEBORAH SUSAN GRECO, DVM, PhD
    Diplomate, ACVIM (Internal Medicine)
    Animal Medical Center
    New York, New York
    Associate Professor

JEAN SWINGLE GREEK, DVM
    Diplomate, ACVD
    Veterinary Specialists
    Overland Park, Kansas

KURT A. GRIMM, DVM, MS
    Visiting Assistant Professor
    Veterinary Clinical Medicine
    University of Illinois
    Urbana, Illinois

AMY M. GROOTERS, DVM
    Diplomate, ACVIM (Internal Medicine)
    Associate Professor and Chief,
    Companion Animal Medicine
    Veterinary Clinical Sciences
    School of Veterinary Medicine
    Louisana State University
    Baton Rouge, Louisiana

SOPHIE ALEXANDRA GRUNDY, BVSc,
MACVSc
    Resident in Internal Medicine
    Veterinary Medical Teaching Hospital
    College of Veterinary Medicine
    University of California—Davis
    Davis, California

NITA KAY GULBAS, DVM
    Owner
    Desert Sage Veterinary Clinic
    Phoenix, Arizona

TIM B. HACKETT, DVM, MS
    Diplomate, ACVECC
    Assistant Professor, Emergency and
    Critical Care Medicine
    Department of Clinical Sciences
    Colorado State University
    College of Veterinary Medicine
    Fort Collins, Colorado

DEBORAH J. HADLOCK, BS, VMD, CVA
    Diplomate, ABVP
    Cardiology Consultant
    Cardiopet, Inc
    Little Falls, New Jersey

KEVIN A. HAHN, DVM, PhD
    Diplomate, ACVIM (Oncology)
    Medical Oncologist
    Gulf Coast Veterinary Oncology
    Gulf Coast Veterinary Specialists
    Houston, Texas

FRASER A. HALE, DVM, FAVD
    Diplomate, AVDC
    Royal City Animal Hospital
    Guelph, Ontario
    Canada

JEFFERY O. HALL, DVM, PhD
Diplomate, ABVT
Assistant Professor, Diagnostic
Veterinary Toxicologist
Utah Veterinary Diagnostic Laboratory
Utah State University
Logan, Utah

BARRON P. HALL, DVM
Veterinary Dental Resident
Dallas Service Animal Clinic
Dallas, Texas

TERRANCE A. HAMILTON, DVM
Diplomate, ACVIM (Oncology)
Veterinary Oncologist
Veterinary Referral Clinic
Cleveland, Ohio

ROBERT L. HAMLIN, DVM, PhD
Diplomate, ACVIM
(Cardiology, Internal Medicine)
Professor
Department of Veterinary Biosciences,
Exercise Physiology and
Biomedical Engineering
The Ohio State University
College of Veterinary Medicine
Columbus, Ohio

SCOTT P. HAMMEL, DVM
Resident in Small Animal Surgery
College of Veterinary Medicine
University of Minnesota
St. Paul, Minnesota

STEVEN R. HANSEN, DVM, MS
Diplomate, ABVT
Senior Vice President / Adjunct Instructor
ASPCA Animal Poison Control Center /
University of Illinois College of
Veterinary Medicine
Urbana, Illinois

ROBERT HARDY, DVM, MS
Diplomate, ACVIM (Internal Medicine)
Professor
Department of Small Animal
Clinical Sciences
College of Veterinary Medicine
University of Minnesota
St. Paul, Minnesota

NEIL K. HARPSTER, VMD
Diplomate, ACVIM (Cardiology)
Department of Cardiology
Angell Memorial Animal Hospital
Boston, Massachusetts

JOHN RICHARD HART, JR., DVM
Diplomate, ACVIM (Internal Medicine)
Staff Internist
Veterinary Specialty Hospital of San Diego
Rancho Santa Fe, California

JOHN W. HARVEY, DVM, PhD
Diplomate, ACVP
Professor and Chair
Department of Physiological Sciences
University of Florida
Gainesville, Florida

ELEANOR C. HAWKINS, DVM
Diplomate, ACVIM (Internal Medicine)
Professor of Internal Medicine
Department of Clinical Sciences
College of Veterinary Medicine
North Carolina State University
Raleigh, North Carolina

KAREN HELTON RHODES, DVM
Diplomate, ACVD
Dermatology Consultations
Goshen, New York

ROSEMARY A. HENIK, DVM, MS
Diplomate, ACVIM (Internal Medicine)
Clinical Associate Professor
Department of Medical Sciences
University of Wisconsin—Madison
Madison, Wisconsin

IAN P. HERRING, DVM, MS
Diplomate, ACVO
Assistant Professor
Department of Small Animal
Clinical Sciences
Virginia-Maryland Regional
College of Veterinary Medicine
Blacksburg, Virginia

KATE E. HILL, BVSc
Small Animal Internal Medicine Resident
Department of Small Animal
Internal Medicine
Purdue University
Veterinary Teaching Hospital
West Lafayette, Indiana

LORA STAHL HITCHCOCK, DVM
Diplomate, ACVIM (Cardiology)
Staff Cardiologist Med Vet
Columbus, Ohio

MARK E. HITT, DVM, MS
Diplomate, ACVIM (Internal Medicine)
Chief of Medicine
Atlantic Veterinary Internal Medicine
Chesapeake Veterinary Referral Center
Annapolis, Maryland

KEITH HNILICA, DVM, MS
Diplomate, ACVD
Assistant Professor of Dermatology
Department of Small Animal
Clinical Sciences
University of Tennessee
Knoxville, Tennessee

WALTER E. HOFFMAN, DVM, PhD
Professor Emeritus Veterinary
Pathobiology and Veterinary Diagnostic
Laboratory University of Illinois
Urbana, Illinois

JUDY HOLDING, RN, BS, DVM
Veterinary Poison Information Specialist
ASPCA—Animal Poison Control Center
Urbana, Illinois

STEVEN B. HOOSER, DVM, PhD
Diplomate, ABVT
Associate Professor
Head, Toxicology Section
Veterinary Pathobiology / Animal Disease
Diagnostic Laboratory
Purdue University
West Lafayette, Indiana

KATE HOPPER BVSC
Diplomate, ACVECC
Resident
Veterinary Surgical and Radiological
Sciences
University of California—Davis
Davis, California

DEBRA F. HORWITZ, DVM
Diplomate, ACVB
Adjunct Clinical Assistant Professor
University of Missouri,
Veterinary Medical Teaching Hospital
Veterinary Behavior Consultations
St. Louis, Missouri

JOHNNY D. HOSKINS, DVM, PhD
Diplomate, ACVIM (Internal Medicine)
Small Animal Consultant
Docutech Services, Inc
Baton Rouge, Louisiana

KATHERINE ALBRO HOUPT, VMD, PhD
Diplomate, ACVB
Animal Behavior Clinic
College of Veterinary Medicine
Cornell University
Ithaca, New York

WAYNE HUNTHAUSEN, DVM
Director
Animal Behavior Consultations
Westwood Animal Hospital
Westwood, Kansas

KAREN DYER INZANA, DVM, PhD
Diplomate, ACVIM (Neurology)
Associate Professor
Department of Small Animal
Clinical Science
Virginia-Maryland Regional College of
Veterinary Medicine Virginia Tech
Blacksburg, Virginia

FRÉDÉRIC JACOB, DVM
Diplomate ACVIM (Internal Medicine)
Department of Small Animal
Clinical Sciences
University of Minnesota
College of Veterinary Medicine
St. Paul, Minnesota

JULIE ANN JARVINEN, DVM, PhD
Associate Professor
Department of Veterinary Pathology
College of Veterinary Medicine—
Iowa State University
Ames, Iowa

CHRISTINE CAROLYN JENKINS, DVM
Diplomate, ACVIM (Internal Medicine)
Technical Services Veterinarian, CAD
Technical Services—Pfizer Adjunct
Associate Professor of Veterinary
Medicine, Department of Small Animal
Clinical Sciences, University of
Tennessee
Companion Animal Division
Pfizer Animal Health
Exton, Pennsylvania

ALBERT E. JERGENS, DVM, PhD
Diplomate, ACVIM (Internal Medicine)
Associate Professor and Staff Internist
Department of Veterinary
Clinical Sciences
College of Veterinary Medicine
Iowa State University
Ames, Iowa

KENNETH A. JOHNSON MVSc, PhD,
FACVSc.
Diplomate, ACVS
Diplomate, ECVS
Professor of Orthopaedics
Department of Veterinary
Clinical Science
The Ohio State University
Columbus, Ohio

LYNELLE R. JOHNSON, DVM, MS
Diplomate, ACVIM (Internal Medicine)
Assistant Professor
Dept of Veterinary Medicine and
Epidemiology
University of California—Davis
Davis, California

SUSAN E. JOHNSON, DVM, MS
Diplomate, ACVIM (Internal Medicine)
Associate Professor
Department of Veterinary
Clinical Sciences
The Ohio State University
Columbus, Ohio

SPENCER A. JOHNSTON, VMD
Diplomate, ACVS
Professor, Small Animal Surgery
Department of Small Animal
Clinical Sciences
Virginia-Maryland Regional
College of Veterinary Medicine
Blacksburg, Virginia

SHIRLEY D. JOHNSTON, DVM, PhD
Diplomate, ACT
Professor and Dean,
College of Veterinary Medicine
Western University of Health Sciences
Pomona, California

RICHARD J. JOSEPH, DVM
Diplomate, ACVIM (Neurology)
Neurologist
Country Animal Specialty Group
Yonkers, New York

BRUCE W. KEENE, DVM, MS
Diplomate, ACVIM (Cardiology)
Associate Professor of Cardiology
College of Veterinary Medicine
North Carolina State University
Raleigh, North Carolina

ROBERT J. KEMPPAINEN, DVM, PhD
Professor
Department of Anatomy,
Physiology and Pharmacology
Auburn University
College of Veterinary Medicine
Auburn, Alabama

MARGARET R. KERN, DVM
Diplomate, ACVIM (Internal Medicine)
Associate Professor
Department of Clinical Sciences
College of Veterinary Medicine
Mississippi State University
Mississippi State, Mississippi

RICHARD D. KIENLE, DVM
Diplomate, ACVIM (Cardiology)
Owner
Mission Valley Veterinary Cardiology
Gilroy, California

LESLEY G. KING MVB, MRCVS
Diplomate, ACVIM (Internal Medicine)
Diplomate, ACVECC
Associate Professor of Critical Care
Department of Clinical Studies
School of Veterinary Medicine
University of Pennsylvania
Philadelphia, Pennsylvania

PETER KINTZER, DVM
Diplomate, ACVIM (Internal Medicine)
Clinical Assistant Professor /
Staff Internist
Department of Medicine
Tufts University School of Veterinary
Medicine / Boston Road Animal Hospital
North Grafton, Massachusetts /
Springfield, Massachusetts

REBECCA KIRBY, DVM
Diplomate, ACVIM (Internal Medicine)
Diplomate, ACVECC
Director of Education
Animal Emergency Center
Glendale, Wisconsin

MARK D. KITTLESON, DVM, PhD
Diplomate, ACVIM (Cardiology)
Professor
Dept of Medicine and Epidemiology
University of California—Davis
Davis, California

JEFFREY S. KLAUSNER, DVM, MS
Diplomate, ACVIM
(Internal Medicine, Oncology)
Dean
College of Veterinary Medicine
University of Minnesota
St. Paul, Minnesota

THOMAS KLEIN, DVM
Adjunct Professor of Dentistry
The Ohio State University
College of Veterinary Dentistry
Owner
East Hilliard Veterinary Services
Hilliard, Ohio

JOYCE S. KNOLL, VMD, PhD
Diplomate, ACVP
Associate Professor
Department of Biomedical Sciences
Tufts University School of
Veterinary Medicine
North Grafton, Massachusetts

GARY J. KOCIBA, DVM, PhD
Diplomate, ACVP
Professor
Department of Veterinary Biosciences
College of Veterinary Medicine
The Ohio State University
Columbus, Ohio

TRACY L. KROLL, DVM
Veterinary Consultant in Behavior
Fair Lawn, New Jersey

JOHN M. KRUGER, DVM, PhD
Diplomate, ACVIM (Internal Medicine)
Associate Professor
Small Animal Clinical Sciences
Michigan State University
East Lansing, Michigan

NED F. KUEHN, DVM, MS
Diplomate, ACVIM (Internal Medicine)
Chief of Internal Medicine Services
Michigan Veterinary Specialists
Southfield, Michigan

KAREN ANN KUHL, DVM
Diplomate, ACVD
Dermatologist
Veterinary Specialty Clinic
Midwest Veterinary Dermatology Center
Buffalo Grove, Illinois

MARY ANNA LABATO, DVM
Diplomate, ACVIM (Internal Medicine)
Clinical Associate Professor /
Staff Veterinarian
Department of Clinical Sciences
Tufts University
School of Veterinary Medicine /
Foster Hospital for Small Animals
North Grafton, Massachusetts

MICHAEL STEVEN LAGUTCHIK, DVM, MS
Chief, Animal Medicine Branch
Department of Veterinary Science
US Army Medical Department
Center and School
Fort Sam Houston, Texas

LEIGH A. LAMONT
Atlantic Veterinary College
University of Prince Edward Island
Charlottetown, Prince Edward Island
Canada

GARY LANDSBERG, DVM
Doncaster Animal Clinic
Thornhill, Ontario
Canada

INDIA F. LANE, DVM, MS
Diplomate, ACVIM (Internal Medicine)
Assistant Professor and Internist
Department of Small Animal
Clinical Sciences
The University of Tennessee
Knoxville, Tennessee

OTTO I. LANZ, DVM
Diplomate ACVS
Assistant Professor
Department of Small Animal
Clinical Sciences
Virginia-Maryland Regional College
of Veterinary Medicine
Blacksburg, Virginia

ROLF E. LARSEN, DVM, PhD
Diplomate, ACT
Associate Professor
Department of Large Animal
Clinical Sciences
College of Veterinary Medicine
University of Florida
Gainesville, Florida

KENNETH S. LATIMER, DVM, PhD
Diplomate, ACVP (Clinical Pathology)
Professor
Veterinary Pathology
College of Veterinary Medicine
The University of Georgia
Athens, Georgia

SUSANNE LAUER, Dr. Med. Vet.
Surgery Resident
Department of Veterinary
Clinical Sciences
College of Veterinary Medicine
Iowa State University
Ames, Iowa

DENNIS F. LAWLER, DVM
Veterinary Scientist
Dept. of Research and Development
Nestle Purina Co. / Animal Hospital
of O'Fallon
St. Louis, Missouri / O'Fallon, Illinois

SUZETTE M. LECLERC, DVM, MVSc
Diplomate, ACVP
Clinical Associate
Prairie Diagnostic Services
Saskatoon, Saskatchewan, Canada

GEORGE E. LEES, DVM, MS
Diplomate, ACVIM (Internal Medicine)
Professor
Small Animal Medicine and Surgery
College of Veterinary Medicine
Texas A&M University
College Station, Texas

ALFRED M. LEGENDRE, DVM, MS
Diplomate, ACVIM (Internal Medicine)
Professor of Medicine
Department of Small Animal
Clinical Sciences
University of Tennessee
Knoxville, Tennessee

MICHAEL B. LESSER, DVM
Diplomate, ACVIM (Cardiology)
Hospital Director
Advanced Veterinary Care Center
Laundale, California

STEVEN A. LEVY, VMD
Hospital Director, Veterinarian
Durham Veterinary Hospital, PC
Durham, Connecticut

DAVID C. LEWIS, BVSc, PhD
Diplomate, ACVIM (Internal Medicine)
Antech Diagnostics
Portland, Oregon

ELLEN M. LINDELL, VMD
Diplomate, ACVB
Pleasant Valley, New York

DAVID LIPSITZ, DVM
Diplomate, ACVIM (Neurology)
Assistant Professor
Department of Veterinary Surgical
and Radiological Sciences
Carlsbad, California

SUSAN E. LITTLE, DVM, PhD
Associate Professor
Department of Medical
Microbiology and Parasitology
University of Georgia College of
Veterinary Medicine
Athens, Georgia

HEIDI B. LOBPRISE, DVM
Diplomate, AVDC
Veterinary Specialty Team
Pfizer Animal Health
McKinney, Texas

DAWN LOGAS, DVM
Diplomate, ACVD
Dermatologist
Veterinary of Dermatology Center
Maitland, Florida

RANDALL CARL LONGSHORE, DVM
Diplomate, ACVIM (Neurology)
Neurologist/Neurosurgeon
Veterinary Neurological Center
Phoenix, Arizona

CARROLL LOYER, DVM
Diplomate, ACVIM
(Cardiology)
Boulder, Colorado

VIRGINIA LUIS FUENTES, MA, VetMB, PhD,
DVC
Diplomate, ACVIM (Cardiology)
Clinical Assistant Professor
Department of Veterinary
Clinical Sciences
The Ohio State University
Columbus, Ohio

JODY P. LULICH, DVM, PhD
Diplomate, ACVIM (Internal Medicine)
Department of Small Animal
Clinical Sciences
College of Veterinary Medicine
University of Minnesota
St. Paul, Minnesota

JOHN E. LUND, DVM, PhD
Diplomate, ACVP
Senior Research Advisor in
Pathology Global Toxicology
Pharmacia Corporation
Kalamazoo, Michigan

PATRICIA J. LUTTGEN, DVM, MS
Diplomate, ACVIM (Neurology)
Neurologist
Neurological Center for Animals
Lakewood, Colorado

SARA K. LYLE, DVM, MS
Diplomate, ACT
Farm Animal Health &
Resource Management
Louisiana State University,
School of Veterinary Medicine
Baton Rouge, Louisiana

PETER S. MACWILLIAMS, DVM, PhD
Diplomate, ACVP
Professor of Clinical Pathology /
Chief of Staff
Pathobiological Sciences /
Veterinary Medical Teaching
Hospital University of
Wisconsin—Madison
Madison, Wisconsin

JILL MADDISON, BVSc, PhD, FACVSc,
MRCVS
The Royal Veterinary College
London, United Kingdom

ORLA M. MAHONY MVB
Diplomate, ACVIM
(Internal Medicine) and ECVIM
Clinical Assistant Professor
Department of Clinical Sciences
Tufts University School of
Veterinary Medicine
North Grafton, Massachusetts

STEVEN L. MARKS, BVSc., MS, MRCVS
Diplomate, ACVIM (Internal Medicine)
Department of Veterinary
Clinical Medicine
University of Illinois Urbana, Illinois

KENNETH V. MASON, BVSc, MVSc, FACVSc
Animal Allergy and Dermatology Service
Albert Animal Hospital
Springwood, Australia

CHRISTIANE MASSICOTTE, DVM, PhD
Diplomate, ACVIM (Neurology)
Assistant Professor of Neurology
Department of Clinical Studies—
Neurology
University of Pennsylvania
School of Veterinary Medicine
Philadelphia, Pennsylvania

ELISA M. MAZZAFERRO, MS, DVM, PhD
Diplomate, ACVECC
Director of Emergency Services
Wheat Ridge Animal Hospital
Wheat Ridge, Colorado

TERRI LORRAINE MCCALLA, DVM
  Diplomate, ACVO
  Animal Eye Care, LLC
  Bellingham, Washington

PATRICK L. MCDONOUGH, MS, PHD
  Assistant Professor of Microbiology
  Assistant Director of Bacteriology—
  Mycology
  Department of Population Medicine and
  Diagnostic Sciences
  Diagnostic Laboratory
  College of Veterinary Medicine
  Cornell University
  Ithaca, New York

BRENDAN C. MCKIERNAN, DVM
  Diplomate, ACVIM (Internal Medicine)
  Staff Internist
  Denver Veterinary Specialists
  Wheat Ridge, Colorado

RON MCLAUGHLIN, DVM, DVSc
  Diplomate, ACVS
  Associate Professor and Chief,
  Small Animal Surgery
  Department of Clinical Sciences
  College of Veterinary Medicine
  Mississippi State University
  Mississippi State, Mississippi

LINDA MEDLEAU, DVM, MS
  Diplomate, ACVD
  Professor of Veterinary Dermatology /
  Chief, Dermatology Service
  Department of Small Animal Medicine
  University of Georgia / UG Veterinary
  Medicine Teaching Hospital
  Athens, Georgia

KATHRYN M. MEURS, DVM, PHD
  Diplomate, ACVIM (Cardiology)
  Associate Professor Veterinary
  Clinical Sciences
  The Ohio State University
  College of Veterinary Medicine
  Columbus, Ohio

VICKI MEYERS-WALLEN, VMD, PhD
  Diplomate, ACT
  Cornell University
  College of Veterinary Medicine
  Ithaca, New York

CARRIE J. MILLER, DVM
  Diplomate, ACVIM (Internal Medicine)
  Wheat Ridge Animal Hospital
  Denver Veterinary Specialists
  Wheat Ridge, Colorado

MATTHEW W. MILLER, DVM, MS
  Diplomate, ACVIM (Cardiology)
  Associate Professor / Staff Cardiologist
  Small Animal Medicine & Surgery /
  Cardiovascular Sciences Section
  Texas A & M University /
  Texas Veterinary Medical Center
  College Station, Texas

PAUL E. MILLER, DVM
  Diplomate, ACVO
  Clinical Associate Professor of
  Ophthalmology
  Department of Surgical Sciences
  School of Veterinary Medicine
  University of Wisconsin—Madison
  Madison, Wisconsin

LISA E. MOORE, DVM
  Diplomate, ACVIM (Internal Medicine)
  Assistant Professor
  Veterinary Medical Teaching Hospital
  Kansas State University
  Manhattan, Kansas

DANIEL O. MORRIS, DVM
  Diplomate, ACVD
  Assistant Professor of Dermatology
  Department of Clinical Studies
  University of Pennsylvania
  Philadelphia, Pennsylvania

JOANN MORRISON, DVM
  Diplomate, ACVIM
  Affiliated Veterinary Specialists, PA
  Resident
  Maitland, Florida

WALLACE B. MORRISON, DVM, MS
  Diplomate, ACVIM (Internal Medicine)
  Professor
  Department of Veterinary
  Clinical Sciences
  Purdue University
  School of Veterinary Medicine
  West Lafayette, Indiana

BRADLEY L. MOSES, DVM
  Diplomate, ACVIM (Cardiology)
  Clinical Assistant Professor
  Department of Clinical Sciences
  Tufts University School of Veterinary
  Medicine
  North Grafton, Massachusetts
  Roberts Animal Hospital
  Hanover, Massachusetts

JOCELYN MOTT, DVM
  Diplomate, ACVIM (Internal Medicine)
  Veterinary Internist
  Affiliated Veterinary Specialists
  Maitland, Florida

KAREN R. MUÑANA, DVM, MS
  Diplomate, ACVIM (Neurology)
  Associate Professor
  Department of Clinical Sciences
  College of Veterinary Medicine
  North Carolina State University
  Raleigh, North Carolina

MICHAEL J. MURPHY, DVM, PhD
  Diplomate, ABVT
  Toxicologist
  Veterinary Diagnostic Laboratory
  College of Veterinary Medicine
  University of Minnesota
  St. Paul, Minnesota

K. MARCIA MURPHY, DVM
  College of Veterinary Medicine
  Veterinary Teaching Hospital
  North Carolina State University
  Raleigh, North Carolina

ANTHONY J. MUTSAERS, DVM
  Diplomate, ACVIM (Oncology)
  Consultant, Medical Oncology
  Animal Cancer Care, P/L
  Veterinary Teaching Hospital
  University of Queensland
  Brisbane, Queensland, Australia

KRISTINA NARFSTRÖM, DVM, PhD
  Diplomate, ECVO
  Professor of Veterinary Ophthalmology
  Department of Medicine and Surgery
  College of Veterinary Medicine
  University of Missouri-Columbia
  Columbia, Missouri

MARK P. NASISSE, DVM
  Diplomate, ACVO
  Staff Ophthalmologist
  Carolina Veterinary Specialists
  Greensboro, North Carolina

T. MARK NEER, DVM
  Diplomate, ACVIM (Internal Medicine)
  Professor of Medicine
  Department of Veterinary
  Clinical Sciences
  Louisiana State University
  Veterinary Teaching Hospital & College
  Baton Rouge, Louisiana

REGG D. NEIGER, DVM, PhD
  Professor
  Department of Veterinary Science
  South Dakota State University
  Brookings, South Dakota

RHETT C.E. NICHOLS, DVM
  Diplomate, ACVIM (Internal Medicine)
  Regional Director of Consulting Services
  Antech Diagnostics
  Farmingdale, New York

GARY D. NORSWORTHY, DVM
  Diplomate, ABVP (Feline)
  Owner
  Alamo Feline Health Center
  San Antonio, Texas

FREDERICK W. OEHME, DVM, PhD
  Diplomate, ABVT, ABT, ATS
  Professor & Director / Clinical
  Toxicologist Comparative Toxicology
  & Veterinary Diagnostic Laboratories /
  Dept of Diagnostic Medicine /
  Pathobiology
  College of Veterinary Medicine
  Kansas State University
  Manhattan, Kansas

NATASHA J. OLBY, VetMB, PhD
  Diplomate, ACVIM (Neurology)
  Assistant Professor of Neurology
  Department of Clinical Sciences
  North Carolina State University
  Raleigh, North Carolina

CARL A. OSBORNE, DVM, PhD
  Diplomate, ACVIM (Internal Medicine)
  Professor
  Department of Small Animal
  Clinical Sciences
  College of Veterinary Medicine
  University of Minnesota
  St. Paul, Minnesota

GARY D. OSWEILER, DVM, PhD
    Diplomate, ABVT
    Professor / Director
    Veterinary Diagnostic &
    Production Animal Medicine /
    Veterinary Diagnostic Laboratory
    Iowa State University
    Ames, Iowa

KAREN L. OVERALL, MA, VMC, PhD
    Diplomate, ACVB
    ABS Certified Applied Animal Behaviorist
    Glen Mills, Pennsylvania

DALE PACCAMONTI, DVM, MS
    Diplomate, ACT
    Professor
    Department of Veterinary
    Clinical Sciences
    School of Veterinary Medicine
    Louisiana State University
    Baton Rouge, Louisiana

MARK PAPICH, DVM, MS
    Diplomate, ACVCP
    College of Veterinary Medicine
    North Carolina State University
    Raleigh, North Carolina

JOANE M. PARENT, DVM, MVSc
    Diplomate, ACVIM (Neurology)
    Professor
    Department of Veterinary Clinical Studies
    Ontario Veterinary College
    University of Guelph
    Guelph, Ontario, Canada

ALLAN J. PAUL, DVM, MS
    Professor
    Department of Veterinary Pathobiology
    College of Veterinary Medicine
    University of Illinois
    Urbana, Illinois

MICHAEL PEAK, DVM
    Diplomate, AVDC
    Tampa Bay Veterinary Dentistry, Inc.
    Largo, Florida

MICHAEL E. PETERSON, DVM, MS
    Staff Veterinarian & Toxicologist
    Reid Veterinary Hospital
    Albany, Oregon

J. PHILLIP PICKETT, DVM
    Diplomate, ACVO
    Associate Professor—Ophthalmology
    Department of Small Animal
    Clinical Sciences
    Virginia-Maryland Regional
    College of Veterinary Medicine
    Blacksburg, Virginia

CARLOS ROBERTO FONTES PINTO,
MedVet, PhD
    Diplomate, ACT
    Department of Veterinary
    Clinical Sciences
    Louisiana State University
    Baton Rouge, Louisiana

JON D. PLANT, DVM
    Diplomate, ACVD
    President
    Animal Dermatology Specialty Clinic
    Marina del Ray, California

KONSTANZE H. PLUMLEE, DVM, MS
    Diplomate, ABVT, ACVIM
    (Internal Medicine)
    Veterinary Toxicologist
    Veterinary Diagnostic Lab
    Arkansas Livestock & Poultry Commission
    Little Rock, Arkansas

DAVID J. POLZIN, DVM, PhD
    Diplomate, ACVIM (Internal Medicine)
    Professor Department of
    Small Animal Clinical Sciences
    College of Veterinary Medicine
    University of Minnesota
    St. Paul, Minnesota

ERIC R. POPE, DVM, MS
    Diplomate, ACVS
    Veterinary Teaching Hospital
    University of Missouri
    Columbia, Missouri

ROBERT H. POPPENGA, DVM, PhD
    Diplomate, ABVT
    Associate Professor of Veterinary
    Toxicology
    Director, Toxicology Laboratory
    at New Bolton Center
    University of Pennsylvania
    Kennett Square, Pennsylvania

KLAAS POST, DVM, M.Vet. Sc.
    Professor and Head
    Department of Small Animal
    Clinical Sciences
    Western College of Veterinary Medicine
    Saskatoon, Saskatchewan, Canada

MICHELLE PRESSEL
    Resident
    College of Veterinary Medicine
    Iowa State University
    Ames, Iowa

JAMES C. PRUETER, DVM
    Diplomate, ACVIM (Internal Medicine)
    Veterinary Consultant
    Prueter & Associates
    Grafton, Ohio

DAVID A. PUERTO, DVM
    Diplomate, ACVS
    Lecturer
    University of Pennsylvania
    Philadelphia, Pennsylvania

BEVERLY J. PURSWELL, DVM, PhD
    Diplomate, ACT
    Professor
    Large Animal Clinical Sciences
    Virginia-Maryland Regional College
    of Veterinary Medicine
    Blacksburg, Virginia

ANDREE D. QUESNEL DMV, DVSc
    Diplomate, ACVIM (Neurology)
    Associate Professor
    Departement des Sciences Cliniques
    Faculte de Medecine Veterinaire
    Universite de Montreal
    St. Hyacinthe, Quebec, Canada

MERL F. RAISBECK, DVM, PHD
    Department of Veterinary Sciences
    University of Wyoming
    Laramie, Wyoming

KENNETH M. RASSNICK, DVM
    Diplomate, ACVIM (Oncology)
    Assistant Professor
    Department of Oncology
    Cornell University
    College of Veterinary Medicine
    Ithaca, New York

CLARENCE A. RAWLINGS, DVM, PhD
    Diplomate, ACVS
    Professor and Head
    Department of Small Animal Medicine
    University of Georgia
    College of Veterinary Medicine
    Athens, Georgia

ALAN H. REBAR, PhD
    Diplomate, ACVP
    Dean
    School of Veterinary Medicine
    Purdue University
    West Lafayette, Indiana

MARSHA R. REICH, DVM
    Diplomate, ACVB
    Veterinary Behaviorist
    Maryland-Virginia
    Veterinary Behavioral Consulting
    Silver Spring, Maryland

KEITH P. RICHTER, DVM
    Diplomate, ACVIM (Internal Medicine)
    Internal Medicine Staff
    Veterinary Specialty Hospital of
    San Diego
    Rancho Santa Fe, California

MARK RISHNIW, BVSc, MS
    Diplomate, ACVIM (Internal Medicine)
    Department of Biomedical Sciences
    Cornell University
    Ithaca, New York

MARGARET V. ROOT-KUSTRITZ, DVM, PhD
    Diplomate, ACT
    Assistant Clinical Specialist
    Small Animal Reproduction
    Department of Small Animal
    Clinical Sciences
    College of Veterinary Medicine
    University of Minnesota
    St. Paul, Minnesota

WAYNE STEWART ROSENKRANTZ, DVM
    Diplomate, ACVD
    Owner-Partner
    Animal Dermatology Clinic
    Tustin/San Diego, California

SHERI J. ROSS
Resident in Clinical Nutrition
and Internal Medicine
Department of Small Animal
Clinical Sciences
College of Veterinary Medicine
University of Minnesota
St. Paul, Minnesota

PHILIP ROUDEBUSH, DVM
Diplomate, ACVIM (Internal Medicine)
Veterinary Fellow Hill's
Science and Technology Center
Topeka, Kansas

ELIZABETH A. ROZANSKI, DVM
Diplomate, ACVECC and ACVIM
(Internal Medicine)
Assistant Professor
Department of Clinical Sciences
Tufts University School of
Veterinary Medicine
North Grafton, Massachusetts

WILSON K. RUMBEIHA, DVM, PhD
Diplomate, ABVT
Assistant Professor
Department of Pathobiology and
Diagnostic Investigations
Michigan State University

JOHN E. RUSH, DVM, MS
Diplomate, ACVIM (Cardiology)
Diplomate, ACVECC
Professor Clinical Sciences
Tufts University School of
Veterinary Medicine
North Grafton, Massachusetts

H. CAROLIEN RUTGERS, DVM
Diplomate, ACVIM (Internal Medicine)
Private Consultant
Brookmans Park, Herts
United Kingdom

CARL D. SAMMARCO, BVSc, MRCVS
Diplomate, ACVIM (Cardiology)
Red Bank Veterinary Hospital
Colts Neck, New Jersey

SHERRY L. SANDERSON, DVM, PhD
Diplomate, ACVIM (Internal Medicine)
Assistant Professor
Department of Small Animal Medicine
University of Georgia
College of Veterinary Medicine
Athens, Georgia

THOMAS SCHERMERHORN
Diplomate, ACVIM (Internal Medicine)
Assistant Professor
Department of Clinical Sciences
Kansas State University
Manhattan, Kansas

CATHRYN CALIA SCHROPE, DVM
Diplomate, ACVIM (Internal Medicine)
Staff Internist
Department of Internal Medicine
Veterinary Referral Center
Little Falls, New Jersey

DONALD PAUL SCHROPE, DVM
Diplomate, ACVIM (Cardiology)
Staff Cardiologist
Cardiology
Oradell Animal Hospital
Oradell, New Jersey

PETER D. SCHWARZ, DVM
Diplomate, ACVS
Veterinary Surgical Specialists of
New Mexico
Albuquerque, New Mexico

FRED W. SCOTT, DVM, PhD
Diplomate, ACVM
Academy of Feline Medicine
Professor Emeritus
Department of Microbiology and
Immunology
College of Veterinary Medicine
Cornell University
Ithaca, New York

J. CATHARINE R. SCOTT-MONCRIEFF, MA,
Vet MB, MS
Diplomate, ACVIM (Internal Medicine)
Diplomate, ECVIM (Internal Medicine)
Associate Professor
Department of Veterinary
Clinical Medicine
Purdue University School of
Veterinary Medicine
West Lafayette, Indiana

LYNNE M. SEIBERT, DVM, PhD
Diplomate, ACVB
Clinical Researcher
Department of Anatomy and Radiology
Animal Emergency and Referral Center
Lynnwood, Washington

KEVIN SHANLEY, DVM
Diplomate, ACVD
Staff Dermatologist
Metropolitan Veterinary Associates &
Delaware Veterinary Specialty Group
Dermatology Clinic for Animals
Valley Forge, Pennsylvania

DARCY H. SHAW, DVM, MVSC
Diplomate, ACVIM (Internal Medicine)
Professor
Department of Companion Animals
Atlantic Veterinary College
University of Prince Edward Island
Charlottetown, Prince Edward Island,
Canada

LINDA G. SHELL, DVM
Diplomate, ACVIM (Neurology)
Professor
Small Animal Clinical Sciences
Virginia-Maryland Regional College of
Veterinary Medicine
Virginia Polytechnical Institute and
State University
Blacksburg, Virginia

G. DIANE SHELTON, DVM, PHD
Diplomate, ACVIM (Internal Medicine)
Adjunct Professor
Department of Pathology
University of California, San Diego
LaJolla, California

PETER K. SHIRES, BVSc, MS
Diplomate, ACVS
Professor
Department of Small Animal Surgery
Virginia-Maryland Regional
College of Veterinary Medicine
Blacksburg, Virginia

DEBORAH C. SILVERSTEIN, DVM
Diplomate, ACVECC
Staff Veterinarian
Department of Emergency and
Critical Care
University of Pennsylvania
Philadelphia, Pennsylvania

BARBARA SHERMAN SIMPSON, DVM, PhD
Diplomate, ACVB
Adjunct Associate Professor /
Veterinary Behaviorist
Department of Clinical Sciences
North Carolina State University
College of Veterinary Medicine /
The Veterinary Behavior Clinic
Raleigh, North Carolina /
South Pines, North Carolina

KENNETH W. SIMPSON, BVM&S, PhD,
MRCVS
Diplomate, ACVIM (Internal Medicine),
Diplomate, ECVIM
Assistant Professor of Medicine
Department of Clinical Sciences
Cornell University College of
Veterinary Medicine
Ithaca, New York

ALLEN FRANKLIN SISSON, DVM, MS
Diplomate, ACVIM (Neurology)
Staff Neurologist
Department of Medicine
Angell Memorial Animal Hospital
Boston, Massachusetts

DAVID D. SISSON
Diplomate, ACVIM (Cardiology)
Veterinary Clinical Medicine
University of Illinois
Urbana, Illinois

STEPHANIE L. SMEDES, DVM
Diplomate, ACVO
Animal Eye Clinic
Seattle, Washington

MARK M. SMITH, VMD
Diplomate, ACVS, AVDC
Professor and Chief of
Small Animal Surgery
Department of Small Animal
Clinical Sciences
Virginia-Maryland Regional
College of Veterinary Medicine
Blacksburg, Virginia

MARY O. SMITH, BVMS, PhD
Diplomate, ACVIM (Neurology)
Department of Clinical Sciences
College of Veterinary Medicine
Colorado State University
Fort Collins, Colorado

PATRICIA J. SMITH, MS, DVM, PhD
Diplomate, ACVO
Adjunct Assistant Professor /
Ophthalmologist
Dept of Small Animal Clinical Sciences
University of Florida
College of Veterinary Medicine /
Animal Eye Care
Gainesville, Florida /
Fremont, California

FRANCIS W.K. SMITH, JR., DVM
Diplomate, ACVIM
(Internal Medicine & Cardiology)
VetMed Consultants
Lexington, Massachusetts
Clinical Assistant Professor
Tufts University School of
Veterinary Medicine
North Grafton, Massachusetts

PATTI S. SNYDER, DVM, MS
Diplomate, ACVIM (Internal Medicine)
North Florida Neurology
Orange Park, Florida

PAUL W. SNYDER, DVM, PhD
Diplomate, ACVP
Associate Professor
Department of Veterinary Pathobiology
Purdue University
West Lafayette, Indiana

JÖERG STEINER
Small Animal Medicine and Surgery
College of Veterinary Medicine
Texas A&M University
College Station, Texas

REBECCA L. STEPIEN, DVM
Diplomate, ACVIM (Cardiology)
Clinical Assistant Professor
Department of Medical Sciences
University of Wisconsin
School of Veterinary Medicine
Madison, Wisconsin

JERRY B. STEVENS, DVM, PhD
Professor, Clinical Pathology
College of Veterinary Medicine
North Carolina State University
Raleigh, North Carolina

ELIZABETH ARNOLD STONE, DVM
Diplomate, ACVS
Professor and Head
Department of Clinical Sciences
North Carolina State University
College of Veterinary Medicine
Raleigh, North Carolina

JUSTIN H. STRAUS, DVM
Diplomate, ACVIM (Internal Medicine)
Animal Emergency & Referral Center
West Caldwell, New Jersey

JAN SUCHODOLSKI
Graduate Assistant
Gastrointestinal Laboratory
Department of Small Animal
Medicine and Surgery
Texas A&M University
College Station, Texas

MARGARET S. SWARTOUT, DVM, MS
Diplomate, ACVIM (Internal Medicine)
Owner
Veterinary Specialty Consultation Service
Knoxville, Tennessee

CHERYL L. SWENSON, DVM, PhD
Diplomate, ACVP (Clinical Pathology)
Associate Professor
Department of Pathobiology and
Diagnostic Investigation
Michigan State University
East Lansing, Michigan

HARRIET M. SYME, BSc, BVetMed, MRCVS
Diplomate, ACVIM (Internal Medicine)
Graduate Student
Veterinary Basic Sciences
Royal Veterinary College
University of London
London, England

JOSEPH TABOADA, DVM
Diplomate, ACVIM (Internal Medicine)
Professor and Director of
Professional Instruction
Department of Veterinary Sciences
School of Veterinary Medicine
Louisiana State University
Baton Rouge, Louisiana

PATRICIA A. TALCOTT, MS, DVM, PhD
Diplomate, ABVT
Associate Professor / Veterinary
Toxicologist
Department of Food Science and
Toxicology / Washington Animal Disease
Diagnostic Laboratory
University of Idaho / Washington State
University, College of Veterinary Medicine
Moscow, Idaho / Pullman, Washington

SUSAN M. TAYLOR, DVM
Diplomate, ACVIM (Internal Medicine)
Professor / Staff Internist
Small Animal Clinical Sciences /
Small Animal Clinic
Western College of Veterinary Medicine /
Veterinary Teaching Hospital
University of Saskatchewan
Saskatoon, Saskatchewan
Canada

WILLIAM B. THOMAS, DVM, MS
Diplomate, ACVIM (Neurology)
Associate Professor
Department of Small Animal
Clinical Sciences
University of Tennessee
Knoxville, Tennessee

MARY F. THOMPSON, BVSc
Diplomate, ACVIM (Internal Medicine)
Visiting Instructor in Small Animal
Medicine
Department of Veterinary
Clinical Sciences
Purdue University
West Lafayette, Indiana

JERRY A. THORNHILL, DVM
Diplomate, ACVIM (Internal Medicine)
Consultant, Veterinary Internal Medicine
& Nephrology
Chicago Veterinary Kidney Center
Franklin Park, Illinois

MARY ANNA THRALL, DVM, MS
Diplomate, ACVP
Professor
Department of Microbiology,
Immunology and Pathology
Colorado State University
Fort Collins, Colorado

LARRY P. TILLEY, DVM
Diplomate, ACVIM (Internal Medicine)
President, VetMed Consultants
Chief Medical Officer, Dr. Tilley &
Associates
Sante Fe, New Mexico

ANDREA TIPOLD, Prof. Dr.
Diplomate, ECVN
Professor
Small Animal Medicine & Surgery
Veterinary
School of Hannover
Hannover, Germany

SHEILA M.F. TORRES, DVM, MS, PhD
Diplomate, ACVD
Assistant Professor
Small Animal Clinical Sciences
University of Minnesota
College of Veterinary Medicine
Minneapolis, Minnesota

WILLIAM J. TRANQUILLI, DVM, MS
Diplomate, ACVA
Professor of Anesthesiology
Department of Veterinary
Clinical Medicine
University of Illinois
College of Veterinary Medicine
Urbana, Illinois

AVENELLE ILENE TURNER, DVM
Oncology Resident
Gulf Coast Veterinary Oncology
Gulf Coast Veterinary Specialists
Houston, TX

DAVID C. TWEDT, DVM
Diplomate, ACVIM (Internal Medicine)
Professor
Clinical Sciences Veterinary
Teaching Hospital
College of Veterinary Medicine
Colorado State University
Fort Collins, Colorado

JOHN WILLIAM TYLER, DVM
Diplomate, ACVIM (Internal Medicine)
Assistant Professor, Small Animal
Internal Medicine
Animal Health Center
Mississippi State University
College of Veterinary Medicine
Mississippi State, Mississippi

LISA L. ULRICH
University of Minnesota
College of Veterinary Medicine
St. Paul, Minnesota

SHELLY L. VADEN, DVM, PhD
Diplomate, ACVIM (Internal Medicine)
Associate Professor
Department of Clinical Sciences
North Carolina State University
College of Veterinary Medicine
Raleigh, North Carolina

MARIA VIANNA, DVM
Department of Clinical Sciences
Department Small Animal
Clinical Sciences
University of Tennessee
Knoxville, Tennessee

VICTORIA VOITH, DVM
Animal Services Division
Albuquerque, New Mexico

MARY ANN VONDERHAAR, DVM, MS
Perrysburg, Ohio

LORI S. WADDELL, DVM
Diplomate, ACVECC
Staff Veterinarian, Critical Care
Department of Clinical Studies
School of Veterinary Medicine
University of Pennsylvania
Philadelphia, Pennsylvania

DON R. WALDRON, DVM
Diplomate, ACVS, ABVP
Professor of Surgery
Department of Small Animal
Clinical Sciences
Virginia-Maryland Regional College of
Veterinary Medicine
Blacksburg, Virginia

MARK WALKER, BVSc, MACVSc
Diplomate, ACVIM (Internal Medicine)
North Florida Veterinary Specialists, P.A.
Jacksonville / Orange Park, Florida

MICHELLE WALL, DVM
Diplomate, ACVIM (Internal Medicine)
Educational Resource Specialist
in Oncology
Small Animal Medicine
College of Veterinary Medicine
University of Georgia
Athens, Georgia

MELISSA S. WALLACE, DVM
Diplomate, ACVIM (Internal Medicine)
Consultant
The E. & M. Bobst Hospital
The Animal Medical Center
New York, New York

JENNIFER WARNOCK
Gulf Coast Veterinary Surgery
Houston, Texas

MICHELLE JOY WASCHAK, DVM, MS
Diplomate, ACVS
Staff Surgeon
South Carolina Surgical Referral Service
Columbia, South Carolina

ROBERT J. WASHABAU, VMD, PhD
Diplomate, ACVIM (Internal Medicine)
Associate Professor and
Section Chief of Medicine
Department of Clinical Studies
College of Veterinary Medicine
University of Pennsylvania
Philadelphia, Pennsylvania

CRAIG B. WEBB, PhD, DVM
Resident
Department of Clinical Sciences
College of Veterinary Medicine
Colorado State University
Fort Collins, Colorado

CYNTHIA R. WEBSTER, DVM
Diplomate, ACVIM (Internal Medicine)
Associate Professor
Department of Clinical Sciences
School of Veterinary Medicine
Tufts University
North Grafton, Massachusetts

GLADE WEISER, DVM
Diplomate, ACVP (Clinical Pathology)
Professor, Special Appointment /
Clinical Pathologist
Department of Pathology
Colorado State University /
Heska Corporation
Fort Collins, Colorado

ALEXANDER HOWARD WERNER, VMD
Diplomate, ACVD
Dermatologist
Valley Veterinary Specialty Services
Studio City, California

ROBERT BRUCE WIGGS, DVM
Diplomate, AVDC
Adjunct Associate Professor / Owner
Department of Biomedical Sciences /
Dallas Dental Service Animal Clinic
Baylor College of Dentistry,
Texas A&M University Systems /
Coit Road Animal Hospital
Dallas, Texas

DAVID ALAN WILLIAMS, MA, Vet MB, PhD,
MRCVS
Diplomate, ACVIM (Internal Medicine)
Diplomate, ECVIM
(Companion Animals)
Professor and Head Department of
Small Animal Medicine and Surgery
College of Veterinary Medicine
Texas A&M University
College Station, Texas

JAMES E. WILLIAMS, JR., DVM,
Carolina Veterinary Specialists
Greensboro, North Carolina

NICOLA L. WILLIAMSON
Veterinary Dermatology of Richmond
Richmond, Virginia

RONALD B. WILSON, DVM
Diplomate, ACVP
Laboratory Director
C.E. Cord Animal Disease
Diagnostic Laboratory
Tennessee Department of Agriculture
Nashville, Tennessee

BRETT C. WOOD, DVM
Department of Small Animal
Clinical Sciences
Virginia-Maryland Regional College of
Veterinary Medicine
Virginia Tech
Blacksburg, Virginia

DARREN WOOD, DVM, DVSC
Diplomate, ACVP
(Clinical Pathology)
Clinical Instructor
Department of Pathobiological Sciences
University of Wisconsin—Madison
Madison, Wisconsin

J. PAUL WOODS, DVM, MS
Diplomate, ACVIM (Internal Medicine),
Certificate of Specialization in
Small Animal Internal Medicine
Canadian Veterinary Medical Association
Associate Professor of Medicine
Department of Clinical Studies
Ontario Veterinary College,
University of Guelph
Guelph, Ontario, Canada

DEANNA WORLEY, DVM
Gulf Coast Veterinary Surgery
Houston, Texas

KAREN M. YOUNG, VMD, PhD
Professor
Department of Pathobiological Sciences
School of Veterinary Medicine
University of Wisconsin—Madison
Madison, Wisconsin

JULIE CORBET PEMBLETON, DVM
Diplomate, ACVIM (Internal Medicine)
Animal Emergency & Referral Center
Fort Pierce, Florida

CONTENTS

CONTENTS *by subject*

CARDIOLOGY

DENTISTRY

DERMATOLOGY

ENDOCRINOLOGY & METABOLISM

HEMATOLOGY/ IMMUNOLOGY

HEPATOLOGY

INFECTIOUS DISEASE

MUSCULOSKELETAL

NEPHROLOGY/UROLOGY

NEUROLOGY

ONCOLOGY

OPHTHALMOLOGY

RESPIRATORY

THERIOGENOLOGY

TOXICOLOGY

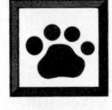

CANINE AND FELINE

ABORTION, SPONTANEOUS, AND PREGNANCY LOSS—CATS

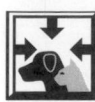

BASICS

DEFINITIONS
• Abortion—expulsion of one or more fetuses that cannot sustain extrauterine life • Pregnancy loss—all pregnancy wastage, including embryonic death, reabsorption of early fetal losses, mummification, abortion, stillbirths, and outcomes of dystocia

PATHOPHYSIOLOGY
• Primary causes—kill the embryo or fetus directly; include lethal genetic defects and most infections • Secondary fetal wastage—fetal life terminated indirectly; includes compromised placentation, inadequate uterine vascular or nutritional support, failure of supportive endocrine function, dam-related events (e.g., dystocia, trauma, extreme stress, metabolic disease) • Possible outcomes—reabsorption during early gestation; abortion or mummification during later gestation; stillbirth at term

SYSTEMS AFFECTED
• Reproductive • Other systems—if pregnancy wastage leads to complications (e.g., toxemia or shock); if pregnancy wastage is secondary to systemic illness

GENETIC
Nonspecific; inbred lines experience pregnancy failure more frequently

INCIDENCE/PREVALENCE
Unknown; early gestational losses are difficult to document, and owners may not recognize later gestational losses

SIGNALMENT
Species Cat

Breed Predilections
Persians and Himalayans—dystocia due to fetal-maternal disproportion

Mean Age and Range
• Noninfectious causes—more common at first parity and in queens >6 years old • Infectious causes—seen in all ages

Predominant Sex Female only

SIGNS
General Comments
• May be asymptomatic, especially early in gestation • **NOTE:** not all signs are seen in every patient; any combination may occur.

Historical Findings
• Failure to litter on time • Decrease in abdominal size • Weight loss • Expulsion of recognizable fetuses or placental structures • Anorexia • Vomiting, diarrhea • Behavioral changes

Physical Examination Findings
• Sanguineous or purulent vulvar discharge—frequently unnoticed in fastidious queens or with early gestational losses • Disappearance of vesicles or fetuses previously documented by palpation, ultrasonography, or radiography • Abdominal straining, discomfort • Depression • Dehydration • Fever in some patients

CAUSES
Infectious
• Viruses—feline panleukopenia virus; feline herpesvirus 1; feline leukemia virus; feline immunodeficiency virus • Bacteria—*Escherichia coli; Streptococcus* spp.; *Staphylococcus* spp.; *Salmonella* spp.; *Mycoplasma* spp.; *Mycobacterium* spp. • *Coxiella burnetii* (Q fever) • *Toxoplasma gondii* (probably uncommon)

Noninfectious—Reproductive
• Early embryonic loss • Dystocia (fetal or maternal)—see Dystocia; Uterine Inertia • Endometrial disease—cystic endometrial hyperplasia (CEH) very common (see Pyometra and Cystic Endometrial Hyperplasia) • Endocrinopathy—hypoluteoidism; indirect evidence, although no documented cases in literature; incidence unknown • Structural or functional placental inadequacy • Fetal defects—genetic or developmental (anatomic, metabolic, and chromosomal abnormalities); possibly gamete aging • Excessive or poorly planned inbreeding and/or poor choices of breeding stock—indirect evidence; difficult diagnoses without thorough family history and test matings • Abortifacient drugs—luteolytics (e.g., $PGF_{2\alpha}$); estrogens; prolactin inhibitors (e.g., cabergoline); glucocorticoids • Abortifacient drugs reported in dogs—bromocriptine; tamoxifen citrate; mifepristone; epostane

Noninfectious—Nonreproductive
• Nutrition—taurine <500 ppm of diet • Severe stress—environmental; physiologic; psychologic • Trauma • Some drugs • Consequence of nonreproductive systemic disease

RISK FACTORS
• Prior history of pregnancy loss or poor reproductive performance • Concurrent acute or chronic disease • Excessive inbreeding • First parity or >6 years of age • High-stress environment (crowding, poor sanitation, noise, temperature or humidity extremes) • Obesity or malnutrition

DIAGNOSIS

DIFFERENTIAL DIAGNOSIS
Differentiate Wastage from Infertility
• Estrus abnormality—confirm estrus with serum estradiol concentration • No mating; mating timed improperly • Failure to ovulate—confirm ovulation with serum progesterone; single matings may cause insufficient LH release in cats • Failure of fertilization or transport; early embryonic losses (difficult differentiation in clinical settings) • Pseudopregnancy

Vulvar Discharge
• Estrus—discharge usually scant; behavioral signs of estrus; vaginal cytologic examination or serum estradiol documents estrus (**NOTE:** sample collection for cytology may induce ovulation) • Impending parturition • Metritis; endometritis • Severe vaginitis • Mucometra, hydrometra—document by ultrasonography or at surgery • Pyometra—**NOTE:** closed pyometra, mucometra, hydrometra are common in cats (see Pyometra and Cystic Endometrial

Hyperplasia). • Uterine trauma or hemorrhage—history of recent injury and clinical signs (bloody discharge, weakness, shock, pallor); acute blood loss noted on CBC; uterine fluid or blood clots seen on ultrasonography; bleeding without inflammation determined from vaginal cytologic examination; intra-abdominal bleeding possible with some uterine injuries • Abnormal vaginal or rectovaginal anatomy—(see Vaginal Malformations and Acquired Lesions) • Uterine or vaginal neoplasia (see Vaginal Tumors) • Uterine stump infection • Ovarian remnant syndrome—(see Ovarian Remnant Syndrome)

Abdominal Signs
• Obstructive uropathy or nonobstructive lower urinary tract disease • Severe renal disease—pyelonephritis • Pancreatitis • Liver disease • Severe gastrointestinal disease • Peritonitis • Abdominal trauma

CBC/BIOCHEMISTRY/URINALYSIS
• Usually normal • Inflammatory or stress leukocyte response—with many infectious causes except panleukopenia • Additional organ involvement possible with complications of primary pregnancy loss, or with pregnancy loss secondary to systemic illness—may be reflected in CBC/biochemistry/urinalysis

OTHER LABORATORY TESTS
Infectious Causes
• Cytologic examination of vulvar discharge—may detect fetal or placental tissue, or other cause • FPLV (see Feline Panleukopenia) • FHV-1 (see Feline Rhinotracheitis Virus Infection) • FeLV (see Feline Leukemia Virus Infection [FeLV]) • FIV (see Feline Immunodeficiency Virus Infection [FIV]) • Bacterial causes—specify potential target organisms to laboratory, especially for *Salmonella, Mycobacterium* • Coxiella—(see Q Fever) • Mycoplasma (see Mycoplasmosis)

Noninfectious Causes
• Hypoluteoidism—serial serum progesterone determinations; begin before time of suspected fetal loss • Hypothyroidism—probably uncommon as a cause of pregnancy loss

IMAGING
• Radiography and palpation—establish existence of fetuses if performed at appropriate intervals of gestation • Ultrasonography—essential for precise evaluation of fetal presence, size, and viability • Radiography and ultrasound—confirm or rule out differential diagnoses other than viable pregnancy

DIAGNOSTIC PROCEDURES
Fetal Defects
• Necropsy—gross and histologic findings vary with cause • Karyotype—submit ear tip of necropsy subject; ship in heparinized dam's blood; contact karyotype laboratory (University of Minnesota: 612-624-4767; save gonad in Bouin's solution for histopathologic evaluation. • Screen for inborn errors of metabolism—submit urine from necropsy subject or live patient; contact laboratory (Medical Genetics Section, University of Pennsylvania: 215-898-3375). • Collect history of involved or related sires and dams.

ABORTION, SPONTANEOUS, AND PREGNANCY LOSS—CATS

Poor Reproductive Planning
• Review production records; calculate inbreeding coefficients of affected and related breeding animals (inbreeding coefficient 5 the probability that the two alleles from a randomly chosen locus are identical by descent; a measure of the effect of relatedness on an individual's genetic constitution); evaluate overall reproductive performance of the cattery.
• Cattery history of neonatal or pediatric mortality, low birth weights, poor growth, susceptibility to infectious diseases—often suggests excessive inbreeding and/or poor choices of breeding stock

PATHOLOGIC FINDINGS
• Dam's reproductive tract—note ovarian activity (follicular phase, luteal phase, inactive); uterus (normal, CEH, endometritis, metritis, hydrometra, mucometra, pyometra) • Fetus (mummified, pre-term, full-term, stillborn, live-born)—necropsy fetus for gross observations; histopathology; culture; virus isolation; karyotype; errors of metabolism.

 TREATMENT

APPROPRIATE HEALTH CARE
• Outpatient medical management—medically stable patients with suspected endocrinopathies or endometrial disease; patients with noninfectious/nonreproductive pregnancy loss
• Inpatient medical management—patients likely to abort; patients aborting visible fetal and placental material; patients with clinical illness; patients with potential zoonoses (unless safe and effective outpatient treatment can be assured); patients being treated with $PGF_{2\alpha}$ to evacuate the uterus • Surgical management—OHE for stable patients with no breeding value • Abortus or discharge—may be infectious; isolate patient

NURSING CARE
• Correct dehydration—Normosol or Lactated Ringer's solution; intravenous, subcutaneous, intramedullary administration, depending on patient cooperation and severity of illness
• Practice strict sanitation for inpatient and outpatient treatment.

ACTIVITY
• No limitations unless an infectious agent is suspected or documented in a cat being treated as an outpatient; specific and clear household or cattery sanitation recommendations should be provided in cases suspected to be infectious in nature. • Hospitalize infectious patients is preferred.

DIET
• No special dietary considerations for uncomplicated cases • Patients with persistent diarrhea may require support with veterinary diet.

CLIENT EDUCATION
• Critical in the case of zoonoses—provide printed explanatory materials if possible, keep careful medical records about discussions. • For catteries—discuss history or possibility of multiple occurrences. • Help client establish a monitoring system—encourage maintaining careful records of reproductive performance.
• For infectious causes—help client establish ongoing surveillance and control measures.
• For primary uterine diseases—OHE is indicated for patients with no breeding value.
• For breeding cats—inform client of risks associated with non-surgical solutions, particularly with infectious or genetic causes of pregnancy loss. • Infertility—may result despite successful immediate treatment. • Prostaglandin treatment—discuss side-effects. • OHE—discuss post-surgical obesity for midlife queens.

SURGICAL CONSIDERATIONS
• Potential contraindications for surgery—serious risk to survival; ability to resolve the problem by less invasive means • OHE—preferred for stable patients with no breeding value

 MEDICATIONS

DRUG(S) OF CHOICE
• Depend on underlying causes • Amoxicillin—11–22 mg/kg PO q8h–q12h, pending results of bacterial culture; other antibiotics if amoxicillin is contraindicated, ineffective, or organism resistance is established • $PGF_{2\alpha}$—no live fetuses but significant uterine contents noted on ultrasonography; 0.10–0.25 mg/kg SC q12–24h for up to 5 days, if needed; obtain informed consent; do not use prostaglandin analogues (safe doses have not been established in the queen).

CONTRAINDICATIONS
• Potential contraindications for $PGF_{2\alpha}$—advanced age; live fetuses; mummified fetuses; closed cervix; sepsis; peritonitis; high risk of uterine rupture; asthma; patient medically unstable • Progesterone/progestogens—endometrial disease; mammary gland tumors

PRECAUTIONS
$PGF_{2\alpha}$ side effects—intense grooming; salivation; defecation; vomiting; urination; tachypnea; vocalization; nervousness; panting; mydriasis; lordosis posture; tail flagging; occasionally hypotension

POSSIBLE INTERACTIONS
Check cautions when administering drugs to manage specific differential diagnoses, especially if patient is pregnant

ALTERNATIVE DRUG(S)
Progesterone/progestogens—safe and effective doses needed to maintain pregnancy have not been established; **CAUTION:** may induce or exacerbate CEH; use only if hypoluteoidism is documented and the endometrium is free of disease

 FOLLOW-UP

PATIENT MONITORING
• Re-evaluate 7–14 days after end of $PGF_{2\alpha}$ treatment • Repeat ultrasonography—document complete uterine evacuation or establish maintenance of live fetuses

PREVENTION/AVOIDANCE
• Genetic problems require attention to breeding program. • Infectious causes require surveillance and control measures. • OHE for cats with no breeding value

POSSIBLE COMPLICATIONS
• Sepsis • Shock • Uterine rupture • Peritonitis • Metritis • Pyometra • Hemorrhage • Infertility • Obesity following OHE in mid-life queens • CEH following progestogen therapy

EXPECTED COURSE AND PROGNOSIS
• Symptomatic retrovirus infection—poor prognosis • Chronic infertility—common after 6 years of age • Queens not bred prior to 3–4 years of age experience higher infertility.
• Severe CEH—recovery of fertility unlikely; pyometra is a common eventual complication.
• Genetic abnormalities causing dystocia or loss of most or all of litter generally have a guarded to poor prognosis for further have reproduction; ethical issues should be discussed. • Dystocias—recurrence depends on cause; guarded prognosis if cause cannot be ascertained • Endocrinopathies—often manageable

 MISCELLANEOUS

AGE-RELATED FACTORS
• Fertility declines naturally after 6 years of age. • OHE—recommended in stable patients >6 years old • Queens greater than 3–4 years of age and never mated—increased incidence.

ZOONOTIC POTENTIAL
• *Coxiella burnetii* • *Toxoplasma gondii* • *Campylobacter upsaliensis*—associated with a human abortion; same strain isolated from a cat in the household

SEE ALSO
• Dystocia • Infertility, Female • Ovarian Remnant Syndrome • Pyometra and Cystic Endometrial Hyperplasia • Uterine Inertia

ABBREVIATIONS
• CEH = cystic endometrial hyperplasia • FeLV = feline leukemia virus • FHV-1 = feline herpesvirus 1 • FIV = feline immunodeficiency virus • FPLV = feline panleukopenia virus • OHE = ovariohysterectomy • $PGF_{2\alpha}$ = prostaglandin $F_{2\alpha}$

Suggested Reading
Little S. Uncovering the cause of infertility in queens. Vet Med 2001;96:557–568.
Johnston SD, Root Kustritz MV, Olson PNS. Feline pregnancy. In: Canine and feline theriogenology. Philadelphia: Saunders, 2001: 414–430.
Papich MG. Effects of drugs on pregnancy. In: Kirk RW, Bonagura JD, eds. Current veterinary therapy X. Philadelphia: Saunders, 1981:1291–1299.
Author Dennis F. Lawler
Consulting Editor Sara K. Lyle

ABORTION, SPONTANEOUS, AND PREGNANCY LOSS—DOGS

 BASICS

DEFINITION
Loss of a fetus because of resorption in early stages or expulsion in later stages of pregnancy

PATHOPHYSIOLOGY
• Direct causes—congenital abnormality, infectious disease, trauma
• Indirect causes—infectious placentitis, abnormal ovarian function, abnormal uterine environment

SYSTEMS AFFECTED
• Reproductive
• Any dysfunction of a major body system can adversely affect pregnancy.

GENETIC
• No genetic basis for most causes of abortion
• Lymphocytic hypothyroidism—single-gene recessive trait in borzois

INCIDENCE/PREVALENCE
• True incidence unknown
• Resorption estimated between 11–13%
• Incidence of stillbirth reported as 2.2–4.4%; increases with dystocia up to 22.3%

GEOGRAPHIC DISTRIBUTION
N/A

SIGNALMENT
Species
Dog

Breed Predilections
Familial lymphocytic hypothyroidism reported in borzois—prolonged interestrus interval, poor conception rates, abortion midgestation, stillbirths

Mean Age and Range
• Infectious causes, pharmacological agents causing abortion, fetal defects—seen in all ages • Cystic endometrial hyperplasia—usually >6 years old

Predominant Sex
• Intact bitches

SIGNS
Historical Findings
• Failure to whelp on time • Expulsion of recognizable fetuses or placental tissues
• Decrease in abdominal size; weight loss
• Anorexia • Vomiting, diarrhea
• Behavioral changes

Physical Examination Findings
• Sanguineous or purulent vulvar discharge
• Disappearance of vesicles or fetuses previously documented by palpation, ultrasonography, or radiography • Abdominal straining, discomfort • Depression
• Dehydration • Fever in some patients

CAUSES
Infectious
• *Brucella canis*
• Canine herpesvirus
• *Toxoplasma gondii, Neospora caninum*
• *Mycoplasma* and *Ureaplasma*
• Miscellaneous bacteria—*E. coli, Streptococcus, Campylobacter, Salmonella*
• Miscellaneous viruses—distemper virus, parvovirus

Uterine
• Cystic endometrial hyperplasia and pyometra
• Trauma—acute and chronic
• Neoplasia
• Embryotoxic drugs
• Chemotherapeutic agents
• Estrogens
• Glucocorticoids—high dosages

Ovarian
• Prostaglandins—lysis of corpora lutea
• Dopamine agonists—lysis of corpora lutea via suppression of prolactin; bromocriptine, cabergoline
• Hypoluteoidism—abnormal luteal function in the absence of fetal, uterine, or placental disease: progesterone concentrations <1–2 ng/ml

Hormonal Dysfunction
• Hypothyroidism
• Hyperadrenocorticism
• Environmental factors—endocrine disrupting contaminants have been documented in human and wildlife instances of fetal loss.

Fetal Defects
• Lethal chromosomal abnormality
• Lethal organ defects

RISK FACTORS
• Exposure of the brood bitch to carrier animals
• Old age
• Hereditary factors

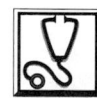 DIAGNOSIS

DIFFERENTIAL DIAGNOSIS
• Differentiate infectious from noninfectious causes—*B. canis* of immediate concern
• Differentiate resorption from infertility—helped by early diagnosis of pregnancy
• History of drug use during pregnancy—particularly during the first trimester, or use of drugs known to cause fetal death
• Vulvar discharges during diestrus—may mimic abortion; evaluate discharge and origin to differentiate uterine from distal reproductive tract disease.
• Necropsy of aborted fetus, stillborn puppies, and placenta—enhances chances of a definitive diagnosis

• History of systemic or endocrine disease—may indicate problems with the maternal environment.

CBC/BIOCHEMISTRY/URINALYSIS
• Usually normal
• Systemic disease, uterine infection, viral infection, or endocrine abnormalities—may produce changes in CBC, biochemistries, or urinalysis

OTHER LABORATORY TESTS
• Serologic testing—*B. canis,* canine herpesvirus, and *Toxoplasma,* neospora; collect serum as soon as possible after abortion; repeat testing for raising titers for canine herpesvirus, *Toxoplasma,* neospora
• Slide test for *B. canis*—very sensitive; negative results reliable; prevalence of false positives as high as 60%; definitive diagnosis made via culture
• Tube agglutination test for *B. canis*—gives titers; titers >1:200 considered positive; titers from 1:50–1:200 considered suspicious
• Agar gel immunodiffusion test for *B. canis*—effectively differentiates between false positives and true positives; detects cytoplasmic and cell surface antigens
• Baseline T_4 serum concentration (when no infectious agents are identified)—hypothyroidism is a common endocrine disease and has been suggested as a cause for fetal wastage; role in pregnancy loss unclear; subnormal T_4 concentrations indicate need for further testing (see Hypothyroidism).
• Progesterone serum concentration (when no infectious agents are identified)—hypoluteoidism may cause fetal wastage; dogs depend on ovarian progesterone production throughout gestation (minimum of 2 ng/mL required to maintain pregnancy); determine as soon as possible after abortion; in subsequent pregnancies, start monitoring at week 3, which may be before pregnancy can be documented with ultrasound.
• Vaginal culture—*B. canis* with positive serologic test; *Mycoplasma, Ureaplasma,* other bacterial agents; all except *B. canis* can be normal flora, therefore diagnosis difficult from vaginal cultures alone

IMAGING
• Radiography—identifies fetal structures after 45 days of gestation; earlier, can determine uterine enlargement but cannot assess uterine contents.
• Ultrasonography—identifies uterine size and contents; assesses fluid and its consistency; assesses fetal remains or fetal viability by noting heartbeats (normal, >200 bpm; stress, <200 bpm).

DIAGNOSTIC PROCEDURES
• Vaginoscopy—identify source of vulvar discharges and vaginal lesions; use a scope of sufficient length (16–20 cm) to examine the entire length of the vagina.

ABORTION, SPONTANEOUS, AND PREGNANCY LOSS—DOGS

• Cytologic examination and bacterial culture—vagina may reveal an inflammatory process (e.g., uterine infection); technique for culture: use a guarded swab culture instrument to ensure an anterior sample (distal reproductive tract is normally heavily contaminated with bacteria).

PATHOLOGIC FINDINGS
Histopathologic examination and culture of fetal and placental tissue—may reveal infectious organisms; tissue culture, particularly of stomach contents, to identify infectious bacterial organisms

 TREATMENT

APPROPRIATE HEALTH CARE
• Most bitches should be confined and isolated pending diagnosis.
• Hospitalization of infectious patients preferred
• *B. canis*—highly infective to dogs; shed in high numbers during abortion; suspected cases should be isolated.
• Outpatient medical management—medically stable patients with noninfectious causes of pregnancy loss, endocrinopathies, or endometrial disease
• Partial abortion—may attempt to salvage the live fetuses; administer antibiotics if a bacterial component is identified.

NURSING CARE
Dehydration—use replacement fluids, supplemented with electrolytes if imbalances are identified by serum biochemistries.

ACTIVITY
Partial abortion—cage rest

DIET
No special dietary considerations for uncomplicated cases

CLIENT EDUCATION
• Critical for *B. canis*—if confirmed, euthanasia recommended owing to lack of successful treatment and to prevent spread of infection; may try OHE and long-term antibiotics; discuss surveillance program for kennel situations; discuss zoonotic potential.
• Primary uterine disease—OHE is indicated in patients with no breeding value; cystic endometrial hyperplasia is an irreversible change.
• Infertility or pregnancy loss—may recur in subsequent estrus cycles despite successful immediate treatment
• Prostaglandin treatment—discuss side-effects.
• Infectious diseases—establish surveillance and control measures.

SURGICAL CONSIDERATIONS
OHE—preferred for stable patients with no breeding value

 MEDICATIONS

DRUG(S) OF CHOICE
• PGF$_{2\alpha}$ (Lutalyse)—uterine evacuation after abortion; 0.1 mg/kg SC q8–24h; not approved for use in dogs, but adequate documentation legitimizes its use; do not substitute analogs (inadequate documentation of safe dosages); use only if all living fetuses have been expelled.
• Antibiotics—for bacterial disease; initially institute broad-spectrum agent; specific agent depends on culture and sensitivity testing of vaginal tissue or necropsy of fetus.
• Progesterone (Regu-mate) at 0.088 mg/kg (1 mL/25 kg PO) or progesterone in oil at 2 mg/kg IM q48h—for documented hypoluteodism only

CONTRAINDICATIONS
Progestogen supplementation—contraindicated in dogs with endometrial or mammary gland disease

PRECAUTIONS
PGF$_{2\alpha}$—metabolized in the lung; side effects are related to smooth muscle contraction, are dose-related, and diminish with each injection; panting, salivation, vomiting, and defecation common; dosing critical (LD$_{50}$ 5 mg/kg)

POSSIBLE INTERACTIONS
N/A

ALTERNATIVE DRUG(S)
Oxytocin—1 U/5 kg SC q6–24h; for uterine evacuation; most effective in the first 24–48 hours after abortion

 FOLLOW-UP

PATIENT MONITORING
• Partial abortion—monitor viability of remaining fetuses with ultrasonography; monitor systemic health of the dam with serial CBC determinations for remainder of pregnancy.
• Vulvar discharges—daily; for decreasing amount, odor, and inflammatory component; for consistency (increasing mucoid content is prognostically good)
• PGF$_{2\alpha}$—continued for 5 days or until most of the discharge ceases (3–15 days)
• *B. canis*—monitor after neutering and antibiotic therapy; yearly serologic testing to identify recrudescence • Hypothyroidism—treat appropriately; neutering recommended (hereditary nature); see Hypothyroidism.

PREVENTION/AVOIDANCE
• Brucellosis and other infectious agents—surveillance programs to prevent introduction to kennel

• OHE—for bitches with no breeding value

POSSIBLE COMPLICATIONS
• Untreated pyometra—septicemia, toxemia, death • Brucellosis—discospondylitis, endophthalmitis, recurrent uveitis

EXPECTED COURSE AND PROGNOSIS
• Pyometra—recurrence rate during subsequent cycle is high (up to 70%) unless pregnancy is established • CEH—recovery of fertility unlikely; pyometra common complication • Hormonal dysfunction—often manageable; familial aspects should be considered • Brucellosis—guarded; extremely difficult to successfully eliminate infection even if combined with neutering

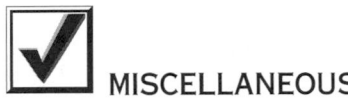 MISCELLANEOUS

ASSOCIATED CONDITIONS
N/A

AGE-RELATED FACTORS
Older bitches more likely to have CEH

ZOONOTIC POTENTIAL
B. canis—can be transmitted to humans, especially when handling the aborting bitch; massive numbers of organisms expelled during abortion

SYNONYMS
N/A

SEE ALSO
• Brucellosis • Hypothyroidism • Infertility, Female • Pyometra and Cystic Endometrial Hyperplasia

ABBREVIATIONS
• CEH = cystic endometrial hyperplasia
• OHE = ovariohysterectomy
• PGF$_{2\alpha}$ = prostaglandin F$_{2\alpha}$

Suggested Reading
Carmichael LE, Green CE. Canine brucellosis. In: Greene CE, ed. Infectious diseases of the dog and cat. Philadelphia: Saunders, 1990:573–584.
Evermann JF. Diagnosis of canine herpetic infections. In: Kirk RW, ed. Current veterinary therapy X. Philadelphia: Saunders, 1989:1313–1316.
Feldman EC, Nelson RW. Canine and feline endocrinology and reproduction. Philadelphia: Saunders, 1987:572–591.
Johnston SD, Root Kustritz MV, Olson PNS. Canine pregnancy. In: Canine and feline theriogenology. Philadelphia: Saunders, 2001:66–104.
Author Beverly J. Purswell
Consulting Editor Sara K. Lyle

ABORTION, TERMINATION OF PREGNANCY

BASICS

DEFINITION
Induced termination of an unwanted pregnancy; may accomplish by drugs that prevent fertilization, prevent implantation, or terminate an established pregnancy

PATHOPHYSIOLOGY
• Corpus luteum—must be functional throughout pregnancy in dogs and most likely in cats; suggested that pituitary rather than uterine or placental influences most important for maintenance
• LH and PRL—principal hormones involved in maintaining corpus luteum; reduced concentration may cause regression of corpus luteum and termination of pregnancy.
• Compounds that inhibit progesterone secretion or compete with progesterone receptors should lead to termination of pregnancy.

SYSTEMS AFFECTED
• Reproductive, Gastrointestinal, Respiratory, Neurologic, and Cardiac—affected by drugs used in treatment

GENETICS
N/A

INCIDENCE/PREVALENCE
N/A

GEOGRAPHIC DISTRIBUTION
N/A

SIGNALMENT
Species
Dogs

Breed Predilections
Unwanted pregnancy in any breed

Mean Age and Range
N/A

Predominant Sex
Female

SIGNS
• Depend on stage of gestation
• May have no visible signs
• Vaginal discharge or expulsion of fetus(es)

CAUSES
• Withdrawing luteotrophic support
• Inhibiting progesterone synthesis
• Using a progesterone receptor antagonist

RISK FACTORS
Causal drugs—undesirable side effects; require a great deal of time and effort for administration and monitoring; many not be approved for use in therapeutic abortions

DIAGNOSIS

DIFFERENTIAL DIAGNOSIS
• Important to establish that a breeding has taken place
• Determine stage of estrous cycle—examine vaginal smears; measure plasma progesterone concentration (see Breeding, Timing)
• Look for sperm—examine vaginal smears; absence of sperm does not mean that breeding did not take place.
• Patient in estrus with very high index of suspicion that she is pregnant—examine vaginal smears daily or every other day; determine day 1 of diestrus and start treatment on day 6.
• Patient in very early diestrus—wait 5 days and start treatment.
• Definitive diagnosis of pregnancy—ultrasound examination after day 20–30 of diestrus; radiographic examination after day 40 of diestrus
• Patient remains pregnant after early diestrus treatment—treat again on day 31–35 of diestrus; usually will accomplish termination

CBC/BIOCHEMISTRY/URINALYSIS
• Before treatment as screening tests in patients
• Normal, unless concurrent underlying disease

OTHER LABORATORY TESTS
• Vaginal cytologic testing—determine stage of estrous cycle and presence of sperm.
• Plasma progesterone concentration—determine stage of estrous cycle; monitor success of luteolysis.

IMAGING
Ultrasound—4–5 weeks after breeding to determine pregnancy; diagnostic test of choice for documenting pregnancy and uterine evacuation

PATHOLOGIC FINDINGS
N/A

TREATMENT

APPROPRIATE HEALTH CARE
• Inpatient—use of off-label drugs; monitor for side effects; if owner insists on taking patient home, wait at least 1 hour after each treatment before discharging the patient.
• Many mismated (accidentally mated) bitches do not become pregnant; therefore, treatment may not be necessary.
• Pregnancy status in early diestrus is unknown, because ultrasound confirmation of pregnancy is not possible until 4–5 weeks after breeding.
• Treat on day 6–10 of diestrus—treatment in midgestation is more unpleasant (more discharge and fetuses may be passed) and may have a psychologic effect on the patient.
• $PGF_{2\alpha}$ and bromocriptine—100% success in a small study (n = 15) in suppressing progesterone concentration below basal concentration

NURSING CARE
N/A

ACTIVITY
• No need to alter patient's activity

DIET
• Delay feedings for at least 1–2 hours after treatments—reduces nausea and vomiting

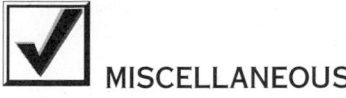

ABORTION, TERMINATION OF PREGNANCY

CLIENT EDUCATION
• Discuss patient's future; if breeding is not a consideration, OHE may be the best alternative.
• Inform client of all options, and come to a mutually agreeable treatment regimen.

SURGICAL CONSIDERATIONS
• OHE—recommended for patients with no breeding value

MEDICATIONS

DRUG(S) OF CHOICE
• $PGF_{2\alpha}$ (Lutalyse)—luteolytic; causes cervical dilation and intense uterine contractions; initiate on day 6 of diestrus; (250 μg/kg SC q12h for 5 days); perform ultrasound examination at day 28–30 diestrus; if patient is pregnant, repeat regimen on day 31–35.
• Bromocriptine mesylate (Parlodel)—a prolactin inhibitor; administer on day 31–35 of diestrus; 30 μg/kg PO q12h or 100 μg/kg PO q24h for 5–6 days; induces abortion
• $PGF_{2\alpha}$ (250 μg/kg SC q12h) and bromocriptine (10 μg/kg PO q12h)—combination produces excellent results; administered on day 6–10 of diestrus; feed patient 2 hours after morning treatment to reduce side effects (vomiting)

CONTRAINDICATIONS
• $PGF_{2\alpha}$—may increase blood pressure and cause bronchoconstriction in some species; do not use in patients with high blood pressure or asthma; do not attempt treatment with synthetic analogues (safe dosages not determined).
• Bromocriptine—some patients are sensitive to ergot alkaloids.
• Estrogens—may cause cystic endometrial hyperplasia, pyometra, and bone marrow suppression leading to pancytopenia.

PRECAUTIONS
• $PGF_{2\alpha}$—side effects are dose-dependent; include hyperpnea, hypersalivation, vomiting, and loose stools; may note mild locomotor incoordination and slight CNS depression with high dosage (440 μg/kg; LD_{50} = 5 mg/kg)
• Bromocriptine—minimal side effects; some vomiting; evacuation of uterus takes longer than with $PGF_{2\alpha}$.

POSSIBLE INTERACTIONS
Bromocriptine—concomitant use of erythromycin may increase plasma concentration of bromocriptine.

ALTERNATIVE DRUG(S)
• Dexamethasone—mode of action not known; may cause endogenous release of $PGF_{2\alpha}$; start on day 30 of diestrus at a dose of 0.1 to 0.2 mg/kg, PO, q12h for 3 doses, then 0.2 mg/kg on days 2–5, then decrease dose from 0.16 to 0.02 for last 5 doses; patients become transiently PU/PD during treatment; option when hospitalization is not an option
• Mifepristone (progesterone and glucocorticoid receptor antagonist) and epostane (inhibitor of progesterone synthesis)—potentially useful; not currently available to veterinarians in North America

FOLLOW-UP

PATIENT MONITORING
Uterine ultrasonography—confirm evacuation of uterine contents.

PREVENTION/AVOIDANCE
• OHE for bitches not intended for breeding
• Confine bitches intended for breeding

POSSIBLE COMPLICATIONS
• May shorten interestrous interval (interval to next estrous cycle)
• Treatment with estrogenic compounds contraindicated

EXPECTED COURSE AND PROGNOSIS
Fertility

☑ MISCELLANEOUS

ASSOCIATED CONDITIONS
N/A

AGE-RELATED FACTORS
N/A

ZOONOTIC POTENTIAL
N/A

PREGNANCY
N/A

SYNONYM
Induced abortion

SEE ALSO
Breeding, Timing

ABBREVIATIONS
• LH = luteinizing hormone
• OHE = ovariohysterectomy
• $PGF_{2\alpha}$ = prostaglandin $F_{2\alpha}$
• PRL = prolactin
• PU/PD = polyuria/polydipsia

Suggested Reading
Braakman A, Okkens AC, van Haaften B. Medical methods to terminate pregnancy in the dog. Compend Contin Educ Pract Vet 1993;15:1505–1512.
Concannon PW, Verstegen J, Wanke P. Pregnancy termination in dogs and cats: use of prostaglandins, dopamine agonists, or dexamethasone. Paper presented at the annual meeting of the Society of Theriogenology, 1997. Montreal, Canada, 240–244.
Johnston SD, Root Kustritz MV, Olson PNS. Prevention and termination of canine pregnancy. In: Canine and feline theriogenology. Philadelphia: Saunders, 2001:168–192.
Olson PN, Johnston SD, Root MV, et al. Terminating pregnancy in dogs and cats. Annu Reprod Sci 1992;28:399–406.
Palmer CW, Post K. Prevention of pregnancy in the dog with a combination of prostaglandin $F_{2\alpha}$ and bromocryptine. Can Vet J 2002;43:460–462.
Author Klaas Post
Consulting Editor Sara K. Lyle

ABSCESSATION

BASICS

DEFINITION
An abscess is a localized collection of purulent exudate contained within a cavity.

PATHOPHYSIOLOGY
• Bacteria are often inoculated under the skin via a puncture wound; the wound surface then seals.
• When bacteria and/or foreign objects persist in the tissue, purulent exudate forms and collects.
• Accumulation of purulent exudate—if not quickly resorbed or discharged to an external surface, stimulates formation of a fibrous capsule; may eventually lead to abscess rupture
• Prolonged delay of evacuation—formation of a fibrous abscess wall; to heal, the cavity must be filled with granulation tissue from which the causative agent may not be totally eliminated; may lead to chronic or intermittent discharge of exudate from a draining sinus tract

SYSTEMS AFFECTED
• Skin/Exocrine—percutaneous (cats > dogs); anal sac (dogs > cats)
• Gastrointestinal—pancreas (dogs > cats)
• Reproductive—prostate gland (dogs > cats); mammary gland
• Ophthalmic—periorbital tissues
• Hepatobiliary—liver parenchyma

GENETICS
N/A

INCIDENCE/PREVALENCE
N/A

GEOGRAPHIC DISTRIBUTION
N/A

SIGNALMENT

Species
Cats and dogs

Breed Predilections
N/A

Mean Age and Range
N/A

Predominant Sex
Mammary glands (female); prostate gland (male)

SIGNS

General Comments
• Determined by organ system and/or tissue affected
• Associated with a combination of inflammation (pain, swelling, redness, heat, and loss of function), tissue destruction, and/or organ system dysfunction caused by accumulation of exudate

Historical Findings
• History of traumatic insult or previous infection
• A rapidly appearing painful swelling with or without discharge, if affected area is visible

Physical Examination Findings
• Determined by the organ system or tissue affected
• A discrete mass may be detectable.
• Inflammation and discharge from a fistulous tract may be visible if the abscess is superficial and has ruptured to an external surface.
• A variably sized, painful mass of fluctuant to firm consistency attached to surrounding tissues may be palpable.
• Fever if abscess is not ruptured and draining
• Sepsis occasionally, especially if abscess ruptures internally

CAUSES
• Foreign objects
• Pyogenic bacteria—*Staphylococcus* spp.; *Escherichia coli;* β-hemolytic *Streptococcus* spp.; *Pseudomonas; Mycoplasma* and *Mycoplasma*-like organisms (L-forms); *Pasteurella multocida; Corynebacterium; Actinomyces* spp.; *Nocardia*
• Obligate anaerobes—*Bacteroides* spp.; *Clostridium* spp.; *Peptostreptococcus; Fusobacterium*

RISK FACTORS
• Anal sac—impaction; anal sacculitis
• Brain—otitis interna sinusitis oral infection
• Liver—omphalophlebitis sepsis
• Lung—foreign object aspiration bacterial pneumonia
• Mammary gland—mastitis
• Periorbital—dental disease; chewing of wood or other plant material
• Percutaneous—fighting
• Prostate gland—bacterial prostatitis
• Immunosuppression—FeLV/FIV infection, immunosuppressive chemotherapy, acquired or inherited immune system dysfunctions, underlying predisposing disease (e.g., diabetes mellitus, chronic renal failure, hyperadrenocorticism)

DIAGNOSIS

DIFFERENTIAL DIAGNOSIS

Mass Lesions
• Cyst—less or only transiently painful; slower growing
• Fibrous scar tissue—firm; nonpainful
• Granuloma—less painful; slower growing; generally firmer without fluctuant center
• Hematoma/seroma—variable pain (depends on cause); nonencapsulated; rapid initial growth but slow increase once full size is attained; unattached to surrounding tissues;

fluctuant and fluid-filled initially but more firm with organization
• Neoplasia—variable growth; consistent; painful

Draining Tracts
• Mycobacterial disease
• Mycetoma—botryomycosis, actinomycotic mycetoma, eumycotic mycetoma
• Neoplasia
• Phaeohyphomycosis
• Sporotrichosis
• Systemic fungal infection—blastomycosis, coccidioidomycosis, cryptococcosis, histoplasmosis, trichosporosis

CBC/BIOCHEMISTRY/URINALYSIS
• CBC—normal or neutrophilia with or without regenerative left shift. Neutropenia and degenerative left shift if sepsis present
• Urinalysis and serum chemistry profile—depend on system affected
• Prostatic—pyuria
• Liver and/or pancreatic—high liver enzymes and/or total bilirubin
• Pancreatic (dogs)—high amylase/lipase
• Diabetes mellitus—persistent hyperglycemia and glucosuria

OTHER LABORATORY TESTS
• FeLV and FIV—for cats with recurrent or slow healing abscesses
• CSF evaluation—increase in cellularity and protein expected with brain abscess
• Adrenal function—evaluate for hyperadrenocorticism

IMAGING
• Radiography—soft tissue density mass in affected area; may reveal foreign body
• Ultrasonography—determine if mass is fluid filled or solid; determine organ system affected; reveal flocculent-appearing fluid characteristic of pus; may reveal foreign object
• Echocardiography—helpful for diagnosis of pericardial abscess
• CT or MRI—helpful for diagnosis of brain abscess

DIAGNOSTIC PROCEDURES

Aspiration
• Reveals a red, white, yellow, or green liquid
• Protein content—> 2.5–3.0 g/dL
• Nucleated cell count—3,000–100,000 (or more) cells/μL; primarily degenerative neutrophils with lesser numbers of macrophages and lymphocytes
• Pyogenic bacteria—may be seen in cells and free within the fluid
• If the causative agent is not readily identified with a Romanovsky-type stain, specimens should be stained with an acid-fast stain to detect mycobacteria or *Nocardia* and PAS stain to detect fungus.

Biopsy
• Sample should contain both normal and abnormal tissue in the same specimen.
• Impression smears—stained and examined
• Tissue—submit for histopathologic examination and culture
• Contact the diagnostic laboratory for specific instructions.

Culture
• Affected tissue and/or exudate—aerobic and anaerobic bacteria and fungus
• Blood and/or urine—isolate bacterium responsible for possible sepsis
• Bacterial sensitivity

PATHOLOGIC FINDINGS
• Pus-containing mass lesion accompanied by inflammation
• Palpable—variably firm or fluctuant mass
• Ruptured—may see pus draining directly from the mass or an adjoining tract
• Exudate—large numbers of neutrophils in various stages of degeneration; other inflammatory cells; necrotic tissue
• Surrounding tissue—congested; fibrin; large number of neutrophils; variable number of lymphocytes; plasma cells; macrophages
• Causative agent variably detectable

TREATMENT
APPROPRIATE HEALTH CARE
• Depends on location of abscess and treatment required
• Outpatient—bite-induced abscesses
• Inpatient—sepsis; extensive surgical procedures; treatment requiring extended hospitalization
• Establish and maintain adequate drainage
• Surgical removal of nidus of infection or foreign object(s) if necessary
• Institution of appropriate antimicrobial therapy

NURSING CARE
• Depends on location of abscess
• Apply hot packs to inflamed area as needed.
• Use protective bandaging and/or Elizabethan collars as needed.
• Accumulated exudate—drain abscess; maintain drainage by medical and/or surgical means.
• Sepsis or peritonitis—aggressive fluid therapy and support

ACTIVITY
Restrict until the abscess has resolved and adequate healing of tissues has taken place.

DIET
• Sufficient nutritional intake to promote a positive nitrogen balance
• Depends on location of abscess and treatment required

CLIENT EDUCATION
• Discuss need to correct or prevent risk factors.
• Discuss need for adequate drainage and continuation of antimicrobial therapy for an adequate period of time.

SURGICAL CONSIDERATIONS
• Appropriate débridement and drainage—may need to leave the wound open to an external surface; may need to place surgical drains
• Early drainage—to prevent further tissue damage and formation of abscess wall
• Remove any foreign objects(s), necrotic tissue, or nidus of infection.

MEDICATIONS
DRUG(S) OF CHOICE
• Antimicrobial drugs—effective against the infectious agent; gain access to site of infection
• Broad-spectrum agent—bactericidal and with both aerobic and anaerobic activity; until results of culture and sensitivity are known; dogs and cats: amoxicillin (11–22 mg/kg PO q8–12h); amoxicillin/clavulanic acid (12.5–25 mg/kg PO q12h); clindamycin (5 mg/kg PO q12h); and trimethoprim/sulfadiazine (15 mg/kg PO IM q12h); cats with *Mycoplasma* and l-forms: doxycycline (3–5 mg/kg PO q12h)
• Aggressive antimicrobial therapy—sepsis or peritonitis

CONTRAINDICATIONS
N/A

PRECAUTIONS
N/A

POSSIBLE INTERACTIONS
N/A

ALTERNATIVE DRUGS
N/A

FOLLOW-UP
PATIENT MONITORING
Monitor for progressive decrease in drainage, resolution of inflammation, and improvement of clinical signs

PREVENTION/AVOIDANCE
• Percutaneous abscesses—prevent fighting
• Anal sac abscesses—prevent impaction; consider anal saculectomy for recurrent cases
• Prostatic abscesses—castration possibly helpful
• Mastitis—prevent lactation (spaying)
• Periorbital abscesses—do not allow chewing on foreign object(s)

POSSIBLE COMPLICATIONS
• Sepsis
• Peritonitis/pleuritis if intra-abdominal or intrathoracic abscess ruptures
• Compromise of organ function
• Delayed evacuation may lead to chronically draining fistulous tracts.

EXPECTED COURSE AND PROGNOSIS
Depend on organ system involved and amount of tissue destruction

MISCELLANEOUS
ASSOCIATED CONDITIONS
• FeLV or FIV infection
• Immunosuppression

AGE-RELATED FACTORS
N/A

ZOONOTIC POTENTIAL
• Minimal for pyogenic bacteria
• Mycobacteria and systemic fungal infections carry some potential.

PREGNANCY
Teratogenic agents—avoid use in pregnant animals.

SEE ALSO
• Actinomycosis
• Anaerobic Infections
• Colibacillosis
• Mycoplasmosis
• Nocardiosis
• Sepsis and Bacteremia

ABBREVIATIONS
• CSF = cerebrospinal fluid
• FeLV = feline leukemia virus
• FIV = feline immunodeficiency virus
• PAS = periodic acid-Schiff

Suggested Reading
Birchard SJ, Sherding RG, eds. Saunders manual of small animal practice. Philadelphia: Saunders, 1994.
DeBoer DJ. Nonhealing cutaneous wounds. In: August JR, ed. Consultations in feline internal medicine. Philadelphia: Saunders, 1991:101–106.
McCaw D. Lumps, bumps, masses, and lymphadenopathy. In: Ettinger SJ, Feldman EC, eds. Textbook of veterinary internal medicine. 4th ed. Philadelphia: Saunders, 1995:219–222.
Author Johnny D. Hoskins
Consulting Editor Stephen C. Barr

ACETAMINOPHEN TOXICITY

BASICS

DEFINITION
Results from owners overdosing the patient with over-the-counter acetaminophen-containing analgesic and antipyretic medications

PATHOPHYSIOLOGY
When the normal biotransformation mechanisms for detoxification (glucuronidation and sulfation) are diminished, cytochrome P450–mediated oxidation produces a toxic metabolite (*N*-acetyl benzoquinoneimine) that is electrophilic, conjugates with glutathione, and toxicologically binds to liver proteins.

Dogs
• Receipt of ≥ 150–200 mg/kg—sufficient electrophilic metabolite generated through the cytochrome P450 pathway that RBC glutathione binding produces methemoglobinemia and attacks liver proteins
• Causes hepatotoxicity in a dose-dependent fashion

Cats
• Lower ability to glucuronidate; more limited capacity for acetaminophen elimination than dogs
• Saturate glucuronidation and sulfation biotransformation routes
• Develop toxic cytochrome P450 metabolite at much lower doses than dogs
• Poisoned by as little as 50–60 mg/kg (often as little as one-half tablet); leads to rapid RBC glutathione depletion that produces rapidly developing methemoglobinemia, because of the unique feline hemoglobin molecule with eight sulfhydryl groups sensitive to oxidation
• Slower-developing hepatotoxicosis may not be fully expressed before development of fatal methemoglobinemia.

SYSTEMS AFFECTED
• Hemic/Lymph/Immune—RBCs are damaged by glutathione depletion allowing oxidation of hemoglobin to methemoglobin
• Hepatobiliary—liver necrosis
• Cardiovascular (cats)—edema of the face, paws, and (to a lesser degree) forelimbs through an undefined mechanism

GENETICS
• Cats—genetic deficiency in the glucuronide conjugation pathway makes them vulnerable.

INCIDENCE/PREVALENCE
• Most common drug toxicity in cats; considerably less frequent in dogs
• Over-the-counter medications—fourth most common cause of poison exposures in small animals

GEOGRAPHIC DISTRIBUTION
N/A

SIGNALMENT
Species
Cats more often than dogs
Breed Predilections
N/A
Mean Age and Range
N/A
Predominant Sex
N/A

SIGNS
General Comments
Relatively common—owing to increasing use in humans
Historical Findings
• Depression
• Rapid breathing
• Darkened mucous membranes
• Owner may recall warnings about acetaminophen in cats after dosing the pet.
Physical Examination Findings
• May develop 1–4 hr after dosing
• Progressive depression
• Salivation
• Vomiting
• Abdominal pain
• Tachypnea and cyanosis—reflect methemoglobinemia
• Edema—face, paws, and possibly forelimbs; after several hours
• Chocolate-colored urine—hematuria and methemoglobinuria; especially in cats
• Death

CAUSES
Acetaminophen overdosing

RISK FACTORS
• Nutritional deficiencies of glucose and/or sulfate
• Simultaneous administration of other glutathione-depressing drugs

DIAGNOSIS

DIFFERENTIAL DIAGNOSIS
• Nitrites
• Phenacetin
• Nitrobenzene
• Phenol and cresol compounds
• Sulfites
• History of exposure—important for differentiating from methemoglobin-forming drugs

CBC/BIOCHEMISTRY/URINALYSIS
• Methemoglobinemia and progressively rising serum activities of liver enzymes—characteristic
• Heinz bodies (cats)—prominent in RBCs
• Hematuria and/or hemoglobinuria

OTHER LABORATORY TESTS
• Acetaminophen serum concentration—maximally elevated 1–3 hr after ingestion; decay dose-dependent in cats (approximately 1/10 the plasma elimination rate of dogs)
• Blood glutathione level—low

IMAGING
N/A

DIAGNOSTIC PROCEDURES
N/A

PATHOLOGIC FINDINGS
• Methemoglobinemia
• Pulmonary edema
• Liver and kidney congestion
• Dogs—centrilobular necrosis of the liver; icterus in chronic cases

TREATMENT

APPROPRIATE HEALTH CARE
• With methemoglobinemia—must evaluate promptly
• With dark or bloody colored urine or icterus—inpatient

NURSING CARE
• Gentle handling—imperative for clinically affected patients
• Emesis and gastric lavage—useful within 4–6 hr of ingestion
• Anemia, hematuria, or hemoglobinuria—may require whole blood transfusion

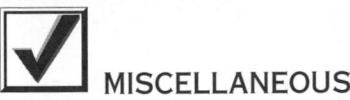
• Fluid therapy—maintain hydration and electrolyte balance
• Drinking water—available at all times
• Food—offered 24 hr after initiation of treatment

ACTIVITY
Restricted

DIET
N/A

CLIENT EDUCATION
• Warn client that treatment in clinically affected patients may be prolonged and expensive.
• Inform client that patients with liver injury may require prolonged and costly management.

SURGICAL CONSIDERATIONS
N/A

MEDICATIONS

DRUG(S) OF CHOICE
• Activated charcoal—2 g/kg PO; immediately after completion of emesis or gastric lavage
• *N*-acetylcysteine (Mucomyst)—140 mg/kg loading dose PO, IV; then 70 mg/kg PO, IV, q4h for five to seven treatments

CONTRAINDICATIONS
Drugs that contribute to methemoglobinemia or hepatotoxicity

PRECAUTIONS
Drugs requiring extensive liver metabolism or biotransformation—use with caution; expect their half-lives to be extended.

POSSIBLE INTERACTIONS
Drugs requiring activation or metabolism by the liver have reduced effectiveness.

ALTERNATIVE DRUG(S)
• Other sulfur donor drugs—if *N*-acetylcysteine not available; sodium sulfate (50 mg 1.6% solution/kg IV q4h for six treatments); effective use requires conscientious management.
• A 1% methylene blue solution—8.8 mg/kg IV q2–3h for two to three treatments;

combats methemoglobinemia without inducing a hemolytic crisis
• Ascorbic acid—125 mg/kg PO q6h for six treatments; only slowly reduces methemoglobinemia

FOLLOW-UP

PATIENT MONITORING
• Continual clinical monitoring of methemoglobinemia—vital for effective management; laboratory determination of methemoglobin percentage every 2–3 hr
• Serum liver enzyme activities (ALT, ALP)—determined every 12 hr; monitor liver damage
• Blood glutathione level—provide evidence of the effectiveness of sulfhydryl-replacement therapy.

PREVENTION/AVOIDANCE
• Never give acetaminophen to cats
• Give careful attention to the acetaminophen dose in dogs.

POSSIBLE COMPLICATIONS
Liver necrosis and resulting fibrosis—may compromise long-term liver function in recovered patients

EXPECTED COURSE AND PROGNOSIS
• Rapidly progressive methemoglobinemia—serious sign
• Methemoglobin concentrations > 50%—grave prognosis
• Progressively rising serum liver enzymes 12–24 hr after ingestion—serious concern
• Expect clinical signs to persist 12–48 hr; death owing to methemoglobinemia possible at any time
• Dogs and cats receiving prompt treatment that reverses methemoglobinemia and prevents excessive liver necrosis—may recover fully
• Dogs—death as a result of liver necrosis may occur in a few days.
• Cats—death as a result of methemoglobinemia occurs 18–36 hr after ingestion.

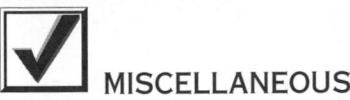
MISCELLANEOUS

ASSOCIATED CONDITIONS
N/A

AGE-RELATED FACTORS
Young and small dogs and cats—greater risk from owner-given single-dose acetaminophen medications

ZOONOTIC POTENTIAL
N/A

PREGNANCY
Imposes additional stress and higher risk on exposed animals.

SYNONYMS
• Paracetamol
• Tylenol

SEE ALSO
Poisoning (Intoxication)

ABBREVIATIONS
• ALP = alkaline phosphatase
• ALT = alanine aminotransferase

Suggested Reading
Hjelle JJ, Grauer GF. Acetaminophen-induced toxicosis in dogs and cats. J Am Vet Med Assoc 1986;188:742–746.
Oehme FW. Aspirin and acetaminophen. In: Kirk RW, ed., Current veterinary therapy IX. Small animal practice. Philadelphia: Saunders, 1986:188–189.
Rumbeiha WK, Oehme FW. Methylene blue can be used to treat methemoglobinemia in cats without inducing Heinz body hemolytic anemia. Vet Hum Toxicol 1992;34:120–122.
Savides MC, Oehme FW, Leipold HW. Effects of various antidotal treatments on acetaminophen toxicosis and biotransformation in cats. Am J Vet Res 1985;46:1485–1489.
Savides MC, Oehme FW, Nash SL, Leipold HW. The toxicity and biotransformation of single doses of acetaminophen in dogs and cats. Toxicol Appl Pharmacol 1984;74:26–34.
Author Frederick W. Oehme
Consulting Editor Gary D. Osweiler

ACIDOSIS, METABOLIC

 BASICS

DEFINITION

Primary decrease in plasma bicarbonate concentration ($[HCO_3^-]$; dogs, <18 mEq/L; cats, <16 mEq/L) with high hydrogen ion concentration ($[H^+]$), low pH, and a compensatory decrease in carbon dioxide tension (PCO_2)

PATHOPHYSIOLOGY

Acidosis results from loss of HCO_3^--rich fluid, addition of acid, acid production by metabolism, or diminished renal excretion of acid. Loss of HCO_3^--rich fluids (which have low chloride concentration) is associated with retention of chloride, which causes hyperchloremic metabolic acidosis. Addition of acids containing chloride (e.g., NH_4Cl, cationic amino acids) and chloride retention by the kidneys (e.g., renal tubular acidosis and administration of carbonic anhydrase inhibitors) also cause hyperchloremic metabolic acidosis. Addition (e.g., ethylene glycol toxicity), excessive production (e.g., lactate produced by prolonged anaerobic metabolism), or renal retention (e.g., renal failure) of anions other than chloride causes metabolic acidosis without increasing chloride concentration (so-called normochloremic or high anion gap metabolic acidosis).

SYSTEMS AFFECTED

• Respiratory—increased $[H^+]$ stimulates peripheral and central chemoreceptors to increase alveolar ventilation; hyperventilation decreases PCO_2, which counters the effects of low plasma $[HCO_3^-]$ on pH. In dogs, a decrease of approximately 0.7 mm Hg in PCO_2 is expected for each 1 mEq/L decrease in plasma $[HCO_3^-]$. Little is known about compensation in cats, but it is less effective than in dogs.
• Renal/Urologic—the kidneys increase net acid excretion, primarily by increasing excretion of NH_4^+.
• Cardiovascular—myocardial contractility is diminished and acidosis may predispose the heart to ventricular arrhythmias and ventricular fibrillation when the pH falls below 7.1.

SIGNALMENT

Any breed, age, or sex of dog and cat

SIGNS

Historical Findings

Chronic disease processes that lead to metabolic acidosis (e.g., renal failure, diabetes mellitus, and hypoadrenocorticism), exposure to toxins (e.g., ethylene glycol, salicylate, and paraldehyde), diarrhea, administration of carbonic anhydrase inhibitors (e.g., acetazolamide and dichlorphenamide)

Physical Examination Findings

• Generally relate to the underlying disease
• Depression in severely acidotic patients
• Tachypnea in some patients results from compensatory increase in ventilation.
• Kussmaul's respiration, typically seen in human beings with metabolic acidosis, is not observed in dogs and cats.

CAUSES

Associated with Hyperchloremia (Hyperchloremic Metabolic Acidosis)

• Diarrhea
• Renal tubular acidosis
• Administration of carbonic anhydrase inhibitors, amiloride, spironolactone, potassium chloride, or NH_4Cl
• Total parenteral nutrition with fluids containing cationic amino acids, lysine, arginine, and histidine
• Rapid correction of hypocapnia (chronic respiratory alkalosis)

Associated with Normochloremia (High Anion-Gap Metabolic Acidosis)

• Uremic acidosis
• Diabetic ketoacidosis
• Lactic acidosis
• Ethylene glycol, salicylate, paraldehyde, and methanol intoxication
• Hyperphosphatemia

RISK FACTORS

• Patients with chronic renal failure, diabetes mellitus, and hypoadrenocorticism are at high risk of developing metabolic acidosis as a complication of the chronic disease process.
• Patients with poor tissue perfusion or hypoxia are at risk of developing lactic acidosis.

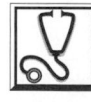 **DIAGNOSIS**

DIFFERENTIAL DIAGNOSIS

Low plasma $[HCO_3^-]$ may also be compensatory in animals with chronic respiratory alkalosis, in which PCO_2 is low and pH is low or near normal, despite decreased $[HCO_3^-]$. Blood gas determination is required to differentiate.

LABORATORY FINDINGS

Drugs That May Alter Laboratory Results

Potassium bromide is measured as chloride in most analyzers, so potassium bromide administration artificially decreases the anion gap.

Disorders That May Alter Laboratory Results

• Too much heparin (>10% of the sample) decreases $[HCO_3^-]$
• Samples stored at room temperature for more than 20 min have low pH because of increased PCO_2.
• Some blood gas analyzers only report pH and PCO_2; $[HCO_3^-]$ must be calculated, which is a potential source of error.

Valid If Run in Human Laboratory?

Yes

CBC/BIOCHEMISTRY/URINALYSIS

• Low total CO_2 (total CO_2 in serum samples handled aerobically) closely approximates the $[HCO_3^-]$ concentration; unfortunately, patients with chronic respiratory alkalosis also have low total CO_2, and the distinction cannot be made without blood gas analysis.
• Metabolic acidoses are traditionally divided into hyperchloremic and high anion gap by means of the anion gap. Anion gap, the difference between the measured cations and the measured anions, is calculated as $AG = [Na^+] - ([HCO_3^-] + [Cl^-])$ or $AG = ([Na^+] + [K^+]) - ([HCO_3^-] + [Cl^-])$, depending on the preference of the clinician or laboratory. Normal values with potassium included in the calculation are usually 12–24 mEq/L in dogs and 13–27 mEq/L in cats. The negative charges of albumin are the major contributors to the normal anion gap; thus estimation of anion gap is not reliable in patients with hypoalbuminemia.
• Normal anion gap (i.e., hyperchloremic metabolic acidosis)—most common cause is diarrhea; also, hypoadrenocorticism
• High anion gap (i.e., normochloremic metabolic acidosis)—most common causes are renal failure, diabetes mellitus, lactic acidosis (caused by tissue hypoperfusion), and hypoadrenocorticism (caused by lactic acidosis)
• Hyperglycemia—consider diabetes mellitus.
• Azotemia—consider renal failure.
• Hyperphosphatemia—consider renal failure, hypertonic sodium phosphate enema toxicity, and toxicity due to urinary acidifiers containing phosphate.

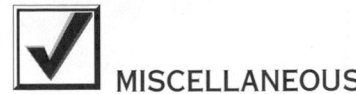

• High lactate concentration—consider lactic acidosis due to poor tissue perfusion or poor metabolism of lactate (e.g., liver disease and lymphoma).
• Hyperkalemia—the only form of metabolic acidosis that can be causative is acute hyperchloremic acidosis; otherwise, it results from the disease process causing the metabolic acidosis (e.g., renal failure and diabetes mellitus), not from the acidosis itself.

OTHER LABORATORY TESTS
Blood gas analysis reveals low $[HCO_3^-]$, low PCO_2, and low pH.

IMAGING
N/A

DIAGNOSTIC PROCEDURES
N/A

TREATMENT
• Acid–base disturbances—secondary phenomena; successful resolution depends on diagnosis and treatment of the underlying disease process.
• Treat patients with blood pH < 7.1 aggressively while pursuing the definitive diagnosis.
• Discontinue drugs that may cause metabolic acidosis.
• Nursing care—lactated Ringer's solution is the fluid of choice for patients with mild metabolic acidosis and normal liver function.

MEDICATIONS

DRUG(S) OF CHOICE
• Patients with metabolic acidosis and pH < 7.2 should receive $NaHCO_3$. Patients with high anion gap metabolic acidosis should receive enough $NaHCO_3$ to bring the pH to 7.2. These patients metabolize organic anions to HCO_3^-, and administration of HCO_3^- may predispose them to metabolic alkalosis. Patients with hyperchloremic acidosis are less likely to develop overshoot metabolic alkalosis.
• Estimation of HCO_3^- dose—dogs, 0.3 × body weight (kg) × (21 − patient $[HCO_3^-]$); cats, 0.3 × body weight (kg) × (19 − patient $[HCO_3^-]$). Give half of this dose slowly IV and reevaluate blood gases before deciding on the need for additional administration. An empirical dose of 2 mEq/kg followed by reevaluation of blood gas status is safe in most patients.

• Potential complications of $NaHCO_3$ administration—volume overload resulting from administered sodium, tetany from low ionized calcium concentration, increased affinity of hemoglobin for oxygen, paradoxical CNS acidosis, overshoot metabolic alkalosis, and hypokalemia

CONTRAINDICATIONS
• Avoid $NaHCO_3$ in patients with respiratory acidosis because it generates CO_2.
• Patients with respiratory acidosis cannot adequately excrete CO_2, and increased PCO_2 will further decrease the pH.
• Avoid diuretics that act in the distal nephron (e.g., spironolactone, triamterene, and amiloride).
• Avoid carbonic anhydrase inhibitors (e.g., acetazolamide, dichlorphenamide).

PRECAUTIONS
Use $NaHCO_3$ cautiously in patients with congestive heart failure because the sodium load may cause decompensation of the heart failure.

POSSIBLE INTERACTIONS
N/A

ALTERNATIVE DRUG(S)
• Carbicarb—an equimolar mixture of Na_2CO_3 and $NaHCO_3$; can use as alternative to bicarbonate; does not generate CO_2 and is especially useful in patients with concurrent respiratory acidosis; appears to be more effective than $NaHCO_3$ in the treatment of hypoxic lactic acidosis
• Dichloroacetate—activates pyruvate dehydrogenase complex; reduces blood lactate levels; can use as alternative to $NaHCO_3$ in patients with lactic acidosis

FOLLOW-UP

PATIENT MONITORING
Recheck acid–base status; frequency dictated by the underlying disease and patient response to treatment

POSSIBLE COMPLICATIONS
• Hyperkalemia
• Myocardial depression and ventricular arrhythmias

✓ MISCELLANEOUS

ASSOCIATED CONDITIONS
• Hyperkalemia
• Hyperchloremia

AGE-RELATED FACTORS
N/A

ZOONOTIC POTENTIAL
N/A

PREGNANCY
N/A

SYNONYMS
• Nonrespiratory acidosis
• Hyperchloremic acidosis—normal anion gap acidosis
• Normochloremic acidosis—high anion gap acidosis
• Hyperphosphatemic acidosis—metabolic acidosis resulting from high phosphate concentration
• Organic acidosis—metabolic acidosis resulting from accumulation of organic anions (e.g., ketoacidosis, uremic acidosis, and lactic acidosis)
• Dilutional acidosis—metabolic acidosis resulting from increased free water in plasma

SEE ALSO
• Diabetes with Ketoacidosis
• Hyperchloremia
• Hyperkalemia

ABBREVIATIONS
• AG = anion gap
• HCO_3^- = bicarbonate
• $NaHCO_3$ = sodium bicarbonate
• PCO_2 = carbon dioxide tension
• H^+ = hydrogen ion
• O_2 = oxygen

Suggested Reading
de Morais HSA, Muir WW. Strong ions and acid-base disorders. In: Bonagura JD, Kirk RW, eds. Kirk's current veterinary therapy XII. Philadelphia: Saunders, 1995:121–127.
DiBartola SP. Metabolic acidosis. In: DiBartola SP, ed. Fluid therapy in small animal practice. Philadelphia: Saunders, 1992: 216–243.
Muir WW, de Morais HSA. Acid-base balance: traditional and modified approaches. In: Thurmon JC, Tranquilli WJ, Benson GJ, eds. Lumb & Jones' veterinary anesthesia. 3rd ed. Baltimore: Williams & Wilkins, 1996:558–571.

Author Helio Autran de Morais
Consulting Editors Larry G. Adams and Carl A. Osborne

ACNE—CATS

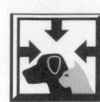

BASICS

OVERVIEW
• Some animals have a single episode; many have a lifelong recurrent problem; for a few, the disease process is continual; frequency and severity of each occurrence vary with the individual.
• Involves the chin and lower lip
• Cause unknown

SIGNALMENT
• Cats
• Any sex, age, and breed

SIGNS
• Comedones, mild erythematous papules, and serous crusts develop on the chin and less commonly on the lips.
• Sometimes swelling of the chin
• More severe cases—nodules, hemorrhagic crusts, pustules, severe erythema, alopecia, and pain
• Pain indicates furunculosis.

CAUSES & RISK FACTORS
• Poor grooming
• Abnormalities in keratinization, sebum production, or immune-barrier function

DIAGNOSIS

DIFFERENTIAL DIAGNOSIS
• Demodicosis
• *Malassezia* infection
• Feline leprosy
• Dermatophytosis
• Neoplasia of the sebaceous glands and other follicular and epidermal neoplasia
• Allergy (including eosinophilic granuloma complex)

CBC/BIOCHEMISTRY/URINALYSIS
N/A

OTHER LABORATORY TESTS
N/A

IMAGING
N/A

DIAGNOSTIC PROCEDURES
• Biopsy—rarely needed but sometimes necessary in selected cases
• Histopathologic examination—differentiate acne from other diseases such as demodicosis, dermatophytosis, and rarely neoplasia

PATHOLOGIC FINDINGS
• Mild disease—follicular distention with keratin (comedo), hyperkeratosis, and follicular plugging
• More severe disease—mild to severe folliculitis and perifolliculitis with follicular pustule formation
• Follicular rupture of keratin and hair into the dermis—leads to furunculosis, which is manifested by neutrophils and numerous macrophages surrounding the keratin debris; bacteria and *Malassezia* in these lesions are considered secondary invaders and not causative agents.

TREATMENT

• Initial treatment—one or a combination of the drugs listed below until all lesions have resolved
• Discontinue treatment by tapering medication over a 2–3-week period.
• Recurrent episodes—once the recurrence rate is determined, an appropriate maintenance protocol can be designed for each individual
• Continual episodes—lifelong treatment twice per week is necessary

MEDICATIONS

DRUG(S)
• Systemic antibiotics—amoxicillin with clavulanate, or cephalosporin alone, or a fluoroquinolone alone
• Oral medication trials—severe cases may warrant trials with isotretinoin (Accutane) or cyclosporine (Neoral)

• Shampoo—one or twice a week with antiseborrheic (sulfur–salicylic acid, benzoyl peroxide, or ethyl lactate) products
• Topical cleansing agents—benzoyl peroxide, salicylic acid
• Topical antibiotic cream—mupirocin
• Other topicals—clindamycin or erythromycin solution or ointment
• Combination topicals—benzoyl peroxide–antibiotic gels (e.g., Benzamycin)
• Topical retinoids (Retin-A 0.01% gel); tretinoin (vitamin A acid, retinoic acid)

CONTRAINDICATIONS/POSSIBLE INTERACTIONS
• Benzoyl peroxide and salicylic acids—can be irritating
• Systemic isotretinoin—use with caution, if animal will not allow application of topical medications; **CAUTION:** inform owners that it can have potential deleterious side effects in humans (drug interactions and teratogenic) if taken by mistake; container should be labeled for animal use only and kept separate from human medications to avoid accidental use.

FOLLOW-UP

• After medication is discontinued, monitor for relapses.
• Maintenance cleansing programs can be used between relapses to extend the time between episodes.

MISCELLANEOUS

PREGNANCY
Systemic isotretinoin should not be used on breeding animals.

Suggested Reading
Scott DW. Feline dermatology 1900–1978. A monograph. J Am Anim Hosp Assoc 1980;16:331–459.

Author David Duclos
Consulting Editor Karen Helton Rhodes

BASICS

OVERVIEW
• Chronic inflammatory disorder of the chin and lips of young animals
• Characterized by folliculitis and furunculosis
• Recognized almost exclusively in short-coated breeds
• Once thought that hormones played a triggering role; now speculated that genetic predisposition plays a more important role

SIGNALMENT
• Dogs
• Predisposed short-coated breeds—boxers, Doberman pinschers, English bulldogs, great Danes, weimaraners, mastiffs, rottweilers, and German short-haired pointers

SIGNS
• The area may be minimally to markedly swollen with numerous erythematous papules.
• Advanced stages—lesions may be exudative and indicate a secondary deep bacterial infection.
• Lesions may be painful on palpation.
• Chronic resolved lesions may be scarred and lichenified.

CAUSES & RISK FACTORS
Some short-coated breeds appear to be genetically predisposed to follicular keratosis and secondary bacterial infection.

DIAGNOSIS

DIFFERENTIAL DIAGNOSIS
• Dermatophytosis
• Demodicosis
• Foreign body
• Contact dermatitis

CBC/BIOCHEMISTRY/URINALYSIS
N/A

OTHER LABORATORY TESTS
N/A

IMAGING
N/A

DIAGNOSTIC PROCEDURES
• Bacterial culture and sensitivity testing—in patients with suppurative folliculitis and furunculosis that are non-responsive to initial antibiotic selection
• Biopsy—histologic confirmation for cases in which diagnosis is in question

PATHOLOGIC FINDINGS
• Clinical signs and histopathologic findings are diagnostic.
• Initial lesions—hairless follicular papules; characterized histopathologically by marked follicular keratosis, plugging, dilatation, and perifolliculitis
• Bacteria—in the early stages: not seen and cannot be isolated from lesions
• As disease progresses: papules enlarge and rupture, promoting a suppurative folliculitis and furunculosis.

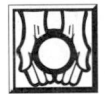

TREATMENT
• Depends on the severity and chronicity of the disease
• Reduce behavioral trauma to the chin (e.g., rubbing on the carpet, chewing bones that increase salivation)
• Frequent cleaning with benzoyl peroxide shampoo or gel or mupirocin ointment to reduce the bacterial numbers on the surface of the skin
• Instruct owners to avoid expressing the lesions, which may cause internal rupture of the papule and massive inflammation.

MEDICATIONS

DRUG(S)
Topical
• Benzoyl peroxide shampoo or gel (antibacterial)
• Mupirocin ointment (antibacterial-staph)
• Isotretinoin (Retin-A) or tretinoin (vitamin A acid, retinoic acid gel)—may reduce follicular keratosis
• Corticosteroids—may be necessary to reduce inflammation

Systemic
• Antibiotics appropriate for deep bacterial infection—especially cephalosporins (Cephalexin, 22 mg/kg PO q8h for 6–8 weeks)
• May need to perform bacterial culture and sensitivity test.

CONTRAINDICATIONS/POSSIBLE INTERACTIONS
• Benzoyl peroxide—may bleach carpets and fabrics; may be irritating
• Mupirocin ointments—greasy
• Topical retinoids—may be drying and irritating
• Topical steroids—may cause adrenal suppression with repeated use

FOLLOW-UP
Long-term topical treatment required

MISCELLANEOUS

Suggested Reading
Scott DW, Miller WH, Griffin CE. Bacterial skin diseases. In: Kirk's small animal dermatology. 5th ed. Philadelphia: Saunders, 1995:304–305.
Author Karen Helton Rhodes
Consulting Editor Karen Helton Rhodes

ACRAL LICK DERMATITIS

BASICS

OVERVIEW
A firm, raised, ulcerative, or thickened plaque that is usually located on the dorsal aspect of the carpus, metacarpus, tarsus, or metatarsus

SIGNALMENT
• Primarily dogs
• Most common in large breeds—especially Doberman pinschers, Labrador retrievers, Great Danes, Irish and English setters, golden retrievers, akitas, Dalmatians, shar peis, and Weimaraners
• Age at onset—varies with the cause
• Sex predilection—some sources suggest more common in males; others indicate no preference

SIGNS
• Excessive licking and chewing of the affected area
• Occasionally a history of trauma to the affected area
• Alopecic, ulcerative, thickened, and raised firm plaques, usually located on the dorsal aspect of the carpus, metacarpus, tarsus, or metatarsus
• Lesions often occur singly, although they may occur in more than one location.

CAUSES & RISK FACTORS
Associated diseases—staphylococcal furunculosis, allergy, endocrinopathy, demodicosis, dermatophytosis, foreign body reaction, neoplasia, arthritis, trauma, and psychogenic and sensory nerve dysfunction

DIAGNOSIS

DIFFERENTIAL DIAGNOSIS
• Allergic animals often have multiple lick granulomas and other areas of pruritus compatible with the specific allergy.
• Endocrinopathies, infectious, neoplasia, demodicosis, and dermatophytosis—determined on the basis of laboratory test results

CBC/BIOCHEMISTRY/URINALYSIS
Normal except in cases of hyper-adrenocorticism

OTHER LABORATORY TESTS
• Low thyroid levels—suggests hypothyroidism
• Abnormal ACTH-stimulation test or abnormal LDDST—suggests hyperadrenocorticism

IMAGING
Radiology—neoplasia; some forms of trauma; radiopaque foreign bodies; bony proliferation may be seen secondary to the chronic irritation.

DIAGNOSTIC PROCEDURES
• Examine skin scrapings, dermatophyte culture, and Tzanck preparations—rule out demodicosis, dermatophytosis, or a bacterial infection
• Bacterial culture and sensitivity (if indicated)—determine appropriate antibiotics
• Food-elimination diet—determine food allergy
• Intradermal allergy testing—helpful for atopic animals
• Biopsy—to rule out neoplasia, if necessary

PATHOLOGIC FINDINGS
Histopathology—ulcerative, hyperplastic epidermis with mild perivascular dermatitis; varying degrees of fibroplasia

TREATMENT
• Affected animal must get plenty of attention and exercise.
• Diet—no modification unless an allergy is suspected
• Difficult to treat, especially if no underlying cause is found; warn owner that patience and time are necessary.
• Surgery—do not consider until all other therapies have been exhausted; will often cause increased licking and attention to the affected area, resulting in poor wound closure; if underlying causes are not addressed, recurrence is likely.

MEDICATIONS

DRUG(S)

Antibiotics
• Based on bacterial culture and sensitivity
• Give until infection is completely resolved, often at least 6 weeks.

Systemic
• Hydroxyzine HCl (1–2 mg/kg PO q8h)
• Chlorpheniramine (4–8 mg/dog q12h PO; maximum of 0.5 mg/kg q12h)
• Naltrexone (2.2 mg/kg PO q12–24h)
• Amitriptyline HCl (1.1–2.2 mg/kg PO q12h); used at the lower dosage for 10 days; if no improvement, use at the higher dosage for 10 days
• Doxepin may also be tried (3–5 mg/kg PO q12h; maximum 150 mg q12h).
• CAUTION: none of these medications should be used concurrently.

Topical
• Flunixin meglumine and fluocinolone in dimethyl sulfoxide (combined), mupirocin, topical 5% benzoyl peroxide, and capsaicin products
• Intralesional corticosteroids have been advocated but are rarely helpful.
• Topical medications should be applied with gloves.

• Animals should be kept from licking the area for 10–15 min.

Other
• After all other underlying diseases have been ruled out or treated, therapies for psychogenic dermatoses may be tried.
• Psychotropic drugs—fluoxetine hydrochloride (1 mg/kg PO q24h) or clomipramine hydrochloride (1–3 mg/kg PO q24h)
• Physical restraints—Elizabethan collars and bandaging; short-term use
• Ablation of the lesion with laser therapy has been proposed but no publications evaluating the efficacy of this modality are currently available.

CONTRAINDICATIONS/POSSIBLE INTERACTIONS
• Doxepin—do not use with monoamine oxidase inhibitors, clonidine, anticonvulsants, oral anticoagulants, steroid hormones, antihistamines, or aspirin.
• Antihistamines—do not use more than one at a time.
• Hydroxyzine may decrease seizure threshold. Avoid in epileptics.

FOLLOW-UP
• Monitor level of licking and chewing closely.
• Treat underlying disease to prevent recurrence.
• If no underlying disease is detected, suspect psychogenic causes (obsessive-compulsive or self-mutilation disorder); prognosis is guarded.
• Cardiotoxicity and hepatoxicity have been reported in rare cases in animals on tricyclics. Select and monitor patients with caution.

MISCELLANEOUS

AGE-RELATED FACTORS
Dogs < 5 years old—strongly consider allergy

ZOONOTIC POTENTIAL
Transmitted to humans only if dermatophytosis is the underlying cause; exceedingly rare

ABBREVIATION
LDDST = low-dose dexamethasone-suppression test

Suggested Reading
Shanley K, Overall K. Psychogenic dermatoses. In: Kirk RW, Bonagura JD, eds. Current veterinary therapy XI. Philadelphia: Saunders, 1992:552–557.

Authors Karen A. Kuhl and Jean S. Greek
Consulting Editor Karen Helton Rhodes

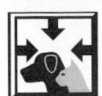

BASICS

OVERVIEW
• A clinical syndrome resulting from growth hormone (somatotropin) hypersecretion by tumorous somatotrophs in the anterior pituitary of adult cats • Clinical signs are a consequence of growth hormone's direct catabolic and indirect anabolic effects. • The anabolic effects are mediated by somatomedin C (insulin-like growth factor I), which is secreted by the liver in response to growth hormone stimulation. Somatomedin C promotes protein synthesis and growth in a variety of tissues. Excessive somatomedin C levels cause abnormal growth of bone (particularly membranous bone), cartilage, soft tissues, and visceral organs. • The bony and soft tissue changes are most prominent in the head and neck region and distal extremities.
• Abnormalities in articular cartilage growth and metabolism alter normal joint biomechanics, which can lead to degenerative joint disease. • Cardiac hypertrophy frequently results in congestive heart failure. The clinical signs and cardiac pathology are very similar to those seen with idiopathic feline hypertrophic cardiomyopathy. • The catabolic actions of growth hormone result from insulin antagonism leading eventually to pancreatic β cell exhaustion. The resultant diabetes mellitus is permanent.

SIGNALMENT
• A rare disease of cats • The average age of affected cats is 10 years; reported range is 8–14 years. • Over 90% of the reported cases have been in males.

SIGNS
Initially signs relate to unregulated diabetes mellitus. As the disease progresses, signs of heart failure, renal failure, or CNS abnormalities caused by tumor expansion frequently develop.
• Polyuria, polydipsia, and polyphagia in all reported cases. • Weight loss is common at presentation; over time many patients gain weight and have increased body size due to increased bone and soft tissue mass, not from increased adipose tissue. Weight gain in an unregulated diabetic cat strongly suggests acromegaly. • Often broadening of the facial features and prognathia inferior develop.
• Abdominal palpation may detect organ enlargement. • Systolic heart murmurs develop commonly; ~50% of acromegalic cats have congestive heart failure • As the pituitary tumor expands, some cats may develop seizures or other CNS signs very late in the disease process.

CAUSES & RISK FACTORS
• Caused by growth hormone hypersecretion by an anterior pituitary acidophil adenoma
• Progesterones, endogenous or exogenous, do not cause growth hormone secretion and acromegaly in cats, unlike in dogs.

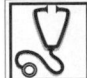

DIAGNOSIS

DIFFERENTIAL DIAGNOSIS
• Diabetes mellitus, hyperthyroidism, hyperadrenocorticism, pancreatic exocrine insufficiency, and renal failure all cause clinical signs resembling those seen in acromegalic cats.
• Insulin-resistant diabetes mellitus (>2.0 U of insulin/kg/dose) was found in all reported cases of feline acromegaly and tends to increase over time. Insulin requirements of 20–130 U/day (average dose, 9.8 U/kg/day) have been reported in acromegalic cats. • A presumptive diagnosis of feline acromegaly is reached by ruling out other causes of insulin-resistant diabetes mellitus.

CBC/BIOCHEMISTRY/URINALYSIS
• Most laboratory abnormalities are caused by unregulated diabetes mellitus. • Laboratory evidence of renal failure may become evident in the later stages of the disease. • Hyperglycemia (100%), hyperproteinemia with normal pattern of distribution on serum electrophoresis (~50%), hyperphosphatemia without azotemia (~50%), hypercholesterolemia (~50%), and azotemia (~50%). • Glucosuria (100%) ketonuria is unusual. • Proteinuria in >50% of affected cats and in all that go on to develop renal failure

OTHER LABORATORY TESTS
• Demonstration of elevated basal serum growth hormone levels in a cat with insulin-resistant diabetes mellitus is diagnostic for acromegaly; unfortunately, no validated growth hormone assay is currently available. • A radioimmunoassay for plasma somatomedin C is available at Michigan State University; a significant elevation in plasma somatomedin C levels in a cat with insulin-resistant diabetes mellitus strongly supports a diagnosis of acromegaly.

IMAGING

Radiography: • Mild-to-moderate cardiomegaly is found in most affected cats; cardiac enlargement tends to worsen over time. • Pulmonary edema in patients that develop left-sided congestive heart failure • Marked vertebral spondylosis is common.
• Degenerative arthropathy is common.

Echocardiography: The interventricular septum and/or left ventricular free wall is usually thickened.

CT or MRI: Identified a pituitary mass in most acromegalic cats that have been scanned

TREATMENT
• Therapy is usually palliative, not curative.
• Aim medical treatment at controlling or ameliorating the secondary diseases (i.e., diabetes mellitus, heart failure, and kidney failure) that develop following prolonged growth hormone hypersecretion. • Cobalt

radiotherapy was used in a small number (7) of acromegalic cats—6 of them showed permanent or transient resolution of insulin resistance following therapy; in 4 cats, insulin therapy was discontinued 4–16 months after cobalt radiotherapy, but 2 of them eventually became diabetic again; 1 cat had resolution of CNS signs following therapy; plasma growth hormone or somatomedin C levels decreased following therapy in 5 of the treated cats.
• Cobalt radiotherapy shows promise as a palliative and, in some instances, a definitive treatment. • Surgical removal of small, noninvasive pituitary adenomas is frequently curative in humans with acromegaly; most affected cats have large tumors, which would markedly decrease the chance for complete surgical removal; surgical removal has not been described in cats. • Cryohypophysectomy was described in one acromegalic cat—plasma somatomedin C slowly returned to normal over a period of months, and the cat's diabetes mellitus resolved ~2 months after cryosurgery. The cat did not develop hypoadrenocorticism, hypothyroidism, or central diabetes mellitus, as occurs when surgical hypophysectomy is performed.

MEDICATIONS
• In humans, dopamine agonists and the long-acting somatostatin analogue octreotide have been used with variable success to inhibit pituitary growth hormone secretion; dopamine agonists have not been used in cats with acromegaly, and octreotide therapy has not been effective. • Diabetes mellitus is treated with insulin; goals are to prevent ketoacidosis and to minimize clinical signs associated with diabetes mellitus. High-dose (>2.2 U/kg/dose), twice-daily insulin therapy is usually required.
• Patients with heart failure have responded well to diuretic therapy; concurrent therapy with diltiazem, atenolol, and/or an angiotensin-converting enzyme inhibitor may be appropriate, based on clinical signs, cardiac ultrasound, or electrocardiogram abnormalities.

FOLLOW-UP
• Patients are usually euthanized or die because of congestive heart failure, renal failure, and/or progressive CNS signs. • Reported survival times following diagnosis vary between 4 and 42 months; median survival time is 20 months.

MISCELLANEOUS

Suggested Reading
Peterson ME, Taylor RS, Greco DS, et al. Acromegaly in 14 cats. JVIM 1990;4:192–201.
Author John W. Tyler
Consulting Editor Deborah S. Greco

ACTINOMYCOSIS

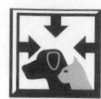 BASICS

OVERVIEW

• An infectious disease caused by gram-positive, branching, pleomorphic, rod-shaped bacteria of the genus *Actinomyces*
• *A. viscosus*—most commonly identified; survives in microaerophilic or anaerobic conditions
• Rarely found as the single bacterial agent in a lesion; more commonly, it is a component of a polymicrobial infection.
• There may be synergism between *Actinomyces* and other organisms.

SIGNALMENT

• Dogs and cats
• Especially common in young male dogs of sporting breeds

SIGNS

• Infections—usually localized; may be disseminated; cervicofacial area commonly involved
• Cutaneous swellings or abscesses with draining tracts—yellow granules ("sulfur granules") may be seen in associated exudates.
• Pain and fever
• Exudative pleural or peritoneal effusions
• Retroperitonitis—in one study, *Actinomyces* was identified in 3 of 34 affected dogs.
• Osteomyelitis of vertebrae or long bones—probably secondary to extension of cutaneous infection; lameness or a swollen extremity may develop.
• Motor and sensory deficits—reported with spinal cord compression by granulomas

CAUSES & RISK FACTORS

• *Actinomyces* spp.—normal inhabitants of the oral cavity of dogs and cats
• Loss of normal protective barriers (mucosa, skin), immunosuppression, or change in the bacterial microenvironment could predispose animals; thought to occur as an opportunistic infection
• Specific risk factors—trauma (bite wound), migrating foreign body (foxtail in the western U.S.), and periodontal disease

 DIAGNOSIS

DIFFERENTIAL DIAGNOSIS

• Nocardiosis—primary differential diagnosis; *Actinomyces* not reliably distinguished from *Nocardia* spp. by gram staining, cytology, or clinical signs • Other causes of chronic draining tracts and pleural or peritoneal effusions must be addressed.

CBC/BIOCHEMISTRY/URINALYSIS

• Leukocytosis with a left shift and monocytosis—common
• Nonregenerative anemia—may develop
• Hypoglycemia and hyperglobulinemia—common

OTHER LABORATORY TESTS

N/A

IMAGING

Radiographs of infected bone—periosteal new bone production, reactive osteosclerosis, and osteolysis

DIAGNOSTIC PROCEDURES
• Pus or osteolytic bone fragments submitted in anaerobic specimen containers for culture (see Anaerobic Infections) provide the only definitive diagnosis; inform the lab to check for actinomycosis.
• Fresh smears—gram staining, cytology, and acid-fast staining; staining does not preclude the need for culture; *Actinomyces* does not stain acid-fast; *Nocardia* is variable.

PATHOLOGIC FINDINGS
Histopathologic examination—not reliable for distinguishing actinomycosis from nocardiosis; useful diagnostic tool, especially with sulfur granules; may demonstrate pyogranulomatous or granulomatous cellulitis with colonies of filamentous bacteria

TREATMENT
• Drain abscesses and lavage for several days; leave lesions open for continued drainage; Penrose drains may be needed.
• Bony involvement—may need to débride or remove bone.
• Surgical resection of tissue—not needed in all cases

MEDICATIONS

DRUG(S)
• Important to distinguish between *Actinomyces* and *Nocardia* for appropriate antimicrobial selection
• Antibiotics—a retrospective study suggests administration for a minimum of 3–4 months after resolution of all signs; may need to be directed against other associated microbes
• Penicillin G—considered to be reliable; specific recommendations for duration of therapy are not determined; try 65,000 U/kg q8h.
• Metronidazole—avoid use; actinomycosis unlikely to respond
• Aminoglycosides—do not use; ineffective against anaerobic infections
• *A. hordeovulneris*—cell-wall deficient variant (L-phase); does not usually respond well to penicillin; consider clindamycin, erythromycin, and chloramphenicol.

CONTRAINDICATIONS/POSSIBLE INTERACTIONS
N/A

FOLLOW-UP
• Redevelopment of infection at the initial site may be expected in about half of all cases.
• Monitor patients closely for recurrence in the months after discontinuation of therapy.

MISCELLANEOUS
Suggested Reading
Edwards DF. Actinomycosis and nocardiosis. In: Greene CE, ed. Infectious diseases of the dog and cat. Philadelphia: Saunders, 1998:303–313.
Author Sharon Fooshee Grace
Consulting Editor Stephen C. Barr

ACUTE ABDOMEN

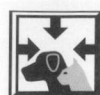

BASICS

DEFINITION
Characterized by historical and physical examination findings of a tense, painful abdomen; cardinal sign is acute abdominal pain; May be life-threatening and should be treated as an emergency.

PATHOPHYSIOLOGY
• A patient with an acute abdomen has pain associated with either distention of an organ, inflammation, traction on the mesentery or peritoneum, or ischemia. • The abdominal viscera are sparsely innervated, and diffuse involvement is often necessary to elicit pain; nerve endings also exist in the submucosa-muscularis of the bowel wall. • Any process that causes fluid or gaseous distension (i.e., intestinal obstruction, gastric dilatation-volvulus, ileus) may produce pain. • Inflammation produces abdominal pain by releasing vasoactive substances that directly stimulate nerve endings. • Many nerves in the peritoneum are sensitive to a diffuse inflammatory response.

SYSTEMS AFFECTED
• Behavioral—trembling, inappetence, crying, lethargy or depression, and abnormal postural changes such as the praying position to achieve comfort • Cardiovascular—severe inflammation, ischemia, and sepsis may lead to acute circulatory collapse (shock). • Gastrointestinal—vomiting, diarrhea, inappetance, generalized functional ileus; pancreatic inflammation, necrosis, and abscesses may lead to cranial abdominal pain, vomiting, and ileus. • Hepatobiliary—jaundice associated with extrahepatic cholestasis from biliary obstructions (including pancreatitis) and bile peritonitis • Renal/Urologic—azotemia can be due to prerenal causes (dehydration, hypovolemia, and shock), renal causes (acute pyelonephritis and acute renal failure), and postrenal causes (urethral obstruction and uroperitoneum from bladder rupture). • Respiratory—increased respiratory rate due to pain or metabolic disturbances.

SIGNALMENT
• Dog and cat • Younger animals tend to have a higher incidence of trauma-related problems, intussusceptions, and acquired diet- and infection-related diseases; old animals have a greater frequency of malignancies. • Male cats and dogs are at higher risk for urethral obstruction. • Male dalmatians in particular have a higher risk of urethral obstruction because of the high incidence of urate urinary calculi. • German shepherds with pancreatic atrophy have a higher risk of mesenteric volvulus.

• Patients treated with corticosteroids and nonsteroidal antiinflammatory drugs (NSAIDs) are at higher risk for gastrointestinal (GI) ulceration and perforation.

SIGNS

General Comments
Clinical signs vary greatly depending on the type and severity of the disease leading to an acute abdomen.

Historical Findings
• Trembling, reluctance to move, inappetance, vomiting, diarrhea, crying, and abnormal postures (tucked up or praying position)—signs that the owner may notice • Question owner carefully to ascertain what system is affected; for example, hematemesis with a history of NSAID treatment suggests GI mucosal disruption.

Physical Examination Findings
• Abnormalities include abdominal pain, splinting of the abdominal musculature, gas- or fluid-filled abdominal organs, abdominal mass, ascites, pyrexia or hypothermia, tachycardia, and tachypnea. • Once abdominal pain is confirmed, attempt to localize the pain to cranial, middle, or caudal abdomen. • Perform a rectal examination to evaluate the colon, pelvic bones, urethra, and prostate, as well as the presence of melena. • Rule out extraabdominal causes of pain by careful palpation of the kidneys and thoracolumbar vertebrae. • Pain associated with intervertebral disk disease often causes referred abdominal splinting and is often mistaken for true abdominal pain.

CAUSES

Gastrointestinal
• Stomach—gastritis, ulcers, perforation, foreign bodies, gastric dilatation-volvulus • Intestine—obstruction (foreign bodies, intussusception, hernias), ulcers, perforations • Rupture after obstruction, ulceration, blunt or penetrating trauma or due to tumor growth • Vascular compromise from infarction, mesenteric volvulus, or torsion

Pancreas
• Pain associated with inflammation, abscess, ischemia. • Pancreatic masses or inflammation obstructing the biliary duct/papilla will cause jaundice.

Hepatic and Biliary System
• Rapid distention of the liver and its capsule can cause pain. • Gall bladder obstructions, ruptures, or necrosis may lead to bile leakage and peritonitis. • Hepatic abscess

Spleen
Splenic torsion, ruptured splenic masses, splenic abscess

Urinary Tract
• Distention is the main cause of pain in the urinary tract. • Lower urinary tract obstruction

can be due to tumors of the trigone area of the bladder or urethra, urinary calculi, or granulomatous urethritis. • Traumatic ruptures of the ureters or bladder are associated with blunt trauma and increased intraabdominal pressure. • Urethral tears can be associated with pelvic fractures from acute trauma. • Free urine in the peritoneal cavity leads to a chemical peritonitis. • Acute pyelonephritis, acute renal failure, nephroliths, and ureteroliths are uncommon causes of acute abdomen.

Genital Tract
• Prostatitis and prostatic abscess, pyometra; a ruptured pyometra or prostatic abscess can cause endotoxemia, sepsis, and cardiovascular collapse. • Infrequent causes include ruptures of the gravid uterus after blunt abdominal trauma, uterine torsion, ovarian tumor or torsion, and intraabdominal testicular torsion (cryptorchid).

Abdominal Wall/Diaphragm
• Umbilical, inguinal, scrotal, abdominal, or peritoneal hernias with strangulated viscera • Trauma or congenital defects leading to organ displacement or entrapment in the hernia will lead to abdominal pain if the vascular supply of the organs involved becomes impaired or ischemic.

RISK FACTORS
• Exposure to NSAIDs or corticosteroid treatment—gastric, duodenal, or colonic ulcers • Garbage or inappropriate food ingestion—pancreatitis • Foreign body ingestion—intestinal obstructions • Abdominal trauma—hollow viscus rupture • Hernias—intestinal obstruction/strangulation

DIAGNOSIS

DIFFERENTIAL DIAGNOSIS
• Renal associated pain, retroperitoneal pain, spinal or paraspinal pain, and disorders causing diffuse muscle pain may mimic abdominal pain; careful history and physical examination are essential in pursuing the appropriate problem. • Parvoviral enteritis can present similarly to intestinal obstructive disease; fecal parvoviral antigen assay and CBC (leukopenia) are helpful differentiating diagnostic tests.

CBC/BIOCHEMISTRY/URINALYSIS
• Inflammation or infection may be associated with leukocytosis or leukopenia. • Anemia may be seen with blood loss associated with GI ulceration. • Azotemia is associated with prerenal, renal, and postrenal causes. • Electrolyte abnormalities can help to evaluate GI disease (i.e., hypochloremic metabolic alkalosis with gastric outflow obstruction) and renal disease (i.e., hyperkalemia with acute renal failure or postrenal obstruction). • Hyperbilirubinemia

and elevated hepatic enzymes help localize a problem to the liver or biliary tract. • Urine specific gravity (before fluid therapy) needed to differentiate prerenal, renal, and postrenal problems. • Urine sediment may be helpful in acute renal failure, ethylene glycol intoxication, and pyelonephritis.

OTHER LABORATORY TESTS

Trypsin-like immunoreactivity (TLI) can be useful in evaluating feline pancreatitis. Canine pancreatic lipase immunoreactivity is useful for canine pancreatitis.

IMAGING

Abdominal Radiography

• May see abdominal masses or changes in shape or shifting of abdominal organs • Loss of abdominal detail with abdominal fluid accumulation is an indication for a peritoneal tap. • Free abdominal gas is consistent with a ruptured GI viscus or infection with gas-producing bacteria and is an indication for emergency surgery. • Use caution when evaluating postoperative radiographs; free gas is a normal finding for a few days postoperatively. • Ileus is a consistent sign with peritonitis. • Contrast in the area of the pancreas can be lost with pancreatic inflammation. • Foreign bodies may be radiopaque. • Characterize ileus as functional (due to metabolic or infectious causes) or mechanical (due to obstruction). • Upper GI barium contrast radiographs are useful in evaluating the GI tract, particularly for determination of GI obstruction.

Abdominal Ultrasound

A sensitive diagnostic tool for the detection of abdominal masses, abdominal fluid, abscesses, cysts, lymphadenopathy, and biliary or urinary calculi

DIAGNOSTIC PROCEDURES

Abdominocentesis/Abdominal Fluid Analysis

• Perform abdominocentesis on all patients presenting with acute abdomen. Fluid can often be obtained for diagnostic evaluation even when only a small amount of free abdominal fluid exists, well before detectable radiographic sensitivity. Although ultrasonography is much more sensitive than radiography for the detection of fluid, the lack of such detection does not preclude abdominocentesis. Abdominal fluid analysis with elevated WBC count, degenerate neutrophils, and intracellular bacteria is consistent with septic peritonitis and is an indication for immediate surgery. • Pancreatitis patients may have an abdominal effusion characterized as a nonseptic (sterile) peritonitis. • Creatinine concentration higher in abdominal fluid than in serum indicates urinary tract leakage. • Similarly, higher bilirubin concentration in abdominal fluid than in serum indicates bile peritonitis.

Sedation and Abdominal Palpation

Because of abdominal splinting associated with pain, a thorough abdominal palpation is often not possible without sedation; this is particularly useful for detecting intestinal foreign bodies that do not appear on survey radiographs.

Exploratory Laparotomy

Surgery may be useful diagnostically (as well as therapeutically) when ultrasonography is not available or when no definitive cause of the acute abdomen has been established with appropriate diagnostics.

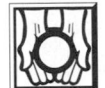

TREATMENT

Inpatient management with supportive care until decision about whether the problem is to be treated medically or surgically.

Supportive Care

• Keep patient NPO if vomiting, until a definitive cause is determined and addressed. • Intravenous fluid therapy is usually required because of the large fluid loss associated with an acute abdomen; the goal is to restore the normal circulating blood volume. • If severe circulatory compromise (shock) exists, supplement initially with isotonic crystalloid fluids (90 mL/kg, dogs; 70 mL/kg, cats) over 1–2 hr; hypertonic fluids or colloids may also be beneficial. • Evaluate hydration and electrolytes (with appropriate treatment adjustments) frequently after commencement of treatment.

Surgical Considerations

• Many different causes of an acute abdomen (with both medical and surgical treatments) exist; make a definitive diagnosis whenever possible prior to surgical intervention. • This can prevent both potentially unnecessary and expensive surgical procedure and associated morbidity and mortality. • It will also allow the surgeon to prepare for the task and to educate the owner on the prognosis and costs involved.

MEDICATIONS

DRUG(S)

Corticosteroids (Soluble Glucocorticoids)

• When indicated for shock treatment; limit to single doses to avoid adverse effects on the GI tract • Dexamethasone sodium phosphate 2–4 mg/kg IV or prednisolone sodium succinate 15–30 mg/kg IV

Histamine H_2 Antagonists

• Reduce gastric acid production. • Cimetidine 5–10 mg/kg IV q8h or ranitidine 0.5–1 mg/kg IV q12h

Sucralfate

• Gastric mucosal protectant, 0.25–1 g PO q8h

Metoclopramide

Antiemetic as needed, 0.2–0.4 mg/kg IV q6–8h (or 24 hr continuous rate infusion)

Antibiotics

• Broad spectrum for gram-positive, gram-negative, and anaerobic bacteria • Gram stain and cultures prior to treatment if possible

CONTRAINDICATIONS

Do not use metoclopramide if GI obstruction is suspected.

PRECAUTIONS

Gentamicin and most NSAIDs can be nephrotoxic and should be used with caution in hypovolemic patients and those with renal impairment.

FOLLOW-UP

PATIENT MONITORING

Patients usually require intensive medical care and frequent evaluation of vital signs and laboratory parameters.

MISCELLANEOUS

SYNONYMS

Colic

SEE ALSO

• Gastric Dilatation and Volvulus Syndrome • Gastrointestinal Obstruction • Gastroduodenal Ulcer Disease • Intussusception • Pancreatitis • Prostatitis and Prostatic Abscess • Urinary Tract Obstruction

Suggested Reading

Bjorling DE. Acute abdomen syndrome. In: Morgan RV, ed. Handbook of small animal practice. New York: Churchill Livingstone, 1992:483–487.

Bjorling DE, Latimer KS, Rawlings CA, et al. Diagnostic peritoneal lavage before and after abdominal surgery in dogs. Am J Vet Res 1983;44:816–819.

Crowe DT, Crane SW. Diagnostic abdominal paracentesis and lavage in the evaluation of abdominal injuries in dogs and cats: Clinical and experimental investigations. J Am Vet Med Assoc 1976;168:700–705.

Strombeck DR, Guilford WG. Small animal gastroenterology. 2nd ed. Davis, CA: Stonegate Publishing, 1990:81–86.

Acknowledgment

The author/editors acknowledge the prior contributions of Dr. Juan Carlos Sardinas, who authored this topic in the previous edition.

Author Albert E. Jergens
Consulting Editor Albert E. Jergens

ACUTE RESPIRATORY DISTRESS SYNDROME

BASICS

DEFINITION
Syndrome of acute onset of respiratory failure typified by diffuse bilateral pulmonary infiltrates on a thoracic radiograph with no evidence of increased hydrostatic pressure, cardiogenic pulmonary edema, or fluid overload. It can be divided into 2 categories based on severity. The less severe form is called acute lung injury (ALI); ALI is defined as a P_aO_2/F_IO_2 ratio of <300.

PATHOPHYSIOLOGY
• Acute respiratory distress syndrome (ARDS) is due to a diffuse inflammatory insult to the lungs resulting in increased permeability of the alveolar-capillary interface. This inflammatory insult can be triggered by primary pulmonary disease or it can be of non-pulmonary origin. Mechanisms may include neutrophil activation, proinflammatory cytokines, and/or ventilator-induced lung injury.
• Acute exudative phase—initially protein-rich edema fluid and white blood cells flood into the interstitium and alveoli. Neutrophils and alveolar macrophages exacerbate the damage by further release of cytokines and inflammatory mediators. The collapse and consolidation of alveoli produces severe hypoxemia and dyspnea. Microthrombi of the pulmonary vasculature, hypoxic pulmonary vasoconstriction, and endogenous vasoconstrictors cause pulmonary hypertension which, if severe, can lead to right-sided heart failure.
• Hyaline membrane phase—hyaline membrane formation in the alveolar spaces 3–7 days after initial insult
• Fibroproliferative phase—if the patient survives the initial 3–7 days, proliferation of type 2 pneumocytes and pulmonary fibrosis occurs.

SYSTEMS AFFECTED
• Respiratory • Cardiovascular—right-sided heart failure secondary to pulmonary hypertension

GENETICS
Some humans may be more prone to developing ARDS than others. Whether this is true in the veterinary population is unknown.

INCIDENCE/PREVALENCE
Unknown

GEOGRAPHIC DISTRIBUTION
N/A

SIGNALMENT
Species
Dogs and cats
Breed Predispositions
N/A
Mean Age and Range
N/A
Predominant Sex
N/A

SIGNS
Historical Findings
• Acute onset of respiratory distress in a patient with a significant underlying disease
• Animal is often hospitalized for its primary disease when it develops ARDS

Physical Examination Findings
• Severe respiratory distress
• Crackles (if present) heard bilaterally on auscultation
• Fever
• Cyanosis in more severe cases
• Signs relevant to the primary disease process

CAUSES
Primary Pulmonary Causes
• Aspiration pneumonia
• Pneumonia
• Pulmonary contusion
• Near drowning
• Smoke inhalation

Non-pulmonary Causes
• Sepsis
• Pancreatitis
• Severe trauma and shock

RISK FACTORS
• Systemic inflammatory response syndrome
• Sepsis
• Severity of illness
• Multiple transfusions

DIAGNOSIS

DIFFERENTIAL DIAGNOSIS
• Left-sided congestive heart failure
• Fluid overload
• Diffuse pneumonia
• Pulmonary hemorrhage

CBC/BIOCHEMISTRY/URINALYSIS
• Leukocytosis or leukopenia
• Other changes dependent on the underlying disease process

OTHER LABORATORY TESTS
• Arterial blood gases—low P_aO_2/F_IO_2 ratio (where P_aO_2 is measured in mmHg and F_IO_2 is 0.21–1.0). Normal P_aO_2/F_IO_2 ratio = 500; comparison with this ratio allows evaluation of severity of lung disease and allows direct comparison of blood gases taken at a different F_IO_2. P_aCO_2 tends to be low; hypercapnia tends to be a late (preterminal) development.
• Total protein of airway edema fluid compared with serum total protein—ratio of edema fluid to serum total protein <0.5 supportive of low-protein, increased hydrostatic pressure pulmonary edema (e.g., heart failure); edema fluid/serum total protein ratio >0.7 supportive of high-protein, increased permeability pulmonary edema (e.g., ARDS)

IMAGING
Thoracic Radiographs
• Bilateral pulmonary infiltrates
• Severity of radiographic signs may lag behind clinical disease by 12–24 hours.
• Can be difficult to distinguish from cardiogenic edema. Cardiac silhouette is usually normal in ARDS.

Echocardiography
• Attempt to rule out cardiogenic cause for pulmonary edema.
• May be able to estimate degree of pulmonary hypertension

DIAGNOSTIC PROCEDURES
Pulmonary artery catheter to measure pulmonary artery occlusion pressure (PAOP) in attempt to rule out cardiogenic cause for edema; by definition, ALI and ARDS are associated with PAOP ≤18 mmHg.

PATHOLOGIC FINDINGS
Gross Pathology
Lungs are dark, heavy, and ooze fluid when cut.

Histopathology
• Acute phase—pulmonary vascular congestion with edema fluid and inflammatory cell accumulation in the interstitium and alveoli; epithelial cell damage, hyaline membrane formation, microthrombi, microatelectasis
• Proliferative phase—hyperplasia of type 2 pneumocytes, interstitial mononuclear infiltration, organization of hyaline membranes and fibroproliferation

TREATMENT

APPROPRIATE HEALTH CARE
• There is no specific therapy. General aims are to maintain tissue oxygenation and to minimize iatrogenic lung injury while treating the underlying disease.

• Oxygen therapy—no more than is required to maintain P_aO_2 >60–80 mmHg in order to minimize oxygen toxicity. Positive-pressure ventilation is used for patients that are hypoxemic despite oxygen therapy, patients requiring high levels of inspired oxygen for prolonged periods, or patients working so hard to breathe that they are at risk of exhaustion. Lung-protective strategies of positive-pressure ventilation with moderate to high peak end-expiratory pressure (PEEP), low tidal volumes, and permissive hypercapnia are used in an attempt to minimize ventilator-induced lung injury. Tidal volumes of 6 ml/kg have been found to significantly increase survival in human ARDS patients compared to tidal volumes of 12 ml/kg. Ventilator maneuvers to recruit collapsed alveoli may be beneficial when using high levels of PEEP.

• Intensive supportive care of the cardiovascular system and other organ systems is vital, as these patients are at high risk for multiple organ dysfunction syndrome.

NURSING CARE

• Monitor temperature closely especially if using an oxygen cage, as dyspneic animals can easily become hyperthermic.

• Ventilator patients require frequent position changes and physiotherapy; regular oral care with a dilute chlorhexidine solution is very important to reduce oral colonization as a source of sepsis, and frequent endotracheal tube suctioning is needed to prevent occlusion. Inflate cuff carefully and change endotracheal cuff position regularly to prevent tracheal damage.

• Blood pressure monitoring, as septic patients are prone to hypotension

• Fluid therapy is important to support the cardiovascular system and to maintain normovolemia.

ACTIVITY

Strict cage confinement monitoring

DIET

Nutritional support is important but challenging. Enteral feeding is desired over parenteral nutrition, but must consider high risk of regurgitation and aspiration in a recumbent patient.

CLIENT EDUCATION

Clients need to be aware of the guarded prognosis and high costs of therapy.

SURGICAL CONSIDERATIONS

The underlying disease may require surgery.

MEDICATIONS

DRUG(S) OF CHOICE

• No specific drug therapy

• Antibiotics for the underlying disease, if necessary

• Positive inotropes to maintain blood pressure

• Anesthetic drugs to allow positive-pressure ventilation

• Analgesia as appropriate

• Corticosteroids may be indicated in late, proliferative phase of ARDS (5–7 days after onset).

CONTRAINDICATIONS

N/A

PRECAUTIONS

N/A

POSSIBLE INTERACTIONS

N/A

ALTERNATIVE DRUG(S)

Furosemide may produce pulmonary venous dilation and improve lung function, as an intermittent bolus or as a CRI of 0.2 mg/kg/h IV.

FOLLOW-UP

PATIENT MONITORING

Arterial blood gases, pulse oximetry, thoracic radiographs, arterial blood pressure, temperature, urine output, CBC, coagulation profiles, serum chemistry, monitoring for other organ dysfunction

PREVENTION/AVOIDANCE

• Aggressive therapy of primary disease processes to maximize lung performance and to reduce the inflammatory insult to the lung

• Intensive cardiovascular monitoring and support of critically ill animals to ensure adequate tissue perfusion

• Careful management of recumbent animals to reduce the chance of aspiration, especially if patient has neurologic disease or upper airway disorders which could reduce the ability to protect the airway

POSSIBLE COMPLICATIONS

Multiorgan dysfunction syndrome—acute renal failure, DIC, and gastrointestinal disease are the more common organ dysfunctions seen

EXPECTED COURSE AND PROGNOSIS

• Mortality in human patients remains at 40–70%.

• Mortality in veterinary patients likely approaches 100%.

MISCELLANEOUS

ASSOCIATED CONDITIONS

Systemic inflammatory response syndrome, multiple organ dysfunction syndrome, sepsis

AGE-RELATED FACTORS

N/A

ZOONOTIC POTENTIAL

N/A

PREGNANCY

N/A

SYNONYMS

• Shock lung

• Adult respiratory distress syndrome

• Acute hypoxemic respiratory failure

• High protein pulmonary edema

SEE ALSO

• Dyspnea, Tachypnea, and Panting

• Pulmonary Edema, Noncardiogenic

• Sepsis and Bacteremia

ABBREVIATIONS

• ALI = acute lung injury

• ARDS = acute respiratory distress syndrome

• CRI = constant rate infusion

• DIC = disseminated intravascular coagulation

• PAOP = pulmonary artery occlusion pressure (formerly pulmonary capillary wedge pressure [PCWP])

• PEEP = positive end-expiratory pressure

• PPV = positive-pressure ventilation

Suggested Reading

Marino PL. Acute respiratory distress syndrome. In: The ICU book. 2nd ed. Baltimore: Williams & Wilkins, 1998: 371–387.

Parent C, King LG, Van Winkle TJ, Walker LM. Respiratory function and treatment in dogs with acute respiratory distress syndrome: 19 cases (1985–1993). J Am Vet Med Assoc 1996;208:1428–1433.

Shoemaker WC. Pathophysiology and management of acute respiratory distress syndrome after surgery, trauma, and other acute illnesses. In: Shoemaker WC et al., eds. Textbook of critical care. 4th ed. Philadelphia: Saunders, 2000:1393–1404.

Ware LB, Matthay MA. The acute respiratory distress syndrome. N Engl J Med 2000;342:1334–1349.

Author Kate Hopper
Consulting Editor Lynelle R. Johnson

ADENOCARCINOMA, ANAL SAC/PERIANAL

BASICS

OVERVIEW
• Uncommon malignant neoplasm derived from apocrine glands of the anal sac
• Locally invasive
• High metastatic rate, often to sublumbar lymph nodes
• Frequently associated with hypercalcemia, thought to be due to PTHrP (parathyroid hormone-related peptide) secretion by tumor cells
• Prognosis guarded to poor

SIGNALMENT
• Older dogs; extremely rare in cats
• Females overrepresented in a few small studies, not in larger studies
• No proven breed predisposition

SIGNS

Historical Findings
May be due to primary tumor (rectal mass, tenesmus), local lymph node metastasis (tenesmus, constipation, stranguria), or hypercalcemia (anorexia, polyuria/polydipsia, lethargy).

Physical Examination Findings
• Mass associated with anal sac; may be quite small despite massive metastatic disease
• Sublumbar lymphadenopathy—on rectal or abdominal palpation

CAUSES & RISK FACTORS
Hormonal role hypothesized

DIAGNOSIS

DIFFERENTIAL DIAGNOSIS
• Anal sac abscess
• Perianal adenoma/adenocarcinoma
• Mast cell tumor
• Lymphoma
• Squamous cell carcinoma
• Perineal hernias

CBC/BIOCHEMISTRY/URINALYSIS
• Hypercalcemia—25–50% of cases
• Secondary renal failure may develop

OTHER LABORATORY TESTS
PTH (parathyroid hormone) and PTHrP levels—elevated PTHrP will help to support neoplasia as the cause of hypercalcemia

IMAGING
• Abdominal radiography—to evaluate sublumbar lymph nodes and lumbar and pelvic bones
• Thoracic radiography—to evaluate for pulmonary metastasis
• Abdominal ultrasonography—may identify mildly enlarged sublumbar lymph nodes not visible radiographically, also nodules in liver/spleen

DIAGNOSTIC PROCEDURES
• Fine needle aspiration of anal sac mass to rule out conditions other than adenocarcinoma; differentiation of benign versus malignant neoplasm of perianal masses is difficult.
• Fine needle aspiration of enlarged lymph nodes, liver, or splenic nodules to confirm metastasis
• Incisional biopsy for histopathology required for definitive diagnosis

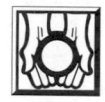

TREATMENT
• Surgical resection—treatment of choice
• Resection of primary tumor and enlarged lymph nodes may prolong survival.

• Surgery often palliative, not curative
• Debulking all disease present may control hypercalcemia until tumor recurrence.
• Saline diuresis (200–300 mL/kg/day) preoperatively if hypercalcemia is severe
• Radiation may help delay local recurrence and control growth of sublumbar metastases—acute and chronic radiation side effects can be moderate to severe

MEDICATIONS

DRUG(S)

Limited reports of partial responses to platinum compounds in dogs—cisplatin (70 mg/m² IV with 6-hour saline diuresis—18.3 mL/kg/hr), carboplatin (300 mg/m² IV as a slow bolus) every 3 weeks

CONTRAINDICATIONS/POSSIBLE INTERACTIONS

• Avoid platinum chemotherapeutic agents in dogs with renal insufficiency
• Do not use cisplatin in cats

FOLLOW-UP

PATIENT MONITORING

• Complete resection—physical examination, thoracic radiography, abdominal ultrasonography, and serum biochemistry at 1, 3, 6, 9, and 12 months post-operatively
• Incomplete resection—monitor tumor size and blood calcium and renal values

EXPECTED COURSE AND PROGNOSIS

• Poor prognosis with both local progression and metastasis occurring
• Growth of the tumor may be slow.
• Presence of hypercalcemia and metastasis were poor prognostic factors in one study—median survival of 6 months if either present, versus 12 months if normocalcemic and 16 months if no metastasis.
• Recent study of 43 dogs found median survival ranged from 7.7–14.4 months, depending on treatment and presence of hypercalcemia; the survival differences were not statistically significant.
• Ultimately, dogs succumb to hypercalcemia-related complications or mass effect from primary tumor or sublumbar nodal metastases.

MISCELLANEOUS

ASSOCIATED CONDITIONS

Hypercalcemia as a paraneoplastic syndrome

ABBREVIATIONS

PTHrP = parathyroid hormone–related peptide

Suggested Reading

Anderson CR, McNeil EA, Gillette EL, et al. Late complications of pelvic irradiation in 16 dogs. Vet Rad US 2002;43:187–192.
Bennett PF, DeNicola DB, Bonney P, et al. Canine anal sac adenocarcinomas: clinical presentation and response to therapy. J Vet Intern Med 2002;16:100–104.
Thomas RC, Fox LE. Tumors of the skin and subcutis. In: Morrison WB, ed. Cancer in dogs and cats: medical and surgical management. Baltimore: Williams & Wilkins, 1998:489–510.

Author Laura D. Garrett
Consulting Editor Wallace B. Morrison

ADENOCARCINOMA, LUNG

BASICS

OVERVIEW
- Makes up 75% of primary pulmonary tumors in dogs and cats
- Primary pulmonary tumors rare in dogs and cats
- Solitary tumors more prevalent than multi-lobed tumors
- May metastasize

SIGNALMENT

Dogs
- Makes up 1% of all tumors
- Mean age of affected animals 10 years
- No sex predilection
- Reports that boxers or brachycephalics predisposed

Cats
- More rare than in dogs
- Mean age of affected animals 11 years
- No breed predilection
- Some studies suggest females are over-represented.

SIGNS

Historical Findings
- Nonproductive cough
- Dyspnea
- Tachypnea
- Lethargy
- Anorexia
- Weight loss
- Hemoptysis
- Pain—pleural involvement
- Lameness—bone metastasis or hypertrophic osteopathy, weight-bearing lytic digit metastasis (cats)
- Polyuria or polydipsia—hypercalcemia or hyperadrenocorticism from ectopic production of ACTH
- Weakness or muscle wasting—polyneuropathy; polymyopathy

Physical Examination Findings
- May be none referable to respiratory system
- Tachypnea and dyspnea
- Fever
- Limb swelling
- Ascites
- Anterior vena cava syndrome

CAUSES & RISK FACTORS
- Some evidence correlates risk to urban environment; controversial • Exposure to passive cigarette smoke unproven

DIAGNOSIS

DIFFERENTIAL DIAGNOSIS
- Granulomatous lesion
- Pulmonary abscess
- Other primary lung tumor—squamous cell carcinoma
- Metastatic lung tumor
- Pneumonia
- Asthma
- Congenital cyst
- Parasitic lesion

CBC/BIOCHEMISTRY/URINALYSIS
No specific abnormalities

OTHER LABORATORY TESTS
N/A

IMAGING
- Thoracic radiography—usually demonstrates a focal, solitary, well-circumscribed mass
- Ultrasonography—may help assess hilar or mediastinal lymphadenopathy; may help with obtaining an aspirate or biopsy specimen

DIAGNOSTIC PROCEDURES
- Thoracocentesis with cytologic examination—if pleural effusion noted
- Transtracheal lavage—limited diagnostic value
- Cytology—transthoracic fine-needle aspiration
- Percutaneous tissue biopsy—use Tru-Cut instrument
- Open lung biopsy—specimen via thoracotomy

PATHOLOGIC FINDINGS
- Adenocarcinoma—classified according to location (bronchial, bronchiolar, bronchiolar-alveolar, or alveolar) and degree of differentiation
- Undifferentiated tumors—more invasive and more likely to metastasize than well-differentiated tumors; sites of metastasis include lymph nodes, bones, pleura, eyes (choroid), and CNS.

TREATMENT
- Surgery—partial or complete lobectomy; mainstay • Radiotherapy—may be of some benefit (mediastinal lymphadenomegaly); reports are only anecdotal.

MEDICATIONS

DRUG(S)
- Chemotherapy—no standard protocol; may be palliative
- Doxorubicin, cisplatin, carboplatin, and/or vindesine—rational choices for palliation
- Chemotherapy can be toxic; seek advice if unfamiliar with cytotoxic drugs.

CONTRAINDICATIONS/POSSIBLE INTERACTIONS
- Doxorubicin—monitor patients with underlying cardiac disease carefully; consider pretreatment and serial echocardiograms and ECG.• Cisplatin—do not give to cats (fatal); do not use in dogs with pre-existing renal disease; never use without appropriate and concurrent diuresis.

FOLLOW-UP

PATIENT MONITORING
- Serial thoracic radiographs—consider every 3 months; administer a minimum of two cycles of chemotherapy before evaluating response to treatment.
- Perform CBC (doxorubicin, cisplatin, carboplatin, and vindesine), biochemical analysis (cisplatin), and urinalysis (cisplatin) before each chemotherapy treatment.

POSSIBLE COMPLICATIONS
- Anemia • DIC • Hemoptysis • Spontaneous pneumothorax • Hypercalcemia
- Hypertrophic osteopathy

EXPECTED COURSE AND PROGNOSIS
- Metastasis to the tracheobronchial lymph nodes—single best prognostic indicator; median survival without metastasis approaches 1 year and with metastasis, 60 days.
- Prognostic factors after surgery—ability to achieve complete cytoreduction; size of the primary tumor; metastasis; degree of cell differentiation (histologic score), lack of preoperable clinical signs
- Patients with well-differentiated adenocarcinomas have a better prognosis that those with undifferentiated tumors.

MISCELLANEOUS

PREGNANCY
Chemotherapy is not advised in pregnant animals.

ABBREVIATIONS
- ACTH = adrenocorticotrophic hormone
- CNS = central nervous system
- DIC = disseminated intravascular coagulation
- ECG = electrocardiogram

Suggested Reading

Fox LE, King RR. Cancers of the respiratory system. In: Morrison WB, ed. Cancer in dogs and cats: medical and surgical management. Baltimore: Williams & Wilkins, 1998:521–536.

McNeil EA, Ogilvie GK, Powers BE, et al. Evaluation of prognostic factors for dogs with primary lung tumors: 67 cases (1985–1992). J Am Vet Med Assoc 1997;211:1422–1427.

Ogilvie GK, Weigel RM, Haschek WM, et al. Prognostic factors for tumor remission and survival in dogs after surgery for primary lung tumor: 76 cases (1975–1985). J Am Vet Med Assoc 1989;195;109–112.

Author Renee Al-Sarraf
Consulting Editor Wallace B. Morrison

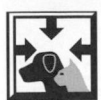

BASICS

OVERVIEW
• Slow, progressive local invasion of the nasal and paranasal sinuses by neoplastic epithelial and glandular epithelial cells
• Most begin as unilateral but progress to bilateral by the time of examination.
• Approximately 20% arise from the frontal sinuses.
• In dogs and cats, more common than fibrosarcoma, squamous cell carcinoma, chondrosarcoma, and others.
• Prevalence of epithelial nasal neoplasia (dogs and cats)—0.3%–8% of all tumors

SIGNALMENT
• Median age (dogs and cats)—10 years (range, 18 months to 18 years)
• Medium to large breeds affected more commonly than are small breeds
• May be more common in male than female dogs

SIGNS

Historical Findings
• Intermittent and progressive history of unilateral to bilateral epistaxis (median duration, 3 months) and/or mucopurulent discharge
• Epiphora
• Sneezing
• Halitosis
• Anorexia
• Seizures secondary to cranial invasion

Physical Examination Findings
• Nasal discharge
• Facial deformity or exophthalmia
• Pain with nasal or paranasal sinus examination
• Obstructed nares (unilateral or bilateral)

CAUSES & RISK FACTORS
Urban environment suspected in dolichocephalic dogs secondary to pollutant exposure

DIAGNOSIS

DIFFERENTIAL DIAGNOSIS
• Bacterial sinusitis—uncommon
• Viral infection—cats
• Aspergillosis, other fungal infections
• Cryptococcosis—cats
• Foreign body
• Trauma
• Tooth root abscess
• Oronasal fistula
• Coagulopathy
• Parasites
• Hypertension

CBC/BIOCHEMISTRY/URINALYSIS
Usually normal

OTHER LABORATORY TESTS
• Cytologic and bacterial examination—rarely helpful
• Coagulation profile

IMAGING
• Survey skull radiography—shows typical pattern of asymmetrical destruction of caudal turbinates with superimposition of a soft tissue mass; may see fluid density in the frontal sinuses secondary to outflow obstruction
• Thoracic radiography—evaluate for lung metastasis (uncommon)
• CT or MRI—best method for observing integrity of cribriform plate or orbital invasion

DIAGNOSTIC PROCEDURES
• Rhinoscopy—visual observation poor; soft, friable, fleshy masses that may be papillary, tubular, or solid and well formed; avoid progressing caudally into the cribriform plate
• Tissue biopsy—necessary for definitive diagnosis
• Bacterial culture—often positive
• Cytologic evaluation of regional lymph nodes—detect metastatic disease

TREATMENT
• Surgery alone ineffective
• Turbinectomy—may do before external (teletherapy) or internal (brachytherapy) irradiation
• Inpatient radiotherapy (with or without surgery)—best clinical control in dogs

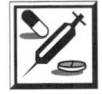

MEDICATIONS

DRUG(S)
• Chemotherapy—good option in some patients
• Cisplatin (dogs)—60–70 mg/m^2 IV once every 3 weeks; median survival after therapy 22 weeks; may provide marked palliation of clinical signs; **caution:** nephrotoxic; use with saline diuresis (18.3 mL/kg/hr IV over 6 hr; give cisplatin after 4 hr)
• Butorphanol—0.4 mg/kg IM; before and after cisplatin to reduce emesis

CONTRAINDICATIONS/POSSIBLE INTERACTIONS
• Chemotherapy can be toxic; seek advice before initiating treatment if unfamiliar with cytotoxic drugs.
• Cisplatin—never use in cats.

FOLLOW-UP
• Untreated—median survival 3–5 months
• Radiotherapy—median disease-free interval 8–23 months in dogs and 1–36 months in cats; 1-year survival rate 20%–57% (dogs and cats); 2-year survival rate 20%–48% (dogs and cats)
• Presence of metastatic disease—poor prognostic indicator
• Brain involvement—poor prognostic sign
• Survey skull radiography, CT, MRI—when clinical signs recur
• Ophthalmic complications of radiotherapy—more likely in dogs than cats

MISCELLANEOUS

Suggested Reading

Cox NR, Brawner WR, Powers RD, Wright JC. Tumors of the nose and paranasal sinuses in cats: 32 cases with comparison to a national database (1977 through 1987). J Am Anim Hosp Assoc 1991;27:339–347.

Hahn KA, Knapp DW, Richardson RC, Matlock CL. Clinical response of nasal adenocarcinoma to cisplatin chemotherapy in 11 dogs. J Am Vet Med Assoc 1992;200: 355–357.

Henry CJ, Brewer WG, Tyler JW, et al. Survival in dogs with nasal adenocarcinoma: 64 cases (1981–1995). J Vet Intern Med 1998;12:436–439.

Theon AP, Peaston AE, Madewell BR, Dungworth DL. Irradiation of nonlymphoproliferative neoplasms of the nasal cavity and paranasal sinuses in 16 cats. J Am Vet Med Assoc 1994;204:78–83.

Authors Kevin A. Hahn and Janet K. Carreras

Consulting Editor Wallace B. Morrison

ADENOCARCINOMA, PANCREAS

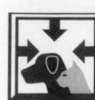 **BASICS**

OVERVIEW
• Malignant tumor of ductal or acinar origin
• Usually metastatic by the time of diagnosis

SIGNALMENT
• Rare in dogs—0.5%–1.8% of all tumors
• Rare in cats—2.8% of all tumors
• Older female dogs and Airedale terriers at higher risk than others
• Median age (dogs)—9.2 years

SIGNS
• Nonspecific—fever; vomiting; weakness; anorexia; icterus; maldigestion; weight loss
• Abdominal pain—variable
• Metastasis to bone and soft tissue common
• Pathologic fractures secondary to metastasis reported
• Diabetes insipidus secondary to pituitary metastasis reported in one dog
• Abdominal mass

CAUSES & RISK FACTORS
Unknown

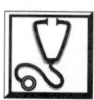 **DIAGNOSIS**

DIFFERENTIAL DIAGNOSIS
• Primary pancreatitis; may be concurrent and complicate or delay early diagnosis
• Pancreatic pseudocyst
• Other causes of vomiting and icterus

CBC/BIOCHEMISTRY/URINALYSIS
• Usually nonspecific changes (e.g., mild anemia and neutrophilia)
• Hyperamylasemia less reliable than hyperlipasemia
• Lipase concentration often markedly high

OTHER LABORATORY TESTS
N/A

IMAGING
• Abdominal radiographs—may reveal a mass or loss of contrast associated with concurrent pancreatitis
• Ultrasonography—may reveal a mass or concurrent pancreatitis (mixed echogenicity, large pancreas, hyperechoic peripancreatic fat)

DIAGNOSTIC PROCEDURES
Surgical biopsy—definitive diagnosis

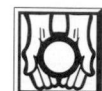 **TREATMENT**

• None reported successfully curative
• Palliation of pain and intestinal and biliary obstruction—surgery, if necessary
• Partial or total pancreatectomy
• Treat concurrent pancreatitis

 **MEDICATIONS**

DRUG(S)
N/A

CONTRAINDICATIONS/POSSIBLE INTERACTIONS
N/A

 FOLLOW-UP

POSSIBLE COMPLICATIONS
• Intestinal obstruction
• Biliary obstruction
• Pancreatic abscess
• Peritonitis

EXPECTED COURSE AND PROGNOSIS
Usually a rapid progression to death, because no successful curative treatment available

 MISCELLANEOUS

ASSOCIATED CONDITIONS
Gastrin-secreting pancreatic carcinoma—reported in dogs and cats; clinical signs also caused by hypergastrinemia, which results in inappropriate HCl secretion by the stomach, leading to gastroduodenitis

ABBREVIATION
HCl = hydrochloric acid

Suggested Reading
Harari J, Lincoln J. Surgery of the exocrine pancreas. In: Slatter D, ed. Textbook of small animal surgery. Philadelphia: Saunders, 1993:678–691.
Morrison WB. Primary cancers and cancer-like lesions of the liver, biliary epithelium, and exocrine pancreas. In: Morrison WB, ed. Cancer in dogs and cats: medical and surgical management. Baltimore: Williams & Wilkins, 1998:559–568.
Author Wallace B. Morrison
Consulting Editor Wallace B. Morrison

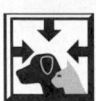

BASICS

OVERVIEW
• A malignant tumor that develops in both neutered and intact male dogs
• Represents <1% of all canine malignancies, but is the most common prostatic disorder in neutered male dogs
• Metastases to regional lymph nodes, lungs, and lumbosacral skeleton common

SIGNALMENT
• Medium to large-breed, intact or neutered male dogs
• Median age, 9–10 years
• Rare in cats

SIGNS

Historical Findings
• Tenesmus—with the production of ribbon-like stool
• Anorexia
• Weight loss
• Stranguria and dysuria
• Rear limb lameness
• Weakness
• Lethargy
• Exercise intolerance

Physical Examination Findings
• Firm, asymmetrical, and immobile prostate gland
• Prostatomegaly common
• Pain—may be elicited in response to abdominal or rectal palpation
• May note caudal abdominal mass, cachexia, pyrexia, and dyspnea

CAUSES & RISK FACTORS
• Hormonal cause theorized
• Castration appears to have no protective effect against the development of this tumor.

DIAGNOSIS

DIFFERENTIAL DIAGNOSIS
• Other primary neoplasia—squamous cell carcinoma
• Metastatic or locally invasive neoplasia—transitional cell carcinoma
• Acute or chronic prostatitis, benign prostatic hypertrophy, and prostatic cysts—possible in intact male dogs; unlikely in neutered dogs

CBC/BIOCHEMISTRY/URINALYSIS
• Inflammatory signs on leukogram possible
• Alkaline phosphatase—may be high
• Postrenal azotemia if urethral obstruction exists
• Evaluate urine samples taken by cystocentesis and free-catch technique—hematuria, pyuria, and malignant epithelial cells may be seen in free-catch samples but are unusual in cystocentesis samples.

OTHER LABORATORY TESTS
Serum and seminal plasma markers (e.g., acid phosphatase, prostate-specific antigen, and canine prostate-specific esterase) are not specific markers of prostatic adenocarcinoma.

IMAGING
• Thoracic radiography—metastasis may appear as pulmonary nodules or increased interstitial markings.
• Abdominal radiography—sublumbar lymphadenomegaly, mineralization of the prostate, and lytic lesions to the lumbar vertebrae or pelvis
• Ultrasonography—focal to multifocal hyperechogenicity with asymmetry and irregular prostatic outline, with or without prostatic mineralization
• Contrast cystography—may help differentiate prostatic from urinary bladder disease

DIAGNOSTIC PROCEDURES
• Examination of prostatic aspirate (percutaneous or transrectal) or prostatic wash
• Prostatic biopsy—take specimen either percutaneously or during surgery.
NOTE: Tumor seeding along needle tract is a rare complication of percutaneous aspirate/biopsy.

TREATMENT
• Prostatectomy—local disease; success depends on the skill of the surgeon and the extent of disease.
• Radiotherapy—some therapeutic benefit; median survival after intraoperative radiotherapy, 114 days
• Castration—however, most tumors are not androgen responsive

MEDICATIONS

DRUG(S)
• Chemotherapy—carboplatin, cisplatin, or doxorubicin; may offer short-term benefit
• Pain relief—NSAID and opioid drugs
• Stool softeners—relieve tenesmus

CONTRAINDICATIONS/POSSIBLE INTERACTIONS
N/A

FOLLOW-UP

PATIENT MONITORING
• Ability to urinate and defecate
• Pain secondary to skeletal metastases
• Quality of life

PREVENTION/AVOIDANCE
Castration does not prevent disease.

POSSIBLE COMPLICATIONS
• Urethral obstruction
• Metastasis to regional lymph nodes, skeleton, and lungs

EXPECTED COURSE AND PROGNOSIS
• Grave prognosis
• Survival 1–3 months

MISCELLANEOUS

ABBREVIATION
NSAID = nonsteroidal antiinflammatory drug

Suggested Reading
Bell FW, Klausner JS, Hayden DW, et al. Clinical and pathologic features of prostatic adenocarcinoma in sexually intact and castrated dogs: 31 cases (1970–1987). J Am Vet Med Assoc 1991;1623–1630.
Cooley DM, Waters DJ. Tumors of the male reproductive system. In: Withrow SJ, MacEwen EG, eds. Small animal clinical oncology. Philadelphia: Saunders, 2001: 478–489.
Morrison WB. Cancers of the reproductive tract. In: Morrison WB, ed. Cancer in dogs and cats: medical and surgical management. Baltimore: Williams & Wilkins, 1998: 581–590.
Author Ruthanne Chun
Consulting Editor Wallace B. Morrison

ADENOCARCINOMA, RENAL

BASICS

OVERVIEW
- Accounts for <1% of all reported neoplasms in dogs
- Tends to be highly metastatic, locally invasive, and often bilateral
- Renal cystadenocarcinoma—German shepherds prone; an apparently heritable syndrome; less aggressive and has a better long-term prognosis than does renal adenocarcinoma

SIGNALMENT
- Adenocarcinoma—old (8–9 years) dogs; male:female ratio, 1.6:1; no breed predilection
- Cystadenocarcinoma—German shepherds, often female
- Cats—rare; lymphoma most common renal tumor

SIGNS
- Adenocarcinoma—may be insidious with nonspecific signs (e.g., weight loss, inappetence, lethargy, hematuria, and pale mucous membranes)
- Cystadenocarcinoma—may be associated with nodular dermatofibrosis (a syndrome of painless, firm, fibrous lesions of the skin and subcutaneous tissues)

CAUSES & RISK FACTORS
- Adenocarcinoma—unknown
- Cystadenocarcinoma—heritable in German shepherds

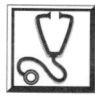

DIAGNOSIS

DIFFERENTIAL DIAGNOSIS
- Other primary neoplasia—lymphosarcoma; nephroblastoma
- Metastatic neoplasia—hemangiosarcoma
- Renal adenoma or cyst, especially in Persian cats
- Pyelonephritis

CBC/BIOCHEMISTRY/URINALYSIS
- CBC—may note paraneoplastic polycythemia, leukocytosis, or anemia
- Biochemistry—may be normal; may reveal azotemia
- Urinalysis—may show hematuria, proteinuria, bacteriuria, or casts; rare to see tumor cells

OTHER LABORATORY TESTS
Urine culture and sensitivity

IMAGING
- Thoracic radiographs—metastatic disease reported in up to 34% of patients
- Abdominal radiographs—mass visualized in 81% of patients
- Intravenous pyelography or abdominal ultrasonography—to identify and stage disease

DIAGNOSTIC PROCEDURES
Renal biopsy—ultrasound-guided or surgical; definitive diagnosis

TREATMENT
- Unilateral adenocarcinoma or cystadeno-carcinoma—aggressive surgical excision is the treatment of choice.
- Renal failure—supportive management may be necessary.

MEDICATIONS

DRUG(S)
Chemotherapeutic management—success has not been described for either disease.

CONTRAINDICATIONS/POSSIBLE INTERACTIONS
N/A

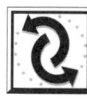

FOLLOW-UP

PATIENT MONITORING
- Renal failure—measure serum urea nitrogen and creatinine; urinalysis
- Metastasis—imaging studies
- Quality of life—for animals with bilateral or otherwise nonsurgical disease

PREVENTION/AVOIDANCE
N/A

POSSIBLE COMPLICATIONS
- Renal failure
- Metastatic disease
- Anemia or polycythemia
- Invasion of local vital structures—vena cava; aorta

EXPECTED COURSE AND PROGNOSIS
- Long-term prognosis—poor, even with apparently localized disease
- Adenocarcinoma—patients who survive the first 21 days postsurgery have a mean survival of 6–10 months.
- Cystadenocarcinoma—better long-term prognosis; survival of 12 months or longer with no definitive treatment

MISCELLANEOUS

ASSOCIATED CONDITIONS
- Paraneoplastic syndromes—hypertrophic osteopathy, polycythemia, and neutrophilic leukocytosis reported in isolated cases
- Renal failure—may develop
- Nodular dermatofibrosis and uterine leiomyoma—commonly associated with cystadenocarcinoma

Suggested Reading
Knapp DW. Tumors of the urinary system. In: Withrow SJ, MacEwen EG, eds. Small animal clinical oncology. Philadelphia: Saunders, 2001:490–499.
Morrison WB. Cancers of the urinary tract. In: Morrison WB, ed. Cancer in dogs and cats: medical and surgical management. Baltimore: Williams & Wilkins, 1998:569–579.

Author Ruthanne Chun
Consulting Editor Wallace B. Morrison

ADENOCARCINOMA, SALIVARY GLAND

BASICS

OVERVIEW
• Tumor arising from major (e.g., parotid, mandibular, sublingual, or zygomatic) or minor glands
• Mandibular or parotid glands constitute 80% of cases.
• Mandibular gland most frequently affected in dogs
• Parotid gland most frequently affected in cats
• Locally invasive
• Cats have more advanced disease than dogs at time of diagnosis.
• Metastasis—regional lymph node in 39% of cats and 17% of dogs at diagnosis; distant metastasis reported in 16% of cats and 8% of dogs at diagnosis but may be slow to develop
• Other salivary gland neoplasms—carcinoma; squamous cell carcinoma; mixed neoplasia
• Epithelial malignancies—constitute roughly 85% of salivary gland tumors
• Fibrosarcomas, lipomas, mast cell tumors and lymphomas have involved the salivary glands by direct extension and invasion.
• Adenomas comprise only 5% of salivary tumors.

SIGNALMENT
• Dogs and cats
• Mean age, 10–12 years
• Siamese cats—may be at relatively higher risk
• Male cats affected twice as often as female cats
• No other breed or sex predilection has been determined.

SIGNS
• Unilateral, firm, painless swelling of the upper neck (mandibular and sublingual), ear base (parotid), upper lip or maxilla (zygomatic), or mucous membrane of lip (accessory or minor salivary tissue)
• Other signs may include halitosis, weight loss, anorexia, dysphagia, exophthalmus, Horner's syndrome, sneezing, and dysphonia.

CAUSES & RISK FACTORS
Unknown

DIAGNOSIS

DIFFERENTIAL DIAGNOSIS
• Squamous cell carcinoma
• Mucocele
• Abscess
• Lymphosarcoma

CBC/BIOCHEMISTRY/URINALYSIS
Results normal

OTHER LABORATORY TESTS
N/A

IMAGING
• Regional radiographs—usually normal; may see periosteal reaction on adjacent bones or displacement of surrounding structures
• Thoracic radiographs—indicate to check for lung metastases.

DIAGNOSTIC PROCEDURES
• Cytologic examination of aspirate—differentiate salivary adenocarcinoma from mucocele and abscess.
• Needle core or wedge biopsy—definitive diagnosis

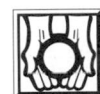

TREATMENT
• Aggressive surgical resection—when possible; most are invasive and difficult to excise
• Radiotherapy—good local control and prolonged survival in three reported cases;
• Aggressive local resection (usually histologically incomplete) followed by adjuvant radiation can achieve local control and long-term survival, but further studies are needed to determine the most effective treatment, including the possible role for chemotherapy.

MEDICATIONS

DRUG(S)
Chemotherapy—largely unreported

CONTRAINDICATIONS/POSSIBLE INTERACTIONS
N/A

FOLLOW-UP

PATIENT MONITORING
Evaluations—dictated by tumor growth; every 3 months reasonable

EXPECTED COURSE AND PROGNOSIS
• Improved survival time in dogs without evidence of nodal or distant metastasis at diagnosis; clinical stage not prognostic for cats
• Median survival 550 days for dogs and 516 days for cats in retrospective study
• Local control through radiation or multiple surgeries remains critical.

MISCELLANEOUS

Suggested Reading
Hammer A, Getzy D, Ogilvie G, et al. Salivary gland neoplasia in the dog and cat: survival times and prognostic factors. J Am Anim Hosp Assoc 2001;37:478–482.

Acknowledgment
The author/editors acknowledge the prior contributions of Dr. J. P. Thompson, who authored this topic in the previous edition.
Author Anthony J. Mutsaers
Consulting Editor Wallace B. Morrison

ADENOCARCINOMA, SKIN (SWEAT GLAND, SEBACEOUS)

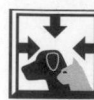

BASICS

OVERVIEW
Malignant growth originating from sebaceous and apocrine sweat glands within the skin

SIGNALMENT
- Sebaceous gland—rare in dogs and cats
- Apocrine sweat gland—rare in dogs and cats; occurs more frequently in cats than does sebaceous gland adenocarcinoma
- Both types—more common in old patients

SIGNS
- May appear as solid, firm, raised lesion
- May be ulcerated and bleeding and accompanied by inflammation of the surrounding tissue
- Apocrine sweat gland—often poorly circumscribed, ulcerates; very invasive into underlying tissue
- Sebaceous gland—may begin in dogs with solitary nodule but then multiple satellite lesions arise due to lymphatic spread; regional lymph node often affected. In cats, metastasis may occur from a primary cutaneous site to multiple digits, resulting in swelling and ulceration of digits.

CAUSES & RISK FACTORS
Unknown

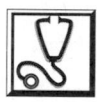

DIAGNOSIS

DIFFERENTIAL DIAGNOSIS
- Any other skin tumor
- Cellulitis

CBC/BIOCHEMISTRY/URINALYSIS
Normal

OTHER LABORATORY TESTS
N/A

IMAGING
Thoracic radiographs and cytologic examination or biopsy of regional lymph nodes—required at the time of diagnosis; rule out metastatic disease

DIAGNOSTIC PROCEDURES
- Histopathologic examination—essential to confirm diagnosis
- Apocrine sweat gland—typically invasive into the underlying stroma and blood vessels; has poorly demarcated borders and a high mitotic index
- Sebaceous gland adenocarcinoma—histopathology typically reveals invasion into lymphatics.

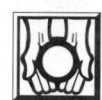

TREATMENT

- Aggressive surgical excision, including resection of draining lymph node, recommended for both types. Histopathologic analysis of lymph nodes assists with determining prognosis and establishing adjuvant treatment plan.
- Entire tissue specimen must be evaluated histologically to assess completeness of resection
- Radiation therapy—recommended for treatment of draining lymph nodes site after resection to prevent recurrence and development of regional metastasis; treatment of primary tumor site recommended when wide and complete resection not possible

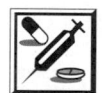

MEDICATIONS

DRUG(S)
Multiple chemotherapy drugs have been used for the treatment of both tumor types, in both species, with some benefit (including cisplatin, carboplatin, mitoxantrone and gemcitabine).

CONTRAINDICATIONS/POSSIBLE INTERACTIONS
None

FOLLOW-UP

- Sebaceous gland adenocarcinoma—little known about the metastatic potential of this malignancy, but rapidly metastatic to regional lymph nodes in author's experience; long-term prognosis seems quite good when aggressive surgery is combined with chemotherapy and radiation therapy.
- Apocrine sweat gland—associated with a very guarded prognosis; aggressive surgical resection required for local tumor control; postoperative chemotherapy recommended to delay or prevent development of metastasis

MISCELLANEOUS

Suggested Reading

Carpenter JL, Andrews LK, Holzworth J. Tumors and tumor like lesions. In: Holzworth J, ed. Diseases of the cat: Medicine and surgery. Philadelphia: Saunders, 1987:406–596.

Thomas RC, Fox LE. Tumors of the skin and subcutis. In: Morrison WB, ed. Cancer in dogs and cats: medical and surgical management. Baltimore: Williams & Wilkins, 1998:489–510.

Author Robyn Elmslie
Consulting Editor Wallace B. Morrison

ADENOCARCINOMA, STOMACH, SMALL AND LARGE INTESTINE, RECTAL

BASICS

OVERVIEW
• Uncommon tumor arising from the epithelial lining of the gastrointestinal tract
• Prognosis usually poor

SIGNALMENT
• Dogs more commonly affected than cats
• Middle-aged to older (> 6 years) animals; age range 3–13 years
• No breed predisposition
• More common in males than females

SIGNS

Historical Findings
• Signs related to gastrointestinal tract
• Stomach—vomiting, anorexia, weight loss, hematemesis, and melena
• Small intestine—vomiting, weight loss, borborygmus, flatulence, and melena
• Large intestine and rectum—mucous and blood-tinged feces and tenesmus

Physical Examination Findings
• Stomach—nonspecific
• Small intestine—may feel midabdominal mass; distended, painful loops of small bowel; melena on rectal exam
• Large intestine and rectum—palpable mass per rectum, forming a "napkin ring," or multiple nodular lesions protruding into the colon; bright red blood on feces

CAUSES & RISK FACTORS
• Unknown
• Nitrosamines—reported as causative agent in experimental literature
• Possible genetic cause—gastric adenocarcinomas in related Belgian shepherds

DIAGNOSIS

DIFFERENTIAL DIAGNOSIS
• Foreign body
• Inflammatory bowel disease
• Lymphoma
• Parasites
• Leiomyoma
• Leiomyosarcoma
• Pancreatitis

CBC/BIOCHEMISTRY/URINALYSIS
• Stomach and small intestine—may see microcytic, hypochromic anemia

• Large intestine and rectum—no characteristic changes

OTHER LABORATORY TESTS
Fecal occult blood—positive after feeding nonmeat diet for 3 days

IMAGING
• Ultrasound—may reveal a thickened stomach or bowel wall; may see mass in the gastrointestinal tract, enlarged lymph nodes
• Positive contrast radiography—filling defect (stomach); intraluminal space-occupying or annular constriction (small bowel); gastric neoplasm most often found in distal two thirds of stomach
• Double contrast radiography—large intestine and rectum; polypoid or annular space-occupying masses

DIAGNOSTIC PROCEDURES
Endoscopic biopsy—may be nondiagnostic because tumors are frequently deep to the mucosal surface; thus surgical biopsy frequently required

TREATMENT
• Surgical resection—treatment of choice; seldom curative
• Gastric—usually nonresectable
• Small intestine—remove by resection and anastomosis; metastasis to regional lymph nodes and the liver common
• Large intestine and rectal—may occasionally be resected by a pull-through surgical procedure; metastasis common; transcolonic debulking may provide palliation of obstruction

MEDICATIONS

DRUG(S)
• Chemotherapy—only anecdotal reports, usually unsuccessful
• Piroxicam—0.3 mg/kg PO once daily can provide palliation for large intestinal and rectal tumors.

CONTRAINDICATIONS/POSSIBLE INTERACTIONS
Seek advice before initiating treatment with cytotoxic drugs.

FOLLOW-UP
Physical examination, thoracic radiographs and abdominal ultrasound—at 1, 3, 6, 9. and 12 months postsurgery

EXPECTED COURSE AND PROGNOSIS

Dogs
• Overall poor; small intestinal adenocarcinomas do best; most cases recur locally, develop metastasis, or both rapidly.
• Median survival gastric—2 months
• Median survival small intestinal—10 months

Cats
• Guarded
• Few reported cases, but may have prolonged survival (> 1 year) even with metastasis in small intestinal cases

MISCELLANEOUS

Suggested Reading
Crawshaw J, Berg J, Sardinas JC, et al. Prognosis for dogs with nonlymphomatous small intestinal tumors treated by surgical excision. J Am Anim Hosp Assoc 1998;34:451–456.
Morrison WB. Nonlymphomatous cancers of the esophagus, stomach, and intestines. In: Morrison WB, ed. Cancer in dogs and cats: medical and surgical management. Baltimore: Williams & Wilkins, 1998:551–558.
Swann HM, Holt DE. Canine gastric adenocarcinoma and leiomyosarcoma: a retrospective study of 21 cases (1986–1999) and literature review. J Am Anim Hosp Assoc 2002;38:157–164.
Takiguchi M, Yasuda J, Hashimoto A, et al. Esophageal/gastric adenocarcinoma in a dog. J Am Anim Hosp Assoc 1997;33:42–44.

Acknowledgment
The author acknowledges the prior contributions of Dr. Ralph Richardson, who authored the topic in the previous edition.

Author Laura D. Garrett
Consulting Editor Wallace B. Morrison

ADENOCARCINOMA, THYROID—DOGS

BASICS

DEFINITION
Malignant neoplasm arising from the thyroid gland

PATHOPHYSIOLOGY
• Tumors rarely produce excess thyroid hormone.
• Locally invasive and moderately to highly metastatic, usually to regional lymph nodes and lungs

SYSTEMS AFFECTED
• Respiratory—dogs may be dyspneic owing to a space-occupying mass adjacent to the trachea; metastasis to the lungs common
• Endocrine/metabolic—affected dogs may be hypothyroid, euthyroid, or hyperthyroid; hypercalcemia may be seen as a paraneoplastic syndrome or secondary to concurrent parathyroid hyperplasia or parathyroid adenocarcinoma.
• Cardiovascular—hyperthyroid dogs are usually tachycardic and may have systemic hypertension; may see anemia and DIC in advanced disease

GENETICS
Unknown

INCIDENCE/PREVALENCE
• Represents 1.2–3.7% of all tumors in dogs
• Represents 10–15% of all primary head and neck tumors

GEOGRAPHIC DISTRIBUTION
May be more common in iodine-deficient areas

SIGNALMENT

Species
Dogs

Breed Predilections
• Beagles, boxers, and golden retrievers—reported to be at higher risk than other breeds
• Any breed may be affected.

Mean Age and Range
• Mean—approximately 9 years
• Range—4–18 years

Predominant Sex
None

SIGNS

General Comments
• Usually not diagnosed until a large mass is palpable
• Approximately 65% are unilateral, 35% are bilateral.

Historical Findings
• Common—dyspnea; large ventral cervical mass; dysphagia; weight loss
• Less common—dysphonia; regurgitation; polydipsia; polyuria
• Hyperthyroid patients—polyphagia; weight loss; polydipsia; polyuria; tachypnea; episodes of collapse
• Hypothyroid patients—poor-quality hair coats; lethargy

Physical Examination Findings
• Firm, nonpainful ventral cervical mass, moveable or fixed
• Usually unilateral
• Hyperthyroid patients—may be tachycardic, perhaps with irregular rhythms; tachypneic; emaciated

CAUSES
Unknown

RISK FACTORS
• Breed predilection
• Iodine deficiency

DIAGNOSIS

DIFFERENTIAL DIAGNOSIS
• Other primary neoplasms—lympho-sarcoma; soft tissue sarcoma; salivary gland adenocarcinoma; parathyroid carcinoma; carotid body tumor
• Secondary tumors—metastatic oral squamous cell carcinoma; oral melanoma
• Inflammatory—abscess or granuloma
• Salivary mucocele

CBC/BIOCHEMISTRY/URINALYSIS
• Usually normal
• May see nonregenerative anemia of chronic disease
• Rare—hypercalcemia; isosthenuria; DIC

OTHER LABORATORY TESTS
• T_4 and/or free T_4 concentration
• Endogenous canine TSH concentration
• TSH stimulation test—with suspected hypothyroidism

IMAGING
• Thoracic radiographs (three views)—rule out pulmonary metastasis
• Cervical radiographs—evaluate displacement of normal structures
• Cervical ultrasound and computed tomography—determine degree of encroachment on adjacent structures
• Thyroid gland scintigraphy—identify location of primary tumor and possible metastatic foci

• Radioiodine studies—may provide information about the tumor's ability to produce thyroid hormone

DIAGNOSTIC PROCEDURES

Biopsy
Tru-Cut not recommended owing to high risk of hemorrhage; open biopsy usually required

Cytology
• Examination of fine–needle aspirate from tumor and palpable regional lymph nodes
• Specimen almost always heavily contaminated with blood owing to highly vascular nature of tumor
• Homogeneous population of epithelial cells, sometimes with colloid—common
• Unable to differentiate malignant from benign thyroid cells; but almost all thyroid neoplasms in dogs are malignant.

PATHOLOGIC FINDINGS

Gross
• Characterized by high vascularity with areas of hemorrhage and necrosis
• Usually poorly encapsulated; often invade adjacent tissues (e.g., trachea and esophagus); may adhere to the jugular vein, carotid artery, and vagosympathetic trunk

Histopathology
• Three main types—follicular, papillary, and compact (solid); mixed follicular and solid tumors most common in dogs
• C-cell (e.g., parafollicular, medullary) carcinomas rare

TREATMENT

APPROPRIATE HEALTH CARE
• Usually outpatient
• Inpatient—hyperthyroid patients after episodes of collapse

NURSING CARE
Varies with signs on examination

ACTIVITY
Restrict activity if dyspneic

DIET
N/A

CLIENT EDUCATION
Warn owners of the importance of controlling heart rate and rhythm in hyperthyroid patients and of the possibility of episodes of collapse.

SURGICAL CONSIDERATIONS
• Complete surgical excision—clearly treatment of choice for nonattached tumors
• Examine regional lymph nodes for staging and prognosis.
• Preoperative radiotherapy—consider for shrinking tumor
• Contralateral gland may be involved.

Risks
• Marked hemorrhage—tumors highly vascular; may need blood transfusion and intensive postoperative care
• Laryngeal paralysis—owing to trauma to recurrent laryngeal nerve
• Damaged parathyroid glands—may occur during surgery

 MEDICATIONS

DRUG(S) OF CHOICE
• Cisplatin (60 mg/m^2 every 3 weeks) and doxorubicin (30 mg/m^2 every 3 weeks)—reported to effect partial remission in approximately 50% of cases
• Cisplatin—nephrotoxic; must use with saline diuresis (18.3 mL/kg/hr IV over 6 hr; give cisplatin after 4 hr)
• Butorphanol—0.4 mg/kg IM before and after cisplatin to reduce emesis
• Thyroxine—maintenance doses to decrease TSH production have been recommended; some tumors contain TSH receptors; value of hormone-replacement therapy in affected dogs not determined
• Methimazole—5 mg PO q8h for medium to large dogs; may be beneficial for hyperthyroid patients
• β-blockers—may be indicated for tachycardia or hypertension

CONTRAINDICATIONS
• Doxorubicin—decreased myocardial function, usually determined by measuring fractional shortening by cardiac ultrasound
• Cisplatin—decreased renal function; monitored via BUN, creatinine, and urine specific gravity

PRECAUTIONS
• Doxorubicin and cisplatin—myelosuppressive
• Chemotherapy can be toxic; consult with an oncologist before initiating treatment.

POSSIBLE INTERACTIONS
Verapamil—may potentiate doxorubicin-induced cardiotoxicity

ALTERNATIVE DRUG(S)
• Radioactive iodine—may be useful for tumors that produce excess thyroid hormone
• External beam radiation therapy—may be beneficial to shrink tumors before surgery or to prevent local tumor recurrence after surgery; may be used palliatively to temporarily relieve signs caused by a space-occupying mass

 FOLLOW-UP

PATIENT MONITORING
• Serum calcium concentration—if bilateral thyroidectomy was performed; signs of hypocalcemia: agitation, panting, muscle tremors, tetany, and seizures; treatment: 10% calcium gluconate (1.0–1.5 mL/kg IV over 10–20 min)
• ECG—during IV administration of calcium; may use subcutaneous injection or intravenous constant-rate infusion until patient is stable enough to start dihydrotachysterol (vitamin D) orally
• Thyroid hormone concentration—treatment with thyroxine may be necessary after bilateral thyroidectomy
• Site of primary tumor—physical examination; thoracic radiographs every 3–4 months to detect pulmonary metastasis

PREVENTION/AVOIDANCE
Unknown

POSSIBLE COMPLICATIONS
• Tumor—anemia; thrombocytopenia; hypercalcemia; DIC; respiratory distress
• Chemotherapy—dilated cardiomyopathy; renal failure; pancreatitis; sepsis
• Surgery—hemorrhage; hypothyroidism; hypoparathyroidism leading to hypocalcemia; laryngeal paralysis
• Radiotherapy—pharyngeal mucositis; esophagitis; hair loss, and skin or coat color change (at radiation site)

EXPECTED COURSE AND PROGNOSIS
• Prognosis—related to size and resectability of primary tumor (small, nonattached tumors have best prognosis), involvement of regional lymph nodes, and occurrence of distant (usually pulmonary) metastases
• Approximately one third of patients have detectable metastasis at the time of diagnosis, usually to the regional lymph nodes or lungs.

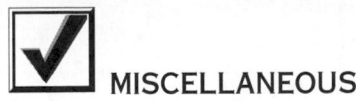 MISCELLANEOUS

ASSOCIATED CONDITIONS
• Nonthyroidal malignancies common
• Multiple endocrine neoplasia reported

AGE-RELATED FACTORS
None

ZOONOTIC POTENTIAL
None

PREGNANCY
Do not use chemotherapy in pregnant animals.

SYNONYMS
Thyroid carcinoma

ABBREVIATIONS
• DIC = disseminated intravascular coagulation
• TSH = thyroid-stimulating hormone

Suggested Reading

Adams WH, Walker MA, Daniel GB, et al. Treatment of differentiated thyroid carcinoma in 7 dogs utilizing ^{131}I. Vet Radiol Ultrasonogr 1994;36:417–424.

Fineman LS, Hamiltion TA, de Gortari A, et al. Cisplatin chemotherapy for treatment of thyroid carcinoma in dogs: 13 cases. J Am Anim Hosp Assoc 1998;34;109–112.

Jeglum KA, Whereat A. Chemotherapy of canine thyroid carcinoma. Compend Contin Educ Pract Vet 1983;5:96–98.

Klein MK, Powers BE, Withrow SJ, et al. Treatment of thyroid carcinoma in dogs by surgical resection alone: 20 cases (1981–1989). J Am Vet Med Assoc 1995;206:1007–1009.

Pack L, Roberts RE, Davson SD, Dookwah HD. Definitive radiation therapy for infiltrative thyroid carcinoma in dogs. Vet Radiol Ultrasound 2001;42:471–474.

Waters CB, Scott-Moncrieff JCR. Cancer of endocrine origin. In: Morrison WB, ed. Cancer in dogs and cats: medical and surgical management. Baltimore: Williams & Wilkins, 1998:599–637.

Author Linda S. Fineman
Consulting Editor Wallace B. Morrison

AGGRESSION, FEAR—CATS

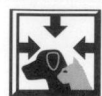

BASICS

OVERVIEW

Fear is characterized by intensive arousal and active avoidance or withdrawal and may lead to aggression. Fear may at times be adaptive. Fear can result from environmental and genetic influences. There are genetically friendly cats and genetically shy cats, influenced by paternal genes. Organ systems affected by fear include nervous, renal/urologic, skin/exocrine, and any organ system that can be affected by stress.

SIGNALMENT

No breed, age, or sex predilection documented

SIGNS

• The most common sign is staring. • Fearful cats withdraw and involute their limbs.
• Fearfully aggressive cats hiss, then swat and, if unable to run away, attack with claws and teeth. Staring, hissing, posturing (including changes in piloerection, tail postures, ear position, pupil shape and dilation, back and rump posture, and facial signs), marking with urine or with scent glands, and attack and fighting may occur.

CAUSES & RISK FACTORS

• Genetic predisposition • Incomplete exposure to cats, people, or other species during ontogeny (2–8 weeks) • Adaptive learning response to abandonment, inappropriate housing in shelters, and abuse

DIAGNOSIS

DIFFERENTIAL DIAGNOSIS

• Aggression due to incomplete socialization
• Intercat aggression • Territorial aggression
• Hyperthyroidism • Lower or upper urinary tract disease • Brain lesions (primarily forebrain)
• Infectious disease (e.g., rabies, feline immunodeficiency virus, feline infectious peritonitis) • Response to the disease state of another housemate

CBC/BIOCHEMISTRY/URINALYSIS

A baseline laboratory examination should be performed. Perform a multi-level urological examination if marking or inappropriate elimination is involved.

OTHER LABORATORY TESTS

Complete thyroid panel, by dialysis method, in older cats

IMAGING

If continued marking or inappropriate elimination, radiography and ultrasonography

DIAGNOSTIC PROCEDURES

• Thorough history taking and a full assessment of the animal's behaviors are necessary. A good history will elicit circumstances that provoke changes in the behavior of the cat. • Videotape the cat in its daily activities. Refrain from videotaping if it makes the animal more fearful.

TREATMENT

• Avoidance of fear-eliciting stimuli to prevent learning associated with further aggression
• The unique neurochemistry of the cat renders cats more reactive, and constrains them to be reactive for long periods of time. Once aggressively aroused, cats are best left alone until sufficiently calm before interaction. • Identify conditions when the cat is calm so active behavior modification can begin. • Identify the stimulus to which the cat reacts (e.g., human, animal, physical, or auditory). • Leashes and harnesses help in desensitization and counter-conditioning. • Food treats, massage, and grooming used as rewards • Keep behavior modification events short; stop if the cat shows any signs of distress. • Pharmacological intervention may allow the behavioral modification program to proceed more smoothly. • No forceful techniques including "punishment," shock, and "flooding"

MEDICATIONS

DRUG(S)

Benzodiazepines

Diazepam or oxazepam (0.2–0.4 mg/kg PO q12–24h) may make the cat more outgoing and friendlier, and increase appetite (helpful for behavior modification using food treats).

Tricyclic Antidepressants (TCAs)

• Amitriptyline: nonspecific anti-anxiety medication (0.5 mg/kg PO q12–24h × 30 days to start) • Nortriptyline: if the cat is sedated when treated with amitriptyline (0.5 mg/kg PO q12–24 h × 30 days to start) • Clomipramine: for cats exhibiting ritualistic behaviors (0.5 mg/kg PO q24h × 60 days to start)

Azapirone

• Buspirone: for very withdrawn cats—renders the cat more outgoing; can result in increased assertiveness that may lead to an aggressive social interaction • 0.5 mg/kg PO q24h × 60 days to start

Selective Serotonin Reuptake Inhibitors (SSRIs)

• Fluoxetine, paroxetine, sertraline: for profound, explosive aggression when cat is frightened; specific anxieties involving outburst (fluoxetine), social anxieties (paroxetine), and true panic (sertraline) • 0.5 mg/kg PO q24h × 60 days to start

Pheromones

Feliway and Felifriend may be helpful, as an adjuvant to other treatment, if routinely applied to areas frequented by cats, but there are no data to support this use.

PRECAUTIONS

• None of the above medications are licensed for use in cats. • Rare rhythm or conduction disturbances have been reported for all TCAs.
• Paradoxical excitement (e.g., serotonin syndrome) is a rare side effect of TCAs and SSRIs. • No SSRI or TCA should ever be used concomitantly with a monoamine oxidase inhibitor (e.g., selegiline, tick collars).
• Buspirone should be given only with the intent of making cats more assertive. There may be changes in social aggression, of which humans can be targets.

FOLLOW-UP

PATIENT MONITORING

• Weekly telephone follow-up to monitor progress • Annual laboratory evaluation for cats maintained on long-term medication is advisable. Weaning is recommended if the clients wish to learn if the cat still needs the medication or can be maintained on a lower dose. • For cats at risk, an ECG if tricyclic antidepressants or some selective serotonin reuptake inhibitors are prescribed

POSSIBLE COMPLICATIONS

• Injury to animals or humans • For safety, children must know how to appropriately respond to a cat that is crouching or withdrawn.

PREVENTION/AVOIDANCE

Clients should be counseled against adding more cats to a household where intercat aggression has already been a problem. Confinement away from fear-eliciting stimuli may be prudent if possible.

EXPECTED COURSE AND PROGNOSIS

• Cats that are aggressive and fearful because of lack of early exposure to humans may never be normal, cuddly pets. They may attach to one person or a small group of people over a period of time. Some cats may become apparently "normal." However, if forced into a situation involving restraint, confinement, or intimate contact, these animals may become extremely aggressive. • Prognosis is improved with reasonable expectations and the ability to protect the cat from any circumstances with which the cat cannot cope, despite behavioral and medical treatment. • The earlier the intervention, the better the prognosis and the shorter the course of medical treatment.

MISCELLANEOUS

ZOONOTIC POTENTIAL

Serious injuries can occur trying to separate actively fighting cats. Use large pieces of cardboard, heavy blankets, and other physical barriers to separate cats. Clients should further be aware that cats could remain highly aroused for more than 24 hours after an attack.

Suggested Reading

Overall KL. Managing an aggressive cat. Vet Med 1998;93:1051–1052.
Author Karen L. Overall
Consulting Editor Debra Horwitz

BASICS

OVERVIEW
Canine fear/defensive aggression occurs when the dog perceives a situation as threatening. May be within range of normal behavior but excessive fearfulness (phobic) behavior also possible. Systems affected include behavioral and signs of sympathetic stimulation (e.g., tachypnea, tachycardia).

SIGNALMENT
• Dog • No gender predilection; not affected by neutering • German shepherds predisposed • Can occur at any age. Signs often develop as puppies leave the peak period for socialization at around 12 weeks of age and again at 6–9 months.

SIGNS
• Aggression (growling, lip-lifting, barking, snapping, lunging, biting) accompanied by fearful or submissive body postures/facial expression (head down, crouching, backing away, ears back, tail tucked, looking away, lip licking) • History may include dog having been hurt or startled in a similar situation. Often directed towards unfamiliar people. • May occur when dog is cornered or cannot escape • May be worse on-leash than off-leash

CAUSES & RISK FACTORS
• May be a normal canine behavior depending on the circumstances • Strongly influenced by previous experience (e.g., inadequate early socialization, painful conditions, rough handling, inappropriate punishment) • Underlying medical conditions, especially those causing pain, may increase level of aggressive response.

DIAGNOSIS

DIFFERENTIAL DIAGNOSIS
• Dominance or social status aggression • Conflict aggression

CBC/BIOCHEMISTRY/URINALYSIS
Usually unremarkable. Abnormalities suggest an underlying or contributing medical condition.

OTHER LABORATORY TESTS
Usually unremarkable

IMAGING
MRI if CNS disease suspected. Other imaging as needed to rule out underlying medical conditions.

TREATMENT

CLIENT EDUCATION
• Treatment is aimed at controlling the problem, not at achieving a "cure." Successful treatment, as measured by a decrease in aggressive incidents, depends upon the owner's understanding basic canine social behavior, the risks involved in living with an aggressive dog, how to follow safety and management recommendations, and correct identification of the fear-eliciting stimuli. • Owners must be aware that the only way to prevent all future injuries is euthanasia. • Safety, preventing human injuries, must be the first concern. This may include confinement and use of headcollars, leashes, and muzzles. Teach the dog to be comfortable wearing a head halter (Gentle Leader) and basket muzzle. Avoid situations that may evoke an aggressive reaction, including situations that have resulted in the dog's being fearful even if not aggressive. The dog must be confined away from potential victims or under the direct physical control of a responsible adult whenever an aggression-provoking situation could arise (e.g., in any public locations, on walks, when visitors arrive at the house).

Affection Control
Used to increase predictability of dog's life and decrease occurrence of fear-provoking situations.

Behavior Modification
• Systematic desensitization and counter-conditioning to specific fear and aggression-provoking stimuli • Basket muzzles recommended • The dog should first be taught to sit and relax on a verbal command in neutral locations using food rewards. • Gradual exposure of the dog to a greatly reduced stimulus is next attempted so no fearful reaction is elicited. The non-fearful behavior is then rewarded. • Level of stimulation is increased gradually, staying below the threshold that would result in fear and/or aggression. • Progress is slow, and careful monitoring of responses is essential. • Relapses are common, and owners must always be vigilant and in control of the dog's behavior.

MEDICATIONS

DRUG(S)
There are no medications licensed for the treatment of canine aggression. Few published studies exist. Owners must be aware that the use of a medication is off-label. Because of liability concerns, note in patient record that owners were informed of potential risks and side effects. A signed informed consent form is advisable. NEVER use medications without behavior modification. Before prescribing medication, be sure that owners understand the risks involved in owning an aggressive dog and will follow safety procedures and not rely on medication to keep others safe. Medication may not be appropriate in some family situations, such as those with small children, family members with disabilities, or immunocompromised individuals.

Selective Serotonin Reuptake Inhibitors (SSRIs)
• Fluoxetine 0.5–1 mg/kg PO q24h, paroxetine 0.5–1 mg/kg PO q24h, sertraline 1–3 mg/kg PO q24h • Side effects: inappetence, irritability

Tricyclic Antidepressants (TCAs)
• Amitriptyline 2.2–4.4 mg/kg q24h or divided q12h, clomipramine 2–4 mg/kg PO q24h or divided q12h (label-restricted for aggression) • Side effects: sedation, anticholinergic, possible cardiac conduction disturbances if predisposed

Benzodiazepines
Alprazolam 0.05–0.1 mg/kg PO q12h or PRN

PRECAUTIONS
• Use caution when prescribing benzodiazepines. They may disinhibit aggression if they reduce fear-based inhibition to biting. • Do not combine SSRIs or TCAs with MAO inhibitors (e.g., amitraz, selegiline). • Avoid combining SSRIs and TCAs—can result in potentially fatal serotonin syndrome.

FOLLOW-UP

PATIENT MONITORING
Clients often need ongoing assistance. They should receive at least one follow-up call within the first 1–3 weeks after the consultation. Provisions for further follow-up should be made at that time. Ongoing communication improves client compliance.

PREVENTION/AVOIDANCE
Treatment recommendations are lifelong—may see recurrence of aggression with treatment lapses and continued exposure to the fear-producing stimuli. Good early socialization and habituation may help avoid fear-based behaviors later in life.

POSSIBLE COMPLICATIONS
Human injuries; euthanasia or relinquishment of patient

EXPECTED COURSE AND PROGNOSIS
There is no cure. Prognosis for improvement is better if aggression is at a low intensity and occurs only in a few predictable situations. Prognosis is highly dependent on owner compliance.

MISCELLANEOUS

ASSOCIATED CONDITIONS
May see other fear- or anxiety-based conditions (e.g., noise phobias, separation anxiety)

ZOONOTIC POTENTIAL
Bite wounds

PREGNANCY
Do not breed dogs with extremely fearful behavior or fear/aggression.

SEE ALSO
Aggression Toward Familiar People—Dogs

Author Laurie Bergman
Consulting Editor Debra F. Horwitz

AGGRESSION, FOOD, POSSESSIVE AND TERRITORIAL—DOGS

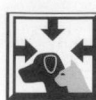

BASICS

OVERVIEW
• Canine food and possessive aggression—aggressively guarding food (e.g., in food bowl, rawhides, real bones, stolen or found items) or objects (e.g., toys, stolen objects). • Territorial aggression—aggressively defending a territory. Territory may be a fixed location (e.g., home, yard, car, bed, or resting area) and aggression may not be evident in other locations. In other cases, the territory is mobile and is an area around the dog, and aggressive responses may occur at any time. Territorial aggression may be exacerbated if the dog is restrained. • Usually within the range of normal behavior but excessive aggression due to learning is also possible • System affected: behavioral

SIGNALMENT
No breed or gender predilections exist for food/possessive aggression. Territorial aggression usually involves intact males.

SIGNS
• Food/Possessive—aggression (growling, lip-lifting, barking, snapping, lunging, biting) towards people or other dogs in the presence of valued food items or objects • Territorial—aggression in defense of a location or space

CAUSES & RISK FACTORS
• May be part of normal canine behavior repertoire • Strongly influenced by previous experiences of successfully defending food, objects, or territory through aggression • Underlying medical conditions, especially those causing polyphagia, may increase level of food aggression.

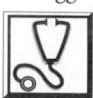

DIAGNOSIS

DIFFERENTIAL DIAGNOSIS
• Social status/dominance aggression • Fear aggression

CBC/BIOCHEMISTRY/URINALYSIS
Usually unremarkable. Abnormalities suggest an underlying or contributing medical condition.

OTHER LABORATORY TESTS
Usually unremarkable

IMAGING
MRI if CNS disease suspected. Other imaging as needed to rule out underlying medical conditions

TREATMENT

CLIENT EDUCATION
• Treatment is aimed at controlling the problem, not at achieving a "cure." Successful treatment, as measured by a decrease in aggressive incidents, depends upon the owner's understanding basic canine social behavior, the risks involved in living with an aggressive dog, and how to follow safety and management recommendations. • Owners must be aware that the only way to absolutely prevent future injuries is euthanasia. • First concern is safety. Avoid situations that may evoke an aggressive reaction. • Feed dogs confined away from people; do not give items that may evoke aggression. • Confine territorial dogs in locations where they cannot see/hear people approaching territory. Confine before the dogs become aggressively aroused. • Teach the dog to be comfortable wearing a head halter (Gentle Leader) and basket muzzle.

Affection Control
Used to help increase owners' leadership over dogs. (See Aggression Toward Familiar People—Dogs)

Behavior Modification
• Systematic desensitization and counter-conditioning to specific aggression-provoking stimuli • Basket muzzles recommended for additional safety • The dog should first be taught to sit and relax on a verbal command in a neutral location using food rewards. Use pea-sized pieces of food to reduce the likelihood of a food-aggressive dog becoming aggressive during behavior modification. • Begin with gradual exposure of the dog to a greatly reduced stimulus so no aggressive reaction is elicited. • The non-aggressive behavior is then rewarded. • Gradually, increase the level of stimulation, staying below the threshold that would result in aggression. • Progress is slow, and careful monitoring of responses is essential.

Counter Commanding
Teaching dogs to perform alternate behaviors (e.g., a "quiet" command, relinquishing objects) on command for rewards

MEDICATIONS

DRUG(S)
There are no medications licensed for the treatment of canine aggression. Few published studies exist. Owners must be aware that the use of a medication is off-label. Because of liability concerns, a note in the patient record is advisable stating that owners were informed of potential risks and potential side effects. Signed informed consent forms are advisable. NEVER use medications without behavior modification. Before prescribing medication be sure that owners will be compliant with safety recommendations and will not rely on medication to ensure public safety.

Selective Serotonin Reuptake Inhibitors (SSRIs)
• Fluoxetine 0.5–1 mg/kg PO q24h, paroxetine 0.5–1 mg/kg PO q24h, sertraline 1–3 mg/kg PO q24h, • Side effects: inappetence, irritability

Tricyclic Antidepressants (TCAs)
• Amitriptyline 2.2–4.4 mg/kg q24h or divided q12h, clomipramine 2–4 mg/kg PO q24h or divided q12h (label-restricted for aggression) • Side effects: sedation, anticholinergic, possible cardiac conduction disturbances if predisposed

Benzodiazepines
Alprazolam 0.05–0.1 mg/kg PO q12h or PRN

CONTRAINDICATIONS/POSSIBLE INTERACTIONS
• Use caution when prescribing benzodiazepines. They may disinhibit aggression if they reduce fear-based inhibition to biting. • Do not combine SSRIs or TCAs with MAO inhibitors (e.g., amitraz, selegiline). • Avoid combining SSRIs and TCAs—can result in potentially fatal serotonin syndrome • Medications that increase appetite (e.g., corticosteroids) and calorie-restricted diets may exacerbate food aggression.

FOLLOW-UP

PATIENT MONITORING
Clients often need ongoing assistance. They should receive at least one follow-up call within the first 1–3 weeks after the consultation. Provisions for further follow-up should be made at that time.

PREVENTION/AVOIDANCE
Treatment recommendations are lifelong. May see recurrence of aggression with treatment lapses or continued exposure to aggressive triggers.

POSSIBLE COMPLICATIONS
Human injuries; euthanasia or relinquishment of patient

EXPECTED COURSE AND PROGNOSIS
There is no cure. Prognosis for improvement is better if aggression is at a low intensity and in a few predictable situations. Prognosis is highly dependent on owner compliance.

MISCELLANEOUS

ASSOCIATED CONDITIONS
Dominance aggression

ZOONOTIC POTENTIAL
Human injury and bite wounds

PREGNANCY
Do not breed dogs with extreme aggression.

SEE ALSO
• Aggression Toward Familiar People—Dogs
• Aggression, Fear/Defensive—Dogs

Suggested Reading
Landsberg G, Hunthausen W, Ackerman L. Handbook of behaviour problems of the dog and cat. Oxford: Butterworth-Heinemann, 1997.
Mertens PA. Canine aggression. In: Horwitz D, Mills D, Heath S, eds. BSAVA manual of canine and feline behavioural medicine. Gloucester, England: British Small Animal Veterinary Association, 2002: 195–215.

Author Laurie Bergman
Consulting Editor Debra F. Horwitz

BASICS

OVERVIEW
Aggression commonly based on conflicts within social hierarchies

SIGNALMENT
• Cat • Most apparent at 2–4 years of age or when the animals become socially mature
• Competition for mates generally involves aggression between males only.

SIGNS
• Primary sign by aggressor—staring and passive displacement of the victim from any environment that the victim occupies • Overt aggression—staring, hissing, posturing (including changes in piloerection, tail postures, ear position, pupil shape and dilation, back and rump posture, and facial signs), marking with urine or with scent glands; attack and fighting may occur • The victim may avoid the aggressor cat.
• Exclusion from the litter box may result in housesoiling. The aggressor may spray; the victim may be involved in non-spraying urine marking.

CAUSES & RISK FACTORS
• Aggression becomes more common with crowding and decreased individual space (both linear and 3-D). • Cats who previously lived in harmony may become destabilized by the addition of another cat or disruption in the household such as moving, illness, or hospitalization of either cat.

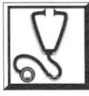

DIAGNOSIS

DIFFERENTIAL DIAGNOSIS
• Aggression due to incomplete socialization
• Fear aggression • Territorial aggression
• Hyperthyroidism • Urinary tract disease
• Brain lesions (primarily forebrain)
• Response to the disease state of another housemate

CBC/BIOCHEMISTRY/URINALYSIS
• Obtain as baseline prior to prescribing medications. • Urological examination if marking or inappropriate elimination involved

OTHER LABORATORY TESTS
Thyroid panel by dialysis method, particularly in senior cats

IMAGING
In continued marking or inappropriate elimination—radiography and ultrasonography

DIAGNOSTIC PROCEDURES
• For cats at risk, an ECG (lead II rhythm strip) should be part of the pre-medication workup if tricyclic antidepressants (TCAs) or some selective serotonin reuptake inhibitors (SSRIs)

are used. • Thorough history-taking and a full assessment of the animals' behaviors: videotapes of the cats in their daily activities and in all spaces where they spend time. Subtle changes in the behavior of one of the cats. Also noted should be changes in the social environment (including the death of another cat), changes in the physical environment, or changes in the health of one of the participants.

TREATMENT

• Separate cats initially. Aggressor is placed behind a locked door in a less desirable room with food, water, and a litter box. Victim is allowed either free range or unconstrained access to favorable areas (e.g., the client's bedroom, the sunny windows).
• Cats are allowed out under supervision only. Client monitors cat's body language. At the first sign of any aggression, the aggressor should be banished. Aggressor should be released only when calm.
• Leashes and harnesses allow client control.
• Desensitize and counter-condition cats to each other using food treats, massage, and grooming as rewards.
• No forceful techniques including "punishment," shock, and "flooding"

MEDICATIONS

DRUG(S)

Benzodiazepines
• Diazepam or oxazepam (0.2–0.4 mg/kg PO q12–24h)
• For the victim, primarily to make more outgoing and friendlier
• For the aggressor if aggression is secondary to anxiety about interaction and increased friendliness will help

Tricyclic Antidepressants
• Amitriptyline—for the victim or aggressor with nonspecific anxiety. Cat: 0.5 mg/kg PO q12–24h × 30 days to start
• Nortriptyline—for the victim or aggressor with nonspecific anxiety and sedation with amitriptyline. Cat: 0.5 mg/kg PO q12–24h × 30 days to start
• Clomipramine—for the victim or aggressor with more specific anxiety. Cat: 0.5 mg/kg PO q24h × 60 days to start

Azapirone
Buspirone—for the victim only; may make more outgoing and situation resolves with some overt aggression. Cat: 0.5 mg/kg PO q24h × 60 days to start

Selective Serotonin Reuptake Inhibitors
Fluoxetine, paroxetine—for more specific anxieties involving outburst (fluoxetine) and social (paroxetine) anxieties. Cat: 0.5 mg/kg PO q24h × 60 days to start

Pheromones
Feliway and Felifriend may help as an adjuvant if routinely applied to areas frequented by both cats, but there are no data to support this use.

CONTRAINDICATIONS/POSSIBLE INTERACTIONS
• None of the above medications are licensed for use in cats in the U.S.
• Rare rhythm or conduction disturbances and tachycardias have been reported for all TCAs.
• Paradoxical excitement (e.g., serotonin syndrome) can be a rare side effect for all TCAs and SSRIs.
• No SSRI or TCA should ever be used concomitantly with a monoamine oxidase inhibitor (MAOI) (e.g., selegiline). Buspirone should be given ONLY to victims: it makes cats more assertive and clients need to be warned that more frank aggression may occur.

FOLLOW-UP

PATIENT MONITORING
• Weekly telephone follow-up to monitor progress is suggested. • Annual laboratory evaluation for cats maintained on long-term medication is advisable.

PREVENTION/AVOIDANCE
Clients should be counseled against adding more cats to a household where intercat aggression has already been a problem.

EXPECTED COURSE AND PROGNOSIS
• Prognosis is excellent if the clients are willing to keep cats separated. • The seriousness of the behaviors of both the victims and aggressors determines prognosis and duration of required treatment with medication. The earlier the intervention, the better the prognosis and the shorter the course of medical treatment. If serious fear or injury has been involved, prognosis is poorer.

MISCELLANEOUS

ZOONOTIC POTENTIAL
Serious injuries can occur trying to separate actively fighting cats. Use large pieces of cardboard, heavy blankets, and other physical barriers to separate cats.

Suggested Reading
Overall KL. Animal behavior case of the month: Intercat aggression associated with spraying and urine marking. J Am Vet Med Assoc 1997;211:1376–1378.
Overall KL. Intercat aggression: Why can't they all just get along? Vet Med 1999;94:688–693.
Author Karen L. Overall
Consulting Editor Debra F. Horwitz

AGGRESSION, INTERDOG AGGRESSION

 BASICS

OVERVIEW
Two basic forms: aggression towards other dog(s) within a household and aggression towards unfamiliar dogs. A variety of different motivations exist, including fear, territoriality, and social status. Usually within the range of normal behavior, but excessive aggression due to learning or genetics (dogs bred for fighting) is also possible.

SYSTEM AFFECTED
Behavioral

SIGNALMENT
• Dog • More common in intact males
• Breed predilection in "fighting breeds" (e.g., pit bull terriers) and terriers
• Signs usually develop at puberty (between 6–9 months of age) or social maturity (between 18–36 months of age).

SIGNS
• Aggression (growling, lip-lifting, barking, snapping, lunging, biting) towards other dogs. This may be accompanied by fearful or submissive body postures/facial expressions (crouching, backing away, ears back, tail tucked, looking away, lip licking) or by confident/dominant body postures (standing straight up, approaching the other dog, direct contact with the other dog, tail up, ears forward).
• History may include dog having been victim of aggression from other dogs (especially if aggression is towards unfamiliar dogs).
• In cases of fighting within a household, the dogs may get along well except in specific triggering situations.

CAUSES & RISK FACTORS
• May be a normal canine behavior; strongly influenced by previous experience (e.g., inadequate early socialization to other dogs, aggressive encounters with other dogs)
• Breed predilections due to selective breeding for interdog aggression
• Aggression is likely to be worse towards dogs of the same gender.
• Underlying medical conditions, especially those causing pain, may increase level of aggression.

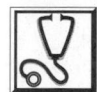 DIAGNOSIS

DIFFERENTIAL DIAGNOSIS
Play behavior or excited non-aggressive arousal

CBC/BIOCHEMISTRY/URINALYSIS
Usually unremarkable. Abnormalities suggest an underlying or contributing medical condition.

OTHER LABORATORY TESTS
Usually unremarkable

IMAGING
MRI if CNS disease suspected; as needed to rule out underlying medical conditions

DIAGNOSTIC PROCEDURES
N/A

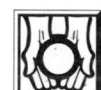 TREATMENT

CLIENT EDUCATION
• Treatment is aimed at controlling the problem, not at achieving a "cure." Successful treatment, as measured by a decrease in aggressive incidents, depends upon the owner's understanding basic canine social behavior, the risks involved in living with an aggressive dog, and how to follow safety and management recommendations.
• Owners must be aware that the only way to absolutely prevent future injuries is rehoming (if aggression is within a household) or euthanasia.
• Preventing human and canine injuries must be the first concern. Owners must be instructed in methods of avoiding and, if needed, safely breaking up dog fights. Avoid situations that may evoke an aggressive reaction. If there is a fear component, avoid situations that have resulted in the dog being fearful even if not aggressive. Dogs within a household may need to be kept separated to prevent contact and fighting. The dog must be confined away from potential victims or under the direct physical control of a responsible adult whenever an aggression-provoking situation could arise (e.g., in any public locations, on walks). Teach the dog(s) to be comfortable wearing a head halter (Gentle Leader) and basket muzzle.
• For aggression within a household, determine which dog is the more dominant individual and reinforce that dominance by providing that dog with priority access to resources (e.g., food, toys, resting areas, human attention) it values. Be aware of "bullies" and that dominance between household dogs can be context-dependent.

Affection Control
Especially for aggression between dogs within a household. To increase owners' leadership over dogs and predictability of dogs' lives (See Aggression, Toward Familiar People—Dogs)

Behavior Modification
• Systematic desensitization and counter-conditioning to specific aggression-provoking stimuli
• Use a basket muzzle if needed for additional safety
• NEVER allow dogs to "fight it out."
• Dog(s) should first be taught to sit and relax on a verbal command using food rewards.
• Expose the dog to a greatly reduced stimulus (the other dog at a distance) so no fearful or aggressive reaction is elicited.
• Reward this non-fearful and/or non-aggressive behavior.
• Gradually, increase the level of stimulation, staying below the threshold that would result in fear and/or aggression. This might mean decreasing distance between dogs as long as no aggressive behaviors are seen.

MEDICATIONS

DRUG(S)
There are no medications licensed for the treatment of canine aggression. Few published studies exist. Owners must be aware that the use of a medication is off-label. Because of liability concerns, a note in the patient record is advisable stating that owners were informed of potential risks and potential side effects. Signed informed consent forms are advisable. NEVER use medications without behavior modification. Medications are most likely to be helpful in situations where there is a strong fear/anxiety component, as opposed to situations where closely-ranked dogs are using aggression to establish dominance.

Selective Serotonin Reuptake Inhibitors (SSRIs)
• Fluoxetine 0.5–1 mg/kg PO q24h, paroxetine 0.5–1 mg/kg PO q24h, sertraline 1–3 mg/kg PO q24h
• Side effects: inappetence, irritability

Tricyclic Antidepressants (TCAs)
• Amitriptyline 2.2–4.4 mg/kg q 24h or divided q12h, clomipramine 2–4 mg/kg PO q24h or divided q12h (label-restricted for aggression)
• Side effects: sedation, anticholinergic, possible cardiac conduction disturbances if predisposed.

Benzodiazepines
Alprazolam 0.05–0.1 mg/kg PO q12h or PRN

CONTRAINDICATIONS/POSSIBLE INTERACTIONS
• Use caution when prescribing benzodiazepines. They may disinhibit aggression if they reduce fear-based inhibition to biting.
• Do not combine SSRIs or TCAs with MAO inhibitors (e.g., amitraz, selegiline).
• Avoid combining SSRIs and TCAs, as potentially fatal serotonin syndrome can result.

FOLLOW-UP

PATIENT MONITORING
Clients often need ongoing assistance. They should receive at least one follow-up call within the first 1–3 weeks after the consultation. Provisions for further follow-up should be made at that time.

PREVENTION/AVOIDANCE
Treatment recommendations are lifelong. There may be recurrence of aggression with treatment lapses.

POSSIBLE COMPLICATIONS
Injuries to dogs involved; human injuries; euthanasia or relinquishment of patient

EXPECTED COURSE AND PROGNOSIS
There is no cure. Prognosis for improvement is better if aggression is at a fairly low intensity and occurs in only a few predictable situations. Prognosis is highly dependent on owner compliance.

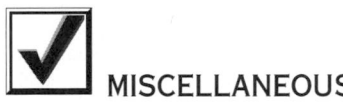

MISCELLANEOUS

ASSOCIATED CONDITIONS
May see other fear- or anxiety-based conditions (e.g., noise phobias, separation anxiety); territorial aggression

ZOONOTIC POTENTIAL
Bite wounds when separating fighting dogs

PREGNANCY
Do not breed dogs with extreme interdog aggression.

SEE ALSO
• Aggression Toward Familiar People—Dogs
• Aggression, Fear/Defensive—Dogs

Suggested Reading
Mertens PA. Canine aggression. In: Horwitz D, Mills D, Heath S, eds. BSAVA Manual of canine and feline behavioural medicine. Gloucester, England: British Small Animal Veterinary Association, 2002:195–215.
Author Laurie Bergman
Consulting Editor Debra F. Horwitz

AGGRESSION, OVERVIEW—CATS

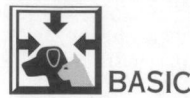

BASICS

DEFINITION
• Can be adaptive and appropriate if it helps the animal protect itself, its resources, or its present or future genetic contribution
• Behavioral medicine—concerned with recognizing when behavior is maladaptive or abnormal

Aggression Owing to Lack of Socialization
• No human contact before 3 months of age—cat misses sensitive period important for development of normal approach responses to people; if not handled until 14 weeks of age, it is fearful and aggressive to people; if handled for only 5 min/day until 7 weeks, it interacts with people, approaches inanimate objects, and plays with toys. • Lack of social interaction with other cats—may result in lack of normal inquisitive response to other cats; negative response may be augmented by suboptimal nutritional conditions for the pregnant queen. • These cats are never normal, cuddly pets; may eventually attach to one person or a small group of people; if forced into a situation involving restraint, confinement, or intimate contact, they may become extremely aggressive.

Play Aggression
• Weaned early and hand-raised by humans—cat may never learn to temper play responses; if not taught as a kitten to modulate responses, it may not learn to sheathe claws or inhibit bite; bottle-fed cats may be overrepresented (no good data).
• Social play—peaks early; replaced by predatory activities by weeks 10–12 and social fighting by week 14

Fearful or Fear-induced Aggression
• Fearful—cat may hiss, spit, arch the back, and piloerect if flight is not possible; combinations of offensive and defensive postures and overt and covert aggressive behaviors are usually involved. • Flight—virtually always a component of fearful aggression • Pursued—if cornered, cat will stop, draw its head in, crouch, growl, roll on its back when approached (not submissive but overtly defensive), and paw at the approacher; if pursuit is continued, cat will strike, then hold the approacher with its forepaws while kicking with the back feet and biting. • If threatened, cat will defend itself; any cat can become fearfully aggressive.

Pain Aggression
Pain may cause aggression; with extended painful treatment, cat may exhibit fearful aggression.

Intercat Aggression
• Male–male aggression associated with mating or hierarchical status within the social group; mating may also involve social hierarchy issues. • Maturity—in peaceful multicat households, problems may occur, regardless of sex composition, when a cat reaches social maturity (2–4 years of age).

Maternal Aggression
• May occur in the periparturient period
• Protection—queens may guard nesting areas and kittens by threatening with long approach distances, rather than attack; usually directed toward unfamiliar individuals; may inappropriately be directed toward known individuals; as kittens mature, aggression resolves.
• Unknown if kittens learn aggressive behavior from an aggressive mother

Predatory Behavior
• Occurs under different behavioral circumstances • Normal predatory behavior develops at 5–7 weeks of age; cat may be proficient hunter by 14 weeks; commonly displayed with field voles, house mice, and birds at feeders; may be learned from mother; more common in cats that have to fend for themselves; if well fed, cat may kill and only behead prey. • Aggression—stealth, silence, heightened attentiveness, body posture associated with hunting (slinking, head lowering, tail twitching, and pounce postures), lunging or springing at prey, exhibiting sudden movement after a quiet period • Free-ranging groups—when a new male enters, he may kill kittens to encourage queen to come into estrus. • Inappropriate context distinctions about prey—potentially dangerous if "prey" is a foot, hand, or infant; cats exhibiting pre-pounce behaviors in these contexts are at risk.

Territorial Aggression
• May be exhibited toward other cats, dogs, or people; owing to transitive nature of social hierarchies, a cat aggressive to one housemate may not be to another if turf is not contested.
• Turf may be delineated by patrol, chin rubbing, spraying, or nonspraying marking; threats and/or fights may occur if a perceived offender enters the area; if the struggle involves social hierarchy, the challenger may be sought out and attacked after the territory is invaded.
• May be difficult to treat, particularly if there is marking; marking problems suggest a possible underlying aggression.

Redirected Aggression
• Difficult to recognize and may be reported as incidental to another form of aggression
• Occurs when a motor pattern appropriate for a specific motivational state is redirected to an accessible target because the primary target is unavailable (e.g., interruption of an aggressive event between two parties by a third party results in redirection of the aggressive behavior to the third party or to an uninvolved individual); cat may remain reactive for some time after being thwarted in an aggressive interaction. • Often precipitated by another inappropriate behavior; important to treat that behavior as well

Assertion or Status-related Aggression
• If unprovoked, most frequently occurs when cat is being petted; a need to control all interactions with humans and when attention starts and ceases; cat may bite and leave or may take hand in teeth but not bite. • May be accompanied by territorial aggression • May best be called impulse control/dyscontrol aggression

Idiopathic Aggression
Rare; poorly understood and poorly defined; unprovoked, unpredictable, toggle-switch aggression

SYSTEMS AFFECTED
• Cardiovascular—signs consistent with sympathetic stimulation • Endocrine/Metabolic—signs consistent with alterations in the HPA axis • Hemic—stress leukogram • Musculoskeletal—damage to teeth and gums, abscesses, abrasions, and lacerations common • Nervous—increased motor activity, repetitive activity, trembling, and prolonged increased reactivity (up to 24h) may accompany or follow outbursts of aggression; OCD may be associated with the victim. • Renal/Urologic—urine marking (spraying and nonspraying); changes in location and substrate preferences for "normal" elimination • Respiratory—tachypnea and the attendant metabolic changes possible in extreme situations • Skin/Exocrine—skin lesions usually secondary and may result from injury; if consistently stressed by aggressive situations, may cease to groom or may overgroom and mutilate

SIGNALMENT
• No breed differences, except for those resulting from a lack of socialization and play
• Appears at onset of social maturity (2–4 years) • Males—may be more prone to intercat aggression (no good data)

SIGNS

General Comments
Elimination behaviors—tightly coupled with aggression; take a thorough behavioral and medical history.

Historical Findings
Abuse—cat may learn aggression as a pre-emptive strategy.

Physical Examination Findings
• Usually nonremarkable except for injuries and a lack of condition associated with increased motor activity and withdrawal
• Continuous anxiety—decreased or increased grooming

CAUSES
Part of the normal feline behavior; greatly influenced by the early social history and exposure to humans and other animals, sex, social context, handling, and many other variables

RISK FACTORS
N/A

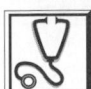

DIAGNOSIS

DIFFERENTIAL DIAGNOSIS
• Conditions that cause similar behavioral changes—seizures; brain disease; metabolic disease (thyroid or adrenal conditions) • Hepatic encephalopathy • Feline ischemic encephalopathy • Lead poisoning • Hyperthyroidism • Epilepsy • Rabies • Behavioral aggression is usually directed towards specific social foci; aggression from organic disease is unexpected, inappropriate, and more continuous, and/or without a social context.

CBC/BIOCHEMISTRY/URINALYSIS
• All should be performed. • Urinalysis—relationship between aggression and elimination disorders • Intercat aggression may be recognized because of attendant elimination problems.

OTHER LABORATORY TESTS
• Hyperthyroidism—test, if indicated • Urine culture and sensitivity—may be indicated when unexplained aggression correlates with urinary tract disease

IMAGING
• CT and MRI—rule out structural brain disease. • Ultrasound—bladder; may be helpful with concomitant stress-related FLUTD attack

DIAGNOSTIC PROCEDURES
• ECG—evaluate for arrhythmia or baseline before treatment with TCAs. • CSF analysis—rule out inflammatory brain disease.

TREATMENT
• Avoid provocation. • Teach client to observe signs (tail flicking, ears flat, pupils dilated, head hunched, claws possibly unsheathed, stillness or tenseness, low growl) and interrupt the behavior by letting the cat fall from his or her lap, abandoning it, and refusing to interact until appropriate behavior is displayed. • Discourage direct physical correction; may intensify aggression • Separate cats; keep the active aggressor in a less favored area to passively reinforce more desirable behavior. • Desensitization, counterconditioning, flooding, and habituation—if subtleties of social systems and communication are understood

MEDICATIONS

DRUG(S)
• Antianxiety medications that increase CNS levels of serotonin—tricyclic antidepressants

(TCAs) and selective serotonin reuptake inhibitors (SSRIs) • Amitriptyline (TCA)—0.5–1 mg/kg (to start) PO q12–24h for 30 days • Imipramine—0.5–1 mg/kg (to start) PO q12–24h for 30 days • Buspirone (a partial 5HT1A agonist)—0.5–1 mg/kg PO q24h; may make some cats more assertive; thus works well for aggressor in anxiety-associated aggression • Clomipramine (TCA)—0.5 mg/kg PO q24h for 60 days • Fluoxetine or paroxetine (SSRI)—0.5 mg/kg PO q24h for 60 days • Buspirone, clomipramine, paroxetine and fluoxetine—may take 3–5 weeks to be fully effective; early effects in cats are seen within 1 week, best for active, overt aggressions • Nortriptyline—active intermediate metabolite of amitriptyline; use instead of amitriptyline or imipramine, at the same dosage, if side effects appear. • Anxious and fearful aggression with concomitant elimination disorders—diazepam (0.2–0.4 mg/kg PO as needed) or other benzodiazepine; use with caution because benzodiazepines can facilitate and worsen inhibited aggressions; may facilitate some behavior modification if food treats used

CONTRAINDICATIONS
• Cats experience more drug-related side effects than do dogs. • Hepatic and renal compromise—some drugs contraindicated; glucuronidated drugs require follow-up. • Cardiac conduction anomalies—give tricyclic antidepressants only with extreme caution and monitoring. • Fat or pre-existing hepatic disease—may develop idiosyncratic, diazepam-induced hepatotoxicity

PRECAUTIONS
• Use of the listed medications is extra-label; Health and Human Services recommendations should be followed. • Tricyclic antidepressants—overdoses can cause profound cardiac conduction disturbances; ECG evaluation before treatment is advised.

POSSIBLE INTERACTIONS
• Benzodiazepines—lipophilic; may be potentiated by other lipophilic drugs; if combination treatment is warranted, use lower dosages. • Medications that impair the glucuronidation of active metabolites into inactive compounds cause increases of the active metabolites.

FOLLOW-UP

PATIENT MONITORING
• CBC, serum biochemistry, and urinalysis—before treatment; semiannually in older

patients; yearly in younger patients if treatment is continuous; adjust dosages accordingly. • As warranted by clinical signs—vomiting; gastrointestinal distress; tachycardia, tachypnea

POSSIBLE COMPLICATIONS
• Early treatment using both behavioral modification and pharmacological intervention crucial • Left untreated, these disorders always progress.

MISCELLANEOUS

ASSOCIATED CONDITIONS
Many occur with elimination disorders—substrate and location aversions and preferences, particularly spraying and nonspraying marking

AGE-RELATED FACTORS
Social maturity—associated with development of intercat aggression, fear aggression, territorial aggression, redirected aggression, and status-related aggression

ZOONOTIC POTENTIAL
• Cat scratch disease (*Bartonella henselae* and *Afipia felis*) • Rabies

PREGNANCY
Listed medications—avoid use of most in pregnant animals.

ABBREVIATIONS
CSF = cerebrospinal fluid
FLUID = feline lower urinary tract disease
HPA = hypothalamic–pituitary–adrenal
OCD = obsessive compulsive disorder
SSRI = selective serotonin reuptake inhibitor
TCA = tricyclic antidepressant

Suggested Reading
Chapman BL. Feline aggression: classification, diagnosis, and treatment. Vet Clin North Am Small Anim Pract 1991;21:315–328.
Frank DF, Erb HN, Houpt KA. Urine spraying in cats: presence of concurrent disease and effects of a pheromone treatment. Appl Anim Behav Sci 1999;61:263–272.
Overall KL. Feline aggression. Part III: The role of social status in hierarchical systems. Feline Pract 1994;22:16–17.
Overall KL. Tracing the roots of feline elimination disorders to aggression. Vet Med 1997;93:363–366.
Pryor PA, Hart BL, CLiff KD, Bain MJ. Effects of a selective serotonin reuptake inhibitor on urine spraying behavior in cats. J Am Vet Med Assoc 2001;219:1557–1561.
Author Karen L. Overall
Consulting Editor Debra Horwitz

AGGRESSION, OVERVIEW—DOGS

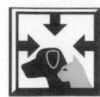 **BASICS**

DEFINITION
• Action by one dog directed against another organism with the result of harming, limiting, or depriving that organism; offensive, defensive, or predatory • Numerous functional types • Offensive—unprovoked attempt to gain some resource at the expense of another; includes social status/dominance, intermale, and interfemale aggression • Defensive—by a victim toward another that is perceived as an instigator or threat; includes fear-induced, territorial defense, protective, irritable (pain-associated or frustration-related), and maternal aggression

PATHOPHYSIOLOGY
• Not necessarily a pathologic condition • Some pathologic states are associated with an increase in aggression because of their effects on the CNS. • Rage—inappropriate offensive aggression; reported to be associated with biochemical abnormalities in the CSF

SYSTEMS AFFECTED
Behavior

SIGNALMENT
• Any age, sex, or breed • Cocker spaniels, springer spaniels, and German shepherds— common; regional differences exist • Pit bulls, rottweilers, German shepherds—most commonly associated with fatal dog bites • Social status/dominance-related offensive aggression—escalates as dog approaches social maturity (1–2 years of age) • Males—intact or castrated; more common

SIGNS
General Comments
• Bites may be preceded by behavioral signs. Offensive—head up, tail up, direct stare, face-on immobility. Defensive—head lowered, tail down, body withdrawn • History—forms the basis for risk analysis and details of the treatment program. Important questions: Under what circumstances does the aggression occur? To whom is the aggression directed? Have injuries occurred that required medical attention?

Historical Findings
Vary according to the situation and the functional type of aggression
Social Status/Dominance Aggression
• Directed toward household members • Head up; tail up; staring; stiff gait • Resents being reached out to, patted on head, and pushed off favored sleeping sites; having its food or stolen objects approached
Intermale and Interfemale Aggression
• Directed toward other dogs • Directed toward humans only when they interfere with fights • Head up; tail up; staring; stiff gait

Fear-Induced Aggression
• Directed to approaching or reaching humans • Certain familiar people may be exempt • Head down; eyes wide; tail tucked
Territorial Aggression
• Directed toward strangers approaching house, yard, or car • May be exacerbated if restrained • Barking; agitation; lunging; baring teeth
Protective Aggression
• Directed toward stranger approaching owner • Escalates with decreasing distance
Irritable (Pain, Frustration) Aggression
• Restricted to specific context associated with pain (e.g., nail trim, injection) • Rule out social status/dominance- and fear-induced aggression.
Maternal Aggression
• Directed toward individuals approaching the whelping area or puppies • Intensity usually inversely related to age of puppies

Physical Examination Findings
• Usually unremarkable • Use extreme care when handling aggressive dogs; use muzzles and other restraints to prevent injury to the examiner. • Dominance-related, fear-related aggression, or irritable aggression—may be evident during the examination • Neurologic examination—abnormalities may suggest an organic disease process (e.g., rabies).

CAUSES
• Part of the normal range of behavior; strongly influenced by breed, sex, early socialization, handling, and other variables • Manifestation of an organic condition— possible but rare • In all cases, rule out medical causes of aggression.

RISK FACTORS
• Poor socialization to certain types of stimuli (e.g., children)—adult dog may display fear-related aggression • Predisposing environmental conditions—associating with other dogs in a pack; barrier frustration or tethering; cruel handling and abuse; and dog baiting and fighting

 DIAGNOSIS

DIFFERENTIAL DIAGNOSIS
• Pathologic conditions associated with aggression must be identified before a purely behavioral diagnosis can be made. • A thorough medical evaluation should be conducted on all cases of aggression. • Rule out developmental abnormalities (hydrocephaly, lissencephaly, hepatic shunts), metabolic disorders (hypoglycemia, hepatic encephalopathy, diabetes), neuroendocrinopathies (hypothyroidism), neurologic conditions (intracranial neoplasm, seizures), toxins, inflammatory diseases (rabies), and pain.

CBC/BIOCHEMISTRY/URINALYSIS
• Usually normal • Abnormalities—may suggest metabolic or endocrine causes

OTHER LABORATORY TESTS
As indicated (e.g., thyroid panel or ACTH-stimulation test)

IMAGING
• May be indicated to identify sources of pain • MRI or CT—if cerebral neoplasia suspected

DIAGNOSTIC PROCEDURES
Postmortem fluorescent antibody test—any aggressive dog for which rabies is a differential diagnosis

RISK ASSESSMENT
General Comments
• Extremely important in cases of aggression • Considered a separate procedure; perform before initiating treatment • Consists of historical questions, observation, and confirmation with supporting data (medical, legal, veterinary records)

Questions
• Has the dog ever broken the skin or otherwise injured a person? If yes, how many times in the past year? • Has anyone sought medical attention for injuries caused by this dog? If yes, describe the circumstances in detail. • Have the injuries by this dog been reported to authorities, resulting in quarantine or citation? If yes, describe. • Is the weight of this dog > 18.2 kg (medium large dog)? • Are there children, elderly people, or others at high risk living in or visiting this household? • Is there any doubt that this dog will be restrained behind a fence, on a leash, fitted with a muzzle, or in other ways effectively controlled by the owner to protect people from injury? • Does this dog ever run free, without being under the owner's strict control? • Does aggression appear to occur unpredictably? • If the owner responds yes to any of these questions, consider the personal and legal liability risks to the owner and the treating veterinarian. Human injury, lawsuits, and loss of home-owners insurance can result. • Euthanasia should be recommended in high-risk cases.

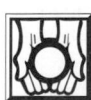 **TREATMENT**

• The first tenet of management is to prevent human injury. • Risk assessment may help the owner objectively evaluate the situation; all parties must understand that aggressive dogs are never cured, although sometimes the behavior can be managed successfully. • Euthanasia—appropriate solution in cases of vicious dogs; offer as the only safe solution. • Recommend techniques to reduce human risk from the aggressive dog until the owner obtains treatment.• Avoid situations that have led to aggression in the past. • Improve physical control of the dog using barriers (fences, baby gates), muzzles, leashes, and head halters. • Avoid the use of punishment, which tends to escalate aggression • Management success—combination of multiple modalities: environmental control, behavior modification, and pharmacotherapy

Social Status/Dominance Aggression

• Environmental—use barriers and restraint to prevent human injury. • Devices—train the dog to a muzzle and head halter. • Behavior modification, step 1—withdraw all attention from the dog for 2 weeks; list situations in which aggression occurs; devise a method of avoiding each situation; daily, list all aggressive incidents and circumstances to avoid in the future. • Behavior modification, step 2—use nonconfrontational means to establish the owner's leadership; teach the dog to reliably sit/stay on command in gradually more challenging situations (dog must acquiesce to the owner to obtain attention and other benefits); no "free" benefits (dog must sit/stay before eating, being petted, going for walk, etc.; the owner initiates all interactions) • Behavior modification, step 3—gain greater control; situations that previously elicited aggression are gradually introduced with the dog controlled in a sit/stay position (muzzle if necessary). • Surgery—neuter males; unless aggression is associated with the heat cycle, OHE will not improve behavior

Intermale and Interfemale Aggression

• Environmental—use barriers to prevent contact between the dogs except when well supervised; note dominance order between dogs; if apparent, comply with dogs' rules (dominant dog is fed first, travels through doorways first, etc.). • Devices—head halter, muzzle • A reduced protein diet may be helpful • Behavior modification, step 1—owner must withdraw all attention to both dogs; teach sit/stay program (as for dominance-related aggression). • Behavior modification, step 2—desensitize or countercondition by gradually decreasing distance between dogs while under leash control; reinforce acceptable behavior. • Surgery—neuter males; OHE recommended only if aggression is associated with heat cycle (otherwise it will not improve behavior)

Fear-Induced Aggression

• Environmental—use barriers and restraint to prevent human injury. • Devices—muzzle • A reduced protein diet may be helpful. • Behavior modification, step 1—list all situations in which the dog appears fearful or exhibits aggression; avoid those situations initially; teach dog basic obedience commands and reinforce under nonfearful conditions (generalize by training in many locations). • Behavior modification, step 2—desensitize and countercondition; subject the dog to mildly fearful conditions with the stimulus (e.g., a stranger) far away; keep the dog

attentive and performing obedience commands; gradually decrease the distance of the stranger; if the dog exhibits fear, the stranger should withdraw and work should continue at an easier level, then gradually progress. • Surgery—castration or OHE probably will not improve the behavior.

Territorial Aggression

• Environmental—use barriers and restraint to prevent human injury; initially, when visitors come, isolate the dog to prevent it from exhibiting the behavior • Devices—head halter, muzzle • Behavior modification, step 1—teach the dog sit/stay, first at neutral locations, then near the door and at other sites of territorial aggression; later, control the dog while a familiar person approaches; reward the dog for calm, obedient behavior. • Behavior modification, step 2—gradually introduce strangers (owner can dress in unfamiliar garb to represent a stranger); increase the difficulty as the dog learns control; move the exercises to the door; add entering the door, ringing the door bell, and other variables. • Surgery—castration or OHE probably will not improve behavior.

MEDICATIONS

DRUG(S) OF CHOICE

• None approved by the FDA for the treatment of aggression • Inform the client of the experimental nature of these treatments and the risk involved; document discussion in the medical record. • Drugs that increase the neurotransmitter serotonin may be helpful. • Amitriptyline—1–2 mg/kg q12h or 2–4 mg/kg q24h; side effects: sedation, anticholinergic effects • Fluoxetine—1–2 mg/kg q24h; side effects: sedation, inappetence • Clomipramine (Clomicalm) is label-restricted for aggression and should not be used for liability reasons.

CONTRAINDICATIONS

Amitriptyline—contraindicated in patients with cardiac conduction disturbances, glaucoma, fecal or urinary incontinence, or liver disease • Fluoxetine is contraindicated in cases of liver disease

PRECAUTIONS

Benzodiazepines (e.g., Diazepam)

• Avoid use in aggressive dogs • Can disinhibit aggression • Dogs can become more aggressive when they lose their fear of the repercussions of biting.

POSSIBLE INTERACTIONS

Do not use listed drugs with monoamine oxidase inhibitors, including amitraz and L-deprenyl.

ALTERNATIVE DRUG(S)

• L-Tryptophan—10 mg/kg PO q12h

• Megestrol acetate—1 mg/kg PO q24h for 2 weeks; then taper to lowest effective dosage; successful with dominance-related and intermale aggression; side effects: obesity, blood dyscrasias, pyometra, polyuria/polydipsia, diabetes mellitus, mammary hyperplasia, and carcinoma

FOLLOW-UP

PATIENT MONITORING

• Weekly to biweekly contact—recommended in the initial phases • Clients frequently need feedback and assistance with behavior modification plans and medication management.

PREVENTION/AVOIDANCE N/A

EXPECTED COURSE AND PROGNOSIS

Aggressive dogs are never cured, although sometimes the behavior can be managed.

POSSIBLE COMPLICATIONS

• Human injury • Social status/dominance aggression—can be directed toward owners • Interdog aggression—humans often seriously injured when interfering with fighting dogs, either by accident or by redirected or irritable aggression; owners should not reach for fighting dogs; pull apart with leashes

MISCELLANEOUS

AGE-RELATED FACTORS

Adult-onset aggression—in the absence of any positive historical findings, suggests a medical cause; carefully evaluate sources of pain and sensory acuity.

ZOONOTIC POTENTIAL

Rabies is a potential cause of aggression.

PREGNANCY

Tricyclic antidepressants—contraindicated in pregnant animals

ABBREVIATIONS

• ACTH = adrenocorticotropic hormone
• CSF = cerebrospinal fluid
• CT = computed tomography
• MRI = magnetic resonance imaging
• OHE = ovariohysterectomy

Suggested Reading

Mertens PA. Canine aggression. In: Horwitz D, Mills D, Heath S, eds. BSAVA Manual of canine and feline behavioural medicine. Gloucester, England: British Small Animal Veterinary Association, 2002:195–215.

Reisner I. An overview of aggression. In: Horwitz D, Mills D, Heath S, eds. BSAVA manual of canine and feline behavioural medicine. Gloucester, England: British Small Animal Veterinary Association, 2002:181–194.

Author Barbara S. Simpson
Consulting Editor Debra F. Horwitz

AGGRESSION TOWARD FAMILIAR PEOPLE—DOGS

 BASICS

DEFINITION
Aggression (growling, lip-lifting, barking, snapping, lunging, biting), usually directed towards household members or familiar people. Context: situations involving access to preferred resources. Also referred to as dominance aggression, status-related aggression, conflict or competitive aggression.

PATHOPHYSIOLOGY
Traditionally thought of as normal canine social behavior directed towards people. However, may be impulsive and unpredictable, with injurious and dangerous consequences.

SYSTEM AFFECTED
Behavioral

GENETICS
Breed predilections exist and pedigree analyses have shown that it may occur more commonly within related dogs. Mode of inheritance is unknown.

INCIDENCE/PREVALENCE
20–40% of behavioral referral case loads

GEOGRAPHIC DISTRIBUTION
Regional breed differences exist.

SIGNALMENT

Species
Dog

Breed Predilections
Spaniels (English springer and cocker), terriers, Lhasa apso, and rottweiler, but may be exhibited by any breed

Mean Age And Range
Usually manifested at the onset of social maturity (12–36 months of age). May be seen in young dogs

Predominant Sex
Males (castrated and intact) more commonly presented than females

SIGNS

General Comments
Careful history-taking is needed to make the diagnosis, assess the risk the dog poses to the owners and public, and formulate a safe and realistic treatment plan. Owners may not recognize or give credence to more mild behavioral signs of aggression such as staring, growling, baring teeth, or snapping, which may have been present for some time. Details of early aggressive episodes are vital for establishing the diagnosis and prognosis. Clinician should be aware that all owner-directed aggression is not motivated by the desire to control, but often is anxiety- or fear-based.

Historical Findings
• Aggression often seen around resting areas, food, toys, handling (including petting and reaching towards) and favored possessions, including people. Aggression is usually directed towards household members or persons that have an established relationship with the dog. Aggressive behaviors may be seen in other contexts, including but not limited to defense of territory, toward other dogs, and toward unfamiliar people. History-taking should attempt to establish aggression triggers, the frequency of aggressive episodes, and their severity. • Aggression may not be seen every time dog is in a certain situation and may not be directed uniformly towards each person within the household. • Stiff body posture, staring, head up, ears up and forward, or tail up usually accompanies aggressive behavior. Owners may report a combination of these postures with more submissive postures (e.g., tail is up but ears are tucked, eyes averted), which may represent an element of conflict, anxiety, or fear in the dog's motivation. • Owners often describe these dogs as "moody" and may be able to judge when the dog is likely to be aggressive in a given situation. Early episodes may show fearful behaviors such as eye aversion, tail tucked, and avoidance that may diminish as the dog becomes more confident that aggression will change the outcome. • Anxiety may be noted in pet-owner interactions and other situations such as owner departure or novel situations. Some dogs control their environment using aggression only because it is effective, but are anxious about every encounter, while other dogs appear confident and secure.

Physical Examination Findings
• Usually unremarkable • Medical conditions, especially painful ones, may contribute to the expression of aggression. These dogs may not show aggression towards a confident but non-threatening examiner. However, extreme caution should be taken when examining dogs that show aggression—including the use of muzzles or other humane restraint devices.

CAUSES
• May actually be part of a normal canine social behavioral repertoire, but its expression influenced by environment, learning, and genetics • The manifestation of aggression may be influenced by underlying medical conditions, early experiences (learning that aggression works to control situations), inconsistent or lack of clear rules and routine within the household and within human-pet interactions. • Rarely a symptom of a medical condition but contributory medical conditions must be ruled out, since illness and/or pain may influence a tendency for aggressive behaviors.

RISK FACTORS
Inconsistent or inappropriate punishment and inconsistent owner interactions may contribute to the development of conflicted and/or aggressive behavior.

 DIAGNOSIS

DIFFERENTIAL DIAGNOSIS
• Pathological disease conditions associated with aggression (e.g., painful musculoskeletal conditions, endocrinopathies) • Fear-based aggression • Anxiety conditions

CBC/BIOCHEMISTRY/URINALYSIS
Usually unremarkable; if abnormalities are found, may indicate underlying metabolic or endocrine diseases

OTHER LABORATORY TESTS
As indicated to rule out underlying diseases

IMAGING
MRI if cerebral disease is suspected; may be useful to rule out sources of pain

DIAGNOSTIC PROCEDURES
N/A

 TREATMENT

APPROPRIATE HEALTH CARE
Outpatient behavior modification and possibly medical management

NURSING CARE
N/A

ACTIVITY
Appropriate physical activity may help decrease incidences of aggression.

DIET
Low protein/high tryptophan diets may help reduce aggression but are unlikely to make a significant difference without behavior modification.

CLIENT EDUCATION

General Comments
• Successful treatment, as measured by a decrease in aggressive incidents, depends upon the owner's understanding of basic canine social behavior, the risks involved in living with an aggressive dog, and how to implement safety and management recommendations.
• Preventing human injuries must be the first concern.
• Treatment is aimed at controlling the problem, not at achieving a "cure."
• Owners must be aware that the only way to prevent future injuries is euthanasia.

Behavioral Therapy
• Avoid situations that might evoke aggression. Do not allow the dog on furniture. Do not give valuable treats or toys (e.g., rawhides). Pick up toys and have owner control playtime and activity. Limit physical contact with the dog, including petting. Do not physically punish or reprimand the dog.

- Teach the dog to comfortably and safely wear a head halter (Gentle Leader) and/or basket muzzle. Have the dog wear the head halter with a lightweight 8–10 foot leash attached whenever in contact with people. Use a long leash to move the dog from situations that may elicit aggression; do not reach for dog directly.
- Behavior Modification—non-confrontational methods to teach the dog to view people as leaders. Use reward-based training techniques to teach the dog to obey commands from people without experiencing conflict or becoming aggressive.
- Affection Control—making the dog follow a command before getting anything it desires from people (also known as "Nothing in life is free" or "Learn to earn"). For example, the dog must sit or lie down before feeding, petting, play, or going for a walk. For initial 2–3 week period, owners should give the dog attention only during brief, structured (e.g., command-response-reward) periods. At other times they must ignore the dog, especially if it is soliciting attention. Owner initiates interaction by giving a command and terminates interaction before the dog is ready.
- Counter Commanding—using positive reinforcement (e.g., food, toys, play, petting) to teach behaviors that are counter to those that have resulted in aggression in the past. For example, teach an "off" command to move off furniture or "drop it" command to release toys.
- Desensitization and Counterconditioning—technique used to decrease responsiveness to situations that have resulted in aggression in the past. Muzzle may be needed for safety. Should not begin until the owner has assumed a greater level of control over the dog through affection control and reward-based training.

SURGICAL CONSIDERATIONS

- Neuter intact males.
- Females that start to show dominance aggression at less than 6 months of age may be less aggressive when mature if not spayed.

MEDICATIONS

DRUG(S) OF CHOICE

- There are no medications licensed for the treatment of canine aggression. Few published studies exist. The only double-blind placebo-controlled study of medication for dominance aggression showed a strong placebo effect and no difference between placebo and medication in reducing aggressive behaviors.
- Owners must be aware that the use of a medication is off-label. Because of liability concerns, a note in the patient record is advisable stating that owners were informed

of potential risks and potential side-effects. Signed informed consent forms are prudent. Before prescribing medication be sure that owners understand the risks involved in owning an aggressive dog and will follow safety procedures and not rely on medication to keep others safe.
- Never use medications without behavior modification.
- Medication may not be appropriate in some family situations such as those with small children, family members with disabilities, or immunocompromised individuals.

Selective Serotonin Reuptake Inhibitors (SSRIs)
- Fluoxetine 0.5–1 mg/kg q24h, paroxetine 0.5–1 mg/kg q24h, sertraline 1–3 mg/kg q24h
- Side effects: inappetence and irritability

Tricyclic Antidepressant (TCA)
- Clomipramine 2–4 mg/kg q24h
- Side effects: sedation, anticholinergic effects, and cardiac conduction disturbances if predisposed; label restrictions on use in aggression

CONTRAINDICATIONS

Benzodiazepines may disinhibit aggression (resulting in increased episodes or intensity of aggression) when fear-based inhibition is diminished.

PRECAUTIONS

Any psychotropic medication may increase rather than decrease aggression. Corticosteroids are contraindicated if the dog is aggressive over food; polyphagia can lead to increased incidents and intensity of aggression.

POSSIBLE INTERACTIONS

TCAs and SSRIs should not be combined with MAO inhibitors (including amitraz and selegiline). Avoid combining SSRIs and TCAs, as this can result in potentially fatal serotonin syndrome.

ALTERNATIVE DRUG(S)

Progestins (DepoProvera 5–10 mg/kg SC, IM q 4 months)

FOLLOW-UP

PATIENT MONITORING

Clients often need ongoing assistance with behavior cases, especially aggression. At least one follow-up call within the first 1–3 weeks after the consultation is advisable. Provisions for further follow-up either by phone or in person should be made at that time.

PREVENTION/AVOIDANCE

Treatment recommendations are lifelong. Owners may see recurrence of aggression with treatment lapses. Continued avoidance of aggression triggers may be necessary.

POSSIBLE COMPLICATIONS

Human injuries; euthanasia of patient

EXPECTED COURSE AND PROGNOSIS

There is no cure. Prognosis for improvement is better if aggression is at a low intensity and in relatively few predictable situations. Prognosis is highly dependent on owner compliance.

MISCELLANEOUS

ASSOCIATED CONDITIONS

Other forms of aggression, most typically territorial aggression and interdog aggression. Underlying anxiety is often a factor in aggression in dogs.

AGE-RELATED FACTORS

Bitches showing dominance aggression when less than 6 months old may show a reduction in the level of aggression if not spayed.

ZOONOTIC POTENTIAL

Injury and infection from bite wounds

PREGNANCY

Do not breed aggressive dogs.

SYNONYMS

- Dominance-related aggression • Conflict aggression • Rage syndrome • Competitive aggression • Status-related aggression

SEE ALSO

Aggression, Food, Possessive and Territorial—Dogs

ABBREVIATIONS

SSRI = selective serotonin reuptake inhibitors
TCA = tricyclic antidepressant

Suggested Reading

Borchelt P, Voith V. Dominance aggression in dogs. In: Voith V, Borchelt P, eds. Readings in companion animal behavior. Trenton, NJ: Trenton Veterinary Learning Systems, 1996.

Luescher AU. Animal behavior case of the month. J Am Vet Med Assoc 2000;217(8): 1143–1145.

Mertens PA. Canine aggression. In: Horwitz D, Mills D, Heath S, eds. BSAVA manual of canine and feline behavioural medicine. Gloucester, England: British Small Animal Veterinary Association, 2002:195–215.

Mills DS, Simpson BS. Psychotropic agents. In: Horwitz D, Mills D, Heath S, eds. BSAVA Manual of canine and feline behavioural medicine. Gloucester, England: British Small Animal Veterinary Association, 2002:237–248.

Overall K. Clinical behavioral medicine for small animals. St. Louis: Mosby—Year Book, 1997.

Author Laurie Bergman
Consulting Editor Debra F. Horwitz

ALANINE AMINOTRANSFERASE (ALT)/ASPARTATE AMINOTRANSFERASE (AST)

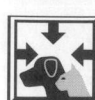

BASICS

DEFINITION

High serum ALT/AST activity usually reflects hepatocellular injury, enzyme induction, or myonecrosis. High enzyme activity may reflect both primary and secondary hepatocellular changes. The magnitude of the enzyme elevation may reflect the activity of underlying disease but cannot discern severity, prognosis, or tissue of origin. Sequential measurements may infer continuation and relative severity of ongoing tissue damage or enzyme induction.

PATHOPHYSIOLOGY

• ALT and AST serve a metabolic role in amino acid metabolism. Both are located in the cytosol and are rapidly dispersed upon cell membrane alteration. They are present in large quantities in liver and striated muscle. AST is also a mitochondrial enzyme. A disproportionate increase in AST relative to ALT suggests release of the mitochondrial isoenzyme. The diagnostic utility of measuring AST isoenzymes has not been demonstrated in companion animals. • Values must be interpreted with knowledge of serum creatinine kinase activity to deduce myonecrosis. • Plasma half-life—ALT: dogs, 4–72 hr; cats, 4–6 hr; AST: dogs, approximately 5 hr; cats, 1.3 hr • Cleared from plasma by enzyme degradation in the monocyte-macrophage system

SYSTEMS AFFECTED

Serum enzyme activity does not contribute directly to clinical signs.

SIGNALMENT

• No breed or sex differences in expression reported • Neonatal enzyme activity— onefold to twofold higher than adult reference range

SIGNS

• Depend on underlying causes of high enzymes • Fulminant hepatic failure owing to diffuse hepatic necrosis—lethargy; jaundice; dehydration; hypoglycemia; hypokalemia; hypocholesterolemia; collapse • Unifocal hepatic necrosis—may find no discernible signs • Hyperthyroidism (cats)—specific induced enzymes and typical clinical signs

CAUSES

• Hepatocellular necrosis—initially associated with only marked transaminase activity; may occur with the following disorders: Idiosyncratic drug toxicity—tetracycline (cats); anticonvulsants (primidone, phenytoin, phenobarbital; dogs); benzimadazole anthelmintics (oxibendizole, mebendazole; dogs); halothane (dogs, cats); diazepam (cats); carparsolate (dogs); carprofen (dogs). Toxin ingestion—

mushroom alkaloids (amatoxin, phylladin); carbon tetrachloride; acetaminophen. Severe acute hypoxia—severe anemia; DIC; cardiac failure; hypovolemia • Endocrinopathies— mild to moderate transaminase activity in dogs and cats (diabetes mellitus, hyperthyroidism, hyperadrenocorticism, sex hormone adrenal hyperplasia, hypothyroidism); high ALP activity; normal total bilirubin • Cholestatic disease—high transaminases; high ALP and GGT activity; high bilirubin, high cholesterol • Vacuolar hepatopathy (dogs)—high ALP and GGT activity, moderate increases in transaminase activity, normal bilirubin • Hepatic lipidosis (cats)—high ALP, normal to slightly high GGT activity unless associated cholangio-hepatitis or pancreatitis (rich sources of GGT); hyperbilirubinemia • Cholangiohepatitis (cats)—high ALP and GGT activity, variable hyperbilirubinemia, high transaminases • Cirrhosis (dogs)—may or may not develop high transaminase activity when at end stage • Chronic hepatitis (dogs)—mild to moderate transaminase activity, greater increase in serum ALP activity; variable bilirubin • Neoplasia (primary or metastatic)—high transaminases may be the only clinicopathologic indicator; inconsistent • Immunologic/infectious (bacterial, viral, parasitic, protozoal, fungal)— variable changes in serum transaminase activity, depending on extent of hepatocellular insult • Myonecrosis—severely high serum creatine kinase activity along with severely high transaminases

RISK FACTORS

• Depend on cause
• Conditions that alter membrane permeability in certain tissues (reversible or irreversible)—may increase activity

DIAGNOSIS

DIFFERENTIAL DIAGOSIS

Generally, no specific aspects of the history or physical examination consistently help differentiate causes of high ALT or AST activity. If either is high, the clinician should first attempt to establish the presence of liver disease, whether it is primary or secondary, and the underlying cause.

LABORATORY FINDINGS

Drugs That May Alter Laboratory Results

• Many drugs and chemicals may cause hepatic transaminase liberation as a result of either hepatocellular damage or induced enzyme synthesis (dogs). • No known drugs that interfere with the biochemical analysis

Disorders That May Alter Laboratory Results

Hemolysis—false-high activity in species other than dogs or cats

Valid If Run in a Human Laboratory?

Yes, if the animal reference range is determined

CBC/BIOCHEMISTRY/URINALYSIS

Adjunctive interpretation of routine screening tests—necessary to deduce liver disease or myonecrosis, to determine the importance of primary or secondary conditions, and to assess the patient's clinical status

CBC

• Poikilocytes (cats)—highly associated with liver disease • Abnormal platelet function and thrombocytopenia—occur with some liver diseases

Serum Biochemistry Profile

• Albumin—low with hepatic failure, high with dehydration • Globulins—high with stimulated acute-phase proteins or reduced hepatic monocyte-macrophage function; high fibrinogen indicates high acute-phase protein production; low fibrinogen suggests synthetic failure • ALP—dogs: increased with many disorders as a result of induction of the glucocorticoid isoenzyme; high with cholestasis and necroinflammatory disorders; gradual and sustained increase • BUN—low with compromised urea cycle function, polyuria/polydipsia, induced high glomerular filtration rate, low protein intake, or protein malnutrition • Glucose—low with portosystemic shunting, severe starvation, fulminant hepatic failure, sepsis; high with diabetes mellitus, hepatocutaneous syndrome, stress (cats), treatment with glucocorticoids (cats) • Cholesterol—low with portosystemic shunting, gut malabsorption, Addison's disease, or pancreatic exocrine insufficiency; high with diabetes mellitus, hepatocutaneous syndrome, nephrotic syndrome, major bile duct occlusion, pancreatitis, hypothyroidism, impaired glomerular filtration rate due to chronic interstitial nephritis (cats) • Potassium—low concentrations in cats may induce myonecrosis, causing significant enzyme release. • Creatine kinase—very high values when transaminase activity derived from myonecrosis • Hyperbilirubinemia— cholestatic disease; severe hemolysis, producing hypoxic liver damage and high transaminase activity

Urinalysis

• Bilirubinuria—cats: always abnormal, indicating hyperbilirubinemia; dogs: may conjugate in renal tubules
• Ammonium urate crystalluria—indicates hyperammonemia with fulminant hepatic failure or portosystemic shunting.
• Hyposthenuria—indicates impaired urine concentration (medullary washout, primary polydipsia in hepatic encephalopathy).

OTHER LABORATORY TESTS

• Bile acids—12-hr fasting and 2-hr postprandial values; sensitive assessment of hepatic function, perfusion, and

ALANINE AMINOTRANSFERASE (ALT)/ASPARTATE AMINOTRANSFERASE (AST)

enterohepatic circulation • Indocyanine green or sulfobromophthalein—cholephilic organic anion water-soluble dyes; assess hepatobiliary function and perfusion • Ammonia tolerance testing—appraises hepatic function and hepatoportal perfusion; documents hyperammonemia; utility impaired in routine practice owing to difficulties associated with test conductance (inability to freeze and mail samples for analysis because of ammonia's lability, spurious values derived from frozen samples, analytic inaccuracies). • Evaluations targeted at underlying disorders—pancreatitis (trypsin-like immunoreactivity, amylase, and lipase); endocrinopathies (thyroid profiles, adrenal function testing, insulin determinations); serologic tests for infectious disorders (FIP, leptospirosis, brucellosis, tick-borne rickettsial disorders, fungal disease) • Coagulation assessments—PT, APTT, or ACT; PIVKA; fibrinogen concentration; platelet count; and mucosal bleeding time; evaluated in patients scheduled for liver aspiration or biopsy

IMAGING

• Abdominal radiography—to evaluate liver size, position, shape, and margins; evaluate parenchyma (mineralization, gas); evaluate other abdominal viscera (position, mass lesions); detect abdominal effusion
• Abdominal ultrasonography—to evaluate echogenic patterns in hepatic parenchyma, biliary tree (wall thickness, lumenal dilation, contents), vascular components (flow, thrombi, relative size of vessels), porta hepatis structures, perihepatic and peripancreatic lymph nodes, pancreatic tissue and peripancreatic fat, and intestinal wall thickness and motility; detect and sample abdominal effusion

OTHER DIAGNOSTIC PROCEDURES

Liver Biopsy

• Needle core—via ultrasound guidance, laparoscopic sampling, or abdominal exploration and wedge biopsies; zonal distribution of lesions requires a minimum of 15 portal triads, necessitating the collection of four to six samples with an 18-gauge needle or three to four samples with a 14-gauge needle; needle sampling from left liver lobes may miss focal lesions; > 50% discordance between 18-gauge needle core and wedge liver biopsy (wedge as gold standard) proven • Wedge (laparotomy) or pinch (laparoscopy) sampling—affords more dependable, definitive diagnosis

 TREATMENT

APPROPRIATE HEALTH CARE

• None specific is advised, unless the underlying cause of high activity is inferred

from the history or diagnosed from liver biopsy. • Removal of inciting cause (e.g., infectious disease, drugs)—most important

Fluids

• If indicated, balanced polyionic solutions are usually safe. • Reduced lactate metabolism—may occur with fulminant hepatic failure or in cats with hepatic lipidosis; avoid lactate in these patients • Ascites—reduced-sodium fluids and diet • Hypoglycemia—supplement with dextrose, to effect • Hypokalemia—correct by judicious administration of supplemental potassium chloride; especially important with hepatic encephalopathy and for cats with hepatic lipidosis • Rate—based on patient hydration status, contemporary losses, and condition

Nutritional Support

• Essential—especially with hepatic encephalopathy • After a necrotizing insult—positive nitrogen balance is important: avoid protein restriction; restricting protein may slow hepatic regeneration • Supplement vitamins and essential trace minerals

 MEDICATIONS

DRUG(S)

• Suspected free radical–induced damage—antioxidants; vitamin E (α-tocopherol: 10 IU/kg/day PO); thiol (glutathione) donors: N-acetylcysteine for oxidant "crisis" (e.g., Heinz body hemolysis, markedly high ALT and AST) (140 mg/kg IV diluted 1:2 in polyionic fluids, given through a nonpyrogenic filter, followed with 70 mg/kg IV q6–12h), followed by S-adenosylmethionine (20 mg/kg/day PO enteric coated tablets) as sources of glutathione • Suspected fulminant hepatic necrosis—broad-spectrum bactericidal antibiotics effective against enteric gram-negative opportunists and anaerobic bacteria • Control of emesis—metoclopramide or ondansetron (use CRI if necessary) • Gastrointestinal ulceration (hematemesis, melena)—H$_2$ blocker famotidine (0.5 mg/kg PO, IM, SC q12–24h) combined with sucralfate (0.25 g/5 kg PO q8–12h) • Fulminant hepatic failure or evidence of bleeding tendencies—vitamin K$_1$ (0.5–1.5 mg/kg IM or SC initially, up to three doses at 12-hr intervals); may require transfusion of whole blood or fresh frozen plasma; DDAVP (0.5–1 μg/kg IV) may control critical hemorrhage on a one-time basis (continued administration ineffectual; mechanism is thought to involve von Willebrand's protein but may involve other mechanisms)

 FOLLOW-UP

PATIENT MONITORING

• Depends on the underlying cause; consult specific disorders; treatment targeted at an underlying condition may require periodic enzyme assessment
• High activity associated with some mild disorders—some patients remain stable; may not require treatment; treatment may consist of outpatient supportive care

POSSIBLE COMPLICATIONS

High activity—may indicate severe hepatobiliary disease, which may lead to severe debilitation or death; may be the only (early) indication of chronic hepatitis; chronic unexplained high liver enzyme activity should not be ignored

 MISCELLANEOUS

ASSOCIATED CONDITIONS N/A

AGE-RELATED FACTORS

Neonatal activity—normally onefold to twofold greater than adult values

ZOONOTIC POTENTIAL

A variety of infectious diseases may involve the liver—leptospirosis, brucellosis, systemic fungal infections, toxoplasmosis, campylobacteriosis; appropriately advise owner to consult a human medical health professional.

SYNONYMS

Serum glutamic pyruvic transaminase = alanine aminotransferase (ALT)
Serum glutamic oxaloacetate transaminase = aspartate aminotransferase (AST)

SEE ALSO

Causes of Liver Disease

ABBREVIATIONS

• ACT = activated clotting time • ALP = alkaline phosphatase • APTT = activated partial thromboplastin time • BUN = blood urea nitrogen • CRI = constant rate infusion • DDAVP = 1 deamino-8-D-arginine vasopressin • DIC = disseminated intravascular coagulation • FIP = feline infectious peritonitis • GGT = γ-glutamyltransferase • PIVKA = proteins invoked by vitamin K absence or antagonism • PT = prothrombin time

Suggested Reading

Center SA. Diagnostic procedures for evaluation of hepatic disease. In: Guilford WG, Center SA, Strombeck DR, et al., eds. Strombeck's small animal gastroenterology. Philadelphia: Saunders, 1996:130–188.

Authors W. E. Hoffman and Sharon A. Center

Consulting Editor Sharon A. Center

ALKALINE PHOSPHATASE (ALP)/γ-GLUTAMYL TRANSFERASE (GGT)

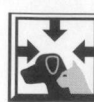

BASICS

DEFINITION
• Both enzymes useful for diagnosis of liver disease
• ALP—also detects other conditions; normal values: 30–150 U/L in dogs; 30–100 U/L in cats
• GGT—serum activity usually 1–7 U/L in healthy dogs and < 2 U/L in healthy cats

PATHOPHYSIOLOGY

ALP
• Found in most organs; highest concentration in kidney, intestine, liver, and bone
• Isoenzymes—only liver (L-ALP), bone (B-ALP), and corticosteroid-induced (C-ALP) in serum; only B-ALP and L-ALP in serum of healthy dogs and cats
• L-ALP—primarily found attached to outer canalicular and sinusoidal surfaces of hepatocytes upon induction; released from sinusoidal surfaces with cholestasis; bile acids are potent enzyme inducers and facilitate membrane release; release during noncholestatic disorders after enzyme induction; release from sinusoidal membrane facilitated by normal bile acid enterohepatic circulation
• B-ALP—found in osteoblasts and matrix vesicles; increases in serum with increased osteogenesis (young animals) and bone remodeling (infection, osteosarcoma) and in cats with hyperthyroidism
• C-ALP—produced in dog liver (not cat liver); influenced by glucocorticoids and other unidentified inducers; release from hepatocyte sinusoidal membrane facilitated by normal bile acid enterohepatic circulation
• Serum activity—lower in cats than in dogs owing to shorter plasma half-life (6 hr vs. 72 hr) and smaller magnitude of enzyme induction in cat liver
• Cats—mild increases in serum activity indicate disease (e.g., cholestasis, hyperthyroidism, hepatic lipidosis)
• Dogs—twofold or greater increases in serum activity often nonspecifically develop with chronic illnesses

GGT
• Membrane-bound enzyme—found primarily on bile ductular epithelium
• Liver and serum—normally lower in dogs and cats than in other species (e.g., horses and humans)
• Release mechanism—in cholestasis requires bile acids; not well understood
• Cats—high serum activity primarily indicates cholestasis; more sensitive than ALP

SYSTEMS AFFECTED
High activity in serum causes no injury

SIGNALMENT
• Newborns—high serum GGT activity develops after colostrum ingestion
• Juveniles—high serum ALP activity common with bone growth and remodeling
• Adult dogs—modest to marked increase in serum ALP activity possible with diseases unrelated to the liver; may be associated with increased cortisol release, or from treatment with glucocorticoids (any route or mode of application)

SIGNS
• Clinical signs compatible with hepatic disease—determine if ALP and GGT activities are indicating cholestasis
• Clinical signs compatible with hyperadrenocorticism (dogs)—determine ALP activity; if not increased, inconsistent with typical hyperadrenocorticism

CAUSES

General Causes of Serum Activity— Dogs
• ALP—modest increases with osteogenic activity; minor to modest increases common with a variety of diseases, reflect induced C-ALP in response to chronic stress and release of endogenous cortisol secondary to the primary disease process
• GGT—minimal increases suggest hepatic disease; higher diagnostic specificity than ALP (fewer false-positives); marked and disproportionate increases > 100 U/L associated with biliary hyperplasia or hepatic cancer (biliary adenocarcinoma); modest increases possible with corticosteroid induction
• Both enzymes—usually increase with cholestasis and vacuolar hepatopathy; induced by some drugs (e.g., anticonvulsants: phenobarbital, primidone, and phenytoin), especially ALP

General Causes of Serum Activity—Cats
• ALP—no drug or glucocorticoid induction likely; mild to marked activity associated with hyperthyroidism (bone isoenzyme shown in one study), cholestasis, and hepatic lipidosis
• GGT—more sensitive to hepatic disorders, except hepatic lipidosis (see below)

Associated Liver Disorders
• High ALP activity—cholestasis; cholangiohepatitis (cats); chronic hepatitis (dogs); vacuolar hepatopathy (dogs); hepatic lipidosis (cats); primary hepatic neoplasia
• High GGT activity—cholestasis; chronic hepatitis (dogs); vacuolar hepatopathy (dogs); primary hepatic neoplasia
• Hepatic lipidosis (cats)—uniquely associated with cholestasis that causes minor or no increase in serum GGT since cholestasis is at level of hepatocyte and unlikely to involve bile ducts and ductules (source of GGT); increased GGT in cats with hepatic lipidosis secondary to pancreatitis or biliary

tree inflammation/obstruction (e.g., cholangiohepatitis, EHBDO)
• Minor increases in ALP—metastatic neoplasia (variable); portosystemic vascular anomaly (young age of patient); cirrhosis (variable)
• Acute disruption of hepatocellular membrane integrity (hepatic necrosis, liver trauma)—because of the relatively low concentration of ALP in normal liver and the absence of increased bile acids in these conditions, ALP displays only minor increases in serum compared with ALT and AST

Glucocorticoid-Induced Vacuolar Hepatopathy (Dogs)
• ALP—minor to marked increases in serum activity after glucocorticoid treatment; initially owing to L-ALP and later to C-ALP isoenzymes; magnitude depends on drug dose, route of administration, duration of treatment, pharmacologic preparation, and biological variation; systemic effects and enzyme increases also noted with ophthalmic and topically administered preparations
• Hyperadrenocorticism—associated with increased C-ALP activity in > 83% of dogs; magnitude ranges from 50 U/L to several thousand U/L; GGT activity increases in approximately 50% of cases

Bone Disease and Remodeling
• Highest activity—newborn; decreases continually until adulthood
• Diseases involving bone—e.g., bone fractures, fungal infections, metabolic disorder, primary or metastatic neoplasia, and chronic renal failure associated with secondary hyperparathyroidism; increased activity up to 200 U/L
• Osteosarcoma—may note normal to high activity; up to 2000 U/L B-ALP activity

RISK FACTORS
N/A

DIAGNOSIS

DIFFERENTIAL DIAGNOSIS
• Significant hepatobiliary disease—high serum ALP and GGT activity in conjunction with high TSBA and/or bilirubin
• Hepatic lipidosis (not associated with pancreatitis, cholangiohepatitis, or EHBDO) or hyperthyroidism (cats)—markedly high serum ALP activity without comparable GGT activity
• Vacuolar hepatopathy (hyperadrenocorticism, adrenal hyperplasia [high sex hormones in neutered dogs], glucocorticoid administration, or stress of primary disease processes) in anicteric dogs—high serum ALP activity with or without high GGT activity; normal or mildly abnormal TSBA; minor increases or normal ALT and AST activity

ALKALINE PHOSPHATASE (ALP)/γ-GLUTAMYL TRANSFERASE (GGT)

• Nonhepatic disease—high serum ALP activity may be associated with both hepatic and nonhepatic disease; must interpret activity along with other liver tests (e.g., TSBA, bilirubin, ALT, AST); increases variable; markedly high ALP activity in absence of markedly high GGT activity or bilirubin usually indicates C-ALP isoenzyme induction, even in the absence of obvious hyperadrenocorticism

• Chronic renal disease (renal azotemia)—mildly to moderately high ALP

LABORATORY FINDINGS

Drugs That May Alter Laboratory Results
ALP (dogs)—numerous drugs and chemicals can induce activity

Valid if Run in Human Laboratory?
Yes

CBC/BIOCHEMISTRY/URINALYSIS

CBC
Not likely to assist in confirming hepatic disease

Serum Biochemistry Profile
• ALP and GGT activity may lack specificity and/or sensitivity for hepatic disease; interpret in conjunction with urinalysis and other tests for hepatic disease (TSBA, bilirubin, albumin, ALT)

• ALT—often secondarily increased in cholestasis; primarily indicates liver necrosis or trauma

• Markedly high ALP (dog) with no or moderate increases of ALT and GGT and normal bilirubin generally indicates the presence of C-ALP isoenzyme

OTHER LABORATORY TESTS
• High ALP activity in dogs with no evidence of cholestasis (normal bilirubin)—rule out hyperadrenocorticism via history, clinical signs, and appropriate adrenal-pituitary axis evaluations (e.g., ACTH response test, low-dose dexamethasone suppression test); consider adrenal hyperplasia syndrome (evaluate ACTH response test measuring sex hormones along with cortisone, before and after ACTH administration); determine C-ALP activity (high sensitivity but low specificity for hyperadrenocorticism); see Vacuolar Hepatopathy

• High ALP activity in cats—evaluate for hepatic lipidosis with abdominal ultrasonography and fine needle hepatic aspiration; measure serum thyroxin to rule out hyperthyroidism

IMAGING

Radiography
Abdominal radiography—microhepatica with cirrhosis or PSVA (may see normal or mildly high ALP and GGT activity, unless an active acquired lesion); hepatomegaly seen with vacuolar hepatopathy, hepatic neoplasia, hepatic lipidosis, or congestion (high ALP with or without high GGT likely)

Ultrasonography
Abdominal ultrasonography—rule out extrahepatic bile duct occlusion, pancreatitis, and focal hepatic mass lesions; may increase suspicion of diffuse hepatopathy; hepatic lipidosis and canine vacuolar hepatopathy associated with hyperechoic parenchyma; irregular liver lobe margin with cirrhosis

DIAGNOSTIC PROCEDURES
• Fine needle aspiration—initial evaluation of suspected hepatic lipidosis (cats), vacuolar hepatopathy (dogs), neoplasia, and septic inflammation; needle aspiration cannot diagnose definitively or rule out other liver disorders; 18-gauge Vim Tru-Cut needle biopsy shows 50% discordance in necroinflammatory liver disorders compared with larger wedge sampling from the same liver lobe; cannot recommend therapy based on aspiration cytology

• Hepatic biopsy—when laboratory findings suggest hepatobiliary disease, ultrasonography rules out extrahepatic bile duct occlusion, and fine needle aspiration cytology fails to ascertain conditions described previously; maintain vigilance to determine definite diagnosis with certainty before recommending costly treatment with potentially adverse side effects.

TREATMENT
Based on underlying disease

MEDICATIONS

DRUG(S) OF CHOICE
Depend on underlying disease

CONTRAINDICATIONS
Depend on underlying disease

PRECAUTIONS
Depend on underlying disease

ALTERNATIVE DRUG(S)
Depend on underlying disease

FOLLOW-UP

PATIENT MONITORING
• Successful treatment of underlying disease—activity generally decreases within a few days to weeks, possibly longer in the case of C-ALP isoenzyme

• Marked biliary hyperplasia—high GGT and ALP may remain sustained

• Hyperadrenocorticism or termination of very long-term corticosteroid therapy—ALP (C-ALP) may normalize only after weeks to months of glucocorticoid drug discontinuation or successful suppression of adrenal hyperfunction

POSSIBLE COMPLICATIONS
N/A

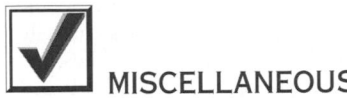

MISCELLANEOUS

ASSOCIATED CONDITIONS
N/A

ZOONOTIC POTENTIAL
N/A

PREGNANCY
Placental ALP not identified in serum of dogs and cats as is reported in human serum

SEE ALSO
• Cirrhosis and Fibrosis of the Liver
• Hepatic Lipidosis
• Hepatitis, Chronic
• Hepatocellular Adenoma
• Hepatocellular Carcinoma
• Hepatotoxins
• Hyperthyroidism
• Hyperadrenocorticism (Cushing's Disease)
• Vacuolar Hepatopathy

ABBREVIATIONS
• ACTH = adrenocorticotropic hormone
• ALT = alanine aminotransferase
• AST = aspartate aminotransferase
• EHBDO = extrahepatic bile duct obstruction
• PSVA = portosystemic vascular anomaly
• TSBA = total serum bile acids

Suggested Reading
Center SA. Diagnostic procedures for evaluation of hepatic disease. In: Guilford WG, Center SA, Strombeck DR, et al., eds. Strombeck's small animal gastroenterology. Philadelphia: Saunders, 1996:130–188.
Kramer JW, Hoffmann WE. Clinical enzymology. In: Kaneko JJ, Harvey JW, Bruss ML, eds. Clinical biochemistry of domestic animals. 5th ed. San Diego: Academic Press, 1997:303–326.
Authors Walter E. Hoffmann and Sharon A. Center
Consulting Editor Sharon A. Center

ALKALOSIS, METABOLIC

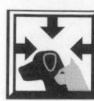

BASICS

DEFINITION
Primary increase in plasma bicarbonate concentration ($[HCO_3^-]$) (dogs, >24 mEq/L; cats, >22 mEq/L) with low hydrogen ion concentration ($[H^+]$), high pH, and a compensatory increase in carbon dioxide tension (P_{CO_2})

PATHOPHYSIOLOGY
Loss of chloride and hydrogen ion-rich fluid via the alimentary tract or kidneys is usually accompanied by volume depletion. Loss of H^+ is associated with an increase in plasma HCO_3^- concentration. With chloride loss and volume depletion, the kidneys reabsorb sodium and HCO_3^- instead of chloride, perpetuating the metabolic alkalosis. Chronic administration of alkali also may result in transient metabolic alkalosis. Renal excretion of exogenously administered alkali is effective, and it is difficult to create metabolic alkalosis by increasing HCO_3^- intake, unless the patient has renal dysfunction.

SYSTEMS AFFECTED
• Respiratory—low $[H^+]$ reduces alveolar ventilation. Hypoventilation increases P_{CO_2} and helps offset the effects of high plasma $[HCO_3^-]$ on pH. In dogs, an increase of approximately 0.7 mm Hg in P_{CO_2} can be expected for each 1 mEq/L increase in plasma $[HCO_3^-]$.
• Renal/Urologic—the kidneys rapidly and effectively excrete excessive alkali. In patients with chloride deficiency (and less importantly, volume depletion), the kidneys cannot excrete the excessive alkali and metabolic alkalosis is maintained.
• Nervous—muscle twitching and seizures occur rarely in dogs.

SIGNALMENT
Any breed, age, or sex of dog and cat

SIGNS

Historical Findings
• Administration of loop diuretics (e.g., furosemide) or thiazides
• Vomiting

Physical Examination Findings
• Signs related to the underlying disease or accompanying potassium depletion (e.g., weakness, cardiac arrhythmias, and ileus)
• Muscle twitching caused by low ionized calcium concentration
• Dehydration in volume-depleted patients
• Muscle twitching and seizures in patients with neurologic involvement (rare)

CAUSES
• Chloride-responsive—diuretic administration, vomiting of stomach contents, and rapid correction of hypercapnia (respiratory acidosis)
• Chloride-resistant—hyperadrenocorticism and primary hyperaldosteronism
• Oral administration of alkali—administration of sodium bicarbonate or other organic anions with sodium (e.g., lactate, acetate, gluconate); administration of cation-exchange resin with nonabsorbable alkali (e.g., phosphorus binders)
• Miscellaneous—hypoalbuminemia, administration of large doses of sodium penicillin or carbenicillin

RISK FACTORS
• Administration of loop or thiazide diuretics
• Vomiting

DIAGNOSIS

DIFFERENTIAL DIAGNOSIS
High plasma $[HCO_3^-]$ in animals can also be compensating for chronic respiratory acidosis, in which P_{CO_2} is high and pH is low despite high $[HCO_3^-]$; blood gas determination required to differentiate.

LABORATORY FINDINGS

Drugs That May Alter Laboratory Results
N/A

Disorders That May Alter Laboratory Results
• Too much heparin (>10% of the sample) decreases $[HCO_3^-]$
• Samples stored at room temperature for more than 20 min have low pH because of increased P_{CO_2}.
• Some blood gas analyzers only report pH and P_{CO_2}; bicarbonate must be calculated, a potential source for error.

Valid If Run in Human Laboratory?
Yes

CBC/BIOCHEMISTRY/URINALYSIS
• High total CO_2 (total CO_2 in samples handled aerobically closely approximates $[HCO_3^-]$)
• Low ionized calcium concentration
• Electrolyte abnormalities vary with underlying cause.
• Hypochloremia—consider hypochloremic metabolic alkalosis, the most common reason for metabolic alkalosis in dogs and cats, which usually results from diuretic administration or vomiting of stomach contents.
• High sodium but normal chloride concentration—consider chloride-resistant metabolic alkalosis (e.g., hyperadrenocorticism or primary hyperaldosteronism) or administration of alkali.
• Hypoalbuminemia—consider hypoalbuminemic metabolic alkalosis; albumin is a weak acid. In human beings, a decrease of 1 g/dL in albumin is associated with a 3.7 mEq/L increase in $[HCO_3^-]$.
• Hypokalemia—hypokalemia likely results from the metabolic alkalosis or the underlying problem (e.g., vomiting of stomach contents or loop diuretic administration); hypokalemia-induced metabolic alkalosis does not occur in dogs and cats.

OTHER LABORATORY TESTS

Blood gas analysis reveals high $[HCO_3^-]$, high PCO_2, and high pH.

IMAGING

N/A

DIAGNOSTIC PROCEDURES

N/A

TREATMENT

• Acid–base disturbances are secondary phenomena. Diagnosis and treatment of the underlying disease process is integral to the successful resolution of acid–base disorders.
• Discontinue drugs that may cause metabolic alkalosis.

NURSING CARE

The fluids of choice contain chloride; give patients with volume depletion an intravenous infusion of 0.9% NaCl supplemented with KCl; patients with hypokalemia may require large doses of KCl (see hypokalemia).

MEDICATIONS

DRUG(S) OF CHOICE

• If the underlying cause cannot be corrected (e.g., chronic heart failure patients receiving diuretics), oral compounds containing chloride without sodium (e.g., KCl, NH_4Cl) can be tried; also consider simultaneous use of distal tubule blocking agents (e.g., spironolactone, triamterene, and amiloride).
• Chloride-resistant metabolic alkalosis can only be corrected by resolution of the underlying disease; metabolic alkalosis is usually mild in these patients.

CONTRAINDICATIONS

• Avoid chloride-free fluids—they may correct volume depletion but will not correct metabolic alkalosis.
• Avoid drugs containing sodium without chloride (e.g., sodium penicillin, sodium

bicarbonate)—they may worsen metabolic alkalosis.
• Avoid using salts of potassium without chloride (e.g., potassium phosphate)—potassium will be excreted in the urine and will correct neither the alkalosis nor the potassium deficit.

PRECAUTIONS

Do not use distal blocking agents (e.g., spironolactone, triamterene, and amiloride) in volume-depleted patients.

POSSIBLE INTERACTIONS

N/A

ALTERNATIVE DRUG(S)

N/A

FOLLOW-UP

PATIENT MONITORING

Acid–base status—frequency dictated by the underlying disease and patient response to treatment

POSSIBLE COMPLICATIONS

• Hypokalemia
• Neurologic signs

✓ MISCELLANEOUS

ASSOCIATED CONDITIONS

• Hypokalemia
• Hypochloremia

AGE-RELATED FACTORS

N/A

ZOONOTIC POTENTIAL

N/A

PREGNANCY

N/A

SYNONYMS

• Nonrespiratory alkalosis
• Chloride-responsive metabolic alkalosis—metabolic alkalosis that responds to chloride administration

• Chloride-resistant metabolic alkalosis—metabolic alkalosis that does not respond to chloride administration
• Hypochloremic metabolic alkalosis—metabolic alkalosis caused by low chloride concentration
• Hypoalbuminemic alkalosis—metabolic alkalosis caused by low albumin concentration
• Concentration alkalosis—metabolic alkalosis caused by high sodium concentration
• Contraction alkalosis—metabolic alkalosis formerly attributed to volume-contraction, but now known to be caused by chloride depletion

SEE ALSO

• Hypochloremia
• Hypokalemia

ABBREVIATIONS

• H^+ = hydrogen ion
• HCO_3^- = bicarbonate
• PCO_2 = carbon dioxide tension

Suggested Reading

de Morais HSA. Chloride ion in small animal practice: the forgotten ion. J Vet Emerg Crit Care 1992;2:11–24

DiBartola SP. Metabolic alkalosis. In: DiBartola SP, ed. Fluid therapy in small animal practice. Philadelphia: Saunders, 1992:244–257.

DiBartola SP, Green RA, de Morais HSA. Electrolytes and acid base disorders. In: Willard MD, Tvedten H, Turnwald GH, eds. Small animal clinical diagnosis by laboratory methods. 2nd ed. Philadelphia: Saunders, 1994:97–113.

Robinson EP, Hardy RM. Clinical signs, diagnosis, and treatment of alkalemia in dogs: 20 cases (1982–1984). J Am Vet Med Assoc 1988;192:943–949.

Authors Helio Autran de Morais and Stephen P. DiBartola
Consulting Editors Larry G. Adams and Carl A. Osborne

ALOPECIA—CATS

BASICS

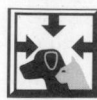

DEFINITION
• Common problem
• Pattern of hair loss—varied or symmetrical
• Causes—multifactorial

PATHOPHYSIOLOGY
Specific and unique for each cause

SYSTEMS AFFECTED
• Skin/Exocrine and associated adnexa
• Endocrine/Metabolic

SIGNALMENT
• No specific age, breed, or sex predilection
• Neoplastic and paraneoplastic associated alopecias—generally recognized in old cats

SIGNS
N/A

CAUSES
• Neurologic/behavioral—obsessive compulsive disorder
• Endocrine—sex hormone alopecia, hyperthyroidism, hyperadrenocorticism, diabetes mellitus
• Immunologic—allergic dermatitis, alopecia areata
• Parasitic—demodicosis, dermatophytosis
• Physiologic—sebaceous adenitis
• Neoplastic—paraneoplastic dermatitis, squamous cell carcinoma in situ, epidermotropic lymphoma
• Idiopathic/inherited—alopecia universalis, hypotrichosis, spontaneous pinnal alopecia, anagen and telogen defluxion

RISK FACTORS
FeLV/FIV—for demodicosis

DIAGNOSIS

DIFFERENTIAL DIAGNOSIS

Endocrine Alopecia/Sex Hormone
• Rarely a hormonal abnormality
• Rare hormonal cases—primarily castrated males; alopecia along the caudal aspect of the hindlimbs, which may extend along the perineum

Obsessive Compulsive Disorder
• Often misdiagnosed as endocrine
• The pattern of alopecia is frequently symmetrical with no associated inflammation.

Allergic Dermatitis
• Varies from mild partial alopecia with little inflammation to severe excoriation and ulceration
• Distribution—varied; often the head and neck region are most severely affected.

• Food allergy and inhalant/percutaneous causes

Hyperthyroidism
• Partial to complete alopecia from self-barbering
• Varied pattern
• Middle-aged to old cats
• Often mistaken for allergic dermatoses, obsessive compulsive disorder, or hormonal

Diabetes Mellitus
• Partial alopecia with an unkempt hair coat
• Poor wound healing
• Increased susceptibility to infections
• Cutaneous xanthomatosis secondary to hyperlipidemia (nodular to linear, yellow-pink alopecic plaques that tend to ulcerate)

Hyperadrenocorticism
• Rare; characterized by alopecia and extreme fragility of the skin
• Truncal alopecia, with or without a rattail and a curling of the pinnal tips
• Extreme skin fragility noted in approximately 70%
• Occurs secondary to pituitary or adrenal tumors
• Iatrogenic form less common in cats than in dogs

Paraneoplastic Alopecia
• Most cases associated with pancreatic exocrine adenocarcinomas
• Middle-aged to old cats (9–16 years)
• Acute onset
• Progresses rapidly
• Bilaterally symmetrical, ventrally distributed (also located along the bridge of the nose and periocular)
• Hair epilates in clumps
• Rare pruritus
• Erythema with dry fissuring footpads
• Glistening appearance to the alopecic skin
• Skin is thin and hypotonic.
• Rapid weight loss

Sebaceous Adenitis
• Slowly progressive partial alopecia associated with scaling along the dorsum of the body and the extremities
• Sebaceous glands are selectively destroyed by toxic intermediate metabolites or immunologic mechanisms.
• Possible dramatic pigment accumulation along the eyelid margins
• Questionable association with systemic disease (e.g., inflammatory bowel disease, lupus-like syndromes, upper respiratory tract infections)

Squamous Cell Carcinoma In Situ
• Multicentric premalignant dermatosis in old cats
• Slightly elevated, plaque-like or papillated lesions with scaling and partially alopecic surfaces

• Often misdiagnosed as seborrhea
• About 25% may convert to squamous cell carcinoma with in situ lesions along the borders (histologically).

Epidermotrophic Lymphoma
• Early stages—varying degrees of alopecia associated with scaling and erythema
• Later stages—plaques and nodules
• Old cats

Alopecia Areata
Rare, complete alopecia in a patchy distribution with no inflammation

Alopecia Universalis (Sphinx Cat)
• Hereditary
• Complete absence of primary hairs; decreased secondary hairs
• Thickened epidermis; normal dermis
• Sebaceous and apocrine ducts open directly onto the skin surface; oily feel to skin
• Wrinkled foreheads; gold eyes; no whiskers; downy fur on paws, tip of tail, and scrotum

Feline Hypotrichosis
• Siamese and Devon Rex cats (autosomal recessive alopecia)
• Poorly developed primary telogen hair follicles
• Born with a normal coat; thin and sparse as young adult

Spontaneous Pinnal Alopecia
• Siamese cats predisposed
• May represent form of alopecia areata or pattern baldness

Anagen and Telogen Defluxion
• Acute loss of hair owing to interference with the growth cycle
• Causes—stress, infection, endocrine disorder, metabolic disorder, fever, surgery, anesthesia, pregnancy, drug therapy

Demodicosis
• Rare; unlike dogs
• Partial to complete multifocal alopecia of the eyelids, periocular region, head, and neck
• Variable pruritus with erythema, scale, and crust, and ceruminous otitis externa
• *Demodex cati* (elongated shape) often associated with metabolic disease (e.g., FIV, systemic lupus erythematosus, diabetes mellitus)
• Short/blunted *D. gatoi* mite is rarely a marker for metabolic disease; this form may be transferable from cat to cat and has been associated with pruritus.

Dermatophytosis
Numerous clinical manifestations; always associated with alopecia of some degree

CBC/BIOCHEMISTRY/URINALYSIS
Abnormalities may be noted with diabetes mellitus, hyperadrenocorticism, and hyperthyroidism.

OTHER LABORATORY TESTS
- FeLV and FIV—risk factors for demodicosis
- Thyroid hormones—document hyperthyroidism
- ANA titer—look for lupus-like syndromes
- ACTH-response test, LDDST, and HDDST—diagnose hyperadrenocorticism

IMAGING
- Abdominal ultrasound—assess adrenals in hyperadrenocorticism and look for cancer in animals with paraneoplastic syndrome
- CT scan—look for pituitary tumors in animals with hyperadrenocorticism

DIAGNOSTIC PROCEDURES
- Skin biopsy
- Skin scraping
- Fungal culture
- T-shirts to prove self-trauma
- Food elimination trials
- Intradermal skin testing

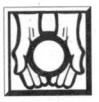

TREATMENT
- Therapy is limited for many of these disorders.
- Behavioral modification or application of a T-shirt may help prevent self-barbering.
- Removal of an offending dietary item may alleviate the symptoms of food allergy.
- If the pet is compliant, shampoo and topical therapy may help secondary problems, such as hyperkeratosis in sebaceous adenitis, crusting in demodicosis, secondary bacterial infections, and malodor for greasy conditions.

MEDICATIONS

DRUG(S) OF CHOICE
- Obsessive compulsive disorder—amitriptyline (10 mg/cat/day for a 21-day trial)
- Endocrine alopecia (males)—testosterone supplementation
- Allergic dermatitis—antihistamines, diet, corticosteroids, hyposensitization vaccine
- Hyperthyroidism—oral medications such as methimazole (tapazole) or radioactive iodine therapy
- Diabetes mellitus—regulation of glucose levels (insulin)

- Hyperadrenocorticism—surgery; no known effective medical therapy
- Paraneoplastic alopecia—no therapy; often fatal
- Epidermotropic lymphoma—retinoids (isotretinoin), corticosteroids, interferon, cyclosporine, lomustine
- Sebaceous adenitis—retinoids, corticosteroids, cyclosporine
- Squamous cell carcinoma in situ—surgical excision, retinoids (topical and oral), topical imiquimod cream
- Alopecia areata—no therapy; possibly counterirritants
- Demodicosis—lime sulfur dips at weekly intervals for 4–6 dips; Mitaban and ivermectin have been tried with variable success (dose and frequency of application are questionable)
- Dermatophytosis—griseofulvin (CAUTION: idiosyncratic toxicity), ketoconazole, itraconazole (best choice), Lufenuron

CONTRAINDICATIONS
N/A

PRECAUTIONS
Toxicity with griseofulvin (see Dermatophytosis)

POSSIBLE INTERACTIONS
N/A

ALTERNATIVE DRUG(S)
N/A

FOLLOW-UP

PATIENT MONITORING
Depends on specific diagnosis

PREVENTION/AVOIDANCE
Depends on specific diagnosis

POSSIBLE COMPLICATIONS
Depend on specific diagnosis

EXPECTED COURSE AND PROGNOSIS
Depend on specific diagnosis

MISCELLANEOUS

ASSOCIATED CONDITIONS
N/A

AGE-RELATED FACTORS
N/A

ZOONOTIC POTENTIAL
Dermatophytosis—can cause skin lesions in humans

PREGNANCY
Retinoids and griseofulvin should not be administered to pregnant animals

SYNONYMS
N/A

SEE ALSO
- Demodicosis
- Dermatophytosis
- Diabetes Mellitus, Uncomplicated
- Feline Paraneoplastic Syndrome
- Hyperthyroidism
- Sebaceous Adenitis

ABBREVIATIONS
- ANA = antinuclear antibody
- FeLV = feline leukemia virus
- FIV = feline immunodeficiency virus
- HDDST = high-dose dexamethasone-suppression test
- LDDST = low-dose dexamethasone-suppression test

Suggested Reading

Baer KE, Helton KA. Multicentric squamous cell carcinoma in situ resembling Bowen's disease in cats. Vet Pathol 1993;30:535–543.

Helton Rhodes KA, Wallace M, Baer KE. Cutaneous manifestations of feline hyperadrenocorticism. In: Ihrke PJ, Mason IS, White SD. Advances in veterinary dermatology. New York: Pergamon, 1993.

Scott DW, Griffin CE, Miller BH. Acquired alopecia. In: Muller & Kirk's small animal dermatology. 5th ed. Philadelphia: Saunders, 1995:720–735.

Scott DW, Griffin CE, Miller BH. Congenital and hereditary defects. In: Muller & Kirk's small animal dermatology. 5th ed. Philadelphia: Saunders, 1995:736–805.

Scott DW, Griffin CE, Miller BH. Endocrine and metabolic diseases. In: Muller & Kirk's small animal dermatology. 5th ed. Philadelphia: Saunders, 1995:627–719.

Author Karen Helton Rhodes
Consulting Editor Karen Helton Rhodes

ALOPECIA—DOGS

 **BASICS**

DEFINITION
- Common disorder
- Characterized by a complete or partial lack of hair in areas where it is normally present
- May be associated with a multifactorial cause
- May be the primary problem or only a secondary phenomenon

PATHOPHYSIOLOGY
- Multifactorial causes
- All of the disorders represent a disruption in the growth of the hair follicle from infection, trauma, immunologic attack, mechanical "plugging," endocrine abnormalities, or blockage of the receptor sites for stimulation of the cycle.

SYSTEMS AFFECTED
- Skin/Exocrine
- Endocrine/Metabolic
- Hemic/Lymphatic/Immune

SIGNALMENT
No specific age, breed, or sex predilection

SIGNS
- May be acute in onset or slowly progressive.
- Multifocal patches of circular alopecia—most frequently associated with folliculitis from bacterial infection and demodicosis
- Large more diffuse areas of alopecia—may indicate a follicular dysplasia or metabolic component.
- The pattern and degree of hair loss are important for establishing a differential diagnosis.

CAUSES

Multifocal
- Localized demodicosis—partial to complete alopecia with erythema and mild scaling; lesions may become inflamed and crusted
- Dermatophytosis—partial to complete alopecia with scaling; with or without erythema; not always ring-like
- Staphylococcal folliculitis—circular patterns of alopecia with epidermal collarettes, erythema, crusting, and hyperpigmented macules
- Injection reactions—inflammation with alopecia and/or cutaneous atrophy from scarring
- Rabies vaccine vasculitis—patch of alopecia observed 2–3 months postvaccination
- Localized scleroderma—well-demarcated, shiny, smooth, alopecic, thickened plaque
- Alopecia areata—noninflammatory areas of complete alopecia
- Sebaceous adenitis (short-coated breeds)—annular to polycyclic areas of alopecia and scaling

Symmetrical
- Hyperadrenocorticism—truncal alopecia associated with atrophic skin, comedones, and pyoderma
- Hypothyroidism—alopecia is an uncommon presentation
- Growth hormone–responsive dermatosis—symmetrical truncal alopecia associated with hyperpigmentation; alopecia often starts along the collar area of the neck
- Hyperestrogenism (females)—symmetrical alopecia of the flanks and perineal and inguinal regions with enlarged vulva and mammary glands
- Hypogonadism in intact females—perineal, flank, and truncal alopecia
- Testosterone-responsive dermatosis in castrated males—slowly progressive truncal alopecia
- Male feminization from Sertoli cell tumor—alopecia of the perineum and genital region with gynecomastia
- Castration-responsive dermatosis—hair loss in the collar area, rump, perineum, and flanks
- Estrogen-responsive dermatosis in spayed female dogs—alopecia of the perineum and genital regions
- Seasonal flank alopecia—serpiginous flank alopecia with hyperpigmentation

Patchy to Diffuse
- Demodicosis—often associated with erythema, folliculitis, and hyperpigmentation
- Bacterial folliculitis—multifocal area of circular alopecia to coalescing large areas of hair loss; epidermal collarettes
- Dermatophytosis—often accompanied by scale
- Sebaceous adenitis—alopecia with a thick adherent scale; predominantly on the dorsum of the body, including the head and extremities
- Color mutant alopecia—thinning of the hair coat with secondary folliculitis
- Follicular dysplasia—slowly progressive alopecia
- Anagen defluxion and telogen defluxion—acute onset of alopecia
- Hypothyroidism—diffuse thinning of the hair coat
- Hyperadrenocorticism—truncal alopecia with thin skin and formation of comedones
- Epidermotropic lymphoma—diffuse, generalized truncal alopecia with scaling and erythema, later nodule and plaque formation
- Pemphigus foliaceus—hair loss associated with scale and crust formation
- Keratinization disorders—alopecia associated with excessive scale and greasy surface texture

Specific Locations
- Pinnal alopecia—miniaturization of hairs and progressive alopecia
- Traction alopecia—hair loss on the top and lateral aspect of the cranium secondary to having barrettes or rubber bands applied to the hair
- Postclipping alopecia—failure to regrow after clipping
- Melanoderma (alopecia of Yorkshire terriers)—symmetrical alopecia of the pinnae, bridge of the nose, tail, and feet
- Seasonal flank alopecia—serpiginous flank alopecia that may connect over the dorsum
- Black hair follicular dysplasia—alopecia of the black-haired areas only

• Dermatomyositis—alopecia of the face, tip of ears, tail, and digits; associated with scale crusting, and scarring

RISK FACTORS
N/A

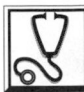

DIAGNOSIS

DIFFERENTIAL DIAGNOSIS
• Pattern and degree—important features for formulating a differential diagnosis
• Inflammation, scale, crust, and epidermal collarettes—important for determining diagnosis

CBC/BIOCHEMISTRY/URINALYSIS
Rule out metabolic causes such as hyperadrenocorticism

OTHER LABORATORY TESTS
• Thyroid testing—diagnose hypothyroidism
• ACTH-response test, LDDST, and HDDST—evaluate for hyperadrenocorticism
• Sex hormone profiles (questionable validity)

IMAGING
Ultrasonography—evaluate adrenal glands for evidence of hyperadrenocorticism

DIAGNOSTIC PROCEDURES
• Response to therapy as a trial
• Fungal culture
• Skin scraping
• Cytology
• Skin biopsy

TREATMENT
• Demodicosis—Amitraz, ivermectin, interceptor
• Dermatophytosis—griseofulvin, ketoconazole, itraconazole, lime sulfur dips, lufenuron
• Staphylococcal folliculitis—shampoo and antibiotic therapy

• Sebaceous adenitis—keratolytic shampoo, essential fatty acid supplementation, retinoids
• Keratinization disorders—shampoos, retinoids, vitamin D
• Endocrine—ovariohysterectomy, castration, Lysodren, adrenalectomy

MEDICATIONS

DRUG(S) OF CHOICE
Varies with specific cause; see Treatment

CONTRAINDICATIONS
N/A

PRECAUTIONS
Toxicity with griseofulvin, retinoids, and ivermectin

POSSIBLE INTERACTIONS
None

ALTERNATIVE DRUG(S)
None

FOLLOW-UP

PATIENT MONITORING
Varies with cause

POSSIBLE COMPLICATIONS
N/A

MISCELLANEOUS

ASSOCIATED CONDITIONS
N/A

AGE-RELATED FACTORS
N/A

ZOONOTIC POTENTIAL
Dermatophytosis can cause skin lesions in people

PREGNANCY
Avoid retinoids and griseofulvin in pregnant animals.

SYNONYMS
None

SEE ALSO
• Demodicosis
• Dermatomyositis
• Dermatophytosis
• Growth Hormone–Responsive Dermatoses
• Hyperadrenocorticism (Cushing's Disease)
• Hypothyroidism
• Pemphigus
• Sebaceous Adenitis
• Sertoli Cell Tumor

ABBREVIATIONS
• HDDST = high-dose dexamethasone-suppression test
• LDDST = low-dose dexamethasone-suppression test

Suggested Reading

Helton-Rhodes KA. Cutaneous manifestations of canine and feline endocrinopathies. Probl Vet Med 1990; 12:617–627.
Schmeitzel LP. Growth hormone responsive alopecia and sex hormone associated dermatoses. In: Birchard SJ, Sherding RG, eds. Saunders manual of small animal practice. Philadelphia: Saunders, 1994:326–330.
Scott DW, Griffin CE, Miller BH. Acquired alopecia. In: Muller & Kirk's small animal dermatology. 5th ed. Philadelphia: Saunders, 1995:720–735.
Scott DW, Griffin CE, Miller BH. Endocrine and metabolic diseases. In: Muller & Kirk's small animal dermatology. 5th ed. Philadelphia: Saunders, 1995:627–719.
Scott DW, Griffin CE, Miller BH. Keratinization defects. In: Muller & Kirk's small animal dermatology. 5th ed. Philadelphia: Saunders, 1995:736–805.

Author Karen Helton Rhodes
Consulting Editor Karen Helton Rhodes

AMELOBLASTOMA

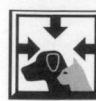

BASICS

OVERVIEW
• Oral tumor of odontogenic (tooth structure) origin
• Called adamantinoma in the older literature
• Most are benign, but rare malignant (highly invasive) forms occur.

SIGNALMENT
• Middle-aged and old dogs
• Uncommon in dogs compared to epulides
• Rare in cats

SIGNS
Smooth, firm, gingival mass that is usually nonulcerated

CAUSES & RISK FACTORS
N/A

DIAGNOSIS

DIFFERENTIAL DIAGNOSIS
• Epulis
• Malignant oral tumor
• Gingival hyperplasia

CBC/BIOCHEMISTRY/URINALYSIS
Unaffected

OTHER LABORATORY TESTS
N/A

IMAGING
Radiographs of skull—often show bone lysis deep to the superficial mass

DIAGNOSTIC PROCEDURES
Deep tissue biopsy—necessary for definitive diagnosis

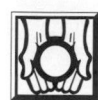

TREATMENT
• Radical surgical excision—andibulectomy/maxillectomy; at least 1–2-cm margins to ensure complete excision
• Radiation therapy may be curative

MEDICATIONS

DRUG(S)
N/A

CONTRAINDICATIONS/POSSIBLE INTERACTIONS
N/A

FOLLOW-UP
Careful oral examination—1, 3, 6, 9, and 12 months after definitive treatment

MISCELLANEOUS
Many histologic subtypes exist and all have similar invasive behavior.

Suggested Reading
Morrison WB. Cancers of the head and neck. In: Morrison WB, ed. Cancer in dogs and cats: medical and surgical management. Baltimore: Williams & Wilkins, 1998:511–519.
Richardson RC, Jones MA, Elliott GS. Oral neoplasms in the dog: a diagnostic and therapeutic dilemma. Compend Contin Educ Small Anim Pract 1983;5:441–446.
Author Wallace B. Morrison
Consulting Editor Wallace B. Morrison

BASICS

OVERVIEW
• Amitraz—formamidine acaricide; applied topically to control ticks, mites, and lice
• Amitraz-containing products (for dogs)—formulated as a 19.9% emulsifiable concentrate in 10.6-mL bottles for dilution and application as a topical pour on and as a 9.0% impregnated 25-in. 27.5-g collar • Systems affected—nervous; endocrine/metabolic (β cells of the pancreas); gastrointestinal • Clinical signs—most associated with α_2-adrenoreceptor agonist
• After high-dose oral administration (dogs)—peak plasma concentration reached at approximately 6 hr; elimination half-life as long as 24 hr; metabolites excreted in the urine
• Ingestion of sustained-release-impregnated collars—constant release and continued systemic exposure until collar segments have passed in the stool • Toxicosis—generally occurs when impregnated collars are ingested, when improperly diluted solutions are applied topically, or when solutions are taken orally
• Idiosyncratic reactions may occur.

SIGNALMENT
• Thorough history—usually identifies use topically or as a collar • Dogs—common, owing to more common use • Cats and other species—rarely reported
• Predilection for old and toy breed animals

SIGNS

Historical Findings
• Develop acutely after exposure

Physical Examination Findings
• Minor to severe depression • Weakness
• Ataxia • Recumbency • Bradycardia
• Hypothermia • Vomiting • Diarrhea
• Polyuria • Abdominal pain • Death

CAUSES & RISK FACTORS
• Ingestion of impregnated collar or pieces of collar
• Inappropriate direct application
• Ingestion of undiluted product
• After application of properly diluted and applied solutions—less common
• Elderly, sick, toy breed, or debilitated animals—may be predisposed

DIAGNOSIS
Depends on clinical signs, history of exposure, or evidence of exposure and elimination of other causes

DIFFERENTIAL DIAGNOSIS
• Recreational and prescription drugs—marijuana; opioids; barbiturates; benzodiazepines; phenothiazines; antihypertensive medications; skeletal muscle relaxants; other depressant drugs or chemicals • Ivermectins, avermectins, milbemycins—generally very high dose or exceptionally sensitive breed
• Alcohols—ethanol; ethylene glycol (antifreeze); methanol (windshield washer fluid); isopropyl alcohol (rubbing alcohol) • Tick paralysis, botulism, cranial trauma, diabetes, hyperadrenocorticism, hypothyroidism, severe anemia, cardiac failure, and anaphylactic shock—marked depression or weakness

CBC/BIOCHEMISTRY/URINALYSIS
• Hyperglycemia—common
• Elevated liver enzymes—uncommon

OTHER LABORATORY TESTS
N/A

IMAGING
Abdominal radiography—may reveal a collar buckle in the gastrointestinal tract

DIAGNOSTIC PROCEDURES
• Identify amitraz on hair or in gastrointestinal contents—analytical methods described; useful only to prove exposure; no data available correlating concentration with clinical signs

PATHOLOGIC FINDINGS
High-dose, prolonged exposure—increased liver weight; slight enlargement of hepatocytes; thinning of the zonae fasciculata and reticularis; slight hyperplasia of the zona glomerulosa of the adrenal glands

TREATMENT
• Inpatient—severely affected patients
• Mild sedation after correctly applied sponge-on solutions—often transient; may require no treatment
• Mild signs after topical application—scrub with a hand dish-washing detergent; rinse with copious amounts of warm water; institute nonspecific supportive therapy (e.g., intravenous fluids, maintenance of normal body temperature, and nutritional support); monitor 1–2 days until improvement is noted.
• Ingestion of collar possible—endoscopic retrieval of the collar—removal of large segments from the stomach may be beneficial; usually numerous small pieces are located throughout the gastrointestinal tract, making removal unrealistic.

MEDICATIONS

DRUG(S)

Collar Ingestion, Asymptomatic Patient
• Emetic—3% USP hydrogen peroxide (2.2 mL/kg PO; maximum 45 mL after feeding a moist meal); apomorphine and especially xylazine not recommended
• Activated charcoal (2 g/kg PO) containing sorbitol as an osmotic cathartic—administer by stomach tube; re-administer every 4 hr until pieces of collar are noted in the stool and the patient is markedly improved.

Marked Depression
• May require pharmacologic reversal of the α_2-adrenergic effects
• Yohimbine (Yobine)—0.11 mg/kg IV, administered slowly; reverses depression and bradycardia within minutes; objective is to keep the patient in a state of low-level depression with normal heart rate, blood pressure, body temperature, and blood glucose concentrations
• Collar ingestions—monitor for recurrence of symptoms; may need additional yohimbine until collar segments appear in the stool
• Atipamezole (Antisedan)—0.05 mg/kg, IM; reported to reverse poisoning within 10 min; repeated as needed; an alternative when yohimbine is unavailable
• Yohimbine and atipamezole—may require initial repeated administration every 4–8 hr, because half-life in dogs is short and elimination half-life of amitraz is longer

CONTRAINDICATIONS/POSSIBLE INTERACTIONS
Yohimbine and atipamezole—excessive administration may result in apprehension, CNS stimulation, and rarely seizures.

FOLLOW-UP
• Body temperature, blood pressure, serum glucose, and heart rate—important parameters • Close observation for recurrence of clinical signs—required for 24–72 hr
• Yohimbine and atipamezole—requires re-administration in severe cases, because reversal effects subside before collar segments have passed or before amitraz has been eliminated from the body
• No long-term adverse effects expected

MISCELLANEOUS
Elderly, sick, or debilitated animals may take longer to fully recover.

Suggested Reading
Grossman MR. Amitraz toxicosis associated with ingestion of an acaricide collar in a dog. J Am Vet Med Assoc 1993:203:55–57.
Hugnet C, Buronfosse F, Pineau X, et al. Toxicity and kinetics of amitraz in dogs. Am J Vet Res 1996;57:1506–1510.
Author Steven R. Hansen
Consulting Editor Gary D. Osweiler

AMYLOIDOSIS

 BASICS

DEFINITION
A group of conditions of diverse cause in which extracellular deposition of insoluble fibrillar proteins (amyloid) in various organs and tissues compromises their normal function

PATHOPHYSIOLOGY
• Patients usually affected by systemic reactive amyloidosis; tissue deposits contain AA, which is a fragment of an acute–phase reactant called SAA • Phases of amyloid deposition

Predeposition phase: SAA concentration is high but without amyloid deposits; colchicine administration during this phase may prevent development of the disease.
Deposition phase (rapid portion): amyloid deposits increase rapidly; colchicine administration delays but does not prevent tissue deposition of amyloid; DMSO may promote resolution of amyloid deposits and a persistent decrease in SAA concentration.
Deposition phase (plateau portion): net deposition of amyloid changes little; neither DMSO or colchicine is beneficial.

• Clinical signs in dogs and cats usually are associated with amyloid deposition in the kidneys. • Dogs—amyloid deposits usually found in the glomeruli leading to proteinuria and nephrotic syndrome. • Cats—amyloid deposits usually found in the medullary interstitium but may occur in glomeruli. • Some Chinese shar pei dogs with familial amyloidosis have medullary amyloidosis without glomerular involvement.

SYSTEMS AFFECTED
Renal/Urologic—predilection for renal AA deposition; liver, spleen, adrenal glands, pancreas, and gastrointestinal tract also may be affected.

GENETICS
No genetic involvement is clearly established; familial amyloidosis occurs in Chinese shar pei, English foxhound, and beagle dogs, and in Abyssinian, Oriental shorthair, and Siamese cats.

INCIDENCE/PREVALENCE
Uncommon disease in domestic animals; occurs most commonly in dogs; rare in cats, except Abyssinians

GEOGRAPHIC DISTRIBUTION
N/A

SIGNALMENT
Species
Dogs and cats
Breed Predilections
• Dogs—Chinese shar pei, beagle, collie, pointer, English foxhound, and walker hound;

German shepherd dog and mixed breeds are at lower risk. • Cats: Abyssinian, Oriental shorthair, and Siamese
Mean Age and Range
• Most affected dogs and cats are more than 5 years old. • Dogs—mean age at diagnosis is 9 years; range, 1–15 years • Cats—mean age at diagnosis 7 years; range, 1–17 years • Prevalence increases with age. • Abyssinian cats—range < 1–17 years • Chinese shar pei dogs—usually <6 years of age when signs of renal failure develop; range, 1.5–6 years • Siamese cats with familial amyloidosis of the liver and thyroid gland usually develop signs of liver disease when 1–4 years old.
Predominant Sex
Dogs and Abyssinian cats—females appear to be at a slightly higher risk (< 2:1).

SIGNS
General Comments
• Depend on the organs affected, the amount of amyloid, and the reaction of the affected organs to amyloid deposits • Usually caused by renal involvement; occasionally, hepatic involvement may cause signs in Chinese shar pei dogs and Oriental shorthair and Siamese cats.
Historical Findings
• No clear history of a predisposing disorder in most (~75%) cases • Anorexia, lethargy, polyuria and polydipsia, weight loss, vomiting, and diarrhea (uncommon) • Ascites and peripheral edema in animals with nephrotic syndrome • Chinese shar pei dogs may have a history of previous episodic joint swelling and high fever that resolves spontaneously within a few days. • Beagle dogs with juvenile polyarteritis may have a history of fever and neck pain that persist for 3–7 days. • Oriental shorthaired and Siamese cats may present with spontaneous hepatic hemorrhage leading to acute collapse and hemoabdomen
Physical Examination Findings
• Related to renal failure—oral ulceration, emaciation, vomiting, and dehydration; kidneys usually small, firm, and irregular in affected cats; they may be small, normal-sized, or slightly enlarged in affected dogs. • Signs of nephrotic syndrome (e.g., ascites, subcutaneous edema) • Related to the primary inflammatory or neoplastic disease process • Thromboembolic phenomena—may occur in up to 40% of affected dogs; signs vary with the location of the thrombus; patients may develop pulmonary thromboembolism (e.g., dyspnea) or iliac or femoral artery thromboembolism (e.g., caudal paresis). • Chinese shar pei dogs and Oriental shorthair and Siamese cats may have signs of hepatic disease (e.g., jaundice, cachexia, and spontaneous hepatic rupture with intraperitoneal bleeding).

CAUSES
• Chronic inflammation—systemic mycoses (e.g., blastomycosis, coccidioidomycosis), chronic bacterial infections (e.g., osteomyelitis, bronchopneumonia, pleuritis, steatitis, pyometra, pyelonephritis, chronic suppurative dermatitis, chronic suppurative arthritis, chronic peritonitis, nocardiosis, chronic stomatitis), parasitic infections (e.g., dirofilariasis, leishmaniasis, hepatozoonosis), and immune-mediated diseases (e.g., systemic lupus erythematosus) • Neoplasia (e.g., lymphosarcoma, plasmacytoma, multiple myeloma, mammary tumors, testicular tumors) • Familial (e.g., Chinese shar pei, English foxhound and beagle dogs; Abyssinian, Siamese, and Oriental shorthair cats) • Others—cyclic hematopoiesis in gray collies; juvenile polyarteritis in beagles

RISK FACTORS
• Chronic inflammation or neoplasia
• Family history in certain breeds

 DIAGNOSIS

DIFFERENTIAL DIAGNOSIS
• Dogs—glomerulonephritis is the main differential diagnosis; proteinuria tends to be more severe in dogs with glomerular amyloidosis than those with glomerulonephritis. • Cats and Chinese shar pei dogs with medullary amyloidosis—consider other causes of medullary renal disease (e.g., pyelonephritis, chronic interstitial disease). • Renal biopsy—necessary for definitive diagnosis

CBC/BIOCHEMISTRY/URINALYSIS
• Nonregenerative anemia is found in some dogs and cats with amyloid-induced renal failure. • Dogs—may see hypercholesterolemia (>85%), azotemia (>70%), hypoalbuminemia (70%), hyperphosphatemia (>60%), hypocalcemia (50%), and metabolic acidosis • Hypercholesterolemia—common finding in cats with renal disorders (>70% of cats with renal disease in one study) but does not reliably predict glomerular disease • Hypoproteinemia—more common than hyperproteinemia (24 vs. 8.5%) in dogs with amyloidosis; hyperglobulinemia common in cats • Proteinuria—with an inactive sediment common in dogs; mild or absent in animals with medullary amyloidosis without glomerular involvement (most mixed-breed cats, at least 25% of Abyssinian cats, and at least 33% of Chinese shar pei dogs). • Isosthenuria, and hyaline, granular, and waxy casts in some patients

OTHER LABORATORY TESTS
Proteinuria—quantify by 24-h urinary protein excretion or urinary protein:creatinine ratio

IMAGING

Abdominal Radiographic Findings
• Kidneys usually small in affected cats • Kidneys small, normal-sized, or large in affected dogs

Abdominal Ultrasonographic Findings
Kidneys usually hyperechoic and small in affected cats; may be small, normal-sized, or large in affected dogs

DIAGNOSTIC PROCEDURES

Renal biopsy needed to differentiate amyloidosis from glomerulonephritis. In dogs other than Chinese shar pei, amyloidosis is primarily a glomerular disease and diagnosis can be obtained by renal cortical biopsy. In most domestic cats, some Abyssinian cats, and some Chinese shar pei dogs, medullary amyloidosis can occur without glomerular involvement; obtain medullary tissue to make the diagnosis.

PATHOLOGIC FINDINGS

• Small kidneys in cats; small, normal, or large kidneys in dogs • Amyloid deposits appear homogeneous and eosinophilic when stained by hematoxylin and eosin and viewed by conventional light microscopy. They demonstrate green birefringence after Congo red staining when viewed under polarized light. Evaluation of Congo red–stained sections before and after permanganate oxidation permits presumptive diagnosis of AA amyloidosis (versus other types) because AA amyloidosis loses its Congo red affinity after permanganate oxidation.
• The liver is very friable and usually contains extensive amyloid deposits in cats presented with acute hepatic hemorrhage.

TREATMENT

APPROPRIATE HEALTH CARE
• Hospitalize patients with chronic renal failure and dehydration for initial medical management. • Can manage stable patients and those with asymptomatic proteinuria as outpatients

NURSING CARE
Correct dehydration with 0.9% NaCl solution or lactated Ringer's solution; patients with severe metabolic acidosis may require bicarbonate supplementation (see Acidosis, Metabolic).

ACTIVITY
Normal

DIET
• Patients with chronic renal failure—restrict phosphorus and moderately restrict protein.
• Patients with hypertension—restrict sodium.

CLIENT EDUCATION
• Discuss progression of the disease.
• Discuss familial predisposition in susceptible breeds.
• Discuss potential complications (e.g., hypertension, thromboembolism).

MEDICATIONS

DRUG(S) OF CHOICE
• Identify underlying inflammatory and neoplastic processes and treat if possible. • Manage renal failure according to the principles of conservative medical treatment (see Renal Failure, Acute and Chronic). • Normalize blood pressure in patients with hypertension (see Hypertension, Systemic). • Patients with thromboembolic syndrome and nephrotic syndrome caused by glomerular amyloidosis usually have a low plasma concentration of antithrombin III; thus heparin is relatively ineffective. Aspirin (0.5 mg/kg q12h) has been suggested for dogs with glomerular disease; this low dosage is as effective in preventing platelet aggregation as is 10 mg/kg q24h. • DMSO—may help patients by solubilizing amyloid fibrils, reducing serum concentration of SAA, and reducing interstitial inflammation and fibrosis in the affected kidneys; may cause lens opacification in dogs. Perivascular inflammation and local thrombosis may occur if undiluted DMSO is administered intravenously. Subcutaneous administration of undiluted DMSO may be painful. The authors have used 90% DMSO diluted 1:4 with sterile water subcutaneously at a dosage of 90 mg/kg three times per week in dogs. Whether or not DMSO treatment benefits renal amyloidosis in dogs remains controversial. • Colchicine—impairs release of SAA from hepatocytes; prevents development of amyloidosis in humans with familial Mediterranean fever (a familial amyloidosis) and stabilizes renal function in patients with nephrotic syndrome but without overt renal failure; no evidence of benefit once the patient develops renal failure; may cause vomiting, diarrhea, and idiosyncratic neutropenia in dogs.

CONTRAINDICATIONS
Avoid use of nephrotoxic drugs (e.g., aminoglycosides).

PRECAUTIONS
• Dosage of drugs excreted by the kidneys may need adjustment in patients with renal failure. • Use nonsteroidal antiinflammatory drugs cautiously in patients with medullary amyloidosis; they can decrease renal blood flow in dehydrated patients.

POSSIBLE INTERACTIONS
None

ALTERNATIVE DRUG(S)
None

FOLLOW-UP

PATIENT MONITORING
• Appetite and activity level daily by the owner; body weight weekly • Serum albumin, creatinine, and BUN concentrations every 2–6 months in stable patients • Can assess degree of proteinuria serially by urine protein: creatinine ratios

PREVENTION/AVOIDANCE
Do not breed affected animals.

POSSIBLE COMPLICATIONS
• Renal failure • Nephrotic syndrome
• Systemic hypertension • Hepatic rupture causing intraperitoneal hemorrhage
• Thromboembolic disease

EXPECTED COURSE AND PROGNOSIS
This is a progressive disease that is usually advanced at the time of diagnosis. Survival for dogs with glomerular amyloidosis varied from 3 to 20 months in one study; some dogs may occasionally live longer. Cats with renal failure because of amyloidosis usually survive < 1 year. Mildly affected cats may not develop renal failure and have an almost normal life expectancy.

MISCELLANEOUS

ASSOCIATED CONDITIONS
• Urinary tract infection • Polyarthritis in Chinese shar pei dogs • Polyarteritis in beagle dogs

AGE-RELATED FACTORS
N/A

ZOONOTIC POTENTIAL
None

PREGNANCY
High risk in affected animals

SYNONYMS
N/A

SEE ALSO
• Glomerulonephritis • Nephrotic Syndrome
• Proteinuria • Renal Failure, Acute and Chronic

ABBREVIATIONS
• AA = amyloid A protein • DMSO = dimethylsulfoxide • SAA = serum amyloid A protein

Suggested Reading

DiBartola SP. Renal amyloidosis. In: Osborne CA, Low D, Finco DR, eds. Canine and feline urology. 2nd ed. Philadelphia: Saunders, 1995:400–415.

DiBartola SP, Tarr MJ, Webb DM, et al. Renal amyloidosis in related Chinese shar pei dogs. J Am Vet Med Assoc 1990;197: 483–487.

Zuber RM. Systemic amyloidosis in Oriental and Siamese cats. Aust Vet Pract 1993;23: 66–70.

Authors Helio Autran de Morais and Stephen P. DiBartola

Consulting Editors Larry G. Adams and Carl A. Osborne

ANAEROBIC INFECTIONS

BASICS

OVERVIEW
• Caused by bacteria requiring low oxygen tension
• Most commonly found genera—*Bacteroides, Fusobacterium, Actinomyces, Clostridium,* and *Peptostreptococcus*
• Individual organisms vary in their potential to withstand oxygen exposure.
• A number of injurious toxins and enzymes may be elaborated by the organisms, leading to extension of the infection into adjacent, healthy tissue.

SIGNALMENT
Dogs and cats

SIGNS

General Comments
• Determined by the body system involved
• Certain areas of the body are more commonly associated with anaerobic infection, perhaps because of proximity to mucosal surfaces.
• It is possible to overlook the potential for anaerobes to be involved in an infectious process, leading to confusion in interpreting culture results and in selecting inappropriate antimicrobials.

Physical Examination Findings
• A foul odor associated with a wound or exudative discharge
• Gas in the tissue or associated exudate
• Peritonitis, pyothorax, or pyometra
• Severe dental disease
• Wounds or deep abscesses that do not heal as anticipated

CAUSES & RISK FACTORS
• Usually caused by normal flora of the body; a break in protective barriers allows bacterial invasion.
• Predisposing factors—bite wounds, dental disease, open fractures, abdominal surgery, and foreign bodies

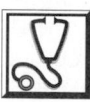

DIAGNOSIS

DIFFERENTIAL DIAGNOSIS
• Wounds that fail to respond to appropriate medical therapy—aerobic cultures may be negative; suspect anaerobic organisms.
• Cats with nonhealing wounds—test for FeLV and FIV.
• Middle-aged and old animals—tumor invasion (e.g., in the gastrointestinal tract) may be responsible for establishing infection.

CBC/BIOCHEMISTRY/URINALYSIS
• Neutrophilic leukocytosis and monocytosis common
• Biochemical abnormalities depend on specific organ involvement.

OTHER LABORATORY TESTS
N/A

IMAGING
None required, except perhaps with bone infection

DIAGNOSTIC PROCEDURES
• Appropriate samples—pus (1–2 mL in stoppered syringe) and tissue (minimum 1g sample)
• Proper handling of samples—minimize exposure to air when collecting and transporting; appropriate transport devices should be on hand before the sample is collected and include screw-top glass vials with media that accept a Culturette swab and syringes evacuated of all air and capped with a rubber stopper.

PATHOLOGIC FINDINGS
N/A

TREATMENT
• Thoracic drainage—important with pyothorax (see specific chapter)
• Hyperbaric oxygen—some potential use; may be limited in availability

SURGERY
• Should not be delayed when anaerobes are suspected
• Generally indicated for all except pyothorax and CNS infections
• Combined with systemic antimicrobial therapy—the best chance of a positive outcome
• Usually indicated when anaerobic organisms complicate pyometra, osteomyelitis, and peritonitis
• Cleanse the wound of toxins and devitalized tissue.
• Enhance drainage of pus.
• Improve local blood flow.
• Increase oxygen tension.

MEDICATIONS

DRUG(S)
• Antimicrobial therapy alone—unlikely to be successful; poor drug penetration into exudates

• Antibiotic selection—largely empiric, owing to the difficulty of isolating anaerobes and the delay in return of culture results; cytology and Gram staining of exudates may aid in selecting the initial antibiotic.
• Although most anaerobic infections are polymicrobial, antibiotic therapy targeted against the anaerobes is more likely to be successful than selecting multiple antibiotics because of the symbiotic nature of the infection.
• Penicillin G—considered the antibiotic of choice (except for *Bacteroides* strains)
• Amoxicillin—comparable to penicillin G in spectrum of activity; convenient and accessible; may be useful to combine with clavulanic acid for *Bacteroides*
• Cefoxitin—the only cephalosporin with reliable activity against anaerobes; expensive
• Clindamycin—may be especially useful for respiratory tract infections
• Chloramphenicol—good tissue penetration, but bacteriostatic
• Metronidazole—useful against all clinically significant anaerobes (except *Actinomyces*)
• Aminoglycosides—uniformly ineffective against anaerobes
• Trimethoprim-sulfa combinations—ineffective; poor penetration into purulent exudates

CONTRAINDICATIONS/POSSIBLE INTERACTIONS
N/A

FOLLOW-UP
Long-term antibiotic therapy may be required.

MISCELLANEOUS

ABBREVIATIONS
• FeLV = feline leukemia virus
• FIV = feline immunodeficiency virus

Suggested Reading
Hirsh DC, Jang SS. Anaerobic infections. In: Greene CE, ed. Infectious diseases of the dog and cat. Philadelphia: Saunders, 1998:258–263.

Author Sharon Fooshee Grace
Consulting Editor Stephen C. Barr

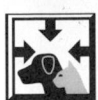

BASICS

OVERVIEW
• Dogs—three types (impaction, sacculitis, and abscess), which are probably stages of the same disease process
• Cats—rare; impaction occasionally noted

SIGNALMENT
• Dogs
• Rarely cats
• Small breeds—miniature poodles, toy poodles, and Chihuahuas reportedly predisposed
• No age or sex predispositions

SIGNS
• Scooting
• Tenesmus
• Perianal pruritus
• Tail chasing
• Perianal discharge, if abscess ruptures
• Behavioral changes
• Pyotraumatic dermatitis

CAUSES & RISK FACTORS
• Unknown
• Possible predisposing factors—chronically soft feces, recent diarrhea, excessive glandular secretions, and poor muscle tone
• Retained secretions may lead to infection and abscess formation.

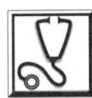

DIAGNOSIS

DIFFERENTIAL DIAGNOSIS
• Erythema and swelling of the perineum—anal sac neoplasia

• Perianal pruritus—food hypersensitivity, flea allergy dermatitis, atopy, tapeworms, tail fold pyoderma, and seborrheic skin disorders affecting the perineum
• Anal sac abscesses must be differentiated from perianal fistulas.

CBC/BIOCHEMISTRY/URINALYSIS
N/A

OTHER LABORATORY TESTS
N/A

IMAGING
N/A

DIAGNOSTIC PROCEDURES
• History and digital palpation examination—establish diagnosis; if easily palpated through the skin, sacs are considered enlarged.
• Normal anal sacs—clear or pale yellow-brown secretion
• Impaction—thick, pasty brown secretion
• Anal sacculitis—creamy yellow or thin green-yellow secretion
• Abscessed—red-brown exudate, fever, swelling, and erythema over the anal sacs
• Ruptured—discharging sinus
• Cytology of anal sac contents—number of leukocytes and bacteria indicate infection
• Bacterial culture and sensitivity—may help for animals with chronic or recurrent anal sac infections

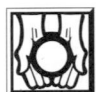

TREATMENT
• Express contents for impaction or sacculitis.
• Instill an antibiotic/corticosteroid ointment for infected anal sacs.
• If necessary, establish drainage in abscesses; clean and flush anal sacs.

• Recurrent abscesses—consider anal sac excision.
• Severe and recurrent cases may require surgical excision.

MEDICATIONS

DRUG(S)
• Abscesses—systemic and topical antibiotics
• Severe cases with fistulation may benefit from oral cyclosporine therapy 5 mg/kg/day.

CONTRAINDICATIONS/POSSIBLE INTERACTIONS
N/A

FOLLOW-UP
Abscesses—examine after 3–7 days of therapy.

MISCELLANEOUS

Suggested Reading
Burrows CF, Ellison GW. Recto-anal diseases. In: Ettinger SJ, ed. Textbook of veterinary internal medicine. 3rd ed. Philadelphia: Saunders, 1989:1570–1572.
Authors Jon D. Plant and Karen Helton Rhodes
Consulting Editor Karen Helton Rhodes

ANAPHYLAXIS

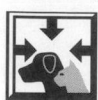 **BASICS**

DEFINITION
• Acute manifestation of a type I hypersensitivity reaction mediated through the rapid introduction of an antigen into a host having antigen-specific antibodies of the IgE subclass
• The binding of antigen to mast cells sensitized with IgE results in the release of preformed and newly synthesized chemical mediators.
• Anaphylactic reactions may be localized (atopy) or systemic (anaphylactic shock).
• Anaphylaxis not mediated by IgE is designated an anaphylactoid reaction and will not be discussed.

PATHOPHYSIOLOGY
• First exposure of the patient to a particular antigen (allergen) causes a humoral response and results in production of IgE, which binds to the surface of mast cells; the patient is then considered to be sensitized to that antigen.
• Second exposure to the antigen results in cross-linking of two or more IgE molecules on the cell surface, resulting in mast cell degranulation and activation; release of mast cell granules initiates an anaphylactic reaction.
• Major mast cell–derived mediators include histamine, eosinophilic chemotactic factor, arachidonic acid, metabolites (e.g., prostaglandins, leukotrienes, and thromboxanes), platelet-activating factor, and proteases, which cause an inflammatory response of increased vascular permeability, smooth muscle contraction, inflammatory cell influx, and tissue damage.
• Clinical manifestations depend on the route of antigen exposure, the dose of antigen, and the level of the IgE response.

SYSTEMS AFFECTED
• Skin/Exocrine—pruritus, urticaria, and edema
• Respiratory (cats)—dyspnea and cyanosis
• Gastrointestinal—salivation, vomiting, and diarrhea
• Hepatobiliary (dogs)—because of portal hypertension and vasoconstriction

GENETICS
Familial basis reported for type I hypersensitivity reaction in dogs

INCIDENCE/PREVALENCE
• Localized type I hypersensitivity reactions not uncommon
• Systemic type I hypersensitivity reactions rare

GEOGRAPHIC DISTRIBUTION
None

SIGNALMENT

Species
Dogs and cats

Breed Predilections
• Dogs—numerous breeds documented as having a predilection for developing atopy
• Cats—no breeds documented as having predilection for atopy

Mean Age and Range
• Dogs—age of clinical onset ranges from 3 months to several years of age; most affected animals 1–3 years old
• Cats—age of clinical onset ranges from 6 months to 2 years.

Predominant Sex
• Dogs—atopy more common in females
• Cats—no reported sex predilection

SIGNS

General Comments
• Initial clinical signs vary depending on the route of exposure to the inciting antigen (allergen).
• Shock—end result of a severe anaphylactic reaction
• Shock organ—dogs, liver; cats, respiratory and gastrointestinal systems
• May be localized to the site of exposure, but may progress to a systemic reaction

Historical Findings
• Onset of signs immediate (usually within minutes)
• Dogs—pruritus, urticaria, vomiting, defecation, and urination
• Cats—intense pruritus about the head, dyspnea, salivation, and vomiting

Physical Examination Findings
• Localized cutaneous edema at the site of exposure
• Hepatomegaly in some dogs
• Hyperexcitability possible in early stages
• Depression and collapse terminally

CAUSES
Virtually any agent; those commonly reported include venoms, blood-based products, vaccines, foods, and drugs.

RISK FACTORS
Previous exposure (sensitization) increases the chance of the animal developing a reaction.

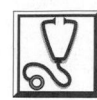 **DIAGNOSIS**

DIFFERENTIAL DIAGNOSIS
• Other types of shock
• Trauma
• Depends on the major organ system involved or if reaction is localized; diagnosis can be made largely on the basis of history and clinical signs.

CBC/BIOCHEMISTRY/URINALYSIS
Because of the acute onset of disease, no tests available that reliably predict individual susceptibility

OTHER LABORATORY TESTS
• Intradermal skin testing to identify allergens
• Radioallergosorbent test to quantify the concentration of serum IgE specific for a particular antigen

IMAGING
N/A

DIAGNOSTIC PROCEDURES
Limited because a severely allergic animal can develop an anaphylactic reaction when exposed to even small quantities of antigen

PATHOLOGIC FINDINGS
• Lesions vary, depending on severity of reaction, from localized cutaneous edema to severe pulmonary edema (in cats) and visceral pooling of blood (in dogs).
• Other nonspecific findings vary and are characteristic of shock.
• Nonspecific characteristics of localized reactions include edema, vasculitis, and thromboembolism.

TREATMENT

APPROPRIATE HEALTH CARE
In an acutely affected animal, the reaction is considered a medical emergency requiring hospitalization.

NURSING CARE
Elimination of inciting antigen, if possible

Systemic Anaphylaxis
• Goal—emergency life support through the maintenance of an open airway, preventing circulatory collapse, and re-establishing physiologic parameters
• Administer fluids intravenously at shock dosages to counteract hypotension.

Localized Anaphylaxis
Goal—limit the reaction and prevent progression to a systemic reaction.

ACTIVITY
N/A

DIET
If a food-based allergen is suspected (uncommon), avoid foods associated with hypersensitivity reaction.

CLIENT EDUCATION
• Discuss the unpredictable nature of the disease.
• Discuss the need to recognize that the animal has an allergic condition that may require immediate medical care.

SURGICAL CONSIDERATIONS
None

MEDICATIONS

DRUG(S) OF CHOICE

Systemic Anaphylaxis
• Epinephrine hydrochloride parenterally (1:1000; 0.01 mL/kg) for shock
• Corticosteroids for shock—prednisolone sodium succinate (2 mg/kg IV q8h) or dexamethasone sodium phosphate (0.25 mg/kg IV q12h)

• Atropine sulfate (0.04 mg/kg IM) to counteract bradycardia and hypotension
• Aminophylline (10 mg/kg IM or slowly IV) in severely dyspneic patients

Localized Anaphylaxis
• Diphenhydramine hydrochloride (1–2 mg/kg IV or IM)
• Prednisolone (2 mg/kg PO)
• Epinephrine hydrochloride (0.15 ml SC at site of initiation)
• If shock develops, initiate treatment for a systemic anaphylaxis.

CONTRAINDICATIONS
None

PRECAUTIONS
Localized reaction can develop into systemic reaction.

POSSIBLE INTERACTIONS
N/A

ALTERNATIVE DRUG(S)
N/A

FOLLOW-UP

PATIENT MONITORING
Closely monitor hospitalized patients for 24–48 hr.

PREVENTION/AVOIDANCE
If inciting antigen (allergen) can be identified, eliminate or reduce exposure

POSSIBLE COMPLICATIONS
None

EXPECTED COURSE AND PROGNOSIS
• If localized reaction is treated early, prognosis is good.
• If the animal is in shock on examination, prognosis guarded to poor

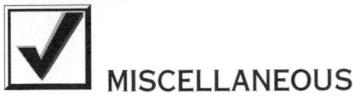
MISCELLANEOUS

ASSOCIATED CONDITIONS
None

AGE-RELATED FACTORS
None

ZOONOTIC POTENTIAL
None

PREGNANCY
N/A

SYNONYMS
None

SEE ALSO
• Atopy
• Shock, Cardiogenic

Suggested Reading
Mueller DL, Noxon JO. Anaphylaxis: pathophysiology and treatment. Compend Contin Ed Pract Vet 1990;12:157–170.
Author Paul W. Snyder
Consulting Editor Stephen A. Kruth

ANEMIA, APLASTIC

 BASICS

OVERVIEW
• A disorder of hematopoietic precursor cells characterized by replacement of normal bone marrow by adipose tissue and decreased production of granulocytes, erythrocytes and platelets, resulting in pancytopenia in the peripheral blood
• In the acute form, neutropenia and thrombocytopenia predominate because of their shorter life spans; in the chronic form, nonregenerative anemia also occurs. In both forms, the bone marrow exhibits variable degrees of panhypoplasia.
• There are many causes of deficient hematopoiesis, including infectious diseases, drug effect, and toxin exposure; immune-mediated mechanisms are often suspected.
• Hemic/lymphatic/immune systems affected

SIGNALMENT
Dogs and cats

SIGNS
• Acute form: signs referable to neutropenia and thrombocytopenia (i.e., fever, petechial hemorrhage, epistaxis, hematuria, melena)
• Chronic form: signs referable to anemia (i.e., pale mucous membranes, weakness, lethargy) in addition to signs observed in acute forms

CAUSES & RISK FACTORS
Often not identified
Infectious Agents
• FeLV, FIV
• Canine and feline parvovirus
• *Ehrlichia* spp.
Drugs and Chemicals
• Estrogen (exogenous administration, Sertoli and interstitial cell tumors)
• Methimazole (cats)
• Chemotherapeutic drugs, including azathioprine, cyclophosphamide, cytosine arabinoside, doxorubicin, vinblastine, and hydroxyurea
• Antibiotics, including trimethoprim-sulfadiazine, cephalosporins, and chloramphenicol
• Griseofulvin
• NSAIDs, including phenylbutazone and meclofenamic acid
• Albendazole
• Captopril
• Quinidine
• Thiacetarsamide
• Ionizing radiation

 DIAGNOSIS

DIFFERENTIAL DIAGNOSIS
Causes of pancytopenia with bone marrow normo- or hypercellularity (e.g., myelodysplastic disorders, leukemias, myelofibrosis)

CBC/BIOCHEMISTRY/URINALYSIS
• Leukopenia characterized by neutropenia with or without lymphopenia
• Normocytic, normochromic, nonregenerative anemia
• Thrombocytopenia

OTHER LABORATORY TESTS
• Immunologic tests for infectious diseases (e.g., serologic titers, ELISA, IFA)
• PCR for infectious agents
• Serologic test for antierythrocyte antibodies (Coombs' test)

IMAGING
N/A

DIAGNOSTIC PROCEDURES
• Bone marrow aspiration—frequently an inadequate or fatty sample is obtained because of decreased hemopoietic tissue and replacement by lipocytes
• Bone marrow core biopsy—allows an evaluation of architecture and reveals hypoplasia of cell lines and replacement by adipose tissue

 TREATMENT

Supportive treatment, antibiotics, blood component therapy, as dictated by clinical condition

 MEDICATIONS

DRUG(S) OF CHOICE
• Cyclosporine A—10–25 mg/kg PO q12h (dogs), 4–5 mg/kg PO q12h (cats)
• Recombinant hematopoietic growth factors (e.g., rhG-CSF: 5 μg/kg/day SC)
• Androgen and corticosteroid administration have been largely unsuccessful.

CONTRAINDICATIONS/POSSIBLE INTERACTIONS
N/A

OTHER DRUGS
• Antibiotics to treat secondary infections if fever and neutropenia present
• Whole or component blood transfusion if indicated

 FOLLOW-UP

PATIENT MONITORING
• Daily physical examination
• CBC every 3–5 days to weekly

PREVENTION/AVOIDANCE
• Castration of cryptorchid males
• Vaccination for infectious diseases
• Frequent monitoring of CBC in cancer patients receiving chemotherapy

POSSIBLE COMPLICATIONS
• Sepsis
• Hemorrhage

EXPECTED COURSE AND PROGNOSIS
• Guarded to poor
• Recovery of hematopoiesis may take weeks to months, if it occurs at all.
• Spontaneous recovery occasionally occurs, especially in young animals.

 MISCELLANEOUS

SEE ALSO
Pancytopenia

ABBREVIATIONS
• ELISA = enzyme-linked immunosorbent assay
• FeLV = feline leukemia virus
• FIV = feline immunodeficiency virus
• IFA = immunofluorescent antibody
• NSAIDs = nonsteroidal anti-inflammatory drugs
• PCR = polymerase chain reaction
• rhG-CSF = recombinant human granulocyte colony-stimulating factor

Suggested Reading
Weiss DJ. Aplastic anemia. In: Feldman BF, Zinkl JG, Jain NC, eds. Schalm's veterinary hematology. 5th ed. Philadelphia: Lippincott Williams & Wilkins, 2000:212–215.

Acknowledgment
The author and editor acknowledge the prior contribution of Dr. Gregory O. Freden, who authored this topic in the previous edition.
Author Darren Wood
Consulting Editor Stephen Kruth

BASICS

OVERVIEW
• Hemolytic anemia is caused by RBC inclusions called Heinz bodies, which are clumps of oxidized, denatured hemoglobin that cause splenic entrapment or lysis of RBCs.
• Caused by ingestion or administration of chemical or dietary oxidants
• New methylene blue stain used to identify Heinz bodies
• Sometimes accompanied by methemoglobinemia
• Treatment includes removing the offending oxidant and providing supportive care.

SIGNALMENT
• Dogs and cats
• More common in cats, which have oxidant-sensitive hemoglobin
• No sex, breed, or age disposition

SIGNS

Historical Findings
• Exposure to oxidant drug, plant, or chemical
• Sudden onset of weakness, anorexia, and fever
• Reddish brown urine (hemoglobinuria), if hemolysis is severe

PHYSICAL EXAMINATION FINDINGS
• Pale or icteric mucous membranes
• Cyanosis, if concurrent methemoglobinemia

CAUSES & RISK FACTORS
• Acetaminophen (cats)
• Phenacetin (cats)
• Phenazopyridine
• Methylene blue
• Onions (i.e., raw, cooked, dehydrated, and powdered)
• Garlic
• Vitamin K_3 (not vitamin K_1)
• Zinc toxicity
• D,L-methionine (cats)
• Benzocaine (topical)
• Naphthalene (moth ball) ingestion
• Propylene glycol, fish-based diets, propofol anesthesia, diabetes mellitus, and other systemic diseases can cause Heinz bodies in cats, but oxidation is not usually severe enough to cause hemolytic anemia.

DIAGNOSIS

DIFFERENTIAL DIAGNOSIS
Other causes of regenerative, hemolytic anemia (e.g., immune-mediated and RBC organisms such as *Haemobartonella*)

CBC/BIOCHEMISTRY/URINALYSIS
• PCV and reticulocyte count indicate regenerative, mild to severe anemia (**REMEMBER:** not all cats with Heinz bodies have hemolytic anemia.)
• Mean corpuscular hemoglobin concentration and automated WBC count—may be falsely high because of interference from Heinz bodies
• Heinz bodies may be visible on a routine blood smear as pale, spherical inclusions that protrude from RBCs.
• Dogs have fragmented RBCs and eccentrocytes.
• Hyperbilirubinemia and bilirubinuria are possible.
• Hemoglobinemia and hemoglobinuria—uncommon but may occur if hemolysis is severe

OTHER LABORATORY TESTS
• Supravital new methylene blue stain—Heinz bodies stain blue for easy visibility and quantitation.
• Heinz bodies—can be present in up to 100% of RBCs; usually small and multiple in dogs; single and large in cats; normal cats have Heinz bodies in <5% of RBCs.
• Methemoglobin test if animal is cyanotic
• Serum zinc concentration if indicated

IMAGING
Abdominal radiographs if zinc toxicity suspected

DIAGNOSTIC PROCEDURES
None

TREATMENT

APPROPRIATE HEALTH CARE
Identify and remove the source of oxidant (may be enough for recovery).

NURSING CARE
Provide supportive care for anemia (e.g., transfusion, oxygen, and quiet).

MEDICATIONS

DRUG(S) OF CHOICE
• Acetaminophen toxicity—*N*-acetylcysteine (140 mg/kg q8h PO or IV, or 140 mg/kg loading dose PO or IV followed by 70 mg/kg q4h for 5 doses)
• Methemoglobinemia—methylene blue (1.0–1.5 mg/kg IV once, slowly)

CONTRAINDICATIONS/POSSIBLE INTERACTIONS
Methylene blue is an oxidant in high doses; use with caution.

ALTERNATIVE DRUG(S)
• Acetaminophen toxicity—sodium sulfate (50 mg/kg q8h IV)
• Dietary antioxidants (vitamin C, vitamin E, bioflavonoids) may be slightly protective against mild oxidative damage.

FOLLOW-UP
• Monitor PCV, reticulocytes, and percentage of Heinz bodies.
• Document disappearance of Heinz bodies and regeneration of RBCs.
• Counsel clients on potential causes of the disorder and how to avoid exposing their pets.
• Prognosis is good once the hemolytic crisis is over.

MISCELLANEOUS

SEE ALSO
• Acetaminophen Toxicity
• Anemia, Regenerative
• Zinc Toxicity

ABBREVIATION
PCV = packed cell volume

Suggested Reading
Desnoyers M. Anemias associated with Heinz bodies. In: Feldman B, Zinkl J, Jain NC, eds. Schalm's veterinary hematology. 5th ed. Philadelphia: Lippincott Williams & Wilkins, 2000:178–184.
Author Mary M. Christopher
Consulting Editor Stephen A. Kruth

ANEMIA, IMMUNE-MEDIATED

BASICS

DEFINITION
Accelerated destruction or removal of RBCs due to anti-RBC antibodies with or without complement

PATHOPHYSIOLOGY
• Anti-RBC antibodies form against normal (primary IMHA) or altered (secondary IMHA) RBC membrane antigens. • Infectious organisms, exposure of previously unexposed antigens, or adsorption of preformed antigen–antibody complexes to the RBC membrane can alter RBC membrane antigens. • Antibodies can be warm type (reactive at body temperature, usually IgG) or cold type (reactive at subnormal body temperature, usually IgM). • Immunoglobulin (IgG or IgM, with or without complement) deposits on the RBC membrane, causing either direct intravascular hemolysis or accelerated removal by the reticuloendothelial system in the spleen and/or liver (extravascular hemolysis). • Intravascular hemolysis occurs when adsorbed antibodies (usually IgG) activate complement. • In vivo agglutination of RBCs occurs when IgM or high titers of IgG molecules cause bridging of RBCs. • Removal of RBCs occurs in the spleen and/or liver and is considered a type of extravascular hemolysis. • A form of nonregenerative IMHA is believed to be caused by immune-mediated destruction of RBC precursors in the bone marrow.

SYSTEMS AFFECTED
• Hemic/Lymphatic/Immune—immune-mediated destruction or removal of RBCs, elaboration of proinflammatory mediators (e.g., cytokines, endothelial-derived substances), DIC • Hepatobiliary—hemolysis leads to hyperbilirubinemia and icterus when hepatic function is overwhelmed; hypoxia may cause centrilobular necrosis. • Cardiovascular—hypoxia leads to tachycardia; low blood viscosity and turbulent blood flow cause low-grade heart murmurs; high-output heart failure occurs with chronic anemia. • Respiratory—hypoxia causes tachypnea. • Renal/Urologic—hypoxia causes renal tubular necrosis. • Skin/Exocrine—cold-type IMHA may cause necrosis of extremities and ear tips because of capillary sludging.

GENETICS
• Isolated families of dogs have been documented to be affected (Viszla, Scottish terrier). • No genetic basis has been established.

GEOGRAPHIC DISTRIBUTION
Secondary IMHA may have a higher prevalence in areas where associated infectious diseases are endemic.

SIGNALMENT
Species
• Dogs • Rarely cats

Breed Predilections
Old English sheepdogs, cocker spaniels, poodles, Irish setters, English springer spaniels, collies
Mean Age and Range
• Mean age, 5–6 years • Reported range, 1–13 years
Predominant Sex
Females

SIGNS
Historical Findings
• Collapse • Weakness • Lethargy • Anorexia • Exercise intolerance • Dyspnea • Tachypnea • Vomiting • Diarrhea • Occasionally polyuria and polydipsia
Physical Examination Findings
• Pale mucous membranes, tachycardia, and tachypnea • Splenomegaly and hepatomegaly • Icterus and pigmenturia (hemoglobin or bilirubin) • Fever and lymphadenomegaly • Systolic murmur and S_3 gallop • Petechiae, ecchymoses, or melena possible in animals with concurrent thrombocytopenia or DIC • Skin lesions possible in animals with cold-type IMHA • Other systemic signs possible (e.g., joint pain and glomerulonephritis) if IMHA is a component of SLE

CAUSES
Primary IMHA (Normal RBC Membrane Antigens)
• Autoimmune hemolytic anemia • SLE • Neonatal isoerythrolysis • Dysregulated immune system (e.g., depressed suppressor T-cell activity, high production of immunoglobulins) • Shared antigenic determinants (e.g., infectious agents and drugs) • Idiopathic
Secondary IMHA
• Infectious causes (e.g., *Haemobartonella, Babesia, Leptospira, Ehrlichia,* FeLV, and other viral agents) • Exposure of previously unexposed antigens • Heartworm disease • Neoplasia • Adsorption of antigen–antibody complexes to RBC membrane • Drugs (e.g., sulfa drugs, cephalosporins, heparin, quinidine, propylthiouracil, and methimazole) • Type III hypersensitivity reactions (e.g., Arthus reaction)

RISK FACTORS
Exposure to infectious agents or drugs known to cause IMHA

DIAGNOSIS

DIFFERENTIAL DIAGNOSIS
Dogs
• Hemorrhage • Pyruvate kinase deficiency • Phosphofructokinase deficiency • Heinz body anemia • Zinc toxicity • Splenic torsion • Chronic progressive hepatitis in Bedlington terriers

Cats
• Hemorrhage • Heinz body anemia • Acetaminophen toxicity • Severe hypophosphatemia • Methemoglobin reductase deficiency • Congenital feline porphyria • Cytauxzoonosis

CBC/BIOCHEMISTRY/URINALYSIS
• CBC—anemia, high MCV (3–5 days posthemolytic episode), spherocytes, anisocytosis, polychromasia, nucleated RBCs leukocytosis with neutrophilic left shift • Serum biochemistry—hyperbilirubinemia, hemoglobinemia, high ALT • Urinalysis—hemoglobinuria, bilirubinuria

OTHER LABORATORY TESTS
• Positive direct antiglobulin (Coombs' test)—positive in 60% of animals with IMHA • Spontaneous autoagglutination in saline • Reticulocytosis—absolute count $>60,000/\mu l$ in dogs and $>50,000/\mu l$ in cats • Thrombocytopenia in animals with Evan's syndrome and DIC • Prolonged APTT and PT in animals with DIC • Positive ANA titer and LE cell test in animals with SLE • Positive serologic titers for infectious causes • Evidence of hematologic parasites in blood smears of capillary blood • Expanded RBC distribution width • High RBC osmotic fragility (may be useful in cats)

IMAGING
• Radiographic findings—hepatomegaly and splenomegaly; thorax usually within normal limits; may see evidence of pulmonary thromboembolism, cardiomegaly, or evidence of heart failure if animal has chronic anemia • Echocardiographic findings—generalized cardiomegaly, eccentric hypertrophy, and hyperdynamic state in animals with chronic anemia • Ultrasonographic findings—hepatomegaly and splenomegaly; liver and spleen can be mottled and hyperechoic or hypoechoic.

DIAGNOSTIC PROCEDURES
• Examination of bone marrow aspirate usually reveals hyperplasia of the erythroid series. • In animals with nonregenerative IMHA, maturation arrest or low numbers of erythroid precursors may be seen. • In animals with chronic IMHA, myelofibrosis may be seen.

PATHOLOGIC FINDINGS
• Hepatosplenomegaly • Splenic and hepatic extramedullary hematopoiesis • Reactive lymphadenomegaly • Signs of congestive heart failure (e.g., pulmonary edema, cardiomegaly, and hepatic congestion), pulmonary thromboembolism, and DIC

TREATMENT

APPROPRIATE HEALTH CARE
• Inpatient during the acute hemolytic crisis; outpatient when PCV has stabilized, ongoing hemolysis has been controlled, and clinical

signs of anemia have resolved • Inpatient if animal has complications such as DIC, pulmonary thromboembolism, thrombocytopenia, gastrointestinal bleeding, and heart failure and/or the need for multiple transfusions • Chronic low-grade extravascular hemolysis can be treated on an outpatient basis if the patient is not exhibiting clinical signs secondary to anemia.

NURSING CARE
Fluid therapy to maintain vascular volume and correct dehydration; exercise caution with chronic anemia patients because volume overload is a concern.

ACTIVITY
Cage rest until stable

DIET
N/A

CLIENT EDUCATION
• IMHA and its complications (e.g., DIC and pulmonary thromboembolism) can be fatal. • Life-long treatment may be needed, and the disease may recur. • Side effects of treatment may be severe.

SURGICAL CONSIDERATIONS
Splenectomy can be considered if medical management fails to control the disease after 4–6 weeks of treatment. Consider blood product administration preoperatively.

MEDICATIONS

DRUG(S) OF CHOICE
• Address underlying cause (e.g., infection and drugs) if secondary IMHA • Cross-matched, packed RBCs (6–10 mL/kg) or oxyhemoglobin (30 mL/kg at 10 mL/kg/hr) for severe anemia • Supportive treatment for animals with DIC • Corticosteroids—prednisone 2 mg/kg/day divided BID for 2–4 weeks; if PCV stable, decrease to 1 mg/kg/day for 2–4 weeks; then, if PCV stable, decrease to 1 mg/kg every other day for 2–4 weeks; then, if PCV stable, gradually discontinue over another 2–4 weeks • Cytotoxic drugs if autoagglutination or peracute hemolysis exists or if there is a poor response to prednisone after 14–21 days • Azathioprine—dogs, 50 mg/m² (2 mg/kg/day) for 1–2 weeks; then 1 mg/kg PO every other day; cats, 1.5– 3.125 mg PO q48h (CAUTION: severe bone marrow suppression may develop.) • Cyclophosphamide—50 mg/m²/day (2 mg/kg/day) for 4 consecutive days; then skip 3 days; repeat up to 6–8 weeks • Studies have shown no increased efficacy with combination therapy of cyclophosphamide and prednisone vs. prednisone alone.

CONTRAINDICATIONS
None

PRECAUTIONS
• Caution with administration of azathioprine to cats; dosage of 2 mg/kg has produced severe bone marrow toxicity. • Check blood type

before any transfusion in cats • Prednisone can cause signs of Cushing's syndrome, pulmonary thromboembolism, pancreatitis, secondary infection, and gastric ulcers (consider misoprostol [2–5 μg/kg PO q8–12h] to prevent ulcers). • Cytotoxic drugs can cause bone marrow suppression, secondary infection, pancreatitis (azathioprine), and cystitis (cyclophosphamide).

POSSIBLE INTERACTIONS
Azathioprine and prednisone can cause pancreatitis.

ALTERNATIVE DRUG(S)
• Dexamethasone (0.3–0.9 mg/kg/day) can be used instead of prednisone; follow similar tapering schedule • Chlorambucil—for cats, 2 mg PO q48–72h • Danazol—5–10 mg/kg PO q12h; taper to 5 mg/kg/day when patient is in remission, then gradually discontinue over 3 to 4 months (studies have shown no less severity of disease or mortality with this drug) • Human γ-globulin—0.5–1.5 g/kg over 12 h, single IV infusion • Cyclosporine—10–20 mg/kg/day IM or PO • Eicosapentaenoic acid • Plasmapheresis

FOLLOW-UP

PATIENT MONITORING
• Monitor heart rate, respiratory rate, and temperature frequently during hospitalization. • Monitor for adverse reactions to treatment (e.g., transfusion reactions and overhydration). • If pulmonary thromboembolism is suspected, monitor thoracic radiographs and arterial blood gases frequently. • During the first month of treatment, check the PCV weekly until stable and then every 2 weeks for 2 months; if still stable, recheck PCV monthly for 6 months and then 2–4 times per year; rechecks may need to be more frequent if patient is on long-term medication. • A CBC should be rechecked at least monthly during treatment, especially if cytotoxic drugs are used; if the neutrophil count falls < 3000 cells/mL, discontinue cytotoxic drugs until the count recovers; reinstitute at a lower dosage. • Reticulocyte count and Coombs tests can be monitored if the PCV is not rising as expected.

PREVENTION/AVOIDANCE
N/A

POSSIBLE COMPLICATIONS
• Pulmonary and multiorgan thromboembolism (up to 44% of all cases) • Portal vein thrombosis • DIC • Cardiac arrhythmias, centrilobular hepatic necrosis, and renal tubular necrosis secondary to hypoxia • Secondary infection and endocarditis

EXPECTED COURSE AND PROGNOSIS
• Peracute disease usually caused by autoagglutination or intravascular hemolysis • Acute disease usually caused by intravascular or extravascular hemolysis

• Chronic disease usually caused by extravascular hemolysis or cold-reacting antibodies • Hyperbilirubinemia >10 mg/dL and low reticulocyte count associated with a poor prognosis • Overall mortality 33.3% • Autoagglutination associated with up to 50% mortality • Peracute, fulminating hemolytic disease associated with up to 80% mortality • Warm-type IMHA has a guarded prognosis; of patients who survive hospitalization (up to 71%), long-term prognosis relatively good • Cold-type IMHA more resistant to immunosuppressive drugs than warm type • Response to treatment may take weeks to months; nonregenerative IMHA may have a more gradual onset than typical IMHA and may be slower to respond to treatment. • Hemolysis may recur despite previous or current therapy.

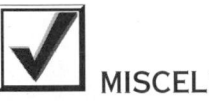

MISCELLANEOUS

ASSOCIATED CONDITIONS
• Evan's syndrome • SLE

PREGNANCY
Cytotoxic drugs should not be used in pregnant animals.

SYNONYMS
• Autoimmune hemolytic anemia • Immune-mediated anemia

SEE ALSO
• Anemia, Regenerative • Chapters on various causes of secondary IMHA • Cold Agglutinin Disease • Disseminated Intravascular Coagulation (DIC)

ABBREVIATIONS
• ALT = alanine aminotransferase • ANA = antinuclear antibody • APTT = activated partial thromboplastin time • DIC = disseminated intravascular coagulation • FeLV = feline leukemia virus • IMHA = immune-mediated hemolytic anemia • LE = lupus erythematosus • MCV = mean cell volume • PCV = packed cell volume • PT = prothrombin time • SLE = systemic lupus erythematosus

Suggested Reading

Bucheler J, Cotter S. Canine immune-mediated hemolytic anemia. In: Bonagura J, Kirk R, eds. Current veterinary therapy XII. Philadelphia: Saunders, 1995:152–157.
Carr A, Panciera D, Kidd L. Prognostic factors for mortality and thromboembolism in canine immune-mediated hemolytic anemia: a retrospective study of 72 dogs. J Vet Intern Med 2002;16:504–509.
Johnson L. Editorial: activation of the immune system and thrombosis. J Vet Intern Med 2002;16:501–503.
Author Cathryn Calia Schrope
Consulting Editor Stephen A. Kruth

ANEMIA, IRON-DEFICIENCY

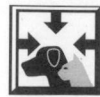 **BASICS**

OVERVIEW
- In adults, caused by hemorrhage
- Develops when erythrocytes are produced under the condition of limited iron availability
- Characteristic changes include erythrocyte microcytosis and hypochromic appearance caused by thin cell geometry.
- Important to recognize—leads clinician to the underlying disease problem, which is chronic external blood loss
- Most common site of related blood loss is the gastrointestinal tract.

SIGNALMENT
- Fairly common in adult dogs
- Rare in adult cats
- Transient, neonatal iron-deficiency anemia occurs at 5–10 weeks of age in about 50% of kittens.

SIGNS
- Signs of anemia (e.g., lethargy, depression, weakness, anorexia, and tachypnea) and underlying disease
- Intermittent melena with gastrointestinal blood loss
- Possible heavy blood-sucking parasite load (e.g., fleas and hookworms)

CAUSES & RISK FACTORS
- Any form of chronic external blood loss
- Blood loss most often occurs through the gastrointestinal tract.
- Common causes—lymphoma,* hookworm infestation,* stomach or intestinal neoplasia
- Less common sites—skin (e.g., flea infestation) and urinary tract
- Overuse of blood donors

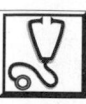 **DIAGNOSIS**

DIFFERENTIAL DIAGNOSIS
- Any cause of anemia, especially hemorrhage
- Specific features of the hemogram used to identify iron deficiency

CBC/BIOCHEMISTRY/URINALYSIS
- PCV usually low, generally 10–40% in dogs
- Anemia, either regenerative or nonregenerative
- Microcytosis—indicated by low normal or low MCV, often accompanied by high-volume heterogeneity, detected by erythrocyte histogram widening or high RBC distribution width value

- Changes in erythrocytes seen on the blood film—hypochromia (indicated by marked central pallor), oxidative lesions (e.g., keratocytes), fragmentation
- Thrombocytosis
- Hypoproteinemia—consistent finding if the blood loss is sustained; both albumin and globulin fractions are low normal or low

OTHER LABORATORY TESTS
- Hypoferremia (serum iron < 70 μg/dL) and low transferrin saturation (< 15%) support the diagnosis.
- Serum iron values may be normal, even in animals with hematologic features of iron deficiency, if blood loss has ceased and the animal is undergoing iron repletion.
- Fecal flotation to rule out hookworms
- Fecal examination for occult blood or gross melena to detect gastrointestinal bleeding

IMAGING
Radiographic or ultrasonographic studies—gastrointestinal disease that accounts for blood loss

DIAGNOSTIC PROCEDURES
- Complete hemogram and iron measurements as detailed above • Cytologic or histologic examination of bone marrow specimen stained with Prussian blue—reveals absence of iron particles (hemosiderin); indicated only when documentation of the diagnosis is difficult; best performed on a core biopsy specimen of marrow

 TREATMENT

- Identify and correct cause of chronic external blood loss.
- Administer iron until hematologic features of iron deficiency resolve.
- If unusually severe (i.e., PCV < 12%), transfusion may be required to treat life-threatening condition; administer whole blood (10–20 mL/kg IV) or packed red blood cells.

 **MEDICATIONS**

DRUG(S)

Iron Supplementation

Parenteral Iron Supplementation
- Iron replacement therapy should be initiated with injectable iron
- Iron dextran—a slowly released form of injectable iron; 1 injection (10–20 mg/kg IM) followed by oral supplementation

Oral Iron Supplementation
- Animals with severe iron deficiency have impaired intestinal absorption of iron, making oral supplementation of little value until partial iron repletion has occurred.
- Follow parenterally injected iron with oral iron supplementation for 1–2 months, or until features of iron deficiency have resolved.
- Kittens undergo spontaneous recovery and iron repletion beginning at 5–6 weeks of age, coinciding with intake of solid food.

Oral Iron Supplements
- Ferrous sulfate powder—place in food or drinking water (100–300 mg PO q24h)
- Ferrous gluconate—1 (325-mg) tablet PO q24h
- Iron and vitamins—Visorbin, liquid iron and multiple vitamin supplement (1 tsp PO q24h)

CONTRAINDICATIONS/POSSIBLE INTERACTIONS
Oral iron supplementation is associated with unexplained death in kittens and should be avoided.

 FOLLOW-UP

- Monitor CBC every 1–4 weeks; if the anemia is severe, monitor more frequently to follow the animal through recovery from a life-threatening illness. • Effectiveness of iron supplementation can be monitored less frequently. • Effective treatment associated with an increase in MCV
- Erythrocyte histogram—effective treatment associated with movement to the right as new, normal cells are produced; subpopulation of microcytes produced under conditions of iron deficiency slowly disappear, as these cells complete their survival time; may take a few months in some animals to establish a normal histogram

 MISCELLANEOUS

ABBREVIATIONS
- MCV = mean cell volume
- PCV = packed cell volume

Suggested Reading

Weiser MG. Erythrocyte responses and disorders. In: Ettinger SJ, Feldman EC, eds. Textbook of veterinary internal medicine. 4th. ed. Philadelphia: Saunders, 1995:1864–1891.

Author Glade Weiser

Consulting Editor Stephen A. Kruth

ANEMIA, METABOLIC (ANEMIAS WITH SPICULATED RED CELLS)

BASICS

OVERVIEW
- Sometimes occurs concomitantly with diffuse diseases of the liver and kidney
- In most animals with liver disease, spiculated cells have 2–10 elongated, blunt, finger-like projections from their surfaces and are classified as acanthocytes.
- Acanthocytic anemias can be associated with renal disease; anemias of renal disease more often have oval red cells with irregular or ruffled membranes (burr cells).
- Pathogenesis not entirely clear; abnormal lipid metabolism with free cholesterol loading of RBC membranes is most frequently implicated as cause.
- Dogs with disseminated abdominal hemangiosarcoma with liver involvement often have acanthocytes.

SIGNALMENT
Dogs and cats (infrequently)

SIGNS
- None in most animals (usually mild to moderate condition)
- Detection of spiculated RBCs on peripheral blood film can be first marker for liver or kidney disease.
- In large-breed dogs with vague signs or large spleen, suggests possibility of splenic or hepatic hemangiosarcoma

CAUSES & RISK FACTORS
- Any disease of the liver or kidneys
- The likelihood of RBC morphologic abnormalities parallels the severity of organ involvement.
- Hemangiosarcoma involving the liver is a frequent cause.
- Observed in cats with fatty liver syndrome

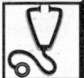

DIAGNOSIS

DIFFERENTIAL DIAGNOSIS
Determination of renal or hepatic causes based on results of biochemistry profile and urinalysis

CBC/BIOCHEMISTRY/URINALYSIS
- Mild to moderately low PCV, RBC count, and hemoglobin
- Normal mean corpuscular volume and mean corpuscular hemoglobin concentration in most animals
- Normocytic, normochromic, and nonregenerative
- Polychromasia on blood films only with accompanying blood loss (as with hepatic hemangiosarcoma)
- WBC changes variable, based on underlying cause of hepatic or renal pathology
- Inflammatory conditions likely to be accompanied by inflammatory leukogram
- Variable findings in liver and kidney function tests (serum biochemistry and urinalysis)

Hepatic Diseases
- High ALT, ALP, and γ-glutamyl transferase
- High bile acids, serum ammonia
- Possibly low albumin and serum urea nitrogen
- Bilirubinuria, bilirubin crystals in urine

Renal Diseases
- High serum urea nitrogen, creatinine, and phosphorus
- Highly variable urinalysis findings, including isosthenuria (urine specific gravity 1.008–1.025 in dogs; 1.008–1.035 in cats)
- Tubular and/or protein casts
- Pyuria
- Proteinuria
- Hematuria

OTHER LABORATORY TESTS
None

IMAGING
Abdominal radiographs and ultrasound—evaluate hepatic and renal structure

DIAGNOSTIC PROCEDURES
Liver or kidney biopsy if indicated

TREATMENT
Focus treatment on diagnosis and treatment of underlying hepatic or renal disease.

MEDICATIONS

DRUG(S)
Variable according to underlying cause

CONTRAINDICATIONS/POSSIBLE INTERACTIONS
Variable according to underlying cause

FOLLOW-UP
Monitor CBC periodically while treating the underlying condition.

MISCELLANEOUS

SEE ALSO
- Anemia of Chronic Renal Disease
- Hemangiosarcoma, spleen and liver

ABBREVIATIONS
- ALP = alkaline phosphatase
- ALT = alanine aminotransferase
- PCV = packed cell volume
- RBC = red blood cell
- WBC = white blood cell

Suggested Reading
Rebar AH. Hemogram interpretation for dogs and cats. Wilmington, DE: The Gloyd Group for Ralston Purina Co., 1998:22–23.
Rebar AH, Lewis HB, DeNicola DB, Halliwell WH, Boon GD. Red blood cell fragmentation in the dog: an editorial review. Vet Pathol 1981;18:415–426.
Weiser EG. Erythrocyte responses and disorders. In: Ettinger SJ, Feldman EC, eds. Textbook of veterinary internal medicine. 4th ed. Philadelphia: Saunders, 1995: 1864–1891.
Author Alan H. Rebar
Consulting Editor Stephen A. Kruth

ANEMIA, NONREGENERATIVE

 BASICS

DEFINITION
Low RBC mass without evidence of a regenerative response (increased polychromasia or reticulocytosis) in the peripheral blood

PATHOPHYSIOLOGY
• Key feature is low or inadequate erythroid production or release • Onset of anemia and its related signs insidious unless RBC survival is concurrently shortened (e.g., hemorrhage and hemolysis) • May be caused by selective alteration in erythropoiesis or generalized bone marrow injury affecting leukocytes and platelets as well • Mechanisms for selectively altered erythropoiesis include deficient hormonal stimulation, deficient or defective nutrition, cytokine-mediated sequestration of iron, and disturbed metabolism in or destruction of precursors; generalized bone marrow injury usually caused by a toxin, infection, or infiltrative process • These distinctions are not absolute; a cat with FeLV infection can have nonregenerative anemia alone, pancytopenia, or leukemia/erythroleukemia.

SYSTEMS AFFECTED
• Cardiovascular—heart murmur associated with low blood viscosity • Hepatobiliary—centrilobular degeneration associated with hypoxic injury

SIGNALMENT
• Varies with primary cause • Giant schnauzers, Border collies, beagles—congenital cobalamin malabsorption

SIGNS

General Comments
• Usually a secondary condition • Signs associated with the primary disease often precede signs directly attributable to the anemia.

Historical Findings
• Lack of energy, exercise intolerance, inappetence, and cold intolerance • Other findings reflect the primary condition, such as polyuria and polydipsia (e.g., chronic renal failure), exposure to paint from remodeling old houses (e.g., lead poisoning), living in multicat households (e.g., FeLV), and treating female dogs for mismating or urinary incontinence and feminization in male dogs (e.g., hyperestrogenism).

Physical Examination Findings
• Pallor, heart murmur (relatively severe anemia), and possibly tachycardia or polypnea • Signs reflecting the primary condition include uremic breath and oral ulcerations (e.g., chronic renal failure), cachexia (e.g., cancer), lymphadenopathy (e.g., lymphoma), gastrointestinal or CNS signs (e.g., lead poisoning), symmetrical alopecia (e.g., hypothyroidism and hyperestrogenism).

CAUSES

Nonregenerative Anemia without Other Cytopenias
• Chronic disease—the most common cause of mild nonregenerative anemia; anemia can be seen within 3 to 10 days of infection (e.g., gingivitis and abscess), inflammation (e.g., dermatologic disease), tissue injury (e.g., fractures), and disseminated neoplasia (e.g., lymphoma and carcinoma); release of IL-1 and TNF causes an acute-phase reaction; subsequent sequestration of iron within bone marrow macrophages, low serum iron and transferrin, and increased concentration of macrophage (and serum) ferritin cause impaired marrow response to anemia; RBC survival shortened • Chronic renal failure—kidneys fail to produce adequate amount of erythropoietin; uremic toxins shorten RBC lifespan and impair the response to erythropoietin. • Chronic liver disease—RBC morphologic changes (target cells and acanthocytes) and shortened RBC survival caused by changes in RBC membrane phospholipid and cholesterol content; mobilization of hepatic iron may be impaired. • Endocrine disease—thyroid hormones and cortisol stimulate erythropoiesis and facilitate the effect of erythropoietin; mild anemia is commonly associated with hypothyroidism and can occasionally be seen in patients with hypoadrenocorticism and hypopituitarism. • Immune-mediated destruction of precursors • Infectious destruction of precursors (although usually > 1 cell line is involved) e.g., FeLV and ehrlichiosis, cytauxzoon felis

Nutritional or Mineral Deficiency
• Iron deficiency—usually caused by chronic blood loss; initially regenerative, but as severity increases, hemoglobin concentration cannot be maintained and anemia becomes nonregenerative. • Cobalamin (vitamin B_{12}) and/or folate deficiency—rare in dogs and cats but can be caused by dietary insufficiency, malabsorption, or chronic drug administration (e.g., methotrexate, sulfas, and anticonvulsants) that inhibits folate; congenital defect in cobalamin absorption reported in giant schnauzers, Border collies and beagles • Disruption of precursor metabolism—chronic lead toxicity and possibly high concentrations of aluminum and cadmium inhibit heme synthesis; cadmium also reported to cause renal toxicity and impaired erythropoietin production

Nonregenerative Anemia with Other Cytopenias
• Toxicities—drugs or chemicals (e.g., cancer chemotherapeutics, chloramphenicol, phenylbutazone, trimethoprim-sulfadiazine, phenobarbital, griseofulvin, methimazole, and benzene), hormones (e.g., estrogen toxicity secondary to abortifacient therapy and Sertoli cell tumor) • Infections—FeLV, FIV, ehrlichiosis, Rocky Mountain spotted fever, and parvoviral infection (although recovery usually precedes development of anemia) • Infiltrative processes—myelodysplasia, myeloproliferative disease, lymphoproliferative disease, metastatic neoplasia, myelofibrosis, and osteosclerosis

RISK FACTORS
• Renal failure • Inflammatory disease • Liver failure • Sertoli cell tumor • Chronic disease process • Cancer • Chronic blood loss • Cats from multicat households (FeLV) • Lead exposure

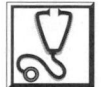 **DIAGNOSIS**

DIFFERENTIAL DIAGNOSIS
Sudden onset of signs more consistent with regenerative than nonregenerative anemia; however, the latter may appear to have an acute onset if associated with a sudden exacerbation of a chronic primary condition.

LABORATORY FINDINGS

Disorders That May Alter Laboratory Results
Factors causing turbidity (lipemia) can falsely elevate hemoglobin and MCHC values.

Valid If Run in Human Laboratory?
• Yes; however, electronic counters used for human RBCs may underestimate counts of small RBCs in most domestic animals other than dogs, which produces a falsely low RBC count and PCV. • A centrifuge is preferable for measuring PCV.

CBC/BIOCHEMISTRY/URINALYSIS

CBC and Blood Smear
• PCV, RBC count, and hemoglobin low • Anemia usually normocytic, normochromic, with normal MCV and MCHC • Macrocytosis (high MCV)—without polychromasia suggests a nuclear maturation defect (cells skip a division); seen in cats with FeLV; caused by vitamin B_{12} or folate deficiency; uncommon in domestic animals • Microcytosis (low MCV)—suggests a cytoplasmic maturation defect (cells undergo an extra division); iron deficiency the most common cause; in late stages, concurrent hypochromasia (low MCHC) common in dogs but not in cats; also seen in approximately one-third of patients with hepatic insufficiency or vascular shunting • Schistocytes commonly associated with iron deficiency • Acanthocytes associated with cholestatic liver disease • Target cells associated with iron deficiency, liver disase, and hypothyroidism • An inflammatory leukogram supports anemia associated with inflammatory disease. • Thrombocytosis often accompanies iron deficiency. • A high number of nucleated RBCs without polychromasia or disproportionate to the degree of anemia and polychromasia seen in animals with lead toxicity; extramedullary hematopoiesis, heat

stroke, and injury to bone marrow stroma by endotoxemia or hypoxia are other sources of circulating nucleated RBCs. • RBC or WBC precursors in the peripheral blood without orderly progression to more mature forms suggests myelodysplasia or myeloproliferative disease (leukemia). • Concurrent cytopenia in other cell lines without evidence of marrow responsiveness (e.g., band neutrophils and macroplatelets) suggests generalized bone marrow injury.

Serum Biochemistry and Urinalysis
• High BUN and creatinine with inadequate urine concentration (dogs, < 1.030; cats, < 1.035) support anemia of renal failure. • High ALT, bilirubinemia, and bilirubinuria suggest liver disease. • High serum cholesterol (> 500 mg/dL) strongly suggests hypo-thyroidism. • Hyponatremia with concurrent hyperkalemia, lymphopenia, and eosinopenia in ill dogs suggests hypoadrenocorticism.

OTHER LABORATORY TESTS
• Reticulocyte count—value of < 60,000/μL in dogs or < 50,000/μL in cats accompanied by a low PCV confirms nonregenerative anemia. • Because it takes the bone marrow 3–5 days to increase erythropoiesis in response to an acute demand, patients in the early stage of acute hemorrhage or hemolysis may appear to be affected with the disease. • Direct anti-globulin test (Coombs')—immune-mediated destruction of erythroid precursors can lead to anemia without reticulocytosis; spherocytosis or autoagglutination may suggest immune-medi-ated hemolytic anemia; positive Coombs' test with species-specific reagents provides support for immune-mediated anemia. • Serum iron profile—indicated for patients with microcytic anemia; in dogs, evaluation of iron stores in a bone marrow aspirate should precede iron assay; iron stores are not readily apparent in normal feline bone marrow; in patients with iron deficiency, serum iron is low, total iron-binding capacity varies, and serum ferritin is low; in patients with anemia associated with inflammatory disease, serum iron is low but serum ferritin is high (MCV and MCHC usually normal). • Bile acids measurement—may be indicated for evaluation of microcytic anemia and confirmation of hepatic insufficiency or vascular shunting • Serum lead measurement—indicated when nucleated red cells are present, especially when the patient has concurrent gastrointestinal or CNS signs; a value > 30 μL/dL (0.3 ppm) strongly supports lead intoxication. • Serologic testing—FeLV test in any cat with nonregenerative anemia; *Ehrlichia canis* and Rocky Mountain spotted fever titers indicated in dogs with unexplained anemia, especially when concurrent with other cytopenias or hyperglobulinemia • Endocrine testing—indicated when clinical signs and laboratory tests suggest a possible endocrine disorder; thyroid: T_4, free T_4, and TSH concentrations and adrenal: low-dose

dexamethasone suppression test, and ACTH-stimulation test

DIAGNOSTIC PROCEDURES
Cytologic Examination of Bone Marrow and Core Biopsy
• Cytologic examination of an aspirate indi-cated in all patients, unless the primary cause is readily apparent (e.g., anemia of inflammatory disease and chronic renal failure) • Erythroid hypoplasia or aplasia confirms the disease. • Myeloid hyperplasia and high iron stores support anemia associated with inflammatory disease. • Absence of canine bone marrow iron stores, which occurs before microcytosis, supports iron deficiency; classically, iron deficiency associated with an expanded erythron and high numbers of metarubricytes • Increased erythrophagocytosis suggests injury to cells (e.g., immune-mediated and toxic disease). • An incomplete maturation sequence suggests injury to a specific maturation stage (e.g., immune-mediated and toxic causes) or possibly incomplete recovery from a previous injury (recheck in 3–5 days). • A disorderly maturation sequence and atypical cellular morphology suggest myelodysplastic syn-drome. • High number of blast cells (> 30% of nucleated cells) indicates hematopoietic neoplasia; morphologic examination of cells, immunophenotyping, and cytochemical stains used to identify the affected cell line(s); circulating neoplastic cells may or may not be seen. • Nonmarrow cells indicate metastatic neoplasia. • If specimens are hypocellular, core biopsy should be done to evaluate bone marrow cellularity and to look for conditions such as myelofibrosis.

TREATMENT
• Nonregenerative anemia usually resolves with resolution of the underlying disease. • Condi-tions associated with severe anemia or pancyto-penia often carry a guarded-to-poor prognosis and may involve long-term treatment without complete resolution. • Metabolic compensation occurs with slowly developing nonregenerative anemia; thus mild to moderately severe anemia (PCV > 15%) generally requires no supportive intervention; for patients with severe anemia (PCV < 10–15%), the degree of hypoxia will probably require restricted exercise, transfu-sions, or both. • If blood volume and tissue perfusion are compromised by concurrent blood loss or shock, administer lactated Ringer's solution or colloids.

MEDICATIONS
DRUG(S)
• Erythropoietin in patients with anemia of chronic renal failure (see Anemia of Chronic

Renal Disease) • Iron supplementation in patients with iron deficiency anemia (see Anemia, Iron-Deficiency) • May supplement with folic acid at a rate of 4–10 mg/kg/day. • May supplement with cobalamin (vitamin B_{12}) at a rate of 100–200 mg/day PO (dogs) or 50–100 mg/day PO (cats); parenteral administration (0.5–1 mg IM weekly to once every few months) needed in giant schnauzers, beagles, or Border collies with inherited cobalamin malabsorption

PRECAUTIONS
Monitor for transfusion reactions in patients receiving multiple transfusions.

FOLLOW-UP
PATIENT MONITORING
• In patients with severe anemia, PCV and blood smear examination every 1–2 days
• In stabilized animals with chronic or slowly improving disease course, re-evaluation every 1–2 weeks

POSSIBLE COMPLICATIONS
N/A

MISCELLANEOUS
PREGNANCY
A mildly low PCV caused by dilution of RBC mass by a high blood volume may be seen in some pregnant animals.

SYNONYMS
Nonresponsive anemia

SEE ALSO
See Causes

ABBREVIATIONS
• ALT = alanine aminotransferase
• FeLV = feline leukemia virus
• FIV = feline immunodeficiency virus
• IL-1 = interleukin-1
• MCHC = mean corpuscular hemoglobin concentration
• MCV = mean cell volume
• PCV = packed cell volume
• TNF = tumor necrosis factor
• TSH = thyroid-stimulating hormone

Suggested Reading
Rogers K. Anemia. In: Ettinger SJ, Feldman EC, eds. Textbook of veterinary internal med-icine: diseases of the dog and cat. Vol. 1. 4th ed. Philadelphia: Saunders, 1995:187–191.
Author Joyce S. Knoll
Consulting Editor Stephen A. Kruth

ANEMIA, NUCLEAR MATURATION DEFECTS (ANEMIA, MEGALOBLASTIC)

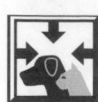

BASICS

OVERVIEW
• Nonregenerative anemia characterized by arrested development of the nuclei of RBC precursors (as a result of interference with DNA synthesis) while the cytoplasm develops normally (nuclear-cytoplasmic asynchrony)
• Affected RBC precursors fail to divide normally and thus are larger than corresponding normal precursors with the same degree of cytoplasmic maturity (hemoglobinization); because their nuclei are deficient in chromatin (DNA), they have a distinctive open and stippled appearance; these giant precursors with atypical, immature nuclei are known as megaloblasts.
• Although these asynchronous changes are most prominent in RBC precursors, WBC and platelet precursors are similarly affected.

SIGNALMENT
• Dogs and cats
• Spontaneous, clinically unimportant occurrence in toy poodles (occasional)
• Breed predilection: Giant schnauzers with inherited cobalamin malabsorption
• Defect usually acquired

SIGNS
• Generally mild, usually not clinically important
• In cats with FeLV-associated nuclear maturation anemia, FeLV-related signs can be anticipated.

CAUSES & RISK FACTORS
• Infectious—FeLV; retroviral infection the most common cause of megaloblastic anemia in cats
• Nutritional—folic acid and vitamin B_{12} deficiencies
• Toxic—phenytoin (Dilantin) toxicity and methotrexate toxicity (folate antagonist)
• Congenital—toy poodles

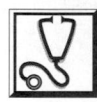

DIAGNOSIS

DIFFERENTIAL DIAGNOSIS
• All other mild to moderate nonregenerative anemias, including anemia of inflammatory disease, renal disease, and lead poisoning
• Differentiation based on the distinctive CBC and bone marrow findings listed

CBC/BIOCHEMISTRY/URINALYSIS
• Mild to moderate anemia (PCV: in dogs, 30–40%; in cats, 25–38%)
• Anemia classically macrocytic (high mean corpuscular volume) and normochromic (normal mean corpuscular hemoglobin concentration)
• Large, fully hemoglobinized RBC; occasional to numerous megaloblasts, particularly at the feather edge; minimal to no polychromasia
• Mild panleukopenia (common)
• Mild thrombocytopenia (common)
• In cats with FeLV, anemia may occur in association with a myelodysplastic syndrome or in conjunction with leukemia of a different cell line.

OTHER LABORATORY TESTS
FeLV

IMAGING
N/A

OTHER DIAGNOSTIC PROCEDURES

Bone Marrow Biopsy
• Hyperplastic, often in all cell lines
• Maturation arrest with nuclear and cytoplasmic asynchrony in all cell lines
• Many megaloblastic RBC precursors may be observed.
• Macrophagic hyperplasia with active phagocytosis of nucleated RBCs and megaloblasts (common)

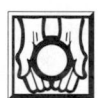

TREATMENT
• Treat by targeting the underlying cause, if possible.
• Except for that occurring with FeLV in cats, megaloblastic anemia is a relatively mild condition.
• Treat most patients on an outpatient basis.

MEDICATIONS

DRUG(S)
• In animals with drug toxicity, discontinue the offending drug.
• In all animals, consider supplementation with folic acid (4–10 mg/kg/day) or vitamin B_{12} (dogs, 100–200 mg/day PO; cats, 50–100 mg/day PO).
• Giant schnauzers with inherited cobalamin malabsorption require parenteral treatment with vitamin B_{12} (0.5–1.0 mg IM weekly to every few months).

CONTRAINDICATIONS/POSSIBLE INTERACTIONS
Drugs known to cause megaloblastic anemia (e.g., methotrexate and phenytoin) should be avoided in patients whose condition results from other causes.

FOLLOW-UP
• Monitor response to treatment by CBC (weekly) and occasional bone marrow collection and evaluation.
• Closely monitor FeLV-positive cats for evidence of onset of other signs of hematopoietic dyscrasia in the peripheral blood and bone marrow.
• Prognosis—depends on underlying cause; in FeLV-positive cats, prognosis guarded; in animals with drug-associated anemia, prognosis good when use of offending drug is interrupted

MISCELLANEOUS

SEE ALSO
• Anemia, Nonregenerative
• Feline Leukemia Virus Infection

ABBREVIATIONS
• DNA = deoxyribonucleic acid
• FeLV = feline leukemia virus
• PCV = packed cell volume
• RBC = red blood cell
• WBC = white blood cell

Suggested Reading
Rebar, AH. Hemogram interpretation for dogs and cats. Wilmington, DE: The Gloyd Group for Ralston Purina Co., 1998:23.
Rebar AH, MacWilliams PS, Feldman BF, et al: Guide to hematology in dogs and cats. Jackson, WY: Teton New Media, 2002:57–58.
Weiser MG. Erythrocyte responses and disorders. In: Ettinger SJ, Feldman EC, eds. Textbook of veterinary internal medicine. Philadelphia: Saunders, 1995:1864–1891.
Author Alan H. Rebar
Consulting Editor Stephen A. Kruth

BASICS

DEFINITION
Low PCV, RBC count, and hemoglobin and hypoplasia of erythroid elements of the bone marrow are associated with progressive or end-stage renal failure. Anemia is normocytic, normochromic, nonregenerative, and proportional to the severity of the renal insufficiency. Principal cause is bone marrow failure secondary to inadequate production of erythropoietin by the kidneys. Shortened RBC life span, uremic inhibitors of erythropoiesis, blood loss, nutritional deficiencies, and marrow fibrosis may contribute.

SIGNALMENT
Middle-aged to old dogs and cats mostly affected; seen in young animals with heritable, congenital, or acquired chronic renal failure

SIGNS
• Anemia contributes to development of anorexia, weight loss, fatigue, lethargy, depression, weakness, apathy, cold intolerance, and behavior and personality changes characterizing chronic renal failure. • Syncope and seizures (rare) • Pallor of the mucous membranes • Tachycardia • Systolic murmur

CAUSES & RISK FACTORS
• Inherited, congenital, and acquired forms of chronic renal failure (e.g., pyelonephritis, glomerulonephritis, amyloidosis, polycystic kidney disease, and lymphoma) • Exacerbated by iron deficiency, inflammatory or neoplastic disease, gastrointestinal blood loss, hemolysis, and myeloproliferative disorder

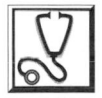

DIAGNOSIS

DIFFERENTIAL DIAGNOSIS
• Anemia of chronic infectious, inflammatory, or neoplastic disease; myeloproliferative disease; chronic blood loss; aplastic anemia; endocrine disease; drug reaction; and chronic immune-mediated toxic, viral, rickettsial, or parasitic anemia • Regenerative anemia excludes diagnosis of anemia of chronic renal failure.

CBC/BIOCHEMISTRY/URINALYSIS
• Normocytic, normochromic, nonregenerative anemia (anemia may be masked by dehydration) • Reticulocytes—low corrected indices and absolute counts • High BUN, creatinine, and phosphorus; variably high calcium; variably low bicarbonate and potassium • High BUN:creatinine ratio may predict concurrent gastrointestinal blood loss. • Impaired urine-concentrating ability, mild to moderate proteinuria, and variably active sediment

OTHER LABORATORY TESTS
• Serum iron—normal or variably low (≤60 mg/dL) • Transferrin saturation—normal or variably low (<20%) • FeLV and FIV testing (cats) or rickettsial titers or PCR (dogs) to exclude agent-induced myelodyscrasia • Serum erythropoietin—normal (inappropriately) or low

IMAGING
Small, irregular kidneys with loss or disruption of renal architecture on radiographs or ultrasound

DIAGNOSTIC PROCEDURES
Cytologic examination of bone marrow—erythroid hypoplasia; myeloid:erythroid ratio normal or high; stainable iron normal or variably low

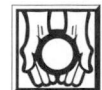

TREATMENT

• Increase RBC mass if patient is symptomatic for anemia (dogs, PCV ≤25%; cats, PCV ≤20). • Stabilize azotemia in patients in uremic crisis. • Establish appropriate nitrogen, caloric, vitamin, and iron intake to reduce uremic inhibitors and bleeding tendency and lengthen life span of RBCs. • Ensure that iron is not deficient. • Correct gastrointestinal ulceration and blood loss by administrating famotidine, ranitidine, omeprazole, or sucralfate. • Correct systemic hypertension.

MEDICATIONS

DRUG(S) AND FLUIDS

Erythropoietin Replacement
• r-HuEPO—a replica of human erythropoietin available as epoetin alfa (Epogen and Procrit); provides consistent, rapid, and long-term correction of anemia in dogs and cats with chronic renal failure • Darbepoetin alfa (Aranesp), a new erythropoiesis-stimulating protein with sustained effects, is available for human patients but has not been evaluated for safety and efficacy in dogs or cats. Species-specific erythropoietins are under development for clinical use in the dog and cat. • Target PCV—dogs, 37–45%; cats, 30–40% • Initial dosage—50–100 U/kg SC thrice weekly until PCV reaches 37% in dogs or 30% in cats (2–8 weeks), then decrease to twice weekly • Maintenance dosage—50–100 U/kg SC once or twice weekly to maintain target PCV; individualize to each patient; life-long treatment required • If PCV exceeds target, discontinue until upper target range is achieved, then decrease previous dosage by 25–50% or increase dosage interval. • Serum iron and transferrin saturation should be normalized before initiating and during r-HuEPO administration. Give ferrous sulfate (dogs, 100–300 mg PO q24h; cats, 50–100 mg PO q24h) if deficiencies are documented. Injectable iron may be required if oral preparations are poorly tolerated or ineffective.

Blood Transfusion
• Short-term or rapid correction (PCV ≤ 20%)—give compatible whole blood or packed RBCs. • Target PCV is 25–30%. • May be given intermittently for prolonged management

Anabolic Steroids
Little or no efficacy or indication for use

FOLLOW-UP

PATIENT MONITORING
• PCV—weekly–semimonthly for 3 months, then monthly to bimonthly • Blood pressure—semimonthly to monthly • Iron and transferrin saturation—at 1, 3, and 6 months, then semiannually • Discontinue erythropoietin if patient develops evidence of polycythemia, local or systemic sensitivity, anti-r-HuEPO antibody formation, or refractory hypertension.

POSSIBLE COMPLICATIONS

Erythropoietin–related
• Development of polycythemia, seizures, hypertension, iron depletion, injection pain, and mucocutaneous reactions • Development of a pure red cell asplasia during the course of r-HuEPO treatment suggests formation of anti-r-HuEPO antibodies, which neutralize r-HuEPO and native erythropoietin, causing severe anemia in 20–30% of animals; reversible with cessation of treatment • Signs associated with production of anti-r-HuEPO antibodies while the patient is receiving erythropoietin include decreasing PCV, erythroid hypoplasia, absolute reticulocyte counts approaching zero, and myeloid:erythroid ratio ≥8. • Use r-HuEPO cautiously or withhold if hypertension or iron deficiency develops; treatment can be reinstituted once hypertension and iron deficiency are corrected.

Transfusion–related
• Incompatibility reaction • Circulatory or iron overload • Transmissible infection

EXPECTED COURSE AND PROGNOSIS
• Disease correction increases appetite, activity, grooming, affection and playfulness, weight gain, and cold tolerance, and decreases sleeping. • Use of r-HuEPO in dogs and cats requires careful assessment of the risks and benefits for individual patients. • Short-term prognosis depends on the severity of the renal failure. Long-term prognosis is guarded to poor because of the underlying chronic renal failure.

MISCELLANEOUS

ABBREVIATIONS
• FeLV = feline leukemia virus • FIV = feline immunodeficiency virus • r-HuEPO = recombinant human erythropoietin

Suggested Reading
Cowgill LD, et al. Use of recombinant human erythropoietin for management of anemia in dogs and cats with renal failure. J Am Vet Med Assoc 1998;212:521–528.
Author Larry D. Cowgill
Consulting Editors Larry G. Adams and Carl A. Osborne

ANEMIA, REGENERATIVE

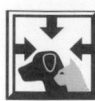 BASICS

DEFINITION
• Characterized by a low circulating RBC mass (as indicated by low PCV, hemoglobin, and total RBC count) accompanied by appropriate, compensatory increase in RBC production by the bone marrow (e.g., reticulocytosis in the peripheral blood and RBC hyperplasia in the bone marrow)
• Regenerative response may not be evident until several days after the onset of anemia.

PATHOPHYSIOLOGY
• Regenerative anemia caused by blood loss or hemolysis • In patients with blood loss anemia, circulating RBC lifespan is normal and RBCs are lost from the body as a result of vascular injury; in patients with hemolytic anemia, vessels are intact but there is excessive intravascular or extravascular destruction of RBCs with shortened circulating RBC life span. • Hemolysis—caused by erythrocyte membrane abnormalities, physical damage, oxidative injury, release of hemolysins, osmotic changes, immune-mediated RBC destruction, and congenital RBC abnormalities
• Intravascular hemolysis may lead to DIC and hemoglobinuria. • Hemolytic anemia usually more regenerative than blood loss anemia; blood loss depletes body of both cells and iron; hemolysis conserves iron, which is readily available for reuse in RBC production; availability of iron makes hemolytic anemia generally more responsive.

SYSTEMS AFFECTED
• Hemic/lymph/immune—marked RBC hyperplasia in the bone marrow; spleno-megaly also can be a feature of extravascular hemolytic anemia. • Cardiovascular—murmurs with marked anemia; tachycardia with severe rapid-onset anemia • Hepatic—anoxia causes centrilobular degeneration of the liver; hemolysis may cause icterus.

SIGNALMENT
• No breed, age, or sex predilections for the broad category of regenerative anemia
• Congenital pyruvate kinase deficiency—basenjis, beagles, West Highland white terriers, Cairn terriers, and Abyssinian cats
• Phosphofructokinase deficiency—English springer spaniels and American cocker spaniels
• Hereditary nonspherocytic hemolytic anemia in some poodles and beagles • Feline congenital porphyria—Siamese and domestic shorthair cats • An uncharacterized hereditary RBC defect described in Abyssinian and Somali cats
• Some breeds of dogs have a genetic predisposition for certain heritable coagulopathies such as factor VIII deficiency and von Willebrand disease. • Middle-aged female dogs, especially German shepherds,

collies, Shetland sheepdogs, and English cocker spaniels, have a predisposition to immune-mediated syndromes, such as immune-mediated hemolytic anemia and SLE.

SIGNS
• Pallor • Weakness • Exercise intolerance
• Anorexia • Possible heart murmur, tachycardia, and jaundice • Clinical signs depend on the degree of anemia and rapidity of onset • Rapid loss of 50–60% of the blood volume or acute hemolysis results in shock and possible death • In patients with chronic anemia, compensatory increases in heart rate, and eventually heart size, lessens the RBC circulation time; hemoglobin can drop to as low as 50% of the minimum normal value without overt signs of hypoxia.

CAUSES

Immune Mediated
• Antibodies and/or complement on the RBC surface shorten RBC lifespan. • Antibodies may target RBC membrane antigens or antibodies may be directed against tumor antigens, infectious agents, or drugs (e.g., trimethoprim-sulfadiazine, penicillins, and methimazole) adherent to RBC surface.
• Hemolysis—depending on the antibody type, may be either intravascular or extra-vascular; may be caused by vaccination or transfusion of incompatible blood. • Neonatal isoerythrolysis seen in kittens born to a blood type B queen mated to a blood type A tom.

Oxidant Injury
• Exposure to oxidants can cause Heinz body formation (aggregates of oxidized hemo-globin), eccentrocytes (oxidative injury to RBC membranes), and methemoglobinemia.
• Changes in RBC morphology results in premature removal of these cells from the circulation (extravascular hemolysis).
• Oxidation and destabilization of membrane lipids causes intravascular hemolysis.
• Oxidants include onions (especially in dogs), acetaminophen (especially in cats), zinc toxicity (from pennies minted after 1982, zinc oxide ointment, and zinc bolts), benzo-caine, vitamin K_3 (dogs), DL-methionine (cats), phenolic compounds (moth balls), and phenazopyridine (cats) • In cats, some systemic diseases (e.g, diabetes mellitus, hyperthyroidism, and lymphoma) enhance Heinz body formation.

Erythrocyte Parasites
• *Haemobartonella felis* (cats); *H. canis* (rare cause of anemia in dogs) • *Babesia canis* and *B. gibsoni* (dogs)

Mechanical RBC Fragmentation
• DIC • Heartworm disease • Cardiac disease
• Liver disease • Vasculitis • Neoplasia (e.g. hemangiosarcoma) • Splenic torsion • Hemo-lytic-uremic syndrome • Renal disease

Inherited RBC Abnormalities
• Pyruvate kinase deficiency—causes impaired erythrocyte glucose use and ATP formation, leading to premature destruction of RBCs.
• Phosphofructokinase deficiency—causes marked alkaline fragility caused by impaired synthesis of 2,3-diphosphoglycerate; hemolytic episodes triggered by hyperventilation-induced alkalemia such as occurs after vigorous exercise
• Hereditary nonspherocytic hemolytic anemia—resembles pyruvate kinase deficiency, but the RBCs have normal glycolytic enzyme activities and the basic defect is undetermined; in poodles, an autosomal dominant mode of inheritance has been described. • Feline congenital porphyria—deficiency in uroporphyrinogen III cosynthetase causes an inability to produce normal amounts of hemoglobin; coproporphyrin and uropor-phyrin accumulate, causing brown-red discoloration of teeth and bones; autosomal dominant trait.

Blood Loss
• Trauma • Bleeding neoplasms (e.g., heman-giosarcoma and intestinal adenocarcinoma or leiomyoma) • Coagulopathies (e.g., warfarin poisoning, hemophilia, and thrombocy-topenia) • Blood sucking parasites (e.g., fleas, ticks, and *Ancylostoma*) • Gastrointestinal ulcers

RISK FACTORS
N/A

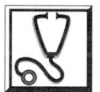 DIAGNOSIS

DIFFERENTIAL DIAGNOSIS
Differentiated from nonregenerative anemia by high reticulocyte count

LABORATORY FINDINGS

Drugs That May Alter Laboratory Results
None

Disorders That May Alter Laboratory Results
Lipemia in the sample can cause in vitro hemolysis, resulting in a falsely low PCV and total RBC count and falsely high MCHC.

Valid If Run in Human Laboratory?
• Dogs, yes • Cats, yes if lab's hematology instrument uses species-specific parameters
• Automated instruments designed strictly for analysis of human specimens may fail to accurately count the small RBCs in cats; reticulocyte counts should be performed manually. • Human labs may be unfamiliar with the punctuate reticulocytes found in cats and may include them in the reticulocyte count, thereby overestimating the regenerative response. • Human labs may be unfamiliar with important RBC parasites such as *Haemobartonella*.

CBC/BIOCHEMISTRY/URINALYSIS
• PCV, RBC count, and hemoglobin low
• RBC indices vary depending on the cause of anemia and degree of regenerative response: MCV, normal to high; MCHC normal to low in most patients
• In patients with intravascular hemolytic anemia with hemoglobinemia, MCHC artifactually may be high.
• Dogs with iron deficiency owing to chronic blood loss may have a low MCV, MCH, and MCHC.
• Cats with iron deficiency often have a low MCV but normal MCH and MCHC.
• Anisocytosis and expanded RBC distribution width associated with increased polychromasia
• In patients with hemolytic anemia, specific morphologic RBC changes suggest cause: marked spherocytosis suggests immune-mediated disease; Heinz bodies suggest oxidant injury; and numerous schistocytes suggest microangiopathy.
• Spherocytes cannot be readily detected in cats because of smallness and lack of central pallor of RBCs.
• Agglutinated RBCs indicate anemia is immune-mediated; autoagglutination must be distinguished from rouleaux by sample dilution with saline.
• Hemolysis may cause neutrophilia with a left shift and monocytosis. Blood loss may be accompanied by either thrombocytopenia or rebound thrombocytosis; iron deficiency is often accompanied by thrombocytosis.
• Total protein normal in patients with hemolytic anemia; may be low in those with blood loss anemia
• Hyperbilirubinemia and bilirubinuria accompany marked hemolysis; hemoglobinemia and hemoglobinuria seen if hemolysis is intravascular

OTHER LABORATORY TESTS
• In an anemic animal, an absolute reticulocyte count (RBC count × reticulocyte %) > 50,000/μL (cats) or > 60,000/μL (dogs) suggests regenerative anemia
• Formula for calculating a corrected reticulocyte count—reticulocyte % × (PCV/normal PCV) (normal PCV: 45, dog; 37, cat); corrected reticulocyte count > 1% suggests a regenerative response.
• If reticulocyte count is low in a patient with suspected regenerative anemia, it may mean that the anemia is in the early stages of response; it takes 3–5 days for the bone marrow to mount a peak regenerative response to anemia.
• Direct antiglobulin test (e.g., DAT and Coombs test) indicated when immune-mediated hemolytic anemia suspected; a

positive test with species-specific reagents and evidence of spherocytosis and polychromasia in the peripheral blood is confirmatory; both false-negatives and false-positives are possible, so the test must be used judiciously and interpreted cautiously.

IMAGING
N/A

DIAGNOSTIC PROCEDURES
• Bone marrow aspirate—cytologic examination of bone marrow reveals RBC hyperplasia; needed only when there is no evidence of RBC responsiveness in the peripheral blood (i.e., no polychromasia and no reticulocytosis); absence of RBC hyperplasia means that the anemia is nonregenerative.
• Bone marrow biopsy—useful in evaluation of bone marrow architecture and overall cellularity; important for confirmation of a nonregenerative process.

 ## TREATMENT
• Emergency if anemia is severe and develops rapidly
• Massive hemorrhage leads to hypovolemic shock and anoxia; acute hemolysis leads to anoxia and systemic toxemia
• Cage rest and careful observation indicated, depending on severity of clinical signs

Blood Loss Anemias
• Fluids to correct hypovolemia may be indicated in animals with acute traumatic blood loss anemia.
• If signs of hypoxia severe (i.e., extremely pale mucous membranes, weakness, tachycardia, and tachypnea), RBC replacement (volume depends on PCV of donor and patient) or oxyhemoglobin (30 mL/kg at rate of 10 mL/kg/hr) indicated

Hemolytic Anemias
• Blood transfusion, packed RBCs, or oxyhemoglobin may be indicated; in patients with an immune-mediated process, RBCs probably survive similarly to the patient's own RBCs, so transfusion should not be withheld if marked signs of anemia are present.

 ## MEDICATIONS

DRUG(S)
• Blood-loss anemias—administration of iron may be of benefit in animals with chronic blood-loss anemia (see Anemia, Iron-Deficiency)
• Hemolytic anemias—varies with cause of hemolysis

 ## FOLLOW-UP

PATIENT MONITORING
• Measurements of RBC mass (e.g., PCV, RBC count, and hemoglobin) and morphologic evaluation of peripheral blood film to monitor effectiveness of treatment and bone marrow responsiveness • Initially, patients should be checked every 24 hr; as regeneration becomes apparent (indicated by rising RBC values and polychromasia), patients should be checked every 3–5 days; return to normal values should occur about 14 days after acute hemorrhage but may take longer with an immune-mediated process.

POSSIBLE COMPLICATIONS
N/A

 ## MISCELLANEOUS

SYNONYMS
Responsive anemias

SEE ALSO
• Acetaminophen Toxicity • Anemia, Heinz Body • Anemia, Immune-Mediated • Anemia, Iron-Deficiency • Babesiosis • Disseminated Intravascular Coagulation (DIC) • Haemobartonellosis • Lupus Erythematosus, Systemic (SLE) • Rodenticide Anticoagulant Toxicity • Zinc Toxicity

ABBREVIATIONS
• DAT = direct antiglobulin (Coombs') test
• DIC = disseminated intravascular coagulation • MCHC = mean corpuscular hemoglobin concentration • MCV = mean cell volume • PCV = packed cell volume • SLE = systemic lupus erythematosus

Suggested Reading
Jain NC. Essentials of veterinary hematology. Philadelphia: Lea & Febiger, 1993.
Weiser MG. Erythrocyte responses and disorders. In: Ettinger SJ, Feldman EC, eds. Textbook of veterinary internal medicine. Diseases of the dog and cat. 4th ed. Philadelphia: Saunders, 1995:1876–1886.
Author Joyce S. Knoll
Consulting Editor Stephen A. Kruth

ANISOCORIA

BASICS

DEFINITION
Inequality of pupil size

PATHOPHYSIOLOGY
• Interruption of sympathetic or parasympathetic innervation of the pupil—causes altered pupil size • Ocular disease

SYSTEMS AFFECTED
• Nervous • Ophthalmic

SIGNALMENT
Dogs and cats

SIGNS N/A

CAUSES

Neurologic
• See Table 1 • Disease affecting optic nerve, optic tract, oculomotor nerve, or cerebellum

Ocular
• See Table 2 • Anterior uveitis • Glaucoma • Iris atrophy or hypoplasia • Posterior synechia • Pharmacologic blockade • Neoplasia • Spastic pupil syndrome

RISK FACTORS N/A

DIAGNOSIS

DIFFERENTIAL DIAGNOSIS
• Must determine which pupil is abnormal— see Algorithm 1. • Distinguish between neurologic and ocular causes.

CBC/BIOCHEMISTRY/URINALYSIS N/A

OTHER LABORATORY TESTS N/A

IMAGING
• See Table 1 • Ultrasound—identifying ocular and retrobulbar lesions • CT and MRI—localizing and identifying CNS lesions

DIAGNOSTIC PROCEDURES
• See Table 1 • CSF tap—evaluate CNS disease • ERG—evaluate retinal function • VEP— evaluate optic nerve function • Pharmacologic testing—see Algorithm 1; postganglionic lesions cause denervation supersensitivity; direct-acting (para)sympathomimetic drugs cause the pupil to constrict or dilate. • Preganglionic lesions—respond to indirect-acting (para)sympathomimetics

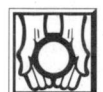

TREATMENT
Depends on underlying disease

MEDICATIONS

DRUG(S) OF CHOICE
Depend on underlying disease

CONTRAINDICATIONS N/A

PRECAUTIONS N/A

POSSIBLE INTERACTIONS N/A

ALTERNATIVE DRUG(S) N/A

FOLLOW-UP

PATIENT MONITORING N/A

POSSIBLE COMPLICATIONS N/A

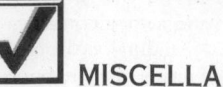

MISCELLANEOUS

ASSOCIATED CONDITIONS N/A

AGE-RELATED FACTORS N/A

ZOONOTIC POTENTIAL N/A

PREGNANCY N/A

SYNONYMS N/A

SEE ALSO
• Anterior Uveitis—Cats • Anterior Uveitis— Dogs • Glaucoma • Horner's Syndrome • Iris atrophy • Optic Neuritis

ABBREVIATIONS
• CSF = cerebrospinal fluid • ERG = electroretinogram • FeLV = feline leukemia virus • PLR = pupillary light reflex • VEP = visual-evoked potential

Suggested Reading
Neer TM, Carter JD. Anisocoria in dogs and cats. Ocular and neurologic causes. Compend Contin Educ Pract Vet 1987; 9:817–824.

Scagliotti RH, Neuro-ophthalmology. In: Birchard SJ, Sherding RG, eds. Saunders manual of small animal practice. Philadelphia: Saunders, 1994:1242–1248.

Author David Lipsitz
Consulting Editor Paul E. Miller

Table 1.

Neurologic Lesions Causing Anisocoria			
Lesion	Neurologic Signs	Differential Diagnosis	Diagnostic Plan
Optic nerve	Ipsilateral mydriasis Ipsilateral monocular anopia (total blindness in one eye) No direct PLR affected eye Consensual PLR affected eye	Optic neuritis Neoplasm	CT/MRI CSF Electroretinogram (ERG)
Optic tract	Contralateral blindness in nasal/temporal visual fields Ipsilateral pupil smaller in light Other neurologic deficits	Neoplasm Infectious/inflammatory disease Trauma	CT/MRI CSF
Oculomotor nerve Parasympathetic nucleus CN III	Ipsilateral dilated pupil Normal vision/no direct PLR No consensual PLR from opposite eye Ptosis upper eyelid Ventrolateral strabismus	Neoplasm Infectious/inflammatory disease Trauma Brain herniation Retrobulbar mass	CT/MRI CSF Ultrasound orbit
Cerebellar disease	Contralateral mydriasis Normal PLR/normal vision Ipsilateral lack of menace response Other cerebellar signs	Neoplasm Infectious/inflammatory disease Trauma	CT/MRI CSF

Table 2.

Ocular Diseases Causing Anisocoria

Lesion	Associated Signs	Causes
Anterior uveitis	Miosis, aqueous flare, Corneal edema, Conjunctival hyperemia	Infectious/inflammatory disease, Trauma, neoplasia
Glaucoma	Mydriasis, Sluggish/absent PLR, Increased intraocular pressure, Corneal edema	Primary glaucoma, Secondary glaucoma
Neoplasm	Miosis/mydriasis, Change in iridial coloration	Lymphoma, Melanoma
Posterior synechia	Variable pupil shape, Sluggish/absent PLR, Anterior uveitis	Secondary to anterior uveitis
Iris atrophy, Iris hypoplasia	Variable pupil shape, iridal thinning, Sluggish/absent PLR, Irregular pupil margin, Other ocular abnormalities	Old age change, Congenital
Pharmacological blockade	Mydriasis, Absent direct/consensual PLR, Normal vision	Atropine
Spastic pupil syndrome	Miosis, Normal vision	FeLV

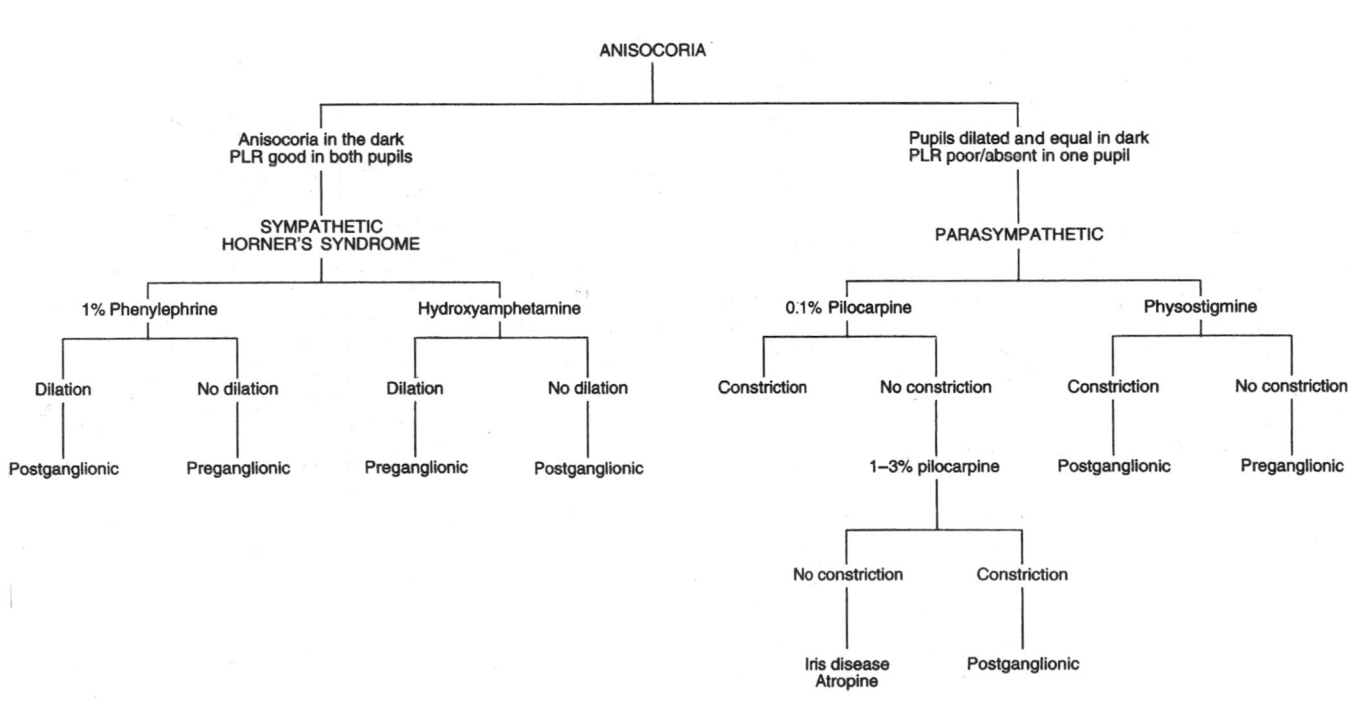

ANOREXIA

 BASICS

DEFINITION
The lack or loss of appetite for food; appetite is psychological and its existence in animals is assumed. Hunger is physiologically aroused by the body's need for food. Anorexia may be partial or complete. Cachexia pertains to dramatic decreases in appetite and increased metabolism of fat and lean body mass.

PATHOPHYSIOLOGY
• The control of appetite is a complex interaction between the central nervous system and the periphery.
• The hypothalamus and brain stem contain peptidergic feeding–regulatory neurons that act as input stations for hormonal and gastrointestinal information. These cell populations project to several brain regions and interconnect extensively.
• Peripheral signals that affect appetite include the palatability, texture, and quantity of recently consumed food.
• Satiety is influenced by gastric and duodenal distention in addition to the presence of nutrients in the gastrointestinal tract.
• Hunger is affected by plasma concentrations of glucose and fatty acids, by interacting with nutrient-specific receptors in the liver and gastrointestinal tract.
• Decreased and increased oxidative metabolism by the liver leads to hunger and satiety, respectively.
• Learned behavior and circadian rhythms modulate appetite and may override other signals for satiety and hunger.
• Leptin is primarily produced by adipocytes and acts on specific hypothalamic receptors to decrease metabolism and decrease appetite.
• Neuropeptide Y released from the gastrointestinal tract induces hunger and hyperphagia, and decreases energy expenditure after food restriction.
• Cholecystokinin (CCK) and bombesin released from the gastrointestinal tract decrease appetite.
• Ghrelin produced by the stomach is a prokinetic and decreases leptin and increases neuropeptide Y production.
• Serotonin is an important and perhaps final mediator of satiety both centrally via a serotonergic tract that passes near the ventromedial hypothalamus (the classical satiety center).
• Dopaminergic tracts in the hypothalamus help regulate food intake and are closely associated with the lateral hypothalamus (classical feeding center).
• Appetite is stimulated by aldosterone and corticosterone and suppressed by glucagons and somatostatin.
• Inflammatory and neoplastic disease can cause anorexia by releasing cytokines such as interleukin-1, tumor necrosis factor, and interferon.
• The expected up-regulation of dietary intake in response to elevated energy expenditure is frequently lost in cancer patients.
• Decreased appetite associated with aging, the so-called anorexia of aging, predisposes older patients to protein-energy malnutrition and is probably mediated by CCK and an enhanced satiating effect of small intestinal carbohydrates.
• Exogenous and endogenous toxins (e.g., renal and liver failure) cause anorexia.
• Any disorder that decreases cerebral arousal will potentially decrease food intake.
• Gastroparesis associated with neoplasia, metabolic disorders, and primary gastrointestinal disease is associated with decreased appetite.
• Fear, pain, and stress may decrease appetite.

SYSTEMS AFFECTED
All body systems

SIGNALMENT
Species
Dogs and cats
Breed Predilections
N/A
Mean Age and Range
N/A
Predominant Sex
N/A

SIGNS
Historical Findings
• Refusal to eat is a common complaint presented by pet owners because poor appetite is strongly associated with illness.
• Patients with disorders causing dysfunction or pain of the face, neck, oropharynx, and esophagus may display an interest in food but cannot eat. These patients are referred to as being pseudoanorectic.
• Animals lacking a sense of smell (anosmia) often show no sniffing behavior.

Physical Examination Findings
• Clinical signs in anorexia vary depending on the underlying cause but include fever, pallor, icterus, pain, changes in organ size, ocular changes, abdominal distention, dyspnea, muffled heart and lung sounds, adventitious lung sounds, cardiac murmurs, and masses. Pseudoanorectic patients commonly display weight loss, halitosis, excessive drooling, difficulty in prehending and masticating food, and odynophagia (painful swallowing).

CAUSES
Anorexia
• Almost any systemic disease process
• Psychological—unpalatable diet, food aversion, stress, alterations in routine and environment
• Acid-base disorders
• Cardiac failure
• Toxicities and drugs
• Pain
• Endocrine and metabolic disease
• Neoplasia
• Infectious disease
• Immune mediated disease
• Respiratory disease
• Gastrointestinal disease
• Musculoskeletal disease
• Neurologic disease
• Anorexia of aging
• Miscellaneous, e.g., motion sickness, high environmental temperature

Pseudoanorexia
• Any disease causing painful or dysfunctional prehension, mastication, and swallowing
• Stomatitis, glossitis, gingivitis, pharyngitis, and esophagitis (e.g., physical agents, caustics, bacterial or viral infections, foreign bodies, immune mediated diseases, uremia)
• Retropharyngeal disorders (e.g., lymphadenopathy, abscess, hematoma, sialocele)
• Dental disease or periodontal disease
• Retrobulbar abscess
• Oral, glossal, pharyngeal, or esophageal neoplasia
• Neurologic disorders (e.g., rabies; neuropathies of cranial nerves V, VII, IX, X, XII; and central nervous system lesions)
• Musculoskeletal lesions (e.g., masticatory myositis, temporomandibular joint disease, fractures, craniomandibular osteopathy, myasthenia gravis, botulism, and cricopharyngeal achalasia)
• Salivary gland neoplasia or inflammation

RISK FACTORS
N/A

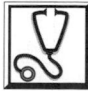 **DIAGNOSIS**

DIFFERENTIAL DIAGNOSIS
• Question owners about the patient's interest in food and ability to prehend, masticate, and swallow food.
• Perform a thorough ophthalmic, dental, oropharyngeal, facial, and cervical examination (sedation or anesthesia may be required) in addition to observing the patient eating to rule out pseudoanorexia.
• Elicit a thorough history regarding the patient's environment, diet, changes in routine, people, or other pets to help identify potential psychological etiologies.

- A complete physical examination is required to determine the presence of systemic disease.
- A database including a complete blood count, serum biochemistry panel, urinalysis, heartworm serology, retrovirus serology, abdominal and thoracic imaging studies, endoscopy, and histologic/cytologic examination of tissue/cell samples are often required make a definitive diagnosis, or at least progress toward one.
- Only if the history, physical examination, and database strongly suggest psychologic anorexia should further diagnostic work-up be forgone; in such cases, daily contact with the pet owner is essential until the anorexia has resolved.

CBC/BIOCHEMISTRY/URINALYSIS
- Abnormalities vary with different underlying diseases and causes of pseudoanorexia and anorexia.
- Can be normal in patients with medical as well as psychologic causes of anorexia

OTHER LABORATORY TESTS
Special diagnostic tests may be necessary to rule out specific diseases suggested by history, physical examination, and preliminary tests.

IMAGING
Thoracic and abdominal imaging (radiographic and ultrasound) studies are often included in the minimum database to detect anatomic abnormalities.

DIAGNOSTIC PROCEDURES
Vary with underlying condition suspected

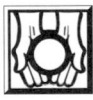

TREATMENT
- Treat underlying disease.
- Symptomatic therapy includes attention to fluid and electrolyte derangements, reduction in environmental stressors, and modification of the diet to improve palatability.
- Palatability can be improved by adding flavored toppings such as chicken and beef broths, seasoning with condiments such as garlic powder, increasing the fat or protein content of the food, and heating the food to body temperature.
- As a general rule, dogs and cats with debilitating disease should not go without food for longer than 3–5 days before enteral or parenteral feeding is used.
- Other factors to consider when deciding whether enteral or parenteral feeding is necessary include ≥ 10 % body weight loss, hypoalbuminemia, lymphopenia, body condition score, and disease process.

- Techniques for providing enteral nutrition include forced feeding and placement of a nasoesophageal, esophagostomy, gastrostomy, or jejunostomy tube.

MEDICATIONS

DRUG(S) OF CHOICE
- Diazepam is a short-acting appetite stimulant with sedative properties dosed at 0.1 mg/kg IV daily or 1 mg PO once daily in cats.
- Oxazepam (2 mg/cat PO q12h) is a short-acting appetite stimulant and sedative.
- Cyproheptadine, an antihistamine with antiserotonergic properties, has been used as an appetite stimulant with mixed success at a dose range of 0.2–0.4 mg/kg PO, 10–20 minutes prior to feeding.
- Analgesics may promote appetite in painful conditions.
- Metoclopramide (0.2–0.4 mg/kg SC or PO), ranitidine (2 mg/kg SC, IV, or PO), or erythromycin (0.5–1.0 mg/kg PO) are useful if anorexia is associated with gastroparesis or ileus.
- Antiemetics such as prochlorperazine (0.1–0.5 mg/kg PO) or metoclopramide are useful to decrease nausea-associated anorexia.

CONTRAINDICATIONS
Avoid antiemetics if gastrointestinal obstruction is present or suspected.

PRECAUTIONS
N/A

POSSIBLE INTERACTIONS
N/A

ALTERNATIVE DRUG(S)
N/A

FOLLOW-UP

PATIENT MONITORING
- Body weight, body condition score assessment, and hydration determination
- Return of appetite

PREVENTION/AVOIDANCE
Feed highly palatable diet.

POSSIBLE COMPLICATIONS
- Dehydration, malnutrition, and cachexia are most likely; these exacerbate the underlying disease.
- A loss of more than 25–30% of body protein compromises the immune system and

muscle strength, and death results from infection and/or pulmonary failure.
- Feline hepatic lipidosis is a possible complication of anorexia in obese cats.
- Breakdown of the intestinal mucosal barrier is a concern in debilitated patients.

EXPECTED COURSE AND PROGNOSIS
Varies with underlying cause

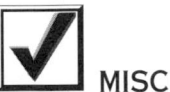

MISCELLANEOUS

ASSOCIATED CONDITIONS
N/A

AGE-RELATED FACTORS
Nutritional support and/or glucose-containing fluids may be necessary to treat or prevent hypoglycemia in anorectic puppies and kittens.

ZOONOTIC POTENTIAL
N/A

PREGNANCY
N/A

SYNONYMS
N/A

SEE ALSO
Causes

ABBREVIATIONS
N/A

Suggested Reading

Guilford WG. Nutritional management of gastrointestinal diseases. In: Guilford WG, Center SA, Strombeck DR, et al., eds. Strombeck's small animal gastroenterology. 3rd ed. Philadelphia: Saunders, 1996:889–910.

Monroe WE. Anorexia and polyphagia. In: Ettinger SJ, Feldman EC., eds. Veterinary internal medicine. 5th ed. Philadelphia: Saunders, 2000:102–104.

Phinney SD, Halstead CH. Obesity, anorexia nervosa, and bulimia. In: Feldman M, Scharschmidt BF, Sleisenger MH, eds. Gastrointestinal and liver disease. 6th ed. Philadelphia: Saunders, 1998:278–297.

Remillard RL, Armstrong PJ, et al. Assisted feeding in hospitalized patients: enteral and parenteral nutrition. In: Hand MS, Thatcher CD, Remillard RL, et al., eds. Small animal clinical nutrition. 4th ed. Topeka, KS: Mark Morris Institute, 2000:351–399.

Author Mark C. Walker
Consulting Editor Albert E. Jergens

ANTEBRACHIAL GROWTH DEFORMITIES

BASICS

DEFINITION
Abnormally shaped forelimbs and/or mal-alignments of the elbow or antebrachial carpal joints that result from abnormal development of the radius or ulna in the growing animal

PATHOPHYSIOLOGY
• Antebrachium—predisposed to deformities resulting from continual growth of one bone after premature growth cessation or decreased growth rate of the paired bone
• Decreased rate of elongation in one bone behaves as a retarding strap; the growing paired bone must twist and bow away from the short bone or overgrow at the elbow or carpus; causes joint malalignment
• Normal growth—bones elongate through the process of endochondral ossification, which occurs in the physis; physis closure occurs when the germinal cell layer stops producing new cartilage and the existing cartilage hypertrophies, ossifies, and is remodeled into bone.
• Hereditary—premature closure of distal ulnar physis reported as recessive trait in Skye terriers; may be a component of common elbow joint malalignment in many chondrodysplastic breeds (basset hounds and Lhasa apsos)
• Osteochondrosis or dietary oversupplementation—possibly associated with retardation of endochondral ossification (retained cartilaginous cores) in giant-breed dogs
• Trauma—most common cause; if chondro-proliferative layer of the physis is crushed (Salter V fracture), new cartilage production and bone elongation are stopped.

SYSTEMS AFFECTED
Musculoskeletal

GENETICS
• Skye terriers—reported as a recessive inheritable trait
• Chondrodysplastic breeds (dogs)—predisposed to elbow malalignment

INCIDENCE/PREVALENCE
• Traumatic—may occur after forelimb injuries in up to 10% of actively growing animals; uncommon in cats
• Elbow malalignment syndrome (chondrodysplastic dog breeds)—fairly common and can be bilateral
• Nutritionally induced—incidence decreasing as nutritional standards are improved
• Congenital agenesis of the radius (cats)—occasionally seen; results in severely bowed antebrachium and carpal subluxation

GEOGRAPHIC DISTRIBUTION
N/A

SIGNALMENT

Species
Dogs and cats

Breed Predilections
• Skye terriers—recessive inheritable form
• Chondrodysplastic and toy breeds (especially basset hounds, dachshunds, Lhasa apsos, Pekingese)—may be predisposed to elbow malalignments
• Giant breeds (e.g., Great Danes, wolfhounds)—may be induced by rapid growth owing to excessive or unbalanced nutrition

Mean Age and Range
• Traumatic—anytime during the active growth phase
• Elbow malarticulations—during growth; may not be recognized until secondary arthritic changes become severe, occasionally at several years of age

Predominant Sex
N/A

SIGNS

General Comments
• Longer-limbed dogs—angular deformities generally more common
• Shorter-limbed dogs—tend to develop more severe joint malalignments
• Age at the time of premature closure—affects relative degree of deformity and joint malarticulation; perhaps because of the variation in stiffness of bone with age and the duration of altered growth until maturity

Historical Findings
• Traumatic—progressive limb angulation or lameness 3–4 weeks after injury; owner may not be aware of causative event.
• Developmental elbow malalignments—insidious onset of lameness in one or both forelimbs; most apparent after exercise

Physical Examination Findings
Premature Distal Ulnar Closure
• Three deformities of the distal radius—lateral deviation (valgus), cranial bowing (curvus), and external rotation (supination)
• Relative shortening of limb length compared to the contralateral normally growing limb
• Caudolateral subluxation of the radial carpal joint and malarticulation of the elbow joint—may occur; causes lameness and painful joint restriction
Premature Radial Physeal Closure
• Affected limb—significantly shorter than the normal contralateral
• Severity of lameness—depends on degree of joint malarticulation

• Complete symmetrical closure of distal physis—may note straight limb with a widened radial carpal joint space; may note caudal bow to radius and ulna
• Asymmetrical closure of medial distal physis—varus angular deformity; occasionally inward rotation
• Closure of lateral distal physis—valgus angular deformity; external rotation
• Closure of proximal radial physis with continued ulnar growth—malarticulation of the elbow joint; widened radial to humeral space and humeral to anconeal space

CAUSES
• Trauma
• Developmental basis
• Nutritional basis

RISK FACTORS
• Forelimb trauma
• Excessive dietary supplementation

DIAGNOSIS

DIFFERENTIAL DIAGNOSIS
• Elbow dysplasia
• Fragmented medial coronoid process
• Un-united anconeal process
• Panosteitis
• Flexor tendon contracture
• Hypertrophic osteodystrophy

CBC/BIOCHEMISTRY/URINALYSIS
N/A

OTHER LABORATORY TESTS
N/A

IMAGING
• Damage to growth potential of the physis—cannot be seen at the time of trauma; usually 2–4 weeks before radiographically apparent
• Standard craniocaudal and mediolateral radiographic views—include entire elbow joint; proximally extend to midmetacarpal level distally; take same series for comparison to normal contralateral limb.
• Degree of angular deformities and relative shortening—determined by comparing relative lengths of radius and ulna within the deformed pair to the normal contralateral pair
• Elbow and carpal joints—evaluate for malalignment (treated surgically) and arthritis (e.g., osteophytes; influences prognosis)
• Elbow joint—evaluate for associated un-united anconeal process and fragmented medial coronoid process

DIAGNOSTIC PROCEDURES
N/A

PATHOLOGIC FINDINGS
Cartilage of prematurely closed physis replaced with bone

TREATMENT

APPROPRIATE HEALTH CARE
• Genetic predisposition—cannot be treated
• Traumatic physeal damage—not seen at time of injury; revealed 2–4 weeks later
• Surgical treatment is recommended as soon as possible following diagnosis.

NURSING CARE
N/A

ACTIVITY
Exercise restriction—reduces joint malalignment damage; slows arthritic progression

DIET
• Decrease nutritional supplementation in giant breed dogs—slows rapid grow; may reduce incidence
• Avoid excess weight—helps control arthritic pain resulting from joint malalignment and overuse

CLIENT EDUCATION
• Discuss heritability in Skye terriers and chondrodysplastic breeds.
• Explain that damage to physeal growth potential is not apparent at time of forelimb trauma and that the diagnosis is often made at 2–4-weeks following an injury.
• Discuss the importance of joint malalignment and resultant arthritis as primary causes of lameness.
• Emphasize that early surgical treatment leads to a better prognosis.

SURGICAL CONSIDERATIONS
• Premature distal ulnar physeal closure in a patient < 5–6 months of age (significant amount of radial growth potential remaining)—treated with a segmental ulnar ostectomy, valgus deformities ≤ 25°—often spontaneously correct and may not require additional surgery, young patients and those with more severe deformities—often require a second definitive correction after maturity
• Radial or ulnar physeal closure in a mature patient (limited or no growth potential) requires deformity correction, joint realignment, or both.
• Deformity correction—may be accomplished with a variety of osteotomy techniques; may be stabilized with several different fixation devices; must correct both rotational and angular deformities; performed at the point of greatest curvature
• Joint malalignment (particularly elbow)—must correct to minimize arthritic

development (primary cause of lameness); obtain optimal joint alignment via dynamic proximal ulnar osteotomy (uses triceps muscle traction and joint pressure).
• Significant limb length discrepancies—distraction osteogenesis; osteotomy of the shortened bone is progressively distracted at the rate of 1 mm/day with an external fixator system to create new bone length.

MEDICATIONS

DRUG(S) OF CHOICE
Anti-inflammatory drugs—symptomatic treatment of arthritis

CONTRAINDICATIONS
Corticosteriods—do not use owing to potential systemic side affects and cartilage damage seen with long-term use.

PRECAUTIONS
Warn client of possible gastrointestinal upset associated with chronic anti-inflammatory therapy.

POSSIBLE INTERACTIONS
N/A

ALTERNATIVE DRUG(S)
Neutraceuticals (e.g., glycosamines)—may help minimize cartilage damage and arthritis development; may be anti-inflammatory and analgesic

FOLLOW-UP

PATIENT MONITORING
• Postoperative—depends on surgical treatment
• Periodic checkups—evaluate arthritic status and anti-inflammatory therapy

PREVENTION/AVOIDANCE
Avoid dietary oversupplementation in rapidly growing giant-breed dogs.

POSSIBLE COMPLICATIONS
Routinely seen with various osteotomy fixation techniques (e.g., infection, nonunion of osteotomy, fixator pin tract inflammation)

EXPECTED COURSE AND PROGNOSIS
• Generally, best results seen with early diagnosis and surgical treatment—minimizes arthritis
• Premature ulnar closure—tends to be easier to manage; yields better results

• Limb lengthening by distraction osteogenesis—requires extensive postoperative management by the veterinarian and owner; high rate of complications

MISCELLANEOUS

ASSOCIATED CONDITIONS
Osteochondrosis

AGE-RELATED FACTORS
The younger the age at the time of traumatically induced physeal closure, the more severe the deformity and malarticulation.

ZOONOTIC POTENTIAL
N/A

PREGNANCY
N/A

SYNONYMS
Radius curvus

Suggested Reading
Forrell EB, Schwarz PD. Use of external skeletal fixation for treatment of angular deformity secondary to premature distal ulnar physeal closure. J Am Anim Hosp Assoc 1993;29:460–465.
Gilson SD, Piermattei DL, Schwarz PD. Treatment of humeroulnar subluxation with a dynamic proximal ulnar osteotomy: a review of 13 cases. Vet Surg 1989;18:114–122.
Henney LH, Gambardella PC. Premature closure of the ulnar physis in the dog: a retrospective clinical study. J Am Anim Hosp Assoc 1989;25:573–581.
Johnson AL. Correction of radial and ulnar growth deformities resulting from premature physeal closure. In: Bojrab MJ, ed. Current techniques in small animal surgery. 3rd ed. Philadelphia: Lea & Febiger, 1990:793–801.
Johnson KA. Retardation of endochondral ossification at the distal ulnar growth plate in dogs. Austral Vet J 1981;57:474–478.
Lau RE. Inherited premature closure of the distal ulnar physis. J Am Anim Hosp Assoc 1978;14:690–697.
Yanoff SR, Hulse DA, Palmer RH, Herron MR. Distraction osteogenesis using modified external fixation devices in five dogs. Vet Surg 1992;21:480–486.
Author Erick L. Egger
Consulting Editor Peter K. Shires

ANTERIOR UVEITIS—CATS

BASICS

DEFINITION
• Inflammation of the anterior uveal tissues, including iris (iritis), ciliary body (cyclitis) or both (iridocyclitis) • May be associated with concurrent posterior uveal and retinal inflammation (choroiditis; chorioretinitis) • May be unilateral or bilateral

PATHOPHYSIOLOGY
• Increased permeability of the blood-aqueous barrier related to infectious, immune-mediated, traumatic or other causes allows entrance of plasma proteins and blood cellular components into aqueous humor. • Disruption of blood-aqueous barrier is initiated and maintained by numerous chemical mediators, including histamine, prostaglandins, leukotrienes, seotonin, kinins, and complement

SYSTEMS AFFECTED
• Ophthalmic • Other systems may also be affected by underlying disease process

GENETICS
N/A

INCIDENCE/PREVALENCE
• Relatively common condition • True incidence/prevalence unknown

GEOGRAPHIC DISTRIBUTION
Geographic location may affect incidence of certain infectious causes of uveitis.

SIGNALMENT
Species
Cats

Breed Predilections
None

Mean Age and Range
• Mean age—7–9 years • Any age may be affected.

Predominant Sex
Males/neutered males more commonly affected than females

SIGNS
Historical Findings
• Cloudy eye—due to corneal edema, aqueous flare, hypopyon, etc. • Painful eye—manifest by blepharospasm, photophobia, or rubbing eye; usually less pronounced than in dogs • Red eye—due to conjunctival hyperemia and ciliary flush; less pronounced than in dogs in most cases • Vision loss—variable

Physical Examination Findings
Importance of a thorough physical examination in cats presenting with uveitis cannot be overstated
Ophthalmic findings
• Ocular discomfort—manifest by blepharospasm and photophobia

• Ocular discharge—usually serous; sometimes mucoid to mucopurulent • Conjunctival hyperemia—bulbar and palpebral conjunctiva both usually affected. • Corneal edema—diffuse; may be mild to severe. • Keratic precipitates—multifocal aggregates of inflammatory cells adherent to corneal endothelium; most notable ventrally • Aqueous flare and cells—cloudiness of aqueous humor due to increased protein content and suspended cellular debris; best visualized with a bright, narrow beam of light shined through anterior chamber. • Ciliary flush—injection of deep perilimbal anterior ciliary vessels • Deep corneal vascularization—circumcorneal distribution (brush border) • Miosis and/or resistance to pharmacologic dilation • Iridal swelling—may be generalized or nodular • Reduced IOP • Posterior synechia—adhesions between posterior iris and anterior lens surface • Fibrin in anterior chamber • Hypopyon or hyphema—accumulations of white blood cells or red blood cells, respectively, in the anterior chamber; usually settles horizontally in ventral aspect of chamber, but may be diffuse. • Chronic changes may include rubeosis iridis, iridal hyperpigmentation, secondary cataract, lens luxation, pupillary seclusion, iris bombé, and secondary glaucoma.

CAUSES
• Infectious—mycotic (*Blastomyces spp., Cryptococcus neoformans; Coccidiodes immitis; Histoplasma capsulatum*); protozoal (*Toxoplasma gondii*); bacterial (any bacterial septicemia); viral (FIV, FeLV, feline coronavirus); parasitic (ophthalmomyiasis; ocular larval migrans) • Idiopathic—lymphocytic plasmacytic uveitis • Immune-mediated—reaction to lens proteins (due to cataract or lens trauma) • Neoplastic—primary ocular tumors (esp. diffuse iris melanoma, ocular sarcoma); metastasis to uveal tract (esp. lymphoma) • Metabolic—hyperlipidemia; hyperviscosity; systemic hypertension • Miscellaneous—trauma; ulcerative keratitis; corneal stromal abscess; toxemia of any cause

RISK FACTORS
None specific; immune suppression and geographic location may increase incidence of certain infectious causes of uveitis.

DIAGNOSIS

DIFFERENTIAL DIAGNOSIS
• Conjunctivitis—redness limited to conjunctival hyperemia (i.e., no ciliary flush); ocular discharge usually thicker and more copious than in uveitis; discomfort less severe than with uveitis and is alleviated with application of topical anesthetic

• Glaucoma—elevated IOP is most consistent distinguishing feature of this disease; others may include dilated pupil, Haab's striae, and buphthalmos. • Ulcerative keratitis—corneal fluorescein staining will detect ulcers; corneal edema associated with ulcers is either localized to or most severe at site of ulcer; ocular discharge often thicker and more copious than with uveitis; discomfort partially alleviated by topical anesthetic. • Horner's syndrome—miosis, enophthalmos, and nictitans protrusion are similar in both conditions, but Horner's is non-painful with no ocular discharge; ptosis with Horner's is distinguished from blepharospasm as the latter is an active process; minor conjunctival hyperemia may be noted with Horner's, but cornea and anterior chamber are clear; clinical signs of Horner's syndrome resolve following application of topical 10% phenylephrine.

CBC/BIOCHEMISTRY/URINALYSIS
• CBC—often normal; changes may be present related to underlying disease. • Biochemistry—often normal; most common abnormality in cats with uveitis is elevated serum proteins (usually due to polyclonal gammopathy). • Urinalysis—often normal; changes may be present related to underlying disease.

OTHER LABORATORY TESTS
• FeLV serum titers • FIV serum titers • Coronavirus titers—not specific for FIP, but may influence the index of suspicion for this disease • *Toxoplasma gondii* IgM and IgG titers performed on serum and/or aqueous humor.

IMAGING
• Thoracic radiography—may show evidence of causative disease process (e.g., infiltrates related to infectious disease; evidence of metastatic neoplastic disease) • Ocular ultrasound—indicated if opacity of ocular media precludes direct examination; may reveal intraocular neoplasm or retinal detachment.

DIAGNOSTIC PROCEDURES
• Tonometry—low IOP consistent with uveitis; elevated IOP indicates glaucoma (primary disease or secondary to uveitis) • Ocular centesis—if retinal detachment is present, cytology of subretinal aspirate may reveal causative agents; anterior chamber centesis may be performed for *Toxoplasma gondii* IgM and IgG titers on aqueous humor

PATHOLOGIC FINDINGS
• Gross—see physical examination findings. • Histopathologic—corneal edema; peripheral corneal deep stromal vascularization; keratic precipitates; preiridal fibrovascular membrane; peripheral anterior synechia; posterior synechia; entropion or ectropion uveae; leukocyte accumulation in iris, ciliary body, sclera, choroid (lymphocytic-plasmacytic, suppurative, or granulomatous

infiltrates, depending on etiology); secondary cataract; with posterior segment involvement in inflammatory process, cyclitic membrane; vitreal traction bands and retinal detachment may be present • Lymphoplasmacytic infiltrate of iris and ciliary body (either diffuse or nodular) is most common histopathologic finding.

TREATMENT

APPROPRIATE HEALTH CARE
Outpatient medical management generally sufficient

NURSING CARE
None

ACTIVITY
No changes indicated in most cases

DIET
No changes indicated

CLIENT EDUCATION
• Inform of potential systemic diseases causing ophthalmic signs and emphasize importance of appropriate diagnostic testing. • In addition to symptomatic uveitis treatment, treatment of underlying disease (when possible) is paramount to a positive outcome. • Inform of potential complications and emphasize compliance with treatment and follow-up recommendations that will reduce the likelihood of complications.

SURGICAL CONSIDERATIONS
• None in most cases • Specific instances requiring surgical intervention include removal of ruptured lenses and surgical management of secondary glaucoma. • Chronic uveitis leading to secondary glaucoma commonly necessitates enucleation of affected globes. • Enucleation is recommended with uveitis related to diffuse iris melanoma.

MEDICATIONS

DRUG(S)

Corticosteroids
Topical
• Prednisolone acetate 1%—apply 2–8 times daily, depending on severity of disease; taper medication as condition resolves. • Dexamethasone 0.1%—apply 2–8 times daily, depending on severity of disease; taper medication as condition resolves. • Other topical corticosteroids (e.g., betamethasone, hydrocortisone) are considerably less effective in the treatment of intraocular inflammation. • Taper treatment frequency as condition improves; stopping topical corticosteroids abruptly may result in rebound of ocular inflammation.

Subconjunctival
• Triamcinolone acetonide—4 mg by subconjunctival injection • Methylprednisolone—4 mg by subconjunctival injection • Often not required • Indicated only in severe cases as one time injection, followed by topical and/or systemic anti-inflammatories
Systemic
• Prednisone—1–3 mg/kg/day initially; taper dose after 7–10 days. • Use only if systemic infectious causes of uveitis have been ruled out.

Nonsteroidal Antiinflammatory Drugs
Topical
• Flurbiprofen—apply 2–4 times daily, depending on severity of disease
• Diclofenac—apply 2–4 times daily, depending on severity of disease
Systemic
• Aspirin—10 mg/kg PO q48 hours. Do not use concurrently with systemic corticosteroids. Avoid in the presence of hyphema.
Topical mydriatic/cycloplegic
• Atropine sulfate 1%—apply 1–4 times daily, depending on severity of disease. Use lowest frequency adequate to maintain dilated pupil and ocular comfort; taper medication as condition resolves. Ointment is preferred over solution in cats, as it causes less salivation.

CONTRAINDICATIONS
• Avoid the use of miotic medications (e.g., pilocarpine), including topical prostaglandins (e.g., latanoprost) in the presence of uveitis. • Topical and subconjunctival corticosteroids are absolutely contraindicated in the presence of ulcerative keratitis. • Corticosteroids (especially systemic) should be avoided in cats with systemic hypertension.

PRECAUTIONS
Owing to concern for secondary glaucoma, topical atropine should be used judiciously and IOP should be monitored periodically.

POSSIBLE INTERACTIONS
Systemic corticosteroids and nonsteroidal anti-inflammatory drugs should not be used concurrently.

FOLLOW-UP

PATIENT MONITORING
Recheck in 3–7 days, depending on severity of disease. IOP should be monitored at recheck to detect secondary glaucoma. Frequency of subsequent rechecks dictated by severity of disease and response to treatment

PREVENTION/AVOIDANCE
N/A

POSSIBLE COMPLICATIONS
Systemic complications
Occur as a result of the systemic etiology of the uveitis

Ophthalmic complications
• Secondary glaucoma—most common complication of chronic uveitis in cats. • Secondary cataract • Lens luxation • Retinal detachment • Phthisis bulbi

EXPECTED COURSE AND PROGNOSIS
• Guarded prognosis for affected eyes. Depends on underlying disease and response to treatment. • Cats with treatable underlying disease (e.g., toxoplasmosis) are more likely to have favorable ophthalmic outcome than those with idiopathic lymphocytic plasmacytic uveitis or untreatable underlying condition (e.g., FIP, FIV).

MISCELLANEOUS

ASSOCIATED CONDITIONS
N/A

AGE-RELATED FACTORS
• Younger cats more likely to be diagnosed with infectious etiology • Older cats at higher risk of idiopathic lymphocytic plasmacytic uveitis and intraocular neoplastic causes

ZOONOTIC POTENTIAL
• None in most cases • Some forms of systemic infection causing uveitis may pose a slight risk to immunocompromised owners.

PREGNANCY
Avoid systemic corticosteroids. Because of systemic absorption, topical corticosteroids may also pose risk, especially with frequent application.

SYNONYM
Iridocyclitis

SEE ALSO
Red Eye

ABBREVIATIONS
• FeLV = feline leukemia virus
• FIP = feline infectious peritonitis
• FIV = feline immunodeficiency virus
• IOP = intraocular pressure

Suggested Reading
Glaze MB, Gelatt KN. Feline ophthalmology. In: Gelatt KN, ed. Veterinary ophthalmology. 3rd ed. Philadelphia: Lippincott Williams & Wilkins, 1999:997–1052.
Slatter D. Uvea. In: Slatter D, ed. Fundamentals of veterinary ophthalmology. 3rd ed. Philadelphia: WB Saunders, 2001:314–349.
Stiles J. Ocular manifestations of systemic disease. Part 2: The cat. In: Gelatt KN, ed. Veterinary ophthalmology. 3rd ed. Philadelphia: Lippincott Williams & Wilkins, 1999:1448–1473.
Author Ian P. Herring
Consulting Editor Paul E. Miller

ANTERIOR UVEITIS—DOGS

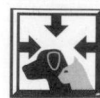 **BASICS**

DEFINITION
• Inflammation of the anterior uveal tissues, including iris (iritis), ciliary body (cyclitis) or both (iridocyclitis) • May be associated with concurrent posterior uveal and retinal inflammation (choroiditis; chorioretinitis) • May be unilateral or bilateral

PATHOPHYSIOLOGY
• Increased permeability of the blood-aqueous barrier related to infectious, immune-mediated, traumatic, or other causes allows entrance of plasma proteins and blood cellular components into aqueous humor. • Disruption of blood-aqueous barrier is initiated and maintained by numerous chemical mediators, including histamine, prostaglandins, leukotrienes, serotonin, kinins, and complement.

SYSTEMS AFFECTED
• Ophthalmic • Other systems may also be affected by underlying disease process.

GENETICS
N/A

INCIDENCE/PREVALENCE
Relatively common condition
True incidence/prevalence unknown

GEOGRAPHIC DISTRIBUTION
Geographic location may affect incidence of certain infectious causes of uveitis.

SIGNALMENT

Species
Dogs

Breed Predilections
• None for most causes • High incidence of pigmentary uveitis in golden retriever. • High incidence of uveodermatologic syndrome in Siberian Husky, Akita, Samoyed, and Shetland sheepdog.

Mean Age and Range
• Any age may be affected. • Mean age in uveodermatologic syndrome—2.8 years

Predominant Sex
None

SIGNS

Historical Findings
Red eye—due to conjunctival hyperemia and ciliary flush
Cloudy eye—due to corneal edema, aqueous flare, hypopyon, etc.
Painful eye—manifest by blepharospasm, photophobia, or rubbing eye
Vision loss—variable

Physical Examination Findings
The importance of a thorough physical examination in dogs presenting with uveitis cannot be overstated.

Ophthalmic Findings
• Ocular discomfort—manifest by blepharospasm, photophobia, and rubbing eye • Ocular discharge—usually serous; sometimes mucoid to mucopurulent • Conjunctival hyperemia—bulbar and palpebral conjunctiva both usually affected • Corneal edema—diffuse • Keratic precipitates—multifocal aggregates of inflammatory cells adherent to corneal endothelium; most notable ventrally • Aqueous flare and cells—cloudiness of aqueous humor due to increased protein content and suspended cellular debris; best visualized with a bright, narrow beam of light shined through anterior chamber • Ciliary flush—injection of deep perilimbal anterior ciliary vessels • Deep corneal vascularization—circumcorneal distribution (brush border) • Miosis and/or resistance to pharmacologic dilation

Iridal Swelling
• Reduced IOP • Posterior synechia—adhesions between posterior iris and anterior lens surface • Fibrin in anterior chamber • Hypopyon or hyphema—accumulations of white blood cells or red blood cells, respectively, in the anterior chamber; usually settles horizontally in ventral aspect of chamber, but may be diffuse. • Chronic changes may include rubeosis iridis, iridal hyperpigmentation, secondary cataract, lens luxation, pupillary seclusion, iris bombé, and secondary glaucoma.

CAUSES
• Infectious—mycotic (*Blastomyces dermatitidis, Cryptococcus neoformans, Coccidiodes immitis, Histoplasma capsulatum*); protozoal (*Toxoplasma gondii, Neospora caninum, Leishmania donovani*); rickettsial (*Ehrlichia canis, Rickettsia rickettsii*); bacterial (*Leptospira* spp., *Brucella canis, Borrelia burgdorferi*, any bacterial septicemia); algal (*Prototheca* spp.); viral (adenovirus, distemper, rabies, herpes); parasitic (ocular filariasis, ocular larval migrans)
• Immune-mediated—reaction to lens proteins (due to cataract or lens trauma); uveodermatologic syndrome; post-vaccinal reaction to canine adenovirus vaccine; vasculitis
• Neoplastic—primary ocular tumors; metastasis to uveal tract
• Metabolic—hyperlipidemia; hyperviscosity; systemic hypertension
• Miscellaneous—idiopathic; trauma; ulcerative keratitis; corneal stromal abscess; scleritis; lens instability/luxation; dental/periodontal disease; toxemia of any cause

RISK FACTORS
None specific; immune suppression and geographic location may increase incidence of certain infectious causes of uveitis.

 DIAGNOSIS

DIFFERENTIAL DIAGNOSIS
• Conjunctivitis—redness limited to conjunctival hyperemia (i.e., no ciliary flush); ocular discharge usually thicker and more copious than in uveitis; discomfort less severe than with uveitis and is alleviated with application of topical anesthetic.
• Glaucoma—elevated IOP is most consistent distinguishing feature of this disease; others may include dilated pupil, Haab's striae, and buphthalmos. • Lens luxation—corneal edema may be localized to site of lens contact with endothelium or may be diffuse as a result of associated uveitis and/or glaucoma; high breed associations for lens luxation
• Ulcerative keratitis—corneal fluorescein staining will detect ulcers; corneal edema associated with ulcers is either localized to or most severe at site of ulcer; ocular discharge often thicker and more copious than with uveitis; discomfort is partially alleviated by topical anesthetic. • Corneal endothelial dystrophy/degeneration—diffuse corneal edema is present, but IOP is normal; conjunctival hyperemia and signs of ocular discomfort are generally absent. • Horner's syndrome—miosis, enophthalmos, and nictitans protrusion are similar in both conditions, but Horner's is non-painful with no ocular discharge; ptosis with Horner's is distinguished from blepharospasm as the latter is an active process; minor conjunctival hyperemia may be noted with Horner's, but cornea and anterior chamber are clear; clinical signs of Horner's syndrome resolve following application of topical 10% phenylephrine.

CBC/BIOCHEMISTRY/URINALYSIS
Often normal; changes related to underlying disease may be present.

OTHER LABORATORY TESTS
• Serology for infectious diseases listed under CAUSES may be appropriate, depending on index of suspicion for infectious etiology. • Clinical signs raising the suspicion of systemic disease including lethargy, pyrexia, weight loss, coughing, lymphadenopathy, etc., warrant serology for infectious diseases.

IMAGING
• Thoracic radiography may show evidence of causative disease process (e.g., systemic mycoses; metastatic neoplasia). • Ocular ultrasound is indicated if opacity of ocular media precludes direct examination, and may reveal intraocular neoplasm or retinal detachment.

DIAGNOSTIC PROCEDURES
Tonometry—low IOP consistent with uveitis; elevated IOP indicates glaucoma (primary disease or secondary to uveitis).

Lymph node aspirates—if enlarged nodes are palpable, aspiration for cytology is indicated. Ocular centesis—if retinal detachment is present, cytology of subretinal aspirate may reveal causative agents; anterior chamber centesis is generally unrewarding.

PATHOLOGIC FINDINGS
• Gross—see physical examination findings.
• Histopathologic—corneal edema; peripheral corneal deep stromal vascularization; keratic precipitates; preiridal fibrovascular membrane; peripheral anterior synechia; posterior synechia; entropion or ectropion uveae; leukocyte accumulation in iris, ciliary body, sclera, choroid (lymphocytic, plasmacytic, suppurative, or granulomatous infiltrates, depending on etiology); secondary cataract; with posterior segment involvement in inflammatory process, cyclitic membrane; vitreal traction bands and retinal detachment may be present.

TREATMENT

APPROPRIATE HEALTH CARE
Outpatient medical management is generally sufficient.

NURSING CARE
None

ACTIVITY
No changes indicated in most cases. Reducing exposure to bright light may alleviate discomfort.

DIET
No changes indicated

CLIENT EDUCATION
• Inform of potential systemic diseases causing ophthalmic signs and emphasize importance of appropriate diagnostic testing.
• In addition to symptomatic uveitis treatment, treatment of underlying disease (when possible) is paramount to a positive outcome. • Inform of potential complications and emphasize compliance with treatment and follow-up recommendations that will reduce the likelihood of complications.

SURGICAL CONSIDERATIONS
None in most cases. Specific instances requiring surgical intervention include removal of ruptured lenses and surgical management of secondary glaucoma.

MEDICATIONS

DRUG(S) OF CHOICE
Corticosteroids
Topical
• Prednisolone acetate 1%—apply 2–8 times daily, depending on severity of disease; taper medication as condition resolves.

• Dexamethasone 0.1%—apply 2–8 times daily, depending on severity of disease; taper medication as condition resolves.
• Other topical corticosteroids (e.g., betamethasone, hydrocortisone) are considerably less effective in the treatment of intraocular inflammation.
• Taper treatment frequency over several weeks as condition improves; stopping topical corticosteroids abruptly may result in rebound of ocular inflammation.
Subconjunctival
• Triamcinolone acetonide—4–6 mg by subconjunctival injection
• Methylprednisolone—3–10 mg by subconjunctival injection
• Often not required
• Indicated only in severe cases as one time injection followed by topical and/or systemic anti-inflammatories
Systemic
• Prednisone—0.5–2.2 mg/kg/day initially; taper dose after 7–10 days. • Use only if systemic infectious causes of uveitis have been ruled out.

Nonsteroidal Antiinflammatory Drugs
Topical
• Flurbiprofen—apply 2–4 times daily, depending on severity of disease.
• Diclofenac—apply 2–4 times daily, depending on severity of disease.
Systemic
(Do not use concurrently with systemic corticosteroids; avoid in the presence of hyphema.)
• Carprofen—2.2 mg/kg PO BID
• Etodolac—10–15 mg/kg PO QD
• Aspirin—10–25 mg/kg PO BID
Topical mydriatic/cycloplegic
Atropine sulfate 1%—apply 1–4 times daily, depending on severity of disease. Use lowest frequency adequate to maintain dilated pupil and ocular comfort; taper medication as condition resolves.

CONTRAINDICATIONS
• Avoid the use of miotic medications (e.g., pilocarpine, demecarium bromide), including topical prostaglandins (e.g., latanoprost) in the presence of uveitis.
• Topical and subconjunctival corticosteroids are absolutely contraindicated in the presence of ulcerative keratitis.
• Corticosteroids should be avoided in dogs with systemic hypertension.

PRECAUTIONS
Out of concern for secondary glaucoma, topical atropine should be used judiciously and IOP should be monitored periodically.

POSSIBLE INTERACTIONS
Systemic corticosteroids and nonsteroidal anti-inflammatory drugs should not be used concurrently.

ALTERNATIVE DRUG(S)
N/A

FOLLOW-UP

PATIENT MONITORING
Recheck in 3–7 days, depending on severity of disease. IOP should be monitored at recheck to detect secondary glaucoma. Frequency of subsequent rechecks dictated by severity of disease and response to treatment.

PREVENTION/AVOIDANCE
N/A

POSSIBLE COMPLICATIONS
• Many systemic complications, including death, may occur due to systemic etiology of uveitis. • Ophthalmic complications include secondary cataract; secondary glaucoma; lens luxation; retinal detachment; phthisis bulbi.

EXPECTED COURSE AND PROGNOSIS
Extremely variable; depends on underlying disease and response to treatment

MISCELLANEOUS

ASSOCIATED CONDITIONS
N/A

AGE-RELATED FACTORS
N/A

ZOONOTIC POTENTIAL
None in most cases. Some forms of systemic infection causing uveitis may pose a slight risk to immune-compromised owners.

PREGNANCY
Avoid systemic corticosteroids. Because of possibility of systemic absorption, topical corticosteroids may also pose risk, especially with frequent application in small dogs.

SYNONYM
Iridocyclitis

SEE ALSO
Red Eye

ABBREVIATION
IOP = intraocular pressure

Suggested Reading
Collins BK, Moore CP. Diseases and surgery of the canine anterior uvea. In: Gelatt KN, ed., Veterinary ophthalmology. 3rd ed. Philadelphia: Lippincott Williams & Wilkins, 1999:755–795.
Martin CL. Ocular manifestations of systemic disease. Part 1: The dog. In: Gelatt KN, ed., Veterinary ophthalmology. 3rd ed. Philadelphia: Lippincott Williams & Wilkins, 1999:1401–1448.
Slatter D. Uvea. In: Slatter D, ed., Fundamentals of veterinary ophthalmology. 3rd ed. Philadelphia: WB Saunders, 2001:314–349.
Author Ian P. Herring
Consulting Editor Paul E. Miller

ANTICOAGULANT RODENTICIDE POISONING

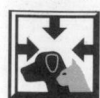

BASICS

DEFINITION
Coagulopathy caused by reduced vitamin K_1–dependent clotting factors in the circulation after exposure to anticoagulant rodenticides

PATHOPHYSIOLOGY
• Inhibits vitamin K_1 epoxide reductase, due to diaphorase, and possibly other enzymes involved in the reduction of vitamin K_1 epoxide to vitamin K_1
• Vitamin K_1—required for carboxylation of clotting factors II, VI, IX, and X; uncarboxylated clotting factors cannot bind calcium and thus are unable to participate in clot formation.

SYSTEMS AFFECTED
Hemic/Lymphatic/Immune—depletion of activated clotting factors, causing hemorrhage

GENETICS
N/A

INCIDENCE/PREVALENCE
Common—many baits are sold over the counter and widely used in homes.

GEOGRAPHIC DISTRIBUTION
None

SIGNALMENT
• Dogs and cats
• No breed, age, or sex predilections

SIGNS

General Comments
• May be slightly more prevalent in the spring and fall when rodenticide products are used

Historical Findings
• Use of anticoagulant rodenticides
• Dyspnea
• Bleeding

Physical Examination Findings
• Hematomas—often ventral and at venipuncture sites
• Muffled heart or lung sounds
• Pale mucous membranes
• Lethargy
• Depression

CAUSES
• Exposure to anticoagulant rodenticide products
• First-generation coumarin anticoagulants (e.g., warfarin, pindone)—largely replaced by more potent second-generation anticoagulants
• Second-generation anticoagulants (e.g., brodifacoum, bromadiolone, diphacinone, and chlorophacinone)—generally more toxic and persist much longer before excretion than are first-generation agents
• Difenthialone (D-Cease)—highly toxic to rats and mice (0.52 mg/kg and 0.47 mg/kg, respectively); less toxic to dogs (LD_{50} 4 mg/kg) than are brodifacoum (LD_{50} 0.25–2.5 mg/kg), bromadiolone (LD_{50} 11–20 mg/kg), chlorophacinone (LD_{50} 50–100 mg/kg), and warfarin (LD_{50} 20–50 mg/kg); similar to diphacinone (LD_{50} 3–7.5 mg/kg); cats, LD_{50} > 16 mg/kg; concentration in baits lower (0.0025%; 25 ppm) than that of other second-generation rodenticide baits (0.005%; 50 ppm), so dogs and cats may tolerate higher intakes.

RISK FACTORS
• Small doses over several days more dangerous than a single large dose; either type of exposure may cause toxicosis.
• Secondary toxicosis by consumption of poisoned rodents—unlikely

DIAGNOSIS

DIFFERENTIAL DIAGNOSIS
• DIC
• Congenital clotting factor deficiencies

CBC/BIOCHEMISTRY/URINALYSIS
Anemia—with marked hemorrhage

OTHER LABORATORY TESTS
• ACT > 150 sec—supports coagulopathy
• Prolonged PT and PTT—support exposure to rodenticide; PT affected earlier than is PTT
• Analysis of blood or liver—confirm exposure to a specific product

IMAGING
Thoracic radiography—may detect hemothorax or hemopericardium

DIAGNOSTIC PROCEDURES
Thoracentesis—dyspneic patients; may confirm hemothorax

PATHOLOGIC FINDINGS
• Free blood in the thoracic cavity, lungs, and abdominal cavity—common
• Hemorrhage into the cranial vault, gastrointestinal tract, and urinary tract—less common; may occur both subcutaneously and intramuscularly

TREATMENT

APPROPRIATE HEALTH CARE
• Inpatient—acute crisis
• Outpatient—consider once the coagulopathy is stabilized

NURSING CARE
Fresh whole blood or plasma transfusion—may be required with hemorrhaging; provides immediate access to vitamin K–dependent clotting factors; whole blood may be preferred with severe anemia from acute or chronic blood loss.

ACTIVITY
Confine patient during the early stages; activity enhances blood loss.

DIET
No recognized effect

CLIENT EDUCATION
Warn client that reexposure could be a serious problem.

SURGICAL CONSIDERATIONS
• Thoracentesis—may be important for removing free thoracic blood, which causes dyspnea and respiratory failure
• Must correct coagulopathy before surgery

MEDICATIONS

DRUG(S) OF CHOICE
Vitamin K_1—2.5–5.0 mg/kg PO q24h 5 days to 6 weeks (depending on the specific product); bioavailability enhanced by the concurrent feeding of a small amount of fat, such as canned dog food
• Vitamin K_1 administration—continued for 3–4 weeks with suspected second-generation anticoagulant toxicosis

CONTRAINDICATIONS
• Vitamin K_3—not efficacious in the treatment of anticoagulant rodenticide toxicosis; contraindicated
• Intravenous vitamin K_1—reported anaphylactic reactions; avoid this route of administration.

PRECAUTIONS
• Avoid unnecessary surgical procedures and parenteral injections.
• Use the smallest possible needle when giving an injection or collecting samples.

POSSIBLE INTERACTIONS
Sulfonamides and phenylbutazone—may displace anticoagulant rodenticides from plasma binding sites, leading to more free toxicant and toxicosis

ALTERNATIVE DRUG(S)
None

FOLLOW-UP

PATIENT MONITORING
ACT and PT—assess efficacy of therapy; monitoring continued 3–5 days after discontinuation of treatment

PREVENTION/AVOIDANCE
Do not allow animals access to anticoagulant rodenticides.

POSSIBLE COMPLICATIONS
May note secondary bacterial pneumonia after intrapulmonary hemorrhage

EXPECTED COURSE AND PROGNOSIS
• Patient survives the first 48 hr of acute coagulopathy—prognosis improves

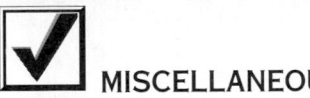

MISCELLANEOUS

ASSOCIATED CONDITIONS
N/A

AGE-RELATED FACTORS
N/A

ZOONOTIC POTENTIAL
N/A

PREGNANCY
Chlorophacinone—may pass into amniotic fluid and on to the fetuses of an exposed pregnant bitch; similar concerns for feeding affected milk to pups

SEE ALSO
Poisoning (Intoxication)

ABBREVIATIONS
• ACT = activated clotting time
• DIC = disseminated intravascular coagulation
• PPT = partial thromboplastin time
• PT = prothrombin time

Suggested Reading
Murphy M, Gerken D. The anticoagulant rodenticides. In: Kirk RW, Bonagura J, eds. Current veterinary therapy X. Philadelphia: Saunders, 1989:143–146.
Author Michael J. Murphy
Consulting Editor Gary D. Osweiler

AORTIC STENOSIS

BASICS

DEFINITION
Narrowing of the left ventricular outflow tract of the heart, most commonly seen as a congenital or perinatal disease. Defect can be valvular, subvalvular (most common in dogs), or supravalvular (most common in cats). As a congenital anomaly in dogs, the obstruction is usually caused by fibrous tissue proximal to the valve, and the disease is referred to as subaortic stenosis (SAS).

PATHOPHYSIOLOGY
Marked aortic obstruction compels the left ventricle to increase intraventricular pressure to maintain forward blood flow and systemic blood pressure. The myocardium compensates by hypertrophy of myocytes leading to thickening of the heart walls. Coronary artery disease, relative cardiac ischemia, arrhythmias, aortic or mitral regurgitation, left-sided congestive heart failure (CHF), and diminished systemic blood flow may result. The mechanism of sudden death is poorly understood.

SYSTEMS AFFECTED
• Cardiovascular—pressure overload of the left ventricle. • Pulmonary—if pulmonary edema develops. • Multisystemic signs may develop secondary to CHF or low cardiac output. If bacterial endocarditis is the cause of the stenosis, the patient may have multisystemic signs due to septic embolization.

GENETICS
Inherited trait in Newfoundland dogs. Polygenic transmission exhibiting pseudodominance; a major dominant gene with modifiers may be involved.

INCIDENCE/PREVALENCE
Approximately 1.5 to 2.0 per 1000 dogs admitted to veterinary teaching institutions; SAS is probably the second most common congenital heart defect in dogs. Approximately 0.2 per 1000 cats admitted to veterinary teaching institutions. In one study, aortic stenosis accounted for 6% of congenital cardiac defects in cats.

SIGNALMENT
Species
Dogs and cats

Breed Predilections
SAS is most common in Newfoundland, German shepherd, golden retriever, Rottweiler, and boxer. Samoyed, English bulldog, and Great Dane also at higher risk than other breeds; bull terriers predisposed to valvular aortic stenosis, typically with concurrent mitral valve dysplasia.

Mean Age and Range
SAS develops postnatally over the first weeks to months of life. Onset of clinical signs can occur at any age depending on the severity of obstruction. Signs may be seen on physical examination without any historical evidence of disease.

SIGNS
Historical Findings
• Related to the severity of obstruction; range from none to CHF, syncope, and sudden death. • Genetic history of affected litters from same sire or bitch.

Physical Examination Findings
• Systolic ejection murmur loudest near the left, fourth intercostal space at the heart base to costochondral junction, which may radiate to the thoracic inlet, carotid arteries, and, if very loud, even to the cranium. Radiation to the left apex and right cranial thorax is common. • Thrill at the left heart base to costochondral junction in some animals. • Diastolic murmur may be heard at the left apex, if aortic regurgitation develops. • Holosystolic murmur at the left apex may be present, if mitral regurgitation develops • Dyspnea, tachypnea, and crackles with the onset of left-sided CHF. • Femoral pulses typically weakened and late rising (pulsus tardus) in animals with disease severe enough to affect hemodynamics. • A left ventricular "heave" (i.e., prolonged and pronounced cardiac impulse palpated on the thorax) in animals with left ventricular hypertrophy. • Arrhythmias.

CAUSES
• Congenital disease • Secondary to bacterial endocarditis of the aortic valve in some dogs. • In cats with hypertrophic cardiomyopathy, functional stenosis (e.g., muscular or subvalvular) is common but significance unknown. • "Dynamic" subaortic stenosis reported in dogs in which muscular hypertrophy can contribute to narrowing of the aortic outflow tract.

RISK FACTORS
• Familial history of subaortic stenosis. • Aortic endocarditis is predisposed by immunosuppression, systemic infection, bacteremia, and abnormal intracardiac blood flow.

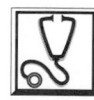

DIAGNOSIS

DIFFERENTIAL DIAGNOSIS
• A systolic ejection murmur may represent an innocent murmur in a young animal; anemia, pain, fever, excitement. Systolic murmurs on the left thorax are commonly caused by patent ductus arteriosus (usually a continuous murmur, but diastolic component may be localized), pulmonic stenosis, mitral regurgitation, ventricular septal defect, atrial septal defect, or tetralogy of Fallot in dogs. Some of these conditions may coexist with SAS. • Weakened pulses may occur in animals with other cardiac conditions in which stroke volume is limited (e.g., pulmonic stenosis and cardiomyopathy) or in animals with aortic obstruction distal to the outflow tract (e.g., aortic coarctation, aortic interruption, and aortic thromboembolism).

CBC/BIOCHEMISTRY/URINALYSIS
Typically normal

IMAGING
Thoracic Radiographic Findings
• May be subtle because myocardial hypertrophy from pressure overload may not increase the size of the cardiac silhouette. • Left-sided heart enlargement, which may appear on lateral radiographs as straightening of the caudal border of the heart. Normal lung fields unless CHF develops causing pulmonary venous distention and interstitial or alveolar pulmonary infiltrates. Mediastinum may be widened and cranial waist of the cardiac silhouette filled as a result of post-stenotic dilation of the aorta.

Echocardiographic Findings
• Spectrum of findings depending on the severity of disease. • Thickening of the left ventricular wall and interventricular septum. • Echogenic ridge and gross narrowing of the left ventricular outflow tract may be visible proximal to the aortic valve in SAS. • Valvular thickening and increased echogenicity for valvular subaortic stenosis, vegetative lesions with endocarditis. • The anterior mitral valve leaflet may also be thickened and echogenic. • Post-stenotic dilation of the aorta in some animals. • Increased echogenicity of the myocardium in some animals, particularly the subendocardial zone and papillary muscles. • "Premature closure" of the aortic valve often seen on M-mode echocardiography.

Doppler Echocardiographic Findings
• High peak ejection velocity (> 2 m/s), which may be delayed to a later time in ejection; flow acceleration proximal to the obstruction, and a jet of turbulent blood flow distal to the valve. • Transvalvular pressure gradient can be estimated from the flow velocity (pressure gradient = 4 × flow velocity squared) with variable accuracy. Color-flow Doppler allows direct visualization of the turbulent jet distal to the obstruction and "flow convergence" proximal.

Angiocardiographic Findings/Cardiac Catheterization
• Contrast radiography shows thickening of the left ventricular wall and septum, narrowing of the left ventricular outflow tract, and post-stenotic dilation of the aorta. Cardiac catheterization allows determination of the transvalvular pressure gradient. Pressure gradients < 50 mm Hg suggest mild disease, 50–75 mm Hg, moderate, 75–100 mm Hg, severe, and > 100 mm Hg, very severe disease. Pressure gradients are greater with increased ejection volume and, therefore, must be interpreted in light of other aspects of cardiac function. Anesthesia depresses myocardial function, so these gradients may underestimate the actual

ones (unanesthetized). • Elevated left ventricular diastolic pressure may accompany loss of ventricular compliance, impending or overt CHF. • Angiocardiography and cardiac catheterization allow characterization of uncommon types of stenosis including valvular, supravalvular, and "tunnel outflow tract" and evaluation of concurrent defects.

DIAGNOSTIC PROCEDURES
Electrocardiographic Findings
• ECG may show signs of left ventricular hypertrophy such as a tall R wave in lead II (> 3.0 mv in dogs), CV6LL (> 3.0 mv in dogs), and others (leads I, III, aVF, CV6LU). • Widening of the QRS complex (> 0.06 sec in dogs) may also be evident. • Mean electrical axis may be shifted to the left (< 40 degrees in dogs) but is typically normal. • Slurring of ST segment consistent with left ventricular hypertrophy or ischemia; ST-segment deviation after mild exercise strongly suggests coronary insufficiency. • Ventricular tachyarrhythmias may occur in severely affected cases and are a potential cause for clinical signs and sudden death. Holter 24 hour ECG monitoring is appropriate in symptomatic or severely affected animals.

TREATMENT

APPROPRIATE HEALTH CARE
Management recommendations for small animals are controversial and vary among experts. Inpatient management appropriate for complications including arrhythmias, episodes of syncope, and CHF

ACTIVITY
Restricted in animals with more than mild disease. Syncope, collapse, or sudden death may be brought on by exertion in animals with severe disease.

DIET
Restricted sodium in animals with overt or impending CHF

CLIENT EDUCATION
• Affected animals should be neutered or otherwise not permitted to breed. • Evaluate closely related dogs for evidence of clinical disease. • Alert owners to potential complications (e.g., sudden death and CHF) in severely affected animals.

SURGICAL CONSIDERATIONS
• Definitive treatment requires open heart surgery with cardiopulmonary bypass to resect, repair (valvuloplasty), or replace (valve replacement) the obstructive lesion. Unfortunately, the risk-to-benefit ratio for open resection of SAS in dogs is not optimal, and dogs still may die suddenly after the procedure. • Balloon dilation of the outflow tract during cardiac catheterization results in acute reduction of transvalvular gradients and

improvement of clinical signs in some symptomatic dogs. Long-term benefits have not been adequately studied in dogs and the procedure is not benign.

MEDICATIONS

DRUG(S) OF CHOICE
• Medical management is, at best, palliative and empirical; no data have been published supporting a specific treatment. • Beta adrenergic blockers have been advocated for dogs with subaortic stenosis with a history of syncope or collapse, a transvalvular pressure gradient > 75 mm Hg, or when ventricular arrhythmias or ST-segment changes are evident on a postexercise ECG. Potential benefits include limitation of myocardial oxygen requirements, protection from ventricular arrhythmias, and slowing of the heart rate. Beta blockers are given to effect; dosage thus depends on the state of the autonomic system. Therapy should be initiated with caution at low dosages and titrated upwards over days to weeks. Propranolol (dogs, 0.2–1.0 mg/kg PO q8h; cats, 2.5–5.0 mg/cat PO q8h–q12h) is the prototype beta blocker. • Specific treatment for ventricular arrhythmias, atrial fibrillation, or left-sided CHF may also be required. Requires careful monitoring (see precautions). • Affected animals are at risk of developing bacterial endocarditis. Meticulous treatment of infections is recommended as is chemoprophylaxis for dental or genitourinary procedures.

CONTRAINDICATIONS
Beta blockers in animals with overt CHF or bronchoconstrictive disorders; discontinue if these complications develop

PRECAUTIONS
• Beta blockers limit the ability of the dysfunctional heart to increase cardiac output, which occurs primarily by an increase in heart rate. • With SAS, the incompliant myocardium is dependent on adequate filling pressure (preload), and overzealous use of diuretics or venodilators may cause a precipitous drop in cardiac output. • Marked reduction of systemic blood pressure by ACE inhibitors, calcium channel blockers, or arteriolar dilators may worsen outflow obstruction or coronary insufficiency. • Digitalis glycosides and positive inotropes may exacerbate outflow obstruction or ventricular arrhythmias. • Anesthetic agents and sedatives with marked hypotensive, arrhythmogenic, or cardiac depressant side effects should be avoided. A narcotic (e.g., butorphanol or oxymorphone) with diazepam for sedation can be combined with low inspired concentrations of isofluorane for anesthesia if necessary.

ALTERNATIVE DRUG(S)
• Metoprolol tartrate (0.5–1.0 mg/kg PO q8–12h for dogs; 2–15 mg/cat PO q8h),

nadolol (0.25–0.5 mg/kg PO q12h), and atenolol (0.25–1.0 mg/kg PO q12h for dogs; 6.25–12.5 mg/cat PO q12–24h) are alternative beta blockers. • Diltiazem (dogs, 0.5–2.0 mg/kg PO q8h for dogs; 7.5–15.0 mg/cat PO q8h) may have similar theoretical benefits in this disease.

FOLLOW-UP

PATIENT MONITORING
Monitor by ECG, thoracic radiography, two-dimensional and Doppler echocardiography. Treatment of complications (e.g., CHF and arrhythmias) necessitates careful monitoring to detect renal/electrolyte, proarrhythmic, negative inotropic, and hypotensive side effects of drugs.

POSSIBLE COMPLICATIONS
CHF, arrhythmias, myocardial infarction, aortic regurgitation, mitral regurgitation, sudden death, bacterial endocarditis

EXPECTED COURSE AND PROGNOSIS
• Mildly affected dogs may live a normal life span without treatment
• Severe disease typically limits longevity.
• CHF suggests severe disease and an ominous prognosis.

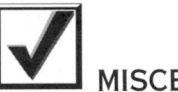

MISCELLANEOUS

ASSOCIATED CONDITIONS
Other cardiac defects

AGE-RELATED FACTORS
Murmur typically not present at birth in SAS; develops in the first weeks to months postnatally along with development of stenotic lesion

PREGNANCY
Contraindicated

SEE ALSO
• Congestive Heart Failure, Left-sided
• Cardiomyopathy, Hypertrophic—Cats
• Cardiomyopathy, Hypertrophic—Dogs
• Endocarditis, Infective

Suggested Reading
Lehmkuhl LB and Bonagura JD. CVT Update: Canine subvalvular aortic stenosis. In: Bonagura JD, Kirk RW, eds. Kirk's current veterinary therapy XII. Philadelphia: Saunders, 1995
Sisson DD, Thomas WP, Bonagura JD. Congenital Heart Disease. In: Ettinger SJ, Feldman EC, eds. Textbook of veterinary internal medicine. 5th ed. Philadelphia: Saunders, 2000:737–787.
Author Donald J. Brown
Consulting Editors Larry P. Tilley and Francis W. K. Smith, Jr.

AORTIC THROMBOEMBOLISM

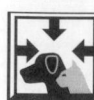 BASICS

DEFINITION

Aortic thromboembolism (ATE) results from a thrombus or blood clot that is dislodged within the aorta, causing severe ischemia to the tissues served by that segment of aorta.

PATHOPHYSIOLOGY

• ATE is most commonly associated with myocardial disease in cats, including hypertrophic, restrictive, and dilated cardiomyopathy. It is theorized that abnormal blood flow (stasis) and a hypercoaguable state contribute to the formation of the thrombus within the left atrium. The blood clot is then embolized distally to the aorta. The most common site of embolization is the caudal aorta trifurcation (hind legs). Other less common sites include the front leg, kidneys, gastrointestinal tract, or cerebrum. • ATE in dogs typically is associated with neoplasia, sepsis, Cushing's disease, protein-losing nephropathy, or other hypercoaguable states.

SYSTEMS AFFECTED

• Cardiovascular—the majority of affected cats have advanced heart disease and left heart failure. • Nervous/musculoskeletal—severe ischemia to the muscles and nerves served by the segment of occluded aorta causes variable pain and paresis. Gait abnormalities or paralysis results in the leg or legs involved.

GENETICS

N/A

INCIDENCE/PREVALENCE

• Prevalence of ATE is not known in the general population of cats. In one study of cats with hypertrophic cardiomyopathy, 12% presented with signs of ATE. In a retrospective study of 100 cats with ATE, only 11% of cats had previous evidence of heart disease. • Rare in dogs.

GEOGRAPHIC DISTRIBUTION

N/A

SIGNALMENT

Species

Cats, rarely dogs

Breed Predilections

None

Mean Age and Range

Age distribution is 1–20 years. The median age is 10.5 years; the mean age is 7.7 years.

Predominant Sex

Males are more commonly affected than females (2:1).

SIGNS

Historical Findings

• Acute onset paralysis and pain are the most common complaints. • Lameness or a gait abnormality • Tachypnea or respiratory distress is common. • Vocalization and anxiety are common.

Physical Examination Findings

• Usually paraparesis or paralysis of the rear legs with signs of lower motor neuron injury. Less commonly, monoparesis of a front leg. • Pain upon palpation of the legs. • Gastrocnemius muscle often becomes firm several hours after embolization. • Absent or diminished femoral pulses • Cyanotic or pale nail beds and foot pads • Cardiac murmur or gallop sound • Tachypnea or dyspnea • Cardiac arrhythmias

CAUSES

• Cardiomyopathy • Neoplasia • Sepsis • Hyperadrenocorticism (dogs) • Protein-losing nephropathy (dogs)

RISK FACTORS

It is theorized that an enlarged left atrium or spontaneous echo contrast (smoke) observed on an echocardiogram may be risk factors.

 DIAGNOSIS

DIFFERENTIAL DIAGNOSIS

Hind limb paresis secondary to other causes such as spinal neoplasia, trauma, myelitis, fibrocartilaginous infarction, or intervertebral disk protrusion. These conditions resulting in spinal cord injury present with signs of upper motor neuron disease, whereas ATE patients present with signs of lower motor neuron disease.

CBC/BIOCHEMISTRY/URINALYSIS

• High creatine kinase as a result of muscle injury. • High aspartate aminotransferase and alanine aminotransferase as a result of muscle and liver injury. • Hyperglycemia secondary to stress. • Mild increases in blood urea nitrogen and creatinine as a result of low cardiac output and renal emboli. • CBC and urinalysis changes are nonspecific.

OTHER LABORATORY TESTS

Coagulation profile typically does not reveal significant abnormalities because the hypercoagulability results from hyperaggregable platelets.

IMAGING

Radiographic Findings

• Cardiomegaly in 85–90% of cats. • Pulmonary edema and/or pleural effusion in approximately 66% of cats.

Echocardiographic Findings

• The majority of cats have hypertrophic cardiomyopathy characterized by left ventricular hypertrophy, nondilated left ventricular lumen, large left atrium, and hypercontractility.

• The second most common echocardiographic diagnosis is restrictive cardiomyopathy. • Dilated cardiomyopathy also can be seen. • Regardless of the type of myocardial disease present, the majority (> 50%) have severe left atrial enlargement, i.e., a left atrial to aortic ratio of 2.0 or greater. • Occasionally, a left atrial thrombus or spontaneous echo contrast (smoke) may be seen.

Abdominal Ultrasonographic Findings

May be able to identify the thrombus in the caudal aorta. This imaging modality typically is not necessary to reach a diagnosis.

Angiographic Findings

Nonselective angiography should identify a negative filling defect in the caudal aorta representing the thrombus. This test usually not necessary to reach a diagnosis.

DIAGNOSTIC PROCEDURES

Electrocardiography

• The most common rhythms are sinus rhythm and sinus tachycardia. Less common rhythms include atrial fibrillation, ventricular arrhythmias, supraventricular arrhythmias, and sinus bradycardia. • Left ventricular enlargement pattern and left ventricular conduction disturbances (left anterior fascicular block) are common.

PATHOLOGIC FINDINGS

• Thrombus typically is identified at the caudal aortic trifurcation. • Occasionally, a left atrial thrombus is seen. • Emboli of the kidneys, gastrointestinal tract, cerebrum, and other organs also may be seen.

 TREATMENT

APPROPRIATE HEALTH CARE

Initially, cats with ATE should be treated as inpatients because most have concurrent congestive heart failure and require injectable drugs.

NURSING CARE

• Fluid therapy is rarely necessary as most cats are in congestive heart failure. • Supplemental oxygen therapy or thoracocentesis may be beneficial if in congestive heart failure. • Initially, the affected legs should be minimally handled. However as reperfusion occurs, physical therapy (passive extension and flexion of the legs) may speed full recovery. • No venipuncture should be performed on the affected legs. • Initially, these cats may have difficulty posturing to urinate and may need to have their bladders expressed to prevent overdistention or urine scald.

ACTIVITY

Activity should be restricted. The cat should be kept quiet and stress-free.

DIET
• Initially, most cats are anorexic. Tempt these cats with any type of diet. It is important to keep these cats eating to avoid hepatic lipodosis.
• Chronic dietary management usually involves sodium restriction.

CLIENT EDUCATION
• Owners should be aware of the poor short- and long-term prognosis.
• Most cats will re-embolize. Most cats that survive an initial episode will be on some type of anticoagulant therapy that may require frequent reevaluations and an indoor lifestyle.
• Most cats that survive an initial episode will recover complete function to the legs; however, if ischemia was severe and prolonged, sloughing of parts of the distal extremities or persistent neurological deficits may result.

SURGICAL CONSIDERATIONS
Surgical embolectomy typically is not recommended because these patients are high risks for surgery as a result of their heart disease.

MEDICATIONS

DRUG(S) OF CHOICE
• Thrombolytic therapy such as streptokinase and tissue plasminogen activator is used extensively in humans and infrequently in cats. These drugs are prohibitively expensive and carry a significant risk for bleeding complications and thus are rarely used in general practice.
• Heparin is the preferred drug in general practice. It has no effect on the established clot; however, it prevents further activation of the coagulation cascade. An initial dose of 100–200 units/kg is given intravenously and then followed with 200–300 units/kg SC q8h. Alternatively, heparin can be administered as a CRI, if there is concern about adequate bioavailability via the SC route of administration, at a dose of 25 units/kg/hr. The dose is then titrated to prolong the activated partial thromboplastin time (APTT) approximately twofold.
• Aspirin is theoretically beneficial during and after an episode of thromboembolism because of its antiplatelet effects. The dose is an 81-mg tablet PO every second or third day.
• Butorphenol may be used for analgesia at a dose of 0.1–0.4 mg/kg SC or IV q6–8h. For stronger analgesia, fentanyl or hydromorphone could be used instead of butorphenol.
• Acepromazine may be used for its sedative and vasodilatory properties at a dose of 0.1–0.5 mg SC q8–12 h.

• Warfarin, a vitamin K antagonist, is the anticoagulant most widely used in humans and has been proposed for prevention of reembolization in cats surviving an initial episode. The initial dose is 0.25–0.5 mg PO q24h. It should be overlapped with heparin therapy for 3 days. The dose is then adjusted to prolong the prothrombin time (PT) approximately two times its baseline value or to attain an international normalized ratio (INR) of 2.0–4.0. Long-term management with warfarin can be challenging because of frequent monitoring and dose adjustments in addition to adverse effects such as bleeding.
• Low molecular weight heparin (LMWH) has recently been proposed for the long-term prevention of feline ATE. LMWH has a more predictable relationship between dose and response than warfarin and does not need monitoring or dose adjustments. It also has a lower risk of bleeding complication. The main disadvantage of LMWH is high drug cost and the injectable route of administration. The two LMWHs that have been used in feline ATE are:
—Dalteparin 100 units/kg SC q24h (can increase to q12h)
—Enoxaparin 1 mg/kg SC q12–24h
• Treatment of the patient's heart disease

CONTRAINDICATIONS
N/A

PRECAUTIONS
• Anticoagulant therapy with heparin, warfarin, or the thrombolytic drugs may cause bleeding complications.
• Avoid a nonselective beta-blocker such as propranolol as it may enhance peripheral vasoconstriction.

POSSIBLE INTERACTIONS
Warfarin may interact with other drugs, which may enhance its anticoagulant effects.

ALTERNATIVE DRUG(S)
N/A

FOLLOW-UP

PATIENT MONITORING
• Examine the legs daily to assess clinical response. Initially, APTT should be performed once daily to titrate the heparin dose.
• If warfarin is used, PT or INR is measured approximately 3 days after initiation of therapy and then weekly until the desired anticoagulant effect is reached. Thereafter, it could be measured 3–4 times yearly or when drug regimen is altered.

PREVENTION/AVOIDANCE
Because of the high rate of re-embolization, prevention with either chronic aspirin, warfarin, or LMWH is strongly recommended.

POSSIBLE COMPLICATIONS
• Bleeding with the anticoagulant therapy
• Permanent neurological deficits or muscular abnormalities in the hind limbs may arise in cats with prolonged ischemia.
• Recurrent congestive heart failure or sudden death

EXPECTED COURSE AND PROGNOSIS
• Expected course is days to weeks for full recovery of function to the legs.
• Prognosis in general is poor. In one study of 100 cats, approximately 60–70% of cats were euthanized or died during the initial thromboembolic episode. Long-term prognosis varies between 2 months to several years; however, the average is approximately a few months with treatment.
• Recurrence of ATE is common.

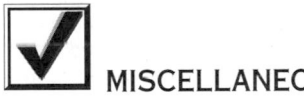

MISCELLANEOUS

ASSOCIATED CONDITIONS
See causes and risk factors.

AGE-RELATED FACTORS
N/A

ZOONOTIC POTENTIAL
N/A

PREGNANCY
N/A

SYNONYMS
Saddle thromboembolism
Systemic thromboembolism

SEE ALSO
Cardiomyopathy, Hypertrophic—Cats
Cardiomyopathy, Restrictive—Cats
Cardiomyopathy, Dilated—Cats

ABBREVIATIONS
• ATE = aortic thromboembolism
• CRI = constant rate infusion
• LMWH = low molecular weight heparin

Suggested Reading

Laste NJ, Harpster NK. A retrospective study of 100 cats with feline distal aortic thromboembolism: 1977–1993. J Am An Hosp Assoc 1995;31:492–500.

Miller WP, Sisson DD. Myocardial diseases. In: Ettinger SJ, Feldman EC, eds. Textbook of Veterinary Internal Medicine. 4th ed. Philadelphia: WB Saunders, 1995.

Author Teresa C. DeFrancesco

Consulting Editors Larry P. Tilley and Francis W. K. Smith, Jr.

APUDOMA

BASICS

OVERVIEW
- Tumors of endocrine cells that are capable of amine precursor uptake and decarboxylation (APUD) and secretion of peptide hormones; the tumors are named after the hormone they secrete.
- APUD cells are generally found in the gastrointestinal tract and CNS.
- Gastrin- and pancreatic polypeptide-secreting tumors are discussed here; insulinoma and glucagonoma are discussed separately.
- Hypergastrinemia from gastrin-secreting tumors causes gastritis and duodenal hyperacidity, which can cause gastric ulceration, esophageal dysfunction from chronic reflux, and intestinal villous atrophy.
- High concentration of pancreatic polypeptide also causes gastric hyperacidity and its consequences.

SIGNALMENT
- Gastrinoma—rare in dogs and cats; age range 3–12 years, mean 7.5 years (dogs)
- Pancreatic polypeptide—extremely rare in dogs

SIGNS
- Vomiting
- Weight loss
- Anorexia
- Diarrhea
- Lethargy, depression
- Polydipsia
- Melena
- Abdominal pain
- Hematemesis
- Hematochezia
- Fever

CAUSES & RISK FACTORS
Unknown

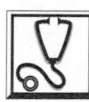

DIAGNOSIS

DIFFERENTIAL DIAGNOSIS
Other conditions associated with hypergastrinemia, gastric hyperacidity, and gastrointestinal ulceration
- Uremia
- Hepatic failure
- Drug-induced ulceration (e.g., NSAIDs or steroids)

- Inflammatory gastritis
- Stress-induced ulceration
- Mast cell disease

CBC/BIOCHEMISTRY/URINALYSIS
- Normal or reflect the chronic effects of general disease
- Iron-deficiency anemia secondary to gastrointestinal bleeding
- Increased BUN secondary to gastrointestinal bleeding
- Hypoproteinemia
- Electrolyte abnormalities with chronic vomiting

OTHER LABORATORY TESTS
- Serum gastrin concentration normal or high normal in patients with gastrinoma
- Provocative test of gastrin secretion—increased gastrin concentration after intravenous calcium gluconate or secretin administration suggests gastrinoma; see Appendix for protocol and interpretation.

IMAGING
Abdominal ultrasound sometimes demonstrates a pancreatic mass but is usually normal.

DIAGNOSTIC PROCEDURES
- Endoscopy with gastric and duodenal biopsy
- Aspirate any detectable masses because of suspicion of mast cell disease.
- If no detectable masses exist, examine a buffy coat smear for mast cells.

PATHOLOGIC FINDINGS
- Endoscopic biopsy reveals gastrointestinal ulceration.
- Histopathologic examination of pancreatic tumors reveals findings consistent with islet cell tumor but not specific for hormone type.
- Immunocytochemical staining can aid in the specific diagnosis.
- Histopathologic examination also can reveal metastasis to liver and regional lymph nodes.

TREATMENT
- Tell owner that most APUDomas are malignant and have metastasized by the time of diagnosis and that long-term control is often difficult.
- Aggressive medical management can sometimes palliate signs for months to years.
- Surgical exploration and excisional biopsy of a pancreatic mass are important both diagnostically and therapeutically.
- Medical management is useful for gastric hyperacidity.

MEDICATIONS

DRUG(S)
- Histamine H_2-receptor antagonists—cimetidine, ranitidine, and famotidine; decrease acid secretion by gastric parietal cells
- Omeprazole—a proton pump inhibitor; the most potent inhibitor of gastric acid secretion available; highly effective and expensive
- Sucralfate—adheres to ulcerated gastric mucosa and protects it from acid; promotes healing by binding pepsin and bile acids and stimulating local prostaglandins

CONTRAINDICATIONS/POSSIBLE INTERACTIONS
None

FOLLOW-UP

PATIENT MONITORING
- Physical examination and clinical signs are the most useful measures of treatment effectiveness and disease progression.
- Gastroscopy can monitor progression of gastritis, but it is not necessary.
- Abdominal radiography or ultrasound may detect development of abdominal masses.

EXPECTED COURSE AND PROGNOSIS
- Difficult to predict
- Patients with gastrinoma have been controlled on medical management for months to years.
- No cure available

MISCELLANEOUS

SEE ALSO
Gastroduodenal Ulcer Disease

ABBREVIATION
APUD = amine precursor uptake and decarboxylation
NSAIDS = nonsteroidal antiinflammatory drugs

Suggested Reading
Zerbe CA. Islet cell tumors secreting insulin, pancreatic polypeptide, gastrin, or glucagon. In: Kirk RW, Bonagura JD, eds. Current veterinary therapy XI. Philadelphia: Saunders, 1992:368–375.
Author Thomas K. Graves
Consulting Editor Deborah S. Greco

BASICS

OVERVIEW
• Caused by herbicides, insecticides, wood preservatives, and treatments for blood parasites
• Leads to disruption of many important metabolic reactions
• Exposure—oral most common; percutaneous exposure may cause systemic toxicosis.

SIGNALMENT
Cats and dogs

SIGNS

Acute Exposure
• Abdominal pain
• Vomiting
• Weakness
• Diarrhea
• Hematochezia
• Rapid weak pulse
• Prostration
• Subnormal temperature
• Collapse
• Death

Subchronic to Chronic Oral Exposure
• Anorexia
• Weight loss

CAUSES & RISK FACTORS
• Oral, percutaneous, or therapeutic exposure to arsenic-containing compounds
• Toxicity varies greatly.
• Weak and debilitated animals more susceptible

DIAGNOSIS

DIFFERENTIAL DIAGNOSIS
• Heavy metal toxicosis
• Ingestion of caustic agents
• Ingestion of irritating plants
• Canine or feline parvovirus

CBC/BIOCHEMISTRY/URINALYSIS
Serum biochemical analysis—liver and renal damage

OTHER LABORATORY TESTS
Arsenic concentration—test urine, vomitus, or stomach contents (acute poisoning), kidney, liver (subacute), hair (chronic); decreases dramatically in urine, kidney, and liver 1–2 days after exposure; unreliable in blood

IMAGING
N/A

DIAGNOSTIC PROCEDURES
N/A

PATHOLOGIC FINDINGS
• Peracute poisoning—death without lesions
• Gastrointestinal tract lesions—common and severe; reddening of the gastric mucosa and proximal small intestine; watery gastrointestinal content; blood and sloughed mucosa in feces
• Liver—soft, yellow liver
• Lungs—congested; edematous
• Skin lesions (cutaneous exposure)—blistering; edema; cracking; bleeding; secondary infections

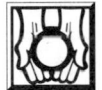

TREATMENT
• Remove arsenic source.
• Gastric lavage—if vomiting has not occurred
• Promote excretion.
• Dialysis in cases of renal failure
• Appropriate fluid therapy
• Kaolin-pectin soothes gastrointestinal tract.
• Keep patient warm and comfortable.
• Diet—when patient is able to keep food down, provide small amounts of high-quality food; increase as tolerated.

MEDICATIONS

DRUG(S)

Dimercaprol (BAL)
• Give 2.5–5 mg/kg in oil by deep IM injection q4h for 2 days; q8h on day 3; q12h for up to 10 days; 5 mg/kg in only acutely affected patients on day 1.

• Signs of toxicosis (vomiting, tremors, convulsions) subside as BAL is excreted over 3–4 hr.
• Releases arsenic, which may worsen signs; give additional BAL.

Other Drugs
• DMSA—less toxic than BAL; effective in laboratory animals and humans
• Emetics
• Strong cathartics
• Parasympathomimetic drugs

FOLLOW-UP
• Prognosis is grave with high-dose exposure, unless the diagnosis is made and treatment is started early.
• Monitor closely for signs of BAL toxicosis.

MISCELLANEOUS

SEE ALSO
Poisoning (Intoxication)

ABBREVIATIONS
• BAL = British anti-Lewisite
• DMSA = 2,3-dimercaptosuccinic acid

Suggested Reading
Hatch RC. Poisons causing abdominal distress of liver or kidney damage. In: Booth NH, McDonald LE, eds. Veterinary pharmacology and therapeutics. 6th ed. Ames: Iowa State University Press, 1988:1102–1125.
Neiger RD. Arsenic. In: Peterson ME, Talcott PA, eds. Small animal toxicology. Philadelphia: Saunders, 2001:420–430.
Author Regg D. Neiger
Consulting Editor Gary D. Osweiler

ARTERIOVENOUS FISTULA

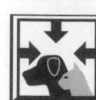

BASICS

OVERVIEW
An abnormal, low resistance connection between an artery and vein. A large arteriovenous fistula allows a significant fraction of the total cardiac output to bypass the capillary bed. The resulting increase in cardiac output may lead to "high output" congestive heart failure (CHF). Location of arteriovenous fistula varies. Reported sites include the head, neck, ear, tongue, limbs, flank, spinal cord, cerebrum, lung, liver, vena cava, and gastrointestinal tract. Usually seen as an acquired lesion.

SIGNALMENT
• Dogs and cats (rare in both).
• No specific age, breed, or sex predilections known

SIGNS

Historical Findings
• Animals with acquired disease often have a history of trauma to the affected area.
• Owner may notice a warm, nonpainful swelling at the site.
• History consistent with impending or overt CHF is possible depending on shunt size and duration.
• Other historical findings depend on the location of the lesion. The shunt may cause local organ dysfunction.

Physical Examination Findings
• Vary and depend on location of the arteriovenous fistula.
• Signs of CHF (e.g., coughing, dyspnea, tachypnea, and exercise intolerance) may develop in animals with long-standing disease and high blood flow.
• Bounding pulses are present in some animals because of high ejection volume and rapid runoff through the arteriovenous fistula.
• Continuous murmur (bruit) at the site caused by blood flow through the lesion.
• Cautious compression of the artery proximal to the lesion abolishes the bruit. When blood flow is high, this compression may also elicit an immediate reflex decrease in heart rate (Branham's sign).
• Edema, ischemia, and congestion of organs and tissues caused by high venous pressure in the proximity of the lesion.
• If the lesion is on a limb, pitting edema, lameness, ulceration, scabbing, and gangrene may result.

• Lesion near vital organs may cause signs associated with organ failure such as ascites (liver), seizures (brain), paresis (spinal cord), and dyspnea (lung).

CAUSES & RISK FACTORS
• Rarely, a congenital lesion
• Acquired arteriovenous fistula typically results from local damage to vasculature secondary to trauma, surgery, venipuncture, perivascular injection (e.g., barbiturates), or tumor.

DIAGNOSIS

DIFFERENTIAL DIAGNOSIS
• The lesion may look like an aneurysm or false aneurysm.
• Bizarre clinical findings, depending on location of arteriovenous fistula, may suggest other disease processes; arteriovenous fistula may be a late diagnostic consideration.

CBC/BIOCHEMISTRY/URINALYSIS
May reflect damage to systems in the vicinity of the lesion, i.e., biochemical abnormalities suggesting hepatic, renal, or other organ dysfunction are possible.

OTHER LABORATORY TESTS
N/A

IMAGING

Thoracic Radiographic Findings
Cardiac enlargement and pulmonary over-circulation in some animals with hemodynamically significant arteriovenous fistula.

Echocardiographic Findings
• May allow imaging of the arteriovenous fistula depicting its cavernous nature.
• Doppler ultrasound may demonstrate high velocity, turbulent flow within the lesion.

Angiography
Selective angiography outlines the lesion, may be necessary for definitive diagnosis, and is highly desirable for presurgical evaluation. Placement of the catheter close to the lesion and rapid injection is necessary; high volume blood flow dilutes the contrast medium quickly.

DIAGNOSTIC PROCEDURES
N/A

TREATMENT
• Definitive treatment requires surgery to divide and remove abnormal vascular connections. Surgery is recommended in animals with clinical signs related to the arteriovenous fistula, since lesions may increase in size.
• Surgery can be difficult and labor intensive and may require blood transfusion; delineation of lesion before surgery by angiography is advised.
• Although surgery is often successful, arteriovenous fistula may recur. In some animals, amputation of the affected part may be necessary.

MEDICATIONS

DRUG(S)
• Concurrent medical treatment depends on the site of the arteriovenous fistula and secondary clinical features.
• Medical treatment for congestive heart failure may be required before surgery.

CONTRAINDICATIONS/POSSIBLE INTERACTIONS
Avoid excessive fluid administration; animals with arteriovenous fistula are volume overloaded.

FOLLOW-UP
Postoperative reevaluation is needed to determine whether arteriovenous fistula recurred.

MISCELLANEOUS

SEE ALSO
Congestive Heart Failure, Left-sided

Suggested Reading
Suter PF, Fox PR. Peripheral vascular disease. In: Ettinger SJ, Feldman EC, eds. Textbook of veterinary internal medicine. 4th ed. Philadelphia: WB Saunders, 1995.

Author Donald J. Brown
Consulting Editors Larry P. Tilley and Francis W. K. Smith, Jr.

ARTERIOVENOUS MALFORMATION OF THE LIVER

BASICS

OVERVIEW
Intrahepatic arteriovenous (AV) fistulae are communications between proper hepatic arteries and intrahepatic portal veins. They create hepatofugal blood flow with retrograde blood flow from hepatic artery to portal system. They are uncommon and are associated with multiple APSS.

SIGNALMENT
• Dogs and, less commonly, cats • Age-related presentation (congenital): < 2 yrs • No sex or breed predilection

SIGNS

General Comments
Development of acute illness and presentation for signs of portal hypertension and APSS

Historical Findings
• Normal transition to growth foods, unlike dogs with PSVA • Acute onset of ascites or hepatic encephalopathy reflects APSS. • Lethargy, anorexia, vomiting, diarrhea, weight loss, polydipsia, dementia, abdominal distention

Physical Examination Findings
• Lethargic, poor body condition, ascites; enlarged liver segment containing AV fistula(e) rarely palpated • Hepatic bruit rarely ausculted

CAUSES & RISK FACTORS
• Usually reflect congenital vascular malformations (multiple vessels); failure of differentiation of common embryologic anlage • May be induced by abdominal trauma, inflammation, neoplasia, surgical interventions, or diagnostic procedures (e.g., liver biopsy) • Portal hypertension due to arterialization of the valveless portal system—results in establishing APSS

DIAGNOSIS

DIFFERENTIAL DIAGNOSIS
• Central nervous system signs—infectious disorders (e.g., distemper); toxicities (e.g., lead); hydrocephalus; idiopathic epilepsy; metabolic disorders (e.g., hypoglycemia, hypo/hyperkalemia); hepatic encephalopathy (e.g., severe liver disease); PSVA; symptomatic MVD; urea cycle enzyme deficiencies • Ascites—pure transudate (protein-losing nephropathy, protein-losing enteropathy, liver disease); modified transudate (congenital cardiac malformations, right-sided heart failure, pericardial tamponade, supradiaphragmatic vena caval obstruction, neoplasia, portal vein thrombosis); hemorrhage • Portal hypertension—chronic hepatic disease, juvenile fibrosing liver disease, noncirrhotic portal hypertension, idiopathic portal hypertension, cirrhosis, portal thrombi

CBC/BIOCHEMISTRY/URINALYSIS
• Erythrocyte microcytosis, target cells • Hypoalbuminemia; serum globulin normal or low; ALP and ALT activity moderately increased; variable low BUN and hypocholesterolemia • Hyposthenuria or isosthenuria; inconsistent ammonium biurate crystalluria

OTHER LABORATORY TESTS
• Coagulation tests—variable abnormalities; prolonged buccal mucosal bleeding times indicate high risk for bleeding • Peritoneal fluid analysis—pure transudate (total protein < 2.5 g/dL) or modified transudate • Total serum bile acids—fasting values increased in most cases; postprandial values always increased • Plasma ammonia concentration—usually abnormal; inconsistent in reliability

IMAGING

Radiography
• Abdominal effusion • Microhepatica or normal size due to large liver lobe associated with AV fistulae • Renomegaly • Normal thorax

Abdominal Ultrasonography
• Abdominal effusion • Liver lobe with AV fistula large compared with other lobes, which are smaller than normal • Diminished portal blood flow in most liver lobes • Tortuous anechoic tubular structures (AV fistulae) display unidirectional or turbulent flow with Doppler interrogation • Hepatic artery and/or portal vein branches may appear tortuous • Hepatofugal portal flow through multiple APSS • Renomegaly • Calculi or sand-like uroliths: urinary bladder or renal pelvis • Rules out portal thrombosis

Contrast Angiography
• Venous portography—demonstrates APSS • Hepatic arteriography—required to demonstrate AV communication (celiac trunk or anterior mesenteric artery contrast injections)

Echocardiography
To rule out right-sided heart disease, pericardial disease, and vena caval occlusion

DIAGNOSTIC PROCEDURES
• Exploratory laparotomy • Liver biopsy—samples from affected and unaffected liver lobes

TREATMENT

APPROPRIATE HEALTH CARE
Inpatient for hepatic encephalopathy and treatment of ascites prior to AV fistula resection

NURSING CARE
• Diet—restrict nitrogen intake to ameliorate hepatic encephalopathy and hyperammonemia; restrict sodium (ascites) • Hepatic encephalopathy—resolve endoparasitism and electrolyte and hydration disturbances, treat infections, initiate treatments to alter enteric uptake and formation of hepatic encephalopathic toxins. • Ascites—mobilize by restricting activity and sodium intake; abdominocentesis for tense ascites impairing ventilation or nutrition

SURGICAL CONSIDERATIONS
• Resection of liver lobe containing AV fistula • Do not ligate APSS.

MEDICATIONS

DRUG(S)

Hepatic Encephalopathy
See Hepatic Encephalopathy

Ascites
• Furosemide (0.5–2 mg/kg PO IM or IV q12–24h)—best used combined with spironolactone • Spironolactone (0.5–2 mg/kg PO q12h)—initiate double dose as loading dose one time • Chronic diuretic therapy individualized to response, 4–7 day intervals

Bleeding Tendencies
See Coagulopathy of Liver Disease

Gastrointestinal Hemorrhage
• Histamine type-2 receptor antagonists (famotidine 0.5 mg/kg PO, IV, or SC q12–24h); give indefinitely, gastrointestinal bleeding and ulceration are common, long-term problems • Gastroprotectant—sucralfate 0.25 g/10 kg PO q8–12h • Eliminate endoparasitism

CONTRAINDICATIONS
Avoid drugs that rely on hepatic biotransformation and drugs that react with GABA-benzodiazepine receptors

FOLLOW-UP

PATIENT MONITORING
Biochemistry—initially bi-monthly to monthly until stabilized, thereafter q4–6 months; monitor for continued hepatic encephalopathy and insufficiency

EXPECTED COURSE AND PROGNOSIS
• Prognosis fair if patient survives surgical resection of AV fistula • May require indefinite nutritional and medical management (hepatic encephalopathy, ascites) • Microscopic vascular lesions may exist in all liver lobes and APSS persist.

MISCELLANEOUS

SEE ALSO
• Ascites • Hepatic Encephalopathy • Hypertension, Portal • Portosystemic Shunting, Acquired • Portosystemic Vascular Anomaly, Congenital

ABBREVIATIONS
• APSS = acquired portosystemic shunt • DDAVP = deamino-8-D-arginine vasopressin • GABA = γ-aminobutyric acid • MVD = microvascular dysplasia • PSVA = portosystemic vascular anomalies
Author Sharon A. Center
Consulting Editor Sharon A. Center

ARTHRITIS (DEGENERATIVE JOINT DISEASE)

 BASICS

DEFINITION
Degenerative joint disease (DJD) is the progressive and permanent deterioration of the articular cartilage of diarthrodial (synovial) joints due to primary (idiopathic) and secondary causes.

PATHOPHYSIOLOGY
• DJD is classified as a noninflammatory joint disease because the initial disease process is not driven by inflammatory mediators; however, inflammation is strongly correlated with the progression of DJD. • Metalloproteinases, serine proteases, and cysteine protease enzymes are released from damaged chondrocytes, causing collagen degradation and loss of collagen cross-linking in cartilage. • Collagen synthesis is altered by production of an abnormal type XI collagen and ratio of type II collagen, resulting in decreased collagen/proteoglycan interaction and weakened collagen structure. • Cartilage matrix is further weakened by increased breakdown of proteoglycans and production of structurally abnormal proteoglycans. • Nitric oxide (NO) is also released, which mediates cartilage breakdown and supports chronic inflammation. Chondrocyte apoptosis is mediated by cyclooxygenase-2 enzymes and inducible NO synthase. • Inflammation causes decreased elasticity and viscosity of the synovial fluid, resulting in increased contact friction and pain. • Subchondral bone becomes sclerotic, reducing bone elasticity and worsening mechanical impact on articular cartilage. • Pain of DJD results from stimulation of Aδ and C fibers in the tendons, ligament, subchondral bone, and joint capsule. Pain is chemically mediated by prostaglandins, leukotrienes, substance P, bradykinin, and cytokines. • The result of these processes is progressive cartilage degradation ranging from fibrillation to deep fissuring of cartilage. Full thickness cartilage loss can eventually occur.

SYSTEMS AFFECTED
Musculoskeletal—diarthrodial joints

GENETICS
• Primary DJD has been associated with a colony of beagles. • Dogs—causes of secondary DJD are likely inheritable, including elbow dysplasia in rottweilers, osteochondrosis dissecans in Bernese mountain dogs, hip dysplasia in large-breed (e.g., German shepherds, Labradors) and small-breed dogs (e.g., cocker spaniels, Shetland sheepdogs), patellar luxation in small and miniature-breed dogs, congenital shoulder luxation and elbow luxation in small-breed dogs. • Cats—causes of secondary DJD are likely inheritable, such as patellar luxation in the Devon rex, hip dysplasia in Siamese and other breeds, and arthropathy in Scottish folds.

INCIDENCE/PREVALENCE
• Dogs—likely the most common skeletal disease; estimated that 20% of dogs older than 1 year have some degree of DJD. Actual incidence unknown. • Cats—one study reported that of 100 cats over 12 years of age presenting for nonmusculoskeletal disease, 90% had evidence of osteoarthritis on radiographs. Actual incidence unknown. • Secondary DJD is much more common than primary DJD.

SIGNALMENT
Species Dogs and cats

Breed Predilections None

Mean Age and Range
• Primary—usually older animals • Hereditary and congenital disorders, such as osteochondrosis, seen in immature animals; hip dysplasia can present bimodally at young and old age • Trauma induced—any age

Predominant Sex None

SIGNS
Historical Findings
Dogs
• Decrease in activity level or willingness to perform certain tasks; intermittent lameness or stiff gait that slowly becomes more severe and frequent • May have a history of previous joint trauma, osteochondral disease, or developmental disorder • May be exacerbated by exercise, long periods of recumbency, and cold weather
Cats
• Overt lameness may not be noted. • May have difficulty grooming, jumping onto furniture, or getting in and out of the litter box; overall increase in irritability

Physical Examination Findings
• Stiffness of gait • Altered gait (e.g., bunny hopping in hip dysplasia) • Lameness • Decreased range of motion • Crepitus • Joint swelling (effusion and thickening of the joint capsule) • Joint pain • Joint instability (ligament tears, subluxation), depending on duration of disease • Gross joint deformity

CAUSES
• Articular cartilage has limited ability to repair and regenerate in response to low-grade wear and tear, trauma, instability, abnormal weight bearing, abnormalities in cartilage structure, or joint incongruity. • Primary—thought to be the result of long-term use combined with aging; no known predisposing cause • Secondary—results from an initiating cause: abnormal wear on normal cartilage (e.g., joint instability, joint incongruity, trauma to cartilage or supporting soft tissues) or normal wear on abnormal cartilage (e.g., osteochondral defects)

RISK FACTORS
• Working, athletic, and obese dogs place more stress on their joints. • Dogs with Cushing's disease, diabetes mellitus, or hypothyroidism may be more prone owing to decreased anabolic capability and increased catabolic processes.

 DIAGNOSIS

DIFFERENTIAL DIAGNOSIS
• Neoplastic (synovial cell sarcoma; rarely, chondrosarcoma; osteosarcoma) • Infectious arthritis (caused by bacteria; spirochetes; L-forms in cats; *Mycoplasma*; *Rickettsia*; *Ehrlichia*; viruses, such as feline calicivirus; fungi, and protozoa) • Immune mediated (erosive vs. nonerosive)

CBC/BIOCHEMISTRY/URINALYSIS N/A

OTHER LABORATORY TESTS
• Coombs' test, ANA, and rheumatoid factor may help to rule out immune-mediated arthritis. • Serum titers for *Borrelia*, *Ehrlichia*, and *Rickettsia* to evaluate for infectious arthritis

IMAGING
• Radiographic changes—include joint capsular distention, osteophytosis, enthesiophytosis, soft tissue thickening, and narrowed joint spaces; in severely affected patients: subchondral sclerosis, subchondral bone cysts, attrition of subchondral bone, mineralization of joint soft tissues, and intra-articular calcified bodies (joint mice). Radiographic severity often does not correlate with clinical severity. • Stress radiography may identify underlying instability and accentuate joint incongruity; e.g., distraction index (passive hip laxity) of the coxofemoral joint is predictive of risk of hip DJD. • Computed tomography can be particularly useful in determining joint incongruence, e.g., elbow dysplasia.
• Ultrasonography can be used to determine ligamentous and tendinous injury (hypoechoic appearance and disruption of normal fibrillar orientation) and has been reported to be useful in identifying soft tissue changes in stifles with cranial cruciate ligament injury. • Three-phase nuclear scintigraphy of bone can assist in localizing subtle DJD via nucleotide uptake at areas of increased perfusion and bone turnover.

DIAGNOSTIC PROCEDURES
• Arthrocentesis and synovial fluid analysis support the diagnosis—cell counts are normal or slightly increased (< 2000–5000 cells/mL) and predominantly mononuclear (macrophages); synovial lining cells or cartilage fragments occasionally observed • Large numbers of neutrophils likely the result of underlying immune-mediated or infectious arthritis • Bacterial culture and sensitivity of synovial fluid—negative • Biopsy of synovial tissue helps rule out neoplasia or other arthritides, such as lymphocytic plasmacytic synovitis. • Force plating allows quantitative determination and analysis of weight bearing; vertical peak force and impulse are decreased in joints affected by osteoarthritis.

PATHOLOGIC FINDINGS
• Fibrillation or erosion of articular cartilage • Eburnation and sclerosis of subchondral bone • Thickening and fibrosis of the joint capsule • Synovial fluid can be grossly normal to thin

ARTHRITIS (DEGENERATIVE JOINT DISEASE)

and watery, usually increased volume
• Synovial villous hypertrophy and hyperplasia
• Osteophytes and enthesiophytes at joint capsule attachments and adjacent to the joint
• Neovascularization or pannus in severe cases over joint surfaces

 TREATMENT

APPROPRIATE HEALTH CARE
• Medical—usually tried initially • Surgical options—if inadequate response to medical management

NURSING CARE
• Physical therapy—very beneficial in enhancing good limb function and general well-being • Passive range of motion exercises
• Massage • Combination cold and heat therapy
• Swimming—increases range of motion of all joints; aerobic exercise with minimal weight bearing • Controlled leash walks up hills or on soft surfaces, such as sand

ACTIVITY
Limited to a level that minimizes aggravation of clinical signs

DIET
• Limited food consumption decreases development of clinical and radiographic evidence of DJD. • Weight reduction for obese patients—decreases stress placed on arthritic joints • Reduced caloric intake—recommended because of decreased activity as a result of disease and aging • Avoid nutrient excess and rapid growth in dogs that may be predisposed to underlying developmental diseases (e.g., hip dysplasia and osteochondrosis). • n-6 and n-3 polyunsaturated fatty acids may decrease the production of certain prostaglandins and modulate inflammation.

CLIENT EDUCATION
• Inform client that medical therapy is palliative and the condition is likely to progress. • Discuss treatment options, activity level, and diet.

SURGICAL CONSIDERATIONS
• Arthrotomy—used to treat underlying causes (e.g., fragmented coronoid process, ununited anconeal process, osteochondral diseases)
• Arthroscopy—allows actual visualization of articular cartilage; used to diagnose and treat underlying causes; has been described for hip, stifle, hock, shoulder, elbow, and carpus; has added benefit of flushing the joint
• Reconstructive procedures—used to eliminate joint instability and correct anatomic deficiencies (e.g., tibial plateau leveling osteotomy for cranial cruciate ligament–deficient stifles) • Corrective procedures—used to alter abnormal weight-bearing forces on joints with incongruity (e.g., corrective ulnar osteotomy in dogs with elbow incongruity)

Arthroplasty Procedures
• Commonly performed for hip • THR—may give excellent results; recommended for dogs that can accommodate the implants • Femoral

head ostectomy—for smaller dogs and cats; selected patients that cannot afford THR
• Total elbow replacement still experimental and offered in select cases

Arthrodesis
• Selected chronic cases and for joint instability
• Complete or partial—based on location of condition or instability • Carpus—generally yields excellent results • Shoulder, elbow, stifle, hock—less predictable results

 MEDICATIONS

DRUG(S) OF CHOICE

NSAIDs
• Work by inhibiting prostaglandin synthesis by the COX enzyme • Deracoxib (3–4 mg/kg PO q24h for 7 days for postoperative pain) (1–2 mg/kg PO q24h for long term treatment over 7 days)—new COX-2 inhibitor (coxib) drug that is selective only for the inducible COX-2 enzyme that causes pain and inflammation; spares the constitutive COX-1 enzyme responsible for gastrointestinal health and kidney function • Carprofen (2.2 mg/kg PO q12h) and etodolac (10–15 mg/kg PO q24h)—more selective for COX-2 and therefore less irritating to the gastrointestinal system; carprofen has also been shown to reduce progression of morphologic changes in cartilage and subchondral bone in canine arthritic joints.
• Buffered aspirin (25 mg/kg PO q12h)
• Meclofenamic acid—0.5 mg/kg PO q12h may also be given • Cats—limited to aspirin (10 mg/kg PO every 3 days)

Chondroprotective Agents
• Inhibits various destructive enzymes and prostaglandins • Chondrostimulation—associated with increased production of proteoglycan, hyaluronate, and collagen
• GAGPs (Adequan)—recent clinical study of dogs with hip dysplasia found the greatest improvement in orthopedic scores at 4.4 mg/kg IM every 3–5 days for eight injections

CONTRAINDICATIONS
• NSAIDs must not be given with steroids or to dogs in which steroid therapy is being considered. • Acetaminophen must not be given to cats. • NSAIDs must not be given to dogs with renal insufficieny or renal failure, dehydration, hypotension, shock, trauma, hemangiosarcoma, disorders of coagulation, or gastrointestinal disorders (especially if there is evidence of gastrointestinal ulceration), or to dogs that may undergo surgery for intervertebral disk disease (increased bleeding at the spinal cord). • NSAIDs and GAGPs—simultaneous use not recommended; potential additive inhibition of hemostasis

PRECAUTIONS
• NSAIDs—decrease platelet function; may cause gastric ulceration; may decrease blood flow to the kidneys; in cases of severe pulmonary disease, may also inhibit bronchiolar

muscle relaxation; COX-2 selective drugs may interfere with liver and placental function
• Naproxen, piroxicam, flunixin meglumine, and ibuprofen—their use is discouraged because of ulcerogenic potential

POSSIBLE INTERACTIONS
None known

ALTERNATIVE DRUG(S)
Nutraceuticals and free-radical scavengers

Corticosteroids
• Glucocorticoids—inhibit inflammatory mediators and cytokines; however, chronic use delays healing and initiates damage to articular cartilage; potential systemic side effects documented; goal is low-dose (dogs, 0.5–2.0 mg/kg; cats, 2.0–4.0 mg/kg), alternate-day therapy • Prednisone—initial dose 1–2 mg/kg PO q24h for dogs and 4 mg/kg PO q24h for cats • Triamcinolone hexacetonide—intra-articular injection of 5 mg in dogs showed a protective and therapeutic effect in one model

 FOLLOW-UP

PATIENT MONITORING
Clinical deterioration—indicates need to change drug selection or dosage; may indicate need for surgical intervention

PREVENTION/AVOIDANCE
Early identification of predisposing causes and prompt treatment to help reduce progression of secondary conditions, e.g., surgical removal of osteochondral lesions

EXPECTED COURSE AND PROGNOSIS
• Slow progression of disease likely • Some form of medical or surgical treatment usually allows a good quality of life.

 **MISCELLANEOUS**

SYNONYMS
• Osteoarthritis • Degenerative joint disease
• Osteoarthrosis • Degenerative arthritis

ABBREVIATIONS
• ANA = antinuclear antibody • COX = cyclooxygenase • DJD = degenerative joint disease • GAGPs = glycosaminoglycan polysulfate esters • NO = nitric oxide
• NSAID = nonsteroidal antiinflammatory drug • THR = total hip replacement

Suggested Readings
Pederson NC. Joint diseases of dogs and cats. In: Ettinger SJ, ed. Textbook of veterinary internal medicine. 5th ed. Philadelphia: Saunders, 2000:1862–1886.
Authors Brian S. Beale & Jennifer J. Warnock
Section Editor Peter K. Shires

ARTHRITIS, SEPTIC

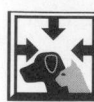 BASICS

DEFINITION
Pathogenic microorganisms within the closed space of one or more synovial joints

PATHOPHYSIOLOGY
• Usually caused by contamination associated with traumatic injury (e.g., a direct penetrating injury such as bite or gunshot wounds), a sequela to surgery, hematogenous spread of microorganisms from a distant septic focus, or the extension of primary osteomyelitis
• Primary sources of hematogenous infection—urogenital, respiratory, integumentary (including ears and anal sacs), respiratory, cardiac, and gastrointestinal systems

SYSTEMS AFFECTED
Musculoskeletal system—usually affects one joint

GENETICS
N/A

INCIDENCE/PREVALENCE
Relatively uncommon cause of monoarticular arthritis in dogs and cats

GEOGRAPHIC DISTRIBUTION
May be an increased incidence in Lyme disease–endemic areas

SIGNALMENT
Species
• Most common in dogs
• Rare in cats

Breed Predilections
Medium to large breeds—most commonly German shepherds, Dobermans, and Labrador retrievers

Mean Age and Range
Any age; usually between 4 and 7 years

Predominant Sex
Male

SIGNS
General Comments
Always consider the diagnosis in patients with monoarticular lameness associated with soft tissue swelling, heat, and pain.

Historical Findings
• Lameness—acute onset most commonly, but can present as a chronic lameness
• Lethargy
• Anorexia
• May report previous trauma—dog bite, penetrating injury

Physical Examination Findings
• Monoarticular lameness, rarely pauciarticular
• Joint pain and swelling—commonly carpus, stifle, hock, shoulder, or cubital joint
• Localized joint heat
• Decreased range of motion
• Fever

CAUSES
• Aerobic bacterial organisms—most common: staphylococci, streptococci, coliforms, and *Pasteurella*
• Anaerobic organisms—most common: *Propionibacterium, Peptostreptococcus, Fusobacterium,* and *Bacteroides*
• Spirochete—*Borrelia burgdorferi*
• Mycoplasma
• Fungal agents—*Blastomyces,* cryptococcus, and *Coccidiodes*
• *Ehrlichia*
• Leishmania

RISK FACTORS
• Predisposing factors for hematogenous infection—diabetes mellitus; Addison disease; immunosuppression
• Penetrating trauma to the joint
• Existing osteoarthritis or other joint damage
• Intra-articular injection, particularly if steroid injected

 DIAGNOSIS

DIFFERENTIAL DIAGNOSIS
• Osteoarthritis
• Trauma
• Immune-mediated arthropathy
• Postvaccinal transient polyarthritis
• Greyhound polyarthritis
• Crystal-induced joint disease
• Synovial cell sarcoma

CBC/BIOCHEMISTRY/URINALYSIS
• Hemogram—inflammatory left shift
• Other results normal

OTHER LABORATORY TESTS
Serologic testing for specific pathogens

IMAGING
Radiography
• Early disease—may reveal thickened and dense periarticular tissues; may see evidence of synovial effusion. Often difficult to diagnose early disease radiographically
• Late disease—reveals bone destruction, osteolysis, irregular joint space, discrete erosions, and periarticular osteophytosis

DIAGNOSTIC PROCEDURES
Synovial Fluid Analysis
• Increased volume
• Turbid fluid
• Decreased mucin clot reaction
• Elevated WBC count—> 80% neutrophils with > $40,000/mm^3$ (normal joint fluid < 10% neutrophils and < $3,000/mm^3$).
• Bacteria in the synovial fluid or within neutrophils—show toxic changes (chromatolysis, nuclear swelling, loss of segmentation). However, toxic neutrophils are not necessary for diagnosis.

Synovial Fluid Culture
• Culture definitive for diagnosis
• Must be collected aseptically; requires heavy sedation or general anesthesia
• Place fluid sample in aerobic and anaerobic Culturettes and in blood culture medium
• Use 1:9 dilution of synovial fluid to blood culture media.
• Culturette samples—cultured immediately upon arrival to the laboratory
• Blood culture medium—re-culturing after 24 hr of incubation increases accuracy by 50% and is the preferred method.

Other
• Synovial biopsy—to rule out immune-mediated joint disease; no more effective than culturing incubated blood culture medium
• Blood and urine cultures if hematogenous source is suspected

PATHOLOGIC FINDINGS
• Synovium—thickened; discolored; often very proliferative
• Histology—evidence of hyperplastic synoviocytes
• Increased numbers of neutrophils, macrophages, and fibrinous debris
• Cartilage—loss of proteoglycan, destruction of articular surface, pannus formation

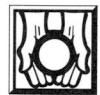 TREATMENT

APPROPRIATE HEALTH CARE
• Inpatient—initial stabilization; initiate systemic antibiotic therapy as soon as fluid is obtained for bacterial culture; initiate joint drainage/lavage as soon as possible to minimize intra-articular injury.
• Identify source if hematogenous spread is suspected.
• Outpatient—long-term management

NURSING CARE
Alternating heat and cold packing—beneficial in promoting increased blood flow and decreased swelling

ACTIVITY
Restricted until resolution of symptoms

DIET
N/A

CLIENT EDUCATION
• Discuss probable cause.
• Warn client about the need for long-term antibiotics and the likelihood of residual degenerative joint disease.

SURGICAL CONSIDERATIONS
• Acute disease with minimal radiogaphic changes—joint drainage and lavage via needle arthrocentesis, arthroscopic lavage, or arthrotomy. An irrigation catheter (ingress/egress) can be placed in larger joints
• Chronic disease—requires open arthrotomy with débridement of the synovium and copious lavage; place an irrigation catheter (ingress/egress) to lavage the joint postoperatively.
• Lavage—use warmed physiologic saline or lactated Ringer's solution (2–4 ml/kg q8h) until effluent is clear. Do not add povidone/iodine or chlorhexidine to lavage fluid.
• Effluent fluid—cytologically monitored daily for existence and character of bacteria and neutrophils
• Removal of catheters—when effluent fluid has no bacteria and the neutrophils are cytologically healthy

 MEDICATIONS

DRUG(S) OF CHOICE
• Pending culture susceptibility data—bactericidal antibiotics, such as first-generation cephalosporin or ampicillin–clavulanic acid, preferred
• Choice of antimicrobial drugs—primarily depends on in vitro determination of susceptibility of microorganisms; toxicity, frequency, route of administration, and expense also considered; most penetrate the synovium well; need to be given for a minimum of 4–8 weeks
• NSAIDs—may help decrease pain and inflammation

CONTRAINDICATIONS
Avoid quinolones in pediatric patients; they induce cartilage lesions experimentally.

PRECAUTIONS
Failure to respond to conventional antibiotic therapy—may indicate anaerobic disease or other unusual cause (fungal, spirochete)

POSSIBLE INTERACTIONS
N/A

ALTERNATIVE DRUG(S)
N/A

 FOLLOW-UP

PATIENT MONITORING
• Drainage and irrigation catheters—may be pulled after 4–6 days or after reassessment of synovial fluid cytology
• Duration of antibiotic therapy—2 weeks following resolution of clinical signs. Total treatment may be 4–8 weeks or longer; depends on clinical signs and pathogenic organism
• Persistent synovial inflammation without viable bacterial organisms (dogs)—may be caused by antigenic bacterial fragments or antigen antibody deposition
• Systemic corticosteroid therapy and aggressive physical therapy—may be needed to maximize normal joint dynamics

PREVENTION/AVOIDANCE
If clinical signs recur, early (within 24–48 hr) treatment provides the greatest benefit.

POSSIBLE COMPLICATIONS
• Chronic disease—severe degenerative joint disease
• Recurrence of infection
• Limited joint range of motion
• Generalized sepsis
• Osteomyelitis

EXPECTED COURSE AND PROGNOSIS
• Acutely diagnosed disease (within 24–48 hr) responds well to antibiotic therapy
• Delayed diagnosis or resistant or highly virulent organisms—guarded to poor prognosis

 MISCELLANEOUS

ASSOCIATED CONDITIONS
N/A

AGE-RELATED FACTORS
N/A

ZOONOTIC POTENTIAL
N/A

PREGNANCY
N/A

SYNONYMS
• Infectious arthritis
• Joint ill

SEE ALSO
• Osteomyelitis
• Polyarthritis, Erosive Immune-Mediated
• Polyarthritis, Nonerosive Immune-Mediated

ABBREVIATION
• NSAIDS = nonsteroidal antiinflammatory drugs

Suggested Reading
Bennett D, Taylor DJ. Bacterial infective arthritis in the dog. J Small Anim Pract 1988;29:207–230.
Ellison RS. The cytologic examination of synovial fluid. Semin Vet Med Surg Small Anim 1988;3.133–139.
Hodgin EC, Michaelson F, Howerth EW. Anaerobic bacterial infections causing osteomyelitis/arthritis in a dog. J Am Vet Med Assoc 1992;201:886–888.
Machevsky Am, Read RA. Bacterial septic arthritis in 19 dogs. Aust Vet J 1999; 77:233–237.
Montgomery RD, Long IR, Milton JL. Comparison of aerobic Culturette, synovial membrane biopsy, and blood culture medium in detection of canine bacterial arthritis. Vet Surg 1989;18:300–303.
Nord KD, Dore DD, Deeney VF, et al. Evaluation of treatment modalities for septic arthritis with histologic grading and analysis of levels of uronic acid, neutral protease, and interleukin-1. J Bone Jt Surg 1995; 77:258–265.

Acknowledgment
The author/editors acknowledge the prior contributions of Dr. Robert A. Taylor, who authored this topic in the previous edition.
Author Spencer A. Johnston
Consulting Editor Peter K. Shires

ASCITES

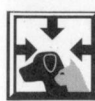 BASICS

DEFINITION
The escape of fluid, either transudate or exudate, into the abdominal cavity between the parietal and visceral peritoneum

PATHOPHYSIOLOGY
Ascites can be caused by the following:
• CHF and associated interference in venous return
• Depletion of plasma proteins associated with inappropriate loss of protein from renal or gastrointestinal disease—protein-losing nephropathy or enteropathy, respectively
• Obstruction of the vena cava or portal vein, or lymphatic drainage due to neoplastic occlusion
• Overt neoplastic effusion
• Peritonitis—infective or inflammatory
• Electrolyte imbalance, especially hypernatremia
• Liver cirrhosis

SYSTEMS AFFECTED
• Cardiovascular
• Gastrointestinal
• Renal/Urologic
• Hemic/Lymph/Immune

SIGNALMENT
• Dogs and cats
• No species or breed predisposition

SIGNS
• Episodic weakness
• Lethargy
• Abdominal fullness
• Abdominal discomfort when palpated
• Dyspnea from abdominal distension or associated pleural effusion
• Anorexia
• Vomiting
• Weight gain
• Scrotal or penile edema
• Groaning when lying down

CAUSES
• Nephrotic syndrome
• Cirrhosis of liver
• Right-sided CHF
• Hypoproteinemia
• Ruptured bladder
• Peritonitis
• Abdominal neoplasia
• Abdominal hemorrhage

RISK FACTORS
N/A

 DIAGNOSIS

DIFFERENTIAL DIAGNOSIS

Differentiating Abdominal Distension Without Effusion
• Organomegaly—hepatomegaly, splenomegaly, renomegaly, and hydrometra
• Abdominal neoplasia
• Pregnancy
• Bladder distension
• Obesity
• Gastric dilatation

Differentiating Diseases
• Transudate—nephrotic syndrome, cirrhosis of liver, right-sided CHF, hypoproteinemia, and ruptured bladder
• Exudate—peritonitis, abdominal neoplasia, and hemorrhage

CBC/BIOCHEMISTRY/URINALYSIS
• Neutrophilic leukocytosis occurs in patients with systemic infection.
• Albumin is low in patients with impaired liver synthesis, gastrointestinal loss, or renal loss.
• Cholesterol is low in patients with impaired liver synthesis.

Liver Enzymes
• Low to normal in patients with impaired liver synthesis
• High in patients with liver inflammation, hyperadrenocorticism, gallbladder obstruction, and chronic passive congestion

Total and Direct Bilirubin
• Low to normal in patients with impaired liver synthesis
• High in patients with biliary obstruction caused by tumor, gallbladder distension, or obstruction

BUN and Creatinine
• High in patients with renal failure
• BUN low in patients with impaired liver synthesis or hyperadrenocorticism

Glucose
Low in patients with impaired liver synthesis

OTHER LABORATORY TESTS
• To detect hypoproteinemia—protein electrophoresis and immune profile
• To detect proteinuria—urinary protein:creatinine ratio (normal < 0.5:1)

IMAGING
• Thoracic and abdominal radiography is sometimes helpful.
• Ultrasonography of the liver, spleen, pancreas, kidney, bladder, and abdomen can often determine cause.

DIAGNOSTIC PROCEDURES

Ascitic Fluid Evaluation
Exfoliative cytologic examination and bacterial culture and antibiotic sensitivity—remove approximately 3–5 mL of abdominal fluid via aseptic technique.

Transudate
• Clear and colorless
• Protein < 2.5 g/dL
• Specific gravity < 1.018
• Cells < 1000/mm^3—neutrophils and mesothelial cells

Modified Transudate
• Red or pink; may be slightly cloudy
• Protein 2.5–5.0 g/dL
• Specific gravity > 1.018
• Cells <5000 /mm^3—neutrophils, mesothelial cells, erythrocytes, and lymphocytes

Exudate (Nonseptic)
• Pink or white; cloudy
• Protein 2.5–5.0 g/dL
• Specific gravity > 1.018
• Cells 5000–50,000/mm^3—neutrophils, mesothelial cells, macrophages, erythrocytes, and lymphocytes

Exudate (Septic)
• Red, white, or yellow; cloudy
• Protein > 4.0 g/dL
• Specific gravity > 1.018
• Cells 5000–100,000/mm^3—neutrophils, mesothelial cells, macrophages, erythrocytes, lymphocytes, and bacteria

Hemorrhage
• Red; spun supernatant clear and sediment red
• Protein > 5.5 g/dL
• Specific gravity 1.007–1.027
• Cells consistent with peripheral blood
• Does not clot

Chyle
• Pink, straw, or white
• Protein 2.5–7.0 g/dL
• Specific gravity 1.007–> 1.040

- Cells < 10,000/mm³—neutrophils, mesothelial cells, and large population of small lymphocytes
- Other—fluid in tube separates into creamlike layer when refrigerated; fat droplets stain with Sudan III

Pseudochyle
- White
- Protein > 2.5 g/dL
- Specific gravity 1.007–1.040
- Cells < 10,000/mm³—neutrophils, mesothelial cells, and small lymphocytes
- Other—fluid in tube does not separate into creamlike layer when refrigerated; does not stain with Sudan III.

Urine
- Clear to pale yellow
- Protein > 2.5 g/dL
- Specific gravity 1.000–> 1.040
- Cells 5000–50,000/mm³—neutrophils, erythrocytes, lymphocytes, and macrophages
- Other—if the urinary bladder ruptured < 12 hr before, urinary glucose and protein could be negative; if bladder ruptured > 12 hr before, urine becomes a dialysis medium with ultrafiltrate of plasma, and urine contains glucose and protein.

Bile
- Slightly cloudy and yellow
- Protein > 2.5 g/dL
- Specific gravity > 1.018
- Cells 5000–750,000/mm³—neutrophils, erythrocytes, macrophages, and lymphocytes
- Other—bilirubin confirmed by urine dipstick; nonicteric patient may have gallbladder rupture, biliary tree leakage, or rupture in the proximal bowel.

TREATMENT
- Can design treatment on an outpatient basis, with follow-up or inpatient care, depending on physical condition and underlying cause
- If patients are markedly uncomfortable when lying down or become more dyspneic with stress, consider removing enough ascites to reverse these signs.
- Dietary salt restriction may help control transudate fluid accumulation due to CHF, cirrhosis, or hypoproteinemia.

- For exudate ascites control, address the underlying cause; corrective surgery is often indicated, followed by specific therapeutic management (e.g., patient with splenic tumor: tumor removed, abdominal bleeding controlled, blood transfusion administered).
- Can recirculate nonseptic ascitic fluid in patients with liver insufficiency or nephrotic syndrome that has become refractory to conservative medical and dietary management; use the LeVeen peritoneovenous shunt concept—a unidirectional shunt conveys ascitic fluid to the jugular vein via a surgically placed one-way catheter from the midabdominal region; this autologous infusion has had limited success in dogs.

MEDICATIONS

DRUG(S) OF CHOICE
- Patients with liver insufficiency or CHF—restrict sodium and give a diuretic combination of hydrochlorothiazide (2–4 mg/kg q12h PO) and spironolactone (1–2 mg/kg q12h PO); if control is inadequate, furosemide (1–2 mg/kg q8h PO) can be substituted for the thiazide with spironolactone continued; must monitor serum potassium concentration to prevent potassium imbalances
- Patients with hypoproteinemia, nephrotic syndrome, and associated ascitic fluid accumulation—can treat as above with the addition of hetastarch (6% hetastarch in 0.9% NaCl); administer an IV bolus (dogs, 20 mL/kg; cats, 10–15 mL/kg) slowly over ~ 1 hr; hetastarch increases plasma oncotic pressure and pulls fluid into the intravascular space for up to 24–48 hr.
- Systemic antibiotic therapy is dictated by bacterial identification and sensitivity testing in patients with septic exudate ascites.

CONTRAINDICATIONS
N/A

PRECAUTIONS
N/A

POSSIBLE INTERACTIONS
N/A

ALTERNATIVE DRUG(S)
N/A

FOLLOW-UP

PATIENT MONITORING
- Varies with the underlying cause
- Check sodium, potassium, BUN, creatinine, and weight fluctuations periodically if the patient is maintained on a diuretic.

POSSIBLE COMPLICATIONS
Aggressive diuretic administration may cause hypokalemia, which could predispose to metabolic alkalosis and exacerbation of hepatic encephalopathy in patients with underlying liver disease; alkalosis causes a shift from NH_4 to NH_3.

MISCELLANEOUS

ASSOCIATED CONDITIONS
N/A

AGE-RELATED FACTORS
N/A

ZOONOTIC POTENTIAL
N/A

PREGNANCY
N/A

SYNONYMS
Abdominal effusion

SEE ALSO
- Cirrhosis and Fibrosis of the Liver
- Congestive Heart Failure, Right-sided
- Nephrotic Syndrome

ABBREVIATION
CHF = congestive heart failure

Suggested Reading
Lewis LD, Morris ML Jr, Hand MS. Small animal clinical nutrition, 3rd ed. Topeka, KS: Mark Morris Associates, 1987.
Porayko MK, Wiesner RH. Management of ascites in patients with cirrhosis. Postgrad Med 1992;2:155.
Author Jerry A. Thornhill
Consulting Editors Larry P. Tilley and Francis W. K. Smith, Jr.

ASPERGILLOSIS

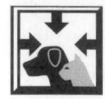

BASICS

OVERVIEW
• An opportunistic fungal infection caused by *Aspergillus* spp., common molds that are ubiquitous in the environment, forming numerous spores in dust, straw, grass clippings, and hay • Two types of infections—diseases localized to the nasal cavity and frontal sinuses and disseminated disease; do not appear to be related, but a report of a dog that developed fungal osteomyelitis 6 months after treatment of nasal aspergillosis raises the possibility • Nasal cavity—*A. fumigatus* most frequently involved; *A. flavus, A. niger,* and *A. nidulans* also isolated; presumed acquired through direct inoculation of the nasal mucosa • Disseminated disease—usually *A. terreus; A. deflectus* and *A. fumigatus* also associated; portal of entry not definitively established, but possibly through the respiratory tract or gastrointestinal tract, with subsequent hematogenous spread

SIGNALMENT
Dogs
• Both forms—more common in dogs than in cats • Nasal—more common in young adult dolichocephalic and mesaticephalic breeds; no sex predilection reported; age range 3 months to 11 years • Disseminated—more common in German shepherds but not confined to this breed; reported average age of affected dogs 3 years, with a range of 1 to 9 years; slight bias toward females

Cats
• Persians—marginally increased incidence • Approximately 40 cases documented in literature; majority involved disseminated disease affecting the lungs and/or gastro-intestinal tract • Nasal—low number of cases with frontal sinus (with or without orbital) involvement reported

SIGNS
Dogs
Nasal
• Chronic unilateral or bilateral serous, mucopurulent, or more commonly profuse sanguinopurulent nasal discharge unresponsive to antibiotics—most common sign • Sneezing • Nasal pain • Epistaxis • Reduced appetite; lethargy • Depigmen-tation or ulceration around the external nares • External nasal distortion or swelling—uncommon • Invasion of the cribriform plate infrequently leads to signs of CNS involvement.
Disseminated
• May develop acutely or slowly over a period of several months • Often associated with spinal pain due to fungal diskospondylitis, or lameness due to fungal osteomyelitis

• Neurologic—spinal cord damage • Polyuria/polydipsia and hematuria—renal involvement • Uveitis—ocular involvement • Nonspecific—fever, weight loss, vomiting, lymphadenopathy, and anorexia

Cats
• Nasal—associated with nasal discharge and stertor • Disseminated—most commonly associated with nonspecific signs (e.g., lethargy and depression or vomiting and diarrhea) • Ocular—exophthalmos

CAUSES & RISK FACTORS
• Nasal—more common in outdoor dogs and farm dogs; young adult dolichocephalic and mesaticephalic dogs • Disseminated—German shepherds most commonly but not exclusively affected • Immune deficiency—may play a factor because the organism is widespread but the disease is uncommon; breed-related immune defect proposed in German shepherds and their crosses • Geographic/environmental conditions—may be a factor because some regions have a higher incidence than others (e.g., California, Louisiana, Michigan, Georgia, Florida, and Virginia in the U.S.; Western Australia; Barcelona; and Milan) • Cats—associated with FIP, FePLV, FeLV, diabetes mellitus, and chronic corticosteroid or antibiotic administration

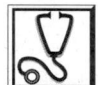

DIAGNOSIS

DIFFERENTIAL DIAGNOSIS
• Nasal—nasal neoplasia; bacterial rhinitis/sinusitis; penicilliosis; foreign body; nasal mites; nasopharyngeal polyps (cats); nasal cryptococcosis (cats) • Disseminated—bacterial osteomyelitis/diskospondylitis; spinal neoplasia; intervertebral disk disease; skeletal neoplasia; bacterial pyelonephritis; bacterial pneumonia; other causes of uveitis (see Uveitis)

CBC/BIOCHEMISTRY/URINALYSIS
Nasal
May see neutrophilic leukocytosis and monocytosis, reflecting chronic inflammation

Disseminated
• Nonspecific • Dogs—often have mature neutrophilic leukocytosis and lymphopenia • Cats—may have nonregenerative anemia and leukopenia • Biochemistry changes—may see high globulins, creatinine, phosphate, and BUN • Urinalysis—may see isosthenuria, hematuria, pyuria, and possible fungal hyphae in the sediment; detection of the fungal hyphae can be improved by allowing the sample to incubate at room temperature for 24–48 hr; sediment samples may be examined unstained as wet preparations or may be air dried and stained with Diff-Quick (the hyphae that branch at 45° stain purple)

OTHER LABORATORY TESTS
• Positive fungal serology (agar gel double diffusion, counterimmunoelectrophoresis, and ELISA)—support the diagnosis; false-positives and cross-reactivity with *Penicillium* spp. reported; useful in making diagnosis in conjunction with radiographs/culture • Cats—test for FeLV and FIV because they affect prognosis

IMAGING
Nasal
• Radiography—open-mouth ventrodorsal view of the nasal cavity and skyline views of the frontal sinuses most useful; reveal an increase in radiolucency on the affected rostral and maxillary nasal turbinate areas owing to turbinate lysis; mixed density may be seen as a result of a combination of turbinate destruction and soft tissue–dense fungal granulomas and/or nasal discharge; fungal disease changes are typically more rostral than those seen in nasal neoplasia; affected frontal sinuses have an increase in opacity owing to soft tissue density of the fungal elements and accumulation of associated inflammatory fluid; may see frontal sinus lysis • CT and MRI—define the extent of the disease more accurately; allow assessment of the integrity of the cribriform plate (which may be of concern before performing nasal flushing in dogs showing CNS signs)

Disseminated
Radiography—spinal views may show end-plate lysis, attempted bony intervertebral bridging, and lysis of vertebral bodies consistent with diskospondylitis; bony proliferation and lysis and periosteal reaction typical of osteomyelitis of the diaphyseal region of long bones; pulmonary involvement reported rarely, mixed interstitial/alveolar pattern

DIAGNOSTIC PROCEDURES
Nasal
• Cytology of nasal swabs and flushes—usually nondiagnostic; findings may reflect an inflammatory process • Rhinoscopy—may allow direct visualization of the fungus on the nasal mucosa (grayish white plaques adherent to the inflamed mucosa); destructive nature can be appreciated (nasal cavity takes on a vast cavernous appearance in more severe cases); excellent tool for collecting samples for culture, cytology, and histology • Fungal cultures of nasal exudates—not accurate for obtaining a definitive diagnosis; may give false-positive or false-negative results; the organism is a common laboratory contaminant; positive culture should be confirmed by histopathology or supported by the history and radiographic and serologic testing • Definitive diagnosis based on histopathology, positive titer plus culture, positive titer plus appropriate radiographic

changes, or identification of fungal plaques at rhinoscopy

PATHOLOGIC FINDINGS

Histopathologic examination of tissue—most likely to render a definitive diagnosis; special stains may be required; granulomas and multiple organ infarcts noted with disseminated disease (kidneys, liver, spleen, and vertebrae)

TREATMENT

Nasal (Dogs)

• Systemic antifungal agents—limited success • If cribriform plate affected, avoid topical therapy and use oral therapy (itraconazole) • Clotrimazole (1%) administered locally for 1 hour via catheters placed in both nasal cavities under general anaesthesia—treatment of choice • Prepare the patient—general anesthesia and placement of a well-fitted, cuffed endotracheal tube • Occlude the caudal nares by placing an appropriate-sized Foley catheter (24-F for average affected dog) in the caudal nasopharynx dorsal to the soft palate and packing around the inflated balloon with moistened, pre-counted laparotomy sponges or gauze to absorb any leakage of antifungal solution; placement assisted by use of curved forceps or by threading heavy suture material (through a red rubber feeding tube) via nostril and attaching suture to the tip of Foley catheter, then drawing catheter forward into the caudal nares • Place a 10-F catheter for infusion of clotrimazole into the dorsal nasal meatus of both nasal cavities to the level of the medial canthus; place two smaller Foley catheters in the tip of both nasal cavities to occlude the nostrils; additional occlusion afforded by cotton tips; place patient in dorsal recumbency. • Fill the nasal passages with 1% clotrimazole for 1 hr; intermittently top off the passages as the solution is absorbed into the gauze and redistributed to the sinuses; average dog requires 50–60 mL for each side (when solution is seen in the Foley catheter tubing, occlude Foley catheters); rotate patient through ventral, dorsal, left, and right lateral recumbency during the 1 hr to aid distribution of clotrimazole. • Then place the patient in sternal recumbency and remove infusion catheters, Foley catheters, and sponges to allow the solution to drain out rostrally. Gently flush the pharynx with saline, and suction to remove any residual solution. • Carefully monitor recovery from anesthesia; some dogs may develop stridor if laryngeal/pharyngeal edema occurs due to irritation from solution (treat with corticosteroids). • More than one treatment may be required. • Surgical placement of catheters into the frontal sinuses is no more effective than nonsurgical placement and is associated with more complications.
• Enilconazole infusion twice daily for 7–14 days via surgically placed frontal sinus catheters may be considered for treatment failures with enilconazole; associated with greater complication rate (discomfort, aspiration, dislodgement of tubes)

Disseminated (Dogs)

• Difficult to eliminate infection; rare cures have been reported • Halt progression of clinical signs rather than eliminate the infection. • Itraconazole—most effective • Combination of flucytosine and subcutaneous amphotericin B in 4.5% saline and 2.5% dextrose—used to successfully treat disseminated cryptococcosis; may prove to have some use in treating aspergillosis (no published reports) • Fluid therapy—indicated by the degree of renal compromise and azotemia

Cats

• Nasal—might be managed successfully using the same techniques used to treat dogs, but no reports are published • Disseminated likely difficult to treat; data are limited

MEDICATIONS

DRUG(S)

Nasal

• 1% clotrimazole in polyethylene glycol base—if possible, avoid formulations in propylene glycol and isopropyl alcohol, but if necessary, use with caution as greater irritation of pharyngeal mucosa and edema may result; 50–60 mL instilled into each nasal cavity for 1 hr is the treatment of choice if cribriform plate is intact • Enilconazole—10% solution diluted 50:50 with water immediately before administration; 5–10 mL q12h instilled into the nasal sinuses via surgically implanted frontal sinus catheters for 7–14 days (NOT appropriate as a 1-hr therapy) • Oral azoles—ketoconazole (10–15 mg/kg q8–12h), fluconazole (10–12 mg/kg per day): much lower rates of cure than with topical treatment (43%–60%); itraconazole (5 mg/kg q24h): 60%–70% response rate reported, but cost a factor

Disseminated

• Itraconazole, 5–10 mg/kg daily (can be divided)—drug of choice; dogs unlikely to be cured, though the disease may be contained with continued use
• Combination therapy with flucytosine and amphotericin B—may prove successful

CONTRAINDICATIONS/POSSIBLE INTERACTIONS

• Amphotericin B—contraindicated in dogs with pre-existing renal compromise or failure
• Oral azoles—nausea, intermittent anorexia, liver enzyme elevation • Pharyngeal irritation/edema from topical antifungals • Prolonged recovery from anesthesia has been reported in a dog treated with topical clotrimazole • Cutaneous drug eruptions in dogs treated with a combination of flucytosine and amphotericin B

FOLLOW-UP

• Nasal—discharge should be well reduced 2 weeks after treatment and eliminated by 4 weeks; if still significant discharge after 2 weeks, consider a treatment failure and re-treat; consider antibiotics because bacterial infection can be a problem owing to damage sustained to nasal mucosa and turbinates; recurrence of discharge after initial resolution is rarely due to recurrence of fungal infection, consider bacteria • Disseminated—monitor serial radiographs every 1–2 months, renal function, and urine cultures

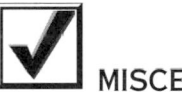

MISCELLANEOUS

ZOONOTIC POTENTIAL

None

ABBREVIATIONS

• BUN = blood urea nitrogen • CT = computed tomography • ELISA = enzyme-linked immunosorbent assay • FeLV = feline leukemia virus • FePLV = feline panleukopenia virus • FIP = feline infectious peritonitis • FIV = feline immunodeficiency virus • MRI = magnetic resonance imaging

Suggested Reading

Davidson A, Pappagianis D. Treatment of nasal aspergillosis with topical clotrimazole. In: Bonagura J, Kirk R, eds. Current veterinary therapy XII. Philadelphia: Saunders, 1995:899–901.

Kelly SE, Shaw SE, Clark WT. Long-term survival of four dogs with disseminated *Aspergillus terreus* treated with itraconazole. Aust Vet J 1995;72:311–313.

Mathews KG, Davidson AP, Koblik PD, et al. Comparison of topical administration of clotrimazole through surgically placed versus nonsurgically placed catheters for treatment of nasal aspergillosis in dogs: 60 cases (1990–1996). J Am Vet Med Assoc 1998;213:501–506.

Russo M, Lamb CR, Jakovljevic S. Distinguishing rhinitis and nasal neoplasia by radiography. Vet Radiol Ultrasound 2000;41:118–124.

Author Tania N. Davey
Consulting Editor Stephen C. Barr

ASPIRIN TOXICITY

 BASICS

OVERVIEW
• Given by owners to relieve minor pain and discomfort; now less commonly used owing to increasing popularity of other over-the-counter pain-relieving drugs
• Gastric irritation and hemorrhage occur in 10%–20% of cases.
• Repeated doses may produce gastro-intestinal ulceration and perforation.
• Toxic hepatitis, suppression of bone marrow activity, and anemia may occur, especially in cats.

SIGNALMENT
Cats and less commonly dogs

SIGNS
• Depression
• Vomiting—vomitus may be blood-tinged.
• Tachypnea
• Fever
• Muscular weakness and ataxia
• Coma and death in 1 or more days

CAUSES & RISK FACTORS
• Owners employing human dosage guidelines to medicate cats—most common
• Deficiency in glucuronide conjugation capability (cats)
• Biological half-life—cats, 44.6 hr; dogs, 7.5 hr; responsible for higher risk in cats

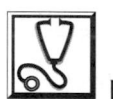 DIAGNOSIS

DIFFERENTIAL DIAGNOSIS
• Clinical signs—uncharacteristic
• History of aspirin ingestion or medication—important; within 5 days of signs should raise concern
• Pre-existing painful condition—question owner about aspirin administration.

CBC/BIOCHEMISTRY/URINALYSIS
• Cats—prone to Heinz body formation
• Hyponatremia and hypokalemia

OTHER LABORATORY TESTS
• Initial respiratory alkalosis followed by metabolic acidosis
• Salicylic acid concentrations in serum or urine
• High ketones and pyruvic, lactic, and amino acid levels
• Decreased sulfuric and phosphoric acid renal clearance

IMAGING
N/A

DIAGNOSTIC PROCEDURES
N/A

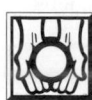 TREATMENT

• Inpatient—following general principles of poisoning management
• Correction of acid–base balance—continuous intravenous fluids
• Induced gastric emptying—gastric lavage or induced emesis
• Peritoneal or hemodialysis or hemo-perfusion—heroic procedures

 MEDICATIONS

DRUG(S)
• No specific antidote available
• Activated charcoal—2 g/kg PO decontaminates gut.
• Sodium bicarbonate 1 mEq/kg IV alkalinizes urine.

CONTRAINDICATIONS/POSSIBLE INTERACTIONS
N/A

 FOLLOW-UP

• Maintaining renal function and acid–base balance is vital.
• Severe acid–base disturbances, severe dehydration, toxic hepatitis, bone marrow depression, and coma are poor prognostic indicators.

 MISCELLANEOUS

Be sure that history of "aspirin" medication does not refer to other available pain medications.

Suggested Reading
Oehme FW. Aspirin and acetaminophen. In: Kirk RW, ed. Current veterinary therapy IX. Small animal practice. Philadelphia: Saunders, 1986:188–189.
Author Frederick W. Oehme
Consulting Editor Gary D. Osweiler

BASICS

DEFINITIONS
• Chronic bronchitis—inflammation in the airways (bronchi and bronchioles); presents clinically as a chronic cough of greater than 2 months' duration
• Asthma—acute or chronic airway inflammation associated with increased responsiveness of the airways to various stimuli, airway narrowing due to smooth muscle hypertrophy/constriction, reversibility of airway constriction, and presence of eosinophils, lymphocytes, and mast cells within the airways
• These criteria are often difficult to determine and/or document, thus the term feline bronchitis or bronchopulmonary disease (FBD) is used more commonly to describe the clinical disease in cats of acute or chronic coughing or wheezing accompanied by lower airway inflammation.

PATHOPHYSIOLOGY
• Noxious or allergic stimuli trigger inflammation within the lower airways. The inflammatory mediators cause mucosal airway damage that releases more inflammatory mediators.
• Bronchiolar smooth muscle constriction—reversible either spontaneously or in response to anti-inflammatory drugs
• Smooth muscle hypertrophy implies chronicity—usually not reversible
• Increase in mucosal goblet cells, mucus production, edema of bronchial wall
• Excessive mucus can cause bronchiolar obstruction and lead to atelectasis or bronchiectasis (dilated airways often obstructed with mucus).
• Chronic inflammation within the airways may lead to fibrosis and lung atelectasis.

SYSTEMS AFFECTED
• Respiratory
• Cardiac—chronic airway disease can lead to pulmonary hypertension and secondary right-sided heart disease.

GENETICS N/A

INCIDENCE/PREVALENCE N/A

GEOGRAPHIC DISTRIBUTION
Worldwide. Parasitic causes of airway inflammation are more common in southern and midwest U.S. states. Heartworm disease is more prevalent in southern U.S. states. *Paragonimus kellicotti* is found in Great Lakes region.

SIGNALMENT

Species
Cats

Breed Predilections
Siamese overrepresented

Mean Age and Range
Any age; more common between 2–8 years

Predominant Sex
One study shows females overrepresented; however this is not a consistent finding.

SIGNS

Historical Findings
• Coughing (80%), sneezing (60%), labored breathing or wheezing (40%)
• Signs are typically episodic and can be acute or chronic.
• Lethargy and inappetence are occasionally reported.

Physical Examination Findings
• Severely affected cats may present with open-mouth breathing, tachypnea, and cyanosis.
• Increased tracheal sensitivity is common.
• Chest auscultation may reveal crackles and/or expiratory wheezes, or may be normal.
• Labored breathing, typically a moderate to severe increase in expiratory effort with an abdominal push on expiration. Inspiratory effort is usually much less affected.
• Heart rate is typically normal to bradycardic, although stress may result in tachycardia.

CAUSES
Triggers of airway inflammation are largely unknown.

RISK FACTORS
• Exposure to cigarette smoke, dusty cat litter, hair sprays, and air fresheners could possibly exacerbate disease in some cats.
• Parasitic lung infections are more common in outdoor cats in certain geographic locations.
• Use of potassium bromide has been implicated as a cause for signs of bronchitis or asthma in some cats.

DIAGNOSIS

DIFFERENTIAL DIAGNOSIS
• Diseases primarily affecting lung parenchyma. Rule out infectious pneumonia (toxoplasmosis, FIP, bacterial pneumonia, histoplasmosis).
• *Dirofilaria immitis* (heartworm) and primary lung parasites (*Aelurostrongylus abstrusus, Capillaria aerophilia,* and *Paragonimus kellicotti*)

• Primary or metastatic neoplasia also similar in clinical, and occasionally radiographic, appearance
• Primary cardiac disease may appear clinically and radiographically similar in certain instances, but these cats typically do not have a history of cough or have tracheal sensitivity on physical exam.

CBC/BIOCHEMISTRY/URINALYSIS
• Frequently normal
• Less than 40% of cats with allergic airway disease have a peripheral eosinophilia. Peripheral eosinophilia is more common with parasitic infection or eosinophilic pulmonary granulomatosis.

OTHER LABORATORY TESTS
• Fecal exams—flotation examination for *Capillaria;* sedimentation for *Paragonimus,* Baermann technique for *Aelurostrongylus.* False negatives occur.
• Heartworm testing—both antigen and antibody test recommended
• Pulmonary lung function testing—available in select academic institutions or specialty practices. Increased airway resistance is the classic finding.
• Radioallergosorbent testing (RAST) or intradermal skin testing—a correlation between skin and respiratory allergies has not been documented at this time.

IMAGING

Radiography
• Classically, diffuse bronchial wall thickening and interstitial pattern
• Patchy alveolar pattern can be seen as well.
• The severity of radiographic changes does not necessarily correlate with clinical severity or duration.
• Hyperinflation of lung fields—characterized by a flattened and caudally displaced diaphragm, an increase in the distance between the heart and diaphragm, or extension of the lungs to the first lumbar vertebrae
• Collapse of the right middle lung lobe has been reported with a frequency of 11%
• Pulmonary lobar arterial enlargement is suspicious for heartworm disease.

Echocardiography
May be useful when evaluating for the possibility of heartworm disease or pulmonary hypertension secondary to chronic lung disease

ASTHMA, BRONCHITIS—CATS

DIAGNOSTIC PROCEDURES

Transoral Tracheal Wash (TTW)
• Use a sterile endotracheal tube and polypropylene catheter for obtaining a cytologic sample; this allows for sampling of airway fluids at the level of the carina.
• Upper airway contamination much more likely with TTW than with bronchoalveolar lavage

Bronchoscopy/Bronchoalveolar Lavage (BAL)
• Allows for visualization of trachea and bronchi. Excessive amounts of thick mucus are common with bronchitis. Mucosa of the airways is typically hyperemic and edematous.
• Biopsy or endoscopic brushing possible, although typically not needed with cases of bronchitis
• BAL should be performed during bronchoscopy; this allows for sampling of airway fluids from areas that appear most affected.

Cytology
• Eosinophils and neutrophils are most prominent cell types. A mixed cell population occurs in about 21% of cats.
• In one study, 22% of cats had normal cytology (macrophages predominated).
• Up to 30% eosinophils on BAL cytology can be found in normal cats. Parasitic and heartworm infections will have high percentages of eosinophils on cytology.

Bacterial Cultures
• Quantitated cultures are recommended. Significant bacterial colony counts are uncommonly obtained in feline bronchopulmonary disease. Significant bacterial growth on a quantitative culture is suggested to be >100–300 cfu/ml.
• Mycoplasma has been isolated from 21–44% of cats with FBD and was not isolated from healthy cats. Its role in bronchitis remains controversial.

Biopsy
Keyhole biopsy typically not indicated because of the invasiveness of the procedure. Rarely will the results alter the course of therapy.

PATHOLOGIC FINDINGS
Histologic findings consistent with FBD include hyperplasia/hypertrophy of goblet cells, airway smooth muscle thickening, epithelial erosion, and inflammatory infiltrates.

TREATMENT

APPROPRIATE HEALTH CARE
• Removal of patient from the inciting environment may help.
• Patient should be hospitalized for an acute crisis of labored breathing and dyspnea.

NURSING CARE
Oxygen therapy and sedatives may help in an acute crisis. Minimize manipulation during a crisis in order to lessen stress and oxygen needs of the animal.

ACTIVITY
Usually self-limited by patient

DIET
Calorie restriction for obese cats

CLIENT EDUCATION
• Most causes of bronchitis are chronic, progressive diseases.
• Do not discontinue medical therapy when clinical signs have resolved—subclinical inflammation within the lungs is common and can lead to progression of disease.
• Life-long medication and environmental changes may be necessary.
• Some clients can be taught to give terbutaline subcutaneously and corticosteroid injections at home for a crisis situation.

SURGICAL CONSIDERATIONS N/A

MEDICATIONS

DRUG(S) OF CHOICE

Emergency Treatment
• Combine the use of oxygen and a parenteral bronchodilator. A short-acting parenteral corticosteroid may also be required. Patient manipulation should be minimized in order to avoid worsening respiratory distress.
• Injectable terbutaline (0.01 mg/kg IV or SC). Can repeat this dose if no clinical improvement (decrease in respiratory rate or effort) in 20–30 minutes.
• Dexamethasone sodium phosphate (2 mg/kg divided by 7, given IV or SC). Can repeat if no improvement visible within 20–30 minutes. Prednisolone sodium succinate (Solu-Delta-Cortef) can also be used (50—100 mg IV).

Long-term Management
Corticosteroids
• Decrease inflammation
• Oral treatment is preferred over injectable because doses and duration can be more closely monitored.
• Prednisone: 0.5–1 mg/kg PO q12h. Begin to taper dose (50% each week) after 2 weeks if clinical signs have improved. If clinical signs resurface, dose should be increased again to 0.5–1 mg/kg PO q12h. Maintenance therapy = 0.5–1 mg/kg PO q24–48h. Some patients may be able to use steroids on a seasonal basis only.
• Dexamethasone sodium phosphate—used mainly for an acute crisis
• Longer-acting parenteral steroids (Vetalog or Depomedrol) should be reserved for situations where owners are unable to administer oral medication on a routine basis.
Inhaled Corticosteroids
• Newer therapy—requires a form-fitting facemask, pediatric spacer, and metered-dose inhaler (MDI)
• The only corticosteroid available as an MDI that has been routinely used in cats is fluticasone propionate (Flovent). The 220-mcg Flovent MDI is recommended (2 actuations, 7–10 breaths q12h) along with other bronchodilators and oral corticosteroids, depending on the severity of clinical signs. The 110-mcg Flovent MDI can be used with the Trudell Aerokat spacer, which allows for sufficient dosing with only 1 actuation q12h (Padrid P. Personal communication, August 2002).
• Flovent is used for long-term control of airway inflammation. Takes 10–14 days to reach peak effect; during this time oral steroids should be used concurrently
• Hypothesized that there is no systemic absorption of inhalant corticosteroids
Bronchodilators
• Methylxanthines (theophylline, aminophylline)—inhibit smooth muscle constriction. The pharmacokinetics of aminophylline would suggest that it is unlikely to be an effective treatment. Other products have not been investigated at this point, although sustained-release theophylline formulations are often recommended (25 mg/kg PO q24h in the evening).
• Beta-2 agonists (terbutaline, albuterol)—inhibit smooth muscle constriction. Injectable terbutaline is most helpful in a distressed animal (0.01 mg/kg SC/IV). Oral terbutaline

dose is 1/4 of a 2.5 mg tablet q12h. Initial albuterol dose is 20 μg/kg PO q12h; can increase to 50 μg/kg PO q8h.

Inhaled Bronchodilators
Albuterol is the preferred inhalant therapy in cats, providing immediate relief of bronchoconstriction—its effect lasts less than 4 hours. Recommended as adjuvant therapy in moderately to severely affected cats (q12–24h) or during respiratory distress.

Anthelminthics
• Routinely recommended for cats with clinical signs of FBD and airway cytology that is predominantly eosinophilic. Parasitic bronchitis can be difficult to diagnose based on airway cytology and fecal examination—empirical therapy is indicated with appropriate clinical signs and geographic location.
• Appropriate medication will depend on specific parasite suspected in the geographic region. Consider fenbendazole, ivermectin, or praziquantel.

Antibiotics
Use should be based on a positive quantitative culture. Choice of antibiotic therapy is based on susceptibility testing.

CONTRAINDICATIONS
Beta-2 antagonists (e.g., propranolol) are contraindicated because of their ability to block sympathetically mediated bronchodilation.

PRECAUTIONS
• Bronchodilators may exacerbate underlying cardiac disease.
• Long-term use of steroids increases risk of development of diabetes mellitus and predisposes to immunosuppression.

POSSIBLE INTERACTIONS
Fluoroquinolones decrease the metabolism of methylxanthines in dogs, although this has not been investigated in cats. Consider decreasing the dose of methylxanthine by 50% when used concurrently with a fluoroquinolone. Watch for toxic side effects of the methylxanthine (e.g., vomiting, diarrhea, tachycardia).

ALTERNATIVE DRUG(S)

Cyproheptadine
Serotonin antagonist. Has been shown in vitro to inhibit airway smooth muscle constriction in cats with experimentally induced asthma. Should be used only in patients refractory to other therapy.

Cyclosporine (Neoral)
• Give 2.5 mg/kg q12h—monitor cyclosporine levels.
• May be helpful in patients refractory to bronchodilator and corticosteroid therapy

Leukotriene Inhibitors or Receptor Blockers
No evidence to support the use of these drugs in FBD

FOLLOW-UP

PATIENT MONITORING
• Owners should watch for and report any increase in coughing, sneezing, wheezing, or respiratory distress. Medications should be increased appropriately if clinical signs recur.
• Follow-up radiographs are helpful in the first weeks after initial diagnosis to evaluate improvement with medical therapy.
• Long-term use of corticosteroids will require blood glucose monitoring every 3–6 months to screen for diabetes mellitus. Urinary tract infections can occur owing to immunosuppression. Owner should watch for signs of PU/PD that may indicate diabetes mellitus or renal disease.

PREVENTION/AVOIDANCE
• Eliminate any environmental factors that may trigger a crisis situation (see Risk Factors).
• Change furnace and air-conditioner filters on a regular basis.

POSSIBLE COMPLICATIONS
• Refractory cases or untreated acute episodes can be life threatening.
• Right-sided heart disease may develop as a result of long-term bronchitis.

EXPECTED COURSE AND PROGNOSIS
• Long-term therapy should be expected.
• Most cats do well if recurrence of clinical signs is carefully monitored and medical therapy appropriately adjusted.
• A few cats will be refractory to treatment; these carry a much worse prognosis.

MISCELLANEOUS

ASSOCIATED CONDITIONS
Cor pulmonale can be a sequela to chronic lower airway disease.

AGE-RELATED FACTORS N/A

ZOONOTIC POTENTIAL
None

PREGNANCY
Glucocorticoids are contraindicated in the pregnant animal. Bronchodilators should be used with caution.

SYNONYMS
Allergic bronchitis, chronic obstructive pulmonary disease, asthmatic bronchitis, feline lower airway disease, extrinsic asthma, eosinophilic bronchitis, immune-mediated airway disease

SEE ALSO
• Heartworm Disease—Cats
• Respiratory Parasites

ABBREVIATIONS
• FBD = feline bronchopulmonary disease
• FIP = feline interstitial pneumonia
• MDI = metered-dose inhaler
• PU/PD = polyuria/polydipsia

Suggested Readings

Dye JA, McKiernan BC, Rozanski EA, et al. Bronchopulmonary disease in the cat: historical, physical, radiographic, clinicopathologic, and pulmonary functional evaluation of 24 affected and 15 healthy cats. J Vet Intern Med 1996;10:385–399.

Moise NS, Wiedenkeller D, Yeager AE, et al. Clinical, radiographic, and bronchial cytologic features of cats with bronchial disease: 65 cases (1980–1986). J Am Vet Med Assoc 1989;194(10):1467–1473.

Padrid PA. Feline asthma. Vet Clin North Am 2000;30(6):1279–1293.

Padrid PA, Koblik PD. The techniques used to diagnose feline respiratory disorders. Vet Med 1990;Sept: 955–985.

Acknowledgment

The author and editors acknowledge the prior contributions of Dr. Kathleen E. Noone, who authored this topic in the previous edition.
Author Carrie J. Miller
Consulting Editor Lynelle R. Johnson

ASTROCYTOMA

BASICS

OVERVIEW
• Glial cell neoplasm of the brain
• Most common primary intracranial neoplasm of dogs; rarely diagnosed in cats
• Biologic behavior depends on the degree of anaplasia (graded I–IV, from best to worst prognosis)

SIGNALMENT
• Dogs—often brachycephalic breeds >5 years of age; no sex predilection reported
• Cats—usually old (>9 years); no sex or breed predilection reported

SIGNS
• Depend on tumor location
• Seizures
• Behavioral changes
• Disorientation
• Loss of conscious proprioception
• Cranial nerve abnormalities
• Upper motor neuron tetraparesis

CAUSES & RISK FACTORS
Unknown

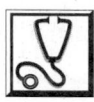

DIAGNOSIS

DIFFERENTIAL DIAGNOSIS
• Other primary or metastatic CNS tumors
• Granulomatous meningoencephalitis
• Trauma
• Cerebrovascular accident
• Meningitis

CBC/BIOCHEMISTRY/URINALYSIS
Usually normal

OTHER LABORATORY TESTS
CSF analysis—may show albuminocytologic dissociation (high protein with few cells)

IMAGING
• MRI or CT (brain)—ideal
• Radionuclide imaging—may show area of increased activity at the tumor site
• Radiography (skull)—rarely aids in detection

DIAGNOSTIC PROCEDURES
EEG—may localize lesion

TREATMENT
Surgery or radiotherapy

MEDICATIONS

DRUG(S)

Seizure Control
• Status epilepticus—diazepam (0.5–1.0 mg/kg IV given up to 3 times to achieve effect); if no response to diazepam, use pentobarbital (5–15 mg/kg IV slowly to effect)
• Long-term management—phenobarbital (1–4 mg/kg PO q12h)

Tumor Control
• Chemotherapy—lomustine (90 mg/m^2 PO every 3 weeks) or carmustine (50 mg/m^2 IV every 6 weeks) reported to achieve partial and complete remissions
• Prednisone—0.5–1.0 mg/kg q24h; may be effective in controlling peritumoral edema

CONTRAINDICATIONS/POSSIBLE INTERACTIONS
• Prednisone and phenobarbital—polyphagia; polydipsia; polyuria
• Phenobarbital—may cause sedation for up to 2 weeks after initiation of treatment; may cause increase in hepatic enzymes on serum biochemical panel
• CBC and platelet count—must perform 7–10 days after chemotherapy and immediately before each dose of chemotherapy to monitor myelosuppression
• Carmustine—cumulative doses of 1400 mg/m^2 may cause pulmonary toxicity.
• Chemotherapy may be toxic; seek advice before initiating treatment if unfamiliar with cytotoxic drugs.

FOLLOW-UP

PATIENT MONITORING
• Blood phenobarbital concentration—after 7–10 days of treatment; modify dosage as needed.
• CT or MRI—after every other chemotherapy treatment; monitor response.

EXPECTED COURSE AND PROGNOSIS
• Long-term prognosis—guarded
• Survival time with no treatment—2 months
• Median survival after chemotherapy plus medical management—up to 7 months
• Median survival after radiotherapy—may be as high as 12 months

MISCELLANEOUS

PREGNANCY
Do not breed animals undergoing chemotherapy.

SEE ALSO
• Seizures (Convulsions, Status Epilepticus)—Cats
• Seizures (Convulsions, Status Epilepticus)—Dogs

ABBREVIATIONS
• CSF = cerebrospinal fluid
• CT= computed tomography
• EEG = electroencephalogram
• MRI = magnetic resonance imaging

Suggested Reading
Frenier SL, Kraft SL, Moore MP, et al. Canine intracranial astrocytomas and comparison with the human counterpart. Compend Contin Educ Pract Vet 1990;12:1422–1433.
Morrison WB. Cancer affecting the nervous system. In: Morrison WB, ed. Cancer in dogs and cats: medical and surgical management. Baltimore: Williams & Wilkins, 1998:655–665.
Author Ruthanne Chun
Consulting Editor Wallace B. Morrison

 BASICS

OVERVIEW

An uncommon intestinal viral infection characterized by enteritis and diarrhea

SIGNALMENT

• Cats
• No known breed, sex, or age predilection

SIGNS

Diarrhea

CAUSES & RISK FACTORS

• A small, nonenveloped, RNA virus of the genus *Astrovirus*
• Details of the incidence, prevalence, and predisposing factors unknown

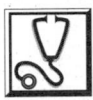 DIAGNOSIS

DIFFERENTIAL DIAGNOSIS

• Many causes of gastroenteritis
• Food allergy
• Toxin ingestion
• Inflammatory bowel disease
• Neoplasia
• Intestinal parasites
• Viral infections—panleukopenia, rotavirus, enteric coronavirus, enteric calicivirus
• Bacterial infections—salmonellosis, coliforms
• Protozoal infections—*Giardia,* cryptosporidiosis

CBC/BIOCHEMISTRY/URINALYSIS

N/A

OTHER LABORATORY TESTS

• Electron microscopy of feces—identify *Astrovirus* particles
• Difficult to isolate in the laboratory

IMAGING

N/A

DIAGNOSTIC PROCEDURES

None

PATHOLOGIC FINDINGS

None described; similar to mild enteritis, rotavirus, or coronavirus enteritis

 TREATMENT

• Control diarrhea.
• Re-establish fluid and electrolyte balance.

 MEDICATIONS

DRUG(S)

No specific antiviral drugs

CONTRAINDICATIONS/POSSIBLE INTERACTIONS

None

 FOLLOW-UP

PATIENT MONITORING

Monitor fluid and electrolytes.

PREVENTION/AVOIDANCE

Isolate infected cats during acute disease.

POSSIBLE COMPLICATIONS

Secondary intestinal viral and bacterial infections

EXPECTED COURSE AND PROGNOSIS

• Illness usually < 1 week
• Mortality—appears low
• Prognosis—good

 MISCELLANEOUS

ZOONOTIC POTENTIAL

• Unknown
• Produces enteritis in many species, including sheep and humans

Suggested Reading

Barr MC, Olsen CW, Scott FW. Feline viral diseases. In: Ettinger SJ, Feldman EC, eds. Veterinary internal medicine. Philadelphia: Saunders, 1995:409–439.

Author Fred W. Scott
Consulting Editor Stephen C. Barr

ATAXIA

 BASICS

DEFINITION

• A sign of sensory dysfunction that produces incoordination of the limbs, head, and/or trunk
• Three clinical types—sensory (proprioceptive), vestibular, and cerebellar; all produce changes in limb coordination, but vestibular and cerebellar ataxia also produce changes in head and neck movement.

PATHOPHYSIOLOGY

Sensory (Proprioceptive)

• Proprioceptive pathways in the spinal cord (i.e., fasciculus gracilis, fasciculus cuneatus, and spinocerebellar tracts) relay limb and trunk position to the brain.
• When the spinal cord is slowly compressed, proprioceptive deficits are usually the first signs observed, because these pathways are located more superficially in the white matter and their larger-sized axons are more susceptible to compression than are other tracts.
• Generally accompanied by weakness owing to early concomitant upper motor neuron involvement; weakness not always obvious early in the course of the disease
• Ataxia can occur with spinal cord, brain stem, and cerebral locations of lesions.

Vestibular

• Changes in head and neck position are relayed through the vestibulocochlear nerve to the brain stem.
• Vestibular receptors or the nerve in the inner ear are considered part of the peripheral nervous system, whereas nuclei in the brain stem are considered part of the central nervous system.
• Localize the vestibular signs to peripheral or central vestibular nervous system because prognosis and rule-outs differ for these two locations.
• Both locations of vestibular disease cause various degrees of disequilibrium with ensuing vestibular ataxia.
• Affected animal leans, tips, falls, or even rolls toward the side of the lesion; accompanied by head tilt
• Central vestibular signs usually have changing types of nystagmus or vertical nystagmus; proprioceptive deficits; quadriparesis or hemiparesis; multiple cranial nerve signs; and somnolence, stupor, or coma (due to involvement of the reticular activating system).

• Peripheral vestibular signs do not include proprioceptive deficits, quadriparesis or hemiparesis, changes in mental status, or vertical nystagmus.

Cerebellar

• The cerebellum regulates, coordinates, and smooths motor activity.
• Proprioception is normal because the ascending proprioceptive pathways to the cortex are intact; weakness does not occur because the upper motor neurons are intact.
• Inadequacy in the performance of motor activity; strength preservation; no proprioceptive deficits
• Affected animal shows uncoordinated motor activity of limbs, head and neck; hypermetria; dysmetria; head tremors; intention tremors; and truncal sway.

SYSTEMS AFFECTED

Nervous—spinal cord (and brain stem and cortex), cerebellum, vestibular system

SIGNALMENT

Any age, breed, or sex

SIGNS

• Important to define the type of ataxia to localize the problem
• Only one limb involved—consider a lameness problem.
• Only hindlimbs affected—likely a spinal cord disorder affecting the spinocerebellar tracts
• All or both ipsilateral limbs affected—cerebellar
• Head tilt—vestibular

CAUSES

Neurologic

Cerebellar
• Degenerative—abiotrophy (Kerry blue terriers, Gordon setters, rough-coated collies, Australian kelpies, Airedales, Bernese mountain dogs, Finnish harriers, Brittany spaniels, border collies, beagles, Samoyeds, wire fox terriers, Labrador retrievers, great Danes, chow chows, Rhodesian ridgebacks, domestic shorthair cats); storage diseases often have cerebellomedullary involvement.
• Anomalous—hypoplasia secondary to perinatal infection with panleukopenia virus (cats); malformed cerebellum due to herpesvirus infection (newborn puppies)
• Neoplastic—any tumor of the CNS (primary or secondary) localized to the cerebellum
• Infectious—canine distemper virus; FIP; and any other CNS infection affecting the cerebellum

• Inflammatory, idiopathic, immune-mediated—granulomatous meningo-encephalomyelitis
• Toxic—metronidazole
Vestibular—CNS
• Infectious—FIP; canine distemper virus; rickettsial diseases
• Inflammatory, idiopathic, immune-mediated—granulomatous meningo-encephalomyelitis
• Toxic—metronidazole
Vestibular—PNS
• Infectious—otitis media interna; *Cryptococcus* granuloma (cats)
• Idiopathic—geriatric vestibular disease (dogs); idiopathic vestibular syndrome (cats); nasopharyngeal (middle ear) polyps (cats)
• Metabolic—hypothyroidism
• Neoplastic—squamous cell carcinoma, bone tumors
• Traumatic
Spinal Cord
• Degenerative—degenerative radiculomyelopathy (old German shepherds)
• Vascular—fibrocartilaginous embolic myelopathy
• Anomalous—hemivertebrae; dens hypoplasia with atlantoaxial subluxation-luxation; other spinal cord and vertebral malformation
• Neoplastic—primary bone tumors; multiple myeloma and metastatic tumors that infiltrate the vertebral body
• Infectious—diskospondylitis; myelitis
• Traumatic—intervertebral disk herniation; fracture or luxation; cervical vertebral instability; atlantoaxial subluxation-luxation

Metabolic

• Anemia
• Electrolyte disturbances—especially hypokalemia and hypoglycemia

Miscellaneous

• Drugs—acepromazine; antihistamines; antiepileptic
• Respiratory compromise
• Cardiac compromise

RISK FACTORS

• Intervertebral disk disease—dachshunds, poodles, cocker spaniels, and beagles
• Cervical cord compression—Doberman pinschers and Great Danes
• Fibrocartilaginous embolism—young, large-breed dogs and miniature schnauzers
• Dens hypoplasia and atlantoaxial luxation—small-breed dogs, poodles

DIAGNOSIS

DIFFERENTIAL DIAGNOSIS
• Differentiate the types of ataxia
• Differentiate from other disease processes that can affect gait—musculoskeletal, metabolic, cardiovascular, respiratory
• Musculoskeletal disorders—typically produce lameness, pain, and a reluctance to move
• Systemic illness and endocrine, cardio-vascular, and metabolic disorders—can cause intermittent ataxia, especially of the pelvic limbs; with fever, weight loss, murmurs, arrhythmias, hair loss, or collapse with exercise, suspect a non-neurologic cause; obtain minimum data from hemogram, biochemistry analysis, and urinalysis
• Head tilt or nystagmus—likely vestibular
• Intention tremors of the head or hypermetria—likely cerebellar
• Only limbs affected: likely spinal cord dysfunction; all four limbs affected: lesion is in the cervical area or is multifocal to diffuse; only pelvic limbs affected: lesion is anywhere below the second thoracic vertebra

CBC/BIOCHEMISTRY/URINALYSIS
Normal unless metabolic cause (e.g., hypoglycemia, electrolyte imbalance, anemia)

OTHER LABORATORY TESTS
• Hypoglycemia—determine serum insulin concentration on the same sample; calculate an amended insulin:glucose ratio (rule out insulinoma)
• Anemia—differentiate as nonregenerative or regenerative on the basis of the reticulocyte count
• Electrolyte imbalance—correct the problem; see if ataxia resolves
• Antiepileptic drugs—if being administered, evaluate serum concentration for toxicity

IMAGING
• Spinal radiography, myelography, or MRI—if spinal cord dysfunction suspected
• Bullae radiography—if peripheral vestibular disease suspected; CT or MRI scans superior but more expensive
• Thoracic radiography—for old patients; identify neoplasia
• CT or MRI—if cerebellar disease suspected; evaluate potential brain disease
• Abdominal ultrasonography—if hepatic, renal, adrenal, or pancreatic dysfunction suspected

DIAGNOSTIC PROCEDURES
• CSF—confirm nervous system causes

TREATMENT
• Usually outpatient, depending on the severity and acuteness of clinical signs
• Exercise—decrease or restrict if spinal cord disease suspected
• Client should monitor gait for increasing dysfunction or weakness; if paresis worsens or paralysis develops, other testing is warranted.
• Avoid drugs that could be contributing to the problem; may not be possible in patients on antiepileptic drugs for seizures

MEDICATIONS

DRUG(S) OF CHOICE
Not recommended until the source or cause of the problem is identified

FOLLOW-UP

PATIENT MONITORING
Periodic neurologic examinations to assess condition

POSSIBLE COMPLICATIONS
• Spinal cord or neuromuscular disease—progression to weakness and possibly paralysis
• Hypoglycemia—seizures
• Cerebellar disease—head tremors and bobbing
• Brain stem disease—stupor, coma, death

MISCELLANEOUS

AGE-RELATED FACTORS
N/A

SEE ALSO
• See specific causes
• Cerebellar Degeneration
• Head Tilt
• Paralysis

ABBREVIATIONS
• CNS = central nervous system
• CSF = cerebrospinal fluid
• CT = computed tomography
• FIP = feline infectious peritonitis
• MRI = magnetic resonance imaging
• PNS = peripheral nervous system

Suggested Reading
Davies C, Shell L. Neurological problems. In: Common small animal medical diagnoses: an algorithmic approach. Philadelphia: Saunders, 2002:36–59.
Oliver JE, Lorenz MD, Kornegay JN. Handbook of veterinary neurology. 3rd ed. Philadelphia: Saunders, 1997:216–239.
Thomas WB. Vestibular dysfunction. Vet Clin North Am Small Anim Pract 2000;30:227–249.
Author Linda G. Shell
Consulting Editor Joane M. Parent

ATHEROSCLEROSIS

BASICS

OVERVIEW
Thickening of the inner arterial wall in association with lipid deposits. Chronic arterial change characterized by loss of elasticity, luminal narrowing, and proliferating and degenerative lesions of the intima and media

SIGNALMENT
- Rare in dogs
- Not described in cats
- Higher prevalence in miniature schnauzer, Doberman pinscher, poodle, and Labrador retriever
- Geriatric patients (> 9 years)

SIGNS

Historical Findings
- None in some animals
- Lethargy
- Anorexia
- Weakness
- Dyspnea
- Collapse
- Vomiting
- Diarrhea

Physical Examination Findings
- Dyspnea
- Irregular rhythm
- Heart failure
- Disorientation
- Blindness
- Circling
- Coma

CAUSES & RISK FACTORS
- Severe hypothyroidism
- Increasing age
- Hyperlipidemia in miniature schnauzers
- Male gender (male dogs may have predisposition)
- High total cholesterol

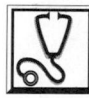

DIAGNOSIS

DIFFERENTIAL DIAGNOSIS
Arteriosclerosis

CBC/BIOCHEMISTRY/URINALYSIS
- Hypercholesterolemia
- Hyperlipidemia
- High BUN and creatinine
- High liver enzymes

OTHER LABORATORY TESTS
- Low T_3 and T_4
- High values for alpha-2 and beta fractions on protein electrophoresis

IMAGING

Radiography
Thoracic and abdominal radiographs may reveal cardiomegaly and hepatomegaly.

DIAGNOSTIC PROCEDURES

Electrocardiography
- Conduction abnormalities and notched QRS complexes
- Atrial fibrillation
- ST segment elevation or depression with myocardial infarction

TREATMENT
- Treat the underlying disorder and clinical signs (e.g., dyspnea if congestive heart failure develops).
- Diet—low-fat diet, weight loss program, and high soluble fiber intake to control hyperlipidemia

MEDICATIONS

DRUG(S)
- Treat conduction disturbances and arrhythmias if clinically indicated
- Thyroid replacement if hypothyroidism is confirmed
- Antihypertensive therapy if hypertension is documented (e.g., enalapril—0.5 mg/kg PO q12–q24h or benazepril—0.5 mg/kg PO q24h)
- Blood cholesterol–reducing medications (e.g., Niacin, Lopid) if hyperlipidemic

CONTRAINDICATIONS/POSSIBLE INTERACTIONS
N/A

FOLLOW-UP
- Monitor T_4 concentration 4–6 hours post-administration after the first 6 weeks of treatment and adjust dosage accordingly.
- Monitor blood triglyceride and cholesterol levels.
- Monitor ECG for conduction disturbances and ST segment changes.

✓ MISCELLANEOUS

ASSOCIATED CONDITIONS
Hypothyroidism

AGE-RELATED FACTORS
Geriatric patients (> 9 years)

SEE ALSO
Myocardial Infarction

Suggested Reading
Drost WT, Bahr RJ, Henay GA, Campbell GA. Aortoiliac thrombus secondary to a mineralized arteriosclerotic lesion. Vet Rad Ultrasound 1999; 40:262–266.

Hamlen HJ. Sinoatrial node arteriosclerosis in two young dogs. J Am Vet Med Assoc 1994;204:751.

Kidd L, Stepien RL, Amrheiw DP. Clinical findings and coronary artery disease in dogs and cats with acute and subacute myocardial necrosis: 28 cases, J Am Anim Hosp Assoc 2000;36:199–208.

Liu SK, Tilley LP, Tappe JP, Fox PR. Clinical and pathologic findings in dogs with atherosclerosis: 21 cases (1970–1983). J Am Vet Med Assoc 1986;189:227–232.

Author Larry P. Tilley
Consulting Editors Larry P. Tilley and Francis W. K. Smith, Jr.

BASICS

OVERVIEW

• Results from malformation or disruption of the articulation between the first two cervical vertebrae (atlas and axis); causes spinal cord compression
• Usually associated with a congenital anomaly of the dens (aplasia, hypoplasia, or deviation of the dens) and its ligamentous attachments
• May be a consequence of traumatic injury, particularly fracture of the dens
• Spinal cord trauma or compression at the junction between the atlas and axis—may cause neck pain and/or upper motor neuron tetraparesis to paralysis

SIGNALMENT

• Congenital—toy-breed dogs (poodles, Chihuahuas, Pekingese)
• Age at onset—usually before 12 months of age
• Uncommon in larger-breed dogs, dogs >1 year old, and cats
• No sex predilection

SIGNS

• Intermittent or progressive tetraparesis, usually with neck pain—most common
• Episodes of collapse—may occur
• May see proprioceptive deficits to complete paralysis, depending on degree of spinal cord compression or trauma
• Spinal reflexes—normal to exaggerated in all four limbs
• May lead to catastrophic acute spinal cord trauma, respiratory arrest, and death

CAUSES & RISK FACTORS

• Usually caused by abnormal formation of the dens
• Fracture of the dens
• Clinical signs—may be exacerbated by activity, especially flexion of the neck
• Toy-breed dogs—at risk for congenital malformation of the dens

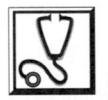

DIAGNOSIS

DIFFERENTIAL DIAGNOSIS

• Disk herniation
• Fibrocartilaginous embolism
• Neoplasia
• Trauma
• Seizures
• With exercise intolerance—myasthenia gravis; hypoglycemia; hypoxia; cardiac abnormalities
• Diagnosis based on thorough physical examination and imaging

CBC/BIOCHEMISTRY/URINALYSIS

Normal

IMAGING

• Cervical spine radiographs—made with patient under general anesthesia; lateral view reveals increase in dorsal atlantoaxial space; lateral and ventrodorsal views reveal absence or fracture of dens.
• Hyperflex the neck only with extreme care during radiography; could cause severe spinal cord trauma and even death
• Myelography—seldom necessary for diagnosis

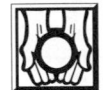

TREATMENT

Conservative—reserved for patients with neck pain alone; includes neck brace and cage confinement for several weeks; recurrence common

Surgery

• Definitive; always indicated for neck pain with neurologic signs; dorsal and ventral approaches
• Dorsal approach—use wire or synthetic suture material to fix the dorsal spinous process of the axis to the dorsal arch of the atlas; common and serious postoperative complication: breakage of the dorsal arch of the atlas by the wire or suture
• Ventral approach—cancellous bone grafting and transarticular pinning; more stable; use polymethyl methacrylate to lock together the ventral tips of the pins to prevent pin migration; may use lag screws instead

MEDICATIONS

DRUG(S)

Methylprednisolone sodium succinate—30 mg/kg; for acute paralysis and perioperatively

CONTRAINDICATIONS/POSSIBLE INTERACTIONS

• Glucocorticoids—use caution when given in conjunction with conservative treatment; may reduce pain, resulting in increased activity and spinal cord trauma
• Avoid NSAIDs in combination with glucocorticoids in all patients—increases risk of life-threatening gastrointestinal hemorrhage

FOLLOW-UP

• Conservative treatment—re-evaluated weekly until clinical signs have resolved; often see recurrence, necessitating surgery
• Surgical treatment—usually no recurrent episodes; success influenced by the expertise and experience of the surgeon; intraoperative and immediately postoperative complications possible
• Untreated—may lead to catastrophic acute spinal cord trauma, respiratory arrest, and death

MISCELLANEOUS

Suggested Reading

Beaver DP, Ellison GW, Lewis DD. Risk factors affecting the outcome of surgery for atlantoaxial subluxation in dogs: 46 cases (1978–1998). J Am Vet Med Assoc 2000; 216(7).

Fossum TW, Hedlund CS, Johnson AL, et al. Small animal surgery. St. Louis: Mosby–Year Book, 1997.

Shires PK. Atlantoaxial instability. In: Slatter D, ed. Textbook of small animal surgery. 3rd ed. Philadelphia: Saunders, 2003.

Acknowledgment

The author and editor acknowledge the prior contributions of Dr. Mary O. Smith, who authored this topic in the previous edition.

Author Peter K. Shires
Consulting Editor Peter K. Shires

ATOPY

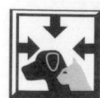

BASICS

DEFINITION
Predisposition to become allergic to normally innocuous substances, such as pollens (grasses, weeds, and trees), molds, house dust mites, epithelial allergens, and other environmental allergens

PATHOPHYSIOLOGY
• Susceptible animals become sensitized to environmental allergens by producing allergen-specific IgE, which binds to receptor sites on cutaneous mast cells; further allergen exposure (inhalation, percutaneous absorption) causes mast cell degranulation, which is a type I immediate hypersensitivity reaction, and results in the release of histamine, proteolytic enzymes, cytokines, chemokines, and many other chemical mediators. • Non-IgE antibodies (IgGd) and a late-phase reaction (8–12 hr) may also be involved.

SYSTEMS AFFECTED
• Skin/Exocrine—pruritus, xerosis, or generalized dryness of the skin; recurrent superficial pyoderma and yeast infections; recurrent bilateral otitis externa • Ophthalmic—recurrent bilateral conjunctivitis • Respiratory, Reproductive, and Gastrointestinal—reported, but not well documented

GENETICS
• Canine—although there is an inherited predisposition, the mode of inheritance is unknown and other factors may also be important. • Feline—unclear

INCIDENCE/PREVALENCE
• Canine—true incidence unknown; estimated at 3%–15% of the canine population; reported to be the second most common allergic skin disease • Feline—unknown; generally believed to be much lower than that for dogs

GEOGRAPHIC DISTRIBUTION
Canine—recognized worldwide; local environmental factors (temperature, humidity, and flora) influence the seasonality, severity, and duration of signs.

SIGNALMENT

Species
Dogs and cats

Breed Predilections
• Canine—any breed, including mongrels; because of genetic predisposition, it may be recognized more frequently in certain breeds or families, which can vary geographically. • In the United States (canine)—Boston terriers, Cairn terriers, dalmatians, English bulldogs, English setters, Irish setters, Lhasa apsos, miniature schnauzers, pugs, Sealyham terriers, Scottish terriers, West Highland white terriers, wire-haired fox terriers, and golden retrievers • Feline—none reported

Mean Age and Range
Canine—mean age at onset 1–3 years; range 3 months–6 years; signs may be so mild the first year that they are not noted but are usually progressive and clinically apparent before 3 years of age.

Predominant Sex
• Both sexes are probably affected equally.

SIGNS

General
• Hallmark sign—pruritus (itching, scratching, rubbing, licking) • Primary lesions may occur, but most cutaneous changes are believed to be produced by self-induced trauma.

Historical Findings
• Facial, pedal, or axillary pruritus • Early onset • Family history of atopy • May be seasonal • Recurring skin or ear infections • Temporary response to glucocorticoids • Symptoms progressively worsen with time

Physical Examination Findings
• Areas most commonly affected—interdigital spaces, carpal and tarsal areas, muzzle, periocular region, axillae, groin, and pinnae • Lesions—vary from none to broken hairs or salivary discoloration to erythema, papular reactions, crusts, alopecia, hyperpigmentation, lichenification, excessively oily or dry seborrhea, and hyperhidrosis (apocrine sweating) • Secondary bacterial and yeast skin infections (common) • Chronic relapsing otitis externa • Conjunctivitis may occur.

CAUSES
• Airborne pollens (grasses, weeds, and trees) • Mold spores (indoor and outdoor) • House dust mite • Animal danders • Insects (controversial)

RISK FACTORS
• Temperate environments with long allergy seasons and high pollen and mold spore levels • Concurrent pruritic dermatoses, such as flea allergy dermatitis and food hypersensitivity (summation effect)

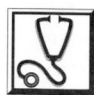

DIAGNOSIS

DIFFERENTIAL DIAGNOSIS
• Food hypersensitivity—may cause identical lesion distribution and physical examination findings but should be nonseasonal; may occur concurrently with atopy; differentiation is made by noting response to hypoallergenic diet. • Flea bite hypersensitivity—most common cause of seasonal pruritus in many geographical regions; may occur concurrently with atopy; differentiation is made by noting lesion distribution, response to flea control, and results of intradermal skin testing. • Sarcoptic mange—often occurs in young or stray dogs; usually causes severe pruritus of the ventral chest, lateral elbows, lateral hocks, and pinnal margins; multiple skin scrapings and/or complete response to a trial of miticidal therapy are indicated to rule out sarcoptic mange. • Secondary pyoderma—usually caused by *Staphylococcus intermedius;* characterized by follicular papules, pustules, crusts, and epidermal collarettes • Secondary yeast infections—usually caused by *Malassezia* pachydermatis; characterized by erythematous, scaly, crusty, greasy, and very malodorous body folds and intertriginous areas; demonstration of numerous budding yeast organisms by skin cytology and obtaining a favorable response to antifungal therapy are diagnostic. • Contact dermatitis (allergic or irritant)—may cause severe erythema and pruritus of the feet and thinly haired areas of the ventral abdomen; history of exposure to a known contact sensitizer or irritant, response to a change of environment, and patch testing may be diagnostic; thought to be rare in dogs and cats.

CBC/BIOCHEMISTRY/URINALYSIS
Eosinophilia—rare in dogs without concurrent flea infections; common in cats

OTHER LABORATORY TESTS

Serologic Allergy Tests
• Tests to measure the amount of allergen-specific IgE antibody in the patient's serum are commercially available. • Advantages over IDST—availability; large areas of hair do not have to be shaved • Disadvantages—frequent false-positive reactions; limited number of allergens tested; inconsistent assay validation and quality control (may vary with the laboratory used) • Reliability in cats is unknown.

DIAGNOSTIC PROCEDURES

IDST
• Small amounts of test allergens are injected intradermally and wheal formation is measured. • Most accurate method of identifying offending allergens for possible avoidance or inclusion in an immunotherapy prescription. • Results are sometimes difficult to interpret in cats owing to the relatively small wheals produced.

PATHOLOGIC FINDINGS
• Gross lesions—see Physical Examination Findings • Skin biopsy—may help rule out other differential diagnoses; results are usually not pathognomonic. • Dermatohistopathologic

changes—acanthosis, mixed mononuclear superficial perivascular dermatitis, sebaceous gland metaplasia, and secondary superficial pyoderma

TREATMENT

APPROPRIATE HEALTH CARE
Outpatient

ACTIVITY
Avoid offending allergens when possible.

DIET
Essential fatty acid supplementation may be beneficial in some cases.

CLIENT EDUCATION
• Explain the progressive nature of the condition. • Inform client that it rarely goes into remission and cannot be cured.
• Inform client that some form of therapy may be necessary for life.

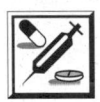

MEDICATIONS

DRUG(S) OF CHOICE

Immunotherapy (Hyposensitization)
• Administration (usually SC injections) of gradually increasing doses of the causative allergens to affected patients in an attempt to reduce their sensitivity
• Allergens selected—based on allergy test results, patient history, and knowledge of local flora
• Indicated when it is desirable to avoid or reduce the amount of corticosteroids required to control signs, when signs last longer than 4–6 months per year, or when nonsteroidal forms of therapy are ineffective
• Successfully reduces pruritus in 60–80% of dogs and cats
• The response is usually slow, often requiring 3–6 months and up to 1 year.

Corticosteroids
• May be given for short-term relief and to break the itch–scratch cycle
• Should be tapered to the lowest dosage that adequately controls pruritus
• Best choices—prednisone suspension (0.5 to 1.0 mg/kg SC or IM); prednisone or methylprednisolone tablets (0.2 to 0.5 mg/kg PO q48h)
• Repository injectable corticosteroids should be avoided in dogs.
• Cats may require methylprednisolone acetate treatment (4 mg/kg SC or IM).

Antihistamines
• Less effective than are corticosteroids
• Efficacy as a sole treatment is probably in the 10%–20% range.
• May act synergistically with essential fatty acid supplements

• Corticosteroid therapy can often be avoided or given at a reduced dosage when used concurrently.
• Dogs—hydroxyzine (1–2 mg/kg PO q8h), chlorpheniramine (0.2–0.4 mg/kg PO q12h), diphenhydramine (2.2 mg/kg PO q8h), and clemastine (0.04–0.10 mg/kg PO q12h)
• Cats—chlorpheniramine (0.5 mg/kg PO q12h); efficacy estimated at 10%–50%

CONTRAINDICATIONS
N/A

PRECAUTIONS
• Corticosteroids—use judiciously in dogs to avoid iatrogenic hyperglucocorticism and associated problems, aggravation of pyoderma, and induction of demodicosis.
• Antihistamines—can produce drowsiness, anorexia, vomiting, diarrhea, and even increased pruritus; use with caution in patients with cardiac arrhythmias.

POSSIBLE INTERACTIONS
The antihistamine astemizole has been associated with life-threatening cardiac arrhythmias in humans when administered concomitantly with imidazole antifungal drugs.

ALTERNATIVE DRUG(S)
• Frequent bathing in cool water with antipruritic shampoos can be beneficial.
• Supplementation with ω-3 and ω-6 fatty acids helps some pruritic patients; some studies have indicated that ω-3 (eicosapentaenoic acid 66 mg/kg/day) may be more effective than ω-6 (linoleic acid 130 mg/kg/day); other studies suggest that a 5:1 ratio of ω-6:ω-3 in the diet is indicated.
• Tricyclic antidepressants (doxepin 1.0–2.0 mg/kg PO q12h; or amitriptyline 1.0–2.0 mg/kg PO q12h) have been given to dogs as antipruritics but their overall effectiveness and mode of action is unclear; not extensively studied in the cat
• Cyclosporine (Neoral 5 mg/kg/day) is quite effective in controlling pruritus associated with allergic dermatitis yet is very expensive. The drug must be administered without food (2 hrs. before and after dosing) to ensure adequate absorption.
• Topical triamcinolone spray .015% (Allerdem, Virbac) can be used over large body surfaces to control pruritus with minimal side effects.

FOLLOW-UP

PATIENT MONITORING
• Examine patient every 2–8 weeks when a new course of therapy is started
• Monitor pruritus, self-trauma, pyoderma, and possible adverse drug reactions
• Once an acceptable level of control is achieved, examine patient every 3–12 months

• CBC, serum chemistry profile, and urinalysis—recommended every 6–12 months for patients on chronic corticosteroid therapy

PREVENTION/AVOIDANCE
• If the offending allergens have been identified through allergy testing, the owner should undertake to reduce the animal's exposure as much as possible. • Minimizing other sources of pruritus (e.g., fleas, food hypersensitivity, and secondary skin infections) may reduce the level of pruritus enough to be tolerated by the animal.

POSSIBLE COMPLICATIONS
Secondary pyoderma and concurrent flea allergy dermatitis

EXPECTED COURSE AND PROGNOSIS
• Not life-threatening unless intractable pruritus results in euthanasia
• If left untreated, the degree of pruritus worsens and the duration of signs last longer each year of the animal's life
• Only rare cases spontaneously resolve.

MISCELLANEOUS

ASSOCIATED CONDITIONS
• Flea allergy dermatitis
• Food hypersensitivity
• Pyoderma
• Otitis externa

AGE-RELATED FACTORS
Severity worsens with age.

ZOONOTIC POTENTIAL
None

PREGNANCY
• Corticosteroids—contraindicated during pregnancy
• Antihistamines—safety during pregnancy has not been established.

SYNONYMS
• Canine allergic inhalant dermatitis
• Canine atopic dermatitis
• Canine atopic disease

SEE ALSO
• Fleas and Flea Control
• Food Reactions (dermatologic)
• Otitis Externa and Media
• Pyoderma

ABBREVIATION
• IDST = intradermal skin test

Suggested Reading
Reedy LM, Miller WH, Willemse T. Allergic skin diseases of dogs and cats. 2nd ed. Philadelphia: Saunders, 1997.
Authors Jon D. Plant and Karen Helton-Rhodes
Consulting Editor Karen Helton-Rhodes

ATRIAL FIBRILLATION AND ATRIAL FLUTTER

BASICS

DEFINITION
• Atrial fibrillation—rapid, irregularly irregular supraventricular rhythm. Two forms recognized: primary atrial fibrillation, an uncommon disease that occurs mostly in large dogs with no or mild underlying cardiac disease, and secondary atrial fibrillation, which occurs in dogs and cats secondary to underlying cardiac disease • Atrial flutter is similar to atrial fibrillation, but the atrial rate is generally slower and is characterized by saw-toothed flutter waves in the baseline of the ECG. The ventricular response is generally rapid but may be regular or irregular.

ECG FEATURES

Atrial Flutter
• Atrial rhythm usually regular; rate approximately 300–400 bpm • P waves usually discerned as either discrete P waves or a "saw-toothed" baseline • Ventricular rhythm and rate generally depend on the atrial rate and AV nodal conduction, but are generally regular or regularly irregular and rapid. • Conduction pattern to the ventricles is variable—in some cases every other atrial depolarization produces a ventricular depolarization (2:1 conduction ratio), giving a regular ventricular rhythm; other times the conduction pattern appears random, giving an irregular ventricular rhythm that can mimic atrial fibrillation.

Secondary Atrial Fibrillation
• No P waves present—baseline may be flat or may have small irregular undulations ("f" waves); some undulations may look like P waves • Ventricular rate high—usually 180–240 bpm in dogs and > 220 bpm in cats. • Interval between QRS complexes is irregularly irregular; QRS complexes usually appear normal.

Primary Atrial Fibrillation
Similar to secondary atrial fibrillation except ventricular rate usually in the normal range.

PATHOPHYSIOLOGY
• Atrial fibrillation—caused by numerous small reentrant pathways creating a rapid (>500 depolarizations/min) and disorganized depolarization pattern in the atria) that results in cessation of atrial contraction. Depolarizations continuously bombard the AV junctional tissue, which acts as a filter and does not allow all depolarizations to conduct to the ventricles. Many atrial depolarizations activate only a part of the atria because the rapid rate renders portions of the atria refractory, and thus they cannot reach the AV junction. Other atrial impulses penetrate into the AV junctional tissue but are not robust enough to penetrate the entire length.

Blocked impulses affect the conduction properties of the AV junctional tissue and alter conduction of subsequent electrical impulses; electrical impulses are conducted through the AV junction irregularly, producing an irregular ventricular rhythm. • Atrial flutter—probably originates from one site of reentry that moves continuously throughout the atrial myocardium and frequently and regularly stimulates the AV node. When the atrial rate becomes sufficiently fast, the refractory period of the AV node exceeds the cycle length (P to P interval) of the SVT, and some atrial depolarizations are blocked from traversing the AV node (functional second-degree AV block).

SYSTEMS AFFECTED

Cardiovascular
Loss of atrial contraction may result in decreased stroke volume and cardiac output depending on heart rate; high heart rate may result in deterioration in myocardial function.

GENETICS
No breeding studies available

INCIDENCE AND PREVALENCE
N/A

GEOGRAPHIC DISTRIBUTION
N/A

SIGNALMENT

Species
Dogs and cats

Breed Predilections
Large and giant-breed dogs are more prone to primary atrial fibrillation.

Mean Age and Range
N/A

Predominant Sex
N/A

SIGNS

General Comments
Generally relate to the underlying disease process and/or CHF rather than the arrhythmia itself, but previously stable animals may decompensate

Historical Findings
• Coughing/dyspnea/tachypnea • Exercise intolerance • Rarely syncope • Dogs with primary atrial fibrillation are typically asymptomatic.

Physical Examination Findings
• On auscultation, patients with atrial fibrillation have an erratic heart rhythm that sounds like "tennis shoes in a dryer." • First heart sound intensity in atrial fibrillation is variable; second heart sound only heard on beats with effective ejection, not on every beat • Third heart sounds (gallop sounds) may be present. • Patients with atrial fibrillation have pulse deficits and variable

pulse quality. • Signs of CHF often present (e.g., cough, dyspnea, cyanosis)

CAUSES
• Chronic valvular disease • Cardiomyopathy • Congenital heart disease • Digoxin toxicity • Idiopathic • Ventricular pre–excitation (atrial flutter)

RISK FACTORS
Heart disease

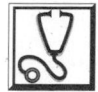

DIAGNOSIS

DIFFERENTIAL DIAGNOSIS
• Frequent atrial (supraventricular) premature depolarizations • Supraventricular tachycardia with AV block

CBC/BIOCHEMISTRY/URINALYSIS
N/A

OTHER LABORATORY TESTS
N/A

IMAGING
• Echocardiography and radiography may characterize type and severity of the underlying cardiac disease; moderate to severe left atrial enlargement common • Typically normal in patients with primary atrial fibrillation, although mild left atrial enlargement may accompany the hemodynamic alterations imposed by the arrhythmia

DIAGNOSTIC PROCEDURES
N/A

PATHOLOGIC FINDINGS
N/A

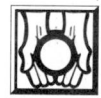

TREATMENT

APPROPRIATE HEALTH CARE
• Patients with fast (secondary) atrial fibrillation are treated medically to slow the ventricular rate. Converting the atrial fibrillation to sinus rhythm would be ideal, but such attempts in patients with severe underlying heart disease or left atrial enlargement are futile because of a low success rate and high rate of recurrence. Consider quinidine or electrical cardioversion to sinus rhythm for a dog with primary atrial fibrillation. • Electrical (DC) cardioversion—application of a transthoracic electrical shock at a specific time in the cardiac cycle; requires special equipment, trained personnel, and general anesthesia. A small (10 joules) electrical shock may suffice, but most require higher power (50–150 joules). Biphasic DC cardioversion consistently cardioverts with lower power (< 50 joules).

NURSING CARE
As indicated for CHF

ATRIAL FIBRILLATION AND ATRIAL FLUTTER

ACTIVITY
Restrict activity until tachycardia is controlled.

DIET
Mild to moderate sodium restriction if CHF

CLIENT EDUCATION
• Secondary atrial fibrillation is usually associated with severe underlying heart disease; goal of therapy is to lower heart rate and control clinical signs • Sustained conversion to sinus rhythm is unlikely with secondary atrial fibrillation.

SURGICAL CONSIDERATIONS N/A

 MEDICATIONS

DRUG(S) OF CHOICE
Digoxin, β-adrenergic blockers, and calcium channel blockers (diltiazem) are frequently used to slow conduction through the AV node; definition of an adequate heart rate response varies among clinicians, but in dogs is generally 140–160 bpm.

Dogs
• Digoxin—maintenance oral dose 0.005–0.01 mg/kg PO q12h; to achieve a therapeutic serum concentration more rapidly, the maintenance dose can be doubled for the first day. If digoxin is administered alone and the heart rate remains high, check the digoxin level and adjust the dose to bring the level into the therapeutic range. If the heart rate remains high, consider adding a calcium channel blocker or a β-adrenergic blocker. • Propranolol—initially administered at a dose of 0.1–0.2 mg/kg PO q8h, then titrated upward until an adequate response is obtained. We do not exceed a dose of 0.5 mg/kg PO q8h. • Diltiazem—initially administered at a dose of 0.5 mg/kg PO q8h, then titrated up to a maximum of 1.5 mg/kg PO q8h or until an adequate response is obtained • Either high-dose oral quinidine or electrical cardioversion can be used to convert primary atrial fibrillation into sinus rhythm. Quinidine doses as high as 20 mg/kg PO q2h can be used safely; doses lower than 12.5 mg/kg q6h are generally ineffective.

Cats
• Diltiazem (1–2.5 mg/kg PO q8h) or atenolol (6.25–12.5 mg/cat PO q12–24h) are the drugs of choice in most cats. • If the heart rate is not sufficiently slowed with these drugs or if myocardial failure is present, digoxin (0.005 mg/kg PO q24–48h) can be added.

CONTRAINDICATIONS
• Digoxin, diltiazem, propranolol, and atenolol should not be used in patients with preexisting AV block. • Use of calcium channel blockers in combination with β-blockers should be avoided because clinically significant bradyarrhythmias and/or AV block can develop.

PRECAUTIONS
• Calcium channel blockers and β-adrenergic blockers, both negative inotropes, should be used cautiously in animals with myocardial failure. • Using high-dose oral quinidine for conversion into sinus rhythm carries a risk of quinidine toxicity (e.g., weakness, ataxia, and seizures)—administration of diazepam intravenously controls seizures; other signs abate within several hours of discontinuing quinidine administration.

POSSIBLE INTERACTIONS
Quinidine raises the digoxin level, generally necessitating a digoxin dose reduction.

ALTERNATIVE DRUG(S)
N/A

 FOLLOW-UP

PATIENT MONITORING
• Monitor heart rate and ECG closely.
• As heart rates in the hospital and those measured on the surface ECG may be inaccurate (due to patient anxiety and other environmental factors), Holter monitoring provides a more accurate means for assessing the need for heart rate control and/or the efficacy of medical therapy.

POSSIBLE COMPLICATIONS
Worsening of cardiac function with onset of arrhythmia

PREVENTION/AVOIDANCE
N/A

EXPECTED COURSE AND PROGNOSIS
• Secondary atrial fibrillation—associated with severe heart disease, so a guarded-to-poor prognosis • Primary atrial fibrillation with normal ultrasound findings—generally a good prognosis

 **MISCELLANEOUS**

ASSOCIATED CONDITIONS
N/A

AGE-RELATED FACTORS
N/A

ZOONOTIC POTENTIAL
N/A

PREGNANCY
N/A

SYNONYMS
N/A

SEE ALSO
N/A

ABBREVIATIONS
• AV = atrioventricular
• DC = direct current
• SVT = supraventricular tachycardia

Suggested Reading
Kittleson MD. Electrocardiography. In: Kittleson MD, Kienle RD, eds. Small animal cardiovascular medicine. St Louis: Mosby, 1998:72–94.
Author Richard D. Kienle
Consulting Editors Larry P. Tilley and Francis W. K. Smith, Jr.

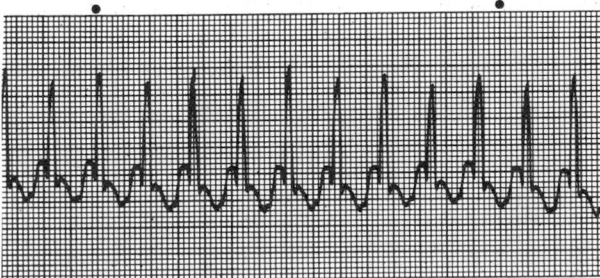

Figure 1.

Atrial flutter with 2:1 conduction at ventricular rate of 330/min in a dog with an atrial septal defect. This supraventricular tachycardia was associated with a Wolff-Parkinson-White pattern. (From: Tilley LP. Essentials of canine and feline electrocardiography, 3rd ed. Baltimore: Williams & Wilkins, 1992, with permission.)

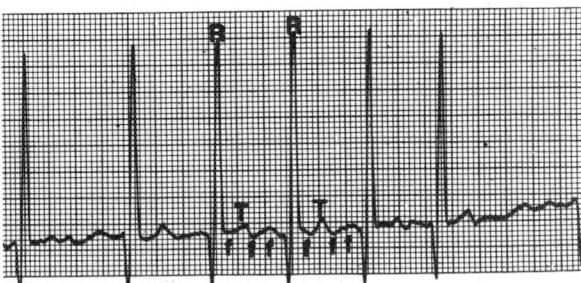

Figure 2.

"Coarse" atrial fibrillation in a dog with patent ductus arteriosus. The f waves are prominent. (From: Tilley LP. Essentials of canine and feline electrocardiography, 3rd ed. Baltimore: Williams & Wilkins, 1992, with permission.)

120   THE 5-MINUTE VETERINARY CONSULT

ATRIAL PREMATURE COMPLEXES

BASICS

DEFINITION
Premature atrial beats that originate outside the sinoatrial node and disrupt the normal sinus rhythm for one or more beats

ECG Features
• Heart rate usually normal; rhythm irregular due to the premature P wave (called a P′ wave) that disrupts the normal P wave rhythm (Fig 1).
• Ectopic P′ wave—premature; configuration differs from that of the sinus P waves and may be negative, positive, biphasic, or superimposed on the previous T wave.
• QRS complex—premature; configuration usually normal (same as that of the sinus complexes). If the P′ wave occurs during the refractory period of the AV node, ventricular conduction does not occur (nonconducted APCs), so no QRS complex follows the P′ wave. If there is partial recovery in the AV node or intraventricular conduction systems, the P′ wave is conducted with a long P′–R interval or with an abnormal QRS configuration (aberrant conduction). The more premature the complex, the more marked the aberration.
• In the P–QRS relationship, the P′–R interval is usually as long as, or longer than, the sinus P–R interval.
• A noncompensatory pause—when the R–R interval of the two normal sinus complexes enclosing an APC is less than the R–R intervals of three consecutive sinus complexes—usually follows an APC (Fig 2). The ectopic atrial impulse discharges the sinus node and resets the cycle.

PATHOPHYSIOLOGY
• Mechanisms—an increase in automaticity of atrial myocardial fibers or a single reentrant circuit

• May be normal finding in aged dogs; commonly seen in dogs with atrial enlargement secondary to chronic mitral valvular insufficiency; may also be observed in dogs or cats with any atrial disease
• May not cause hemodynamic problems; the clinical significance relates to their frequency, timing relative to other complexes, and to the underlying clinical problems.
• Can presage more serious rhythm disturbances (e.g., atrial fibrillation, atrial flutter, or atrial tachycardia)

SYSTEMS AFFECTED
Cardiovascular

GENETICS
N/A

INCIDENCE/PREVALENCE
Not documented

GEOGRAPHIC DISTRIBUTION
N/A

SIGNALMENT

Species
Dogs and cats

Breed Predilections
Small breed dogs

Mean Age and Range
Geriatric animals, except those with congenital heart disease

Predominant Sex
N/A

SIGNS

Historical Findings
• No signs
• CHF
• Coughing and dyspnea
• Exercise intolerance
• Syncope

Physical Examination Findings
• Irregular heart rhythm
• Cardiac murmur
• Gallop rhythm
• Signs of CHF

CAUSES & RISK FACTORS
• Chronic valvular disease
• Congenital heart disease
• Cardiomyopathy
• Atrial myocarditis
• Electrolyte disorders
• Neoplasia
• Hyperthyroidism
• Toxemias
• Drug toxicity (e.g., digitalis)
• Normal variation in aged animals

Risk Factors
Same as causes

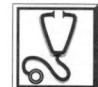

DIAGNOSIS

DIFFERENTIAL DIAGNOSIS
• Marked sinus arrhythmia
• Ventricular premature complexes when aberrant ventricular conduction follows an APC

CBC/BIOCHEMISTRY/URINALYSIS
N/A

OTHER LABORATORY TESTS
N/A

IMAGING
Echocardiography and Doppler ultrasound may reveal the type and severity of the underlying heart disease.

DIAGNOSTIC PROCEDURES
Electrocardiography

PATHOLOGIC FINDINGS
Atrial enlargement; other features vary depending on underlying cause.

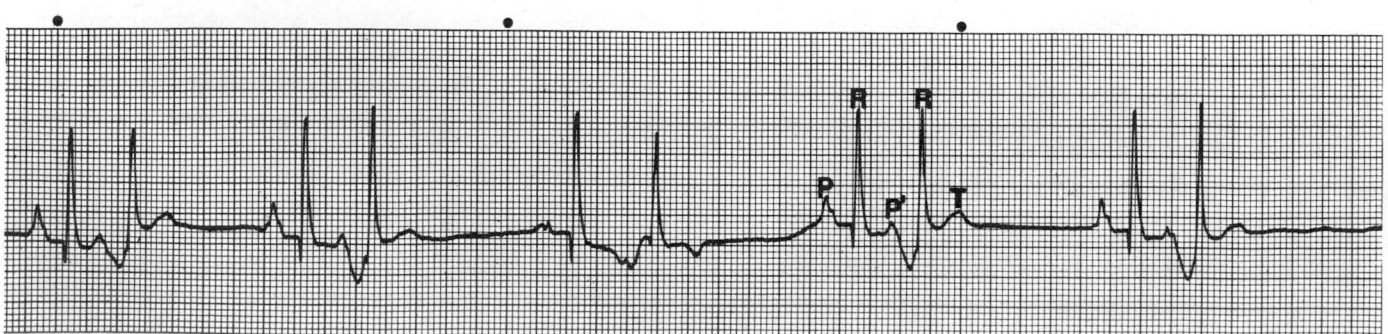

Figure 1.

APCs in a dog. P′ represents the premature complex. The premature QRS resembles the basic QRS. The upright P′ wave is superimposed on the T wave of the preceding complex. (From: Tilley LP. Essentials of canine and feline electrocardiography. 3rd ed. Baltimore: Williams & Wilkins 1992, with permission.)

ATRIAL PREMATURE COMPLEXES

TREATMENT

APPROPRIATE HEALTH CARE
• Treat animal as inpatient or outpatient.
• Treat the underlying CHF, cardiac disease, or other causes.

NURSING CARE
Usually not necessary; varies with underlying cause

ACTIVITY
Restrict if symptomatic.

DIET
No modifications unless required for management of underlying condition (i.e., low-salt diet)

CLIENT EDUCATION
APCs may not cause hemodynamic abnormalities; may be precursors of serious arrhythmias

SURGICAL CONSIDERATIONS
N/A

MEDICATIONS

DRUG(S) OF CHOICE
Treat CHF and correct any electrolyte or acid/base imbalances.

Dogs
• Digoxin (0.005–0.01 mg/kg PO q12h, maintenance dosage), diltiazem (0.5–1.5 mg/kg PO q8h), propranolol (0.2–1 mg/kg PO q8h), or atenolol (0.25–1 mg/kg PO q12h) are used to treat clinically significant arrhythmias
• Digoxin—treatment of choice; also indicated to treat the cardiac decompensation that is usually present

• CHF is treated with appropriate dosage of diuretic and angiotensin converting enzyme inhibitor; appropriate management of CHF may reduce APC frequency.

Cats
• Cats with hypertrophic cardiomyopathy—diltiazem (1–2.5 mg/kg PO q8h) or atenolol (6.25–12.5 mg PO q12–24h)
• Cats with dilated cardiomyopathy—digoxin (1/4 of a 0.125 mg digoxin tablet q24h or q48h)

CONTRAINDICATIONS
Negative inotropic agents (e.g., propranolol) should be avoided in animals with CHF.

PRECAUTIONS
Use digoxin, diltiazem, atenolol, or propranolol cautiously in animals with underlying atrioventricular block or hypotension.

POSSIBLE INTERACTIONS
N/A

ALTERNATIVE DRUG(S)
N/A

FOLLOW-UP

PATIENT MONITORING
Monitor heart rate and rhythm with serial ECG.

PREVENTION/AVOIDANCE
N/A

POSSIBLE COMPLICATIONS
Frequent APCs may further diminish cardiac output in patients with underlying heart disease and worsen clinical symptoms.

EXPECTED COURSE AND PROGNOSIS
Even with optimal antiarrhythmic drug therapy some animals have an increased frequency of APCs or deteriorate to more severe arrhythmia as the underlying disease progresses.

MISCELLANEOUS

ASSOCIATED CONDITIONS
None

AGE-RELATED FACTORS
Typically occurs in geriatric dogs

ZOONOTIC POTENTIAL
N/A

PREGNANCY
N/A

SYNONYMS
Atrial extrasystoles, atrial premature contractions, atrial premature impulses

SEE ALSO
Supraventricular Tachycardia

ABBREVIATIONS
• APCs = atrial premature complexes
• AV = atrioventricular
• CHF = congestive heart failure

Suggested Reading
Goodwin JK. Electrocardiography. In: Tilley LP, Goodwin, J. eds. Manual of canine and feline cardiology. 3rd ed. Philadelphia: WB Saunders, 2000:43–70.
Authors Larry P. Tilley and Naomi L. Burtnick
Consulting Editors Larry P. Tilley and Francis W. K. Smith, Jr.

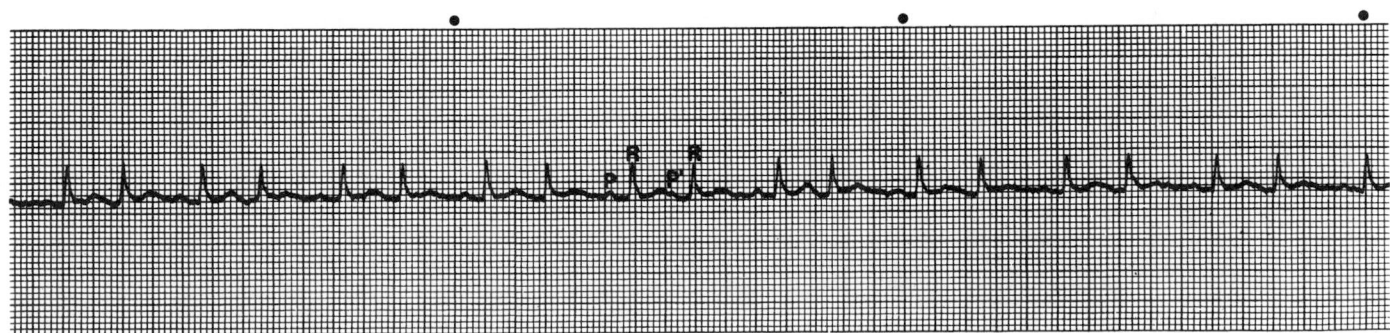

Figure 2.

APCs in bigeminy in a cat under general anesthesia. The second complex of each pair is an APC, where the first is a sinus complex. The abnormality in rhythm disappeared after the anesthetic was stopped. (From: Tilley L.P. Essentials of canine and feline electrocardiography. 3rd ed. Baltimore: Williams & Wilkins, 1992, with permission.)

ATRIAL SEPTAL DEFECT

BASICS

OVERVIEW
• Congenital cardiac anomaly allowing communication between the atria through a defect in the interatrial septum (Figure 1)
• Defects occur in one of three locations: ostium primum defect, lower atrial septum; ostium secundum defect, near fossa ovalis; and sinus venous defect, craniodorsal to fossa ovalis.
• Blood usually shunts into the right atrium, causing volume overload to the right atrium, right ventricle, and pulmonary vasculature, sometimes leading to pulmonary hypertension.
• If right-sided pressures are high, shunting may occur right to left, causing generalized cyanosis.
• Comprises 0.7% of congenital heart defects in dogs and 9% of congenital heart defects in cats

SIGNALMENT
• Dogs and cats
• Genetic basis suggested for Old English sheepdog
• Doberman pinscher, boxer, and Samoyed may be overrepresented.

SIGNS

General
If defect is small, maybe none

Historical Findings
Variable degrees of exercise intolerance, syncope, and dyspnea the first year of life

Physical Examination Findings
• Soft systolic murmur over the pulmonic valve due to relative pulmonic stenosis
• Rarely a diastolic murmur over tricuspid valve due to relative tricuspid stenosis
• Systolic mitral murmur may be heard if endocardial cushion defect and cleft mitral valve are present.
• Cyanosis if right-to-left shunt
• Ascites if right heart failure develops
• Splitting of the second heart sound

CAUSES & RISK FACTORS
Unknown; genetic basis not documented

DIAGNOSIS

DIFFERENTIAL DIAGNOSIS
• Pulmonic stenosis—murmur of pulmonic stenosis usually harsh and loud
• Anomalous pulmonary venous return to the right atrium

CBC/BIOCHEMISTRY/URINALYSIS
Polycythemia in some patients with right-to-left shunt

OTHER BLOOD TESTS
N/A

IMAGING

Radiographic Findings
• None in patients with small defects
• Right-sided heart and pulmonary vessel enlargement in patients with large defects

Echocardiographic Findings
• Right atrial and right ventricular dilation

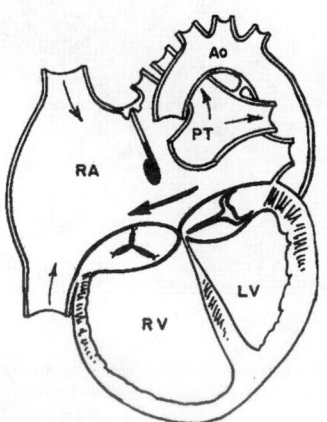

Figure 1.

Atrial septal defect. Defect involves the lowermost part of the atrial septum, known as ostium primum defect. Note the left dominant left-to-right shunt. RV = right ventricle, LV = left ventricle, RA = right atrium, Ao = aorta, PT = pulmonary trunk. (From: Roberts W. Adult congenital heart disease. Philadelphia: FA Davis Co., 1987, with permission.)

• May reveal the defect—septal dropout
• Doppler useful in documenting flow through the defect and high ejection velocity through the pulmonary artery

OTHER DIAGNOSTIC PROCEDURES

Electrocardiography
• Right ventricular enlargement pattern on ECG in some patients with large defects
• Arrhythmias and intraventricular conduction disturbances possible

 TREATMENT

• Hospitalize patients with congestive heart failure (CHF) until stable.
• Restrict activity.
• A low-sodium diet may be of value.
• Surgical correction is prohibitively expensive for most owners.
• Pulmonary artery banding may be palliative in patients with severe disease.

 MEDICATIONS

DRUG(S) AND FLUIDS
• CHF—diuretics; furosemide, 1–2 mg/kg PO q6–12h
• Vasodilators may help reduce signs (e.g., enalapril, 0.5 mg/kg PO q12–24h, or benazepril 0.25–0.5 mg/kg PO q24h).

CONTRAINDICATIONS/POSSIBLE INTERACTIONS
N/A

 FOLLOW-UP

PATIENT MONITORING
Recheck when decompensation or other clinical signs develop.

EXPECTED COURSE AND PROGNOSIS
• Depend on size of the defect and coexisting abnormalities; small, isolated defects unlikely to cause signs or to progress
• Progressive, right-sided CHF expected if the defect is large or associated with an endocardial cushion defect

 MISCELLANEOUS

ASSOCIATED CONDITIONS
Pulmonic stenosis and tricuspid dysplasia

SEE ALSO
Congestive Heart Failure, Right-sided

ABBREVIATIONS
CHF = congestive heart failure

Suggested Reading
Bonagura JD, Lehmkuhl LB. Congenital heart disease. In: Fox PR, Sisson D, Moise ND, eds. Textbook of canine and feline cardiology. 2nd ed. Philadelphia: Saunders, 1999:471–535.

Acknowledgment
The author and editors acknowledge the prior contributions of Dr. John-Karl Goodwin, who authored this topic in the previous edition.
Author Francis W. K. Smith, Jr.
Consulting Editors Larry P. Tilley and Francis W. K. Smith, Jr.

ATRIAL STANDSTILL

 BASICS

DEFINITION

ECG rhythm characterized by absence of P waves; condition can be temporary (e.g., associated with hyperkalemia or drug-induced), terminal (e.g., associated with severe hyperkalemia or dying heart), or persistent.

ECG Features

Persistent Atrial Standstill
• P waves absent (Figure 1)
• Heart rate usually slow (<60 bpm)
• Rhythm regular with supraventricular type QRS complexes
• Heart rate does not increase with atropine administration.

Hyperkalemic Atrial Standstill
• Heart rate normal or slow
• Rhythm regular or irregular
• QRS complexes tend to be wide and become wider as the potassium level rises; with severe hyperkalemia (potassium >10 mEq/mL), the QRS complexes are replaced by a smooth biphasic curve.
• Heart rate may increase slightly with atropine.

PATHOPHYSIOLOGY

Persistent Atrial Standstill

Caused by an atrial muscular dystrophy; skeletal muscle involvement common

Hyperkalemic Atrial Standstill

Generally occurs with serum potassium levels > 8.5 mEq/L; value influenced by serum sodium and calcium levels and acid–base status. Hyperkalemic patients with atrial standstill have sinus node function, but impulses do not activate atrial myocytes; thus, the associated rhythm is termed a sinoventricular rhythm. Since the sinus node is functional, an irregular rhythm may be due to sinus arrhythmia.

SYSTEMS AFFECTED

Cardiovascular

GENETICS

N/A

INCIDENCE/PREVALENCE

Rare rhythm disturbance

GEOGRAPHIC DISTRIBUTION

N/A

SIGNALMENT

Species

Dog and cat

Breed Predisposition

Persistent atrial standstill—most common in English springer spaniels; other breeds occasionally affected

Mean Age and Range

Most animals with persistent atrial standstill are young; animals with hypoadrenocorticism are usually young to middle–aged.

Predominant Sex

Hypoadrenocorticism more common in females

SIGNS

Historical Findings

• Vary with underlying cause
• Lethargy common; syncope may occur.
• Patients with persistent atrial standstill may show signs of congestive heart failure (CHF).

Physical Examination Findings

• Vary with underlying cause
• Bradycardia common
• Patients with persistent atrial standstill may have skeletal muscle wasting of the antebrachium and scapula.

CAUSES

• Hyperkalemia
• Atrial disease, often associated with atrial distension (e.g., cats with cardiomyopathy)
• Atrial myopathy (persistent atrial standstill)

RISK FACTORS

Hyperkalemic Atrial Standstill

• Hypoadrenocorticism
• Conditions leading to obstruction or rupture of the urinary tract
• Oliguric or anuric renal failure

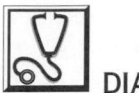 DIAGNOSIS

DIFFERENTIAL DIAGNOSIS

• Slow atrial fibrillation
• Sinus bradycardia with small P waves lost in the baseline

CBC/BIOCHEMISTRY/URINALYSIS

Persistent Atrial Standstill

Normal

Hyperkalemic Atrial Standstill

• Hyperkalemia
• Hyponatremia and sodium:potassium ratio <27 if atrial standstill secondary to hypoadrenocorticism
• Azotemia and hyperphosphatemia with hypoadrenocorticism, renal failure, and rupture or obstruction of the urinary tract

OTHER LABORATORY TESTS

ACTH stimulation test if hypoadreno-corticism suspected

IMAGING

Echocardiogram and electromyography if persistent atrial standstill suspected—cardiomegaly and depressed contractility may be seen.

DIAGNOSTIC PROCEDURES

Skeletal muscle biopsy in animals with persistent atrial standstill

PATHOLOGIC FINDINGS

Persistent Atrial Standstill

• Greatly enlarged and paper-thin atria; usually biatrial involvement, although one case of only left atrial involvement was reported

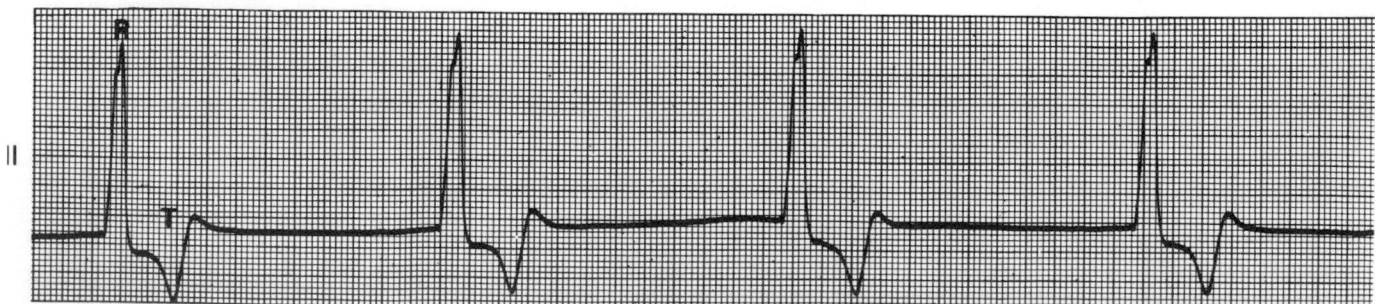

Figure 1.

Persistent atrial standstill in English springer spaniel. No P waves are present on any of the leads (also including chest leads and intracardiac electrocardiogram, not shown here). The regular bradycardia is either junctional in origin, with pathologic involvement of the left bundle branch block (wide positive QRS complexes), or ventricular. (From: Tilley LP: Essentials of canine and feline electrocardiography. 3rd ed. Baltimore: Williams & Wilkins, 1992, with permission.)

- Severe scapular and brachial muscle wasting in some dogs
- Marked fibrosis, fibroelastosis, chronic mononuclear cell inflammation, and steatosis throughout the atria and interatrial septum

TREATMENT

APPROPRIATE HEALTH CARE

Persistent Atrial Standstill
Not life-threatening condition; animal can be treated as an outpatient

Hyperkalemic Atrial Standstill
Potentially life-threatening; often requires aggressive treatment

NURSING CARE
Aggressive fluid therapy with 0.9% saline often required to correct hypovolemia and lower serum potassium levels (see Hyperkalemia) in patients with hyperkalemic atrial standstill

ACTIVITY
Restrict activity in patients with persistent atrial standstill and signs of CHF or syncope.

DIET
N/A

CLIENT EDUCATION

Persistent Atrial Standstill
Clinical signs generally improve after pacemaker implantation; signs of CHF may develop, and weakness and lethargy may persist even after heart rate and rhythm are corrected with the pacemaker.

SURGICAL CONSIDERATIONS

Persistent Atrial Standstill
Implant permanent ventricular pacemaker to regulate rate and rhythm.

Hyperkalemic Atrial Standstill
Hyperkalemia secondary to urinary tract obstruction or rupture may require surgery.

MEDICATIONS

DRUG(S) OF CHOICE

Persistent Atrial Standstill
Treat with diuretics, digoxin (after pacemaker is implanted), and ACE inhibitor if CHF develops.

Hyperkalemic Atrial Standstill
- Treat the underlying cause (e.g., oliguric renal failure, hypoadrenocorticism).
- Aggressive fluid therapy with 0.9% saline and possibly insulin; dextrose or sodium bicarbonate as discussed under Hyperkalemia.
- Calcium gluconate—counters the effects of hyperkalemia; can be used in life-threatening situations to reestablish a sinus rhythm while instituting treatment to lower potassium concentration

CONTRAINDICATIONS
Avoid potassium-containing fluids or medications that increase potassium concentration in hyperkalemic patients.

PRECAUTIONS
Diuretics lower preload and may worsen weakness in dogs with persistent atrial standstill and CHF unless a pacemaker has been implanted.

POSSIBLE INTERACTIONS
N/A

ALTERNATIVE DRUG(S)
N/A

FOLLOW-UP

PATIENT MONITORING
- Monitor ECG during treatment of hyperkalemia and periodically in animals with a permanent ventricular pacemaker.
- Monitor electrolytes in patients with hyperkalemic atrial standstill.
- Monitor patients with persistent atrial standstill for signs of CHF.

PREVENTION/AVOIDANCE
N/A

POSSIBLE COMPLICATIONS
CHF in patients with persistent atrial standstill

EXPECTED COURSE AND PROGNOSIS

Persistent Atrial Standstill
Clinical signs generally improve after pacemaker implantation. Signs of CHF may develop, and weakness and lethargy persist even after heart rate and rhythm are corrected with the pacemaker. There may be persistence of signs related to muscular dystrophy.

Hyperkalemic Atrial Standstill
Long-term prognosis is excellent if underlying cause can be corrected and hyperkalemia reversed.

MISCELLANEOUS

ASSOCIATED CONDITIONS
Diseases causing hyperkalemia (e.g., hypoadrenocorticism, urethral obstruction or urinary tract tear, acidosis, and drugs)

AGE-RELATED FACTORS
Persistent atrial standstill—usually diagnosed in young animals; hypoadrenocorticism—usually diagnosed in young to middle-aged animals

ZOONOTIC POTENTIAL
None

PREGNANCY
N/A

SYNONYMS
Silent atrial

SEE ALSO
- Digoxin Toxicity
- Hyperkalemia
- Hypoadrenocorticism (Addison's Disease)
- Urinary Tract Obstruction

ABBREVIATIONS
- ACE = angiotensin-converting enzyme
- CHF = congestive heart failure

Suggested Reading
Tilley LP. Essentials of canine and feline electrocardiograph. 3rd ed. Philadelphia: Lea & Febiger, 1992.
Author Francis W. K. Smith, Jr.
Consulting Editors Larry P. Tilley and Francis W. K. Smith, Jr.

ATRIAL WALL TEAR

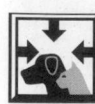 **BASICS**

OVERVIEW

• Split in the endocardial surface or complete tear (rupture) in the atrial wall when the left atrium is distended beyond its elastic limits; if the split is incomplete, fibrin may seal the defect temporarily; this either heals as a depression in the atrial surface or subsequently ruptures completely.
• When a tear is complete, bleeding occurs into the pericardial sac and cardiac tamponade quickly ensues; if the interatrial wall is affected, an acquired atrial septal defect may form.
• Death occurs quickly in most patients.

SIGNALMENT

• Dogs and rarely cats
• Predisposition—same as endocardiosis breeds
• Older, small-breed male dogs may be predisposed.
• Cocker spaniels and dachshunds may be overrepresented.

SIGNS

Historical Findings

• Acute onset of weakness and collapse that may progress quickly to death
• Long-standing cardiac disease in most patients, so other signs of congestive heart failure may have been observed

Physical Examination Findings

• Pale mucous membranes
• Tachycardia
• Weak arterial pulses
• Collapse
• Signs of right heart failure (e.g., ascites and jugular venous distension) in some patients
• Some patients show other signs of cardiac disease (e.g., murmur, gallop rhythm, arrhythmia, and dyspnea).
• If a murmur was heard before the atrial wall tear occurred, it may not be as loud.
• Muffled heart sounds

CAUSES & RISK FACTORS

• Mitral valve endocardiosis—chronic valvular heart disease
• Dilated cardiomyopathy
• Patent ductus arteriosus
• Cardiac neoplasia
• Chest trauma

 DIAGNOSIS

DIFFERENTIAL DIAGNOSIS

• Other causes of acute cardiovascular collapse
• Pericardial effusion from other causes (e.g., neoplastic and idiopathic)
• Severe cardiac arrhythmias
• Myocardial infarction
• Pulmonary thromboembolism
• Other causes of hypotension

CBC/BIOCHEMISTRY/URINALYSIS

• Anemia is uncommon since volume of blood loss is relatively small.
• Prerenal azotemia in some patients

IMAGING

Radiographic Findings

• Comparison with previous thoracic radiographs may show rounding of cardiac silhouette; however, the spherical cardiac silhouette seen in patients with pericardial effusion is often not observed.
• Ascites and large caudal vena cava in some patients

Echocardiographic Findings
• Pericardial effusion is seen as a hypoechoic space between the heart and pericardial sac; the heart may swing in the pericardial sac.
• Left atrium often remains large; may see a clot in the left atrium or pericardial sac

DIAGNOSTIC PROCEDURES

Electrocardiographic Findings
• Arrhythmias
• Tachycardia
• Dampened QRS complex
• Electrical alternans
• ST-segment abnormalities
• May reveal heart enlargement pattern

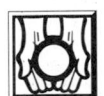 TREATMENT

• If a left atrial tear is strongly suspected, perform pericardiocentesis only if the effusion is considered life-threatening; further hemorrhage into the pericardial sac or exsanguination may occur.
• If a fibrin clot forms over the defect, the patient may stabilize; if pericardiocentesis is performed, remove only enough fluid to improve clinical signs.

• Strict cage rest
• Surgical exploration may be considered if hemorrhage persists or recurs.
• Administer IV fluids or blood products to expand the intravascular space and maintain cardiac output.

 MEDICATIONS

DRUG(S)
Combination of IV fluids and dobutamine has improved hemodynamic status in models of cardiac rupture.

CONTRAINDICATIONS/POSSIBLE INTERACTIONS
Preload (e.g., diuretics and venous dilators) and afterload reducers (e.g., arterial vasodilators) are not indicated in the treatment of left atrial rupture, because they may further diminish cardiac output; if necessary to treat concomitant congestive heart failure, use sparingly.

 FOLLOW-UP

• Prognosis is poor; even if the tear seals, the patient is prone to further tears because of underlying cardiac disease.
• If the patient survives, follow-up examination with echocardiography helps determine resolution of pericardial effusion and resorption of an atrial or pericardial clot.

 MISCELLANEOUS

SEE ALSO
Pericardial Effusion

Suggested Reading
Fox PR, Sisson D, Moise S. Textbook of canine and feline cardiology. Philadelphia: Saunders, 1999.
Author Patti S. Snyder
Consulting Editors Larry P. Tilley and Francis W. K. Smith, Jr.

ATRIOVENTRICULAR BLOCK, COMPLETE (THIRD DEGREE)

BASICS

DEFINITION
• All atrial impulses are blocked at the AV junction; atria and ventricles beat independently. A secondary "escape" pacemaker site (junctional or ventricular) stimulates the ventricles.
• Atrial rate normal
• Idioventricular escape rhythm slow

ECG Features
• Ventricular rate slower than the atrial rate (more P waves than QRS complexes)—ventricular escape rhythm (idioventricular) usually <40 bpm; junctional escape rhythm (idiojunctional) 40–60 bpm in dogs and 60–100 bpm in cats
• P waves—usually normal configuration (Figure 1)
• QRS complex—wide and bizarre when pacemaker located in the ventricle, or in the lower AV junction in a patient with bundle branch block; normal when escape pacemaker in the lower AV junction (above the bifurcation of the bundle of His) in a patient without bundle branch block
• No conduction between the atria and the ventricles; P waves have no constant relationship with QRS complexes; P-P and R-R intervals relatively constant (except for a sinus arrhythmia)

PATHOPHYSIOLOGY
Slow ventricular escape rhythms (<40 bpm) result in low cardiac output and eventual heart failure, often when animal is excited or exercised, since demand for greater cardiac output is not satisfied. As the heart fails, signs increase with mild activity.

SYSTEMS AFFECTED
Cardiovascular

GENETICS
Can be an isolated congenital defect

INCIDENCE/PREVALENCE
Not documented

GEOGRAPHIC DISTRIBUTION
N/A

SIGNALMENT

Species
Dogs and cats

Breed Predilections
• Cocker spaniels—can have idiopathic fibrosis
• Pugs and Doberman pinschers—can have associated sudden death, AV conduction defects, and bundle of His lesions.

Mean Age and Range
Geriatric animals, except congenital heart disease patients

Predominant Sex
N/A

SIGNS

Historical Findings
• Exercise intolerance
• Weakness or syncope
• Occasionally, CHF

Physical Examination Findings
• Bradycardia
• Variable third and fourth heart sounds
• Variation in intensity of the first heart sounds
• Signs of CHF
• Intermittent "cannon" A waves in jugular venous pulses

CAUSES
• Isolated congenital defect
• Idiopathic fibrosis
• Infiltrative cardiomyopathy (amyloidosis or neoplasia)
• Hypertrophic cardiomyopathy in cats
• Digitalis toxicity
• Myocarditis
• Endocarditis
• Electrolyte disorder
• Myocardial infarction
• Other congenital heart defects
• Lyme disease
• Chagas' disease

RISK FACTORS
Same as Causes

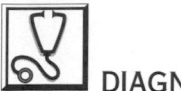

DIAGNOSIS

DIFFERENTIAL DIAGNOSIS
• Advanced second-degree AV block
• Atrial standstill
• Accelerated idioventricular rhythm

CBC/BIOCHEMISTRY/URINALYSIS
• Abnormal serum electrolytes (e.g., hyperkalemia, hypokalemia) possible
• High WBC with left shift in animals with bacterial endocarditis

OTHER LABORATORY TESTS
• High serum digoxin concentration if AV block is due to digoxin toxicity
• Lyme titer and accompanying clinical signs if AV block due to Lyme disease

IMAGING
Echocardiography and Doppler ultrasound to assess cardiac structure and function

DIAGNOSTIC PROCEDURES
• Electrocardiography
• His bundle electrogram to determine the site of the AV block
• Long-term (Holter) ambulatory recording if AV block is intermittent

PATHOLOGIC FINDINGS
Degeneration or fibrosis of the AV node and its bundle branches, associated with endocardial and myocardial fibrosis and organized endomyocarditis

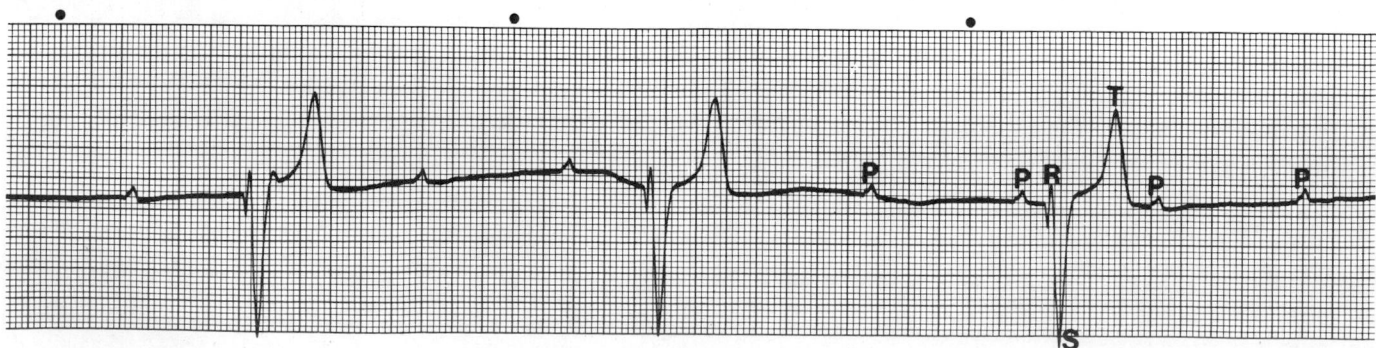

Figure 1.

Complete heart block. The P waves occur at a rate of 120 bpm, independent of the ventricular rate of 50 bpm. The QRS configuration is a right bundle branch block pattern. The regular rate and stable QRS indicate that the rescuing focus is probably near the AV junction. (From: Tilley LP: Essentials of canine and feline electrocardiography. 3rd ed. Baltimore: Williams & Wilkins, 1992, with permission.)

ATRIOVENTRICULAR BLOCK, COMPLETE (THIRD DEGREE)

 TREATMENT

APPROPRIATE HEALTH CARE
• Temporary or permanent cardiac pacemaker—only effective treatment in symptomatic patients
• Carefully monitor asymptomatic patients without a pacemaker for development of clinical signs.

NURSING CARE
Cage rest prior to pacemaker implantation; when the pulse generator is put into a subcutaneous pocket, a nonconstricting bandage is required around the ventral neck or abdomen for 3–5 days to prevent seroma formation or pacemaker movement.

ACTIVITY
Restrict if symptomatic

DIET
No modifications unless required to manage underlying condition (e.g., low-salt diet)

CLIENT EDUCATION
• Temporary or permanent cardiac pacemaker—only effective treatment in symptomatic patients
• Asymptomatic patients without a pacemaker—must be carefully monitored for development of clinical signs

SURGICAL CONSIDERATIONS
• Most patients—at high anesthetic cardiopulmonary risk; usually paced preoperatively with a temporary external pacemaker system
• The small size of cats makes pacemaker implantation more difficult than in dogs.

 MEDICATIONS

DRUG(S) OF CHOICE
• Treatment with drugs—usually of no value. Traditionally used to treat complete AV block: atropine, isoproterenol, theophylline, and corticosteroids
• Intravenous isoproterenol infusion may help increase the rate of the ventricular escape rhythm to stabilize hemodynamics.
• If CHF—diuretic and vasodilator therapy may be needed before pacemaker implantation

CONTRAINDICATIONS
Avoid digoxin, xylazine, acepromazine, β-blockers (e.g., propranolol and atenolol), and calcium channel blockers (e.g., verapamil and diltiazem); ventricular antiarrhythmic agents are dangerous because they suppress lower escape foci.

PRECAUTIONS
Vasodilators—may cause hypotension in animals with complete AV block; monitor closely if used, especially prior to pacemaker implantation.

POSSIBLE INTERACTIONS
N/A

ALTERNATIVE DRUG(S)
N/A

 FOLLOW-UP

PATIENT MONITORING
• Monitor—pacemaker function with serial ECGs
• Radiographs—following pacemaker implantation, to confirm the position of the lead and generator

PREVENTION/AVOIDANCE
N/A

POSSIBLE COMPLICATIONS
Pulse generators—broad range of clinical life; pacemaker replacement necessary when battery is depleted, pulse generator malfunction occurs, or exit block develops; pacemaker leads can become dislodged and infected.

EXPECTED COURSE AND PROGNOSIS
Poor long-term prognosis if no cardiac pacemaker implanted, especially when the animal has clinical signs.

 MISCELLANEOUS

ASSOCIATED CONDITIONS
None

AGE-RELATED FACTORS
N/A

ZOONOTIC POTENTIAL
N/A

PREGNANCY
N/A

SYNONYMS
None

SEE ALSO
Atrioventricular Dissociation

ABBREVIATIONS
• AV = atrioventricular
• bpm = beats per minute
• CHF = congestive heart failure

Suggested Reading
Tilley LP, Goodwin J, eds. Manual of canine and feline cardiology. 3rd ed. Philadelphia: WB Saunders, 2000.
Authors Larry P. Tilley and Naomi L. Burtnick
Consulting Editors Larry P. Tilley and Francis W. K. Smith, Jr.

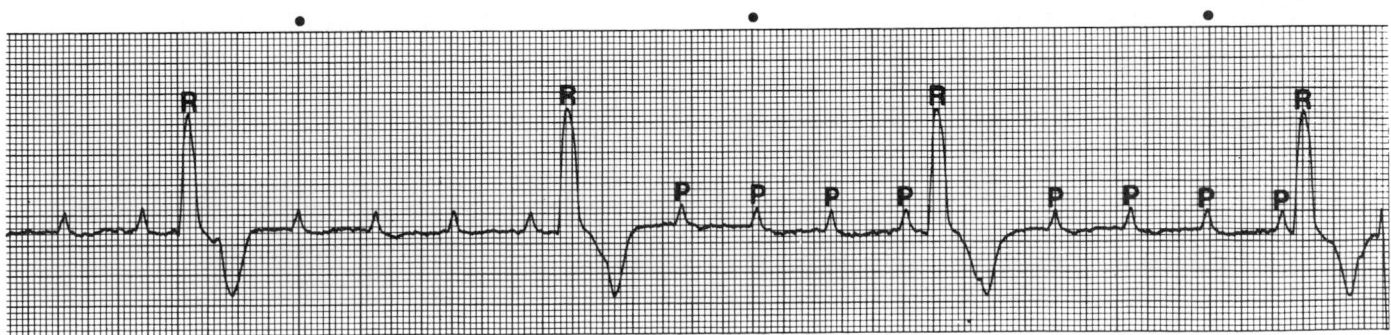

Figure 2.

Complete heart block in a cat. The P waves rate is 240/min, independent of the ventricular rate of 48/min. QRS configuration is a left bundle branch block pattern. (From: Tilley LP: Essentials of canine and feline electrocardiography. 3rd ed. Baltimore: Williams & Wilkins, 1992, with permission.)

ATRIOVENTRICULAR BLOCK, FIRST DEGREE

 BASICS

DEFINITION
Refers to a delay in conduction that occurs between atrial and ventricular activation

ECG Features
• Rate and rhythm—usually normal
• Regularly occurring normal P waves and QRS complexes (Figures 1 and 2)
• Prolonged, consistent PR intervals—dogs, >0.13 sec; cats, >0.09 sec (Figures 1 and 2)

PATHOPHYSIOLOGY
• Virtually never causes clinical signs
• May become a more severe AV conduction disturbance in some animals
• PR interval tends to shorten with rapid heart rates.

SYSTEMS AFFECTED
Cardiovascular

GENETICS
N/A

INCIDENCE/PREVALENCE
Common

GEOGRAPHIC DISTRIBUTION
N/A

SIGNALMENT

Species
Dogs and cats

Breed Predilections
American cocker spaniels, dachshunds

Mean Age and Range
• May occur in young, otherwise healthy dogs as a manifestation of high vagal tone

• May be noted in aged patients with degenerative conduction system disease, particularly cocker spaniels and dachshunds
• Also seen in cats with hypertrophic cardiomyopathy

SIGNS

Historical Findings
• Most animals are asymptomatic.
• If drug-induced, may see signs of drug toxicity—anorexia, vomiting, and diarrhea with digoxin; weakness with calcium channel blockers or β-adrenergic antagonists

Physical Examination Findings
Normal—unless also signs of more generalized myocardial disease or extracardiac disease

CAUSES
• May occur in normal animals
• Enhanced vagal stimulation resulting from noncardiac diseases—usually accompanied by sinus arrhythmia, sinus arrest, and/or Mobitz type I second degree AV block
• Pharmacologic agents (e.g., digoxin, β-adrenergic antagonists, calcium channel blocking agents, α_2-adrenergic agonists, or severe procainamide or quinidine toxicity)
• Degenerative disease of the conduction system
• Hypertrophic cardiomyopathy
• Myocarditis (especially *Trypanosoma cruzi*, *Borrelia burgdorferi*, *Rickettsia rickettsii*)
• Infiltrative diseases (tumors, amyloid)
• Atropine administered intravenously may briefly prolong the PR interval

RISK FACTORS
Any condition or intervention that raises vagal tone

 DIAGNOSIS

DIFFERENTIAL DIAGNOSIS
• P waves superimposed upon preceding T waves because of first degree AV block should be differentiated from bifid T waves.
• Hypokalemia may predispose to first degree block

OTHER LABORATORY TESTS
• Serum digoxin concentration—may be high
• *T. cruzi, B. burgdorferi, R. rickettsii* titers—may be high

IMAGING
Echocardiographic examination—may reveal hypertrophic or infiltrative myocardial disorder

DIAGNOSTIC PROCEDURES
May be needed to identify causes of high vagal tone—upper airway disease, cervical and thoracic masses, gastrointestinal disorders, and high intraocular pressure

PATHOLOGIC FINDINGS
Variable—depend on underlying cause

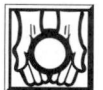 TREATMENT

APPROPRIATE HEALTH CARE
• Remove or treat underlying cause(s)
• Hospitalization may be necessary to manage the underlying cause (e.g., cardiomyopathy, gastrointestinal disease, airway disease)

NURSING CARE
N/A

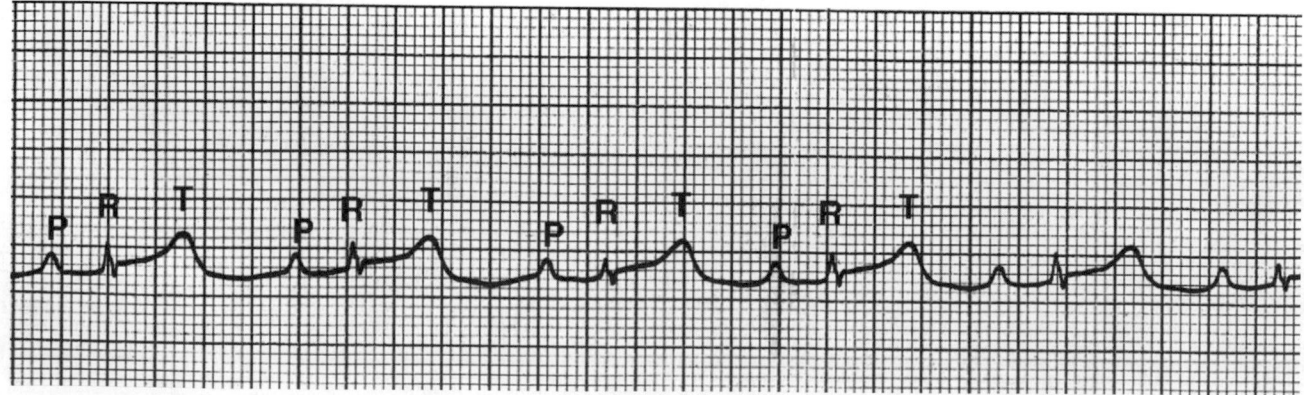

Figure 1.

Lead II ECG rhythm strip recorded from a cat with hypertrophic cardiomyopathy. There is sinus bradycardia (120 beats/minute) and first degree atrioventricular conduction block. The PR interval is 0.12 second (paper speed 50 mm/s).

ACTIVITY
Unrestricted

DIET
No modifications or restrictions unless required to manage an underlying condition

CLIENT EDUCATION
Generally unnecessary

SURGICAL CONSIDERATIONS
None unless required to manage an underlying condition

 MEDICATIONS

DRUG(S) OF CHOICE
Medications used only if needed to manage an underlying condition

CONTRAINDICATIONS
Hypokalemia—increases sensitivity to vagal tone; may potentiate AV conduction delay

PRECAUTIONS
Drugs with vagomimetic action (e.g., digoxin, bethanechol, physostigmine, pilocarpine) may potentiate first degree block.

POSSIBLE INTERACTIONS
N/A

ALTERNATIVE DRUG(S)
N/A

 FOLLOW-UP

PATIENT MONITORING
Except in healthy young animals, monitor ECG to detect any progression in conduction disturbance.

PREVENTION/AVOIDANCE
N/A

POSSIBLE COMPLICATIONS
N/A

EXPECTED COURSE AND PROGNOSIS
N/A

 MISCELLANEOUS

ASSOCIATED CONDITIONS
N/A

AGE-RELATED FACTORS
PR interval—tends to lengthen with advancing age

ZOONOTIC POTENTIAL
None

PREGNANCY
N/A

SYNONYMS
None

SEE ALSO
• Atrioventricular Block, Complete (Third Degree)
• Atrioventricular Block, Second Degree—Mobitz Type I
• Atrioventricular Block, Second Degree—Mobitz Type II

ABBREVIATION
AV = atrioventricular

Suggested Reading
Miller MS, Tilley LP, Smith FWK, Fox PR. Electrocardiography. In: Fox PR, Sisson D, Moise NS, eds. Textbook of canine and feline cardiology. Philadelphia: Saunders, 1999:67–106.
Podrid PJ, Kowey PR. Cardiac arrhythmia—mechanisms, diagnosis, and management. Baltimore: Williams & Wilkins, 1995.
Smith FWK, Hadlock DJ. Electrocardiography. In: Miller MS, Tilley LP, eds. Manual of canine and feline cardiology. 2nd ed. Philadelphia: Saunders, 1995:47–74.
Tilley LP. Essentials of canine and feline electrocardiography. 3rd ed. Baltimore: Williams & Wilkins, 1992.
Author Janice McIntosh Bright
Consulting Editors Larry P. Tilley and Francis W. K. Smith, Jr

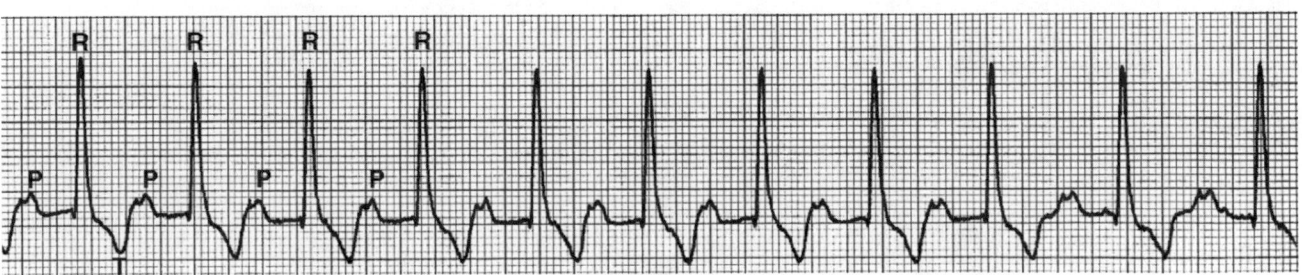
Figure 2.

Lead II ECG rhythm strip recorded from a dog showing sinus tachycardia (175 beats/minute) and first degree atrioventricular conduction block. Because the heart rate is rapid, P waves are superimposed on the upslope of the preceding T waves. The PR interval exceeds 0.16 second (paper speed = 50 mm/s).

ATRIOVENTRICULAR BLOCK, SECOND DEGREE—MOBITZ TYPE I

BASICS

DEFINITION
Occurs when AV transmission is progressively delayed prior to a nonconducted P wave

ECG Features
• PR interval—becomes progressively longer prior to the appearance of a P wave not followed by a QRS complex (Figure 1)
• Heart rate and QRS morphology—usually normal
• Often cyclical

PATHOPHYSIOLOGY
• Frequently associated with high resting vagal tone and sinus arrhythmia in dogs
• Generally not hemodynamically significant

SYSTEMS AFFECTED
Cardiovascular

GENETICS
N/A

INCIDENCE/PREVALENCE
Studies using radiotelemetry found that this arrhythmia occurs in 64% of healthy adult dogs and 100% of healthy puppies 8–12 weeks of age

GEOGRAPHIC DISTRIBUTION
N/A

SIGNALMENT

Species
Dogs; uncommon in cats

Breed Predilections
May be hereditary in pugs

Mean Age and Range
• May occur in young, otherwise healthy dogs as a manifestation of high vagal tone
• Rarely noted in old dogs with degenerative conduction system disease

SIGNS

Historical Findings
• Most animals are asymptomatic.
• If drug-induced, may see signs of drug toxicity—anorexia, vomiting, and diarrhea with digoxin; weakness with calcium channel blockers or β-adrenergic antagonists
• If heart rate is abnormally slow, syncope or weakness may occur.

Physical Examination Findings
• May be normal unless signs of more-generalized myocardial disease or extracardiac disease are present.
• First heart sound may become progressively softer, followed by a pause.

CAUSES
• Occasionally noted in normal animals
• Enhanced vagal stimulation resulting from noncardiac diseases—usually accompanied by sinus arrhythmia, sinus arrest
• Pharmacologic agents—digoxin, β-adrenergic antagonists, calcium channel blocking agents, α₂-adrenergic agonists, opioids

RISK FACTORS
Any condition or intervention that enhances vagal tone

DIAGNOSIS

DIFFERENTIAL DIAGNOSIS
• Nonconducted P waves from supraventricular premature impulses or supraventricular tachycardias should be distinguished from pathologic AV block.
• Type II second degree AV block (no variation in PR intervals)

CBC/BIOCHEMISTRY/URINALYSIS
Hypokalemia may predispose to AV conduction disturbances.

OTHER LABORATORY TESTS
Serum digoxin concentration—may be high

IMAGING
N/A

DIAGNOSTIC PROCEDURES
• May be needed to identify causes of enhanced vagal tone (e.g., upper airway disease, cervical and thoracic masses, gastrointestinal disorders, and high intraocular pressure)
• Atropine response test—administer 0.04 mg/kg atropine IM and repeat ECG in 20–30 min; may be used to determine whether AV block is due to vagal tone; loss of AV block with atropine supports vagal cause.

PATHOLOGIC FINDINGS
• Generally, no gross or histopathologic findings

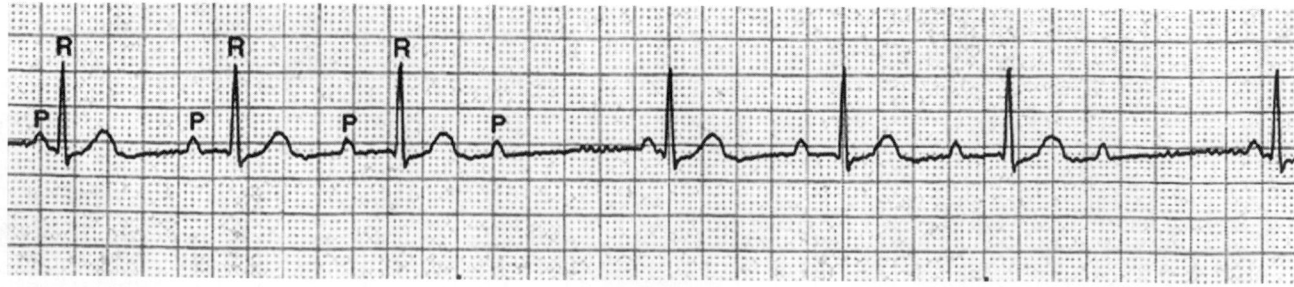

Figure 1.

Lead II ECG rhythm strip recorded from a dog with Mobitz type I, second degree AV block. The PR intervals become progressively longer, with the longest PR intervals preceding nonconducted P waves (typical Wenkebach phenomenon) (paper speed = 50 mm/s).

ATRIOVENTRICULAR BLOCK, SECOND DEGREE—MOBITZ TYPE I

• Old dogs may have focal mineralization of the interventricular septal crest visible grossly, with chondroid metaplasia of the central fibrous body and increased fibrous connective tissue in the AV bundle noted microscopically.

 TREATMENT

APPROPRIATE HEALTH CARE
• Treatment usually unnecessary
• Treat or remove underlying cause(s)

NURSING CARE
Generally unnecessary

ACTIVITY
Unrestricted

DIET
Modifications or restrictions only to manage an underlying condition

CLIENT EDUCATION
Explain that any treatment is directed toward reversing or eliminating an underlying cause.

SURGICAL CONSIDERATIONS
N/A except to manage an underlying condition

 MEDICATIONS

DRUG(S)
Only as needed to manage an underlying condition

CONTRAINDICATIONS
Drugs with vagomimetic action (e.g., digoxin, bethanechol, physostigmine, pilocarpine) may potentiate block.

PRECAUTIONS
Hypokalemia increases the sensitivity to vagal tone and may potentiate AV conduction delay.

POSSIBLE INTERACTIONS
N/A

ALTERNATIVE DRUG(S)
N/A

 FOLLOW-UP

PATIENT MONITORING
Unless the conduction disturbance resulted from normal vagal tone, the ECG should be monitored to detect progression to a more significant conduction disturbance.

PREVENTION/AVOIDANCE
N/A

POSSIBLE COMPLICATIONS
N/A

EXPECTED COURSE AND PROGNOSIS
N/A

 **MISCELLANEOUS**

ASSOCIATED CONDITIONS
N/A

AGE-RELATED FACTORS
N/A

ZOONOTIC POTENTIAL
N/A

PREGNANCY
N/A

SYNONYMS
Wenckebach phenomenon

SEE ALSO
• Atrioventricular Block, Complete (Third Degree)
• Atrioventricular Block, First Degree
• Atrioventricular Block, Second Degree—Mobitz Type II

ABBREVIATION
AV = atrioventricular

Suggested Reading

Branch CE, Robertson BT, Williams JC. Frequency of second-degree atrioventricular heart block in dogs. Am J Vet Res 1975;36:925–929.

Mangrum JM, DiMarco JP. The evaluation and management of bradycardia. N Engl J Med 2000; 342:703–709.

Miller MS, Tilley LP. Electrocardiography in canine and feline cardiology. In: Fox PR, ed. New York: Churchill Livingstone, 1988.

Podrid PJ, Kowey PR. Cardiac arrhythmia—mechanisms, diagnosis, and management. Baltimore: Williams & Wilkins, 1995.

Tilley LP. Essentials of canine and feline electrocardiography. 3rd ed. Baltimore: Williams & Wilkins, 1992.

Author Janice McIntosh Bright
Consulting Editors Larry P. Tilley and Francis W. K. Smith, Jr.

ATRIOVENTRICULAR BLOCK, SECOND DEGREE—MOBITZ TYPE II

 BASICS

DEFINITION

Occurs when one or more P waves are blocked without a preceding progressive delay in AV transmission.

ECG Features

• One or more P waves not followed by a QRS complex, and PR intervals of conducted beats are consistent (Figure 1)
• Ventricular rate—usually slow
• Fixed ratio of P waves to QRS complexes may occur (e.g., 2:1, 3:1, 4:1 AV block).
• In second degree AV block with a 2:1 conduction ratio or higher, it is impossible to observe prolongation of the PR interval before the block, so a designation of Mobitz is not appropriate (Figure 1).
• QRS complexes may appear normal but are often wide or have an abnormal morphology due to aberrant intraventricular conduction or to ventricular enlargement.
• Abnormally wide QRS complexes (type B) generally indicate serious, extensive cardiac disease.

PATHOPHYSIOLOGY

• Rare in healthy animals
• May be hemodynamically important when ventricular rate is abnormally slow
• Frequently progresses to complete AV block, particularly when accompanied by wide QRS complexes

SYSTEMS AFFECTED

• Cardiovascular
• Central nervous system if inadequate cerebral blood flow

GENETICS

May be heritable in pugs

INCIDENCE/PREVALENCE

Unknown

GEOGRAPHIC DISTRIBUTION

N/A

SIGNALMENT

Species

Dogs and cats

Breed Predilections

• American cocker spaniels and dachshunds
• Pugs
• Dachshunds

Mean Age and Range

Often occurs in older animals

Predominant Sex

N/A

SIGNS

Historical Findings

• Presenting complaint may be syncope, collapse, weakness, or lethargy
• Some animals are asymptomatic.

Physical Examination Findings

• May be weakness
• Bradycardia common
• May be intermittent pauses in the cardiac rhythm

• An S4 may be audible in lieu of the normally expected heart sounds (i.e., S1,S2) when the block occurs.
• If associated with digoxin intoxication, there may be vomiting, anorexia, and diarrhea.

CAUSES

• Heritable in pugs
• Enhanced vagal stimulation from noncardiac diseases
• Degenerative change within the cardiac conduction system—replacement of AV nodal cells and/or Purkinje fibers by fibrotic and adipose tissue in old cats and dogs
• Pharmacologic agents (e.g., digoxin, β-adrenergic antagonists, calcium channel blocking agents, α_2-adrenergic agonists, muscarinic cholinergic agonists, or severe procainamide or quinidine toxicity)
• Infiltrative myocardial disorders (neoplasia, amyloid)
• Endocarditis (particularly involving the aortic valve)
• Myocarditis (viral, bacterial, parasitic, idiopathic)
• Atropine administered intravenously may cause a brief period of first or second degree heart block before increasing the heart rate.

RISK FACTORS

Any condition or intervention that enhances vagal tone

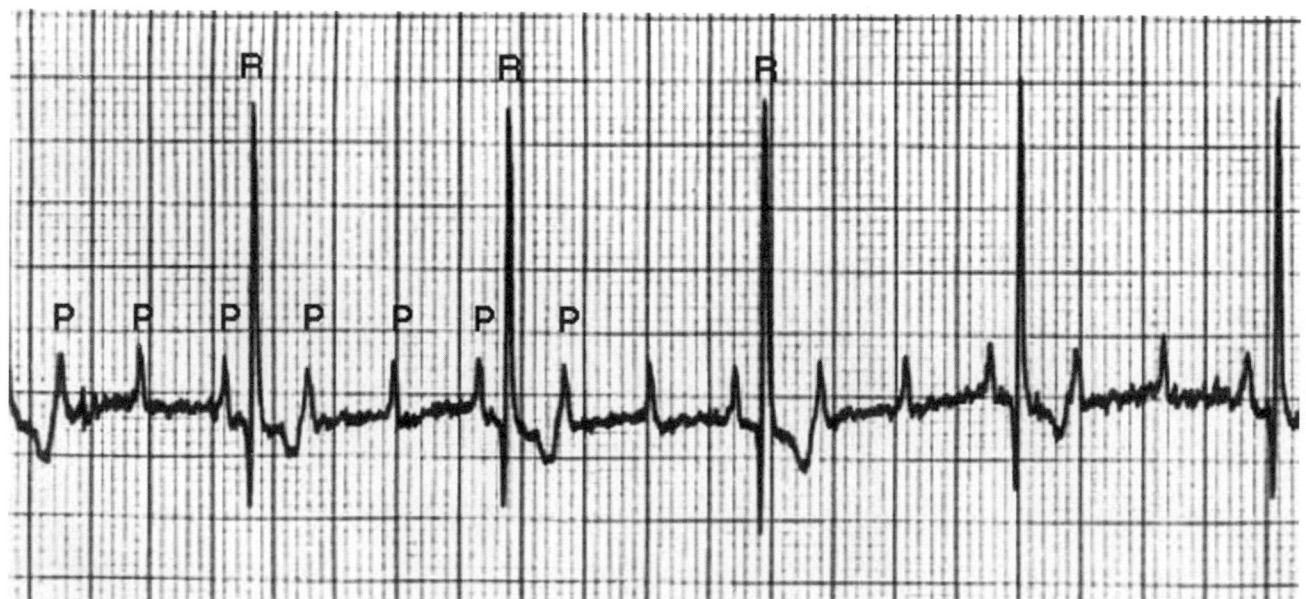

Figure 1.

Lead II ECG rhythm strip recorded from a dog with 3:1, second degree AV block. The PR interval for the conducted beats is constant (0.10 second) (paper speed = 25 mm/s).

ATRIOVENTRICULAR BLOCK, SECOND DEGREE—MOBITZ TYPE II

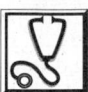

DIAGNOSIS

DIFFERENTIAL DIAGNOSIS
• Advanced form (i.e., persistent block of two or more consecutive P waves) distinguished from complete AV block
• Nonconducted P waves arising from refractoriness of the conduction system during supraventricular tachycardias differentiated from pathologic conduction block

CBC/BIOCHEMISTRY/URINALYSIS
Electrolyte abnormalities (e.g., severe hypokalemia or hypercalcemia) may predispose to AV block.

OTHER LABORATORY TESTS
• Serum digoxin concentration—may be high
• High T_4 in cats—if associated with hyperthyroidism
• High arterial blood pressure in cats—if associated with hypertensive heart disease
• Positive *Borrelia*, *Rickettsia*, or *Trypanosoma cruzi* titers—if associated with one of these infectious agents
• Blood cultures may be positive in patients with vegetative endocarditis.

IMAGING
Echocardiographic examination may reveal structural heart disease (e.g., endocarditis, neoplasia, or left ventricular hypertrophy)

DIAGNOSTIC PROCEDURES
Atropine response test—administer 0.04 mg/kg atropine IM and repeat ECG in 20–30 min; may be used to determine whether AV block is due to high vagal tone

PATHOLOGIC FINDINGS
• Variable—depend on underlying cause
• Old animals with degenerative change of the conduction system may have focal mineralization of the interventricular septal crest visible grossly; chondroid metaplasia of the central fibrous body and increased fibrous connective tissue in the AV bundle is noted histopathologically.

TREATMENT

APPROPRIATE HEALTH CARE
• Treatment—may be unnecessary if heart rate maintains adequate cardiac output
• Positive chronotropic interventions indicated for symptomatic patients
• Treat or remove underlying cause(s)

NURSING CARE
Generally unnecessary

ACTIVITY
Cage rest advised for symptomatic patients

DIET
Modifications or restrictions only to manage an underlying condition

CLIENT EDUCATION
• Need to seek and specifically treat underlying cause
• Pharmacologic agents may not be effective long term.

SURGICAL CONSIDERATIONS
Permanent pacemaker may be required for long term management of symptomatic patients.

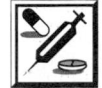

MEDICATIONS

DRUG(S) OF CHOICE
• Atropine (0.02–0.04 mg/kg IV, IM) or glycopyrrolate (0.005–0.01 mg/kg IV, IM) may be used short term if positive atropine response
• Chronic anticholinergic therapy (propantheline 0.5–2 mg/kg PO q8–12h or hyoscyamine 0.003–0.006 mg/kg q8h)—indicated for symptomatic patients if improved AV conduction with atropine response test
• Isoproterenol (0.04–0.09 μg/kg/min IV to effect) or dopamine (2–5 μg/kg/min IV to effect) may be administered in acute, life-threatening situations to enhance AV conduction and/or accelerate an escape focus.

CONTRAINDICATIONS
• Drugs with vagomimetic action (e.g., digoxin, bethanechol, physostigmine, pilocarpine) may potentiate block
• Avoid drugs likely to impair impulse conduction further or depress a ventricular escape focus (e.g., procainamide, quinidine, lidocaine, calcium channel blocking agents, β-adrenergic blocking agents)

PRECAUTIONS
Hypokalemia—increases sensitivity to vagal tone; may potentiate AV conduction delay

POSSIBLE INTERACTIONS
N/A

ALTERNATIVE DRUG(S)
N/A

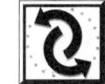

FOLLOW-UP

PATIENT MONITORING
Frequent ECG because often progresses to complete (third degree) AV block

PREVENTION/AVOIDANCE
N/A

POSSIBLE COMPLICATIONS
Prolonged bradycardia may cause secondary congestive heart failure or inadequate renal perfusion.

EXPECTED COURSE AND PROGNOSIS
• Variable—depends on cause
• If degenerative disease of the cardiac conduction system, often progresses to complete (third degree) AV block

MISCELLANEOUS

ASSOCIATED CONDITIONS
May be noted in cats with primary or secondary left ventricular hypertrophy

AGE-RELATED FACTORS
N/A

ZOONOTIC POTENTIAL
N/A

PREGNANCY
N/A

SYNONYMS
None

SEE ALSO
• Atrioventricular Block, Complete (Third Degree)
• Atrioventricular Block, Second Degree—Mobitz Type I

ABBREVIATION
AV = atrioventricular

Suggested Reading
Edwards NJ. Bolton's handbook of canine and feline electrocardiography. 2nd ed. Philadelphia: Saunders, 1987.
Kittleson MD. Electrocardiography. In: Kittleson MD, Kienle RD, eds. Small animal cardiovascular medicine. St. Louis: Mosby, 1998:72–94.
Mangrum JM, DiMarco JP. The evaluation and management of bradycardia. N Engl J Med 2000;342:703–709.
Podrid PJ, Kowey PR. Cardiac arrhythmia—mechanisms, diagnosis, and management. Baltimore: Williams & Wilkins, 1995.
Tilley LP. Essentials of canine and feline electrocardiography. 3rd ed. Baltimore: Williams & Wilkins, 1992.
Author Janice McIntosh Bright
Consulting Editors Larry P. Tilley and Francis W. K. Smith, Jr.

ATRIOVENTRICULAR VALVE DYSPLASIA

BASICS

DEFINITION
A congenital malformation of the mitral or tricuspid valve apparatus

PATHOPHYSIOLOGY
• Atrioventricular valve dysplasia (AVVD) can result in valvular insufficiency, valvular stenosis, or dynamic outflow tract obstruction depending on the anatomic abnormality. AVVD may occur alone or in association with abnormalities of the ipsilateral outflow tract, e.g., valvular or subvalvular aortic or pulmonic stenosis. • Valvular insufficiency results in dilation of the ipsilateral atrium, eccentric hypertrophy of the associated ventricle and, if sufficiently severe, signs of congestive heart failure. Cardiomyopathy of chronic volume overload and elevated atrial pressures are the end result culminating in pulmonary congestion if the mitral valve is affected and systemic congestion if the tricuspid valve is affected. • Valvular stenosis results in atrial dilation and hypertrophy and, when severe, hypoplasia of the receiving ventricle. Tricuspid valve stenosis results in elevated right atrial pressure and systemic congestion if pressures exceed 15 to 20 mmHg. Right to left shunting may occur if there is an atrial septal defect or patent foramen ovale. Mitral valve stenosis results in elevated pulmonary capillary pressure and pulmonary edema if pressures exceed 25 to 30 mmHg. Pulmonary hypertension is common in animals with mitral valve stenosis. • Outflow tract obstruction may develop from valvular malformations, causing elongation of the anterior leaflet of the mitral valve or which translocate the anterior leaflet to a position closer to the interventricular septum. Concentric left ventricular hypertrophy develops in proportion to the severity of the obstruction.

SYSTEMS AFFECTED
• Cardiovascular—inflow obstruction due to valvular stenosis and chronic volume overload from valvular insufficiency result in elevated pulmonary (left AV valve) or systemic (right AV valve) venous pressures and signs of low cardiac output if sufficiently severe. Pressure overload and concentric left ventricular hypertrophy develop secondary to dynamic outflow obstruction. • Respiratory—pulmonary edema may develop secondary to mitral stenosis or mitral valve insufficiency. Pulmonary hypertension is also common in animals with mitral stenosis. • Neurologic—collapse and loss of consciousness may occur with severe valvular stenosis due to hypotension, most often during physical exertion. Collapse in animals with dynamic outflow obstruction is most often due to arrhythmia.

GENETICS
Tricuspid valve dysplasia is inherited as an autosomal recessive trait in Labrador retrievers. Heritability and pattern of inheritance not established in other breeds

INCIDENCE/PREVALENCE
One of the most common congenital cardiac anomalies in cats (17% of reported congenital cardiac defects in one study). Less frequently diagnosed in dogs

GEOGRAPHIC DISTRIBUTION
N/A

SIGNALMENT

Species
Dogs and cats

Breed Predilections
• Tricuspid valve dysplasia—increased risk for Labrador retrievers, German shepherd dogs, Great Pyrenees, possibly Old English sheepdogs. Also common in cats • Mitral valve dysplasia—increased risk in bull terriers, Newfoundland retrievers, Great Danes, Golden retrievers, possibly Dalmatians and Siamese cats. Perhaps the most common congenital heart defects of cats. Mitral valve malformations also common in cats with hypertrophic cardiomyopathy.

Mean Age and Range
Variable. Signs are most often manifest within the first few years after birth.

Predominant Sex
Males are more likely to evidence heart failure.

SIGNS

Historical Findings
• Exercise intolerance most common problem in dogs and cats with AV valve dysplasia. • Abdominal distention, weight loss, and stunting may be observed with severe tricuspid valve dysplasia. • Labored respiration common in dogs or cats with mitral valve dysplasia • Syncope and collapse if severe mitral or tricuspid valve stenosis or if there is concurrent outflow tract obstruction or an associated arrhythmia.

Physical Examination Findings
Mitral Valve Dysplasia
• A holosystolic murmur is heard over the cardiac apex on the left. With severe disease the murmur is accompanied by a thrill or gallop heart sounds. A soft diastolic murmur may be present in the same location in animals with mitral stenosis but many affected animals have no audible murmur. A systolic ejection murmur that intensifies with exercise or excitement is audible in animals with dynamic outflow tract obstructions. • Evidence of left heart failure—tachypnea, increased respiratory efforts, pulmonary crackles and cyanosis in animals with severe defects

Tricuspid Valve Dysplasia
• A holosystolic murmur is heard over the cardiac apex on the right. With severe disease the murmur is accompanied by a thrill or gallop heart sounds. Silent tricuspid regurgitation is well documented in cats and is attributable to a very large regurgitant orifice. Distention and pulsation of the external jugular vein may be evident. • Evidence of right heart failure—ascites and, more rarely, peripheral edema with severe malformations.

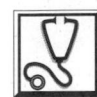

DIAGNOSIS

DIFFERENTIAL DIAGNOSIS
• With the noted exception of the age of onset, congenital AV valvular insufficiency resembles acquired degenerative AV valve insufficiency with respect to historical findings, physical examination abnormalities, and clinical sequelae. • The right-sided murmur of tricuspid insufficiency is sometimes confused with the right-sided murmur of a ventricular septal defect. • Ascites caused by silent tricuspid regurgitation or tricuspid valve stenosis is often attributed to pericardial effusion, hepatic disease, or obstruction of the caudal vena cava. • There is no certain way to distinguish mitral valve dysplasia producing outflow tract obstruction and the obstructive form of cardiomyopathy. If the obstruction can be abolished with beta blocker and left ventricular hypertrophy resolves, it is likely that the primary abnormality was mitral valve dysplasia.

CBC/CHEMISTRY/URINALYSIS
Usually normal

OTHER LABORATORY TESTS N/A

IMAGING

Radiographic Findings
Mitral Valve Dysplasia
• Left atrial and left ventricular enlargement with valvular insufficiency. Isolated left atrial enlargement with valvular stenosis. Mild left atrial enlargement with dynamic outflow obstruction • Evidence of left heart failure—distended pulmonary veins, interstitial or alveolar edema in severe cases.
Tricuspid Valve Dysplasia
• Right atrial and right ventricular enlargement with valvular insufficiency. Cardiac silhouette may appear globoid with pronounced enlargement. Isolated right atrial enlargement with valvular stenosis. • Evidence of right heart failure—dilated caudal vena cava, hepatosplenomegaly or ascites in severe cases.

Echocardiography
Mitral Valve Dysplasia
• Valvular insufficiency results in left atrial dilation and eccentric hypertrophy of the left

ventricle. The papillary muscles are typically small and displaced dorsally. Chordae tendineae are often short and thickened. Doppler echocardiography demonstrates a high velocity retrograde systolic transmitral jet and modestly increased transmitral inflow velocities. • Mitral stenosis results in left atrial dilation while the left ventricular dimensions are normal or small. The valve leaflets are often thickened, relatively immobile and often fused. Doppler echocardiography demonstrates a high velocity transmitral diastolic jet with a reduced EF slope. There may also be evidence of mitral insufficiency and/or secondary pulmonary hypertension. • Dynamic left ventricular outflow obstruction is characterized by systolic motion of the anterior mitral valve leaflet towards the interventricular septum, increased LV outflow tract velocities and concentric left ventricular hypertrophy.

Tricuspid Valve Dysplasia
• Valvular insufficiency results in right atrial dilation and eccentric hypertrophy of the right ventricle. The papillary muscles and chordae tendineae may be fused, creating a curtain-like appearance of the tricuspid valve. Doppler echocardiography demonstrates a high velocity retrograde systolic trans-tricuspid jet and modestly increased trans-tricuspid inflow velocities. • Tricuspid stenosis results in right atrial dilation with normal or small right ventricular dimensions. The valve leaflets do not open completely. Doppler echocardiography demonstrates a high velocity diastolic trans-tricuspid jet. There may be evidence of concurrent tricuspid valve insufficiency and/or right-to-left shunting across a patent foramen ovale or associated atrial septal defect.

Cardiac Catheterization
• Indicated only in those cases where the diagnosis cannot be confirmed by echocardiography or if surgical correction is anticipated • Mitral dysplasia—hemodynamic measurements should include left ventricular pressures, pulmonary capillary wedge pressure or direct measurement of LA pressure, pulmonary artery pressures; and, in cases of dynamic obstruction, simultaneous recording of aortic and left ventricular pressures with medical provocation. Contrast studies are best accomplished with a left ventricular injection in cases of valvular insufficiency and direct left atrial injection via trans-septal catheterization in cases of valvular stenosis. • Tricuspid dysplasia—hemodynamic measurements should include right ventricular and right atrial pressures. Contrast studies are best accomplished with a right ventricular injection in cases of valvular insufficiency and right atrial injection in cases of valvular stenosis.

DIAGNOSTIC PROCEDURES
Electrocardiographic Findings
Usually reflect pattern of chamber enlargement. Severe defects may be accompanied by a variety of arrhythmias, particularly atrial premature beats, supraventricular tachycardia, or atrial fibrillation.

TREATMENT
APPROPRIATE HEALTH CARE
Inpatient treatment required for CHF

CLIENT EDUCATION
Owners should be informed of heritability and advised against breeding.

ACTIVITY
Restricted in accordance with severity

DIET
Sodium-restricted if overt or pending heart failure.

SURGICAL CONSIDERATIONS
Available in a few centers. Expensive

MEDICATIONS
DRUG(S) OF CHOICE
• Mitral or tricuspid dysplasia with insufficiency—diuretics, angiotensin converting enzyme inhibitors, and digoxin for patients with imminent or overt congestive heart failure. Furosemide (2.0–4.0 mg/kg q12–24h), enalapril (0.5 mg/kg q12h), and digoxin (0.003–0.004 mg/kg q12h) are typical dosages that must be adjusted to meet unique circumstances of each patient.
• Mitral or tricuspid stenosis—diuretics to control edema. Furosemide (2.0–4.0 mg/kg q12–24h) dose adjusted to resolve congestion. Heart rate should be maintained near to 150 bpm using digoxin (0.003–0.004 mg/kg q12h), a calcium channel blocker such as diltiazem (1.0–1.5 mg/kg q8h), or a beta-receptor blocking drug, such as atenolol (0.5–1.5 mg/kg q12–24h).
• Dynamic outflow tract obstruction—titrate a beta-receptor blocking drug, such as atenolol (0.5–1.5 mg/kg q12–24h), to abolish or diminish severity of outflow obstruction. Furosemide if evidence of CHF

CONTRAINDICATIONS
N/A

PRECAUTIONS
Standard patient monitoring for cardiac medication side-effects (e.g., digitalis toxicity, azotemia)

POSSIBLE INTERACTIONS
N/A

ALTERNATIVE DRUG(S)
N/A

FOLLOW-UP
PATIENT MONITORING
Recheck yearly if no signs of heart failure. Recheck at a minimum of every 3 months if signs of CHF. Thoracic radiographs, ECG, and echocardiography advisable

PREVENTION/AVOIDANCE
Do not breed affected animals.

POSSIBLE COMPLICATIONS
• Congestive heart failure: left-sided with mitral valve dysplasia; right-sided with tricuspid valve dysplasia • Collapse or syncope with exercise • Paroxysmal supraventricular tachycardia or atrial fibrillation with severe disease

EXPECTED COURSE
Depends on severity of underlying defect. Guarded to poor with serious defects

MISCELLANEOUS
ASSOCIATED CONDITIONS
• Mitral valve dysplasia commonly accompanies valvular or subvalvular aortic stenosis. • Tricuspid valve dysplasia commonly accompanies pulmonic stenosis.

PREGNANCY
Should be avoided—heritable defect and possibility of causing decompensated or worsening heart failure

SEE ALSO
• Congestive Heart Failure, Left-sided
• Congestive Heart Failure, Right-sided

ABBREVIATIONS
AVVD = atrioventricular valve dysplasia
MS = mitral valve stenosis
MVD = mitral valve dysplasia
TS = tricuspid valve stenosis
TVD = tricuspid valve dysplasia

Suggested Reading
Bonagura JD and Lehmkuhl LB. Congenital heart disease. In Fox PR, Sisson D, and Moise NS. Textbook of canine and feline cardiology. Principles and clinical practice. 2nd Edition. Philadelphia, Saunders, 1999:520–526
Sisson D, Thomas WP, Bonagura JD. Congenital Heart Disease. In Ettinger SJ, and Feldman EC. Textbook of veterinary internal Medicine. 5th Edition. Philadelphia, Saunders, 2000:774–778.
Author David Sisson
Consulting Editors Larry P. Tilley and Francis W. K. Smith, Jr.

ATRIOVENTRICULAR VALVE ENDOCARDIOSIS

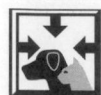

BASICS

DEFINITION
A chronic degenerative disease affecting the mitral and tricuspid valves, leading to valvular insufficiency and heart failure

PATHOPHYSIOLOGY
• Proliferation and deposition of mucopolysaccharide within the subendothelial spongiosa layer leads to thickening, distortion, and stiffening of the AV valves; initially, swellings are nodular, but coalescence occurs until the entire valve and often the attached chordae are involved.
• AV valve incompetence causes regurgitation, high atrial pressure, reduced cardiac output, activation of compensatory mechanisms (sympathetic nervous system, renin-angiotensin-aldosterone system, and atrial natriuretic factor), and CHF. • Volume overload leads to progressive ventricular dilation, advancing ventricular stiffness, and impaired ventricular function; congestive and low-output (forward) failure result.
• With atrial tear, acute cardiac tamponade may result. • Degenerative changes in the chordae tendineae lead to distortion, weakening, and rupture, causing valvular instability and increased regurgitation.

SYSTEMS AFFECTED
• Cardiovascular—both AV valves are affected, but one study found the distribution in necropsy specimens to be mitral alone, 62%; tricuspid alone, 1%; and both, 33%.
• Respiratory—if edema develops
• Renal/Urologic—prerenal azotemia
• Hepatobiliary—passive congestion

GENETICS
Not established

INCIDENCE/PREVALENCE
Chronic valvular disease increases from about 5% in middle-aged dogs (5–7 years) to >35% in old dogs (12 years).

SIGNALMENT

Species
Mainly dogs, but may be seen in old cats

Breed Predilections
• Typically small breeds • Highest prevalence—Cavalier King Charles spaniel, Chihuahua, miniature schnauzer, Maltese, Pomeranian, cocker spaniel, Pekingese, fox terrier, Boston terrier, miniature poodle, toy poodle, miniature pinscher, and whippet

Mean Age and Range
Heart failure onset at 10–12 years, although may detect a murmur several years earlier; Cavalier King Charles spaniels typically affected much earlier (6–8 years)

Predominant Sex
Males—male:female ratio, 1.5:1

SIGNS

Asymptomatic Valve Disease
• Systolic murmur is heard best at the left fifth intercostal space (mitral) or right fourth intercostal space (tricuspid). • Murmurs may vary from a low-frequency, holosystolic, band-shaped sound to a shorter, high-frequency, midsystolic murmur; occasionally only a midsystolic click is detected. • As the disease progresses, the murmur typically gets louder and radiates more widely; with severe disease, the volume of regurgitation becomes so large that the murmur may decrease in frequency and loudness.

Mild Heart Failure
Coughing, exercise intolerance, and dyspnea with exercise

Moderate Heart Failure
Coughing, exercise intolerance, and dyspnea at all times

Severe Heart Failure
Severe dyspnea, profound weakness, abdominal distention, productive coughing (i.e., pink, frothy fluid), orthopnea, cyanosis, and syncope; occasionally, syncope may be the only owner complaint.

CAUSES
Idiopathic

RISK FACTORS N/A

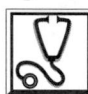

DIAGNOSIS

DIFFERENTIAL DIAGNOSIS
• Dilated cardiomyopathy • Congenital heart disease • Chronic airway or interstitial lung disease • Pneumonia • Pulmonary embolism • Pulmonary neoplasia • Heartworm disease

CBC/BIOCHEMISTRY/URINALYSIS
• Prerenal azotemia secondary to impaired renal perfusion; urinary specific gravity is high unless complicated by underlying renal disease or previous diuretic administration.
• High liver enzyme activity in many patients with passive congestion

IMAGING

Radiographic Findings
• Heart size ranges from normal to left-sided or generalized cardiomegaly. • Left atrial enlargement in the lateral projection exhibits elevation of the distal fourth of the trachea and splitting of the mainstem bronchi; dorsoventral projection shows accentuation of the angle between the mainstem bronchi, a double shadow at the six o'clock position, where the caudal edge of the atrium extends beyond the left ventricle, and bulging of the left atrial appendage in the one to three o'clock position. • Left-sided heart failure—the pulmonary vein is larger than the associated pulmonary artery; air bronchograms are typical of, but not

pathognomonic for, cardiogenic pulmonary edema; initially, congestion and edema are perihilar, with all lung fields eventually showing changes. The right lung may be affected before the left.

Echocardiographic Findings
• Thickening and distortion of the mitral valve; septal leaflet is most severely affected.
• Elongation and rupture of the chordae tendineae, causing mitral valve prolapse
• Large left atrium • The left ventricle may be distended and is hyperdynamic if the regurgitant flow is high and myocardial function intact; as the ventricle becomes more grossly distended, it may become hypodynamic because of myocardial failure.
• Pericardial effusion in some patients
• Doppler studies document a jet of regurgitation into the left atrium and the area of the regurgitant jet on color flow.
• Doppler has been used to assess severity.

Diagnostic Procedures
• Abdominocentesis/pleurocentesis—a modified transudate is characteristic of CHF.
• Arterial/venous blood gases have been used to quantify hypoxemia and monitor treatment response.

Electrocardiographic Findings
• Sinus tachycardia is common in animals with CHF. • May show evidence of left atrial enlargement (P mitrale) or left ventricular enlargement (tall and wide R waves)
• Atrioventricular arrhythmias may develop.

PATHOLOGIC FINDINGS
• Gross valvular changes are divided into four types—type I shows only a few discrete nodules at the line of closure; type IV shows gross distortion of the valve by gray-white nodules and plaques causing contraction of the cusps and rolling of the free edge; the chordae are irregularly thickened, with regions of tapering and rupture. • Jet lesions—irregular thickening and opacity of the atrial endocardium • Recent and healed left atrium splits or tears in some patients; full-thickness tears lead to hemopericardium (free wall) or acquired atrial septal defect (septum). • Left atrium and left ventricle dilation in many patients • The degree of left ventricular hypertrophy may be apparent only on weighing the heart. • Small thrombi in the left atrium rare in dogs—more common and extensive in cats.

TREATMENT

APPROPRIATE HEALTH CARE
Treat patients that need oxygen support as inpatients; if stable, patients may be less stressed at home.

NURSING CARE
Oxygen therapy as needed for hypoxemia

ATRIOVENTRICULAR VALVE ENDOCARDIOSIS

ACTIVITY
• Absolute exercise restriction for symptomatic patients • Stable patients receiving medical treatment—restrict exercise to leash walking; avoid sudden, explosive exercise.

DIET
• A salt-restricted diet is recommended, if tolerated, for a patient in heart failure; monitor sodium concentration closely. • Hyponatremia may develop as CHF progresses and in patients fed severely sodium–restricted diets in conjunction with loop diuretics and angiotensin-converting enzyme (ACE) inhibitors. • If hyponatremia develops, switch to a less sodium-restricted diet (e.g., renal or geriatric diet).

CLIENT EDUCATION
• Discuss the progressive nature of the disease. • Emphasize the importance of consistent dosing of all medications and diet and exercise management. • Highlight the signs of digoxin toxicity, and advise the owner to stop treatment and notify the veterinarian immediately should any develop.

SURGICAL CONSIDERATIONS
Surgical valve replacement and purse-string suture techniques to reduce the area of the mitral valve orifice have been used; experience with these techniques is limited, but surgical repair may be an option when access to a cardiovascular surgeon and cardiopulmonary bypass are available.

MEDICATIONS

DRUG(S) OF CHOICE
Recommended treatment depends on the stage of the disease; these recommendations follow the guidelines set by the ISACHC.

Asymptomatic Patients
• If no cardiac enlargement, no treatment is recommended. • Administering ACE inhibitors to asymptomatic patients showing progressive cardiomegaly may slow progression; this hypothesis is, as yet, unsubstantiated.

Mild or Moderate CHF
• Diuretics—furosemide (1–2 mg/kg q8–12h) • ACE inhibitors enalapril (0.5 mg/kg q12–24h), benazepril (0.25–0.5 mg/kg q24h) • Spironolactone, while typically used for its diuretic effect in combination with other diuretics, has been shown to have a positive influence on deleterious remodeling that occurs as heart disease progresses. It is used initially at 0.5–1 mg/kg PO q24h. The dose can be raised to 1–2 mg/kg PO q12h for refractory heart failure. • Nitroglycerin—2% percutaneous ointment (0.125–1 inch q6h until patient is stable) • Digoxin—especially if supraventricular arrhythmias, including atrial

fibrillation, are documented (0.005 mg/kg or 0.22 mg/m² PO q12h) • Sodium restriction if tolerated • Antiarrhythmics—as needed • Calcium channel blockers—to treat atrial arrhythmias • β-Blockers—to treat atrial and ventricular arrhythmias • Class 1 antiarrhythmics—procainamide, quinidine, mexiletine, and tocainide; to treat ventricular arrhythmias • Class III antiarrhythmics—sotalol, amiodarone for intractable arrhythmias

Severe Congestive Heart Failure
• Oxygen—40% in O_2 cage (can go as high as 100%) up to 24h; use nasal O_2 in large-breed dogs, 50–100 mL/kg/min through humidifier • Diuretics—furosemide (Lasix, 2–4 mg/kg IV q4–8h)

Vasodilators
• Benazepril (0.25–0.5 mg/kg q24h) • Enalapril (0.5 mg/kg q12h—q24h) • Hydralazine (0.5 mg/kg q12h titrated up to 2 mg/kg if necessary)—used in acute stages to decrease afterload rapidly; may cause hypotension • Nitroglycerin—ointment (1/4 inch/5 kg up to 2 inches percutaneously) or injectable (1–5 μg/kg/min CRI) • Sodium nitroprusside (1–10 μg/kg/min)—monitor blood pressure.

Positive Inotropes
• Digoxin (0.005 mg/kg or 0.22 mg/m² PO q12h) • Dobutamine (dogs, 1–10 μg/kg/min; cats, 1–5 μg/kg/min)—may cause seizures • Dopamine (1–10 μg/kg/min) • Agents with β-blocking properties (e.g., carvedilol) are being investigated for their ability to up-regulate β-receptors in patients with severe myocardial dysfunction. Carvedilol (0.1–0.4 mg/kg PO q12h) is an alpha- and beta-blocker with antioxidant activity. Start at the low end of the dose range and gradually raise dose if tolerated.

PRECAUTIONS
• Use digoxin, diuretics, and ACE inhibitors with caution in patients with renal disease. • Nitrate tolerance may develop if appropriate 12-h nitrate-free intervals are omitted from the dosing schedule. • Beta blockers are negative inotropes and may have an acute adverse effect on myocardial function, although their long-term use may improve myocardial function.

POSSIBLE INTERACTIONS
Monitor digoxin concentration in patients receiving concurrent calcium channel blockers or quinidine.

ALTERNATIVE DRUG(S)
• Diuretics—add thiazide and potassium-sparing diuretic (e.g., spironolactone) in refractory animals. • Bumetanide is an alternative to furosemide. • Vasodilators—other ACE inhibitors include lisinopril; isosorbide dinitrate can be used in place of nitroglycerin ointment in patients requiring long-term nitrate administration.

FOLLOW-UP

PATIENT MONITORING
• Take a baseline radiograph when a murmur is first detected and every 6–12 months thereafter to document progressive cardiomegaly. • After an episode of CHF, check patients weekly during the first month of treatment; may repeat thoracic radiographs and an ECG at the first weekly checkup and on subsequent visits if any changes are seen on physical examination. • Monitor BUN and creatinine when diuretics and ACE inhibitors are used in combination. Monitor serum potassium levels when spironolactone and ACE inhibitors are used concurrently.

PREVENTION/AVOIDANCE N/A

POSSIBLE COMPLICATIONS
Endocarditis because of bacterial colonization of the diseased mitral valve

EXPECTED COURSE AND PROGNOSIS
Progressive degeneration of both valve changes and myocardial function occurs, necessitating increasing drug dosages; long-term prognosis depends on response to treatment and stage of heart failure.

MISCELLANEOUS

SYNONYMS
• Degenerative valve disease • Chronic valve disease • Acquired valvular insufficiency • Valve fibrosis

SEE ALSO
• Atrial Wall Tear • Congestive Heart Failure, Left-Sided • Congestive Heart Failure, Right-Sided

ABBREVIATIONS
• ACE = angiotensin-converting enzyme • AV = atrioventricular • CHF = congestive heart failure

Suggested Reading
Abbott J. Acquired valvular disease. In: Tilley LP, Goodwin J-K, eds. Manual of canine and feline cardiology. Philadelphia: Saunders, 2001:113–136.
Kvart C, Haggstrom J, Pedersen HD, et al. Efficacy of enalapril for prevention of congestive heart failure in dogs with myxomatous valve disease and asymptomatic mitral regurgitation.J Vet Intern Med 2002 Jan–Feb;16(1):80–88.
Author Andrew Beardow
Consulting Editors Larry P. Tilley and Francis W.K. Smith, Jr.

ATRIOVENTRICULAR VALVULAR STENOSIS

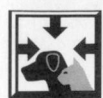 BASICS

OVERVIEW
• AV valvular stenosis is a pathologic narrowing of the mitral or tricuspid valve orifice; ventricular filling in clinically significant disease requires a persistent diastolic pressure gradient between atrium and ventricle.
• Rarely diagnosed in dogs and cats
• Concomitant valvular regurgitation is common.
• The increased atrial pressure can lead to atrial dilation, venous congestion, and CHF.
• The foramen ovale may remain patent in patients with tricuspid stenosis, allowing right-to-left shunting with signs of cyanotic heart disease.
• Cardiac output and exercise capacity are limited; with mitral stenosis, exertional dyspnea and left-sided CHF are common.

SIGNALMENT
• Mitral stenosis is a condition of uncertain genetic basis; bull terriers and Newfoundlands may be overrepresented, but the condition is also seen in other breeds.
• Of the three reported cats with mitral stenosis, two were Siamese.
• Tricuspid stenosis has been reported most often in Old English sheepdogs and Labrador retrievers.
• Most patients are presented at a young age, though exceptions do occur, especially in cats.

SIGNS

Historical Findings
• Exercise intolerance
• Syncope
• Exertional dyspnea or tachypnea
• Cough—mitral stenosis
• Cyanosis—tricuspid stenosis
• Abdominal distention—tricuspid stenosis
• Acute posterior paresis—cats with mitral stenosis
• Stunted growth

Physical Examination Findings
• Soft diastolic murmur with point of maximal intensity over the left apex (mitral stenosis) or right hemithorax (tricuspid stenosis)
• Holosystolic murmur of mitral or tricuspid regurgitation is common, especially with mitral stenosis.
• Crackles, dyspnea with mitral stenosis
• Jugular distention, jugular pulses, ascites, hepatomegaly with tricuspid stenosis
• Cyanosis from right to left shunt with tricuspid stenosis

CAUSES & RISK FACTORS
• AV valvular stenosis is most likely due to congenital valve dysplasia; supravalvular lesions (a membrane with central perforation or a fibrous ring) have been described.
• Bacterial endocarditis and intracardiac neoplasia are potential causes of acquired AV valvular stenosis.

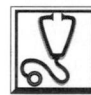 DIAGNOSIS

DIFFERENTIAL DIAGNOSIS
Must differentiate from the more common causes of mitral and tricuspid regurgitation in the absence of stenosis

CBC/BIOCHEMISTRY/URINALYSIS
May be normal or reflect changes related to CHF or drug therapy for heart failure

OTHER LABORATORY TESTS
N/A

IMAGING

Thoracic Radiography
• Atrial enlargement is the most consistent and outstanding feature.
• May see generalized cardiomegaly
• If the patient is in left-sided CHF, may see patchy alveolar opacities of pulmonary edema
• Tricuspid stenosis—may be hepatomegaly; diameter of the caudal vena cava may be increased.

Echocardiography
• Diagnostic test of choice
• Two-dimensional echocardiography reveals a markedly dilated atrium with attenuated valve excursion during diastole, often with thickened irregular AV valve leaflets evident; mobile, but fused, valve leaflets may appear to "dome" during diastole.
• May see shortened chordae tendineae or an anomalous papillary muscle; may see some subtle tethering of the mitral valve in some asymptomatic breeds at risk (e.g., bull terrier, mastiff)
• M-mode studies show an enlarged atrium with concordant motion of the AV valve leaflets; both leaflets move together during diastole, indicating commissural fusion; the E-to-F slope is decreased.
• Color-flow imaging reveals a turbulent diastolic jet that originates at the stenotic valve and projects toward the apex of the ventricle; a turbulent jet of AV valve regurgitation is often present as well.
• Pulsed-wave and continuous-wave Doppler studies show increased diastolic transvalvular flow velocities; prolonged calculated pressure half-time is a hallmark feature; E-wave/A-wave amplitude reversal may be seen.

Angiography
• Atrial injection demonstrates a markedly dilated atrium; with tricuspid stenosis and a patent foramen ovale, opacification of the left atrium may be observed following right atrial injection.
• Often see delayed opacification of the ventricle and great vessels; one may visualize thickened, irregular valve leaflets or a stenotic valve funnel; ventricular injection typically reveals valvular regurgitation.

Cardiac Catheterization
• A diastolic pressure gradient exists between the atrium and ventricle.
• High left atrial, pulmonary capillary wedge, and pulmonary artery pressures occur in mitral stenosis.
• High right atrial and central venous pressures are present in tricuspid stenosis.

• Ventricular pressure may be normal in the absence of concurrent defects.

DIAGNOSTIC PROCEDURES

Electrocardiography

May be variable enlargement patterns (atrial and ventricular); ectopic rhythms, especially of atrial origin, are often observed.

PATHOLOGIC FINDINGS

• Usually the atrioventricular valve is abnormal, with thickened leaflets and fused commissures.

• Many patients also have evidence of valve dysplasia with abnormal chordae tendineae and papillary muscles.

• Atrial dilation and hypertrophy are common.

• Concurrent cardiac defects are not uncommon, especially a patent foramen ovale in tricuspid stenosis (due to increased right atrial pressure) and subaortic stenosis in cases of mitral stenosis.

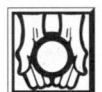

TREATMENT

• Hospitalization and diuresis for patients in overt CHF

• Surgical valve replacement or repair is the therapy of choice; this requires cardiopulmonary bypass or hypothermia; cost and availability are limiting factors.

• Balloon valvuloplasty is an alternative referral treatment to decrease the diastolic gradient between the atrium and ventricle.

• Use medical therapy for CHF; feed a low-sodium diet to patients with overt CHF.

• The diastolic pressure gradient increases exponentially at higher heart rates, and the ability to increase cardiac output is limited; exercise restriction is recommended for patients with exercise intolerance, exertional dyspnea, and CHF.

MEDICATIONS

DRUG(S)

CHF

• Digoxin—dogs, 0.003–0.005 mg/kg q12h; cats, 1/4 of a 0.125-mg tablet q48h

• Furosemide—dogs, 2–6 mg/kg IV, IM, SC, PO q8–24h; cats, 1–4 mg/kg IV, IM, SC, PO q8–24h

• Enalapril—dogs, 0.25–0.5 mg/kg PO q12–24h; cats, 0.25–0.5 mg/kg PO q12–48h; see below under Follow-Up for patient monitoring.

• Might consider use of B-blockers (propanolol: dogs, 0.2–1 mg/kg PO q8h; atenolol: dogs, 6.25–25 mg/dog q12h; cats, 6.25–12.5 mg/cat q12–24h; start low and titrate to effect) to blunt heart rate response and/or nitroglycerin paste (1/4″–1″ topically q8–12h) to reduce pulmonary venous pressures, but these have not been evaluated critically.

Atrial Tachyarrhythmias

• Digoxin as above

• β-Blocker (see above) or calcium channel blocker (diltiazem: dogs, 0.5–1.5 mg/kg PO q8h; Dilacor XR or Cardizem CD: cats, 10 mg/kg q24h) for heart rate control

CONTRAINDICATIONS/POSSIBLE INTERACTIONS

Use ACE inhibitors or other vasodilators judiciously in patients with AV valvular stenosis and CHF; cardiac output is limited and vasodilation may induce hypotension; monitor arterial blood pressure.

FOLLOW-UP

PATIENT MONITORING

• Digoxin level—check 7–10 days following institution of therapy; 8- to 12-hour trough should be 0.8–1.5 ng/mL.

• Renal function, electrolyte status (especially potassium), and arterial blood pressure when on diuretic and/or ACE inhibitor

POSSIBLE COMPLICATIONS

• CHF

• Atrial fibrillation

• Syncope

• Aortic thromboembolism—cats

EXPECTED COURSE AND PROGNOSIS

• Morbidity is high; except for mild cases, prognosis is generally poor.

• Surgical intervention or balloon valvuloplasty may alter course of disease, but data are limited.

MISCELLANEOUS

ASSOCIATED CONDITIONS

Concurrent congenital defects are common (e.g., subaortic stenosis in mitral stenosis, patent foramen ovale in tricuspid stenosis).

SEE ALSO

• Atrioventricular Valve Dysplasia

• Endocarditis, Infective

ABBREVIATIONS

• ACE = angiotensin converting enzyme

• AV = atrioventricular

• CHF = congestive heart failure

Suggested Reading

Sisson DD, Thomas WP, Bonagura JD. Congenital heart disease. In: Ettinger SJ, Feldman EC, eds. Textbook of veterinary internal medicine. 5th ed. Philadelphia: Saunders, 2000;737–787.

Authors Lora S. Hitchcock and John D. Bonagura

Consulting Editors Larry P. Tilley and Francis W. K. Smith, Jr.

AZOTEMIA AND UREMIA

 BASICS

DEFINITION
Azotemia is an excess of urea, creatinine, or other nonprotein nitrogenous substances in blood, plasma, or serum. Uremia is the polysystemic toxic syndrome that results from abnormal renal function in animals with azotemia. Uremia occurs simultaneously in animals with increased quantities of urine constituents in blood.

PATHOPHYSIOLOGY
• Azotemia can be caused by 1) high production of nonprotein nitrogenous substances, 2) low glomerular filtration rate, or 3) reabsorption of urine that has escaped from the urinary tract into the bloodstream. High production of nonprotein nitrogenous waste substances may result from high intake of protein (diet or gastrointestinal bleeding) or accelerated catabolism of endogenous proteins. Glomerular filtration rate may decline because of reduced renal perfusion (prerenal azotemia), renal insufficiency or failure due to primary renal disease (renal azotemia), or urinary obstruction (postrenal azotemia). Reabsorption of urine into the systemic circulation may result from leakage of urine from the excretory pathways (also termed postrenal azotemia). • Pathophysiology of uremia—incompletely understood; may be related to 1) metabolic and toxic systemic effects of waste products retained because of renal excretory failure, 2) deranged renal regulation of fluids, electrolytes, and acid–base balance, and 3) impaired renal production and degradation of hormones and other substances (e.g., erythropoietin and 1,25-dihydroxycholecalciferol)

SYSTEMS AFFECTED
• Gastrointestinal—anorexia, nausea, vomiting, diarrhea, uremic stomatitis, xerostomia, uremic breath, constipation • Neuromuscular—dullness, drowsiness, lethargy, fatigue, irritability, tremors, gait imbalance, flaccid muscle weakness, myoclonus, behavioral changes, dementia, isolated cranial nerve deficits, seizures, stupor, coma • Endocrine/Metabolic—renal secondary hyperparathyroidism, inadequate production of 1,25-dihydroxycholecalciferol and erythropoietin, hypergastrinemia, weight loss • Cardiovascular—arterial hypertension, left ventricular hypertrophy, heart murmur, cardiomegaly, cardiac rhythm disturbances • Hemic/Lymph/Immune—nonregenerative anemia (normocytic, normochromic) and immunodeficiency • Ophthalmic—scleral and conjunctival injection, retinopathy, acute-onset blindness • Respiratory—dyspnea • Skin/Exocrine—pallor, bruising, increased shedding, unkempt appearance, loss of normal sheen to coat

SIGNALMENT
Dogs and cats

SIGNS

General Comments
Azotemia may or may not be associated with historical or physical abnormalities. Unless patient has uremia, clinical findings are limited to the disease responsible for azotemia. Findings described here are those of uremia.

Historical Findings
• Weight loss • Declining appetite or anorexia • Reduced activity • Depression • Fatigue • Weakness • Vomiting • Diarrhea • Halitosis • Constipation • Poor haircoat or unkempt appearance

Physical Examination Findings
• Cachexia • Depression • Dehydration • Weakness • Pallor • Petechiae and ecchymoses • Dull and unkempt haircoat • Uremic breath • Uremic stomatitis • Scleral and conjunctival injection

CAUSES

Prerenal Azotemia
• Reduced renal perfusion due to low blood volume or low blood pressure • Accelerated production of nitrogenous waste products because of enhanced catabolism of tissues in association with infection, fever, trauma, corticosteroid excess, or burns • Increased gastrointestinal digestion and absorption of protein sources (diet or gastrointestinal hemorrhage)

Renal Azotemia
Acute or chronic renal failure (primary renal disease affecting glomeruli, renal tubules, renal interstitium, or renal vasculature) that impairs at least 75% of renal function

Postrenal Azotemia
Urinary obstruction; rupture of the excretory pathway

RISK FACTORS
• Medical conditions—renal disease, hypoadrenocorticism, low cardiac output, hypotension, fever, sepsis, polyuria, liver disease, pyometra, hypoalbuminemia, dehydration, acidosis, exposure to nephrotoxic chemicals, gastrointestinal hemorrhage, urolithiasis, urethral plugs in cats, urethral trauma and neoplasia • Advanced age may be a risk factor. • Drugs—potentially nephrotoxic drugs, nonsteroidal antiinflammatory drugs, diuretics, antihypertensive medications

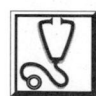 DIAGNOSIS

DIFFERENTIAL DIAGNOSIS
• Dehydration, poor peripheral perfusion, low cardiac output, history of recent fluid loss, high protein diet, or black, tarry stools—rule out prerenal azotemia. • Recent onset of altered urine output (high or low), clinical signs consistent with uremia, exposure to possible nephrotoxicants or ischemic renal injury, or kidney size normal or enlarged—rule out acute renal failure. • Progressive weight loss, polyuria, polydipsia, small kidneys, pallor, and signs of uremia that have developed over several weeks to months—rule out chronic renal failure. • Abrupt decline in urine output and onset of signs of uremia; occasionally dysuria, stranguria, and hematuria; large urinary bladder or fluid-filled abdomen—rule out postrenal azotemia.

LABORATORY FINDINGS

Drugs That May Alter Laboratory Results
N/A

Disorders That May Alter Laboratory Results
N/A

Valid if Run in Human Laboratory?
Yes

CBC/BIOCHEMISTRY/URINALYSIS

CBC
• Nonregenerative anemia—often present with chronic renal failure • Hemoconcentration—often present with prerenal azotemia; can also be seen with acute renal failure and postrenal azotemia

Biochemistry
• Serial determinations of serum urea nitrogen and creatinine concentrations may help differentiate the cause of azotemia. Appropriate therapy to restore renal perfusion typically yields a dramatic reduction in azotemia in patients with prerenal azotemia (typically within 24–48 hr). Correcting obstruction to urine flow or a rent in the excretory pathway typically gives a rapid reduction in the magnitude of azotemia in patients with postrenal azotemia. • Concurrent hyperkalemia may be consistent with postrenal azotemia, primary renal azotemia due to oliguric renal failure, or prerenal azotemia associated with hypoadrenocorticism.

Urinalysis
• A urine specific gravity value ≥ 1.030 in dogs and ≥ 1.035 in cats supports a diagnosis of prerenal azotemia. Administration of fluid therapy before urine collection may interfere with interpretation of low specific gravity values. • Azotemia patients that have not been treated with fluids and have urine specific gravity < 1.030 in dogs and < 1.035 in cats typically have primary renal azotemia. A notable exception to this rule is dogs and cats with glomerular disease. Glomerulopathy is sometimes characterized by glomerulotubular imbalance in which urine-concentrating ability may persist despite sufficient renal glomerular damage to cause primary renal azotemia; these patients are recognized by moderate to marked proteinuria in the absence of hematuria and pyuria. Urine

specific gravity does not help differentiate postrenal azotemia from prerenal or primary renal azotemia.

OTHER LABORATORY TESTS
Endogenous or exogenous creatinine clearance tests or other specific tests of glomerular filtration rate may be used to confirm that azotemia is caused by reduced glomerular filtration rate.

IMAGING
• Abdominal radiographs—used to determine kidney size (small kidneys consistent with chronic renal failure; mild-to-moderate enlargement of kidneys may be consistent with acute renal failure or urinary obstruction) and to rule out urinary obstruction (marked dilation of the urinary bladder or mineral densities within the excretory pathway) • Ultrasonography—may detect changes in echogenicity of the renal parenchyma and size and shape of kidneys that support a diagnosis of primary renal azotemia; useful to rule out postrenal azotemia characterized by distension of the excretory pathway and uroliths or masses within or impinging on the excretory pathway and intraabdominal fluid accumulation (with rupture of the excretory pathway) • Excretory urography or cystourethrography—may help establish the diagnosis of postrenal azotemia due to urinary obstruction or rupture of the excretory pathway

DIAGNOSTIC PROCEDURES
Renal biopsy can be used to confirm the diagnosis of primary renal failure, to differentiate acute from chronic renal failure, and to attempt to establish the underlying disease process responsible for primary renal failure.

TREATMENT
• Prerenal azotemia caused by impaired renal perfusion—direct at correcting the underlying cause of renal hypoperfusion; aggressiveness of treatment depends on the severity of the underlying condition and the probability that persistent renal hypo–perfusion will lead to primary renal injury or failure.
• Primary renal azotemia and associated uremia—1) specific therapy directed at halting or reversing the primary disease process affecting the kidneys, and 2) symptomatic, supportive, and palliative therapies that ameliorate clinical signs of uremia; minimize the clinical impact of deficits and excesses in fluid, electrolyte, acid–base balances; minimize the effects of inadequate renal biosynthesis of hormones and other substances, and maintain adequate nutrition.

• Postrenal azotemia—direct at eliminating urinary obstruction or repairing rents in the excretory pathway; supplemental fluid administration is often required to prevent dehydration that may develop during the solute diuresis that follows correction of postrenal azotemia.
• Fluid therapy—indicated for most azotemic patients; preferred fluid selections include 0.9% saline or lactated Ringer's solution. Estimate the quantity of fluid to be administered on the basis of severity of dehydration or volume depletion. If no clinical dehydration is evident, cautiously assume that the patient is less than 5% dehydrated and administer a corresponding volume of fluid. Generally provide the bulk of volume replacement over 2–6 h, except in patients with overt or suspected cardiac failure.
• Treat patients in shock appropriately.

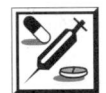

MEDICATIONS
DRUG(S) OF CHOICE
N/A

CONTRAINDICATIONS
Administration of nephrotoxic drugs

PRECAUTIONS
• Use caution when administering drugs requiring renal excretion. Consult appropriate references concerning dose-reduction schedules or adjustments of maintenance intervals.
• Use caution in administering fluids to patients that are oliguric or anuric. Monitor urine production rates and body weight during fluid therapy to minimize the likelihood of inducing overhydration.
• Use caution in administering drugs that may promote hypovolemia or hypotension (e.g., diuretics); carefully monitor the response to such drugs by assessing hydration status, peripheral perfusion, and blood pressure, with serial evaluation of renal function tests.
• Corticosteroids may worsen azotemia by increasing catabolism of endogenous proteins.

POSSIBLE INTERACTIONS
N/A

ALTERNATIVE DRUG(S)
N/A

FOLLOW-UP
PATIENT MONITORING
Serum urea nitrogen and creatinine concentrations 24 h after initiating fluid administration; also urine production, body weight, and hydration status

POSSIBLE COMPLICATIONS
• Failure to correct prerenal azotemia caused by renal hypoperfusion rapidly could result in ischemic primary renal failure. • Primary renal azotemia can progress to uremia. • Failure to restore normal urine flow in patients with postrenal azotemia can result in progressive renal damage or death due to hyperkalemia and uremia.

MISCELLANEOUS
ASSOCIATED CONDITIONS
An association may exist between hypokalemia and azotemia in cats. Preliminary findings suggest that hypokalemia may be associated with functional or structural renal changes leading to azotemia.

AGE-RELATED FACTORS
Primary renal failure may occur in animals of any age, but geriatric dogs and cats appear to be at substantially higher risk for both acute and chronic renal failure. However, do not assume that azotemia in geriatric dogs and cats indicates primary renal failure, because these patients are also at higher risk for prerenal and postrenal causes for azotemia.

ZOONOTIC POTENTIAL
Leptospirosis

PREGNANCY
• Data on azotemia and pregnancy in dogs and cats are very limited. Humans may tolerate minimal renal disease well during pregnancy; however, ability to sustain a viable pregnancy declines as renal function declines.
• Pregnant azotemic animals—pharmacologic agents excreted by nonrenal pathways are preferred

SYNONYMS
N/A

SEE ALSO
• Renal Failure, Acute • Renal Failure, Chronic • Urinary Tract Obstruction

Suggested Reading
Osborne CA, Polzin DJ. Azotemia: a review of what's old and what's new. Part I. Definition of terms and concepts. Compend Cont Educ 1983;5:497–508.
Osborne CA, Polzin DJ. Azotemia: a review of what's old and what's new. Part II. Localization. Compend Cont Educ 1983; 5:561–574.
Author David J. Polzin
Consulting Editors Larry G. Adams and Carl A. Osborne

BABESIOSIS

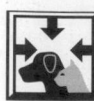 **BASICS**

OVERVIEW

• Babesiosis is the disease caused by the protozoal parasites of the genus *Babesia*. Merozoites or piroplasms are the stage that infects mammalian red blood cells.
• *B. canis*—A large (4–7 μm) piroplasm that infects dogs, *B. canis* is distributed worldwide, and there are three subspecies based on genetic, biologic, and geographic data. *B. canis vogeli* has been reported in the United States, Africa, Asia, and Australia. *B. canis rossi* is the most virulent and is present in Africa. *B. canis canis* has been reported in Europe.
• Recent studies have identified at least three genetically distinct small (2–5 μm) piroplasms that can infect dogs.
• *B. gibsoni* (Asia)—small piroplasm that infects dogs; worldwide distribution; emerging disease in the United States
• *B. gibsoni* (California)—small piroplasm that infects dogs; only reported in California
• *Theileria annae* (Spanish dog piroplasm)— small piroplasm that infects dogs; reported in Spain and other parts of Europe
• *B. felis*—small (2–5 μm) piroplasm that infects cats; reported in Africa
• *Cytauxzoon felis*—small piroplasm that infects cats; reported in the United States
• Infection may occur either by tick transmission, direct transmission via blood transfer/transfusion, or transplacental transmission.
• Incubation period averages about 2 weeks, but some cases are not diagnosed for months to years.
• Piroplasms infect and replicate in red blood cells, resulting in both direct and immune-mediated hemolytic anemia.
• Immune-mediated hemolytic anemia is likely to be more clinically important than parasite-induced RBC destruction, since the severity of signs is not dependent on the degree of parasitemia.

SYSTEMS AFFECTED

• Hemic/lymphatic/immune—anemia, thrombocytopenia (bleeding tendencies appear rare), fever, splenomegaly, lymphadenomegaly, vasculitis
• Hepatobiliary—increased liver enzymes
• Nervous—cerebral babesiosis, weakness, disorientation, collapse
• Renal/urologic—renal failure (*B. canis rossi*)

SIGNALMENT

• Any age or breed of dog can be infected.
• *B. canis* infections are more prevalent in greyhounds.
• *B. gibsoni* (Asia) infections are more prevalent in American pit bull terriers.
• Any age or breed of cat can be infected, but to date, only *C. felis* has been reported in the United States.

SIGNS

• Signs are similar in dogs and cats.
• Signs can be peracute, acute, or chronic.
• Some carrier animals have no detectable clinical signs.
• Dogs—lethargy, anorexia, pale mucous membranes, fever, splenomegaly, lymphadenomegaly, pigmenturia, icterus, weight loss, discolored stool
• Cats—lethargy, anorexia, pale mucous membranes, icterus

CAUSES & RISK FACTORS

• History of tick attachment
• Splenectomized animals develop more severe clinical disease.
• Immune suppression may cause clinical signs and increased parasitemia in chronically infected dogs.
• History of a recent dog-bite wound may be a risk for *B. gibsoni* (Asia) infection.

 DIAGNOSIS

DIFFERENTIAL DIAGNOSIS

• Any cause of immune-mediated hemolytic anemia or thrombocytopenia, including idiopathic immune-mediated hemolytic anemia or thrombocytopenia, ehrlichiosis, Rocky Mountain spotted fever, systemic lupus erythematosus, neoplasia, endocarditis, haemobartonellosis, and cytauxzoonosis
• A positive Coombs' test does not rule out babesiosis since many animals with babesiosis are also Coombs' positive.
• Non–immune-mediated hemolytic anemia, including microangiopathic anemia, caval syndrome, splenic torsion, DIC, Heinz body anemia, pyruvate kinase deficiency, phosphofructokinase deficiency
• Hepatic and posthepatic jaundice

CBC/BIOCHEMISTRY/URINALYSIS

• Anemia—mild to severe; usually regenerative (reticulocytosis) unless signs are very acute; can be severe in some cases (PCV < 10%), but anemia is not present in all cases
• Thrombocytopenia—usually moderate to severe; some animals have thrombocytopenia without anemia
• Leukocyte responses are variable, with both leukocytosis and leukopenia reported.
• Hyperbilirubinemia may be present depending on the rate of hemolysis.
• Hyperglobulinemia is common in chronic infections and may be the only biochemical abnormality in chronically infected animals.
• Mildly elevated liver enzymes from anemia/hypoxia
• Renal failure and metabolic acidosis have been reported with *B. canis rossi*.
• Bilirubinuria is common.
• Hemoglobinuria is detected less commonly in the United States than in Africa.

OTHER LABORATORY TESTS

• Microscopic examination of stained thin or thick blood smears—can provide a definitive diagnosis; sensitivity is dependent on microscopist experience and staining technique; we have had the most success using a quick modified Wright's stain; capillary blood may enhance sensitivity; microscopy may not accurately differentiate the species or subspecies
• IFA—tests for antibodies in serum that react with *Babesia* organisms; cross-reactive antibodies can prevent the differentiation of species and subspecies; some infected animals, particularly young dogs, may have no detectable antibodies

• PCR—tests for the presence of *Babesia* DNA in a biological sample (usually EDTA anticoagulated whole blood); can differentiate subspecies and species; more sensitive than microscopy

TREATMENT
• May require inpatient or outpatient care, depending on the severity of disease
• Hypovolemic animals should receive aggressive fluid therapy.
• Severely anemic animals may require blood transfusion.

MEDICATIONS
DRUG(S) OF CHOICE
• Imidocarb diproprionate (FDA approved; 6.6 mg/kg SC or IM every 1–2 weeks) and diminazine aceturate (not FDA approved; 3.5–7 mg/kg SC or IM every 1–2 weeks) decrease morbidity and mortality in affected animals. They may completely clear *B. canis* infections but not *B. gibsoni* (Asia).
• Metronidazole (25–50 mg/kg PO q24h for 7 days), clindamycin (12.5–25 mg/kg PO b.i.d. for 7–10 days), and doxycycline (10 mg/kg PO b.i.d. for 7–10 days) have been reported to decrease clinical signs but not to clear infections.
• Combination therapy of azithromycin (10 mg/kg PO q24h for 10 days) and atovaquone (13.3 mg/kg PO t.i.d for 10 days) was effective in clearing *Babesia* infections in humans and mice and is currently under investigation for the treatment of *B. gibsoni* (Asia) infections in dogs.
• Primaquine phosphate (1 mg/kg IM, single injection) is the treatment of choice for *B. felis.*

• Since the anemia and thrombocytopenia are often immune mediated, immunosuppressive agents, such as prednisone (2.2 mg/kg/day PO), may be indicated in some cases.
• The use of a polymerized bovine hemoglobin solution may improve oxygen-carrying capacity in severely anemic animals.
• Antibabesial drugs can cause cholinergic signs that can be minimized by administering atropine (0.02 mg/kg SC, 30 minutes prior to imidocarb or diminazine administration).

CONTRAINDICATIONS
High doses of anti-babesial drugs have resulted in liver and kidney failure.

FOLLOW-UP
• Recheck the CBC and biochemistry as needed to monitor for resolution of anemia, thrombocytopenia, icterus, and other signs.
• Most patients have a clinical response within 1–2 weeks of treatment.
• Microscopy and PCR may be better for post-treatment follow-up, as IFA titers may persist for years.
• Dogs infected with *B. gibsoni* (Asia) remain persistently infected and can act as carrier animals even after treatment.
• Dogs infected with *B. canis* may be cured after treatment.
• Long-term follow-up of *B. gibsoni* (California), *T. annea,* or *B. felis* after treatment has not been reported.
• When a dog housed in a multi-dog kennel is diagnosed with babesiosis, all dogs in that kennel should be screened since there is a high percentage of carrier animals in kennel situations.
• Coinfection with other vector-transmitted pathogens (e.g., *Erhlichia, Haemobartonella, Leishmania*) should be considered, especially in animals that fail to respond to treatment.

PREVENTION/AVOIDANCE
A vaccine for *B. canis canis* is available in Europe, but this vaccine does not confer protection against *B. canis vogeli, B. canis rossi,* or *B. gibsoni.* Tick control is important for disease prevention. All attached ticks should be removed within 24 hours of attachment.

MISCELLANEOUS
All potential blood donors should test negative for the disease (preferably by microscopy, IFA, and PCR) prior to use as a donor animal.

ZOONOTIC POTENTIAL
May be a concern for *B. gibsoni* (California)

PREGNANCY
Transplacental transmission

ABBREVIATIONS
• DIC = disseminated intravascular coagulation
• EDTA = ethylenediaminetetra-acetic acid
• FDA = Food and Drug Administration (U.S.)
• IFA = indirect fluorescent antibody
• PCR = polymerase chain reaction
• PCV = packed cell volume

Suggested Reading
MacIntire DK, Boudreaux MK, West GD, et al. *Babesia gibsoni* infection among dogs in the southeastern United States. J Am Vet Med Assoc 2002;220:325–329.
Taboada J. Babesiosis. In: Greene CE, ed. Infectious diseases of the dog and cat. 2nd ed. Philadelphia: Saunders, 1998:473–481.
Author Adam J. Birkenheuer
Consulting Editor Stephen C. Barr

BARTONELLOSIS

 BASICS

OVERVIEW
• Human syndrome—typified by regional lymphadenopathy after a cat scratch or bite distal to the involved lymph node
• Agents—small curved, argyrophilic, gram-negative rod *Bartonella henselae* (formerly *Rochalimaea henselae*) in majority of cases; *B. clarridgeiae* and *Afipia felis* also reported
• Worldwide occurrence
• Estimated >25,000 cases/year in U.S.; >2,000 cases require hospitalization; almost no fatalities

SIGNALMENT
• More males than females (1.2:1)
• Majority of human patients (80%) <21 years of age
• Seasonal; more cases reported between July and January

SIGNS

Human
• Erythematous papule at inoculation site (scratch, bite); then unilateral regional lymphadenopathy (painful, often suppurative) in 3–10 days (>90% of cases)
• Mild fever
• Chills—infrequent
• Malaise
• Anorexia
• Myalgia
• Nausea
• Atypical manifestations (in up to 25% of cases)—encephalopathy (1–7%); palpebral conjunctivitis (3–5%); meningitis; osteolytic lesions; granulomatous hepatitis; pneumonia

Cats
• No signs of illness
• Between 5 and 60% seropositive, depending on geographical area
• Lymphoid hyperplasia—sometimes

CAUSES & RISK FACTORS
• Contact with domestic kittens and cats (>90%), particularly young cats with fleas
• Scratched by cat—up to 83%
• Up to 95% of cats residing in households of affected humans are seropositive
• Other members of household likely exposed to *B. henselae*

 DIAGNOSIS

DIFFERENTIAL DIAGNOSIS
• Benign adenopathy in human children and young adults—most common cause
• History of contact with a cat
• Formation of a papule at the site of primary inoculation (scratch or bite)
• Compatible clinical picture—unilateral regional lymphadenitis
• Exclusion of other identifiable causes
• Characteristic histopathological findings
• Serologic tests—indirect fluorescent antibody for *B. henselae*
• Positive skin test no longer used
• Other causes of lymphadenopathy—lymphogranuloma venereum; syphilis; typical or atypical tuberculosis; other forms of bacterial adenitis; sporotrichosis; tularemia; brucellosis; histoplasmosis; sarcoidosis; toxoplasmosis; infectious mononucleosis; and benign or malignant tumors

CBC/BIOCHEMISTRY/URINALYSIS
Noncontributory

OTHER LABORATORY TESTS
• Indirect fluorescent antibody test
• Enzyme immunoassay—IgG antibodies to *B. henselae* (Specialty Laboratories, Santa Monica, CA)
• Culture—on enriched (blood-containing) media in presence of 5% carbon dioxide at 35–37°C; fastidious and slow growing; requires 14–30 days
• PCR amplification of bacterial DNA from lesions

DIAGNOSTIC PROCEDURES
N/A

IMAGING
N/A

PATHOLOGIC FINDINGS
• Histopathology of lymph nodes—nonspecific inflammatory reaction, including granuloma, microabscess, and necrosis
• Warthin-Starry silver stain—bacilli

 TREATMENT

• Supportive treatment—bed rest; heat on swollen lymph nodes; needle aspiration of suppurative nodes
• Thoroughly cleanse all cat scratches or bites.
• Prevent cats from contacting open wounds.

 MEDICATIONS

DRUG(S)
• Specific antimicrobials—not efficacious
• Most cases spontaneously resolve in a few weeks or months.
• Severe cases—antibiotic therapy (gentamicin, doxycycline, erythromycin, azithromycin) based on the antimicrobial susceptibility of *B. henselae* may be appropriate.

CONTRAINDICATIONS/POSSIBLE INTERACTIONS
N/A

 FOLLOW-UP

PREVENTION/AVOIDANCE
Immunocompromised persons should avoid young cats.

POSSIBLE COMPLICATIONS
Uncommon

 MISCELLANEOUS

• One episode appears to confer lifelong immunity.
• Bacillary angiomatosis—vascular proliferative disease of the skin; may also be caused by *B. henselae;* responds to antimicrobial drugs (bartonellosis rarely does)
• Natural host of *B. henselae* is unknown; a related species, *B. quintana,* is spread by lice and causes trench fever in humans.

ZOONOTIC POTENTIAL
Uncertain for *Bartonella* infections in dogs and cats

ABBREVIATION
• PCR = polymerase chain reaction

Suggested Reading
Windsor JJ. Cat-scratch disease: epidemiology, aetiology and treatment. Br J Biomed Sci 2001;58:101–110.
Author J. Paul Woods
Consulting Editor Stephen C. Barr

BASICS

OVERVIEW
• Tumor that originates from the basal epithelium of the skin
• Includes benign (e.g., basal cell epithelioma and basaloid tumor) and malignant (e.g., basal cell carcinoma) tumors

SIGNALMENT
• Common—makes up 3%–12% and 15%–18% of all skin tumors in dogs and cats, respectively
• Age—dogs: 6–9 years; cats: 5–18 years (mean, 10.8 years)
• Cocker spaniels, poodles, and Siamese cats—more commonly affected than other breeds

SIGNS
• Solitary, well-circumscribed, formed, hairless, intradermal raised mass, typically located on the head, neck, or shoulders
• Variable in size—0.2–10 cm in diameter
• Masses (cats)—often heavily pigmented, cystic, and occasionally ulcerated

CAUSES & RISK FACTORS
Unknown

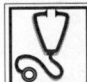 DIAGNOSIS

DIFFERENTIAL DIAGNOSIS
• Other skin tumors—mast cell tumor; melanoma; hemangioma; hemangiosarcoma
• Intradermal cysts

CBC/BIOCHEMISTRY/URINALYSIS
Normal

OTHER LABORATORY TESTS
N/A

IMAGING
N/A

DIAGNOSTIC PROCEDURES
Histopathologic examination—definitive diagnosis

PATHOLOGIC FINDINGS
• Histologic cellular patterns—vary from solid to cystic to ribbon appearance
• Tumor cells—may contain melanin pigmentation; may have a fine eosinophilic stroma

 TREATMENT

Surgical excision—treatment of choice; generally curative

 MEDICATIONS

DRUG(S)
N/A

CONTRAINDICATIONS/POSSIBLE INTERACTIONS
N/A

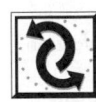 FOLLOW-UP

• Tumors—< 10% malignant
• Complete surgical excision—usually curative

 MISCELLANEOUS

Suggested Reading
Carpenter JL, Andrews LK, Holzworth J. Tumors and Tumor-like lesions.
Holzworth J, ed. Diseases of the cat: medicine and surgery. Philadelphia: Saunders, 1987:406–596.
Thomas RC, Fox LE. Tumors of the skin and subcutis. In: Morrison WB. ed. Cancer in dogs and cats: medical and surgical management. Baltimore: Williams & Wilkins, 1998:489–510.
Author Robyn Elmslie
Consulting Editor Wallace B. Morrison

BAYLISASCARIASIS

BASICS

OVERVIEW
• Two forms of baylisascariasis have been reported in dogs: an intestinal infestation occurring in adults and a larval form resulting in visceral disease caused by larval migration in puppies.
• The disease is caused by the raccoon roundworm *Baylisascaris procyonis*. Infection of raccoons occurs by ingestion of eggs or by ingestion of larvae in tissues of mammalian paratenic host.
• Dogs probably are infected by the ingestion of paratenic hosts and develop patent infections with adult worms in their small intestine. Puppies, probably infected by the ingestion of eggs, develop visceral disease like most other mammals.
• Dogs with intestinal infestation are typically without signs. Puppies with larval baylisascariasis show signs of neurologic disease.

SIGNALMENT
• Dogs
• Intestinal form—reported from adult animals
• Larval form—reported in two puppies; suspected that only severe cases have been reported; infection with only a few larvae probably does not cause severe disease in most puppies

SIGNS
• Intestinal form—none
• Larval form—weakness, ataxia, dysphagia, circling, recumbency

CAUSES & RISK FACTORS
Sharing space with areas frequented by raccoons

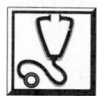

DIAGNOSIS

DIFFERENTIAL DIAGNOSIS
• Intestinal form—eggs in feces can be distinguished from those of either *Toxocara* or *Toxascaris*

• Larval form—rabies, canine distemper, congenital neurologic defect

CBC/BIOCHEMISTRY/URINALYSIS
Usually normal

OTHER LABORATORY TESTS
N/A

IMAGING
N/A

DIAGNOSTIC PROCEDURES
• Intestinal form—direct fecal smear or fecal flotation
• Larval form—ophthalmoscopic examination may show migratory tracks in retina

TREATMENT

• Intestinal form—may want to treat as inpatient to prevent environmental contamination with eggs and to insure proper disposal (as biohazard) or destruction (incineration) of fecal material and worms after treatment
• Larval form—no treatment to date

MEDICATIONS

DRUG(S)

Intestinal Form
• Pyrantel pamoate (5 mg/kg) (Nemex)
• Febantel (25–35 mg/kg), pyrantel pamoate (5–7 mg/kg), praziquantel (5–7 mg/kg) (Drontal Plus)
• Ivermectin (0.005 mg/kg), pyrantel pamoate (5 mg/kg) (Heartgard Plus)
• Milbemycin (0.5 mg/kg) (Interceptor)

Larval Form
Corticosteroids and long-term albendazole (25–50 mg/kg/day for 10 days) may prove beneficial.

CONTRAINDICATIONS/POSSIBLE INTERACTIONS
N/A

FOLLOW-UP

• Intestinal form—check feces two weeks after deworming and again one month later
• Larval form—disease has proven fatal

MISCELLANEOUS

ZOONOTIC POTENTIAL
• Intestinal form—eggs are not infectious when passed but can develop in the environment in several days; ingestion of eggs containing infective larvae by humans can cause severe disease, i.e., larval baylisascariasis
• Larval form—infected puppies pose no zoonotic threat; puppy in one case represented the typical presentation of larval baylisascariasis wherein animals are held in areas that have previously housed a raccoon
• Alert owner of potential risk to people who may frequent similar habitats as raccoons

Suggested Reading
Kazacos KR. *Baylisascaris procyonis* and related species. In: Samuel WM, Pybus MJ, Kocan AA, eds. Parasitic diseases of wild mammals. 2nd ed. Ames: Iowa State University Press, 2001:301–341.
Rudmann DG, Kazacos KR, Storandt ST, et al. *Baylisascaris procyonis* larva migrans in a puppy: a case report and update for the veterinarian. J Am Anim Hosp Assoc 1996;32:73–76.
Author Dwight D. Bowman
Consulting Editor Stephen Barr

BENIGN PROSTATIC HYPERPLASIA

BASICS

OVERVIEW
- Age-related pathologic change in the prostate gland making it nonpainfully large
- Occurs in two phases, glandular and complex
- Glandular phase characterized by high number of large prostatic cells and a symmetrically large prostate gland
- Complex phase characterized by glandular hyperplasia, glandular atrophy, small cyst formation, chronic inflammation, and squamous metaplasia of epithelium

SIGNALMENT
- Observed initially in intact male dogs 1–2 years old
- Prevalence increases linearly; 60% of male dogs are affected by 6 years of age and 95% of male dogs are affected by 9 years of age

SIGNS

Historical Findings
- None in most dogs
- Bloody urethral discharge
- Hematuria
- Blood in ejaculate
- Straining to defecate
- Ribbon-like stools
- Dysuria

Physical Examination Findings
- Symmetric, nonpainfully large prostate gland
- Prostatic pain in dogs with complication of bacterial infection or prostatic carcinoma

CAUSES & RISK FACTORS
- Testosterone and 5-α-dihydrotestosterone
- Estrogens
- Prostatic stroma
- Aging
- Risk eliminated by castration

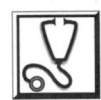

DIAGNOSIS

DIFFERENTIAL DIAGNOSIS
- Acute bacterial prostatitis—typically associated with fever, depression, pain on rectal palpation, neutrophilia, pyuria, and bacteriuria; may occur concurrently with benign prostatic hyperplasia
- Chronic bacterial prostatitis—typically associated with recurrent lower urinary tract infections; may occur concurrently with benign prostatic hyperplasia
- Prostatic adenocarcinoma—typically associated with poor appetite, weight loss, hind limb weakness, dysuria, hematuria, and dyschezia; may see carcinoma cells in urine sediment
- Prostatic and paraprostatic cysts—can cause palpable abdominal cystic mass filled with yellow to orange fluid

CBC/BIOCHEMISTRY/URINALYSIS
- CBC and biochemistry—normal
- Urinalysis—may be normal or reveal hematuria; pyuria and bacteriuria are absent unless dog has concurrent bacterial infection

OTHER LABORATORY TESTS
- Prostatic fluid obtained by ejaculation or prostatic massage is clear or hemorrhagic; RBC count high; WBC count normal; culture reveals <100,000 bacteria/mL unless the dog has concurrent bacterial infection
- Serum concentration of prostatic esterase is high in some dogs.

IMAGING

Radiography
- Abdominal radiographs reveal prostatomegaly.
- Retrograde urethrocystography may be normal or reveal narrowing of prostatic urethra or reflux of contrast media into the prostate gland.

Ultrasonography
Reveals large prostate gland with uniform prostatic parenchymal echogenicity; small, fluid-filled cysts in some dogs

DIAGNOSTIC PROCEDURES
N/A

TREATMENT
- Frequently not required
- Castration—most effective and prevents recurrence; if benign prostatic hyperplasia is complicated by acute bacterial prostatitis, delay surgery until the infection is resolved.

MEDICATIONS

DRUG(S)
If castration is not acceptable, the following drugs may temporarily shrink the prostate gland:
- Finasteride (0.1–0.5 mg/kg/day for up to 4 months)
- Megestrol acetate (0.11 mg/kg PO daily for 3 weeks)
- Medroxyprogesterone (3 mg/kg SC)

CONTRAINDICATIONS/POSSIBLE INTERACTIONS
- Avoid estrogens because of possible hematologic toxicity and development of squamous metaplasia of the prostate.
- Long-term administration of megestrol acetate or medroxyprogesterone may result in development of diabetes mellitus.

FOLLOW-UP
- Castration will result in rapid involution of the enlarged prostate.
- BPH will recur after withdrawal of finasteride; time until clinical signs recur is variable.

MISCELLANEOUS

ASSOCIATED CONDITIONS
- Bacterial prostatitis and prostatic carcinoma
- Prostatomegaly in a castrated dog strongly suggests prostatic carcinoma.

SEE ALSO
- Prostatic Cysts
- Prostatitis and Prostatic Abscess
- Prostatomegaly

Suggested Reading
Barsanti JA, Finco DR. Prostatic diseases. In: Ettinger SJ, Feldman EC, eds. Textbook of veterinary internal medicine. Philadelphia: Saunders, 1995:1662–1685.
Authors Jeffrey S. Klausner and Margaret V. Root-Kustritz
Consulting Editors Larry G. Adams and Carl A. Osborne

BILE DUCT CARCINOMA

BASICS

DEFINITION
Malignancy of the biliary tissues

PATHOPHYSIOLOGY
Develops from the epithelial cells lining the biliary ducts

SYSTEMS AFFECTED
• Intrahepatic bile duct origin more frequently reported than extrahepatic bile duct or gall bladder
• Common metastatic sites include the lungs, hepatic lymph nodes, and peritoneum.
• Other metastatic sites include other lymph nodes, diaphragm, intestine, pancreas, spleen, kidney, urinary bladder, and bone.

GENETICS
None

INCIDENCE/PREVALENCE
• Most common hepatic neoplasia in cats
• Second most common hepatic neoplasia in dogs

GEOGRAPHIC DISTRIBUTION
None

SIGNALMENT

Species
Dogs and cats

Breed Predilections
None

Mean Age and Range
> 10 years of age

Predominant Sex
Female predisposition may exist

SIGNS

Historical Findings
• Anorexia
• Lethargy
• Polydipsia and polyuria
• Vomiting
• In advanced disease, icterus and abdominal distention

Physical Examination Findings
• Hepatomegaly
• Ascites
• Abdominal distention
• Icterus
• Palpable abdominal mass

CAUSES
Possible association with liver fluke and other parasitic infestations

RISK FACTORS
Environmental exposure to carcinogens implicated

DIAGNOSIS

DIFFERENTIAL DIAGNOSIS
• Gross pathology—hepatocellular adenoma, hepatocellular adenocarcinoma, cholangio-cellular adenoma, nodular hyperplasia, cirrhosis, chronic active hepatitis, hepatic myelolipoma, hepatobiliary cystadenoma
• Histopathology—easily distinguished from hepatocellular adenocarcinoma

CBC/BIOCHEMISTRY/URINALYSIS
• High serum enzyme (e.g., ALP, ALT, and AST) activity is not specific for neoplastic disease.
• High ALP is less common in cats because of the enzyme's short half-life.
• Leukocytosis and bilirubinemia are inconsistent findings.

OTHER LABORATORY TESTS
• α-Fetoprotein concentration may differentiate neoplastic from non-neoplastic lesions in dogs.
• Coagulation profile should be performed before biopsy or any surgical procedure.
• FeLV has no known association in cats.

IMAGING
• Abdominal radiography may localize a mass to the liver or may show loss of detail in patients with ascites.
• Thoracic radiography may identify pulmonary metastasis.
• Use abdominal ultrasonography to assess location of lesion, echogenicity of remaining liver, and presence of effusion, and to guide biopsy.

DIAGNOSTIC PROCEDURES
• Abdominocentesis and cytologic evaluation if ascites present
• Biopsy sample obtained by percutaneous biopsy, laparoscopy, or laparotomy for definitive diagnosis

PATHOLOGIC FINDINGS
• Massive (most common), nodular, or diffuse
• Benign lesions—usually cystic and multinodular
• Malignant lesions often involve multiple lobes.
• Histologic classification is not prognostic.

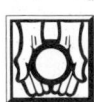 TREATMENT
Surgical excision is treatment of choice.

NURSING CARE
Provide supportive care and appropriate antibiotics as needed.

CLIENT EDUCATION
Guarded to poor prognosis because of high metastatic rate

SURGICAL CONSIDERATIONS
Up to 80% of the liver can be resected if the remaining liver tissue is functional.

 MEDICATIONS

DRUG(S)
No reported effective chemotherapy

PRECAUTIONS
• Medications requiring metabolism by the liver should be used with caution.

• Hepatotoxicity caused by chemotherapeutics appears to be of little or no importance in small animals.

 FOLLOW-UP

PATIENT MONITORING
• Liver enzyme activity and physical examination every 2 months.
• Abdominal ultrasonography and thoracic radiography every 2 months

PREVENTION/AVOIDANCE
None

POSSIBLE COMPLICATIONS
• Hemorrhage—transfusion rarely necessary

EXPECTED COURSE AND PROGNOSIS
• Aggressive; high rate of metastasis (67%–88%)
• Complete surgical resection—unlikely, owing to multifocal or diffuse involvement of the liver

 MISCELLANEOUS

ASSOCIATED CONDITIONS
Unlike in humans, no association with biliary calculi reported

AGE-RELATED FACTORS
None

PREGNANCY
Chemotherapy drugs may be carcinogenic and mutagenic

SYNONYMS
• Biliary carcinoma
• Cholangiocellular carcinoma
• Cholangiocarcinoma

SEE ALSO
• Hepatocellular Carcinoma

ABBREVIATIONS
• ALP = alkaline phosphatase
• ALT = alanine aminotransaminase
• AST = aspartate aminotransaminase
• FeLV = feline leukemia virus

Suggested Reading
Morrison WB. Primary cancers and cancer-like lesions of the liver, biliary epithelium, and exocrine pancreas. In: Morrison WB, ed. Cancer in dogs and cats: medical and surgical management. Baltimore: Williams & Wilkins, 1998:559–568.
Thamm, DH. Hepatobiliary tumors. In: Withrow SJ, MacEwen EG, eds. Small animal clinical oncology. Philadelphia: Saunders, 2001:327–334.
Author Sue Downing
Consulting Editor Wallace B. Morrison

BILE DUCT OBSTRUCTION

BASICS

DEFINITION
Cholestasis caused by obstruction of the biliary tree at the level of the common bile duct (EHBDO) or at the level of the hepatic ducts (may involve one, several, or all, depending on the disorder in the porta hepatis)

PATHOPHYSIOLOGY
• Serious hepatobiliary injury—may occur within weeks; derived from inflammatory mediators, noxious bile acids and bile constituents, mechanical effect of duct distention; oxidative damage considered a major pathomechanism
• Bile—may become colorless (white bile) owing to reduced secretion of bilirubin and increased production of mucin if cystic duct occluded
• Bacterial infection of biliary structures—increased risk due to impairment of the normal biliary-enteric bacterial circulation and normal clearance mechanisms

SYSTEMS AFFECTED
Hepatobiliary

SIGNALMENT

Species
Dogs and cats

Breed Predilection
Animals predisposed to pancreatitis—hyperlipidemic breeds (e.g., miniature schnauzers, Shetland sheepdogs)

Mean Age and Range
Middle-aged to old animals

Predominant Sex
None

SIGNS

Historical Findings
• Depend on underlying disorder
• Progressive lethargy • Intermittent illness
• Jaundice • Pale (acholic) stools
• Polyphagia—if complete obstruction and nutrient malassimilation • Bleeding tendencies within 10 days

Physical Examination Findings
• Depend on underlying disorder • Weight loss • Severe jaundice • Hepatomegaly
• Cranial mass effect—extrahepatic biliary structures (small dogs and cats) • Acholic feces—unless melena (pigment source)
• Bleeding tendencies • Orange urine

CAUSES
• Associated with diverse disorders
• Cholelithiasis • Choledochitis • Neoplasia
• Malformation of ducts (choledochal cysts, polycystic hepatobiliary disease [cats])
• Parasitic infestation (flukes; cats) • Extrinsic compression (lymph nodes, pancreatitis, entrapment in diaphragmatic hernia)
• Duct fibrosis (trauma, peritonitis,

pancreatitis; some cats with cholangitis/cholangiohepatitis) • Duct stricture (blunt trauma, iatrogenic from surgical handling or procedures)

RISK FACTORS
See Causes

DIAGNOSIS

DIFFERENTIAL DIAGNOSIS
• Mass lesions—primary or metastatic hepatic tumors; tumors in adjacent viscera • Diffuse infiltrative liver disease—inflammatory, neoplastic, amyloid, hepatic lipidosis (cats)
• Infectious hepatitis—bacterial, viral, flukes
• Decompensated chronic "active" hepatitis
• Copper storage hepatopathy—acute crisis
• End-stage cirrhosis • Fulminant hepatic failure • Biliary cysts—cystadenoma, duct dysplasia, choledochal cyst, hepatobiliary polycystic disease (cats) • Pancreatitis
• Hepatic lipidosis—cats • Cholangitis/cholangiohepatitis—cats (especially sclerosing form)

CBC/BIOCHEMISTRY/URINALYSIS

CBC
• Anemia—mild nonregenerative (anemia of chronic disease) or regenerative (significant gastrointestinal bleeding due to high propensity for enteric ulcerations and coagulopathy)
• Microcytosis—uncommon • Leukogram—may show a neutrophilic leukocytosis
• Plasma—markedly jaundiced

Biochemistry
• Liver enzymes—variable; marked increases in ALP and GGT typical; high transaminases
• Serum total bilirubin—moderately to markedly high; often lower than observed with hemolysis or hepatic lipidosis
• Albumin—usually in the normal range except when EHBDO > 6 weeks' duration (established biliary cirrhosis); values decline with chronicity owing to synthetic failure
• Globulins—usually normal • Glucose—usually normal unless biliary cirrhosis (may note hypoglycemia) or sepsis (acquired biliary tree infection) • Hypercholesterolemia—common

Urinalysis
• Bilirubinuria and bilirubin crystals
• Absence of urobilinogen—unless enteric bleeding; unreliable test

OTHER LABORATORY TESTS
• Serum bile acids—always markedly increased; do not add diagnostic information
• Coagulation abnormalities—develop within 10 days of EHBDO due to vitamin K deficiency (PIVKA and PT clotting times most sensitive); may develop DIC
• Fecal examination—acholic stools suggest EHBDO; masked by small-volume melena; trematode eggs suggest fluke infestation

IMAGING
• Abdominal radiography—hepatomegaly; may suggest mass lesion in area of gallbladder; may demonstrate signs of pancreatitis (e.g., duodenal ileus, mass lesion in right cranial abdominal quadrant, ill-defined right kidney silhouette, cranial displacement of the transverse colon, saponification of peripancreatic fat); rarely, mineralized cholelith(s) • Cholecystography—rarely provides additional information because contrast competes with bilirubin for entry into bile • Abdominal ultrasonography—evidence of obstruction within 72 hours (distended, tortuous extrahepatic bile duct, distended intrahepatic bile ducts); may note evidence of underlying or primary disease (e.g., pancreatitis, cystic lesions, mass lesions, choleliths) Caution: Feline extrahepatic ducts are serpiginous compared with those of the dog; always interrogate liver for evidence of distended intrahepatic bile ducts, suggesting EHBDO. • Biliary scintigraphy—may assist in diagnosis when biliary tree leakage suspected but elusive

DIAGNOSTIC PROCEDURES
• Hepatic aspiration cytology—indicated when imaging reveals mass lesions to rule out neoplasia • Needle biopsy—strongly contraindicated; may lead to iatrogenic bile peritonitis
• Laparotomy—best approach; allows tissue biopsy; biliary decompression: mass excision, cholelith or inspissated bile removal; creation of biliary-enteric anastomosis

PATHOLOGIC FINDINGS
• Gross—distended and tortuous bile duct; distended gall bladder: cause usually obvious; obstruction > 2 weeks old: large, dark green or mahogany-colored liver; chronic complete obstruction of cystic duct produces white or clear gallbladder bile • Microscopic—early: biliary epithelial hyperplasia and bile ductule proliferation; chronic distention of the biliary structures: devitalized biliary epithelium; necrotic debris and suppurative inflammation in bile ducts; mixed periportal inflammation and edema; and multifocal parenchymal necrosis

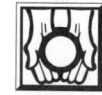

TREATMENT

APPROPRIATE HEALTH CARE
Inpatient—surgical intervention for suspected obstruction

NURSING CARE
• Fluid therapy—depends on underlying conditions (see Pancreatitis); rehydrate and provide maintenance fluids before general anesthesia and surgical intervention; supplement polyionic fluids with potassium chloride and phosphate, depending on electrolyte status • Water-soluble vitamins—

in intravenous fluids; B complex (2 mL/L polyionic fluids)

ACTIVITY
Depends on patient's condition and bleeding tendencies

DIET
• Maintain nitrogen balance: avoid protein-restricted diets. • Restrict fat—fat malassimilation caused by lack of enteric bile acids • Supplement fat-soluble vitamins parenterally (vitamins E and K most urgent; others [vitamins D and A] can lead to toxicity).

CLIENT EDUCATION
• Inform client that surgical biliary decompression is essential; obstruction will progress to biliary cirrhosis within 6 weeks; exception is pancreatitis causing EHBDO that may self-resolve within 2–3 weeks. • Warn client that surgical success is contingent on underlying cause and results of liver biopsy and specimen cultures.

SURGICAL CONSIDERATIONS
• Surgical exploration—imperative for treating and determining underlying cause • Excise masses; remove choleliths and inspissated bile. • Resect gallbladder—if necrotizing cholecystitis • Biliary-enteric anastomosis—for uncorrectable occlusion, fibrosing pancreatitis, or neoplasia; anastomotic stoma at least 2.5 cm wide • Hypotension and bradycardia (vasovagal reflex)—may occur with biliary tree manipulation; ensure intravenous catheter access and volume expansion; use colloids if necessary; be prepared for hemorrhage; ensure availability of emergency drugs (anticholinergics) to avert vasovagal reflex • Surgical biopsies/samples—submit tissue and bile samples for aerobic and anaerobic bacterial cultures; submit tissue for histology; make cytology preps from tissue imprints and bile smears; cytologically inspect for bacterial infection and fluke eggs • Bacterial organisms—observed only on Wright-Giemsa–type stained slides; Gram stain used to characterize organisms and guide antimicrobial selection • Sclerosing cholangitis (cats)—may clinically emulate EHBDO since disease may involve extrahepatic biliary structures; will not respond to biliary tree decompression; liver biopsy essential for diagnosis

 MEDICATIONS

DRUG(S) OF CHOICE
Vitamin K₁
Provide 12–36 hr before surgery (0.5–1.5 mg/kg IM or SC). Administer 3 doses at 12 hour intervals. **Caution:** IV may cause anaphylaxis.

Antibiotics
Before surgery—broad-spectrum antimicrobials must be administered for potential biliary infections as surgical manipulations may open biliary drainage, damage microcirculation, and facilitate bacteremia; initially select antibiotics empirically for enteric gram-negative opportunists and anaerobic flora

Antioxidants
• Vitamin E (α-tocopherol acetate)—10–30 IU/kg; larger-than-normal dose needed in chronic EHBDO when given PO because of fat malabsorption (lack of enteric bile acids) • *S*-Adenosylmethionine (SAMe)—thiol donor; 20 mg/kg enteric-coated tablet PO q24h 2 hours before feeding; other advantageous benefits

Ursodeoxycholic Acid
10–15 mg/kg PO per day—for postsurgical choleresis; adequate hydration essential for choleretic effect; inappropriate before biliary decompression; will not improve fat assimilation

Gastrointestinal Protectants
Agents reducing gastric acidity—famotidine (H₂-blocker) or omeprazol (pump inhibitor) combined with sucralfate for local cytoprotection if PO medications tolerated; stagger sucralfate administration from other oral medications to avoid drug interactions

CONTRAINDICATIONS
Ursodeoxycholic acid—provide biliary decompression before treatment

PRECAUTIONS
See "Hypotension and bradycardia (vasovagal reflex)" under Surgical Considerations.

ALTERNATIVE DRUG(S) N/A

 FOLLOW-UP

PATIENT MONITORING
• Depends on underlying condition—special monitoring based on underlying disease causing EHBDO; see information regarding appropriate conditions • Total bilirubin values—assess biliary decompression efficacy; decline to near normal within 10 days if successful • Liver enzyme activities—decline more slowly than total bilirubin values • CBC—repeat every few days initially; characterizes systemic response • Bile peritonitis—evaluate abdominal girth and abdominal fluid accumulation (e.g., by palpation, ultrasonography [preferred], appropriate abdominocentesis) • Determine necessity for pancreatic enzyme supplementation based on site of biliary-enteric anastomosis; patients with cholecystojejunostomies may benefit from exogenous enzyme supplementation; cannot rely on trypsin-like immunoreactive substance

to estimate pancreatic exocrine adequacy; evaluate body weight and condition, and feces; steatorrhea suggests fat malassimilation (suspend feces in a small amount of water, examine microscopically for lipid globules; relevant only if fed a normal, fat-containing diet); if steatorrheic, reduce dietary fat and supplement pancreatic enzymes

PREVENTION/AVOIDANCE N/A

POSSIBLE COMPLICATIONS
• Bile peritonitis • Restenosis of bile duct—if not bypassed • Stenosis of biliary-enteric anastomosis • Severe enteric hemorrhage with EHBDO—hypertensive portal vasculopathy and coagulopathy due to vitamin K deficiency • Hemorrhage during surgery • Vasovagal reflex—biliary tree manipulations

EXPECTED COURSE AND PROGNOSIS
• Depend on underlying disease • Prognosis good if fibrosing pancreatitis and pancreatic inflammation resolve; bile duct patency may return and biliary-enteric anastomosis spontaneously close • Be aware that biliary tree will appear distended on subsequent ultrasonographic evaluations • Permanent peribiliary fibrosis from EHBDO • Cats with sclerosing cholangitis can appear to have EHBDO; do not respond as appropriate for biliary decompression; liver biopsy essential for diagnosis

CONSIDERATIONS/PRECAUTIONS
• Anticipate bleeding tendencies and vasovagal reflex during surgical procedures • Always submit samples for histology and for aerobic and anaerobic culture.

 MISCELLANEOUS

ASSOCIATED CONDITIONS
• See Causes and Risk Factors • Sclerosing cholangitis (cats) confused with EHBDO

SEE ALSO
• Cholangitis/Cholangiohepatitis Syndrome • See Causes

ABBREVIATIONS
• DIC = disseminated intravascular coagulation • EHBDO = extrahepatic bile duct obstruction • PIVKA = proteins invoked by vitamin K absence • PT = prothrombin time

Suggested Reading
Center SA. Diseases of the gallbladder and biliary tree. In: Guilford WG, Center SA, Strombeck DR, et al., eds. Strombeck's small animal gastroenterology. 3rd ed. Philadelphia: Saunders, 1996:860–888.
Author Sharon A. Center
Consulting Editor Sharon A. Center

BILE PERITONITIS

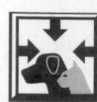

BASICS

OVERVIEW
Chemical peritonitis associated with rupture of the biliary tree and expulsion of free bile; focal or diffuse peritoneal inflammation, depending on chronicity and causal factors

SIGNALMENT
• More common in dogs than in cats • No age, breed, or sex predilection

SIGNS

Historical Findings
• Acute presentation if septic peritonitis • May have chronic illness if nonseptic • Abdominal discomfort • Lethargy • Anorexia • Weight loss • Vomiting • Diarrhea • Abdominal distention • Variable jaundice • Collapse, if septic

Physical Examination Findings
• Lethargy • Variable cranial abdominal pain • Jaundice • Abdominal effusion • Fever • Endotoxic shock, if septic

CAUSES & RISK FACTORS
• Trauma to biliary structures—automobile injuries, surgical manipulations, animal bites, gunshot wounds; poorly vascularized gallbladder fundus most common site of rupture; common bile duct is most common site of ductal rupture • Cholecystitis/choledochitis—sepsis more commonly associated with necrotizing cholecystitis • Gallbladder mucocele—leads to necrotizing cholecystitis • Biliary tree obstruction—neoplasia, cholelithiasis, pancreatitis • Focal, small-volume, idiopathic biliary peritonitis—associated with cholecystitis; may reflect leakage of bile without biliary tree rupture and with omental entrapment and localization of fluid • Chemical peritonitis due to bile—augments development of septic peritonitis

DIFFERENTIAL DIAGNOSIS
• Conditions causing EHBDO (e.g., neoplasia, choleliths, pancreatitis) • Conditions causing abdominal effusion and jaundice • Conditions causing inflammation/devitalization of biliary structures (e.g., cholecystitis/choledochitis, neoplasia, EHBDO) • Conditions impairing arterial blood supply to the gallbladder (e.g., blunt abdominal trauma, surgical manipulations, fight-related injuries) • Conditions causing sepsis and endotoxemia

CBC/BIOCHEMISTRY/URINALYSIS
CBC: Inflammatory leukogram—left shift and toxic neutrophils if necrotizing cholecystitis or sepsis; nonregenerative anemia if chronic disease

Biochemistry: • High liver enzymes, especially ALP; hyperbilirubinemia; hypoalbuminemia; prerenal azotemia • Electrolyte, fluid, and acid-base disturbances; hyponatremia most common

Urinalysis: No specific features

OTHER LABORATORY TESTS
Coagulation assays—abnormal if sepsis syndrome, DIC, or EHBDO

IMAGING
• Abdominal radiography—poor abdominal detail, usually generalized, may be focal in area of gallbladder; mass effect in region of liver; rare mineralized cholelith or gas • Thoracic radiography—rare pleural effusion, traumatic injury indicated (e.g., fractured rib) • Abdominal ultrasonography—effusion; distended gallbladder or common bile duct and thick gallbladder or duct wall suggest cholecystitis/choledochitis; segmental gallbladder wall hyperechogenicity or necrotic slough appearing as intraluminal membrane parallel to the wall (necrotizing cholecystitis); fluid interface surrounding gallbladder enhances image; perihepatic/pancreatic mass effect, choleliths or biliary mucocele ("kiwi fruit sign"), gas in biliary structures (gas-forming organism); gallbladder may be difficult to image if ruptured; liver normal size, variable parenchymal echogenicity depending on pathology and presence of ascending cholangitis

DIAGNOSTIC PROCEDURES
• Abdominocentesis—physicochemical and cytologic evaluations and cultures; use ultrasound guidance for sampling fluid as close as possible to, but without penetrating, biliary structures • Cytology—at surgery impression smears of gallbladder, liver, and bile for immediate determination of septic inflammation and neoplasia; modified transudate or exudate; high WBC count (> 9000/μL) predominated by neutrophils; bile debris/bilirubin may be found in macrophages and neutrophils or free in effusion • Effusion bilirubin:serum bilirubin ratio—commonly 2–3:1; important diagnostic feature • Bacterial culture and sensitivity—effusion, gallbladder, liver, and gallbladder contents; request aerobic and anaerobic cultures; gram-negative enteric opportunists and anaerobes most common; polymicrobial infections possible • Exploratory laparotomy—for diagnosis and treatment; as indicated: cholecystectomy, cholecystoenterostomy, duct or gallbladder repair • Liver biopsy—evaluates coexistent disease in the biliary tree and liver

PATHOLOGIC FINDINGS
Depend on underlying cause and site of rupture

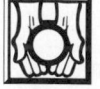

TREATMENT
• Inpatient—expediency of surgery depends on patient condition; achieve euhydration and correct electrolyte and acid-base status for best survival • Abdominal lavage to reduce peritoneal bile content if surgery delayed; use warmed polyionic fluids • Surgical experience important for best outcome as complicated resections and anastomoses may be required • Need for cholecystectomy decided by surgeon; dark discolored gallbladder wall indicates ischemic injury.

MEDICATIONS

DRUG(S)
• Antimicrobials—in all patients, initiate broad-spectrum antimicrobials *before* surgical intervention; enteric gram-negative and anaerobic organisms most common pathogens (good initial choices: ticarcillin, piperacillin, third-generation cephalosporins, or enrofloxacin combined with metronidazole); continue for no less than 8 weeks if sepsis confirmed; adjust medications based on culture and sensitivity findings • Vitamin K_1 (0.5–1.5 mg/kg IM or SC q12h for up to 3 doses)—provide if patient is jaundiced • Prepare for blood component and synthetic colloid therapy. • Antiemetics (metoclopramide, 0.2–0.5 mg/kg PO, SC q6–8h or 1–2 mg/kg/24h IV by CRI; ondansetron, 0.5–1.0 mg/kg PO q12h 30 minutes before feeding)—if patient is vomiting • H_2-receptor antagonists (e.g., famotidine 0.5 mg/kg PO, IV, SC q12–24h) and sucralfate (0.25–1.0 g PO q8–12h)—if enteric bleeding • Ursodeoxycholic acid—give indefinitely (10–15 mg/kg PO daily) if gallbladder muco-cele, choleliths, or associated cholangiohepatitis • Antioxidants—give vitamin E (10 IU/kg daily) and *S*-adenosylmethionine (20 mg/kg PO daily 2 hr before feeding) until enzymes normalize, indefinitely if chronic hepatitis

FOLLOW-UP

PATIENT MONITORING
• Repeat sequential hematologic, biochemical, and imaging evaluations—may be useful • Repeat abdominocentesis may be necessary to assess continued infection and/or bile leakage • Rarely, cholescintigraphic studies required to document continued bile leakage

POSSIBLE COMPLICATIONS
• Cholangitis/cholangiohepatitis • Pancreatitis

EXPECTED COURSE AND PROGNOSIS
• Good if surgery successful and infection eliminated • High mortality if infectious bile peritonitis (up to 75%) • Anticipate protracted clinical recovery and slow normalization of liver enzymes

MISCELLANEOUS

SEE ALSO
• Cholecystitis • Cholelithiasis • Gallbladder mucocele • Hepatitis, Chronic

ABBREVIATIONS
EHBDO = extrahepatic bile duct obstruction
Author Sharon A. Center
Consulting Editor Sharon A. Center

BASICS

OVERVIEW
• Clinical entity associated with chronic intermittent vomiting of bile caused by bile reflux into the stomach. Normal gastric motility and pressure gradients normally prevent or quickly remove any refluxed bile into the stomach before gastric mucosal irritation occurs. The presence of bile in the gastric lumen subsequently causes gastric mucosal damage. Bile reflux is suspected to be secondary to alterations in normal gastrointestinal motility.
• Clinical signs often occur early in the morning, suggesting that prolonged fasting or gastric inactivity may modify normal motility patterns, resulting in duodenal reflux.

SIGNALMENT
• Commonly observed in dogs, rarely in cats
• Most animals are middle-aged or older
• No breed, age or sex predisposition

SIGNS
• Chronic intermittent vomiting of only bile associated with an empty stomach. Signs generally occur late at night or early in the morning. Signs may occur daily but are usually more intermittent. Between episodes, the animal appears normal in all other respects. • Results of physical examination are usually unremarkable.

CAUSES & RISK FACTORS
• Cause unknown
• Primary gastric hypomotility suspected as the underlying cause
• Conditions causing gastritis or duodenitis may also be responsible for altered proximal gastrointestinal motility and may cause bile reflux. Investigate *Giardia* or inflammatory bowel disease as possible etiologies.

DIAGNOSIS

DIFFERENTIAL DIAGNOSIS
• Any number of gastrointestinal and non-gastrointestinal disorders can cause chronic vomiting. *Giardia* should be excluded since the signs of this disease may mimic those of bilious vomiting. • Inflammatory bowel disease can result in bile reflux. • Intestinal

obstruction or partial obstructions should be ruled out.

CBC/BIOCHEMISTRY/URINALYSIS
Results usually normal

OTHER LABORATORY TESTS
Fecal examination to detect *Giardia* or other parasites

IMAGING
Liquid barium contrast study may reveal delayed gastric emptying. Barium meals or radiopaque markers may demonstrate delayed gastric motility.

DIAGNOSTIC PROCEDURES
Endoscopic findings are frequently normal. Evidence of bile in the stomach or gastritis in the antral region may be observed in some patients. Endoscopy is useful to rule out structural or inflammatory disease of the stomach or duodenum.

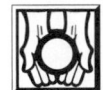

TREATMENT

• It is not a serious debilitating disorder and the patient should be treated symptomatically on an outpatient basis.
• Feeding the animal a late evening meal often resolves clinical signs. Food possibly acts as a buffer to the refluxed bile or may enhance gastric motility.
• If diet modification fails, medical treatment should be considered.

MEDICATIONS

DRUG(S)
• Choices include agents for gastric mucosal protection against the refluxed bile or the use of gastric prokinetic agents to improve motility. Often a single evening dose of a medication may be all that is required to prevent clinical signs.
• Drugs for gastric mucosal protection include various antacids or carafate (1 gm/25 kg).
• Drugs that block gastric acid production including cimetidine (5 mg/kg q8h), ranitidine (2 mg/kg q8h), nizatidine (5 mg/kg q24h) may be beneficial. Both ranitidine and nizatidine also have significant prokinetic effects on gastric motility.
• Specific gastric prokinetic agents include metoclopramide (0.2 to 0.4 mg/kg PO

q6–8h) and cisapride (0.1 mg/kg PO q8–12h). Cisapride is now available only through compounding pharmacies. Newer prokinetic tegaserod (0.3 mg/kg q12h) has similar prokinetic effects as cisapride but there is as yet limited clinical experience.
• Erythromycin (0.5–1 mg/kg q8h) also promotes gastric motility and may resolve signs. A benefit of this drug is that it is inexpensive.

CONTRAINDICATIONS/POSSIBLE INTERACTIONS
• Gastric prokinetic agents should not be administered in patients with gastrointestinal obstruction.
• Metoclopramide is contraindicated with concurrent phenothiazine and narcotic administration and in animals with epilepsy. Metoclopramide can cause nervousness, anxiety, or depression.
• Cisapride can cause vomiting, diarrhea, or abdominal cramping.
• Erythromycin can cause vomiting.

FOLLOW-UP

Most patients respond to one of the above treatments and a clinical response supports the diagnosis. Failure to respond suggests another underlying or causative factor.

MISCELLANEOUS

ASSOCIATED CONDITIONS
Gastroesophageal reflux

SEE ALSO
• Gastric or Gastrointestinal Motility Disorders
• Gastroesophageal Reflux

Suggested Reading
Hall JA, Twedt DC, Burrows CF. Gastric motility in dogs. Part 2. Disorders of gastric motility. Compend Small Anim Med Pract Vet 1990;12:1373–1390.
Hall JA, Washabau RJ. Diagnosis and treatment of gastric motility disorders. Vet Clin North Am Small Anim Pract 1999; 29:377–395.
Author David C. Twedt
Consulting Editor Albert E. Jergens

BLASTOMYCOSIS

BASICS

DEFINITION
A systemic, mycotic infection caused by the soil organism *Blastomyces dermatitidis*

PATHOPHYSIOLOGY
• A small spore (conidia) is shed from the mycelial phase of the organism growing in the soil and inhaled, entering the terminal airway
• At body temperature, the spore becomes a yeast, which initiates the infection in the lungs.
• From this focus of mycotic pneumonia, the yeast disseminates hematogenously throughout the body.
• The immune response to the invading organism produces a pyogranulomatous infiltrate to control the organism.
• The result is organ dysfunction.

SYSTEMS AFFECTED
• Respiratory—85% of affected dogs have lung disease
• Eyes, skin, lymphatic system, and bones—commonly affected
• Brain, testes, prostate, mammary gland, nasal cavity, gums, and vulva—less commonly affected

GENETICS
• No genetic predisposition identified
• Large breeds of dogs most often affected

INCIDENCE/PREVALENCE
• Depends on environmental and soil conditions that favor growth of *Blastomyces*
• Some areas of Wisconsin—incidence in dogs reaches 1,420/100,000 annually

GEOGRAPHIC DISTRIBUTION
Most common along the Mississippi, Ohio, and Tennessee River basins

SIGNALMENT
Species
• Dogs
• Occasionally cats

Breed Predilection
Large breed dogs weighing ≤ 25 kg, especially sporting breeds; may reflect exposure rather than susceptibility

Mean Age and Range
• Dogs—most common 2–4 years of age; uncommon after 7 years of age
• Cats—young to middle-aged

Predominant Sex
Dogs—males in most studies

SIGNS
Historical Findings
• Weight loss
• Depressed appetite
• Cough and dyspnea

• Eye inflammation and discharge
• Lameness
• Draining skin lesions

Physical Examination Findings
Dogs
• Fever up to 104.0°F (40°C)—approximately 50% of patients
• Harsh, dry lung sounds associated with increased respiratory effort—common
• Generalized or regional lymphadenopathy with or without skin lesions
• Uveitis with or without secondary glaucoma and conjunctivitis, ocular exudates, and corneal edema
• Lameness—common because of fungal osteomyelitis
• Testicular enlargement and prostatomegaly—occasionally seen

Cats
• Increased respiratory effort
• Granulomatous skin lesions

CAUSES
Inhaling fungal spores

RISK FACTORS
• Wet environment—fosters growth of the fungus; banks of rivers, streams, and lakes or in swamps; most affected dogs live within 400 m of water.
• Exposure to recently excavated areas

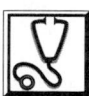

DIAGNOSIS

DIFFERENTIAL DIAGNOSIS
• Respiratory signs—bacterial pneumonia, neoplasia, heart failure, or other fungal infection
• Lymph node enlargement—similar to lymphosarcoma
• The combination of respiratory disease with eye, bone, or skin involvement in a young dog suggests the diagnosis.

CBC/BIOCHEMISTRY/URINALYSIS
• CBC changes reflect mild to moderate inflammation.
• High serum globulins with borderline low albumin concentrations in dogs with chronic infections
• Hypercalcemia in some dogs secondary to the granulomatous changes
• *Blastomyces* yeasts can be found in the urine of dogs with prostatic involvement.

OTHER LABORATORY TESTS
AGID—useful for making a diagnosis if organisms cannot be found on cytology or histopathology; positive test strongly supports diagnosis, with a specificity of > 90%; negative tests common in dogs with early infection

IMAGING
Radiographs
• Lungs—essential for diagnosis and prognosis
• Generalized interstitial to nodular infiltrate
• Tracheobronchial lymphadenopathy—common
• Changes—inconsistent with bacterial pneumonia; may resemble metastatic tumors, especially hemangiosarcoma
• Chylothorax secondary to blastomycosis can occur in dogs.
• Focal bone lesions—lytic and proliferative; can be mistaken for osteosarcoma

DIAGNOSTIC PROCEDURES
• Cytology of lymph node aspirates, lung aspirates, tracheal wash fluid, or impression smears of draining skin lesions—best method for diagnosis
• Histopathology of bone biopsies or enucleated blind eyes—identify the organism
• Organisms—usually plentiful in the tissues; may be scarce in tracheal washes if there is no productive cough

PATHOLOGIC FINDINGS
• Lesions—pyogranulomatous with many thick walled, budding yeast; occasionally very fibrous with few organisms found
• Lungs with large amounts of inflammatory infiltrate do not collapse when the chest is opened.
• Special fungal stains—facilitate finding the organisms

TREATMENT

APPROPRIATE HEALTH CARE
Usually outpatient with oral itraconazole treatment

NURSING CARE
Severely dyspneic dogs—require an oxygen cage for a minimum of 1 week before lung improvement is sufficient for comfort in room air; many have worsening of lung disease during the first few days of treatment, owing to an increase in the inflammatory response after the *Blastomyces* organisms die and release their contents.

ACTIVITY
Patients with respiratory compromise must be restricted.

DIET
Palatable and high-quality to stimulate the appetite

CLIENT EDUCATION
Inform owner that treatment is costly and requires a minimum of 60–90 days.

SURGICAL CONSIDERATIONS

Removal of an abscessed lung lobe may be required when medical treatment cannot resolve the infection.

 MEDICATIONS

DRUG(S) OF CHOICE

Itraconazole
• Dogs—5 mg/kg PO q12h with a fat-rich meal, such as canned dog food, for the first 3 days to achieve a therapeutic blood concentration as soon as possible; then reduce to 5 μg/kg once a day.
• Cats—5 mg/kg PO q12h; open the 100-mg capsules containing pellets and mix with palatable food.
• Treat for a minimum of 60 days or for 1 month after all signs of disease have disappeared.
• Dogs with neurologic signs should be treated with amphotericin B.

CONTRAINDICATIONS

Corticosteroids—usually contraindicated because the antiinflammatory effects allow uninhibited proliferation of the organisms; patients with previous steroid therapy require a longer duration of treatment; for dogs with life-threatening dyspnea, dexamethasone (0.2 mg/kg daily) for 2–3 days may be lifesaving when given in conjunction with itraconazole treatment; discontinue steroids as soon as possible.

PRECAUTIONS

Itraconazole Toxicity
• Anorexia—most common sign; attributed to liver toxicity; monitor serum ALT monthly for duration of treatment or when anorexia occurs; temporarily discontinue drug for patients with anorexia and ALT activities > 200; after appetite improves, restart at half the previously used dose.
• Ulcerative dermatitis—seen in some dogs; the result of vasculitis; dose-related condition; temporarily discontinue drug; when ulcers have resolved, restart at half the previously used dose.

POSSIBLE INTERACTIONS

For humans, itraconazole is contraindicated with terfenadine and cisapride.

ALTERNATIVE DRUG(S)

• Amphotericin B—0.5 mg/kg IV every other day in dogs that cannot take oral medication or that do not respond to itraconazole (see Histoplasmosis); use the lipid complex for dogs with renal dysfunction that cannot take itraconazole

• Ketoconazole—10 mg/kg PO q12h; cheaper alternative to itraconazole; lower response rate and higher recurrence rate

 FOLLOW-UP

PATIENT MONITORING

Serum chemistry—monthly to monitor for hepatic toxicity or if anorexia develops

Thoracic Radiographs
• Determine duration of treatment
• Considerable permanent changes in the lungs may occur after the infection has resolved, making determination of persistent active disease difficult.
• At 60 days of treatment—if active lung disease is seen, continue treatment for 30 days. • If lungs are normal, stop treatment and do radiographs again in 30 days.
• At 90 days of treatment—if the same as day 60, changes are residual. Fibrosis—inactive disease; if better than day 60, continue treatment for 30 more days, if lesions are significantly worse than at 60 days, change treatment to amphotericin B and then re-radiograph.
• At 120 days of treatment—re-radiograph. Continue treatment as long as there is improvement in the lungs. If there is no further improvement and no indication of active disease, the lesions are probably scarring.

PREVENTION/AVOIDANCE

• Location of environmental growth of *Blastomyces* organisms unknown; thus difficult to avoid exposure; restricting exposure to lakes and streams could be done but is not very practical.
• Dogs that recover from the infection are probably immune to reinfection.

POSSIBLE COMPLICATIONS

Death

EXPECTED COURSE AND PROGNOSIS

• Death—25% of dogs die during the first week of treatment; early diagnosis improves chance of survival.
• Severity of lung involvement and invasion into the brain affect prognosis
• Recurrence—about 20% of dogs; usually within 3–6 months after completion of treatment, even with 60–90 days of treatment; may occur up to 15 months after treatment; a second course of itraconazole treatment will cure most patients; drug resistance to itraconazole has not been observed

 MISCELLANEOUS

ASSOCIATED CONDITIONS
N/A

AGE-RELATED FACTORS
N/A

ZOONOTIC POTENTIAL

• Not spread from animals to people, except through bite wounds; inoculation of organisms from dog bites has occurred.
• Avoid cuts during necropsy of infected dogs and avoid needle sticks when aspirating lesions.
• Warn clients that blastomycosis is acquired from an environmental source and that they may have been exposed at the same time as the patient; common source exposure has been documented in duck and coon hunters; the incidence in dogs is 10 times that in humans.
• Encourage clients with respiratory and skin lesions to inform their physicians that they may have been exposed to blastomycosis.

PREGNANCY

No teratogenic effects of itraconazole at therapeutic doses in rats and mice; embryotoxicity found at high doses; no dog or cat studies; one dog started on itraconazole halfway through her pregnancy delivered a normal litter.

SYNONYMS
N/A

SEE ALSO
N/A

ABBREVIATIONS
• AGID = agar gel immunodiffusion
• ALT = alanine transferase

Suggested Reading
Arceneaux KA, Taboada J, Hosgood G. Blastomycosis in dogs: 115 cases (1980–1995). J Am Vet Med Assoc 1998;213:658–664.
Krawiec DR, McKiernan BC, Twardock AR, et al. Use of amphotericin B lipid complex for treatment of blastomycosis in dogs. J Am Vet Med Assoc 1996;209:2073–2075.
Legendre AM, Rohrbach BW, Toal RL, et al. Treatment of blastomycosis with itraconazole in 112 dogs. J Vet Intern Med 1996;10:365–371.
Legendre AM. Blastomycosis. In: Greene CE, ed. Infectious diseases of the dog and cat. Philadelphia: Saunders, 1998:371–377.

Author Alfred M. Legendre
Consulting Editor Stephen C. Barr

BLEPHARITIS

BASICS

DEFINITION
• Inflammation of the outer (skin) and middle portion (muscle, connective tissue, and glands) of the eyelid, usually with secondary inflammation of the palpebral conjunctiva • Chronic—anterior or posterior, based on the site of predominant involvement • Anterior—most commonly associated with bacterial infection or self-trauma • Posterior—disorders of the meibomian glands

PATHOPHYSIOLOGY
• Same as virtually every condition that affects the skin in general • Mechanisms of inflammation—immune mediated, infectious, endocrine mediated, self- and external trauma, parasitic, radiation, and nutritional • Inflammatory response often exaggerated because eyelid conjunctiva is rich in mast cells and densely vascularized • Meibomian gland dysfunction—common; bacterial lipases alter meibomian lipids so they plug the gland; they also produce irritating fatty acids, enhance bacterial growth and destabilize the tear film.

SYSTEMS AFFECTED
Ophthalmic

SIGNALMENT
See Causes

SIGNS
• Serous, mucoid, or mucopurulent ocular discharge • Blepharospasm • Eyelid hyperemia, edema, and thickening • Pruritus • Excoriation • Depigmentation—skin; hair • Alopecia • Swollen, cream-colored meibomian glands • Elevated, pinpoint meibomian gland orifices • Abscesses • Scales and crusts • Papules or pustules • Single or multiple nodular hyperemic swellings • Concurrent conjunctivitis and/or keratitis

CAUSES
Congenital
• Eyelid abnormalities—may promote self-trauma or moist dermatitis • Prominent nasal folds, medial trichiasis, and lower lid entropion—shih tzus, Pekingese, English bulldogs, lhasa apsos, pugs, Persian and Himalayan cats • Distichia— shih tzus, pugs, golden retrievers, Labrador retrievers, poodles, English bulldogs • Ectopic cilia • Lateral lid entropion—shar peis, chow chows, Labrador retrievers, rottweilers; adult cats (rare) • Lagophthalmos—brachycephalic dogs; Persian, Himalayan, and Burmese cats • Deep medial canthal pockets—dolichocephalic dogs • Dermoids—rottweilers, dachshunds, and others; Burmese cats

Allergic
• Type I (immediate)—atopy; food; insect bite; inhalant; *Staphylococcus* hypersensitivity • Type II (cytotoxic)—pemphigus; pemphigoid; drug eruption • Type III (immune complex)—SLE; *Staphylococcus* hypersensitivity; drug eruption • Type IV (cell mediated)—contact and flea bite hypersensitivity; drug eruption

Bacterial
• Hordeolum—localized abscess of eyelid glands, usually staphylococcal; may be external (sty in young dogs, involving glands of Zeis) or internal (in old dogs, involves one or more meibomian glands) • Generalized bacterial blepharitis and meibomianitis—usually *Staphylococcus* or *Streptococcus* • Pyogranulomas • *Staphylococcus* hypersensitivity—young and old dogs

Neoplastic
• Sebaceous adenomas and adenocarcinomas—originate from meibomian gland • Squamous cell carcinoma—white cats • Mast cell—may masquerade as swollen, hyperemic lesion

Other
• External trauma—eyelid lacerations; thermal or chemical burns • Mycotic—dermatophytosis; systemic fungal granulomas • Parasitic—demodicosis; sarcoptic mange; *Cuterebra* and *Notoedres cati* • Chalazia (singular, chalazion)—sterile, yellow-white, painless meibomian gland swellings caused by a granulomatous inflammatory response to escape of meibum into surrounding eyelid tissue • Nutritional—zinc-responsive dermatosis (Siberian huskies, Alaskan malamutes, puppies); fatty acid deficiency • Endocrine—hypothyroidism (dogs); hyperadrenocorticism (dogs); diabetic dermatosis • Viral—chronic blepharitis in cats secondary to FHV-1 • Irritant—topical ocular drug reaction; nicotine smoke in environment; after parotid duct transposition • Familial canine dermatomyositis—collies and Shetland sheepdogs • Nodular granulomatous episclerokeratitis—fibrous histiocytoma and collie granuloma in collies; may affect the eyelids, cornea, or conjunctiva • Eosinophilic granuloma—cats; may affect eyelids, cornea, or conjunctiva • Eyelid contact with purulent exudate (tear burn) • Conjunctivitis • Keratitis • Dry eye • Dacryocystitis • Orbital disease • Radiotherapy • Drug contact irritant—any drug, often neomycin • Idiopathic—particularly in cats with chronic idiopathic conjunctivitis

RISK FACTORS
• Breed predisposition to congenital eyelid abnormalities, e.g., entropion, ectropion, etc. • Outdoor animals—traumatic • Hypothyroidism—may promote chronic bacterial disease in dogs

• Canine seborrhea—may promote chronic generalized meibomianitis

DIAGNOSIS

DIFFERENTIAL DIAGNOSIS
Clinical signs are diagnostic.

CBC/BIOCHEMISTRY/URINALYSIS
Usually nondiagnostic unless metabolic cause (e.g., diabetic dermatosis)

OTHER LABORATORY TESTS
• Indicated for suspected systemic disorder • Consider tests for hypothyroidism.

DIAGNOSTIC PROCEDURES
If possible, avoid topical anesthetic or fluorescein before obtaining culture. • Cytology—deep skin scrapings; conjunctival scrapings; expressed exudate from meibomian glands and pustules • Dermatophyte culture—deep skin scrapings • Wood's light evaluation—skin • KOH preparation—skin scrapings • Aerobic bacterial culture and sensitivity—exudate from skin; conjunctiva; expressed exudate from meibomian glands and pustules; often will not recover *Staphylococcus* from patients with chronic meibomianitis and suspected *Staphylococcus* hypersensitivity • IFA or PCR for FHV-1 and *Chlamydia*—conjunctival scrapings from cats with primary conjunctivitis or keratitis • Eye examination—potential inciting cause; corneal ulcer; foreign body; distichia; ectopic cilia; dry eye • Ancillary ocular tests—fluorescein application; Schirmer tear test • Thorough medical history and dermatologic examination—help identify generalized dermatologic disease • Full-thickness wedge biopsy of eyelid—histologic evaluation • Direct immunofluorescence for autoimmune disease; Intradermal skin testing, RAST, ELISA, and food elimination diet for hypersensitivity induced disease.

PATHOLOGIC FINDINGS
• Routine histopathology often nondiagnostic in chronic disease • Wedge biopsy—may be unrewarding; carefully select patients based on history, ophthalmic exam, and response to medical therapy.

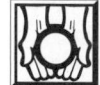

TREATMENT

APPROPRIATE HEALTH CARE
See Nursing Care

NURSING CARE
• Secondary disease—treat primary disease • Suspected self-trauma—Elizabethan collar • Topical gentamicin, neomycin, terramycin, antiviral medication (e.g., trifluridine

solution), and most ointments—may cause an irritant blepharoconjunctivitis (rare); withdrawal of agent may resolve condition • Cleanse eyelids—to remove crusts; warm compresses applied for 5–15 min 3–4 times daily avoiding ocular surfaces; saline, lactated Ringer's solution, or a commercial ocular cleansing agent (e.g., Eye Scrub); must clip periocular hair short

DIET
Only with food allergy–induced disease

CLIENT EDUCATION
• Warn client that most patients cannot be cured but that the condition often can be controlled medically. • Inform client that there is no cure for FHV-1 and that clinical signs often recur when the animal is stressed. • Instruct owner to keep the Elizabethan collar on at all times.

SURGICAL CONSIDERATIONS
• Temporary everting eyelid sutures—spastic entropion; or in puppies before permanent surgical correction • Repair eyelid lacerations • Lancing—large abscesses only; lance and curette hordeola that are resistant to medical treatment and chalazia that have hardened and come to a point, causing keratitis; manually express infected meibomian secretions.

MEDICATIONS

DRUG(S)

Antibiotics
• Systemic—generally required for effective treatment of bacterial eyelid infections; may try amoxicillin–clavulanic acid, or cephalexin; 20 mg/kg q8h • Topical—may try neomycin, polymyxin B, and bacitracin combination or chloramphenicol. Avoid neomycin if suspected of being irritating.

Congenital
• Topical antibiotic ointment—q6–12h; until surgery is performed to prevent frictional rubbing of eyelid hairs or cilia on the ocular surface • Saline, lactated Ringer's solution, or ocular irrigant—regularly flush deep medial canthal pocket debris

External Trauma
• Topical antibiotic ointment—q6–12h; for spastic entropion secondary to pain and blepharospasm to reduce friction until entropion is surgically relieved • Systemic antibiotics indicated

Allergic
• *Staphylococcus* hypersensitivity blepharitis—systemic broad-spectrum antibiotics and systemic corticosteroids (prednisolone, 0.5

mg/kg q12h for 3–5 days, then taper); many patients respond to systemic corticosteroids alone. • Affected meibomian glands—oral tetracycline (15–20 mg/kg PO q8h) or doxycycline (3–5 mg/kg PO q12h) for at least 3 weeks (lipophilic and cause decreased production of bacterial lipases and irritating fatty acids); topical polymyxin B and neomycin with 0.1% dexamethasone (q6–8h to the eye) • Failure of treatment—may try injections of homologous or commercial *Staphylococcus aureus* bacterin (*Staphylococcus* Lysate) • *Propionibacterium acnes* immunotherapy—investigational; of unknown value • Eyelid lesions associated with puppy strangles—usually benefit from treatment of the generalized condition

Bacterial
• Based on culture and sensitivity testing • While results are pending—topical polymyxin B and neomycin with 0.1% dexamethasone ointment (q4–6h); plus a systemic broad-spectrum antibiotic

Mycotic
Microsporium canis infection—usually self-limiting; treatment includes 2% miconazole cream, 1% clotrimazole cream, or diluted povidone-iodine solution (1 part to 300 parts saline) applied q12–24h for at least 6 weeks; do not use lotions.

Parasitic
• Demodicosis—localized disease, diluted amitraz (1 part amitraz to 9 parts mineral oil; Mitaban) once every 3 days for 4–8 weeks; fairly safe around the eyes (see Demodicosis) • Notoedres infection—lime sulfur dips • Sarcoptic mange—same as for generalized disease

Idiopathic
Clinical signs often controlled with topical polymyxin B and neomycin with 0.1% dexamethasone (q8–24h or as needed); occasionally may also need systemic prednisolone (0.5 mg/kg q12h for 3–5days, then taper) and/or a systemic antibiotic

CONTRAINDICATIONS
• Topical corticosteroids—do not use with corneal ulceration. • Cats—many patients with presumed idiopathic blepharoconjunctivitis actually have FHV-1 infection; topical and systemic corticosteroids may exacerbate the infection. • Oral tetracycline and doxycycline—do not use in puppies and kittens. • Neomycin—avoid topical use if suspect it is causing the blepharitis.

PRECAUTIONS
Ectoparasitism—wear gloves; do not contact ocular surfaces with the drug; apply artificial tear ointment to the eyes for protection.

POSSIBLE INTERACTIONS
Staphylococcal bacterin for *Staphylococcus* hypersensitivity—anaphylactic reaction (rare)

FOLLOW-UP

PATIENT MONITORING
• Depends on cause • Bacterial—treated with systemic and topical treatment for at least 3 weeks; should notice improvement within 10 days • Most common causes of treatment failure—use of subinhibitory antibiotic concentrations; failure to correct one or more predisposing factors; stopping medications too soon

PREVENTION/AVOIDANCE
Depend on cause

POSSIBLE COMPLICATIONS
• Cicatricial lid contracture—results in trichiasis, ectropion, or lagophthalmos • Spastic entropion—because of blepharospasm and pain • Inability to open eyelids—owing to matting of discharge and hair • Qualitative tear film deficiency—result of loss of proper meibum secretion • Recurrence of bacterial infection or FHV-1 blepharoconjunctivitis

EXPECTED COURSE AND PROGNOSIS
Depends on cause

MISCELLANEOUS

ZOONOTIC POTENTIAL
• Dermatophytosis • Sarcoptic mange

SEE ALSO
• Conjunctivitis—Cats • Conjunctivitis—Dogs • Epiphora • Keratitis, Nonulcerative • Keratitis, Ulcerative • Red Eye

ABBREVIATIONS
• ELISA = enzyme-linked immunoadsorbent assay • FHV-1 = feline herpesvirus type 1 • PCR = polymerase chain reaction • RAST = radioallergosorbent test • SLE = systemic lupus erythematosus

Suggested Reading
Bedford PCG. Diseases and surgery of the canine eyelid. In: Gelatt KN, ed. Veterinary ophthamology, 3rd ed. Philadelphia: Lippincott Williams & Wilkins 1999:535–568.
Gelatt KN. Diseases and Surgery of the canine eyelids. In: Essentials of veterinary Ophthalmology. Philadelphia: Lippincott Williams & Wilkins 2000:67–72.
Author Terri L. McCalla
Consulting Editor Paul E. Miller

BLIND QUIET EYE

 BASICS

DEFINITION
Loss of vision in one or both eyes without ocular vascular injection or other externally apparent signs of ocular inflammation

PATHOPHYSIOLOGY
Results from abnormalities in focusing images on the retina, retinal image detection, optic nerve transmission, or CNS interpretation

SYSTEMS AFFECTED
• Ophthalmic
• Nervous

SIGNALMENT
• Dogs and cats
• Any age, breed, or sex
• Many causes (e.g., cataracts and progressive retinal atrophy) have a genetic basis and are often highly breed- and age-specific.
• SARDS—tends to occur in old dogs
• Optic nerve hypoplasia—congenital

SIGNS

Historical Findings
• Depend on underlying cause
• Bumping into objects
• Clumsy behavior
• Reluctance to move
• Impaired vision in dim light

Physical Examination Findings
• Depend on underlying cause
• Decreased or absent menace response
• Impaired visual placing responses

CAUSES
• Cataracts—generally, entire lens must become opaque to produce complete blindness; incomplete opacification may reduce performance of visually demanding tasks
• Loss of focusing power of the lens—rarely completely blinding; substantial hyperopia (far-sightedness) occurs when the optical power of the lens is not replaced after lens extraction or if the lens luxates posteriorly out of the pupillary plane and into the vitreous
• Retina—SARDS; PRA; retinal detachment; taurine deficiency (cats), enrofloxacin toxicity (cats); ivermetin toxicity (dogs, cats) • Optic nerve—optic neuritis; neoplasia of the optic nerve or adjacent tissues; trauma; optic nerve hypoplasia; lead toxicity; excessive traction on the optic nerve during enucleation resulting in trauma to the contralateral optic nerve or optic chiasm (especially cats and brachycephalic dogs) • CNS (amaurosis)—lesions of the optic chiasm or tract; optic radiation; visual cortex

RISK FACTORS
• Poorly regulated diabetes mellitus—cataracts
• Related animals with genetic cataracts or PRA
• Systemic hypertension—retinal detachment
• CNS hypoxia—blindness may become apparent after excessively deep anesthesia or revival from cardiac arrest.

 DIAGNOSIS

DIFFERENTIAL DIAGNOSIS

Signs
• Anterior segment inflammation and glaucoma—conjunctiva typically injected
• Young patients—may lack menace responses; usually successfully navigate a maze or visually track hand movements or cotton balls
• Postictal period—transient vision loss
• Abnormal mentation—may be difficult to determine whether an animal is visual; other neurologic abnormalities help localize the lesion.

Causes
• Optic neuritis, retinal detachment, SARDS, or visual cortex hypoxia—sudden vision loss (over hours to weeks)
• SARDS—often preceded by polyuria, polydipsia, polyphagia and weight gain
• PRA—gradual vision loss, especially in dim light; apparently acute vision loss with sudden change in environment
• Cataract—history of either gradual or rapidly increasing opacification and vision loss in a quiet eye
• Optic nerve hypoplasia—congenital; may be unilateral or bilateral
• Optic neuropathy or CNS disease—signs of other neurologic abnormalities
• Pupillary light responses—usually normal with cataracts or visual cortex lesions; sluggish to absent with retinal or optic nerve diseases
• Ophthalmoscopy—normal with SARDS, retrobulbar optic neuritis, and higher visual pathway lesions; abnormal with retinal detachment and neuropathies of the optic nerve head

CBC/BIOCHEMISTRY/URINALYSIS
• Usually normal, unless underlying systemic disease
• Hyperglycemia or glucosuria—may note with diabetic cataracts
• Elevated ALP and changes consistent with hyperadrenocorticism (Cushing syndrome)—suggest SARDS
• Retinal detachment secondary to systemic hypertension (cats)—mildly high BUN or serum creatinine; changes consistent with hyperthyroidism

OTHER LABORATORY TESTS
• Blood lead and serology for deep fungal or viral infections—consider for suspected optic neuritis (see Optic Neuritis).
• LDDST—may help rule out Cushing syndrome with SARDS

IMAGING
• Ocular ultrasound—may demonstrate a retinal detachment (especially if the ocular media are opaque) or optic nerve mass lesion
• Plain skull radiographs—seldom informative
• CT or MRI—often helpful with orbital or CNS lesions

DIAGNOSTIC PROCEDURES
• Ophthalmic examination with a penlight—usually permits diagnosis of cataracts or retinal detachments severe enough to cause blindness
• Ophthalmoscopy—may reveal PRA or optic nerve disease; normal examination suggests SARDS, retrobulbar optic neuritis, or a CNS lesion.
• Systemic blood pressure—determine in retinal detachments
• Electroretinography—differentiates retinal from optic nerve or CNS disease when the diagnosis is in doubt
• CSF tap—may be of value with a neurogenic cause of vision loss

 TREATMENT

• Try to obtain a definitive diagnosis on an outpatient basis before initiating treatment.
• Consider referral before attempting empirical therapy.
• Most causes are not fatal, but must perform a workup to rule out potentially fatal diseases.
• Reassure client that most causes of a blind quiet eye are not painful and that blind animals can lead a relatively normal and functional life.
• Warn client that the environment should be examined for potential hazards to a blind animal.
• Advise client that patients with progressive retinal atrophy or genetic cataracts should not be bred and that related animals should be examined.
• Retinal detachment—recommend severely restricted exercise until the retina is firmly reattached.
• Calorie-restricted diet—to prevent obesity; owing to reduced activity level
• Cats with nutritionally induced retinopathy—ensure diet has adequate levels of taurine.
• SARDS, progressive retinal atrophy, optic nerve atrophy, and optic nerve hypoplasia—no effective treatment
• Cataracts, luxated lenses, and some forms of retinal detachment—best treated surgically

MEDICATIONS

DRUG(S) OF CHOICE
• Depend on cause
• Workup is declined, infectious disease is unlikely, and the likely diagnosis is SARDS or retrobulbar optic neuritis—consider systemic prednisolone (1–2 mg/kg/day for 7–14 days, then taper); may concurrently administer oral chloramphenicol or other systemic broad-spectrum antibiotic

CONTRAINDICATIONS
Do not use systemic corticosteroids and other immunosuppressive drugs with optic neuritis and retinal detachments that are infectious in origin.

PRECAUTIONS
Pretreatment with corticosteroids may mimic or mask liver enzyme changes in SARDS.

POSSIBLE INTERACTIONS
N/A

ALTERNATIVE DRUG(S)
• Flunixin meglumine (dogs)—may try a single dose (0.5 mg/kg IV) in place of corticosteroids if infectious causes have not been ruled out • Oral azathioprine—1–2 mg/kg/day for 3–7 days, then taper; may be used to treat immune-mediated retinal detachments if systemic corticosteroids are not effective; perform a CBC, platelet count, and liver enzyme every 1–2 weeks for the first 8 weeks, then periodically.

FOLLOW-UP

PATIENT MONITORING
• Repeat ophthalmic examinations—as required to ensure that ocular inflammation is controlled, and, if possible, vision is maintained
• Recurrence of vision loss—common in optic neuritis; may occur weeks, months, or years after initial presentation

POSSIBLE COMPLICATIONS
• Death
• Permanent vision loss
• Loss of the eye
• Chronic ocular inflammation and pain
• Obesity from inactivity or as a sequela of SARDS

MISCELLANEOUS

ASSOCIATED CONDITIONS
• SARDS (dogs)—signs similar to those of hyperadrenocorticism
• Neurologic disease—may note seizures, behavior or personality changes, circling or other CNS signs
• Cardiomyopathy (cats)—taurine deficiency

AGE-RELATED FACTORS
• PRA and many cataracts—breed-specific ages of onset

• SARDS—tend to occur in older dogs
• Optic nerve hypoplasia—congenital

ZOONOTIC POTENTIAL
N/A

PREGNANCY
Corticosteroids and immunosuppressive drugs may complicate pregnancy.

SEE ALSO
See Causes

ABBREVIATIONS
ALP = alkaline phosphatase
CSF = cerebrospinal fluid
LDDST = low-dose dexamethasone-suppression test
PRA = progressive retinal atrophy
SARDS = sudden acquired retinal degeneration syndrome

Suggested Reading
Gelatt KN, ed. Veterinary ophthalmology. 3rd ed. Baltimore: Lippincott Williams & Wilkins 1999.
Rubin LF. Inherited eye disease in purebred dogs. Baltimore: Williams & Wilkins, 1989.
Slatter DS. Fundamentals of veterinary ophthalmology. 3rd ed. Philadelphia: Saunders, 2001.
Author Paul E. Miller
Consulting Editor Paul E. Miller

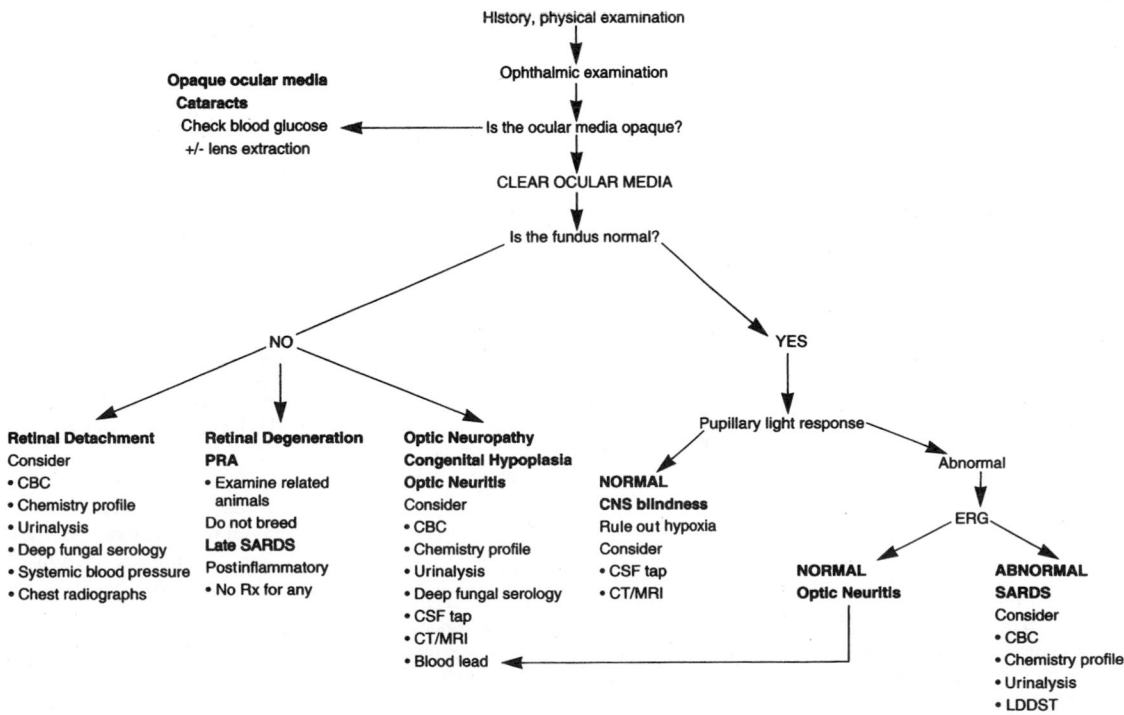

BLOOD TRANSFUSION REACTIONS

BASICS

OVERVIEW
• Classified as acute or delayed, immune mediated or not immune-mediated
• Severe reactions usually occur during or shortly after transfusion.
• Can occur with any blood product, including hemoglobin-based oxygen-carrying solutions.

SIGNALMENT
• Dogs and cats
• No sex predilection
• All ages affected

SIGNS

Acute Hemolytic Reaction
• Restlessness
• Fever
• Tachycardia
• Vomiting
• Tremors
• Weakness
• Incontinence
• Collapse
• Shock
• Oliguria
• Loss of transfusion efficacy

Delayed Hemolytic Reaction
Loss of transfusion efficacy—usually no clinical signs

Acute Nonhemolytic Reaction
• Anaphylactic reaction—fever, urticaria, erythema, and pruritus
• Transfusion of contaminated blood—acute septicemia, fever, and shock
• Circulatory overload/rapid transfusion—vomiting, distended jugular veins, dyspnea, cough, cyanosis, and congestive heart failure
• Citrate toxicity—hypocalcemia, myocardial depression, and weakness
• Hyperammonemia—encephalopathy
• Hypothermia—shivering and impaired platelet function

CAUSES & RISK FACTORS
Purebred cats and previously transfused dogs have a higher risk of severe transfusion reaction than other animals.

Acute Hemolysis
• Blood group mismatch
• Transfusion of damaged and hemolyzed RBCs (after excessive heating, freezing, or mechanical damage)

Delayed Hemolysis
Immune reaction to minor red cell antigens; occurs after 3–14 days

Acute Nonhemolytic Reaction
• Anaphylaxis and immune reaction to donor leukocytes, major histocompatibility complex antigens, or plasma antigens, resulting in release of inflammatory mediators and pyrogens
• Transfusion of contaminated blood—lack of aseptic collection and storage conditions
• Circulatory overload—rapid transfusion; excessive volume of blood in small animal or in animal with heart failure or oliguric renal failure
• Citrate toxicity—after circulatory overload, particularly in small animal or in animal with hepatopathy
• Hyperammonemia—high ammonia concentration in stored blood; important only for animal with hepatopathy
• Hypothermia—rapid transfusion of refrigerated blood to small or already hypothermic animal

Delayed Nonhemolytic Reaction
Transmission of blood-borne disease—use of infected donor

DIAGNOSIS

DIFFERENTIAL DIAGNOSIS
• Hemolysis—rule out ongoing fulminant hemolytic disease and use of hemolyzed blood
• Fever, hypotension—rule out underlying infectious and inflammatory diseases

CBC/BIOCHEMISTRY/URINALYSIS
Hemoglobinemia, leukocytosis, bilirubinemia, hemoglobinuria, and bilirubinuria

OTHER LABORATORY TESTS
• Repeat cross-match to confirm incompatibility.
• Bacterial culture or gram staining of contaminated blood may reveal organism.

IMAGING
N/A

DIAGNOSTIC PROCEDURES
N/A

TREATMENT
• Immediately discontinue transfusion.
• Administer fluids to maintain blood pressure and renal blood flow; for hypotension, use lactated Ringer's solution (50–90 mL/kg/h to effect).
• Additional supportive therapy for DIC, shock, or thromboembolism (see appropriate chapters)

MEDICATIONS

DRUG(S)
• For hemolysis—rapid-acting corticosteroid, such as prednisolone sodium succinate (10–30 mg/kg once) or dexamethasone sodium phosphate (6–15 mg/kg once); heparin (75 U/kg SC q6h; not for use in bleeding animals)
• For urticaria, fever—diphenhydramine (1–2 mg/kg); prednisolone (2–4 mg/kg); continue transfusion afterward, if clinically indicated.
• For septicemia—broad-spectrum IV antibiotics while bacterial culture results are pending (e.g., cephalothin/gentamycin); heparin

CONTRAINDICATIONS/POSSIBLE INTERACTIONS
None

FOLLOW-UP

PATIENT MONITORING
• Check attitude, temperature, vital signs, lung sounds, PCV/total solids, and plasma color before, during, and after transfusion.
• If pulmonary thromboembolism is suspected, check chest radiographs and arterial blood gases frequently.

PREVENTION/AVOIDANCE
• Carefully record any transfusion reaction in the patient's medical file.
• Adhere to standard transfusion protocols (e.g., blood typing; cross-matching; use of healthy donors; and appropriate collection, storage, and administration techniques).

POSSIBLE COMPLICATIONS
• Fulminant hemolysis may cause acute renal failure, pulmonary thromboembolism, multiorgan thromboembolism, DIC, and cardiac arrhythmias.
• Volume overload may cause heart failure.
• Cardiac arrest

EXPECTED COURSE AND PROGNOSIS
• Acute course in most animals
• Prognosis good in stable animals, guarded in severely ill animals or when not recognized early
• Cats with type B blood receiving mismatched blood have the worst prognosis.

MISCELLANEOUS

ABBREVIATIONS
• DIC = disseminated intravascular coagulation • PCV = packed cell volume

Suggested Reading
Gibson GR, Callan MB, Hoffman V, Giger U. Use of a hemoglobin-based oxygen-carrying solution in cats: 72 cases (1998–2000). J Am Vet Med Assoc 2002;221:96–102.
Harrell KA, Kristensen AT. Canine transfusion reactions and their management. Vet Clin North Am Small An Pract 1995;25:1333–1364.
Author Jörg Bücheler
Consulting Editor Stephen A. Kruth

BASICS

OVERVIEW
A contagious bacterial disease of cats that primarily causes respiratory abnormalities

SIGNALMENT
• Most severe in kittens <6 weeks old and kittens living in less than ideal hygienic conditions
• Occurs at all ages and often with pre-existing, subclinical airway disease (e.g., feline herpesvirus and calicivirus infections)
• No breed or gender predilection recognized

SIGNS
• May be nonexistent, mild, or severe (e.g., kittens with life-threatening pneumonia); usually begin about 5 days after exposure to infecting agent
• Bacterial agent—spreads rapidly from seemingly healthy cats to others in the same environment
• Fever, sneezing, nasal discharge, mandibular lymphadenopathy, and spontaneous or induced cough characteristic of uncomplicated disease

Severe Disease
• May note constant, low-grade, or fluctuating fever (39.4–40°C; 103–104°F)
• Cough—may be noted; moist and productive
• Nasal discharge
• Lethargy
• Anorexia
• Dyspnea
• Lung sounds—often normal; may detect increased intensity of normal sounds, crackles, or (less frequently) wheezes

CAUSES & RISK FACTORS
• *Bordetella bronchiseptica*—a small, aerobic gram-negative coccobacillus
• Coexisting subclinical airway disease—congenital anomalies; chronic bronchitis

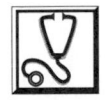

DIAGNOSIS

DIFFERENTIAL DIAGNOSIS
• Specific diagnosis difficult; clinical signs mimic those seen with other respiratory disease agents.
• Several agents may be involved concurrently, which adds to the confusion of signs.
• See Cough

CBC/BIOCHEMISTRY/URINALYSIS
• Neutrophilic leukocytosis with a left shift—frequently found with severe pneumonia
• Serum chemistry profile and urinalysis—usually normal

OTHER LABORATORY TESTS
• Oropharyngeal swab specimens—identify *B. bronchiseptica* infection
• Isolation of the bacterium—with active clinical disease, relatively easy; with chronic carrier state, often few organisms are shed.

IMAGING
Thoracic radiographs—unremarkable with uncomplicated disease; useful for ruling out noninfectious causes; may demonstrate an interstitial and alveolar lung pattern with a cranioventral distribution typical of bacterial pneumonia, a diffuse interstitial lung pattern typical of viral pneumonia, or a mixed lung pattern (combination of alveolar, interstitial, and peribronchial lung patterns)

DIAGNOSTIC PROCEDURES
Endotracheal wash or tracheobronchial lavage via bronchoscopy for suspected severe disease; identify antimicrobial sensitivity pattern—helps develop an effective treatment plan

TREATMENT
• Outpatient—strongly recommended for uncomplicated disease
• Inpatient—strongly recommended for complicated disease and/or pneumonia
• Fluid therapy—with complicated disease and/or pneumonia
• Enforced rest—for at least 14–21 days with uncomplicated disease; for at least the duration of radiographic evidence of pneumonia

MEDICATIONS

DRUG(S)
• Tetracycline (10 mg/kg PO q8h), doxycycline (3–5 mg/kg PO, IV q12h or 10 mg/kg PO q24h), or amoxicillin/clavulanic acid (62.5 mg/cat PO q12h) for 10–14 days
• Antimicrobial therapy—may continue for at least 10 days beyond radiographic resolution

CONTRAINDICATIONS/POSSIBLE INTERACTIONS
Tetracycline and related drugs—may induce a drug fever

FOLLOW-UP

PATIENT MONITORING
• Uncomplicated disease—should respond to treatment in 10–14 days; question diagnosis of uncomplicated disease if respiratory signs exist 14 days or more after initiating treatment
• Severe disease—repeat thoracic radiography until at least 14 days beyond resolution of all clinical signs

PREVENTION/AVOIDANCE
• Shedding of *B. bronchiseptica* in respiratory secretions of asymptomatic carriers—accounts for the persistence of disease in catteries, animal shelters, boarding facilities, and veterinary hospitals
• Vaccine available

POSSIBLE COMPLICATIONS
N/A

EXPECTED COURSE AND PROGNOSIS
• Uncomplicated disease without treatment—natural course, 10–14 days
• Severe disease—typical course, 2–6 weeks
• Death—severe pneumonia that affects multiple lung lobes
• Seroconversion of kittens in infected environments—at 7–10 weeks of age
• Affected cats may shed *B. bronchiseptica* for at least 19 weeks after infection.

MISCELLANEOUS

Suggested Reading

Coutts AJ, Dawson S, Binns S, et al. Studies on natural transmission of *Bordetella bronchiseptica* in cats. Vet Microbiology 1996;48:19–27.
Hoskins JD, Williams J, Rohde KR, et al. The prevalence of feline *Bordetella bronchiseptica* in the respiratory tract. (abst) J Vet Intern Med 1997;11:133.
Jacobs AA, Chalmers WS, Pasman J, et al. Feline bordetellosis: challenge and vaccine studies. Vet Rec 1993;133:260–263.
Author Johnny D. Hoskins
Consulting Editor Lynelle R. Johnson

BOTULISM

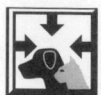

BASICS

OVERVIEW
• Botulism usually results from the ingestion of the preformed *Clostridium botulinum* type C neurotoxin contained in carrion and spoiled foodstuff (e.g., raw meat).
• Botulinal neurotoxin inhibits acetylcholine release at neuromuscular junctions and autonomic cholinergic synapses, resulting in diffuse neuromuscular blockade and autonomic dysfunction.

SIGNALMENT
• Dogs • Cats—susceptible experimentally; no natural cases reported

SIGNS

Historical Findings
• Onset of signs appears a few hours to 6 days after toxin ingestion. • Other dogs of the household, neighborhood, or kennel may be affected. • Acute hindlimb weakness that rapidly ascends to the trunk, front limbs, neck, and muscles innervated by the cranial nerves • Gait—may appear stiff and short-strided (but not ataxic) until recumbence develops (usually within 12–24 hr)

Physical Examination Findings
• Generalized lower motor neuron weakness to tetraplegia—hypotonia or atonia; hyporeflexia or areflexia • Tail—tone and movements (wagging) preserved • Patient remains alert with normal pain perception.
• Cranial nerve dysfunction—dysphagia with pseudoptyalism; weak voice; droopy face with poor eyelid closure; poor jaw and tongue tone; megaesophagus with regurgitation
• Autonomic—mydriasis with decreased pupillary light reflexes; ileus or constipation; urine retention or frequent voiding of small volumes; decreased lacrimation • Muscle atrophy—may be marked after 5–7 days

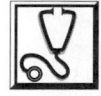

DIAGNOSIS

DIFFERENTIAL DIAGNOSIS
• Coonhound paralysis (acute idiopathic polyradiculoneuritis)—may follow a raccoon bite, systemic illness, or vaccination; cause often unknown; cranial nerve involvement usually limited to facial and pharyngeal/laryngeal paresis; no autonomic signs; diffuse hyperesthesia may be present; CSF protein may be elevated; diffuse denervation potentials on EMG (after 5–7 days) • Tick bite paralysis—in U.S.: cranial nerve involvement unusual or mild; no autonomic signs; rapid recovery after tick removal or insecticide treatment (within 24–72 hr); in Australia: cranial nerve and autonomic involvement; more severe signs that may continue after tick removal; cats may be affected • Myasthenia gravis—

exercise-induced weakness (stiffening gait) leading to collapse; rapid improvement after a short period of rest; megaesophagus common, but other cranial nerve involvement usually limited to moderate facial and pharyngeal/laryngeal paresis; normal spinal reflexes except with the most severe fulminating form in dogs (mimics severe botulism, acute polyradiculoneuritis, and tick bite paralysis); response to IV injection of edrophonium may be mitigated or negative in severe disease (when patient is nonambulatory); elevated antiacetylcholine receptor antibodies are diagnostic in 98% of the canine cases (2% false-negative)

CBC/BIOCHEMISTRY/URINALYSIS
Usually normal

OTHER LABORATORY TESTS
Identify botulinal toxin—in ingested material, serum, vomit, and feces; by neutralization test in small rodents, or in vitro tests (measure toxin antigenicity rather than toxicity).

DIAGNOSTIC PROCEDURES
EMG—usually no or few denervation potentials (more numerous during the recovery phase); reduced amplitude of evoked motor unit potentials

TREATMENT
• Respiratory difficulties—intensive care with maximal capabilities • Swallowing difficulties or regurgitation (megaesophagus)—alimentation by nasogastric or gastrostomy tube • Bladder care (expression or catheterization), if necessary • Turn patient frequently, and provide good bedding to prevent decubital sores. • Passive and active physiotherapy—minimize tendon contraction and muscle atrophy

MEDICATIONS

DRUG(S)
• Type C antitoxin (10,000 to 15,000 U IV or IM twice at 4-hr interval) or polyvalent containing type C antitoxin (5 mL IV or IM; Statens Serum Institute, Copenhagen, Denmark)—may not be available; may cause anaphylaxis; intradermal testing recommended (0.1 mL 20 min prior to systemic administration); not effective after toxin has penetrated the nerve endings but could prevent further binding if absorption is still occurring • Laxative and enemas—if recent ingestion or constipation
• Ophthalmic ointment—prevents exposure corneal ulceration and keratoconjunctivitis sicca • Antibiotics—no benefits (gastrointestinal colonization usually does not occur) if no secondary infections (respiratory,

urinary); potentially detrimental (disturbances of enteric microflora may favor colonization, *Clostridium* organism lysis may lead to further neurotoxin release)
• Neuromuscular potentiators (e.g., 4-aminopyridine, diaminopyridine, guanidine) and anticholinesterase (e.g., neostigmine) have not proven effective or safe.

CONTRAINDICATIONS/POSSIBLE INTERACTIONS
Aminoglycosides, procaine penicillin, tetracyclines, phenothiazines, antiarrhythmic agents, and magnesium—may potentiate neuromuscular blockade

FOLLOW-UP

PATIENT MONITORING
• Monitor intensively during initial progressive phase to assist patient with developing respiratory difficulties (tachypneic, superficial, diaphragmatic breathing). • Meticulously manage the airway in patients with ventilatory support.

PREVENTION/AVOIDANCE
• Prevent access to carrion. • Thoroughly cook food fed to dogs, especially spoiled raw meat stuff from slaughterhouses; freezing does not inactivate botulinal toxin.

POSSIBLE COMPLICATIONS
• Respiratory failure and death in severe cases • Aspiration pneumonia from regurgitation or false deglutition • Keratoconjunctivitis sicca and corneal ulceration • Prolonged recumbence—pulmonary atelectasia and infection; decubital sores; urine scalding

EXPECTED COURSE AND PROGNOSIS
• Maximum severity of signs usually reached within 12–24 hr • Signs disappear in the reverse order in which they appeared • Complete recovery usually occurs within 1–3 weeks, and requires the formation of new nerve terminals and functional neuromuscular junctions.

MISCELLANEOUS

SEE ALSO
• Coonhound Paralysis (Idiopathic Polyradiculoneuritis) • Myasthenia Gravis • Tick Bite Paralysis

ABBREVIATIONS
CSF = cerebrospinal fluid
EMG = electromyography

Suggested Reading
Barsanti JA. Botulism. In: Greene CE, ed. Infectious diseases of the dog and cat. 2nd ed. Philadelphia: Saunders, 1998:263–267.
Author Andrée D. Quesnel
Consulting Editor Joane M. Parent

BASICS

OVERVIEW
• Trauma with traction and/or abduction of the forelimb causes avulsion of nerve rootlets from their spinal cord attachment. • Ventral (motor) roots are more susceptible than are dorsal (sensory) roots. • Rule out nerve root avulsion in traumatized animals not able to bear weight on a forelimb, especially before surgical repair of orthopedic injuries.

SIGNALMENT
• Dogs and cats
• No age, sex, or breed predilection

SIGNS
• Depend on the extent and distribution of rootlet damage • Motor signs—weakness to paralysis (ventral root avulsion)
• Sensory signs—decreased to absent pain perception (dorsal root avulsion)
• Muscle atrophy—begins within a week of injury • Complete avulsion—spinal nerves C5 to T2; most common; combines cranial and caudal avulsion deficits
• Cranial avulsion—spinal nerves C5 to C7; causes loss of shoulder movements, elbow flexion (dropped elbow), and analgesia of the craniodorsal scapula and medial forearm; if roots C8 to T2 preserved: weight-bearing remains almost normal; hemiplegia of the diaphragm may be seen by fluoroscopy (phrenic nerve roots C5 to C7).
• Caudal avulsion—spinal nerves C7 to T2; causes inability to bear weight, with knuckling over dorsum of paw; if C5 to C7 spared: limb held in a flexed position and analgesia distal to the elbow (except for a small area on medial aspect of forearm); T1 to T2 involvement: causes an ipsilateral partial Horner syndrome (anisocoria only) and lack of ipsilateral contraction of the cutaneous trunci reflex (contraction present contralaterally)
• Bilateral—rarely encountered after a significant fall with sternal landing

CAUSES & RISK FACTORS
Trauma—road accident; hung by foot; fall

DIAGNOSIS

DIFFERENTIAL DIAGNOSIS
• Brachial plexus trauma without avulsion—rare; temporary deficit owing to root contusion • Brachial plexus tumor—usually chronic onset • Brachial plexus neuritis—rare, bilateral deficits. Acute onset but no trauma
• Fibrocartilaginous emboli myelopathy—mild deficits of the ipsilateral and contralateral hindlimbs and mild deficits of contralateral forelimb

• Pure radial nerve paralysis caused by fracture of the humerus or first rib—no nerve root sign

CBC/BIOCHEMISTRY/URINALYSIS
Usually normal

OTHER LABORATORY TESTS
N/A

IMAGING
High-definition CT or MRI scan—visualize lesion; rarely needed for diagnosis

DIAGNOSTIC PROCEDURES
• Clinical—history of trauma with sudden onset of typical neurologic deficits
• Define involved spinal nerve roots—map motor and sensory deficits; note signs of Horner syndrome; determine cutaneous trunci reflex
• Electrophysiology (EMG)—shows denervation in affected muscles 5–7 days post-injury; with nerve conduction studies, may help further define deficits and detect signs of recovery

PATHOLOGIC FINDINGS
• Ventral and dorsal root avulsions—intradurally at the level of root–spinal cord junction (most fragile area, because it lacks protective perineurium)
• Neuroma formation—on the pial surface of the spinal cord

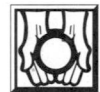

TREATMENT

APPROPRIATE HEALTH CARE
• No specific treatment
• Outcome depends on initial damage.
• Amputation of limb—advisable for patients showing complications and no improvement
• Carpal fusion (arthrodesis) and transposition of the biceps muscle tendon—consider only with adequate function of the triceps muscle and musculocutaneous

NURSING CARE
• Use protective wrapping or boot when patient walks on rough surfaces, because of increased skin fragility and lack of protective reflexes in the affected limb.
• Physical therapy—crucial for keeping joints and muscles mobile during recovery of reversible injuries
• Monitor noncomplicated cases for 4–6 months before considering amputation.

MEDICATIONS

DRUG(S)
Prednisolone (prednisone)—initial anti-inflammatory course for 1 week; may decrease edema and favor healing of reversible components of injury

CONTRAINDICATIONS/POSSIBLE INTERACTIONS
N/A

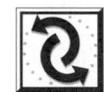

FOLLOW-UP

PATIENT MONITORING
Serial clinical and electrophysiologic monitoring—assess improvement

PREVENTION/AVOIDANCE
Avoid free roaming.

POSSIBLE COMPLICATIONS
• Skin excoriation with secondary infection of the digit(s)—from rubbing the paw on the ground • Trophic ulcers—on thin, traumatized skin, especially over arthrodesis sites • Self-mutilation—often devastating; result of paresthesia

EXPECTED COURSE AND PROGNOSIS
• Preserved pain sensation (dorsal roots intact)—suggests less severe injury to the ventral nerve roots • Cranial avulsion—better prognosis because sensation to the distal limb and ability to bear weight are spared
• Complete avulsion—poor prognosis for recovery, amputation likely • Rarely, mild cases may resolve after 2–3 months.

MISCELLANEOUS

SEE ALSO
Peripheral Neuropathies (Polyneuropathies)

ABBREVIATIONS
• CT = computed tomography
• EMG = electromyography
• MRI = magnetic resonance imaging

Suggested Reading

Bailey CS. Patterns of cutaneous anesthesia associated with brachial plexus avulsions in the dog. J Am Vet Med Assoc 1984; 185:889–899.

Cuddon PA, Delauche AJ, Hutchison JM. Assessment of dorsal nerve root and spinal cord dorsal horn function in clinically normal dogs by determination of cord dorsum potentials. Am J Vet Res 1999;60(2): 222–226.

Moissonnier P, Duchossoy Y, Lavieille S, Horvat JC. Lateral approach of the dog brachial plexus for ventral root reimplantation. Spinal Cord 1998;36(6):391–398.

Platt SR, Graham J, Chrisman CL, et al. Magnetic resonance imaging and ultrasonography in the diagnosis of a malignant peripheral nerve sheath tumor in a dog. Vet Radiol Ultrasound 1999;40(4):367–371.

Author Christine Berthelin-Baker
Consulting Editor Joane M. Parent

BRACHYCEPHALIC AIRWAY SYNDROME

 BASICS

DEFINITION
Partial upper airway obstruction caused by any combination of the following: stenotic nares, overlong soft palate, everted laryngeal saccules, and hypoplastic trachea in brachycephalic breeds of dogs and cats.

PATHOPHYSIOLOGY
• In normal dogs the upper airway accounts for 50–70% of total airway resistance, but congenital conditions (stenotic nares, overlong soft palate, and hypoplastic trachea) cause this to be a higher percentage in brachycephalic breeds. • Skull bones of brachycephalic breeds are shortened in length but are of normal width. Soft tissues are not proportionately reduced, resulting in narrowed air passages and redundant tissue that may cause obstruction of the glottis. • Increased airway resistance causes increased negative airway pressures that may result in eversion of laryngeal saccules, further elongation of palate, and laryngeal collapse. • Analysis of respiratory patterns has shown that brachycephalic dogs often have a combination of fixed and dynamic airway obstruction. • Recruitment of pharyngeal dilator muscles (sternohyoid) becomes necessary to maintain airway patency. Sleep apnea (sleep disordered breathing) may occur secondary to relaxation of muscles of pharyngeal dilation. • Severe upper airway obstruction can result in development of non-cardiogenic pulmonary edema.

SYSTEMS AFFECTED
• Respiratory—respiratory distress, hypoxemia, hypercarbia, hyperthermia, aspiration pneumonia • Cardiovascular—cardiovascular collapse if complete airway obstruction or severe hyperthermia occurs. • Musculoskeletal—exercise intolerance, collapse • Gastrointestinal—if severe, may result in reluctance to eat or drink, and increased airway resistance may exacerbate hiatal hernia.

GENETICS
• No specific genes have been identified. • Brachycephalic head shape inherited defect of development of skull bones perpetuated by selective breeding.

INCIDENCE/PREVALENCE
• Common in brachycephalic breeds of dogs • Cats—uncommonly severe enough to require treatment

SIGNALMENT

Species
Dogs and cats

Breed Predilections
• Dogs—English bulldogs (most common), pugs, Boston terriers, boxers, Pekingese, Cavalier King Charles spaniels, Shih Tzu, Sharpei, and others. • Cats—Persians and Himalayans

Mean Age and Range
• Young adults, most diagnosed by 2–3 years.

• If diagnosed later than 4 years look for concurrent disease or exacerbating circumstances. Older dogs have poorer outcome postoperatively.

Predominant Sex
No sex predilection.

SIGNS

Historical Findings
• Snoring, stridor, stertorous breathing • Tachypnea, frequent panting • Coughing and gagging, or difficulty eating and swallowing • Inability to perform physical activity and worsening of condition during warm and humid weather • Occasionally, syncope and episodes of collapse

Physical Examination Findings
• Stridor and stertorous breathing • Stenotic nares—diagnosed if medial collapse of lateral nasal cartilage is present and there is a failure of the nares to dilate on inspiration • Increased respiratory effort—retraction of the commissures of the lips, open-mouth breathing or constant panting, increased respiratory rate, abduction of forelimbs, increased abdominal component of respiration, recruitment of the secondary muscles of respiration • If in severe distress, may see paradoxical abdominal movement, inward collapse of intercostals, orthopnea, and cyanosis. • Hyperthermia may be present. • May appear anxious and resent restraint.

CAUSES
• Inherited or congenital defects in conformation • Elongated soft palate—reported in up to 100% of cases in dogs • Stenotic nares—reported in about 50% of cases in dogs. Most common defect in cats • Laryngeal disease—everted laryngeal saccules and/or laryngeal collapse reported in about 30% of cases • Hypoplastic trachea

RISK FACTORS
• Breed • Obesity—worsens airway obstruction, associated with poorer outcome postoperatively, and may contribute to gastroesophageal reflux and development of aspiration pneumonia. • Hypoplastic trachea results in decreased mucociliary clearance, worsens aspiration pneumonia, and increases airway resistance. • Warm, humid weather—increased panting can lead to edema of the airway, further compromise of the airway, and hyperthermia. • Exercise—dogs are often exercise-intolerant owing to airway compromise and hypoxia. Forced exercise may lead to rapid development of hyperthermia and collapse. • Excitement—can cause increased panting, resulting in edema, increased airway obstruction, and hyperthermia • Sedation—relaxation of muscles of pharynx, palate, and pharyngeal dilators may cause complete airway obstruction. • Sleep—decreased activity of pharyngeal dilators can result in airway obstruction and reduction in arterial PO_2. • Allergic reactions—acute allergic reactions causing airway edema may cause airway obstruction. • Pulmonary disease (pneumonia, pulmonary edema)—will cause further respiratory compromise. • Endocrine

disease (hypothyroidism and hyperadrenocorticism)—could worsen weight gain and cause excessive panting.

 DIAGNOSIS

DIFFERENTIAL DIAGNOSES
• Foreign bodies of nasopharynx, larynx or trachea • Infection—upper respiratory infection, nasopharyngeal abscesses • Neoplasia obstructing the nasopharynx, glottis, larynx or trachea • Laryngeal paralysis • Tracheal collapse • Pharyngeal mucocele • Allergic reaction causing upper airway swelling

CBC/BIOCHEMISTRY/URINALYSIS
• CBC—usually normal, but polycythemia can occur with chronic hypoxia, and leukocytosis if concurrent infection or severe stress. • Chemistry screen—usually normal, but an increase in total protein and pre-renal azotemia (increased BUN, creatinine) may be present if dehydrated. An elevated T_{CO_2} may be seen with respiratory acidosis. • Urinalysis—N/A

OTHER LABORATORY TESTS
• Arterial blood gas—to determine degree of hypercarbia, presence of a respiratory acidosis, and degree of hypoxia and response to oxygen supplementation. Also can assess presence of metabolic acidosis. • Venous blood gas—less stressful to obtain than arterial sample, and can provide information about pH and metabolic derangements.

IMAGING

Radiographic Findings
• If animal can tolerate radiography, cervical and thoracic radiographs recommended. • Cervical radiographs may reveal thickened, elongated soft palate and possible tracheal collapse. • Thoracic radiographs may reveal aspiration pneumonia, pulmonary edema, heart failure, air in the esophagus, and hypoplastic trachea (TD/TI = tracheal diameter at the level of thoracic inlet/Thoracic inlet distance which is the distance from the sternum to the ventral surface of T1. A ratio < 0.13 in bulldogs and < 0.16 in non-bulldog brachycephalics suggests hypoplastic trachea).

Fluoroscopy
Can give information about degree of dynamic pharyngeal obstruction by palate and concurrent disease such as collapsing trachea, but is not essential, especially in patients in respiratory distress.

DIAGNOSTIC PROCEDURES

Pulse Oximetry
Rapid and non-invasive, gives measure of SpO_2 (percent oxygen saturation of hemoglobin).

Laryngoscopy/pharyngoscopy
• Performed under general anesthesia, and because of risk of airway obstruction, owner should be prepared to proceed with surgical intervention if deemed necessary. • An overlong soft palate extends more than just a few millimeters beyond tip of epiglottis and hangs

down into glottis. • The palate is often thickened and inflamed and there may be inflammation and edema of the arytenoid cartilages. • Dorsally displacing the soft palate improves visualization of the larynx. • Everted laryngeal saccules are diagnosed by visualizing two smooth, round, glistening masses in the ventral half of the laryngeal opening—they often obscure visualization of the vocal folds. • There are 3 stages of laryngeal collapse: stage 1 is the development of laryngeal saccule eversion, stage 2 is medial deviation of the cuneiform cartilage and aryepiglottic fold or aryepiglottic fold collapse, and stage 3 is characterized by medial deviation of corniculate process of the arytenoids and medial flattening of cuneiform processes allowing overlap of the arytenoid cartilages. Stage 2 and 3 laryngeal collapse are severe.

Tracheoscopy
• May reveal hypoplastic trachea with overlap of dorsal tracheal rings and dorsal tracheal membrane. • Collapsing trachea may also be diagnosed and location and severity assessed.

TREATMENT

APPROPRIATE HEALTH CARE
• No treatment necessary for patients without clinical signs. Avoidance of risk factors recommended. • Surgery recommended for patients with significant clinical signs. • Emergency presentation in severe respiratory distress requires rapid intervention. • Oxygen supplementation • If hyperthermic, should be cooled with cool water and by directing a fan to blow over the patient (increase convective heat loss). IV fluids should be administered, up to a shock rate if extremely hyperthermic (T > 106). • If complete airway obstruction, orotracheal intubation and/or temporary tracheostomy • Dexamethasone can be administered IV at a dose of 0.1 mg/kg to reduce inflammation.

NURSING CARE
• Patients require 24-hour monitoring because of risk of acute airway obstruction and death. • Respiratory rate, effort, heart rate, pulse quality, mucous membrane color, capillary refill time, temperature, and other physical parameters should be monitored. • Pulse oximetry and arterial blood gases may be monitored, depending on severity of condition. • Intravenous fluids are administered at maintenance rate and handling and stress are minimized. • Oxygen therapy and cooling as necessary

ACTIVITY
• Usually self-limited • Dogs should not be forced to exercise, especially in warm weather.

DIET
• Weight loss is recommended for all overweight dogs. • For obese, stable patients, weight loss is recommended prior to surgery.

CLIENT EDUCATION
• Education about avoidance of risk factors is critical. • Client should be informed that dogs with brachycephalic airway syndrome are at increased anesthetic risk, and an even higher risk occurs with concurrent obesity, cardiac disease, and aspiration pneumonia. • Owner should be made aware that corrective surgery often improves but does not result in a completely normal airway. • Owners of show dogs should be informed that the American Kennel Club will not allow a dog that has had surgery for stenotic nares or elongated soft palate to compete.

SURGICAL CONSIDERATIONS
• Evaluation for elongated soft palate generally performed under general anesthesia when patient stable. • Temporary tracheostomy can be placed to facilitate exposure or to treat airway obstruction. • Stenotic nares are corrected by resection of a wedge of the dorsolateral nasal cartilage and planum. Hemorrhage is temporarily controlled with pressure followed by closure of the surgical wound with 3 or 4 sutures of 3-0 or 4-0 absorbable suture material. • Elongated soft palate is resected using scissors or carbon dioxide laser from caudal to midpoint of the tonsil to a length that allows contact with the tip of the epiglottis and the center of the soft palate. • Permanent tracheostomy may be necessary if severe laryngeal collapse. • Dexamethasone given for 12–24 hours post-operatively at 0.1 mg/kg IV q12h to reduce edema and inflammation

MEDICATIONS

DRUG(S)
• Dexamethasone given for 12–24 hours pre- or post-operatively at 0.1 mg/kg IV q12h to reduce edema and inflammation • Broad spectrum antibiotics are indicated if aspiration pneumonia present until culture and sensitivity results are obtained.

PRECAUTIONS
Sedation for relief of anxiety, excitement or fear should be used with extreme caution because of the risk of upper airway obstruction with muscle relaxation.

FOLLOW-UP

PATIENT MONITORING
• Post-operatively, require 24 hour monitoring to observe for airway swelling and obstruction, requiring temporary tracheostomy.
• Respiratory rate, effort, heart rate, pulse quality, mucous membrane color, capillary refill time, temperature, and other physical parameters should be monitored. • Owner needs to be educated about clinical signs to monitor at home such as open-mouth breathing

or constant panting, increased respiratory rate, abduction of forelimbs, restlessness, and increased noise of breathing.

PREVENTION/AVOIDANCE
• Selection by breeders for dogs without severe conformational changes—may be difficult because breed standards encourage these structural abnormalities. • Avoid risk factors

POSSIBLE COMPLICATIONS
• Hyperthermia and heat stroke • Aspiration pneumonia • Death in about 10% of patients as a result of airway disease. • The most common post-operative complication is airway swelling and obstruction within the first 24 hours, may necessitate temporary tracheostomy. • Continued respiratory difficulty after corrective surgery • Excessive resection of palate resulting in nasal aspiration of food contents due to inability to close nasopharynx during swallowing

EXPECTED COURSE AND PROGNOSIS
• Prognosis is good for improvement in breathing (about 60% have good to excellent results) but airway is still far from normal. • Prognosis better for dogs other than English Bulldogs and for dogs that had concurrent correction of stenotic nares and elongated soft palate. • Without surgery, prognosis is poor due to continued progression of acquired components of brachycephalic airway syndrome. • Lifelong avoidance of risk factors recommended to reduce chance of decompensation or worsening of disease.

MISCELLANEOUS

ASSOCIATED CONDITIONS
• Aspiration pneumonia • Heat Stroke

AGE-RELATED FACTORS
Without surgical therapy, disease process will worsen as patient develops acquired components of brachycephalic airway disease.

PREGNANCY
Enlarged abdomen may further compromise respiratory function of the pregnant bitch by decreasing tidal volume from pressure on the diaphragm.

SEE ALSO
Stertor and Stridor

Suggested Reading
Davidson EB, Davis MS, Campbell KK, et al. Evaluation of carbon dioxide laser and conventional incisional techniques for resection of soft palates in brachycephalic dogs. J Am Vet Med Assoc 2001;219:776–781.
Lorinson D, Bright RM, and White RA. Brachycephalic airway obstruction syndrome—a review of 118 cases. Canine Pract 1997;22:18–21.
Authors David A. Puerto and Lori S. Waddell
Consulting Editor Lynelle R. Johnson

BRAIN INJURY

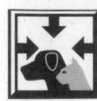 BASICS

DEFINITION

• Primary—direct result of the initial insult; complete at the time of presentation; cannot be altered • Secondary—alteration of brain tissue; anatomic or physiologic; occurs after a primary injury; can be prevented or ameliorated with optimal supportive care

PATHOPHYSIOLOGY

• Brain—high oxygen and glucose requirements; minimal storage of oxygen; few recruitable capillaries; consumes oxygen at a constant rate; stage is set for hypoxic injury • Secondary—from bleeding, cerebral edema, or vasospasms; causes elevation in ICP • Elevated ICP—vicious circle occurs when high ICP leads to low cerebral perfusion and blood flow, leading to further ischemia and brain swelling; may result in brain shift or herniation; slow, progressive rise in ICP better tolerated than a small acute increase • Hypotension and hypoxia—the major contributors to ICP elevation and secondary brain injury; at the cellular level: high energy substrates depleted and anaerobic glycolysis results in lactic acid production and intracellular acidosis

SYSTEMS AFFECTED

• Nervous—secondary brain injury and interruption of function • Ophthalmic—potential changes in eye position, eye movements, pupillary light reflexes, and vision • Cardiovascular—arrhythmias caused by dysfunction of central cardiovascular centers • Respiratory—abnormal breathing patterns caused by dysfunction of regulatory centers • Musculoskeletal—possible postural and/or gait abnormalities caused by lesions of the central motor pathways

GENETICS N/A

SIGNS

Historical Findings

• Determine possible cause—trauma; cardiac arrest; prolonged syncopal episodes; severe heart failure; thromboembolic episodes; coagulopathies with intracranial bleeding; prolonged severe respiratory compromise • Decline in the level of consciousness—implies progression of secondary brain injury from intracranial bleeding or cerebral edema • Seizure activity—localizes lesion to the cerebral cortex or diencephalon • Trauma—associated with secondary brain injury from either bleeding or cerebral edema • Ischemia—associated with secondary brain injury from cerebral edema

Physical Examination Findings

• Look for external and internal evidence of trauma. • Hypoxia or cyanosis, ecchymosis or petechiations, or cardiac or respiratory insufficiency—metabolic causes • Retinal hemorrhages or distended vessels—hypertension or coagulopathy • Papilledema—cerebral edema • Retinal detachment—infectious, neoplastic, or hypertensive causes • Sustained bradycardia with normal potassium—midbrain, pontine, or medullary lesion • Blood from the ears or nose—severe trauma with intracranial bleeding • Palpation of the skull—reveals fractures that require surgical decompression • Ischemic causes—examine carefully for cardiovascular, respiratory, or hemorrhagic problems.

Neurologic Examination Findings

• Can worsen dramatically during resuscitative efforts owing to hypertension and intracranial bleeding • Determine level of consciousness and whether patient is arousable. • Oculocephalic reflex—perform if cervical manipulation is possible; loss of physiologic vestibular nystagmus indicates brainstem involvement. • Postural changes—decerebrate rigidity: midbrain lesion • Absence of lateralizing signs suggests diffuse cerebrocortical involvement.

Pupillary Light Reflexes

• Miotic responsive pupils—cerebral or diencephalic lesion • Dilated unresponsive pupils (unilateral or bilateral) or midpoint fixed unresponsive pupils—midbrain lesion • Miotic or normal pupils—pontine or medullary lesion

Respiratory Patterns

• Cheyne-Stokes—severe diffuse cerebral or diencephalic pathology • Hyperventilation—midbrain pathology • Ataxic or apneustic—pontine or medullary pathology

Cranial Nerves

• Normal—cerebrum-diencephalon lesion • Cranial nerve III deficit—midbrain lesion • Cranial nerves V–XII—pons or medulla lesion

CAUSES

• Head trauma • Prolonged hypoxia or ischemia • Severe hypoglycemia or hyperthermia

RISK FACTORS

• Free roaming—trauma • Coexisting cardiac or respiratory disease

 DIAGNOSIS

DIFFERENTIAL DIAGNOSIS

• Other causes of brain disease—neoplasia; inflammation; immune-mediated processes; infection; congenital problems • Systemic causes of altered states of consciousness—narcolepsy; syncope; metabolic disease; toxins; drugs; infection; nutrition • Other causes of brainstem signs—tentorial herniation after progression of cerebral edema

CBC/BIOCHEMISTRY/URINALYSIS

Reflect systemic effects of trauma or hypoxemia

OTHER LABORATORY TESTS

• Arterial blood gases—hypoxemia; severe pH changes; hypercarbia • Coagulogram—when intracranial bleeding or thrombosis may be cause

IMAGING

• Skull radiographs—fractures in trauma patients • CT scan—excellent for detecting acute hemorrhage within the calvaria; depressed fractures; penetrating foreign bodies

DIAGNOSTIC PROCEDURES

• Measure intracranial pressure—determine severity of ICP elevation and response to therapy • Evaluate brainstem auditory evoked potentials—determine brainstem function • ECG—detect arrhythmias • Blood pressure—determine perfusion.

PATHOLOGIC FINDINGS

• Brain edema • Herniation • Hemorrhage • Laceration • Contusion • Hematomas • Skull fracture

 TREATMENT

APPROPRIATE HEALTH CARE

• Head position—level with the body or elevated to a 20° angle; never lower than the body to avoid significant elevations in ICP • $PaCO_2$—maintain at 35–45 mm Hg; with suspected elevated ICP, hyperventilation to 25–30 mm Hg may reduce cerebral blood flow and ICP. • PaO_2—must be >50 mm Hg to maintain cerebral blood flow autoregulation • Avoid cough or sneeze reflex during intubation or oxygen supplementation by nasal cannula—may severely elevate ICP; give lidocaine (dogs, 0.75 mg/kg IV) before intubation to blunt the gag and cough reflexes—use peripheral veins, leaving the jugular vein blood flow unobstructed; shifting of blood volume into the jugular veins is an important compensatory mechanism during ICP elevation.

NURSING CARE

• Meticulous nursing care prevents secondary complications of recumbency. • Maintain unobstructed airways; use suction and humidify if intubated. • Lubricate the eyes. • Turn the patient every 2 hr to avoid hypostatic pulmonary congestion. • Prevent fecal or urine soiling. • Maintain core body temperature at normal or mild hypothermia; avoid hyperthermia. • Maintain hydration with a balanced electrolyte crystalloid solution • Maintain normal head position.

ACTIVITY

Restricted

DIET
Initiate nutritional support as soon as possible, compensating for elevated metabolic demands of brain injury.

CLIENT EDUCATION
• Inform client that the extent of neurologic recovery may not be evident for several days in the acute phase, and possibly for >6 months for residual neurologic deficits. • Inform client that there may be serious systemic abnormalities that could contribute to the instability of the nervous system.

SURGICAL CONSIDERATIONS
Worsening of neurologic signs, increased ICP not responsive to medical therapy, midbrain signs with history of cerebral trauma or bleed, depressed skull fracture, or penetrating foreign body—seriously consider surgical decompression and exploration

MEDICATIONS
DRUG(S) OF CHOICE
Poor Perfusion
• Resuscitate with a minimal amount of crystalloids, because these contribute to brain edema. • Small-volume resuscitation—combination of crystalloids with large-molecular-weight colloids (hetastarch at 5 mL/kg increments over 5–8 min; use minimal amount to maintain systolic blood pressure >90 mm Hg)
• Do not use colloids with intracranial hemorrhage.

Systolic Arterial Blood Pressure
• Raise rapidly and maintain >90 mm Hg using crystalloids and/or colloids. • Avoid hypertension.

Elevated Intracranial Pressure (ICP)
• Lower by hyperventilation, drug therapy, drainage of CSF from the ventricles, or surgical decompression.
• Mannitol—0.1–0.5 g/kg IV bolus repeated at 2-hr intervals 3–4 times in dogs and 2–3 times in cats; repeated doses must be given on time; improves brain blood flow and lowers ICP; most commonly used in patients with hypoxic, ischemic, or traumatic brain injury and declining neurologic status or if surgical decompression is imminent; may exacerbate hemorrhage
• Furosemide—0.75 mg/kg IV; decreases CSF production; lowers ICP; preferably used in patients with hemorrhage, congestive heart failure, volume overload, and hyperosmolar diseases or anuric renal failure; use before mannitol or as sole diuretic.
• High-dose methylprednisolone—no benefit in the acute management of brain injury in

humans; no effect on reducing ICP; no effect on the volume–pressure response (a measure of brain elastance); no improvement on long-term outcome
• Prevent thrashing, seizures, or any other form of uncontrolled motor activity that may elevate ICP; diazepam infusion (0.5–1.0 mg/kg/hr) may be required.
• Barbiturate coma—for refractory ICP elevation; administer loading dose of pentobarbital to effect (up to 10 mg/kg IV over 30 min; maintain at 1 mg/kg/hr by constant rate infusion); must intubate patient and support blood pressure, oxygenation, and ventilation

Other
• Cooling the patient down to 32–33°C (89–91°F) may provide cerebral protection when administered within 6 hr of global ischemia or severe brain injury.
• Glucose supplementation—as required for hypoglycemia
• Tube-feeding may be required for early nutritional support; cisapride (0.5 mg/kg q8–12h) may be necessary to promote GI motility.

CONTRAINDICATIONS
• Drugs that cause hypertension
• Drugs that cause hyperexcitability
• Do not use colloids when there is intracranial hemorrhage.

PRECAUTIONS
• Avoid hypertension.
• Avoid intravascular volume overload.
• Do not allow head to lie below plane of body.
• Do not use the jugular veins.
• Mannitol and hypertonic saline—may worsen neurologic status when there is intracranial hemorrhage
• Hyperventilation—maintain PCO_2 >25 mm Hg; do not perform for extended periods (>48 hr).

POSSIBLE INTERACTIONS N/A
ALTERNATIVE DRUG(S) N/A

FOLLOW-UP
PATIENT MONITORING
• Neurologic examinations—detect deterioration of function that warrants aggressive therapeutic intervention. • Blood pressure—keep fluid therapy adequate for perfusion but avoid hypertension. • Blood gases—assess need for oxygen supplementation or ventilation; monitor PCO_2 when hyperventilation is required. • Blood glucose—ensure adequate blood level to maintain brain functions and avoid hyperosmolality from high amounts.

• ECG—detect arrhythmias that may affect perfusion, oxygenation, and cerebral blood flow. • ICP—to detect significant elevations; monitor success of therapeutics.

PREVENTION/AVOIDANCE
Keep pets in a confined area with supervised activity.

POSSIBLE COMPLICATIONS
• Increasing ICP • Brain herniation
• Intracranial hemorrhage • Progression from cerebrocortical to midbrain signs • Seizures
• Malnutrition • Hypostatic pulmonary congestion • Corneal desiccation • Urine scalding • Airway obstruction from mucus
• Cardiac arrhythmias—usually bradyarrhythmias • Hypotension
• Hypernatremia • Hypokalemia • Respiratory failure • Death

EXPECTED COURSE AND PROGNOSIS
• Minimal primary brain injury and secondary injury consisting of cerebral edema—best prognosis • No deterioration of neurologic status for 48 hr—better prognosis • Rapid resuscitation of systolic blood pressure to >90 mm Hg—better neurologic outcome

MISCELLANEOUS
ASSOCIATED CONDITIONS N/A
AGE-RELATED FACTORS N/A
ZOONOTIC POTENTIAL N/A
PREGNANCY N/A
SYNONYMS
• Head trauma • Traumatic brain injury

SEE ALSO
Stupor and Coma

ABBREVIATIONS
• CSF = cerebrospinal fluid
• ICP = intracranial pressure

Suggested Reading
Bullock R. Mannitol and other diuretics in severe neurotrauma. N Horizons 1995;3:448–452.
Hayek DA, Veremakis C. Therapeutic options in brain resuscitation. In: Veremakis C, ed. Problems in critical care: resuscitation following acute brain injury. Philadelphia: Lippincott, 1991:156–186.
Kelly DF. Steroids in head injury. N Horizons 1995;3:453–455.
Wilberger JE, Cantella D. High-dose barbiturates for intracranial pressure control. N Horizons 1995;3:469–473.
Author Rebecca Kirby
Consulting Editor Joane M. Parent

BREEDING, TIMING

BASICS

DEFINITION
Timing of inseminations during estrus to maximize fertility

PATHOPHYSIOLOGY
Dogs
• Multiple breedings—mate every other day during estrus to maximize fertility.
• Fresh, cooled, or frozen semen—usually limited to one or two inseminations; requires insemination to be timed with ovulation for maximum fertility
• Precise estimation of day of ovulation—variations in time of ovulation in relation to onset of behavioral or cytologic estrus; reduced longevity of semen; bitch that refuses to allow natural mating
• Luteinizing hormone (LH)—controls ovulation; peaks on same day or up to 2 days after full cornification is observed; ovulation occurs approximately 2 days after the surge; 2–3 days more required for oocyte maturation; mature oocytes viable for another 2–3 days; thus fertile period is 4–8 days after the surge, and fertility peaks 5–6 days after the surge; assay is a precise method for determining the day of the surge.
• Physical signs alone—may be unreliable for precise determination of fertile period
• Onset of estrus—usually associated with a change in the vaginal discharge from sanguinous to straw-colored and a reduction of vulvar swelling; sanguinous discharge may continue during estrus and cease only at the onset of diestrus (fertile period has passed; bitch no longer receptive)
• Receptivity—may be detected by stroking near the tailhead; if receptive, female will flag by elevating the tail to one side
• Vaginal cytologic examination—better indicator of fertile period than behavioral or physical signs; cornification of the vaginal epithelium controlled by estrogen; full cornification usually coincides with sexual receptivity; estimation of the day of ovulation, which is controlled by LH, on the basis of vaginal cytologic examination is imprecise.
• Serum progesterone—increase closely associated with the LH peak; useful for predicting the surge and estimating ovulation, and thus the fertile period; concentration <1 ng/ml (3.18 nmol/L) before the surge, 1.5–2.0 ng/ml (4.8–6.4 nmol/L) on the day of the surge, approximately 4–10 ng/mL (12.7–31.8 nmol/L) at ovulation; continues to rise during diestrus or pregnancy; consider pattern of rise as well as actual values.

Cats
• Ovulation—induced; timing of breeding is not as critical as with dogs; depends on adequate LH release, which is triggered by stimulation of the vagina and cervix

• Inadequate stimulation—characterized by lack of both a copulatory cry and a postcoital reaction; may fail to induce ovulation; frequency of coital stimuli important in determining adequacy of coital contact
• LH—peak concentration and duration of the elevation determine ovulation; higher plasma concentration with multiple copulations (more likely to result in ovulation than single mating); response to copulation depends on the day of estrus (greater release on estrus day 3 than on estrus day 1); release partially depends on duration of exposure to estrogen

SYSTEMS AFFECTED
• Renal
• Reproductive

GENETICS
N/A

INCIDENCE/PREVALENCE
N/A

GEOGRAPHIC DISTRIBUTION
N/A

SIGNALMENT
N/A

SIGNS
General Comments
Dogs
• Normal bitch—sanguinous discharge during proestrus becomes straw-colored during estrus; vulvar swelling of proestrus decreases slightly during estrus; receptive to male during estrus
• Limited number of available breedings—must know ovulation day
Cats
• LH response to a single mating—may vary substantially
• Neither single nor multiple copulations ensure ovulation.

Historical Findings
Dogs
• Refusal to accept male at the expected time
• Sanguinous vulvar discharge during estrus
Cats
• Return to estrus in <30 days—indicates failure to ovulate; interestrus (postestrus) usually 8–10 days during reproductive cycling

Physical Examination Findings
Dogs
• Fully cornified vaginal epithelium
• Interest shown by male
• Swollen vulva
• Vaginal discharge
• Flagging
Cats
• Fully cornified vaginal epithelium
• Interest shown by male
• No changes in external genitalia
• Vocalizes, rubs objects
• Lordotic posture ("dragster posture")

CAUSES
Dogs
• Limited number of breedings
• Female unreceptive to male
• Breeding by artificial insemination (fresh, cooled, or frozen semen)

Cats
• Coitus—too early or too late in estrus; too few times
• Breeding by artificial insemination (fresh, cooled, or frozen semen)

RISK FACTORS
N/A

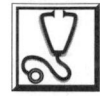

DIAGNOSIS

DIFFERENTIAL DIAGNOSIS
• Vaginal discharge—proestrus or estrus; vaginitis; neoplasia
• Refused to allow intromission—vaginal stricture

CBC/BIOCHEMISTRY/URINALYSIS
N/A

OTHER LABORATORY TESTS
Dogs
• In-house semiquantitative progesterone testing—as an adjunct to vaginal cytologic examination; to establish a baseline, begin when vaginal cytologic examination reveals 60–75% cornified epithelial cells; with no cytologic examination, begin early in proestrus (day 3 or 4); perform every other day.
• Quantitative progesterone testing—more accurate; preferred with frozen semen use
• In-house LH testing—must run samples daily to observe the LH peak

Cats
Submit samples for progesterone testing to verify ovulation.

IMAGING
Ultrasonographic imaging of the ovaries—may help determine ovulation; not reliable as the sole method of verifying ovulation

DIAGNOSTIC PROCEDURES
Dogs
• Vaginal cytologic examination—at the onset of proestrus, most epithelial cells appear noncornified (nucleus appears stippled like a normal viable cell); percentage of cornified epithelial cells (cells with angular cytoplasm and pyknotic nuclei or nuclei that fail to take up stain) increases by approximately 10% per day during proestrus, reaching 90% or more by estrus. At the onset of diestrus, an abrupt decline in the percentage of cornified epithelial cells (usually 20–30%, often as great as 50%) occurs in a single day; the first day of noticeable decline in cornification is defined as Day 1 of diestrus (D1); normal to see neutrophils on days 2–4 of diestrus

• Vaginoscopy—hyperplastic and wrinkled vaginal epithelium from proestrus to estrus

PATHOLOGIC FINDINGS
N/A

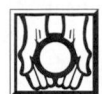

TREATMENT

APPROPRIATE HEALTH CARE

Dogs
• Multiple breedings—inseminate every other day after the initial rise in progesterone is observed until D1
• Two breedings—inseminate either on days 3 and 5 or on days 4 and 6 after the LH peak or initial rise in progesterone (day 0); use fresh chilled semen (viability lower than fresh semen)
• Frozen semen—less viable than fresh chilled, thus timing is more critical; inseminate vaginally on days 4, 5, and 6 after the LH rise; a single surgical insemination more common: inseminate surgically on day 5 or 6 after the LH peak or initial rise in progesterone (day 0) or 3 days after progesterone ≥5 ng/mL (16 nmol/L); transcervical intrauterine insemination via endoscopy is an alternative to surgery
• May treat as outpatient—every-other-day visits for blood collection and vaginal cytologic examination

NURSING CARE
N/A

ACTIVITY
No alteration in activity necessary

DIET
No modification of diet necessary

CLIENT EDUCATION
Client education on the physical, vaginal cytologic, and endocrinologic changes that occur during the estrous cycle, and how variable the timing of these changes can be from animal to animal, can improve owner compliance and satisfaction.

SURGICAL CONSIDERATIONS
Surgical artificial insemination requires standard postoperative care.

Cats
• Increase the likelihood of ovulation by maximizing the number of matings; breed on successive days during estrus.
• Breed four times a day spaced at least 2–3 hr apart on days 2 and 3 of estrus to maximize LH release
• May induce ovulation by administration of exogenous hormones—GnRH or hCG after mating

MEDICATIONS

DRUG(S) OF CHOICE
Cats—hCG (100–500 IU IM); GnRH (25–50 μg IM or IV)

CONTRAINDICATIONS
N/A

PRECAUTIONS
N/A

POSSIBLE INTERACTIONS
N/A

ALTERNATIVE DRUG(S)
N/A

FOLLOW-UP

PATIENT MONITORING
• Follow-up pregnancy examination
• Dogs—continue to obtain vaginal specimens after breeding throughout estrus to determine Day 1 of diestrus (D1), retrospective estimation of the day of ovulation is 6 days before D1. For frozen semen: repeat quantitative progesterone 3 days after initial progesterone rise or LH surge to verify >5 ng/mL (16 nmol/L); for fresh, cooled semen: repeat quantitative or semiquantitative progesterone test 3–4 days after the initial rise is recommended to verify a continued rise.
• Cats—use progesterone assay to verify ovulation.

PREVENTION/AVOIDANCE
N/A

POSSIBLE COMPLICATIONS

Dogs
• Vaginal cytologic examination—determine Day 1 of diestrus; allows retrospective estimation of the day of ovulation (6 days before Day 1 of diestrus); compare with the prospective estimation based on progesterone; if the estimates differ, pregnancy rates are reduced.
• Semiquantitative progesterone kits—must come to room temperature before use; false high values common when using a cold kit
• Serum progesterone—allow blood to clot at a cool temperature; separate cells from serum or plasma as soon as possible (within 20 min of collection); false low values occur when using serum mixed with RBCs (progesterone will be bound).
• A hemolyzed or lipemic specimen—may give a false low progesterone value
• Quantitative progesterone—more accurate when performed by a commercial laboratory than by semi-quantitative kits; preferable in cases of questionable fertility; turn-around

times may make it difficult to use for prospective timing of breeding.
• Serum LH—unidentified factors in the serum of some bitches interfere with the LH kits, causing the positive control line and test result to be obscured; must rely on serum progesterone

MISCELLANEOUS

ASSOCIATED CONDITIONS
Vaginal stricture

AGE-RELATED FACTORS
Split heats in young bitches—typified by a period of proestrus, followed by cessation of signs, and subsequent resumption of the estrus cycle (1–3 weeks later); no initial rise in progesterone or LH occurs with the first proestrus/estrus; subsequent estrus is usually normal with an LH peak and progesterone rise; fertility should be normal if breeding is based on LH peak or initial progesterone rise (must confirm continued rise 3–4 days later) rather than on vaginal bleeding or cytology.

ZOONOTIC POTENTIAL
N/A

PREGNANCY
Examine for pregnancy at appropriate time

SEE ALSO
• Infertility, Female
• Vaginal Discharge

ABBREVIATIONS
• D1 = day 1 of diestrus
• GnRH = gonadotropin-releasing hormone
• hCG = human chorionic gonadotropin
• LH = luteinizing hormone

Suggested Reading
Eilts BE, Paccamonti DL, Causey RC. Reproductive disorders. In: Norsworthy GD ed. Feline practice. Philadelphia: Lippincott, 1993:458–476.
Johnston SD, Root-Kustritz MV, Olson PN. Breeding management and artificial insemination of the bitch. In: canine and feline theriogenology. Philadelphia: Saunders, 2001:49–63.
Johnston SD, Root-Kustritz MV, Olson PN. Vaginal cytology. In: Canine and feline theriogenology. Philadelphia: Saunders, 2001:32–40.
Johnston SD, Root-Kustritz MV, Olson PN. Breeding management, artificial insemination, in vitro fertilization, and embryo transfer in the queen. In: Canine and feline theriogenology. Philadelphia: Saunders, 2001:406–413.
Author Dale Paccamonti
Consulting Editor Sara K. Lyle

BRONCHIECTASIS

 BASICS

OVERVIEW
• Condition seen primarily in dogs, characterized by an irreversible dilatation of the bronchi with accumulation of pulmonary secretions; also occurs in cats as a sequela to long-standing inflammatory lung disease
• Diseases that lead to condition—those associated with ciliostasis, which disrupts the normal defense mechanisms within the lung and delays clearance of bacteria and mucus
• Production of cytokines and destructive enzymes by WBCs or bacteria and prolonged contact of inflammatory mediators with pulmonary tissue lead to damage of supporting structures within the lung.
• The airways are pulled open by surrounding lung tissue; further pooling of secretions occurs, which perpetuates lung damage and colonization by bacteria.

SIGNALMENT
• Primarily dogs and rarely cats
• Cocker spaniels—seem predisposed
• In the U.K.—reported higher incidence in large-breed dogs
• Young animals (<1 year)—secondary to primary ciliary dyskinesia
• Middle-aged to old dogs with chronic pulmonary disease

SIGNS
• Chronic cough—usually moist and productive; observant owners may notice hemoptysis.
• Recurrent fever
• Exercise intolerance
• Tachypnea or dyspnea
• Moist, harsh inspiratory crackles and moist rales; loud expiratory lung sounds or wheezes
• Tracheal hypersensitivity
• Chronic nasal discharge or sinusitis, particularly with primary ciliary dyskinesia

CAUSES & RISK FACTORS
• Primary ciliary dyskinesia
• Inadequately treated infectious or inflammatory lung conditions—may lead to severe inflammation, tissue destruction, and irreversible lung damage
• Smoke inhalation, aspiration pneumonia, radiation injury, and inhalation of environmental toxins—may predispose animal to airway injury and colonization by bacteria
• Chronic bronchial obstruction or foreign body pneumonia—development of bronchiectasis distal to the obstructed region common, owing to accumulation of inflammatory mediators and bacterial colonization

 DIAGNOSIS

DIFFERENTIAL DIAGNOSIS
• Recurrent bacterial bronchopneumonia
• Fungal pneumonia
• Chronic bronchitis
• Infectious or parasitic bronchitis
• Congestive heart failure
• Neoplasia
• Tracheal collapse

CBC/BIOCHEMISTRY/URINALYSIS
• Neutrophilia and monocytosis
• Hyperglobulinemia owing to chronic antigenic stimulation
• Proteinuria—may be seen with secondary amyloidosis, glomerulonephritis, or sepsis

OTHER LABORATORY TESTS
Arterial blood gas analysis—hypoxemia; widened alveolar–arterial oxygen gradient

IMAGING
• Radiography—dilatation of the lobar bronchi with lack of normal tapering in the periphery; mixed bronchial, interstitial, and alveolar pattern; diffuse thickening of bronchial walls
• CT—abnormally dilated bronchi near the lung periphery; cystic dilatations of the bronchi with or without fluid

DIAGNOSTIC PROCEDURES
• Bronchoscopy—saccular or tubular dilatation of the airways; loss of the cylindrical shape to the lumen; airway hyperemia with or without mucosal irregularity and nodule formation; trapped secretions
• Airway sampling—cytologic examination of bronchoalveolar lavage fluid or transtracheal wash specimens; culture for aerobic and anaerobic bacteria; typically find suppurative inflammation with high numbers of neutrophils and monocytes; may culture a mixed population of bacteria; may appear to be sterile inflammation

PATHOLOGIC FINDINGS
• Diffuse peribronchial and alveolar inflammation and fibrosis
• Squamous metaplasia of bronchial epithelium
• Bronchiolar obliteration

TREATMENT

• Inpatient—severe condition: intravenous fluids and antibiotics; oxygen administration
• Most patients benefit from airway humidification and coupage to facilitate removal of viscid pulmonary secretions.
• Encourage gentle activity, as much as the patient's condition allows; enhance clearance of secretions.
• Long-term antibiotic administration (2 months to lifelong)—may be needed; stress to owner importance of appropriate follow-up care.
• Single affected lung lobe or bronchial obstruction—may require lung lobectomy

MEDICATIONS

DRUG(S)

• Intravenous antibiotics—may be required initially; good choices: ampicillin (10–20 mg/kg IV q6–8h) and gentamicin (2–4 mg/kg IV q8–12h) or enrofloxacin
• Broad-spectrum agents with efficacy against both aerobes and anaerobes and that offer good penetration of pulmonary tissue—preferred; combination of enrofloxacin (2.5–10 mg/kg PO q12h) and clindamycin (5–11 mg/kg PO q12h) often effective
• Long-term use of antibiotics—based on bacterial culture and sensitivity testing; may be required even if culture of airway specimens yields no growth

• Bronchodilators—may be beneficial, although animals usually have irreversible airflow limitation; extended-release theophylline (10 mg/kg PO q12h), terbutaline (1.25–5.0 mg/dog PO q12h), or albuterol (0.03–0.05 mg/kg PO q8–12h)

CONTRAINDICATIONS/POSSIBLE INTERACTIONS

• Theophylline derivatives and fluoroquinolones—concurrent use causes high and possibly toxic plasma theophylline concentration.
• Furosemide—avoid; dries out airway secretions
• Cough suppressants—avoid

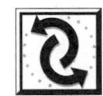

FOLLOW-UP

PATIENT MONITORING

• Body temperature—outpatient; by owner
• Serial CBC, blood gas analysis, and thoracic radiographs

PREVENTION/AVOIDANCE

Antibiotics—complete a full course of therapy in patients that appear to have parenchymal infection; short course (10–14 days) may predispose patient to infection with resistant bacteria.

POSSIBLE COMPLICATIONS

Chronic recurrent pulmonary infection likely

EXPECTED COURSE AND PROGNOSIS

• Patient may succumb to respiratory failure.
• Pulmonary hypertension and cor pulmonale may develop.

• Other organs may fail if bacteremia or glomerulonephritis develops.

MISCELLANEOUS

ASSOCIATED CONDITIONS

• Primary ciliary dyskinesia
• Chronic sinusitis
• Chronic bronchitis
• Bacterial pneumonia
• Aspiration pneumonia
• Smoke inhalation

AGE-RELATED FACTORS

Evaluate young patients for primary ciliary dyskinesia.

SEE ALSO

• Pneumonia, Bacterial
• Primary Ciliary Dyskinesia
• Smoke Inhalation

Suggested Reading

Nicotra MB. Bronchiectasis. Semin Respir Infect 1994;9:31–40.
Norris CR, Samii VF. Clinical, radiographic and pathologic features of bronchiectasis in cats: 12 cases (1987–1999). J Am Vet Med Assoc 2000;216:530–534.

Author Lynelle R. Johnson
Consulting Editor Lynelle R. Johnson

BRONCHITIS, CHRONIC (COPD)

 BASICS

DEFINITION
• Chronic coughing for 2 consecutive months that is not attributable to another cause (e.g., neoplasia and congestive heart failure) • Non-reversible and often slowly progressive condition, owing to the accompanying pathologic airway changes

PATHOPHYSIOLOGY
• Specific cause rarely determined. • Recurrent airway inflammation suspected • Persistent tracheobronchial irritation—causes chronic coughing; leads to changes in the tracheo-bronchial epithelium and submucosal structures
• Airway inflammation, epithelial edema, thickening, and metaplasia—prominent
• Excess mucus production is a hallmark.
• Net effect of changes—narrowed airways; increased lung resistance; decreased expiratory air flow rates

SYSTEMS AFFECTED
• Respiratory • Cardiovascular—pulmonary hypertension, cor pulmonale • Nervous—syncope

SIGNALMENT

Species
Dogs and cats

Breed Predilections
• Dogs—small and toy breeds common; also observed in large breeds • West Highland white terriers—develop a progressive disorder characterized by chronic coughing, respira-tory distress, and crackles • Cocker spaniels—bronchiectasis common after a long history of chronic bronchitis

Mean Age and Range
Most often affects middle-aged and old animals

Predominant Sex
N/A

SIGNS

Historical Findings
• Coughing—hallmark of tracheobronchial irritation; usually dry; posttussive gagging common (owners may misinterpret it as vomiting) • Exercise intolerance • Cyanosis and even syncope may be noted.

Physical Examination and Findings
• Patients usually bright, alert, and afebrile
• Tracheal palpation—typically results in coughing because of tracheal sensitivity
• Small airway disease—assumed when an expiratory abdominal push (during quiet breathing) or end-expiratory wheezing is detected • Bronchovesicular lung sounds, end-inspiratory crackles, and wheezing (result of airways obstructed by secretions) may be

heard • Cardiac auscultation—murmurs secondary to valvular insufficiency common but not always associated with congestive heart failure; chronic bronchitis usually results in a normal or slower than normal resting heart rate and pronounced sinus arrhythmia. • Obesity—common; important complicating factor • Severe dental disease may predispose to lower airway infection and sepsis.

CAUSES
Chronic airway inflammation initiated by multiple causes

RISK FACTORS
• Recurrent bacterial infection
• Long-term exposure to inhaled irritants
• Obesity
• Dental disease and laryngeal disease—result in bacterial showering of the lower airways

 DIAGNOSIS

DIFFERENTIAL DIAGNOSIS
• Bacterial or fungal pneumonia
• Bronchiectasis
• Allergic lung disease
• Foreign bodies
• Heartworm disease
• Neoplasia—metastatic more than primary
• Pulmonary parasites or parasitic larval migration
• Pulmonary fibrosis
• Pulmonary granulomatosis
• Congestive heart failure–typically associated with a high resting heart rate and left atrial enlargement causing collapse of the left principal bronchus

CBC/BIOCHEMISTRY/URINALYSIS
• Rarely diagnostic
• Absolute eosinophilia—suggests but not diagnostic for allergic bronchitis; noted in < 50% of confirmed cases
• Polycythemia secondary to chronic hypoxia—may be seen
• SAP and ALT—may be high owing to passive congestion

OTHER LABORATORY TESTS
• Run routine fecal and heartworm tests.
• Arterial blood gas analysis—collect, ice, and have analyzed at a local hospital; low PaO_2 but not high $PaCO_2$ common with severe condition; aids in prognosis

IMAGING

Thoracic Radiography
• Common features (in descending order of frequency)—bronchial thickening (classically doughnuts and tram lines); interstitial pattern; middle lung lobe consolidation; atelectasis; hyperinflation and diaphragmatic flattening (primarily cats)

Echocardiography
• May reveal right heart enlargement
• Helps rule out congestive heart failure as a cause of coughing
• Estimate pulmonary hypertension via Doppler echocardiography.

DIAGNOSTIC PROCEDURES

ECG
• Wandering atrial pacemaker, marked sinus arrhythmia, P pulmonale, occasionally evidence of right ventricular hypertrophy

Evaluation of Airway Secretions
• Must be from lower airways—helps to establish underlying cause
• Throat swab cultures—are *not* representative of lower airway flora
• Transtracheal aspiration biopsy or bronchoalveolar lavage (BAL)—collect specimens for cytologic examination and bacterial culture.
• Quantitated BAL cultures help differentiate infection vs. airway colonization; reported cut off is $\geq 1.7 \times 10^3$ CFU for infection.
• Cytology—inflammation primary finding; most cells neutrophils, eosinophils, or macrophages; evaluate for bacteria, parasites, and neoplastic cells.
• Recurrent infections—implicated pathogenesis; positive cultures are not frequently reported; *Mycoplasma* discussed but rarely confirmed as a cause

Bronchoscopy
• Preferred test for assessing the lower airways
• Allows direct visualization of the structural as well as functional (dynamic) changes encountered; allows selected airway sampling (e.g., biopsy and lavage)
• Gross changes—excess mucoid to mucopurulent secretions; epithelial edema or thickening with blunting of bronchial bifurcations; irregular or granular mucosa; mucosal polypoid proliferations are pathognomonic
• Large airway caliber changes (e.g., dynamic airway collapse and bronchiectasis)—may detect as complicating problems

PATHOLOGIC FINDINGS
See Diagnostic Procedures—Bronchoscopy

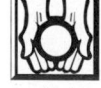 TREATMENT

APPROPRIATE HEALTH CARE
• Usually outpatient—oxygen may be given at home.
• Inpatient—requires oxygen therapy, parenteral medication, or aerosol therapy; patients that owners cannot keep calm at home during recovery

NURSING CARE N/A

ACTIVITY

• Exercise—moderate (not forced) useful in clearing secretions; assists with weight loss
• Limit if exertion results in coughing.
• Use a harness instead of a collar.

DIET

Weight loss critical—improves PaO_2, cough frequency, attitude, and exercise tolerance in obese patients

CLIENT EDUCATION

• Warn client that chronic bronchitis is an incurable disease and complete suppression of all coughing is an unattainable goal.
• Stress that aggressive treatment—including weight control, avoiding risk factors, and medical treatment—minimizes the severity of the coughing and slows disease progression in most patients.

SURGICAL CONSIDERATIONS

Treat severe dental disease to minimize secondary bacterial complications.

MEDICATIONS

DRUG(S) OF CHOICE

Corticosteroids

• Diminish airway inflammation and coughing regardless of the underlying cause
• Indicated for noninfectious condition
• With allergic or hypersensitivity reactions—require long-term administration; attempt to wean off steroids or determine lowest effective dosage.

Bronchodilators

• Beneficial effects (depend on drug)—bronchodilation; heightened mucociliary clearance; improvement in diaphragmatic contractility; lowered pulmonary artery pressure; increased CNS sensitivity to $PaCO_2$; and stabilization of mast cells
• β-agonists—terbutaline (1.25–5 mg/dog q8–12h; 0.625 mg/cat q12h) and albuterol (0.02–0.05 mg/kg q8–12h in dogs)
• Sustained-release theophylline—oral administration; previously proven SRT products (Theo-Dur and Slo-Bio Gyrocaps) no longer available. A recent study showed Inwood Labs brand of SRT to have acceptable pharmacokinetics in dogs (10 mg/kg PO q12h).
• Aminophylline—immediate-release tablets or injectable; not recommended

Antibiotics

• Select on the basis of quantitated culture sensitivity test results
• Bacterial culture results unavailable—choose an agent with a good gram-negative

spectrum, with good tissue and secretion penetration, and that is bactericidal with minimal toxicity (e.g., potentiated sulfa/trimethoprim, amoxicillin/clavulanic acid, or enrofloxacin).
• Associated chronic aspiration or dental disease—may prefer an anaerobic and gram-positive spectrum antibiotic

Antitussives

• Indicated for nonproductive, paroxysmal, continuous, or debilitating cough
• Dogs—butorphanol (0.55 mg/kg PO q6–12h; 0.055–0.11 mg/kg SC); hydrocodone (2.5–5 mg/dog q6–24h PO); codeine (0.1–0.3 mg/kg q6–8h PO)

CONTRAINDICATIONS

Lasix and atropine—do not use because of drying effects on tracheobronchial secretions.

PRECAUTIONS

• β-agonists (e.g., terbutaline and albuterol)—may cause tachycardia, nervousness, and muscle tremors; typically transient
• Methylxanthines (e.g., theophylline)—may cause tachycardia, restlessness, excitability, vomiting, and diarrhea; evaluate EDTA plasma sample for peak plasma concentration (ideally achieve 5–20 μg/mL)

POSSIBLE INTERACTIONS

Enrofloxacin decreases theophylline clearance in dogs and can result in theophylline toxicity.

ALTERNATIVE DRUG(S)

• Metered dose inhalers (steroids—Flovent, and bronchodilators—albuterol) are being used in many cases
• Serotonin blockers (not leukotriene blockers)—shown to effectively block airway hyper-responsiveness in muscle from cats with experimentally induced airway disease
• Cyclosporine-induced immune suppression—shown to block changes associated with experimental asthma in cats

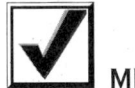

FOLLOW-UP

PATIENT MONITORING

• Follow abnormalities revealed by physical examination and selected diagnostic tests—determine response to treatment • Monitor weight; arterial blood gases usually improve after marked weight loss.

PREVENTION/AVOIDANCE

Avoid and address risk factors (see Risk Factors).

POSSIBLE COMPLICATIONS

• Syncope—frequent complication of chronic coughing, particularly in toy breed dogs

• Pulmonary hypertension and cor pulmonale—most serious complications

EXPECTED COURSE AND PROGNOSIS

• Progressive airway changes—syncopal episodes, chronic hypoxia, right ventricular hypertrophy, and pulmonary hypertension common • Acute exacerbations—common with seasonal changes, air quality changes, worsened inflammation, and potentially the development of secondary infection

✓ MISCELLANEOUS

ASSOCIATED CONDITIONS

• Syncope—secondary to chronic coughing
• Increased susceptibility to airway infection, chronic hypoxia, pulmonary hypertension, and cor pulmonale

PREGNANCY

Safety in pregnant animals not established for most of the recommended drugs

SYNONYMS

• Bronchiolitis • Chronic bronchitis • Chronic obstructive lung disease (COLD) • Chronic obstructive pulmonary disease (COPD)
• Small airway disease

SEE ALSO

• Asthma, Bronchitis—Cats • Bronchiectasis
• Cough • Hypoxia • Tracheal Collapse—Dogs • Tracheobronchitis, Infectious—Dogs

ABBREVIATIONS

• ALT = alanine aminotransferase • BAL = bronchoalveolar lavage • SAP = serum alkaline phosphatase • SRT = sustained-release theophylline

Suggested Reading

Dye JA, McKiernan BC, Rozanski EA, et al. Bronchopulmonary disease in the cat. Historical, physical, radiographical, clinico-pathologic and pulmonary functional evaluation of 24 diseased and 15 healthy cats. J Vet Intern Med 1996;10:385–400.
Johnson L. Bronchial disease. In: August JR, ed. Consultations in feline internal medicine. 3rd ed. Philadelphia: Saunders, 1997:303–309.
Padrid PA, Hornoff WJ, Kurpershoek CJ, Cross CE. Canine chronic bronchitis. J Vet Intern Med 1990;4:172–180.
Peelers DE, McKiernan BC, Weisiger RM et al. Quantitative bacterial cultures and cytological examination of bronchoalveolar lavage specimens in dogs. J Vet Intern Med 2000;14:534–541.

Author Brendan C. McKiernan
Consulting Editor Lynelle R. Johnson

BRUCELLOSIS

 BASICS

DEFINITION
• Contagious disease of dogs caused by *Brucella canis,* a small, intracellular, gram-negative organism
• Characterized by abortion and infertility in females and epididymitis and testicular atrophy in males

PATHOPHYSIOLOGY
B. canis—an intracellular parasite; has a propensity for growth in lymphatic, placental, and male genital (epididymis and prostate) tissues

SYSTEMS AFFECTED
• Reproductive—target tissues of gonadal steroids (gravid uterus, fetus, testes [epididymides], prostate gland)
• Hemic/Lymph/Immune—lymph nodes and spleen; bone marrow; mononuclear leukocytes
• Other tissues—intervertebral disks, anterior uvea, meninges (uncommon)

GENETICS
• No known genetic predisposition
• Occurs most commonly in beagles

INCIDENCE/PREVALENCE
• Incidence unknown
• Seroprevalence rates—not accurately defined; false-positive results common with agglutination tests
• Prevalence—relatively low (1–18%) in the U.S. and Japan; in the U.S., higher in rural areas of the south; in Mexico and Peru, 25–30% in stray dogs

GEOGRAPHIC DISTRIBUTION
Stray dogs, pets, and kennels—U.S. (mostly beagles), Mexico, Japan, and several South American countries; seen in Spain, Tunisia, China, and Bulgaria; individual outbreaks in Germany and the former Czechoslovakia (some traced to the importation of dogs)

SIGNALMENT

Species
Dogs and, infrequently, humans

Breed Predilections
• No evidence of breed susceptibility, but exceptionally high prevalence in beagles
• Infected Labrador retrievers and several other breeds found in commercial kennels ("puppy mills")

Mean Age and Range
• No age preference
• Most common in sexually mature dogs

Predominant Sex
• Both sexes are affected
• More common in females

SIGNS

General Comments
Suspect whenever female dogs experience abortions or reproductive failures or males have genital disease

Historical Findings
• Affected animals, especially females, may appear healthy or have vague signs of illness.
• Lethargy
• Loss of libido
• Swollen lymph nodes
• Back pain
• Abortion—commonly at 6–8 weeks after conception, although pregnancy may terminate at any stage

Physical Examination Findings
• Males—swollen scrotal sacs, often with scrotal dermatitis; enlarged and firm epididymides
• Chronic infection—unilateral or bilateral testicular atrophy; cloudy eyes (anterior uveitis with corneal edema); spinal pain; posterior weakness; ataxia
• Fever rare
• Enlarged superficial lymph nodes (e.g., retropharyngeal, external inguinal) common
• Vaginal discharge may last for several weeks after an abortion

CAUSES
B. canis—gram-negative coccobacillus; morphologically indistinguishable from other members of the genus; unlike other *Brucella* spp. (e.g., *B. abortus, B. suis,* and *B. melitensis*), can result in a high rate (50%) of false-positive reactions with commonly used tests

RISK FACTORS
• Breeding kennels and pack hounds
• Risk increases when popular breeding animals become infected.
• Contact with strays in endemic areas

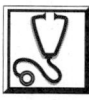 **DIAGNOSIS**

DIFFERENTIAL DIAGNOSIS
• Abortions—maternal, fetal, or placental abnormalities
• Systemic infections—canine distemper, canine herpesvirus infection, *B. abortus* infection, hemolytic streptococci, *E. coli,* leptospirosis, and toxoplasmosis
• Inguinal hernias—may be provoked by epididymitis and scrotal edema; also caused by blastomycosis and other granulomatous infections, and Rocky Mountain spotted fever
• Diskospondylitis—fungal infections, actinomycosis, staphylococcal infections, nocardiosis, streptococci, or *Corynebacterium diphtheroids*

CBC/BIOCHEMISTRY/URINALYSIS
Generally normal in uncomplicated cases

OTHER LABORATORY TESTS
Serologic testing—most commonly used diagnostic method; subject to error; false-positive reactions to lipopolysaccharide antigens of several species of bacteria common with the RSAT and mercaptoethanol tube agglutination tests

RSAT
• Commercially available; simple and rapid
• Detects infected dogs 3–4 weeks after infection; accurate in identifying noninfected ("negative") dogs
• Suffers a high rate (50%) of false-positive reactions
• Results must be confirmed by other tests.

Mercaptoethanol Tube Agglutination Test
• Semiquantitative
• Generally performed by commercial diagnostic laboratories
• Provides information similar to the RSAT
• Suffers from lack of specificity; good screening test

AGID Tests
• Cell wall antigen test—employs a lipopolysaccharide antigen derived from the cell walls of *B. canis;* highly sensitive; test conditions not standardized; frequent false positives; not recommended
• Soluble antigen test—employs soluble antigens that consist of proteins extracted from the bacterial cytoplasm; antigens highly specific for antibodies against *Brucella* spp. (including *B. canis, B. abortus,* and *B. suis*); reactive antibodies appear 4–12 weeks after infection and persist for a long time; may give precipitin lines after other tests become equivocal or negative; highly recommended.

IMAGING
Radiographic evidence of diskospondylitis—test for brucellosis

DIAGNOSTIC PROCEDURES

Isolation of Organism
• Blood cultures—when clinical and serologic findings suggest the diagnosis; *Brucella* are readily isolated from the blood of infected dogs if they have not received antibiotics; onset of bacteremia occurs 2–4 weeks after oral-nasal exposure and may persist for 8 months to 5.5 years.
• Cultures of vaginal fluids—after an abortion; usually give positive results
• Cultures of semen or urine—not practical for routine diagnosis, because overgrowth of contaminants is common
• Contaminated samples—media that contain antibiotics (e.g., Thayer-Martin medium) have proven useful.

Semen Quality
• Sperm motility, immature sperm, inflammatory cells (neutrophils)—with epididymitis
• Abnormalities—usually evident by 5–8 weeks postinfection; conspicuous by 20 weeks
• Aspermia without inflammatory cells—common with bilateral testicular atrophy

Lymph Node Biopsy
• Reveal lymphoid hyperplasia with large numbers of plasma cells
• If done in a sterile manner, tissues should be cultured on appropriate media.
• Intracellular bacteria—may be observed in macrophages with special stains (e.g., Brown-Brenn stain)
• Histopathological examination of the testes—often reveals necrotizing vasculitis, infiltration of inflammatory cells, and granulomatous lesions

PATHOLOGIC FINDINGS
• Gross findings—lymph node enlargement; splenomegaly; males: enlarged and firm epididymides, scrotal edema, or atrophy of one or both testes; chronic infection: anterior uveitis and diskospondylitis
• Microscopic changes—relatively consistent; diffuse lymphoreticular hyperplasia; chronic infection: lymph node sinusoids with abundant plasma cells and macrophages that contain bacteria diffuse lymphocytic infiltration and granulomatous lesions in all genitourinary organs (especially prostate, epididymis, uterus, and scrotum); may be extensive inflammatory cell infiltration and necrosis of the prostate parenchyma and seminiferous tubules
• Ocular changes—granulomatous iridocyclitis; exudative retinitis; leukocytic exudates in the anterior chamber

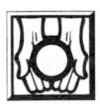
TREATMENT

APPROPRIATE HEALTH CARE
Outpatient

NURSING CARE
N/A

ACTIVITY
Restrict working dogs

DIET
N/A

CLIENT EDUCATION
• Client should be aware that the goal of treatment is the eradication of *B. canis* from the animal (seronegative status and no bacteremia for at least 3 months), but sometimes the result is persistent low antibody titers with no systemic infection.

• Inform client that antibiotic treatment, especially minocycline and doxycycline, is expensive, time-consuming, and controversial (because outcomes are uncertain).
• Treatment is not recommended for breeding or commercial kennels; it is recommended only for nonbreeding dogs or those who have been spayed or castrated.
• Before treatment is attempted for an intact household pet or breeding dog, the client must clearly agree that the animal must be neutered or destroyed if treatment fails.

SURGICAL CONSIDERATIONS
Neutering/spaying plus treatment—when euthanasia is unacceptable to an owner

MEDICATIONS

DRUG(S) OF CHOICE
• Several therapeutic regimens have been evaluated, but results have been equivocal.
• Most successful—combination of a tetracycline (tetracycline hydrochloride, chlortetracycline, or minocycline at 25mg/kg PO q8h for 4 weeks) or doxycycline (10 mg/kg PO q12h for 4 weeks) and dihydrostreptomycin (10 mg/kg IM q8h during weeks 1 and 4)

CONTRAINDICATIONS
• Tetracyclines—do no use in immature pups
• Gentamicin—contraindicated with kidney disease

PRECAUTIONS
Gentamicin—monitor renal function closely.

POSSIBLE INTERACTIONS
N/A

ALTERNATIVE DRUG(S)
Gentamicin—3 mg/kg q12h; limited success; insufficient data on the efficacy combined with tetracycline

FOLLOW-UP

PATIENT MONITORING
• Serologic tests—monthly for at least 3 months after completion of treatment; continuous, persistent decline in antibodies to negative status indicates successful treatment.
• Recrudescent infections (rise in antibody levels and recurrence of bacteremia after therapy)—re-treat, neuter and re-treat, or euthanize
• Blood cultures—negative for at least 3 months after completion of treatment

PREVENTION/AVOIDANCE
• Vaccine—none; would complicate serologic testing

• Testing—all brood bitches, before they come into estrus if a breeding is planned; males used for breeding, at frequent intervals
• Quarantine and test all new dogs twice at monthly intervals before allowing them to enter a breeding kennel.

POSSIBLE COMPLICATIONS
• Owners may be reluctant to neuter or destroy valuable dogs, regardless of treatment failure.
• Remind owners of ethical considerations and their obligation not to sell or distribute infected dogs.

EXPECTED COURSE AND PROGNOSIS
• Prognosis guarded
• Infected for < 3–4 months—likely to respond to treatment
• Chronic infections—males may fail to respond to therapy.
• Successfully treated (seronegative) dogs—fully susceptible to reinfection

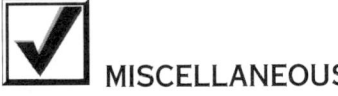
MISCELLANEOUS

ASSOCIATED CONDITIONS
N/A

AGE-RELATED FACTORS
N/A

ZOONOTIC POTENTIAL
Human infections—reported; usually mild; respond readily to tetracyclines

PREGNANCY
• Abortions at 45–60 days of gestation typical
• Pups from infected bitches may be infected or normal.

SYNONYMS
Contagious canine abortion

SEE ALSO
N/A

ABBREVIATIONS
• AGID = agar gel immunodiffusion
• RSAT = rapid 2-mercaptoethanol slide agglutination test

Suggested Reading
Carmichael LE. Brucella canis. In: Nielsen K, Duncan JR, eds. Animal brucellosis. Boca Raton, FL: CRC, 1990:335–350.
Carmichael LE, Greene CE. Canine brucellosis. In: Greene CE, ed. Infectious diseases of the dog and cat. Philadelphia: Saunders, 1990:573–585.
Johnson CA, Walker RD. Clinical signs and diagnosis of *Brucella canis* infection. Comp Contin Educ Prac Vet 1992;14:763–772.
Author Leland Carmichael
Consulting Editor Stephen C. Barr

BULLOUS PEMPHIGOID

 BASICS

OVERVIEW
• Very rare, autoimmune vesiculobullous severe ulcerative dermatosis of the skin and/or oral mucosa in dogs
• Forms—bullous (commonly identified) and chronic (rare)

SIGNALMENT
• Dogs
• Breed predilection—collies, Shetland sheepdogs, and (possibly) Doberman pinschers
• No age or sex predisposition

SIGNS

Bullous
• Cutaneous lesions—transient blisters, crusts, epidermal collarettes, and ulcerations
• Widespread distribution—mucous membranes, head, neck, axillae, ventral abdomen, groin, and feet (nailbed involvement or footpad ulceration); oral cavity and skin of the axillae and groin most frequently involved
• Onset often acute with severe signs
• Severely affected dogs—anorexia, depression, and pyrexia
• Pain and pruritus variable
• Signs similar to pemphigus vulgaris

Chronic Pemphigoid
• Clinically benign
• Lesions—confined to the axillae, groin, or isolated mucocutaneous areas
• Slow and chronic course

CAUSES & RISK FACTORS
• Deposit of an autoantibody ("pemphigoid antibody") directed against the antigen at the basement membrane zone of skin and mucosa; results in blister formation below the epidermis
• Sunlight may exacerbate lesions.

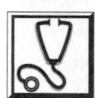 **DIAGNOSIS**

DIFFERENTIAL DIAGNOSIS
• Pemphigus vulgaris
• Systemic lupus erythematosus
• Erythema multiforme
• Toxic epidermal necrolysis
• Drug eruption
• Mycosis fungoides
• Lymphoreticular neoplasia
• Hidradenitis suppurativa
• Ulcerative stomatitis

CBC/BIOCHEMISTRY/URINALYSIS
Leukocytosis, neutrophilia, mild nonregenerative anemia, hypoalbuminemia, and hyperglobulinemia may be seen.

OTHER LABORATORY TESTS
• Antinuclear antibody titer normal
• Lupus erythematosus test negative

IMAGING
N/A

DIAGNOSTIC PROCEDURES
• Biopsies of lesions—subepidermal vesicle formation with inflammatory infiltrates of granulocytes and mononuclear cells; no acantholysis
• Direct immunofluorescence usually negative if positive, dermoepidermal junction pattern
• Bacteriologic culture—identification and drug sensitivity of secondary bacteria

 TREATMENT

• Supportive inpatient care if serious systemic signs or secondary infections occur
• Subsequent outpatient treatment; frequent hospital rechecks and monitoring every 1–4 weeks
• Low-fat diet—avoids pancreatitis secondary to corticosteroid and possible azathioprine therapy
• Avoid sunlight—UV light may exacerbate lesions.

Bullous
• Immunosuppressive agents
• Antibiotics for common secondary bacterial infections
• Gentle soaks/cleansing with antibacterial shampoos or povidone-iodine and water

Chronic
• Immunosuppressive therapy
• Topical or intralesional corticosteroids

MEDICATIONS

DRUG(S)

Corticosteroids
• Prednisone or prednisolone—1.1–3.3 mg/kg PO q12h
• Higher doses are probably necessary, but side effects are likely and need to be monitored.

Cytotoxic Agents
• Required by many patients to achieve control, owing to intolerable side effects of high-dose corticosteroids or failure to achieve or maintain remission with corticosteroids alone
• Work synergistically with corticosteroids to reduce side effects
• Azathioprine—2.2 mg/kg PO q24h; then q48h
• Chlorambucil—0.1 mg/kg PO q24h; then q48h
• Cyclophosphamide—50 mg/m² BSA q48h
• 6-Mercaptopurine—2.2 mg/kg PO q24h; then q48h
• Dapsone—1 mg/kg PO q8h; then as needed; rarely used

Chrysotherapy with Prednisone
• Aurothioglucose—administer a test dose of 1 mg IM (animals < 25 kg) or 5 mg IM (animals > 25 kg) 1st week; 2 mg IM (animals < 25 kg) or 10 mg IM (animals > 25 kg) 2nd week; then 1 mg/kg IM weekly until a clinical response is noted (usually a lag phase of 6–8 weeks); then 1 mg/kg IM every 2–4 weeks for maintenance
• Auranofin—0.1–0.2 mg/kg PO q12–24h

CONTRAINDICATIONS/POSSIBLE INTERACTIONS
• Corticosteroids—polyuria, polydipsia, polyphagia, temperament changes, hepatotoxicity
• Corticosteroid and azathioprine—pancreatitis
• Cytotoxic drugs—leukopenia, thrombocytopenia, nephrotoxicity, hepatotoxicity
• Chrysotherapy—nephrotoxicity, dermatitis, stomatitis, and allergic reactions
• Cyclophosphamide—hemorrhagic cystitis
• Immunosuppression—may predispose patient to *Demodex,* cutaneous and systemic fungal and bacterial infections

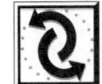

FOLLOW-UP

PATIENT MONITORING
Monitor often for signs of immunosuppression or progression of disease and medication side effects (reported, hematologic studies, and serum biochemistry).

EXPECTED COURSE AND PROGNOSIS
Bullous
• May be fatal if untreated
• Treatment must be aggressive; side effects may affect quality of life.
• Lifelong treatment and monitoring of side effects are usually necessary.
• Secondary infections cause morbidity and possible mortality.
• Some patients may not respond to therapy.

Chronic
• Fair prognosis
• Mild, chronic disease treated with relatively low doses of systemic glucocorticoids; some patients can be treated with topical glucocorticoids alone.

MISCELLANEOUS

Suggested Reading
Scott DW, Miller WH, Griffin CE. Bullous pemphigoid. In: Muller & Kirk's small animal dermatology. 5th ed. Philadelphia: Saunders, 1995:573–578.
Author Margaret S. Swartout
Consulting Editor Karen Helton Rhodes

CAMPYLOBACTERIOSIS

 BASICS

OVERVIEW

• *Campylobacter jejuni*—fastidious, micro-aerophilic, gram-negative curved bacteria; often isolated from the gastrointestinal tract of healthy dogs, cats, and other mammals; may cause a superficial erosive enterocolitis • Infection—fecal–oral route from contamination of food, water, fresh meat (poultry, beef), and the environment; localized in mucus-filled crypts of the intestine; darting motility (flagella) essential for colonization; produces enterotoxin, cytotoxin, cytolethal-distending toxin, and invasin • Invasion of mucosa of gastrointestinal—hematochezia; leukocytes in feces; ulceration; edema; congestion of intestine; bacteremia; occasionally septicemia; bacteria shed in feces for weeks to months • Up to 49% of dogs without diarrhea and 45% of normal cats carry *C. jejuni* and shed it in feces • In younger dogs, more animals with diarrhea shed *Campylobacter* than in diarrheic controls; this age difference is *not* seen in *cats*.

SIGNALMENT

• Dogs and less commonly cats • Prevalence—higher in puppies and kittens from birth to 6 months • Can result in chronic disease in dogs and cats

SIGNS

• Diarrhea—ranges from mucous-like and watery to bloody or bile streaked; common; may be chronic • Tenesmus common • Fever (mild or absent), anorexia, and intermittent vomiting (3–15 days' duration) may accompany diarrhea. • Young animals (up to 6 months of age)—clinical signs most severe; attributable to enterocolitis/diarrhea • Adults—usually asymptomatic carriers

CAUSES & RISK FACTORS

• *C. jejuni* • Kennels with poor sanitation and hygiene and fecal buildup in the environment • Young animals—debilitated, immuno-suppressed, or parasitized (e.g., *Giardia, Toxocara, Isospora*) • Nosocomial infection may develop in hospitalized patients. • Adults—concurrent gastrointestinal infections (e.g., *Salmonella,* parvovirus, hookworms)

 DIAGNOSIS

DIFFERENTIAL DIAGNOSIS

• Signalment, history, physical examination, and fecal examination (direct smear and bacterial culture) enable diagnosis in most cases. • Distinguish from other causes of acute enterocolitis. • Bacterial enterocolitis—*Salmonella, Yersinia enterocolitica, Clostridium difficile,* and *Clostridium perfringens* • Parasitic enterocolitis—helminths (particularly whipworms) and protozoa (e.g., *Giardia* and *Isospora*) • Viral enterocolitis—enteric coronavirus and parvovirus; signs often more severe than with *Campylobacter* • Dietary indiscretion or intolerance • Drugs and toxins • Acute pancreatitis • Severely affected patients—also consider viral gastroenteritis, intussusception, and other causes of abdominal pain. • Distinguish from other causes of chronic diarrhea. • Primary intestinal disease

CBC/BIOCHEMISTRY/URINALYSIS

• Leukocytosis—if the strain is invasive and bacteremia develops • Biochemistry abnormalities—effects of diarrhea and dehydration (e.g., azotemia, electrolyte disturbances)

DIAGNOSTIC PROCEDURES

• Fecal leukocytes—in gastrointestinal tract and stool • Fecal culture—microaerophilic at about 42°C for 48 hr on special *Campylobacter* blood agar plates

Direct Examination of Feces

• Gram stain—make a smear of watery stool on a glass slide; heat fix; use gram stain; leave counterstain (safranin) on for longer than usual. • Wet mount—drop a small amount of stool (if not watery, mix with a small amount of saline or broth) on a glass slide; add a cover slip; view on phase or dark-field objective (40×); note large numbers of curved, highly motile bacteria (characteristic darting motility)

PATHOLOGIC FINDINGS

Gross—diffuse colon thickening and congestion/edema; hyperemia of small intestine; enlarged mesenteric lymph nodes

 TREATMENT

Mild Enterocolitis

• Outpatient • Usually self-limiting

Severe Enterocolitis

• Inpatient, especially neonatal and immature patients • Severe neonatal disease—isolate; confine to cage; monitor; encourage rest • NPO for 24 hr; then bland diet • Mild dehydration—oral fluid therapy with an enteric fluid replacement solution • Severe dehydration—intravenous fluid therapy with balanced polyionic isotonic solution (e.g., lactated Ringer's) • Plasma transfusion may be required if serum albumin < 2.0 g/dL • Locally acting intestinal adsorbents and protectants

 MEDICATIONS

DRUG(S)

• Antibiotics—recommended for signs of systemic illness (e.g., high fever or dehydration) when diarrhea or abnormal clinical signs persist > 7 days and in immune-suppressed patients • Erythromycin—10–20 mg/kg PO q8h for 5 days; drug of choice • Tylosin—11 mg/kg PO q8h for 7 days; may be effective • Neomycin—10–20 mg/kg PO q6–12h for 5 days; may be effective • Penicillins and ampicillin—potentially ineffective • Septicemia—parenteral antibiotics with an aminoglycoside (e.g., amikacin) and a cephalosporin may be initiated

CONTRAINDICATIONS/POSSIBLE INTERACTIONS

Antidiarrheal drugs that reduce intestinal motility are contraindicated.

 FOLLOW-UP

PATIENT MONITORING

Repeat fecal culture after completion of treatment.

PREVENTION/AVOIDANCE

• Good hygiene (hand washing) • Routinely clean and disinfect runs, food, and water bowls.

POSSIBLE COMPLICATIONS

Bacteremia and septicemia

EXPECTED COURSE AND PROGNOSIS

• Adults—usually self-limiting • Juveniles with severe or persistent enterocolitis—treat with antibiotics

 MISCELLANEOUS

ASSOCIATED CONDITIONS

Concurrent infection with *Campylobacter* and other pathogenic bacteria, enteric parasites, or viruses

AGE-RELATED FACTORS

Young animals at greatest risk

ZOONOTIC POTENTIAL

High potential to infect humans

PREGNANCY

• Erythromycin—safe to use in early pregnancy • Chloramphenicol and gentamicin—do not use in pregnant animals

Suggested Reading

Fox JG. Enteric bacterial infections. In: Greene CE, ed. Infectious diseases of the dog and cat. Philadelphia: Saunders, 1998:226–229.

Authors Patrick L. McDonough and Kenneth W. Simpson

Consulting Editor Stephen C. Barr

BASICS

OVERVIEW
• *Candida*—part of the normal flora of the mouth, nose, ears, and gastrointestinal and genital tracts of dogs and cats; recovery from mucosal surfaces does not imply disease; opportunistic, colonizing damaged tissues or invading normal tissues of immuno-suppressed animals; pathogenic role determined by identifying a fungemia, infiltration of organisms into the tissues, or signs of organisms in presumed sterile sites (e.g., urinary bladder)
• Isolation—conditions that suppress the immune system increase the likelihood of isolation in asymptomatic animal; isolated from throat cultures five times more often in FIV-infected cats than in asymptomatic, non-FIV-infected cats of a similar age and sex
• Infection—rare; associated with neutropenia, diabetes mellitus, retrovirus-induced immunosuppression, chronic glucocorticoid treatment, prolonged antibiotic treatment, and incomplete emptying of the bladder.

SIGNALMENT
Cats and less commonly dogs

SIGNS
• Urinary bladder involvement—cystitis
• Ear infection—head shaking and scratching
• Oral cavity involvement—drooling

CAUSES & RISK FACTORS
• Skin damaged by burns, trauma, or necrotizing dermatitis
• Urinary tract—preferred site in diabetic cats and cats that have urinary retention due to strictures secondary to urethrostomy; indwelling catheters
• Neutropenia secondary to parvovirus infection, FeLV, FIV, or bone marrow suppression from chemotherapy

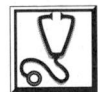

DIAGNOSIS

DIFFERENTIAL DIAGNOSIS
Considered whenever the primary condition does not respond as expected

CBC/BIOCHEMISTRY/URINALYSIS
• Reflect the underlying condition
• Urinalysis—may show yeast form or clumps of mycelial elements (pseudohyphae) accompanied by an increase in inflammatory cells; normal fat globules in cat urine may adhere, giving the appearance of budding yeast
• Neutropenic patients—inflammatory response may be absent

OTHER LABORATORY TESTS
• Pyuria without bacterial growth—culture for fungi and *Mycoplasma*.

IMAGING
N/A

DIAGNOSTIC PROCEDURES
• Lesions—culture for histopathologic study to determine if *Candida* is truly a pathogen; requires demonstration of organisms penetrating the tissues
• Urine sample—obtain by cystocentesis; culture of a number of colonies of *Candida* strongly supports the diagnosis.
• Otitis (dogs)—culture of *Candida* or identification of yeast or mycelial elements on ear cytology suggests the diagnosis.

PATHOLOGIC FINDINGS
• White cheesy foci in the infected tissue may be noted.
• Usually large numbers of both yeast and pseudohyphae in the tissues surrounded by necrosis and a suppurative inflammatory reaction
• Response may be pyogranulomatous in more chronic sites of infection.

TREATMENT
• Regulate diabetes mellitus.
• Remove indwelling catheters.
• Improve immune suppression, if possible.

MEDICATIONS

DRUG(S)
• Fluconazole—5 mg/kg PO q12h (dogs and cats); very effective; excreted unchanged in the urine, achieving a high concentration in commonly infected sites
• Itraconazole—effective; use if the organism becomes resistant to fluconazole; not recommended for urinary tract infection because it is not excreted in the urine
• In urinary tract *Candida* infections resistant to fluconazole, infuse 10 to 30 mLs of 1% clotrimazole into the bladder every other day for 3 treatments.

CONTRAINDICATIONS/POSSIBLE INTERACTIONS
N/A

FOLLOW-UP

PATIENT MONITORING
• Fluconazole and itraconazole—hepatic toxicity; monitor serum ALT monthly and check if patient becomes anorexic; withdraw drug if ALT > 200 U or with anorexia.
• After signs have resolved—reculture sites of infection; continue treatment for 2 weeks more; repeat cultures 2 weeks after completion of treatment and again if signs recur.

EXPECTED COURSE AND PROGNOSIS
• Should resolve within 2–4 weeks of treatment
• Control of the underlying disease is necessary to prevent recurrence.

MISCELLANEOUS

ZOONOTIC POTENTIAL
None

ABBREVIATIONS
• ALT = alanine transferase
• FeLV = feline leukemia virus
• FIV = feline immunodeficiency virus

Suggested Reading
Forward ZA, Legendre AM, Khalsa HDS. Use of intermittent bladder infusion with clotrimazole for treatment of candiduria in a dog. J Am Vet Med Assoc 2002;220:1496–1498.
Greene CE, Chandler FW. Candidiasis, torulopsosis, rhodotorulosis. In: Greene CE, ed. Infectious diseases of the dog and cat. Philadelphia: Saunders, 1998:414–417.
Lulich JP, Osborne CA. Fungal infections of the feline lower urinary tract. Vet Clin North Am 1996;26:309–315.
Author Alfred M. Legendre
Consulting Editor Stephen C. Barr

CANINE DISTEMPER

BASICS

DEFINITION
• An acute to subacute contagious febrile and often fatal disease with respiratory, gastrointestinal, and CNS manifestations
• Caused by CDV, a morbillivirus in the Paramyxoviridae family
• Affects many different species of the order Carnivora; mortality rate varies greatly among species.

PATHOPHYSIOLOGY
• Natural route of infection—airborne and droplet exposure; from the nasal cavity, pharynx, and lungs, macrophages carry the virus to local lymph nodes, where virus replication occurs; within 1 week, virtually all lymphatic tissues become infected; spreads via viremia to the surface epithelium of respiratory, gastrointestinal, and urogenital tracts and to the CNS
• Fever for 1–2 days and lymphopenia may be the only findings during initial period; further development depends on the virus strain and the immune response.
• Strong cellular and humoral immune response—may remain subclinical
• Weak immune response—subacute infection; may survive longer
• Failure of immune response—acute death within 2–4 weeks after infection; convulsions and other CNS disturbances frequent causes of death

SYSTEMS AFFECTED
• Multisystemic—all lymphatic tissues; surface epithelium in the respiratory, alimentary, and urogenital tracts; endocrine and exocrine glands
• Nervous—skin; gray and white matter in the CNS

GENETICS
N/A

INCIDENCE/PREVALENCE
• Dogs—restricted to sporadic outbreaks
• Wildlife (raccoons, skunks, fox)—fairly common

GEOGRAPHIC DISTRIBUTION
Worldwide

SIGNALMENT

Species
• Most species of the order Carnivora—Canidae, Hyaenidae, Mustelidae, Procyonidae, Viverridae
• Felidae families—recent; large cats in Californian zoos and in Tanzania

Breed Predilection
None

Mean Age and Range
Young animals are more susceptible than are adults.

Predominant Sex
None

SIGNS
• Fever—first peak 3–6 days after infection, may pass unnoticed; second peak several days later (and intermittent thereafter), usually associated with nasal and ocular discharge, depression, and anorexia
• Gastrointestinal and/or respiratory signs—follow, often enhanced by secondary bacterial infection
• CNS—many infected dogs; often, but not always, after systemic disease; depends on the virus strain; either acute gray matter disease (seizures and myoclonus with depression) or subacute white matter disease (incoordination ataxia, paresis, paralysis, and muscle tremors); meningeal signs of hyperesthesia and cervical rigidity may be seen in both.
• Optic neuritis and retinal lesions not uncommon; sometimes infected scleral blood vessels from anterior uveitis
• Hardening of the footpads (hyperkeratosis) and nose—some virus strains; now much less common than it once was
• Enamel hypoplasia of the teeth after neonatal infection common

CAUSES
• CDV, a morbillivirus within the Paramyxoviridae family; closely related to measles virus, rinderpest virus of cattle, and phocine (seal) and dolphin distemper viruses
• Secondary bacterial infections frequently involve the respiratory and gastrointestinal systems.

RISK FACTORS
Contact of nonimmunized animals with CDV-infected animals (dogs or wild carnivores)

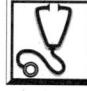

DIAGNOSIS

DIFFERENTIAL DIAGNOSIS
• Kennel cough—can mimic the respiratory disease
• Enteric signs—differentiate from canine parvovirus and coronavirus infections, parasitism (giardiasis), bacterial infections, gastroenteritis from toxin ingestion, inflammatory bowel disease
• CNS form—confused with granulomatous meningoencephalomyelitis, protozoal encephalitis (toxoplasmosis, neosporosis), cryptococcosis or other infections (meningitis, ehrlichiosis, Rocky Mountain spotted fever), pug dog encephalitis, and lead poisoning
• Considered in any young unvaccinated dog with multifocal CNS disease with other organ involvement

CBC/BIOCHEMISTRY/URINALYSIS
Lymphopenia during early infection

OTHER LABORATORY TESTS
• Serology—limited value; positive antibody tests do not differentiate between vaccination and exposure to virulent virus; patient may die from acute disease before neutralizing antibody can be produced; IgM responses may be seen for up to 3 months after exposure to virulent virus and for up to 3 weeks after vaccination.
• CDV antibody in CSF—indicative, but not always diagnostic, of distemper encephalitis

IMAGING
• Radiographs—determine the extent of pneumonia
• Computed tomography (CT) and magnetic resonance imaging (MRI)—cannot typically detect brain changes

DIAGNOSTIC PROCEDURES
• Viral antigen or viral inclusions—in buffy coat cells and conjunctival or vaginal imprints; negative results do not rule out the diagnosis.
• PCR—on buffy coat and urine sediment cells; more sensitive
• CSF—test for cell and protein content, CDV-specific antibody, interferon, and viral antigen early in disease course.
• Postmortem diagnosis—histopathology, immunofluorescence and/or immunocytochemistry, virus isolation, and/or PCR; preferred tissues from lungs, stomach, urinary bladder, lymph nodes, and brain

PATHOLOGIC FINDINGS

Gross
• Thymus—in young animals greatly reduced in size; sometimes gelatinous
• Lungs—patchy consolidation as a result of interstitial pneumonia
• Footpads and nose—rarely hyperkeratosis
• Mucopurulent discharges—from eyes and nose, bronchopneumonia, catarrhal enteritis, and skin pustules; probably caused by secondary bacterial infections; commonly seen

Histologic
• Intracytoplasmic eosinophilic inclusion bodies—frequently found in epithelium of the bronchi, stomach, and urinary bladder; also seen in reticulum cells and leukocytes in lymphatic tissues
• Inclusion bodies in the CNS—glial cells and neurons; frequently intranuclear; can also be found in cytoplasm
• Staining by fluorescent antibody or immunoperoxidase may detect viral antigen where inclusion bodies are not seen.

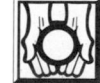

TREATMENT

APPROPRIATE HEALTH CARE
Inpatients and in isolation, to prevent infection of other dogs

NURSING CARE
• Symptomatic
• Intravenous fluids—with anorexia and diarrhea
• Once fevers and secondary bacterial infections are controlled, patients usually begin to eat again.
• Clean away ocular discharges.

ACTIVITY
Limited

DIET
Depends on the extent of gastrointestinal involvement

CLIENT EDUCATION
• Inform client that mortality rate is about 50%.
• Inform client that dogs that appear to recover from early catarrhal signs may later develop fatal CNS signs.

SURGICAL CONSIDERATIONS
N/A

 MEDICATIONS

DRUG(S) OF CHOICE
• Antiviral drugs—none known to be effective
• Antibiotics—to reduce secondary bacterial infection, because CDV is highly immunosuppressive
• Anticonvulsant therapy—phenobarbital, potassium bromide; to control less severe neurologic manifestations (e.g., myoclonus, seizures)

CONTRAINDICATIONS
Corticosteroids—do not use, because they augment the immunosuppression and may enhance viral dissemination; may provide short-term control of signs

PRECAUTIONS
Tetracycline and fluorinated quinolones—do not use for young and growing animals

POSSIBLE INTERACTIONS
N/A

ALTERNATIVE DRUG(S)
N/A

 FOLLOW-UP

PATIENT MONITORING
• Monitor for signs of pneumonia or dehydration from diarrhea in the acute phase of the disease.
• Monitor for CNS signs, because seizures generally follow.

PREVENTION/AVOIDANCE
• Avoid infection of pups by isolation to prevent infection from wildlife (e.g., raccoons, fox, skunks) or from CDV-infected dogs
• Recovered dogs are not carriers.

Vaccines
• MLV-CD—prevents infection and disease; two types available, each with advantages and disadvantages
• Canine tissue culture–adapted vaccines (e.g., Rockborn strain)—induce complete immunity in virtually 100% of susceptible dogs; rarely a postvaccinal fatal encephalitis develops 7–14 days after vaccination, especially in immunosuppressed animals
• Chick embryo–adapted vaccines (e.g., Onderstepoort, Lederle strain)—safer; postvaccinal encephalitis does not occur; only about 80% of susceptible dogs seroconvert
• Other species—chick embryo can safely be used in a variety of zoo and wildlife species (e.g., gray fox); Rockborn type fatal in these animals
• Killed vaccines—useful for species for which either type of MLV-CD is fatal (e.g., red panda, black-footed ferret)
• Canarypox recombinant CDV vaccine—recently available; being tested in other species

Maternal Antibody
• Important
• Most pups lose protection from maternal antibody at 6–12 weeks of age; give 2–3 vaccinations during this period.
• Heterotypic (measles virus) vaccination—recommended for pups that have maternal antibody; induces protection from disease but not from infection

POSSIBLE COMPLICATIONS
Possibility of occurrence of CNS signs for 2–3 months after catarrhal signs have subsided

EXPECTED COURSE AND PROGNOSIS
• Depend on the strain and the individual host response—subclinical, acute, subacute, fatal, or nonfatal infection
• Mild CNS signs (e.g., myoclonus)—patient may recover; myoclonus may continue for several months.
• Death—2 weeks to 3 months after infection; mortality rate approximately 50%
• Euthanasia—owner may elect if or when neurologic signs develop; indicated when repeated seizures occur
• Fully recovered dogs do not shed CDV.

✓ MISCELLANEOUS

ASSOCIATED CONDITIONS
• Persistent or latent toxoplasma infections—reactivated because of the immunosuppressive state
• Respiratory infections with *Bordetella bronchiseptica* (a major cause of kennel cough)

AGE-RELATED FACTORS
• Young pups—more susceptible; mortality rate is higher
• Nonimmunized old dogs—highly susceptible to infection and disease

ZOONOTIC POTENTIAL
• Possible that humans may become subclinically infected with CDV; immunization against measles virus also protects against CDV infection
• Speculated that CDV may cause MS; several studies have refuted this proposition; most compelling evidence: canine distemper became rare in dogs after the introduction of MLV-CD vaccines in the early 1960s, although the incidence of MS remained unchanged; incubation period of MS is usually < 30 years; thus CDV cannot be a factor.

PREGNANCY
In utero infection of fetuses—occurs in antibody-negative bitches; rare; may lead to abortion or to persistent infection; infected neonates appear but may develop fatal disease by 4–6 weeks of age

SYNONYMS
• Canine distemper
• Hard pad disease
• Hundestaupe
• Maladie de Carré

SEE ALSO
Myoclonus

ABBREVIATIONS
• CDV = canine distemper virus
• CSF = cerebrospinal fluid
• MLV-CD = modified live virus of canine distemper
• MS = multiple sclerosis
• PCR = polymerase chain reaction

Suggested Reading
Appel MJG, Summers BA. Pathogenicity of morbilliviruses for terrestrial carnivores. Vet Microbiol 1995;44:187–191.
Greene CE, Appel MJ. Canine distemper. In: Greene CE, ed. Infectious diseases of the dog and cat. Philadelphia: Saunders, 1998:9–22.
Author Max J. G. Appel
Consulting Editor Stephen C. Barr

CANINE PARVOVIRUS INFECTION

 BASICS

DEFINITION
• CPV causes a systemic illness with primarily gastrointestinal and immunologic effects. CPV is characterized clinically by inappetence, vomiting, diarrhea, and weight loss. Severe disease results in sepsis, endotoxemia, DIC, and acute respiratory distress syndrome.
• The original CPV underwent genetic alterations, developing into CPV-1 and CPV-2. CPV-2 developed further into CPV-2a (1980) and CPV-2b (1984). The most severe disease is associated with CPV-2b. CPV-1 may cause intractable, usually fatal diarrhea in neonatal puppies.

PATHOPHYSIOLOGY
• CPV has a fecal-oral route of infection. Lymphoid proliferation within tonsils, mesenteric lymph nodes, and other lymphoid tissue follows. Viremia is seen by day 3–5 post infection and precedes clinical signs.
• Viremic animals will show fecal shedding prior to clinical signs. Fecal shedding is typically not longer than 10 days.
• The incubation period is 7–14 days.
• CPV targets the crypt cells of the distal duodenum initially, then extends to the jejunum.
• Clinical signs begin to manifest by day 6–10 post infection.
• Affected animals will have concurrent leukopenia and neutropenia. This is primarily due to increased tissue demand, shift from circulating to marginating pool, and depletion of marrow stores.
• A myocardial form of CPV is rarely seen. This virus is due to in utero or neonatal infection with CPV-2 and typically causes acute death.
• Severe cases develop sepsis and endotoxemia from gram-negative enteric bacteria. Gnotobiotic dogs show minimal signs of sepsis. The cytokine response seen in parvovirus is equivalent to that seen with sepsis. Sepsis causes circulatory collapse, multiorgan failure, and death.

SYSTEMS AFFECTED
• Gastrointestinal—intestinal crypt destruction; inappetence; vomiting; osmotic, secretory, hemorrhagic, small bowel diarrhea
• Hemic/lymphatic/immune—lymphoid depletion; bone marrow depletion; destruction of thymus, Peyer's patches, and GALT leading to immunosuppression
• Behavioral—lethargy, depression from dehydration, sepsis, hypoglycemia
• Cardiovascular—myocarditis causing sudden death; hypovolemic shock causing circulatory collapse; bacteremia, septicemia,

endotoxemia, hypercoagulability; hypercoagulability is an early change; hypocoagulability is seen with DIC and significant losses of antithrombin III
• Nervous—mental depression; coma due to hypoglycemia, shock, intracranial hemorrhage
• Hepatobiliary—icterus; high liver enzymes from cholestasis; endotoxemia
• Renal/urologic—prerenal azotemia; renal azotemia due to multiorgan failure
• Respiratory—acute respiratory distress syndrome in severe cases

GENETICS
Unknown

INCIDENCE/PREVALENCE
• Incidence has decreased dramatically with vaccination.
• Still seen in breeding kennels, pounds, shelters, and areas with high numbers of immunocompromised or inadequately vaccinated puppies

GEOGRAPHIC DISTRIBUTION
Worldwide

SIGNALMENT

Species
• Dogs
• Cats—can be infected with CPV-2b

Breed Predilections
• Rottweilers, Doberman pinschers, pit bulls, Labrador retrievers, German shepherds, English springer spaniels, Alaskan sled dogs

Mean Age and Range
• Most cases are seen between 6 weeks and 6 months of age.
• More severe disease is seen in younger puppies.

Predominant Sex
N/A

SIGNS

General Comments
Pups with signs of lethargy, inappetence, vomiting, or diarrhea should be viewed as suspicious for CPV.

Historical Findings
Owners report loss of energy, lethargy, inappetence, vomiting, and profuse diarrhea with rapid, severe weight loss.

Physical Examination Findings
• Tachycardia
• Mucous membranes may be pale, injected, or icteric.
• Dehydration
• Pain or discomfort on abdominal palpation
• Intestines may be fluid filled, or rarely, there may be a palpable intussusception.
• Pups may be febrile or hypothermic.
• Pups may exhibit vomiting/diarrhea in the examination room.

CAUSES
CPV-2

RISK FACTORS
• Breed predisposition as above
• Possible concurrent immunosuppressive conditions (e.g., heavy parasitism)
• Incomplete vaccination protocol, vaccine failure, or interference with maternal antibodies

 DIAGNOSIS

DIFFERENTIAL DIAGNOSIS
• Foreign body or toxin ingestion, dietary indiscretion
• Gastrointestinal parasitism (hookworm, *Cryptosporidia*)
• *Clostridium perfringens* infection
• *Campylobacter* infection
• Coronavirus
• Hemorrhagic gastroenteritis
• Intussusception

CBC/ BIOCHEMISTRY/ URINALYSIS
• Neutropenia (typically severe) and lymphopenia
• Leukocytosis may be seen during recovery phase.
• Elevated liver enzymes, hypoglycemia, panhypoproteinemia, azotemia, electrolyte imbalances, and evidence of multiorgan involvement may be seen on chemistry.

OTHER LABORATORY TESTS
N/A

IMAGING
• Survey abdominal radiographs to evaluate the gastrointestinal tract for possible foreign body or intestinal obstruction; generalized ileus may be seen.
• Abdominal ultrasonography may show enlarged mesenteric lymph nodes (rarely) and distended, fluid-filled intestinal loops.

DIAGNOSTIC PROCEDURES
• Fecal ELISA—for parvoviral antigen; false-negatives may be seen due to relatively short time of viral shedding; false-positives may be seen with recent vaccination (5–15 days after vaccine)
• Other, less commonly used tests—virus isolation, PCR, electron microscopy, tissue culture, and serology for hemagglutination inhibition

PATHOLOGIC FINDINGS

Gross
• Inspection of the intestinal walls shows edema and hemorrhage.
• Intestines may contain watery, hemorrhagic fluid with necrotic, sloughed mucosa.
• Lymphadenomegaly is not typically seen.
• The thymus may be atrophied.
• In myocardial cases, there may be pale streaks in the myocardium.

Histologic
• Microscopic intestinal lesions include necrosis of the crypt epithelium; shortened, blunted villi; and collapse of the lamina propria.
• Lymphoid tissue and Peyer's patches may be necrotic.
• Viral inclusion bodies may be seen with various methods.
• Microscopic cardiac lesions include lymphocytic and plasmacytic infiltration around myocytes.
• Lesions may be seen in various organs with concurrent endotoxemia and shock.

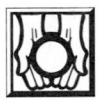

TREATMENT

APPROPRIATE HEALTH CARE
• Hospitalization for intensive therapy and supportive treatment significantly improves survival. Hospitalized cases must be kept isolated from other patients. Hospital personnel must be educated on proper cleaning and disinfecting to prevent spread of the virus.
• Less severely affected puppies may be managed on an outpatient basis with subcutaneous and/or intraperitoneal therapy if owner has financial constraints.

NURSING CARE
• Intravenous crystalloid fluid therapy is a mainstay of treatment. Fluid rates must account for maintenance needs plus ongoing losses, which may be profound.
• Colloid therapy may be necessary in hypoalbuminemic patients.
• Transfusions with plasma or hyperimmune serum may be used.

ACTIVITY
Activity should be restricted until pups are recovering.

DIET
• Food and water should be withheld if vomiting is protracted.
• Small amounts of water may be introduced after 24 hours with no vomiting.
• Enteral or microenteral nutrition should be considered in cases with anorexia of 3–4 days' duration.
• Parenteral nutrition may be required in severe cases.
• Glutamine supplementation has been shown to improve enterocyte health.
• A bland, easily digestible diet (e.g., Hill's i/d, Purina EN) should be fed initially, with gradual transition to the normal ration.

CLIENT EDUCATION
• The virus is stable in the environment but may be destroyed by 1:30 bleach solution.
• Vaccine does not produce an immediate immunity, so susceptible puppies should be kept isolated.

SURGICAL CONSIDERATIONS
The only surgical indication is the rare development of intestinal intussusception due to hypermotility. Careful, daily abdominal palpation is mandatory.

MEDICATIONS

DRUG(S) OF CHOICE
• Antiemetics—very frequently needed due to protracted vomiting; metoclopramide (0.2–0.4 mg/kg SC q6–8h or constant rate infusion of 1–2 mg/kg/day IV); phenothiazines may worsen depression (promethazine, 0.2–0.4 mg/kg IV, IM q 6–8h); serotonin receptor antagonists (ondansetron 0.5–1.0 mg/kg IV q12–24h)
• H$_2$-blockers—may reduce nausea; cimetidine (4–10 mg/kg SC, IM, IV q6h); ranitidine (1–2 mg/kg IV q12h); famotidine (0.5–1.0 mg/kg SC, IM, IV q12–24h)
• Antibiotics (see precautions)—to combat sepsis; should have spectrum to include gram-negative organisms; combination protocols are commonly utilized
• Anthelmintics—may be used to eradicate concurrent parasites
• Analgesics—may be needed in severe cases
• There are anecdotal reports describing the use of equine endotoxin antiserum. At this time, there have been no controlled studies demonstrating a survival benefit with this therapy.
• Recent studies have shown no survival benefit in using granulocyte colony-stimulating factor, anti-TNF, or recombinant bactericidal/permeability–increasing protein (rBPI$_{21}$).
• Activated protein C and IFNΣ may be promising future treatment options.

CONTRAINDICATIONS
N/A

PRECAUTIONS
• Fluoroquinolones should not be used because of the risk of cartilage defects.
• Aminoglycosides should only be used if puppies are well hydrated.
• Nonsteroidal antiinflammatory drugs (including flunixin meglumine [Banamine]) should be used with extreme caution because of renal toxicity.

POSSIBLE INTERACTIONS
N/A

ALTERNATIVE DRUG(S)
N/A

FOLLOW-UP

PATIENT MONITORING
Recovery is typically complete. Immunity is long term and may be lifelong.

PREVENTION/AVOIDANCE
• Vaccination has been effective at drastically reducing disease incidence. • Modified live (high-titer) vaccines are recommended to minimize interference from maternal antibodies. • Interference from maternal antibody is the main reason for vaccine failure. Some pups may have maternal antibody up to 18 weeks. • Protocols recommend vaccinating at 6, 9, and 12 weeks of age. • High-risk breeds may require longer initial protocol, extending up to 22 weeks.

POSSIBLE COMPLICATIONS
• Sepsis • Endotoxemia • Shock
• Intussusception • DIC
• Acute respiratory distress syndrome

EXPECTED COURSE AND PROGNOSIS
• Mortality is primarily due to endotoxemia.
• Aggressive therapy improves survival, but mortality rates may still approach 30%.

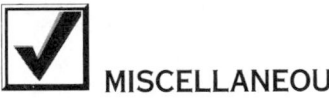

MISCELLANEOUS

ASSOCIATED CONDITIONS
N/A

AGE-RELATED FACTORS
Younger pups have more severe illness.

ZOONOTIC POTENTIAL
None

PREGNANCY
N/A

SYNONYMS
N/A

SEE ALSO
• Diarrhea, Acute • Sepsis and Bacteremia
• Shock, Septic • Vomiting, Acute

ABBREVIATIONS
• CPV = canine parvovirus • DIC = disseminated intravascular coagulation
• ELISA = enzyme-linked immunosorbent assay • GALT = gut-associated lymphoid tissue • IFNΣ = interferon omega • PCR = polymerase chain reaction • TNF = tumor necrosis factor

Suggested Reading
Hoskins JD. Canine viral enteritis. In: Greene CE, ed. Infectious diseases of the dog and cat. 2nd ed. Philadelphia: Saunders, 1998:40–45.
Rewerts JM, Cohn LA. CVT update: diagnosis and treatment of parvovirus. In: Bonagura J, ed. Kirk's current veterinary therapy XIII. Philadelphia: Saunders, 2000:629–632.
Author Jo Ann Morrison
Consulting Editor Albert E. Jergens

CAPILLARIASIS

 **BASICS**

OVERVIEW
- *Capillaria plica* is a parasite that invades the mucosa or submucosa of the bladder or (rarely) the renal pelvis and ureter, causing a mild inflammatory response.
- *C. plica* in dogs and cats and *C. feliscati* in cats have been uncommonly associated with signs of lower urinary tract disease.
- *C. plica* passes ova with bipolar plugs in urine. After earthworms ingest embryonated ova, the parasite develops into the infective stage. Ingestion of infective earthworm results in a patent infection in dogs in 58–88 days.
- Details of life cycle of *C. feliscati* are poorly understood.

SIGNALMENT
- Dogs—no predilection reported
- Cats—affected cats almost always >8 months old

SIGNS
- Usually none
- Pollakiuria, hematuria, stranguria, and dysuria in some animals, particularly those heavily infected

CAUSES & RISK FACTORS
Dogs
- High prevalence of infection (up to 50%) in the natural hosts (foxes and raccoons) in the southeastern United States may predispose animals in this geographic region.
- In kennels, high infection rates are associated with the use of soil surfaces.

Cats
Rare in United States; infection prevalence of 18–34% is reported in Australia.

 DIAGNOSIS

DIFFERENTIAL DIAGNOSES
Consider other more common causes of lower urinary tract disease, such as urolithiasis, urinary tract infection, trauma, and neoplasia.

CBC/BIOCHEMISTRY/URINALYSIS
- Ova with bipolar plugs in urine sediment are diagnostic.
- Consider the possibility of fecal contamination of urine with *Trichuris vulpis* or other *Capillaria* spp. ova if free-catch urine specimens are used or if inadvertent rectal puncture occurs during cystocentesis.
- Alternatively, in an affected animal, urine contamination of feces can produce false fecal examination findings.

OTHER LABORATORY TESTS
N/A

IMAGING
N/A

DIAGNOSTIC PROCEDURES
N/A

 TREATMENT

- Infection is usually self-limiting in both species; ova are no longer detectable in the urine sediment of infected dogs in 10–12 weeks if isolated.
- Replacing soil surfaces with sand, gravel, or concrete may reduce prevalence of infection in kennels.

 MEDICATIONS

DRUG(S)
- Consider anthelmintic therapy if clinical signs are present; monitor therapeutic success by examining urine sediment for ova and observing clinical signs.
- Fenbendazole (50 mg/kg PO q24h for 5 days) has been reported to result in disappearance of ova from urine sediment in dogs and cats.
- Ivermectin (0.2 mg/kg SC once) has been suggested as an alternative therapy, but objective information on its efficacy in this disease is limited.

CONTRAINDICATIONS/POSSIBLE INTERACTIONS
N/A

 FOLLOW-UP

Monitor treatment success by examining urine sediment for ova and observing clinical signs.

 MISCELLANEOUS

Suggested Reading
Brown SA, Prestwood KA. Parasites of the urinary tract. In: Kirk RW, ed. Current veterinary therapy IX. Philadelphia: Saunders, 1986:1153–1155.
Authors Susan E. Little and Scott A. Brown
Consulting Editors Larry G. Adams and Carl A. Osborne

CARBON MONOXIDE POISONING

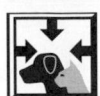 BASICS

OVERVIEW
Carbon monoxide—odorless, colorless, nonirritating gas produced by inefficient combustion of carbonaceous fuels; absorbed into the blood, forming carboxyhemoglobin and reducing oxygen, which causes hypoxia of the brain and heart

SIGNALMENT
All animals

SIGNS
Historical Findings
Exposure to automobile exhaust or fumes from carbon-based fuel heating devices

Physical Examination Findings
Acute
- Drowsiness
- Lethargy
- Weakness
- Deafness
- Incoordination
- Reduced heart excitability
- Cherry red skin and mucous membranes
- Dyspnea
- Coma
- Terminal clonic spasms
- Acute death
Chronic
- Low exercise tolerance
- Disturbance of postural and position reflexes and gait

CAUSES & RISK FACTORS
- Incomplete combustion of carbon fuels
- Poor ventilation
- Automobile exhaust in a closed garage or faulty exhaust system
- Unvented or faulty furnaces, gas water heaters, or gas or kerosene space heaters
- Fires—carbon monoxide concentration may reach 10% in the atmosphere of a burning building.
- Animals with impaired cardiac or pulmonary function—at higher risk than clinically normal animals

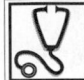 DIAGNOSIS

DIFFERENTIAL DIAGNOSIS
Similar clinical signs—barbiturate, ethanol, cyanide, or hydrogen sulfide gas toxicosis

CBC/BIOCHEMISTRY/URINALYSIS
Creatine kinase—high because of muscle ischemia

OTHER LABORATORY TESTS
- Carboxyhemoglobin in whole blood—expressed as a percent of hemoglobin in the carboxyhemoglobin form; most useful for acute cases; may return to normal levels within a few hours after carbon monoxide exposure stops
- Blood pH—lower than normal secondary to metabolic acidosis
- PAO_2—normal; percent oxygen saturation low

IMAGING
N/A

DIAGNOSTIC PROCEDURES
ECG—consistent with anoxia and necrosis of single heart muscle fibers

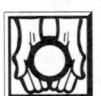 TREATMENT
- Restore adequate oxygen to brain and heart.
- Provide fresh air, maintain patent airway, and provide artificial respiration if necessary.
- Supplemental oxygen or hyperbaric oxygen—promotes recovery
- Supportive fluids

 MEDICATIONS

DRUG(S)
None

CONTRAINDICATIONS/POSSIBLE INTERACTIONS
Avoid respiratory depressants.

 FOLLOW-UP
- Significant response to therapy—should be observed in 1–4 hr, depending on cellular damage owing to hypoxia.
- Monitor cardiac, pulmonary, and neurologic function and limit physical activity for 2 weeks.
- Neurologic signs—may appear within a few days to as long as 6 weeks after apparent recovery
- Eliminate source of carbon monoxide; prevent re-exposure by using in-home carbon monoxide detectors.

 MISCELLANEOUS

PREGNANCY
Carbon monoxide—reduces oxygen-carrying ability of maternal blood; crosses the placenta, producing fetal hypoxia, abortion, or neurologic impairment of the fetus, even when the dam is asymptomatic

ZOONOTIC POTENTIAL
Humans in the same carbon monoxide–contaminated environment are at risk.

Suggested Reading
Ellenhorn MJ, Schonwald S, Ordog G, Wasserberger J . Ellenhorn's medical toxicology: diagnosis and treatment of human poisoning. 2nd ed. Baltimore: Williams & Wilkins, 1997:1465–1474.
Fitzgerald KT. Carbon monoxide poisoning. In: Peterson ME, Talcot PA, eds. Small animal toxicology. Philadelphia: Saunders, 2001:445–451.
Author Thomas L. Carson
Consulting Editor Gary D. Osweiler

CARCINOID TUMOR

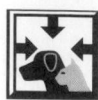

BASIC

OVERVIEW
• Carcinoid tumors are rare, slow-growing, neuroendocrine tumors that arise from amine precursor uptake and decarboxylation (APUD) cells, most commonly the enterochromaffin cells of the gastrointestinal tract. These tumors can secrete a variety of amines, such as serotonin and histamine, and peptides such as bradykinins and tachykinins. In humans, these secretory substances can cause a well-recognized "carcinoid syndrome" once metastasis has occurred in the liver and hepatic degradation is bypassed. The human carcinoid syndrome is most commonly characterized by flushing and diarrhea. Domestic small animals have not been reported to show these clinical signs. Instead, morbidity and mortality are often a function of tumor size and impedance. Clinical signs vary with the location of the primary tumor and metastasis.
• Primary carcinoid tumors have been reported in the stomach, small intestine, colon, lung, and liver in dogs. In cats, carcinoids have been found in the stomach, small intestine, liver, and heart.

SIGNALMENT
• Dog—rare, >9 years of age
• Cat—rare, >7 years of age

SIGNS
Clinical signs are generally dependent on the location of the primary tumor and the metastasized lesions. They have ranged from anorexia and vomiting, dyschezia and weight loss to hepatic failure or heart disease.

CAUSES & RISK FACTORS
N/A

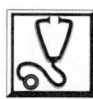

DIAGNOSIS

DIFFERENTIAL DIAGNOSIS
Differentials will vary depending on presenting complaint. May include primary gastrointestinal diseases such as other neoplasias, infections, inflammation, and parasites, foreign body ingestion or dietary indiscretion, or secondary gastrointestinal signs such as liver disease.

CBC/BIOCHEMISTRY/URINALYSIS
• Results can appear normal except for a mild anemia that is generally nonregenerative.
• Electrolyte abnormalities and liver enzymes can be present depending on the clinical signs.

OTHER LABORATORY TESTS
Serotonin metabolites are measured in humans suspected of carcinoid tumors. This is purportedly more accurate than direct measurement of serum amine and peptide levels. Neither of these diagnostics has been reported in the diagnosis of carcinoid tumors in small animals.

IMAGING
• Ultrasound has been used to identify both primary tumors and metastasis in both the abdomen and the thorax of dogs and cats.
• CT scans, MR imaging, and radiolabeled octreotide nuclear scans have also been used for localization of carcinoids in humans.

DIAGNOSTIC PROCEDURES
Biopsy of affected tissue will confirm the diagnosis. Immunohistochemical stains are used to determine the amines and peptides actively secreted by these tumor cells.

PATHOLOGIC FINDINGS
In general, these tumors have a fine fibrovascular stroma. Cells can be pleiomorphic or isomorphic. Cytoplasm is eosinophilic and often contains fine secretory granules. They can stain argyrophilic or argentaffin-positive. Many different immunohistochemical stains can be considered, as secretory substances are variable.

TREATMENT

In some cases, surgical excision can be curative. Debulking can decrease hormone secretion in humans, and it may relieve gastrointestinal signs in animals that are obstructed because of tumor size.

MEDICATIONS

DRUG(S)
Octreotide, a somatostatin analog, is often used in people for palliative therapy when surgery is not an option. This drug will inhibit hormone secretion from the tumor cells. Since this is not the primary mechanism of disease in the animals that have been reported with carcinoid tumors, this would likely be of little benefit in veterinary medicine.

CONTRADICTIONS/POSSIBLE INTERACTIONS
N/A

FOLLOW-UP

• Blood work should be monitored routinely to detect destructive hepatic metastasis if the initial tumor burden was not completely excised.
• Annual ultrasound may also help to detect further metastasis before the liver or other organs are functionally affected.

MISCELLANEOUS

Suggested Reading

Albers TM, et al. A poorly differentiated gastric carcinoid in a dog. J Vet Diagn Invest 1998:10:116–118.

Alexander RW, Kock RA. Primary hepatic carcinoid (APUD cell carcinoma) in the cat. J Small Anim Pract 1982:23:767–771.

Churcher, RK. Hepatic carcinoid, hypercortisolism and hypokalemia in a dog. Aust Vet J. 1999:77(10):641–645.

Feldman EC, Nelson RW. Gastrinoma, glucagonoma and other APUDomas. In: Feldman EC, Nelson RW. Canine and feline endocrinology and reproduction, 2nd ed. Philadelphia: Saunders, 1996:452.

Kipnis RM. A canine carcinoid tumor. Canine Practice 1998:23(6):20–22.

Author Nicole Bennett
Consulting Editor Deborah Greco

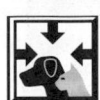

BASICS

OVERVIEW
A myocardial disease most commonly characterized by ventricular tachyarrhythmias (i.e., ventricular premature complexes, ventricular tachycardia) that can be accompanied by syncope or sudden cardiac death. A small percentage (<5%) of patients develop congestive heart failure with systolic dysfunction, which is comparable to the dilated car-diomyopathy observed in other canine breeds.

SIGNALMENT
• Dog • Specific to the boxer, although a similar clinical presentation has been infrequently observed in the English bulldog • Usually observed in mature dogs, at least 2 years of age. Dogs as young as 6 months have been reported. Some affected individuals may not develop clinical signs until over 10 years of age.

SIGNS
Clinical signs are variable but are usually one of three presentations:
• Asymptomatic dog with ventricular premature complexes (VPCs) detected on routine examination • Syncope in a dog with VPCs detected on an ECG or Holter monitor (ambulatory ECG) • Signs of left heart failure (e.g., coughing, tachypnea) or biventricular failure (e.g., ascites, tachypnea, coughing) with VPCs. This presentation is the least common and is characterized by ventricular dilation and systolic dysfunction. • Sudden death may occur before development of obvious clinical signs.

CAUSES & RISK FACTORS
• Believed to be inherited (autosomal dominant); however, a specific genetic defect has not been identified. • At least one family of boxers with VPCs, ventricular dilation, and systolic dysfunction was found to have decreased myocardial L-carnitine levels and demonstrated some clinical improvement when supplemented with L-carnitine. The cause and effect of this relationship is unclear, and response to this supplementation does not occur in all dogs with myocardial dysfunction.

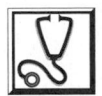

DIAGNOSIS

DIFFERENTIAL DIAGNOSIS
• Aortic stenosis is common in the boxer and can be associated with VPCs. • Uncommon forms of acquired cardiac disease (neoplasia, endocarditis) • Abdominal disease (especially splenic disease) can be associated with the development of VPCs. • Echocardiography and abdominal ultrasonography can be used to differentiate boxer cardiomyopathy from other causes of VPCs.

CBC/BIOCHEMISTRY/URINALYSIS
N/A

OTHER LABORATORY TESTS
Plasma L-carnitine levels may be evaluated in boxers with ventricular dilation and systolic dysfunction. However, plasma levels are not always reflective of myocardial levels. If plasma levels are not low, it is still possible to have low myocardial levels, and supplementation with L-carnitine might be considered.

IMAGING
Thoracic Radiography
• Normal in most affected dogs • Dogs with ventricular dilation and systolic dysfunction may have cardiac enlargement and evidence of heart failure (e.g., pulmonary edema).

Echocardiography
• Normal in most affected dogs • A small percentage of dogs have ventricular dilation and systolic dysfunction.

DIAGNOSTIC PROCEDURES
Electrocardiogram
Many dogs will not have VPCs on an ECG of brief duration, since the arrhythmia can be intermittent. Some dogs will have one or more upright VPCs on a brief lead II ECG. In either case, if suspicion of disease is present, Holter monitoring is recommended to determine the severity and complexity of the arrhythmia and to have a baseline for comparison once treatment is started. If Holter monitoring is not available and the dog is symptomatic with upright VPCs on an ECG, therapy should be considered.

PATHOLOGIC FINDINGS
• Gross pathology is nonspecific in most cases. In a small percentage of cases, left and right ventricular dilation may be observed. • Histopathologic abnormalities include a fatty and fibrous infiltrate into the right ventricular (and sometimes left ventricular) free wall.

TREATMENT
• The goals of therapy include reduction of the number of VPCs, reduction of clinical signs, and reduction of the risk of sudden cardiac death. Unfortunately, there is no evidence that therapy can reduce the risk of sudden death. The decision to start therapy in the asymptomatic boxer with VPCs is controversial, since all antiarrhythmics have the potential to make the arrhythmia worse. However, dogs with as few as 300 VPCs/24 hr have been observed to die suddenly. In general, we prescribe ventricular antiarrhythmic drugs if there are >1000 VPCs/24 hr, significant runs of ventricular tachycardia or other signs of complexity (e.g., bigeminy, couplets), or clinical signs related to the VPCs. • Episodes of syncope and sudden cardiac death are more frequently (but not always) associated with

stress and excitement. Attempt to reduce stress and effort when possible.

MEDICATIONS

DRUG(S)
• The two best choices for treating the ventricular arrhythmia are sotalol (1.5–3.5 mg/kg PO q12h) or a combination of mexiletine (5–8 mg/kg PO q8h) and atenolol (0.3–0.6 mg/kg PO q12h). There appears to be some individual dog variability as to which option works better, so if an appropriate response is not observed, it is reasonable to switch to the other. • In dogs with systolic dysfunction and heart failure, consider treatment with furosemide (1–2 mg/kg PO q12h), enalapril (0.5 mg/kg PO q12h), spironolactone (1–2 mg/kg PO q12–24h) and L-carnitine (50 mg/kg PO q8–12h).

CONTRAINDICATIONS/POSSIBLE INTERACTIONS
Any antiarrhythmic drug has the potential to make an arrhythmia worse.

FOLLOW-UP
• If possible, repeat the Holter monitor 2 weeks after starting therapy to evaluate for a response. A good response to therapy would be an 85% reduction in VPC number. If clinical signs increase while dog is on therapy, or if the results of the Holter monitor do not show improvement, switch to the other drug choice. • Annual Holter monitoring and echocardiography are suggested. • Owners should be advised that dogs are always at risk of sudden death. However, many dogs can be maintained on antiarrhythmics for years. Dogs with systolic dysfunction and dilation have the worst prognosis, although some of these dogs do show improvement and a decreased rate of progression on L-carnitine supplementation.

MISCELLANEOUS

SYNONYM
Boxer familial ventricular arrhythmia

ABBREVIATIONS
ECG = electrocardiogram
VPC = ventricular premature complex

Suggested Reading
Harpster NK. Boxer cardiomyopathy. A review of the long-term benefits of anti-arrhythmic therapy. Vet Clin North Am Small Anim Pract 1991;21:989–1004.
Author Kathryn M. Meurs
Consulting Editors Larry P. Tilley and Francis W. K. Smith Jr.

CARDIOMYOPATHY, DILATED—CATS

BASICS

OVERVIEW
• Dilated cardiomyopathy is a disease of the ventricular muscle characterized by systolic myocardial failure and an enlarged, volume overloaded heart that leads to signs of congestive heart failure or low cardiac output.
• Before 1987, dilated cardiomyopathy was one of the most commonly diagnosed heart diseases in cats. Most cats probably had secondary cardiomyopathy as a result of taurine deficiency. Primary idiopathic dilated cardiomyopathy is now an uncommon cause of heart disease in cats.

SIGNALMENT
Siamese, Abyssinian, and Burmese cats have a reported increased incidence. Familial patterns have been identified in some families of cats.

SIGNS

Historical Findings
Signs related to low cardiac output—
• Anorexia
• Weakness
• Depression
Signs related to congestive heart failure—
• Dyspnea
• Tachypnea
Signs related to thromboembolism—
Sudden-onset pain and paraparesis

Physical Examination Findings
• Heart rate can be fast, normal, or slow.
• Soft systolic heart murmur
• Weak left cardiac impulse
• Gallop rhythm
• Possible arrhythmia
• Hypothermia

• Prolonged capillary refill time
• Tachypnea
• Quiet lung sounds (pleural effusion)
• Crackles (pulmonary edema)
• Hypokinetic femoral pulses
• Possibly posterior paresis and pain as a result of aortic thromboembolism

CAUSES & RISK FACTORS
The underlying etiology of idiopathic dilated cardiomyopathy remains unknown, although a genetic predisposition has been identified in some families of cats. Taurine deficiency was a common cause of secondary myocardial failure before 1987.

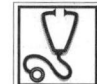

DIAGNOSIS

DIFFERENTIAL DIAGNOSIS
• Taurine deficiency dilated cardiomyopathy. Because primary idiopathic dilated cardiomyopathy and taurine deficiency have similar clinical presentations, cats with myocardial failure should be assumed to have taurine deficiency until shown to be unresponsive to taurine.
• Myocardial failure secondary to longstanding congenital or acquired left ventricular volume overload diseases.

CBC/BIOCHEMISTRY/URINALYSIS
Many cats will have pre-renal azotemia related to low cardiac output.

OTHER LABORATORY TESTS
Plasma taurine concentrations less than 40 nmoles/L or whole blood taurine concentrations less than 250 nmoles/L are subnormal and suggestive of taurine-deficiency dilated cardiomyopathy. Taurine assays are performed at a limited number of institutions and require special handling.

IMAGING

Radiographic Findings
• Radiography often shows pleural effusion or pulmonary edema.
• Generalized cardiomegaly

Echocardiographic Findings
• Diagnostic modality of choice
• Characteristic findings include thin ventricular walls, enlarged left ventricular end systolic and end diastolic dimensions, left atrial enlargement, and low fractional shortening.

DIAGNOSTIC TESTS

Electrocardiography
• Electrocardiography may be normal or may show left atrial or ventricular enlargement patterns.
• Both ventricular and supraventricular arrhythmias can be seen.

Pleural Effusion Analysis
Pleural effusion typically is a modified transudate with total protein less than 4.0 g/dl and nucleated cell counts of less than 2500/ml. Chylous effusion may also be present. Analysis of the pleural effusion is important to rule out other causes of pleural effusion such as pyothorax, infectious peritonitis, or lymphosarcoma.

PATHOLOGIC FINDINGS
• Heart to body ratio is increased.
• Ventricle walls are thin and the lumen is enlarged.
• Valve anatomy is normal.
• Histopathology shows myocyte atrophy and myocardial fibrosis.

CARDIOMYOPATHY, DILATED—CATS

TREATMENT

- These cats usually are in congestive heart failure and should be treated as inpatients.
- Thoracocentesis is both therapeutic and diagnostic.
- Supplemental oxygen therapy is beneficial for cats in congestive heart failure.
- If hypothermic, external heat (incubator or heating pad) is recommended.
- These cats typically are anorexic, thus tempting their appetite with many types of food may be necessary. Eventually, a low-sodium diet is recommended.

MEDICATIONS

DRUG(S)

- Furosemide is recommended at the lowest effective dose to eliminate pulmonary edema and pleural effusion. Recommended dose range is 1–3 mg/kg q8–12h. Initially, furosemide should be administered parenterally.
- Nitroglycerin (2% ointment) 0.25–0.5 inch applied topically can be used in conjunction with diuretics in the acute management of congestive heart failure to further reduce preload. Nitroglycerin will lower the dose of furosemide and is particularly useful in patients with hypothermia or dehydration.

- Enalapril at a dose of 0.25 to 0.5 mg/kg PO q24h is recommended to reduce afterload and preload.
- Digoxin is recommended to strengthen contractility and for its positive neurohumoral effects at a dose of 0.03 mg/cat (one quarter of a 0.125-mg tablet) or 0.01 mg/kg PO q48h.
- Taurine supplementation is recommended at 250 mg PO q12h until it is demonstrated that the patient is unresponsive to taurine.
- Dobutamine at extremely low dosages can be given to a patient with severe signs of congestive heart failure and low cardiac output. Dose varies from 1–5 mcg/kg/min.
- Because thromboembolic disease is a concern, many will recommend either aspirin 81 mg PO q72h (with food) or low molecular weight heparin (e.g., Daltaperin 100 units/kg SC q24h or Enoxaparin 1 mg/kg SC q24h).
- Beta-blockers are useful in the long term management of dilated cardiomyopathy in humans because of their positive myocardial effects and survival benefit. Clinical experience is limited in feline dilated cardiomyopathy and they must be used cautiously as they acutely decrease contractility.
- See aortic thromboembolism chapter for therapeutic recommendations.

CONTRAINDICATIONS/POSSIBLE INTERACTIONS

- Unless needed for acute cardiac rhythm control, drugs such as calcium channel blockers or beta-adrenergic blockers may reduce contractility and lower cardiac output.

- Overzealous diuretic therapy may cause dehydration and hypokalemia.
- Digoxin dose should be reduced if renal insufficiency is documented or suspected.
- Dobutamine may cause seizures and cardiac arrhythmias.

FOLLOW-UP

- Repeat thoracic radiographs within 1 week to determine efficacy of therapy.
- Periodically monitor electrolyte and renal parameters.
- Digoxin concentrations should be measured 2 weeks after initiating therapy. Therapeutic range is between 1–2 ng/dl 8–12 hours post-pill.
- Repeat echocardiogram in 3–6 months after initiating taurine supplementation to determine response to therapy.
- These cats have a poor prognosis despite intensive therapy.

MISCELLANEOUS

Suggested Reading

Pion PD, Kittleson MD, Rogers QR, et al. Myocardial failure in cats associated with low plasma taurine: A reversible cardiomyopathy. Science 1987; 237:764–768.

Author Teresa C. DeFrancesco

Consulting Editors Larry P. Tilley and Francis W. K. Smith, Jr.

CARDIOMYOPATHY, DILATED—DOGS

 BASICS

DEFINITION
Characterized by left- and right-sided dilation, normal coronary arteries, normal (or minimally diseased) atrioventricular valves, significantly decreased inotropic state, and myocardial dysfunction occurring primarily during systole

PATHOPHYSIOLOGY
• Myocardial failure leads to reduced cardiac output and CHF. • A-V anulus dilation and altered papillary muscle function promote valvular insufficiency.

SYSTEMS AFFECTED
• Cardiovascular • Respiratory—pulmonary edema • Renal/Urologic—pre-renal azotemia • All organ systems are affected by reductions in cardiac output.

GENETICS
Genetic cause or heritable susceptibility strongly suspected but as yet unproven

INCIDENCE/PREVALENCE
Estimated at 0.5–1.1%

GEOGRAPHIC DISTRIBUTION
N/A with the exception of Chagas' cardiomyopathy, which is limited to the Southern United States

SIGNALMENT

Species
Dogs

Breed Predilections
• Doberman pinscher, boxer • "Giant" breeds: Scottish deerhound, Irish wolfhound, Great Dane, Saint Bernard, Afghan hound, Burmese mountain dog • Cocker spaniel

Mean Age and Range
4–10 years

Predominant Sex
Males > females in most but not all breeds

SIGNS

Historical Findings
• Respiratory—tachypnea, dyspnea, coughing • Weight loss • Weakness, lethargy, anorexia • Abdominal distention • Syncope • Some dogs are asymptomatic, having what is termed "occult dilated cardiomyopathy."

Physical Examination Findings
• Weakness, depression, possibly cardiogenic shock • Hypokinetic femoral pulse from low cardiac output • Pulse deficits with atrial fibrillation, ventricular premature contractions, and paroxysmal ventricular tachycardia • Jugular pulses from tricuspid regurgitation, arrhythmias, or right-sided CHF • Breath sounds—muffled with pleural effusion; crackles with pulmonary edema • S_3 or summation gallops • Mitral regurgitation and/or tricuspid regurgitation murmurs are common but usually soft. • Auscultatory evidence of cardiac arrhythmia • Slow capillary refill time, possible cyanosis • Hepatomegaly with or without ascites

CAUSES
• Primary mechanism yet to be identified and is idiopathic in the vast majority of cases. Most authors believe that the majority of cases represent familial abnormalities of structural or contractile cardiac proteins. • Nutritional deficiencies (taurine and/or carnitine) have been documented in several breeds including golden retrievers, boxers, Doberman pinschers, and cocker spaniels. • Viral, protozoal, and immune-mediated mechanisms have been proposed. • Hypothyroidism may cause reversible myocardial failure.

RISK FACTORS
N/A

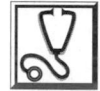 DIAGNOSIS

DIFFERENTIAL DIAGNOSIS
• Endocardiosis • Congenital heart disease • Heartworm disease • Bacterial endocarditis • Cardiac tumors and pericardial effusion • Airway obstruction: foreign body, neoplasm, laryngeal paralysis • Primary pulmonary disease: bronchial disease, pneumonia, neoplasia, aspiration, vascular disease (e.g., heartworms) • Pleural effusions (e.g., pyothorax, hemothorax, chylothorax) • Trauma resulting in diaphragmatic hernia, pulmonary hemorrhage, pneumothorax

CBC/BIOCHEMISTRY/URINALYSIS
Routine hematologic tests and urinalysis are usually normal unless altered by severe heart failure (e.g., prerenal azotemia, high ALT, hyponatremia), therapy for heart failure (e.g. hypokalemia, hypochloremia, and metabolic alkalosis from diuresis), or concurrent disease

OTHER LABORATORY TESTS
N/A

IMAGING

Radiographic Findings
• Generalized cardiomegaly and signs of CHF are common. • Left ventricular enlargement and left atrial enlargement may be most evident in early cases. • Doberman pinschers—marked LAE is a major finding; pulmonary edema is often patchy and diffuse. • Pleural effusion, hepatomegaly, ascites

Echocardiographic Findings
• "Gold standard" for diagnosis • Ventricular and atrial dilation • Reduced myocardial systolic function (low FS%) • Doppler studies may confirm low velocity and/or acceleration of transaortic flow as well as mitral regurgitation and/or tricuspid regurgitation.

DIAGNOSTIC TESTS

Electrocardiography
• Sinus rhythm or sinus tachycardia with isolated atrial or ventricular premature complexes • Atrial fibrillation is common. • Ventricular tachycardia is very common in Doberman pinschers and boxers. • Prolonged QRS (> 0.06 sec), possible increased voltages (R > 3.0 mV lead II), suggesting LV enlargement • May have "sloppy" R wave descent with ST-T coving, suggesting myocardial disease or LV ischemia • May have low voltages (pleural or pericardial effusion, concurrent hypothyroidism).

PATHOLOGIC FINDINGS
• Dilation of all chambers with thinning of the chamber walls • Slightly thickened endocardium with pale areas within the myocardium (necrosis, fibrosis) • Two histologically distinct forms; (1) fatty infiltration—degenerative type seen in boxers and Doberman pinschers and (2) an attenuated wavy fiber type seen in many giant, large-, and medium-sized breeds, including some boxers and Doberman pinschers

 TREATMENT

APPROPRIATE HEALTH CARE
With the exception of severely affected dogs, most therapy can be administered on an outpatient basis.

ACTIVITY
Allow the dog to choose its own level of activity

DIET
• Goal: reduce dietary sodium intake to < 12–15 mg/kg/day • Severe sodium restriction is not necessary when using potent vasodilators and diuretics. • Best to use commercially prepared diets

CLIENT EDUCATION
Emphasize potential signs associated with progression of disease and adverse side effects of medication.

 MEDICATIONS

DRUG(S) OF CHOICE
First identify patient problems: CHF (left or right-sided), arrhythmia, hypothermia, renal failure, shock.

Initial Stabilization
• Treat hypoxemia with oxygen administration; prevent heat loss if hypothermic (warm environment); administer IV or SQ fluids (D_5W or 0.45% NaCl with 2.5% dextrose) only after pulmonary edema is controlled or pleural effusion has been aspirated. • If there is pulmonary edema:

furosemide (2–4 mg/kg IM or IV, then 1–2 mg/kg q8–12h for the first 2–3 days) • 2% topical nitroglycerin for the first 24–48 hr for severe pulmonary edema—apply 1″–2″ q8h.
• Aminophylline (initial 24 hr) for bronchodilation (4–6 mg/kg, slowly IV q8h)
• If there is significant pleural effusion, drain each hemithorax with an 18–20 gauge butterfly catheter. • If there is severe heart failure and cardiogenic shock, digoxin and dobutamine are indicated. These may predispose to malignant arrhythmias, particularly in the hypoxic dog. • Digoxin—oral therapy (see below) • Dobutamine—5–10 µg/kg/min infused for 24–72 hr with care • If paroxysmal ventricular tachycardia is present, administer lidocaine slowly in 2 mg/kg boluses (up to 8 mg/kg total) to convert to sinus rhythm. Follow with lidocaine infusion (40–75 µg/kg/min).
• If lidocaine is ineffective administer procainamide slowly in 2 mg/kg/IV boluses (up to 20 mg/kg total) to convert to sinus rhythm. Follow with a 20–50 µg/kg/min infusion or 8–20 mg/kg IM q6h.

Maintenance Therapy
• Vasodilators, especially the ACE inhibitors (enalapril, benazepril, lisinopril), are considered a cornerstone of therapy for DCM. • Enalapril (0.25–0.5 mg/kg PO q12h), benazepril (0.5 mg/kg PO q24h), or lisinopril (0.5 mg/kg PO q24h) should be initiated early in the therapeutic regimen.
• A daily maintenance dose of 0.375 to 0.75 mg of digoxin (divided q12h) is given to most giant-breed dogs. Do not exceed 0.015 mg/kg/day and do not exceed 0.375 mg per day in Doberman pinschers. If necessary, an oral loading dose (2× maintenance dose) can be given the first 24–48 hr to dogs with atrial fibrillation or cardiogenic shock (uncommonly needed). • Furosemide (0.5–1 mg/kg/ PO q8–24h) is used to control pulmonary edema, pleural effusion, or ascites.
• Spironolactone (0.5–1 mg/kg PO q24h) reduces mortality in humans with heart failure by blocking aldosterone. Higher doses can be used for refractory heart failure (1–2 mg/kg PO q12h). • Beta blockers can be used cautiously once heart failure is controlled with other drugs (see precautions). If tolerated, may improve myocardial function with chronic use. Carvedilol (0.1–0.4 mg/kg PO q12h) is an alpha and beta blocker with antioxidant activity. Start at the low end of the dose range and gradually raise dose over 6-week period if tolerated. Consult with a cardiologist before using beta blockers in DCM patients. • Pimobendan (0.1–0.3 mg/kg PO q12h) is a calcium-sensitizing drug that is a vasodilating positive inotrope that when added to furosemide, ACE inhibitor, and digoxin improves functional heart failure class and in Doberman pinschers increases survival time. • The role of carnitine and taurine in the therapy of DCM remains

controversial. However, American cocker spaniels with dilated cardiomyopathy generally respond favorably to taurine supplementation. Those not responding to taurine will often respond to the addition of L-carnitine.

Arrhythmias
• In the case of atrial fibrillation, slowing of the ventricular rate response is achieved with chronic administration of digitalis combined with atenolol (0.75–1.5 mg/kg PO q12h) or diltiazem (1–1.5 mg/kg PO q8h).
• Therapeutic goal is obtaining a ventricular rate between 100–140 bpm at rest.
• The above therapy merely controls the ventricular rate, by depressing AV nodal conduction; it generally does not convert the rhythm from atrial fibrillation to sinus rhythm. • Chronic oral therapy for ventricular tachycardia includes procainamide (8–20 mg/kg PO q6–8h), mexiletine (5–8 mg/kg PO q8h) or sotalol (2 mg/kg PO q12h).
• Procainamide and mexiletine can be combined with a beta blocker if necessary.

CONTRAINDICATIONS
Digoxin should be avoided in severe uncontrolled paroxysmal ventricular tachycardia.

PRECAUTIONS
• Beta blockers and calcium channel blockers are negative inotropes and may have an acute adverse effect on myocardial function, although recent human studies have suggested that chronic administration of beta blockers may be of benefit in DCM.
• The combination of diuretics and ACE inhibitors my result in azotemia, especially in patients with severe heart failure or pre-existing renal dysfunction.

POSSIBLE INTERACTIONS
• Both quinidine and verapamil will increase serum digoxin levels and predispose to digitalis intoxication. • Propranolol will decrease lidocaine excretion and predispose to toxicity. • Renal dysfunction, hypothyroidism, and hypokalemia predispose to digitalis intoxication.

ALTERNATIVE DRUG(S)
• Other vasodilators, including hydralazine and amlodipine, may be used instead of or in addition to an ACE inhibitor (beware of hypotension). • Propranolol can be used instead of diltiazem or atenolol to help control ventricular response rate in atrial fibrillation. • The role of co-enzyme Q10 remains to be determined.

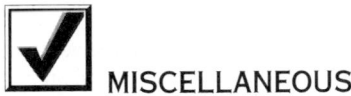

FOLLOW-UP

PATIENT MONITORING
• Serial clinical examinations, thoracic radiographs, and ECG are most helpful.

• Repeat echocardiography is rarely informative. • Serial evaluation of serum digoxin levels (therapeutic range = 0.5–1 ng/mL) taken 6–8 hr post-pill and serum biochemistries may help prevent iatrogenic problems.

POSSIBLE COMPLICATIONS
• Sudden death due to arrhythmias
• Iatrogenic problems associated with medical management (see above)

EXPECTED COURSE AND PROGNOSIS
• Always fatal • Death usually occurs 6–24 months following diagnosis. • Dobermans typically have a worse prognosis, with survival generally less than 6 months from the time of diagnosis. • Atrial fibrillation, paroxysmal ventricular tachycardia, and markedly decreased FS% are probably markers for short survival and sudden death.

✓ MISCELLANEOUS

AGE-RELATED FACTORS
Prevalence increases with age.

SYNONYMS
• Congestive cardiomyopathy
• Giant breed cardiomyopathy

SEE ALSO
• Atrial Fibrillation and Atrial Flutter
• Carnitine Deficiency • Taurine Deficiency
• Ventricular Tachycardia

ABBREVIATIONS
• ACE = angiotensin converting enzyme
• AV = atrioventricular • CHF = congestive heart failure • DCM = dilated cardiomyopathy • FS% = percent fractional shortening • LAE = left atrial enlargement

Suggested Reading
Calvert CA. Canine cardiomyopathy. In Tilley LP, Goodwin J-K, eds. Manual of canine and feline cardiology, 3rd ed. Philadelphia:Saunders, 2001:137.
Fuentes VL, Corcoran B, French A, et al. A double-blind, randomized, placebo-controlled study of pimobendan in dogs with dilated cardiomyopathy J Vet Intern Med 2002;16:(3) 255–261.
Sisson DD, O'Grady MR. Myocardial diseases of dogs. In Fox PR, Sisson DD, Moise NS, eds. Canine and feline cardiology, 2nd ed. Philadelphia: Saunders, 1999:581–620.
Author Matthew W. Miller
Consulting Editors Larry P. Tilley and Francis W. K. Smith Jr.

CARDIOMYOPATHY, HYPERTROPHIC—CATS

BASICS

DEFINITION
Hypertrophic cardiomyopathy is characterized by inappropriate concentric hypertrophy of the ventricular free wall or the intraventricular septum of the nondilated left ventricle. The disease occurs independently of other cardiac or systemic disorders.

PATHOPHYSIOLOGY
• Diastolic dysfunction results from a thickened, noncompliant left ventricle. • High left ventricular filling pressure develops, causing left atrial enlargement. • Pulmonary venous hypertension causes pulmonary edema. Some cats develop biventricular failure (i.e., pulmonary edema, pleural effusion, and, rarely, ascites). • Stasis of blood in the large left atrium predisposes the patient to aortic thromboembolism. • Dynamic aortic outflow obstruction and systolic anterior mitral motion (SAM) with secondary mitral insufficiency occurs in some cats.

SYSTEMS AFFECTED
• Cardiovascular—congestive heart failure (CHF), aortic thromboembolism, and arrhythmias • Pulmonary—dyspnea if CHF develops • Renal/urologic—azotemia due to poor perfusion

GENETICS
Some families of cats have been identified with a high prevalence of the disease, and the disease appears to be inherited as an autosomal dominant trait in Maine coon cats, but the genetics have not been definitively determined.

INCIDENCE/PREVALENCE
Unknown, but relatively common

GEOGRAPHIC DISTRIBUTION
N/A

SIGNALMENT
Species
Cats

Breed Predilections
A familial association has been documented in Maine coon cats, American shorthairs, and Persians.

Mean Age and Range
5–7 years with reported ages of 3 months to 17 years

Predominant Sex
Male

SIGNS
Historical Findings
• Dyspnea • Anorexia • Exercise intolerance • Vomiting • Collapse • Sudden death • Coughing is uncommon in cats with cardiomyopathy and usually suggests pulmonary disease.

Physical Examination Findings
• Gallop rhythm (S3 or S4) • Systolic murmur in many animals • Apex heart beat may be exaggerated. • Muffled heart sounds, lack of chest compliance, and dyspnea characterized by rapid shallow respirations may be associated with pleural effusion. • Dyspnea and crackles if pulmonary edema is present • Weak femoral pulse • Acute pelvic limb paralysis with cyanotic pads and nailbeds, cold limbs, and absence of femoral pulse in animals with aortic thromboembolism. Emboli rarely affect thoracic limbs. • Arrhythmia in some animals

CAUSES
Unknown—probably multiple causes exist

Possible Causes
• Abnormality of the contractile protein myosin or other sarcomeric proteins (e.g., troponin, myosin binding proteins, tropomyosin) • Abnormality affecting catecholamine-influenced excitation-contraction coupling • Abnormal myocardial calcium metabolism • Collagen or other intercellular matrix abnormality • Growth hormone excess • Dynamic left ventricular outflow obstruction leading to secondary left ventricular hypertrophy

RISK FACTORS
Offspring of animals with familial HCM

DIAGNOSIS

DIFFERENTIAL DIAGNOSIS
• Hyperthyroidism • Aortic stenosis • Systemic hypertension • Acromegaly • Noncardiac causes of pleural effusion (e.g., pyothorax, chylothorax, neoplasia, diaphragmatic hernia)

CBC/BIOCHEMISTRY/URINALYSIS
• Results usually normal • Prerenal azotemia in some animals

OTHER LABORATORY TESTS
• In cats over 6 years old, check thyroid concentration to rule out hyperthyroidism. Hyperthyroidism causes myocardial hypertrophy that might be confused with HCM. • A validated growth hormone assay for cats is not currently available. Some cats with HCM have high growth hormone concentration.

IMAGING
Radiography
• Dorsal ventral radiographs often reveal a valentine-appearing heart because of biatrial enlargement and a left ventricle that comes to a point. • Pulmonary edema, pleural effusion, or both in some animals • Radiographs may be normal in asymptomatic cats. • The different forms of cardiomyopathy can not be differentiated by radiography.

Echocardiography
• Hypertrophy of the interventricular septum (IVS) or the left ventricular posterior wall (diastolic wall thickness > 6 mm) • Hypertrophy may be symmetric (affecting IVS and posterior wall) or asymmetric (affecting IVS or posterior wall, but not both) • Hypertrophy of the papillary muscles • Normal or high fractional shortening • Normal or reduced left ventricular lumen • Left atrial enlargement • Systolic anterior motion of the mitral valve (some animals) • Left ventricular outflow obstruction (some animals) • Thrombus in the left atrium (rare) • Note: There is some overlap between normal cats (especially ketaminized and dehydrated) and cats with mild HCM. Correlate echo findings with physical findings. Presence of left atrial enlargement favors HCM.

DIAGNOSTIC PROCEDURES
Electrocardiography
• Sinus tachycardia (HR > 240) is common with heart failure; however, some cats with severe heart failure and hypothermia are bradycardic. • Atrial premature complexes and ventricular premature complexes occasionally seen • Atrial fibrillation is uncommon. • A left axis deviation is seen in many cats. • ECG cannot differentiate different forms of cardiomyopathy or distinguish cardiomyopathy from hyperthyroidism. • Cats with HCM may have a normal ECG.

Systemic Blood Pressure
• Normotensive or hypotensive • Evaluate blood pressure in all patients with myocardial hypertrophy to rule out systemic hypertension as the cause or contributing factor.

PATHOLOGIC FINDINGS
• Nondilated left ventricle with hypertrophy of intraventricular septum or left ventricular free wall • Hypertrophy of papillary muscles • Left atrial enlargement • Mitral valve thickening • Myocardial hypertrophy with disorganized alignment of myocytes (myofiber disarray) • Interstitial fibrosis • Myocardial scarring • Hypertrophy and luminal narrowing of intramural coronary arteries

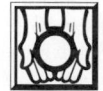

TREATMENT

APPROPRIATE HEALTH CARE
Cats with CHF should be hospitalized for initial medical management.

NURSING CARE
• Minimize stress • Oxygen if dyspneic • Warm environment if hypothermic

ACTIVITY
Restricted

DIET
Sodium restriction in animals with CHF

CLIENT EDUCATION
• Many cats diagnosed while asymptomatic eventually develop CHF and may develop aortic thromboembolism and die suddenly.
• If cat is receiving warfarin, minimize potential for trauma and subsequent hemorrhage.

SURGICAL CONSIDERATIONS
N/A

 MEDICATIONS

DRUG(S) OF CHOICE

Diltiazem
• Dosage—7.5–15 mg/cat PO q8h or 10 mg/kg PO q24h (Cardizem CD) or 30 mg/cat q12h (Dilacor XR) • Beneficial effects may include slower sinus rate, resolution of supraventricular arrhythmias, improved diastolic relaxation, coronary vasodilation, peripheral vasodilation, platelet inhibition.
• Reduces hypertrophy and left atrial dimensions in some cats with HCM • Superior to propranolol and verapamil according to one small study • Role in asymptomatic patients unresolved

Beta Blockers
• Dosage—Atenolol (6.25–12.5 mg/cat PO q12h) • Beneficial effects may include slowing of sinus rate, correcting atrial and ventricular arrhythmias, platelet inhibition. • More effective than diltiazem in controlling sinus tachycardia and dynamic outflow tract obstruction
• Role in asymptomatic patients unresolved, but authors generally use if dynamic outflow obstruction and hypertrophy present

Aspirin
• Dosage—81 mg/cat q 2–3 days if severe atrial enlargement • Depresses platelet aggregation, hopefully minimizing the risk of thromboembolism • Warn owners that thrombi can still develop despite aspirin administration.

Furosemide
• Dosage—1–2 mg/kg PO, IM, IV q8h–q24h
• Critically dyspneic animals often require high dosage (4 mg/kg IV) to stabilize. This dose can be repeated in 1 hour if the cat is still severely dyspneic. Indicated to treat pulmonary edema, pleural effusion, and ascites. • Cats are sensitive to furosemide and prone to dehydration, prerenal azotemia, and hypokalemia. • Once pulmonary edema resolves, taper the dosage to the lowest that controls edema.

Nitroglycerin Ointment
• Dosage—0.25–0.5 in/cat topically applied q6h–q8h or 2.5 mg/24-hr patch • Often used in the acute stabilization of cats with severe pulmonary edema or pleural effusion
• When used intermittently, it may be useful for long-term management of refractory cases.

ACE Inhibitors
• Dosage—Enalapril or benazepril 0.25–0.5 mg/kg q24 h • Indications in cats with HCM not well-defined—authors currently use for CHF • Potential benefits include lowered angiotensin II concentration, lowered catecholamine concentration, minimizing of diuretic-induced potassium depletion.
• Angiotensin II is a potent stimulator of myocardial hypertrophy.

CONTRAINDICATIONS
Avoid beta blockers in cats with emboli; these agents cause peripheral vasoconstriction. If beta blockers must be used in this setting for arrhythmia control, choose a beta-1 selective blocker like atenolol.

PRECAUTIONS
Use ACE inhibitors cautiously if the cat has renal disease or dynamic outflow obstruction.

POSSIBLE INTERACTIONS
N/A

ALTERNATIVE DRUG(S)

Spirinolactone
• Dosage—1 mg/kg q12–24h
• Used in conjunction with furosemide in cats with CHF

Warfarin
Used sometimes in cats at high risk for thromboembolism (see chapter on aortic thromboembolism for appropriate dosing and monitoring)

Dalteparin (Fragmin)
Dosage—100 units/kg SC q24h. Alternative to warfarin that eliminates need for patient monitoring for those at high risk of aortic thromboembolism.

Beta Blocker Plus Diltiazem
• Cats that remain tachycardic on a single agent can be treated cautiously with a combination of a beta blocker and diltiazem.
• Monitor closely for bradycardia and hypotension.

 FOLLOW-UP

PATIENT MONITORING
• Observe closely for signs of dyspnea, lethargy, weakness, anorexia, and posterior paralysis.
• If treating with warfarin, monitor prothrombin time • If treating with an ACE inhibitor or spironolactone, monitor renal function and electrolytes. • Repeat echocardiogram in 4 months to assess efficacy of treatment for hypertrophy. If a beta blocker or diltiazem was prescribed in an asymptomatic animal and there is no evidence of improvement, consider discontinuing treatment or switch to another class of medications and recheck the patient 4 months later.

PREVENTION/AVOIDANCE
Avoid stressful situations that might precipitate CHF.

POSSIBLE COMPLICATIONS
• Left heart failure • Aortic thromboembolism and paralysis • Cardiac arrhythmias

EXPECTED COURSE AND PROGNOSIS
• Prognosis varies considerably, probably because there are multiple causes. Some animals have complete resolution and remain normal after medications are withdrawn. Others show poor response to medications and die shortly after examination. • In one study:
—Cats that were asymptomatic at the time of diagnosis lived from 1 day to 6 years
—Median survival for cats with aortic thromboembolism was 61 days
—Median survival for cats with heart failure was 92 days
—Cats with a resting heart rate < 200 live longer than cats with rates > 200.

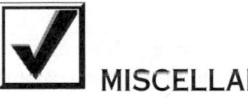 MISCELLANEOUS

ASSOCIATED CONDITIONS
Aortic thromboembolism

AGE-RELATED FACTORS
N/A

ZOONOTIC POTENTIAL
N/A

PREGNANCY
• High risk of complications • Avoid aspirin

SYNONYMS
N/A

SEE ALSO
• Acromegaly—Cats • Aortic Thromboembolism • Congestive Heart Failure, Left-sided • Hypertension, Systemic • Hyperthyroidism • Murmurs, Heart

ABBREVIATIONS
ACE = angiotensin converting enzyme
HCM = hypertrophic cardiomyopathy
IVS = intraventricular septum

Suggested Reading
Atkins CE, Gallo AM, Kurman ID. A retrospective study of risk factors, presenting signs, and survival in 74 cases of feline idiopathic hypertrophic cardiomyopathy. J Vet Intern Med 1991;5:122.

Fox PR. Feline Cardiomyopathies. In Fox PR, Sisson D, Moise NS, eds. Textbook of Canine and Feline Cardiology. Principles and Clinical Practice. Philadelphia; Saunders. 1999:621–678.

Authors Francis W. K. Smith, Jr. and Bruce W. Keene

Consulting Editors Larry P. Tilley and Francis W. K. Smith, Jr.

CARDIOMYOPATHY, HYPERTROPHIC—DOGS

BASICS

OVERVIEW
Hypertrophic cardiomyopathy (HCM) is a rare disease in dogs characterized by left ventricular concentric hypertrophy (increased wall thickness). The primary disease process is confined to the heart and only affects other organ systems when congestive heart failure is present. Increased LV wall thickness leads to impaired ventricular filling (due to lack of compliance and abnormal relaxation) with a resultant increase in LV end-diastolic pressure and left atrial pressure. The left atrium usually enlarges in response to increased LV end-diastolic pressure. Mitral insufficiency and/or dynamic LV outflow tract obstruction commonly occur secondary to structural and/or functional changes of the mitral valve apparatus caused by papillary muscle mal-alignment secondary to the hypertrophy.

SIGNALMENT
The incidence of HCM in dogs is very low, such that accurate accounts of signalment are lacking. Some authors have suggested that German shepherd dogs may be predisposed, and recent reports suggest an increased incidence in the Dalmatian and pointer dogs.

SIGNS

Historical Findings
• May be asymptomatic
• Left heart failure
• Syncope
• Sudden death

Physical Examination Findings
• Systolic heart murmur
• Cardiac gallop rhythm
• Signs of left heart failure (e.g., cough, dyspnea, cyanosis, exercise intolerance)

CAUSES & RISK FACTORS
The cause of hypertrophic cardiomyopathy is unknown. Genetic abnormalities in genes coding for myocardial contractile proteins have been documented in humans and in cats but not in dogs.

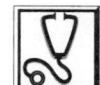

DIAGNOSIS

DIFFERENTIAL DIAGNOSIS
• Systemic hypertension
• Infiltrative cardiac disorders
• Other causes of heart failure
• Thyrotoxicosis
• Congenital mitral dysplasia

CBC/BIOCHEMISTRY/URINALYSIS
N/A

OTHER LABORATORY TESTS
N/A

IMAGING

Radiography
• May be normal
• May show LA or LV enlargement
• Pulmonary edema is present in dogs with left congestive heart failure.

Echocardiography
• Dogs with severe HCM usually have markedly thickened left ventricular walls, papillary muscle hypertrophy, and an enlarged left atrium. The hypertrophy can be global, affecting all areas of the left ventricular wall, or can be more regional or segmental (asymmetric). Milder forms may have subtle LV hypertrophy.
• Systolic anterior motion of the mitral valve, suggesting dynamic LV outflow tract obstruction, is common in dogs with HCM.

OTHER DIAGNOSTIC PROCEDURES

Electrocardiography
• May be normal
• ST segment and T wave abnormalities have been reported.
• Atrial or ventricular ectopic arrhythmias may rarely occur.

Blood Pressure
Usually normal. Should be evaluated to rule out systemic hypertension as the cause of LV hypertrophy

PATHOLOGIC FINDINGS
Abnormal heart:body weight ratio. Left ventricular concentric hypertrophy. Left atrial enlargement

 TREATMENT
Outpatient management unless in congestive heart failure. Exercise restriction and sodium restriction are beneficial.

 **MEDICATIONS**

DRUG(S)
• Treatment is generally only pursued if there is evidence of congestive heart failure.

• In patients with left congestive heart failure, diuretics and ACE inhibitor therapy are advocated.
• In dogs with high LV-aorta pressure gradients due to dynamic LV outflow obstruction, administration of a beta adrenergic blocker or calcium channel blocker has been advocated; however, benefit has not been proven.
• Beta adrenergic blockers or calcium channel blockers may also improve myocardial oxygenation, reduce heart rate, improve LV diastolic function, and control arrhythmias and therefore may also be beneficial in dogs with left congestive heart failure.

CONTRAINDICATIONS/POSSIBLE INTERACTIONS
• Positive inotropic drugs should be avoided as they may worsen dynamic LV outflow obstruction.
• The use of a calcium channel blocker in combination with a beta blocker should be avoided as clinically significant bradyarrhythmias can develop.
• The use of potent arteriolar dilators should be avoided in patients with dynamic LV outflow tract obstruction. However, the use of milder vasodilators such as ACE inhibitors in patients with congestive heart failure is generally well tolerated.

 FOLLOW-UP
• Reevaluation depends on the severity of the clinical signs. Reevaluation with radiography and echocardiography may be useful to characterize disease progression and make appropriate medication adjustments.
• Due to the rarity of this condition in dogs, information regarding prognosis is lacking. In dogs with severe congestive heart failure or other complications, prognosis is generally guarded.

 **MISCELLANEOUS**

ABBREVIATIONS
• ACE = angiotensin converting enzyme
• HCM = hypertrophic cardiomyopathy
• LV = left ventricle

Suggested Reading
Kittleson MD, Kienle RD. eds. Small animal cardiovascular medicine. St Louis: Mosby, 1998.
Author Richard D. Kienle
Consulting Editors Larry P. Tilley & Francis W. K. Smith Jr.

CARDIOMYOPATHY, RESTRICTIVE—CATS

 BASICS

OVERVIEW

• A poorly defined feline myocardial disease resulting from regional or diffuse ventricular myocardial or subendocardial fibrosis, sometimes referred to as "intermediate" or "intergrade" cardiomyopathy
• Myocardial fibrosis results in both systolic (pumping) and diastolic (filling) dysfunction, leading to congestive heart failure (CHF), arrhythmias, and arterial thromboembolism
• May be "final common pathway" of more than one myocardial disease
• Usually diagnosed by recognition of "typical" clinical, radiographic, and echocardiographic findings

SIGNALMENT

Cats

SIGNS

Historical Findings

If cat does not have CHF:
• Lethargy
• Poor appetite and weight loss
• Syncope (rare; usually indicates serious arrhythmia)
• Paresis or paralysis (i.e., signs of arterial thromboembolism)
• Some cats are asymptomatic.
If cat has CHF, above signs plus the following:
• Dyspnea
• Tachypnea
• Open mouth breathing
• Cyanosis
• Abdominal distention

Physical Examination Findings

If cat does not have CHF:
• Depression
• Cachexia
• Tachycardia
• Arrhythmias
• Gallop rhythm
• May have systolic heart murmur
If cat has CHF, above signs plus the following:
• Tachypnea
• Dyspnea
• Panting
• Cyanosis
• Hepatomegaly or ascites with jugular venous distention
• Pulmonary crackles
• Muffled cardiac or respiratory sounds if cat has pleural effusion

• Paralysis or paresis with loss of femoral pulses; one or more extremities cold and painful (arterial thromboembolism)

CAUSES & RISK FACTORS

• True cause(s) unknown; often no "predisposing" disease can be documented.
• Suspected initiating causes include myocarditis, endomyocarditis, eosinophilic myocardial infiltration, hypertrophic cardiomyopathy with myocardial infarction, diffuse "small vessel disease," and other causes of myocardial ischemia.

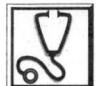 DIAGNOSIS

DIFFERENTIAL DIAGNOSIS

Other causes of signs of CHF (e.g. pulmonary edema, ascites, exercise intolerance):
• Hypertrophic cardiomyopathy
• Dilated cardiomyopathy
• Decompensated congenital cardiac abnormalities (e.g., aortic stenosis, ventricular septal defect, atrioventricular canal defect, or excessive left ventricular moderator bands)
• CHF secondary to thyrotoxicosis or hypertensive heart disease
Other causes of syncope, collapse, weakness, and lethargy:
• Arrhythmias associated with any other form of cardiac disease
• Arrhythmias associated with metabolic or neurologic disease
• Neurologic or musculoskeletal abnormality
• Metabolic disease or electrolyte disturbance
Other causes of paralysis or paresis (arterial thromboembolism):
• Any form of cardiac disease
• Neurologic or musculoskeletal abnormality

CBC/BIOCHEMISTRY/URINALYSIS

• Most laboratory testing does not contribute to diagnosis of restrictive cardiomyopathy
• Routine chemistry panel (with electrolytes) and urinalysis helpful to document concurrent or complicating conditions (e.g., pre-renal azotemia and potassium abnormalities)

OTHER LABORATORY TESTS

Plasma taurine levels low in some cats

IMAGING

Thoracic Radiographic Findings

• Cardiomegaly with disproportionate atrial enlargement

• Interstitial or alveolar infiltrates or pleural effusion with pulmonary venous distention if cat has CHF

Echocardiographic Findings

Note—"Typical" findings controversial; diagnosis of restrictive cardiomyopathy usually based on the following echocardiographic findings (see references):
• Mild or moderate right atrial and ventricular enlargement
• Left atrial enlargement inappropriate to the magnitude of hypertrophy, myocardial failure, or mitral insufficiency
• Normal to slightly thickened left ventricular wall
• Small left ventricular lumen size or narrowing in midventricle caused by fibrosis or fibrous bands
• Dilation of the left ventricle immediately distal to the mitral valve
• Regional wall motion abnormalities or hypertrophy, hyperechoic subendocardial foci, moderator bands
• Normal to slightly decreased shortening fraction
• No or mild atrioventricular valve insufficiency by Doppler echocardiography
• Pericardial effusion of variable severity
• Echodense intracardiac thrombi in atria or attached to atrial or ventricular wall in some cats

DIAGNOSTIC PROCEDURES

Electrocardiographic Findings

• Sinus tachycardia common
• Intraventricular conduction defects, including bundle branch blocks
• Isolated ectopy, paroxysmal or sustained supraventricular or ventricular tachycardias, and atrial fibrillation
• Atrial or ventricular enlargement patterns

 TREATMENT

• Patients with acute, severe CHF are hospitalized for emergency care.
• Mildly symptomatic or asymptomatic animals can be treated with outpatient medical management.
• Severely dyspneic animals should receive oxygen via oxygen cage, nasal cannula, or mask (beware of stress to patient).
• Life-threatening pleural effusions are reduced via thoracocentesis.

• Low sodium fluids administered cautiously if dehydration occurs (beware of worsening CHF)
• Maintain a low stress environment to decrease patient anxiety (e.g., cage rest, minimize handling).
• Heating pad may be necessary for hypothermic patients.
• Low salt diet chronically may decrease fluid retention but strict adherence to dietary changes should be avoided in acute CHF to maintain oral intake; handfeed as necessary.

 MEDICATIONS

DRUG(S)

Acute Congestive Heart Failure
• Parenteral administration of furosemide (0.5–2 mg/kg IV, IM, SC q1–6h)
• Dermal application of nitroglycerin ointment (2%, 1/8–1/4 inch q12h)
• Oxygen delivered by cage, mask, nasal tube
• Thoracocentesis as necessary to relieve dyspnea due to pleural effusion
• Severe supraventricular arrhythmias may be treated with diltiazem (1.5–2.5 mg/kg PO q8h) or long-acting diltiazem (10 mg/kg PO q24h).
• Ventricular tachycardia may resolve with resolution of CHF.
• Acute therapy of ventricular tachycardia may include lidocaine (0.25–0.5 mg/kg IV SLOWLY); monitor closely for neurologic signs of toxicity.
• Beta blockers (propranolol [2.5–7.5 mg PO q8h] or atenolol [6.25–12.5 mg PO q12h]) may be used to treat supraventricular or ventricular arrhythmias, but not until CHF is treated (see contraindications).

Chronic Therapy
• Furosemide gradually decreased to lowest effective dose
• Chronic therapy with diltiazem decreases heart rate and improves supraventricular arrhythmias and may improve diastolic function.
• Beta blockers may be used to slow heart rate and treat supraventricular or ventricular arrhythmias.
• Angiotensin-converting enzyme inhibitors (ACEIs) may reduce fluid retention and decrease need for diuretics (enalapril 0.25–0.5 mg/kg PO q24–48h; benazepril 0.25–0.5 mg/kg PO q24h)

• Digoxin (0.007 mg/kg PO q48h) may be used if systolic function is impaired or atrial fibrillation is present.
• Treat associated conditions (e.g., dehydration, hypothermia).
• Aspirin (80 mg PO q72h) may be administered to prevent thromboembolism, but efficacy is questionable.
• Warfarin (0.5 mg PO q24 h) may be administered to prevent thromboembolism but is not recommended unless close monitoring and repeated measurement of prothrombin time are feasible.

CONTRAINDICATIONS/POSSIBLE INTERACTIONS

Contraindications
• Beta-blocking drugs—atrioventricular block, untreated CHF, bradycardia, myocardial failure, and asthma (especially non-selective beta blockers, e.g., propranolol)
• Diltiazem—bradycardia, atrioventricular block, myocardial failure, and hypotension
• Digoxin—azotemia, atrioventricular block, and severe ventricular arrhythmias
• Furosemide—dehydration, hypokalemia, and azotemia
• Nitroglycerin ointment—hypotension
• ACEIs—azotemia, hypotension, and hyperkalemia

POSSIBLE INTERACTIONS
• Beta blockers and diltiazem should not be used together; combination may lead to bradycardia, hypotension, and severe atrioventricular block.
• Use of ACEIs in dehydrated or hyponatremic animals may result in hypotension, azotemia, and hyperkalemia.
• Chronic aspirin therapy may increase risk of renal side effects of ACEIs.

 FOLLOW-UP

PATIENT MONITORING
• Frequent serial physical examinations (minimal stress to patient) to assess response to treatment and resolution of pulmonary edema and effusions
• Frequent assessment of hydration and renal function is important in first few days of therapy to avoid overdiuresis and azotemia.
• Repeated thoracocentesis may be necessary to maintain effusions at level compatible with comfort.

• Radiographs may be repeated in 12–24 hours to monitor pulmonary infiltrate resolution.
• Electrolytes (especially creatinine and potassium) should be monitored closely during the first 3–5 days of therapy to detect dehydration, renal failure, and hypokalemia (caused by diuretic administration and anorexia) or hyperkalemia (if ACEI is administered).
• Repeat physical examination and electrolyte analysis after approximately 10–14 days of treatment
• ECG and radiographs repeated at clinician's discretion
• Stable patients are reevaluated every 2–4 months, or more frequently if problems occur.

EXPECTED COURSE AND PROGNOSIS
• Most cats with restrictive cardiomyopathy and CHF live 3–12 months, some 2 years.

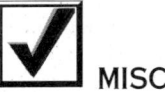 **MISCELLANEOUS**

ASSOCIATED CONDITIONS
Aortic thromboembolism

SYNONYMS
• Intermediate cardiomyopathy
• Intergrade cardiomyopathy

SEE ALSO
• Aortic Thromboembolism
• Congestive Heart Failure, Left-sided
• Congestive Heart Failure, Right-sided

ABBREVIATIONS
ACEI = angiotensin-converting enzyme inhibitor

Suggested Reading
Bonagura JD, Fox PR. Restrictive cardiomyopathy. In: Bonagura JD, ed. Kirk's current veterinary therapy XII. Small animal practice. Philadelphia: Saunders, 1995:863–867.
Pion PD, Kienle RD. Feline cardiomyopathy. In: Miller MS, Tilley LP, eds. Manual of canine and feline cardiology. 2nd ed. Philadelphia: Saunders, 1995.
Author Rebecca L. Stepien
Consulting Editors Larry P. Tilley and Francis W. K. Smith, Jr.

CARDIOPULMONARY ARREST

 BASICS

DEFINITION
• Cessation of effective perfusion and ventilation because of the loss of coordinated cardiac and respiratory function
• Cardiac arrest invariably follows respiratory arrest if not recognized and corrected.

PATHOPHYSIOLOGY
• Generalized or cellular hypoxemia may be the cause or effect of sudden death.
• After 1–4 min of airway obstruction, breathing efforts stop while circulation remains intact.
• If obstruction continues for 6–9 min, severe hypotension and bradycardia lead to dilated pupils, absence of heart sounds, and lack of palpable pulse.
• After 6–9 min, myocardial contractions cease even though the ECG may look normal—electrical mechanical dissociation
• Ventricular fibrillation, ventricular asystole, and electrical mechanical dissociation are rhythms indicating cessation of myocardial contractility.

SYSTEMS AFFECTED
• All systems are affected, but those requiring the greatest supply of oxygen and nutrients are affected first.
• Cardiovascular
• Renal/Urologic
• Neurologic

SIGNALMENT
• Dogs and cats
• Any age, breed, or sex

SIGNS
• Loss of consciousness
• Dilated pupils
• Cyanosis
• Agonal gasping or absence of ventilation
• Absence of peripheral pulses
• Hypothermia
• Absence of audible heart sounds
• Lack of response to stimulation

CAUSES
• Hypoxemia caused by ventilation perfusion mismatch, diffusion barrier impairment, hypoventilation, or shunting
• Poor oxygen delivery due to anemia or vasoconstriction
• Myocardial disease—infectious, inflammatory, infiltrative, traumatic, neoplastic, or embolic
• Acid–base abnormalities
• Electrolyte derangements—hyperkalemia, hypocalcemia, and hypomagnesemia
• Hypovolemia
• Shock

• Anesthetic agents
• Toxemia
• CNS trauma
• Electrical shock

RISK FACTORS
• Cardiovascular disease
• Respiratory
• Trauma
• Anesthesia
• Septicemia
• Endotoxemia
• Ventricular arrhythmias—ventricular flutter, R on T phenomenon, multiform
• Increased parasympathetic tone—gastrointestinal disease, respiratory disease, manipulation of eyes, larynx, or abdominal viscera
• Prolonged seizing
• Invasive cardiovascular manipulation—pericardiocentesis, surgery, angiography

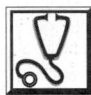 DIAGNOSIS

• Sudden cardiovascular collapse associated with inadequate cardiac output can lead to severe consequences.
• Quick assessment and diagnosis are critical.
• Assess the ABCs—airway, breathing, circulation.

DIFFERENTIAL DIAGNOSIS
• Severe hypovolemia and absence of palpable pulses
• Pericardial effusion, decreased cardiac output, and muffled heart sounds
• Pleural effusion with respiratory arrest
• Respiratory arrest can be confused with CPA.
• Upper airway obstruction can rapidly progress to CPA.

CBC/BIOCHEMISTRY/URINALYSIS
May help identify an underlying cause for CPA but should not be part of initial triage

OTHER LABORATORY TESTS
Blood gas evaluation may be useful during or after resuscitative procedures, but is not part of initial emergency management.

IMAGING
• Thoracic radiographs may help identify underlying disease processes but only consider after the patient has been stabilized.
• Echocardiography may confirm pericardial effusion or underlying myocardial disease but should not interfere with resuscitative procedures.

DIAGNOSTIC PROCEDURES
Once CPA has developed, continuous ECG monitoring, blood pressure monitoring, pulse oximetry, and capnography may be useful in monitoring effectiveness of resuscitative procedures.

 TREATMENT

Institute cardiopulmonary resuscitation (CPR) immediately upon diagnosing CPA; can divide CPR into basic cardiac life support and advanced cardiac life support

BASIC CARDIAC LIFE SUPPORT

A—Airway
• Assessment—Visualize the airway by extending the patient's head and neck and pulling the tongue forward; clear any debris (e.g., secretions, blood, or vomitus), manually or with suction.
• Establish an airway by either oral endotracheal intubation or, if complete obstruction exists, emergency tracheostomy.

B—Breathing
• Assessment—make sure animal is not breathing.
• Institute artificial ventilation—administer two short breaths of ~2-sec duration each and reassess; if no spontaneous respiration occurs continue ventilations at a rate suitable for this animal (normal respiratory rate).
• Techniques for ventilation include mouth to mouth, mouth to nose, or mouth to endotracheal tube; these techniques provide ~16% oxygen; use of an Ambu bag and room air provides 21% oxygen.
• The preferred technique is endotracheal intubation and ventilation with 100% oxygen using an Ambu bag or an anesthesia machine.
• The suggested rate of oxygen administration is 150 mL/kg/min.

C—Circulation
• Assessment—palpate peripheral pulses and auscultate heart to confirm CPA.
• External cardiac massage provides at best ~30% of normal cardiac output; internal cardiac massage is two to three times more effective in improving cerebral and coronary perfusion.
• Hemodynamic studies in animal models suggest that several different mechanisms exist for generation of blood flow (artificial systole) during chest compressions; during external cardiac massage the cardiac pump theory takes advantage of direct compression of the heart in patients weighing < 7 kg; in patients > 7 kg the thoracic pump theory is used; this technique uses increases in intrathoracic pressures to increase cardiac output via the major arteries.

Compression/Ventilation Techniques
• Perform chest compressions rapidly, at a rate of between 80 and 100 compressions/min; the chest should be displaced ~30%.
• Use the cardiac pump in patients weighing < 7 kg body weight; with the patient in right

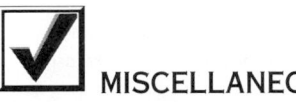
lateral recumbency, perform compressions directly over the heart (intercostal spaces 3–5); this can be done using one or two hands.
• Use the thoracic pump for patients weighing > 7 kg body; with the patient in right lateral or dorsal recumbency, apply thoracic compressions at the widest portion of the thorax.
• If ventilation is provided without an endotracheal tube in place, one breath is given for every five compressions.
• If ventilation is provided via an endotracheal tube, one breath is given simultaneously with every compression or every other on compression.
• Interposing abdominal compressions between chest compressions enhances cerebral and coronary blood flow by increasing aortic diastolic pressure.

OPEN-CHEST CPR
• Indicated if closed-chest CPR is ineffective or preexisting conditions such as flail chest, obesity, diaphragmatic hernia, or pericardial effusion preclude closed-chest techniques
• Perform through a left thoracotomy at the fifth or sixth intercostal space.
• Perform a pericardectomy.
• The palmar surface of the fingers and thumb are used to push the ventricular blood toward the great vessel; digital compression of the descending aorta may help cranial perfusion.

ADVANCED CARDIAC LIFE SUPPORT

D—Drugs
• Base drug selection on the arrhythmia present.
• Atropine and epinephrine are most often correct selections.

E—ECG
• Accurate ECG interpretation is imperative.
• Check ECG leads.

F—Fibrillation Control and Fluids
• Defibrillation is time-dependent; perform immediately.
• Administer fluids cautiously.

 MEDICATIONS

DRUG(S) OF CHOICE
• Base drug selection on the arrhythmia present.
• Administer drugs via central vein, intratracheal, intraosseous, or peripheral vein,

in descending order of preference.
• Use intracardiac drug administration only as a last resort unless open-chest CPR is being performed.

CONTRAINDICATIONS
N/A

PRECAUTIONS
Only use high rates of fluid administration if there is a known history of hypovolemia; excessive fluid administration may lead to decreased coronary perfusion.

POSSIBLE INTERACTIONS
N/A

ALTERNATIVE DRUG(S)
N/A

 FOLLOW-UP

PATIENT MONITORING
• Maintain normal heart rate and blood pressure with fluids and inotropic agents.
• Arterial blood pressure
• Central venous pressure
• Blood gas analysis
• Support respiration with artificial ventilation and supplemental oxygen.
• Neurologic status—if signs of increased intracranial pressure develop, consider mannitol, corticosteroids, and furosemide
• ECG—continuously
• Urine output
• Body temperature
• Radiograph thorax to assess resuscitative injury.
• Diagnose and correct factors that led to initial CPA.

PREVENTION/AVOIDANCE
Careful monitoring of all critically ill patients

POSSIBLE COMPLICATIONS
• Vomiting
• Aspiration pneumonia
• Fractured ribs or sternebrae
• Pulmonary contusions and edema
• Pneumothorax
• Acute renal failure
• Neurologic deficits
• Cardiac arrhythmias

EXPECTED COURSE AND PROGNOSIS
• Prognosis depends on underlying disease process.

• Rapid return to spontaneous cardiac and respiratory function improves the prognosis.
• Overall prognosis is poor; < 10% of patients are discharged.

MISCELLANEOUS

ASSOCIATED CONDITIONS
N/A

AGE-RELATED FACTORS
N/A

ZOONOTIC POTENTIAL
N/A

PREGNANCY
N/A

SYNONYMS
• Cardiac arrest
• Heart attack

SEE ALSO
• Ventricular Fibrillation
• Ventricular Asystole

ABBREVIATIONS
CPA = cardiopulmonary arrest
CPR = cardiopulmonary resuscitation

Suggested Reading
American Heart Association. Guidelines for cardiopulmonary resuscitation and emergency cardiovascular care. Circulation 2000:102 (supplement)I1–I384.
Borde DJ, Dhupa N. Cardiopulmonary arrest and resuscitation. In Tilley LP, Goodwin JK, eds. Manual of canine and feline cardiology, 3rd ed. Philadelphia: Saunders, 2001:407.
Hackett TB, Van Pelt DR. Cardiopulmonary resuscitation. In: Bonagura JD, Kirk RW, eds. Kirks current veterinary therapy XII. Philadelphia: Saunders, 1995:167.
Kass PH, Haskins SC. Survival following cardiopulmonary resuscitation in dogs and cats. Vet Emerg Crit Care 1992;2:57.
Van Pelt DR, Wingfield WE. Controversial issues in drug treatment during cardiopulmonary resuscitation. J Am Vet Med Assoc 1992;200:1938.
Authors Andrew W. Beardow and Steven L. Marks
Consulting Editors Larry P. Tilley and Francis W. K. Smith, Jr.

CARNITINE DEFICIENCY

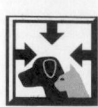 BASICS

OVERVIEW

L-carnitine is a quaternary amine that is an important part of the enzymes that transport fatty acids into mitochondria so that they can be oxidized to make energy available to the cell. In the heart and other organs that depend on the oxidation of fatty acids to supply their high energy requirements for contraction or other work, L-carnitine deficiency results in inadequate production of energy to meet those needs. Carnitine deficiency appears to complicate approximately 40% of cases of dilated cardiomyopathy in dogs. The presence of L-carnitine deficiency in association with cardiomyopathy does not mean that the deficiency is the sole cause of the myopathy, although correcting the deficiency (if possible) makes medical and physiologic sense. L-carnitine is not synthesized in heart or skeletal muscle and must therefore be transported into those cells from plasma. In the dog, dietary carnitine intake influences plasma concentrations significantly, and oral carnitine supplementation is usually an effective means of raising plasma and subsequently muscle carnitine levels. The FDA has approved the addition of physiologic amounts of carnitine to commercial dog foods for the prevention of plasma (and subsequently muscle) carnitine deficiency. This action is prudent based on current knowledge regarding the lack of L-carnitine in most commercial dog food and the effect of those diets on canine carnitine plasma levels. It is not known whether this action will affect the prevalence of dilated cardiomyopathy or other manifestations of carnitine deficiency.

SIGNALMENT

Dogs

• Boxers, Doberman pinschers, Great Danes, Irish wolfhounds, and other large- and giant-breed dogs appear to be most commonly affected with dilated cardiomyopathy.
• At least some American cocker spaniels with DCM are carnitine deficient, and a blinded, placebo-controlled trial suggests showed that L-carnitine supplementation combined with taurine supplementation is beneficial in the medical management of these patients.

SIGNS

• Clinical signs of carnitine deficiency can be diverse; mitochondria in all tissues utilize L-carnitine to produce energy from fatty acids.
• Signs range from heart muscle failure and dilated cardiomyopathy (most frequently recognized) to skeletal muscle pain, weakness, exercise intolerance, and/or lethargy.
• See Cardiomyopathy, Dilated—Dogs

CAUSES & RISK FACTORS

• Some dogs with cardiomyopathy have been documented to have carnitine transport defects, where muscle carnitine is low even in the face of adequate plasma carnitine concentrations. In order to transport fatty acids or other compounds (such as acetyl Co-A) into or out of the mitochondria, free L-carnitine is esterified to the substance, forming a carnitine ester. In cases where a mitochondrial enzyme defect causes the accumulation of a metabolite to toxic levels within the mitochondria (e.g., multiple Co-A dehydrogenase defects), free L-carnitine is used to "scavenge" the potentially toxic excess metabolites, which appear harmlessly in the plasma and eventually the urine as carnitine esters. In these cases, the total amount of carnitine (free carnitine plus that esterified to other molecules) in the plasma or muscle may be normal or even high, but the ratio of free carnitine to esterified carnitine is decreased. This situation is known as carnitine insufficiency (because even though the concentration of free carnitine may be within the normal range, it is insufficient to meet the body's pathologically increased need for free carnitine).
• Certain families of Boxers appear to be at especially high risk of developing symptomatic dilated cardiomyopathy in association with and probably caused by carnitine deficiency. A known first-degree relative with cardiomyopathy should increase the index of suspicion.

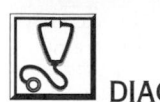

DIAGNOSIS

DIFFERENTIAL DIAGNOSIS
See Cardiomyopathy, Dilated–Dogs

CBC/BIOCHEMISTRY/URINALYSIS
Normal

OTHER LABORATORY TESTS
Plasma carnitine concentrations appear to be a specific but insensitive indicator of myocardial or skeletal muscle carnitine deficiency. Plasma free carnitine concentrations of less than 8 micromoles/L are considered diagnostic of systemic carnitine deficiency. Plasma concentrations in the normal or supernormal range do not rule out myocardial carnitine deficiency or insufficiency.

IMAGING
See Cardiomyopathy, Dilated—Dogs

DIAGNOSTIC TESTS
Endomyocardial biopsy specimens must be blotted dry and snap frozen in liquid nitrogen. Measurement of free and esterified L-carnitine concentrations normalized to the amount of noncollagenous protein in the biopsy remains the only definitive diagnostic test. Myocardial free carnitine concentrations of less than 3.5 nanomoles/mg of non-collagenous protein are considered diagnostic of myocardial carnitine deficiency. Ratios of esterified to free carnitine greater than 0.4 are considered diagnostic of carnitine insufficiency.

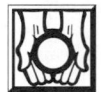

TREATMENT
Treatment with L-carnitine does not replace conventional treatment for DCM, even in most dogs with carnitine deficiency. Some dogs, including some families of carnitine deficient Boxers, fail to respond clinically to supplementation. While supplementation dramatically improves a small percentage (about 5% in the author's experience) of dogs with dilated cardiomyopathy, the overall efficacy of L-carnitine supplementation for the treatment of dilated cardiomyopathy is untested.

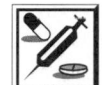

MEDICATIONS

DRUG(S)

Carnitine Supplementation
• Large-breed dogs, 2 g (approximately 1 tsp. L-carnitine powder) q8–12h
• American cocker spaniels (in combination with taurine) 1 g (approximately 1/2 tsp L-carnitine powder) q8–12h

CONTRAINDICATIONS/POSSIBLE INTERACTIONS
• None have been identified • Mild diarrhea has been associated with high doses of carnitine in some people.

FOLLOW-UP
Repeat echocardiogram 3–6 months after initiating L-carnitine supplementation to assess the efficacy of treatment

MISCELLANEOUS

Suggested Reading
Keene BW, Panciera DP, Atkins CE, et al.: Myocardial L-carnitine deficiency in a family of dogs with dilated cardiomyopathy. J Am Vet Med Assoc 1991;201:647–650.
Keene BW, Kittleson MD, Rush JE, et al.: Myocardial carnitine deficiency associated with dilated cardiomyopathy in Doberman pinschers. J Vet Intern Med 1989, 3.126 (Abstract)
Author Bruce W. Keene
Consulting Editors Larry P Tilley and Francis W. K. Smith Jr.

CATARACT

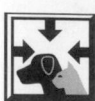

BASICS

DEFINITION
• Opacification of the lens
• Term *cataract*—may refer to an entire lens that is opaque or to an opacity within the lens; does not imply cause

PATHOPHYSIOLOGY
• Basic mechanism—thought to be cross-linking of lens protein
• Specific causes—genetic defects; nutritional deficiency; focal disruption of normal lens metabolism by adhesion to uveal tissue (synechia); radiation; elevated blood glucose; hypocalcemia; toxins; faulty embryogenesis; altered composition of the aqueous humor caused by uveitis
• Traditional terminology—immature (only part of the lens is involved); mature (entire lens is opaque); hypermature (lens liquefaction has occurred); implies progressive condition
• Liquefaction—occurs more readily in young patients; with time will eventually occur to some degree in all patients

SYSTEMS AFFECTED
Ophthalmic

GENETICS
• Most are inherited.
• Most common mode of inheritance—simple autosomal recessive
• Some breeds—dominantly inherited

INCIDENCE/PREVALENCE
• Dogs—common; exact prevalence unknown; one of the most important causes of vision loss
• Cats—uncommon

GEOGRAPHIC DISTRIBUTION
N/A

SIGNALMENT

Species
Dogs and cats

Breed Predilection
• Many dog breeds are affected by hereditary cataracts; refer to general reference texts.
• Cataracts that typically progress to blindness—miniature poodles; American cocker spaniels; miniature schnauzers
• Other commonly affected breeds—golden retrievers; Boston terriers; Siberian huskies
• Cats—Persians; Birmans; Himalayans

Mean Age and Range
• Depend on cause
• Hereditary (dogs)—may be congenital; may be acquired anytime from several months to many years of age, depending on breed
• Hereditary (cats)—all reported to date have been congenital.

Predominant Sex
None

SIGNS

Historical Findings
• Related to the degree of vision impairment
• Occupy <30% of the lens or affect only one eye—often go unnoticed
• Occupy >60% of the lens—usually reported
• Caused by diabetes mellitus—polyuria, polydipsia, and weight loss
• Cloudiness noticed before vision impairment—usually sclerosis
• Associated progressive retinal degeneration (dogs)—difficulty seeing in dimly lighted conditions (nyctalopia)

Physical Examination Findings
• Opacification of lens
• Slit lamp biomicroscope—determine exact location (e.g., nuclear, cortical)
• Hypermature—minute crystals within the lens
• Liquefied lens material leaking from the lens—wrinkling of the lens capsule
• Associated with uveitis—typically see aqueous flare, synechiae, and low intraocular pressure

Tapetal Reflection
• Easiest method of detection
• Obstruction of light by lenticular opacities (retroillumination)
• Appear as black or gray spots
• Cloudiness owing to sclerosis—will not detect discrete foci of tapetal obstruction

CAUSES
• Heredity
• Diabetes mellitus
• Spontaneous—age-related
• Advanced retinal degeneration—response to toxic dialdehydes
• Uveitis—secondary to synechia formation or altered aqueous humor composition
• Toxic substances—dinitrophenol; naphthalene
• Nutrition—milk-replacer diet
• Hypocalcemia
• Radiation
• Electric shock

RISK FACTORS
• Faulty genetics
• Multiple congenital ocular defects
• Any disease capable of causing uveitis
• Advanced retinal degeneration
• Systemic metabolic diseases—diabetes; diseases capable of causing hypocalcemia

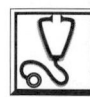

DIAGNOSIS

DIFFERENTIAL DIAGNOSIS
• Lenticular sclerosis—normal aging phenomenon; often mistaken for cataracts; does not cause vision loss; easily distinguished by retroillumination (see Physical Examination Findings)

• Uveitis (dogs)—may cause or be caused by cataracts; distinction made on the basis of signalment, history, extent of cataract formation, and appearance of the cataract; assumed to be lens-induced until proven otherwise in purebreds with concurrent complete cataracts; assumed to be secondary to the inflammation (especially in non-purebreds) with concurrent incomplete cataracts
• Chronic uveitis (cats)—focal cataracts frequent sequelae

CBC/BIOCHEMISTRY/URINALYSIS
• Not routinely necessary; condition usually hereditary
• Routine hematology—screen for infectious diseases when associated with uveitis.
• Blood chemistry profiles—rule out systemic metabolic disease (e.g., diabetes mellitus, hypocalcemia).

OTHER LABORATORY TESTS
Serologic Testing
• Non–lens-induced and associated with uveitis—routine
• Dogs—rule out systemic mycoses (e.g., histoplasmosis, coccidioidomycosis, blastomycosis, cryptococcosis), rickettsial disease (e.g., *Ehrlichia canis, Borrelia burgdorferi, Rickettsia rickettsii*), and brucellosis.
• Cats with chronic uveitis and secondary cataracts—rule out toxoplasmosis, FeLV infection, and FIV infection.

IMAGING
• Ophthalmic ultrasonography—indicated for hypermature cataracts if surgery anticipated (associated retinal detachment)
• Also indicated for complete congenital cataracts to rule out other intraocular defects (e.g., persistent hyaloid artery, persistent primary vitreous, lenticonus)

DIAGNOSTIC PROCEDURES
Electroretinography—always done if surgery anticipated; evaluate the retina; rule out concurrent retinal degeneration.

PATHOLOGIC FINDINGS
• Lens fiber swelling
• Posterior migration of lens epithelium
• Liquefaction of lens material
• Lens epithelial fibrous metaplasia
• Lens mineralization

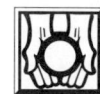

TREATMENT

APPROPRIATE HEALTH CARE
• Dogs undergoing surgery—inpatient or outpatient
• Hospitalization—rarely required for >48 hr

NURSING CARE
N/A

ACTIVITY
N/A

DIET
N/A

CLIENT EDUCATION
• Inform client that surgery can normally be done on any hereditary cataract that is causing or is anticipated to cause vision loss.
• Warn client that the prognosis for surgery is better if it is done early in the course of cataract development, before hypermaturity, lens-induced uveitis, and retinal detachment occur.
• It is not advisable to delay surgery until the patient is blind in both eyes.
• Discuss that surgery may or may not be indicated for nonhereditary cataracts.
• Point out that because of the high success rate of phacoemulsification, it is no longer appropriate to observe cataracts for possible resorption, even in young dogs.

SURGICAL CONSIDERATIONS
• Phacoemulsification—ultrasonic lens fragmentation; procedure of choice
• Prognosis for successful surgery—generally >90%; depends on the stage of the cataract and other concurrent findings
• Intraocular lenses—may be safely implanted at the time of surgery, so patient will not suffer extreme farsightedness

MEDICATIONS

DRUG(S) OF CHOICE
1% prednisolone acetate q6h to prevent and control lens-induced uveitis; indicated for progressing condition for which surgery is planned

CONTRAINDICATIONS
Chronic topical atropine therapy—avoid in dogs that will be undergoing surgery; causes parasympathetic receptor hyperplasia, thereby contributing to intraoperative miosis

PRECAUTIONS
N/A

POSSIBLE INTERACTIONS
N/A

ALTERNATIVE DRUG(S)
N/A

FOLLOW-UP

PATIENT MONITORING
• All patients—monitor carefully for progression.
• Hereditary—condition may progress very quickly in young dogs.

PREVENTION/AVOIDANCE
Do not breed patients with known or suspected inherited conditions.

POSSIBLE COMPLICATIONS
Complete cataracts—potential to cause lens-induced uveitis, secondary glaucoma, and retinal detachment

EXPECTED COURSE AND PROGNOSIS
• Rate of progression—depends on location within the lens and patient's age
• Nuclear—may appear to become smaller because the nucleus compresses with age
• Cortical—almost always progress, except for specific hereditary types (e.g., posterior triangular cataracts in golden retrievers)
• Normal lens aging—lens protein becomes insoluble and sclerotic, inhibiting cataract progression; thus a small cataract in a 1-year-old cocker spaniel may enlarge and cause blindness within several months, whereas the same size cataract in a 10-year-old poodle may cause blindness only after several years.
• Diabetes mellitus–induced—usually very rapid progress
• Surgical intervention—for hereditary or diabetes-caused cataracts, prognosis for good vision excellent; for other types of cataracts, depends on cause

MISCELLANEOUS

ASSOCIATED CONDITIONS
See Causes.

AGE-RELATED FACTORS
• Development of nonhereditary cataracts in senile dogs—subject of debate, but seems to occur
• Age by itself is not a consideration when recommending surgery.

ZOONOTIC POTENTIAL
N/A

PREGNANCY
N/A

SEE ALSO
• Anterior Uveitis—Cats
• Anterior Uveitis—Dogs
• Blind Quiet Eye
• Diabetes Mellitus Without Complication—Dogs
• Retinal Degeneration

ABBREVIATIONS
• FeLV = feline leukemia virus
• FIV = feline immunodeficiency virus

Suggested Reading
Beam S, Correa MT, Davidson MG. A retrospective-cohort study on the development of cataract in dogs with diabetes mellitus: 200 cases. Vet Ophthalmol 1992;2:169–172.
Davidson MG, Nasisse MP, Jamieson VE, et al. Phacoemulsification and intraocular lens implantation: a study of results in 182 dogs. Prog Vet Compend Ophthalmol 1991;1:233–238.
Geraldi JG, Colitz CMH, Dubielzig RR, et al. Immunohistochemical analysis of lens epithelial-derived membranes following cataract extraction in the dog. Vet Ophthalmol 1999;2:163–168.
Glover TL, Constantinescu GM. Surgery for cataracts. Vet Clin North Am 1997;27:1143–1173.
Nasisse MP, Davidson MG, Jamieson VE, et al. Phacoemulsification and intraocular lens implantation: a study of technique in 182 dogs. Prog Vet Compend Ophthalmol 1991;1:225–232.
Nasisse MP. Innovations in cataract surgery. In: Kirk RW, ed. Current veterinary therapy XII. Philadelphia, Saunders, 1994:1261–1264.
van der Woerdt A, Wilkie DA, Myer W. Ultrasonic abnormalities in the eyes of dogs with cataracts. J Am Vet Med Assoc 1993;203:838–841.
Author Mark P. Nasisse
Consulting Editor Paul E. Miller

CECOCOLIC INTUSSUSCEPTION

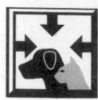 **BASICS**

OVERVIEW
Cecal inversion or cecocolic intussusception causes partial-to-complete, intermittent obstruction of the ileocolic junction.

SIGNALMENT
• Reported more frequently in dogs, but has been reported in one cat.
• No age, sex, or breed predilection
• Age range, 1–15 years

SIGNS

Historical Findings
• Possibly weight loss
• Chronic intermittent hematochezia and soft stools
• Nonresponsive to administration of anthelmintics, protectants, and antibiotics, dietary adjustment, and motility modification

Physical Examination Findings
• Usually unremarkable
• Acute vomiting, depression, dehydration in patients with complete obstruction
• Painful midabdominal mass may be palpable.

CAUSES & RISK FACTORS
• Cause unknown
• Possible causes include parasitism (whipworms) and neoplasia.
• Intestinal lymphoma has been seen in patients with intussusception.

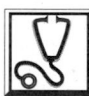 **DIAGNOSIS**

DIFFERENTIAL DIAGNOSIS
• Consider diseases characterized by hematochezia and intermittent soft stool (e.g., intestinal parasitism, neoplasia, inflammatory bowel disease, ileocolic intussusception, infectious bowel diseases).
• Consider diseases that cause midabdominal palpable masses (e.g., neoplasia, abdominal lymphadenopathy).

CBC/BIOCHEMISTRY/URINALYSIS
• Usually normal or nonspecific
• Anemia or hypoalbuminemia associated with chronic blood loss is uncommon.

OTHER LABORATORY TESTS
Fecal flotation and direct examination are indicated.

IMAGING

Abdominal Radiography
Usually nonspecific unless the patient has gastrointestinal obstruction

Contrast Radiography
• Upper or lower gastrointestinal positive-contrast study—the inverted cecum may be seen in the proximal colon surrounded by contrast material.
• Pneumocolonography (negative-contrast study)—the inverted cecum may be seen in the proximal colon.

Abdominal Ultrasonography
Multiple intestinal wall layering may be seen in the area of the cecum/proximal colon.

DIAGNOSTIC PROCEDURES
• Flexible colonoscopy—allows direct visualization of a fingerlike projection protruding into the colon through the ileocolic junction
• Exploratory celiotomy on the basis of imaging or colonoscopic findings

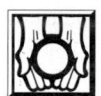 **TREATMENT**

• Inpatient surgical management
• Restore/address dehydration and any electrolyte abnormalities.
• Exploratory celiotomy and typhlectomy are indicated.
• If reduction can be achieved, perform the typhlectomy from the serosal surface.
• If reduction cannot be achieved, make an incision opposite the lesion on the antimesenteric border of the colon, and remove the cecum from the mucosal surface; in general, a two-layer closure is recommended for colonotomy and typhlectomy; surgical stapling has been described as appropriate for use in typhlectomy.

• Treat any underlying conditions (e.g., intestinal parasitism).

 MEDICATIONS

DRUG(S)
• Standard anesthetic protocols should be adequate.
• Perioperative antibiotics appropriate for colonic surgery (e.g., cefazolin sodium, 20–35 mg/kg IV or cefoxitin sodium, 30 mg/kg IV q6–8h) can be used as prophylaxis (during surgery q1.5–2.0h and for 12 h postoperatively).

CONTRAINDICATIONS/POSSIBLE INTERACTIONS
N/A

 FOLLOW-UP

PATIENT MONITORING
• Standard postoperative care for abdominal/GI surgery
• Suture removal 10–14 days

POSSIBLE COMPLICATIONS
• Potential for fecal staining with blood from typhlectomy site for 10–14 days
• Potential for colonic dehiscence in 5–7 days
• Potential for colonic stricture formation if colonotomy is required

 MISCELLANEOUS

SYNONYM
Cecal inversion

Suggested Reading
Aronsohn M. Large intestine. In: Slatter DH, ed. Textbook of small animal surgery. 2nd ed. Philadelphia: Saunders, 1993:613–627.
Author Michelle J. Waschak
Consulting Editor Albert E. Jergens

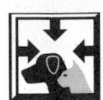 BASICS

OVERVIEW
• Progressive, breed-specific, and apparently genetically induced defect of unknown cause and pathogenesis; neonatal, postnatal, and (rare) adult onset; premature aging and death of cerebellar cortical neurons
• Occurs after in utero or neonatal viral infection in cats (feline panleukopenia) and dogs (canine herpesvirus)

SIGNALMENT
Nonprogressive
• Dogs and cats
• Irish setters, wire-haired fox terriers, Samoyeds, chow chows, rough-coated collies, border collies, bullmastiffs, Labrador retrievers, beagles—common; may be seen in other breeds of dogs and cats.
• Signs appear when patient is 3–5 weeks old.

Progressive
• Dogs and cats
• Kerry blue terriers (signs at 12–16 weeks), rough-coated collies in Australia, Finnish harriers, Bern running dogs, Irish setters, English pointers, Gordon setters (signs at 6–36 months), Brittany spaniels (signs at 7–13 years)—common, American Staffordshire Terriers (2.5–6 years) and English bulldogs (5–8 months)
• Autosomal recessive mode of inheritance—probable in Gordon setters, Kerry blue terriers, rough-coated collies, Old English sheepdogs and possibly in cats
• X-linked mode of inheritance—probable in English pointers because only males affected
• Cerebellar degeneration and coat color dilution—reported in a family of Rhodesian ridgebacks
• Coton de Tulear—onset 2–6 weeks, likely genetic
• Adult-onset cerebellar cortical abiotropy and retinal degeneration was described in a domestic shorthair cat.

SIGNS
• Dysmetria—frequently as hypermetria
• Broad-based stance
• Swaying of body
• Intention tremors
• Lack of menace responses with normal vision and facial muscle strength
• Head tilt and episodes of vestibular ataxia with resting or positional nystagmus
• Diffuse tapetal hyper-reflectivity on funduscopic exam
• Decerebellate posture—opisthotonos with extensor rigidity of the forelimbs and flexed hind limbs
• Alterations of mentation, proprioceptive deficits, and paresis are not features of this condition.
• Progression of signs varies

CAUSES & RISK FACTORS
• Feline panleukopenia or canine herpesvirus infection in utero or neonatally
• Poor vaccination history or exposure to modified live virus during gestation
• Breeding affected animals or those with a familial history and predisposition to cerebellar degeneration
• A syndrome of hepatocerebellar degeneration was described in a litter of Bernese mountain dogs.
• Paraneoplastic cerebellar degeneration has been reported in humans.

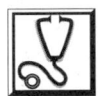 DIAGNOSIS

DIFFERENTIAL DIAGNOSIS
• Lysosomal storage diseases—diffuse diseases of the CNS; differentiate by signs related to other parts of the CNS besides the cerebellum
• Toxicity (e.g., hexachlorophene)—differentiate by history of exposure
• Inflammatory diseases (e.g., canine distemper and FIP)—frequently accompanied or preceded by systemic signs of illness; differentiate by CSF analysis
• Cerebellar cyst—differentiate by imaging (MRI and CT)
• Medulloblastoma (cerebellar tumor)—reported in dogs and cats < 1 year old; differentiate by imaging (MRI and CT) and CSF analysis
• Other primary and metastatic tumors in adult dogs—differentiate by imaging (MRI and CT) and CSF analysis

CBC/BIOCHEMISTRY/URINALYSIS
Usually normal

OTHER LABORATORY TESTS
N/A

IMAGING
MRI—cerebellum may be smaller than normal.

DIAGNOSTIC PROCEDURES
• CSF analysis—normal with nonprogressive disease; normal or high protein concentration and normal cell counts with progressive disease
• Cerebellar biopsy—may be only definitive means of antemortem diagnosis

 TREATMENT
• None available that will alter the course of the disease.
• Outpatient—unless severe deficits preclude nursing care at home
• Restrict activity to safe areas; avoid stairs, swimming pools, etc.
• Diet—normal; restrict intake if vestibular episodes are accompanied by emesis (to avoid aspiration pneumonia).
• Nonprogressive disease—patient may show some improvement as animal learns to compensate for disabilities.

 MEDICATIONS

DRUG(S)
N/A

CONTRAINDICATIONS/POSSIBLE INTERACTIONS
N/A

 FOLLOW-UP
• Neurologic status—examine at weekly to monthly intervals if progression of signs is uncertain; consider videotaping the patient to determine progression more objectively.
• Progression of signs—rate varies; depends on signalment; ranges from days to years
• Do not vaccinate pregnant animals with MLV.
• Do not breed animals with a familial history of cerebellar disease.

 MISCELLANEOUS

ABBREVIATIONS
• CNS = central nervous system
• CSF = cerebrospinal fluid
• CT = computed tomography
• FIP = feline infectious peritonitis
• MLV = modified-live virus
• MRI = magnetic resonance imaging

Suggested Reading

Summers BA, Cummings JF, de Lahunta A. Veterinary neuropathology. St. Louis: Mosby, 1995:301–305.
van der Merwe LL, Lane E. Diagnosis of cerebellar cortical degeneration in a Scottish terrier using magnetic resonance imaging. J Small Anim Pract 2001;42(8):409–412.
Author Richard J. Joseph
Consulting Editor Joane M. Parent

CEREBELLAR HYPOPLASIA

BASICS

OVERVIEW
Caused by incomplete development of parts of the cerebellum owing to intrinsic (inherited) or extrinsic (infectious, toxic, or nutritional) factors

SIGNALMENT
• Symptoms visible when puppies and kittens begin to stand and walk (by age 6 weeks)
• Hereditary in Airedales, chow chows, Boston terriers, and bull terrier breeds

SIGNS
• Nonprogressive cerebellar disorder—head bobbing; limb tremors; aggravated by movement or eating (intention tremors); disappear during sleep.
• Cerebellar ataxia with a wide-base stance
• Dysmetria and disequilibrium—falling, flipping over
• Slight improvement may occur as patient accommodates for its deficits.

CAUSES & RISK FACTORS
• Cats—usually transplacental or perinatal infection with panleukopenia virus (wild parvovirus or modified live virus), which selectively attacks rapidly dividing cells (e.g., external germinal layer of the cerebellum at birth and for 2 weeks postnatal)
• Dogs—hereditary in some breeds (see Signalment)

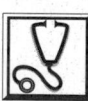

DIAGNOSIS

DIFFERENTIAL DIAGNOSIS
• Age, breed, history, and typical nonprogressive symptoms—usually sufficient for tentative diagnosis
• Cerebellar abiotrophy—postnatal degeneration after normal development; slow progression of signs over weeks to months; neonatal onset (beagles, Samoyeds)

or postnatal onset (Australian kelpies at 5–6 weeks; Kerry blue terriers at 9–16 weeks; rough-coated collies at 4–8 weeks; bull mastiff at 4–9 weeks)
• Neuroaxonal dystrophy—slowly progressive cerebellar signs starting around 5 weeks of age in cats and 7 weeks in Chihuahuas
• Cerebellar sequels of systemic canine herpesvirus infection—follow systemic illness
• Concomitant seizures or other cerebral symptoms—suggest multiple malformations, such as lissencephaly (wire-haired fox terriers and Irish setters) or hydrocephalus
• Final diagnosis possible only at necropsy

CBC/BIOCHEMISTRY/URINALYSIS
Usually normal

OTHER LABORATORY TESTS
N/A

IMAGING
MRI scan—cerebellar atrophy or malformation (incomplete or asymmetrical filling of the caudal cranial fossa by the cerebellum); other malformations

PATHOLOGIC FINDINGS
• Cerebellum—normally very small in the newborn kitten or puppy, because development continues for up to 10 weeks postnatal; subtle to marked atrophy noted at necropsy performed weeks to months after birth; no sign of active inflammation
• Transverse fibers of the pons—decrease in size associated with marked cortical cerebellar atrophy
• Hydrocephalus—may be noted; result from multifocal inflammation or multiple malformations (e.g., Dandy-Walker syndrome)
• Microscopic—cellular depletion of cerebellar cortex

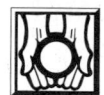

TREATMENT
None

MEDICATIONS

DRUG(S)
N/A

CONTRAINDICATIONS/POSSIBLE INTERACTIONS
N/A

FOLLOW-UP

PATIENT MONITORING
N/A

PREVENTION/AVOIDANCE
N/A

POSSIBLE COMPLICATIONS
N/A

EXPECTED COURSE AND PROGNOSIS
• Some patients may be acceptable pets.
• Deficits—permanent; do not progress; usually compatible with a normal life span

CARE
• Restrict environment to prevent injuries and road accidents—no climbing, falling, or escaping
• Euthanasia—severely affected animals that are unable to feed, groom, or be toilet trained

MISCELLANEOUS

Suggested Reading
Summers BA, Cummings JF, de Lahunta A. Veterinary neuropathology. St. Louis: Mosby, 1997.
Author Christine Berthelin-Baker
Consulting Editor Joane M. Parent

CERUMINOUS GLAND ADENOCARCINOMA, EAR

BASICS

OVERVIEW
• Primary malignant tumor of the external auditory meatus arising from coiled tubular apocrine sweat glands (e.g., ceruminous glands)
• May be locally invasive but has a low rate of distant metastasis

SIGNALMENT
• Rare but the most common malignant tumor of the ear canal in dogs and cats
• Cocker spaniel may be predisposed.
• Mean age—dogs, 8–11 years; cats, 10.5–13 years
• No known sex predisposition

SIGNS
• Similar to otitis externa
• Early appearance—pale pink, friable, ulcerative, bleeding nodular mass(es)
• Late appearance—large mass(es) filling the canal and invading through canal wall into surrounding structures
• Local lymphadenomegaly
• May see vestibular signs

CAUSES & RISK FACTORS
Chronic inflammation may play a role in tumor development.

DIAGNOSIS

DIFFERENTIAL DIAGNOSIS
• Nodular hyperplasia
• Pedunculated inflammatory polyps (cats)
• Squamous cell carcinoma
• Basal cell tumor
• Papilloma
• Sebaceous gland tumor
• Ceruminous gland adenoma

CBC/BIOCHEMISTRY/URINALYSIS
Usually normal

OTHER LABORATORY TESTS
N/A

IMAGING
• Skull radiography—determine involvement of tympanic bulla
• Thoracic radiography—evaluate for lung metastasis
• CT—useful before radiotherapy

DIAGNOSTIC PROCEDURES
• Cytologic examination of aspirate from large lymph nodes
• Biopsy

PATHOLOGIC FINDINGS
• Histopathologic characteristics—apocrine type differentiation from ceruminous glands and local invasion into stroma
• Tumor cells—show moderate to marked nuclear atypia with frequent mitosis

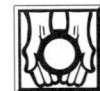

TREATMENT
• Ear canal ablation and lateral bulla osteotomy—preferred over lateral ear resection
• Radiotherapy—large or incompletely excised masses

MEDICATIONS

DRUG(S)
Chemotherapy not evaluated

CONTRAINDICATIONS/POSSIBLE INTERACTIONS
N/A

FOLLOW-UP

PATIENT MONITORING
Physical examination and thoracic radiography—at 1, 3, 6, 9, 12, 18, and 24 months after treatment

POSSIBLE COMPLICATIONS
Permanent or transient Horner syndrome

EXPECTED COURSE AND PROGNOSIS
• Median survival after lateral ear resection (cats)—10 months (1-year survival, 33.3%), (dogs)—9 months
• Median survival after ear ablation and lateral bulla osteotomy (cats)—42 months (1-year survival 75%), (dogs)—36 months
• Median survival after radiotherapy (cats)—39.5 months (1-year survival 56%)
• Poor prognosis associated with extensive tumor involvement and neurologic signs

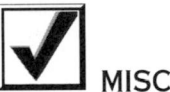

MISCELLANEOUS

ASSOCIATED CONDITIONS
• Otitis externa
• Peripheral vestibular disease

ABBREVIATIONS
CT = computed tomography

Suggested Reading
Marino DJ, MacDonald JM, Matthisen DT, et al. Results of surgery in cats with ceruminous gland adenocarcinoma. J Am Anim Hosp Assoc 1994;30:54–58.
Morrison WB. Cancers of the head and neck. In: Morrison WB, ed. Cancer in dogs and cats: medical and surgical management. Philadelphia: Lippincott Williams & Wilkins, 1998:511–519.

Author Joanne C. Graham
Consulting Editor Wallace B. Morrison

CHAGAS DISEASE (AMERICAN TRYPANOSOMIASIS)

BASICS

OVERVIEW
• Caused by the zoonotic hemoflagellate protozoan parasite *Trypanosoma cruzi*
• Infection—infected feces of a vector (Triatominae, commonly called kissing or assassin bugs) are deposited in a wound (bite site of vector) or mucous membrane; dog eats an infected vector or infected host (opossum, raccoon, armadillo) in which the organism is sequestered in muscle; transmission by contaminated blood transfusion • After local multiplication at site of entry (5 days postinfection), hematogenous spread occurs to most organs but mainly the heart and brain. • Organisms become intracellular, multiply, then rupture out into the circulation to produce maximal parasitemias, associated particularly with acute myocarditis and less commonly with diffuse encephalitis (14 days postinfection). • Parasitemias wane (subpatent 30 days postinfection). • Antibody titers rise (detectable by 26 days postinfection). • Dog enters a protracted asymptomatic period (can last for months to years) if it survives the acute myocarditis; progressive and insidious development of myocardial degeneration; eventual dilative cardiomyopathy of unknown pathogenesis • South and Central America—endemic (in both humans and pets) • United States—mostly in Texas; also Louisiana, Oklahoma, South Carolina, and Virginia; infected vectors and reservoir hosts reported in the west (California, New Mexico), south (Florida, Georgia, North Carolina), and east (Maryland)

SIGNALMENT
• Young dogs—most common • Acute—dogs usually <2 years • Chronic—old dogs • Hunting breeds—likely to contact vectors or reservoir hosts • More often males • Cats—no cases reported in North America

SIGNS
General Comments
• Two syndromes—acute (myocarditis or encephalitis in young dogs) and chronic (dilative cardiomyopathy in old dogs)

Historical Findings
Acute
• Sudden death • Lethargy • Depression • Anorexia • Diarrhea • Weakness • Exercise intolerance • Mild to severe CNS dysfunction (like distemper) • Ataxia, seizures
Chronic
• Weakness • Exercise intolerance • Syncope • Sudden death

Physical Examination Findings
Acute
• Generalized lymphadenopathy • Both left- and right-sided heart failure • Tachycardia with or without arrhythmias • Neurologic—weakness; ataxia; chorea; seizures (indistinguishable from distemper)
Chronic
Tachycardia—sustained or paroxysmal

CAUSES & RISK FACTORS
T. cruzi

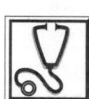

DIAGNOSIS

DIFFERENTIAL DIAGNOSIS
• Cardiomyopathy • Congenital cardiac defects • Traumatic myocarditis • Distemper • Toxoplasmosis • Neosporosis

CBC/BIOCHEMISTRY/URINALYSIS
Generally normal

OTHER LABORATORY TESTS
• Serology—positive titer confirms diagnosis available from the CDC's parasitology unit • Organism isolation—LIT culture; collect 50 mL heparinized blood • Examination above the buffy coat in a microhematocrit tube (spun down to read PCV) using 40× microscope objective—organisms during period of high parasitemia • Elevated troponin I—acute disease

IMAGING
• Radiography—acute: cardiomegaly, pulmonary edema, and (rarely) mild pleural effusion; chronic: cardiomegaly • Echocardiography—acute: rarely shows chamber or wall abnormalities; chronic: reduced ejection fraction, fractional shortening, and thinning of right and left ventricular free wall

DIAGNOSTIC PROCEDURES
Electrocardiography
• Acute—atrioventricular block; depression of R wave and QRS amplitude; right bundle branch block
• Chronic—low QRS amplitude; right bundle branch block; ventricular arrhythmias (initially unifocal VPC, becomes multiform, then degenerates into various forms of ventricular tachycardia)

TREATMENT
• Medical therapy does not produce clinical cure.
• With poor prognosis and zoonotic potential, euthanasia is an option.

CLIENT EDUCATION
• Alert owner to possible zoonotic risk and potential for sudden death.
• Acute—usually develops into the chronic form, which is often fatal.
• Infected intact female—can transfer infection to offspring.

MEDICATIONS

DRUG(S)
• Several drugs have limited efficacy during the acute stage; none produces a clinical cure; even treated animals progress to chronic disease.
• Nifurtimox (Lampit)—investigational drug available only from the Communicable Disease Center; 30 mg/kg PO q12h for 90–120 days
• Allopurinol—some efficacy in humans; use not reported in dogs; try 30 mg/kg PO q12h for 100 days
• Benzimidazole (Ragonil)—5 mg/kg PO q12h for 60 days; markedly improves acute disease in humans
• Ketoconazole—little efficacy
• Verapamil (calcium channel blocker)—improves acute cardiac pathology and survival of *T. cruzi*–infected mice; use of the drug in dogs has not been as successful.
• Cythioate (Proban)—3.3 mg/kg PO every other day; effective in reducing vector populations
• Supportive treatment of dilated cardiomyopathy (right and left cardiac failure) and ventricular arrhythmias

FOLLOW-UP
• Cardiac disease—prognosis always guarded
• Chronic—prognosis guarded to hopeless

MISCELLANEOUS

ZOONOTIC POTENTIAL
Exists; essentially incurable in humans, thus euthanasia of infected dogs is an option.

ABBREVIATIONS
• LIT = liver infusion tryptose • PCV = packed cell volume • VPC = ventricular premature complex

Suggested Reading
Barr SC. American trypanosomiasis. In: Greene CE, ed. Infectious diseases of the dog and cat. 2nd ed. Philadelphia: Saunders, 1998:445–449.
Author Stephen C. Barr
Consulting Editor Stephen C. Barr

BASICS

OVERVIEW
• Autosomal recessive inherited disorder of Persian cats characterized by abnormalities in cellular morphology and pigment formation
• Large intracytoplasmic granules in circulating leukocytes and melanocytes formed by fusion of pre-existing granules
• Storage pool deficiency of ADP, ATP, magnesium, and serotonin results from lack of platelet-dense granules.
• Prolonged bleeding from trauma, venipuncture, or minor surgery occurs because of impaired platelet aggregation and release reaction.
• Normal coagulation times
• Depressed chemotaxis
• No change in rates of infection
• Mildly depressed neutrophil count but within reference range

SIGNALMENT
• Persian cats with dilute smoke-blue coat color and yellow-green irises (and white tigers)
• Does not occur in dogs
• Some Arctic foxes with blue or pearl hair coat color

SIGNS
Historical Findings
Prolonged bleeding from trauma, venipuncture, or minor surgery
Physical Examination Findings
• Red fundic reflex (lack of choroidal pigment)
• Dilute smoke-blue coat color and yellow-green irises

• Photophobia (blepharospasm and epiphora) in bright light

CAUSES & RISK FACTORS
Genetic disease

DIAGNOSIS

DIFFERENTIAL DIAGNOSIS
Dilute hair coat color

CBC/BIOCHEMISTRY/URINALYSIS
Romanowsky-stained blood smear—leukocytes, especially neutrophils, that contain pink to magenta cytoplasmic inclusions 2 μm in diameter

OTHER LABORATORY TESTS
None

IMAGING
N/A

DIAGNOSTIC PROCEDURES
None

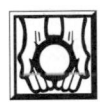
TREATMENT
Provide ascorbic acid (vitamin C) to increase cGMP concentration and to improve cell and platelet function (no controlled studies in cats).

MEDICATIONS

DRUG(S)
Ascorbic acid (100 mg PO q8h)

CONTRAINDICATIONS/POSSIBLE INTERACTIONS
None

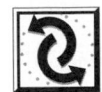
FOLLOW-UP

PATIENT MONITORING
None

PREVENTION/AVOIDANCE
• Advise owner of potential for prolonged bleeding after trauma, venipuncture, or minor surgery.
• Provide genetic counseling to eliminate Chediak-Higashi syndrome from animals used for breeding.
• Neuter affected and carrier animals or advise owner not to breed.

POSSIBLE COMPLICATIONS
Prolonged bleeding time

EXPECTED COURSE AND PROGNOSIS
Normal life span

MISCELLANEOUS

ABBREVIATIONS
• ADP = adenosine diphosphate
• ATP = adenosine triphosphate

Suggested Reading
August JR. Consultations in feline internal medicine. 2nd ed. Philadelphia: Saunders, 1994.
Author Kenneth S. Latimer
Contributing Editor Stephen A. Kruth

CHEMODECTOMA

 BASICS

OVERVIEW
Aortic body tumor in the heart-base region and carotid body tumor in the neck—two most common

SIGNALMENT
• Rare in cats
• Dogs—uncommon; 80%–90% are aortic body; age, 10–15 years old
• Boxers and Boston terriers—most commonly affected
• Aortic body—males predisposed
• Carotid body—no sex predilection

SIGNS
Aortic Body
• Similar to congestive heart failure
• Coughing
• Dyspnea

Carotid Body Tumor
• Regurgitation
• Dysphagia
• Neck mass
• Arteriovenous fistula in the neck

Both Types
• Acute hemorrhage from invaded blood vessels—may cause sudden death
• Distant metastasis with associated signs of organ dysfunction—up to 20% of patients
• Local invasion of blood vessels—up to 50% of patients

CAUSES & RISK FACTORS
Chronic hypoxemia—suspected risk factor; may explain predisposition of brachycephalic breeds

 DIAGNOSIS

DIFFERENTIAL DIAGNOSIS
• Congestive heart failure
• Megaesophagus
• Mediastinal lymphosarcoma
• Thyroid carcinoma
• Pericardial effusion

CBC/BIOCHEMISTRY/URINALYSIS
• Anemia from bleeding
• May see nucleated RBCs without anemia
• High liver enzymes, BUN, and creatinine—with metastasis to liver or kidneys

OTHER LABORATORY TESTS
N/A

IMAGING
• Thoracic radiography (aortic body)—identify heart-base mass, lung metastasis, or vertebral invasion
• Cardiac ultrasound

DIAGNOSTIC PROCEDURES
Histopathologic examination—differentiate from other tumors

 TREATMENT

• Surgical removal—difficult because highly invasive
• Debulking—may be treatment of choice, especially if the masses are somewhat freely movable
• Partial pericardectomy—average survival about 19 months
• Radiotherapy—successful as adjuvant treatment to surgery in two dogs with carotid body tumor

 MEDICATIONS

DRUG(S)
• Chemotherapy—treatment not reported
• Doxorubicin and cyclophosphamide—for metastatic carotid body tumor; partial remission in one dog treated by the author; patient survived 15 months

CONTRAINDICATIONS/POSSIBLE INTERACTIONS
Doxorubicin—do not use with congestive heart failure

 FOLLOW-UP

• Thoracic radiography and physical examination—every 3 months; monitor for recurrence and metastasis
• Median survival time after surgery (dogs; carotid body)—23 months
• Survival after surgery and radiotherapy for two dogs—6 and 27 months

 MISCELLANEOUS

Suggested Reading

Morrison WB. Nonpulmonary intrathoracic cancer. In: Morrison WB, ed. Cancer in dogs and cats: medical and surgical management. Jackson, Wyoming: Teton New Media, 2002:513–526.
Obradovich JE, Withrow SJ, Powers BE, et al. Carotid body tumors in the dog: eleven cases (1978–1988). J Vet Intern Med 1992;6:96–101.
Author Terrance A. Hamilton
Consulting Editor Wallace B. Morrison

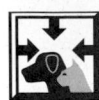

BASICS

OVERVIEW
• A highly contagious parasitic skin disease of dogs, cats, and rabbits, caused by infestation with *Cheyletiella* spp. mites
• Signs of scaling and pruritus can mimic other more common diseases.
• Often referred to as "walking dandruff," because of the large mite size and excessive scaling
• Prevalence varies by geographic region owing to mite susceptibility to common flea-control insecticides.
• Human (zoonotic) lesions can occur.

SIGNALMENT
• Dogs and cats
• More common in young animals
• Cocker spaniels, poodles, and long-haired cats are frequent asymptomatic carriers

SIGNS
Historical Findings
• Cats may exhibit bizarre behavioral signs or excessive grooming.
• Pruritus—none to severe, depending on the individual's response to infestation
• Infestation may be suspected after lesions in humans have developed.

Physical Examination Findings
• Scaling—most important clinical sign; diffuse or plaque-like; most severe in chronically infested and debilitated animals
• Lesions—dorsal orientation is commonly noted
• Underlying skin irritation may be minimal.
• Cats may exhibit bilaterally symmetrical alopecia.

CAUSES & RISK FACTORS
• Young animals and those in frequent contact with others are most at risk.
• Common sources of infestation—animal shelters, breeders, and grooming establishments.

DIAGNOSIS

DIFFERENTIAL DIAGNOSIS
• Cheyletiellosis should be considered in every animal that has scaling, with or without pruritus.
• Also consider—seborrhea, flea allergic dermatitis, *Sarcoptes* spp. mite infestation, atopy, food hypersensitivity, and idiopathic pruritus

CBC/BIOCHEMISTRY/URINALYSIS
N/A

OTHER LABORATORY TESTS
N/A

IMAGING
N/A

DIAGNOSTIC PROCEDURES
• Examination of epidermal debris—very effective in diagnosing infestation
• Collection of debris—flea combing (most effective), skin scraping, and acetate tape preparation
• *Cheyletiella* mites are large and can be visualized with a simple handheld magnifying lens; scales and hair may be examined under low magnification; staining is not necessary.
• Response to insecticide preparations may be required to definitively diagnose suspicious cases in which mites cannot be identified.

TREATMENT
• Must treat all animals in the household
• Clip long coats to facilitate treatment.
• Mainstay—6–8 weekly baths to remove scale, followed by rinses with an insecticide
• Lime-sulfur and pyrethrin rinses—cats, kittens, puppies, and rabbits
• Pyrethrin or organophosphates—dogs
• Routine flea sprays and powders—not always effective
• Environmental treatment with frequent cleanings and insecticide sprays—important for eliminating infestation
• Combs, brushes, and grooming utensils—discard or thoroughly disinfect before reuse
• Zoonotic lesions—self-limiting after eradication of the mites from household animals

MEDICATIONS

DRUG(S)
• Alternatives (or additions) to topical therapy—amitraz and ivermectin
• Amitraz (Mitaban)—use on dogs (4 rinses at 2-week intervals)
• Ivermectin—highly effective (300 μg/kg SC 3 times at 2-week intervals); dogs, cats, and rabbits > 3 months old; pour-on forms have shown efficacy in cats (500 μg/kg 2 times at 2-week intervals).
• Selanectin (Revolution®)—apply every 2 weeks for 3 applications (non–FDA-approved usage).

CONTRAINDICATIONS/POSSIBLE INTERACTIONS
Ivermectin—not FDA-approved for this use in dogs, cats, or rabbits; client disclosure and consent are paramount before administration; several dog breeds (e.g., collies, shelties, Australian shepherds) have shown increased sensitivity and should not be treated.

FOLLOW-UP
• Treatment failure necessitates reevaluation for other causes of pruritus and scaling.
• Reinfestation may indicate contact with an asymptomatic carrier or the presence of an unidentified source of mites (e.g., untreated bedding).

MISCELLANEOUS

ZOONOTIC POTENTIAL
A pruritic papular rash may develop in areas of contact with the pet.

Suggested Reading
Moriello KA. Cheyletiellosis. In: Griffin CE, Kwochka KW, MacDonald JM, eds. Current veterinary dermatology: the science and art of therapy. St. Louis: Mosby, 1993.
Author Alexander H. Werner
Consulting Editor Karen Helton Rhodes

BASICS

DEFINITION
A chronic respiratory infection of cats caused by an intracellular bacterium, characterized by conjunctivitis, mild upper respiratory signs, and mild pneumonitis

PATHOPHYSIOLOGY
• *Chlamydia psittaci*—an obligate intracellular bacterium; replicates on the mucosa of the upper and lower respiratory epithelium; produces a persistent commensal flora that causes a local irritation with resulting mild upper and lower respiratory signs; can also colonize the mucosa of the gastrointestinal and reproductive tracts
• Incubation period—7–10 days; longer than that for other common respiratory pathogens of the cat

SYSTEMS AFFECTED
• Respiratory—mild rhinitis, bronchitis, and bronchiolitis
• Ophthalmic—chronic conjunctivitis, often unilateral but may be bilateral
• Gastrointestinal—cat: infection without clinical disease; other species: may have clinical gastroenteritis
• Reproductive—infection without clinical disease

GENETICS
None

INCIDENCE/PREVALENCE
• Incidence of clinical disease—sporadic; outbreaks of respiratory disease may occur, especially in multicat facilities
• Prevalence of *C. psittaci* in the feline population—not uncommon, 5–10% chronically infected

GEOGRAPHIC DISTRIBUTION
Worldwide

SIGNALMENT

Species
• Cats
• Humans

Breed Predilections
None

Mean Age and Range
Usually kittens 2–6 months of age; any age cat possible

Predominant Sex
None

SIGNS

General Comments
• Infection often subclinical
• Clinical disease—only as a co-infection by other organisms

Historical Findings
• Upper respiratory infection, with some sneezing, watery eyes, and coughing
• Sometimes difficult breathing
• Varying degrees of anorexia

Physical Examination Findings
• Conjunctivitis—often granular; initially unilateral, sometimes becoming bilateral
• Lacrimation, photophobia, and blepharospasm
• Rhinitis with nasal discharge—usually mild
• Pneumonitis—with the inflammatory process in the alveoli; bronchiolar tubes and airways give audible rales

CAUSE
C. psittaci

RISK FACTORS
• Concurrent infections with other respiratory pathogens
• Lack of vaccination
• Multicat facilities, especially adoption shelters and breeding catteries

DIAGNOSIS

DIFFERENTIAL DIAGNOSIS
• Feline viral rhinotracheitis—short incubation period (4–5 days); rapid bilateral conjunctivitis; severe sneezing; and ulcerative keratitis
• Feline calicivirus infection—short incubation period (3–5 days); ulcerative stomatitis; and severe pneumonia
• Feline reovirus infection—very mild upper respiratory infection; short incubation and duration
• Bronchial pneumonia caused by bacteria such as *Bordetella bronchiseptica*—localized areas of density within the lungs on radiographs

CBC/BIOCHEMISTRY/URINALYSIS
Leukocytosis

OTHER LABORATORY TESTS
None

IMAGING
Radiographs of lungs—helpful with pneumonitis

DIAGNOSTIC PROCEDURES
• Conjunctival scrapings stained with Giemsa stain—characteristic intracytoplasmic inclusions
• Swab samples taken from conjunctiva—isolation of the causative organism in cell cultures
• Smear samples taken from conjunctiva—immunofluorescence assay to detect chlamydial antigen

PATHOLOGIC FINDINGS
• Gross—evidence of chronic conjunctivitis with mucopurulent ocular discharge; minor rhinitis with nasal discharge; sometimes lung changes indicative of pneumonitis
• Histopathologic (conjunctiva)—an early intense infiltration of neutrophils; inflamma-

tory response changes to lymphocytes and plasma cells; inclusions detected with special stains; inclusions invisible with routine H&E stains

TREATMENT

APPROPRIATE HEALTH CARE
Generally as outpatient

NURSING CARE
• Keep nostrils and eyes clean of discharge.
• Generally does not require other supportive therapy (e.g., fluids), unless complicated by concurrent infections

ACTIVITY
• Quarantine affected cats from contact with other cats.
• Do not allow affected cats to go outside.

DIET
Normal

CLIENT EDUCATION
Inform clients of the causative organism, the anticipated chronic course of disease, and the need to vaccinate other cats before exposure.

SURGICAL CONSIDERATIONS
None

MEDICATIONS

DRUG(S) OF CHOICE
• Systemic—tetracycline (22 mg/kg PO q8h for 3–4 weeks); doxycycline 10 mg/kg PO daily
• Ocular—ophthalmic ointments containing tetracycline (q8h)

CONTRAINDICATIONS
Tetracycline—may affect growing teeth of young kittens

PRECAUTIONS
Colonies—the entire colony may have to be treated; treatment may have to be continued for as long as 6 weeks.

POSSIBLE INTERACTIONS
None

ALTERNATIVE DRUG(S)
Other antibiotics are generally less effective than is tetracycline.

FOLLOW-UP

PATIENT MONITORING
Monitor for improved health as treatment proceeds.

PREVENTION/AVOIDANCE

Vaccines
• Both inactivated and modified live vaccines are available to reduce the severity of infection.
• Vaccines do not prevent infection; rather, they reduce severity and duration.
• American Association of Feline Practitioners—classifies as noncore; give a single vaccination the initial visit; revaccinate 1 year later; then give annual revaccinations.

POSSIBLE COMPLICATIONS
Adverse vaccine reactions—mild clinical disease; small percentage of vaccinated cats

EXPECTED COURSE AND PROGNOSIS
• Tends to be chronic, lasting for several weeks or months, unless successful antibiotic treatment is given
• Prognosis good

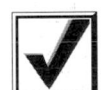

MISCELLANEOUS

ASSOCIATED CONDITIONS
None

AGE-RELATED FACTORS
Primarily a disease of young cats

ZOONOTIC POTENTIAL
C. psittaci can infect humans; limited number of reports of mild conjunctivitis in humans transmitted from infected cats

PREGNANCY
Role of *C. psittaci* as a pathogen during pregnancy—unclear; can colonize the reproductive mucosa; severe conjunctivitis neonatorum can occur in neonatal kittens infected at or shortly after birth.

SYNONYMS
Feline pneumonitis

ABBREVIATION
• H&E = hematoxylin and eosin

Suggested Reading
Elston T, Rodan I, Flemming D, et al. 1998 report of the American Association of Feline Practitioners and Academy of Feline Medicine Advisory Panel on Feline Vaccines. J Am Vet Med Assoc 1998;212:227–241.
Ford RB, Levy JK. Infectious diseases of the respiratory tract. In: Sherding RG, ed. The cat: diseases and clinical management. New York: Churchill Livingstone, 1994:489–500.
Ford RB. Role of infectious agents in respiratory disease. Vet Clin North Am Small Anim Pract 1993;23:17–35.
Gaskell RM. Upper respiratory disease in the cat (including *Chlamydia*): control and prevention. Feline Pract 1993;21:29–34.
Greene CE. Chlamydial infections. In: Greene CE, ed. Infectious diseases of the dog and cat. 2nd ed. Philadelphia: Saunders, 1998:172–174.
Hoover EA. Viral respiratory diseases and chlamydiosis. In: Holzworth J, ed. Diseases of the cat. Philadelphia: Saunders, 1987:214–237.

Author Fred W. Scott
Consulting Editor Stephen C. Barr

CHOCOLATE TOXICITY

BASICS

DEFINITION
Acute gastroenteric, neurologic, and cardiac toxicosis caused by excessive intake of methylxanthine alkaloids, present in chocolate

PATHOPHYSIOLOGY
• Methylxanthine alkaloids—primarily theobromine and caffeine; inhibit adenosine receptors, leading to vasoconstriction, tachycardia, and CNS stimulation
• Inhibition of phosphodiesterase—increases cAMP, which potentiates catecholamine effects (increases its release)
• Combined effects—result in cerebral vasoconstriction, cardiac muscle contraction, and CNS stimulation and seizures

SYSTEMS AFFECTED
• Gastrointestinal—early onset of vomiting and diarrhea; may be mediated centrally; may result even from parenteral administration of methylxanthine alkaloids
• Nervous—stimulation; enhanced alertness and reflex hyperactivity; tremors; seizures
• Cardiovascular—increased myocardial contractility and tachyarrhythmias

GENETICS
N/A

INCIDENCE/PREVALENCE
• Dogs—among the 20 most common poisonings reported in recent literature, by the National Animal Poison Control Center, and by the Hennepin County (Minneapolis) Poison Control Center
• More common at holiday times—chocolate products and candies readily available
• Caffeine-containing stimulant tablets—occasional source

GEOGRAPHIC DISTRIBUTION
• Urban and indoor dogs—may be more at risk owing to close proximity to chocolate products

SIGNALMENT
Species
Dogs and rarely cats

Breed Predilection
Small dogs—may be more at risk (amount of chocolate available relative to body weight)

Mean Age and Range
Puppies and young dogs—may be more likely to ingest large amounts of unusual foods

Predominant Sex
N/A

SIGNS
Historical Findings
• Recent chocolate ingestion
• Vomiting and diarrhea—often the first reported; 2–4 hr after ingestion
• Early restlessness and enhanced activity
• Polyuria—may result from diuretic action
• Advanced signs—stiffness; excitement; seizures; hyperreflexia

Physical Examination Findings
• Hyperthermia
• Hyperreflexia
• Muscle rigidity
• Tachypnea
• Tachycardia
• Hypotension
• Advanced signs—lead to cardiac failure, weakness, coma, and death
• Death—12–36 hr after ingestion

CAUSES
• Usually some form of processed chocolate (used for candies and baking)—contain high concentrations of theobromine and caffeine

PRODUCTS WITH HIGH METHYLXANTHINE CONCENTRATIONS

Product	Methylxanthines (mg/g)
Cacao bean	14–53
Baking chocolate	16
Semisweet chocolate	9
Milk chocolate	2
Hot chocolate	0.4
White chocolate	0.05

• Minimum lethal dosage for caffeine and theobromine (dogs)—100–200 mg/kg
• Potentially lethal (dogs)—7.0 g baking chocolate or 60 g milk chocolate per kilogram of body weight; 420 g milk chocolate or 49 g baking chocolate in a 7-kg dog

RISK FACTORS
• Dogs—most commonly affected because they consume large amounts of unusual foods quickly
• Chocolate—highly palatable and attractive; often readily available and unprotected in homes and kitchens
• Methylxanthine alkaloids—readily and rapidly absorbed; only slightly bound (20%) to plasma proteins

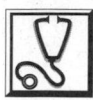

DIAGNOSIS

DIFFERENTIAL DIAGNOSES
• Convulsant or excitatory alkaloids—strychnine; amphetamine; nicotine; 4-aminopyridine
• Convulsant pesticides—cyclodiene-chlorinated hydrocarbons (e.g., chlordane, toxaphene, and lindane)
• Tremorogenic mycotoxins–penitrem A; aflatrem
• Acute psychogenic drugs—LSD; morning glory
• Fluoroacetate toxicosis
• Cardioactive glycosides—*Digitalis* spp.; *Nerium oleander*
• Hypomagnesemia and hypocalcemia

CBC/BIOCHEMISTRY/URINALYSIS
• Hypoglycemia—may note secondary to increased muscular activity
• Low urine specific gravity and proteinuria—occasionally

OTHER LABORATORY TESTS
• Stomach contents, plasma, and urine—analyzed chemically for methylxanthines
• Elimination half-life (dogs)—17.5 hr (theobromine); detectable plasma or serum concentration should persist 3–4 days.

IMAGING
N/A

DIAGNOSTIC PROCEDURES
ECG—confirm tachycardia and ventricular tachyarrhythmia

PATHOLOGIC FINDINGS
• Stomach contents—may note small or large amounts of chocolate
• Microscopic renal lesions—reported; characterized by hyaline droplet degeneration, pyknosis, and karyorrhexis

TREATMENT

APPROPRIATE HEALTH CARE
Reported by phone—attempt to determine type and amount of exposure; if not possible, recommend referral to hospital as a potential toxicologic emergency.

NURSING CARE
Fluid therapy—correct electrolyte disturbances caused by vomiting, as necessary.

ACTIVITY
Avoid stress and excitement—could precipitate hyperreflexia or seizures

DIET
• Acutely affected patient—do not feed.
• Convalescence—bland diet for several days to allow recovery from gastroenteritis

CLIENT EDUCATION
Warn client of the hazards of chocolate ingestion.

SURGICAL CONSIDERATIONS
N/A

MEDICATIONS

DRUG(S) OF CHOICE
• Induce emesis—*only if patient is not already seizing;* apomorphine (0.03 mg/kg IV); syrup of ipecac (1–2 mL/kg PO); hydrogen peroxide (1–5 mL/kg PO)
• Gastric lavage—only before onset of vomiting and other clinical signs, if emetics are not effective
• Vomiting controlled—activated charcoal (0.5–1.0 g/kg PO); adsorbs remaining alkaloids in the gastrointestinal tract
• Osmotic cathartic—sodium sulfate (1 g/kg PO); promotes gastrointestinal elimination of chocolate

• Hyperactivity and seizures—controlled with diazepam (0–5 mg/kg IV q10–20 min up to four times)
• Ventricular tachycardia (dogs)—lidocaine (without epinephrine), 1–2 mg/kg IV followed by 0.03–0.05 mg/kg/min IV drip
• Serious refractory arrhythmias—metoprolol or propranolol (0.04–0.06 mg/kg IV; rate not > 1 mg/min); metoprolol preferred but may be difficult to obtain; may use oral therapy once patient is stable (metoprolol at 0.2–1.0 mg/kg PO q12h; propranolol at 0.2–1.0 mg/kg PO q8h); monitor ECG for hypotension (a sequela to this treatment).

CONTRAINDICATIONS
• Do not use epinephrine concurrent with lidocaine.
• Avoid erythromycin and corticosteroids—these reduce the excretion of methylxanthines.
• Do not use lidocaine in affected cats.

PRECAUTIONS
• Effects may persist longer than the effective life of therapeutic drugs.
• Keep patient under observation until drug administration is no longer needed.
• Methylxanthines—cross the placenta; excreted in milk

POSSIBLE INTERACTIONS
N/A

ALTERNATIVE DRUG(S)
• If response to diazepam inadequate—consider phenobarbital (30 mg/kg IV administered over 5–10 min)
• Refractory seizures—pentobarbital (3–15 mg/kg IV slowly, as needed)

FOLLOW-UP

PATIENT MONITORING
• ECG—arrhythmias
• Watch for mild to moderate nephrosis in convalescent patients.

PREVENTION/AVOIDANCE
Warn owners about the toxicologic hazards of chocolate.

POSSIBLE COMPLICATIONS
Pregnant or nursing animals—risk for teratogenesis of newborns or stimulation of nursing neonates

EXPECTED COURSE AND PROGNOSIS
• Expected course—12–36 hr, depending on dosage and effectiveness of decontamination and treatment
• Successfully treated patients—usually recover completely
• Prognosis—good if oral decontamination occurs within 2–4 hr of ingestion; guarded with advanced signs of seizures and arrhythmias

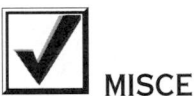

MISCELLANEOUS

ASSOCIATED CONDITIONS
N/A

AGE-RELATED FACTORS
N/A

ZOONOTIC POTENTIAL
Not transmissible, but humans and dogs may access similar sources.

PREGNANCY
Methylxanthines—teratogens in laboratory animals

SEE ALSO
• Metaldehyde Poisoning
• Poisoning (Intoxication)
• Strychnine Poisoning

Suggested Reading
Carson T. Methylxanthines. In: Peterson M, Talcott P, eds. Small animal toxicology. Philadelphia: Saunders, 2001:563–570.

Drolet P, Arendt TD, Stowe CM. Cacao bean shell poisoning in 2 dogs. J Am Vet Med Assoc 1984;185:902–904.

Glauberg A, Blumenthal HP. Chocolate toxicosis in a dog. J Am Anim Hosp Assoc 1983;19:246–248.

Hooser SB, Beasley VR. Methylxanthine poisoning (chocolate and caffeine toxicosis) In: Kirk RW, ed. Current veterinary therapy IX. Small animal practice. Philadelphia: Saunders, 1986.

Author Gary D. Osweiler
Consulting Editor Gary D. Osweiler

CHOLANGITIS/CHOLANGIOHEPATITIS SYNDROME

BASICS

DEFINITION
• Cholangitis—inflammation of the biliary tree • Cholangiohepatitis—inflammation of biliary structures and surrounding hepatocellular parenchyma • CCHS—occur together in cats; histologically classified as suppurative or nonsuppurative (lymphoplasmacytic, lymphocytic), granulomatous, or lymphoproliferative (transition to lymphosarcoma)

PATHOPHYSIOLOGY
• Preceding or coexisting conditions—inflammation or obstruction of the extrahepatic biliary tree, pancreatitis, IBD, CIN (cats) • Bacterial cholangitis—stasis of bile flow may aid development; may result in mineralized biliary structures; initiates biliary epithelial hyperplasia • Suppurative disease—usually positive bacterial culture • Nonsuppurative disease—immune mediated • Immune-mediated bile duct destruction—results in a ductopenia of small- and medium-sized bile ductules (sclerosing cholangitis) • Pyogranulomatous CCHS—secondary to infection or immune mechanisms (dogs) • Lymphoproliferative disease—transition stage: inflammation/neoplasia (speculative)

SYSTEMS AFFECTED
• Hepatobiliary—liver and biliary system
• Gastrointestinal—pancreas and intestines

INCIDENCE/PREVALENCE
Nonsuppurative CCHS—most common chronic liver disorder of the cat

SIGNALMENT
Species
Cats and dogs (uncommon)

Breed Predilections
Possibly Himalayan, Persian, and Siamese cats

Mean Age and Range
• Suppurative CCHS—range, 0.4–16 years; mostly young to middle-aged cats • Nonsuppurative CCHS—range, 2–17 years; mostly middle-aged cats

Predominant Sex
• Suppurative CCHS—male cats predisposed
• Nonsuppurative CCHS—none

SIGNS
General Comments
• Suppurative CCHS—most severe clinical illness, acute abdomen, acute febrile illness often < 5 days; associated with EHBDO
• Nonsuppurative—illness > 3 weeks (months to years)

Historical Findings
• Suppurative CCHS—acute illness; fever; anorexia; vomiting; collapse • Nonsuppurative CCHS—cyclic illness; chronic vague signs, including lethargy, vomiting, anorexia, and weight loss; ductopenia (cats)—

polyphagic owing to reduced bile flow compromising nutrient assimilation; chronic vitamin K depletion

Physical Examination Findings
• Suppurative CCHS—fever; painful abdomen; anicteric to jaundiced; dehydrated; shock • Nonsuppurative CCHS—few physical abnormalities other than hepatomegaly; thickened intestines with IBD; abdominal effusion rare; jaundice variable • Ductopenia (cats)—unkempt coat; intermittent acholic feces

CAUSES
Suppurative CCHS
• Bacterial infection—most common in cats: *E. coli, Enterobacter, Enterococcus,* β-hemolytic *Streptococcus, Klebsiella, Actinomyces, Clostridia,* and *Bacteroides;* may also be associated with toxoplasmosis; in dogs: enteric organisms, *Campylobacter, Salmonella,* and *Leptospirosis*
• Highly associated with EHBDO and bile stasis

Nonsuppurative CCHS
Concurrent disorders—cholecystitis; cholelithiasis; pancreatitis; EHBDO; IBD; CIN; infections elsewhere

RISK FACTORS
• Suppurative CCHS—EHBDO; cholestasis
• Nonsuppurative CCHS—IBD, pancreatitis, EHBDO

DIAGNOSIS

DIFFERENTIAL DIAGNOSES
• HLS—may co-exist; similar enzyme abnormalities and jaundice; if not associated with biliary tree or pancreatic inflammation, have minimal GGT activity
• EHBDO—marked jaundice and high ALP, GGT, and transaminase activities; high cholesterol; ultrasonographic evidence of EHBDO • Pancreatitis—may initiate CCHS; lipemia; high cholesterol and bilirubin; inconsistently high TLI, lipase, and amylase; ultrasonographic features • Lymphoproliferative disease and lymphosarcoma—may involve intestines or stomach; periportal infiltrates and same clinical features as CCHS; may have circulating blast cells; hepatic lesions may be histologically defined by immunohistochemical staining; thick bowel • Jaundice associated with septicemia—high liver enzymes; sepsis • Polycystic disease (Himalayan and Persian cats)—normal to modest increase in liver enzymes; progressive, severe peribiliary fibrosis; multifocal but minor nonsuppurative inflammation

CBC/BIOCHEMISTRY/URINALYSIS
CBC
• Poikilocytes common with severe liver disease in cats; nonregenerative anemia in chronic disease; Heinz body hemolysis in

severely ill cats • Suppurative CCHS—leukocytosis, left shift, toxic neutrophils
• Nonsuppurative CCHS—lymphoproliferative disorders may have high circulating lymphocyte count; cell morphology not convincingly neoplastic

Serum Biochemistry
• Consistent findings—high ALP, GGT, AST, ALT; higher enzymes with nonsuppurative disease • Variable findings—high bile acids, bilirubin, and cholesterol, depending on associated illness; functional liver impairment; and cholestasis

OTHER LABORATORY TESTS
• TLI—may be high with pancreatitis and enteritis • Vitamin B_{12}—low value indicates severe malabsorption (small bowel disease)
• Coagulation tests—normal or increased PT, APTT, ACT, PIVKA (PIVKA most sensitive for vitamin K–induced coagulopathy)
• Aerobic and anaerobic bacterial cultures—hepatic and biliary samples • Thyroxine—rules out hyperthyroidism as cause of liver enzyme elevation

IMAGING
• Thoracic radiography—sternal lymphadenopathy with abdominal disease
• Abdominal radiography—hepatomegaly in nonsuppurative CCHS; may find no abnormalities • Abdominal ultrasonography—hepatomegaly; echogenic changes in biliary structures; cholelithiasis; sludged bile; thick gallbladder wall suggests possible cholecystitis; focal lesions suggest parenchymal abscess; lymphadenopathy (peripancreatic, perihilar hepatic, or mesenteric) indicates pancreatic, liver, or intestinal inflammation; hepatic echogenicity confused by concurrent HLS; cysts (polycystic disease); no ultrasound lesions in some cats with severe CCHS

OTHER DIAGNOSTIC PROCEDURES
Fine-needle Aspiration Cytology
• Hepatic aspiration—culture sample if suppurative CCHS suspected; cytology reveals bacteria not visualized on histopathology; cytology unreliable for diagnosis of nonsuppurative CCHS; hepatocellular vacuolation common in ill cats before full HLS
• Cholecystocentesis—may reveal suppuration, bacteria, trematode eggs, or neoplasia

Percutaneous Biopsy
• Ultrasound-directed core-needle biopsy—may misdiagnose CCHS • Requires minimum of 15 portal triads for accurate diagnosis • Using an 18-gauge needle, collect a minimum of four samples • Inaccuracy reflects differential liver lobe involvement
• Postbiopsy complications and unintentional sampling of nonhepatic tissues may occur with ultrasound guidance in cats (small size).

Laparoscopy
• Permits visualization of gallbladder, porta hepatis, pancreas, and perihepatic and

peripancreatic lymph nodes, and biopsy of liver and pancreas • In EHBDO—not recommended; pursue laparotomy • If nonsuppurative CCHS suspected, also sample bowel for IBD and pancreas for pancreatitis

Laparotomy
• Suspected EHBDO—recommended • Permits inspection of biliary structures; removal of obstructions; biliary enteric anastomosis; and biopsy of liver, biliary structures, pancreas, intestines, and large lymph nodes

PATHOLOGIC FINDINGS
• Suppurative CCHS—swollen liver with blunt edges and focal discolorations; may note erythematous, necrotic, or thick-walled gallbladder (cholecystitis); peripancreatic steatonecrosis and fat saponification (pancreatitis); perihepatic and peripancreatic lymphadenopathy; verification of EHBDO • Nonsuppurative CCHS—large, firm liver (small in very chronic disease); blunt margins; variable surface irregularity; yellow or pale and friable if concurrent HLS

TREATMENT
APPROPRIATE HEALTH CARE
Inpatient Management
• Suppurative CCHS with acute febrile illness, painful abdomen, left-shifted leukogram—hydration support, "best guess" bactericidal antimicrobials (based on aspiration cytology and gram stain initially); evaluate for EHBDO or cholecystitis requiring surgery; continue antibiotic therapy for at least 8 weeks; provide choleretic therapy (ursodeoxycholic acid) to thin bile secretions until enzymes are normalized
• Nonsuppurative symptomatic cats—fluid therapy; diagnostic evaluations; liver biopsy (24 hr before biopsy, administer vitamin K_1 at 0.5–1.5 mg/ kg IM) • Both forms CCHS (cats)—may require blood transfusion in association with surgery or biopsy
• Polyionic fluids—supplement with B-soluble vitamins (2 ml/L), KCl, and K phosphate as needed; avoid dextrose supplementation without full caloric support (promotes HLS)

Outpatient Management
• Suppurative—after acute crisis is managed
• Nonsuppurative—after resolution of acute crisis, provide chronic (lifelong) immunomodulatory, antioxidant, and hepatoprotective therapy

ACTIVITY
Restricted while symptomatic

DIET
Nutritional support—essential to avoid HLS; balanced high-protein, high-calorie feline diet with water-soluble vitamin supplements; antigen-restricted diet with concurrent IBD; fat-restricted diet with severe ductopenia, fat malabsorption, or chronic pancreatitis

causing maldigestion; may initially require PPN transitioned to enteral support or TPN; feeding tubes may be required (usually esophagostomy or gastrostomy, but jejunal with pancreatitis)

CLIENT EDUCATION
Emphasize chronic nature of nonsuppurative CCHS and requirement for lifelong therapy

SURGICAL CONSIDERATIONS
• Cholecystectomy—with severe cholecystitis
• Cholecystoenterostomy—with EHBDO
• Cholelith removal

MEDICATIONS
DRUG(S)
Antibiotics for Suppurative CCHS
• Bactericidal—directed at enteric opportunists; Clavamox (62.5 PO q12h) or enrofloxacin (2.5 mg/kg/q12h) combined with metronidazole (7.5 mg/kg PO q12h)
• Resistant enterococci—vancomycin (10 mg/kg q12hr IV slow infusion for 7–10 days)
• Modify initial empiric drug selection based on culture and sensitivity reports

Immunomodulation for Nonsuppurative CCHS
• Glucocorticoids—prednisolone (dogs: 2 mg/kg/day; cats: 4 mg/kg/day) for 14–21 days; slowly taper to lowest effective alternate-day dose; chronic therapy advised • Metronidazole—in combination with prednisolone for cell-mediated immunomodulation (dose above), especially with IBD • Cats with confirmed ductopenia—require more aggressive therapy; poor response to and toxicity from azathioprine or chlorambucil; clinical experience suggests combination of prednisolone, metronidazole with pulsed methotrexate (0.4 mg *total dose* given in three divided doses on 1 day [0.13 mg total at 0, 12, and 24 hr] and repeated at 1-week intervals); may be given PO, IV, IM (parenteral routes require 50% dose reduction); concurrently provide folate (folinic acid) at 0.25 mg/kg daily • Some cats require chemotherapy protocols developed for lymphoma.

Antioxidants
• Vitamin E (α-tocopherol acetate, 10–30 IU/kg)—high dose for chronic EHBDO when given PO because of fat malabsorption
• S-adenosylmethionine, 20 mg/kg enteric-coated tablet PO q24h, 2 hr before feeding

Other
• Ursodeoxycholic acid—immunomodulatory, hepatoprotectant, choleretic, antifibrotic, and antioxidant effects; 10–15 mg/kg/day PO q24h or divided q12h, capsule or aqueous solution • B vitamin supplementation with thiamine (B_1) and B_{12}—thiamine 50–100 mg PO q24h for at least 3 days, then as water-soluble vitamin supplement; B_{12} (1 mg SC, single injection);

if suspect gut malabsorption rechecking plasma B_{12} concentration determines strategy; some cats require weekly injections until vitamin restored, then require monthly injections based on serum B_{12}

CONTRAINDICATIONS
Adjust drug dosages with regard to liver function and cholestasis.

FOLLOW-UP
PATIENT MONITORING
Nonsuppurative CCHS—initially, monitor enzymes and bilirubin at 7- to 14-day intervals; with remission, assess quarterly; serum bile acid measurements complicated by ursodeoxycholic acid (detected by assay)

PREVENTION/AVOIDANCE
Control IBD

POSSIBLE COMPLICATIONS
• Suppurative CCHS may progress to nonsuppurative CCHS and immune-mediated duct injury. • Diabetes mellitus in 30% of cats with sclerosing CCHS when treated with prednisolone • HLS with inadequate nutrition

EXPECTED COURSE AND PROGNOSIS
• Suppurative CCHS—may be cured • Nonsuppurative CCHS—chronic, long-term remission possible (> 8 years documented)

MISCELLANEOUS
ASSOCIATED CONDITIONS
• Pancreatitis • Hepatic lipidosis • Polycystic liver disease • Lymphosarcoma • Lymphoproliferative disease • Cholangiocarcinoma—may develop in some cats with chronic nonsuppurative CCHS

SEE ALSO
• Bile Duct Obstruction • Cholecystitis
• Cholelithiasis • Hepatic Lipidosis
• Inflammatory Bowel Disease • Pancreatitis

ABBREVIATIONS
• ACT = activated clotting time • APTT = activated partial thromboplastin time
• CCHS = cholangitis/cholangiohepatitis syndrome • CIN = chronic interstitial nephritis • EHBDO = extrahepatic bile duct obstruction • HLS = hepatic lipidosis syndrome • IBD = inflammatory bowel disease • PIVKA = proteins invoked by vitamin K absence • PPN = partial parenteral nutrition • PT = prothrombin time • TLI = trypsin-like immunoreactivity • TPN = total parenteral nutrition

Suggested Reading
Center SA. Cholangitis/cholangiohepatitis in the cat. Proc Annual Meeting ACVIM 1997.
Author Sharon A. Center
Consulting Editor Sharon A. Center

CHOLECYSTITIS

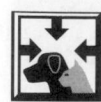 BASICS

OVERVIEW
• Inflammation of the gallbladder, sometimes associated with cholelithiasis; often associated with obstruction and/or inflammation of the common bile duct and/or intrahepatic biliary system
• Severe cases result in rupture of the gallbladder and subsequent bile peritonitis, necessitating combined surgical and medical treatment.
• Bile peritonitis enhances trans-mural migration of enteric bacteria across the bowel wall and increased permeability of the microvasculature to bacteria causing septic peritonitis.

SIGNALMENT
• Dogs and cats
• No breed, sex, or age predilection
• Necrotizing cholecystitis (dogs)—usually middle-aged or older
• Hyperlipidemic dogs—predisposed to biliary mucocele; leading to cholestasis and cholecystitis; (see Gallbladder Mucocele)

SIGNS
• Sudden onset of inappetence, depression, vomiting, and abdominal pain
• Severe disease—shock due to endotoxemia and hypovolemia
• Mild to moderate jaundice and fever are common.
• Soft tissue mass in right cranial abdominal quadrant—palpable in small dogs and cats; develops subsequent to inflammation of the gallbladder and surrounding tissues

CAUSES & RISK FACTORS
• Impaired bile flow in cystic duct or gallbladder, dysmotility, or ischemic insult to the gallbladder wall may precede cholecystitis.
• Irritants in bile (e.g., sludged bile, lysolecithin, choleliths, liver flukes) or retrograde flow of pancreatic enzymes may initiate and promote inflammation.
• Previous gastrointestinal disorders, trauma, or abdominal surgery—may be contributing factors
• Anomalous development of the gallbladder—rarely implicated
• Bacterial infection—common; retrograde invasion from the intestine or hematogenous spread
• Toxoplasmosis and biliary coccidiosis—rarely reported causes
• Necrotizing cholecystitis (dogs)—ruptured gallbladder common; cholelithiasis common; *Escherichia coli* common bacterial isolate
• Emphysematous cholecystitis/choledochitis—associated with diabetes mellitus, traumatic ischemia of the gallbladder, and acute cholecystitis (with or without cholelithiasis); gas-forming organisms (e.g., *Clostridia*) and *E. coli* often cultured

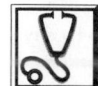 DIAGNOSIS

DIFFERENTIAL DIAGNOSIS
• Pancreatitis
  Focal to diffuse peritonitis
• Gastroenteritis with secondary biliary tract involvement
• Bile peritonitis
• Cholelithiasis
• Cholangiohepatitis
• Hepatic necrosis
• Hepatic abscessation
• Septicemia
• EHBDO

CBC/BIOCHEMISTRY/URINALYSIS
• Variable leukocytosis with toxic neutrophils and inconsistent left shift
• High bilirubin; bilirubinuria
• High ALT, AST, ALP, and GGT
• Low albumin with peritonitis
• High cholesterol if EHBDO

OTHER LABORATORY TESTS
• Abdominocentesis—inflammatory cytology noted in abdominal effusion; bile indicates a ruptured biliary tract
• Bile culture (dogs)—*E. coli, Klebsiella* spp., *Pseudomonas* spp., and *Clostridium* spp. reported
• Coagulation tests—abnormal with severe disease due to vitamin K deficiency (from EHBDO) or DIC

IMAGING
• Abdominal radiography—may reveal focal to diffuse peritonitis, ileus, choleliths, or gas accumulation in biliary structures; may note radiodense gallbladder if dystrophic mineralization (porcelain gallbladder)
• Ultrasonography—bilayer appearance of the gallbladder wall indicates inflammation, edema, ascites, adjacent hepatic inflammation or congestion; necrotic slough appears as an intraluminal membrane parallel to the wall and is associated with irregular texture; pericystic fluid suggests necrotizing cholecystitis and surgical urgency; failure to image the gallbladder may indicate rupture of biliary structures

PATHOLOGIC FINDINGS
Gross appearance—erythematous gallbladder; may appear green-black if necrotizing cholecystitis; tenacious "inspissated" biliary material common

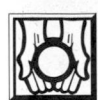

TREATMENT

• Inpatient—required for critical care during diagnostic and presurgical evaluations
• Place intravenous catheter in peripheral vein for fluid, colloid, and blood component delivery
• Restore fluid and electrolyte balance; monitor electrolytes frequently
• Polyionic fluids—combined with colloids
• Plasma—preferred colloid; indicated if hypoalbuminemia
• Whole blood—for surgical cases with bleeding tendencies
• Hetastarch—preferred over dextran 70 (higher rate of iatrogenic coagulopathy); 10–20 mL/kg/day slow drip as a constant rate infusion
• Monitor urine output
• Remain vigilant for vasovagal reflex (abrupt pathologic bradycardia, hypotension, cardiac arrest) when biliary structures manipulated; be prepared with anticholinergics (atropine)
• Gallbladder resection—based on gross evaluation

MEDICATIONS

DRUG(S)
• Antibiotics—before surgery; broad spectrum; surgical manipulations facilitate bacteremia; select antibiotics for enteric gram-negative and anaerobic flora; refine treatment using culture and sensitivity results; good initial choices: combination of aminoglycoside and metronidazole, or clindamycin and imipenem or ticarcillin or a fluorinated quinolone. Reduce standard dose for metronidazole and clindamycin by 50% in the circumstance of cholestasis and jaundice.
• Ursodeoxycholic acid—10–15 mg/kg PO q24h
• Antioxidants: vitamin E (α-toco-pherol acetate)—10 IU/kg, larger-than-normal dose needed in chronic EHBDO when given PO because of fat malabsorption (lack of enteric bile acids); S-adenosylmethio-nine (SAMe)—thiol donor (20 mg/kg PO q24h), 2 hours before feeding
• Vitamin K₁—0.5–1.5 mg/kg SC or IM to a maximum of three doses over 36 hr; **Caution:** never administer intravenously because of danger of anaphylactoid reaction; treat early to allow response time before surgical manipulations

CONTRAINDICATIONS
Ursodeoxycholic acid—contraindicated if biliary tree obstruction or bile peritonitis uncorrected

FOLLOW-UP

PATIENT MONITORING
Physical examination and pertinent diagnostic testing—repeat every 2–4 weeks until signs and clinicopathologic abnormalities resolve

POSSIBLE COMPLICATIONS
Anticipate a protracted clinical course with ruptured biliary tract or peritonitis.

MISCELLANEOUS

ASSOCIATED CONDITIONS
• Cholelithiasis
• EHBDO
• Choledochitis
• Gallbladder mucocele
• Bile peritonitis

AGE-RELATED FACTORS
Congenital malformations of biliary structures do not predispose patients to cholecystitis

ZOONOTIC POTENTIAL
Campylobacter and *Salmonella* may cause cholecystitis in dogs; advise owner if diagnosed

ABBREVIATIONS
ALP = alkaline phosphatase
ALT = alanine aminotransferase
AST = aspartate aminotransferase
DIC = disseminated intravascular coagulation
EHBDO = extrahepatic bile duct obstruction
GGT = γ-glutamyltransferase

Suggested Reading
Center SA. Diseases of the gallbladder and biliary tree. In: Guilford WG, Center SA, Strombeck DR, et al., eds. Strombeck's small animal gastroenterology. Philadelphia: Saunders, 1996:860–888.
Author Sharon A. Center
Consulting Editor Sharon A. Center

CHOLELITHIASIS

BASICS

OVERVIEW
• Radiopaque or radiolucent calculi in the biliary tree or gallbladder
• May be asymptomatic or associated with signs attributed to sludged bile, OBTD, cholecystitis, cholangiohepatitis, or bile peritonitis
• Primary constituents of choleliths—mucin, calcium, and bilirubin; in dogs, usually lower cholesterol and calcium than in humans and cats
• Surgical and/or medical treatment—not recommended in the absence of clinical or clinicopathologic signs

SIGNALMENT
• Cats and dogs
• Particularly miniature schnauzers and poodles
• Hyperlipidemic dogs—seemingly predisposed to developing thick mucinous biliary sludge, which may behave as choleliths (see Gallbladder Mucocele)

SIGNS
• May be asymptomatic
• When accompanied by infection or OBTD (with or without peritonitis)—vomiting; abdominal pain; fever; jaundice

CAUSES & RISK FACTORS
• Predisposing factors—conditions that cause stasis of bile flow (gallbladder dysmotility), stone nidus formation (inflammatory debris, infection, tumor exfoliation), and supersaturation of bile (pigment, cholesterol); anatomic union of the pancreatic and biliary ducts (cats) may promote duct inflammation and bile stasis
• Bile sludging and/or gallbladder distention—stimulate increased mucin production and coalescence of bile particles
• Inflammatory mediators and bacterial enzymes associated with cholecystitis—aggravate the condition; mucin production; subsequent stone formation
• Low-protein and low-taurine diets—considered lithogenic

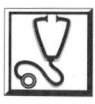

DIAGNOSIS

DIFFERENTIAL DIAGNOSIS
• OBTD—attributed to inflammatory, infectious, or neoplastic conditions involving the liver or adjacent extrahepatic tissues in the porta hepatis; suggested by marked increases in cholesterol, ALP, and bilirubin
• Cholangiohepatitis
• Pancreatitis
• Bile peritonitis
• Biliary mucocele

CBC/BIOCHEMISTRY/URINALYSIS
• CBC—may be normal; abnormalities reflect bacterial infection, endotoxemia, biliary obstruction, or underlying causal factors; inflammatory leukogram in some cases
• Biochemistry—hyperbilirubinemia, variable increases in serum ALP, GGT, ALT, and AST

OTHER LABORATORY TESTS
• Bacterial culture—bile: aerobic and anaerobic bacteria common in symptomatic patients
• Coagulation profile—prolonged clotting time (especially PIVKA and PT); responsive to parenteral vitamin K administration; bleeding may develop with chronic OBTD (see Bile Duct Obstruction)

IMAGING
• Abdominal radiography—limited value in delineating gallbladder structure and content; choleliths often radiolucent
• Ultrasonography—may detect cholelith as small as 2 mm in diameter, thickening of the gallbladder wall, distention of the biliary tract, hepatic parenchymal lesions (change in echogenicity due to inflammation, lipid, or glycogen) and extrahepatic tissue involvement; may facilitate collection of specimens for culture, cytology, and histopathology; may detect evidence of OBTD within 72 hr;
Caution: sludged bile and a full gallbladder are common ultrasonographic findings in anorectic patients: do not mistake for cholelithiasis

DIAGNOSTIC PROCEDURES
Histopathologic evaluation for underlying liver disease to determine prognosis

TREATMENT
• Not indicated without clinical and clinicopathologic signs
• Supportive fluids—according to hydration status, electrolyte depletion, and acid–base balance
• Hyperlipidemia as a predisposing factor—prescribe a fat-restricted diet, diagnostic evaluation for cause
• Exploratory surgery, choledochotomy, cholecystotomy, and possibly cholecystectomy or biliary-enteric anastomosis—indicated in symptomatic cases according to circumstances
• Warn client that cholelithiasis is a chronic problem and that new stones may form even after surgical removal.

MEDICATIONS

DRUG(S)
• Antibiotics—based on biliary culture or directed against enteric organisms; initial treatment with Timentin, metronidazole, or clindamycin (anaerobic spectrum) combined with a fluoroquinolone, or ampicillin/gentamicin
• Ursodeoxycholic acid—10–15 mg/kg/day PO; induces choleresis, blunts hepatobiliary inflammation and fibrogenesis; possibly assists in dissolving non–cholesterol-rich stones; known to dissolve cholesterol-rich stones; must be used in the context of normal hydration; continued therapy usually for life
• Vitamin K—parenterally; 0.5–1.5 mg/kg to a maximum of three doses in 36 hr. Never administer IV because of risk of anaphylaxis.

CONTRAINDICATIONS/POSSIBLE INTERACTIONS
Ursodeoxycholic acid—contraindicated with OBTD until biliary decompression

FOLLOW-UP

PATIENT MONITORING
• Physical examination and pertinent diagnostic testing—every 2–4 weeks until clinical signs and clinicopathologic abnormalities resolve postoperatively
• Periodic ultrasonography—assess cholelith status, integrity of biliary tract, hepatic parenchymal change

POSSIBLE COMPLICATIONS
Sudden onset of fever, abdominal pain, and depression—may signify bile peritonitis and/or sepsis from a breakdown in bile containment

EXPECTED COURSE AND PROGNOSIS
• May be asymptomatic • Symptomatic disease—depends on existing infection, OBTD, cholecystitis, or bile peritonitis

MISCELLANEOUS

ASSOCIATED CONDITIONS
• Cholecystitis • Choledochitis
• Biliary tree obstruction

ABBREVIATIONS
ALP = alkaline phosphatase
ALT = alanine aminotransferase
AST = aspartate aminotransferase
GGT = γ-glutamyltransferase
OBTD = obstructed biliary tract disease
PIVKA = proteins invoked by vitamin K absence or antagonism
PT = prothrombin time

Suggested Reading
Center SA. Diseases of the gallbladder and biliary tree. In: Guilford WG, Center SA, Strombeck DR, et al., eds. Strombeck's small animal gastroenterology. Philadelphia: Saunders, 1996:860–888.
Author Sharon A. Center
Consulting Editor Sharon A. Center

BASICS

OVERVIEW
• An uncommon form of epidermoid cyst found within the middle ear cavity of dogs. The term is a misnomer because it is not a granuloma or neoplasm and it does not contain fat. The cystic structure is lined by stratified squamous keratinizing epithelium that rests on a fibrous stroma of inflammatory granulation tissue and slowly enlarges due to the shedding of keratin into the lumen, which also incites the inflammatory response. Can be either congenital or acquired as a complication of otitis media. The congenital form develops from embryonic cells within the middle ear cavity and has not been recognized in dogs. The acquired form develops out of stratified squamous epithelium from the tympanic membrane or external ear and may also involve metaplasia of the respiratory epithelium. The acquired form may be either primary, as a result of chronic auditory tube dysfunction from otitis media, or secondary to a perforated tympanum, caused iatrogenically or as a result of trauma.

SIGNALMENT
• The condition has not been described in cats. • There is no apparent breed, age, or sex predisposition, although few cases have been reported. • Dogs predisposed to otitis may be at increased risk, but this is unproven.
• Cholesteatoma has been described in dogs as young as 13 months and as old as 9.5 years.

SIGNS
• Dogs present with signs of chronic (often > 1 year) unilateral or bilateral aural disease, usually otitis externa with scratching/pawing at ears and head shaking.
• Discomfort during eating, yawning, or manipulation of the jaw may be present.
• Neurologic abnormalities, such as head tilt or ataxia, may occur but are relatively rare. Signs of decreased hearing or deafness may also rarely be present.
• Otoscopic examination often reveals a heavy accumulation of debris and stenosis in the ear canal. Detailed inspection of the tympanic membrane is often not possible due to either ear canal stenosis or obstruction by the mass.

CAUSES & RISK FACTORS
• Chronic otitis
• Congenital (not yet reported in the dog)

DIAGNOSIS

DIFFERENTIAL DIAGNOSIS
• Inflammatory polyp or cyst
• Chronic otitis media
• Ceruminous gland carcinoma or adenoma
• Squamous cell carcinoma

CBC/BIOCHEMISTRY/URINALYSIS
No specific abnormalities

OTHER LABORATORY TESTS
Aerobic and anaerobic cultures from the ear canal are indicated but may not yield growth. Animals have often been previously or currently treated with antibiotics and/or antifungals.

IMAGING
• Radiography shows stenosis of the ipsilateral ear canal and often calcification/ossification of the auricular and annular cartilages. Increased density of the middle ear and/or disruption of the wall of the tympanic bulla are also present. Radiographic evidence of involvement of the temporomandibular joint may also be seen.
• Computed tomography is considered to be superior to traditional radiography because it provides increased resolution and more accurate information about the status of the middle ear cavity and bone thickness. The extent of the soft tissue mass, decrease in aeration, sclerosis of the tympanic bulla, and involvement of the tympanic membrane and ear canal can be determined.

DIAGNOSTIC PROCEDURES
Fine-needle aspiration cytology and incisional biopsy are not likely to confirm the diagnosis because a superficial sample may not reveal all the layers of the lesion.

PATHOLOGIC FINDINGS
• Grossly, a cystic structure (0.5–1.5 cm) is found occupying part of the mesotympanum of the middle ear cavity.
• Histologic analysis of an excised specimen or a specimen obtained at necropsy reveals a squamous epithelial cystic structure with a core of keratin lamellae enclosed by the tympanic membrane. Granulation tissue is evident, and adhesions may be found between the granulation tissue and the tympanic membrane. Alterations in the respiratory epithelium may also be present.

TREATMENT

Surgical extirpation of the diseased tissues within the middle ear and external ear cavity is the treatment of choice. This is usually accomplished via total ear canal ablation with lateral bulla osteotomy or ventral bulla osteotomy, depending on the extent of the lesion. A successful caudal auricular surgical approach has also been described, with preservation of hearing and external appearance.

MEDICATIONS

DRUG(S)
Medical therapy is targeted to the accompanying infection. Antibiotic and antifungal treatment is ideally based on culture and sensitivity testing. Perioperative antibiotic treatment is indicated.

CONTRAINDICATIONS/POSSIBLE INTERACTIONS
Aminoglycoside antibiotic use in the ears of dogs should be approached with caution.

FOLLOW-UP

PATIENT MONITORING
Evaluate the surgical site until healing is adequate.

PREVENTION/AVOIDANCE
Early successful management of otitis externa may decrease the chance of otitis media and therefore cholesteatoma development; however, this is unproven.

POSSIBLE COMPLICATIONS
• Neurologic signs may occur and progress if the disease is left untreated.
• Surgical complications include partial hearing loss and possibly facial nerve damage.

EXPECTED COURSE AND PROGNOSIS
Cure is expected with complete surgical excision using the appropriate technique. Although cholesteatoma is an uncommon complication of otitis media, it is considered to confer a worse prognosis for management of this disease.

MISCELLANEOUS

ASSOCIATED CONDITIONS
N/A

PREGNANCY
Surgery can likely be delayed until after whelping.

SEE ALSO
Otitis Media

Suggested Reading
Davidson EB, Brodie HA, Breznock EM. Removal of a cholesteatoma in a dog, using a caudal auricular approach. J Am Vet Med Assoc 1997;211:1549–1553.
Little CJL, Lane JG, Gibbs LC, et al. Inflammatory middle ear disease of the dog: the clinical and pathological features of cholesteatoma, a complication of otitis media. Vet Rec 1991;128:319–322.
Author Anthony J. Mutsaers
Consulting Editor Wallace B. Morrison

CHONDROSARCOMA, BONE

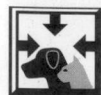 BASICS

OVERVIEW
- Malignant neoplasm arising from cartilage and characterized histologically by anaplastic cartilage cells
- Second most common primary bone tumor in dogs; represents 5%–10% of all primary bone tumors
- More common in the axial skeleton
- Most common primary rib tumor
- Must differentiate from chondroblastic osteosarcoma
- Histologic grade and tumor location helpful for predicting survival
- High-grade tumors similar to osteosarcoma in respect to metastatic potential

SIGNALMENT
- Most common in large (not giant) dog breeds
- Uncommon in cats
- Mean age—8.7 years

SIGNS

Historical Findings
- Lameness
- Pain in affected limb
- Visible swelling at tumor site
- Nasal discharge

Physical Examination Findings
- Long-bone tumors
- Monostotic swelling in metaphyseal site
- Pain on palpation of tumor site
- May see pathologic fracture
- Rib tumors
- Asymptomatic palpable mass in thoracic wall
- May see pleural effusion secondary to intrathoracic extension of tumor

CAUSES & RISK FACTORS
Multiple cartilaginous exostosis

 DIAGNOSIS

DIFFERENTIAL DIAGNOSIS
- Osteosarcoma, fibrosarcoma, and hemangiosarcoma
- Metastatic bone lesion from another primary site
- Osteomyelitis—fungal or bacterial

CBC/BIOCHEMISTRY/URINALYSIS
Usually normal

OTHER LABORATORY TESTS
N/A

IMAGING
- Radiographs of primary lesion (lytic and/or productive lesions)—impossible to differentiate from other types of primary bone tumors; lesions in long bones usually located in metaphyseal sites
- Thoracic radiography—detects metastasis
- CT scan—may help determine local extent of disease in patients with rib tumor
- Nuclear bone scan or radiographic scan of entire skeleton—useful for staging

DIAGNOSTIC PROCEDURES
- Biopsy and histopathologic examination of bone tumor—as described for osteosarcoma
- Small specimens of osteosarcoma may be misdiagnosed as chondrosarcoma.

 TREATMENT

- Amputation or limb salvage—remove primary long-bone tumor
- Chest wall resection—with rib tumor
- Hemipelvectomy—with tumor involving bones of the pelvis
- Radiotherapy—consider for palliation in patients with inoperable tumor

 MEDICATIONS

DRUG(S)
- Chemotherapy (dogs)—cisplatin; post-surgery for high-grade tumors, as recommended for osteosarcoma
- Doxorubicin-based protocols—may be useful

CONTRAINDICATIONS/POSSIBLE INTERACTIONS
- Cisplatin—contraindicated in cats; do not use with compromised renal function
- Doxorubicin—do not use with congestive heart failure

 FOLLOW-UP

- Thoracic radiography—monthly for 3 months and every 3rd month thereafter
- Low-grade tumor of long bones—prognosis excellent
- High-grade tumor of long bones—prognosis guarded to poor

 MISCELLANEOUS

Suggested Reading
Waters DJ, Cooley DM. Skeletal neoplasms. In: Morrison WB, ed. Cancer in dogs and cats: medical and surgical management. Jackson, Wyoming: Teton, New Media, 2002:611–626.
Author Terrance A. Hamilton
Consulting Editor Wallace B. Morrison

CHONDROSARCOMA, LARYNX AND TRACHEA

BASICS

OVERVIEW
• Malignant, cartilage-producing tumors with progressive local invasion of the surrounding tissues
• Uncommon; slowly progressive (weeks)

SIGNALMENT
• Dogs and cats
• Middle-aged to old animals (5–15 years)
• No breed predilection
• Males affected slightly more than females

SIGNS

Historical Findings
• Change in voice; loss of bark or purr; or harsh, noisy breath
• Exercise intolerance
• Severe respiratory distress; open-mouth breathing; cyanosis; and acute collapse
• Dysphagia

Physical Examination Findings
• Inspiratory stridor
• Laryngeal mass
• Aspiration pneumonia secondary to laryngeal dysfunction

CAUSES & RISK FACTORS
None known

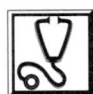

DIAGNOSIS

DIFFERENTIAL DIAGNOSIS
• Laryngeal paralysis
• Laryngeal spasm and collapse
• Laryngeal trauma and secondary inflammation
• Other laryngeal or tracheal malignancies—squamous cell carcinoma; oncocytoma (rhabdomyoma); mast cell tumor; lymphoma, fibrosarcoma, osteosarcoma, adenocarcinoma

CBC/BIOCHEMISTRY/URINALYSIS
Usually normal

OTHER LABORATORY TESTS
• Cytologic examination—tissue obtained by endoscopic bronchial brushing or fine-needle aspiration
• Biopsy—usually nondiagnostic

IMAGING
• Survey radiography—often not helpful
• Thoracic radiography—detect pulmonary metastasis

DIAGNOSTIC PROCEDURES
• Tissue biopsy—definitive diagnosis
• Careful cervical examination—regional lymphadenopathy

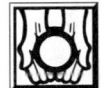

TREATMENT
• Inpatient
• Benign laryngeal cancers can be removed surgically with preservation of function.
• Tracheal tumors should be treated with resection—full-thickness removal with end-to-end anastomosis can be performed on up to 3–4 tracheal rings
• Complete laryngectomy with a permanent tracheostomy—rarely performed in animals; does not offer any significant long-term palliation of clinical signs (< 15 weeks)
• Radiotherapy (with or without surgery)—rarely reported as effective

MEDICATIONS

DRUG(S)
Chemotherapeutic agent for local or systemic control—effective agent not reported

CONTRAINDICATIONS/POSSIBLE INTERACTIONS
N/A

FOLLOW-UP

PATIENT MONITORING
Survey radiography of the laryngeal region or laryngoscopy—may perform when clinical signs recur

EXPECTED COURSE AND PROGNOSIS
• Guarded prognosis because of advanced infiltrative disease at the time of diagnosis
• Local recurrence—common; with extension to regional lymph nodes
• Aspiration pneumonia—may occur secondary to laryngeal dysfunction or via tracheostomy site

MISCELLANEOUS

Suggested Reading
Flanders JA, Castleman W, Carberry CA, et al. Laryngeal chondrosarcoma in a dog. J Am Vet Med Assoc 1987;190:68–70.
Hahn KA, Anderson TA. Tumors of the respiratory tract. In: Bonagura JD, ed. Kirk's current veterinary therapy XIII. Philadelphia: Saunders, 1998:500–505.
Authors Kevin A. Hahn and Avenelle Turner
Consulting Editor Wallace B. Morrison

CHONDROSARCOMA, NASAL AND PARANASAL SINUS

BASICS

OVERVIEW
• Slow, progressive invasion of neoplastic mesenchymal cells within the nasal and paranasal sinuses
• Usually begins as unilateral but progresses slowly to bilateral by the time the patient is examined
• Prevalence of nonepithelial nasal neoplasia in dogs and cats—0.3%–4.7% of all tumors

SIGNALMENT
• More common in dogs than cats (rare)
• Median age (dogs and cats)—7 years (range, 2–11 years)
• Tends to develop at a younger age than other nasal tumors (64% occur in dogs < 8 years old)
• May be more common in male than female dogs

SIGNS

Historical Findings
• Intermittent and progressive history of unilateral to bilateral epistaxis and/or mucopurulent discharge (median duration, 3 months)
• Epiphora
• Sneezing
• Halitosis
• Anorexia
• Seizures secondary to cranial invasion

Physical Examination Findings
• Nasal discharge
• Facial deformity or exophthalmia
• Pain on nasal or paranasal sinus examination
• Obstruction of nasal air flow (unilateral or bilateral)

CAUSES & RISK FACTORS
Unknown

DIAGNOSIS

DIFFERENTIAL DIAGNOSIS
• Bacterial sinusitis—uncommon
• Viral infection (cats)
• Aspergillosis, penicillium, rhinosporidiosis, sporotrichosis (dogs)
• Parasites
• Hypertension
• Allergic rhinitis
• Cryptococcosis (cats)
• Foreign body
• Trauma
• Tooth root abscess
• Oronasal fistula
• Coagulopathy

CBC/BIOCHEMISTRY/URINALYSIS
Usually normal

OTHER LABORATORY TESTS
Cytologic and bacterial examination—rarely helpful
• Coagulation profile

IMAGING
• Survey radiography (skull)—shows typical pattern of asymmetrical destruction of caudal turbinates with superimposition of a soft tissue mass; may see fluid density in the frontal sinuses secondary to outflow obstruction
• Thoracic radiography—detect lung metastasis (uncommon)
• CT or MRI—best for observing integrity of cribriform plate or orbital invasion

DIAGNOSTIC PROCEDURES
• Rhinoscopy (visual observation poor)—chondrosarcoma may be firm, hard mass or soft, friable, fleshy mass; avoid progressing caudally into the cribriform plate
• Tissue biopsy—necessary for definitive diagnosis
• Bacterial culture—often positive
• Lymph node cytology—detect metastatic disease (uncommon)

TREATMENT
• Surgery alone—ineffective
• Turbinectomy—may be done before external (teletherapy) or internal (brachytherapy) irradiation
• Inpatient radiotherapy (with or without surgery)—36–60 Gy; best clinical control in dogs

MEDICATIONS

DRUG(S)
Chemotherapy—good option in some animals; doxorubicin (30 mg/m^2 IV once every 2 weeks for 5 treatments in dogs

weighing > 10 kg; 1 mg/kg for dogs < 10 kg and for cats); median survival (dogs) 18 weeks; may provide marked palliation of clinical signs

CONTRAINDICATIONS/POSSIBLE INTERACTIONS
Chemotherapy can be toxic; seek advice before initiating treatment if you are unfamiliar with cytotoxic drugs.

FOLLOW-UP

PATIENT MONITORING
Survey radiography (skull) and/or CT or MRI—may be performed when clinical signs recur

EXPECTED COURSE AND PROGNOSIS
• Median survival if left untreated—3 months
• Median disease-free interval after radiotherapy—dogs, 8–23 months; cats, 1–36 months
• Survival with radiotherapy (dogs and cats)—1-year survival, 20%–60%; 2-year survival, 20%–40%; some reports of shorter survival times with nonepithelial nasal tumors (8–16 months); also reports of longer survival times with chondrosarcoma vs. epithelial nasal tumors
• Brain involvement—poor prognostic sign

MISCELLANEOUS

Suggested Reading

Frazier DL, Hahn KA. Cancer chemotherapeutics. In: Hahn KA, Richardson RC, eds. Cancer chemotherapy—a veterinary handbook. Baltimore: Williams & Wilkins, 1995:77–150.

Patnaik AK. Canine sinonasal neoplasms: soft tissue tumors. J Am Anim Hosp Assoc 1989;25:491–497.

Theon AP. Megavoltage irradiation of neoplasms of the nasal and paranasal cavities in 77 dogs. J Am Vet Med Assoc 1993; 202:1469–1475.

Authors Kevin A. Hahn and Janet K. Carreras
Consulting Editor Wallace B. Morrison

BASICS

OVERVIEW
• Malignant, cartilage-producing tumor with progressive local invasion of the surrounding tissues
• Slowly progressive (months); adherent to bone; generally nonencapsulated with a smooth to slightly nodular surface (commonly mistaken as benign)
• Slow to metastasize; lung more common site than regional lymph nodes
• Death usually secondary to local recurrence and cachexia
• Uncommon in dogs and cats

SIGNALMENT
• Dogs and cats
• Dogs—usually middle-aged; more common in large breeds

SIGNS
Historical Findings
• Excessive salivation
• Halitosis
• Dysphagia
• Bloody oral discharge
• Weight loss

Physical Examination Findings
• Oral mass, most commonly located on the maxilla
• Loose teeth
• Facial deformity
• Occasional cervical lymphadenomegaly (reactive hyperplasia)

CAUSES & RISK FACTORS
None identified

DIAGNOSIS

DIFFERENTIAL DIAGNOSIS
Oral Malignancies
• Multilobular osteochondrosarcoma—appears radiographically as an osteoma arising from flat bones of the skull; highly metastatic; complete surgical excision uncommon
• Osteoma
• Multiple cartilaginous exostoses (osteochondromatosis)—condition of growing dogs; cartilage-capped bony growths from the surface of flat bones; growth ceases upon skeletal maturity; sessile or pedunculated painful bony mass; excise if growth continues beyond maturity; may transform to osteosarcoma or chondrosarcoma
• Undifferentiated oral malignancy

Oral Masses
• Epulis
• Abscess
• Benign polyp

CBC/BIOCHEMISTRY/URINALYSIS
Usually normal

OTHER LABORATORY TESTS
Cytologic evaluation—impression smear obtained by incisional biopsy (wedge); may yield diagnosis

IMAGING
• Skull radiography—evaluate for bone involvement deep to the mass.
• Thoracic radiographs—evaluate lungs for metastasis.

DIAGNOSTIC PROCEDURES
• A large, deep-tissue biopsy (down to bone)—required to sufficiently differentiate from other oral malignancies
• Carefully palpate regional lymph nodes (mandibular and retropharyngeal).

TREATMENT

SURGERY
• Radical excision—required (e.g., hemimaxillectomy); well-tolerated; margins of at least 2 cm necessary; survival rates after surgery limited, but the metastatic behavior of most chondrosarcomas is low (< 15%); survival improves when excisional margins are free of neoplastic cells.
• Cryosurgery—not indicated owing to invasive bony involvement

RADIATION
• Results unreported; most chondrosarcomas poorly responsive

• Soft foods—may recommend to prevent ulceration of tumor or after radical oral excision
• Pain management—radiation therapy may be considered. Oral pain medication

MEDICATIONS

DRUG(S)
• Chemotherapy—efficacy unreported; many mesenchymal-origin tumors poorly responsive
• Cisplatin—intralesionally administered; local control (palliation) reported

CONTRAINDICATIONS/POSSIBLE INTERACTIONS
Chemotherapy may be toxic; seek advice before initiating treatment if you are unfamiliar with cytotoxic drugs.

FOLLOW-UP
• Lymph node metastasis on examination common (dogs)
• Euthanasia—most dogs within 30 days of diagnosis; tumor growth progressive and uncontrolled, resulting in dysphagia and cachexia
• Survival rates after surgery limited

MISCELLANEOUS

Suggested Reading
Frazier DL, Hahn KA. Cancer chemotherapeutics. In: Hahn KA, Richardson RC, eds. Cancer chemotherapy—a veterinary handbook. Baltimore: Williams & Wilkins, 1995:77–150.
Oakes MG, Lewis DD, Hedlund CS, Hosgood G. Canine oral neoplasia. Compend Contin Educ Small Anim Pract 1993;15:15–31.
Authors Kevin A. Hahn and Kimberly P. Freeman
Consulting Editor Wallace B. Morrison

CHORIORETINITIS

 BASICS

DEFINITION
• Inflammation of the choroid and retina
• Choroid is also called posterior uvea.
• Diffuse inflammation may result in frank retinal detachment (see Retinal Detachment).

PATHOPHYSIOLOGY
• Caused by infectious agents, neoplastic or immune cells, or immune complexes (immune-mediated diseases); hematogenous pathogenic factors inducing choroidal inflammation, most common
• Choroid and retina—closely apposed; physiologically interdependent; inflammation of one usually results in inflammation of the other.
• May also occur as a retinochoroiditis—retinal inflammation preceding and inducing choroidal inflammation

SYSTEMS AFFECTED
• Ophthalmic
• Nervous
• Other systems if disease is systemic

GENETICS
N/A

INCIDENCE/PREVALENCE
• Fairly common
• Exact incidence unknown.

GEOGRAPHIC DISTRIBUTION
Depends on the prevalence of infectious cause (e.g., systemic mycoses, rickettsial disease)

SIGNALMENT
Species
Dogs and cats

Breed Predilections
• Systemic mycoses—more common in large hunting breed dogs
• Uveodermatologic syndrome—akitas, chows, and Siberian huskies are predisposed

Mean Age and Range
Depend on underlying cause

Predominant Sex
Uveodermatologic syndrome—more common in young male dogs

SIGNS
• Not usually painful, except when anterior uvea is affected
• Vitreous abnormalities—may note exudates, hemorrhage, or syneresis (liquefaction)
• Interruption or alteration of the course of retinal blood vessels—owing to retinal elevation
• Ophthalmomyiasis (cats)—curvilinear tracts from migrating larvae
• Others—related to underlying systemic disease

Lesions
• Active—indistinct margins; tapetal hyporeflectivity; white-gray color; alter course of retinal blood vessels
• Few, small—may note no apparent visual deficits
• Extensive, involving larger areas of the retina—blindness or reduced vision
• Inactive (scars)—discrete margins; hyper-reflective in the tapetum sometimes with hyperpigmented central areas; depigmented in the nontapetum and may have some surrounding or central hyperpigmentation

CAUSES
Dogs
• Viral—canine distemper; herpesvirus (rare, usually neonates); rabies
• Bacterial or rickettsial—septicemia or bacteremia; leptospirosis; brucellosis; pyometra (toxic uveitis); *Borrelia;* ehrlichiosis; Rocky Mountain spotted fever
• Fungal—aspergillosis; blastomycosis; coccidioidomycosis; histoplasmosis; cryptococcosis
• Algal—geotrichosis; protothecosis
• Parasitic—ocular larval migrans (*Strongyles, Ascarids, Baylisascaris*); toxoplasmosis; leishmaniasis; *Neospora;* ophthalmomyiasis interna (Diptera larval migrans more common in cats)
• Autoimmune—target of Vogt-Koyanagi-Harada-like (uveodermatologic) syndrome is melanin pigment granule (abundant in uveal tissue), leading to severe anterior and posterior inflammation (affected dogs may also exhibit depigmentation of the skin, especially at mucocutaneous junctions); target of SLE is nuclear antigen

Cats
• Viral—FeLV; FIV; FIP
• Bacterial—septicemia or bacteremia
• Fungal—cryptococcosis; histoplasmosis; blastomycosis; others
• Parasitic—toxoplasmosis; ophthalmomyiasis interna (Diptera); ocular larval migrans
• Protozoal—toxoplasmosis
• Autoimmune—periarteritis nodosa; SLE

Dogs and Cats
• Exogenous infection—trauma (perforating wound); intraocular surgery
• Endogenous or hematogenous infection—ocular manifestation of systemic disease; may extend from the CNS via the optic nerve
• Septicemia or bacteremia—diskospondylitis; endocarditis; pyometra; may result from primary infection or associated immune complex disease
• Neoplasia—primary or metastatic; with granulomatous meningoencephalitis, peripapillary chorioretinal inflammation (around an inflamed optic nerve); lymphosarcoma most common; with early multiple myeloma, may

note multifocal chorioretinitis before frank bullous retinal detachment can be ruled out
• Immune mediated—may cause vasculitis or inflammation, resulting in exudative retinal detachment or chorioretinitis; exact cause usually undetermined; with thrombocytopenia, may see small multifocal or large retinal and/or vitreal hemorrhages with associated inflammation
• Idiopathic—common
• Toxicity—ethylene glycol; idiosyncratic drug reactions (e.g., trimethoprim-sulfa)
• Trauma

RISK FACTORS
FeLV or FIV infection—may predispose cat to ocular toxoplasmosis and chorioretinitis/uveitis

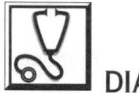 DIAGNOSIS

DIFFERENTIAL DIAGNOSIS
• Ophthalmic examination—usually sufficient for diagnosis; may note a slow pupillary light reflex if large areas of the retina are affected
• Blindness or impaired vision—optic neuritis; CNS disease; diffuse retinal inflammation
• See Causes
• Retinal dysplasia—similar to inactive disease; bilateral, symmetrical folds or geographic clumps of pigment or altered fundus reflectivity; no associated signs of inflammation in the eye; Labrador retrievers and springer spaniels predisposed but occurs in many breeds

CBC/BIOCHEMISTRY/URINALYSIS
• Normal—if problem confined to the eye
• Abnormal—depend on underlying systemic disease

OTHER LABORATORY TESTS
• Depend on suspected systemic problem
• Protein electrophoresis
• Documentation of Bence-Jones protein in urine
• Skin biopsy—SLE; uveodermatologic syndrome
• Coagulation profile
• Bacterial culture of ocular or body fluids
• Serologic testing—infectious disease (see Causes)

IMAGING
• Thoracic radiography—lymphadenopathy; metastatic disease; infiltrates consistent with infectious agents
• Spinal radiography—bony changes consistent with diskospondylitis or multiple myeloma
• Ocular ultrasound—retinal detachments; intraocular masses; especially helpful if the ocular media are not clear

DIAGNOSTIC PROCEDURES
• Indirect ophthalmoscopy—screens a large area of the retina
• Direct ophthalmoscopy—facilitates examination of suspicious areas
• CSF tap—indicated for signs of CNS disease or optic neuritis
• Vitreocentesis or subretinal fluid aspirate—may perform if other diagnostic tests fail to yield a causal agent or for suspected infectious agent or neoplasia; vitreocentesis may aggravate inflammation or induce hemorrhage, lessening the chance for retinal reattachment and restoration of vision.

PATHOLOGIC FINDINGS
• Masses or retinal or choroidal exudates
• Fungal organisms—in exudates and inflammatory cells
• Perivascular inflammation—vasculitis; FIP
• Inactive lesions—retinal and choroidal atrophy (thinning); may note RPE hyperpigmentation and tapetal destruction

 TREATMENT

APPROPRIATE HEALTH CARE
• Depends on physical condition of patient
• Usually outpatient

NURSING CARE
Fluid or other therapy for systemic disease

ACTIVITY
N/A

DIET
N/A

CLIENT EDUCATION
• Inform client that chorioretinitis may be a sign of systemic disease, so diagnostic testing is important.
• Warn client that immune-mediated disease requires lifelong therapy for controlling inflammation.
• Inform client that dogs with uveodermatologic syndrome may also have anterior uveitis and secondary glaucoma, which require treatment. Dermatitis may also require management.

SURGICAL CONSIDERATIONS
N/A

 MEDICATIONS

DRUG(S) OF CHOICE
• Identify and treat any underlying systemic disease (e.g., itraconazole for systemic mycosis).

• Topical medications—not effective in dogs with intact lenses
• Systemic therapy—required
• Feline toxoplasmosis—clindamycin 12.5 mg/kg PO BID for 14–21 days
• Systemic prednisone at antiinflammatory doses—0.5 mg/kg PO, then taper; when systemic mycosis has been ruled out or is being treated with appropriate systemic antifungal therapy; avoid use, unless large areas of the retina are affected and vision is severely threatened
• Prednisone at immunosuppressive doses—2 mg/kg divided q12 for 3–10 days (ideal), then taper very slowly over months; for immune-mediated disease; may facilitate retinal reattachment
• Topical corticosteroids (1% prednisolone acetate or 0.1% dexamethasone given TID to QID) and parasympatholytics (1% atropine given at a frequency that dilates the pupil and reduces pain)—for panuveitis (concurrent anterior uveitis)
• Anti-glaucoma therapy—as appropriate for secondary glaucoma

CONTRAINDICATIONS
Systemically administered corticosteroids—do not use unless systemic mycosis is ruled out or is being definitively treated.

PRECAUTIONS
With prednisone treatment consider concurrent oral antacids such as ranitidine

POSSIBLE INTERACTIONS
N/A

ALTERNATIVE DRUG(S)
• Neoplastic conditions (lymphosarcoma, GME, or multiple myeloma)—chemotherapeutic agents
• Uveodermatologic syndrome—may require azathioprine (see Retinal Detachment) and steroids to control inflammation

 FOLLOW-UP

PATIENT MONITORING
• As appropriate for underlying cause and type of medical treatment
• CBC platlet count and liver enzymes—if giving azathioprine
• IOP—for anterior uveitis

PREVENTION/AVOIDANCE
N/A

POSSIBLE COMPLICATIONS
• Permanent blindness
• Cataracts

• Glaucoma
• Chronic ocular pain
• Death—secondary to systemic disease

EXPECTED COURSE AND PROGNOSIS
• Prognosis for vision—guarded to good, depending on amount of retina affected; visual deficits or blindness if large areas of the retina were destroyed; focal and multifocal disease do not markedly impair vision but do leave scars
• Prognosis for life—guarded to good, depending on underlying cause

 MISCELLANEOUS

ASSOCIATED CONDITIONS
Several systemic diseases

AGE-RELATED FACTORS
N/A

ZOONOTIC POTENTIAL
Toxoplasmosis—may be transmitted to humans if patient is shedding oocysts in feces

PREGNANCY
N/A

SYNONYMS
Retinochoroiditis

SEE ALSO
• Retinal Degeneration
• Retinal Detachment

ABBREVIATIONS
• CSF = cerebrospinal fluid
• FeLV = feline leukemia virus
• FIP = feline infectious peritonitis
• FIV = feline immunodeficiency virus
• GME = granulomatous meningoencephalitis
• IOP = intraocular pressure
• RPE = retinal pigment epithelium
• SLE = systemic lupus erythematosus

Suggested Reading
Narfström K, Eketsen B. Diseases of the canine ocular fundus. In: Veterinary ophthalmology 3rd ed. Philadelphia: Lippincott Williams and Wilkins, 1999:869–993.
Millichamp NJ, Dziezyc J. Small animal ophthalmology. Vet Clin North Am Small Anim Pract 1990;20:564–877.
Stiles, J. Infectious diseases and the eye. Vet Clin North Am Small Anim Pract 2000;30:971–1167.
Author Patricia J. Smith
Consulting Editor Paul E. Miller

CHYLOTHORAX

BASICS

DEFINITION
• A collection of chyle in the pleural space
• Chyle—lymphatic fluid arising from the intestine and, therefore, containing a high quantity of fat
• Thoracic lymphangiectasia—the tortuous, dilated lymphatics found in many animals with chylothorax
• Fibrosing pleuritis—condition in which pleural thickening leads to constriction of the lung lobes; when severe, results in marked restriction of ventilation; may be caused by any chronic pleural exudate but is most commonly associated with chylothorax and pyothorax

PATHOPHYSIOLOGY
• Abnormal flows or pressures within the thoracic duct are thought to lead to exudation of chyle from intact, but dilated, thoracic lymphatic vessels in most animals.
• Lymphangiectasia—may result from increased lymphatic flows, decreased lymphatic drainage into the venous system because of high venous pressures, or both factors acting simultaneously
• May be caused by any disease or process that increases systemic venous pressures, including right heart failure, mediastinal neoplasia, and cranial vena cava thrombi or granulomas
• Thoracic duct rupture, as from trauma—uncommon cause in dogs and cats

SYSTEMS AFFECTED
Respiratory—chylous effusion or fibrosing pleuritis interferes with the ability of the lungs to expand.

GENETICS
Unknown

INCIDENCE/PREVALENCE
Unknown

GEOGRAPHIC DISTRIBUTION
Worldwide

SIGNALMENT

Species
Dogs and cats

Breed Predilections
• Dogs—Afghan hounds and Shiba Inus
• Cats—Asian breeds (e.g., Siamese and Himalayan) appear to have a higher prevalence than other breeds.

Mean Age And Range
• Any age may be affected
• Cats—old animals may be more likely to develop condition than young cats; may indicate an association with neoplasia
• Afghan hounds—develop when middle-aged
• Shiba Inus—develop when young (< 1–2 years of age)

Predominant Sex
None identified

SIGNS

General Comments
• Vary, depending on the underlying cause, rapidity of fluid accumulation, and volume of fluid
• Usually not exhibited until there is marked impairment of ventilation
• Many patients appear to have condition for prolonged periods before diagnosis; they probably reabsorb chyle at a rate that prevents obvious respiratory impairment.

Historical Findings
• Usually examined because of evaluation of dyspnea or coughing
• Coughing—may have been present for months before examination
• Many patients will have been treated with antibiotics for presumed respiratory infection before diagnosis.
• Tachypnea
• Depression
• Anorexia and weight loss
• Exercise intolerance

Physical Examination Findings
• Muffled heart and lung sounds
• Increased bronchovesicular sounds, particularly in the dorsal lung fields
• Cyanosis
• Pale mucous membranes
• Arrhythmia
• Murmur
• Jugular pulses in association with right-sided heart failure
• Decrease in the compressibility of the anterior chest—common in cats with a cranial mediastinal mass and pleural effusion

CAUSES
• Anterior mediastinal masses—mediastinal lymphosarcoma; thymoma
• Heart disease—cardiomyopathy; pericardial effusion; heartworm infection; tetralogy of Fallot; tricuspid dysplasia; cor triatriatum dexter
• Fungal granuloma
• Venous thrombus
• Congenital abnormality of the thoracic duct
• Idiopathic—most patients

RISK FACTORS
Unknown

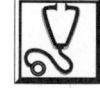

DIAGNOSIS

DIFFERENTIAL DIAGNOSIS
• Consider any cause of respiratory distress or coughing.
• Once pleural effusion has been identified—diseases causing exudative pleural effusion (e.g., pyothorax, FIP, and neoplastic effusion)

• Pseudochylous effusion—misused in the veterinary literature to describe an effusion that looks like chyle but in which a ruptured thoracic duct is not found; reserve term for effusions in which fluid cholesterol is higher than serum cholesterol and fluid triglyceride is lower than serum triglyceride

CBC/BIOCHEMISTRY/URINALYSIS
• Often normal
• Lymphopenia and hypoalbuminemia—may be found

OTHER LABORATORY TESTS

Fluid Analysis
• Characteristics—usually milky white and opaque, may range from yellow to pink, depending on diet and the occurrence of concurrent hemorrhage
• Protein content—inaccurate owing to interference of the refractive index by the high lipid content of the fluid
• Total nucleated cell count—usually < 10,000 cells/μL

Cytology
• Primarily small lymphocytes or neutrophils
• Nondegenerative neutrophils—may predominate with prolonged loss of lymphocytes, with chronicity, or when multiple therapeutic thoracocenteses have induced inflammation
• Abnormal lymphocytes—may indicate underlying neoplasia

OTHER LABORATORY TESTS
• Compare fluid and serum triglyceride concentrations—true chyle if higher in the fluid
• Sudan III stain—lipid droplets
• Ether clearance test—not quantitative

IMAGING

Thoracic Radiography
• Dyspnea—dorsoventral and standing lateral views
• No dyspnea—ventrodorsal and lateral recumbent views
• Pleural effusion—repeat studies after removal of most of the pleural fluid; if collapsed lung lobes do not appear to re-expand after pleural fluid is removed; suspect underlying pulmonary parenchymal or pleural disease (e.g., fibrosing pleuritis); if dyspnea persists with only minimal fluid, consider fibrosing pleuritis

Ultrasonography
• Perform before removing fluid—fluid acts as an acoustic window, enhancing visualization of thoracic structures.
• Detect abnormal cardiac structure and function, pericardial disease, and mediastinal masses

PATHOLOGIC FINDINGS
• Lymphatics (including the thoracic duct)—difficult to identify at necropsy

- Fibrosing pleuritis—lungs appear shrunken; pleura (visceral and parietal) are diffusely thickened.
- Fibrosing pleuritis—characterized histologically by diffuse, moderate to marked thickening of the pleura by fibrous connective tissue with moderate infiltrates of lymphocytes, macrophages, and plasma cells

TREATMENT

APPROPRIATE HEALTH CARE
- Dyspneic patients with suspected pleural effusion—immediate thoracentesis; removal of even small amounts of pleural effusion may markedly improve ventilation.
- Identify and treat the underlying cause, if possible.
- Medical management—usually outpatient with intermittent thoracentesis as necessary to prevent dyspnea
- Chest tubes—place only in patients with suspected chylothorax secondary to trauma (very rare), with rapid fluid accumulation, or after surgery
- Unsuccessful medical management (try 2–3 months)—consider surgery (see Surgical Considerations)

NURSING CARE
- Patients may become debilitated if thoracentesis is performed frequently; attention to diet (see below) is important.
- Chest taps—perform under aseptic conditions to reduce the risk of iatrogenic infection; antibiotic prophylaxis generally unnecessary if proper technique is used

ACTIVITY
Patients will usually restrict their own exercise as the pleural fluid volume increases or if they develop fibrosing pleuritis.

DIET
- Low-fat—may decrease the amount of fat in the effusion, which may improve the patient's ability to resorb fluid from the thoracic cavity; not a cure; may help in management by facilitating reabsorption
- Medium-chain triglycerides—once thought to be absorbed directly into the portal system, bypassing the thoracic duct; actually transported via the thoracic duct of dogs; thus less useful than previously believed; no longer recommended by the author

CLIENT EDUCATION
- Inform client that no treatment will stop the effusion in all patients with the idiopathic form of the disease.
- Inform client that the condition may spontaneously resolve in some patients after several weeks or months

SURGICAL CONSIDERATIONS
Thoracic Duct Ligation and Pericardectomy
- Recommended initially in patients who do not respond to medical management
- The duct usually has multiple branches in the caudal thorax where ligation is performed; failure to occlude all branches results in continued pleural effusion.
- Always perform in conjunction with catheterization of a mesenteric lymphatic for lymphangiography or injection of dye; methylene blue injected in the mesenteric catheter greatly facilitates visualization and complete occlusion of all branches.
- Thickening of the pericardium may prevent formation of lymphaticovenous communications—perform pericardectomy simultaneously with thoracic duct ligation.

Other
- Thoracic duct ligation not successful—may consider pleuroperitoneal or pleurovenous shunts
- Extensive fibrosing pleuritis—poor surgical candidate; very grave prognosis

MEDICATIONS

DRUG(S) OF CHOICE
Rutin—50–100 mg/kg PO q8h; preliminary findings by the author suggest that complete resolution of effusion was achieved 2 months after initiation in at least 25% of patients; further study is required to determine whether resolution occurred spontaneously or in response to drug therapy.

CONTRAINDICATIONS
Severe fibrosing pleuritis—poor prognosis; medical or surgical treatment unlikely to offer benefit

PRECAUTIONS
N/A

POSSIBLE INTERACTIONS
N/A

ALTERNATIVE DRUG(S)
N/A

FOLLOW-UP

PATIENT MONITORING
- Monitor closely for dyspnea; perform thoracentesis as needed.
- Resolution (spontaneously or postsurgery)—periodically re-evaluate for several years to detect recurrence

PREVENTION/AVOIDANCE
N/A

POSSIBLE COMPLICATIONS
- Fibrosing pleuritis—most common serious complication of chronic disease
- Immunosuppression—caused by lymphocyte depletion; may develop in patients undergoing repeated and frequent thoracentesis
- Hyponatremia and hyperkalemia—documented in affected dogs undergoing multiple thoracentesis

EXPECTED COURSE AND PROGNOSIS
- May resolve spontaneously or after surgery
- Untreated or chronic disease—may result in severe fibrosing pleuritis and persistent dyspnea
- Euthanasia—frequently performed in patients that do not respond to surgery or medical management

MISCELLANEOUS

ASSOCIATED CONDITIONS
Diffuse lymphatic abnormalities (e.g., intestinal lymphangiectasia, hepatic lymphangiectasia, pulmonary lymphangiectasia, and chylous ascites)—may be noted; may worsen the prognosis

AGE-RELATED FACTORS
Young patients may have a better prognosis than old animals because of the association of neoplasia with advanced age.

ZOONOTIC POTENTIAL
N/A

PREGNANCY
N/A

ABBREVIATION
FIP = feline infectious peritonitis

Suggested Reading

Fossum TW. Feline chylothorax, what treatments work? J Feline Med Surg 2001; 3:73–79.

Fossum TW, Birchard SJ, Jacobs RM. Chylothorax in thirty-four dogs. J Am Vet Med Assoc 1986;188:1315–1318.

Fossum TW, Evering WN, Miller MW, et al. Severe bilateral fibrosing pleuritis associated with chronic chylothorax in dogs and cats. J Am Vet Med Assoc 1992;201:317–324.

Fossum TW, Miller MW, Rogers KS, et al. Chylothorax associated with right-sided heart failure in 5 cats. J Am Vet Med Assoc 1994;204:84–89.

Kerpsack SJ, McLoughlin MA, Birchard SJ, et al. Evaluation of mesenteric lymphangiography and thoracic duct ligation in cats with chylothorax: 19 cases (1987–1992). J Am Vet Med Assoc 1994;205:711–715.

Author Theresa W. Fossum
Consulting Editor Lynelle R. Johnson

CIRRHOSIS AND FIBROSIS OF THE LIVER

BASICS

DEFINITION
• Hepatic fibrosis—replacement of normal hepatic parenchyma by ECM • Cirrhosis—diffuse hepatic fibrosis; regenerative nodules; irreparably altered hepatic architecture

PATHOPHYSIOLOGY
• Fibrosis—develops subsequent to chronic injury, chronic inflammation, and/or oxidant damage causing soluble cytokine release that stimulates excess ECM deposition; may be idiopathic in young dogs • Cirrhosis—consequence of chronic fibrogenesis combined with attempted hepatic regeneration forming regenerative nodules; loss of functional hepatic mass and collagen deposition in hepatic sinusoids • Cirrhosis/ fibrosis—leads to generalized hepatic dysfunction and portal hypertension • Portal hypertension—leads to (1) APSS and HE, (2) splanchnic pooling of blood, decreased effective blood volume, renal sodium and water retention, and (3) portal hypertensive gastroenteropathy predisposing to enteric ulceration • Generalized hepatic dysfunction—coagulopathy; inability to maintain euglycemia; hypoalbuminemia; decreased hepatic macrophage function predisposing to infection • Chronic liver conditions usually lead to cirrhosis. Rarely, single episode of massive hepatic necrosis causes postnecrotic cirrhosis.

SYSTEMS AFFECTED
• GI—portal hypertension leads to ascites and propensity for enteric ulceration; rare fat malabsorption • Neurologic—HE • Hemic—RBC microcytosis with APSS; bleeding tendencies: failure to synthesize or activate coagulation factors or insufficient vitamin K; DIC; mild thrombocytopenia • Renal/urologic—ammonium biurate urolithiasis; isosthenuria; polyuria/polydipsia; hepatorenal syndrome (rare) • Endocrine/metabolic—hypoglycemia with end stage (provoked on fasting) • Respiratory—tachypnea due to tense ascites; pulmonary edema (rare) • Skin—superficial necrolytic dermatitis

GENETICS
• Familial predisposition for chronic active hepatitis—Doberman pinschers, cocker spaniels, Labrador retrievers • Copper storage hepatopathy—Bedlington terriers • Juvenile idiopathic hepatic fibrosis—German shepherds, standard poodles • Uncertain disorders—West Highland white terriers, Skye blue terriers, and dalmatians

INCIDENCE/PREVALENCE
High in dogs with chronic liver disease

SIGNALMENT
Species Dogs and cats (biliary cirrhosis)

Breed Predilection
• Any breed • Some breeds predisposed

Mean Age and Range
• Cirrhosis (dogs)—any age; common in middle to old age; copper storage hepatopathy (Bedlington terriers) and idiopathic hepatic fibrosis—young adults • Cirrhosis, biliary (cats) with chronic cholangiohepatitis—> 7 years old

Predominant Sex
• Cocker spaniels—2–8 times more common in males • Doberman pinschers and Labrador retrievers—more common in females

SIGNS

General Comments
• Initially—vague and nonspecific • Later—relate to complications of portal hypertension (e.g., HE, ascites, gastroduodenal ulcerations), or to loss of hepatic function

Historical Findings
• Chronic history of waxing and waning lethargy, anorexia, and loss of body condition • Vomiting • Diarrhea or constipation • Melena • Polydipsia and polyuria • Late onset—ascites, jaundice, bleeding tendencies, hepatic encephalopathy • Cats—ascites uncommon until very advanced disease; ptyalism with HE

Physical Examination Findings
• Lethargy • Poor body condition • Ascites • Jaundice • HE • Obstructive uropathy due to ammonium urate calculi • Anasarca—initially rare; may develop with overzealous fluid therapy • Liver size—often normal to hepatomegalic in cats; microhepatica in dogs • Rare bleeding tendencies • Rare cutaneous lesions

CAUSES
• Chronic inflammatory or idiopathic immune-mediated hepatitis • Chronic inflammatory bowel disease • Drug- or toxin-induced liver injury—copper (familial); anticonvulsants; azole antifungals; oxibendazole; trimethoprim-sulfamethoxazole; NSAIDs • Infections—leptospirosis (rare), canine adenovirus I (rare); acidophil hepatitis (rare, suspected infectious cause) • Chronic cholangiohepatitis (cats) • Chronic EHBDO (> 6 weeks) • Single episode of massive hepatic necrosis—postnecrotic cirrhosis (rare)

RISK FACTORS
• Breed associations • Chronic hepatobiliary inflammation • Hepatic copper or iron accumulation • EHBDO

DIAGNOSIS

DIFFERENTIAL DIAGNOSIS
• Chronic hepatitis—common in dogs • Cholangiohepatitis—common in cats • Noncirrhotic portal hypertension • Chronic EHBDO • Chronic pancreatitis • Hepatic neoplasia • Metastatic neoplasia or carcinomatosis • Congenital portosystemic shunt • Right-sided heart failure • Cats—hepatic lipidosis; FIP; toxoplasmosis • Hemolytic anemia (cause of jaundice mistaken)

CBC/BIOCHEMISTRY/URINALYSIS
CBC: • Microcytic or normocytic, normochromic nonregenerative anemia • Mild thrombocytopenia

Biochemistry: • Hyperbilirubinemia • Liver enzyme activities—high (mostly ALP and ALT); noted before clinical signs appear; with end-stage disease, may be normal or only mildly high • Hypoalbuminemia • Normal to hyper-globulinemia • Hypocholesterolemia—end-stage liver disease or APSS • Low BUN—with reduced urea cycle activity, APSS, protein-restricted diet. • Hypoglycemia—dogs, rarely in cats • Hypokalemia—may predispose to hepatic encephalopathy • Hyponatremia—end-stage

Urinalysis
• Isosthenuria—with polyuria and polydipsia • Ammonium biurate crystalluria

OTHER LABORATORY TESTS
• Ascitic fluid—pure or modified transudate • Coagulation tests—prolonged PT, APTT, ACT, and/or buccal mucosal bleeding time • Serum bile acids—high • Hyperammonemia

IMAGING

Radiography
Abdominal—small liver (dogs); normal to large liver (cats); ascites may obscure abdominal detail; radiolucent urate calculi visible if complexed with calcium mineral

Ultrasonography
• Abdominal—hepatic image may be hyperechoic or have mixed echogenicity; may note nodular pattern, abdominal effusion (ascites), splenomegaly, and APSS; in some cases, there is no parenchymal change • Doppler interrogation of portal vasculature—may reveal hepatofugal blood flow

DIAGNOSTIC PROCEDURES
• Fine-needle aspiration cytology—helps rule out neoplasia; detects bacterial infection; will not define fibrosis or nonsuppurative inflammation • Liver biopsy—necessary for definitive diagnosis; needle core biopsies often inaccurate owing to small sample size • Laparoscopy—relatively noninvasive gross visualization and biopsy of all liver lobes

PATHOLOGIC FINDINGS

Gross
• Fibrosis—small, firm liver with an irregular to finely nodular contour • Cirrhosis—firm liver with an irregular contour and prominent nodules

Histopathology
• Inflammatory fibrosis—fibrosis starts periportally and breaks through limiting plate interconnecting portal areas (bridging fibrosis); often associated with lymphoplasmacytic infiltrates, necrosis, and bile ductule hyperplasia • Noninflammatory fibrosis—fibrosis may focus on sinusoids, portal triads, or hepatic venules • Cirrhosis—diffuse fibrosis; nodular regeneration with marked architectural distortion of hepatic lobules; may be accompanied by inflammatory infiltrate

TREATMENT

APPROPRIATE HEALTH CARE
• Outpatient—patients that appear normal and are eating • Inpatient—diagnostic tests; treatment for dehydration, anorexia, neurologic signs of HE, or enteric bleeding due to portal hypertensive gastroenteropathy

NURSING CARE
• Fluids—avoid lactate with severe hepatic failure; avoid 0.9% NaCl with ascites • B complex vitamins (cats)—2 mL/L fluid advised • Glucose—for hypoglycemia; 2.5% dextrose in polyionic solution; if persistent hypoglycemia, increase glucose to avert neuroglycopenia; must administer into central vein • Potassium chloride—as needed • Avoid alkalosis—worsens HE • Therapeutic abdominocentesis for tense ascites

ACTIVITY Limit

DIET
• Withhold food if there is acute HE with stupor or coma, acute persistent vomiting associated with enteric ulceration, or concurrent pancreatitis • Vegetable or dairy protein sources (dogs) with fermentable fiber for chronic HE combined with medical interventions to increase nitrogen tolerance (See Hepatic Encephalopathy); do not restrict dietary protein unless HE is not controlled with medication; dietary protein individualized to maintain body condition and albumin while minimizing hepatic encephalopathy • Sodium restriction if ascites present • Fat restriction rarely needed

CLIENT EDUCATION
• Warn client that treatment is palliative and symptomatic once cirrhosis is established. • Conditions predisposing to HE—dehydration; infection; catabolism; hypokalemia; alkalemia; high-protein meals; enteric parasitism; enteric bleeding; and certain catabolic drugs

SURGICAL CONSIDERATIONS
• Cirrhosis—high anesthetic risk; avoid certain drugs or use with special consideration (e.g., barbiturates, phenothiazines, benzodiazepines) • Gas anesthetics—isoflurane best • Coagulopathy—may lead to severe hemorrhagic complications from even minor surgeries • Postoperative intensive care—critical for avoiding HE; to maintain hydration and euglycemia • Predisposition to bacterial infection—administer antibiotics as necessary

MEDICATIONS

DRUG(S) OF CHOICE
• Focus treatment on specific etiology; chelate copper if copper storage hepatopathy (see Copper Storage Hepatopathy); withdraw potentially hepatotoxic drugs • Immune modulation—see Hepatitis, Chronic • Prednisolone/prednisone—1–4 mg/kg daily PO; taper to lowest effective dose (e.g., 0.25 mg/kg PO q48h) • Azathioprine—in combination with prednisone in dogs: 1 mg/kg PO q48h; toxic to cats • Nonspecific antifibrotic agents—see Hepatitis, Chronic; no controlled studies; colchicine, especially if noninflammatory fibrotic disease: 0.03 mg/kg PO q24h; polyunsaturated phosphatidyl-choline: 50–100 mg/kg PO q24h (not to exceed 3 g; dose extrapolated from human studies); elemental zinc: 1.5–3 mg PO daily, adjust dose using sequential plasma zinc concentrations (avoid plasma values > 800 μg/dL); prednisone is also antifibrotic as it decreases inflammation driving fibrogenesis • Hepatoprotectants—see Hepatitis, Chronic; ursodeoxycholate: 10–15 mg/kg PO q24h; *Silybum marianum* (milk thistle): 20–50 mg/kg/day (dose extrapolated from human clinical studies) • Gastroprotectants (sucralfate) or gastric acid inhibitors—see Hepatitis, Chronic; enteric bleeding can precipitate HE; eliminate enteric parasites

Specific Conditions
• Ascites—diuretics (see Hepatitis, Chronic); combine furosemide (0.5–2 mg/kg IV, SC, PO q12h) and spironolactone (0.5–2 mg/kg PO q12h); combine diuretics with dietary sodium restriction and restricted activity to slowly mobilize ascites; adjust dose using recheck intervals every 4–7 days; perform therapeutic abdominocentesis if failure to respond within 7–14 days of titrated diuretic therapy • Coagulopathy—see Coagulopathy of Liver Disease. • Hepatic encephalopathy—see Hepatic Encephalopathy; ameliorate signs • Oxidative damage—see Hepatitis, Chronic; vitamin E: 10 IU/kg PO q24h; S-adenosylmethionine: 20 mg/kg enteric-coated tablet PO q24h on empty stomach, daily for 3–6 weeks then treat every 2–3 days.

CONTRAINDICATIONS
NSAIDs—avoid; potentiate gastroduodenal ulceration; inhibit natriuresis; may worsen ascites; potentially hepatotoxic

PRECAUTIONS
• Diuretics—may cause dehydration or metabolic alkalosis that can worsen HE • Glucocorticoids—increase susceptibility to infections; promote sodium and water retention (prednisone); increase protein catabolism; predispose to enteric ulceration • Avoid drugs that depend on first-pass hepatic extraction and drugs that rely solely on hepatic conjugation or biotransformation for elimination; if use is necessary, empirically reduce the dose • Tetracycline, NSAIDs, barbiturates, lidocaine, theophylline, propranolol, captopril, benzodiazepines, and methionine—avoid if possible • Metronidazole—reduce conventionally recommended dose; use 7.5 mg/kg PO q12h for HE

ALTERNATIVE DRUG(S)
Dexamethasone—if ascites present; use instead of prednisone to avoid mineralocorticoid effect; divide prednisone dose by 8–10 and administer every 2–4 days; taper to lowest effective dose

FOLLOW-UP

PATIENT MONITORING
• Liver enzymes, albumin, BUN, and cholesterol—monthly or quarterly, depending on patient's condition • Serial monitoring of bile acid values—does not add prognostic or diagnostic information • Body condition score and muscle mass—prognostic indicators of nutritional adequacy and nitrogen balance • Abdominal girth with ascites • Azathioprine—monitor for possible bone marrow toxicity via sequential CBC.

POSSIBLE COMPLICATIONS
• HE, septicemia, and bleeding—may be life threatening • DIC—may be a terminal event

EXPECTED COURSE AND PROGNOSIS
• Natural history of fibrotic/cirrhotic hepatic disease is poorly characterized; severity of fibrosis and presence of bridging fibrosis related to significantly shorter survival time in one retrospective study • Juvenile idiopathic fibrosis (dogs)—survival up to 6 years • Cirrhosis—survival > 5 years with aggressive interventional and supportive care and therapy

MISCELLANEOUS

ZOONOTIC POTENTIAL
Dogs with leptospirosis-associated chronic liver disease (rare) may shed organisms.

SEE ALSO
• Copper Storage Hepatopathy • Diabetic Hepatopathy • Hepatic Encephalopathy • Hepatitis, Chronic • Hypertension, Portal • Juvenile Fibrosing Liver Disease • Superficial Necrolytic Dermatitis

ABBREVIATIONS
• ACT = activated clotting time • APSS = acquired portosystemic shunt(s) • APTT = activated partial thromboplastin time • ECM = extracellular matrix • EHBDO = extrahepatic bile duct occlusion • HE = hepatic encephalopathy • PT = prothrombin time

Suggested Reading
Leveille CR, Arias IM. Pathophysiology and pharmacologic modulation of hepatic fibrosis. J Vet Intern Med 1993;7:73–84.

Acknowledgment
The author and editors acknowledge the contributions of Dr. David Twedt, who authored this topic in the previous edition.
Author Cynthia R. L. Webster
Consulting Editor Sharon A. Center

CLOSTRIDIAL ENTEROTOXICOSIS

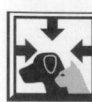

BASICS

DEFINITION
A complex syndrome characterized by diarrhea in dogs and cats associated with *Clostridium perfringens* (CP). The presence of CP enterotoxin and enterotoxogenic fecal isolates appears to provide the best evidence of CP-associated diarrhea.

PATHOPHYSIOLOGY
Clostridium perfringens is a common enteric inhabitant generally found in the vegetative form living in a symbiotic relationship with the host. It appears that there are certain strains of CP (generally Type A based on PCR analysis) capable of producing an enterotoxin that binds to the enteric mucosa, alters cell permeability, and results in cell damage and/or subsequent cell death. CP enterotoxin production is thought to be associated with enteric sporulation. CP enterotoxin does not cause systemic illness. There appear to be a number of intrinsic host-related factors that influence enterotoxin production and pathogenicity of CP.

SYSTEM AFFECTED
Gastrointestinal

GENETICS
N/A

INCIDENCE AND PREVALENCE
Incidence is unknown, but it is suspected that up to 15–20% of cases of chronic large bowel diarrhea in dogs is CP-related. Less common in cats

GEOGRAPHIC DISTRIBUTION
N/A

SIGNALMENT
Species
Dogs and cats

Breed Predilections
N/A

Mean Age and Range
Disease may occur in any age animal. Most animals that develop chronic clinical signs tend to be middle-aged or older.

Predominant Sex
N/A

SIGNS
General Comments
• Clinical syndromes are associated with either an acquired acute self-limiting bowel diarrhea lasting for 5–7 days, chronic intermittent diarrhea, or signs associated with other gastrointestinal or non-gastrointestinal disease.

• Chronic signs are often characterized by intermittent episodes occurring every 2–4 weeks that may persist for months to years. The syndrome may result as a nosocomial (hospital-acquired) disease with signs precipitated during or shortly following hospitalization or boarding at a kennel.
• CP has also been associated with some cases of parvovirus and acute hemorrhagic gastroenteritis.

Historical Findings
• Most common sign is large bowel diarrhea having fecal mucus, small amounts of fresh blood, small scant stools, tenesmus with an increased frequency of stools.
• Occasionally dogs will have signs of small bowel diarrhea characterized by a large volume of watery stool.
• Other signs include vomiting, flatulence, abdominal discomfort, or a generalized unthriftiness.

Physical Examination Findings
Evidence of systemic illness or debilitation is rare. Abdominal discomfort may be detected on palpation. There may be evidence of blood or mucus in the feces. Fever is uncommon.

CAUSES
It is unknown if enterotoxigenic CP is a true acquired infection or an opportunistic pathogen. There are only certain strains of CP genetically capable of producing enterotoxin, and only certain animals are affected clinically. The disease may be associated with small intestinal bacterial overgrowth.

RISK FACTORS
• Stress factors to the gastrointestinal tract, dietary change, concurrent disease, or hospitalization may precipitate signs.
• The pathogenicity of CP may depend on the metabolic, mucosal, and immunologic integrity of the gastrointestinal tract.
• Possibly IgA deficiency
• An alkaline intestinal luminal environment promotes CP sporulation and enterotoxin production.
• Primary intestinal bacterial overgrowth

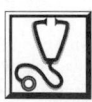

DIAGNOSIS

Cases having chronic intermittent clinical signs suspected of being caused by CP should always be evaluated during the onset of clinical episodes.

DIFFERENTIAL DIAGNOSIS
• All causes of diarrhea, including systemic or metabolic disease as well as specific intestinal disorders, should be considered.

• Gastrointestinal parasites, inflammatory bowel disease, chronic idiopathic colitis, and nervous or irritable bowel syndrome may resemble CP enterotoxicosis.

CBC/BIOCHEMISTRY/URINALYSIS
Usually normal

OTHER LABORATORY TESTS
Diagnostic confirmation of CP enterotoxicosis is as yet controversial and no test appears to be completely accurate.

Microbiology
• Anaerobic fecal cultures will generally identify high concentrations of CP organisms but occasionally will be negative. • Specific fecal spore cultures will detect high concentrations of clostridial spores ($> 10^6$ spores per gram of feces) in affected animals and correlate well with clinical disease, but are rarely performed.

Enterotoxin Assay
• Identification of positive fecal CP enterotoxin in conjunction with clinical signs, fecal culture, and a response to antibiotic therapy supports CP as a contributing pathogen.
• Enterotoxin analysis is performed using a fecal ELISA (Tech Labs, Blacksburg, VA). The reverse passive latex agglutination assay is considered inaccurate. The assay requires one gram (small pea-size sample) of feces. The enterotoxin is quite stable, and feces can be refrigerated or frozen prior to analysis.
• Assay findings do not always correlate with clinical disease. False positive results have been observed in a number of asymptomatic dogs, suggesting inherent resistance to pathogenicity of the enterotoxin. False negative results may occur from interfering substances in the feces or from samples taken during the recovery period. PCR identifying the CP enterotoxin gene correlates well with clinical disease but is uncommonly performed.

Fecal Cytology
• Identification of high numbers of CP endospores in the feces does not always correlate with clinical disease or fecal enterotoxin assay. The presence or lack of endospores is variable; some CP endospores are not pathogenic, some endospores are from other spore forming bacteria, and the presence of pathogenic CP endospores occurs early in disease and may not be seen if feces are evaluated later in the course of disease. Greater than 5 spores per high power oil immersion is considered abnormal.
• Cytology involves making a thin fecal smear on a microscope slide, air-drying or heat-

fixing and staining with Diff-Quick or Wright's stain. Specific spore stain malachite green can also be used to identify spores.
• CP spores will have a "safety-pin" appearance with an oval structure and a dense body at one end of the spore wall.
• Detection of spores should be performed shortly following onset of clinical signs.
• Presence of spores should be evaluated in context of other laboratory and clinical findings.

IMAGING
N/A

DIAGNOSTIC PROCEDURES
Colonoscopy will help rule out concurrent intestinal disease.

PATHOLOGIC FINDINGS
• Colon biopsies taken during asymptomatic periods are usually normal.
• Patients with CP enterotoxicosis may have colonoscopic evidence of hyperemic or ulcerated mucosa.
• Histology may show catarrhal or suppurative colitis. Occasionally mild inflammatory bowel disease is present.

TREATMENT

APPROPRIATE HEALTH CARE
• Most treated as outpatients
• When diarrhea or vomiting is severe, and resulting in dehydration and electrolyte imbalance, hospitalization may be required.

NURSING CARE
Fluid and electrolyte therapy may be required to replace losses occurring from diarrhea (uncommon).

ACTIVITY
Restricted during acute disease

DIET
• Dietary manipulation plays an important role in the treatment and management of cases with chronic recurring disease. Diets formulated high in fiber, either soluble (or fermentable) and insoluble fiber, often result in clinical improvement by reducing enteric clostridial numbers and by acidifying the distal intestine, thus limiting CP sporulation and enterotoxin production.
• Commercial high-fiber diets can be supplemented with psyllium (1/2–2 tsp./day) as a source of soluble fiber.
• Diets low in fiber should be supplemented with fiber (coarse bran [1–3 tbs./day]) as a source of insoluble fiber or psyllium added as a source of soluble fiber.

CLIENT EDUCATION
Acute disease is often self-limiting, while chronic cases may require prolonged therapy.

SURGICAL CONSIDERATIONS
N/A

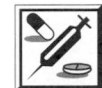

MEDICATIONS

DRUG(S) OF CHOICE
Antibiotics
• Acute self-limiting disease usually requires a 5–7 day antibiotic course. Most patients respond well to appropriate antibiotic therapy (e.g., oral ampicillin or amoxicillin, clindamycin, metronidazole, or tylosin).
• Chronic reoccurring cases often require prolonged antibiotic therapy. Tylosin (Tylan Soluble) given at a dose of 7–15 mg/kg q12–24h mixed with the food or formulated in capsules is suggested for long-term management.
• It appears that high doses of antibiotics may not be necessary to prevent recurrence in chronic cases. Administration of oral antibiotics at submicrobial inhibitory concentrations may be effective in chronic cases. Low antibiotic levels may not actually reduce enteric CP numbers but may change the ecologic microenvironment, preventing sporulation and enterotoxin production.

CONTRAINDICATIONS
N/A

PRECAUTIONS
N/A

POSSIBLE INTERACTIONS
N/A

ALTERNATIVE DRUG(S)
Chronic cases may respond well to high-fiber diets (see Diet), and dietary manipulation may be attempted as the sole therapy following resolution of signs.

FOLLOW-UP

PATIENT MONITORING
The patient's response to therapy supports the diagnosis, and rarely are repeated diagnostics necessary.

PREVENTION/AVOIDANCE
• Infection is associated with environmental contamination, and disinfection is difficult.
• Feeding high-fiber diets may decrease the incidence of nosocomial acquired diarrhea.

POSSIBLE COMPLICATIONS
N/A

EXPECTED COURSE AND PROGNOSIS
• Most animals respond well to therapy. Chronic cases may require lifelong therapy to control clinical signs.
• A failure in response suggests concurrent disease, and further diagnostic evaluation is indicated.

MISCELLANEOUS

ASSOCIATED CONDITIONS
CP enterotoxicosis is frequently associated with other enteric disease such as parvovirus, acute hemorrhagic gastroenteritis, or inflammatory bowel disease.

AGE-RELATED FACTORS
N/A

ZOONOTIC POTENTIAL
Unknown.

PREGNANCY
Antibiotic therapy may be contraindicated.

SYNONYM
Idiopathic chronic colitis

SEE ALSO
• Colitis and Proctitis
• Small Intestinal Bacterial Overgrowth

ABBREVIATIONS
• CP = *Clostridium perfringens*
• tbs = tablespoon
• tsp = teaspoon

Suggested Reading
Foley J, Hirsh DC, Pedersen NC: An outbreak of *Clostridium perfringens* enteritis in a cattery of Bengal cats and experimental transmission to specific pathogen free cats. Feline Practice 1996;24(6):31–35.
Kirth SA, Prescott JF, Welch MK, et al. Nosocomial diarrhea associated with enterotoxigenic *Clostridium perfringens* infection in dogs. J Am Vet Med Assoc 1989; 195:331–334.
Marks SL, Kather EJ, Kass PH, Melli AC. Genotypic and phenotypic characterization of *Clostridium perfringens* and *Clostridium difficile* in diarrheic and healthy dogs. J Vet Intern Med 2002;16:533–540.
Twedt DC. *Clostridium perfringens* associated enterotoxicosis in dogs. In: Kirk RW, Bonagura JD. Current veterinary therapy XI. Philadelphia: Saunders, 1992:602–604.
Weese JS, Staempfli HR, Prescott JF et al. The roles of *Clostridium difficile* and enterotoxigenic *Clostridium perfringens* in diarrhea in dogs. J Vet Intern Med 2001; 15:374–378.
Author David C. Twedt
Consulting Editor Albert E. Jergens

COAGULATION FACTOR DEFICIENCY

BASICS

DEFINITION
Hemostatic defects characterized by deficient activity of one or more coagulation factors

PATHOPHYSIOLOGY
• Coagulation mechanism involves a series of sequential enzyme activations leading to the generation of thrombin, which converts fibrinogen to fibrin monomers, and subsequent polymerization of the monomers into fibrin strands, which stabilize the platelet plugs at sites of vessel injury
• Severe deficiency or defective function of coagulation factors causes defective hemostasis.

SYSTEMS AFFECTED
• Coagulation defects can cause hemorrhage in any tissue or organ and anemia.
• Hemorrhage—most commonly in and around the joints and major muscle masses (causing large swellings) and into the body cavities; region of the larynx or pleural cavity of special concern because of the risk of asphyxia; brain or spinal cord of major concern because the rigid bony case limits expansion, and the risk for permanent damage is high

SIGNALMENT
• Factor VIII and factor IX deficiencies—severe defects usually recognized as spontaneous hemorrhages before 10 weeks of age; X-linked defects; males are clinically affected, whereas females are carriers and usually clinically normal. Females can have these deficiencies though relatively rarely.
• von Willebrand disease—autosomal defect; both males and females are affected clinically; the most common inherited coagulation defect with high prevalence in many breeds
• Factor X deficiency—rare defect in American cocker spaniels and Jack Russell terriers; manifests as stillborn puppies or neonatal deaths related to internal hemorrhage; autosomal trait: homozygotes severely affected; heterozygotes may be clinically normal or have only a mild bleeding tendency.
• Factor XI deficiency—rare defect described in the English springer spaniels, great Pyrenees, and Kerry blue terriers; mild autosomal defect with bleeding after surgery or injury
• Factor XII deficiency—fairly common in cats but rarely detected because no bleeding tendency is associated with the defect

SIGNS
• Inactivity
• Swollen joints
• Subcutaneous swellings
• Abnormal bleeding from cuts or mucous membranes
• Hemorrhages in deeper tissues or body cavities

CAUSES
• True deficiency of clotting factors (e.g., genetic defect, liver disease, rodenticide anticoagulant toxicity, and vitamin K deficiency)
• Synthesis of defective factors
• Exposure to inhibitors (e.g., heparin)

RISK FACTORS
• NSAIDs can potentiate a bleeding defect.
• Environmental exposure to rodenticide anticoagulants
• Liver disease

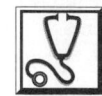

DIAGNOSIS

DIFFERENTIAL DIAGNOSIS
• Factor VIII or factor IX deficiency—spontaneous bleeding noticed in young males but not female litter mates
• von Willebrand disease or factor XI deficiency—usually detected as abnormal bleeding after injury or surgery in males or females
• Factor XII deficiency—no clinical bleeding defect
• DIC is secondary to severe systemic disease and may be associated with thrombocytopenia or platelet function defects causing petechiae.
• Rodenticide anticoagulants often cause major bleeding into body cavities.

LABORATORY FINDINGS

Drugs That May Alter Laboratory Results
Heparin and other anticoagulants used in treatment or from samples collected through heparinized catheters cause abnormal coagulation test results.

Disorders That May Alter Laboratory Results
• Shortening or prolonging of coagulation test results can be caused by contamination of blood with tissue fluid during problems with venipuncture; evidence of hemolysis should raise concern about possible tissue fluid contamination or prolonged time before testing.
• Extreme lipemia may interfere with clot detection by some automated coagulation analyzers.
• Because of the lability of some coagulation factors, especially factor VIII, plasma should be separated from the rest of the sample and sent on ice or frozen to the laboratory.

Valid if Run in Human Laboratory?
• Coagulation assays vary in sensitivity but generally should yield valid data; it is important to interpret results in relation to concurrent data from samples of normal plasma from the same species.
• Some of the activators used in the APTT are not as effective on domestic animal samples as they are on human samples.

• Some tests for fibrin degradation products are species-specific.

CBC/BIOCHEMISTRY/URINALYSIS
• Regenerative anemia is proportional to the blood loss caused by bleeding episodes.
• Platelet count is normal unless the patient has DIC or massive bleeding.
• Resorption of blood from large hematoma may cause high bilirubin.

OTHER LABORATORY TESTS
• Measurement of PT the test of choice for screening for extrinsic mechanism defects
• Measurement of APTT the test of choice for screening for intrinsic mechanism defects; although not as sensitive or precise, ACT is a practical substitute for the APTT test.
• Specific assays for coagulation factors required for diagnosis of most inherited defects; these assays can be run with human deficient plasma as substrate, but the assays must be performed with dilutions of species-specific normal plasma for the activity curves.

IMAGING
N/A

DIAGNOSTIC PROCEDURES
• Bleeding time with a gauze tourniquet on the folded lip over the maxilla prolonged in patients with von Willebrand disease
• Bleeding time normal in patients with most other coagulation defects, except DIC

TREATMENT
• Most bleeding episodes in animals with inherited coagulation defects can be effectively treated by transfusion of fresh blood, fresh plasma, cryoprecipitate, or fresh frozen plasma.
• Because repeated transfusions may be required in the future, cryoprecipitate or plasma is recommended unless the need for RBC replacement is severe.
• In patients with factor VIII deficiency, the short half-life of this factor (10–12 hr) may necessitate repeat transfusions at 12–24-hr intervals.

MEDICATIONS

DRUG(S) OF CHOICE
Vitamin K_1 an effective treatment for patients with anticoagulant rodenticide poisoning or vitamin K deficiency; if PT is normal, no rationale for vitamin K_1 administration

CONTRAINDICATIONS
Aspirin and NSAIDs should be avoided because of adverse effects on platelet function.

PRECAUTIONS
• Intramuscular injections should be avoided because of the risk of inducing additional bleeding.

• Intravenous administration of vitamin K not recommended because of the risk of anaphylaxis

POSSIBLE INTERACTIONS
None

ALTERNATIVE DRUG(S)
Desmopressin acetate (1 µg/kg SC) just before surgery may increase the concentration of von Willebrand factor and shorten the bleeding time in dogs with von Willebrand disease.

 FOLLOW-UP

PATIENT MONITORING
• PT can be used to monitor effectiveness of vitamin K administration in animals with anticoagulant toxicity; with appropriate treatment, prolonged PT should be corrected within 24 hr; persistence after this time suggests incorrect diagnosis or undertreatment of poisoning.
• ACT a less-sensitive but reasonable substitute for monitoring response to vitamin K
• Most inherited defects can be monitored by clinical arrest of bleeding and improvement in results of coagulation screening tests.

POSSIBLE COMPLICATIONS
Animals with inherited defects at continual risk for repeated hemorrhagic episodes

 MISCELLANEOUS

ASSOCIATED CONDITIONS
None

AGE-RELATED FACTORS
None

ZOONOTIC POTENTIAL
None

PREGNANCY
May cause fluctuations in clotting factor activity, which generally do not lead to bleeding episodes

SYNONYMS
• Coagulation defects
• Coagulopathies

SEE ALSO
• Disseminated Intravascular Coagulation (DIC)
• von Willebrand Disease

ABBREVIATIONS
• ACT = activated clotting time
• APTT = activated partial thromboplastin time

• DIC = disseminated intravascular coagulation
• NSAID = nonsteroidal antiinflammatory drug
• PT = prothrombin time
• RBC = red blood cell

Suggested Reading
Brooks M. Coagulopathies and Thrombosis. In: Ettinger SJ, Feldman EC, ed. Textbook of veterinary internal medicine. Philadelphia: Saunders, 2000:1829–1841.
Dodds WJ. Hemostasis. In: Kaneko JJ, Harvey JW, Bruss ML, eds. Clinical biochemistry of domestic animals. New York: Academic Press, 1997:241–283.
Jain NC. Coagulation and its disorders. In: Jain NC, ed. Essentials of veterinary hematology. Philadelphia: Lea & Febiger, 1993:82–104.
Parry BW. Laboratory evaluation of hemorrhagic coagulopathies in small animal practice. Vet Clin North Am Small Anim 1989; 19:729–742.
Author Gary J. Kociba
Consulting Editor Stephen A. Kruth

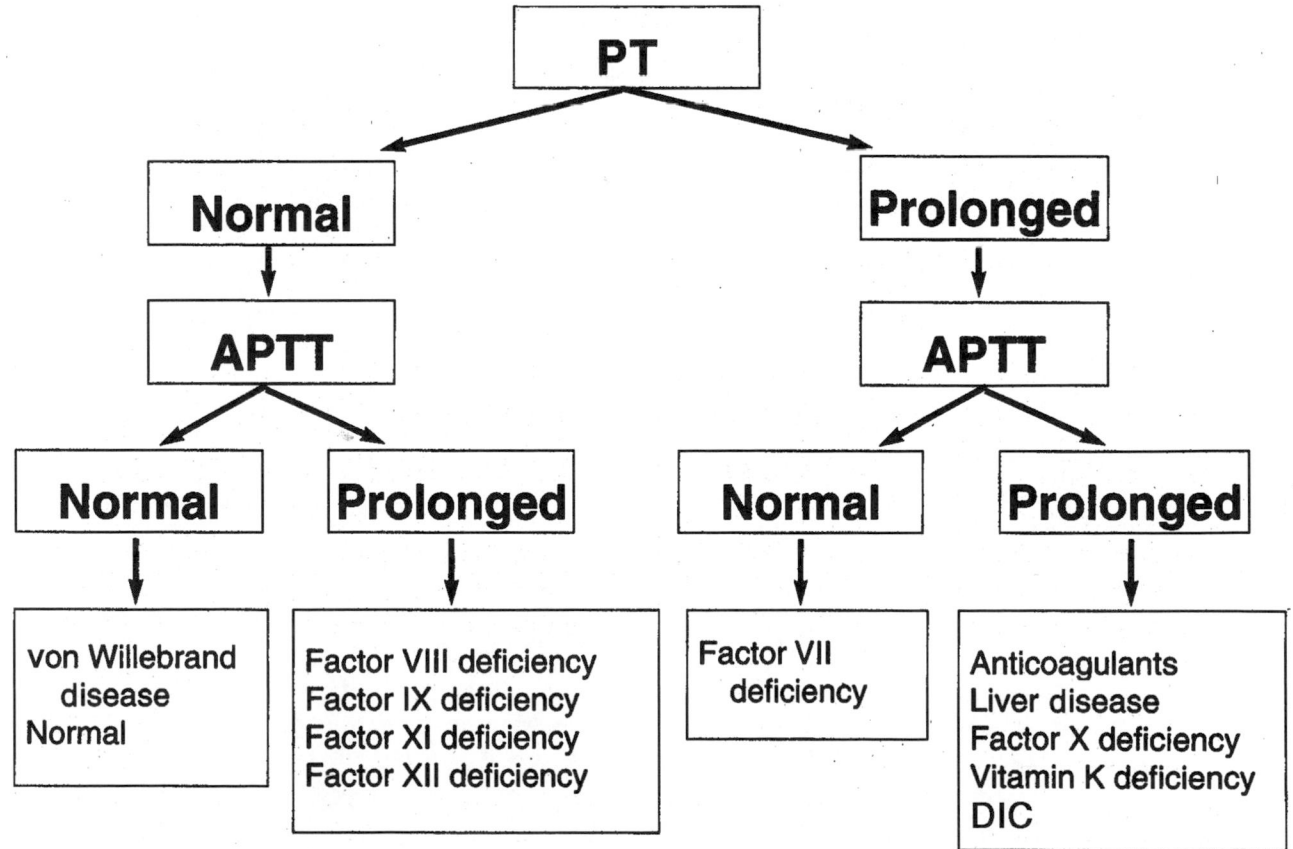

COAGULOPATHY OF LIVER DISEASE

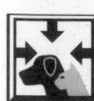 BASICS

OVERVIEW
• Patients with liver disease may have a measurable hemostatic defect, but few exhibit spontaneous bleeding.
• The liver is the sole or primary site of synthesis of most coagulation factors, anticoagulants, and fibrinolytic proteins; exceptions: factors V and VIII, vWF, TF, and tPA
• Causes of impaired hemostasis—reduced synthesis of clotting factors and other hemostatic proteins; vitamin K deficiency; high concentrations of FDPs and anticoagulants; thrombocytopenia or thrombocytopathy; and enhanced fibrinolysis
• DIC often accompanies sepsis, neoplasia, and advanced liver disease.
• Vitamin K deficiency may occur with intra- or extrahepatic obstruction to bile flow or fat malabsorption.

SIGNALMENT
Dogs and cats of any age, breed, or sex

SIGNS
• Usually no obvious signs of bleeding; requires careful inspection of body surfaces (especially venipuncture sites), mucous membranes, urine, and feces
• Melena; hematemesis; hematochezia
• Prolonged bleeding—venipuncture; biopsy sites; surgical wound
• Spontaneous bruising or hematomas—uncommon unless severe vitamin K deficiency or fulminant DIC

CAUSES & RISK FACTORS
• Severe hepatic failure of any etiology
• Acute viral liver disease
• Cirrhosis
• EHBDO

• Chronic liver disease—usually no bleeding until cirrhosis develops
• Concurrent small bowel disease (e.g., in cats with cholangiohepatitis complex)—may predispose the patient to vitamin K deficiency
• PSVA (rare)

 DIAGNOSIS

DIFFERENTIAL DIAGNOSIS
• Toxicities—vitamin K antagonism (rodenticide); NSAID-induced gastrointestinal bleeding; gastrointestinal irritants
• Hereditary hemostatic defects
• Immune and infectious thrombocytopenia
• DIC
• Gastrointestinal infiltrative disorders
• Hepatic amyloidosis (factor deficiency, spontaneous liver lobe fractures)
• Abdominal trauma

CBC/BIOCHEMISTRY/URINALYSIS
• CBC—may be normal; regenerative anemia if severe bleeding lasts several days; microcytosis if portosystemic shunting; thrombocytopenia (rare, unless DIC noted)
• Biochemistry—high liver enzyme activities; bilirubinemia; low albumin with synthetic failure, accompanied by hypoglobulinemia with extracorporeal blood loss
• Urinalysis—microhematuria; gross blood; bilirubinuria

OTHER LABORATORY TESTS
Hemostatic tests—low platelet count; prolonged APTT (ACT), PT, TCT, and PIVKA; low activity of coagulation factors and anticoagulants (ATIII, protein C); dysfibrinogenemia; high FDPs; D-dimers

IMAGING
Abdominal Ultrasonography
• Abdominal effusion (hemorrhage)—may be seen
• Change in liver variable

• Abnorma gastrointestinal motility, thickening in area of ulceration, or perforation associated with portal hypertensive vasculopathy and bleeding

 TREATMENT

• Not necessary unless invasive procedures are planned or spontaneous hemorrhage occurs
• Spontaneous bleeding—indicates severe liver dysfunction; initiate treatment
• Fresh whole blood—for anemia, coagulation factors, functional platelets
• Fresh frozen plasma—for coagulation factors in case of spontaneous bleeding; for long in vitro clotting times and invasive procedures
• Cryoprecipitate—only for severe fibrinogen deficiency or bleeding with coexistent vWD
• Platelet-rich plasma—rarely beneficial

Biopsy
• Increased likelihood of bleeding—PIVKA, PT, APTT, or ACT prolonged by > 50%; thrombocytopenia < 50,000/μL; or prolonged mucosal bleeding time
• Iatrogenic hemorrhage—grave risk with spontaneous bleeding for which a cause cannot be identified and eliminated
• Liver—provide hemostasis for postprocedure hemorrhage
• Ultrasound-guided needle core—high risk; observe site for 15 minutes and again several hours after procedure
• Laparoscopy—affords visibility and hemostasis (cautery, Gelfoam)
• Laparotomy—wedge biopsy; ill-advised with overt bleeding

 MEDICATIONS

DRUG(S)
• Specific and supportive care based on cause of hepatic disease

• Vitamin K deficiency—parenteral vitamin K_1 (0.5–1.5 mg/kg q12h SC up to 3 doses in 24-hr interval one time); oral vitamin K_1 (mephyton, 1 mg/kg q24h) if enteric bile acids and their uptake are adequate
• DIC—correct primary disease; heparin for thrombotic DIC (unfractionated heparin: 100–200 U/kg q8–12h; or low molecular weight heparin [enoxaparin]: 100 U/kg [1 mg/kg] q12–24h)
• Blood products—fresh whole blood (red cells, platelets, hemostatic proteins): 12–20 mL/kg q24h; fresh frozen plasma (all hemostatic proteins): 10–20 mL/kg q12h; plasma cryosupernatant (albumin, vitamin K–dependent factors, ATIII): 10–20 mL/kg q12h; cryoprecipitate (fibrinogen, vWF, factor VIII): 1 U/10 kg or dose to effect; platelet-rich plasma (platelets and hemostatic proteins): 6–10 mL/kg
• DDAVP—0.5–1.0 μg/kg IV in saline; may increase coagulation factors, shorten mucosal bleeding time, and reduce bleeding tendencies (mechanism has not been fully explained, but is effective clinically and has been reported beneficial in humans with liver disease–associated coagulopathies actively bleeding from biopsy sites)

CONTRAINDICATIONS
• Whole blood transfusion—may precipitate hepatic encephalopathy, especially if using high-volume stored blood
• Vitamin K (cats)—too much causes Heinz body hemolytic anemia and oxidant liver injury
• Aspirin and other NSAIDs—may reduce renal prostaglandin synthesis, worsen ascites, and predispose patient to renal failure, gastrointestinal ulceration, and spontaneous bleeding
• Citrated blood—large volume (especially in animals < 5 kg) may result in citrate overload and hypocalcemia (may cause signs of hypocalcemia and bleeding tendency since ionized hypocalcemia impairs procoagulant activation); treat with 10% calcium chloride

0.1 mL/kg diluted in 10 to 20 mL of 0.9% saline and given over 10 to 20 minutes
• Jugular venipuncture, jugular vein catheter placement, and cystocentesis—avoid in patients with bleeding tendencies

FOLLOW-UP

PATIENT MONITORING
• Optimized PT test, PIVKA, factor VII—most sensitive to vitamin K deficiency; if no improvement within 48 hr of vitamin K_1 injection, it is unlikely subsequent vitamin K_1 will be beneficial
• Heart rate, blood pressure, mucous membrane color and refill, PCV, and total solids—with suspected active bleeding
• Biopsy site—observe immediately and sequentially (ultrasonography) for evidence of hemorrhage
• Sample abdominal effusion—determine if there is hemorrhage

PREVENTION/AVOIDANCE
• Well-balanced diet replete with vitamins
• Consider possibility of impaired vitamin K availability or synthesis due to chronic oral antimicrobial therapy
• Invasive procedures—anticipate bleeding; be prepared for blood component therapy (intravenous catheter, blood components); pretreat patient with vitamin K_1; administer DDAVP within 20 min of anticipated iatrogenic trauma (biopsy) if persistent bleeding tendencies exist despite vitamin K_1 therapy; administer fresh frozen plasma as definitive treatment; repeated DDAVP of no use
• Eliminate enteric parasitism

POSSIBLE COMPLICATIONS
Hemorrhage, anemia, hypovolemia, hepatic encephalopathy

EXPECTED COURSE/PROGNOSIS
Spontaneous hemorrhage, refractory coagulopathy, and DIC—poor prognosis

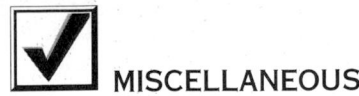
MISCELLANEOUS

ABBREVIATIONS
• ACT = activated clotting time
• APTT = activated partial thromboplastin time
• ATIII = antithrombin III
• DDAVP = 1 deamino-8-D-arginine vasopressin
• DIC = disseminated intravascular coagulation
• EHBDO = extrahepatic bile duct obstruction
• FDPs = fibrin/fibrinogen degradation products
• NSAIDs = nonsteroidal anti-inflammatory drugs
• PCV = packed cell volume
• PIVKA = proteins invoked by vitamin K absence or antagonism
• PSVA = portosystemic vascular anomaly
• PT = prothrombin time
• TCT = thrombin clotting time
• TF = tissue factor
• tPA = tissue plasminogen activator
• vWD = von Willebrand's disease
• vWF = von Willebrand factor

Suggested Reading

Amitrano L, Guardascione MA, Brancaccio V, Balzano A. Coagulation disorders in liver disease. Semin Liver Dis 2002;22:83–96.

Acknowledgment

The author and editor acknowledge the prior contributions of Dr. Joseph Taboada, who authored this topic in the previous edition

Author Marjory Brooks
Consulting Editor Sharon A. Center

COBALAMIN MALABSORPTION IN GIANT SCHNAUZERS AND BORDER COLLIES

BASICS

OVERVIEW
• Congenital anomaly involving selective malabsorption of cobalamin (vitamin B_{12})
• Occurs secondary to absence of the receptor for intrinsic factor–cobalamin complex in the ileal brush border in giant schnauzers; very rare

SIGNALMENT
• Inherited as a simple autosomal recessive trait in the giant schnauzer
• Signs appear at 6–12 weeks of age in giant schnauzers but at 4–6 months of age in border collies.

SIGNS
• Anorexia
• Lethargy
• Failure to gain weight

CAUSES & RISK FACTORS
The disease is inherited.

DIAGNOSIS

DIFFERENTIAL DIAGNOSIS
• Other congenital metabolic diseases
• Gastrointestinal parasitism

CBC/BIOCHEMISTRY/URINALYSIS
• Mild-to-severe neutropenia (1760–$4440/mm^3$)
• Chronic nonregenerative anemia (PCV 21–33%)

OTHER LABORATORY TESTS
• Serum cobalamin concentrations are very low (< 100 ng/L; normal, > 225 ng/L).
• Serum and urinary methylmalonic acid concentrations are above normal.

IMAGING
Not useful

DIAGNOSTIC PROCEDURES
N/A

COBALAMIN MALABSORPTION IN GIANT SCHNAUZERS AND BORDER COLLIES

TREATMENT

Outpatient medical treatment is warranted (long-term parenteral administration of cobalamin).

MEDICATIONS

DRUG(S)

Cyanocobalamin (0.5–1.0 mg IM q24h for 7 days, then q3–6 months).

CONTRAINDICATIONS/POSSIBLE INTERACTIONS

N/A

FOLLOW-UP

Periodic parenteral administration of cobalamin

MISCELLANEOUS

Suggested Reading

Fyfe JC, Giger U, Hall CA, et al. Inherited selective intestinal cobalamin malabsorption and cobalamin deficiency in dogs. Pediatr Res 1991;29:24–31.

Outerbridge CA, Myers SL, Giger U. Hereditary cobalamin deficiency in collie dogs. J Vet Intern Med 996; (Abstract) 10.

Author David A. Williams

Consulting Editor Albert E. Jergens

COCCIDIOIDOMYCOSIS

BASICS

DEFINITION
A systemic mycosis caused by the inhalation of infective arthroconidia of the soil-borne fungus *Coccidioides immitis.*

PATHOPHYSIOLOGY
• Inhalation of infective arthroconidia is the primary route of infection. Fever, lethargy, inappetence, coughing, and joint pain or stiffness may be noticed. Dissemination may occur within 10 days, resulting in signs related to the organ system involved. Asymptomatic infections may occur, and some animals develop immunity without onset of clinical signs. • Skin lesions are usually associated with dissemination, but penetrating wounds have rarely been associated with skin lesions. • Fewer than 10 inhaled arthrospores are sufficient to cause disease in susceptible animals. "Susceptible" refers to the animals in which extrapulmonary dissemination occurs. Signs of dissemination may not be evident for several months after the initial infection.

SYSTEMS AFFECTED
• Respiratory—the site of initial infection
• Extrapulmonary spread may occur to long bones and joints, eyes, skin, liver, kidneys, CNS, cardiovascular system (pericardium and myocardium), and testes.

GENETICS
N/A

INCIDENCE/PREVALENCE
An uncommon disease, even in endemic areas. It occurs more commonly in dogs, and rarely in cats.

GEOGRAPHIC DISTRIBUTION
Coccidioides immitis is found in the southwestern United States in the geographic Lower Sonoran life zone. It is more common in Southern California, Arizona, and southwest Texas, and is less prevalent in New Mexico, Nevada, and Utah.

SIGNALMENT

Species
Dogs and cats

Breed Predilections
None

Mean Age and Range
Most patients are young animals (< 4 years of age).

Predominant Sex
None

SIGNS

Historical Findings
• Anorexia • Coughing • Fever unresponsive to antibiotics • Lameness • Weakness, paraparesis, back and neck pain • Seizures • Visual changes • Weight loss

PHYSICAL EXAMINATION FINDINGS

Dogs
Signs with Pulmonary Involvement
• Coughing • Dyspnea • Fever
Signs with Disseminated Disease
• Bone swelling, joint enlargement, and lameness • Cachexia • Lethargy
• Lymphadenomegaly • Neurologic dysfunction caused by dissemination to both the central and peripheral nervous systems
• Skin ulcers and draining tracts • Uveitis, keratitis, iritis

Cats
• Cachexia • Draining skin lesions • Dyspnea
• Lameness caused by bone involvement
• Uveitis

CAUSE
Coccidioides immitis grows several inches deep in the soil, where it survives high ambient temperatures and low moisture. After a period of rainfall, the organism returns to the soil surface where it sporulates, releasing many arthroconidia that are disseminated by wind and dust storms.

RISK FACTORS
• Aggressive nosing about in soil and underbrush may expose susceptible animals to large doses of the fungus in contaminated soil. • Dust storms after the rainy season. Increased incidences are noted after earthquakes. • Land development where much earth disruption occurs may lead to increased exposure.

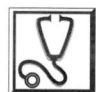

DIAGNOSIS

DIFFERENTIAL DIAGNOSIS
• Pulmonary lesions may resemble those of other systemic mycoses (e.g., histoplasmosis, blastomycosis). • Lymphadenomegaly may be seen in lymphosarcoma, other systemic mycoses, and localized bacterial infections.
• Bone lesions may resemble those caused by primary or metastatic bone tumors or bacterial osteomyelitis. • Skin lesions must be differentiated from routine abscesses or other bacterial disease processes.

CBC/BIOCHEMISTRY/URINALYSIS
• Hemogram—mild nonregenerative anemia, neutrophilic leukocytosis, monocytosis
• Serum chemistry profile—hyperglobulinemia, hypoalbuminemia, azotemia with renal involvement
• Urinalysis—low urine specific gravity and proteinuria with inflammatory glomerulonephritis

OTHER LABORATORY TESTS
Serologic tests for antibody to *C. immitis* by a laboratory proficient in handling the tests may provide a presumptive diagnosis and aid in monitoring response to therapy.

IMAGING
Radiography of lung (interstitial infiltrates) and bone lesions (osteolysis) may aid in diagnosis.

DIAGNOSTIC PROCEDURES
• Microscopic identification of the large spherule form of *C. immitis* in lesion or biopsy material is the definitive method of diagnosis. Lymph node aspirates and impression smears of skin lesions or draining exudate may, in some patients, yield organisms. • Caution should be used if culturing draining lesions suspected of being infected with *C. immitis,* as the mycelial form is highly contagious. Cultures should be performed by trained laboratory personnel using protective hoods. • Biopsy of infected tissue often is preferred to avoid false-negative results. Tissues involved, however, may not be readily accessible, and serologic testing is a more logical approach.

PATHOLOGIC FINDINGS
• Granulomatous, suppurative, or pyo-granulomatous inflammation present in many tissues • Presence of the characteristic spherule forms in affected tissues. In some patients, the numbers of spherules present may be small.

TREATMENT

APPROPRIATE HEALTH CARE
Generally treated as outpatients. Concurrent clinical symptoms (e.g., seizures, pain, coughing) should be treated appropriately.

NURSING CARE
N/A

ACTIVITY
Restrict activity until clinical signs begin to subside.

DIET
Feed a high-quality palatable diet to maintain body weight.

CLIENT EDUCATION
The necessity and expense of long-term therapy of a serious illness with the possibility of treatment failure should be reviewed. In addition, the client should be made aware of the possible side effects of the drugs used.

SURGICAL CONSIDERATIONS
In cases of focal granulomatous organ involvement (e.g., consolidated pulmonary lung lobe, eye, kidney) surgical removal of the affected organ may be indicated.

MEDICATIONS

DRUG(S) OF CHOICE

Coccidioidomycosis is considered one of the most severe and life-threatening of the systemic mycoses. Treatment of disseminated disease often requires at least one year of aggressive antifungal therapy.

Dogs

Several oral medications in the azole family of drugs are currently available for the treatment of coccidioidomycoses.
• Ketoconazole (KTZ) is dosed at 5–10 mg/kg PO q12h. May be given with food: some belief that co-administration of high doses of vitamin C may improve the absorption of the drug. Treatment should be continued for 1 year. • Fluconazole (FCZ) is dosed at 5 mg/kg PO q12h; it has been noted to greatly increase the success of treatment. Neurologists recommend 10 mg/kg to increase penetration in neurologic infections. The drug is extremely expensive, However, veterinary compounding pharmacies in Arizona and California have made the drug available for significantly less, thus making treatment with this drug more feasible. After extended use, the frequency of dosing in some cases may be lowered to once a day.
• Itraconazole (ITZ) is dosed at 5 mg/kg PO q12h. The drug is administered similarly as KTZ. It has been reported to have a higher penetration rate than ketoconazole, but a better clinical response has not been observed.
• Amphotericin B (AMB) is rarely recommended because of the high risk of renal damage and the availability of effective oral medications. Amphotericin B can be administered at a dosage of 0.5 mg/kg IV 3 times a week, for a total cumulative dosage of 8–10 mg/kg. It is given IV either as a slow infusion (in dogs that are gravely ill) or as a rapid bolus (in fairly healthy dogs). For slow infusion, add AMB to 250–500 mL of 5% dextrose solution and administer as a drip over a period of 4–6 hours. For a rapid bolus, add AMB to 30 mL of 5% dextrose solution and administer over a period of 5 minutes through a butterfly catheter. To lessen the adverse renal effects of AMB, give 0.9% NaCl (2 mL/kg/hr) for several hours before initiating AMB therapy.

Cats

• Any of the following azoles may be used in cats:
Ketoconazole 50 mg total dose PO q12h
Itraconazole 25–50 mg total dose PO q12h
Fluconazole 25–50 mg total dose PO q12h

CONTRAINDICATIONS

• Drugs metabolized primarily by the liver should not be administered along with KTZ.
• Drugs metabolized primarily by the kidneys should not be administered along with AMB.

PRECAUTIONS

• Side effects of azoles include inappetence, vomiting, and hepatotoxicity. The drugs may be stopped until signs abate, and restarted at a lower dose, which may be slowly increased to the recommended dose if the animal is able to tolerate the drug. The newer azoles (ITZ and FCZ) have fewer side effects. • Side effects of AMB therapy can be severe and include renal dysfunction, fever, inappetence, vomiting, and phlebitis.

POSSIBLE INTERACTIONS

N/A

ALTERNATIVE DRUG(S)

N/A

FOLLOW-UP

PATIENT MONITORING

• Serologic titers should be monitored every 3–4 months. Animals should be treated until their titers fall to less than 1:4. Animals displaying poor response to therapy should have a 2–4 hour post-pill drug level measured to assure adequate absorption of the drug.
• BUN and urinalysis should be monitored in all animals treated with AMB. Treatment should be temporarily discontinued if the BUN rises above 50 mg/dL or if granular casts are noted in the urine.

PREVENTION/AVOIDANCE

• No vaccine is available for dogs or cats.
• Contaminated soil in endemic areas should be avoided, particularly during dust storms after the rainy season.

POSSIBLE COMPLICATIONS

• Pulmonary disease resulting in severe coughing may temporarily worsen after therapy is begun owing to inflammation in the lungs. Low-dose short-term oral prednisone and cough suppressants may be required to alleviate the respiratory signs.
• Hepatotoxicity may result from KTZ therapy. • Nephrotoxicity may result from AMB therapy.

EXPECTED COURSE AND PROGNOSIS

• The prognosis is guarded to grave. Many dogs will improve following oral therapy; however, relapses may be seen, especially if therapy is shortened. The overall recovery rate has been estimated at 60%, but some report a 90% response to fluconazole therapy. • The prognosis for cats is not well documented, but rapid dissemination requiring long-term

therapy should be anticipated. • Serologic testing every 3–4 months after completion of therapy is recommended to monitor the possibility of relapse. • Spontaneous recovery from disseminated coccidioidomycosis without treatment is extremely rare.

MISCELLANEOUS

ASSOCIATED CONDITIONS

N/A

AGE-RELATED FACTORS

N/A

ZOONOTIC POTENTIAL

The spherule form of the fungus, as found in animal tissues, is not directly transmissible to people or other animals. Under certain rare circumstances, however, there could be reversion to growth of the infective mold form of the fungus on or within bandages placed over a draining lesion or in contaminated bedding. Draining lesions can lead to contamination of the environment with arthrospores. Care should be exercised whenever handling an infected draining lesion. Special precautions should be recommended to households where the owners may be immunosuppressed.

PREGNANCY

• KTZ should be used in pregnant animals only if the potential benefit justifies the potential risk to offspring. • Teratogen identified

SYNONYMS

• San Joaquin Valley fever • Valley fever
• Desert rheumatism (in humans)

ABBREVIATIONS

• AMB = amphotericin B
• BUN = blood urea nitrogen
• CNS = central nervous system
• FCZ = fluconazole
• ITZ = itraconazole
• KTZ = ketoconazole

Suggested Reading

Armstrong PJ, DiBartola SP. Canine coccidioidomycosis: a literature review and report of eight cases. J Am Anim Hosp Assoc 1983;19:937–945.
Greene RT. Coccidioidomycosis. In: Greene CE, ed. Infectious diseases of the dog and cat. 2nd ed. Philadelphia: Saunders, 1998: 391–398.
Legendre AM. Coccidioidomycosis. In: Sherding RG, ed. The cat: diseases and clinical management. 2nd ed. New York: Churchill Livingstone, 1994:561.
Author Nita Kay Gulbas
Consulting Editor Stephen C. Barr

COCCIDIOSIS

 **BASICS**

OVERVIEW
• An enteric infection, traditionally associated with *Isospora canis* (dogs) and *Isospora felis* (cats) as potential pathogens; other species of *Isospora* may be present
• Strictly host-specific (i.e., no cross-transmission)
• *Eimeria* spp. are not parasitic for dogs or cats.
• *Toxoplasma gondii* in cats and *Cryptosporidium parvum* in neonatal pups and kittens are coccidians in a nontraditional sense.
• *Toxoplasma* infection in cats may cause clinical signs similar to those with *Isospora* infections; oocysts shed in the environment may potentially cause a public health problem
• *Cryptosporidium* is still being assessed as an acute, life-threatening coccidiosis (cryptosporidiosis) of neonatal pups and kittens.
• Voluminous watery diarrhea is characteristic; autoinfection and continuing recycling within the intestinal tract result in a rapid loss of mucosal lining with cryptosporidiosis.

SIGNALMENT
Dogs and cats (especially pups and kittens)

SIGNS
• Watery-to-mucoid, sometimes blood-tinged, diarrhea
• Weak pups and kittens

CAUSES & RISK FACTORS
• Infected dogs or cats contaminating environment with oocysts of *Isospora* spp. or *Cryptosporidium*
• Stress

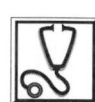 **DIAGNOSIS**

DIFFERENTIAL DIAGNOSIS
Enteric viral infections and other intestinal parasites

CBC/BIOCHEMISTRY/URINALYSIS
Usually normal; may be hemoconcentrated if dehydrated

OTHER LABORATORY TESTS
N/A

IMAGING
N/A

DIAGNOSTIC PROCEDURES
• Fecal examination for oocysts: (distinguish from pseudoparasitic *Eimeria* sp.); use sucrose α-flotation solution (s.g., 1.33) or special staining such as acid fast for *Cryptosporidium*
• *Isospora* oocysts should be 40 μm long; cysts of *Cryptosporidium* approximately 5 μm diameter

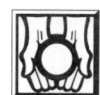 **TREATMENT**

• Usually treated as an outpatient
• Inpatient if debilitated
• Fluid therapy if dehydrated

MEDICATIONS

DRUG(S)
• Sulfadimethoxine—55 mg/kg PO on the first day, then 27.5 mg/kg for 4 days or until dog is asymptomatic for *Isospora* and fecal examination is negative for oocysts
• Sulfadiazine/trimethoprim 30 mg/kg sulfadiazine PO daily up to 14 days.
• Amprolium (extra-label) for prevention or treatment; dogs, 100–200 mg/kg q24h PO in food or water for 7 days; cats, 20–40 mg/kg PO for 10 days, 110–220 mg/kg for 7–12 days, or 300–400 mg/kg for 5 days
• On an extra-label use basis, albendazole for *Isospora*—25 mg/kg PO q12h for 2 days
• No effective or approved treatment for *Cryptosporidium*; paromomycin 165 mg/kg q12h for 5 days suggested (extra-label).

CONTRAINDICATIONS/POSSIBLE INTERACTIONS
N/A

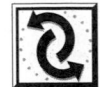

FOLLOW-UP
Fecal examination for oocysts 1–2 weeks following treatment

MISCELLANEOUS

AGE-RELATED FACTORS
More severe disease in young patients

SEE ALSO
• Toxoplasmosis
• Cryptosporidiosis

ABBREVIATION
s.g. = specific gravity

Suggested Reading
Bowman DD, Lynn RC, Eberhard ML. Georgi's parasitology for veterinarians, 8th ed. St. Louis: Saunders (Elsevier Science), 2003:92–100.
Bowman DD, Hendrix CM, Lindsay DS, Barr SC. Feline clinical parasitology. Ames: Iowa State University Press, 2002:5–14.

Acknowledgment
The author and editors acknowledge the prior contributions of Dr. Robert M. Corwin, who authored this topic in the previous edition.

Author Julie Ann Jarvinen
Consulting Editor Albert E. Jergens

COGNITIVE DYSFUNCTION SYNDROME

 BASICS

DEFINITION

Syndrome associated with brain aging. Leads to alterations in awareness, decreased responsiveness to stimuli, and deficits in learning and memory. Subtle signs are seen in early stages, referred to as cognitive decline.

PATHOPHYSIOLOGY

• Unclear which changes are associated with the clinical signs of cognitive decline
• Decline in neurons, increase in ventricular volume, and neurotoxic deposits including lipofuscin, ubiquitin, and beta-amyloid
• Possible correlations between the amount of beta-amyloid in the cerebral cortex and decline in cognitive ability • Toxic free radicals (reactive oxygen species) increase with age as a result of chronic illness and stressors, age-related decline in mitochondrial efficiency, and decreased clearance mechanisms. • Increased toxic free radicals appear to be correlated to cognitive decline.
• Compromised cerebral vascular blood flow may be contributory.
• Neurotransmission is compromised as toxins accumulate, blood flow is reduced, and neurons degenerate.

SYSTEMS AFFECTED

• Behavioral • Nervous

GENETICS

Genetic correlation with respect to the distribution of beta-amyloid and the age at which it begins to accumulate

INCIDENCE/PREVALENCE

• In different studies approximately 50% of dogs and cats >11 years of age may display at least one sign of cognitive decline. • 28% of dogs age 11 to 12 and 68% of dogs between the ages of 15 and 16 may show at least one sign. • Progressive—over 50% of dogs with at least one clinical sign show additional signs after 12 months.

SIGNALMENT

Species
Dogs and cats

Breed Predilection
None

Mean Age and Range
• Increased prevalence with increasing age
• Neuropsychological testing in dogs can identify a decline in cognitive function as early as 7 to 8 years of age. • Clinical signs in cats may develop at a slightly older age; neuropsychological testing has not been done in cats. • Deficits may not be noticed by pet owners until several years later except in dogs trained to perform more specialized tasks (e.g., hearing ear, seeing eye, drug detection, agility).

Predominant Sex
Neutered dogs may be at slightly higher risk.

SIGNS

Historical Findings
Using the acronym DISHA, most clinical signs can be placed in 5 categories:
• **D**isorientation, including getting lost in familiar environments, confusion, or inability to navigate through familiar routes (e.g., goes to the wrong side of door) • **I**nteractions with humans or other animals may be altered (possible decline in play, increased/decreased interest in affection, or an increase in irritability). • **S**leep-wake cycle alterations (temporal disorientation), including night waking or vocalization and perhaps an increase in sleep during the day
• **H**ousetraining and other previously learned behaviors might deteriorate. Housesoiling, lack of response to previously learned commands, or becoming less adept at performing learned tasks (e.g., agility, flyball, working ability) may occur. • **A**ctivity may be altered—inactivity, less interest in exploration, self-care, or even eating. As the condition progresses, the pet may become restless with pacing, aimless wandering, or compulsive activity disorders such as excessive licking.

Physical Examination
No specific abnormalities

CAUSES

• Exact cause is unknown and not all animals are affected. • Genetic factors may predispose pets to developing cognitive decline.
• See Pathophysiology.

RISK FACTORS

• Chronic or recurrent illness or stress might lead to increased accumulation of reactive oxygen species • Conditions that affect the cerebral vascular blood supply (e.g., systemic hypertension, anemia)

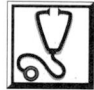 DIAGNOSIS

DIFFERENTIAL DIAGNOSIS

• Any medical condition or disease process that affects the pet's mental attitude or behavior must be ruled out. • Painful conditions (e.g., arthritis, dental disease) can lead to increased irritability or fear of being handled.
• If mobility is affected, the pet may become increasingly aggressive rather than retreat, and may be less able to access its elimination area.
• Impaired sight or hearing might lead to a decreased responsiveness or increased reactivity to stimuli. • Diseases of the urinary tract can cause or contribute to inappropriate urination. • Organ failure, tumors, and immune diseases can also affect behavior.

• Endocrinopathies such as hypothyroidism can lead to behavior changes ranging from lethargy to aggression, while dogs with hyper-adrenocorticism may exhibit altered sleep-wake cycles, lethargy, housesoiling, panting, and polyphagia. Hyperthyroidism in cats can lead to increased irritability, increased activity, and alterations in appetite. • Diseases that affect the central nervous system or its circulation, whether directly (tumors) or indirectly (e.g., anemia), can affect behavior.

CBC/BIOCHEMICAL/URINALYSIS

• Normal with CDS
• Used to screen for other diseases in senior pet with behavioral signs

OTHER LABORATORY TESTS

Normal with CDS

IMAGING

• Used to rule out primary organic/structural cause • Most important when there are abnormalities on the neurological examination or when the onset is sudden, and less likely to be of diagnostic value when the signs have been slowly progressive • Pets with cognitive dysfunction may have increased ventricular volume and an overall decline in brain mass, but these findings alone are not diagnostic.

DIAGNOSTIC PROCEDURES

• Endoscopy, radiography, ultrasound, and other specialized diagnostic procedures may be necessary to rule out other causes of the clinical signs. • Additional tests such as BAER testing or ophthalmologic referral might be indicated if sensory dysfunction is a suspected cause of the signs. • A therapeutic trial might be another diagnostic aid, for example, to determine the effects of pain management on the resolution of clinical signs.

PATHOLOGIC FINDINGS

• Evaluation of amyloid deposition might be indicative of the degree of cognitive dysfunction. This type of assessment is available only on postmortem samples in specialized laboratories.

 TREATMENT

APPROPRIATE HEALTH CARE
Outpatient care

NURSING CARE
Depends on the type and severity of the clinical signs of cognitive dysfunction

ACTIVITY AND TRAINING
• Maintain as much exercise, play, training, work, and other daily routines as is practical for the pet's age and health.
• Maintaining mental and physical stimulation has been shown to reduce the chance of cognitive decline.

DIET
- Selected based on the pet's health assessment
- If the pet's health does not require the need for a special therapeutic diet, then an antioxidant-fortified senior diet (e.g., Hill's Prescription Diet b/d™) should be utilized.
- Hill's Prescription Diet b/d has been shown to improve memory, learning ability, and clinical signs of cognitive dysfunction syndrome. Diet is supplemented with antioxidants such as vitamins E and C, selenium, beta carotene, and flavonoids and carotenoids in the form of fruits and vegetables, omega-3 fatty acids EPA and DHA to promote cell membranes, and carnitine and lipoic acid, which are purported to improve mitochondrial health.

CLIENT EDUCATION
- Lifelong therapy is required, and concurrent medications may be necessary if the pet has multiple problems. • Any changes in the pet's health or behavior should be reported immediately, as this may be due to the progression of previously diagnosed problems such as cognitive dysfunction or the emergence of new health problems.
- Considering the pet's health and cognitive status, the owner must be advised on any limitations on what might be achieved.

MEDICATIONS

DRUG(S) OF CHOICE

Selegiline
- Licensed for use in dogs in North America
- Monoamine oxidase (MAO) B inhibitor, in dogs, may contribute to improved dopamine transmission, lead to a decrease in free radicals, and have a neuroprotective effect.
- Dog dose: 0.5 to 1 mg/kg PO daily in the morning and maintained if effective
- Reevaluate clinical signs for improvement after 1 to 2 months.
- Side effects might include occasional gastrointestinal upset and restlessness, and repetitive behavior at higher doses.

Nicergoline
- Not licensed for use in dogs in North America, but is licensed in other countries
- Alpha-1 and alpha-2 adrenergic antagonists
- Used in elderly dogs with decreased activity, sleep disorders, decreased exercise tolerance, housesoiling (including incontinence), reduced appetite, and decreased awareness
- May increase cerebral blood flow, enhance neuronal transmission, have a neuroprotective effect on neural cells, increase dopamine and noradrenaline turnover, and inhibit platelet aggregation
- Dog dose: 0.25–0.5 mg/kg/PO daily each morning for 30 days and maintained if effective

Propentofylline
- Not licensed for use in dogs in North America, but is licensed in other countries
- Methylxanthine • Purported to inhibit platelet aggregation and thrombus formation, make the red cells more pliable, and increase blood flow • For use in the treatment of dullness and lethargy in old dogs
- May increase oxygen supply to the CNS without increasing glucose demand
- Dog dose: 3 mg/kg PO q12h

General Comment Regarding Cats
- No therapeutic agents licensed for treatment of CDS • Selegiline has been used off-label (0.5–1 mg/kg/day) and might be effective in cats with anxiety, decreased responsiveness to stimuli, nocturnal activity and vocalization, and decreased grooming and appetite.

CONTRAINDICATIONS
- Selegiline should not be used concurrently with MAO inhibitors such as amitraz, narcotics, or alpha-adrenergic agents such as phenylpropanolamine or ephedrine or selective serotonin reuptake inhibitors (e.g., fluoxetine) or tricyclic antidepressants (e.g., clomipramine or amitriptyline).
- A two-week washout is needed following most tricyclic antidepressants and 5 weeks following fluoxetine before starting selegiline.

PRECAUTIONS
- Choose medications that are least sedating and least anticholinergic. • Potential drug interactions must be considered since older pets may require multiple medications.

POSSIBLE INTERACTIONS
See Contraindications

ALTERNATIVE DRUG(S)
- Enhancement of the noradrenergic system with drugs such as adrafanil and modafinil to improve alertness and exploration
- Anti-inflammatory medication, hormone replacement therapy, phosphatidylserine, and gingko extract might be considered based on preliminary work in other species.
- Medication used in humans for Alzheimer's disease to enhance cholinergic transmission might be considered in refractory cases. Potential side effects include nausea, vomiting, diarrhea, and sleep-wake disturbances.
- Anxiolytics (e.g., buspirone), drugs to help induce sleep (e.g., benzodiazepines), or antidepressants (e.g., fluoxetine) might also be considered to treat generalized anxiety and apathy (but not in conjunction with selegiline).
- Homeopathic and natural supplements are also a consideration to help normalize sleep-wake cycles or reduce anxiety in the elderly pet (melatonin, valerian, Bach's flower remedies).

FOLLOW-UP

PATIENT MONITORING
- If a drug or diet is dispensed, then response to therapy should be evaluated after 30 to 60 days and the dose adjusted or treatment changed if there is insufficient improvement.
- If the pet is stable, twice-yearly checkups are recommended for senior pets unless new problems arise before a reassessment is due.

PREVENTION/AVOIDANCE
- Maintaining a stimulating environment and as much activity as is practical for the pet's age and health may help to prevent or delay the onset of cognitive decline.
- Early intervention is the best way to slow the progress or prevent complications.

EXPECTED COURSE AND PROGNOSIS
- Diet and medication should control the clinical signs and slow progression in a majority of cases. • Because of the pet's increasing age, cognitive decline may advance and other concurrent health problems are likely to arise despite medical intervention.

MISCELLANEOUS

ASSOCIATED CONDITIONS
None

SYNONYMS
- Senility • Dementia • Age-related cognitive and affective disorders, including confusional syndrome, involutive depression, dysthymia

ABBREVIATIONS
CDS = cognitive dysfunction syndrome

Suggested Reading
Bain MJ, Hart BL, Cliff KD, Ruehl WW. Predicting behavioral changes associated with age-related cognitive impairment in dogs. J Am Vet Med Assoc 218;1792–1795, 2001.

Landsberg GM, Hunthausen W, Ackerman L. Handbook of behaviour problems of the dog and cat. 2nd ed. Philadelphia: Saunders (in press for 2003).

Landsberg GM, Ruehl WW. Geriatric behavioral problems. Vet Clin N Am Sm Anim Pract 27;1537–1559, 1997.

Nielson JC, Hart BL, Cliff KD, Ruehl WW. Prevalence of behavioral changes associated with age-related cognitive cognitive impairment in dogs. J Am Vet Med Assoc 218 (11);1787–1791, 2001.

Author Gary Landsberg
Consulting Editor Debra F. Horwitz

COLD AGGLUTININ DISEASE

BASICS

OVERVIEW
• A rare type II autoimmune disorder in which antierythrocyte antibodies have enhanced activity at temperatures < 99°F (37.2°C) and usually < 88°F (31.1°C)
• Cold agglutinins are typically IgM, although IgG and IgG-IgM mixed have been reported.
• Cold agglutinins with low thermal amplitude usually associated with direct erythrocyte agglutination at low body temperatures in the peripheral microvasculature and with acrocyanotic disease or other peripheral vaso-occlusive phenomena, all initiated or intensified by cold exposure
• Fixation of complement and hemolysis is a warm reactive process occurring at high body temperatures; therefore, patients may have very high titers of cold agglutinins, but these antibodies may be unable to hemolyze erythrocytes at temperatures achieved in the bloodstream.
• Most cold agglutinins cause little or no shortening of erythrocyte life span.
• High thermal amplitude cold agglutinins (rare)—may cause sustained hemolysis; resulting anemia is often mild and stable, but exposure to cold may greatly augment binding of cold agglutinins and complement-mediated intravascular hemolysis.

SIGNALMENT
• Rare disorder in dogs and cats
• Low titer of naturally occurring cold agglutinins (usually 1:32 or less) may be found in healthy dogs and cats; this is without clinical significance.
• Genetic basis, mean age and range, breed and sex predilections unknown
• More likely to occur in colder climates

SIGNS
• Often a history of cold exposure
• Acrocyanosis associated with sludging of erythrocyte agglutinates in cutaneous microvasculature
• Erythema
• Skin ulceration with secondary crusting
• Dry, gangrenous necrosis of ear tips, tail tip, nose, and feet
• Affected areas may be painful.
• Anemia may or may not be an important feature; clinical signs include pallor, weakness, tachycardia, tachypnea, icterus, pigmenturia, mild splenomegaly, and soft heart murmur.

CAUSES & RISK FACTORS
• Primary disease—idiopathic
• Secondary disease—associated with upper respiratory infection (cats), neonatal isoerythrolysis, and lead intoxication (dogs)
• Cold exposure a risk factor

DIAGNOSIS

DIFFERENTIAL DIAGNOSIS
• Diagnosis made by historical findings (cold exposure), results of physical examination, demonstrating cold agglutination in vitro
• Skin lesions—cutaneous vasculitis, hepatocutaneous syndrome, erythema multiforme, toxic epidermic necrolysis, dermatomyositis, DIC, SLE, lymphoreticular neoplasms, frostbite, lead poisoning, and pemphigus
• Anemia—warm antibody hemolytic anemia; other causes of anemia
• Macroscopic hemagglutination in vitro—dysproteinemias may lead to rouleaux formation, mimicking erythrocyte agglutination on a glass slide.

CBC/BIOCHEMISTRY/URINALYSIS
• Autoagglutination at room temperature
• Laboratory abnormalities secondary to hemolysis

OTHER LABORATORY TESTS
• Cold agglutinins should be suspected when blood in heparin or EDTA on a glass slide agglutinates spontaneously at room temperature with enhancement at 39°F (3.9°C), and the erythrocytes disperse again upon warming to 99°F (37.2°C)
• If no agglutination can be induced in vitro, it is inconceivable for it to occur in vivo in extremities.

• Doubtful cases can be confirmed by Coombs test at 39°F and 99°F
• Coombs test at 99°F—cold agglutinins usually not detected because they may be eluted off the erythrocytes during washing; thus test requires the use of anti-complement factor serum.
• Coombs test at 39°F—incidence of a positive result in healthy dogs has been reported to be > 50%, which may be caused by unspecific binding of the reagent itself or by binding of naturally occurring nonpathogenic low-titer cold agglutinins
• The globulin class can be established by immunoelectrophoresis of a concentrated eluate of the patient's erythrocytes, which is important for prognosis and treatment.

PATHOLOGIC FINDINGS
• Dermal necrosis
• Ulceration with secondary features of opportunistic infections
• Vascular thrombosis with evidence of ischemic necrosis

TREATMENT
• The patient should be hospitalized in a warm environment until the disease is nonprogressive.

• Supportive care and wound management depend on clinical signs; if necrosis involving the tail tip or feet is severe, amputation may be required.
• Splenectomy of little assistance in patients with IgM-mediated hemolytic disorders, but may be helpful in those with therapy-resistant IgG-mediated hemolytic anemia
• Inform the client to keep the patient in a warm environment at all times to prevent relapse.

MEDICATIONS

DRUG(S)

IgM Cold Agglutinins
• Immunosuppressive therapy is not very effective against IgM-mediated disorders but should be tried (i.e., corticosteroids, cyclophosphamide, or azathioprine).
• Plasmapheresis

IgG Cold Agglutinins
Immunosuppressive therapy

CONTRAINDICATIONS/POSSIBLE INTERACTIONS
• Monitor patient for signs of infection secondary to immunosuppressive therapy.
• Do not use cold IV fluids.

FOLLOW-UP
• A patient with known cold agglutinin disease should be kept in warm environments at all times.
• Cold agglutinin disease usually characterized by acute onset and rapid progression
• Prognosis guarded to fair
• Recovery may take weeks.

MISCELLANEOUS

SEE ALSO
Anemia, Immune-mediated

ABBREVIATIONS
• DIC = disseminated intravascular coagulation
• EDTA = ethylene diamine tetraacetic acid
• SLE = systemic lupus erythematosus

Suggested Reading
Dickson NJ. Cold agglutinin disease in a puppy associated with lead intoxication. J Small Anim Pract 1990;31:105–108.
Author Jörg Bücheler
Consulting Editor Stephen A. Kruth

COLIBACILLOSIS

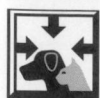 BASICS

DEFINITION
• *Escherichia coli*—gram-negative member of the Enterobacteriaceae; normal inhabitant of the intestine of most mammals; along with other infectious agents, may increase the severity of parvovirus infections
• Acute infection of puppies and kittens in the first week of life; characterized by septicemia and multiple organ involvement
• Isolation from stool of young animals—inconclusive evidence of pathogenic potential because it is normal flora
• Isolation from blood cultures or internal organs—good evidence of causality
• Infection of old dogs and cats—documented; individual strains poorly characterized in regard to virulence attributes

Pathophysiology
• Virulence factors—not well defined; likely *E. coli* as a cause of septicemia in neonatal dogs and cats has more to do with the immunologic immaturity of the host than with the virulence of a particular strain
• ETEC, EPEC, uropathogenic *E. coli,* and CNF+ *E. coli* strains—recovered from dogs
• EPEC, VTEC, and uropathogenic *E. coli* strains—isolated from cats
• Intestinal strains colonize and multiply in the small intestine; ETEC then elaborates *E. coli* K99 or other uncharacterized adhesins and enterotoxins; the attaching and effacing factor of ETEC (EAE+) or VTEC (EAE+) produces SLT.
• Many strains of *E. coli* from dogs and cats are hemolytic.

SYSTEMS AFFECTED
• Neonates—small intestine (enteritis); multiple body systems (septicemia)
• Puppies/kittens and adults—small intestine (enteritis); urogenital (cystitis, endometritis, pyelonephritis, prostatitis); mammary gland (mastitis)

GENETICS
N/A

INCIDENCE/PREVALENCE
• Few statistics available
• More common in neonatal puppies and kittens < 1 week old that have not received any or adequate amounts of colostrum
• Problem in overpopulated kennels and catteries
• Sporadic accounts in old dogs and cats (mainly diarrhea and urogenital problems)
• Purulent skin disease and otitis and meningoencephalomyelitis

Dogs
• ETEC—2.7–29.5% of diarrheic dogs; strains: K99+/−, Sta/STb+/−, and CNF+ isolated from diarrheic dogs along with hemolysin
• *E. coli* (usually β-hemolytic)—major cause of septicemia in newborn puppies exposed in utero, during birth, or from mastitic milk

Cats
EPEC/VTEC—diarrheic cats; strains: EAE+, SLT+, hemolytic, aerobactin+, serum resistant, and CNF+

GEOGRAPHIC DISTRIBUTION
Worldwide

SIGNALMENT

Species
Dogs and cats

Breed Predilections
None

Mean Age and Range
• Neonatal infections common (diarrhea, septicemia) up to 2 weeks of age
• Puppies/kittens and adult animals—sporadic disease often associated with other infectious agents

Predominant Sex
None

SIGNS

General Comments
E. coli—one of the most common causes of septicemia and death in puppies and kittens

Historical Findings
• Neonates—sudden-onset vomiting, weakness/lethargy, diarrhea, cold skin; one or more animals affected in a litter
• Puppies/kittens and adults—vomiting and diarrhea

Physical Examination Findings
• Neonates—acute depression, anorexia, vomiting, tachycardia, weakness, hypothermia, cyanosis, watery diarrhea
• Puppies/kittens and adults—ETEC associated with acute vomiting, diarrhea, anorexia, rapid dehydration, fever

CAUSES
• *E. coli*—member of the endogenous microbial flora of the adult's gastrointestinal tract, prepuce, and vagina
• Many strains isolated from case material are poorly characterized in regard to virulence factors.
• Often found in old dogs and cats concurrently with other infectious agents

RISK FACTORS

Neonates
• Bitch/queen in poor health and nutritional status—unable to provide good care and colostrum to offspring

• Lack of colostrum or insufficient colostrum
• Dirty birthing environment
• Difficult or prolonged labor and birth
• Crowded facilities—build up of feces in environment, greater chance for fecal–oral spread of infection

Puppies/Kittens and Adults
• Concurrent disease—parvovirus; heavy parasitism
• Antimicrobial drugs—upset microbial flora of gastrointestinal tract
• Immunosuppression
• Post-parturient mastitis
• Venous catheterization

 DIAGNOSIS

DIFFERENTIAL DIAGNOSIS
• Infectious enteritis—viral: feline panleukopenia, FeLV, FIV, enteric coronavirus, canine parvovirus, rotavirus, canine distemper; bacterial: *Salmonella, E. coli, Campylobacter jejuni, Yersinia enterocolitica;* bacterial overgrowth syndrome, *Clostridium difficile, Clostridium perfringens;* parasitic: hookworms, ascarids, whipworms, *Strongyloides, Giardia,* coccidia, *Cryptosporidia; Rickettsiae* (salmon poisoning)
• Dietary-induced enteritis—overeating; abrupt changes; starvation; thirst; food intolerance or allergy; indiscretions (e.g., foreign material or garbage)
• Drug- or toxin-induced enteritis—antimicrobial agents; antineoplastic agents; anthelmintics; heavy metals; organophosphates
• Extraintestinal disorders or metabolic diseases—acute pancreatitis; hypoadrenocorticism; liver or kidney disease; pyometra; peritonitis
• Functional or mechanical ileus—gastricdilatation volvulus; intussusception; electrolyte disorder; gastrointestinal foreign body
• Neurologic disorders—vestibular disease; psychogenic such as fear, excitement, pain
• Fading neonates

CBC/BIOCHEMISTRY/URINALYSIS
• Few abnormalities noted, owing to rapidity of death in puppies
• Adults with enteritis may show chemistry abnormality, depending on the state of dehydration.

OTHER LABORATORY TESTS
N/A

IMAGING
N/A

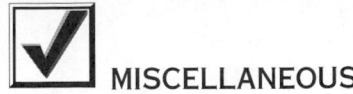

DIAGNOSTIC PROCEDURES

• Antimicrobials—produce false-negative results if used before obtaining bacterial cultures
• Routine bacterial culture and identification of *E. coli* from blood (antemortem) or necropsy tissue (bone marrow, heart blood, liver/spleen, brain, mesenteric lymph node) required
• Appropriate testing of strains—identify adhesins and toxins (by DNA colony hybridization, PCR) in ETEC and VTEC strains.

PATHOLOGIC FINDINGS

• Acute enteritis
• Mucosal inflammation of small intestine
• Petechiae and hemorrhagic lesions on serosal surface of gastrointestinal mucosae and all body cavities
• Fibrin on abdominal wall
• Necrosis of liver/spleen

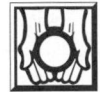 TREATMENT

APPROPRIATE HEALTH CARE

Acutely ill puppies/kittens—inpatients; good nursing care

NURSING CARE

• Balanced parenteral polyionic isotonic solution (lactated Ringer's)—restore fluid balance
• Oral hypertonic glucose solution—for secretory diarrhea, as required

ACTIVITY

Acutely ill immature puppies/kittens (bacteremic/septicemic)—restricted activity, cage rest, monitoring, and warmth

DIET

Puppies—likely to still be nursing when affected; good nursing care needed with bottle-feeding and/or IV nutrients

CLIENT EDUCATION

Neonates—life-threatening with poor prognosis

SURGICAL CONSIDERATIONS

N/A

 MEDICATIONS

DRUG(S) OF CHOICE

• Antimicrobial therapy—septicemia
• Guided by culture and susceptibility (MIC) testing of *E. coli;* empiric therapy until results available
• Trimethoprim-sulfa—dogs, 30 mg/kg PO q12–24h; cats, 30 mg/kg PO or SC q12–24h

• Chloramphenicol—dogs, 50 mg/kg PO, IM, IV, or SC q8h; cats, 12.5–20 mg/kg PO, IV, IM, or SC q12h
• Amoxicillin—dogs and cats, 10–20 mg/kg PO q8–12h

CONTRAINDICATIONS

Fluoroquinolones—do not use in immature dogs and cats

PRECAUTIONS

Chloramphenicol and trimethoprim-sulfa—use with caution in neonates; monitor

POSSIBLE INTERACTION

N/A

ALTERNATIVE DRUG(S)

• Adult—fluoroquinolones: in dogs only (enrofloxacin, 2.5–5 mg/kg PO q12h); avoid use in pregnant, neonatal, or growing animals (medium-sized dogs < 8 months of age; large or giant breeds < 12–18 months of age) because of cartilage lesions
• Immature—third-generation cephalosporin class drugs

 FOLLOW-UP

PATIENT MONITORING

• Blood culture—puppies/kittens with fever and/or diarrhea
• Monitor temperature—with signs of lethargy and/or depression
• Monitor behavior—eating, drinking, and/or nursing; adequate weight gain

PREVENTION/AVOIDANCE

• Bitch/queen—good health; vaccinated; good nutritional status
• Clean and disinfect parturition environment (1:32 dilution of bleach); clean bedding after birth frequently.
• Ensure adequate colostrum intake of all litter mates.
• Separate mother with nursing litter from other cats or dogs.
• Keep the density low in kennel or cattery rooms.
• Wash hands and change clothes and shoes after handling other cats/dogs and before dealing with neonates.

POSSIBLE COMPLICATIONS

N/A

EXPECTED COURSE AND PROGNOSIS

• Neonates—life-threatening; prognosis often poor; neonate may rapidly succumb; quick treatment with supportive care essential for survival
• Adults—self-limiting with supportive care, depending on the degree of dehydration and existence of other diseases

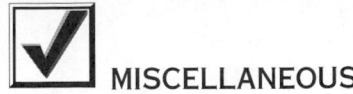 MISCELLANEOUS

ASSOCIATED CONDITIONS

N/A

AGE-RELATED FACTORS

Neonates—greatest risk of infection and subsequent septicemia

ZOONOTIC POTENTIAL

• Little documented information of the virulence potential of *E. coli* strains from dogs or cats for humans, although recently, similarities have been found between canine UTI *E. coli* and human extraintestinal *E. coli.*
• Always wash hands after handling animals (especially patients with diarrhea) because of the risk of acquiring other infectious agents (e.g., salmonellae, *Giardia*)
• **CAUTION:** keep children and immuno-suppressed persons away from pets with diarrhea

PREGNANCY

N/A

SYNONYMS

• Neonatal enteritis
• *E. coli* septicemia

ABBREVIATIONS

• CNF = cytotoxic necrotizing factor
• DNA = deoxyribonucleic acid
• EAE = experimental autoimmune encephalomyelitis
• EPEC = enteropathogenic *E. coli*
• ETEC = enterotoxigenic *E. coli*
• FeLV = feline leukemia virus
• FIV = feline immunodeficiency virus
• MIC = minimal inhibitory concentration
• PCR = polymerase chain reaction
• SLT = Shiga-like toxin
• UTI = urinary tract infection
• VTEC = verocytotoxigenic *E. coli*

Suggested Reading

Gyles CL. *Escherichia coli.* In: Gyles CL, Thoen CO, eds. Pathogenesis of bacterial infections in animals. 2nd ed. Ames: Iowa State University Press, 1993:164–187.
Kruth SA. Gram-negative bacterial infections. In: Greene CE, ed. Infectious diseases of the dog and cat. Philadelphia: Saunders, 1998:217–222.
Peeters JE. *Escherichia coli* infections in rabbits, cats, dogs, goats and horses. In: Gyles CL, ed. *Escherichia coli* in domestic animals and humans. United Kingdom: Wallingford: Commonwealth Agricultural Bureaux, 1994:261–283.
Authors Patrick L. McDonough and Kenneth W. Simpson
Consulting Editor Stephen C. Barr

COLITIS AND PROCTITIS

BASICS

DEFINITION
- Colitis—inflammation of the colon
- Proctitis—inflammation of the rectum

PATHOPHYSIOLOGY
- Inflammation of the colon causes accumulation of inflammatory cytokines, disrupts tight junctions between epithelial cells, stimulates colonic secretion, stimulates goblet cell secretion of mucus, and disrupts motility.
- These mechanisms reduce the ability of the colon to absorb water and store feces, which causes frequent diarrhea, often with mucus or blood.

SYSTEMS AFFECTED
Gastrointestinal

GENETICS
Breed predisposition to histiocytic ulcerative colitis in young boxers

INCIDENCE/PREVALENCE
Approximately 30% of dogs with chronic diarrhea examined at the University of Florida Veterinary Medical Teaching Hospital; prevalence not well documented

GEOGRAPHIC DISTRIBUTION
- Generally N/A, but pythiosis is seen in Gulf Coast and southeast United States
- Histoplasmosis is seen in the Midwest and, to a lesser extent, the eastern United States.

SIGNALMENT
Species
Dogs and cats

Breed Predilections
Boxer (histiocytic ulcerative colitis)

Mean Age and Range
Any age; boxers usually symptomatic by 2 years old

Predominant Sex
None

SIGNS
Historical Findings
- Feces vary from semiformed to liquid
- High frequency of defecation with small fecal volume
- Often demonstrate prolonged tenesmus after defecation
- Chronic diarrhea often with mucus or blood; cats may have formed feces with hematochezia.
- Vomiting in some (~30%) dogs
- Weight loss is rare.

Physical Examination Findings
- Usually normal
- Dogs with histiocytic ulcerative colitis may show systemic signs of weight loss and anorexia.

CAUSES
- Infectious—*Trichuris vulpis, Ancylostoma caninum, Entamoeba histolytica, Balantidium coli, Giardia spp., Trichomonas spp., Cryptosporidium spp., Salmonella spp., Clostridium spp., Campylobacter spp., Yersinia enterocolitica, Escherichia coli, Prototheca, Histoplasma capsulatum,* and pythiosis/phycomycosis
- Traumatic—foreign body and abrasive material
- Uremia
- Segmental—secondary to chronic pancreatitis (transverse colitis)
- Allergic—dietary protein and possibly bacterial protein
- Inflammatory/immune—lymphoplasmacytic, eosinophilic, granulomatous, and histiocytic

RISK FACTORS
N/A

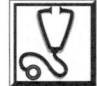
DIAGNOSIS

DIFFERENTIAL DIAGNOSIS
- Neoplasia—lymphoma and adenocarcinoma
- Irritable bowel syndrome
- Rectocolonic polyps
- Cecal inversion
- Ileocecocolic intussusception

CBC/BIOCHEMISTRY/URINALYSIS
- Results usually normal; neutrophilia with a left shift is possible; eosinophilia occasionally observed in eosinophilic colitis, parasitism, and pythiosis/phycomycosis
- Mild microcytic, hypochromic anemia may occur in some patients with persistent bleeding.
- Rare hyperglobulinemia in some patients (especially cats) with chronic disease

OTHER LABORATORY TESTS
- Examination of fecal flotation, direct fecal smear, bacterial culture, or fungal culture (*Pythium*) may reveal an infectious cause.
- Feces may test positive for *Clostridium perfringens* toxin.
- Budding organisms (spores) may support clostridial toxin.
- Rectal cytology for *Histoplasma* organisms

IMAGING
- Abdominal radiographs—usually normal
- Barium enema—may reveal mucosal irregularities or filling defects in severely affected patients, but this procedure is time-consuming and not cost-effective
- Abdominal ultrasonography—may reveal masses, diffuse thickening, or altered architecture.

OTHER DIAGNOSTIC PROCEDURES
- Colonoscopy with biopsy—technique of choice for diagnosis; may see disappearance of submucosal blood vessels, granular appearance of mucosa, hyperemia, excessive mucus, ulceration, pinpoint hemorrhage (small ulcerations), or mass
- Always take multiple biopsy specimens because the extent of mucosal change does not necessarily reflect severity or absence of disease.

PATHOLOGIC FINDINGS
- Gross findings as described
- Histopathologic findings depend on the histologic type of colitis—lymphoplasmacytic, eosinophilic, granulomatous, or histiocytic; hyperplastic mucosa may be seen with irritable bowel syndrome; various infectious agents may be seen with special stains.

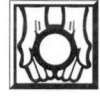
TREATMENT

APPROPRIATE HEALTH CARE
Outpatient medical management unless diarrhea is severe enough to cause dehydration

NURSING CARE
Give dehydrated patients balanced electrolyte solution with potassium, intravenously, subcutaneously, or orally.

ACTIVITY
N/A

DIET
- Patients with acute colitis can be fasted for 24–48 h.
- Try a hypoallergenic diet in patients with inflammatory colitis; use a commercial or home-prepared diet that contains a protein to which the dog or cat has not been exposed.
- Fiber supplementation with poorly fermented fiber (e.g., bran and α-cellulose) is recommended to increase fecal bulk, improve colonic muscle contractility, and bind fecal water to produce formed feces.
- Some fermentable fiber (e.g., psyllium or a diet containing beet pulp or fructooligosaccharides) may be beneficial—short-chain fatty acids produced by fermentation may help the colon heal and restore normal colonic bacterial flora.

CLIENT EDUCATION
- Treatment may be intermittent and long-term in patients with inflammatory/immune colitis, and repeated recurrence is seen in some cases, especially those with the histiocytic and granulomatous forms.
- Granulomatous and histiocytic colitis, pythiosis/phycomycosis, and protothecal colitis respond poorly to medical treatment; surgery may be necessary.

SURGICAL CONSIDERATIONS
Segments of colon severely affected by fibrosis from chronic inflammation and subsequent stricture formation may need surgical excision,

especially in patients with the granulomatous form of the disease; cecal inversion and ileocecocolic intussusception require surgical intervention; pythiosis/phycomycosis often requires surgical excision or debulking.

MEDICATIONS

DRUG(S) OF CHOICE

Antimicrobial Drugs
• *Trichuris, Ancylostoma,* and *Giardia*—fenbendazole (50 mg/kg PO q24h for 3 days, repeat in 3 months)
• *Entamoeba, Balantidium, Giardia,* and *Trichomonas*—metronidazole (25 mg/kg PO q12h for 5–7 days)
• *Salmonella*—treatment is controversial because a carrier state can be induced; in patients with systemic involvement, choose the antibiotic on the basis of bacterial culture and sensitivity testing (e.g., enrofloxacin, chloramphenicol, or trimethoprim-sulfa).
• *Clostridium*—metronidazole (10–15 mg/kg PO q12h for 5–14 days) or tylosin (10–15 mg/kg PO q12h for 7 days)
• *Campylobacter*—erythromycin (30–40 mg/kg PO q24h for 5 days) or tylosin (45 mg/kg PO q24h for 5 days)
• *Yersinia* and *E. coli*—choose the drug on the basis of bacterial culture and sensitivity testing
• *Prototheca*—no known treatment
• *Histoplasma*—itraconazole (dogs, 5 mg/kg PO q24h; cats, 5 mg/kg PO q12 h; several months of therapy is necessary); amphotericin B (0.25–0.5 mg/kg slow IV q48h up to cumulative dose of 4–8 mg/kg) in advanced cases
• Pythiosis/phycomycosis—ABLC (dilute in 5% dextrose to 1 mg/mL, give 3 mg/kg IV Monday-Wednesday-Friday for 9 treatments)

Antiinflammatory and Immunosuppressive Drugs for Inflammatory/Immune Colitis
• Sulfasalazine (dogs, 25–40 mg/kg PO q8h for 2–4 weeks; cats, 20 mg/kg PO q12h for 2 weeks)
• Corticosteroids—prednisone (dogs, 1–2 mg/kg PO q24h; cats, 2–4 mg/kg PO q24h; taper dosage slowly over 4–6 months once clinical remission is achieved)
• Azathioprine (dogs, 1 mg/kg PO q24h for 2 weeks followed by alternate-day administration; cats, 0.3 mg/kg PO q24h for 3–4 months)
• Sulfasalazine—drug of choice for plasmacytic lymphocytic colitis
• Prednisone and azathioprine are indicated only in eosinophilic colitis and *severe* plasmacytic lymphocytic colitis that does not respond to sulfasalazine.
• Histiocytic ulcerative colitis in boxer dogs may respond to treatment with a triple antibiotic combination of metronidazole at 15–20 mg/kg PO q12h, amoxicillin-

clavulanate (Clavamox) at 25 mg/kg PO q12h, and enrofloxacin at 5 mg/kg PO q24h for a minimum period of 6 weeks.
• Reexamine the diagnosis carefully in dogs that do not respond to sulfasalazine treatment in 4 weeks; the need for chronic maintenance therapy means that an underlying cause (e.g., *C. perfringens* infection) may have been missed.

Motility Modifiers (Symptomatic Relief Only)
• Loperamide (0.1 mg/kg PO q8–12h)
• Diphenoxylate (0.1–0.2 mg/kg PO q8h)
• Propantheline bromide (0.25–0.5 mg/kg PO q8h) if colonic spasm is contributing to clinical signs

CONTRAINDICATIONS
Anticholinergics

PRECAUTIONS
• Monitor patients on sulfasalazine for signs of keratoconjunctivitis sicca.
• Monitor patients on azathioprine for bone marrow suppression—CBC every 2–3 weeks; stop treatment or go to alternate-day if WBC count falls below 3000 cells/µL.
• Amphotericin B and ABLC are nephrotoxic and require renal assessment and monitoring.

POSSIBLE INTERACTIONS
N/A

ALTERNATIVE DRUG(S)
Albendazole (25 mg/kg PO q12h for 2 days) to treat giardiasis if fenbendazole or metronidazole is ineffective

FOLLOW-UP

PATIENT MONITORING
Infrequent recheck examinations or client communication by phone

PREVENTION/AVOIDANCE
• Avoid exposure to infectious agents (e.g., other dogs, contaminated foods, moist environments).
• Avoid abrupt dietary changes.

POSSIBLE COMPLICATIONS
• Recurrence of signs without treatment, when treatment is tapered, and with progression of disease
• Stricture formation due to chronic inflammation

EXPECTED COURSE AND PROGNOSIS
• Most infections—excellent with treatment (cure)
• *Prototheca*—grave; no known treatment except excision
• *Histoplasma*—poor in moderate-to-advanced or disseminated disease; mild cases generally respond to therapy

• Pythiosis/phycomycosis—guarded to poor; poorly responsive to treatment; some dogs have fair results with excision and ABLC
• Traumatic, uremic, and segmental—good, if underlying cause is treatable
• Cecal inversion, ileocecocolic intussusception, and polyps—good with surgical removal
• Inflammatory—good with treatment in patients with lymphoplasmacytic and eosinophilic disease; most patients with lymphoplasmacytic colitis respond to sulfasalazine therapy within 2–4 weeks of treatment.
• Reexamine the diagnosis if signs persist; prognosis is poor in patients with granulomatous and histiocytic disease in the short term and worsens with recurrence or poor response to treatment.

MISCELLANEOUS

ASSOCIATED CONDITIONS
Inflammatory/immune disease and infectious agents may also affect the small intestine.

AGE-RELATED FACTORS
N/A

ZOONOTIC POTENTIAL
Entamoeba, Balantidium, Giardia, Salmonella, Clostridium, Campylobacter, Yersinia, and *E. coli; Prototheca, Histoplasma* in immunosuppressed individuals

PREGNANCY
Caution with drug use—corticosteroids, azathioprine, antifungals, and antibiotics

SYNONYMS
• Large bowel diarrhea
• Inflammatory bowel disease

SEE ALSO
• Colitis, Histiocytic Ulcerative
• Individual infectious and parasitic agents
• Inflammatory Bowel Disease

ABBREVIATION
ABLC = Amphotericin B lipid complex

Suggested Reading
Burrows CF. Canine colitis. Comp Cont Ed Pract Vet 1992;10:1347–1354.
Leib MS, Matz ME. Diseases of the large intestine. In: Ettinger SJ, Feldman EC, eds., Textbook of veterinary internal medicine. Philadelphia: Saunders, 1995:1232–1260.
Sherding RG, Burrows CF. Diarrhea. In: Anderson NV, ed., Veterinary gastroenterology. Philadelphia: Lea & Febiger, 1992:455–477.
Authors Colin F. Burrows and Lisa E. Moore
Consulting Editors Albert E. Jergens

COLITIS, HISTIOCYTIC ULCERATIVE

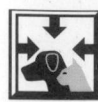

BASICS

OVERVIEW
• Rare disease characterized by colonic mucosal ulceration and inflammation with periodic acid–Schiff (PAS) positive histiocytes
• Etiologic and pathogenic mechanism unknown

SIGNALMENT
• Dogs; primarily affects young boxers, usually less than 2 years of age
• Reported in a French bulldog, a mastiff, an Alaskan malamute, and a Doberman pinscher
• Possible genetic basis, but unknown

SIGNS
• Bloody, mucoid diarrhea with increasing frequency of defecation
• Tenesmus
• Weight loss and debilitation may develop late in the disease process

CAUSES & RISK FACTORS
No known cause or predisposing factors

DIAGNOSIS

DIFFERENTIAL DIAGNOSIS
• Other causes of colitis—nonhistiocytic IBD, infectious colitis, parasitic colitis, allergic colitis
• Cecal inversion
• Ileocolic intussusception
• Neoplasia—lymphoma, adenocarcinoma
• Foreign body
• Rectocolonic polyps
• Irritable bowel syndrome
• Differentiate by examination of fecal flotations, direct smears, bacterial culture for pathogens, abdominal imaging, and colonoscopy and biopsy

CBC/BIOCHEMISTRY/URINALYSIS
• Usually normal
• Neutrophilia and mild anemia in some patients

OTHER LABORATORY TESTS
N/A

IMAGING
N/A

DIAGNOSTIC PROCEDURES
Colonoscopy reveals patchy red foci (pinpoint ulcerations), overt ulceration, thick mucosal folds, areas of granulation tissue, and strictures; take multiple biopsy specimens.

PATHOLOGIC FINDINGS
• Thickening of the lamina propria and infiltration of the mucosa and submucosa with histiocytes, lymphocytes, and plasma cells; ulceration with neutrophil infiltration in some animals
• Histiocytes are PAS positive.

TREATMENT
• Outpatient medical management
• Change diet to include fiber supplementation.
• Advise owner of progressive nature, possibility of recurrence, and ultimate inability to control disease.

MEDICATIONS

DRUGS
Antiinflammatory/Immunosuppressive Drugs
• Corticosteroids—prednisone (1–2 mg/kg PO q24h until clinical remission, then taper slowly over 4–6 months)
• Sulfasalazine (25–40 mg/kg PO q8h)
• Azathioprine (2 mg/kg q24h for 2 weeks followed by alternate-day administration)

Antimicrobials
• Metronidazole (15 mg/kg PO q12h)
• Tylosin (45 mg/kg PO q24h)

CONTRAINDICATIONS/POSSIBLE INTERACTIONS
• Avoid anticholinergics.
• Monitor for keratoconjunctivitis sicca, sometimes seen with sulfasalazine therapy.
• Monitor for immunosuppression (CBCs), sometimes seen with azathioprine.

FOLLOW-UP

PATIENT MONITORING
Clinical signs and body weight every week to 2 weeks initially

PREVENTION/AVOIDANCE
N/A

POSSIBLE COMPLICATIONS
• Progressive, uncontrollable disease
• Colonic stricture

EXPECTED COURSE AND PROGNOSIS
Patient may initially respond to treatment if begun early in course of disease; eventually, the disease usually progresses over months; prognosis is guarded.

MISCELLANEOUS

PREGNANCY
• Cautions with drug use—corticosteroids, azathioprine
• Patients probably should not be bred, because of the potential for inheritance.

SEE ALSO
Colitis and Proctitis

ABBREVIATIONS
• IBD = inflammatory bowel disease
• PAS = periodic acid–Schiff

Suggested Reading
Churcher RK, Watson ADJ. Canine histiocytic ulcerative colitis. Aust Vet J 1997;75:710–713.
Hall EJ, Rutgers HC, et al. Histiocytic ulcerative colitis in boxer dogs in the U.K. J Small Anim Pract 1994;35:509–515.
Sherding RG, Burrows CF. Diarrhea. In: Anderson NV, ed. Veterinary gastroenterology. Philadelphia: Lea & Febiger, 1992:465–466.
Author Lisa E. Moore
Consulting Editor Albert E. Jergens

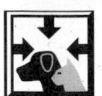

BASICS

OVERVIEW
• Congenital, autosomal recessive condition minimally consisting of temporal to superotemporal choroidal hypoplasia and excessive tortuosity of primary retinal vessels
• Possible accompanying defects indicating more severe manifestations—optic nerve coloboma; staphyloma; retinal detachment; intraocular hemorrhage
• Always bilateral; may note disparate severity between the eyes
• Potential for blindness because of retinal detachment
• Associated anomalies not directly part of syndrome—enophthalmia; microphthalmia; retinal folds; mineralization of the anterior corneal stroma
• Approximately 85% of collies in North America are homozygously affected or heterozygous carriers.
• Up to 30% of collies in Europe are affected or carriers.

SIGNALMENT
• Dogs
• Present at birth
• Seen in both smooth- and rough-coated collies
• Similar condition affects Shetland sheepdogs, Australian shepherds, and border collies

SIGNS
• None to partial or complete blindness
• Minimal ophthalmoscopic findings necessary for diagnosis—increased retinal vessel tortuosity and choroidal hypoplasia
• Vessels tortuous and disorganized (radiating pattern normal)
• Choroidal hypoplasia—a focal to diffuse area of anomalous choroidal vasculature; reduced number of vessels; temporal or superotemporal to the optic disk; may extend more nasally with severe disease
• Overlying tapetum—usually focally absent; allows visualization of the underlying choroid
• Underlying sclera—may be seen between choroidal vessels

• May note optic nerve coloboma (pitting of the optic nerve head), retinal detachment, and intraocular hemorrhage

CAUSES & RISK FACTORS
• Autosomal recessive trait; occurs only from mating between affected or carrier animals

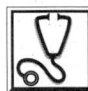

DIAGNOSIS

DIFFERENTIAL DIAGNOSIS
• Excessive tortuosity of retinal vessels with no choroidal hypoplasia—not classified as collie eye anomaly
• Merling of the coat—usually associated with lack of pigment in the pigmented epithelial layer of the retina, allowing visualization of normal choroidal vasculature; differentiated by normal, regular, radiating choroidal vessels
• Optic nerve colobomas and retinal detachment not accompanied by choroidal hypoplasia—not classified as collie eye anomaly

CBC/BIOCHEMISTRY/URINALYSIS
N/A

OTHER LABORATORY TESTS
N/A

IMAGING
N/A

DIAGNOSTIC PROCEDURES
N/A

TREATMENT
• None for reversal of condition
• Cryosurgery or laser surgery around the area of the optic nerve coloboma—may prevent retinal detachment; may be used to help reattach a retina

MEDICATIONS

DRUG(S)
None

CONTRAINDICATIONS/POSSIBLE INTERACTIONS
N/A

FOLLOW-UP

PATIENT MONITORING
Patients with colobomas—monitor during first year of life for secondary retinal detachment; after 1 year, retinal detachments rarely occur.

PREVENTION/AVOIDANCE
• Breed only genotypically normal dogs
• Breeding of minimally affected dogs to other minimally affected or carrier dogs may result in minimally affected offspring; however, any level of severity can be produced by such breedings. Breeding of more severely affected dogs is highly likely to produce severely affected offspring.

EXPECTED COURSE AND PROGNOSIS
• Does not progress, except when a coloboma leads to retinal detachment after birth.
• Some patients with minor areas of choroidal hypoplasia may develop pigment across the affected area but appear phenotypically normal; thus early examination (in the first 6–8 weeks of life) is highly recommended.

MISCELLANEOUS

ASSOCIATED CONDITIONS
• Microphthalmia
• Enophthalmia
• Retinal folds
• Anterior corneal stromal mineralization

SYNONYM
Scleral ectasia syndrome

Suggested Reading
Roberts SR. The collie eye anomaly. J Am Vet Med Assoc 1969;155:859–864.
Author Stephanie L. Smedes
Consulting Editor Paul E. Miller

COMPULSIVE DISORDERS—CATS

BASICS

DEFINITION
• Repetitive, relatively invariant exaggerated behavior patterns without apparent function
• Controversial in their classification and interpretation; behaviors such as psychogenic alopecia, compulsive pacing, repetitive vocalizing, and sucking or fabric chewing may be included under this heading when other causes cannot be identified.

PATHOPHYSIOLOGY
• Diagnosis of exclusion; must rule out pathophysiologic causes before the diagnosis may be made
• May be a behavioral response to confinement or undefined environmental conditions (e.g., stress, anxiety, frustration); over time, may become fixed and independent of the environment
• Species, breed, and family lines may be predisposed.
• Behaviors may be self-reinforcing, possibly caused by the release of endogenous opioids in the CNS; may allow some animals to cope with conditions that do not meet their species-specific needs
• Owner may reinforce by feeding or giving attention to cat in response to compulsive behavior

SYSTEMS AFFECTED
• Behavior
• Skin/Exocrine—psychogenic alopecia
• Musculoskeletal—repetitive vocalization, compulsive pacing
• Gastrointestinal—fabric chewing

SIGNALMENT
• Any age, sex, or breed
• Siamese and other Asian breeds and crosses—may be overrepresented for repetitive vocalization and fabric chewing

SIGNS

General Comments
• These behaviors, once started, may quickly increase in frequency if they are reinforced in some way by the owner, as with feeding or attention
• Client's response to the behavior is an important part of the history.

Historical Findings
• Psychogenic alopecia—excessive grooming to the exclusion of other activities; behavior may occur secretly in order to avoid owner's negative response; duration of the problem variable; onset may be coincident with an environmental change (e.g., move or new household member)

• Compulsive pacing—behavior may begin intermittently and increase in frequency; initiation may occur at a time of confinement (e.g., restricted from going outdoors)
• Repetitive vocalization
• Sucking may be directed at a person or object, often spontaneously appears; patients weaned early may suck in a manner reminiscent of suckling.
• Fabric chewing—some patients show preference for a specific fabric type or texture such as wool; may chew and ingest fabric; patient may become adept at detecting opportunities for engaging in the behavior.

Physical Examination Findings
• Psychogenic alopecia—focal, partial, and bilateral; most commonly in the groin, ventrum, and medial or caudal thigh regions; appearance of skin variable (normal or abnormal; erythematous to abraded)
• Compulsive pacing—typically within normal limits; rule out neurologic abnormalities
• Repetitive vocalization—typically within normal limits
• Fabric sucking/chewing—typically within normal limits; secondary gastrointestinal inflammation or obstruction may occur.

CAUSES
• Unidentified
• Rule out organic causes before a psychogenic basis is presumed.

RISK FACTORS
• Changes in surroundings predispose cat.
• More commonly reported in indoor cats; may be an artifact of the higher level of attention such pets receive or may be related to the stress of confinement or social isolation, as the pacing and other forms of barrier frustration seen in felids in zoologic parks

DIAGNOSIS

DIFFERENTIAL DIAGNOSIS
Rule out medical differentials before a behavioral diagnosis is made.

Psychogenic Alopecia
• Skin conditions—especially those associated with pruritus
• External parasites
• Fungal dermatitis
• Bacterial dermatitis
• Allergic dermatitis—including food allergy
• Cutaneous neoplasia
• Eosinophilic granuloma complex
• Nervous system disorders
• Disk rupture and associated neuritis
• Feline hyperesthesia syndrome
• Pain

Compulsive Pacing
• Normal sexual behavior
• Nervous system disorders
• Chronic pain
• Focal brain lesions—tumor; vascular accident
• Postictal seizure disorder
• Metabolic and endocrine disorders
• Biotin deficiency
• Hepatic encephalopathy
• Hyperthyroidism
• Lead intoxication
• Renal failure
• Thiamin deficiency
• Hyperesthesia syndrome

Repetitive Vocalization
• Normal sexual behavior
• Deafness
• Hyperthyroidism
• Lead intoxication

Fabric Sucking/Chewing
• Lead intoxication
• Hyperthyroidism
• Thiamin deficiency

CBC/BIOCHEMISTRY/URINALYSIS
Rule out metabolic abnormalities.

OTHER LABORATORY TESTS

Psychogenic Alopecia
• Microscopic examination of hairs—typically shafts are cleanly broken off at variable length as a result of trauma from the tongue.
• Skin scraping, fungal culture, bacterial culture, skin biopsy, and intradermal allergy testing—rule out dermatologic condition.

Compulsive Pacing
• CSF analysis—if indicated by abnormal neurologic examination
• Serum T_4

Repetitive Vocalization
• CSF analysis—if indicated by abnormal neurologic examination
• Serum T_4

Fabric Sucking/Chewing
• Serum lead level—if indicated for pica
• Serum T_4

IMAGING
• CT or MRI—if indicated by abnormalities on the neurologic examination
• Thyroid imaging—if indicated by questionable serum thyroid levels

DIAGNOSTIC PROCEDURES
Psychogenic alopecia—skin scrape or other dermatologic tests; examine for fleas and their products; may attempt an elimination diet

TREATMENT

ENVIRONMENTAL AND SURGICAL CONTROL

• Reduce environmental stress—increase the predictability of household events (feeding, play, exercise, and social time with the client); eliminate unpredictable events as much as possible; confinement contraindicated
• Psychogenic alopecia—topical agents as deterrents usually ineffective
• Compulsive pacing—allowing the patient to go outside after the start of this behavior may reinforce it; if possible, let the patient out before the behavior begins.
• Repetitive vocalizations—breed or spay an intact female; castrate an intact male.
• Fabric chewing/sucking—keep fabrics of interest out of the patient's reach; increase dietary roughage.

BEHAVIOR MODIFICATION

• Do not reward the behavior.
• Instruct client to ignore the behavior as much as possible.
• Advise client to note details of the time, place, and social milieu so that an alternative behavior (play or feeding) may be scheduled then.
• Inform client that punishment associated with his or her voice, movement, and touch increases the unpredictability of the patient's environment, may increase the patient's fear or aggressive behavior, and may disrupt the human/animal bond.

MEDICATIONS

DRUG(S) OF CHOICE

• Environmental control—preferred method of management; psychoactive drugs may be needed concurrently.
• Goal—use the drugs until control is achieved for 2 months; then attempt gradual withdrawal.
• Drugs are listed with dosage used to manage behavior, the latency, and common side effects.
• Tricyclic antidepressant—amitriptyline: 2.5–7.5 mg/cat PO q12–24h; 3–4 weeks; sedation, anticholinergic effects; or clomipramine: 1–5 mg/cat PO q12–24h; 3–4 weeks; sedation, anticholinergic effects, cardiac conduction disturbances in predisposed cats
• Selective serotonin re-uptake inhibitor—fluoxetine: 1–5 mg/cat PO q24h; 3–4 weeks; inappetence, irritability, sedation, constipation

CONTRAINDICATIONS

• Tricyclic antidepressants—potent antihistamine and anticholinergic (atropine-like) side effects; contraindicated with cardiovascular abnormalities (cardiac conduction disturbances) glaucoma, and urinary and fecal retention
• Selective serotonin re-uptake inhibitors—poor appetite, constipation, sedation

PRECAUTIONS

• Drug abuse—psychotropic drugs have human abuse potential; take sensible precautions to ensure that prescriptions for pets are not abused by humans
• Tricyclic antidepressants—overdose (e.g., ingesting a bottle of pills) by pets or humans can cause fatal cardiac disturbances; no antidote; dispense in small quantities (not more than a 4-week supply) with refills to decrease the risk of fatalities; generally well tolerated but numerous potential side effects, including anticholinergic (atropine-like) and antihistaminic effects; use with caution in patients with urinary or fecal retention
• Extralabel drug use—no drugs are approved by the FDA for the treatment of these disorders in cats; inform client of the experimental nature of these treatments and the risks involved; document the discussion in the medical record or with a dedicated release form.
• Side effects—provide written instructions along with common side effects (e.g., tricyclic antidepressants may cause sedation until drug tolerance develops); initiate psychotropic drugs and monitor the patient in the presence of the owner

POSSIBLE INTERACTIONS

Do not use tricyclics listed drugs with monoamine oxidase inhibitors, including amitraz and L-deprenyl.

ALTERNATIVE DRUG(S)

Phenobarbital (although most cases are nonresponsive to this treatment)
Deponyl (seligeline) if cognitive dysfunction

FOLLOW-UP

PATIENT MONITORING

• Successful treatment requires a schedule of follow-up examinations.
• Environmental modification program and/or psychoactive medications must be adjusted according to patient response.
• If a medication is not effective after dosage adjustment, select an agent from another drug class.

POSSIBLE COMPLICATIONS

• Realistic expectations must be made; immediate control of a long-standing problem is unlikely.
• Before initiating treatment, record the frequency of stereotypic bouts that occur each week so that progress can be monitored.

MISCELLANEOUS

ASSOCIATED CONDITIONS

Avoidance behavior or aggression toward the owner—if the owner punishes the patient when it exhibits a stereotypic behavior

ZOONOTIC POTENTIAL

N/A

PREGNANCY

Tricyclic antidepressants—contraindicated in pregnant animals

SYNONYMS

• Compulsive behavior
• Obsessive–compulsive behavior
• Psychogenic alopecia
• Neurodermatitis
• Psychic eczema
• Pacing
• Repetitive vocalizations
• Crying
• Vocalizing
• Fabric chewing/sucking
• Wool chewing/sucking

ABBREVIATIONS

• CNS = central nervous system
• CSF = cerebrospinal fluid
• CT = computed tomography
• MRI = magnetic resonance imaging
• T$_4$ = thyrosine

Suggested Reading

Luescher AU. Compulsive behavior. In: Horwitz D, Mills D, Heath S, eds. BSAVA manual of canine and feline behavioural medicine. Gloucester, England: British Small Animal Veterinary Association, 2002:229–236.
Simpson BS, Papich MG. Pharmacologic management in veterinary behaviorial medicine. Vet Clin NA: Sm Anim Pract 2003;33:365–404.
Author Barbara S. Simpson
Consulting Editor Debra F. Horwitz

COMPULSIVE DISORDERS—DOGS

BASICS

DEFINITION
• A repetitious, relatively unvaried sequence of movements that has no obvious purpose or function, usually derived from contextually normal maintenance behaviors (e.g., grooming, eating, walking); inherent is that the behavior interferes with normal behavioral functioning. • Also called OCD • An American Psychiatric Association classification of abnormal behavior characterized by recurrent, frequent thoughts or actions that are out of context to the situations in which they occur; may involve cognitive or physical rituals and are deemed excessive (given the context) in duration, frequency, and intensity • One hallmark distinguishing it from motor tics (humans)—behaviors follow a set of rules created by the patient; veterinary clients also recognize this • Condition in domestic animals—probably similar and analogous through descent; probably includes stereotypies, self-directed behaviors, etc.; behavior must be sufficiently pronounced to interfere with normal functioning to be labeled OCD • Most common—spinning; tail chasing; self-mutilation; hallucinating ("fly biting"); circling; fence running; hair/air biting; pica; pacing; staring and vocalizing; self-directed vocalization; potentially some aggressions

PATHOPHYSIOLOGY
• Unclear; clinical signs consistent with alterations in CNS transmitter functions; caudate nucleus function may be affected. • Main neurotransmitters implicated in stereotypic behavior—dopamine; serotonin; endorphins, for conditions involving mutilation; serotonin effects may predominate. • Humans—basal nuclei, particularly the putamen and the caudate nuclei, are the regions most commonly implicated in aberrant neurochemistry. • Pet brought to the clinic because the client perceives changes in the patient's behavior or because the client believes patient has never been normal

SYSTEMS AFFECTED
• Cardiovascular—tachycardia • Endocrine/Metabolic—signs caused by alterations in the HPA axis • Gastrointestinal—inappetence; aberrant appetite (including pica and coprophagia); gastrointestinal distress (salivation, vomiting, diarrhea, tenesmus, hematochezia); aerophagia • Hemic/Lymphatic/Immune—stress leukogram common • Musculo-skeletal—poor condition attributable to increased motor activity and self-injury; weight loss, injured pads, damage to teeth and gums, and abrasions and lacerations common • Nervous—increased

motor activity, repetitive activity, trembling, and self-injury common • Respiratory—tachypnea and the attendant metabolic changes possible in extreme situations

Skin/Exocrine
• Skin lesions—usually secondary; may be a result of self-injury, overgrooming, barbering, sucking, or abrasion from repetitive activity • Lick granulomas—not uncommon; may be a dermatologic manifestation; mild type usually not the only sign; type associated with deep tissue damage may occur; almost all behaviors associated with lick granulomas of sudden violent onset will meet criteria for OCD

SIGNALMENT
• No age, breed, or sex overrepresented, although type of OCD (e.g., spinning vs. self-mutilation) may be affected by breed. • Begin to develop at onset (12–24 months) of social maturity (12–36 months), like other anxiety disorders • Bull terriers—tail chasing not uncommon and seems to run in families • German shepherds—reported to be over-represented for spinning and tail chasing • Great Danes and German short-haired pointers—some lines display self-mutilation, stereotypic motor behavior (fence running), or hallucinations; prevalence only recently appreciated, so likely more widespread than now thought; may be more familial than breed-associated • Breed vs. familial association—confounded in dogs; not all family members show the same manifestation (e.g., spinning, grooming, or hallucinating) and, in fact, the opposite may be true; humans: occurrence of any one characteristic behavior is associated with an increased risk of another manifestation in first-degree relatives. If client sees signs developing in a dog derived from a line where other dogs are affected, early intervention is critical; treat all nonspecific vitalistic behaviors with increased exercise, behavior modification, and, minimally, nonspecific TCAs

SIGNS

General Comments
• May be nonspecific • One hallmark—immutable rule structure that specifies how and when the patient is to perform the activity • The behavior may be a manifestation of an OCD if the client cannot interrupt it and if it intensifies over time, increases in frequency or duration, and interferes with normal functioning. • Have clients videotape dogs in all circumstances where they see the behavior. Pattern will be clear.

Historical Findings
• Patient may have begun to chase its tail as part of play but now the tip is missing and even physical restraint does not stop the behavior. • May be seen in young dogs, but its onset is more common during social

maturity; play decreases with age, OCD increases. • A solitary focus may have seemed to spur the behavior (e.g., chasing a mouse that the patient could not catch), but usually no provocative stimulus is noted. • One hallmark—behavior worsens with time.

Physical Examination Findings
• Usually unremarkable • May see self-induced injuries and the lack of condition that may be associated with increased motor activity and the repetitive behaviors; may note self-mutilation with a focus on the tail, forelimbs, and distal extremities

CAUSES
• Illness or painful physical condition—may increase an animal's anxieties and contribute to these problems; few of these conditions actually cause OCD • Kenneling and incarceration—may be associated with spinning • Degenerative (e.g., aging and concomitant neurologic changes), anatomic, infectious (primarily CNS viral conditions), and toxic (lead toxicosis) causes—may be causal, but abnormal behavior likely rooted in primary or secondary aberrant neurochemical activity

DIAGNOSIS

DIFFERENTIAL DIAGNOSIS
• Conditions that cause similar behavioral changes—seizures; brain disease; metabolic disease (e.g., thyroid or pancreatic conditions) • Some behavioral conditions (play and attention seeking) may look like the early stages of OCD.

CBC/BIOCHEMISTRY/URINALYSIS
Perform; results within the laboratory's reference range

OTHER LABORATORY TESTS
Thyroid or liver profile—rule out hypo-thyroidism and hepatic encephalopathy if there is any doubt that the signs are behavioral

IMAGING
CT and MRI—rule out structural brain disease

DIAGNOSTIC PROCEDURES
• Biopsies of skin lesions ± plain radiography—confirm if they are primary (underlying abnormality) or secondary (first-degree • infections) • CSF analysis—rule out inflammatory CNS disease • Endoscopy—evaluate primary bowel disease • ECG—diagnostic; premedication precaution; cardiac disease may produce physical signs of anxiety. • Aberrant endorphin metabolism—evaluate by administering naloxone (11–22 μg/kg IV); if behavior does not decrease dramatically in intensity or frequency within 15–20 min, endorphin metabolism unlikely to be the main driving mechanism

TREATMENT

• Most patients respond to a combination of behavior modification and pharmacologic treatment with antianxiety medication.
• Pharmacologic intervention—implement early; may be a prerequisite to effecting any behavioral therapy • Usually outpatient
• Inpatient—patients with severe self-mutilation and self-induced injury; patients that must be protected from the environment until the antianxiety medications reach effective plasma and CSF levels (days to weeks); constant monitoring, stimulation, and care
• Sedation—profound cases; only a stop-gap measure, but necessary if serious and acute mutilation involved. • Behavior modification—geared toward teaching the patient to relax in a variety of environmental settings and to substitute a calm, competitive behavior for the stereotypic one • Discourage the client from reassuring the patient that it does not have to spin, chew, etc.; this inadvertently rewards the repetitive behavior; have them reward dog only when not engaged in behavior and relaxed
• Desensitization and counterconditioning—most effective if instituted early; may be coupled to a verbal cue that signals the patient to execute a behavior that is competitive with the abnormal one (e.g., instead of circling, the patient is taught to relax and lie down with its head and neck stretched prone on the floor when the client says "Head down") • Help client understand the subtlety of the signs and learn to recognize the outward physical signs associated with the underlying physiologic state characterized by sympathetic stimulation. • Punishment—contraindicated; may make the behavior worse and render the patient more secretive • Atopic and painful conditions—diagnose and control (including the use of dietary management); pruritus and pain neurochemically related to anxiety and its perception • All infections must be treated for 2–4 months. • Amputation—avoid; eliminates the outward signs but does nothing to alleviate the condition • Incarceration/physical restraint—avoid bandages, collars, braces, and crates; all serve to focus animal more on nidus of distress and will make the dog worse • Have clients monitor behaviors via weekly videos and written logs; will provide unbiased assessments of change and help with alterations in treatment plans

MEDICATIONS

DRUG(S)
• TCAs and SSRIs—increase CNS levels of serotonin • Mild—amitriptyline (1–2 mg/kg PO q12h for 30 days, to start); imipramine (1–2 mg/kg PO q12h for 30 days); only useful for nonspecific ritualistic behaviors that may be associated with OCD • Severe or long-standing—clomipramine (1 mg/kg PO q12h for 14 days; then 2 mg/kg PO q12h for 14 days; then 3 mg/kg PO q12h for 28 days; if successful, this will be the maintenance dosage); fluoxetine (1 mg/kg PO q24h for 2 months); some combination of the above; these drugs may take 3–5 weeks to be effective. • May take months to get real effect
• Self-mutilation—narcotic antagonists (naltrexone 2.2 mg/kg PO q8–12–24h) may be useful, but expensive and short $t_{1/2}$ in dog.
• Unlikely to work if the behavior was not first blocked by intravenous administration.
• Thioridazine—occasionally used as an adjuvant treatment; newer more specific treatments appear more effective. Some antipsychotics (risperidone, olanzepine, clozapine) • Treatment is lifelong; any attempt to withdraw medication should be gradual; recurrence is common.

CONTRAINDICATIONS
• Hepatic and renal compromise medications for which these are the main routes of metabolism • Cardiac conduction anomalies—give TCA with extreme caution; monitor closely.

PRECAUTIONS
• All listed medications are extralabel in the U.S.; recommendations from Health and Human Services should be followed.
• TCA overdose (human and animal)—profound cardiac conduction disturbances; perform a cardiac evaluation with an ECG before treatment.

POSSIBLE INTERACTIONS
• Medications that impair the glucuronidation of active metabolites into inactive compounds—may increase the active metabolites • TCAs and SSRIs—most have active intermediate metabolites; pharmacokinetics may differ from that of the parent compound • Combination therapy with two antianxiety agents—may potentiate either or both medications; lower the dosages.

FOLLOW-UP

PATIENT MONITORING
• CBC, biochemistry and urinalysis—semiannually or yearly if the patient is on chronic treatment; adjust dosages accordingly.
• Advise client to observe for vomiting, gastrointestinal distress, and tachypnea.

POSSIBLE COMPLICATIONS
Early intervention, using both behavioral modification and pharmacologic inter

vention, is crucial; if left untreated, these conditions always progress.

MISCELLANEOUS

ASSOCIATED CONDITIONS
• Irritable bowel syndrome • Lick granulomas

AGE-RELATED FACTORS
• Appears most frequently at social maturity
• Little is known about contributory and developmental factors, but any condition that contributes to the patient's underlying anxiety or to its perception of it can worsen the condition.

ZOONOTIC POTENTIAL
N/A

PREGNANCY
Most of the drugs used to treat these conditions either are not evaluated in or are contraindicated in pregnant animals; their use should be avoided.

SYNONYMS
Obsessive–compulsive disorder

ABBREVIATIONS
• CNS = central nervous system
• CT = computed tomography
• CSF = cerebrospinal fluid
• ECG = electrocardiogram
• HPA = hypothalamic–pituitary–adrenal
• MRI = magnetic resonance imaging
• OCD = obsessive–compulsive disorder
• TCA = tricyclic antidepressant
• SSRI = selective serotonin reuptake inhibitor

Suggested Reading
Hewsan CJ, Luescher UA, Parent JM, et al. Efficacy of clomipromine in the treatment of canine compulsive disorders. J Am Vet Med Assoc 1998;213:1760–1766.
Luescher UA, McKeown DB, Halip J. Stereotypic or obsessive-compulsive disorders in dogs and cats. Vet Clin North Am Small Anim Pract 1991;21:401–414.
Overall KL. Recognition, diagnosis, and management of obsessive-compulsive disorders. Part I. Canine Pract 1992;17:40–44.
Overall KL. Use of clomipramine to treat ritualistic stereotypic motor behavior in three dogs. J Am Vet Med Assoc 1994;205:1733–1741.
Overall KL, Dunham AE. Clinical features and outcome in dogs and cats with obsesive-compulsive disorder: 126 cases (1989–2000). J Am Vet Med Assoc 2002;221:1445–1452.
Author Karen L. Overall
Consulting Editor Debra F. Horwitz

CONGENITAL AND DEVELOPMENTAL RENAL DISEASES

BASICS

DEFINITIONS

• Functional or morphologic abnormalities resulting from heritable (genetic) or acquired disease processes affecting differentiation and growth of the developing kidney before or shortly after birth • Renal agenesis—complete absence of one or both kidneys • Renal dysplasia—disorganized renal parenchymal development • Renal ectopia—congenital malposition of one or both kidneys; ectopic kidneys may be fused. • Glomerulopathy—glomerular disease of any type • Tubulointerstitial nephropathy—a noninflammatory disorder of renal tubules and interstitium • Polycystic renal disease—characterized by formation of multiple, variable-sized cysts throughout the renal medulla and cortex • Renal telangiectasia—characterized by multifocal vascular malformations involving the kidneys and other organs • Renal amyloidosis—the extracellular deposition of amyloid in glomerular capillaries, glomeruli, and interstitium • Nephroblastoma—a congenital renal neoplasm arising from the pluripotent metanephric blastema • Multifocal renal cystadenocarcinoma—a hereditary renal neoplasm in dogs • Fanconi's syndrome—a generalized renal tubular functional anomaly characterized by impaired reabsorption of glucose, phosphate, electrolytes, amino acids, and uric acid • Primary renal glucosuria—an isolated functional defect in renal tubular reabsorption of glucose • Cystinuria—excessive urinary excretion of cystine because of an isolated functional defect in renal tubular reabsorption of cystine and other dibasic amino acids • Hyperuricuria—excessive urinary excretion of uric acid, sodium urate, or ammonium urate caused by impaired hepatic conversion of uric acid to allantoin and enhanced renal tubular secretion of uric acid • Primary hyperoxaluria—a disorder characterized by intermittent hyperoxaluria, L-glyceric aciduria, oxalate nephropathy, and acute renal failure • Congenital nephrogenic diabetes insipidus—a disorder of renal concentrating ability, caused by diminished renal responsiveness to antidiuretic hormone

PATHOPHYSIOLOGY

• Many congenital and developmental renal disorders are caused by genetic abnormalities that disrupt the normal sequential and coordinated development and interaction of multiple embryonic tissues involved in formation of the mature kidney. • Congenital and developmental renal disorders may also be caused by nongenetic factors affecting the developing kidney before or shortly after birth.

SYSTEMS AFFECTED

Renal/Urologic

GENETICS

Familial renal disorders have been reported in the following breeds of dogs and cats:
• Renal agenesis in beagle and Doberman pinscher dogs • Renal dysplasia in Alaskan malamate, boxer, chow chow, golden retriever, keeshond, Lhasa apso, miniature schnauzer, shih tzu, soft-coated wheaten terrier, and standard poodle dogs • Glomerulopathy in beagle, Brittany spaniel, English cocker spaniel, samoyed, Doberman pinscher, cocker spaniel, rottweiler, soft-coated wheaten terrier, and Bernese mountain dogs • Tubulointerstitial nephropathy in Norwegian elkhound dogs • Polycystic renal disease in beagle, bull terrier, West Highland white terrier, and Cairn terrier dogs and Persian and domestic longhaired cats • Renal telangiectasia in Welsh corgi dogs • Renal amyloidosis in Abyssinian, oriental shorthaired, and Siamese cats and in English foxhound and shar-pei dogs • Renal cystadenocarcinoma in German shepherd dogs • Fanconi's syndrome in basenji and border terrier dogs • Primary renal glucosuria in Norwegian elkhound dogs • Cystinuria in basset hound, bulldog, dachshund, Irish terrier, and Newfoundland dogs and in domestic cats • Hyperuricuria in Dalmatians and English bulldogs • Primary hyperoxaluria in domestic shorthaired cats and in Tibetan spaniel dogs

INCIDENCE/PREVALENCE

Uncommon, but disorders caused by genetic factors occur more frequently in related animals from more than one generation than in the general population.

GEOGRAPHIC DISTRIBUTION

N/A

SIGNALMENT

Species

Dogs and cats

Breed Predilections

Sporadic cases of congenital/developmental renal disease can occur without a familial predisposition in any breed of dog or cat.

Mean Age and Range

Most patients are <5 years old at time of diagnosis

Predominant Sex

• Familial cystinuria primarily in male dogs • Samoyed hereditary glomerulopathy more common in males than females; Newfoundlands have both genders affected. • Familial glomerulonephropathy of Bernese mountain dogs more in females than males

SIGNS

General Comments

Most congenital and developmental disorders cannot be distinguished from noncongenital/ developmental renal diseases on the basis of history or physical examination.

Historical Findings

• Indicate chronic renal failure • Some glomerulopathies associated with abdominal distension, edema, or other signs of the nephrotic syndrome • Abdominal distension in some patients with polycystic kidneys or renal neoplasms • Hematuria in some patients with renal telangiectasia or renal neoplasms • Apparent abdominal pain in some patients with renal telangiectasia • Patients with unilateral renal agenesis, ectopic kidneys, and isolated renal tubular transport defects are frequently asymptomatic.

Physical Examination Findings

• Those associated with chronic renal failure • Ascites or pitting edema in some patients with protein-losing glomerulopathies or amyloidosis • Renomegaly or abdominal mass lesions in some patients with polycystic kidneys, renal neoplasms, or fused ectopic kidneys • Renal pain in some patients with renal telangiectasia

CAUSES

Nonhereditary

• Infectious agents—feline panleukopenia virus and canine herpesvirus infection associated with renal dysplasia • Drugs—corticosteroids, diphenylamine, and biphenyls associated with polycystic kidneys; chlorambucil and sodium arsenate associated with renal agenesis • Dietary factors—hypo- or hypervitaminosis A associated with renal ectopia

RISK FACTORS

See factors listed under Causes.

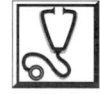

DIAGNOSIS

DIFFERENTIAL DIAGNOSIS

• Rule out noncongenital and nondevelopmental causes of primary renal disease. • Rule out nonrenal causes of hematuria, proteinuria, glucosuria, abdominal distention, or ascites.

CBC/BIOCHEMISTRY/URINALYSIS

• Nonregenerative anemia in patients with chronic renal failure • Azotemia and urine specific gravity <1.030 in dogs and <1.035 in cats if renal failure develops • Proteinuria, hypoalbuminemia, and hypercholesterolemia in patients with the nephrotic syndrome • Normoglycemic glucosuria in animals with Fanconi's syndrome or primary renal glucosuria • Hematuria in patients with congenital renal neoplasia or renal telangiectasia • Cystine crystalluria in patients with cystinuria • Urate crystalluria in patients with hyperuricuria

OTHER LABORATORY TESTS

See chapters describing specific renal diseases or clinical syndromes

CONGENITAL AND DEVELOPMENTAL RENAL DISEASES

IMAGING
Survey abdominal radiography, renal ultrasonography, and excretory urography are important means of identifying and characterizing congenital and developmental renal disorders.

DIAGNOSTIC PROCEDURES
Consider light microscopic evaluation of kidney biopsy specimens from patients with morphologic or functional abnormalities of the kidney for which a definitive diagnosis has not been established by other, less invasive means.

PATHOLOGIC FINDINGS
• Congenital and developmental renal disorders may be associated with various combinations of primary, compensatory, and degenerative lesions. Conversely, some functional disorders may not be associated with alterations in renal morphology. • Renal dysplasia—end-stage kidneys; primary lesions include immature ("fetal") glomeruli, persistent mesenchyme, persistent metanephric ducts, atypical tubular epithelium, and dysontogenic metaplasia; primary lesions usually associated with, and may be obscured by, secondary degenerative, inflammatory, and compensatory lesions
• Glomerulopathies—usually normal-to-small kidneys; most hereditary glomerulopathies are characterized by a primary membrano-proliferative glomerulonephritis with variable degrees of tubulointerstitial disease, but cystic atrophic membranous glomerulopathy is the characteristic lesion in affected rottweilers.
• Tubulointerstitial nephropathy—end-stage kidneys; renal lesions include periglomerular fibrosis, parietal epithelial cell hyperplasia and hypertrophy, interstitial fibrosis, and interstitial mononuclear cell infiltrate. • Polycystic renal disease—see specific chapter • Renal amyloidosis—see specific chapter • Renal telangiectasia—lesions include multiple, variable-sized, red-black, blood-filled nodules in the renal cortex and medulla, interstitial fibrosis, interstitial mononuclear cell infiltrate, and hydronephrosis. • Nephroblastoma—unilateral renal mass; microscopically characterized by both embryonic mesenchymal and epithelial tissue components • Multifocal renal cyst-adenocarcinoma—bilaterally large kidneys with irregular protruding cystic structures or multifocal neoplastic renal tubular epithelial cell proliferations; often associated with cutaneous nodular dermatofibrosis and multiple uterine leiomyomas • Renal ectopia—kidneys may be located in the retroperitoneal space of the pelvic canal, iliac fossa, or abdomen; fused kidneys assume a variety of shapes; horseshoe kidneys are symmetrically fused along the medial border of either pole. • Fanconi's syndrome—inconsistent microscopic findings of tubular

atrophy, interstitial fibrosis, tubular cell karyomegaly, and acute papillary necrosis • Primary hyperoxaluria—large, irregularly-shaped kidneys; microscopic lesions include renal tubular deposition of calcium oxalate crystals and variable interstitial and periglomerular fibrosis.

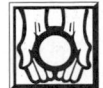

TREATMENT
• The nature of congenital and developmental renal disorders often precludes specific treatment.
• Supportive or symptomatic treatment may improve quality of life and minimize progression in patients with renal dysfunction.
• Base treatment options on clinical signs and appropriate laboratory evaluations.
• Refer to chapters describing specific renal diseases or clinical syndromes.

MEDICATIONS

DRUG(S) OF CHOICE
Refer to chapters describing specific renal diseases or clinical syndromes.

CONTRAINDICATIONS
Avoid potentially nephrotoxic drugs (e.g., gentamicin) or anesthetic agents that decrease renal function (e.g., methoxyflurane) when possible.

PRECAUTIONS
Avoid drugs requiring renal excretion in patients with renal failure; if necessary, modify dosage regimens to compensate for decreased renal clearance of drugs and other metabolites.

POSSIBLE INTERACTIONS
N/A

ALTERNATIVE DRUG(S)
N/A

FOLLOW-UP

PATIENT MONITORING
Refer to chapters describing specific renal diseases or clinical syndromes.

PREVENTION/AVOIDANCE
Congenital and developmental renal disorders are irreversible, so control lies in preventing breeding of affected animals. Always consider early identification and correction of predisposing factors (genetic and nongenetic) that may affect future offspring.

POSSIBLE COMPLICATIONS
• Acute or chronic renal failure • Nephrotic syndrome • Urolithiasis • Hydronephrosis • Urinary tract infection

EXPECTED COURSE AND PROGNOSIS
• Highly variable; depends on the specific disorder, the extent of primary lesions, and the severity of renal dysfunction • Most congenital and developmental disorders are irreversible and may result in advanced chronic renal failure, but some patients with mild-to-moderate renal dysfunction may remain stable for long periods. • Patients with some disorders (e.g., unilateral renal agenesis, renal ectopia, cystinuria, hyperuricuria, primary renal glucosuria) may remain asymptomatic unless the disorder is complicated by urolithiasis, urinary tract infection, or other disease processes that promote progressive renal dysfunction.

MISCELLANEOUS

ASSOCIATED CONDITIONS
• Polycystic renal disease associated with hepatic biliary cysts • Cystinuria and hyperuricuria associated with formation of uroliths • Amyloidosis in Chinese shar peis associated with intermittent pyrexia or swelling of the hocks • Renal neoplasms associated with hypertrophic osteoarthropathy, polycythemia, or other paraneoplastic syndromes

PREGNANCY
N/A

SYNONYMS
Familial renal disease, juvenile renal disease

SEE ALSO
• Amyloidosis • Anemia of Chronic Renal Disease • Fanconi's Syndrome • Hematuria • Hyperparathyroidism, Renal Secondary • Nephrotic Syndrome • Oliguria/Anuria • Polycystic Kidneys • Polyuria and Polydipsia • Renal Failure, Acute • Renal Failure, Chronic • Renal Tubular Acidosis • Renomegaly • Urolithiasis, Cystine

Suggested Reading

Finco DR. Inherited and congenital renal disorders. In: Osborne CA, Finco DR, eds. Canine and feline nephrology and urology. 2nd ed. Baltimore: Williams & Wilkins, 1995: 471–483.
Kruger JM, Osborne CA, Lulich JP, et al. The urinary system. In: Hoskins JD, ed. Veterinary pediatrics. 3rd ed. Philadelphia: Saunders, 2001:371–401.
Authors John M. Kruger, Carl A. Osborne, and Scott D. Fitzgerald
Consulting Editors Larry G. Adams and Carl A. Osborne

CONGENITAL OCULAR ANOMALIES

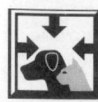

BASICS

DEFINITION
Solitary or multiple abnormalities that affect the globe or its adnexa that may be observed in young dogs and cats at birth or within the first 6–8 weeks of life

PATHOPHYSIOLOGY
• Breed-related inherited defects—most common; include colobomas (segmental areas that fail to develop properly) of the fundus in collie eye anomaly • Spontaneous malformations—colobomas of the anterior segment, resulting in notch-like defects of the iris or lens • In utero systemic infections and inflammations, exposure to toxic compounds, and lack of specific nutrients in pregnant dams or bitches

SYSTEMS AFFECTED
Ophthalmic—entire eye or any part; unilateral or bilateral

GENETICS
• Suspected genetic background for several causal diseases, some with a unknown mode of inheritance • PPM in basenjis—simple autosomal dominant trait • PHTVL and PHPV in Doberman pinschers—autosomal dominant allele with variable expression • Multifocal retinal dysplasia in English springer spaniels—autosomal simple recessive trait • Collie eye anomaly—autosomal recessive trait • Retinal dystrophy in briards—simple autosomal recessive allele • Photoreceptor dysplasia in collies, Irish setters, and Cardigan Welsh Corgi dogs—autosomal recessive trait; nonallelic disease • Other photoreceptor dysplasias in dogs—recessively inherited • Photoreceptor dysplasia in Abyssinians, Persian and domestic shorthair cats—postulated autosomal dominant trait

INCIDENCE/PREVALENCE
• Incidence in dogs and cats—low in the general population; somewhat higher in dogs than cats • Collie eye anomaly—affects collies and Shetland sheepdogs; most common; worldwide prevalence > 50%

SIGNALMENT
• Dogs and cats • See Genetics.

SIGNS

General Comments
• Depend on defect • May cause no signs of disease and may be an incidental finding in a thorough ophthalmic examination

Historical Findings
• Ranges from none to severe visual impairment or blindness

Physical Examination Findings
• Microphthalmos—a congenitally small eye; found in different degrees; easily noted by comparing the eyes; more difficult to detect if bilateral; often associated with other hereditary defects (e.g., corneal opacities, PPM, cataract, retinal detachment, and dysplasia) • Anophthalmos—congenital lack of the globe; often associated with other hereditary defects (e.g., corneal opacities, PPM, cataract, retinal detachment, and dysplasia) • Cryptophthalmos—a small globe that is concealed by other adnexal defects; often associated with other hereditary defects (e.g., corneal opacities, PPM, cataract, retinal detachment, and dysplasia) • Eyelid agenesis or colobomas of the eyelids—often result in congenitally open eyelids; considered hereditary in Burmese cats; usually affect the temporal portion of the upper eyelid; may note blepharospasm and epiphora • Dermoids—congenital, tumor-like, islands of aberrant skin tissue involving either eyelids, conjunctiva, or cornea; sometimes affect more than one structure; may note blepharospasm and epiphora • Congenital atresia and imperforate puncta of the lacrimal system—affects cats and dogs; imperforate puncta: common in several dog breeds (e.g., cocker spaniels); results in a tear streak at the nasal canthus and on the side of the nose; usually not associated with other ocular findings • Congenital KCS—may occur sporadically in any dog or cat breed; may be hereditary in Yorkshire terriers; usually unilateral; affected eye often appears smaller than the normal eye; results in a thick mucoid discharge from a red and irritated eye • PPM—remnants of the pupillary membrane that extend from the iris collarette to the corneal endothelium, the anterior lens capsule, or just across the pupil; may coexist with a variety of iris defects, cataracts, and uveal colobomas; affects any species; recorded in numerous dog breeds; shown to be hereditary in basenjis • Iris cysts—circular, pigmented or nonpigmented ball-like structures that float freely in the anterior chamber or are attached to the iris or corneal endothelium • Congenital glaucoma with buphthalmos—affects dogs and cats; rare; often note increased tearing and an enlarged, red, and painful eye • Congenital pupillary abnormalities—polycoria (more than one pupil); ancoria (no pupil); aniridia (lack of iris); dyscoria (abnormally shaped pupil) • Congenital cataracts—primary, often inherited (e.g., cavalier King Charles spaniels) or secondary to other developmental defects; often associated with other congenital anomalies of the lens, including microphakia (a small lens), lenticonus or lentiglobus (a protrusion of the lens capsule, most often posteriorly), and coloboma (notching of the lens equator, which may also include defects in the zonules and ciliary body); associated leukocoria common • PHTVL and PHPV—hereditary defect; affects Doberman pinschers and Staffordshire bull terriers; persistence of parts of the hyaloid vasculature; developmental aberrations of the vitreous, lens, and lens capsule; may note a cataract and leukocoria or a reddish sheen from the pupillary area in conjunction with intralenticular bleeding (unusual) or vascular abnormalities on the posterior lens capsule • Retinal dysplasia—affects a variety of dog breeds; occurs sporadically in cats; effect on neural retinal structure depends on severity; ranges from focal folds to geographic focal detachment to complete retinal detachment • Coloboma of the posterior segment—found in conjunction with hereditary collie eye anomaly; occurs sporadically in other dog breeds; typically seen in the optic nerve head, usually at the 6 o'clock position; may also be noted in other locations in the fundus, usually in the vicinity of the optic nerve head • Photoreceptor dysplasia—hereditary anomaly in dogs and cats; rods, cones, or both may be affected from birth; direct and indirect pupillary light reflexes may be abnormal and may react sluggishly when the patient opens its eyes • Rod and cone dysplasias of dogs—rod and cone dysplasia affects Irish setters (rcd1) and collies (rcd2); rod dysplasia and early rod degeneration affect the Norwegian elkhound; cone degeneration or hemeralopia affects Alaskan malamutes • Rod–cone dysplasia of cats—affects Persians, Abyssinians, and American mixed-breeds; may show pupillary dilatation at 2–3 weeks, nystagmus at 4–5 weeks, ophthalmoscopic signs of retinal degeneration at 8 weeks, and night and day blindness some weeks later • Retinal dystrophy—in briards; RPE65 null mutation, causes congenital night blindness, nystagmus, abnormally large pupils although the fundus is normal until middle age; affects retinal pigment epithelium and photoreceptors • Retinal detachment—seen in conjunction with the hereditary diseases (e.g., retinal dysplasia); mainly found in Labrador retrievers, Bedlingtons, and Sealyham terriers and with collie eye anomaly; may be seen with other ocular syndromes in which several other eye defects are involved; may note a widely dilated pupil that is unresponsive to light stimuli; may be seen in the pupil as a funnel-shaped curtain; complete detachment results in blindness. • Optic nerve hypoplasia—occurs sporadically as a congenital ocular defect in dogs and cats; believed to have a hereditary background in miniature and toy poodles; often results in blindness

CAUSES
• Genetic • Spontaneous malformations • Infections and inflammations during pregnancy—congenital cataracts; syndromes with multiple defects • Toxicity during pregnancy • Nutritional deficiencies

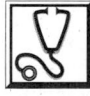

DIAGNOSIS

DIFFERENTIAL DIAGNOSIS
• Early-onset infectious and inflammatory processes of the adnexal structures—may mimic and even mask congenital abnormalities, such as congenital KCS • Cataracts induced at an early age and especially those that progress quickly (e.g., after trauma or with diabetes mellitus)—may seem to be congenital • Postinflammatory ophthalmic lesions resulting in synechia—may be confused with PPM • Tumors of the anterior segment of the eye—may be confused with iris cysts • Generalized retinopathy of inflammatory origin—may appear to be photoreceptor dysplasia with retinal atrophy; usually unilateral • Retinal detachment as result of trauma or uveitis in

young dogs—may appear to be a congenital abnormality of the neural retina (e.g., postin-flammatory neuroretinal folding as opposed to multifocal retinal dysplasia) • Optic nerve atrophy owing to an inflammatory process—may be difficult to differentiate from congenital optic nerve hypoplasia

IMAGING

Ultrasound—diagnosis of abnormalities of the lens and the posterior segment of the eye, abnormalities of the position of the lens or configuration of its capsule, and abnormalities in the vitreous and retina (e.g., congenital retinal detachment)

DIAGNOSTIC PROCEDURES

• Penlight examination—usually permits the diagnosis of complete cataract or retinal detach-ment • Evaluation of tear production (using Shirmer tear strips)—perform routinely with chronic adnexal inflammatory and infectious processes • Direct and/or indirect ophthalmoscope and slitlamp biomicroscopy—necessary to diagnose most abnormalities of the internal structures (e.g., multifocal retinal dysplasia and PHTVL/PHPV); examine after pupil dilation (check pupillary light reflexes before dilating); difficult to perform in patients younger than 5 weeks • Electroretinography and visually evoked potentials—objective evaluation and differentiation of retinal and optic nerve function; usually performed in patients aged 7–12 weeks; electroretinography diagnostic for photoreceptor dysplasias and retinal dystrophy of briards

PATHOLOGIC FINDINGS

• Depend on type and severity of defect; range from solitary defects of specific structures to involvement of the whole globe, such as severe microphthalmos • Congenital KCS—usually a severe keratitis with corneal neovascularization, scarring, and pigmentation; inflammatory changes of the conjunctiva; may note abnor-mally developed or atrophied lacrimal glands • Congenital glaucoma—buphthalmos com-mon, sometimes with secondary lens luxation and always neuroretinal thinning; collapse of the iridocorneal filtration angle • PHTVL and PHPV—range of defects; retrolental darkly pigmented dots and plaques to complete strands of vascular tissue passing from the optic nerve head to the posterior lens capsule; often malformations of the posterior lens capsule (e.g., lenticonus) and some degree of cataract formation • Retinal dysplasia—some degree of abnormality and folding of the retina; with multifocal defect, often see rosettes of abnormal neuroretinal tissue along the major blood vessels in the central tapetal fundus; with geographic defect, usually find a large, abnormal area where the retina is slightly elevated and the surrounding tissue is hyperpigmented and scarred; may note an abnormal and completely detached retina • Photoreceptor dysplasia—abnormalities in the rods and/ or cones; thin inner and outer segment layers; dropout of photoreceptor nuclei in the outer nuclear layer • Retinal dystrophy (briards)—large lipoid-like inclusions in the retinal pigment epithelium

and degeneration and dropout of photoreceptors with time • Colobomas—a notch in the tissue with anterior defect (e.g., lens or iris); thinning of the neural retina, either in the region of the optic nerve head or near its border with posterior defect; may be rather large and extend far back as an outpouching of the sclera • Retinal detachment—neural retina detached from the retinal pigment epithelium; usually attached only around the optic nerve head • Optic nerve hypoplasia—avascular, dark, abnormally small, and circular optic nerve head

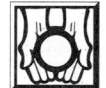

TREATMENT

APPROPIATE HEALTH CARE

• Patients are usually referred to an ophthal-mologist for a complete evaluation, especially if abnormality affects the internal structures of the eye or vision is impaired. • No medical treatment for most congenital abnormalities, except possibly symptomatic treatment (e.g., congenital KCS)

NURSING CARE

Inhibit self-mutilation after surgical procedures by using an Elizabethan collar or by directly bandaging the paws or eye.

ACTIVITY

Usually unaltered

CLIENT EDUCATION

• Discuss visual capacity, possible progression, and sequelae. • Inform client that blind animals may need direct supervision when exposed to a potentially hazardous environment. • Congenital KCS—discuss medical treatment versus surgical intervention; inform client that if the eye is medicated on a regular basis, the patient will do fine, especially if there is some tear production; if client cannot or will not medicate, recommend surgery.

SURGICAL CONSIDERATIONS

• Depend on specific abnormality • If undesirable sequelae will not result, wait until the patient has reached adult size to avoid overcorrecting the defect. • Adnexal abnormalities (e.g., dermoids or severe malfor-mations of the eyelids)—surgery as soon as possible • Imperforate puncta—surgically correct as soon as anesthesia is safe • Congenital KCS—parotid duct transposition • Cataract extraction—congenital cataract may have other anomalies that cause surgical complications • Congenital glaucoma—enucleation or intrascleral prosthesis usually treatments of choice; consider euthanasia if bilateral

MEDICATIONS

DRUG(S)

• Congenital KCS—tear substitutes (Tears Naturale and Visco-Tears), possibly in combi-nation with antibiotics (drops or gel); cyclo-sporin ophthalmic (Optimmune) ointment

BID • Congenital cataracts—when involving the nuclear region of the lens only, mydriatics may be used to increase visual capability. • When larger—cataract surgery

FOLLOW-UP

PATIENT MONITORING

• Depends on defect • Congenital KCS—requires frequent monitoring of tear production and the status of the external eye structures • Congenital cataracts and severe PHTVL and PHPV—regular checkups, usually on a 6-month basis, to monitor possible progression • Large colobomatous defects of the fundus and geographic retinal dysplasia—yearly checkups to monitor possible complete retinal detachment

PREVENTION/AVOIDANCE

• Depend on type and severity of defect • Re-strict breeding of affected animals and of known carriers of documented hereditary defects.

POSSIBLE COMPLICATIONS

• Depend on defect • Untreated eyelid agenesis, dermoids, and congenital KCS—recurrent problems with conjunctivitis and keratitis • Congenital glaucoma—painful, blind eye in conjunction with buphthalmos; often a dry, pigmented cornea • Large colobomas of the optic nerve head—may cause retinal detach-ment • Retinal detachment—may cause intraocular primarily vitreal hemorrhage

EXPECTED COURSE AND PROGNOSIS

• Depend on defect and type of medical and/or surgical treatment provided • Adnexal abnor-malities—good prognosis with surgical treat-ment • Congenital KCS—rather poor prognosis with medical treatment only; somewhat better prognosis with surgical treatment • Congenital cataract—usually good prognosis with surgical treatment

MISCELLANEOUS

ASSOCIATED CONDITIONS

Retinal dysplasia—described with chondrodysplastic skeletal abnormalities in field-trial Labradors

Suggested Reading

Narfström K, Ekesten B. Diseases of the canine ocular fundus. In: Gelatt KN, ed. Veterinary Ophthalmology. 3rd ed. Philadelphia: Lippin-cott Williams & Wilkins, 1999;869–933.

Peiffer RL, Petersen-Jones SM. Small animal ophthalmology: a problem-oriented approach. London: Saunders, 1997.

Petersen-Jones SM, Crispin SM. Manual of small animal ophthalmology. Gloucestershire, UK: British Small Animal Veterinary Associa-tion, 1993.

Author Kristina Narfström
Consulting Editor Paul E. Miller

CONGENITAL SPINAL AND VERTEBRAL MALFORMATIONS

 BASICS

DEFINITION
Anomalous development of spinal structures, which are apparent at birth or within the first weeks of life

PATHOPHYSIOLOGY
• Malformation of the occipital bones, atlas, and axis; malformation of the odontoid process; occipitoatlantoaxial malformation; and occipital dysplasia—may cause atlantoaxial subluxation with secondary compression and trauma to the first segments of the cervical spinal cord
• Other embryonic or developmental anomalies of the vertebrae—hemivertebra, transitional vertebra, block vertebra, and butterfly vertebra; these defects cause deformity and instability of the vertebral canal and, in rare occasions, compression of the associated spinal cord or nerve roots
• Sacrococcygeal dysgenesis—characterized by absence or partial development of the sacrocaudal spinal cord segments; often associated with additional malformations (e.g., spina bifida)
• Spina bifida—caused by failure of fusion of the vertebral arches; may be associated with protrusion of the spinal cord and meninges; other malformations often linked to this syndrome include spinal dysplasia, dysraphism, syringomyelia/hydromyelia, and myelodysplasia
• Congenital spinal stenosis—can occur when vertebral malformations cause segmental or diffuse narrowing of the spinal cord; inborn errors in skeletal growth, hypertrophy of ligamentum flavum, and bony proliferation may also contribute to the stenosis

SYSTEMS AFFECTED
Nervous—spinal cord; spinal nerve roots; and spinal column (vertebrae)

GENETICS
• A genetic background, with unknown mode of inheritance, is suspected in most congenital spinal diseases.
• Sacrococcygeal dysgenesis—autosomal dominant
• Thoracic hemivertebra of German shorthaired pointers—autosomal recessive

GEOGRAPHIC DISTRIBUTION
N/A

SIGNALMENT
Species and Breed Predilections
• Malformation of the occipital bones, atlas, and axis—most common in small-breed dogs

• Hemivertebra, transitional vertebra, block vertebra, and butterfly vertebra—most common in brachycephalic, "screw-tailed" breeds (e.g., French and English bulldogs, pugs, Boston terriers)
• Sacrococcygeal dysgenesis—Manx cats
• Spina bifida—bulldogs, Manx cats, and other screw-tailed breeds
• Myelodysplasia—weimaraners
• Congenital spinal stenosis—Doberman pinschers; chondrodystrophic breeds

Mean Age Range
• Often silent, vertebral malformation may cause clinical disease during the rapid growth of the animal (e.g., 5–9 months of age).
• Spinal cord anomalies cause clinical disease from birth on.

SIGNS
• Distortion of the spinal column—lordosis; kyphosis; and scoliosis in cases of vertebral malformations
• Ataxia and paresis associated with spinal cord compression and trauma
• Signs vary with spinal cord segment(s) involved.

CAUSES
Breed-related inherited defects are suspected for most congenital spinal abnormalities, although interactions between several genes and environmental factors (e.g., teratogenic compounds, nutritional deficiencies) are likely involved and would explain some of these complex pathologic changes.

RISK FACTORS
• Teratogenic compounds
• Toxins
• Nutritional deficiencies
• Stress

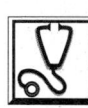 DIAGNOSIS

DIFFERENTIAL DIAGNOSIS
• Metabolic disease (e.g., storage diseases)
• Nutritional disease (e.g., hypovitaminosis and hypervitaminosis A, thiamine deficiency)
• Early-onset inflammatory or infectious processes (e.g., viral, protozoal, and rarely bacterial)
• Toxin exposure (e.g., lead, organo-phosphates, hexachlorophene, organochlorine)
• Trauma

CBC/BIOCHEMISTRY/URINALYSIS
Usually within normal limits

OTHER LABORATORY TESTS
N/A

IMAGING
• Survey radiography—in most cases can reveal vertebral malformation(s) and deviation of the spinal column
• Myelography—essential to determine with precision the level(s) of spinal cord compression when neurologic signs are observed; flexed and extended views can be performed with great caution under fluoroscopy
• Advanced imaging, including CT and MRI—may be useful to further characterize surrounding structures involved (e.g., spinal nerve root compression, ligament hypertrophy, hypoplasia of the odontoid process)

DIAGNOSTIC PROCEDURES
N/A

PATHOLOGIC FINDINGS
• Multiple congenital malformations—often present concomitantly; pathologic changes reflect several disease processes
• Acute compression of the spinal cord secondary to congenital malformation(s)—may result in spinal cord ischemia, hemorrhage, ballooning of the myelin sheath at the point of compression or trauma, and axonal swelling or loss; in chronic spinal cord compression, myelin degeneration, astrocytosis, and fibrosis are more prominent; at spinal sites cranial and caudal to the primary injury, wallerian degeneration can be observed in ascending or descending pathways, respectively
• Chronic changes—may result from vertebral malformations secondary to bony proliferation, thickening of the joint capsule, hypertrophy of articular processes, and thickening of the ligaments surrounding the spinal cord
• Atlantoaxial subluxation—congenital aplasia or hypoplasia of the odontoid process and surrounding ligaments
• Occipitoatlantoaxial malformations—fusion of the atlas to the occipital bone (cats) and dorsal angulation of the dens (dogs)
• Occipital dysplasia—anomaly of the foramen magnum in which the occipital bone is incompletely formed and fibrous tissue membrane covers the caudal cerebellum
• Sacrococcygeal dysgenesis—caudal vertebral aplasia or hypoplasia
• Spina bifida—incomplete fusion of the dorsal vertebral arches where the meninges or spinal cord can protrude; most commonly seen in the caudal lumbar or sacral area; a dimple can be observed in few cases secondary to the lack of separation between the neuroectoderm and other ectodermal structures, leaving a small attachment

CONGENITAL SPINAL AND VERTEBRAL MALFORMATIONS

between the spinal cord or meninges and the skin; often seen with myelodysplasia, central canal defects, syringomyelia or hydromyelia, and abnormal gray-matter differentiation
• Spinal stenosis—pathologic changes observed within the spinal cord are most commonly chronic and are caused by focal or diffuse narrowing of the spinal canal

TREATMENT

APPROPRIATE HEALTH CARE
• Depends on severity of neurologic deficits
• Outpatient—if animal is ambulatory
• Inpatient—if animal is nonambulatory or requires emergency surgical treatment (e.g., for atlantoaxial subluxation)

NURSING CARE
• Restricted activity combined with physical therapy–may help neurologically disabled patients in their postoperative period; a cart may be necessary for severely affected patients
• Management of urination—may be essential for cases in which disorders of micturition accompany the spinal injury

ACTIVITY
Restricted, especially if vertebral subluxation is present

DIET
N/A

CLIENT EDUCATION
Many congenital vertebral malformations are clinically silent. Perform a thorough work-up when a congenial malformation results in neurologic abnormalities. In addition, heritability is suspected and breeding must be performed only with serious consideration. Many neurologically affected dogs and cats left untreated are euthanized. Therefore, early surgical intervention is often necessary to alleviate compression of the spinal cord and prevent further damage.

SURGICAL CONSIDERATIONS
• In general, surgical decompression is required when congenital malformation(s) cause narrowing of the spinal canal and compression of the spinal cord. In cases of chronic or diffuse spinal cord compression, therapeutic responses following surgery are minimal.
• Atlantoaxial subluxation—surgical ventral decompression combined with stabilization of the atlantoaxial joint with pins or screws is the treatment of choice

• Spina bifida—meningoceles can be closed surgically to prevent leakage of cerebrospinal fluid and infections; surgery usually is not attempted when the spinal cord parenchyma is involved

MEDICATIONS

DRUG(S) OF CHOICE
Corticosteroids may be used in some cases, with questionable results.

CONTRAINDICATIONS
Avoid steroids with concomitant infections.

PRECAUTIONS
Steroids may cause ulcerations of the gastrointestinal tract and inhibit bone growth.

POSSIBLE INTERACTIONS
Steroids reduce immune response following vaccination.

ALTERNATIVE DRUG(S)
N/A

FOLLOW-UP

PATIENT MONITORING
• Frequent neurologic examinations—often required to monitor the progression of clinical signs (e.g., every 4–6 months)
• Radiography—repeat as needed.

PREVENTION/AVOIDANCE
Avoid breeding affected animals.

POSSIBLE COMPLICATIONS
• Depend on the type and severity of neurologic signs. In cases of subluxation of the atlantoaxial joint, acute death may occur. Acute paralysis can also be seen with vertebral subluxation, with further trauma and spinal cord compression.
• Implant failure may be observed after surgical decompression/stabilization.

EXPECTED COURSE AND PROGNOSIS
• Prognosis varies depending on the type of malformation, degree of spinal cord compression or injury, and surgical decompression or stabilization techniques.
• Vertebral malformation without compression of the spinal cord—prognosis is good
• Atlantoaxial subluxation following surgical decompression or stabilization—prognosis is fair to good

• Spinal cord compression treated surgically—prognosis is fair
• Spina bifida associated with spinal cord malformation, chronic neurologic disease despite surgical treatment, and lower motor neuron incontinence—prognosis is poor
• Medical treatment usually is insufficient to alleviate moderate to severe neurologic signs caused by spinal cord compression secondary to congenital vertebral malformation(s).

MISCELLANEOUS

ASSOCIATED CONDITIONS
N/A

AGE-RELATED FACTORS
N/A

ZOONOTIC POTENTIAL
N/A

PREGNANCY
N/A

SEE ALSO
• Ataxia
• Atlantoaxial Instability
• Spinal Dysraphism
• Paralysis
• Wobbler Syndrome (Cervical Vertebral Instability)

ABBREVIATIONS
CT = computed tomography
MRI = magnetic resonance imaging

Suggested Reading
Bailey SC, Morgan JP. Congenital spinal malformations. Vet Clin North Am 1992;22:985–1015.
Jeffrey ND. Handbook of small animal spinal surgery. Philadelphia: Saunders, 1995.
Oliver JE, Lorenz MD, Kornegay JN. Handbook of veterinary neurology. 3rd ed. Philadelphia: Saunders, 1997.
Sande RD. Radiology, myelography, computed tomography and magnetic resonance imaging of the spine. Vet Clin North Am 1992;22:811–831.
Summer BA, Cummings JF, de Lahunta A. Veterinary pathology. Philadelphia: Mosby-Year Book, 1995.
Author Christiane Massicotte
Consulting Editor Joane M. Parent

CONGESTIVE HEART FAILURE, LEFT-SIDED

 **BASICS**

DEFINITION
Failure of the left side of the heart to advance blood at a sufficient rate to meet the metabolic needs of the patient or to prevent blood from pooling within the pulmonary venous circulation

PATHOPHYSIOLOGY
• Low cardiac output causes lethargy, exercise intolerance, syncope, and prerenal azotemia. • High hydrostatic pressure causes leakage of fluid from pulmonary venous circulation into pulmonary interstitium and alveoli. When fluid leakage exceeds ability of lymphatics to drain the affected areas, pulmonary edema develops.

SYSTEMS AFFECTED
• All organ systems can be affected by poor delivery of blood. • Respiratory because of edema • Cardiovascular

GENETICS
Some congenital heart defects have a genetic basis in certain breeds.

INCIDENCE/PREVALENCE
Common

GEOGRAPHIC DISTRIBUTION
Seen everywhere, but prevalence of causes varies with location.

SIGNALMENT
Species
Dogs and cats

Breed Predilections
Varies with cause

Mean Age and Range
Varies with cause

Predominant Sex
Varies with cause

SIGNS
General Comments
Signs vary with underlying cause and between species

Historical Findings
• Weakness, lethargy, exercise intolerance. • Coughing (dogs) and dyspnea; respiratory signs often worsen at night and can be relieved by assuming a standing, sternal, or "elbows abducted" position (orthopnea). • Cats rarely cough.

Physical Examination Findings
• Tachypnea • Coughing, often soft in conjunction with tachypnea • Inspiratory and expiratory dyspnea when animal has pulmonary edema • Pulmonary crackles and wheezes • Prolonged capillary refill time • Possible murmur or gallop • Weak femoral pulses

CAUSES
Pump (Muscle) Failure of Left Ventricle
• Idiopathic dilated cardiomyopathy (DCM) • Trypanosomiasis (rare) • Doxorubicin cardiotoxicity (dogs) • Hypothyroidism (rare) • Hyperthyroidism (rarely causes pump failure; more commonly causes high output failure)

Pressure Overload of Left Heart
• Systemic hypertension • Subaortic stenosis • Coarctation of the aorta (rare; airdales predisposed) • Left ventricular tumors (rare)

Volume Overload of Left Heart
• Mitral valve endocardiosis • Mitral valve dysplasia • PDA • Ventricular septal defect

Impediment to Filling of Left Heart
• Pericardial effusion with tamponade • Restrictive pericarditis • Restrictive cardiomyopathy • Hypertrophic cardiomyopathy • Left atrial masses (e.g., tumors and thrombus) • Pulmonary thromboembolism • Mitral stenosis (rare)

Rhythm Disturbances
• Bradycardia (AV block) • Tachycardia (e.g., atrial fibrillation, atrial tachycardia, and ventricular tachycardia)

RISK FACTORS
Conditions causing high cardiac output (e.g., hyperthyroidism, anemia, and pregnancy)

 DIAGNOSIS

DIFFERENTIAL DIAGNOSIS
Must differentiate from other causes of coughing, dyspnea, and weakness

CBC/BIOCHEMISTRY/URINALYSIS
• CBC usually normal; may be stress leukogram • Mild to moderate liver enzyme elevation; bilirubin generally normal • Prerenal azotemia in some animals

OTHER LABORATORY TESTS
Thyroid disorders may be detected.

IMAGING
Radiographic Findings
• Left heart and pulmonary veins enlarged • Pulmonary edema, often hilar, initially; may be patchy, especially in cats; usually symmetrical, but may begin in right caudal lung lobe

Echocardiography
• Findings vary markedly with cause, but left atrial enlargement a relatively consistent finding in congested animals • Diagnostic test of choice for documenting congenital defects, cardiac masses, and pericardial effusion

DIAGNOSTIC PROCEDURES
Electrocardiographic Findings
• Atrial or ventricular arrhythmias • Evidence of left heart enlargement (e.g., wide P waves, tall and wide QRS complexes, and left axis orientation) • May be normal

PATHOLOGIC FINDINGS
Cardiac findings vary with disease

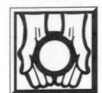 **TREATMENT**

APPROPRIATE HEALTH CARE
• Usually treat as outpatient unless animal is dyspneic or severely hypotensive. • Identify and correct underlying cause whenever possible. • Minimize handling of critically dyspneic animals. Stress can kill!

NURSING CARE
Oxygen is life saving in critically dyspneic patients.

ACTIVITY
Restrict activity.

DIET
Initiate moderately sodium-restricted diet. Severe sodium restriction is indicated in animals with advanced disease.

CLIENT EDUCATION
With few exceptions (e.g., animals with thyroid disorders, arrhythmias, nutritionally responsive heart disease), left congestive heart failure (L-CHF) is not curable.

SURGICAL CONSIDERATIONS
• Surgical intervention or balloon valvuloplasty may benefit selected patients with congenital defects such as PDA and subaortic stenosis. Response to these interventions varies. • Pericardiocentesis in animals with pericardial effusion

 MEDICATIONS

DRUG(S) OF CHOICE
Diuretics
• Furosemide (1–2 mg/kg q8–24h) or other loop diuretic is the initial diuretic of choice; diuretics are indicated to remove pulmonary edema. Critically dyspneic animals often require high doses (4–8 mg/kg) given IV to stabilize; this dose can be repeated in 1 hour if animal is still severely dyspneic. Once edema resolves, taper to the lowest effective dosage.
• Spironolactone (0.5–2 mg/kg PO q12–24h) increases survival in humans with heart failure because of its ability to block aldosterone. Use in combination with furosemide.
• Thiazide diuretics can be added to furosemide and spironolactone in refractory heart failure cases.

Digoxin

• Digoxin (dogs, 0.22 mg/M^2 q12h; cats, 0.01 mg/kg q48h) is used in animals with myocardial failure (e.g., dilated cardiomyopathy). • Digoxin is also indicated to treat supraventricular arrhythmias (e.g., sinus tachycardia, atrial fibrillation, and atrial or junctional tachycardia) in patients with CHF. • In humans, digoxin has no effect on mortality but decreases hospitalization due to heart failure.

Venodilators

• Nitroglycerin ointment (0.25 in/5 kg q6–8h) causes venodilation, lowering left atrial filling pressures. • Use for acute stabilization of patients with severe pulmonary edema and dyspnea. • May be useful in animals with chronic L-CHF when used intermittently; to avoid tolerance, use intermittently and with 12-hour dose-free interval between the last dose of one day and the first dose of the next day.

ACE Inhibitors

• ACE inhibitor such as enalapril (0.5 mg/kg q12–24h) indicated in most animals with L-CHF • Use in L-CHF secondary to degenerative mitral valve disease • ACE inhibitors improve survival and quality of life in dogs with L-CHF secondary to degenerative valve disease and DCM.

Positive Inotropes

• Dopamine (dogs, 2.5–10 mcg/kg/min; cats, 1–5 μg/kg/min) and dobutamine (dogs, 2.5–10 μg/kg/min; cats, 2–10 μg/kg/min) are potent positive inotropic agents that may provide valuable short-term support of a heart failure patient with poor cardiac contractility. • These agents are arrhythmogenic, and dopamine can cause hypertension at high infusion rates. Careful monitoring is required.

Antiarrhythmic Agents

Treat arrhythmias if clinically indicated.

CONTRAINDICATIONS

Avoid vasodilators in patients with pericardial effusion or fixed outflow obstruction.

PRECAUTIONS

• ACE inhibitor and arterial dilators must be used with caution in patients with possible outflow obstruction. • Patients with pulmonary hypertension and hypoxia are at high risk for digoxin toxicity. • ACE inhibitor and digoxin must be used cautiously in patients with renal disease. • Use dobutamine cautiously in cats. • Hypothyroidism predisposes animal to digoxin toxicity, while hyperthyroidism diminishes effects of digoxin.

POSSIBLE INTERACTIONS

• Combination of high-dose diuretics and ACE inhibitor may cause azotemia, especially in animals with severe sodium restriction. • Combination diuretic therapy adds to risk of dehydration and electrolyte disturbances.

• Combination vasodilator therapy predisposes animal to hypotension.

ALTERNATIVE DRUG(S)

Arterial Dilators

• Hydralazine (1–2 mg/kg PO q12h) or amlodipine (0.05–0.2 mg/kg PO q24h) can be substituted for an ACE inhibitor in patients that do not tolerate the drug or have advanced renal failure. Monitor for hypotension and tachycardia; can be cautiously added to an ACE inhibitor in animals with refractory L-CHF. • Nitroprusside (1–10 μg/kg/min) is a potent arterial dilator that is usually reserved for short-term support of patients with life-threatening edema.

Calcium Channel Blockers

Diltiazem (0.5–1.5 mg/kg PO q8h) is frequently used in L-CHF patients for rate control in animals with supraventricular arrhythmias not controlled by digoxin and in cats with hypertrophic cardiomyopathy.

Beta Blockers

•Atenolol and metoprolol are used for rate control in animals with supraventricular tachycardia, hypertrophic cardiomyopathy, and hyperthyroidism. • Used alone or with a class 1 antiarrhythmic drug for control of ventricular arrhythmias; these drugs depress contractility (negative inotropes), so use cautiously in patients with myocardial failure. • On basis of human studies, may enhance survival in animals with idiopathic DCM; treatment is best initiated under the guidance of a cardiologist, starting with very low dosage and gradually increasing the dosage. Carvedilol is often used for this purpose, starting at 0.1 mg/kg q24h and titrating to 0.4 mg/kg q12h.

Nutritional Supplements

• Potassium supplementation if hypokalemia is documented; use potassium supplements cautiously in animals receiving an ACE inhibitor or spironolactone. • Taurine supplementation in cats with DCM and dogs with DCM and taurine deficiency (e.g., American cocker spaniels) • L-carnitine supplementation may help some dogs with DCM. • Coenzyme Q$_{10}$ is of potential value based on the results of small trials in humans with DCM.

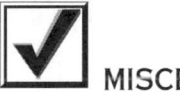

FOLLOW-UP

PATIENT MONITORING

• Monitor renal status, electrolytes, hydration, respiratory rate and effort, heart rate, body weight, and abdominal girth (dogs). • If azotemia develops, reduce the dosage of diuretic. If azotemia persists and the animal is also on an ACE inhibitor, reduce or discon-

tinue the ACE inhibitor. Use digoxin with caution if azotemia develops. • Monitor ECG if arrhythmias are suspected. • Check digoxin concentration periodically. Normal range is 0.5–1.5 ng/ml, 8–10 hours after a dose.

PREVENTION/AVOIDANCE

• Minimize stress, exercise, and sodium intake in patients with heart disease. • Prescribing an ACE inhibitor early in the course of heart disease in patients with DCM may slow the progression of heart disease and delay onset of CHF. Their role in asymptomatic animals with mitral valve disease remains controversial.

POSSIBLE COMPLICATIONS

• Syncope • Aortic thromboembolism (cats) • Arrhythmias • Electrolyte imbalances • Digoxin toxicity • Azotemia and renal failure

EXPECTED COURSE AND PROGNOSIS

Prognosis varies with underlying cause

✓ MISCELLANEOUS

ASSOCIATED CONDITIONS

N/A

AGE-RELATED FACTORS

• Congenital causes seen in young animals • Degenerative heart conditions and neoplasia generally seen in old animals

ZOONOTIC POTENTIAL

None

PREGNANCY

N/A

SEE ALSO

• Diseases Causing L-CHF • Pulmonary Edema

ABBREVIATIONS

• ACE = angiotensin-converting enzyme • DCM = dilated cardiomyopathy • L-CHF = left-sided congestive heart failure • PDA = patent ductus arteriosus

Suggested Reading

Sisson D. Medical management of refractory congestive heart failure in dogs. In: Bonagura JD, ed. Current Veterinary Therapy XIII. Philadelphia: Saunders, 2000;752–756.

Ware WA, Keene BW. Outpatient management of chronic heart failure. In: Bonagura JD, ed. Current Veterinary Therapy XIII. Philadelphia: Saunders, 2000;748–752.

Authors Francis W. K. Smith, Jr., and Bruce W. Keene

Consulting Editors Larry P. Tilley and Francis W. K. Smith, Jr.

CONGESTIVE HEART FAILURE, RIGHT-SIDED

 BASICS

DEFINITION
Failure of the right side of the heart to advance blood at a sufficient rate to meet the metabolic needs of the patient or to prevent blood from pooling within the systemic venous circulation

PATHOPHYSIOLOGY
• High hydrostatic pressure leads to leakage of fluid from venous circulation into the pleural and peritoneal space and interstitium of peripheral tissue.
• When fluid leakage exceeds ability of lymphatics to drain the affected areas, pleural effusion, ascites, and peripheral edema develop.

SYSTEMS AFFECTED
All organ systems can be affected by either poor delivery of blood or the effects of passive congestion from backup of venous blood.

GENETICS
Some congenital cardiac defects have a genetic basis in certain breeds.

INCIDENCE/PREVALENCE
Common

GEOGRAPHIC DISTRIBUTION
Syndrome seen everywhere, but prevalence of various causes varies with location

SIGNALMENT

Species
Dogs and cats

Breed Predilection
Varies with cause

Mean Age and Range
Varies with cause

Predominant Sex
Varies with cause

SIGNS

General Comments
• Signs vary with underlying cause and between species.
• Pleural effusion without ascites and hepatomegaly is rare in dogs with R-CHF (right-sided congestive heart failure).
• Ascites without pleural effusion is rare in cats with R-CHF.

Historical Findings
• Weakness
• Lethargy
• Exercise intolerance.
• Abdominal distension
• Dyspnea, tachypnea

Physical Examination Findings
• Jugular venous distention
• Hepatojugular reflex
• Jugular pulse in some animals
• Hepatomegaly
• Ascites common in dogs and rare in cats with R-CHF
• Possible regurgitant murmur in tricuspid valve region or ejection murmur at left heart base (pulmonic stenosis)
• Muffled heart sounds if animal has pleural or pericardial effusion
• Weak femoral pulses
• Rapid, shallow respiration if animal has pleural effusion or severe ascites
• Peripheral edema (infrequent)

CAUSES

Pump (Myocardial) Failure of Right Ventricle
• Idiopathic dilated cardiomyopathy (DCM)
• Trypanosomiasis
• Doxorubicin cardiotoxicity

Pressure Overload to Right Ventricle
• Heartworm disease
• Chronic obstructive pulmonary disease
• Pulmonary thromboembolism
• Pulmonic stenosis
• Tetralogy of Fallot
• Right ventricular tumors
• Primary pulmonary hypertension

Impediment to Right Ventricular Filling
• Pericardial effusion
• Restrictive pericarditis
• Right atrial or caval masses (caval syndrome)
• Tricuspid stenosis
• Cor triatriatum dexter

Rhythm Disturbances
• Bradycardia, generally atrioventricular block
• Tachyarrhythmias, generally supraventricular tachycardia

RISK FACTORS
• No heartworm prophylaxis
• Offspring of animal with right-sided congenital cardiac defect
• Conditions that augment demand for cardiac output (e.g., hyperthyroidism, anemia, pregnancy)

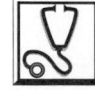 DIAGNOSIS

DIFFERENTIAL DIAGNOSIS
• Must differentiate from other causes of pleural effusion and ascites; generally requires a complete diagnostic work-up that includes CBC, biochemistry profile, heartworm test, thoracentesis or abdominocentesis with fluid analysis and cytologic examination, and, sometimes, thoracic and abdominal ultrasound

• Animals with ascites or pleural effusion due to heart failure should have jugular venous distension.

CBC/BIOCHEMISTRY/URINALYSIS
• CBC usually normal; animals with heartworm disease may have eosinophilia
• Mild to moderately high alanine aminotransferase, aspartate aminotransferase, serum alkaline phosphatase because of passive congestion of the liver; bilirubin generally normal
• Prerenal azotemia in some animals

OTHER LABORATORY TESTS
Heartworm test may be positive

IMAGING

Thoracic Radiographic Findings
• Right heart enlargement in some animals
• Dilated caudal vena cava (diameter greater than the length of the vertebra directly above the heart)
• Pleural effusion (especially cats)
• Hepatosplenomegaly and possible ascites (especially dogs)

Echocardiography
• Findings vary with underlying cause. Especially useful for documenting congenital defect, cardiac mass, and pericardial effusion
• Abdominal ultrasound reveals hepatomegaly with hepatic vein dilation and, possibly, ascites.

DIAGNOSTIC PROCEDURES

Electrocardiographic Findings
• Small complexes if animal has pericardial or pleural effusion
• Electrical alternans or elevated ST segment in animal with pericardial effusion
• Evidence of right heart enlargement (e.g., tall P waves in lead II, deep S waves in leads I, II, aVF, and right axis deviation)
• Atrial or ventricular arrhythmias; NOTE: ECG may be normal in patients with R-CHF.

Abdominocentesis
• Analysis of ascitic fluid in patients with R-CHF generally reveals modified transudate with a total protein >2.5 mg/dl.

Thoracentesis
• Cats with pleural effusion associated with R-CHF may have transudate, modified transudate, or chylous effusion.
• Dogs with pleural effusion and R-CHF may have transudate or modified transudate.

Central Venous Pressure
Central venous pressure is high (> 9 cm H_2O)

PATHOLOGIC FINDINGS
• Cardiac findings vary with disease
• Hepatomegaly in animals with centrolobular necrosis (chronic condition)

CONGESTIVE HEART FAILURE, RIGHT-SIDED

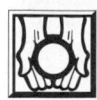

TREATMENT

APPROPRIATE HEALTH CARE
Most animals treated as outpatients unless dyspneic

NURSING CARE
Thoracentesis and abdominocentesis may be required periodically for patients no longer responsive to medical management or for those with severe dyspnea due to pleural effusion or ascites.

ACTIVITY
Restrict activity.

DIET
Restrict sodium moderately; severe sodium restriction is indicated for animals with advanced disease.

CLIENT EDUCATION
• With few exceptions (e.g., in heartworm disease, arrhythmias, and idiopathic pericardial effusion), R-CHF is not curable.
• Most patients improve with initial treatment but often have recurrent failure.

SURGICAL CONSIDERATIONS
• Surgical intervention or balloon valvuloplasty is indicated to treat certain congenital defects such as pulmonic stenosis.
• Pericardiocentesis or pericardectomy is done if animal has pericardial effusion.

MEDICATIONS

DRUG(S) OF CHOICE
Drugs should be administered only after a definitive diagnosis is made.

Diuretics
• Furosemide (1–2 mg/kg q8–24h) or another loop diuretic is the initial diuretic of choice. Diuretics are indicated to remove excess fluid accumulation.
• Spironolactone (0.5–2 mg/kg PO q12–24h) increases survival in humans with heart failure. Use in combination with furosemide.

Digoxin
• Digoxin (dogs, 0.22 mg/M^2 q12h; cats, 0.01 mg/kg q48h) is used in animals with myocardial failure (e.g., dilated cardiomyopathy).
• Digoxin is also indicated in animals with CHF that have supraventricular arrhythmias (e.g., sinus tachycardia, atrial fibrillation, and atrial or junctional tachycardia).

ACE Inhibitors
ACE inhibitors such as enalapril (0.5 mg/kg q12–24h) or benazepril (0.25–0.5 mg/kg q24h) may be helpful.

CONTRAINDICATIONS
Avoid vasodilators in patients with pericardial effusion or fixed outflow obstructions.

PRECAUTIONS
• ACE inhibitors and arterial dilators must be used with caution in patients with possible outflow obstructions.
• Patients with pulmonary hypertension and hypoxia are at higher risk than others for digoxin toxicity.
• ACE inhibitors and digoxin must be used cautiously in patients with renal disease.
• Animals with hypothyroidism are predisposed to digoxin toxicity, while hyperthyroidism diminishes digoxin effects.

POSSIBLE INTERACTIONS
• Combination of high-dose diuretics and ACE inhibitor may alter renal perfusion and cause azotemia.
• Combination diuretic therapy promotes risk of dehydration and electrolyte disturbances.

ALTERNATIVE DRUG(S)
• Patients unresponsive to furosemide, spironolactone, vasodilator, and digoxin (if indicated) may benefit from triple diuretic therapy by adding a thiazide diuretic.
• Potassium supplementation if animal has hypokalemia; use potassium supplements cautiously in animals receiving ACE inhibitor or spironolactone.
• Treat arrhythmias if clinically indicated.
• Taurine supplementation in cats with DCM and dogs with DCM and taurine deficiency
• Carnitine supplementation may help some dogs with DCM (e.g., cocker spaniels and boxers).

FOLLOW-UP

PATIENT MONITORING
• Monitor renal status, electrolytes, hydration, respiratory rate and effort, body weight, and abdominal girth (dogs).
• If azotemia develops, reduce the diuretic dosage. If azotemia persists and the animal is also on an ACE inhibitor, reduce or discontinue this drug. If azotemia develops, reduce the digoxin dosage to avoid toxicity.
• Monitor ECG periodically to detect arrhythmias.
• Monitor digoxin concentrations. Normal values are 0.5–1.5 ng/ml for a serum sample obtained 8–10 hours after a dose is administered.

PREVENTION/AVOIDANCE
N/A

POSSIBLE COMPLICATIONS
• Pulmonary thromboembolism
• Arrhythmias
• Electrolyte imbalances
• Digoxin toxicity
• Azotemia and renal failure

EXPECTED COURSE AND PROGNOSIS
Prognosis varies with underlying cause.

MISCELLANEOUS

ASSOCIATED CONDITIONS
N/A

AGE-RELATED FACTORS
• Congenital causes seen in young animals
• Degenerative heart conditions and neoplasia generally seen in old animals

ZOONOTIC POTENTIAL
None

PREGNANCY
N/A

SEE ALSO
• Ascites
• Chylothorax
• Diseases causing R-CHF
• Pleural Effusion

ABBREVIATIONS
• ACE = angiotensin-converting enzyme
• DCM = dilated cardiomyopathy
• L-CHF = left-sided congestive heart failure
• R-CHF = right-sided congestive heart failure

Suggested Reading
International Small Animal Cardiac Health Council. Recommendations for the diagnosis of heart disease and the treatment of heart failure in small animals. In: Miller MS, Tilley LP, eds. Manual of canine and feline cardiology. 2nd ed. Philadelphia: Saunders, 1995.
Sisson D. Medical management of refractory congestive heart failure in dogs. In: Bonagura JD, ed. Current veterinary therapy XIII. Philadelphia: Saunders, 2000, 752–756.
Ware WA, Keene BW. Outpatient management of chronic heart failure. In: Bonagura JD, ed. Current veterinary therapy XIII. Philadelphia: Saunders, 2000, 748–752.
Authors Francis W. K. Smith, Jr., and Bruce W. Keene
Consulting Editors Larry P. Tilley and Francis W. K. Smith, Jr.

CONJUNCTIVITIS—CATS

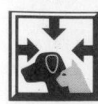 BASICS

DEFINITION
Inflammation of the conjunctiva, the vascularized mucous membrane that covers the anterior portion of the globe (bulbar portion) and lines the lids and third eyelid (palpebral portion)

PATHOPHYSIOLOGY
May be primary (e.g., infectious) or secondary to an underlying ocular or systemic disease (e.g., glaucoma, uveitis, immune-mediated disease, neoplasia)

SYSTEMS AFFECTED
Ophthalmic—ocular with occasional lid involvement (e.g., blepharoconjunctivitis)

GENETICS
N/A

INCIDENCE/PREVALENCE
Common

GEOGRAPHIC DISTRIBUTION
N/A

SIGNALMENT
Species
Cats

Breed Predilections
Infectious—purebred cats seem predisposed

Mean Age and Range
Infections—most commonly affects young animals

Predominant Sex
N/A

SIGNS
• Blepharospasm • Conjunctival hyperemia • Ocular discharge—serous, mucoid, or mucopurulent • Chemosis • Bulbar or palpebral conjunctiva—may be primarily involved • Upper respiratory infection—possible

CAUSES
Viral
• FHV—most common infectious cause; only one that leads to corneal changes (e.g., dendritic or geographic ulcers) • Calicivirus

Bacterial
• Primary condition (i.e., not secondary to another condition such as KCS)—rare, except for chlamydia and mycoplasma • Neonatal—accumulation of exudates, often with a bacterial or viral component; seen before lid separation

Immune-mediated
• Eosinophilic • Related to systemic immune-mediated diseases—pemphigus

Neoplastic, Pseudoneoplastic
Rare; lymphosarcoma and squamous cell carcinoma most common

Secondary to Adnexal Disease
• Aqueous tear film deficiency • May develop KCS as a result of scarring (see Keratoconjunctivitis Sicca) • Lid diseases (e.g., entropion)—may lead to clinical signs of conjunctivitis • Secondary to obstruction of the outflow portion of the nasolacrimal system—obstructed nasolacrimal duct

Secondary to Trauma or Environmental Causes
• Conjunctival foreign body • Irritation from dust, chemicals, or ophthalmic medications

Secondary to Other Ocular Diseases
• Ulcerative keratitis • Anterior uveitis • Glaucoma

RISK FACTORS
N/A

 DIAGNOSIS

DIFFERENTIAL DIAGNOSIS
• Primary—must distinguish from condition that is secondary to other ocular diseases • Intraocular disease—involvement of the bulbar conjunctiva with minimal or no involvement of the palpebral conjunctiva • Primary or allergic—involvement of mainly the palpebral conjunctiva, sparing the bulbar conjunctiva; consider primary and secondary causes if both surfaces are involved. • Must differentiate between conjunctival vessels (freely mobile and will blanch with sympathomimetics) and episcleral (deep) vessels (immobile and do not blanch with sympathomimetics)—episcleral congestion indicates intraocular disease; conjunctival hyperemia may be a sign of primary conjunctivitis or intraocular disease.

CBC/BIOCHEMISTRY/URINALYSIS
Normal, except with systemic disease

OTHER LABORATORY TESTS
• Infectious—consider serologic tests for FeLV and FIV; rule out underlying immunocompromise.

IMAGING
N/A

DIAGNOSTIC PROCEDURES
• Complete ophthalmic examination—rule out underlying intraocular diseases (e.g., uveitis and glaucoma). • Thorough adnexal examination—rule out lid abnormalities and foreign bodies in cul-de-sacs or under nictitans. • Nasolacrimal flush—considered to rule out nasolacrimal disease • Aerobic bacterial culture and sensitivity—with mucopurulent discharge; specimens ideally taken before anything is placed in the eye (e.g., topical anesthetic, fluorescein, and flush) to prevent inhibition or dilution of bacterial growth • Conjunctival cytology—

may reveal a cause (rare); eosinophils and basophils may help diagnose allergic and eosinophilic conjunctivitis but are rarely seen with allergic conjunctivitis except on biopsy; may see degenerate neutrophils and intracytoplasmic bacteria, which indicate bacterial infection; may see inclusion bodies with chlamydial or mycoplasmal infection; rarely see FHV inclusions • Conjunctival scrapings for FHV—use PCR or an IFA technique; but may note false-positive results with chronic disease; PCR more sensitive and test of choice; may note false-positive result if fluorescein staining is done before IFA testing • Conjunctival scrapings for *Chlamydia*—use special stains, which are fairly reliable • Viral culture—not widely available but may help diagnose FHV • Conjunctival biopsy—may be useful with mass lesions and immune-mediated disease; may help with chronic disease for which a definitive diagnosis has not been made

PATHOLOGIC FINDINGS
• Biopsy—typical signs of inflammation (e.g., neutrophils and lymphocytes); possibly infectious agents • Histopathologic features of mass lesions (e.g., squamous cell carcinoma and lymphosarcoma)—consistent with similar lesions elsewhere

 TREATMENT

APPROPRIATE HEALTH CARE
• Primary—often outpatient • Secondary to other diseases (e.g., uveitis and ulcerative keratitis)—may need hospitalization while the underlying problem is diagnosed and treated

ACTIVITY
• Primary—no restriction for most patients • Suspected contact irritant or acute allergic disease—prevent (if possible) contact with the offending agent. • Suspected FHV—minimizing stress recommended • Do not expose patients to susceptible animals.

DIET
Suspected underlying skin disease and/or food allergy—food elimination diet recommended

CLIENT EDUCATION
• If copious discharge is noted, instruct the client to clean the eyes before giving treatment. • If solutions and ointments are both prescribed, instruct the client to use the solution(s) before the ointment(s). • If several solutions are prescribed, instruct the client to wait several minutes between treatments.

• Instruct the client to call for instructions if the condition worsens, which indicates that the condition may not be responsive or may be progressing or that the animal may be having an adverse reaction to a prescribed medication.

SURGICAL CONSIDERATIONS
• Nasolacrimal duct obstruction—difficult; treatment often not recommended (see Epiphora)
• Conjunctival neoplasia—may require only local resection; may involve excision followed by β-irradiation, cryotherapy, radiofrequency hyperthermia, enucleation, or exenteration, depending on the type of tumor and the extent of involvement
• Symblepharon—may require surgical resection once active conjunctival infection is controlled
• Corneal sequestration—keratectomy may be required

MEDICATIONS
DRUG(S) OF CHOICE
Herpetic
• Condition usually mild and self-limiting
• Antiviral treatment—indicated for herpetic keratitis, before keratectomy for corneal sequestrums suspected to be related to FHV, and for severe intractable conjunctivitis; drug penetration into the conjunctiva (vs. the cornea) poor; optional; treatment may be directed at controlling secondary bacterial infection only.
• 0.1% Idoxuridine solution (available from compounding pharmacies)—topical q6h initially
• Vidarabine 3% ointment—topical q6h initially
• Trifluridine—recommended hourly for the first day, then 5 times a day
• Lysine 250–500 mg PO BID for adult cat

Chlamydial or Mycoplasmal
• Tetracycline—topical q6h; continue for several days past resolution of all clinical signs; recurrence or reinfection common; systemic treatment recommended by some authors for difficult cases
• Azithromycin 5 mg/kg PO every other day

Bacterial
Based on bacterial culture and sensitivity results

Neonatal
• Carefully open the lid margins (medial to temporal), establish drainage, and treat with topical antibiotic and an antiviral for suspected FHV.

• Symblepharon (adhesions between the conjunctival surfaces and possibly the cornea)—common sequela; may require surgical intervention

Eosinophilic
• Topical corticosteroids—usual treatment; 0.1% dexamethasone generally effective when used three or four times daily; taper to the lowest effective dose
• Oral megestrol acetate—may help resistant condition; consider possible systemic side effects

CONTRAINDICATIONS
• Topical corticosteroids—avoid with known or suspected herpetic conjunctivitis; evidence shows that agents predispose the patient to corneal sequestrum formation; avoid if corneal ulceration is noted
• Topical cyclosporine—best to avoid with known or suspected herpetic conjunctivitis, unless a topically administered antiviral is used concurrently

PRECAUTIONS
• Topical aminoglycosides and antiviral medication may be irritating.
• Monitor all patients treated with topical corticosteroids for signs of corneal ulceration; discontinue agent immediately if corneal ulceration occurs.

POSSIBLE INTERACTIONS
N/A

ALTERNATIVE DRUG(S)
• Other corticosteroids—1% prednisolone acetate; betamethasone; hydrocortisone

FOLLOW-UP
PATIENT MONITORING
Recheck shortly after beginning treatment (at 5–7 days); then recheck as needed.

PREVENTION/AVOIDANCE
• Treat any underlying disease that may be exacerbating the ocular disease—allergic or immune-mediated skin disease; KCS.
• Prevent re-exposure to source of infection.
• Minimize stress for patients with herpetic conjunctivitis. • Isolate patients with infectious conjunctivitis to prevent spread.
• Vaccination against viral causes—recommended; infection is still possible if the cat was exposed to an infectious agent before being vaccinated (e.g., FHV infection from an infected queen).

POSSIBLE COMPLICATIONS
• Corneal sequestration • Symblepharon
• KCS

EXPECTED COURSE AND PROGNOSIS
• FVH—most patients become chronic carriers; episodes less common as patient matures; may see repeated exacerbations; tend to note more severe clinical signs at times of stress or immunocompromise
• Bacterial conjunctivitis—usually resolves with appropriate administration of antibiotics; if an underlying disease is found (e.g., KCS), resolution may depend on appropriate treatment and resolution of the disease.
• Immune-mediated diseases (e.g., eosinophilic)—control not cure; may require chronic treatment at the lowest level possible

MISCELLANEOUS
ASSOCIATED CONDITIONS
FeLV and FIV—may predispose patient to the chronic carrier state of FHV conjunctivitis

AGE-RELATED FACTORS
FHV—tends to be more severe in kittens and in old cats with waning immunity

ZOONOTIC POTENTIAL
Chlamydia psittaci—low

PREGNANCY
• Use systemic antibiotics and corticosteroids with caution, if at all, in pregnant animals.
• Absorption of topically applied medications should be considered a possibility, and the benefits of treatment should be weighed against the possible complications.

SEE ALSO
Keratoconjunctivitis Sicca (KCS)

ABBREVIATIONS
• FeLV = feline leukemia virus
• FHV = feline herpesvirus
• FIV = feline immunodeficiency virus
• IFA = immunofluorescent antibody test
• KCS = keratoconjunctivitis sicca
• PCR = polymerase chain reaction

Suggested Reading
Glazè MB, Gelett KN. Feline ophthalmology. In Gelatt KN, ed. Veterinary ophthalmology 3rd ed. Philadelphia: Lippincott Williams and Wilkins, 1999:997–1052.
Nasisse MP. Manifestations, diagnosis, and treatment of ocular herpesvirus infection in the cat. Compend Contin Educ Pract Vet 1982;4:962–971.
Nasisse MP, Weigler BJ. The diagnosis of ocular feline herpesvirus infection. Vet Comp Ophthalmol 1997;7:44–51.
Author Erin S. Champagne
Consulting Editor Paul E. Miller

CONJUNCTIVITIS—DOGS

 BASICS

DEFINITION
Inflammation of the conjunctiva, the vascularized mucous membrane that covers the anterior portion of the globe (bulbar portion) and lines the lids and third eyelid (palpebral portion)

PATHOPHYSIOLOGY
• Primary—allergic; infectious; environmental; KCS
• Secondary to an underlying ocular or systemic disease—glaucoma; uveitis; immune-mediated disease; neoplasia

SYSTEMS AFFECTED
Ophthalmic—ocular with occasional lid involvement (e.g., blepharoconjunctivitis)

GENETICS
N/A

INCIDENCE/PREVALENCE
Common

GEOGRAPHIC DISTRIBUTION
N/A

SIGNALMENT

Species
Dogs

Breed Predilection
Breeds predisposed to allergic or immune-mediated skin diseases (e.g., atopy) tend to have more problems with allergic conjunctivitis or KCS.

Mean Age and Range
N/A

Predominant Sex
N/A

SIGNS
• Blepharospasm
• Conjunctival hyperemia
• Ocular discharge—serous, mucoid, or mucopurulent
• Chemosis
• Follicle formation
• Bulbar or palpebral conjunctiva—may be primarily involved

CAUSES

Bacterial
• Primary condition (i.e., not secondary to another condition such as KCS)—rare
• Neonatal—an accumulation of exudates, often with a bacterial or viral component; seen before lid separation

Viral
Canine distemper virus

Immune-mediated
• Allergic—especially in atopic patients
• Follicular conjunctivitis
• Plasma cell conjunctivitis—especially in German shepherds
• Related to systemic immune-mediated diseases (e.g., pemphigus)

Neoplastic, Pseudoneoplastic
• Tumors involving conjunctiva—rare; include melanoma, hemangioma, hemangiosarcoma, lymphosarcoma, papilloma, and mast cell
• Pseudoneoplastic—nodular episcleritis (also called fibrous histiocytoma, ocular nodular granuloma, and conjunctival pseudotumor); most commonly seen in collies and mixed collies; believed to be immune-mediated; pink mass, usually located at the temporal limbus

Secondary to Adnexal Disease
• Aqueous tear film deficiency (see Kerato-conjunctivitis Sicca)
• Lid diseases (e.g., entropion, ectropion, exaggerated cul-de-sac) and lash diseases (e.g., distichiasis, ectopic cilia)—may lead to clinical signs of conjunctivitis
• Secondary to obstruction of the outflow portion of the nasolacrimal system (e.g., obstructed nasolacrimal duct and imperforate punctum)

Secondary to Trauma or Environmental Causes
• Conjunctival foreign body
• Irritation—dust, chemicals, or ophthalmic medications

Secondary to Other Ocular Diseases
• Ulcerative keratitis
• Anterior uveitis
• Glaucoma

RISK FACTORS
N/A

 DIAGNOSIS

DIFFERENTIAL DIAGNOSIS
• Primary—must distinguish from condition that is secondary to other ocular diseases
• Intraocular disease—involvement of the bulbar conjunctiva with minimal or no involvement of the palpebral conjunctiva
• Primary or allergic—involvement of mainly the palpebral conjunctiva sparing the bulbar conjunctiva; consider primary and secondary causes if both surfaces are involved.
• Must differentiate between conjunctival vessels (freely mobile and will blanch with sympathomimetic) and episcleral (deep) vessels (immobile and do not blanch with sympatho-mimetics), because episcleral congestion indicates intraocular disease, whereas conjunctival hyperemia may be a sign of primary conjunctivitis or intraocular disease

CBC/BIOCHEMISTRY/URINALYSIS
Normal, except with systemic disease

OTHER LABORATORY TESTS
N/A

IMAGING
N/A

DIAGNOSTIC PROCEDURES
• Complete ophthalmic examination (Schirmer tear test)—rule out KCS.
• Fluorescein stain—rule out ulcerative keratitis.
• Intraocular pressures—rule out glaucoma.
• Examine for signs of anterior uveitis (e.g., hypotony, aqueous flare, and miosis).
• Thorough adnexal examination—rule out lid abnormalities, lash abnormalities, and foreign bodies in cul-de-sacs or under nictitans
• Consider a nasolacrimal flush—rule out nasolacrimal disease.
• Aerobic bacterial culture and sensitivity—consider with mucopurulent discharge; ideally, specimens are taken before anything is placed in the eye (e.g., topical anesthetic, fluorescein, and flush) to prevent inhibition or dilution of bacterial growth; not routinely indicated for KCS and a mucopurulent discharge (secondary bacterial overgrowth almost certain)
• Conjunctival cytology—may reveal a cause (rare); eosinophils and basophils may help diagnose allergic and eosinophilic conjunctivitis but are rarely seen with allergic conjunctivitis except on biopsy; may see degenerate neutrophils and intracytoplasmic bacteria, which indicate bacterial infection; may see inclusion bodies (intracytoplasmic with distemper virus)
• Conjunctival biopsy—may be useful with mass lesions and immune-mediated disease; may help with chronic disease for which a definitive diagnosis has not been made
• Intradermal skin testing—may be helpful with suspected allergic conjunctivitis

PATHOLOGIC FINDINGS
• Biopsy—typical signs of inflammation (e.g., neutrophils and lymphocytes); may note infectious agents

• Histopathologic features of mass lesions (e.g., papilloma and mast cell tumor)—consistent with similar lesions elsewhere

 TREATMENT

APPROPRIATE HEALTH CARE
• Primary—often outpatient
• Secondary to other diseases (e.g., uveitis and ulcerative keratitis)—may require hospitalization while the underlying problem is diagnosed and treated

ACTIVITY
• Primary—usually no restriction
• Suspected contact irritant or acute allergic disease—prevent (if possible) contact with the offending agent.
• Do not expose patients to susceptible animals

DIET
Suspected underlying skin disease and/or food allergy—food elimination diet recommended

CLIENT EDUCATION
• If copious discharge is noted, instruct the client to clean the eyes before giving treatment.
• If solutions and ointments are both prescribed, instruct the client to use the solution(s) before the ointment(s).
• If several solutions are prescribed, instruct the client to wait several minutes between treatments.
• Instruct the client to call for instructions if the condition worsens, which indicates that the condition may not be responsive or may be progressing or that the animal may be having an adverse reaction to a prescribed medication.
• Inform the client that an Elizabethan collar should be placed on the patient if self-trauma occurs.

SURGICAL CONSIDERATIONS
• Nasolacrimal duct obstruction—difficult; treatment often not recommended (see Epiphora)
• Conjunctival neoplasia—may require only local resection; may involve excision followed by β-irradiation, cryotherapy, radiofrequency hyperthermia, enucleation, or exenteration, depending on the type of tumor and the extent of involvement

 MEDICATIONS

DRUG(S) OF CHOICE
Bacterial
• Based on bacterial culture and sensitivity results
• Initial treatment—broad-spectrum topical antibiotic or specific agent based on results of cytologic examination while waiting for culture results; may try empirical treatment, performing a culture only if patient is refractory to treatment
• Topical triple antibiotic or chloramphenicol—if cocci seen on cytologic examination
• Gentamicin or tobramycin—if rods seen on cytologic examination
• Ciprofloxacin—q6–12h, depending on severity; limited bacterial resistance (some streptococci are resistant); may be useful for severe bacterial conjunctivitis
• Systemic antibiotics—occasionally indicated, especially for more generalized disease (e.g., pyoderma)
Neonatal
Carefully open the lid margins (medial to temporal), establish drainage, and treat with topical antibiotic.
Immune-mediated
• Depends on severity
• Topical corticosteroids—0.1% dexamethasone; improve clinical signs of allergic, follicular, and plasma cell conjunctivitis; improvement often temporary
• Treatment of any underlying disease (e.g., atopy) often improves clinical signs.

CONTRAINDICATIONS
Topical corticosteroids—avoid if corneal ulceration is noted.

PRECAUTIONS
• Topical aminoglycosides—may be irritating
• Topical corticosteroids—monitor all patients carefully for signs of corneal ulceration; discontinue agent immediately if corneal ulceration occurs.

POSSIBLE INTERACTIONS
N/A

ALTERNATIVE DRUG(S)
Other corticosteroids—1% prednisolone acetate; betamethasone; hydrocortisone

 FOLLOW-UP

PATIENT MONITORING
Recheck shortly after beginning treatment (i.e., 5–7 days); then recheck as needed.

PREVENTION/AVOIDANCE
Treat any underlying disease that may be exacerbating the condition (e.g., allergic or immune-mediated skin disease; KCS).

POSSIBLE COMPLICATIONS
N/A

EXPECTED COURSE AND PROGNOSIS
• Bacterial—usually resolves with appropriate antibiotics; may depend on resolution of underlying disease (e.g., KCS)
• Immune-mediated diseases—tend to be controlled and not cured; may require chronic treatment at the lowest level possible

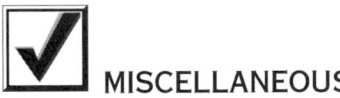 **MISCELLANEOUS**

ASSOCIATED CONDITIONS
• Atopy
• Pyoderma

AGE-RELATED FACTORS
N/A

ZOONOTIC POTENTIAL
N/A

PREGNANCY
• Use systemic antibiotics and corticosteroids with caution, if at all, in pregnant animals.
• Consider absorption of topically applied medications; weigh benefits of treatment against possible complications.

SEE ALSO
• Epiphora
• Keratoconjunctivitis Sicca
• Red Eye

ABBREVIATION
KCS = keratoconjunctivitis sicca

Suggested Reading
Hendrix DVH, Diseases and surgery of the canine conjunctiva. In: Gelatt KN, ed. Veterinary ophthalmology. 3rd ed. Philadelphia: Lippincott Williams & Wilkins, 1999: 619–634.
Author Erin S. Champagne
Consulting Editor Paul E. Miller

CONSTIPATION AND OBSTIPATION

 BASICS

DEFINITION
• Constipation—infrequent, incomplete, or difficult defecation with passage of hard or dry feces
• Obstipation—intractable constipation caused by prolonged retention of hard, dry feces; defecation is impossible in the obstipated patient.

PATHOPHYSIOLOGY
• Constipation can develop with any disease that impairs the passage of feces through the colon.
• Delayed fecal transit allows removal of additional salt and water, producing drier feces.
• Peristaltic contractions may increase during constipation, but eventually motility diminishes because of smooth muscle degeneration secondary to chronic overdistention.

SYSTEMS AFFECTED
Gastrointestinal

GENETICS
N/A

INCIDENCE/PREVALENCE
Common clinical problem

GEOGRAPHIC DISTRIBUTION
N/A

SIGNALMENT

Species
• Dogs and cats
• More common in cats

Breed Predilection
N/A

Mean Age and Range
N/A

Predominant Sex
N/A

SIGNS

Historical Findings
• Straining to defecate with small or no fecal volume
• Hard, dry feces
• Infrequent defecation
• Small amount of liquid, mucoid stool—sometimes with blood present produced after prolonged tenesmus
• Occasional vomiting, inappetence, and/or depression

Physical Examination Findings
• Colon filled with hard feces
• Other findings depend on cause.
• Rectal examination may reveal mass, stricture, perineal hernia, anal sac disease, foreign body or material, prostatic enlargement, or narrowed pelvic canal.

CAUSES

Dietary
• Bones
• Hair
• Foreign material
• Excessive fiber
• Inadequate water intake

Environmental
• Lack of exercise
• Change of environment—hospitalization, dirty litter box
• Inability to ambulate

Drugs
• Anticholinergics
• Antihistamines
• Opioids
• Barium sulfate
• Sucralfate
• Antacids
• Kaopectolin
• Iron supplements
• Diuretics

Painful Defecation
• Anorectal disease—anal sacculitis, anal sac abscess, perianal fistula, anal stricture, anal spasm, rectal foreign body, rectal prolapse, pseudocoprostasis, proctitis
• Trauma—fractured pelvis, fractured limb, dislocated hip, perianal bite wound or laceration, perineal abscess

Mechanical Obstruction
• Extraluminal—healed pelvic fracture with narrowed pelvic canal, prostatic hypertrophy, prostatitis, prostatic neoplasia, intrapelvic neoplasia, pseudocoprostasis, sublumbar lymphadenopathy
• Intraluminal and intramural—colonic or rectal neoplasia or polyp, rectal stricture, rectal foreign body, rectal diverticulum, perineal hernia, rectal prolapse, and congenital defect (atresia ani)

Neuromuscular Disease
• Central nervous system—paraplegia, spinal cord disease, intervertebral disk disease, cerebral disease (lead toxicity, rabies)
• Peripheral nervous system—dysautonomia, sacral nerve disease, sacral nerve trauma (e.g., tail fracture/pull injury)

• Colonic smooth muscle dysfunction—idiopathic megacolon in cats

Metabolic and Endocrine Disease
• Impaired colonic smooth muscle function—hyperparathyroidism, hypothyroidism, hypokalemia (chronic renal failure), hypercalcemia
• Debility—general muscle weakness, dehydration, neoplasia

RISK FACTORS
• Drug therapy—anticholinergics, narcotics, barium sulfate
• Metabolic disease causing dehydration
• Intact male—perineal hernia, prostatic disease
• Perianal fistula
• Pica—foreign material
• Excessive grooming—hair ingestion
• Decreased grooming/inability to groom—long-haired cats, pseudocoprostasis
• Pelvic fracture

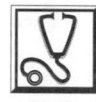 DIAGNOSIS

DIFFERENTIAL DIAGNOSIS
• Dyschezia and tenesmus (e.g., caused by colitis)—unlike constipation, associated with increased frequency of attempts to defecate, and frequent production of small amounts of liquid feces containing blood and/or mucus; rectal examination reveals diarrhea and lack of hard stool.
• Stranguria (e.g., caused by cystitis)—unlike constipation, can be associated with hematuria and abnormal findings on urinalysis (pyuria, crystalluria, bacteriuria).

CBC/BIOCHEMISTRY/URINALYSIS
• Usually normal
• May detect hypokalemia, hypercalcemia
• High packed cell volume (PCV) and total protein in dehydrated patients
• High WBC in patients with abscess, perianal fistula, prostatic disease
• Pyuria and hematuria with prostatitis

OTHER LABORATORY TESTS
• If patient (dog) is hypercholesterolemic, consider T_4 and TSH assay to rule out hypothyroidism.
• If patient is hypercalcemic, consider parathyroid hormone assay.

IMAGING
• Abdominal radiography may reveal colonic or rectal foreign body, colonic or rectal mass, prostatic enlargement, fractured pelvis, dislocated hip, or perineal hernias.

• Barium enema (after enemas to clean colon) may better define an intraluminal mass or stricture.

• Ultrasonography may help define extraluminal mass and prostatic disease.

DIAGNOSTIC PROCEDURES

Colonoscopy may be needed to identify a mass, stricture, or other colonic or rectal lesion; biopsy specimens can also be obtained.

TREATMENT

APPROPRIATE HEALTH CARE

• Remove or ameliorate any underlying cause if possible.

• Discontinue any medications that may cause constipation.

• May need to treat as inpatient if obstipation and/or dehydration present

NURSING CARE

Dehydrated patients should receive IV (preferably) or SC balanced electrolyte solutions (with potassium supplementation if indicated).

ACTIVITY

Encourage activity.

DIET

Dietary supplementation with a bulk-forming agent (bran, methylcellulose, canned pumpkin, psyllium) is often helpful, though they can sometimes worsen colonic fecal distension; in this case, feed a low-residue-producing diet.

CLIENT EDUCATION

Feed appropriate diet and encourage activity.

SURGICAL CONSIDERATIONS

• Manual removal of feces with the animal under general anesthesia (after rehydration) may be required if enemas and medications are unsuccessful.

• Subtotal colectomy may be required with recurring obstipation that responds poorly to assertive medical therapy.

MEDICATIONS

DRUG(S) OF CHOICE

• Emollient laxatives—docusate sodium or docusate calcium (dogs, 50–100 mg PO q12–24h; cats, 50 mg PO q12–24h)

• Stimulant laxatives—bisacodyl (5 mg/animal PO q8–24h)

• Saline laxatives—isosmotic mixture of polyethylene glycol and poorly absorbed salts; usually used to prepare the colon for colonoscopy (GoLytely, 30–50 mL/ kg PO once or twice 6–12 hr prior to procedure)

• Disaccharide laxative—lactulose (1 mL/4.5 kg PO q8–12h to effect)

• Warm water enemas may be needed; a small amount of mild soap or docusate sodium can be added but is usually not needed; sodium phosphate retention enemas (e.g., Fleet, C.B. Fleet Co., Inc.) are contraindicated because of their association with severe hypocalcemia.

• Suppositories can be used as a replacement for enemas; use glycerol, bisocodyl, or docusate sodium products.

• Motility modifiers can be tried—cisapride (dogs, 0.1–0.5 mg/kg PO q8–12h; cats, 2.5–10.0 mg/cat PO q8–12h) may stimulate motility; indicated with early megacolon

CONTRAINDICATIONS

• Lubricants such as mineral oil and white petrolatum are NOT recommended because of the danger of fatal lipoid aspiration pneumonia due to their lack of taste.

• Fleet enemas

• Anticholinergics

• Diuretics

PRECAUTIONS

Metoclopramide, cisapride, and cholinergics—can be used with caution; contraindicated in obstructive processes

POSSIBLE INTERACTIONS

N/A

ALTERNATIVE DRUG(S)

• Ranitidine causes contraction of colonic smooth muscle in vitro.

• Newer generation cisapride-like drugs may be available soon.

FOLLOW-UP

PATIENT MONITORING

Monitor frequency of defecation and stool consistency at least twice a week initially, then weekly or biweekly.

PREVENTION/AVOIDANCE

Keep pet active and feed appropriate diet.

POSSIBLE COMPLICATIONS

• Chronic constipation or recurrent obstipation can lead to acquired megacolon.

• Overuse of laxatives and enemas can cause diarrhea.

• Colonic mucosa can be damaged by improper enema technique, repeated rough mechanical breakdown of feces, or ischemic necrosis secondary to pressure of hard feces.

• Perineal irritation and ulceration can lead to fecal incontinence.

EXPECTED COURSE AND PROGNOSIS

Varies with underlying cause

MISCELLANEOUS

ASSOCIATED CONDITIONS

Vomiting—with severe/prolonged obstipation

AGE-RELATED FACTORS

N/A

ZOONOTIC POTENTIAL

N/A

PREGNANCY

N/A

SYNONYMS

• Fecal impaction

• Colonic impaction

SEE ALSO

Megacolon

ABBREVIATIONS

TSH = thyroid-stimulating hormone

Suggested Reading

Bright RM. Management of constipation and megacolon in cats. In: Proceedings of 17th Annual Waltham/OSU Symposium, 1993: 73–78.

Burrows CF. Medical diseases of the colon. In: Jones BD, ed. Canine and feline gastroenterology. Philadelphia: Saunders, 1986:221–256.

Burrows CF, Sherding RG. Constipation and dyschezia. In: Anderson NV, ed. Veterinary gastroenterology. Philadelphia: Lea & Febiger, 1992:484–503.

Hoskins JD. Management of fecal impaction. Compend Cont Ed Pract Vet 1990;12:1579–1585.

Authors Lisa E. Moore and Colin F. Burrows

Consulting Editor Albert E. Jergens

CONTACT DERMATITIS

 BASICS

OVERVIEW

• Irritant contact dermatitis (ICD) and allergic contact dermatitis (ACD)—two rare and possibly different pathophysiologic syndromes with similar clinical signs
• ICD—results from direct damage to keratinocytes by exposure to a particular compound; damaged keratinocytes induce an inflammatory response directed at the skin
• ACD—an immunologic event requiring sensitization, memory, and elicitation: Langerhans cells process antigens that penetrate the skin and present them to naive T cells within lymph nodes; sensitized T cell clones (memory cells) then proliferate and circulate throughout the body; Langerhans cells encounter the antigens again and present them to sensitized T cells, resulting in an immunologic response.

SIGNALMENT

• Dogs and cats
• ICD—occurs at any age as a direct result of the irritant nature of the offending compound
• ACD—rare in young animals; most animals are chronically exposed to the antigen; extremely rare in cats, except when exposed to D-limonene-containing insecticides
• Predisposed to ACD—German shepherds
• Increased risk of ACD (unsubstantiated)—French poodles, wire-haired fox terriers, Scottish terriers, West Highland white terriers, and golden retrievers

SIGNS

Lesions

• Location depends on the way in which the antigen is contacted; commonly limited to glabrous skin and regions frequently in contact with the ground (chin, ventral neck, sternum, ventral abdomen, inguinum, perineum, scrotum, and ventral contact regions of the tail and interdigital areas)
• The thick hair coat of dogs is an effective barrier against contactants.
• In classic cases, extreme erythroderma stops abruptly at the hairline.
• Initially consist of erythema and swelling, leading to papules and plaques; vesicles are uncommon.

Others

• Reactions to topical medications (most often otic preparations) are usually localized; generalized reactions, resulting from shampoos or insecticide sprays, are less common.
• Pruritus—moderate to severe; severe is most common. • A seasonal incidence may indicate that the offending antigen is a plant or outdoor compound.

CAUSES & RISK FACTORS

• Inflammatory dermatitis—may increase the penetration of antigens through the skin; thus may facilitate ACD
• Reported offending substances—plants, mulch, cedar chips; fabrics, rugs and carpets, plastics, rubber, leather, metal, concrete; soaps, detergents, floor waxes, carpet and litter deodorizers; herbicides, fertilizers, insecticides (including newer topical flea treatments), flea collars; topical preparations and medications

• Increased incidence of ACD in atopic animals

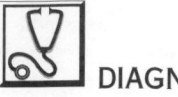 DIAGNOSIS

DIFFERENTIAL DIAGNOSIS

• Atopy
• Food allergy
• Drug eruptions
• Parasite hypersensitivity or infestation
• Insect bites
• Pyoderma
• *Malassezia* dermatitis
• Dermatophytosis
• Demodicosis
• Lupus erythematosus
• Seborrheic dermatitis
• Solar dermatitis
• Thermal injuries
• Trauma from rough surfaces

DIAGNOSTIC PROCEDURES

• Closed-patch testing—sometimes helpful (corticosteroids and NSAIDs must be discontinued 3–6 weeks before testing); use materials directly from the environment or a standard patch test kit for humans (Hermal, Oak Hill, NY) applied to the skin under a bandage for 48 hr.
• Best diagnostic test—eliminate contact irritant or antigen, follow with provocative exposure testing
• Bacterial cultures to define secondary pyoderma may be performed, if needed.

• Because the hair coat can protect the skin from contact with antigen, clipping a patch of hair in a nonaffected region should result in development of a local reaction.

PATHOLOGIC FINDINGS
• Skin biopsies—intraepidermal vesiculation and spongiosis; superficial dermal edema with perivascular mononuclear cell infiltrate in ICD and ACD; polymorphonuclear cell infiltrate in ICD; leukocyte exocytosis common. Lymphocytic spongiotic or eosinophilic and lymphocytic spongiotic infiltrate with intraepidermal eosinophilic pustules in canine ACD.

 TREATMENT
• Eliminate offending substance(s).
• Bathe with hypoallergenic shampoos to remove antigen from the skin.
• Create mechanical barriers, if possible—socks, T-shirts, restriction from environment

 MEDICATIONS
DRUG(S)
• Systemic corticosteroids—prednisone (0.25–0.5 mg/kg PO q24h for 3–5 days; then q48h for 2 weeks)

• Topical corticosteroids for focal lesions
• Pentoxifylline 10 mg/kg BID to TID initially may be reduced to q24h to maintain.

CONTRAINDICATIONS/POSSIBLE INTERACTIONS
Pentoxifylline—do not administer with alkylating agents, cisplatin, and amphotericin B; cimetidine may increase serum levels of pentoxifylline. Hemograms suggested for monitoring

 FOLLOW-UP
PREVENTION/AVOIDANCE
Remove offending substances from the environment.

EXPECTED COURSE AND PROGNOSIS
ICD
• Acute condition—may occur after only one exposure; can be manifested within 24 hr of exposure
• Steroids are rarely helpful.
• Lesions resolve 1–2 days after irritant removal.

ACD
• Requires months to years of exposure for the hypersensitivity to develop

• Re-exposure results in the development of clinical signs 3–5 days following exposure; signs may persist for several weeks.
• Responds well to corticosteroids; but the pruritus returns after discontinuation if the antigenic stimulus has not been removed.
• Hyposensitization is disappointing.
• Prognosis—good if the allergen is identified and removed; poor if the allergen is not identified, which may then require lifelong treatment

 MISCELLANEOUS
ABBREVIATIONS
• ACD = allergic contact dematitis
• ICD = irritant contact dermatitis
• NSAID = nonsteroidal antiinflammatory drug

Suggested Reading
Walder EJ, Conroy JD. Contact dermatitis in dogs and cats: pathogenesis, histopathology, experimental induction, and case reports. Vet Dermatol 1994;5:149–162.
Authors Alexander H. Werner and Margaret Swartout
Consulting Editor Karen Helton Rhodes

COONHOUND PARALYSIS (IDIOPATHIC POLYRADICULONEURITIS)

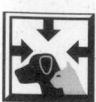 BASICS

DEFINITION
• Acute inflammation of multiple nerve roots and peripheral nerves in dogs, with or without a previous history of contact with a raccoon
• Proposed animal model for Guillain-Barré syndrome in humans

PATHOPHYSIOLOGY
• Largely unknown
• Suspected immune-mediated disease

SYSTEMS AFFECTED
Nervous
• PNS—most severe involvement in the ventral nerve roots and ventral root components of the spinal nerves
• Cranial nerves—in some patients; primarily nerves VII and X
• Respiratory paralysis—secondary to intercostal and phrenic nerve involvement in some patients

GENETICS
No proven basis

INCIDENCE/PREVALENCE
• Most commonly recognized polyneuropathy in dogs in North America
• Incidence low

GEOGRAPHIC DISTRIBUTION
• Coonhound paralysis—relative to the distribution of raccoons (e.g., North and Central America; parts of South America)
• ACIP—worldwide

SIGNALMENT
Breed Predilections
• Coonhound paralysis—coonhounds; any breed in contact with raccoons susceptible
• ACIP—none

Mean Age and Range
N/A

Predominant Sex
N/A

SIGNS
General Comments
ACIP—neurologic signs and progression of disease same as listed, except for initial encounter with a racoon

Historical Findings
• Appear 7–14 days after contact with a raccoon
• Stiff-stilted gait in all four limbs—initially

• Rapid progression to a flaccid lower motor neuron tetraparesis to tetraplegia
• Appetite and water consumption—usually normal
• Urination and defecation—normal
• Initial progression—usually occurs over 4–5 days; maximum progression can take up to 10 days.

Neurologic Examination Findings
• Usually symmetrical
• Generalized hyporeflexia to areflexia, hypotonia to atonia, and severe neurogenic muscle atrophy
• Pelvic limbs more severely affected than are thoracic limbs in a few patients
• Respiration—labored in severely affected dogs; occasional progression to respiratory paralysis; aphonia or dysphonia common
• Facial paresis—in a few patients
• Pain—sensation intact; hyperesthesia common, because of variable dorsal nerve root involvement
• Motor dysfunction—always predominates; even tetraplegic patient can usually wag its tail

CAUSES
• Coonhound paralysis—contact with a raccoon; perhaps more important, contact with raccoon saliva
• ACIP—none proven; possibly previous respiratory or gastrointestinal viral or bacterial infection, or vaccination

RISK FACTORS
• Coonhound paralysis—coonhounds tend to be predisposed primarily because of the nature of their activities; previous disease does not confer immunity and may increase risk of redevelopment; multiple bouts not uncommon
• ACIP—unknown

 DIAGNOSIS

DIFFERENTIAL DIAGNOSIS
Other acute polyneuropathy
• Distal denervating disease
• Botulism
• Tick paralysis
• Generalized (diffuse) or multifocal myelopathy (involving both cervical and lumbosacral intumescences)

CBC/BIOCHEMISTRY/URINALYSIS
Usually normal

OTHER LABORATORY TESTS
• Serum immunoglobulins—high serum IgG but not IgM in some patients

• Immunologic—serum reaction to raccoon saliva on ELISA; dogs with coonhound paralysis have a strong positive reaction that decreases in intensity over time; dogs without disease but with racoon contact have a strong positive reaction; dogs with ACIP but with no raccoon contact have a negative reaction.

IMAGING
N/A

DIAGNOSTIC PROCEDURES
CSF Analysis
• Lumbar—high protein without an increase in leukocytes at all stages of disease
• Cerebellomedullary—mildly high protein in patients examined after the acute stages of disease
• Albumin leakage across a suspected disrupted blood–brain barrier is the primary cause of the protein increase.
• Most patients have no intrathecal production of immunoglobulin.

Electrodiagnostics
• Generalized spontaneous activity, the severity of which depends on the time of examination after disease onset and the severity of neurologic signs
• Markedly low compound muscle action potential amplitudes after motor nerve stimulation
• F waves—late waves that indicate proximal motor nerve and ventral nerve root function; common abnormalities: increased minimum latencies, increased ratio, low amplitudes
• Motor nerve conduction velocities—usually within normal range; severely affected patients may have mildly low values.
• Sensory nerve function—usually normal
• These abnormalities provide evidence of severe peripheral axonopathy, along with axonal involvement and demyelination in the ventral nerve roots.

PATHOLOGIC FINDINGS
• Ventral nerve roots and the ventral root components of the spinal nerves—develop the most severe lesions, consisting of various degrees of axonal degeneration, paranodal and segmental demyelination, and leukocyte infiltration (predominantly monocytes and macrophages, with scattered groups of lymphocytes and plasma cells)
• Peripheral nerves—similarly affected, although to a lesser degree
• Dorsal nerve roots—much less severely affected

COONHOUND PARALYSIS (IDIOPATHIC POLYRADICULONEURITIS)

 TREATMENT

APPROPRIATE HEALTH CARE
• Inpatient—closely monitor patients in the progressive stage of the disease (especially during the first 4 days) for respiratory problems.
• Severe respiratory compromise—intensive care; ventilatory support, as required
• Intravenous fluid therapy—lactated Ringer's solution; necessary only if patient is dehydrated because of an inability to reach water
• Outpatient—stabilize patient, after initial diagnostic confirmation of disease.

NURSING CARE
• Patients are usually able to eat and drink if they can reach the food and water; often must be hand fed because of paralysis
• Intensive physiotherapy—important to decrease muscle atrophy
• Frequent turning and excellent padding—essential to prevent pressure sores

ACTIVITY
Encourage as much movement as possible, many patients are tetraplegic.

DIET
• No restrictions
• Make sure patient is able to reach food and water.
• Cervical weakness—may need to hand feed patient

CLIENT EDUCATION
• Inform client that good nursing care is essential.
• Discuss the importance of preventing pressure sores and urine scalding and of limiting the degree of muscle atrophy by diligent physiotherapy (e.g., passive limb movement and swimming as the patient's strength begins to improve).
• Inform client that the patient needs soft, resilient bedding (straw is excellent) that must be kept clean and free of urine and feces, frequent turning (every 3–4 hr), frequent bathing, and adequate nutrition.

SURGICAL CONSIDERATIONS
N/A

 MEDICATIONS

DRUG(S) OF CHOICE
• None proven effective
• Immunoglobulin—1 g/kg IV daily for 2 consecutive days or 0.4 g/kg IV daily for 4–5 consecutive days; given early may decrease severity and/or shorten recovery time

CONTRAINDICATIONS
Corticosteroids—do not improve clinical signs or shorten course of disease; may reduce survival in humans with Guillain-Barré syndrome

PRECAUTIONS
N/A

POSSIBLE INTERACTIONS
N/A

ALTERNATIVE DRUG(S)
N/A

 FOLLOW-UP

PATIENT MONITORING
• Outpatient—keep in close contact with client regarding complications or changes in the patient's condition.
• Urinalysis—perform periodically to check for cystitis in tetraplegic or severely tetraparetic patients.
• Ideally, re-evaluate at least every 2–3 weeks.

PREVENTION/AVOIDANCE
• Coonhound paralysis—avoid contact with raccoons; often not feasible because of coonhounds' environment and primary use as raccoon hunters
• ACIP—none

POSSIBLE COMPLICATIONS
• Respiratory paralysis—in progressive stage of the disease
• Pressure sores, urine scalding, and cystitis—common in chronically recumbent dogs

EXPECTED COURSE AND PROGNOSIS
• Most recover fully.
• Mild residual neurologic deficits—duration of several weeks in mildly to moderately affected dogs; duration of 3–4 months with severe disease

 MISCELLANEOUS

ASSOCIATED CONDITIONS
N/A

AGE-RELATED FACTORS
N/A

ZOONOTIC POTENTIAL
N/A

PREGNANCY
Unknown effect on the fetuses of an affected bitch

SYNONYM
• Coondog paralysis

SEE ALSO
• Botulism
• Peripheral Neuropathies (Polyneuropathies)
• Tick Bite Paralysis

ABBREVIATIONS
• ACIP = acute canine idiopathic polyradiculoneuritis
• CSF = cerebrospinal fluid
• ELISA = enzyme-linked immunosorbent assay
• PNS = peripheral nervous system

Suggested Reading
Cuddon PA. Acute canine idiopathic polyradiculoneuropathy—electrophysiology, CSF analysis, and immunology. Paper presented at the eighth annual symposium of the European Society of Veterinary Neurologists, Limoges, France, 1994.
Cummings JF, Hass DC. Coonhound paralysis: an acute idiopathic polyradiculoneuritis resembling the Landry-Guillain-Barré syndrome. J Neurol Sci 1967;4:51–81.
Cummings JF, de Lahunta A, Holmes DF, Schultz RD. Coonhound paralysis: further clinical studies and electron microscopic observations. Acta Neuropathol 1982;56:167–178.
Northington JW, Brown MJ. Acute canine idiopathic polyneuropathy: a Guillain-Barré-like syndrome in dogs. J Neurol Sci 1982;56:259–273.
Author Paul A. Cuddon
Consulting Editor Joane M. Parent

COPPER STORAGE HEPATOPATHY

 BASICS

DEFINITION
The abnormal hepatic accumulation of copper causing acute hepatitis or chronic hepatitis and eventually cirrhosis. Primary disease is thought to be the result of genetic-based abnormal copper metabolism. Most of the following information is based on studies from affected Bedlington terriers.

PATHOPHYSIOLOGY
• Abnormal hepatic copper concentrations can occur from either a primary metabolic defect in hepatic metabolism or as a secondary event due to abnormal copper retention secondary to cholestatic liver disease. • Copper is normally absorbed from the small intestine, stored in the liver, and excess copper is excreted through the biliary system. • Secondary cholestatic copper accumulation rarely exceeds 1000 µg/g dry weight liver while inherited copper metabolism disorders generally exceed 1000–2000 µg/g dry weight liver. Copper results in hepatocellular damage occurring in part as a result of oxidative mitochondrial damage. • Focal hepatitis progressing to chronic hepatitis and eventually cirrhosis occurs in the primary disease. • Severe acute hepatic necrosis may release hepatic copper into the blood, causing copper-generated hemolysis.

SYSTEMS AFFECTED
• Hepatobiliary—focal hepatitis leading to chronic hepatitis and eventually cirrhosis
• Hemic/lymphatic—serum copper and ceruloplasm concentrations are normal; hemolytic anemia is a rare sequela to hepatic necrosis, with abnormal copper release due to increased serum copper levels.

GENETICS
• Autosomal recessive trait in Bedlington terriers thought to be due to an abnormal hepatic biliary excretion of copper • The mode of inheritance in West Highland white or Skye terriers and other breeds affected is unknown.
• Dalmatians and Doberman pinschers also have breed-related chronic hepatitis with copper accumulation due to suspected genetic transmission.

INCIDENCE/PREVALENCE
• Bedlington terrier—possibly as many as two thirds of Bedlingtons in the United States may be either carriers or affected. • The prevalence in certain lines of West Highland white terrier is high but the overall incidence of clinical disease is low. • The incidence in other breeds is unknown.

SIGNALMENT

Species
Dogs

Breed Predilection
Bedlington terrier, West Highland white terrier, Skye terrier, Doberman pinschers, Dalmatians, Keeshonds, Labrador retrievers, and other breeds may have increased hepatic copper concentrations; the etiology, primary or secondary, is unknown for most.

Mean Age and Range
• Bedlington terrier—copper accumulates over time to a maximum level about 6 years of age
• Dogs can be clinically affected at any age though most present as middle-aged to older dogs having chronic hepatitis. • West Highland white terrier—maximum copper accumulation is observed by 6 months of age but clinical disease can occur at any time • Skye terrier—all ages can be affected • Doberman pinscher and Dalmatians are generally middle-aged when clinical.

Predominant Sex
Doberman pinscher—females

SIGNS

General Comments
• Primary copper hepatopathies (i.e., Bedlington terriers and West Highland white terriers) can fall in one of three categories: subclinical disease, acute signs observed most frequently in young dogs associated with acute hepatic necrosis, or chronic progressive signs in middle-aged and older dogs having chronic hepatitis and cirrhosis. • Secondary copper hepatopathies present with chronic progressive signs of liver disease due to chronic hepatitis or cirrhosis.

Historical Findings
• Acute signs—sudden onset of lethargy, anorexia, depression, and vomiting. Many of these dogs have a rapid course and die despite intensive supportive treatment • Chronic signs—history of waxing and waning lethargy, depression, anorexia, and weight loss. Vomiting, diarrhea, and polydipsia and polyuria may be seen. Later signs may include abdominal distention, jaundice, spontaneous bleeding, and hepatic encephalopathy.

Physical Examination Findings
• Acute signs—depression, weakness, and jaundice. Pale membranes (anemia) and dark urine (bilirubinuria and hemoglobinuria) in some dogs • Chronic signs—evidence of weight loss, ascites, and jaundice. Microhepatica is characteristic. Melena or petechial or ecchymotic hemorrhages in some dogs

CAUSES
• Primary—unknown in all but the Bedlington terrier but suspected to be the result of abnormal hepatic copper metabolism or excretion defect • Secondary—cholestatic liver disease results in secondary copper retention

RISK FACTORS
Primary—feeding high-copper diets, or stress factors that may precipitate acute disease

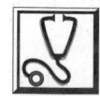 DIAGNOSIS

DIFFERENTIAL DIAGNOSIS
• Acute diseases—infectious diseases (e.g., infectious canine hepatitis, leptospirosis, and bacterial septicemia), acute hepatic necrosis, hepatic abscessation, drug- or toxin-induced hepatic injury, acute pancreatitis, hepatic lymphosarcoma, autoimmune hemolytic anemia, or zinc intoxication • Chronic diseases—chronic hepatitis, cholangiohepatitis of inflammatory or immune-mediated origin, drug- or toxin-induced hepatic injury, infectious hepatitis, chronic obstructive biliary disease, chronic fibrosing pancreatitis, congenital portosystemic shunt, hepatic neoplasia, or metastatic neoplasia

CBC/BIOCHEMISTRY/URINALYSIS
• CBC—results may be normal. Regenerative anemia, leukocytosis, neutrophilia in some animals with acute copper-associated hemolytic crisis. Microcytic or normocytic, normochromic nonregenerative anemia in some dogs with chronic progressive disease • Biochemistry—high liver enzyme activities (i.e., ALT, AST, GGT and SAP) and hyperbilirubinemia in some. Abnormal liver enzymes without clinical signs in predisposed breeds should raise a high index of suspicion for copper hepatopathy. As hepatic function deteriorates, hypoalbuminemia, hyperglobulinemia, low BUN, hypoglycemia, or hypokalemia may occur.
• Urinalysis—results usually normal or positive for bilirubinuria

OTHER LABORATORY TESTS
High fasting and postprandial bile acid concentration. Prolonged PT, APTT, ACT, and buccal mucosal bleeding time in advanced cases. Serum copper concentrations may be increased with acute hepatic necrosis in Bedlington terriers. Hepatic copper determination with histopathologic examination of liver is diagnostic. Genetic testing for homozygous affected Bedlington terriers is available.

IMAGING

Radiography
Small liver in some chronically affected dogs. Poor abdominal detail if dog has ascites. Abdominal radiographs unremarkable in most dogs

Ultrasonography
Early, the appearance of the liver is normal. Later, the liver may have a hyperechoic to mixed nodular echogenic pattern.

DIAGNOSTIC PROCEDURES
A liver biopsy is required to determine copper concentrations. Normal hepatic copper concentrations range from 200–400 µg/g DW liver. Affected Bedlington terriers range from 850–12,000 µg/g DW and affected West Highland white terriers up to 3,500 µg/g DW. Secondary copper retention concentrations generally range less than 1000 µg/g DW. Hepatic copper determination can be performed on fresh (preferred) or formalin-fixed liver tissue. Some laboratories need a minimum of a full needle biopsy sample; however some may require a "pea size" amount of tissue.
• Both biopsy and copper determination should be performed on any liver specimen from breeds predisposed to hepatic copper toxicosis

or any animal having evidence of chronic liver disease. Rhodanine or rubeanic acid histochemical stains identify copper within hepatocytes. • DNA genetic marker is available for diagnosis of Bedlington terrier copper hepatopathy, with a reported 95% accuracy rate in detecting both affected and carrier dogs.

PATHOLOGIC FINDINGS
• Grossly, in dogs having end-stage disease the liver will appear small, nodular, and cirrhotic. • Histologically, copper accumulates in hepatic lysosomes most often in the centrilobular location. Histochemical staining, a semiquantitative evaluation for copper, demonstrates copper-positive lysosomal granules when stained with rhodanine or rubeanic acid. Histologic chronic inflammatory changes first occur as focal hepatic necrosis that progresses over time to chronic hepatitis and finally to cirrhosis.

TREATMENT

APPROPRIATE HEALTH CARE
Most dogs are treated as outpatients. Inpatient evaluation and treatment are needed for dogs with signs of hepatic failure. Refer to treatment sections on chronic hepatitis or fibrosis and cirrhosis for detailed management of liver disease.

NURSING CARE
Animals in liver failure will require appropriate fluid and electrolyte correction.

ACTIVITY
Normal

DIET
• Low-copper diets should be fed to affected animals; however, almost all commercially available diets contain an excess of copper. Balanced homemade diets avoiding copper-rich foods (e.g., organ meats) may be used. Avoid mineral supplements containing copper. Frequently, feeding a low-copper diet is generally not feasible, and commercial diets must be used. Chelation therapy in conjunction with commercial diets has been successful in management of Bedlington terriers. • A high-quality, protein-sufficient, moderate-fat–containing diet should be fed to meet caloric needs. Protein content should be reduced only when the patient exhibits protein intolerance (i.e., signs of hepatic encephalopathy). • Water-soluble vitamins should be supplemented.

CLIENT EDUCATION
• All Bedlington terriers should be screened by using either DNA markers or liver biopsy. Other breeds should be monitored for abnormal liver enzymes or liver biopsy. • Therapy is needed for life. • Affected animals should not be bred.

SURGICAL CONSIDERATIONS
Animals with hepatic failure are surgical and anesthetic risks.

MEDICATIONS

DRUG(S) OF CHOICE
• See other sections for other specific treatments of chronic hepatitis and cirrhosis. • D-Penicillamine (10–15 mg/kg PO q12h) chelates copper and promotes urinary excretion and is suspected to also have other copper-protective effects. Treatment should be initiated in affected Bedlington, West Highland white, and Skye terriers or dogs having abnormal hepatic copper concentrations (> 1000–2000 μg/g DW). Reductions of about 1000 μg/g DW per year of treatment can be expected. Administer 1 hour before feeding. Drug may be associated with vomiting. • Trientine hydrochloride (10–15 mg/kg PO q12h) is an alternative copper chelator that appears to be as effective as penicillamine. Administer 1 hour before meals. Few if any side effects noted • Zinc (100 mg of elemental zinc PO q12h as loading dose for 2 months, then 50 mg PO q 12h given as zinc acetate) should be administered 1 hour before feeding. Mechanism of action is by reducing intestinal absorption of copper. Studies have demonstrated lowered hepatic copper concentrations in treated Bedlington and West Highland white terriers. May be beneficial in all affected dogs having early or lower hepatic copper concentrations. The author has found zinc not effective in Bedlingtons with high copper concentrations and evidence of hepatitis. In these dogs chelation therapy should be used first to reduce the level of toxic copper and should then be followed with zinc therapy. Vomiting is a frequent side effect of zinc.

CONTRAINDICATIONS
Ascorbic acid (vitamin C) has been recommended to reduce intestinal absorption of copper but in the presence of high copper vitamin C becomes a potent pro-oxidant and is therefore not recommended.

POSSIBLE INTERACTIONS
Penicillamine or trientine may not be effective when given with zinc orally.

ALTERNATIVE DRUG(S)
• 2,3,2 tetramine (15 mg/kg PO q12h) is a more potent copper chelator but not commercially available. • D-alpha tocopherol (vitamin E 200–600 IU q24h) may protect the liver from oxidative damage caused by copper and is suggested as an adjunct therapy.

FOLLOW-UP

PATIENT MONITORING
• Liver enzymes every 4–6 months. Body weight. Measure hepatic copper concentration within 1 year and thereafter as required by clinical findings. • When using zinc therapy assess serum zinc concentration every 2–3 weeks until stable in desired range (200–600

μg/dL) and then every 4–6 months. Discontinue if >1000 mcg/dL to avoid hemolytic crisis

PREVENTION/AVOIDANCE
Breed only Bedlington terrier dogs that do not carry the gene causing the disease. A liver registry is available for Bedlington terriers that are proven unaffected on the basis of hepatic copper concentration < 400 μg/g DW at 1 year of age or DNA gene evaluation.

POSSIBLE COMPLICATIONS
• D-Penicillamine can cause anorexia and vomiting. Starting at the low end of the dosage for the first week may reduce adverse effects. Give 1 hour before meals. A small amount of food may be included, but drug effect is reduced when given with meals. D-Penicillamine may, in rare cases, cause an autoimmune-like vesicular disease of the mucocutaneous junctions that resolves on withdrawal of the drug. • Excess zinc (oral dose of > 200 mg/day or blood concentration of > 1000 μg/dL) can cause hemolytic anemia.

EXPECTED COURSE AND PROGNOSIS
The prognosis is poor in acutely affected young dogs with fulminant hepatic failure or older dogs with cirrhosis. Young dogs with mild to moderate acute hepatic failure usually respond to chelation therapy. The prognosis is fair for these animals. The prognosis is good if the disease is detected before hepatic inflammatory changes are noted, and the dog is started on appropriate therapy.

MISCELLANEOUS

AGE-RELATED FACTORS
Determining hepatic copper concentrations at greater than one year of age aids in diagnosing affected animals. Affected West Highland white terriers have the highest concentration at 6 months of age.

PREGNANCY
Do not breed affected animals and carriers.

SYNONYMS
• Bedlington hepatitis • Chronic active hepatitis • Chronic copper toxicity • Copper toxicosis

SEE ALSO
Hepatitis, Chronic Active

ABBREVIATION
DW = dry weight

Suggested Reading

Rolfe DS, Twedt DC: Copper-associated hepatopathies in dogs. Vet Clin N Amer Small Anim Pract 25(2):399–417, 1995.
Thornburg LP. A perspective on copper and liver disease in the dog. J Vet Diagn Invest 2000;12:101–110.

Author David C. Twedt
Consulting Editor Sharon A. Center

COPROPHAGIA AND PICA

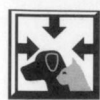 BASICS

DEFINITION
Ingestion of nonfood items including ingestion of feces (coprophagia)

PATHOPHYSIOLOGY
Most cases not caused by disease, but anemia and gastrointestinal or hepatic disease may lead to ingestion of nonfood items. Dogs and cats with polyphagia secondary to drug administration, an underlying endocrinopathy, or a disease causing malassimilation of nutrients may exhibit coprophagia; the benefit of this behavior to dogs is unknown.

SYSTEMS AFFECTED
Gastrointestinal—obstruction from foreign objects, vomiting, and/or diarrhea can occur. Parasites possible with coprophagia

SIGNALMENT
Species
Dogs and cats

Breed Predilections
Oriental breeds if fabric ingested

Mean Age and Range
N/A

Predominant Sex
Nursing bitches frequently eat the feces of their pups; females, whether intact or spayed, are more likely to exhibit coprophagia.

SIGNS
Historical Findings
Ingestion of nonfood items (e.g., dogs—rocks and feces; cats—fabrics and plastics)

Physical Examination Findings
• Halitosis if problem is coprophagia
• Pallor and weakness if anemic
• Thin body condition if signs accompanied by maldigestion or malabsorption
• Neurologic signs if behavior caused by neurologic disease

CAUSES
Behavioral Causes
• Nest cleaning
• Displacement activity from unavailable herbivore feces
• Responding to punishment, by removing evidence of soiling
• Imitating owners' behavior—cleaning the nest
• Compulsive
• Attention seeking

Medical Causes
• Exocrine pancreatic insufficiency
• Inflammatory bowel disease
• Small intestinal bacterial overgrowth
• Megaesophagus and/or esophageal stricture
• Intestinal parasitism
• Hyperthyroidism
• Diabetes mellitus
• Hyperadrenocorticism
• Dietary deficiencies—unproven
• Drug induced (e.g., glucocorticoids, progestins, phenobarbital)
• Anemia—iron deficiency, other
• Maldigestion/malabsorption (e.g., exocrine pancreatic insufficiency)
• Hunger
• Neurologic disease—primary central nervous system, portosystemic shunt

RISK FACTORS
• Confinement of dogs in barren yards with no environmental stimulation or enrichment—especially predisposes to coprophagia
• Early weaned oriental-breed cats fed low-roughage diets with no access to prey or grass are most at risk for wool eating.
• Underlying disease predisposing to anemia, maldigestion, or malabsorption

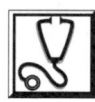 DIAGNOSIS

DIFFERENTIAL DIAGNOSIS
• The diagnosis is based on the owners' history.
• Must distinguish medical and behavioral causes
• A thorough evaluation of the animal's diet, environment, appetite, and handling is essential
• Licking behaviors may indicate nausea; differentiate by observation.
• A complete physical examination is necessary to evaluate for underlying diseases.

CBC/BIOCHEMISTRY/URINALYSIS
• May see anemia, hypoproteinemia (maldigestion/malabsorption), or changes representative of a portosystemic shunt (microcytosis, target cells, hypoalbuminemia, low BUN, ammonium biurate crystalluria)
• Peripheral eosinophilia may occur with gastrointestinal parasitism or eosinophilic inflammatory bowel disease.
• Results may suggest diabetes mellitus, hyperthyroidism, hyperadrenocorticism, or drug-induced causes of polyphagia.

OTHER LABORATORY TESTS
• Multiple fecal flotations or a treatment trial with fenbendazole (dogs: 50 mg/kg PO q24h for 3 days; cats: 25 mg/kg PO q24h for 3 days), to evaluate for gastrointestinal parasitism
• Trypsin-like immunoreactivity (TLI) to evaluate for exocrine pancreatic insufficiency
• Cobalamin and folate levels to evaluate for small intestinal bacterial overgrowth and severe small intestinal mucosal disease
• ACTH stimulation test or low-dose dexamethasone suppression test to evaluate for hyperadrenocorticism
• Serum total T_4 or T_3 suppression test to evaluate for hyperthyroidism
• Test any anemic cat for feline leukemia virus (FeLV) and feline immunodeficiency virus (FIV).
• Test fasting and 2-hour postprandial serum bile acids if a portosystemic shunt is suspected.

IMAGING
• Survey abdominal radiography and abdominal ultrasonography—may help rule

out some foreign bodies in the gastro-intestinal tract; may demonstrate microhepatica if a portosystemic shunt exists.
• Thoracic radiographs to evaluate for megaesophagus
• Swallowing studies (via contrast radiography or contrast fluoroscopy) to evaluate for megaesophagus or esophageal stricture

DIAGNOSTIC PROCEDURES
• Esophagoscopy to evaluate for foreign body, megaesophagus, or esophageal stricture
• Small intestinal biopsy specimens obtained at surgery or via endoscopy to evaluate for infiltrative small bowel disease
• Quantitative cultures of the small intestine to evaluate for small intestinal bacterial overgrowth

 TREATMENT

GENERAL COMMENTS
• Varies depending on whether the cause is medical or behavioral
• Treat any underlying disease (e.g., endocrinopathies, gastrointestinal disease, or pancreatic disorders) and withdraw any drugs that could cause polyphagia.
• Correct any dietary deficiencies.
• When no pathologic cause exists—(1) limit access to nonfood items to prevent ingestion; (2) find a safe substitute that the animal can ingest with impunity; and (3) change the animal's motivation to ingest the nonfood item.

TREATMENT OF PICA
• If pica is attention-getting, muzzle dog to prevent ingestion and ignore attempts to obtain nonfood items.
• Fabric chewing in cats can be treated by: (1) removing plastic and woolen clothes from the cat's environment; (2) applying a pungent or bitter taste to objects, which may discourage consumption; (3) feeding a high-roughage diet or tough meat to chew, or providing a garden of grass or catnip to graze on.

TREATMENT OF COPROPHAGIA
• Can treat coprophagia in a number of ways—can decrease access to feces by prompt disposal; walk dogs on a leash to facilitate removal from vicinity of feces.

• Can use a muzzle or head halter on walks. Can give the dog a food reward when it defecates, thereby counterconditioning it to expect food rather than search for feces. Other recommendations, although unsupported by any published data, include feeding a less digestible diet; use of a meat tenderizer or pancreatic enzymes; and sprinkling noxious tasting/smelling substances on feces.
• Bitter and hot substances such as quinine, cayenne pepper, and commercial products (e.g., FOR-BID, Alpar Laboratories, Inc., La Grange, IL) have yielded variable results.
• Taste aversion learning is another potentially effective method. Treat feces with an emetic agent that has a short duration of action; after a few experiences of coprophagy followed by nausea and malaise, the dog may learn to avoid feces.

 MEDICATIONS

DRUG(S) OF CHOICE
The animal's motivation can be changed by administering psychoactive drugs or punishment.

Clomipramine
• A tricyclic antidepressant, serotonin reuptake blocker for compulsive behavior
• Dogs: 1–3 mg/kg PO q24h
• Cats: 0.25–1 mg/kg PO q24h

CONTRAINDICATIONS
N/A

PRECAUTIONS
N/A

POSSIBLE INTERACTIONS
Do not use clomipramine with monoamine oxidase inhibitors.

ALTERNATIVE DRUG(S)
Cyproheptadine (4 mg/cat PO q24h)—an appetite stimulant, serotonin antagonist

 FOLLOW-UP

PATIENT MONITORING
• Contact the owner in 10–14 days to confirm compliance and determine if pica has abated.

• If dietary management changes did not markedly improve the problem, prescribe further diagnostic work and/or medication.

POSSIBLE COMPLICATIONS
Gastrointestinal complications—foreign bodies, diarrhea, vomiting, halitosis

 MISCELLANEOUS

ASSOCIATED CONDITIONS
N/A

AGE-RELATED FACTORS
Chewing and sometimes swallowing objects is normal puppy behavior; the mouth is the best instrument the dog can use to feel and taste its environment during its exploratory period.

ZOONOTIC POTENTIAL
N/A

PREGNANCY
Coprophagia of puppies' feces is normal.

SYNONYMS
• Depraved appetite
• Wool chewing
• Wool sucking

SEE ALSO
Gastrointestinal Obstruction

ABBREVIATION
BUN = blood urea nitrogen

Suggested Reading
Bradshaw JWS. The behavior of the domestic cat. Oxon, UK: C.A.B. International, 1992:200–203.
Houpt KA. Domestic animal behavior for veterinarians and animal scientists. Ames: Iowa State University Press, 1991:310–312.
Houpt KA. Feeding and drinking behavior problems. Vet Clin North Am Small Anim Pract 1991;21:288–289.
Voith VL. Feeding behaviors. In Wills JM, Simpson KW, eds. The Waltham book of clinical nutrition. Oxford: Pergamon, 1994: 121–129.
Author Katherine A. Houpt
Consulting Editor Debra F. Horwitz

CORNEAL AND SCLERAL LACERATIONS

 BASICS

DEFINITION
• Penetrating—a wound or foreign body enters but does not completely pass through the cornea or sclera • Perforating—a wound or foreign body completely passes through the cornea or sclera; greater risk of vision loss than penetrating • Simple—involve only the cornea or sclera; may be penetrating or perforating; other ocular structures intact • Complicated—perforating; involves other structures besides the cornea or sclera; uveal, vitreal, or retinal incarceration or prolapse through the wound; traumatic cataract; hyphema; lid lacerations

PATHOPHYSIOLOGY
• Sharp trauma—wounds by an outside-in mechanism • Blunt trauma—wounds by an inside-out mechanism; eye undergoes sudden changes in its equatorial and axial dimensions and IOP; actual wound may be at a site other than the point of impact; often more damaging than sharp trauma • All or a portion of the foreign object initiating the injury may be retained in the wound or eye.

SYSTEMS AFFECTED
• Ophthalmic • Musculoskeletal—surrounding skull or orbital tissue • Nervous—unconsciousness or brain injury

INCIDENCE/PREVALENCE
Common

SIGNALMENT
Species
Dogs and cats

SIGNS
Historical Findings
• Usually acute onset • History of running through heavy vegetation, being hit by gunshot pellets or other projectiles, or being scratched by a cat common • Trauma may not be observed.

Physical Examination Findings
• Depend on tissues affected • Common—corneal, scleral, or eyelid deformity; edema; hemorrhage • May see a retained foreign body • Often rapidly seal; may appear only as a subconjunctival hematoma • May also see iris defects, pupil distortion, hyphema, cataract, vitreal hemorrhage, retinal detachment, and exophthalmia

CAUSES
Blunt or sharp trauma

RISK FACTORS
• Pre-existing visual impairment • Young, naive, or highly excitable animals • Hunting or running through heavy vegetation • Fighting

 DIAGNOSIS

DIFFERENTIAL DIAGNOSIS
• History or a retained foreign body usually diagnostic • Traumatic event not observed and no foreign body found—consider non-traumatic corneal ulcer, hyphema, etc. • Traumatic ulcerative keratitis—acute onset; linear, stellate or V-shaped; possibly multiple • Traumatic hyphema—almost invariably accompanied by corneal or scleral lesions and subconjunctival or periocular hemorrhage • Traumatic cataracts—disrupted lens capsule common • Traumatic retinal detachment—almost invariably accompanied by intraocular hemorrhage

CBC/BIOCHEMISTRY/URINALYSIS
• Usually noncontributory • Consider as a preanesthesia screen or when nontraumatic cause is possible.

OTHER LABORATORY TESTS
• Cytologic examination and aerobic culture and sensitivity testing of the wound and foreign body—recommended even if infection is not apparent; may need to collect specimen under general anesthesia at the time of surgery • Consider other tests (platelet count, coagulation profile, etc.) if nontraumatic causes are possible.

IMAGING
• Ocular ultrasonography—if the ocular media are opaque; may clarify the extent and nature of intraocular disease; may detect foreign body • Orbital radiographs or CT—may help determine projectile's course; may detect foreign body

DIAGNOSTIC PROCEDURES
• Determine the nature, force, and direction of impact of the object—help identify which tissues may be involved • Do not put pressure on the eye until rupture or laceration of the globe has been ruled out. • Assess vision—menace response; aversion to bright light • Periocular skin and orbit—examine for lacerations or deformities; suspect globe involvement if a lid laceration crosses the eyelid margin or penetrates the orbital septum; entry sites are often small and quickly seal. • Abnormal ocular motility—suggests extraocular muscle trauma, orbital hemorrhage or edema, retained foreign bodies or peripheral nerve or CNS damage • Scleral rupture—consider with subconjunctival hemorrhage, especially if the anterior chamber is abnormally deep or shallow, there is vitreal hemorrhage, or the eye is abnormally soft. • Pupils—size; shape; symmetry; direct and consensual light reflexes • Detailed ophthalmoscopy—assess clarity of ocular media and fundus integrity; rule out intraocular foreign body • Seidel test—if any question of corneal or scleral leaking; use a dry or slightly moist fluorescein strip to paint a thin coat of fluorescein over the surface of the defect; leaking aqueous combines with the orange fluorescein, forming a bright green rivulet (seen best with cobalt illumination)

PATHOLOGIC FINDINGS
• Depend on wound and affected tissues • Usually correlate closely with clinical examination findings • Vitreal hemorrhage—may organize into a fibrous band that applies traction to the retina, causing it to detach • Post-traumatic sarcoma (cats)—may occur months to years after severe ocular trauma

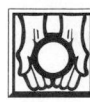 TREATMENT

APPROPRIATE HEALTH CARE
• Depends on severity • Outpatient—if integrity of the globe is ensured

NURSING CARE
• Sedation—considered for excited or fractious patients • When walking—apply an E-collar and put ipsilateral foreleg through the leash to avoid increasing intraocular pressure in affected eye • Avoid third eyelid flaps in patients with perforations or deep or long penetrating wounds.

Injuries Considered for Medical Treatment
• Nonperforating wounds with no wound edge override or gape—apply an E-collar; give topical antibiotic or atropine ophthalmic solutions • Nonperforating wounds with mild wound gape or shelved edges—apply a therapeutic soft contact lens Bausch & Lomb (Plano T) and an E-collar; give topical antibiotic or atropine ophthalmic solutions • Simple full-thickness, pinpoint corneal perforation with a negative Seidel test that has a formed anterior chamber and no uveal prolapse—sedentary patients; use a therapeutic soft contact lens and an E-collar; give topical antibiotic or atropine ophthalmic solutions; re-examine a few hours after applying the lens and at 24 and 48 hr.

ACTIVITY
Usually confined indoors (cats) or limited to leash walks until healing is complete

CLIENT EDUCATION
Warn client that the full extent of the injury (cataracts, retinal detachment, infection) may not be apparent until several days or weeks after the injury and that long-term follow-up is necessary.

SURGICAL CONSIDERATIONS
Injuries Requiring Surgical Exploration or Repair
• Full-thickness corneal lacerations with a positive Seidel test • Full-thickness wounds with iris incarceration or prolapse • Full-thickness scleral or corneoscleral lacerations

• Suspected retained foreign body or a posterior scleral rupture • Simple nonperforating wound with edges that are moderately or overtly gaping and that are long or more than two-thirds the corneal thickness

Injuries Considered for Surgical Exploration or Repair

• Small full-thickness corneal lacerations with a negative Seidel test and no uveal incarceration or prolapse • Large conjunctival lacerations • Partial-thickness corneal or scleral lacerations in an active patient

MEDICATIONS

DRUG(S) OF CHOICE

Antibiotics

• Complicated wounds, those with retained plant material, and those caused by blunt trauma with tissue devitalization—infection common • Bacterial endophthalmitis—5%–7% of perforations; very rare in penetrating wounds • Penetrating—topical antibiotics alone (e.g., neomycin, polymyxin B, and bacitracin) or gentamicin solution q6–8h; usually sufficient • Perforating wounds with negative Seidel test—systemic ciprofloxacin (dogs, 10–20 mg/kg PO SID); topical cefazolin (33 mg/mL by adding injectable cefazolin to artificial tears) and fortified gentamicin or tobramycin (add injectable aminoglycoside to the commercial ophthalmic solution to achieve a final concentration of 14 mg/mL) both drugs q4–6h • Perforating wounds with positive Seidel test—systemic ciprofloxacin (dogs, 10–20 mg/kg PO SID); topical cefazolin and fortified gentamicin or tobramycin as noted above, only after defect has been made watertight

Antiinflammatories

• Topical 1% prednisolone acetate or 0.1% dexamethasone solution—q6–12h; as soon as the wound is sutured or epithelialized if there is no infection • Systemic prednisone—0.5–1.0 mg/kg SID to BID; for sutured or epithelialized wounds when inflammation is severe; when the lens or more posterior structures are involved; when the wound is infected or not epithelialized and control of inflammation is mandatory to preserve the eye • Topical NSAIDs—suprofen or flurbiprofen; may be used if topical corticosteroids are contraindicated and control of inflammation is mandatory to preserve the eye

Mydriatics

1% atropine ophthalmic solution—q6–12h; when there is significant miosis or anterior chamber reaction

Analgesics

• Topical atropine or oral aspirin (dogs, 10–15 mg/kg PO BID to TID)—may provide sufficient pain relief • Butorphanol—dogs, 0.2–0.4 mg/kg; cats, 0.1–0.2 mg/kg IV, SC, or IM q2–4h or as needed; acute mild pain; sedation not required • Oxymorphone—dogs, 0.05–0.1 mg/kg; cats, 0.05 mg/kg IV, SC, or IM q4–6h or as needed; acute severe pain; sedation required • Naloxone—0.04 mg/kg IV, SC, or IM; to reverse narcotics

CONTRAINDICATIONS

• Topical ophthalmic preparations—avoid for perforations with positive Seidel test. • Ciprofloxacin—avoid in small and medium dog breeds aged 2–8 months; avoid in large dog breeds aged 2–12 months; avoid in giant dog breeds aged 2–18 months; potential for damaging rapidly growing articular cartilage

PRECAUTIONS

• Aminoglycosides—topical application may be irritating and may impede re-epithelization if used frequently or at high concentrations; possibility of toxicity when given to very small patients or when giving by more than one route • Topical solutions may be preferable to ointments if corneal perforation is possible. • Atropine—may exacerbate KCS and glaucoma • Topical or systemic NSAIDs—use cautiously with hyphema; safety of topical NSAIDs in cats unknown

POSSIBLE INTERACTIONS

Systemic NSAIDs—may potentiate the nephrotoxicity of aminoglycosides; ensure good hydration and adequate renal function, especially in small dogs

ALTERNATIVE DRUG(S)

Topical ciprofloxacin ophthalmic solution—may be used instead of the combination of topical cefazolin and a fortified aminoglycoside; some streptococci are resistant

FOLLOW-UP

PATIENT MONITORING

• Deep or long penetrating wounds that have not been sutured and perforating wounds—rechecked every 24–48 hr for the first several days to ensure integrity of the globe, to monitor for infection, and to check control of ocular inflammation • Superficial penetrating wounds—usually rechecked at 3–5-day intervals until healed • Antibiotic therapy—altered according to culture and sensitivity results

PREVENTION/AVOIDANCE

• Take care when introducing new puppies to households with cats that have front claws.

• Minimize running through dense vegetation or the owner should consider having a bottle of saline eyewash to irrigate foreign debris from the eye. • Minimize visually impaired or blind dogs' exposure to dense vegetation.

POSSIBLE COMPLICATIONS

• Loss of the eye or vision • Chronic ocular inflammation or pain • Post-traumatic sarcoma—may develop in blind cat eyes that have been severely traumatized; consider enucleation for all blind, traumatized feline eyes to prevent post-traumatic sarcoma.

EXPECTED COURSE AND PROGNOSIS

• Most eyes with corneal lacerations or a retained corneal foreign body are salvageable. • The more posterior the injury, the poorer the prognosis for retention of vision. • Poor prognosis—scleral or uveal involvement; no light perception; perforating injuries involving the lens, or with significant vitreal hemorrhage, or retinal detachment • Penetrating injuries usually better prognosis than perforating injuries • Blunt trauma carries a poorer prognosis than sharp trauma.

MISCELLANEOUS

ASSOCIATED CONDITIONS

Depends on nature and extent of injury

AGE-RELATED FACTORS

N/A

ZOONOTIC POTENTIAL

N/A

PREGNANCY

• Systemic corticosteroids—may complicate pregnancy • Systemic ciprofloxacin—probably should be avoided during pregnancy

SEE ALSO

• Cataracts • Hyphema • Keratitis, Ulcerative • Proptosis • Retinal Detachment

ABBREVIATIONS

• IOP = intraocular pressure • KCS = keratoconjunctivitis sicca

Suggested Reading

Gilger BC, Whitley RO. Surgery of the cornea and sclera. In: Gerlatt KN, ed. Veterinary ophthalmology 3rd ed. Baltimore: Lippincott Williams & Wilkins, 1999:675–700.

Kuhn F, Morris R, Witherspoon D, et al. A standardized classification of ocular trauma. Ophthalmology 1996;103:240–243.

Pieramici DJ, Sternberg P, Aaberg TM, et al. A system for classifying mechanical injuries of the eye (globe). Am J Ophthalmol 1997;123:820–831.

Author Paul E. Miller

Consulting Editor Paul E. Miller

CORNEAL DEGENERATIONS AND INFILTRATIONS

 **BASICS**

OVERVIEW
• Corneal degeneration—unilateral or bilateral non-inherited condition secondary to other ocular or systemic disorders. Characterized by lipid or calcium deposition within the corneal stroma and/or epithelium

SIGNALMENT
• Lipid deposition—Dogs, rare in cats; can occur secondary to systemic hyper-lipoproteinemia
• Calcium deposition—Dogs, rare in cats. Seen less frequently than lipid deposition

SIGNS
• Lipid—gray or white; can be band-shaped, irregular, or circular. When secondary to systemic hyperlipoproteinemia—can be complete annular ring with clear zone between affected cornea and limbus; bilateral involvement to different degrees
• Calcium—white to crystalline; irregular, band-shaped
• Neovascularization, pigmentation may be present
• Roughened appearance to cornea, distinct margins
• Can have fluorescein stain stippling around margin of deposit if raised
• Associated ocular conditions—corneal scars, KCS, exposure keratitis, chronic uveitis, episcleritis, phthisis bulbi, chronic topical steroid therapy

CAUSES & RISK FACTORS
• Lipid—hyperlipoproteinemia: may increase risk, may worsen already existing deposits; can be secondary to hypothyroidism, diabetes mellitus, hyperadrenocorticism, pancreatitis, nephrotic syndrome, liver disease, primary disease of miniature schnauzers
• Calcium—hypercalcemia, hypo-phosphatemia, hypervitaminosis D, hyperadrenocorticism
• Both—Above-listed ocular conditions

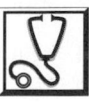 **DIAGNOSIS**

DIFFERENTIAL DIAGNOSIS
• Other causes of corneal opacities
• Corneal scar—gray to white depending on severity; negative fluorescein stain retention; relatively smooth corneal surface
• Corneal stromal dystrophies—bilateral, often symmetrical foci of deposition, gray to white in appearance, distinct margins;

heritable, not associated with ocular inflammation; do not retain fluorescein
• Edema—Bluish to gray; usually more homogeneous; can vary in size depending on severity; indistinct margins; can retain fluorescein stain if corneal erosion/ulceration also present
• Corneal ulcer—retains fluorescein stain, varying degrees of edema
• Inflammatory cell infiltrates—appear gray to white with indistinct margins; cytologic examination of cornea reveals white blood cells, organisms present

CBC/BIOCHEMISTRY/URINALYSIS
• Lipid—evaluate fasting cholesterol, triglyceride levels.
• Calcium—evaluate serum calcium levels.

OTHER LABORATORY TESTS
• Lipid—hypothyroidism: low thyroid hormone concentrations and depressed response to TSH
• Cushing's—ACTH stimulation test

IMAGING
N/A

DIAGNOSTIC PROCEDURES
May retain fluorescein around margins of deposit if raised

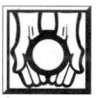 **TREATMENT**

• Treat primary ocular disease if present.
• Usually benefit from low-fat diet if hyperlipoproteinemia; treat primary systemic disease if present; both may help slow or stop progression of the disease
• Lipid and calcium deposits that impair vision or create ocular discomfort either from a roughened surface or by disrupting the corneal epithelium and causing ulceration may benefit from vigorous corneal scraping or su-perficial keratectomy followed by medical treatment; they are likely to recur following treatment.

 MEDICATIONS

DRUG(S)
• Topical antibiotics (i.e., triple antibiotic) indicated for ulcerated cornea; frequency depends on severity; usually uncomplicated ulcers treated BID–TID
• Topical nonsteroidal antiinflammatory BID to TID—indicated to treat secondary uveitis if noted
• Topical 1% atropine q8–24h—indicated to reduce pain if signs associated with secondary uveitis noted

• Topical EDTA solution 0.4%–1.38% q6h; may help minimize calcium deposits; usually used after a procedure has been performed to remove most of the deposits to improve efficacy
• Artificial tear ointment q6–12h; may prevent or reduce frequency of secondary corneal ulceration; may lubricate eye to provide comfort if corneal surface rough.

CONTRAINDICATIONS/POSSIBLE COMPLICATIONS
• Topical corticosteroids—questionable benefit and may worsen severity; contraindicated with corneal ulceration
• Topical atropine—contraindicated with KCS, glaucoma, lens luxations

 **FOLLOW-UP**

PATIENT MONITORING
Monitor serum cholesterol and triglycerides to assess efficacy of dietary management; monitor treatment of primary disease if present.

EXPECTED COURSE AND PROGNOSIS
• Corneal ulceration—may be associated with worsening of disease
• Vision—may be affected in advanced disease; may be severe if primary ocular disease present (e. g., uveitis)
• Deposits may recur in patients following superficial keratectomy surgery.

 **MISCELLANEOUS**

SEE ALSO
• Corneal Dystrophies
• Keratitis, Ulcerative

ABBREVIATIONS
• ACTH = adrenocorticotropic hormone
• EDTA = ethylene diamine tetra-acetate
• KCS = keratoconjunctivitis sicca
• TSH = thyroid stimulating hormone

Suggested Reading
Crispin SM, Barnett KC. Dystrophy, degen-eration and infiltration of the canine cornea. J Small Anim Pract 1983;24:63–83.

Acknowledgment
The author wishes to acknowledge the contributions made by B. Keith Collins in preparing this chapter.

Author George A. Abrams
Consulting Editor Paul E. Miller

 BASICS

OVERVIEW
• Primary, inherited (or familial), bilateral, and often symmetrical condition of the cornea that is not associated with other ocular or systemic diseases
• Three types based on anatomic location: epithelial—associated with dyskeratotic and necrotic epithelial cells, focal absence of epithelial basement membrane, and increased cells in anterior corneal stroma; stromal—lipid deposition within the corneal stroma; endothelial—characterized by abnormal, dystrophic endothelial cells

SIGNALMENT
Usually dogs; rare in cats

Epithelial
• Shetland sheepdogs—age of onset 6 months to 6 years; slow progression

Stromal
• Usually young adult dogs at age of onset
• Affected breeds—Afghan hound, Airedale terrier, Alaskan malamute, American cocker spaniel, beagle, bearded collie, bichon frise, cavalier King Charles spaniel, German shepherd, Lhasa apso, mastiff, miniature pinscher, rough collie, Siberian husky, Samoyed, Weimaraner, whippet, and others; inheritance pattern identified in only a few breeds

Endothelial
• Dogs—primarily affects Boston terriers, Chihuahuas, and dachshunds; may affect other breeds; typically middle-aged or older at onset of clinical signs; female predilection suggested
• Cats—affects young animals; described most often in domestic shorthairs; a similar condition that occurs without endothelial disease is inherited in Manx as an autosomal recessive disorder.

SIGNS
All cause some degree of opacity in the cornea.

Epithelial
• Can be asymptomatic or have blepharospasm; multifocal white or gray circular to irregular opacities or rings; sometimes associated with multifocal corneal erosions
• Vision—usually not affected

Stromal
• Usually asymptomatic with no associated inflammation
• Central—most common; gray, white, or silver oval to circular opacity of the central or paracentral cornea; with magnification may note multiple fibrillar to coalescing opacities that have a crystalline or ground-glass appearance (crystalline corneal dystrophy)

• Diffuse—affects Airedales; more diffuse, dense opacity than with central dystrophy
• Annular—affects Siberian Huskies most commonly; doughnut-shaped opacity of the paracentral or peripheral cornea
• Vision—usually not affected; visual deficit possible with advanced or diffuse disease

ENDOTHELIAL
• Asymptomatic in early stages
• Edema of lateral or ventrolateral cornea that usually progresses to involve the entire cornea after months to years
• Corneal epithelial bullae (bullous keratopathy) and subsequent corneal erosion ulceration may develop; erosions or ulceration may cause blepharospasm due to pain.
• Vision—may be impaired with advanced disease

CAUSES & RISK FACTORS
• Epithelial—result of degenerative or innate abnormalities of the corneal epithelium and/or basement membrane
• Stromal—innate abnormality or localized error in corneal lipid metabolism; may be affected by hyperlipoproteinemia (may increase opacity).
• Endothelium—degeneration of the endothelial cell layer; subsequent loss of endothelial cell pump function results in corneal edema.

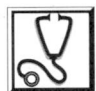 DIAGNOSIS

DIFFERENTIAL DIAGNOSIS
• Epithelial, stromal—other causes of corneal opacity: corneal degenerations, ulcers, scars, inflammatory cell infiltrates
• Endothelial—other causes of diffuse corneal edema: uveitis and glaucoma

CBC/BIOCHEMISTRY/URINALYSIS
Epithelial, stromal—high concentrations of cholesterol and triglyceride levels may modify the course of the disease but are not the cause

OTHER LABORATORY TESTS
N/A

IMAGING
N/A

DIAGNOSTIC PROCEDURES
• Stromal—usually does not retain fluorescein stain.
• Epithelial or endothelial—may retain fluorescein stain, often in multifocal areas, particularly with advanced disease.
• Tonometry—to eliminate glaucoma as cause of corneal edema

TREATMENT
• Advanced epithelial or endothelial disease with ulceration—may require treatment for ulcerative keratitis
• Stromal—usually none required; may

perform superficial keratectomy to remove lipid deposits if severe, but usually unnecessary and deposits may recur
• Inform client that some corneal dystrophies are inherited.
• Advanced endothelial dystrophy—may use therapeutic soft contact lens with or without debridement of redundant corneal epithelial tags; conjunctival flap surgery; thermo-keratoplasty; penetrating keratoplasty (corneal transplant) may be of benefit but success rates vary (fair to good for cats, poor for dogs).

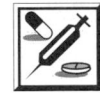 MEDICATIONS

DRUG(S)
• Corneal ulceration—topical antibiotics and possibly atropine (see Keratitis, Ulcerative)
• Epithelial—1% to 2% cyclosporine in oil or 0.2% ointment q8h–q24h as needed to relieve clinical signs
• Endothelial—topical 5% sodium chloride ointment; palliative treatment; does not markedly clear cornea but may prevent progression and rupture of corneal epithelial bullae.

CONTRAINDICATIONS/POSSIBLE INTERACTIONS
Topical corticosteroids—no benefit to lipid (stromal) dystrophy; of questionable benefit to other forms of dystrophy

 FOLLOW-UP

• Reexamination—necessary only if ocular pain or corneal ulceration develops
• Corneal opacity—may wax and wane with lipid dystrophy; unlikely to resolve
• Corneal ulceration—may accompany progression of epithelial or endothelial dystrophy
• Vision—not substantially affected except in advanced cases

 MISCELLANEOUS

SEE ALSO
• Corneal Degenerations and Infiltrations
• Keratitis, Ulcerative

Suggested Reading
Crispin SM, Barnett KC. Dystrophy, degeneration and infiltration of the canine cornea. J Small Anim Pract 1983;24:63–83.

Acknowledgment
The author would like to acknowledge the contributions of B. Keith Collins in preparing this chapter.
Author Ellison Bentley
Consulting Editor Paul E. Miller

CORONAVIRUS INFECTION—DOGS

 BASICS

OVERVIEW
• CCV—sporadic outbreaks of vomiting and diarrhea in dogs; widely distributed throughout the world, including wild canids
• Infection—inapparent usual; mild to severe enteritis may occur, from which most dogs recover; death reported in young pups; restricted to the upper two-thirds of the small intestine and associated lymph nodes; unlike CPV-2 infection, crypt cells spared
• Simultaneous infection with CPV-2 may occur; more severe; often fatal
• No viremia or other manifestation of systemic disease

SIGNALMENT
• Only wild and domestic dogs are known to be susceptible to disease.
• CCV may cause inapparent infections in cats.
• All ages and breeds

SIGNS
• Vary greatly
• Adults—most infections inapparent
• Puppies—may develop severe, fatal enteritis
• Incubation period—1–3 days
• Sudden onset of vomiting, usually only once
• Diarrhea—may be explosive; yellow-green or orange; loose or liquid; typically malodorous (characteristic); may persist for a few days up to > 3 weeks; may recur later
• Young pups—may suffer severe, protracted diarrhea and dehydration
• Anorexia and depression common
• Fever rare
• Mild respiratory effects

CAUSES & RISK FACTORS
• CCV—closely related to FIP virus, feline enteric coronavirus, and transmissible gastro-enteritis virus of swine; pig and cat viruses not known to cause natural illness in dogs; readily inactivated by common disinfectants
• Stress (e.g., intensive training, crowding)—greatest risk; sporadic outbreaks have occurred in dogs attending shows and in kennels where introductions of new dogs are frequent; crowding and unsanitary conditions promote clinical illness
• Feces—primary source of infection; virus shed for about 2 weeks

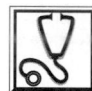 DIAGNOSIS

DIFFERENTIAL DIAGNOSIS
• Infections caused by enteric bacteria, protozoa, or other viruses
• Food intoxication or intolerance

CBC/BIOCHEMISTRY/URINALYSIS
Normal

OTHER LABORATORY TESTS
• Serologic tests—available; not standardized
• Antibody titers—generally low; may not indicate recent infection because of high rate of asymptomatic infection

IMAGING
N/A

DIAGNOSTIC PROCEDURES
• Viral isolation—from feces in feline cell cultures at onset of diarrhea
• Immunofluorescent staining of frozen sections of the small intestine—fatal cases; may reveal viral antigen in cells lining the villous epithelium
• Electron microscopy—typical CCV particles; interpretation requires expertise

PATHOLOGIC FINDINGS
• Necropsy reports limited, except experimental infections
• May be dilated loops of small intestine filled with gas and watery green-yellow material
• Gross—restricted to the small intestinal mucosa, which may be congested or hemor-rhagic; mesenteric lymph nodes usually enlarged and edematous
• Typical microscopic changes—atrophy and fusion of intestinal villi; deepening of the crypts; increased cellularity of the lamina

propria; flattening of epithelial cells with increased goblet cells
• Lesions—commonly obscured by postmortem autolysis

TREATMENT

• Most affected dogs recover without treatment.
• Supportive fluid and electrolyte treatment—indicated, especially in severe infections with dehydration

MEDICATIONS

DRUG(S)
Antibiotics—not usually indicated, except with enteritis, sepsis, or respiratory illness

CONTRAINDICATIONS/POSSIBLE INTERACTIONS
N/A

FOLLOW-UP

PATIENT MONITORING
Not usually required

PREVENTION/AVOIDANCE
• Vaccines—controversial; inactivated and live viral vaccines available; appear to be safe; efficacy unknown, except for brief periods (2–4 weeks) after vaccination. Not recommended
• Strict isolation and sanitation are essential in kennels.
• CCV—highly contagious; spreads rapidly

POSSIBLE COMPLICATIONS
Diarrhea—may persist 10–12 days; may recur

EXPECTED COURSE AND PROGNOSIS
• Prognosis—normally good, except severe infections of young pups
• Majority recover after a few days of illness.
• Fluid or soft stools may persist for several weeks.

MISCELLANEOUS

ASSOCIATED CONDITIONS
• Infection with canine parvovirus or other agent may occur concurrently.
• Infections by other enteric pathogens are believed to augment the disease.

AGE-RELATED FACTORS
• Young pups seem to be at risk.

ZOONOTIC POTENTIAL
N/A

ABBREVIATIONS
• CCV = canine coronavirus
• CPV = canine parvovirus
• FIP = feline infectious peritonitis

Suggested Reading
Hoskins JD. Canine viral enteritis. In: Greene, CE. Infectious diseases of the dog and cat. Philadelphia: Saunders, 1998.
Author Leland E. Carmichael
Consulting Editor Stephen C. Barr

COUGH

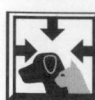

BASICS

DEFINITION
A sudden forceful expiration of air through the glottis, usually accompanied by an audible sound, which is preceded by an exaggerated inspiratory effort

PATHOPHYSIOLOGY
• One of the most powerful reflexes in the body
• Induced by stimulation of either afferent fibers of the pharyngeal distribution of the glossopharyngeal nerves or sensory endings of the vagus nerves located in the larynx, trachea, and larger bronchi
• Begins with an inspiratory phase followed in sequence by an inspiratory pause, glottis closure, increased intrathoracic pressure, and glottis opening
• Serves as an early warning system for the pharynx and respiratory system and as a protective mechanism; cough is predominant manner by which upper respiratory tract and the passageways of the lungs are maintained free of foreign material.

SYSTEMS AFFECTED
• Respiratory—at all levels except, perhaps, the respiratory bronchioles and alveoli
• Musculoskeletal—because of the role played in the reflex by inspiratory and expiratory muscles of respiration
• Cardiovascular—severe or prolonged coughing may result in Mobitz type II or complete AV block, or even obstructive cardiomyopathy, thereby contributing to cough syncope.
• Nervous—this component of cough syncope is felt to be the combined effect of decreased cardiac output and high intravascular pressures in the cranium, which reduce cerebral blood flow, resulting in syncope.

SIGNALMENT
Dogs and cats of all ages and breeds

SIGNS
• The classic cough as spelled out in the definition may not always be present, but may be supplanted by a softer, less forceful expiratory effort.

CAUSES

Upper Respiratory Tract Diseases
• Nasopharyngeal—rhinitis; sinusitis; nasopharyngeal foreign body or tumor; tonsillitis; tonsillar tumor
• Laryngeal—inflammation; foreign body; injuries; tumors
• Tracheal—inflammation (inhalation of irritating substances and heat); infections (viral and bacterial); foreign body; tracheal collapse; tumor

Lower Respiratory Tract Diseases
• Bronchial—inflammation; infection (viral, bacterial, and parasitic); allergy; foreign body; tumor
• Pulmonary—inflammation; infection (viral, bacterial, and fungal); aspiration pneumonia; pulmonary edema; tumor
• Pulmonary/vascular—heartworm disease; thrombosis or embolism; CHF; pulmonary hypertension; tumor

Other Diseases
• Esophageal—inflammation; foreign body; tumor
• Pleural—inflammation; infection (bacterial and fungal); hernia; tumor

RISK FACTORS
• Congenital and acquired esophageal, gastroesophageal, and upper gastrointestinal disorders—predispose the patient to aspiration pneumonia
• Hyperadrenocorticism and chronic administration of corticosteroids—may increase incidence of pulmonary thromboembolism, and decrease resistance to respiratory infections
• Genetic predisposition to certain cardiac disorders—increases risk of pulmonary edema secondary to CHF
• Environmental factors—exposure to certain viral, bacterial, fungal, and parasitic diseases; exposure of dogs or cats to mosquitoes without effective heartworm prophylaxis
• Complications of the cough—disseminate respiratory infections, complicate inflammatory conditions in the airways, or even result in emphysema, or pneumothorax, by causing rupture of focal areas of lung tissue

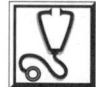

DIAGNOSIS

DIFFERENTIAL DIAGNOSIS

Similar Signs
• Sneezing and coughing—expiratory events that may occur together in certain conditions (e.g., rhinitis, sinusitis, and regurgitation); may confuse both the owner and the history; forceful expiration of a sneeze: mouth usually closed; cough: mouth usually open
• Reverse sneeze—commonly misinterpreted as a cough by owners; associated with both an audible inspiratory and an expiratory component without the forceful expiratory event that characterizes both the sneeze and the cough; nasopharyngeal irritation usual cause; some of the same conditions that cause sneezing and coughing may be responsible

Causes
• Patterns and characteristics—frequently suggest underlying cause
• Nocturnal—commonly associated with early stages of left-sided CHF and tracheal collapse
• Precipitated by exercise or excitement—frequently the result of inflammation or irritation involving the larynx, trachea, and bronchi
• Harsh and prolonged—suggests involvement of the large airways
• Soft and infrequent—likely the result of alveolar disease or CHF
• Productive—suggests fluid or mucus in the expectorated material
• Hemoptysis—can be the result of a number of different conditions, including pulmonary neoplasia, foreign body, granuloma, or secondary to a coagulopathy
• Dry—indicates lack of mucus or fluid production

CBC/BIOCHEMISTRY/URINALYSIS
• CBC—may suggest possible causes: neutrophilia with a left shift (e.g., infection and inflammation) or eosinophilia (e.g., hypersensitivity response)
• High liver enzymes with exaggerated SAP elevation—suggests hyperadrenocorticism
• Mild to moderate elevations in SAP—suggest liver congestion secondary to pulmonary disease or right heart failure
• Proteinuria—may be associated with pulmonary thromboembolism in patients with glomerulonephritis, amyloidosis, or hyperadrenocorticism

OTHER LABORATORY TESTS
• Filter test for microfilaria and/or filaria serologic test—evaluate for heartworm disease
• Low-dose dexamethasone suppression test or ACTH-response test—further evaluate elevations in liver enzymes
• Coagulation profile—for any patient that presents with a cough associated with either epistaxis or hemoptysis

IMAGING
• Radiographs—particularly useful for evaluating patients with nasal, sinus, tracheal, and lower respiratory tract disorders
• Fluoroscopy—especially beneficial in establishing a definitive diagnosis in dynamic conditions such as tracheal collapse and swallowing disorders; false negative evaluation possible
• Thoracic ultrasound—useful for patients with primary cardiac disease, right heart disease secondary to a pulmonary condition, consolidated lung lesions, and pleural effusion

DIAGNOSTIC PROCEDURES
• Direct, flotation, Baermann, and sedimentation fecal tests—detect respiratory parasites and ova
• Transtracheal aspirate with cytologic examination and culture—evaluate lower respiratory tract disorders
• Laryngoscopy, tracheoscopy, and bronchoscopy—evaluate suspected foreign body, tumor, or other disorders in these regions; combine endoscopy with biopsy and bronchoalveolar lavage.
• Thoracocentesis—with pleural effusion
• Barium swallow—for more thorough evaluation of suspected aspiration pneumonia secondary to swallowing disorders
• CT scan—better evaluate nasal and sinus disorders

TREATMENT
• Outpatient—unless CHF is diagnosed or marked alteration in pulmonary function or hemoptysis noted
• Exercise restriction—best enforced until a cause is established and corrected, especially when activity aggravates the condition
• Inform client that a wide variety of conditions can be responsible for the cough, and a fairly extensive workup may be required to define and treat the underlying cause.
• Surgical intervention—primary indications include tracheal collapse, laryngeal paralysis, and tumors involving the respiratory tract at various levels

MEDICATIONS

DRUG(S) OF CHOICE
• Symptomatic treatment without other abnormalities—broad-spectrum antibiotics; bronchodilator-expectorant; appropriate follow-up evaluations
• Collect airway specimens for bacterial culture and sensitivity testing before administering antibiotics
• Broad-spectrum antibiotics—for suspected infection when results of bacterial culture and sensitivity testing are pending
• Bronchodilators (e.g., theophylline and terbutaline) with or without the use of expectorants—may be beneficial for a variety of diseases affecting the trachea and lower respiratory airways
• Corticosteroids may be the only effective therapy in the long-term management of chronic bronchitis in dogs and asthma in domestic cats.

• Cough suppressants (e.g., hydrocodone and torbutrol)—avoid in patients with coughs secondary to bacterial respiratory infection and CHF; frequently beneficial for coughs of other origin
• Therapeutic thoracentesis—perform on any patient in which the pleural effusion is felt to be contributing to any respiratory discomfort or distress

CONTRAINDICATIONS
• Corticosteroids—do not use until a definitive inflammation is defined in the absence of infection, parasitic infestation, or cardiac disease; may potentiate the development of pulmonary thromboembolism; may reduce the efficacy of caparsolate in the treatment of heartworm disease
• Cough suppressants—do not use in any patient in which either a respiratory infection or clinically important heart disease is suspected.

PRECAUTIONS
• Cough suppressants—indiscriminate use may obscure the warning signs of serious cardiac and pulmonary disorders and predispose the patient to serious complications or even death.
• Bronchodilator therapy—intravenous use of aminophylline may cause tachyarrhythmias.
• Corticosteroids—the key to avoiding adverse drug reactions (i.e., such as diabetes mellitus) is to use the lowest effective dose on an alternate day or every third day regimen, and to use in combination with other beneficial therapeutic agents (e.g., bronchodilators, cough suppressants).
• Diuretics—do not use in patients with primary airway disease; drying of secretions decreases clearance of mucus and exudate.

POSSIBLE INTERACTIONS
Theophylline bronchodilators—clearance may be inhibited by other drugs (e.g., enrofloxacin and chloramphenicol); signs of toxicity may develop with the addition of such drugs.

ALTERNATIVE DRUG(S)
N/A

FOLLOW-UP

PATIENT MONITORING
• Communicate with client concerning control of the cough.
• Follow-up thoracic radiographs in 3–7 days with cardiovascular disease, in 10–14 days with bronchopulmonary disease; in 3–4 weeks to monitor potential tumors

POSSIBLE COMPLICATIONS
• Resolution or medical control of the cough does not ensure complete elimination of the inciting cause.
• Serious respiratory dysfunction and even death may be caused by underlying disease.

MISCELLANEOUS

ASSOCIATED CONDITIONS
• Heavy breathing
• Dyspnea

AGE-RELATED FACTORS
N/A

ZOONOTIC POTENTIAL
N/A

PREGNANCY
N/A

SEE ALSO
• Chronic Bronchitis
• Congestive Heart Failure
• Feline Asthma
• Hypoxemia
• Nasal Discharge (Sneezing, Reverse Sneezing, Gagging)
• Pneumonia, Bacterial
• Pneumonia, Eosinophilic
• Respiratory Parasites
• Tracheal Collapse

ABBREVIATIONS
• ACTH = adrenocorticotropic hormone
• AV = atrioventricular
• CHF = congestive heart failure
• CT = computed tomography
• SAP = serum alkaline phosphatase

Suggested Reading

Ettinger SJ. Coughing. In: Ettinger ST, Feldman EC, eds. Textbook of veterinary internal medicine. 5th ed. Philadelphia: Saunders 2000:162–166.

Johnson L. Tracheal collapse, diagnosis and medical and surgical treatment. Vet Clin North Am 2000;30:1253–1266.

Kopos J, Tomori Z. Cough and other respiratory reflexes. Prog Respir Res 1979; 12:15–188.

Langlands T. The dynamics of cough in health and in chronic bronchitis. Thorax 1967;22:88–96.

Yanagihara N, von Ledan H, Werner-Kukuk E. The physical parameters of cough: the larynx in a normal single cough. Acta Otolaryngol (Stockh) 1965;495–510.

Author Neil K. Harpster
Consulting Editor Lynelle R. Johnson

CRANIOMANDIBULAR OSTEOPATHY

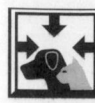

BASICS

OVERVIEW
• A nonneoplastic, noninflammatory proliferative disease of the bones of the head
• Primary bones affected—mandibular rami; occipital and parietal; tympanic bullae; zygomatic portion of the temporal
• Bilateral symmetric involvement most common
• Affects musculoskeletal system

SIGNALMENT
• Scottish, cairn, and West Highland white terrier breeds—most common
• Labrador retrievers, Great Danes, Boston terriers, Doberman pinschers, Irish setters, English bulldogs, and boxers—may be affected
• Usually growing puppies 4–8 months of age
• No gender predilection
• Neutering may increase incidence.

SIGNS

Historical Findings
• Usually relate to pain around the mouth and difficulty eating
• Angular processes of the mandible affected—jaw movement progressively restricted
• Difficulty in prehension, mastication, and swallowing—may lead to starvation
• Lameness or limb swelling—may precede cranial involvement

Physical Examination Findings
• Temporal and masseter muscle atrophy—common
• Palpable irregular thickening of the mandibular rami and/or TMJ region
• Inability to fully open jaw, even under general anesthesia
• Intermittent pyrexia—40°C
• Bilateral exophthalmos

CAUSES & RISK FACTORS
• Believed to be hereditary—occurs in certain breeds and families
• West Highland white terriers—autosomal recessive trait
• Scottish terriers—possible predisposition
• Possible link to infection—pyrexia; histologic evidence of inflammation only at the periphery of the lesion
• Young terrier with periosteal long bone disease—monitor for disease.

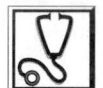

DIAGNOSIS

DIFFERENTIAL DIAGNOSIS
• Osteomyelitis—bones not symmetrically affected; generally not as extensive; lysis; lack of breed predilection; history of penetrating wound
• Traumatic periostitis—bones not symmetrically affected; generally not as extensive; history of trauma
• Neoplasia—mature patient; not symmetrically affected; more lytic bone reaction; metastatic disease

CBC/BIOCHEMISTRY/URINALYSIS
• Serum ALP and inorganic phosphate—may be high
• May note hypogammaglobulinemia or α_2-hyperglobulinemia

OTHER LABORATORY TESTS
Serology—rule out fungal agents; indicated in atypical cases

IMAGING
• Skull radiography—reveals uneven, bead-like osseous proliferation of the mandible or tympanic bullae (bilateral); extensive, periosteal new bone formation (exostoses) affecting one or more bones around the TMJ; may show fusion of the tympanic bullae and angular process of the mandible
• CT—may help evaluate osseous involvement of the TMJ

DIAGNOSTIC PROCEDURES
Bone biopsy and culture (bacterial and fungal)—necessary only in atypical cases; rule out neoplasia and osteomyelitis

PATHOLOGIC FINDINGS
• Bone biopsy—reveals normal lamellar bone being replaced by an enlarged coarse-fiber bone and osteoclastic osteolysis of the periosteal or subperiosteal region
• Bone marrow—replaced by a vascular fibrous-type stroma
• Inflammatory cells—occasionally seen at the periphery of the bony lesion

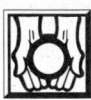

TREATMENT
• Palliative only
• Surgical excision of exostoses—results in regrowth within weeks
• High-calorie, protein-rich gruel diet—helps maintain nutritional balance
• Surgical placement of a pharyngostomy, esophagostomy, or gastrostomy tube—considered to help maintain nutritional balance

MEDICATIONS
DRUG(S)
• Analgesics and antiinflammatory drugs—palliative use warranted

• NSAIDs—may be used to minimize pain and decrease inflammation; may try buffered or enteric-coated aspirin (10–25 mg/kg PO q8–12h), caroprofen (2.2 mg/kg PO q12h), etodolac (10–15 mg/kg, PO, once daily), phenylbutazone (3–7 mg/kg PO q8h, total dose < 800 mg/day), meclofenamic acid (0.5 mg/kg PO q12h), or piroxicam (0.3 mg/kg PO q24h for 3 days, then q48h)

CONTRAINDICATIONS/POSSIBLE INTERACTIONS
N/A

FOLLOW-UP
PATIENT MONITORING
Frequent re-examinations—mandatory to ensure adequate nutritional balance and pain control

PREVENTION/AVOIDANCE
• Do not repeat dam–sire breedings that resulted in affected offspring.
• Discourage breeding of affected animals.

EXPECTED COURSE AND PROGNOSIS
• Pain and discomfort may diminish at skeletal maturity (10–12 months of age); the exostoses may regress.

• Prognosis—depends on involvement of bones surrounding the TMJ
• Elective euthanasia may be necessary.

MISCELLANEOUS
SYNONYMS
Lion jaw

ABBREVIATIONS
• ALP = alkaline phosphatase
• NSAIDS = nonsteroidal antiinflammatory drugs
• TMJ = temporomandibular joint

Suggested Reading
Watson ADJ, Adams WM, Thomas CB. Craniomandibular osteopathy in dogs. Compend Contin Educ Pract Vet 1995;17:911–921.
Author Peter D. Schwarz
Consulting Editor Peter K. Shires

CRUCIATE LIGAMENT DISEASE, CRANIAL

BASICS

DEFINITION
The acute or degenerative injury of the CrCL, which results in partial to complete instability of the stifle joint

PATHOPHYSIOLOGY
• Function of the CrCL—constrain the stifle joint by limiting internal rotation and cranial displacement of the tibia relative to the femur; prevents hyperextension
• CrCL injury—from trauma (acute) or degenerative causes (chronic); breaking strength approximately equal to four times the body weight of the dog
• Acute rupture—< 20% caused by exceeding the strength of the ligament in dogs; usually caused by hyperextension and excessive internal rotation with the stifle in partial flexion (20–50°); trauma most common cause in cats; a ligament weakened by degeneration is more easily ruptured than is a normal ligament.
• Degeneration—aging, conformational abnormalities, disuse related to sedentary habits or limb immobilization, and immune-mediated
• Aging and degeneration—related to size; dogs > 15 kg show more changes and have a more significant change in CrCL strength than do smaller dogs; degenerative changes and a decrease in material properties have been shown consistently in dogs > 5 years of age
• Conformational abnormalities—genu varum (bowlegged), genu valgum (knock-kneed), straight stifles and hock, caudal sloping of the tibial plateau, patella luxation, and narrowing of the intercondylar notch—may predispose patient to rupture.
• Immune-mediated arthritis, lymphocytic–plasmocytic synovitis, and septic arthritis—may predispose patient to rupture
• Immune complexes—found in dogs with unilateral and bilateral rupture; unknown if they are a cause or a result of the rupture
• Partial rupture—accounts for 25–30% of stifle lameness cases
• Untreated rupture—degenerative changes within a few weeks; severe changes within a few months
• Medial meniscal (caudal horn) damage—from abnormal joint mechanics after CrCL injury; occurs in > 50% of cases
• Cranial tibial thrust—may play an important role in CrCL rupture; theoretically, a cranially directed force is generated during weight bearing, based on the caudal slope of the tibial plateau and the tibial compression mechanism

SYSTEMS AFFECTED
Musculoskeletal

GENETICS
• Unknown
• May be important in predisposing patient to DJD, degeneration of the CrCL, or conformation abnormalities

INCIDENCE/PREVALENCE
CrCL rupture—one of the most common causes of hindlimb lameness in dogs; major cause of DJD in the stifle joint

GEOGRAPHIC DISTRIBUTION
N/A

SIGNALMENT

Species
• Dogs
• Uncommon in cats

Breed Predilections
• All susceptible
• Rottweilers and Labrador retrievers—increased incidence of CrCL rupture when < 4 years of age

Mean Age and Range
• Dogs > 5 years of age
• Large breed dogs—between 1 and 2 years of age

Predominant Sex
Possibly female dogs

SIGNS

General Comments
Related to the degree of rupture (partial vs. complete), the mode of rupture (acute vs. chronic), the occurrence of meniscal injury, and the severity of inflammation and DJD

Historical Findings
• Athletic or traumatic events—generally precede acute injury, resulting in non-weight-bearing lameness with the affected limb held in flexion
• Normal activity resulting in acute lameness—suggests degenerative rupture
• Subtle to marked intermittent lameness (for weeks to months)—consistent with partial tears that are progressing to complete rupture

Physical Examination Findings
• Demonstration of cranial drawer motion—diagnostic for rupture; often dramatic after acute injury; subtle, almost imperceptible motion that ends gradually as a result of tissue stretching consistent with chronic rupture or partial tears; tested in flexion, normal standing angle, and extension
• Cranial movement of tibia relative to the femur during the tibial compression test
• Joint effusion

• Palpable thickening of the joint capsule—especially on the medial aspect (medial buttress)
• Hindlimb muscle atrophy—especially the quadriceps muscle group
• No cranial drawer sign (or negative tibial compression test)—does not rule out rupture; may see false-negative results with chronic or partial tears and in painful or anxious patients that are not sedated or anesthetized

CAUSES
• Trauma
• Degenerative changes
• Conformation abnormalities
• Immune-mediated

RISK FACTORS
• Obesity
• Patella luxation
• Poor conformation
• Excessive caudal slope of tibial plateau
• Narrowed intercondylar notch

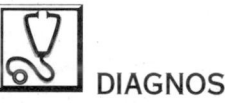

DIAGNOSIS

DIFFERENTIAL DIAGNOSIS
• Skeletally immature dogs and dogs with significant muscle atrophy—slight drawer motion that stops abruptly as the CrCL is stretched taut common
• Caudal cruciate ligament rupture—uncommon as an isolated occurrence
• Palpation—distinguish cranial from caudal rupture
• Patella luxation (medial or lateral)—alone or with CrCL rupture
• Stifle joint trauma
• Osteochondritis dissecans of the femoral condyle or patella
• Neoplasia (e.g., synovial cell sarcoma)—generally more painful than rupture

CBC/BIOCHEMISTRY/URINALYSIS
N/A

OTHER LABORATORY TESTS
N/A

IMAGING

Radiography
• Rarely diagnostic for rupture
• Extremely helpful in confirming intra-articular disease
• Common findings—joint effusion with capsular distention and compression of the infrapatellar fat pad; periarticular osteophytes; enthesiophytes; CrCL avulsion fractures; calcification of the CrCL

Magnetic Resonance Imaging
Graphically shows cruciate ligament and meniscal pathology

DIAGNOSTIC PROCEDURES
• Arthrocentesis—joint cytology to identify intra-articular disease and rule out sepsis and immune-mediated disease
• Arthroscopy—directly visualize the cruciate ligaments, menisci, and other intra-articular structures

PATHOLOGIC FINDINGS
• Varying degrees of cartilage fibrillation and erosion
• Periarticular osteophyte formation
• Meniscal damage
• Synovitis
• Ruptured fibers of the CrCL—hyalinization; fibrous tissue invasion; necrosis; loss of the parallel orientation of ligament bundles

TREATMENT

APPROPRIATE HEALTH CARE
• Dogs < 15 kg—may treat conservatively as outpatients; 85% improve or are normal by 6 months
• Dogs > 15 kg—treated with surgery; only 20% improve or are normal by 6 months
• Surgery—recommended for all dogs; speeds rate of recovery; prevents degenerative changes; enhances function

NURSING CARE
Postsurgery—physical therapy (e.g., ice packing, range-of-motion exercises, massage, and muscle electrical stimulation); important for improving mobility and strength

ACTIVITY
Restricted—with conservative treatment and after surgical stabilization; duration depends on method of treatment and progress of patient.

DIET
Weight control—important for decreasing the load and thus stress on the stifle joint

CLIENT EDUCATION
• Warn client that, regardless of the method of treatment, DJD is common.
• Inform client that return to complete athletic function is uncommon.
• Warn client that 20%–40% of dogs with unilateral CrCL rupture will experience rupture of the contralateral ligament within 17 months.

SURGICAL CONSIDERATIONS
No one technique has proven superior to the others.

Extra-articular Methods
• A wide variety of techniques that use a heavy-gauge implant to imbricate the joint and restore stability
• Implant material—placed in the approximate plane of the CrCL origin and insertion

Intra-articular Methods
• Designed to replace the CrCL anatomically
• Autografts (patella ligament, fascia), allografts (bone-tendon-bone), and synthetic materials—commonly used
• Femoral intercondylar notchplasty—recommended to minimize graft injury
• Arthroscopic replacement—recently described; long-term benefits unknown

Modified Extra-articular Methods
• Fibular head transposition or popliteal tendon transposition
• Realign and tension the lateral collateral ligament or popliteal tendon to restrict internal rotation and cranial drawer

Tibial Plateau Leveling Osteotomy
• Rotational osteotomy of the proximal tibia
• Levels tibial plateau and neutralizes cranial tibial thrust

MEDICATIONS

DRUG(S) OF CHOICE
NSAIDs and analgesics—symptomatically treat associated synovitis and DJD; may use buffered or enteric-coated aspirin (10–25 mg/kg PO q8–12h), caroprofen (2.2 mg/kg PO q12h), etodolac (10–15 mg/kg PO q24h), phenylbutazone (3–7 mg/kg PO q8h, total dose < 800 mg/day), meclofenamic acid (0.5 mg/kg PO q12h), piroxicam (0.3 mg/ kg PO q24h for 3 days, then q48h), or deracoxib (3–4 mg/kg PO q24h for 7 days for postoperative pain) (1–2 mg/kg PO q24h for long-term treatment over 7 days)

CONTRAINDICATIONS
Avoid corticosteroids—potential side effects; articular cartilage damage associated with long-term use

PRECAUTIONS
NSAIDs—may cause gastrointestinal irritation; may preclude use in some patients

POSSIBLE INTERACTIONS
N/A

ALTERNATIVE DRUG(S)
Chondroprotective drugs (polysulfated glycosaminoglycans, glucosamine, and chondroitin sulfate)—may help limit cartilage damage and degeneration

FOLLOW-UP

PATIENT MONITORING
• Depends on method of treatment
• Most techniques require 2–4 months of rehabilitation

PREVENTION/AVOIDANCE
Avoid breeding animals with conformation abnormalities.

POSSIBLE COMPLICATIONS
Second surgery—required in 10–15% of cases because of subsequent meniscal damage

EXPECTED COURSE AND PROGNOSIS
Regardless of surgical technique, the success rate is approximately 85%.

MISCELLANEOUS

ASSOCIATED CONDITIONS
Meniscal damage

AGE-RELATED FACTORS
See Pathophysiology

ZOONOTIC POTENTIAL
N/A

PREGNANCY
N/A

SEE ALSO
• Arthritis (Osteoarthritis)
• Patellar Luxation

ABBREVIATIONS
• CrCL = cranial cruciate ligament
• DJD = degenerative joint disease
• NSAID = nonsteroidal antiinflammatory drug

Suggested Reading
Brinker WO, Piermattei DL, Flo GL. Rupture of the cranial cruciate ligament. In: Brinker WO, Piermattei DL, Flo GL, eds. Handbook of small animal orthopedics and fracture repair. 3rd ed. Philadelphia: Saunders, 1997:534–563.
Johnson JM, Johnson AL. Cranial cruciate ligament rupture: pathogenesis, diagnosis, and postoperative rehabilitation. Vet Clin North Am 1993;23:717–733.
Slocum B, Slocum TD. Treatment of the stifle for cranial cruciate ligament rupture. In: Bojrab MJ, ed. Current techniques in small animal surgery. 4th ed. Philadelphia: Lea & Febiger, 1998:1187–11215.
Author Peter D. Schwarz
Consulting Editor Peter K. Shires

CRYPTOCOCCOSIS

 BASICS

DEFINITION
A localized or systemic fungal infection caused by the environmental yeast *Cryptococcus neoformans*

PATHOPHYSIOLOGY
• *C. neoformans*—grows in bird droppings and decaying vegetation
• Dogs and cats inhale the yeast and a foci of infection is established, usually in the nasal passages; smaller dried, shrunken organisms may reach the terminal airways (uncommon)
• Stomach and intestinal infections suggest that primary GI entry occurs.
• Dissemination—hematogenously from the nasal passages to the brain, eyes, lungs, and other tissues; by extension to the skin of the nose, the eye, retro-orbital tissues, and draining lymph nodes

SYSTEMS AFFECTED
• Cats—mainly the nose and sinuses; facial skin; nasal planum; nasopharynx; brain; eyes
• Dogs—mainly the head and brain, nasal passages, and sinuses; skin over the nose and sinuses; mucous membranes; draining lymph nodes; eyes; periorbital areas; occasionally lungs and abdominal organs

GENETICS
No known influence

INCIDENCE/PREVALENCE
• Dogs—rare in U.S.; prevalence 0.00013%
• Cats—7–10 times more common than in dogs

GEOGRAPHIC DISTRIBUTION
• Worldwide
• Some areas of southern California and Australia have an increased incidence
• Some *Cryptococcus* spp. grow well on eucalyptus trees.

SIGNALMENT

Species
Cats and dogs

Breed Predilection
• Dogs—American cocker spaniels, Great Danes, Doberman pinschers, and Labrador retrievers over-represented
• Cats—Siamese at increased risk

Mean Age and Range
• Most common 2–7 years of age (dogs and cats)
• May occur at any age

Predominant Sex
• Dogs—none
• Cats—males over-represented

SIGNS

Historical Findings
• Lethargy
• Vary depending on organ systems involved
• May have a history of problems for weeks to months
Dogs
• Neurologic—seizures, ataxia, paresis, blindness
• Skin ulceration
• Lymphadenopathy
Cats
• Nasal discharge
• Neurologic signs—seizures, disorientation, and vestibular signs
• Granulomatous tissue seen at the nares
• Firm swellings over the bridge of the nose

Physical Examination Findings
• Mild fever—< 50% of patients
• Dogs—anorexia; nasal discharge
• Cats—increased respiratory noise; ulcerated crusty skin lesions on the head; lymphadenopathy; neurologic; ocular

CAUSES
Exposure to cryptococcal organisms and inability of the immune system to prevent colonization and invasion into tissues

RISK FACTORS
Cats concurrently infected with FeLV or FIV—higher risk; more extensive disease

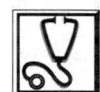 DIAGNOSIS

DIFFERENTIAL DIAGNOSIS

Dogs
• Other causes of focal or diffuse neurologic disease—distemper; bacterial meningo-encephalitis; brain tumors; rickettsial diseases; granulomatous meningoencephalomyelitis; other fungal diseases
• Nasal lesions, especially at the muco-cutaneous junction—considered immune-mediated
• Lymphosarcoma—possible cause of the lymphadenopathy
• With chorioretinitis and optic neuritis—consider other fungal infections, distemper, and neoplasia

Cats
• Nasal lesions—similar to nasal tumors, chronic rhinitis, and chronic sinusitis
• Ulcerative skin changes—may be the result of bacterial infection, fights, or tumor (especially squamous cell carcinoma of the nasal planum)
• Ocular and brain signs—may be attributed to lymphosarcoma, FIP, and toxoplasmosis

CBC/BIOCHEMISTRY/URINALYSIS
• Mild anemia in some cats
• Eosinophilia occasionally seen
• Chemistries usually normal

OTHER LABORATORY TESTS
Latex agglutination or ELISA—detect cryptococcal capsular antigen in serum; few false-positive tests; most infected animals have measurable capsular antigen titers; magnitude of titer correlates with extent of infection

IMAGING
• Lateral radiographs of the nasopharynx—cryptococcal granuloma behind the soft palate
• Nasal radiographs (cats)—soft tissue–density material filling the nasal passage; occasional bone destruction of the nasal dorsum
• Contrast-enhanced CT or MRI may identify brain granulomas.
• Thoracic radiographs—not indicated, unless signs of lower respiratory tract disease

DIAGNOSTIC PROCEDURES
Dogs with neurologic disease—additional procedures: cytologic examination and culture of CSF and measurement of CSF capsular antigen often make the diagnosis.

Cats
• Definitive diagnosis—aspirates of the mucoid material in the nasal passages or biopsy of the granulomatous tissue that protrudes from the nares. Flushing the nose with saline may dislodge granulomatous tissue.
• Patients with upper respiratory obstruction or severe respiratory noise—granuloma in the nasopharynx; identify by pulling the soft palate forward with a spay hook to expose the mass or retroflexion of endoscope in nasopharynx to examine and biopsy mass in the choanal area
• Biopsy—skin lesions of the head; aspirates of involved lymph nodes; usually identifies organisms
• Cultures—confirm the diagnosis; determine drug susceptibility if poorly responsive infection
• One study found that 14% of normal dogs and 7% of normal cats have cryptococcal organisms in the nasal passages.

Pathologic Findings
• Gross lesions—gray, gelatinous mass produced by the polysaccharide capsule; usually found in the nose, sinuses, and nasopharynx of cats. Skin lesions are usually ulcerative.
• Neurologic lesions—usually seen in dogs; diffuse or fungal granulomas producing a mass in the brain
• Chorioretinitis with or without retinal detachment or optic neuritis—dogs and cats
• Histologic response—usually pyogranulo-

matous; inflammatory cell infiltrate may be mild because the polysaccharide capsule interferes with neutrophil migration.

 TREATMENT

APPROPRIATE HEALTH CARE
• Outpatient if stable
• Neurologic signs—may require inpatient supportive care until stable

NURSING CARE
Cats—nasal obstruction influences appetite; encourage patients to eat by offering palatable food

ACTIVITY
No restrictions in most cases

DIET
• No special foods
• Patients treated with itraconazole—give medication in fatty food (e.g., canned food) to improve absorption

CLIENT EDUCATION
• Inform client that this is a chronic disease that requires months of treatment.
• Reassure client that the infection is not zoonotic.

SURGICAL CONSIDERATIONS
Remove granulomatous masses in the nasopharynx to reduce respiratory difficulties.

 MEDICATIONS

DRUG(S) OF CHOICE
• Triazole antifungal agents—expensive; itraconazole somewhat more economical
• Fluconazole—preferred for ocular or CNS involvement because it is water-soluble and penetrates the nervous system better; cats, 50 mg PO q12h; dogs, 5 mg/kg PO q12h
• Itraconazole—give with a fatty meal to maximize absorption; cats, 10–15 mg/kg PO daily; dogs, 5 mg/kg PO q12h; pellets in the capsule can be mixed with food; no apparent adverse taste
• Terbinafine at a dose of 5 mg/kg q12h has been effective in treatment of cats with resistant infections.

CONTRAINDICATIONS
Avoid steroids

PRECAUTIONS
• Triazoles—hepatic toxicity; anorexia signals problems; monitor liver enzymes monthly.
• Terbinafine–monitor for hepatic toxicity and anorexia.

• Itraconazole—ulcerative dermatitis (differentiate from the skin lesions of cryptococcosis); new skin lesions after the disease is much improved should be considered a drug reaction.

POSSIBLE INTERACTIONS
Itraconazole—do not give with the antihistamines terfenadine and astemizole or with cisapride.

ALTERNATIVE DRUG(S)
Cryptococcal organisms are prone to become resistant to antifungal treatment. Amphotericin B (intravenous)—dogs and cats that do not respond to a triazole; monitor BUN closely to avoid permanent renal damage

 FOLLOW-UP

PATIENT MONITORING
• Monitor liver enzymes monthly in patients receiving a triazole antifungal agent
• Improvement in clinical signs, resolution of lesions, improvement in well-being, and return of appetite measure the response to treatment.
• Capsular antigen titers—determine response to and duration of treatment; after 2 months of treatment, the titers should decrease substantially if effective; if ineffective, try the other triazole or terbinafine, because organism can become resistant.

PREVENTION/AVOIDANCE
The organism is ubiquitous and cannot be avoided.

POSSIBLE COMPLICATIONS
Patients with neurologic disease may have seizures and permanent neurologic changes.

EXPECTED COURSE AND PROGNOSIS
• Treatment—anticipated duration 3 months to 1 year; patients with CNS disease may require lifelong maintenance.
• Cats concurrently infected with FeLV or FIV—have a worse prognosis
• Capsular antigen titers—measure every 2 months until 6 months after completion of treatment; continue treatment for 2 months after antigen is nondetectable, if possible; if patient maintains low titers for months after all signs of disease have resolved, continue treatment for at least 3 months after reduction in antigen levels and resolution of clinical signs; if titers then rise significantly, resume therapy

 MISCELLANEOUS

ASSOCIATED CONDITIONS
N/A

AGE-RELATED FACTORS
N/A

ZOONOTIC POTENTIAL
• Not considered zoonotic, but possibility of transmission through bite wounds
• Inform client that the organism was acquired from the environment and that he or she could be at increased risk, especially if immunosuppressed.

PREGNANCY
N/A

ABBREVIATIONS
• CNS = central nervous system
• CSF = cerebrospinal fluid
• ELISA = enzyme-linked immunoadsorbent assay
• FeLV = feline leukemia virus
• FIP = feline infectious peritonitis
• FIV = feline immunodeficiency virus

Suggested Reading

Beaty JA, Barrs VR, Swinney GR, et al. Peripheral vestibular disease associated with cryptococcosis in three cats. J Fel Med Surg 2000;2:29–34.

Berthelin CF, Bailey CS, Kass PH, et al. Cryptococcosis of the nervous system in dogs. Part 1, Epidemiologic, clinical and neuropathologic features. Prog Vet Neurol 1994;5:88–97.

Berthelin CF, Legendre AM, Bailey CS, et al. Cryptococcosis of the nervous system in dogs. Part 2, Diagnosis, treatment, monitoring and prognosis. Prog Vet Neurol 1994;5:136–146.

Jacobs GJ, Medleau L, Clavert C, et al. Cryptococcal infection in cats: factors influencing treatment outcome, and results of sequential serum antigen titers in 35 cats. J Vet Intern Med 1997;11:1–4.

Malik R, Dill-Macky E, Maring P, et al. Cryptococcosis in dogs: a retrospective study of 20 consecutive cases. J Med Vet Mycol 1995;33:291–297.

Malik R, Hunt GB, Bellenger CR, et al. Intra-abdominal cryptococcosis in two dogs. J Small Anim Pract 1999;40:387–391.

Malik R, Wigney DI, Muir DB, Love DN. Asymptomatic carriage of *Cryptococcus neoformans* in the nasal cavity of dogs and cats. J Med Vet Mycol 1997;35:27–31.

Malik R, Wigney DI, Muir DB, et al. Cryptococcosis in cats: clinical and mycological assessment of 29 cases and evaluation of treatment using orally administered fluconazole. J Med Vet Mycol 1992;30:133–144.

Medleau L, Jacobs GJ, Marks A. Itraconazole for the treatment of cryptococcosis in cats. J Vet Intern Med 1995;9:39–42.

Author Alfred M. Legendre
Consulting Editor Stephen C. Barr

CRYPTORCHIDISM

BASICS

OVERVIEW
• The incomplete descent of one or both testes into the scrotum
• Inguinal—retained testis often palpable
• Abdominal—testis difficult to palpate or identify by radiology; may be imaged with ultrasound
• Descent to final scrotal position—expected to be complete by 2 months postpartum; may occur later in some breeds, but rarely after 6 months in any individual; presume the diagnosis if no palpable testes at 2 months
• Beagles—testes at the exterior inguinal ring by day 5 postpartum, between the inguinal ring and scrotum by day 15, and in the scrotum by day 40

SIGNALMENT
• Dogs—reported in almost all breeds; toy poodles, Pomeranians, Yorkshire terriers (especially toy and miniature breeds) at significantly higher risk; unilateral more common than bilateral (75:25); right testis retained twice as often as left in dogs; right and left testis retained at equal frequency in cats
• Prevalence—dogs, 1.2%; cats, 1.7%
• Genetics (dogs)—thought to be heritable as a sex-limited autosomal recessive trait; exact mode of inheritance unknown (number and penetrance of genes involved)
• Genetics (cats)—may be inherited, but no data documents hereditary defect; Persians over-represented in surveys

SIGNS
• Rarely associated with pain or other signs of disease
• Acute onset of abdominal pain—spermatic cord of retained testes at increased risk for torsion; 36% of retained testes with torsion of the spermatic cord were neoplastic
• Feminizing paraneoplastic syndrome—estrogen-secreting Sertoli cell tumors in retained testes produce feminizing signs: gynecomastia, symmetrical alopecia of trunk and flanks, hyperpigmentation of inguinal skin, pendulous preputial sheath, prostatic squamous metaplasia

CAUSES & RISK FACTORS
• Removal of affected males from breeding lines—believed to cause a reduction in frequency; heritability thought to involve more than one gene

• Nonhereditary predisposing factors (e.g., birth weight)—identified in humans; not reported in dogs

DIAGNOSIS

DIFFERENTIAL DIAGNOSIS
• Castration—differentiate bilateral condition from previous castration, previous castration of single scrotal testis with retained abdominal testis, or anorchidism (rare)
• Bilaterally cryptorchid cats may have urine odor and behavior of intact cats

CBC/BIOCHEMISTRY/URINALYSIS
N/A

OTHER LABORATORY TESTS
hCG stimulation—doubles blood testosterone with bilateral condition; doubles blood testosterone with unilateral condition in which only the scrotal testis has been removed; differentiates between cryptorchidism and castration; administration of 750 IU hCG IV or 50 μg GnRH IM with blood sample collection pre- and 2–3 hr post injection; castrated dogs have testosterone concentrations < 0.1 ng/ml and do not stimulate with hCG or GnRH administration

IMAGING
Ultrasound—locate testes

DIAGNOSTIC PROCEDURES
N/A

TREATMENT

• None except castration of both retained and scrotal testes generally recommended
• Orchiopexy—surgical placement of a retained testis into the scrotum; considered unethical
• hCG or GnRH—anecdotal evidence of causing descent when given to dogs < 4 months old
• Warn client of the increased risk of testicular neoplasia in dogs with retained testes; encourage client to have dog castrated by 4 years of age; 53% of Sertoli cell tumors and 36% of seminomas occur in retained testes

MEDICATIONS

DRUG(S)
hCG (dogs)—100–1000 IU IM four times in a 2-week period before 16 weeks of age (dogs); after 16 weeks, generally unsuccessful
• GnRH (dogs)—50–750 μg 1–6 times betwen 2 and 4 months of age

CONTRAINDICATIONS/POSSIBLE INTERACTIONS
N/A

FOLLOW-UP

• Descent after 4 months is rare; after 6 months, unlikely
• Risk of testicular neoplasia thought to be approximately 10 times greater in affected dogs than in normal dogs

MISCELLANEOUS

ASSOCIATED CONDITIONS
• Inguinal hernia, umbilical hernia
• Hip dysplasia
• Patellar luxation
• Penile and preputial defects (e.g., hypospadias)

ABBREVIATIONS
• GnRH = gonadotropin-releasing hormone
• hCG = human chorionic gonadotropin

Suggested Reading
England GCW, Allen WE, Porter DJ. Evaluation of the testosterone response to hCG and the identification of a presumed anorchid dog. J Sm Anim Pract 1989:441–443.
Feldman EC, Nelson RW. Canine and feline endocrinology and reproduction. Philadelphia: Saunders, 1987:697–699.
Johnston SD, Root Kustritz MV, Olson PNS. Disorders of the canine testes and epididymes. In: Canine and feline theriogenology. Philadelphia: Saunders, 2001:312–332.
Romagnoli SE. Canine cryptorchidism. Vet Clin North Am Small Anim Pract 1991;21:533–544
Authors Carlos R.F. Pinto and Rolf E. Larsen
Consulting Editor Sara K. Lyle

BASICS

OVERVIEW
• *Cryptosporidium* spp.—coccidian protozoan; causes gastrointestinal disease in dogs, cats, humans, calves, and rodents; ubiquitous in nature; worldwide distribution; enteric life cycle
• Infection—when sporulated oocysts are ingested, sporozoites are released and penetrate intestinal epithelial cells; after asexual reproduction, merozoites are released to infect other cells.
• Prepatent period—cats, 5–10 days
• Immunocompetent animals—intestinal disease
• Immunocompromised animals—intestinal, liver, gallbladder, pancreatic, and respiratory infection

SIGNALMENT
• Dogs and cats
• No sex or breed predilection
• Dogs—virtually all clinical cases have occurred in animals ≤ 6 months of age; old dogs can excrete oocysts without clinical signs.
• Cats—no age predilection

SIGNS
• Most infections subclinical
• Principally small bowel diarrhea
• Large bowel diarrhea reported

CAUSES & RISK FACTORS
• *C. parvum, C. canis, C. felis*—acquired by ingestion of contaminated water or feces
• Immunosuppression—major risk factor; common causes are FeLV (cats), canine distemper virus (dogs), canine parvovirus, and intestinal lymphosarcoma (cats and dogs).

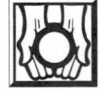

DIAGNOSIS

DIFFERENTIAL DIAGNOSIS
• Dietary indiscretion or intolerance
• Drugs—antibiotics
• Toxins—lead
• Parasites—giardiasis, trichuriasis
• Infectious agents—parvovirus, coronavirus, FIP, salmonella, *Campylobacter,* rickettsia, *Histoplasma*
• Organ disease—cardiac, renal, hepatic, and pancreatic exocrine insufficiency

• Metabolic—hypoadrenocorticism, hyperthyroidism (cats)
• Neoplasia—intestinal lymphoma
• Infiltrative diseases—e.g., inflammatory bowel disease

CBC/BIOCHEMISTRY/URINALYSIS
Usually normal, unless an underlying immunosuppressive disease

OTHER LABORATORY TESTS
N/A

IMAGING
N/A

DIAGNOSTIC PROCEDURES
• Fecal antigen detection test (ProSpecT Cryptosporidium Microtiter Assay; Color-Vue Cryptosporidium) available but not extensively evaluated using cat or dog feces
• Sugar and zinc sulfate flotation—specific gravity = 1.18; concentrates fecal oocysts (oocysts are 5 μm, so routine salt flotation often fails); oocysts best visualized after staining with modified acid-fast stain
• Fluorescent antibody techniques—available in some laboratories (Meridian Diagnostics)
• Submitting feces to a laboratory—mix one part 100% formalin with nine parts feces to inactivate oocysts and decrease health risk to laboratory personnel.
• Intestinal biopsy—cytologic and histopathologic identification of intracellular organisms; diagnostic but impractical; can produce false-negative results

PATHOLOGIC FINDINGS
• Gross lesions—enlarged mesenteric lymph nodes; hyperemic intestinal (particular ileum) mucosa; fix specimens in Bouin or formalin solution within hours of death because autolysis causes rapid loss of the intestinal surface containing the organisms
• Microscopic lesions—villous atrophy; reactive lymphoid tissue; inflammatory infiltrates (neutrophils, macrophages, lymphocytes) in the lamina propria; parasites may be found throughout the intestines but are usually most numerous in the distal small intestine.

TREATMENT
• Outpatient
• Food—may withhold 24–48 hr until diarrhea is under control
• Mild diarrhea—oral glucose–electrolyte solution (Entrolyte, SmithKline)

• Severe diarrhea with dehydration—parenteral fluids (isotonic with potassium added)

MEDICATIONS

DRUG(S)
• Paromomycin (Humatin), 125–165 mg/kg PO q12h for 5 days, is an aminoglycoside antibiotic effective in treating acute intestinal patients. It may cause nephropathy in young animals with a damaged gastrointestinal barrier.
• Tylosin—11 mg/kg PO q12h for 28 days; effective in treating an affected cat that also had lymphocytic duodenitis

CONTRAINDICATIONS/POSSIBLE INTERACTIONS
N/A

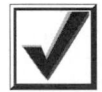

FOLLOW-UP
• Monitor clinical improvement for treatment efficacy.
• Monitor oocyst shedding in the feces 2 weeks after completion of treatment or if signs persist.
• Prognosis excellent if cause of immunosuppression can be overcome

MISCELLANEOUS

ZOONOTIC POTENTIAL
Warn clients of potential zoonotic transmission from organisms in feces and that immunocompromised people (e.g., HIV patients or those on chemotherapy or systemic corticosteroids) are at great risk

ABBREVIATIONS
• FeLV = feline leukemia virus
• FIP = feline infectious peritonitis

Suggested Reading
Barr SC. Cryptosporidiosis. In: Greene CE, ed. Infectious diseases of the dog and cat. Philadelphia: Saunders, 1998:518–523.
Fayes R, Trout JM, Xiao L, et al. *Cryptosporidium canis* n. sp. from domestic dogs. J Parasitol 2001;87:1415–1422.
Author Stephen C. Barr
Consulting Editor Stephen C. Barr

CRYSTALLURIA

 BASICS

DEFINITION
Appearance of crystals in urine

PATHOPHYSIOLOGY
• Crystals form only in urine that is, or recently has been, supersaturated with crystallogenic substances; thus crystalluria represents a risk factor for urolithiasis. However, detection of urine crystals is not synonymous with uroliths and clinical signs associated with them, nor is detection of urine crystals irrefutable evidence of a stone-forming tendency.
• Certain crystal types indicate an underlying disease. Proper identification and interpretation of urine crystals is also important in formulation of medical protocols to dissolve uroliths. Evaluation of urine crystals may aid in 1) detection of disorders predisposing animals to urolith formation, 2) estimation of the mineral composition of uroliths, and 3) evaluation of the effectiveness of medical protocols initiated to dissolve or prevent uroliths.
• Crystalluria in individuals with anatomically and functionally normal urinary tracts is usually harmless because the crystals are eliminated before they grow large enough to interfere with normal urinary function. However, they represent a risk factor for urolithiasis.
• Crystals that form following elimination or removal of urine from the patient often are of little clinical importance. Identification of crystals that have formed in vitro does not justify therapy.
• Detection of some types of crystals (e.g., cystine and ammonium urate) in clinically asymptomatic patients, frequent detection of large aggregates of crystals (e.g., calcium oxalate or magnesium ammonium phosphate) in apparently normal individuals, or detection of any form of crystals in fresh urine collected from patients with confirmed urolithiasis may have diagnostic, prognostic, or therapeutic importance.

SYSTEMS AFFECTED
Renal/Urologic

SIGNALMENT
• Calcium oxalate in miniature schnauzer, Yorkshire terrier, Lhasa apso, and miniature poodle dogs and Burmese, Himalayan, and Persian cats
• Cystine in dachshund, English bulldog, and Newfoundland
• Ammonium urate in Dalmatian and English bulldogs
• Xanthine uroliths in Cavalier King Charles spaniels

SIGNS
None or those caused by concomitant urolithiasis

CAUSES
In vivo variables
• Concentration of crystallogenic substances in urine (which in turn is influenced by their rate of excretion and urine concentration of water)
• Urine pH (struvite and calcium phosphate are most common in neutral-to-alkaline urine; ammonium urate, sodium urate, calcium oxalate, cystine, and xanthine crystals are most common in acid-to-neutral urine)
• Solubility of crystallogenic substances in urine
• Excretion of diagnostic agents (e.g., radiopaque contrast agents) and medications (e.g., sulfonamides)
• Dietary influence—hospital diet may differ from home diet; timing of sample collection (fasting vs. postprandial) may influence evidence of crystalluria.

In vitro variables
• Temperature
• Evaporation
• pH changes following sample collection
• Technique of specimen preparation—centrifugation vs. noncentrifugation, volume of urine examined
• Important in vitro changes that occur following urine collection may enhance formation or dissolution of crystals. When knowledge of in vivo urine crystal type and quantity is especially important, examine fresh specimens, ideally at body temperature. If this is not possible, they should be at room temperature, not refrigeration temperature.

RISK FACTORS
See preceding discussion about in vivo and in vitro variables in crystalluria.

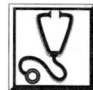 **DIAGNOSIS**

DIFFERENTIAL DIAGNOSIS
Ammonium Urate, Sodium Urate, and Amorphous Urate Crystalluria
• Uncommonly observed in apparently healthy dogs and cats
• Frequently observed in dogs and occasionally observed in cats with portal vascular anomalies, with or without concomitant ammonium urate uroliths
• Observed in some dogs and cats with urate uroliths caused by disorders other than portal vascular anomalies

Bilirubin Crystalluria
• Observed in highly concentrated urine from some healthy dogs
• Large numbers in serial samples should arouse suspicion of an abnormality in bilirubin metabolism.
• Usually associated with underlying diseases in cats

Calcium Oxalate Monohydrate and Calcium Oxalate Dihydrate Crystalluria
• May be observed in apparently healthy dogs and cats and in dogs and cats with uroliths primarily composed of calcium oxalate
• Calcium oxalate dihydrate observed in some cats and dogs intoxicated with ethylene glycol, but calcium oxalate monohydrate crystals more common (ethylene glycol toxicity may also occur without crystalluria)

Calcium Phosphate Crystalluria
• Large numbers of crystals presumed to be composed of calcium phosphate have been observed in apparently healthy dogs, dogs with persistently alkaline urine, dogs with calcium phosphate uroliths, and dogs with uroliths composed of a mixture of calcium phosphate and calcium oxalate.
• Small numbers of calcium phosphate crystals may occur in association with infection-induced struvite crystalluria.

Struvite Crystalluria
• Observed in dogs and cats that are apparently healthy
• Observed in dogs and cats with infection-induced struvite uroliths, sterile struvite uroliths, nonstruvite uroliths, and uroliths of mixed composition (e.g., a nucleus composed of calcium oxalate and a shell composed of struvite)
• Observed in dogs and cats with urinary tract disease without uroliths

Uric Acid Crystalluria
• Uncommon in dogs and cats
• Importance as described for ammonium and amorphous urates

Xanthine Crystalluria
• Suggests administration of excessive dosages of allopurinol in conjunction with consumption of relatively high amounts of dietary purine precursors
• Primary xanthinuria has been observed in Cavalier King Charles spaniels.
• Primary xanthinuria and xanthine uroliths occur in cats.

Miscellaneous Crystalluria
• Cholesterol crystals—observed in humans with excessive tissue destruction, nephrotic syndrome, and chyluria; observed in apparently healthy dogs
• Cystine uroliths—develop in some dogs and cats with cystinuria
• Hippuric acid crystals—apparently rare in dogs and cats; importance unknown

• Leucine crystals in dogs—importance not determined; may occur in association with cystinuria
• Tyrosine crystals—occur in association with severe liver disease in humans; uncommonly observed in dogs and cats with liver disorders

Drug-induced Crystalluria
• May be observed following administration of radiopaque contrast agents
• May be observed following treatment with sulfadiazine, fluoroquinolones, primidone, and tetracycline

LABORATORY FINDINGS

Drugs That May Alter Laboratory Results
• Urinary acidifiers (e.g., d,l-methionine and ammonium chloride)
• Urinary alkalinizers (e.g., sodium bicarbonate and potassium citrate)

Disorders That May Alter Laboratory Results
N/A

Valid If Run in Human Laboratory?
Yes

CBC/BIOCHEMISTRY/URINALYSIS
• Bilirubin crystals may be associated with bilirubinemia and other laboratory abnormalities of hepatic disorders.
• Most dogs and cats with calcium oxalate and calcium phosphate crystalluria are normocalcemic; some are hypercalcemic.
• Some dogs and cats with calcium oxalate crystalluria may be acidemic.
• Serially examine fresh specimens when knowledge of in vivo urine crystal type is especially important; evaluate the number, size, and structure of crystals and their tendency to aggregate.
• Microscopic evaluation of the appearance of urine crystals gives only a tentative indication of their composition; variable conditions associated with their formation, growth, and dissolution may alter their appearance. Definitive identification of crystal composition depends on optical crystallography, infrared spectrophotometry, thermal analysis, x-ray diffraction, electron microprobe analysis, or a combination of these.
• To confirm the composition of microscopic crystalluria, prepare a large pellet of crystals by centrifuging an appropriate volume of urine in a cone-tipped centrifuge tube. Evaluate the pellet by methods designed for quantitative urolith analysis. The type of crystals identified by this method may reflect only the outer portions of uroliths.

OTHER LABORATORY TESTS
• Cystine crystalluria is usually associated with a positive urine cyanide-nitroprusside reaction.

• Sulfonamide crystalluria may be associated with a positive lignin test.
• Ammonium urate and amorphous urate crystals are insoluble in acetic acid; addition of 10% acetic acid to urine sediment containing these crystals often yields uric acid and sometimes sodium urate crystals.
• Most dogs and a few cats with struvite crystalluria have urinary tract infections caused by urease-producing bacteria (especially staphylococci and sometimes *Proteus* spp.).
• Dogs and cats with ammonium urate crystalluria and portosystemic shunts often have high serum bile acid levels and hyperammonemia.
• Dogs and cats with calcium oxalate crystalluria secondary to ethylene glycol poisoning have detectable levels of ethylene glycol in serum and urine up to 48 hr after ingestion.

IMAGING
Crystalluria may be associated with radiographically or ultrasonographically detectable uroliths

DIAGNOSTIC PROCEDURES
Voiding urohydropropulsion or aspiration through a transurethral catheter to retrieve small urocystoliths

 TREATMENT
• Manage clinically important in vivo crystalluria by eliminating or controlling the underlying cause(s) or associated risk factors.
• Minimize clinically important crystalluria by increasing urine volume, by encouraging complete and frequent voiding, by dietary modification, in some instances by appropriate drug therapy, and, in some instances, by modifying pH.

 MEDICATIONS

DRUG(S) OF CHOICE
N/A

CONTRAINDICATIONS
N/A

PRECAUTIONS
N/A

POSSIBLE INTERACTIONS
N/A

ALTERNATIVE DRUG(S)
N/A

 FOLLOW-UP

PATIENT MONITORING
• Recheck urinalysis to determine if crystalluria is present.
• See chapters on specific urolith types for monitoring urolithiasis.

POSSIBLE COMPLICATIONS
• Persistent crystalluria may contribute to formation and growth of uroliths.
• Crystalluria may solidify crystalline-matrix plugs, resulting in urethral obstruction.

 MISCELLANEOUS

ASSOCIATED CONDITIONS
N/A

AGE-RELATED FACTORS
N/A

ZOONOTIC POTENTIAL
None

PREGNANCY
N/A

SEE ALSO
• Nephrolithiasis
• Urolithiasis, Calcium Phosphate
• Urolithiasis, Cystine
• Urolithiasis, Struvite—Cats
• Urolithiasis, Struvite—Dogs
• Urolithiasis, Urate
• Urolithiasis, Xanthine

Suggested Reading
Osborne CA, Davis LS, Sanna J, et al. Identification and interpretation of crystalluria in domestic animals. A light and scanning electron microscopic study. Vet Med 1990;85:18–37.
Osborne CA, Lulich JP, Bartges JW, et al. Drug-induced urolithiasis. Vet Clin North Am 1999;29:251–266.
Osborne CA, Lulich JP, Ulrich LK, et al. Feline crystalluria. Detection and interpretation. Vet Clin North Am 1996;26:369–391.
Osborne CA, Stevens B. Urinalysis: a clinical guide to compassionate patient care. Shawnee Mission, KS: Bayer Corp., 1999.

Authors Carl A. Osborne and Lisa K. Ulrich
Consulting Editors Larry G. Adams and Carl A. Osborne

CUTANEOUS ASTHENIA

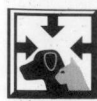 BASICS

OVERVIEW
• Group of hereditary diseases characterized by abnormal skin hyperextensibility and fragility
• Also known as Ehlers-Danlos syndrome and dermatosparaxis
• Abnormal collagen synthesis or fiber formation is responsible for the skin fragility in most syndromes; however, the biochemical defects have been elucidated in only a few dogs and cats.
• Varying modes of inheritance have been suspected.

SIGNALMENT
• Congenital syndrome—patients are usually presented quite young.
• Dogs—beagles, dachshunds, boxers, St. Bernards, German shepherds, English springer spaniels, greyhounds, Manchester terriers, Welsh corgis, red kelpies, soft-coated wheaten terriers, Irish setters, Keeshonds, English setters, and mongrels
• Cats—domestic shorthairs, domestic long-hairs, and Himalayans

SIGNS
• Skin hyperextensibility
• Easily torn skin
• Diminished skin elasticity
• Scars from previous trauma
• Widening of the bridge of the nose
• Joint laxity
• Elbow hygromas
• Lens luxation
• Cataracts

CAUSES & RISK FACTORS
Even minor trauma to the skin can produce large skin tears.

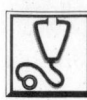 DIAGNOSIS

DIFFERENTIAL DIAGNOSIS
Clinically characteristic syndrome

CBC/BIOCHEMISTRY/URINALYSIS
N/A

OTHER LABORATORY TESTS
N/A

IMAGING
N/A

DIAGNOSTIC PROCEDURES
Skin extensibility index—identifies affected animals; calculated by dividing the maximal height of a dorsal lumbar skin fold by the body length (from the base of the tail to the occipital crest) and converting to a percentage; affected dogs >14.5% and affected cats > 19%

PATHOLOGIC FINDINGS
• Histopathologic examination of the skin—either normal dermal architecture or collagen abnormalities (disoriented, fragmented, abnormal tinctorial properties or abnormal organization)
• Electron microscopy—ascertain collagen abnormalities more precisely

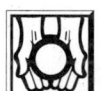 TREATMENT

• Because of poor prognosis, affected animals may be euthanatized.

• If the owner chooses to keep the animal—keep environment free of sharp corners and other animals; handle and restrain affected animal carefully to prevent large skin tears; keep resting areas well padded to prevent elbow hygromas.

 MEDICATIONS

DRUG(S)
No proven medical therapy.

CONTRAINDICATIONS/POSSIBLE INTERACTIONS
N/A

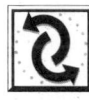 FOLLOW-UP

Lacerations should be surgically repaired as they occur.

 MISCELLANEOUS

Suggested Reading
Scott DW, Miller WH, Griffin CE, eds. Congenital hereditary defects. In: Muller & Kirk's small animal dermatology, 5th ed. Philadelphia: Saunders, 1995:785–789.
Author Jon D. Plant
Consulting Editor Karen Helton Rhodes

BASICS

OVERVIEW
• A spectrum of diseases and clinical signs that vary markedly in clinical appearance and pathophysiology
• Likely that many mild drug reactions go unnoticed or unreported; thus incidence rates for specific drugs are unknown and most of the facts available on drug-specific reactivities have been extrapolated from reports in the human literature.

SIGNALMENT
• Dogs and cats
• Age, breed, and sex predispositions—unknown
• Some types of drug reactions appear to have a familial basis (e.g., rabies vaccine reactions in dogs have been diagnosed in litter mates).

SIGNS
• Pruritus—can be activated by a wide variety of compounds; most common symptom of drug eruption in humans
• Macular and papular rashes—commonly accompany pruritus as a nonspecific sign of inflammation
• Exfoliative erythroderma—a diffuse erythematous response caused by vasodilation; often leads to exfoliation (diffuse scaling)
• Urticaria/angioedema—results from an immediate (type I) hypersensitivity; requires prior sensitization; increased vascular permeability leads to fluid leakage into the interstitium.
• Hypersensitivity vasculitis—inflammation of cutaneous vasculature; results in poor blood flow and anoxic injury to recipient tissue; in most cases, thought to represent a type III hypersensitivity response
• EM—erythremic macules or plaques expand peripherally and may clear in the center, producing a bull's-eye appearance; multiple shapes/forms can be seen.
• TEN—extensive necrosis and sloughing of the epidermis in sheets; results in a moist and intensely inflamed skin surface
• Drug-induced pemphigus/pemphigoid—least common drug reaction in animals; can closely mimic the autoimmune (spontaneous) forms of these diseases

CAUSES & RISK FACTORS
• Drugs of any type
• Exfoliative erythroderma—most often associated with shampoos and dips
• Can occur after the first dose after weeks to months of administration of the same drug

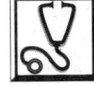

DIAGNOSIS

DIFFERENTIAL DIAGNOSIS
• Pruritus, macular/papular rashes, and urticaria/angioedema—allergic diseases (atopy, food allergy, contact allergy) and reactions to ectoparasites (scabies, flea-bite allergy, stinging insects)
• Exfoliative erythroderma—rule out cutaneous T cell lymphoma in old dogs and cats.
• Vasculitis—infectious, neoplastic, and autoimmune diseases; many cases of vasculitis are idiopathic.
• EM—rule out respiratory infections and internal neoplasms.
• Pemphigus/pemphigoid—consider drug reaction whenever these diseases are diagnosed; however, spontaneously occurring autoimmune disease is much more common.

CBC/BIOCHEMISTRY/URINALYSIS
When cutaneous vasculitis is suspected or diagnosed—potential for concurrent hepatic, renal, and gastrointestinal disease

OTHER LABORATORY TESTS
• Dogs with vasculitis—rickettsial serology, ANA
• Cats with vasculitis—FIV and FeLV serology
• Bacterial and fungal cultures and sensitivity testing—for vasculitis with pyogranulomatous inflammation

IMAGING
N/A

DIAGNOSTIC PROCEDURES
Skin biopsy for histopathology—mandatory for diagnosis of most drug-induced diseases (vasculitis, EM, TEN, pemphigus/pemphigoid)

PATHOLOGIC FINDINGS
Vary according to the specific disease process

TREATMENT
• Discontinue use of the offending drug.
• TEN—intensive supportive care and fluid/nutritional support because of fluid and protein exudation and risk of sepsis

MEDICATIONS

DRUG(S)
Varies according to the disease process if withdrawal of the offending drug alone is insufficient

CONTRAINDICATIONS/POSSIBLE INTERACTIONS
The offending drug or any other drug in the same class or family should be strictly avoided.

FOLLOW-UP

PATIENT MONITORING
• Inpatient—if debilitated
• Outpatient—regular rechecks, depending on physical condition

EXPECTED COURSE AND PROGNOSIS
• Some reactions appear to activate self-perpetuating immune responses.
• Some drug metabolites may persist for days to weeks and provoke a continued response.
• TEN—prognosis poor
• Vasculitis—prognosis guarded when there are systemic complications

MISCELLANEOUS

ASSOCIATED CONDITIONS
Cutaneous vasculitis—arthropathy, hepatitis, glomerulonephritis, and neuromuscular disorders, among others

SEE ALSO
• Pemphigus
• Vasculitis, Cutaneous

ABBREVIATIONS
• ANA = antinuclear antibody
• EM = erythema multiforme
• FeLV = feline leukemia virus
• FIV = feline immunodeficiency virus
• TEN = toxic epidermal necrolysis

Suggested Reading
Scott DW, Miller WH, Griffin GE, eds. In: Muller & Kirk's small animal dermatology. 6th ed. Philadelphia: Saunders, 2001:720–756.
Author Daniel O. Morris
Consulting Editor Karen Helton-Rhodes

CUTEREBROSIS

 BASICS

OVERVIEW
• Flies of the genus *Cuterebra* are found in the Americas where they are obligatory parasites of rodents and lagomorphs. Adult flies lay eggs on blades of grass or in nests, and they hatch and crawl onto the skin of the passing host. The small maggots enter a body orifice, migrate through various internal tissues, and, ultimately, make their way to the skin where they establish a warble. The mature maggots, which may be an inch long, then drop out of the rodent or rabbit host and then pupate in the soil.
• Dogs and cats become infected when they walk past a blade of grass with an egg containing an infective maggot that is stimulated to hatch and to jump onto the passing animal. The maggots then crawl around on the cat or dog until they find an orifice in which to enter.
• Dogs and cats can develop maggots in warbles or can develop signs associated with the larvae migrating within their tissues.
• Dogs and cats can present with respiratory signs, neurologic signs, ophthalmic lesions, or maggots in their skin.

SIGNALMENT
Dogs and cats—all ages

SIGNS
• Respiratory—eosinophilic respiratory disease
• Neurologic—ataxia, circling, paralysis, blindness, recumbency
• Ophthalmic lesions—larvae in conjunctiva
• Dermatologic—warble containing bot with protruding spiracles

CAUSES & RISK FACTORS
• Dogs and cats with access to outdoors where they contact the eggs and larvae
• Neonatal cats have been infected, presumably with larvae being brought home on queen's fur.

 DIAGNOSIS

DIFFERENTIAL DIAGNOSIS
• Respiratory—allergies, lungworms, migrating ascarids or hookworms
• Neurologic—rabies, distemper, angiostrongylosis
• Ophthalmic lesions—larval *Hypoderma* or *Oestrus*
• Dermatologic—mature warble unmistakable; young warble may present as a pustule or papule

CBC/BIOCHEMISTRY/URINALYSIS
May have elevated eosinophils

OTHER LABORATORY TESTS
N/A

IMAGING
CT scan has shown lesions in cranial images of cats.

TREATMENT

• Can remove maggots from subcutaneous lesions, eyes, or nares.
• Manifestations of lung migration may be alleviated by corticosteroids.
• Neurologic disease may have a poor prognosis; euthanasia is an option.

MEDICATIONS

DRUG(S)

Ivermectin—0.2 mg/kg SC should kill migrating maggots; may want to begin corticosteroid treatment before administering the ivermectin. The ivermectin can be administered either to alleviate the signs caused by maggots suspected of migrating in the lungs or to kill larvae in other tissues, including the CNS.

FOLLOW-UP

Good return of function following ivermectin treatment possible

MISCELLANEOUS

• In northern US, disease is very seasonal with most cases occurring in late summer and early fall when the adult flies are active. Seasonality is less demarcated in areas where warmer temperatures and active flies occur through longer periods of the year.
• Does not seem to be any prolonged immunity; the same cat can develop skin lesions several years in a row.
• Application of monthly heartworm preventatives (ivermectini-containing products), flea development control products (lufenuron-containing products) or topical flea and tick treatments may either prevent the maggots from developing in the dog or cat or may kill them before they have time to gain access to an orifice for entry.

ZOONOTIC POTENTIAL

The maggots in the dog or cat pose no zoonotic threat.

Suggested Reading

Bowman DD, ed. Georgi's parasitology for veterinarians, 8th ed. Philadelphia: Saunders, 2003: 95–97.
Bowman DD. Feline clinical parasitology. Ames: Iowa State University Press, 430–439.

Author Dwight D. Bowman
Consulting Editor Stephen C. Barr

CYANOSIS

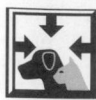 BASICS

DEFINITION
A bluish discoloration of the skin and mucous membranes owing to an increase in the amount of reduced, or deoxygenated, hemoglobin within the blood

PATHOPHYSIOLOGY
• Concentration of deoxygenated hemoglobin—must be > 5 g/dL to detect condition; thus anemia (PCV < 15%) may obscure detection. • Central—associated with systemic arterial hypoxemia or hemoglobin abnormalities • Peripheral—limited to one or more extremities of the body; associated with diminished peripheral blood flow; arterial oxygen tension and saturation typically normal

Arterial Hypoxemia
• Decreased fraction of inspired oxygen—high altitude • Hypoventilation—upper airway obstructive disorders; restrictive or obstructive lung disease; pleural space disorders; neuromuscular failure • Ventilation–perfusion mismatching—pulmonary parenchymal or thromboembolic diseases • Diffusion impairment—thickening of the alveolar barrier through which oxygen must pass to reach the RBCs • Addition of venous blood to the arterial circulation—congenital right-to-left shunting cardiac defects (e.g., tetralogy of Fallot, transposition of the great vessels); reversed shunting cardiac defects caused by high pulmonary vascular resistance (e.g., right-to-left shunting PDA, ASD, VSD) • Anatomic shunts—distinguished from other causes of hypoxemia by the failure to respond to supplemental oxygen

Abnormal Hemoglobin
• Methemoglobin—most common abnormal heme pigment; unable to bind oxygen; normally formed at a low rate in erythrocytes • NADH-MR—intracellular reductive enzyme; maintains the methemoglobin: hemoglobin ratio at < 2%; deficiency and/or exposure to oxidizing agents causes methemoglobinemia. • Hypoxia—when >20%–40% of hemoglobin has been oxidized to methemoglobin

Other
• Peripheral—results from increased oxygen extraction from the arterial supply to an area, e.g., a limb; caused by severe vasoconstriction, poor peripheral blood flow, obstruction to flow associated with arterial thromboembolism, or stagnation or obstruction of venous blood flow • Differential—with reverse shunting PDA, the head and neck receive oxygenated blood via the brachiocephalic trunk and left subclavian artery, which arise from the aortic arch; the rest of the body receives desaturated blood through the ductus located in the descending aorta.

SYSTEMS AFFECTED
• Central—all systems affected • Peripheral—may diminish or abolish the neuromuscular function of the affected limb(s)

SIGNALMENT
• Right-to-left cardiac shunts in association with high pulmonary vascular resistance and pulmonary hypertension (Eisenmenger physiology)—dogs: Keeshonds, English bulldogs, and beagles; some cats; generally young animals • Tracheal collapse—usually young or middle-aged small-breed dogs (e.g., Pomeranians, Yorkshire terriers, poodles) • Congenital laryngeal paralysis—young animals; reported in Dalmatians, Bouvier des Flandres, and Siberian huskies • Acquired laryngeal paralysis—most common in old large-breed dogs (e.g., Labrador retrievers, Afghans, setters, and greyhounds) • Hypoplastic trachea—identified in young English bull terriers; occasionally other breeds • Asthma (cats)— higher incidence reported in Siamese

SIGNS

Historical Findings
• Central—stridor; dyspnea; cough; voice change; episodic weakness; syncope; exposure to oxidizing substances or drugs causing methemoglobinemia • Peripheral—limb paresis or paralysis

Physical Examination Findings
• Heart murmur or splitting of the second heart sound—with cardiac disease or pulmonary hypertension • Pulmonary crackles or wheezes—with pulmonary edema or respiratory disease • Muffled heart sounds—owing to pleural space or pericardial disease • Upper airway stridor with laryngeal paralysis • Honking cough—typical of tracheal collapse; may be induced by tracheal palpation • Dyspnea—may be inspiratory, expiratory, or a combination (see Differential Diagnosis) • Limbs—may be cyanotic, cool, pale, painful, and edematous; may pulse in conditions causing peripheral cyanosis • Weakness—may be generalized and persistent with severe cardiac diseases; may be episodic and especially noticeable with exercise or excitement • Posterior paresis or paralysis—may be seen with distal aorta arterial thromboembolism; differentiated from primary neuromuscular disease by absence (or near absence) of pulses

CAUSES

Respiratory System
• Larynx—paralysis (acquired or congenital); collapse; spasm; edema; trauma; neoplasia; granulomatous disease • Trachea—collapse; neoplasia; foreign body; trauma; hypoplasia • Lower airway and parenchyma—pneumonia (viral, bacterial, fungal, allergic, mycobacteria, aspiration); chronic bronchitis; hypersensitivity bronchial disease (allergic, asthma); bronchiectasis; neoplasia; foreign body; parasites (filarioidea, *Paragonimus,* protozoa); pulmonary contusion or hemorrhage; noncardiogenic edema (inhalation, snake bite, electric shock); near drowning • Pleural space—pneumothorax; infectious (bacterial, fungal, FIP); chylothorax; hemothorax; neoplasia; trauma • Thoracic wall or diaphragm—congenital (pericardial, diaphragmatic hernia); trauma (diaphragmatic hernia, fractured ribs, flail chest); neuromuscular disease (tick paralysis, coonhound paralysis)

Cardiovascular System
• Congenital defects—Eisenmenger physiology (right-to-left shunting PDA, VSD, ASD); tetralogy of Fallot; truncus arteriosis; double outlet right ventricle; anomalous pulmonary venous return; atresia of aortic or tricuspid or pulmonary valves • Acquired disease—mitral valve disease; cardiomyopathy • Pericardial effusion—idiopathic disease; neoplasia • Pulmonary thromboembolic disease—hyperadrenocorticism; immune-mediated hemolytic anemia; protein-losing nephropathy; dirofilariasis • Pulmonary hypertension—idiopathic; right-to-left cardiac shunts • Peripheral vascular disease—arterial thromboembolism (feline cardiomyopathies); venous obstruction; reduced cardiac output; shock, arteriolar constriction

Neuromusculoskeletal System
• Brainstem dysfunction—encephalitis; trauma; hemorrhage; neoplasia; drug-induced depression of respiratory center (morphine, barbiturates) • Spinal cord dysfunction—edema; trauma; vertebral fractures; disk prolapse • Neuromuscular dysfunction—overdose of paralytic agents (succinylcholine, pancuronium); tick paralysis; botulism; acute polyradiculoneuritis (coonhound paralysis); dysautonomia; myasthenia gravis

Methemoglobinemia
• Congenital—NADH-MR deficiency (dogs) • Ingestion of oxidant chemicals—acetaminophen; nitrates; nitrites; phenacetin; sulfonamides; benzocaine; aniline dyes; dapsone

RISK FACTORS
N/A

DIAGNOSIS

DIFFERENTIAL DIAGNOSIS
• Generalized—systemic hypoxemia or heme abnormality • Peripheral only—reduced blood flow to extremities • Caudal body—right-to-left shunting PDA • Cardiac versus respiratory causes—differentiation may be difficult; cardiac murmur may suggest cardiac disease; murmurs may be heard in old patients with primary respiratory disease; thoracic radiography and echocardiography useful for differentiation
• Central or peripheral neurologic signs—should prompt concern of arterial hypoxemia owing to primary neuromuscular disease

Breathing Pattern
• May help define cause
• Inspiratory dyspnea—often associated with obstructive upper airway or pleural space disease; stridor frequently localizes problem to the larynx.
• Expiratory dyspnea—generally seen with obstructive lower airway disease
• Rapid shallow (restrictive)—may be associated with pleural space disease or neuromuscular abnormalities of the thoracic wall

CBC/BIOCHEMISTRY/URINALYSIS
• Color of blood—often noticeably darkened with condition; chocolate brown with methemoglobinemia
• Polycythemia—often accompanies congenital heart disease; may occur with chronic hypoxemia owing to severe respiratory disease
• Proteinuria—accompanies protein-losing nephropathies, which may cause pulmonary thromboembolism

OTHER LABORATORY TESTS
• Methemoglobin concentrations—measure through a laboratory; alternatively, shake a blood sample in air 15 min: red, reduced hemoglobin with cardiac or respiratory disease; chocolate brown, methemoglobin
• Arterial blood gas analysis
• Urine protein:creatinine ratio—with suspected pulmonary thromboembolism secondary to a protein-losing nephropathy

IMAGING
• Radiography—essential for determining cause
• Echocardiography with Doppler—aids in diagnosis of congenital or acquired cardiac disease, pulmonary hypertension, and pulmonary thromboembolism

DIAGNOSTIC PROCEDURES
• Pulse oximetry—determine oxygen saturation
• Laryngoscopic examination—evaluate laryngeal structure and arytenoid function
• Bronchoscopy—may be used in the diagnosis of tracheal and pulmonary diseases

• Transtracheal wash, bronchoalveolar lavage, or fine-needle lung aspirate—may be required to characterize bronchopulmonary diseases
• Thoracocentesis—required for diagnosis and treatment of pleural space disorders
• Electrocardiography—may reveal heart enlargement changes; unreliable; echocardiography better

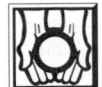

TREATMENT

• Inpatient—immediate diagnostic testing and treatment
• Stabilization therapy (e.g., oxygen, thoracocentesis, tracheostomy)—usually instituted before aggressive diagnostics
• Specific therapy—depends on the ultimate diagnosis; usually exercise restriction and dietary modification required
• Surgical treatment—depends on primary disease process and the extent of cardiac or respiratory involvement
• Warn client when admitting the patient that diseases associated with cyanosis can have dire outcomes.

MEDICATIONS

DRUG(S) OF CHOICE
• Depends on final diagnosis
• Oxygen therapy—provide as soon as possible
• Diuretics (furosemide)—aggressive use indicated with suspected cardiogenic pulmonary edema
• Methemoglobinemia as a result of ingestion of oxidizing substances (acetaminophen)—give acetylcysteine as soon as possible (140 mg/kg PO or IV; then 70 mg/kg q4h for 3–5 treatments); cimetidine (10 mg/kg PO; then 5 mg/kg PO q6h for 48 hr) is a useful adjunct to acetylcysteine; ascorbic acid (30 mg/kg PO q6h for 7 treatments) may be of some value but do not use as the sole agent.
• Plasminogen activators (alteplase, streptokinase)—may use for thrombolysis in cats with aortic thromboembolism; best administered by experienced clinicians

CONTRAINDICATIONS
Avoid using paralytic agents (succinylcholine, pancuronium) and agents that cause profound depression of the respiratory center (morphine, barbiturates).

PRECAUTIONS
N/A

POSSIBLE INTERACTIONS
N/A

ALTERNATIVE DRUG(S)
N/A

FOLLOW-UP

PATIENT MONITORING
• Patients in an oxygen cage should be disturbed as infrequently as possible for monitoring. • Assess efficacy of therapy—changes in depth and rate of respiration; color of mucous membranes (should return to a normal pink color if the cause is not an anatomic shunt and patient has adequate reserves); pulse oximetry or arterial blood analysis • Instruct client to monitor mucous membrane color and respiratory effort and advise immediate veterinary care if cyanotic condition returns.

POSSIBLE COMPLICATIONS
Advanced pulmonary or airway disease and severe cardiac disease—poor long-term prognosis

MISCELLANEOUS

ASSOCIATED CONDITIONS
Obesity—may complicate or exacerbate underlying respiratory or cardiac diseases

AGE-RELATED FACTORS
Congenital cardiac abnormalities—usually the cause in young patients

ZOONOTIC POTENTIAL
N/A

PREGNANCY
• Advanced pregnancy may exacerbate symptoms because of pressure on the diaphragm and reduced lung expansion. • Fetuses are likely to be harmed or aborted by the hypoxemia associated with cyanosis.

SEE ALSO
• Dyspnea, Tachypnea, and Panting • Stertor and Stridor • See also Causes.

ABBREVIATIONS
• ASD = atrial septal defect • FIP = feline infectious peritonitis • MR = methemoglobin reductase • PCV = packed cell volume • PDA = patent ductus arteriosus • VSD = ventricular septal defect

Suggested Reading
Krotje LJ. Cyanosis: physiology and pathogenesis. Compend Contin Educ Pract Vet 1987;9:271–278.
Stepien RL. Cyanosis. In: Ettinger SJ, Feldman EC, eds. Textbook of veterinary internal medicine. 5th ed. Philadelphia: Saunders, 2000:206–210.
Author Ned F. Kuehn
Consulting Editor Lynelle R. Johnson

CYCLIC HEMATOPOIESIS—DOGS

BASICS

OVERVIEW
• Cyclic hematopoiesis in color-dilute gray collie pups is characterized by frequent episodes of infection with failure to thrive and early death; clinically, pups have diarrhea, conjunctivitis, gingivitis, pneumonia, skin infections, and carpal joint pain accompanied by fever; intussusception is a common cause of death.
• Episodes of illness, varying from inactivity accompanied by fever to life-threatening infection, repeat at 11–14-day intervals
• The pups are smaller than litter mates at birth, are weak, and are often abandoned by the bitch.
• The condition has been observed in many collie bloodlines throughout the U.S.; however, experienced collie breeders do not attempt to raise the pups; therefore, gray collie pups are not commonly seen.

SIGNALMENT
• Cyclic hematopoiesis in collies is present only in the color-dilute pups.

• In the collie breed, cyclic hematopoiesis is inherited as an autosomal recessive trait; thus it is possible to observe similar color-dilute pups with the disease in any mongrel litter from parents with collie parentage in their background.
• Clinical signs occur as early as 1–2 weeks of age and are always apparent by 8–12 weeks of age.
• An apparently similar disease was reported in normal-colored pups in two Border collie litters in the United Kingdom (UK). Single cases of cyclic hematopoiesis have been reported in Pomeranians and cocker spaniels; the disease is not well characterized in these breeds.

SIGNS

Historical Findings
• Weakness
• Failure to thrive
• Conjunctivitis
• Gingivitis
• Diarrhea
• Pneumonia
• Skin infections
• Carpal joint pain

Physical Examination Findings
• Dilute coat color
• Color dilution on skin of the nose
• Smaller and weaker than normal-colored litter mates
• Fever
• Watery eyes, reddened gums, and diarrhea nearly always present during the phase of the hematopoietic cycle when clinical signs are evident; other signs vary depending on the site of sepsis.
• Painful carpal joints observed during the initial recovery phase of the disease cycle

CAUSES & RISK FACTORS
Inherited disease

DIAGNOSIS

DIFFERENTIAL DIAGNOSIS
• Coat color dilution pathognomonic for the disease in collies or collie mixed breeds
• Color dilution not associated with cyclic hematopoiesis also observed in collie pups
• Collie pups with other color variants—normal size; do not develop frequent episodes of infection; may attain normal coat color

intensity by 6 months of age; normal color intensity on the nose
• Collie pups with cyclic hematopoiesis always have color dilution on the skin of the nose.

CBC/BIOCHEMISTRY/URINALYSIS
• Severe neutropenia, lasting 2–5 days and occurring at 11–14-day intervals with marginal normocytic to microcytic anemia
• Important to recognize that signs of infection are often minimal during the neutropenic episodes
• Local swelling, redness, and systemic signs of infection usually occur during the first days of the neutrophilic phase of the disease cycle; therefore, on initial examination, neutrophilia with moderate monocytosis is observed.
• CBC should be repeated at 2–3-day intervals to confirm the diagnosis.

OTHER LABORATORY TESTS
None

IMAGING
N/A

DIAGNOSTIC PROCEDURES
None

TREATMENT
• Advise clients not to attempt to raise the pup(s).
• Antibiotics and supportive therapy may extend the life of the pups for several years but at considerable cost.
• The disease cycle has been interrupted experimentally by bone marrow transplantation and by daily treatment with endotoxin, lithium carbonate (10 mg/kg PO q12h), or recombinant human or canine colony-stimulating factor.

MEDICATIONS

DRUG(S)
Antibiotics and fluids as required

CONTRAINDICATIONS/POSSIBLE INTERACTIONS
None

MISCELLANEOUS

Suggested Reading

DiGiacomo RF, Hammond WP, Kunz LL, Cox PA. Clinical and pathologic features of cyclic hematopoiesis in grey collie dogs. Am J Pathol 1983;111:224–233.

Hammond WP, Boone TC, Donahue RE, et al. A comparison of treatment of canine cyclic hematopoiesis with recombinant human granulocyte-macrophage colony-stimulating factor (GM-CSF), G-CSF interleukin-3, and canine G-CSF. Blood 1990:76:523–532.

Yang, TJ. Pathobiology of canine cyclic hematopoiesis (review). In Vivo 1987;5:297–302.

Author John E. Lund
Consulting Editor Stephen A. Kruth

CYLINDRURIA

BASICS

DEFINITION
Abnormally high number of casts (>2 casts/lpf) in urine sediment

PATHOPHYSIOLOGY
• May develop in animals with primary renal disease or systemic disorder that secondarily affects the kidneys
• High number of casts indicates accelerated renal cellular degeneration, glomerular leakage of protein, hemorrhage, or exudation into renal tubular lumens.

SYSTEMS AFFECTED
Renal/Urologic

SIGNALMENT
Dogs and cats

SIGNS
None

CAUSES

Nephrotoxicosis
• Toxin (e.g., ethylene glycol)
• Nephrotoxic drug (e.g., aminoglycoside, intravenously administered tetracycline, amphotericin B, cisplatin, thiacetarsamide, nonsteroidal antiinflammatory drug, angiotensin-converting enzyme inhibitor)
• Diagnostic agent (e.g., intravenously administered radiocontrast agent)

Renal Ischemia
• Dehydration
• Hypovolemia
• Low cardiac output (e.g., congestive heart failure, cardiac arrhythmia, or pericardial disease)
• Renal vessel thrombosis (e.g., emboli from bacterial endocarditis or DIC)

• Hemoglobinuria (e.g., intravascular hemolysis)
• Myoglobulinuria (e.g., rhabdomyolysis)

Renal Inflammation
Infectious diseases (e.g., pyelonephritis, leptospirosis, feline infectious peritonitis, Rocky Mountain spotted fever, or ehrlichiosis)

Glomerular Disease
• Glomerulonephritis
• Amyloidosis

RISK FACTORS
• Any disorder that impairs renal perfusion
• Exposure to nephrotoxins

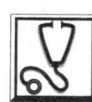

DIAGNOSIS

DIFFERENTIAL DIAGNOSIS
• History of potential exposure to toxins or nephrotoxic drugs—rule out acute tubular necrosis.
• Recent onset of vomiting or diarrhea—rule out renal ischemia caused by dehydration.
• Recent inhalation anesthesia—rule out tubular necrosis caused by ischemia.
• Potential for exposure to infectious diseases—rule out nephritis.
• Fever—rule out infectious, inflammatory, and neoplastic disease.
• Cardiac murmur, especially if diastolic and of recent onset—rule out bacterial endocarditis.
• Petechiae and ecchymoses—rule out systemic thrombosis.

LABORATORY FINDINGS

Drugs That May Alter Laboratory Results
N/A

Disorders That May Alter Laboratory Results
• Waiting longer than 2 hours to perform urinalysis may result in disappearance of casts.

• Alkaline urine causes dissolution of casts.
• Dilute urine (specific gravity < 1.003) causes dissolution of casts; interpret numbers of casts in light of urine specific gravity.

Valid If Run in Human Laboratory?
Yes

CBC/BIOCHEMISTRY/URINALYSIS
• Anemia, hemoconcentration, leukocytosis, or thrombocytopenia in some patients
• High serum concentrations of urea nitrogen, creatinine, and phosphorus in patients with dehydration or renal failure
• Epithelial, granular, or waxy casts indicate diseases that cause degeneration and necrosis of renal tubular epithelial cells.
• RBC casts indicate severe glomerular disease or hemorrhage into renal tubules.
• WBC casts indicate renal inflammation, most often caused by pyelonephritis; most patients with pyelonephritis do not have WBC casts.
• Hyaline casts—commonly associated with disorders that cause proteinuria; also may be observed during diuresis and after dehydration

Laboratory Test Patterns
• Cylindruria plus azotemia and adequately concentrated urine (specific gravity 1.030 in dogs and 1.040 in cats)—consider prerenal disorders such as dehydration.
• Cylindruria plus azotemia and inadequately concentrated urine (specific gravity < 1.030 in dogs and < 1.035 in cats)—consider renal failure.
• Cylindruria plus leukocytosis—consider infectious and inflammatory disorders.
• Cylindruria plus thrombocytopenia—consider DIC.
• Cylindruria plus glucosuria and proteinuria—consider renal tubular necrosis.

OTHER LABORATORY TESTS

• If the patient has thrombocytopenia or RBC casts, perform coagulation studies (e.g., PTT, PT, FDP, D-dimers) to rule out consumptive coagulopathy such as DIC.
• If the patient has proteinuria, determine urine protein:creatinine ratio to evaluate the magnitude of proteinuria.
• If the patient has pyuria or WBC casts, perform urine culture to rule out urinary tract infection.
• If systemic infectious diseases are suspected, submit serum for appropriate titers.

IMAGING
N/A

DIAGNOSTIC PROCEDURES

Consider renal biopsy if renal disease persists and progresses and the cause cannot be determined from routine and special laboratory tests.

TREATMENT

• Treat as outpatient unless the patient is dehydrated or has decompensated renal failure.
• If the patient is healthy otherwise, feed normal diet and allow normal exercise.
• If the patient cannot maintain hydration, administer lactated Ringer's solution or a maintenance fluid either intravenously or subcutaneously.
• If the patient has dehydration or continuing fluid losses such as vomiting or diarrhea, administer fluids intravenously to correct hydration deficits, maintain daily fluid requirements, and replace ongoing losses.

MEDICATIONS

DRUG(S) OF CHOICE
N/A

CONTRAINDICATIONS
Avoid nephrotoxic drugs.

PRECAUTIONS
N/A

POSSIBLE INTERACTIONS
N/A

ALTERNATIVE DRUG(S)
N/A

FOLLOW-UP

PATIENT MONITORING
Physical examination including patient's weight to assess hydration status

POSSIBLE COMPLICATIONS
Renal failure depending on underlying cause of cylindruria

MISCELLANEOUS

ASSOCIATED CONDITIONS
N/A

AGE-RELATED FACTORS
N/A

ZOONOTIC POTENTIAL
N/A

PREGNANCY
N/A

SYNONYMS
N/A

SEE ALSO
N/A

ABBREVIATIONS
• DIC = disseminated intravascular coagulation
• FDP = fibrin degradation products
• PT = prothrombin time
• PTT = partial thromboplastin time

Suggested Reading

Barsanti JA, Lees GE, Willard MD, et al. Urinary disorders. In: Willard MD, Tvedten H, Turnwald GH, eds. Small animal clinical diagnosis by laboratory methods. 3rd ed. Philadelphia: Saunders, 1999:108–135.

Chew DJ, DiBartola, SP. Diagnosis and pathophysiology of renal disease. In: Ettinger SJ, ed. Textbook of veterinary internal medicine. Philadelphia: Saunders, 1994:1893–1961.

Chew DJ, DiBartola SP. Interpretation of canine and feline urinalysis. St. Louis. Ralston Purina Company, 1998:24–29.

Osborne CA, Stevens JB. Urinalysis: a clinical guide to compassionate patient care. Shawnee Mission, KS: Bayer Corporation, 1999:136–141.

Author S. Dru Forrester
Consulting Editors Larry G. Adams and Carl A. Osborne

CYSTICERCOSIS

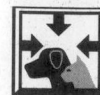 **BASICS**

OVERVIEW
• Rare disease of dogs caused by the larvae of *Taenia crassiceps*, the adults of which are found in foxes, coyotes, and sometimes domestic dogs
• Eggs shed by foxes are consumed by rabbits (or other rodents) where they develop into a cysticercal stage in the abdominal and subcutaneous tissues.
• The cysticercus is capable of undergoing asexual multiplication, so very large numbers of cysticerci can develop in the tissues of the intermediate hosts.
• Infected dogs (with cysticercal stage) may develop large masses of cysticerci in the abdominal cavity, lungs, muscles, and subcutaneous tissues.
• Rare cases reported from Europe and USA

SIGNALMENT
• Dogs—older, and in young immunocompromised animals

SIGNS
• Subcutaneous masses
• Signs associated with masses in other organs—respiratory insufficiency (lungs), icterus (abdominal cavity), anemia (of chronic disease), and anorexia.

CAUSES & RISK FACTORS
• Mode of infection not clear, but 3 hypothesized:
   • Ingestion of parasite eggs in feces of infected fox
   • Autoinfection with eggs from an intestinal infection with the adult stages
   • Ingestion of cysticercal stage

 DIAGNOSIS

DIFFERENTIAL DIAGNOSIS
• Larval *Mesocestoides* spp. infection.
• Neoplasia, especially in older animals

CBC/BIOCHEMISTRY/URINALYSIS
• Not described

OTHER LABORATORY TESTS
• N/A

IMAGING
• Radiographs—determine degree of spread to internal organs.
• Ultrasound—delineates cystic nature of mass (in cutaneous or abdominal cavity) as opposed to solid mass of a neoplasm

DIAGNOSTIC PROCEDURES
• Aspirate cytology
• Surgical biopsy

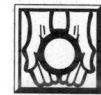 **TREATMENT**

• Inpatient if debilitated.
• Treat signs as needed.
• Surgically remove as many of the masses as possible.

 MEDICATIONS

DRUG(S)
• Praziquantel (5 mg/kg, PO, initially, then progressively increase dose over several weeks to 50 mg/kg if appears tolerated. Concern is that dog may react to dying cysticerci).

• Albendazole (50 mg/kg, PO, q24h for 10 to 20 days after the termination of praziquantel therapy may aid in preventing recurrence). NOTE: Albendazole may be myelosuppressive at this dose–check CBC.
• Fenbendazole (50 mg/kg, PO, q24h for 30 days may be used also with some hope of success for long term prevention of recurrence)

 FOLLOW-UP

• Lesions very often recur. Thus, necessary to carefully follow the dog to monitor with abdominal ultrasound the potential spread of lesions and the development of new lesions in different sites.

 MISCELLANEOUS

ZOONOTIC POTENTIAL
• Stages causing clinical signs in dogs pose no zoonotic threat.

SEE ALSO
• Coenurosis
• Mesocestoides
• Tetrathyridia

Suggested Reading
Hoberg EP, Ebinger W, Render JA. Fatal cysticercosis by *Taenia crassiceps* (Cyclophyllidea: Taeniidae) in a presumed immuno-compromised canine host. J Parasitol 2000;85:1174–1180.
Author Dwight D. Bowman
Consulting Editor Stephen C. Barr

BASICS

OVERVIEW
• Infection with the protozoan *Cytauxzoon felis*
• Affects vascular system of lungs, liver, spleen, kidneys, and brain; bone marrow; developmental stages of RBCs
• Uncommon
• Affects feral and domestic cats in south-central and southeastern U.S.

SIGNALMENT
• Feral and domestic cats of all ages
• No breed or sex predilection

SIGNS
• Severe illness at presentation
• Pale mucous membranes
• Depression
• Anorexia
• Dehydration
• High fever
• Icterus
• Splenomegaly
• Hepatomegaly

CAUSES & RISK FACTORS
• Bite of infected ixodid tick
• Roaming in areas shared by reservoir hosts (bobcat, Florida panther)

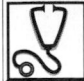 **DIAGNOSIS**

DIFFERENTIAL DIAGNOSIS
Other causes of anemia—marked decrease in packed red cell volume beginning 5–6 days after infection

CBC/BIOCHEMISTRY/URINALYSIS
Reflect changes associated with the severe anemia, caused by combination of hemolysis and hemorrhage

OTHER LABORATORY TESTS
• Fresh blood smear—*Cytauxzoon* erythrocytic form; 1–2 μm in diameter; shape of a signet ring or safety pin or looks like tiny dots
• Splenic and bone marrow aspirate—best suited to demonstrate extraerythrocytic form

IMAGING
N/A

DIAGNOSTIC PROCEDURES
N/A

PATHOLOGIC FINDINGS
Organisms inside mononuclear cells in bone marrow aspirate and in dramatically enlarged endothelial cells of venules of lung, liver, spleen, kidney, and brain

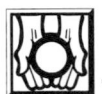 **TREATMENT**

• Inpatient with supportive therapy
• Euthanasia

 MEDICATIONS

DRUG(S)
No known chemotherapy—suggest supportive therapy or euthanasia

CONTRAINDICATIONS/POSSIBLE INTERACTIONS
N/A

 FOLLOW-UP

EXPECTED COURSE AND PROGNOSIS
• Unfortunately, diagnosis is usually made at postmortem.
• All known infected cats have died within 2 weeks of presentation.

 **MISCELLANEOUS**

ZOONOTIC POTENTIAL
• No known risk to humans
• Cannot be directly transmitted to another cat except by blood or tissue inoculation

Suggested Reading
Kier AB, Greene CE. Cytauxzoonosis. In: Greene CE, ed. Infectious diseases of the dog and cat. 2nd ed. Philadelphia: Saunders, 1998:470–473.
Author Johnny D. Hoskins
Consulting Editor Stephen C. Barr

DANCING DOBERMAN DISEASE

BASICS

OVERVIEW
• Syndrome characterized by the flexion of one rear limb when standing, progressing over months to years to involve the opposite pelvic limb
• Affected dog flexes and extends the limbs alternatively, as in a dancing motion.
• A mixed sensorimotor autonomic neuropathy is suspected.

SIGNALMENT
• Doberman pinschers
• Age of onset 6 months to 7 years
• Males and females

SIGNS
• Affected dog holds one pelvic limb flexed while standing; the alternate limb usually becomes affected in 3–6 months.
• Hyperactive tendon reflexes with gastrocnemius muscle atrophy—early
• More extensive pelvic limb muscle atrophy—with progression
• Proprioceptive deficits—occasionally

CAUSES & RISK FACTORS
• Unknown
• Autosomal recessive inheritance probable

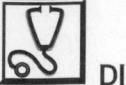

DIAGNOSIS

DIFFERENTIAL DIAGNOSIS
• Lumbosacral stenosis, intervertebral disk disease, and discospondylitis of the lower lumbar spine—usually painful
• Neoplasia of the lumbar spinal cord or nerve roots—progresses more rapidly; can be painful

CBC/BIOCHEMISTRY/URINALYSIS
• Usually normal

OTHER LABORATORY TESTS
N/A

IMAGING
N/A

DIAGNOSTIC PROCEDURES
• Electromyography—prolonged insertion activity; positive sharp waves; fibrillation potentials
• Motor and sensory nerve conduction velocity—normal
• Biopsy—gastrocnemius muscles; findings vary: some consistent with primary muscle disease, others suggest denervation

 TREATMENT
None effective at controlling clinical signs or altering progression

 MEDICATIONS

DRUG(S)
N/A

CONTRAINDICATIONS/POSSIBLE INTERACTIONS
N/A

 FOLLOW-UP
Several patients have been followed for > 5 years; all remain acceptable pets.

 MISCELLANEOUS

Suggested Reading
Braund KG. Neuropathic disorders. In: Clinical neurology in small animals—Localization, diagnosis and treatment, Ithaca: International Veterinary Information Service (www.ivis.org), 2002; B0241.0502
Chrisman CL. Dancing Doberman disease: clinical findings and prognosis. Prog Vet Neurol 1990;1:83–90.
Author Karen Dyer Inzana
Consulting Editor Joane M. Parent

DEAFNESS

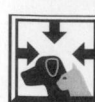 **BASICS**

DEFINITION
Lack or loss of sense of hearing, complete or partial

PATHOPHYSIOLOGY
• Either conduction deafness or nerve deafness
• Conduction—caused by diseases that obliterate the external ear canal, rupture the tympanum, or interfere with the function of the ear ossicles in the middle ear
• Nerve—acquired or congenital disease
• Acquired—caused by destruction of the normal inner ear structures; **NOTE:** for brainstem disease to cause deafness, extensive damage to auditory pathways is necessary, and such lesions would produce severe neurologic deficits from interference with the other systems adjacent to the auditory pathways.
• Congenital—caused by degeneration, hypoplasia, or aplasia of the spiral organ

SYSTEMS AFFECTED
Nervous—inner ear

SIGNALMENT
• Congenital—very young age; > 30 dog breeds known to be predisposed (Table 1); white cats with blue irises
• Acquired—any age; more common in geriatric dogs

SIGNS
General Comments
• Unilateral deafness difficult for most owners to ascertain; thus most animals brought to clinics for hearing problems have bilateral deafness.
• Conduction—usually relatively small hearing losses

Historical Findings
• Animal no longer responds to everyday sounds, does not respond to its name, or cannot be aroused from sleep by a loud noise.
• Puppy does not respond to the sounds of squeaky toys.

CAUSES
Conduction
• Otitis externa and other external ear canal disease (e.g., stenosis of canal, neoplasia, or ruptured tympanum)
• Otitis media

Nerve
• Degenerative changes in the cochlea of an old dog
• Anatomic—hypoplasia or aplasia of the spiral organ; hydrocephalus with damage to auditory cortex
• Neoplastic—acoustic neuroma; neurofibroma; neurofibrosarcoma
• Inflammatory and infectious—otitis interna; canine distemper virus (may cause alterations in hearing, not complete deafness); naso-pharyngeal polyps invading middle ear (cats)
• Trauma

Toxins and Drugs
• Antibiotics—aminoglycosides; polymixin B; erythromycin; vancomycin; chloramphenicol
• Antiseptics—ethanol; chlorhexidine; cetrimide
• Antineoplastics—cisplatin
• Diuretics—furosemide
• Heavy metals—arsenic; lead; mercury
• Miscellaneous—ceruminolytic agents; propylene glycol; salicylates

RISK FACTORS
• Chronic otitis externa, media, or interna
• Merle, piebald gene, or white coat color
• Use of certain drugs

 DIAGNOSIS

DIFFERENTIAL DIAGNOSIS
• Attempt to differentiate causes.
• Early age onset—usually suggests congenital causes in predisposed breeds
• History—use of ototoxic drugs; chronic ear disease
• Evaluate for presence of brain disease—with slowly progressive disease of the cerebral cortex (e.g., senility, neoplasia), the brain may not be able to register what the ear can hear.
• Assess status of external ear canal and tympanum.

CBC/BIOCHEMISTRY/URINALYSIS
Usually normal

Table 1

Breeds with Reported Congenital Deafness	
Akita	Ibizan hound
American Staffordshire terrier	Jack Russell terrier
Australian heeler	Kuvasz
Australian shepherd	Maltese
Beagle	Miniature pinscher
Border collie	Miniature poodle
Boston terrier	Mongrel
Boxer	Norwegian dunkerhound
Bull terrier	Old English sheepdog
Catahoula leopard dog	Papillon
Cocker spaniel	Pointer
Collie	Rhodesian ridgeback
Dalmatian	Rottweiler
Dappled dachshund	St. Bernard
Doberman pinscher	Schnauzer
Dogo Argentino	Scottish terrier
English bulldog	Sealyham terrier
English setter	Shetland sheepdog
Fox terrier	Shropshire terrier
Foxhound	Siberian husky
German shepherd	Toy poodle
Great Dane	Walker American foxhound
Great Pyrenees	West Highland white terrier

OTHER LABORATORY TESTS
Bacterial culture and sensitivity testing of ear canal—with otitis externa, media, or interna

IMAGING
• Tympanic bullae and skull radiographs—detect otitis media or otitis interna
• CT more sensitive for middle-inner ear disease

DIAGNOSTIC PROCEDURES
BAER—objectively assess hearing; essential for determining unilateral hearing loss and selecting breeding dogs

 TREATMENT
• Directed toward acquired causes; congenital deafness irreversible
• Otitis externa, media, or interna—medical or surgical approaches depend on culture and sensitivity test results and radiographic findings. • Conduction—may improve as otitis externa or media resolves
• Hearing aids—have been used; apparatus must be modified for practical use.

 MEDICATIONS

DRUG(S) OF CHOICE
• None specific for deafness
• To treat otitis externa, media, and interna accordingly

CONTRAINDICATIONS
N/A

PRECAUTIONS
• Aminoglycosides or other ototoxic drugs—use with caution to prevent additional damage or damage to the normal side, if one exists.
• Topical treatment of external ear canal—avoid if tympanic membrane is ruptured.

POSSIBLE INTERACTIONS
N/A

ALTERNATIVE DRUG(S)
N/A

 FOLLOW-UP

PATIENT MONITORING
• Weekly to assess treatment of ear disease until resolved
• BAER—assess response to treatment of otitis interna

POSSIBLE COMPLICATIONS
Environment—may need to control for patient's protection

 MISCELLANEOUS

ASSOCIATED CONDITIONS
N/A

AGE-RELATED FACTORS
N/A

ZOONOTIC POTENTIAL
N/A

PREGNANCY
N/A

SYNONYMS
N/A

SEE ALSO
Otitis Media and Interna

ABBREVIATION
BAER = brainstem auditory-evoked response
CT = computed tomography

Suggested Reading

Braund KG. Clinical syndromes in veterinary neurology. 2nd ed. St. Louis: Mosby, 1994.
Hayes HM, et al. Canine congenital deafness: epidemiologic study of 272 cases. J Am Anim Hosp Assoc 1981;17:473–476.
Mansfield PD. Ototoxicity in dogs and cats. Compend Contin Educ Pract Vet 1990;112:331–337.
Marshall AE. Hearing loss in aged dogs. Adv Small Anim Med Surg 1990;2:6–.
Strain GM. Congenital deafness in dogs and cats. Compend Contin Educ Pract Vet 1991;13:245–254.
Strain GM, Kearney MT, Gignac IJ, et al. Brainstem auditory-evoked potential assessment of congenital deafness in Dalmatians: associations with phenotypic markers. J Vet Intern Med 1992;5:175–182.
Author T. Mark Neer
Consulting Editor Joane M. Parent

DECIINUOUS TEETH, RETAINED

BASICS

OVERVIEW
• Permanent teeth are formed by 11 weeks of age.
• Root and alveolar bone development, continued growth of the pulp tissue, and the driving force of the periodontal ligament all facilitate the movement of the crown through the gingiva.
• Pressure from the erupting crown on the root of a deciduous tooth causes resorption of root.
• Normally, loss of the primary tooth makes a pathway for the erupting permanent tooth.

SIGNALMENT
• Dogs and cats
• More common in small-breed dogs than in cats or large-breed dogs

SIGNS

Initial signs
• Two teeth of the same type (deciduous and permanent) occupying the same space (in the alveolus) at the same time

• Canine teeth—mandibular permanent canine tooth erupts lingual (medial) to the retained deciduous tooth; maxillary permanent canine tooth erupts mesial (rostral) to the retained deciduous canine tooth
• Incisors—permanent maxillary and mandibular incisors erupt palatal and lingual (respectively) to the retained deciduous incisors
• Premolars—permanent premolars erupt lingual (mandible) and palatal (maxilla) to the retained deciduous teeth, except the maxillary fourth premolar, which erupts buccal and slightly caudal (distal) to the last deciduous premolar

Halitosis
• Localized gingivitis
• Gingival recession and bone loss possible
• Sign when left untreated

Malocclusion
• Localized gingivitis
• Periodontal disease
• Oronasal fistula possible
Permanent lower canines erupt lingual to the retained deciduous teeth and will assume a vertical position in the mouth, resulting in impingement on the hard palate, which creates pain, inflammation, and, long term, an oronasal fistula if the teeth continue to erupt.

CAUSES & RISK FACTORS
• Cause unknown
• Small-breed dogs predisposed

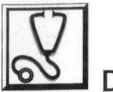

DIAGNOSIS

DIFFERENTIAL DIAGNOSIS
N/A

CBC/BIOCHEMISTRY/URINALYSIS
N/A

OTHER LABORATORY TESTS
N/A

IMAGING
Intraoral radiographs to identify dental abnormalities prior to extraction; to identify retained root where crown is missing but opposite side retained; to confirm absence of deciduous root after extraction; to determine if permanent tooth is present but not erupted; to determine if permanent tooth is retained or missing

DIAGNOSTIC PROCEDURES
N/A

PATHOLOGIC FINDINGS
Evidence of root resorption of the apex of the deciduous root

 TREATMENT

SURGICAL CONSIDERATIONS
• Ideally, perform extraction as soon as the permanent tooth has erupted through the gingiva.
• Buprenorphine HCl (0.007 mg/kg SC or IM)
• Analgesia—butorphanol (0.22 mg/kg SC)
• General anesthesia with endotracheal tube in place and cuff inflated to prevent a foreign body (e.g., extracted tooth, dislodged piece of tartar) from entering upper airway

Extraction
• Sever epithelial attachment in gingival sulcus with a sharp blade (No. 15 or 15C); elevate gingiva with a small surgical periosteal elevator.

• Sever periodontal ligament by placing a luxator or elevator in the periodontal ligament space (between the tooth and the bone of the socket) and gently move the instrument around the tooth.
• Advance the elevator as space allows, and apply even pressure for 30 sec to weaken the fibers and produce bleeding in the socket; the hemorrhage is space-occupying and facilitates extraction.

Extraction with Other Surgical Procedures
Extract the retained deciduous teeth of any patient undergoing anesthesia (e.g., spay/neuter).

Fractured and Retained Root Tips
If a fracture occurs during extraction, the retained root can deflect the permanent tooth's eruption and should be extracted; it may be necessary to make a full-thickness gingival flap and remove enough buccal bone to get good visualization. With any elevation force, it is essential to avoid direct contact with the permanent tooth or permanent tooth bud.

 MEDICATIONS

DRUG(S)
N/A

CONTRAINDICATIONS/POSSIBLE INTERACTIONS
N/A

 **FOLLOW-UP**
Recheck patient within 1 week of surgery.

 MISCELLANEOUS

Suggested Reading
Wiggs R, Lobprise H. Veterinary dentistry, principles and practice. Philadelphia: Lippincott-Raven, 1997.
Author Randi Diane Brannan
Consulting Editor Heidi B. Lobprise

DEGENERATIVE MYELOPATHY

 **BASICS**

DEFINITION
Syndrome characterized by slow, progressive degeneration of axons and myelin in the spinal cord

Pathophysiology
Vitamin B_{12} deficiency, vitamin E deficiency, progressive increase in circulating suppressor T lymphocytes, an autoimmune response to a neural antigen, and dying-back neuropathy—examined as possible links; none is established as an important factor

Systems Affected
Nervous

Genetics
Suspected, but not proven, hereditary basis—German shepherds, German shepherd mixed breeds, and Siberian huskies

Incidence/Prevalence
• Data unavailable
• Most common cause of pelvic limb paresis in middle-aged German shepherds and German shepherd mixed breeds
• Rare in other breeds of dogs and in cats

Geographic Distribution
N/A

SIGNALMENT

Species
Dogs and cats

Breed Predilections
• Most commonly affected—German shepherds and German shepherd mixed breeds
• Other large and medium breeds occasionally affected—collies and collie crosses, Labrador retrievers, Siberian huskies, Chesapeake Bay retrievers, Kerry blue terriers, and Welsh corgis

Mean Age and Range
• Mean age of onset—9.6 years
• Range—4–14 years
• German shepherds—two cases reported at 6 and 7 months old

Predominant Sex
Males

SIGNS

Historical Findings
• Insidious onset
• Bilateral but not necessarily symmetrical
• Initially—mild ataxia and paresis of the pelvic limbs; thoracic limbs not affected
• Owners often bring their dog in for examination several months after onset of clinical signs, suspecting arthritis.
• Knuckling and scuffing of the toes of the pelvic limbs—most common complaint
• Crossing over and swaying of the rear quarters—often occur when patient is turning
• Urination and defecation—voluntary control retained until extremely late in the disease
• Caudal paraspinal and pelvic limb muscles—often atrophy from disuse late in the disease
• Pain or discomfort—not evident

Neurologic Examination Findings
• Deficits limited to the pelvic limbs
• Ataxia and upper motor neuron paresis—localized to the T3-L3 spinal cord segments
• Proprioception deficits—worse than expected for the mild degree of paresis observed early in the disease; may be considerably asymmetric
• Withdrawal reflexes—normal to exaggerated; may see a crossed extensor reflex
• Anal sphincter tone, perineal reflex, and tail tone—normal
• Patellar reflexes—usually normal to exaggerated; sometimes impaired or absent unilaterally or bilaterally because of degeneration of the dorsal root ganglia or dorsal gray matter of the spinal cord; ventral motor roots not affected, so this is not a true lower motor neuron sign but indicates the disease
• Pain perception—preserved

CAUSES
Unknown

RISK FACTORS
N/A

 DIAGNOSIS

DIFFERENTIAL DIAGNOSIS
• Hansen type II intervertebral disk protrusion and spinal neoplasia—most likely to resemble degenerative myelopathy; back pain at the lesion site is common but may not be observed; differentiated by survey radiography and myelography
• Myelitis—usually more acute and progressive; ruled out by CSF analysis at the time of myelography
• Diskospondylitis—differentiated by occurrence of back pain; survey radiography helpful
• Lumbosacral stenosis—generally causes pain; to rule out, may need electromyography and epidurography
• Vertebral spondylosis and dural ossification—common radiographic findings in old, large-breed dogs; almost never cause clinical signs

CBC/BIOCHEMISTRY/URINALYSIS
Usually normal

OTHER LABORATORY TESTS
Abnormal cell-mediated immune studies—depressed responses to concanavalin A, phytohemagglutinin P, and pokeweed mitogens in most affected dogs; tests are not readily available; diagnostic accuracy not confirmed by double-blind studies

IMAGING
• Thoracic and abdominal radiography—screen for metastatic disease; consider the age of the patient and the possibility of spinal neoplasia.
• Spinal survey radiography—generally normal; may reveal dural ossification or spondylosis; findings are generally of no clinical significance.
• Myelography—normal
• CT—normal
• MRI—normal

DIAGNOSTIC PROCEDURES
CSF analysis—may contain a high protein concentration (40–100 mg/dL) with a normal WBC count; unfortunately, these findings are also seen with type II disk protrusion, the main differential

PATHOLOGIC FINDINGS
• Gross necropsy findings—normal
• Histologic examination—demyelination, axonal degeneration, and astrocytosis of the white matter
• Lesions—most severe in the thoracic spinal cord in dorsolateral and ventromedial funiculi; bilateral but not necessarily symmetrical; lesions discontinuous
• May see marked degeneration in the lumbar dorsal nerve roots but not the ventral nerve roots

 TREATMENT

APPROPRIATE HEALTH CARE
• Outpatient
• Inpatient—for diagnostic workup only

NURSING CARE
• Dog should be encouraged to be active as long as possible to delay onset of a nonambulatory state.
• Nonambulatory patients—prevent pressure sores; provide good bedding.
• A cart may be beneficial.

ACTIVITY
Encourage exercise to prevent muscle atrophy; the stronger and more active the patient is, the longer it will stay ambulatory as the paresis progresses.

DIET
Avoid excess weight.

CLIENT EDUCATION
• Inform client that this is a nontreatable disease that progresses slowly and steadily.
• Inform client that euthanasia is recommended once a nonambulatory state is reached.

SURGICAL CONSIDERATIONS
• No effective surgery available
• It is possible for a dog to have concurrent type II disk protrusion; unless the spinal cord compression is significant, surgery should not be done until a therapeutic trial of corticosteroids is completed; if marked improvement is seen, then decompressive surgery is warranted; CAUTION: surgery to remove a type II disk protrusion in a patient with clinical signs that are actually the result of degenerative myelopathy often causes irreversible neurologic deterioration.

MEDICATIONS

DRUG(S) OF CHOICE
• No proven effective treatment available
• Proposed treatment—suggested by one author; combination of exercise, vitamin supplements, and epsilon aminocaproic acid (Amicar, Lederle, NY; 500 mg PO q8h mixed with a hematinic compound); apparently slows the progression in 50% of patients; 15%–20% of patients do not deteriorate further if treatment is maintained; no controlled trials have been done.

CONTRAINDICATIONS
• Corticosteroids—do not use; not beneficial in the treatment of this disease
• Steroid myopathy—may worsen muscle atrophy and pelvic limb weakness, hastening the onset of a nonambulatory state

PRECAUTIONS
N/A

POSSIBLE INTERACTIONS
N/A

ALTERNATIVE DRUG(S)
N/A

FOLLOW-UP

PATIENT MONITORING
• Epsilon aminocaproic acid administration—if effective, improvement should be seen within 8 weeks; perform a neurologic examination at that time to assess therapeutic response; if patient has deteriorated, discontinue treatment because it is expensive.
• Reevaluate patient on a regular basis to monitor progression and avoid complications.

PREVENTION/AVOIDANCE
N/A

POSSIBLE COMPLICATIONS
Pressure sores and urine scalding once a nonambulatory state is reached

EXPECTED COURSE AND PROGNOSIS
• Most affected dogs gradually lose function in the pelvic limbs, reaching a nonambulatory state within 6 months to 2 years after onset.
• Nonambulatory patients eventually lose thoracic limb function and may develop urinary and fecal incontinence.

MISCELLANEOUS

ASSOCIATED CONDITIONS
• Enteropathy—seen in some patients; leads to subnormal serum vitamin B_{12} and vitamin E concentrations; speculated cause is degenerative myelopathy that leads to autonomic nerve dysfunction, which, in turn, leads to impaired intestinal motility and intestinal bacterial overgrowth.
• Depressed cell-mediated immunity—seen in some patients; may be a response to the lesion or may indicate that the disease has an immunologic basis.

AGE-RELATED FACTORS
• Clinical signs develop in dogs > 4 years old.
• A few cases of a similar nature have been reported in dogs < 1 year old.

ZOONOTIC POTENTIAL
N/A

PREGNANCY
Because the disease is slowly progressive, an ambulatory affected dog should reach term normally; important to discuss with the client the probable heritability of the disease.

SYNONYMS
Degenerative radiculomyelopathy of the aged German shepherd

SEE ALSO
Intervertebral Disk Disease, Thoracolumbar

ABBREVIATIONS
CSF = cerebrospinal fluid
CT = computed tomography
MRI = magnetic resonance imaging

Suggested Reading
Clemmons RM. Degenerative myelopathy. In: Kirk RW, ed. Current veterinary therapy X. Philadelphia: Saunders, 1989.830–833.
Coates J. Canine degenerative myelopathy. Proceedings. 19th Annual Veterinary Medical Forum. pp 405–407, 2001.
Kornegay JN. Congenital and degenerative diseases of the central nervous system: axonal and myelin lesions—degenerative myelopathy. In: Kornegay JN, ed. Neurologic disorders. New York: Churchill Livingstone, 1986:120–122.
LeCouteur RA, Grandy L. Diseases of the spinal cord: degenerative myelopathy. In: Ettinger SJ, Feldman EC, eds. Textbook of veterinary internal medicine. 5th ed. Philadelphia: Saunders, 2000:622–623.
Oliver JE, Lorenz MD. Handbook of veterinary neurology. 3rd ed. Philadelphia: Saunders, 1997.
Author Allen Sisson
Consulting Editor Joane M. Parent

DEMODICOSIS

 BASICS

DEFINITION
• An inflammatory parasitic disease of dogs and rarely cats that is characterized by an increased number of mites in the hair follicles, which often leads to furunculosis and secondary bacterial infection
• May be localized or generalized in dogs

PATHOPHYSIOLOGY

Dogs
• *Demodex canis*—a mite; part of the normal fauna of the skin; typically present in small numbers; resides in the hair follicles and sebaceous glands of the skin
• Pathology develops when numbers exceed that tolerated by the immune system.
• The initial proliferation of mites may be the result of a genetic or immunologic disorder.

Cats
• Poorly understood disorder
• Mites have been identified on the skin and within the otic canal.
• Two species: *D. cati* and *D. gatoi*

SYSTEMS AFFECTED
Skin/Exocrine—dead and degenerate *D. canis* mites may be found in noncutaneous sites (e.g., lymph node, intestinal wall, spleen, liver, kidney, urinary bladder, lung, thyroid gland, blood, urine, and feces) and are considered to represent drainage to these areas by blood and/or lymph.

GENETICS
The initial proliferation of mites may be the result of a genetic disorder.

INCIDENCE/PREVALENCE
• Dogs—common
• Cats—rare

GEOGRAPHIC DISTRIBUTION
None

SIGNALMENT

Species
Dogs and rarely cats

Breed Predilections
Potential increased incidence in Siamese and Burmese cat breeds

Mean Age and Range
• Localized—usually in young dogs; median age 3–6 months
• Generalized—both young and old animals

Predominant Sex
None

SIGNS

Dogs
Localized
• Lesions—usually mild; consist of erythema and a light scale
• Patches—several may be noted; most common site is the face, especially around the perioral and periocular areas; may also be seen on the trunk and legs
Generalized
• Can be widespread from the onset, with multiple poorly circumscribed patches of erythema, alopecia, and scale
• As hair follicles become distended with large numbers of mites, secondary bacterial infections are common, often with resultant rupturing of the follicle (furunculosis).
• With progression, the skin can become severely inflamed, exudative, and granulomatous.

Cats
• Often characterized by partial to complete multifocal alopecia of the eyelids, periocular region, head, and neck
• Lesions—variably pruritic with erythema, scale, and crust; those caused by the un-named species are often quite pruritic.
• Ceruminous otitis externa has been reported.

CAUSES
• *Demodex canis*
• *Demodex cati* and *D. gatoi*

RISK FACTORS

Dogs
• Exact immunopathologic mechanism unknown
• Studies indicate that dogs with generalized demodicosis have a subnormal percentage of IL-2 receptors on their lymphocytes and subnormal IL-2 production.
• Genetic factors, immunosuppression, and/or metabolic diseases may predispose animal.

Cats
• Often associated with metabolic diseases (e.g., FIV, systemic lupus erythematosus, diabetes mellitus)
• *D. gatoi*—short and blunted; rarely a marker for metabolic disease; individual reports indicate that it may be transferable from cat to cat within the same household

 DIAGNOSIS

DIFFERENTIAL DIAGNOSIS

Dogs
• Bacterial folliculitis/furunculosis
• Dermatophytosis
• Contact dermatitis
• Pemphigus complex
• Dermatomyositis
• Systemic lupus erythematosus

Cats
• Allergic dermatitis
• Scabies
• Dermatophyte

CBC/BIOCHEMISTRY/URINALYSIS
• Nondiagnostic for *Demodex* spp.
• May be useful for identifying underlying metabolic diseases in cats

OTHER LABORATORY TESTS
FeLV and FIV serology—identify underlying metabolic diseases in cats

IMAGING
N/A

DIAGNOSTIC PROCEDURES
• Skin scrapings—diagnostic for finding large numbers of mites in the majority of cases
• Cutaneous biopsy—may be needed when lesions are chronic, granulomatous, and fibrotic (especially on the paw)

PATHOLOGIC FINDINGS
N/A

 TREATMENT

APPROPRIATE HEALTH CARE
• Outpatient
• Localized—conservative; most cases (90%) resolve spontaneously with no treatment.
• Evaluate the general health status of dogs with either the localized or the generalized form.

NURSING CARE
N/A

ACTIVITY
N/A

DIET
N/A

CLIENT EDUCATION
• Localized—most cases resolve spontaneously
• Generalized (adult dog)—frequent management problem; expense and frustration with the chronicity of the problem are issues; many cases are medically controlled, not cured.

SURGICAL CONSIDERATIONS
N/A

 MEDICATIONS

DRUG(S) OF CHOICE

Amitraz (Mitaban; Taktic-EC)
• A formamidine, which inhibits monoamine oxidase and prostaglandin synthesis; an α_2-adrenergic agonist
• Use weekly until resolution of clinical signs and no mites are found on skin scrapings; do not rinse off; let air-dry.
• Treat for one month following negative skin scrape.
• Apply a benzoyl peroxide shampoo before application of the dip as a bactericidal therapy and to increase exposure of the mites to the miticide through follicular flushing activity.
• The efficacy is proportional to the frequency of administration and the concentration of the dip.
• Success with the 9% amitraz collar has not been established, although there are positive anecdotal reports.
• Between 11% and 30% of cases will not be cured; may need to try an alternative therapy or control with maintenance dips every 2–8 weeks.
• The small animal formulation Mitaban is no longer available.

Ivermectin (Ivomec; Eqvalan Liquid), DVM
• A macrocyclic lactone with GABA agonist activity
• Daily oral administration of 0.3–0.6 mg/kg very effective, even when amitraz fails
• Treat for 30–60 days beyond negative skin scrapings (average 3–8 months).

Milbemycin (Interceptor)
• A macrocyclic lactone with GABA agonist activity
• Dosage of 1 mg/kg PO q24h cures 50% of cases; 2 mg/kg PO q24h cures 85% of cases.

• Treat for 30–60 days beyond multiple negative skin scrapings.

Cats
• Exact protocols are not defined.
• Topical lime-sulfur dips or amitraz solutions applied weekly for 4 treatments often lead to good resolution of clinical signs.

CONTRAINDICATIONS
Ivermectin—contraindicated in collies, Shetland sheepdogs, old English sheepdogs, other herding breeds, and crosses with these breeds; sensitive breeds appear to tolerate the acaricidal dosages of milbemycin (see above).

PRECAUTIONS

Amitraz
• Most common side effects—somnolence, lethargy, depression, anorexia seen in 30% of patients for 12–36 hr after treatment
• Other side effects—vomiting, diarrhea, pruritus, polyuria, mydriasis, bradycardia, hypoventilation, hypotension, hypothermia, ataxia, ileus, bloat, hyperglycemia, convulsions, death
• The incidence and severity of side effects do not appear to be proportional to the dose or frequency of use.
• Humans can develop dermatitis, headaches, and respiratory difficulty after exposure.
• Yohimbine at 0.11 mg/kg IV is an antidote.

Ivermectin and Milbemycin
Signs of toxicity—salivation, vomiting, mydriasis, confusion, ataxia, hypersensitivity to sound, weakness, recumbency, coma, and death

POSSIBLE INTERACTIONS
• Amitraz—may interact with heterocyclic antidepressants, xylazine, benzodiazepines, and macrocyclic lactones
• Ivermectin and milbemycin—cause elevated levels of monoamine neurotransmitter metabolites, which could result in adverse drug interactions with amitraz and benzodiazepines

ALTERNATIVE DRUG(S)
None

 FOLLOW-UP

PATIENT MONITORING
Multiple skin scrapings and evidence of clinical resolution are used to monitor progress.

PREVENTION/AVOIDANCE
Avoid breeding animals with generalized form

POSSIBLE COMPLICATIONS
Secondary bacterial infections

EXPECTED COURSE AND PROGNOSIS
• Prognosis (dogs)—depends heavily on genetic, immunologic, and underlying diseases
• Localized—most cases (90%) resolve spontaneously with no treatment; < 10% progress to the generalized form
• Adult-onset (dogs)—often severe and refractory to treatment

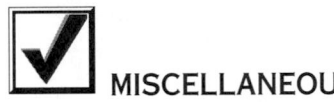 MISCELLANEOUS

ASSOCIATED CONDITIONS
Adult-onset—sudden occurrence is often associated with internal disease, malignant neoplasia, and/or immunosuppressive disease; approximately 25% of cases are idiopathic over a follow-up period of 1–2 years.

AGE-RELATED FACTORS
Young dogs are often predisposed.

ZOONOTIC POTENTIAL
None

PREGNANCY
Do not breed animals with the generalized form.

SYNONYMS
Mange

SEE ALSO
• Amitraz Toxicity
• Ivermectin Toxicity

ABBREVIATIONS
• FeLV = feline leukemia virus
• FIV = feline immunodeficiency virus
• GABA = γ-aminobutyric acid
• IL = interleukin

Suggested Reading
Scott DW, Miller WH, Griffin CE, eds. Parasitic skin diseases. In: Muller & Kirk's small animal dermatology. 5th ed. Philadelphia: Saunders, 1995:417–432.

Author Karen Helton Rhodes
Consulting Editor Karen Helton Rhodes

DENTAL CARIES (CAVITIES)

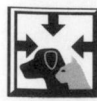

BASICS

OVERVIEW
• Caries is the decay of the dental hard tissues (enamel, cementum, and dentin) due to the effects of oral bacteria on fermentable carbohydrates on the tooth surface.
• Caries is very common in humans in "westernized" society, where diets rich in highly refined carbohydrates are the norm.
• For various reasons (e.g., diet lower in carbohydrates, higher salivary pH, lower salivary amylase, conical crown shape, different indigenous oral flora), caries is not common in the domestic dog, but it does occur and should be looked for.
• A study published in the *Journal of Veterinary Dentistry* in 1998 (see Suggested Reading) reported that 5.3% of dogs 1 year of age or older had one or more caries lesions, with 52% having bilaterally symmetrical lesions.
• Caries can affect the crown or roots of the teeth and is classified as pit-and-fissure, smooth-surface, or root caries.

SIGNALMENT
• Caries occurs in dogs.
• Reported in cats; feline odontoclastic resorptive lesions have sometimes been misnamed feline caries
• There is no known breed, age, or gender predilection.

SIGNS
• Incipient smooth-surface caries—appears as an area of dull, frosty-white enamel
• Clinical caries—appears as a structural defect on the surface of the crown or root
• The defect is frequently filled with or lined by dark, soft necrotic dentin.
• Affected dentin will yield to a dental explorer and can be removed with a dental excavator or curette.

CAUSES & RISK FACTORS
• Caries is caused by oral bacteria fermenting carbohydrates on the tooth surface, leading to the production of acids (acetic, lactic, propionic) that demineralize the enamel and dentin, followed by digestion of the organic matrix of the tooth by oral bacteria and/or leukocytes.
• There is a constant exchange of minerals between enamel and oral fluids; if there is a net loss of mineral, caries develops.
• Early (incipient) caries may be reversible through remineralization.
• Once the protein matrix collapses, the lesion is irreversible.
• Any factors that allow prolonged retention of fermentable carbohydrates and bacterial plaque on the tooth surface predispose to the development of caries.
• A deep occlusal pit on the maxillary first molar is the most common place for caries to develop.
• Dental surfaces in close contact with an established caries are at risk of developing a lesion.
• Deep occlusal pits and developmental grooves on the crown surface predispose to pit and fissure caries.
• Tight interdental contacts predispose to smooth-surface caries.
• Deep periodontal pockets predispose to root caries.
• Animals with poorly mineralized enamel, lower salivary pH, diets high in fermentable carbohydrates, and poor oral hygiene are at risk of developing caries.

DIAGNOSIS

DIFFERENTIAL DIAGNOSIS
• Crown fracture, abrasive wear, attrition with exposed tertiary dentin, or extrinsic staining
• Enamel hypocalcification with exposed and stained dentin
• Feline odontoclastic resorptive lesions have been misnamed feline caries in the past.
• Sound dentin is hard and will not yield to a dental explorer, whereas carious dentin is soft and will yield to a sharp instrument.
• Root caries may be confused with external root resorption, though the distinction would often be academic as either usually indicates extraction.
• The lesion should be staged as to the depth of the pathology.

Stage 1	defect involves enamel only
Stage 2	defect extends into dentin; pulp canal not involved
Stage 3	defect extends into pulp canal
Stage 4	significant structure damage of crown
Stage 5	majority of crown lost; roots remaining

CBC/BIOCHEMISTRY/URINALYSIS
N/A

IMAGING
Intraoral dental radiography—to examine the affected tooth carefully; areas of demineralization and tissue loss will appear as lucent areas contrasted against radiodense normal dental tissues; if the lesion has penetrated into the pulp chamber, there will be endodontic disease and there may be periapical disease evident radiographically

DIAGNOSTIC PROCEDURES
• Visual examination—clean, dry tooth surface under good light and magnification
• Exploration with a sharp dental explorer—the explorer will sink into carious dentin and stick, providing the sensation of "tug-back" upon withdrawal
• Subgingival exploration—reveals irregularities in the root surface

 TREATMENT
• Deep pits on the occlusal surface of the maxillary first molar—fill with a pit-and-fissure sealant to prevent caries development
• Incipient caries—can be arrested and possibly reversed by application of a fluoride varnish or fluoride-releasing dentin bonding agent and modification of the risk factors

• Lesions that result in mild to moderate coronal tissue loss (stage 1 or 2)—remove carious dentin and unsupported enamel, then restore the coronal anatomy with amalgam (traditional), bonded composite restorations, or prosthetic restorations
• Lesions that extend into pulp canal (stage 3)—endodontic treatment must precede restorative treatment
• Lesions that result in extensive coronal tissue loss (stage 4 or 5)—extraction may be the only treatment option
• Root caries—if the periodontal disease can be managed and the restoration placed supragingivally, restoration may be possible; however, for most teeth with root caries, extraction will be the treatment of choice
• If only one root of a multirooted tooth is carious—extraction of the affected root with endodontic treatment of the remaining root(s) is also an option
• High-risk patients—application of a pit-and-fissure sealant on remaining teeth with occlusal surfaces may be considered

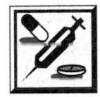 **MEDICATIONS**

DRUG(S)
• Postoperative broad-spectrum antibiotics—may be indicated if there is pulp involvement necessitating endodontic treatment or extraction

• Postoperative analgesia with nonsteroidal anti-inflammatory drugs—indicated following endodontic or exodontic treatment or extensive restorative work

 FOLLOW-UP
• Examine and radiograph treated teeth 6 months postoperatively, then annually or as the opportunity presents
• As affected individuals frequently have more than one caries, examine all teeth carefully at any opportunity to monitor for new lesions.

 MISCELLANEOUS

Suggested Reading
Hale FA. Dental caries in the dog. J Vet Dent 1998;15:79–83.
Author Fraser A. Hale
Consulting Editor Heidi Lobprise

DERMATOMYOSITIS

 BASICS

DEFINITION
• An inherited inflammatory disease of the skin, muscles, and vasculature that usually occurs in young dogs
• Occurs primarily in collies, Shetland sheepdogs, and their related crossbreeds but has been reported in Beauceron shepherds, Welsh corgis, Lakeland terriers, chow chows, German shepherds, and kuvaszes.

PATHOPHYSIOLOGY
• The exact pathogenesis of dermatomyositis is unknown.
• A familial predisposition has been reported in Collies and Shetland sheepdogs; however, possible triggers for the disease include infectious agents (especially viral), vaccines, and other drugs.
• Based on the clinical and histopathologic evidence, an immune-mediated or autoimmune process may be involved.

SYSTEMS AFFECTED
• Skin—alopecic, erythematous dermatitis on the face, ears, and tail tip, and over the bony prominences of the distal extremities is the most common clinical sign; cutaneous erosions and ulcerations may develop
• Musculoskeletal—myositis, which can be subtle to severe, develops after the dermatitis; usually the temporal and masseter muscles are involved, affecting mastication; in more severe cases, there may be generalized muscle disease and involvement of the esophageal muscles (megaesophagus)

GENETICS
Collies and Shetland sheepdogs—studies suggest that dermatomyositis is inherited in an autosomal dominant manner, with variable expression

INCIDENCE/PREVALENCE
Exact prevalence is unknown.

GEOGRAPHIC DISTRIBUTION
Probably worldwide

SIGNALMENT
Species
Dogs

Breed Predilection
Collies, Shetland sheepdogs, and their crossbreeds; Beauceron shepherds; Welsh corgis; Lakeland terriers; chow chows; German shepherds; and kuvaszes

Mean Age and Range
• Cutaneous lesions usually develop when the dog is between 7 weeks and 6 months of age.
• The lesions usually resolve as the dog ages (within 3–6 months).
• In severely affected dogs, lesions may persist throughout life.
• Adult-onset dermatomyositis can occur, but is rare.

Predominant Sex
None

SIGNS
General Comments
The clinical signs vary from subtle skin lesions and subclinical myositis to severe skin lesions and generalized muscle atrophy with megaesophagus.

Historical Findings
• Waxing and waning skin lesions around the eyes, lips, face, inner ear pinnae, tip of the tail, and bony prominences—usually seen in affected dogs before they are 6 months old
• Scarring—may occur as a sequela to the initial skin lesions
• Muscle atrophy of the masseter and temporal muscles—may be evident
• More severely affected dogs may have difficulty eating, drinking, and swallowing.
• Several littermates may be affected, but the severity of the disease often varies significantly among affected dogs.

Physical Examination Findings
• Skin lesions—characterized by variable degrees of alopecia, erythema, scaling, crusting, ulceration, and scarring on the face, around the lips and eyes, in the inner ear pinnae, on the tip of the tail, and over bony prominences on the distal extremities
• Foot pad and oral ulcers—rarely
• Myositis—signs may be absent or vary from subtle decrease in the mass of the temporalis muscles to generalized symmetric muscle atrophy and lameness
• Dogs with megaesophagus may present with aspiration pneumonia.

CAUSES
• Hereditary
• Infectious agents
• Immune mediated

RISK FACTORS
Mechanical pressure and trauma, and ultraviolet light exposure may induce cutaneous lesions.

 DIAGNOSIS

DIFFERENTIAL DIAGNOSIS
• Demodicosis
• Dermatophytosis
• Bacterial folliculitis
• Juvenile cellulitis
• Discoid lupus erythematosus
• Systemic lupus erythematosus
• Polymyositis

CBC/BIOCHEMISTRY/URINALYSIS
Serum creatine kinase may be slightly high.

OTHER LABORATORY TESTS
Antinuclear antibody titers are negative.

IMAGING
N/A

DIAGNOSTIC PROCEDURES
• Skin biopsy—may be diagnostic for dermatomyositis, although this disease can be difficult to definitively diagnose; avoid infected and scarred lesions
• Muscle biopsy—proper muscle selection can be difficult because pathologic changes may be mild.
• EMG—ideally, is used to select affected muscles for biopsy; if EMG is not available, atrophied muscles should be biopsied; EMG abnormalities are present in affected muscles; findings include fibrillation potentials, bizarre high-frequency discharges, and positive sharp waves.

PATHOLOGIC FINDINGS
Skin Biopsy
• Scattered necrosis or vacuolation of individual basal cells—may be seen; may lead to intrabasal or subepidermal clefting
• Superficial, mild, diffuse dermal and perivascular cellular infiltrates—composed of lymphocytes, plasma cells, and histiocytes
• Follicular atrophy and fibrosis—usually seen
• Secondary epidermal ulceration and dermal scarring—may be present
• The histopathologic features may be subtle and consist mostly of atrophic changes; however, the combination of epidermal and follicular cell degeneration, perivascular

inflammation, and follicular atrophy with fibrosis is highly suggestive of dermatomyositis.

Muscle Biopsy
• Variable multifocal accumulations of inflammatory cells, including lymphocytes, plasma cells, macrophages, and neutrophils
• Myofibril degeneration—characterized by fragmentation, vacuolation, atrophy, fibrosis, and regeneration

 TREATMENT

APPROPRIATE HEALTH CARE
• Most dogs can be treated as outpatients.
• Dogs with severe myositis and megaesophagus may need to be hospitalized for supportive care.

NURSING CARE
N/A

ACTIVITY
• Avoid activities that may traumatize the skin.
• Keep indoors during the day to avoid exposure to intense sunlight.

DIET
N/A

CLIENT EDUCATION
• Discuss the hereditary nature of the disease.
• Note that affected dogs should not be bred.
• Inform the owner that the disease is not curable, although spontaneous resolution can occur.
• Discuss prognosis and possible complications, especially in severely affected dogs.

 MEDICATIONS

DRUG(S) OF CHOICE
• Nonspecific symptomatic therapy includes hypoallergenic shampoo baths, treating secondary pyoderma and demodicosis, and avoiding trauma and sunlight.
• Vitamin E—200–800 IU PO q24h
• Essential fatty acid supplements
• Prednisone—1–2 mg/kg PO q12–24h until remission, then alternate-day administration using the lowest dosage possible for long-term control

• Pentoxifylline—10–25 mg/kg q8–12h
• The therapeutic efficacy of medical treatment can be difficult to assess because the disease tends to be cyclic in nature and is often self-limiting.

CONTRAINDICATIONS
Pentoxifylline should not be used in dogs that are sensitive to methylxanthine derivatives.

PRECAUTIONS
• Pentoxifylline—may cause gastric irritation; dogs with prolonged clotting times and dogs receiving anticoagulant therapy should be monitored carefully when treated with this drug.
• Glucocorticoids—discuss possible side effects with the owner.

ALTERNATIVE DRUG(S)
N/A

 FOLLOW-UP

PATIENT MONITORING
N/A

PREVENTION/AVOIDANCE
• Do not breed affected animals.
• Neuter intact animals.
• Minimize trauma and exposure to sunlight.

POSSIBLE COMPLICATIONS
• Secondary pyoderma and demodicosis
• Mildly to moderately affected dogs may have residual scarring.
• Severely affected dogs may have trouble chewing, drinking, and swallowing if the masticatory and esophageal muscles are involved.
• Megaesophagus may develop, predisposing the dog to aspiration pneumonia.

EXPECTED COURSE AND PROGNOSIS
• Long-term prognosis—variable, depending on severity of disease
• Minimal disease—prognosis good; tends to spontaneously resolve with no evidence of scarring
• Mild to moderate disease—tends to resolve spontaneously, but residual scarring is common
• Severe disease—prognosis for long-term survival is poor as the dermatitis and myositis may be lifelong

✓ MISCELLANEOUS

ASSOCIATED CONDITIONS
Idiopathic ulcerative dermatosis of Shetland sheepdogs and collies—poorly understood disease; described in adult collies and Shetland sheepdogs; characterized by well-demarcated serpiginous ulcers in the intertriginous areas of the groin and axillae; may occur alone or concurrently with dermatomyositis; may represent a subgroup of dermatomyositis

AGE-RELATED FACTORS
• Clinical signs usually occur in dogs younger than 6 months
• Adult onset—rare; more commonly seen in dogs that had subtle lesions as puppies

ZOONOTIC POTENTIAL
N/A

PREGNANCY
• Do not breed affected dogs.
• Pregnancy may exacerbate clinical symptoms.

SYNONYMS
• Familial canine dermatomyositis
• Canine familial dermatomyositis

SEE ALSO
• Lupus Erythematosus, Cutaneous
• Lupus Erythematosus, Systemic

ABBREVIATIONS
EMG = electromyography, electromyographic

Suggested Reading
Gross TL, Ihrke PJ, Walder E. Veterinary dermatopathology: a macroscopic and microscopic evaluation of canine and feline skin disease. St. Louis: Mosby, 1992:34–36.
Hargis AM, Mundell AC. Familial canine dermatomyositis. Comp Cont Ed 1992;14:855–864.
Scott DW, Miller WH, Griffin CE. Muller & Kirk's small animal dermatology. 6th ed. Philadelphia: Saunders, 2001:940–946.
Authors Keith A. Hnilica and Linda Medleau
Consulting Editor Karen Helton Rhodes

DERMATOPHILOSIS

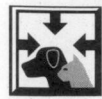 **BASICS**

OVERVIEW
• A crusting skin disease in dogs and cats and a nodular subcutaneous and oral disease in cats
• Reported infrequently
• *Dermatophilus congolensis*—causative agent; gram-positive, branching filamentous bacterium classified as an Actinomycete; common cause of crusting dermatoses in hoofed animals, causing crusted skin lesions of affected large animals, and persists in their environment within crusts and other debris shed from infected hoof stock
• Dogs, cats, and humans can rarely be secondarily infected.

SIGNALMENT
• Dogs and cats
• No age, breed, or sex predilection

SIGNS

Historical Findings
• Association with farm animals or free-roaming lifestyle often reported
• Cats with subcutaneous disease—episode of trauma; existence of a foreign body; lesions generally chronic; no systemic clinical signs, except when internal organs or large oral lesions develop

Physical Examination Findings
• Dogs—lesions: papular; crusted; mainly on the skin of the trunk or head; circular to coalescent; similar to those in superficial pyoderma caused by *Staphylococcus intermedius;* resemble dermatophilosis in horses (adherent thick, gray-yellow crusts that incorporate hair and leave a circular glistening shallow erosion when removed); pruritus variable

• Cats—subcutaneous, oral, or internal ulcerated and fistulated nodules or abscesses similar to lesions caused by other actinomycetes in this species; superficial pyogenic crusting disease of the face is recently reported.

CAUSES & RISK FACTORS
• Dogs, cats, and humans can be exposed directly from lesions on large animals or from environmental exposure.
• Infectious stage—requires wetting for activation; probably cannot penetrate intact epithelium, thus antecedent minor trauma or mechanical transmission by biting ectoparasites required
• Deeper infections—presumably acquired by traumatic inoculation of infectious material

 DIAGNOSIS

DIFFERENTIAL DIAGNOSIS

Dogs
• Staphylococcal pyoderma
• Acute moist dermatitis
• Dermatophytosis
• Pemphigus foliaceus
• Keratinization disorder

Cats
• Actinomycosis and nocardiosis
• Atypical mycobacterial granuloma
• Sporotrichosis
• Other subcutaneous fungal infection
• Deep mycotic infection, especially *Cryptococcosis*

• Foreign body
• Chronic bite/wound abscess
• Bacterial L-form infection
• *Rhodococcus equi* infection
• Cutaneous or mucosal neoplasm, especially squamous cell carcinoma

CBC/BIOCHEMISTRY/URINALYSIS
Usually normal or neutrophilic leucocytosis in cats

OTHER LABORATORY TESTS N/A

IMAGING N/A

DIAGNOSTIC PROCEDURES

Dogs
• Cytologic examination of crusts—most important procedure; differentiates from more typical bacterial pyodermas
• Organism—distinctive morphology in cytologic and histologic preparations; resembles "railroad tracks" as the bacterium forms chains of small diplococci; chains often branching
• Cytologic diagnosis—from impression smears made of exudate from under crusts or by preparation of minced crusts; mince crusts finely in a drop of water and allow to macerate several minutes; then dry the preparation and stain with any Wright-Giemsa stain.
• Histopathologic specimens—from crusts

Cats
• Histopathologic examination—biopsy of ulcerated nodules; procedure of choice
• Cytologic examination—exudate obtained from aspiration or swabbing of a draining tract

• Culture of biopsy specimens—may yield the organism; facilitated if the laboratory is alerted to the possible presence of *Dermatophilus* (aerobic, relatively slow growing, and easily obscured by contamination)
• Culture from crusts—requires the use of special selective medium; generally employed to corroborate cytologic findings

PATHOLOGIC FINDINGS
• Dogs—crusting and superficial pustular dermatitis; palisading of the crusts with orthokeratotic and parakeratotic hyperkeratosis; organism visualized within the crusts, generally without the use of special bacterial stains
• Cats—pyogranulomatous inflammation; central necrosis; fistulous tract formation; organism visualized near the necrotic center of granulomas, especially with Gram stain

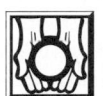 **TREATMENT**
• Dogs—antibacterial shampoo and gentle removal (and disposal) of crusts; shampoo may contain benzoyl peroxide, ethyl lactate, chlorhexidine, or selenium disulfide; one or two applications suffice in most cases
• Cats—for pyogranulomas and abscesses: surgical débridement; exploration for foreign body; establishment of drainage for exudate; maintain effective drainage and postoperative wound care.

 MEDICATIONS

DRUG(S)
• Penicillin V—10 mg/kg PO q12h for 10–20 days; drug of choice
• Tetracycline, doxycycline, or minocycline—standard dosage
• Ampicillin—10–20 mg/kg PO q12h for 10–20 days; some isolates resistant in vitro
• Amoxicillin—10–20 mg/kg PO q12h for 10–20 days; some isolates resistant in vitro

CONTRAINDICATIONS/POSSIBLE INTERACTIONS
Penicillin and ampicillin—allergy

 FOLLOW-UP

PATIENT MONITORING
• Dogs—reexamine after 2 weeks of treatment to ensure complete resolution of symptoms; give an additional 7 days of systemic therapy
• Cats—monitor biweekly for 1 month after apparent resolution of lesions, depending on their location

EXPECTED COURSE AND PROGNOSIS
• Dogs—excellent

• Cats—varies with the location of lesions and extent of surgical débridement; complete resolution can be achieved with timely diagnosis and appropriate surgical and medical therapy.

 MISCELLANEOUS

ZOONOTIC POTENTIAL
• Veterinarians and animal care workers—very seldom infected, even after traumatic exposure when working with farm animals known to be infected
• Dogs and cats—very unlikely to serve as a source for human infection; caution is warranted for exposure of immuno-compromised individuals.

Suggested Reading
Greene CE. Dermatophilosis. In: Greene CE, ed. Infectious diseases of the dog and cat. Philadelphia: Saunders, 1998:326–327.
Kaya O, Kirkan S, Unal B. Isolation of *Dermatophilus congolensis* from a cat. J Vet Med B 47:155–157, 2000.
Scott DW, Miller WH, Jr., Griffin CE. Bacterial Skin Diseases. In: Muller and Kirk's Small Animal Dermatology. 6th ed. Philadelphia: Saunders 2001; 274–335.
Author Carol S. Foil
Consulting Editor Stephen C. Barr

DERMATOPHYTOSIS

 BASICS

DEFINITION
• A cutaneous fungal infection affecting the cornified regions of hair, nails, and occasionally the superficial layers of the skin
• Most commonly isolated organisms—*Microsporum canis, Trichophyton mentagrophytes,* and *M. gypseum*

PATHOPHYSIOLOGY
• Exposure to or contact with a dermatophyte does not necessarily result in an infection.
• Infection may not result in clinical signs.
• Dermatophytes—grow in the keratinized layers of hair, nail, and skin; do not thrive in living tissue or persist in the presence of severe inflammation; incubation period: 1–4 weeks
• An affected animal that does not show signs may remain in this inapparent carrier state for a prolonged period of time; some animals never become symptomatic.
• Corticosteroids can modulate inflammation and prolong the infection.

SYSTEMS AFFECTED
Skin/Exocrine—keratinized layers of the hair, nails, and skin may harbor the hyphae and spores.

GENETICS
N/A

INCIDENCE/PREVALENCE
• Reliance on clinical signs and incorrectly interpreted Wood's lamp examination results in overdiagnosis.
• Infection rates vary widely, depending on the population studied.

GEOGRAPHIC DISTRIBUTION
Although ubiquitous, the incidence is higher in hot and humid regions.

SIGNALMENT
Species
Dogs and cats

Breed Predilections
Cats—more common in long-haired breeds

Mean Age and Range
Clinical signs—more common in young animals

Predominant Sex
None

SIGNS
Historical Findings
• Lesions may begin as alopecia or a poor hair coat.
• A history of previously confirmed infection or exposure to an infected animal or environment (e.g., a cattery) is a useful but not consistent finding.

Physical Examination Findings
• Vary from an inapparent carrier state to a patchy or circular alopecia
• Classic circular alopecia—common in cats; often misinterpreted in dogs
• Scales, erythema, hyperpigmentation, and pruritus—variable
• Paronychosis, granulomatous lesions, or kerions may occur.

CAUSES
• Cats—*M. canis* is by far the most common agent.
• Dogs—*M. canis, M. gypseum,* and *T. mentagrophytes;* incidence of each agent varies geographically.

RISK FACTORS
• Immunocompromising diseases or immunosuppressive medications
• High population density
• Poor nutrition
• Poor management practices
• Lack of an adequate quarantine period

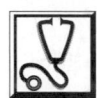 DIAGNOSIS

DIFFERENTIAL DIAGNOSIS
• Cats—miliary dermatitis and almost any other dermatitis
• Dogs—folliculitis, furunculosis, and most cases of alopecia
• Demodicosis and bacterial skin infection—epidermal collarettes more typical of a bacterial infection; grossly enlarged follicular ostia with furunculosis suggest demodicosis; these characteristics are not consistent; concurrent bacterial or mite infections can be seen with dermatophytosis; all three diseases can cause focal hyperpigmentation
• Immune-mediated skin diseases—severe inflammation associated with dermatophytosis affecting the face or feet

CBC/BIOCHEMISTRY/URINALYSIS
Not useful for diagnosis

OTHER LABORATORY TESTS
N/A

IMAGING
N/A

DIAGNOSTIC PROCEDURES
Fungal Culture with Macroconidia Identification
• Best means of confirming diagnosis
• Hairs that exhibit a positive apple-green fluorescence under Wood's lamp examination are considered ideal candidates for culture.
• Pluck hairs from the periphery of an alopecic area; do not use a random pattern.
• Use a sterile toothbrush to brush the hair coat of an asymptomatic animal to yield better results.
• Test media—change to red when they become alkaline; dermatophytes typically produce this color during the early growing phase of their culture; saprophytes, which also produce this color, do so in the late growing phase; thus it is important to examine the media daily.
• Microscopic examination of the macroconidia—necessary to confirm pathogenic dermatophyte and to identify genus and species; helps identify source of infection
• Positive culture—indicates existence of a dermatophyte; however, it may have been there only transiently, as commonly occurs when the culture is obtained from the feet, which are likely to come in contact with a geophilic dermatophyte.

Microscopic Examination of Hair
• Examination after using a clearing solution can help provide a rapid diagnosis.
• Time-consuming and often produces false-negative results
• Use hairs that fluoresce under Wood's lamp illumination to increase the likelihood of identifying the fungal hyphae associated with the hair shaft.
• Wood's lamp examination—not a very useful screening tool; many pathogenic dermatophytes do not fluoresce; false fluorescence is common; lamp should warm up for a minimum of 5 min and then be exposed to suspicious lesions for up to 5 min; a true positive reaction associated with *M. canis* consists of apple-green fluorescence of the hair shaft; keratin associated with epidermal scales and sebum will often produce a false-positive fluorescence.

Skin Biopsy
• Not usually needed
• Can be helpful in confirming true invasion and infection

PATHOLOGIC FINDINGS
• Folliculitis, perifolliculitis, or furunculosis
• Hyperkeratosis
• Intraepidermal pustules
• Pyogranulomatous reaction pattern
• Fungal hyphae may be observed in H&E-stained sections; special stains allow easier visualization of the organism.

TREATMENT

APPROPRIATE HEALTH CARE
• Most animals are treated as outpatients.
• Consider quarantine owing to the infective and zoonotic nature of the disease.

NURSING CARE
N/A

ACTIVITY
N/A

DIET
• A fatty meal improves absorption of griseofulvin.
• An acid meal (add tomato juice) enhances the absorption of ketoconazole.

CLIENT EDUCATION
• Inform owner that many short-haired cats in a single-cat environment and many dogs will undergo spontaneous remission.
• Advise that treatment can be both frustrating and expensive, especially in multianimal households or recurrent cases.
• Inform owner that environmental treatment, including fomites, is important, especially in recurrent cases; dilute bleach (1:10) is a practical and relatively effective means of providing environmental decontamination; concentrated bleach and formalin (1%) are more effective at killing spores, but their use is not as practical in many situations; chlorhexidine was ineffective in pilot studies.
• Inform owner that in a multianimal environment or cattery situation, treatment and control can be very complicated; referral to a veterinarian with expertise in this type of situation should be considered.

SURGICAL CONSIDERATIONS
N/A

MEDICATIONS

DRUG(S) OF CHOICE
• Griseofulvin—most widely prescribed systemic drug; microsized formulation: 25–60 mg/kg PO q12h for 4–6 weeks; ultra-microsized formulation: 2.5–5.0 mg/kg PO q12–24h; pediatric suspension: 10–25 mg/kg PO q12h; gastrointestinal upset is the most common side effect; alleviate by reducing the dose or dividing the dose for more frequent administration
• Ketoconazole—not labeled for use in dogs or cats in the U.S.; dose: 10 mg/kg PO q24h or divided twice per day for 3–4 weeks; anorexia is the most common side effect.
• Lufenuron (Program) @ 100 mg/kg for 2 doses at 2-week intervals and then treat monthly. Response is variable.

• Vaccination—product literature claims are based on clinical signs and Wood's lamp findings; may be useful as an adjuvant to systemic therapy; may be valuable for treating asymptomatic carriers, which can be frustrating to the client and veterinarian and can complicate the diagnosis and management; studies involving dermatophyte cultures as a measure of achieving a cure or prevention are necessary to ensure true efficacy.
• Topical therapy and clipping—once strongly advocated; may help prevent environmental contamination; often associated with an initial exacerbation of signs after the procedures are initiated; lime sulfur (1:16), enilconazole (bottle dilution), and miconazole shampoo are the most effective agents; lime sulfur is odoriferous and can stain; enilconazole is not available in the U.S.

CONTRAINDICATIONS
Corticosteroids

PRECAUTIONS

Griseofulvin
• Bone marrow suppression (anemia, pancytopenia, and neutropenia) can occur as an idiosyncratic reaction or with prolonged therapy.
• Neutropenia—most common fatal reaction in cats; can persist after discontinuation of drug; weekly or biweekly CBC is recommended; can be life-threatening in cats with FIV infection
• Neurologic side effects
• Do not use during the first two trimesters of pregnancy; it is teratogenic.

Ketoconazole
• Hepatopathy has been reported and can be quite severe.
• Inhibits endogenous production of steroidal hormones in dogs

POSSIBLE INTERACTIONS
N/A

ALTERNATIVE DRUG(S)
Itraconazole—similar to ketoconazole but with fewer side effects; probably more effective; expensive; supplied as 100-mg capsules; dose: 10 mg/kg PO q24h or 5 mg/kg PO q12h

FOLLOW-UP

PATIENT MONITORING
• Dermatophyte culture is the only means of truly monitoring response to therapy; many animals will clinically improve, but remain culture positive.
• Repeat fungal cultures toward the end of the treatment regimen and continue treatment until at least one culture result is negative.

• In resistant cases, the culture may be repeated weekly, using the toothbrush technique; continue treatment until 2–3 consecutive culture results are negative.

PREVENTION/AVOIDANCE
• Initiate a quarantine period and obtain dermatophyte cultures of all animals entering the household to prevent reinfection from other animals.
• Consider the possibility of rodents aiding in the spread of the disease.
• Avoid infective soil, if a geophilic dermatophyte is involved
• Consider using griseofulvin for 10–14 days as a prophylactic treatment of exposed animals.

POSSIBLE COMPLICATIONS
False-negative dermatophyte cultures

EXPECTED COURSE AND PROGNOSIS
• Many animals will "self-clear" a dermatophyte infection over a period of a few months.
• Treatment for the disease hastens clinical cure and helps reduce environmental contamination.
• Some infections, particularly in long-haired cats or multianimal situations, can be very persistent.

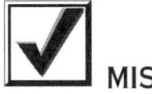

MISCELLANEOUS

ASSOCIATED CONDITIONS
N/A

AGE-RELATED FACTORS
N/A

ZOONOTIC POTENTIAL
Dermatophytosis is zoonotic.

PREGNANCY
• Griseofulvin is teratogenic.
• Ketoconazole can affect steroidal hormone synthesis, especially testosterone.

SYNONYMS
Ringworm

ABBREVIATIONS
• FIV = feline immunodeficiency virus
• H&E = hematoxylin and eosin

Suggested Reading
Moriello KA, DeBoer DJ. Dermatophytosis. In: August JR, ed. Consultations in feline internal medicine 2. Philadelphia: Saunders, 1994:219–225.
Scott DW, Miller WH, Griffin CE, eds. Fungal skin diseases. In: Muller & Kirk's small animal dermatology. 5th ed. Philadelphia: Saunders, 1995:332–350.
Author W. Dunbar Gram
Consulting Editor Karen Helton Rhodes

DERMATOSES, DEPIGMENTING DISORDERS

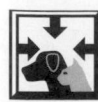 BASICS

DEFINITION
Pathologic or cosmetic condition involving depigmentation of the skin and/or hair coat

SYSTEMS AFFECTED
Skin/Exocrine

SIGNALMENT
• SLE and DLE—collies, Shetland sheepdogs, German shepherds
• DLE—may occur more often in females
• Pemphigus foliaceus—chow chows, akitas
• Uveodermatologic syndrome—akitas, Samoyeds, Siberian huskies
• Vitiligo—Dobermans and Rottweilers, typically < 3 years old
• Seasonal nasal hypopigmentation—Siberian huskies, Alaskan malamutes, Labrador retrievers
• Cutaneous T cell lymphoma (mycosis fungoides)—typically dogs > 10 years old

SIGNS
• Leukotrichia
• Leukoderma
• Erythema
• Erosion and ulcerations

CAUSES
• Nasal solar dermatitis
• DLE
• SLE
• Pemphigus foliaceus
• Pemphigus erythematosus
• Uveodermatologic syndrome
• Contact hypersensitivity
• Vitiligo
• Seasonal nasal depigmentation
• Albinism
• Schnauzer gilding syndrome
• Drug reaction

RISK FACTORS
• Sun exposure—nasal solar dermatitis, DLE, SLE, pemphigus foliaceus, and pemphigus erythematosus
• Poorly pigmented nose—nasal solar dermatitis

 DIAGNOSIS

DIFFERENTIAL DIAGNOSIS

Nasal Solar Dermatitis
• Lesions confined to nose and precipitated by heavy sunlight exposure
• Begins in poorly pigmented skin at the junction of the nasal planum and dorsal muzzle
• Negative for direct immunofluorescence

DLE
• Primarily affects nasal area
• Exacerbated by sunlight
• Positive direct immunofluorescence at basement membrane zone
• Biopsy—interface dermatitis

SLE
• Multisystemic disease
• Skin lesions—often involve nose, face, and mucocutaneous junctions; multifocal or generalized
• ANA—positive
• Positive direct immunofluorescence at basement membrane zone

Pemphigus Foliaceus
• Lesions—usually start on face and ears; commonly involve footpads; eventually generalized
• Biopsy—subcorneal pustules with acantholysis
• Positive direct immunofluorescence in intercellular spaces of epidermis

Pemphigus Erythematosus
• Lesions—primarily confined to face and ears
• Biopsy—intraepidermal pustules with acantholysis and interface dermatitis
• Positive direct immunofluorescence at basement membrane zone and intercellular spaces
• ANA—positive

Uveodermatologic Syndrome
• Typical breed
• Uveitis and cutaneous macular depigmentation with inflammation on nose, lips, and eyelids
• Biopsy of early lesions—interface dermatitis, pigmentary incontinence

Others
• Plastic or rubber dish dermatitis—depigmentation and erythema of the rostral nasal planum and lips; no ulceration and minimal crusting; history of exposure
• Vitiligo—cutaneous macular depigmentation without inflammation on nose, lips, eyelids, footpads, and nails; leukotrichia may be present with leukoderma.
• Seasonal nasal hypopigmentation—normal black coloration of nasal planum fades to light tan or pink; usually seasonal or slowly progressive with age
• Albinism—hereditary lack of pigment of the skin, hair coat, and irises
• Schnauzer gilding syndrome—young miniature schnauzers may develop idiopathic golden hair coat coloration, primarily of the trunk.

• Drug reaction—may resemble various cutaneous disorders such as DLE, SLE, pemphigus foliaceus, and pemphigus erythematosus; pruritus is variable; onset of signs is usually within 2 weeks of administration.

CBC/BIOCHEMISTRY/URINALYSIS
• Usually normal
• SLE—may see hemolytic anemia, thrombocytopenia, or evidence of glomerulonephritis

OTHER LABORATORY TESTS
N/A

IMAGING
N/A

DIAGNOSTIC PROCEDURES
• Cytology—acantholytic cells (pemphigus)
• Joint tap—evidence of polyarthritis in SLE
• ANA—positive in most cases of SLE
• Ocular examination—uveitis in uveodermatologic syndrome
• Direct immunofluorescence—deposition of immunoglobulin at the basement membrane zone with DLE, SLE, and pemphigus erythematosus, and in the intercellular spaces of the epidermis with pemphigus foliaceus and pemphigus erythematosus
• Skin biopsy

PATHOLOGIC FINDINGS
• Interface dermatitis—DLE, SLE, uveodermatologic syndrome
• Intraepidermal pustules with acantholysis—pemphigus foliaceus and pemphigus erythematosus
• Hypomelanosis—vitiligo, uveodermatologic syndrome, seasonal nasal hypopigmentation, and Schnauzer gilding syndrome
• Apoptosis—drug reaction (individual cell necrosis of keratinocytes)

TREATMENT
• Outpatient, except for SLE when severe multiorgan dysfunction is present
• Reduce exposure to sunlight—DLE, SLE, pemphigus erythematosus, and nasal solar dermatitis
• Avoid contact with topical drugs.
• Replace plastic or rubber dishes.
• Application of water-resistant ointments or gels with a SPF > 15 to depigmented areas

MEDICATIONS
DRUG(S) OF CHOICE
• Nasal solar dermatitis—topical corticosteroids; sunscreens (SPF > 15); tattoo hypopigmented skin
• SLE—immunosuppressive therapy with prednisolone, azathioprine (dogs), chlorambucil, or gold salts (cats)
• Vitiligo and nasal depigmentation—no treatment

CONTRAINDICATIONS
• Avoid chrysotherapy in patients with renal disease.
• Azathioprine therapy—not recommended in cats; may cause fatal leukopenia or thrombocytopenia

PRECAUTIONS
Ketoconazole—may cause anorexia, gastric irritation, hepatotoxicity, lightening of the hair coat, or lethargy and inappetence owing to decreased glucocorticoid levels

POSSIBLE INTERACTIONS
N/A

ALTERNATIVE DRUG(S)
N/A

FOLLOW-UP
PATIENT MONITORING
Varies with specific disease and treatment prescribed

POSSIBLE COMPLICATIONS
SLE—associated scarring with ulcerative dermatitis

MISCELLANEOUS
ZOONOTIC POTENTIAL
None

SYNONYMS
None

SEE ALSO
• Cutaneous Drug Eruptions
• Lymphosarcoma, Epidermotropic
• Lupus Erythematosus, Cutaneous (Discoid)
• Lupus Erythematous, Systemic (SLE)
• Pemphigus
• Uveodermatologic syndrome (VKH)

ABBREVIATIONS
• ANA = antinuclear antibody
• DLE = discoid lupus erythematosus
• SLE = systemic lupus erythematous

Suggested Reading
Scott DW, Miller WH, Griffin CE. Muller & Kirk's small animal dermatology. 5th ed. Philadelphia: Saunders, 1995.
Author John G. Gordon
Consulting Editor Karen Helton Rhodes

DERMATOSES, EROSIVE OR ULCERATIVE

 BASICS

DEFINITION
A heterogenous group of skin disorders characterized by disruption of the epidermis (erosions) or, if the basement membrane is compromised, the epidermis and dermis (ulcers).

PATHOPHYSIOLOGY
Varies widely, depending on the cause; may include congenital or developmental disorders that compromise tissue cohesion; cell-mediated (inflammatory or neoplastic) injury; anoxic injury; destruction by trauma, toxins, irritants, contactants, microbial organisms, or parasitic migration; and antigen-specific autoimmune disorders.

SYSTEMS AFFECTED
Skin/Exocrine

SIGNALMENT
Age, breed, and sex predispositions vary according to the disease in question.

SIGNS
N/A

CAUSES

Autoimmune
- Pemphigus foliaceus
- Pemphigus vulgaris
- Bullous pemphigoid
- Systemic or discoid lupus erythematosus
- Cold agglutinin disease

Immune-Mediated
- Erythema multiforme and toxic epidermal necrolysis (usually drug-induced or idiopathic)
- Vasculitis
- Canine eosinophilic furunculosis of the face (may be insect-related)
- Canine juvenile cellulitis (puppy strangles)
- Cutaneous histiocytosis
- Feline indolent ulcer (rodent ulcer)
- Feline hypereosinophilic syndrome

Infectious
- Superficial or deep staphylococcal pyoderma
- Deep fungal (e.g., sporotrichosis, coccidiodomycosis)
- Superficial fungal (malasseziasis, dermatophytosis)
- Atypical mycobacteriosis
- Actinomycetic bacteria (e.g., *Nocardia* spp., *Actinomyces* spp., *Streptomyces* spp.)
- Pythiosis
- Prototheosis
- Leishmaniasis
- Feline cow pox
- FIV/FeLV-related

Parasitic
- Demodicosis
- Sarcoptic/notoedric and demodectic acariases
- Flea bite allergy
- Feline mosquito bite hypersensitivity
- Pelodera and hookworm migration

Congenital/Hereditary
- Canine juvenile dermatomyositis
- Junctional epidermolysis bullosa
- Cutaneous asthenia (Ehlers-Danlos syndrome)
- Aplasia cutis (epitheliogenesis imperfecta)

Metabolic
- Necrolytic migratory erythema (hepatocutaneous syndrome)
- Hyperadrenocorticism (especially when complicated by secondary infections or calcinosis cutis)
- Uremia (mucous membranes)

Neoplastic
- Squamous cell carcinoma
- Squamous cell carcinoma in situ (Bowen's disease)
- Mast cell tumors
- Cutaneous T cell lymphoma (mycosis fungoides)

Nutritional
- Zinc-responsive dermatosis
- Generic dog food dermatosis

Physical/Conformational Dermatoses
- Pressure point ulcers
- Intertrigo
- Self-trauma as a result of pruritic dermatoses

Idiopathic
- Ulcerative dermatosis of collies and shelties
- Feline ulcerative dermatosis with linear subepidermal fibrosis
- Lupoid dermatosis of German short-haired pointers
- Canine and feline acne
- Feline plasma cell pododermatitis

Miscellaneous
- Thermal, electrical, solar, or chemical burns
- Frost bite
- Chemical irritants
- Venomous snake and insect bites
- Thallium toxicosis

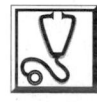 **DIAGNOSIS**

DIFFERENTIAL DIAGNOSIS
- History and physical examination—especially important owing to the extensive differential list (see Causes)
- Ascertain history of pruritus (self-induced ulcers or erosions), exposure to infectious organisms, travel history (for some fungal diseases), diet, and signs of systemic disease.
- Many of the causes have subtle differences in appearance and distribution of lesions.

CBC/BIOCHEMISTRY/URINALYSIS
Most helpful when metabolic disease is suspected or in any patient with signs of systemic disease

OTHER LABORATORY TESTS
Fungal serology and tests for immune-mediated diseases (e.g., ANA titer) may be indicated on a case-by-case basis.

IMAGING
- Rarely indicated
- Thoracic radiographs—for deep/systemic fungal disease
- Thoracic or abdominal radiographs—identify calcinosis associated with hyperadrenocorticism

DIAGNOSTIC PROCEDURES
- Skin scrapings—suspected parasitism
- Direct impression cytology (Tzanck prep)—identify acantholytic cells if pemphigus is suspected
- Fine needle aspirate with cytology—indurated or nodular lesions
- Bacterial (aerobic and anaerobic), mycobacterial, and/or fungal cultures—suspected infectious disease (especially in cats with ulcers or draining tracts)
- Skin biopsy for histopathology—most informative test; for cavitary lesions, the leading edge should be harvested with a scalpel blade if the defect is too large to be excised in total; punch biopsy sufficient for diffuse erosive lesions

 TREATMENT
- Outpatient for most diseases
- Varies widely according to the cause
- Supportive therapy with fluid and nutritional supplementation is indicated in cases with severe fluid and protein loss through transepidermal exudation.

 MEDICATIONS

DRUG(S) OF CHOICE
Vary widely according to cause

CONTRAINDICATIONS
A definitive diagnosis can be imperative, because some immune-mediated cases that require immunosuppression may mimic infectious diseases that require specific antimicrobial chemotherapy (and for which immunosuppression could be fatal).

PRECAUTIONS
Side effects—associated with many antimicrobial, immunosuppressive, and antineoplastic drugs; consult a veterinary drug text.

POSSIBLE INTERACTIONS
Case-by-case basis

ALTERNATIVE DRUGS
N/A

 FOLLOW-UP

PATIENT MONITORING
Case-by-case basis, depending on the disease process, concurrent systemic disease(s), drugs used, and potential side effects expected

POSSIBLE COMPLICATIONS
- Depend on cause
- Some diseases are potentially life-threatening.
- Some diseases have zoonotic potential.
- Superinfections and drug side effects are possible in cases requiring immunosuppression.
- Some infectious diseases (nocardiosis, atypical mycobacteriosis) may be controlled but not cured.

 MISCELLANEOUS

ASSOCIATED CONDITIONS
N/A

AGE-RELATED FACTORS
N/A

ZOONOTIC POTENTIAL
- Sarcoptic acariasis
- Dermatophytosis
- Sporotrichosis
- Mycelial phase of some fungi (e.g., *Coccidioides immitis, Blastomyces dermatitidis*), when grown on culture media, can be infectious to humans through inhalation.
- In-clinic fungal culturing (other than for dermatophytes) is not advised.

PREGNANCY
N/A

SYNONYMS
N/A

SEE ALSO
Specific chapters devoted to diseases listed under Causes

ABBREVIATIONS
- ANA = antinuclear antibody
- FeLV = feline leukemia virus
- FIV = feline immunodeficiency virus

Suggested Reading
Angarano DW. Erosive and ulcerative skin disease. In: Kunkle GA, ed. Veterinary clinics of North America: small animal practice. Feline dermatology. Philadelphia: Saunders, 1995:871–885.
Beale KM. Nodules and draining tracts. In: Kunkle GA, ed. Veterinary clinics of North America: small animal practice. Feline dermatology. Philadelphia: Saunders, 1995:887–900.
Scott DW, Miller WH, Griffin CE, eds. Muller & Kirk's small animal dermatology. 6th ed. Philadelphia: Saunders, 2001.
Author Daniel O. Morris
Consulting Editor Karen Helton-Rhodes

DERMATOSES, EXFOLIATIVE

 BASICS

DEFINITION
Excessive or abnormal shedding of epidermal cells resulting in the clinical presentation of cutaneous scaling

PATHOPHYSIOLOGY
• An increase in the production, an increase in the desquamation, or a decrease in the cohesion of keratinocytes results in abnormal shedding of epidermal cells individually (fine scale) and in sheets (coarse scale). • Primary exfoliative disorders—keratinization defects, in which the genetic control of epidermal cell proliferation and maturation is abnormal • Secondary exfoliative disorders—from the effects of disease states on the normal maturation and proliferation of epidermal cells

SYSTEMS AFFECTED
• Skin/Exocrine—epidermal tissues, including nails

SIGNALMENT
• Primary—apparent by 2 years of age; characteristic in affected breeds (see Causes) • Secondary—any age; any breed of dog or cat

SIGNS

Historical Findings
• Excessive scaling • Malodorous skin • Pruritus

Physical Examination Findings
• Dry or greasy accumulations of fine scale or coarse rafts of epidermal cells located diffusely throughout the hair coat or focally in keratinaceous plaques • "Rancid fat" odor common • Comedones • Follicular casts (accumulation of adherent debris around the hair shaft) • Alopecia • Pruritus • Secondary pyoderma • *Malassezia* overgrowth

CAUSES

Primary
• Primary idiopathic seborrhea (primary keratinization disorder)—primary cellular defect; accelerated epidermopoiesis and hyperproliferation of the epidermis, follicular infundibulum, and sebaceous gland identified in some breeds; breeds at highest risk: cocker and springer spaniels, West Highland white terriers, basset hounds, Doberman pinschers, Irish setters, and Labrador retrievers; dry (sicca) and greasy (oleosa) forms exist, but determination of type has little prognostic value. • Vitamin A–responsive dermatosis—nutritionally responsive; seen primarily in young cocker spaniels; clinical signs similar to severe idiopathic seborrhea; distinguished by the response to dietary vitamin A supplementation • Zinc-responsive dermatosis—nutritionally responsive; results in alopecia,

scaling, crusting, and erythema around the eyes, ears, feet, lips, and other external orifices; two syndromes: young adult dogs (especially Siberian huskies and Alaskan malamutes) and rapidly growing, large-breed puppies • Ectodermal defects—follicular dysplasias; seen as color mutant or dilution alopecia; represent abnormalities in melanization of the hair shaft and structural hair growth; keratinization defects theorized as causative for several syndromes; breeds commonly affected: blue and fawn Doberman pinschers, Irish setters, dachshunds, chow chows, Yorkshire terriers, poodles, great Danes, whippets, salukis, and Italian greyhounds; signs include the failure to regrow blue or fawn hair with normal "point" hair growth, excessive scaliness, comedone formation, and secondary pyoderma • Idiopathic nasodigital hyperkeratosis—excessive accumulation of scale and crusts on the nasal planum and footpad margins; common in middle-aged spaniels; lesions generally asymptomatic, unless severe enough to result in cracking and secondary bacterial infection • Sebaceous adenitis—inflammatory disease; breeds: middle-aged standard poodles, akitas, and Samoyeds; characteristic diffuse hair loss and excessive scaling; tightly adherent follicular casts; most dogs are generally healthy and asymptomatic; akitas: frequently develop severe and deep bacterial pyoderma; Vizslas: disease appears distinctly different and granulomatous • Epidermal dysplasia and ichthyosis—rare and severe congenital disorder of keratinization; reported in West Highland white terriers; generalized accumulations of scale and crusts at an early age; secondary infections (bacterial and yeast) common; prognosis in severe cases is poor

Secondary
• Cutaneous hypersensitivity—atopy, flea allergic dermatitis, food allergy, and contact dermatitis; pruritus and resultant skin trauma and irritation • Ectoparasitism—scabies, demodicosis, and cheyletiellosis; inflammation and exfoliation • Pyoderma—skin infection; bacterial enzymatic dyshesion and increased exfoliation of keratinocytes in the attempt to shed pathogenic organisms • Dermatophytosis—commonly exfoliative; increased shedding of affected keratinocytes is a primary skin mechanism in resolving fungal infection. • Endocrinopathy—hypothyroidism and hyperadrenocorticism commonly produce excessive scaling; hypothyroidism: abnormalities in keratinization, failure to regrow hair, and excessive sebum production; hyperadrenocorticism: abnormal keratinization and decreased follicular activity; secondary pyoderma common in both

syndromes; other hormonal abnormalities (e.g., sex hormone abnormalities, hyperthyroidism, and diabetes mellitus) may also be associated with excessive scaling. • Age—geriatric animals may have a dull, brittle, and scaly hair coat; changes may be caused by natural alterations in epidermal metabolism associated with age; no specific defect identified • Nutritional disorders—malnutrition and generic dog food dermatosis; result in scaling from abnormalities in keratinization • Autoimmune skin diseases—pemphigus complex: may appear exfoliative owing to rupturing of fragile vesicles and secondary pyoderma; cutaneous and systemic lupus erythematosus: cutaneous signs frequently appear as regions of alopecia and scaling. • Neoplasia—primary epidermal neoplasia (epidermotropic lymphoma): may produce alopecia and scaling as epidermal structures are damaged; preneoplastic conditions (alopecia mucinosis, actinic keratosis): initially appear exfoliative • Miscellaneous—any disease process may result in excessive scale formation owing to metabolic dyscrasia or cutaneous inflammation.

RISK FACTORS
N/A

 DIAGNOSIS

DIFFERENTIAL DIAGNOSIS
• Signalment and history—paramount in distinguishing the possible causes of exfoliation • Occurrence of pruritus—assists in determining the possibility of a cutaneous hypersensitivity; primary keratinization defects are often nonpruritic, unless secondary pyoderma develops. • Concurrent signs (e.g., lethargy, weight gain, polyuria/polydipsia, reproductive failure, change in body conformation, and lack of hair regrowth), with or without inflammation, can assist in differentiation.

CBC/BIOCHEMISTRY/URINALYSIS
• Normal with primary keratinization disorders • Mild, nonregenerative anemia and hypercholesteremia are consistent with hypothyroidism. • Neutrophilia, monocytosis, eosinopenia, lymphopenia, elevated serum alkaline phosphatase, hypercholesterolemia, and hyposthenuria suggest hyperadrenocorticism.

OTHER LABORATORY TESTS
Thyroid hormone levels and adrenal function tests if an endocrinopathy is suspected; see specific chapters for test recommendations.

IMAGING
N/A

DIAGNOSTIC PROCEDURES

- Skin scrapings—diagnose ectoparasitism
- Skin biopsy—rule out particular differential diagnoses; strongly recommended for most cases
- Intradermal skin testing—identify atopy
- Food-elimination trial—identify food allergy
- Epidermal exudate preparations—determine type of microflora on the skin

TREATMENT

- Frequent and appropriate topical therapy—cornerstone of proper treatment
- Underbathing, rather than overbathing, is a common error.
- Diagnose and control all treatable primary and secondary diseases.
- Recurrence of secondary pyoderma may require repeated therapy and further diagnostics.
- Maintaining control is often lifelong.

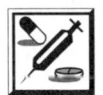

MEDICATIONS

DRUG(S) OF CHOICE

Shampoos

- Contact time—5–15 min required; > 15 min discouraged, because it results in epidermal maceration, loss of barrier function, and excessive epidermal drying
- Hypoallergenic (soap free)—useful only in mild cases of dry scale and to maintain secondary exfoliation after the primary disease has been controlled
- Sulfur/salicylic acid—keratolytic, keratoplastic, and bacteriostatic; an excellent first choice for the moderately scaly patient; not overly drying
- Benzoyl peroxide—strongly keratolytic, antimicrobial, and follicle flushing; may cause irritation and severe dryness; benzoyl peroxide best for recurrent bacterial infection and/or extreme greasiness
- Ethyl lactate—less effective than benzoyl peroxide for follicular flushing and antimicrobial activity, but not as irritating or drying; most useful for moderate pyoderma and dry scale
- Tar—keratolytic, keratoplastic, and antipruritic; degreasing, but less so than benzoyl peroxide; use for moderate scale associated with pruritus

Moisturizers

- Excellent for restoring skin hydration (frequent shampooing may result in excessive dryness and discomfort) and increasing effectiveness of subsequent shampoos
- Humectants—encourage hydration of the stratum corneum by attracting water from the dermis; at high concentrations may be keratolytic

- Microencapsulation—recent advances may improve the residual activity of moisturizers by permitting sustained release after bathing.
- Emollients—coat the skin; smooth the roughened surfaces produced by excessive scaling; usually combined with occlusives to encourage hydration of the epidermis

Systemic Therapy

- Specific causes require specific treatments (i.e., thyroxine replacement for hypothyroidism; zinc supplements for zinc-responsive dermatosis).
- Systemic antibiotics—always indicated for secondary pyoderma
- Retinoid drugs—varied success for idiopathic or primary seborrhea; reports of individual response to retinoids (especially cocker spaniels with a primary keratinization defect); generally, topical therapy provides more benefits for dogs than does retinoid administration; vitamin A analogs (soriatane and isotretinoin) used in limited studies
- Cyclosporine (Neoral®)–5 mg/kg/day until controlled, then decreased to minimal effective maintenance dosage effective for individual cases of keratinization disorder associated with hypersensitivity and/or *Malassezia* dermatitis
- Ketoconazole—10 mg/kg/day for severe *Malassezia* dermatitis

CONTRAINDICATIONS

N/A

PRECAUTIONS

- Corticosteroids—may be used judiciously to control the inflammation resulting from many exfoliative disorders; will mask signs of pyoderma and prevent accurate diagnosis of primary disease
- Vitamin A and D analogs—side effects can be severe; thus, patients should be referred to a dermatologist before being treated with these experimental drugs.

POSSIBLE INTERACTIONS

N/A

ALTERNATIVE DRUG(S)

N/A

FOLLOW-UP

PATIENT MONITORING

- Antibiotics and topical therapy—recheck every 3 weeks to monitor response; patients may respond differently to the various topical therapies. • Seasonal changes, development of additional diseases (especially cutaneous hypersensitivity), and recurrence of pyoderma—may cause previously controlled patients to worsen; re-evaluation critical for determining if new factors are involved and if changes in therapy are necessary

- Endocrinopathies—after pill administration, routine 4–6-hr thyroid monitoring or ACTH-stimulation tests should be used for proper management
- Selective autoimmune disorders—re-evaluate frequently during the initial phase of induction; less often after remission; clinical evaluation and laboratory data required
- Immunosuppressive therapy—frequent hemograms, serum chemistries, and urinalyses with culture to monitor for complications
- Retinoid drugs—serum chemistries, including triglycerides, and Schirmer tear tests • Ketoconazole—serum chemistries

POSSIBLE COMPLICATIONS

N/A

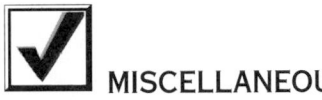

MISCELLANEOUS

ASSOCIATED CONDITIONS

N/A

AGE-RELATED FACTORS

N/A

ZOONOTIC POTENTIAL

Dermatophytosis and several ectoparasites have either zoonotic potential or the ability to produce human lesions.

PREGNANCY

- Sulfonamide antibiotics and chloramphenicol—do not use in pregnant animals.
- Systemic retinoids and vitamin A in therapeutic dosages—do not use in intact females, because of severe and predictable teratogenicity and the extremely long withdrawal period

SYNONYMS

Keratinization disorders—seborrhea, idiopathic seborrhea, keratinization defect, dyskeratinization, and incorrect human terms (eczema and psoriasis); sebopsoriasis: correct term to describe the similarities between some human and canine keratinization defects

SEE ALSO

- Atopy • Demodicosis
- Hyperadrenocorticism (Cushing Disease)
- Hypothyroidism • *Malassezia* Dermatitis
- Pyoderma • Sarcoptic Mange

ABBREVIATION

- ACTH = adrenocorticotropic hormone

Suggested Reading

Griffin CE, Kwochka KW, Macdonald JM. Current veterinary dermatology: the science and art of therapy. St. Louis: Mosby, 1993.

Author Alexander H. Werner
Consulting Editor Karen Helton Rhodes

DERMATOSES, PAPULONODULAR

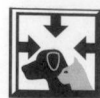 **BASICS**

DEFINITION
Diseases whose primary lesions may manifest as papules and nodules, which are solid, elevated lesions of the skin

PATHOPHYSIOLOGY
• Papules—usually the result of tissue infiltration by inflammatory cells; accompanying intraepidermal edema or epidermal hyperplasia and dermal edema
• Nodules—larger than papules; usually the result of a massive infiltration of inflammatory cells into the dermis or subcutis

SYSTEMS AFFECTED
Skin/Exocrine

SIGNALMENT
Any age, breed, or sex

CAUSES
• Superficial and deep bacterial folliculitis
• Dermatophytosis
• Sebaceous adenitis
• Sterile eosinophilic pustulosis
• Canine and feline acne
• Kerions
• Demodicosis
• Rhabditic dermatitis
• Actinic conditions
• Sterile idiopathic periadnexal pyogranulomatous dermatitis
• Cutaneous histiocytosis

RISK FACTORS
• Folliculitis, dermatophytosis, and demodicosis—any disease or medication that causes immune compromise predisposes animals
• Rhabditic dermatitis—may be associated with contact with decaying organic debris (straw or hay) containing *Pelodera strongyloides*

• Actinic conditions—seen more frequently in outdoor, short-haired dogs living in areas with ample sunlight

 DIAGNOSIS

DIFFERENTIAL DIAGNOSIS
• See Causes
• These diseases can be most easily differentiated by diagnostic tests (see below).

CBC/BIOCHEMISTRY/URINALYSIS
• Should be within normal range in most patients
• A circulating eosinophilia may be present with sterile eosinophilic pustulosis.

OTHER LABORATORY TESTS
N/A

IMAGING
N/A

DIAGNOSTIC PROCEDURES
• Skin scrapings—identify possible *Demodex* mites or rhabditiform larvae
• Dermatophyte cultures—identify possible dermatophytosis
• Tzanck preparations—determine if bacteria and degenerative neutrophils are present; compatible with bacterial folliculitis; eosinophils indicate eosinophilic pustulosis or furunculosis is more likely
• Skin biopsy—if none of these tests has revealed a definitive diagnosis

 TREATMENT

• For nearly all causes, animal can be treated as an outpatient.
• Generalized demodicosis and secondary sepsis require hospitalization.
• Alteration of activity or diet should not be necessary.

 MEDICATIONS

DRUG(S) OF CHOICE
Bacterial Folliculitis
• Superficial pyoderma—appropriate antibiotics based on bacterial culture and sensitivity should be given for 3–4 weeks
• Deep pyoderma—appropriate antibiotics based on bacterial culture and sensitivity should be given for 6–8 weeks or more

Sebaceous Adenitis
• A 50%–75% mixture of propylene glycol and water once daily as a spray to affected areas or bathing and soaking in baby oil weekly
• Essential fatty acid dietary supplements (PO q12h) in addition to evening primrose oil (500 mg PO q12h)
• Refractory cases—isotretinoin (1 mg/kg PO q12–24h); if response is seen, taper dosage (1 mg/kg q48h or 0.5 mg/kg q24h)
• Cyclosporine has also been used (5 mg/kg PO q12h).
• Most cases are refractory to corticosteroids.

Canine Acne
• May resolve without therapy in mild cases
• More severe cases—benzoyl peroxide shampoos and gels every 24 hr until lesions resolve; then as needed
• Mupirocin—topical antibiotic; apply every 24 hr or alternate with the benzoyl peroxide therapies
• Recurrent or very deep infection (furunculosis)—systemic antibiotics and warm water soaks
• Very refractory cases—topical tretinoin (every 12 hr) or isotretinoin (1–2 mg/kg PO q24h)
Feline Acne
• Underlying cause should be sought and treated accordingly
• No underlying cause found—Stri-Dex pads or benzoyl peroxide gels used daily or alternated daily

- Cats can be sensitive to the irritant effects of benzoyl peroxide.
- Refractory cases—try systemic antibiotics

Rhabditic Dermatitis
- Remove and destroy bedding.
- Wash kennels, beds, and cages and treat with a premise insecticide or flea spray.
- Bathe affected animal and remove crusts.
- Parasiticidal dip—at least 2 times at weekly intervals
- Severe infection—antibiotics may be necessary

Actinic Conditions
- Sunlight—avoid between 10 A.M. and 4 P.M; apply sunscreen with an SPF ≥ 15 every 12 hr
- Severe inflammation—topical or systemic corticosteroids may provide comfort; topical, 1%–2.5% hydrocortisone usually sufficient; systemic, prednisone (initially, 1 mg/kg PO for 3–5 days)
- Secondary infection—antibiotics may be necessary
- Squamous cell carcinoma—prognosis is guarded to poor, depending on the stage of the disease; therapy includes synthetic retinoids, hyperthermia, cryosurgery, photochemotherapy, radiation therapy, and surgical excision

Sterile Nodular Dermatoses
- Cyclosporine (Neoral) @ 5mg/kg PO once daily (no food 2 hr before or after dosing)
- Tetracycline and niacinamide combinations
- Corticosteroids at immunosuppresive doses
- Chemotherapeutic drugs (chlorambucil or azathioprine)

Other
- Dermatophytosis—see specific chapter
- Sterile eosinophilic pustulosis—prednisolone/prednisone (2.2–4.4 mg/kg q24h; then taper to an alternate-day low dosage)
- Kerion—see Dermatophytosis
- Demodicosis—see specific chapter

CONTRAINDICATIONS
Corticosteroids and other immune suppressants should be avoided with folliculitis, dermatophytosis, kerions, and demodicosis.

PRECAUTIONS
- Fatty acids—use with caution in dogs with inflammatory bowel disease or recurrent bouts of pancreatitis
- Isotretinoin—may cause keratoconjunctivitis sicca, hyperactivity, ear pruritus, erythematous mucocutaneous junction, lethargy with vomiting, abdominal distension and erythema, anorexia with lethargy, collapse, and swollen tongue; CBC and chemistry screen abnormalities include high platelet count, hypertriglyceridemia, hypercholesterolemia, and high alanine transaminase.
- Cyclosporine—may cause vomiting and diarrhea, gingival hyperplasia, B lymphocyte hyperplasia, hirsutism, papillomatous skin lesions, and high incidence of infection; potential toxic reactions include nephrotoxicity and hepatotoxicity.

POSSIBLE INTERACTIONS
N/A

ALTERNATIVE DRUG(S)
N/A

 **FOLLOW-UP**

PATIENT MONITORING
- CBC, chemistry screen, and urinalysis—monitor monthly for 4–6 months in patients receiving cyclosporine and synthetic retinoid therapy
- Tear production—monitor monthly for 4–6 months, then every 6 months in patients receiving synthetic retinoid therapy
- Skin scrapings—monitor therapy in patients with demodicosis (see Demodicosis)
- Repeat fungal cultures—monitor therapy in patients with dermatophytosis (see Dermatophytosis)

- Resolution of lesions—monitor progress of sebaceous adenitis, actinic conditions, and all other diseases.

POSSIBLE COMPLICATIONS
Actinic conditions may progress to squamous cell carcinoma.

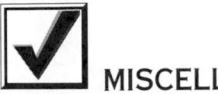 **MISCELLANEOUS**

ASSOCIATED CONDITIONS
N/A

AGE-RELATED FACTORS
N/A

ZOONOTIC POTENTIAL
Dermatophytosis—contagious to humans in 30%–50% of cases of *Microsporum canis*

PREGNANCY
- Synthetic retinoids—very teratogenic; do not use in pregnant animals, animals intended for reproduction, or intact animals; should not be used by women of childbearing age
- Corticosteroids—do not use in pregnant animals

SYNONYMS
N/A

SEE ALSO
- Demodicosis
- Dermatophytosis
- Pyoderma

Suggested Reading
Griffin CE, Kwochka KW, MacDonald JM, eds. Current veterinary dermatology. St. Louis: Mosby, 1993.
Gross TL, Ihrke PJ, Walder EJ. Veterinary dermatopathology. St. Louis: Mosby, 1992.
Scott DW, Miller WH, Griffen CE. Mueller & Kirk's Small Animal Dermatology. 6th ed, Philadelphia: Saunders, 2001.
Authors Karen A. Kuhl and Jean Swingle Greek
Consulting Editor Karen Helton Rhodes

DERMATOSES, STERILE NODULAR/GRANULOMATOUS

BASICS

DEFINITION
Diseases whose primary lesions are nodules that are solid, elevated, and > 1 cm in diameter

PATHOPHYSIOLOGY
• Nodules—usually result from an infiltration of inflammatory cells into the dermis and subcutis; may be secondary to endogenous or exogenous stimuli
• Inflammation is typically, but not always, granulomatous to pyogranulomatous.

SYSTEMS AFFECTED
• Skin/Exocrine
• Several of these conditions may affect internal organs.

SIGNALMENT
• Nodular dermatofibrosis—German shepherds, 3–5 years old
• Calcinosis circumscripta—German shepherds, < 2 years old
• Malignant histiocytosis—Bernese mountain dogs
• May affect any age, breed, or sex, although Bernese mountain dogs are at higher risk for malignant histiocytosis and German shepherds are at higher risk for nodular dermatofibrosis

CAUSES
• Amyloidosis
• Foreign body reaction
• Spherulocytosis
• Idiopathic sterile granuloma and pyogranuloma
• Canine eosinophilic granuloma
• Calcinosis cutis
• Calcinosis circumscripta
• Malignant histiocytosis
• Cutaneous histiocytosis
• Sterile panniculitis
• Nodular dermatofibrosis
• Cutaneous xanthoma

RISK FACTORS
• Foreign body reaction—induced by exposure to any irritating material (e.g., concrete dust or fiberglass)
• Hair foreign bodies—increased risk for large dogs that rest on very hard surfaces
• Calcinosis cutis—increased risk with exposure to high doses of exogenous glucocorticoids
• Panniculitis—increased risk with vitamin E–deficient diet

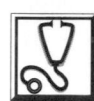

DIAGNOSIS

DIFFERENTIAL DIAGNOSIS
• See Causes
• Sterile nodular dermatoses—must be differentiated from deep bacterial and fungal infections and dermal neoplasias
• All of these diseases can be diagnosed by histopathology and deep tissue cultures.

CBC/BIOCHEMISTRY/URINALYSIS
• Normal in most conditions causing sterile nodules
• Amyloidosis—possible changes in biochemistry and/or urinalysis if internal organs are affected
• Malignant histiocytosis—pancytopenia
• Calcinosis cutis—changes characteristic of hyperglucocorticoidism (e.g., stress leukogram, high ALP, hyperglycemia, low urine specific gravity)
• Cutaneous xanthomas—may be glucosuria, hyperglycemia, and/or lipid profile abnormalities

OTHER LABORATORY TESTS
Serum ferritin levels—may be high with malignant histiocytosis but not with cutaneous histiocytosis

IMAGING
• Radiology and ultrasonography—delineate involvement of internal organs in amyloidosis and histiocytosis
• Radiology—identify other areas of dystrophic calcification in dogs with calcinosis cutis
• Ultrasonography—identify cystadenocarcinomas in dogs with nodular dermatofibrosis

DIAGNOSTIC PROCEDURES
Skin biopsies for histopathology and cultures (fungal, aerobic, and mycobacterial) are essential for nodular dermatoses.

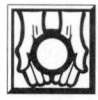

TREATMENT
• Most of these disorders can be treated on an outpatient basis.
• A few of these disorders (e.g., malignant histiocytosis, amyloidosis, and nodular dermatofibrosis) are almost always fatal.
• Dogs with calcinosis cutis may need to be hospitalized for sepsis and intense topical therapy.

MEDICATIONS

DRUG(S)
• Amyloidosis—no known therapy, unless the lesion is solitary and can be surgically removed
• Sperulocytosis—only effective treatment is surgical removal
• Idiopathic sterile granuloma and pyogranuloma—prednisone (2.2–4.4 mg/kg

DERMATOSES, STERILE NODULAR/GRANULOMATOUS

divided PO q12h) is the first line of therapy; continue steroids for 7–14 days after complete remission; then taper dose; for cases that are refractory to glucocorticoids, azathioprine (2.2 mg/kg PO q48h) in combination with prednisone or sodium iodide may be tried
• Foreign body reactions—best treated by removal of the offending substance if possible; for hair foreign bodies, the dog should be placed on softer bedding and topical therapy with keratolytic agents should be initiated; many dogs with hair foreign bodies also have secondary deep bacterial infections that need to be treated with both topical and systemic antibiotics.
• Canine eosinophilic granuloma— prednisone (1.1–2.2 mg/kg PO q24h) produces a good response
• Malignant histiocytosis—no effective therapy; it is rapidly fatal.
• Cutaneous histiocytosis—high-dose glucocorticoids and cytotoxic drugs result in remission; recurrences are common; L-asparaginase has been helpful in some cases.
• Calcinosis cutis—underlying disease must be controlled if possible; most cases require antibiotics to control secondary bacterial infections; hydrotherapy and frequent bathing in antibacterial shampoos minimize secondary problems; topical DMSO is useful (applied to no more than one-third of the body once daily until lesions resolve); if lesions are extensive, serum calcium levels should be monitored closely.
• Calcinosis circumscripta—surgical excision is the therapy of choice in most cases.
• Sterile panniculitis—single lesions can be removed surgically; prednisone (2.2 mg/kg

PO q24h or divided PO q12h) is the treatment of choice; administered until lesions regress; then tapered; some dogs remain in long-term remission, but others require prolonged alternate-day therapy; a few cases respond to oral vitamin E (400 IU q12h).
• Nodular dermatofibrosis—no therapy for most cases, because the cystadenocarcinomas are usually bilateral; for rare unilateral case of cystadenocarcinoma or a cystadenoma, removal of the single affected kidney may be helpful.
• Cutaneous xanthoma—correction of the underlying diabetes mellitus or hyperlipoproteinemia is usually curative.

CONTRAINDICATIONS
Corticosteroids and other immunosuppressive drugs should be avoided, if possible, in any animal with a secondary infection.

PRECAUTIONS
DMSO—handle with care; monitor serum calcium levels if used to treat calcinosis cutis.

POSSIBLE INTERACTIONS
N/A

ALTERNATIVE DRUGS
N/A

 FOLLOW-UP

PATIENT MONITORING
• Patients on long-term glucocorticoids should have a CBC, chemistry screen, urinalysis, and urine culture done every 6 months.
• Dogs being treated with DMSO for calcinosis cutis should have calcium levels checked every 7–14 days, starting at the beginning of therapy.

POSSIBLE COMPLICATIONS
Systemic amyloidosis, malignant histiocytosis, and nodular dermatofibrosis—invariably fatal

 **MISCELLANEOUS**

ASSOCIATED CONDITIONS
• Calcinosis cutis—hyperglucocorticoidism, chronic renal failure, and diabetes mellitus
• Calcinosis circumscripta—(occasionally) hypertrophic osteodystrophy and idiopathic polyarthritis
• Nodular dermatofibrosis—cystadeno-carcinomas
• Cutaneous xanthoma—diabetes mellitus and hyperlipoproteinemia

SEE ALSO
• Adenocarcinoma, Renal
• Amyloidosis
• Hyperadrenocorticism (Cushing's Disease)

ABBREVIATIONS
• ALP = alkaline phosphatase
• DMSO = dimethyl sulfoxide

Suggested Reading

Griffin CE, Kwochka KW, MacDonald JM, eds. Current veterinary dermatology. St Louis: Mosby, 1993.
Gross TL, lhrke PJ, Walder EJ. Veterinary dermatopathology. St Louis: Mosby, 1992.
Scott DW, Miller BH, Griffin CE, eds. Muller & Kirk's small animal dermatology. 5th ed. Philadelphia: Saunders, 1995.
Author Dawn E. Logas
Consulting Editor Karen Helton Rhodes

DERMATOSES, VESICULOPUSTULAR

 BASICS

DEFINITION
• Pustule—small, circumscribed elevation of the epidermis filled with pus
• Vesicle—small, circumscribed elevation of the epidermis filled with clear fluid

PATHOPHYSIOLOGY
Pustules and vesicles—produced by edema, acantholysis (pemphigus), ballooning degeneration (viral infections), proteolytic enzymes from neutrophils (pyoderma), degeneration of basal cells (lupus), or dermoepidermal separation (bullous pemphigoid)

SYSTEMS AFFECTED
• Multiple systems with SLE
• Skin/Exocrine—integument and muscle with dermatomyositis

SIGNALMENT
• Lupus—collies, shelties, and German shepherds may be predisposed
• Pemphigus erythematosus—collies and German shepherds may be predisposed
• Pemphigus foliaceus—akitas, chow chows, dachshunds, bearded collies, Newfoundlands, Doberman pinschers, and schipperkes may be predisposed
• Bullous pemphigoid—collies and Doberman pinschers may be predisposed
• Dermatomyositis—young collies and shelties
• Subcorneal pustular dermatosis—schnauzers affected most frequently
• Linear IgA dermatosis—dachshunds exclusively
• Dermatophytosis—young animals

SIGNS
N/A

CAUSES
Pustules
• Superficial pyoderma—impetigo, superficial spreading pyoderma, superficial bacterial folliculitis, acne
• Pemphigus complex—pemphigus foliaceus, pemphigus erythematosus, pemphigus vegetans
• Subcorneal pustular dermatosis
• Dermatophytosis
• Sterile eosinophilic pustulosis
• Linear IgA dermatosis

Vesicles
• SLE
• DLE

• Bullous pemphigoid
• Pemphigus vulgaris
• Dermatomyositis

RISK FACTORS
• Drug exposure—SLE and bullous pemphigoid
• Pyodermas are usually secondary to a predisposing factor (e.g., demodicosis, hypothyroidism, allergy, or steroid administration)
• Sunlight—pemphigus erythematosus, bullous pemphigoid, SLE, DLE, and dermatomyositis

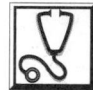 DIAGNOSIS

DIFFERENTIAL DIAGNOSIS
Pustular
Superficial Pyodermas
• Most common cause
• Readily respond to appropriate antibiotic therapy if the underlying cause is effectively managed
• Intact pustule—direct smear reveals neutrophils engulfing bacteria; culture usually yields *Staphylococcus intermedius;* biopsy shows intraepidermal neutrophilic pustules or folliculitis.

Pemphigus Complex
• A group of immune-mediated diseases characterized histologically by acantholytic cells
• Direct smears—many acantholytic cells, nondegenerate neutrophils, and no bacteria
• Culture of an intact pustule negative
• Direct immunofluorescence—deposits in the intercellular spaces of the epidermis in approximately 50% of the cases
• Tends to wax and wane irrespective of antibiotic therapy; responds to immunosuppressive therapy

Subcorneal Pustular Dermatosis
• A rare idiopathic pustular dermatosis of dogs
• Tends to wax and wane
• Intact pustules—direct smears reveal numerous neutrophils, no bacteria, and occasional acantholytic cells; cultures negative
• Direct immunofluorescence negative
• Poor response to glucocorticoids and antibiotics

Dermatophytosis
• Common disease of both dogs and cats
• Dermatophyte culture positive
• Secondary bacterial infection common
• Biopsy—folliculitis with fungal elements

Sterile Eosinophilic Pustulosis
• A rare idiopathic dermatosis of dogs
• Direct smears—numerous eosinophils, nondegenerate neutrophils, occasional acantholytic cells, and no bacteria
• Biopsy—eosinophilic intraepidermal pustules, folliculitis, and furunculosis
• Direct immunofluorescence negative
• Rapid response to glucocorticoids

Linear IgA Dermatosis
• A rare idiopathic dermatosis of dachshunds
• Tends to wax and wane
• Pustules—sterile and subcorneal
• Direct immunofluorescence positive for IgA at the basement membrane zone

Vesicles/Ulceration
SLE
• A multisystemic disease with variable clinical signs and cutaneous manifestations, including mucocutaneous ulceration
• Direct immunofluorescence positive at the basement membrane zone
• ANA positive

DLE
• Affects only the skin; lesions usually confined to the face
• Depigmentation, erythema, and ulceration of the nasal planum common
• Biopsy—interface dermatitis
• Direct immunofluorescence positive at the basement membrane zone
• ANA negative

Bullous Pemphigoid
• Ulcerative disorder of the skin and/or mucous membranes
• Biopsy—subepidermal cleft formation
• Direct immunofluorescence positive at the basement membrane zone
• Acantholysis is not seen.

Pemphigus Vulgaris
• Most severe form of pemphigus
• Characterized by ulceration of the oral cavity, mucocutaneous junction, and skin
• Biopsy—suprabasal acantholysis and cleft formation
• Direct immunofluorescence positive at the intercellular spaces of the epidermis

Dermatomyositis
• An idiopathic inflammatory disease of the skin and muscle of young collies and shelties
• Lesions affect the face, ear tips, tail tip, and pressure points of the extremities.
• Characterized by alopecia, crusting, pigmentation disturbances, erosions/ulceration, and scarring

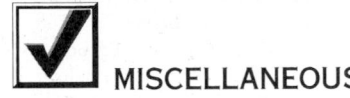

- Biopsy—follicular atrophy, perifolliculitis, and hydropic degeneration of the basal cells
- Direct immunofluorescence negative
- Muscle biopsy and EMG—evidence of inflammation

CBC/BIOCHEMISTRY/URINALYSIS
- Results usually unremarkable
- SLE—anemia, thrombocytopenia, or glomerulonephritis may develop.
- Eosinophilic pustular dermatosis—most affected dogs have peripheral eosinophilia.

OTHER LABORATORY TESTS
N/A

IMAGING
N/A

DIAGNOSTIC PROCEDURES
- Direct smear from intact pustule
- Culture of intact pustule
- Biopsy for histopathology
- Direct immunofluorescence, including IgA
- ANA titer
- EMG
- Muscle biopsy

TREATMENT
- Periodic bathing with an antimicrobial shampoo—helps remove surface debris and control secondary bacterial infections
- Usually treated as an outpatient
- SLE, pemphigus vulgaris, and bullous pemphigoid may be life-threatening and require inpatient intensive care.

MEDICATIONS

DRUG(S) OF CHOICE

Pemphigus Complex/Bullous Pemphigoid
- Chemotherapeutic drugs: azathioprine or chlorambucil
- Tetracycline and niacinamide combination
- Cyclosporine (Neoral)

Subcorneal Pustular Dermatosis
- Dapsone—1 mg/kg PO q8h until remission (usually 1–4 weeks); then tapered to 1 mg/kg q24h or twice weekly
- Sulfasalazine (Azulfidine)—10–20 mg/kg PO q8h until remission; then as needed

Linear IgA Dermatosis
- Prednisolone—2.2–4.4 mg/kg PO q24h until remission; then taper to alternate-day therapy
- Dapsone—1 mg/kg PO q8h until remission; then taper and give as needed; individual patients may respond to one drug and not the other.

Sterile Eosinophilic Pustulosis
- Prednisolone: 2.2–4.4 mg/kg PO q24h until remission (usually 5–10 days); then as needed to prevent relapses (usually long-term, alternate-day therapy required)

See specific diseases.

CONTRAINDICATIONS
N/A

PRECAUTIONS

Prednisolone
- Secondary infections
- Iatrogenic Cushing disease
- Muscle wasting
- Steroid hepatopathy
- Behavioral changes
- Polydipsia, polyuria
- Polyphagia

Dapsone
- Dogs—mild anemia, mild leukopenia, and mild elevation of ALT, which are not associated with clinical signs, are frequently noted; usually return to normal when dosage is reduced for maintenance
- Occasionally, fatal thrombocytopenia or severe leukopenia
- Occasional vomiting, diarrhea, or pruritic skin eruption
- Cats—more susceptible to dapsone toxicity; hemolytic anemia and neurotoxicity reported

Sulfasalazine
Keratoconjunctivitis sicca

POSSIBLE INTERACTIONS
N/A

ALTERNATIVE DRUG(S)
N/A

FOLLOW-UP

PATIENT MONITORING
- Dapsone—monitor hemogram, platelet count, and ALT every 2 weeks initially and if any clinical side effects develop.

- Long-term sulfasalazine therapy—monitor tear production.
- Immunosuppressive therapy—monitor every 1–2 weeks initially; then every 3–4 months during maintenance therapy.

POSSIBLE COMPLICATIONS
N/A

✓ MISCELLANEOUS

ASSOCIATED CONDITIONS
N/A

AGE-RELATED FACTORS
N/A

ZOONOTIC POTENTIAL
Dermatophytosis

PREGNANCY
N/A

SYNONYMS
None

SEE ALSO
- Acne—Cats; Acne—Dogs
- Dermatomyositis
- Dermatophytosis
- Lupus Erythematosus, Cutaneus (Discoid)
- Lupus Erythematosus, Systemic (SLE)
- Pemphigoid, Bullous
- Pemphigus
- Pyoderma

ABBREVIATIONS
- ALT = alanine aminotransferase
- ANA = antinuclear antibody
- DLE = discoid lupus erythematosus
- EMG = electromyography
- SLE = systemic lupus erythematosus

Suggested Reading
Muller GH, Kirk RW, Scott DW. Small animal dermatology. 4th ed. Philadelphia: Saunders, 1989.
Authors Ellen C. Codner and Karen Helton Rhodes
Consulting Editor Karen Helton Rhodes

DESTRUCTIVE BEHAVIORS

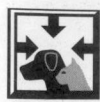

BASICS

OVERVIEW
Behavior that causes damage to an owner's home or belongings. Primary destructive behavior is a normal behavior that includes exploratory and play-based behavior, scratching of surfaces during feline grooming, and marking. Secondary destructive behavior is a clinical sign reflecting any of several behavioral conditions and other disease states. Behavior can affect the following organ systems:
• Gastrointestinal—damage to teeth; vomiting and diarrhea, obstruction if target items are ingested
• Musculoskeletal—traumatic damage caused by intense scratching
• Ingestion of toxic material could affect any organ system.

SIGNALMENT
• Dogs and cats
• Any breed or gender; probable genetic basis in Oriental breeds of cats that present for sucking or chewing fabric
• Primary destructive behavior most often seen in dogs and cats less than 1 year of age; secondary destructive behavior more often seen in mature animals

SIGNS

Primary Destructive Behavior
• Initially occurs in the presence or absence of the owner
• Not preceded by a specific environmental trigger
• Absence of anxiety or aggression
• Usual targets are small items, malleable items, edges of furniture, and houseplants.

Secondary Destructive Behavior
• Attention-seeking behavior (dogs and cats)—destructive behavior occurs in the presence of the owner.
• Obsessive-compulsive behavior (dogs and cats)—licking, chewing, and/or ingesting non-food items; occurs in the presence or absence of the owner; time spent engaged in the behavior is excessive
• Separation-related anxiety (dogs)—destructive behavior occurs in the absence of the owner and is exhibited during a majority of departures; target items may include personal belongings, furniture, or points of egress.
• Storm phobia, noise phobia (dogs)—destructive behavior and/or anxiety-related behavior (pace, pant, tremble) is observed in the presence of the owner; destructive behavior is intermittent and dependent upon presence of relevant trigger; points of egress are frequently targeted. May also occur during owner absence
• Territorial aggression (dogs)—reactivity to external stimuli is observed in presence of owner; destructive behavior is intermittent based on presence of triggers; window frames and doorways are damaged.

CAUSES & RISK FACTORS
• Primary destructive behavior represents normal behavior; inadequate supervision and insufficient access to appropriate chew toys or scratching posts or other activities may predispose pets to exhibit destructive behavior.
• Risk factors for anxiety-based conditions are not clearly identified.
• Territorial aggression may have genetic and learned components.

DIAGNOSIS

DIFFERENTIAL DIAGNOSIS
• Pathological conditions must be identified before a purely behavioral diagnosis is assigned.
• If pica accompanies destructive chewing—rule out conditions affecting digestion, absorption, and appetite.
• For sudden onset of destructive behavior in a mature pet in the absence of significant environmental changes—rule out medical conditions associated with pain or anxiety.
• For late-onset destructive behavior in senior dogs: rule out cognitive dysfunction syndrome.

CBC/BIOCHEMISTRY/URINALYSIS
Usually normal

OTHER LABORATORY TESTS
As indicated to rule out medical condition (thyroid panel, ACTH response test)

IMAGING
May be indicated if sudden onset in mature pet

DIAGNOSTIC PROCEDURES
May be indicated if sudden onset in mature pet

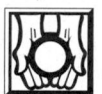

TREATMENT
Treat any underlying disease.

PRIMARY DESTRUCTIVE BEHAVIOR
• Supervise/confine; assure access to acceptable chew toys/scratching substrate (place posts in prominent locations, select suitable substrate); reward appropriate behavior; interrupt inappropriate behavior—apply non-toxic bitter-tasting product to

target items to deter chewing, apply double-sided sticky tape to furniture to deter cats from scratching. Provide adequate alternative exercise and activity.
• Remote activated devices designed to startle pets may be used with caution—counsel clients to assure that these devices are used in a humane manner. Appropriate outlet must also be provided for normal behaviors.
• Declawing should not be considered a first-line therapy for normal feline scratching; while behavior modification is being implemented, plastic claw covers may be applied to prevent further damage.

SECONDARY DESTRUCTIVE BEHAVIOR

• Attention-seeking behavior—provide owner-initiated interactions; review principles of learning and reinforcement.
• Obsessive-compulsive behavior—identify and reduce sources of anxiety in environment; offer interactive play and appropriate chewable items; prevent access to target items to assure safety of pet. See Compulsive Disorders—Dogs; Compulsive Disorders—Cats.
• Separation-related anxiety—behavior modification to reduce anxiety related to separation, including desensitization to separation; punishment is contraindicated. See Separation Anxiety Syndrome.
• Storm phobia/noise phobia—behavior modification (desensitization and counterconditioning) to reduce reactivity to relevant triggers. See Thunderstorm Phobias.
• Territorial aggression—behavior modification (desensitization and counterconditioning); dogs: low-protein diet. See Aggression, Food, Possessive, and Territorial—Dogs.

 MEDICATIONS

DRUGS

Medication complements behavior modification and may provide a more rapid resolution of clinical signs when treating anxiety-based conditions (obsessive-compulsive behavior, separation anxiety, phobias). Medication is not usually needed or advisable for primary destructive behaviors. Informed consent should be obtained when prescribing medication that has not been approved for use in dogs or cats.

Tricyclic Antidepressants (TCAs)
Clomipramine: (dogs, 1–3 mg/kg q12h; cats, 0.5 mg/kg q24h)

Selective Serotonin Reuptake Inhibitors (SSRIs)
Fluoxetine: dogs, 0.5–1 mg/kg q24h; cats, 0.5 mg/kg q24h

Benzodiazepines
Alprazolam: dogs, 0.02–0.04 mg/kg q12h (to reduce situational anxiety)

CONTRAINDICATIONS/POSSIBLE INTERACTIONS

• Psychotropic medication is not indicated for the treatment of primary destructive behavior.
• TCAs and SSRIs should not be used with monamine oxidase inhibitors, including products that contain amitraz and selegiline.
• TCAs and SSRIs can interfere with the metabolism of other medications.
• Benzodiazepines may disinhibit aggression; use with caution in dogs and cats with a history of aggressive behavior.

 FOLLOW-UP

PATIENT MONITORING

Weekly follow-up communication during initial phase of treatment

EXPECTED COURSE AND PROGNOSIS

Resolution of normal exploratory behavior is usually rapid. Anxiety-based conditions often require long-term management including the long-term use of psychotropic medication.

 **MISCELLANEOUS**

AGE-RELATED FACTORS

Age of presentation may not be equivalent to age of onset.

PREGNANCY

Preparturient destructive behavior (nesting)

Suggested Reading

Lindell EL. Diagnosis and treatment of destructive behavior in dogs. In: Vet Clin N Am. Philadelphia: Saunders, 1997:533–547.

Author Ellen M. Lindell
Consulting Editor Debra F. Horwitz

DIABETES INSIPIDUS

BASICS

DEFINITION
Diabetes insipidus (DI) is a disorder of water metabolism characterized by polyuria, urine of low specific gravity or osmolality (so-called insipid, or tasteless, urine), and polydipsia.

PATHOPHYSIOLOGY
• Central DI—deficiency in the secretion of ADH
• Nephrogenic DI—renal insensitivity to ADH

SYSTEMS AFFECTED
• Endocrine/Metabolic
• Renal/Urologic

GENETICS
N/A

INCIDENCE/PREVALENCE
• Central DI—rare
• Nephrogenic—rare

GEOGRAPHIC DISTRIBUTION
N/A

SIGNALMENT

Species
Dog and cat

Breed Predilections
None

Mean Age and Range
• Congenital forms <1 year
• Acquired forms (e.g., neoplastic, traumatic, and idiopathic), any age

Predominant Sex
None

SIGNS
• Polyuria
• Polydipsia
• Incontinence—occasional

CAUSES

Inadequate Secretion of ADH
• Congenital defect
• Idiopathic
• Trauma
• Neoplasia

Renal Insensitivity to ADH
• Congenital
• Secondary to drugs (e.g., lithium, demeclocycline, and methoxyflurane)
• Secondary to endocrine and metabolic disorders (e.g., hyperadrenocorticism, hypokalemia, pyometra, and hypercalcemia)
• Secondary to renal disease or infection (e.g., pyelonephritis, chronic renal failure, pyometra)

RISK FACTORS
N/A

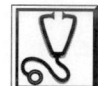

DIAGNOSIS

DIFFERENTIAL DIAGNOSIS

Polyuric Disorders
• Hyperadrenocorticism
• Diabetes mellitus
• Liver disease—portosystemic shunt
• Hyperadrenocorticism
• Pyometra
• Pyelonephritis
• Hyperthyroidism—cats
• Hypercalcemia
• Psychogenic polydipsia
• Renal failure

CBC/BIOCHEMISTRY/URINALYSIS
• Usually normal, hypernatremia in some patients
• Urinary specific gravity low (usually <1.012, often <1.008)

OTHER LABORATORY TESTS
Plasma ADH

IMAGING
MRI or CT scan if a pituitary tumor is suspected

DIAGNOSTIC PROCEDURES
• Modified water deprivation test (see Appendix for protocol)
• ADH supplementation trial—therapeutic trial with synthetic ADH (DDAVP); a positive response (water intake decreases by 50% in 3–5 days)
• Rule out all other causes of PU/PD before conducting an ADH trial.

PATHOLOGIC FINDINGS
Degeneration and death of neurosecretory neurons in the neurohypophysis (CDI)

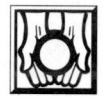

TREATMENT

APPROPRIATE HEALTH CARE
Patients should be hospitalized for the modified water deprivation test; the ADH trial is often performed as an outpatient procedure.

ACTIVITY
Not restricted

DIET
Normal, with free access to water

CLIENT EDUCATION
• Review dosage of DDAVP and administration technique.
• Importance of having water available at all times

SURGICAL CONSIDERATIONS
N/A

 MEDICATIONS

DRUG(S) OF CHOICE
• CDI—DDAVP (1–2 drops of the intranasal preparation in the conjunctival sac q12–24h to control PU/PD); alternatively, the intranasal preparation may be given SC (2–5 µg q12–24h).
• NDI—chlorothiazide (10–40 mg/kg PO q12h)

CONTRAINDICATIONS
None

PRECAUTIONS
Overdose of DDAVP can cause water intoxication.

ALTERNATIVE DRUGS
Chlorpropamide (Diabinese; 125–250 mg/day may reduce PU/PD in CDI)

 FOLLOW-UP

PATIENT MONITORING
• Adjust treatment according to the patient's signs; the ideal dosage and frequency of DDAVP administration is based on water intake.
• Laboratory tests such as PCV, total solids, and serum sodium concentration to detect dehydration (inadequate DDAVP replacement)—usually not necessary

PREVENTION/AVOIDANCE
Circumstances that might markedly increase water loss

POSSIBLE COMPLICATIONS
Anticipate complications of primary disease (pituitary tumor).

EXPECTED COURSE AND PROGNOSIS
• The condition is usually permanent, except in rare patients in which the condition was trauma induced.
• Prognosis is generally good, depending on the underlying disorder.
• Without treatment, dehydration can lead to stupor, coma, and death.

 MISCELLANEOUS

ASSOCIATED CONDITIONS
N/A

AGE-RELATED FACTORS
• Congenital CDI and NDI usually manifest before 6 months of age
• CDI related to pituitary tumors is usually seen in dogs >5 years old.

ZOONOTIC POTENTIAL
N/A

PREGNANCY
N/A

SYNONYMS
• Central diabetes insipidus
• Cranial diabetes insipidus
• ADH-responsive diabetes insipidus
• Nephrogenic diabetes insipidus

SEE ALSO
Hyposthenuria

ABBREVIATIONS
• ADH = antidiuretic hormone
• CDI = central diabetes insipidus
• DDAVP = brand name of desmopressin
• DI = diabetes insipidus
• MRI = magnetic resonance imaging
• NDI = nephrogenic diabetes insipidus
• PCV = packed cell volume
• PU/PD = polyuria/polydipsia

Suggested Reading
Feldman EC, Nelson RW. Canine and feline endocrinology and reproduction. Philadelphia: Saunders, 1996:2–37.
Author Rhett Nichols
Consulting Editor Deborah S. Greco

DIABETES MELLITUS WITHOUT COMPLICATION—CATS

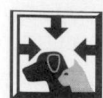

BASICS

DEFINITION
• Disorder of carbohydrate, fat, and protein metabolism caused by an absolute or relative insulin deficiency • Type II (non-insulin-dependent DM) is characterized by inadequate or delayed insulin secretion relative to the needs of the patient; many of these patients live without exogenous insulin and are less prone to ketoacidosis; most common form in cats.

PATHOPHYSIOLOGY
• Insulin deficiency impairs the ability of tissues (especially muscle, adipose tissue, and liver) to use carbohydrates, fats, and proteins. • Impaired glucose use and ongoing gluco-neogenesis cause hyperglycemia. • Glucosuria develops, causing osmotic diuresis, polyuria, and compensatory weight loss; mobilization of free fatty acids to the liver causes both hepatic lipidosis and ketogenesis.

SYSTEMS AFFECTED
• Endocrine/Metabolic—electrolyte depletion and metabolic acidosis • Hepatobiliary—hepatic lipidosis; liver failure may develop, • Renal/Urologic—urinary tract infection and osmotic diuresis • Nervous—peripheral neuropathy

INCIDENCE/PREVALENCE
Prevalence in cats is 1:200.

GEOGRAPHIC DISTRIBUTION
N/A

SIGNALMENT
Species
Cats

Breed Predilections
None

Mean Age and Range
• 75% are 8–13 years; range, 1–19 years

Predominant Sex
• Male

SIGNS
• Early signs—polyuria and polydipsia (PU/PD), polyphagia, and weight loss • Later signs—anorexia, lethargy, depression, and vomiting • Obesity with recent weight loss is typical. • Dorsal muscle wasting and an oily coat with dandruff common in cats • Hepatomegaly, but jaundice more prevalent in cats • Less common findings—a plantigrade stance in cats (diabetic neuropathy)

CAUSES
• Genetic susceptibility • Amyloid • Pancreatitis • Predisposing diseases (e.g., hyper-adrenocorticism and acromegaly) • Drugs (e.g., glucocorticoids and progestogens)

RISK FACTORS
• Obesity for type II DM • See Causes.

DIAGNOSIS

DIFFERENTIAL DIAGNOSIS
• Renal glucosuria—usually does not cause PU/PD, weight loss, or hyperglycemia • Stress hyperglycemia in cats—no PU/PD or weight loss; blood glucose concentration normal if sample taken when cat is not stressed.

CBC/BIOCHEMISTRY/URINALYSIS
• Results of hemogram usually normal • Glucose > 200 mg/dL • High SAP, alanine aminotransferase (ALT), and aspartate aminotransferase (AST) activities, and hypercholesterolemia and lipemia common • Electrolytes vary, but hypernatremia, hypokalemia, and hypophosphatemia indicate severe decompensation. • Total CO_2 or HCO_3 is low if the patient has ketoacidosis or severe dehydration. • Glucosuria is a consistent finding. • Ketonuria is common. • Urinary specific gravity often is low.

OTHER LABORATORY TESTS
• Anion gap—high in patients with ketoacidosis • Fructosamine >350 micromol/L

IMAGING
• Radiography—useful to evaluate for concurrent or underlying disease (e.g., cystic or renal calculi, emphysematous cystitis or cholecystitis, and pancreatitis) • Ultrasonography—indicated in selected patients, particularly those with jaundice, to evaluate for hepatic lipidosis, cholangiohepatitis, and pancreatitis

DIAGNOSTIC PROCEDURES
Liver biopsy (percutaneous)—indicated in some jaundiced patients

PATHOLOGIC FINDINGS
• Usually no gross necropsy changes • Histopathologic findings may be normal or reveal vacuolar degeneration of the islets of Langerhans or low numbers of islet cells; usually see amyloid deposits in the islets

TREATMENT

APPROPRIATE HEALTH CARE
• Compensated cats can be managed as outpatients; they are alert, hydrated, and eating and drinking without vomiting. • For management of decompensated patients, see Diabetes with Ketoacidosis.

NURSING CARE
Fluid therapy—see Diabetes with Ketoacidosis.

ACTIVITY
Strenuous activity may lower insulin requirement; a consistent amount of activity each day is helpful.

DIET
• Avoid soft, moist foods because they cause severe postprandial hyperglycemia. • Nonobese cats—feed a consistent diet that the pet will eat reliably; keep daily caloric intake constant. • Obese cats—gradual weight reduction improves insulin sensitivity and reverses diabetes in some cats with type II DM; either reduce the caloric intake to 70% of the requirement for the animal's ideal body weight (technique 1) or feed a high-fiber, low-calorie food in an amount similar to what the pet is accustomed (technique 2); try to achieve the target weight over 2–4 months; rapid weight loss is inadvisable, especially in obese cats with DM, because they are prone to hepatic lipidosis. • Thin cats—avoid reduced-calorie diet; starvation exacerbates ketoacidosis and poor immune function. • Role of fiber—key role is in weight loss and obesity prevention. In diabetic cats, low-carbohydrate, protein-replete canned foods are recommended. • Special considerations for feline diabetics: cats evolved as obligate carnivores with metabolic pathways adapted for efficient utilization of protein but not well suited for large-carbohydrate loads (cats have normal hepatic hexokinase enzyme activity, but virtually no hepatic glucokinase enzyme activity); preliminary studies suggest that low-carbohydrate canned diets may lower insulin requirements in diabetic cats; most dry pet food is manufactured with a higher carbohydrate content than the equivalent wet form, and simply switching from dry to wet food may reduce percentage of body fat and improve glycemic control in obese, diabetic cats; monitor closely for change in insulin requirement following any adjustment in diet.

DIABETES MELLITUS WITHOUT COMPLICATION—CATS

CLIENT EDUCATION
• Discuss daily feeding and medication schedule, home monitoring, signs of hypoglycemia and what to do, and when to call or visit veterinarian.
• Clients are encouraged to keep a chart of pertinent information about the pet, such as urine dipstick results, daily insulin dose, and weekly body weight.

SURGICAL CONSIDERATIONS
Intact females should have an ovariohysterectomy when stable; progesterone secreted during diestrus makes management of DM difficult.

 ## MEDICATIONS

DRUG(S) OF CHOICE
• Insulin—treatment of choice for most cats
• Regular crystalline insulin—rapid bioavailability and short duration of action; can be given by any parenteral route; used for patients with anorexia, vomiting, or ketoacidosis; can mix with other insulins
• NPH (Isophane) insulin—intermediate duration; given SC q12h in all cats, 0.25–0.5 unit/kg; adjust the dosage according to individual response.
• Lente insulin—intermediate duration; given SC; initial dosage same as for NPH
• Ultralente insulin—long-acting insulin; given SC, usually q24h; some cats require injections q12h.
• Species of origin of the insulin may affect pharmacokinetics; beef, beef/pork, human recombinant insulin are options; Beef preferred for cats
• Oral administration of hypoglycemic agent—glipizide is useful with dietary therapy in cats with type II DM; the cat should have uncomplicated DM and no history of ketoacidosis; initial dosage, 2.5 mg PO q12h; monitoring is the same as for patients on insulin; if hyperglycemia is not controlled, 5 mg q12h may be tried; potential side effects are hypoglycemia, hepatic enzyme alterations, icterus, and vomiting.

CONTRAINDICATIONS
N/A

PRECAUTIONS
• Glucocorticoids, megestrol acetate, and progesterone cause insulin resistance.
• Hyperosmotic agents (e.g., mannitol and radiographic contrast agents) if the patient is already hyperosmolar from hyperglycemia

POSSIBLE INTERACTIONS
Many drugs (e.g., NSAIDs, sulfonamides, miconazole, chloramphenicol, monoamine oxidase inhibitors, and β-blockers) potentiate the effect of hypoglycemic agents given orally; consult the product insert.

ALTERNATIVE DRUGS
Acarbose 12.5 mg PO q12h

 ## FOLLOW-UP

PATIENT MONITORING
• Glucose curve—not helpful in cats
• Urinary glucose monitoring—urine is tested for glucose and ketones before the meal and insulin injection; to use this as a regulatory method, the pet must be allowed to have trace to 1/4% glucosuria to avoid hypoglycemia. Animals regulated by urine monitoring alone may be more hyperglycemic than ideal, and insulin overdose with rebound hyperglycemia is an inherent risk with this method. It is best to combine urine monitoring with intermittent glucose determinations; owners should seek veterinary attention if ketonuria is detected.
• Fructosamine—maintain <400 micromol/L. Recheck q4wk during initial regulation, then q3 months.
• Clinical signs—owner can assess degree of PU/PD, appetite, and body weight; if these are normal, the disease is well regulated.

PREVENTION/AVOIDANCE
Prevent or correct obesity; avoid unnecessary use of glucocorticoids or megestrol acetate.

POSSIBLE COMPLICATIONS
• Seizure or coma with insulin overdose
• Anemia and hemoglobinemia with severe hypophosphatemia, which can occur after initial insulin therapy
• Diabetic neuropathy

EXPECTED COURSE AND PROGNOSIS
• Some cats recover but may relapse at a later time.
• Prognosis with treatment is good; most animals have a normal life span.

 ## MISCELLANEOUS

ASSOCIATED CONDITIONS
Urinary tract infection

AGE-RELATED FACTORS
Juvenile DM is rare and may be more difficult to manage.

ZOONOTIC POTENTIAL
N/A

SYNONYMS
N/A

SEE ALSO
Diabetes with Ketoacidosis

ABBREVIATIONS
• ALT = alanine aminotransferase
• AST = aspartate aminotransferase • DM = diabetes mellitus • NSAID = nonsteroidal antiinflammatory drug • PU/PD = polyuria and polydipsia • SAP = serum alkaline phosphatase

Suggested Reading
Crenshaw KL, Peterson ME, Heeb LA, et al. Pretreatment clinical and laboratory evaluation of cats with diabetes mellitus: 104 cases (1992–1994). J Am Vet Med Assoc 1996;209:943–949.
Goosens MMC, Nelson RW, Feldman EC, et al. Response to treatment and survival in 104 cats with diabetes mellitus (1985–1995). J Vet Intern Med 1998;12:1–6.
Rand JS, Martin GJ. Management of feline diabetes mellitus. Vet Clin North Am Small Anim Pract 2001;31:881–913.

Author Deborah S. Greco
Consulting Editor Deborah S. Greco

DIABETES MELLITUS WITHOUT COMPLICATION—DOGS

BASICS

DEFINITION
• Fasted hyperglycemia with glucosuria
• Disorder of carbohydrate, fat, and protein metabolism caused by an absolute or relative insulin deficiency • Type I diabetes mellitus is characterized by autoimmune destruction of insulin-secreting pancreatic β cells and results in a dependence on exogenous insulin (insulin-dependent DM or IDDM). • Type II diabetes mellitus is characterized by a relative insulin deficiency and peripheral insulin resistance, and may result in IDDM, non–insulin dependent DM (NIDDM), or both through the course of the disease.
• "Other specific types of diabetes" is characterized by a loss of β cell function secondary to disease such as pancreatic neoplasia, hyperadrenocorticism, and acromegaly. • IDDM patients are prone to developing diabetic ketoacidosis. • NIDDM patients may be amenable to treatment with oral hypoglycemic agents.

PATHOPHYSIOLOGY
• Absolute or relative insulin deficiency shifts insulin:glucagon ratio and alters cellular carbohydrate, lipid, and protein metabolism.
• Hypoinsulinemia, peripheral insulin resistance, and continued hepatic gluconeogenesis result in persistent hyperglycemia and glucosuria, osmotic diuresis, and polyuria/polydipsia. • Loss of insulin-dependent glucose-mediated hypothalamic satiation signal results in polyphagia. • Decreased insulin-dependent utilization of glucose for energy results in catabolic protein breakdown with weight loss and increased lipid mobilization (hyperlipidemia, hepatic lipidosis, ketone production).

SYSTEMS AFFECTED
• Endocrine/Metabolic—electrolyte depletion and metabolic acidosis • Hepatobiliary—hepatic lipidosis • Ophthalmic—cataracts
• Renal/Urologic—urinary tract infection and osmotic diuresis

GENETICS
Familial associations in some breeds of dog

INCIDENCE/PREVALENCE
Prevalence in dogs varies between 1:400 and 1:500.

GEOGRAPHIC DISTRIBUTION
N/A

SIGNALMENT
Species
Dogs

Breed Predilections
• Higher risk than other breeds—keeshond, puli, miniature pinscher, and Cairn terrier
• Possibly higher risk than other breeds—poodle, dachshund, miniature schnauzer, and beagle

Mean Age and Range
Mean, ~8 years; range, 4–14 years (excluding rare juvenile form)

Predominant Sex
Female

SIGNS
• Early signs—polyuria and polydipsia (PU/PD), polyphagia, and weight loss • Later signs—anorexia, lethargy, depression, and vomiting • Obesity with recent weight loss is typical. • Hepatomegaly • Less common findings—cataracts

CAUSES
• Genetic susceptibility • Infectious (viral) diseases • Immune-mediated β-cell destruction
• Pancreatitis • Predisposing diseases (e.g., hyperadrenocorticism and acromegaly) • Drugs (e.g., glucocorticoids and progestogens)

RISK FACTORS
• Obesity for type II DM • Diestrus in the bitch • See Causes.

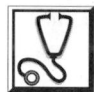

DIAGNOSIS

DIFFERENTIAL DIAGNOSIS
Renal glucosuria—usually does not cause PU/PD, weight loss, or hyperglycemia

CBC/BIOCHEMISTRY/URINALYSIS
• Results of hemogram usually normal
• Glucose > 200 mg/dL in dogs • High SAP, alanine aminotransferase (ALT), and aspartate aminotransferase (AST) activities, and hypercholesterolemia and lipemia common
• Electrolytes vary, but hypernatremia, hypokalemia, and hypophosphatemia indicate severe decompensation.
• Total CO_2 or HCO_3 is low if the patient has ketoacidosis or severe dehydration.
• Glucosuria is a consistent finding.
• Ketonuria is common. • Urinary specific gravity often is low.

OTHER LABORATORY TESTS
• Anion gap—high in patients with ketoacidosis • Plasma insulin—may help to differentiate type I from type II DM • Normal or high insulin concentration with hyperglycemia is found in patients with type II DM; low insulin concentration suggests type I DM but may be an incorrect diagnosis because persistent hyperglycemia can impair insulin secretory activity, even if functional β cells are present.

IMAGING
• Radiography—useful to evaluate for concurrent or underlying disease (e.g., cystic or renal calculi, emphysematous cystitis or cholecystitis, and pancreatitis) • Ultrasonography—indicated in selected patients, particularly those with jaundice, to evaluate for hepatic lipidosis, cholangiohepatitis, and pancreatitis

DIAGNOSTIC PROCEDURES
Liver biopsy (percutaneous)—indicated in some jaundiced patients

PATHOLOGIC FINDINGS
• Usually no gross necropsy changes
• Histopathologic findings may be normal or reveal vacuolar degeneration of the islets of Langerhans or low numbers of islet cells; immunohistochemical staining is necessary to show low numbers of β cells.

TREATMENT

APPROPRIATE HEALTH CARE
• Compensated dogs can be managed as outpatients; they are alert, hydrated, and eating and drinking without vomiting.
• For management of decompensated patients, see Diabetes with Ketoacidosis.

NURSING CARE
• Fluid therapy—see Diabetes with Ketoacidosis.

ACTIVITY
Strenuous activity may lower insulin requirement; a consistent amount of activity each day is helpful.

DIET
• Avoid soft, moist foods because they cause severe postprandial hyperglycemia.
• Nonobese dogs—feed a consistent diet that the pet will eat reliably; keep daily caloric intake constant.
• Obese dogs—reduce the caloric intake to 60% of the requirement for the animal's ideal body weight (technique 1) or feed a high-fiber, low-calorie food in an amount similar to what the pet is accustomed (technique 2); try to achieve the target weight over 2–4 months.
• Thin dogs—avoid reduced-calorie diet; starvation exacerbates ketoacidosis and poor immune function.
• Role of fiber—key role is in weight loss and obesity prevention; another benefit may be improved glycemic control; recommended diet is high in fiber, low in fat, and high in complex carbohydrates.
• Feed the pet half its daily food every 12 h to coincide with twice-daily insulin injections or orally administered hypoglycemic agent; give animals on once-daily insulin injections half the food with the injection and the remainder in 8–10 h or at the time of peak insulin

DIABETES MELLITUS WITHOUT COMPLICATION—DOGS

activity, if that is known; nibblers can be fed dry food ad libitum and given two small meals of canned food as described.

CLIENT EDUCATION
• Discuss daily feeding and medication schedule, home monitoring, signs of hypoglycemia and what to do, and when to call or visit veterinarian.
• Clients are encouraged to keep a chart of pertinent information about the pet, such as urine dipstick results, daily insulin dose, and weekly body weight.

SURGICAL CONSIDERATIONS
Intact females should have an ovariohysterectomy when stable; progesterone secreted during diestrus makes management of DM difficult.

MEDICATIONS

DRUG(S) OF CHOICE
• Insulin—required for IDDM; frequently utilized as part of management of NIDDM
• Lente insulin-intermediate duration; given SC q12h in most cases; q24h injections rarely achieve adequate glycemic control; dosage same as for NPH
• Ultralente insulin-long-acting insulin; given SC; despite reported duration of action q12h dosing often required for adequate control
• Species of origin of the insulin may affect pharmacokinetics; most available insulin is recombinant human insulin, which is most similar to canine amino acid sequence.
• Oral administration of hypoglycemic agents are generally not recommended in canine diabetes.

CONTRAINDICATIONS
N/A

PRECAUTIONS
• Glucocorticoids, megestrol acetate, and progesterone cause insulin resistance.
• Hyperosmotic agents (e.g., mannitol and radiographic contrast agents) if the patient is already hyperosmolar from hyperglycemia

POSSIBLE INTERACTIONS
N/A

ALTERNATIVE DRUG(S)
N/A

FOLLOW-UP

PATIENT MONITORING
• Glucose curve—"gold standard"; can provide information on insulin effectiveness, duration of action, nadir (lowest blood glucose level achieved during dosing interval), and Somogyi effect; results subject to outside influences; stress of hospitalization and multiple blood draws; used most frequently when establishing initial control, changing insulin type, dose, or frequency, or problem solving the difficult diabetic; duration of curve ideally matches dosing interval (12 or 24 hours) but often abbreviated; identification of nadir is most important aspect of curve (to avoid iatrogenic hypoglycemia, determine need for dose adjustment); mimic "normal" conditions as closely as possible; can have owner feed and administer insulin at home prior to hospitalization; measure blood glucose q2h; goal is effective insulin dose (decline in blood glucose to 100–200 mg/dL) for appropriate duration (majority of 12- or 24-hour dosing interval) with a nadir >80 mg/dL and <150 mg/dL
• Glycated proteins—glycosylated hemoglobin or fructosamine; nonenzymatic, irreversible binding of glucose to hemoglobin (glycosylated hemoglobin) or albumin (fructosamine); extent of glycosylation directly related to blood glucose concentration over lifespan of protein in blood (5–9 weeks for hemoglobin, 1–3 weeks for fructosamine); not affected by stress of hospitalization or dietary intake day of sample acquisition; requires single blood draw, best used for ongoing management of stable diabetic patient; fructosamine of 400 mg/dL is consistent with adequate glycemic control
• At-home monitoring—urine glucose and/or blood glucose (lancet device for capillary blood from pinna) requires significant owner commitment, compliance, and competence; most useful as early indicator of need for reduction in dose with persistent absence of glucosuria; should never be used as sole criterion for owner adjustment of insulin, especially an increase in dose; removes physical examination, adjunct laboratory data (i.e., evidence of concurrent disease), and "hands-on" veterinarian involvement from decision-making process; minimal evidence supports the need for the extent of monitoring, frequency of dose adjustments, or exactness of control in pets as is required in the management of human diabetics.
• Clinical signs—owner can assess degree of PU/PD, appetite, and body weight; if these are normal, the disease is well regulated.

PREVENTION/AVOIDANCE
Prevent or correct obesity; avoid unnecessary use of glucocorticoids or megestrol acetate.

POSSIBLE COMPLICATIONS
• Cataracts with poor glycemic control
• Seizure or coma with insulin overdose
• Anemia and hemoglobinemia with severe hypophosphatemia, which can occur after initial insulin therapy

EXPECTED COURSE AND PROGNOSIS
• Dogs have permanent disease.
• Prognosis with treatment is good; most animals have a normal life span.

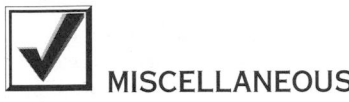

MISCELLANEOUS

ASSOCIATED CONDITIONS
Urinary tract infection

AGE-RELATED FACTORS
Juvenile DM is rare and may be more difficult to manage.

ZOONOTIC POTENTIAL
None

PREGNANCY
• Diabetes mellitus can develop during pregnancy, in which case the pregnancy is difficult to maintain. • Exogenous insulin administration may cause fetal oversize and dystocia.
• Insulin resistance develops, making hyperglycemia difficult to control. • The pregnant bitch is prone to ketoacidosis; an emergency ovariohysterectomy may be necessary.
• Do not breed dogs with DM.

SYNONYMS
N/A

SEE ALSO
Diabetes with Ketoacidosis

ABBREVIATIONS
• ALT = alanine aminotransferase • AST = aspartate aminotransferase • DM = diabetes mellitus • IDDM = insulin-dependent diabetes mellitus • NIDDM = non–insulin dependent diabetes mellitus • NSAID = nonsteroidal antiinflammatory drug
• PU/PD = polyuria and polydypsia
• SAP = serum alkaline phosphatase

Suggested Reading

Fleeman LM, Rand JS. Management of canine diabetes mellitus. Vet Clin N Amer Small Anim Pract 2001;31:855–880.
Hess RS, Ward CR. Effect of insulin dosage on glycemic response in dogs with diabetes mellitus: 221 cases (1993–1998) J Amer Vet Med Assoc 2000;216:217–221.
Nelson RW. Diabetes mellitus. In: Ettinger SJ, Feldman EC, eds. Textbook of veterinary internal medicine. Philadelphia: Saunders, 1995:1510–1537.
Wallace MS, Kirk CA. The diagnosis and treatment of insulin-dependent and non-insulin-dependent DM in the dog and the cat. Probl Vet Med 1990;2:573–590.
Author Craig Webb
Consulting Editor Deborah S. Greco

DIABETES WITH HYPEROSMOLAR COMA

BASICS

DEFINITION
Disease characterized by severe hyperglycemia, hyperosmolarity, severe dehydration, lack of urine or serum ketones, lack of or mild-to-moderate metabolic acidosis, and CNS depression

PATHOPHYSIOLOGY
• Insulin deficiency causes reduced use of glucose and excessive glucose production.
• The resultant high extracellular blood glucose concentration causes a hyperosmolar state with a reduced extracellular fluid volume.
• Intracellular dehydration, azotemia, and uremia develop, and intracellular dehydration becomes more pronounced as the glomerular filtration rate decreases; tissue hypoxia ensues.
• Azotemia, hyperglycemia, and hyperosmolarity worsen as a result of glucose retention and glucose-induced osmotic diuresis.
• Although ketonemia and ketonuria usually are not features of this syndrome, anorexia (especially when prolonged) may cause mild ketoacidosis in some patients, but increased lactic acid is a major contributor to the metabolic acidosis that may develop in these patients.

SYSTEMS AFFECTED
• Renal/Urologic—prerenal and primary renal azotemia develop because of reduced extracellular fluid volume, reduced tissue perfusion, or diabetic glomerulonephropathy; urinary specific gravity is low because of osmotic diuresis, diabetic glomerulonephropathy, or concurrent renal insufficiency.
• Cardiovascular—hypotension because of low extracellular fluid volume, vascular collapse, and depressed myocardial contractility
• Nervous—depression, disorientation or mental confusion, seizures, and coma are caused by intracellular dehydration and hyperosmolarity; CNS dysfunction worsens as serum osmolarity rises.

GENETICS
N/A

INCIDENCE/PREVALENCE
Uncommon

GEOGRAPHIC DISTRIBUTION
N/A

SIGNALMENT

Species
Dogs and cats

Breed Predilection
N/A

Mean Age and Range
• Dogs—peak prevalence, 7–9 years of age
• Cats—any age; most >6 years old

Predominant Sex
• Dogs—female
• Cats—neutered males

SIGNS

Historical Findings
• Early signs—polydipsia, polyuria, polyphagia, and weight loss
• Late signs—weakness, vomiting, anorexia, depression, stupor, and coma

Physical Examination Findings
Dehydration, hypothermia, prolonged capillary refill time, cataracts, lethargy, depression, seizures (severe hyperosmolarity), and stupor or coma (severe hyperosmolarity)

CAUSES
Diabetes mellitus associated with severe hyperosmolarity, severe hyperglycemia, and severe dehydration

RISK FACTORS
• Concurrent problems such as heart disease, renal insufficiency, pneumonia, acute pancreatitis, and other severe diseases
• Drugs—anticonvulsants, glucocorticoids, and thiazide diuretics may precipitate or aggravate this syndrome.

DIAGNOSIS

DIFFERENTIAL DIAGNOSIS
• Uncomplicated diabetes mellitus—mentally alert with fasting hyperglycemia and glucosuria
• Ketoacidotic diabetes mellitus—fasting hyperglycemia with glucosuria, ketonuria, and metabolic acidosis
• Extreme lethargy and depression with severe hyperosmolarity, severe hyperglycemia, severe dehydration without ketonemia and ketonuria usually differentiate diabetes mellitus non-ketotic hyperosmolar syndrome from uncomplicated and ketoacidotic diabetes mellitus.

CBC/BIOCHEMISTRY/URINALYSIS
• Severe hyperglycemia—usually >600 mg/dL
• High BUN and creatinine concentration
• Normokalemia (despite total body potassium depletion) or hypokalemia
• Hyperkalemia is expected in patients with anuric or oliguric renal failure.
• Low TCO_2
• High anion gap
• Glucosuria
• Low urinary specific gravity

OTHER LABORATORY TESTS
• Severe hyperosmolarity—usually >350 mOsm/L
• Estimated serum osmolarity may be calculated from serum chemistries as follows:

$$2\,(Na) + \frac{BUN}{2.8} + \frac{glucose}{18}$$

• High plasma lactate concentration may help confirm metabolic lactic acidosis in the absence of ketonemia and ketonuria.

IMAGING
N/A

DIAGNOSTIC PROCEDURES
N/A

PATHOLOGIC FINDINGS
Pancreatic islet cell atrophy

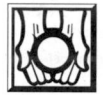

TREATMENT

APPROPRIATE HEALTH CARE
A life-threatening medical emergency requiring inpatient treatment

NURSING CARE
• Fluid therapy is a major component of medical management.
• Replace one-half the fluid deficits in the first 12 hours and the remainder during the next 24 hours.
• Administer normal saline (0.9%) IV if the patient is hypotensive or hyponatremic.
• Add potassium (20 mEq/L) to the initial fluids unless the patient has hyperkalemia.
• Switch to IV administration of 0.45% saline after restoration of normal blood pressure and urine output.
• Switch to 2.5%–5% dextrose plus 0.45% saline when blood glucose < 250 mg/dL, and continue until the patient is eating and drinking on its own.

ACTIVITY
N/A

DIABETES WITH HYPEROSMOLAR COMA

DIET
A low-fat, high-fiber, high-complex carbohydrate diet is recommended once the patient is stabilized.

CLIENT EDUCATION
• Poor-to-guarded prognosis
• Intensive care and frequent monitoring are required during hospitalization.

SURGICAL CONSIDERATIONS
N/A

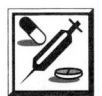 MEDICATIONS

DRUGS OF CHOICE
• Administer regular insulin 2–4 hours after initiating IV fluid therapy.
• Regular insulin for patients < 10 kg—initial dose is 2 U IM followed by 1 U IM hourly until blood glucose is < 250 mg/dL.
• Regular insulin for patients >10 kg—initial dose is 0.25 U/kg IM followed by 0.1 U/kg IM, hourly until blood glucose is < 250 mg/dL.
• Monitor blood glucose hourly; aim is to drop concentration by 50–100 mg/dL/h; adjust insulin dosage accordingly.
• Discontinue hourly IM regular insulin when blood glucose is <250 mg/dL; switch to regular insulin (0.5 U/kg) IM q4–6h or SC q6–8h if blood glucose concentration remains between 150 and 250 mg/dL.
• Alternatively, an IV constant-rate infusion of regular insulin may be used at a dosage of 1.1 U/kg/24h. Add 1.1 U/kg regular insulin to 250 ml 0.9% NaCl and administer at 10 ml/hr (0.045 U/kg/h) in a separate line. Discard the first 50 ml of the solution to compensate for insulin binding to the plastic tubing.
• Reduce the dosage/rate of the constant-rate infusion when the blood glucose is <. 250 mg/dL.
• Once the patient is stabilized (eating and drinking on its own without vomiting), discontinue fluids and regular insulin; NPH PZI, or Lente insulin can then be administered SC in a routine manner.
• Other concurrent diseases must be treated appropriately.

CONTRAINDICATIONS
N/A

PRECAUTIONS
Avoid rapid reduction of serum osmolarity and glucose because the brain will become hyperosmolar compared with serum; fluid may then shift from extracellular to intracellular spaces, resulting in cerebral edema and worsening of neurologic status.

POSSIBLE INTERACTIONS
N/A

ALTERNATIVE DRUGS
Once stable, oral hypoglycemics (e.g., glipizide, Glucotrol) may be tried; these agents are more likely to be efficacious in cats with type II (non–insulin-dependent diabetes mellitus) than in dogs.

 FOLLOW-UP

PATIENT MONITORING
• Blood glucose concentrations, closely, to avoid hypoglycemia and abrupt, precipitous decreases
• Ideally, the blood glucose should drop 50–100 mg/dL/h until a concentration of 250 mg/dL is reached.
• Blood glucose hourly before administering the next dose of regular insulin IM during initial stabilization
• Urine output for early detection of acute renal failure
• Hydration status, ECG, CVP, serum electrolytes, BUN, and urine glucose every 2 hours during the initial stabilization period
• Long-term glucose control by determining serum glycosylated hemoglobin and serum fructosamine concentrations
• Watch for return of clinical signs such as polydipsia, polyuria, and polyphagia.

PREVENTION/AVOIDANCE
• Avoid inappropriate insulin therapy.
• Avoid hypoglycemia, hypokalemia, and hyponatremia.

POSSIBLE COMPLICATIONS
• Irreversible coma and death are possible, especially in patients with renal insufficiency.
• Acute renal failure

EXPECTED COURSE AND PROGNOSIS
Clinical signs and laboratory values may improve within the initial 24 hours of treatment, but these patients have a guarded prognosis.

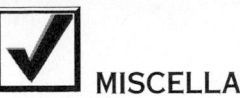 MISCELLANEOUS

ASSOCIATED CONDITIONS
Congestive heart failure, renal disease, infection, gastrointestinal hemorrhage, and other serious illnesses

AGE-RELATED FACTORS
N/A

ZOONOTIC POTENTIAL
N/A

PREGNANCY
May encounter insulin resistance and thus poor glycemic control in pregnant animals

SYNONYMS
• Diabetic coma
• Hyperosmolar coma

SEE ALSO
• Diabetes Mellitus Without Complication—Cats
• Diabetes Mellitus Without Complication—Dogs
• Diabetes with Ketoacidosis
• Hyperosmolarity
• Hyperglycemia

ABBREVIATION(S)
• BUN = blood urea nitrogen
• CVP = central venous pressure
• TCO_2 = total carbon dioxide

Suggested Reading
Brody GM. Diabetic ketoacidosis and hyperosmolar hyperglycemic nonketotic coma. Topics Emerg Med 1992;14:12–22.
Chastain CB, Nichols CE. Low dose intramuscular insulin therapy for diabetic ketoacidosis in dogs. J Am Vet Med Assoc 1981;178:561–564.
MacIntire DK. Emergency therapy of diabetic crises: insulin overdose, diabetic ketoacidosis, and hyperosmolar coma. Vet Clin N Am 1995;25:639–650.
Melendez LD. Diabetes mellitus. In: Wingfield W, ed. Veterinary emergency medicine secrets. Philadelphia: Hanley and Belfus, 1997:253–258.
Author Margaret R. Kern
Consulting Editor Deborah S. Greco

DIABETES WITH KETOACIDOSIS

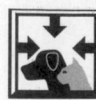 BASICS

DEFINITION
A true medical emergency secondary to absolute or relative insulin deficiency, characterized by hyperglycemia, ketonemia, metabolic acidosis, dehydration, and electrolyte depletion

PATHOPHYSIOLOGY
• Insulin deficiency causes an increase in lipolysis, which results in excessive ketone body production and acidosis; an inability to maintain fluid and electrolyte homeostasis causes dehydration, prerenal azotemia, electrolyte disorders, obtundation, and death.
• Many diabetic ketoacidosis patients have underlying conditions such as infection, inflammation, or heart disease that cause stress hormone (e.g., glucagon, cortisol, growth hormone, and epinephrine) secretion; this probably contributes to the development of insulin resistance and diabetic ketoacidosis by promoting lipolysis, ketogenesis, gluconeogenesis, and glycogenolysis.
• Dehydration and electrolyte abnormalities result from osmotic diuresis promoting the loss of total body water and electrolytes.

SYSTEMS AFFECTED
• Endocrine/Metabolic
• Hematologic (cats)

GENETICS
N/A

INCIDENCE/PREVALENCE
Unknown

GEOGRAPHIC DISTRIBUTION
N/A

SIGNALMENT
Species
Dogs and cats
Breed Predilections
• Dogs—miniature poodle and dachshund
• Cats—none
Mean Age and Range
• Dogs—mean age, 8.4 years
• Cats—median age, 11 years (range, 1–19 years)
Predominant Sex
• Dogs—females 1.5 times males
• Cats—males 2 times females

SIGNS
• Polyuria
• Polydipsia or adipsia
• Diminished activity
• Anorexia
• Weakness
• Vomiting
• Lethargy and depression
• Muscle wasting and weight loss
• Unkempt haircoat
• Tachypnea
• Dehydration
• Thin body condition
• Hypothermia
• Dandruff
• Thickened bowel loops
• Hepatomegaly
• Ketone odor on breath
• Icterus

CAUSES
• Insulin-dependent diabetes mellitus
• Infection (e.g., skin, respiratory, urinary tract, prostate gland, pyelonephritis, pyometra, and pneumonia)
• Concurrent disease (e.g., heart failure, pancreatitis, renal insufficiency, or failure, asthma, neoplasia, acromegaly and estrus)
• Idiopathic
• Medication noncompliance
• Stress
• Surgery

RISK FACTORS
• Any condition that leads to an absolute or relative insulin deficiency
• History of corticosteroid or β-blocker administration

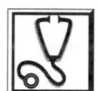 DIAGNOSIS

DIFFERENTIAL DIAGNOSIS
• Hyperosmolar nonketotic coma
• Acute hypoglycemic coma
• Uremia
• Lactic acidosis

CBC/BIOCHEMISTRY/URINALYSIS
• Leukocytosis with mature neutrophilia
• Hyperglycemia—blood glucose usually >250 mg/dL
• High liver enzyme activity
• Hypercholesterolemia and lipemia
• Azotemia
• Hypochloremia
• Hypokalemia
• Hyponatremia
• Hypophosphatemia
• High anion gap—anion gap = (sodium + potassium) − (chloride + bicarbonate); normal is 16 ± 4.
• Glucosuria and ketonuria
• Variable urinary specific gravity with active or inactive sediment
• Hyperproteinemia
• Heinz body anemia (cats)

OTHER LABORATORY TESTS
• Metabolic acidosis—venous TCO_2 < 15 mEq/L caused by ketosis
• Hyperosmolarity (>330 mOsm/kg)
• Bacterial culture of urine and blood

DIAGNOSTIC PROCEDURES
ECG may help evaluate potassium status; prolonged Q-T interval in some patients with hypokalemia; tall, tented T waves in some patients with hyperkalemia

PATHOLOGIC FINDINGS
Pancreatic islet cell atrophy

 TREATMENT

APPROPRIATE HEALTH CARE
• If the animal is bright, alert, and well hydrated, intensive care and intravenous fluid administration are not required; start subcutaneous administration of insulin (short- or intermediate-acting insulin), offer food, and supply constant access to water; monitor closely for signs of illness (e.g., anorexia, lethargy, vomiting).
• Treatment of "sick" diabetic ketoacidotic dog or cat requires inpatient intensive care; this is a life-threatening emergency; goals are to correct the depletion of water and electrolytes, reverse ketonemia and acidosis, and increase the rate of glucose use by insulin-dependent tissues.

NURSING CARE
• Fluids—necessary to ensure adequate cardiac output and tissue perfusion and to maintain vascular volume; also reduce blood glucose concentration.
• IV administration of 0.9% saline supplemented with potassium is the initial fluid of choice.
• Volume determined by dehydration deficit plus maintenance requirements; replace over 24–48 h.

ACTIVITY
N/A

DIET
A low-fat, high-fiber, high-complex-carbohydrate diet recommended once the patient is stabilized

CLIENT EDUCATION
Serious medical condition requiring lifelong insulin administration in most patients

SURGICAL CONSIDERATIONS
N/A

 MEDICATIONS

DRUG(S) OF CHOICE
Insulin
• Necessary to inhibit lipolysis, inhibit hepatic gluconeogenesis, and promote peripheral glucose uptake
• Regular insulin is the insulin of choice.
• Initial dosage—0.2 U/kg IM (or SC if hydration is normal)

- Subsequent dosage 0.1–0.2 U/kg given 3–6 h later—may be given hourly if patient is closely monitored; response to previous insulin dosage should be considered when calculating subsequent dosages. Ideally, glucose concentration should drop to 50–100 mg/dL/h.
- Regular insulin can also be administered as a continuous-rate infusion via a designated catheter. For dogs, place 2.2 units/kg into 250 mL of 0.9% NaCl fluid. For cats, place 1.1 units/kg into 250 mL 0.9% NaCl fluid. Then, allow 50 mL of the dilute insulin to flow through the IV tubing and discard. If blood glucose is >250 mg/dL, administer at 10 mL/hour. If blood glucose is between 200 mg/dL and 250 mg/dL, administer at 7 mL/hour. If blood glucose is between 150 mg/dL and 200 mg/dL, administer at 5 mL/hour. If blood glucose is between 100 mg/dL and 150 mg/dL, administer at 5 mL/hour and add 2.5% dextrose to the IV crystalloid fluids. If blood glucose is <100 mg/dL, discontinue IV insulin infusion and continue 2.5%–5% dextrose in IV crystalloid infusion.
- Check blood glucose every 1–3 h with Chemstrip BG reagent strips and an automated test strip analyzer (Accu-Chek III, Boehringer Mannheim).
- Monitor urine glucose and ketones daily.
- Start administering longer-acting insulin (e.g., NPH, lente, and ultralente) when the patient is eating, drinking, and no longer receiving IV fluids and ketosis is resolved or greatly diminished; the dosage is based on that of short-acting insulin given in hospital.

Potassium Supplementation
- Total body potassium is depleted and treatment (e.g., fluids and insulin) will further lower serum potassium; potassium supplementation is always necessary.
- If possible, check potassium concentration before initiating insulin therapy, to guide supplementation dosage; if it is extremely low, insulin therapy may need to be delayed (hours) until serum potassium concentration increases.
- Refractory hypokalemia may indicate magnesium depletion, requiring magnesium replacement at 0.75–1.0 mEq/kg/day as magnesium chloride or magnesium sulfate as a continuous-rate infusion.
- If potassium concentration is unknown, add potassium (40 mEq/L) to the IV fluids, obtain results of pretreatment biochemical analysis ASAP, and draw blood for follow-up biochemical analysis 24 h after treatment is initiated.

Dextrose Supplementation
- Must give insulin, regardless of the blood glucose concentration, to correct the ketoacidotic state

- Whenever blood glucose is < 200–250 mg/dL, 50% dextrose should be added to the fluids to produce a 2.5% dextrose solution (increase to 5% dextrose if needed). Discontinue dextrose once glucose is maintained above 250 mg/dL.
- Do not stop insulin therapy.

Bicarbonate Supplementation
- Controversial; consider if patient's venous blood pH is <7.0 or total CO_2 is <11 mEq/L; bicarbonate is of no benefit if the pH is >7.0.
- Dosage—body weight (kg) × 0.3 × base deficit (base deficit = normal serum bicarbonate − patient's serum bicarbonate); *slowly* administer one-quarter to one-half of the dose IV and give the remainder in fluids over 3–6 h.
- Recheck blood gas or serum TCO_2 before further supplementation.

Phosphorus Supplementation
- Pretreatment serum phosphorus usually is normal; however, treatment of ketoacidosis reduces phosphorus, and serum concentrations should be checked every 12–24 h once supplementation is initiated.
- Dosage—0.01–0.03 mmol/kg/h for 6–12 h in IV fluids (may need to increase dose to 0.03–0.06)

CONTRAINDICATIONS
If the patient is anuric or oliguric or if potassium is >5 mEq/L, do not supplement potassium until urine flow is established or potassium concentration decreases.

PRECAUTIONS
Use bicarbonate with caution in patients without normal ventilation because of their inability to excrete carbon dioxide created during treatment.

POSSIBLE INTERACTIONS
N/A

ALTERNATIVE DRUG(S)
N/A

 FOLLOW-UP

PATIENT MONITORING
- Attitude, hydration, cardiopulmonary status, urine output, and body weight
- Blood sugar q1–3h initially; q6h once stable
- Electrolytes q4–8h initially; q24h once stable
- Acid–base status q8–12h initially; q24h once stable

PREVENTION/AVOIDANCE
Appropriate insulin administration

POSSIBLE COMPLICATIONS
- Hypokalemia
- Hypoglycemia

- Hypophosphatemia
- Cerebral edema
- Pulmonary edema
- Renal failure
- Heart failure

EXPECTED COURSE AND PROGNOSIS
Guarded

 MISCELLANEOUS

ASSOCIATED CONDITIONS
- Pancreatitis
- Hyperadrenocorticism
- Diestrus
- Bacterial infection
- Electrolyte depletion

AGE-RELATED FACTORS
N/A

ZOONOTIC POTENTIAL
N/A

PREGNANCY
- Risk of fetal death may be relatively high.
- Glucose regulation is often difficult.

SYNONYMS
N/A

SEE ALSO
Diabetes Mellitus without Complication—Cats
Diabetes Mellitus without Complication—Dogs

ABBREVIATIONS
TCO_2 = total carbon dioxide

Suggested Reading
Feldman EC, Nelson RW. Diabetic ketoacidosis. Canine and feline endocrinology and reproduction. 2nd ed. Philadelphia: Saunders, 1996:392–421.
Greco DS. Endocrine emergencies: part I. endocrine pancreatic disorders. Compendium Contin Educ Pract Vet 1997;19:15–23.
MacIntire DK. Emergency treatment of diabetic crisis: insulin overdose, diabetic ketoacidosis and hyperosmolar coma. Vet Clin North Am Small Anim Pract 1995;25:639.
Nichols R, Crenshaw KL. Complications and concurrent disease associated with diabetic ketoacidosis and other severe forms of diabetes mellitus. In: Bonagura JB, ed. Small animal practice current veterinary therapy XII. Philadelphia: Saunders, 1995:384–386.
Wheeler SL. Emergency management of the diabetic patient. Sem Vet Med Surg Small Anim 1988;3:265–273.
Author Elisa M. Mazzaferro
Consulting Editor Deborah S. Greco

DIABETIC HEPATOPATHY

BASICS

OVERVIEW
• Liver lesion characterized by vacuolar degenerative hepatopathy and stromal collapse resulting in marked hepatic nodularity; associated with an uncommon dermatosis and diabetes mellitus • Liver lesions may precede development of cutaneous lesions and diabetes mellitus.

SIGNALMENT
• Middle-aged to older dogs • Males may have greater predilection • No breed predilection

SIGNS

Historical Findings
• Acute onset • Common signs—weight loss; lethargy; polyuria and polydipsia; jaundice; anorexia; diarrhea; vomiting; sometimes lameness • May be few signs

Physical Examination Findings
• Lethargy, skin lesions, poor body condition • Cutaneous lesions—see Superficial Necrolytic Dermatitis. • Normal to large hepatic size—rarely, may palpate irregular liver margin

CAUSES & RISK FACTORS
• Etiology—undetermined; hypoaminoacidemia role in cutaneous lesions. • Remains unclarified whether unique liver lesion mediates skin lesions or another metabolic abnormality initiates changes in each organ system • Secondary etiopathogenic role—suggested for ill-defined zinc, fatty acid, or niacin deficiencies • Hyperglucagonemia—originally proposed as causal mechanism; inconsistent (only 30%–40% of dogs demonstrate high plasma glucagon); may reflect specificity of assays or high hepatic glucagon extraction rather than lack of association; pancreatic mass representing a glucagon-producing tumor demonstrated in < 25% of dogs • Insulin—high concentration suggests insulin resistance • Cutaneous lesions occasionally associated with other primary hepatic injuries: anticonvulsant or mycotoxin ingestion; cirrhosis

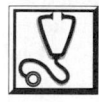

DIAGNOSIS

DIFFERENTIAL DIAGNOSIS
• Cirrhosis—regenerative nodular hyperplasia with connective tissue deposition and loss of architectural organization • Chronic hepatitis—inflammatory cell infiltrates; periportal piecemeal necrosis • Copper storage hepatopathy—high tissue copper associated with acquired necroinflammatory lesion • Diffuse nodular hyperplasia

CBC/BIOCHEMISTRY/URINALYSIS
• CBC—mild to moderate nonregenerative to mildly regenerative anemia; with advanced liver lesion microcytosis; neutrophilic leukocytosis reflects cutaneous infections • Biochemistry—high liver enzymes (especially ALP and ALT); hypoproteinemia; hypoalbuminemia; fasting hyperglycemia; variable cholesterol and BUN • Urinalysis—no consistent findings; ammonium biurate crystalluria consistent with severe hepatic insufficiency

OTHER LABORATORY TESTS
• Total serum bile acids—abnormally increased in most cases • Plasma glucagon—inconsistently high • Plasma amino acids—30%–50% of normal concentrations for most amino acids (dogs with cutaneous lesions); intermediate reductions in dogs with liver lesions preceding skin lesions

IMAGING
• Abdominal radiography—normal to large liver; often no abnormalities; rare effusion • Abdominal ultrasonography—may see irregular liver margin; characteristic nodular pattern: hypoechoic foci in hyperechoic parenchyma, referred to as Swiss cheese pattern; although suggested as pathognomonic, other severe vacuolar hepatopathies also may demonstrate this pattern; occasional diffuse nodularity unexplainably cannot be imaged; pancreatic mass imaged in < 20% of dogs

DIAGNOSTIC PROCEDURES
• Aspiration sampling—hepatocytes show vacuolation typical of glycogen and lipid • Liver biopsy—needle biopsy may compromise definitive diagnosis by limiting evaluation for regenerative nodules and fibroplasia; laparoscopic sampling preferred over laparotomy as affected dogs do not heal well • If pancreatic mass found, resect for histology and immunohistochemical staining for glucagon and other products. • Skin biopsy—see Superficial Necrolytic Dermatitis.

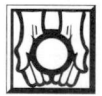

TREATMENT
Diet—high in good-quality protein; enteral or parenteral feeding may be required; improve nitrogen tolerance with lactulose and metronidazole (see Hepatic Encephalopathy)

MEDICATIONS

DRUG(S)
• Manage diabetes • Cutaneous or nail bed infections—systemic antimicrobials or antifungals; germicidal baths • Amino acid supplementation—egg yolk (3–6 yolks per day) or anabolic protein supplements (health food store products for muscle accretion) of some benefit; better response to 10% crystalline amino acid solution (Aminosyn, Abbott Laboratories; 100 mL contains total of 10 g amino acids), 500 mL per dog given slowly over 8–12 hr via a large central vein (i.e., jugular vein, unless coagulopathy is present, then use long jugular catheter threaded deeply into a peripheral vein); rare hepatic encephalopathy induction; cutaneous lesions resolve with prolonged remission in some dogs after only one amino acid treatment; if little response, repeat treatments (at 7–10 day intervals for four treatments); if no response, grave prognosis • Essential fatty acid supplementation—omega-3 fatty acids; double normal dose; use high-potency supplement • Zinc supplementation—2 mg/kg q24h with zinc methionine (or zinc acetate with hepatic encephalopathy) • Niacinamide—used in some dogs; 250–500 mg/dog q8–12h (500 mg for dogs > 10 kg); watch for toxic effects • Topical glucocorticoids—for unresponsive inflammatory skin lesions, after infection managed (Caution: systemic glucocorticoids may promote hepatic encephalopathy, enteric ulceration, and infection) • Ketoconazole—to clear secondary yeast infection; antiinflammatory and antipruritic effects • Somatostatin—long-acting octreotide theorized as possible improved treatment; based on speculated involvement of hormonal and metabolic interactions • Ursodeoxycholic acid—10–15 mg/kg PO daily • Antioxidants—vitamin E (10 IU/kg daily) and optionally, S-adenosylmethionine (20 mg/kg PO daily)

POSSIBLE INTERACTIONS
• Hepatic encephalopathy with high protein intake and amino acid infusions • Toxic effects of ketoconazole and interference in drug metabolism, and toxic effects of niacinamide and zinc.

FOLLOW-UP

PATIENT MONITORING
• Monthly physical exam to determine need for amino acid infusion and treatment for secondary infection • Quarterly CBC, biochemistry, and urinalysis to monitor liver function and secondary infection • Diabetes management

POSSIBLE COMPLICATIONS
• Ketoacidosis—uncommon • Hepatic encephalopathy • Sepsis—due to diabetes and skin lesions • Pain—from skin lesions

EXPECTED COURSE AND PROGNOSIS
Some dogs achieve cutaneous remission > 1 year with described therapies; others have unremitting progression, necessitating euthanasia; anecdotal report of improved liver lesions with treatment

MISCELLANEOUS

SYNONYMS
• Superficial necrolytic dermatitis • Necrolytic migratory erythema • Metabolic epidermal necrosis • Glucagonoma syndrome • Hepatocutaneous syndrome

Suggested Reading
Rosychuk RAW. Superficial necrolytic dermatitis (hepatocutaneous syndrome). Seattle: Proc 18th ACVIM, 2000:651–653.

Author Sharon A. Center
Consulting Editor Sharon A. Center

BASICS

OVERVIEW
• Protrusion of an abdominal organ through an abnormal opening in the diaphragm either as an acquired injury or as a congenital defect
• Traumatic—most common acquired cause; usually the result of automobile trauma but also any forceful blow; sudden increase of pressure results in an abdominal–thoracic pressure gradient, causing a tear in the diaphragm, usually at a muscular portion.
• Congenital—pleuroperitoneal or peritoneopericardial; may note other congenital defects (e.g., ventricular septal defect, aortic stenosis, portal caval shunt, and cranioventral abdominal wall defects)
• Mechanical and organic factors contribute to clinical signs.
• Impaired normal lung expansion—because of lack of lung contact with parietal pleura
• Rib fractures—may contribute to hypoventilation because of pain or mechanical (flail chest) factors
• Accumulation of fluid or air or organ entrapment—prevents lung expansion and contributes to hypoventilation; fluid may be blood from a lung laceration or intercostal vessel tear, chyle from thoracic duct trauma, or transudate from abdominal organ entrapment, leading to transudation of fluid from venous stasis and increased hydrostatic pressure.
• Intrapulmonary changes (e.g., lung contusion, atelectasis, and capillary permeability changes causing edema)—contribute to poor gas exchange
• Myocardial trauma may result in various dysrhythmias—ventricular tachyarrhythmias: most common; may in turn cause low cardiac output and tissue hypoxia; dysrhythmias: most commonly seen within 24–72 hr after trauma; difficult to control with conventional treatment; commonly resolve within 5 days
• Various stages of shock—may cause multiple organ system failure

SIGNALMENT
• Dogs and cats
• Acquired—no breed predilection
• Congenital—Weimeraners and cocker spaniels may be predisposed; may be diagnosed at any age because clinical signs are variable and intermittent
• Young animals at higher risk

SIGNS
Traumatic
• May be acute, subacute, or chronic (with no history of trauma)
• Low-grade respiratory signs
• Vague history of gastrointestinal problems
• May be progressive

• Dyspnea—most common; acutely affected patients frequently in shock
• Arrhythmias—may be detected
• Muffled heart and lung sounds along with intestinal sounds—may be auscultated in the thorax
• Abdomen—may feel empty on palpation
• Acute incarceration of bowel—may cause vomiting, diarrhea, retching, bloating, pain, and acute collapse

Congenital
• May be asymptomatic; may become symptomatic late in life
• Referable to the respiratory, cardiac, or gastrointestinal system
• Dyspnea, muffled heart sounds, murmurs, and concurrent ventral abdominal wall defects—most common
• May be acute from strangulation of incarcerated bowel, liver, or spleen or rapid formation of pericardial effusions

CAUSES & RISK FACTORS
Traumatic—lack of confinement and exposure to automobiles; any blunt trauma; roaming animals and male dogs at higher risk than others

DIAGNOSIS

DIFFERENTIAL DIAGNOSIS
• See Dyspnea, Tachypnea, and Panting
• See Pleural Effusion

CBC/BIOCHEMISTRY/URINALYSIS
Nonspecific changes due to ischemia or shock may be noted.

OTHER LABORATORY TESTS
N/A

IMAGING
• Radiography—most useful diagnostic test; may need prior thoracentesis for pleural effusion
• Positive-contrast celiography and/or ultrasonography—if definitive diagnosis not made

DIAGNOSTIC PROCEDURES
N/A

TREATMENT

TRAUMATIC
• Inpatient—treat shock; improve ventilation and cardiac output; manage concurrent injury; stabilize patient before surgery.
• Surgery—intervention in the first 24 hr historically has resulted in a higher mortality rate; early intervention indicated with persistent hypotension despite adequate fluid therapy (including transfusion when needed), severe respiratory failure from excessive lung

compression, severe liver failure secondary to organ entrapment, bowel rupture, or enlarging gas-filled bowel seen on radiographs; if patient cannot be stabilized, surgical repair will not necessarily improve cardiovascular and respiratory status.
• Intrathoracic gastric dilation—requires immediate decompression; use methods other than immediate surgery.

CONGENITAL
• Surgical repair—perform as early as possible to avoid adhesion formation and organ entrapment.
• Stabilize symptomatic patients before surgery.

MEDICATIONS

DRUGS
Antiarrhythmic agents—as indicated; cardiac arrhythmias often difficult to control

CONTRAINDICATIONS/POSSIBLE INTERACTIONS
Take care when treating for shock with concurrent severe pulmonary contusion; products such as hetastarch (Hespan) may be beneficial.

FOLLOW-UP
• Pneumothorax—may develop from excessive pressure on damaged lung tissue during anesthetic bagging or from failure to remove air from the chest cavity after diaphragmatic closure
• Pulmonary edema—may develop from excessive fluid administration in the face of low oncotic pressure from blood loss, capillary permeability changes secondary to inflammation in response to pulmonary contusion, or re-expansion
• Frequent electrocardiographic monitoring—advised; evaluate for arrhythmias
• Prognosis—always initially guarded; favorable after successful control of shock, elimination of any cardiac arrhythmias, successful surgery, and the lack of re-expansion pulmonary edema

MISCELLANEOUS

Suggested Reading
Boudrieau RJ, Muir WW. Pathophysiology of traumatic diaphragmatic hernia in dogs. Compend Contin Educ Pract Vet 1987;9:379–385.
Author Justin H. Straus
Consulting Editor Lynelle R. Johnson

DIARRHEA, ACUTE

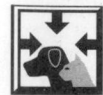

BASICS

DEFINITION
Abrupt or recent onset of abnormally frequent discharge and fluid content of fecal matter

PATHOPHYSIOLOGY
• Caused by imbalance in the absorptive, secretory, and motility actions of the intestines
• May or may not be associated with osmotic diarrhea inflammation of the intestinal tract (enteritis) • Osmotic diarrhea—Ingestion of osmotically active foodstuffs that are poorly digestible, dietary malassimilation, malabsorption, or osmotically active medications (e.g., lactulose or magnesium sulfate) can increase intestinal lumen osmotic force, which holds and draws fluid into the gut lumen. • Fiber content contributes to the osmotic force exerted by a diet.
• The clinical signs of osmotic diarrhea often abate or resolve with fasting.
• In secretory diarrhea, the intestinal epithelium secretes fluid and electrolytes to aid in the digestion, absorption, and propulsion of foodstuffs. • In disease states this secretion can overwhelm the absorptive activity • Stimulation of the parasympathetic nervous system or exposure to a variety of secretogogues can increase intestinal secretion.
• Many of the infectious causes of diarrhea are related to increased secretion and abnormal motility. • Forward intestinal motility propels intestinal chyme toward the colon and out of the body; segmental motility tends to slow forward progression and increase time for digestion and absorption of food; increased forward propulsion or decreased segmental contractions can produce diarrhea due to motility changes and secondary decreases in absorption. • Diarrhea can result from a combination of factors. • Inflammatory and infectious diarrhea—often produced by changes in secretion, motility, and absorptive ability • Abnormal permeability—various diseases cause mucosal inflammatory ulceration and/or necrosis, resulting in leaky tight functions between cells. Mild cases end in fluid loss. Severe cases result in the loss of large molecules (albumin, red blood cells, globulin).

SYSTEMS AFFECTED
• Endocrine/Metabolic • Gastrointestinal

SIGNALMENT
• Dogs and cats • Any animal can suffer from acute diarrhea; kittens and puppies are most frequently affected.

SIGNS

General Comments
• Acute diarrhea is usually self limiting
• Diarrhea can occur with or without systemic illness. • Signs can vary from diarrhea in an apparently healthy patient to severe systemic signs. • The choice of diagnostic and therapeutic measures depends on the severity of illness. • Patients that are not systemically ill have normal hydration and minimal systemic signs. • Signs of more severe illness (e.g., concurrent vomiting, abdominal pain, blood in the diarrhea or vomit, severe dehydration, and depression) should prompt more-aggressive diagnostic and therapeutic measures.

Historical Findings
• Increased fecal fluidity and frequency of short duration • Owner may report fecal accidents, vomiting, changes in fecal consistency and volume, blood or mucus in the feces, or straining to defecate. • A period of listlessness and anorexia may precede the onset of viral enteritis. • Owners may be able to report exposure to toxins, dietary changes, or dietary indiscretion.

Physical Examination Findings
• Vary with the severity of disease
• Dehydration, depression, or lethargy often present to some degree • Abdominal pain, abdominal discomfort, fever, signs of hypotension, nausea, and weakness may occur in more severely affected individuals.

CAUSES
• Systemic illness may also result in diarrhea as a secondary event. • Dietary indiscretion—ingestion of garbage, nonfood material, or spoiled food • Dietary changes—abrupt changes in amount or type of foodstuffs
• Dietary intolerance—maldigestion or malassimilation of foodstuffs, dietary hypersensitivity • Metabolic diseases—hypoadrenocorticism (Addison's disease), liver disease, renal diseases, and pancreatic disease can cause acute or chronic diarrhea. • Obstruction or foreign bodies—ingestion of foreign bodies, intussusception, or intestinal volvulus • Idiopathic—hemorrhagic gastroenteritis • Infectious
—Viral—parvovirus (CPV and feline panleukopenia), coronavirus, rotavirus, canine distemper virus
—Bacterial—*Salmonella, Campylobacter, Clostridium* spp., *Escherichia coli*, etc.
—Parasitic—verminous (hookworms, ascarids, whipworms, strongyles, and cestodes) or protozoal (*Giardia,* coccidia, and *Entamoeba*)
—Rickettsial—salmon poisoning (*Neorickettsia*)
• Drugs and toxins—heavy metals (i.e., lead), organophosphates, nonsteroidal antiinflammatories, steroids, antimicrobials, anthelmintic, antineoplastic agents, lawn and garden products, etc.

RISK FACTORS
Young dogs and cats present for diarrhea from dietary indiscretion, intussusception, foreign bodies, and infectious causes more often than older patients.

DIAGNOSIS

DIFFERENTIAL DIAGNOSIS
• Patients should have a complete physical examination, fecal examination, and a minimal database to assess their hydration status. • Further diagnostic tests depend on the extent of illness and other clinical signs.

CBC/BIOCHEMISTRY/URINALYSIS
• Generally normal; not necessary with mild illness • More-severe illness should prompt a more complete evaluation. • Can see leukopenia (especially neutropenia) with parvoviral enteritis • Electrolytes are commonly abnormal because of intestinal losses (hypokalemia, hypochloremia, hyponatremia). • Altered protein levels because of intestinal loss (decreased) or dehydration (increased)
• Altered renal values with dehydration or gastrointestinal hemorrhage (prerenal azotemia) or with renal disease • Liver and pancreatic enzymes can be elevated with disease in these organ systems.

OTHER LABORATORY TESTS
N/A

IMAGING
• Abdominal radiographs can help identify or rule out intestinal foreign bodies or obstruction.
• Ileus—commonly seen with acute diarrhea, regardless of cause
• Radiographs—generally not necessary in patients with mild illness
• More-severe signs (i.e., abdominal pain or persistent vomiting) may increase the likely diagnostic benefit of radiology.
• Contrast abdominal radiography and ultrasonography may be useful with some patients.

DIAGNOSTIC PROCEDURES
• Perform fecal analysis for parasites on all patients.
• Because helminth ova and *Giardia* oocytes can be shed in low numbers or intermittently, multiple fecal analyses are recommended, and empiric treatment may be advisable.
• Can perform fecal ELISA tests for parvovirus antigen in dogs
• Endoscopy and biopsy—useful in select cases; more commonly needed in chronic diarrhea

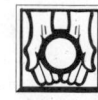

TREATMENT
• Depends largely on the severity of illness; patients with mild illness can most often be handled as outpatients with symptomatic therapy; patients with more-severe illness or that fail to respond to therapy should be treated more aggressively.

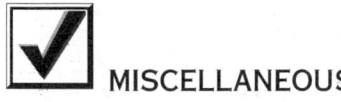

• Fluid therapy and correction of electrolyte imbalances is the mainstay of treatment in most cases.
• Can give crystalloid fluid therapy orally, subcutaneously, or intravenously, as required; can give oral fluids (water or carbohydrate- and electrolyte-containing fluids) to patients that are not vomiting
• Aim to return the patient to proper hydration status (over 12–24 hr) and replace any ongoing losses.
• Severe volume depletion can occur with acute diarrhea; aggressive shock fluid therapy may be necessary.
• Fluid choice for intravenous or subcutaneous use should take into consideration the electrolyte and hydration status.
• Use potassium supplementation (potassium chloride 20–40 mEq/L) in most patients, but not during shock fluid therapy.
• Patients with severe hypokalemia may require more-aggressive potassium supplementation.
• Patients with mild illness that are not vomiting—a period of fasting (12–24 hr) is often followed by a bland diet such as boiled rice and chicken or a prepared diet.
• Limiting exposure to garbage, foods other than the patient's normal diet, and potential foreign bodies is also recommended.
• Patients with obstruction or foreign bodies may require surgery to evaluate the intestine and remove the foreign objects.

MEDICATIONS

DRUG(S) OF CHOICE
• Antidiarrheal drugs can be classified as motility-modifying drugs, antisecretory drugs, or intestinal protectants.
• Motility-modifying drugs generally operate by increasing segmental motility and thus increasing transit time (i.e., narcotic antidiarrheals such as loperamide; 0.1 mg/kg PO q8–12h in dogs; 0.08 mg/kg PO q12h in cats) or by decreasing forward motility (i.e., anticholinergics); these medications are not necessary in mild disease, as it is generally self-limiting.
• In severe disease, give proper fluid therapy and seek underlying problems; do not use these medications longer than 1–2 days because of adverse effects.
• Acute diarrhea that does not resolve with antidiarrheal drugs merits further investigation.
• Anticholinergics (i.e., atropine, propantheline) can produce a generalized ileus because they decrease segmental and peristaltic motion; this decrease in tone can increase the severity of diarrhea in some patients.

• Antisecretory drugs are used to decrease the volume of fluid in the feces; opiates, anticholinergics, chlorpromazine, and salicylates may decrease secretion into the intestinal lumen.
• Intestinal protectants are generally not helpful in patents with acute diarrhea and have not been shown to change intestinal fluid or electrolyte loss.
• Bismuth subsalicylate may be of some benefit because of the antisecretory properties of salicylate.
• Anthelmintics (i.e., fenbendazole 50 mg/kg PO q24h for 3 days) and antiprotozoal drugs (i.e., metronidazole 30–60 mg/kg PO q24h for 5 days) are recommended as empiric treatment for patients with acute diarrhea or those with positive fecal analyses.
• Can use coccidiostatic (i.e., sulfadimethoxine) drugs if fecal analysis warrants
• Antibiotic therapy is probably unnecessary for most cases of mild illness and may actually cause diarrhea.
• Patients with bacterial enteritis, severe illness, concomitant leukopenia, or suspected breakdown of the gastrointestinal mucosal barrier (as evidenced by blood in the feces) should be treated with broad-spectrum antimicrobial agents.

CONTRAINDICATIONS
• Anticholinergics in patients with suspected intestinal obstruction, glaucoma, or intestinal ileus
• Narcotic analgesics—can cause CNS depression; undesirable in patients with more-severe illness that are already depressed or lethargic
• Narcotic analgesics in patients with liver disease and bacterial or toxic enteritis

PRECAUTIONS
• Most cases of acute mild diarrhea resolve with minimal treatment; be cautious of excessive diagnostics and overtreating these patients.
• Almost any drug can produce adverse effects (often including diarrhea and vomiting); these may be more severe than the initial problem.

POSSIBLE INTERACTIONS
N/A

ALTERNATIVE DRUG(S)
N/A

FOLLOW-UP

PATIENT MONITORING
• Most acute diarrhea resolves within a few days. • If clinical signs persist, additional diagnostics and treatments may be necessary.
• Upon completion of medication, recheck patients that exhibited parasites by fecal analysis.

POSSIBLE COMPLICATIONS
• Intussusception is thought to be associated with increased intestinal motility.
• Monitor for this complication in patients with acute diarrhea due to other causes, especially young dogs with parvoviral enteritis and parasitism.

MISCELLANEOUS

ASSOCIATED CONDITIONS
Acute vomiting commonly occurs concurrently with acute diarrhea.

AGE-RELATED FACTORS
• Young dogs and cats present for diarrhea from dietary indiscretion, intussusception, foreign bodies, and infectious causes more often than older patients. • Younger and smaller animals are also more prone to dehydration and may require more-aggressive fluid therapy.

ZOONOTIC POTENTIAL
• *Campylobacter* enteritis is contagious to people. • Some strains of *Giardia* may be contagious to people. • Parasitic larvae can cause visceral larval migrans (ascarids) and cutaneous larval migrans (hookworms) in people, particularly children.

PREGNANCY
N/A

SEE ALSO
See Causes.

ABBREVIATIONS
• CNS = central nervous system
• CPV = canine parvovirus • ELISA = enzyme-linked immunosorbent assay

Suggested Reading
Burrows CF, Batt RM, Sherding RG. Disease of the small intestine. In: Ettinger SJ, Feldman EC, eds. Textbook of veterinary internal medicine. Philadelphia: Saunders, 1995:1169–1232.
Jergens AE. Acute diarrhea. In: Bonagura JD, ed. Kirk's current veterinary therapy XII. Philadelphia: Saunders, 1995:701–705.
Lewis LD, Morris ML, Hand MS. Gastrointestinal, pancreatic and hepatic diseases. In: Small animal clinical nutrition III. Topeka, KN: Mark Morris Associates, 1989.

Acknowledgment
The author/editors acknowledge the prior contributions of Dr. Derek S. Duval, who authored this topic in the previous edition.
Author Michelle Pressel
Consulting Editors Albert E. Jergens

DIARRHEA, CHRONIC—CATS

 BASICS

DEFINITION
• A change in the frequency, consistency, and volume of feces for more than 3 weeks or with a pattern of episodic recurrence
• Can be either small bowel or large bowel in origin

PATHOPHYSIOLOGY
• High solute and fluid secretion—secretory diarrhea
• Low solute and fluid absorption—osmotic diarrhea
• High intestinal permeability
• Abnormal GI motility

SYSTEMS AFFECTED
• Gastrointestinal
• Endocrine/metabolic/fluid, electrolyte, and acid–base
• Nutritional
• Lymphatic
• Exocrine

SIGNALMENT
Cats

SIGNS

General Comments
Underlying disease process determines extent of clinical signs.

Historical Findings
Small Bowel
• Larger volume of feces than normal
• Frequency of defecation is mild to moderately above normal (2–4 times per day)
• Weight loss
• Polyphagia with malabsorption/maldigestion and hyperthyroidism
• May be melena; no hematochezia and mucus
• No tenesmus or dyschezia
• Vomiting is common.
Large Bowel
• Smaller volume of feces per defecation than normal
• Frequency of defecation significantly higher than normal (>4 times per day)
• No weight loss
• Melena absent; usually hematochezia and mucus
• Tenesmus and urgency; dyschezia with rectal or distal colonic disease
• Vomiting in some cats

Physical Examination Findings
• Poor body condition associated with infiltrative bowel diseases, chronic obstruction, and metabolic disorders

• Diffuse intestinal thickening suggests infiltrative disease (lymphoma, IBD)
• Segmental thickening caused by neoplasia (especially lymphoma), foreign body, mesenteric lymphadenopathy, and eosinophilic or granulomatous enteritis (both rare)
• Aggregation of bowel loops may be palpated in a cat with a linear foreign body.
• A palpable thyroid nodule suggests hyperthyroidism.
• Small kidneys may indicate chronic renal disease.
• Hepatomegaly or icterus may indicate hepatic lipidosis, feline infectious peritonitis (FIP), hepatic neoplasia, or biliary disease.
• Rectal palpation may reveal abnormal rectal mucosa, intraluminal or extraluminal rectal mass, or rectal stricture; small or large bowel diarrhea
• Fundic examination may reveal lesions suggestive of toxoplasmosis, FIP, histoplasmosis, or feline leukemia virus (FeLV)

CAUSES
• IBD—lymphoplasmacytic enterocolitis, granulomatous enteritis, eosinophilic enteritis/hypereosinophilic syndrome, and idiopathic inflammatory colitis
• Neoplasia—lymphoma, adenocarcinoma, mast cell tumor, and polyps
• Obstruction—neoplasia, foreign body, IBD, intussusception, and stricture
• Parasitic—*Giardia, Toxoplasma gondii, Toxocara cati, Toxascaris leonina, Cryptosporidium* spp., *Cystoisospora* spp, *Tritrichomonas foetus*
• Metabolic disorders—hyperthyroidism, renal disease, hepatobiliary disease, diabetes mellitus, toxins, and drug administration
• Bacterial—*Campylobacter jejuni, Salmonella* spp., *Yersinia pseudotuberculosis,* and *Clostridium perfringens*
• Viral—FeLV, FIV, and FIP
• Mycotic—histoplasmosis and aspergillosis
• Noninflammatory malabsorption—lymphangiectasia, small intestinal bacterial overgrowth, short bowel syndrome, villous atrophy, and duodenal ulcers
• Maldigestion—hepatobiliary disease and exocrine pancreatic insufficiency (uncommon in cats)
• Dietary—dietary sensitivity, dietary indiscretion, and diet changes
• Congenital anomalies—short colon, portosystemic shunt, and persistent pancreaticomesojejunal ligament

RISK FACTORS
Dietary changes and feeding poorly digestible or high-fat diet

 DIAGNOSIS

DIFFERENTIAL DIAGNOSIS
First localize the origin of the diarrhea to the small or large bowel or both on the basis of historical signs.

CBC/BIOCHEMISTRY/URINALYSIS
• Eosinophilia in some cats with parasitism, eosinophilic enterocolitis/hypereosinophilic syndrome, or mast cell tumor
• Macrocytosis in some cats with hyperthyroidism or FeLV infection
• Anemia and microcytosis suggest chronic GI bleeding and iron deficiency
• Leukopenia in some cats with FeLV or FIV infection
• Biochemical and urinalysis abnormalities may suggest renal disease, hepatobiliary disease, or endocrinopathy.
• Panhypoproteinemia caused by protein-losing enteropathy is uncommon in cats with intestinal disease.

OTHER LABORATORY TESTS

Fecal and/or Rectal Scraping Examination
• Direct fecal examination, routine fecal flotation, and zinc sulfate centrifugation (for *Giardia*) may reveal GI parasites.
• Cytologic examination of rectal scrapings may reveal specific organism (e.g., *Histoplasma*).
• Sudan stain for fecal fats may indicate steatorrhea, suggesting malabsorption or maldigestion.
• Culture feces if *Campylobacter* or *Salmonella* is suspected—special media required; check with your laboratory prior to submission.

Thyroid Function Tests
• High serum total T_4 concentration indicates hyperthyroidism.
• If hyperthyroidism is suspected but the total T_4 is normal, perform a T_3 suppression test, TRH response test, or technetium thyroid scan; free T_4 by dialysis can also be used but some false-positive results can occur.

Serologic Testing
Test for FeLV and FIV—especially if hematologic abnormalities are present.

Test for Exocrine Pancreatic Function
• Feline-specific TLI—fasted serum TLI <8 μg/L is diagnostic of exocrine pancreatic insufficiency.
• Can measure fecal proteolytic activity in fecal samples from 3 consecutive days

IMAGING

• Survey abdominal radiography may indicate intestinal obstruction, mass, organomegaly, foreign body, small kidneys, hepatobiliary disease, or abdominal effusion.
• Contrast radiography (upper GI series or barium enema) may indicate bowel wall thickening, mucosal irregularity, mass, radiolucent foreign body, or stricture.
• Abdominal ultrasonography may demonstrate bowel wall thickening, abnormal bowel wall layering, GI or extra-GI masses, intussusception, foreign body, ileus, abdominal effusion, hepatobiliary disease, renal disease, or mesenteric lymphadenopathy.

DIAGNOSTIC PROCEDURES

If maldigestive (EPI), metabolic, parasitic, dietary, and infectious causes have been excluded, endoscopy and mucosal biopsy or GI ultrasound and fine-needle aspiration or microcore biopsy are indicated for definitive diagnosis and treatment.

Endoscopy

• Upper GI endoscopy allows examination and biopsy of the gastric and duodenal mucosa; always obtain multiple mucosal specimens from both duodenum and stomach.
• Flexible colonoscopy allows examination of the entire colon, cecum, and often the distal ileum; rigid colonoscopy limits examination to the descending colon and rectum; always obtain multiple mucosal specimens from all areas examined.

Ultrasound-guided GI Biopsy

Can use ultrasound-guided fine-needle aspiration on most GI lesions and guided microcore (true-cut) biopsy on noncystic lesions >2 cm in diameter

TREATMENT

APPROPRIATE HEALTH CARE

• Often must be specific for the underlying cause to be successful
• When no definitive diagnosis is possible, empirical treatment with dietary management and metronidazole sometimes results in clinical improvement.

NURSING CARE

• Give fluid therapy with balanced electrolyte solution (e.g., normal saline or lactated Ringer's solution) for dehydration.
• Correct electrolyte and acid–base imbalances.

SURGICAL CONSIDERATIONS

Pursue exploratory laparotomy and surgical biopsy if there is evidence of obstruction, an intestinal mass, mid–small bowel disease unreachable via ultrasound-guided procedure, or if a diagnosis based on endoscopic biopsy or ultrasound-guided procedure is questioned because of poor response to therapy.

MEDICATIONS

DRUGS OF CHOICE

• A bland or hypoallergenic diet may be beneficial.
• A therapeutic trial with fenbendazole (25 mg/kg PO q24h for 3 days) or metronidazole (10–20 mg/kg PO q12h for 10–14 days) is often used to rule out occult *Giardia* infection. Fenbendazole has the additional benefit of anthelmintic therapy; metronidazole may have nonspecific antiinflammatory GI effects and is effective in treating small intestinal bacterial overgrowth.

CONTRAINDICATIONS

Anticholinergics exacerbate most types of chronic diarrhea and should not be used for empirical treatment.

PRECAUTIONS

Opiate antidiarrheals such as diphenoxylate and loperamide can cause hyperactivity and respiratory depression in cats and should not be used for more than 3 days.

POSSIBLE INTERACTIONS

N/A

ALTERNATIVE DRUGS

N/A

FOLLOW-UP

PATIENT MONITORING

• Fecal volume and character, frequency of defecation, and body weight
• Resolution usually occurs gradually with treatment; if diarrhea does not resolve, consider reevaluating the diagnosis.

POSSIBLE COMPLICATIONS

• Dehydration
• Abdominal effusion with intestinal adenocarcinoma

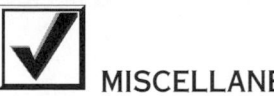

MISCELLANEOUS

ASSOCIATED CONDITIONS

N/A

AGE-RELATED FACTORS

N/A

ZOONOTIC POTENTIAL

• *Toxoplasma*
• *Giardia*
• *Cryptosporidium*
• *Salmonella*
• *Campylobacter*

PREGNANCY

N/A

SYNONYMS

N/A

SEE ALSO

See Causes.

ABBREVIATIONS

• EPI = exocrine pancreatic insufficiency
• FeLV = feline leukemia virus
• FIP = feline infectious peritonitis
• FIV = feline immunodeficiency virus
• GI = gastrointestinal
• IBD = inflammatory bowel disease
• TLI = trypsin-like immunoreactivity

Suggested Reading

Gookin JL, Breitschwerdt EB, Levy MG, et al. Diarrhea associated with trichomonosis in cats. J Am Vet Med Assoc 1999;215:1450–1454.

Jergens AE. Inflammatory bowel disease. Current perspectives. Vet Clin North Am Small Anim Pract 1999;29:501–521.

Lappin MR. Diagnosis and management of cryptosporidiosis in dogs and cats. In: Proceedings of the 20th American College of Veterinary Internal Medicine Forum; Dallas, TX, 2002.

Steiner JM, Medinger TL, Williams DA. Feline trypsin-like immunoreactivity in feline exocrine pancreatic disease. Comp Contin Educ Pract Vet 1996;18:543–547.

Willard MD. Feline inflammatory bowel disease: a review. J Feline Med Surg 1999; 3:155–164.

Zajac AM. Giardiasis. Comp Contin Educ Pract Vet 1992;14:604–611.

Author Amy M. Grooters
Consulting Editor Albert E. Jergens

DIARRHEA, CHRONIC—DOGS

BASICS

DEFINITION
• A change in the frequency, consistency, and volume of feces for more than 3 weeks or with a pattern of episodic recurrence • Can be either small bowel or large bowel in origin

PATHOPHYSIOLOGY
• High solute and fluid secretion—secretory diarrhea • Low solute and fluid absorption—osmotic diarrhea • High intestinal permeability • Abnormal GI motility

SYSTEMS AFFECTED
• Gastrointestinal • Endocrine/Metabolic
• Lymphatic
• Exocrine

SIGNALMENT
Dogs

SIGNS

General Comments
Underlying disease process determines extent of clinical signs

Historical Findings
Small Bowel
• Larger volume of feces than normal
• Frequency of defecation—mildly to moderately above normal (2–4 times per day)
• Weight loss • Polyphagia with malabsorption/maldigestion • May be melena; no hematochezia or mucus • No tenesmus or dyschezia • May be flatulence and borborygmus • Vomiting in some dogs
Large Bowel
• Smaller volume of feces per defecation than normal • Frequency of defecation is significantly higher than normal (>4 times per day)
• No weight loss • No melena; usually hematochezia and mucus • Tenesmus and urgency; dyschezia with rectal or distal colonic disease
• Flatulence and borborygmus—variable
• Vomiting—uncommon

Physical Examination Findings
Small Bowel
• Poor body condition associated with malabsorption, maldigestion, and PLE
• May be dehydration
• Abdominal palpation may reveal thickened small bowel loops associated with infiltrative small bowel disease, abdominal effusion as a result of hypoproteinemia from PLE, or an abdominal mass such as a foreign body, neoplastic mass, intussusception, or enlarged mesenteric lymph node.
• Rectal palpation normal aside from small bowel diarrhea
Large Bowel
• Body condition typically normal
• Dehydration—uncommon
• Abdominal palpation may reveal thickened large bowel loops or an abdominal mass such

as a foreign body, neoplastic mass, intussusception, or enlarged mesenteric lymph node.
• Rectal palpation may reveal irregularity and thickening of the rectal mucosa, intraluminal or extraluminal rectal masses, rectal stricture, or sublumbar lymphadenopathy; large bowel diarrhea

CAUSES

Small Bowel
Primary Small Intestinal Disease
• Inflammatory bowel disease (e.g., lymphoplasmacytic enteritis, eosinophilic enteritis, granulomatous enteritis, immunoproliferative enteropathy of basenjis, and sprue),
• Lymphangiectasia
• Neoplasia (e.g., lymphoma and adenocarcinoma)
• Infection (e.g., histoplasmosis, *Salmonella* spp., *Clostridium perfringens,* and pythiosis)
• Parasites (e.g., *Giardia, Toxocara* spp., *Ancylostoma caninum,* and *A. strongyloides*)
• Partial obstruction (e.g., foreign body, intussusception, and neoplasia)
• Small intestinal bacterial overgrowth
• Short bowel syndrome
• Gastroduodenal ulcers
Maldigestion
• EPI (e.g., juvenile pancreatic acinar atrophy and chronic pancreatitis)
• Hepatobiliary disease
Dietary
• Dietary intolerance or allergy
• Gluten-sensitive enteropathy in Irish setters
Metabolic Disorders
• Hepatobiliary disease, hypoadrenocorticism, uremia, toxins, and drug administration (e.g., anticholinergics and antibiotics)
• Apudoma (rare)

Large Bowel
Primary Large Intestinal Disease
• Inflammatory bowel disease (e.g., lymphoplasmacytic colitis, eosinophilic colitis, histiocytic ulcerative colitis, and granulomatous colitis)
• Neoplasia (e.g., benign polyp, lymphoma, adenocarcinoma, leiomyoma, and leiomyosarcoma)
• Infection (e.g., histoplasmosis, *Clostridium perfringens, Salmonella* spp., *Campylobacter jejuni, Prototheca,* and pythiosis)
• Parasites (e.g., *Trichuris vulpis, Giardia, Ancylostoma caninum, Entamoeba histolytica,* and *Balantidium coli*)
• Noninflammatory causes (e.g., ileocolic intussusception and cecal inversion)
Dietary
• Diet—dietary indiscretion, diet changes, and foreign material (e.g., bones and hair)
• Fiber—responsive large bowel diarrhea
• Idiopathic—irritable bowel syndrome
• Metabolic disorders—uremia, hypoadrenocorticism, toxins, drug administration

RISK FACTORS
Small Bowel
• Dietary changes and feeding poorly digestible or high-fat diets
• Large-breed dogs, especially German shepherds, have the highest incidence of EPI.
• Pythiosis occurs most often in young, large-breed dogs living in states bordering the Gulf of Mexico.

Large Bowel
• Dietary changes or indiscretion, stress, and psychologic factors may play a role.
• Histiocytic ulcerative colitis occurs most often in boxers < 3 years old.
• Pythiosis occurs most often in young, large-breed dogs living in states bordering the Gulf of Mexico.

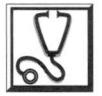

DIAGNOSIS

DIFFERENTIAL DIAGNOSIS
First localize the origin of the diarrhea to the small or large bowel or both on the basis of historical signs.

CBC/BIOCHEMISTRY/URINALYSIS
• Eosinophilia may be associated with parasitism, eosinophilic enterocolitis, hypoadrenocorticism, or pythiosis.
• Lymphopenia and hypocholesterolemia may be associated with lymphangiectasia.
• Anemia and microcytosis suggest chronic GI bleeding and iron deficiency.
• Panhypoproteinemia resulting from PLE is associated with infiltrative small bowel disorders and lymphangiectasia.
• Biochemical and urinalysis abnormalities may suggest renal disease, hepatobiliary disease, or endocrinopathy.

OTHER LABORATORY TESTS
Fecal and/or Rectal Scraping Examination
• Direct fecal examination, routine fecal flotation, and zinc sulfate centrifugation (for *Giardia*) may indicate GI parasites.
• Cytologic examination of rectal scrapings may reveal specific organisms, such as *Histoplasma* or *Prototheca*.
• Sudan stain for fecal fats may indicate steatorrhea, suggesting malabsorption or maldigestion.
• Culture feces if *Campylobacter* or *Salmonella* is suspected—special media required; check with your laboratory prior to submission.

Tests of Exocrine Pancreatic Function
• TLI—test of choice for confirming EPI in dogs; fasted serum TLI < 2.5 μg/L is diagnostic.
• Oral bentiromide (BT-PABA) test—a negligible rise in plasma PABA is consistent with a diagnosis of EPI.

Tests for Malabsorption
• Xylose absorption test—an insensitive and nonspecific test of intestinal malabsorption; peak plasma xylose concentration <45 mg/dL indicates malabsorption, but a normal value does not rule it out.
• Serum folate and B_{12} (cobalamin)—low serum B_{12} may be associated with EPI or distal small bowel malabsorption; low serum folate may be associated with proximal small bowel malabsorption; small intestinal bacterial overgrowth may increase serum folate and decrease serum B_{12}.

Tests for Metabolic Disease
• ACTH stimulation test—if hypoadreno-corticism is suspected; subnormal results indicate hypoadrenocorticism.
• Fasting and 2-hour postprandial serum bile acids—test if hepatobiliary disease is suspected; significantly increased values suggest hepatic dysfunction, cholestasis, or portosystemic shunting.

IMAGING
• Survey abdominal radiography may indicate intestinal obstruction, organomegaly, mass, foreign body, hepatobiliary disease, renal disease, or abdominal effusion
• Contrast radiography (upper GI series or barium enema) may indicate bowel wall thickening, intestinal ulcers, mucosal irregularities, mass, radiolucent foreign body, or stricture.
• Abdominal ultrasonography may demonstrate bowel wall thickening, abnormal bowel wall layering, GI or extra-GI masses, intussusception, foreign body, ileus, abdominal effusion, hepatobiliary disease, renal disease, or mesenteric lymphadenopathy.

DIAGNOSTIC PROCEDURES
If maldigestive (EPI), metabolic, parasitic, dietary, and infectious causes have been excluded, perform endoscopy and mucosal biopsy or ultrasound and fine-needle aspiration or microcore biopsy for definitive diagnosis and treatment.

Endoscopy
• Upper GI endoscopy allows examination and biopsy of the gastric and duodenal mucosa; always obtain multiple mucosal specimens from both duodenum and stomach.
• Flexible colonoscopy allows examination of the entire colon, cecum, and often the distal ileum; rigid colonoscopy limits examination to the descending colon and rectum; always obtain multiple mucosal specimens from all areas examined.

Ultrasound-guided GI Biopsy
Can perform ultrasound-guided fine-needle aspiration on most GI lesions and guided microcore (true-cut) biopsy on noncystic lesions > 2 cm in diameter.

TREATMENT

APPROPRIATE HEALTH CARE
• Treat the underlying cause—symptomatic or empirical therapy rarely resolves chronic diarrhea.
• Inform the owner that complete resolution of signs is not always possible despite a correct diagnosis and proper treatment; this is especially true for lymphangiectasia, intestinal neoplasia, pythiosis, and histoplasmosis.
• Fecal examinations are often negative in whipworm-infested dogs because of intermittent shedding of ova; because parasites are a common cause of diarrhea, perform therapeutic deworming with fenbendazole before pursuing extensive diagnostic tests.
• Feeding a low-fat, highly digestible diet for 3–4 weeks may resolve diarrhea due to dietary intolerance or allergy.

NURSING CARE
• Give fluid therapy with balanced electrolyte solution such as normal saline or lactated Ringer solution if patient is dehydrated.
• Consider colloids for hypoproteinemic patients requiring fluid therapy.
• Correct electrolyte and acid–base imbalances.

SURGICAL CONSIDERATIONS
Pursue exploratory laparotomy and surgical biopsy if there is evidence of obstruction, an intestinal mass, or mid–small bowel disease unreachable via ultrasound-guided procedure or if a diagnosis based on endoscopic biopsy or ultrasound-guided procedure is questioned because of poor response to therapy.

MEDICATIONS

DRUG(S) OF CHOICE
In dogs with signs of colitis, perform therapeutic deworming with fenbendazole (50 mg/kg PO q24h for 3 days; repeat in 3 weeks and 3 months) before pursuing extensive diagnostic testing.

CONTRAINDICATIONS
Anticholinergics exacerbate most types of chronic diarrhea; they are sometimes used to relieve cramping associated with irritable bowel syndrome; do not use them for empiric treatment of diarrhea.

PRECAUTIONS
N/A

POSSIBLE INTERACTIONS
N/A

ALTERNATIVE DRUG(S)
N/A

FOLLOW-UP

PATIENT MONITORING
• Fecal volume and character, frequency of defecation, and body weight
• In dogs with PLE—serum proteins and clinical signs (ascites, subcutaneous edema, pleural effusion) • Resolution of diarrhea is usually gradual after treatment; if it does not resolve with treatment, consider reevaluating the diagnosis.
• Some dogs with inflammatory bowel disease or EPI have secondary small intestinal bacterial overgrowth, which must be treated along with the primary disorder.

POSSIBLE COMPLICATIONS
• Dehydration
• Ascites, subcutaneous edema and/or pleural effusion with hypoalbuminemia from PLEs

MISCELLANEOUS

ASSOCIATED CONDITIONS
N/A

AGE-RELATED FACTORS
N/A

ZOONOTIC POTENTIAL
• *Giardia*
• *Salmonella*
• *Campylobacter*

PREGNANCY
N/A

SEE ALSO
See Causes.

ABBREVIATIONS
• B_{12} = vitamin B_{12}, cobalamin
• EPI = exocrine pancreatic insufficiency
• GI = gastrointestinal
• PABA = para-aminobenzoic acid
• PLE = protein-losing enteropathy
• TLI = trypsin-like immunoreactivity

Suggested Reading
Jergens AE. Inflammatory bowel disease. Current perspectives. Vet Clin North Am Small Anim Pract 1999;29:501–521.
Moore LE. Protein-losing enteropathies. In: Bonagura JD, ed. Current veterinary therapy XIII. Philadelphia: Saunders, 2000: 641–643.
Lieb MS. Chronic colitis in dogs. In: Bonagura JD, ed. Current veterinary therapy XIII. Philadelphia: Saunders, 2000: 643–648.
Author Amy M. Grooters
Consulting Editor Albert E. Jergens

DIETARY INTOLERANCE

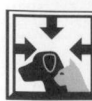 BASICS

DEFINITION
- Nonimmunologic reaction to food
- A syndrome in which adverse clinical signs are associated with the inability to digest, absorb, and/or utilize a foodstuff or with an untoward reaction to a diet
- Dietary allergies or allergic reactions to food are differentiated from dietary intolerance by the prominent immune component in the allergies.
- In a practical sense, dietary allergy and dietary intolerance may have similar signs, causes, diagnostics, and treatments and may not be easily distinguishable.

PATHOPHYSIOLOGY
- Dietary intolerance may be due to idiosyncratic reactions to dietary ingredients or additives, pharmacologic reactions to compounds in the diet, defects or deficiencies in the metabolic pathways needed to utilize the food, or a toxicity reaction to food ingredients or spoiled foodstuffs.
- Idiosyncratic reactions can produce local irritation to the intestinal lining and subsequent enteritis or such systemic signs as pruritus or urticaria.
- Pharmacologically active food ingredients can also produce local or systemic effects.
- Metabolic defects generally produce maldigestion of a dietary constituent and subsequent malabsorption, fermentation, and osmotic diarrhea.
- Toxic reactions to food may occur when a foodstuff is ingested in large amounts (e.g., onion poisoning).
- Food that is spoiled or that contains microorganisms or their toxins can produce a wide range of clinical signs and severity.

SYSTEMS AFFECTED
- Dermatologic
- Gastrointestinal
- Endocrine/Metabolic

GENETICS
- In general, no genetic basis has been shown.
- Gluten-sensitive enteropathy has been seen primarily in Irish setters.
- The specifics of a genetic basis are not well defined.

INCIDENCE/PREVALENCE
More common in cats than dogs

GEOGRAPHIC DISTRIBUTION
N/A

SIGNALMENT
- Cats and dogs of any age or breed and either sex can be affected.
- Irish setters seem predisposed to develop gluten-sensitive enteropathy; they tend to display clinical signs by 4–7 months of age.
- Juvenile dogs and cats have higher lactase activity and are less likely to display lactose intolerance, which is common in adults of both species.

SIGNS

General Comments
- Dietary intolerance commonly produces diarrhea (small or large bowel), vomiting, flatulence, anorexia, and abdominal discomfort.
- Dermatologic changes, poor weight gain, and failure to thrive may be seen in chronic dietary intolerance.

Historical Findings
- Acute dietary intolerance may accompany feeding a novel foodstuff, a new food source, or dietary change.
- The client may report cessation of clinical signs in the fasted state or within days of a dietary change.

Physical Examination Findings
The physical examination is generally nonspecific but may show abdominal discomfort, flatulence, gaseous bloating, or a poor body condition and evidence of weight loss.

CAUSES
- Idiosyncratic reactions to food additives—colorings, preservatives (BHA, monosodium glutamate, sodium nitrate, sulfur dioxide, etc.), spices, propylene glycol, etc.
- Pharmacologic reactions—vasoactive substances (i.e., histamine), psychoactive agents, stimulants (i.e., theobromine, caffeine), etc.
- Metabolic defects or deficiencies—brush border enzyme defects (i.e., lactase deficiency), inborn errors of metabolism, aminopeptidase N (in gluten-sensitive enteropathy)
- Toxic reactions to foods or spoiled foods—spices, oxalate toxicity, lectin toxicity, N-propyl disulfide aflatoxicosis, ergotism, botulism, dietary indiscretion, etc.

RISK FACTORS
Young Irish setters susceptible to gluten-sensitive enteropathy may be at greater risk to develop the disease if exposed to gluten at an early age.

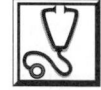 DIAGNOSIS

DIFFERENTIAL DIAGNOSIS
- Dietary allergies, inflammatory bowel disease, parasitism, exocrine pancreatic insufficiency, small intestinal bacterial overgrowth, and partial gastrointestinal obstruction can produce signs similar to those of dietary intolerance.
- Some of these disorders may occur with dietary intolerance, complicating diagnosis and treatment.
- Can make a presumptive diagnosis of dietary intolerance when dietary manipulation controls the clinical signs and other differentials are eliminated
- More-rigorous diagnosis requires demonstrating dietary sensitivity, with gastrointestinal histopathologic evaluation before and after a dietary challenge.
- Exclusion diet trials should use a novel protein source and not contain gluten (no wheat, barley, rye, buckwheat, or oats).
- Dietary trials should initially use home-cooked diets, or diets with minimal ingredients or additives.
- Clinical signs often improve within days, especially as seen in cats with gastrointestinal signs; dietary allergies may require weeks to months of feeding before seeing improvement.
- Weight gain typically lags behind the resolution of other clinical signs.

CBC/BIOCHEMISTRY/URINALYSIS
No specific changes

OTHER LABORATORY TESTS
- Few diagnostic tests are specific.
- Diagnostics mostly aim to eliminate other differentials and treat complicating factors.
- Fasting serum folate and cobalamin levels are useful in evaluating for SIBO and small intestinal malabsorption.
- Rule out exocrine pancreatic insufficiency by a fasting serum trypsin-like immunoreactivity assay.
- In select patients, gastrointestinal permeability can be assessed with a differential sugar absorption test.
- Some specific enzyme activity assays are available in the research setting.
- The use of intradermal skin testing or RAST is generally not recommended because of their low accuracy rates.

IMAGING
Abdominal radiographs or ultrasound may be useful in eliminating differential diagnoses, but specific findings are not seen in dietary intolerance.

DIAGNOSTIC PROCEDURES
- Do fecal evaluation for parasites and empiric broad-spectrum deworming (e.g., fenbendazole 50 mg/kg PO q24h for 3 consecutive days; repeat in 3 weeks and 3 months) and anti-*Giardia* therapy (e.g., metronidazole 30–60 mg/kg PO q24h for 5 days) to rule out parasitism.
- Use dietary manipulation with an exclusion diet as outlined above when intolerance is suspected.

- Following improvement on an exclusion diet, use rigorous challenge exposure to sequential single ingredients to specifically identify a dietary intolerance.
- Practically, continuing an exclusion diet or avoiding suspected problem ingredients is often undertaken instead.
- Can use gastrointestinal endoscopy to assess the mucosa of the intestinal tract; can examine biopsy specimen and histopathology before and after a dietary challenge
- Evaluate for SIBO by bacterial quantification of samples of duodenal juice.
- Gastroscopic food sensitivity testing is not considered useful in the cat and may not be helpful in the dog.

PATHOLOGIC FINDINGS

Villous atrophy and lymphoplasmacytic enteritis can be seen with dietary intolerance, but are not specific; thus pathologic evaluation must be done before and after provocation, to be useful.

TREATMENT

APPROPRIATE HEALTH CARE
- Patients with extreme and acute cases may need hospitalization for intravenous fluid therapy, antibiotics, and supportive care.
- Generally can treat on an outpatient basis

NURSING CARE
N/A

ACTIVITY
No restrictions

DIET
- Feed a diet free of the offending ingredient(s).
- Cats are generally sensitive to more than one ingredient
- If no specific ingredient has been identified, feed a nutritionally complete exclusion diet.
- Can use trial and error to find a commercial diet that does not cause dietary intolerance.
- If this approach is used, examination of the ingredients of the various diets is recommended to determine if any patterns exist that might help identify the offending ingredient(s).

CLIENT EDUCATION
Caution against feeding any scraps or varying from a set diet.

SURGICAL CONSIDERATIONS
N/A

MEDICATIONS

DRUG(S) OF CHOICE
- Generally no medications are used.
- Associated problems (e.g., bacterial overgrowth or inflammatory bowel disease) may require medical therapy as suggested in the sections specific to these problems.

CONTRAINDICATIONS
N/A

PRECAUTIONS
N/A

POSSIBLE INTERACTIONS
N/A

ALTERNATIVE DRUG(S)
N/A

FOLLOW-UP

PATIENT MONITORING
- Assess efficacy of treatment by observing improvement in clinical signs.
- Consider repeating evaluation for bacterial overgrowth or endoscopy and biopsy following dietary therapy.

PREVENTION/AVOIDANCE
- Avoiding the offending food ingredient(s) is recommended.
- If no specific ingredient has been identified, adherence to a set exclusion diet is recommended.

POSSIBLE COMPLICATIONS
SIBO and inflammatory bowel disease

EXPECTED COURSE AND PROGNOSIS
- Prognosis for a full recovery is excellent in most cases if diet is found that the patient tolerates.
- Rarely, severe reactions are produced that require short-term, aggressive in-hospital therapy.

MISCELLANEOUS

ASSOCIATED CONDITIONS
SIBO and inflammatory bowel disease are frequently associated with chronic dietary intolerance.

AGE-RELATED FACTORS
The severity of gluten-sensitive enteropathy in susceptible Irish setter puppies may be reduced by avoiding gluten-containing cereals.

ZOONOTIC POTENTIAL
N/A

PREGNANCY
N/A

SYNONYMS
Food intolerance

SEE ALSO
- Diarrhea, Chronic
- Diarrhea, Acute
- Exocrine Pancreatic Insufficiency
- Gastroenteritis, Eosinophilic
- Gastroenteritis, Lymphocytic Plasmacytic
- Gluten Enteropathy
- Inflammatory Bowel Disease
- Small Intestinal Bacterial Overgrowth

ABBREVIATIONS
- BHA = butylated hydroxyanisole
- RAST = radioallergosorbent test
- SIBO = small intestine bacterial overgrowth

Suggested Reading

Batt RM. Wheat-sensitive enteropathy in Irish setters. In: Kirk RW, ed. Current veterinary therapy IX. Philadelphia: Saunders, 1986:893–896.

Burrows CF, Batt RM, Sherding RG. Disease of the small intestine. In: Ettinger SJ, Feldman EC, eds. Textbook of veterinary internal medicine. Philadelphia: Saunders, 1995:1169–1232.

Guilford WG. Adverse reactions to food. In: Kirk RW, Bonagura JD, eds. Current veterinary therapy XI. Philadelphia: Saunders, 1992:587–592.

Guilford WG. Food sensitivity in cats with chronic idiopathic gastrointestinal problems. J Vet Intern Med 2001;15:7–13.

Acknowledgment

The author and editors acknowledge the prior contributions of Dr. Derek S. Duval, who authored this topic in the previous edition.

Author Michelle Pressel
Consulting Editor Albert E. Jergens

DIGOXIN TOXICITY

BASICS

OVERVIEW
Common in veterinary practice because of digoxin's narrow therapeutic index and prevalence of renal impairment in elderly patients with cardiac disease

SIGNALMENT
- Dogs and cats
- More common in geriatric patients

SIGNS

Historical Findings
- Anorexia
- Vomiting
- Diarrhea
- Lethargy
- Depression

Physical Examination Findings
Heart rate may range from severe bradycardia to severe tachycardia.

CAUSES & RISK FACTORS
- Renal disease—impairs digoxin elimination
- Chronic pulmonary disease—results in hypoxia and acid–base disturbances
- Obesity—if dosage not calculated on lean body weight
- Hypokalemia, hypercalcemia, hypomagnesemia, and hypoxia predispose to arrhythmias.
- Drugs and conditions that alter digoxin metabolism or elimination (e.g., quinidine and hypothyroidism)
- Rapid IV digitalization
- Overdosage or accidental ingestion of owner's medication
- Administration of diuretic leading to hypokalemia

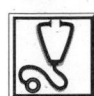

DIAGNOSIS

DIFFERENTIAL DIAGNOSIS
- Arrhythmias and conduction disturbances—may reflect structural heart disease, not digoxin toxicity
- Anorexia—common in animals with heart failure

CBC/BIOCHEMISTRY/URINALYSIS
Animals with hypokalemia, hypercalcemia, hypomagnesemia, and renal failure are predisposed to toxicity.

OTHER LABORATORY TESTS
- Consider checking thyroid status.
- Obtain digoxin serum concentration 8–10 hours after an oral dose—therapeutic range is 0.5–1.5 ng/mL. A recent study in humans found digoxin levels greater than 1 mg/ml were associated with increased mortality; not all patients with concentrations >1.5 ng/mL have signs of toxicity; some with values in the normal range have signs of toxicity, especially if hypokalemic.

IMAGING
N/A

DIAGNOSTIC PROCEDURES

Electrocardiographic Findings
- Conduction disturbances—atrioventricular (AV) block, arrhythmias, and ST segment depression in some patients
- Digoxin—can cause any arrhythmia

TREATMENT
- Discontinue digoxin until signs of toxicity resolve (24–72 hours); reevaluate need for the medication; if necessary, resume treatment at a dosage based on the serum digoxin concentration.
- Maintain hydration and correct any electrolyte disturbance (especially hypokalemia) with parenteral fluid administration.

• Discontinue drugs that slow digoxin metabolism or elimination (e.g., quinidine, verapamil, amiodarone).
• Severe arrhythmias (ventricular tachycardia) and conduction disturbances—can be life threatening; require hospitalization for treatment and monitoring

MEDICATIONS

DRUGS
• Treat clinically important bradyarrhythmias with atropine or a temporary transvenous pacemaker.
• Treat clinically important ventricular arrhythmias with lidocaine or phenytoin; phenytoin also reverses high-degree AV block.
• Digoxin-binding antibodies (e.g., Digibind) rapidly drop digoxin concentration in critically ill animals; the use of these products is limited in veterinary practice by their exorbitant cost.
• Thyroxin supplementation if hypothyroidism confirmed

CONTRAINDICATIONS/POSSIBLE INTERACTIONS
• Avoid or discontinue drugs that slow digoxin elimination or metabolism (e.g., quinidine, verapamil, and diltiazem).
• Avoid drugs that could worsen conduction disturbances (e.g., β-blockers and calcium channel blockers).
• Class 1A antiarrhythmic drugs (e.g., quinidine and procainamide) may worsen AV block.

FOLLOW-UP
• Monitor renal function and electrolytes frequently in patients receiving digoxin; lower digoxin dose if renal disease develops.
• Monitor serum digoxin concentration periodically.
• Monitor ECG periodically to assess for arrhythmias or conduction disturbances that may suggest digoxin toxicity.
• Monitor body weight frequently; alter digoxin dosage accordingly; patients with congestive heart failure (CHF) often lose weight.

✓ MISCELLANEOUS

SEE ALSO
• AV Block, Complete
• AV Block, First Degree
• AV Block, Second Degree, Mobitz Type I
• AV Block, Second Degree, Mobitz Type II
• Ventricular Tachycardia

ABBREVIATIONS
• AV = atrioventricular
• CHF = congestive heart failure

Suggested Reading
Opie LH, Gersh BJ. Digitalis, acute inotropes, and inotropic dilators. In Opie LH, Gersh BJ, eds. Drugs for the heart. 5th ed. Philadelphia: Saunders, 2001:154–186.
Author Francis W. K. Smith, Jr.
Consulting Editors Larry P. Tilley and Francis W. K. Smith, Jr.

DISCOLORED TOOTH/TEETH

BASICS

DEFINITION
• Any change from the norm—the normal color varies and depends on the shade, translucency, and thickness of enamel.
• Extrinsic—from surface accumulation of exogenous pigment
• Intrinsic—secondary to endogenous factors discoloring the underlying dentin

PATHOPHYSIOLOGY

Extrinsic Discoloration
• Bacterial stains—chromogenic bacteria give a green to black-brown to orange color.
• Plaque-related—a black-brown stain; usually secondary to the formation of ferric sulfide from the interaction of bacterial ferric sulfide and iron in the saliva
• Foods—charcoal biscuits and similar products penetrate the pits and fissures of the enamel; food that contains abundant chlorophyll can produce a green discoloration.
• Gingival hemorrhage—gives a green staining; results from the breakdown of hemoglobin into green biliverdin
• Dental restorative materials—amalgam gives a black-gray discoloration
• Medications—products containing iron or iodine give a black discoloration; those containing sulfides, silver nitrate, or manganese give a gray-to-yellow to brown-to-black discoloration; those containing copper or nickel give a green discoloration; products containing cadmium give a yellow-to-golden brown discoloration (e.g., 8% stannous fluoride combines with bacterial sulfides, giving a black stain; chlorhexidine gives a yellowish-brown discoloration)
• Metals—wear from chewing on cages or food dishes

Intrinsic Discoloration
• Hyperbilirubinemia—affects all teeth; occurs during the developmental stages of the dentition (during dentin formation); bilirubin accumulation in the dentin occurs from excess red blood cell breakdown; extent of tooth discoloration depends on the length of hyperbilirubinemia (one can see lines of resolution on the teeth once the condition has been resolved); gives a green discoloration
• Localized red blood cell destruction, usually one tooth—usually follows a traumatic injury to the tooth; discoloration comes from hemo-globin breakdown within the pulp from a pulpitis and secondary release into adjacent dentinal tubules; discoloration goes from pink (pulpitis) to gray (pulpal necrosis or resolution) to black (liquefactive necrosis); blood factors that cause tooth discoloration are hemoglobin, methemoglobin, hematoidin, hemosiderin, hematin, hemin, and sulfmethemoglobin
• Amelogenesis imperfecta—developmental alteration in the structure of enamel affecting all teeth; teeth have a chalky appearance and a pinkish hue; can be a problem in the formation of the organic matrix, mineralization of the matrix, or the maturation of the matrix
• Dentinogenesis imperfecta—developmental alteration in the dentin formation; enamel separates easily from the dentin, resulting in grayish discoloration
• Infectious agents (systemic)—parvovirus, distemper virus, or any infectious agent that causes a sustained body temperature rise; affects the formation of enamel; a distinct line of resolution is visible on the teeth; affects all teeth; results in enamel hypoplasia where the pitted areas have black edges and the dentin is brownish
• Dental fluorosis—affects all teeth; excess fluoride consumption affects the maturation of enamel, resulting in pits (enamel hypoplasia) with black edges; the enamel is a lusterless, opaque white, with yellow brown zones of discoloration

Internal/External Resorption
• Internal—follows pulpal injury (trauma) causing vascular changes with increased oxygen tension and a decreased pH, resulting in destruction (resorption) of the tooth from within the pulp from dentinoclasts; tooth has pinkish hue; usually one tooth affected
• External—many factors cause this, such as trauma, orthodontic treatment, excessive occlusal forces, periodontal disease, tumors, and periapical inflammation; reabsorption can occur anywhere along the periodontal ligament and can extend to the pulp; osteoclasts resorb the tooth structure.

Medications and Discoloration
• Tetracycline—binds to calcium, forming a calcium orthophosphate complex that is laid down into the collagen matrix of enamel; occurs on all teeth; occurs only when the enamel is being formed; results in a yellow-brown discoloration
• Amalgam (as with extrinsic stains)
• Iodine/essential oils

• From endodontically treated teeth with the mendicants penetrating the dentinal tubules

SYSTEMS AFFECTED
N/A

GENETICS
• Both amelogenesis imperfecta and dentinogenesis imperfecta in humans are inherited conditions that have many modes of inheritance: X-linked dominant, X-linked recessive, autosomal dominant, autosomal recessive.
• The mode of inheritance in animals has not been studied.

INCIDENCE/PREVALENCE
• Discoloration of the teeth or a tooth is extremely common in all animals.
• Extrinsic staining is very common, especially bacterial stains; others are less common.
• Intrinsic staining is likewise very common, especially internal and external resorption, followed by localized red blood cell destruction; the other causes are rare.

GEOGRAPHIC DISTRIBUTION
N/A

SIGNALMENT
• Dog and cat
• Affects all species, breeds
• No sex predilections
• The reported age range varies—when the condition affects the maturing enamel or dentin it can be first noted after 6 months.

SIGNS

Historical Findings
Owner reports a variation in color of a tooth or teeth

Physical Examination
• Abnormal coloration to tooth or teeth
• Pitted enamel with staining
• Fractured tooth
• Rings or lines of discoloration around tooth or teeth

CAUSES & RISK FACTORS
• Extrinsic discoloration—bacterial stains from plaque and calculus; foods; gingival hemorrhage; dental restorative materials, medications (chlorhexidine, 8% stannous fluoride), metal
• Intrinsic discoloration—internal (trauma); external (feline osteoblastic resorptive lesions) resorption; localized red blood cell destruction in the tooth (trauma); systemic infections; medications (tetracycline); fluorosis; hyperbilirubinemia; amelogenesis imperfecta; dentinogenesis imperfecta

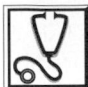
DIAGNOSIS

DIFFERENTIAL DIAGNOSIS
• Calculus on the teeth
• Normal tooth aging—increased translucence

CBC/BIOCHEMISTRY/URINALYSIS
N/A

OTHER LABORATORY TESTS
N/A

IMAGING
Dental radiography is extremely useful in identifying internal or external resorption, restorative materials, or bacterial stain from coronal percolation.

DIAGNOSTIC PROCEDURES
• If many teeth are affected, one tooth can be extracted and sent for histologic evaluation.
• Transillumination with a strong fiberoptic light can benefit the clinician by distinguishing between a vital and necrotic pulp.

PATHOLOGIC FINDINGS
• Tooth or teeth are discolored; enamel and/or dentin can be pitted or broken with staining.
• Extrinsic discoloration—all stain is in the enamel or exposed dentin, otherwise the tooth structure is normal.
• Intrinsic discoloration—hyperbilirubinemia; enamel hypoplasia; lines of resolution on the tooth; all teeth affected
• Localized red blood cell destruction—stain in dentinal tubules; pulpitis/liquefactive necrosis of the pulp
• Internal resorption—well-circumscribed enlargement of an area of the endodontic system with granulation tissue containing many odontoclasts
• External resorption—moth-eaten loss of tooth structure anywhere along the periodontal ligament; can extend into the endodontic system; areas of tooth resorption have granulation tissue with many osteoclasts
• Fluorosis—enamel hypoplasia; enamel hypocalcification; medications; systemic (e.g., tetracycline has irregular matrix formation to the enamel and dentin), all teeth affected
• Amelogenesis imperfecta—irregular formation of the enamel matrix, mineralization, or maturation
• Dentinogenesis imperfecta—irregular formation of dentin; enamel may be separated from the dentin

TREATMENT

APPROPRIATE HEALTH CARE
• Nonemergency
• Extrinsic stain removal—mainly cosmetic
• Intrinsic stain treatment—functional and pain relieving

NURSING CARE
• Extrinsic stain—remove inciting cause.
• Intrinsic stain—soft food; remove chew toys.

ACTIVITY
N/A

DIET
Intrinsic stain—soft food

CLIENT EDUCATION
• To prevent it in future animals or litters
• Intrinsic causes—if untreated the tooth or teeth are more likely to accumulate plaque and calculus, leading to subsequent periodontal disease; tooth fracture is more prevalent, which could result in tooth abscessation.

SURGICAL CONSIDERATIONS
• Extrinsic stain (cosmetic)—internal and/or external bleaching; veneers or crowns
• Intrinsic stain (functional and pain relief)—possible endodontic treatment (internal resorption and localized red blood cell destruction)
• Restorative procedures such as crowns or veneers to protect both tooth and pulp

MEDICATIONS

DRUG(S) OF CHOICE
N/A

CONTRAINDICATIONS
N/A

PRECAUTIONS
N/A

POSSIBLE INTERACTIONS
N/A

ALTERNATIVE DRUG(S)
N/A

FOLLOW-UP

PATIENT MONITORING
N/A

PREVENTION/AVOIDANCE
See Pathophysiology

POSSIBLE COMPLICATIONS
See Client Education

EXPECTED COURSE AND PROGNOSIS
N/A

MISCELLANEOUS

ASSOCIATED CONDITIONS
Juvenile purpura

AGE-RELATED FACTORS
Most common in young dogs and cats

SYNONYMS
• Intrinsic staining
• Tetracycline staining
• Extrinsic staining
• Chlorhexidine staining

Suggested Reading
Harvey CE, Emily PP. Small animal dentistry. Philadelphia: Mosby, 1993.
Wiggs RB, Lobprise HB. Veterinary dentistry: principles and practice. Philadelphia: Lippincott-Raven, 1997.
Author James M. G. Anthony
Consulting Editor Heidi B. Lobprise

DISKOSPONDYLITIS

BASICS

DEFINITION
A bacterial or fungal infection of the intervertebral disks and adjacent vertebral bodies

PATHOPHYSIOLOGY
• Hematogenous spread of bacterial or fungal organisms—most common cause
• Neurologic dysfunction—may occur; usually the result of spinal cord compression caused by proliferation of bone and fibrous tissue; less commonly owing to luxation or pathologic fracture of the spine, epidural abscess, or extension of infection to the meninges and spinal cord

SYSTEMS AFFECTED
• Musculoskeletal—infection and inflammation of the spine
• Nervous—compression of the spinal cord

GENETICS
• No definite predisposition identified
• An inherited immunodeficiency has been detected in a few cases.

INCIDENCE/PREVALENCE
Approximately 0.2% of dog hospital admissions

GEOGRAPHIC DISTRIBUTION
Grass awn migration and coccidiomycosis—more common in certain regions

SIGNALMENT
Species
Dogs; rare in cats

Breed Predilection
Large and giant breeds, especially German shepherds and Great Danes

Mean Age and Range
• Mean age —4–5 years
• Range—5 months to 12 years

Predominant Sex
Males outnumber females by ~2:1

SIGNS
Historical Findings
• Onset usually relatively acute; some patients have mild signs for several months before examination.
• Pain—difficulty rising, reluctance to jump, and stilted gait are most common signs.
• Ataxia or paresis
• Weight loss and anorexia
• Lameness
• Draining tracts

Physical Examination Findings
• Focal or multifocal areas of spinal pain in >80% of patients
• Any disk space may be affected; lumbosacral space is most commonly involved.
• Paresis or paralysis, especially in chronic, untreated cases
• Fever in ~30% of patients
• Lameness

CAUSES
• Bacterial—*Staphylococcus intermedius* is the most common. Others include *Streptococcus, Brucella canis,* and *E. coli,* but virtually any bacteria can be causative.
• Fungal—*Aspergillus, Paecilomyces,* and *Coccidioides immitis*
• Grass awn migration is often associated with mixed infections, especially *Actinomyces;* tends to affect the L2–L4 disk spaces and vertebrae
• Other causes—surgery, bite wounds

RISK FACTORS
• Urinary tract infection
• Periodontal disease
• Bacterial endocarditis
• Dermatitis
• Immunodeficiency

DIAGNOSIS

DIFFERENTIAL DIAGNOSIS
• Intervertebral disk protrusion—may cause similar clinical signs; differentiated on the basis of radiography and myelography
• Vertebral fracture or luxation—detected on radiographs
• Vertebral neoplasia—usually does not affect adjacent vertebral end plates
• Spondylosis deformans—rarely causes clinical signs; has similar radiographic features, including sclerosis, ventral spur formation, and collapse of the disk space; rarely causes lysis of the vertebral end plates
• Focal meningomyelitis—often identified by CSF analysis

CBC/BIOCHEMISTRY/URINALYSIS
• Hemogram—often normal; may see leukocytosis
• Urinalysis—may reveal pyuria and/or bacteriuria with concurrent urinary tract infections

OTHER LABORATORY TESTS
• Aerobic, anaerobic, and fungal blood cultures identify the causative organism in up to 75% of cases; obtain if available.
• Sensitivity testing—indicated if cultures are positive
• Urine cultures—indicated; positive in about 25% of patients
• Organisms other than *Staphylococcus* spp.—may not be the cause
• Serologic testing for *Brucella canis*—indicated

IMAGING
• Spinal radiography—usually reveals lysis of vertebral end plates adjacent to the affected disk, collapse of the disk space, and varying degrees of sclerosis of the end plates and ventral spur formation; may not see lesions until 3–4 weeks after infection
• Myelography—indicated with substantial neurologic deficits; determine location and degree of spinal cord compression, especially if considering decompressive surgery; spinal cord compression caused by diskospondylitis typically displays an extradural pattern.
• Computed tomography or magnetic resonance imaging—more sensitive than radiography; indicated when radiographs are normal or inconclusive

DIAGNOSTIC PROCEDURES
• CSF analysis—occasionally indicated to rule out meningomyelitis; usually normal or reveals mildly high protein
• Bone scintigraphy—occasionally useful for detecting early lesions; helps clarify if radiographic changes are infectious or degenerative (spondylosis deformans)
• Fluoroscopically guided fine-needle aspiration of the disk—valuable for obtaining tissue for culture when blood and urine cultures are negative and there is no improvement with empiric antibiotic therapy

PATHOLOGIC FINDINGS
• Gross—loss of normal disk space; bony proliferation of adjacent vertebrae
• Microscopic—fibrosing pyogranulomatous destruction of the disk and vertebral bodies

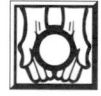

TREATMENT

APPROPRIATE HEALTH CARE
• Outpatient—mild pain
• Inpatient—severe pain or progressive neurologic deficits

NURSING CARE
Nonambulatory patients—keep on a clean, dry, well-padded surface to prevent decubitus ulcers.

ACTIVITY
Restricted

DIET
Normal

CLIENT EDUCATION
• Explain that observation of response to treatment is very important in determining the need for further diagnostic or therapeutic procedures.
• Instruct the client to immediately contact the veterinarian if clinical signs progress or recur or if neurologic deficits develop.

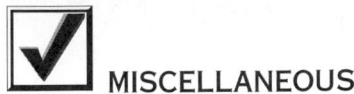

SURGICAL CONSIDERATIONS

• Curettage of a single affected disk space—occasionally necessary for patients that are refractory to antibiotic therapy
• Goals—remove infected tissue; obtain tissue for culture and histologic evaluation
• Decompression of the spinal cord by hemilaminectomy or dorsal laminectomy—indicated for substantial neurologic deficits and spinal cord compression evident on myelography when there is no improvement with antibiotic therapy; also perform curettage of the infected disk space; it may be necessary to perform surgical stabilization if more than one articular facet is removed.

 MEDICATIONS

DRUGS OF CHOICE

Antibiotics

• Selection based on results of blood cultures and serology
• Negative culture and serology—assume causative organism is *Staphylococcus* spp.; treat with a cephalosporin (e.g., cefadroxil; dogs: 22 mg/kg PO q12h; cats: 22 mg/kg PO q24h).
• Acutely progressive signs or substantial neurologic deficits—initially treated with parenteral antibiotics (e.g., cefazolin; dogs and cats: 20–35 mg/kg IV q8h); continued for at least 6 weeks
• Brucellosis—treated with tetracycline (dogs: 15 mg/kg PO q8h) and streptomycin (dogs: 3.4 mg/kg IM q24h) or enrofloxacin (dogs: 2.5–5.0 mg/kg PO q12h)

Analgesics

• Signs of severe pain—treated with an analgesic (e.g., oxymorphone; dogs: 0.05–0.2 mg/kg IV, IM, SC q4–6h)
• Taper dosage after 3–5 days to gauge effectiveness of antibiotic therapy.

CONTRAINDICATIONS

Glucocorticoids

PRECAUTIONS

Use NSAIDs and other analgesics cautiously—may cause a temporary resolution of clinical signs even when infection is progressing; when used, discontinue after 3–5 days to assess efficacy of antibiotic therapy.

POSSIBLE INTERACTIONS

None

ALTERNATIVE DRUGS

• Initial therapy—cephradine (dogs: 20 mg/kg PO q8h); cloxacillin (dogs: 10 mg/kg PO q8h)
• Refractory patients—clindamycin (dogs and cats: 10 mg/kg PO q12h), enrofloxacin (dogs: 5–20 mg/kg PO q24h; cats: 5 mg/kg PO q24h), orbifloxacin (dogs and cats: 2.5–7.5 mg/kg PO q24h)

 FOLLOW-UP

PATIENT MONITORING

• Reevaluate after 5 days of therapy
• No improvement in pain, fever, or appetite—reassess therapy; consider a different antibiotic, percutaneous aspiration of the affected disk space, or surgery.
• Improvement—evaluate clinically and radiographically every 2–4 weeks.

PREVENTION/AVOIDANCE

Early identification of predisposing causes and prompt diagnosis and treatment—help reduce progression of clinical symptoms and neurologic deterioration

POSSIBLE COMPLICATIONS

• Spinal cord compression owing to proliferative bony and fibrous tissue
• Vertebral fracture or luxation
• Meningitis or meningomyelitis
• Epidural abscess

EXPECTED COURSE AND PROGNOSIS

• Recurrence is common if antibiotic therapy is stopped prematurely (before 6 weeks of treatment).
• Prognosis—depends on causative organism and degree of spinal cord damage
• Mild or no neurologic dysfunction (dogs)—usually respond within 5 days of starting antibiotic therapy
• Substantial paresis or paralysis (dogs)—prognosis guarded; may note gradual resolution of neurologic dysfunction after several weeks of therapy; treatment warranted
• *Brucella canis*—signs usually resolve with therapy; infection may not be eradicated; recurrence common

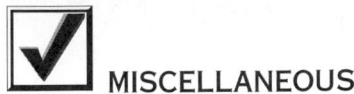 MISCELLANEOUS

ASSOCIATED CONDITIONS

See Risk Factors.

AGE-RELATED FACTORS

N/A

ZOONOTIC POTENTIAL

Brucella canis—human infection uncommon but may occur

PREGNANCY

N/A

SYNONYMS

• Intradiskal osteomyelitis
• Intervertebral disk infection
• Vertebral osteomyelitis
• Diskitis

SEE ALSO

Brucellosis

ABBREVIATION

CSF = cerebrospinal fluid

Suggested Reading

Davis MJ, Dewey CW, Walker MA, et al. Contrast radiographic findings in canine bacterial discospondylitis: A multicenter, retrospective study of 27 cases. J Am Anim Hosp Assoc 2000;36:81–85
Fischer A, Mahaffey MB, Oliver JE. Fluoroscopically guided percutaneous disk aspiration in 10 dogs with diskospondylitis. J Vet Intern Med 1997;11:284–287.
Johnson RG, Prata RG. Intradiskal osteomyelitis: a conservative approach. J Am Anim Hosp Assoc 1983;19:743–750.
Kerwin SC, Lewis DD, Hribernik TN, et al. Diskospondylitis associated with *Brucella canis* infection in dogs: 14 cases (1989–1991). J Am Vet Med Assoc 1992;201:1253–1257.
Kornegay JN. Diskospondylitis. In: Kirk RW, ed. Current veterinary therapy IX. Philadelphia: Saunders, 1986:810–814.
Thomas WB. Diskospondylitis and other vertebral infections. Vet Clin North Am Small Anim Pract 2000;30:169–182.
Author William B. Thomas
Consulting Editor Peter K. Shires

DISSEMINATED INTRAVASCULAR COAGULATION

 BASICS

DEFINITION
A complex hemostatic defect with enhanced coagulation and fibrinolysis secondary to severe systemic disease

PATHOPHYSIOLOGY
• Occurs secondary to activation of coagulation and fibrinolysis; changes are induced in animals with diseases characterized by stasis of blood flow, vascular damage, activation and consumption of coagulation factors, reduced clearance of activated clotting factors by the liver, or release of tissue factors from damaged cells, tumors, or other tissues.
• Activation of fibrinolysis is a secondary response to clear fibrin thrombi in capillaries.
• Bleeding defect is complicated by thrombocytopenia related to consumption at sites of damaged endothelium and thrombi and by a platelet function defect induced by coating of platelets with FDP from the action of the fibrinolytic mechanism on fibrin or fibrinogen.

SYSTEMS AFFECTED
• Multisystemic
• Hemorrhages in many tissues
• Organ dysfunction related to obstruction of capillaries

GENETICS
N/A

INCIDENCE/PREVALENCE
• Associated with severe systemic disease
• Common in the terminal stages of several fatal diseases

GEOGRAPHIC DISTRIBUTION
N/A

SIGNALMENT

Species
Dogs and cats, but more commonly recognized in dogs

Breed Predilections
None

Mean Age and Range
Correlate with those of the severe systemic disease

Predominant Sex
None

SIGNS
• Usually relate to the primary disease
• Petechiae, abnormal bleeding from venipuncture sites, and other abnormal bleeding

CAUSES
• Malignancies, especially hemangiosarcoma
• Shock
• Pancreatitis
• Hemolysis
• Heat stroke
• Leishmaniasis
• Other systemic infectious diseases (including gram-negative septicemia)
• Heart failure
• Hemorrhagic gastroenteritis
• Chronic active liver disease
• Gastric dilatation-volvulus
• Splenic torsion
• Heartworm disease
• Snake venom

RISK FACTORS
Vary with cause

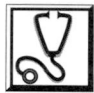 DIAGNOSIS

DIFFERENTIAL DIAGNOSIS
• Immune-mediated or idiopathic thrombocytopenia
• Anticoagulant toxicity
• Coagulation factor deficiency
• Deficient production of clotting factors in severe liver disease
• Paraproteinemia
• Characterized by marked variation; diagnosis is usually based on the combination of at least three of the following: petechiae or abnormal bleeding from venipuncture sites, thrombocytopenia, prolonged PT, prolonged APTT, low antithrombin III, and high FDP.

CBC/BIOCHEMISTRY/URINALYSIS
• Thrombocytopenia is common, and macroplatelets provide evidence of enhanced thrombopoiesis.
• Schistocytes are produced by mechanical fragmentation of erythrocytes on intraluminal fibrin strands.
• Biochemical analysis may reveal azotemia, acidosis, and high enzyme activities related to the primary disease and organ dysfunction or necrosis related to capillary obstruction.

OTHER LABORATORY TESTS
• PT and APTT may be prolonged secondary to the anticoagulant effects of FDP and consumption of coagulation factors, especially antithrombin III, factor VIII, and fibrinogen.
• Latex agglutination test for FDP or D-dimers
• Practical assays to demonstrate depletion of clotting factors include fibrinogen and antithrombin III.

IMAGING
N/A

DIAGNOSTIC PROCEDURES
None

PATHOLOGIC FINDINGS
• Usually relate to the primary disease
• Petechiae common
• Fibrin thrombi may be dissolved by fibrinolysis during the postmortem interval.

 TREATMENT

APPROPRIATE HEALTH CARE
Associated with severe disease, requiring intensive and inpatient treatment

NURSING CARE
• Most important is intensive treatment of the primary disease.
• Fluid therapy to correct deficits in plasma volume or acid–base imbalance reduces the potential for activation of clotting factors and enhances clearance of activated clotting factors by the mononuclear phagocyte system.

ACTIVITY
Not an issue because of the severity of the primary disease

DIET
N/A

CLIENT EDUCATION
• Inform the owner of the life-threatening nature of the associated processes.
• Prognosis is usually that associated with the primary disease.

SURGICAL CONSIDERATIONS
Related to primary disease

MEDICATIONS

DRUGS OF CHOICE
• The role of heparin or low-molecular-weight heparin treatment is controversial. Heparin may be used to inhibit proteolytic activation of coagulation, preferably by continuous IV infusion sufficient to prolong the APTT to $1^{1}/_{2}$–2 times normal; low-dose heparin is safer and has been reported to produce beneficial results in some dogs when infused at 5–10 IU/kg/h IV or at 75 IU/kg SC q8h.
• The anticoagulant effect of heparin is achieved by binding to antithrombin III, which may be depleted in these patients; therefore, it may be beneficial to transfuse with heparinized blood or heparinized plasma.

CONTRAINDICATIONS
• The long-term use of corticosteroids should be considered carefully because of the inhibition of mononuclear phagocyte function, which might be important in clearance of activated coagulation factors.
• Inhibitors of fibrinolysis should not be used, because fibrinolysis is important in the clearance of thrombi.

PRECAUTIONS
High doses of heparin may cause bleeding episodes that could be life-threatening. If there is active bleeding, clotting factors should be replaced by plasma transfusion.

POSSIBLE INTERACTIONS
None

ALTERNATIVE DRUGS
None

FOLLOW-UP

PATIENT MONITORING
• Clinical improvement and the arrest of bleeding are indications of a positive response to treatment.
• Diminishing concentration of FDP is a positive sign.
• Platelet counts usually increase slowly over a period of days.

PREVENTION/AVOIDANCE
Related to primary disease

EXPECTED COURSE AND PROGNOSIS
Because of the serious nature of the primary diseases, these animals have a high rate of mortality.

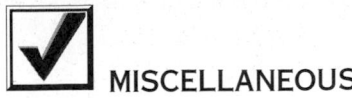

MISCELLANEOUS

ASSOCIATED CONDITIONS
See Causes.

AGE-RELATED FACTORS
N/A

ZOONOTIC POTENTIAL
N/A

PREGNANCY
Associated obstetric complications (e.g., dystocia, eclampsia, and retained fetuses) have been demonstrated in humans but are not well documented in dogs and cats.

SYNONYMS
• Consumption coagulopathy
• Intravascular coagulation-fibrinolysis syndrome
• DIC

SEE ALSO
• Clotting Factor Deficiencies
• Thrombocytopenia

ABBREVIATIONS
• APTT = activated partial thromboplastin time
• FDP = fibrin degradation products
• PT = prothrombin time

Suggested Reading

Dodds WJ. Hemostasis. In: Kaneko JJ, Harvey JW, Bruss ML, eds. Clinical biochemistry of domestic animals. New York: Academic Press, 1997:241–283.

Feldman BF, Kirby R, Caldin M. Recognition and treatment of disseminated intravascular coagulation. In: Bonagura JD, ed. Current veterinary therapy XIII. Philadelphia, Saunders, 2000:190–194.

Feldman BF, Madewell BR, O'Neil S. Disseminated intravascular coagulation: antithrombin, plasminogen, and coagulation abnormalities in 41 dogs. J Am Vet Med Assoc 1981;179:151–154.

Author Gary J. Kociba
Consulting Editor Stephen A. Krath

DROWNING (NEAR DROWNING)

BASICS

DEFINITION
Water submersion followed by survival for at least 24 hours (near drowning)

PATHOPHYSIOLOGY
Following submersion, elevations in carbon dioxide levels in the bloodstream stimulate respiration, and subsequent aspiration of water occurs. In rare cases, hyperventilation prior to submersion or laryngospasm may prevent aspiration of water ("dry drowning"). The four phases of a typical drowning in experimental dogs include: (1) breath holding and swimming motion; (2) water aspiration, choking, and struggling; (3) vomition; and (4) cessation of movement followed by death. The mammalian diving reflex may occur, leading to bradycardia, apnea, and vasoconstriction to nonessential capillary beds. Large volumes of water are not typically aspirated. Fresh water aspiration dilutes pulmonary surfactant and leads to alveolar collapse ± infectious pneumonia. Hypertonic seawater aspiration leads to diffusion of interstitial water into the alveoli. Regardless of the type of water aspirated, ventilation-perfusion mismatch commonly occurs, leading to hypoxemia and a metabolic acidosis. Submersion time, temperature of the water, and type of water (fresh versus salt versus chemical water) will significantly affect development of organ damage.

SYSTEMS AFFECTED
• Respiratory • Nervous • Cardiovascular • Gastrointestinal • Hemic

GEOGRAPHIC DISTRIBUTION
Greater near bodies of water, although indoor drowning common (buckets, bathtubs)

SIGNALMENT
Dogs and cats. Approximately half of the animals involved in immersion accidents are less than 4 months of age.

SIGNS
• Cyanosis • Coughing ± clear to frothy red sputum • Apnea • Dyspnea • Crackles or wheezes auscultated over chest • Tachycardia or bradycardia • Vomiting • Obtunded to comatose • Asystole

CAUSES & RISK FACTORS
• Owner negligence • Inadequate safety precautions • Young (<4 months of age) • Animals who are in or near water at the time of a seizure, head trauma, hypoglycemic event, cardiac arrhythmia, or syncopal episode are at risk of drowning.

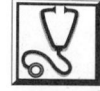

DIAGNOSIS

DIFFERENTIAL DIAGNOSIS
• Hypothermia, neck trauma, and meningitis should be ruled out • In the event of drowning secondary to a seizure, head trauma, hypoglycemic event, cardiac arrhythmia, or syncopal episode, appropriate diagnostics should be performed. The history at the time of presentation is often informative.

CBC/BIOCHEMISTRY/URINALYSIS
• Inhalation or ingestion of large amounts of fresh water can lead to hemodilution, hemolysis, and decreases in sodium, chloride, and urine specific gravity. • Inhalation or ingestion of hypertonic salt water can lead to hemoconcentration as well as increases in sodium, chloride, and urine specific gravity.

OTHER LABORATORY TESTS
Arterial blood gas reveals hypoxemia (PaO_2 < 80 mmHg), hypoventilation ($PaCO_2$ > 50 mmHg), and acid-base derangements such as a respiratory or metabolic acidosis (HCO_3 < 18 mEq/L).

IMAGING

Thoracic Radiography
• Radiographic changes may not be detectable for 24–48 hours. • Focal or diffuse alveolar pattern due to aspiration pneumonia or noncardiogenic pulmonary edema • Mixed bronchial, alveolar, and interstitial patterns may be present, and a radiopaque material filling the airways ("sand bronchogram") has been described. • Foreign body inhalation may produce segmental atelectasis. • Progression of pulmonary injury to ARDS is possible and may appear as bilateral, diffuse, symmetrical alveolar infiltrates.

DIAGNOSTIC PROCEDURES
• Endotracheal or transtracheal wash with cytologic evaluation and culture with sensitivities is indicated. • Electrocardiographic monitoring • Cervical radiographs, CT or MRI of the brain, and BAER assessment may be helpful in select cases.

TREATMENT
• Initiate mouth-to-muzzle resuscitation on site. • Emergent inpatient care is required. • Airway clearance, if obstructed, is the first priority. • Cardiopulmonary resuscitation may be necessary. • Oxygen supplementation should be provided. • Intubation and mechanical ventilation with positive end-expiratory pressure may be required in animals with severe hypoxemia, hypercapnia, or imminent respiratory fatigue. • Gravitational drainage or abdominal thrusts (Heimlich maneuver) are not recommended in the absence of airway obstruction owing to high risk of regurgitation and subsequent aspiration of stomach contents. • Fluid therapy and acid-base/electrolyte management are crucial. • Gradually rewarm (over 2–3 hours) hypothermic animals. • Prolonged parenteral nutrition may be required in animals with severe neurologic or pulmonary injury.

MEDICATIONS

DRUGS OF CHOICE
• Mannitol therapy, 0.5 g/kg IV over 20 minutes, may be beneficial in animals with suspected cerebral edema and high intracranial pressures. • Broad-spectrum antibiotics (e.g., ampicillin, 22 mg/kg IV q8h, and enrofloxacin, 5–10 mg/kg IV divided over 24 hours in the dog or 5 mg/kg IV q24h in the cat) may be necessary for aspiration pneumonia.

CONTRAINDICATIONS
• Corticosteroid therapy is not indicated in near-drowning victims, and use of this drug could be detrimental in animals with aspiration pneumonia. • The use of enrofloxacin in young animals may cause cartilage erosion.

FOLLOW-UP

PATIENT MONITORING
• Frequent or continuous monitoring of heart rate and rhythm, respiratory rate, mucous membrane color and capillary refill time, urine output, arterial blood pressure, rectal temperature, neurologic status, +/− central venous pressure • Arterial blood gas, complete blood count, biochemical profile, coagulogram, and acid-base status should be rechecked as needed.

PREVENTION/AVOIDANCE
Close monitoring of animals (especially young animals) near bodies of water

POSSIBLE COMPLICATIONS
• Aspiration pneumonia, non-cardiogenic pulmonary edema, ARDS, gastrointestinal bleeding, diarrhea, vomiting, acute renal failure, permanent neurologic derangements, DIC, central diabetes insipidus • Owner—may have feelings of guilt and remorse and may require counseling.

EXPECTED COURSE AND PROGNOSIS
Directly related to animal's status at time of admission: animals who present comatose, severely acidotic (pH <7.0), or requiring cardiopulmonary resuscitation or mechanical ventilation have a poor prognosis. Animals who present conscious have a good prognosis if no complications ensue.

MISCELLANEOUS

ABBREVIATIONS:
ARDS = acute respiratory distress syndrome
BAER = brainstem auditory evoked response

Suggested Reading:
Farrow CS. Near-drowning (water inhalation). In: Kirk RW, ed. Current veterinary therapy VIII. Philadelphia: Saunders, 1983:167–173.
Author Deborah C. Silverstein
Consulting Editor Lynelle R. Johnson

DYSAUTONOMIA (KEY-GASKELL SYNDROME)

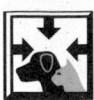 BASICS

OVERVIEW
• Dysfunction of the autonomic nervous system
• Etiopathogenesis unknown

SIGNALMENT
• Mainly cats in Great Britain
• Mainly dogs in rural environments
• Endemic in dogs in Kansas and Missouri
• Rare in dogs and cats worldwide
• Most affected dogs and cats < 3 years old
• No breed or sex predilection—although some studies show Labrador Retrievers are most commonly affected, all breeds have been reported.
• No genetic basis

SIGNS
• Generally acute
• Depression
• Anorexia
• Constipation
• Dry external nares and mouth
• Reduced tear production
• Regurgitation owing to megaesophagus
• Dilated pupils with absent or depressed pupillary light reflexes
• Prolapsed third eyelids
• Bradycardia
• Less common—anal areflexia; fecal incontinence; dysuria or urinary incontinence
• Dog—diarrhea more common than constipation, and absent anal tone is common

CAUSES & RISK FACTORS
Unknown

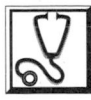 DIAGNOSIS

DIFFERENTIAL DIAGNOSIS
• Dehydration secondary to a primary gastrointestinal disorder
• Most primary gastrointestinal diseases—differentiate by dilated, poorly responsive pupils, no tear production on Schirmer tear test, poor esophageal motility on contrast radiography

CBC/BIOCHEMISTRY/URINALYSIS
• Normal or indicate dehydration
• Heinz body anemia in some cats

OTHER LABORATORY TESTS
N/A

IMAGING
• Survey radiography of the thorax—often reveals megaesophagus
• Barium contrast radiography or fluoroscopy—demonstrates esophageal dysfunction; delayed gastric emptying and contrast retention in the colon common

DIAGNOSTIC PROCEDURES
• Schirmer tear test—usually < 5 mm/min
• Ophthalmic pharmacologic testing—phospholine iodide 0.06% has no miotic effect; pilocarpine 0.1% has an exaggerated miotic effect because of denervation hypersensitivity; testing is not 100% reliable: some patients do not respond as expected
• Low plasma or urinary catecholamine concentration—confirms sympathetic insufficiency
• Intradermal histamine (1:1000) response test—fails to demonstrate the normal wheal and flare reaction because of the defect in sympathetic innervation of blood vessels

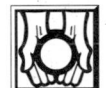 TREATMENT

• Inpatient—initial treatment
• Warm isotonic fluids—intravenous administration; correct hypovolemia, hypothermia, hypoglycemia, and other electrolyte abnormalities
• Oral intake—temporarily withhold (especially dogs) to prevent aspiration pneumonia secondary to regurgitation.
• Nutrition—almost all patients require nasogastric tube, percutaneous gastrostomy tube, or total parenteral nutrition for weeks to months until regurgitation has subsided; percutaneous gastrostomy tube is generally best, because client can easily feed the patient at home
• Outpatient—extensive nursing care; several months to 1 year for recovery; even with the best management, relapse and death common

 MEDICATIONS

DRUG(S)
• Cisapride (dogs: 0.1–0.5 mg/kg PO q8–12h; cats: 2.5–5.0 mg/cat PO q8–12h) or metoclopramide (0.2–0.5 mg/kg IV, IM, PO q6–8h or 1–2 mg/kg continuous IV infusion daily) may reduce vomiting and improve gastrointestinal motility.
• Parasympathomimetic eye drops—pilocarpine (0.1%–1%) q8–12h; improve lacrimation
• Bethanechol—2.5–7.5 mg PO divided q8–12h; may improve gastrointestinal motility and bladder emptying

CONTRAINDICATIONS/POSSIBLE INTERACTIONS
Pilocarpine and bethanechol—use carefully; start with the lowest possible dosage; denervation hypersensitivity can cause arrhythmias and bradycardia

 FOLLOW-UP

• Prognosis poor
• Only 20%–50% survive after several months to 1 year of slow recovery.
• Megaesophagus, constipation, fecal incontinence, and pupil dilation may persist.
• Aspiration pneumonia may cause death.

 MISCELLANEOUS

Suggested Reading
Harkin KR, Andrews GA, Nietfeld JC. Dysautonomia in dogs: 65 cases (1993–2000). JAVMA 2002;220:633–639.
Sharp NJH. Feline dysautonomia. Semin Vet Med Surg Small Anim 1990;5:67–71.
Author Allen Franklin Sisson
Consulting Editor Joane M. Parent

DYSCHEZIA AND HEMATOCHEZIA

 BASICS

DEFINITION
• Dyschezia—painful or difficult defecation
• Hematochezia—bright red blood in the feces

PATHOPHYSIOLOGY
• Result from various causes of inflammation or irritation of the rectum or anus
• Hematochezia may also occur with diseases of the colon.

SYSTEMS AFFECTED
Gastrointestinal

SIGNALMENT
• Dogs and cats
• No breed or sex predilection

SIGNS

Historical Findings
• Crying and whimpering during defecation
• Tenesmus common
• Lack of defecation with obstipation may occur if pain is severe.
• Mucoid, bloody diarrhea in patients with colonic disease

Physical Examination
• Rectal examination may reveal hard feces (constipation or obstipation), diarrhea (colorectal disease), polyps, masses, rectoanal thickening, anal gland enlargement/pain, prostatomegaly, or perineal hernias.

• Fistulous tracts or wounds occur with perianal fistulas.
• Anal occlusion with matted hair and feces occurs with pseudocoprostasis.

CAUSES

Rectal/Anal Disease
• Stricture or spasm
• Anal sacculitis or abscess
• Perianal fistulas
• Rectal or anal foreign body
• Pseudocoprostasis
• Rectal prolapse
• Trauma—bite wounds, etc.
• Neoplasia—adenocarcinoma, lymphoma, and anal sac tumors
• Rectal polyps

Colonic Disease
• Neoplasia—adenocarcinoma, lymphoma
• Idiopathic megacolon—cats
• Inflammation—IBD, infectious or parasitic agents, allergic colitis (see Colitis and Proctitis)
• Constipation (see Constipation and Obstipation)

Extraintestinal Disease
• Fractured pelvis or hind limb
• Prostatic disease
• Perineal hernia
• Intrapelvic neoplasia

RISK FACTORS
• Ingestion of hair, bone, foreign material may contribute to constipation and subsequent dyschezia.
• Environmental factors such as a dirty litter pan and infrequent outside walks may contribute to constipation and subsequent dyschezia.

 DIAGNOSIS

DIFFERENTIAL DIAGNOSIS
• Dysuria, stranguria, or hematuria—abnormal findings on urinalysis, such as pyuria, crystalluria, bacteriuria
• Dystocia—differentiate with history and imaging

CBC/BIOCHEMISTRY/URINALYSIS
• Usually normal
• Neutrophilia with infection or inflammation

OTHER LABORATORY TESTS
Fecal examination to rule out infectious/parasitic causes of colitis

IMAGING
• Pelvic radiographs may reveal intrapelvic disease, foreign body, or fracture.
• Ultrasonography may demonstrate prostatic disease or caudal abdominal masses.

DIAGNOSTIC PROCEDURES
Colonoscopy/proctoscopy to evaluate for inflammatory or neoplastic disease

TREATMENT
- Usually outpatient
- Consider laxatives to ease defecation if rectoanal disease.
- Balloon dilation of strictures
- Rectoanal diseases may need surgical correction—perineal hernias, rectoanal polyps

MEDICATIONS

DRUG(S) OF CHOICE
- Antibiotics—if bacterial infection (e.g., anal sac abscess); amoxicillin/clavulanic acid 15 mg/kg PO q12h
- Antiinflammatory drugs—sulfasalazine or prednisone if colitis is present (see Colitis)
- Laxatives—lactulose, 1 ml per 4.5 kg PO q8–12h to effect; docusate sodium or docusate calcium, dogs 50–100 mg PO q12–24h, cats 50 mg PO q12–24h

CONTRAINDICATIONS
Avoid agents that cause increased fecal bulk (fiber), unless specifically indicated (colitis).

PRECAUTIONS
N/A

POSSIBLE INTERACTIONS
N/A

ALTERNATIVE DRUGS
N/A

FOLLOW-UP

PATIENT MONITORING
Clinical signs every 2–3 weeks initially

POSSIBLE COMPLICATIONS
May see fecal incontinence if aggressive surgical therapy is needed

MISCELLANEOUS

ASSOCIATED CONDITIONS
N/A

AGE-RELATED FACTORS
N/A

ZOONOTIC POTENTIAL
N/A

PREGNANCY
Caution with corticosteroids, antibiotics

SYNONYMS
None

SEE ALSO
- Constipation and Obstipation
- Colitis and Proctitis

ABBREVIATION
IBD = inflammatory bowel disease

Suggested Reading
Burrows CF, Sherding RG. Constipation and dyschezia. In: Anderson NV, ed. Veterinary gastroenterology. Philadelphia: Lea & Febiger, 1992:484–503.

Authors Lisa E. Moore and Colin F. Burrows
Consulting Editor Albert E. Jergens

DYSPHAGIA

 **BASICS**

DEFINITION
• Difficulty swallowing, resulting from the inability to prehend, form, and move a bolus of food through the oropharynx into the esophagus
• Esophageal dysphagia is discussed under the topics Megaesophagus and Regurgitation.

PATHOPHYSIOLOGY
• Swallowing difficulties can be caused by mechanical obstruction of the oral cavity or pharynx, neuromuscular dysfunction resulting in weak or uncoordinated swallowing movements, or pain associated with prehension, mastication, or swallowing.
• Oral dysphagia refers to difficulty with the voluntary components of swallowing—prehending and forming a bolus of food at the base of the tongue.
• Pharyngeal dysphagia occurs when there is a malfunction of the involuntary movement of the food bolus through the oropharynx.
• Cricopharyngeal dysphagia refers to abnormal movement of the food bolus from the pharynx through the cricopharyngeus muscle, caused by either failure of the cricopharyngeus to relax (cricopharyngeal achalasia) or asynchrony between pharyngeal contractions and cricopharyngeus opening (cricopharyngeal asynchrony).
• Deglutition is coordinated by the swallowing center in the brain stem; sensory afferents are transmitted to the swallowing center by CNs V and IX.
• Motor efferents responsible for swallowing are carried by CN V, VII, XII (prehension and mastication) and IX and X (pharyngeal contraction); disorders in any of these areas may result in dysphagia.

SYSTEMS AFFECTED
• Neuromuscular
• Nervous
• Gastrointestinal
• Respiratory

SIGNALMENT
• Dogs and cats
• Congenital disorders that cause dysphagia (e.g., cricopharyngeal achalasia and cleft palate) are usually diagnosed in animals < 1 year old.
• Acquired pharyngeal dysphagias are more common in older patients.

SIGNS
Historical Findings
• Drooling, gagging, weight loss, ravenous appetite, repeated attempts at swallowing, swallowing with the head in an abnormal position, coughing (due to aspiration), regurgitation, painful swallowing, and occasionally anorexia are all possible.
• Ascertain onset and progression.
• Foreign bodies cause acute dysphagia; pharyngeal dysphagia may be chronic and intermittent.

Physical Examination Findings
• A thorough oral examination, with the patient sedated or anesthetized, if necessary, is most important.
• Observe for asymmetry, anatomic defect, foreign body, inflammation, tumor, edema, abscessed teeth, and loose teeth.
• Must observe the patient eating; this may localize the abnormal phase of swallowing.
• Perform a complete neurologic examination, with emphasis on the cranial nerves.

Oral Dysphagia
• Modified eating behavior (e.g., eating with head tilted to one side and throwing head back while eating) may compensate for oral dysphagia.
• Mandibular paralysis, tongue paralysis, dental disease, masticatory muscle swelling or atrophy, inability to open the mouth, and food packed in the buccal folds without retention of saliva suggest oral dysphagia.

Pharyngeal Dysphagia
• Prehension of food is normal.
• Repeated attempts at swallowing while repeatedly flexing and extending the head and neck, excessive chewing, and gagging suggest pharyngeal dysphagia.
• Saliva-coated food retained in the buccal folds, a diminished gag reflex, and nasal discharge from aspiration may also exist.

Cricopharyngeal Dysphagia
• Patients make repeated, nonproductive efforts to swallow, gag, and cough, then forcibly regurgitate immediately after swallowing.
• Gag reflex and prehension are normal.
• Emaciation is more common with this form of dysphagia than others.

CAUSES
• Anatomic or mechanical lesions include pharyngeal inflammation (e.g., abscess, inflammatory polyps, and oral eosinophilic granuloma), retropharyngeal lymphadeno-megaly, neoplasia, pharyngeal and retropharyngeal foreign body, sialocele, temporomandibular joint disorders (e.g., luxation, fracture, and craniomandibular osteopathy), mandibular fracture, cleft palate, lingual frenulum disorder, and pharyngeal trauma.
• Pain due to dental disease (e.g., tooth fractures and abscess), mandibular trauma, stomatitis, glossitis, and pharyngeal inflammation may also disrupt normal prehension, bolus formation, and swallowing.
• Neuromuscular disorders that impair prehension and bolus formation include cranial nerve deficits (e.g., idiopathic trigeminal neuropathy CN V, lingual paralysis CN XII) and masticatory muscle myositis.
• Pharyngeal weakness, paresis, or paralysis can be caused by infectious polymyositis (e.g., toxoplasmosis and neosporosis), immune-mediated polymyositis, muscular dystrophy, polyneuropathies, and myoneural junction disorders (e.g., myasthenia gravis, tick paralysis, and botulism).
• Rabies can cause dysphagia by affecting both the brain stem and peripheral nerves.
• Other CNS disorders, especially those involving the brain stem

RISK FACTORS
Many of the causative neuromuscular conditions have breed predispositions.

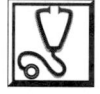 **DIAGNOSIS**

DIFFERENTIAL DIAGNOSIS
• Must be differentiated from vomiting and regurgitation from esophageal disease
• Exaggerated or repeated efforts to swallow—characteristic of dysphagia; most useful means of distinguishing it from vomiting or regurgitation
• Vomiting is associated with abdominal contractions; dysphagia is not.

CBC/BIOCHEMISTRY/URINALYSIS
• Inflammatory conditions often cause a leukocytosis, sometimes with a left shift.
• High serum creatine phosphokinase activity is usually found in patients with muscular disorders resulting in dysphagia.
• May find evidence of renal disease (e.g., azotemia and low urine concentration) in patients with oral and lingual ulcers

OTHER LABORATORY TESTS
• Type 2M muscle antibody serology (masticatory muscle myositis)

- Acetylcholinesterase receptor antibody serology (acquired myasthenia gravis)
- Antinuclear antibody serology (immune-mediated diseases)
- Low-dose dexamethasone suppression test or ACTH stimulation test (hyperadreno-corticism—patients with chronic infections or myopathy)

IMAGING
- Obtain survey radiographs of the skull and neck, including the hyoid apparatus; give particular attention to the mandibles and temporomandibular joint, teeth, pharyngeal and retropharyngeal area, and position of the hyoid apparatus.
- Ultrasonography of the pharynx may be useful in patients with mass lesions and for obtaining ultrasound-guided biopsy specimens.
- Fluoroscopy, with or without positive contrast, is useful in evaluating pharyngeal movement in patients with suspected pharyngeal or cricopharyngeal dysphagia.
- Computed tomography (CT) and/or magnetic resonance imaging (MRI) for a suspected intracranial mass

DIAGNOSTIC PROCEDURES
- Excisional or incisional biopsies of a mass lesion
- Pharyngoscopy
- Electromyography of the pharyngeal musculature to confirm the presence of a neuro-muscular disorder; also evaluate the patient for systemic neuromuscular disease.
- Repetitive nerve stimulation and edrophonium chloride (0.1–0.2 mg/kg IV) test for suspected myasthenia gravis
- Cerebrospinal fluid analysis in patients with a CNS disorder
- Cricopharyngeal manometry if cricopharyngeal achalasia is suspected

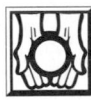 TREATMENT
- Determine the underlying cause to develop a treatment plan and accurate prognosis.
- Direct primary treatment at the underlying cause.
- Nutritional support is important for all dysphagic patients.
- Patients with oral dysphagia may be able to swallow if a bolus of food is place in the caudal pharynx; other patients may find a gruel that can be lapped easier to swallow; take care to avoid aspiration when feeding orally.

- Elevating the head and neck may make swallowing easier for patients with pharyngeal or cricopharyngeal dysphagia and help prevent aspiration of food.
- If nutritional requirements cannot be met orally, a gastrotomy may be necessary.
- Surgical excision of a mass lesion and foreign body may be curative or temporarily improve the signs of dysphagia.
- Cricopharyngeal myotomy may benefit patients with cricopharyngeal dysphagia; a correct diagnosis is essential before surgery, because cricopharyngeal myotomy will exacerbate dysphagia of patients with oropharyngeal dysphagia.

 MEDICATIONS

DRUG(S) OF CHOICE
- Dysphagia is not immediately life-threatening; direct drug therapy at the underlying cause.
- Empirical treatment may consist of a broad-spectrum antibiotic (e.g., cephalexin 22 mg/kg PO q8h).

CONTRAINDICATIONS
NA

PRECAUTIONS
- Use barium sulfate with caution in patients with evidence of aspiration.
- Use corticosteroids with caution or not at all in patients with evidence of, or at risk for, aspiration.

POSSIBLE INTERACTIONS
N/A

ALTERNATIVE DRUG(S)
NA

 FOLLOW-UP

PATIENT MONITORING
- Daily for signs of aspiration pneumonia (e.g., depression, fever, mucopurulent nasal discharge, coughing, and dyspnea)
- Body condition and hydration status daily; if oral nutrition does not meet requirements, use gastrostomy tube feeding

POSSIBLE COMPLICATIONS
- Aspiration pneumonia is a common complication with swallowing disorders.

- Feeding multiple small meals with the patient in an upright position and maintaining this position for 10–15 min after feeding help prevent aspiration of food.

 MISCELLANEOUS

ASSOCIATED CONDITIONS
- Megaesophagus
- Aspiration pneumonia

AGE-RELATED FACTORS
- Young dogs are more likely to ingest foreign objects and suffer facial trauma.
- Young cats are more likely to form inflammatory polyps.

ZOONOTIC POTENTIAL
- Consider rabies in any patient with dysphagia, especially if the animal's rabies vaccination status is unknown or questionable or it has been exposed to a potentially rabid animal.
- If a dysphagic animal dies of rapidly progressive neurologic disease, submit the head to a qualified laboratory designated by the local or state health department for rabies examination.

PREGNANCY
N/A

SYNONYMS
N/A

SEE ALSO
- Megaesophagus
- Pneumonia, Bacterial
- Regurgitation

ABBREVIATION
CNs = cranial nerves
CT = computed tomography
MRI = magnetic resonance imaging

Suggested Reading

Niles JD, Williams JM, Sullivan M, et al. Resolution of dysphagia following cricopharyngeal myectomy in six young dogs. J Small Anim Pract 2001;42(1):32–35.

Watrous BJ. Clinical presentation and diagnosis of dysphagia. Vet Clin North Am 1983;13:437–459.

Willard MD. Dysphagia and swallowing disorders. In: Kirk's current veterinary therapy XI. Philadelphia: Saunders, 1992:572–577.

Author Randall C. Longshore
Consulting Editors Albert E. Jergens

DYSPNEA, TACHYPNEA, AND PANTING

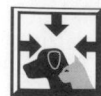 BASICS

DEFINITION
• Dyspnea—a subjective term that in human medicine means "an uncomfortable sensation in breathing" or a sensation of air hunger; in veterinary medicine, it means difficulty breathing or respiratory distress. • Tachypnea is increased respiratory rate. • Panting is rapid, shallow, open-mouth breathing.

PATHOPHYSIOLOGY
Respiratory rate, rhythm, and and effort are controlled by the respiratory center in the brain stem in response to numerous afferent pathways, both central and peripheral in origin. These include the cerebral cortex; central chemoreceptors; peripheral chemoreceptors; stimulation of mechanoreceptors in the airways that sense lung inflation and deflation; stimulation of irritant receptors of the airways; stimulation of C-fibers in the alveoli and pulmonary blood vessels, which sense interstitial congestion; and baroreceptors, which sense changes in blood pressure.

SYSTEMS AFFECTED Respiratory

SIGNALMENT
Dogs and cats; no breed, age, or sex predilection

SIGNS

Historical Findings
• Patients with primary respiratory disease—coughing, tachypnea, exercise intolerance
• Nonrespiratory causes—signs associated with the primary disease

Physical Examination Findings
• General signs of dyspnea—increased abdominal effort, nasal flaring (esp. cats), open mouth breathing, neck extension, elbow abduction; other signs depend on underlying cause.
• Nasal disease—stertor, lack of airflow through nostrils; dyspnea improves with open-mouth breathing. • Upper airway disease—stridor, hyperthermia • Dynamic obstruction such as laryngeal paralysis—dyspnea on inspiration
• Fixed obstruction such as a mass or foreign body—dyspnea on inspiration and expiration.
• Tracheal collapse—honking cough • Lower airway disease—cough, expiratory wheezes on auscultation • Pulmonary parenchymal disease—expiratory dyspnea; may have crackles on auscultation; may be normal auscultation.
• Pneumonia—fever • Cardiogenic pulmonary edema—heart murmur, hypothermia, pale mucous membranes, poor capillary refill time
• Pleural space disease—diminished breath sounds: ventrally—fluid; dorsally—air
• Prominent abdominal effort • Thoracic wall disease—visible trauma • Abdominal distention—evident • Nonrespiratory diseases—findings will depend on the other diseases, e.g., pale mucous membranes if anemic. • PTE—may have clinical signs of the underlying disease predisposing to thrombosis
• Other signs will pertain to the underlying disease, e.g., animals with traumatic pneumothorax may be in shock or have other signs of trauma.

CAUSES & RISK FACTORS

Panting
Pain, anxiety, drug therapy (opioids), heat regulation; can also be a normal behavioral pattern in some dogs

Tachypnea
• Hypoxemia, hypercapnia, hypotension, fever, anemia, acidosis, inflammatory mediators (TNFα) • Airway pathology—inhaled irritant, allergic disease, bronchoconstriction, airway compression, airway infection • Interstitial pathology—edema, hemorrhage, inflammation, neoplasia;

Dyspnea
• **Upper Airway Disease:** Nasal obstruction—stenotic nares; infection; inflammation; neoplasia; trauma; coagulopathy. Pharynx—elongated soft palate; pharyngeal polyp (cat); everted laryngeal saccules; foreign body; neoplasia. Larynx—laryngeal paralysis; edema; collapse; foreign body; neoplasia; trauma; webbing. Cervical trachea—collapse; stenosis; trauma; foreign body; neoplasia; parasites
• **Lower Airway Disease:** Thoracic trachea—see cervical trachea; extraluminal compression—lymphadenopathy; enlarged left atrium; heart-based tumors. • **Small Airway Disease,** allergic; inflammatory; infectious (*Mycoplasma*); parasitic; neoplastic (bronchogenic carcinoma)
• **Pulmonary Parenchymal Disease:** Edema—cardiogenic edema; non-cardiogenic edema (neurogenic, upper airway obstruction, electrocution) • Pneumonia—infectious; parasitic; aspiration • Neoplasia (primary or metastatic) • Inflammatory—allergic; infiltrative eosinophilia; acute respiratory distress syndrome; uremic pneumonitis
• Hemorrhage—trauma; coagulopathy
• PTE—Immune-mediated hemolytic anemia; heartworm disease; hyperadrenocorticism; DIC
• **Pleural Space Disease:** Pneumothorax—traumatic; secondary to pulmonary parenchymal disease; ruptured bulla; migrating foreign body; spontaneous • Pleural effusion—transudates seen with CHF; neoplasia; lung lobe torsion; exudates seen with pyothorax; neoplasia.
• Hemothorax—trauma; coagulopathy; lung lobe torsion; spontaneous thymic hemorrhage.
• Chylothorax—idiopathic; CHF; traumatic
• Soft tissue—neoplasia; diaphragmatic hernia
• **Thoracic Wall Disease:** Open pneumothorax—trauma; flail segment—trauma; neoplasia; paralysis due to botulism, polyradiculoneuritis, tick paralysis
• **Abdominal Distention:** Organomegaly—hyperplasia; neoplasia; pregnancy; obesity; ascites; gastric dilatation, torsion

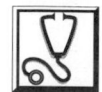 DIAGNOSIS

DIFFERENTIAL DIAGNOSIS
• Tachypnea without dyspnea—may be suggestive of a non-respiratory problem
• Inspiratory dyspnea—suggestive of upper airway disease • Expiratory dyspnea—suggests intrathoracic disease such as pulmonary parenchymal or small airway disease • Dyspnea on inspiration and expiration can occur with fixed upper airway obstructions and severe intrathoracic disease. • Stertor and stridor are features of upper airway disease—auscultation over the trachea can help delineate upper airway noises from lower airway noises. • Congestive heart failure—murmur, tachycardia, poor pulse quality, jugular pulses, hypothermia, crackles on auscultation, fluid dripping from nose

CBC/BIOCHEMISTRY/URINALYSIS
• Anemia—can cause non-respiratory dyspnea • Polycythemia—chronic hypoxia
• Inflammatory leukogram—pneumonia, pyothorax • Eosinophilia—allergic or parasitic disease • Thrombocytosis—hyperadrenocorticism predisposes to PTE
• Sodium:potassium ratio < 27—can be seen with pleural or abdominal chylous effusions
• High alkaline phosphatase—hyperadrenocorticism predisposes to PTE • Azotemia—if severe may lead to uremic pneumonitis
• Multiple organ dysfunction—ARDS
• Proteinuria—can predispose to PTE

OTHER LABORATORY TESTS
• Heartworm testing • Pleural fluid analysis
• Blood gases—can help determine the etiology and severity of a patient's respiratory distress
• PaO_2—partial pressure of oxygen dissolved in arterial blood; normoxemia: PaO_2 80–120 mmHg (room air, sea level), hypoxemia: PaO_2 < 80 mmHg (room air, sea level) hyperoxemia: PaO_2 > 120 mmHg; F_iO_2—fraction of inspired oxygen ranges from 0.21 (room air) to 1.0; PaO_2/F_iO_2 ratio—measure of lung efficiency; PaO_2/F_iO_2 ≥500—normal lung efficiency; 300–500—mild inefficiency; 200–300—moderate inefficiency; <200—severe inefficiency. Reduction in lung efficiency is most commonly due to pulmonary parenchymal disease (exceptions are anatomical right to left vascular shunts). • PvO_2—partial pressure of oxygen dissolved in venous blood; a central blood sample (jugular) most reliable; PvO_2 is determined by oxygen delivery and oxygen consumption by tissues; normal PvO_2 on room air = 40–60 mmHg; PvO_2 < 30 mmHg is clinically concerning; PvO_2 < 20 mmHg is life-threatening. • $PaCO_2$—partial pressure of CO_2 dissolved in arterial blood; measure of ventilation; normal $PaCO_2$ = 40 mmHg (dog); 31 mmHg (cat). Hypercapnia = hypoventilation = decreased alveolar minute ventilation (MV). Hypocapnia = hyperventilation = increased MV. Hypoventilation can be due to upper airway obstruction, pleural space disease, thoracic wall disease and abdominal distention; Respiratory muscle fatigue from a prolonged period of dyspnea can lead to hypoventilation. • $PvCO_2$—partial pressure of CO_2 dissolved in venous blood; when correlation with $PaCO_2$ is good, $PvCO_2$ tends to be 4 mmHg < $PaCO_2$; central blood samples are the most representative.

IMAGING

• **Thoracic Radiography:** Upper airway disease—large airway narrowing, lymphadenopathy, intraluminal abnormalities. *Pneumonia*—alveolar infiltrates; aspiration pneumonia tends to have cranioventral distribution. *Cardiogenic pulmonary edema*—enlarged cardiac shadow, pulmonary venous distention, enlarged left atrium with perihilar pulmonary infiltrates in dogs; infiltrates can be of any distribution in cats. *Non-cardiogenic pulmonary edema*—caudodorsal distribution. ARDS—diffuse, symmetrical alveolar infiltrates. *Pulmonary vascular abnormalities*—PTE. *Pleural space disease*—pneumothorax, pleural effusion, mass lesions, diaphragmatic hernias. *Thoracic wall disease*—rib fractures
• **Thoracic Ultrasound:** Evaluation of distribution of pleural effusion (excellent as guide for thoracocentesis). Pulmonary mass identification—guide fine needle aspiration; mediastinal evaluation
• **Echocardiography:** Evaluate cardiac function if cardiogenic pulmonary edema or pleural effusion suspected; elevated pulmonary artery pressure and right ventricular overload can support diagnosis of PTE; visualize heart-based masses.
• **Abdominal Radiographs:** Evaluation of abdominal distention
• **Fluoroscopy:** Evaluate tracheal and/or large airway collapse.
• **Computed Tomography:** Airway, pulmonary parenchymal, and pleural space disease can be evaluated; can detect lesions not as clearly defined on radiographs
• **Pulmonary Vascular Angiography:** Gold standard for diagnosis of PTE
• **Ventilation-Perfusion Scintigraphy:** Ventilation perfusion mismatching is suggestive of PTE but is rarely performed; abnormal perfusion scan is considered supportive of the diagnosis.

DIAGNOSTIC PROCEDURES

• Pulse oximetry—SpO_2—percentage of hemoglobin saturated with oxygen as measured by a pulse oximeter. The relationship between PaO_2 and SpO_2 is defined by the oxygen hemoglobin dissociation curve; PaO_2 of 60 mmHg = SpO_2 of 90%; PaO_2 of 80 mmHg = SpO_2 of 95%; PaO_2 of > 100 mmHg = SpO_2 of 100%. Small changes in SpO_2 signify large changes in PaO_2; SpO_2 measurements in animals on high inspired oxygen (e.g., under anesthesia) are not a sensitive monitor since PaO_2 needs to fall below 100 mm Hg before the pulse oximeter will register a change; pulse oximetry is prone to inaccuracy and must be interpreted in light of the patient's clinical condition. • Thoracocentesis—fluid analysis and culture • Laryngopharyngoscopy—to evaluate laryngeal function and visualize foreign bodies and masses; with spay hook and dental mirror, visualize caudal nasopharyngeal region.
• Rhinoscopy—visualize abnormalities; biopsy.
• Bronchoscopy—evaluate large and small airways; take biopsies; perform bronchoalveolar lavage for cytology and culture. • Transtracheal wash—obtain sample from lower airways for cytology and culture; be careful to avoid contamination by airwawy inhabitants, which, of course, will render the results inaccurate.

TREATMENT

APPROPRIATE HEALTH CARE
• Inpatient care until the cause is identified and treated or determined not to be life-threatening; therapy dependent on underlying cause
• ALWAYS administer oxygen until patient's ability to oxygenate is determined. • Keep patient in sternal recumbency until stabilized.
• Upper airway disease—patient with mild to moderate upper airway obstruction may benefit from sedation to reduce inspiratory effort. Actively cool patients as necessary since hyperthermia will increase respiratory effort. Severe upper airway disease requires intubation to stabilize; if the problem cannot be immediately cured, placement of a temporary tracheostomy tube is indicated. Remove foreign bodies; perform surgical excision/biopsy of masses, surgical correction for laryngeal paralysis and brachycephalic syndrome; give anti-inflammatory medications for laryngeal edema. • Lower airway disease—bronchodilators (terbutaline, theophylline); systemic corticosteroids often required to stabilize cats with acute bronchoconstriction, oxygen therapy until stable • Pulmonary parenchymal disease—oxygen therapy, antibiotics if pneumonia; treat coagulation disorders accordingly; cardiogenic edema requires furosemide +/− vasodilators. Noncardiogenic edema requires oxygen therapy; single dose of furosemide may be beneficial; pulmonary parenchymal disease may require positive-pressure ventilation with positive-end-expiratory pressure if oxygen therapy alone is not adequate to stabilize the patient. • Pleural space disease—thoracocentesis for air and fluid; remove as much as possible. Place a chest tube if repeated chest taps are needed to keep patient stable. Surgery for diaphragmatic hernias or spontaneous pneumothorax. • Thoracic wall disease—surgery as indicated, particularly if open chest wound is present; flail chest may require surgery, although it is usually the ensuing pleural space disease that is life-threatening following chest wall trauma. Thoracic wall paralysis—positive-pressure ventilation if severely hypercapnic • Abdominal distention—drain ascites as needed to keep the patient comfortable; relieve gastric distention.
• Nonrespiratory diseases—treat primary problem.

NURSING CARE
• Oxygen therapy via cage, nasal cannula, E-collar covered in plastic wrap, mask, or flow-by. Humidify oxygen source if giving oxygen therapy for more than a few hours. • Maintain in sternal recumbency and turn hips every 3–4 hours if patient cannot tolerate lateral recumbency. Monitor temperature regularly, as dyspneic animals often become hyperthermic, and hyperthermia in turn will worsen dyspnea.

ACTIVITY
Strict cage confinement until dyspnea is resolved

DIET
Weight reducing diet if obesity is a contributing cause

CLIENT EDUCATION N/A

SURGICAL CONSIDERATIONS
Anesthesia must be carefully tailored to the patient. Securing an airway is essential and the ability to positive-pressure–ventilate patients is often required. Avoid positive-pressure ventilation in patients with a closed pneumothorax.

MEDICATIONS

DRUGS
Vary with underlying cause (see Appropriate Health Care)

CONTRAINDICATIONS N/A

PRECAUTIONS N/A

POSSIBLE INTERACTIONS N/A

FOLLOW UP

PATIENT MONITORING
• Patients receiving oxygen therapy can be monitored by assessing the degree of dyspnea; measure arterial blood gases. • Pulse oximetry is an effective tool for monitoring patients on room-air. A room air trial evaluating degree of dyspnea, blood gases, etc., can be a useful assessment. • Repeat radiographs are often indicated in assessing pulmonary parenchymal disease and pleural space disease.

MISCELLANEOUS

SEE ALSO
• Laryngeal Disease • Brachycephalic Airway Syndrome • Asthma, Bronchitis—Cats
• Congestive Heart Failure • Pneumonia
• Pulmonary Edema, Noncardiogenic • Acute Respiratory Distress Syndrome • Pneumothorax

ABBREVIATIONS
• ARDS = acute respiratory distress syndrome
• CHF = congestive heart failure
• CNS = central nervous system
• DIC = disseminated intravascular coagulation
• MV = minute ventilation
• PTE = pulmonary thromboembolism

Suggested Reading

Turnwald GH. Dyspnea and tachypnea. In: Ettinger SJ, Feldman EC, eds. Textbook of small animal internal medicine. 3rd ed. Philadelphia: Saunders, 2000:166–169.
Author Kate Hopper
Consulting Editor Lynelle R. Johnson

DYSTOCIA

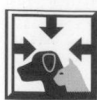 BASICS

DEFINITION
Difficult birth

PATHOPHYSIOLOGY
• Occurs with a small or deformed birth canal, fetal oversize, or uterine weakness (e.g., insufficient uterine force to propel fetus through birth canal)
• Three stages of labor:

Stage 1
• Begins with onset of uterine contractions; ends when cervix is fully dilated; averages 6–12 hr • Bitches—may be restless, nervous, and anorectic; may shiver, pant, vomit, or pace; near end will usually seek a place to nest • Queens—tend to vocalize initially; purr as delivery approaches

Stage 2
• Begins with full dilation of cervix, entry of the first fetus into the cervical canal, and rupture of the chorioallantois; ends with delivery of the last of the litter • Bitch—obvious abdominal contractions in attempt to deliver; from beginning of stage to delivery of first offspring usually < 4 hr; time between delivery of subsequent offspring usually 20–60 min (may be as long as 2–3 hr in bitches) • Queen—average length of parturition is 16 hr, with a range of 4–42 hr; important to consider this variability when intervening

Stage 3
• Begins after delivery of the offspring; ends with passage of all placentae
• Bitch with multiple puppies—may alternate between stage 2 and 3

SYSTEMS AFFECTED
• Reproductive
• Cardiovascular

GENETICS
N/A

INCIDENCE/PREVALENCE
• Dog—incidence unknown; difficult to estimate due to breed variability and breeder intervention
• Cat—reported average ranges from 3.3–5.8%; mixed-breed cats, 0.4%; increased with pedigreed cats, to a high of 18.2% in the Devon rex

GEOGRAPHIC DISTRIBUTION
N/A

SIGNALMENT

Species
Dogs and cats

Breed Predilection
Dogs
• Higher incidence with miniature and small breeds; occasionally noted in large breeds with large litters • Brachycephalic—bulldogs, Boston terriers; broad head and narrow pelvis • Large fetal head:maternal pelvis ratio—Sealyham terrier, Scottish terrier • Uterine inertia—Scottish terrier, dachshund, border terrier, Aberdeen terrier • Miscellaneous breeds with overall increased incidence of dystocia—Chihuahua, dachshund, Pekingese, Yorkshire terrier, miniature poodle, Pomeranian
Cats
• Brachycephalic—Persian, Himalayan
• Dolichocephalic—Devon rex

Mean Age and Range
Prevalence increases with age

Predominant Sex
N/A

SIGNS

Historical Findings
• Female undergoes 30 min of persistent, strong, abdominal contractions without expulsion of offspring. • More than 4 hr from the onset of stage 2 to delivery of first offspring • More than 2 hr between delivery of offspring • Failure to deliver 24 hr after rectal temperature falls < 37.2°C (99°F) or within 36 hr of serum progesterone < 2 ng/mL (dogs) • Female cries, displays signs of pain, and constantly licks the vulvar area when delivering • Prolonged gestation—> 70 days from day of first mating; > 59 days from the first day of cytologic diestrus (dogs); > 66 days from LH peak (dogs)

PHYSICAL EXAMINATION FINDINGS
• Greenish-black discharge (uteroverdin)—precedes birth of first pup • Determine relationship between offspring and maternal birth canal. Presentation: relationship of fetal spinal axis to maternal pelvis—longitudinal is normal; transverse is abnormal. Position: relationship of dorsum of fetus (or head in a transverse presentation) to maternal pelvic quadrants. Posture: relationship of fetal extremities or head to the fetal body.
• Determine strength of Ferguson reflex (stimulation or pressure to dorsal vaginal wall elicits abdominal straining [feathering])—absent or diminished with uterine inertia

CAUSES

Fetal
• Oversize—one-pup litter; monster, anasarcous fetus; hydrocephalus; prolonged gestation • Abnormal presentation, position, or posture of fetus in the birth canal

Maternal
• Abnormal pelvic canal from previous pelvic fracture • Congenitally small pelvis—Welsh corgis; brachycephalic breeds • Pelvic immaturity • Abnormality of the vaginal vault—stricture; septate; hyperplasia; intraluminal or extraluminal cyst; neoplasia; hypoplastic vagina • Insufficient cervical dilation • Lack of adequate lubrication • Uterine torsion; uterine rupture • Poor uterine contractions—myometrial defect; biochemical imbalance; psychogenic disturbance; exhaustion (see Uterine Inertia) • Ineffective abdominal press—pain; debility (exhaustion); diaphragmatic hernia; age; perforated trachea

RISK FACTORS
• Age
• Brachycephalic and toy breeds
• Persian and Himalayan breeds
• Obesity
• Abrupt changes in environment peripartum
• Previous history of dystocia

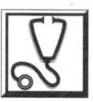 DIAGNOSIS

DIFFERENTIAL DIAGNOSIS
• Uterine inertia—distinguished from obstructive dystocia by previously diagnosed pelvic or vaginal anomaly and type of breed
• Complete physical examination—essential; determine concurrent or contributing problems (e.g., hypoglycemia, hypocalcemia, dehydration, and fever); perform careful abdominal palpation to confirm the existence of fetuses.
• Detailed and meticulous digital vaginal examination—identify a fetus engaged in the vaginal canal; find abnormalities of the maternal pelvic canal or vaginal vault; determine the strength of abdominal press in response to stimulation of the roof of the vagina.
• Bitches that fail to produce abdominal contractions in response to feathering or oxytocin—more likely to have uterine inertia than obstructive dystocia, unless the obstruction is of several hours' duration

CBC/BIOCHEMISTRY/URINALYSIS
• Minimum database—PCV, total protein, BUN, serum glucose, and calcium concentrations
• Depend on duration of condition—may be normal; may note hypoglycemia, dehydration, and hypocalcemia
• Perform analyses, although results might not be available until after resolution of the condition.

OTHER LABORATORY TESTS
N/A

IMAGING
• Radiography (abdomen and pelvic area)—paramount; determine state of pregnancy, pelvic structure, number and malposition of fetuses, fetal oversize, and fetal death
• Ultrasonography—recommended for monitoring fetal viability; detects fetal stress (e.g., fetal heart rate < 200 bpm)

DIAGNOSTIC PROCEDURES
N/A

PATHOLOGIC FINDINGS
N/A

TREATMENT

APPROPRIATE HEALTH CARE
• Inpatient—until delivery of all offspring and mother has stabilized
• Uterine inertia—initiate treatment if no evidence of fetal stress; administer balanced electrolyte solution (adjusted to correct for any identified electrolyte imbalance).

Manual Delivery
• To deliver a fetus lodged in vaginal vault
• Apply lubrication liberally; place patient in a standing position
• Use of fingers—safest and most reliable approach
• Instrument delivery (dogs)—if vaginal vault too small for digital manipulations; use with adequate lubrication; always place a finger in the vaginal vault to direct the instrument; spay hook or nonratcheted forceps recommended; apply traction in a posterior and ventral direction.
• Use extreme caution; undesirable sequelae include mutilation of the fetus and laceration of the dam.
• Traction on a distal extremity—definitely contraindicated
• Cats—use of instruments not recommended because of the small size of the vaginal vault
• Failure to deliver the fetus within 25–30 minutes—cesarean section indicated
• Severely depressed queen—fluid and electrolyte balance must be restored before induction of anesthesia

NURSING CARE
Fluid replacement—balanced electrolyte solutions; for clinical dehydration

ACTIVITY
N/A

DIET
N/A

CLIENT EDUCATION
N/A

SURGICAL CONSIDERATIONS
• Indications for cesarean section—uterine inertia unresponsive to oxytocin; pelvic or vaginal obstruction; uncorrectable fetal malposition; fetal oversize; fetal stress; in utero fetal death
• Elective cesarean section—breeds highly prone to dystocia; bitches with a history of dystocia

Anesthesia
• Healthy or depressed bitch—premedication with diazepam (0.2–0.4 mg/kg IM) and butorphanol (0.2–0.4 mg/kg IM) with or without anticholinergics; isoflurane and mask for induction; then intubate to maintain; provide intravenous fluids.
• Healthy queen—premedication with diazepam (0.4 mg/kg IV) and ketamine (6 mg/kg IV); administer intravenous fluids; 0.5% lidocaine spray for intubation; isoflurane preferred but may use halothane
• Severely depressed queen (exhausted from prolonged labor)—premedication with diazepam or midazolam (0.2–0.4 mg/kg IV, IM) with either butorphanol (0.4 mg/kg IV, IM) or oxymorphone (0.2 mg/kg IM); low-dose ketamine (1–2 mg/kg IV) for intubation; etomidate or propofol for induction
• After surgery, effects of drugs can be reversed.

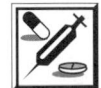

MEDICATIONS

DRUG(S) OF CHOICE
Oxytocin—for uterine inertia

CONTRAINDICATIONS
Oxytocin—contraindicated with obstructive dystocia of fetal or maternal cause, fetal stress, and longstanding in utero fetal death

PRECAUTIONS
N/A

POSSIBLE INTERACTIONS
N/A

ALTERNATIVE DRUG(S)
N/A

FOLLOW-UP

PATIENT MONITORING
Ultrasonography—recommended; monitor fetal heart rate during medical management of uterine inertia

PREVENTION/AVOIDANCE
• Scheduled elective cesarean section—abnormal pelvic canal; small pelvis; vaginal vault abnormalities; breeds predisposed to dystocia; dams with previous history of obstructive dystocia
• Scheduling of surgery—extremely important that either D1 diestrus or the LH peak is identified during breeding; significantly improves fetal survivability; see Breeding, Timing.

POSSIBLE COMPLICATIONS
• Increased risk in future pregnancies
• Neonatal loss if treatment is not begun promptly

EXPECTED COURSE AND PROGNOSIS
• If dystocia is identified promptly and intervention is successful—good to fair for life of the dam; fair for survival of offspring
• If dystocia unrecognized or untreated for 24–48 hours (dogs)—poor to guarded for life of the dam; unlikely that any offspring will survive
• If dystocia unrecognized or untreated for 24–48 hours (cats)—prognosis highly variable depending on cause

MISCELLANEOUS

ASSOCIATED CONDITIONS
N/A

AGE-RELATED FACTORS
Old, obese bitches—increased risk of uterine inertia

ZOONOTIC POTENTIAL
N/A

PREGNANCY
N/A

SYNONYMS
N/A

SEE ALSO
Uterine Inertia
Breeding, Timing

ABBREVIATIONS
• LH = luteinizing hormone
• PCV = packed cell volume

Suggested Reading
Johnston SD, Root Kustritz MV, Olson PNS. Canine parturition—eutocia and dystocia. In: Canine and feline theriogenology. Philadelphia: Saunders, 2001:105–128.
Johnston SD, Root Kustritz MV, Olson PNS. Feline parturition. In: Canine and feline theriogenology. Philadelphia: Saunders, 2001:431–437.
Paddleford RR. Anesthetic management of the cesarean section. In: Manual of small animal anesthesia. Churchill Livingstone, 1988:290–296.
Shille VM. Diagnosis and management of dystocia in the bitch and queen. In: Bojrab MJ, ed. Current techniques in small animal surgery. Philadelphia: Lea & Febiger, 1983:338–346.
Tranquilli WJ. Anesthesia for cesarean section in the cat. Vet Clin North Am Small Anim Pract 1992;22:484–486.
Author Louis F. Archbald
Consulting Editor Sara K. Lyle

DYSURIA AND POLLAKIURIA

 **BASICS**

DEFINITION
• Dysuria—difficult or painful urination
• Pollakiuria—voiding small quantities of urine with increased frequency

PATHOPHYSIOLOGY
The urinary bladder and urethra normally serve as a reservoir for storage and periodic release of urine. Inflammatory and non-inflammatory disorders of the lower urinary tract may decrease bladder compliance and storage capacity by damaging structural components of the bladder wall or by stimulating sensory nerve endings located in the bladder or urethra. Sensations of bladder fullness, urgency, and pain stimulate premature micturition and reduce functional bladder capacity. Dysuria and pollakiuria are caused by lesions of the urinary bladder and/or urethra and provide unequivocal evidence of lower urinary tract disease; these clinical signs do not exclude concurrent involvement of the upper urinary tract or disorders of other body systems.

SYSTEMS AFFECTED
Renal/Urologic—bladder, urethra, and prostate gland

SIGNALMENT
Dogs and Cats

SIGNS
N/A

CAUSES

Urinary Bladder
• Urinary tract infection—bacterial, viral, fungal, parasitic, or mycoplasmal
• Urocystolithiasis
• Neoplasia—e.g., transitional cell carcinoma
• Trauma
• Anatomic abnormalities—e.g., ureterocele, persistent uterus masculinus, perineal hernias containing the urinary bladder, and spay granulomas
• Detrusor atony—e.g., chronic partial obstruction and dysautonomia
• Chemicals/drugs—e.g., cyclophosphamide
• Iatrogenic—e.g., catheterization, palpation, reverse flushing, overdistension of the bladder during contrast radiography, urohydro-propulsion, urethrocystoscopy, and surgery
• Idiopathic—e.g., idiopathic feline lower urinary tract disease

Urethra
• Urinary tract infection—see previous section.
• Urethrolithiasis—see previous section.
• Urethral plugs—e.g., matrix and matrix-crystalline
• Neoplasia—see previous section; local invasion by malignant neoplasms of adjacent structures
• Trauma
• Anatomic anomalies—e.g., congenital or acquired strictures, urethrorectal fistulas, and pseudohermaphrodites
• Urethral sphincter hypertonicity—e.g., upper motor neuron spinal cord lesions, reflex dyssynergia, and urethral spasm
• Iatrogenic—see previous section.
• Idiopathic—see previous section.

Prostate Gland
• Prostatitis or prostatic abscess
• Neoplasia—adenocarcinoma and transitional cell carcinoma
• Cystic hyperplasia
• Paraprostatic cysts

RISK FACTORS
• Diseases, diagnostic procedures, or treatments that (1) alter normal host urinary tract defenses and predispose to infection, (2) predispose to formation of uroliths, or (3) damage the urothelium or other tissues of the lower urinary tract
• Mural or extramural diseases that compress the bladder or urethral lumen

 DIAGNOSIS

DIFFERENTIAL DIAGNOSIS

Differentiating from Other Abnormal Patterns of Micturition
• Rule out polyuria—increased frequency and volume of urine > 50 mL/kg/day
• Rule out urethral obstruction—stranguria, anuria, overdistended urinary bladder, signs of postrenal uremia
• Rule out urinary incontinence—involuntary urination, urine dribbling, enuresis, incomplete bladder emptying
• Rule out urine spraying or marking—voiding small amounts of urine on vertical surfaces or other socially significant places

Differentiate Causes of Dysuria and Pollakiuria
• Rule out urinary tract infection—hematuria; malodorous or cloudy urine; small, painful, thickened bladder
• Rule out urolithiasis—hematuria; palpable uroliths in urethra or bladder
• Rule out neoplasia—hematuria; palpable masses in urethra or bladder
• Rule out neurogenic disorders—flaccid bladder wall; residual urine in bladder lumen after micturition; other neurologic deficits to hind legs, tail, perineum, and anal sphincter
• Rule out prostatic diseases—urethral discharge, prostatomegaly, pyrexia, depression, tenesmus, caudal abdominal pain, stiff gait
• Rule out cyclophosphamide cystitis—history
• Rule out iatrogenic disorders—history of catheterization, reverse flushing, contrast radiography, urohydropropulsion, urethro-cystoscopy, or surgery

CBC/BIOCHEMISTRY/URINALYSIS
• Results often normal. Lower urinary tract disease complicated by urethral obstruction may be associated with azotemia, hyperphos-phatemia, acidosis, and hyperkalemia. Patients with concurrent pyelonephritis may have impaired urine-concentrating capacity, leukocytosis, and azotemia. Patients with acute prostatitis or prostatic abscesses may have leukocytosis. Dehydrated patients may have elevated total plasma protein.
• Disorders of the urinary bladder are best evaluated with a urine specimen collected by cystocentesis. Urethral disorders are best evaluated with a voided urine sample or by comparison of results of analysis of voided and cystocentesis samples. (Caution: cystocentesis may induce hematuria.)
• Pyuria, hematuria, and proteinuria indicate urinary tract inflammation, but these are nonspecific findings that may result from infectious and noninfectious causes of lower urinary tract disease.
• Identification of bacteria, fungi, or parasite ova in urine sediment suggests, but does not prove, that urinary tract infection is causing or complicating lower urinary tract disease. Consider contamination of urine during collection and storage when interpreting urinalysis results.
• Identification of neoplastic cells in urine sediment indicates urinary tract neoplasia. Use caution in establishing a diagnosis of neoplasia based on urine sediment examination. Urinary tract inflammation or extremes in urine pH or osmolality can cause epithelial cell atypia that is difficult to differentiate from neoplasia.
• Crystalluria occurs in normal patients, patients with urolithiasis, or patients with lower urinary tract disease unassociated with uroliths. Interpret the significance of crystal-luria cautiously.
• Hematuria, proteinuria, and variable crys-talluria occur in cats with nonobstructive idiopathic lower urinary tract disease. Significant pyuria is rare in these patients.

OTHER LABORATORY TESTS

• Quantitative urine culture—the most definitive means of identifying and characterizing bacterial urinary tract infection; negative urine culture results suggest a noninfectious cause (e.g., uroliths and neoplasia) or inflammation associated with urinary tract infection caused by fastidious organisms (e.g., mycoplasmas or viruses).

• Cytologic evaluation of urine sediment, prostatic fluid, urethral or vaginal discharges or biopsy specimens obtained by catheter or needle aspiration—may help in evaluating patients with localized urinary tract disease; may establish a definitive diagnosis of urinary tract neoplasia, but cannot rule it out

IMAGING

Survey abdominal radiography, contrast urethrocystography and cystography, urinary tract ultrasonography, and excretory urography are important means of identifying and localizing causes of dysuria and pollakiuria.

DIAGNOSTIC PROCEDURES

• Use urethrocystoscopy in patients with persistent lesions of the lower urinary tract for which no definitive diagnosis has been established by other, less-invasive, means.

• Use light microscopic evaluation of tissue biopsy specimens from patients with persistent lesions of the urinary tract for which no definitive diagnosis has been established by other, less-invasive, means. Tissue specimens may be obtained by catheter biopsy, urethrocystoscopy and forceps biopsy, or surgery.

 TREATMENT

• Patients with nonobstructive lower urinary tract diseases are typically managed as outpatients; diagnostic evaluation may require brief hospitalization.

• Dysuria and pollakiuria associated with systemic signs of illness (e.g., pyrexia, depression, anorexia, vomiting, and dehydration) or laboratory findings of azotemia or leukocytosis warrant aggressive diagnostic evaluation and initiation of supportive and symptomatic treatment.

• Treatment depends on the underlying cause and specific sites involved. See specific chapters describing diseases listed in section on causes.

• Clinical signs of dysuria and pollakiuria often resolve rapidly following specific treatment of the underlying cause(s).

 MEDICATIONS

DRUG(S) OF CHOICE

• Patients with urge incontinence, severe or persistent signs, or untreatable lower urinary tract disease may benefit from symptomatic therapy with propantheline or oxybutynin, anticholinergic agents that may reduce the force and frequency of uncontrolled detrusor contractions.

• Patients with transitional cell carcinoma of the urinary bladder or urethra may be symptomatically managed with the nonsteroidal antiinflammatory drug piroxicam, which reduces the severity of clinical signs, improves quality of life, and in some cases, induces tumor remission.

CONTRAINDICATIONS

• Glucocorticoids or other immunosuppressive agents in patients suspected of having urinary or genital tract infection.

• Potentially nephrotoxic drugs (e.g., gentamicin) in patients that are febrile, dehydrated, or azotemic or that are suspected of having pyelonephritis, septicemia, or preexisting renal disease.

PRECAUTIONS
N/A

POSSIBLE INTERACTIONS
N/A

ALTERNATIVE DRUGS
N/A

 FOLLOW-UP

PATIENT MONITORING

• Response to treatment by clinical signs, serial physical examinations, laboratory testing, and radiographic and ultrasonic evaluations appropriate for each specific cause

• Refer to specific chapters describing diseases listed, under Causes.

POSSIBLE COMPLICATIONS

• Dysuria and pollakiuria may be associated with formation of macroscopic vesicourachal diverticula.

• Refer to specific chapters describing diseases listed, under Causes.

 MISCELLANEOUS

ASSOCIATED CONDITIONS

• Hematuria, pyuria, and proteinuria
• Disorders predisposing to urinary tract infection
• Disorders predisposing to formation of uroliths
• Macroscopic vesicourachal diverticula

AGE-RELATED FACTORS
N/A

ZOONOTIC POTENTIAL
N/A

PREGNANCY
N/A

SYNONYMS
• Feline urological syndrome (FUS)
• Lower urinary tract disease

SEE ALSO
• Lower Urinary Tract Infection
• Urolithiasis
• Urinary Retention, Functional
• Urinary Tract Obstruction
• Feline Idiopathic Lower Urinary Tract Disease
• Vesicourachal Diverticula

Suggested Reading

Hammer AS, LaRue S. Tumors of the urinary tract. In: Ettinger SJ, Feldman EC, eds. Textbook of veterinary internal medicine. 4th ed. Philadelphia: Saunders, 1995: 1788–1796.

Ling GV. Bacterial infections of the urinary tract. In: Ettinger SJ, Feldman EC, eds. Textbook of veterinary internal medicine. 5th ed. Philadelphia: Saunders, 2000:1678–1686.

Osborne CA, Kruger JM, Lulich JP, et al. Feline lower urinary tract diseases. In: Ettinger SJ, Feldman EC, eds. Textbook of veterinary internal medicine. 5th ed. Philadelphia: Saunders, 2000:1710–1747.

Authors John M. Kruger and Carl A. Osborne

Consulting Editors Larry G. Adams and Carl A. Osborne

EAR MITES

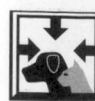

BASICS

OVERVIEW
• *Otodectes cynotis* mites cause a hypersensitivity reaction that results in intense irritation of the external ear of dogs and cats.

SIGNALMENT
• Common in young dogs and cats, although it may occur at any age
• No breed or sex predilection

SIGNS
• Pruritus primarily located around the ears, head, and neck; occasionally generalized
• Thick, red-brown or black crusts—usually seen in the outer ear
• Crusting and scales may occur on the neck, rump, and tail.
• Excoriations on the convex surface of the pinnae often occur, owing to the intense pruritus.

CASES & RISK FACTORS
O. cynotis

DIAGNOSIS

DIFFERENTIAL DIAGNOSIS
• Flea bite hypersensitivity
• Pediculosis
• *Pelodera* dermatitis
• Sarcoptic mange
• Chiggers
• Allergic otitis

CBC/BIOCHEMISTRY/URINALYSIS
Normal

OTHER LABORATORY TESTS
N/A

IMAGING
N/A

DIAGNOSTIC PROCEDURES
• Skin scrapings—identify mites, if signs are generalized
• Ear swabs placed in mineral oil—usually a very effective means of identification
• Mites may be visualized otoscopically.
• In hypersensitive animals, diagnosis may be made by response to treatment.

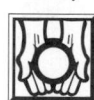

TREATMENT

• Outpatient
• Diet and activity—no alteration necessary
• Very contagious; important to treat all incontact animals
• Thoroughly clean and treat the environment.

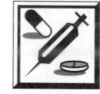

MEDICATIONS

DRUG(S)
• Ears should be thoroughly cleaned with a commercial ear cleaner.
• Otitic parasiticides should be used for 7 to 10 days to eradicate mites and eggs. Topical commercial products containing pyrethrins, thiabendazole, ivermectin, rotenone as well as other parasiticides have been effective.
• Selamectin (Revolution®, Pfizer) applied topically to the base of the neck.
• Ivermectin—300 ug/kg SC every 1 to 2 weeks for 4 treatments is an off label but effective treatment.
• Flea treatments should be applied to animal for elimination of ectopic mites.
• Mites can persist in the environment, unless it is thoroughly cleaned.

CONTRAINDICATIONS/POSSIBLE INTERACTIONS
• Ivermectin—do not use in collies, shelties, their crosses, or other herding breeds; use only if absolutely necessary in animals < 6 months of age; an increasing number of toxic reactions have been reported in kittens.

FOLLOW-UP

• An ear swab and physical examination should be done 1 month after therapy commences.
• For most patients, prognosis is good.
• Rarely, the infestation will be cleared only to find an underlying allergy that keeps the otitis externa active.

MISCELLANEOUS

ZOONOTIC POTENTIAL
The mites will also bite humans (rare).

Suggested Reading
Scott DW, Miller WH, Griffin CE. Muller & Kirk's small animal dermatology. 6th ed. Philadelphia: Saunders, 2001.

Authors Karen A. Kuhl and Jean S. Greek
Consulting Editors Karen Helton Rhodes

BASICS

OVERVIEW
• Atrialization of the right ventricle—an apical displacement of the tricuspid valve complex into the right ventricle
• Accompanied by various degrees of tricuspid insufficiency
• Major pathophysiology related to the degree of tricuspid insufficiency
• An abnormal accessory pathway may lead to supraventricular tachycardias.

SIGNALMENT
• Very rare—occasionally encountered in dogs and cats
• No breed or sex predilection
• Murmur auscultated at a young age

SIGNS
• Animals with mild tricuspid insufficiency are asymptomatic.
• Animals with severe insufficiency have R-CHF with pleural effusion and/or ascites.

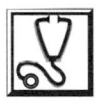

DIAGNOSIS

DIFFERENTIAL DIAGNOSIS
Tricuspid dysplasia

CBC/BIOCHEMISTRY/URINALYSIS
Results usually normal

OTHER LABORATORY TESTS
N/A

IMAGING
Thoracic Radiography
• Right atrial and ventricular enlargement
• Hepatomegaly

Echocardiography
Two-dimensional echocardiography reveals apically displaced tricuspid valve.

OTHER DIAGNOSTIC PROCEDURES
Electrocardiography
• Simultaneous intracardiac pressure and ECG tracings may be needed to verify the diagnosis.
• Accessory conduction pathway (ventricular pre-excitation) or supraventricular tachycardia

TREATMENT
• Medical management currently the only practical approach
• Restrict sodium intake if right heart failure develops.

MEDICATIONS

DRUG(S)
• Patients with R-CHF—institute furosemide (2–4 mg/kg q6–12h) and enalapril (0.5 mg/kg q12h)
• Patients with supraventricular tachycardia (WPW syndrome)—start procainamide (15 mg/kg q8h)
• If WPW syndrome persists, consider a calcium channel blocker (i.e., verapamil or diltiazem) or a β-blocker (i.e., propranolol or atenolol).

CONTRAINDICATIONS/POSSIBLE INTERACTIONS
Do not use calcium channel blockers and β-blockers concurrently.

FOLLOW-UP
Monitor with serial echocardiography, ECG, and radiography.

MISCELLANEOUS

SEE ALSO
Tricuspid Valve Dysplasia

ABBREVIATIONS
• ECG = electrocardiography
• R-CHF = right-sided congestive heart failure
• WPW = Wolff-Parkinson-White (syndrome)

Suggested Reading

Bonagura JD, Lehmkuhl LB. Congenital heart disease. In: Fox PR, Sisson D, Moise NS, eds. Textbook of canine and feline cardiology. 2nd ed. Philadelphia: Saunders, 1999:471–535.
Friedman WF. Congenital heart disease in infancy and childhood. In: Braunwald F., ed. Heart disease. 4th ed. Philadelphia: Saunders, 1992.

Author Carroll Loyer
Consulting Editors Larry P. Tilley and Francis W. K. Smith, Jr.

ECLAMPSIA

 BASICS

OVERVIEW
• Postparturient hypocalcemia
• Usually develops 1–4 weeks postpartum; may occur at term, prepartum, or during late lactation
• Alters cell membrane potentials, causing spontaneous discharge of nerve fibers and tonoclonic contraction of skeletal muscles
• Life-threatening tetany and convulsions, leading to hyperthermia
• Cerebral edema possible

SIGNALMENT
• Dogs—postpartum bitch; most common in toy breeds; higher incidence with first litter
• Breeds at increased risk: Chihuahua, miniature pinscher, Shih Tzu, miniature poodle, Mexican hairless, Pomeranian
• Cats—rare

SIGNS
Historical Findings
• Poor mothering
• Restlessness, nervousness
• Panting, whining
• Vomiting, diarrhea
• Ataxia, stiff gait
• Muscle tremors, tetany, convulsions
• Recumbency, extensor rigidity—usually seen 8–12 hours after onset of signs

Physical Examination Findings
• Hyperthermia
• Rapid respiratory rate
• Dilated pupils, sluggish pupillary light responses
• Muscle tremors, muscular rigidity, convulsions

CAUSES & RISK FACTORS
• Calcium supplementation during gestation
• Low body weight–to–litter size ratio
• Poor prenatal nutrition
• First litter

 DIAGNOSIS

DIFFERENTIAL DIAGNOSIS
• Hypoglycemia—may be concurrent; muscular rigidity does not occur with hypoglycemia alone.
• Toxicosis—distinguished by signalment and history
• Epilepsy or other neurologic disorder—differentiated by signalment; calcium concentration diagnostic

CBC/BIOCHEMISTRY/URINALYSIS
• Serum calcium < 7 mg/dL
• Hypoglycemia—may be concurrent
• Hypomagnesemia has been reported in 44% of affected bitches; significance unknown

IMAGING
N/A

OTHER LABORATORY TESTS
N/A

DIAGNOSTIC PROCEDURES
ECG shows prolonged QT interval, bradycardia, tachycardia, or PVCs.

 TREATMENT

• Emergency inpatient
• Hyperthermia—cool with cool water soak and fans; use caution with cool water enemas.
• Puppies—remove from dam to hand-raise; if owner refuses, remove pups from dam for 24 hours to spare her, and provide supplementation for remainder of lactation.

 MEDICATIONS

DRUGS
• Calcium gluconate—10% solution 1 mL/kg IV given slowly to effect over 5 min; monitor heart rate or ECG during administration; may give additional drug intramuscularly or subcutaneously
• Correct hypoglycemia.
• Diazepam—5 mg IV; for unresponsive seizures

• Cerebral edema—treat, if indicated.
• Calcium lactate, carbonate, or gluconate—30–100 mg/kg/day PO until lactation ends
• Magnesium supplementation may be helpful in hypomagnesemic bitches.

CONTRAINDICATIONS/POSSIBLE INTERACTIONS
Corticosteroids—avoid; cause decreased intestinal absorption of and increased renal excretion of calcium

 FOLLOW-UP

PATIENT MONITORING
• Serum calcium concentration—monitor until it stabilizes in the normal range.
• Avoid calcium supplementation during gestation.
• Diet—maternal: ensure a calcium:phosphorus ratio of 1:1 or 1.2:1; avoid high-phytate foods (e.g., soybeans); puppies: supplement feeding for large litters

POSSIBLE COMPLICATIONS
• Cerebral edema
• Death
• Hand-raising of puppies

EXPECTED COURSE AND PROGNOSIS
• Probably will recur with subsequent litters
• Prognosis—good with immediate treatment; poor with delayed treatment

 MISCELLANEOUS

Suggested Reading
Aroch I, Srebro H, Shpigel NY. Serum electrolyte concentration in bitches with eclampsia. Vet Rec 1999;145:318–320.
Drobatz KJ, Casey KK. Eclampsia in dogs: 31 cases (1995–1998). J Am Vet Med Assoc 2000;217(2):216–219.
Kaufman J. Eclampsia in the bitch. In: Morrow DA, ed. Current therapy in theriogenology. 2nd ed. Philadelphia: Saunders, 1986:511–512.
Author Joni L. Freshman
Consulting Editor Sara K. Lyle

BASICS

OVERVIEW
• Congenital abnormality in which one or both ureters open into the urethra or vagina
• Dogs—the ureter may enter the bladder in the normal location, tunnel through the bladder wall, and bypass the trigone (intramural type).
• Less frequently, the ureter opens into the trigone and continues as a trough into the urethra.
• Cats—the ureter completely bypasses the bladder and enters the urethra (extramural type); this rarely occurs in dogs.

SIGNALMENT
• The following dog breeds are predisposed—Siberian husky, Newfoundland, bulldog, West Highland white terrier, fox terrier, and miniature and toy poodles
• Infrequently diagnosed in cats and male dogs

SIGNS
• Intermittent or continuous incontinence
• Normal voiding in some animals
• Vaginitis from urine scalding

CAUSES & RISK FACTORS
• Apparent breed predisposition
• Unknown mode of inheritance; bitches with ectopic ureters have had litters of puppies with no observed incontinence.

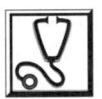

DIAGNOSIS

DIFFERENTIAL DIAGNOSIS
• Inappropriate urination—wrong place or time, but under voluntary control
• Urethral sphincter mechanism incompetence—use excretory urogram to exclude possibility of ectopic ureter; some dogs have ectopic ureters and urethral sphincter mechanism incompetence.
• Patent urachus—moist abdomen; radiographic contrast studies identify opening in ventral abdomen.
• Paradoxical incontinence—occurs secondary to urethral obstruction; pass catheter to identify calculi, stricture, or mass.

• Urinary tract infection—can cause pollakiuria that mimics incontinence
• Severe polyuria associated with renal failure caused by either congenital kidney disease or severe pyelonephritis—measure urine specific gravity to determine ability to concentrate urine; polyuria and polydipsia associated with low urine specific gravity

CBC/BIOCHEMISTRY/URINALYSIS
Urine specific gravity and serum creatinine or urea nitrogen concentration should be normal.

OTHER LABORATORY TESTS
Urine bacteriologic culture—collect by cystocentesis; often reveals concurrent urinary tract infection

IMAGING
• Excretory urography and a positive contrast cystogram or a pneumocystogram, followed by a vaginourethrogram (female) or urethrogram (male)—may be used to identify ectopic ureter(s); may also diagnose hydroureter; absent, small, or misshapen kidneys; hydronephrosis; and tortuous or obstructed ureters
• Ultrasonographic examination may reveal the ureter(s) alongside the urethra

DIAGNOSTIC PROCEDURES
• Urethrocystoscopy—use for direct visualization of the opening of the ectopic ureter(s) into the urethra or vagina
• Urethral pressure profilometry—can detect concurrent urethral sphincter mechanism incompetence

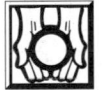

TREATMENT
• Surgically create a new ureteral opening into the bladder or excise a hydronephrotic or severely infected kidney.
• Warn owners that incontinence may continue if dog also has urethral sphincter mechanism incompetence; some puppies with urethral sphincter mechanism incompetence become continent after their first heat cycle.
• Incontinent dogs should not be spayed before their first heat.

MEDICATIONS

DRUG(S)
N/A

CONTRAINDICATIONS/POSSIBLE INTERACTIONS
N/A

FOLLOW-UP
• Incontinence may persist after surgery.
• Incontinent dogs need repeat evaluation including excretory urogram, pneumocystogram, and vaginourethrogram.
• An intrapelvic bladder neck may contribute to urinary incontinence in dogs with urethral sphincter mechanism incompetence. Surgically advancing the bladder neck into an intraabdominal position using the colposuspension technique may correct the incontinence.
• If incontinence persists, try phenylpropanolamine (1.5 mg/kg PO q8h), an α-blocker, or imipramine (0.5–1 mg/kg PO q8h), a tricyclic antidepressor agent. Reproductive hormone therapy may increase the sensitivity of urethral α-adrenergic receptors to α-agonists.
• Diethylstilbestrol (1.0 mg q24h for 3–5 days, then no more than 1.0 mg/week) is administered orally to spayed bitches. In some dogs, a combination of estrogen therapy and phenylpropanolamine may be more effective.
• In incontinent male dogs, testosterone propionate (2.2 mg/kg IM q2–3 days) is administered initially to see if replacement therapy will be effective. For longer action, testosterone cypionate (2.2 mg/kg IM q30 days) is used. Reproductive hormone therapy is not advised in immature animals.

MISCELLANEOUS

Suggested Reading
Stone EA, Barsanti JA. Urologic surgery of the dog and cat. Philadelphia: Lea & Febiger, 1992:201–211.
Author Elizabeth Arnold Stone
Consulting Editors Larry G. Adams and Carl A. Osborne

ECTROPION

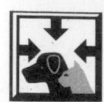

BASICS

OVERVIEW
• Eversion or rolling out of the eyelid margin, resulting in exposure of the palpebral conjunctiva
• Exposure and poor tear distribution—may predispose patient to sight-threatening corneal disease

SIGNALMENT
• Dogs, seldom cats
• Breeds with higher than average prevalence—sporting breeds (e.g., spaniels, hounds, and retrievers); giant breeds (e.g., St. Bernards and mastiffs); any breed with loose facial skin (especially bloodhounds)
• Developmental—genetic predisposition in listed breeds; may occur in dogs < 1 year old
• Acquired—noted in other breeds; occurs late in life secondary to age-related loss of facial musculature and developing skin laxity
• Intermittent—caused by fatigue; may be observed after strenuous exercise or when drowsy

SIGNS
• Eversion of the lower eyelid with lack of contact of the lower lid to the globe and exposure of the palpebral conjunctiva and third eyelid—usually obvious
• Facial staining caused by poor tear drainage—tears spill over onto the face instead of passing from the eye to the nose via the nasolacrimal ducts
• History of mucoid to mucopurulent discharge owing to conjunctival exposure
• Recurrent foreign body irritation
• History of bacterial conjunctivitis

CAUSES & RISK FACTORS
• Usually secondary to breed-associated alterations in facial conformation and eyelid support
• Marked weight loss or muscle mass loss about the head and orbits—may result in acquired disease
• Tragic facial expression in hypothyroid dogs
• Scarring of the eyelids secondary to injury or after overcorrection of entropion—may result in cicatricial disease

DIAGNOSIS

DIFFERENTIAL DIAGNOSIS
• Usually clinically obvious
• Look for any underlying disorder in non-predisposed breeds and patients with late-age onset.
• Loss of orbital or periorbital mass—may cause condition in patients with masticatory myositis
• Palpebral nerve paralysis—condition associated with lack of muscle tone of the orbicularis oculi muscles

CBC/BIOCHEMISTRY/URINALYSIS
N/A

OTHER LABORATORY TESTS
• Possible masticatory myositis—test for autoantibodies against type 2M muscle fibers.
• Palpebral nerve paralysis or tragic facial expression—consider testing for hypothyroidism.

IMAGING
N/A

DIAGNOSTIC PROCEDURES
• Palpebral nerve paralysis—full neurologic evaluation; potential for hypothyroidism
• Secondary conjunctivitis—consider bacterial culture or cytologic examination to help select an appropriate topical antibiotic
• Fluorescein or rose bengal staining of the cornea and conjunctiva—may document corneal ulcerations; may reveal severity of the exposure problem

 TREATMENT
• Supportive care and good ocular and facial hygiene—sufficient for most mild disease
• Surgical treatment—eyelid shortening or radical facelift; necessary for severely affected patients that have chronic ocular irritation
• Intermittent, fatigue-induced condition—do not treat surgically.

 MEDICATIONS

DRUG(S)
• Topical broad-spectrum ophthalmic antibiotics—bacterial conjunctivitis or corneal ulceration
• Lubricant eye drops and ointments—reduce conjunctival and corneal desiccation secondary to exposure
• Hypothyroid and masticatory myositis–induced conditions—may respond well to appropriate medical treatment of the underlying disease

CONTRAINDICATIONS/POSSIBLE INTERACTIONS
N/A

 FOLLOW-UP
• May become more severe as patient ages
• Nonsurgically treated patient—monitor for signs of infectious conjunctivitis, exposure keratopathy, corneal ulceration, and facial dermatitis.

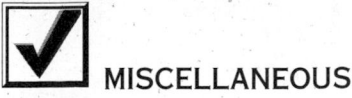 **MISCELLANEOUS**

ASSOCIATED CONDITIONS
• Hypothyroidism
• Masticatory myositis

AGE-RELATED FACTORS
Old animals more likely to have ectropion secondary to loss of facial muscle tone

SEE ALSO
• Hypothyroidism
• Myopathy, Masticatory Muscle Myositis

Suggested Reading
Slatter D. Eyelids. In: Fundamentals of veterinary ophthalmology. 2nd ed. Philadelphia: Saunders, 1990:147–203.
Author J. Phillip Pickett
Consulting Editor Paul E. Miller

EHRLICHIOSIS

BASICS

DEFINITION
Ehrlichia spp.—cause tick-borne rickettsial disease

Dogs
• Species divided into three groups
(1) *E. canis* (ehrlichiosis found intracytoplasmically in circulating leukocytes), *E. ewingii* (canine granulocytic ehrlichiosis), and *E. chaffeensis*
(2) *E. equi* and *E. phagocytophilia*
(3) *E. risticii* and *E. sennetsu* (not in the U.S.)
• *E. platys*—not fully characterized; causes infectious cyclic thrombocytopenia found in platelets
• Recent evidence suggests other as yet unidentified *Ehrlichia* species infect dogs.

Cats
• Extremely rare
• *E. risticii* and *E. equi*
• Serologic evidence suggests a species that cross-reacts with *E. canis* can cause illness

PATHOPHYSIOLOGY
E. canis
• *Rhipicephalus sanguineus*—brown dog tick; transmits disease to dogs in saliva; 1–3-week incubation period; 3 stages of disease
• *Dermacentor variabilis* also capable of transmitting *E. canis.*
• Acute—spreads from bite site to the spleen, liver, and lymph nodes (causes organomegaly); then subclinical with mild thrombocytopenia; mainly endothelial cells affected; vasculitis; antiplatelet antibodies may exacerbate thrombocytopenia; variable leukopenia; mild anemia; severity depends on organism
• Subclinical—organism persists; antibody response increases (hyperglobulinemia); thrombocytopenia persists.
• Chronic—impaired bone marrow production (platelets, erythroid suppression); marrow hypercellular with plasma cells

SYSTEMS AFFECTED
• Multisystemic
• Bleeding tendencies—thrombocytopenia and vasculitis
• Lymphadenopathy
• Splenomegaly
• CNS, eyes (anterior uveitis), and lungs—rarely affected by vasculitis

INCIDENCE/PREVALENCE
• Occurs throughout the year; insidious
• Average duration from onset to presentation—usually >2 months
• Prevalence varies, depending on geographic locality.

GEOGRAPHIC DISTRIBUTION
• Worldwide
• North America—mainly Gulf Coast and eastern seaboard; also the Midwest and California

SIGNALMENT
Species
• Dogs—can be infected with a number of species; *E. canis, E. platys, E. ewingii,* and *E. chaffeensis* produce main disease entities.
• Cats—*E. risticii;* also serologic evidence suggests a species similar to *E. canis*

Breed Predilection
Chronic (*E. canis*)—seems more severe in Doberman pinschers and German shepherds

Mean Age and Range
• Average age—5.22 years
• Range—2 months to 14 years

Predominant Sex
None

SIGNS
General Comments
Duration of clinical signs from initial acute illness to presentation—usually > 2 months

Historical Findings
• Lethargy
• Depression
• Anorexia and weight loss
• Fever
• Spontaneous bleeding—sneezing, epistaxis
• Respiratory distress
• Ataxia
• Head tilt
• Ocular pain (uveitis)

Physical Examination Findings
Acute
• Bleeding diathesis (petechiation of mucous membranes as a result of thrombocytopenia) associated with fever (with depression, anorexia, weight loss) and generalized lymphadenopathy should raise suspicions.
• Ticks—found in 40% of cases
• Respiratory—dyspnea (even cyanosis); increased bronchovesicular sound
• Diffuse CNS disease (meningitis)
• Ataxia with upper motor neuron dysfunction
• Vestibular dysfunction
• Generalized or local hyperesthesia
• Most dogs recover without treatment and enter a subclinical state.
Chronic
• In nonendemic areas
• Spontaneous bleeding
• Anemia
• Generalized lymphadenopathy
• Scrotal and limb edema
• Splenomegaly
• Hepatomegaly
• Uveitis
• Hyphema
• Retinal hemorrhages and detachment with blindness
• Corneal edema
• Arthritis (rare)
• Seizures (rare)

RISK FACTORS
Concurrent infection with *Babesia, Haemobartonella, E. platys,* and *Hepatozoon canis*—worsens clinical syndrome

DIAGNOSIS

DIFFERENTIAL DIAGNOSIS
• Rocky Mountain spotted fever (*Rickettsia rickettsii*)—usually seasonal between March and October; serologic testing for diagnosis; responds to same treatment as ehrlichiosis
• Immune-mediated thrombocytopenia—not usually associated with fever or lymphadenopathy; serologic testing best distinguishes; may treat for both until results are known
• Systemic lupus erythematosus—ANA test usually negative with ehrlichiosis; serologic testing for diagnosis
• Multiple myeloma—serologic testing to differentiate and determine cause of hyperglobulinemia
• Chronic lymphocytic leukemia—differentiate by lymphocytosis and cytology of bone marrow
• Brucellosis—serologic testing for diagnosis and to determine cause of scrotal edema

CBC/BIOCHEMISTRY/URINALYSIS
Acute
• Thrombocytopenia—before onset of clinical signs
• Anemia
• Leukopenia—from lymphopenia and eosinopenia
• Leukocytosis and monocytosis—as disease becomes more chronic
• Morulae—intracytoplasmic inclusions in leukocytes rare
• Nonspecific changes—mild increases in ALT, ALP, BUN, creatinine, and total bilirubin (rare)
• Hyperglobulinemia—progressively increases 1–3 weeks postinfection
• Hypoalbuminemia—usually from renal loss
• Proteinuria—with or without azotemia; about half of patients

Chronic
• Pancytopenia—typical; monocytosis and lymphocytosis may be present.
• Hyperglobulinemia—magnitude of globulin increase correlates with duration of infection; usually polyclonal gammopathy, but monoclonal (IgG) gammopathies occur.
• Hypoalbuminemia
• High BUN and creatinine—from primary renal disease, owing to glomerulonephritis and renal interstitial plasmacytosis

OTHER LABORATORY TESTS
Serologic Testing
• Most clinically useful and reliable method
• IFA highly sensitive; poor specificity with cross-reactivity between *E. canis* and *E. equi,* but not between *E. canis* and *E. platys*

- More specific tests being developed
- Titers—reliable 3 weeks after infection; > 1:10 diagnostic
- Coombs-positive anemia—may be seen; may confuse the diagnosis
- PCR—proving to be more sensitive than IFA; not commercially available
- Test for other accompanying pathogens—*Babesiosis, Hemobartonellosis, E. platys,* and *Hepatozoon canis*

DIAGNOSTIC PROCEDURES

Bone Marrow Aspirate
- Acute—hypercellularity of megakaryocytic and myeloid series
- Chronic—often erythroid hypoplasia with increased M:E ratios and plasmacytosis
- Increased numbers of mast cells are occasionally seen on marrow smears.

PATHOLOGIC FINDINGS
- Acute—petechial hemorrhages on serosal and mucosal surfaces of most organs; generalized lymphadenopathy (brownish discoloration), splenomegaly, hepatomegaly, and red bone marrow (hypercellularity)
- Chronic—pale marrow (hypoplastic); subcutaneous edema; histologically, perivascular plasma cell infiltrate in numerous organs most characteristic; multifocal nonsuppurative meningoencephalitis with lymphoplasmacytic cell infiltrate into the meninges common

TREATMENT

APPROPRIATE HEALTH CARE
- Inpatient—initial medical stabilization for anemia and/or hemorrhagic tendency resulting from thrombocytopenia
- Outpatient—stable patients; monitor blood and response to medication frequently.

NURSING CARE
- Balanced electrolyte solution is indicated for dehydration.
- Blood transfusion is indicated for anemia.
- Platelet-rich plasma or a blood transfusion is indicated for hemorrhage resulting from thrombocytopenia.

ACTIVITY
Restricted

CLIENT EDUCATION
- Acute—prognosis excellent with appropriate therapy
- Chronic—response may take 1 month; prognosis poor if the bone marrow is severely hypoplastic
- Progression from acute to chronic can be easily prevented by early, effective treatment; but many dogs remain seropositive and may relapse (even years later).
- German shepherds and Doberman pinschers—more chronic and severe form of disease

SURGICAL CONSIDERATIONS
If surgery is needed for other reasons, blood transfusion may be needed to correct anemia and/or thrombocytopenia.

MEDICATIONS

DRUG(S) OF CHOICE
- Doxycycline—5 mg/kg PO q12h or 10 mg/kg PO q24h for 14 to 28 days; give intravenously for 5 days if the dog is vomiting.
- Imidocarb dipropionate—5 mg/kg IM for 2 doses 14 days apart; effective against both *E. canis* and babesiosis; reasonable alternative to doxycycline
- Glucocorticoids—prednisolone or prednisone; 1–2 mg/kg PO q12h for 5 days; may be indicated when thrombocytopenia is life-threatening (thought to be a result of immune-mediated mechanisms); because immune-mediated thrombocytopenia is a principal differential diagnosis, may be indicated until results of serologic tests are available
- Androgenic steroids—to stimulate bone marrow production in chronically affected dogs with hypoplastic marrows; oxymetholone (2 mg/kg q24h PO until response) or nandrolone decanoate (1.5 mg/kg IM weekly)

CONTRAINDICATIONS
Tetracycline (and derivatives)—do not use in dogs < 6 months old (permanent yellowing of teeth occurs); do not use with renal insufficiency (try doxycycline because it can be excreted via the gastrointestinal tract).
- Enrofloxacin not effective against *E. canis.*

PRECAUTIONS
Glucocorticoids—prolonged use at immunosuppressive levels may interfere with the clearance and elimination of *E. canis* after use of tetracycline

ALTERNATIVE DRUGS
- Oxytetracycline and tetracycline—22 mg/kg PO q8h for 21 days; effective and less expensive
- Chloramphenicol—20 mg/kg PO q8h for 14 days; for puppies < 6 months of age; avoids yellow discoloration of erupting teeth caused by tetracyclines; warn client of public health risks, because it directly interferes with heme and bone marrow synthesis; avoid in dogs with thrombocytopenia, pancytopenia, or anemia.

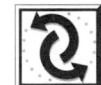

FOLLOW-UP

PATIENT MONITORING
- Platelet count—every 3 days after initiating antirickettsial agent until normal; improvement is rapid in acute cases.

- Serologic testing—repeat in 9 months; most dogs will become seronegative; positive titer suggests reinfection (prior infection does not imply protective immunity) or ineffective treatment (reinstitute treatment regimen)

PREVENTION/AVOIDANCE
- Control tick infestation—dips or sprays containing dichlorvos, chlorfenvinphos, dioxathion, propoxur, or carbaryl; flea and tick collars may reduce reinfestation but reliability unproven; avoid tick-infested areas.
- Removing ticks by hand—use gloves (see Zoonotic Potential); ensure mouth parts are removed to avoid a foreign body reaction

EXPECTED COURSE AND PROGNOSIS
- Acute—excellent prognosis with appropriate treatment
- Chronic—may take 4 weeks for a clinical response; prognosis poor with hypoplastic marrow

MISCELLANEOUS

ASSOCIATED CONDITIONS
- *Babesia* • *Haemobartonella* • *E. platys*

ZOONOTIC POTENTIAL
- Serologic evidence indicates that *E. canis* (or possibly a related species) occurs in people; probably not directly infected from dogs; tick exposure thought to be necessary; *R. sanguineus* probably not the vector in humans
- Most cases in the southern and south-central U.S. • Major clinical signs in humans—fever, headache, myalgia, ocular pain, and gastrointestinal upset • Treatment with tetracyclines results in rapid recovery.

SYNONYMS
- Tropical canine pancytopenia • Canine rickettsiosis • Canine hemorrhagic fever
- Lahore canine fever • Canine typhus
- Tracker dog disease • Nairobi bleeding disease

ABBREVIATIONS
- ALP = alkaline phosphatase • ALT = alanine transferase • ANA = antinuclear antibody • IFA = indirect fluorescent antibody • M:E = myeloid:erythroid ratio • PCR = polymerase chain reaction

Suggested Reading

Frank JR, Breitschwerdt EB. A retrospective study of ehrlichiosis in 62 dogs from North Carolina and Virginia. J Vet Intern Med 1999;13:194–201.

Greig B. Granulocytic ehrlichiosis. In: Bonagura JD, Kirk RW, eds. Current veterinary therapy XIII. Philadelphia: Saunders, 2000:298–300.

Author Stephen C. Barr
Consulting Editor Stephen C. Barr

ELBOW DYSPLASIA

 BASICS

DEFINITION
A series of four developmental abnormalities that lead to malformation and degeneration of the elbow joint

PATHOPHYSIOLOGY
• Four abnormalities—UAP, OCD, FMCP, and incongruity; may occur alone or in combination; may be seen in one or both elbows; bilateral disease common (50% of cases)
• UAP—characterized by failure of the anconeal process (which contains a separate ossification center) to unite with the proximal ulnar metaphysis (olecranon) by 5 months of age; may be the result of abnormal mechanical stress on the anconeal process
• OCD—affects the medial aspect of the humeral condyle; retention of articular cartilage due to a disturbance in endochondral ossification and mechanical stress; leads to formation of a cartilage flap lesion; may be the result of abnormal mechanical stress on the medial aspect
• FMCP—chondral or osteochondral fragmentation or fissure of the medial coronoid process of the ulna; not considered a traumatic injury; a manifestation of osteochondrosis of the coronoid process; differs from the related pathology of the anconeal process because the coronoid does not have a separate ossification center; may be the result of abnormal mechanical stress on the medial coronoid process
• Incongruity—manifestation of malalignment and malformation of the elbow joint; asynchronous proximal growth between the radius and ulna may lead to abnormal load and to wear and erosion of cartilage in the humeroulnar compartment; may be the result of malformation of the trochlear notch of the ulna; a slightly elliptical trochlear notch with a decreased arc of curvature is too small to articulate with the humeral trochlea, which results in major points of contact in areas of the anconeal process, coronoid process, and medial humeral condyle and little or no contact in other areas of the trochlea

SYSTEMS AFFECTED
Musculoskeletal

GENETICS
• Inherited disease
• High heritability—heritability index ranges between 0.25 and 0.45.

INCIDENCE/PREVALENCE
• Most common cause for elbow pain and lameness
• One of the most common causes for forelimb lameness in large-breed dogs

GEOGRAPHIC DISTRIBUTION
N/A

SIGNALMENT

Species
Dogs

Breed Predilections
Large and giant breeds—Labrador retrievers; Rottweilers; golden retrievers; German shepherds; Bernese mountain dogs; chow chows; bearded collies; Newfoundlands

Mean Age and Range
• Age at onset of clinical signs—typically 4–10 months
• Age at diagnosis—generally 4–18 months
• Onset of symptoms related to DJD—any age

Predominant Sex
• FMCP—males predisposed
• UAP, OCD, incongruity—none established

SIGNS

General Comments
• Lameness—if no distinct abnormalities noted on physical examination or radiographs, repeat examination 4–8 weeks later.
• Not all patients are symptomatic when young.
• Acute episode of elbow lameness due to advanced DJD changes in a mature patient—common

Historical Findings
Intermittent or persistent forelimb lameness—exacerbated by exercise; progressed from a stiffness seen only after rest

Physical Examination Findings
• Pain—elicited on elbow hyperflexion or extension; elicited when holding the elbow and carpus at 90° while pronating and supinating the carpus
• Affected limb—tendency to be held in abduction and supination
• Joint effusion and capsular distension—especially noted between the lateral epicondyle and olecranon
• Crepitus—may be palpated with advanced DJD
• Diminished range of motion

CAUSES
• Genetic
• Developmental
• Nutritional

RISK FACTORS
• Rapid growth and weight gain
• High-calorie diet

 DIAGNOSIS

DIFFERENTIAL DIAGNOSIS
• Trauma
• Septic arthritis
• Panosteitis
• Avulsion or calcification of the flexor muscles
• Synovial cell sarcoma

CBC/BIOCHEMISTRY/URINALYSIS
N/A

OTHER LABORATORY TESTS
N/A

IMAGING

Radiography
• May need four views for diagnosis—mediolateral; mediolateral hyperflexed; 25° craniocaudal-lateromedial oblique; craniocaudal
• Image both elbows—high incidence of bilateral disease
• UAP—best diagnosed from the mediolateral hyperflexed view; may easily see lack of bony union
• OCD—best diagnosed from the craniocaudal and craniocaudal-lateromedial oblique views; reveals a radiolucent defect or flattening of the medial aspect of the humeral condyle
• FMCP—seldom visualized; diagnosis is presumptive based on DJD and the absence of UAP or OCD lesions; commonly see osteophyte formation on the proximal rim of the anconeal process, medial coronoid process, and cranial margin of the radial head and epicondyles (medial and lateral); also commonly see sclerosis of the ulna caudal to the coronoid process and trochlear notch and stairstep between the joint surface of the radius and lateral coronoid; may also see these changes with UAP, OCD, and incongruity

Other
CT, MRI, and linear tomography—accurately diagnose FMCP

DIAGNOSTIC PROCEDURES
• Joint tap and analysis of synovial fluid—confirm involvement of joint
• Synovial fluid—should be straw colored with normal to decreased viscosity; cytology reveals < 10,000 nucleated cells/μL (> 90% are mononuclear cells); normal results do not necessarily rule out the diagnosis.

• Arthroscopy—may use to diagnose UAP, FMCP, and OCD

PATHOLOGIC FINDINGS
• UAP—fibrous union between anconeal process and proximal ulnar metaphysis; fibrous tissue invasion and degeneration of the anconeal process; DJD
• OCD—chondral flap on medial humeral condyle; sclerosis of underlying subchondral bone with fibrous tissue invasion; erosive lesion on apposing coronoid cartilage; DJD
• FMCP—chondral or osteochondral fragmentation of the cranial tip or lateral margin of the medial coronoid; erosive lesion on cartilage of the apposing medial aspect of the humeral condyle; DJD
• Incongruity—erosive lesions involving part or all of medial coronoid process and the apposing articular cartilage of the medial aspect of the humeral condyle; DJD; linear striations in the articular cartilage

TREATMENT

APPROPRIATE HEALTH CARE
Surgery—controversial but recommended for all patients

NURSING CARE
• Cold packing the elbow joint—perform immediately postsurgery to help decrease swelling and control pain; perform at least 15–20 min q8h for 3–5 days.
• Range-of-motion exercises—beneficial until the patient can bear weight on the limb(s)

ACTIVITY
Restricted for all patients postoperatively

DIET
• Weight control—important for decreasing the load and stress on the affected joint(s)
• Restricted weight gain and growth in young dogs—may decrease incidence and severity

CLIENT EDUCATION
• Discuss the heritability of the disease.
• Discuss the potential for DJD progression.
• Discuss the influence of excessive intake of nutrients that promote rapid growth.

SURGICAL CONSIDERATIONS
• Severity of DJD and age of patient—negatively influence outcome
• UAP—four options: removal, lag screw fixation, dynamic proximal ulnar osteotomy, and lag screw fixation plus dynamic proximal osteotomy; base decision on degree of DJD, patient's age, and surgical expertise.

• OCD and FMCP—medial approach to elbow (diagnostic differentiation not necessary); removal of loose fragment(s)
• Incongruity—controversial; four options: no surgery, coronoidectomy, dynamic proximal ulnar osteotomy, intra-articular osteotomy; base decision on type of incongruity, degree of DJD, patient's age, and surgical expertise.
• Arthroscopic diagnosis and treatment—excellent option for FMCP, OCD, and incongruity; benefits: superior diagnostic capabilities, minimal invasiveness, decreased postoperative discomfort, and decreased postoperative morbidity

MEDICATIONS

DRUG(S) OF CHOICE
• None that promotes healing of osteochondral or chondral fragments
• NSAIDs—minimize pain, decrease inflammation, symptomatically treat associated DJD; may try buffered or enteric-coated aspirin (10–25 mg/kg PO q8–12h), caroprofen (2.2 mg/kg PO q12h), etodolac (10–15 mg/kg PO q24h), phenylbutazone (3–7 mg/kg PO q8h, dose < 800 mg/day), meclofenamic acid (0.5 mg/kg PO q12h), and piroxicam (0.3 mg/kg PO q24h for 3 days then q48h), deracoxib (3–4 mg/kg PO q24h for 7 days for postoperative pain) (1–2 mg/kg PO q24h for long-term treatment over 7 days)

CONTRAINDICATIONS
Avoid corticosteroids—potential side effects; articular cartilage damage associated with long-term use

PRECAUTIONS
NSAIDs—gastrointestinal irritation may preclude use in some patients.

POSSIBLE INTERACTIONS
N/A

ALTERNATIVE DRUG(S)
Chondroprotective drugs (e.g., polysulfated glycosaminoglycans, glucosamine, and chondroitin sulfate)—may help limit cartilage damage and degeneration; may help alleviate pain and inflammation

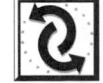

FOLLOW-UP

PATIENT MONITORING
• Postsurgery—limit activity for a minimum of 4 weeks; encourage early, active movement of the affected joint(s).

• Yearly examinations—recommended to evaluate progression of DJD

PREVENTION/AVOIDANCE
• Discourage breeding of affected animals.
• Do not repeat dam–sire breedings that result in affected offspring.

POSSIBLE COMPLICATIONS
N/A

EXPECTED COURSE AND PROGNOSIS
• Progression of DJD—expected
• Prognosis—fair to good for all forms

MISCELLANEOUS

ASSOCIATED CONDITIONS
N/A

AGE-RELATED FACTORS
Middle-aged to old dogs with advanced DJD are not candidates for surgical intervention.

ZOONOTIC POTENTIAL
N/A

PREGNANCY
N/A

SYNONYMS
Elbow osteochondrosis

SEE ALSO
Osteochondrosis

ABBREVIATIONS
• CT = computed tomography
• DJD = degenerative joint disease
• FMCP = fragmented medial coronoid process
• MRI = magnetic resonance imaging
• NSAIDs = nonsteroidal antiinflammatory drugs
• OCD = osteochondritis dissecans
• UAP = un-united anconeal process

Suggested Reading
Olsson SE. Pathophysiology, morphology, and clinical signs of osteochondrosis in the dog. In: Bojrab MJ, ed. Disease mechanisms in small animal surgery. Philadelphia: Lea & Febiger, 1993:777–779.
Schwarz PD. Elbow dysplasia. In: Bonagura JD, Kersey R, eds. Current veterinary therapy XIII: Small animal practice. Philadelphia: Saunders, 2000:1004–1014.
Wind AP. Elbow incongruity and developmental elbow diseases in the dog: parts I and II. J Am Anim Hosp Assoc 1986; 22:711–724.
Author Peter D. Schwarz
Consulting Editor Peter K. Shires

ELECTRIC CORD BITE INJURY

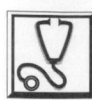

BASICS

OVERVIEW
• Electric cord bite injury is an uncommon event that occurs when an animal bites an electric cord. • Other causes of electrocution are uncommon in dogs and cats but can occur. • Household electrical currents are alternating (60 Hz) and dangerous. • Injury can be due to thermal injury or due to disruption of normal electrophysiologic activity of excitable tissue. • Pulmonary edema can be a sequela to electrocution; the pathophysiology is thought to be neurogenic and centrally mediated, leading to pulmonary hypertension. • Cataract formation is reported following electrocution.

SIGNALMENT
• Dogs and, less commonly, cats. • Most commonly seen in dogs. • Most commonly seen in young animals. In published reports, ages ranged from 5 months to 1.5 years. • No breed or sex predilection

SIGNS
• Burns of gingiva, tongue, and palate • Singed hair or whiskers • The most common clinical signs are related to acute dyspnea. • Coughing • Tachypnea • Orthopnea • Increased respiratory effort • Cyanosis • Crackles during pulmonary auscultation • Tachycardia • Muscle tremors • Tonic-clonic activity • Collapse

CAUSES & RISK FACTORS
• Chewing electric cord • Young age

DIAGNOSIS

DIFFERENTIAL DIAGNOSIS
• Left-sided congestive heart failure—may be due to congenital or acquired heart disease; presence of cardiac murmur or dysrhythmia may help differentiate, but dysrhythmias may also be seen with electric cord injury • Vitamin K antagonist—rodenticide intoxication history, coagulation tests (e.g., PT, PTT, PIVKA) • Thoracic trauma—history, thoracic radiographs • Pleural space disease—muffled lung sounds during auscultation, thoracic radiographs • Thermal or chemical injuries—history, physical examination, thoracic radiographs • Exposure to fire and smoke inhalation—history, physical examination • Atypical pneumonia—history, physical examination, thoracic radiographs

CBC/BIOCHEMISTRY/URINALYSIS
N/A

OTHER LABORATORY TESTS
N/A

IMAGING
• Thoracic radiographs may help distinguish between cardiogenic and non-cardiogenic causes of pulmonary edema. With non-cardiogenic pulmonary edema there is no pulmonary venous congestion and heart size is normal, unless there is concurrent cardiac disease. • The radiographic pattern is usually a generalized, mixed alveolar bronchial pattern. The edema is often most notable in the diaphragmatic lung lobes. • Echocardiography may help identify underlying cardiac disease.

DIAGNOSTIC PROCEDURES
ECG may help distinguish cardiogenic disease from non-cardiogenic disease, however, dysrhythmias may also be seen with electrocution.

PATHOLOGIC FINDINGS
• Pink, frothy fluid in airways
• Fluid-filled, congested lungs
• Subendocardial and subepicardial petechiae
• Circumscribed pale gray or tan oral lesions

TREATMENT
• If patient is close to live wire, turn off electricity and or remove patient to safe area. • Establish patent airway if patient is unconscious. • Oxygen supplementation • Mechanical ventilation may be required. • Establish venous access.

MEDICATIONS

DRUG(S)
• If in shock, treat with intravenous crystalloids (90 ml/kg/h in dog, 45–60 ml/kg/h in cat) or colloids (20 ml/kg in dog, 5–10 ml/kg in cat) • If pulmonary edema is present, administer furosemide (2–4 mg/kg IV). • Corticosteroids have been employed but are controversial and of unknown value. • Inotropic support if required • Antiarrhythmic therapy if required • Treat oral and cutaneous burns symptomatically.

CONTRAINDICATIONS/POSSIBLE INTERACTIONS
N/A

FOLLOW-UP

PATIENT MONITORING
• Patient should be monitored until stable. • Physical examination • Oral lesion should be monitored (may prevent the animal from eating). • Electrocardiography

• Central venous pressure • Blood pressure • Arterial blood gases • Thoracic radiographs

PREVENTION/AVOIDANCE
• Damaged electric cords should be discarded. • Avoid animal exposure to electric cords. • Follow child safety rules for a safe home.

POSSIBLE COMPLICATIONS
• Infected burn wounds can occur but are uncommon. • Oral-nasal fistula due to severe burns

EXPECTED COURSE AND PROGNOSIS
• The prognosis is based on the response to therapy. • Pulmonary edema can develop as soon as 1 hour and as late as 36 hours after incident. • Pulmonary edema associated with electrocution is associated with high mortality (38.5%). • If patient survives first 24 hours the prognosis improves. • Resolution of pulmonary edema may take 3–5 days. • Most oral lesions resolve. • Inappetence related to oral lesions resolves.

MISCELLANEOUS

ASSOCIATED CONDITIONS
Cataracts have been reported in one dog 18 months after electrocution.

SYNONYMS
Electrocution

ABBREVIATIONS
PT = prothrombin time
PTT = partial thromboplastin time
PIVKA = proteins invoked by vitamin K antagonism

Suggested Reading
Atkins CE. Cardiac manifestations of systemic and metabolic disease. In: Fox PR, Sisson D, Moise NS. Textbook of canine and feline cardiology. Philadelphia: Saunders, 1999:757–780.
Brightman AH, Brogdon JD, Helper LC, Everds N. Electrical cataracts in the canine: a case report. J Am An Hosp Assoc 1984:20:895–898.
Kolata RJ, Burrows CF. The clinical features of injury by chewing electrical cords in dogs and cats. J Am An Hosp Assoc 1981:17:219–222.
Author Steven L. Marks
Consulting Editors Larry P. Tilley and Francis W.K. Smith, Jr.

BASICS

OVERVIEW
• Apparent defect in enamel surfaces, often pitted and discolored; focal or generalized
• Defects due to disruption of normal enamel formation
• Influences during enamel formation (distemper, fever, etc.) over an extended time may cause generalized changes; during a short time (focal, local; e.g., trauma, even from deciduous tooth extraction) they cause specific patterns or bands.
• Most cases are primarily esthetic; some patients can have extensive structural damage, even root involvement.
• A more correct description would be enamel hypocalcification, since the amount of enamel is adequate (not hypoplastic), but it has defects in calcification that lead to enamel defect.
• Teeth may be more sensitive with exposed dentin, and occasionally fractures of severely compromised teeth occur; usually they remain fully functional.

SIGNALMENT
• Dogs and cats (less common)
• Often apparent at time of tooth eruption (after 6 months of age) or shortly thereafter (with signs of wear)

SIGNS
Historical Findings
Discolored teeth

Physical Examination Findings
• Irregular, pitted enamel surface with discoloration of diseased enamel and potential exposure of underlying dentin (light brown)
• Early or rapid accumulation of plaque and calculus on roughened tooth surface; possible gingivitis and/or accelerated periodontal disease

CAUSES & RISK FACTORS
• Insult during enamel formation
• Canine distemper virus, fever, trauma (e.g., accidents, excessive force during deciduous tooth extraction)

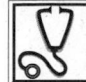

DIAGNOSIS

DIFFERENTIAL DIAGNOSIS
• Enamel staining—discolored but smooth surface (tetracycline)
• Carious lesions—cavities with decay
• Amelogenesis imperfecta—genetic enamel disorder
• Erosive lesions—similar to those found in cats

CBC/BIOCHEMISTRY/URINALYSIS
Usually normal

OTHER LABORATORY TESTS
N/A

IMAGING
• Intraoral radiographs are necessary to determine viability of roots.
• Cases reported of abnormal root formation, no root formation, or separated crown and root

DIAGNOSTIC PROCEDURES
N/A

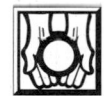

TREATMENT
• Treatment depends upon extent of lesions and equipment and materials available.
• Goal is to provide the smoothest surface possible.

Optimal Treatment
• Ideal treatment is to gently remove diseased enamel (enamel scrub) with white stone burs or finishing disks on high-speed handpiece (adequate water coolant); rotary burs can cause excessive damage and heat—handle with care!
• Take care not to damage the tooth—excess enamel/dentin removal; hyperthermic damage to pulp
• Focal defects may be amenable to composite or glass ionomer restoration, but long-term success is poor; metallic crown restoration is preferred; many restorative materials (bonding agents, composites) require use of light-curing units and appropriate skill levels.
• Bonding agent recommended to seal exposed dentinal tubules and protect surface

Alternative Treatment
• Without a high-speed handpiece and appropriate attachments, treatment can be more challenging.
• The soft, diseased enamel can sometimes be removed with ultrasonic scalers, but take care to avoid damage and hyperthermia.
• A strong fluoride treatment (in-hospital, on a dry tooth surface; varnish or strong sodium fluoride paste) can be used to decrease sensitivity and enhance enamel strength.

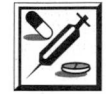

MEDICATIONS

DRUG(S)
N/A

CONTRAINDICATION/POSSIBLE INTERACTIONS
N/A

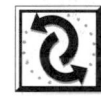

FOLLOW-UP

PATIENT MONITORING
Inform the owner that further degeneration of remaining enamel may occur, necessitating additional therapy in the future.

PREVENTION/AVOIDANCE
• Recommend regular professional dental cleaning and a routine home-care program (brushing); may include weekly application of stannous fluoride at home (minimize ingestion because of toxicity).
• Avoid excessive chewing on hard objects.

MISCELLANEOUS

Suggested Reading
Wiggs BW, Lobprise HB. Veterinary dentistry: principles and practice. Philadelphia: Lippincott-Raven, 1997.
Author Heidi B. Lobprise
Consulting Editor Heidi B. Lobprise

ENCEPHALITIS

 BASICS

DEFINITION
Inflammation of the brain that may be accompanied by spinal cord and/or meningeal involvement

Pathophysiology
• Inflammation—caused by an infectious agent or by the patient's own immune system • Immune-mediated—cause of immune system derangement generally unknown

SYSTEMS AFFECTED
• Nervous • Multisystemic signs—may be noted in patients with infectious diseases

GENETICS
N/A

INCIDENCE/PREVALENCE
Unknown

GEOGRAPHIC DISTRIBUTION
Varies with the cause or agent implicated

SIGNALMENT

Species
Dogs and cats

Breed Predilections
• GME—mostly small-breed dogs, especially terriers and miniature poodles; large-breed dogs also affected • Pug encephalitis—pugs • PME—German short-haired pointers • Maltese encephalitis—Maltese • YNE—Yorkshire terriers

Mean Age and Range
N/A

Predominant Sex
N/A

SIGNS

Historical Findings
• Usually a peracute to acute onset of clinical signs that rapidly progresses • GME, fungal and protozoal encephalitis—sometimes signs are more chronically progressive

Physical Examination Findings
• Fever, lung disease, and/or gastrointestinal disturbances—usually precede encephalitis • With mycotic, rickettsial, viral, and protothecal organisms—fundic lesions frequently seen

Neurologic Examination Findings
• Determined by the portion of the brain most affected • Rostral fossa—seizures; circling; pacing; personality change; decreasing level of responsiveness • Caudal fossa—abnormalities related to the brainstem (e.g., somnolence, head tilt, facial paresis/ paralysis, incoordination) • Progression (e.g., anisocoria, pinpoint pupils, decreasing level of consciousness, and poor physiologic nystagmus)—suggests tentorial herniation

CAUSES

Dogs
• Idiopathic, immune-mediated—GME; pug encephalitis; Maltese encephalitis; YNE; EME • Viral—canine distemper virus; rabies; herpes; parvovirus; adenovirus; pseudorabies; Eastern and Venezuelan equine encephalomyelitis virus • Postvaccinal encephalo-myelitis—canine distemper virus; rabies; canine coronavirus-parvovirus • Rickettsial—Rocky Mountain spotted fever; ehrlichiosis • Mycotic—cryptococcosis; blastomycosis; histoplasmosis; coccidioidomycosis; aspergillosis; phaeohyphomycosis • Bacterial—anaerobic and aerobic • Protozoal—toxoplasmosis; neosporosis; encephalitozoonosis • Spirochetes—borreliosis • Parasite migration—*Dirofilaria immitis; Toxocara canis; Ancylostoma caninum; Cuterebra;* cysticercosis • Migrating foreign body—plant awn; others • Prototheocosis • PME

Cats
• Idiopathic, immune-mediated—GME; EME • Idiopathic polioencephalomyelitis • Viral—FIP; rabies; FIV; pseudorabies; panleukopenia; rhinotracheitis • Mycotic— cryptococcosis; blastomycosis; phaeohypho- mycoses • Bacterial—anaerobic and aerobic • Protozoal—toxoplasmosis • Parasite migration—*Dirofilaria immitis; Cuterebra*

RISK FACTORS
• Immunosuppressive drugs and FIV or FeLV infection—infectious encephalitides • Tick-infected areas—rickettsial and *Borrelia* infections • Travel history—mycotic infections

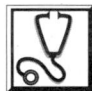 DIAGNOSIS

DIFFERENTIAL DIAGNOSIS
• Fungal encephalitides—frequently accompanied by systemic signs • Protozoal diseases—systemic; may have a chronic history • Rickettsial diseases—hemogram abnormalities common • FIP—patients usually < 3 years of age; protracted course; characteristic CSF analysis • Canine distemper virus—commonly seen as acute encephalitis with systemic signs in patients < 1 year old; can be difficult to confirm antemortem • Primary CNS neoplasia—signs may be similar to encephalitis • Degenerative disorders—usually slow, insidiously progressive onset • Metabolic or toxic encephalopathy— bilateral, symmetrical neurologic abnor-malities that relate to the cerebrum; confirm toxins by laboratory tests or serum assay

CBC/BIOCHEMISTRY/URINALYSIS
• Hemogram—frequently normal; leuko-cytosis may be seen in diseases that produce systemic signs; may be lymphopenia in the early stages of canine distemper virus and rickettsial infection; rickettsial encephalitis may be accompanied by thrombocytopenia and anemia • Serum chemistry—frequently normal; hyperproteinemia with polyclonal gammopathy often seen with FIP and chronic systemic infections; creatine kinase may be moderately high with *Neospora* infection (dogs)

OTHER LABORATORY TESTS
• Serology—available for fungal, protozoal, rickettsial, and viral diseases; helpful but must be interpreted with caution because a positive titer does not always indicate active disease (e.g., toxoplasma in cats) and a negative titer does not always rule out active disease (e.g., FIP) • Indirect fluorescent antibody—a single positive titer of 1:10 or greater confirms ehrlichiosis • ELISA—a fourfold rise between acute and convalescent IgG titers when the first titer is > 1:128 confirms Rocky Mountain spotted fever; an IgM titer of > 1:256 suggests infection within the previous 16 weeks by *Toxoplasma gondii* and may indicate exacerbation of chronic infection • Latex agglutination antigen—a single positive titer from serum or CSF confirms cryptococcus • Agar-gel immunodiffusion—diagnose blastomycosis with a high degree of accuracy • Local production of canine distemper virus–specific antibody (IgG and IgM)—in CSF after virus infects the CNS • Positive *Neospora caninum* titer—correlates well with active disease • Positive FIP titer—indicates only infection with a coronavirus; may not be pathogenic • Positive *Borrelia burgdorferi* titer—indicates exposure to the organism, not necessarily active disease

IMAGING
• Thoracic radiographs—may confirm lung abnormalities • Skull radiographs—may confirm sinusitis/rhinitis in some cats with cryptococcosis • CT or MRI of the brain— may detect multifocal or single mass lesions

DIAGNOSTIC PROCEDURES
• CSF analysis—perform on all animals with clinical signs that suggest encephalitis; results almost always abnormal; normal results do not rule out acute viral encephalitis that is limited to the parenchyma; with pleocytosis, culture for bacteria (aerobic and anaerobic). • CNS reaction—neutrophils indicate an acute active inflammatory process; small lymphocytes indicate an antigenic response; eosinophils indicate an allergic response or a reaction to foreign material (tumor, parasite).

PATHOLOGIC FINDINGS
The lesions are a function of the brain response to the infectious agent or other cause.

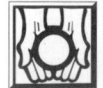 TREATMENT

APPROPRIATE HEALTH CARE
Inpatient—diagnosis and initial therapy

NURSING CARE
• Symptomatic treatment—control brain edema and seizure activity as necessary.
• Cerebral edema—give 20% mannitol (2.2 g/kg IV over 30–45 min); may repeat within 1–2 hr to achieve maximum response; limit parenteral fluids to prevent rebound cerebral edema; with mannitol, short-term (72 hr) corticosteroid treatment indicated for further control (dexamethasone sodium phosphate at 0.5 mg/kg IV q12h for 24 hr; then reduce to 0.25 mg/kg q12h for 48 hr) • Seizures—treat with antiepileptic drugs; control may be erratic until the encephalitis is treated; with boluses or constant-rate infusions, monitor closely for respiratory depression because the blood–brain barrier is altered.

ACTIVITY
As tolerated

DIET
With severe depression or vomiting—nothing by mouth until condition improves, to prevent aspiration

CLIENT EDUCATION
• Inform client that the condition is life-threatening if left untreated. • Inform client that relapse is possible with an idiopathic or immune-mediated encephalitis when therapy is discontinued.

SURGICAL CONSIDERATIONS
Brain biopsy—may be needed for specific diagnosis

 MEDICATIONS

DRUG(S) OF CHOICE
• Apply specific therapy once diagnosis is reached or highly suspected. • Idiopathic and immune-mediated—respond to immuno-suppressive dosage of prednisone • Rickettsial and borreliosis—doxycycline • Protozoal—clindamycin • Mycotic—requires treatment for 1–2 years; use itraconazole (5 mg/kg PO q12h with food) or fluconazole (6.25–12.5 mg/kg PO or IV q12h); corticosteroids often needed during the first 4–6 weeks to control cerebral edema • Viral and postvaccinal—none definitive; treat symptomatically
• Bacterial—broad-spectrum antibiotics that penetrate the blood–brain barrier; if agent is unknown, try a combination of enrofloxacin (5 mg/kg PO or IV q12h) and ticarcillin-clavulanate (50 mg/kg IV q8h) or amoxicillin-clavulanate (13.75 mg/kg PO q8h).

CONTRAINDICATIONS
• Bacterial and Rocky Mountain spotted fever—corticosteroids contraindicated
• Puppies < 6 months of age with a rickettsial disease—use chloramphenicol (doxycycline-induced tooth discoloration)
• Puppies < 8 months of age—enrofloxacin contraindicated (cartilage damage); use amoxicillin-clavulanate or ticarcillin-clavulanate alone. • CNS infections—do not use aminoglycosides and first-generation cephalosporins because CNS penetration is poor

PRECAUTIONS
• Administer mannitol intravenously 10 min before giving anesthesia for CSF collection, to decrease intracranial pressure. • Cortico-steroids—observe closely for worsening signs that suggest an infectious cause.

POSSIBLE INTERACTIONS
• Chloramphenicol and cimetidine—do not use concurrently with phenobarbital, to avoid toxic serum phenobarbital levels secondary to interference with liver metabolism.
• Corticosteroids alter the CSF analysis if used for 12 hr or more.

ALTERNATIVE DRUG
• Lomustine (CCNU)—60 mg/m² PO q 3–4 weeks may be effective in causing remission in dogs with immune-mediated encephalitis that are not prednisone-responsive. Adverse effects are bone marrow depression, GI effects, hepatotoxicity. Nadirs are in 1–3 weeks. CBC should be done at 1 and 3 weeks post therapy. Serum chemistry profile and serum bile acids should be done at 3 weeks and q 2 months. (Personal communication March, P, Ohio State University)

 FOLLOW-UP

PATIENT MONITORING
• Frequent neurologic evaluations in the first 48–72 hr to monitor progress • Relapse as medication is withdrawn—repeat CSF analysis • Measure serum titer of cryptococcus capsular antigen every 3 months until negative.

PREVENTION/AVOIDANCE
• A method of effective tick control should be used on animals that live in endemic areas.
• Avoid vaccination of dogs that have had GME.

POSSIBLE COMPLICATIONS
• Long-term corticosteroid therapy—signs of iatrogenic hyperadrenocorticism • CSF collection or natural course of the disease—tentorial herniation and death

EXPECTED COURSE AND PROGNOSIS
• Resolution of signs—generally gradual (2–8 weeks) • Prototothecal—almost always progresses to death • Immune-mediated—fair prognosis for complete remission with aggressive immunosuppression • Rickettsial, mycotic, bacterial, protozoal, and spirochete infections—fair chance of survival • Parasite migration, migrating foreign bodies, PME, YNE, and polioencephalomyelitis—usually fatal • Pug and Maltese encephalitis—may be fatal; course varies greatly; some patients respond to steroid treatment for long periods.
• Postvaccinal encephalomyelitis—may resolve on its own; often permanent damage and death

 MISCELLANEOUS

ASSOCIATED CONDITIONS
N/A

AGE-RELATED FACTORS
• Young (< 2 years) and old (> 8 years) animals—at more risk for infectious diseases
• Dogs < 6 years of age—immune-mediated and idiopathic encephalitides

ZOONOTIC POTENTIAL
• Rabies—consider in endemic areas if the patient is an outdoor animal that has rapidly progressive encephalitis • Humans may be infected by the same vector tick that affected the patient. • Exudates from animals with mycosis can revert to the spore-forming, infectious mycelial stage. • Cultures are highly contagious and should be handled with great care.

PREGNANCY
N/A

SYNONYMS
N/A

SEE ALSO
• Causes • Seizures (Convulsions, Status Epilepticus—Cats) • Seizures (Convulsions, Status Epilepticus—Dogs) • Stupor and Coma

ABBREVIATIONS
• CSF = cerebrospinal fluid • CT = computed tomography • ELISA = enzyme-linked immunosorbent assay • EME = eosinophilic meningoencephalitis • FeLV = feline leukemia virus • FIP = feline infectious peritonitis • FIV = feline immunodeficiency virus • GME = granulomatous meningo-encephalitis • MRI = magnetic resonance imaging • PME = pyogranulomatous meningoencephalitis • YNE = Yorkshire terrier necrotizing encephalitis

Suggested Reading
Braund KG. Clinical syndromes in veterinary neurology. 2nd ed. St. Louis: Mosby, 1994.
Greene CE, ed. Infectious diseases of the dog and cat. Philadelphia: Saunders, 1990.
Summers BA, Cummings JF, de Lahunta A. Veterinary neuropathology. Baltimore: Mosby, 1995.

Author Allen Sisson
Consulting Editor Joane M. Parent

ENCEPHALITIS SECONDARY TO PARASITIC MIGRATION

BASICS

OVERVIEW
• Aberrant migration of worms (helminthiasis) or fly larvae (myiasis) into the CNS
• Parasites may normally affect another organ system of the same host (e.g., *Dirofilaria immitis, Taenia, Ancylostoma caninum, Angiostrongylus,* or *Toxocara canis*), or a different host species (e.g., raccoon roundworm, *Baylisascaris procyonis;* skunk roundworm, *B. columnaris; Coenurus* spp., or *Cysticercus cellulosae*).
• Access to CNS—generally: hematogenously (dirofilariasis) or through adjacent tissues; *Cuterebra* fly larvae: various routes, including through the middle ear, skull foramina, cribriform plate, or open fontanelles

SIGNALMENT
• Dogs and cats—rare and sporadic
• Dirofilariasis—adult animals
• Other parasites—young animals exposed to an outside environment

SIGNS
• Vary with the portion of CNS affected
• Likely asymmetrical
• May suggest a mass lesion or multifocal disease process
• Rat parasite, *Angiostrongylus cantonensis*
• (Australia)—lumbosacral syndrome (hindlimbs, tail, and bladder paralysis/paresis) in puppies that may ascend to thoracic limbs and cranial nerves

CAUSES & RISK FACTORS
Housing in a cage previously occupied by wildlife (raccoons, skunks)

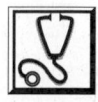

DIAGNOSIS

DIFFERENTIAL DIAGNOSIS
• Other causes of (focal) encephalopathy—infectious diseases (viral, bacterial, protozoan, or fungal); idiopathic granulomatous meningoencephalomyelitis; brain tumor; ischemic encephalopathy (cats) • CSF analysis and brain imaging—often inconclusive
• Diagnosis is usually made on necropsy.

CBC/BIOCHEMISTRY/URINALYSIS
Normal unless the parasite also affects non-neural tissues

OTHER LABORATORY TESTS
CSF—may show an eosinophilic, neutrophilic, or mononuclear pleocytosis (also found in protozoal, fungal, and prototthecal encephalitides); may be normal in strictly intraparenchymal lesions

IMAGING
CT or MRI—brain; focal lesion and/or cerebral infarction from occlusion of cerebral vessels

PATHOLOGIC FINDINGS
• Local to extensive necrosis, malacia, vascular rupture and hemorrhage, vascular emboli, granulomatous proliferation, or obstructive hydrocephalus
• *Dirofilaria immitis*—intravascular or extra-vascular
• Adult worms produce focal infarction or inflammation.

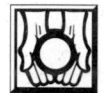

TREATMENT
None effective

MEDICATIONS

DRUG(S)
• Dirofilariasis and neural angiostrongylosis—anthelmintic treatments may cause worsening of signs and sometimes death.
• Mild neural angiostrongylosis—puppies may recover with supportive care and corticosteroid therapy.

CONTRAINDICATIONS/INTERACTIONS
N/A

FOLLOW-UP

PATIENT MONITORING
N/A

PREVENTION/AVOIDANCE
N/A

POSSIBLE COMPLICATIONS
N/A

EXPECTED COURSE AND PROGNOSIS
Usually progressive after acute or insidious onset

MISCELLANEOUS

SEE ALSO
• Encephalitis
• Encephalitozoonosis
• Heartworm Disease—Cats
• Heartworm Disease—Dogs

ABBREVIATION
CNS = central nervous system
CSF = cerebrospinal fluid
CT = computed tomography
MRI = magnetic resonance imaging

Suggested Reading
Braund KG. Clinical syndromes in veterinary neurology. 2nd ed. St. Louis: Mosby, 1994.
Author Christine Berthelin-Baker
Consulting Editor Joane M. Parent

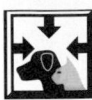

BASICS

OVERVIEW
- Infection with the protozoan *Encephalitozoon cuniculi*
- Involves lungs, heart, kidneys, and brain
- Uncommon in the U.S.

SIGNALMENT
- Dogs and cats
- No age, sex, or breed predilection

SIGNS

Neonates
- Appears a few weeks postpartum
- Stunted growth
- Unthriftiness
- Progress to renal failure
- Neurologic abnormalities

Adults
- Same as neonates
- May exhibit aggressive behavior, seizures, or blindness

CAUSES & RISK FACTORS
- Most likely route is oronasal from spore contaminated urine
- Kennel housing is a risk factor.

DIAGNOSIS

DIFFERENTIAL DIAGNOSIS
- Rabies
- Canine distemper
- Neosporosis
- Toxoplasmosis

CBC/BIOCHEMISTRY/URINALYSIS
- Normochromic, normocytic anemia
- Lymphocytosis and monocytosis
- High serum ALT and ALP expected

OTHER LABORATORY TESTS
Serology—blood and CSF

IMAGING
May be contributory but not diagnostic

DIAGNOSTIC PROCEDURES
- Urinalysis—sediment stained with Gram or Ziehl-Neelsen; Gram-positive spores; birefringent
- Positive identification requires immunologic procedures.

PATHOLOGIC FINDINGS
- Nonsuppurative interstitial nephritis—consistent finding
- Hepatomegaly and petechiae throughout surfaces of multiple organs
- Swollen kidneys, hemorrhagic cystitis, renal cortical cysts, or infarcts
- Brain—if lesions present, thrombosis and encephalomalacia, cystic spaces in parenchyma

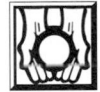

TREATMENT
- Inpatient with supportive therapy
- Euthanasia—when severe neurologic signs occur

MEDICATIONS

DRUG(S)
Chemotherapy—no known for dogs and cats; try benzimidazoles, particularly albendazole (50 mg/kg q8h for 7 days), because they work in mice and humans.

CONTRAINDICATIONS/POSSIBLE INTERACTIONS
N/A

FOLLOW-UP

PREVENTION/AVOIDANCE
Sanitation—important; accomplish with 70% ethanol

EXPECTED COURSE AND PROGNOSIS
A number of patients recover without further signs if neither the renal nor the cerebral manifestation becomes severe.

MISCELLANEOUS

ZOONOTIC POTENTIAL
Potential risks to humans, especially the immunosuppressed

ABBREVIATIONS
- ALP = alkaline phosphatase
- ALT = alanine transferase
- CSF = cerebrospinal fluid

Suggested Reading
Didier PJ, Didier ES, Snowden K, Shadduck JA. Encephalitozoonosis. In: Greene CE, ed., Infectious diseases of the dog and cat. 2nd ed. Philadelphia: Saunders, 1998:465–470.

Author Johnny D. Hoskins
Consulting Editor Stephen C. Barr

ENDOCARDITIS, INFECTIVE

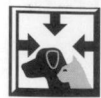

BASICS

DEFINITION
The invasion of the cardiac endothelium, usually the valves, by infectious agents. Usually gram-positive bacteria, especially coagulase-positive staphylococci. Occasionally rickettsia or *Bartonella* in dogs. Rarely fungi in dogs. Culture-negative cases may be due to *Bartonella*. Less likely due to *Brucella, Coxiella,* and *Chlamydia*.

PATHOPHYSIOLOGY
• Bacteremia develops from various portals of entry; bacteria invade and colonize the heart valves—usually the aortic, occasionally the mitral, and rarely the tricuspid and pulmonic valves. • Endocardial ulceration exposes collagen, causing platelet aggregation and clot formation. • Vegetations on heart valves are composed of an inner layer of platelets, fibrin, RBCs, and bacteria; a middle layer of bacteria; and an outer layer of fibrin. • Valvular insufficiency develops in virtually all patients; aortic insufficiency almost invariably leads to intractable left-sided CHF within weeks to several months. • CHF is less frequent and latent when only the mitral valve is affected.

SYSTEMS AFFECTED
• Cardiovascular—bacteremia • Respiratory—pulmonary edema • Renal/urologic—renal infarction • Musculoskeletal—septic or immune-mediated polyarthropathy

GENETICS
Genetic predisposition unlikely

INCIDENCE/PREVALENCE
Vary by geographic region and habitus

GEOGRAPHIC DISTRIBUTION
No well-documented patterns published; bacteremia and hence bacterial endocarditis may be more common in tropical and semitropical regions.

SIGNALMENT

Species
Dogs; rarely cats

Breed Predilection
• Middle-sized to large breeds
• Those predisposed to subaortic stenosis

Mean Age and Range
Most affected dogs are 4–6 years of age; infection can occur at any age.

Predominant Sex
Most studies report male predominance—may be as great as 2:1

SIGNS

General Comments
• Depend on whether infection is subacute or chronic, and if CHF, renal failure, metastatic abscessation, or secondary immune complications are present • Most prevalent when associated with sepsis and CHF

Historical Findings
• Infectious disease within the past few weeks to several months in some patients • CHF (e.g., coughing, dyspnea, and exercise intolerance)

Physical Examination Findings
• Usually diverse and misleading—"the great imitator" • Fever and general malaise
• Dyspnea caused by CHF • Multiple single or shifting leg lameness in some patients
• Systolic heart murmur • Diastolic heart murmur associated with aortic insufficiency—difficult to detect without careful auscultation of the right cranioventral precordium • Hyperdynamic femoral arterial pulses strongly suggest advanced aortic valve endocarditis. • Volume overload produces high systolic arterial pressure followed by a rapid, accentuated drop in diastolic pressure associated with blood "runoff" back into the left ventricle.

CAUSES
• Bacterial infection associated with the oral cavity, bone, prostate, skin, and other sites
• Invasive diagnostic or surgical procedures forcing bacteria into the bloodstream

RISK FACTORS
• Congenital subaortic stenosis
• Immunosuppression from long-term or high-dose corticosteroids, neoplasia, or cytotoxic drug administration

DIAGNOSIS

DIFFERENTIAL DIAGNOSIS
• Bacteremia of any cause produces identical hematologic abnormalities and similar clinical signs. • Polysystemic, immune-mediated disorders are often difficult to differentiate from bacteremia and rickettsemia. • Left-sided CHF caused by dilated cardiomyopathy or congenital subaortic stenosis

CBC/BIOCHEMISTRY/URINALYSIS
• Active, severe infection associated with an inflammatory leukogram (i.e., neutrophilia, left shift, and monocytosis)—patients with chronic, relatively inactive, or walled-off infection may have normal or nearly normal leukogram; those with chronic infection may have mature neutrophilia with monocytosis.
• Anemia • Thrombocytopenia—variable severity; depends on duration and severity of infection, vasculitis, and DIC • Low-normal or low albumin, low-normal or low glucose, and high SAP activity are inconsistently associated with sepsis. • Proteinuria caused by bacteremia and septic embolization or infarction of the kidneys; hematuria, pyuria, and casts associated with pyelonephritis and glomerulonephritis

OTHER LABORATORY TESTS
• Blood culturing—three samples taken at least one hour apart over 24 hours; at least two should yield the same microbe; both aerobic and anaerobic cultures recommended; antibiotic removal systems available for diagnosis of patients given antibiotics
• Catheter tips—culture • Urine cultures—easy; often yield positive results; do not necessarily incriminate the urinary tract as the source of infection, but are not a substitute for blood cultures • Tests for prostate, kidney, and bone infection may be warranted.
• Positive antinuclear antibody, lupus erythematosus, rheumatoid factor, and Coombs' test results occasionally found—nonspecific; tend to confound the diagnosis

IMAGING

Radiographic Findings
Left heart enlargement; rarely, calcification of one or more heart valves

Echocardiography
• Best test: Vegetative endocarditis of the aortic valve is easily discerned; mitral valve infection is difficult to differentiate from myxomatous degeneration.

DIAGNOSTIC PROCEDURES
Joint taps for cytologic examination and culture—cytologic examination may not differentiate septic from immune-mediated arthritis; either can exist with infective endocarditis. Neutrophils are usually nondegenerate regardless of cause; bacterial culture is usually negative because the condition usually is immune mediated.

Electrocardiographic Findings
• ECG—may be normal; occasionally reflects left heart enlargement; often detects ventricular tachyarrhythmias; occasionally reveals heart block of variable severity • Heart block suggests aortic valve involvement with infection or infarction of the adjacent septum. • Intermittent heart rhythm disturbances often require extended ECG monitoring (Holter or cageside) for detection.

PATHOLOGIC FINDINGS
• Cardiac enlargement • Vegetative lesions and blood clots on one or more valves
• Infection, hemorrhage, and infarction of adjacent myocardium • Renal infarcts
• Primary or secondary sites of infection
• Pulmonary hemorrhage or edema

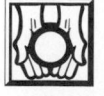

TREATMENT

APPROPRIATE HEALTH CARE
Virtually all animals with suspected infective endocarditis should be hospitalized.

NURSING CARE
• Good hydration for septic patients, particularly those receiving an aminoglycoside
• Aggressive fluid therapy—at least twice

maintenance level for patients with renal failure
• Overt or impending CHF limits fluid volumes that can be administered; this problem is virtually insurmountable in patients with concomitant renal failure.
• Imminent CHF—provide no more than maintenance volumes of fluid; alternate D5W with LRS (or 2.5% dextrose in half-strength LRS); potassium supplementation usually required

ACTIVITY
Variable—depends on whether or not CHF is present or imminent

DIET
Sodium restriction if CHF is present or imminent

CLIENT EDUCATION
Guarded prognosis if only mitral valve involved; grave prognosis if aortic valve involved

SURGICAL CONSIDERATIONS
Aortic valve endocarditis—almost always results in intractable left-sided CHF; aortic valve replacement indicated; procedure routinely performed in human medicine but rarely attempted in veterinary medicine because of lack of expertise and facilities, and high cost

 MEDICATIONS

DRUGS OF CHOICE
Treatment variable—depends on severity of sepsis and presence or absence of CHF

Antibiotics
• Backbone of treatment but usually don't eradicate infection before irreversible valve damage occurs; more than minimal damage to the aortic valve is life-threatening because aortic insufficiency tends to be a lethal complication.
• High-dose IV administration of bactericidal antibiotics is imperative and recommended for as long as feasible, followed by SC administration.
• Oral administration—recommended only after at least 4 weeks of injectable therapy and at least 1 week after hematologic and clinical signs of infection and inflammation have disappeared; long-term (2–4 months) treatment required to eradicate the infection from the vegetations
• Selection determined by both the urgency of septic complications and results of bacterial culture; coagulase-positive staphylococci and streptococci are most often incriminated, so choices can be logically made before culture results are obtained.
• Coagulase-positive staphylococci—usually resistant to penicillin and ampicillin

• Streptococci—often resistant to aminoglycosides and fluoroquinolones
• Gram-negative bacteria—often sensitive to third-generation cephalosporins, fluoroquinolones, and aminoglycosides
• First-generation cephalosporins—reasonable choice for stable patients until culture results are obtained
• Treat life-threatening sepsis immediately with drug combinations. Pending culture results, one of three regimens is recommended: (1) Penicillin, ampicillin, ticarcillin, or a first-generation cephalosporin is combined with an aminoglycoside. High doses of the latter cannot be administered, and fluid support with monitoring for nephrotoxicity is required; thus aminoglycosides are not good choices for animals with overt or impending CHF. Gentamicin (2 mg/kg q8h) is recommended for only 5–10 days because of renal toxicity. A fluoroquinolone may be substituted for an aminoglycoside. (2) Clindamycin (2 to 10 mg/kg IV q8h) plus enrofloxacin (6 mg/kg q12h given diluted 1:1 in sterile water and injected slowly over 15–20 minutes) (3) Advanced-generation cephalosporins or ticarcillin-clavulanic acid (Timentin)—high dosages, but only normal dosages if patient has renal failure

Treatment of CHF
• Digoxin, angiotensin-converting enzyme inhibitor, amlodipine, and furosemide indicated for patients with chronic CHF
• Oxygen, nitroglycerin, high-dose furosemide (2–8 mg/kg IV), and hydralazine (1–2 mg/kg q12h) for patients with acute, severe pulmonary edema

CONTRAINDICATIONS
• Avoid antibiotics that cannot penetrate fibrin (e.g., sulfonamides).
• Corticosteroids

PRECAUTIONS
Renal disease and digoxin, enalapril, and aminoglycoside administration

POSSIBLE INTERACTIONS
Concurrent use of aminoglycoside and furosemide raises the risk of nephrotoxicity and ototoxicity.

ALTERNATIVE DRUGS
N/A

 FOLLOW-UP

PATIENT MONITORING
• Emergence of antibiotic resistance—relapsing fever and inflammatory leukogram; imperative to adjust treatment on the basis of culture results • Weekly examination and CBC after discharge • Repeat blood cultures 1 week after antibiotics are discontinued or if fever recurs.

PREVENTION/AVOIDANCE
• Indwelling catheters—restrict to appropriate indications; aseptic placement; replace within 3–5 days. • Administer antibiotics to animals undergoing dentistry—controversial except in animals with congenital heart defects and oral infections • Avoid careless use of corticosteroids.

POSSIBLE COMPLICATIONS
• CHF • Renal failure • Septic embolization of many tissues and organs • Persistent or latent immune-mediated polyarthropathy

EXPECTED COURSE AND PROGNOSIS
• Best prognosis associated with short history of bacteremia, rapid diagnosis, and aggressive treatment • Mortality relatively higher in animals recently given corticosteroids.
• Grave prognosis for most patients with aortic valve endocarditis • Latent CHF may develop (months to years later) with mitral valve endocarditis.

 MISCELLANEOUS

ASSOCIATED CONDITIONS
Congenital heart defects (usually subaortic stenosis) in some animals

AGE-RELATED FACTORS
N/A

ZOONOTIC POTENTIAL
None

PREGNANCY
N/A

SYNONYMS
• Infective endocarditis
• Vegetative endocarditis

SEE ALSO
• Congestive Heart Failure, Left-sided
• Septicemia and Bacteremia
• Diskospondylitis • Prostatitis and Prostatic Abscess • Renal Failure, Acute • Bartonellosis

ABBREVIATIONS
• CHF = congestive heart failure
• IE = infective endocarditis

Suggested Reading
Kittleson MD. In: Kittleson MD, Krenle RD, eds. Small animal cardiovascular medicine. St. Louis: Mosby, 1998; 402–412.
Miller MW, Sisson D. In: Fox PR, Sisson D, Moise NS, eds. Textbook of canine and feline cardiology. Philadelphia, Saunders, 1999: 567–580.
Authors Clay A. Calvert and Michelle Wall
Consulting Editors Larry P. Tilley and Francis W. K. Smith, Jr.

ENDOMYOCARDIAL DISEASES—CATS

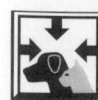

BASICS

OVERVIEW
• Endomyocarditis—acute cardiopulmonary disease that typically develops following a stressful event; characterized by interstitial pneumonia and endomyocardial inflammation; pneumonia is usually severe and commonly causes death; one report recorded the incidence of endomyocarditis at postmortem to be equivalent to that of hypertrophic cardiomyopathy.
• Endocardial fibroelastosis—congenital heart disease in which severe fibrous endocardial thickening leads to heart failure secondary to diastolic and systolic failure
• Excessive moderator bands (EMBs)–This is a rare and unique pathologic disease. Moderator bands are normal muscular bands in the right ventricle, but can sometimes occur in the left ventricle.

SIGNALMENT
• Cats
• Endomyocarditis—predominantly males (62%) age 1–4 years
• Endocardial fibroelastosis—early development of biventricular or left heart failure, usually prior to 6 months of age
• EMBs—can be seen in any age cat

SIGNS
Historical Findings
Endomyocarditis
• Dyspnea following a stressful event in a young, healthy cat
• Respiratory signs usually occur 5–21 days after the stressor.
• In one report, 73% of cases presented between August and September.
Endocardial Fibroelastosis and EMBs
• Lethargy, weakness, collapse, syncope
• Poor appetite and weight loss
• Dyspnea
• Tachypnea
• Cyanosis
• Abdominal distention
• Paresis or paralysis; signs of thromboembolic disease

Physical Examination Findings
Endomyocarditis
• Severe dyspnea
• Occasional crackles
• May be murmur or gallop; murmur may vary in intensity.
• May be evidence of thromboembolic disease
• Typically no significant abnormalities prior to the stressful event
Endocardial Fibroelastosis and EMB
• Gallop
• Systolic murmur, possible mitral regurgitation
• Dyspnea and increased lung sounds or crackles
• Paresis or paralysis with weak or absent femoral pulses
• Arrhythmias possible

CAUSES & RISK FACTORS
• Cause unknown for all three diseases
• Risk factors for endomyocarditis include stressful incidents such as anesthesia (commonly associated with neutering or declawing), vaccination, relocation, or bathing.
• Endocardial fibroelastosis may be familial in Burmese and Siamese cats.
• The appearance of EMBs in a young cat would suggest a congenital malformation.

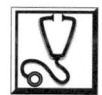

DIAGNOSIS

DIFFERENTIAL DIAGNOSIS

Other Causes of Cardiac Disease
Hypertrophic cardiomyopathy, restrictive cardiomyopathy, dilated cardiomyopathy, congenital heart malformations

Other Causes of Dyspnea
• Other forms of cardiac disease, hypertrophic cardiomyopathy, restrictive cardiomyopathy, dilated cardiomyopathy, congenital malformations
• Primary respiratory disease
• Pleural space disease
• Mediastinal disorders, infection, trauma, neoplasia
• Hemoglobin disorders, anemia, methemoglobinemia, causes of central cyanosis

Other Causes of Collapse, Weakness, or Syncope
• Arrhythmias
• Neurologic or musculoskeletal disease
• Metabolic disease or electrolyte disorders
• Other forms of paresis or paralysis
• Arterial thromboembolism secondary to any form of cardiac disease or neoplasia
• Neurologic or musculoskeletal disease
• Neoplasia

CBC/BIOCHEMISTRY/URINALYSIS
Not diagnostic

OTHER LABORATORY TESTS
N/A

IMAGING

Thoracic Radiographic Findings for All Three Diseases
• Cardiomegaly
• Interstitial or alveolar infiltrates or pleural effusion if congestion has developed

Echocardiographic Findings
Endomyocarditis
• Normal to mildly large left atrium
• Left ventricular wall thickness can be normal to mildly thick (0.6–0.7 cm).
• Hyperechoic endomyocardium reported—incidence seems to vary and is subjective; in one report it was as high as 86%.
Endocardial Fibroelastosis
• Limited data available
• Reduced left ventricular function and enlarged left atrium
Excessive Moderator Bands
Many findings can overlap restrictive cardiomyopathy. A network of false tendons can sometimes be imaged with two-dimensional echocardiography.

DIAGNOSTIC PROCEDURES

Electrocardiographic Findings
• Endomyocarditis—sinus tachycardia common; ventricular premature complexes, atrial premature complexes, bundle branch block, and complete AV block reported
• Endocardial fibroelastosis—evidence for left-sided enlargement; sinus rhythm typically present, but various arrhythmias possible
• EMBs—various electrocardiographic findings have been reported: AV block, sinus

bradycardia, right bundle branch block, and left axis deviation.

PATHOLOGIC FINDINGS

Endomyocarditis
• Interstitial pneumonia
• Left heart enlargement and opacity of the left ventricular endomyocardium with foci of hemorrhage; fibroplasia of the endocardium is striking.
• Varying degrees of endomyocardial inflammation with infiltrates of neutrophils, lymphocytes, plasma cells, histiocytes, and macrophages seen histologically

Endocardial Fibroelastosis
• Left ventricular and atrial dilation with severe diffuse white opaque thickening of the endocardium
• Diffuse hypocellular, fibroelastic thickening of the endomyocardium; prominent endomyocardial edema with dilation of lymphatics

Excessive Moderator Bands
Changes typically include an irregular left ventricular endocardial contour with a rounded apex and numerous irregular left ventricular false tendons. Heart weights can be greater then normal. The moderator bands are composed of central Purkinje fibers and collagen.

TREATMENT

Endomyocarditis
• No one therapy protocol to date
• Small percentage of cats have survived; these cats are on long-term therapy.
• Supportive care with oxygen and possibly ventilation

Endocardial Fibroelastosis and EMBs
• Oxygen therapy via cage delivery is least stressful.
• Thoracocentesis if pleural effusion

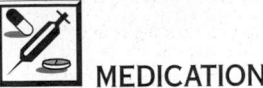

MEDICATIONS

DRUGS OF CHOICE

Endomyocarditis
Steroids, furosemide, and vasodilators have been tried, but efficacy is still unknown.

Endocardial fibroelastosis and EMB
Acute CHF
• Parenteral administration of furosemide, 0.5–1.0 mg/kg IV or IM, q1–6h
• Dermal application of 2% nitroglycerin ointment, 1/8 to 1/4 inch q4–6h
• Arrhythmias may resolve with stabilization. If there is rapid atrial fibrillation (heart rate > 200), a calcium channel blocker or β-blocker can be given to help control the ventricular response. If there is dilated cardiomyopathy, digoxin may be a better choice for controlling the atrial fibrillation rate. For other supraventricular arrhythmias and ventricular arrhythmias, waiting for a response to heart failure therapy may be wise before starting antiarrhythmic therapy.
• Intractable edema—nitroprusside, 1–5 μg/kg/min, may be helpful.
Chronic CHF
• Treat as other CHF, with furosemide and enalapril
• Digoxin can be added when patient is stable and eating.

CONTRAINDICATIONS/POSSIBLE INTERACTIONS
N/A

FOLLOW-UP

EXPECTED COURSE AND PROGNOSIS
• Endomyocarditis—Poor, although some animals survive; consider the suggestion that endomyocarditis may progress to left ventricular endocardial fibrosis.

• Endocardial fibroelastosis and EMBs—medical treatment of CHF may prolong life, but recovery is unlikely.

MISCELLANEOUS

ASSOCIATED CONDITIONS
• Aortic thromboembolism
• May be a relationship between endomyocarditis and left ventricular endocardial fibrosis

SEE ALSO
• Aortic Thromboembolism
• Congestive Heart Failure, Left-sided
• Congestive Heart Failure, Right-sided
• Myocarditis

ABBREVIATIONS
• CHF = congestive heart failure
• EMB = excessive moderator band

Suggested Reading
Bossbaly MB, Stalis I, Knight D, Van Winkle T. Feline endomyocarditis: a clinical/pathological study of 44 cases. Proceedings of the 12th ACVIM Forum, 1994:975.
Liu S, Tilley LP. Excessive moderator bands in the left ventricle of 21 cats. J Am Vet Med Assoc 1982;180:1215–1219.
Stalis IH, Bossbaly MJ, Van Winkle TJ. Feline endomyocarditis and left ventricular endocardial fibrosis. Vet Pathol 1995;32(2):122–126.
Authors Carl D. Sammarco and Maribeth J. Bossbaly
Consulting Editors Larry P. Tilley and Francis W. K. Smith, Jr.

ENTROPION

BASICS

OVERVIEW
• Inversion of part or all of the eyelid margin
• Frictional irritation of the cornea—because of contact by the eyelash or eyelid hair; may result in corneal ulceration or perforation or pigmentary keratitis
• Vision may be threatened.

SIGNALMENT
• Common in dogs; occasional in cats
• Cats—usually seen in brachycephalic breeds (e.g, Persian and Himalayan)
• Dogs—seen in chow chows, shar peis, Norwegian elkhounds, sporting breeds (e.g., spaniels, retrievers), brachycephalic breeds (e.g., English bulldogs, pugs, Pekingese), toy breeds (e.g., poodles, Yorkshire terriers), and giant breeds (e.g., mastiffs, St. Bernards, Newfoundlands)
• Age—seen in puppies 2–6 weeks old (especially chow chows and shar peis); usually identified in dogs < 1 year old

SIGNS
• Depend on type and degree of condition
• Mild, medial—chronic epiphora and medial pigmentary keratitis (toy dogs and brachycephalic dogs and cats)
• Mild, lateral—chronic mucoid to mucopurulent ocular discharge (giant-breed dogs)
• Upper lid, lower lid, or lateral canthal—severe blepharospasm, purulent discharge, pigmentary or ulcerative keratitis, and potential cornea rupture (chow chows, shar peis, and sporting breeds)

CAUSES & RISK FACTORS
• Primarily genetic predisposition in facial conformation and eyelid support
• Brachycephalic breeds (dogs and cats)—excessive tension on the ligamentous structures of the medial canthus coupled with nasal folds and facial conformation defects results in rolling inward of the medial aspects of the upper and lower eyelids and the medial canthus
• Giant breeds and breeds with heavy facial skin (bloodhounds) or excessive facial folds (chow chows, shar peis)—laxity of the lateral canthal ligamentous structures allows for entropion of the upper and lower eyelids and the lateral canthus.

• Chronic infectious conjunctivitis or keratitis (cats)—may lead to functional entropion caused by chronic blepharospasm (spastic entropion)
• Predisposed breeds (dogs)—spastic entropion, if ocular irritation (e.g., distichia, ectopic cilia, trichiasis, foreign body, and irritant conjunctivitis) leads to excessive blepharospasm.
• Nonpredisposed breeds—may be the result of a primary irritant causing secondary spastic entropion
• Severe weight loss or muscle atrophy caused by masticatory muscle myositis (dogs)—loss of orbital fat or periorbital musculature may lead to enophthalmos and entropion.

DIAGNOSIS

DIFFERENTIAL DIAGNOSIS
• Usually obvious clinically—underlying causes of spastic entropion should be ruled out and corrected, if possible, before an attempt at surgical correction is made.
• Puppies—common for first-time breeders of chows and shar peis to mistakenly think that

the eyelids have not opened at 4–5 weeks of age, when puppies actually have severe blepharospasm and entropion

CBC/BIOCHEMISTRY/URINALYSIS
N/A

OTHER LABORATORY TESTS
N/A

IMAGING
N/A

DIAGNOSTIC PROCEDURES
N/A

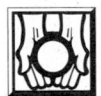 TREATMENT

PUPPIES
• Young (especially shar peis and chows)—do not initially perform skin resection surgery.
• Eyelid eversion suture technique—attempted to temporarily evert the eyelid margins to break the spasm-irritation-spasm cycle; if successful, permanent procedure is unnecessary.
• Permanent skin resection technique—postponed until patient's facial conformation matures (increases success)

DOGS AND CATS
Toy dog breeds and brachycephalic dogs and cats—medial canthal reconstruction, if medial condition and trichiasis cause pigmentary keratitis, chronic epiphora, or corneal scarring

MATURE DOGS
• Chronic entropion—requires some type of eyelid margin–everting surgery; simple Hotz-Celsus procedure or more radical lateral canthoplasty
• No history of previous entropion and clinical signs of acute condition—examine meticulously for cause of spastic condition and correct; may attempt a temporary eversion suture technique before performing permanent skin resection, if necessary

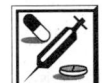 MEDICATIONS

DRUG(S)
Topical ophthalmic ointment—triple-antibiotic or antibiotic based on culture and sensitivity testing; q12–24h; may use postoperatively or as a presurgical lubricant

CONTRAINDICATIONS/POSSIBLE INTERACTIONS
N/A

 FOLLOW-UP

Temporary eversion suture technique—may revert when sutures are removed or spontaneously pull through the skin; repeated as necessary until the patient is mature enough to undergo a more permanent form of skin resection repair (approximately 6 months of age)

 MISCELLANEOUS

Suggested Reading
Severin GA. Eyelids. In Severin's veterinary ophthalmology notes. 3rd ed. Ft. Collins, CO: DesignPointe Communications, Inc., 1996:188–195.
Author J. Phillip Pickett
Consulting Editor Paul E. Miller

EOSINOPHILIA AND BASOPHILIA

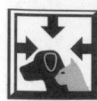 **BASICS**

DEFINITION
• Peripheral blood eosinophil count > 750–1500/μL (reference interval may vary regionally) • Peripheral blood basophil count > 200/μL or a minimum of 3–6% of the differential count

PATHOPHYSIOLOGY

Eosinophilia
• Develops in response to a primary disease process; highest counts seen in patients with hypereosinophilic syndrome, disseminated mast cell tumor, flea allergy, asthma, and some parasitic diseases • The level does not predict the degree of eosinophilic infiltration of tissues, which can be marked even in the absence of eosinophilia and occurs in response to mast cell/basophil products, immune complexes, cytokines, chemotactic factors, and vasoactive amines. • Results from heightened bone marrow production mediated by T cell elaboration of IL-5 in response to specific stimuli (e.g., allergens, parasitic antigens, and products of tumor cells); repeated exposure to an antigen produces more rapid and dramatic eosinophilia. • Eosinophils can kill parasites and may contribute to host defense against tumors, but eosinophil-derived products can also cause destruction of host tissue. • Whether eosinophilic inflammation is beneficial or harmful varies according to the situation.

Basophilia
• Basophils play a role in immune-mediated inflammation, especially anaphylaxis and cutaneous hypersensitivity, but specific stimuli are not well characterized. • Basophils may participate in host rejection of parasites (especially ticks) and may play a role in tumor cytotoxicity. • May play roles in plasma lipolysis and hemostasis. • Often accompanies eosinophilia, especially in patients with ectoparasites (mites) and dirofilariasis. • Basophil numbers may increase in the face of sustained lipemia or altered lipid metabolism.

SYSTEMS AFFECTED
• Skin • Respiratory • Gastrointestinal • Reproductive—during estrus • Hemolymphatic • Patients with hypereosinophilic syndrome or eosinophilic leukemia—gastrointestinal tract, liver, spleen, and lymph nodes, especially mesenteric lymph nodes

SIGNS

General Comments
Signs usually relate to underlying disease process.

Historical Findings
• Skin—pruritus, flea infestation, alopecia, and crusty lesions • Respiratory tract—coughing and dyspnea • Gastrointestinal tract—vomiting, diarrhea, anorexia, and weight loss • Lethargy and depression

PHYSICAL EXAMINATION FINDINGS
• Skin—pruritus, alopecia, miliary dermatitis, oral lesions, other cutaneous lesions, regional lymphadenopathy, plaques, granulomas, and indolent ulcers • Respiratory—abnormal lung sounds, coughing, tachypnea, dyspnea, and pleural effusion • Gastrointestinal—thickened intestines, mesenteric lymphadenopathy, and abdominal effusion • Reproductive—estrus or vaginal discharge • Neoplasia—mass lesions and lymphadenopathy

CAUSES

Eosinophilia
• Causes are associated with tissue infiltrates of eosinophils with or without accompanying basophilic infiltration.
• Circulating eosinophilia is a variable finding.

Parasitism
• Especially parasites that invade tissues • Migrating helminthic parasites—particularly *Toxocara* spp., *Strongyloides stercoralis*, and *Ancylostoma* spp. • *Dirofilaria immitis* and *Dipetalonema reconditum* • Respiratory helminths—*Capillaria aerophila*, *Paragonimus kellicotti* (dogs and cats); *Aelurostrongylus abstrusus* (cats); *Oslerus osleri*, *Filaroides hirthi*, *Crenosoma vulpis*, and *Andersonstrongylus milksi* (dogs) • Ectoparasites—mites and fleas • Protozoa—*Giardia*, *Coccidia*, *Toxoplasma*, and *Neospora* • *Trichinella spiralis* • *Cuterebra*

Hypersensitivity Reactions and Other Inflammatory Conditions
• Skin—hypersensitivity to fleas and mites, reaction to insect bites/stings (e.g., *Hymenoptera*), food allergy, inhalant allergic dermatitis (e.g., atopy), eosinophilic granuloma complex (e.g., indolent ulcer, plaque, and granuloma) in cats, eosinophilic granuloma in dogs, sterile eosinophilic folliculitis in cats, sterile eosinophilic pustulosis in dogs, chronic inflammation of skin • Respiratory—chronic upper respiratory infection and rhinitis or sinusitis in cats, allergic bronchopulmonary disease (e.g., asthma, bronchitis, pneumonitis) in cats, less commonly seen in dogs as part of chronic obstructive pulmonary disease, parasitic pneumonia, granulomatous disease in dogs (mostly dirofilariasis), pulmonary infiltrates with eosinophilia (PIE—nonspecific term that includes pulmonary eosinophilic granulomatosis; eosinophilic pneumonia; bronchitis; bronchiolitis; and alveolitis caused by parasitism, allergic disease, dirofilariasis, drug reactions, bacterial and fungal infection, neoplasia, and idiopathic disease), focal pneumonia, interstitial pneumonia, pneumothorax, foreign body, chronic inflammation of the lung, *Mycoplasma* pneumonia in cats, and lymphomatoid granulomatosis

• Gastrointestinal—endoparasitism, oral or gastrointestinal eosinophilic granuloma, eosinophilic gastroenterocolitis (caused by dietary, bacterial, toxic, parasitic, and altered mucosal antigens) in dogs may be isolated to one segment of the GI tract; eosinophilic gastroenteritis in cats may be part of the hypereosinophilic syndrome and bacterial infection (including *Helicobacter*) • Urogenital tract—estrus (occasionally in dogs), chronic inflammation of the reproductive tract, and urologic syndrome in cats • Musculoskeletal (dogs)—eosinophilic myositis, panosteitis, immune-mediated polyarthritis, idiopathic eosinophilic polyarthritis, diskospondylitis (Airedales) • Other inflammatory conditions—chronic fungal (e.g., gastric phycomycosis, disseminated coccidioidomycosis, and crypto-coccosis of the CNS) and protozoal (e.g., hepatozoonosis and granulomatous meningo-encephalitis) infections • Tumor-associated eosinophilia (paraneoplastic syndrome)—most commonly observed in patients with mast cell tumor (visceral or disseminated) and lymphoma and occasionally other neoplasms (e.g., carcinoma and sarcoma); usually mediated by IL-5 or IL-2 • Hypereosinophilic syndrome • Myeloproliferative disease (dogs and cats)—FeLV-associated eosinophilia (Rickard strain) and eosinophilic leukemia (rare) • Miscellaneous—hypoadrenocorticism, eosinophilic meningoencephalitis (e.g., idiopathic steroid-responsive, protozoal, and migrating helminths), immune-mediated disease (e.g., SLE and IMHA), vaccine reaction (e.g., SC rabies vaccine inoculation with granulomatous response), drug-associated eosinophilia (e.g., cyclophosphamide and tetracycline), administration of IL-2 or GM-CSF • Miscellaneous (cats)—eosinophilic keratitis and conjunctivitis, hyperthyroidism, panleukopenia, infectious peritonitis, chronic gingivitis, infections with *Staphylococcus* and *Streptococcus* spp., and cardiac disease • Most common diseases (cats)—flea allergy dermatitis, eosinophilic granuloma complex, allergic bronchitis and asthma, chronic upper respiratory infection, chronic rhinitis and sinusitis, and gastrointestinal disease with endoparasitism

Basophilia
• Parasitism—dirofilariasis (especially occult), tick infestation, other ectoparasites, and tracheal parasites • Often accompanies eosinophilia (e.g., caused by chronic inflammation of mucosal and skin surfaces, disseminated mast cell tumor, and PIE) • Lymphomatoid granulomatosis • Basophilic leukemia; occasionally chronic granulocytic leukemia, polycythemia vera, essential thrombocythemia, and thymoma • Possibly in animals with altered lipid metabolism that have sustained lipemia (e.g., chronic liver

disease; nephrotic syndrome; genetic hyperlipoproteinemia; and endocrinopathy such as hyperadrenocorticism, diabetes mellitus, and hypothyroidism); not confirmed to result from lipemia

RISK FACTORS
• Parasitism • Hypersensitivity disorder • Inflammation • Neoplasia

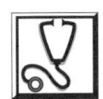

DIAGNOSIS

DIFFERENTIAL DIAGNOSIS
• Pruritus, alopecia, dermatitis, ulcer/plaque/granuloma, flea infestation—rule out atopy, flea or food allergy, eosinophilic granuloma complex, other disorders of hypersensitivity, and other inflammatory disorders of the skin.
• Coughing, dyspnea, tachypnea—rule out allergic diseases of respiratory tract (e.g., bronchitis and asthma), parasitic diseases (e.g., dirofilariasis and lungworm), PIE, and chronic inflammation. • Nodular lung lesions with eosinophilia—rule out mycotic infection, idiopathic eosinophilic granuloma, primary or metastatic neoplasia, and lymphomatoid granulomatosis. • Vomiting, diarrhea, weight loss—rule out eosinophilic gastroenterocolitis, parasitism, and hypereosinophilic syndrome.
• Lymphadenopathy or mass lesion—rule out mast cell tumor, lymphoma, other neoplasms, and hypereosinophilic syndrome.

LABORATORY FINDINGS

Drugs That May Alter Laboratory Results
Corticosteroid-induced eosinopenia can mask eosinophilia.

Disorders That May Alter Laboratory Results
None

Valid If Run in Human Laboratory?
Yes; laboratory should be informed that eosinophil granules vary in size, shape, and number depending on species; basophils in cats have beige-gray or mauve, round granules.

CBC/BIOCHEMISTRY/URINALYSIS
• Eosinophilia and basophilia • Biochemical analysis may detect organ dysfunction.

OTHER LABORATORY TESTS
• Fecal flotation test to identify parasitic ova • Baermann fecal sedimentation test to identify parasite larvae, especially nematode lungworms • Heartworm test • Cytologic examination of tracheobronchial fluid to identify eosinophilic inflammation, ova, and larvae • Cytologic examination of skin, mucosal (e.g., oral and rectal), and corneal or conjunctival scrapings or fine-needle aspirates of masses for eosinophilic infiltrates and possible cause of eosinophilia • Examination of buffy coat for mast cells, presence of which may indicate disseminated mast cell tumor; positive buffy coats also found in many other diseases • Examination of bone marrow to rule out neoplasia

IMAGING
• Survey radiography of thorax to detect thoracic disease (e.g., diffuse, peribronchial, interstitial, or alveolar lung patterns, pleural fluid, and pneumothorax) and of abdomen to detect mass lesions or abdominal fluid • Contrast studies of gastrointestinal tract to identify mucosal irregularities and wall thickenings • Ultrasonography of thoracic or abdominal mass

DIAGNOSTIC PROCEDURES
• Intradermal skin testing (atopy) • Transtracheal wash or bronchoalveolar lavage (respiratory disease) • Thoracocentesis or abdominocentesis • Examination of fine-needle aspirate or biopsy of mass lesion, skin, gastrointestinal tract, lung, lymph nodes, or bone marrow to rule out neoplasia • Endoscopy (gastrointestinal disease) • Laparotomy • Exclusion diet • Medical trial of corticosteroids or other medications

TREATMENT
• Treatment varies with the primary cause. • Because eosinophils can cause damage to host cells, treatment aimed at decreasing or eliminating eosinophilic infiltrates may be required.

MEDICATIONS

DRUG(S)
• Specific medications for the primary disease • If not contraindicated, corticosteroids are the most effective anti-inflammatory drug for treating eosinophil-related disorders (e.g., prednisolone, 1 mg/kg q12h, then taper by giving q24h, then alternate days to lowest dose that is still effective). • For some conditions, cytotoxic drugs such as hydroxyurea may be required. • Cyclosporine may prove useful in controlling eosinophilic infiltrates induced by activated T cells.

CONTRAINDICATIONS
Corticosteroids are generally contraindicated in patients with infectious diseases.

PRECAUTIONS
• Corticosteroids are associated with hepatopathy and pancreatitis and affect the pituitary-adrenal axis. • Chemotherapeutic and immunosuppressive agents have toxic effects (e.g., myelosuppression).

FOLLOW-UP

PATIENT MONITORING
• Monitor primary disease as indicated. • Recheck eosinophil and basophil counts.

POSSIBLE COMPLICATIONS
Eosinophilic infiltrates can cause severe tissue damage.

MISCELLANEOUS

ASSOCIATED CONDITIONS
Basophilia is often associated with eosinophilia.

ZOONOTIC POTENTIAL
Some parasitic diseases

SEE ALSO
Hypereosinophilic Syndrome

ABBREVIATIONS
• FeLV = feline leukemia virus • GM-CSF = granulocyte-macrophage colony-stimulating factor • IL-2 = interleukin 2 • IL-5 = interleukin 5 • IL-12 = interleukin 12 • IMHA = immune-medated hemolytic anemia • PIE = pulmonary infiltrates with eosinophilia • SLE = systemic lupus erythematosus

Suggested Reading
Cowell RL, Decker LS. Interpretation of feline leukocyte responses. In: Feldman B, Zinkl J, Jain NC, eds. Schalm's veterinary hematology. 5th ed. Philadelphia: Lippincott Williams & Wilkins, 2000:382–390.
Schultze AE. Interpretation of canine leukocyte responses. In: Feldman B, Zinkl J, Jain NC, eds. Schalm's veterinary hematology. 5th ed. Philadelphia: Lippincott Williams & Wilkins, 2000:366–381.
Scott MA, Stockham SL. Basophils and mast cells. In: Feldman B, Zinkl J, Jain NC, eds. Schalm's veterinary hematology. 5th ed. Philadelphia: Lippincott Williams & Wilkins 2000:308–317.
Young KM. Eosinophils. In: Feldman B, Zinkl J, Jain NC, eds. Schalm's veterinary hematology. 5th ed. Philadelphia: Lippincott Williams & Wilkins, 2000:297–307.
Author Karen M. Young
Consulting Editor Stephen A. Kruth

EOSINOPHILIC GRANULOMA COMPLEX

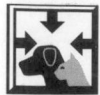

BASICS

DEFINITION
• Cats—often confusing term for three distinct syndromes: eosinophilic plaque, eosinophilic granuloma, and indolent ulcer; grouped primarily according to their clinical similarities, their frequent concurrent development, and their positive response to corticosteroids
• Dogs—eosinophilic granulomas in dogs (EGD) rare; not part of disease complex; specific differences from cats are listed separately.

PATHOPHYSIOLOGY
• Eosinophilic plaque—hypersensitivity reaction, most often to insects (fleas, mosquitos); less often to food or environmental allergens
• Eosinophilic granuloma—multiple causes, including hypersensitivity and genetic predisposition
• Indolent ulcer—may have both hypersensitivity and genetic causes
• Eosinophil—major infiltrative cell for eosinophilic granuloma and eosinophilic plaque; leukocyte located in greatest numbers in epithelial tissues; most often associated with allergic or parasitic conditions, but has a more general role in the inflammatory reaction
• EGD—may have both a genetic predisposition and a hypersensitivity cause

SYSTEMS AFFECTED
• Skin/Exocrine—the integument is most often affected.
• Oral cavity—eosinophilic granuloma can affect the tongue, palatine arches, and palate
• EGD—most often affects the tongue and palatine arches; reported cutaneous lesions on the prepuce and flanks

GENETICS
• Unknown
• Several reports of related affected individuals and a study of disease development in a colony of specific pathogen-free cats indicate that, in at least some individuals, genetic predisposition (perhaps resulting in a heritable dysfunction of eosinophilic regulation) is a significant component of the disease.

INCIDENCE/PREVALENCE
Unknown

GEOGRAPHIC DISTRIBUTION
Seasonal incidence in some geographic locations may indicate insect or environmental allergen exposure.

SIGNALMENT

Species
• Restricted to cats
• Eosinophilic granulomas occur in dogs and other species, but are not considered part of this disease complex.

Breed Predilections
• Cats—none
• EGD—Siberian huskies (76% of cases)

Mean Age and Range
• Eosinophilic plaque—2–6 years of age
• Genetically initiated eosinophilic granuloma—< 2 years of age
• Allergic disorder—> 2 years of age
• Indolent ulcer—no age predisposition reported
• EGD—usually < 3 years of age

Predominant Sex
• Cats—predilection for females has been reported only for the indolent ulcer.
• EGD—males (72% of cases)

SIGNS

General Comments
• Distinguishing among the syndromes depends on both clinical signs and histopathologic findings.
• Lesions of more than one syndrome may occur simultaneously.

Historical Findings
• Lesions of all three syndromes may develop spontaneously and acutely.
• Development of eosinophilic plaques can be preceded by periods of lethargy.
• A seasonal incidence is common.
• Waxing and waning of clinical signs is common in all three syndromes.

Physical Examination Findings
• Eosinophilic plaques—alopecic, erythematous, erosive patches and plaques; usually occur in the inguinal, perineal, lateral thigh, and axillary regions; frequently moist or glistening
• Eosinophilic granulomas—occur in a distinctly linear orientation (linear granuloma) on the caudal thigh, or as individual or coalescing plaques located anywhere on the body; ulcerated with a "cobblestone" or coarse pattern; white or yellow, possibly representing collagen degeneration; lip margin and chin swelling ("pouting"); footpad swelling, pain, and lameness; oral cavity ulcerations (especially on the tongue, palate, and palatine arches); cats with oral lesions may be dysphagic, have halitosis, and may drool.
• Lesion development may stop spontaneously in some cats, especially with the heritable form of eosinophilic plaque.
• Indolent ulcers—classically raised and indurated ulcerations confined to the upper lips adjacent to the philtrum
• EGD—ulcerated plaques and masses; dark or orange color

CAUSES
• Allergy—flea or insect, food hypersensitivity, and atopy
• A heritable dysfunction of eosinophil regulation has been proposed.

• EGD—unknown; a hypersensitivity reaction is often suspected (insect bite).

RISK FACTORS
N/A

DIAGNOSIS

DIFFERENTIAL DIAGNOSIS
• Includes the other diseases in the complex
• Unresponsive lesions—exclude pemphigus foliaceus, dermatophytosis and deep fungal infection, demodicosis, pyoderma, and neoplasia (especially metastatic adenocarcinoma and cutaneous lymphosarcoma)

CBC/BIOCHEMISTRY/URINALYSIS
• CBC—mild to moderate eosinophilia
• Biochemistry and urinalysis—usually normal

OTHER LABORATORY TESTS
FeLV and FIV—pruritic diseases have been associated with these viruses

IMAGING
N/A

DIAGNOSTIC PROCEDURES
• Impression smears from lesions—large numbers of eosinophils
• Comprehensive flea and insect control—assist in excluding flea or mosquito bite hypersensitivity
• Food-elimination trial—for all cases; feed a protein (e.g., lamb, pork, venison, or rabbit) to which the cat has never been exposed; use exclusively for 8–10 weeks; then reinstitute previous diet and observe for development of new lesions.
• Environmental allergy (atopy)—identified by intradermal skin testing (some cases); inject small amounts of dilute allergens intradermally; positive reaction (allergy) is indicated by the development of a hive or wheal at the injection site.
• In vitro serum tests—available for identifying allergy-specific serum in cats; tests have not been validated and are not recommended over intradermal testing.

PATHOLOGIC FINDINGS
• Histopathologic diagnosis—required for distinguishing the syndromes
• Biopsy samples from indolent ulcers frequently fail to reveal eosinophils.
• Eosinophilic plaque—severe epidermal and follicular acanthosis with eosinophilic exocytosis and spongiosis; intense eosinophilic dermal infiltrate common; epidermis commonly eroded or ulcerated
• Eosinophilic granuloma—distinct foci of eosinophilic degranulation and collagen degeneration similar to granuloma formation; epidermis may be eroded or ulcerated.
• Indolent ulcer—early lesions may be indistinguishable from those of eosinophilic granuloma (eosinophilic infiltration and

collagen degeneration); late-stage lesions characterized by fibrosis with perivascular neutrophilic and mononuclear infiltration
• EGD—foci of collagen degeneration with palisading granulomas; eosinophilic and histiocytic infiltration

 TREATMENT

APPROPRIATE HEALTH CARE
• Most patients can be treated as outpatients unless severe oral disease prevents adequate fluid intake.
• Try to identify and eliminate offending allergen(s) before providing medical intervention.
• Hyposensitization of intradermal skin test–positive cats—may be successful in 60%–73% of cases; preferable to long-term corticosteroid administration

NURSING CARE
Discourage client from damaging lesions by excessive grooming.

ACTIVITY
No restrictions

DIET
No restrictions unless a food allergy is suspected

CLIENT EDUCATION
• Inform clients about the possible allergic or heritable causes.
• Discuss the waxing and waning nature of these diseases.
• Responsible clients may choose to postpone medical intervention, unless severe lesions develop.

SURGICAL CONSIDERATIONS
None

 MEDICATIONS

DRUG(S) OF CHOICE
Eosinophilic Plaque
• Injectable methylprednisolone—20 mg/cat, repeat in 2 weeks (if needed); most common treatment
• Corticosteroids—ongoing treatment with prednisone (3–5 mg/kg q48h) required to control lesions; steroid tachyphylaxis may occur and may be specific to the drug administered; may be useful to changing the formulation; other drugs: dexamethasone (0.1–0.2 mg/kg q24–72h) and triamcinolone (0.1–0.2 mg/kg q24–72h); higher induction dosages may be required but should be tapered as quickly as possible.

Eosinophilic Granuloma
• Injectable or oral corticosteroids—see Eosinophilic Plaque (above); most common treatment

• Combination of oral corticosteroids and selective immunosuppressive agents—for severe lesions; e.g., chlorambucil (0.1–0.2 mg/kg q24–48h)
• Chrysotherapy with aurothioglucose—1 mg/kg IM every 7 days; mixed results
• Cyclophosphamide—1 mg/kg q24h for 4 out of every 7 days; another alternative
• Antibiotics—may be beneficial if oral lesions are secondarily infected

Indolent Ulcer
• Injectable or oral corticosteroids—see Eosinophilic Plaque (above)
• α-interferon—30–60 U daily in cycles of 7 days on, 7 days off; limited success; side effects rare; no specific treatment monitoring required
• Antibiotics—clindamycin 5.5 mg/kg BID PO, cephalexin (22 mg/kg PO q12h), or amoxicillin trihydrate-clavulanate (12.5 mg/kg PO q12h); effective in some cases; preferable to long-term corticosteroid administration; response may be the result of the anti-inflammatory activity of these drugs rather than their primary bactericidal properties

Alternate Therapies
• Radiation, surgical excision, and immuno-modulation (e.g., levamisole, bacterin injections)—occasional reports of success
• CO_2 laser—may offer relief from individual or painful lesions, especially those in the mouth
• Topical—application of potent cortico-steroid ointments may help with isolated lesions but is rarely practical.
• Doxycycline 5 mg/kg BID; cyclosporine (Neoral) 5 mg/kg/day

EGD
• Oral prednisone—0.5–2.2 mg/kg/day initially; then taper gradually
• Cessation of therapy without recurrence is common.

CONTRAINDICATIONS
N/A

PRECAUTIONS
N/A

POSSIBLE INTERACTIONS
N/A

ALTERNATIVE DRUG(S)
Megestrol acetate—2.5–5 mg every 2–7 days; can be effective in rare cases; not recommended because of the severity of possible side effects

 FOLLOW-UP

PATIENT MONITORING
• Corticosteroids—baseline and frequent hemograms, serum chemistry profiles, and urinalyses with culture
• Selective immunosuppressant drugs—frequent hemograms (biweekly at first, then monthly or bimonthly as therapy continues) to monitor for bone marrow suppression;

routine serum chemistry profiles and urinalyses with culture (monthly at first, then every 3 months) to monitor for complications (renal disease, diabetes mellitus, and urinary tract infection)

PREVENTION/AVOIDANCE
N/A

POSSIBLE COMPLICATIONS
N/A

EXPECTED COURSE AND PROGNOSIS
• If a primary cause (allergy) can be determined and controlled, lesions should resolve permanently, unless the animal re-encounters the offending allergen.
• Most lesions wax and wane, with or without therapy; thus an unpredictable schedule of recurrence should be anticipated.
• Drug dosages should be tapered to the lowest possible level (or discontinued, if possible) once the lesions have resolved.

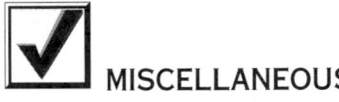 MISCELLANEOUS

ASSOCIATED CONDITIONS
N/A

AGE-RELATED FACTORS
N/A

ZOONOTIC POTENTIAL
N/A

PREGNANCY
Systemic glucocorticoids and immuno-suppressive drugs should not be used during pregnancy.

SYNONYMS
• Eosinophilic granuloma—feline collagenolytic granuloma; feline linear granuloma
• Indolent ulcer—eosinophilic ulcer; rodent ulcer; feline upper lip ulcerative dermatitis

SEE ALSO
• Atopy
• Food Reactions (Dermatologic)

ABBREVIATION
• FeLV = feline leukemia virus
• FIV = feline immunodeficiency virus
• EGD = eosinophilic granulomas in dogs

Suggested Reading
Power HT, Ihrke PJ. Selected feline eosinophilic skin diseases (eosinophilic granuloma complex). In: Kunkle G, ed. Feline dermatoses. Vet Clin North Am Sm Anim Pract 1995;25:833–850.
Rosenkrantz WS. Feline eosinophilic granu-loma complex. In: Griffin CE, Kwochka KW, MacDonald JM, eds. Current veteri-nary dermatology: the science and art of therapy. St. Louis: Mosby, 1993.
Author Alexander H. Werner
Consulting Editor Karen Helton Rhodes

EPIDIDYMITIS/ORCHITIS

 BASICS

OVERVIEW
• Epididymitis—inflammation of the epididymis
• Orchitis—inflammation of the testis
• May be acute or chronic
• Direct trauma to the scrotum—most common cause of acute form

SIGNALMENT
• Not uncommon in dogs; rare in cats
• No genetic basis or breed predilections
• Mean age 3.7 years; range 11 months to 10 years

SIGNS
• Swollen testis
• Pain (acute)
• Licking of the scrotum—may lead to dermatitis
• Listlessness
• Anorexia
• Reluctance to walk
• Open wound or abscess
• Infertility
• Pyrexia

CAUSES & RISK FACTORS
• *Brucella canis*—predilection for infecting the tail of the epididymis
• Distemper
• Ascending infection—associated with prostatitis and cystitis
• Retrograde urine contamination of the ductus deferens—sequel to high intra-abdominal pressure as caused by automobile trauma
• Bite wounds and other puncture wounds—isolated from infected testes: *Staphylococcus, Streptococcus, Escherichia coli, Protcus,* and *Mycoplasma*
• Lymphocytic autoimmune thyroiditis and orchitis—familial in beagles

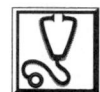 DIAGNOSIS

DIFFERENTIAL DIAGNOSIS
• Inguinoscrotal hernia
• Scrotal dermatitis
• Torsion of the spermatic cord
• Hydrocele
• Sperm granuloma
• Testicular neoplasia
• Prostatitis
• Cystitis

CBC/BIOCHEMISTRY/URINALYSIS
• Leukocytosis—may be found with acute or infectious orchitis
• Pyuria, hematuria, proteinuria—may be found if epididymitis/orchitis is secondary to prostatitis or cystitis

OTHER LABORATORY TESTS
• *B. canis* antibodies—perform immediate testing in any dog with scrotal enlargement.

IMAGING
• Ultrasonographic evaluation of the prostate—guided aspiration for cytologic examination and bacterial culture
• Ultrasonographic evaluation of the testes and epididymides—inflamed testes have patchy hypoechoic areas; inflamed epididymides have irregular contours and hypoechoic or hyperechoic areas; obtain measurements for future comparisons.

DIAGNOSTIC PROCEDURES
• Semen—collect if possible; cytological evaluation; bacterial culture
• Cytology (semen)—leukocytes; bacteria; spermatozoa with coiled tails, detached heads, and retained proximal and distal cytoplasmic droplets; head-to-head agglutination (*B. canis*)
• Prostatic massage—cytologic examination; bacterial culture; sample collected aseptically by urethral catheter
• Open wounds—bacterial culture
• Fine needle aspirate—sample enlarged testes/epididymes for cytology and culture; leukocytes vary from numerous neutrophils (suppurative) to minimal inflammatory cells (granulomatous).

 TREATMENT
• Fertility not a concern—culture appropriate specimen; administer needed antibiotics; medically stabilize; castrate
• Fertility a concern (unilateral orchitis)—unilateral castration when the patient's future as a sire must be maintained

 MEDICATIONS

DRUG(S)
Antibiotics—continue for at least 3 weeks; initially oxacillin, trimethoprim-sulfonamide, aminoglycoside, or enrofloxacin; changed when results of culture and sensitivity testing are available; antibiotic therapy without unilateral or bilateral castration unlikely to be successful

CONTRAINDICATIONS/POSSIBLE INTERACTIONS
N/A

 FOLLOW-UP
• Prognosis for fertility—guarded to poor, especially with bilateral orchitis
• Testicular heating causes testicular degeneration—degeneration in contralateral testis can result from primary disease or following unilateral castration.

• Trauma or inflammation can cause obstruction of efferent tubules or epididymal duct, leading to spermatoceles or sperm granuloma
• Semen (dogs)—evaluate characteristics 3 months after treatment for orchitis is completed

 MISCELLANEOUS

Suggested Reading
Feldman EC, Nelson RW. Canine and feline endocrinology and reproduction. Philadelphia: Saunders, 1987:705–709.
Johnston SD, Root Kustritz MV, Olson PNS. Disorders of the canine testis and epididymes. Canine and feline theriogenology. Philadelphia: Saunders, 2001:313–317.
Authors Carlos R. F. Pinto and Rolf E. Larsen
Consulting Editor Sara K. Lyle

EPILEPSY, IDIOPATHIC, GENETIC, PRIMARY

BASICS

DEFINITION
• A brain disorder characterized by recurrent seizures in the absence of morphologic brain lesion • The brain is structurally normal but not functionally normal.

PATHOPHYSIOLOGY
• Exact mechanism unknown
• Dysfunction may be biochemical or the animal may have an intrinsic propensity to have seizures.
• Likely different mechanisms between breeds

SYSTEMS AFFECTED
Nervous

GENETICS
• Genetic in many breeds • Mode of inheritance unknown (several have been suggested) • Primary generalized epilepsy—likely genetic. Seizures generalized from onset
• Idiopathic epilepsy—may be genetic in some breeds. Seizures often partial at onset (aura) but have frequent rapid secondary generalization

INCIDENCE/PREVALENCE
• Between 0.5% and 2.3% of all dogs; higher for dogs in research colonies • Highly prevalent; 40%–80% of dogs with seizure activity • Cats—rare; poorly documented

GEOGRAPHIC DISTRIBUTION
Widespread

SIGNALMENT

Species
Dogs and rarely cats

Breed Predilections
Beagles; all shepherds (German, Australian, Belgian Tervuren); border collies; boxers; cocker spaniels; collies; dachshunds; golden retrievers; Irish setters; keeshonds; Labrador retrievers; poodles (all sizes); St. Bernards; Shetland sheepdogs; Siberian huskies; springer spaniels; Welsh corgis; wire-haired fox terriers

Mean Age and Range
• Range—6 months to 5 years
• Prevalence—6 months to 3 years

Predominant Sex
Male

SIGNS

General Comments
• Seizures are generalized (bilateral and symmetrical) and usually convulsive.
• In idiopathic epilepsy, there is frequently an aura (animal appears frightened, dazed, seeks attention, or hides, etc.) preceding the convulsion.

Historical Findings
• Seizures—most occur while the patient is resting or asleep; often at night or in early morning; frequency tends to increase if left untreated; affected animal becomes stiff, chomps its jaw, salivates profusely, urinates, defecates, vocalizes, and paddles with all four limbs in varying combinations. • Postseizure behavior—periods of confusion and disorientation; aimless, compulsive, blind, pacing; frequent polydipsia and polyphagia; recovery immediate or may take up to 24 hr
• Dogs with established epilepsy experience cluster seizures at regular intervals of 1–4 weeks; particularly prevalent in large-breed dogs

Physical Examination Findings
• None; patient usually recovered
• Patient may be in the postictal phase of the seizure at presentation

CAUSES
Likely genetic in some breeds, idiopathic in others

RISK FACTORS
Acepromazine—may cause seizures in otherwise normal dogs by lowering seizure threshold

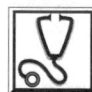

DIAGNOSIS

DIFFERENTIAL DIAGNOSIS
• Two most important factors—age at onset and pattern of seizures (type and frequency)
• First seizure—between 6 months and 5 years; the younger the animal, the more severe the epilepsy; as a rule, with an onset < 2 years, the condition frequently becomes refractory to medication. • Acute onset of cluster seizures or status epilepticus—unusual; rule out toxicity or structural brain disease • More than two seizures within the first week at onset—consider a diagnosis other than idiopathic or genetic epilepsy.
• Seizures at < 6 months or > 5 years of age—may be metabolic or intracranial and structural in origin • Partial seizures or neurologic deficits—indicate structural intracranial disease

CBC/BIOCHEMISTRY/URINALYSIS
• Usually normal
• Perform before initiation of antiepileptic medication, to obtain baseline data.

OTHER LABORATORY TESTS
• Bile acids unnecessary in dogs that have seizures without accompanying episodic abnormal behavior

IMAGING
MRI and CT—only for suspected structural intracranial diseases

DIAGNOSTIC PROCEDURES
CSF analysis—for suspected structural intracranial diseases

PATHOLOGIC FINDINGS
• No primary lesion

• Secondary neuronal loss and gliosis from prolonged or repeated seizures

TREATMENT

APPROPRIATE HEALTH CARE
• Initiate treatment at the second generalized seizure or if there are acute cluster seizures, or acute status epilepticus. • Inpatient—cluster seizures (> 1 seizure/24 hr) or status epilepticus; treat early and aggressively.
• Outpatient—recurrence of isolated seizures

NURSING CARE
• Inpatients with a seizure disorder require constant monitoring.

ACTIVITY
Avoid swimming to prevent drowning.

DIET
• Most dogs on chronic antiepileptic drugs become overweight; monitor closely; add a weight-reducing program as necessary.
• KBr treatment—patients should have steady levels of salt in their diet; an increase in salt causes an increase in bromide excretion preferentially over chloride, with subsequent decreased serum KBr levels; S/D prescription diets have higher chloride contents than do most diets.

CLIENT EDUCATION
• Inform client that animals do not die after a seizure; however, severe cluster seizures and status epilepticus are life-threatening emergencies that require immediate and aggressive medical attention. • Advise client that he or she should prevent the patient from injuring itself on surrounding objects during a seizure. • Encourage client to keep a calendar of the seizures, because it is the only objective way to assess response to treatment.
• Inform client that once treatment is instituted, the patient will require medication for life in most cases.

SURGICAL CONSIDERATIONS
Corpus callosum section—selected refractory patients

MEDICATIONS

DRUG(S) OF CHOICE

Phenobarbital and KBr
• Steady state—phenobarbital requires 12–15 days; KBr requires 3–4 months and varies with salt concentration in diet; if necessary, give both drugs at loading dosages to reach therapeutic levels rapidly (seizures may continue until steady state is reached). • Both drugs combined—may produce a beneficial and synergistic effect • **Phenobarbital**—traditional first-line drug; initial dosage: 2–5 mg/kg PO q12h; evaluate serum levels 12–15

days after onset of treatment and after changes in dosage; levels decrease significantly in the first few weeks owing to activation of the lysosomal enzymes; evaluate levels again 4 weeks after initiation; optimal serum levels: 100–120 μmol/L or 23–28 μg/mL; increase dosage if needed and recheck levels until optimal therapeutic range is reached • **KBr**— alternative first-line drug; initial dosage: 30 mg/kg PO q24h or divided q12h; use same dosage as a substitute for or added to phenobarbital for patients started on PB that continue to have seizures at a frequency of more than one every 6–8 weeks; optimal serum levels: 15–20 mmol/L or 1.2–1.6 mg/mL; if KBr used as sole antiepileptic agent, serum level of 20–30 mmol/L can be safely used. Loading Doses
• Sometimes desirable to reach the therapeutic range rapidly • Phenobarbital— intravenous loading dose (total mg) = desired serum level (μg/mL) × body weight (kg) × 0.8 L/kg; oral loading dose: 5–10 mg/kg q12h for 2 days • KBr—orally only; in principle, 600 mg/kg necessary to reach optimal range; but acute large doses lead frequently to vomiting, diarrhea, profound longstanding sedation. We advocate to treat with lower loading doses twice daily (30 mg–60 mg/kg q12h) to minimize side effects.

Diazepam
• To treat ongoing seizures; dogs with cluster seizures or status epilepticus • Inpatient treatment—0.5–1.0 mg/kg IV bolus; repeat in 5 min if gross motor seizure activity persists; follow immediately with 0.5–1.0 mg/kg constant-rate infusion added to the maintenance fluids in an in-line burette (prepare only 1–2 hr of infusion at a time to avoid adsorption to the plastic tubing); if seizures continue, add phenobarbital at 2–12 mg/dog/hr; once seizures have been controlled for at least 4–6 hr, slowly decrease the infusion rate, discontinuing over 4–12 hr • Reinstate oral medications as soon as possible; increase the oral dosage of KBr and/or phenobarbital to optimal ranges if the serum drug levels before emergency treatment were inadequate. • Outpatient treatment—for cluster seizures; on the seizing day, insert 0.5–1.0 mg/kg injectable drug in the rectum via a teat cannula as soon as a seizure occurs; repeat 20 and 40 min later for a total of three insertions within 40 min; mimics intravenous infusion; given early in the course of ongoing seizures, increases the chance to abort subsequent seizures

CONTRAINDICATIONS
Acepromazine, xylazine—do not administer; may cause seizure activity

PRECAUTIONS
• Phenobarbital and diazepam—use caution when combining for status epilepticus; they act synergistically; cardiac and respiratory depression may ensue.

• Phenobarbital—polyphagia; polydipsia,
• KBr—polyuria/polydipsia; polyphagia

POSSIBLE INTERACTIONS
• Cimetidine and chloramphenicol—interfere with the metabolism of phenobarbital; may lead to toxic levels of phenobarbital
• Whenever drugs must be given to affected animals on lifetime medication, refer to the manufacturer's drug profile or a pharmacist for interaction information.

ALTERNATIVE DRUG(S)
• Human antiepileptic drugs—phenytoin, valproic acid, and carbamazepine cannot be used in dogs because of unsuitable pharmacokinetics. • If phenobarbital and KBr fail, contact a veterinary neurologist. • Other treatments—gabapentin, felbamate, clorazepate, clonazepam, vigabatrin, zonisamide • Acupuncture, vagal nerve stimulation

 FOLLOW-UP

PATIENT MONITORING
• Serum drug levels—essential to monitor; blood is usually drawn at trough and, if possible, at the same time for each sampling.
• Phenobarbital—measure 2 and 4 weeks after initiating therapy; adjust oral dose as needed; repeat until the optimal serum levels are reached; at these levels, hepatotoxicity is not as likely and the patients that are going to respond will have; with chronic use perform hemogram, serum chemistry profile, and drug levels every 6–12 months to monitor side effects; keep records of albumin, liver enzymes, and serum drug levels; drug essentially hepatotoxic and most dogs eventually develop hepatotoxicity if serum levels > 140 μmol/L for a long time (> 1 yr)
• KBr—elimination rate depends on concentration of salt in the food; measure serum levels (along with phenobarbital levels) 4–6 weeks after initiating (should be 8–12 mmol/L or 0.5–1.0 mg/mL); seems to enhance excretion or metabolism of phenobarbital, causing levels to drop
• Monitor particularly well older dogs with renal insufficiency and on KBr treatment.

PREVENTION/AVOIDANCE
• Discuss with the client the possibility of inheritance and, for this reason, consider neutering. • For humans and animals, unknown if estrogens decrease seizure threshold; unlikely • Abrupt discontinuation of oral medication may precipitate seizures.

POSSIBLE COMPLICATIONS
• Phenobarbital-induced high SAP (isoenzyme-steroid band)—occurs frequently; may be an early sign of hepatotoxicity but is of less concern if ALT is within reference range

• Phenobarbital-induced hepatotoxicity— occurs after chronic treatment at serum levels in the middle to upper therapeutic range (> 140 μmol/L or > 33 μg/mL); may be insidious in onset; the only biochemical abnormality may be a decrease in albumin.
• Rare bone marrow suppression with neutropenia may develop after onset of phenobarbital; discontinue drug.
• KBr—when levels are > 22 mmol/L or > 1.8 mg/mL, owners may complain of patients' unsteadiness while managing stairs.
• Higher incidence of pancreatitis in patients treated with phenobarbital and KBr; once dog develops pancreatitis, recurrence is frequent

EXPECTED COURSE AND PROGNOSIS
• Antiepileptic treatment—decreases frequency, severity, and length of seizures; perfect control rarely achieved
• In many young, large-breed dogs, seizures may continue despite adequate treatment.
• Refractoriness may develop.
• Patient may develop status epilepticus and die.

 MISCELLANEOUS

ASSOCIATED CONDITIONS
N/A

AGE-RELATED FACTORS
• If onset is < 2 years of age, seizures are more likely to be difficult to control.
• If onset is > 3 years of age, generally seizures have more chances to be adequately controlled.

ZOONOTIC POTENTIAL
N/A

PREGNANCY
Avoid breeding affected animals.

SYNONYMS
Primary generalized epilepsy

SEE ALSO
Seizures (Convulsions, Status Epilepticus)— Dogs

ABBREVIATIONS
• ALT = alanine aminotransferase • CSF = cerebrospinal fluid • CT = computed tomography • KBr = potassium bromide • MRI = magnetic resonance imaging • SAP = serum alkaline phosphatase

Suggested Reading
Oliver JE, Lorenz MD, Kornegay JN. Handbook of veterinary neurology, 3rd ed. Philadelphia: Saunders, 1997.
Podell M. Canine epilepsy. In: Standards of care: emergency and critical care medicine. Vol. 1. Standards of Care 1999:1–8.
Author Joane M. Parent
Consulting Editor Joane M. Parent

EPIPHORA

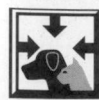 **BASICS**

DEFINITION
Abnormal overflow of the aqueous portion of the precorneal tear film

PATHOPHYSIOLOGY
Caused by overproduction of the aqueous portion of tears (usually in response to ocular irritation), poor eyelid function secondary to malformation or deformity, or blockage of the nasolacrimal drainage system

SYSTEMS AFFECTED
Ophthalmic

SIGNALMENT
See Causes

SIGNS
N/A

CAUSES

Overproduction of Tears Secondary to Ocular Irritants
Congenital
• Distichiasis or trichiasis—young shelties; shih tzus; lhasa apsos; cocker spaniels; miniature poodles
• Entropion—shar peis; chow chows
• Eyelid agenesis—domestic shorthaired cats
Acquired
• Corneal or conjunctival foreign bodies—usually young, large-breed, active dogs
• Eyelid neoplasms—old dogs (all breeds)
• Blepharitis—infectious or immune-mediated
• Conjunctivitis—infectious or immune-mediated
• Ulcerative keratitis
• Anterior uveitis
• Glaucoma

Eyelid Abnormalities or Poor Eyelid Function
Tears never reach the nasolacrimal puncta but instead spill over the eyelid margin.
Congenital
• Macropalpebral fissures—brachiocephalic breeds
• Ectropion—Great Danes; bloodhounds; spaniels
• Entropion—especially of the medial lower lid
Acquired
• Post-traumatic eyelid scarring
• Facial nerve paralysis

Obstruction of the Nasolacrimal Drainage System
Congenital
• Imperforate nasolacrimal puncta—cocker spaniels; bulldogs; poodles
• Ectopic nasolacrimal openings—extra openings along the side of the face ventral to the medial canthus
• Nasolacrimal atresia—lack of distal openings into the nose
Acquired
• Rhinitis or sinusitis—causes swelling adjacent to the nasolacrimal duct
• Trauma or fractures of the lacrimal or maxillary bones
• Foreign bodies—grass awns; seeds; sand; parasites
• Neoplasia—of the third eyelid, conjunctiva, medial eyelids, nasal cavity, maxillary bone, or periocular sinuses
• Dacryocystitis—inflammation of the canaliculi, lacrimal sac, or nasolacrimal ducts

RISK FACTORS
• Breeds prone to congenital eyelid abnormalities (see Causes)
• Active outdoor dogs—at risk for foreign bodies

 DIAGNOSIS

DIFFERENTIAL DIAGNOSIS
• Other ocular discharges (e.g., mucous or purulent)—epiphora is a watery, serous discharge.
• Eye—usually red when caused by overproduction of tears; quiet when secondary to impaired outflow
• Irritative causes and some congenital causes of obstruction—thorough ocular examination
• Acute onset, unilateral condition with ocular pain (blepharospasm)—usually indicates a foreign body or corneal injury
• Chronic, bilateral condition—usually indicates a congenital problem
• Facial pain, swelling, nasal discharge, or sneezing—may indicate nasal or sinus infection; may indicate obstruction from neoplasm
• With mucous or purulent discharge at the medial canthus—may indicate dacryocystitis

CBC/BIOCHEMISTRY/URINALYSIS
N/A

OTHER LABORATORY TESTS
N/A

IMAGING
• Skull radiographs—may show a nasal, sinus, or maxillary bone lesion
• Dacryocystorhinography—radiopaque contrast material to help localize obstruction
• MRI or CT—may help localize obstruction and characterize associated lesions

DIAGNOSTIC PROCEDURES
• Bacterial culture and sensitivity testing and cytologic examination of the material—with purulent material at the medial canthus (e.g., dacryocystitis); performed before instilling any substance into the eye
• Topical fluorescein dye application to the eye—most physiologic test for nasolacrimal function; should be performed first; dye flows through the nasolacrimal system and reaches the external nares in approximately 10 sec in normal dogs.
• Rhinoscopy—with or without biopsy or bacterial culture; may be indicated if previous tests suggest a nasal or sinus lesion
• Surgical exploratory—may be the only way to obtain a definitive diagnosis
• Temporary tacking out of the lower medial eyelid with suture—may help determine whether repair of medial lower entropion or repositioning of the eyelid would reduce epiphora secondary to eyelid conformational abnormalities

Nasolacrimal Flush
• Confirms obstruction
• May dislodge foreign material
• A nasolacrimal cannula is inserted into the upper nasolacrimal punctum
• Eyewash is flushed through the cannula—if fluid does not exit the lower nasolacrimal punctum, the obstruction is in the upper or lower canaliculi, the nasolacrimal sac, or the lower punctum (imperforate).
• Lower punctum is manually obstructed—if flushed fluid does not exit the external nares, the obstruction is in the nasolacrimal duct or at its distal opening (atresia or blockage from a nasal sinus lesion).

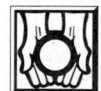 **TREATMENT**

• Remove cause of ocular irritation—removal of a conjunctival or corneal foreign body; treatment of the primary ocular disease (e.g., conjunctivitis, ulcerative keratitis, and uveitis); cryosurgery or electroepilation for distichiasis, entropion correction; medial or

lateral canthoplasty (for medial trichiasis and macropalpebral fissures); correction of cicatricial eyelid abnormalities
• Treat primary obstructing lesion (e.g., third eyelid mass, nasal or sinus mass, and infection)—do initially; successful management may allow normal nasolacrimal flow to resume.
• Warn client that patient is predisposed to nasolacrimal obstruction and that recurrence is common.
• Inform client that early detection and intervention provide a better long-term prognosis.

SURGICAL CONSIDERATIONS

Imperforate Puncta
• Surgical opening of the puncta is indicated.
• If one of the puncta is patent (usually the upper punctum), flushing eyewash through the upper opening will cause "tenting" of the conjunctiva at the site of the lower punctum.
• Place patient under topical or general anesthesia.
• Grasp conjunctiva overlying the lower canaliculi with forceps and cut with scissors to leave a patent punctum.
• Puncta closed by conjunctival scarring (symblepharon) caused by severe conjunctivitis (e.g., herpesvirus conjunctivitis in cats)—use same procedure.
• Recurrent disease—may be necessary to suture Silastic tubing in place to prevent stricture formation.

Obstructed or Obliterated Distal Nasolacrimal Duct
• Dacryocystorhinotomy or conjunctivorhinostomy—create an opening to drain the tears into the nasal cavity
• See Suggested Reading for surgical technique.

 MEDICATIONS

DRUG(S) OF CHOICE
• Topical broad-spectrum antibiotic ophthalmic solutions—while waiting for results of diagnostic tests (e.g., bacterial culture and sensitivity testing; diagnostic radiographs); q4–6h; may try neomycin, gramicidin, polymyxin B triple ophthalmic antibiotic solutions, or ophthalmic chloramphenicol solution
• Dacryocystitis—based on bacterial culture and sensitivity test results; continued for at least 21 days

CONTRAINDICATIONS
• Topical corticosteroids or antibiotic–corticosteroid combinations—avoid unless a definitive diagnosis has been made.
• Topical corticosteroids—never use if the cornea retains fluorescein stain.

PRECAUTIONS
N/A

POSSIBLE INTERACTIONS
N/A

ALTERNATIVE DRUG(S)
Tetracycline—5 mg/kg PO q24h; may help reduce idiopathic tear staining of the periocular facial hair; staining recurs when the drug is discontinued.

 FOLLOW-UP

PATIENT MONITORING

Dacryocystitis
• Reevaluate every 7 days until the condition is resolved.
• Continue treatment for at least 7 days after resolution of clinical signs to help prevent recurrence.
• Problem persists more than 7–10 days with treatment or recurs soon after cessation of treatment—indicates a foreign body or nidus of persistent infection; requires further diagnostics (e.g., dacryocystorhinography)
Nasolacrimal Catheter
• Commonly required for persistent dacryocystitis
• Maintains patency of the duct and prevents stricturing
• Catheter—Silastic or polyethylene (PE90) tubing; left in place 2–4 weeks
• Procedure—pass 2-0 nylon via the upper punctum and thread it through the nasolacrimal duct to exit the external nares; pass tubing retrograde over the suture; suture the upper and lower portions of the tubing to the face.
• Most dogs tolerate the tubing well.
• Continue topical antibiotics as before.

Dacryocystorhinotomy/Conjunctivorhinostomy
• Tubing—reevaluate every 7 days to ensure it remains intact; may need to resuture if it becomes loosened or dislodged
• After tubing has been removed—reevaluate in 14 days; for this and future examinations,

place fluorescein on the eye and check nasolacrimal patency by examining the external nares for fluorescein; may evaluate the nasolacrimal system further by cannulating and flushing with eyewash
• Dacryocystorhinography contrast study—repeated 3–4 months after surgery to evaluate size of the nasal opening; repeated for recurrence or with no nasolacrimal fluorescein drainage

POSSIBLE COMPLICATIONS
• Recurrence—most common complication; caused by recurrence of ocular irritation (e.g., corneal ulceration, distichiasis, entropion), recurrence of dacryocystitis, or closure of the dacryocystorhinotomy or conjunctivorhinostomy openings into the nasal cavity

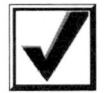 **MISCELLANEOUS**

ASSOCIATED CONDITIONS
• Chronic conjunctivitis—Cats
• Chronic conjunctivitis—Dogs
• Recurrent eye "infections"
• Moist dermatitis (hot spots) ventral to the medial canthus
• Nasal discharge

AGE-RELATED FACTORS
N/A

ZOONOTIC POTENTIAL
N/A

PREGNANCY
N/A

SEE ALSO
• Conjunctivitis—Cats
• Conjunctivitis—Dogs
• Eyelash Disorders (Trichiasis/Distichiasis/Ectopic Cilia)
• Keratitis, Ulcerative
• Third Eyelid Protrusion

Suggested Reading
Grahn BH. Diseases and surgery of the canine nasolacrimal system. In: Gelatt KN, ed. Veterinary ophthalmology. 3rd ed. Philadelphia: Lippincott Williams & Wilkins, 1999; 569–581.
Author Brian C. Gilger
Consulting Editor Paul E. Miller

EPISCLERITIS

BASICS

OVERVIEW
• Focal or diffuse infiltration of the episclera and/or scleral stroma by a varying mix of inflammatory cells and fibroblasts
• Primary—affects only the eye; probably immune mediated; appears either as a peri-limbal episcleral/scleral nodule (nodular episcleritis) or as a diffuse thickening of the episclera (diffuse episcleritis); nodular form may affect cornea and third eyelid with similar appearing nodules
• Secondary—usually diffuse; from the spillover of inflammatory cells into the episclera from other ocular disorders (e.g., endophthal-mitis and panophthalmitis); may affect virtually any other organ system

SIGNALMENT
• Dogs
• Young to middle-aged collies, Shetland sheepdogs

SIGNS
• Nodular—typically appears as a smooth, painless, localized, raised, pink-tan, firm episcleral/scleral mass.
• Diffuse—less common; appears as a diffuse reddening and thickening of the entire episclera/sclera; accompanied by variable amounts of ocular pain
• Secondary—uveitis often pronounced
• Conjunctiva—usually moves freely over the surface of the lesion
• Nodules—tend to be slowly progressive, bilateral, and prone to recurrence

CAUSES & RISK FACTORS
• Nodular and diffuse primary—idiopathic; believed to be immune mediated
• Secondary—may result from deep fungal or bacterial ocular infection, lymphosarcoma, systemic histiocytosis in Bernese mountain dogs, chronic glaucoma, and ocular trauma

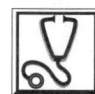

DIAGNOSIS

DIFFERENTIAL DIAGNOSIS
• Other causes of a red eye—differentiated by careful ophthalmic examination and tonometry
• Other mass-like lesions—differentiated by biopsy or cytologic examination
• Neoplasia—lymphosarcoma; squamous cell carcinoma; extension of an intraocular mass; other tumors
• Granuloma—deep fungal infection; retained foreign body
• Granulation tissue—trauma; healing corneal ulcer; globe perforation with uveal prolapse

CBC/BIOCHEMISTRY/URINALYSIS
• Usually normal if the lesion is confined to eye or adnexa
• Secondary—may see abnormalities consist-ent with other systemic diseases (e.g., deep fungal or systemic histiocytosis)

OTHER LABORATORY TESTS
• Rheumatoid factor, antinuclear antibody, and lupus erythematosus cell preparations—usually not helpful
• Serologic testing—may help rule out deep fungal infection

IMAGING
• Thoracic and abdominal radiographs or abdominal ultrasound—may help rule out deep fungal infection or disseminated neoplasia
• Ocular ultrasound—may help reveal other ocular abnormalities if ocular media opacities prevent a thorough ocular examination

DIAGNOSTIC PROCEDURES
• Incisional biopsy and histopathologic examination of affected tissue
• Nodular—typified by varying numbers of histiocytes, lymphocytes, plasma cells, and fibroblasts
• If uveitis prominent—perform a uveitis workup (see Anterior Uveitis—Dogs).

TREATMENT

• Try to verify the diagnosis histologically or cytologically before treatment.
• Primary nodular—tends to have a benign course; observation alone may be appropriate with mild disease
• Outpatient—if ocular pain, diffuse scleral involvement, disruption of eyelid function, corneal encroachment, or threat to vision

MEDICATIONS

DRUG(S)

• Progress down the list only if the previous modality was ineffective.
• Topically applied 1% prednisolone acetate—q4h for 1 week; then q6h for 2 weeks; then tapered
• Systemically administered prednisolone—1–2 mg/kg/day; tapered with improvement
• Systemically administered azathioprine—1–2 mg/kg/day for 3–7 days; then tapered to as low a dosage as possible
• Cryosurgery or attempt excision
• Alternative to listed drugs or surgery—may try a combination of tetracycline and niacinamide (q8h PO); 250 mg each for dogs < 10 kg; 500 mg each for dogs > 10 kg; may not observe good clinical response for at least 8 weeks; side effects uncommon and primarily the result of gastrointestinal upset by niacinamide

CONTRAINDICATIONS/POSSIBLE INTERACTIONS

• Avoid systemic immunosuppressive drugs with deep fungal infections.
• Systemically administered prednisolone or azathioprine—may precipitate pancreatitis; potentially hepatotoxic
• Azathioprine—may induce potentially fatal myelosuppression
• Niacin—do not substitute for niacinamide.

FOLLOW-UP

PATIENT MONITORING

• Primary—monitor for nodule regression or reduction in episcleral thickening or reddening every 2–3 weeks for 6–9 weeks and then as needed; prognosis usually good; may require therapy for months to life
• Secondary—follow-up, prognosis, and complications usually depend on the primary disease.
• Azathioprine—repeat CBC, platelet count, and measurement of liver enzymes every 1–2 weeks for the first 8 weeks, then periodically.

POSSIBLE COMPLICATIONS

• Vision loss
• Chronic ocular pain
• Uveitis
• Secondary glaucoma

MISCELLANEOUS

SYNONYMS

• Collie granuloma
• Nodular granulomatous episcleritis
• Nodular fasciitis
• Fibrous histiocytoma
• Necrogranulomatous sclerouveitis
• Proliferative keratoconjunctivitis
• Limbal granuloma

Suggested Reading

Murphy CJ. Disorders of the cornea and sclera. In Kirk RW, ed., Current veterinary therapy XI. Philadelphia: Saunders, 1992:1101–1111.

Rothstein E, Scott DW, Riis RC. Tetracycline and niacinamide for the treatment of sterile pyogranuloma/granuloma syndrome in a dog. J Am Anim Hosp Assoc 1997;33:540–543.

Author Paul E. Miller
Consulting Editor Paul E. Miller

EPISTAXIS

 BASICS

DEFINITION
Bleeding from the nose

PATHOPHYSIOLOGY
Results from one of three abnormalities—coagulopathy; space-occupying lesion; vascular or systemic disease

SYSTEMS AFFECTED
• Respiratory—hemorrhage; sneezing
• Hemic/Lymphatic/Immune—anemia
• Gastrointestinal—melena

SIGNALMENT
Depends on underlying cause

SIGNS

Historical Findings
• Nasal hemorrhage
• Sneezing
• With coagulopathy—hematochezia, melena, hematuria, or hemorrhage from other areas of the body
• Melena

Physical Examination Findings
• Melena—may be from swallowing blood
• Nasal hemorrhage
• With coagulopathy—possibly petechiae, ecchymosis, hematomas, hematochezia, melena, and hematuria
• With coagulopathy or hypertension—possibly retinal hemorrhages

CAUSES

Coagulopathy
Thrombocytopenia
• Immune-mediated disease—idiopathic disease; SLE; drug reaction; MLV reaction
• Rickettsial disease—ehrlichiosis; Rocky Mounted spotted fever
• Bone marrow disease—neoplasia; aplastic anemia; infectious (fungal, rickettsial, or viral)
• DIC
Thrombopathia
• Congenital—von Willebrand disease; thrombasthenia; thrombopathia
• Acquired—NSAIDs; hyperglobulinemia (*Ehrlichia,* multiple myeloma); uremia; DIC
• Coagulation factor defects—congenital: hemophilia A (factor VIIIc deficiency) and hemophilia B (factor IX deficiency); acquired: anticoagulant rodenticide (warfarin) intoxication, hepatobiliary disease, and DIC

Space-occupying Lesion
• Foreign body
• Trauma
• Infection—fungal (aspergillus, cryptococcus, and *Rhinosporidium*); viral or bacterial. Usually blood tinged mucopurulent exudate rather than frank hemorrhage

• Neoplasia—adenocarcinoma; carcinoma; chondrosarcoma; squamous cell carcinoma; fibrosarcoma; lymphoma; transmissible venereal tumor

Vascular or Systemic Disease
• Hypertension—renal disease; hyperthyroidism; hyperadrenocorticism; idiopathic disease
• Hyperviscosity—multiple myeloma; *Ehrlichia;* polycythemia
• Vasculitis—immune-mediated and rickettsial diseases

RISK FACTORS

Coagulopathy
• Immune-mediated disease—young to middle-aged, small to medium female dogs
• Rickettsial disease—dogs living in or traveling to endemic areas
• Thrombasthenia—otter hounds
• Thrombopathia—basset hounds
• von Willebrand disease—Doberman pinschers, Airedales, German shepherds, Scottish terriers, Chesapeake Bay retrievers, and many other breeds; cats
• Hemophilia A—German shepherds and many other breeds; cats
• Hemophilia B—Cairn terriers, coonhounds, St. Bernards, and other breeds; cats

Space-occupying Lesions
• Aspergillosis—German shepherds
• Neoplasia—dolicephalic breeds

 DIAGNOSIS

DIFFERENTIAL DIAGNOSIS
See Causes.

CBC/BIOCHEMISTRY/URINALYSIS
• Anemia—if enough hemorrhage has occurred
• Thrombocytopenia—possible
• Neutrophilia—infection; neoplasia
• Pancytopenia—bone marrow disease
• Hypoproteinemia—if enough hemorrhage has occurred
• High BUN with normal creatinine—possible, owing to gastrointestinal blood
• Hyperglobulinemia—ehrlichiosis, multiple myeloma
• Azotemia—renal failure–induced hypertension
• High ALT, AST, and total bilirubin—severe hepatic disease with coagulopathy possible
• Urinalysis usually normal
• Hematuria (coagulopathy), isosthenuria, renal failure–induced hypertension, and proteinuria (SLE) possible

OTHER LABORATORY TESTS
• Coagulation profile—prolonged times with coagulation factor defects; normal with thrombocytopenia and thrombopathia

• Antinuclear antibody test—for suspected SLE
• Platelet function testing (e.g., bleeding time, von Willebrand factor analysis)—for suspected coagulopathy despite normal platelet count and coagulation profile
• *Ehrlichia* and Rocky Mountain spotted fever titers—with possible exposure
• Thyroid hormone assay—in old cats when coagulopathies and space-occupying lesions have been ruled out

IMAGING
• Thoracic radiograph—screen for metastasis with suspected neoplasia
• Nasal series—under anesthesia, including open-mouth ventrodorsal and skyline sinus views when space-occupying lesion is suspected; osteolysis noted with neoplasia and fungal sinusitis; foreign bodies usually not seen
• CT scan—more sensitive than radiographs for some diseases

DIAGNOSTIC PROCEDURES
• Rhinoscopy, nasal lavage, nasal biopsy (blind or via rhinoscopy)—indicated for suspected space-occupying disease; aimed at removing foreign bodies and evaluating and sampling nasal tissue for a causal diagnosis (e.g., neoplasia and infection)
• Cytologic and histopathologic examination and bacterial and fungal culture and sensitivity testing—nasal tissue sample
• Bone marrow aspiration biopsy—with pancytopenia
• Blood pressure evaluation—when coagulopathies and space-occupying lesions have been ruled out and azotemia is noted

 TREATMENT

• Coagulopathy—usually inpatient
• Space-occupying lesion or vascular or systemic disease—outpatient or inpatient, depending on the disease and its severity
• Minimize activity or stimuli that precipitate hemorrhage episodes.
• Inform client about the disease process.
• Teach client how to recognize a serious hemorrhage (e.g., weakness, collapse, pallor, and blood loss > 30 mL/kg of body weight).
• Whole blood or packed RBC transfusion—may be needed with severe anemia

Coagulopathy
• von Willebrand disease—plasma or cryoprecipitate for acute bleeding
• Hemophilia A—plasma or cryoprecipitate for acute bleeding; no long-term treatment
• Hemophilia B—plasma for acute bleeding; no long-term treatment
• Anticoagulant rodenticide intoxication—plasma for acute bleeding; vitamin K

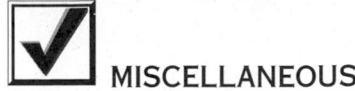
• Liver disease and DIC—treat and support the underlying cause; plasma may be beneficial.
• Discontinue all NSAIDs.
• Hyperglobulinemia—plasmapheresis

Space-occupying lesion
• Radiotherapy—nasal tumors, various response rates, depending on tumor type
• Surgery—foreign body unremovable by rhinoscopy or blind attempt; fungal rhinitis (e.g., aspergillus and *Rhinosporidium*) can be treated (also see Medications, below).

MEDICATIONS

DRUGS OF CHOICE

Coagulopathy
• Immune-mediated disease—prednisone (1.1 mg/kg q12h; taper over 4–6 months); other drugs may be used in addition to prednisone for refractory cases: azathioprine, 2.2 mg/kg PO q24h for 14 days; then q48h—dogs only; cyclosporine, 5–10 mg/kg PO q12h; danazol, 5 mg/kg PO q12h
• Rickettsial disease—doxycycline (5 mg/kg PO q12h for 2–3 weeks)
• Bone marrow neoplasia—see Myeloproliferative Disorders.
• Thrombopathia and thrombasthenia—no treatment unless lymphoproliferative disease
• Thyroid supplementation for chronic management of hypothyroidism
• DDAVP—1 µg/kg SC or IV diluted in 20 mL of 0.9% NaCl given over 10 min; may help control hemorrhage owing to von Willebrand disease; intranasal formulation (less expensive) may be used if first passed through a bacteriostatic filter
• Anticoagulant rodenticide intoxication—plasma for acute bleeding; vitamin K at 5.0 mg/kg loading dose followed by 1.25 mg/kg q12h for 1 week (if warfarin formulation) to 4 weeks (longer-acting formulation)

Space-occupying Lesion
• Serious hemorrhage—control with cage rest and acepromazine (0.05–0.1 mg/kg SC, IV) to lower blood pressure and promote clotting if the patient is not hypovolemic; intranasal instillation of Neosynephrine or dilute epinephrine may help (promotes vasoconstriction).
• Bacterial infection—antibiotics; based on culture and sensitivity testing
• Fungal infection—topical treatment with 1-hr nonsurgical soaking throughout the nasal cavity and frontal sinuses with 1% clotrimazole effective (see Aspergillosis for protocol); topical treatment with clotrimazole or enilconazole administered by surgical tubes (either q12h for 7–10 days or for 1-hr soaks)

reported; dapsone (1 mg/kg PO q8h for 2 weeks, then 1 mg/kg PO q12h for 4 months) following surgery for rhinosporidiosis

Vascular or Systemic Disease
• Hyperviscosity—treat underlying disease (e.g., ehrlichiosis and multiple myeloma); plasmapheresis for hyperglobulinemia; phlebotomy for polycythemia
• Vasculitis—doxycycline for rickettsial disease (5 mg/kg q12h for 2–3 weeks); prednisone for immune-mediated disease (1.1 mg/kg q12h; taper over 4–6 months)

Hypertension
• Treat underlying disease—renal disease, hyperthyroidism, hyperadrenocorticism
• Reduce weight.
• Restrict sodium.
• ACE inhibitors—benazepril (0.25–0.5 mg/kg q24h); enalapril (0.25–0.5 mg/kg q12–24h)
• β-blockers—propranolol (0.5–1.0 mg/kg q8h); atenolol (2.0 mg/kg q24h)
• Calcium channel blockers—amlodipine (dogs: 0.1 mg/kg PO q12–24 h; cats: 0.625 mg/cat PO q12–24h)—treatment of choice; diltiazem (dogs: 0.5–1.5 mg/kg q8h; cats: 1.75–2.5 mg/kg q8h)
• Diuretics—hydrochlorothiazide (2–4 mg/kg q12h); furosemide (0.5–2.0 mg/kg q8–12h)

CONTRAINDICATIONS
• Avoid drugs that may predispose patient to hemorrhage—NSAIDs; heparin; phenothiazine tranquilizers
• Topical antifungals—do not use in dogs with disruption of the cribriform plate

PRECAUTIONS
• Chemotherapeutic drugs (e.g., azathioprine)—monitor neutrophil counts weekly until a pattern has been established that shows that the patient is tolerating the drug.
• Enalapril and/or diuretics—closely monitor patient with renal failure; avoid severe salt restriction when using enalapril.

POSSIBLE INTERACTIONS
N/A

ALTERNATIVE DRUGS
N/A

FOLLOW-UP

PATIENT MONITORING
• Platelet count with thrombocytopenia
• Coagulation profile with coagulation factor defects
• Blood pressure with hypertension
• Monitor clinical signs

POSSIBLE COMPLICATIONS
Anemia and collapse rare

MISCELLANEOUS

ASSOCIATED CONDITIONS
N/A

AGE-RELATED FACTORS
N/A

ZOONOTIC POTENTIAL
N/A

PREGNANCY
Avoid teratogenic drugs (e.g., itraconazole)

SEE ALSO
See Causes.

ABBREVIATIONS
ACE = angiotensin-converting enzyme
ALT = alanine transferase
AST = aspartate aminotransferase
DDAVP = 1-deamino-8-D-arginine vasopressin
DIC = disseminated intravascular coagulation
MLV = modified live virus
SLE = systemic lupus erythematosus

Suggested Reading
Breit Schwerdt EB, Castellano MC. Rhinosporidiosis. In: Greene CE, ed. Infectious diseases of the dog and cat. 2nd ed. Philadelphia: Saunders, 1998:402–404.
Brooks M. Coagulopathies and thrombosis. In: Ettinger SJ, Feldman EC, eds. Textbook of veterinary internal medicine. 5th ed. Philadelphia: Saunders, 2000:1829–1841.
Brown SA, Henik RA, Finco DR. Diagnosis of systemic hypertension in dogs and cats. In: Bonagura JD, ed. Kirk's current veterinary therapy XIII. Philadelphia: Saunders, 2000:835–838.
Brown SA, Henik RA. Therapy for systemic hypertension in dogs and cats. In: Bonagura JD, ed. Kirk's current veterinary therapy XIII. Philadelphia: Saunders, 2000: 838–841.
Davidson AP, Mathews KG. CVT update: therapy for nasal aspergillosis. In: Bonagura JD, ed. Kirk's current veterinary therapy XIII. Philadelphia: Saunders, 2000:315–317.
Ruiz de Gopegui R, Feldman BF. Platelets and von Willebrand's disease. In: Ettinger SJ, Feldman EC, eds. Textbook of veterinary internal medicine. 5th ed. Philadelphia: Saunders, 2000:1817–1828.
Author Mitchell A. Crystal
Consulting Editor Lynelle R. Johnson

EPULIS

BASICS

OVERVIEW
• Categories of epulides are fibromatous, ossifying, and acanthomatous.
• Tumors of nonodontogenic origin that arise from periodontal connective tissue stroma and do not metastasize
• Most tumors adhere to bone and are nonencapsulated, with a smooth to slightly nodular surface.

SIGNALMENT
• Dogs—fourth most common oral malignancy
• Cats—rare
• Most common in brachycephalic breeds
• Boxers have a higher incidence of fibromatous epuli.
• Mean age, 7 years

SIGNS

Historical Findings
• Often none—incidental finding detected on routine physical examination
• Excessive salivation
• Halitosis
• Dysphagia
• Bloody oral discharge
• Weight loss

Physical Examination Findings
• Oral mass—in early cases, may appear as small pedunculated masses
• Acanthomatous epuli are most commonly found on the rostral mandible.
• Displacement of tooth structures due to the expansile nature of the mass
• Possible facial deformity due to asymmetry of the maxilla or mandible
• Occasionally cervical lymphadenopathy

CAUSES & RISK FACTORS
None identified

DIAGNOSIS

DIFFERENTIAL DIAGNOSIS
• Fibroma
• Benign polyp
• Ameloblastoma
• Malignant oral tumor
• Gingival hyperplasia
• Abscess
• Differentiated from other types of masses by excisional biopsy coupled with radiographic appearance

CBC/BIOCHEMISTRY/URINALYSIS
Results usually normal

OTHER LABORATORY TESTS
Cytologic preparations are rarely diagnostic.

IMAGING
• Determine tumor borders by intraoral radiographs.
• Radiographs of acanthomatous epuli typically demonstrate a well-defined area of lysis with margins that are distinct, smooth, and sclerotic; fibromatous epuli do not have well-defined borders on radiographs; tooth structures are usually displaced, and resorption may occur unidirectionally along the lesion's edge in any epulis; ossifying epuli may have bony margins because of their osteoid component.
• CT scan may be necessary to detail the invasiveness of an acanthomatous epulis.

DIAGNOSTIC PROCEDURES
A large, deep tissue biopsy (down to bone) is required to differentiate from other oral malignancies—fibroma, fibrosarcoma, or low-grade fibrosarcoma

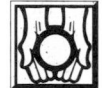

TREATMENT

DIET
Soft foods may be recommended to prevent tumor ulceration or after conservative or radical oral excision.

SURGICAL CONSIDERATIONS
• Fibromatous epulis—surgical excision with at least 1-cm margins is usually curative; these tumors are of periodontal ligament stromal origin, so extraction of affected teeth and curettage of the alveolar socket are indicated; more advanced cases may require en bloc tooth and bone excision; cryosurgery may be indicated for small lesions minimally adherent to bone.
• Ossifying epuli—characteristically have a bony matrix and excision is often more difficult; techniques are similar to those for the fibromatous epuli
• Acanthomatous epuli—because of the aggressiveness of this tumor, at least 2-cm margins are recommended; partial mandibulectomy or maxillectomy is often indicated by the location of the tumor.
• Radiotherapy offers long-term control in dogs with an acanthomatous epulis deemed inoperable; most radiotherapy plans attempt 40–60 Gy over 3–6 weeks.

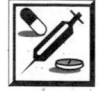

MEDICATIONS

DRUG(S)
• Efficacy of outpatient chemotherapy is unreported; most tumors of mesenchymal origin respond poorly.
• Local control (palliation) with intralesionally administered cisplatin has been reported.
• Bleomycin injected locally has been successful in treating acanthomaotus epuli.

CONTRAINDICATIONS/POSSIBLE INTERACTIONS
Chemotherapy can be toxic; seek advice before initiating treatment if you are unfamiliar with cytotoxic drugs.

FOLLOW-UP

PATIENT MONITORING
• Thorough oral, head, and neck examination 1, 2, 3, 6, 9, 12, 15, 18, and 24 months after treatment
• Periodic intraoral radiographs, especially for acanthomatous epuli

EXPECTED COURSE AND PROGNOSIS
• Epuli do not metastasize.
• Most epulides are cured when excisional margins are free of neoplastic cells; recurrence is likely if surgical margins do not include periodontal structures (i.e., excision includes normal bone).
• Mean survival time after surgery of acanthomatous epuli is 43 months (range, 6–134 months); mean survival times for patients with acanthomatous, ossifying, and fibromatous epulides are 52, 29, and 47 months, respectively.
• Mean survival after radiotherapy in dogs with acanthomatous epulis ranges from 1–102 months (median, 37 months); the 1-year survival rate is 85%; the 2-year survival rate is 67%.
• Malignant transformation of an acanthomatous epulis has been reported in up to 20% of irradiated patients years after treatment, suggesting that an acanthomatous epulis may be a precancerous lesion.
• Acanthomatous epulides are highly invasive to bone.

MISCELLANEOUS

SEE ALSO
Oral Masses

ABBREVIATION
CT = computed tomography

Suggested Reading
Bjorling DE, Chambers JN, Mahaffey EA. Surgical treatment of epulides in dogs: 25 cases (1974–1984). J Am Vet Med Assoc 1987;190:1315–1318.
Thrall DE. Orthovoltage radiotherapy of acanthomatous epulides in 39 dogs. J Am Vet Med Assoc 1984;184:826–829.
Wiggs RB, Lobprise HB. Veterinary dentistry: principles and practice. Philadelphia: Lippincott-Raven, 1997.
Author Thomas Klein
Consulting Editor Heidi B. Lobprise

BASICS

OVERVIEW
- Large pouch-like sacculations of the esophageal wall that accumulate ingesta
- Diverticula may be congenital or acquired, and are rare.
- Pulsion diverticula occur as a consequence of increased intraluminal pressure, as seen with obstruction or focal motility disturbance.
- Traction diverticula occur secondary to periesophageal inflammation, where fibrosis and contraction pull out the wall of the esophagus into a pouch.
- Diverticuli most commonly occur at the thoracic inlet or near the hiatus.
- Organ systems affected include the gastrointestinal (regurgitation), musculoskeletal (weight loss), and respiratory (aspiration pneumonia).

SIGNALMENT
- Rare; more common in dogs than cats
- Congenital or acquired (no genetic basis proven)
- No important breed or sex predisposition

SIGNS
- Postprandial regurgitation, dysphagia, anorexia, coughing
- Weight loss, respiratory distress

CAUSES & RISK FACTORS
Pulsion Diverticulum
- Embryonic developmental disorders of the esophageal wall
- Esophageal foreign body or focal motility disturbance

Traction Diverticulum
Inflammatory process associated with the trachea, lungs, hilar lymph nodes, or pericardium; causes fibrous tissue formation around the esophagus

DIAGNOSIS

DIFFERENTIAL DIAGNOSIS
Esophageal Redundancy
Contrast accumulation in the region of the thoracic inlet can occur normally in young dogs (especially brachycephalic breeds).

Periesophageal Mass
Esophagram or esophagoscopy should differentiate.

CBC/BIOCHEMISTRY/URINALYSIS
Usually within normal limits

OTHER LABORATORY TESTS
N/A

IMAGING
- Thoracic radiography—may show air or soft tissue opacity cranial to the diaphragm or cranial to the thoracic inlet
- Contrast esophagram—shows contrast accumulation in the diverticulum
- Fluoroscopy—useful to evaluate esophageal motility

DIAGNOSTIC PROCEDURES
Esophagoscopy confirms ingesta/debris outpouchings of the esophagus.

TREATMENT
- If the diverticulum is small and not causing significant clinical signs, treat conservatively with elevated feedings of a soft, bland diet followed by copious liquids.
- If the diverticulum is large or associated with significant clinical signs, surgical resection is recommended.
- Client education should include the importance of dietary management and the potential for aspiration pneumonia.
- Fluid therapy, antibiotics, and aggressive nursing, if concurrent aspiration pneumonia is present; alternative enteral nutrition via PEG or PEJ tube may be necessary in patients with aspiration pneumonia.
- Treat for esophagitis if present.

MEDICATIONS
DRUGS
- Drug therapy for esophagitis, if present
- Give H$_2$ histamine antagonists (e.g., cimetidine (10 mg/kg PO q6–8h) or ranitidine (2 mg/kg PO q12h) if the patient has concurrent esophagitis.
- Give broad-spectrum antibiotics if the patient has concurrent aspiration pneumonia; if severe pneumonia is present, base specific antibiotic selection on culture and sensitivity of samples obtained by transtracheal or bronchoalveolar lavage.

CONTRAINDICATIONS/POSSIBLE INTERACTIONS
N/A

FOLLOW-UP
PATIENT MONITORING
- Evaluate for evidence of infection or aspiration pneumonia.
- Maintain positive nutritional balance throughout disease process.

POSSIBLE COMPLICATIONS
Patients with diverticula and impaction are predisposed to perforation, fistula, stricture, and postoperative incisional dehiscence.

EXPECTED COURSE AND PROGNOSIS
Prognosis is guarded in patients with large diverticula and overt clinical signs.

MISCELLANEOUS
ABBREVIATIONS
- PEG = percutaneous endoscopic gastrotomy
- PEJ = percutaneous endoscopic jejunostomy

Suggested Reading
Fingeroth J. Surgical diseases of the esophagus. In: Slatter D, ed. Textbook of small animal surgery. 2nd ed. Philadelphia: Saunders, 1993:534–561.
Author Albert E. Jergens
Consulting Editor Albert E. Jergens

ESOPHAGEAL FOREIGN BODIES

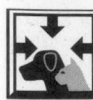

BASICS

DEFINITION
Ingestion of foreign material or foodstuffs too large to pass through the esophagus, causing intraluminal obstruction

PATHOPHYSIOLOGY
Esophageal foreign bodies cause mechanical obstruction, and possibly mucosal inflammation with edema and ischemic necrosis.

SYSTEMS AFFECTED
• Gastrointestinal
• Respiratory—if aspiration pneumonia

GENETICS
N/A

INCIDENCE/PREVALENCE
Unknown

GEOGRAPHIC DISTRIBUTION
N/A

SIGNALMENT
Species
Due to the indiscriminate eating habits of many dogs, they have a higher incidence than cats.

Breed Predilection
More common in small-breed dogs; terrier breeds often overrepresented

Mean Age and Range
More common in young to middle-aged animals

Predominant Sex
N/A

SIGNS
General Comments
The pet may have been observed ingesting a foreign body.

Historical Findings
Most common include retching, gagging, lethargy, anorexia, ptyalism, regurgitation, restlessness, dysphagia, and persistent gulping.

Physical Examination Findings
• Most often unremarkable
• Occasionally discomfort when palpating the neck or cranial abdomen

CAUSES
Occurs most often with an object whose size, shape, or texture does not allow free movement through the esophagus, causing it to become lodged before it can pass

RISK FACTORS
N/A

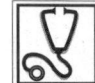

DIAGNOSIS

DIFFERENTIAL DIAGNOSIS
• Esophagitis
• Esophageal stricture
• Esophageal neoplasia
• Megaesophagus
• Other esophageal disorders

CBC/BIOCHEMISTRY/URINALYSIS
• Usually normal
• Occasionally, electrolyte abnormalities, an inflammatory leukogram, and/or hemoconcentration, depending upon the severity of signs and degree of dehydration

OTHER LABORATORY TESTS
N/A

IMAGING
Thoracic Radiography
• Radiopaque foreign bodies are readily visualized.
• Esophageal distension with air may be visualized cranial to the foreign body.

• A contrast esophagram is required to identify radiolucent objects. Use iohexol (Omnipaque) rather than barium sulfate if perforation is a possibility.
• Air and/or fluid in the mediastinum or pleural space suggests esophageal perforation; depending on severity, this can be an indication for surgery instead of esophagoscopy.
• Pulmonary infiltrates suggest aspiration pneumonia.

DIAGNOSTIC PROCEDURES
Esophagoscopy affords direct visualization of both the foreign object and the esophageal mucosa, allowing assessment of the extent of esophageal injury.

PATHOLOGIC FINDINGS
N/A

TREATMENT

APPROPRIATE HEALTH CARE
• Emergencies—treat as inpatients and perform endoscopy as soon as possible after diagnosis.
• If endoscopic retrieval of the foreign body succeeds *and* esophageal damage is minimal, the patient may be discharged the same day.

NURSING CARE
• If the procedure to remove the foreign body is atraumatic and the esophagus has sustained minimal damage, no special aftercare is needed.
• Severe mucosal trauma may require placing a gastrostomy tube for enteral nutritional support during esophageal healing.

ACTIVITY
The patient may resume normal activity after a foreign body has been routinely removed.

DIET
No change needed

CLIENT EDUCATION
Discuss the possibility of complications and repeat offenders.

SURGICAL CONSIDERATIONS
• Endoscopy is much less traumatic and invasive than surgery.
• Surgery is indicated when endoscopy fails to retrieve the foreign body; when endoscopy enables advancement of the object into the gastric lumen, but it is too large to pass through the gastrointestinal tract; or when a large esophageal perforation or area of necrosis requires resection.
• It is often less traumatic to advance a bone foreign body into the stomach than to attempt retrieval.
• Most bone foreign bodies can be safely left to dissolve in the stomach without need for surgical removal.

 MEDICATIONS

DRUGS OF CHOICE
If there is significant mucosal injury and esophageal ulceration, recommendations include:
• Broad-spectrum antibiotics such as amoxicillin or Clavamox for 10–14 days.
• Sucralfate slurry (0.5–1 g/dog PO q8h) for mucosal cytoprotection and healing
• Short-term corticosteroids (prednisone, 1 mg/kg PO q24h) decrease the risk of stricture formation by inhibiting fibroblasts; contraindicated if there is aspiration pneumonia
• H_2-antagonists (e.g., ranitidine, 2 mg/kg PO, IV, SC q12h) for reflux esophagitis
• Metoclopramide (0.2–0.5 mg/kg IV, SC, PO q8h) for reflux esophagitis
• Percutaneous gastrostomy tube placement for enteral nutrition during mucosal healing

CONTRAINDICATIONS
N/A

PRECAUTIONS
N/A

POSSIBLE INTERACTIONS
N/A

ALTERNATIVE DRUGS
N/A

 FOLLOW-UP

PATIENT MONITORING
• Examine the esophagus closely for mucosal damage.
• Mild erythema/erosions are not uncommon, and tend to heal uneventfully.
• If an esophageal laceration/perforation—parenteral nutrition or gastrostomy tube feedings allow esophageal rest and healing.
• Advise postprocedural survey thoracic radiographs to assess for pneumomediastinum/pneumothorax.
• Monitor at least 2–3 weeks for evidence of stricture formation.
• Esophageal stricture—most common clinical sign is regurgitation; esophagram and/or esophagoscopy may be indicated.

PREVENTION/AVOIDANCE
Carefully monitor the environment and what is fed to the pet.

POSSIBLE COMPLICATIONS
• Approximately 25% of patients with foreign bodies develop complications.
• Complications most frequently encountered include esophageal perforation, esophageal strictures, esophageal fistulas, and severe esophagitis. Focal, transient esophageal motility disturbances can occur secondary to esophageal trauma.

• Pneumomediastinum, pneumothorax, pneumonia, pleuritis, mediastinitis, and bronchoesophageal fistulas can all occur secondarily to perforation.

EXPECTED COURSE AND PROGNOSIS
• Most of these patients do well and recover uneventfully.
• With complications, the prognosis is guarded.

 MISCELLANEOUS

ASSOCIATED CONDITIONS
None

AGE-RELATED FACTORS
N/A

ZOONOTIC POTENTIAL
None

PREGNANCY
N/A

SYNONYMS
N/A

SEE ALSO
• Regurgitation
• Esophageal Diverticula

Suggested Reading
Gualtieri M. Esophagoscopy. Vet Clin North Am Small Anim Pract 2001;31:605–630.
Spielman BL, Shaker EH, Garvey MS. Esophageal foreign body in dogs: a retrospective study of 23 cases. J Am Anim Hosp Assoc 1992;28:570–574.
Tams TR. Endoscopic removal of gastrointestinal foreign bodies. In: Tams TR, ed. Small animal endoscopy. 2nd ed. Philadelphia: Mosby, 1999:247–295.
Author Albert E. Jergens
Consulting Editor Albert E. Jergens

ESOPHAGEAL STRICTURE

 BASICS

DEFINITION
An abnormal narrowing of the esophageal lumen

PATHOPHYSIOLOGY
• Can occur secondary to severe esophagitis when the inflammation extends beyond the mucosa and into the submucosa and muscle layers, resulting in fibrosis
• Ingestion of acid or alkali, gastroesophageal reflux (especially secondary to general anesthetic procedures), or trauma from esophageal foreign bodies can result in severe esophagitis and consequent stricture formation.
• Can also be associated with esophageal surgery, esophageal neoplasia, and *Spirocerca lupi* granulomas

SYSTEMS AFFECTED
• Gastrointestinal—esophagus affected segmentally or diffusely
• Respiratory—aspiration pneumonia may develop secondary to regurgitation

GENETICS
No apparent genetic basis

INCIDENCE/PREVALENCE
Unknown; believed to be low

GEOGRAPHIC DISTRIBUTION
• *Spirocerca lupi* granulomatous strictures—occasionally seen in the southeastern United States
• Other causes—no specific geographic distribution

SIGNALMENT
Species
Dogs and cats

Breed Predilections
None reported

Mean Age and Range
Any age; neoplastic strictures tend to occur in middle-aged to older animals

Predominant Sex
None

SIGNS
General Comments
• Usually involve the entire circumference of the esophagus; can occur at any location or over any length of the esophagus
• Clinical signs are related to the severity and extent of stricture.

Historical Findings
• Regurgitation—usually of solid foods; observed shortly after feeding
• Affected animals may reingest the regurgitated meal.
• Liquid meals often tolerated better than solid meals

• Dysphagia—with proximal esophageal strictures
• Salivation
• Howling, crying, or yelping during swallowing (odynophagia) with active esophagitis
• Good appetite initially; eventually, anorexia with progressive esophageal narrowing and inflammation
• Weight loss and malnutrition as the disease progresses
• May see aspiration pneumonia with progressive regurgitation and dysphagia

Physical Examination Findings
• Usually unremarkable
• Weight loss and cachexia—in animals with chronic or advanced stricture
• Hypersalivation and/or pain on palpation of neck and esophagus—may be seen in animals with concurrent esophagitis
• Pulmonary wheezes and coughing—may be detected in animals with aspiration pneumonia

CAUSES
• Gastroesophageal reflux during anesthesia—most common
• Ingestion of chemical irritants
• Gastroesophageal reflux disease
• Esophageal foreign body
• Esophageal surgery
• Malignancies—intramural and extramural
• *Spirocerca lupi* granuloma

RISK FACTORS
• Poor preparation (not fasted) and positioning during anesthesia (abdomen positioned above thorax) place some patients at risk for gastroesophageal reflux, esophagitis, and subsequent stricture formation.
• Use of certain drugs prior to anesthesia (e.g., diazepam, atropine, pentobarbital, phenothiazine-derivative tranquilizers)—decreases the pressure of the gastroesophageal sphincter and can result in gastroesophageal reflux

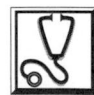 DIAGNOSIS

DIFFERENTIAL DIAGNOSIS
• Vascular ring anomaly—important differential diagnosis in a young animal with midesophageal stricture and proximal esophageal dilation; these animals are usually presented shortly after weaning
• Esophagitis—patient may have clinical signs identical to those of esophageal stricture; differentiation requires barium contrast radiography and endoscopy
• Esophageal foreign body—clinical signs may be identical to those of esophageal stricture; survey radiography may identify an esophageal foreign body, although barium

contrast radiography or endoscopy may be necessary
• Intraluminal mass—rare; may be detected by radiography, but many require endoscopy; leiomyoma, squamous cell carcinoma, fibrosarcoma, and osteosarcoma are the most common esophageal malignancies
• Extraluminal periesophageal mass—often detected by radiography, but may require thoracic ultrasonography; lymphoma, heart base tumors, and mediastinal abscess are the most common causes of extraluminal esophageal compression

CBC/BIOCHEMISTRY/URINALYSIS
• Usually normal
• Patients with ulcerative esophagitis or aspiration pneumonia may have leukocytosis and neutrophilia.

OTHER LABORATORY TESTS
N/A

IMAGING
• Survey thoracic radiography; usually normal; rarely, demonstrates dilation of the esophagus cranial to the stricture (retention of food may be seen in the dilated portion of the esophagus) or an intraluminal or extraluminal mass; aspiration pneumonia may be evident in patients with frequent regurgitation
• Barium contrast radiography—often diagnostic; depending on stricture severity, liquid barium may pass unimpeded; barium paste or barium mixed with food is often necessary to identify the stricture; may see segmental or diffuse narrowing of the esophagus with some dilation proximal to the stricture
• Ultrasonography—not proven useful, unless an extramural compressive mass lesion is suspected

DIAGNOSTIC PROCEDURES
• Endoscopy—perform in all patients to confirm the site and severity of stricture and to exclude intraluminal malignancy
• Histopathology—sometimes necessary to differentiate neoplasia from non-neoplastic (i.e., fibrotic) stricture

PATHOLOGIC FINDINGS
• Esophageal stricture
• Esophagitis in some patients
• Dilation and muscular hypertrophy proximal to the stricture
• Aspiration pneumonia

 TREATMENT

APPROPRIATE HEALTH CARE
• Inpatient management initially
• May discharge patients from the hospital after addressing hydration needs, achieving dilation of the affected segment, and initiating any needed treatment for aspiration pneumonia and esophagitis

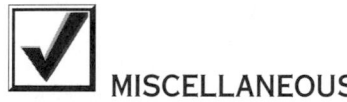

NURSING CARE
• Intravenous fluids—may be needed to correct hydration status
• Medications—give parenterally following dilation procedures, to facilitate healing
• Oxygen—may be needed for patients with severe concurrent aspiration pneumonia

ACTIVITY
Unrestricted

DIET
• Withhold oral feedings in patients with severe esophagitis and following dilation procedures.
• May place a temporary gastrostomy tube at the time of esophageal dilation as a means of providing continual nutritional support
• Give liquid meals when reinstituting oral feedings.

CLIENT EDUCATION
• Animals generally do not recover from untreated esophageal stricture.
• Benign strictures are best treated by esophageal dilation.
• Patients with malignant stricture have a poor prognosis.
• Discuss the high probability of recurrence and common need for multiple dilation procedures.
• Discuss the possibility of improvement (e.g., decreased to absent regurgitation, ability to eat softened canned foods but not dry food) but not cure.

SURGICAL CONSIDERATIONS
• Bougienage tube dilation
• Mechanical dilation via balloon catheter under endoscopy or fluoroscopy—best management option; superior to bougienage because applying radial forces rather than shearing forces results in less chance of esophageal perforation; perform endoscopy after dilation to assess esophageal mucosal damage; redilation at 1- to 2-week intervals may be necessary until stricture is resolved
• Resection of esophageal stricture—reportedly has a < 50% success rate and is often associated with substantial postoperative complications
• Other surgical methods—esophagotomy; esophagectomy with anastomosis; jejunal interposition; and creation of a traction diverticulum

 MEDICATIONS

DRUG(S) OF CHOICE
• Administer medications parenterally following dilation procedures and if severe esophagitis is present.
• When oral therapy is resumed, dissolve medications in water and give by syringe or give directly via gastrostomy tube to ensure that they reach the stomach.

• Anti-inflammatory dosage of corticosteroids (e.g., prednisone 0.5–1.0 mg/kg PO q12h)—may help prevent fibrosis and restricture during the healing phase
• Sucralfate suspension—0.5–1.0 g PO q8h
• Gastric acid antisecretory agents—famotidine 0.5 mg/kg PO, IV q12–24h; ranitidine 1–2 mg/kg PO, IV, SC q8–12h; cimetidine 5–10 mg/kg PO, SC, IV q8h; omeprazole 0.7 mg/kg PO q24h
• Prokinetic agent (i.e., cisapride)—0.1–0.5 mg/kg PO q8–12h to increase gastro-esophageal sphincter tone after resolution of the stricture
• Lidocaine solution—0.5 mg/kg PO q4–6h; to manage severe esophageal pain

CONTRAINDICATIONS
Emetic agents

PRECAUTIONS
None

POSSIBLE INTERACTIONS
• Cimetidine and ranitidine bind to hepatic cytochrome P-450 enzyme and may interfere with metabolism of other drugs.
• H$_2$-receptor antagonists prevent uptake of omeprazole by oxyntic cells.
• Sucralfate may inhibit the gastrointestinal absorption of other drugs (e.g., cimetidine, ranitidine, omeprazole); this may not be clinically important.

ALTERNATIVE DRUGS
N/A

 FOLLOW-UP

PATIENT MONITORING
Repeat barium contrast radiography or endoscopy every 2–4 weeks until clinical signs have resolved and adequate esophageal lumen size has been achieved.

PREVENTION/AVOIDANCE
• Proper patient preparation prior to anesthesia (12-hr preoperative fast) and proper patient positioning during anesthesia (prevent elevation of abdomen above thorax)
• Avoid certain drugs (e.g., diazepam, atropine, pentobarbital, morphine, phenothiazine-derivative tranquilizers) prior to anesthesia
• If gastroesophageal reflux is present, advise owner to avoid late-night feedings as they tend to diminish gastroesophageal sphincter pressure during sleep.
• Prevent animal from ingesting caustic substances and foreign bodies.

POSSIBLE COMPLICATIONS
• Esophageal perforation—a life-threatening complication of esophageal stricture dilation; usually occurs at the time of dilation, although it has been observed several days to weeks later

• Patients are at risk for aspiration pneumonia.

EXPECTED COURSE AND PROGNOSIS
• Generally, the longer the stricture, the more guarded the prognosis.
• Fibrosing esophageal strictures—generally, fair to guarded prognosis; many recur despite repeated esophageal dilation; improvement without cure is a more realistic goal (see Client Education)
• Malignant stricture—poor prognosis

☑ MISCELLANEOUS

ASSOCIATED CONDITIONS
N/A

AGE-RELATED FACTORS
N/A

ZOONOTIC POTENTIAL
None

PREGNANCY
Esophageal stricture and malnutrition—pregnancy may be difficult

SYNONYMS
• Esophageal narrowing
• Esophageal obstruction

SEE ALSO
• Esophagitis
• Gastroesophageal Reflux
• Megaesophagus
• Regurgitation
• Esophageal Foreign Bodies
• Dysphagia

Suggested Reading
Burk RL, Zawie DA, Garvey MS. Balloon catheter dilation of intramural esophageal strictures in the dog and cat: a description of the procedure and a report of six cases. Semin Vet Med Surg 1987;2:241–247.
Harai BH, Johnson SE, Sherding RG. Endoscopically guided balloon dilation of benign esophageal strictures in 6 cats and 7 dogs. J Vet Intern Med 1995;9:332–335.
Leib MS. Endoscopic balloon dilation of esophageal strictures in dogs and cats. J Vet Intern Med 2001;15:547–552.
Melendez L, Twedt D, Weyrauch E, et al. Conservative therapy using balloon dilation for intramural, inflammatory esophageal strictures in dogs and cats. Eur J Comp Gastroenterol 1998;3:31–36.
Washabau RJ. Diseases of the esophagus. In: Ettinger SJ, Feldman EC, eds. Textbook of veterinary internal medicine. 5th ed. Philadelphia: Saunders, 2000:1142–1153.
Author Robert J. Washabau
Consulting Editor Albert E. Jergens

ESOPHAGITIS

 BASICS

DEFINITION
• Inflammation of the esophagus—typically the esophageal body and gastroesophageal sphincter; occasionally the cricopharyngeal sphincter
• Varies from mild inflammation of the superficial mucosa to severe ulceration involving the submucosa and muscularis

PATHOPHYSIOLOGY
• The esophageal mucosa has several important barrier mechanisms to withstand caustic substances, including stratified squamous epithelium with intracellular tight junctions, mucous gel, and surface bicarbonate ions.
• Rapid esophageal clearance by peristalsis and neutralization of acid by bicarbonate-rich saliva are important defense mechanisms to prevent reflux esophagitis.
• Disruption of these barrier and defense mechanisms causes inflammation, erosion, and/or ulceration of the underlying structures.

SYSTEMS AFFECTED
• Gastrointestinal—esophageal body (most common); gastroesophageal sphincter; occasionally, the cricopharyngeal sphincter
• Respiratory—aspiration pneumonia may develop with concurrent laryngitis and pharyngitis if regurgitation is severe

GENETICS
N/A

INCIDENCE/PREVALENCE
Unknown; believed to be low

GEOGRAPHIC DISTRIBUTION
Esophagitis caused by *Pythium* spp.—usually regionally distributed in states that border the Gulf of Mexico

SIGNALMENT
Species
Dogs and cats

Breed Predilections
None reported

Mean Age and Range
Any age; young animals with congenital esophageal hiatal hernia may be at higher risk for reflux esophagitis

Predominant Sex
None

SIGNS
General Comments
• Related to the type of chemical injury, severity of inflammation, and involvement of structures underlying the esophageal mucosa (e.g., muscularis)
• May be intermittent and often more prominent during or after feeding
• Patients with mild esophagitis may show subtle or no clinical signs.

Historical Findings
• Regurgitation
• Hypersalivation
• Howling, crying, or yelping during swallowing (odynophagia)
• Extension of the head and neck during swallowing (odynophagia)
• Dysphagia
• Avoidance of food
• Weight loss
• Coughing in animals with concurrent aspiration pneumonia

Physical Examination Findings
• Often unremarkable
• General debilitation with severe esophagitis
• Oral and pharyngeal inflammation and/or ulceration if caustic or irritating substances have been ingested
• Fever and hypersalivation in some patients with severe ulcerative esophagitis
• Pain on palpation of neck and esophagus
• Cachexia and weight loss with prolonged disease
• Pulmonary wheezes and coughing in patients with aspiration pneumonia

CAUSES
• Gastroesophageal reflux of gastric and/or intestinal fluids
• Anesthesia resulting in gastroesophageal reflux
• Ingestion of chemical irritants
• Infectious agents—calicivirus, pythiosis, *Candida*
• Esophageal and/or thoracic surgery
• Nasogastric, esophagostomy, or pharyngostomy feeding tube
• Chronic vomiting
• Esophageal retention of pills or capsules
• Esophageal foreign body

RISK FACTORS
• Hiatal hernia—increases risk for gastroesophageal reflux
• Anesthesia—use of certain drugs, such as diazepam, atropine, pentobarbital, and phenothiazine-derivative tranquilizers, prior to anesthesia decreases the pressure of the gastroesophageal sphincter and can result in gastroesophageal reflux
• Poor preparation and poor positioning during anesthesia places some patients at risk for gastroesophageal reflux and esophagitis.

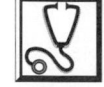 DIAGNOSIS

DIFFERENTIAL DIAGNOSIS
• Esophageal foreign body—usually detected by survey radiography or esophagoscopy
• Esophageal stricture—segmental narrowing revealed by barium contrast radiography or esophagoscopy
• Oropharyngeal dysphagia—diagnosed by evaluating swallowing of barium under fluoroscopy
• Hiatal hernia—congenital form is usually recognized as a caudodorsal gas-filled opacity in the thoracic cavity; contrast studies may be required to document acquired hiatal hernia
• Megaesophagus—survey radiography usually reveals diffuse dilation of the esophageal body
• Esophageal diverticula—focal pouches detected by survey or contrast radiography or esophagoscopy
• Vascular ring anomaly—usually revealed by barium contrast radiography as a focal dilation of the proximal esophageal body

CBC/BIOCHEMISTRY/URINALYSIS
Usually normal; patients with ulcerative esophagitis or aspiration pneumonia may have leukocytosis and neutrophilia

OTHER LABORATORY TESTS
N/A

IMAGING
• Survey thoracic radiography—usually unremarkable; in patients with hiatal hernia, may show increased density in the caudal esophagus; aspiration pneumonia may be evident in the dependent portions of the lung; rarely, demonstrates dilation of the esophagus cranial to the stricture (retention of food may be seen in the dilated portion of the esophagus) or an intraluminal or extraluminal mass
• Barium contrast radiography—may reveal an irregular mucosal surface, segmental narrowing, esophageal dilation, or diffuse esophageal hypomotility; stricture formation may be apparent in severely affected patients
• Ultrasonography—generally not useful

DIAGNOSTIC PROCEDURES
• Endoscopy and biopsy—most reliable means of diagnosis; in patients with severe esophagitis, the mucosa appears hyperemic and edematous, with areas of ulceration and active bleeding
• Mild cases of esophagitis may appear endoscopically normal and require mucosal biopsy for confirmation of the diagnosis.
• Transtracheal aspiration for cytology, and culture and sensitivity testing if aspiration pneumonia is suspected

PATHOLOGIC FINDINGS
• Esophageal inflammation and/or ulceration
• Aspiration pneumonia

 TREATMENT

APPROPRIATE HEALTH CARE
Mildly affected animals can be managed as outpatients; those with more severe esophagitis (e.g., complete anorexia,

dehydration, and aspiration pneumonia) require hospitalization.

NURSING CARE
• Intravenous fluids to maintain hydration—more severe cases
• Medications—give parenterally during hospitalization
• Oxygen therapy—may be necessary in patients with severe aspiration pneumonia

ACTIVITY
N/A

DIET
• Mild esophagitis—withhold oral intake of food for 1–2 days
• Severe esophagitis—withhold food and water for 3–5 days; maintain with gastrostomy tube feedings (preferably) or total parenteral nutrition
• Patients that can ingest food orally—give small, frequent, low-fat, high protein meals of liquid or soft consistency

CLIENT EDUCATION
• Discuss need to restrict food intake in patients with severe esophagitis.
• Discuss potential complications, including aspiration pneumonia, esophageal stricture, esophageal perforation, and/or esophageal motility abnormalities.

SURGICAL CONSIDERATIONS
• Percutaneous endoscopic gastrostomy or surgical gastrostomy tube placement is indicated in severe cases.

MEDICATIONS

DRUG(S) OF CHOICE
• Usually given parenterally (except for sucralfate) in severe cases; when administered enterally, dissolve in water and use oral (e.g., via syringe, dropper) or gastrostomy tube delivery.
• Sucralfate suspension (0.5–1.0 g PO q8h)—more therapeutic than intact sucralfate tablets
• Antibiotics—indicated with concurrent aspiration pneumonia or severe esophageal ulceration or esophageal perforation
• Gastric acid antisecretory agent (e.g., famotidine 0.5 mg/kg PO, SC, IV q12–24h, ranitidine 1–2 mg/kg PO, SC, IV, q8–12h, cimetidine 5–10 mg/kg PO, SC, IV q8h, omeprazole 0.7 mg/kg PO q24h)—to prevent occurrence of further irritation by gastroesophageal reflux
• Lidocaine solution (0.5 mg/kg PO q4–6h)—to manage severe esophageal pain
• Anti-inflammatory dosage of corticosteroids (e.g., prednisone 0.5–1.0 mg/kg PO q12h)—to decrease the possibility of esophageal stricture formation in severe cases

• Gastrointestinal prokinetic drugs (cisapride 0.1–0.5 mg/kg PO q8–12h, metoclopramide 0.2–0.5 mg/kg PO, SC q8h)—may help decrease gastroesophageal reflux but are without effect on esophageal motility

CONTRAINDICATIONS
None

PRECAUTIONS
None

POSSIBLE INTERACTIONS
• Cimetidine and ranitidine bind to hepatic cytochrome P-450 enzyme and may interfere with metabolism of other drugs.
• H_2-receptor antagonists prevent uptake of omeprazole by oxyntic cells.
• Sucralfate may interfere with gastrointestinal absorption of other drugs (e.g., cimetidine, ranitidine, omeprazole); may not be clinically important

ALTERNATIVE DRUG(S)
• Fentanyl analgesic patches—may be useful in severe cases of painful esophagitis
• Analogues of erythromycin—may be useful in treating cats with esophagitis secondary to gastroesophageal reflux disease.

FOLLOW-UP

PATIENT MONITORING
• Patients with mild esophagitis do not necessarily require follow-up endoscopy; tracking of clinical signs may be sufficient.
• Consider endoscopy in patients with ulcerative esophagitis and those at risk for esophageal stricture.

PREVENTION/AVOIDANCE
• Prevent animals from ingesting caustic substances and foreign bodies.
• If gastroesophageal reflux is the cause of esophagitis, owners should avoid late-night feedings; this tends to diminish gastroesophageal sphincter pressure during sleep.
• Proper patient preparation prior to anesthesia (fasting) and proper patient positioning during anesthesia (abdomen should not be elevated above thorax) decreases the risk of gastroesophageal reflux.

POSSIBLE COMPLICATIONS
• Stricture formation
• Esophageal perforation
• Aspiration pneumonia
• Permanent esophageal motility dysfunction

EXPECTED COURSE AND PROGNOSIS
• Best results when patients are treated with a diffusion barrier (e.g., sucralfate) and gastric acid secretory inhibitor (e.g., famotidine, ranitidine, cimetidine, omeprazole)

• Mild esophagitis—generally favorable prognosis
• Severe or ulcerative esophagitis—guarded prognosis
• Complete recovery is possible if the disorder is recognized and treated before serious complications develop.

MISCELLANEOUS

ASSOCIATED CONDITIONS
N/A

AGE-RELATED FACTORS
N/A

ZOONOTIC POTENTIAL
None

PREGNANCY
H_2-receptor antagonists (e.g., cimetidine, ranitidine, famotidine), proton pump inhibitors (e.g., omeprazole), and glucocorticoids should all be used with caution during pregnancy.

SYNONYMS
Esophageal inflammation

SEE ALSO
• Esophageal Stricture
• Esophageal Diverticula
• Megaesophagus
• Hiatal Hernia
• Dysphagia
• Regurgitation
• Gastroesophageal Reflux
• Esophageal Foreign Bodies

Suggested Reading
Eastwood CL, Beck BD, Castell DO, et al. Beneficial effect of indomethacin on acid-induced esophagitis in cats. Dig Dis Sci 1981;26:601–608.
Eastwood CL, Castell DO, Higgs RH. Experimental esophagitis in cats impairs lower esophageal sphincter pressure. Gastroenterology 1975;69:146–153.
Greenwood B, Dieckman D, Kirst H, et al. Effects of LY267108, an erythromycin analogue derivative, on lower esophageal sphincter function in the cat. Gastroenterology 1994;106:624–628.
Katz PD, Geisinger KR, Hassan M, et al. Acid-induced esophagitis in cats is prevented by sucralfate but not synthetic prostaglandins. Dig Dis Sci 1988;33:217–224.
Washabau RJ. Diseases of the esophagus. In: Ettinger SJ, Feldman EC, eds. Textbook of veterinary internal medicine. 5th ed. Philadelphia: Saunders, 2000:1142–1153.
Author Robert J. Washabau
Consulting Editor Albert E. Jergens

ESTROGEN TOXICITY

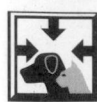 ## BASICS

OVERVIEW
• Dogs more sensitive to estrogen than other species but vary widely in their sensitivity
• Can cause pancytopenia, feminization of male animals, and estrus and pyometra in female animals
• In dogs, pancytopenia may result from the induction of a thymic stromal, myelopoiesis inhibitory factor.

SIGNALMENT
• Dogs
• Old, intact male and female animals at greater risk for developing estrogen-producing tumors, although cryptorchid males may be comparatively younger

SIGNS
• Exercise intolerance and pale mucous membranes because of anemia
• Hemorrhage—petechiae, hematuria, and melena caused by thrombocytopenia
• Fever associated with infection resulting from leukopenia
• Alopecia
• Estrus in females and feminization of males in some animals
• Abdominal masses, testicular masses, cryptorchidism in some animals

CAUSES & RISK FACTORS
• Endogenous estrogen from testicular (especially Sertoli cell) tumors and ovarian granulosa cell tumors
• Exogenous estrogen used in the management of benign prostatic hyperplasia, perianal adenoma, pregnancy prevention, urinary incontinence, and infertility
• Cryptorchid males at greater risk of developing Sertoli cell tumor

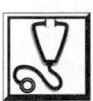 ## DIAGNOSIS

DIFFERENTIAL DIAGNOSIS
• Other causes of pancytopenia include toxins, drugs, infection, neoplasia, immune-mediated diseases, myelodysplasia, bone marrow necrosis, osteosclerosis, and myelofibrosis.
• Important factors in the diagnosis include history of administration of estrogen, testicular or ovarian tumor, thin hair coat, evidence of estrus, and signs of feminization.

CBC/BIOCHEMISTRY/URINALYSIS
After Estrogen Overdosage
• Thrombocytosis occurs within 1 week, followed by thrombocytopenia within 2 weeks.
• Leukocytosis develops and persists until week 3.
• Normocytic, normochromic anemia develops insidiously.
• Pancytopenia occurs within 4 weeks.

OTHER LABORATORY TESTS
Blood culture may be considered in febrile, leukopenic patients.

IMAGING
Radiography and ultrasonography—locate and stage potential estrogen-producing tumors and help diagnose pyometra

DIAGNOSTIC PROCEDURES
• Examination of bone marrow aspirate ± core biopsy—5–7 days after estrogen overdosage: suppression of megakaryo-cytopoiesis and erythropoiesis with concurrent stimulation of granulopoiesis; by day 10: all cell lines are affected; by day 20: granulopoiesis ceases completely while the other cell lines start to recover.
• Hematologic recovery can take 3 months; signs of marrow improvement are seen 3 days later in the peripheral blood.
• Abdominal laparotomy or laparoscopy and/or biopsy to locate and identify estrogen-producing tumors

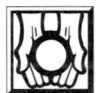 ## TREATMENT
• Remove source of estrogen if possible.
• Severely affected animals may require extensive and prolonged supportive care, including transfusions of blood and platelet-rich plasma.
• Care should be taken with venipuncture and other invasive procedures to avoid bruising in severely thrombocytopenic patients.

 ## MEDICATIONS
• Broad-spectrum antibiotics necessary in febrile, leukopenic patients; choice of antibiotic should be based on bacterial culture if possible.
• Although no reports have been published of their use to treat estrogen toxicity, growth factors such as recombinant human erythro-poietin (100 IU/kg SC 3 times weekly) and rhG-CSF (2.5–5 µg/kg SC q24h) may be useful.

• Lithium carbonate (10 mg/kg PO q12h) has been used to treat estrogen-induced pancytopenia.

CONTRAINDICATIONS/POSSIBLE INTERACTIONS
Consider avoiding sulfonamides and cephalosporins, because they are occasionally associated with blood dyscrasias.

 ## FOLLOW-UP
• Monitor the bleeding or febrile estrogen toxicity patient closely, including checking PCV 1–2 times daily; monitoring temperature, heart rate and rhythm, and respiratory rate; and checking for bleeding
• When PCV has stabilized or the temperature normalized, the patient may be monitored as an outpatient.
• CBC—biweekly or weekly, depending on the patient's progress; weekly in patients who have undergone surgical excision of an estrogen-producing tumor to check for progression of hematologic abnormalities
• The patient may require changes of antibiotics, multiple blood or platelet transfusions, and intermittent hospitalization.
• Complications include sepsis and hemorrhage into vital organs, such as the heart and CNS.
• Recovery may take as long as 3 months.
• Prognosis guarded

 ## MISCELLANEOUS

SEE ALSO
• Anemia, Aplastic
• Anemia, Nonregenerative
• Leukopenia
• Ovarian Tumors
• Sertoli Cell Tumor

ABBREVIATIONS
• PCV = packed cell volume
• rhG-CSF = recombinant human granulocyte colony-stimulating factor

Suggested Reading
Hall EJ. Use of lithium for treatment of estrogen-induced bone marrow hypoplasia in a dog. J Am Vet Med Assoc 1992;200: 814–816.
Author Orla M. Mahony
Consulting Editor Stephen A. Kruth

BASICS

OVERVIEW
• Ethanol (CH_2OH)—short-chain aliphatic alcohol; highly miscible with water; soluble in aqueous systems; less volatile than comparable hydrocarbons (e.g., ethane); solvent for medications; major component of alcoholic beverages; metabolized to acetaldehyde

ALCOHOL CONTENT OF COMMON BEVERAGES

Beer	3–5%
Wines	9–12%
Whiskey	50–90%

• Alcohol concentration—expressed as proof (twice the percentage concentration)
• Acute toxicity—5–8 mL/kg as pure alcohol; to calculate beverage volume that will cause toxicosis, consider the percentage of alcohol.
• Mechanism of action—affects lipids and proteins of the cell membrane; then reduces sodium and potassium conduction in nerve membranes

SIGNALMENT
• Most common in dogs
• No breed or sex predilections

SIGNS
• CNS—predominate; develop within 15–30 min after ingestion on an empty stomach or 1–2 hr on full stomach.
• High dosages—ataxia; reduced reflexes; behavioral changes; excitement or depression
• Polyuria and/or incontinence
• Advanced signs—depression or narcosis; slowed respiratory rate; cardiac arrest; death

CAUSES & RISK FACTORS
• Accidental—access to spilled beverages or medications containing alcohol
• Intentional—given by owners or others; dogs may readily consume beer if offered.
• Fermented products—bread dough
• Dermal exposure—alcohol-containing products

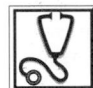

DIAGNOSIS

DIFFERENTIAL DIAGNOSIS
• Other alcohols—methanol; isopropanol; butanol
• Abused drugs—marijuana
• Early stages of ethylene glycol (antifreeze) toxicosis
• Halogenated or aliphatic hydrocarbon solvents

CBC/BIOCHEMISTRY/URINALYSIS
Monitor for hypoglycemia.

OTHER LABORATORY TESTS
• Osmolal gap—increased
• Blood ethanol concentrations—clinical signs of toxicosis in puppies at > 0.6 mg/mL and in adults at > 1–4 mg/mL; available at human laboratories
• Blood gases and anion gap—evaluate potential acidosis.

IMAGING
N/A

DIAGNOSTIC PROCEDURES
N/A

TREATMENT

• Depressed respiratory function—artificial ventilation
• Acidosis—treat
• Cardiac arrest—cardiac therapy (see Cardiopulmonary Arrest)

MEDICATIONS

DRUG(S)
• Activated charcoal—2 g/kg PO; as soon as possible after exposure; gastrointestinal detoxication
• 4-Methyl pyrazole—possible inhibition of alcohol metabolism (see Ethylene Glycol Toxicity)
• Epinephrine and bicarbonate—cardiac arrest (see Cardiopulmonary Arrest)

CONTRAINDICATIONS/POSSIBLE INTERACTIONS
Do not administer other CNS depressive drugs.

FOLLOW-UP

• Monitor blood pH, blood gases, urine pH, and anion gap—evidence of acidosis
• Recovery from clinical signs—usually within 8–12 hr

MISCELLANEOUS

Suggested Reading
Valentine WM. Short chain alcohols. Vet Clin North Am 1990;20:515–523.
Author Gary D. Osweiler
Consulting Editor Gary D. Osweiler

ETHYLENE GLYCOL POISONING

 BASICS

DEFINITION
Results from ingesting substances containing ethylene glycol (e.g., antifreeze)

PATHOPHYSIOLOGY
• Ethylene glycol—rapidly absorbed from the gastrointestinal tract; food in the stomach delays absorption.
• Toxicity—initially causes CNS depression, ataxia, gastrointestinal irritation, and polyuria or polydipsia; rapidly metabolized by the liver enzyme ADH to glycoaldehyde, glycolic acid; glyoxalic acid, and oxalic acid; leads to severe metabolic acidosis and renal epithelial damage
• Minimum lethal dose—cats, 1.4 mL/kg; dogs, 6.6 mL/kg

SYSTEMS AFFECTED
• Nervous—inebriation from ethylene glycol and glycoaldehyde owing to inhibition of respiration, glucose metabolism, and serotonin metabolism and alteration of amine concentrations
• Gastrointestinal—irritated mucosa
• Renal/Urologic—initially, osmotic diuresis; later, metabolites, especially glycoaldehyde and glyoxylate, are directly cytotoxic to renal tubular epithelium, resulting in renal failure; very minor role for oxalate crystal deposition in causing renal tubular damage

GENETICS
N/A

INCIDENCE/PREVALENCE
• Common in small animals
• Highest fatality rate of all poisons; fatality rates higher for cats than dogs
• Incidence similar in cats and dogs

GEOGRAPHIC DISTRIBUTION
Higher incidence in colder areas where antifreeze is more commonly used

SIGNALMENT

Species
Dogs, cats, and many other species, including birds

Breed Predilections
N/A

Mean Age and Range
• Any age susceptible (3 months to 13 years)
• Mean—3 years

Predominant Sex
N/A

SIGNS

General Comments
• Dose-dependent
• Almost always acute
• Caused by unmetabolized ethylene glycol and its toxic metabolites (frequently fatal)

Physical Examination Findings
• Early—seen from 30 min to 12 hr post-ingestion in dogs; nausea and vomiting; mild to severe depression; ataxia and knuckling; muscle fasciculations; nystagmus; head tremors; decreased withdrawal reflexes and righting ability; polyuria and polydipsia
• Dogs—with increasing depression, patient drinks less but polyuria continues, resulting in dehydration; CNS signs abate transiently after approximately 12 hr, but recur later.
• Cats—usually remain markedly depressed; do not exhibit polydipsia
• Oliguria (dogs, 36–72 hr; cats, 12–24 hr) and anuria (72–96 hr postingestion)—often develop if untreated
• May note severe hypothermia
• Severe lethargy or coma
• Seizures
• Anorexia
• Vomiting
• Oral ulcers
• Salivation
• Kidneys—often swollen and painful, particularly in cats

CAUSES
Ingestion of ethylene glycol, the principal component (95%) of most antifreeze solutions

RISK FACTORS
Access to ethylene glycol—widespread availability; somewhat pleasant taste; small minimum lethal dose; lack of public awareness of toxicity

 DIAGNOSIS

DIFFERENTIAL DIAGNOSIS
• Acute (30 min to 12 hr postingestion)—ethanol toxicosis; ketoacidotic diabetes mellitus; pancreatitis; gastroenteritis
• Renal stage—acute renal failure by nephrotoxins (e.g., aminoglycoside antibiotics, amphotericin B, cancer chemotherapeutic drugs, cyclosporin, and heavy metals); tubulointerstitial nephritis; glomerular and vascular disease; renal ischemia (hypoperfusion)

CBC/BIOCHEMISTRY/URINALYSIS
• PCV and total protein—often high owing to dehydration
• Stress leukogram—common
• High BUN and creatinine—dog, 36–48 hr postingestion; cat, 12 hr postingestion
• Hyperphosphatemia may occur transiently 3–6 hr postingestion, owing to phosphate rust inhibitors in the antifreeze; hyperphosphatemia is also seen with azotemia owing to decreased glomerular filtration.
• Hyperkalemia if oliguric or anuric
• Hypocalcemia—occurs in approximately half of patients, owing to chelation of calcium by oxalic acid; clinical signs infrequently observed because of acidosis
• Hyperglycemia—occurs in half of patients, owing to inhibition of glucose metabolism by aldehydes, increased epinephrine and endogenous corticosteroids, and uremia
• Isosthenuria—by 3 hr postingestion, owing to osmotic diuresis and serum hyper-osmolality–induced polydipsia; continues in the later stages of toxicosis because of renal dysfunction
• Calcium oxalate crystalluria—consistent finding; as early as 3 hr postingestion in cats and 6 hr in dogs; monohydrate form is more common
• Urine pH—consistently decreases
• Inconsistent findings—hematuria; proteinuria; glucosuria
• May note granular and cellular casts, WBCs, RBCs, and renal epithelial cells

OTHER LABORATORY TESTS

Blood Gases
• Metabolites cause severe metabolic acidosis.
• Total CO_2, plasma bicarbonate concentration, and blood pH—low by 3 hr postingestion; markedly low by 12 hr
• PCO_2—decreases, owing to partial respiratory compensation
• Anion gap—increased by 3 hr postingestion; peaks at 6 hr postingestion; remains increased for approximately 48 hr (ethylene glycol metabolites are unmeasured anions)

Other
• Serum osmolality and osmolal gap—high by 1 hr postingestion, in parallel with serum ethylene glycol concentrations; dose-related; usually remain high for approximately 18 hr postingestion; ethylene glycol toxicosis most common cause of a high osmolal gap
• Ethylene glycol serum concentration—peaks 1–6 hr postingestion; usually not detectable in the serum or urine by 72 hr; commercial kits (EGT Test Kit) measure concentrations at > 50 mg/dL; estimate by multiplying the osmolal gap by 6.2.

IMAGING
Ultrasound—renal cortices may be hyperechoic as a result of crystals.

DIAGNOSTIC PROCEDURES
• Kidney biopsy—with anuria; confirm diagnosis
• Cytologic examination of kidney imprints—often diagnostic; numerous calcium oxalate crystals

PATHOLOGIC FINDINGS
Kidneys—often swollen

TREATMENT

APPROPRIATE HEALTH CARE
• Cats—usually inpatient
• Dogs—usually outpatient if < 5 hr postingestion and treated with fomepizole; inpatient if > 5 hr for intravenous fluids to correct dehydration, increase tissue perfusion, and promote diuresis

NURSING CARE
• Goals—prevent absorption; increase excretion; prevent metabolism
• Induction of vomiting and gastric lavage with activated charcoal—may not be beneficial due to the rapid absorption of ethylene glycol
• Intravenous fluids—correct dehydration, increase tissue perfusion, and promote diuresis; accompanied by bicarbonate given slowly intravenously to correct metabolic acidosis
• Monitor serial plasma bicarbonate concentrations—$0.3 - 0.5 \times$ body weight (kg) $\times$ (24 − plasma bicarbonate) − sodium bicarbonate needed (mEq)
• Monitor urine pH in response to therapy.
• Azotemia and oliguric renal failure (dogs)—most of the ethylene glycol has been metabolized; little benefit from inhibition of ADH; correct fluid, electrolyte, and acid–base disorders; establish diuresis; diuretics (particularly mannitol) may help; peritoneal dialysis may be useful; may need extended treatment (several weeks) before renal function is reestablished

SURGICAL CONSIDERATIONS
Kidney transplantation—successfully employed in cats with ethylene glycol–induced renal failure

MEDICATIONS

DRUG(S) OF CHOICE
Dogs
• Fomepizole (4-methyl pyrazole; Antizol-Vet)—effective and nontoxic liver ADH inhibitor; more expensive than ethanol (initial cost offset by less time in intensive care); 5% (50 mg/mL) at 20 mg/kg IV initially; then 15 mg/kg IV at 12 and 24 hr; then 5 mg/kg IV at 36 hr

Cats
• Fomepizole—ineffective; not recommended, at least with dosage schedules used in dogs; clinical trials suggest much larger doses may be effective.

• Ethanol—therapy of choice; 20% at 5 mL/kg diluted in fluids and given in a IV drip over 6 hr for five treatments; then over 8 hr for four more treatments

CONTRAINDICATIONS
Avoid drugs that cause CNS depression.

PRECAUTIONS
• Competitive substrates (alcohols, such as ethanol)—contribute to CNS depression; monitor respiration
• Cats—usually become hypothermic; require an external heat source
• Other pyrazoles—may be toxic to the marrow and liver; do not substitute for fomepizole.

POSSIBLE INTERACTIONS
• Fomepizole—none
• Ethanol—contributes to CNS depression; further increases serum osmolality

ALTERNATIVE DRUG(S)
Ethanol, propylene glycol, and 1,3-butanediol—higher affinity for ADH than does ethylene glycol; effectively to inhibit ethylene glycol metabolism; may cause CNS depression and increase serum osmolality; constant serum ethanol concentrations of 100 mg/dL will inhibit most ethylene glycol metabolism.
• Ethanol—even in early stages requires hospitalization for approximately 3 days; constant intravenous infusion (ethanol and fluids); continuous monitoring for respiratory and acid–base status

FOLLOW-UP

PATIENT MONITORING
BUN, acid–base status, and urine output—monitored daily for the first few days

PREVENTION/AVOIDANCE
• Increasing client awareness of the toxicity—help prevent exposure; earlier treatment of patients
• Use of new antifreeze products containing propylene glycol (relatively nontoxic)

POSSIBLE COMPLICATIONS
• Without azotemia—usually no complications
• Urine concentrating ability—may be impaired with azotemia; patients recover.

EXPECTED COURSE AND PROGNOSIS
• Untreated—oliguric renal failure (dogs, 36–72 hr; cats, 12–24 hr); anuria by 72–96 hr postingestion
• Dogs treated < 5 hr postingestion—prognosis excellent with fomepizole treatment
• Dogs treated up to 8 hr postingestion—most recover
• Dogs treated up to 36 hr postingestion—may be of benefit to prevent metabolism of any remaining ethylene glycol

• Cats treated within 3 hr postingestion—prognosis good with ethanol treatment • If a large quantity of ethylene glycol is ingested, prognosis is poor, unless treated within 4 hours of ingestion
• Patients with azotemia and oliguric renal failure—prognosis poor; almost all of the ethylene glycol will have been metabolized.

MISCELLANEOUS

AGE-RELATED FACTORS
Patients < 6 months of age with oliguric renal failure sometimes fully recover.

SYNONYMS
Antifreeze poisoning

SEE ALSO
• Osmolarity, Hyperosmolarity
• Renal Failure, Acute

ABBREVIATIONS
• ADH = alcohol dehydrogenase
• BUN = blood urea nitrogen
• CVS = cardiovascular system
• PCV = packed cell volume
• RBC = red blood cell
• WBC = white blood cell

Suggested Reading
Connally HE, Thrall MA, Forney SD, et al. Safety and efficacy of 4-methylpyrazole as treatment for suspected or confirmed ethylene glycol intoxication in dogs: 107 cases (1983–1995). J Am Vet Med Assoc 1996; 209:1880–1883.
Dial SM, Thrall MA, Hamar DW. Comparison of ethanol and 4-methylpyrazole as therapies for ethylene glycol intoxication in the cat. Am J Vet Res 1994;55:1771–1782.
Dial SM, Thrall MA, Hamar DW. Efficacy of 4-methylpyrazole for treatment of ethylene glycol intoxication in dogs. Am J Vet Res 1994;55:1762–1770.
Poldelski V, Johnson A, Wright S, et al. Ethylene glycol–mediated tubular injury; identification of critical metabolites and injury pathways. Am J Kidney Dis 2001; 38:239–248.
Thrall MA, Grauer GF, Dial SM. Antifreeze poisoning. In: Bonagura JD, ed. Kirk's current veterinary therapy XII. Philadelphia: Saunders, 1995:232–237.
Thrall MA, Grauer GF, Connally HE, et al. Ethylene glycol. In: Talcott P, Peterson M, eds. Small animal toxicology. Philadelphia: Saunders, 2000:484–504.
Authors Mary Anna Thrall, Gregory F. Grauer, and Sharon M. Dial
Consulting Editor Gary D. Osweiler

EXCESSIVE VOCALIZATION

BASICS

OVERVIEW
• Vocalization that is uncontrollable, excessive, or occurs at inappropriate times of day or night or that disrupts owners, neighbors, or other pets
• Pain or illness can lead to distress or care-soliciting vocalization. Cognitive dysfunction syndrome (CDS) can lead to excessive vocalization and night waking. Hearing decline may be associated with excessive vocalization.

SIGNALMENT
• Dogs and cats
• Oriental breeds of cats may be more prone.
• Dog breeds that are bred for work, high energy, and stamina may be prone to excess barking.
• Senior pets more prone to hearing loss and CDS
• Intact cats during estrus and mating

SIGNS
Subjective—related to intensity, duration, time of day, or environment

CAUSES & RISK FACTORS
• Medical—disease, pain, CDS
• Anxiety or conflict
• Alarm barking—territorial or response to novel stimuli
• Territorial—warning or guarding response
• Social or attention-seeking behavior that is reinforced
• Distress vocalization (e.g., howling/whining)—separation from mother, family, or social group
• Growl—may be associated with agonistic displays
• Hyperactivity disorders (hyperkinesis)—dogs
• Stereotypical behaviors or compulsive disorders—dogs
• Mating—sexual (cats)

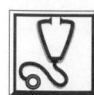

DIAGNOSIS

DIFFERENTIAL DIAGNOSIS
• Barking due to anxiety conditions occurs primarily during owner absence.
• Barking due to territorial behaviors occurs when the owner is present or absent.

CBC/BIOCHEMISTRY/URINALYSIS
To rule out underlying disorders

OTHER LABORATORY TESTS
T_4—cats

IMAGING
If medical/neurological disorder suspected

DIAGNOSTIC PROCEDURES
• BAER testing if auditory deficiency suspected
• Behavioral diagnosis to determine inciting stimuli based on detailed and accurate history; observation of pet, owner, and interactions between the two; video if available.

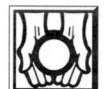

TREATMENT

General Comments
• Must be individualized for the pet, household, and type of problem
• Design a program that addresses the underlying cause and any aggravating factors.

• Products such as head halters, bark-activated alarms, bark-activated citronella collars, and disruptive devices such as alarms or water sprayers can be used to achieve a quiet response, which can then be reinforced, and are best used when the owner is present.
• Devocalization (illegal in some countries) can be used as a last option but does not address the underlying cause and may not sufficiently reduce vocalization, since some vocalization may recur postoperatively.

Behavior Modification
• Avoid reinforcement. If the stimulus retreats before the vocalization ceases, the pet is reinforced. If the owner gives any form of attention, including insufficiently aversive punishment, the vocalization may be reinforced.
• Reward-based training—teach pets to respond to basic commands.
• Train dogs to be quiet on command (consider head halter control).
• Owners must remain calm and in control. Owner anxiety, verbal reprimands, and punishment can increase the pet's anxiety and potentiate barking.
• Response substitution—teach an appropriate response to the stimulus (e.g., sitting quietly).
• Desensitize and countercondition—expose the pet to the inciting stimulus at a low level (under the response threshold) and pair a favored reinforcer such as a food treat with the stimulus to change the emotional response to one that is calm or positive. Then progress to gradually more intense stimulus.

• Punishment is not recommended except for devices that disrupt or inhibit vocalization so that the pet can be quieted and reinforced.

Environmental Modification
Make adjustments to limit or prevent exposure to the stimuli that incite vocalization.

 MEDICATIONS

DRUG(S)
• Might be indicated if there is anxiety, conflict, excessive responsiveness to stimuli or a compulsive disorder
• Benzodiazepines on a short-term or as-needed basis when situations of anxiety might be expected or for inducing sleep (dog: diazepam, 0.5–2.2 mg/kg PO as needed up to q8h; cat: oxazepam, 0.2–.05 mg/kg PO as needed up to q12h)
• Sedatives such as acepromazine (0.5–2.2 mg/kg PO as needed) may be effective for tranquilizing the pet prior to exposure to stimuli (e.g., car rides, fireworks) but do not decrease anxiety and may increase noise sensitivity and vocalization in some dogs.
• Tricyclic antidepressants or selective serotonin reuptake inhibitors (SSRIs) for long term or ongoing therapy for excessive and chronic anxiety; combine with behavior modification. Clomipramine—dog: 1–3 mg/kg PO q12h; cat: 0.5 mg/kg PO q24h.

• SSRIs or clomipramine combined with behavior therapy for compulsive disorders
• Selegiline and Hills Prescription Diet b/d (dogs) for vocalization and night waking related to CDS

CONTRAINDICATIONS/POSSIBLE INTERACTIONS
Review contraindications for any drug utilized

 FOLLOW-UP

PATIENT MONITORING
• Modify the program based on response.
• Drugs, bark-activated collars, disruptive devices, and devocalization might be added if not previously utilized.

PREVENTION/AVOIDANCE
• Obedience training, head halter training, training the quiet command (dogs)
• Avoid reinforcement of inappropriate behavior.
• Habituate pet to a variety of stimuli and environments throughout development.
• Socialize pet to a variety of people and other pets throughout development.

POSSIBLE COMPLICATIONS
• Owner anxiety and verbal reprimands may aggravate problem.
• Intermittent reinforcement will aggravate problem.

EXPECTED COURSE AND PROGNOSIS
• Variable—based on diagnosis, environment, pet and owner expectations
• Most can be sufficiently improved over time.
• It is impractical to expect to eliminate all vocalization.

 MISCELLANEOUS

SEE ALSO
• Cognitive Dysfunction Syndrome
• Compulsive Disorders—Dogs
• Compulsive Disorders—Cats
• Separation Anxiety Syndrome

ABBREVIATIONS
• BAER = brainstem auditory evoked response
• CDS = cognitive dysfunction syndrome

Suggested Reading
Juarbe-Diaz SV. Assessment and treatment of excessive barking in the domestic dog, Vet Clin North Am Small Anim Pract; 27(3):1997, 515–532.
Landsberg G, Hunthausen W, Ackerman L. Handbook of behaviour problems of the dog and cat. 2nd ed. Philadelphia: Saunders, published 2003.
Authors Gary Landsberg and Sagi Denenberg
Consulting Editor Debra F. Horwitz

EXOCRINE PANCREATIC INSUFFICIENCY

 BASICS

DEFINITION
Progressive loss of exocrine pancreatic acinar cells, causing failure of absorption because of inadequate production of digestive enzymes

PATHOPHYSIOLOGY
• Idiopathic pancreatic acinar atrophy—the most common cause in dogs
• Chronic pancreatitis, with resultant destruction of acinar tissue—much less common cause in dogs; most common cause in cats
• May rarely develop with pancreatic adenocarcinoma and pancreatic duct obstruction
• Deficient exocrine pancreatic secretion results in maldigestion, nutrient malabsorption, and osmotic diarrhea.
• Malabsorption contributes to small intestinal bacterial overgrowth (SIBO), which may cause secretory diarrhea.

SYSTEMS AFFECTED
• Gastrointestinal—duodenal mucosal disease (villus atrophy, inflammatory cellular infiltrates, abnormal mucosal enzyme activities), and SIBO
• Nutritional—protein-calorie malnourishment

GENETICS
Assumed to be hereditary in the German shepherd dog and transmitted by an autosomal recessive trait

INCIDENCE/PREVALENCE
• Relatively common in the German shepherd dog; may be seen in all canine breeds
• Rare in cats

GEOGRAPHIC DISTRIBUTION
• Dogs—N/A
• Cats—may be seen with pancreatic fluke infestation (southeast United States)

SIGNALMENT

Species
Dogs and cats

Breed Predilection
German shepherd dogs

Mean Age and Range
• Pancreatic acinar atrophy in young dogs
• Chronic pancreatitis in old dogs
• Chronic pancreatitis or pancreatic fluke infestation in middle-aged and older cats

Predominant Sex
N/A

SIGNS

General Comments
• Consider in young German shepherd dogs with chronic diarrhea suggesting malassimilation.
• Severity—varies; depends on the time elapsed prior to diagnosis and therapy

Historical Findings
• Weight loss with a normal to increased appetite
• Chronic watery diarrhea of small bowel origin is common.
• Diarrhea—often resembles cow feces; may be continuous or intermittent
• Fecal volumes larger than normal; steatorrhea present
• Diarrhea may decrease with a low-fat, highly digestible diet
• Flatulence and borborygmus—common
• May be coprophagia and pica
• May see polyuria/polydipsia with diabetes mellitus caused by chronic pancreatitis

Physical Examination Findings
• Thin body
• Decreased muscle mass
• "Unthrifty" appearance with a poor-quality haircoat
• Cats with steatorrhea may have greasy "soiling" of the haircoat around the rectum.

CAUSES
• Pancreatic acinar atrophy
• Chronic relapsing pancreatitis
• Pancreatic adenocarcinoma
• Pancreatic fluke *(Eurytrema procyonis)* infection in cats

RISK FACTORS
• Breed—German shepherd dogs
• Any condition predisposing patients to recurrent pancreatitis

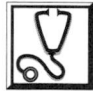 DIAGNOSIS

DIFFERENTIAL DIAGNOSIS
• Exclude causes of malabsorption (small intestinal mucosal disease, lymphangiectasia) by intestinal mucosal biopsy.
• Rule out SIBO or antibiotic-responsive diarrhea with a therapeutic trial of oxytetracyclines administered for 14–21 days.
• Exclude chronic parasitism by performing multiple fecal examinations +/− anthelmintic therapy.
• Exclude diabetes mellitus and feline hyperthyroidism by appropriate laboratory testing.

CBC/BIOCHEMISTRY/URINALYSIS
Usually normal

OTHER LABORATORY TESTS

Direct/Indirect Fecal Examinations
Negative for parasites

Exocrine Pancreatic Function Tests— Trypsin-like Immunoreactivity (TLI)
• Diagnostic test of choice in both dogs and cats
• Theory of test—serum TLI can be detected by an assay that measures trypsinogen leaked directly into the blood from pancreatic acinar tissue; serum TLI is detected in all normal dogs and cats with a functional exocrine pancreatic mass.
• Serum TLI concentrations—dramatically reduced with EPI
• Canine and feline TLI tests—differ; species-specific
• Advantages—simple; quick; single serum specimen (fasted) required; highly sensitive

Exocrine Pancreatic Function Tests— Others
Assays of fecal proteolytic activity using casein-based substrates are an accurate means of diagnosing EPI in both dogs and cats; disadvantages include the need for collecting multiple fecal specimens over days and the lack of availability of the test.

Screening Tests for Malassimilation
Microscopic examination of feces for undigested food, assessment of fecal proteolytic activity by x-ray film digestion, and the plasma turbidity test are unreliable and *not* recommended.

Cobalamin and Folate
• Often run as a panel with TLI
• Used to assess for SIBO and as a nonspecific indicator of moderate-to-advanced small intestinal malabsorption

IMAGING
Abdominal radiography and ultrasonography are unremarkable.

DIAGNOSTIC PROCEDURES
N/A

PATHOLOGIC FINDINGS
• Pancreatic acinar atrophy—marked atrophy/absence of pancreatic acinar tissue on gross inspection
• Pancreatitis—microscopically, acini and possibly islets are depleted and replaced by fibrous tissue.

TREATMENT

APPROPRIATE HEALTH CARE
• Outpatient medical management
• Patients with concurrent diabetes mellitus may initially require hospitalization for insulin regulation of hyperglycemia.

NURSING CARE
N/A

ACTIVITY
N/A

DIET
• Modification is a cornerstone of therapy in dogs.
• Ideally is highly digestible, low in fat, low in fiber, and nutritionally balanced
• High digestibility reduces nutrient availability for bacterial overgrowth
• Avoid high-fat diets—fat absorption remains impaired despite appropriate enzyme therapy.
• Avoid high-fiber diets—fiber inhibits the activity of pancreatic enzymes.
• Severely malnourished dogs may require supplementation with cobalamin, tocopherol, and fat-soluble vitamins A, D, E, and K.

CLIENT EDUCATION
• Discuss hereditary nature in German shepherd dogs.
• Discuss expense of pancreatic enzymes and need for lifelong therapy.
• Discuss the possibility of diabetes mellitus in patients with recurrent pancreatitis.

SURGICAL CONSIDERATIONS
Mesenteric torsion reported in German shepherd dogs in Scandinavia but not North America.

MEDICATIONS

DRUGS OF CHOICE
• Powdered, non–enteric-coated pancreatic enzyme concentrates—therapy of choice
• Initially—mix enzyme powder in food at a dosage of 1 teaspoon with each meal per 10 kg body weight; feed two meals daily to promote weight gain.
• Preincubation of enzymes with food does *not* improve the effectiveness of oral enzyme therapy.

• Administration of bicarbonate or histamine blockers (famotidine, ranitidine, cimetidine) does *not* improve the effectiveness of enzyme therapy.
• Most dogs respond to therapy within 5–7 days; then the amount of daily pancreatic supplement may be gradually reduced to a dose that prevents return of clinical signs.
• Oral antibiotic therapy (metronidazole, 10–15 mg/kg PO q12h, oxytetracycline, 20 mg/kg PO q12h) may be required for 14–21 days in dogs with concurrent SIBO.

CONTRAINDICATIONS
Avoid enteric-coated pancreatic enzyme tablets; dissolution of their protective coating is unpredictable, and poor responses may be seen.

PRECAUTIONS
• Avoid tetracycline antibiotics in very young animals.
• Tetracycline antibiotics may cause fever, abdominal pain, hair loss, and depression in cats.

POSSIBLE INTERACTIONS
N/A

ALTERNATIVE DRUGS
N/A

FOLLOW-UP

PATIENT MONITORING
• Weekly for first month of therapy
• Diarrhea improves markedly—fecal consistency typically normalizes within 1 week.
• Gain in body weight
• Dogs that fail to respond after 1 week of enzyme therapy—place on antibiotics for SIBO.
• Once body weight and conditioning normalize, gradually reduce the daily dosage of enzyme supplements to a level that maintains normal body weight.

PREVENTION/AVOIDANCE
Do not breed animals with pancreatic acinar atrophy.

POSSIBLE COMPLICATIONS
• 20% of dogs fail to respond to pancreatic enzymes.
• SIBO

EXPECTED COURSE AND PROGNOSIS
• Most causes are irreversible, and lifelong therapy will be required.

• Dogs with EPI alone—prognosis is good with appropriate enzyme therapy and dietary management.
• Prognosis is more guarded in patients with EPI and diabetes mellitus due to chronic pancreatitis.

MISCELLANEOUS

ASSOCIATED CONDITIONS
• SIBO
• Diabetes mellitus
• Associated vitamin K–responsive coagulopathy has been reported in a cat.

AGE-RELATED FACTORS
Consider EPI in young adult dogs with chronic diarrhea.

ZOONOTIC POTENTIAL
None

PREGNANCY
• Do not breed animals with EPI from pancreatic acinar atrophy.
• Do not use tetracycline antibiotics or metronidazole in pregnant animals.

SYNONYMS
• Juvenile pancreatic atrophy
• Pancreatic acinar atrophy

SEE ALSO
• Diarrhea, Chronic—Dogs
• Diarrhea, Chronic—Cats
• Small Intestinal Bacterial Overgrowth
• Pancreatitis

ABBREVIATIONS
• EPI = exocrine pancreatic insufficiency
• SIBO = small intestinal bacterial overgrowth
• TLI = trypsin-like immunoreactivity

Suggested Reading
Dennis HG, Stocker R. Exocrine pancreatic insufficiency. Vet Rec 1996;138:192.
Williams DA. Sensitivity and specificity of serum trypsin-like immunoreactivity for the diagnosis of canine exocrine pancreatic insufficiency. J Am Vet Med Assoc 1988;192;195–201.
Williams DA. Exocrine pancreatic disease. In: Ettinger SJ, Feldman EC, eds. Textbook of veterinary internal medicine. 5th ed. Philadelphia: Saunders, 2000:1345–1367.
Author Albert E. Jergens
Consulting Editor Albert E. Jergens

EYELASH DISORDERS (TRICHIASIS/DISTICHIASIS/ECTOPIC CILIA)

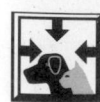

BASICS

OVERVIEW
• Trichiasis—when hair arising from normal sites contacts the corneal or conjunctival surfaces
• Distichiasis—when cilia emerge from or near the meibomian gland orifices on the lid margin and may or may not contact the cornea.
• Ectopic cilia—single or multiple hairs that arise from the palpebral conjunctival surface several millimeters from the lid margin, most commonly near the middle of the superior lid

SIGNALMENT
• Common in dogs; rare in cats
• Most common in young dogs
• Any breed may be affected
• Facial-fold trichiasis—breeds with prominent facial folds (e.g., Pekingese, pugs, and bulldogs)
• Distichiasis—found in some degree in most cocker spaniels
• Ectopic cilia—more common than average in dachshunds, lhasa apsos, and Shetland sheepdogs

SIGNS
Facial-fold Trichiasis
• Nasal corneal vascularization and pigmentation
• Blepharospasm
• Epiphora

Distichiasis
• Usually asymptomatic
• Stiff, stout cilia contacting the cornea—may note blepharospasm, epiphora, corneal vascularization, pigmentation, and ulceration

Ectopic Cilia
• Ocular pain
• Severe blepharospasm
• Epiphora
• Superficial corneal ulcers with a linear appearance (corresponding to lid movement) on the superior cornea—common; resistant to healing until the underlying problem is diagnosed and corrected

CAUSES & RISK FACTORS
Usually related to facial conformation or breed predisposition or is idiopathic

DIAGNOSIS

DIFFERENTIAL DIAGNOSIS
• Other adnexal abnormalities—entropion
• Keratoconjunctivitis sicca
• Conjunctival foreign body
• Infectious conjunctivitis
• Diagnosis based on direct observation of abnormal cilia

CBC/BIOCHEMISTRY/URINALYSIS
N/A

OTHER LABORATORY TESTS
N/A

IMAGING
N/A

DIAGNOSTIC PROCEDURES
N/A

EYELASH DISORDERS (TRICHIASIS/DISTICHIASIS/ECTOPIC CILIA)

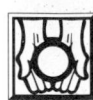

TREATMENT

TRICHIASIS
• May be managed conservatively in some patients
• Keeping the periocular hair short may help; however, clipping the hair on facial folds may make it stiffer and more irritating.
• Surgical correction of adnexal abnormalities—indicated; entropion correction
• May resect facial folds
• Medial canthal closure—often a better procedure; also eliminates lagophthalmos and medial entropion

DISTICHIASIS
• Usually asymptomatic and requires no treatment
• Symptomatic—may treat surgically by cryotherapy, electrocautery or electroepilation, or resection from the conjunctival surface
• Lid splitting techniques—avoid; postoperative scarring may predispose patient to cicatricial entropion and impaired lid function.

ECTOPIC CILIA
• May be treated surgically—en-bloc resection of the cilia and associated meibomian gland
• Cryotherapy—may be used as the sole treatment or as an adjunct after surgical resection
• Warn client that patient is at risk for developing ectopic cilia at other locations.
• Advise client to have patient rechecked if clinical signs recur.

MEDICATIONS

DRUG(S)
• Rarely indicated
• Lubricant ointments—sometimes valuable to soften cilia and lessen irritation before surgical correction
• Topical antibiotics—perioperative; recommended for patients undergoing surgery to minimize conjunctival flora in the surgical sites

CONTRAINDICATIONS/POSSIBLE INTERACTIONS
N/A

FOLLOW-UP
Distichia—regrowth common because destructive procedures (cryotherapy and electroepilation) must be done conservatively to minimize lid damage.

MISCELLANEOUS

Suggested Reading
Gelatt KN. Veterinary ophthalmology, 3rd ed. Baltimore: Lippincott Williams & Wilkins, 1999.
Slatter D. Fundamentals of veterinary ophthalmology. 3rd ed. Philadelphia: Saunders, 2001.
Author Erin S. Champagne
Consulting Editor Paul E. Miller

FACIAL NERVE PARESIS AND PARALYSIS

BASICS

DEFINITION
Dysfunction of the facial nerve (seventh cranial nerve), causing paralysis or weakness of the muscles of the ears, eyelids, lips, and nostrils

PATHOPHYSIOLOGY
Weakness or paralysis caused by impairment of the facial nerve or the neuromuscular junction peripherally or the facial nucleus in the brainstem

SYSTEMS AFFECTED
• Nervous—facial nerve peripherally or its nucleus in the brainstem
• Ophthalmic—if parasympathetic preganglionic neurons that supply the lacrimal glands and course with the facial nerve are involved, keratoconjunctivitis sicca develops because of lack of tear secretion.

GENETICS
N/A

INCIDENCE/PREVALENCE
More common in dogs than cats

GEOGRAPHIC DISTRIBUTION
N/A

SIGNALMENT

Species
Dogs and cats

Breed Predilections
Idiopathic paralysis—cocker spaniels, Pembroke Welsh corgis, boxers, English setters, and domestic longhair cats

Mean Age and Range
Adults

Predominant Sex
N/A

SIGNS

General Comments
• Assess strength of the palpebral closure; there should be full eyelid closure when a finger is gently passed over both eyelids simultaneously.
• Paresis—unilateral and idiopathic in most animals; not infrequently, unaffected facial nerve becomes affected within a few weeks to months; idiopathic paresis may rarely occur bilaterally.

• Most patients with bilateral nerve involvement have a systemic disease.
• Unilateral paresis or paralysis—may accompany other clinical signs; may indicate focal or systemic disease

Historical Findings
• Messy eating; food left around mouth
• Excessive drooling
• Facial asymmetry
• Eye—inability to close; rubbing; ocular discharge

Physical Examination Findings
• Ipsilateral ear and lip drooping
• Excessive drooling
• Food falling from the side of mouth
• Collapse of the nostril
• Inability to close the eyelids
• Wide palpebral fissure
• Decreased or absent menace response and palpebral reflex
• Chronic—patient may have deviation of the face toward the affected side.
• Mucopurulent discharge from the affected eye and exposure conjunctivitis or keratitis—may be noted
• When secondary to brainstem disease—altered mentation (e.g., somnolence or stupor); other cranial nerve and gait abnormalities may be noted.

CAUSES

Unilateral Peripheral
• Idiopathic*
• Metabolic—hypothyroid
• Inflammatory—otitis media or interna* (dogs and cats); nasopharyngeal polyps (cats)*
• Neoplasia
• Trauma—fracture of the petrous temporal bone; injury to the facial nerve external to the stylomastoid foramen or secondary to surgical ablation of external ear canal

Bilateral Peripheral
• Idiopathic—rare
• Inflammatory and immune mediated—polyradiculoneuritis, including coonhound paralysis;* polyneuropathies;* myasthenia gravis*
• Metabolic—paraneoplastic polyneuropathy* (e.g., insulinoma)
• Toxic—botulism
• Pituitary neoplasm—unknown cause
• Infectious—Lyme borreliosis in humans not proven in dogs at this time

CNS
• Most unilateral
• Inflammatory—infectious (e.g., viral, bacterial, fungal, rickettsial, protozoal) and noninfectious (e.g., granulomatous meningoencephalomyelitis)
• Neoplastic—primary brain tumor; metastatic tumor

RISK FACTORS
Chronic ear disease

DIAGNOSIS

DIFFERENTIAL DIAGNOSIS
• Differentiate unilateral from bilateral.
• Look for other neurologic deficits.
• Idiopathic—likely if patient has no historical or physical signs of ear disease and no other neurologic deficits
• Hypothyroidism—with clinical evidence (e.g., lethargy and poor hair coat)
• Middle or inner ear disease—if Horner's syndrome and/or head tilt and/or deafness and/or KCS simultaneously present
• CNS disease—suspect if the patient is somnolent and displays neurologic signs related to the brainstem

CBC/BIOCHEMISTRY/URINALYSIS
• Usually normal in idiopathic facial paralysis
• Hypercholesterolemia and/or nonregenerative anemia—may be seen with hypothyroidism-associated facial paralysis
• Hypoglycemia—with insulinoma

OTHER LABORATORY TESTS
• Mainly indicated for patients with bilateral weakness
• Insulin:glucose determined simultaneously—detect insulinoma
• Acetylcholine receptor antibodies—detect myasthenia gravis
• ELISA—detect coonhound paralysis
• Hypothyroidism tests

FACIAL NERVE PARESIS AND PARALYSIS

IMAGING
• Bullae radiographs—(i.e., oblique, open mouthed) not sensitive for middle-inner ear diseases
• CT—sensitive test to define middle-inner ear; MRI preferable for brainstem disease

DIAGNOSTIC PROCEDURES
• Schirmer tear test—evaluate tear production
• Electromyography and evaluation of motor nerve conduction velocity—detect poly-radiculoneuritis and polyneuropathy
• CSF examination—detect brainstem disease

PATHOLOGIC FINDINGS
• Idiopathic—may see degeneration of large and small myelinated fibers without evidence of inflammation

TREATMENT

APPROPRIATE HEALTH CARE
• Outpatient—idiopathic facial paralysis
• Inpatient—initial medical work up and management of systemic or CNS disease

NURSING CARE
N/A

ACTIVITY
N/A

DIET
No change required

CLIENT EDUCATION
• Advise client that the clinical signs may be permanent, but as muscle fibrosis develops, there is a natural "tuck up" that reduces asymmetry; drooling usually stops within 2–4 weeks.
• Inform client that the other side can become affected.
• Discuss eye care: the cornea on the affected side may need lubrication; extra care may be needed if the animal is a breed with natural exophthalmos; client must regularly check for corneal ulcers.

• Inform client that most animals tolerate this nerve deficit well.

SURGICAL CONSIDERATIONS
Bulla osteotomy—may be necessary in patients with disorders of the middle ear

MEDICATIONS

DRUG(S) OF CHOICE
• Treat specific disease if possible
• Idiopathic disease—none specific; efficacy of steroids unknown, although used very commonly in people to treat Bell's palsy
• Tear replacement—if Schirmer tear test value low; with ectropion or exophthalmic globes

CONTRAINDICATIONS
N/A

PRECAUTIONS
N/A

POSSIBLE INTERACTIONS
N/A

ALTERNATIVE DRUG(S)
N/A

FOLLOW-UP

PATIENT MONITORING
• Reevaluate early for evidence of corneal ulcers.
• Assess monthly for menace responses, palpebral reflexes, and lip and ear movements to evaluate return of function and condition of affected eye, although damage is usually permanent.

PREVENTION/AVOIDANCE
N/A

POSSIBLE COMPLICATIONS
• Keratoconjunctivitis sicca
• Corneal ulcers
• Severe contracture on side of lesion

EXPECTED COURSE AND PROGNOSIS
• Depend on cause
• Idiopathic disease—prognosis guarded for recovery
• Improvement may take weeks or months or may never occur.
• Lip contracture sometimes develops.

MISCELLANEOUS

ASSOCIATED CONDITIONS
N/A

AGE-RELATED FACTORS
N/A

ZOONOTIC POTENTIAL
N/A

PREGNANCY
N/A

SYNONYMS
Idiopathic facial paresis and paralysis

SEE ALSO
• Hypothyroidism
• Keratitis, Ulcerative
• Keratoconjunctivitis Sicca (KCS)
• Otitis Media and Interna

ABBREVIATIONS
• CSF = cerebrospinal fluid
• CT = computed tomography
• ELISA = enzyme-linked immunosorbent assay
• KCS = Keratoconjunctivitis sicca
• MRI = magnetic resonance imaging

Suggested Reading
Braund KG, Luttgen PJ, Sorjonen DC, et al. Idiopathic facial paralysis in the dog. Vet Rec 1979;105:297–299.
Kern TJ, Hollis NE. Facial neuropathy in dogs and cats: 95 cases (1975–1985). J Am Vet Med Assoc 1987;191:1604–1609.
Author T. Mark Neer
Consulting Editor Joane M. Parent

FALSE PREGNANCY

 BASICS

DEFINITION
Display of maternal behavior and physical signs of pregnancy in middle to late diestrus by a nonpregnant bitch

PATHOPHYSIOLOGY
• Underlying endocrinologic mechanism—poorly understood; all bitches that ovulate produce functional corpora lutea and remain under progesterone influence for 2–3 months.
• Serum progesterone concentrations—similar in pregnant, nonpregnant, and false-pregnant animals, except for a sharp decline 1–2 days before parturition
• Thought that the falling serum progesterone concentration causes a marked increase in prolactin (expressed as a percentage change in the serum prolactin concentration), which may be responsible for initiating the changes seen in false-pregnant animals
• Mating during the preceding estrus—no influence on occurrence
• Future fertility not affected

SYSTEMS AFFECTED
• Reproductive
• Behavioral

GENETICS
N/A

INCIDENCE/PREVALENCE
Unknown

GEOGRAPHIC DISTRIBUTION
N/A

SIGNALMENT
Species
• Common in dogs
• Rare in cats

Breed Predilection
None

Mean Age and Range
Any age

Predominant Sex
Nonpregnant females that were in estrus 2–3 months earlier and that are experiencing a decline in serum progesterone concentration

SIGNS
General Comments
Severity variable among individuals and from one occurrence to the next within the same individual

Historical Findings
• Behavior changes—nesting, mothering activity, restlessness, and self-nursing
• Abdominal distention and mammary gland enlargement
• Vomiting, depression, and anorexia
• Signs of labor (rare)

Physical Examination Findings
Large mammary glands that secrete a brownish serous fluid or milk

CAUSES
• Progesterone and prolactin—inverse relationship; drop in progesterone concentration in late diestrus causes prolactin concentration to rise.
• Treatment with progestin for conditions not related to false pregnancy—may develop signs after drug withdrawal
• Oophorectomy or ovariohysterectomy during diestrus (when progesterone is high)—may develop signs postsurgery
• Hypothyroidism with high TSH concentration (stimulates prolactin secretion)—may note some associated clinical signs

RISK FACTORS
• Not thought to be influenced by previous pregnancy
• Does not cause predisposition to other reproductive diseases

 DIAGNOSIS

DIFFERENTIAL DIAGNOSIS
• Diagnosis—made by a history of estrus within the preceding 2–3 months and clinical signs
• Other causes of mammary gland enlargement—neoplasia; mastitis
• Other causes of abdominal enlargement—ascites; organomegaly
• Closed pyometra—usually associated with more severe systemic signs than false pregnancy
• Pregnancy

CBC/BIOCHEMISTRY/URINALYSIS
Usually normal; if not, suspect other reproductive tract or systemic disease.

OTHER LABORATORY TESTS
N/A

IMAGING
Radiography or ultrasonography—recommended to rule out pyometra and normal pregnancy

DIAGNOSTIC PROCEDURES
N/A

PATHOLOGIC FINDINGS
N/A

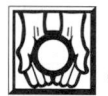 TREATMENT

APPROPRIATE HEALTH CARE
• May discharge immediately if medical treatment is tried
• Inpatient—planned surgery
• Treatment usually unnecessary—all pregnant, nonpregnant, and false-pregnant ovulating dogs go through a similar diestrus stage.
• Progestins and androgens for suppression of prolactin secretion
• Ovariohysterectomy during anestrus—prevents recurrence

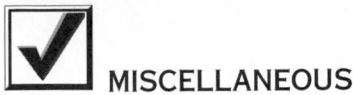

NURSING CARE
• Mammary glands—minimize stimuli that promote lactation (e.g., cold and warm packs).
• Elizabethan collar—prevent self-nursing or licking; but even rubbing of the collar on the mammary glands may be sufficient to prolong lactation.

ACTIVITY
N/A

DIET
Reduction of food over 3–4 days—may reduce lactation

CLIENT EDUCATION
• Inform client that false pregnancy is a normal phenomenon in ovulatory bitches.
• Assure client that there is no association between false pregnancy and reproductive abnormalities.
• If a litter is desired, encourage client to breed bitch during the next estrus.

SURGICAL CONSIDERATIONS
Ovariohysterectomy—if fertility not an issue; recommended during the next anestrus; do not perform while patient has clinical signs of false pregnancy, because surgery will not alleviate signs and medical treatment may be required.

 MEDICATIONS

DRUG(S) OF CHOICE
Bromocriptine—10 μg/kg PO q12h for 5 days; not approved for veterinary use in U.S. and Canada; will reduce lactation

CONTRAINDICATIONS
Bromocriptine induces abortion in pregnant animals.

PRECAUTIONS
Bromocriptine—with vomiting, give half the dosage for the next two doses; then give the full dosage again.

POSSIBLE INTERACTIONS
Concomitant use of erythromycin may increase bromocriptine plasma concentration.

ALTERNATIVE DRUG(S)
• Testosterone—1 mg/kg IM once; may cause virilizing effects (e.g., clitoral hypertrophy); contraindicated with hepatic or nephritic conditions; causes masculinization of female fetuses if given during pregnancy
• Mibolerone (Cheque)—40 μg/kg PO q24h for 5 days; same side effects as testosterone
• Megestrol acetate (Ovaban)—1–2 mg/kg PO q24h for 8 days; may cause mammary hyperplasia, pyometra, diabetes mellitus, increased appetite, weight gain, and atrophy of the adrenal cortex; signs of pseudopregnancy may recur after discontinuation.
• Mild tranquilizers may reduce behavioral signs; do not use phenothiazines, which may increase prolactin concentration.

 **FOLLOW-UP**

PATIENT MONITORING
N/A

PREVENTION/AVOIDANCE
Ovariohysterectomy during anestrus—prevents recurrence

POSSIBLE COMPLICATIONS
N/A

EXPECTED COURSE AND PROGNOSIS
• Usually resolves in 2–3 weeks without treatment
• Bromocriptine—may resolve condition in 1 week
• May develop during subsequent estrus cycles

✓ **MISCELLANEOUS**

ASSOCIATED CONDITIONS
N/A

AGE-RELATED FACTORS
N/A

ZOONOTIC POTENTIAL
N/A

PREGNANCY
Do not treat pregnant animals.

SYNONYMS
• Pseudopregnancy
• Pseudocyesis
• Phantom pregnancy

SEE ALSO
N/A

ABBREVIATIONS
TSH = thyroid-stimulating hormone

Suggested Reading
Arbeiter K, Brass W, Ballabio R, et al. Treatment of pseudopregnancy in the bitch with cabergoline, an ergoline derivative. J Small Anim Pract 1988;29:781–788.
Gobello C, Baschar H, Castex G, et al. Diestrous ovariectomy: a model to study the role of progesterone in the onset of canine pseudopregnancy. J Reprod Fert Suppl 2001;57:55–60.
Johnston SD, Root-Kustritz MV, Olsen PN. Disorders of the mammary glands of the bitch. In: Canine and feline theriogenology. Philadelphia: Saunders, 2001;243–256.
Author Klaas Post
Consulting Editor Sara K. Lyle

FAMILIAL SHAR-PEI FEVER

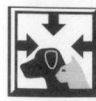 **BASICS**

DEFINITION
A familial immunoreactive disorder in the Chinese shar-pei dog characterized by episodic fever and swollen hocks, and associated with progressive systemic amyloidosis

PATHOPHYSIOLOGY
• Shar-pei dogs have a predisposition to reactive systemic amyloid deposition. The exact mechanism is unknown; however, it is suggested to be secondary to increased levels of IL-6, possibly along with other inflammatory mediators. • IL-6 can induce increased levels of serum amyloid A (an acute-phase reactant). Excessive production of serum amyloid A results in the extracellular deposition of amyloid. Amyloid deposition leads to organ failure, depending on the site of deposition. • Amyloid is deposited throughout the tissues; however, the most clinically important sites are the kidneys and liver. • Hepatic amyloidosis can lead to a friable liver susceptible to rupture and secondary hemoabdomen. • Renal amyloidosis and secondary nephrotic syndrome predispose shar-peis to states of hypercoagulability. • Similar to familial Mediterranean fever in people, these inflammatory mediators cause fever and serosal inflammation, affecting the pleura, peritoneum, and synovial membranes.

SYSTEMS AFFECTED
• Skin/exocrine—periarticular edematous soft tissue swelling, especially involving the tibiotarsal joint region; swollen muzzle; icterus • Musculoskeletal—joint effusion, especially of the tibiotarsi; lameness • Endocrine/metabolic—fever; weakness; lethargy • Renal/urologic—proteinuria; low specific gravity; polyuria; polydipsia • Hemic/lymphatic/immune—anemia; leukocytosis, with or without left shift; coagulation defects; hypercoagulable states; decreased immunoglobulin levels • Gastrointestinal—abdominal pain; vomiting; diarrhea; hemoabdomen; ascites • Hepatobiliary—hepatomegaly; hepatic rupture; elevated liver enzymes; impaired hepatic function • Cardiovascular—venous thrombosis (e.g., PTE); systemic hypertension • Respiratory—tachypnea or dyspnea • Nervous—vascular accident; acute-onset neurologic signs (e.g., head tilt, vestibular ataxia, seizures) • Ophthalmic—retinal detachment

GENETICS
Hypothesized to be an autosomal recessive inherited disorder

INCIDENCE/PREVALENCE
• An estimated 23% of shar-peis are affected by this disorder. • An estimated 53% of shar-peis with fever have shar-pei fever.

SIGNALMENT
• Mean age—4 years • Range—19 weeks to 9 years • Sex predisposition—none

SIGNS

General Comments
• Historical and physical examination findings may vary depending on the organ affected and the severity of amyloidosis. • Some cases may have only a few of the following findings.

Historical Findings
• Episodic anorexia, lethargy, and swollen hocks—self-limiting or responsive to NSAIDs • Intermittent bouts of abdominal pain, vomiting, and/or diarrhea • Polyuria and polydipsia • Weight loss

Physical Examination Findings
• Marked fever (103°–107° F) of 24–36 hr duration • Lethargy and dehydration • Edematous periarticular soft tissue swellings involving one or more joints • Joint effusion • Abdominal pain • Reluctance to move • Hunched posture • Tachypnea • Hepatomegaly, ascites, and icterus • Pale mucous membranes secondary to chronic renal failure or, in rare cases, hemoabdomen

CAUSES
• Dysregulation of immune and inflammatory processes in the shar-pei are thought to predispose the breed to development of secondary or reactive amyloidosis. • Any chronic infection, inflammation, immune-mediated disease, or neoplasia can cause reactive or secondary amyloidosis.

RISK FACTORS
N/A

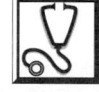 **DIAGNOSIS**

DIFFERENTIAL DIAGNOSIS
• Infectious or immune-mediated causes of polyarthritis—e.g., *Ehrlichia*, Lyme disease, systemic lupus erythematosus, idiopathic polyarthritis • Icterus (see chapter) • Chronic renal failure (see chapter) • Polyuria and polydipsia (see chapter) • Fever of unknown origin

CBC/BIOCHEMISTRY/URINALYSIS
• Nonregenerative anemia—secondary to chronic renal failure or acute hemoabdomen • Leukocytosis with or without left shift • Changes compatible with renal failure—e.g., elevations in urea, creatinine, and phosphorus levels, and increased anion gap • Hypoalbuminemia—secondary to proteinuria or hepatic failure • Hypercholesterolemia—consistent with nephrotic syndrome (hypoalbuminemia, proteinuria, ascites, and elevated cholesterol) • Elevations in ALP and ALT activity; elevated bilirubin level • Proteinuria—in cases where the amyloid is deposited in the renal cortex; note: the majority of dogs have medullary amyloid deposition, thus proteinuria may be absent • Isosthenuria—with renal involvement or hepatic failure • Bilirubinuria—secondary to liver involvement

OTHER LABORATORY TESTS
• *Ehrlichia* and *Borrelia* serology • Heartworm tests—to rule out glomerulonephritis secondary to heartworm induced antigen-antibody complexes • Coombs' test, ANA, and rheumatoid factor—to identify concurrent, underlying immune-mediated disease • PT and PTT—factors IX and X may be lost through the glomerulus and prolong PTT; liver failure can cause prolongation of both PT and PTT; organ thrombosis may cause DIC and concurrent prolongation of PT and PTT • Antithrombin III level—may be low secondary to loss through the glomerulus; thought to fall in direct relationship with the degree of hypoalbuminemia; possibly predicts the risk of thrombus formation • IgA or IgG levels—may be low in some cases; low level thought to lead to increased risk of inflammation or infection • Urine protein:creatinine ratio—elevated with deposition of amyloid in the glomeruli; typically > 13 with amyloidosis (normal: < 1)

IMAGING
• Abdominal radiography—abnormalities may include hepatomegaly or decreased detail secondary to peritoneal effusion; abdominal effusion may be secondary to hypo-albuminemia, portal hypertension, or hemorrhage • Thoracic radiography—abnormalities may include pleural effusion secondary to severe hypoalbuminemia or pleural inflammation • Joint radiography—typically shows periarticular swelling of the soft tissues without bony involvement • Abdominal ultrasonography—may reveal a diffuse homogeneous hypoechoic appearance to the hepatic parenchyma; the kidneys may appear hyperechoic

DIAGNOSTIC PROCEDURES
• Synovial fluid analysis—may or may not reveal evidence of acute synovitis (i.e., the presence of PMNs and decreased joint fluid viscosity); inflammation may be limited to the lower supporting structures of the synovium
• Kidney and/or liver biopsy (pending normal PT, PTT, platelet number, and buccal mucosal bleeding time)—amyloid deposition

PATHOLOGIC FINDINGS
• Systemic deposition of amyloid in multiple organs, e.g., the kidneys, liver, gastrointestinal tract, spleen, lymph node, adrenal glands, heart, lungs, thyroid gland, prostate gland, and pancreas • Amyloid deposition may be associated primarily with vessels or within the parenchyma, e.g., the space of Disse in the liver.

TREATMENT

APPROPRIATE HEALTH CARE
• Outpatient—during minor episodes of pain and fever that respond to NSAIDs
• Inpatient—required during periods of anorexia, fever, marked lameness or nonspecific pain, vomiting or diarrhea, ascites, or episodes of cholestasis • Intensive care management—required during organ failure or thromboembolic events
• Emergency surgery—indicated for hemoabdomen or if splenic, portal, or renal vein thrombosis is suspected

NURSING CARE
• Balanced polyionic fluids—if patient is dehydrated or anorexic, or if vomiting and/or diarrhea are present. • Oxygen—in suspected cases of pulmonary thromboembolism
• Abdominocentesis—may be required if ascites is causing respiratory compromise
• Blood transfusions—may be indicated if anemia is severe • Fresh frozen plasma—may be considered for DIC or other coagulopathies • Human serum albumin transfusions—may be considered for ascites secondary to profound hypoalbuminemia
• Antibiotics—if sepsis is suspected or concurrent infection is diagnosed; broad spectrum should be used if sepsis is suspected; otherwise, antibiotic choice should be guided by a sensitivity panel • NSAIDs or other analgesics (e.g., opioids)—may be required for fever and pain; NSAIDs are

contraindicated in cases with concurrent renal disease or gastrointestinal signs
• Gastroprotectants—if gastric ulcer secondary to renal or hepatic disease is suspected

ACTIVITY
Limit during febrile episodes; otherwise, depends on the severity and extent of the underlying systemic disorder

DIET
• Protein-restricted diet—may be indicated in renal failure to decrease the clinical signs of uremia; dogs showing evidence of hepatic encephalopathy should be fed a protein-restricted diet once they are stable
• Omega-3 fatty acids—may be beneficial for glomerular disease

CLIENT EDUCATION
• There is no cure for familial shar-pei amyloidosis; therapy is palliative.
• Therapy may decrease the deposition of amyloid, but often the condition has progressed beyond the stage at which medication is of benefit.
• Diagnostics should be performed to ensure that there is no underlying or concurrent problem that may be treatable.
• Affected dogs should not be bred.

MEDICATION

DRUG(S)
• Colchicine—0.03 mg/kg PO q12–24h; to delay amyloid deposition; unknown if colchicine has any beneficial effect once amyloid has been deposited • DMSO—80 mg/kg SC three times per week or 125 mg PO q12h; controversial, generally doubted to have significant clinical effect • Steroids—only if a concurrent immune-mediated disease is present • Low-dose aspirin therapy—0.5–5 mg/kg PO q12–24h; if concerned about hypercoagulability

CONTRAINDICATIONS
NSAIDs are contraindicated in renal disease and gastrointestinal ulcers.

PRECAUTIONS
• Steroid use may accelerate amyloid deposition. • Colchicine can cause gastrointestinal upset; chronic use can be associated with bone marrow suppression.
• DMSO has a very strong odor.

FOLLOW-UP

PATIENT MONITORING
• Urine protein:creatinine ratios—to monitor glomerular disease • Biochemistry panel—to monitor renal and hepatic parameters, including hypoalbuminemia • Hematocrit monitoring—for anemia • Blood pressure monitoring and fundic examination—for hypertensive patients

PREVENTION/AVOIDANCE
• Avoid puppies from lines that have a history of shar-pei fever.

POSSIBLE COMPLICATIONS
Death—due to hepatic rupture or pulmonary thromboembolism

EXPECTED COURSE AND PROGNOSIS
• Waxing and waning, progressive disorder with a guarded to poor prognosis, depending on the time of diagnosis • Inevitably fatal due to chronic renal or hepatic failure • Time course may be weeks to years

AGE-RELATED FACTORS
Tends to be more severe in cases diagnosed at an early age

ZOONOTIC POTENTIAL
None

PREGNANCY
Do not breed affected dogs.

SYNONYMS
Swollen hock syndrome

ABBREVIATIONS
• ALP = alkaline phosphatase • ALT = alanine aminotransferase • ANA = antinuclear antibody • DIC = disseminated intravascular coagulation • DMSO = dimethyl sulfoxide • IL-6 = interleukin-6
• NSAID = nonsteroidal antiinflammatory drug • PMN = polymorphonuclear neutrophil • PT = prothrombin time
• PTT = partial thromboplastin time
• PTE = pulmonary thromboembolism

Suggested Reading

DiBartola SP, Tarr MJ, Webb DM, Giger U. Familial renal amyloidosis in Chinese Shar Pei dogs. J Am Vet Med Assoc 1990; 197:483–487.

May C, Hammill J, Bennett D. Chinese shar pei fever: a preliminary report. Vet Rec 1992;26:586–587.

Rivas AL, Tintle L, Kimball ES, et al. A canine febrile disorder associated with elevated interleukin-6. Clin Immunol Immunopathol 1992;64:36–45.

Author Julie Armstrong
Editor Stephen Kruth

FANCONI SYNDROME

BASICS

OVERVIEW
A collection of abnormalities arising from defective renal tubular transport of water, sodium, potassium, glucose, phosphate, bicarbonate, and amino acids; impaired tubular reabsorption causes excessive urinary excretion of these solutes.

SIGNALMENT

Species
Dogs

Breed Predilections
• Approximately 75% of the reported cases have occurred in the Basenji breed; estimates of the prevalence within the Basenji breed in North America range from 10 to 30%; it is presumed to be inherited in this breed, but the mode of inheritance is unknown.
• Idiopathic Fanconi syndrome reported sporadically in several different breeds, including border terriers, Norwegian elkhounds, a whippet, a Yorkshire terrier, a Labrador retriever, a Shetland sheepdog, and a mixed-breed dog.

Mean Age and Range
Age at diagnosis ranges from 10 weeks to 11 years; most develop clinical signs from 2–4 years.

Predominant Sex
No sex predilection

SIGNS

General Comments
• Vary depending on the severity of specific solute losses and whether renal failure has developed
• Loss of amino acids and glucose—usually not associated with clinical signs other than polyuria and polydipsia

Historical Findings
• Polyuria
• Polydipsia
• Weight loss
• ± Lethargy
• ± Reduced appetite

Physical Examination Findings
• Poor body condition
• Reduced and/or abnormal growth (rickets) in young, growing animals

CAUSES & RISK FACTORS
• Inherited in most cases; particularly in Basenjis
• Acquired Fanconi syndrome—reported in dogs treated with gentamicin, streptozotocin, and amoxicillin; also reported secondary to primary hypoparathyroidism

DIAGNOSIS

DIFFERENTIAL DIAGNOSIS
Primary renal glucosuria—both cause glucosuria in the absence of hyperglycemia; documentation of aminoaciduria, mild proteinuria, or a normal anion gap metabolic acidosis (indicating bicarbonate loss) suggests Fanconi syndrome

CBC/BIOCHEMISTRY/URINALYSIS
• CBC usually normal
• Hypokalemia in about one-third
• Azotemia if patient has renal failure
• Hypophosphatemia and hypocalcemia may occur in young, growing animals.
• Urine specific gravity usually low (1.005–1.018); mild proteinuria common
• Glucosuria in the absence of hyperglycemia—found frequently; often the first suggestion of Fanconi syndrome

OTHER LABORATORY TESTS
Blood gas analysis may reveal normal anion gap metabolic acidosis, which develops because of urinary bicarbonate loss (referred to as proximal renal tubular acidosis); urine remains acidic, and bicarbonate does not appear in the urine unless a bicarbonate load is administered.

IMAGING

Young, growing dogs may exhibit radiographic findings consistent with rickets (decreased bone density, wide irregular growth plates) and angular limb deformities; adult patients may exhibit decreased bone density.

DIAGNOSTIC PROCEDURES

Urinary clearance studies to document excessive excretion of solutes such as amino acids may be needed for confirmation.

PATHOLOGIC FINDINGS

Renal papillary necrosis in many patients

TREATMENT

• Discontinue any drug that may cause Fanconi syndrome or treat for a specific intoxication.
• No treatment will reverse the transport defects in dogs with inherited or idiopathic disease.
• Because the number and severity of transport defects vary markedly between animals, treatments for hypokalemia, metabolic acidosis, renal failure, or rickets must be individualized. Treatments for hypokalemia, renal failure, and rickets are discussed elsewhere in this publication.
• Institute treatment for metabolic acidosis if blood bicarbonate concentration is < 12

mEq/L; large doses of bicarbonate may be required because reduced tubular resorptive capacity results in marked urinary bicarbonate loss; the goal of bicarbonate therapy is to maintain blood bicarbonate concentration from 12 to 18 mEq/L.
• Young, growing dogs may require vitamin D and/or calcium and phosphorus supplementation.

MEDICATIONS

DRUG(S)

Sodium bicarbonate (10–50 mg/kg q8–12h) or potassium citrate (40–75 mg/kg q12h) as required (based on blood gas and electrolyte measurements) in patients with metabolic acidosis

CONTRAINDICATIONS/POSSIBLE INTERACTIONS

Avoid drugs that are nephrotoxic or have the potential to cause Fanconi syndrome (see Causes and Risk Factors).

FOLLOW-UP

• Monitor serum biochemistry at 10- to 14-day intervals to assess the effect of treatment and any change in parameters

(especially BUN, creatinine, and potassium concentration); because bicarbonate therapy may aggravate renal potassium loss, monitor serum potassium concentration regularly; once stable, monitor serum chemistry at 2- to 4-month intervals. • Clinical course—varies; some dogs remain stable for years; others develop rapidly progressive renal failure over a few months; the cause of death is usually acute renal failure, often associated with severe metabolic acidosis.

MISCELLANEOUS

SEE ALSO

• Hypokalemia
• Renal Failure, Acute
• Renal Failure, Chronic

Suggested Reading

Bartges JW. Disorders of renal tubules. In: Ettinger SJ, Feldman EC, eds. Textbook of veterinary internal medicine, 5th ed. Philadelphia: Saunders, 2000:1704–1710.
Author Darcy H. Shaw
Consulting Editors Larry G. Adams and Carl A. Osborne

FEARS, PHOBIAS, AND ANXIETIES—CATS

 BASICS

DEFINITION
• Fear is the feeling of apprehension resulting from the nearness of some situation or object presenting an external threat. The response of the autonomic nervous system prepares the body for "freeze, fight, or flight." As such, it is a normal behavior.
• Anxiety is the anticipation of dangers from unknown or imagined origins that results in physiologic reactions associated with fear. Anxiety may occur in the aftermath of a fear-producing event or as a result of unrelated environmental changes that are unpredictable.
• A phobia is a persistent and excessive fear of a specific stimulus, such as a thunderstorm or separation from an attachment figure.

PATHOPHYSIOLOGY
Chronic anxiety or fear can lead to secondary behavior problems, such as overgrooming, spraying, or intercat aggression, or predispose the cat to health problems owing to a compromised immune system.

SYSTEMS AFFECTED
• Behavioral—hypervigilance, avoidance behaviors, possible aggression if handling or restraint attempted
• Cardiovascular—increased heart rate and blood flow to internal organs during fear-provoking incidents
• Endocrine/Metabolic—glucose release into the bloodstream, release of glucocorticoids
• Gastrointestinal—decreased appetite
• Hemic/Lymphatic/Immune—chronic stress effects on immune function
• Musculoskeletal—weight loss over time as response to chronic stress effects on appetite, decreased food intake due to hiding behavior
• Neuromuscular—may see a decrease in activity due to avoidance and hiding. Fearful/anxious reaction may also include pacing, trembling, repetitive activity.
• Ophthalmic—Dilated pupils in response to autonomic nervous system stimulation
• Respiratory—increased respiratory rate when anxious or frightened
• Skin/Exocrine—may show signs of secondary problem behavior such as overgrooming

GENETICS
Genetic component unknown, but possible

INCIDENCE/PREVALENCE
N/A

GEOGRAPHIC DISTRIBUTION
N/A

SIGNALMENT
Any age, sex, or breed.

SIGNS

General Comments
• Signs of fear or anxiety can vary between individuals and may vary to different environmental stimuli.
• In mild cases of anxiety or fear, the cat may become tense and more reactive to environmental stimuli. At the other extreme, cats in a panic can become very aggressive or destructive in their attempts to get away from the thing they fear.

Historical Findings
• Obtain a clear description of the cat's body language and behavior and any events or situations that consistently trigger anxiety or fear. Information about specific triggers associated with fearful behavior is helpful in setting up a behavioral modification program.
• Hiding and avoidance are commonly seen in anxious or fearful cats.
• Body postures associated with fearful behavior include ears flattened to the back or to the side of the head, crouched body posture when resting or moving, lowered head, tail tucked alongside the body or held low.
• Pupils are often dilated, and the cat may be panting, shaking, drooling, or shedding hair.
• If the fear is intense, the cat may lose bladder and bowel control and may express its anal sacs.
• Vocalizations are usually minimal, unless the cat is showing defensive behavior in response to a perceived threat.
• The cat may pace, vocalize, and solicit attention from the owner.
• Urine spraying and possibly some types of destructive scratching may be seen in anxious cats.
• Details of the cat's early life, if known, may indicate a history of poor socialization and environmental exposure or point out possible genetic influences, such as unfriendly parents or feral ancestry.

Physical Examination Findings
Usually unremarkable unless the cat has injured itself trying to escape or while seeking shelter during its fright

CAUSES & RISK FACTORS
Fearful behavior in cats can be related to the following factors:
• Genetic influences on temperament
• Early experience and socialization. Cats who did not have the chance to be around other cats or around humans during the first few weeks of life are more likely to be uncomfortable and fearful around them.
• Later learning through negative experiences.

 DIAGNOSIS

DIFFERENTIAL DIAGNOSIS
In cases in which cats show social withdrawal and resistance to handling not associated with a particular situation or stimulus, and in which the behavior occurred suddenly, there may be an underlying medical reason. A thorough medical history and physical will help delineate physical causes from a problem behavior.

CBC/BIOCHEMISTRY/URINALYSIS
Laboratory testing may be indicated by information obtained in the history and physical examination.

OTHER LABORATORY TESTS
As indicated if physical causes are suspected

IMAGING
Imaging of the brain or other body organs may be indicated if history, physical, and laboratory tests strongly suggest an organic cause for the cat's behavior.

OTHER DIAGNOSTIC PROCEDURES
N/A

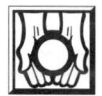 **TREATMENT**

APPROPRIATE HEALTH CARE
N/A

NURSING CARE
N/A

ACTIVITY
Normal interactions with owners encouraged

DIET
Normal dietary routine

CLIENT EDUCATION

General Comments
• Discuss behavioral expectations. Animals with shy personalities or poor socialization histories may show a minimal response to treatment after many months.
• A realistic "end point" would depend on the animal's background (socialization history, genetic and individual differences in personality), the home situation, and other confounding factors such as the frequency of natural exposure to fear-producing stimuli.

Behavioral Therapy
• Identify the specific stimulus that provokes the fearful behavior.
• Avoid exposure or close proximity to the fear-producing stimuli, if possible. Provide ways for the cat itself to manage the situation, by noting its "hideout" preferences and creating a "safe place" for the cat to go to if the situation cannot be avoided.

• Desensitization and counterconditioning to the fear-provoking stimulus. Systematic desensitization is a program of slowly increasing exposure to the object or situation the cat fears. Counterconditioning consists of enhancing an internal and external environment counter to one of fear usually accomplished with food rewards.
• Address secondary problems such as defensive aggression directed towards humans or other cats, or eliminate problems that may be the result of fears or anxieties.

SURGICAL CONSIDERATIONS
N/A

 MEDICATIONS

DRUG(S)
• Medication can be a helpful adjunct to behavioral modification, if the animal's fearful or anxious behavior is so intense that it interferes with learning or other normal behavioral activities.
• Drug classes most often suggested for fearful behavior focus primarily on increasing the available amount of the neurotransmitters serotonin and GABA (gamma aminobutyric acid) in the CNS; however, levels of other neurotransmitters are also affected.
• No drug is approved by the FDA for use in cats for fearful behavior, and so clients must be advised that information concerning efficacy, contraindications, and side effects is limited and often extrapolated from human literature.

Selective Serotonin Reuptake Inhibitors (SSRIs)
• Fluoxetine (Prozac)—0.5–1.0 mg/kg PO q24h. Side effects: decreased appetite and irritability
• Paroxetine (Paxil)—0.5–1.0 mg/kg PO q24h. Side effects: decreased appetite, irritability, constipation

Tricyclic Antidepressants (TCAs)
• Clomipramine—2.5–5.0 mg/cat PO q24h. Side effects: sedation, anticholinergic effects, possible cardiac conduction disturbances in predisposed animals
• Amitriptyline–2.5–10 mg/cat PO q24h. Side effects: sedation, anticholinergic effects, possible cardiac conduction disturbances in predisposed animals

Azapirone
• Buspirone—2.5–7.5 mg/cat PO q12h
• Side effects: GI upset, mild sedation, disinhibition of aggressive behavior

Benzodiazepines
• Alprazolam—0.125–0.25 mg/cat q12h
• Side effects: sedation, disinhibition of aggression, increased appetite

CONTRAINDICATIONS
• Use of buspirone, tricyclic antidepressants, and the selective serotonin reuptake inhibitors is not recommended in animals with seizures.
• Owing to reported cases of fatal idiopathic hepatic necrosis linked to short-term use of diazepam (Valium) in cats, its use is not currently recommended.

PRECAUTIONS
Animals with compromised hepatic or renal function may not be able to metabolize or clear medications normally, and so caution should be taken when treating those patients. Basic laboratory tests are also strongly suggested before placing an animal on a psychotropic medication, to make sure that liver and kidney functions are sufficient to metabolize the medication, and to check for any physical condition that may be a contraindication to specific drugs.

POSSIBLE INTERACTIONS
The reader is urged to discuss any questions on possible drug interactions with a veterinary behaviorist or a pharmacist. Information on the subject is limited and usually extrapolated from human literature.

ALTERNATIVE DRUG(S)
While alternative medications such as herbal preparations have been suggested for fearful behaviors in animals, these substances have not yet been scientifically studied for these conditions in this species.

 FOLLOW-UP

PATIENT MONITORING
Frequent follow-up either in person or by telephone is necessary especially during the first few months of treatment, in order to motivate the client and monitor the effectiveness of any adjunct drug treatment.

PREVENTION/AVOIDANCE
• Frequent early exposure to new and novel people, places, and things during the first 3–9 weeks of life may be helpful in avoiding later fear-based reactions. Continued exposure throughout the first year of life may also be helpful.
• Calm interactions and positive associations with fear-producing stimuli may keep fear-based reactions to a minimum.

POSSIBLE COMPLICATIONS
Secondary behavior problems may arise or persist after the fearful or anxious behavior has diminished and will need specific treatment.

EXPECTED COURSE AND PROGNOSIS
• Animals with shy personalities or poor socialization histories may show a minimal response to treatment.

• A realistic "end point" would depend on the animal's background (socialization history, genetic and individual differences in personality), the home situation, and other confounding factors such as the frequency of natural exposure to fear-producing stimuli.
• Medication may help improve response to behavior modification but not totally ameliorate signs.

 MISCELLANEOUS

ASSOCIATED CONDITIONS
• Chronic anxiety can lead to other expressions of stress, such as stereotypic or compulsive disorders, urine-marking behavior, or inappropriate elimination.
• Anxious and fearful animals may show defensive aggression if interactions are forced on them by humans or other animals.
• Fearful, defensive, reactive behavior by one cat may make it a target for aggression from other cats and create an intercat aggression problem within the household.

AGE-RELATED FACTORS
N/A

ZOONOTIC POTENTIAL
N/A

PREGNANCY
Drug use in pregnant animals should be avoided.

SEE ALSO
• Aggression, Overview—Cats
• Compulsive Disorders—Cats
• Housesoiling—Cats

Suggested Reading
Askew HR. Treatment of behavior problems in dogs and cats, a guide for the small animal veterinarian. Oxford, U.K.: Blackwell Science, 1996:304–317.
Crowell-Davis SL, Barry K, Wolfe R. Social behavior and aggressive problems of cats. Vet Clin North Am Small Anim Pract 1997; 27:549–568.
Landsberg G, Hunthausen W, Ackerman L. Handbook of behaviour problems of the dog and cat. Oxford U.K.: Butterworth-Heinemann, 1997:119–128.
Mendl M, Harcourt R. Individuality in the domestic cat: origins, development and stability. In: Turner DC, Bateson P, eds. The domestic cat, the biology of its behaviour, 2nd ed. Cambridge U.K.: The Cambridge University Press, 2000:48–64.
Voith VL, Borchelt PL. Fears and phobias in companion animals. In: Voith VL, Borchelt, PL. Readings in companion animal behavior. Trenton, NJ: Veterinary Learning Systems, 1996:140–152.
Author Leslie Larson Cooper
Consulting editor Debra F. Horwitz

FEARS, PHOBIAS, AND ANXIETIES—DOGS

 BASICS

DEFINITION

Fear
• A feeling of apprehension associated with the presence or proximity of an object, individual, social situation, or class of these
• Part of normal behavior; can be an adaptive response • Context determines whether response is abnormal or inappropriate.
• Normal and abnormal—usually manifests as graded responses; intensity of the response proportional to the perceived or actual proximity of the stimulus • Reactions develop relatively gradually; within a bout of fearful behavior, animal may display some variation in response. • Most reactions are learned and can be unlearned with gradual exposure.

Phobias
• Sudden, all-or-nothing, profound, abnormal responses that result in extremely fearful behaviors (catatonia, mania). Animals may lose all sensitivity to pain or to social stimuli. • Do not extinguish with gradual exposure to the object or with no exposure over time • Immediate, excessive anxiety response is characteristic; little change among bouts • It has been postulated that once a phobic event has been experienced, any event associated with it or the memory of it is sufficient to generate the response; without reinforcement, response can remain at or exceed its former high level for years.
• Origin—extremely scary and traumatic event; dog may have profound problems with internal fear (the fear itself acts as a reinforcer) • Animal avoids trigger situation at all costs or, if unavoidable, endures it with intense anxiety or distress. • Most common—associated with noises (e.g., thunderstorms or firecrackers) • May co-occur or co-vary with separation anxiety; it is prudent to question the owner of a dog with separation anxiety about the animal's response to loud noises.

Anxiety
• Apprehensive anticipation of future danger or misfortune accompanied by a feeling of dysphoria (humans) and/or somatic signs of tension (vigilance and scanning, autonomic hyperactivity, increased motor activity, tension)
• Focus of the reaction can be internal or external; internal focus is almost always under-appreciated.
• Separation anxiety—most common specific anxiety in companion dogs; when alone, the animal exhibits anxiety or excessive distress.
• Most common visible behaviors—elimination, destruction, and excessive vocalization; drooling, panting, and cognitive signs are not often observed but probably occur.

PATHOPHYSIOLOGY
• Unclear • Clinical signs—consistent with alterations in CNS transmitter levels and/or increases in ACTH levels (primary or secondary) • Animal is usually brought to the clinic because the client becomes concerned about perceived changes in the animal's behavior or believes that the animal has never been normal.

SYSTEMS AFFECTED
• Cardiovascular—tachycardia
• Endocrine/Metabolic—alterations in the HPA axis
• Gastrointestinal—inappetence; aberrant appetite; gastrointestinal distress (salivation, vomiting, diarrhea, tenesmus, hematochezia)
• Hemic/Lymphatic/Immune—stress leukogram
• Musculoskeletal—poor condition attributable to increased motor activity and self-injury (weight loss, injured pads, damage to teeth and gums, and abrasions and lacerations)
• Nervous—increased motor activity; repetitive activity; trembling; self-injury
• Respiratory—tachypnea and the attendant metabolic changes
• Skin/Exocrine—lesions, usually secondary to self-injury (lick granulomas)

SIGNALMENT
• No age, breed, or sex is over-represented.
• Most develop at the onset of social maturity (12–36 months of age).
• Old-age onset idiopathic separation anxiety—may be a variant of cognitive dysfunction; reported in elderly dogs
• Profound form of idiopathic fear and withdrawal—occurs at 8–10 months of age; noted in Siberian huskies, German shorthaired pointers, Chesapeake Bay retrievers, Bernese mountain dogs, Great Pyrenees, border collies, and standard poodles among others; appears to be a strong familial component with genetic liability

SIGNS

General Comments
• Fears and anxieties—variable; diagnosis may be made only on the basis of nonspecific signs for which no discrete, identifiable stimulus is present
• The extent to which the animal is experiencing the fear or phobia may affect the presentation.
• Mild fears—trembling, tail tucked, withdrawal, and hiding; reduced activity and passive escape behaviors
• Panic—active escape behavior; increased, out-of-context, and potentially injurious motor activity
• Classic signs of sympathetic autonomic nervous system activity

Historical Findings
• Fear—from a horrific experience; may have been forced into an unfamiliar experience
• Uncommon for a dog to be fearful, anxious, or phobic because of lack of exposure early in puppyhood (neophobia)
• Dogs that are absolutely deprived of variable social and environmental exposure until 14 weeks of age may become pathologically fearful; can be avoided with only little exposure
• With phobias and panic—may have history of incarceration or inability to escape stimulus (e.g., locked in crate)
• Separation anxiety—history of abandonment, multiple owners, rehoming, or prior neglect common; often abandoned/rehomed because of separation anxiety

Physical Examination Findings
• Usually nonremarkable, except for self-induced injuries and the lack of condition that may be associated with increased motor activity and withdrawal, especially if panic is a co-morbid diagnosis
• Anxieties—lesions such as lick granuloma may be more common than has generally been appreciated.

CAUSES
• Any illness or painful physical condition increases anxiety and contributes to the development of fears, phobias, and anxieties.
• Degenerative (e.g., associated with aged concomitant neurologic changes), anatomic, infectious (primarily CNS viral conditions) and toxic (lead toxicosis) conditions—may lead to behavioral problems through primary or secondary aberrant neurochemical activity

 DIAGNOSIS

DIFFERENTIAL DIAGNOSIS
Rule out conditions that cause similar behavioral changes—seizures; brain disease, metabolic disease (e.g., thyroid or adrenal).

CBC/BIOCHEMISTRY/URINALYSIS
• Should be normal
• Perform before initiating drug treatment.

OTHER LABORATORY TESTS
Thyroid or adrenal tests—depending on clinical signs and serum biochemistry results

IMAGING
CT or MRI—rule out structural brain disorder.

DIAGNOSTIC PROCEDURES
• Biopsy of dermatologic lesions—determine if primary or secondary.
• CSF analysis—rule out inflammatory CNS disease
• Endoscopy—evaluate primary bowel disease
• ECG—rule out cardiac disease that may produce physical signs mimicking anxiety.

TREATMENT

- Usually outpatient
- Inpatient—patients with profound panic and separation anxiety who need to be protected until antianxiety medications reach effective plasma and CSF levels (days to weeks); patients who must be treated for or protected from physical injury (e.g., throwing itself from a window); constant daycare, dog-sitting, or inpatient monitoring and stimulation may be best
- Affected animals respond to some extent to a combination of behavior modification and pharmacologic treatment with antianxiety medication.
- Diagnose and control any atopic and painful condition because pruritus and pain are both neurochemically related to anxiety and its perception; may include dietary management
- Some profound, idiopathically fearful patients may need to live in a protected environment with as few social stressors as possible; these animals do not do well in dog shows.

Behavior Modification

- Gear toward teaching the dog to relax in a variety of environmental settings.
- Client may reassure the dog when it is experiencing fear or panic; inform client that the dog may interpret this as a reward for its behavior.
- Client must encourage calmness but not reinforce the fear reaction. Clients need to remember that not all dogs are calmer when crated; some dogs panic when caged and will injure themselves if forced to be confined.
- Client must absolutely avoid punishment.
- Desensitization and counterconditioning—most effective if the fear, anxiety, or phobia is treated early; goal is to decrease the reaction to a specific stimulus (e.g., being left alone in the dark).
- Help client understand the subtlety of the signs involved and learn to recognize physical signs associated with the underlying physiologic state characterized by sympathetic stimulation.

MEDICATIONS

DRUG(S)

Anxiety

- Antianxiety medications that increase CNS levels of serotonin—tricyclic antidepressants and selective serotonin reuptake inhibitors
- Amitriptyline—1–2 mg/kg PO q12h for 30 days to start
- Imipramine—1–2 mg/kg PO q12h for 30 days

- Clomipramine—1 mg/kg PO q12h for 14 days; then 2 mg/kg PO q12h for 14 days; then 3 mg/kg PO q12h for 28 days (if successful, use as maintenance level); takes 3–5 weeks to begin to be effective; best drug for repetitive behaviors and for separation anxiety involving repetitive barking, motor activity, or elimination
- Sertraline 1 + mg/kg PO q24h for 2 months, minimum; start at 1 mg/kg or below and work up q2wk to minimally effective dose, not to exceed 3 mg/kg.
- Fluoxetine—1 mg/kg PO q24h for 2 months; takes 3–5 weeks to be effective, and dog will continue to improve with time.
- Most treatment will be long-term, possibly years; treatment duration will depend on number and intensity of signs and duration of condition.
- Minimum treatment will be 4–6 mos.

Phobias and True Panic Disorders

- Respond to benzodiazepines; work best if administered before any signs of anxiety, fear, or panic; must be given minimally 30–60 min before the anticipated provocative stimulus
- Diazepam—0.5–2.2 mg/kg PO as needed
- Clorazepate—0.55–2.2 mg/kg PO q8–12h or as needed (phobias)
- Alprazolam—0.01–1.0 mg/kg as needed q4–6h, not to exceed 4 mg/day for small to medium dogs; best initial dosage range—0.02–0.04 mg/kg for medium dog (25 kg)
- Severe separation anxiety (e.g., dog breaks out of crates or throw itself from windows) and thunderstorm phobia that is accompanied by panic—alprazolam can be used concomitantly with other medications on an as-needed basis

CONTRAINDICATIONS

- Hepatic and renal compromise—some listed drugs contraindicated because of their main route of metabolism
- Use caution when prescribing drugs to old patients that have generally diminished volume of distribution and decreased metabolism.
- Cardiac conduction anomalies—use extreme caution and monitoring when giving tricyclic antidepressants

PRECAUTIONS

- All listed medications are extra-label—follow Health and Human Services recommendations. • Overdose of tricyclic antidepressants—may cause profound cardiac conduction disturbances; perform a cardiac evaluation (preferably with ECG) before treatment. Clients can take pulse and report any extreme increase

POSSIBLE INTERACTIONS

- Benzodiazepines—lipophilic and may be potentiated by other lipophilic drugs; if combination treatment is warranted, use lower doses of either medication

- Medication that impairs the glucuronidation of active metabolites into inactive compounds may cause increases of the active metabolites.

FOLLOW-UP

PATIENT MONITORING

- Chronic treatment—CBC, biochemistry, and urinalysis: as indicated by clinical signs, annually for young patients, and semiannually for old patients; adjust dosages accordingly.
- Advise clients to observe for vomiting, gastrointestinal distress, and tachypnea.

POSSIBLE COMPLICATIONS

Early treatment with both behavioral modification and pharmacologic intervention is key; if left untreated, these disorders always progress.

MISCELLANEOUS

ASSOCIATED CONDITIONS

Irritable bowel syndrome and lick granulomas—common; may indicate underlying anxiety-related conditions

AGE-RELATED FACTORS

Idiopathic separation anxiety in old dogs—frequently undiagnosed because it is insidious and not associated with social or environmental changes; changes appear to be in the dog's perception. Early cognitive dysfuction can present as nonspecific fear.

PREGNANCY

Most of the listed drugs are either not evaluated in or contraindicated in pregnant animals.

SYNONYMS

Generalized anxiety, neophobia, noise phobia, and thunderstorm phobia—not synonymous but are frequently discussed under the same heading.

ABBREVIATIONS

- CSF = cerebrospinal fluid
- HPA = hypothalamic–pituitary–adrenal

Suggested Reading

King J, Simpson B, Overall KL, et al. Treatment of separation anxiety in dogs with clomipramine. Results from a prospective, randomized, double-blinded, placebo-controlled clinical trial. Appl Anim Beh Sci 2000;67:255–275.

Overall, KL, Dunham AE, Frank DF. Frequency of nonspecific clinical signs in dog with separation anxiety, thunderstorm phobia, and noise phobia, alone or in combination. J Am Vet Med Assoc 2001; 219:467–473.

Author Karen L. Overall
Consulting Editor Debra F. Horwitz

FELINE CALICIVIRUS INFECTION

 **BASICS**

DEFINITION
A common viral respiratory disease of domestic and exotic cats characterized by upper respiratory signs, oral ulceration, pneumonia, and occasionally arthritis

PATHOPHYSIOLOGY
Rapid cytolysis of infected cells with resulting tissue pathology and clinical disease

SYSTEMS AFFECTED
• Respiratory—rhinitis; interstitial pneumonia; ulceration of the tip of the nose
• Ophthalmic—acute serous conjunctivitis without keratitis or corneal ulcers
• Musculoskeletal—acute arthritis
• Gastrointestinal—ulceration of the tongue common; occasional ulceration of the hard palate and lips; infection occurs in intestines; usually no clinical disease

GENETICS
None

INCIDENCE/PREVALENCE
• Persistent infection common
• Clinical disease—common in multicat facilities and breeding catteries
• Routine vaccination—reduced incidence of clinical disease; has not decreased the prevalence of the virus

GEOGRAPHIC DISTRIBUTION
Worldwide

SIGNALMENT

Species
Cats

Breed Predilections
None

Mean Age and Range
• Young kittens > 6 weeks old—most common
• Cats of any age may show clinical disease.

Predominant Sex
None

SIGNS

General Comments
May present as an upper respiratory infection with eye and nose involvement, as an ulcerative disease primarily of the mouth, as pneumonia, as an acute arthritis, or any combination of these

Historical Findings
• Sudden onset
• Anorexia
• Ocular or nasal discharge, usually with little or no sneezing
• Ulcers on the tongue, hard palate, lips, tip of nose, or around claws
• Dyspnea from pneumonia
• Acute, painful lameness

Physical Examination Findings
• Generally alert and in good condition
• Fever
• Ulcers may occur without other signs.

CAUSES
• A small, nonenveloped single-stranded RNA virus
• Numerous strains exist in nature, with varying degrees of antigenic cross-reactivity.
• More than one serotype
• Relatively stable and resistant to many disinfectants

RISK FACTORS
• Lack of vaccination or improper vaccination
• Multicat facilities
• Concurrent infections with other pathogens (e.g., FHV-1 or FPV)
• Poor ventilation

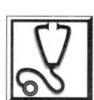 **DIAGNOSIS**

DIFFERENTIAL DIAGNOSIS
• Feline viral rhinotracheitis
• Chlamydiosis
• *Bordetella bronchiseptica*

CBC/BIOCHEMISTRY/URINALYSIS
No characteristic or consistent findings

OTHER LABORATORY TESTS
Serologic testing on paired serum samples—detect a rise in neutralizing antibody titers against the virus

IMAGING
Radiographs of the lungs—a consolidation of lung tissue in cats with pneumonia

DIAGNOSTIC PROCEDURES
• Cell cultures to isolate the virus—oral pharynx; lung tissue; feces; blood; secretions from the nose and conjunctiva
• Immunofluorescent assays of lung tissue—viral antigen

PATHOLOGIC FINDINGS
• Gross—upper respiratory infection; ocular and nasal discharge; pneumonia with consolidation of large portions of individual lung lobes; possible ulcerations on the tongue, lips, and hard palate
• Histopathologic—interstitial pneumonia of large portions of individual lung lobes; ulcerations on epithelium of the tongue, lips, and hard palate; mild inflammatory reactions in the nose and conjunctiva

 TREATMENT

APPROPRIATE HEALTH CARE
Outpatient, unless severe pneumonia occurs

NURSING CARE
• Clean eyes and nose as indicated
• Provide soft foods
• Oxygen—with severe pneumonia

ACTIVITY
Patients should be restricted from contact with other cats to prevent transmission of the disease.

DIET
• No restrictions
• Special diets—perhaps to entice anorectic cats to resume eating
• Soft foods—if ulcerations restrict eating

CLIENT EDUCATION
Discuss the need for proper vaccination and the need to modify the vaccination protocol in breeding catteries to include kittens before they become infected (often at 6–8 weeks of age) from a carrier queen.

SURGICAL CONSIDERATIONS
None

MEDICATIONS

DRUG(S) OF CHOICE
• No specific antiviral drugs that are effective
• Broad-spectrum antibiotics—usually indicated (e.g., amoxicillin at 22 mg/kg PO q12h)
• Secondary bacterial infections of affected cats are not nearly as important as with FHV-1 infections.
• Antibiotic eye ointments—to reduce secondary bacterial infections of the conjunctiva
• Appropriate pain medication—for transient arthritis pain

CONTRAINDICATIONS
None

PRECAUTIONS
None

POSSIBLE INTERACTIONS
None

ALTERNATIVE DRUG(S)
None

FOLLOW-UP

PATIENT MONITORING
• Monitor for sudden development of dyspnea associated with pneumonia.
• No specific laboratory tests

PREVENTION/AVOIDANCE
• All cats should be vaccinated at the same time they are vaccinated against FHV-1; routine vaccination with either MLV or inactivated vaccines should be done at 8–10 weeks of age and repeated 3–4 weeks later.
• Breeding catteries—respiratory disease is a problem; vaccinate kittens at an earlier age, either with an additional vaccination at 4–5 weeks of age or with intranasal administration at 10–14 days of age; follow-up vaccinations at 6, 10, and 14 weeks of age
• Annual vaccines recommended; immunity undoubtedly lasts > 1 year
• American Association of Feline Practitioners—classifies FHV, FPV, and calicivirus as core vaccines; recommends vaccination of all cats with these three agents on the initial visit, after 12 weeks of age, and 1 year later; boosters for calicivirus should be given every 3 years.
• Vaccination will not eliminate infection in a subsequent exposure but will prevent clinical disease caused by most strains.

POSSIBLE COMPLICATIONS
• Interstitial pneumonia—most serious complication; can be life-threatening
• Secondary bacterial infections of the lungs or upper airways
• Oral ulcers and the acute arthritis usually heal without complications.

EXPECTED COURSE AND PROGNOSIS
• Clinical disease—usually appears 3–4 days after exposure
• Once neutralizing antibodies appear, about 7 days after exposure, recovery is usually rapid.
• Prognosis excellent, unless severe pneumonia develops
• Recovered cats—persistently infected for long periods; will continuously shed small quantities of virus in oral secretions

MISCELLANEOUS

ASSOCIATED CONDITIONS
Affected cats may also be concurrently infected with FHV-1, especially in multicat and breeding facilities.

AGE-RELATED FACTORS
Usually occurs in young kittens whose maternally derived immunity has waned

ZOONOTIC POTENTIAL
None

PREGNANCY
Generally no problem, because most cats have been exposed or vaccinated before becoming pregnant

SYNONYMS
Feline picornavirus infection—originally classified as a picornavirus; older literature refers to the infection by this name; no known picornavirus that infects cats

SEE ALSO
• Bordetellosis—Cats
• Chlamydiosis—Cats
• Feline Rhinotracheitis Virus

ABBREVIATIONS
• FHV = feline herpesvirus
• FPV = feline parvovirus
• MLV = modified live vaccine
• RNA = ribonucleic acid

Suggested Readings

Barr MC, Olsen CW, Scott FW. Feline viral diseases. In: Ettinger SJ, Feldman EC, eds. Veterinary internal medicine. 4th ed. Philadelphia: Saunders, 1995:409–439.

Elston T, Rodan I, Flemming D, et al. 1998 report of the American Association of Feline Practitioners and Academy of Feline Medicine Advisory Panel on Feline Vaccines. J Am Vet Med Assoc 1998;212:227–241.

Ford RB, Levy JK. Infectious diseases of the respiratory tract. In: Sherding RG, ed. The cat: diseases and clinical management. New York: Churchill Livingstone, 1994: 489–500.

Ford RB. Role of infectious agents in respiratory disease. Vet Clin North Am Sm Anim Pract 1993;23:17–35.

Pedersen NC. Feline calicivirus infection. In: Pratt PW, ed. Feline infectious diseases. Goleta, CA: American Veterinary, 1988:61–67.

Author Fred W. Scott
Consulting Editor Stephen C. Barr

FELINE HYPERESTHESIA SYNDROME

BASICS

DEFINITION
• An idiopathic disorder of cats characterized by paroxysmal agitation, focal spasms of the epaxial muscles, vocalization, and intense biting or licking of the back, tail, and pelvic limbs
• Has also been called neurodermatitis, twitchy-skin syndrome, neuritis, psycho-motor epilepsy, and pruritic dermatosis of Siamese cats

PATHOPHYSIOLOGY
Unknown

SYSTEM AFFECTED
• Behavioral
• Nervous
• Neuromuscular
• Skin

SIGNALMENT

Species
Cats

Breed Predilections
Siamese cats, but described in other breeds as well

Mean Age and Range
Signs may occur at any age; one report cited a peak onset at 1–4 years of age, another at 5–8 years of age.

SIGNS
• Episodes of twitching of the skin on the dorsum, violent swishing of the tail, vocalizing, and biting or licking of the flank and pelvic region
• Pupils are often widely dilated, and the cat often appears disoriented and runs wildly about the environment.
• Episodes are several seconds to several minutes in length. Cats are typically normal between episodes. Some cats appear slightly agitated between episodes and may be intolerant of being petted along the back.
• General physical examination often reveals no abnormalities aside from possible alopecia and broken hair over the lumbar area from self-mutilation. An apparent zone of hyperpathia in the thoracolumbar musculature is present in some cats, and palpation of the area may elicit an episode. No neurologic deficits have been noted.

CAUSES & RISK FACTORS
• It is not known whether this syndrome is a manifestation of an underlying behavioral problem, an atypical seizure disorder, or a localized sensory neuropathy or myopathy causing hyperesthesia. It has been speculated that the cause is multifactorial, or that the syndrome is not a distinct entity with a single cause but rather can develop from a variety of different factors.
• Cats that tend to be nervous or hyper-excitable have been described as having an increased risk; environmental stresses may serve as a trigger.

DIAGNOSIS

DIFFERENTIAL DIAGNOSIS
• Dermatologic conditions causing pruritus—parasitic (e.g., flea, *Notoedres*, *Cheyletiella*), fungal (e.g., dermatophytosis), or allergic (e.g., parasitic, inhalant, dietary); evaluate for evidence of underlying dermatitis; skin scrapings and fungal cultures may help confirm diagnosis
• Diseases of the vertebral column causing spinal hyperpathia—degenerative (inter-vertebral disk disease), inflammatory (diskospondylitis, local meningitis), neoplastic, or traumatic; radiography of the vertebral column is helpful in evaluating for abnormalities that may cause localized pain; further diagnostics (e.g., myelography, serologic testing for infectious agents, CSF analysis) may be necessary
• Forebrain disease causing behavioral changes and/or seizures—metabolic (hepatic encephalopathy), neoplastic, infectious/inflammatory (feline leukemia virus, feline immunodeficiency virus, feline infectious peritonitis, cryptococcosis, toxoplasmosis), vascular (feline ischemic encephalopathy); complete diagnostic evaluation including bile acid tolerance, serologic testing for infectious causes of encephalitis, CSF analysis, and brain imaging may be indicated to assess for underlying brain disease

CBC/BIOCHEMISTRY/URINALYSIS
• Frequently normal
• An increased globulin level has been reported in some cats.

OTHER LABORATORY TESTS
None required

IMAGING
None required aside from the imaging necessary to exclude differential diagnoses

DIAGNOSTIC PROCEDURES
• Diagnosis of exclusion—currently there is no test or group of tests that support a definitive diagnosis
• EEG—abnormalities have been reported in some affected cats
• EMG—revealed evidence of abnormal spontaneous activity in the thoracolumbar epaxial muscles in one study of affected cats
• Muscle biopsy—in cats with EMG changes; may reveal numerous vacuoles within the epaxial muscles, with antibody labeling characteristics similar to those described with inclusion body myositis/myopathy in humans

TREATMENT
• Outpatient
• Eliminate environmental changes that may precipitate episodes.
• Behavioral modification has been successful in reducing clinical manifestations in some cats.
• In severe cases of self-mutilation, an E-collar or tail bandaging may be necessary.

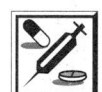

MEDICATIONS

DRUG(S)
• Several pharmacologic agents have been used, depending on cause—prednisolone, phenobarbital, primidone, diazepam, progestational compounds, amitriptyline, carnitine, and coenzyme Q10
• Phenobarbital (1–2 mg/kg PO q12 h)—most effective, but does not successfully control the episodes in all cats
• Therapy is often lifelong as attacks typically resume after medication is discontinued.

CONTRAINDICATIONS/POSSIBLE INTERACTIONS
N/A

FOLLOW-UP

PATIENT MONITORING
Cats placed on phenobarbital—check serum drug concentrations in 2–3 weeks; repeat minimum database (CBC, biochemistry profile, urinalysis) at 6–12-month intervals to monitor for adverse effects

PREVENTION/AVOIDANCE
Avoid any known environmental stresses.

AGE-RELATED FACTORS
N/A

ABBREVIATIONS
• CSF = cerebrospinal fluid
• EEG = electroencephalography
• EMG = electromyography

Suggested Reading

March PA, Fischer JR, Potthoff A, et al. Electromyographic and histological abnormalities in epaxial muscles of cats with feline hyperesthesia syndrome. Proceedings of the 17th annual veterinary medical forum, Chicago, Illinois, June 1999. J Vet Intern Med 1999;13:238.

Scott DW. The skin. In: Holzworth J. Diseases of the cat. Medicine & surgery. Philadelphia: Saunders, 1987:654–655.

Author Karen R. Muñana
Consulting Editor Joane M. Parent

FELINE IDIOPATHIC LOWER URINARY TRACT DISEASE

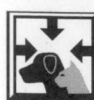 BASICS

DEFINITION

The terms *feline urologic syndrome* and *FUS* are used commonly by the veterinary profession as diagnostic terms to describe disorders of domestic cats characterized by hematuria, dysuria, pollakiuria, periuria, and partial or complete urethral obstruction, because varying combinations of these signs may be associated with any cause of feline lower urinary tract disease. The similarity of clinical signs with diverse causes is not surprising since the feline urinary tract responds to various diseases in a limited and predictable fashion. When used, the term *FUS* should be redefined as feline urologic *signs;* in this context, FUS is no more a diagnosis than is vomiting or pruritus. Idiopathic feline urinary tract disease (iLUTD) is an exclusionary diagnosis established only after known causes have been eliminated.

PATHOPHYSIOLOGY

• Refer to specific chapters describing diseases listed in section on Differential Diagnosis.
• Experimental and clinical studies have implicated calicivirus, feline syncytia-forming virus, and a gamma herpesvirus (bovine herpesvirus 4) as potential etiologic agents in some cats.
• Initial episodes of idiopathic lower urinary tract diseases usually occur in the absence of significant numbers of detectable bacteria and pyuria. Prospective diagnostic studies of male and female obstructed and nonobstructed cats identified bacterial urinary tract infections in <3% of young to middle-age adults and approximately 10% of geriatric adults.
• Some cats with lower urinary tract diseases exhibit findings similar to those observed in humans with interstitial cystitis, an idiopathic inflammatory disorder—decreased urine concentrations of glycosaminoglycans, increased urinary bladder permeability, associated with damage to the glycosaminoglycan layer that covers the luminal surface of the urinary tract, and similar gross and light microscopic changes. These similarities prompted the hypothesis that some lower urinary tract diseases are analogous to human interstitial cystitis; further studies are essential to prove or disprove this hypothesis.

SYSTEMS AFFECTED

• Renal/Urologic—lower urinary tract
• Persistent urethral outflow obstruction results in postrenal azotemia.

GENETICS

N/A

INCIDENCE/PREVALENCE

• The incidence of hematuria, dysuria, and/or urethral obstruction in domestic cats in the United States and Great Britain has been previously reported to be approximately 0.5–1.0% per year.
• The hospital proportional morbidity rate for iLUTD in cats admitted with lower urinary tract signs is approximately 65%.

SIGNALMENT

Species
Cats, both male and female

Breed Predilection
None

Mean Age and Range
• May occur at any age, but is most commonly recognized in young to middle-aged adults (mean age, 3.5 years).
• Uncommon in cats <1 year old and >10 years old

SIGNS

Historical Findings
• Dysuria
• Hematuria
• Pollakiuria
• Periuria—urinating in inappropriate locations
• Outflow obstruction

Physical Examination Findings
• Thickened, firm, contracted bladder wall
• May detect urethral plugs or uroliths by examination of the distal penis and penile urethra

CAUSES
• See Pathophysiology.
• Noninfectious diseases, including interstitial cystitis
• Viruses implicated

RISK FACTORS
Stress—may play a role in precipitating or exacerbating signs; an unlikely primary cause

 DIAGNOSIS

DIFFERENTIAL DIAGNOSIS
• Metabolic disorders including various types of uroliths and urethral plugs
• Infectious agents including bacteria, mycoplasma/ureaplasma, fungal agents, and parasites
• Trauma
• Neurogenic disorders including reflex dys-synergia, urethral spasm, and hypotonic or atonic bladder (primary or secondary)
• Iatrogenic disease including reverse flushing solutions, urethral catheters, indwelling urethral catheters (especially open systems), postsurgical urethral catheters, and ureth-rostomy complications
• Anatomic abnormalities including urachal anomalies and acquired urethral strictures
• Neoplasia (benign and malignant)

• Clinical signs may be confused with constipation, which can be ruled out by abdominal palpation.

CBC/BIOCHEMISTRY/URINALYSIS
• Hematuria and proteinuria—usually present
• If urethral obstruction persists, serum chemistry profiles reveal azotemia, hyper-phosphatemia, hyperkalemia, and reduced TCO_2.

OTHER LABORATORY TESTS
• Absence of bacteriuria—verify by quantitative urine culture; collect urine specimens by cystocentesis to avoid contamination with organisms that normally inhabit the distal urinary tract.
• Indirect fluorescent antibody test may reveal serum antibodies against bovine herpesvirus type 4 in some cats.
• Transmission electron microscopy may reveal calicivirus-like particles in some urethral plugs.

IMAGING
• Survey radiography—may exclude uroliths or urethral plugs
• Positive-contrast retrograde urethrocystography or antegrade cystography—may exclude urethral strictures, vesicourachal diverticula, and neoplasia
• Double-contrast cystography—may exclude small or radiolucent uroliths, blood clots, and thickening of the bladder wall due to inflammation or neoplasia
• Ultrasonography—may exclude uroliths

DIAGNOSTIC PROCEDURES
• Cystoscopy—may exclude uroliths and diverticula
• Biopsies obtained with urinary catheters, cystoscopes, or via surgery—may permit morphologic characterization of inflammatory or neoplastic lesions; not routinely needed

PATHOLOGIC FINDINGS
• Cystoscopy may reveal petechial hemorrhages (also called glomerulations) of the mucosal surface of the urinary bladder.
• Mucosal ulceration, congestion, submucosal edema, hemorrhage, and fibrosis; inflammatory cells may not be prominent, unless secondary bacterial urinary tract infections have resulted from catheterization or perineal urethrostomy.

 TREATMENT

APPROPRIATE HEALTH CARE
• Patients with nonobstructive lower urinary tract diseases—typically managed as outpatients; diagnostic evaluation may require brief hospitalization.
• Patients with obstructive lower urinary tract diseases—usually hospitalized for diagnosis and management

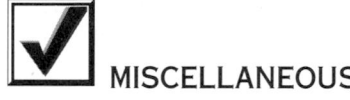

FELINE IDIOPATHIC LOWER URINARY TRACT DISEASE

NURSING CARE
N/A

ACTIVITY
N/A

DIET
• Management recommended for persistent crystalluria associated with matrix-crystalline urethral plugs
• Empirical observations suggest that recurrence of signs may be minimized by feeding moist rather than dry foods. The goal is to promote the flushing action of increased urine volume, and increased dilution of toxins, chemical irritants, inflammatory mediators, and urolith-promoting constituents.

CLIENT EDUCATION
• Hematuria, dysuria, and pollakiuria—often self-limiting; subside within 4–7 days, but signs often recur unpredictably
• Lack of controlled studies that demonstrate efficacy of most drugs used to treat symptomatically
• Males should be monitored for signs of urethral obstruction.
• Reduce environmental stress by minimizing changes in the home, maintaining a constant diet, and providing safe places to hide.
• Provide proper litter box hygiene.

SURGICAL CONSIDERATIONS
• We do not recommend cystotomy to lavage and debride the bladder mucosa as a form of treatment.
• Do not perform perineal urethrostomies to minimize recurrent urethral obstruction without localizing obstructive disease to the penile urethra by contrast urethrography.

MEDICATIONS

DRUG(S) OF CHOICE
• Propantheline may be considered as an anticholinergic to minimize hyperactivity of the bladder detrusor muscle and urge incontinence; because the smallest available tablet is 7.5 mg, suggested empirical dose is 0.25–0.5 mg/kg PO q12–24h.
• Amitriptyline, a tricyclic antidepressant and anxiolytic drug (with anticholinergic, antihistaminic, anti-α-adrenergic, antiinflammatory, and analgesic properties)—empirically advocated to treat cats with persistent signs; suggested empirical dosage is 5–10 mg/cat q24h given at night. We do not recommend amitriptyline for treatment of acute, self-limiting episodes of iLUTD.
• Butorphanol—empirically recommended to reduce pain associated with lower urinary tract inflammation; suggested dosage is 1 mg/cat PO q12h.

• Phenoxybenzamine—may be used to minimize reflex dyssynergia and functional urethral outflow obstruction; suggested empirical dosage is 0.5 mg/kg PO q12h.
• Pentosan polysulfate sodium, a semisynthetic glycosaminoglycan—empirically recommended to help repair the glycosaminoglycan coating of the mucosa of the urinary tract; results of a controlled clinical trial are not yet available.
• Corticosteroids—no detectable effect on remission of clinical signs demonstrated; predispose to bacterial urinary tract infections, especially in cats with indwelling transurethral catheters
• Dimethylsulfoxide (DMSO)—no detectable effect on remission of clinical signs demonstrated
• Antibiotics and methenamine—no detectable effect on remission of clinical signs in cats demonstrated

CONTRAINDICATIONS
• Phenazopyridine—a urinary tract analgesic used alone or in combination with sulfa drugs; may result in methemoglobinemia and irreversible oxidative changes in hemoglobin resulting in formation of Heinz bodies and anemia
• Methylene blue—a weak antiseptic agent; may cause Heinz bodies and severe anemia
• Bethanechol—a cholinergic drug used to manage hypotonic urinary bladders; do not use in patients with urethral obstruction.

PRECAUTIONS
• Cats with urethral obstruction and postrenal azotemia are at increased risk for adverse drug events, especially with drugs and anesthetics that depend on renal elimination or metabolism.
• Indwelling transurethral catheters, especially when associated with fluid-induced diuresis, predispose patients to bacterial urinary tract infections.

POSSIBLE INTERACTIONS
N/A

ALTERNATIVE DRUG(S)
N/A

FOLLOW-UP

PATIENT MONITORING
Monitor hematuria by urinalysis; cystocentesis may cause iatrogenic hematuria, so naturally voided samples are preferred.

PREVENTION/AVOIDANCE
• Empirical observations suggest that recurrence of signs may be minimized by feeding moist rather than dry foods.
• Reduce environmental stress.

POSSIBLE COMPLICATIONS
• Indwelling transurethral catheters—often cause trauma; predispose to ascending bacterial urinary tract infections • Perineal urethrostomies—may predispose to bacterial urinary tract infections and urethral strictures

EXPECTED COURSE AND PROGNOSIS
Hematuria, dysuria, and pollakiuria often are self-limiting in patients with most idiopathic lower urinary tract diseases, subsiding within 4 to 7 days. These signs often recur unpredictably; the frequency of recurrence appears to decline with advancing age.

✓ MISCELLANEOUS

ASSOCIATED CONDITIONS
N/A

AGE-RELATED FACTORS
Frequency of recurrence appears to decline with advancing age.

ZOONOTIC POTENTIAL
N/A

PREGNANCY
N/A

SYNONYMS
• FUS (see section on definition) • Feline urological disease • Feline urinary tract inflammation • Feline interstitial cystitis • Feline idiopathic cystitis

SEE ALSO
• Urolithiasis, Struvite—Cats • Dysuria and Pollakiuria • Lower Urinary Tract Infection • Hematuria

ABBREVIATIONS
iLUTD = idiopathic lower urinary tract disease

Suggested Reading

Lekcharoensuk C, Osborne CA, Lulich JP. Epidemiologic study of risk factors for lower urinary tract diseases in cats. J Am Vet Med Assoc 2001;218:1429–1435.

Osborne CA, Kruger JM, Lulich JP, eds. Disorders of the feline lower urinary tract. I. Etiology and pathophysiology. Vet Clin North Am 1996;26:169–421.

Osborne CA, Kruger JM, Lulich JP, eds. Disorders of the feline lower urinary tract. II. Diagnosis and therapy. Vet Clin North Am 1996;26:423–665.

Osborne, CA, Kruger, JM, Lulich JP, et al. Feline lower urinary tract diseases. In: Ettinger SJ, Feldman EC, eds. Textbook of veterinary internal medicine. 5th ed. Philadelphia: Saunders, 2000:1710–1747.

Authors Carl A. Osborne, John M. Kruger, Jody P. Lulich, and David J. Polzin
Consulting Editors Larry G. Adams and Carl A. Osborne

FELINE IMMUNODEFICIENCY VIRUS INFECTION (FIV)

BASICS

DEFINITION
A retrovirus that causes an immunodeficiency disease in domestic cats; same genus (Lentivirus) as HIV, the causative agent of AIDS in humans

PATHOPHYSIOLOGY
• Infection disrupts immune system function; feline lymphocytes and macrophages serve as the main target cells for virus replication
• Acute infection—virus spreads from the site of entry to the lymph tissues and thymus, first infecting T lymphocytes then macrophages
• CD4+ and CD8+ cells—both can be infected lytically in culture; virus selectively and progressively decreases CD4+ (T helper) cells; inversion of the CD4+:CD8+ ratio (from ~ 2:1 to < 1:1) develops slowly; an absolute decrease of CD4+ T cells is seen after several months of infection; patients are clinically asymptomatic until cell-mediated immunity is disrupted.
• Humoral immune function—perturbed in advanced stages of infection
• Macrophages—main reservoir of virus in affected cats; transport virus to tissues throughout the body; defects in function (e.g., increased production of TNF)
• Astrocyte and microglial cells in the brain and megakaryocytes and mononuclear bone marrow cells may be infected.
• Co-infection with FeLV may increase the expression of FIV in many tissues, including kidney, brain, and liver.

SYSTEMS AFFECTED
• Hemic/Lymphatic/Immune—loss of CD4+ T cells
• Renal/Urologic—nephropathy
• Nervous—alterations in sleep patterns and changes in visual, auditory, and spinal-evoked potentials; peripheral neuropathies
• Behavioral—repetitive movements, anxiety, or increased aggression may be seen.
• Other body systems—result of immuno-suppression and secondary infections

GENETICS
• No predisposition for infection
• May play a role in progression and severity

INCIDENCE/PREVALENCE
U.S. and Canada—1.5–3% in the healthy cat population; 9–15% in cats with signs of clinical illness

GEOGRAPHIC DISTRIBUTION
Worldwide; seroprevalence rates vary greatly

SIGNALMENT

Species
Cats

Breed Predilections
None

Mean Age and Range
• Prevalence of infection increases with age
• Mean age—5 years at time of diagnosis

Predominant Sex
Male—more aggressive; roaming

SIGNS

General Comments
• Diverse owing to immunosuppressive nature of infection
• Associated disease cannot be clinically distinguished from FeLV-associated immunodeficiencies.

Historical Findings
Recurrent minor illnesses, especially with upper respiratory and gastrointestinal signs

Physical Examination Findings
• Depend on occurrence of opportunistic infections
• Lymphadenomegaly—mild to moderate
• Gingivitis, stomatitis, periodontitis—25–50% of cases
• Upper respiratory tract—rhinitis; conjunctivitis; keratitis (~ 30% of cases); often associated with feline herpesvirus and calicivirus infections
• Chronic renal insufficiency
• Persistent diarrhea—10–20% of cases; bacterial or fungal overgrowth, parasite-induced inflammation; direct effect of FIV infection on the gastrointestinal epithelium
• Chronic, nonresponsive, or recurrent infections of the external ear and skin—from bacterial infections or dermatophytosis
• Fever and wasting—especially in later stage; possibly from high levels of TNF
• Ocular disease—anterior uveitis; pars planitis; glaucoma
• Lymphosarcoma or other neoplasia
• Neurologic abnormalities—disruption of normal sleep patterns; behavioral changes (pacing and aggression); peripheral neuropathies

CAUSES
• Cat-to-cat transmission; usually by bite wounds
• Occasional perinatal transmission

RISK FACTORS
• Male
• Free-roaming

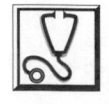

DIAGNOSIS

DIFFERENTIAL DIAGNOSIS
• Primary bacterial, parasitic, viral, or fungal infections

• Toxoplasmosis—neurologic and ocular manifestations may be the result of Toxoplasma infection, FIV infection, or both
• Nonviral neoplastic diseases

CBC/BIOCHEMISTRY/URINALYSIS
• Hemogram may be normal.
• Anemia, lymphopenia, or neutropenia—may be seen; neutrophilia may occur in response to secondary infections.
• Urinalysis and serum chemistry profile—high serum protein from hypergamma-globulinemia; otherwise usually normal unless secondary infections are present

OTHER LABORATORY TESTS

Serologic Testing
• Detects antibodies to FIV
• ELISA—routine screening test; kits for in-house use to microtiter plates for diagnostic laboratory use; confirm positive results with additional testing, especially in healthy, low-risk cats or when diagnosis would result in euthanasia.
• Western blot (immunoblot)—confirmatory testing of ELISA-positive samples
• Kittens—when < 6 months old may test positive owing to passive transfer of anti-bodies from an FIV-positive queen; a positive test does not indicate infection; retest at 8–12 months to determine infection.

Others
• Virus isolation or detection—other methods occasionally available on an experimental basis
• RT-PCR—useful in vaccinated cats or kittens with maternal antibody
• CD4+:CD8+ evaluation—helps determine extent of immunosuppression

IMAGING
N/A

DIAGNOSTIC PROCEDURES
N/A

PATHOLOGIC FINDINGS
• Lymphadenopathy—associated with follicular hyperplasia and massive paracortical infiltration of plasmacytes; later, may see a mixture of follicular hyperplasia and follicular depletion or involution; in terminal stages, lymphoid depletion is predominant finding.
• Lymphocytic and plasmacytic infiltrates—gingiva, lymph nodes and other lymphoid tissues, spleen, kidney, liver, and brain
• Perivascular cuffing, gliosis, neuronal loss, white matter vacuolization, and occasional giant cells in the brain
• Intestinal lesions similar to those seen with feline parvovirus infection (feline panleukopenia-like syndrome)

FELINE IMMUNODEFICIENCY VIRUS INFECTION (FIV)

TREATMENT

APPROPRIATE HEALTH CARE
• Outpatient sufficient for most patients
• Inpatient—with severe secondary infections until condition is stable

NURSING CARE
• Primary consideration—manage secondary and opportunistic infections
• Supportive therapy—parenteral fluids and nutritional supplements, as required

ACTIVITY
Normal

DIET
• Normal
• Diarrhea, kidney disease, or chronic wasting—special food, as needed

CLIENT EDUCATION
• Inform client that the infection is slowly progressive and healthy antibody-positive cats may remain healthy for years.
• Advise client that cats with clinical signs will have recurrent or chronic health problems that require medical attention.
• Discuss the importance of keeping cats indoors to protect them from exposure to secondary pathogens and to prevent spread of FIV.

SURGICAL CONSIDERATIONS
• Oral treatment or surgery—frequently required; dental cleaning, tooth extraction, gingival biopsy
• Biopsy or removal of tumors

MEDICATIONS

DRUG(S) OF CHOICE
• Zidovudine (Retrovir)—5–15 mg/kg PO, q12h–direct antiviral agent; most effective against acute infection; monitor for bone marrow toxicity
• Immunomodulatory drugs—alleviate some clinical signs; hrα-interferon (Roferon) diluted in saline at 30 units/day PO for 7 days every other week; may increase survival rates and improve clinical status; also try *Propionibacterium acnes* (Immunoregulin) at 0.5 mL/cat IV, once or twice weekly, or acemannan (Carrisyn) at 100 mg/cat PO daily.
• Gingivitis and stomatitis—may be refractory to treatment
• Antibacterial or antimycotic drugs—useful for overgrowth of bacteria or fungi; prolonged therapy or high dosages may be required; for anaerobic bacterial infections use metronidazole (Flagyl) at 7–15 mg/kg PO q8h or q12h or clindamycin (Antirobe) at 11 mg/kg PO q12h.

• Corticosteroids or gold salts—judicious but aggressive use may help control immune-mediated inflammation.
• Anorexia—short-term appetite stimulation: diazepam (Valium) at 0.2 mg/kg IV or oxazepam (Serax) at 2.5 mg/cat PO; more prolonged appetite stimulation and reversal of cachexia: anabolic steroids or megestrol acetate; efficacy in FIV-positive cats unknown
• Topical corticosteroids—for anterior uveitis; long-term response may be incomplete or poor; pars planitis often regresses spontaneously and may recur.
• Glaucoma—standard treatment
• Yearly vaccination for respiratory and enteric viruses with inactivated vaccines is recommended.

CONTRAINDICATIONS
• Griseofulvin—avoid or use with extreme caution in FIV-positive cats; may induce severe neutropenia; neutropenia is reversible if the drug is withdrawn early enough but secondary infections associated with the condition can be life-threatening.
• MLV vaccines—may cause disease in immunosuppressed cats

PRECAUTIONS
Systemic corticosteroids—use with caution; may lead to further immunosuppression

POSSIBLE INTERACTIONS
See Contraindications

ALTERNATIVE DRUG(S)
N/A

FOLLOW-UP

PATIENT MONITORING
Varies according to secondary infections and other manifestations of disease

PREVENTION/AVOIDANCE
• Prevent contact with FIV-positive cats.
• Quarantine and test incoming cats before introducing into multicat households.

Vaccine
• Dual subtype (A&D), inactivated whole virus vaccine (Fel-O-Vax FIV, Fort Dodge Animal Health)
• 60–80% efficacy after 3 doses
• Cannot distinguish between vaccinated and FIV-infected cats with antibody assays

POSSIBLE COMPLICATIONS
N/A

EXPECTED COURSE AND PROGNOSIS
• Within the first 2 years after diagnosis or 4.5–6 years after the estimated time of infection, about 20% of cats die but > 50% remain asymptomatic.
• In late stages of disease (wasting and frequent or severe opportunistic infections), life expectancy is ≤ 1 year.

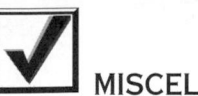

MISCELLANEOUS

ASSOCIATED CONDITIONS
• Secondary bacterial, viral, fungal, and parasitic disease
• Lymphoid tumors
• Immune-mediated disease

AGE-RELATED FACTORS
Kittens may test positive because of passive antibody transfer.

ZOONOTIC POTENTIAL
• None known; evidence against FIV transmission to humans is compelling but cannot be considered conclusive owing to the relatively short time the virus has been studied.
• Potential transmission of secondary pathogens (e.g., *Toxoplasma gondii*) to immunocompromised humans

PREGNANCY
FIV-positive queens—reported abortions and stillbirths; transmission to kittens is infrequent if the queen is antibody-positive before conception; rate of transmission may be subtype or strain-dependent.

SYNONYMS
Feline immunodeficiency syndrome

SEE ALSO
Individual topics on secondary infectious diseases, ocular disease, gingivitis, and stomatitis

ABBREVIATIONS
• ELISA = enzyme-linked immunosorbent assay
• FeLV = feline leukemia virus
• HIV = human immunodeficiency virus
• hrα-interferon = human recombinant α-interferon
• MLV = modified live virus
• TNF = tumor necrosis factor

Suggested Reading

Barr MC, Phillips TR. FIV and FIV-related diseases. In: Ettinger SJ, Feldman EC, eds., Textbook of veterinary internal medicine, 5th ed. Philadelphia: Saunders, 2000:433–438.

Levy JK. CVT update: feline immunodeficiency virus. In: Bonagura JD, ed., Kirk's current veterinary therapy XIII: small animal practice. Philadelphia: Saunders, 2000:284–288.

Author Margaret C. Barr
Consulting Editor Stephen C. Barr

FELINE INFECTIOUS PERITONITIS (FIP)

BASICS

DEFINITION
A systemic, viral disease characterized by insidious onset, persistent nonresponsive fever, pyogranulomatous tissue reaction, accumulation of exudative effusions in body cavities, and high mortality

PATHOPHYSIOLOGY
• FIP virus replicates locally in epithelial cells of the upper respiratory tract or oropharynx.
• Antiviral antibodies are produced, and the virus is taken up by macrophages.
• The virus is transported within monocytes/macrophages throughout the body; localizes at various vein wall and perivascular sites
• Local perivascular viral replication and subsequent pyogranulomatous tissue reaction produce the classic lesion.

SYSTEMS AFFECTED
• Multisystemic—pyogranulomatous or granulomatous lesions in the omentum, on the serosal surface of abdominal organs (e.g., liver, kidney, and intestines), within abdominal lymph nodes, and in the submucosa of the intestinal tract
• Respiratory—lesions on lung surfaces; pleural effusion in the wet form
• Nervous—vascular lesions can occur throughout the CNS, especially in the meninges.
• Ophthalmic—lesions may include uveitis and chorioretinitis.

GENETICS
N/A

INCIDENCE/PREVALENCE
• Prevalence of antibodies against FCoV—high in most populations, especially in multicat facilities
• Incidence of clinical disease—low in most populations, especially in single-cat households
• Because of the difficulty in diagnosis, control, and prevention, outbreaks within breeding catteries may be catastrophic; in endemic catteries, the risk of a FCoV antibody-positive cat eventually developing FIP is usually < 10%.

GEOGRAPHIC DISTRIBUTION
Worldwide

SIGNALMENT

Species
Cats—domestic and exotic

Breed Predilections
Some families or lines of cats appear more susceptible.

Mean Age and Range
• Highest incidence—in kittens 3 months to 3 years of age
• Incidence decreases sharply after cats reach 3 years of age.

Predominant Sex
N/A

SIGNS

General Comments
• A wide range, depending on the virulence of the strain, effectiveness of the host immune response, and organ system affected
• Two classic forms—wet or effusive form, targets the body cavities; dry or noneffusive form, targets a variety of organs

Historical Findings
• Insidious onset
• Gradual weight loss and decrease in appetite
• Stunting in kittens
• Gradual increase in the size of the abdomen, giving a potbellied appearance
• Persistent fever—fluctuating; antibiotic unresponsive

Physical Examination Findings
• Depression
• Poor condition
• Stunted growth
• Weight loss
• Dull, rough hair coat
• Icterus
• Abdominal and/or pleural effusion
• Palpation of the abdomen—abdominal masses (granulomas or pyogranulomas) within the omentum, on the surface of viscera (especially the kidney), and within the intestinal wall; mesenteric lymph nodes may be enlarged.
• Ocular—anterior uveitis; keratic precipitates; color change to the iris; and irregularly shaped pupil
• Neurologic—brain stem, cerebrocortical, or spinal cord

CAUSES
• Two genomic types of FCoV—FCoV-1 (causes perhaps 85% of infections) and FCoV-2
• Distinguishing between forms—there has been great effort to distinguish between the low virulent or avirulent enteric strains (FECV) and the virulent strains; but FECV and FIP virus occur in both type 1 and type 2 forms; within each type is a spectrum from avirulent viruses that produce asymptomatic infections to those that produce fatal FIP.

RISK FACTORS
• Contact with an FCoV antibody-positive cat
• Breeding catteries or multicat facilities
• Less than 3 years of age
• FeLV infection

DIAGNOSIS
• Wet form—relatively easy to diagnose clinically
• Dry form—difficult to diagnose accurately
• No single diagnostic laboratory test

DIFFERENTIAL DIAGNOSIS
• Fever of unknown origin—when other causes of fever are ruled out
• Cardiac disease causing pleural effusion—effusion has low specific gravity and cell count
• Lesions of lymphoma, especially in the kidney, on palpation
• CNS tumors—most cats test positive for FeLV; for FeLV-negative cats, biopsy the lesion (if accessible) for histopathology and immunohistochemistry for FCoV
• Respiratory disease—FCV, FHV, chlamydiosis, or various bacteria
• Pansteatitis (yellow fat disease)—classic feel and appearance of fat within the abdominal cavity; pain on abdominal palpation; often a fish-only diet
• Panleukopenia producing enteritis—leukopenia; positive fecal canine parvovirus antigen assay

CBC/BIOCHEMISTRY/URINALYSIS
• Leukopenia—common early in the infection; later leukocytosis with neutrophilia and lymphopenia
• Mild to moderate anemia may occur.
• High total plasma globulin common
• Often hyperbilirubinemia and hyperbilirubinuria

OTHER LABORATORY TESTS
• Serum antibody tests—immunoassays, viral neutralization assays; detect antibodies against FCoV; positive tests not diagnostic, indicate only previous infection; correlation between height of titer and eventual confirmation of infection not high
• PCR assays—detect viral antigen; accuracy of positive tests correlating with clinical disease is still being evaluated.
• Immunohistochemistry (immunoperoxidase) assays detect FCoV within specific cells of biopsy samples or histopathologic sections of tissues from cats with fatal diseases; excellent for confirming cause of specific lesions, especially inflammatory abdominal disease, which is often is not diagnosed as FIP

IMAGING
• Generally not required
• May confirm abdominal and pleural effusions
• May detect granulomatous lesions

DIAGNOSTIC PROCEDURES
• Fluid obtained via thoracocentesis and abdominocentesis—pale to straw colored; viscous; flecks of white fibrin often seen; will clot upon standing; specific gravity usually high (1.030–1.040)

- Laparoscopy—to observe specific lesions of the peritoneal cavity; to obtain a biopsy sample for histopathology or immuno-histochemistry confirmation
- Exploratory laparotomy—may be indicated for difficult-to-diagnose patients if laparoscopy is not available

PATHOLOGIC FINDINGS

Gross
- Vary depending on the organs or tissues involved
- Patient will be emaciated, with a rough hair coat.

Wet Form
- Abdomen and/or thoracic cavity—may contain a thick, viscous exudate
- White, rough, pyogranulomatous plaques—may be on serosal surface of abdominal organs and the omentum
- Granulomatous lumps—may protrude from the surface of the kidney
- Granulomas—may be in the intestinal wall
- Fibrous strands—may extend between organs
- Liver—may have focal, pale lesions
- Iris—may be discolored
- Cornea—may see keratic precipitates
- Neurologic signs—may see lesions in the brain and/or the spinal cord

Histopathologic
- Granulomas or pyogranulomas in any affected tissue
- Lesions—start around veins; increase in size, involving large portions of tissue; microscopic appearance suggests the diagnosis.

TREATMENT

APPROPRIATE HEALTH CARE
Inpatient or outpatient, depending on stage and severity of disease and owner's willingness and ability to provide good supportive care

NURSING CARE
- Therapeutic paracentesis—to relieve pressure from excessive ascites or pleural effusions
- Important to encourage the affected cat to eat

ACTIVITY
Restrict to prevent exposure of other cats, although greatest degree of virus shed occurs before the patient shows signs

DIET
Any food that will entice the patient to eat

CLIENT EDUCATION
- Discuss the various aspects of disease, including the grave prognosis.
- Inform client of the high prevalence of FCoV infection but low incidence of actual clinical disease; < 10% of FCoV antibody–positive cats < 3 years of age eventually develop clinical disease.

SURGICAL CONSIDERATIONS
- Generally none
- Rarely, inflammatory abdominal disease from FCoV may present with intestinal obstruction; abdominal surgery may be required.

MEDICATIONS

DRUG(S) OF CHOICE
- No treatment routinely effective
- Patients with generalized and typical signs almost invariably die
- Most FCoV-positive cats have subclinical infection or mild, localized granulomatous disease that is not diagnosed as FIP
- Immunosuppressive drugs (e.g., prednisolone and cyclophosphamide)—limited success
- Corticosteroids (subconjunctival injection)—may help ocular involvement
- Interferons—effective in vitro; limited success; a recombinant interferon reported to have some success in Japan
- Antibiotics—ineffective because generally not associated with secondary bacterial infections

CONTRAINDICATIONS
N/A

PRECAUTIONS
N/A

POSSIBLE INTERACTIONS
N/A

ALTERNATIVE DRUG(S)
No antiviral drugs proven to be efficacious

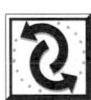

FOLLOW-UP

PATIENT MONITORING
Monitor for development of large quantities of pleural effusion.

PREVENTION/AVOIDANCE
- MLV intranasal vaccine—available against FIP virus; efficacy low; cannot rely on vaccination alone for control; may produce antibody-positive cats, complicating monitoring in catteries or colonies
- Mother/offspring—main method of transmission appears to be from asymptomatic carrier queens to their kittens at 5–7 weeks of age, after maternally derived immunity wanes; break cycle of transmission by early weaning at 4–5 weeks of age and isolating litter from direct contact with other cats, including the queen
- Routine disinfection—premise, cages, and water/food dishes; readily inactivates virus; reduces transmission • Introduce only FCoV antibody–negative cats to catteries or colonies that are free of virus • Restrict household cats to indoor environments.

POSSIBLE COMPLICATIONS
- Pleural effusion may require thoracocentesis.
- Intestinal obstruction from inflammatory abdominal disease
- Neurologic disease from CNS lesions

EXPECTED COURSE AND PROGNOSIS
- Clinical course—a few days to several months • Prognosis grave once typical signs occur; mortality nearly 100%

MISCELLANEOUS

ASSOCIATED CONDITIONS
- FeLV-positive cats—more prone to develop clinical disease

AGE-RELATED FACTORS
N/A

ZOONOTIC POTENTIAL
None

PREGNANCY
FIP virus can infect fetuses, resulting in fetal death or neonatal disease.

SYNONYMS
- Feline coronavirus infection
- Feline coronaviral polyserositis

ABBREVIATIONS
- CNS = central nervous system
- FCoV = feline coronavirus
- FCV = feline calicivirus
- FECV = feline enteric coronavirus
- FeLV = feline leukemia virus
- FHV = feline herpes virus
- MLV = modified live virus
- PCR = polymerase chain reaction

Suggested Reading

Barr MC, Olsen CW, Scott FW. Feline viral diseases. In: Ettinger SJ, Feldman EC, eds. Veterinary internal medicine, 4th ed. Philadelphia: Saunders, 1995:409–439.

Horzinek MC, Lutz H. An update on feline infectious peritonitis. Veterinary sciences tomorrow Jan. 2001;1–11 http://roquade.library.uu.nl/cgi-bin/vst/pw.exe/reviews/txt_index_0800.htm

Olsen CW. A review of feline infectious peritonitis virus: molecular biology, immunopathogenesis, clinical aspects, and vaccination. Vet Microbiol 1993;36:1–37.

Report from the International FIP/FECV Workshop. Feline Pract 1995;23:2–111.

Sparkes AH, Gruffydd-Jones TJ, Harbour DA. An appraisal of the value of laboratory tests in the diagnosis of feline infectious peritonitis. J Am Anim Hosp Assoc 1994; 30:345–350.

Author Fred W. Scott
Consulting Editor Stephen C. Barr

FELINE ISCHEMIC ENCEPHALOPATHY

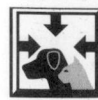 **BASICS**

DEFINITION
Naturally occurring neurologic syndrome characterized by acute ischemic necrosis of brain tissue

PATHOPHYSIOLOGY
• Recent histopathology has demonstrated parts of *Cuterebra* larvae in affected brain parts of some cats.
• Main lesion—often involves the middle cerebral artery on one side of the brain
• Unilateral lesions near the frontal lobe or rostral thalamus—often cause the patient to circle or turn toward the affected side; referred to as adversive syndrome
• Limbic system—involvement may cause behavioral changes and seizure activity
• Vascular abnormalities (e.g., vascular thrombosis, vasculitis)—not consistently found

SYSTEMS AFFECTED
Nervous—specifically the cerebrum; occasionally the brain stem; rarely the cerebellum

GENETICS
N/A

INCIDENCE/PREVALENCE
Unknown

GEOGRAPHIC DISTRIBUTION
N/A

SIGNALMENT

Species
Cats

Breed Predilections
N/A

Mean Age and Range
• Any age
• Kittens seem to be spared.

Predominant Sex
N/A

SIGNS

General Comments
Related to the severity and location of the ischemia

Historical Findings
• Acute onset
• Generalized or partial seizures—common
• Behavioral changes—aggression; depression; dementia; polyphagia; stupor
• Many affected cats are ambulatory but ataxic; may circle toward the side of the lesion (adversive syndrome)
• Blindness—may be present

Physical Examination Findings
• Initially, the neurologic signs might be generalized, but as the edema subsides, a more focal effect is usually found on the neurologic examination.
• Focal neurologic examination changes are consistent with a unilateral cerebral lesion—circling to the side of the lesion with contralateral motor and/or sensory deficits (e.g., reduced eyelid closure and lip retraction, reduced facial sensation, reduced menace response, impaired proprioceptive positioning, hemiwalking and hopping)
• Behavioral changes (e.g., mental dullness, dementia, aggression, stupor) may be evident during examination.
• Blindness—normal pupillary light reflexes imply a cerebral lesion; dilated, unresponsive pupils suggest an optic chiasm or midbrain lesion.

CAUSES
• *Cuterebra* larvae migration may cause a vasospasm, resulting in ischemia, or it may be toxic to the host tissue or elicit an inflammatory response from the host tissue.
• *Cuterebra* larvae migration may explain the prevalence of suspected ischemic encephalopathy cases in the summer months, but there may be other causes of brain ischemia to explain cases seen at other times of the year.

RISK FACTORS
• History of recent upper respiratory infection has been observed in a few affected cats, suggesting that the larvae might enter via the cribriform plate.

• Generally nonseasonal, but one report of a higher prevalence in summer

 DIAGNOSIS

DIFFERENTIAL DIAGNOSIS
Distinguish by skull radiography (trauma), CSF analysis (encephalitis), and CT or MRI scans (neoplasia, trauma, and vascular disease); if tests are unavailable or nondiagnostic, note that clinical signs are usually nonprogressive with ischemia and trauma but progressive with neoplasia and encephalitis.

CBC/BIOCHEMISTRY/URINALYSIS
Usually normal

OTHER LABORATORY TESTS
FeLV and FIV tests—negative

IMAGING
• Radiography (skull)—normal; may reveal head trauma or bony neoplasia, if these are causing the clinical signs
• CT and MRI—may show edema and disruption of the blood–brain barrier in the acute stages; may reveal asymmetry of cerebral hemispheres, excessive CSF filling of subarachnoid space, and compensatory hydrocephalus in chronic stages

DIAGNOSTIC PROCEDURES

CSF Analysis
• Normal results or high protein and/or WBC count
• Primary cell type often mononuclear (e.g., lymphocytes and macrophages)
• Xanthochromia or erythrophagocytosis in some patients, especially in the acute stage
• Cytology findings—may differ according to time of sampling in relation to onset of signs

Electroencephalography
• May confirm brain dysfunction or help confirm a specific location
• Cannot distinguish among vascular disease, neoplasia, trauma, and infection

PATHOLOGIC FINDINGS
• With long duration of clinical signs—widened sulci and atrophy of the affected side

• Histologic—atrophy; degeneration; necrosis; astrocytosis; gliosis; phagocytic macrophages

 TREATMENT

APPROPRIATE HEALTH CARE
• Inpatient—at least 2 days for observation and treatment
• Hyperventilation (oxygen therapy)—may help reduce cerebral edema associated with ischemia
• Outpatient—if seizures are controlled and patient is able to eat and drink

NURSING CARE
Intravenous fluid administration—conservative, to reduce risk of overhydration and worsening of cerebral edema

ACTIVITY
N/A

DIET
N/A

CLIENT EDUCATION
• About one-half of affected cats remain functional pets.
• Secondary (acquired) epilepsy—may develop as a result of ischemia

SURGICAL CONSIDERATIONS
N/A

 MEDICATIONS

DRUG(S) OF CHOICE
• Dexamethasone (0.5–1 mg/kg IV) or methylprednisolone sodium succinate (30 mg/kg IV bolus followed by 15 mg/kg IV 2 and 6 hr after initial dose) have been used for suspected edema and inflammation, but they have no proven efficacy in these cases
• Diazepam—0.5–1.0 mg/kg IV; only if there is seizure activity or agitation

• Chronic oral administration of phenobarbital or diazepam—recommended for patients with seizures because of potential for acquired epilepsy; if patient remains seizure free for 6 months, wean from drug slowly (over 12 weeks)

CONTRAINDICATIONS
• Drugs that raise intracranial pressure
• Drugs that lower seizure threshold (e.g., acepromazine, amphetamines)

PRECAUTIONS
Overhydration can contribute to cerebral edema and worsen the clinical signs.

POSSIBLE INTERACTIONS
N/A

ALTERNATIVE DRUG(S)
N/A

 FOLLOW-UP

PATIENT MONITORING
Daily neurologic examination—determine if signs are stabilizing or improving

PREVENTION/AVOIDANCE
N/A

POSSIBLE COMPLICATIONS
• Status epilepticus
• Death—uncommon

EXPECTED COURSE AND PROGNOSIS
• Until it can be determined that the clinical signs are improving, prognosis is guarded.
• Steadily improving signs over 1–2 weeks—associated with favorable prognosis
• Permanent behavioral changes (especially aggression) and seizures—common sequelae

 **MISCELLANEOUS**

ASSOCIATED CONDITIONS
N/A

AGE-RELATED FACTORS
N/A

ZOONOTIC POTENTIAL
N/A

PREGNANCY
N/A

SYNONYMS
• Feline cerebral infarct
• Feline stroke

SEE ALSO
• Brain Injury
• Seizures (Convulsions, Status Epilepticus)—Cats

ABBREVIATIONS
• CSF = cerebrospinal fluid
• CT = computed tomography
• FeLV = feline leukemia virus
• FIV = feline immunodeficiency virus
• MRI = magnetic resonance imaging
• WBC = white blood cell

Suggested Reading
Bernstein NM, Fiske RA. Feline ischemic encephalopathy in a cat. J Am Anim Hosp Assoc 1986;22:205–206.
De Lahunta A. Upper motor neuron system. In: Veterinary neuroanatomy and clinical neurology, 2nd ed. Philadelphia: Saunders, 1983:130–155.
Glass EN, Cornetta AM, DeLahunta A, et al. Clinical and clinicopathologic features in 11 cats with *Cuterebra* larvae myiasis of the central nervous system. J Vet Intern Med 1998;12:365–368.
Summers BA, Cummings JF, de Lahunta A. Veterinary neuropathology. St. Louis: Mosby, 1995.
Williams KJ, Summers BA, DeLahunta A. Cerebrospinal cuterebriasis in cats and its association with feline ischemic encephalopathy. Vet Pathol 1998;35:330–343.
Zaki FA, Nafe LA. Ischemic encephalopathy and focal granulomatous meningoencephalitis in the cat. J Small Anim Pract 1980;21:429–438.

Author Linda G. Shell
Consulting Editor Joane M. Parent

FELINE LEUKEMIA VIRUS INFECTION (FeLV)

 BASICS

DEFINITION
A retrovirus (Gammaretrovirus genus) that causes immunodeficiency and neoplastic disease in domestic cats

PATHOPHYSIOLOGY
• Early infection consists of five stages—(1) viral replication in tonsils and pharyngeal lymph nodes; (2) infection of a few circulating B lymphocytes and macrophages that disseminate the virus; (3) replication in lymphoid tissues, intestinal crypt epithelial cells, and bone marrow precursor cells; (4) release of infected neutrophils and platelets from the bone marrow into the circulatory system; and (5) infection of epithelial and glandular tissues, with subsequent shedding of virus into the saliva and urine.
• An adequate immune response stops progression at stage 2 or 3 (4–8 weeks after exposure) and forces the virus into latency.
• Persistent viremia (stages 4 and 5) usually develops 4–6 weeks after infection, but may take 12 weeks.
Tumor Induction
• Occurs when the DNA provirus integrates into cat chromosomal DNA in critical regions (oncogenes)
• Virus integration near the cellular gene c-*myc* or near genes influencing the expression of c-*myc*—often results in thymic lymphosarcoma
• Changes in the virus's *env* gene—owing to mutations or recombinations with endogenous retroviral *env* sequences
• Feline sarcoma viruses—mutants of FeLV; arise by recombination between the genes of FeLV and host; virus–host fusion proteins are responsible for the efficient induction of fibrosarcomas

SYSTEMS AFFECTED
• Hemic/Lymphatic/Immune—anemia; blood cell dyscrasias; neoplasias originating in the bone marrow; immunosuppression, possibly resulting from neuroendocrine dysfunction; absolute decrease in CD4+ and CD8+ subsets of T cells; decreased CD4+:CD8+ ratio
• Nervous—degenerative myelopathy, neoplasias
• All other body systems—immunosuppression with secondary infections or development of neoplastic disease

GENETICS
No genetic predisposition

INCIDENCE/PREVALENCE
Prevalence in U.S.—2–3% in the healthy cat population; three to four times greater in cats exhibiting signs of clinical illness

GEOGRAPHIC DISTRIBUTION
Worldwide

SIGNALMENT
Species
Cats
Breed Predilections
None
Mean Age and Range
• Prevalence highest between 1 and 6 years of age
• Mean—3 years
Predominant Sex
Male:female ratio—1.7:1

SIGNS
General Comments
• Onset of FeLV-associated disease—usually occurs over a period of months to years after infection
• Associated diseases—nonneoplastic or neoplastic; most of the nonneoplastic or degenerative diseases result from immunosuppression.
• Clinical signs of FeLV-induced immunodeficiency cannot be distinguished from those of FIV-induced immunodeficiency.
Historical Findings
• Patient allowed outdoors
• Member of a multicat household
Physical Examination Findings
• Depend on the type of disease (neoplastic or nonneoplastic) and occurrence of secondary infections
• Lymphadenomegaly—mild to severe
• Upper respiratory tract—rhinitis, conjunctivitis, and keratitis
• Persistent diarrhea—bacterial or fungal overgrowth; parasite-induced inflammation; direct effect of infection on crypt cells
• Gingivitis; stomatitis; periodontitis
• Chronic, nonresponsive or recurrent infections of the external ear and skin
• Fever and wasting
• Lymphoma (lymphosarcoma)—most common associated neoplastic disease; thymic and multicentric lymphomas highly associated; miscellaneous lymphomas (extranodal origin) most frequently involve the eye and nervous system.
• Erythroid and myelomonocytic leukemias—predominant nonlymphoid leukemias
• Fibrosarcomas—in patients co-infected with mutated sarcoma virus; most frequently in young cats
• Peripheral neuropathies; progressive ataxia

CAUSES
• Cat-to-cat transmission—bites; close casual contact (grooming); shared dishes or litter pans
• Perinatal transmission—fetal and neonatal death of kittens from 80% of affected queens; transplacental and transmammary transmission in at least 20% of surviving kittens from infected queens

RISK FACTORS
• Male—result of behavior
• Free roaming
• Multicat household

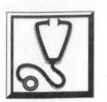 DIAGNOSIS

DIFFERENTIAL DIAGNOSIS
• FIV
• Other infections—bacterial, parasitic, viral, or fungal
• Nonviral neoplastic diseases

CBC/BIOCHEMISTRY/URINALYSIS
• Anemia—often severe
• Lymphopenia
• Neutropenia—may be in response to secondary infections
• Thrombocytopenia and immune-mediated hemolytic anemia—may occur secondary to immune complexes
• Urinalysis and serum chemistry profile findings—depend on system affected and type of disease

OTHER LABORATORY TESTS
• IFA—identify FeLV p27 antigen in leukocytes and platelets in fixed smears of whole blood or buffy coat preparations; positive result indicates a productive infection in bone marrow cells; 97% IFA-positive cats remain persistently infected and viremic for life; p27 antigen can usually be detected by 4 weeks after infection, but may take up to 12 weeks to develop a positive test; for leukopenic cats, use buffy coat smears rather than whole blood smears.
• ELISA—detect soluble FeLV p27 antigen in whole blood, serum, plasma, saliva, or tears; more sensitive than IFA at detecting early or transient infections; a single positive test cannot predict which cats will be persistently viremic; retest in 12 weeks (many veterinarians test with IFA at this point); false-positive results more common when whole blood rather than serum or plasma is used; positive tests with saliva or tears should be checked with whole blood (IFA) or serum (ELISA).
• A few cats are persistently ELISA-positive and IFA-negative; recently, FeLV proviral genetic material has been detected in circulating blood cells from some of these cats; demonstrates infection despite no detectable viremia.
• Neither test detects FeLV-vaccinated cats, because the vaccine induces antibodies against gp70 antigen, not p27 antigen.

IMAGING
Thymic atrophy (fading kittens)

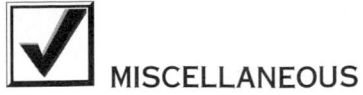

DIAGNOSTIC PROCEDURES

Bone marrow aspiration or biopsy—with erythroblastopenia (nonregenerative anemia), bone marrow often hypercellular owing to an arrest in differentiation of erythroid cells; true aplastic anemia with hypocellular bone marrow may be seen; some cases of anemia result from myeloproliferative disease.

PATHOLOGIC FINDINGS

• Lesions—depend on type of disease; bone marrow hypercellularity often accompanies neoplastic disease.
• Lymphocytic and plasmacytic infiltrates of the gingiva, lymph nodes, other lymphoid tissues, spleen, kidney, and liver
• Intestinal lesions similar to those seen with feline parvovirus infection (feline panleukopenia-like syndrome)

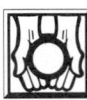

TREATMENT

APPROPRIATE HEALTH CARE

• Outpatient for most cats
• Inpatient—may be required with severe secondary infections, anemia, or cachexia until condition stable
• Blood transfusions—emergency support; multiple transfusions may be necessary; passive antibody transfer reduces level of FeLV antigenemia in some cats; thus immunization of blood donor cats with FeLV vaccines is useful.

NURSING CARE

• Management of secondary and opportunistic infections—primary consideration
• Supportive therapy (e.g., parenteral fluids and nutritional supplements) may be useful.

ACTIVITY

Normal

DIET

• Normal
• Diarrhea, kidney disease, or chronic wasting—may require special diet

CLIENT EDUCATION

Discuss importance of keeping cats indoors and separated from FeLV-negative cats, to protect them from exposure to secondary pathogens and to prevent spread of FeLV.

SURGICAL CONSIDERATIONS

• Biopsy or removal of tumors
• Oral treatment or surgery—dental cleaning, tooth extraction, gingival biopsy

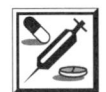

MEDICATIONS

DRUG(S) OF CHOICE

• Zidovudine (retrovir) 5–15 mg/kg PO q12h—clinical improvement but does not clear virus

• Immunomodulatory drugs—may alleviate some clinical signs; hrα-interferon (Roferon, diluted in saline, 30 U/day PO for 7 days every other week) may increase survival rates and improve clinical status; *Propionibacterium acnes* (Immunoregulin, 0.5 mL/cat IV once or twice weekly); acemannan (Carrasyn, 100 mg/cat/day PO)
• *Haemobartonella* infection—suspect in all cats with regenerative hemolytic anemias; oxytetracycline (Terramycin, 15 mg/kg PO q8h or Liquamycin 7 mg/kg IM or IV q12h) or doxycycline (5 mg/kg PO q12h) for 3 weeks; short-term use of oral glucocorticoids in severe cases
• Lymphosarcoma—managed successfully with standard combination chemotherapy protocols; periods of remission average 3–4 months; some cats may remain in remission for much longer
• Myeloproliferative disease and leukemias—more refractory to treatment
• Yearly vaccination for respiratory and enteric viruses with inactivated vaccines recommended

CONTRAINDICATIONS

Modified live vaccines may cause disease in immunosuppressed cats.

PRECAUTIONS

Systemic corticosteroids—use with caution because of the potential for further immunosuppression.

POSSIBLE INTERACTIONS

N/A

ALTERNATIVE DRUG(S)

N/A

FOLLOW-UP

PATIENT MONITORING

Varies according to the secondary infections and other manifestations of disease

PREVENTION/AVOIDANCE

• Prevent contact with FeLV-positive cats.
• Quarantine and test incoming cats before introduction into multiple cat households.
• Vaccines—most commercial vaccines induce virus-neutralizing antibodies specific for gp70; reported efficacy ranges from < 20% to almost 100%, depending on the trial and challenge system; test cats for FeLV before initial vaccination; if pre-vaccination testing is not done, clients should be aware that the cat may already be infected.

POSSIBLE COMPLICATIONS

N/A

EXPECTED COURSE AND PROGNOSIS

Persistently viremic cats—> 50% succumb to related diseases within 2–3 years after infection

☑ **MISCELLANEOUS**

ASSOCIATED CONDITIONS

• Secondary bacterial, viral, fungal, and parasitic disease
• Lymphoid tumors
• Fibrosarcomas
• Immune-mediated disease

AGE-RELATED FACTORS

• Neonatal kittens—most susceptible to persistent infection (70–100%)
• Older kittens—< 30% susceptible by 16 weeks of age

ZOONOTIC POTENTIAL

Probably low, but controversial—studies report conflicting results of antibodies to FeLV in humans and of correlation between certain human leukemias and exposure to cats.

PREGNANCY

• Abortions, stillbirths, and fetal resorptions common in FeLV-positive queens
• Transmission from queen to kittens—in at least 20% of live births

SYNONYMS

FeLV-AIDS—a mutated FeLV that causes immunodeficiency disease to develop rapidly

SEE ALSO

Individual topics on neoplasia, secondary infectious diseases, ocular disease, and gingivitis/stomatitis

ABBREVIATIONS

• ELISA = enzyme-linked immunosorbent assay
• FIV = feline immunodeficiency virus
• hrα-interferon = human recombinant interferon
• IFA = immunofluorescent antibody

Suggested Reading

Levy JK. FeLV and non-neoplastic FeLV–related disease: In: Ettinger SJ, Feldman EC, eds., Textbook of veterinary internal medicine, 5th ed. Philadelphia: Saunders, 2000:424–432.

Wolf AM. CVT update: feline leukemia virus. In: Bonagura JD, ed., Kirk's current veterinary therapy XIII: small animal practice. Philadelphia: Saunders, 2000: 280–284.

Sparkes AH. Feline leukemia virus: a review of immunity and vaccination. J Small Anim Pract 1997;38:187–194.

Author Margaret C. Barr

Consulting Editor Stephen C. Barr

FELINE PANLEUKOPENIA

 BASICS

DEFINITION
An acute, enteric, viral infection of cats characterized by sudden onset, depression, vomiting and diarrhea, severe dehydration, and a high mortality

PATHOPHYSIOLOGY
The causative virus, feline parvovirus (FPV), infects only mitotic cells, causing acute cell cytolysis of rapidly dividing cells.

SYSTEMS AFFECTED
• Hemic/Lymphatic/Immune—severe panleukopenia; atrophy of the thymus
• Gastrointestinal—intestinal crypt cells of the jejunum and ileum destroyed; acute enteritis with vomiting and diarrhea; shortened blunt villi with poor absorption of nutrients, dehydration, and secondary bacteremia
• Reproductive—in utero infection leading to fetal death, fetal resorption, abortion, stillbirth, or fetal mummification
• Nervous and Ophthalmic—in neonatal kittens rapidly dividing granular cells of the cerebellum and retinal cells of the eye destroyed; cerebellar hypoplasia with ataxia and retinal dysplasia

GENETICS
N/A

INCIDENCE/PREVALENCE
• Unvaccinated populations—the most severe and important feline infectious disease
• Routine vaccination—almost total control of this disease
• Extremely contagious
• Extremely stable virus, surviving for years on contaminated premises

GEOGRAPHIC DISTRIBUTION
Worldwide in unvaccinated populations

SIGNALMENT
Species
• Felidae—all, domestic and exotic
• Canidae—susceptible to the closely related canine parvovirus; some exotic canids may be susceptible to FPV infection.
• Mustelidae—especially mink; may be susceptible
• Procyonidae—raccoon and coatimundi; susceptible

Breed Predilections
None

Mean Age and Range
• Unvaccinated and previously unexposed cats of any age can become infected once passively transferred maternal immunity has been lost.
• Kittens 2–6 months of age—most susceptible to develop severe disease
• Adults—often mild or subclinical infection

Predominant Sex
N/A

SIGNS
Historical Findings
• History of recent exposure (e.g., adoption shelter)
• Newly acquired kitten
• Kitten 2–4 months old from a premise with a history of FP
• No vaccination history or last vaccinated when < 12 weeks of age
• Sudden onset, with vomiting, diarrhea, depression, and complete anorexia
• Owner may suspect poisoning.
• Cat may have disappeared or hid for 1 day or more before being found.
• Owner may report cat hangs head over water bowl or food dish but does not eat or drink.

Physical Examination Findings
• Depression—may be mild to severe
• Typical "panleukopenia posture"—sternum and chin resting on floor, feet tucked under body, and top of scapulae elevated above the back
• Dehydration—appears rapidly; may be severe
• Vomiting and diarrhea may occur.
• Body temperature—usually mild to moderately elevated or depressed in the early stages of disease; becomes severely subnormal as affected cat becomes moribund
• Abdominal pain—may be elicited on palpation
• Small intestine—either turgid and hose-like or flaccid
• Subclinical or mild infections with few or no clinical signs common, especially in adults
• Ataxia from cerebellar hypoplasia—kittens infected in utero or neonatally; signs evident at 10–14 days of age and persist for life: hypermetria; dysmetria; incoordination with a base-wide stance and an elevated "rudder" tail; alert, afebrile, and otherwise normal; retinal dysplasia sometimes seen

CAUSES
Feline Parvovirus (FPV)
• Small, single-stranded DNA virus
• Single antigenic serotype
• Considerable antigenic cross-reactivity with canine parvovirus (CPV) type 2 and mink enteritis virus
• Extremely stable against environmental factors, temperature, and most disinfectants
• Requires a mitotic cell for replication

Canine Parvovirus (CPV) Types 2a and 2b
• Recent isolates of CPV-2a and CPV-2b have been made from cats with FP.
• Prevalence of CPV-2a and 2b infection in a wide range of cat populations
• Properties of CPV like those for FPV

RISK FACTORS
• Anything that increases the mitotic activity of the small intestinal crypt cells—intestinal parasites; pathogenic bacteria
• Secondary or co-infections—viral upper respiratory infections
• Age—kittens 2–6 months of age tend to be more severely affected.

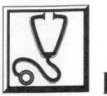 **DIAGNOSIS**

DIFFERENTIAL DIAGNOSIS
• Panleukopenia-like syndrome of FeLV infection—chronic infection; chronic enteritis; chronic panleukopenia; often anemia; patient positive for FeLV antigen in the blood and/or saliva
• Salmonellosis—usually subclinical infection; severe gastroenteritis; total WBC counts usually high
• Acute poisoning—similar to acute or fulminating disease; severe depression; subnormal temperature; total WBC count not severely depressed
• Many diseases of cats can cause mild clinical signs that are hard to differentiate from mild FP; total WBC count is always low during the acute infection with FP, even in subclinical infections.

CBC/BIOCHEMISTRY/URINALYSIS
• Panleukopenia—most consistent finding; leukocyte counts usually between 500 and 3,000 cells/dL during the acute disease
• Biochemical findings usually nonspecific

OTHER LABORATORY TESTS
• CPV antigen fecal immunoassay (CITE[R] Canine Parvovirus Test Kit, IDEXX Labs)—not licensed for feline panleukopenia; will detect FPV antigen in feces
• Chromatographic test strip—feces for FPV and CPV
• Serologic testing—paired serum samples (acute and convalescent); detects rising antibody titer

DIAGNOSTIC PROCEDURES
• Viral isolation from feces or affected tissues (e.g., thymus, small intestine, spleen)
• Electron microscopy of feces—detects parvovirus particles, presumably FPV

PATHOLOGIC FINDINGS
Gross
• Rough hair coat
• Severe dehydration
• Evidence of vomiting and diarrhea
• Weight loss
• Edematous and turgid small intestine
• Petechial or ecchymotic hemorrhages on the serosal and/or mucosal surfaces of the jejunum and ileum

- Thymic atrophy
- Gelatinous or liquid bone marrow
- In utero infection—gross hypoplasia of the cerebellum

Microscopic
- Dilated small intestinal crypts with sloughing of epithelial cells
- Shortened and blunt intestinal villi
- Absence of lymphocytic infiltrates in all tissues
- Lymphocytic depletion of follicles of lymph nodes, Peyer's patches, and spleen
- Neonatal and fetal infection—disorientation and depletion of the granular and Purkinje's cells of the cerebellum
- Eosinophilic intranuclear inclusions in affected tissues during early stages of infection; not usually observed on routine histopathologic examination of formalin-fixed tissues

 TREATMENT

APPROPRIATE HEALTH CARE
- Main principles of treatment—rehydration; reestablishment of electrolyte balance; supportive care until the patient's immune system produces antiviral antibodies that neutralize the virus
- Inpatient—severe cases; hydration and replacement electrolyte therapy
- Outpatient—mild cases

NURSING CARE
- Fluid therapy—essential in severe cases; with electrolyte replacement and intravenous nutrient support may well make the difference between survival and death
- Whole blood transfusions—if plasma protein falls < 4 g/dL or if total WBC counts fall < 2000 cells/dL

ACTIVITY
Keep patient indoors during the acute disease—prevent contamination of the environment; prevent the cat from going into hiding.

DIET
Temporarily withhold food until the acute gastroenteritis is controlled.

CLIENT EDUCATION
- Inform client that all current and future cats in the household must be vaccinated against FPV before exposure
- Inform client that the virus will remain infectious on the premise for years unless environment can be adequately disinfected with household bleach

SURGICAL CONSIDERATIONS
None

 MEDICATIONS

DRUG(S) OF CHOICE
Broad-spectrum antibiotics—counter secondary bacteremia from intestinal bacteria

CONTRAINDICATIONS
Oral medications until gastroenteritis has been controlled

PRECAUTIONS
N/A

POSSIBLE INTERACTIONS
None known

ALTERNATIVE DRUG(S)
None

 FOLLOW-UP

PATIENT MONITORING
- Monitor hydration and electrolyte balance closely.
- Monitor CBC daily or at least every 2 days until recovery.
- Recovered cats are immune against FPV infection for life and do not require further vaccination.

PREVENTION/AVOIDANCE
- Contaminated environments (e.g., cages, floors, food and water dishes) should be disinfected with a 1:32 dilution of household bleach.
- FPV resistant to most commercial disinfectants

Vaccines
- Completely preventable by routine vaccination of kittens
- MLV or inactivated parenteral vaccines
- MLV intranasal vaccine
- Immunity—long duration, perhaps even for life
- Kittens—vaccinate at 8–10 weeks of age; then after 12 weeks of age, when maternally derived immunity has waned.
- Boosters—after 1 year; repeat every 3 years to provide excellent immunity.

POSSIBLE COMPLICATIONS
- Chronic enteritis—fungal or other cause
- Teratogenic effects (cerebellar hypoplasia resulting in ataxia for life)—virus infection of fetus
- Shock and other complications—severe dehydration and electrolyte imbalance

EXPECTED COURSE AND PROGNOSIS
- Most cases acute, lasting only 5–7 days
- If death does not occur during the acute disease, recovery is usually rapid and uncomplicated; it may take several weeks for the patient to regain weight and body condition.

- Prognosis is guarded during the acute disease, especially if the total WBC count is < 2000 cells/dL.

 MISCELLANEOUS

ASSOCIATED CONDITIONS
Viral upper respiratory diseases, including feline viral rhinotracheitis and feline calicivirus infection

AGE-RELATED FACTORS
- Clinical—generally a disease of kittens
- Subclinical—usually adults

ZOONOTIC POTENTIAL
None

PREGNANCY
- Unvaccinated pregnant cats are at great risk of infection.
- Fetuses almost always become infected with fatal or teratogenic effects, even when the dam has a subclinical infection.
- Fetal resorption, abortion, fetal mummification, stillbirth, or birth of weak, fading kittens
- Kittens may show ataxia from cerebellar hypoplasia when they become ambulatory.

SYNONYMS
- Feline distemper
- Feline viral enteritis
- Feline parvovirus infection

ABBREVIATIONS
- CPV = canine parvovirus
- FeLV = feline leukemia virus
- FPV = feline parvovirus
- MLV = modified live virus
- WBC = white blood cell

Suggested Reading
Barr MC, Olsen CW, Scott FW. Feline viral diseases. In: Ettinger SJ, Feldman EC, eds. Veterinary internal medicine. Philadelphia: Saunders, 1995:409–439.

Elston T, Rodan I, Flemming D, et al. 1998 Report of the American Association of Feline Practitioners and Academy of Feline Medicine Advisory Panel on Feline Vaccines. J Am Vet Med Assoc 1998; 212:227–241.

Greene CE, Scott FW. Feline panleukopenia. In: Greene CE, ed. Infectious diseases of the dog and cat. 2nd ed. Philadelphia: Saunders, 1998:52–57.

Pollock RVH, Postorino NC. Feline panleukopenia and other enteric viral diseases. In: Sherding RG, ed. The cat: diseases and clinical management. New York: Churchill Livingstone, 1994:479–487.

Scott FW. Panleukopenia. In: Holzworth J, ed. Diseases of the cat. Philadelphia: Saunders, 1987:182–193.

Author Fred W. Scott
Consulting Editor Stephen C. Barr

FELINE PARANEOPLASTIC SYNDROME

BASICS

OVERVIEW
• Rare
• Characterized by cutaneous lesions, which serve as markers of internal neoplasia

PATHOPHYSIOLOGY
• Most affected cats have had pancreatic adenocarcinomas with metastases to liver, lungs, pleura, and/or peritoneum; also reports of bile duct carcinomas.
• The link between internal malignancies and cutaneous lesions is unknown; may involve cytokines producing atrophy of the hair follicles.

SYSTEMS AFFECTED
• Skin/Exocrine—alopecia
• Gastrointestinal—weight loss, anorexia
• Other systems—result of metastasis of the pancreatic or biliary tumor (e.g., liver, lungs, pleura, and/or peritoneal cavity)

SIGNALMENT
• All affected animals were mixed-breed or domestic shorthair cats.
• Mean age 12.5 years; range of 9–16 years

SIGNS

Historical Findings
• Decrease in appetite followed by rapid weight loss and excessive shedding
• Pruritus—variable; sometimes with excessive grooming
• Hair loss—rapidly progressive
• Some affected cats may be reluctant to walk, owing to painful fissuring of the footpads.

Physical Examination Findings
• Hairs epilate easily
• Severe alopecia—ventral neck, abdomen, and medial thighs
• The stratum corneum may "peel," leading to a glistening appearance to the skin.
• Gray lentigines may develop in alopecic areas.
• Footpads may be fissured and/or scaly.

CAUSES & RISK FACTORS
• The majority of cases are associated with an underlying pancreatic adenocarcinoma.
• Other internal carcinomas, such as bile duct carcinomas, may be involved.

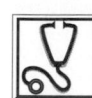

DIAGNOSIS

DIFFERENTIAL DIAGNOSIS
• Hyperadrenocorticism—polyuria, polydipsia, and skin fragility
• Hyperthyroidism—polyphagia
• Hypothyroidism—spontaneous condition rare in cats; not associated with glistening skin
• Feline symmetrical alopecia—hair loss self-induced; not associated with easy epilation
• Demodicosis—mites are not associated with paraneoplastic alopecia.
• Dermatophytosis—hair loss often associated with breakage, not spontaneous shedding; inappetence and weight loss rare
• Alopecia areata—rarely involves the entire ventral surface; inappetence and weight loss rare
• Telogen effluvium—not associated with miniaturization of hair follicles
• Skin fragility syndrome—fragile skin not associated with paraneoplastic alopecia

• Superficial necrolytic dermatitis—not associated with marked exfoliation and miniaturization of hair follicles

CBC/BIOCHEMISTRY/URINALYSIS
Results usually unremarkable

OTHER LABORATORY TESTS
• Endocrine (thyroid profiles and a dexamethasone suppression test)—rule out endocrine disease
• Skin scrapings—rule out demodicosis
• KOH examination of hairs and/or fungal culture—rule out dermatophytosis

IMAGING
• Ultrasonography—pancreatic mass and/or nodular lesions in the liver or peritoneal cavity; failure to demonstrate nodules does not exclude the diagnosis, because they may be too small for detection.
• Thoracic radiographs—metastatic lesions in the lungs or pleural cavity

DIAGNOSTIC PROCEDURES
• Skin biopsies
• Laparoscopy or exploratory laparotomy—identify primary and metastatic tumors.

PATHOLOGIC FINDINGS
• Histopathologic examination of the skin—nonscarring alopecia; severe atrophy of hair follicles and adnexa; miniaturization of hair bulbs; mild acanthosis; variable absence of stratum corneum; variable mixed superficial perivascular infiltrates of neutrophils, eosinophils, and mononuclear cells
• Primary tumor—usually pancreatic adenocarcinoma, rarely primary bile duct carcinomas
• Metastatic nodules—common in the liver, lungs, pleura, and peritoneum

TREATMENT

• Removal of tumor via partial pancreatectomy may be curative; however, prognosis is guarded, as majority of cats have metastatic disease.
• Chemotherapy or other—no reported response
• Affected animals rapidly deteriorate; euthanasia should be suggested as a humane intervention.
• Supportive care—only if owners refuse to consider euthanasia; feed highly palatable, nutrient-dense foods and/or tube feed

MEDICATIONS

DRUG(S)
N/A

CONTRAINDICATIONS/POSSIBLE INTERACTIONS
N/A

FOLLOW-UP

• Progressive deterioration
• Supportive care—ultrasonography and thoracic radiographs may demonstrate progression of metastatic disease
• Expect death to occur within 2–20 weeks after onset of skin lesions.

MISCELLANEOUS

SYNONYMS
• Pancreatic paraneoplastic alopecia
• Paraneoplastic alopecia associated with internal malignancies
• Paraneoplastic alopecia associated with visceral neoplasia

SEE ALSO
Adenocarcinoma, Pancreas

Suggested Reading
Brooks DG, Campbell KL, Dennis JS, et al. Pancreatic paraneoplastic alopecia in three cats. J Am Anim Hosp Assoc 1994;30: 557–562.
Pascal-Tenorio A, Olivry T, Gross TL, et al. Paraneoplastic alopecia associated with internal malignancies in the cat. Vet Dermatol 1997;8:47–52.
Tasker S, Griffon D, Nutall T, et al. Resolution of paraneoplastic alopecia following surgical removal of a pancreatic carcinoma in a cat. J Small Anim Pract 1999; 40:16–19.
Author Karen L. Campbell
Consulting Editor Karen Helton Rhodes

FELINE RHINOTRACHEITIS VIRUS INFECTION

BASICS

DEFINITION
Causes an acute disease in domestic and exotic cats, which is characterized by sneezing, fever, rhinitis, conjunctivitis, and ulcerative keratitis

PATHOPHYSIOLOGY
FHV-1—causes an acute cytolytic infection of respiratory or ocular epithelium after oral, intranasal, or conjunctival exposure

SYSTEMS AFFECTED
• Respiratory—rhinitis with sneezing and serous to purulent nasal discharge; tracheitis may occur; chronic sinusitis may be a sequela.
• Ophthalmic—often conjunctivitis with serous or purulent ocular discharge; ulcerative keratitis or panophthalmitis can occur
• Reproductive—in utero infection owing to infection of pregnant queens may result in severe herpetic infections in neonates.
• Integumentary—herpes dermatitis may occur near the nasal openings.

GENETICS
N/A

INCIDENCE/PREVALENCE
• Common, especially in multicat households or facilities
• Perpetuated by latent carriers that harbor the virus in nerve ganglia, especially in the trigeminal ganglion

GEOGRAPHIC DISTRIBUTION
Found worldwide

SIGNALMENT
Species
Affects all domestic and many exotic felines

Breed Predilections
None

Mean Age and Range
• Cats of all ages
• Kittens most susceptible

Predominant Sex
N/A

SIGNS

Historical Findings
• Acute onset of paroxysmal sneezing
• Blepharospasm and ocular discharge
• Anorexia—from high fever, general malaise, or inability to smell
• Recurrent signs—carriers
• Abortion

Physical Examination Findings
• Fever—up to 106°F (41°C)
• Rhinitis—serous, mucopurulent, or purulent nasal discharge
• Conjunctivitis—serous, mucopurulent, or purulent nasal discharge
• Chronic rhinitis/sinusitis—chronic purulent nasal discharge
• Keratitis—ulceration, descemetocele, or panophthalmitis

CAUSES
FHV-1, of which there is only one serotype

RISK FACTORS
• Lack of vaccination for FHV-1
• Multiple cat facilities with overcrowding, poor ventilation, poor sanitation, poor nutrition, or physical or psychological stress
• Pregnancy and lactation
• Concomitant disease, especially owing to immunosuppressive organisms or other respiratory organisms
• Kittens born to carrier queens—infected about 5 weeks of age

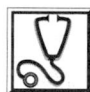

DIAGNOSIS

DIFFERENTIAL DIAGNOSES
• Feline calicivirus infection—less sneezing, conjunctivitis, ulcerative keratitis; may cause ulcerative stomatitis, pneumonia
• Feline chlamydiosis—more chronic conjunctivitis, which may be unilateral; pneumonitis; intracytoplasmic inclusions in conjunctival scrapings; responds to tetracyclines or chloramphenicol
• Bacterial infection (*Bordetella, haemophilus,* or *Pasteurella*)—less nasal and ocular involvement; often respond to antibiotics

CBC/BIOCHEMISTRY/URINALYSIS
• Not diagnostic
• Transient leukopenia followed by leukocytosis may occur.

OTHER LABORATORY TESTS
• Immunofluorescent assay—nasal or conjunctival scrapings; viral detection
• Viral isolation—pharyngeal swab sample
• Stained conjunctival smears—detect intranuclear inclusion bodies

IMAGING
Radiography—open mouth and skyline views of the skull reveal presence of chronic disease in the nasal cavity and frontal sinuses; infection cannot be reliably distinguished from neoplasia and inflammatory polyps; no abnormal radiographic findings with acute disease

DIAGNOSTIC PROCEDURES
N/A

PATHOLOGIC FINDINGS
• Gross—ocular and nasal discharge; mucosal edema of upper airway epithelium; tracheitis; sinusitis; ulcerative keratitis; and panophthalmitis
• Microscopic—submucosal edema; inflammatory cell infiltrates of upper respiratory and conjunctival tissues; chronic sinusitis; and intranuclear inclusion bodies in epithelial cells

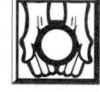

TREATMENT

APPROPRIATE HEALTH CARE
Inpatient—nutritional and fluid support to anorectic cats; prevent contagion

NURSING CARE
• Outpatient—keep patient indoors to prevent environmentally induced stress, which may lengthen the course of the disease.
• Fluids—intravenous or subcutaneous; to correct and prevent dehydration; to keep nasal secretions thin

ACTIVITY
Isolate affected cats during the acute phase, because they are contagious.

DIET
• Outpatient—entice food consumption to avoid anorexia, which induces a cascade of negative consequences; offer foods with appealing tastes and smells.
• Inpatients—forced enteral feeding for anorectic cats; remove nasal secretions (so nasal breathing can occur) before starting orogastric tube feeding; avoid nasoesophageal tubes because of rhinitis.

CLIENT EDUCATION
• Inform client of the contagious nature of the disease.
• Discuss proper vaccination protocols and early vaccination to cats in multicat facilities and households.
• Inform client that early weaning and isolation from all other cats except litter mates may prevent infections.

SURGICAL CONSIDERATIONS
Surgically implanted feeding tubes (esophagostomy tube, gastrostomy tube) may be needed when prolonged anorexia occurs.

 MEDICATIONS

DRUG(S) OF CHOICE
• Broad-spectrum antibiotics—amoxicillin (22 mg/kg PO q12h) for secondary bacterial infections
• Antibiotic combinations—amoxicillin and enrofloxacin (2.5–5.0 mg/kg PO q12h) for secondary bacterial infections
• Lysine (250 mg q12h) may have some virusidal effect.
• Ophthalmic antibiotics—for keratitis
• Ophthalmic antivirals—Herplex, Vira-A; for herpetic ulcers; must be instilled every 2 hours for significant effect
• Conjunctival vaccination with an intranasal FHV-1 vaccine—may help chronic keratitis

CONTRAINDICATIONS
• Systemic corticosteroids—may induce relapse in chronically infected cats
• Ophthalmic corticosteroids—may predispose to ulcerative keratitis
• Nasal decongestant drops—0.25% oxymetazoline HCl; decrease nasal discharge;

contraindicated because some cats object and some experience rebound rhinorrhea

PRECAUTIONS
Death is usually the result of inadequate nutritional and fluid support.

POSSIBLE INTERACTIONS
None

ALTERNATIVE DRUG(S)
α-Interferon—Roferon; 30 units PO q24h; some efficacy in controlling the viral aspect of chronic infectious nasal discharge; for kittens: 2 units PO q24h when 3–8 weeks old to help prevent the effects of early exposure to FHV-1

 FOLLOW-UP

PATIENT MONITORING
Monitor appetite closely; hospitalize for forced enteral feeding if anorexia develops.

PREVENTION/AVOIDANCE
Vaccines
• Routine vaccination with an MLV or inactivated virus vaccine—prevents development of severe disease; does not prevent infection and local viral replication with virus shedding
• Vaccinate at 8–10 weeks of age; at 12–14 weeks of age; and with annual boosters
• Endemic multicat facilities or households—vaccinate kittens with a dose of an intranasal vaccine at 10–14 days of age; then parenterally at 6, 10, and 14 weeks of age; isolate the litter from *all* other cats at 3–5 weeks of age; then use kitten vaccination protocol to prevent early infections

POSSIBLE COMPLICATIONS
• Chronic rhinosinusitis with lifetime sneezing and nasal discharge
• Herpetic ulcerative keratitis
• Permanent closure of the nasolacrimal duct with chronic ocular discharge

EXPECTED COURSE AND PROGNOSIS
• Usually 7–10 days before spontaneous remission, if secondary bacterial infections do not occur

• Prognosis generally good, if fluid and nutritional therapy are adequate

 **MISCELLANEOUS**

ASSOCIATED CONDITIONS
Simultaneous viral or bacterial respiratory diseases

AGE-RELATED FACTORS
Primarily a disease of young kittens

ZOONOTIC POTENTIAL
None

PREGNANCY
Pregnant cats that develop disease may transmit FHV-1 to kittens in utero, resulting in abortion or neonatal disease

SYNONYMS
• Feline herpesvirus infection
• Rhino
• Coryza

SEE ALSO
• Bordetellosis—Cats
• Feline Calicivirus Infection

ABBREVIATIONS
• FHV-1 = feline herpesvirus type 1
• MLV = modified live virus

Suggested Reading
Barr MC, Olsen CW, Scott FW. Feline viral diseases. In: Ettinger SJ, Feldman EC, eds. Veterinary internal medicine. Philadelphia: Saunders, 1995:409–439.
Ford RB, Levy JK. Infectious diseases of the respiratory tract. In: Sherding RG, ed. The cat: diseases and clinical management. New York: Churchill Livingstone, 1994: 489–500.
Ford RB. Role of infectious agents in respiratory disease. Vet Clin North Am Small Anim Pract 1993:23;17–35.
Gaskell R, Dawson S. Feline respiratory disease. In: Greene CE, ed. Infectious diseases of the dog and cat. Philadelphia: Saunders, 1998:97–106.
Author Gary D. Norsworthy
Consulting Editor Stephen C. Barr

FELINE SKIN FRAGILITY SYNDROME

BASICS

OVERVIEW
• A disorder of multifactorial causes characterized by extremely fragile skin
• Tends to occur in old cats that may have concurrent hyperadrenocorticism, diabetes mellitus, or excessive use of megestrol acetate or other progestational compounds
• A small number of cats have had no biochemical alterations.

SIGNALMENT
• Naturally occurring disease tends to be recognized in old cats.
• Iatrogenic cases have no age predilection.
• No breed or sex predilection

SIGNS

Historical Findings
• Gradual onset of clinical signs
• Progressive alopecia (not always present)
• Often associated with weight loss, lusterless coat, poor appetite, and lack of energy

Physical Examination Findings
• The skin becomes markedly thin and tears with normal handling.
• The skin rarely bleeds upon tearing.
• Multiple lacerations (both old and new) may be noted on close examination.
• Partial to complete alopecia of the truncal region may be noted.
• Sometimes associated with rat tail, pinnal folding, pot-belly appearance

CAUSES & RISK FACTORS
• Hyperadrenocorticism—pituitary or adrenal dependent
• Iatrogenic—secondary to excessive cortico-steroid or progestational drug use
• Diabetes mellitus—rare, unless associated with hyperadrenocorticism
• Possibly idiopathic

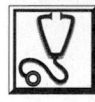

DIAGNOSIS

DIFFERENTIAL DIAGNOSIS
• Cutaneous asthenia
• Feline paraneoplastic syndrome—pancreatic neoplasia, hepatic lipidosis, cholangio-carcinoma
• Progestogen administration

CBC/BIOCHEMISTRY/URINALYSIS
• Of little diagnostic significance in most cases
• Approximately 80% of cats with hyperadrenocorticism have concurrent diabetes mellitus (hyperglycemia, glucosuria).

OTHER LABORATORY TESTS
• ACTH-stimulation test—70% of cats with hyperadrenocorticism have an exaggerated response.
• LDDST—15%–20% of normal cats may fail to decrease cortisol levels; typically unsuppressed with hyperadrenocorticism and nonadrenal illness
• HDDST—normal cats show decreases in cortisol concentrations; typically decreased with nonadrenal illnesses; considered by many clinicians to be the best screening test for hyperadrenocorticism; unreliable for discriminating between adrenal tumors and pituitary-dependent causes of hyperadreno-corticism, because both conditions fail to show suppression
• Endogenous ACTH levels—normal range for most labs is 20–100 pg/mL.

IMAGING
• Abdominal ultrasonography—adrenal masses are often small until end-stage disease.
• CT and MRI—small pituitary tumors may be difficult to visualize; MRI may be more successful.

DIAGNOSTIC PROCEDURES
N/A

PATHOLOGIC FINDINGS
Histopathology—suggestive, not diagnostic; epidermis and dermis are thin; attenuated collagen fibers are evident.

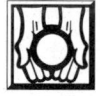

TREATMENT
• Underlying metabolic disease should be ruled out.
• Many patients are debilitated and require supportive care.
• Surgical correction of the lacerations—not helpful because the tissue cannot withstand any pressure from the sutures
• Hyperadrenocorticism—adrenalectomy is the preferred treatment.
• Cobalt 60 radiation therapy—variable success in the treatment of pituitary tumors

MEDICATIONS

DRUG(S)
• Medical management—may be useful for preparing patient for surgery and for minimizing postoperative complications (e.g., infections and poor wound healing)
• No known effective medical therapy for feline hyperadrenocorticism
• o,p′-DDD (mitotane)—12.5–50 mg/kg PO q12h; response has been equivocal; side effects include anorexia, vomiting, and diarrhea.
• Ketoconazole (Nizoral)—10–15 mg/kg PO q12h; variable response
• Metyrapone—65 mg/kg PO q12h; clinical improvement noted more often with this drug than the others

CONTRAINDICATIONS/POSSIBLE INTERACTIONS
Hyperadrenocorticism—closely monitor diabetic cat; adjust insulin to prevent hypoglycemia when the cortisol levels fall.

FOLLOW-UP
Patients are often quite debilitated, making any form of treatment risky; close monitoring is required in all cases.

MISCELLANEOUS

ABBREVIATIONS
• HDDST = high-dose dexamethasone-suppression test
• LDDST = low-dose dexamethasone-suppression test
• o,p′-DDD = 1,1-(o,p′-dichlorodiphenyl)-2,2-dichloroethane

Suggested Reading
Gross TL, Ihrke PJ, Walder EJ. Veterinary dermatopathology. Philadelphia: Mosby, 1992.

Helton Rhodes K. Cutaneous manifestations of hyperadrenocorticism. In: August JR, ed. Consultations in feline internal medicine. Philadelphia: Saunders, 1997:191–198.

Author Karen Helton Rhodes
Contributing Editor Karen Helton Rhodes

BASICS

OVERVIEW
• Alopecia in a symmetrical pattern with no gross changes in the skin
• Common clinical presentation in cats
• Manifestation of several underlying disorders

SIGNALMENT
No age, breed, or sex predilection

SIGNS
• Total to partial hair loss; most often symmetrical but can occur in a patchy distribution
• Areas of the trunk most commonly affected are the ventrum, caudal dorsum, and lateral and caudal thighs.
• Sometimes patchy areas of hair loss (unsymmetrical) on the distal extremities or trunk

CAUSES & RISK FACTORS
• Hypersensitivity reactions—fleas, food, atopy
• Parasites—fleas, *Cheyletiella*
• Infections—dermatophytosis
• Neurologic/behavioral—psychogenic
• Stress/metabolic—telogen effluvium
• Neoplasia—pancreatic neoplasia (paraneoplastic alopecia)
• Hyperadrenocorticism
• Alopecia areata
• Hyperthyroid (early sign)

DIAGNOSIS

DIFFERENTIAL DIAGNOSIS
See Causes & Risk Factors

CBC/BIOCHEMISTRY/URINALYSIS
Eosinophilia in some allergic cats

OTHER LABORATORY TESTS
T_4-hyperthyroid

IMAGING
N/A

DIAGNOSTIC PROCEDURES
• Flea combing—identify fleas, flea excrement, or both
• Microscopic examination of hair—self-induced hair loss results in broken ends, whereas endogenous hair loss results in tapered ends.
• Fecal examination—excess hair, mites and ova (*Cheyletiella*), tapeworm, or fleas
• Food elimination diet trial—see Food Reactions (Dermatologic)
• Intradermal skin test—see Atopy
• Histopathologic examination—see below

PATHOLOGIC FINDINGS
• Biopsies—help confirm underlying cause (e.g., allergic dermatitis, psychogenic, or rarely, systemic disease)
• Histopathologic findings—vary depending on the cause
• Feline psychogenic alopecia—hair follicles and skin normal
• High numbers of mast cells, eosinophils, lymphocytes, or macrophages suggest allergic dermatitis.
• Alopecia areata—lymphocytic inflammation that encircles the bulb portions of the hair follicles; rare

TREATMENT
• Effective management of the underlying causes is important.
• Inform the owner of the diagnostic plan and the time it could take to see a response (e.g., fleas, 4–6 weeks; diet, 3–12 weeks).

MEDICATIONS

DRUG(S)
• Antihistamines—e.g., chlorpheniramine, 0.5 mg/kg PO q8h
• Glucocorticoids—0.5 mg/kg PO, alternate-day therapy
• Amitriptyline—1–2 mg/kg PO daily

CONTRAINDICATIONS/POSSIBLE INTERACTIONS
• Glucocorticoids—can cause alopecia, diabetes mellitus, polydipsia, polyuria, polyphagia, and weight gain; can suppress pruritus, making it difficult to determine the underlying cause
• Withdraw antipruritic medications (including glucocorticoids) as the diagnostic tests near completion (e.g., food hypersensitivity reactions)

FOLLOW-UP
• Frequent examinations are essential in confirming the differential diagnoses.
• Successful identification of the underlying cause offers the best prognosis, if the cause can be controlled (e.g., flea bites or food hypersensitivity).

MISCELLANEOUS

Suggested Reading
O'Dair HA, Foster AP. Focal and generalized alopecia. Vet Clin North Am Small Anim Pract 1995;25:851–870.
Author David Duclos
Consulting Editor Karen Helton Rhodes

FELINE SYNCYTIUM-FORMING VIRUS INFECTION (FeSFV)

 BASICS

OVERVIEW
• A retrovirus in the Spumavirus genus that infects cats, apparently with little or no pathogenic effect
• Found worldwide; estimated prevalences, 10-70% or greater
• Present in some nondomestic feline populations
• Infection linked statistically with chronic progressive polyarthritis; disease has not been reproduced by experimental infection.
• Research—disease potential low; nuisance when using feline-origin tissue culture cells; test cats and remove from study if FeSFV-positive

SIGNALMENT
• Cats
• The prevalence of virus—low in kittens; increases with age

• Males—more likely than females to be infected; chronic progressive polyarthritis occurs predominantly in males aged 1.5–5 years.

SIGNS
• Most affected cats healthy
• Co-infections with FIV and FeLV—fairly common, probably because of shared transmission modes and risk factors
• Statistical links with myeloproliferative disease and chronic progressive polyarthritis—may actually reflect co-infection with FIV
• Chronic progressive polyarthritis—swollen joints; abnormal gait; lymphadenopathy

CAUSES & RISK FACTORS
• Transmission—primarily by biting; free-roaming cats at greater risk of infection
• Transmitted efficiently from infected queens to their offspring, probably in utero
• The high prevalence of infection in some cat populations suggests casual contact may play a role in transmission; this has not been demonstrated experimentally.

 DIAGNOSIS

DIFFERENTIAL DIAGNOSIS
Signs of chronic progressive polyarthritis—test for FIV, FeLV, and septic joint disease

CBC/BIOCHEMISTRY/URINALYSIS
Usually normal

OTHER LABORATORY TESTS
Serologic testing—for FeSFV antibodies and virus isolation; not readily available; not particularly useful because correlation between FeSFV infection and disease is so tenuous.

IMAGING
N/A

DIAGNOSTIC PROCEDURES
Joint fluid cytology—with chronic progressive polyarthritis; may reveal high numbers of neutrophils and large mononuclear cells

FELINE SYNCYTIUM-FORMING VIRUS INFECTION (FESFV)

 TREATMENT

None, except for chronic progressive polyarthritis

 MEDICATIONS

DRUG(S)
Chronic progressive polyarthritis—immunosuppressive doses of prednisolone (10–15 mg/cat/day) and cyclophosphamide (7.5 mg/cat/day for 4 days each week)

CONTRAINDICATIONS/POSSIBLE INTERACTIONS
Immunosuppressive drugs—take care when using in patients co-infected with FIV or FeLV.

 FOLLOW-UP

EXPECTED COURSE AND PROGNOSIS
• Infection with FeSFV alone—adverse consequences unlikely
• Chronic progressive polyarthritis—often difficult to control; poor prognosis for long-term recovery

 **MISCELLANEOUS**

ASSOCIATED CONDITIONS
• Chronic progressive polyarthritis
• Co-infections with FIV and FeLV

SYNONYMS
• Feline syncytial virus
• Feline foamy virus

SEE ALSO
• Polyarthritis, Erosive Immune-mediated
• Polyarthritis, Nonerosive Immune-mediated

ABBREVIATIONS
• FeLV = feline leukemia virus
• FIV = feline immunodeficiency virus

Suggested Reading

Greene CE. Syncytium-forming virus infection. In: Greene CE, ed. Infectious diseases of the dog and cat. Philadelphia: Saunders, 1998:106–107.

Author Margaret C. Barr
Consulting Editor Stephen C. Barr

FEVER

 BASICS

DEFINITION
Higher than normal body temperature because of a changed thermoregulatory set point in the hypothalamus; normal body temperature in dogs and cats is 100.2–102.8°F (37.8–39.3°C). Fever of unknown origin (FUO)—at least 103.5°F (39.7°C) on at least four occasions over a 14-day period and illness of 14 days' duration without an obvious cause

PATHOPHYSIOLOGY
Exogenous or endogenous pyrogens cause release of endogenous substances (e.g., interleukin-1 and prostaglandins) that reset the hypothalamic thermoregulatory center to a higher temperature, activating appropriate physiologic responses to raise the body temperature to this new set point. Physiologic consequences include increased metabolic demands, muscle catabolism, bone marrow suppression, heightened fluid and caloric requirements, and possibly disseminated intravascular coagulation (DIC) and shock.

SYSTEMS AFFECTED
• Cardiovascular—tachycardia • Nervous—cerebral edema • Hemic/Lymph/Immune—bone marrow depression and DIC

SIGNALMENT
• Dog and cat • Any age, breed, and sex

SIGNS

General Comments
• Fever itself is beneficial: the increased body temperature lowers bacterial division and increases immune competence.
• Prolonged fever > 105°F (> 40.5°C) leads to dehydration, anorexia, and depression.
• Fevers > 106°F (> 41.1°C) may lead to cerebral edema, bone marrow depression, and DIC.

Physical Examination Findings
• Hyperthermia • Lethargy • Inappetence
• Tachycardia • Hyperpnea • Dehydration
• Shock

CAUSES

Infectious Agents (Most Common)
• Viruses—feline leukemia (FeLV), feline immunodeficiency (FIV), parvovirus, distemper, herpes, and calicivirus
• Bacteria—gram-positive and gram-negative endotoxins, *Mycoplasma, Haemobartonella*
• Systemic fungi—*Histoplasma, Blastomyces, Coccidioidomyces,* and *Cryptococcus*
• Rickettsia—*Ehrlichia, Rickettsia rickettsii* (Rocky Mountain spotted fever)
• Parasites and protozoa—*Babesia, Toxoplasma,* aberrant larva migrans, *Dirofilaria thromboemboli, Leishmania*
• *Borrelia burgdorferi* (Lyme disease)

Immune-mediated Processes
Systemic lupus erythematosus, immune-mediated hemolytic anemia, immune-mediated thrombocytopenia, pemphigus, polyarthritis, polymyositis, vasculitis, hypersensitivity reactions, transfusion reaction, and infection secondary to inherited or acquired immune defects

Endocrine and Metabolic
Hyperthyroidism, hypoadrenocorticism (rare), pheochromocytoma, hyperlipidemia, and hypernatremia

Neoplasia
Lymphoma, myeloproliferative disease, plasma cell neoplasm, mast cell tumor, metastatic disease, and solid tumor, particularly in liver, kidney, bone, lungs, and lymph nodes

Other Inflammatory Conditions
Cholangiohepatitis, hepatic lipidosis, toxic hepatopathy, cirrhosis, inflammatory bowel disease, pancreatitis, peritonitis, pleuritis, granulomatous diseases, thrombophlebitis, infarctions, pansteatitis, panniculitis, hypertrophic osteodystrophy, blunt trauma, cyclic neutropenia, intracranial lesions (encephalitis, trauma), and pulmonary thromboembolism

Drugs and Toxins
Tetracycline, sulfonamide, penicillins, nitrofurantoin, amphotericin B, barbiturates, iodine, atropine, cimetidine, salicylates (high dosages), antihistamines, procainamide, and heavy metals

FUO—Dogs
• Recurrent bacteremia caused by endocarditis or localized abscess of organ or tissue—liver, pancreas, prostate, retroperitoneal and pleural space (pyothorax), lungs, kidneys and genitourinary system (chronic pyelonephritis and prostatitis), osteomyelitis, arthritis, discospondylitis, and meningitis
• Systemic infection—particularly early, chronic, or latent infection, including brucellosis, systemic mycoses, ehrlichiosis, Rocky Mountain spotted fever, toxoplasmosis
• Neoplasia—as above
• Immune disorders—as above
• Other causes—chronic hepatic diseases and chronic granulomatous disease

FUO—Cats
• Most are virally mediated (e.g., FeLV, FIV, FIP, less commonly parvovirus, herpes, and calicivirus)
• Persistent occult bacterial infection with atypical bacteria, sometimes secondary to bite wounds (e.g., *Yersinia, Mycobacteria, Nocardia, Actinomyces,* and *Brucella*
• Pyothorax common
• Additional causes—pyelonephritis, blunt trauma, penetrating intestinal lesion, dental abscess, systemic mycoses (e.g., *Histoplasma,*

Blastomyces, Coccidioides), lymphoma, and solid tumors
• Immune disorders are rare, as are prostatitis, endometritis, discospondylitis, pneumonia, and endocarditis.

RISK FACTORS
• Recent travel
• Exposure to biologic agents
• Immunosuppression
• Very young or old animals

 DIAGNOSIS

DIFFERENTIAL DIAGNOSIS
• Good clinical history (e.g., contact with infectious agents, recent vaccination, drug administration, insect bites, allergies) and thorough physical examination may help identify an underlying disease condition.
• Elucidation of patterns of fever (e.g., sustained, intermittent) is rarely helpful.
• True fever must be differentiated from hyperthermia. Stress and anxiety in the hospital may cause a mild temperature rise. Temperatures up to 103°F (39.4°C) may be caused by stress or illness. Temperatures > 104°F (> 40°C) are almost always important. Temperatures > 107°F (> 41.7°C) are usually not fever, more likely to be primary hyperthermia.

CBC/BIOCHEMISTRY/URINALYSIS
• CBC—leukopenia or leukocytosis, left shift, monocytosis, lymphocytosis, thrombo-cytopenia, or thrombocytosis
• Biochemistry profile and urinalysis vary with the organ system involved

OTHER LABORATORY TESTS
• Additional laboratory testing depends on history, physical examination findings, and abnormalities in CBC, serum biochemistry profile, and urinalysis.
• If infectious disease is suspected, attempt to culture an organism—urine culture, blood cultures (i.e., three anaerobic and three aerobic cultures, taken during a rise in temperature or 30 min apart), fungal culture, and cultures of CSF, synovial fluid, and biopsy specimens, if clinically indicated
• FeLV and FIV test, serologic tests for *Toxoplasma,* Lyme disease, systemic mycoses, and rickettsial infection
• Fecal examination if gastrointestinal signs
• Tracheal wash or bronchoalveolar lavage if respiratory involvement
• Occult heartworm test if pulmonary embolism suspected
• If immune disorders suspected—cytologic examination of synovial fluid; Coombs', antinuclear antibody, and rheumatoid factor tests; serum protein electrophoresis
• T4 to rule out hyperthyroidism

IMAGING

Radiography
• Abdominal radiographs to scan for tumors
• Thoracic radiographs to rule out pneumonia, neoplasia, and pyothorax
• Survey skeletal radiographs for bone tumors, multiple myeloma, osteomyelitis, discospondylitis, panosteitis, and hypertrophic osteodystrophy
• Dental and skull radiographs to look for tooth root abscess, sinus infections, and neoplasia
• Contrast radiography (e.g., gastrointestinal and excretory urography) to look for evidence of neoplasia or infection

Ultrasonography
• Abdominal (plus directed biopsy, if indicated) to look for abdominal neoplasia and abscess or other site of infection (e.g., pyelonephritis and pyometra)
• Echocardiography if endocarditis suspected

Nuclear Imaging
Radionuclide scanning procedures to evaluate for bone tumors, osteomyelitis, and pulmonary embolism

DIAGNOSTIC PROCEDURES
• Endoscopy and biopsy if gastrointestinal signs
• Bone marrow aspirate and biopsy if malignancy suspected
• Lymph node, skin, or muscle biopsy if clinically indicated
• Examination of fine-needle aspirate of any mass or large organ
• CSF tap if neurologic signs suggest brain tumor or meningitis
• Exploratory laparotomy—last resort if all other diagnostic tests fail to determine the cause and the patient is not improving

TREATMENT
• Restrict activity. • Febrile patients are in a hypercatabolic state and require high caloric intake. • Explain to the owner that the diagnostic workup of patients with fever of unknown origin (FUO) is often extensive, expensive, and invasive and does not always provide a definitive diagnosis.
• Surgery may be necessary in some animals with underlying infectious (e.g., pyometra, peritonitis, pyothorax, and liver abscess) or localized neoplastic cause of fever.

MEDICATIONS

DRUG(S) OF CHOICE
• Goal of treatment—reset the thermoregulatory set point to a lower level.
• Selection depends on the diagnosis and specific cause.

• Do not use broad-spectrum (i.e., "shotgun") treatment in place of a thorough diagnostic workup unless the patient's status is critical and deteriorating rapidly.
• Only use antipyretic treatment when fever is prolonged and life-threatening (> 106°F, > 41.1°C) and topical cooling is unsuccessful. Impaired patients (e.g., those with heart failure, seizures, or respiratory disease) require antipyretic treatment earlier. Antipyretic treatment may preclude elucidation of the cause, delay correct treatment, and complicate patient monitoring (e.g., reduction of fever is an important indication of response to treatment).
• Fluid administration often lowers body temperature.
• If the patient is dehydrated, initiate isotonic fluids (i.e., lactated Ringer's or 0.9% saline).

Antibiotics
• Based on results of bacterial culture
• In emergency situations, combination antibiotic therapy can be started after culture specimens have been obtained (e.g., cephalothin, 20 mg/kg IV q6–8h; gentamicin 2 mg/kg IV q8h).
• Do not give antibiotics longer than 1–2 weeks if the response is not favorable.

Antipyretics
• Salicylates—dogs, 10 mg/kg PO q12h; cats, 6 mg/kg PO q48h
• Flunixin meglumine—dogs, 0.5–1 mg/kg IV or IM once

Glucocorticoids
• Do not use unless infectious causes have been ruled out.
• May mask clinical signs, may lead to immunosuppression, and are not recommended for use as antipyretics; administration of corticosteroids to cats with intractable FUO after ruling out infectious diseases may promote a favorable response.
• Primarily indicated for fever associated with immune-mediated disease and certain steroid-responsive tumors (e.g., lymphoma)

CONTRAINDICATIONS
N/A

PRECAUTIONS
Side effects of antipyretics include emesis, diarrhea, gastrointestinal ulceration, renal damage, hemolysis, hepatotoxicity (acetaminophen, particularly dangerous in cats), and muscle stiffness (flunixin meglumine).

POSSIBLE INTERACTIONS
Combination of nonsteroidal antiinflammatory drugs (NSAIDS) and steroids raises the risk of gastrointestinal hemorrhage

ALTERNATIVE DRUG(S)
N/A

FOLLOW-UP

PATIENT MONITORING
• Patient's temperature at least q12h. • If the cause of the fever continues to elude the clinician, repeat the history and physical examination along with screening laboratory tests. • If fever develops or worsens during hospitalization, consider nosocomial infection or superinfection.

PREVENTION/AVOIDANCE
N/A

POSSIBLE COMPLICATIONS
Depend on cause

EXPECTED COURSE AND PROGNOSIS
Vary with cause; in some patients (more commonly in cats), an underlying cause cannot be determined.

MISCELLANEOUS

ASSOCIATED CONDITIONS
N/A

AGE-RELATED FACTORS
• Young animals—infectious disease more likely than other causes; prognosis better than in old animals • Old animals—common causes are neoplasia and intraabdominal infection; signs tend to be more nonspecific; prognosis often guarded

ZOONOTIC POTENTIAL
Depends on cause

PREGNANCY
N/A

SYNONYMS
Pyrexia

SEE ALSO
Heatstroke and Hyperthermia

ABBREVIATIONS
N/A

Suggested Reading
Couto CG. Fever of undetermined origin. In: Nelson RW, Couto CG, eds. Essentials of small animal internal medicine. Philadelphia: Mosby Year Book, 1992:974–977.
Lagutchik MS. Fever in the ICU patient. In: Wingfield WE, Raffe MR, eds. The veterinary ICU book. Jackson, WY: Teton New Media, 2002:671–684.
Authors Maria Vianna and Jörg Bücheler
Consulting Editors Larry P. Tilley and Francis W. K. Smith, Jr.

FIBROCARTILAGINOUS EMBOLIC MYELOPATHY

BASICS

DEFINITION
Acute ischemic necrosis of the spinal cord caused by fibrocartilaginous emboli

PATHOPHYSIOLOGY
• Emboli—found in spinal cord arteries, veins, or both; source is possibly intervertebral disk material or marrow of vertebral body.
• Exact mechanism of entry into the spinal vasculature unknown

SYSTEMS AFFECTED
Nervous

GENETICS
N/A

INCIDENCE/PREVALENCE
• Common cause of spinal cord disease in nonchondrodystophic breeds of dogs
• Not reported in chondrodystrophic breeds
• Rare in cats

GEOGRAPHIC DISTRIBUTION
N/A

SIGNALMENT

Species
Dogs and cats

Breed Predilections
• Giant- and large-breed dogs—highest prevalence
• Miniature schnauzers and Shetland sheepdogs—over-represented; hyperlipo-proteinemia and resultant hyperviscosity common in these breeds; may contribute to spinal cord infarction without fibrocartilaginous emboli.

Mean Age and Range
• Most patients 3–5 years old
• Range 16 weeks to 10 years

Predominant Sex
Slight male predominance

SIGNS

Historical Findings
• Mild trauma or vigorous exercise at the onset of signs common
• Sudden onset
• Affected dog typically cries in pain; pain subsides in minutes to hours (at most).
• Signs of paresis or paralysis develop over a matter of seconds, minutes, or hours.
• Condition stabilizes within 12–24 hr.

Physical Examination Findings
N/A

Neurologic Examination Findings
• Deficits—usually lateralized; unaffected side usually mildly affected or normal; symmetrically distributed in a few patients
• Pain—at onset of signs and then generally absent; usually subsided by the time the patient is being examined; may be felt for a few hours in severely affected patients
• Any level of the spinal cord can be affected, depending on the distribution of the embolic material.
• Mild ataxia to paralysis
• Upper or lower motor neuron deficits
• Spinal cord injury—unilateral; or only the dorsal or ventral aspect of the spinal cord, causing an ipsilateral limb with sensory loss but muscle tone and motor function preserved (or vice versa); or other odd combinations are possible in patients with focal quadrant injuries
• If signs progress beyond 24 hr, consider other diseases that cause ascending and descending myelomalacia.

CAUSES
Unknown

RISK FACTORS
• Vigorous exercise may trigger the incident.
• Hyperlipoproteinemia

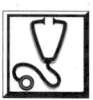

DIAGNOSIS

DIFFERENTIAL DIAGNOSIS
• Acute nonprogressive, asymmetric, and nonpainful—characteristic; greatly helps in the diagnosis
• Back and neck pain with symmetrical signs—intervertebral disk disease; diskospondylitis; vertebral tumor; fracture and luxation; survey radiography and myelography help confirm the diagnosis.
• Parenchymal spinal cord hemorrhage secondary to a bleeding diathesis (e.g., caused by anticoagulant rodenticide ingestion, thrombocytopenia, or DIC)—rule out by carefully examining for evidence of hemorrhage, performing a platelet count, and determining blood clotting times.
• Focal myelitis—differentiate by progressive history and CSF analysis

CBC/BIOCHEMISTRY/URINALYSIS
Usually normal

OTHER LABORATORY TESTS
N/A

IMAGING
• Survey spinal radiograph—usually normal
• Myelography—in acute stage often demonstrates focal intramedullary swelling at the embolic site; later often normal or shows an area of cord atrophy

MRI of the Spine
• Most diagnostic technique in both acute and chronic stages
• Degenerative disk that was the source of the emboli—decreased signal intensity on T2 images
• Area of spinal cord infarction—increased signal intensity on T2 images

DIAGNOSTIC PROCEDURES

CSF Analysis
• Results depend on the location (e.g., lumbar vs. cerebellomedullary) and the time fluid was collected in relation to the onset of clinical signs.
• Acute stage—high RBC count and mildly high neutrophil count may be seen; a few days later, may see only mildly high protein
• Sometimes normal

PATHOLOGIC FINDINGS
• Gross—focal spinal cord swelling with hemorrhage
• Microscopic—emboli of fibrocartilage in arteries and veins of the spinal cord and meninges; hemorrhagic necrosis and malacia in gray and white matter

TREATMENT

APPROPRIATE HEALTH CARE
Inpatient—for immediate medical treatment and diagnostic procedures

NURSING CARE
• Keep recumbent patients on a padded surface; turn frequently to prevent pressure sores.
• Assist and encourage patients to ambulate as soon as possible.

ACTIVITY
Restrict until diagnosis is made.

DIET
Normal

CLIENT EDUCATION
• Inform client that recovery from paresis or paralysis is slow and gradual, when it occurs.
• Inform client that most patients need considerable supportive care at home during recovery.

SURGICAL CONSIDERATIONS
N/A

FIBROCARTILAGINOUS EMBOLIC MYELOPATHY

MEDICATIONS

DRUG(S) OF CHOICE
Methylprednisolone sodium succinate—may be beneficial if given within the first 8 hr after the onset of signs according to studies of acute spinal cord injury caused by spinal cord impact; 30 mg/kg IV as first treatment; then 15 mg/kg at 2 and 6 hr and every 6 hr thereafter for a total treatment period of 24–48 hr; give each dose slowly over 10–15 min; too rapid of an injection can cause vomiting.

CONTRAINDICATIONS
Nonsteroidal analgesics—do not administer with methylprednisolone sodium succinate; increases probability of gastrointestinal ulceration

PRECAUTIONS
• Methylprednisolone sodium succinate—no benefit with treatment for longer than 24–48 hr and dramatically increases adverse effects (e.g., gastrointestinal ulceration)
• High-fiber diet during and after steroid treatment reduces gastrointestinal ulceration.

POSSIBLE INTERACTIONS
N/A

ALTERNATIVE DRUG(S)
N/A

FOLLOW-UP

PATIENT MONITORING
• Sequential neurologic evaluations—during the first 12–24 hr after examination
• Neurologic status—2, 3, and 4 weeks after onset of clinical signs
• Urinary incontinence—urinalysis and bacterial culture and sensitivity to detect urinary tract infection

PREVENTION/AVOIDANCE
• Recurrence highly unlikely
• No known method of prevention

POSSIBLE COMPLICATIONS
• Fecal and urinary incontinence
• Urinary tract infection
• Urine scalding and pressure sores

EXPECTED COURSE AND PROGNOSIS
• Pain perception and upper motor neuron signs—prognosis for marked improvement generally good
• Loss of pain perception—prognosis poor
• Areflexia of limbs or sphincters—almost no chance of recovery; reduced purposeful movements and reflexes—functional recovery common; some degree of permanent deficit likely
• Progression of clinical signs from upper to lower motor neuron and an enlarging area of sensory loss indicate ascending or descending myelomalacia and a hopeless prognosis; consider euthanasia.
• Neurologic status—little change in the first 14 days after onset; most improvement occurs between days 21 and 42; remyelination is complete in most patients within 6–12 weeks after onset; if no improvement after 21–30 days, recovery is highly unlikely

MISCELLANEOUS

ASSOCIATED CONDITIONS
Disorders that lead to a compromise in circulatory function may predispose or mimic fibrocartilaginous embolic myelopathy—hyperadrenocorticism; hypothyroidism; high systemic blood pressure; hyperviscosity syndrome; hyperlipidemia; bleeding diathesis; bacterial endocarditis

AGE-RELATED FACTORS
N/A

ZOONOTIC POTENTIAL
N/A

PREGNANCY
High-dose corticosteroid administration—may cause premature delivery

ABBREVIATIONS
• CSF = cerebrospinal fluid
• DIC = disseminated intravascular coagulation
• MRI = magnetic resonance imaging

Suggested Reading
Abramson C. Tetraparesis in a cat with fibro-cartilaginous emboli. J Am Anim Hosp Assoc 2002;38:153–156.
Braughler JM, Hall ED. Current application of "high-dose" steroid therapy for CNS injury: a pharmacological perspective. J Neurosurg 1985;62:806–810.
Cauzinille L. Fibrocartilaginous embolism of the spinal cord. Paper presented at the 11th annual forum of the American College of Veterinary Internal Medicine, Washington, DC, 1993.
Cook JR. Fibrocartilaginous embolism. Vet Clin North Am Small Anim Pract 1988;18:581–592.
Summers BA, Cummings JF, de Lahunta A. Veterinary neuropathology. St. Louis: Mosby, 1995:246–249.
Author Allen Sisson
Consulting Editor Joane M. Parent

FIBROSARCOMA, BONE

BASICS

OVERVIEW
- Usually develops in the axial skeleton
- Characterized histologically by well-to-poorly differentiated spindle-shaped cells
- Tends to be locally invasive but late to metastasize
- Metastasizes to lymph nodes, heart, pericardium, skin, and other bones
- Primary tumor uncommon in cats
- Less than 5% of all primary bone tumors

SIGNALMENT
- Dogs and cats
- Breed predilections not reported
- More common in mature male dogs

SIGNS

Historical Findings
- Lameness
- Palpable mass

Physical Examination Findings
- Long-bone tumor—monostotic swelling at a metaphyseal site
- Pain on palpation of tumor site
- Pathologic fracture
- Axial tumor—palpable mass

CAUSES & RISK FACTORS
Unknown

DIAGNOSIS

DIFFERENTIAL DIAGNOSIS
- Other primary bone neoplasms—osteo-sarcoma; hemangiosarcoma; chondrosarcoma
- Metastatic neoplasia from another primary site
- Osteomyelitis—fungal or bacterial

CBC/BIOCHEMISTRY/URINALYSIS
Usually normal

OTHER LABORATORY TESTS
N/A

IMAGING
- Radiography—impossible to differentiate primary lesion from other primary bone tumors; lesions typically in metaphyseal sites of long bones and can be lytic, productive, or both (see Osteosarcoma)
- Thoracic radiography—detect metastasis
- CT—determine extent of local disease in patients with an axial tumor

DIAGNOSTIC PROCEDURES
Biopsy and histopathology of tumor—as described for osteosarcoma; take care to differentiate between fibrosarcoma and fibroblastic osteosarcoma.

TREATMENT
- Aggressive surgical resection—amputation; limb salvage; hemipelvectomy; maxillectomy; mandibulectomy
- Radiotherapy—as an adjuvant to surgery

MEDICATIONS

DRUGS
Chemotherapy—investigate, because late metastasis can be a problem

CONTRAINDICATIONS/POSSIBLE INTERACTIONS
N/A

FOLLOW-UP
- Thoracic radiography—monthly for 3 months; then every 3rd month
- Believed to be less aggressive than osteosarcoma
- Metastatic sites include heart, pericardium, skin, and other bones.

MISCELLANEOUS

Suggested Reading
Waters DJ, Cooley DM. Skeletal neoplasms. In: Morrison WB, ed. Cancer in dogs and cats: medical and surgical management. Jackson, Wyoming: Teton NewMedia, 2002:611–626.
Author Terrance A. Hamilton
Consulting Editor Wallace B. Morrison

BASICS

OVERVIEW
• Slowly progressive (months) and locally invasive mesenchymal malignancy in the oral cavity of dogs and cats
• Third most common oral malignancy in dogs; second most common oral malignancy in cats
• Gingiva most commonly involved site
• Highly invasive to surrounding bone
• Metastasis—uncommon
• Death usually secondary to local recurrence, dysphagia, and cachexia
• A subset of histologically low-grade, yet biologically high-grade fibrosarcomas has been described.

SIGNALMENT
• Dogs and cats
• Breed predilections—none known; medium to large breeds more commonly affected; golden retrievers may be predisposed.
• Mean age—7.6 years (range, 0.5–15 years)
• Slight male predilection

SIGNS
Historical Findings
• Excessive salivation
• Halitosis
• Dysphagia
• Bloody oral discharge
• Weight loss

Physical Examination Findings
• Oral mass
• Loose teeth
• Facial deformity
• Occasional cervical lymphadenomegaly

CAUSES & RISK FACTORS
None identified

DIAGNOSIS

DIFFERENTIAL DIAGNOSIS
• Other oral malignancy
• Epulis
• Abscess
• Benign polyp

CBC/BIOCHEMISTRY/URINALYSIS
Usually normal

OTHER LABORATORY TESTS
Cytologic evaluation—rarely diagnostic

IMAGING
• Skull radiography—evaluate for bone involvement deep to the mass
• Thoracic radiography—evaluate lungs for metastasis

DIAGNOSTIC PROCEDURES
• Large, deep-tissue biopsy (down to the bone)—required to sufficiently differentiate from other oral malignancies
• Carefully palpate regional lymph nodes (mandibular and retropharyngeal).
• CT scan or MRI may help evaluate degree of invasiveness.

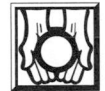
TREATMENT

SURGERY
• Radical excision—required (e.g., hemi-mandibulectomy); well tolerated by most patients; at least 2-cm margins necessary
• Cryosurgery—indicated for small lesions (< 2 cm diameter) minimally adherent to bone

RADIATION
• Inpatient radiotherapy—offers considerable long-term control if the tumor is deemed inoperable
• Most radiotherapy plans attempt 40–60 Gy over 3–6 weeks.
• Soft foods—may recommend to prevent tumor ulceration and after radical oral excision
• Pain medication

MEDICATIONS

DRUG(S)
• Chemotherapy—good option for some patients; doxorubicin (Adriamycin, 25–30 mg/m² IV once every 2 weeks for 5 treatments); median survival (dogs), 18 weeks; may provide marked palliation of clinical signs
• Cisplatin—intralesionally administered; local control (palliation) reported

CONTRAINDICATIONS/POSSIBLE INTERACTIONS
Chemotherapy may be toxic; seek advice before initiating treatment if you are unfamiliar with cytotoxic drugs.

FOLLOW-UP

EXPECTED COURSE AND PROGNOSIS
• Survival after excision—1-year, 25%–45%; 2-year, 20%–35%; median (dogs), 7–11 months; improves when excisional margins are free of neoplastic cells
• Survival after radiotherapy treatment—0–27 months; median, 7 months
• Survival after doxorubicin (dogs)—median, 18 weeks
• Cause of death—related to local recurrence and secondary anorexia and cachexia

MISCELLANEOUS

Suggested Reading
Ciekot PA, Powers BE, Withrow SJ, et al. Histologically low-grade, yet biologically high-grade, fibrosarcomas of the mandible and maxilla in dogs: 25 cases (1982–1991). J Am Vet Med Assoc 1994;204:610–615.
Oakes MG, Lewis DD, Hedlund CS, Hosgood G. Canine oral neoplasia. Compend Contin Educ Small Anim Pract 1993;15:15–31.
Author Kevin A. Hahn and Kimberly P. Freeman
Consulting Editor Wallace B. Morrison

FIBROSARCOMA, NASAL AND PARANASAL SINUS

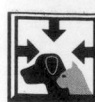

BASICS

OVERVIEW
• Slow, progressive invasion of neoplastic mesenchymal cells within the nasal and paranasal sinuses
• Usually begins unilateral but progresses slowly to bilateral by the time the patient is examined
• Second most common nonepithelial histologic tumor type in dogs; prevalence of nonepithelial nasal neoplasia (dogs and cats), 0.3–4.7% of all tumors

SIGNALMENT
• More common in dogs than cats
• Median age (dogs and cats)—9–12 years (range, 1–16 years)
• Male predilection (2:1)

SIGNS

Historical Findings
• Intermittent and progressive history of unilateral to bilateral epistaxis and/or mucopurulent discharge (median duration, 3 months)
• Epiphora
• Sneezing
• Halitosis
• Anorexia
• Seizures secondary to brain invasion

Physical Examination Findings
• Nasal discharge
• Facial deformity or exophthalmia
• Pain on examination of nasal or paranasal sinuses

CAUSES & RISK FACTORS
N/A

DIAGNOSIS

DIFFERENTIAL DIAGNOSIS
• Bacterial sinusitis—uncommon
• Viral infection (cats)
• Aspergillosis, other fungal infections
• Hypertension
• Parasites
• Cryptococcosis (cats)
• Foreign body
• Trauma
• Tooth root abscess
• Oronasal fistula
• Coagulopathy

CBC/BIOCHEMISTRY/URINALYSIS
Usually normal

OTHER LABORATORY TESTS
Cytologic and bacterial examination—rarely helpful

IMAGING
• Survey radiography (skull)—shows typical pattern of asymmetrical destruction of caudal turbinates with superimposition of a soft tissue mass; may find fluid density in the frontal sinuses secondary to outflow obstruction
• Thoracic radiography—detect lung metastasis (uncommon)
• CT or MRI—best method to observe integrity of cribriform plate or orbital invasion

DIAGNOSTIC PROCEDURES
• Rhinoscopy (visual observation is poor)—firm, fleshy masses; avoid progressing caudally into the cribriform plate.
• Tissue biopsy—necessary for definitive diagnosis
• Bacterial culture—often positive
• Cytology of regional lymph nodes—to detect metastatic disease (uncommon)

FIBROSARCOMA, NASAL AND PARANASAL SINUS

TREATMENT
• Surgery alone—ineffective; turbinectomy may be done before external (teletherapy) or internal (brachytherapy) irradiation.
• Inpatient radiotherapy (with or without surgery)—36–60 Gy; provides the best clinical control in dogs

MEDICATIONS

DRUG(S)
Chemotherapy—good option for some patients; doxorubicin (30 mg/m² IV once every 2 weeks for 5 treatments in dogs weighing > 10 kg; 1 mg/kg for dogs < 10 kg and for cats); median survival (dogs) 18 weeks; may provide marked palliation of clinical signs

CONTRAINDICATIONS/POSSIBLE INTERACTIONS
Chemotherapy may be toxic; seek advice before initiating treatment if you are unfamiliar with cytotoxic drugs.

FOLLOW-UP

PATIENT MONITORING
Survey radiography and/or CT or MRI (skull)—may be performed when clinical signs recur

EXPECTED COURSE AND PROGNOSIS
• Median survival if left untreated—3–5 months
• Median disease-free interval after radiotherapy—dogs, 8–23 months; cats, 1–36 months
• Survival rates with radiotherapy (dogs and cats)—1-year survival, 20% to 60%; 2-year survival, 30%–48%; reports of shorter survival times with nonepithelial nasal tumors (8–16 months)
• Median survival after doxorubicin (dogs)—18 weeks
• Brain involvement—poor prognostic sign

MISCELLANEOUS

ABBREVIATIONS
• CT = computed tomography
• MRI = magnetic resonance imaging

Suggested Reading

Evans SM, Goldschmidt M, McKee LJ, Harvey CE. Prognostic factors and survival after radiotherapy for intranasal neoplasms in dogs: 70 cases (1974–1985). J Am Vet Med Assoc 1989;194:1460–1463.

LaDue TA, Dodge R, Page RL, et al. Factors influencing survival after radiotherapy of nasal tumors in 130 dogs. Vet Radiol Ultrasound 1999;40:312–317.

Northrup NC, Etue SM, Ruslander DM, et al. Retrospective study of orthovoltage radiation therapy for nasal tumors in 42 dogs. J Vet Intern Med 2001;15:183–189.

Patnaik AK. Canine sinonasal neoplasms: soft tissue tumors. J Am Anim Hosp Assoc 1989;25:491–497.

Authors Kevin A. Hahn and Janet K. Carreras
Consulting Editor Wallace B. Morrison

FLATULENCE

BASICS

DEFINITION
Excessive formation of gases in the stomach or intestine; flatus refers to the gas released through the anus

PATHOPHYSIOLOGY
• Often results from a diet change or indiscretion but may herald a more serious gastrointestinal disease, especially in cats
• Swallowed air (aerophagia) and the bacterial fermentation of nutrients are the main sources of gastrointestinal gas; less significant sources include the interaction of gastric acid and pancreatic/salivary bicarbonate and diffusion of gases from the blood.
• Poorly digestible diets that escape intestinal assimilation, and are therefore available for colonic fermentation, and diets that liberate odiferous gases are associated with flatulence; these include nonabsorbable oligosaccharides (soybeans, beans, and peas), spoiled food, high-fat diets, milk products, and spices.
• Fiber-containing foods contribute to flatus indirectly through reduced dry-matter digestibility.
• Dogs and cats are lactose intolerant; a dietary concentration of 1.5 g/kg/day (11g lactose in 1 cup of milk) may produce flatus and diarrhea.
• A rapid change in diet or an increase in the concentration of a dietary component, especially carbohydrate or fiber, may cause flatus during a period of intestinal adaptation.
• As much as 99% of flatus is composed of nitrogen, oxygen, hydrogen, carbon dioxide and methane, all of which are odorless.
• Malodorous gases, including ammonia, hydrogen sulfide, indole, skatole, volatile amines, and short-chain fatty acids, compose the residual 1%.
• Disease states causing malassimilation of nutrients, making them available for colonic fermentation, can cause flatus.

SIGNALMENT

Species
Common complaint in dogs; rare in cats

Breed Predilection
Excessive aerophagia is seen in brachycephalic breeds, sporting dogs, and those with gluttonous/competitive eating behavior.

Mean Age and Range
Any age

Predominant Sex
None

SIGNS

Historical Findings
Increased frequency and possibly volume of flatus detected by the pet owner

Physical Examination Findings
• Mild abdominal discomfort caused by gastrointestinal distention possible
• Concurrent gastrointestinal signs—diarrhea, vomiting, borborygmus, and weight loss—may be present.

CAUSES

Increased Aerophagia
• Gluttony or competitive eating
• Respiratory disease
• Feeding shortly after exercise
• Brachycephalic breeds

Diet-Related
• Diets high in nonabsorbable oligosaccharides—soybeans, peas, beans
• Diets high in fermentable fiber—lactulose, fibrim, psyllium, oat bran
• Spoiled diets
• Milk products
• Abrupt changes in diet
• Spices and food additives/supplements

Disease Conditions
• Acute and chronic intestinal disease—inflammatory bowel, small intestinal bacterial overgrowth, neoplasia, irritable bowel syndrome, parasitism, bacterial enteritis, and viral enteritis
• Exocrine pancreatic insufficiency

RISK FACTORS
• Nervous, gluttonous, or competitive eating
• Eating soon after exercise
• Brachycephalic breeds
• Abrupt dietary changes
• Inappropriate or spoiled foods
• Sedentary lifestyle. A 1998 study (Jones, et al) reported that 43% of randomly chosen dog owners detected flatulence, most commonly in sedentary pets, with no association to a particular diet.

DIAGNOSIS

DIFFERENTIAL DIAGNOSIS
• Distinguish dietary and behavioral causes of flatus from gastrointestinal disease by thorough evaluation of the patient history; this allows the clinician to ascertain the type of diet, amount fed, frequency of feeding, frequency of dietary changes or additions, and the environment in which the patient is fed.
• Investigate feeding method—frequency, amount, relationship to exercise, how offered, and incidence of competitive eating. Observation of the patient while eating may be required to identify gluttony.
• Perform a complete physical examination with a focus on gastrointestinal evaluation. Palpate the abdomen for gassy bowel loops, pain, and distention, and auscultate the abdomen for bowel sounds, absence of which indicates ileus. Rectal examination for evaluation of rectal and pelvic anatomy.
• Assess body condition score; if low, this may indicate concurrent gastrointestinal disease or inadequate food intake.

CBC/BIOCHEMISTRY/URINALYSIS
Usually normal

OTHER LABORATORY TESTS
• Rectal cytology to evaluate presence of neoplasia, parasites, clostridial spores, neutrophils
• Zinc sulfate flotation tests (×3) or fecal ELISA to evaluate giardiasis
• Fecal cultures to evaluate salmonellosis or campylobacteriosis
• Serum trypsin-like immunoreactivity (TLI) to evaluate exocrine pancreatic insufficiency
• Serum cobalamin and folate concentrations to test for small intestinal bacterial overgrowth or severe mucosal disease
• Serum unconjugated cholic acid concentration or quantitative duodenal cultures (procured at endoscopy) to detect small intestinal bacterial overgrowth

IMAGING
• Abdominal ultrasonography to diagnose gastrointestinal masses or mural thickening
• Radiopaque marker study to detect changes in gastrointestinal motility or partial gastrointestinal obstruction

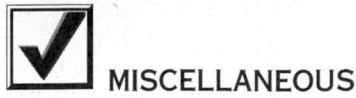

DIAGNOSTIC PROCEDURES

Gastrointestinal biopsy specimens obtained at surgery or via endoscopy to detect infiltrative gastrointestinal disease

TREATMENT

APPROPRIATE HEALTH CARE

Outpatient. Treat any underlying gastrointestinal disease.

NURSING CARE

None

ACTIVITY

Encourage an active lifestyle so flatus and feces can be expelled during exercise.

DIET

• Feed smaller meals more frequently in an isolated, quiet environment.
• Change diet to one that is highly digestible, with low fiber and fat concentrations (e.g., Eukanuba Low Residue Formula, Hill's i/d Diet, Innovative Veterinary Diet Select Care Neutral or Sensitive Formula, Purina EN Formula), or feed homemade diets containing boiled white rice (dogs) or baby cereal (cats) with skinned chicken or cottage cheese (balanced with vitamins and minerals).
• A change in the protein or carbohydrate source benefits some individuals.

CLIENT EDUCATION

Discourage dietary indiscretions (e.g., garbage ingestion or coprophagia).

SURGICAL CONSIDERATIONS

None

MEDICATIONS

DRUG(S) OF CHOICE

• Carminitives are medications that relieve flatulence.
• Zinc acetate binds sulfhydryl compounds.
• *Yucca schidigera* binds ammonia and is added to pet foods as a flavoring agent.
• Dry activated charcoal absorbs virtually all odiferous gases when mixed directly with human feces and flatus; however, the number of flatus events, gas volume, or odor were not decreased in people.

• Inclusion of activated charcoal, *Y. schidigera,* and zinc acetate in a treat reduced the frequency of highly odiferous episodes in dogs.
• Bismuth subsalicylate (dogs, 1 mL/kg PO initially then 0.25 mL/kg q6h) adsorbs hydrogen sulfide and has antibacterial properties; however, long-term, multiple daily dosing precludes its practicality.
• Simethicone is an antifoaming agent that reduces the surface tension of gas bubbles, allowing easier coalescence and release of intestinal gas; however, gas production is unaltered.
• Pancreatic enzyme supplements may reduce flatulence in some patients.

CONTRAINDICATIONS

Avoid bismuth subsalicylate in cats, and dogs with gastroduodenal ulceration and bleeding disorders.

PRECAUTIONS

N/A

POSSIBLE INTERACTIONS

N/A

ALTERNATIVE DRUG(S)

More than 30 herbal and botanical preparations are available; however, the dosage, safety, and efficacy are unknown.

FOLLOW-UP

PATIENT MONITORING

Response to therapy

PREVENTION/AVOIDANCE

• Avoid diets high in nonabsorbable oligosaccharides and high in fermentable fiber.
• Avoid milk products, spoiled diets, and abrupt changes in diet.
• Do not feed shortly after exercise.

POSSIBLE COMPLICATIONS

None

EXPECTED COURSE AND PROGNOSIS

N/A

✓ MISCELLANEOUS

ASSOCIATED CONDITIONS

Gastrointestinal disease

AGE-RELATED FACTORS

N/A

ZOONOTIC POTENTIAL

N/A

PREGNANCY

N/A

SYNONYMS

N/A

SEE ALSO

• Exocrine Pancreatic Insufficiency
• Inflammatory Bowel Disease
• Small Intestinal Bacterial Overgrowth
• Salmonellosis
• Campylobacteriosis
• Irritable Bowel Syndrome

ABBREVIATIONS

None

Suggested Reading

Davenport DJ, Remillard RL, Simpson KW, et al. Gastrointestinal and exocrine pancreatic disease. In: Hand MS, Thatcher CD, Remillard RL, et al., eds. Small animal clinical nutrition. 4th ed. Topeka, KS: Mark Morris Institute, 2000:725–810.

Giffard CJ, Collins SB, Stoodley N, et al. Ability of an antiflatulence treat to reduce the hydrogen sulfide content of canine flatulence. Proc. 18th ACVIM 2000:726.

Guilford WG. New ideas for management of gastrointestinal tract disease. J Small Anim Pract 1994;35:620–624.

Guilford WG. Approach to problems in gastroenterology. In: Guilford WG, Center SA, Strombeck DR, et al., eds. Strombeck's small animal gastroenterology. 3rd ed. Philadelphia: Saunders, 1996:50–76.

Jones BR, Jones KA, Turner K, et al. Flatulence in pet dogs. N Z Vet J 1998;46:191–193.

Roudebush P. Flatulence: what do we know about intestinal gas? Proc. 19th ACVIM 2001:592–594.

Author Mark C. Walker

Consulting Editor Albert E. Jergens

FLEA BITE HYPERSENSITIVITY AND FLEA CONTROL

 BASICS

DEFINITION
• Flea allergy dermatitis—hypersensitivity reaction to antigens in flea saliva with or without evidence of fleas and flea dirt
• Flea infestation—large number of fleas and a large amount of flea dirt with or without a flea allergy dermatitis

PATHOPHYSIOLOGY
• Flea bite hypersensitivity (FBH)—caused by a low molecular weight hapten and two high molecular weight allergens that help initiate the allergic reaction
• High molecular weight allergens—increased binding to dermal collagen; when bound, form a complete antigen necessary for eliciting FBH
• Flea saliva—contains histamine-like compounds that irritate skin
• Intermittent exposure favors FBH; continuous exposure is less likely to result in hypersensitivity
• Both IgE and IgG antiflea antibodies have been noted.
• Immediate and delayed hypersensitivity reactions have been noted.
• Late-phase IgE-mediated response—part of FBH reaction; occurs 3–6 hr after exposure
• Cutaneous basophil hypersensitivity—part of FBH reaction; an infiltration of basophils into the dermis; mediated by either IgE or IgG; subsequent exposures cause the basophils to degranulate; manifests as immediate and delayed hypersensitivity

SYSTEMS AFFECTED
Skin/Exocrine

GENETICS
FBH—unknown inheritance pattern; more common in atopic breeds

INCIDENCE/PREVALENCE
Varies with climatic conditions and flea population

GEOGRAPHIC DISTRIBUTION
• FBH—may occur anywhere; nonseasonal only in climates that are warm and humid year round and in animals housed indoors

SIGNALMENT

Species
Dogs and cats

Breed Predilection
FBH—any breed; most common in atopic breeds

Mean Age and Range
FBH—rare < 6 months of age; average age range, 3–6 years, but may be seen at any age

Predominant Sex
N/A

SIGNS

Historical Findings
• Compulsive biting
• Chewing (corncob nibbling)
• Licking, primarily in the back half of the body but may include the antebrachial regions
• Cats—scratching around the head and neck
• Signs of fleas and flea dirt

Physical Examination Findings
• Depends somewhat on the severity of the reaction and the degree of exposure to fleas (i.e., seasonal vs. year-round)
• Finding fleas and flea dirt is beneficial, although not essential, for the diagnosis of FBH; sensitive animals require a low exposure and tend to overgroom, making identification of the parasites difficult.
• Dogs—lesions concentrated in a triangular area of the caudal-dorsal-lumbosacral region; caudal aspect of the thighs, lower abdomen, inguinal region, and cranial forearms usually involved; primary lesions are papules; secondary lesions (e.g., hyperpigmentation, lichenification, alopecia, and scaling) common in uncontrolled FBH; secondary folliculitis and furunculosis may be seen.
• Cats—several patterns are seen; most common is a miliary crusting dermatitis in a wedge-shaped pattern over the caudal dorsal lumbosacral region and often around the head and neck; other presentations are alopecia of the inguinal region with or without inflammation or eosinophilic plaques and other forms of eosinophilic granuloma complex.
• Exposure to other animals and previous flea treatment should be ascertained.

CAUSES
See Pathophysiology

RISK FACTORS
FBH—intermittent exposure to fleas increases the likelihood of development; commonly seen in conjunction with atopy

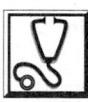 DIAGNOSIS

DIFFERENTIAL DIAGNOSIS
• Food allergy
• Atopy
• Sarcoptic mange
• Cheyletiellosis
• Primary keratinization defects
• Diagnosis is best based on the history and laboratory tests.

CBC/BIOCHEMISTRY/URINALYSIS
• Usually normal
• Cats—hypereosinophilia may be detected

OTHER LABORATORY TESTS
• Skin scrapings—negative
• Flea combings—fleas or flea dirt, but often nothing is found
• RAST and ELISA—variable accuracy; both false-positive and false-negative results reported

IMAGING
N/A

DIAGNOSTIC PROCEDURES
• Diagnosis usually based on historical information and distribution of lesions
• Fleas or flea dirt is supportive but is often quite difficult to find, especially in cats.
• Identification of *Dipylidium caninum* segments is supportive.
• Intradermal allergy testing with flea antigen—reveals positive immediate reactions in 90% of flea-allergic animals; delayed reactions (24–48 hr) may sometimes be observed in allergic animals that show no immediate reaction.
• The most accurate test may be response to appropriate treatment.

PATHOLOGIC FINDINGS
• Superficial perivascular dermatitis
• Eosinophilic intraepidermal micro-abscesses—strongly suggest FBH
• Eosinophils as a major cellular component of the dermis—supportive of FBH
• Histopathologic evaluation—cannot accurately differentiate FBH from atopy, food allergy, or other hypersensitivities

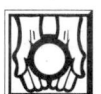 TREATMENT

APPROPRIATE HEALTH CARE
Outpatient therapy

NURSING CARE
N/A

ACTIVITY
N/A

DIET
N/A

CLIENT EDUCATION
• Inform owners that there is no cure for FBH.
• Advise owners that flea-allergic animals often become more sensitive to flea bites as they age.
• Inform owners that controlling exposure to fleas is currently the only means of therapy; hyposensitization has not worked satisfactorily.

SURGICAL CONSIDERATIONS
N/A

FLEA BITE HYPERSENSITIVITY AND FLEA CONTROL

MEDICATIONS

DRUG(S) OF CHOICE
• Corticosteroids—antiinflammatory dosages for symptomatic relief while the fleas are being controlled
• Antihistamines—symptomatic relief
• Fipronil (GABA antagonist)—monthly spot treatment for cats and dogs and spray treatment for dogs; activity against fleas and ticks; resistant to removal with water; excellent safety and efficacy profile
• Imidacloprid—monthly spot treatment for cats and dogs; excellent safety and efficacy profile
• Systemic treatments—limited benefit because they require a flea bite that has already initiated FBH; may help animals with flea infestation; primarily licensed for use in only dogs; lufenuron, a chitin inhibitor, available as an oral formulation for cats and dogs and as an injection for cats; permethrin available as a spot treatment and reputed to have some repellent activity; imidacloprid (flea adulticide) available as a spot treatment for cats and dogs
• Sprays—usually contain pyrethrins and pyrethroids (synthetic pyrethrins) with an insect growth regulator or synergist; generally effective < 48–72 hr; advantages are low toxicity and repellent activity; disadvantages are frequent applications and expense.
• Indoor treatment—fogs and premises sprays; usually contain organophosphates, pyrethrins, and/or insect growth regulators; apply according to manufacturer's directions; treat all areas of the house; can be applied by the owner; advantages are weak chemicals and generally inexpensive; disadvantage is labor intensity; premises sprays concentrate the chemicals in areas that most need treatment.
• Professional exterminators—advantages are less labor-intensive; relatively few applications; sometimes guaranteed; disadvantages are strength of chemicals and cost; specific recommendations and guidelines must be followed.
• Inert substances—boric acid, diatomaceous earth, and silica aerogel; treat every 6–12 months; follow manufacturer's recommendations; very safe and effective if applied properly
• Outdoor treatment—concentrated in shaded areas; sprays usually contain pyrethroids or organophosphates and an insect growth regulator; powders are usually organophosphates; product containing nematodes (*Steinerma carpocapsae*) is very safe and chemical-free.

CONTRAINDICATIONS
N/A

PRECAUTIONS
• Insecticidal sprays and dips should not be used on dogs and cats ≤ 3 months, unless otherwise specified on the label.
• Pyrethrin/pyrethroid-type flea products—adverse reactions include depression, hypersalivation, muscle tremors, vomiting, ataxia, dyspnea, and anorexia.
• Organophosphates—adverse reactions include hypersalivation, lacrimation, urination, defecation, vomiting, diarrhea, miosis, fever, muscle tremors, seizures, coma, and death
• All pesticides must be applied according to label directions.
• Toxicity—if any signs are noted, the animal should be bathed thoroughly to remove any remaining chemicals and treated appropriately
• Rodents and fish are very sensitive to pyrethrins.

POSSIBLE INTERACTIONS
• Organophosphate treatments—do not use more than one form at a time.
• Topical organophosphates—avoid in cats, very young animals (< 3 months of age), and sick or debilitated animals.
• Straight permethrin sprays or spot-ons—do not use in cats.
• Cythioate—contraindicated in heartworm-positive dogs and greyhounds
• Piperonyl butoxide—do not use in concentrations > 1% in cats.

ALTERNATIVE DRUG(S)
• Powders—usually contain organophosphates or carbamates; advantage is high residual effectiveness; disadvantages are dry skin and toxicity; organophosphates and carbamates should be avoided in cats.
• Dips, sprays, powders, and foams—dips usually contain organophosphates and synthetic pyrethrins and should not be used more than once per week; follow manufacturer's instructions for safest and best results; after repeated use, these agents can be drying or irritating; newer, safer spot treatments have essentially replaced these products.

FOLLOW-UP

PATIENT MONITORING
• Pruritus—a decrease means the FBH is being controlled.

• Fleas and flea dirt—absence is not always a reliable indicator of successful treatment in very sensitive animals.

PREVENTION/AVOIDANCE
• See Medications
• Year-round warm climates—year-round flea control
• Seasonally warm climates—begin flea control in May or June

POSSIBLE COMPLICATIONS
• Secondary bacterial infections
• Acute moist dermatitis
• Acral lick dermatitis

EXPECTED COURSE AND PROGNOSIS
Prognosis is good, if strict flea control is instituted.

MISCELLANEOUS

ASSOCIATED CONDITIONS
Approximately 80% of atopic dogs are also allergic to flea bites.

AGE-RELATED FACTORS
Organophosphates—use with utmost caution in old animals; not recommended for use in very young animals (< 3 months)

ZOONOTIC POTENTIAL
In areas of moderate to severe flea infestation, people can be bitten by fleas; usually papular lesions are located on the wrists and ankles.

PREGNANCY
• Corticosteroids and organophosphates—do not use in pregnant bitches and queens
• Carefully follow the label directions of each individual product to determine its safety.

SYNONYM
• Flea bite allergy

ABBREVIATIONS
• ELISA = enzyme-linked immunosorbent assay
• GABA = γ-aminobutyric acid
• RAST = radioallergosorbent test

Suggested Reading
Bevier-Tournay DE. Fleas and flea control. In: Kirk RW, Bonagura JD, eds. Current veterinary therapy X. Philadelphia: Saunders, 1989:586–591.
Griffin CE, Kwochka KW, MacDonald JM. Current veterinary dermatology. St. Louis: Mosby, 1993.
Authors Karen A. Kuhl and Jean S. Greek
Consulting Editor Karen Helton Rhodes

FOOD REACTIONS (DERMATOLOGIC)

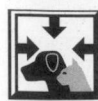

BASICS

DEFINITION
Pruritic, nonseasonal reactions associated with ingestion of one or more substances in the animal's food

PATHOPHYSIOLOGY
• Pathogenesis not completely understood
• Immediate and delayed reactions to specific ingredients—documented in the veterinary literature; immediate reactions presumed to be type I hypersensitivity reactions; delayed owing to type III or IV
• Food intolerance—nonimmunologic, idiosyncratic reaction; involves metabolic, toxic, or pharmacologic effects of offending ingredients
• Adverse food reaction is the most common term used, because it is not easy to distinguish between immunologic and idiosyncratic reactions.

SYSTEMS AFFECTED
• Skin/Exocrine—pruritus in any location on the body; otitis externa
• Gastrointestinal—vomiting; diarrhea; more frequent bowel movements
• Nervous—very rare; seizures have been documented with adverse food reaction/intolerance

GENETICS
N/A

INCIDENCE/PREVALENCE
• Approximately 5% of all skin diseases and 10–15% of all allergic skin diseases in dogs and cats are the result of adverse food reactions.
• Third-most-common pruritic skin disease in the dog; second-most-common in the cat
• Percentages vary greatly with clinicians and geographic location.

GEOGRAPHIC DISTRIBUTION
N/A

SIGNALMENT

Species
Dogs and cats

Breed Predilections
None

Mean Age and Range
Any age

Predominant Sex
None

SIGNS

General Comments
A wide range of signs that can mimic any of the other hypersensitivity reactions

Historical Findings
• Nonseasonal pruritus of any body location
• Poor response to antiinflammatory doses of glucocorticoids suggests a food hypersensitivity.
• Vomiting
• Diarrhea
• Excessive borborygmus, flatulence, and frequent bowel movements

Physical Examination Findings
• *Malassezia* dermatitis, pyoderma, and otitis externa
• Plaques
• Pustules
• Erythema
• Crusts
• Scale
• Self-induced alopecia
• Excoriation
• Lichenification
• Hyperpigmentation
• Urticaria
• Angioedema
• Pyotraumatic dermatitis

CAUSES
• Immune-mediated reactions—result of the ingestion and subsequent presentation of one or more glycoproteins (allergens) either before or after digestion; sensitization may occur at the gastrointestinal mucosa, after the substance is absorbed, or both.
• Nonimmune (food intolerance) reactions—result of ingestion of foods with high levels of histamine or substances that induce histamine either directly or through histamine-releasing factors

RISK FACTORS
• Unknown

• It is speculated that in juvenile animals intestinal parasites or intestinal infections may cause damage to the intestinal mucosa, resulting in the abnormal absorption of allergens and subsequent sensitization.

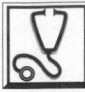

DIAGNOSIS

DIFFERENTIAL DIAGNOSIS
• Flea bite hypersensitivity—usually confined to the caudal half of the body; often seasonal
• Atopy—associated with pruritus on the face, ventrum, and feet; often seasonal; if pruritus first occurs at < 6 months or > 6 years of age, then food hypersensitivity may be more likely than inhalant allergy.
• Drug reactions—history of drug administration before the development of signs and improvement after withdrawal of the suspected drug confirms the diagnosis.
• Scabies—pruritus often very specific in the location (ears, elbows and hocks); mites in skin scrapings and response to specific therapy confirm the diagnosis.

CBC/BIOCHEMISTRY/URINALYSIS
No important changes

OTHER LABORATORY TESTS
N/A

IMAGING
N/A

DIAGNOSTIC PROCEDURES

Food Elimination Diet
• Definitive test for adverse food reactions
• Tailored to the individual patient
• The diet must be restricted to one protein and one carbohydrate to which the animal has had limited or no previous exposure.
• It may take up to 13 weeks for maximum improvement of the clinical signs.
• If the patient is sensitive to one or more foods, noticeable improvement will be seen by the 4th week of the diet.

Challenge and Provocation Diet Trials
• Used if the patient improves on the elimination diet
• Challenge—feed the patient with the original diet; a return of the signs confirms that something in the diet is causing the signs; the challenge period should last until the signs return but no longer than 10 days.

FOOD REACTIONS (DERMATOLOGIC)

• Provoke (provocation diet trial)—if the challenge confirmed the presence of adverse food reaction, add single ingredients to the elimination diet; test ingredients include a full range of meats (beef, chicken, fish, pork, lamb), a full range of grains (corn, wheat, soybean, rice), eggs, and dairy products; the provocation period for each ingredient should last up to 10 days or less if signs develop sooner (dogs usually develop signs within 1–2 days); results guide the selection of commercial foods that do not contain the offending substance(s).

PATHOLOGIC FINDINGS
• Skin biopsies—not diagnostic; help confirm other differentials
• Histopathologic findings—variable; common findings suggest hypersensitivity; a secondary pyoderma or *Malassezia* infection may be seen.

TREATMENT

APPROPRIATE HEALTH CARE
Outpatient management

NURSING CARE
N/A

ACTIVITY
No change

DIET
Avoid any food substances that caused the clinical signs to return during the provocation phase of the diagnosis.

CLIENT EDUCATION
• Make sure the client understands the principles involved in each phase of the diagnostic test diets.
• Inform client to eliminate treats, chewable toys, vitamins, and other chewable medications (e.g., heartworm preventive), which may contain ingredients from the patient's previous diet.
• Outdoor pets must be confined to prevent foraging and hunting, which might alter the test diet.
• Provide handouts for clients to take home.
• Advise client that all family members must be aware of the test protocol and must help keep the test diet clean and free of any other food sources.

SURGICAL CONSIDERATIONS
N/A

MEDICATIONS

DRUG(S) OF CHOICE
• Systemic antipruritic drugs—may be useful during the first 2–3 weeks of diet trial to control self-mutilation
• Antibiotics or antifungal medications—useful for secondary pyodermas or *Malassezia* infections

CONTRAINDICATIONS
• Antibiotics that are known to have anti-inflammatory effects (e.g., tetracycline, erythromycin, and trimethoprim-potentiated sulfas)
• Glucocorticoids and antihistamines must be discontinued for at least 10–14 days while on the diet trial to allow correct assessment of the animal's response.

PRECAUTIONS
N/A

POSSIBLE INTERACTIONS
Chewable vitamins and heartworm medications may contain offending food substances.

ALTERNATIVE DRUG(S)
None

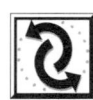

FOLLOW-UP

PATIENT MONITORING
Examine patient and evaluate and document the pruritus and clinical signs every 3–4 weeks.

PREVENTION/AVOIDANCE
• Avoid intake of any of the proteins included in the previous diet.
• Treats and chewable toys should be limited to known safe substances (e.g., apples, vegetables).

POSSIBLE COMPLICATIONS
Other causes of pruritus (e.g., flea bite hypersensitivity; atopy; and external parasites such as sarcoptic, *Notoedres,* and *Cheyletiella* mites) can mask the response to the food elimination diet trial.

EXPECTED COURSE AND PROGNOSIS
• Prognosis is good, if food ingredients are the only cause of the pruritus and offending ingredients are avoided.
• Rarely a dog or cat may develop hypersensitivity to new substances, which may require a new elimination diet trial.
• Any other hypersensitivities (flea or atopy) must also be treated.

MISCELLANEOUS

ASSOCIATED CONDITIONS
• Superficial pyoderma
• *Malassezia* dermatitis
• Otitis externa

AGE-RELATED FACTORS
Animals who develop pruritus for the first time at < 6 months or > 6 years of age are more likely to have adverse food reaction than atopy.

ZOONOTIC POTENTIAL
None

PREGNANCY
N/A

SYNONYMS
• Food allergy
• Food intolerance

SEE ALSO
• Atopy
• Contact Dermatitis
• Flea and Flea Control
• Malassezia Dermatitis
• Otitis Externa and Media
• Pyoderma

Suggested Reading
Jeffers JG, Shanley KJ. Diagnostic testing of dogs for food hypersensitivity. J Am Vet Med Assoc 1991;198:245–250.
MacDonald JM. Food allergy. In: Griffin CE, Kwochka KW, MacDonald JM, eds. Current veterinary dermatology. St. Louis: Mosby, 1993:121.
Rosser EJ. Diagnosis of food allergy in dogs. J Am Vet Med Assoc 1993:203:259.
White SD. Food hypersensitivity in 30 dogs. J Am Vet Med Assoc 1986:188:695–698.
Author David Duclos
Consulting Editor Karen Helton Rhodes

GALLBLADDER MUCOCELE

 BASICS

OVERVIEW
• Formation of a tenacious, thick, mucoid conglomerate in the gallbladder, obstructing its storage capacity and function
• Inspissated biliary sludge expands the gallbladder, leading to necrotizing cholecystitis.

SIGNALMENT
• Dogs
• Shetland sheepdogs, miniature schnauzers, cocker spaniels—overrepresented
• Middle-aged to older adults
• No sex predilection

SIGNS

General Comments
• Symptomatic or asymptomatic
• Asymptomatic discovered on abdominal ultrasonography for other health concerns

Historical Findings
Symptomatic
• Episodic abdominal discomfort
• Anorexia
• Polyuria and polydipsia
• Lethargy
• Vomiting
• Collapse

Physical Examination Findings
• Lethargy
• Cranial abdominal pain
• Jaundice
• Dehydration
• Fever

CAUSES & RISK FACTORS
• Inborn errors of lipid metabolism, as noted in miniature schnauzer and Shetland sheepdogs
• Medical conditions associated with hypercholesterolemia, especially hypothyroidism
• Gallbladder dysmotility—may play a causal role
• Cystic hypertrophy of the mucus-producing gallbladder glands—common in older dogs; may play a causal or permissive role

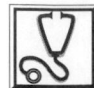 **DIAGNOSIS**

DIFFERENTIAL DIAGNOSIS
Conditions causing bile stasis—gallbladder dysmotility; neoplasia; choleliths; pancreatitis

CBC/BIOCHEMISTRY/URINALYSIS

CBC
• Inflammatory leukogram—if necrotizing cholecystitis present
• Nonregenerative anemia—if chronic inflammation or hypothyroidism

Biochemistry
• High liver enzyme activity—chronic or noted only on acute presentation; ALP, GGT, ALT, and AST
• Variable hyperbilirubinemia
• Ruptured biliary tree and peritonitis—low albumin
• Prerenal azotemia—causing high BUN and creatinine
• Electrolyte abnormalities with fluid and acid-base disturbances—due to biliary tree rupture or extensive vomiting

Urinalysis
No specific features

OTHER LABORATORY TESTS
• Triglyceride concentrations—may be markedly increased
• Coagulation assays—usually normal, unless EHBDO, biliary tree rupture, bile peritonitis, sepsis, or DIC

IMAGING
• Abdominal radiography—normal or large liver; loss of detail in cranial abdomen with focal peritonitis in necrotizing cholecystitis; presence of gas indicates septic inflammation with gas-producing organism (rare)
• Abdominal ultrasonography—liver may be large, with rounded margins; diffuse to multifocal hyperechoic hepatic parenchyma common; distended gallbladder and sometimes distended common bile duct and cystic duct; fluid interface surrounding gallbladder enhances wall image; diffusely thick gallbladder wall with segmental hyperechogenicity; double-rimmed wall (also can be seen with acute cholecystitis, hepatitis, cholangiohepatitis, hypoproteinemia, right heart failure, renal failure, pyelonephritis, and abdominal effusion); necrotic slough may appear as intraluminal membrane parallel to the wall; gallbladder lumen filled with amorphous echogenic stellate or finely striated pattern, resembling a sliced kiwi fruit ("kiwi sign"); discontinuation of gallbladder wall consistent with rupture; pericholecystic fluid or hyperechogenicity of surrounding fat with rupture; intrahepatic bile ducts may be difficult to visualize or may appear prominent (ascending cholangitis or EHBDO); biliary tree rupture associated with effusion

DIAGNOSTIC PROCEDURES
• Aspiration sampling—fluid adjacent to biliary structures or free in abdominal cavity; clarifies biliary tree rupture and suppurative septic inflammation; **Caution:** do not perform cholecystocentesis, may cause bile peritonitis; mucocele difficult to sample owing to its thick, tenacious nature
• Exploratory laparotomy—for diagnosis and cholecystectomy; be prepared for chole-cystoenterostomy
• Liver biopsy—evaluates coexistent ascending disease in the biliary tree
• Bacterial culture and sensitivity—effusion, gallbladder, liver, and gallbladder contents taken at surgery; request aerobic and anaerobic bacteria
• Cytology—impression smears of gallbladder, liver, and bile for immediate determination of suppurative septic inflammation and neoplasia

PATHOLOGIC FINDINGS

• Gross—gallbladder distended, wall may be erythematosus with focal areas of necrosis; focal peritonitis may be evident; liver and extrahepatic biliary structures usually appear normal; gallbladder contents: dark green-black, tenacious, firm, or organized solid yellow-green on cut surface
• Microscopic—mixed inflammatory infiltrate and fibrosis in lamina propria of gallbladder wall, with focal areas of necrosis if necrotizing cholecystitis present; gallbladder mucosal hyperplasia; ascending cholangitis and cholangiohepatitis; hepatocytes may demonstrate vacuolation consistent with glycogen and discrete lipid inclusions

TREATMENT

• Outpatient management with ursodeoxycholic acid—not reliable
• Inpatient—treatment depends on whether patient presents with severe acute necrotizing cholecystitis or syndrome determined incidentally on ultrasound examination
• If patient is hyperlipidemic, investigate cause and restrict dietary fat.
• Symptomatic patients require exploratory surgery for cholecystectomy and treatment for potential bile peritonitis.
• Removal of biliary contents and retention of gallbladder likely will lead to recrudescence.
• Fluid therapy—balanced polyionic solutions to correct hydration and electrolyte abnormalities; judiciously supplement with potassium chloride
• Prepare for blood component therapy
• Abdominal lavage—at surgery if bile peritonitis present

MEDICATIONS

DRUG(S)

• Antimicrobials—initiate broad-spectrum antimicrobials *before* surgery in all patients: enteric gram-negative and anaerobic organisms most likely to cause infection; continue for no less than 8 weeks if septic complications; adjust drugs based on culture and sensitivity testing
• Vitamin K_1 (0.5–1.5 mg/kg IM or SC q12h for three doses)—if jaundice present
• Antiemetics (e.g., metoclopramide 0.2–0.5 mg/kg PO, IV, or SC q6–8h or 1–2 mg/kg/day by CRI; ondansetron 0.5–1.0 mg/kg PO 30 min before feeding, maximum q8h or 0.1–0.2 mg/kg slow IV push q6–12h)—if patient is vomiting
• H_2-receptor antagonists (e.g., famotidine 0.5 mg/kg PO, IV, SC q12–24h; sucralfate 0.25–1.0 g PO q8–12h)—for gastrointestinal bleeding
• Ursodeoxycholic acid (10–15 mg/kg PO daily)—choleretic and hepatoprotectant; give indefinitely
• Antioxidants—vitamin E (α-tocopherol 10 IU/kg PO daily); S-adenosylmethionine (20 mg/kg PO daily 2 hr before feeding); give until liver enzymes normalize or indefinitely with chronic hepatitis

CONTRAINDICATIONS/POSSIBLE INTERACTIONS

N/A

FOLLOW-UP

PATIENT MONITORING

Repeat sequential hematology, biochemistry, and imaging to monitor response.

POSSIBLE COMPLICATIONS

• Cholangitis or cholangiohepatitis
• Bile peritonitis
• EHBDO

EXPECTED COURSE AND PROGNOSIS

• Good with successful surgery, chronic choleretic therapy, and diet modification
• Anticipate a protracted clinical course with ruptured biliary tract or peritonitis.
• Recrudescence may occur even if gallbladder removed and medical therapy chronically administered

MISCELLANEOUS

SEE ALSO

• Bile Peritonitis
• Cholecystitis
• Cholelithiasis
• Hepatitis, Chronic

ABBREVIATIONS

• ALP = alkaline phosphatase
• ALT = alanine aminotransferase
• AST = aspartate aminotransferase
• BUN = blood urea nitrogen
• CRI = constant rate infusion
• DIC = disseminated intravascular coagulation
• EHBDO = extrahepatic biliary duct obstruction
• GGT = γ-glutamyltransferase

Suggested Reading

Besso JG, Wrigley RH, Gliatto JM, et al. Ultrasonographic appearance and clinical findings in 14 dogs with gallbladder mucocele. Vet Radiol Ultrasound 2000;41(3): 261–271.
Newell SM, Selcer BA, Mahaffey MB, et al. Gallbladder mucocele causing biliary obstruction in two dogs: Ultrasonographic, scintigraphic and pathologic findings. J Am Anim Hosp Assoc 1995;31(6):467–472.
Author Sharon A. Center
Consulting Editor Sharon A. Center

GASTRIC DILATION AND VOLVULUS SYNDROME

 BASICS

DEFINITION

A syndrome of dogs in which the stomach dilates and twists around its central axis, which results in complex local and systemic pathologic and physiologic changes

PATHOPHYSIOLOGY

• Fluid or ingesta accumulates in the stomach in conjunction with a mechanical or functional obstruction of the gastroesophageal and pyloric orifices. • Dilation of the stomach may progress, adding to functional obstruction and potentiating volvulus. • Twisting of the stomach may occur without dilation. • When viewing the dog in dorsal recumbency from caudal to cranial, the stomach may twist in a clockwise or counterclockwise direction. • The most common presentation is clockwise, with the duodenum passing ventrally from right to left; the rotation is around the long axis from the cardia to the pylorus; rotation varies from 90° to 360°. • Direct gastric damage and multiple systemic abnormalities occur secondary to ischemia and reperfusion injury. Ischemia results from rising intragastric pressures, decreased cardiac return as the stomach compresses the portal vein and caudal vena cava, direct outflow obstruction of gastric and splanchnic vessels due to twisting, infarction of the gastric mucosa due to neutrophil accumulation and margination, and edema due to multiple cell damage and inflammatory mediator release. • These changes account for the acute clinical signs, which include hypovolemic shock and cardiovascular failure. • Reperfusion injury is a complex entity involving the formation of oxygen free radicals and multiple inflammatory mediators following appropriate surgical intervention.

SYSTEMS AFFECTED

• Gastrointestinal—fundus of the stomach is most severely compromised by occlusion of its blood supply during torsion • Cardiovascular—low venous return to the right side of the heart results in severe hypoxia to other organ systems and hypovolemic shock; arrhythmias occur secondary to the effects of hypoxia, inflammatory mediators, and other cardiogenic factors. • Respiratory—direct impedance of volume expansion caused by gastric distension and decreased cardiac output to the lungs • Hemic/Lymphatic/Immune—splenic infarction • Hepatobiliary—multiple factors including inflammatory mediators, hypoxia, endotoxemia, and potentially reperfusion injury of the liver

GENETICS

No direct genetic predisposition confirmed

INCIDENCE/PREVALENCE

• Vary • Metropolitan emergency clinics see these cases frequently.

SIGNALMENT

Species
Dog

Breed Predilections
• German shepherds • Great Danes • Saint Bernards • Rottweilers • Labrador retrievers • Alaskan malamutes • Any large, deep-chested breed • Rarely reported in dachshunds and Pekingese

Mean Age And Range
Any age; most commonly in middle-aged to older dogs

Predominant Sex
N/A

SIGNS

Historical Findings
• Nonproductive retching • Ptyalism • Progressive abdominal distension • Weakness or collapse • Depression • Frequent belching

Physical Examination Findings
• Tympanic cranial abdomen • Tachycardia • Tachypnea • Rectal body temperature may vary widely. • Signs of hypovolemic shock (e.g., pale mucous membranes, decreased capillary refill time, weak pulses)

CAUSES

Theories of interest include pyloric outflow obstruction, gastric myoelectric abnormalities, dynamic movement of the stomach following ingestion of food or water, and aerophagia.

RISK FACTORS

• Activity following ingestion of large quantities of food or water • Any intense activity or stress (including hospitalization and surgery)

 DIAGNOSIS

DIFFERENTIAL DIAGNOSIS

• Gastric dilation without torsion—due to overdistension, usually from ingesting excessive quantities of food • Other diseases that cause acute abdominal distension (e.g., intestinal volvulus, splenic torsion, abdominal effusion or hemorrhage) • Differentiate non-GDV conditions via examination and imaging.

CBC/BIOCHEMISTRY/URINALYSIS

• Expect hemogram abnormalities consistent with acute inflammation and hemoconcentration/shock • Electrolyte abnormalities and acid–base alterations are common. • Urinalysis generally reflects hypovolemia—high urine specific gravity due to prerenal azotemia

OTHER LABORATORY TESTS
N/A

IMAGING

• Abdominal radiography—a right lateral abdominal radiograph is the imaging modality of choice; a "double bubble" compartmentalized stomach is considered pathognomonic;

the pylorus is air filled on this view; a left lateral radiograph may help to determine if a volvulus is present; the pylorus is fluid-filled on this view. • Dorsoventral view—the pylorus may be shifted toward, or located in, the left cranial abdomen. • Stabilization may be necessary prior to imaging procedures.

DIAGNOSTIC PROCEDURES

Abdominocentesis and cytology may help determine if perforation has occurred.

PATHOLOGIC FINDINGS

• Gastric distension with resultant gastric edema, hyperemia, congestion, infarction, and necrosis, depending on the duration of the condition • Splenic torsion may also be present with similar changes.

 TREATMENT

APPROPRIATE HEALTH CARE

• Emergency inpatient medical and surgical management • Patients require immediate medical therapy with special attention to establishing improved cardiovascular function and then gastric decompression. • Shock/fluid therapy should precede gastric decompression; give isotonic fluids at the rate of 90 mL/kg within the first 30–60 min, the general treatment of choice for hypovolemic (shock) patients; delivery of this volume may require placing two large-gauge intravenous catheters. • Use of colloid solutions is advocated to restore cardiovascular function rapidly. • Supportive fluids on the basis of hydration status are recommended for animals not in shock. • Postoperative fluid support is needed until the patient is stable and able to eat and drink. • First try gastric decompression by orogastric intubation; light sedation with narcotics may facilitate this process. • Decompression by other techniques such as trocarization and indwelling catheters is described. • Maintain gastric decompression either by a pharyngogastric tube or an indwelling catheter until definitive treatment or surgical derotation and gastropexy. • Surgery is indicated in all cases of GDV, though the time interval from presentation to surgery may vary depending on response or lack of response to treatment. • Immediate surgery is indicated in patients unresponsive to cardiorespiratory stabilization and in all patients following successful stabilization.

NURSING CARE

• Maintain blood pressure with ample fluid support following volume replacement/shock therapy. • Electrolyte and acid–base management are indicated; often potassium supplementation is necessary. • Monitor patients closely for recurrence of dilation or cardiorespiratory decompensation. Supplemental nasal oxygen (O_2) therapy may assist antiarrhythmic therapy and tissue hypoxemia

GASTRIC DILATION AND VOLVULUS SYNDROME

ACTIVITY
Severely restrict activity prior to surgery and for a minimum of 10–14 days postsurgery

DIET
• Begin oral alimentation as soon as appropriate on the basis of gastric integrity at surgery. • Placing a jejunostomy feeding tube at the time of surgery when prolonged gastric healing is expected may allow early enteral supplementation. • Small multiple feedings of a high-quality, easily digested, easily assimilated diet is recommended during surgical recovery to prevent gastric distension. • Soaking dry food in water for 15–20 min prior to feeding helps prevent rapid expansion of food in the stomach. • Institute dietary changes on a permanent basis to prevent future dilatory episodes.

CLIENT EDUCATION
• Discuss potential risks of surgery and the potential for recurrence of the dilation. • Explain signs of recurrence of gastric dilation, so the client may detect the condition early.

SURGICAL CONSIDERATIONS
• Definitive treatment—exploratory celiotomy with gastric derotation and permanent right-sided gastropexy • Timing of surgery—controversial; based on the patient's cardiovascular condition, gastric decompression, and other physical parameters • Prolonged delay may result in death of the patient. • Derotation without gastropexy results in an 80% recurrence rate. • Multiple techniques for gastropexy are appropriate and are described in detail in surgical texts. • Partial gastrectomy may be required on the basis of gastric wall integrity, especially in the fundic region. • Thromboses of short gastric vessels, blue-to-black persistent serosal discoloration after derotation, and lack of hemorrhage from cut surfaces indicate nonviable tissue and necessitate excision. • Supplemental alimentation may be indicated with partial gastrectomies, depending on the remaining gastric integrity; a jejunostomy tube may be placed at the time of surgery for postoperative enteral support. • Splenic vasculature infarction is an indication for splenectomy. • Surgical exploration should be thorough and yet efficient to minimize surgical time. • Decreased survival time is associated with prolonged surgery and anesthesia in a hemodynamically unstable patient.

MEDICATIONS

DRUG(S) OF CHOICE
• Corticosteroids such as dexamethasone sodium phosphate (5 mg/kg slow IV) or prednisolone sodium succinate (22 mg/kg slow IV)—used to stabilize membranes, aid in cardiovascular support, and potentially help with treatment and prevention of reperfusion injury • Antibiotics effective against gastrointestinal flora are often recommended because of the potential for endotoxemia associated with shock, gastric compromise, and potential abdominal contamination at the time of surgery. • Effective antibiotic choices include cefazolin sodium (20–35 mg/kg IV q8h or every 2 h interoperatively) or cefoxitin sodium (30 mg/kg IV q6–8h). • Additional antibiotics may be necessary, depending on cultures of abdominal contents at the time of surgery. • H_2-receptor antagonists may ameliorate or prevent gastric ulceration (e.g., famotidine 0.5 mg/kg IV or PO q12–24h; ranitidine 1.0 mg/kg IV or PO q12h).

CONTRAINDICATIONS
• Avoid drugs that may exacerbate hypovolemia (e.g., acetylpromazine). • Avoid drugs that may lead to renal compromise, until shock and hypovolemia are corrected (e.g., aminoglycosides). • Reserve drugs for correction of acid–base abnormalities until the patient is stabilized.

PRECAUTIONS
• Choose anesthetic agents for their cardiovascular supportive effects. • Pay special attention to maintaining the mean arterial pressure at or above 60 mm Hg. • Rapid administration of prednisolone sodium succinate may cause vomiting.

POSSIBLE INTERACTIONS
N/A

ALTERNATIVE DRUG(S)
• Hypertonic saline (7% NaCl solution) in 6% Dextran 70—5 mL/kg given over 5 min and followed with lactated Ringer's solution at 20 mL/kg/h • Colloids (e.g. hydroxylethyl starch [Hetastarch], 10–20 mL/kg IV administered slowly to effect; 6% dextran 70 in 0.9% sodium chloride [Dextran 70], 10–20 mL/kg IV administered slowly to effect; polymerized bovine hemoglobin glutamer-200 [Oxyglobin] 30 mL/kg IV given at 10 mL/kg/h) followed by lactated Ringer's solution at 20 mL/kg/h

FOLLOW-UP

PATIENT MONITORING
• Cardiorespiratory function for at least 24 h after surgery; blood pressure and perfusion • Electrocardiographic monitoring • Splenectomy frequently results in multifocal intermittent-to-continuous premature ventricular contractions. • Administer antiarrhythmics only when necessary. • Institute general supportive care with special attention to electrolyte and acid–base status. • Base treatment on serial laboratory analyses.

PREVENTION/AVOIDANCE
• Avoid ingestion of excessive amounts of food or fluids. • Feed small meals multiple times daily. • Avoid postprandial exercise.

POSSIBLE COMPLICATIONS
• Postoperative gastric ulceration may occur within 5–7 days if severe mucosal defects remain. • Rupture of gastric ulcers may result in septic peritonitis and its sequelae. • Other complications reported following gastropexy include belching and intermittent vomiting. • Gastric dilation may recur.

EXPECTED COURSE AND PROGNOSIS
• Based on surgical assessment and postoperative recovery • Patients recovering well after 7 days appear to have a good prognosis for complete recovery. • Gastropexy appears to be the most significant factor preventing recurrence; recurrence rates are as high as 80% without gastropexy and 3–5% with various gastropexy procedures.

MISCELLANEOUS

ASSOCIATED CONDITIONS
N/A

AGE-RELATED FACTORS
N/A

ZOONOTIC POTENTIAL
N/A

PREGNANCY
• No specific considerations aside from hemodynamic support • Associated hypoxia may be detrimental to the fetuses.

SYNONYMS
• Bloat • Gastric dilation—volvulus • Gastric torsion

SEE ALSO
• Shock • Sepsis and Bacteremia

ABBREVIATION
GDV = gastric dilation and volvulus syndrome

Suggested Reading
Guilford WG. Gastric dilatation, gastric dilatation-volvulus, and chronic gastric volvulus. In: Guilford WG, Center SA, Stombeck DR, et al., eds. Strombeck's small animal gastroenterology. 3rd ed. Philadelphia: Saunders, 1996:303–317.
Matthiesen DT. Gastric dilation-volvulus syndrome. In: Slatter D, ed. Textbook of small animal surgery. 2nd ed. Philadelphia: Lea & Febiger, 1993:580–593.
Matthiesen DT. Pathophysiology of gastric dilatation volvulus. In: Bojrab MJ, ed. Disease mechanisms in small animal surgery. 2nd ed. Philadelphia: Lea & Febiger, 1993: 220–231.
Schertel ER, Allen DA, Muir WW, et al. Evaluation of a hypertonic saline-dextran solution for treatment of dogs with shock induced by gastric dilatation-volvulus. J Am Vet Med Assoc 1997;210:226–230.
Author Michelle Joy Waschak
Consulting Editor Albert E. Jergens

GASTRIC OR GASTROINTESTINAL MOTILITY DISORDERS

BASICS

DEFINITION
Gastric motility disorders result from conditions that directly or indirectly disrupt normal gastric emptying, which in turn may cause abnormal gastric retention, gastric distention, and subsequent gastric signs associated with anorexia, nausea, and vomiting.

PATHOPHYSIOLOGY
The stomach has two distinct motor regions. The proximal region relaxes to accommodate food and regulates expulsion of liquids. Intrinsic slow contractions of this region push liquids through the pylorus. The distal stomach mechanically breaks down and expels solids through strong peristaltic contractions. Distal gastric motility and emptying are regulated by a gastric pacemaker, an area of intrinsic electrical activity found in the greater curvature. Gastric electrical activity, dietary composition, and extrinsic factors all influence emptying. During fasting, indigestible solids are expelled from the stomach by migrating myoelectric complexes. These complexes produce strong contractions that sweep through the stomach and intestine every 2 hours in the fasted state. This motility is under the regulation of the hormone motilin. Dysrhythmias in normal gastric electrical activity may be fundamental in the pathophysiology of disorders affecting gastric motility.

SYSTEM AFFECTED
Gastrointestinal

GENETICS
N/A

INCIDENCE AND PREVALENCE
Unknown. Many factors can alter gastric emptying although they may not result in clinical disease.

GEOGRAPHIC DISTRIBUTION
N/A

SIGNALMENT

Species
Dogs and cats

Breed Predilections
Unknown

Mean Age and Range
Symptoms occur at any age though it is uncommon to observe primary motility disorders in young animals.

Predominant Sex
N/A

SIGNS

General Comments
Clinical signs are often secondary to the primary etiology causing the gastric motility disorder.

Historical Findings
• The major clinical sign is chronic postprandial vomiting of food. The stomach should be empty after an average size meal in approximately 6–8 hours (cats 4–6 hours). Vomiting of undigested food greater than 10 hours following the meal suggests a gastric motility disorder or outflow obstruction. Vomiting can occur, however, anytime following eating.
• Other signs include gastric distention, nausea, anorexia, belching, pica, and weight loss.

Physical Examination Findings
• Normal or findings associated with the underlying cause of the disorder
• Palpation of a large, distended stomach
• Decreased gastric sounds on abdominal auscultation

CAUSES
• Primary idiopathic gastric motility disorders may arise from defects in normal myoelectric activity. Most motility disorders occur secondary to other primary conditions.
• Metabolic disorders include hypokalemia, uremia, hepatic encephalopathy, and hypothyroidism.
• Nervous inhibition as the result of stress, fear, pain or trauma
• Drugs such as the anticholinergics, beta-adrenergic agonists, and narcotics
• Primary gastric disease such as outflow obstructions, gastritis, gastric ulcers, parvovirus, and gastric surgery
• Gastric dilatation-volvulus syndrome (GDV) is suspected to result from a primary motility disorder of abnormal myoelectric and mechanical activity. Dogs may continue to have signs of gastric hypomotility following surgical gastropexy.
• Gastroesophageal reflux and enterogastric reflux (see Bilious Vomiting Syndrome) may result from gastric hypomotility.
• Dysautonomia syndromes have gastric hypomotility as part of a generalized disease.

RISK FACTORS
Any potential gastric disease may result in secondary hypomotility.

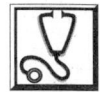

DIAGNOSIS

DIFFERENTIAL DIAGNOSIS
The differential diagnosis is extensive and should include any condition causing vomiting. Gastric outflow obstructions must always be ruled out.

CBC/BIOCHEMISTRY/URINALYSIS
Routine hemogram, serum chemistry profile, urinalysis, and fecal flotation must be performed to rule out the potential cause of gastric hypomotility. Continued vomiting may result in dehydration, electrolyte abnormalities, or acid-base imbalance. Hypokalemia is a common electrolyte abnormality associated with abnormal gastrointestinal motility.

OTHER LABORATORY TESTS
Specialized testing may be required to determine a specific cause of gastric hypomotility, and is individualized for each patient.

IMAGING

Survey Radiographs
Abdominal radiographs may reveal a gas-, fluid-, or ingesta-distended stomach.

Liquid Barium Contrast Study
May be evidence of delayed gastric emptying and decreased gastric contractions if evaluated using fluoroscopy. Some cases may have normal emptying of liquids but abnormal emptying of solids.

Food Barium Contrast Study
Barium mixed with a standard meal may demonstrate delayed gastric emptying of solids. Normal patients should empty their stomachs by approximately 6–8 hours. Abnormal gastric retention is associated with longer gastric emptying times.

Food-marker Contrast Study
Barium-impregnated small markers (Bips®) or other radiopaque markers mixed with a standard meal will have delayed passage similar to the food barium contrast study.

Radionuclide Emission Imaging
Radionuclide markers mixed with a meal give the most clinically accurate measurement of emptying. Gastric emptying times (time for a standard meal to leave the stomach) ranges from 4–8 hours.

Ultrasonography
Ultrasound can be used to evaluate antral and pyloric motility.

DIAGNOSTIC PROCEDURES

Endoscopy
Endoscopic findings are frequently normal in idiopathic conditions. Food may be found in the stomach when it should be empty following a 10–12 hour pre-endoscopic fasting period. Endoscopy will detect obstructive or inflammatory diseases of the stomach.

PATHOLOGIC FINDINGS
Idiopathic conditions have normal gastric mucosa. Histology may identify inflammatory or neoplastic causes of gastric hypomotility.

GASTRIC OR GASTROINTESTINAL MOTILITY DISORDERS

TREATMENT

APPROPRIATE HEALTH CARE
Most patients are treated as outpatients. With severe vomiting or dehydration and electrolyte imbalance, hospitalization and specific therapy are required.

NURSING CARE
Dehydration with fluid and electrolyte imbalance requires appropriate fluid replacement.

ACTIVITY
Restrictions are based on the underlying disease.

DIET
• Dietary manipulation is important in the management of primary gastric motility disorders.
• Diets should be formulated that are liquid or a semi-liquid consistency and low in fat and fiber content.
• Small-volume meals with frequent feeding should be given.
• Often dietary manipulation alone is successful in managing patients with delayed gastric emptying from a motility disorder.

CLIENT EDUCATION
Discuss possible underlying etiologies of altered gastric motility and that the response to therapy will vary with individual cases.

SURGICAL CONSIDERATIONS
• Dogs with chronic GDV syndrome and gastric retention should have a surgical gastropexy.
• Following any gastric surgery it may take as long as 14 days for motility to return to normal.
• Patients with gastric outflow obstructions require surgical correction.

MEDICATIONS

DRUGS(S) OF CHOICE

Gastric Prokinetic Agents
• Metoclopramide (Reglan) increases the amplitude of antral contractions, inhibits fundic receptive relaxation, and coordinates duodenal and gastric motility. It also has antiemetic effects, blocking the chemoreceptor trigger zone in the brain stem in dogs but not cats. Oral dosage is 0.2–0.4 mg/kg q6–8h given 30 minutes before meals (use lower dose in cats). Metoclopramide is considered to be a weak prokinetic agent.
• Cisapride (Propulsid) works directly by cholinergic neurotransmission of gastrointestinal smooth muscle, stimulating motility. Cisapride increases lower esophageal sphincter pressure, improves gastric emptying, and promotes increased motility of both the small and large intestine. A suggested dose is 0.1 mg/kg PO q8–12h given before meals. Cisapride has recently been taken off the market but is still available through compounding pharmacies. Newer prokinetic agent tegaserod (Zelnorm 0.3 mg/kg q12h) has similar prokinetic effects as cisapride but there is as yet limited clinical experience in the dog and cat.
• Erythromycin given at low (sub-microbiologic) doses acts as a motilin agonist, promoting acetylcholine release, which in turn promotes gastric emptying. Suggested dose of erythromycin for specific motility effects is 0.5–1 mg/kg PO q8–12h, given 30 minutes before meals. Erythromycin appears to be more effective than metoclopramide.
• The H_2 receptor antagonists ranitidine (2 mg/kg q8h) and nizatidine (5 mg/kg q24h) have significant prokinetic effects on gastric motility similar to cisapride. Neither cimetidine nor famotidine affects gastric emptying.

CONTRAINDICATIONS
Gastric prokinetic agents should not be administered in patients having a gastric outflow obstruction. Metoclopramide is contraindicated with concurrent phenothiazine and narcotic administration or in animals with epilepsy.

PRECAUTIONS
• Metoclopramide may cause nervousness, anxiety, or depression.
• Cisapride may cause depression, vomiting, diarrhea, or abdominal cramping.
• Erythromycin may cause vomiting.

POSSIBLE INTERACTIONS
N/A

ALTERNATIVE DRUG(S)
N/A

FOLLOW-UP

PATIENT MONITORING
Response to therapy varies according to the underlying cause. Failure to respond medically necessitates further investigation for mechanical obstruction.

PREVENTION/AVOIDANCE
N/A

POSSIBLE COMPLICATIONS
N/A

EXPECTED COURSE AND PROGNOSIS
• The length of treatment depends on ability to resolve the underlying disorder or on the response to therapy. • It may take gastric surgery or parvovirus cases 10 to 14 days to regain normal gastric function. • Generalized dysautonomia has a grave prognosis.

MISCELLANEOUS

ASSOCIATED CONDITIONS
Gastric hypomotility may be associated with both reflux esophagitis and reflux gastritis (bilious vomiting syndrome).

AGE-RELATED FACTORS
N/A

ZOONOTIC POTENTIAL
N/A

PREGNANCY
Avoid gastric prokinetic agents in pregnant animals.

SYNONYMS
• Gastric hypomotility
• Gastric atony

SEE ALSO
• Bilious Vomiting Syndrome
• Gastric Dilatation and Volvulus Syndrome
• Gastritis, Atrophic
• Gastritis, Chronic
• Gastroesophageal Reflux

ABBREVIATIONS
GDV= Gastric dilatation-volvulus syndrome

Suggested Reading

Hall JA. Diseases of the stomach. In: Ettinger SJ, Feldman EC, eds. Textbook of veterinary internal medicine, 5th ed. Philadelphia: Saunders, 2000;1154–1181.

Hall JA, Burrows CF, Twedt DC. Gastric motility in dogs. Part 1. Normal gastric function. Comp Small Anim 1988; 10:1282–1291.

Hall JA, Twedt DC, Burrows CF. Gastric motility in dogs. Part 2. Disorders of gastric motility. Comp Small Anim 1990; 12:1373–1390.

Hall JA, Washabau RJ. Diagnosis and treatment of gastric motility disorders. Vet Clin North Am Small Anim Pract 1999; 29:377–395.

Twedt DC. Diseases of the stomach. The cat diseases and clinical management. 2nd ed. New York: Churchill Livingstone, 1994; 1181–1210.

Wise LA, Lappin MR: Canine dysautonomia. Semin Vet Med Surg (Sm Anim) 5:72, 1990

Author David C. Twedt
Consulting Editor Albert E. Jergens

GASTRITIS, ATROPHIC

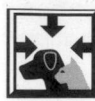 BASICS

OVERVIEW
A class of chronic gastritis characterized histologically by a focal or diffuse reduction in size and depth of gastric glands

SIGNALMENT
• Probably highly variable
• Not reported in cats
• A high prevalence reported in the Norwegian lundehunde

SIGNS
• Vomiting—usually intermittent
• Anorexia, lethargy, pica, weight loss

CAUSES & RISK FACTORS
• Unknown
• May reflect chronic gastritis due to any cause

• Immunization of dogs with their own gastric juice can induce chronic gastritis.
• *Helicobacter* spp. may be important in the development of canine and feline gastritis.
• May be a genetic predisposition in the Norwegian lundehunde

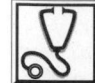 DIAGNOSIS

DIFFERENTIAL DIAGNOSIS
Other forms of chronic gastritis and chronic enteritis

CBC/BIOCHEMISTRY/URINALYSIS
Generally unremarkable

OTHER LABORATORY TESTS
N/A

IMAGING
Survey radiographs, contrast radiography, and ultrasonography are useful only to rule out other causes of chronic vomiting.

DIAGNOSTIC PROCEDURES
• Definitive diagnosis via gastroscopy and biopsy
• Gastroscopy may reveal prominent mucosal blood vessels caused by mucosal thinning.

PATHOLOGIC FINDINGS
• Histologic examination of gastric biopsy specimens reveals glandular atrophy.
• Urease activity in gastric biopsy specimens indicates infection with *Helicobacter* spp.

 TREATMENT

• Typically, outpatient medical treatment
• Dietary elimination studies—warranted if underlying dietary sensitivity is suspected

MEDICATIONS

DRUG(S)
• Histamine type-2 receptor antagonists (e.g., famotidine 0.5 mg/kg PO q12–24h) or proton pump inhibitors (e.g., omeprazole 0.7 mg/kg PO q24h) to inhibit gastric acid secretion
• Antibiotic treatment (e.g., amoxicillin at 10–20 mg/kg PO q12h for 3 weeks) if infection with *Helicobacter* spp. is confirmed.
• If vomiting persists, prokinetic agents such as metoclopramide (0.2–0.5 mg/kg PO q8h) or cisapride (0.1–0.5 mg/kg PO q8–12h) may be indicated.

CONTRAINDICATIONS/POSSIBLE INTERACTIONS
Be cautious with medications known to exacerbate gastritis, such as corticosteroids and nonsteroidal antiinflammatory drugs.

FOLLOW-UP
• Long-term intermittent antacid therapy may be required.
• Associated with a high prevalence of gastric carcinoma in the Norwegian lundehunde.

MISCELLANEOUS
With severe atrophy, gastric acid secretion may be impaired; this will likely be a subclinical abnormality.

ASSOCIATED CONDITIONS
Chronic enteritis

SEE ALSO
• Gastritis, chronic
• Vomiting, chronic

Suggested Reading
Twedt DC. Vomiting. In: Anderson NV, ed. Veterinary gastroenterology. Philadelphia: Lea & Febiger, 1992:336–367.
Williams DA, Melgarejo T. Gastroenteropathy in Norwegian Lundehunds in the USA. J Vet Int Med 1997;11:114.
Author David A. Williams
Consulting Editor Albert E. Jergens

GASTRITIS, CHRONIC

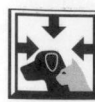 BASICS

DEFINITION
• Intermittent vomiting of >1–2 weeks duration secondary to gastric inflammation
• Presence of gastric erosions or ulcers dependent on the inciting cause and duration

PATHOPHYSIOLOGY
• Chronic irritation of the gastric mucosa by chemical irritants, drugs, foreign bodies, infectious agents, or hyperacidity syndromes resulting in an inflammatory response in the mucosal surface that may extend to involve submucosal layers
• Chronic allergen exposure or immune-mediated disease may also produce chronic inflammation.

SYSTEMS AFFECTED
• Gastrointestinal—esophagitis may result from chronic vomiting or gastroesophageal reflux.
• Respiratory—aspiration pneumonia is infrequently seen secondary to chronic vomiting; it is more likely if concurrent esophageal disease exists or if patient is debilitated.

GENETICS
N/A

INCIDENCE/PREVALENCE
Relatively common

GEOGRAPHIC DISTRIBUTION
N/A

SIGNALMENT
Species
Dogs and cats

Breed Predilections
• Old, small-breed dogs (i.e., Lhasa apso, shih tzu, miniature poodle) are more commonly affected with antral mucosal hyperplasia and hypertrophy.
• Basenjis and the Drentse patrijshond breed can develop chronic hypertrophic gastritis.

Mean Age and Range
Varies with underlying cause

Predominant Sex
Varies with underlying cause

SIGNS
Historical Findings
• Vomit is frequently bile stained and may contain undigested food, flecks of blood, or digested blood ("coffee grounds").
• Frequency varies from daily to every few weeks and increases as gastritis progresses.
• Vomiting may be stimulated by eating or drinking.

• Early morning vomiting before eating may indicate bilious vomiting syndrome.
• May see weight loss with chronic anorexia
• May see melena with ulceration
• Diarrhea

Physical Examination Findings
• Often normal
• May be thin with persistent anorexia
• May have pale mucous membranes with anemia from chronic blood loss

CAUSES
• Inflammatory—immune-mediated, dietary allergy or intolerance, idiopathic
• Dietary indiscretion—plant material, foreign objects, chemical irritants
• Toxins—fertilizers, herbicides, cleaning agents, heavy metals
• Metabolic/endocrine disease—uremia, chronic liver disease, hypoadrenocorticism
• Neoplastic—gastrinoma
• Parasitism—*Ollulanus tricuspis* and *Gnathostoma* spp. (cats); *Physaloptera* spp. (dogs)
• Drugs—NSAIDs, glucocorticoids
• Infectious—*Helicobacter* spp., viral (distemper in dogs, feline leukemias virus [FeLV] in cats)
• Miscellaneous—duodenogastric reflux (bilious vomiting syndrome), stress, achlorhydria

RISK FACTORS
• Medications—NSAIDs, glucocorticoids
• Environmental—unsupervised/free-roaming pets are more likely to ingest inappropriate foods or materials, intentionally or unintentionally.
• Ingestion of a dietary antigen to which an allergy or intolerance has been acquired

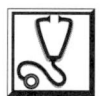 DIAGNOSIS

DIFFERENTIAL DIAGNOSIS
• Must differentiate chronic vomiting from chronic regurgitation
• Small intestinal inflammation and gastric or small intestinal neoplasia often present with signs and physical exam findings similar to those of gastric inflammation.
• All the causes listed above are included in the differential diagnosis of chronic gastritis; commonly no identifiable cause exists for the gastric inflammation.
• Idiopathic gastritis—diagnosis of exclusion; often characterized by a predominantly lymphoplasmacytic infiltrate (superficial or diffuse)
• Eosinophilic gastritis, hypertrophic gastritis, granulomatous/histiocytic gastritis, and atro-

phic gastritis are less common; often overlap of histologic changes exists in the types of inflammatory infiltrates.
• Atrophic gastritis differs on endoscopic examination—visualization of the submucosal vessels secondary to thinning of the gastric mucosa
• Hypertrophic gastritis—prominent mucosal folds that do not flatten with gastric insufflation

CBC/BIOCHEMISTRY/URINALYSIS
• Hemogram usually unremarkable unless systemic disease present
• Hemoconcentration if severe dehydration
• With ulceration—microcytic, hypochromic anemia associated with iron deficiency if prolonged, severe blood loss
• May see eosinophilia with eosinophilic gastroenteritis
• Azotemia with low urine specific gravity in uremic gastritis
• Increased serum hepatic enzyme activities, total bilirubin, or hypoalbuminemia with chronic hepatic disease
• Hyperkalemia and hyponatremia suggest Addison's disease.
• Hyponatremia, hypokalemia, hypochloremia, and an elevated bicarbonate level with an acidotic urine suggest a gastric outflow obstruction (hypochloremic metabolic alkalosis).

OTHER LABORATORY TESTS
Elevated serum gastrin level without azotemia suggests a gastrinoma.

IMAGING
• Survey abdominal radiographs—usually normal, but may reveal radiodense foreign objects, a thickened gastric wall, or gastric outlet obstruction with persistent gastric distension
• Contrast radiography—may detect foreign objects, gastric outlet obstruction, delayed gastric emptying, or gastric wall defects or thickening
• Ultrasonography—may detect gastric wall thickening and gastric foreign objects

DIAGNOSTIC PROCEDURES
• Gastroscopy—usually adequate for visualization of the gastric mucosa and for biopsy
• Gastric biopsy and histopathology is required for diagnosis; should biopsy, even if gastric mucosa appears normal
• Foreign objects can be identified and retrieved via endoscopy.
• Exploratory celiotomy is indicated if a perforated ulcer or submucosal lesion of the gastric wall is suspected and partial gastrectomy or full-thickness biopsy is required.
• Fecal flotation may reveal intestinal parasites

PATHOLOGIC FINDINGS
• Idiopathic gastritis—inflammatory infiltrates vary; can be lymphocytes, plasma cells, neutrophils, eosinophils, and/or histiocytes
• Mucosal changes can be degenerative, hyperplastic, or atrophic.
• May be varying levels of edema and fibrous tissue; may be *Helicobacter* spp.; special stains can be requested for fungal hyphae
• If hyperplastic changes are noted, a gastrin level should be obtained before institution or after discontinuation of antacids, H_2 blockers, or proton pump blockers.

TREATMENT

APPROPRIATE HEALTH CARE
• Most patients are stable at presentation unless vomiting is severe enough to cause dehydration.
• Can typically manage as outpatient, pending diagnostic testing or undergoing clinical trials of special diets or medications
• If patient is dehydrated or if vomiting becomes severe, hospitalize and institute appropriate intravenous crystalloid fluid therapy (see Vomiting, Acute).

NURSING CARE
N/A

ACTIVITY
N/A

DIET
• NPO for 12–24 hr if vomiting frequently
• Soft, low-fat food ideally from a single carbohydrate and protein source
• Non-fat cottage cheese, skinless white meat chicken, or tofu as a protein source, and rice, pasta, or potato as a carbohydrate source, in a ratio of 1:3
• Frequent, small meals
• Can use novel protein source or hydrolyzed protein diet if dietary allergy is suspected
• Feed diets for a minimum of 3 weeks to assess adequacy of response.

CLIENT EDUCATION
• Gastritis has numerous causes.
• Diagnostic workup—may be extensive; usually requires a biopsy for a definitive diagnosis

SURGICAL CONSIDERATIONS
• Surgical management if a granulomatous mass or hypertrophy is causing a gastric outflow obstruction
• Gastrotomy for removal of foreign objects if endoscopic retrieval is unsuccessful or is not available

MEDICATIONS

DRUG(S) OF CHOICE
• Treat any gastric erosions and ulcers (see Gastroduodenal Ulcer Disease).
• Give glucocorticoids (prednisone 1–2 mg/kg PO q12h; taper every 2–3 weeks over 2–3 months) for chronic gastritis secondary to suspected immune-mediated mechanisms if no clinical response to dietary management.
• Antiemetics for fluid and electrolyte disorders caused by frequent or profuse vomiting (see Vomiting, Acute)
• Metoclopramide (0.4 mg/kg PO q6–8h), cisapride (0.5–1 mg/kg PO q8h), or low-dose erythromycin (0.5–1 mg/kg PO q8h) to increase gastric emptying and normalize intestinal motility if gastric emptying is delayed or gastroduodenal reflux is present

CONTRAINDICATIONS
• Do not use prokinetics, metoclopramide, or cisapride if gastric outlet obstruction is present.
• Antacids are not indicated with atrophic gastritis and achlorhydria.

PRECAUTIONS
Steroids are immunosuppressive, making close monitoring for secondary infections important. Steroids may also inhibit the normal gastric mucosal barrier, leading to ulceration.

POSSIBLE INTERACTIONS
N/A

ALTERNATIVE DRUG(S)
• Synthetic prostaglandin E (misoprostol 1–3 μg/kg PO q6–8h) to prevent gastric mucosal ulcers with NSAID toxicity
• Immunosuppressive drugs such as azathioprine (50 mg/M² PO q24h, tapering to every other day after 2–3 weeks) if an immune-mediated mechanism is suspected and response to dietary management and glucocorticoid administration is inadequate

FOLLOW-UP

PATIENT MONITORING
• Resolution of clinical signs indicates a positive response.
• Electrolytes and acid–base status if initially abnormal
• Complete blood counts should be obtained initially at 3-week intervals for patients on myelosuppressive drugs (i.e., azathioprine)
• Repeat biopsy if signs decrease but do not resolve.

PREVENTION/AVOIDANCE
• Avoid medications (e.g., corticosteroids, NSAIDs) and foods that cause gastric irritation or allergic response in the patient.
• Prevent free roaming and potential for dietary indiscretion.

POSSIBLE COMPLICATIONS
• Progression of gastritis from superficial to atrophic gastritis
• Gastric erosions and ulcers with progressive mucosal damage
• Aspiration pneumonia
• Electrolyte or acid–base imbalances

EXPECTED COURSE AND PROGNOSIS
Varies with underlying cause

MISCELLANEOUS

ASSOCIATED CONDITIONS
N/A

AGE-RELATED FACTORS
Young animals are more likely to ingest foreign objects.

ZOONOTIC POTENTIAL
N/A

PREGNANCY
Do not administer misoprostol to pregnant animals.

SYNONYMS
N/A

SEE ALSO
• Gastritis, Atrophic
• Gastroduodenal Ulcer Disease
• Gastroenteritis, Eosinophilic
• Gastroenteritis, Lymphocytic-Plasmacytic
• Hypertrophic Pyloric Gastropathy, Chronic
• Physalopterosis
• Vomiting, Chronic

ABBREVIATIONS
• FeLV = feline leukemia virus
• NPO = nothing per os
• NSAIDs = nonsteroidal antiinflammatory drugs

Suggested Reading

Guilford WG, Strombeck DR. Chronic gastric diseases. In: Guilford WG, Center SA, Strombeck DR, et al., eds. Small animal gastroenterology. Philadelphia: Saunders, 1996:275–302.

Hall JA. Diseases of the stomach. In: Ettinger SJ, Feldman EC, eds., Textbook of veterinary internal medicine. Philadelphia: Saunders, 2000:1154–1181.

Author John Richard Hart, Jr.
Consulting Editor Albert E. Jergens

GASTRODUODENAL ULCER DISEASE

 BASICS

DEFINITION
Gastroduodenal ulcers are lesions that extend through the mucosa and into the muscularis mucosae.

PATHOPHYSIOLOGY
• Gastroduodenal ulcers result from single or multiple factors altering, damaging, or overwhelming the normal defense and repair mechanisms of the gastric mucosal barrier. • Factors that comprise the gastric mucosal barrier and protect the stomach from ulcer formation include the mucous-bicarbonate layer over the epithelial cells, the gastric epithelial cells, gastric mucosal blood flow, epithelial cell restitution and repair, and prostaglandins produced by the gastrointestinal tract. • Factors that cause mucosal barrier damage and predispose to gastroduodenal ulcer formation include inhibition of the epithelial cells' ability to repair themselves, decrease in the mucosal blood supply, and/or increase in gastric acid secretion. • The risk of gastroduodenal ulcer formation increases with the number of insults to the gastric mucosal barrier.

SYSTEMS AFFECTED
• Gastrointestinal—gastric fundus and antrum are most common sites of ulceration; gastrinomas (rare) usually cause ulcer formation in the proximal duodenum • Cardiovascular/ hemic— acute hemorrhage may result in anemia and subsequent tachycardia, systolic heart murmur, and/or hypotension • Respiratory—rarely, aspiration pneumonia secondary to vomiting; tachypnea may be present with anemia

INCIDENCE/PREVALENCE
True incidence unknown, but probably more common than clinically recognized

GEOGRAPHIC DISTRIBUTION
Pythiosis has a regional distribution—states that border the Gulf of Mexico

SIGNALMENT
Species
Dogs and, less commonly, cats
Mean Age and Range
All ages
Predominant Sex
Male dogs have increased incidence of gastric carcinoma.

SIGNS
General Comments
Some animals may be asymptomatic despite significant gastroduodenal ulcer disease.
Historical Findings
• Vomiting: most common clinical sign • Hematemesis may be present. • Melena may be present. • Cranial abdominal pain—patient may stand hunched in the back or assume the "praying position." • Anorexia • Weakness, pallor, lethargy, and/or collapse if severe anemia or perforation/peritonitis develops

Physical Examination Findings
• Pale mucous membranes and weakness if significant anemia is present • Weight loss and cachexia if disease is chronic • Systolic heart murmur if anemia is acute and severe • Tachycardia, hypotension, and prolonged capillary refill time if hypovolemic shock or perforation and septic peritonitis; hyperthermia and abdominal distention may be present with perforation and septic peritonitis • Edema—from blood/plasma loss causing hypoproteinemia • May be cutaneous or subcutaneous mass, splenomegaly, and/or hepatomegaly if mast cell disease • May be icterus if liver disease • May be oral ulceration and uremic breath if renal failure

CAUSES
Drugs
NSAIDS, glucocorticoids
Gastrointestinal Diseases
• Inflammatory bowel disease • Oral, esophageal, gastric, or duodenal neoplasia • Oral, esophageal, gastric, or duodenal foreign body • Correction of chronic diaphragmatic hernia
Infectious Diseases
• Gastrointestinal parasitism • Pythiosis • *Helicobacter* infection • Viral, fungal, or bacterial gastroenteritis
Metabolic Diseases
• Renal failure • Liver failure • Hypoadrenocorticism • Pancreatitis
Neoplasia
• Mastocytosis • Gastrinoma
Neurologic Diseases
• Head trauma • Spinal cord disease
Stress/Major Medical Illness
• Sepsis • Shock • Severe illness • Burns • Heat stroke • Major surgery • Trauma • Hypotension • Thromboembolic disease
RISK FACTORS
• Administration of ulcerogenic drugs—NSAIDs or glucocorticoids • Critically ill patients • Hypovolemic or septic shock

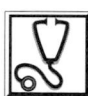 DIAGNOSIS

DIFFERENTIAL DIAGNOSIS
• Esophageal disease (neoplasia, esophagitis, foreign body)—differentiate by radiography, contrast radiography, and/or endoscopy • Thrombocytopenia (immune mediated, paraneoplastic, infectious)—identified on complete blood cell count • Coagulopathies (DIC, anticoagulant rodenticide poisoning)—detected by coagulation panel • Hemoptysis—physical examination findings may differentiate hemoptysis from hematemesis; thoracic radiographs may reveal presence of airway or pulmonary disease • Regurgitation or vomiting of swallowed blood from extra gastrointestinal diseases (e.g., oropharyngeal, nasopharyngeal, cutaneous, urogenital tract, and anal sac disease)—physical examination findings may differentiate; may need observation of patient for ingestion of blood

and thorough examination with or without imaging under sedation or anesthesia • Administration of oral iron may stain vomitus; Pepto-Bismol may cause black and tarry stools.

CBC/BIOCHEMISTRY/URINALYSIS
• If acute (3–5 days) blood loss, nonregenerative anemia (normocytic, normochromic, minimal reticulocytosis) • If blood loss > 5 days duration—regenerative anemia (macrocytic, hyperchromic, reticulocytosis) • If chronic blood loss—iron deficiency anemia (microcytic, hypochromic, poor reticulocytosis, with or without thrombocytopenia) • May be thrombocytopenia • May be panhypoproteinemia with alimentary hemorrhage • May be mature neutrophilia or left shift neutrophilia with sepsis and/or gastroduodenal ulcer perforation • Blood urea nitrogen (BUN):creatinine ratio may be elevated with gastrointestinal hemorrhage • Elevated BUN and creatinine, and hyperphosphatemia and isosthenuria if ulcers due to renal failure • High liver enzymes, hyperbilirubinemia, and/or hypoalbuminemia if ulcers due to liver disease or failure • Hyperkalemia, hyponatremia, and azotemia if ulcers due to hypoadrenocorticism—atypical hypoadrenocorticism will not have electrolyte abnormalities • Elevated lipase and amylase may be present if ulcers are due to pancreatitis

OTHER LABORATORY TESTS
• Fecal occult blood test may be positive—test is accurate if dog is eating dry food • Fecal flotation—to screen for gastrointestinal parasitism • Bile acids—if liver disease is suspected • ACTH stimulation—if hypoadrenocorticism is suspected • Buffy coat—if systemic mast cell disease is suspected • Gastrin levels—if more common causes excluded

IMAGING
• Abdominal radiography may identify a gastric or duodenal foreign body or mass, pancreatitis, or changes consistent with kidney or liver disease. • Contrast radiography (preferably double-contrast gastrogram) may identify a gastroduodenal ulcer or neoplastic disease. • Thoracic radiographs may reveal pulmonary metastasis. • Abdominal ultrasonography may identify a gastric or duodenal mass, gastric or duodenal wall thickening, gastroduodenal ulcer, and/or abdominal lymphadenopathy.

DIAGNOSTIC PROCEDURES
• Endoscopy—most definitive method for diagnosing; allows removal of foreign bodies and collection of biopsy specimens from the gastric and/or duodenal ulcerations • If an infectious etiology is suspected, submit biopsies for culture. • If abdominal ultrasonography shows the presence of a gastric or duodenal mass or gastroduodenal wall thickening, an abdominal ultrasound-guided biopsy can also be obtained. Occasionally the ultrasound-guided gastroduodenal biopsy may yield different or additional information compared with that from endoscopic biopsies. • Abdominocentesis may be used to identify septic peritonitis and gastro-

duodenal ulcer perforation. • Urease testing of gastric biopsy specimens may reveal *Helicobacter* organisms. • Pythiosis—requires biopsies; samples should be submitted unrefrigerated in saline for culture and in formalin for histopathology with special stains; serologic testing and PCR-based assay are available • Obtain fine-needle aspirates or biopsy specimens of cutaneous or intraabdominal masses to identify mast cell tumor.

PATHOLOGIC FINDINGS
• Gastroduodenal inflammation and hemorrhage • Ulcers may have more necrosis, microthrombi, and hemorrhage and have deeper penetration than do erosions • May identify *Helicobacter* spp. in gastric biopsies • May need special stains to identify presence of pythiosis

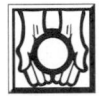
TREATMENT

APPROPRIATE HEALTH CARE
• Treat any underlying causes • Treat on an outpatient basis if the cause is identified and removed, vomiting is not excessive, and gastroduodenal bleeding is minimal. • Inpatients—those with severe gastroduodenal bleeding and/or ulcer perforation, excessive vomiting, and/or undetermined cause • May need emergency management of hemorrhage or septic peritonitis

NURSING CARE
• Intravenous fluids to maintain hydration, gastric mucosal perfusion, and/or treatment of shock • May need transfusions (whole blood or packed red blood cells) or oxygen-carrying hemoglobin solution infusions in patients with severe gastroduodenal hemorrhage • Severe hypoproteinemic patients may require colloids and/or plasma to increase vascular oncotic pressure. • In severe cases of hematemesis—to stop the gastrointestinal bleeding, ice water lavage (10–20 mL/kg remaining in stomach for 15–30 minutes) or lavage with norepi-nephrine (8 mg/500 mL) diluted in ice water can be attempted

ACTIVITY
Restricted

DIET
• Discontinue oral intake if vomiting.
• When feeding is resumed, feed small amounts in multiple feedings: low fat and fiber diet with primarily an easily digestible starch, such as rice.
• Protein should be added gradually to the diet in small amounts, and it is preferable that it be a vegetable (tofu) or milk protein (low fat cottage cheese).

CLIENT EDUCATION
• NSAIDs should be administered to pets only under the guidance of a veterinarian.
• Administration of NSAIDs can result in gastroduodenal ulcerations and perforations.
• Adverse effects of NSAIDs can be reduced by giving drug with food and concurrent adminis-

tration of a synthetic prostaglandin analogue (e.g., misoprostol).

SURGICAL CONSIDERATIONS
Surgical treatment is indicated if medical treatment fails after 5–7 days, hemorrhage is uncontrolled and severe, gastroduodenal ulcer perforates, and/or potentially resectable tumor is identified.

MEDICATIONS

DRUG(S) OF CHOICE
• Histamine (H_2) receptor antagonists competitively inhibit gastric acid secretion and are the initial drug of choice (cimetidine 5–10 mg/kg PO, SC, IV q8h, ranitidine 1–4 mg/kg SC, PO, IV q8–12h, famotidine 0.5 mg/kg PO, IV q12–24h). Treat for at least 6–8 weeks.
• Antacids neutralize gastric acid but must be given at least six times per day to be effective.
• Sucralfate suspension (0.5–1 g PO q8h) protects ulcerated tissue (cytoprotection) by binding to ulcer sites. • Antibiotic(s) with activity against enteric gram-negative and anaerobes parenterally if a break in gastrointestinal mucosal barrier is suspected or aspiration pneumonia is present • Antiemetics (chlorpromazine 0.5–4 mg/kg q6–8h SC, IM, IV; prochlorperazine 0.1–0.5 mg/kg q6–8h SC, IM, IV, PO) are administered if vomiting occurs frequently or results in significant fluid losses.
• Omeprazole (0.7 mg/kg PO q24h)—most potent inhibitor of gastric acid secretion; treatment of choice for gastrinomas with evidence of metastasis or nonresectable disease
• Appropriate therapy (metronidazole, colloidal bismuth, tetracycline, or amoxicillin) if *Helicobacter* spp. infection

CONTRAINDICATIONS
Do not administer phenothiazine derivatives to hypovolemic patients or those at risk for hypotension.

POSSIBLE INTERACTIONS
• Cimetidine binds to hepatic cytochrome P-450 enzyme and may interfere with metabolism of other drugs. • H_2 blockers prevent uptake of omeprazole by oxyntic cells. • Sucralfate may alter absorption of other drugs.

ALTERNATIVE DRUG(S)
Misoprostol, synthetic prostaglandin analogue (2–5 μg/kg PO q8–12h), prevents or decreases severity of NSAID-induced ulcers.

FOLLOW-UP

PATIENT MONITORING
• Improvement in some cases may be assessed on resolution of clinical signs; can use the packed cell volume, total protein, fecal occult blood, and BUN to detect continued blood loss. • Repeat endoscopic evaluation is recommended for advanced cases to help determine

duration of therapy. • Depending on the underlying cause, specific laboratory or imaging tests may be necessary to monitor response to therapy.

PREVENTION/AVOIDANCE
• Avoid gastric irritants (e.g., NSAIDs, corticosteroids). • Concurrent use of misoprostol with NSAIDs • Administer NSAIDs with food.

POSSIBLE COMPLICATIONS
• Severe blood loss requiring transfusion
• Sepsis • Ulcer perforation • Death secondary to ulcer perforation, sepsis, hemorrhage
• Aspiration pneumonia—rare

EXPECTED COURSE AND PROGNOSIS
• Varies with underlying causes • Patients with malignant gastric neoplasia, renal failure, liver failure, pythiosis, systemic mastocytosis, sepsis, and/or gastric perforation—prognosis is poor.
• Gastroduodenal ulcers secondary to NSAID administration, *Helicobacter* infection, inflammatory bowel disease, or hypoadrenocorticism—prognosis may be good to excellent, depending on severity of disease

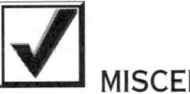
MISCELLANEOUS

ASSOCIATED CONDITIONS
Anemia

AGE-RELATED FACTORS
Neoplasia more common in older animals

ZOONOTIC POTENTIAL
Zoonotic potential of *Helicobacter* spp. is controversial.

PREGNANCY
Synthetic prostaglandins (e.g., misoprostol) cause abortion.

SEE ALSO
• Gastritis, Chronic • *Helicobacter*
• Hematemesis • Inflammatory Bowel Disease
• Melena • Pancreatitis • Pythiosis • Vomiting, Acute • Vomiting, Chronic

ABBREVIATIONS
• ACTH = adrenocorticotropic hormone
• DIC = disseminated intravascular coagulation
• NSAIDs = nonsteroidal antiinflammatory drugs • PCR = polymerase chain reaction

Suggested Reading
Guilford WG, Center SA, Strombeck DR, et al., eds. Strombeck's small animal gastroenterology. 3rd ed. Philadelphia: Saunders, 1996.
Washabau R. Acute gastrointestinal hemorrhage. Part I. Compend Contin Educ Pract Vet 1996;18:1317–1325.
Washabau R. Acute gastrointestinal hemorrhage. Part II. Compend Contin Educ Pract Vet 1996;18:1327–1337.
Author Jocelyn Mott
Consulting Editor Albert E. Jergens

GASTROENTERITIS, EOSINOPHILIC

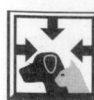

BASICS

DEFINITION
An inflammatory disease of the stomach and intestine, characterized by an infiltration of eosinophils, usually into the lamina propria, but occasionally involving the submucosa and muscularis

PATHOPHYSIOLOGY
• Antigens bind to IgE on the surface of mast cells, resulting in mast cell degranulation.
• Some of the products released are potent eosinophil chemotactants.
• Eosinophils contain granules with substances that directly damage the surrounding tissues.
• Eosinophils also can activate mast cells directly, setting up a vicious cycle of degranulation and tissue destruction.

SYSTEMS AFFECTED
• Gastrointestinal—the large intestine may also be affected.
• In the cat, hypereosinophilic syndrome can involve the gastrointestinal tract, liver, spleen, kidney, adrenal glands, and heart.

GENETICS
N/A

INCIDENCE/PREVALENCE
• Eosinophilic gastroenteritis is reportedly more common in dogs than in cats.
• Less common than lymphocytic-plasmacytic gastroenteritis; occasionally, a mixed cellular infiltrate is present.

GEOGRAPHIC DISTRIBUTION
N/A

SIGNALMENT
Species
Dog and cat

Breed Predilections
German shepherd, rottweiler, soft-coated wheaten terrier, and shar pei may be predisposed.

Mean Age and Range
• Dogs—most common in animals < 5 years of age, although any age may be affected
• Cats—median age, 8 years; range, 1.5–11 years reported

Predominant Sex
None reported

SIGNS

Historical Findings
• Intermittent vomiting, small bowel diarrhea, anorexia, and weight loss are the most common client complaints.
• One report states that 50% of cats with eosinophilic gastritis/enteritis had hematochezia or melena.

Physical Examination Findings
• Cats—thickened bowel loops may be palpated.
• May be evidence of weight loss
• If hypereosinophilic syndrome is the cause of the gastrointestinal disease, enlarged peripheral lymph nodes, mesenteric lymphadenopathy, hepatomegaly, and splenomegaly may be noted.

CAUSES
• Idiopathic eosinophilic gastroenteritis
• Parasitic
• Immune-mediated—food allergy; adverse drug reaction; associated with other forms of inflammatory bowel disease
• Systemic mastocytosis
• Hypereosinophilic syndrome
• Eosinophilic granuloma

RISK FACTORS
N/A

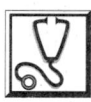

DIAGNOSIS

DIFFERENTIAL DIAGNOSIS
• All of the above-listed causes are included in the differential diagnosis of eosinophilic infiltrates in the stomach and small bowel.
• Idiopathic eosinophilic gastroenteritis is a diagnosis of exclusion.
• Multiple fecal flotations and direct smears are imperative to rule in or out intestinal parasitism.
• Intestinal biopsy differentiates the other causes of inflammatory bowel disease from eosinophilic gastroenteritis.
• Dietary trial will rule in or out food allergy or hypersensitivity.

CBC/BIOCHEMISTRY/URINALYSIS
• Hemogram may reveal a peripheral eosinophilia—more common in cats than dogs
• Panhypoproteinemia or hypoalbuminemia may be present if a protein-losing enteropathy is also present.
• Urinalysis is usually normal.

OTHER LABORATORY TESTS
Buffy-coat smear to rule out systemic mastocytosis

IMAGING
• Plain abdominal radiographs provide little information.
• Barium contrast radiography may demonstrate thick intestinal walls and mucosal irregularities but does not provide any information about etiology or the nature of the thickening.
• Ultrasonography—may be used to measure stomach and intestinal wall thickness, and to rule out other diseases; can be used to examine the liver, spleen, and mesenteric lymph nodes in cats with hypereosinophilic syndrome

DIAGNOSTIC PROCEDURES
• Definitive diagnosis requires biopsy and histopathology, usually obtained via endoscopy.
• Bone marrow aspirates are recommended if systemic mastocytosis is suspected.
• Exploratory laparotomy may be indicated when portions of the gastrointestinal tract, unapproachable by endoscopy, are involved, or abdominal organomegaly is present.

PATHOLOGIC FINDINGS
• Thickened rugal folds, erosions, ulcers, and increased mucosal friability may be present in the stomach, although grossly it can appear normal.
• Ulcerations and erosions may also be seen in the intestine.
• Eosinophilic infiltrates can be patchy in the intestine; multiple biopsies may be necessary to obtain a diagnostic sample.
• Histopathology reveals a diffuse infiltrate of eosinophils into the lamina propria; the submucosa and muscularis can also be involved (reportedly more common in cats with this disease).

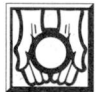

TREATMENT

APPROPRIATE HEALTH CARE
• Most can be successfully treated on an outpatient basis.
• Patients with systemic mastocytosis, protein-losing enteropathies, or other concurrent illnesses may require hospitalization until they are stabilized.

GASTROENTERITIS, EOSINOPHILIC

NURSING CARE
• If the patient is dehydrated or must be NPO because of vomiting, any balanced fluid such as lactated Ringer's solution is adequate (for a patient without other concurrent disease); otherwise, select fluids on the basis of secondary diseases.
• If severe hypoalbuminemia from protein-losing enteropathy, consider colloids such as dextrans, plasma, or hetastarch.

ACTIVITY
No need to restrict unless severely debilitated.

DIET
• Manipulation—usually a critical component of therapy; may take several forms
• In patients with severe intestinal involvement and protein-losing enteropathy, total parenteral nutrition (TPN) may be indicated until remission is obtained. It is rare that TPN is necessary.
• Monomeric diets (e.g., elemental diet)—have nonallergenic components; can be used in patients who are not vomiting but have moderate-to-severe gastrointestinal inflammation; useful if a food allergy is suspected
• Highly digestible diets with limited nutrient sources—extremely useful for eliciting remission; can be used as maintenance diets once the patient is stabilized
• Dog—examples include Hill's prescription diets d/d, z/d, and i/d, Purina HA or LA, Select Care Innovative Veterinary Diets, Eukanuba Low Residue Diet, Canine Response Formula FP or KO, ANF, Hill's Science diets Maximum Stress and Canine Growth, or homemade diets
• Cat—examples include Iams Feline and Eukanuba Low Residue Diet, Tender Vittles, Hill's prescription diets i/d, z/d, and d/d
• Once the patient is stabilized, may institute an elimination diet trial if food allergy or intolerance is the suspected cause

CLIENT EDUCATION
Explain the waxing and waning nature of the disease, the necessity for lifelong vigilance regarding inciting factors, and the potential for long-term therapy.

SURGICAL CONSIDERATIONS
N/A

MEDICATIONS

DRUG(S) OF CHOICE
• Corticosteroids—mainstay of treatment; prednisone used most frequently (1–2 mg/kg PO q12h in dogs; 2–3 mg/kg PO q12h in cats)
• Gradually taper corticosteroids; relapses are more common in patients that are taken off corticosteroids too quickly.
• Budesonide, a new oral glucocorticoid, has been used successfully to treat cats and dogs with inflammatory bowel disease; it has been recently approved in the United States but must be compounded.
• Occasionally other immunosuppressive drugs can be used to allow a reduction in corticosteroid dose and avoid some of the adverse effects of steroid therapy.
• Azathioprine (1–1.5 mg/kg q24h PO in dogs) is the most common adjunctive immunosuppresive therapy.

CONTRAINDICATIONS
If secondary problems are present, avoid therapeutic agents that might be contra-indicated for those conditions.

PRECAUTIONS
• Azathioprine rarely causes bone marrow suppression, usually more of a problem in cats than dogs.
• All patients on azathioprine—perform a complete blood count 10–14 days after the start of treatment, with rechecks monthly and then bimonthly thereafter; usually the condition is reversible when the drug is discontinued
• Pancreatitis, hepatic damage, and anorexia are other potential side effects of this drug.

POSSIBLE INTERACTIONS
N/A

ALTERNATIVE DRUG(S)
N/A

FOLLOW-UP

PATIENT MONITORING
• Initially frequent for some more severely affected patients; peripheral eosinophil counts may be helpful; the corticosteroid dosage is usually adjusted during these visits
• Patients with less severe disease—may be checked 2–5 weeks after the initial evaluation; monthly to bimonthly thereafter until corticosteroid therapy is completed
• Patients receiving azathioprine—monitor as mentioned above; patients usually do not require long-term follow-up unless the problem recurs.

PREVENTION/AVOIDANCE
If a food intolerance or allergy is suspected or documented, avoid that particular item and adhere strictly to dietary changes.

POSSIBLE COMPLICATIONS
• Weight loss, debilitation in refractory cases
• Adverse effects of prednisone therapy
• Bone marrow suppression, pancreatitis, hepatitis, or anorexia caused by azathioprine

EXPECTED COURSE AND PROGNOSIS
• The vast majority of dogs with eosinophilic gastroenteritis respond to a combination of dietary manipulation and steroid therapy.
• Cats often have a more severe form of the disease, with a poorer prognosis than in dogs.
• Cats often require higher doses of corticosteroids for longer periods of time to elicit remission.

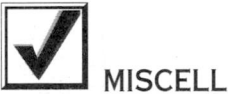

MISCELLANEOUS

ASSOCIATED CONDITIONS
None

AGE-RELATED FACTORS
None

ZOONOTIC POTENTIAL
A consideration only when eosinophilic infiltrates are secondary to parasites (e.g., *Ancylostoma, Giardia* and ascarids)

PREGNANCY
• Prednisone has been used safely in pregnant women; corticosteroids have been associated with increased incidence of congenital defects, abortion, and fetal death.
• Azathioprine has been used safely in pregnant women and may be a good substitute for corticosteroids in pregnant animals.

SYNONYMS
N/A

SEE ALSO
• Gastroenteritis, Lymphocytic-Plasmacytic
• Gastrointestinal Parasites
• Inflammatory Bowel Disease
• Mast Cell Tumors

ABBREVIATIONS
• IgE = immunoglobulin E
• NPO = nothing per os

Suggested Reading
Strombeck DR, Guilford WG. Idiopathic inflammatory bowel diseases. In: Guilford WG, Center SA, Strombeck DR, et al., eds. Strombeck's small animal gastroenterology. 3rd ed. Philadelphia: Saunders, 1996.
Tarris TR. Feline inflammatory bowel disease. Vet Clin North Am 1993;23:569–586.
Author Kelly J. Diehl
Consulting Editor Albert E. Jergens

GASTROENTERITIS, HEMORRHAGIC

 BASICS

DEFINITION
A peracute hemorrhagic enteritis of dogs characterized by a sudden onset of severe bloody diarrhea that is often explosive with vomiting and hypovolemia and a dramatic loss of water and electrolytes into the intestinal lumen.

PATHOPHYSIOLOGY
Many conditions result in hemorrhagic diarrhea, but the acute hemorrhagic gastroenteritis (HGE) syndrome of dogs appears to have unique clinical features that distinguish it as a clinical entity separate from other causes. HGE is characterized as a peracute loss of intestinal mucosal integrity with the rapid movement of blood, fluid, and electrolytes into the gut lumen. Dehydration and hypovolemic shock occur quickly. Translocation of bacteria or toxins through the damaged intestinal mucosa may result in septic or endotoxic shock.

SYSTEMS AFFECTED
• Gastrointestinal
• Cardiovascular

GENETICS
Unknown; however, there appear to be specific breeds overrepresented.

INCIDENCE AND PREVALENCE
A common clinical condition

GEOGRAPHIC DISTRIBUTION
N/A

SIGNALMENT

Species
Dogs

Breed Predilections
All breeds can be affected but the incidence is greater in small-breed dogs. Breeds most represented include miniature Schnauzers, dachshunds, Yorkshire terriers, and miniature poodles.

Mean Age and Range
Usually in adult dogs with a mean age of 5 years

Predominant Sex
N/A

SIGNS

General Comments
• Clinical findings are variable in both the course and severity of the disease. The disease is usually peracute and associated with concurrent hypovolemic shock.
• Most animals affected have been healthy, with no historical environmental changes.

Historical Findings
• The signs usually begin with acute vomiting, anorexia, and depression that is then followed with bloody diarrhea.
• Signs progress rapidly and become severe within a period of hours (usually 8–12 h) and are the result of hypovolemic shock and hemoconcentration.

Physical Examination Findings
• The patient is generally depressed and weak and has prolonged capillary refill time and weak pulse pressure.
• Skin turgor as a reflection of dehydration is normal owing to the peracute nature of the disease and the lag time in fluid compartmental shifts.
• Abdominal palpation may be painful and fluid-filled bowel detected.
• Rectal examination will identify bloody diarrhea, and later in the course of disease a "raspberry jam" characteristic stool develops.
• Occasionally fever, but often the temperature is normal or even subnormal.

CAUSES
• The etiology is unknown.
• Type 1 hypersensitivity reaction directed against host enteric mucosa
• Cultures of some dogs with HGE yield mostly pure cultures of *Clostridium perfringens* and enterotoxin but the significance is unknown.
• Searches for toxigenic *E. coli* strains have been unrewarding.

RISK FACTORS
• Unknown
• Most dogs are previously healthy with no major concurrent illness.

 DIAGNOSIS

DIFFERENTIAL DIAGNOSIS
• Parvovirus
• Bacterial enteritis such as salmonellosis or *Campylobacter*
• Conditions resulting in endotoxic or hypovolemic shock

• Intestinal obstruction or intussusception
• Hypoadrenocorticism
• Pancreatitis
• Coagulopathy

CBC/BIOCHEMISTRY/URINALYSIS
• Hemoconcentration with the PCV generally greater than 60% and sometimes as high as 75%. Usually a stress leukogram
• Biochemistry profile may reveal secondary hepatic enzyme elevations and high BUN due to prerenal causes. Total protein may be normal or low because of protein loss into the GI tract.

OTHER LABORATORY TESTS

Fecal Tests
• The stool is negative for parasites.
• ELISA for parvovirus is negative.
• Fecal cytology will show many RBCs and occasional WBCs.
• *Clostridium* may be cultured in high concentration but cultures are negative for other enteric pathogens.

Coagulogram
Usually normal but occasionally secondary DIC is a complication

IMAGING
Abdominal radiographs show fluid- and gas-filled small and large intestine.

DIAGNOSTIC PROCEDURES

Electrocardiogram
Cardiac arrhythmias such as ventricular premature contractions and ventricular tachycardia may be noted.

Endoscopy
• Colonoscopic examination is not indicated or helpful in the diagnosis.
• May show diffuse mucosal hemorrhage, ulceration and hyperemia

PATHOLOGIC FINDINGS
Changes in the intestine include gross congestion and microscopic evidence of autolysis that is devoid of marked inflammation.

 TREATMENT

APPROPRIATE HEALTH CARE
Patients suspected of having acute HGE should be hospitalized and treated aggressively because clinical deterioration is often rapid and can be fatal.

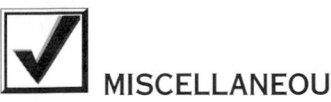

GASTROENTERITIS, HEMORRHAGIC

NURSING CARE
• Rapid volume replacement is required in all cases.
• Balanced electrolyte solutions are given up to the rate of 40–60 mL/kg/hour IV until the PCV is less than 50%.
• A moderate rate of maintenance fluids is given to maintain circulatory function and to correct any potassium or other electrolyte deficits during the recovery period.
• Continued GI fluid losses should be estimated and that volume added to the fluid requirements.
• Hypoproteinemic animals may require colloids or plasma.

ACTIVITY
Restricted

DIET
• NPO during acute disease
• During recovery period a bland, low-fat, low-fiber diet should be fed for several days before returning to the normal diet.

CLIENT EDUCATION
• Discuss the need for immediate and aggressive medical management. With appropriate therapy, mortality is usually low.
• Recurrence is reported in about 10% of the cases.

SURGICAL CONSIDERATIONS
N/A

 MEDICATIONS

DRUG(S) OF CHOICE
• Parenteral antibiotics are given because of the potential for septicemia and possible implications of *Clostridium perfringens*. Ampicillin is recommended.
• Alternate choices include trimethoprimsulfa or cephalosporins. Ampicillin in combination with gentamicin or a fluoroquinolone (Enrofloxacin) is suggested in cases of suspected septicemia.
• Short-acting glucocorticoids are given to dogs in shock using dexamethasone sodium phosphate 0.5–1.0 mg/kg IV.
• Excessive blood loss may require a blood transfusion (rare).

CONTRAINDICATIONS
N/A

PRECAUTIONS
Gentamicin should be used with great care and not given to patients with dehydration or renal compromise because of potential for nephrotoxicity.

POSSIBLE INTERACTIONS
N/A

ALTERNATIVE DRUG(S)
• Oral antibiotics and intestinal protectants are of little benefit and generally not administered.
• Rectal administration of mucosal protectants is of questionable value.
• Antiemetics may be given to control severe vomiting. Intestinal motility modifiers are not considered necessary and are not recommended.

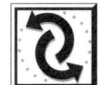 **FOLLOW-UP**

PATIENT MONITORING
• Monitor the PCV and total solids frequently (at least every 4–6 hours).
• Modify the fluid replacement–based PCV, continued GI fluid losses, and circulatory function.
• If there is a failure of clinical improvement in 24–48 hours, reevaluate the patient, as other causes of hemorrhagic diarrhea are probable.

PREVENTION/AVOIDANCE
N/A

POSSIBLE COMPLICATIONS
• Occasionally DIC may develop. Neurologic signs or even seizures secondary to the hemoconcentration may occur.
• Cardiac arrhythmias occur from suspected myocardial reperfusion injury.
• A hemolytic-uremic syndrome may occur (rare).

EXPECTED COURSE AND PROGNOSIS
• The course of the disease is generally short, lasting from 24–72 hours. The prognosis is good, and most patients recover with no complications.
• Sudden death is uncommon.

✔️ **MISCELLANEOUS**

ASSOCIATED CONDITIONS
N/A

AGE-RELATED FACTORS
N/A

ZOONOTIC POTENTIAL
Unknown.

PREGNANCY
N/A

SYNONYMS
Acute hemorrhagic enterocolitis

SEE ALSO
• Diarrhea, Acute
• Vomiting, Acute

ABBREVIATIONS
• DIC = disseminated intravascular coagulation
• ELISA = enzyme-linked immunosorbent assay
• HGE = hemorrhagic gastroenteritis
• NPO = nothing by mouth
• PCV = packed cell volume
• RBC = red blood cells
• WBC = white blood cells

Suggested Reading
Burrows CF. Canine hemorrhagic gastroenteritis. J Am Anim Hosp Assoc 1977; 13:451–458.
Hall JH, Simpson KW. Diseases of the small intestine. In: Ettinger SJ, Feldman EC eds. Textbook of veterinary internal medicine, 5th ed. Philadelphia: Saunders, 2000: 1214–1215.
Sasaki J, Goryo M, Asahina M et al. Hemorrhagic enteritis associated with *Clostridium perfringens* type A in a dog. J Vet Med Sci 1999;61:175–177.
Spielman BL, Garvey MS. Hemorrhagic gastroenteritis in dogs. JAAHA 1993; 29:341–344.
Strombeck DR, Guilford WG. In: Guilford WG, Center SA, et al, eds. Strombeck's small animal gastroenterology. Philadelphia: Saunders, 1996:433–435.
Author David C. Twedt
Consulting Editor Albert E. Jergens

GASTROENTERITIS, LYMPHOCYTIC-PLASMACYTIC

 BASICS

DEFINITION
• A form of inflammatory bowel disease characterized by lymphocyte and/or plasma cell infiltration into the lamina propria of the stomach and intestine • Less commonly the infiltrates may extend into the submucosa and muscularis.

PATHOPHYSIOLOGY
• An abnormal immune response to environmental stimuli is most likely responsible for initiating gastrointestinal inflammation. Evidence in people suggests that intestinal bacteria may be the trigger. • Continued exposure to antigen, coupled with self-perpetuating inflammation, results in disease. • The exact mechanisms, antigens, and patient factors involved in initiation and progression remain unknown.

SYSTEMS AFFECTED
• Gastrointestinal—seldom is the stomach affected alone; the large bowel can also be affected • Hemic/Lymphatic/Immune, Ophthalmic, Skin/Exocrine—other immune-mediated diseases frequently affect the hematopoietic system (autoimmune hemolytic anemia [AIHA], coagulopathies), eyes, and integument in humans with IBDs; animals may also develop these complications, although to date they are not as well characterized

GENETICS
Basenjis and lundehunds have particular familial forms of IBD.

INCIDENCE/PREVALENCE
A common problem in both cats and dogs; represents most of the cases of IBD

GEOGRAPHIC DISTRIBUTION
N/A

SIGNALMENT

Species
Dogs and cats

Breed Predilections
• Lundehunds and basenjis have particular forms of IBD; gluten-sensitive enteropathy affects Irish setters. • German shepherds and shar peis are reportedly predisposed to lymphocytic-plasmacytic gastroenteritis. • No breed predilection reported in cats

Mean Age And Range
• Most common in middle-aged to old animals • Dogs as young as 8 months and cats as young as 5 months of age with IBD have been reported.

Predominant Sex
None reported

SIGNS

Historical Findings
• Signs associated with lymphocytic-plasmacytic gastritis with or without enteritis can vary greatly in type, severity, and frequency. • Generally have an intermittent, chronic course, but increase in frequency over time. • Cats—intermittent, chronic vomiting is the most common; chronic small bowel diarrhea is second. • Dogs—chronic small bowel diarrhea is the most common; if only the stomach is involved, vomiting is the most common. • Dogs and cats—anorexia (sometimes alternating with periods of ravenous appetite) and chronic weight loss are common; hematochezia, hematemesis, and melena are occasionally noted.

Physical Examination Findings
• Can vary from perfectly normal animal to a dehydrated, cachectic, and depressed patient • If only the stomach is involved, may be no discernible abnormalities

CAUSES
• Pathogenesis is most likely multifactorial. • Several causative factors have been identified.

Infectious Agents
Giardia, Salmonella, Campylobacter, and normal resident gastrointestinal flora have been implicated but not documented.

Dietary Agents
Meat proteins, food additives, artificial coloring, preservatives, milk proteins, and gluten (wheat) have all been proposed.

Genetic Factors
• Certain forms of IBD are more common in some breeds of dogs (see above). • Certain major histocompatibility genes, which are important components of normal immune responses, may render an individual susceptible to development of IBD.

RISK FACTORS
See Causes

 DIAGNOSIS

DIFFERENTIAL DIAGNOSIS
• Other infiltrative inflammatory bowel conditions (e.g., eosinophilic gastroenteritis, granulomatous IBD) • Neoplastic conditions • Infectious diseases (e.g., histoplasmosis, giardiasis, salmonellosis, *Campylobacter* enteritis, and bacterial overgrowth) • Miscellaneous diseases (e.g., lymphangiectasia, gastrointestinal motility disorders, and exocrine pancreatic insufficiency) • In the cat, consider hyperthyroidism, systemic viral infection (e.g., FeLV, FIV, FIP), and chronic pancreatitis.

CBC/BIOCHEMISTRY/URINALYSIS
• Often normal • Mild nonregenerative anemia and mild leukocytosis without a left shift—sometimes seen in cats • Neutrophilic leukocytosis, often with a left shift—frequently seen in dogs • Hypoproteinemia is more common in dogs than cats with IBD. • Cobalamin deficiency may be present in cats with IBD.

OTHER LABORATORY TESTS
• Useful to eliminate other differentials • Dogs—tests include fasting serum TLI to evaluate exocrine pancreatic function, and fasting serum cobalamin and folate assays to evaluate for small intestinal function and bacterial overgrowth • Cats—T_4 and FeLV/FIV serology are recommended; fasting serum TLI (if exocrine pancreatic insufficiency suspected); cobalamin assay

IMAGING
• Survey abdominal radiographs—usually normal • Barium contrast studies—occasionally reveal mucosal abnormalities and thickened bowel loops; generally not helpful in establishing a definitive diagnosis; can be normal even in individuals with severe disease

DIAGNOSTIC PROCEDURES
• May first initiate a hypoallergenic diet trial to rule in or rule out dietary allergy or intolerance • Occasionally, certain forms of IBD respond to dietary manipulations alone. • If signs resolve completely, a diagnosis of dietary allergy or intolerance is likely, and no further workup is necessary. • Always perform fecal examination for parasites. • Definitive diagnosis requires biopsy and histopathology, usually obtained via endoscopy. • Duodenal aspirates for *Giardia* spp. may be collected during endoscopy. • Intestinal fluid obtained during endoscopy can also be submitted for quantitative culture if bacterial overgrowth is suspected. • Exploratory laparotomy may be indicated when portions of the gastrointestinal tract, unapproachable by endoscopy, are involved or if abdominal organomegaly is present.

PATHOLOGIC FINDINGS
• Grossly, stomach and intestinal appearance can range from normal to edematous, thickened, and ulcerated. • The hallmark histopathologic finding is an infiltrate of lymphocytes and plasma cells in the lamina propria. • The distribution may be patchy, so several biopsy specimens are necessary to make the diagnosis.

 TREATMENT

APPROPRIATE HEALTH CARE
Outpatient, unless the patient is debilitated from dehydration, hypoproteinemia, or cachexia

NURSING CARE
• If the patient is dehydrated or must be NPO because of vomiting, any balanced fluid such as lactated Ringer's solution is adequate (for a patient without other concurrent disease); otherwise, select fluids on the basis of secondary diseases. • If severe hypoalbuminemia from protein-losing enteropathy, consider colloids (e.g., dextrans or hetastarch).

ACTIVITY
No restrictions

DIET
• Dietary therapy is an essential component of patient management. • Patients with severe intestinal involvement and protein-losing enteropathy may require total parenteral nutrition until remission. • Can feed monomeric diets such as elemental diets with nonallergenic components to patients that are not vomiting but have moderate-to-severe gastrointestinal inflammation; useful if a food allergy is suspected • Highly digestible diets with limited nutrient sources are extremely useful in eliciting remission and, after the patient is stabilized, can be used as maintenance diets • Dog—examples include Hill's prescription diets d/d, i/d, and z/d; Purina HA and LA, Select Care Innovative Veterinary Diets, Eukanuba Low Residue Diet, Canine Response Formula FP or KO, ANF, Hill's Science diets Maximum Stress and Canine Growth, or homemade diets • Cat—examples include Iams Feline and Eukanuba Low Residue Diet, Tender Vittles, and Hill's prescription diets i/d, d/d, and z/d • Once the patient is stabilized, an elimination diet or food trial may be instituted if food allergy or intolerance is the suspected cause.

CLIENT EDUCATION
• IBD is not necessarily cured as much as controlled. • Relapses are common. • Patience is required during the various food and medication trials that are often necessary.

SURGICAL CONSIDERATIONS
N/A

MEDICATIONS

DRUG(S) OF CHOICE
• Corticosteroids—the mainstay of treatment for idiopathic lymphocytic-plasmacytic enteritis; prednisone used most frequently (1–2 mg/kg PO q12h in dogs; 2–3 mg/kg PO q12h in cats); cats may require a higher dose to control their disease; when signs resolve, gradually taper the corticosteroid dose; a new oral glucocorticoid, budesonide, has been used successfully to treat cats and dogs with IBD; the drug is not readily available in the United States, but is available at some referral institutions; relapses are more common in individuals who are taken off corticosteroids

too quickly. • Azathioprine (1–1.5 mg/kg q24h PO in dogs; 0.3 mg/kg q48h PO in cats)—an immunosuppressive drug that can be used to allow a reduction in corticosteroid dose and avoid some of the adverse effects of chronic steroid therapy • Metronidazole—has antibacterial and antiprotozoal properties; some evidence that it also has immune-modulating effects; the dosage for IBD in dogs and cats is 10 mg/kg PO q8–12h

CONTRAINDICATIONS
If secondary problems are present, avoid therapeutic agents that might be contraindicated for those conditions.

PRECAUTIONS
• Azathioprine—causes bone marrow suppression rarely; usually more of a problem in cats than dogs • Perform a CBC on all individuals placed on azathioprine, 10–14 days after the start of treatment; recheck monthly and then bimonthly thereafter; usually the condition is reversible when the drug is discontinued. Pancreatitis, hepatic damage, and anorexia are other potential adverse effects of this drug. • Metronidazole—can cause reversible neurotoxicity at high dosages; carcinogenic and mutagenic in laboratory animals; discontinuing the drug usually reverses the neurologic signs • Cyclosporine—can cause gastrointestinal irritation, gingival hyperplasia, and papillomatosis. Associated with the development of lymphoma in people.

POSSIBLE INTERACTIONS
• Cyclosporine can interfere with the metabolism of phenobarbital and phenytoin. • Ketoconazole, erythromycin, and cimetidine can decrease hepatic metabolism of cyclosporin. • Any drugs that are potentially nephrotoxic should be used with caution in conjunction with cyclosporine.

ALTERNATIVE DRUG(S)
• Cyclosporine— may be useful in the therapy of refractory cases of lymphocytic-plasmacytic gastroenteritis; a wide dose range, 0.5–8.5 mg/kg PO q12h, has been reported; initiate therapy at a high dose and taper as signs resolve; cost prohibits routine use of this drug. • Recommend measuring blood levels of drug. • Cyclosporine can be used in place of azathioprine.

FOLLOW-UP

PATIENT MONITORING
• Resolution of clinical signs • Severely affected patients require frequent monitoring; adjust medications during these visits. • Check patients with less severe disease 2–3 weeks after their initial evaluation and then monthly to bimonthly until immunosuppressive therapy is discontinued.

• Monitor patients receiving azathioprine or cyclophosphamide as mentioned above.

PREVENTION/AVOIDANCE
When a food intolerance or allergy is suspected or documented, avoid that particular item and adhere strictly to dietary changes.

POSSIBLE COMPLICATIONS
• Weight loss, debilitation in refractory cases • Side effects of prednisone therapy • Bone marrow suppression, pancreatitis, hepatitis, or anorexia caused by azathioprine

EXPECTED COURSE AND PROGNOSIS
• Dogs and cats with mild inflammation—good-to-excellent prognosis for full recovery • Patients with severe infiltrates, particularly if other portions of the GI tract are involved—more-guarded prognosis • Often the initial response to therapy sets the tone for a given individual's ability to recover.

MISCELLANEOUS

ASSOCIATED CONDITIONS
N/A

AGE-RELATED FACTORS
N/A

ZOONOTIC POTENTIAL
N/A

PREGNANCY
• Corticosteroids have been associated with increased incidence of congenital defects, abortion, and fetal death. • Azathioprine has been used safely in pregnant women, and may be a good substitute for corticosteroids in pregnant animals. • Metronidazole is mutagenic in laboratory animals; avoid

SYNONYMS
N/A

SEE ALSO
• Gastroenteritis, Eosinophilic • Inflammatory Bowel Disease

ABBREVIATIONS
• AIHA = autoimmune hemolytic anemia • FeLV = feline leukemia virus • FIP = feline infectious peritonitis • FIV = feline immunodeficiency virus • IBD = inflammatory bowel disease • NPO = nothing per os • TLI = trypsin-like immunoreactivity

Suggested Reading
Strombeck DR, Guilford WG. Idiopathic inflammatory bowel diseases. In: Guilford WG, Center SA, Strombeck DR, et al., eds. Strombeck's small animal gastroenterology. 3rd ed. Philadelphia: Saunders, 1996: 451–486.
Author Kelly J. Diehl
Consulting Editor Albert E. Jergens

GASTROESOPHAGEAL REFLUX

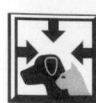 BASICS

OVERVIEW
• Reflux of gastric or intestinal fluid into the esophageal lumen
• Incidence unknown; probably more common than clinically recognized
• Transient relaxation of the gastroesophageal sphincter or chronic vomiting may permit reflux of gastrointestinal juices into the esophageal lumen.
• Gastric acid, pepsin, trypsin, bicarbonate, and bile salts are all injurious to the esophageal mucosa.
• Esophagitis resulting from reflux may vary from mild inflammation of the superficial mucosa to severe ulceration involving the submucosa and muscularis.

SIGNALMENT
• Dogs and cats; male or female
• No breed predilections reported
• May be associated with congenital hiatal hernia seen in Chinese shar-peis
• Occurs at any age; younger animals may be at increased risk because of developmental immaturity of the gastroesophageal sphincter
• Young animals with congenital hiatal hernia may also be at increased risk.

SIGNS

Historical Findings
• Regurgitation
• Hypersalivation
• Howling or crying during swallowing— odynophagia
• Anorexia
• Weight loss

Physical Examination Findings
• Often unremarkable
• Fever and hypersalivation—with severe ulcerative esophagitis

CAUSES & RISK FACTORS
• Anesthesia
• Failure to fast an animal prior to anesthesia
• Poor patient positioning during anesthesia
• Hiatal hernia
• Chronic vomiting
• Young age

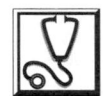 DIAGNOSIS

DIFFERENTIAL DIAGNOSIS
• Oral or pharyngeal disease
• Ingestion of caustic agent
• Esophageal foreign body
• Esophageal tumor
• Megaesophagus—idiopathic; myasthenia gravis; vascular ring anomaly
• Hiatal hernia
• Gastroesophageal intussusception

CBC/BIOCHEMISTRY/URINALYSIS
Usually normal

OTHER LABORATORY TESTS
N/A

IMAGING
• Survey thoracic radiography—usually unremarkable; may be air in the distal esophagus (nonspecific finding)
• Barium contrast radiography—reveals gastroesophageal reflux in some, but not all, animals; aspiration pneumonia may be evident in the dependent portions of the lung; barium paste may be more useful than liquid barium for evaluating esophageal function

DIAGNOSTIC PROCEDURES
• Endoscopy and biopsy—probably the best means of documenting mucosal changes consistent with reflux esophagitis; patients may have an irregular mucosal surface with hyperemia or active bleeding in the distal esophagus
• Esophageal manometry and pH-metry— may help document this disorder in veterinary referral centers

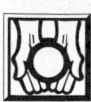

TREATMENT

• Generally, managed as outpatient
• Not necessary to restrict activity
• Moderate to severe cases—may withhold food for 1–2 days; thereafter, feed low-fat, low-protein meals in small, frequent feedings; dietary fat decreases gastroesophageal sphincter pressure and delays gastric emptying; protein stimulates gastric acid secretion

MEDICATIONS

DRUG(S)

• Oral sucralfate suspension (0.5–1.0 g PO q8h)
• Gastric acid antisecretory agents—cimetidine (5–10 mg/kg PO q8h); ranitidine (1.0–2.0 mg/kg PO q12h); famotidine (0.5 mg/kg PO, SC, IV q12–24h); omeprazole (0.7 mg/kg PO q24h)
• Prokinetic agents—cisapride (0.1–0.5 mg/kg PO q12h); ranitidine (1–2 mg/kg PO, IV, SC q8–12h); low-dose erythromycin (0.5–1.0 mg/kg IV q8–12h)

CONTRAINDICATIONS/POSSIBLE INTERACTIONS

Sucralfate suspension may interfere with the absorption of other drugs (e.g., cimetidine, ranitidine, omeprazole, cisapride); may not be clinically important

FOLLOW-UP

• Patients do not necessarily require follow-up endoscopy.
• It may be appropriate in many patients to simply monitor clinical signs.
• Consider endoscopy for patients that do not respond to medical therapies.
• Clients should avoid feeding high-fat foods; they might exacerbate reflux.
• The most important complications are esophagitis and stricture formation.

MISCELLANEOUS

ASSOCIATED CONDITIONS

Hiatal hernia

AGE-RELATED FACTORS

May be worse in younger animals because of developmental immaturity of the gastroesophageal sphincter mechanism

ZOONOTIC POTENTIAL

N/A

PREGNANCY

N/A

Suggested Reading

Callan MB, Washabau RJ, Saunders HM, et al. Congenital esophageal hiatal hernia in the Chinese shar-pei dog. J Vet Intern Med 1993;7:210–215.

Evander A, Little AG, Riddell RH, et al. Composition of the reflux material determines the degree of reflux esophagitis in the dog. Gastroenterology 1987;93:280–286.

Washabau RJ. Diseases of the esophagus. In: Ettinger SJ, Feldman EC, eds. Textbook of veterinary internal medicine. 5th ed. Philadelphia: Saunders, 2000:1142–1153.

Author Robert J. Washabau
Consulting Editor Albert E. Jergens

GASTROINTESTINAL OBSTRUCTION

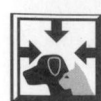

BASICS

DEFINITION
The partial or complete physical impedance to the flow of ingesta and/or secretions in an aboral direction through the pylorus into the duodenum (gastric outlet obstruction) or through the small intestine. Obstructions in the pharynx, esophagus, large intestine, and rectum, and motility disorders are addressed in separate chapters (refer to "See Also").

PATHOPHYSIOLOGY
Gastric Outflow Obstruction
• Ingesta and fluids accumulate in the stomach. • Vomiting often results in loss of fluids rich in hydrochloric acid (from gastric secretions) with subsequent hypochloremic metabolic alkalosis. • Varying degrees of dehydration, tissue compromise, malaise, and weight loss occur, depending on underlying etiology, severity, and chronicity.

Small Intestinal Obstruction
• Ingesta and fluids accumulate proximal to the obstruction. • Vomiting often results in significant dehydration and electrolyte imbalances (particularly hypokalemia), depending on location (proximal vs. distal), partial or complete obstruction, and chronicity. • Mucosal damage and bowel ischemia can result in endotoxemia and sepsis.

SYSTEMS AFFECTED
• Behavioral—associated with abdominal discomfort or pain (praying position, change in temperament) • Cardiovascular—hypovolemic shock • Gastrointestinal—anorexia; vomiting; diarrhea; and malaise • Respiratory—aspiration pneumonia

GENETICS
Unknown (see "Breed Predilections")

INCIDENCE/PREVALENCE
Common

GEOGRAPHIC DISTRIBUTION
N/A

SIGNALMENT
Species
• Dogs and cats • Foreign bodies more common in dogs due to indiscriminate ingestion

Breed Predilections
• Congenital pyloric stenosis—more common in brachycephalic breeds (e.g., boxers, Boston terriers) and Siamese cats • Acquired CHPG—more common in Lhasa apsos, shih tzus, Pekingeses, and poodles • Gastric dilation and volvulus—more common in large-breed dogs (e.g., German shepherds, Great Danes).

Mean Age and Range
• Foreign bodies—more common in young animals, but can occur at any age

• Pyloric stenosis—occurs most often in young animals • CHPG—more common in middle-aged and older animals • Intussusceptions—most common in young animals

Predominant Sex
None

SIGNS
Historical Findings
• Vomiting—hallmark sign; important to differentiate vomiting (forceful abdominal contractions) from regurgitation (passive); may occur soon after eating, especially with gastric outlet obstruction; vomiting food ingested > 8 hours after ingestion is consistent with delayed gastric emptying; usually more severe with gastric and proximal small intestinal obstructions; may be characterized as projectile • Other variable clinical signs—anorexia; lethargy; malaise; ptyalism; diarrhea; melena; and weight loss • Even if the animal is continuing to have bowel movements, this does not rule-out intestinal obstruction. • Clients should be questioned about access to potential foreign bodies and tendency of the animal to ingest them.

Physical Examination Findings
• The physical examination is often the most useful diagnostic procedure for intestinal obstruction. • Findings can vary from normal to animal in life-threatening crisis—include dehydration, shock, presence of a foreign body, abdominal discomfort or pain, and abdominal mass (intussusception or tumor) • Linear foreign bodies—careful sublingual examination essential for detection; although more common in cats, linear foreign bodies occur in dogs also; sedation or anesthesia for oral examination and abdominal palpation is often very helpful in diagnosis

CAUSES
Gastric Outflow Obstruction
• Foreign bodies • Pyloric stenosis • CHPG • Neoplasia • GDV • Granulomatous gastritis or gastroenteritis (e.g., pythiosis)

Small Intestinal Obstruction
• Foreign bodies • Intussusception • Hernias (with incarceration) • Mesenteric torsion or volvulus • Neoplasia • Granulomatous enteritis • Stricture

RISK FACTORS
• Exposure to and tendency to ingest foreign bodies • Intussusception—associated with intestinal parasitism and viral enteritis

DIAGNOSIS

DIFFERENTIAL DIAGNOSIS
• Metabolic disease (e.g., renal failure, hepatic disease, ketoacidotic diabetes mellitus,

hypoadrenocorticism) • Infectious gastroenteritis (e.g., viral, bacterial, parasitic) • Pancreatitis • Peritonitis • Toxicity • Gastroduodenal ulcer disease • Nonspecific gastroenteritis • CNS disease

CBC/BIOCHEMISTRY/URINALYSIS
• These diagnostic tests are useful to rule out other causes (e.g., renal failure, pancreatitis, liver disease, hypoadrenocorticism, diabetic ketoacidosis) and to evaluate overall status of the patient. • Hemogram—may reveal anemia from gastrointestinal blood loss, stress leukocytosis, or possibly a degenerative left-shifted leukocytosis or leukopenia with severe mucosal injury or intestinal perforation and subsequent septic peritonitis • Chemistry profile and blood gases—often reveal hypochloremic metabolic alkalosis with gastric outlet obstruction; hypokalemia and prerenal azotemia are variable findings

OTHER LABORATORY TESTS
N/A

IMAGING
Survey Abdominal Radiography
• May reveal a foreign body in the stomach or intestine, severe gastric distention, or obstructed loops of intestine with dilation due to fluid and/or gas • It is important to differentiate adynamic ileus (usually diffuse) from obstruction (usually segmental). • Interpreting radiographs must be done within the context of the history, physical examination, and other laboratory data to avoid misdiagnosis and unnecessary surgery.

Contrast Radiography
• Positive contrast studies—may reveal delayed gastric emptying (> 4 hrs with liquid contrast and > 8–10 hrs with liquid contrast mixed with food), foreign bodies, complete obstruction, and masses • Barium impregnated spheres—can also be used for radiographic evaluation • Barium enemas—may be useful when ileocolic intussusception is suspected

Abdominal Ultrasonography
May be useful in detecting foreign bodies and obstructions (especially intestinal intussusception)

DIAGNOSTIC PROCEDURES
• Endoscopy—may be useful for confirming gastric and proximal intestinal obstruction and for obtaining biopsies of masses; particularly useful with some types of foreign bodies as retrieval may be possible • Abdominal paracentesis and cytology/fluid analysis—more sensitive than physical examination and radiography (i.e., can detect small amounts of abdominal effusion); may reveal nonseptic inflammation associated with intestinal vascular compromise (prior to perforation) or septic peritonitis; can be an additional indication for exploratory laparotomy

PATHOLOGIC FINDINGS

Histopathology of gastrointestinal masses causing obstruction—can reveal granulomatous inflammation, fungal infection (e.g., pythiosis), and neoplasia

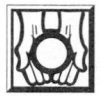

TREATMENT

APPROPRIATE HEALTH CARE

• Inpatient—for diagnosis, initial supportive medical care, and relief of the obstruction (usually with surgery) • Surgery—acute intestinal obstructions are emergencies, and surgery should be performed as soon as possible after immediate supportive medical care; intestines do not tolerate vascular compromise well; intestinal resection and anastomosis frequently required (with associated increased morbidity and potential complications), but enterotomy may be successful if earlier diagnosis is made • Delay in diagnosis may result in intestinal necrosis, perforation, and septic peritonitis

NURSING CARE

• Intravenous crystalloid fluids—necessary for rehydration, circulatory support, and to correct acid–base and electrolyte abnormalities; for severe circulatory compromise (shock), administer isotonic crystalloid fluids at 90 mL/kg (dogs) or 70 mL/kg (cats) over 1–2 hrs. • Colloids (dextran or hetastarch)—may also be beneficial; frequent evaluation of hydration and electrolytes (with appropriate treatment adjustments) is necessary; for gastric outlet obstruction causing hypochloremic metabolic alkalosis, fluid of choice is 0.9% saline; otherwise, lactated Ringer's solution or other balanced electrolyte solution is adequate • Appropriate potassium supplementation—important

ACTIVITY

Restricted

DIET

Nothing by mouth until relief of obstruction and resolution of vomiting; then feed bland diet for 1–2 days, with gradual return to normal diet

CLIENT EDUCATION

Warn that animals with the tendency to ingest foreign bodies are often repeat offenders; all reasonable efforts to prevent access to foreign bodies should be made.

SURGICAL CONSIDERATIONS

Gastric Outflow Obstruction

• Pyloroplasty or pyloromyotomy—for pyloric stenosis or CHPG • Gastrotomy—for foreign bodies not able to be removed with endoscopy • Resection (e.g., Billroth I

gastroduodenostomy, Billroth II gastrojejunostomy)—for granulomatous or neoplastic masses • Gastropexy—for GDV

Intestinal Obstruction

• Enterotomy • Resection and anastomosis—with bowel ischemia and necrosis • Open peritoneal lavage—with perforation and septic peritonitis • Prophylactic enteropexy—with intussusception

MEDICATIONS

DRUG(S)

• Broad-spectrum parenteral antibiotics—with significant mucosal injury or sepsis; ampicillin (20 mg/kg IV q8h) or ticarcillin/clavulanate (50 mg/kg IV q8h) and an aminoglycoside (gentamicin 6.6 mg/kg IV q24h) or a fluoroquinolone (enrofloxacin 5 mg/kg IV or IM q24h) • Short-acting soluble glucocorticoids—for shock; dexamethasone sodium phosphate (0.5–1.0 mg/kg IV) or prednisolone sodium succinate (5 mg/kg IV) • Antiemetics—metoclopramide (0.2–0.5 mg/kg SC or IV q6–8h or 1–2 mg/kg/24h as a CRI); may be given *after* the obstruction has been relieved • H_2-receptor antagonists (e.g., ranitidine 1–2 mg/kg PO, SC, IV q12h) and/or the gastric mucosal protectant sucralfate (250 mg/cat PO q8–12h or 250–1000 mg/dog PO q8–12h)—may be used in patients with mucosal ulceration

CONTRAINDICATIONS

Prokinetic agents (e.g., metoclopramide and cisapride)

PRECAUTIONS

Aminoglycoside antibiotics should be not used with shock, dehydration, or renal compromise because of their potential nephrotoxicity.

FOLLOW-UP

PATIENT MONITORING

• Monitor hydration, PCV/TS, and electrolyte status closely; adjust fluid therapy accordingly. • Monitor postoperatively for signs of peritonitis.

PREVENTION/AVOIDANCE

• Clients should be cautioned that some pets with tendencies to ingest foreign bodies may do so repeatedly. • Efforts to prevent ingestion of foreign bodies are important.

POSSIBLE COMPLICATIONS

• Aspiration pneumonia • Septic peritonitis (intestinal necrosis and perforation, dehiscence) • Adynamic ileus and/or gastroparesis

EXPECTED COURSE AND PROGNOSIS

• Uncomplicated cases—prognosis good to excellent • Intestinal perforation and septic peritonitis—prognosis guarded initially • Obstructive granulomatous gastroenteritis—prognosis guarded to poor, especially with pythiosis • Mesenteric torsion or volvulus—prognosis poor to grave (most patients die despite surgery)

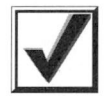

MISCELLANEOUS

ASSOCIATED CONDITIONS

N/A

AGE-RELATED FACTORS

See Signalment

ZOONOTIC POTENTIAL

N/A

PREGNANCY

N/A

SEE ALSO

• Acute Abdomen • Constipation and Obstipation • Dysphagia • Esophageal Foreign Bodies • Esophageal Stricture • Gastric Dilation and Volvulus Syndrome • Gastric or Gastrointestinal Motility Disorders • Hiatal Hernia • Hypertrophic Pyloric Gastropathy, Chronic • Intussusception • Megacolon • Megaesophagus • Pythiosis • Rectal Stricture • Regurgitation • Vomiting, Acute • Vomiting, Chronic

ABBREVIATIONS

• CHPG = chronic hypertrophic pyloric gastropathy • CNS = central nervous system • CRI = constant rate infusion • GDV = gastric dilation and volvulus • PCV/TS = packed cell volume/total solids

Suggested Reading

Bjorling DE. Acute abdomen syndrome In: Morgan RV, ed. Handbook of small animal practice. New York: Churchill Livingstone, 1992:483–487.

Slatter D. Textbook of small animal surgery. 2nd ed. Philadelphia: Saunders, 1993.

Strombeck DR, Guilford WG. Small animal gastroenterology. 2nd ed. Davis, CA: Stonegate, 1990:219–223, 391–401.

Tams TR. Small animal endoscopy. St. Louis: Mosby, 1990.

Author Brett M. Feder

Consulting Editor Albert E. Jergens

GIARDIASIS

BASICS

OVERVIEW
• Enteric infection of dogs with *Giardia canis,* a protozoan parasite; occasionally cats
• Water-borne transmission of cysts
• Motile (flagellated) organisms attach to surface of enterocytes in small intestine, especially duodenum through jejunum.
• Malabsorption syndrome with soft voluminous stools
• Importance as a reservoir for human infections not known

SIGNALMENT
• Dogs—up to 50% for pups, up to 100% in kennels
• Cats—up to 11%

SIGNS
• May be acute, intermittent, or chronic
• Soft, frothy diarrhea, usually with rancid odor
• Persistence may lead to chronic debilitation.

CAUSES & RISK FACTORS
Giardia canis is transmitted by oral ingestion of cysts, usually from water supplies.

DIAGNOSIS

DIFFERENTIAL DIAGNOSIS
Other causes of maldigestion and malabsorption (e.g., pancreatic exocrine insufficiency, inflammatory bowel disease)

CBC/BIOCHEMISTRY/URINALYSIS
Usually normal

OTHER LABORATORY TESTS
N/A

IMAGING
N/A

DIAGNOSTIC PROCEDURES
• Motile organisms, tear-drop–shaped, 15 × 8 μm; "falling leaf" appearance in fresh fecal smear
• Cysts—seen as crescent shapes with fecal flotation; 12 μm
• Zinc sulfate flotation best
• Fecal ELISA not superior to zinc sulfate flotation
• Duodenal aspirates obtained via endoscopy

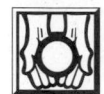

TREATMENT
Treat as outpatients unless debilitated or dehydrated.

MEDICATIONS

DRUG(S)
• All drug use is extra-label.
• Albendazole 25 mg/kg PO q12h for 2 days 90% effective; 50× more effective than metronidazole; second 5-day course may be necessary.
• Fenbendazole 50 mg/kg PO q24h for 3 days effective; second 5-day course may be necessary.
• Metronidazole 25 mg/kg q12h for 5 days in dogs; 12–25 mg/kg PO for 5 days in cats
• Quinacrine hydrochloride 6.6 mg/kg q12h for 5 days

CONTRAINDICATIONS/POSSIBLE INTERACTIONS
• Metronidazole only 67% effective in dogs; bitter taste; anorexia; vomiting
• Quinacrine HCl may cause lethargy, fever; do not use in pregnant dogs or cats.
• Albendazole may cause myelosuppression, anorexia, depression, ataxia, vomiting, or diarrhea; teratogenic; may cause abortion.

FOLLOW-UP
• Serial fecal examinations to confirm efficacy of treatment
• May lead to chronic debilitation

MISCELLANEOUS

ZOONOTIC POTENTIAL
• *Giardia* is the most common intestinal parasite in humans residing in North America.
• *Giardia* spp. may not be highly host-specific; no conclusive evidence indicates that cysts shed by dogs and cats are infective for humans.

PREGNANCY
Do not use quinacrine HCl or albendazole in pregnant dogs or cats.

Suggested Reading
Bowman DD, Lynn RC, Eberhard ML. Georgi's parasitology for veterinarians, 8th ed. St. Louis: Saunders (Elsevier Science), 2003:88–89.
Bowman DD, Hendrix CM, Lindsay DS, Barr SC. Feline clinical parasitology. Ames: Iowa State University Press, 2002:53–59.

Acknowledgment
The authors/editors acknowledge the prior contributions of Dr. Robert M. Corwin, who authored this topic in the previous edition.
Author Julie Ann Jarvinen
Consulting Editor Albert E. Jergens

GINGIVAL HYPERPLASIA

BASICS

DEFINITION
Enlargement of gingival tissue due to proliferation of its elements (abnormal multiplication or increase in the normal number of cells in normal arrangement)

SYSTEMS AFFECTED
Gastrointestinal—oral cavity

GENETICS
Probable familial tendency—boxers

SIGNALMENT
Breed predilections—boxers; Great Danes; collies; Doberman pinschers; dalmatians

SIGNS
• Thickening and increase in height of attached gingiva and gingival margin—sometimes completely covers tooth surface
• Resultant formation of "pseudopockets"—increase in pocket depth due to increased gingival height; not due to loss of attachment, unless untreated and progresses to concurrent periodontal disease
• Gingival margin may be symmetrically enlarged, especially at incisors.
• Locally affected areas possible (Shelties), but typically more generalized pattern found
• May form as protuberant masses (grape cluster) at gingival margins—biopsy necessary to rule out neoplasia

CAUSES
Chronic inflammatory response to presence of bacteria in plaque associated with periodontal disease

RISK FACTORS
• Breed predilection (see Signalment)
• Chronic drug administration—diphenylhydantoin; cyclosporine; nitrendipine; nifedipine

DIAGNOSIS
• Presumptive diagnosis based on clinical appearance, especially if generalized and found in breed with high predilection
• Focal areas or areas that do not respond to standard therapy should be biopsied.
• Histologic evaluation is only way to confirm.

DIFFERENTIAL DIAGNOSIS
• Oral neoplasia—e.g., epulides; usually not generalized; sometimes osseous changes present
• Oral papillomatosis—papilloma usually on mucosal surfaces
• Operculum—seen in young animals during eruption phase of teeth; incomplete loss of gingival tissue covering erupting tooth

CBC/BIOCHEMISTRY/URINALYSIS
N/A

IMAGING
• Intraoral radiology—to rule out any underlying osseous changes (more common with epulides or tumors)

DIAGNOSTIC PROCEDURES
• Histopathology—to rule out neoplasia and other causes

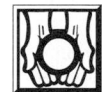

TREATMENT

APPROPRIATE HEALTH CARE
• Regular dental cleanings and home care—to minimize effects of plaque and bacterial accumulation

CLIENT EDUCATION
• Chronic, recurring problem that often needs repeated therapy
• Encourage the highest level of home care and regular professional cleaning

SURGICAL CONSIDERATIONS
Gingivoplasty (Re-contouring)
• To remove excess gingival tissue and return pocket depths to normal
• Local anesthetic injections or topical gels
• Periodontal probe—to determine depth of pseudopocket; can mark pocket depth on outside of pocket with end of probe ("dots")
• Excise excess tissue and re-shape gingival margin
• Cold steel—sharp, stout scissors or scalpel blade
• Connect the dots made by probe with blade to approximate normal gingival margin or use scissors, following pocket depth to remove bulk tissue
• 12-fluted bur on high-speed handpiece—contour margin to feather angle; assists in hemostasis
• Electrocautery—use fully or partially rectified current; avoid damage to underlying bone or tissue
• Excessive thickness (incisor and canine region)—modified Widman technique; envelop flap to lift gingiva off tooth surfaces; excise tissue wedge to remove gingiva at the inside of the pocket to provide a more narrow width of attached gingiva; suture interdentally to secure gingiva; use digital pressure to reposition
• Tincture of myrrh and benzoin—use dropper; coat cut margins and dry; 4 to 5 layers
• Hemostatic solutions—to aid in hemorrhage control as needed

MEDICATIONS

DRUG(S)
• Oral antimicrobials—chlorhexidine; zinc ascorbate gel
• Postoperative pain management

CONTRAINDICATIONS/POSSIBLE INTERACTIONS
Patients on chronic administration of diphenylhydantoin or cyclosporine—may be predisposed to hyperplastic changes

FOLLOW-UP

PATIENT MONITORING
• Postoperative comfort—give pain medication as needed
• Regular examinations and professional cleaning and treatment—to avoid recurrence, which is common

PREVENTION/AVOIDANCE
Regular professional cleaning, meticulous home care

POSSIBLE COMPLICATIONS
• Possible exacerbation of periodontal disease in pseudopockets if left untreated; deeper pockets are more susceptible to anaerobic bacterial infections.
• Excessive heat with electrosurgical treatment may result in damaged teeth (pulpitis, pulpal death) and alveolar bone.

EXPECTED COURSE AND PROGNOSIS
• Good prognosis with regular care
• Recurrence common

MISCELLANEOUS

SEE ALSO
Oral Masses

Suggested Reading
Lobprise HB, Wiggs RB. The veterinarian's companion for common dental procedures. Lakewood, CO: AAHA Press, 2000.
Wiggs RB, Lobprise HB. Veterinary dentistry principles & practice. Philadelphia: Lippincott-Raven, 1997.
Author Heidi B. Lobprise
Consulting Editor Heidi B. Lobprise

GINGIVITIS

 BASICS

DEFINITION
A reversible inflammatory response of the marginal gumline; the earliest phase of periodontal disease

PATHOPHYSIOLOGY
• The gingiva covers the alveolar processes of the mandible and maxilla and conforms closely to the neck of the tooth.
• The gingiva is divided into attached and free, or marginal, portions—the attached gingiva is tightly bound to the periosteum overlying the alveolar processes; the marginal gingiva extends above the crest of the alveolar bone and tapers to a knifelike edge that lies in contact with surface of the tooth.
• The gingival sulcus—the narrow cleft between the inner wall of the marginal gingiva and the tooth; in dogs, normally < 3 mm but may be deeper around the canine teeth in large-breed dogs; in cats, normally = 1 mm
• The junction between the gingiva and oral mucosa appears as a distinct line or furrow called the mucogingival line.
• The connective tissue of the gingiva (lamina propria) contains an extensive array of blood vessels, lymphatics, nerves, and collagen fibers; plasma cells, lymphocytes, and neutrophils are also abundant and are important in local defense mechanisms.
• Crevicular fluid—plasma-derived; passes from the gingival connective tissue through the crevicular epithelium to lavage the gingival sulcus; flow occurs in response to bacteria (plaque) in the gingival sulcus; contains immunoglobulins, other nonspecific antibacterial substances, and neutrophils as the predominant cells; important in controlling the bacterial population
• In healthy animals, gram-positive aerobic cocci and rods predominate in supragingival plaque; anaerobes are more abundant subgingivally, and spirochetes are found tightly packed in the apical region of the gingival sulcus.

• As gingivitis develops, anaerobes and spirochetes become increasingly more abundant in the subgingival sulcus.
• In dogs the bacteroides organisms (*Bacteroides, Prevotella, Porphyromonas* spp.) and *Fusobacterium* spp. appear to be important pathogens; *Porphyromonas* and *Peptostreptococcus* spp. are common in samples from cats with gingivitis.
• Gram-negative organisms—increase in number as gingivitis develops; invade tissues and elaborate endotoxins that can result in tissue destruction
• The fact that these bacteria are present in disease and health and that periodontal disease does not progress in linear fashion (i.e., periods of active disease are followed by quiescent periods) indicates that host–bacteria interaction is important in the pathogenesis of periodontal disease.
• Plaque—composed of bacteria, PMNs, and salivary glycoproteins; forms within 24 hr on clean tooth surfaces; the gingiva's inflammatory response to plaque consists of vasculitis, edema, and collagen loss.
• Gingivitis of different severity can exist in one patient's mouth, based on the host's immunocompetency and local oral factors.
• Stage 1—early gingivitis; a small amount of plaque, mild gumline erythema, and smooth gingival surfaces
• Stage 2—advanced gingivitis; subgingival plaque and calculus, moderate-to-severe erythema, and irregular gingival surfaces

SYSTEMS AFFECTED
Oral cavity

SIGNALMENT
• Dogs and cats
• Over 80% of pets 3 years old and older have gingivitis.
• Higher prevalence earlier in life in toy breeds
• Cats generally are affected later in life than dogs.

SIGNS

Historical Findings
• Usually detected during routine wellness examinations
• Gingival swelling or bleeding
• Halitosis

Physical Examination Findings
• Halitosis
• Erythremic or edematous gingiva, especially buccal maxillary surfaces
• Variable degrees of plaque and calculus formation
• Gingival surfaces bleed easily on contact.

CAUSES
Plaque accumulation

RISK FACTORS
• Age
• Head shape and occlusive pattern; crowding of teeth reduces natural cleaning mechanisms (toy and brachycephalic breeds).
• Toy breeds affected earlier in life
• Soft foods
• Open-mouth breathing
• Chewing habits
• Lack of oral health care
• Metabolic diseases such as uremia and diabetes mellitus predispose to more pathogenic oral bacteria.
• Autoimmune disease—pemphigus vulgaris, systemic lupus erythematosus

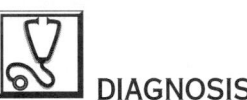 **DIAGNOSIS**

DIFFERENTIAL DIAGNOSIS
• Periodontitis
• Stomatitis
• FeLV
• FIV

CBC/BIOCHEMISTRY/URINALYSIS
May help identify risk factors

OTHER LABORATORY TESTS
FeLV and FIV testing in cats

IMAGING
N/A

DIAGNOSTIC PROCEDURES
• Anesthetized oral examination allows more thorough visual examination of all dental surfaces; use of a periodontal probe helps distinguish between gingivitis (normal sulcal depths of < 3 mm in dogs and < 1 mm in cats) and periodontitis.
• The use of plaque-disclosing agents helps identify plaque and bacterial accumulations on enamel surfaces.
• Biopsy and histopathology

TREATMENT

• Modify behavior to avoid chewing hard objects such as rocks and sticks and eliminate repetitive trauma, if possible.
• Stress the importance of home care and regular dental prophylaxis before lesions develop; daily or at least twice-weekly brushing is recommended, using an enzymatic toothpaste or zinc-ascorbic acid solution to remove and retard plaque accumulation; if the owner is unwilling to brush the teeth but the patient is manageable, the owner might possibly bring the pet to the clinic for brushing.
• Rawhide chew strips help to clean the teeth mechanically and exercise the attachment apparatus but should not be relied upon as the sole method of home care.
• Hard food leaves less substrate on the teeth than soft food; chewing also helps to clean teeth mechanically; Prescription Diet t/d (Hill's Pet Nutrition, Inc., Topeka, KS) is formulated to reduce plaque and tartar accumulation and reduce staining; IAMS Dental Formula is also formulated to reduce tartar (IAMS Company Inc, Dayton, OH.)
• Professional periodontal therapy followed by postoperative home care completely reverses gingivitis.
• Proper dental cleaning—complete oral examination; supragingival removal of plaque and calculus; subgingival scaling and root planing (if needed); polishing; subgingival irrigation; postcleaning examination; home care instructions; and follow-up examinations
• Eliminate predisposing factors such as retained deciduous teeth and crowded teeth.

MEDICATIONS

DRUG(S) OF CHOICE

• Lactoperoxidase- and chlorhexidine-containing dentifrices are effective in retarding plaque.
• Topically applied chlorhexidine, 0.4% stannous fluoride gel, and zinc ascorbate also reduce the inciting plaque formation.

• Antibiotics are generally not necessary at this stage.

CONTRAINDICATIONS
N/A

PRECAUTIONS
N/A

POSSIBLE INTERACTIONS
N/A

ALTERNATIVE DRUG(S)
N/A

FOLLOW-UP

PATIENT MONITORING

Regular oral reexaminations are necessary so the clinician can determine the proper interval between periodontal therapies and assess the effectiveness of oral home care; these steps can cure gingivitis and help to avoid the progression to periodontitis.

POSSIBLE COMPLICATIONS

• Gingivitis begins when bacteria invade the sulcular epithelium and connective tissue; the inflammatory response results in swelling and reddening of the marginal gingiva, which also becomes friable and bleeds easily; these lesions are reversible with dental prophylaxis and home care; if not controlled at this point, the attached gingiva and attachment apparatus (alveolar bone, periodontal ligament, and tooth root cementum) become involved, signifying the transition to periodontitis.
• Once periodontitis is established the lesions are generally considered controllable but not reversible.
• Uncontrolled periodontitis invariably leads to tooth loss.

MISCELLANEOUS

ASSOCIATED CONDITIONS

Always look for dental resorptive lesions (neck lesions) in cats, especially if gingivitis is focal or has the appearance of granulation tissue.

AGE-RELATED FACTORS

Transient gingivitis is a common, self-limiting problem in teething animals; if inflammation persists after adult tooth eruption, the cause should be determined.

ZOONOTIC POTENTIAL
None

PREGNANCY

Dental prophylaxis for simple gingivitis can be delayed until the puppies or kittens are weaned.

SYNONYMS
None

SEE ALSO

• Periodontal Disease
• Stomatitis

ABBREVIATIONS

• FeLV = feline leukemia virus
• FIV = feline immunodeficiency virus
• PMN = polymorphonuclear neutrophil leukocytes

Suggested Reading

Bojrab MJ, Tholen M, eds. Small animal medicine and oral surgery. Philadelphia: Lea & Febiger, 1990.
Colmery B, Frost P. Periodontal disease: etiology and pathogenesis. Vet Clin North Am Small Anim Pract 1986;16:817–834.
Harvey CE, Emily PP. Small animal dentistry. St. Louis, MO: Mosby, 1993.
West-Hyde L, Floyd M. Dentistry. In: Ettinger SJ; Feldman EC, eds. Textbook of veterinary internal medicine. 4th ed. Philadelphia: Saunders, 1995:1097–1121.
Wiggs RB, Lobprise HB. Veterinary dentistry: principles and practice. Philadelphia: Lippincott-Raven, 1997.

Author Thomas Klein
Consulting Editor Heidi B. Lobprise

GLAUCOMA

 BASICS

DEFINITION
• High IOP that causes characteristic degenerative changes in the optic nerve and retina with subsequent loss of vision
• Diagnosis—IOP > 25–30 mm Hg (dogs) or > 31 mm Hg (cats) as determined via applanation tonometry or Schiotz tonometry (using the 1955 Friedenwald human conversion chart that accompanies the instrument) with changes in vision or the appearance of the optic nerve or retina

PATHOPHYSIOLOGY
• Develops when the normal outflow of aqueous humor is impaired
• May be result of primary eye disease (narrow or closed filtration angles and goniodysgenesis, which have a genetic predisposition)
• May be secondary to other eye diseases (primary lens luxation, anterior uveitis, intraocular tumor or hyphema)

SYSTEMS AFFECTED
Ophthalmic

GENETICS
Dogs—predisposing anomalous configuration of the filtration angles is thought to be inherited; mode of inheritance uncertain

INCIDENCE/PREVALENCE
Dogs—more common in some breeds; overall incidence is 0.5% of all hospital admissions to the veterinary teaching hospitals of the colleges of veterinary medicine of North America.

GEOGRAPHIC DISTRIBUTION
N/A

SIGNALMENT
Species
• Dogs—primary and secondary
• Cats—primary rare; secondary seen in patients with signs of long-standing uveitis or with lens luxation

Breed Predilections
• Goniodysgenesis—Arctic circle breeds (e.g., Norwegian elkhounds, Siberian huskies, malamutes, akitas, Samoyeds); Bouvier des Flanders; basset hounds; chow chows; shar peis; spaniels (e.g., American and English cockers, English and Welsh springers)
• Narrow filtration angles—spaniels; chow chows; shar peis; toy breeds (e.g., poodles, Maltese, and shih tzus)
• Secondary to lens luxations—terriers (e.g., Boston, cairns, Manchesters, dandie dinmonts, Norfolks, Norwich, Scottish, Sealyhams, West Highland whites, and fox)

Mean Age and Range
• Primary (dogs)—any age; predominantly affects middle-aged (4–9 years of age)

• Secondary to lens luxations (dogs)—usually affects young (2–6 years of age)
• Secondary with chronic uveitis (cats)—usually affects older cats (> 6 yrs)

Predominant Sex
N/A

SIGNS
General Comments
• Cannot be accurately diagnosed without instrument tonometry
• All well-equipped small animal hospitals should have at least a Schiotz tonometer.

Historical Findings
• Acute angle closure—apparent pain (blepharospasm, tenderness about the head, serous to seromucoid discharge); may note a cloudy or red eye; unless bilateral, vision loss usually not noticed
• Secondary—depends on primary disease
• Uveitis—may note pain (for many days), scleral injection, and corneal edema
• Anterior lens luxation—may note acute pain, scleral injection, and corneal edema; may see lens in the anterior chamber (if corneal edema is not severe)
• Chronic uveitis (cats)—may note no signs of pain; enlarged, seemingly painless eye or a dilated pupil common
• Globe enlargement—may be noticed first by owners

Physical Examination Findings
Acute Primary
• High IOP
• Blepharospasm
• Enophthalmos
• Episcleral injection
• Corneal edema
• Dilated pupil
• Vision loss—may be detected by lack of a menace or dazzle response and/or lack of a direct or consensual pupillary light reflex
• Optic nerve may be depressed or cupped.

Chronic (End Stage)
• Globe enlargement (buphthalmos)
• Descemet streaks
• Subluxated lens with an aphakic crescent
• Optic nerve head atrophy
• Retinal necrosis—detected by peripapillary tapetal hyperreflectivity

Uveitis-induced
• Elevated IOP
• Episcleral injection
• Corneal edema
• Inflammatory debris in the anterior chamber
• Miotic pupil
• Posterior synechia
• Iris bombé

CAUSES
• Primary—filtration angle anomalies
• Secondary—impediment to aqueous humor outflow (e.g., uveitis: inflammatory cells or debris; lens luxation: lens or attached vitreous;

hyphema: RBCs; ocular tumors: neoplastic cells)

RISK FACTORS
• Anterior uveitis
• Lens luxation
• Hyphema
• Intraocular neoplasia
• Topically applied mydriatics—may precipitate acute glaucoma in predisposed animals
• Primary (dogs)—consider all cases to be bilateral, even if one eye is normotensive; evaluation of the unaffected eye by a veterinary ophthalmologist for filtration angle anomalies is indicated to determine the risk for future glaucoma in that eye

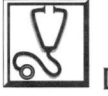 DIAGNOSIS

DIFFERENTIAL DIAGNOSIS
• See Red Eye.
• Conjunctivitis—IOP not high; pupil not dilated; conjunctival hyperemia a more diffuse, red discoloration instead of episcleral vessel engorgement
• Uveitis—initially IOP is subnormal or hypotensive; usually results in a miotic pupil
• Tonometry—usually differentiates other causes of a red eye

CBC/BIOCHEMISTRY/URINALYSIS
• Primary—typically normal
• Secondary—abnormalities consistent with the primary systemic disease (e.g., thrombocytopenia with hyphema)

OTHER LABORATORY TESTS
Serologic testing for infectious diseases—may help diagnose cause of uveitis

IMAGING
• Radiography or ultrasonography (secondary disease)—may demonstrate lesions consistent with fungal or neoplastic dissemination to the eye
• Ocular ultrasound (secondary disease)—may facilitate evaluation of the eye if the ocular media is opaque

DIAGNOSTIC PROCEDURES
• Instrument tonometry—essential
• Acute disease—refer to a veterinary ophthalmologist for a detailed ocular examination of both eyes, including evaluation of the filtration angles (gonioscopy).
• ERG—may help determine if affected eye is capable of vision restoration with medical and/or surgical treatment; normal tracing does not necessarily indicate that the eye will be visual; decreased amplitude or flat tracing guarantees that vision will not return.

PATHOLOGIC FINDINGS
• Collapse of the filtration apparatus
• Loss of retinal ganglion cells
• Photoreceptor disruption
• Gliosis of the optic nerve head

TREATMENT

APPROPRIATE HEALTH CARE
• Acute (dogs)—inpatient
• After discharge—reevaluate every 1–2 days for 1 week to monitor for return of increased IOP.

NURSING CARE
N/A

ACTIVITY
N/A

DIET
N/A

CLIENT EDUCATION
• Warn client that primary glaucoma is a bilateral disease; 50% develop glaucoma in the other eye in 8 months without prophylactic therapy.
• Warn client that 40% or more of dogs will be blind in the affected eye within the first year no matter what is done medically or surgically.

SURGICAL CONSIDERATIONS
• Most forms are best treated surgically.
• Primary (dogs)—< 10% of patients undergoing medical treatment alone will be visual at the end of the first year.
• Procedures—enhance aqueous humor outflow (filtration devices); decrease production of aqueous humor (e.g., Nd:YAG or diode laser cyclophotocoagulation; cyclocryosurgery to cause ciliary body ablation); equally effective in maintaining normal IOP and vision
• Blind, painful eyes—enucleate; evisceration and intraocular prosthesis implantation (with no intraocular infection or neoplasia), or procedure to minimize long-term medical therapy

MEDICATIONS

DRUG(S) OF CHOICE
• Use multiple agents to lower IOP into the normal range as quickly as possible in an attempt to salvage vision.

Acute Primary (Dogs)
• Emergency medical treatment may include one or more of the following:
• Topical miotic—2% pilocarpine solution (q6–12h) or 0.25% demecarium bromide (Humorsol; q12h); enhance aqueous outflow.
• Topical β-adrenergic antagonist—0.5% timolol maleate (Timoptic; q8–12h); reduce aqueous humor production.
• Oral carbonic anhydrase inhibitor methazolamide (Neptazane; 2–4 mg/kg

q8–12h); reduce production of aqueous humor.
• Topical carbonic anhydrase inhibitor—dorzolamide 2% (TruSopt; q8h); reduce aqueous humor production
• Hyperosmotic agent—mannitol (1–2 g/kg IV over 20 min) or glycerin (1–2 mL/kg PO q8–12h); dehydrate the vitreous humor.
• Prostaglandin analog—latanoprost 0.005% (Xalatan; q12–24h); enhance aqueous outflow

Uveitis-induced (Dogs)
• Treated like primary disease
• Miotic agents—do not use.
• Prostaglandin analogs—do not use.
• Topical corticosteroids—used to reduce primary disease

Chronic Smoldering Uveitis (Cats)
• Topical corticosteroids
• Topical β-blockers
• Carbonic anhydrase inhibitor diuretics and topical carbonic anhydrase inhibitors

CONTRAINDICATIONS
• Topical atropine—do not use.
• Miotic agents—do not use with primary anterior lens luxation or uveitis
• Prostaglandin analogs—do not use with primary anterior lens luxations or uveitis.

PRECAUTIONS
• Topical pilocarpine—irritating; may cause conjunctivitis and painful brow ache; may worsen uveitis
• Systemic absorption of topical β-adrenergic antagonists—may cause bronchoconstriction and bradycardia in small dogs and cats
• Systemic carbonic anhydrase inhibitors—cause metabolic acidosis and electrolyte imbalances seen as panting, weakness, disorientation, and/or behavioral change
• Osmotic diuretics—may initiate acute pulmonary edema in patients with compromised cardiovascular-pulmonary disease
• Glycerin—do not use with diabetes; causes hyperglycemia

POSSIBLE INTERACTIONS
Demecarium bromide—cholinesterase inhibitor; may lead to organophosphate poisoning if used in conjunction with organophosphate products

ALTERNATIVE DRUG(S)
• Other diuretics (furosemide, thiazides, etc.)—will not reduce IOP

FOLLOW-UP

PATIENT MONITORING
• IOP—monitored often and regularly after starting initial therapy; if a hypotensive level is maintained for many weeks, *slowly* taper drug therapy. • Monitor for drug reactions.

PREVENTION/AVOIDANCE
• Primary—bilateral disease; recommend that a veterinary ophthalmologist examine the unaffected eye to determine its risk of developing glaucoma. • Prophylactic therapy for the predisposed, unaffected eye—0.25% demecarium bromide (1 drop SID at bedtime); delays onset of acute angle closure glaucoma so median time to an attack is 31 months; 0.5% timolol maleate (1 drop BID); delays onset of glaucoma in second predisposed eye.

POSSIBLE COMPLICATIONS
• Blindness
• Chronic ocular pain

EXPECTED COURSE AND PROGNOSIS
• Chronic disease that requires constant medical treatment
• With medical treatment only—most patients ultimately go blind.
• Surgical treatment—better chance of retaining vision longer; most patients do not remain visual for more than 2 years after initial diagnosis.
• Secondary to lens luxation—may carry a fair prognosis with successful removal of the luxated lens

MISCELLANEOUS

ASSOCIATED CONDITIONS
N/A

AGE-RELATED FACTORS
N/A

PREGNANCY
• All listed drugs may affect pregnancy
• Primary—inherited; do not breed affected animals.

SEE ALSO
• Anterior Uveitis—Cats
• Anterior Uveitis—Dogs
• Red Eye

ABBREVIATIONS
• ERG = electroretinography
• IOP = intraocular pressure

Suggested Reading
Miller PE. Glaucoma. In: Bonagura JD, ed. Kirk's current veterinary therapy XII. Philadelphia: Saunders, 1995:1265–1272.
Miller PE, Schmidt GM, Vainisi SJ, et al. The efficacy of topical prophylactic antiglaucoma therapy in primary closed angle glaucoma in dogs: A multicenter clinical trial. J Am Anim Hosp Assoc, 2000;36:431–438.
Author J. Phillip Pickett
Consulting Editor Paul E. Miller

GLOMERULONEPHRITIS

BASICS

DEFINITION
Pathology associated with the presence of intraglomerular immune complexes even though inflammatory cells are not always present.

PATHOPHYSIOLOGY
Soluble, circulating antigen–antibody complexes may be deposited or trapped in the glomerulus. Alternatively, immune complexes can be formed in situ within the glomerular capillary wall when circulating antibodies react with "planted" antigens there. Following the formation or deposition of glomerular immune complexes, several factors, including activation of the complement system, infiltration of neutrophils and macrophages, platelet aggregation, activation of the coagulation system, and fibrin deposition, can contribute to glomerular damage. The glomerulus responds to these various insults by cellular proliferation (proliferative glomerulonephritis), thickening of the glomerular basement membrane (membranous glomerulonephritis), and, if the injury persists, hyalinization and sclerosis that can lead to nephron loss and eventually chronic renal insufficiency and failure.

SYSTEMS AFFECTED
• Renal/Urologic—proteinuria initially; often the disease is progressive, resulting in irreversible glomerular damage, nephron loss, azotemia, and chronic renal failure.
• Cardiovascular (with severe proteinuria)—hypoalbuminemia and sodium retention (edema and ascites), hypercholesterolemia, hypertension, hypercoagulability, and thromboembolic disease

GENETICS
Familial glomerular disease has been reported in Bernese mountain dogs, samoyeds, dobermans, cocker spaniels, rottweilers, greyhounds, soft-coated wheaten terriers, and cats.

INCIDENCE/PREVALENCE
• In some studies, 90% of random-source dogs have histologic evidence of disease.
• Thought to be a leading cause of chronic renal failure in dogs

SIGNALMENT
Species
Dogs; less commonly, cats
Breed Predilection
• See Genetics above. • In some studies golden retrievers, miniature schnauzers, and long-haired dachshunds, in addition to those breeds listed above, appear to be overrepresented. • Labrador and golden retrievers appear to be predisposed to developing glomerulonephritis, acute tubular necrosis,

and interstitial inflammation associated with *Borrelia burgdorferi* infection.

Mean Age and Range
• Dogs—mean age, 6.5–7.0 years; range, 0.8–17 years • Cats—mean age at presentation, 4.0 years

Predominant Sex
• Dogs—N/A • Cats—75% are males

SIGNS
General Comments
• Presenting complaint depends on the severity and duration of the proteinuria.
• Abnormal proteinuria is often discovered on yearly health screens or while working up other problems. • Occasionally, signs associated with an underlying infectious, inflammatory, or neoplastic disease may be why owners seek veterinary care.

Historical and Physical Examination Findings
• If protein loss is mild to moderate, nonspecific signs may include weight loss and lethargy, but the animal may also appear to be normal. • If protein loss is severe (serum albumin concentration < 1.5–1.0 g/dL), there is often edema and/or ascites.
• If disease leads to renal failure, polyuria–polydipsia, anorexia, nausea, and vomiting may occur. • Acute dyspnea or severe panting in dogs caused by a pulmonary thromboembolism (rare) • Acute blindness due to retinal hemorrhage or detachment associated with systemic hypertension (rare)

CAUSES
• True autoimmune or primary glomerulonephritis has not been documented in dogs or cats. • Several infectious and inflammatory diseases have been associated with glomerular deposition or in situ formation of immune complexes. In many cases no antigen source or underlying disease process is identified, and the disease is referred to as idiopathic. The following diseases have been associated with glomerulonephritis: • Dogs—infectious (e.g., infectious canine hepatitis, bacterial endocarditis, brucellosis, dirofilariasis, ehrlichiosis, leishmaniasis, pyometra, borreliosis, chronic bacterial infection, Rocky Mountain spotted fever, trypanosomiasis, and septicemia); neoplastic or inflammatory (e.g., pancreatitis, systemic lupus erythematosus, polyarthritis, and prostatitis); idiopathic, familial, endocrine (e.g., hyperadrenocorticism, diabetes mellitus, and long-term administration of corticosteroids) • Cats—infectious (e.g., FeLV, FIP, and mycoplasma polyarthritis), neoplastic or inflammatory (e.g., pancreatitis, systemic lupus erythematosus, other immune-mediated diseases, and chronic skin disease); idiopathic, familial, and possibly endocrine (e.g., diabetes mellitus)

RISK FACTORS
See diseases/conditions listed above.

DIAGNOSIS

DIFFERENTIAL DIAGNOSIS
• Proteinuria—most common cause is inflammation of the urinary tract (e.g., bacterial cystitis/pyelonephritis, urolithiasis, and neoplasia); urinary tract inflammation is usually associated with active urine sediment (i.e., increased numbers of RBCs, WBCs, epithelial cells, and bacteria/hpf). Like glomerulonephritis, renal amyloidosis often causes severe proteinuria with inactive urine sediment (hyaline casts may be present). Renal biopsy is the only accurate way to distinguish amyloidosis from glomerulonephritis.
• Hypoalbuminemia—can be associated with decreased albumin production (severe liver disease) and increased albumin loss (protein-losing enteropathies and protein-losing nephropathies)

CBC/BIOCHEMISTRY/URINALYSIS
• Hypoalbuminemia and hypercholesterolemia in severe cases. • Persistent, significant proteinuria with an inactive urine sediment (hyaline casts may be observed)
• Microalbuminuria often precedes overt proteinuria and may become an important early diagnostic tool.

OTHER LABORATORY TESTS
Urine Protein:Creatinine Ratio
• Used to confirm and quantify abnormal proteinuria • Magnitude of proteinuria roughly correlates with the severity of glomerular lesions, making the urine protein:creatinine ratio a useful parameter to assess response to therapy or progression of disease.

Protein Electrophoresis
• Urine and serum protein electrophoresis may help identify the source of the proteinuria and establish a prognosis. • Proteinuria associated with hemorrhage into the urinary tract may have an electrophoretic pattern similar to that of the serum. • Light chain immunoglobulins (Bence Jones proteins) may be present in the urine in cases of lymphoid malignancy. • Early glomerular damage usually results principally in albuminuria; with disease progression, an increasing amount of globulin may be lost as well. • Marked decreases in serum albumin and increased concentrations of large-molecular-weight proteins, such as IgM, in the serum suggest severe glomerular proteinuria and the nephrotic syndrome. As the glomerular disease progresses and causes loss of three-quarters of the nephrons, the decreased glomerular filtration usually results in decreased proteinuria.

IMAGING
• No specific changes on abdominal radiographs or renal ultrasound, but these tests are useful in ruling out other concurrent condi-

tions. • Can use ultrasonography to guide percutaneous renal biopsy

DIAGNOSTIC PROCEDURES

• Renal biopsy—if significant and persistent proteinuria with inactive urine sediment; histopathologic evaluation of renal tissue will establish a diagnosis (e.g., glomerulonephritis vs. amyloidosis) and aid in formulation of a prognosis; consider only after performing less invasive tests (e.g., CBC, serum biochemistry profile, urinalysis, quantitation of proteinuria) and assessing blood clotting ability.
• Contraindications to renal biopsy—a solitary kidney, thrombocytopenia or other coagulopathy, and renal lesions associated with fluid accumulation (e.g., hydronephrosis and renal cysts and abscesses); renal biopsy should not be attempted by inexperienced clinicians or in patients that are not adequately restrained.

PATHOLOGIC FINDINGS

• Usually classified by histologic findings because the underlying cause is often unknown: glomerular basement membrane thickening—referred to as membranous glomerulonephritis; increased cellularity referred to as proliferative glomerulonephritis; a combination of membrane-thickening and increased cellularity—referred to as membranoproliferative glomerulonephritis; glomerular scarring associated with increases in mesangial matrix—referred to as glomerulosclerosis • Whenever possible, use immunofluorescent and/or immunocytochemical staining and electron microscopy to maximize the information gained from the biopsy specimen. • Request a Congo red stain in addition to routine stains since small amyloid deposits can be missed. Amyloid deposits appear green and birefringent when stained with Congo red and viewed under a polarized light source.

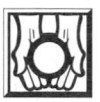 TREATMENT

APPROPRIATE HEALTH CARE

Most patients can be treated as outpatients; exceptions include severely azotemic and/or hypertensive patients and patients with thromboembolic disease.

ACTIVITY

Restrict because of the possibility of thromboembolic disease.

DIET

Sodium-reduced, high-quality, low-quantity protein diets

CLIENT EDUCATION

If the underlying cause cannot be identified and corrected, the disease is often progressive, resulting in chronic renal failure.

 MEDICATIONS

DRUG(S) OF CHOICE

• Since most glomerulonephritis is mediated by immunopathogenic mechanisms, the most specific and perhaps the most effective therapy is elimination of the source of antigenic stimulation. Unfortunately, this is often difficult because the disease process or antigen source is not identified or is impossible to eliminate (e.g., neoplasia).
• Immunosuppressive drugs are often used in dogs and cats as a second line of treatment. Corticosteroids, azathioprine, chlorambucil, cyclophosphamide, and cyclosporine have been used clinically or experimentally to prevent immunoglobulin production by B cells or to alter the function of T-helper or T-suppressor cells. Despite widespread use of immunosuppressive agents, no controlled clinical trials in veterinary medicine have demonstrated their efficacy. • The third type of treatment is aimed at reducing glomerular inflammation. Thromboxane is a major cause of glomerular inflammation associated with immune complexes; thus low-dose aspirin has been recommended to decrease thromboxane production. Aspirin also decreases platelet aggregation and resultant thromboembolic disease. Low-dose aspirin (5–10 mg/kg PO q24–48h) reportedly decreases platelet aggregation in dogs more effectively than 10 mg/kg once daily and may have less effect on the production of beneficial prostaglandins.
• In one study, enalapril (0.5 mg/kg q12–24h), an angiotensin-converting enzyme inhibitor, had antihypertensive and antiproteinuric effects and decreased progression of renal disease in dogs with idiopathic glomerulonephritis.

CONTRAINDICATIONS

Do not use corticosteroids in azotemic patients.

PRECAUTIONS

• Exercise caution with the use of immunosuppressive drugs. • Dosages of highly protein bound drugs (e.g., aspirin) may need to be adjusted; serum albumin concentrations change with treatment or progression of disease. • Use angiotensin-converting enzyme inhibitors cautiously in azotemic patients.

POSSIBLE INTERACTIONS

See Precautions above.

ALTERNATIVE DRUG(S)

N/A

 FOLLOW-UP

PATIENT MONITORING

• Follow the urine protein:creatinine ratio closely. Immunosuppressive therapy may worsen proteinuria; if this happens, discontinue immunosuppressive therapy.
• Also follow serum urea nitrogen, creatinine, albumin, and electrolyte concentrations, blood pressure, and body weight.
• Magnitude of proteinuria will decrease as more nephrons are lost to progressive disease; therefore, always interpret changes in the urine protein: creatinine ratio in light of changes in serum creatinine concentration.
• Ideally, reexamine 1, 3, 6, 9, and 12 months after initiation of treatment.

PREVENTION/AVOIDANCE

Do not breed affected animals of breeds with suspected familial glomerular disease.

POSSIBLE COMPLICATIONS

• Nephrotic syndrome • Chronic renal insufficiency or failure

EXPECTED COURSE AND PROGNOSIS

• Long-term prognosis is guarded.
• Often progresses to chronic renal insufficiency or failure despite treatment

 MISCELLANEOUS

ASSOCIATED CONDITIONS

See associated diseases/conditions, nephrotic syndrome, and possible complications.

PREGNANCY

High risk for patients with severe hypoalbuminemia and/or hypertension

SYNONYMS

• Glomerular disease • Glomerulopathy
• Protein-losing nephropathy

SEE ALSO

• Nephrotic Syndrome • Amyloidosis
• Proteinuria

ABBREVIATIONS

• FeLV = feline leukemia virus
• FIP = feline infectious peritonitis
• GN = glomerulonephritis

Suggested Reading

Cook AK, Cowgill LD. Clinical and pathologic features of protein-losing glomerular disease in the dog. A review of 137 cases (1985–1992). J Am Anim Hosp Assoc 1996;32:313–322.

Dambach DM, Smith CA, Lewis RM, Van Winkle TJ. Morphologic, immunohistochemical, and ultrastructural characterization of a distinctive renal lesion in dogs putatively associated with *Borrelia burgdorferi* infection: 49 cases (1987–1992). Vet Pathol 1997;34:85–96.

Grauer GF. Glomerulonephritis. Semin Vet Med Surg (Small Animal) 1992;7:187–197.

Grauer GF, Greco DS, Getsy DM, et al. Effects of enalapril versus placebo as a treatment for canine idiopathic glomerulonephritis. J Vet Intern Med 2000;14:526–533.

Author Gregory F. Grauer
Consulting Editors Larry G. Adams and Carl A. Osborne

GLUCAGONOMA

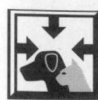

BASICS

OVERVIEW
• Glucagonoma is a rare neoplasm of alpha-pancreatic islet cells that actively secrete glucagon. Many will secrete other hormones as well, such as insulin, gastrin, and pancreatic polypeptide. Excess circulating glucagon results in increased protein catabolism, increased lipolysis, gluconeogenesis, and glycogenolysis. Glucagon can also exert a secretory effect on the small intestine.
• Glucagonomas can affect musculoskeletal, integumentary, endocrine, gastrointestinal, nervous, behavioral, and hepatobiliary organ systems.

SIGNALMENT
• Dogs—rare; older animals
• No known incidence in cats

SIGNS
• The hallmark sign of glucagonomas reported in both humans and dogs is a characteristic dermatitis. The dermatopathy has been referred to as metabolic epidermal necrosis, superficial necrolytic dermatitis, necrolytic migratory erythema, diabetic dermatopathy, and hepatocutaneous syndrome in the veterinary literature.
• This skin pathology is also seen with liver disease and hypoaminoacidemia.
• Skin lesions include erythema, crusting, and erosions generally located around muco-cutaneous junctions on the face, perineum, and genitalia as well as along distal extremities and footpads. Lesions can be pruritic and the footpads are characteristically hyperkeratotic and painful. Often, the feet are the only affected area.
• Secondary pyodermas and yeast infections are common.
• Other systemic signs may include lethargy, polyuria/polydipsia, diarrhea, and weight loss.

CAUSES & RISK FACTORS
Both solitary pancreatic glucagonomas and hepatic metastases have been reported in dogs. Glucagonomas can also be seen in multiple endocrine neoplasia syndrome.

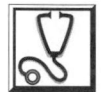

DIAGNOSIS

DIFFERENTIAL DIAGNOSIS
• Metabolic epidermal necrosis (MEN) has been associated with diabetes, pancreatic tumors, and hepatic disease. Other dermatopathy differentials include pemphigus foliaceus, systemic lupus erythematosus, vasculitis, and zinc deficiency dermatopathy.
• Hyperglucagonemia secondary to islet cell tumors, liver disease, pancreatic disease, chronic renal failure, starvation, bacteremia, diabetic ketoacidosis, hyperadrenocorticism

CBC/BIOCHEMISTRY/URINALYSIS
• CBC—mild normocytic, normochromic anemia, neutrophilia
• Chemistry—mild liver enzyme elevations and total bilirubin, mild hyperglycemia, hypoalbuminemia; may be within normal limits
• Urinalysis—may show decreased urine specific gravity, glucosuria if diabetes is present

OTHER LABORATORY TESTS
• Plasma glucagon levels—normal glucagon levels do not rule out glucagonoma.
• Plasma amino acid levels—hypoamino-acidemia is thought to be associated with the development of metabolic epidermal necrolysis.
• Zinc levels—low levels of zinc may contribute to dermatologic changes.
• Fructosamine—hyperglucagonemia can result in overt diabetes mellitus.

IMAGING
Ultrasound has been used to detect both pancreatic masses and hepatic metastases. Computed tomography (CT) scans are also used for tumor localization in humans. Selective visceral angiography is considered to be the gold standard in localization of glucagonomas in humans.

DIAGNOSTIC PROCEDURES
Biopsy and immunohistochemical staining for glucagon is necessary for definitive diagnosis. Immunohistochemical staining for other pancreatic and gastrointestinal hormones is recommended. Malignancy is generally determined by the presence of metastasis.

PATHOLOGIC FINDINGS
• Skin histology—severe superficial to mid-epidermal edema, diffuse parakeratotic hyperkeratosis, irregular epidermal hyperplasia

• Tumor histopathology—pleiomorphic islet cells with occasional mitoses and fine cytoplasmic granules. Immunohistochemical stains positive for glucagon and often other secretory hormones

TREATMENT

• Surgical excision is the only chance for cure. However, there is a high rate of postoperative morbidity and mortality reported in dogs. Glucagonoma syndrome is associated with thromboembolic disease, which can occur postoperatively, as well as pancreatitis.
• In humans, palliative tumor debulking to reduce circulating glucagon levels is not sufficient. Combined debulking and octreotide medical therapy can, however, resolve skin lesions and provide symptomatic relief. This palliative therapy will not prolong survival time.
• High-protein diet and egg whites (approx. 2–3 egg whites/day for a 25-kg dog) may improve hypoaminoacidemia to some extent and thereby relieve skin symptoms.
• Zinc and fatty acid supplementation may improve skin signs even in the face of normal measured zinc levels.
• Secondary infections must be treated.

MEDICATIONS

• Octreotide is a somatostatin analog that inhibits the conversion of preproglucagon to glucagon. Many side effects have been reported with human use of this drug, including injection site pain, cholestasis, vomiting, and diarrhea.
• Various chemotherapeutics have also been used in human glucagonoma syndrome; 5-FU and streptozotocin is currently the recommended combination.
• Glucocorticoids may help improve skin lesions, but they can also exacerbate hyperglycemia.
• Intravenous amino acids (500 ml of essential amino acids added to saline or lactated Ringer's solution given over 12 hours) has shown variable improvement in skin lesions in dogs. Some dogs resolve completely, others not at all. Treatments can be repeated every 1–2 weeks if effective.
• Sulfur/salicylic acid shampoos or very mild shampoos may help remove crusts, soften skin, and improve pain or pruritus associated with skin and footpad lesions.
• Anti-yeast formulations or antibiotics are necessary if secondary infections are found.

CONTRAINDICATIONS/POSSIBLE INTERACTIONS

Glucocorticoids can exacerbate diabetes mellitus if present.

FOLLOW-UP

• Monitoring of blood work should be done regularly to alleviate developing symptoms early on.
• Follow-up ultrasounds should be performed to monitor for metastasis.

MISCELLANEOUS

Suggested Reading

Allenspach K, et al. Glucagon-producing neuroendocrine tumour associated with hypoaminoacidemia and skin lesions. J Small Anim Pract 2000:41:402–406.
Chastain MA. The glucagonoma syndrome: a review of its features and discussion of new perspectives. The American Journal of the Medical Sciences 2001:321(5):306–320.
Gross TL, et al. Glucagon-producing pancreatic endocrine tumours in two dogs with superficial necrolytic dermatitis. JAVMA 1990;197(12):1619–1622.

Author Nicole Bennett
Consulting Editor Deborah Greco

GLUCOSURIA

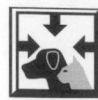 BASICS

DEFINITION
Urinary glucose concentration detectable by routine laboratory tests. The small quantity of glucose normally present in urine is not detected by routine laboratory tests; persistent glucosuria is abnormal.

PATHOPHYSIOLOGY
• Should be categorized as hyperglycemic or normoglycemic, and subcategorized as transient or persistent. • Glucose passes readily through glomerular capillary walls and has the same concentration in glomerular filtrate and blood. It is reabsorbed at the luminal membrane of proximal renal tubular cells by secondary active transport coupled with sodium reabsorption. In this way, glucose attains a high intracellular concentration. It is then transported into renal interstitium through basolateral membranes by a sodium-independent mechanism and returned to the peripheral circulation via renal peritubular capillaries.

Hyperglycemic Glucosuria
Occurs when the concentration of glucose in glomerular filtrate exceeds the transport maximum of tubular epithelial cells; the renal tubular threshold for glucose in dogs is 170–220 mg/dL; for cats, 260–310 mg/dL as measured in venous blood. When hyperglycemia is observed, the next step is to determine whether it is transient or persistent.

Transient Glucosuria
• Physiologic glucosuria—typically transient; associated with increases of "stress" hormones (glucagon, catecholamines, glucocorticoids), particularly in cats • Pharmacologic (iatrogenic) glucosuria—transient; results from administration of parenteral solutions (e.g., dextrose, total parenteral nutrition solutions) that contain sufficient glucose; parenteral administration of glucocorticoids is an uncommonly recognized cause of glucosuria in dogs and cats. • Adrenocorticotropic hormone, glucagon, epinephrine, morphine, and phenothiazines also have the potential to cause transient glucosuria.

Persistent (or Pathologic) Glucosuria
• Patient may be normoglycemic or hyperglycemic. • Normoglycemic glucosuria—includes renal tubular dysfunction associated with generalized and specific reabsorptive defects of proximal nephrons; can be further subdivided into congenital or acquired proximal renal tubular defects • Primary renal glucosuria—a congenital disorder in Scottish terriers and mixed-breed dogs; associated with specific reabsorptive defects for glucose in proximal renal tubular cells • Fanconi's

syndrome (aminodiabetes)—characterized by generalized proximal renal tubular defects associated with glucosuria, phosphaturia, and aminoaciduria; dogs may also have varying degrees of hypercalciuria, hyperbicarbonaturia, hypernatriuria, hyperkalluria, and hyperuricuria. See section entitled "Fanconi's syndrome." • A congenital (juvenile) renal disease associated with renal tubular transport dysfunction has been reported in Norwegian elkhounds.
• Congenital glomerular diseases reported in Doberman pinschers, cocker spaniels, and Samoyed dogs are typically not associated with proximal renal tubular defects and glucosuria. • Acquired normoglycemic glucosuria may also be associated with some forms of acute renal failure but is not commonly observed in association with chronic renal failure. • Etiologic agents include heavy metal poisons (e.g., lead, mercury), drugs (e.g., gentamicin, cisplatin), and chemicals (e.g., Lysol, maleic acid). In humans, multiple myeloma may lead to development of acquired Fanconi's syndrome.

SYSTEMS AFFECTED
• Renal/Urologic—in normoglycemic glucosuria, renal tubular cell function is abnormal. Dogs with Fanconi's syndrome commonly develop CRF and secondary multisystem involvement. Glucosuria may also predispose to a bacterial urinary tract infection and associated manifestations.
• Endocrine—diabetes mellitus and hyperadrenocorticism cause hyperglycemic glucosuria.

SIGNALMENT
• Persistent hyperglycemic glucosuria is usually caused by adult-onset diabetes mellitus. • Onset of clinical disease in dogs with Fanconi's syndrome typically occurs after they reach maturity. Defective reabsorption of glucose and amino acids is recognized at 4–5 years of age. There is no sex predilection for the disease. • Primary renal glucosuria is an incidental finding that can be recognized at an early age. • Familial tubular disorders have been reported in Basenjis, border terriers, and Scottish terriers, and in Norwegian elkhounds with generalized familial (juvenile) nephropathies.

SIGNS

General Comments
Clinical signs—vary; depend on the primary cause

Historical Findings
• If glucosuria is of sufficient magnitude, polyuria secondary to osmotic diuresis and compensatory polydipsia develop.
• The frequency of occurrence of polyuria and polydipsia with primary renal glucosuria is unknown; there have been too few docu-

mented cases to formulate generalities. However, dogs with primary renal glucosuria may form less concentrated urine. • Urinary tract infections that develop secondary to disease associated with glucosuria show signs typical of lower and/or upper urinary tract disease. • Breed and drug history are important.

Physical Examination Findings
• Hyperglycemic glucosuria may be associated with systemic signs. • Body systems are often normal in patients with normoglycemic glucosuria. • Dogs with Fanconi's syndrome may develop signs of renal failure.

CAUSES

Hyperglycemic Glucosuria
• Transient physiologic—stress hyperglycemia is common in cats. • Transient pharmacologic—parenteral solutions (e.g., dextrose, total parenteral nutrition solutions), xylazine in cats, glucocorticoids, ACTH, glucagon, epinephrine, morphine, phenothiazine, diazoxide, l-asparaginase • Persistent hyperglycemic glucosuria—diabetes mellitus (100%), hyperadrenocorticism (5–10%), acute pancreatitis, CNS lesions, pheochromocytoma, progesterone-associated hyperglycemia, acromegaly, sepsis, glucagonoma, chronic liver failure (failure to metabolize glucagon)

Normoglycemic Glucosuria
• Congenital normoglycemic glucosuria—primary renal glucosuria (Scottish terriers and mixed-breed dogs); congenital Fanconi's syndrome (basenji, Norwegian elkhound, Shetland sheepdog, miniature schnauzer); congenital diseases associated with renal dysfunction (Norwegian elkhound) • Acquired normoglycemic glucosuria—acute renal failure associated with significant proximal tubular lesions; CRF (rare); acquired Fanconi's syndrome due to heavy metal poisoning (lead, mercury, cadmium, uranium), drugs (gentamicin, cephalosporins, outdated tetracycline, cisplatin, streptozotocin, amoxicillin), and chemicals (Lysol, maleic acid)

RISK FACTORS
Vary with causes

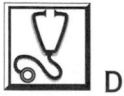 DIAGNOSIS

DIFFERENTIAL DIAGNOSIS
• Fasted, persistent, hyperglycemic glucosuria is most often associated with endocrinopathies (e.g., diabetes mellitus, hyperadrenocorticism). • Normoglycemic glucosuria is associated with renal tubular reabsorptive dysfunctions. • Further diagnostic procedures are required to find the cause of glucosuria. • Expect mild transient hyperglycemia in stressed animals.

LABORATORY FINDINGS

Screening Tests

• Normally too little glucose is present in urine to be detected by routine laboratory tests.
• Dipsticks and reagent tapes impregnated with glucose oxidase, peroxidase, and other reagents that result in color changes when glucose is present involve interrelated sequential bienzymatic reactions. Glucose oxidase reacts specifically with glucose; the enzyme will not react with nonglucose-reducing substances. Drugs containing azo dyes, nitrofurantoin, and riboflavin, or other causes of severe pigmenturia (hemoglobinuria, bilirubinuria) may affect the readability of the reagent pad and lead to misinterpretation. • False-negative results—(1) Ascorbic acid concentration as low as 50 mg/dL can prevent detection of low concentrations (50 or 100 mg/dL) of urine glucose by the glucose oxidase test. Ascorbic acid concentrations as high as 90 mg/dL have been detected in urine samples collected from dogs and as high as 50 mg/dL in cats with diabetes mellitus. Consumption of large amounts of ascorbic acid or salicylates (e.g., vitamin C supplements, tetracycline drugs because of ascorbic acid in formulation) may yield false-negative results. (2) Moderately high ketonuria (40 mg/dL) may cause false-negative results for specimens containing small amounts of glucose (75–125 mg/dL). (3) Refrigerated urine may reduce the rate of enzymatic activity in glucose oxidase/peroxidase tests. (4) Reactivity of the glucose test area for Multistix reagents may decrease with increasing specific gravity. (5) Outdated reagents or reagents exposed to sunlight may also give erratic results. • Colorimetric copper reduction methods are based on the change from cupric acid (blue) to cuprous oxide (orange-red). The color change (blue to green to orange) depends on the concentration of reducing compounds (including glucose) in urine. Copper reduction methods are not specific for glucose and are less sensitive than glucose oxidase methods.
• False-positive results may be caused by contamination of the sample or test system with small quantities of hydrogen peroxide (0.006%), hydrochlorite, chlorine, or other strong oxidizing agents. False-positive results may also be caused by (1) sufficient concentrations of nonglucose-reducing substances, including fructose, lactose, galactose, pentose, and maltose; (2) sufficient quantities of glucuronic acids (e.g., conjugated bilirubin); penicillin, salicylates, and chloral hydrate act as reducing substances; and (3) formaldehyde. *Note:* No ascorbic acid concentrations high enough to cause false-positive results with copper reduction techniques have been observed at the University of Minnesota.

Confirmation Testing

When unsuspected results or unusual test pad colors from highly pigmented urine occur, results can be confirmed by measuring glucose in the urine. Hexokinase- or glucose dehydrogenase–based techniques are recommended for quantitation of urinary glucose.

Drugs That May Alter Laboratory Results

See Laboratory Findings—Screening Tests.

Disorders That May Alter Laboratory Results

See Laboratory Findings—Screening Tests.

Valid If Run in Human Laboratory?

Yes

CBC/BIOCHEMISTRY/URINALYSIS

Hyperglycemic Glucosuria

• Detection of ketonuria, hyperglycemia, and glucosuria indicates diabetic ketoacidosis.
• Mild hyperglycemia with concomitant transient glucosuria is physiologic in stressed animals. • Inflammatory leukogram, high serum lipase, and amylase activity in glucosuric dogs with adequate renal function supports a diagnosis of acute pancreatitis.
• High serum ALP activity in dogs with hyperglycemic glucosuria should prompt consideration of hyperadrenocorticism.

Normoglycemic Glucosuria

• Glucosuria is typically the only abnormal finding in dogs with normoglycemic primary renal glucosuria. • In other conditions associated with normoglycemic glucosuria, high serum urea nitrogen, creatinine, and phosphorus with impaired urine-concentrating ability suggests renal tubular dysfunction. Hyperchloremic metabolic acidosis may occur secondary to decreased bicarbonate resorption by proximal renal epithelial cells (renal tubular acidosis type 2). If progressive renal failure develops, characteristic clinical and laboratory findings will result.

OTHER LABORATORY TESTS

• Normoglycemic glucosuria—measurement of phosphorus, glucose, and amino acid concentrations in timed urine collections permits differentiation of Fanconi's syndrome and renal primary glucosuria.
• Hyperglycemic glucosuria—ACTH response test or low-dose dexamethasone suppression test if suspect hyperadrenocorticism; see chapters related to specific causes.

IMAGING

Ultrasonography may be helpful in diagnosis of hyperadrenocorticism.

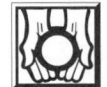 **TREATMENT**

• Discontinue any drugs associated with acquired tubular transport defects.
• Treatment varies with cause; see relevant chapters.

 MEDICATIONS

DRUG(S) OF CHOICE

• No specific drugs for glucose transport defects
• Treat underlying disease when possible.

CONTRAINDICATIONS

Diabetogenic drugs (e.g., corticosteroids) or dextrose-containing fluids

 **FOLLOW-UP**

PATIENT MONITORING

Varies with cause

POSSIBLE COMPLICATIONS

• Persistent glucosuria is predisposing for development of cystitis, ascending pyelonephritis, and sepsis. • Osmotic diuresis with obligatory polyuria and secondary polydipsia

 **MISCELLANEOUS**

ASSOCIATED CONDITIONS

Urinary tract infections

PREGNANCY

Diestrus in bitches may induce diabetes mellitus (non–insulin-dependent) caused by high progesterone concentration.

SEE ALSO

• Diabetes Mellitus, Uncomplicated
• Fanconi's Syndrome
• Hyperadrenocorticism
• Renal Disease, Congenital and Developmental

ABBREVIATIONS

• ACTH = adrenocorticotropic hormone
• ALP = alkaline phosphatase
• CRF = chronic renal failure

Suggested Reading

Brown SA. Fanconi's syndrome; inherited and acquired. In: Kirk RW, Current veterinary therapy X. Philadelphia: Saunders, 1989:1163–1165.

Finco DR. Congenital, inherited, and familial renal diseases. In: Osborne CA, Finco DR, eds. Canine and feline nephrology and urology. Baltimore: Williams & Wilkins, 1995: 1471–1483.

Meyers DJ, Harvey JW. Veterinary laboratory medicine interpretation and diagnosis. 2nd ed. Philadelphia: Saunders, 1998:221–237.

Authors Frédéric Jacob and Carl A. Osborne
Consulting Editors Larry G. Adams and Carl A. Osborne

GLUTEN ENTEROPATHY IN IRISH SETTERS

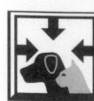 ## BASICS

OVERVIEW
A rare inherited disease in which there is a predisposition to develop a sensitivity to dietary gluten present in wheat and other grains

SIGNALMENT
• Only reported in the Irish setter breed in the United Kingdom
• Mode of inheritance not known
• Signs develop in young to middle-aged dogs.

SIGNS
• Poor weight gain (or weight loss)
• Mild diarrhea

CAUSES & RISK FACTORS
The enteropathy and clinical signs are exacerbated by gluten-containing diet.

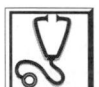 ## DIAGNOSIS

DIFFERENTIAL DIAGNOSIS
Other chronic small intestinal diseases

CBC/BIOCHEMISTRY/URINALYSIS
Unremarkable

OTHER LABORATORY TESTS
• Serum folate concentrations are subnormal in some patients, reflecting chronic malabsorption.
• Serum trypsin-like immunoreactivity and cobalamin concentrations are usually normal.

IMAGING
Not useful

DIAGNOSTIC PROCEDURES
Intestinal biopsy specimens (jejunal) obtained via endoscopy or laparotomy

PATHOLOGIC FINDINGS
• Histologic examination of jejunal biopsy specimens from affected dogs reared on a wheat-containing diet reveals partial villus atrophy and accumulation of intraepithelial lymphocytes.
• Jejunal abnormalities improve following gluten withdrawal but recur with gluten challenge.

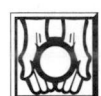 ## TREATMENT
Avoid diets containing gluten.

 ## MEDICATIONS

DRUG(S)
Folate (0.5–2.0 mg PO q24h for 2–4 weeks) if serum folate concentration is markedly subnormal (< 4 µg/L)

CONTRAINDICATIONS/POSSIBLE INTERACTIONS
N/A

 ## FOLLOW-UP
Consider periodic assay of serum folate (q6–12 months)

 ## MISCELLANEOUS

Suggested Reading
Hall EJ, Batt RM. Dietary modulation of gluten sensitivity in a naturally occurring enteropathy of Irish setter dogs. Gut 1992;33:198–205.
Author David A. Williams
Consulting Editor Albert E. Jergens

BASICS

OVERVIEW
• Also known as glycogenoses: rare inherited disorders characterized by abnormal glycogen metabolism owing to defective or deficient enzyme activity controlling glycogen metabolism • Tissue glycogen accumulation—leads to organ enlargement and dysfunction; primarily affects liver, heart, skeletal muscle, kidney, and CNS • Impaired hepatic glycogen mobilization—produces symptomatic hypoglycemia • Classification—according to type of enzymatic defect and primary organ(s) involved: more than 12 types in humans, four types in dogs (Ia, II, III, and VII), 1 type in cats (IV)

SIGNALMENT
• Clinical signs manifest in juveniles—days to several months after birth in most disorders • Type Ia (von Gierke's disease)—Maltese puppies • Type II (Pompe's disease)—Lapland dogs; onset beginning at 6 months of age • Type III (Cori's disease)—young female German shepherds • Type IV—Norwegian forest cats; may be stillborn; may fade shortly after birth; may manifest signs at 5–7 months of age • Type VII—English springer spaniels 2–9 years of age • No known sex predilection • Autosomal recessive inheritance—Norwegian forest cats, English springer spaniels, Lapland dogs, and Maltese dogs; suspected for German shepherds

SIGNS
• Depend on enzymatic defect • Type Ia (Maltese puppies)—failure to thrive; mental depression; hypoglycemia; abdominal distention; hepatomegaly; death or euthanization by 60 days of age • Type II (Lapland dogs)—vomiting and regurgitation related to megaesophagus; progressive muscle weakness; cardiac changes; death before 2 years of age • Type III (German shepherds)—depression; weakness; failure to grow; abdominal distention from hepatomegaly; mild hypoglycemia • Type IV (Norwegian forest cats)—death occurs often in the perinatal period; intermittent fever; generalized muscle tremors; muscle atrophy and weakness progressing to tetraplegia; sudden death from myocardial degeneration and terminal dysrhythmia • Type VII (English springer spaniels)—compensated hemolytic anemia; episodic intravascular hemolysis; hemoglobinuria; one patient developed a progressive myopathy at 11 years of age

CAUSES & RISK FACTORS
Deficiencies
• Type Ia—glucose-6-phosphatase • Type II—acid-α-glucosidase • Type III—amylo-1,6-glucosidase • Type IV—glycogen branching enzyme (α-1,4-D-glucan) • Type VII—phosphofructokinase

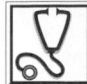

DIAGNOSIS

DIFFERENTIAL DIAGNOSIS
• High index of suspicion for diagnosis • Breed affiliation • Differentiate other causes of juvenile hypoglycemia—malnutrition; endoparasitism; transient fasting hypoglycemia; portosystemic vascular anomaly • Other causes of muscular weakness—infectious diseases; endocrinopathy; immune-mediated causes; hypokalemia; other neuromyopathy

CBC/BIOCHEMISTRY/URINALYSIS
• Types I and III—hypoglycemia; type I: recent work in laboratory-reared affected dogs demonstrates hyperlactacidemia, hypercholesterolemia, hypertriglyceridemia, and hyperuricemia • Type VII—anemia; reticulocytosis; pigmenturia

OTHER LABORATORY TESTS
• Type I—genetic characterization in Maltese dogs • Type IV—PCR carrier test (developed for Norwegian forest cats), available through Michigan State University • Type VII—in vitro erythrocyte testing; genetic characterization accomplished

IMAGING
• Type II—thoracic radiography; may show cardiomegaly and megaesophagus • Types Ia and III—abdominal radiography; may reveal hepatomegaly • Abdominal ultrasonography—may reveal hepatomegaly and echogenic changes suggesting hepatic glycogen deposition (hyperechogenicity) • Types II and IV—echocardiography; may reveal cardiac changes

DIAGNOSTIC PROCEDURES
• Tissue enzyme analysis and glycogen determination—definitive diagnosis • Electromyography • Electrocardiography

PATHOLOGIC FINDINGS
• Type Ia—emaciation; massive hepatomegaly; glycogen and lipid accumulation (vacuolation) in hepatocytes and renal tubule epithelial cells • Type II—glycogen accumulation in skeletal, smooth, and cardiac muscle • Type III—hepatomegaly owing to hepatic glycogen accumulation; also in skeletal muscle • Type IV—generalized muscle atrophy; glycogen accumulation: skeletal muscle, CNS, and peripheral nervous system • Type VII—polysaccharide deposits in skeletal muscle

TREATMENT

NURSING CARE
• Supportive care • Types I and III—may require intravenous dextrose for management of hypoglycemic crisis; long-term management is futile.

DIET
Control hypoglycemia (types I and III) with frequent feedings of a high-carbohydrate diet until diagnosis is confirmed.

CLIENT EDUCATION
• Advise that specimens be sent to specialty laboratories for genetic/enzyme characterizations • Discuss known mechanisms of inheritance to modify breeding programs.

MEDICATIONS

DRUG(S) N/A

CONTRAINDICATIONS/POSSIBLE INTERACTIONS N/A

FOLLOW-UP
• Monitor for hypoglycemia • Cull parents from breeding programs • Prognosis—poor; most patients die or are euthanized owing to progressive deterioration, exception is in Springer spaniels with hematologic manifestations

MISCELLANEOUS

SEE ALSO
• Lysosomal Storage Disease • Mucopolysaccharidosis • Portosystemic Vascular Anomaly, Congenital

ABBREVIATIONS
• CNS = central nervous system • PCR = polymerase chain reaction

Suggested Reading
Brix AE, Howerth EW, et al. Glycogen storage disease type Ia in two littermate maltese puppies. Vet Pathol 1995;32:460–465.
Harvey JW, Calderwood MB. Polysaccharide storage myopathy in canine phosphofructokinase deficiency (type VII glycogen storage disease). Vet Pathol 1990;27:1–8.
Kishnani PS, Bao Y, Wu JY, et al. Isolation and nucleotide sequence of canine glucose-6-phosphatase mRNA: identification of mutation in puppies with glycogen storage disease type Ia. Biochem Mol Med 1997;61:168–177.
Walvoort HC. Glycogen storage disease type II in the lapland dog. Vet Q 1985; 7:187–190.
Author Angelyn M. Cornetta
Consulting Editor Sharon A. Center

GROWTH HORMONE-RESPONSIVE DERMATOSES

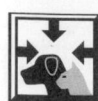 BASICS

OVERVIEW

• Uncommon dermatoses resulting from a growth hormone deficiency or dermatoses responding to growth hormone therapy
• Pituitary dwarfism—the result of a primary growth hormone deficiency
• Adult-onset growth hormone–responsive dermatosis—a clinical syndrome that responds to growth hormone therapy; patients may be strictly growth hormone–deficient; may have one or more of a plethora of hormonal abnormalities, including possible imbalances of adrenal sex hormones

SIGNALMENT

• Pituitary dwarfism—most commonly seen in German shepherds; also reported in spitzes, toy pinschers, and Carnelian bear dogs; noted at 2–3 months of age
• Adult-onset—reported in the chow chows, Pomeranians, poodles, keeshonds, Samoyeds, and American water spaniels; generally noted at 1–2 years of age; primarily affects males, although seen in both sexes (neutered and intact) and at all ages

SIGNS

Pituitary Dwarfism

• Patients appear normal at birth; by 2–3 months, bilaterally symmetrical alopecia begins to be apparent; trunk, neck, and caudal thighs severely affected
• Primary hair growth over face and distal extremities only; retained puppy coat is easily epilated.
• Skin—thin, hypotonic, scaly, and hyperpigmented; comedones noted

Adult-onset Growth Hormone–responsive Dermatosis

• Alopecia—bilaterally symmetrical; involves trunk, neck, caudomedial thighs, tail, ventral abdomen, perineum, and pinnae; the head and legs are spared.
• Primary hairs are lost first; then loss of secondary hairs in the affected areas; hair readily epilates; tufts of regrowth at trauma or biopsy sites
• Skin—thin and hyperpigmented; secondary seborrhea and pyoderma uncommon

CAUSES & RISK FACTORS

• Pituitary dwarfism—mediated by an autosomal recessive trait, which results in a developmental abnormality of the pituitary and lack of growth hormone production
• Adult-onset—unknown; breed predisposition suggests a hereditary influence; pituitary neoplasia has been suggested
• Although an absolute growth hormone deficiency may be noted, other causes may lead to a similar clinical syndrome that responds to growth hormone supplementation (e.g., castration-responsive dermatosis, congenital adrenal hyperplasia–like syndrome).

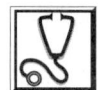 DIAGNOSIS

DIFFERENTIAL DIAGNOSIS

• Pituitary dwarfism—hypothyroidism, malnutrition, and metabolic disorders
• Adult-onset—hypothyroidism, hyperadrenocorticism, castration-responsive dermatosis, cyclic flank alopecia, estrogen/testosterone-responsive dermatosis, follicular dysplasia, and congenital adrenal hyperplasia–like syndrome

CBC/BIOCHEMISTRY/URINALYSIS

Results usually unremarkable

OTHER LABORATORY TESTS

• Growth hormone–stimulation test—dubious value; not currently available
• Somatomedin C (insulin-like growth factor 1)—growth hormone dependent; concentrations parallel body size; release may be impaired by glucocorticoids and estrogens; an indirect assay of growth hormone levels; expected to be low in growth hormone–deficient states (performed at Michigan State University Animal Health Diagnostic Laboratory, Lansing, MI)
• Pituitary dwarfism—low thyroid-stimulating hormone, ACTH, gonadotropin-releasing hormone, and human chorionic gonadotropin response test results
• Insulin response test—may aid diagnosis; causes severe hypoglycemia
• Adrenal reproductive hormone testing—ACTH-stimulation test with evaluation of adrenocortical hormones and their precursors (performed at the University of Tennessee College of Veterinary Medicine Endocrinology Laboratory, Nashville, TN).

IMAGING N/A

DIAGNOSTIC PROCEDURES

• Skin biopsy—general endocrinopathy; orthokeratotic hyperkeratosis; epidermal atrophy; follicular keratosis, dilation, and atrophy; telogenization of hair follicles; atrophy of sebaceous glands; amounts and sizes of dermal elastin fibers are small
• Castration-responsive or growth hormone–responsive dermatoses (dogs)—hypereosinophilic tricholemmal keratinization of hair follicles ("flame follicles")

GROWTH HORMONE–RESPONSIVE DERMATOSES

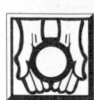

TREATMENT

Outpatients

MEDICATIONS

DRUG(S)

• L-Thyroxine—0.02 mg/kg PO q12h for a 6-week trial; recommended if the baseline total T_4 is low or low normal
• o,p'-DDD (Lysodren)—15–25 mg/kg PO q24h for 2–7 days; an ACTH-stimulation test to evaluate the response should demonstrate suppression of the baseline cortisol to a low-normal range; poststimulation range is 30–50 ng/mL (3.0–5.0 μg/dL); conduct ACTH-stimulation testing quarterly
• Methyltestosterone—1 mg/kg (maximum dose, 30 mg/dog) PO q48h for a maximum of 3 months; after hair regrowth, maintain at 1 mg/kg (maximum dose, 30 mg/dog) PO every 4–7 days
• Bovine, porcine, or synthetic human growth hormone—0.15 IU/kg SC twice weekly for 6 weeks; may repeat if no response within 3 months

CONTRAINDICATIONS/POSSIBLE INTERACTIONS

Intact male dogs—neuter to rule out castration-responsive dermatosis.

FOLLOW-UP

PATIENT MONITORING

• Growth hormones—monitor blood glucose before each treatment; growth hormone is diabetogenic
• Methyltestosterone—cholangiohepatitis, seborrhea, and behavioral changes; monitor liver enzymes and clinical status
• If post-ACTH stimulation blood cortisols are too low, evaluate serum electrolytes to determine the need for mineralocorticoid treatment.

POSSIBLE COMPLICATIONS

Growth hormone therapy—anaphylaxis with repeated dosing; diabetes mellitus (transient or permanent)

EXPECTED COURSE AND PROGNOSIS

• Pituitary dwarfism—hair regrowth will begin within 4–8 weeks of beginning therapy and lasts 6 months to 2 years; re-treatment is usually necessary.
• Adult-onset—hair regrowth is usually observed in 2–12 weeks after therapy and lasts 6 months to 3 years; re-treatment is often necessary.
• o,p'-DDD—gives a good prognosis for hair regrowth if imbalance of adrenal sex hormone concentrations is suspected; may be a transient increase in epilation, but hair regrowth may be noted 4–12 weeks after beginning therapy
• Signs are confined to the skin, so treatment is not mandatory; owners may decline therapy because of the possible side effects.

MISCELLANEOUS

ABBREVIATIONS

• ACTH = adrenocorticotropic hormone
• o,p'-DDD = 1,1-(o,p'-dichlorodiphenyl)-2,2-dichloroethane
• T_4 = thyroxine

Suggested Reading

Schmeitzel LP. Sex hormone–related and growth hormone-related alopecias. Vet Clin North Am Small Anim Pract 1990;20: 1579–1601.

Author Margaret S. Swartout
Consulting Editor Karen Helton Rhodes

HAEMOBARTONELLOSIS (ERYTHROCYTIC MYCOPLASMA INFECTIONS)

BASICS

OVERVIEW
Red blood cell destruction and anemia caused by parasite attachment to the external surface of RBCs and immune response by the host

SIGNALMENT
• Dogs and cats • Most common in adults • In cats, more common in males • No sex prevalence in dogs

SIGNS

Cats
• Variable disease severity ranging from inapparent infection to marked depression and death • Intermittent fever (only 50% of the time) during the acute phase, depression, weakness, anorexia, pale mucous membranes, splenomegaly, and (occasionally) icterus

Dogs
Mild or inapparent signs (e.g., pale mucous membranes and listlessness)—except when dogs have been splenectomized

CAUSES & RISK FACTORS
• Caused by organisms previously classified as rickettsial bacteria *Haemobartonella felis* (cats) and *Haemobartonella canis* (dogs), but these organisms were recently recognized to be mycoplasmal bacteria based on genetic determinations • Proposed new names include *Mycoplasma haemofelis* for a large form of *H. felis*, *Mycoplasma haemominutum* for the small form of *H. felis*, and *Mycoplasma haemocanis* for *H. canis* (dogs).
• The large species of mycoplasmal organisms infecting cats generally causes more severe disease than does the small species.
• Cats—anemia more severe if FeLV infected
• Dogs—likelihood of severe anemia greatly increased if splenectomized or with pathologic changes in the spleen

DIAGNOSIS

DIFFERENTIAL DIAGNOSIS
• Other causes of hemolytic anemia, including AIHA, babesiosis (not in cats in the U.S.), cytauxzoonosis (cats only), Heinz body hemolytic anemia, microangiopathic hemolytic anemia, pyruvate kinase deficiency, and phosphofructokinase deficiency (dogs only) • Differentiated from AIHA only by recognition of parasites in blood (stained blood film or PCR-based assays)—both disorders may be Coombs' test–positive.
• *Babesia* and *Cytauxzoon* species are protozoal organisms that differ in morphology from these mycoplasmal organisms. • New methylene blue stains used to identify Heinz bodies • Enzyme assays or

specialized DNA tests used to diagnose pyruvate kinase and phosphofructokinase deficiencies

CBC/BIOCHEMISTRY/URINALYSIS
• Anemia, most often present with reticulocytosis in animals with clinically important haemobartonellosis—may appear poorly regenerative if a precipitous decrease in PCV has occurred early in the disease or if there are other concurrent disorders (e.g., FeLV or FIV infections in cats)
• Autoagglutination may be seen in feline blood samples after they cool to below body temperature. • Variable total and differential leukocyte counts of little diagnostic assistance
• Slight hemoglobinemia rarely observed; no hemoglobinuria reported • Hyperbilirubinemia may be measured at times but is seldom severe. • Substantial bilirubinuria seen in some dogs • Abnormalities related to anemic hypoxia may be shown by clinical chemistry profiles, but profile can be normal.
• Hypoglycemia possible in moribund cats or if slow to separate blood cells from plasma or serum • Plasma protein concentrations usually normal but may be increased

OTHER LABORATORY TESTS
• Routine blood stains (e.g., Giemsa-Wright) to identify organisms in blood films, which must be examined for organisms before treatment is begun • Reticulocyte stains cannot be used because punctate reticulocytes in cats appear similar to the parasites.
• Organisms must be differentiated from precipitated stain, refractile drying or fixation artifacts, poorly staining Howell-Jolly bodies, and basophilic stippling. • Feline organisms—small blue-staining cocci, rings, or rods on RBCs • Canine organisms—commonly form chains of organisms that appear as filamentous structures on the surface of RBCs
• Parasitemia is cyclic and thus organisms not always identifiable in blood (especially in cats)
• PCR-based assays can detect parasites in blood below the number required to make a diagnosis by a stained blood film.
• Direct Coombs' test may be positive.

DIAGNOSTIC PROCEDURES
In patients with nonregenerative anemia, bone marrow biopsy should be performed to detect other disorders (e.g., myeloproliferative disorders).

TREATMENT
• Without therapy, mortality with the larger form may reach 30% in cats. • Outpatient treatment unless severely anemic or moribund
• Blood transfusions required when the anemia is considered life-threatening
• IV administration of glucose-containing fluid recommended in moribund animals

MEDICATIONS

DRUG(S)
• Doxycycline (5 mg/kg PO q12h), tetracycline/oxytetracycline (20 mg/kg PO q8h), or oxytetracycline (20 mg/kg PO q8h) should be given for 3 weeks. • Preliminary findings indicate that enrofloxacin (10 mg/kg PO q24h) may be an efficacious alternative for cats that do not tolerate tetracycline antibiotics. • Glucocorticoids, such as prednisolone (1–2 mg/kg PO q12h), may be given to severely anemic animals; gradually decrease dosage as the PCV increases.

CONTRAINDICATIONS/POSSIBLE INTERACTIONS
• Tetracycline antibiotics may produce fever or evidence of gastrointestinal disease in cats; use a lower dosage or a different drug, or discontinue drug therapy altogether.
• Chloramphenicol should not be used to treat cats because it causes dose-dependent erythroid hypoplasia.

FOLLOW-UP
• Examine animal after 1 week of treatment to confirm that PCV has risen. • Alert owners that cats may remain carriers even after completion of treatment but seldom relapse with disease once PCV returns to normal.

MISCELLANEOUS

ASSOCIATED CONDITIONS
FELV

ABBREVIATIONS
AIHA = autoimmune hemolytic anemia
FeLV = feline leukemia virus
FIV = feline immunodeficiency virus
PCR = polymerase chain reaction
PCV = packed cell volume
RBCs = red blood cells

Suggested Reading
Harvey JW. Haemobartonellosis. In: Greene CE, ed. Infectious diseases of the dog and cat. 2nd ed. Philadelphia: Saunders, 1998:166–171.
Harvey JW. *Haemobartonella* infection in cats. Proc Am Assoc Feline Pract 2001;18–22.
Jensen WA, Lappin MR, Kamkar S, Reagan WJ. Use of a polymerase chain reaction assay to detect and differentiate two strains of *Haemobartonella felis* in naturally infected cats. Am J Vet Res 2001;62:604–608.
Author John W. Harvey
Consulting Editor Stephen A. Kruth

HAIR FOLLICLE TUMORS

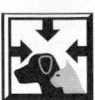

BASICS

OVERVIEW
• Two main types—trichoepithelioma, which arises from keratinocytes in the outer root sheath of the hair follicle or from both the sheath and the hair matrix; pilomatricoma, which arises from the hair matrix
• Both types—generally benign; a few published reports of malignant pilomatricoma

SIGNALMENT

Dogs and Cats
• Age—usually > 5 years
• No sex predisposition
• Trichoepithelioma—common in dogs; rare in cats; golden retrievers, basset hounds, German shepherd dogs, cocker spaniels, Irish setters, English springer spaniels, miniature schnauzers and standard poodles may be predisposed; Persian cats
• Pilomatricoma—uncommon in dogs and cats; Kerry blue terriers and poodles may be predisposed; no known breed predisposition in cats

SIGNS
• Usually a solitary mass
• Trichoepithelioma—common on the back and head (cats)
• Pilomatricoma—common on the back, shoulders, flanks, and limbs
• Firm, round, elevated, well-circumscribed, hairless, or ulcerated dermoepithelial masses; cut surface gray (trichoepithelioma) or lobulated with white chalky areas (pilomatricoma)

CAUSES & RISK FACTORS
Unknown

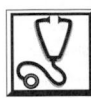

DIAGNOSIS

DIFFERENTIAL DIAGNOSIS
Histopathologic examination—distinguish from basal cell tumor and squamous cell carcinoma

CBC/BIOCHEMISTRY/URINALYSIS
Usually normal

OTHER LABORATORY TESTS
N/A

IMAGING
N/A

DIAGNOSTIC PROCEDURES
Tissue biopsy

PATHOLOGIC FINDINGS
• Trichoepithelioma—varies in degree of differentiation and site of origin (root sheath or hair matrix); horn cysts, lack of desmosomes, and differentiation toward hair follicle-like structures and formation of hair common
• Pilomatricoma—characterized by a variable proliferation of basophilic cells resembling hair matrix cells and fully keratinized, faintly eosinophilic cells with a central unstained nucleus (shadow cells); calcification common

TREATMENT
Complete excision—curative

MEDICATIONS

DRUG(S)
N/A

CONTRAINDICATIONS/POSSIBLE INTERACTIONS
N/A

FOLLOW-UP
• Monitor for local recurrence.
• Prognosis usually excellent

MISCELLANEOUS

Suggested Reading
Scott DW, Miller WM, Griffin CE. Neoplastic and nonneoplastic tumors. In: Muller & Kirk's small animal dermatology. 5th ed. Philadelphia: Saunders, 1995:1008–1016.
Thomas RC, Fox LE. Tumors of the skin and subcutis. In: Morrison WB, ed. Cancer in dogs and cats: medical and surgical management. Philadelphia: Lippincott Williams & Wilkins, 1998:489–510.
Author Joanne C. Graham
Consulting Editor Wallace B. Morrison

HALITOSIS

BASICS

DEFINITION
An offensive odor emanating from the oral cavity

PATHOPHYSIOLOGY
• The sour milk odor accompanying periodontal disease may result from bacterial populations associated with plaque, calculus, unhealthy tissues, decomposing food particles retained within the oral cavity, or from the rotten meat odor from tissue necrosis.
• Contrary to common belief, neither normal lung air or stomach aroma contribute.
• The most common cause is periodontal disease caused by plaque—bacteria are attracted to an acellular film formed from the precipitation of salivary glycoproteins (the pellicle).
• This biofilm forms over a freshly cleaned and polished tooth as soon as the patient starts to salivate; bacteria attach to the pellicle within 6–8 h; within days, the plaque becomes mineralized, producing calculus; as plaque ages and gingivitis develops into periodontitis (bone loss), the bacterial flora changes from a predominantly nonmotile gram-positive aerobic coccoid flora to a more motile, gram-negative anaerobic population including *Bacteroides, Fusobacterium,* and *Actinomyces* spp.
• The rough surface of calculus attracts more bacteria while irritating the free gingiva; as the inflammation continues, the gingival sulcus is pathologically transformed into a periodontal pocket; the pocket accumulates putrefied food debris, bacterial breakdown products, and resorbing bone, leading to halitosis.
• The primary cause of malodor is gram-negative anaerobic bacterial putrefaction that generates volatile sulfur compounds, such as hydrogen sulfide, methyl mercaptan, dimethyl sulfide, and volatile fatty acids.
• Volatile sulfur compounds may also play a role in periodontal disease affecting the integrity of the tissue barrier, allowing endotoxins to produce periodontal destruction, endotoxemia, and bacteremia.

SYSTEMS AFFECTED
N/A

SIGNALMENT
• Dog and cat
• Small breeds and brachycephalic breeds are more prone to oral disease because the teeth are closer together, smaller animals live longer, and their owners tend to feed softer food.
• Older animals are predisposed.

SIGNS
• If due to oral disease, ptyalism, pawing at mouth, anorexia, may occur.
• In most cases, no clinical signs other than the odor

CAUSES
• Multiple causes
• Eating malodorous food
• Metabolic—diabetes, uremia
• Respiratory—rhinitis, sinusitis, neoplasia
• Gastrointestinal—megaesophagus, neoplasia, foreign body
• Dermatologic—lip-fold pyoderma
• Dietary—fetid foodstuffs, coprophagy
• Oral disease—periodontal disease and ulceration, orthodontic, pharyngitis, tonsillitis, neoplasia, foreign bodies
• Trauma—electric cord injury, open fractures, caustic agents
• Infectious—bacterial, fungal, viral
• Autoimmune diseases
• Eosinophilic granuloma complex

RISK FACTORS
N/A

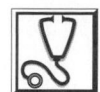

DIAGNOSIS

CBC/BIOCHEMISTRY/URINALYSIS
N/A

OTHER LABORATORY TESTS
N/A

IMAGING
N/A

DIAGNOSTIC PROCEDURES
• Hydrogen sulfide, mercaptans, and volatile fatty acids are the primary components of halitosis; an industrial sulfide monitor can be used to measure sulfide concentration in peak parts per billion.
• Other diagnostic procedures to evaluate periodontal disease include intraoral radiography, probing pocket depths, attachment levels, and tooth mobility.

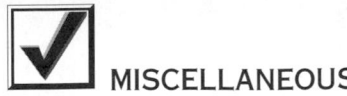

 TREATMENT

- Once the specific cause of halitosis is known, direct therapy at correcting existing pathology.
- Topical treatment with zinc ascorbate cysteine gel usually reduces halitosis within 30 min because of cysteine's effect on sulfur compounds in the mouth.
- Clean the teeth when physical examination reveals gingivitis and/or when calculus exists on the maxillary fourth premolar; cleaning removes plaque and calculus above and below the gumline (with the help of hand instruments or scaler tips designed to be used subgingivally), irrigates debris from the mouth, and polishes the teeth.

 MEDICATIONS

DRUG(S) OF CHOICE
- Clindamycin—destroys most periodontal pathogens; can be used as pulse therapy, administering the label dose the first 5 days of each month.
- Controlling periodontal pathogens helps control dental infections and accompanying malodor.
- The use of oral care products that contain metal ions, especially zinc, inhibits odor formation because of the affinity of the metal ion to sulfur; zinc complexes with hydrogen sulfide to form insoluble zinc sulfide; zinc interferes with microbial proliferation and calcification of microbial deposits (by interfering with the crystal development of calculus).
- Chlorhexidine used as a rinse or paste also helps control plaque, decreasing eventual odor; supplied as CHX Guard, CHX Guard LA, CET Oral Hygiene Spray (VRx Products, Harbor City, CA); DentiVet toothpaste and Hexarinse (Virbac, Fort Worth, TX); zinc ascorbate plus amino acid (Maxi/Guard Oral Cleansing Gel-Addison Biologicals)
- DentTreats (VRx Products)—a breath tablet for dogs; contains zinc citrate, sodium copper chlorophyllin, and essential oils (parsley seed, mint, and rosemary); does not treat a specific disease but neutralizes odor.

CONTRAINDICATIONS
N/A

PRECAUTIONS
N/A

POSSIBLE INTERACTIONS
N/A

ALTERNATIVE DRUG(S)
N/A

 FOLLOW-UP

PATIENT MONITORING
Daily brushing to remove plaque and control dental disease and odor; periodic examinations to monitor care

POSSIBLE COMPLICATIONS
N/A

✔ **MISCELLANEOUS**

ASSOCIATED CONDITIONS
N/A

AGE-RELATED FACTORS
N/A

ZOONOTIC POTENTIAL
N/A

PREGNANCY
N/A

SYNONYMS
- Bad breath
- Foul breath
- Malodor
- Fetor ex ore
- Fetor oris

ABBREVIATIONS
N/A

Suggested Reading
Harvey CE, Emily PP. Small animal dentistry. Philadelphia: Mosby, 1993.
Wiggs RB, Lobprise HB. Veterinary dentistry: Principles and practice. Philadelphia: Lippincott-Raven, 1997.
Author Jan Bellows
Consulting Editor Heidi B. Lobprise

HEAD PRESSING

 BASICS

DEFINITION
Compulsive pressing of the head against a wall or other object for no apparent reason

PATHOPHYSIOLOGY
• Alterations in behavior—caused by lesions in the prosencephalon (i.e., forebrain: cerebrum, limbic system, thalamus, and hypothalamus), particularly those affecting the limbic system and frontal and temporal cortex
• Lesions may result in compulsive pacing; when an obstacle (e.g., a wall) is reached, the animal may press its head against it for long periods of time, apparently unable to turn and move away.
• Apparent inability to voluntarily move away—may reflect impaired integration of sensory information, leading to inappropriate behavior

SYSTEMS AFFECTED
Nervous—specifically the cerebrum, limbic system, thalamus, and hypothalamus

SIGNALMENT
Dogs and cats of any age, breed, and sex

SIGNS
• Head pressing—just one sign of prosencephalon disease
• Compulsive pacing and circling
• Change in learned behavior
• Seizures
• Postural reaction deficits
• Visual deficits

CAUSES & RISK FACTORS
• Anatomic—hydrocephalus, most commonly in young toy breed dogs
• Metabolic—hepatic encephalopathy as a result of a portosystemic shunt or severe hepatic disease; severe hyper- or hyponatremia
• Nutritional—very unusual now since most pets are fed compounded diets; thiamine deficiency can occur in cats fed a diet of raw fish or in cats with severe malabsorptive syndromes; however, vestibular signs predominate

• Neoplastic—primary (e.g., glioma, meningioma) or metastatic (e.g., hemangiosarcoma) tumors affecting the brain; more common in older animals (> 6 years)
• Immune-mediated/inflammatory—GME; necrotizing encephalitides (Maltese encephalitis, Pug encephalitis)
• Infectious (dogs)—viral (rabies virus, canine distemper virus), rickettsial (*Ehrlichia canis*, Rocky mountain spotted fever), protozoal, or fungal (*Blastomyces, Cryptococcus*); rabies is of particular importance because neurons in the limbic system are frequently infected in carnivores
• Infectious (cats)—viral (rabies, feline infectious peritonitis, feline leukemia virus [associated immunosuppression predisposes to other encephalitides and neoplasia], feline immunodeficiency virus [can cause encephalopathy primarily and can predispose to other encephalitides and neoplasia due to immunosuppression]); *Bartonella henselae*; *Cuterebra* migration; toxoplasmosis; *Cryptococcus* and other fungal infections
• Toxic—e.g., lead poisoning
• Trauma
• Vascular—intracranial hemorrhage as a result of hypertension (consider in older cats with hyperthyroidism or chronic renal insufficiency); bleeding disorder (either primary or secondary to rodenticide toxicity)

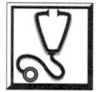 DIAGNOSIS

CBC/BIOCHEMISTRY/URINALYSIS
CBC
• May reflect a metabolic or toxic cause
• Hepatic encephalopathy—decreased serum albumin, blood urea nitrogen, cholesterol, and glucose concentrations, with or without elevated ALP, ALT, and bilirubin concentrations; microcytic anemia may be present; ammonium biurate crystals may be present in the urine
• Lead toxicity—basophilic stippling of erythrocytes; presence of reticulocytes and nucleated RBCs in the absence of anemia

• Encephalitis—findings often unremarkable, but may reflect an inflammatory process (e.g., with fungal infection)
• CNS lymphoma—may see evidence of bone marrow involvement

OTHER LABORATORY TESTS
• Bile acid tolerance—to diagnose hepatic encephalopathy; blood ammonia concentrations may also be elevated
• Acute and convalescent serologic titers—to diagnose rickettsial, protozoal, fungal, and viral diseases; for some infections (e.g., canine distemper virus, *Toxoplasma, Cryptococcus*), also measure CSF antibody or antigen (*Cryptococcus*) titers
• Blood lead concentration—to diagnose lead toxicity

IMAGING
• Thoracic radiography—recommended for older patients to identify metastatic disease
• Abdominal ultrasonography—recommended for older patients if intra-abdominal neoplasia is suspected; indicated if a portosystemic shunt or other hepatic disease is suspected
• Rectal scintigraphy—may be used to definitively diagnose a portosystemic shunt
• Brain CT or MRI—to identify intracranial masses, malformations, skull fractures, and hemorrhage
• Ultrasonography of the brain via persistent fontanelles—may be used to diagnose hydrocephalus in dogs

DIAGNOSTIC PROCEDURES
• Fundic examination—to identify chorioretinitis (evidence of infectious/inflammatory disease) and vascular lesions
• CSF analysis—to diagnose encephalitis

PATHOLOGIC FINDINGS
Findings at necropsy will reflect the etiology.

 TREATMENT

• Severe clinical signs—hospitalization for diagnostic work-up and treatment; in patients with severe prosencephalic syndrome, intravenous fluids may be necessary

• Suspected hepatic encephalopathy—appropriate low-protein diet
• Suspected rabies—quarantine outdoor animal with no vaccination or unknown vaccination history when rapidly progressive neurologic signs are present and animal lives in a rabies-endemic area; minimize the number of people in contact with the animal, and maintain a contact log; if neurologic signs deteriorate rapidly, euthanize the animal and send it to a public health laboratory to be tested for rabies

MEDICATIONS

DRUG(S)
Different causes require different treatment; do not initiate therapy until a diagnosis has been established.

FOLLOW-UP

PATIENT MONITORING
• Periodic repeat neurologic examinations to monitor progress
• See specific diseases for specific instructions.

MISCELLANEOUS

ZOONOTIC POTENTIAL
• Rabies should be considered in endemic areas.
• Fungal infections may be zoonotic if spores are released; most likely to occur if exudative skin lesions are present

SEE ALSO
• Brain Injury
• Encephalitis
• Hepatic Encephalopathy
• Hydrocephalus

ABBREVIATIONS
• ALP = alanine phosphatase
• ALT = alanine aminotransferase
• CNS = central nervous system
• CSF = cerebrospinal fluid
• CT = computed tomography
• GME = granulomatous meningoencephalitis
• MRI = magnetic resonance imaging

Suggested Reading
Braund KG. Clinical syndromes in veterinary neurology. 2nd ed. Baltimore: Mosby, 1994.
Author Natasha J. Olby
Consulting Editor Joane M. Parent

HEAD TILT

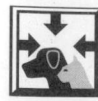 **BASICS**

DEFINITION
Tilting of the head away from its normal orientation with the trunk and limbs; usually associated with disorders of the vestibular system

PATHOPHYSIOLOGY
• Vestibular system—coordinates position and movement of the head with that of the eyes, trunk, and limbs by detecting linear acceleration and rotational movements of the head; includes vestibular nuclei in the rostral medulla of the brain stem, vestibular portion of the vestibulocochlear nerve (cranial nerve VIII), and receptors in the semicircular canals of the inner ear • Head tilt—most consistent sign of diseases affecting the vestibular system and its projections to the cerebellum, spinal cord, cerebral cortex, reticular formation, and extraocular eye muscles via the medial longitudinal fasciculus; usually directed toward the same side as the lesion

SYSTEMS AFFECTED
Nervous—peripheral or CNS

SIGNALMENT N/A

SIGNS
• Be sure that abnormal head posture is a true head tilt and is not head turning (i.e., turning the head and neck to the side as if to turn in a circle), which is of thalamocortical origin and is not associated with other vestibular signs (e.g., abnormal nystagmus). • Head tilt may be not be present if disease is bilateral.

CAUSES

Peripheral Disease
• Anatomic—congenital head tilt
• Metabolic—hypothyroidism; pituitary chromophobe adenoma; paraneoplastic disease
• Neoplastic—nerve sheath tumor of cranial nerve VIII; neoplasia of the bone and surrounding tissue (e.g., osteosarcoma, fibrosarcoma, chondrosarcoma, and squamous cell carcinoma) • Inflammatory—otitis media and interna; primarily bacterial but also parasitic (e.g., *Otodectes*), mycotic, and fungal origins; foreign body; nasopharyngeal polyps
• Idiopathic—canine geriatric vestibular disease; feline idiopathic vestibular disease
• Immune mediated—cranial nerve neuropathy • Toxic—aminoglycosides, lead, hexachlorophene
• Traumatic—tympanic bulla or petrosal bone fracture; ear flush

Central Disease
• Degenerative—storage disease; demyelinating disease; vascular event
• Anatomic—hydrocephalus • Neoplastic—glioma, choroid plexus papilloma, meningioma, lymphosarcoma, nerve sheath tumor, medulloblastoma, skull tumor (e.g., osteosarcoma); metastasis (e.g., hemangiosarcoma and melanoma)
• Nutritional—thiamine deficiency
• Inflammatory, infectious—viral (e.g., FIP, canine distemper virus); protozoal (e.g., toxoplasmosis, neospora); fungal (e.g., cryptococcosis, blastomycosis, histoplasmosis, coccidioidomycosis, nocardiosis); bacterial (e.g., central extension from otitis media and interna); parasitic (e.g., *Cuterebra* larvae); rickettsial (e.g., ehrlichiosis); algae (prototheocosis) • Inflammatory, noninfectious—granulomatous meningoencephalomyelitis • Trauma—petrosal bone fracture with brain stem injury
• Toxic—metronidazole

RISK FACTORS
• Hypothyroidism • Administration of ototoxic drugs • Thiamine-deficient diet (e.g., exclusively fish diet) • Otitis externa, media, and interna

 DIAGNOSIS

DIFFERENTIAL DIAGNOSIS

Vestibular Disease
• Unilateral disease—head tilt usually directed toward the side of the lesion; may be accompanied by other vestibular signs; abnormal nystagmus (resting, positional) with fast phase usually in the direction opposite the tilt; mild ventral deviation of the eye (vestibular strabismus) ipsilateral to the tilt that is exacerbated by elevation of the head; ataxia and disequilibrium with a tendency to fall, lean, or circle toward the side of the tilt
• Bilateral disease—head tilt may be absent or mild in the direction of the more severely affected side; abnormal nystagmus may be seen; physiologic nystagmus (e.g., normal vestibular nystagmus or conjugate eye movements) may be depressed or absent with wide side-to-side swaying movements of the head (especially evident in cats); may note a wide-based stance, especially in the thoracic limbs, or a crouched posture with reluctance to move • Head tilt—localizes to the peripheral (e.g., vestibular portion of cranial nerve VIII or receptors in the inner ear) or central (e.g., vestibular nuclei and their neuronal pathways) nervous system
• Peripheral deficits—horizontal or rotatory nystagmus with fast phase always in the direction opposite the head tilt; patient may have concomitant ipsilateral facial nerve paresis or paralysis or Horner's syndrome, because of the close association of cranial nerve VII in the petrosal bone and the sympathetic nervous system in the tympanic bulla • Central deficits—vertical, horizontal, or rotatory nystagmus that can change with the position of the head; altered mentation; ipsilateral paresis or proprioceptive deficits; other signs related to the cerebellum, rostral medulla, and caudal pons; in some patients, multiple cranial nerve involvement other than cranial nerve VII. • Paradoxical vestibular syndrome—caused by lesions in the cerebellar peduncles, cerebellar medulla, or flocculonodular lobes of the cerebellum; vestibular signs (e.g., head tilt and nystagmus) are opposite the side of the lesion, whereas the cerebellar signs and the proprioceptive deficits are ipsilateral to the lesion.

Nonvestibular Head Tilt and Head Posture
• Uncommon • Must be differentiated from vestibular head tilt • Unilateral lesions of the midbrain can cause severe rotation of the head of > 90° toward the side opposite the lesion; no other vestibular signs; tilt corrects when the patient is blindfolded.
• Adversive syndrome (secondary to rostral thalamic lesions)—the head turn, lean, or neck curvature and/or circling can be misinterpreted as a vestibular tilt; no vestibular signs; contralateral postural, menace, or sensory deficits reflect a thalamic lesion; compulsive turning, usually in large circles and without the disequilibrium of vestibular circling

CBC/BIOCHEMISTRY/URINALYSIS
• Usually normal • Mild anemia—hypothyroidism • Leucocytosis with neutrophilia—otitis media or interna
• Thrombocytopenia—ehrlichiosis
• Hypercholesterolemia—hypothyroidism
• High serum globulin concentration—FIP

OTHER LABORATORY TESTS
• T_4, free T_4, FT_4 E_9D, and endogenous TSH levels—when hypothyroidism is suspected on the basis of physical examination findings and unilateral or bilateral involvement of cranial nerve VIII and possibly VII • Bacterial culture and sensitivity testing—sample from myringotomy or surgical drainage of tympanic bulla if otitis media or interna is suspected • Microscopic examination of ear swab—parasites (e.g., ear mites) • Serologic testing—infectious causes (e.g., canine distemper; FIP; and protozoal, fungal, and rickettsial diseases)

IMAGING
• Tympanic bullae and skull radiography—normal radiographs do not rule out bulla disease • CT and MRI—valuable for confirming bulla lesions, CNS extension from peripheral disease, localizing tumor, granuloma, and documenting extent of inflammation

DIAGNOSTIC PROCEDURES
• CSF analysis—sample from the cerebellomedullary cistern; valuable for evaluating central vestibular disease; detect inflammatory process; protein electrophoresis

and titers to match with serologic testing may be indicated; sample collection may put the patient at risk for herniation if there is a mass or high intracranial pressure. • BAER—assess cochlear portion of cranial nerve VIII and brain stem auditory pathways; particularly valuable for evaluating peripheral vestibular disease, because some diseases may cause ipsilateral deafness (e.g., otitis media and interna), whereas other diseases (e.g., canine geriatric vestibular disease and hypothyroidism) affect only the vestibular portion of cranial nerve VIII • Biopsy—bone: when a tumor or osteomyelitis is suspected; brainstem masses (e.g., cerebellomedullary angle): difficult to approach and to remove surgically

TREATMENT

• Inpatient vs. outpatient—depends on severity of the signs (especially vestibular ataxia), size, and age of the patient, and need for supportive care
• Supportive fluids—replacement or maintenance fluids (depend on clinical state); may be required in the acute phase when disorientation, nausea, and vomiting preclude oral intake; especially important in geriatric patients
• Activity—restrict (e.g., avoid stairs and slippery surfaces) according to the degree of disequilibrium
• Diet—usually no need for modification unless the cause is thiamine deficiency (e.g., exclusively fish diet without vitamin supplementation); oral intake may need to be restricted with nausea and vomiting; CAUTION: be aware of aspiration secondary to abnormal body posture in patients with severe head tilt and vestibular disequilibrium or brain stem dysfunction.
• Advise client that the prognosis for central vestibular disorders is usually poorer than that for peripheral disorders.
• Inform client of the risks associated with biopsy, surgery, and radiation of a brain stem mass.
• Surgical treatment—may be required to drain bulla with otitis media, to remove nasopharyngeal polyps in cats, and to resect tumor, if accessible

MEDICATIONS

DRUG(S) OF CHOICE
• Otitis media and interna—broad-spectrum antibiotic (parenteral or oral) that penetrates

bone while awaiting culture results; trimethoprim-sulfa (15 mg/kg PO q12h or 30 mg/kg PO q12–24h); first-generation cephalosporins, such as cephalexin (10–30 mg/kg PO q6–8h) or amoxicillin/clavulanic acid (12.2–25 mg/kg PO q12h for dogs or 62.5 mg/cat PO q12h); treatment often required for 4–6 weeks • Hypothyroidism—T_4 replacement (dogs, levothyroxine 22 μg/kg PO q12h) should be introduced gradually in geriatric patients, especially with cardiac disease; response varies, partly depending on the duration of signs (e.g., in some patients, neuropathy is not reversible)
• Drug affecting vestibular function—discontinue offending agent; signs are usually, but not always, reversible • Infectious—specific treatment, if indicated; for bacterial diseases, antibiotic that penetrates the blood–brain barrier (e.g., trimethoprim-sulfa, 15 mg/kg PO q12h); for protozoal diseases, clindamycin (12.5–25 mg/kg PO q12h); for fungal diseases, itraconazole (dogs, 2.5 mg/kg PO q12h or 5 mg/kg PO q24h; cats, 5 mg/kg PO q12h); prognosis usually grave for protozoal, fungal, and viral diseases (e.g., canine distemper and FIP) • Granulomatous meningoencephalomyelitis—usually initially treated with steroids: dexamethasone (dogs, 0.25 mg/kg PO, IM q12h for 3 days; then 0.25 mg/kg PO q24h for 3 days), followed by prednisone (1 mg/kg PO q24h for 1–2 weeks; then decrease slowly); depending on progress, may need stronger immunosuppression—azathioprine (dogs, 2 mg/kg PO q24h initially; then 0.5–1 mg/kg PO q48h)—or radiation • Trauma—supportive care (e.g., antiinflammatory drugs, antibiotics, intravenous fluid administration); specific fracture repair or hematoma removal is difficult, considering the location. • Canine geriatric and feline idiopathic vestibular disease—supportive care only • Cranial nerve polyneuropathy—response to prednisone usually good if the patient has a primary immune disorder • Thiamine deficiency—diet modification and thiamine replacement

CONTRAINDICATIONS
Drugs potentially toxic to the vestibular system—aminoglycoside antibiotics; prolonged high-dose metronidazole

PRECAUTIONS
• Trimethoprim-sulfa administration—keratoconjunctivitis sicca (dry eye)
• Avoid topical drugs (especially oil based) if the tympanic membrane is ruptured.

POSSIBLE INTERACTIONS N/A

ALTERNATIVE DRUG(S) N/A

FOLLOW-UP

PATIENT MONITORING
• Repeat the neurologic examination at a frequency dictated by the underlying cause.
• Head tilt may persist.
• Hypothyroidism—measure T_4 concentration 6 hr after treatment at 4–6 weeks after initiation of hormone replacement therapy to evaluate dosage
• Repeat CSF and brain imaging—with some central vestibular disorders • Monitor tear production (Schirmer tear test) with trimethoprim-sulfa administration.

POSSIBLE COMPLICATIONS
• Progression of disease with deterioration of mental status • Brain herniation

MISCELLANEOUS

ASSOCIATED CONDITIONS
• Facial nerve (cranial nerve VII) paresis or paralysis • Horner's syndrome

AGE-RELATED FACTORS
Canine geriatric vestibular syndrome affects only old dogs.

ZOONOTIC POTENTIAL N/A

PREGNANCY N/A

SYNONYMS N/A

SEE ALSO
• Encephalitis • Meningoencephalomyelitis, Granulomatous • Nasal and Nasopharyngeal Polyps • Otitis Media and Interna
• Vestibular Disease, Geriatric—Dogs
• Vestibular Disease, Idiopathic—Cats

ABBREVIATIONS
• BAER = brain stem auditory-evoked response
• CNS = central nervous system
• CSF = cerebrospinal fluid
• CT = computed tomography
• FIP = feline infectious peritonitis
• MRI = magnetic resonance imaging
• TSH = thyroid-stimulating hormone
• $FT_4 E_9D$ = free T_4 by equilibrium dialysis

Suggested Reading
de Lahunta A. Veterinary neuroanatomy and clinical neurology. 2nd ed. Philadelphia: Saunders, 1983.
Oliver JE, Lorenz MD. Handbook of veterinary neurologic diagnosis. 2nd ed. Philadelphia: Saunders, 1993.
Parent JM, Cochrane SM. Head tilt. In: Allen DG, ed. Small animal medicine. Philadelphia: Lippincott, 1991:753–759.
Author Susan M. Cochrane
Consulting Editor Joane M. Parent

HEARTWORM DISEASE—CATS

BASICS

OVERVIEW
• Disease caused by infection with *Dirofilaria immitis*
• Microfilaremia uncommon (< 20%)
• Prevalence one-tenth that of unprotected dogs
• Low average worm burden
• Worms are physically smaller and have a shorter life span in cats.

SIGNALMENT
• Cats
• No age or breed predisposition
• Males more commonly infected

SIGNS

Historical Findings
• Coughing
• Dyspnea
• Vomiting
• PTE frequently results in acute respiratory failure and death.
• Vomiting and respiratory signs predominate in chronic disease.

Physical Examination Findings
• Usually normal
• Increased bronchovesicular sounds
• Murmur or gallop rhythm should increase suspicion of primary cardiac disease.

CAUSES & RISK FACTORS
• Outdoor cats at increased risk (2:1)
• FeLV infection is not a predisposing factor.

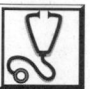

DIAGNOSIS

DIFFERENTIAL DIAGNOSIS
• Asthma
• Cardiomyopathy
• Chylothorax
• *Aelurostrongylus abstrusus* infection
• *Paragonimus kellicotti* infection

CBC/BIOCHEMISTRY/URINALYSIS
• Mild nonregenerative anemia
• Eosinophilia inconsistent
• Basophilia should increase suspicion.
• Hyperglobulinemia

OTHER LABORATORY TESTS

Heartworm Concentration Tests
Low sensitivity, high specificity

Heartworm Antigen Tests
• ELISA or immunochromatographic tests
• Tests that detect circulating HWAg are more specific than antibody tests; a positive antigen test result is strong evidence of heartworm disease.
• Low worm burdens (fewer than 5 worms) and single-sex infections commonly result in false-negative results.
• Negative result does not rule out heartworm disease; more than 40% of cats with adult infection are antigen-negative.

Heartworm Antibody Tests
• ELISA or immunochromatographic tests
• Tests that detect circulating antibodies to immature and adult heartworm antigen are the most sensitive tests for feline heartworm disease.
• A positive result simply documents exposure to heartworms.
• The more intense the antibody response (higher titer or antibody unit [ABU] level), the more likely is an adult infection.

IMAGING

Radiography/Angiography
• Enlarged (> pulmonary vein, > 1.6 times the width of the 9th rib), blunted, tortuous pulmonary arteries
• Patchy perivascular pulmonary infiltrates
• Pulmonary arterial obstruction and linear filling defects seen on nonselective angiography

Echocardiography
• Dilated main pulmonary artery
• Identification of worms in heart or main pulmonary artery; most commonly seen in the right pulmonary artery
• Excludes or confirms other primary cardiac diseases (cardiomyopathy)

DIAGNOSTIC TESTS
N/A

 TREATMENT
• Asymptomatic cats should not receive adulticide therapy; perhaps no cats should.
• Symptomatic cats should be stabilized.
• Spontaneous "cure" is probably much more common in cats than dogs (shorter heartworm life span).

 MEDICATIONS

DRUG(S)
Initial Stabilization
• Supplemental oxygen
• Theophylline (sustained release formulation) 25 mg/kg PO q24h in the evening
• Prednisolone 1–2 mg/kg PO q24h for 10–14 days; then reduce gradually
• Cautiously balanced fluid therapy if indicated

Adulticide/Thromboembolism
• Thiacetarsamide: 2.2 mg/kg IV q12h for 2 days
• 30% mortality should be expected from adulticide therapy and subsequent PTE
• Supportive care for PTE the same as initial stabilization
• PTE complications most severe 5–10 days after adulticide therapy; commonly fatal

CONTRAINDICATIONS/POSSIBLE INTERACTIONS
• Aspirin therapy—no documented benefit
• Current information does not support the use of melarsomine (Immiticide) in cats.

 FOLLOW-UP

PATIENT MONITORING
Serial evaluation of clinical response, thoracic radiographs, and heartworm antigen and antibody tests are most informative.

PREVENTION/AVOIDANCE
• Ivermectin (Heartgard for Cats)—24 µg/kg PO every 30 days
• Milbemycin oxime—0.5–0.1 mg/kg PO every 30 days (not currently approved for use in cats)

 MISCELLANEOUS

SYNONYMS
Dirofilariasis

ABBREVIATIONS
• ABU = antibody unit
• HWAg = adult heartworm antigen
• PTE = pulmonary thromboembolism

Suggested Reading
Miller MW. *Feline dirofilariasis.* Clin Tech Small Anim Pract 1998;13(2):99–108.
Dillon R. Feline heartworm disease. In Tilley LP, Goodwin J-K (Eds). Manual of canine and feline cardiology. 3rd ed. Philadelphia: Saunders, 2001:235.
Author Matthew W. Miller
Consulting Editors Larry P. Tilley and Francis W. K. Smith, Jr.

HEARTWORM DISEASE—DOGS

BASICS

DEFINITION
Disease caused by infection with *Dirofilaria immitis*

PATHOPHYSIOLOGY
Disease is directly related to the number of worms, duration of infection, and host response. Endothelial damage leads to myo-intimal proliferation. Lobar arterial enlargement, tortuosity, and obstruction cause impaired compliance, loss of collateral recruitment, pulmonary hypertension, and thrombosis. Pulmonary damage exacerbated after the death of adult worms.

SYSTEMS AFFECTED
• Cardiovascular—high right ventricular afterload causes myocardial hypertrophy and, in some animals, congestive heart failure (CHF)
• Respiratory—pulmonary hypertension, embolization, allergic pneumonitis, eosinophilic granulomatous
• Renal/urologic—immune complex glomerulopathy

GENETICS
None

INCIDENCE/PREVALENCE
• Varies with geographic location, but widespread
• Virtually 100% in unprotected dogs living in highly endemic regions

GEOGRAPHIC DISTRIBUTION
• Most common in tropical and semitropical zones
• Common along the Atlantic and Gulf coasts and Ohio and Mississippi River basins
• Gradually extending across the United States
• Numerous pockets of infection in otherwise low prevalence regions
• Ubiquitous—mosquito vector

SIGNALMENT

Species
Dogs

Breed Predilection
• Medium- to large-breed dogs that spend a lot of time outdoors
• All unprotected dogs at risk in endemic regions

Mean Age and Range
Infection can occur at any age; most affected animals are 3–8 years old.

Predominant Sex
None

SIGNS

Historial Findings
• Animals often asymptomatic or exhibit minimal signs such as occasional coughing (Class I)

• Coughing and exercise intolerance associated with moderate pulmonary damage
• Cachexia, exercise intolerance, syncope, and ascites (right-sided CHF [R-CHF]) in severely affected dogs (Class III)

Physical Examination Findings
• No abnormalities—animals with mild infection (Class I) and some with moderately severe infection (Class II)
• Labored breathing or crackles—dogs with severe pulmonary hypertension (Class III) or pulmonary thromboembolic complications
• Tachycardia, ascites, and hepatomegaly indicate R-CHF (Class III).
• Hemoptysis—occasionally occurs; indicates severe pulmonary thromboembolic complications

CAUSE
Infection with *D. immitis*

RISK FACTORS
• Residence in endemic regions
• Outside habitus
• Lack of prophylaxis
• Greater than 64°F all day, every day for at least 1 month.
• Greater than 80° every day for 10–14 days.

DIAGNOSIS

DIFFERENTIAL DIAGNOSIS
• Other causes of pulmonary hypertension and thrombosis (e.g., hyperadrenocorticism)
• Allergic lung disease
• Other causes of ascites (e.g., dilated cardiomyopathy)

CBC/BIOCHEMISTRY/URINALYSIS
• Anemia—absent, mild, or moderate depending on chronicity and severity of disease and thromboembolic complications
• Eosinophilia and basophilia—vary
• Inflammatory leukogram and thrombocytopenia associated with thromboembolism
• Hyperglobulinemia—inconsistent finding
• Proteinuria—common in animals with severe and chronic infection; may be caused by immune-complex glomerulonephritis or amyloidosis

OTHER LABORATORY TESTS
• Highly specific, sensitive serologic tests that identify adult female *D. immitis* antigen are widely available.
• Test 7 months after the end of the previous transmission season.
• Microfilaria identification tests include the modified Knott's test, filter tests, and direct smear.

IMAGING

Radiographic Findings
• Main pulmonary artery segment enlargement and lobar arterial enlargement and tortuosity vary from absent (Class I) to severe (Class III).

• Parenchymal lung infiltrates of variable severity—surround lobar arteries; may extend into most or all of one or multiple lung lobes when thromboembolism occurs
• Diffuse, symmetrical, alveolar, and interstitial infiltrates occasionally occur because of an allergic reaction to microfilaria.

Echocardiographic Findings
• Often unremarkable; may reflect right ventricular dilation and wall hypertrophy
• Parallel, linear echodensities produced by heartworms may be detected in the right ventricle, right atrium, and pulmonary arteries.

Angiography
Little practical clinical importance

DIAGNOSTIC PROCEDURES

Electrocardiographic Findings
• Usually normal
• May reflect right ventricular hypertrophy in dogs with severe (Class III) infection
• Heart rhythm disturbances—occasionally seen (atrial fibrillation most common) in severe infection

PATHOLOGIC FINDINGS
• Large right heart
• Pulmonary arterial myointimal proliferation
• Pulmonary thromboembolism
• Pulmonary hemorrhage
• Hepatomegaly and congestion in animals with R-CHF

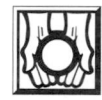

TREATMENT

APPROPRIATE HEALTH CARE
• Most patients hospitalized during adulticide administration
• Appropriate patients should be given microfilaricide in the morning and discharged in the evening.
• Hospitalization recommended for dogs experiencing thromboembolic complications

ACTIVITY
• Severe restriction of activity required for 4–6 weeks after adulticide administration
• Cage confinement recommended for 3–4 weeks after adulticide administration for severe (Class III) disease
• Cage confinement for 7 days recommended for dogs experiencing pulmonary thromboembolic complications

DIET
Restricted sodium diet recommended for dogs with CHF

CLIENT EDUCATION
• Good prognosis for animals with mild-to-moderate infection
• Postadulticide pulmonary complications likely in patients with moderate-to-severe infection
• Reinfection can occur unless appropriate prophylaxis administered

SURGICAL CONSIDERATIONS

• Treatment of choice for vena cava syndrome
• Worm removal from right heart and pulmonary artery via jugular vein by use of fluoroscopy and a long, flexible, alligator forceps is highly effective for treating high worm burden when employed by an experienced operator.

MEDICATIONS

DRUG(S) OF CHOICE

• Stabilize animals with R-CHF with diuretics, cage rest, and sodium restriction before adulticide treatment.
• Stabilize pulmonary failure with antithrombotic agents (e.g., aspirin or heparin) or antiinflammatory dosages of corticosteroid, depending on the clinical and radiographic findings.
• Melarsomine dihydrochloride (Immiticide, 2.5 mg/kg IM)—an adulticide drug with the advantage of IM administration and less hepatotoxicity, and better efficacy against both sexes of adult worms of all ages than thiacetarsamide sodium
• Class I infection—two injections 24 h apart are given into the epaxial muscles (first on one side, then on the opposite side, using 22-gauge needles); apply pressure over the injection site during and after needle withdrawal. A positive antigen test result 4 months later usually indicates repeat treatment; with a weakly positive antigen test result, repeat test in 1–2 months before deciding to repeat adulticide treatment.
• Class III infections—one injection administered 1 month later, two injections 24 h apart are recommended. This alternate dosage spreads the adulticide killing effect and thromboembolism over 2 treatments. The overall kill rate is also improved as compared to the standard two-injection treatment.
• Many veterinarians use the alternate protocol for all infections.
• Microfilaricide administration indicated for most dogs with circulating microfilariae, 4–6 weeks after adulticide. Interceptor, at the preventive dosage, is administered in the morning, and the patient observed for the day and discharged in the evening.

CONTRAINDICATIONS

Adulticide treatment with icterus or hepatic failure

PRECAUTIONS

• Adulticide treatment—not indicated in patients with renal failure, hepatic failure, or nephrotic syndrome
• Standard adulticide therapy in dogs with severe infection is associated with high mortality due to subsequent pulmonary thromboembolism.

POSSIBLE INTERACTIONS

None

ALTERNATIVE DRUG(S)

• Heparin (75 units/kg SC q8h) or aspirin (5–7 mg/kg PO q24h) for 1–3 weeks before and during, and for 3 weeks after, adulticide administration is a controversial recommendation for the most severe cases of Class III disease; therapy is combined with strict, extended cage confinement.
• Heparin (75 units/kg SC q8h) is recommended for dogs with pulmonary thrombosis, thrombocytopenia, or hemoglobinuria.
• Ivermectin (Heartgard Plus) administered monthly for at least 32 months kills some adult heartworms.

FOLLOW-UP

PATIENT MONITORING

• Perform a microfilaria concentration test in appropriate patients 4 months after microfilaricide administration. Initiate prophylaxis 1 month following melarsomine treatment.
• Perform an antigen test—4 to 5 months after adulticide treatment; if positive, must decide whether or not to repeat the adulticide treatment. If a weakly positive test result; repeat in 1–3 months. Some dogs with persistent adult infection may not require retreatment—determined by age, severity of infection, degree of improvement since the first treatment, strength of the positive antigen test result, and concomitant disease.

PREVENTION/AVOIDANCE

Heartworm prophylaxis should be provided for all dogs at risk:
• Antigen test prior to starting preventive treatment • Antigen test 7 months after end of previous season • Ivermectin (Heartgard)—a highly effective, monthly preventive that, when combined with pyrantel pamoate (Heartgard Plus), also controls hookworm and roundworm infection; can be given safely to microfilaremic dogs • Milbemycin oxime (Interceptor)—a highly effective, monthly prophylaxis that also controls hookworms, roundworms, and whipworms; the preventive dosage is microfilaricidal; acute reactions may occur when given to microfilaremic dogs.
• Moxidectin (ProHeart)—a monthly prophylactic drug that can be given to microfilaremic dogs. • Oral macrocyclic lactone preventives such as Milbemycin Oxime, ivermectin, Selamactin, and Moxidectin provide retroactive efficacy of 100% for 1 month and at least 75% for 2 months. • Moxidectin (ProHeart-6)—prophylactic effective for at least 6 months after injection. • Selamectin (Revolution) is available for monthly topical administration
• All of the prophylactic drugs can be administered safely to collies at the

appropriate dosages. • Macrocyclic lactones all eliminate microfilariae by 6–12 months.

POSSIBLE COMPLICATIONS

• Postadulticide pulmonary thromboembolic complications—may occur up to 4–6 weeks after treatment; usually more severe in dogs with severe heartworm infection (Class III) and those not properly confined
• Thrombocytopenia, disseminated intravascular coagulation
• Melarsomine adverse effects—pulmonary thromboembolism (usually 7–30 days after therapy); anorexia (13% incidence); injection site reaction (myositis) 32% incidence but mild and only lasts 1–2 days; lethargy or depression (15% incidence); causes elevations of hepatic enzymes

EXPECTED COURSE AND PROGNOSIS

• Usually uneventful with excellent prognosis in asymptomatic and mildly symptomatic animals (Class I)
• Guarded prognosis with higher risk of complications in dogs with severe infection (Class III)

MISCELLANEOUS

ASSOCIATED CONDITIONS

N/A

AGE-RELATED FACTORS

Old dogs may not require treatment, since heartworm infection may not be the life-limiting factor.

ZOONOTIC POTENTIAL

N/A

PREGNANCY

• Adulticide treatment should be delayed.
• Transplacental infection by microfilaria can occur. Dead-end infection

SYNONYMS

N/A

SEE ALSO

• Congestive Heart Failure, Right-sided
• Disseminated Intravascular Coagulation
• Hepatotoxins
• Hypertension, Pulmonary
• Nephrotic Syndrome
• Pulmonary Thromboembolism

ABBREVIATIONS

CHF = congestive heart failure

Suggested Reading

Dillon R. Dirofilariosis in dogs and cats. In: Ettinger SJ, Feldman EC, eds. Textbook of canine and feline veterinary internal medicine. 5th ed. Philadelphia: Saunders, 2000:937–963.
Authors Clay A. Calvert and Clarence A. Rawlings
Consulting Editors Larry P. Tilley and Francis W. K. Smith, Jr.

HEAT STROKE AND HYPERTHERMIA

 BASICS

DEFINITION
• Hyperthermia is an elevation in body temperature above the normal range. Although published normal values for dogs and cats vary slightly, it is generally accepted that body temperatures >103° F (39° C) are abnormal. • Hyperthermia can be categorized into pyrogenic hyperthermia (pyrexia or fever) and non-pyrogenic hyperthermia. • Heat stroke is a form of non-pyrogenic hyperthermia that occurs when heat-dissipating mechanisms of the body cannot accommodate excessive heat. This can lead to multisystemic organ dysfunction. Temperatures of 106° F (41° C) without signs of inflammation are suggestive of non-pyrogenic hyperthermia. • Malignant hyperthermia is an uncommon familial non-pyrogenic hyperthermia that can occur secondary to some anesthetic agents. • Other causes of non-pyrogenic hyperthermia include excessive exercise, thyrotoxicosis, and hypothalamic lesions.

PATHOPHYSIOLOGY
• The hypothalamic set point is changed with true fever. This is most likely mediated via the endogenous pyrogen interleukin I.
• Non-pyrogenic hyperthermia does not change the hypothalamic set point.
• The critical temperature leading to multiple organ dysfunction is 109° F (42.7° C).
• The primary pathophysiologic processes of heat stroke are related to thermal damage, which can lead to cellular necrosis, hypoxemia, and protein denaturalization.
• Heat stroke and its sequelae can lead to systemic inflammatory response syndrome (SIRS).

SYSTEMS AFFECTED
• Nervous—neuronal damage, parenchymal hemorrhage, cerebral edema
• Cardiovascular—hypovolemia, cardiac arrhythmias, myocardial ischemia and necrosis
• Gastrointestinal—mucosal ischemia and ulceration, bacterial translocation and endotoxemia
• Hepatobiliary—hepatocellular necrosis
• Renal/Urologic—acute renal failure
• Hemic/Lymphatic/Immune—hemoconcentration, thrombocytopenia, disseminated intravascular coagulopathy
• Musculoskeletal—rhabdomyolysis

GENETICS
N/A

GEOGRAPHIC DISTRIBUTION
May be seem in any climate but more common in warm and or humid environments

SIGNALMENT

Species
Dogs and uncommonly cats

Breed Predilection
• May occur in any breed • Long-haired animals • Brachycephalic breeds

Mean Age and Range
• All ages but often age extremes • Young dogs may tend to overexert. • Old dogs with preexisting disease

Predominant Sex
None

SIGNS

Historical Findings
• Identifiable underlying cause (hot day, locked in car or other confined area without adequate ventilation, grooming accident associated with drying cages, excessive exercise, restricted access to water)
• Predisposing underlying disease: laryngeal paralysis, cardiovascular disease, neuromuscular disease, previous history of heat-related disease

Physical Examination Findings
• Panting • Hypersalivation • Hyperthermia
• Hyperemic mucous membranes
• Tachycardia • Cardiac dysrhythmias
• Shock • Respiratory distress
• Hematemesis • Hematochezia • Melena
• Petechiation • Changes in mentation
• Seizures • Muscle tremors • Ataxia
• Coma • Oliguria/anuria • Respiratory arrest
• Cardiopulmonary arrest

CAUSES
• Excessive environmental heat and humidity (may be due to weather conditions, or accidents such as being enclosed in unventilated room, car, or grooming dryer cages) • Upper airway disease • Exercise
• Toxicosis (some compounds that lead to seizures, i.e., strychnine and metaldehyde)
• Anesthesia (malignant hyperthermia)

RISK FACTORS
• Previous history of heat-related disease
• Age extremes • Heat intolerance due to poor acclimatization • Obesity
• Poor cardiopulmonary conditioning
• Hyperthyroidism • Underlying cardiopulmonary disease • Brachycephalic breeds • Thick hair coat • Dehydration

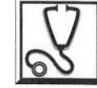 DIAGNOSIS

DIFFERENTIAL DIAGNOSIS
• If temperatures exceed 106° F (41° C) without evidence of inflammation, consider heat stroke.
• Panting and hypersalivation may not be seen with true fever, as hypothalamic set point is raised with fever.

CBC/BIOCHEMISTRY/URINALYSIS
• May help to identify underlying disease process
• May be beneficial in identifying sequelae to hyperthermia
• CBC abnormalities may include stress leukogram, leukopenia, anemia, nucleated RBCs, thrombocytopenia, or hemoconcentration.
• Biochemistry profile may show azotemia, hyperalbuminemia, elevations in serum enzymes (ALT, AST, CK), hypernatremia, hyperchloremia, hyperglycemia, hypoglycemia, hyperphosphatemia, hyperkalemia, hypokalemia, hyperbilirubinemia
• Urinalysis may show hypersthenuria, proteinuria, cylindruria, hemoglobinuria, myoglobinuria

OTHER LABORATORY TESTS
• Blood gas analysis may show mixed acid/base disorder, respiratory alkalosis, or metabolic acidosis.
• Coagulation profile may indicate prolonged activated clotting time (ACT), prothrombin time (PT), or partial thromboplastin time (PTT). Fibrin degradation products (FDPs) or D-dimer may be positive. Disseminated intravascular coagulopathy (DIC) may be present if PT and PTT are prolonged along with positive FDPs or D-dimers and thrombocytopenia. If available, the measurement of antithrombin III may be valuable.

IMAGING
• Thoracic radiographs may help identify underlying cardiopulmonary disease or predisposing factors.
• Abdominal radiographs and/or ultrasound may help identify underlying disease process.
• Computed tomography or magnetic resonance imaging may help identify hypothalamic lesion.

DIAGNOSTIC PROCEDURES
N/A

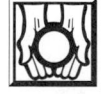 TREATMENT

APPROPRIATE HEALTH CARE
• Early recognition is key.
• Immediately correct hyperthermia.
• Patients should be hospitalized until temperature is stabilized.
• Most patients need intensive care for several days.
• Treat complications, DIC, renal failure, cerebral edema.
• Treat underlying disease or correct predisposing factors.

HEAT STROKE AND HYPERTHERMIA

NURSING CARE

External Cooling Techniques
• Spray with water or immerse in water prior to transport to veterinary facility.
• Convection cooling with fans
• Evaporative cooling such as isopropyl alcohol on foot pads, axilla, and groin
• Stop cooling procedures when temperature reaches 103° F to avoid hypothermia.
• Avoid ice, as this may cause peripheral vasoconstriction and impede heat dissipation. Shivering response is also undesirable, as this creates heat.

Other Care
• Continuous temperature monitoring
• Fluid therapy: Isotonic crystalloids can be administered at shock rates (90 ml/kg/h for dogs; 45–60 ml/kg/h for cats) based on clinical assessment. Synthetic colloids may also be used to treat shock (20 ml/kg in dogs, 5–10 ml/kg in cats).
• Provide oxygen supplementation via mask, cage, or nasal catheter.
• Ventilatory support if required

ACTIVITY
Restricted

DIET
Nothing per os until animal is stable

CLIENT EDUCATION
• Be aware of clinical signs.
• Know how to cool off animals.
• An episode of heat stroke may predispose pets to additional episodes.

SURGICAL CONSIDERATIONS
Tracheostomy may be required if upper airway obstruction is an underlying cause or a contributing factor.

MEDICATIONS

DRUG(S) OF CHOICE
• There are no specific drugs that are required for hyperthermia or heat stroke; therapy is dependent on clinical presentation.
• Prophylactic broad-spectrum antimicrobials may decrease the incidence of bacterial translocation. First-generation cephalosporins in combination with fluoroquinolones provide excellent four-quadrant coverage.
• Acute renal failure—dopamine, continuous rate intravenous infusion (2–5 µg/kg/min); furosemide intravenously (2–4 mg/kg PRN)
• Cerebral edema—mannitol (1g/kg IV over 15–30 minutes); furosemide (1 mg/kg IV), 30 minutes following mannitol infusion; corticosteroids (dexamethasone sodium phosphate [1–2 mg/kg IV]; prednisone sodium succinate [10–20 mg/kg IV]; or methyl prednisolone [15 mg/kg IV]). The use of corticosteroids is considered controversial due to adverse side effects in these patients.

• Ventricular arrhythmia—lidocaine bolus (2 mg/kg IV) followed by continuous rate intravenous infusion (25–75 µg/kg/min) or procainamide (6–8 mg/kg IV)
• Metabolic acidosis—sodium bicarbonate (0.3 × body weight [kg] × base excess); give half as IV bolus.
• Disseminated intravascular coagulopathy—fresh frozen plasma (20 ml/kg) and heparin (50–200 U/kg SC q6–8h). The first dose of heparin can be placed into the unit of plasma.
• Thrombocytopenia—severe thrombocytopenia can be treated with newly available frozen platelet concentrates.
• Hemorrhagic vomiting or diarrhea—broad-spectrum antibiotic as well as a histamine-2 (H2) antagonist (e.g., famotidine) in combination with sucralfate
• Seizures—diazepam (0.5–1 mg/kg IV); phenobarbital (6 mg/kg IV as needed)

CONTRAINDICATIONS
Nonsteroidal antiinflammatory agents are not indicated in non-pyrogenic hyperthermia because the hypothalamic set point is not altered.

PRECAUTIONS
The use of corticosteroids is considered controversial in heat stroke owing to side effects.

POSSIBLE INTERACTIONS
N/A

ALTERNATIVE DRUG(S)
N/A

FOLLOW-UP

PATIENT MONITORING
Patients should be closely monitored during cooling down period and for a minimum of 24 hours post episode. Most animals must be monitored for several days depending on clinical presentation and sequelae. A thorough physical examination should be performed daily. In addition, the following parameters should be given consideration:
• Body temperature • Body weight • Blood pressure • Central venous pressure
• Coagulation status (e.g., ACT, PT, PTT, FDP) • Electrocardiogram • Thoracic auscultation • Urinalysis and urine output
• PCV, total protein • CBC, biochemical profile

PREVENTION/AVOIDANCE
Avoid risk factors

POSSIBLE COMPLICATIONS
• Cardiac dysrhythmias • Organ failure
• Coma • Seizures • Acute renal failure
• Disseminated intravascular coagulation
• Systemic inflammatory response syndrome

• Pulmonary edema–acute respiratory distress
• Rhabdomyolysis • Hepatocellular necrosis
• Respiratory arrest • Cardiopulmonary arrest

EXPECTED COURSE AND PROGNOSIS
• Prognosis is dependent on underlying cause or disease process. • Prognosis is guarded, depending on complications that occur and duration of episode. • One episode predisposes animal to further episodes because of damage to the thermoregulatory center.

MISCELLANEOUS

ASSOCIATED CONDITIONS
N/A

AGE-RELATED FACTORS
N/A

PREGNANCY
N/A

SYNONYMS
• Heat stroke • Heat exhaustion • Heat prostration • Heat-related disease

SEE ALSO
Fever

ABBREVIATIONS
• ACT = activated clotting time
• ALT = alanine aminotransferase
• AST = aspartate aminotransferase
• CK = creatine kinase
• DIC = disseminated intravascular coagulopathy
• FDP = fibrin degradation product
• PT = prothrombin time
• PTT = partial thromboplastin time
• SIRS = systemic inflammatory response syndrome

Suggested Reading
Bouchama A, Knochel JP. Heatstroke. N Engl J Med 2002:346:1978–1988.
Drobatz KJ, MacIntire DK. Heat-induced illness in dogs: 42 cases (1976–1993). J Am Vet Med Assoc 1996:209:1894–1899.
Miller JB. Hyperthermia and hypothermia. In: Ettinger SJ, Feldman EC, eds. Textbook of veterinary internal medicine. 5th ed. Philadelphia: Saunders, 2000:6–10.
Rushlander D. Heat stroke. In: Kirk RW, Bonagura JD, eds. Current veterinary therapy. 11th ed. Philadelphia: Saunders, 1992:143–146.
Waters JM. Hyperthermia. In: Wingfield WE, Raffe MR, eds. The veterinary ICU book. Jackson Hole: Teton NewMedia, 2002:1130–1136.

Author Steven L. Marks
Consulting Editors Larry P. Tilley and Francis W. K. Smith, Jr.

HELICOBACTER INFECTION

 BASICS

DEFINITION
Helicobacter spp. are microaerophilic, Gram-negative, urease-positive bacteria ranging from coccoid to curved to spiral.

PATHOPHYSIOLOGY
Gastric Helicobacter
• The discovery of the association of *Helicobacter pylori* with gastritis, peptic ulcers, and gastric neoplasia has fundamentally changed the understanding of gastric disease in human beings. • Putative mechanisms by which *H. pylori* alters gastric physiology in human beings include disruption of the gastric mucosal barrier (due to secretion of phospholipases and vacuolating cytotoxins) and alterations in the gastric secretory activity (e.g., decreased somatostatin secretion leading to hypergastrinemia). • *H. pylori* infection in human beings is also associated with increased secretion of proinflammatory cytokines, tumor necrosis factor-α, and nitric oxide. • *Helicobacter* spp. isolated from stomachs of dogs and cats include *H. felis, H. bizzozeronii, H. salomonis,* and *Flexispira rappini*. To date *H. pylori*, the most important species affecting human beings, has only been identified in a single colony of laboratory cats. • The cause-effect relationship of *Helicobacter* spp. with gastric inflammation in cats and dogs is unresolved; inflammation or glandular degeneration accompanies infection in some but not all subjects. • The presence of multiple species complicates the investigation of pathogenicity. • Experiments to determine the pathogenicity of *H. pylori* in SPF cats and *H. pylori* and *H. felis* in gnotobiotic dogs demonstrated gastritis, lymphoid follicle proliferation, and humoral immune responses after infection.

Intestinal and Hepatic Helicobacter
• The role of *Helicobacter* spp. in intestinal and hepatic disease in dogs and cats is unclear. • *H. canis* has been isolated from dogs and cats with diarrhea but also in clinically healthy dogs and cats. • *H. canis* has also been isolated from the liver of a dog with active, multifocal hepatitis. • *H. fennelliae* has been isolated from dogs and *H. cinaedi* from dogs and cats; neither has been associated with clinical signs.

SYSTEMS AFFECTED
• Gastrointestinal—stomach: gastric infection with *Helicobacter* spp. may lead to gastritis; intestines: diarrhea observed in some dogs with *H. canis* infection. • Hepatobiliary—acute hepatitis has been associated with *H. canis* infection.

INCIDENCE/PREVALENCE
Gastric Helicobacter spp.
• Gastric Helicobacter-like organisms (HLOs) are highly prevalent in dogs and cats—86% of random-source cats, 90% of clinically healthy pet cats, 67–86% of clinically healthy pet dogs, and almost 100% of laboratory beagles and shelter dogs infected. • HLOs demonstrated in gastric biopsy specimens from 57–76% of cats and 61–82% of dogs presented for investigation of recurrent vomiting. • To date *H. pylori* has been identified only in a colony of laboratory cats.

Intestinal and Hepatic Helicobacter spp.
• *H. canis* was isolated from 4% of 1000 dogs. • Only one case of *H. canis*–associated hepatitis has been reported. • Prevalence of *H. fennelliae* and *H. cinaedi* is undetermined.

GEOGRAPHIC DISTRIBUTION
• *H. pylori* infection in human beings has a higher prevalence in less-developed countries. • No information available for dogs and cats.

SIGNALMENT
Species
Dogs and cats
Breed Predilections
None known
Mean Age and Range
• Infection with gastric *Helicobacter* spp. appears to be acquired at a young age. • The dog with *H. canis*–associated hepatitis was 2 months old.
Predominant Sex N/A

SIGNS
Historical Findings
• Asymptomatic *Helicobacter* infection is common • Vomiting, anorexia, abdominal pain, weight loss, and/or borborygmus in dogs and cats with gastric *Helicobacter* spp. • Diarrhea in dogs may be associated with *H. canis* infection. • Vomiting, weakness, and sudden death in a dog with hepatic *H. canis*

Physical Examination Findings
• Usually unremarkable • May have signs of dehydration from fluid and electrolyte loss due to vomiting or diarrhea

CAUSES
Gastric Helicobacter spp.
• *H. felis, H. pylori, H. heilmannii* have been found in cats. • *H. felis, H. heilmannii, H. bizzozeronii, H. salomonis, H. bilis,* and *Flexispira rappini* have been found in dogs.

Intestinal and Hepatic Helicobacter spp.
• *H. fennelliae*—dog (significance unknown) • *H. cinaedi*—dogs and a cat (significance unknown) • *H. canis*—normal and diarrheic dogs and cats; one dog with acute hepatitis

RISK FACTORS
Potentially poor sanitary conditions and overcrowding may facilitate the spread of infection.

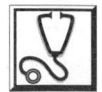 DIAGNOSIS

DIFFERENTIAL DIAGNOSIS
General Comments
High *Helicobacter* spp. prevalence rates exist in dogs and cats. Therefore, exclusion of other causes of gastric disease and a positive test for *Helicobacter* infection are necessary before a conclusive diagnosis of gastrointestinal disease due to *Helicobacter* spp. infection can be made.
Gastric Helicobacteriosis
Distinguish from other causes of vomiting (both gastrointestinal and non-gastrointestinal).
Intestinal Helicobacteriosis
Distinguish from other causes of diarrhea (both gastrointestinal and non-gastrointestinal).
Hepatic Helicobacteriosis
Distinguish from other causes of hepatobiliary disease.

CBC/BIOCHEMISTRY/URINALYSIS
• May reflect fluid and electrolyte abnormalities secondary to vomiting and/or diarrhea • May reflect changes consistent with hepatic disease in *H. canis*–associated hepatitis

OTHER LABORATORY TESTS
• Examination of impression smears from the gastric mucosa using May-Grünwald-Giemsa, Gram, or Diff-Quik stain is a sensitive test and can easily be performed. • Rapid-urease test—requires gastric biopsy specimen; easy to perform in animals that undergo gastroduodenoscopy. • ^{13}C-urea breath or blood test has been shown to be reliable in identifying infected dogs. • Bacterial culture—requires special techniques and media; success rate is low. • PCR of DNA extracted from biopsy specimens or from gastric juice • Serologic tests (ELISA) measure circulating IgG in serum—cannot distinguish between different HLOs. • Histopathology enables the definitive diagnosis of gastric *Helicobacter* infection.

IMAGING
Radiography and ultrasonography—usually normal

DIAGNOSTIC PROCEDURES
Gastric Helicobacteriosis
• Endoscopy may reveal superficial nodules that suggest lymphoid follicle hyperplasia. • Other endoscopic findings include diffuse gastric rugal thickening, mucosal flattening, punctate hemorrhages, and erosions.

Hepatobiliary Helicobacteriosis
Hepatic biopsy/histopathology (Warthin-Starry staining) and culture

PATHOLOGIC FINDINGS
• Requires histopathological examination of gastric or hepatic biopsy specimens along with special staining of tissue samples with Warthin-Starry or modified-Steiner stain; routine H&E staining may reveal larger *Helicobacter* organisms, smaller organisms are often missed. • Stomach—gastric spiral organisms on silver-stained sections; lymphocytic plasmacytic gastritis and lymphoid follicle hyperplasia; rarely neutrophilic infiltrations; no ulcers reported in dogs and cats • *H. canis*–associated hepatitis—hepatocellular necrosis, mononuclear cells, and neutrophils; spiral to curved bacteria predominantly in biliary canaliculi

TREATMENT

APPROPRIATE HEALTH CARE
• The pathogenicity of *Helicobacter* spp. in dogs and cats is still unclear; therefore, there are no unanimously accepted guidelines for treatment of *Helicobacter* spp. infections in dogs and cats.
• Currently there is no indication for treating asymptomatic animals with *Helicobacter* spp. infection. • The authors attempt to eradicate gastric *Helicobacter* spp. in infected dogs and cats that have compatible clinical signs that cannot be attributed to another disease process.

NURSING CARE
Fluid therapy for dehydration from vomiting

ACTIVITY N/A

DIET
Diets that facilitate gastric emptying—high in digestible carbohydrates

CLIENT EDUCATION
Explain the difficulty of establishing a diagnosis, the high prevalence rates of infections with HLOs in normal dogs and cats, the potential for recurrence, and the zoonotic potential of the disease.

SURGICAL CONSIDERATIONS N/A

MEDICATIONS

GENERAL COMMENTS
• A triple therapy (combination of two antibiotics and one antisecretory drug) is effective in people with *H. pylori* infection—cure rates approach/exceed 90%. • Combination therapy may eliminate *Helicobacter* spp. infections in dogs and cats less effectively than in humans.
• Treat for 2–3 weeks.

DRUG(S) OF CHOICE

Antibiotics (Two with One Antisecretory Agent)
• Amoxicillin (20 mg/kg PO q12h)
• Azithromycin (5 mg/kg PO q24h)
• Bismuth subsalicylate (17–20 mg/kg PO q12h or 1 mL/kg of regular strength preparation [262 mg/15 mL] PO q12h)
• Clarithromycin (5 mg/kg PO q12h)
• Metronidazole (dogs, 15–20 mg/kg PO q12h; cats, 12.5 mg/kg PO q12h)
• Tetracycline (20 mg/kg PO q8h)

Antisecretory Agents (One with Two Antibiotics)
• Famotidine (0.5 mg/kg PO q12–24h)
• Omeprazole (0.7 mg/kg PO q24h)
• Ranitidine (1.0 mg/kg PO q12h)
• Cimetidine (10 mg/kg PO q8h)

Intestinal and Hepatic Helicobacter spp. *in Dogs*
The combination of amoxicillin and metronidazole may be effective.

CONTRAINDICATIONS
Previously established hypersensitivity to one of the antibiotics

ALTERNATIVE DRUG(S)
Patients with HLO infections and gastritis that do not respond to antibiotic therapy usually are given immunosuppressive therapy (prednisolone, or others) for inflammatory bowel disease with gastric involvement.

FOLLOW-UP

PATIENT MONITORING
• Serologic tests are not useful to confirm eradication of gastric HLOs—serum IgG titers may not decrease for up to 6 months after cleared infection. • ^{13}C-urea breath and blood test has been evaluated to monitor the eradication of HLOs in dogs and cats—shows promise for routine application. • If vomiting persists or recurs after cessation of combination therapy, a repeat endoscopic biopsy to determine whether the infection has been successfully eradicated may be necessary.

PREVENTION/AVOIDANCE
Avoid overcrowding and unsanitary conditions.

POSSIBLE COMPLICATIONS
• Recurrence • Zoonotic potential

EXPECTED COURSE AND PROGNOSIS
• The efficacy of therapeutic regimens currently employed in dogs and cats for eradicating *Helicobacter* spp. infections is questionable.
• Metronidazole (20 mg/kg PO q12h), amoxicillin (20 mg/kg PO q12h), and famotidine (0.5 mg/kg PO q12h) for 14 days effectively eradicated *Helicobacter* in 6 of 8 dogs evaluated 3 days post-treatment, but all dogs were recolonized by day 28 after completion of treatment.
• Clarithromycin (30 mg/cat PO q12h), metronidazole (30 mg/cat PO q12h), ranitidine (20 mg/cat PO q12h), and bismuth (40 mg PO q12h) for 4 days was effective in eradicating *H. heilmannii* in 11 of 11 cats by 10 days, but 2 cats were re-infected 42 days post-treatment.
• Amoxicillin (20 mg/kg PO q8h), metronidazole (20 mg/kg PO q8h), and omeprazole (0.7 mg/kg PO q24h) for 21 days transiently eradicated *H. pylori* in 6 cats, but all were reinfected 6 weeks post-treatment (*Note:* this dose of metronidazole has the potential for toxicity).
• It is unclear if recurrent infection following therapy is due to reinfection or recrudescence of infection.

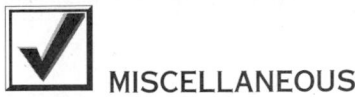
MISCELLANEOUS

ASSOCIATED CONDITIONS
Gastrointestinal erosions

AGE-RELATED FACTORS
Gastric HLOs appear to be acquired at a young age.

ZOONOTIC POTENTIAL
• The high prevalence of *Helicobacter* spp. in dogs and cats raises the possibility that household pets may serve as a reservoir for the transmission of *Helicobacter* spp. to human beings.
• *H. pylori, H. heilmannii,* and *H. felis* have been isolated from humans with gastritis.
• *H. fennelliae* and *H. cinaedi* have been isolated from immunocompromised people with proctitis and colitis. • *H. cinaedi* has also been associated with septicemia in people. • *H. canis* has also been isolated from human beings.

PREGNANCY
Avoid metronidazole and tetracycline in pregnant animals.

SYNONYMS
• Gastric spiral bacteria • Gastrospirillum

SEE ALSO
• Gastritis, Chronic • Gastroduodenal Ulcer Disease • Inflammatory Bowel Disease
• Vomiting, Chronic

ABBREVIATIONS
• HLO = *Helicobacter*-like organism
• PCR = polymerase chain reaction

Suggested Reading
Crystal MA. Helicobacter Infection. In: Norsworthy GD, Crystal MA, Fooshee Grace SK, Tilley LP, eds. The feline patient. Essentials of diagnosis and treatment. 2nd ed. Baltimore: Williams & Wilkins, 2003:254–258.
Fox JG. Helicobacter-associated gastric disease in ferrets, dogs and cats. In: Bonagura JD, ed. Kirk's current veterinary therapy XII small animal practice. Philadelphia: Saunders, 1995:720–723.
Fox JG, Lee A. The role of *Helicobacter* species in newly recognized gastrointestinal tract disease of animals. Lab Anim Sci 1997;47:222–255.
Neiger R, Simpson KW. *Helicobacter* infection in dogs and cats: Facts and Fiction. J Vet Intern Med 2000;14:125–133.
Simpson KW, Neiger R, DeNovo RC, Sherding RG. The relationship of *Helicobacter* spp infection to gastric disease in dogs and cats, ACVIM Consensus Statement. J Vet Intern Med 2000;14:223–227.

Acknowledgment
The authors and editors acknowledge the prior contribution of Dr Kenneth W. Simpson, who authored this topic in the previous edition.
Authors Jan S. Suchodolski and Jörg M. Steiner
Consulting Editor Albert E. Jergens

HEMANGIOPERICYTOMA

BASICS

OVERVIEW
• A soft tissue sarcoma arising from pericytes, which are cells surrounding capillaries in subcutaneous tissue
• Locally invasive, often extending far beyond visible margins
• Metastasizes in up to 20% of patients
• Local growth can interfere with limb function.

SIGNALMENT
• More common in large-breed than in small-breed dogs
• Rare in cats

SIGNS

Historical Findings
• Typically, slow-growing mass (weeks to months)
• Rapid growth uncommon unless high-grade variant

Physical Examination Findings
• Soft tissue mass, usually located on extremity; less commonly found on trunk
• Soft, fluctuant, or firm
• Generally adhered to underlying tissue
• Regional lymph node metastasis uncommon

CAUSES & RISK FACTORS
Unknown

DIAGNOSIS

DIFFERENTIAL DIAGNOSIS
• Other soft tissue sarcomas—nerve sheath tumor; fibrosarcoma
• Lipoma and other tumors—benign and malignant
• Biopsy—essential to confirm diagnosis

CBC/BIOCHEMISTRY/URINALYSIS
N/A

OTHER LABORATORY TESTS
N/A

IMAGING
• Thoracic radiographs—recommended before treatment, although metastasis uncommon
• CT or MRI—may be required to determine extent of disease and to optimize surgical treatment

DIAGNOSTIC PROCEDURES
• Biopsy—essential to confirm diagnosis and determine grade of the tumor
• Regional lymph node evaluation—appropriate for high-grade tumors

TREATMENT
• Early, aggressive surgical excision—treatment of choice
• Local recurrence, metastasis, and overall survival time—greatly affected by surgical margin width as determined by a pathologist
• Radiotherapy—good option when complete surgical excision is not possible

Surgical Technique
• Microscopically, cancer cells extend far beyond gross tumor borders.
• Pseudocapsule composed of cancer cells common
• Excise tumor en bloc; if it is peeled out, a healthy bed of cancer cells is left behind.
• Submit the entire sample to a pathologist for surgical margin evaluation; mark two edges of the tissue with suture material to orient the pathologist and allow for proper margin evaluation.
• Toe or limb amputation may be necessary.
• Rib resection or abdominal wall resection—may be required for tumors of the trunk

MEDICATIONS

DRUG(S)
Chemotherapy—not consistently reported as beneficial; recommended after excision of a high-grade (grade III) tumor; doxorubicin is drug of choice.

CONTRAINDICATIONS/POSSIBLE INTERACTIONS
N/A

FOLLOW-UP

PATIENT MONITORING
Incomplete surgical excision—perform a second surgery or start radiotherapy as soon as possible.

EXPECTED COURSE AND PROGNOSIS
• Cure—possible when surgery is aggressive and surgical margins are tumor free
• Recurrence—inevitable if treatment is not aggressive; increased risk for metastatic disease
• Long-term tumor control—radiotherapy after surgically debulking the tumor gives 1- to 5-year control rates of 60%–85%.

MISCELLANEOUS

Suggested Reading

Kuntz CA, Dernell WS, Powers BE, et al. Prognostic factors for surgical treatment of soft tissue sarcomas in dogs: 75 cases (1986–1996). J Am Vet Med Assoc 1997;211:1147–1151.

Mazzei M, Millante F, Ati S, et al. Haemangiopericytoma: histological spectrum, immunohistochemical characterization and prognosis. Vet Dermatol 2002;13:15–21.

Salisbury SK. Aggressive cancer surgery and aftercare. In: Morrison WB, ed. Cancer in dogs and cats: medical and surgical management. Baltimore: Williams & Wilkins, 1998:265–321.

Author Robyn Elmslie
Consulting Editor Wallace B. Morrison

BASICS

OVERVIEW
• A highly metastatic malignant tumor of vascular endothelial cells
• Primary disease rare
• Incidence rates—3%–8% of all bone tumors
• May be difficult to distinguish primary from metastatic lesions

SIGNALMENT
• Mean age—dogs, 6 years; cats, 17–18 years
• Boxers, Great Danes, and German shepherds predisposed
• Male dogs have higher incidence

SIGNS

Historical Findings
• Tumor on limb—lameness; swelling; pathologic fracture
• Tumor on rib—thoracic wall swelling; dyspnea if patient has pleural effusion

Physical Examination Findings
• Soft tissue swelling at tumor site
• Palpable fracture
• Quiet or absent ventral lung sounds (if pleural effusion present)
• Pale mucous membranes

CAUSES & RISK FACTORS
Unknown

DIAGNOSIS

DIFFERENTIAL DIAGNOSIS
• Other primary or metastatic bone tumors
• Osteomyelitis (bacterial or fungal)

CBC/BIOCHEMISTRY/URINALYSIS
• Regenerative anemia
• Nucleated RBC
• Poikilocytosis—acanthocytes; schistocytes; spherocytes
• Anisocytosis
• Thrombocytopenia
• Leukocytosis
• Hypoproteinemia

OTHER LABORATORY TESTS
High fibrin degradation products, PT, PTT, and low fibrinogen concentration—may indicate DIC

IMAGING
• Radiology of bone—reveals poorly marginated osteolytic lesion with minimal periosteal reaction; pathologic fractures possible
• Thoracic radiography—evaluate lungs for metastasis
• Abdominal and cardiac ultrasound—look for primary tumor or metastasis
• CT scan—may help determine extent of bone tumor before surgery

DIAGNOSTIC PROCEDURES
Biopsy—incisional may be helpful, but because of the vascular nature of the tumor, blood contamination of specimen may preclude a diagnosis; excisional may be preferred.

PATHOLOGIC FINDINGS
• Dark, friable mass within the medullary cavity of the bone
• Histopathologic—vascular spaces and clefts filled with RBCs, thrombi, and necrotic debris; spaces lined by pleomorphic tumor cells with round, ovoid, or pleomorphic nuclei

TREATMENT
• Aggressive surgical excision of tumor sites
• Amputation—required if limbs affected
• Axial tumors—may be more difficult to remove
• Adjunctive chemotherapy—indicated in all cases

MEDICATIONS

DRUG(S)
Doxorubicin—30 mg/m^2 dogs > 10 kg; 1 mg/kg dogs < 10 kg and cats day 1; cyclophosphamide—50 mg/m^2 PO days 3, 4, 5, 6; repeat cycle every 3 weeks for 4–6 cycles

CONTRAINDICATIONS/ POSSIBLE INTERACTIONS
Doxorubicin—cardiotoxic; do not use with pre-existing heart disease

FOLLOW-UP

PATIENT MONITORING
• Thoracic radiography, cardiac and abdominal ultrasound, and physical examination—1, 3, 6, 9, 12, 18, and 24 months after treatment
• Creatinine—monitor in small dogs and cats receiving doxorubicin because of potential nephrotoxicity.

POSSIBLE COMPLICATIONS
• Pathologic fractures
• Tumors and metastatic lesions may rupture causing serious acute blood loss.

EXPECTED COURSE AND PROGNOSIS
• Mean survival—unknown
• Less than 10% of patients survive 1 year following surgery.
• Median survival (all locations) after surgery and chemotherapy—180 days

MISCELLANEOUS

ASSOCIATED CONDITIONS
High incidence of DIC

ABBREVIATIONS
• CT = computed tomography
• DIC = disseminated intravascular coagulation
• PT = prothrombin time
• PTT = partial thromboplastin time

Suggested Reading
Dernell WS, Straw RC, Withrow SJ. Tumors of the skeletal system. In: Withrow JJ, MacEwen EG, eds. Small animal clinical oncology. 3rd ed. Philadelphia: Saunders, 2001:378–417.
Waters DJ, Cooley DM. Skeletal neoplasms. In: Morrison WB, ed. Cancer in dogs and cats: medical and surgical management. Baltimore: Williams & Wilkins, 1998: 639–654.
Author Joanne C. Graham
Consulting Editor Wallace B. Morrison

HEMANGIOSARCOMA, HEART

 BASICS

OVERVIEW
- The most common cardiac tumor in dogs
- The heart can be a primary or metastatic site in dogs and cats.
- Most tumors involve the right atrium or right auricular appendage, or both.
- Rarely involves the right ventricular wall or heart valve

SIGNALMENT
- Dogs and rarely cats
- Most commonly reported in German shepherds and golden retrievers

SIGNS

General Comments
Most relate to the development of pericardial effusion and right-sided congestive heart failure rather than to the tumor itself.

Physical Examination Findings
- Abdominal effusion
- Quiet or absent ventral lung sounds—with pleural effusion
- Dyspnea
- Weight loss
- Muffled heart sounds with pericardial effusion
- Syncope
- Arrhythmia
- Pulse deficits
- Pulsus paradoxus
- Exercise intolerance
- Hepatomegaly
- Jugular distention

CAUSES & RISK FACTORS
Unknown

 DIAGNOSIS

DIFFERENTIAL DIAGNOSIS
- Other causes of right heart failure—heartworm disease
- Other cardiac neoplasia
- Idiopathic hemorrhagic pericardial effusion
- Other causes of pericardial effusion

CBC/BIOCHEMISTRY/URINALYSIS
- May find anemia and nucleated RBCs
- Prerenal azotemia with congestive heart failure

OTHER LABORATORY TESTS
N/A

IMAGING
- Radiographs—often reveal evidence of pericardial and/or pleural effusion; rarely detect cardiac mass
- Ultrasound (heart)—useful for identifying cardiac location of tumor

DIAGNOSTIC PROCEDURES
Biopsy of mass—required for definitive diagnosis

 TREATMENT

- Surgery and chemotherapy—primary choices
- Periodic centesis of pericardial and pleural effusion—may provide symptomatic relief

 MEDICATIONS

DRUG(S)
Chemotherapy—doxorubicin; may be effective in providing palliation for varying periods of time

CONTRAINDICATIONS/POSSIBLE INTERACTIONS
N/A

 FOLLOW-UP

PATIENT MONITORING
Physical examination, thoracic radiographs, and cardiac ultrasound—monthly intervals

PREVENTION/AVOIDANCE
N/A

POSSIBLE COMPLICATIONS
Relate to centesis of pericardial and pleural space (e.g., arrhythmia, pneumothorax, and infection) or from primary treatment by surgery and/or chemotherapy

EXPECTED COURSE AND PROGNOSIS
Prognosis—guarded to poor

 MISCELLANEOUS

ASSOCIATED CONDITIONS
- Concurrent hemangiosarcoma at other sites (e.g., liver and spleen)
- Clinical signs of congestive heart failure secondary to pericardial effusion

ABBREVIATION
RBC = red blood cell

Suggested Reading
Morrison WB. Nonpulmonary intrathoracic cancer. In: Morrison WB, ed. Cancer in dogs and cats: medical and surgical management. Baltimore: Williams & Wilkins, 1998:537–550.

Author Wallace B. Morrison

Consulting Editor Wallace B. Morrison

BASICS

OVERVIEW
• Malignant tumor arising from endothelial cells
• Primary tumor develops within dermal or subcutaneous tissues
• Accounts for 14% of all hemangiosarcoma in dogs
• Prevalence (dogs)—0.3%-2.0%

SIGNALMENT
• Dogs and rarely cats
• Pit bulls, boxers, and German shepherds—affected more commonly than other breeds
• Multicentric dermal hemangiosarcoma—whippet dogs and related breeds
• Median age, 9 year; range, 4.5–15 years

SIGNS
• Usually solitary mass; may see multiple masses
• Dermal—firm, raised, dark nodules primarily on the limbs, prepuce, and ventral abdomen
• Subcutaneous—firm or soft, fluctuant masses with or without associated bruising; masses may appear to change size quickly because of intratumoral bleeding; typically larger than dermal; often found on the pelvic limbs, but may arise in any location

CAUSES & RISK FACTORS
• Vascular stasis, radiotherapy, trauma, and sun exposure—predisposing factors in humans; may be risk factors in dogs
• Pit bulls, boxers, and German shepherds—may have genetic predisposition
• Whippets—may be genetically predisposed to multicentric dermal hemangiosarcoma

DIAGNOSIS

DIFFERENTIAL DIAGNOSIS
• Trauma—subcutaneous hematoma
• Other benign or malignant tumors

CBC/BIOCHEMISTRY/URINALYSIS
• Usually normal
• May see laboratory abnormalities compatible with DIC—prolonged bleeding times, thrombocytopenia, low fibrinogen, and high fibrin split products

OTHER LABORATORY TESTS
N/A

IMAGING
• Thoracic radiographs—detect pulmonary metastasis
• CT or MRI—delineate extent of disease; often required to determine feasibility of surgery

DIAGNOSTIC PROCEDURES
Skin biopsy—required to confirm diagnosis; differentiate between dermal and subcutaneous

PATHOLOGIC FINDINGS
• Dermal—well circumscribed; confined to the dermis
• Subcutaneous—poorly circumscribed; very invasive

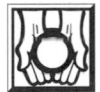

TREATMENT
• Aggressive surgical excision—treatment of choice; complete surgical excision of subcutaneous tumor difficult
• DIC and bleeding—important intraoperative and postoperative concerns

MEDICATIONS

DRUG(S)
• Chemotherapy (subcutaneous tumor)—recommended after excision; may be administered to patients before surgery to cytoreduce tumor and increase the likelihood of successful surgical outcome; treatment with doxorubicin, cyclophosphamide, and vincristine shown to improve survival time in dogs
• Multicentric dermal—etretinate (0.75–1 mg/kg q24h) and vitamin E (400 IU PO q12h); author successfully induced partial remission in whippets with nonresectable disease

CONTRAINDICATIONS/POSSIBLE INTERACTIONS
Aspirin and other NSAIDs—avoid because of associated increased potential for bleeding

FOLLOW-UP

EXPECTED COURSE AND PROGNOSIS
• Dermal—median survival, 780 days
• Subcutaneous—median survival, > 6 months; depends on the degree of invasion
• Metastasis—may occur

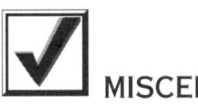

MISCELLANEOUS

ABBREVIATIONS
DIC = disseminated intravascular coagulation
NSAIDs = nonsteroidal antiinflammatory drugs

Suggested Reading
Clifford CA, Mackin AJ, Henry CJ. Treatment of canine hemangiosarcoma: 2000 and beyond. J Vet Intern Med 2000; 14:479–485.
Sorenmo K, Duda L, Barber L, et al. Canine hemangiosarcoma treated with standard chemotherapy and menocycline. J Vet Intern Med 2000:14:395–398.
Ward H, Fox LE, Calderwood-Mays MB, et al. Cutaneous hemangiosarcoma in 25 dogs: a retrospective study. J Vet Intern Med 1994:8:345–348.
Author Robyn Elmslie
Consulting Editor Wallace B. Morrison

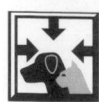 BASICS

DEFINITION
Highly metastatic malignant vascular neoplasm arising from endothelial cells

PATHOPHYSIOLOGY
• A large mass develops in the liver or spleen.
• Metastasis—rapidly via hematogenous routes; most frequently to the liver (from the spleen) and lungs (from the spleen and liver)
• Can rupture, leading to acute hemorrhage, collapse, and sudden death

SYSTEMS AFFECTED
• Hepatobiliary
• Hemic/Lymphatic/Immune—spleen
• Possible metastasis—lungs; kidneys; muscle; peritoneum; omentum; lymph nodes; mesentery; adrenal glands; spinal cord; brain; subcutaneous tissue; diaphragm

GENETICS
N/A

INCIDENCE/PREVALENCE
• Dogs—0.3%–2.0% of recorded necropsies; 7% of all malignancies; about 50% hemangiosarcomas splenic and 5% hepatic
• Cats—18 affected cats out of 3145 necropsies; liver most common site

GEOGRAPHIC DISTRIBUTION
N/A

SIGNALMENT
Species
Dogs and cats

Breed Predilections
• Dogs—German shepherds, boxers, Great Danes, English setters, golden retrievers, pointers
• Cats—domestic shorthair

Mean Age and Range
• Dogs—mean age, 8–10 years; can be seen < 1 year old
• Cats—mean age, 10 years

Predominant Sex
• Dogs—possible male predilection
• Cats—none

SIGNS
General Comments
• Related to the organs involved
• Also caused by bleeding secondary to rupture of the mass or DIC

Historical Findings
• Sudden death because of acute blood loss
• Weight loss
• Weakness
• Intermittent collapse
• Ataxia
• Lameness
• Seizures
• Dementia
• Paresis

Physical Examination Findings
• Pale mucous membranes
• Tachycardia
• Peritoneal fluid
• Palpable cranial abdominal mass

CAUSES
• Dogs and cats—unknown
• Humans—arsenicals; vinyl chloride; thorium dioxide
• Minks—methyl nitrosamine

RISK FACTORS
N/A

 DIAGNOSIS

DIFFERENTIAL DIAGNOSIS
• Other causes of splenic and hepatic masses—lymphosarcoma; leiomyosarcoma; liposarcoma; hematoma; hemangioma; splenic cyst; hepatoma; hepatocellular carcinoma; hepatic cyst
• One study reported 43 of 100 splenic masses as hemangiosarcoma.

CBC/BIOCHEMISTRY/URINALYSIS
• Regenerative anemia with polychromasia, reticulocytosis, anisocytosis, and nucleated RBCs

• Leukocytosis—caused by mature neutrophilia
• Thrombocytopenia
• High liver enzyme activity—with liver involvement

OTHER LABORATORY TESTS
• High PT, PTT, and fibrin degradation products—with DIC
• Evaluate clotting cascade—evidence of spontaneous hemorrhage; considering surgery

IMAGING
Radiography
• Abdominal—reveals cranial abdominal mass; possible evidence of abdominal fluid
• Thoracic radiography—detects metastasis
• Area of any lameness—pain from metastasis to bone possible; bone lysis with little to no proliferation common

Ultrasonography
• Reveals splenic masses with multiple cavitations
• Hepatic involvement—usually appears as multiple hypoechoic nodules

Echocardiography
• Perform in patients with evidence of pericardial effusion.
• May detect cardiac masses—primary cardiac (often right atrial location) or metastasis

DIAGNOSTIC PROCEDURES
Peritoneocentesis—with evidence of abdominal effusion; usually obtain serosanguinous fluid or frank blood that does not clot; may see spindle-shaped neoplastic cells

PATHOLOGIC FINDINGS
• Spleen—a large hemorrhagic, friable mass; usually some degree of abdominal hemorrhage
• Liver—multiple, variable-sized, hemorrhagic nodules in many patients
• Spleen and liver—widespread abdominal metastasis in many patients
• Histopathologic examination—necessary for definitive diagnosis; three patterns predominate: large blood spaces lined by endothelial cells, numerous small capillary structures, and solid areas of endothelial cells without apparent vascular structure

TREATMENT

APPROPRIATE HEALTH CARE
Inpatient—initial medical and surgical management

NURSING CARE
• Balanced isotonic electrolyte solutions—correct dehydration
• Fresh whole blood transfusion—with severe anemia
• Manage DIC as necessary.

ACTIVITY
Restricted until after initial surgical management; spontaneous hemorrhage may occur.

DIET
No change

CLIENT EDUCATION
• Inform client that emergency surgery may be indicated.
• Warn client that sudden death is possible.
• Discuss the importance of follow-up chemotherapy.

SURGICAL CONSIDERATIONS
Initial treatment of choice

MEDICATIONS

DRUG(S) OF CHOICE
Chemotherapy Cycle
• Day 1—doxorubicin (30 mg/m^2 IV for dogs > 10 kg; 1 mg/kg for dogs and cats < 10 kg) and cyclophosphamide (100–150 mg/m^2 IV); diphenhydramine (2.2 mg/kg IM) 20 min before the doxorubicin to prevent anaphylactoid reaction
• Days 8 and 15—vincristine (0.75 mg/m^2 IV)
• Repeat every 21 days; generally, four cycles are given after surgery.
• Mitoxantrone, carboplatin, and doxorubicin have been used successfully in cats.

CONTRAINDICATIONS
• Doxorubicin—do not use with arrhythmias or reduced fractional shortening of the heart.
• Chemotherapy may cause gastrointestinal, bone marrow, and cardiac toxicity; seek advice before treatment if unfamiliar with cytotoxic drugs.

PRECAUTIONS
• Monitor WBC count—delay chemotherapy if neutrophil count < 2,000/µL
• Monitor platelets—delay chemotherapy if platelets < 100,000/µL

POSSIBLE INTERACTIONS
None

ALTERNATIVE DRUG(S)
None

FOLLOW-UP

PATIENT MONITORING
Thoracic and abdominal radiography and abdominal ultrasound—every 3 months after treatment; monitor for recurrence or metastasis.

PREVENTION/AVOIDANCE
N/A

POSSIBLE COMPLICATIONS
• Sepsis—because of neutropenia
• Doxorubicin-induced cardiomyopathy
• Skin sloughs—caused by extravasation of doxorubicin or vincristine
• Vomiting and diarrhea

EXPECTED COURSE AND PROGNOSIS
• Mean time to recurrence (cats)—4–5 months
• Median survival time with surgery alone (dogs)—19–65 days
• Median survival time with surgery plus chemotherapy (dogs)—145 days (mean survival, 271 days)

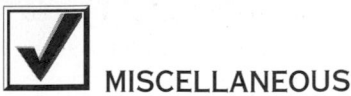

MISCELLANEOUS

ASSOCIATED CONDITIONS
DIC

AGE-RELATED FACTORS
None

ZOONOTIC POTENTIAL
None

PREGNANCY
Do not use chemotherapy in pregnant animals.

SYNONYMS
• Malignant hemangioendothelioma
• Angiosarcoma

SEE ALSO
• Hemangiosarcoma, bone
• Hemangiosarcoma, heart
• Hemangiosarcoma, skin

ABBREVIATIONS
• DIC = disseminated intravascular coagulation
• PT = prothrombin time
• PTT = partial thromboplastin time

Suggested Reading

Hammer AS, Couto G, Filppi J, et al. Efficacy and toxicity of VAC chemotherapy (vincristine, doxorubicin, and cyclophosphamide) in dogs with hemangiosarcoma. J Vet Intern Med 1991;5:160–166.

Johnson KA, Powers BE, Withrow SJ, et al. Splenomegaly in dogs: predictors of neoplasia and survival after splenectomy. J Vet Intern Med 1989;3:160–166.

Morrison WB. Blood vascular, lymphatic, and splenic cancer. In: Morrison WB, ed. Cancer in dogs and cats: medical and surgical management. Jackson, Wyoming: Teton New Media, 2002:679–688.

Prymak C, McKee LJ, Goldschmidt MH, et al. Epidemiologic, clinical, pathologic, and prognostic characteristics of splenic hemangiosarcoma and splenic hematoma in dogs: 217 cases (1985). J Am Vet Med Assoc 1988;193:706–712.

Scavelli TD, Patnaik AK, Melhaff CJ, et al. Hemangiosarcoma in the cat: retrospective evaluation of 31 surgical cases. J Am Vet Med Assoc 1985;187:817–819.

Author Terrance A. Hamilton
Consulting Editor Wallace B. Morrison

HEMATEMESIS

 BASICS

DEFINITION
The vomiting of blood

PATHOPHYSIOLOGY
A disruption in the esophageal, gastric, or upper small intestinal mucosal barrier leading to inflammation and bleeding. Coagulopathies can also present with hematemesis. An animal may vomit blood that originated in the oral cavity or respiratory system (upper or lower) and was swallowed.

SYSTEMS AFFECTED
• Gastrointestinal—inflammation, trauma, ulceration, neoplasia and/or foreign body in the oral cavity, pharyngeal area, esophagus, stomach and/or duodenum • Cardiovascular—acute, severe hemorrhage may result in tachycardia, systolic heart murmur, and/or hypotension • Respiratory—respiratory hemorrhage with ingestion can lead to hematemesis; tachypnea may occur with severe hemorrhage; rarely, aspiration pneumonia may occur with severe vomiting • Hematologic—coagulopathy with gastrointestinal hemorrhage can lead to hematemesis

INCIDENCE/PREVALENCE
True incidence unknown, but probably more common than clinically recognized

GEOGRAPHIC DISTRIBUTION
Pythiosis has a regional distribution—states that border the Gulf of Mexico

SIGNALMENT
Species: Dogs and, less commonly, cats

Breed Predilection: N/A

Mean Age and Range: All ages

Predominant Sex: Male dogs have increased incidence of gastric carcinoma.

SIGNS
Historical Findings
• Vomiting with blood—blood in the vomitus may appear as fresh flecks of blood, blood clots, or digested blood, which looks like coffee grounds. • Melena may be present. • Anorexia • Abdominal pain (may assume the praying position) • If coagulopathy—hematochezia, melena, petechiation, ecchymoses, epistaxis, and/or hematuria • If patient is anemic—pallor, weakness, lethargy, and/or collapse • If respiratory disease—dyspnea, epistaxis, hemoptysis, and/or coughing • If oral, pharyngeal, or esophageal disease—excessive salivation

Physical Examination Findings
• Abdominal pain • Melena • If coagulopathy—hematochezia, melena, petechiation, ecchymoses, epistaxis, and/or retinal hemorrhage • If respiratory disease—dyspnea, epistaxis, hemoptysis, and/or coughing • If patient is anemic—tachycardia, heart murmur, pallor, weakness, and/or collapse • If esophageal disease—dysphagia, painful swallowing, regurgitation, and/or salivation • Edema—from blood/plasma loss

CAUSES
Coagulopathies
• Thrombocytopenia • Thrombocytopathia—von Willebrand's disease, NSAIDs, hyperviscosity syndrome • Disseminated intravascular coagulopathy • Anticoagulant rodenticide toxicity • Coagulation factor deficiency • Liver failure • Polycythemia

Drugs
• NSAIDs, glucocorticoids

Gastrointestinal Diseases
• Inflammatory bowel disease • Oral, esophageal, gastric, or duodenal neoplasia • Oral, esophageal, gastric, or duodenal foreign body • Hemorrhagic gastroenteritis • Ingestion of blood from anal sac infection • Esophagitis • Gastroduodenal ulcers

Heavy Metal Poisoning
• Arsenic, zinc, thallium, or lead poisoning

Infectious Diseases
• Gastrointestinal parasitism • Pythiosis • *Helicobacter* infection • Viral, fungal, or bacterial gastroenteritis

Metabolic Diseases
• Renal failure • Liver failure • Hypoadrenocorticism • Pancreatitis

Neoplasia
• Mastocytosis • Gastrinoma • Oral, nasal, respiratory, or gastrointestinal tumors

Neurologic Diseases
• Head trauma • Spinal cord disease

Respiratory Diseases
• Nasal disease—neoplasia, fungal infection, foreign body • Pulmonary and airway disease—neoplasia, severe pneumonia, fungal infection, foreign body, heartworm disease

Stress/Major Medical Illness
• Septic or hypovolemic shock • Severe illness • Burns • Heat stroke • Major surgery • Trauma • Systemic hypertension • Hypotension

RISK FACTORS
• Administration of ulcerogenic drugs—NSAIDs or glucocorticoids • Critically ill patients • Hypovolemic or septic shock • Thrombocytopenia

 DIAGNOSIS

DIFFERENTIAL DIAGNOSIS
• Hemoptysis—physical examination findings may differentiate hemoptysis from hematemesis; thoracic radiographs may reveal presence of airway or pulmonary disease • Regurgitation or vomiting of swallowed blood from extragastrointestinal diseases (e.g., oropharyngeal, nasopharyngeal, cutaneous, urogenital tract, and anal sac disease)—physical examination findings may differentiate; may need observation of patient for ingestion of blood and thorough examination with or without imaging under sedation or anesthesia • Ingestion and vomiting of foreign materials or foods that look like fresh or digested blood (e.g., oral iron)

CBC/BIOCHEMISTRY/URINALYSIS
• If acute (3–5 days) blood loss—nonregenerative anemia (normocytic, normochromic, minimal reticulocytosis) • If blood loss > 5 days duration—regenerative anemia (macrocytic, hyperchromic, reticulocytosis) • If chronic blood loss—iron deficiency anemia (microcytic, hypochromic, poor reticulocytosis, with or without thrombocytosis) • May have thrombocytopenia • May have panhypoproteinemia with alimentary hemorrhage • May have mature neutrophilia or left shift neutrophilia with sepsis, gastroduodenal ulcer perforation, pancreatitis, neoplasia, and/or inflammatory disease • Blood urea nitrogen (BUN):creatinine ratio may be elevated with gastrointestinal hemorrhage • If renal failure—elevated BUN and creatinine, and hyperphosphatemia and isosthenuria • If liver disease or failure—elevated liver enzymes, hyperbilirubinemia, and/or hypoalbuminemia • If hypoadrenocorticism—hyperkalemia, hyponatremia, and azotemia; atypical hypoadrenocorticism will not have electrolyte abnormalities • Elevated lipase and amylase may be present with pancreatitis

OTHER LABORATORY TESTS
• Fecal occult blood test may be positive (test is accurate if dog is eating dry food). • Fecal flotation—to screen for gastrointestinal parasitism • Coagulation profile—if bleeding disorder suspected • Bile acids—if liver disease suspected • ACTH stimulation—if hypoadrenocorticism suspected • Buffy coat—if systemic mast cell disease suspected • Gastrin levels—if more common causes ruled out

IMAGING
• Abdominal radiography may identify a gastric or duodenal foreign body or mass, pancreatitis, or changes consistent with kidney or liver disease • Contrast radiography (preferably double-contrast gastrogram) may identify a gastroduodenal ulcer or neoplastic disease • Thoracic radiographs may reveal esophageal foreign body or mass, gastroesophageal intussusception and/or pulmonary metastasis • Abdominal ultrasonography may identify a gastric or duodenal mass, gastric or duodenal wall thickening, and/or abdominal lymphadenopathy. • Abdominal ultrasound can also screen for abnormalities in the pancreas, liver, kidneys, and other abdominal organs as source of hematemesis.

DIAGNOSTIC PROCEDURES
• Endoscopy to evaluate esophagus, stomach, and upper small intestinal tract if extragastrointestinal causes are ruled out • Biopsy the lesions for histopathology to determine the nature of the underlying gastrointestinal disease. • If an infectious etiology is suspected, submit biopsies for culture. • If abdominal ultrasonography shows the presence of a gastric or duodenal mass or gastroduodenal wall thickening, an abdominal ultrasound-guided biopsy can also be obtained. Occasionally the ultrasound-guided gastroduodenal biopsy may yield different or additional information compared with that obtained from endoscopic biopsies • Abdominocentesis may identify septic peritonitis and gastroduodenal ulcer perforation. • Urease testing

of gastric biopsy specimens may reveal *Helicobacter* organisms. • Pythiosis—requires biopsies; samples should be submitted unrefrigerated in saline for culture and in formalin for histopathology with special stains; serologic testing and PCR-based assay are available
• Obtain fine needle aspirates or biopsy specimens of cutaneous or intraabdominal masses to identify mast cell tumor.

PATHOLOGIC FINDINGS
• Gastroduodenal inflammation and hemorrhage • Ulcers may have more necrosis, microthrombi, and hemorrhage, and have deeper penetration than do erosions • May identify *Helicobacter* sp. in gastric biopsies • May need special stains to identify presence of pythiosis

TREATMENT

APPROPRIATE HEALTH CARE
• Treat any underlying causes. • Treat on an outpatient basis if the cause is identified and removed, vomiting is not excessive, and gastroduodenal bleeding is minimal.
• Inpatients—those with severe hemorrhage and/or ulcer perforation, excessive vomiting, and/or undetermined cause • May need emergency management of hemorrhage or septic peritonitis

NURSING CARE
• Intravenous fluids to maintain hydration
• May need aggressive intravenous fluid treatment for shock—crystalloids and/or colloids
• Severe hypoproteinemic patients may require colloids and/or plasma to increase vascular oncotic pressure. • May need transfusions (whole blood or packed red blood cells) or oxygen-carrying hemoglobin solution infusions in patients with severe gastroduodenal hemorrhage
• Patients with underlying coagulopathies may need whole blood, fresh plasma, or fresh frozen plasma to replace clotting factors. • In severe cases of hematemesis—to stop the gastrointestinal bleeding, ice water lavage (10–20 ml/kg remaining in stomach for 15–30 minutes) or lavage with norepinephrine (8 mg/500 mL) diluted in ice water can be attempted.

ACTIVITY
Restricted

DIET
• Discontinue oral intake if vomiting • When feeding is resumed, feed small amounts in multiple feedings. • Recommended diet depends on the underlying disease.

CLIENT EDUCATION
• NSAIDs should be administered to pets only under the guidance of a veterinarian.
• Administration of NSAIDs can result in gastroduodenal ulcerations and perforations.
• Adverse effects of NSAIDs can be reduced by giving drug with food and concurrent administration of a synthetic prostaglandin analogue (e.g., misoprostol).

SURGICAL CONSIDERATIONS
Surgical treatment is indicated if medical treatment fails after 5–7 days, hemorrhage is uncontrolled and severe, gastroduodenal ulcer perforates, and/or potentially resectable tumor is identified.

MEDICATIONS

DRUG(S) OF CHOICE
• Histamine (H_2) receptor antagonists competitively inhibit gastric acid secretion and are the initial drug of choice (cimetidine 5–10 mg/kg PO, SC, IV q8h; ranitidine 1–4 mg/kg SC, PO, IV q8–12h; famotidine 0.5 mg/kg PO, IV q12–24h). Treat for at least 6–8 weeks.
• Antacids neutralize gastric acid but must be given at least six times per day to be effective.
• Sucralfate suspension (0.5–1 g PO q8h) protects ulcerated tissue (cytoprotection) by binding to ulcer sites.
• Antibiotic(s) with activity against enteric gram-negative and anaerobes parenterally if a break in gastrointestinal mucosal barrier is suspected or aspiration pneumonia is present
• Antiemetics (chlorpromazine 0.5–4 mg/kg q6–8h SC, IM, IV; prochlorperazine 0.1–0.5 mg/kg q6–8h SC, IM, IV, PO) are administered if vomiting occurs frequently or results in significant fluid losses.
• Omeprazole (0.7 mg/kg PO q24h)—most potent inhibitor of gastric acid secretion; treatment of choice for gastrinomas with evidence of metastasis or nonresectable disease
• Appropriate therapy (metronidazole, colloidal bismuth, tetracycline, or amoxicillin) if *Helicobacter* sp. infection
• See Gastritis, Acute; Gastritis, Chronic; and/or Gastroduodenal Ulcer Disease for specific drug therapy.

CONTRAINDICATIONS
• Do not administer phenothiazine derivatives to hypovolemic patients or those at risk for hypotension. • Avoid drugs that might damage the gastroduodenal mucosal barrier (e.g., NSAIDs and corticosteroids).

POSSIBLE INTERACTIONS
• Cimetidine binds to hepatic cytochrome P-450 enzyme and may interfere with metabolism of other drugs. • H_2 blockers prevent uptake of omeprazole by oxyntic cells. • Sucralfate may alter absorption of other drugs.

ALTERNATIVE DRUG(S)
Misoprostol, synthetic prostaglandin analogue (2–5 µg/kg PO q8–12h) prevents or decreases severity of NSAID-induced ulcers.

FOLLOW-UP

PATIENT MONITORING
• Improvement in some cases may be assessed on resolution of clinical signs; can use the packed cell volume, total protein, fecal occult

blood, and BUN to detect continued blood loss. • Depending on the underlying cause of the hematemesis, specific laboratory or imaging tests may be necessary to monitor response to therapy.

POSSIBLE COMPLICATIONS
• Severe blood loss requiring transfusion
• Sepsis • Ulcer perforation • Death—secondary to ulcer perforation, sepsis, hemorrhage
• Aspiration pneumonia—rare

EXPECTED COURSE AND PROGNOSIS
• Varies with underlying causes • Patients with malignant gastric neoplasia, renal failure, liver failure, pythiosis, systemic mastocytosis, sepsis, and/or gastric perforation—prognosis poor
• Gastroduodenal ulcers secondary to NSAID administration, *Helicobacter* infection, inflammatory bowel disease, or hypoadrenocorticism—prognosis may be good to excellent, depending on severity of disease

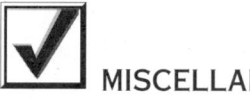

MISCELLANEOUS

ASSOCIATED CONDITIONS
Anemia

AGE-RELATED FACTORS
Neoplasia more common in older animals

ZOONOTIC POTENTIAL
Zoonotic potential of *Helicobacter* spp. is controversial.

PREGNANCY
Synthetic prostaglandins (e.g., misoprostol) cause abortion.

SYNONYMS N/A

SEE ALSO
• Gastroduodenal Ulcer Disease • Helicobacter
• Inflammatory Bowel Disease • Melena
• Pancreatitis • Pythiosis

ABBREVIATIONS
• ACTH = adrenocorticotropic hormone
• DIC = disseminated intravascular coagulation • NSAIDs = nonsteroidal antiinflammatory drugs • PCR = polymerase chain reaction

Suggested Reading
Davenport D. Hematemesis: diagnosis and treatment. In: Kirk RW, Bonagura J, eds. Current veterinary therapy XI. Philadelphia: Saunders, 1992:132–137.
Washabau R. Acute gastrointestinal hemorrhage. Part I. Compend Contin Educ Pract Vet 1996;18:1317–1325.
Washabau R. Acute gastrointestinal hemorrhage. Part II. Compend Contin Educ Pract Vet 1996;18:1327–1337.
Author Jocelyn Mott
Consulting Editor Albert E. Jergens

HEMATURIA

 BASICS

DEFINITION
The presence of blood in the urine

Pathophysiology
Secondary to loss of endothelial integrity in urinary tract, clotting factor deficiency, or thrombocytopenia

Systems Affected
- Renal/Urologic
- Reproductive

SIGNALMENT
- Dogs and cats
- Familial hematuria in young animals, neoplasia in older animals
- Females at greater risk for UTI

SIGNS

Historical Findings
Red-tinged urine with or without pollakiuria

Physical Examination Findings
- Palpable mass in patients with neoplasia
- Abdominal pain in some patients
- Painful prostate gland in males
- Petechiae or ecchymoses in patients with coagulopathy

CAUSES

Systemic
- Coagulopathy
- Thrombocytopenia
- Vasculitis

Upper Urinary Tract
- Anatomic—e.g., cystic kidney disease and familial
- Metabolic—e.g., nephrolithiasis
- Neoplastic—e.g., renal lymphoma, adenocarcinoma, and hemangiosarcoma
- Infectious—e.g., leptospirosis, feline infectious peritonitis (FIP), and bacteria
- Inflammatory—e.g., glomerulonephritis
- Idiopathic
- Trauma

Lower Urinary Tract
- Anatomic—e.g., bladder malformations
- Metabolic—e.g., uroliths
- Neoplasia—e.g., transitional cell carcinoma and lymphosarcoma
- Infectious—e.g., bacterial, fungal, and viral disease
- Idiopathic—cats
- Trauma
- Cyclophosphamide-induced hemorrhagic cystitis

Genitalia
- Metabolic—e.g., estrus
- Neoplastic—e.g., transmissible venereal tumor, leiomyoma, and prostatic adenocarcinoma
- Infectious—e.g., bacterial and fungal disease

- Inflammatory—e.g., benign prostatic hyperplasia
- Trauma

RISK FACTORS
Breed predisposed to urolithiasis and coagulopathy

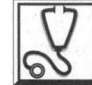 DIAGNOSIS

DIFFERENTIAL DIAGNOSIS
- Other causes of discolored urine (e.g., myoglobinuria, hemoglobinuria, and bilirubinuria)

LABORATORY FINDINGS

Drugs That May Alter Laboratory Results
Substantial doses of vitamin C (ascorbic aid) may cause false-negative reagent test strip results; newer generations of reagent strips are more resistant to interference by reducing substances such as ascorbic acid.

Disorders That May Alter Laboratory Results
- Common urine reagent strip tests for blood are designed to detect red blood cells, hemoglobin, or myoglobin.
- Low specific urine gravity (polyuric syndromes) lyses RBCs.
- Bacteriuria (bacterial peroxidase) causes false-positive reagent test strip results.
- Formalin preservative causes false-negative reagent test strip results.

Valid if Run in a Human Laboratory?
Yes

CBC/BIOCHEMISTRY/URINALYSIS
- Thrombocytopenia and severe anemia in some patients
- Azotemia in some patients with bilateral renal disease
- RBCs and possibly infectious agents may be seen in urine sediment.
- Crystalluria in some patients with urolithiasis

OTHER LABORATORY TESTS
- Activated clotting time (ACT) or clotting profile to rule out coagulopathy
- Bacterial culture of urine to identify urinary tract infection
- Examination of an ejaculate to identify prostatic disease

IMAGING
Ultrasonography, radiography, and possibly contrast radiography may be useful in obtaining a diagnosis.

DIAGNOSTIC PROCEDURES
- Biopsy of mass lesion
- Vaginoscopy in females or cystoscopy

 TREATMENT

- Hematuria may indicate a serious disease process.

- Urolithiasis and renal failure may require diet modification.
- Urinary tract infection may be caused by another disease, local (e.g., neoplasia and urolithiasis) or systemic (e.g., hyperadrenocorticism and diabetes mellitus), that also requires treatment.

 MEDICATIONS

DRUG(S) OF CHOICE
- Blood transfusion may be necessary if patient is severely anemic.
- Crystalloids to treat dehydration
- Antibiotics to treat urinary tract infection and septicemia
- Heparin for disseminated intravascular coagulation (DIC)

CONTRAINDICATIONS
Immunosuppressive drugs, except to treat immune-mediated disease

PRECAUTIONS
N/A

POSSIBLE INTERACTIONS
Intravenous contrast media can cause acute renal failure.

ALTERNATIVE DRUG(S)
N/A

 FOLLOW-UP

PATIENT MONITORING
Depends on primary or associated diseases

POSSIBLE COMPLICATIONS
- Anemia
- Hypovolemia if severe hemorrhage
- Ureteral or urethral obstruction due to blood clots

 MISCELLANEOUS

ASSOCIATED CONDITIONS
N/A

AGE-RELATED FACTORS
- Neoplasia tends to occur in older animals.
- Immune-mediated diseases tend to occur in young adult animals.

ZOONOTIC POTENTIAL
Leptospirosis

PREGNANCY
N/A

SEE ALSO
- Coagulation Factor Deficiency
- Crystalluria
- Cylindruria
- Dysuria and Pollakiuria
- Feline Idiopathic Lower Urinary Tract Disease

- Glomerulonephritis
- Hemoglobinuria and Myoglobinuria
- Lower Urinary Tract Infection
- Nephrolithiasis
- Prostatitis and Prostatic Abscess
- Prostatomegaly
- Proteinuria
- Pyelonephritis
- Thrombocytopenia
- Urolithiasis

ABBREVIATIONS
- ACT = activated clotting time
- FIP = feline infectious peritonitis
- IVP = intravenous pyelography
- TVT = transmissible venereal tumor
- UTI = urinary tract infection

Suggested Reading

Bartges JW. Discolored urine. In: Ettinger SJ, Feldman EC, ed. Textbook of veterinary internal medicine. 5th ed. Philadelphia: Saunders, 2000:96–99.

Lage AL. Diagnostic approach to canine and feline hematuria. In: Kirk RW, ed. Current veterinary therapy X. Philadelphia: Saunders, 1989:1117–1123.

Author Joseph W. Bartges
Consulting Editors Larry G. Adams and Carl A. Osborne

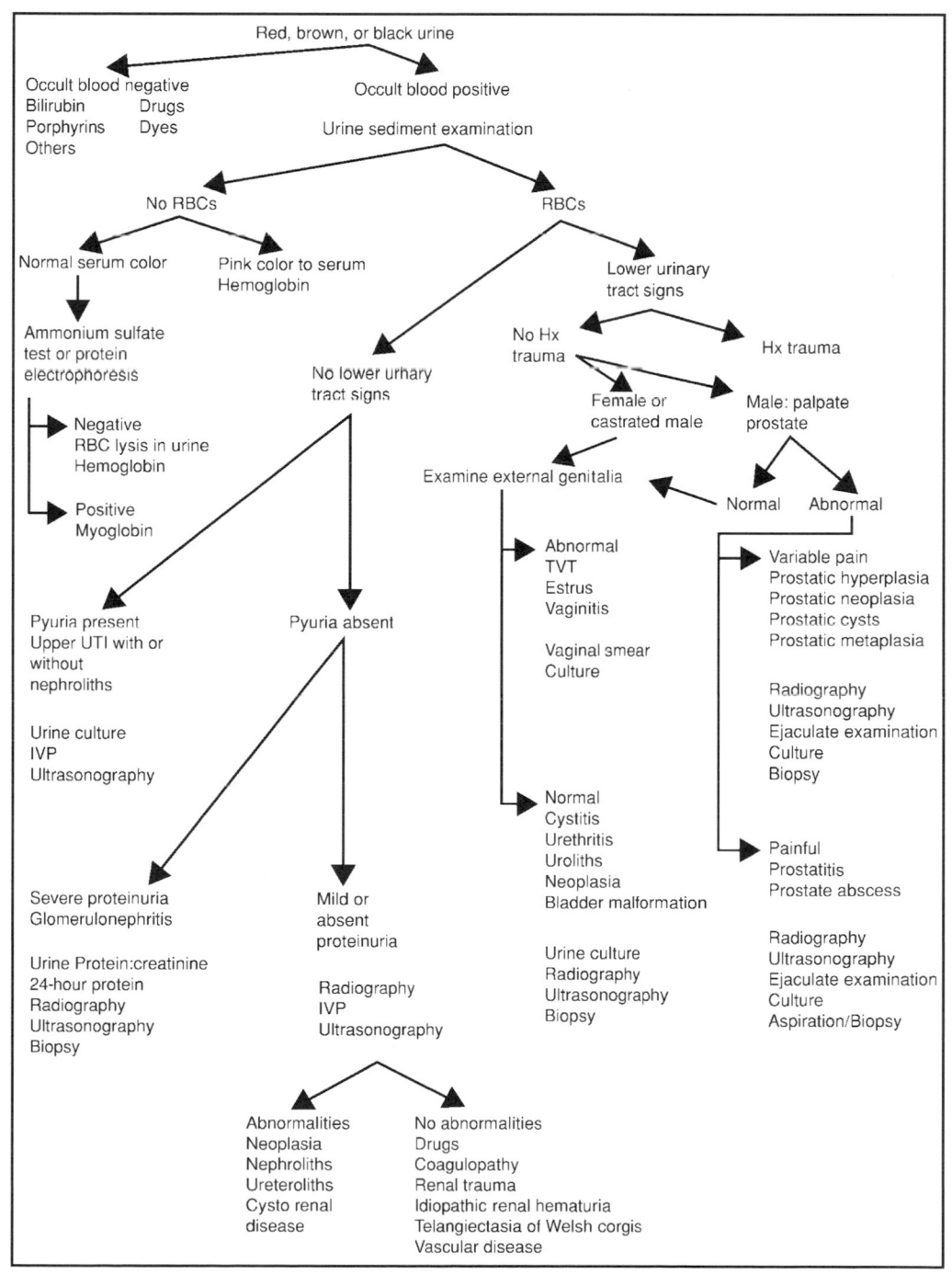

Figure 1.

Algorithm for the diagnosis of red, brown, or black urine.

HEMOGLOBINURIA AND MYOGLOBINURIA

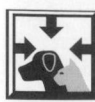

BASICS

DEFINITION
Loss of sufficient hemoglobin or myoglobin through the glomeruli to cause a positive reaction to a test for blood in the urine when tested by the pseudophosphatase-orthotoluidine method

PATHOPHYSIOLOGY
• Intravascular hemolysis causes release of free hemoglobin into plasma. Hemoglobin forms a complex with haptoglobin. Once haptoglobin is saturated, free hemoglobin appears in the blood, divides into subunits, and is cleared from the blood by the kidneys. Some unbound plasma hemoglobin releases ferriheme, which binds reversibly to either albumin (methemalbumin) or a plasma protein called hemopexin. Free hemoglobin, hemoglobin–haptoglobin complex, hemoglobin subunits, methemalbumin, ferriheme–hemopexin complex, and bilirubin all contribute to the color of plasma. Hemoglobin complexes in concentrations over about 50 mg/dL of plasma are detectable as pink plasma.
• Myoglobin released from damaged muscle is not associated with pink plasma because it does not bind to serum proteins and so is rapidly cleared by the liver and kidneys.
• Both hemoglobin and myoglobin are reabsorbed and metabolized by proximal renal tubule cells; these proteins appear in urine only after the renal tubular uptake mechanism is saturated.

SYSTEMS AFFECTED
• Renal/Urologic—hemoglobin and myoglobin can be nephrotoxic, particularly when renal perfusion is compromised.
• Hemic/Lymph/Immune—intravascular hemolysis, extensive muscle damage, and hypoxia can precipitate disseminated intravascular coagulopathy (DIC).
• Low oxygen-carrying capacity (acute) can lead to secondary central lobular liver cell damage, lactic acid acidosis, and shock, which in turn exacerbates hypoxia.

SIGNALMENT
• Copper-associated liver disease in the Bedlington and West Highland white terriers
• Exertional lactic acidosis in the Old English sheepdog—hemoglobinuria

• Exertional myopathy in the racing greyhound; hematuria should clear within 6–12 hours; if it doesn't, suspect myoglobinuria from muscle damage.
• Neonatal isoerythrolysis (blood type B queen with type A or AB kitten) in the British shorthair, Cornish rex, Devon rex, Abyssinian, Birman, Himalayan, Persian, Scottish fold, and Somali breeds; neonates die within 2 days of birth.
• Phosphofructokinase deficiency in the male English springer spaniel
• Pyruvate kinase deficiency in the basenji and beagle; affected dogs <3 years old
• Red cell osmotic fragility syndrome in Somoli and Abyssinian cats

SIGNS

General Comments
A wide variety of clinical signs are associated with specific causes; see Causes.

Historical Findings
Breed and drug treatment history are particularly important. See Signalment.

Physical Examination Findings
• Signs associated with anemia, such as tachycardia, lethargy, pale mucous membranes, fever, and icterus, are not seen in patients with muscle damage or hematuria.
• Fever may be associated with intravascular hemolysis.
• DIC secondary to intravascular hemolysis or muscle trauma may induce hematuria.
• Patients with muscle damage have muscle tenderness or bruising.

CAUSES

Hemoglobinuria
• Genetic associated—pyruvate kinase deficiency, phosphofructokinase deficiency, exertional lactic acidosis in the Old English sheepdog; copper-associated liver disease, malignant hyperthermia, red cell osmotic fragility syndrome in Somoli and Abyssinian cats
• Toxins and drugs—chlorates, benzocaine, copper, DMSO, menadione (vitamin K_3), mercury, methylene blue, nitrates, methionine, phenazopyridine, paracetamol (acetaminophen), phenylhydrazine, propylene glycol, propylthiouracil, snake venom (Elapidae), zinc
• Plants—onions
• Physical agents—burns (severe), crush injury, electric shock, extreme exercise, heat stroke,

hypoosmotic solution, microangiopathy (e.g., caval syndrome and DIC)
• Infectious agents—babesiasis (i.e., B. canis but usually not B. gibsoni or B. vogeli), Mycoplasma felis (formerly feline hemobartonellosis; rarely causes intravascular hemolysis), leptospirosis (i.e., L. icterohemorrhagica), Cytauxzoon felis—cause hemolytic uremic syndrome.
• Immune-mediated—idiopathic immune-mediated hemolytic anemia, incompatible blood transfusion, isoerythrolysis in blood type B queen with type A or AB kittens, systemic lupus erythematosus
• Deficiencies—hypophosphatemia (induced by hyperalimentation or diabetes mellitus)

Myoglobinuria
• Acute myositis (e.g., toxoplasmosis)
• Compartment syndrome
• Crush injury
• Extreme exercise
• Tourniquet syndrome
• Prolonged seizures

RISK FACTORS
• Genetic predisposition (see Signalment)
• Exposure to selected drugs and toxins (e.g., zinc cage bolts and copper and zinc coins)
• Extreme physical exertion

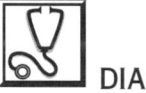

DIAGNOSIS

DIFFERENTIAL DIAGNOSIS
• Common urine reagent strip tests for blood are designed to detect RBCs, hemoglobin, or myoglobin that is not visible to the human eye.
• RBCs or ghost cells in the sediment suggest hematuria.
• Clear plasma suggests myoglobinuria or hematuria.
• Pink plasma with urine positive for occult blood suggests intravascular hemolysis.
• Chocolate-colored whole blood and urine positive for occult blood suggest hemolyzing, methemoglobin-producing toxins (oxidants).
• Hemoglobinuria without icterus suggests acute hemolytic anemia; both findings suggest chronic hemolytic anemia.
• Icterus without hemoglobinuria suggests extravascular hemolysis or liver disease.
• False-positive results (see below, under Laboratory Findings)

HEMOGLOBINURIA AND MYOGLOBINURIA

LABORATORY FINDINGS

Drugs That May Alter Laboratory Results
• Administration of substantial doses of vitamin C (ascorbic aid) may cause false-negative results with reagent test strips; newer generations of reagent strips are more resistant to interference by reducing substances such as ascorbic acid.
• Resuscitation fluids containing polymerized hemoglobin may give false-positive results.

Disorders That May Alter Laboratory Results
• Low urinary specific gravity (polyuric syndromes) lyses RBCs.
• Bacteriuria (bacterial peroxidase) causes false-positive test results.
• Formalin preservative causes false-negative results.
• Urine contaminated with residues of oxidizing agents in disinfectants used to clean table tops may cause false-positive reactions.
• Free hemoglobin in transfused blood

Valid If Run in Human Laboratory?
Yes

CBC/BIOCHEMISTRY/URINALYSIS
• Intravascular hemolysis
• Low and falling PCV, often accompanied by leukocytosis
• Blood smear evaluation—possibly spherocytes, parasites, and Heinz bodies
• Bilirubinemia and high alanine ALT activity
• Bilirubinuria
• Rhabdomyolysis
• High creatine kinase activity
• High aspartate transaminase (AST) activity

OTHER LABORATORY TESTS
• Ammonium sulfate precipitation test—mix 5 mL of urine well with 2.8 mg of ammonium sulfate and centrifuge. Hemoglobin precipitates, myoglobin does not. If the supernatant remains dark after centrifugation, suspect myoglobinuria.
• New methylene blue–stained blood film to detect Heinz bodies
• Methemoglobin in RBCs helps identify toxin as an oxidant.
• Haptoglobin concentration is low if the patient has acute or chronic progressive intravascular hemolysis.
• Serum copper and zinc concentrations

IMAGING
• Abdominal radiography or ultrasonography may reveal coins or cage bolts or nuts in the gastrointestinal tract.
• Abnormal liver size and conformation in patients with copper-associated liver disease

DIAGNOSTIC PROCEDURES
• Forced exercise (Old English sheepdog)
• Liver biopsy for copper concentration (copper-associated liver disease)
• Bone marrow biopsy (pyruvate kinase and phosphofructokinase deficiencies)

TREATMENT
• Copious amounts of fluids to maintain renal function, especially in the face of shock; lactated Ringer's solution or isotonic saline if the patient is dehydrated; maintenance fluids if not
• Exercise-induced hematuria has a benign, self-limiting course.
• Avoid stress and excitement if the patient has anemia or copper-associated liver disease.
• Avoid hyperventilation if the patient has phosphofructokinase deficiency.
• See suspected causes for specific treatment.

MEDICATIONS

DRUG(S) OF CHOICE
Vary with underlying cause

CONTRAINDICATIONS
See list of causes for contraindicated drugs.

PRECAUTIONS
N/A

POSSIBLE INTERACTIONS
N/A

ALTERNATIVE DRUG(S)
N/A

FOLLOW-UP

PATIENT MONITORING
PCV, pO₂, urinalysis, serum creatinine, and ALT (copper-associated liver disease)

POSSIBLE COMPLICATIONS
Renal damage (failure) can develop, especially in association with shock.

MISCELLANEOUS

ASSOCIATED CONDITIONS
N/A

AGE-RELATED FACTORS
Neonatal isoerythrolysis

ZOONOTIC POTENTIAL
• Leptospirosis
• Toxoplasmosis

PREGNANCY
N/A

SYNONYMS
• Hemosiderinuria
• Pigmenturia

SEE ALSO
See Causes.

ABBREVIATIONS
• ALT = alanine aminotransferase
• AST = aspartate aminotransferase
• DIC = disseminated intravascular coagulopathy
• DMSO = dimethyl sulfoxide
• PCV = packed cell volume

Suggested Reading
Ettinger S, ed. Textbook of veterinary internal medicine: diseases of the dog and cat. 4th ed. Philadelphia: Saunders, 1995.
Jain NC, ed. Schalm's veterinary hematology. 4th ed. Philadelphia: Lea & Febiger, 1986.
Kaneko JJ, ed. Clinical biochemistry of domestic animals. 4th ed. San Diego: Academic Press, 1989.
Osborne CA, Stevens JB: Urinalysis: a clinical guide to compassionate patient care. Shawnee Mission, KS: Bayer, 1999.
Sherding RG, ed. The cat: diseases and clinical management. 2nd ed. New York: Churchill Livingstone, 1994.

Authors Carl A Osborne, Sheri J. Ross, and Jerry B. Stevens
Consulting Editors Carl A. Osborne and Larry G. Adams

HEMOTHORAX

 BASICS

OVERVIEW
• Collection of blood in the pleural space
• May range from peracute to chronic
• Cardiovascular and respiratory systems commonly affected

SIGNALMENT
Any age, breed, or sex of dogs and cats

SIGNS
• Peracute to acute onset—hypovolemic signs usually occur before sufficient blood volume accumulates in the pleural space to impair respiration.
• Respiratory distress
• Pale membranes
• Weakness and collapse
• Weak, rapid pulse
• Ventral thoracic dullness; dorsal hyperresonance if concurrent pneumothorax
• Associated with causative factor—trauma or coagulopathy

CAUSES & RISK FACTORS
• Trauma—bleeding from any artery or vein of the thoracic wall, mediastinum, or thoracic spine; damaged heart, lungs, thymus, and diaphragm; herniated abdominal viscera (liver or spleen)
• Neoplasia—involving any structure adjacent to the pleural cavity
• Coagulopathies—congenital or acquired; rodenticide ingestion common; liver failure; cholangiohepatitis with concurrent small bowel disease
• Lung lobe torsion
• Acute thymic hemorrhage in young animals

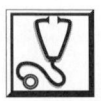 **DIAGNOSIS**

DIFFERENTIAL DIAGNOSIS
• Pulmonary contusion
• Pneumothorax
• Diaphragmatic hernia
• Flail chest
• Nonhemorrhagic pleural effusions—chylothorax; pyothorax; modified transudates; transudates

CBC/BIOCHEMISTRY/URINALYSIS
• PCV and hemoglobin—reflect blood loss after initial fluid compartment shifts have occurred
• Chemistry panel may reveal low glucose, low albumin, low BUN, and low cholesterol in animals with liver failure.

OTHER LABORATORY TESTS
Fluid Analysis
• Hemorrhage-produced effusion—PCV and protein content similar to that of the peripheral blood; platelets commonly seen on cytology
• Inflammation- or vascular congestion–produced effusion—PCV < 8%
• Cytologic examination—often fails to identify malignant causes

Coagulation Tests
• ACT and blood smear evaluation—may provide rapid diagnostic information
• PIVKA—especially useful in cats
• PT, APTT, and platelet count—may be mildly to moderately abnormal with DIC
• Specific tests—may diagnose congenital defect or acquired coagulopathy
• D-dimer to detect DIC
• Mucosal bleeding time

IMAGING
• Radiology—reveals pleural effusion varying from a diffuse increase in radiopacity to ventral leafing, interlobar fissures, and localized pleural densities; may see associated lesions (e.g., rib fractures, pneumothorax, pulmonary contusions, diaphragmatic lesions, and masses)
• Ultrasound—confirm pleural effusion; look for masses, lung lobe torsion, and herniation of liver, gallbladder, spleen, or bowel

DIAGNOSTIC PROCEDURES
• Thoracentesis
• Surgical exploration—may be necessary to establish a diagnosis; if imaging does not suggest the appropriate side to enter, the left side is recommended.

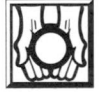 **TREATMENT**

• Acute—fluids to treat hypovolemia
• Coexisting pneumothorax—generally requires needle thoracentesis or tube thoracostomy
• Pulmonary contusion—may require ventilator support
• Drain large volumes of hemorrhaged blood to relieve dyspnea; may leave small volumes of blood unassociated with contamination or extensive tissue devitalization
• Severe or recurrent thoracic hemorrhage—may require surgical exploration in conjunction with appropriate medications
• Oxygen therapy
• Maintenance of body heat
• Plasma or blood transfusion—may be needed to restore clotting factors or provide RBC for oxygen transport

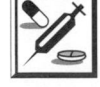 **MEDICATIONS**

DRUG(S)
• Hypovolemia—see Shock, Hemorrhagic.
• Vitamin K or specific factor replacement—if indicated
• Analgesics—systemically or as nerve blocks
• Broad-spectrum antibiotics—when indicated

CONTRAINDICATIONS/POSSIBLE INTERACTIONS
Avoid aspirin and other NSAIDs.

 FOLLOW-UP

PATIENT MONITORING
• Clinical signs
• Temperature
• Urine production
• Relief from pain
• Follow-up radiographs at 48-hour intervals

POSSIBLE COMPLICATIONS
• Pyothorax
• Sepsis
• Entrapment and constriction of lungs by scar tissue and fibrosis

 MISCELLANEOUS

ASSOCIATED CONDITIONS
• Peritonitis—with penetrating wounds (e.g., gunshot) into the abdomen
• Esophageal perforation

SEE ALSO
• Anticoagulant Rodenticide Toxicity
• Disseminated Intravascular Coagulation
• Lung Lobe Torsion
• Pleural Effusion
• Pulmonary Contusions

ABBREVIATIONS
• ACT = activated clotting time
• APTT = activated partial thromboplastin time
• BUN = blood urea nitrogen
• DIC = disseminated intravascular coagulation
• PCV = packed cell volume
• PIVKA = proteins invoked by vitamin K absence
• PT = prothrombin time

Suggested Reading
Center SA, Warner K, Corbett J, et al. Proteins invoked by vitamin K absence and clotting times in clinically ill cats. J Vet Intern Med 2000;14:292–297.
Glaus TM, Rawlings CA, Mahaffey EA, Mahaffey MB. Acute thymic hemorrhage and hemothorax in a dog. J Am Anim Hosp Assoc 1993;29:481–491.

Author Bradley L. Moses
Consulting Editor Lynelle R. Johnson

BASICS

OVERVIEW
• Amyloidosis—disorders that share the common feature of pathologic deposition of an extracellular insoluble fibrillar proteinaceous matrix • Amyloid—accumulates secondary to inflammatory or lymphoproliferative disorders or as a familial tendency • Dogs and cats—usually reactive or secondary amyloidosis; underlying primary inflammatory disorder common • Associated familial disorders—certain kindreds of dogs and cats • Multiple organs commonly involved; clinical signs usually due to renal or liver involvement • Liver involvement—may be insidious; may lead to high liver enzymes, severe hepatomegaly, coagulopathy, liver rupture leading to hemoabdomen, and/or liver failure

SIGNALMENT
• Dogs—certain Chinese shar-pei dogs with cyclic fevers (shar-pei fever syndrome), Akitas with cyclic fever and polyarthropathy, and collies with "gray collie syndrome" are predisposed; usually develop renal signs, although some develop signs of liver failure • Cats—Oriental shorthair and Siamese cats predisposed; also reported in Devon rex and domestic shorthair cats; usually < 5 years of age (hepatic signs predominant); familial disorder in Abyssinian cats (renal signs)

SIGNS
Historical Findings
• Episodic fever and swollen hocks—shar-pei • Episodic polyarthropathy, pain, and signs of meningitis—Akitas • Acute lethargy • Anorexia • Polyuria and polydipsia • Vomiting

Physical Examination Findings
• Pallor • Abdominal effusion—hemorrhage or ascites • Jaundice • Hepatomegaly • Edema • Joint pain • Nonlocalized pain, meningeal pain, and abdominal discomfort

CAUSES & RISK FACTORS
• Familial immunoregulatory disorders—kindreds of predisposed dogs and cats • Chronic infection—coccidioidomycosis; blastomycosis; tick-borne diseases • Cyclic neutropenia—gray collie syndrome • Bacterial endocarditis • Chronic inflammation (e.g., SLE) • Neoplasia

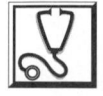

DIAGNOSIS

DIFFERENTIAL DIAGNOSIS
• Chronic hepatic inflammation • Hepatic neoplasia • Primary coagulopathy • Rodenticide-associated coagulopathy • Glomerulonephritis • Pyelonephritis • SLE • Abdominal trauma • Peritonitis • Meningitis

CBC/BIOCHEMISTRY/URINALYSIS
• Anemia secondary to hepatic hemorrhage or rupture or chronic inflammation • Leukocytosis with a left shift during febrile episodes in shar-peis and Akitas • Normal to high liver enzymes, total bilirubin, and serum bile acids • Azotemia • Proteinuria • Dilute urine—with renal involvement or failure

OTHER LABORATORY TESTS
• Coagulation tests—normal to prolonged • Synovial fluid—with joint swelling or pain, shows suppurative, nonseptic inflammation • CSF—with meningeal pain, shows increased protein and neutrophilic inflammation

IMAGING
• Abdominal radiography—hepatomegaly; renomegaly to normal kidney size; effusion • Abdominal ultrasonography—hepato-megaly; hypoechoic parenchyma with diffuse amyloid; enlarged or normal kidney with normal or equivocally hypoechoic parenchyma; occasional mesenteric lymphadenopathy; thickened gut wall due to amyloid deposition; abdominal effusion

DIAGNOSTIC PROCEDURES
• Fine-needle aspiration cytology—may suggest the presence of hepatic amyloid (rare) • Liver or kidney biopsy • Abdominocentesis—may reveal hemorrhagic effusion or transudate

PATHOLOGIC FINDINGS
Gross
Liver—normal color to pale; large, firm to friable; hemorrhages (subcapsular hematomas, capsular tears) or overt parenchymal fractures

Microscopic
• Liver—acellular amorphous material diffusely deposited in the space of Disse, associated with hepatic cord atrophy; may note primarily involved blood vessels in the portal triad (often observed in Abyssinian cats) • Cats may show amyloid deposition in most organs • Amyloid stained with Congo red and viewed with polarized light appears birefringent and apple green

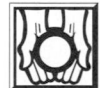

TREATMENT
• Dictated by the severity of clinical signs • No curative treatment; manage underlying disease when identified • Fluids—for dehydration • Blood transfusion—for acute blood loss; notably involved in care for cats with amyloid • Diet—individually tailored to patient's organ function • Liver failure—consider measures appropriate for hepatic encephalopathy • Pathologic proteinuria—see Nephrotic Syndrome • Warn client that this syndrome is difficult to treat and has a guarded to poor prognosis. • Surgical

considerations—hepatic lobe resection as an emergency measure for catastrophic bleeding from a fractured liver lobe in feline patients

MEDICATIONS

DRUG(S)
• Colchicine—dogs: 0.03 mg/kg PO q24h; may block formation of amyloid in early disease; recent experimental work suggests mechanism may involve modified expression of cell membrane receptor(s) involved with signaling inflammatory response and amyloid production; side effects include vomiting, diarrhea (bloody), and bone marrow suppression (rare); use colchicine without added probenecid • DMSO—use medical grade only; dogs: 80 mg/kg as an 18% solution in sterile water given SC three times a week; may promote dissolution of amyloid fibrils or provide a unique antiinflammatory or antiamyloid effect; side effects include garlic smell and objectionable taste

POSSIBLE INTERACTIONS
Colchicine combined with probenecid may cause vomiting; probenecid prolongs residence time of drug.

FOLLOW-UP
• Shar-peis—may survive > 2 years; most will have episodes of fever and cholestasis; some have resolved clinical signs and diminished hepatic amyloid on colchicine therapy • Akitas with cyclic clinical signs—grave prognosis • Cats that survive liver hemorrhage eventually succumb to renal failure

MISCELLANEOUS

SEE ALSO
Amyloidosis

ABBREVIATIONS
• CSF = cerebrospinal fluid • DMSO = dimethylsulfoxide • SLE = systemic lupus erythematosus

Suggested Reading
Beatty JA, Barrs VR, Martin PA. Spontaneous hepatic rupture in six cats with systemic amyloidosis. J Small Anim Pract 2002; 43:355–363.
Loevan KO. Hepatic amyloidosis in two Chinese Shar Pei dogs. J Am Vet Med Assoc 1994;204:1212–1216.
Author Susan E. Johnson
Consulting Editor Sharon A. Center

HEPATIC ENCEPHALOPATHY

 **BASIC**

DEFINITION
Metabolic disorder affecting the CNS, developing secondary to hepatic disease

PATHOPHYSIOLOGY
• Complex pathophysiologic state with a multifactorial origin • Gut-derived substances of bacterial and protein metabolism—important in the pathogenesis • Current theories concerning pathogenesis—ammonia as the putative neurotoxin with or without other synergistic toxins; alteration in the monoamine or catecholamine neurotransmitters as a result of perturbed aromatic amino acid metabolism; alteration in amino acid neurotransmitters, GABA, and/or glutamate; increase in cerebral levels of endogenous benzodiazepine-like substances; neuroglycopenia; altered blood–brain barrier

SYSTEMS AFFECTED
• Nervous—generally a decrease in neuronal function; seizures, particularly in cats • GI—presumably as a result of liver dysfunction, vomiting, diarrhea, and anorexia • Renal/urologic—ammonium biurate crystalluria; renal pelvic and cystic calculi

GENETICS
Congenital PSVA—inherited in some breeds

INCIDENCE/PREVALENCE
Uncommon in small animal practice

SIGNALMENT
Species Dogs and cats

Breed Predilections
PSVA—usually in purebred dogs; apparent increased occurrence in some breeds in different geographic locations (e.g., Yorkshire terriers [USA], Australian cattle dogs [Australia], Maltese terriers [USA, Australia], and Irish wolfhounds [Europe]

Mean Age and Range
• PSVA—usually young animals • Acquired liver disease resulting in APSS—any age

Predominant Sex None

SIGNS
General Comments
• Neurologic—may relate to meal ingestion • Dramatic temporary resolution may occur with antibiotic or lactulose therapy. • Prolonged recovery from sedation or anesthesia

Historical Findings
• Episodic abnormalities • Lethargy • Anorexia • Vomiting • Disorientation—aimless wandering; compulsive pacing; head pressing • Polyuria and polydipsia • Amaurotic blindness • Seizures • Coma • More frequent in cats than in dogs—ptyalism; seizures; aggression; disorientation; ataxic stupor • More frequent

in dogs than in cats—compulsive behavior (head pressing, circling, aimless wandering); vomiting; diarrhea; polyuria and polydipsia; hematuria, pollakiuria, and dysuria associated with ammonium biurate uroliths

Physical Examination Findings
• PSVA—cats may appear normal size, but most have stunted stature; microhepatica • Hepatic encephalopathy—golden or copper irises in non—blue-eyed and non-Persian cats; ascites and edema (rare) • Acquired liver disease—depends on chronicity of underlying disorder and formation of APSS; ascites and edema common (wax and wane in severity) • May develop ammonium biurate urolithiasis and associated signs

CAUSES
• PSVA—congenital malformations; • APSS—occurs with diseases that induce portal hypertension (cirrhosis, intrahepatic AV fistula, fibrosis) • Acute hepatic failure—induced by drugs, toxins, or infection

RISK FACTORS
• Alkalosis • Hypokalemia • Certain anesthetics and sedatives • Certain drugs (e.g., methionine, tetracycline, antihistamines) • Enteric bleeding—most common precipitating cause • Transfusion—stored blood products containing high concentrations of ammonia; incompatible blood transfusions • Infections • Constipation • Catabolism—disorders causing muscle wasting; large amounts of ammonia normally stored temporarily in muscle tissue

 DIAGNOSIS

DIFFERENTIAL DIAGNOSIS
• Lead toxicity • Urinary tract infection—urolithiasis • Intestinal parasitism • Primary gastrointestinal disease • Hypoglycemia • Toxoplasmosis • Congenital CNS disease or malformation—hydrocephalus; storage diseases • Acute ethylene glycol toxicity • Infectious diseases—rabies; canine distemper • CNS neoplasia • Thiamine deficiency—Wernicke's encephalopathy (especially in cats) • Drug intoxication

CBC/BIOCHEMISTRY/URINALYSIS
CBC
PSVA and APSS—microcytosis; mild nonregenerative anemia; poikilocytosis (cats); target cells (dogs)

Biochemistry
• Low BUN and creatinine—values reflect polyuria and polydipsia, high GFR, and reduced synthesis of each substance in the liver • Hypoglycemia—young toy breed dogs with PSVA; fulminant hepatic failure; cirrhosis • Low cholesterol—common • Liver enzymes—activity variable with APSS; ALP

usually high in young patients with PSVA owing to bone isoenzyme • Bilirubin—normal with PSVA but may be high with APSS • Hypoalbuminemia—common with APSS but inconsistent and mild with PSVA

Urinalysis
• Low concentration—common with PSVA • Ammonium urate crystalluria—causing hematuria, pyuria, and proteinuria due to mechanical inflammation and infection secondary to metabolic calculi

OTHER LABORATORY TESTS
• Blood ammonia—sensitive indicator of hepatic encephalopathy; fasting hyperammonemia common but hepatic encephalopathy may occur without hyperammonemia owing to its multifactorial complex cause; less reliable than TSBA owing to analytic/methodologic issues and because samples cannot be mailed for analysis • Ammonia tolerance testing—most reliable demonstration of ammonia intolerance; **Caution:** may induce hepatic encephalopathy • TSBA—confirm hepatic insufficiency • Coagulation tests—PSVA: abnormalities usually not associated with bleeding; APSS: increased PT, APTT, PIVKA, and fibrinogen reflect severity of liver dysfunction, synthetic failure, DIC, and vitamin K adequacy • Abdominal effusion—acquired liver disease; hepatoportal AV fistula; pure or modified transudate • Liver zinc values—usually low

IMAGING
See Portosystemic Vascular Anomaly, Congenital and Portosystemic Shunting, Acquired

DIAGNOSTIC PROCEDURES
• Hepatic aspiration—cannot differentiate among disorders causing portosystemic shunting • Liver biopsy—open surgical wedge biopsy or laparoscopic sampling (cup biopsy forceps) obtaining tissue from several liver lobes; tissue sampling with needle biopsy procedures inadequate in defining many disorders

PATHOLOGIC FINDINGS
• Gross—none specific; brain herniation may occur in acute fulminant hepatic failure • Microscopic—CNS vacuolation of glial cells and cerebral edema with severe disease (usually acute); hepatic: depends on primary liver disease

 TREATMENT

APPROPRIATE HEALTH CARE
• Depends on underlying condition • PSVA—surgical correction for many

NURSING CARE
• Depends on underlying condition; eliminate factors promoting hepatic encephalopathy • Improve dietary protein

tolerance by concurrent treatment with fermentable carbohydrates (see Medications) • If hepatic coma—discontinue oral medications • Avoid risk factors • Fluids—0.9% saline or lactated Ringer's solution with 2.5%–5.0% dextrose and 20–30 mEq/L potassium chloride (not to exceed 0.5 mEq/kg/h), titrate according to needs; avoid lactate with fulminant hepatic failure (rare); sodium-restricted fluids with acquired liver disease, ascites, and/or marked hypoalbuminemia • B-soluble vitamins (2mL/L fluids)

ACTIVITY
Keep patient warm, inactive, and hydrated

DIET
• Adequate calories—avoid catabolism and maintain muscle mass (attenuates hyper-ammonemia) • Dietary protein restriction—cornerstone of medical management; use commercially formulated diet specific for liver disease or moderate renal insufficiency; dogs: dairy and soy protein best sources; cats: pure carnivore must have meat-derived protein • Good-quality vitamin supplements (without methionine)—vitamin metabolism perturbed with liver disease and losses in urine • Ensure thiamine repletion—to avoid Wernicke's encephalopathy; 50–100 mg daily for 3 days, then with water-soluble vitamins in fluids; **Caution:** anaphylactoid reactions may occur with injectable thiamine • Partial parenteral nutrition—recommended for short-term inappetence to minimize catabolic mobilization of muscle; total parenteral nutrition if > 5 days inappetence; use of branched-chain amino acid solutions remains controversial

CLIENT EDUCATION
• Hepatic encephalopathy—often episodic and relapsing if underlying disorder cannot be cured • PSVA—surgical ligation may be curative; surgical/anesthetic risk of intraoperative or postoperative death: 10%–29% reported, depending on surgeon experience and ICU facility; clinical signs may persist, requiring chronic nutritional and medical management • APSS—depends on underlying cause

SURGICAL CONSIDERATIONS
• See Portosystemic Vascular Anomaly, Congenital • APSS—do not ligate

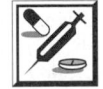 MEDICATIONS

DRUG(S)
• Medications that increase dietary protein tolerance alter enteric flora or conditions, reducing production or availability of substances provoking hepatic encephalopathy. • Antibiotics—spectrum altering intestinal flora (aerobic and anaerobic) or their

products; nonabsorbable (neomycin 10–22 mg/kg PO q12h): **Caution:** chronic neomycin treatment can result in renal and otic toxicity; approximately 3% absorbed systemically; local antimicrobials (enema); systemic (metronidazole 7.5 mg/kg q12h or amoxicillin, especially in cats, 12.5–25 mg/kg PO q8–12h); combined use with lactulose • Nonabsorbable-fermented carbohydrates—lactulose, lactitol, or lactose (if lactase deficient); decrease production or absorption of ammonia; increase rate of stool transit (catharsis); trap nitrogen in bacteria; lactulose most commonly used (start at 0.5–1.0 mL/kg q8–12h); therapeutic goal is passage of two to three soft stools daily; may also administer as enema for acute hepatic encephalopathy and coma • Enemas—*cleansing enemas* (warmed polyionic fluids) mechanically clean colon (10–15 mL/kg); *retention enemas* directly deliver fermentable substrates or directly alter colonic pH and organisms: diluted lactulose, lactitol, or lactose (1:2 in water); neomycin in water (do not exceed PO dose, do not dose PO and rectally); diluted Betadine (1:10 in water, rinse well in 15 min); diluted vinegar (1:10 in water) • Zinc supplementation—two urea cycle enzymes require zinc; measure baseline plasma zinc, dose 1–3 mg/kg elemental zinc PO (zinc acetate); titrate dose based on sequential plasma zinc measurements; avoid values > 800 µg/dL • Cerebral edema—complicates acute hepatic encephalopathy; mannitol (1 g/kg diluted in saline, over 30 min); nasal oxygen; *N*-acetylcysteine (140 mg/kg IV diluted 1:2 in saline given through nonpyrogenic filter; then 70 mg/kg q8h); glucocorticoids not beneficial, may induce enteric bleeding • Salvage therapy for intractable hepatic encephalopathy (experimental)—L-ornithine—L-aspartate (humans, rats: 180–300 mg/kg/day divided into three doses); L-carnitine (100 mg/kg PO or IV), may attenuate hepatic encephalopathy-associated hyperammonemia • If epileptic seizure activity—potassium bromide preferred anticonvulsant after ruling out hepatic encephalopathy mechanisms

CONTRAINDICATIONS
Avoid drugs metabolized by the liver.

PRECAUTIONS
• Use anesthetics, sedatives, tranquilizers, potassium-wasting diuretics, analgesics, and highly protein-bound drugs cautiously. • If possible, avoid drugs that rely on hepatic metabolism, biotransformation, or excretion • Consider altered pharmacokinetics; reduced first-pass extraction with portosystemic shunting; low albumin reduces protein binding

POSSIBLE INTERACTIONS
Drugs that affect or depend on hepatic metabolism—e.g., cimetidine, chlor-amphenicol, barbiturates, ketoconazole

 FOLLOW-UP

PATIENT MONITORING
• Reevaluate patient's at-home behavior, body condition, and weight • Monitor albumin and glucose—in patients with noncorrectable disorders; adjust nutrition • Monitor electrolytes—especially potassium; avoid hypokalemia as it aggravates hyperammonemia

PREVENTION/AVOIDANCE
Avoid dehydration, azotemia, hemolysis, constipation, enteric bleeding, infusion of stored blood, ammonium challenge, urinary tract infections (especially with urease-producing organisms, e.g., *Staphylococcus*), hypokalemia, hypomagnesemia, and alkalemia.

POSSIBLE COMPLICATIONS
Permanent neurologic damage (rare)

EXPECTED COURSE AND PROGNOSIS
• Depends on underlying disorder • Acute or chronic hepatic failure—may be fully or partially reversible, or patient may die

 MISCELLANEOUS

AGE-RELATED FACTORS
PSVA—surgical outcome may be good in young and old patients; treat hepatic encephalopathy medically first

SYNONYMS
• Hepatic coma • Portosystemic encephalopathy

SEE ALSO
• Arteriovenous Malformation of Liver • Hepatic Failure, Acute • Portosystemic Shunting, Acquired • Portosystemic Vascular Anomaly, Congenital

ABBREVIATIONS
• APSS = acquired portosystemic shunt • APTT = activated partial thromboplastin time • AV = arteriovenous • CNS = central nervous system • GABA = γ-aminobutyric acid • GFR = glomerular filtration rate • PIVKA = proteins invoked by vitamin K absence or antagonism • PT = prothrombin time • PSVA = portosystemic vascular anomaly • TSBA = total serum bile acids

Suggested Reading
Maddison JE. Medical management of chronic hepatic encephalopathy. In: Kirk RW, Bonagura J, eds. Current veterinary therapy XII. Philadelphia: Saunders, 1995;1153–1158.
Authors Sharon A. Center & Jill E. Maddison
Consulting Editor Sharon A. Center

HEPATIC FAILURE, ACUTE

BASICS

DEFINITION
Sudden loss of > 75% of functional hepatic mass; occurs primarily because of acute, massive hepatic necrosis

PATHOPHYSIOLOGY
• Necrosis follows insults caused by poor perfusion, hypoxia, hepatotoxic drugs or chemicals, heat excess, or infectious agents; consequences to hepatic function depend on insult type and zonal distribution within the hepatic lobule; accompanied by enzyme leakage and impairment in multiple hepatic functions, resulting in organ failure • Events that decrease perfusion or cause hypoxia commonly affect zone 3 of the hepatic acinus, corresponding to the pericentral or centrilobular region. • Ingested toxins affect the zone where agent is metabolized and toxic moiety generated, often zone 1 of the acinus, located periportally. • Hepatic failure is associated with a myriad of metabolic derangements, including alterations in glucose homeostasis, protein synthesis (albumin, transport proteins, procoagulants, and anticoagulant factors), and detoxification; may result in death.

SYSTEMS AFFECTED
• Hepatobiliary—hepatocellular necrosis; hepatic failure • Nervous—hepatic encephalopathy • Gastrointestinal—vomiting; diarrhea; melena; hematochezia • Hemic/lymphatic/immune—pro- and anticoagulant factor imbalances; DIC • Renal/urologic—renal tubules may undergo concurrent injury from toxin or its metabolite

INCIDENCE/PREVALENCE
• Mild to moderate hepatic necrosis is common with many primary and secondary hepatobiliary diseases. • Severe hepatic necrosis resulting in acute hepatic failure is less common; prevalence difficult to assess

GEOGRAPHIC DISTRIBUTION
N/A

SIGNALMENT
Species
More common in dogs than in cats

Breed Predilections N/A

Mean Age and Range N/A

Predominant Sex N/A

SIGNS
• Acute onset • Vomiting • Small intestinal diarrhea—may be bloody • Tender hepatomegaly • Bleeding • Jaundice • Hepatic encephalopathy • Seizures

CAUSES

Drugs
• See Hepatotoxins • Any drug, administered acutely, may be associated.

Biologic Toxins
See Hepatotoxins

Infectious Agents
See Hepatotoxins

Thermal Injury
• Heatstroke • Post–whole-body hyperthermia treatment for cancer

Hepatic Hypoxia
• Thromboembolic disease • Shock • DIC • Acute circulatory failure from any cause

RISK FACTORS
• Administration of any potentially hepatotoxic drug • Exposure to environmental toxins (e.g., *Amanita phylloides* mushroom) • Treatment with enzyme inducers—increased toxin production from some xenobiotics • Indiscriminant substance ingestion

DIAGNOSIS

DIFFERENTIAL DIAGNOSIS
• Severe acute pancreatitis or gastroenteritis—differentiated via laboratory data • Acute decompensation of chronic hepatobiliary disease—distinguished by review of prior medical record and results of blood tests, abdominal ultrasonography, and liver biopsy

CBC/BIOCHEMISTRY/URINALYSIS
• Anemia and panhypoproteinemia—associated with bleeding • Thrombocytopenia—owing to bleeding, DIC, or portal hypertension • Liver enzyme activity—dramatically high ALT and AST; less strikingly acute increase in ALP activity • Hypoglycemia—low glucose portends a grave prognosis in cats • Normal to low BUN concentration • Hyperbilirubinemia • Bilirubinuria—always abnormal in cats; ammonium urate crystalluria signifies hyperammonemia and hepatic insufficiency; granular casts and renal glucosuria indicate proximal tubule injury from toxicity (e.g., carprofen toxicity in dogs)

OTHER LABORATORY TESTS
• TSBA—high values confirm hepatic dysfunction; redundant with hepatic or posthepatic jaundice • Plasma ammonia concentration—high values coincide with high TSBA; confirms hepatic insufficiency; hyperammonemia inconsistent • Coagulation tests—identify coagulation factor deficiencies, platelet dysfunction, and DIC

IMAGING
• Abdominal radiography—may identify a normal to slightly large liver • Abdominal ultrasonography—may disclose evidence of nonhepatic disease (e.g., pancreatitis) and/or overt changes in liver tissue consistent with chronic liver injury and remodeling (e.g., heterogeneous liver texture, multiple nodules, hepatofugal portal blood flow); rules out biliary obstruction

OTHER DIAGNOSTIC PROCEDURES
Liver biopsy—required to confirm necrosis and characterize acinar zone involvement

PATHOLOGIC FINDINGS
• Gross—may note slightly large and mottled liver • Microscopic—reveals necrosis; identifies zonal involvement that may assist in determining underlying cause: hypoxia commonly leads to pericentral and toxin to periportal necrosis

TREATMENT

APPROPRIATE HEALTH CARE
Inpatient—intensive care required

NURSING CARE
• **Caution:** Do not insert central catheters until bleeding diathesis is controlled with vitamin K_1, fresh frozen plasma, and/or fresh whole blood transfusion. • Fluids—non–lactate-containing; initially at a resuscitation rate; monitor peripheral blood pressure and pulse oximetry • Colloid replacement—with low oncotic pressure from bleeding and protein loss; plasma preferred; hetastarch next best alternative; avoid dextran 70; human albumin may induce allergic reactions and is expensive • Potassium and glucose—supplement as appropriate; may mitigate severity of hepatic encephalopathy when corrected • Fluid regimen—adjust for maintenance and rate needs after achieving normovolemia; typically one-third of normal maintenance rate with polyionic fluids if administered concurrent with slow CRI of synthetic colloid • Phosphate—supplement judiciously; low phosphate may aggravate hepatic encephalopathy and cause constitutional signs, making critical care support difficult • Supplemental oxygen—if pulse oximetry ≤ 80% saturation

ACTIVITY
Restricted activity promotes healing and regeneration of the liver.

DIET
• Intractable vomiting—withhold PO food until controlled; use antiemetics (see below) • When enteric nutrition is contraindicated, provide partial parenteral nutrition until balanced feeding is instituted; no more than 5 days. • If enteric nutrition is chronically compromised, establish total parenteral nutrition feeding catheter; use total parenteral nutritional formula with normal nitrogen content; value of supplemented branched

amino acid formulations remains controversial. • Enteral feeding—small volume, frequent meals to optimize digestion and absorption and minimize formation of enteric toxins contributing to hepatic encephalopathy • Diet composition—use normal protein (nitrogen) content if patient is tolerant; moderate protein restriction with hepatic encephalopathy; positive nitrogen balance essential for hepatic regeneration • Supplemental vitamins essential—water-soluble (twofold normal); vitamin K_1 (0.5–1.5 mg/kg SC or IM, three doses at 12-hr intervals, then once weekly); vitamin E (10 IU/kg PO or by injection q24h)

CLIENT EDUCATION
• Inform client that acute hepatic failure is a serious condition. • Warn client that some patients die even with optimal treatment. • Inform client that an underlying cause for the necrosis (e.g., exposure to a drug or toxin) should be investigated but that often an underlying cause is not identified.

SURGICAL CONSIDERATIONS
N/A

 MEDICATIONS

DRUG(S) OF CHOICE

Drugs for Vomiting
• Metoclopramide—1–2 mg/kg/day CRI for mild or infrequent vomiting; contraindicated if spironolactone used for ascites mobilization • Chlorpromazine—0.5 mg/kg SC, IM, or rectally, q8–24h) for severe vomiting; ensure volume expansion first • Ondansetron—0.5–1.0 mg/kg IV q24h • Histamine H_2-blockers—famotidine (0.5 mg/kg IM or SC q12–24h) for enteric bleeding; reserve cimetidine (0.5 mg/kg q8–12h) for circumstances in which P-450 cytochrome inhibition may be useful in reducing toxin production from xenobiotic (e.g., acetaminophen toxicity)

Drugs for Hepatic Encephalopathy
• Lactulose—0.5 mL/kg PO q8h; may also be given rectally if PO hazardous • Metronidazole—7.5 mg/kg PO q12h; may also be given rectally if PO hazardous

Drugs for Cerebral Edema Associated with Hepatic Encephalopathy
• Mannitol—1 g/kg over 10–20 min, administered via a blood filter; if brisk diuresis does not occur within 1 hr, check plasma osmolality (measured) and blood pressure for excessive volume expansion • Furosemide—0.5–1.0 mg/kg IV q8–24h to increase free water excretion and reduce CSF production; monitor hydration and serum potassium to avoid dehydration and hypokalemia

Drugs for Coagulopathy
Fresh whole blood or fresh frozen plasma—for clinically significant bleeding

Free Radical Scavengers and Antioxidants
• For ongoing damage (membrane injury), reperfusion injury, and hypoxia • Vitamin E—10 IU/kg PO q24h • Vitamin C—100–500 mg q24h • N-acetylcysteine—140 mg/kg IV or PO; IV use 10% solution diluted 1:2 in saline, administer via 0.25 μm nonpyrogenic filter; follow with 70 mg/kg q6–12h • S-adenosylmethionine—20 mg/kg PO q24h on empty stomach, enteric-coated tablets; may assist importantly in intermediary metabolism, provide glutathione, and promote hepatocyte regeneration

Hepatoprotectants
• Silymarin (milk thistle extract, 60%–80% potency)—proven useful in Amanita toxicity and other hepatotoxins (20–50 mg/kg PO q24h) • Ursodeoxycholic acid—if chronic liver injury or very high bile acids persist (10–15 mg/kg q24h PO)

CONTRAINDICATIONS
Ideally, drugs that are biotransformed primarily by the liver, or that alter liver blood flow or metabolic enzyme activity should be avoided. This may be impractical since metabolism of many drugs in clinical use involves the liver in some way.

PRECAUTIONS
Administration of stored whole blood or packed RBCs may precipitate or exacerbate hepatic encephalopathy because of high ammonia concentrations

POSSIBLE INTERACTIONS N/A

ALTERNATIVE DRUG(S) N/A

 FOLLOW-UP

PATIENT MONITORING
• Temperature, pulse, respiration, and mental status—q1–2h for the first 24 hr • High vigilance for infection, especially iatrogenic catheter-associated nosocomial organisms • Body weight—twice daily to guide fluid therapy; body weight and condition scoring once weekly to appraise nitrogen balance and energy adequacy • Acid–base, electrolyte balances (especially potassium and phosphate), and glucose—q12–24h for the first 72 hr • Liver enzyme activities and serum bilirubin concentration—every 2–3 days until marked improvement

PREVENTION/AVOIDANCE
• Vaccinate dogs against infectious canine hepatitis virus. • Avoid indiscriminant ingestion of drugs or toxins associated with hepatotoxicity. • Remove potential toxins

from environment. • Scrutinize all chronic medications as potential toxin.

POSSIBLE COMPLICATIONS
• Hypoglycemia • DIC • Uncontrolled gastrointestinal bleeding • Hepatic encephalopathy • Chronic hepatic insufficiency • Hepatic cirrhosis/fibrosis from postnecrotic scarring • Acute renal failure • Death

EXPECTED COURSE AND PROGNOSIS
• Prognosis—depends on quantity of liver mass destroyed and proficiency of clinical support • Adequate critical care may permit hepatic regeneration and recovery.

 **MISCELLANEOUS**

ASSOCIATED CONDITIONS
• Pancreatitis • Sepsis/endotoxemia • Shock • Bleeding diathesis; severe enteric hemorrhage; DIC • Renal failure

ZOONOTIC POTENTIAL N/A

SYNONYMS
• Acute hepatic necrosis • Fulminant hepatic failure

SEE ALSO
• Alanine Aminotransferase (ALT)/Aspartate Aminotransferase (AST) • Alkaline Phosphatase (ALP) and Gamma Glutamyl Transpeptidase (GGT) • Ascites • Coagulopathy of Liver Disease • Hepatic Encephalopathy • Hepatitis, Infectious Canine • Hepatotoxins • Hyperbilirubinemia • Renal Failure, Acute

ABBREVIATIONS
• ALP = alkaline phosphatase • ALT = alanine aminotransferase • AST = aspartate aminotransferase • BUN = blood urea nitrogen • CRI = constant rate infusion • CSF = cerebrospinal fluid • DIC = disseminated intravascular coagulation • GGT = γ-glutamyltransferase • TSBA = total serum bile acids

Suggested Reading
Center SA. Acute hepatic injury: hepatic necrosis and fulminant hepatic failure. In: Guilford GW, Center SA, Strombeck DR, et al. Small animal gastroenterology. Philadelphia: Saunders, 1996:654–704.
Center SA, Elston TH, Rowland PH, et al. Fulminant hepatic failure associated with oral administration of diazepam in 11 cats. J Am Vet Med Assoc 1996;209:618–625.
Hughes D, King LG. The diagnosis and management of acute liver failure in dogs and cats. Vet Clin North Am Small Anim Pract 1995;25:437–460.
Authors Susan E. Bunch and Sharon A. Center
Consulting Editor Sharon A. Center

HEPATIC LIPIDOSIS

 BASICS

DEFINITION
• Feline hepatic lipidosis syndrome occurs when > 50% of hepatocytes accumulate excessive triglycerides, resulting in severe cholestasis and liver dysfunction. • Untreated—progressive metabolic dysregulation and death • May be secondary (most common) or idiopathic condition

PATHOPHYSIOLOGY
• Cats have an unusual propensity for accumulation of hepatocyte lipid vacuoles • Energy and protein deprivation leads to excess accumulation of hepatic triglycerides; protein deficiency may play a leading role, limiting exportation of triglycerides from the liver • Causal factors—increased peripheral fat mobilization; increased *de novo* hepatic triglyceride synthesis; impaired hepatic β-oxidation of fatty acids; reduced hepatocellular triglyceride exportation • Triglyceride vacuoles—hepatocyte distention; displacement of organelles to cell periphery; organelle dysfunction; canalicular compression • Hepatic failure may lead to hepatic encephalopathy

SYSTEMS AFFECTED
• Hepatobiliary—severe intrahepatic cholestasis; hepatic dysfunction or failure • Gastrointestinal—anorexia; vomiting • Musculoskeletal—peripheral tissue wasting • Nervous—hepatic encephalopathy • Hemic/lymphatic/immune—abnormal RBC shapes (poikilocytes), Heinz bodies leading to hemolysis • Renal/urologic—potassium wasting may be associated with tubule triglyceride accumulation

INCIDENCE/PREVALENCE
Most common severe feline hepatopathy in North America causing jaundice

GEOGRAPHIC DISTRIBUTION
Worldwide

SIGNALMENT

Species
Cats and rarely dogs (puppies, especially with storage disease as in Malteses; see Glycogen Storage Disease)

Breed Predilection
None

Mean Age and Range
• Mean—8 years • Range—1–16 years • Primarily middle-aged adults

Predominant Sex
Inconsistent predilection for obese females

SIGNS

Historical Findings
• Anorexia • Weight loss • Jaundice • Lethargy • Vomiting • Diarrhea or constipation • Weakness • Ptyalism • Hepatic encephalopathy • Collapse • Abnormalities due to an underlying disease (common)

Physical Examination Findings
• Jaundice • Hepatomegaly • Dehydration • Weakness—neck ventroflexion, recumbency • Ptyalism • Obtunded • Others, depending on underlying or primary disease

CAUSES

Idiopathic Hepatic Lipidosis
No underlying disease or cause for anorexia

Secondary Hepatic Lipidosis
• More than 85% of affected animals have a disease promoting anorexia or malassimilation. • Primary liver disease—PSVA; CCHS; EHBDO; cholelithiasis; neoplasia • Small intestinal disease—obstruction; neoplasia; IBD • Pancreatitis • Urogenital disease—chronic interstitial nephritis; renal failure (acute or chronic); feline lower urinary tract disease • Neurologic conditions • Infectious diseases—toxoplasmosis; FIP; FIV- or FeLV-related • Hyperthyroidism • B₁₂ deficiency • Other systemic conditions, including toxins

RISK FACTORS
• Obesity • Anorexia • Negative nitrogen balance; catabolism • Rapid weight loss

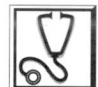 DIAGNOSIS

DIFFERENTIAL DIAGNOSIS
• Primary underlying liver disease—CCHS, cholelithiasis, EHBDO, and neoplasia most important differentials; differentiate by abdominal ultrasonography, liver aspiration, and definitively by liver biopsy • PSVA—rarely confused; differentiated by abdominal ultrasonography or colorectal scintigraphy • Hepatic toxoplasmosis or FIP—differentiated by liver biopsy • Pancreatitis—differentiated by abdominal ultrasonography, serum tests (high TLI, amylase, lipase [none of these tests are consistently reliable]), pancreatic aspiration cytology, laparoscopic or surgical inspection, and biopsy • Gastrointestinal disease—IBD differentiated by endoscopic or full-thickness bowel biopsy; obstruction: differentiated by abdominal survey or contrast radiography and ultrasonography • Toxicities—suspected based on history (e.g., oral diazepam, acetaminophen, methimazole) • Hyperthyroidism differentiated via serum thyroid panel

CBC/BIOCHEMISTRY/URINALYSIS
• Hematology—poikilocytes common; mild nonregenerative anemia; hemolytic anemia with severe hypophosphatemia; Heinz body anemia reflects GSH depletion; leukogram reflects underlying disorder • Biochemistry—hyperbilirubinemia; high ALP, ALT activity; normal or mildly high GGT if there is no primary necroinflammatory disorder involving biliary tree or pancreas; low BUN; normal creatinine; variable glucose (hypoglycemia rare); variable cholesterol and albumin; globulins usually normal (may be high with underlying inflammatory disease); hypokalemia (associated with failure to survive); may note severe hypophosphatemia (< 2 mg/dL) during initial 72 hr

(before and after initiation of feeding; causes hemolysis) • Urinalysis—lipiduria and unconcentrated urine common; ammonium biurate crystalluria extremely uncommon; high potassium loss in urine (some cats)

OTHER LABORATORY TESTS
• Prolonged coagulation times—PT, APTT, ACT, and especially PIVKA in 50% of cats; fibrinogen usually normal; vitamin K deficient • Hyperammonemia—rare • Serum bile acids—high before hyperbilirubinemia; determination redundant once jaundiced • B₁₂ deficiency—thought to increase susceptibility; may compromise recovery

IMAGING

Survey Abdominal Radiography
• Hepatomegaly • May note features of underlying disorder

Abdominal Ultrasonography
• Diffuse hepatic parenchymal hyperechogenicity—reflects triglyceride content; renal tubule triglyceride vacuolation compromises comparison between kidney and liver • Cannot differentiate idiopathic from secondary hepatic lipidosis unless underlying condition discovered

DIAGNOSTIC PROCEDURES
• Fine-needle aspiration—liver tissue: confirms vacuolation; > 80% of hepatocytes show cytosolic vacuolation • Aspiration cytology—based on history, clinical features, high ALP, and diffuse hepatic parenchymal echogenicity; cannot rule out underlying primary hepatic disorders (e.g., CCHS, EHBDO, PSVA) or other primary disorders • Liver biopsy—provides definitive diagnosis; done primarily to rule out a more primary liver disease if response to therapy is atypical (i.e., persistently high enzyme activity and hyperbilirubinemia); **Caution:** cat must be stabilized before anesthesia and biopsy to reduce risks • Give vitamin K₁ (0.5–1.5 mg/kg SC or IM) at least 12 hr before aspiration or biopsy to reduce iatrogenic hemorrhage; three doses at 12-hr intervals recommended; corrects PIVKA prolongation in many cats

PATHOLOGIC FINDINGS
• Gross—diffuse hepatomegaly, smooth surface; friable, greasy, yellow/pale in color, and reticulated in appearance; biopsy sample floats in formalin • Microscopic—diffuse, severe vacuolation of hepatocytes; few and large (macrovesicular) or many small (microvesicular) hepatocellular vacuoles

 TREATMENT

APPROPRIATE HEALTH CARE
• Inpatient—supportive care for severe disease; neck ventroflexion suggests severe electrolyte disturbance (potassium or phosphate) or thiamine deficiency; discharge home after stabilization and institution of feeding route • Frequent reevaluations—imperative • Outpatient—reduces stress and thereby facilitates recovery

NURSING CARE

• Balanced polyionic fluids—avoid lactate and dextrose supplementation; potassium chloride supplementation is important, use sliding scale (see Hypokalemia)

Correct Hypophosphatemia

• Serum phosphate < 2.0 mg/dL causes pathologic signs; weakness, myonecrosis, ileus, hemolysis, and neurologic signs confused with hepatic encephalopathy and anorexia • Low phosphate common as re-feeding phenomenon • Treatment—potassium phosphate initial dose of 0.01–0.03 mmol/kg/hr IV (commercial parenteral phosphate = 3 mmol/mL phosphate = 93 mg/mL elemental phosphorus); monitor serum phosphate q3–6h; discontinue when concentrations > 2 mg/dL; reduce potassium chloride supplement appropriately to avoid hyperkalemia

Correct Hepatic GSH Depletion

• Recently shown in hepatic lipidosis; suggests risk for oxidant injury from primary disease or hypophosphatemia-induced energy deprivation • Crisis intervention for Heinz body anemia—use NAC (140 mg/kg IV, then 70 mg/kg IV, 10% solution diluted 1:2 in saline; administer through 0.22 micron nonpyrogenic filter); when enteral feeding is established, change to SAMe (200 mg/cat PO q24h)

ACTIVITY

Most patients limit activity because of weakness; activity may augment gastric motility when gastroparesis complicates feeding

DIET

• Nutritional support—cornerstone of recovery • High-protein, high-calorie diets recommended

Tube Feeding

• Forced alimentation usually required; forced PO feeding may cause food aversion • Initiate food intake via nasogastric intubation; then establish a more substantial and comfortable route (i.e., esophageal or gastric intubation) after animal is stabilized • Avoid laparotomy for feeding tube insertion • Cautiously offer PO food daily to assess response

Food Content

• High-protein, high-energy, balanced cat food • Energy—60–90 kcal/kg ideal body weight/day • Supplements—controversial; seem to accelerate recovery but have not been rigorously evaluated; L-carnitine (250 mg/day); taurine (250–500 mg/day); thiamine (50–100 mg/day); vitamin B_{12} (initially, 1 mg IM or SC in a single injection): appraise continued need by sequential comparison to initial concentration; water-soluble vitamins (twice normal dose); vitamin E (10 IU/kg/day); thiol donors (NAC, SAMe): as above; potassium gluconate (to abate hypokalemia) will reduce fluid potassium supplementation; marine oil in food (2000 mg q24h) • Human stress formulas—require arginine (or citrulline) and taurine supplementation • Vitamin K_1 (as above); avoid overdosage (oxidant hemolysis and liver injury)

CLIENT EDUCATION

• Instruct client to perform tube feedings. • Warn client that feeding tubes may be retained for 4–6 months. • Inform client that recurrence is unlikely.

SURGICAL CONSIDERATIONS

• Exploratory laparotomy and liver biopsy (if indicated)—carefully inspect for underlying disorder, and biopsy pancreas, stomach, and/or small bowel, as indicated • Avoid surgical interventions until hydration is stable, electrolyte depletions are corrected, Heinz body anemia is alleviated, and coagulopathy is abated.

MEDICATIONS

DRUG(S)

• Drugs to ameliorate hepatic encephalopathy (see Hepatic Encephalopathy) • Metoclopramide—for vomiting, nausea, and gastroparesis; 0.2–0.5 mg/kg SC q8h, 30 min before feeding, or as a CRI IV drip at 0.01–0.02 mg/kg/hr or 1–2 mg/kg/day • Systemic antibiotics—as appropriate for concurrent infections

CONTRAINDICATIONS/PRECAUTIONS

• Adjust dosages for medications relying on hepatic metabolism or excretion • Avoid benzodiazepines and barbiturates—interact with neuroreceptors provoking hepatic encephalopathy • Appetite stimulants (e.g., diazepam, oxazepam, cyproheptadine)—do not initiate dependable energy intake; may produce sedation • Avoid drugs containing propylene glycol carrier (e.g., etomidate, diazepam)—lead to hemolysis in animals with hepatic lipidosis • Ursodeoxycholic acid—use in hepatic lipidosis is controversial • Dextrose supplements—may increase hepatic triglyceride deposition • Avoid tetracyclines—can promote triglyceride deposition • Avoid stanozolol—may augment development of hepatic lipidosis • Avoid propofol—phenol derivative may provoke hemolysis

FOLLOW-UP

PATIENT MONITORING

• Body weight, condition, hydration—judicious adjustment in energy and fluid provision important • Serum bilirubin—improves after 5–7 days of adequate management • Liver enzyme activity—slow to normalize • Discharge for home care—when vomiting is controlled, gastroparesis is resolved, total bilirubin values are declining, patient is ambulatory, and tube-feeding apparatus is problem-free • Tube feeding—discontinue only after proven ability and willingness to eat normally for 1 week

PREVENTION/AVOIDANCE

• Obesity—prevent; weight reduction must not exceed 2.0% body weight per week • Caution owner to verify food intake during weight loss regimen and during at-home stress (e.g., moved household, new housemates, home construction)

POSSIBLE COMPLICATIONS

• Feeding tube malfunction or obstruction—obstruction of gastrostomy tube relieved by papaya juice, carbonated soft drink, or pancreatic enzyme slurry; 15-min dwell time, then warm water flush • Hepatic encephalopathy after dietary support introduced • DIC (rare) • Hepatic failure leading to death • Untreatable underlying causal condition or disease

EXPECTED COURSE AND PROGNOSIS

• Optimal response to tube feeding and nutritional supplements—recovery of strength and vigor within 1–2 weeks • Complete recovery—14–21 days; sometimes longer • Therapy described herein results in 85% recovery in very severely affected animals • Underlying disease causing hepatic lipidosis influences outcome. • Hepatic lipidosis rarely recurs.

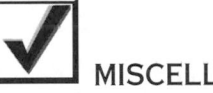

MISCELLANEOUS

ASSOCIATED CONDITIONS

• Primary liver disorders • Pancreatitis • Diabetes mellitus • Neoplasia—hepatic and systemic • Hepatic encephalopathy • Systemic illness limiting nutrition intake

SYNONYMS

• Fatty liver syndrome • Hepatosteatosis • Feline hepatic vacuolation • Vacuolar hepatopathy • Vacuolar degeneration

SEE ALSO

• Cholangitis/Cholangiohepatitis Syndrome • Hepatic Encephalopathy

ABBREVIATIONS

• CCHS = cholangitis/cholangiohepatitis syndrome • EHBDO = extrahepatic bile duct obstruction • GSH = glutathione • IBD = inflammatory bowel disease • NAC = *N*-acetylcysteine • PIVKA = proteins invoked by vitamin K absence or antagonism • PSVA = portosystemic vascular anomaly • SAMe = *S*-adenosylmethionine • TLI = trypsin-like immunoreactivity

Suggested Reading

Center SA. Hepatic lipidosis, glucocorticoid hepatopathy, vacuolar hepatopathy, storage disorders, amyloidosis, and iron toxicity. In: Guilford WG, Center SA, Strombeck DR, et al., eds. Strombeck's small animal gastroenterology. 3rd ed. Philadelphia: Saunders, 1996:766–801.

Author Sharon A. Center
Consulting Editor Sharon A. Center

HEPATIC NODULAR HYPERPLASIA

BASICS

OVERVIEW
• Hepatic nodular hyperplasia—common, benign lesion observed in the liver of middle-aged to old dogs, consisting of discrete accumulations of hyperplastic hepatocytes
• Clinically old dogs, either healthy or sick, having high biochemical liver enzymes must have nodular hyperplasia included in their differential diagnosis
• Clinical concern derived from associated high liver enzyme (especially ALP) activity and detection of nodules by imaging (ultrasonography) or grossly during exploratory surgery
• Because of the varied ultrasonographic appearance and the need for larger wedge biopsy samples to make the diagnosis, this common condition in older dogs may be easily misdiagnosed as regeneration secondary to chronic hepatitis or as hepatocellular neoplasia on needle core biopsy

SIGNALMENT
• Age-related lesion
• Nodules may be present by 6 or 8 years of age; one study documented lesions in all dogs > 14 years of age

SIGNS

Physical Examination Findings
• Nodular hyperplasia does not appear to cause clinical illness.
• May be no abnormalities
• Hepatomegaly; may palpate irregular hepatic margin (rarely)
• Findings reflecting another health problem

CAUSES & RISK FACTORS
• Etiology—unknown; metabolic factors and prior injurious events may play a factor
• Associations—considered a benign neoplasm in man; may reflect potential carcinogenicity in other species used for drug toxicity studies (e.g., rodents); no evidence that this is premalignant in dogs

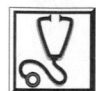

DIAGNOSIS

DIFFERENTIAL DIAGNOSIS
• Cirrhosis—regenerative nodular hyperplasia involves the entire liver; formation of irregular nodules that vary in size and are separated by fibrous tissue; loss of architectural organization involves the entire organ
• Neoplasia—single or multifocal large nodules may be mistaken for primary or secondary hepatic neoplasia; highest confusion with primary hepatocellular neoplasia: hepatocellular adenoma or carcinoma, differentiated based on hepatocyte dysplasia, nuclear atypia, pseudoglandular formation, loss or reduction of reticulin fibers, and architectural integration with normal surrounding hepatic tissue
• Vacuolar hepatopathy—hepatocyte vacuolation in lesions; consider adequacy of tissue sampling before undergoing extensive tests indicated for diffuse vacuolar hepatopathy

CBC/BIOCHEMISTRY/URINALYSIS
• CBC—no consistent associations
• Biochemistry profile—increased serum ALP common (range 2.5- to 16-fold normal); may be associated with increases in other liver enzymes; ALP activity surmised to reflect intralesional cholestasis or mechanical compression of adjacent normal hepatic tissue; high ALT activity may reflect compression and relative hypoxia of adjacent normal hepatocytes or increased cell replication within lesions; usually no change in total protein, albumin, total bilirubin, or cholesterol
• Urinalysis—no consistent findings

OTHER LABORATORY TESTS
TSBA—usually normal, unless hyperplasia is severe (may be associated with moderately increased TSBA concentrations, e.g., 50–80 μmol/L)

IMAGING
• Abdominal radiography—usually no abnormalities; rarely irregular hepatic margins suspected on lateral view
• Abdominal ultrasonography—variable echogenicity relating to varied histologic features and nodule size; echogenicity may be hypoechoic, hyperechoic, or mixed; nodules with echogenicity identical to adjacent normal parenchyma are overlooked

DIAGNOSTIC PROCEDURES
• Aspiration sampling—may yield normal hepatocytes; hepatocytes with cytosolic rarification and fragility consistent with vacuolar hepatopathy (glycogen retention), or discrete vacuoles suggesting lipid retention, and occasional binucleate hepatocytes

• Liver biopsy—collection of a needle biopsy may not differentiate lesion clearly because small dimension of the specimen compromises accurate histologic characterization; definitive diagnosis requires targeted sampling of large-enough tissue specimen including lesion and adjacent normal hepatic parenchyma

• Recommended biopsy methods—laparoscopic or open wedge biopsy by laparotomy

• Special stains—Masson's trichrome verifies absence of excess collagen deposition and remodeling typical of regenerative nodules associated with chronic liver disease; reticulin stain delineation of hyperplastic nodule and normal architecture of adjacent hepatic tissue; PAS stain (with and without diastase) demonstrates glycogen in hepatocyte cytosol

PATHOLOGIC FINDINGS

• Gross—single or multiple mass lesions, rarely > 3 cm in diameter; color similar to adjacent normal hepatic tissue; extensive lesions may mimic macronodular cirrhosis

• Microscopic—well-demarcated, expansive lesion where hepatocytes compress adjacent parenchyma; nodules seldom > 3 cm in diameter, with variable hepatocellular appearance including cytoplasmic changes consistent with lipidosis, hydropic degeneration, or glycogen accumulation (vacuolar hepatopathy) as compared to adjacent normal tissue; hyperplastic foci of hepatocytes form disorganized cords with decreased numbers of portal tracts and hepatic venules and occasional dilated sinusoids; occasional mitotic figures and binucleate hepatocytes; lipogranulomas may be observed; definitive diagnosis compromised by inadequate tissue samples (e.g., needle biopsy technique)

TREATMENT

N/A

MEDICATIONS

DRUG(S)

Nodular hyperplasia has a benign course and can be treated conservatively.

FOLLOW-UP

PATIENT MONITORING

• Quarterly biochemical profiles

• Sequential ultrasonography to evaluate enlargement of individual nodules

POSSIBLE COMPLICATIONS

• Nodular hyperplasia lesions—may initiate laboratory, imaging, gross, and microscopic hepatic changes that distract clinical attention from appropriate medical issues (e.g., significant clinical disease unrelated to the liver)

• Distinction from neoplasia not possible based only on clinical or laboratory data or imaging

EXPECTED COURSE AND PROGNOSIS

More extensive nodules may develop; rarely, necrotic foci or serious hemorrhage develops.

MISCELLANEOUS

SEE ALSO

• Cirrhosis and Fibrosis of the Liver
• Hepatitis, Chronic Active
• Hepatocellular Adenoma
• Hepatocellular Carcinoma
• Vacuolar Hepatopathy

ABBREVIATIONS

• PAS = periodic acid-Schiff
• TSBA = total serum bile acids

Suggested Reading
Stowater JL, Lamb CR, Schelling SH. Ultrasonographic features of canine hepatic nodular hyperplasia. Vet Radiol 1990; 31:268–272.

Author Sharon A. Center
Consulting Editor Sharon A. Center

HEPATITIS, CHRONIC ACTIVE

BASIC

DEFINITION
Ongoing hepatic inflammation associated with accumulation of inflammatory cells and progressive fibrosis in the liver

PATHOPHYSIOLOGY
• Caused by any event that alters normal hepatic architecture and activates cell-mediated immune mechanisms to interact with hepatic components • Infectious agents and toxins are inciting causes • Inflammatory cells (predominantly lymphocytes and plasma cells) appear initially in periportal area; eventually bridge hepatic lobules with chronicity, resulting in development of fibrosis • Cirrhosis and hepatic failure—late stage

SYSTEMS AFFECTED
• Hepatobiliary—inflammation; necrosis; cholestasis; fibrosis • Nervous—hepatic encephalopathy • Gastrointestinal—vomiting; diarrhea; anorexia • Urinary—polyuria and polydipsia; ammonium urate crystalluria (advanced stage) • Hemic/lymph/immune—coagulopathy

GENETICS
• Inheritable copper hepatotoxicity—Bedlington terriers; others (see Copper Storage Hepatopathy) • May play a role—cocker spaniels, Doberman pinschers, Labrador retrievers

INCIDENCE/PREVALENCE
Exact incidence unknown

SIGNALMENT
Species Dogs

Breed Predilections
• Bedlington terriers • Doberman pinschers • Cocker spaniels • Labrador retrievers • Skye terriers • Standard poodles • West Highland white terriers (controversial)

Mean Age and Range
• Mean age—6 years • Range—2–10 years

Predominant Sex
• Many breeds—females may be at risk • Cocker spaniels—more common in males

SIGNS
Historical Findings
• Lethargy • Anorexia • Weight loss • Vomiting • Polyuria and polydipsia • Jaundice • Ascites

Physical Examination Findings
• Lethargy • Poor body condition • Jaundice • Ascites • Hepatic encephalopathy

CAUSES
• Infectious—canine hepatitis virus; leptospirosis; canine acidophil cell hepatitis (viral infection hypothesized but may be initiated by other infectious agents) • Immune-mediated—autoimmune with positive ANA titer; nonsuppurative inflammation • Toxic—copper storage disease; drugs (e.g., anticonvulsants, trimethoprim sulfate, dimethylnitrosamine, oxibendazole); environmental

RISK FACTORS
• Breed • Age • Gender • Drugs—especially anticonvulsants that induce microsomal enzymes

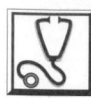

DIAGNOSIS

DIFFERENTIAL DIAGNOSES
• Acute hepatitis—history; liver biopsy • Portosystemic shunting (congenital or late-onset acquired)—abdominal ultrasonography; contrast venography; colorectal scintigraphy; liver biopsy • Hepatic neoplasia—radiography or ultrasonography; cytology; biopsy • Other causes of ascites—hypoalbuminemia; right heart failure; carcinomatosis • Other causes of portal hypertension—see Hypertension, Portal • Other causes of jaundice—EHBDO; hemolysis

CBC/BIOCHEMISTRY/URINALYSIS
• CBC—nonregenerative anemia; RBC microcytosis with APSS; variable leukogram; variable thrombocytopenia; low total protein; icteric plasma • Biochemistry—high liver enzymes; variable total bilirubin, albumin, BUN, glucose, and cholesterol; hepatic failure suggested by low albumin, BUN, glucose, and cholesterol, in the absence of other explanations • Urinalysis—variable urine concentration; bilirubinuria; ammonium biurate crystalluria

OTHER LABORATORY TESTS
• TSBA—normal or high fasting and high postprandial • Ammonia intolerance—ammonia values less reliable as a diagnostic test than is TSBA • Coagulation tests—may note prolonged PT, APTT, and PIVKA, low fibrinogen, and increased FDP (D-dimer test is very sensitive); coagulation tests reflect severity of liver dysfunction, synthetic failure, DIC, and vitamin K adequacy (see Coagulopathy of Liver Disease) • Abdominal effusion—chronic liver disease or portal hypertension: pure or modified transudate • Liver zinc values—low with chronic disease and especially with APSS; • Serologic tests (e.g., leptospirosis with expanded serovar titers, rickettsial diseases, *Borrelia*, *Bartonella*, endemic fungal agents, ANA titer); immunohistochemical staining for infectious agents

IMAGING
Abdominal Radiography
• Microhepatica—late-stage disease • Abdominal effusion—obscures image • Ammonium urate calculi—radiolucent unless combined with radiodense minerals

Abdominal Ultrasonography
• Liver size depends on stage of disease; microhepatica in late-stage disease • Normal to variably altered parenchymal and biliary tract echogenicity; may note nodularity and irregular liver margins • Portosystemic collaterals—tortuous vessels confirmed by Doppler interrogation • Abdominal effusion • Uroliths (very small or large) may be noted in renal pelvis or urinary bladder • Rules out EHBDO as cause of jaundice and chronic liver disease

Colorectal Scintigraphy
• Sensitive and noninvasive • Confirms portosystemic shunting

DIAGNOSTIC PROCEDURES
Fine-needle Aspiration Cytology
Hepatic aspiration—cannot differentiate chronic hepatitis; cannot be used to recommend therapy

Liver Biopsy
• Open surgical for wedge biopsy or laparoscopic sampling (cup biopsy forceps)—recommended; obtain tissue from several liver lobes; inadequate tissue sampling with needle biopsy procedures (18-gauge Vim TruCut: > 50% discordance with matched wedge sample) • Bacterial culture and sensitivity of liver with or without bile • Metal analysis—determines copper, iron, and zinc concentrations; copper and iron contribute to oxidant damage; zinc values used to determine need for oral zinc supplementation

PATHOLOGIC FINDINGS
• Gross—early: no gross change; late stage: microhepatica with irregular surface (fine or coarse nodules) or edge, tortuous APSS • Microscopic—nonsuppurative periportal (zone 1) inflammation; variable cholestasis and biliary hyperplasia; piecemeal and/or bridging necrosis with disruption of limiting plate; with cirrhosis: periportal fibrosis with bridging between portal areas and regenerative nodules

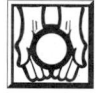

TREATMENT

APPROPRIATE HEALTH CARE
• Inpatient—for diagnostic testing and initiation of medical therapy in overtly ill dogs • Outpatient—if condition is stable at diagnosis; slowly titrated onto medical therapy

NURSING CARE
• Depends on underlying condition • Fluid therapy—balanced polyionic fluids supplemented appropriately with potassium and dextrose; restrict sodium if ascites is present • B-soluble vitamins (2 mL/L fluids) • Abdominocentesis—aseptic procedure for tense ascites compromising food intake and ventilation or impairing sleep; diuretics are the first option for ascites mobilization

ACTIVITY
Keep patient warm, inactive, and hydrated; inactivity may promote hepatic regeneration, euglycemia, and ascites mobilization

DIET
• Adequate calories—avoid catabolism and maintain muscle mass (attenuates hyperammonemia); record body condition score • Dietary protein—restrict only if signs of hepatic encephalopathy (see Hepatic Encephalopathy); feed balanced diet; with hepatic encephalopathy, avoid fish, meat, and egg-quality protein (dogs); cats are true carnivores and require meat source protein • Meal frequency—feeding several small meals per day optimizes

nutrient assimilation • Sodium restriction—with ascites or severe hypoalbuminemia • Good-quality vitamin supplement (without methionine)—vitamin metabolism perturbed with liver disease and losses in urine • Thiamine—ensure repletion to avoid Wernicke's encephalopathy; 50–100 mg PO daily; **Caution:** anaphylactoid reactions may occur with injectable thiamine • Partial parenteral nutrition—recommended for short-term inappetence to minimize catabolic mobilization of muscle; give total parenteral nutrition if inappetence lasts > 5 days; use of branched-chain amino acid solutions remains controversial in animals with liver dysfunction

CLIENT EDUCATION
• Medication is required for life; disease is cyclic; quarterly or biannual evaluations are needed • Inform client of the lack of long-term veterinary studies proving efficacy of single or polypharmacy approaches; recommendations derived from (1) broad clinical experience, (2) retrospective and prospective studies in human beings, and (3) animal disease models.

SURGICAL CONSIDERATIONS
APSS—do not ligate

MEDICATIONS

DRUG(S)

Diuretics
For ascites—combination of furosemide (0.5–2 mg/kg IV, SC, PO q12h) and spironolactone (0.5–2 mg/kg PO q12h; loading spironolactone is important, use doubled dose once); recheck and adjust dose at 4–7-day intervals by 25–50%.

Drugs for Hepatic Encephalopathy
(see Hepatic Encephalopathy)

Antioxidants
• Vitamin E—α-tocopherol, 10 IU/kg PO daily • S-adenosylmethionine—20 mg/kg enteric-coated tablet PO q24hr on empty stomach • Avoid vitamin C (ascorbate) with high tissue copper or iron concentration—augments oxidant injury associated with transition metals

Zinc (Zinc Acetate)
• Antioxidant; antifibrotic • Blocks enteric copper uptake • Optimizes two urea cycle enzymes • Elemental zinc 1.5–3 mg PO daily; adjust dose using sequential plasma zinc concentrations (avoid plasma values > 800 μg/dL)

Copper Chelation
• See Copper Storage Hepatopathy • If tissue copper > 1500 μg/g dry liver • D-penicillamine (first choice) or trientine • Follow chelation therapy with chronic zinc supplementation

Immunomodulation
• Prednisolone or prednisone—2–4 mg/kg daily PO; with ascites: use dexamethasone to avoid mineralocorticoid effect (divide prednisone dose by 8 to 10), administer every 2–4 days • Azathioprine—adjunctive therapy for immune-mediated inflammation; 0.5–2 mg/kg PO q24h for 3–5 days, then every other day; titrate by 25%–50% dose reduction after 2–6 months based on sequential biochemistries showing improvements (e.g., declining total bilirubin and liver enzyme activity); monitor CBC and biochemistry profile every 7–10 days for first month to ensure absence of hematopoietic, hepatic, and pancreatic toxicity; if acute hematopoietic toxicity occurs, stop therapy, allow recovery, then reintroduce at 25% dose reduction; if insidious chronic hematopoietic toxicity (after many months) or acute cholestatic liver or pancreatic injury occurs, discontinue therapy permanently • Mycophenolate mofetil (very limited experience)—surrogate drug for patients intolerant to azathioprine; suggested dose: 5–10 mg/kg PO q24–48h; depends on hepatic glucuronidation and renal excretion for elimination; monitor for hematopoietic toxicity (rare at recommended dose) • Microemulsified cyclosporine—option but limited long term experience • Other immunomodulatory drugs listed below

Ursodeoxycholic Acid
• Immunomodulatory, hepatoprotectant, antifibrotic, choleretic, antiendotoxic, antioxidant effect • 10–15 mg/kg PO daily; divided dose may be better assimilated; may prepare as aqueous solution; safe; therapy can be maintained indefinitely

Antifibrotics
• Polyunsaturated phosphatidylcholine (phosphatidylcholine lecithin)—50–100 mg/kg PO daily with food; maximum dose is 3 g in humans; as potent as colchicine in some models tested; corticosteroid-sparing effect allows downward titration of prednisolone for disease management; other effects: immunomodulatory, antioxidant, hepatoprotectant; routinely prescribed • Colchicine—inhibits collagen production, may suppress cell receptors involved with perpetuated inflammation; 0.03 mg/kg PO daily; toxic effects include hemorrhagic diarrhea and bone marrow suppression; avoid form complexed with probenecid (prolongs drug retention time); selected as therapy when fibroplasia is a more overriding feature histologically than inflammation • Silibinin—hepatoprotectant (numerous toxins), antifibrotic, and antioxidant effects; promotes hepatocellular regeneration; 20–50 mg/kg PO daily; use source with 60%–80% potency silymarin extract; especially if toxin- or drug-mediated injury suspected

CONTRAINDICATIONS
Avoid drugs requiring hepatic metabolism whenever possible.

PRECAUTIONS
• Glucocorticoids—may precipitate hepatic encephalopathy, enteric bleeding, vomiting, and/or ascites • Zinc overdose may cause hemolysis.

POSSIBLE INTERACTIONS
Avoid medications that alter hepatic biotransformation or excretion pathways (e.g., cimetidine, quinidine, ketoconazole)

FOLLOW-UP

PATIENT MONITORING
• At-home behavior • Body condition and weight—adjust intake to nitrogen tolerance and energy needs • CBC, biochemistry, and urinalysis—look for signs of drug toxicity, disease remission, synthetic capacity, ammonium biurate crystalluria, and urinary tract infection

PREVENTION/AVOIDANCE
Maintain high vigilance for early signs of hepatitis in predisposed breeds (e.g., high liver enzyme activity); ascertain diagnosis and initiate therapy early

POSSIBLE COMPLICATIONS
• Sepsis secondary to immunosuppression • Hepatic encephalopathy • DIC • Enteric ulceration • Hepatic failure and death

EXPECTED COURSE AND PROGNOSIS
• Depends on underlying disorder • Chronic disease, jaundice, and ascites—poorer prognosis • Polypharmacy and nutritional support extend quality survival compared with untreated cases, but no long term studies yet available • Early diagnosis in Doberman pinschers, Bedlington terriers, and Cocker spaniels appear to suspend disease progression for years

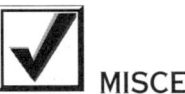

MISCELLANEOUS

ZOONOTIC POTENTIAL
• Leptospirosis; *Bartonella*; rickettsial agents (if vector) • Inform client; inspect titers of housemate pets.

SYNONYMS
• Doberman hepatitis • Cocker spaniel hepatitis • Copper storage hepatopathy

SEE ALSO
• Ascites • Hepatic Failure, Acute • Portosystemic Shunting, Acquired

ABBREVIATIONS
• APSS = acquired portosystemic shunt • EHBDO = extrahepatic bile duct obstruction • FDP = fibrin degradation products • PIVKA = proteins invoked by vitamin K absence or antagonism • PSVA = portosystemic vascular anomaly • TSBA = total serum bile acids

Suggested Reading
Center SA. Chronic liver disease. In: Guilford WG, Center SA, Strombeck DR, et al., eds. Strombeck's small animal gastroenterology. 3rd ed. Philadelphia: Saunders, 1996: 705–765.

Acknowledgment
The author/editors acknowledge the prior contributions of Dr. Robert M. Hardy, who authored this topic in the previous edition.

Author Sharon A. Center
Consulting Editor Sharon A. Center

HEPATITIS, GRANULOMATOUS

 **BASICS**

OVERVIEW

• Occurs secondary to infection by specific bacterial, viral, parasitic, protozoal, or fungal organisms resulting in granuloma formation or mononuclear phagocyte infiltration and inflammation of the liver
• May be localized to the liver or may be part of a multisystemic disease (spleen, lymph nodes), which may mask the underlying hepatic disease
• Rarely, reflects an immunoregulatory disorder or reticuloendothelial neoplasia

SIGNALMENT

• Cats and dogs
• No breed, sex, or age predilection
• Suspicion that immunoregulatory or reticuloendothelial neoplasia may cause a granulomatous hepatic reaction—more common in golden retrievers

SIGNS

General Comments
Depend on cause

Historical Findings
• Anorexia
• Lethargy
• Weight loss
• Vomiting
• Diarrhea
• Polyuria or polydipsia

Physical Examination Findings
• Severe hepatomegaly
• Abdominal pain
• Jaundice
• Abdominal distention—ascites; marked hepatomegaly
• Splenomegaly—coexisting granulomatous reaction or reticuloendothelial hyperplasia
• Lymphadenopathy
• Fever
• Tachypnea

CAUSES & RISK FACTORS

• Systemic fungal infection—most common; histoplasmosis; blastomycosis; coccidioidomycosis; pythiosis
• Bacterial infection—brucellosis; mycobacterial disease; *Bartonella*
• Rickettsial infection
• Parasitism—visceral larval migrans; liver flukes; dirofilariasis
• Virus—FIP
• Protozoal disease—toxoplasmosis; leishmaniasis
• Miscellaneous—intestinal lymphangiectasia; neoplasia (malignant histiocytosis); immune-mediated disorders (hemophagocytic syndrome); idiopathic

 DIAGNOSIS

DIFFERENTIAL DIAGNOSIS

Degree of suspicion needed to make the diagnosis; multisystemic nature

CBC/BIOCHEMISTRY/URINALYSIS

• CBC—inflammatory or stress leukogram; nonregenerative anemia (chronic inflammation); spherocytes with microangiopathic anemia or immune-mediated anemia; monocytosis in some samples
• Biochemistry—high liver enzymes; hyperbilirubinemia, hypoglycemia; hypoalbuminemia; low BUN; high or low total serum proteins; hypergammaglobulinemia; may note electrolyte abnormalities with fluid and acid–base disturbances
• Urinalysis—may be normal; may note nonspecific abnormalities, proteinuria, RBCs, WBCs, cellular casts, other casts, and bilirubinuria

OTHER LABORATORY TESTS

• Serum bile acid concentrations—high
• Coagulation assays—normal, except with end-stage liver failure
• Serologic tests—high fungal titer (fungal disease); must evaluate with caution and procure convalescent titers; increased IgM titers to toxoplasmosis support active infection
• Antinuclear antibody titer—positive with SLE; **Caution:** nonspecificity of low positive titers
• Bacterial cultures—including mycobacterium

IMAGING

• Abdominal radiography—hepatomegaly; abdominal mass; loss of detail owing to ascites
• Abdominal ultrasonography—assesses liver size and parenchymal change (diffuse vs. focal); defines mass lesions; other visceral lesions; mesenteric lymphadenopathy; enables diagnostic aspiration sampling

DIAGNOSTIC PROCEDURES

• Aspiration sampling—hepatic parenchyma; other visceral lesions; abdominal effusion
• Bacterial culture and sensitivity tests and cytology—useful

- Liver biopsy—definitive diagnosis
- Blood, liver aspirates, and liver biopsy—fungal stain; Gram stain; bacterial and fungal cultures and sensitivity

PATHOLOGIC FINDINGS
- Gross—hepatomegaly; normal appearance; firm texture; blunted margins; finely irregular surface
- Microscopic—pyogranulomatous reaction with no consistent zonal orientation

 TREATMENT

- Inpatient vs. outpatient—dictated by severity of clinical signs
- Fluid therapy—with balanced polyionic solution for dehydration; may require dextrose (2.5%–5%); judicious potassium supplements
- Nutritional support (enteral or parenteral)—if patient is unwilling or unable to eat; positive nitrogen balance essential; do not restrict protein intake if there is no evidence of hepatic encephalopathy
- Inform client that the causes of the syndrome (e.g., FIP) are often difficult to treat

 MEDICATIONS

DRUG(S)
- Depend on the initiating cause; see specific chapters

- Idiopathic disease (no underlying cause or possible markers of immune-mediated process)—glucocorticoids combined with azathioprine proven successful; risky if undetected infectious condition is present
- Immunomodulation—if immune-mediated mechanisms are suspected and survey for infectious etiologies is negative
- Vomiting—antiemetics (e.g., metoclopramide 0.2–0.5 mg/kg PO or SC q6–8h; ondansetron 0.5–1.0 mg/kg 30 min before feeding, up to q12h)
- Gastrointestinal bleeding—H_2-receptor antagonists (e.g., famotidine 0.5 mg/kg PO, IM, SC q12–24h) and sucralfate

POSSIBLE INTERACTIONS
- Important to consider possible drug interactions because of the broad spectrum of possible causes
- May need to adjust medications that require hepatic activation, biotransformation, or elimination
- Glucocorticoids and azathioprine—may worsen clinical signs when an underlying infectious agent exists

 FOLLOW-UP

PATIENT MONITORING
- Routine monitoring of fluids, acid–base balance, electrolytes, and general response to treatment
- Repeat sequential hematologic, biochemical, and imaging evaluations—may be useful

POSSIBLE COMPLICATIONS
- Chronic hepatitis
- Fibrosis or cirrhosis
- Hepatic failure
- Coagulopathy

EXPECTED COURSE AND PROGNOSIS
- Depends on primary cause
- Prognosis usually guarded at best, owing to multisystemic nature of the syndrome

 MISCELLANEOUS

ZOONOTIC POTENTIAL
- Brucellosis—main causal agent of concern
- Blastomycosis and coccidioidomycosis—not contagious; may be contracted when humans and pets share common environment
- Leishmaniasis—if no plausible origin is obvious, as this may indicate presence of transmission vector

SEE ALSO
- Bartonellosis
- Blastomycosis
- Coccidioidomycosis
- Feline Infectious Peritonitis (FIP)
- Histoplasmosis
- Lupus Erythematosus, Systemic (SLE)
- Pythiosis

Suggested Reading

Center SA. Chronic liver disease In: Guilford WG, Center SA, Strombeck DR, et al., eds. Strombeck's small animal gastroenterology. Philadelphia: Saunders, 1996, pp. 705–765.
Authors Robert M. Hardy and Sharon Center
Consulting Editor Sharon A. Center

HEPATITIS, INFECTIOUS CANINE

BASICS

OVERVIEW
• Viral disease of dogs and other Canidae caused by CAV-1, which is serologically homogeneous but antigenically distinct from respiratory CAV-2 • Infection—targets parenchymal organs (especially liver), eyes, and endothelium • Oronasal exposure—leads to viremia (4–8 days); virus shed in saliva and feces; initial dispersal to hepatic macrophages (Kupffer cells) and endothelium; replicates in Kupffer cells; damage to adjacent hepatocytes and massive viremia when released • Adequate antibody response clears organs in 10–14 days; persists in renal tubules and may be shed in urine for 6–9 months • Chronic hepatitis—follows infection in dogs, with only partial neutralizing antibody response • Cytotoxic ocular injury—anterior uveitis; leads to classic "hepatitis blue eye"

SIGNALMENT
• Dogs • No breed or sex predilections • Most common in dogs < 1 year of age

SIGNS
• Depend on immunologic status of host and degree of initial cytotoxic injury • Peracute—fever; CNS signs; vascular collapse; DIC; death within hours • Acute—fever; anorexia; lethargy; vomiting; diarrhea; hepatomegaly; abdominal pain; abdominal effusion; vasculitis (petechia, bruising); DIC; lymphadenopathy; rarely, nonsuppurative encephalitis • Uncomplicated—lethargy; anorexia; transient fever; tonsillitis; vomiting; diarrhea; lymphadenopathy; hepatomegaly; abdominal pain • Late—20% of cases develop anterior uveitis and corneal edema 4–6 days postinfection; recover within 21 days; may progress to glaucoma and corneal ulceration

CAUSES & RISK FACTORS
• CAV-1 • Unvaccinated dogs susceptible

DIAGNOSIS

DIFFERENTIAL DIAGNOSIS
• Other infectious hepatopathies • Leptospirosis • Granulomatous hepatitis • Toxic hepatitis • Fulminant infectious disease—e.g., parvovirus, canine distemper

CBC/BIOCHEMISTRY/URINALYSIS
• CBC—schistocytes; leukopenia during acute viremia, followed by leukocytosis with reactive lymphocytosis and nucleated RBCs • Biochemistry—liver enzyme activity high initially, begins declining within 14 days; low glucose and albumin reflect fulminant hepatic failure, vasculitis, and endotoxemia; low sodium and potassium levels reflect GI losses; hyperbilirubinemia • Urinalysis—proteinuria reflects glomerular injury; granular casts reflect renal tubule damage; bilirubinuria

OTHER LABORATORY TESTS
• Coagulation tests—reflect severity of liver injury and DIC • Serology for antibodies to CAV-1—fourfold rise in IgM and IgG; vaccine-induced antibodies confuse interpretation • Viral isolation—anterior segment of eye, kidney, tonsil, and urine; difficult in parenchymal organs (especially liver) unless first week of infection

IMAGING
• Abdominal radiography—normal or large liver; poor detail due to effusion • Abdominal ultrasonography—may observe hepatomegaly, hypoechoic parenchyma (multifocal or diffuse pattern), and effusion

DIAGNOSTIC PROCEDURES
Liver biopsy

PATHOLOGIC FINDINGS
• Acute—edema and hemorrhage of lymph nodes; abdominal effusion; serosal hemorrhages; liver large, dark, and mottled; gallbladder edematous; fibrinous exudate on liver, gallbladder, and other viscera; splenomegaly; renal infarcts • Chronic—small, fibrotic or cirrhotic liver

TREATMENT

• Usually inpatient • Fluid therapy—balanced polyionic fluids; carefully monitor fluids to avoid overhydration in context of increased vascular permeability • In fulminant hepatic failure (acute/peracute presentation)—lactate may be contraindicated (inability to metabolize) • Judicious potassium and magnesium supplementation since electrolyte depletion may augment hepatic encephalopathy • Avoid neuroglycopenia—supplement fluids with dextrose (2.5%–5.0%) as necessary • Blood component or synthetic colloids for coagulopathy and low colloidal osmotic pressure • With overt DIC—fresh blood products and low molecular weight heparin (e.g., enoxaparin 100 U/kg [1 mg/kg] q24h) • Nutritional support—frequent small meals as tolerated; optimize nitrogen intake to patient; inappropriate protein restriction may impair tissue repair and regeneration • If oral feeding is not tolerated, provide partial parenteral nutrition (maximum of 5 days) or, preferably, total parenteral nutrition

MEDICATIONS

DRUG(S)
• Prophylactic antimicrobials—for anticipated transmural migration of enteric flora and endotoxemia in the context of hepatic failure; e.g., ticarcillin (33–50 mg/kg q6–8h) combined with metronidazole (reduce conventional dose to 7.5 mg/kg IV q8–12h) • Antiemetics—for vomiting; e.g., metoclopramide (0.2–0.5 mg/kg PO or SC q6–8h or by CRI), ondansetron (0.5–1.0 mg/kg PO q12h) • H_2-receptor antagonists (e.g., famotidine 0.5 mg/kg PO, IV, SC q12–24h) and sucralfate (0.25–1.0 g PO q8–12h)—for gastrointestinal bleeding • Drugs for hepatic encephalopathy (see Hepatic Encephalopathy) • Ursodeoxycholic acid—choleretic and hepatoprotectant (10–15 mg/kg daily); give indefinitely for chronic hepatitis • Antioxidants—vitamin E (10 IU/kg daily), S-adenosylmethionine (20 mg/kg PO daily) until liver enzymes normalize and dog fully recovers, indefinitely with chronic hepatitis

CONTRAINDICATIONS
Consider severity of hepatic injury, protein depletion, and age when calculating dosages.

FOLLOW-UP

PATIENT MONITORING
• Routinely monitor fluid, electrolyte, acid–base, and coagulation status to adjust supportive measures • Monitor for acute renal failure

PREVENTION/AVOIDANCE
• MLV vaccination—at 6–8 weeks of age; two boosters 3–4 weeks apart until 16 weeks of age; booster at 1 year; highly effective vaccine; boosters may not be needed

POSSIBLE COMPLICATIONS
• Fulminant hepatic failure • Acute renal failure • DIC • Glaucoma • Chronic hepatitis • Septicemia • Hepatic encephalopathy

EXPECTED COURSE AND PROGNOSIS
• Peracute—poor prognosis; death within hours • Acute—guarded to good prognosis • Poor antibody response (titer 1:16–1:50)—chronic hepatitis may develop • Good antibody response (titer > 1:500 IgG)—complete recovery in 5–7 days possible • Recovered patients—may develop chronic liver or renal disease

MISCELLANEOUS

AGE-RELATED FACTORS
• Maternal antibody—may protect some pups for first 8 weeks; depends on antibody concentration in bitch and on effective passive transfer • Vaccination of pups with high levels of passively acquired antibodies—successful at 14–16 weeks of age

SEE ALSO
• Disseminated Intravascular Coagulation • Hepatic Encephalopathy • Hepatic Failure, Acute • Renal Failure, Acute

ABBREVIATIONS
• CAV-1 = canine adenovirus-1 • MLV = modified live virus

Suggested Reading
Greene CE. Infectious canine hepatitis and canine acidophil cell hepatitis. In: Greene CE, ed. Infectious diseases of the dog and cat. 2nd ed. Philadelphia: Saunders, 1998;22–28.

Author Sharon A. Center
Consulting Editor Sharon A. Center

BASICS

OVERVIEW
Bacterial infections restricted to the hepatobiliary system—uncommon; consist of multifocal microabscessation, diffuse cholangitis or cholangiohepatitis, cholecystitis, and choledochitis or discrete unifocal suppurative, necrotic lesions; usually associated with pyogenic organisms

SIGNALMENT
• Dogs and cats • No breed, sex, or age predilections • Hepatic abscesses—most common in old dogs; may develop subsequent to omphalitis in neonates; subsequent to diabetes mellitus • Suppurative cholangitis or cholangiohepatitis—most common in young to middle-aged male cats

SIGNS

Historical Findings
• Anorexia • Lethargy • Weight loss • Vomiting • Diarrhea • Polyuria and polydipsia • Trembling • Fever

Physical Examination Findings
• Fever • Abdominal pain • Dehydration • Tachycardia • Tachypnea • Hepatomegaly • Coagulopathy • Abdominal distention or fluid wave • Jaundice • Signs of endotoxemia • Collapse associated with hypoglycemia

CAUSES & RISK FACTORS
• Ascending biliary tract infection • Hematogenous infection via the portal vein, hepatic artery, or umbilical vein • Penetrating wounds • Complication of hepatic biopsy • Diabetes mellitus • Glucocorticoid administration or hyperadrenocorticism • Immunosuppressive therapy for cancer or immune-mediated disease • Preexisting disease of the liver, biliary tree, or pancreas

DIAGNOSIS

DIFFERENTIAL DIAGNOSIS
• Infectious or necroinflammatory disease—most patients are febrile • Hepatic abscess—fever, abdominal pain, and/or hepatomegaly (especially with a risk factor) • Pancreatitis or pancreatic abscess • Hepatobiliary neoplasia • Gastrointestinal obstruction or perforation • Peritonitis or other intra-abdominal abscess • Cholelithiasis and biliary colic

CBC/BIOCHEMISTRY/URINALYSIS
• CBC—neutrophilic leukocytosis with a left shift; toxic changes in WBCs; monocytosis; thrombocytopenia; nonregenerative anemia • Biochemistry—may note high ALP, ALT, and AST activity; hypoalbuminemia, hyperglobulinemia, inconsistent hyperbilirubinemia, and hypoglycemia; may note features of endotox-

emia owing to infection with gram-negative organisms • Urinalysis—usually normal; bilirubinuria; culture usually negative but may disclose hematogenously dispersed organisms

OTHER LABORATORY TESTS
• Serum bile acids—may be high; depends on the degree of hepatic involvement or cholestasis • Coagulation assessments and RBC morphology (schistocytes)—consistent with DIC

IMAGING

Abdominal Radiography
• Hepatomegaly or hepatic mass effect (abscess) • Loss of abdominal detail (effusion) • Gas within the hepatic parenchyma or biliary tree (gas-producing organisms)

Ultrasonography
• Abscess—most noninvasive method of detection (> 0.5 cm); solitary, variably echogenic, cavitated lesions • Dystrophic tissue mineralization or entrapped gas—may appear hyperechoic • Multiple masses—occasionally have mixed echogenicity • Highly echogenic interface in a cavitated mass—may be gas; combination with an abdominal effusion and highly echogenic perilesional area supports an abscess • Miliary abscesses—cannot discern from other parenchymal hepatic disorders

DIAGNOSTIC PROCEDURES

Cytology
• Histologic specimens rarely disclose bacterial organisms • Cytologic evaluation essential • Samples—paracentesis; abdominocentesis of effusion; sampling of discrete lesions by ultrasound guidance; hepatic parenchymal aspiration; cholecystocentesis • Stains—Wright-Giemsa; Gram stain if bacteria are seen • Look for bacterial organism within WBCs and for signs of a primary disease process (e.g., neoplasia)

Culture and Sensitivity Testing
• Specimens with a suppurative or pyogranulomatous reaction—culture for aerobic and anaerobic bacteria and fungus • Blood (aerobic and anaerobic cultures)—more likely to be positive if multiple abscesses • Polymicrobial infections—common (40%) • Gram-negative bacteria—common; *E. coli* (most common); *Enterobacter* spp.; *Klebsiella* spp.; *Proteus* spp. • Gram-positive bacteria—*Staphylococcus* spp. • Anaerobic organisms—less common; *Bacteroides* spp. suggests polymicrobial infection

TREATMENT
• Inpatient—if there are signs of sepsis • Intravenous fluid and antibiotics—aggressive therapy essential • Fluid support—correct dehydration deficits; rectify acid–base and electrolyte disturbances; potassium chloride supplementation as appropriate • Abscess—drain via hepatic lobectomy during laparotomy or under ultrasound guidance; after drainage,

monitor body temperature and liver enzymes and repeat ultrasonographic assessment (look for generalized or loculated abdominal fluid); repeat drainage if required; may use an indwelling catheter directly inserted into the area of suppuration for continued extracorporeal drainage • Bile duct occlusion—biliary decompression essential; antimicrobials must be administered intravenously before performing biliary tree manipulations to avoid septicemia

MEDICATIONS

DRUG(S)
• Antibiotics—based on culture and sensitivity results; continue for a minimum of 3–4 months • Initial treatment—combine antibiotics to eliminate common aerobic and anaerobic pathogens; first-generation cephalosporins (e.g., cefazolin 20 mg/kg IV q8h) combined with either metronidazole (15 mg/kg IV q12h if no hepatic dysfunction or severe cholestasis; reduce dose by 50% if hepatic function compromised) or clindamycin (10–16 mg/kg SC per day); or penicillins (e.g., ampicillin 20 mg/kg IV q8h) combined with an aminoglycoside (e.g., gentamicin dog: 6–10 mg/kg IV q24h; cat: 5–8 mg/kg IV q24h) or enrofloxacin (2.5 mg/kg PO or SC q12h)

CONTRAINDICATIONS
• Aminoglycosides—do not give until hydration status is normalized; may not penetrate abscess capsule • Avoid drugs metabolized or excreted by the liver or those known to be hepatotoxic

FOLLOW-UP

PATIENT MONITORING
• Assess vital signs and physical condition • Ultrasound examination—determine abscess recurrence.

POSSIBLE COMPLICATIONS
• DIC • Septicemia • Fulminant hepatic failure • Septic peritonitis • Endotoxemia

EXPECTED COURSE AND PROGNOSIS
• Favorable prognosis—early detection and aggressive treatment • Worst prognosis—concurrent diseases; surgery required

MISCELLANEOUS

Suggested Reading
Center SA. Chronic liver disease. In: Guilford WG, Center SA, Strombeck DR, et al., eds. Strombeck's small animal gastroenterology. Philadelphia: Saunders, 1996, pp. 705–765.
Author Cynthia R. L. Webster
Consulting Editor Sharon A. Center

HEPATOCELLULAR ADENOMA

BASICS

OVERVIEW
• A benign tumor of epithelial origin • More common than primary malignant liver tumors

SIGNALMENT
• Rare in dogs and very rare in cats
• Affected dogs commonly > 10 years of age
• Breed predispositions unknown

SIGNS
• Usually clinically silent • Rupture may lead to hemoperitoneum, resulting in weakness.
• Single or multiple, well-circumscribed liver masses that may be pedunculated
• Occasionally, cranial abdominal pain, vomiting, and inappetence

CAUSES & RISK FACTORS
• Unknown • May be associated with chronic inflammation or hepatotoxicity

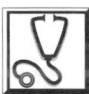

DIAGNOSIS

DIFFERENTIAL DIAGNOSIS
• Hepatic adenocarcinoma • Hepatic abscess
• Abdominal mass • Splenomegaly
• Nodular hyperplasia

CBC/BIOCHEMISTRY/URINALYSIS

CBC
• Usually normal • Anemia—rarely unexplained; regenerative anemia if tumor is bleeding • Leukocytosis with a left shift—tumors with necrotic centers

Biochemistry
• Liver enzymes variable • ALP, ALT, AST—normal or mild to markedly high • Serum total bilirubin values—usually normal

Urinalysis
No significant abnormalities

OTHER LABORATORY TESTS
• Serum bile acids—normal unless tumor strategically impairs hepatic perfusion and bile flow in the porta hepatis
• Coagulation—abnormalities consistent with DIC (rare) associated with necrotic tumors and bleeding

IMAGING

Radiography
• May demonstrate a single mass lesion or apparent asymmetry of hepatic silhouette
• Rarely, gas in necrotic center of tumor

Abdominal Ultrasonography
• Discrete mass lesion with variable echogenicity, depending on intratumor necrosis, hemorrhage, gas, or cystic cavities
• A mixed echogenic pattern—most common

DIAGNOSTIC PROCEDURES
• Hepatic aspiration cytology—use a 23- or 25-gauge 1–1.5-inch needle under ultrasono-graphic guidance; may find normal hepatocytes or cells with mild atypia, making differentiation from hepatocellular adenocarcinoma impossible • Hepatic biopsy—with needle biopsy, several core biopsies necessary to provide enough tissue for histopathologic characterization, so not recommended (insufficient tissue may impair accurate characterization); often confused with regenerative or hyperplastic nodules; histopathology of resected mass preferred method of diagnosis; wide resection recommended because mass may be hepatocellular carcinoma

PATHOLOGIC FINDINGS

Gross
• Usually well-circumscribed single nodules < 10 cm in diameter • May be yellow brown
• Often soft, highly vascular, and friable
• Occasionally multiple • Occasionally very large (> 20 cm)

Microscopic
• May be difficult to distinguish from nodular hyperplasia or normal liver tissue; misdiagnosis of hepatocellular carcinoma may occur
• Usually well-defined trabecular pattern; not necessarily encapsulated • Compression of adjacent hepatic parenchyma common
• Mitotic figures infrequent • Affected liver cells resemble normal hepatocytes but often are larger and have a clear cytosol. • Conspicuous absence of portal tracts • Normal reticulin pattern helps differentiate adenomas from regenerative nodules and hepatocellular carcinoma

TREATMENT
• Symptomatic care to minimize discomfort
• Outpatient—appropriate unless surgical intervention requires postoperative critical care • Bleeding tumor—requires blood transfusion; surgical excision advised
• Activity—normal, unless massive liver lobe enlargement causes discomfort or hemorrhage; confine to cage if actively bleeding.

SURGICAL CONSIDERATIONS
• Excision recommended for large single mass lesions • Between 60% and 70% of the liver lobes can be resected if the patient is given appropriate critical care. • Biopsy local lymph nodes and normal liver for histologic evaluation.

MEDICATIONS

DRUG(S)
N/A

CONTRAINDICATIONS/POSSIBLE INTERACTIONS
N/A

FOLLOW-UP

PATIENT MONITORING
• Abdominal palpation—every 3–4 months; evaluate for recurrence (low-yield method of evaluation) • Liver enzymes—sequential evaluation; assess recurrence of mass-associated enzyme liberation • Abdominal ultrasonography—every 3–4 months for the first year; preferred method of reappraisal

POSSIBLE COMPLICATIONS
• Avoid making a definitive diagnosis on the basis of aspiration cytology; solid tissue biopsy best for accurate diagnosis; resection better than needle biopsy for definitive diagnosis
• Risk of tumor necrosis and massive abdominal hemorrhage if unresected

EXPECTED COURSE AND PROGNOSIS
Usually good

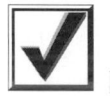

MISCELLANEOUS

SYNONYMS
Hepatoma—a confusing term that should be avoided; refers to hepatocellular carcinoma in human medicine although considered synonymous with hepatocellular adenoma in veterinary medicine

SEE ALSO
Hepatocellular Carcinoma

ABBREVIATIONS
• ALP = alkaline phosphatase
• ALT = alanine aminotransferase
• AST = aspartate aminotransferase
• DIC = disseminated intravascular coagulation

Suggested Reading
Guilford WG, Strombeck DR. Hepatic neoplasms. In: Guilford WG, Center SA, Strombeck DR, et al., eds. Strombeck's small animal gastroenterology. 3rd ed. Philadelphia: 1996:847–859.
Morrison WB. Primary cancers and cancer-like lesions of the liver, biliary epithelium, and exocrine pancreas. In: Morrison WB, ed. Cancer in dogs and cats: medical and surgical management. Baltimore: Williams & Wilkins, 1998:559–568.
Author Wallace B. Morrison
Consulting Editor Wallace B. Morrison

BASICS

OVERVIEW
• A malignant tumor of epithelial origin
• Less common than benign liver tumors in dogs, but accounts for > 50% of malignant hepatic tumors

SIGNALMENT
• Rare in dogs and very rare in cats
• Affected dogs commonly > 10 years of age
• No breed predispositions

SIGNS
• Typically absent until disease is advanced
• Lethargy • Weakness • Anorexia • Weight loss • Polydipsia • Diarrhea • Vomiting
• Hepatomegaly (asymmetric)—consistent; precedes development of overt clinical signs
• Abdominal hemorrhage

CAUSES & RISK FACTORS
• Unknown • May be associated with chronic inflammation or hepatotoxicity
• Toxins—induce tumor in experimental animals (e.g., aflatoxins, dimethylnitrosamine, CCl_4) and in humans (e.g., chronic hepatitis viruses)

DIAGNOSIS

DIFFERENTIAL DIAGNOSIS
• Hepatic adenoma • Hepatic abscess
• Abdominal mass • Splenomegaly • Nodular hyperplasia • Biliary cystadenoma • Bile duct adenoma/carcinoma • Metastatic carcinoma
• Polycystic liver disease—less common form; fibrous stroma hyperplasia with anaplastic duct cells; few cysts • Hepatic lymphosarcoma • Hepatic hemangiosarcoma • Hepatic carcinoid

CBC/BIOCHEMISTRY/URINALYSIS
CBC
• Usually normal • Anemia—rarely unexplained anemia; may develop a regenerative anemia if tumor is a bleeding tumor
• Leukocytosis with a left shift—tumors with necrotic centers

Biochemistry
• Liver enzymes variable • ALT, AST, ALP, and GGT—usually very high; suggests a pathologic process more severe than indicated by the clinical signs • Serum total bilirubin values—usually normal • May note hypoalbuminemia, hyperglobulinemia, hypoglycemia, and hypercholesterolemia

OTHER LABORATORY TESTS
• Serum bile acids—normal unless tumor strategically impairs hepatic perfusion and bile flow in the porta hepatis
• Coagulation—may see abnormalities consistent with DIC in patients with necrotic tumors and abdominal bleeding

IMAGING
Radiography
• May demonstrate a single mass lesion or apparent asymmetry of hepatic silhouette associated with a single lobe • Caudolateral displacement of stomach owing to marked hepatomegaly • Rarely, gas in necrotic center of tumor • Thoracic—may reveal pulmonary metastases

Abdominal Ultrasonography
• Discrete mass lesion with variable echogenicity, depending on the intratumor necrosis, hemorrhage, gas, or cystic cavities
• Mixed echogenic pattern—most common
• Target lesions may develop.

DIAGNOSTIC PROCEDURES
• Hepatic aspiration cytology—often reflects dysplasia and overt malignant features; occasionally only necrotic cells; discordant findings between cytology and histopathology; use histologic features to make a definitive diagnosis. • Hepatic biopsy for confirmation—needle biopsy not recommended

PATHOLOGIC FINDINGS
Gross
• Usually a discrete mass; sometimes multiple nodules or infiltrative tumor into adjacent liver lobes • May be friable • Color varies from almost white to normal liver color • Necrotic core may be obvious
• Diffusely infiltrated tumors may not be grossly apparent other than hepatomegaly (of involved lobes).

Microscopic
Varies from well differentiated and closely resembling the cell of origin to severely anaplastic

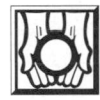

TREATMENT
Outpatient, unless surgical intervention requires postoperative critical care during recuperation or bleeding tumors require blood component or whole blood transfusion

NUTRITION
• Consider strategies appropriate for neoplasia—frequent small meals; increased calorie intake; shift balance of energy intake to protein and fat rather than from carbohydrate (if fat assimilation normal)
• Supplement with ω-3 fatty acids, water-soluble vitamins (twice normal), and vitamin E • Administer vitamin K_1—with EHBDO

SURGICAL CONSIDERATIONS
• Excision recommended • Between 60% and 70% of the liver lobes can be resected if the patient is given appropriate critical care.
• Resect primary or metastatic focal lesions.
• Biopsy local lymph nodes and normal-appearing liver.

MEDICATIONS

DRUG(S)
• Chemotherapy—none generally effective
• Mitoxantrone—one of four treated dogs had a complete remission for 65 days

FOLLOW-UP

PATIENT MONITORING
• Abdominal palpation—every 2–4 months; evaluate recurrence (low-yield method of evaluation) • Abdominal ultrasonography—every 2–4 months for the first year; preferred method of reappraisal monitor liver enzymes

POSSIBLE COMPLICATIONS
• Risk of tumor necrosis and massive abdominal hemorrhage if unresected

EXPECTED COURSE AND PROGNOSIS
• Prognosis is variable; histologic classification is not prognostic
• Mean survival with surgical resection (lobectomy or partial hepatectomy)—> 300 days • Metastatic rate—61%; lungs, hepatic lymph nodes, and peritoneum common metastatic sites

MISCELLANEOUS

ASSOCIATED CONDITIONS
• Chronic hepatitis • Cholangiohepatitis
• Polycystic liver disease • Chronic toxin ingestion

SEE ALSO
Hepatocellular Adenoma (Hepatoma)

ABBREVIATIONS
• ALP = alkaline phosphatase
• ALT = alanine aminotransferase
• AST = aspartate transaminase
• CCl_4 = carbon tetrachloride
• DIC = disseminated intravascular coagulation
• EHBDO = extrahepatic bile duct obstruction
• GGT = γ-glutamyltransferase

Suggested Reading
Hammer AS, Sikkema DA. Hepatic neoplasia in the dog and cat. Vet Clin North Am Small Anim Pract 1995;25:419–435.
Author Wallace B. Morrison
Consulting Editor Wallace B. Morrison

HEPATOMEGALY

BASICS

DEFINITION
Large liver detected on physical examination, abdominal radiography, ultrasonography, or direct visualization; liver is normally 1.3–5.0% of body weight

PATHOPHYSIOLOGY
Normal size is determined by hepatotropic factors (produced in the gut and pancreas and delivered in portal blood); enlargement due to sinusoidal capacitance or parenchymal or sinusoidal accumulation of cells, substrates, or storage products

Diffuse or Generalized
• Inflammatory—immune-mediated or infectious hepatitis; classified according to cell type • Lymphoreticular hyperplasia—response to antigens or accelerated erythrocyte destruction • Congestion—impaired venous drainage • Infiltration—cellular (usually neoplastic) invasion or accumulation of abnormal substances (glycogen, lipid, amyloid, storage disease) • Cystic lesions • Cholestasis—EHBDO; intrahepatic cholestasis • Extramedullary hematopoiesis

Nodular, Focal, or Asymmetric
• Neoplasia • Hemorrhage • Infection or inflammation • Nodular hyperplasia • Arteriovenous fistula—involved lobe larger than other lobes • Asymmetric regeneration after large-volume hepatic resection • Cystic lesions

SYSTEMS AFFECTED
• Gastrointestinal—gastric compression or displacement • Pulmonary—compromised ventilatory space (rare)

SIGNALMENT
• Dogs and cats • Old animals more commonly affected • Puppies and kittens normally have a larger liver:body mass ratio than do adults.

SIGNS

Historical Findings
• Abdominal distention or palpable mass • Depend on underlying cause

Physical Examination Findings
• Dogs—liver palpable beyond costal margin (normal liver may be palpable in certain conformations; small liver not palpable) • Cats—liver palpable > 1.5 cm beyond costal margin (normal liver palpable in some cats) • May remain undetected in obese animals

CAUSES

Inflammation
• Infectious hepatitis—chronic active hepatitis (early) • Acute hepatic necrosis—toxins; drug; ischemia; other • Feline CCHS • Biliary cirrhosis • Lymphoreticular hyperplasia—immune-mediated disease (rickettsial, hemolytic anemia, systemic lupus erythematosus, idiopathic)

Venous Outflow Occlusion
• High central venous pressure—right-sided congestive heart failure secondary to tricuspid valve disease; cardiomyopathy; congenital anomaly (cor triatriatum dexter); neoplasia; pericardial disease; heartworm disease; pulmonary hypertension; severe arrhythmia • High vena caval or hepatic venous resistance—venous occlusion secondary to thrombosis; tumor invasion or extramural occlusion; heartworm vena cava syndrome; vena caval stenosis or congenital kink; diaphragmatic hernia; intrahepatic hepatic vein occlusion (Budd-Chiari syndrome; venoocclusive disease); liver lobe torsion

Infiltration
• Neoplasia • Metabolic abnormalities—amyloid; glycogen (vacuolar hepatopathy in dogs); lipid (hepatic lipidosis in cats): neonatal cats and dogs, dogs with diabetes mellitus or hyperlipidemia syndromes; metabolic products of storage disease • Lymphoreticular hyperplasia—infectious disease, hemolytic anemia, antigenic stimulation

Extramedullary Hematopoiesis
Regenerative anemias—hemolytic (immune-mediated, congenital or metabolic, infectious); chronic oxidant injury; erythroparasitemia; bone marrow failure; idiopathic

Neoplasia
• Infiltrative, diffuse, or large focal tumors • Primary hepatic—lymphoma; hepatocellular adenoma or carcinoma; cholangiocarcinoma (bile duct carcinoma) • Hemangioma or hemangiosarcoma • Fibroma or fibrosarcoma • Leiomyoma or leiomyosarcoma • Osteosarcoma • Various metastatic tumors

Biliary Obstruction
• Pancreatitis; pancreatic neoplasia; other neoplasms in porta hepatis (bile duct carcinoma); granuloma of common bile duct • Inspissated bile • Cholelithiasis • Abscess • Proximal duodenitis; duodenal foreign body • Fluke migration (cats)

Cystic Lesions
• Hepatic or biliary cysts • Cystadenoma • Polycystic diseases—may be associated with renal cysts (common in Persian cats) • Acquired cysts—tumors • Hepatic abscesses (cystic cavitation)

Other
• Drugs—corticosteroids, phenobarbital • Nodular hyperplasia

RISK FACTORS
• Cardiac disease • Heartworm disease • Neoplasia • Primary hepatic disease—inflammatory, neoplastic, or cystic • Corticosteroids—exogenous or endogenous • Phenobarbital • Poorly controlled diabetes mellitus • Obesity complicated by anorexia (cats)—hepatic lipidosis • EHBDO • Certain anemias

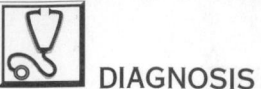

DIAGNOSIS

DIFFERENTIAL DIAGNOSIS

Similar Signs
Distinguished from gastric, splenic, or other cranial abdominal masses or effusions via radiography and ultrasonography

Differential Causes
• Cardiac disorders (e.g., heart murmur, weak femoral pulses, hepatojugular reflex, jugular distention and pulses, muffled heart sounds); significant anemia (pallor with or without jaundice); tachycardia; tachypnea; exercise intolerance; bounding pulses • Parenchymal liver disease—characterized by lethargy, anorexia, vomiting, diarrhea, weight loss, jaundice, bleeding tendency, hepatic encephalopathy, polyuria and polydipsia, and ascites • Vacuolar hepatopathy (dog)—Signs of hyperadrenocorticism or adrenal hyperplasia • Hepatic lipidosis—suggested by jaundice in obese anorectic cat or poorly controlled diabetes mellitus (dog or cat)

CBC/BIOCHEMISTRY/URINALYSIS

CBC
• Identify anemia and cause; spherocytes (immune-mediated hemolytic anemia, microangiopathic anemia); schistocytes (vascular shearing-microangiopathic, vena cava syndrome, hemangiosarcoma, DIC, *Haemobartonella*, *Babesia*) • Circulating blast cells—myeloproliferative or lymphoproliferative disease • Nucleated red cells—extramedullary hematopoiesis • Macrocytosis and nonregenerative anemia—FIV, FeLV • Thrombocytopenia—increased consumption; increased destruction; reduced production • Thrombocytosis—neoplasia; inflammation; hyperadrenocorticism; splenic disease

Biochemistry
• Inflammatory disorders—usually have high liver enzyme activity; variable hyperglobulinemia; variable bilirubin and albumin concentrations • Lymphoreticular hyperplasia—mild to moderately high liver enzymes • Primary hepatic neoplasia—moderate to markedly high liver enzymes (ALT, ALP, GGT) • Metastatic neoplasia—normal to moderately high liver enzymes; may see hypercalcemia or hyperglobulinemia • Infiltrative disorders—minor liver enzyme changes; hyperbilirubinemia • Vacuolar hepatopathy (dogs)—markedly high ALP; high cholesterol with glucocorticoids • Hepatic lipidosis (cats)—markedly high ALP, AST, and ALT; minor increase in GGT unless concurrent pancreatitis, CCHS, or EHBDO • Storage diseases—few abnormalities • EHBDO—markedly high ALP and other enzymes; severe hyperbilirubinemia and hypercholesterolemia • Cystic lesions—normal, except with hepatic abscess (markedly high ALT and

AST) • Phenobarbital associated—high liver enzymes (especially ALP) • Nodular hyperplasia—normal or moderately high ALP

OTHER LABORATORY TESTS
• FeLV and FIV testing • Buffy coat smears—circulating blast cells (neoplasia) • Coagulation panel—DIC common with hemangiosarcoma or diffuse lymphoma; prolonged coagulation times common with EHBDO (especially on PIVKA test) • TSBA—high with diffuse disorders and EHBDO; redundant if hemolysis ruled out as cause of jaundice • Pituitary-adrenal axis testing (dogs)—vacuolar hepatopathy • Heartworm testing—in endemic areas • Fungal serology—in endemic areas

IMAGING

Abdominal Radiography
• Hepatomegaly—extension of a rounded liver margin caudal to the costal arch; caudal-dorsal displacement of stomach; caudal displacement of cranial duodenal flexure, right kidney, and transverse colon • May suggest cause

Thoracic Radiography
• Three views (right and left lateral and dorsal-ventral views)—screen for metastasis and underlying disorders • Cardiac, pulmonary, pericardial, and vena caval disorders • Sternal lymphadenopathy—reflects abdominal inflammation or neoplasia • Puppies, kittens, and deep inspirations—spurious hepatomegaly

Abdominal Ultrasonography
• Liver size and contour • Diffuse enlargement with normal echogenicity—congestion; cellular infiltration (lymphoma); inflammation; extramedullary hematopoiesis; reticuloendothelial hyperplasia • Diffuse enlargement with hypoechoic parenchyma—normal variation; congestion, lymphoma, and diffuse sarcoma; amyloidosis • Diffuse enlargement with hyperechoic parenchymal (minor nodularity)—lipid or glycogen accumulation; inflammation; diffuse fibrosis • Diffuse enlargement with hypoechoic nodules—neoplasia; abscesses; vacuolar hepatopathy (dog); glycogen • Distinguish intrahepatic from posthepatic cholestasis—EHBDO • Identify concurrent abdominal disease—liver; kidneys; intestines; lymph nodes; effusion; interrogate the porta hepatis • Cannot differentiate benign from malignant disease • Abdominal effusions—distribution and echogenic patterns

OTHER DIAGNOSTIC PROCEDURES

Electrocardiography and Echocardiography
Discern abnormalities in cardiac conduction and structure

Fine-needle Aspiration
• Procedure—22- or 25-gauge, 2.5–3.75-cm (1–1.5-in) needle; diffusely large liver directly aspirated without ultrasonography; focal lesions aspirated with ultrasound guidance

• Cytology—may reveal infectious agents, vacuolar change, neoplasia, inflammation, or extramedullary hematopoiesis; definitive diagnosis seldom confidently confirmed • Hepatic biopsy—if ultrasonography rules out EHBDO, cytology does not indicate septic inflammation, and there are no other obvious diagnoses; percutaneous ultrasound-guided needle for suspected neoplasia and amyloid (avoid if abscess or EHBDO present); otherwise, best sampling with laparoscopic or surgical exploratory approaches • Microbial culture—aerobic and anaerobic bacterial; fungal as appropriate • Staining—trichrome (fibrosis); rhodanine (copper); PAS (glycogen); acid-fast stain (mycobacterial if granulomatous reactions appear); Congo red (amyloid); oil red O (lipid, frozen section) • Coagulation testing—before liver sampling, measure PT, APTT or ACT, fibrinogen, PIVKA, and buccal mucosal bleeding time; lack of dependable association of test findings with bleeding and low predictive capabilities of tests for iatrogenic hemorrhage recognized • Abdominal effusion—cytology; protein content; cultures; collect and evaluate before tissue sampling • Pericardiocentesis—with pericardial tamponade

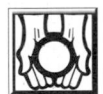

TREATMENT

APPROPRIATE HEALTH CARE
• Outpatient—except with cardiac or hepatic failure • General supportive goals—eliminate or manage inciting cause; prevent complications; reverse derangements associated with hepatic failure • Important derangements—dehydration and hypovolemia; hepatic encephalopathy; hypoglycemia; acid–base and electrolyte abnormalities; coagulopathies; enteric ulcerations; sepsis; endotoxemia

NURSING CARE
• Heart failure or ascites—avoid sodium-rich fluids and food • Supplement potassium chloride in maintenance fluids—20 mEq/L fluid • Supplement B-soluble vitamins

ACTIVITY
Restricted; cage rest during diagnostic and primary therapy

DIET
• Dietary protein—restrict only with hepatic encephalopathy • Well-balanced with adequate energy; positive nitrogen balance essential; adequate vitamins and micronutrients • Sodium—restrict with cardiac failure or ascites

CLIENT EDUCATION
• Treatment depends on underlying cause. • Many causes are life threatening, although others are less serious and are amenable to treatment. • A thorough evaluation is essential for attaining a definitive diagnosis.

SURGICAL CONSIDERATIONS
• Resection of primary or focal hepatic mass lesions (neoplasia, abscess, compromising cyst)—indicated for EHBDO • Pericardectomy (thoracoscopic procedure)—if effusion recurs after initial pericardiocentesis

MEDICATIONS

DRUG(S)
Varies with underlying cause

CONTRAINDICATIONS
• Avoid hepatotoxic drugs • Vacuolar hepatopathy (dogs)—avoid glucocorticoids • Hepatic lipidosis (cats)—avoid catabolism or drugs that promote catabolism; avoid fasting

FOLLOW-UP

PATIENT MONITORING
• Physical assessment and hepatic imaging—reassess liver size • CBC, biochemistry, TSBA—assess progression of hepatic dysfunction; reticulocyte count with anemia • Thoracic radiography, electrocardiography, and echocardiography—assess previous abnormalities • Pituitary-adrenal axis—with adrenal disorders • Fructosamine with or without glucose profiling—with diabetes mellitus • Adjust drug dosages according to status of liver function, body condition, and weight.

POSSIBLE COMPLICATIONS
Many causes are life threatening.

MISCELLANEOUS

ZOONOTIC POTENTIAL
Certain infectious agents of concern

SEE ALSO
• Amyloidosis • Anemia, Immune-Mediated • Bile Duct Obstruction • Congestive Heart Failure, Right-Sided • Hepatitis, Granulomatous • Hepatitis, Suppurative and Hepatic Abscess • Hepatocellular Adenoma • Hepatocellular Carcinoma • Vacuolar Hepatopathy

ABBREVIATIONS
• ACT = activated clotting time • APTT = activated partial thromboplastin time • CCHS = cholangitis/cholangiohepatitis syndrome • EHBDO = extrahepatic bile duct obstruction • PAS = periodic acid-Schiff • PIVKA = proteins invoked by vitamin K absence or antagonism • PT = prothrombin time • TSBA = total serum bile acids

Authors Keith P. Richter & Sharon A. Center
Consulting Editor Sharon A. Center

HEPATOPORTAL MICROVASCULAR DYSPLASIA

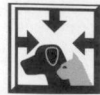 **BASICS**

DEFINITION
• An intrahepatic vascular abnormality causing intrahepatic shunting between the portal and systemic circulation.
• Clinicopathologic hallmark is increased TSBA concentration • Suspected association with PSVA; coexists with irreversible MVD in many small dogs; explains failure of TSBA to normalize after PSVA ligation in many dogs despite complete PSVA occlusion

PATHOPHYSIOLOGY
• Vascular defect not precisely known; suspected abnormal microperfusion between intrahepatic portal and hepatic venules
• Hepatic encephalopathy—seen in a small number of dogs (rare)

SYSTEMS AFFECTED
• Nervous—hepatic encephalopathy; seizures; may observe slow anesthetic recovery and adverse drug reactions • Gastrointestinal—vomiting; diarrhea • Behavioral—various abnormalities but rare compared with PSVA
• Renal/urologic—ammonium biurate crystalluria/urolithiasis (rare)

GENETICS
• Inherited in cairn terriers
• Compelling clinical evidence of inheritance in Yorkshire terriers and Maltese dogs
• Inheritance—complex; not recessive; not sex linked; may be autosomal dominant with variable expression or polygenic with complex expression • Unaffected parents may produce affected progeny

INCIDENCE/PREVALENCE
• Estimates of prevalence not available
• Clinical impression consistent with common occurrence in certain small breed dogs: Yorkshire terriers, cairn terriers, Maltese dogs, shih tzus, and bichons frises

GEOGRAPHIC DISTRIBUTION
Worldwide

SIGNALMENT

Species
Dogs

Breed Predilections
• Usually small breeds • Well described in cairn terriers • Commonly affected: Yorkshire terriers, Maltese dogs, shih tzus, bichons frises. • Clinically documented in dachshunds, miniature schnauzers, Pekinese, Tibetan terriers, border terriers, toy and miniature poodles, and Lhasa apsos
• Rare in large breed dogs.

Mean Age and Range
Congenital; patients detected as juveniles (by 4–6 months of age), as early as 6 weeks

Predominant Sex
N/A

SIGNS

General Comments
• Two groups—asymptomatic (diagnosed in the course of routine screening or diagnostic evaluations for an unrelated health problem) and symptomatic (patients manifest subtle or severe signs related to hepatic encephalopathy, gastrointestinal problems, and renal/urologic problems); symptomatic cases are rare
• Care must be taken to rule out other possible causes before clinical signs or increased TSBA are ascribed to MVD; concurrent illnesses complicate interpretation of TSBA.

Historical Findings
• Asymptomatic dogs—usually unremarkable history; occasionally, delayed anesthetic recovery or drug intolerance
• Symptomatic dogs (no concurrent illness)—nonspecific complaints (anorexia, lethargy, vomiting, or diarrhea); complaints related to a specific body system (abnormal behavior, acute seizure activity, dysuria, or hematuria); may note slow recovery from anesthesia or sedation; some of these dogs may have PSVA missed on radiographic contrast imaging studies (see Imaging; caution)

Physical Examination Findings
• Usually unremarkable • Hepatic encephalopathy—diffuse cerebral abnormalities (e.g., altered behavior, aggression, stupor), blindness, or seizures (See Hepatic Encephalopathy)

CAUSES
Congenital and likely inheritable disorder

RISK FACTORS
Pure bred, terrier lineage

 DIAGNOSIS

DIFFERENTIAL DIAGNOSIS
• PSVA—any asymptomatic young dog with increased TSBA values or in any young dog with hepatic encephalopathy • Symptomatic (> 2 years of age)—APSS owing to acute or chronic inflammatory, infiltrative, neoplastic, toxic, or cirrhotic hepatopathies

CBC/BIOCHEMISTRY/URINALYSIS
• CBC—usually normal • Biochemistry—generally unremarkable; hepatic enzyme activities usually normal (expect high ALP in young patients due to bone growth; confuses significance of ALP activity); mild hypoglobulinemia or hypoalbuminemia noted in approximately 50% of young patients • Urinalysis—rarely may find ammonium biurate crystalluria; urine specific gravity usually normal

OTHER LABORATORY TESTS

TSBA
• Preprandial and postprandial measurements—recommended diagnostic test
• Shunting pattern—common (postprandial TSBA concentrations several-fold higher than preprandial); also seen with PSVA and APSS
• Generally, magnitude of increase is lower than with PSVA but markedly high TSBA in same range as PSVA is occasionally seen; impossible to distinguish between MVD and PSVA on the basis of TSBA values
• Quantitative variations in abnormal TSBA values—cannot be used to judge "severity" of MVD histologic lesion

Clearance Studies
• Affected cairn terrier studies—prove impaired clearance of organic anions (ICG, an indicator/dilution dye used to evaluate liver perfusion and function)
• Findings complement TSBA abnormalities; ICG test does not have clinical utility

IMAGING
• Abdominal radiography—usually normal; microhepatica and renomegaly not noted as in PSVA • Abdominal ultrasonography—no macroscopic shunting vessel as in PSVA; liver size usually normal; experienced ultrasonographer may suspect a hypovascular liver
• Mesenteric portography—routine technique documents lack of PSVA; prolonged parenchymal contrast retention observed with MVD dogs; some liver lobes lack perfusion; **Caution:** in PSVA, shunting vessel may be missed if portography completed only in a single recumbency
• Colorectal scintigraphy—normal or slightly increased shunt fractions in MVD; rules out macroscopic shunting (as in PSVA)

DIAGNOSTIC PROCEDURES
• Liver biopsy—important to sample several liver lobes as lesion may not affect all liver lobes similarly • Microscopic examination of liver tissue—required for definitive diagnosis and to rule out other liver disorders that cause increased TSBA • Needle biopsies—may not demonstrate enough tissue for definitive diagnosis • Wedge or laparoscopically retrieved samples (cup biopsy forceps)—reliably diagnostic • Cannot discriminate between MVD and PSVA in all samples owing to similar histologic features; must consider histologic changes in light of history, clinical and laboratory findings, and results of diagnostic imaging • Some liver lobes show portal veins with lumenal blood—unusual for PSVA

PATHOLOGIC FINDINGS

Gross
Normal appearance and liver size

Microscopic
• Lesions nearly identical to those typical for PSVA but less pronounced; no hepatic

atrophy; unusual apparent apposition of hepatic venules and portal veins without intercalated hepatic parenchyma; increased hepatic arteriole cross-sections in portal triads; juvenile-appearing portal structures distributed in zone 2 of the hepatic lobule; increased number of ill-defined vascular spaces at margin of portal triad (thought to represent lymphatics) • Multifocal lipogranulomas—inconsistent • Some dogs develop lesions characterized by vacuolation of hepatocytes (lipid) and nonsuppurative inflammatory infiltrate in zone 3; consistent with an ongoing degenerative/nonsuppurative inflammatory reaction adjacent to hepatic venules; may progressively lead to a veno-oclusive influence and clinical signs of such.

TREATMENT

APPROPRIATE HEALTH CARE
• Asymptomatic—no specific medical care recommended; watch for adverse reactions to drugs dependent on hepatic first-pass extraction or conjugation • Hepatic encephalopathy and protracted vomiting or diarrhea—hospitalize for supportive care and diagnostic evaluation (rare) • Mild hepatic encephalopathy—controlled with protein-restricted diet and medical treatment of hepatic encephalopathy (see Hepatic Encephalopathy); rare that medical intervention or dietary adjustments are required • Rarely, some dogs with zone 3 degenerative changes develop a progressive decline in hepatic function; manage as with any dog with hepatic insufficiency and ascites

NURSING CARE
N/A

ACTIVITY
N/A

DIET
• Hepatic encephalopathy—restricted quantity-modified quality protein diet; combine with medical management to improve nitrogen tolerance (see Hepatic Encephalopathy)• Asymptomatic—no modification

CLIENT EDUCATION
• Counsel breeder that MVD trait cannot be culled from a kindred. • Counsel breeder that TSBA values cannot be used to grade severity of MVD. • Warn breeder that proven nonaffected parents have produced affected progeny. • Inform client that the value of the TSBA test in detecting disease is to identify affected dogs; results will help avoid future confusion in test interpretation when the dog is presented for other, nonhepatic health problems.

SURGICAL CONSIDERATIONS
N/A

MEDICATIONS

DRUG(S) OF CHOICE
For hepatic encephalopathy—consult Hepatic Encephalopathy

CONTRAINDICATIONS
N/A

PRECAUTIONS
Beware of rare adverse reactions to drugs reliant on hepatic first-pass extraction or metabolism for elimination

POSSIBLE INTERACTIONS
N/A

ALTERNATIVE DRUG(S)
N/A

FOLLOW-UP

PATIENT MONITORING
• Asymptomatic dogs—no specific recommendations; long-term follow-up of dogs lacking the hepatic venule–associated lesion (described above) has shown no progressive deterioration in liver function or shortening of life span.
• Some dogs with MVD develop a progressive increase in TSBA values during the first year of life.

PREVENTION/AVOIDANCE
• Specific recommendations to eliminate MVD from a particular genetic line or breed are not possible—mode of inheritance remains unclarified but is likely polygenic.
• Cairn terriers—seems unlikely that simply breeding unaffected parents can eliminate MVD from a kindred.
• Extending observations in cairn terriers to include all breeds remains speculative; however, the very high clinical incidence in Yorkshire terriers and Maltese dogs suggests that similar recommendations are appropriate.
• In high-incidence kindreds—remain vigilant for the vaguely ill dog that may have a PSVA; surgical exploration can miss PSVA as can portovenography if only done in a single recumbency; colorectal scintigraphy is a good method for definitively detecting portosystemic shunting (hepatofugal blood flow)

POSSIBLE COMPLICATIONS
N/A

EXPECTED COURSE AND PROGNOSIS
• Most affected dogs remain asymptomatic.
• Progressive increase of TSBA values with age (juvenile to adult) has been documented in some asymptomatic dogs.

• Mild to marked progressive increases in TSBA values in an adult likely indicate the presence of an acquired hepatobiliary disorder and should be investigated with appropriate clinical tests.
• Dogs with the zone 3 lesion described above may develop a progressive hepatopathy associated with clinical signs of hepatic encephalopathy, portal hypertension, APSS, ascites, and rarely portal thromboembolism

MISCELLANEOUS

ASSOCIATED CONDITIONS
Breeds most frequently diagnosed with PSVA are also most frequently affected by MVD

AGE-RELATED FACTORS
• TSBA screening of young cairn terriers (prototype for MVD characterization)—majority of dogs diagnosed by 4 months of age
• A few puppies with normal TSBA at 4 months of age had abnormally increased TSBA by 9 months, suggesting a developmental component.

ZOONOTIC POTENTIAL
N/A

PREGNANCY
Affected bitches can carry litters to term.

SYNONYMS
• Hepatic microvascular dysplasia • Hepatic portal hypoplasia (controversial, MVD not proven to be only a portal venous aberration) • Microscopic portovascular dysplasia

SEE ALSO
• Hepatic Encephalopathy
• Portosystemic Vascular Anomaly, Congenital
• Juvenile Fibrosing Liver Disease

ABBREVIATIONS
• ALP = alkaline phosphatase
• APSS = acquired portosystemic shunt
• ICG = indocyanine green
• MVD = microvascular dysplasia
• PSVA = portosystemic vascular anomaly
• TSBA = total serum bile acids

Suggested Reading
Phillips L, Tappe J, Lyman R, et al. Hepatic microvascular dysplasia in dogs. Prog Vet Neurol 1996;7:88–96.
Schermerhorn T, Center SA, Dykes NL, Rowland PH, et al. Characterization of hepatoportal microvascular dysplasia in a kindred of cairn terriers. J Vet Intern Med 1996;10:219–230.
Authors Thomas Schermerhorn and Sharon A. Center
Consulting Editor Sharon A. Center

HEPATOTOXINS

BASICS

DEFINITION
• Endogenous or exogenous substances (drugs, xenobiotics, toxins) that cause dysfunction or clinical or overt pathologic changes in the liver • Direct—cause predictable injury • Idiosyncratic—unpredictable

PATHOPHYSIOLOGY
• The liver is targeted by a wide array of substances because of its location and central role in metabolic and detoxification pathways. • May cause cytopathic injury (necrosis, induced apoptosis, marked hepatocellular injury), cholestasis, or mixed histopathologic patterns of injury • Susceptibility and severity of injury—affected by age, species, nutrition, concurrent drug administration, coexistent disease, hereditary factors, and current or prior exposure to the same or similar compounds

SYSTEMS AFFECTED
• Hepatobiliary—injury depends on factors listed above, toxin concentration, and duration and intermittence of exposure; effects range from high serum enzyme activity and absence of clinical signs to fulminant hepatic failure • Nervous—Hepatic encephalopathy • Renal—hepatorenal syndrome (rare)

GENETICS
Some breeds of dogs may have predisposition to drug-associated hepatotoxicity.

INCIDENCE/PREVALENCE
Not uncommon

GEOGRAPHIC DISTRIBUTION
N/A

SIGNALMENT

Species
• Dogs and cats • Cats may be more susceptible than dogs owing to their lower endogenous detoxification abilities and possibly greater susceptibly to GSH depletion.

Breed Predilections
• Siamese cats—some kindreds suspected to have higher risk because of lower concentrations of glucuronides • Dogs at greater risk for certain drug toxicities—Doberman pinschers and Samoyeds for trimethoprim sulfate; Doberman pinschers for oxibendazole; Labrador retrievers possibly for carprofen, German shepherd dogs for phenobarbital

Mean Age and Range
Young animals (< 16 weeks of age)—immature hepatic drug and toxin metabolism and excretion; less discriminating about substances ingested

Predominant Sex
N/A

SIGNS

General Comments
• Symptoms may reflect chronic long-term exposure or single acute exposure to a toxin • Detailed history—important: include environment, drug, and past medical history

Historical Findings
• Severe malaise to moribund state • Anorexia • Vomiting • Diarrhea • Jaundice

Physical Examination Findings
• Variable fever • Icterus—may develop later (e.g., 48–96 hours postexposure) • Ascites—rare (grave sign) • Severe hepatic failure—hepatic encephalopathy or coma • DIC secondary to liver necrosis—hemorrhage; petechia; ecchymosis

CAUSES

Most Commonly Reported Drugs
• Azole antifungals • Amoxicillin • Azathioprine • Carprofen (dogs) • Diazepam (cats) • Danacrine HCl (dogs) • Acetaminophen (dogs and cats) • Diethylcarbamazine (*Dirofilaria immitis* microfilaria–positive dogs) • Diethylcarbamazine-oxibendazole (dogs) • Galactosamine • Glucocorticoids (dogs) • Griseofulvin (cats) • Halothane (dogs) • Mebendazole (dogs) • Methimazole (cats) • Methoxyflurane (dogs) • Mitotane (dogs) • Phenytoin (dogs) • Primidone (dogs) • Phenobarbital (dogs) • Stanozolol (cats) • Sulfa-type antibiotics (dogs) • Tetracycline (cats, dogs) • Thiacetarsamide (dogs) • Trimethoprim-sulfadiazine (dogs)

Commonly Reported Toxins
• *Amanita* mushrooms • Aflatoxins/mycotoxins • Blue-green algae • Cycad (sago palm nuts) • Chlorinated compounds • Dimethylnitrosamine • Dinitrophenol • Heavy metals (Pb, Zn, Mn, Ar, Fe, Cu) • Phenols (especially cats)

Endotoxins
• Enteric organisms—*Clostridium perfringens*; *Clostridium difficile* • Food poisoning—*Staphylococcus; E. coli; Salmonella*

RISK FACTORS
• Medications influencing hepatic metabolism (phenobarbital: enzyme induction; chloramphenicol, halothane, ranitidine, cimetidine, ketoconazole: enzyme inhibition) • Primary liver disease

DIAGNOSIS

DIFFERENTIAL DIAGNOSIS
• Must distinguish from other disorders affecting the liver • Infectious canine hepatitis • FIP • Toxoplasmosis • Suppurative cholangitis/cholangiohepatitis • DIC • Rocky Mountain spotted fever • Acute hemorrhagic necrotizing pancreatitis • Leptospirosis • Trauma to the liver • Any drug is a potential idiosyncratic hepatotoxin

CBC/BIOCHEMISTRY/URINALYSIS
• PCV and total solids—normal or high in acute hepatotoxicoses (shock or dehydration) • Serum ALT and AST—may be extremely high without trauma; proportionately higher than serum ALP activity; monitor for peak values (often in the thousands) that quickly decline within 7–14 days (many hepatotoxins associated with acute exposure only); no prognostic importance to a single high value; markedly high values may reflect myonecrosis • Creatine kinase—must determine; high activity associated with myonecrosis; some hepatotoxins also concurrently damage muscle (e.g., diazepam toxicity in cats) • Hyperbilirubinemia—may be marked • Albumin, BUN, and glucose—variable • Urinalysis—may note glucosuria and granular casts if renal tubular damage also incurred (e.g., carprofen toxicity)

OTHER LABORATORY TESTS
• Coagulation profile—PT, APTT, FDP, and platelets; AT III variable; monitor for DIC (coagulation tests, RBC morphology: schistocytes) • Nonicteric—TSBA to assess hepatic function • Drug assays—costly; results often delayed

IMAGING
• Abdominal radiography—acute toxicity: normal to large liver; chronic injury: small, normal, or large liver • Abdominal ultrasonography—variable echogenicity and hepatic margins (from normal to overtly abnormal)

DIAGNOSTIC PROCEDURES
Needle biopsy (liver)—may confirm or support the diagnosis; assesses severity if sampled tissue contains enough hepatic lobules to demonstrate zone of injury; if needle biopsies are collected, multiple samples will be necessary to ensure an accurate diagnosis; laparoscopic sampling more dependable for accurate description of hepatobiliary injury

PATHOLOGIC FINDINGS
Variable, depends on toxin

TREATMENT

APPROPRIATE HEALTH CARE
Inpatient—critical care setting required

NURSING CARE
• Prevention or correction of shock • Fluid therapy—maintain hepatic microvascular perfusion and improve oxygen delivery and waste removal; administer 1.5-

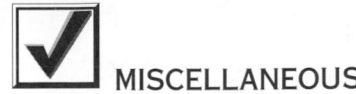

fold maintenance; pay attention to oncotic pressure and avoid overhydration; administer colloid if albumin ≤ 1.5 g/dL
• Colloid administration—plasma preferred for delivery of clotting and anticoagulant precursor proteins • Bleeding tendencies—provide appropriate dose of vitamin K_1 (0.5–1.5 mg/kg SC, up to three doses in 24 hr at 12-hr intervals; administer whole blood or fresh frozen plasma as needed • Nasal oxygen—if problems maintaining blood pressure or evidence of endotoxic shock; may importantly influence delivery of oxygen to the hepatic tissue • Suspect oxidant damage as a component of most hepatotoxic events—administer thiol or GSH donors (see below); GSH important for direct conjugation of certain toxins, facilitates metabolic detoxification of others, and provides important antioxidant function; influences cell resistance to apoptosis, as well as cell repair and regeneration • Monitor urine output—initiate diuretics and dopamine (low-dose CRI) as appropriate; see Renal Failure, Acute • Hypoglycemia—administer dextrose-containing solutions to achieve euglycemia

ACTIVITY
Quiet and rest

DIET
• Protein—normal, unless overt hepatic encepalopathy exists • Initial nutritional support—PPN; phase to TPN if inappetence lasts longers than 5 days; placement of feeding catheter for TPN in central vein problematic if bleeding tendencies exist; later phase to nasogastric or esophageal feeding tube for enteral nutrition • Energy—must be accurately calculated and delivery ensured • Water-soluble vitamins—administered at twofold normal recommendations • Vitamin K_1—0.5–1.5 mg/kg per day for three doses, then weekly

CLIENT EDUCATION
• Discuss the potential for 3–10 days in intensive care. • Warn client that fibrosis or cirrhosis may develop in some patients with fulminant hepatic injury; others may develop chronic hepatitis; others will recover completely.

 MEDICATIONS

DRUG(S) OF CHOICE
• Fluid therapy—non–lactate-containing replacement fluids with fulminant hepatic failure
• Electrolyte supplementation: judicious use of KCl and K phosphate as indicated
• Short-acting glucocorticoids—may be given for endotoxic shock (prednisolone sodium succinate)

• Ampicillin, metronidazole, imipenem or ticarcillin (intravenous)—for infection derived from transmural migration of enteric flora (aerobic and anaerobic bacteria), along with parenteral aminoglycoside or enrofloxacin
• Antioxidant therapy—for crisis intervention: N-acetylcysteine for acute or fulminant hepatic necrosis (140 mg/kg IV load, followed by 70 mg/kg IV q6–8h), dilute in saline and administer through a nonpyrogenic 0.25 μm filter; when stable, use oral route: S-adenosylmethionine, based on experimental work, functions as a hepatoprotectant against a variety of hepatotoxins, dose based on studies in dogs and cats (20 mg/kg enteric-coated tablet PO q24h, on an empty stomach); vitamin E (α-tocopherol acetate): oral or injectable forms (10 IU/kg PO q24h)
• Hepatoprotectants—silymarin (milk thistle extract, 60%–80% potency); proven useful in Amanita and other hepatotoxins (20–50 mg/kg PO q24h)
• Ursodeoxycholic acid—not justified unless liver injury becomes chronic (10–15 mg/kg PO q12–24h)

CONTRAINDICATIONS
Avoid or assess risk for drugs known to lead to hepatotoxicosis or that require or inhibit hepatic metabolism

PRECAUTIONS
• Drugs listed as hepatotoxins—use with caution • Catheterization of large vessels—use caution if overt signs of coagulopathy exist

POSSIBLE INTERACTIONS N/A

ALTERNATIVE DRUG(S) N/A

 FOLLOW-UP

PATIENT MONITORING
• Prevent hypothermia.
• Blood glucose, electrolytes, and PCV—monitor daily; fluctuations may occur rapidly
• Serum biochemical analysis—repeat every 48 hr

PREVENTION/AVOIDANCE
Close scrutiny of environment and future medications

POSSIBLE COMPLICATIONS
• DIC
• Hepatic encephalopathy
• Progressive hepatic failure

EXPECTED COURSE AND PROGNOSIS
• 3–5 days are needed to estimate prognosis
• Progressive worsening of status: intractable emesis and hematemesis, intolerance to supportive treatments, oliguria, DIC, and hepatic encephalopathy—negative indicators
• Postnecrotic cirrhosis is possible.

✓ **MISCELLANEOUS**

ASSOCIATED CONDITIONS
• Hepatitis • Fibrosis • Hepatic encephalopathy • Hepatic lipidosis (cats) • Icterus • Ascites • Hypoglycemia

AGE-RELATED FACTORS
• Young animals—may have greater exposure and risk for toxin ingestion • Older animals—may have diseases requiring drug therapy that increases their risk (e.g., phenobarbital)

ZOONOTIC POTENTIAL
N/A

PREGNANCY
N/A

SYNONYMS
N/A

SEE ALSO
• Cirrhosis and Fibrosis of the Liver
• Hepatic Encephalopathy
• Hepatic Failure, Acute
• Poisoning (Intoxication)
• Acetaminophen Toxicity

ABBREVIATIONS
• APTT = activated partial thromboplastin time • ALP = alkaline phosphatase • ALT = alanine aminotransferase • AST = aspartate aminotransferase • AT III = antithrombin III • BUN = blood urea nitrogen • CRI = constant rate infusion • DIC = disseminated intravascular coagulation • FDP = fibrin degradation products • FIP = feline infectious peritonitis • GSH = glutathione • PCV = packed cell volume • PPN = partial parenteral nutrition • PT = prothrombin time • TPN = total parenteral nutrition

Suggested Reading
Center SA. Acute hepatic injury: hepatic necrosis and fluminant hepatic failure. In: Guilford WG, Center SA, Strombeck DR, et al., eds. Strombeck's small animal gastroenterology. 3rd ed. Philadelphia: Saunders, 1996:654–704.
Chitturi S, Farrell GC. Drug-induced liver disease. Curr Treat Options Gastroenterol 2000;3:457–462.
George CF, George RH. The liver and response to drugs. In: Wright R, Alberti KG, Karran S, eds. Liver and biliary diseases. Philadelphia: Saunders, 1985:415–452.
Jaeschke H, Gores GJ, Cederbaum AI, et al. Mechanisms of hepatotoxicity. Toxicol Sci 2002;65:166–176.
Author Mark E. Hitt
Consulting Editor Sharon A. Center

HEPATOZOONOSIS

 BASICS

OVERVIEW
• Systemic infection with the protozoan *Hepatozoon americanum*
• May involve bone, liver, spleen, muscles, capillaries of the myocardium, and small intestinal epithelium
• Dogs—more common in the southern and southwestern U.S.
• Cats—uncommon in the U.S.; one reported case from Hawaii

SIGNALMENT
• Dogs and rarely cats
• No age, breed, or sex predilections

SIGNS
• Usually subclinical infection
• May be intermittent and recurrent
• Severe clinical disease—fever; inappetence; weight loss; bloody diarrhea; neurologic (hyperesthesia over the paralumbar regions)

CAUSE & RISK FACTORS
Amblyomma maculatum—tick; bite or ingestion

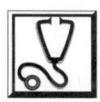 **DIAGNOSIS**

DIFFERENTIAL DIAGNOSIS
• Neoplasia
• Endocarditis
• Immune-mediated polyarthritis or polymyositis
• Chagas disease
• Leishmaniasis
• Babesiosis
• Ehrlichiosis
• Diskospondylitis

CBC/BIOCHEMISTRY/URINALYSIS
• Neutrophilic leukocytosis, sometimes with a left shift
• Anemia—mild to moderate
• High serum ALP activity

OTHER LABORATORY TESTS
Blood films—identify organisms in circulating neutrophils and monocytes

IMAGING
Radiographs—pelvis, lumbar vertebrae, and long bones; reveal periosteal proliferation

DIAGNOSTIC PROCEDURES
Muscle biopsy

PATHOLOGIC FINDINGS
• Cachexia
• Muscle atrophy
• Enlarged liver and spleen—may contain schizont stages on histopathology
• Periosteal proliferation of bone

 TREATMENT

• Inpatient—for severe pain; provide symptomatic relief
• Pain management—as for any musculoskeletal disease
• General activity level and appetite—depend on pain level
• Not possible to predict responsiveness to drug therapy (except pain management) because data are limited

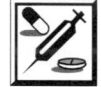 **MEDICATIONS**

DRUG(S)
• Mostly palliative
• Glucocorticoids—may give temporary relief
• NSAIDs
• Combination therapy initially:
Trimethoprim = sulfadiazine—15 mg/kg PO q12h for 14 days
Clindamycin—10 mg/kg PO q8h for 14 days
Pyrimethamine—0.25 mg/kg PO q24h for 14 days

• Followed with long-term therapy:
Desoquinate 10–20 mg/kg PO q12h for up to 33 months

CONTRAINDICATIONS/POSSIBLE INTERACTIONS
None

 FOLLOW-UP

PATIENT MONITORING
• Difficult to monitor organisms in chronically infected dogs
• Best to monitor for improvement

PREVENTION/AVOIDANCE
Control ticks within the household or kennel

POSSIBLE COMPLICATIONS
• Glucocorticoids—may exacerbate clinical disease
• Radiographic changes may never occur.

EXPECTED COURSE AND PROGNOSIS
• Infection often asymptomatic
• Long-term quality of life may not be satisfactory, even with good therapeutic results.

 MISCELLANEOUS

ZOONOTIC POTENTIAL
No reported risk to humans

ABBREVIATIONS
ALP = alkaline phosphatase
NSAIDS = nonsteroidal antiinflammatories

Suggested Reading
Craig TM. Hepatozoonosis. In: Greene CE, ed., Infectious diseases of the dog and cat. Philadelphia: Saunders, 1998:458–465.
Macintire DK, Vincent-Johnson NA, Kane CW, et al. Treatment of dogs infected with *Hepatozoon americanum*: 53 cases (1989–1998). J Am Vet Med Assoc 2001;218:77–82.
Author Johnny D. Hoskins
Consulting Editor Stephen C. Barr

BASICS

OVERVIEW
• A systemic, usually fatal disease in young pups caused by CHV • CHV—common in the worldwide dog population but disease is infrequent; remains latent in several tissues after primary infection; latent in the trigeminal nerve ganglia; may be excreted in nasal secretions at unpredictable intervals; recrudescence can be provoked by stress or corticosteroid treatment; isolated from dogs with respiratory illness, but no causal link demonstrated • Litter mortality high; poor regulation of body temperature and immature immune response mechanisms believed responsible for the exceptional susceptibility of pups < 2–3 weeks of age • All organ systems are affected. • Clinical disease rare in dogs older than 3–4 weeks of age • Mature nonpregnant animals usually have inapparent, localized infections in the nasopharynx or external genitalia. • Transplacental infections during the last 3–4 weeks of gestation—fetal deaths, often with mummification; abortions; birth of dead or dying pups • Localized genital infections have been reported in both sexes.

SIGNALMENT
• Only members of the canine family (dogs, coyotes, and wolves) are susceptible. • Death usually occurs between 9 and 14 days after birth; range is from 1 day (prenatal infection) to about 1 month (neonatal infection). • Most commonly reported in purebred dogs, although there is no breed predilection.

SIGNS
• Dyspnea • Serous to mucopurulent nasal discharge • Anorexia • Grayish yellow or green, soft, odorless stool • Persistent, agonizing crying • Encephalitic signs • Severe gasping before death • Petechial hemorrhages on the mucous membranes occasionally seen • The incubation period in neonatal pups 4–6 days • Onset sudden; death occurs 12–36 hr later. • Some pups are found dead without premonitory signs. • Occasionally, pups with mild signs survive but often later develop ataxia, persistent vestibular signs, ataxia, or blindness. • Mature females may have lymphofollicular or hemorrhagic lesions in the vagina. • Conjunctivitis—observed on rare occasions • CHV keratitis—reported but not confirmed

CAUSES & RISK FACTORS
• CHV—typical herpesvirus; only one serotype described; an atypical virus was isolated in Great Britain from dog-pox–like lesions on the genital tract that was associated with male genital lesions, abortions, and stillbirths.

• Young, susceptible females and their newborn pups at greatest risk
• Closed breeding kennels—CHV endemic; infection is less common and most adults are immune; newly introduced susceptible breeding bitches at high risk
• Abortion storms with massive pup losses have occurred when pregnant bitches maintained in private homes were assembled for whelping.

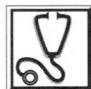

DIAGNOSIS

DIFFERENTIAL DIAGNOSIS
• Bacteria (brucellosis, coliform bacteria, or streptococci), toxoplasmosis, toxic substances—no typical gross lesions of CHV
• MVC (canine parvovirus type 1)—causes enteric or respiratory disease; no characteristic CHV lesions
• Distemper and canine adenovirus type 1 (canine hepatitis)—uncommon; no characteristic CHV renal lesions

CBC/BIOCHEMISTRY/URINALYSIS
Thrombocytopenia may occur.

OTHER LABORATORY TESTS
Serologic testing of little value

DIAGNOSTIC PROCEDURES
• Frozen tissue sections—immuno-fluorescence or immunoperoxidase staining; reveal viral antigen in most organs, especially in the lesion areas
• Cell cultures—viral isolation readily accomplished from several tissues, especially lung and kidney; refrigerate, do not freeze, samples.

PATHOLOGIC FINDINGS
Gross
• Characteristic lesions—disseminated focal necrosis; hemorrhage in several organs
• Kidneys—diffuse hemorrhagic areas, necrotic foci, and hemorrhagic infarcts pathognomonic
• Lungs, liver, adrenal glands—diffuse foci of hemorrhage and necrosis
• Small intestine variably affected
• Lymph nodes and spleen—generalized enlargement; consistent finding

Histopathologic
• Foci of perivascular necrosis—with or without mild cellular infiltration; kidney, lung, liver, spleen, small intestine, and brain
• Lesions in the CNS of recovered pups—nonsuppurative ganglioneuritis; meningo-encephalitis; necrotic changes in the cerebellum and retina; acidophilic intra-nuclear inclusions may be observed but are not abundant.
• Necrotizing lesions—may be seen in fetal placentas

TREATMENT
• Not recommended
• Antiviral drug therapy—generally unsuccessful
• Immune sera from recovered bitches—beneficial in reducing pup deaths when antiserum is given before onset of illness

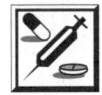

MEDICATIONS
DRUG(S) N/A
CONTRAINDICATIONS/POSSIBLE INTERACTIONS N/A

FOLLOW-UP
• Normal litters can be expected from bitches that have suffered pup losses or abortions.
• No vaccine • Isolate pregnant dams, especially young bitches, when introduced into a kennel; adults commonly shed latent CHV in nasal secretions for 1–2 weeks after encountering newly introduced dogs.
• Surviving pups may suffer deafness, blindness, encephalopathy, or renal damage.

MISCELLANEOUS
AGE-RELATED FACTORS
• Dogs of all ages susceptible • Fatal illness occurs only in pups infected during the neonatal period (1–10 days after birth).

ZOONOTIC POTENTIAL
None

PREGNANCY
Infection of dams during last 3 weeks of gestation—fetal infections with death and mummification, or ill pups that die shortly after birth

ABBREVIATIONS
• CHV = canine herpesvirus
• MVC = minute virus of canines

Suggested Reading
Carmichael LE, Greene CE. Canine herpesvirus infection. In: Greene CE, ed. Infectious diseases of the dog and cat. Philadelphia: Saunders, 1998:28–32.
Author Leland Carmichael
Consulting Editor Stephen C. Barr

HIATAL HERNIA

BASICS

OVERVIEW
• Protrusion of abdominal contents into the thoracic cavity through the esophageal hiatus of the diaphragm; can be intermittent or persistent
• Three basic types—(1) sliding: gastroesophageal junction moves cranially to the diaphragm (most common); (2) paraesophageal: gastroesophageal junction remains in the normal position but the gastric fundus moves cranial to the diaphragm (rare); (3) combination of sliding and paraesophageal

SIGNALMENT
• Dogs and cats
• Congenital in most patients (< 1 year old), but can be acquired from trauma
• Possible predilection for males
• Chinese shar-pei breed may be over-represented.

SIGNS
• Vomiting
• Regurgitation
• Hypersalivation—ptyalism
• Hematemesis
• Dyspnea

CAUSES & RISK FACTORS
• Congenital
• Traumatic
• May be concurrent gastroesophageal reflux and subsequent esophagitis—depends on the amount of functional intraabdominal esophagus remaining

DIAGNOSIS

DIFFERENTIAL DIAGNOSIS
• Megaesophagus
• Esophageal obstruction
• Gastroesophageal intussusception—characterized by a highly fatal acute onset of severe vomiting, hematemesis, abdominal pain, and dyspnea in young, large-breed dogs with concurrent esophageal disease (usually megaesophagus); German shepherd breed appears to be overrepresented; rare

CBC/BIOCHEMISTRY/URINALYSIS
Generally within normal limits

OTHER LABORATORY TESTS
N/A

IMAGING

Thoracic Radiography
May show a dilated esophagus, soft tissue opacity in the caudal thorax dorsal to the vena cava, absence of the right crus of the diaphragm, or an alveolar pattern indicating aspiration pneumonia; because of the dynamic nature, false-negative results are often obtained

Contrast Esophagram
Evaluates esophageal size and gastric fundus location

Contrast Fluoroscopy
Best way to evaluate gastric motility and intermittent herniation

DIAGNOSTIC PROCEDURES
Esophagoscopy may reveal evidence of inflammation (erythema, erosions) consistent with reflux esophagitis in the distal esophagus.

TREATMENT
• Best initial approach is conservative medical treatment to control esophagitis and clinical signs.
• A low-fat, high-protein diet and elevated feedings
• Lack of response warrants surgical intervention.
• Untreated animals are predisposed to developing chronic esophagitis with mucosal ulceration, aspiration pneumonia, strictures, and strangulation of abdominal organs.

• Surgical intervention consists of anatomic replacement of herniated organs, reduction in size of the esophageal hiatus, phrenicoesophageal pexy, and a left-sided fundic gastropexy.
• Use of an antireflux surgical procedure (fundoplication) is controversial and is indicated for patients with documented primary incompetence of the lower esophageal sphincter (rare).
• Client education should include the importance of dietary management and the potential for aspiration pneumonia.
• Parenteral fluids and aggressive nursing care are needed if concurrent aspiration pneumonia exists.

 MEDICATIONS

DRUG(S)
• Histamine H_2-antagonist (e.g., cimetidine 10 mg/kg PO q6–8h or ranitidine 2 mg/kg PO q12h) to reduce gastric acid production and treat gastroesophageal reflux; an alternative antisecretory drug is the proton pump inhibitor omeprazole (0.7 mg/kg PO q24h).
• Prokinetic agent (e.g., metoclopramide 0.2–0.5 mg/kg PO q8h) to increase lower esophageal sphincter pressure
• Appropriate antibiotics on the basis of culture and sensitivity results as needed to treat concurrent aspiration pneumonia

CONTRAINDICATIONS/POSSIBLE INTERACTIONS
Avoid anticholinergic agents because of their negative effects on gastric motility.

 FOLLOW-UP

• Postoperative megaesophagus has been reported.
• Aspiration pneumonia—common secondary complication
• Prognosis guarded; postsurgical complications include recurrent herniation, gastric dilatation (without volvulus), and gastroesophageal reflux.

 MISCELLANEOUS

Suggested Reading

Ellison G, Lewis D, Phillips L, et al. Esophageal hiatal hernia in small animals: literature review and a modified surgical technique. J Am Anim Hosp Assoc 1987;23:391–399.
Prymak C, Saunders M, Washabau R. Hiatal hernia repair by restoration and stabilization of normal anatomy. Vet Surg 1989;18(5):386–391.
Waldron D, Leib M. Hiatal hernia. In: Bojrab MJ, ed. Disease mechanisms in small animal surgery. 2nd ed. Philadelphia: Lea & Febiger, 1993:210–213.

Authors Albert E. Jergens and James E. Williams, Jr.
Consulting Editor Albert E. Jergens

BASICS

DEFINITION
The malformation and degeneration of the coxofemoral joints

PATHOPHYSIOLOGY
• Developmental defect initiated by a genetic predisposition to subluxation of the immature hip joint
• Poor congruence between the femoral head and acetabulum—creates abnormal forces across the joint; interferes with normal development (leading to irregularly shaped acetabula and femoral heads); overloads the articular cartilage (causing microfractures and DJD)

SYSTEMS AFFECTED
Musculoskeletal

GENETICS
• Complicated, polygenetic transmission
• Expression—determined by an interaction of genetic and environmental factors
• Heritability index—depends on breed

INCIDENCE/PREVALENCE
• One of the most common skeletal diseases encountered clinically in dogs
• Actual incidence—unknown; depends on breed

GEOGRAPHIC DISTRIBUTION
N/A

SIGNALMENT

Species
Dogs

Breed Predilection
• Large breeds—St. Bernards; German shepherds; Labrador retrievers; golden retrievers; rottweilers
• Smaller breeds—may be affected; less likely to demonstrate clinical signs

Mean Age and Range
• Begins in the immature dog
• Clinical signs—may develop after 4 months of age; may develop later with DJD

Predominant Sex
None

SIGNS

General Comments
• Depend on the degree of joint laxity, degree of DJD, and chronicity of the disease
• Early—related to joint laxity
• Later—related to joint degeneration

Historical Findings
• Decreased activity
• Difficulty rising
• Reluctance to run, jump, or climb stairs
• Intermittent or persistent hind limb lameness—often worse after exercise
• Bunny-hopping or swaying gait
• Narrow stance in the hind limbs

Physical Examination Findings
• Pain
• Joint laxity (positive Ortolani sign)—characteristic of early disease; may not be seen in chronic cases owing to periarticular fibrosis
• Crepitus
• Decreased range of motion in the hip joints
• Atrophy of thigh muscles
• Hypertrophy of shoulder muscles

CAUSES
• Genetic predisposition for hip laxity
• Rapid weight gain, nutrition level, and pelvic muscle mass—influence expression and progression

RISK FACTORS
N/A

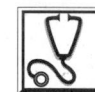 DIAGNOSIS

DIFFERENTIAL DIAGNOSIS
• Degenerative myelopathy
• Lumbosacral instability
• Bilateral stifle disease
• Panosteitis
• Polyarthropathies

CBC/BIOCHEMISTRY/URINALYSIS
N/A

OTHER LABORATORY TESTS
N/A

IMAGING
• Ventrodorsal hip-extended radiographs—commonly used for diagnosis; may need sedation or general anesthesia for accurate positioning
• Early radiographic signs—subluxation of the hip joint with poor congruence between the femoral head and acetabulum; initially normally shaped acetabulum and femoral head; with disease progression, shallow acetabulum, and flattened femoral head
• Radiographic evidence of DJD—flattening of the femoral head; shallow acetabulum; periarticular osteophyte production; thickening of the femoral neck; sclerosis of the subchondral bone; periarticular soft tissue fibrosis

• Distraction radiographs—quantify joint laxity; may accentuate the laxity for more accurate diagnosis
• PennHIP registry uses distraction radiography method. Dorsolateral subluxation (DLS) is another available distraction radiography method.
• Dorsal acetabular rim view radiographs—evaluate acetabular rim; assess dorsal coverage of the femoral head

DIAGNOSTIC PROCEDURES
N/A

PATHOLOGIC FINDINGS
• Early—normal femoral head and acetabulum; may note joint laxity and excess synovial fluid
• With progression—malformed acetabulum and femoral head; synovitis; articular cartilage degeneration
• Chronic—may note full-thickness cartilage erosion

 TREATMENT

APPROPRIATE HEALTH CARE
• May treat with conservative medical therapy or surgery
• Outpatient unless surgery is performed
• Depends on the patient's size, age, and intended function; severity of joint laxity; degree of DJD; clinician's preference; and financial considerations of the owner

NURSING CARE
• Physiotherapy (passive joint motion)—decreases joint stiffness; helps maintain muscle integrity
• Swimming (hydrotherapy)—excellent nonconcussive form of physical therapy; encourages joint and muscle activity without exacerbating joint injury

ACTIVITY
• As tolerated
• Swimming—recommended to maintain joint mobility while minimizing weight-bearing activities

DIET
Weight control—important; decrease the load applied to the painful joint; minimize weight gain associated with reduced exercise

CLIENT EDUCATION
- Discuss the heritability of the disease.
- Explain that medical therapy is palliative, because the joint instability is not corrected.
- Warn the client that joint degeneration often progresses unless a corrective osteotomy procedure is performed early in the disease.
- Explain that surgical procedures can salvage joint function once severe joint degeneration occurs.

SURGICAL CONSIDERATIONS

Triple Pelvic Osteotomy
- Corrective procedure; designed to reestablish congruity between the femoral head and the acetabulum
- Immature patient (6–12 months of age)
- Rotate acetabulum—improve dorsal coverage of the femoral head; correct the forces acting on the joint; minimize the progression of DJD; may allow development of a more normal joint if performed early (before severe degeneration develops)

Juvenile Pubic Symphysiodesis
- Newly developed technique still under evaluation
- Pubic symphysis is fused at an early age (using electrocautery).
- Causes ventroversion of the acetabulum to better cover the femoral head
- Improves joint congruence and stability—similar effects as TPO without surgical implants
- Minimal morbidity; easy to perform—must be performed very early (3–4 months of age) to achieve effect; minimal effect achieved if performed after 6 months of age

Total Hip Replacement
- Indicated to salvage function in mature dogs with severe degenerative disease that is unresponsive to medical therapy
- Pain-free joint function—reported in >90% of cases
- Unilateral joint replacement—provides acceptable function in ~80% of cases
- Complications—luxation; sciatic neuropraxia; infection

Excision Arthroplasty
- Removal of the femoral head and neck to eliminate joint pain
- Primarily a salvage procedure—for significant DJD; when pain cannot be controlled medically; when total hip replacement is cost-prohibitive
- Best results—small, light dogs (< 20 kg); patients with good hip musculature
- A slightly abnormal gait often persists.
- Postoperative muscle atrophy—common, particularly in large dogs

MEDICATIONS

DRUG(S) OF CHOICE
- Analgesics and anti-inflammatory drugs—minimize joint pain (and thus stiffness and muscle atrophy caused by limited usage); decrease synovitis
- Medical therapy—does not correct biomechanical abnormality; degenerative process likely to progress; often provides only temporary relief of signs
- Agents—carprofen (2.2 mg/kg PO q12h or 4.4 mg/kg PO q24h); etodolac (10–15 mg/kg PO q24h); deracoxib (3–4 mg/kg PO q24h for 1 week for postoperative pain) (1–2 mg/kg PO q24h for long-term treatment over 7 days)

CONTRAINDICATIONS
Avoid corticosteroids—potential side effects; articular cartilage damage associated with long-term use

PRECAUTIONS
- NSAIDs—gastrointestinal upset may preclude use in some patients.
- Carprofen—reported to cause acute hepatotoxicity in some dogs

POSSIBLE INTERACTIONS
N/A

ALTERNATIVE DRUG(S)
Polysulfated glycosaminoglycans, glucosamine, and chondroitin sulfate—may have a chondroprotective effect in DJD; not fully evaluated for treatment of hip dysplasia

FOLLOW-UP

PATIENT MONITORING
- Clinical and radiographic monitoring—assess progression.
- Medical treatment—clinical deterioration suggests an alternative dosage or medication or surgical intervention.
- Triple pelvic osteotomy—monitored radiographically; assess healing, implant stability, joint congruence, and progression of DJD.
- Hip replacement—monitored radiographically; assess implant stability.

PREVENTION/AVOIDANCE
- Best prevented by not breeding affected dogs
- Pelvic radiographs—may help identify phenotypically abnormal dogs; may not identify all dogs carrying the disease
- Do not repeat dam–sire breedings that result in affected offspring.
- Special diets designed for rapidly growing large-breed dogs—may decrease the severity

POSSIBLE COMPLICATIONS
N/A

EXPECTED COURSE AND PROGNOSIS
Joint degeneration usually progresses—most patients lead normal lives with proper medical or surgical management.

MISCELLANEOUS

ASSOCIATED CONDITIONS
N/A

AGE-RELATED FACTORS
N/A

ZOONOTIC POTENTIAL
N/A

PREGNANCY
Do not breed affected dogs; added weight owing to pregnancy may exacerbate clinical signs.

ABBREVIATIONS
DJD = degenerative joint disease
TPO = triple pelvic osteotomy
NSAIDs = nonsteroidal antiinflammatory drugs

Suggested Reading
Manley PA. The hip joint. In: Slatter D, ed. Textbook of small animal surgery. 2nd ed. Philadelphia: Saunders, 1993:1786–1804.
McLaughlin RM, Tomlinson J. Alternative surgical treatments for canine hip dysplasia. Vet Med 1996;91:137–143.
McLaughlin RM, Tomlinson J. Radiographic diagnosis of canine hip dysplasia. Vet Med 1996;91:36–47.
McLaughlin RM, Tomlinson J. Treating canine hip dysplasia with triple pelvic osteotomy. Vet Med 1996;91:126–136.
Rettenmaier JL, Constantinescu GM. Canine hip dysplasia. Compend Contin Educ Pract Vet 1991;13:643–653.
Swainson SW, Conzemius MG, Riedesel EA, Smith GK, Riley CB. Effect of pubic symphysiodesis on pelvic development in the skeletally immature greyhound. Vet Surg 29:178–190, 2000.
Tomlinson J, McLaughlin RM. Canine hip dysplasia: developmental factors, clinical signs and initial examination steps. Vet Med 1996;91:26–33.
Tomlinson J, McLaughlin RM. Medically managing canine hip dysplasia. Vet Med 1996;91:48–53.
Tomlinson J, McLaughlin RM. Total hip replacement. Vet Med 1996;91:118–124.
Wallace LJ. Canine hip dysplasia: past and present. Semin Vet Med Surg 1987;2:92–106.
Author Ron M. McLaughlin
Consulting Editor Peter K. Shires

HISTIOCYTOMA

 BASICS

OVERVIEW
Benign skin tumor arising from Langerhans cells (e.g., histiocytes) of the skin

SIGNALMENT
• Common in dogs but extremely rare in cats
• More than 50% of patients are dogs < 2 years old.
• Flat-coated retrievers, bull terriers, boxers, dachshunds, cocker spaniels, Great Danes, and Shetland sheepdogs—may be predisposed
• No breed predilection in cats
• No sex predilection in cats or dogs

SIGNS
• Small, firm, dome- or button-shaped, dermoepithelial mass that may be ulcerated
• Fast growing, nonpainful, usually solitary
• Common sites—head, ear pinna, and limbs
• Occasionally multiple cutaneous nodules or plaques

CAUSES & RISK FACTORS
Unknown

 DIAGNOSIS

DIFFERENTIAL DIAGNOSIS
Histopathologic examination and immuno-histochemical stains—distinguish from focal granulomatous inflammation, transmissible venereal tumor, lymphosarcoma, and mast cell tumor (latter stains positive with tolui-dine blue; histiocytoma does not)

CBC/BIOCHEMISTRY/URINALYSIS
Usually normal

OTHER LABORATORY TESTS
N/A

IMAGING
N/A

OTHER DIAGNOSTIC PROCEDURES
• Cytologic examination—fine-needle aspirate; reveals pleomorphic round cells, 12–24 μm in diameter; variable-sized and -shaped nuclei; variable amounts of pale blue cytoplasm that resemble monocytes
• Mitotic index usually high
• May see substantial lymphocyte, plasma cell, and neutrophil infiltration

PATHOLOGIC FINDINGS
• Histopathologic—characterized by uniform sheets of histiocytes that penetrate the dermis and subcutis; cells may be densely packed in deeper layers of the dermis.
• Collagen fibers and skin adnexa—may be displaced
• Immunophenotyping—confirms cell origin

 TREATMENT

• May spontaneously regress within 3 months
• Surgical excision or cryosurgery—generally curative
• Important to differentiate histiocytoma from malignant tumor if client elects the wait-and-see approach

MEDICATIONS

DRUG(S)
N/A

CONTRAINDICATIONS/POSSIBLE INTERACTIONS
N/A

 FOLLOW-UP

PATIENT MONITORING
Surgical excision—recommended if mass has not spontaneously regressed within 3 months

EXPECTED COURSE AND PROGNOSIS
• Prognosis—excellent with surgical removal
• Spontaneous regression possible within 3 months

 MISCELLANEOUS

Suggested Reading
Thomas RC, Fox LE. Tumors of the skin and subcutis. In: Morrison WB, ed. Cancer in dogs and cats: medical and surgical management. Baltimore: Williams & Wilkins, 1998:489–510.
Author Joanne C. Graham
Consulting Editor Wallace B. Morrison

HISTIOCYTOSIS—DOGS

 BASICS

OVERVIEW
• Uncommon disorder resulting from proliferation of cells from the monocyte/macrophage and Langerhans/dendritic cell lineages
• Organ systems affected—skin; lymphatic; hemic; nervous; ophthalmic; musculoskeletal; and respiratory
• Many authors have attempted to differentiate systemic and cutaneous histiocytosis from malignant histiocytosis based on cytologic appearance of the histiocytes and tissue distribution.
• Malignant histiocytosis—also referred to as disseminated histiocytic sarcoma
• Combinations of immunohistochemical markers may be needed to confirm histiocytic origin and to differentiate these diseases from each other as well as from histiocytic inflammation.

SIGNALMENT

Systemic/Cutaneous
• Young to middle-aged dogs (mean age 5 years)
• No apparent gender predilection
• Systemic disease has been reported predominantly in Bernese mountain dogs, but it has been reported in other breeds.
• Cutaneous disease is not restricted to particular breeds.

Malignant
• Older dogs (mean age 7 years)
• Reported in a variety of breeds but most commonly in Bernese mountain dogs
• Has been documented in cats

SIGNS

General Comments
• Systemic histiocytosis—chronic and fluctuating debilitating disease; multiple clinical episodes and asymptomatic periods may occur • Cutaneous histiocytosis—often a fluctuating, chronic course; spontaneous regression of lesions may occur • Malignant histiocytosis—rapidly progressive and fatal

Historical Findings
• Lethargy • Anorexia • Weight loss
• Respiratory stertor • Coughing • Dyspnea
• Signs of systemic illness may not be present in dogs with cutaneous histiocytosis and in some dogs with systemic histiocytosis

Physical Examination Findings
Systemic Histiocytosis
• Marked predilection for skin, lymph nodes
• Cutaneous masses—multiple; nodular; well-circumscribed and often ulcerated, crusted or alopecic; occur commonly on the muzzle, nasal planum, eyelids, flank, and scrotum
• Moderate to severe peripheral lymphadenomegaly is often present.

• Ocular manifestations—conjunctivitis; chemosis; scleritis; episcleritis; episcleral nodules; corneal edema; anterior and posterior uveitis; retinal detachment; glaucoma; and exophthalmos • Abnormal respiratory sounds and/or nasal mucosa infiltration • Organomegaly occurs with systemic involvement.
Cutaneous Histiocytosis
• Lesions involve skin and subcutis; multiple nodules or plaques on the head and neck, trunk, extremities, and scrotum
• No cases involving the eye have been reported. • No systemic organ involvement
Malignant Histiocytosis
• Pallor, weakness, dyspnea with abnormal lung sounds, and neurologic signs (e.g., seizures, central disturbances, posterior paresis)—common • Moderate to severe lymphadenomegaly and hepatosplenomegaly
• Masses—occasionally palpated in the liver and/or spleen
• Eyes and skin—rarely affected

CAUSES & RISK FACTORS
• Systemic and cutaneous histiocytosis—reactive (inflammatory), non-neoplastic diseases arising from expansion of activated dermal Langerhans cells; the absence of infectious agents and responses to immunomodulating drugs suggest immune dysregulatory mechanisms may be involved
• Malignant histiocytosis (disseminated histiocytic sarcoma)—neoplastic histiocytic disease; origin of proliferating dendritic cells is unknown • Familial disease of Bernese mountain dogs—polygenic mode of inheritance; heritability is 0.298; accounts for up to 25% of all tumors in this breed • Flat-coated retrievers, Golden retrievers, and rottweilers appear to be predisposed, suggesting genetic factors.

 DIAGNOSIS

DIFFERENTIAL DIAGNOSIS
• Histiocytic lymphoma—histiocytosis may be difficult to differentiate from the histiocytic variation of lymphoma; definitive diagnosis often requires special staining and immunohistochemical markers
• Cutaneous histiocytoma—common benign skin tumor of young dogs derived from epitheliotropic, CD4 and Thy-1 (CD90) negative Langerhans cells; solitary, alopecic, frequently ulcerated masses; lymph nodes may be rarely involved; regression without treatment often occurs
• Malignant fibrous histiocytoma—locally aggressive soft tissue sarcoma composed of histiocytes and fibroblasts; no breed predilection; distant metastases are rare; in the spleen, biologic behavior is more aggressive (see Fibrohistiocytic Splenic

Nodules below); histopathology may be similar to malignant histiocytosis and histiocytic sarcomas; immunohistochemical staining is positive for actin and vimentin and negative for CD18, indicating a mesenchymal origin
• Localized histiocytic sarcoma—tumors of dendritic cell origin that often occur in the subcutis on limbs; other subcutaneous sites are possible; metastases are possible; when these tumors arise in other primary locations, such as the spleen and joints, they are frequently associated with a very high rate of metastases to lungs, lymph nodes, and other organs
• Fibrohistiocytic splenic nodules—nodular splenomegaly resulting from proliferation of fibrohistiocytic cells within splenic lymphoid nodules; retrievers, German shepherds, and possibly cocker spaniels appear to be overrepresented; a spectrum of splenic lesions occurs: grade I: fibrous and histiocytoid cells proliferating as a component of lymphoid nodular hyperplasia (≥ 70% lymphoid cells), grade II: hyperplastic lymphoid nodules containing equal proportions of lymphoid (40%–69%) cells and fibrohistiocytic cells, and grade III: pleomorphic sarcoma with < 40% lymphoid cells; lymphoid-to-histiocytic proportion is predictive of survival; prognosis for grade III is poor; metastases may occur to lungs, lymph nodes, omentum, and organs
• Splenic histiocytosis—splenomegaly with distinctive microscopic changes, including myeloid metaplasia (diffuse hematopoiesis), histiocytosis, erythrophagocytosis, and thrombosis with infarction; multicentric organ involvement is common; prognosis is grave, and the presence of giant cells may be predictive of a fatal outcome; currently the disease is descriptive but may represent part of the spectrum of histiocytic diseases including malignant histiocytosis and histiocytic sarcoma; immune-mediated diseases and systemic infections may also be underlying causes of this pathology
• Fibrous histiocytoma—lesion involving the eye(s), generally appearing as an elevated limbal mass; involvement of the cornea, conjunctiva, nictitans, eyelid, and periocular areas is possible
• Periadnexal multinodular granulomatous dermatitis—well-demarcated cutaneous nodules; commonly on muzzle and may affect the eye; histologically distinct granulomas and variable numbers of inflammatory cells; aside from periadnexal association, may be indistinguishable from cutaneous histiocytosis; disease is benign and idiopathic and may regress without treatment or respond to corticosteroids
• Lymphomatoid granulomatosis—extensive pulmonary infiltrate composed of lymphocytes, plasma cells, histiocytes, and atypical lymphoreticular cells; affects young

to middle-aged dogs, with respiratory disease as the chief complaint; lack of lymph node, organ, or bone marrow involvement
• Granulomatous diseases—dogs with infectious diseases such as nocardiosis, actinomycosis, and mycotic diseases may have nodular pulmonary opacities; cytology and histopathology of associated macrophages may appear atypical and bizarre
• Hemophagocytic syndrome (histiocytosis)—benign histiocytic proliferation secondary to infectious, neoplastic, or metabolic disease; histiocytes are well differentiated and may affect bone marrow, lymph nodes, liver, and spleen; causes cytopenias of at least two cell lines
• Anaplastic carcinomas or sarcomas—histopathologic findings in dogs with histiocytosis may resemble a poorly differentiated tumor; histochemical stains for tissue-specific markers will differentiate

CBC/BIOCHEMISTRY/URINALYSIS

• Dogs with cutaneous histiocytosis do not have systemic abnormalities.
• Mild to severe anemia (regenerative or nonregenerative) and thrombocytopenia are common in dogs with systemic and malignant histiocytosis and vary from mild to severe; anemia may be regenerative or nonregenerative; cytopenias are believed to initially be due to phagocytosis by histiocytes and later to impaired production due to bone marrow involvement.
• Biochemistry results vary and may reflect the degree of organ involvement.

OTHER LABORATORY TESTS

Serum ferritin—may be a tumor marker for malignant histiocytosis; one affected dog had a very high serum ferritin concentration, suggesting secretion by neoplastic mononuclear phagocytes

IMAGING

• Thoracic radiography—well-defined, nodular pulmonary opacities (single or multiple); pleural effusion; lung lobe consolidation; diffuse interstitial infiltrates; mediastinal masses; sternal and tracheobronchial lymphadenomegaly
• Abdominal radiography and ultrasonography—hepatomegaly; splenomegaly; abdominal effusion
• Other imaging modalities, such as vertebral radiography and cerebrospinal fluid analysis, should be performed as indicated.

DIAGNOSTIC PROCEDURES

• Biopsy of affected organs and/or lymph nodes
• Cytologic examination of bone marrow aspiration or biopsy—may show histiocytic infiltration

• Immunohistochemistry—diagnosis of histiocytosis may be difficult because results of cytologic/histologic examinations are not always definitive; immunohistochemical staining may be useful in verifying the histiocytic origin of cells

PATHOLOGIC FINDINGS

Gross

• Skin masses • Mildly enlarged lymph nodes
• Ill-defined white foci in the spleen, lung, kidney, testes, skeletal muscles of the head, liver, and pancreas • Splenomegaly and/or hepatomegaly with possible mass lesions

Histopathologic

Systemic/Cutaneous Histiocytosis
• Histiocytic infiltrates fail to demonstrate the bizarre cytologic characteristics of the cells of malignant histiocytosis.
• Histiocytes appear to target small blood vessels (angiocentric). • Multinucleated giant cells rarely seen • Varying numbers of other inflammatory cells are intermixed. • In the skin, lack of epithelial involvement distinguishes the disease from benign cutaneous histiocytomas.
Malignant Histiocytosis
• Cytologic atypia is the hallmark characteristic; histiocytes are large and pleomorphic with foamy cytoplasm.
• Mitotic index is generally high, and abnormal mitotic figures may be present.
• Multinucleated giant cells are often seen.
• Classically, erythrophagocytosis by neoplastic histiocytes is evident.
• Occasionally, leukophagocytosis and thrombophagocytosis may be demonstrated.
• Histopathology of histiocytosis may resemble an anaplastic tumor or even lymphoma. • Lack of expression of lymphoid markers, such as CD3 and CD79a, rules out lymphoma. • Special stains for histiocytic markers, such as lysozyme or α_1-antitrypsin, may be helpful. • Given the complexity of histiocytic diseases, additional studies to confirm myeloid dendritic origin may be needed for a definitive diagnosis. • Malignant, systemic, and cutaneous histiocytosis stain positively using markers for cells of dendritic origin, including CD1, major histocompatibility complex class II, CD11c adhesion molecule, and ICAM-1, and stain positively for surface markers expressed by leukocytes such as CD45, CD18, and CD11a.
• Systemic and cutaneous histiocytosis are positive for Thy-1 (CD90; normal dermal perivascular dendritic cells) and are positive for CD4 (consistent with activated antigen-presenting cells).
• Malignant histiocytosis is negative for CD4 and inconsistently positive for Thy-1.

TREATMENT

Fluid therapy or blood transfusions may be required, depending on clinical findings.

MEDICATIONS

DRUG(S)

No definitive treatment

Systemic/Cutaneous Histiocytosis

• Dogs have episodes of clinical disease followed by periods when they are asymptomatic, without any therapy.
• Responses to corticosteroids, including complete and partial remission, have been reported, primarily in dogs with cutaneous histiocytosis. • Relapses often occur, and continuous therapy may be required.
• Therapeutic success seen using other immunosuppressive drugs, such as azathioprine, cyclosporine, and leflunomide

Malignant Histiocytosis

Responses to corticosteroids, cyclophosphamide, vincristine, and doxorubicin-based protocols have been reported; optimal choice of drugs is unknown.

FOLLOW-UP

• Effectiveness of treatment is determined by repeated physical examinations, CBC and biochemistry profiles, and diagnostic imaging.
• The prognosis for dogs with malignant histiocytosis is extremely poor; death usually occurs within a few months of diagnosis.

MISCELLANEOUS

Suggested Reading

Affolter VK, Moore PF. Canine cutaneous and systemic histiocytosis: reactive histiocytosis of dermal dendritic cells. Am J Dermatopathol 2000;22:40–48.
Affolter VK, Moore PF. Localized and disseminated histiocytic sarcoma of dendritic cell origin in dogs. Vet Pathol 2002; 39:74–83.
Author Kenneth M. Rassnick
Consulting Editor Stephen A. Kruth

HISTOPLASMOSIS

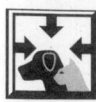 BASICS

DEFINITION
A systemic fungal infection cause by *Histoplasma capsulatum*

PATHOPHYSIOLOGY
• Mycelial form grows in bird manure or organically enriched soil.
• Mycelium—produces infectious spores (microconidia); inhaled into the terminal airways
• Spores—germinate in the lungs; develop into yeasts, which are phagocytized by macrophages
• Macrophages—distribute the organisms throughout the body
• Ingested organisms may directly infect the intestinal tract.
• Immune response—determines whether disease develops; affected animals often develop transient, asymptomatic infection

SYSTEMS AFFECTED
• Cats—respiratory tract main site of infection; bone, bone marrow, liver, spleen, skin, and lymph nodes also affected; intestinal tract, eyes, kidneys, adrenals, and brain less frequently involved
• Dogs—intestinal tract most frequently involved site; liver, lung, spleen, and lymph nodes often involved; bones, bone marrow, kidneys, adrenals, oral cavity, tongue, eyes, and testes less frequently affected

GENETICS
N/A

INCIDENCE/PREVALENCE
Prevalence of clinically relevant histoplasmosis relatively low in cats and dogs; an active practice, even in endemic areas, would see 3–4 cases a year.

GEOGRAPHIC DISTRIBUTION
• Endemic areas—Ohio, Missouri, Mississippi, Tennessee, and St. Lawrence River basins
• Also seen in Texas, the southeastern U.S., and the Great Lakes region

SIGNALMENT
Species
Cats and dogs

Breed Predilection
N/A

Mean Age and Range
• Cats—predominantly young; many < 1 year of age; all ages can be infected.
• Dogs—most often middle-aged; all ages can be infected

Predominant Sex
N/A

SIGNS
Historical Findings
Cats
• Insidious onset over days to weeks
• Anorexia, weight loss, and dyspnea—most common
• Coughing
• Lameness
• Ocular discharges
• Diarrhea
Dogs
• Weight loss, depression, and diarrhea—most common
• Coughing
• Dyspnea
• Exercise intolerance
• Lymphadenopathy
• Lameness and eye and skin changes—less common

Physical Examination Findings
Cats
• Fever to 40°C (104.0°F)
• Increased respiratory effort and harsh lung sounds
• Mucous membranes pale
• Enlarged lymph nodes
• Lameness and ocular changes may be found.
Dogs
• Thin to emaciated
• Fever to 40°C (104.0°F)
• Hepatosplenomegaly
• Mucous membranes often pale
• Icterus occasionally seen
• Coughing and dyspnea associated with harsh lung sounds

CAUSES
H. capsulatum

RISK FACTORS
• Bird roosts where the soil is enriched with bird or bat droppings are high-risk environments; old chicken coops and cones have been implicated.
• Exposure to airborne dust contaminated with fungal spores coming from sites of fungal growth (especially cats)
• Tissue samples from nearly half of stray dogs and cats from an endemic area were positive for *Histoplasma,* supporting the theory that many people and animals are infected but few develop clinically significant disease.

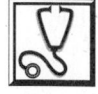 DIAGNOSIS

DIFFERENTIAL DIAGNOSIS
Cats
• Dyspnea from fungal pneumonia—differentiate from heart failure, feline asthma, lymphosarcoma, pneumonia, pyothorax, and other fungal pneumonias.
• Lameness—differentiate from trauma.
• Ocular changes—differentiate from lymphosarcoma, toxoplasmosis, and feline infectious peritonitis.

Dogs
• Severe chronic diarrhea and weight loss—consider lymphocytic plasmacytic enteritis, eosinophilic enteritis, lymphosarcoma, chronic parasitism, and pancreatic exocrine insufficiency.
• Diarrhea and anemia—consider severe hookworm infection.
• Hepatosplenomegaly and peripheral lymphadenopathy—consistent with lymphosarcoma
• Respiratory signs—distemper, bacterial pneumonia, and heart disease

CBC/BIOCHEMISTRY/URINALYSIS
• Moderate to severe nonregenerative anemia common
• Leukocyte counts—usually normal; some patients have a leukocytosis; patients with bone marrow involvement may be leukopenic.
• *Histoplasma* organisms—may be found in circulating neutrophils and monocytes
• Severe liver involvement—may see hyperbilirubinemia and high ALT activity
• Dogs with severe intestinal histoplasmosis often have low total protein.

OTHER LABORATORY TESTS
• AGID test—for antibodies; supports diagnosis; positive results indicate active disease; previous infections may produce false-positive results; many animals with active disease are negative on serology.
• Coombs test—may be positive because antibodies to *Histoplasma* may cross-react with RBCs; steroid therapy contraindicated

IMAGING
Thoracic Radiography
• Dogs—diffuse interstitial to nodular pneumonia; enlarged tracheobronchial lymph nodes compressing the tracheal bifurcation; old lung lesions may be calcified, coin-like opacities that suggest metastatic tumors.
• Cats—usually a diffuse interstitial pattern of lung involvement; calcification and tracheobronchial lymphadenopathy uncommon

Abdominal and Bone Radiography
• Dogs—splenic, mesenteric lymph node, and hepatic enlargement
• Cats and less often dogs—bone lesions predominantly osteolytic and usually occur distal to the elbows and stifles

DIAGNOSTIC PROCEDURES
• Identification of organisms on cytology, histopathology, or culture—definitive diagnosis
• Tissue samples—enlarged lymph nodes, liver, and spleen are good sites; rectal scrapings may be rich in organisms; bone marrow; lung aspirates (when less-invasive procedures are not diagnostic); tracheal washes inconsistent

PATHOLOGIC FINDINGS
• Multifocal, granulomatous lesions in organs rich in reticuloendothelial cells (e.g., spleen, liver, lymph nodes, lungs, and bone marrow)
• Dogs—gut prime site of involvement; tracheobronchial lymph node enlargement common
• Cats—predominantly respiratory involvement

TREATMENT

APPROPRIATE HEALTH CARE
• Usually outpatient with oral itraconazole
• Inpatient with intravenous amphotericin B—dogs with severe intestinal disease and malabsorption

NURSING CARE
• Dogs on amphotericin B therapy—keep well hydrated with a balanced electrolyte solution to decrease potential for renal toxicity
• Emaciated animals with malabsorption—give total parenteral nutrition to reverse wasting until the intestinal disease is resolved enough for adequate food absorption
• Animals with severe dyspnea—oxygen supplementation

ACTIVITY
Dogs with dyspnea—reduce

DIET
Good-quality, easily absorbed, palatable food required

CLIENT EDUCATION
• Discuss possible areas of exposure in the home environment.
• Inform client that both pets and family members may have been exposed to the same source and that the animal is not a hazard to the family.

SURGICAL CONSIDERATIONS
N/A

MEDICATIONS

DRUG(S) OF CHOICE

Itraconazole
• Drug of choice if adequate intestinal function for drug absorption exists.
• Dogs and cats—5mg/kg PO q12h; give with a high-fat meal.
• Duration depends on the clinical response; minimum treatment is 90 days.

Intravenous Amphotericin B
Dogs
• With severe inflammatory bowel disease and malabsorption—use until patient begins to gain weight; then start on itraconazole.
• Patient must be well hydrated before starting treatment; do not give amphotericin

B in electrolyte solutions that may precipitate the drug.
• BUN—check before each dose; discontinue if level approaches 50 mg/dL and maintain hydration; resume when level < 30 mg/dL
• Usual dose—0.5 mg/kg IV q48h
• Reconstitute in 5% dextrose and dilute for administration
• Normal renal function—dilute in 60–120 mL 5% dextrose and give over 15 min
• Some renal compromise—dilute in 0.5–1 L 5% dextrose and give over 3–4 hr to reduce renal toxicity
Cats
• Use cautiously
• Usual dose—0.25 mg/kg IV in 5% dextrose over 3–4 hr
• More sensitive to the drug than are dogs

Fluconazole
• Use for dogs that cannot be given amphotericin B.
• Usual dose (intravenous form)—5 mg/kg IV q12h until intestinal absorption allows oral itraconazole treatment

CONTRAINDICATIONS
Amphotericin B—renal failure precludes use

PRECAUTIONS
• Steroids—use with caution; will allow proliferation of *Histoplasma;* life-threatening respiratory distress due to infiltrative lung disease or hilar lymphadenopathy justifies use of dexamethasone 0.2 mg/kg IV daily for 2 to 3 days, but treatment time with antifungal drugs is likely to be increased
• Itraconazole and fluconazole—hepatic toxicity; temporarily discontinue if patient becomes anorexic or if serum ALT activity > 300 U/L; restart at half dose after appetite improves.

POSSIBLE INTERACTIONS
Itraconazole—contraindicated with terfenadine and cisapride in humans

ALTERNATIVE DRUG(S)
None

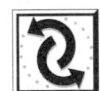

FOLLOW-UP

PATIENT MONITORING
• Serum ALT—with itraconazole treatment; check monthly or if the patient becomes anorexic
• Chest radiographs—with pulmonary involvement; check after 60 days of treatment to assess improvement; repeat at 30-day intervals and stop treatment when infiltrates are clear or remaining lung lesions fail to improve, indicating residual scarring; may be difficult to differentiate between residual fibrotic lesions and active disease; continue treatment for at least 1 month after all signs of active disease have resolved.

PREVENTION/AVOIDANCE
• Avoid suspected areas of exposure (e.g., bird roosts).
• Recovered dogs are probably immune.

POSSIBLE COMPLICATIONS
Recurrence possible; requires a second course of treatment

EXPECTED COURSE AND PROGNOSIS
• Treatment—duration is usually about 4 months; drugs are expensive, especially for large dogs.
• Prognosis—good for stable patients without severe dyspnea; influenced by severity of lung involvement and debility of patient

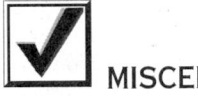

MISCELLANEOUS

ASSOCIATED CONDITIONS
• No apparent predisposing conditions

AGE-RELATED FACTORS
N/A

ZOONOTIC POTENTIAL
• Not spread from animals to people
• Care must be taken to avoid needlesticks when collecting aspirates.
• Infection can occur from cuts when doing necropsies on infected animals.

PREGNANCY
Itraconazole—no teratogenic effects in rats and mice at therapeutic doses; embryotoxicity found at high doses; no dog or cat studies; one dog given the drug halfway through her pregnancy delivered a normal litter.

ABBREVIATIONS
• AGID = agar gel immunodiffusion
• ALT = alanine aminotransferase
• BUN = blood urea nitrogen
• RBC = red blood cell

Suggested Reading
Clinkenbeard KD, Cowell RL, Tyler RD. Disseminated histoplasmosis in cats: 12 cases. J Am Vet Med Assoc 1987; 190:1445–1448.
Hodges RD, Legendre AM, Adams LG, et al. Itraconazole for the treatment of histoplasmosis in cats. J Vet Intern Med 1994; 8:409–413.
Schulman RL, McKiernan BC, Schaeffer DJ. Use of corticosteroids for treating dogs with airway obstruction secondary to hilar lymphadenopathy caused by chronic histoplasmosis: 16 cases (1979–1997). J Am Vet Med Assoc 1999;214:1345–1448.
Wolf AM. Histoplasmosis. In: Greene CE, ed. Infectious diseases of the dog and cat. Philadelphia: Saunders, 1998:378–383.
Author Alfred M. Legendre
Consulting Editor Stephen C. Barr

HOOKWORMS (ANCYLOSTOMIASIS)

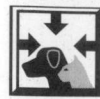

BASICS

OVERVIEW
- Nematode parasites of the species *Ancylostoma caninum* in the small intestine of dogs, *A. tubaeforme* of cats, and *A. braziliense* and *Uncinaria stenocephala* in both dogs and cats
- *A. braziliense* is found in southern states; the others are in the temperate zone as well.
- Voracious blood-sucking adults and fourth-stage larvae of *A. caninum* and *A. tubaeforme* cause blood-loss anemia and enteritis; active worms leave bite sites with continuing seepage of blood.
- Of special concern is infection in neonates with acute to peracute disease; infections may be acute to chronic compensatory at weaning or chronic noncompensatory in those immunosuppressed or debilitated.
- *Uncinaria* is of little clinical concern.
- *A. braziliense* is the major cause of CLM.
- Coughing may result from larval migration following skin penetration.
- *A. caninum* is transmitted via colostrum to pups; all species are transmitted by ingestion of infective larvae or by skin penetration.

SIGNALMENT
Acute disease in young; chronic disease in mature dogs and cats.

SIGNS

Historical Findings
- Pale mucous membranes
- Dark, tarry stools (melena); diarrhea; constipation
- Loss of condition
- Poor appetite
- Dry cough
- Sudden death

Physical Examination Findings
- Poor condition
- Pale mucous membranes

CAUSES & RISK FACTORS
- Infected bitch or queen
- Contaminated environment
- Concurrent enteric infections
- Other compromising conditions (e.g., pregnancy)

DIAGNOSIS

DIFFERENTIAL DIAGNOSIS
- Toxocariasis—large roundworm infection
- Coccidiosis
- Strongyloidosis
- *Uncinaria* eggs, 70 μm; *A. caninum*, 60 μm

CBC/BIOCHEMISTRY/URINALYSIS
- Eosinophilia
- Anemia—may be microcytic, hypochromic due to chronic iron deficiency

OTHER LABORATORY TESTS
N/A

IMAGING
N/A

DIAGNOSTIC PROCEDURES
- Fecal flotation; fecal egg examination—*A. caninum, A. tubaeforme* at 60 × 40 μm
- Necropsy of sibling pups, kittens that have died following appearance of similar clinical signs

PATHOLOGIC FINDINGS
Eosinophilic enteritis due to larval activity in wall of small intestine

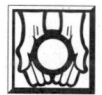

TREATMENT
- Pups in an environment with a history of hookworm infections—routinely treat at 2-week intervals to weaning
- Acute, severe cases—inpatients for fluid therapy and blood transfusion (as indicated by severity of anemia and clinical signs)
- Alert owner to potential for sudden death.
- Chronic compensatory cases, including breeding females—deworming program to eliminate intestinal and somatic infections

MEDICATIONS

DRUG(S)

A/L Antihelmintic Activity
- Fenbendazole—50 mg/kg PO q24h for 3 consecutive days in dogs
- Milbemycin oxime—0.5 mg/kg (dogs) or 2 mg/kg (cats) PO q30d

Adulticide Activity
- Pyrantel pamoate—15 mg/kg PO in dogs; 20–30 mg/kg PO in cats (extra-label)
- Praziquantel/pyrantel pamoate/febantel tablets for dogs; praziquantel/pyrantel pamoate tablets for cats

- Ivermectin—6 μg/kg PO for dogs and 24 μg/kg for cats (with pyrantel pamoate)
- Dichlorvos packets/tablets biweekly
- Selamectin: 6 mg/kg topically once for treatment of *A. tubaeforme* in cats

Adulticide Activity—Dogs
- A/L dewormer (fenbendazole) during third trimester of pregnancy to kill migrating larvae in somatic tissue and adults
- A/L dewormer on daily or monthly basis for pups and mature dogs
- Treat pup biweekly until weaning if at risk

Adulticide Activity—Cats
- A/L dewormer for queen prior to breeding and after littering
- Adulticide dewormer by 4 weeks for kitten

CONTRAINDICATIONS/POSSIBLE INTERACTIONS
- Do not give organophosphates to heartworm-positive dogs or cats.
- Do not give dichlorvos concurrently with other organophosphates such as insecticides.

FOLLOW-UP
- Monitor fecal egg counts posttreatment.
- Hematocrit if infection resulted in blood loss

MISCELLANEOUS

AGE-RELATED FACTORS
Disease more acute in young animals and chronic in adults

ZOONOTIC POTENTIAL
CLM, especially with *A. braziliense;* infective larvae penetrate skin

SYNONYMS
Ancylostomiasis

ABBREVIATIONS
- A/L = adulticide/larvicide
- CLM = cutaneous larva migrans

Suggested Reading

Bowman DD, Lynn RC, Eberhard ML. Georgi's parasitology for veterinarians, 8th ed. St. Louis: Saunders (Elsevier Science), 2003:183–188.

Bowman DD, Hendrix CM, Lindsay DS, Barr SC. Feline clinical parasitology. Ames: Iowa State University Press, 2002:242–257.

Acknowledgment

The author/editors acknowledge the prior contributions of Dr. Robert Corwin, who authored this topic in the previous edition.

Author Julie Ann Jarvinen
Consulting Editor Albert E. Jergens

BASICS

OVERVIEW
• Sympathetic denervation of the eye
• Anatomic pathway very important

Hypothalamus
↓
brain stem/cervical cord
T1-T3 spinal cord segments
and nerve roots
↓
vagosympathetic trunk
↓
cranial cervical ganglion
↓
middle ear
↓
ophthalmic branch (cranial nerve V)
↓
long ciliary nerve
↓
iris dilator muscle
↓
other fibers: smooth muscle in periorbita
upper and third eyelid
• Affects the ophthalmic and nervous systems

SIGNALMENT
• Idiopathic—one study suggests male
Golden retrievers 4–13 years of age.
• Idiopathic—dogs, 50–93%; cats, 45%
• Other causes—N/A

SIGNS
• Miosis • Protruding third eyelid • Ptosis
(drooping) of upper eyelid • Enophthalmia
• See Table 1 • Otitis—possible • Other
neurologic abnormalities—possible

CAUSES & RISK FACTORS
See Table 1

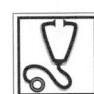

DIAGNOSIS

DIFFERENTIAL DIAGNOSIS
Anterior uveitis—IOP abnormal; aqueous
flare

CBC/BIOCHEMISTRY/URINALYSIS
N/A

OTHER LABORATORY TESTS
N/A

IMAGING
• See Table 1 • Vertebral column radiographs
and myelogram—may reveal spinal cord
lesion • Thoracic radiographs—may reveal
cause of injury to the sympathetic trunk (e.g.,
trauma and mediastinal tumor) • Skull
radiographs—may reveal middle ear problem
• CT and MRI—may help identify brain stem
lesion, retrobulbar mass, or middle ear problem
• Ultrasonography—orbit; may reveal
retrobulbar mass

DIAGNOSTIC PROCEDURES
• See Table 1 • CSF tap—investigate brain
and spinal cord disease
• Electromyography—look for brachial plexus
avulsion • Pharmacologic testing—see
Anisocoria

TREATMENT
• Treat underlying disease

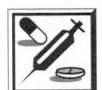

MEDICATIONS

DRUG(S)
• Depend on underlying disease • Idiopathic—
none

CONTRAINDICATIONS/POSSIBLE INTERACTIONS
N/A

FOLLOW-UP
• Depends on severity of underlying disease
• Idiopathic—may take up to 4 months for a
partial or complete recovery

MISCELLANEOUS

ABBREVIATIONS
• CSF = cerebrospinal fluid • FCE = fibrocartilaginous embolism • LMN = lower motor
neuron • UMN = upper motor neuron

Suggested Reading
Scagliotti RH. Comparative neuro-ophthalmology. In: Gelatt KN, ed. Veterinary ophthalmology. 3rd ed. Philadelphia: Lippincott Williams & Wilkins, 1999:1307–1400.
Author David Lipsitz
Consulting Editor Paul E. Miller

Table 1.

Summary of Lesions Resulting in Horner's Syndrome

Location	Causes	Associated Neurologic Signs	Diagnostic Plan
brain stem	trauma; neoplasm; infectious; inflammatory; vascular	altered mental status; ipsilateral motor defects; ipsilateral cranial nerve deficits	CT or MRI; CSF analysis
cervical spinal cord	trauma; disk; neoplasm; FCE	ipsilateral hemiparesis/paralysis; tetraparesis/paralysis; UMN; thoracic/pelvic limbs	spinal films; CSF analysis; myelogram, MRI
T1-T3 spinal cord	trauma; disk; neoplasm; FCE	LMN: thoracic limb(s); UMN: pelvic limb(s)	spinal films; CSF analysis; myelogram, MRI
T1-T3 ventral roots	brachial plexus avulsion; nerve sheath tumor	ipsilateral brachial plexus injury; ipsilateral loss of panniculus reflex	neurologic examination; EMG, MRI
sympathetic trunk, cranial cervical ganglion	trauma; mediastinal neoplasm; iatrogenic-surgical trauma	unilateral: none; bilateral: laryngeal/pharyngeal dysfunction	thoracic radiographs ultrasound neck, MRI
middle ear	trauma; neoplasm; otitis media/interna; nasopharyngeal polyp (cat)	ipsilateral peripheral vestibular disease; ipsilateral facial nerve paralysis	otic examination; bullae radiographs or CT; MRI myringotomy
retrobulbar	trauma; neoplasm; abscess	variable: none or involvement of cranial nerves II, III, IV, VI, V	CT or MRI; ultrasound orbit

BASICS

DEFINITION
Includes inappropriate urination, characterized by simple (squat) urination on horizontal surfaces outside the litter box, and urine marking, most commonly on vertical surfaces outside the litter box

PATHOPHYSIOLOGY
• Urine marking—a normal behavior observed in feral and domestic cats; behavior may have a heritable component
• Inappropriate urination—behavior may be a normal response to dissatisfaction with litter box environment or specific preference for an alternative location or substrate or may reflect an underlying pathophysiologic state such as a negative (pain) association with the litter box

SYSTEMS AFFECTED
• Behavior • Renal/urologic

SIGNALMENT
• Inappropriate urination can occur in any age, breed, or sex. • Urine spraying is more common in intact and neutered males than in females.

SIGNS

Inappropriate Urination
• Acute or chronic problem • History of lower urinary disease or systemic illness may suggest an underlying medical problem. • History may suggest dissatisfaction with features of the litter box, preference for specific substrate, or location or change in environment. • Presence of abnormal physical findings depends on whether problem is pathophysiologic or behavioral.

Urine Marking
• Usually manifest as spraying—the cat orients caudally to a vertical surface, stiffens its posture, raises and quivers its tail, and directs a small burst of urine caudally.
• The owner may detect urine marks at prominent vertical sites such as around doorways or windows or selectively sprayed on new objects brought into the house. • Horizontal urine marks may be found on clothing or bedding associated with a particular person. • Spraying around doors or windows suggests a marking response to the presence of an outdoor cat.
• Marking may be a response to another cat in the home or outside the home. Spraying on grocery bags or new furniture suggests olfactory marking associated with arousal in response to new stimuli. Urine marking on clothing or bedding associated with specific humans or visitors may occur.

CAUSES

Medical Abnormalities Associated with Inappropriate Urination
• Lower urinary tract disease including interstitial cystitis • Diabetes mellitus

• Urolithiasis • Hyperthyroidism • Iatrogenic—administration of fluids, corticosteroids, diuretics • FeLV • FIV • Liver disease • Senility • Cognitive dysfunction

Environmental Factors Contributing to Inappropriate Urination
Litter Box Characteristics
• Soiled box • Inadequate number of boxes or locations (one box per cat plus one is recommended) • Box located in remote or unpleasant surrounding • Inappropriate type of box—a covered litter box may maintain odors at an offensive level or may be too small to allow large cats to move around comfortably; a covered litter box allows other cats, pet dogs, and young children to target the cat as it exits • Time factors—daily or weekly temporal patterns of inappropriate urination suggest an environmental cause; acute onset in a cat that has previously used the litter box reliably suggest a medical problem. • Substrate—unacceptable litter type; preference tests indicate that most cats prefer unscented, fine-grained (clumping) litter; coincident change in litter box habits with new litter type suggests an association; a sudden shift from one substrate (e.g., litter) to an unusual substrate (e.g., a porcelain sink) suggests a lower urinary tract disorder • Location—urination outside the litter box may suggest a location preference or influential social factors • Social dynamics—consider social conflicts between cats and any concomitant changes in the social world of the cat at the time the problem started (e.g., addition of a new cat)

Environmental Factors Contributing to Urine Marking
• Probability of urine spraying is directly proportional to the number of cats in the household. • The presence of outdoor cats may elicit spraying around doorways and windows.

RISK FACTORS

Inappropriate Urination
• Infrequently changed litter box (or boxes)
• Frequent travel by owner (separation anxiety)

Urine Marking
• History of urine marking by a parent
• Multiple-cat households

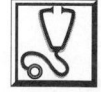 DIAGNOSIS

DIFFERENTIAL DIAGNOSIS
• *Must* differentiate inappropriate urination from urine marking • Inappropriate urination—most common behavioral cause is dissatisfaction with the litter box • Urine marking—most commonly in response to presence of other cats

CBC/BIOCHEMISTRY/URINALYSIS
Usually normal when urine marking and inappropriate urination are strictly behavioral

problems; urinalysis is the minimum database in any cat examined because of inappropriate urination; collect serial samples from cats whose behavioral signs wax and wane; CBC and biochemistry are recommended prior to administration of medication.

OTHER LABORATORY TESTS
Cats with refractory inappropriate urination or progressive signs should be tested for hyperthyroidism, FeLV, and FIV.

IMAGING
Abdominal radiographs to rule out urolithiasis as an underlying cause for inappropriate urination

DIAGNOSTIC PROCEDURES
In multicat households it may be difficult to determine which cat is responsible for inappropriate elimination. Identify the offending cat in one of two ways:
1. Isolate each cat, one at a time, in a small room to identify the culprit by process of elimination; however, this protocol may alter the social milieu enough to stop inappropriate elimination during the serial confinement.
2. Administer the dye fluorescein (4 fluorescein test strips in a gel capsule PO) sequentially to each cat. Urine outside the litter box fluoresces under a Wood's light for approximately 24 hr; if negative after 36 hr, the test can be repeated on another cat. Negative results are common in households in which the frequency of spraying is low.

 TREATMENT

• Treat any underlying medical condition.
• Use environmental and behavioral therapies before or with pharmacologic treatment.
• If the owner requires immediate cessation of the problem, it is helpful to confine the cat to one room in the owner's absence. Provide a litter box, water, food, and resting sites. The cat can be let out of the room when the owner returns and is available for strict supervision of the cat. Initiate other, more permanent treatments.
• To monitor progress, the owner should keep a daily record of urinations and their location.

Inappropriate Urination
Environmental Management Techniques
• Scoop out the litter box daily and clean thoroughly weekly. • Avoid deodorizers or other strong odors in the vicinity of the litter box. • Provide at least one litter box per cat, distributed in more than one location, and avoid high traffic or noisy areas. • Move food bowls away from the litter box. • If the litter box is covered, provide an additional large, plain, uncovered litter box filled with unscented, fine-grained, clumping litter, with no liner. • If one site in the home is preferred for inappropriate urination, place another litter

box over this site. After it is in regular use, move it several inches a day to a site more acceptable to the owner. • If numerous sites outside the litter box are used, use tactile (e.g., aluminum foil, plastic drop cloths) or olfactory (e.g., citrus odor eliminator or mothballs) deterrents at those sites.

Behavior Modification
• Some owners have sufficient patience to monitor the cat and take it to the litter box at an appropriate time (e.g., first thing in the morning). The cat is then rewarded with a favored treat for using the litter box. • Punishment (e.g., a water pistol or sound alarm) is generally not effective. Punishment associated with sounds or movements by the owner will condition the cat to avoid the owner. • Feeding or playing with the cat at inappropriate elimination sites may countercondition the unacceptable behavior.

Urine Marking
• Neuter intact animals—this curbs spraying behavior in up to 90% of males and 95% of females. • If there are signs that the cat is spraying in response to cats outside, prevent visual or olfactory access to those cats. An environmental product (Feliway, Veterinary Product Laboratories), a concentrate of synthesized feline facial pheromone, is commercially available as a treatment for urine marking. The product is sprayed regularly or diffused in the environment. • Block inside cat's ability to see outside cats. • To focus the affected cat's attention away from other cats, the owner should spend time interacting with the cat daily. • Pharmacotherapy plays an important role in the control of urine marking.

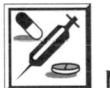

MEDICATIONS

DRUG(S) OF CHOICE

Inappropriate Urination
Usually are not indicated, except in treatment-resistant cases or when associated with generalized anxiety

Urine Marking
Drugs from a number of drug classes may be used. All have the general effect of decreasing arousal and anxiety. Side effects can be seda-

tion and/or altered social behavior. (See Appendix IX—Formulary). Options are listed in Table 1.

CONTRAINDICATIONS
• Benzodiazepines in cats with hepatic disease, because of the potential for fatal idiopathic hepatic necrosis • Tricyclic antidepressants in cats with a history of cardiac conduction disturbances, megacolon, lower urinary tract blockages, and glaucoma

PRECAUTIONS
• All drugs listed are used in an extra-label fashion. Explain to the client the experimental nature of these treatments and common side effects; document the discussion by a notation in the medical record or use a release form. Start using psychotropic drugs when the owner is present to monitor the patient. • Some psychotropic drugs have human abuse potential. Dispense not more than a 4-week supply, with refills available. • Benzodiazepines rarely cause idiopathic hepatic necrosis (a total condition) in apparently healthy cats. • Use tricyclic antidepressants or selective serotonin reuptake inhibitors with caution in patients with urinary or fecal retention.

POSSIBLE INTERACTIONS
• Benzodiazepine drugs can interact with cimetidine. • Do not use monoamine oxidase inhibitors (including amitraz and L-deprenyl) concurrently with tricyclic antidepressants or selective serotonin reuptake inhibitors.

ALTERNATIVE DRUG(S)
Synthetic progestins—the risk of serious side effects, including blood dyscrasias, pyometra, mammary hyperplasia, mammary carcinoma, diabetes mellitus, and obesity, has diminished their once-common use; dosage: 5 mg q24h 1–2 weeks, then taper gradually to 2.5 mg 2×/week.

FOLLOW-UP

PATIENT MONITORING
The owner should keep a daily log of elimination pattern so that treatment success can be evaluated and appropriate adjustments in therapy can be made. Regular follow-up is essential.

POSSIBLE COMPLICATIONS
Client expectations must be realistic. Immediate control of a longstanding problem of housesoiling is unlikely; the goal is gradual improvement over time. Treatment failure may result in the cat being euthanized, dropped at an animal shelter, or released outside.

MISCELLANEOUS

ZOONOTIC POTENTIAL
Pregnant women should not clean up cat urine because of the risk of toxoplasmosis.

PREGNANCY
Tricyclic antidepressants are contraindicated in pregnant animals.

SYNONYMS
Feline inappropriate elimination (FIE), feline housesoiling, squat urination, urination outside the litter box, urine marking, urine spraying

ABBREVIATIONS
• FeLV = feline leukemia virus • FIE = feline inappropriate elimination • FIV = feline immunodeficiency virus

Suggested Reading
Horwitz DF. Housesoiling by cats. In: Horwitz D, Mills D, Heath S, eds. BSAVA Manual of Canine and Feline Behavioural Medicine. Gloucester, England: British Small Animal Veterinary Association, 2002:97–108.
Pryor PA, Hart BL, Bain MJ, Cliff CK. Causes of urine marking in cats and the effects of environmental management on the frequency of marking. J Am Vet Med Assoc 2001;1709–1713.
Simpson BS. Feline housesoiling. Part I. Inappropriate elimination. Comp Cont Educ 1998;20:1319–1329.
Simpson BS. Feline housesoiling. Part II. Inappropriate elimination. Comp Cont Educ 1998;20:1331–1340.
Author Barbara S. Simpson
Consulting Editor Debra F. Horwitz

Table 1

Drugs and Dosages Used to Manage Feline Urine Housesoiling				
Drug Class	*Drug*	*Dosage in Cats (mg/cat; PO)*	*Frequency*	*Latency to Effect*
Benzodiazepine	Diazepam	1–2	q12h	Immediate
Azaperone	Buspirone	2.5–7.5	q12h	1–3 weeks
Tricyclic antidepressant	Amitriptyline	2.5–10	q12–24h	1–4 weeks
Tricyclic antidepressant	Clomipramine	1–5	q12–24h	1–4 weeks
Selective serotonin reuptake inhibitor	Fluoxetine	1–5	q24h	1–4 weeks

HOUSESOILING—DOGS

 BASICS

DEFINITION
Urination and/or defecation, for the means of eliminating or marking territory, in a location that the owner finds inappropriate

PATHOPHYSIOLOGY
• Improper housetraining • Submissive or excitement urination • Testosterone, leading to marking behavior • Marking behavior • Anxiety (separation anxiety, noise phobia) • Cognitive dysfunction

SYSTEMS AFFECTED
• Behavioral—shelter relinquishment, leading to euthanasia or rehoming
• Neurologic if cognitive dysfunction syndrome

GENETICS
Some dog breeds appear to be more easily housetrained.

INCIDENCE/PREVALENCE
• In surveys of dog owners, between 6.4 and 7.4% mentioned some form of housesoiling problem. • 37% of owners that reported talking to their veterinarian about a behavior problem reported that their dog was housesoiling. • Of dogs referred to a behavior specialist for a behavior problem, housesoiling represented between 5.5 and 16.8% of the cases. • The incidence of inappropriate elimination, including marking behavior, in intact male dogs is higher than that seen in castrated male dogs and intact or spayed female dogs, at almost 60%.

GEOGRAPHIC DISTRIBUTION
None seen

SIGNALMENT

Species
Dogs

Breed Predilections
Potential genetic breed predisposition for ease of housetraining and submissive or excitement urination

Mean Age and Range
• Inappropriate elimination due to improper housetraining seen at a younger age
• Submissive and excitement urination seen primarily in younger dogs • Urine marking starts to be displayed as the dog begins to reach sexual maturity.

Predominant Sex
• Female dogs are generally easier to housetrain than male dogs. • Intact male dogs are more likely to urine-mark than castrated male dogs and intact or spayed female dogs.

SIGNS

General Comments
• Inappropriate elimination is the most common individual reason for relinquishment of a pet to a shelter. • Proper housetraining should be stressed with clients from the very beginning.

Historical Findings
• History of urinating in inappropriate areas (according to the owners), usually inside a home • May be associated with signs of other behavioral disorders (such as separation anxiety) • May be associated with lack of time spent on owner's part to properly teach housetraining • May be associated with inappropriate punishment of a dog that has submissive urination
• Determine potential triggers, via a complete behavioral history, including when, where, and how often the elimination occurs and reliability of outdoor elimination.

Physical Examination Findings
• If there are no abnormal physical examination findings, the housesoiling is probably due to a behavioral cause.
• Abnormal physical examination findings would be related to an underlying medical cause of inappropriate elimination.

CAUSES
The causes of canine inappropriate elimination can be primarily due to a behavioral problem or secondary to/concurrent with a medical disorder.

Behavioral
• Lack of or incomplete housetraining
• Marking behavior • Submissive urination
• Excitement urination • Separation anxiety
• Cognitive dysfunction • Noise phobia
• Fear-induced • Psychogenic polydipsia

Medical Causes
Degenerative
• Hip dysplasia/osteoarthritis/degenerative joint disease • Renal failure
Anatomic
• Ectopic ureters
Metabolic
• Estrogen-responsive incontinence
• Diabetes mellitus • Diabetes insipidus
• Hepatic insufficiency
• Hyperadrenocorticism • Hypercalcemia
• Hypoadrenocorticism • Hypokalemia
• Seizures • Neurogenic incontinence
Neoplastic
• Renal neoplasia • Bladder neoplasia
• Other neoplastic diseases causing weakness
Infectious/Inflammatory
• Urinary tract infection
• Crystalluria/urolithiasis

RISK FACTORS
• Intact male • Owners poorly informed or motivated to properly housetrain their dog

 DIAGNOSIS

DIFFERENTIAL DIAGNOSIS
Differentiate behavioral causes of inappropriate elimination from medical causes with a proper medical workup.

CBC/BIOCHEMISTRY/URINALYSIS
• Indicated to rule out medical causes
• Normal if inappropriate elimination is due to behavioral causes

OTHER LABORATORY TESTS
None, other than to rule out medical causes

IMAGING
Not indicated, other than to rule out medical causes, primarily urolithiasis or ectopic ureters

DIAGNOSTIC PROCEDURES
• Videotaping the dog when the owner is present to view the household interactions with the dog • Journal to monitor potential causal factors for inappropriate elimination, as well as to monitor improvement of the problem • Videotaping the dog when the owner is gone from the home to rule in/rule out separation anxiety

PATHOLOGIC FINDINGS
None for behavioral causes

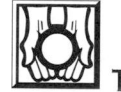 TREATMENT

APPROPRIATE HEALTH CARE
Any appropriate measures to assure continued good health of the dog

NURSING CARE
None

ACTIVITY
• Take dog outside often to ensure that the dog has enough access to eliminate outside, or provide acceptable access to the outside, for example via a dog door. • Increase activity level to help in the treatment of separation anxiety, as well as to improve the dog's health.

DIET
• If the dog is inappropriately eliminating, feeding meals (as opposed to free feeding) may help in maintaining the dog on a schedule of elimination for defecation.
• Feeding a diet of higher caloric density may help decrease the urge to defecate as often.

CLIENT EDUCATION

General Comments
• Counsel the owner as to the cause(s) of the inappropriate elimination, as well as the potential long-term management of the problem. • Treat underlying/contributing medical problems. • Treat other underlying/contributing behavioral problems.

• Clean the soiled areas with an enzymatic cleaner, to help eliminate any odor that may attract the dog to eliminate there again. If the object soiled is a piece of clothing, wash it in the washing machine.

Incomplete Housetraining
• Keep the dog completely supervised or confined at all times. • Take the dog outside frequently to eliminate. • Reward the elimination when it occurs at the appropriate time and place; requires the owner to go outside with the pet.
• Thoroughly clean soiled areas.

Submissive Urination
• Do not punish the behavior, since this may make problem worse. • Have the owners ignore the dog when they come into the house (no verbal or physical interactions or eye contact). • The dog should go outside to eliminate before being greeted. • The dog should be greeted in a non-confrontational and quiet manner; do not lean over the dog or institute interactive play at the time of greeting. • Alternate activities at homecoming, such as asking for a toy or requesting a "sit," may help in mild cases. • For excitement urination, much the same recommendations are applicable as for submissive urination, especially concentrating on not getting the dog overexcited.

Urine-marking Behavior
• Determine by the history any possible triggers to the behavior including anxiety-provoking stimuli. • Address those triggers with desensitization and counterconditioning and/or avoidance of the trigger as appropriate. • Educate the owners on the effectiveness of neutering to decrease urine marking. • Make the areas marked aversive to the dog by use of "booby traps" such as upside-down plastic carpet runners or mousetraps, or by use of remote punishment at the very beginning of each and every urine marking episode if the owner is able to catch the dog in the act of marking. • Prevent access to the preferred marking locations.
• Alternatively, the owner can change the significance of the area to a positive place, by feeding the dog in the area marked.

SURGICAL CONSIDERATIONS
Neutering an intact male dog decreases urine marking rapidly in 30% of dogs, with a gradual decline in 20% of dogs, and no change in 50% of them. The results are the same regardless of the age of neutering.

 MEDICATIONS

DRUG(S) OF CHOICE
• Behavioral modification should always be used in conjunction with psychotropic medications.

• If the dog is urine marking or inappropriately eliminating owing to anxiety, medications may be helpful, but only in conjunction with behavior modification.
• Selective serotonin reuptake inhibitors (SSRIs) or tricyclic antidepressants/antianxiety medications (TCAs) may be helpful. An example of an SSRI is fluoxetine at a dose of 1 mg/kg PO q24h. An example of a TCA is clomipramine at a dose of 1–2 mg/kg PO q12h.
• The full onset of action of these medications can be four to six weeks after initiation of treatment, and owners should be made aware of this.
• Side effects of the TCAs can include nausea, vomiting, diarrhea, lethargy, cardiac arrhythmias, and potentiation of seizure activity.
• Side effects of the SSRIs can include nausea, vomiting, diarrhea, and lethargy.
• Rarely effective if anxiety not part of the problem. Will have negligible effect in animals that are not house trained or in submissive urination.

CONTRAINDICATIONS N/A

PRECAUTIONS N/A

POSSIBLE INTERACTIONS
Do not use an SSRI and TCA together, or in conjunction with a monoamine oxidase inhibitor (MAO-I) such as L-deprenyl or amitraz.

ALTERNATIVE DRUG(S)
Progestins have been used in the past to control urine marking, but are rarely recommended because of the potential severe side effects.

 FOLLOW-UP

PATIENT MONITORING
Patients should be monitored with owner follow-up visits or telephone calls. The owner should keep a journal of incidents, inciting factors, and treatments instituted to give an objective view of improvement. Follow-up is necessary to help ensure client compliance.

PREVENTION/AVOIDANCE
• Properly housetrain the dog. • Neuter male and female dogs. • Treat any underlying behavioral condition. • Treat any underlying medical condition.

POSSIBLE COMPLICATIONS
Recurrence if owner relapses in treatment

EXPECTED COURSE AND PROGNOSIS
• Prognosis for any behavioral problem is highly dependent on the owner's ability to fully follow instructions. Also, rarely are animals with behavioral problems considered "cured," but, instead, are "managed." The

following estimations of prognosis are based on the owner's following your instructions for behavior modification. • Prognosis for decreasing submissive and excitement urination is good. • Prognosis for managing incomplete housetraining is good.
• Prognosis for marking in previously intact male: 50% improve (30% quickly, 20% more slowly) with neutering, even without complementary behavior modification.
• Prognosis for managing urine marking in spayed or neutered dogs is good if the triggers can be identified and managed with avoidance or other forms of behavior modification. • Some animals with a history of a medical cause of inappropriate elimination can still eliminate inappropriately after the medical cause has been properly treated.

 **MISCELLANEOUS**

ASSOCIATED CONDITIONS
N/A

AGE-RELATED FACTORS
• Puppies are more likely to present for lack of or incomplete housetraining, as well as for submissive and excitement urination.
• Cognitive dysfunction becomes more likely as the dog ages.

ZOONOTIC POTENTIAL
Low zoonotic potential, unless the dog has leptospirosis in its urine or parasites or bacteria, such as *Salmonella,* in its feces

SYNONYMS
• Urine marking • Inappropriate urination
• Inappropriate defecation • Inappropriate elimination

SEE ALSO
• Cognitive Dysfunction Syndrome
• Separation Anxiety Syndrome

Suggested Reading
Beaver BV. Canine behavior: a guide for veterinarians. Philadelphia: Saunders, 1999.
Hart BL, Hart LA. The perfect puppy: how to choose your dog by its behavior. New York: WH Freeman, 1988.
Landsberg G, Hunthausen W, Ackerman L. Handbook of behaviour problems of the dog and cat. Oxford: Butterworth Heinemann, 1997.
Overall KL. Clinical behavioral medicine for small animals. St. Louis: Mosby, 1997.
Author Melissa Bain
Consulting Editor Debra F. Horwitz

HYDROCEPHALUS

 BASICS

DEFINITION
• Abnormal dilation of the ventricular system from an increased volume of CSF
• May be symmetrical or asymmetrical
• May involve the entire ventricular system or only elements proximal to a site of ventricular system obstruction

PATHOPHYSIOLOGY
• Two types—compensatory and obstructive
• Compensatory—CSF fills the space where the nervous parenchyma was destroyed and/or failed to develop; intracranial pressure normal; ventricular dilation incidental to the primary disease
• Obstructive—CSF accumulates in front of an obstruction along the normal CSF circulatory pattern (noncommunicating) or at its resorption site by the meningeal arachnoid villi (communicating); intracranial pressure high or normal; clinical signs may be noted when intracranial pressure is normal.
• Congenital obstruction—primary obstructive hydrocephalus; most common site is at the level of the mesencephalic aqueduct; prenatal infections (especially parainfluenza virus) may cause aqueductal stenosis with subsequent hydrocephalus; may result in considerable disruption of the architecture of the brain
• Acquired obstruction—secondary obstructive hydrocephalus; caused by tumors, abscesses, and inflammatory diseases (including inflammation resulting from hemorrhage caused by traumatic injuries or other causes of bleeding); sites include the interventricular foramina, mesencephalic aqueduct, or lateral apertures of the fourth ventricle.
• Overproduction of CSF—rare; caused, for example, by a choroid plexus tumor

SYSTEMS AFFECTED
Nervous

GENETICS
Siamese cats—autosomal recessive

INCIDENCE/PREVALENCE
Unknown

GEOGRAPHIC DISTRIBUTION
N/A

SIGNALMENT
Species
Dogs and cats

Breed Predilections
• Congenital—small and brachycephalic dogs: bulldogs, Chihuahuas, Maltese, Pomeranians, toy poodles, Yorkshire terriers, Lhasa apsos, cairn terriers, Boston terriers, pugs, and Pekingese
• Inherited—Siamese cats and Yorkshire terrier. High incidence of clinically asymptomatic ventriculomegaly in normal adult beagles
• Acquired—any breed of cat or dog

Mean Age and Range
• Congenital—usually becomes apparent at a few weeks up to 1 year of age. Acute onset of signs can occur in dogs with previously undiagnosed congenital hydrocephalus. The exact cause of this decompensation is uncertain.
• Acquired—any age

Predominant Sex
None

SIGNS
General Comments
• Congenital—may occur without clinical signs, especially in dogs of toy breeds; other malformations or anomalies of the CNS may be noted (e.g., malformations of the cerebellum or syringomyelia), which may further contribute to the constellation of signs.
• Acquired—signs attributable to the underlying disease may be as or more prominent than the signs attributable to the hydrocephalus.
• Severity of the clinical signs may not correspond to the degree of ventricular enlargement.

Historical Findings
• Behavioral—decreased awareness; lack of or loss of training ability (including housetraining); excessive sleepiness; vocalization; sometimes hyperexcitability
• Blindness
• Seizures—may be noted

Physical Examination Findings
Head—may appear large and dome-shaped with an exaggerated "stop"; open sutures and/or fontanelles. Bilaterally divergent strabismus is present in some dogs with severe congenital hydrocephalus.

Neurologic Examination Findings
• Cerebral disease—abnormal behavior (especially dullness and sleepiness), cortical blindness (loss of vision with normal eyes and pupillary light reflexes), inappropriate vocalization, sometimes hyperexcitable
• Gait abnormalities—incoordination, ataxia, and decreased postural reactions
• Seizures—may occur
• Congenital form—malformation of the orbit during growth may result in a ventrolateral strabismus with normal oculocephalic eye movements.
• Severely increased intracranial pressure—stupor or coma, pinpoint or dilated fixed pupils, abnormal respiratory patterns, and decerebrate posture; may lead to fatal tentorial herniation

CAUSES
• Congenital—unclear
• Acquired—intracranial inflammatory diseases or mass lesions

RISK FACTORS
Animals with compensated hydrocephalus may decompensate in the face of an insult such as infection or trauma.

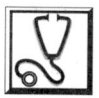 DIAGNOSIS

DIFFERENTIAL DIAGNOSIS
• Other congenital brain anomalies
• Metabolic or toxic diseases resulting in cerebral dysfunction
• Brain mass lesions or infectious diseases resulting in high intracranial pressure (hydrocephalus may coexist)
• Traumatic injury to the brain (hydrocephalus may coexist)

CBC/BIOCHEMISTRY/URINALYSIS
• Usually normal

OTHER LABORATORY TESTS
N/A

IMAGING
• Skull radiography (congenital)—reveals an enlarged domed cranium with sutures and fontanelles open past their normal closure time; cranial vault may have a ground-glass appearance. Skull radiographs also may reveal calvarial thinning.
• CT and MRI—provide definite diagnosis
• Ultrasound scan through open fontanelle may reveal enlarged ventricles.

DIAGNOSTIC PROCEDURES

• CSF analysis—use caution when collecting sample if patient has high intracranial pressure (may lead to fatal brain herniation through the foramen magnum and/or beneath the tentorium cerebelli); composition normal if no other intracranial disease (e.g., neoplasia, inflammation)
• EEG—congenital: usually characteristic, including hypersynchrony, high amplitude (25–300 μV), and low frequency (1–7 Hz); acquired: varies

PATHOLOGIC FINDINGS

• Brain—may be large with loss of the normal pattern of sulci and gyri; may see distortion of the parenchyma, including thinning of the cerebral cortex, rupture of the septum pellucidum, and atrophy of other adjacent structures; with severe disease, brain herniation may occur, either of the cerebrum and midbrain under the tentorium cerebelli or of the cerebellum and caudal medulla oblongata through the foramen magnum.
• Ventricular system—mildly to severely distended (either entirely or only the part rostral to the obstructive lesion); with noncommunicating form, narrowing or blockage of the ventricular system due to inflammation or mass lesions

 TREATMENT

APPROPRIATE HEALTH CARE

• Inpatient—intensive care for patients with severe signs or when undergoing surgical therapy
• Outpatient—patients with mild to moderate signs that can be treated medically

NURSING CARE

Prevent secondary complications of recumbency for stuporous or comatose patients—avoid pressure sores; drying eyes; and hypostatic lung congestion.

ACTIVITY
N/A

DIET
N/A

CLIENT EDUCATION

Advise client to observe for deterioration in mental alertness, vision, and behavior, which may signal worsening of the problem.

SURGICAL CONSIDERATIONS

• Surgical shunting of the CSF from the ventricles to the peritoneal cavity—definitive treatment
• Complications—infection and shunt blockage common; shunt revision commonly needed
• Clinical signs may not resolve completely; residual signs usually indicate irreversible brain damage.
• Surgery for a brain tumor or other mass lesion—consider if it is the underlying cause.

 MEDICATIONS

DRUG(S) OF CHOICE

• Reduce CSF production—corticosteroids: prednisone (0.25–0.5 mg/kg PO q12h) or dexamethasone (0.25 mg/kg PO q12h, tapered to an alternate-day regimen); or carbonic anhydrase inhibitors: acetazolamide (10 mg/kg PO q6h)
• Reduce intracranial pressure—osmotic diuretics: mannitol (1 g/kg slow IV infusion over 20 min; may repeat twice at 6-hr intervals); and/or loop diuretics: furosemide (dogs, 2–8 mg/kg IV, IM, SC q12h; cats, 1–2 mg/kg IV, IM, SC q12h)
• Treat underlying cause—administer specific drugs when possible (e.g., antibiotics for bacterial infection).

CONTRAINDICATIONS

Fluid therapy—use with caution with severe disease; do not overhydrate.

PRECAUTIONS

• Corticosteroids—long-term treatment may cause iatrogenic hyperadrenocorticism or hypoadrenocorticism if drug is suddenly withdrawn.
• Diuretics—may cause shock or electrolyte imbalances, especially hypokalemia with furosemide administration

POSSIBLE INTERACTIONS
N/A

ALTERNATIVE DRUG(S)
N/A

 FOLLOW-UP

PATIENT MONITORING

• Monitor for exacerbation of the hydrocephalus and for signs attributable to an underlying cause (e.g., intracranial neoplasia).

PREVENTION/AVOIDANCE
N/A

POSSIBLE COMPLICATIONS

• Brain herniation and death
• Infection and blockage when ventriculoperitoneal shunting is carried out; shunt revision and specific treatment for bacterial infection are then indicated

EXPECTED COURSE AND PROGNOSIS

• Depend on cause and severity
• Mild congenital form—good prognosis; may require only occasional medical treatment

 MISCELLANEOUS

ASSOCIATED CONDITIONS

Cerebellar hypoplasia in kittens congenitally infected with feline panleukopenia virus

AGE-RELATED FACTORS

Congenital—usually seen in animals < 1 year old

ZOONOTIC POTENTIAL
N/A

PREGNANCY
N/A

SYNONYMS
N/A

SEE ALSO
Stupor and Coma

ABBREVIATIONS

• CNS = central nervous system
• CSF = cerebrospinal fluid
• CT = computed tomography
• EEG = elecroencephalogram
• MRI = magnetic resonance imaging

Suggested Reading

Harrington ML, Bagley RS, Moore MP. Hydrocephalus. Vet Clin North Am Small Anim Pract 1996;26:4:843–856.
Oliver JE, Lorenz MD, Kornegay JN. Handbook of veterinary neurology, 3rd ed. Philadelphia: Saunders, 1997.
Summers BA, Cummings JF, de Lahunta A. Veterinary neuropathology. St. Louis: Mosby, 1995:75–77.
Vullo T, Korenman E, Manzo RP, et al. Diagnosis of cerebral ventriculomegaly in normal adult beagles using quantitative MRI. Vet Radiol & US 1997;38(4):277–281.
Author Mary O. Smith
Consulting Editor Joane M. Parent

HYDRONEPHROSIS

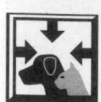

BASICS

OVERVIEW
• Causes progressive distention of the renal pelvis and diverticula, with atrophy of the renal parenchyma secondary to obstruction in most patients; the disease is usually unilateral and occurs secondary to complete or partial obstruction of the kidney or ureter by uroliths, neoplasia, retroperitoneal disease, trauma, radiotherapy, and accidental ligation of the ureter during ovariohysterectomy and after ectopic ureter surgery.
• Bilateral hydronephrosis—rare; usually secondary to trigonal, prostatic, or urethral disease

SIGNALMENT
Dogs affected more often than cats

SIGNS

Historical Findings
• None in some animals
• Anorexia
• Restlessness
• Polydipsia and polyuria
• Hematuria
• Signs of uremia in patients with bilateral hydronephrosis or if the contralateral kidney has compromised function
• May be referable to the cause of the obstruction

Physical Examination Findings
• Normal in some patients
• Renomegaly
• Renal, abdominal, or lumbar pain
• Abdominal mass—bladder or prostate
• Trigonal, prostatic, vaginal, or urethral mass palpable on rectal examination

CAUSES & RISK FACTORS
Any cause of ureteral obstruction including uroliths, ureteral stenosis, atresia, fibrosis (cats), or neoplasia; trigonal mass; prostatic disease; vaginal mass; retroperitoneal abscess, cysts, hematoma, or other mass; inadvertent ureteral ligation during ovariohysterectomy; postoperative complication from ectopic ureter surgery; perineal hernia

DIAGNOSIS

DIFFERENTIAL DIAGNOSIS
• Other causes of renomegaly—e.g., amyloidosis, neoplasia, granuloma, cysts, and perinephric pseudocysts (cats)
• Other causes of abdominal pain—e.g., pancreatitis and peritonitis
• Intervertebral disk disease leading to lumbar pain
• Pyelonephritis without obstruction

CBC/BIOCHEMISTRY/URINALYSIS
• Normal in some patients
• Loss of urine-concentrating ability (first abnormality detected), hematuria, pyuria
• Azotemia, hyperphosphatemia, hyperkalemia, and acidemia in patients with severe, bilateral hydronephrosis resulting in renal failure

OTHER LABORATORY TESTS
N/A

IMAGING
• Abdominal radiographs may be normal or show renomegaly, prostatomegaly, uroliths, reduced retroperitoneal contrast, or urinary bladder distension.

• Excretory urography, cystography, or injection of radiographic contrast by nephropyelocentesis may be required to determine the location and cause of obstruction.
• Ultrasonography reveals dilation of the renal pelvis and diverticula, with thinning of the renal parenchyma; dilation of one or both ureters is detected in some animals.

DIAGNOSTIC PROCEDURES
Transurethral urethocystoscopy or vaginoscopy may help determine the cause and location of some obstructions.

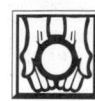

TREATMENT
• Treat as an inpatient and start supportive care (e.g., fluids ± antibiotics) while performing diagnostic tests. Correct fluid and electrolyte deficits with intravenous fluid therapy (0.9% NaCl or lactated Ringer's solution) over 4–6 hr, followed by maintenance fluids as needed. Some patients may be extremely polyuric, necessitating higher maintenance fluid rates.
• Relieve lower urinary tract obstruction as soon as possible by catheterization, serial cystocentesis, or tube cystostomy, pending surgical correction.
• Discuss renal disease versus failure and possible need for surgery with the owner.
• Specific treatment (usually surgical) depends on the cause and whether there is concurrent renal failure or other disease process (e.g., metastatic neoplasia).
• Emergency surgery rarely required; treat metabolic and electrolyte abnormalities prior to surgery.
• Kidney removal may not be necessary unless infected or neoplastic.

• If mild disease is secondary to nephroliths or ureteroliths, extracorporeal shock wave lithotripsy may be used as an alternative to surgery.

 MEDICATIONS

DRUG(S)
• Administer sodium bicarbonate to treat severe metabolic acidemia. For a measured acid deficit, give one-quarter of the calculated dose (weight in kg × 0.3 × base deficit) of bicarbonate as a slow intravenous bolus and the remainder with intravenous fluids. If the base deficit is not known, give bicarbonate at a dosage of 2–4 mEq/kg, depending on the severity of signs.
• Hyperkalemia (mild to moderate) often resolves with fluid replacement and/or bicarbonate administration. Severe, symptomatic hyperkalemia requires more-aggressive medical management such as regular insulin (0.5 u/kg IV) and 50% dextrose (2.0 g/kg IV). Some veterinary literature implies that potassium-containing solutions (e.g., lactated Ringer's solution) should be avoided in hyperkalemic patients, but current data do not support this.

• See chapters on acute or chronic renal failure for additional treatment principles for patients with bilateral hydronephrosis.

CONTRAINDICATIONS/POSSIBLE INTERACTIONS
• Do not add or mix sodium bicarbonate with calcium-containing fluids.
• Many contraindications and potential complications are associated with the use of sodium bicarbonate; consider them before administering bicarbonate.
• Do not give radiographic contrast material intravenously until the patient is rehydrated.

 FOLLOW-UP

PATIENT MONITORING
• Ultrasonography—can repeat at 2- to 4-week intervals after relief of obstruction, to assess improvement; often some signs of resolution appear by 3 months after relief of obstruction
• BUN, creatinine, and electrolytes
• After relief of obstruction—polyuria and postobstructive diuresis leading to hypokalemia, weight loss, dehydration, and possibly renal failure

POSSIBLE COMPLICATIONS
Rupture of the excretory system and irreversible renal damage

EXPECTED COURSE AND PROGNOSIS
Depends on the cause, duration of obstruction, and presence or absence of concurrent infection. Irreversible damage to the kidney usually begins 15–45 days after obstruction. If the obstruction is relieved within 1 week, renal damage is reversible; some function may be regained with relief of obstruction present for as long as 4 weeks. Concurrent infection accelerates the severity of renal damage.

 **MISCELLANEOUS**

Suggested Reading
Christie BA, Bjorling DE. Kidneys. In: Slatter D, ed. Textbook of small animal surgery. 2nd ed. Philadelphia: Saunders, 1993: 1428–1442.
Author Marc G. Bercovitch
Consulting Editors Larry G. Adams and Carl A. Osborne

HYPERADRENOCORTICISM (CUSHING'S DISEASE)

BASICS

DEFINITION
• Spontaneous hyperadrenocorticism (HAC) is a disorder caused by excessive production of cortisol by the adrenal cortex. • Iatrogenic HAC results from excessive exogenous administration of glucocorticoids. • In either instance, clinical signs are due to the deleterious effects of the elevated circulating cortisol concentrations on multiple organ systems.

PATHOPHYSIOLOGY
• Approximately 85–90% of cases of naturally occurring HAC are due to bilateral adrenocortical hyperplasia resulting from pituitary corticotroph tumors or hyperplasia with oversecretion of ACTH • In the remaining 10–15% of cases, cortisol-secreting adrenocortical neoplasia is present; approximately one-half of these are malignant. • Iatrogenic HAC results from excessive exogenous administration of glucocorticoids.

SYSTEMS AFFECTED
• HAC is a multisystemic disorder. • The degree to which each system is involved varies considerably; in some patients signs referable to one system may predominate; others have several systems involved to a comparable degree. • Signs referable to the urinary tract or skin often predominate.

INCIDENCE/PREVALENCE
• No exact figures available • Considered one of the most common endocrine disorders in dogs; rare in cats

SIGNALMENT
Dogs and cats

Breed Predilections
• Dogs—poodles, dachshunds, Boston terriers, boxers, and beagles are reportedly at increased risk • Cats—no apparent predilection

Predominant Sex
• No predilection for pituitary-dependent hyperadrenocorticism (PDH) in dogs; possible predilection for female dogs to have adrenal tumors • No apparent predilection in cats

Mean Age and Range
HAC is generally a disorder of middle-aged to old animals; PDH can be seen in dogs as young as 1 year.

SIGNS

General Comments
• Severity may vary greatly, depending on the duration and severity of cortisol excess. • In some cases, the physical presence of the neoplastic process (pituitary or adrenal) contributes.

Historical and Physical Examination Findings
Polyuria and polydipsia, polyphagia, pendulous abdomen, hepatomegaly, hair loss, lethargy, muscle weakness, anestrus, obesity, muscle atrophy, comedones, increased panting, testicular atrophy, hyperpigmentation, calcinosis cutis, facial nerve palsy, thin skin, bruising

CAUSES
• Pituitary-dependent—adenoma most common; corticotroph hyperplasia and adenocarcinomas rare; anterior pituitary involved in approximately 80% of cases, intermediate lobe of pituitary in the remaining cases • Adrenal tumor (AT)—adenoma or carcinoma • Iatrogenic—due to glucocorticoid administration

DIAGNOSIS

DIFFERENTIAL DIAGNOSIS
• Depends on the clinical and laboratory abnormalities displayed • Includes hypothyroidism, sex hormone dermatoses, sex hormone–secreting tumors, acromegaly, diabetes mellitus, hepatopathies, renal disease, and other causes of polyuria/polydipsia

CBC/BIOCHEMISTRY/URINALYSIS
• Hemogram may show eosinopenia, lymphopenia, leukocytosis, and erythrocytosis. • In dogs and cats, serum chemistry may show high liver enzymes, cholesterol, and total CO_2; alkaline phosphatase activity is high in approximately 90% of dogs with HAC but only 1/3 of cats with HAC; hyperglycemia is common but only about 10% of dogs with HAC will have concurrent diabetes mellitus as compared with about 80% of cats with HAC.
• Urinalysis may reveal low specific gravity, proteinuria, hematuria, pyuria and/or bacteriuria.

OTHER LABORATORY TESTS
• Endocrine testing in dogs with history, clinical signs, and laboratory abnormalities suggestive of HAC • Do not perform testing for HAC in sick dogs unless clinical signs are present consistent with HAC. • Screening tests are designed to determine if HAC is present or not. • Once a diagnosis of HAC is made, a differentiation test should be performed to determine if PDH or AT is present; differentiation provides information crucial to therapeutic decisions and to provision of an accurate prognosis.
• Differentiation tests should never be performed before a diagnosis of HAC is made via use of screening tests. • See Appendix for table of endocrine test protocols.
• The value used below to indicate suppression in response to dexamethasone is 1.5 μg/dL; check with your own laboratory for its normal ranges and cut-off values

Screening Tests
Urine Cortisol:Creatinine Ratio (UCCR)
• Urine cortisol excretion increases as a reflection of augmented adrenal secretion of the hormone, whether PDH or AT is present. • An elevated UCCR is a sensitive marker of HAC, being present in 90–100% of affected dogs and cats. • False-positive results are common; only about 25–30% of dogs with an elevated UCCR actually have HAC; similarly, in cats the UCCR is of high sensitivity and a false-positive result is likely in a cat with non-adrenal illness. • A normal ratio makes the diagnosis of HAC very unlikely (≤ 10% chance). • An elevated ratio is consistent with a diagnosis of HAC, but since the chance of a false-positive result is great, an ACTH stimulation test or low-dose dexamethasone suppression test must always be done to confirm the presence of HAC.
Low-dose Dexamethasone Suppression Test (LDDST)
• Lack of suppression 8 hours after an injection of a low dose of dexamethasone is consistent with a diagnosis of HAC. • The dose of dexamethasone used is different for dogs and cats. • The sensitivity of the LDDST is approximately 95% in dogs; in cats, approximately 80%. • In dogs, there is a relatively high chance of a false-positive result, about 50%, if non-adrenal illness is present. • In cats, the chance of a false-positive result is unknown. • With certain results, the LDDST can serve as a differentiation test as well as a screening test; if the 8-hour sample is > 1.5 μg/dL, the result is consistent with PDH; if, in addition, there is suppression at 4-hour post-dexamethasone (i.e. an "escape" at 8 hours post-dexamethasone) or the 4- and/or 8-hour post-dexamethasone samples are <50% of baseline, the results are consistent with PDH.
ACTH Stimulation Test
• A response greater than normal would be consistent with a diagnosis of HAC. • In dogs, the overall sensitivity of the ACTH stimulation test is approximately 80%. For HAC due to pituitary disease, the sensitivity is approximately 87%, while for HAC due to an adrenal tumor the sensitivity is approximately 61%. • In cats, the overall sensitivity of the ACTH stimulation test is approximately 81%. • The ACTH stimulation test is more specific in dogs than the LDDST (only a 15% chance of a false-positive result with non-adrenal illness).
• How large a chance of a false-positive result exists in cats is unknown. • The ACTH stimulation test can never differentiate between PDH and an AT.

Differentiating Tests
High-dose Dexamethasone Suppression Test (HDDST)
• The dose of dexamethasone used is different between dogs and cats. • Two responses are

consistent with PDH; if there is suppression to <1.5 μg/dL at 4 and/or 8 hours post-dexamethasone or the 4- and/or 8-hour post-dexamethasone samples are <50% of baseline, PDH is present. • When baseline values are close to 1.5 μg/dl or when suppression is just at 50%, the results may be suspect, and presence of PDH should be confirmed by other means.
• The HDDST can never confirm the presence of an AT; if the criteria for diagnosis of PDH are not met, there is a 50/50 chance the patient has PDH or an AT.
Endogenous ACTH Concentration
• A single blood sample is used (special handling required). • In patients with PDH, ACTH concentration should be normal to increased as a result of secretion from the pituitary tumor; with AT, endogenous ACTH concentration should be below normal. • This test can be used to confirm the presence of AT. • A gray zone exists in the results; if the patient's endogenous ACTH concentration falls into this zone, the results are not diagnostic. • In dogs, with repeat testing when the original concentration measured was in the gray zone, approximately 96% had definitive differentiation; similar results have been achieved in cats. • There is no way to predict when endogenous ACTH concentration will be in the gray zone.

IMAGING
• Abdominal radiographs may differentiate PDH from AT; approximately 50% of canine AT are visualized; adrenal mineralization is highly suspicious for the presence of a tumor in dogs, but can occur in up to 30% of normal cats. • Chest radiographs are indicated in patients with an AT to check for metastases. • Ultrasonography, CT, and MR—useful for differentiating PDH from AT and for staging AT • CT and MR—often useful for demonstrating macroadenomas

DIAGNOSTIC PROCEDURES
N/A

PATHOLOGIC FINDINGS
• PDH—gross examination reveals normal-sized pituitary to pituitary macroadenoma and bilateral adrenocortical enlargement
• Microscopically, pituitary adenoma, adenocarcinoma, or corticotroph hyperplasia of pars distalis or pars intermedia and adrenocortical hyperplasia
• AT—gross examination reveals variable-sized adrenal mass, atrophy of contralateral gland (rarely bilateral tumors), and metastasis in some patients with adrenal carcinoma; invasion into the vena cava or vena caval thrombosis may be seen with malignant tumors.
• Microscopically, see adrenocortical adenoma or carcinoma

TREATMENT

APPROPRIATE HEALTH CARE
Dictated by the severity of clinical signs, the patient's overall condition, and any complicating factors (e.g., diabetes mellitus, pulmonary embolism)

ACTIVITY
No alteration of activity necessary.

DIET
Usually no need to alter; use appropriate diet if there is concurrent diabetes mellitus.

CLIENT EDUCATION
• If using medical therapy, lifelong therapy required
• If adverse reaction to mitotane occurs—discontinue drug, give prednisone, and have veterinarian reevaluate next day; if no response to prednisone is noted in a few hours, veterinarian should evaluate immediately.

SURGICAL CONSIDERATIONS
Hypophysectomy—described, but generally not available
• Bilateral adrenalectomy is the treatment of choice for PDH in cats, but not used for treatment of PDH in dogs; appropriate personnel and facilities are required as this is a technically demanding surgery and intensive postoperative management is required.
• Surgery is the treatment of choice in dogs and cats with adrenocortical adenomas and small carcinomas unless the patient is a poor surgical risk or the client refuses surgery.
• Medical control of HAC is recommended prior to surgery, if possible.

MEDICATIONS

DRUG(S) OF CHOICE
Mitotane
• Mitotane (*o,p'*-DDD, Lysodren) remains the drug of choice for medical management of both PDH and AT in dogs; selectively destroys the glucocorticoid secreting cells of the adrenal cortex
• PDH—give an initial loading dose of 40–50 mg/kg divided daily until both basal and post-ACTH cortisol levels are in the normal resting range (1–5 μg/dL); then 50 mg/kg/week divided; dosage adjustments are based on ACTH response testing (maintain basal and post-ACTH cortisol levels between 1 and 5 μg/dL); if relapse occurs, as indicated by cortisol levels outside the normal resting range, reload for 5–7 days and increase weekly maintenance dose by approximately 50%; give prednisone (0.2 mg/kg/day) during initial and subsequent loading periods

• AT—goal of mitotane use is low-to-nondetectable (i.e. < 1 μg/dL) basal and post-ACTH cortisol levels; starting dose is 50–75 mg/kg divided daily; induction typically requires higher doses and is of longer duration than for treatment of PDH; dose should be increased by 50 mg/kg/day every 10–14 days if control has not been achieved as judged by an ACTH stimulation test; if adverse effects develop due to mitotane, administration should continue at the highest tolerable dose; once control is achieved, maintenance therapy should begin at 75–100 mg/kg divided weekly; if cortisol levels pre- and post-ACTH rise into the normal resting range (i.e., 1–5 μg/dl), increase the maintenance dose by 50%; if cortisol levels rise above the normal resting range pre- and post-ACTH, reload until control is achieved and increase weekly maintenance dose by approximately 50%; during induction and maintenance, since the goal is to create glucocorticoid insufficiency, give prednisone at 0.2 mg/kg/day.

l-*Deprenyl*
• *l*-Deprenyl (selegiline hydrochloride; Anipryl)—may be used as an alternative treatment for PDH; decreases pituitary ACTH secretion by increasing dopaminergic tone to the hypothalamic-pituitary axis, thus decreasing serum cortisol concentrations; indicated only for the treatment of uncomplicated PDH; not recommended for treatment of PDH in dogs with concurrent illnesses such as diabetes mellitus; cannot be used to treat cortisol-secreting adrenocortical neoplasia; initiate therapy with 1 mg/kg daily and increase to 2 mg/kg/day after 2 months if the response is inadequate; if this dose is also ineffective, give alternative therapy
• The multicenter trial performed by Deprenyl Animal Health, Inc., reported that 75–80% of dogs had a good response to therapy as assessed by resolution of clinical signs and monthly low-dose dexamethasone suppression testing; other investigators reported lower efficacy rates (as low as 20%); further independent clinical trials are necessary to assess the efficacy of this medication in controlling PDH; adverse effects such as anorexia, lethargy, vomiting and diarrhea are uncommon (<5% of dogs) and usually mild; disadvantages include the need for lifelong daily administration and the expense of the medication

Ketoconazole
Ketoconazole (10 mg/kg q12h initially; up to 20 mg/kg q12h in some dogs) inhibits enzymes responsible for cortisol synthesis—indicated for dogs unable to tolerate mitotane at doses necessary to control HAC; may be useful for palliation of clinical signs of HAC in dogs with AT; efficacy is approximately 50% or less; adverse effects include anorexia, vomiting, diarrhea, lethargy, and an idiosyncratic hepatopathy

HYPERADRENOCORTICISM (CUSHING'S DISEASE)

Feline HAC

• The drug of choice for medical management is controversial; further studies are needed; mitotane at 50 mg/kg/day, then 50 mg/kg week with dosage adjustments based on ACTH stimulation testing has been reported, but higher doses may be required; metyrapone (65 mg/kg BID to TID, with dosage adjustments based on ACTH stimulation testing) may be the treatment of choice if the medication can be obtained; success with ketoconazole (5 mg/kg BID for 7 days followed by 10 mg/kg BID, with dosage adjustments based on ACTH stimulation testing) has had mixed success; L-deprenyl is an alternative for therapy of canine PDH, but its use has not been described in cats with HAC; a short-term safety study in normal cats revealed no significant adverse effects.

PRECAUTIONS

• Side effects of mitotane—not uncommon; mild in most dogs; include lethargy, weakness, anorexia, vomiting, diarrhea, ataxia, and iatrogenic hypoadrenocorticism
• Side effects are more common in dogs with AT given high doses of mitotane.
• Side effects of ketoconazole—seem to be less common; include anorexia, vomiting, diarrhea, and hepatopathy
• Side effects of L-deprenyl are uncommon.

ALTERNATIVE DRUG(S)

• Consider radiation therapy for animals with pituitary macroadenomas.
• ACTH levels may take several months to decrease; control HAC with above drugs in the interim.

FOLLOW-UP

PATIENT MONITORING

• Response to therapy—use periodic ACTH stimulation testing (see references) to assess mitotane, ketoconazole, or metyrapone efficacy; test after the initial 8 days if treating PDH and 10–14 days if treating AT, or sooner if decreased appetite, vomiting, diarrhea, listlessness or decreased water intake (<60 ml/kg/day) is noted. Continue induction with repeat testing as necessary until adequate response is seen; once on maintenance, test at 1, 3, and 6 months and every 6–12 months thereafter; adequacy of any necessary mitotane reloading period is checked with an ACTH stimulation test before higher maintenance mitotane dose initiated; adequacy of ketoconazole or metyrapone dose checked with an ACTH stimulation test after any dose alteration; depending on the problem, clinical signs of HAC resolve several days to months after control achieved; current label recommendations are to evaluate the efficacy of L-deprenyl therapy solely on the basis of resolution of clinical signs of HAC; the ACTH stimulation test is not indicated for assessing the response to treatment.

EXPECTED COURSE/PROGNOSIS

• Untreated HAC—generally a progressive disorder with a poor prognosis • Treated PDH—usually a good prognosis; median survival time for a dog with PDH treated with mitotane is 1.7 years; at least 10% survive 4 years; dogs living longer than 6 months tend to die of causes unrelated to their HAC.
• Macroadenomas and neurologic signs—poor to grave prognosis; macroadenomas with no or mild neurologic signs—fair to good prognosis with radiation and medical therapy • Adrenal adenomas—usually a good to excellent prognosis; small carcinomas (not metastasized) have a fair to good prognosis.
• Large carcinomas and AT with widespread metastasis—generally a poor to fair prognosis, but impressive responses to high doses of mitotane are occasionally seen.

MISCELLANEOUS

ASSOCIATED CONDITIONS

Neurologic signs in dogs with large pituitary tumors; glucose intolerance or concurrent diabetes mellitus; pulmonary thromboembolism; increased incidence of urinary tract and skin infections; hypertension; proteinuria/glomerulopathy

AGE-RELATED FACTORS

N/A

PREGNANCY

N/A

SYNONYMS

Cushing's disease; Cushing's syndrome

ABBREVIATIONS

• AT = adrenal tumor • ACTH = adrenocorticotrophic hormone • HAC = hyperadrenocorticism • HDDST = high-dose dexamethasone suppression test • LDDST = low-dose dexamethasone suppression test • PDH = pituitary-dependent hyperadrenocorticism • UCCR = urine cortisol:creatinine ratio

Suggested Reading

Behrend EN, Kemppainen RJ. Adrenocortical disease. In: August J, ed. Consultations in feline internal medicine, 4th ed. Philadelphia: Saunders, 2001:159–168.

Behrend EN, Kemppainen RJ. Diagnosis of canine hyperadrenocorticism. Vet Clin North Am 2001;31:985–1003.

Feldman EC, Nelson RW. Hyperadrenocorticism (Cushing's syndrome). In: Feldman EC, Nelson RW, eds. Feline and Canine Endocrinology and Reproduction, 2nd ed. Philadelphia: Saunders, 1996:187–265.

Kintzer PP, Peterson ME. Mitotane treatment of cortisol secreting adrenocortical neoplasia: 32 cases (1980–1992). J Am Vet Med Assoc 1994;205:54–61.

Kintzer PP, Peterson ME. Mitotane (o, p'-DDD) treatment of 200 dogs with pituitary-dependent hyperadrenocorticism. J Vet Intern Med 1991;5:182–190.

Peterson ME. Medical treatment of canine pituitary-dependent hyperadrenocorticism (Cushing's disease). Vet Clin North Am 2001;31:1005–1014.

Reusch CE, Steffen T, Hoerauf A. The efficacy of L-deprenyl in dogs with pituitary-dependent hyperadrenocorticism. J Vet Intern Med 1999;13:291–301.

Acknowledgment

The authors and editors acknowledge the prior contributions of Dr. Peter Kintzer, who authored this topic in a previous edition.

Authors Ellen N. Behrend and Robert J. Kemppainen
Consulting Editor Deborah Greco

BASICS

OVERVIEW
• Hyperandrogenism is a rare syndrome in dogs characterized by absolute or relative elevations in serum concentrations of masculinizing sex hormones, such as testosterone and its derivatives. It has not been reported in the cat.
• In males, androgens (testosterone and dihydrotestosterone) are produced by the interstitial cells of the testes and are responsible for normal sexual development, behavior, and spermatogenesis. Androgens are also produced by the adrenal cortex, and by the ovary in females
• Hyperandrogenism may occur as a result of excessive production by the testes, ovaries, or adrenal cortex, but more commonly occurs secondary to administration of exogenous synthetic androgens. • Hyperandrogenism may result in behavioral changes, abnormalities of the reproductive tract, and dermatologic problems.

Hyperandrogenism and Alopecia
• The endocrine and metabolic causes of truncal alopecia have confusing nomenclature. There are many different names that are used to describe truncal alopecia that is thought to be related to a relative sex hormone imbalance, or elevated circulating serum concentrations of sex hormones such as testosterone. • Sex hormone imbalance may occur secondary to excessive production, as seen in association with adrenal hyperplasia or adrenal tumors. It may be seen in association with testicular tumors or oversexed dogs (true hyperandrogenism); or it may be seen with altered adrenal steroidogenesis as occurs with adrenal hyperplasia–like syndrome (also referred to as congenital adrenal hyperplasia–like syndrome, growth hormone–responsive alopecia, adrenal sex hormone imbalance, sex-hormone alopecia). The most recent terminology refers to these conditions as alopecia X of the Nordic breeds. These terms are used to refer to the syndrome in Pomeranians, the chow chow, keeshonden, and Samoyed breeds that is thought to result from an adrenal cortical 21-hydroxylase deficiency, resulting in hyperandrogenism and a secondary decrease in growth hormone
• Owing to differing etiologies of the hyperandrogenic state, success of treatment with castration, mitotane administration, or growth hormone administration will vary with each condition. With respect to the animals with altered adrenal steroidogenesis, why dogs have varying responses to the same therapy is not well understood.

SIGNALMENT
Dogs—Pomeranians, chow chows, poodles, keeshonden, Samoyeds

SIGNS

Historical Findings
• Aggression • Stunted growth (secondary to premature closure of epiphyseal growth plates)
• Irregular estrous cycles • Anestrus
• Virilization

Physical Examination Findings
General
• Endocrine alopecia (bilaterally symmetrical involving the neck, trunk, caudal thighs, pinnae, and tail) • Dry, brittle hair • Hyperpigmentation of the skin • Seborrhea oleosa
Female
• Clitoral hypertrophy (in association with prolonged exposure) • Vaginitis • Virilization
• Abnormal sexual differentiation (with exposure in utero)
Male
• Prostatomegaly • Abnormalities of sperm morphology • Circumanal gland hyperplasia
Prepubertal
Premature epiphyseal growth plate closure

CAUSES & RISK FACTORS
• Exogenous administration of androgens
• Increased endogenous androgen secretion
• Testicular tumor (most commonly secondary to interstitial testicular tumors) • Exposure in utero of female fetus to androgens

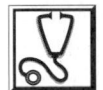

DIAGNOSIS

DIFFERENTIAL DIAGNOSIS

Nonpruritic, Symmetrical Alopecia (Endocrine Alopecia)
• Hypothyroidism • Hyperadrenocorticism
• Hyperestrogenism

Clitoral Hypertrophy
• Abnormalities of gonadal sex (pseudohermaphroditism, true hermaphroditism)
• Hyperadrenocorticism

Aggression
• Neurologic disease • Behavioral

CBC/BIOCHEMISTRY/URINALYSIS
Usually normal

OTHER LABORATORY TESTS
• Karyotype—to detect intersex/gonadal sex abnormalities • Growth hormone stimulation test—this test is completed using xylazine or clonidine, may be used to demonstrate lack of increase in serum growth hormone concentrations after administration. This test is unreliable in documenting hyperandrogenism; some dogs have normal growth hormone response yet respond well to growth hormone supplementation. • Serum testosterone concentrations—single serum concentrations may be within normal limits owing to fluctuations in serum concentrations. Multiple measurements are more indicative of serum concentration as compared to single measurements. • ACTH stimulation test—submit serum samples for evaluation of sex hormones. Results may be variable.

IMAGING
Abdominal radiography or ultrasound—used as a screening test for intraabdominal masses or gonadal tissue as a source of hyperandrogenism

DIAGNOSTIC PROCEDURES
Skin biopsy may reveal nonspecific changes associated with endocrine alopecia

TREATMENT
• Surgical neutering of intact animals • Surgical excision of testosterone-secreting masses, neoplastic tissue

MEDICATIONS

DRUG(S)
• Progestogens—such as megestrol acetate are anti-androgenic and can be used to decrease serum concentrations of testosterone; however their use may be associated with serious side effects (see contraindications) and risk versus benefit must be considered prior to use in dogs.
• Inhibitors of steroidogenesis—such as ketoconazole • Controlled destruction of the adrenal cortex (zona reticularis)—via administration of mitotane • Melatonin—this is experimental at present • Growth hormone administration—0.1 IU (0.05 mg/kg) SC three times a week for 4–6 weeks

CONTRAINDICATIONS/POSSIBLE INTERACTIONS
• Progestogens—use may be associated with elevated levels of growth hormone, diabetes mellitus, and adrenocortical suppression
• Melatonin—regulates light-mediated reproductive events and its use should be avoided in breeding animals. • Growth hormone and megestrol acetate are both potentially diabetogenic and increase risk of mammary cancer. Serum blood glucose or urine dipsticks should be monitored during therapy. Diabetes may not be reversible upon discontinuing therapy. • 5-alpha-reductase inhibitors—such as finasteride inhibit the conversion of testosterone to dihydrotestosterone only in the prostate.

FOLLOW-UP
• Repeat ACTH stimulation with evaluation of serum samples for sex hormones post therapy
• Physical examination for response to therapy
• Recheck serum testosterone concentrations post therapy if initially high.

MISCELLANEOUS

ASSOCIATED CONDITIONS
• Interstitial cell tumors • Adrenal hyperplasia–like syndrome • Hyperadrenocorticism
• Benign prostatic hyperplasia • Clitoral hypertrophy

Suggested Reading
Endocrine and metabolic diseases. In Scott DW, Miller WH, Griffin CE. Muller and Kirk's small animal dermatology. Philadelphia: Saunders, 2001:780–885.

Authors Sophie A. Grundy and Autumn P. Davidson

Consulting Editor Deborah S. Greco

HYPERBILIRUBINEMIA

 BASICS

DEFINITION
Serum total bilirubin concentration higher than reference range

PATHOPHYSIOLOGY
• Bilirubin—originates from degradation of heme-containing proteins; most (80%) comes from senescent erythrocytes; remainder comes from heme-containing proteins.
• Unconjugated bilirubin—transported in plasma bound to albumin after hepatocellular uptake is conjugated with glucuronic acid
• Conjugated bilirubin—transported (with other components of bile) into the biliary system; expelled into the intestines, where most is converted to other products; formed urobilinogen can undergo enterohepatic circulation • Hyperbilirubinemia—caused by increased production (RBC destruction; hemolysis) in excess of the liver's ability to take up and process it, or impaired clearance (disturbed handling by hepatocytes or interference with discharge into the intestines) causing cholestasis
• Nonhemolytic jaundice (dogs and cats)—caused by hepatobiliary disease

SYSTEMS AFFECTED
• Skin/Exocrine—discoloration of the skin (jaundice) when serum bilirubin > 2.5 mg/dL • Hepatobiliary—retained bile acids and possibly bilirubin may contribute to hepatocellular injury • Renal/urologic—very high concentration may cause renal tubular injury • Nervous—very high unconjugated bilirubin may cause degenerative brain lesions (rare)

SIGNALMENT
Species
Dogs and cats

Breed Predilections
• All breeds affected • Familial hepatic diseases—described in certain breeds (e.g., Doberman pinschers, Bedlington terriers)

Mean Age and Range
• Most causes—diseases of adult animals
• Young, unvaccinated dogs—at risk for infectious canine hepatitis

Predominant Sex
Adult female pure-bred dogs—at risk for immune-mediated hemolytic anemia

SIGNS
Historical Findings
Increased Formation—Hemolysis
• Lethargy • Anorexia • Weakness • Jaundice
• Recent blood transfusion • Severe trauma: bleeding into muscle or hematoma formation
Decreased Elimination—Cholestasis
• Lethargy • Anorexia • Jaundice

• Change in color of urine and feces
• Abdominal enlargement • Altered mentation • Vomiting • Diarrhea • Polyuria and polydipsia

Physical Examination Findings
Increased Formation—Hemolysis
• Pallor • Jaundice • Hepatomegaly
• Splenomegaly • Bleeding tendencies—thrombocytopenia • Orange feces
• Lymphadenopathy • Fever • "Gelatinous" feel to skin (vasculopathy)
Decreased Elimination—Cholestasis
• Weight loss • Jaundice • Hepatomegaly
• Splenomegaly • Abdominal effusion
• Abdominal pain • Cranial abdominal mass
• Melena • Fever • Acholic feces

CAUSES
Prehepatic Jaundice
• Hemolytic disorders causing RBC destruction • Immune-mediated hemolysis—certain drugs; SLE; infectious disorders
• Infections—FeLV; *Mycoplasma haemofelis*; heartworm; *Babesia; Ehrlichia; Cytauxzoon*
• Oxidative injury—onions; phenolic compounds; zinc; hypophosphatemia
• Resorption of blood—large hematoma

Hepatic Jaundice
• Chronic idiopathic or familial hepatitis
• Adverse drug reactions—e.g., anti-convulsants; acetaminophen; trimethoprim sulfate; carprofen; stanozolol (cats); benzodiazepines (cats)
• Cholangitis/cholangiohepatitis • Infiltrative neoplasia—lymphoma • Cirrhosis (dogs)
• Hepatic lipidosis (cats) • Massive hepatic necrosis • Systemic illnesses with a hepatic component—certain serovars of leptospirosis (dogs); histoplasmosis; FIP; hyperthyroidism (cats); toxoplasmosis (cats) • Bacterial sepsis—originating anywhere in the body; may elaborate bacterial products impairing hepatic bilirubin processing

Posthepatic Jaundice
• Transient or persistent mechanical interference with the excretion of bilirubin and other bile elements: (1) pancreatitis (usually transient); (2) neoplasia—bile duct, pancreas, duodenum; (3) intraluminal duct occlusion—cholelithiasis, sludged bile, liver flukes (cats), immune-mediated duct destruction (sclerosing cholangitis in cats; controversial); (4) ruptured gallbladder or bile duct causing bile peritonitis

RISK FACTORS
• Young unvaccinated dogs—infectious disease • Breed predisposition for familial hepatic disease—Doberman pinschers, Bedlington terriers, cocker spaniels, and dalmatians • Middle-aged, obese dogs—pancreatitis • Anorectic, obese cats—hepatic lipidosis • Hepatotoxic drugs • Blunt abdominal trauma, chronic biliary tract disease, bile mucocele—bile peritonitis
• Hemolytic anemia

 DIAGNOSIS

DIFFERENTIAL DIAGNOSIS
• Prehepatic jaundice—usually abrupt onset; mucous membrane pallor; mild to moderate jaundice; weakness; tachypnea; cardiac murmur with severe anemia
• Hepatic jaundice—breed risk for familial hepatitis; variable jaundice; otherwise normal mucous membranes; alteration in liver size (large or small); abdominal effusion (pure or modified transudate); polyuria and polydipsia; behavioral abnormalities; bleeding
• Posthepatic jaundice—chronic and/or recurrent bouts of apparent gastroenteritis or pancreatitis; moderate or marked jaundice; otherwise normal mucous membranes; diffuse abdominal pain; cranial abdominal pain or mass; abdominal effusion (septic or nonseptic exudates); bleeding; acholic feces

LABORATORY FINDINGS
Drugs That May Alter Laboratory Results
Bovine hemoglobin for anemia (Oxyglobin; Biopure, Cambridge, MA) results in high bilirubin concentrations.

Disorders That May Alter Laboratory Results
• Bilirubin assay—based on the diazo reaction; assesses direct-reacting and total serum bilirubins; most yield reasonable total bilirubin results; values for direct bilirubin vary • Sample management—important; total bilirubin may decrease by 50% per hour with direct exposure to sunlight or artificial lighting • Hemolysis—variable effects on total bilirubin measured by spectrophotometry.
• Lipemia—falsely increases total bilirubin values measured by endpoint assays
• Fractionation into conjugated and unconjugated—unable to define causes of jaundice, contrary to dogma

Valid if Run in Human Laboratory? Yes

CBC/BIOCHEMISTRY/URINALYSIS
Prehepatic Jaundice
• CBC—severe anemia (usually regenerative); RBC morphology may reveal evidence of autoagglutination, spherocytes, Heinz bodies, or parasites; hemoglobinemia with intravascular hemolysis, normal to low platelets, and normal to high WBCs, with a left shift • Biochemistry—Normal to high ALT and ALP activity and BUN concentration; normal to low albumin; normal to high globulin; normal glucose and cholesterol; high bilirubin

Hepatic Jaundice
• CBC—mild nonregenerative anemia; low MCV with chronic liver disease and portosystemic shunting

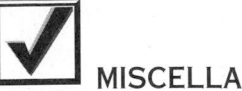
• Biochemistry—mildly to markedly high ALT and ALP; normal to low albumin, BUN, glucose, and cholesterol
• Urinalysis—normal to dilute urine; bilirubinuria precedes hyperbilirubinemia

Posthepatic Jaundice
• CBC—mild nonregenerative anemia
• Biochemistry—mildly high ALT and moderate to markedly high ALP; usually normal albumin, BUN, and glucose concentrations; normal to high cholesterol

OTHER LABORATORY TESTS
• Saline autoagglutination or dispersion slide test—with suspected RBC agglutination; high MCV on automated analyzers • Direct Coombs test—submit if no evidence of autoagglutination or spherocytes
• Osmotic fragility test • Blood smears—for hemoparasites • ANA—with hemolytic anemia • Serum bile acids—no need if prehepatic causes for jaundice are eliminated
• Serology—for infectious diseases (e.g., FeLV, leptospirosis, mycoses) with signs of multisystemic illness and hepatic jaundice
• Abdominal effusion—characterize cells and protein content • Coagulation tests—prolonged values, especially PIVKA and PT, with bile duct occlusion • Microbial culture and sensitivity—blood and/or other specimens; with an inflammatory leukon and potential focus of bacterial infection (e.g., urinary tract, biliary tract)

IMAGING
• Abdominal radiography—details obscured by effusion; may reveal hepatomegaly, a mass effect, or mineral or gas interfaces in liver; splenomegaly (hemolytic anemia, portal hypertension, abdominal neoplasia); metallic foreign body with zinc-induced hemolysis
• Thoracic radiography—may reveal metastatic disease; sternal lymphadenopathy (reflects inflammatory abdominal disease or neoplasia) • Abdominal ultrasonography—may distinguish parenchymal liver disease from extrahepatic biliary obstruction; characterizes hepatic parenchymal lesions; may disclose neoplasm causing immune-mediated or microangiopathic hemolysis; may determine cause of abdominal effusion; may be used to direct lesion sampling (aspirates or needle biopsy)

OTHER DIAGNOSTIC PROCEDURES
• Fine-needle aspiration—cytology of mass, lymph node, or parenchymal tissue lesions
• Liver biopsy—bacterial culture of liver tissue, bile, and specimens obtained via celiotomy, blind percutaneous, keyhole, laparoscopic, or ultrasound-guided technique
• Surgical intervention—required for diagnosis and treatment of most posthepatic disorders

TREATMENT
• Depends on underlying cause
• Inpatient—for initial medical care
• Cage rest—to facilitate liver regeneration
• Diet—important for hepatic and posthepatic jaundice; nutritionally balanced with maximum protein tolerated by patient; carbohydrate based (dogs) with moderately restricted protein for hepatic encephalopathy; restricted sodium for ascites
• Vitamin supplementation—water-soluble vitamins in all patients; parenteral vitamin K$_1$ for bile duct obstruction or severe cholestasis

MEDICATIONS
DRUG(S)
• Prehepatic jaundice—eliminate inciting cause; see Anemia, Immune-mediated; whole blood transfusion for life-threatening anemia
• Hepatic/posthepatic jaundice—treat specific disorder defined by biopsy and cultures

CONTRAINDICATIONS
• Avoid known hepatotoxic drugs. • Avoid tetracyclines unless clearly indicated—suppress hepatic protein synthesis promoting hepatic lipidosis • Avoid analgesics, anesthetics, barbiturates—with hepatic failure

PRECAUTIONS
• Sedatives—avoid; may precipitate hepatic encephalopathy • Corticosteroids—use carefully for nonseptic inflammatory hepatobiliary disease; increases risk for intercurrent infection; may aggravate ascites by promoting water and sodium retention

POSSIBLE INTERACTIONS
• Use all drugs cautiously—the liver is the most important organ involved in drug metabolism; duration and intensity of action of many drugs requiring hepatic biotransformation may be increased; others may not be transformed to their effective form; with low albumin, highly protein-bound drugs unbound in the circulation

FOLLOW-UP
PATIENT MONITORING
• Prehepatic jaundice—recheck PCV as needed; may require repeat transfusions; gradually taper immunosuppressive drugs
• Hepatic and posthepatic jaundice—recheck serum biochemical profile as dictated by underlying disease; continue symptomatic and specific treatment

POSSIBLE COMPLICATIONS
Diseases causing jaundice may cause death.

MISCELLANEOUS
ASSOCIATED CONDITIONS
• Patients with immune-mediated hemolysis that are treated with immunosuppressive doses of corticosteroids are predisposed to thromboembolism, possible gastrointestinal ulceration, and infections. • Patients with hepatic failure are susceptible to infection and gastrointestinal bleeding. • Patients that have had reconstructive biliary surgery are at risk for recurrent ascending bacterial cholangitis.

ZOONOTIC POTENTIAL
Certain serovars of leptospirosis

SYNONYMS
• Icterus • Jaundice

SEE ALSO
• Anemia, Heinz Body • Anemia, Immune-mediated • Anemia, Regenerative • Babesiosis • Blood Transfusion Reactions • Cholangitis/Cholangiohepatitis Syndrome • Cholelithiasis • Cirrhosis and Fibrosis of the Liver • Copper Storage Hepatopathy • Gallbladder Mucocele • Haemobartonellosis • Hepatic Failure, Acute • Hepatic Lipidosis • Hepatitis, Chronic • Hepatitis, Infectious Canine • Hepatitis, Suppurative and Hepatic Abscess • Hepatotoxins • Liver Fluke Infestation • Lupus Erythematosus, Systemic (SLE) • Pancreatitis • Zinc Toxicity

ABBREVIATIONS
• ALP = alkaline phosphatase
• ALT = alanine aminotransferase
• ANA = antinuclear antibodies
• BUN = blood urea nitrogen
• FeLV = feline leukemia virus
• FIP = feline infectious peritonitis
• MCV = mean corpuscular volume
• PCV = packed cell volume
• PIVKA = proteins invoked by vitamin K absence or antagonism
• PT = prothrombin time
• RBC = red blood cell
• SLE = systemic lupus erythematosus
• WBC = white blood cell

Suggested Reading
Bunch SE. Acute hepatic disorders and systemic disorders that involve the liver. In: Ettinger SJ, Feldman EC, eds. Textbook of veterinary internal medicine. 5th ed. Philadelphia: Saunders, 2000:1326–1340.
Leveille-Webster CR. Laboratory diagnosis of hepatobiliary disease. In: Ettinger SJ, Feldman EC, eds. Textbook of veterinary internal medicine. 5th ed. Philadelphia: Saunders, 2000:1277–1293.
Author Susan E. Bunch
Consulting Editor Sharon A. Center

HYPERCALCEMIA

BASICS

DEFINITION
• Serum total calcium > 11.5 mg/dL (dogs)
• Serum total calcium > 10.5 mg/dL (cats)

PATHOPHYSIOLOGY
• Control of calcium is complex and is influenced by the actions of PTH and vitamin D and the interaction of these hormones with the gut, bone, kidneys, and parathyroid glands.
• Derangement in the function of these can lead to hypercalcemia.
• Secretory productions of some neoplastic cells can also disturb calcium homeostasis.

SYSTEMS AFFECTED
• Renal/Urologic—high levels of calcium are toxic to the renal tubules and can cause polyuria and polydipsia (PU/PD) and renal failure; can also lead to urolithiasis and associated lower urinary tract disease
• Gastrointestinal—reduces excitability of smooth muscle and can alter gastrointestinal function
• Neuromuscular—depressed skeletal muscle contractility causes weakness.
• Cardiovascular—hypertension and altered cardiac contractility

SIGNALMENT
• Dog and cat
• Primary hyperparathyroidism in the keeshond and Siamese cat

SIGNS

General Comments
• Depend on the cause of hypercalcemia
• Patients with underlying neoplasia, renal failure, or hypoadrenocorticism generally appear ill.
• Patients with primary hyperparathyroidism show mild clinical signs, if any, due solely to the effects of hypercalcemia.
• Signs become apparent when hypercalcemia is severe and chronic.

Historical Findings
• PU/PD—most common in dogs
• Anorexia
• Lethargy—most common in cats
• Vomiting
• Constipation
• Weakness
• Stupor and coma—severe cases

Physical Examination Findings
• Lymphadenopathy or abdominal organomegaly in patients with lymphosarcoma
• Usually unremarkable in dogs with primary hyperparathyroidism
• Parathyroid gland adenoma—not palpable in dogs; often palpable in cats with primary hyperparathyroidism

CAUSES
• Neoplasia—lymphosarcoma (most common in dogs, less common in cats), anal sac apocrine gland adenocarcinoma (dogs), multiple myeloma, lymphocytic leukemia, metastatic bone tumor, fibrosarcoma (cats), various types of carcinoma
• Primary hyperparathyroidism
• Renal failure—acute or chronic
• Blastomycosis
• Hypoadrenocorticism
• Vitamin D rodenticide intoxication—no longer marketed in the United States

RISK FACTORS
• Keeshond breed—hyperparathyroidism
• Renal failure
• Neoplasia
• Use of calcium supplements or calcium-containing intestinal phosphate binders
• Use of calcitriol or other vitamin D preparations

DIAGNOSIS

DIFFERENTIAL DIAGNOSIS
• History should include exposure to rat poison and any previous response to steroids.
• History of waxing/waning illness suggests hypoadrenocorticism.
• Complete lymph node, rectal, and abdominal palpation may raise index of suspicion for lymphosarcoma and other neoplasia.
• Assessment of hydration status, renal palpation, and urinary history points toward lower urinary tract disease or renal failure.

LABORATORY FINDINGS

Drugs That May Alter Laboratory Results
• Oxalate, citrate, and EDTA anticoagulants bind calcium and falsely lower calcium measurement.
• Vitamin D preparations and thiazide diuretics can raise serum calcium concentrations.

Disorders That May Alter Laboratory Results
• Hemolysis and lipemia can falsely raise calcium concentrations.
• Hypoalbuminemia can falsely lower total calcium concentration.

Valid if Run in Human Laboratory?
Yes

CBC/BIOCHEMISTRY/URINALYSIS
• Serum calcium—total calcium concentration depends on binding proteins; adjusted (corrected) calcium can be estimated by the following formulas:

$$\text{Corrected Ca} = \text{Ca (mg/dL)} - \text{albumin (g/dL)} + 3.5$$

or

$$\text{Corrected Ca} = \text{Ca (mg/dL)} - [0.4 \times \text{total protein (g/dL)}] + 3.3$$

• Azotemia and isosthenuria help define degree of renal impairment.
• Serum phosphorus is usually low or low-normal in patients with primary hyperparathyroidism or hypercalcemia associated with malignancy.
• Hyperphosphatemia in the absence of azotemia suggests a nonparathyroid cause of hypercalcemia.
• Combination of hyperphosphatemia and azotemia is difficult to interpret, since renal failure can be the cause or effect of hypercalcemia.

- Hyperkalemia and hyponatremia suggest hypoadrenocorticism.
- Hyperglobulinemia is associated with multiple myeloma.
- Cytopenias are seen in patients with myelophthisic disease.

OTHER LABORATORY TESTS
- Serum ionized calcium is high in patients with primary hyperparathyroidism or hypercalcemia associated with malignancy; usually normal or low in patients with hypercalcemia associated with renal failure
- Serum PTH measurement—intact molecule and two-site assay methods have the greatest specificity; high-normal or high concentration suggests primary hyperparathyroidism; low concentration suggests neoplasia.
- Serum PTH-rp measurement is often high in patients with hypercalcemia associated with malignancy.
- Vitamin D assays are not readily available.

IMAGING
- Radiography is useful for assessing renal size and shape, urolithiasis, bone lysis, and occult neoplasia.
- Ultrasonography valuable for assessing renal architecture, abdominal lymphadenopathy, and urolithiasis

DIAGNOSTIC PROCEDURES
- Cytologic examination of fine-needle aspirate of lymph nodes to confirm lymphosarcoma
- Examination of bone marrow aspirate to confirm occult hematopoietic neoplasia
- ACTH stimulation testing to confirm hypoadrenocorticism

 TREATMENT
- Inpatient care because of the deleterious effects of hypercalcemia and the need for fluid therapy
- Consider severe hypercalcemia a medical emergency.

 MEDICATIONS

DRUG(S) OF CHOICE
- Normal saline—fluid of choice
- Avoid calcium-containing fluids.
- Diuretics (furosemide) and corticosteroids can be useful.

CONTRAINDICATIONS
- Do not use glucocorticoids until the diagnosis of lymphoma is excluded; they can obfuscate the diagnosis; if hypoadrenocorticism is suspected, do not give glucocorticoids until after ACTH stimulation testing.
- Thiazide diuretics can cause calcium retention.

PRECAUTIONS
N/A

POSSIBLE INTERACTIONS
Avoid the use of calcium- or phosphorus-containing compounds; they can cause soft tissue mineralization in severely hypercalcemic and hyperphosphatemic patients.

ALTERNATIVE DRUG(S)
- Sodium bicarbonate (1–4 mEq/kg) may be useful in combination with other treatments.
- Mithramycin has been used in severe hypercalcemic crises; avoid its use if possible, because of associated nephrotoxicity and hepatotoxicity.
- Calcitonin may be useful in the treatment of hypervitaminosis D.
- Pamidronate is a potentially useful drug for the treatment of hypervitaminosis D and other causes of hypercalcemia associated with increased bone resorption.

 FOLLOW-UP

PATIENT MONITORING
- Serum calcium every 12 hr
- Renal function tests—the first sign of tubular damage may be casts in the urine sediment.
- Must monitor urine output, particularly if oliguric renal failure is suspected, in which case urine output should be measured carefully; oliguria cannot be determined unless the patient is fully hydrated.
- Hydration status must be monitored; indicators of overhydration include increased body weight, increased central venous pressure, and edema (pulmonary or subcutaneous).

POSSIBLE COMPLICATIONS
- Irreversible renal failure
- Soft tissue mineralization

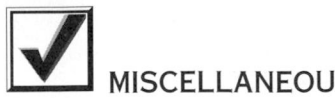 MISCELLANEOUS

ASSOCIATED CONDITIONS
Calcium-containing urolithiasis

AGE-RELATED FACTORS
- Mild elevations in calcium and phosphorus may be normal in growing animals.
- Middle-aged and older dogs and cats are at increased risk for cancer.

ZOONOTIC POTENTIAL
N/A

PREGNANCY
A fetus is at the same risk as the dam; do not alter treatment because of pregnancy.

SYNONYMS
N/A

SEE ALSO
- Hyperparathyroidism
- Paraneoplastic syndromes
- Renal Failure (Chronic or Acute)
- Vitamin D Toxicity

ABBREVIATIONS
- ACTH = adrenocorticotropic hormone
- Ca = calcium
- EDTA = ethylenediamine tetraacetic acid
- PTH = parathyroid hormone
- PTH-rp = parathyroid hormone–related peptide
- PU/PD = polyuria and polydipsia

Suggested Reading

Chew DJ, Nagode LA, Carothers M. Disorders of calcium: hypercalcemia and hypocalcemia. In: DiBartola SP, ed. Fluid therapy in small animal practice. Philadelphia: Saunders 1992:116–176.

Feldman EC, Nelson RW. Hypercalcemia and primary hyperparathyroidism. In: Canine and feline endocrinology and reproduction. 2nd ed. Philadelphia: Saunders, 1996; 455–496.

Rumbeiha WK, Kruger JM, Fitzgerald SF, et al. Use of pamidronate to reverse vitamin D3–induced toxicosis in dogs. Am J Vet Res 1999;60(9):1092–1097.

Savary KC, Price GS, Vaden SL. Hypercalcemia in cats: a retrospective study of 71 cases (1991–1997). J Vet Intern Med 2000;14(2):184–189.

Author Thomas K. Graves
Consulting Editor Deborah S. Greco

HYPERCAPNIA

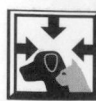 BASICS

DEFINITION
• An increase in the partial pressure of carbon dioxide in the arterial blood
• Normal $PaCO_2$ values—35–45 mm Hg

PATHOPHYSIOLOGY
• CO_2—end product of aerobic cellular metabolism; considered the primary drive to ventilation by stimulation of central chemoreceptors in the medulla oblongata; carried in the blood in three forms: bicarbonate (65%), bound to hemoglobin (30%), and dissolved in plasma (5%; the source of $PaCO_2$ values); constantly being added to alveolar gas from the pulmonary circulation and removed by alveolar ventilation
• Uncommon in nonanesthetized, clinically normal patient; result of alveolar hypoventilation

SYSTEMS AFFECTED
• Nervous—the brain is primary affected organ; cerebral blood flow related to $PaCO_2$ in a linear fashion; hypercapnia results in increased cerebral blood flow and intracranial pressure; $PaCO_2 > 90$ mm Hg may lead to CO_2 narcosis and unconsciousness.
• Hemic/Lymphatic/Immune—may alter acid–base balance; acute increase results in production of excess hydrogen ions and a decrease in pH (respiratory acidosis).
• Cardiovascular—may result in endogenous catecholamine release, which may induce cardiac arrhythmias; may cause vasodilation leading to hypotension

SIGNALMENT
Any breed, age, and sex of dogs and cats

SIGNS

Historical Findings
• Abnormal breathing pattern
• Weakness—secondary to concurrent hypoxemia or primary neuromuscular disease

Physical Examination Findings
• Anesthetized patients—usually no obvious signs; severe condition may lead to tachypnea
• Hypoventilation owing to muscle weakness or neuropathy—weak respiratory efforts; decreased thoracic excursion; possibly generalized weakness
• Upper airway obstruction—marked, prolonged inspiratory efforts with variable expirations, depending on whether the obstruction is fixed (e.g., mass) or nonfixed (e.g., laryngeal paralysis); stertor or stridor common
• Pleural effusion—may have shallow rapid respirations; may note a marked abdominal component; lung sounds normal to decreased
• Pulmonary parenchymal disease—increased bronchovesicular sounds; crackles (edema, infection, contusions)

CAUSES
• Hypoventilation—an increase in $PaCO_2$ that results from a decrease in alveolar ventilation; may result from anesthesia, muscular paralysis, upper airway obstruction, air or fluid in the pleural space, restriction in movement of the thoracic cage, diaphragmatic hernia, pulmonary parenchymal disease, and CNS disease
• May occur in spontaneously breathing patients during inhalation anesthesia (isoflurane or sevoflurane)
• Increased inspired CO_2—rebreathing of expired gases because of exhausted CO_2 absorbent in an anesthesia machine most common cause; also inadequate fresh gas flow in a nonrebreathing anesthesia circuit (e.g., Bain and Ayres T-piece)
• Exogenous administration of sodium bicarbonate, which dissociates into CO_2, with inadequate ventilation

RISK FACTORS
• Deep planes of inhalation anesthesia
• Inadequate fresh flow of oxygen with nonrebreathing anesthesia circuits
• Bronchial or alveolar disease
• Upper airway obstruction
• Pleural disease
• Inadequate ventilation during administration of sodium bicarbonate

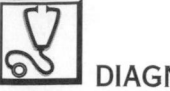 DIAGNOSIS

DIFFERENTIAL DIAGNOSIS
• Conscious patient with tachypnea—excitement or anxiety; hyperthermia; hypoxemia; head trauma; pain
• Anesthetized patient with tachypnea—light plane of anesthesia; hypoxemia

LABORATORY FINDINGS

Drugs That May Alter Laboratory Results
N/A

Disorders That May Alter Laboratory Results
Air bubbles in the arterial blood sample and/or improper packaging of the arterial blood sample—falsely low $PaCO_2$ values after approximately 30 min

Valid If Run in Human Laboratory?
Yes

CBC/BIOCHEMISTRY/URINALYSIS
N/A

OTHER LABORATORY TESTS
• Arterial blood gas analysis—diagnosis determined from a blood sample collected in an anaerobic manner, as follows: Use enough heparin to coat the needle and the inside of the syringe; place a rubber stopper on the needle or cover the hub of the syringe to prevent room air from entering the sample.
• Analyze sample within 15 min if left at room temperature; place sample on ice to extend time for safe and accurate analysis to 2–4 hours.
• Bedside or portable blood gas analyzers—several models available; make analysis more convenient

IMAGING
Thoracic radiography—may reveal bronchial, alveolar, or pleural space disease

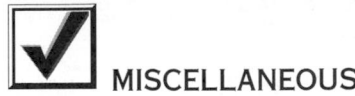

OTHER DIAGNOSTIC PROCEDURES
• Alternative method of analysis—capnometer
• End tidal gas is almost entirely alveolar gas and provides nearly the same value as $PaCO_2$, which closely approximates the mean value of perfused alveoli.
• Exception—during conditions of pulmonary thromboembolism, $PaCO_2$ much higher than $PETCO_2$; need to open thoracic cavity (surgery)
• Advantage of capnometry—may monitor $PaCO_2$ on a breath-by-breath basis, whereas a blood gas sample is a finite value at a finite time except during open chest procedures

 TREATMENT
• Provide adequate alveolar ventilation—most important
• Anesthesia—ventilation accomplished manually or mechanically
• Nonanesthetized patient with severe pulmonary or CNS disease—mechanical ventilation may require heavy sedation, muscle relaxants, or general anesthesia.
• Supplemental oxygen—need determined by primary disease
• Definitive treatment—treat primary cause (e.g., discontinuing inhalation anesthesia is the definitive treatment for anesthesia-induced hypoventilation).

 MEDICATIONS

DRUG(S) OF CHOICE
• Respiratory stimulants (e.g., doxapram) may be administered but are rarely indicated.

• Doxapram—nonspecific stimulant of the respiratory center; does not provide definitive treatment; administer only as an infusion (just 1 bolus will increase ventilation and lower $PaCO_2$, decreasing the drive of ventilation and causing apnea).

CONTRAINDICATIONS
Anesthetic drugs or other respiratory depressants—contraindicated with CNS disease if adequate ventilatory support cannot be provided; increased $PaCO_2$ may result in dangerous elevations of intracranial pressure and predispose patient to herniation of the brainstem.

PRECAUTIONS
N/A

POSSIBLE INTERACTIONS
N/A

ALTERNATIVE DRUG(S)
N/A

 **FOLLOW-UP**

PATIENT MONITORING
• Assess effectiveness of supportive (ventilation) and definitive treatment—should result in decrease in respiratory effort
• Re-evaluate the arterial blood gas or capnometry—determine improvement; assess adequacy of ventilation

POSSIBLE COMPLICATIONS
Concurrent CNS disease may cause high intracranial pressure and predispose the patient to herniation of the brainstem and death.

✓ **MISCELLANEOUS**

ASSOCIATED CONDITIONS
N/A

AGE-RELATED FACTORS
N/A

ZOONOTIC POTENTIAL
N/A

PREGNANCY
N/A

SYNONYMS
Hypercarbia

SEE ALSO
Dyspnea, Tachypnea, and Panting

ABBREVIATION
$PETCO_2$ = end tidal carbon dioxide
$PaCO_2$ = partial pressure of carbon dioxide in arterial blood

Suggested Reading
Martin L. All you really need to know to interpret arterial blood gases. Philadelphia: Lippincott Williams & Wilkins, 1999:27–47.
West JB. Pulmonary physiology and pathophysiology. Philadelphia: Lippincott Williams & Wilkins, 2001:84–111, 125–144.
West JB. Respiratory physiology: the essentials. 6th ed. Philadelphia: Lippincott Williams & Wilkins, 2000:11–21, 103–115.
Author Thomas Kevin Day
Consulting Editor Lynelle R. Johnson

HYPERCHLOREMIA

 BASICS

DEFINITION
Serum chloride concentration >122 mEq/L in dogs and >129 mEq/L in cats

PATHOPHYSIOLOGY
• Chloride is the most abundant anion in the extracellular fluid.
• Hyperchloremia is associated with similar conditions to those that cause hypernatremia—water loss in excess of sodium and chloride or excessive NaCl intake
• Chloride concentration varies inversely to bicarbonate concentration; high bicarbonate loss (i.e., GI or renal wasting), followed by low renal chloride resorption in excess of bicarbonate, can cause hyperchloremia.

SYSTEMS AFFECTED
Relates to underlying cause

GENETICS
N/A

INCIDENCE
N/A

GEOGRAPHIC DISTRIBUTION
N/A

SIGNALMENT

Species
Dogs and cats

Breed Predilection
None

Predominant Sex
None

Mean Age and Range
N/A

SIGNS

General Comments
• Related to concurrent hypernatremia or the underlying disorder or both
• Severity of neurologic signs is related to the degree of hypernatremia and the rate at which it develops.

History and Physical Examination Findings
• Polydipsia
• Disorientation
• Coma
• Seizures

CAUSES

High Total Body Chloride
• Oral ingestion—rare
• NaCl administered IV during cardiovascular resuscitation

Normal Total Body Chloride with Water Deficit
• Low intake (e.g., no access to water)
• High urinary water loss (e.g., diabetes insipidus)
• High insensible water loss (e.g., panting)

Low Total Body Chloride with Hypotonic Fluid Loss
Urinary loss—diabetes mellitus, osmotic diuresis, and diuresis after urinary obstruction

Hyperchloremic Metabolic Acidosis
• Renal tubular acidosis—renal tubular disorders that cause renal wasting of bicarbonate or low hydrogen ion secretion
• Diarrhea associated with gastrointestinal loss of bicarbonate and renal resorption of chloride

RISK FACTORS
N/A

 DIAGNOSIS

DIFFERENTIAL DIAGNOSIS
• Normal anion gap metabolic acidosis (e.g., renal tubular acidosis and gastrointestinal bicarbonate loss)
• Diabetes insipidus
• Hypertonic dehydration
• Severe forms of diabetes mellitus (e.g., diabetic ketoacidosis and hyperosmolar nonketotic syndrome)
• Salt ingestion—rare

LABORATORY FINDINGS

Drugs That May Alter Laboratory Results
• A wide variety of drugs can interfere with renal capacity to concentrate urine, leading to water loss in excess of sodium, and high sodium and chloride concentrations; these drugs include lithium, demeclocycline, and amphotericin.
• Other drugs that may increase chloride concentration include acetazolamide, ammonium chloride, androgens, and cholestyramine.
• A falsely high chloride concentration can occur with a high serum concentration of iodide or bromide—most commonly seen in patients with epilepsy treated with potassium bromide.

Disorders That May Alter Laboratory Results
Hemoglobin and bilirubin cause falsely high chloride readings if colorimetric tests are used.

Valid If Run in Human Laboratory?
Yes

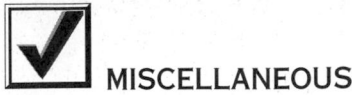

CBC/BIOCHEMISTRY/URINALYSIS
• High chloride, often coupled with high sodium
• Diabetes insipidus—low urinary specific gravity, polyuria, and low urinary sodium
• Diabetic ketoacidosis and hyperosmolar nonketotic syndrome—high blood glucose
• Hypertonic dehydration—low urinary sodium and high urinary specific gravity (usually >1.030)
• Renal tubular acidosis—hyperchloremic acidosis, urine pH > 5.3, serum potassium often low, and other causes of metabolic acidosis have been ruled out

OTHER LABORATORY TESTS
Renal tubular acidosis—response to $NaHCO_3$ or NH_4Cl.

IMAGING
CT scan or MRI in patients with diabetes insipidus to rule out pituitary tumor

OTHER DIAGNOSTIC PROCEDURES
N/A

 TREATMENT

Hyperchloremia with hypernatremia—hypotonic fluids (5% dextrose in water); decrease sodium by 0.5 mEq/h or by no more than 20 mEq/L/day.

 MEDICATIONS

DRUG(S) OF CHOICE
• Hypovolemia—isotonic saline (normal saline or lactated Ringer's solution) or isotonic fluid (5% dextrose with half-normal saline)

• Central diabetes insipidus—DDAVP (1–2 drops in the conjunctival sac q12–24h)
• Nephrogenic diabetes insipidus—chlorothiazide (10–40 mg/kg PO q12h)
• Hyperchloremic metabolic acidosis—treat underlying cause; consider bicarbonate and potassium replacement if needed.

CONTRAINDICATIONS
N/A

PRECAUTIONS
• Rapid correction of hyperchloremia with hypernatremia can cause pulmonary edema.
• Hypocalcemia may develop during correction of hyperchloremia.

POSSIBLE INTERACTIONS
N/A

ALTERNATIVE DRUG(S)
N/A

 FOLLOW-UP

PATIENT MONITORING
Electrolytes, body weight, and hydration status

POSSIBLE COMPLICATIONS
• Related to associated hypernatremia or the underlying disorder
• Neurologic complications include CNS thrombosis or hemorrhage; seizures; and hyperactivity

✓ MISCELLANEOUS

ASSOCIATED CONDITIONS
N/A

AGE-RELATED FACTORS
N/A

ZOONOTIC POTENTIAL
N/A

PREGNANCY
N/A

SYNONYMS
N/A

SEE ALSO
Hypernatremia

ABBREVIATIONS
• DDAVP = brand name for desmopressin, a synthetic antidiuretic hormone preparation
• GI = gastrointestinal

Suggested Reading
DiBartola SP. Fluid therapy in small animal practice. Philadelphia: Saunders, 1992.
Ross DB. Clinical physiology of acid-base and electrolyte disorders. 3rd ed. New York: McGraw-Hill, 1989.
Author Rhett Nichols
Editor Deborah S. Greco

HYPERCOAGULABILITY

BASICS

OVERVIEW
• An imbalance between procoagulants and anticoagulants that shifts the balance toward clot formation, resulting in predisposition to thrombosis • Hypercoagulability may result from platelet hyperaggregability; excessive activation or decreased removal of coagulation factors; deficiencies of natural anticoagulants, such as antithrombin; or defective fibrinolysis. • Hypercoagulability is most often recognized when an animal suffers an episode of thrombosis. • In the majority of veterinary cases, the hypercoagulable state is acquired in association with an underlying disease. • Thrombosis reported to involve pulmonary arteries, distal aorta, cranial or caudal vena cava, intestinal or mesenteric vessels, portal vein, and peripheral arteries

SIGNS
• Signs depend on site and organs involved; thrombosis may be subclinical. • Patients with pulmonary thromboembolism may present with acute severe dyspnea and tachypnea or have a more chronic history of labored breathing and lethargy; possible physical examination findings include fever, jugular distention, cardiac murmurs, and hepatosplenomegaly. • Patients with aortic thromboembolism often suffer acute paresis or paralysis and have limb pain, absent or weak femoral pulses, cold limbs, cyanotic nail beds, and peripheral neuropathy on examination. • Canine distal aortic thromboembolism may be more insidious in comparison with the feline type; dogs may show mild neuromuscular signs for days to months prior to paraparesis and paresthesia. • Primary disease process often causes clinical signs unrelated to thrombosis.

CAUSES & RISK FACTORS
• Protein-losing nephropathy • IMHA • DIC or sepsis • Hyperadrenocorticism • Pancreatitis • Dirofilariasis • Hypothyroidism • Neoplasia

DIAGNOSIS

DIFFERENTIAL DIAGNOSIS
• PTE may mimic pulmonary parenchymal diseases such as bacterial or fungal pneumonia, pulmonary edema, and dirofilariasis. • Distal aortic thromboembolism requires differentiation from other causes of paraparesis and paraplegia; absence of femoral pulses and cold limbs is supportive of a thrombus.

CBC/BIOCHEMISTRY/URINALYSIS
• Typically reflect underlying disease • Thrombocytopenia and schistocytosis in some animals with DIC, sepsis, and neoplasia

OTHER LABORATORY TESTS
• APTT, PT, fibrin(ogen) degradation products—abnormal in some animals with DIC, IMHA, sepsis, or pancreatitis • Antithrombin activity—may be decreased in protein-losing nephropathies, protein-losing enteropathies, DIC, sepsis, and IMHA • D-dimer concentration—elevations associated with DIC or subsequent to thrombus formation • Arterial blood gas—hypoxemia and hypocapnea (occasional hypercapnea) supportive of PTE

IMAGING
• Thoracic radiography—may reveal few abnormalities despite severe dyspnea in some cases of PTE; most common abnormalities include regional oligemia, alveolar pulmonary infiltrates, pulmonary vascular changes, and pleural effusion • Abdominal ultrasonography—may confirm aortic occlusion in many patients with aortic thromboembolism • Echocardiography—to identify intracardiac thrombi and gain evidence for pulmonary hypertension associated with PTE (dilation of right ventricle and pulmonary artery)

DIAGNOSTIC PROCEDURES
• Angiography—may be necessary to localize and confirm a thrombus. • Nuclear perfusion scintigraphy—noninvasive study used to gain support for a diagnosis of PTE

TREATMENT
• Inpatient—necessary for initial management of thrombosis and initiation of anticoagulant therapy • Surgical intervention—rarely indicated • Supportive care—to ensure adequate hydration to maintain perfusion and minimize vascular stasis, correction and monitoring of acid–base and electrolyte abnormalities, and appropriate use and handling of venous catheters • Severe restriction of activity—recommended; exercise compounds the effects of poor tissue perfusion in areas supplied by thrombosed vessels • Oxygen therapy—indicated in many cases of PTE • Owners should be informed that animals with conditions associated with a hypercoagulable state have a risk of future thrombotic episodes if the underlying disease cannot be resolved.

MEDICATIONS

DRUG(S)
Anticoagulants
• Heparin—most commonly used initial anticoagulant in veterinary patients; dose is titrated to achieve a 1.5–2.0-fold increase in APTT; appropriate starting doses: 150–200 IU/kg SC q6h (dogs) and 200 IU/kg q8h (cats); check APTT once daily (2 hr postheparin administration) • Warfarin—vitamin K antagonist; may be used for long-term oral anticoagulation; therapy is adjusted to prolong the PT to approximately twice the baseline or to attain an INR of 2.0–3.0 (used to minimize the effects of test kit variability on measurements of PT); appropriate starting doses: 0.1–0.2 mg/kg PO q24h (dogs) and 0.5 mg per cat q24h

CONTRAINDICATIONS/POSSIBLE INTERACTIONS
• Do not treat with warfarin initially or exclusively; effect on anticoagulant proteins C and S and on vitamin K–dependent factors leads to initial hypercoagulability; overlap with adequate heparin anticoagulation for 4 days • High rate of interaction between warfarin and other drugs; reassess INR with any changes in medication • Bleeding is the major risk with anticoagulation; discontinue anticoagulant and administer protamine (with heparin overdose) or vitamin K (warfarin) and plasma as necessary to treat bleeding.

FOLLOW-UP
PT—monitor daily for 4–5 days and discontinue heparin when appropriate INR is achieved; check PT 6–8 hr after last heparin dose as it may decrease; following discharge, check PT twice weekly, then weekly for several weeks, then every 2 months

MISCELLANEOUS

SEE ALSO
• Amyloidosis • Aortic Thromboembolism • Disseminated Intravascular Coagulation • Glomerulonephritis • Nephrotic Syndrome • Pulmonary Thromboembolism

ABBREVIATIONS
• APTT = activated partial thromboplastin time • DIC = disseminated intravascular coagulation • IMHA = immune-mediated hemolytic anemia • INR = international normalized ratio • PT = prothrombin time • PTE = pulmonary thromboembolism

Suggested Reading
Bick RL. Hypercoagulability and thrombosis. Med Clin North Am 1994;78:635–664.
Author Mary F. Thompson
Consulting Editor Stephen Kruth

BASICS

OVERVIEW

• Idiopathic persistent eosinophilia caused by sustained overproduction of eosinophils in the bone marrow • Hypothesized to be caused by severe reaction to an undefined antigen or dysregulation of immunologic control of eosinophil production • Multisystemic syndrome with invasion of tissues by eosinophils and subsequent organ damage and dysfunction, leading to death • Organ damage caused by effects of eosinophil granule products and eosinophil-derived cytokines that are released in the tissues from activated or necrotic cells • Probably includes a heterogeneous group of disorders • Common sites of infiltration—gastrointestinal tract (especially intestine and liver), spleen, and lymph nodes (especially mesenteric nodes) • Less common sites of infiltration—skin, muscle, kidney, heart, thyroid, lung, adrenal glands, and pancreas

SIGNALMENT

• Cats—may occur more frequently in female, middle-aged, domestic shorthair animals than others • Dogs—rare and incompletely described

SIGNS

Historical Findings

• Lethargy • Anorexia • Intermittent vomiting and diarrhea • Weight loss • Less frequently—fever, pruritus, and seizures

PHYSICAL EXAMINATION FINDINGS

• Fever • Emaciation • Hepatosplenomegaly • Thickened (diffuse or segmental) intestine that is nonpainful • Mesenteric, and possible peripheral, lymphadenopathy • Mass lesions caused by eosinophilic granulomatous inflammation involving lymph nodes or organs • Pruritic erythroderma

CAUSES & RISK FACTORS

• Unknown, but believed to be a severe reaction to an underlying, but unidentifiable, antigenic stimulus • Cats—eosinophilic enteritis may be an early form.

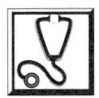

DIAGNOSIS

DIFFERENTIAL DIAGNOSIS

• Identifiable causes of eosinophilia—parasitism, hypersensitivity disorder, infectious disease, immune-mediated disease, and neoplasia; with these conditions, eosinophilia is usually limited in degree and remains confined to a specific organ, such as the lungs in feline asthma.
• Eosinophilic leukemia—distinction is controversial; differentiating criteria of this leukemia: (1) immature eosinophils seen in higher numbers in the circulation and constitute a higher percentage of the leukocyte differential; (2) anemia more common; (3) myeloid:erythroid ratio in bone marrow is higher (> 10:1) and blast forms are more numerous; (4) tissue infiltrates consist of immature eosinophils and may show a sinusoidal pattern in the liver without fibrosis; (5) in cats, chloroma-like masses in the kidneys reported; (6) serum IgE concentrations not increased.

CBC/BIOCHEMISTRY/URINALYSIS

• Leukocytosis with eosinophilia (usually marked), possibly with a left shift in the eosinophil series; eosinophil count range: 3,200–130,000 cells/μL • Basophilia • Anemia in some animals • In animals with organ dysfunction, biochemical abnormalities may be seen.

OTHER LABORATORY TESTS

• Rule out identifiable causes of eosinophilia—fecal flotation, heartworm test, fungal culture, and biopsy to detect neoplasm • Serum IgE concentrations may be increased.

IMAGING

Intestinal mucosal irregularities and thickened intestine seen on radiographic contrast studies

DIAGNOSTIC PROCEDURES

• Bone marrow—hypercellularity, eosinophilic hyperplasia (up to 40% of nucleated cells consist of eosinophils), lack of morphologic abnormalities (usually), and high myeloid:erythroid ratio (mean 7.27:1) • Biopsy of affected organ or mass

PATHOLOGIC FINDINGS

• Spleen—eosinophilic infiltrates in red pulp, sometimes in white pulp • Gastrointestinal tract—mucosal and submucosal eosinophilic infiltrates in small intestine, sometimes in colon and stomach • Lymph nodes—reactive hyperplasia and infiltration of cords and sinuses with eosinophils • Heart—eosinophilic infiltrates in the myocardium and endocardium; fibrosis and thrombus formation • Less frequently—eosinophilic infiltrates in the skin, liver, lung, pancreas, kidney, adrenal, muscle, and thyroid gland

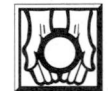

TREATMENT

• Use long-term maintenance therapy to control or reduce the eosinophilia and organ damage.
• Massive tissue infiltration impedes treatment and usually signifies a poor prognosis.
• High serum IgE concentration predicts a good response to treatment with prednisone and a better prognosis.

MEDICATIONS

DRUG(S)

• Corticosteroids—prednisolone, 1–3 mg/kg/day initially; then taper to alternate-day administration if eosinophilia is suppressed; if eosinophilia returns, resume higher daily dose.
• Chemotherapeutic agents—try if eosinophilia is steroid-resistant, but the paucity of case reports describing these therapies precludes recommending their use
• Hydroxyurea (inhibits DNA synthesis)—administer to reduce the eosinophil count if not normal or near normal after 7–14 days of treatment with steroids; most likely would be used long-term if effective in conjunction with steroids
• Cyclosporine—suppresses production of eosinophilopoietic factors by T cells
• Vincristine and alkylating agents, such as chlorambucil, effective in humans
• Reduce dosage or discontinue drug if bone marrow suppression or thrombocytopenia develops.

CONTRAINDICATIONS/POSSIBLE INTERACTIONS

Aggressive cytotoxic therapy has been deleterious in some human patients.

FOLLOW-UP

• Monitor eosinophil count (not always indicative of tissue infiltrates) and myelosuppression if chemotherapeutic drugs are used.
• Monitor clinical signs (e.g., anorexia, lethargy, vomiting, and diarrhea) and any physical abnormalities.

MISCELLANEOUS

SEE ALSO

Eosinophilia and Basophilia

Suggested Reading

Huibregtse BA, Turner JL. Hypereosinophilic syndrome and eosinophilic leukemia: a comparison of 22 hypereosinophilic cats. J Anim Hosp Assoc 1994;30:591–599.
Perkins M, Watson A. Successful treatment of hypereosinophilic syndrome in a dog. Austral Vet J 2001;79:686–689.
Sykes JE, Weiss DJ, Buoen LC, et al. Idiopathic hypereosinophilic syndrome in 3 Rottweilers. J Vet Int Med 2001;15:162–166.
Author Karen M. Young
Consulting Editor Stephen A. Kruth

HYPERESTROGENISM

BASICS

OVERVIEW
• A syndrome characterized by high serum concentration of estrogens (estradiol, estriol, and estrone)
• May occur as a result of excessive estrogen secretion or administration of exogenous estrogens, such as diethylstilbestrol
• Sites of endogenous estrogen production include ovarian follicles, Leydig cells, and the adrenal cortex (zona glomerulosa and fasciculata); may also occur as a result of peripheral conversion of excessive androgens.
• Endogenous estrogens in the female are responsible for normal sexual behavior and development and function of the female reproductive tract; in the male, estrogens are responsible for Leydig cell function.
• Estrogens potentiate the stimulatory effect of progesterone in the endometrium and permit cervical relaxation; these two effects increase the risk of cystic endometrial hyperplasia and pyometra. Estrogens also increase osteoblastic activity, retention of calcium and phosphorus, and total body protein and metabolic rate.
• High serum concentration of estrogens—provides a source of negative feedback at the hypothalamic-pituitary axis and result in suppression of gonadotropin secretion; interferes with stem cell differentiation in the bone marrow and erythrocyte iron metabolism.

SIGNALMENT
Endogenous Hyperestrogenism
• Estrus ferrets
• Older male dogs (secondary to testicular tumors)
• Older female dogs (secondary to granulosa cell tumors and other ovarian tumor types)
• Young female dogs (follicular cysts)

Exogenous Hyperestrogenism
All species and ages in association with estrogen administration

SIGNS
Historical Findings
• Attractive to male dogs
• Infertility
• Prolonged proestrus and estrus
• Decreased libido
• Nymphomania
• Vulvar bleeding
• Hematuria (in association with thrombocytopenia)

Physical Examination Findings
• Skin/endocrine—nonpruritic, symmetric alopecia (endocrine alopecia); stud dog tail; hyperpigmentation
• Reproductive (male)—testicular mass; testicular asymmetry (in association with a tumor mass or testicular atrophy); testicular atrophy: may be unilateral in the non–tumor-containing testicle, as seen in association with a functional estrogen-producing testicular tumor, or bilateral, as seen in association with exogenous hyperestrogenism; cryptorchidism; prostatomegaly (secondary to squamous metaplasia); gynecomastia
• Reproductive (female)—vulvar edema; vulvar discharge; gynecomastia
• Hemic/lymphatic/immune—pale mucous membranes; thrombocytopenic hemorrhage; petechia; fever (due to secondary bacterial infection in association with neutropenia); depression

CAUSES & RISK FACTORS
• Follicular ovarian cysts
• Functional ovarian tumor (granulosa cell tumor and other ovarian tumors)
• Testicular tumor (specifically Sertoli cell tumor, but also occurs secondary to Leydig and interstitial cell tumors) • Exogenous estrogen administration—iatrogenic

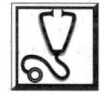

DIAGNOSIS

DIFFERENTIAL DIAGNOSIS
Nonpruritic, Symmetric Alopecia (Endocrine Alopecia)
• Hypothyroidism—diagnosis based on appropriate clinical signs in conjunction with typical hematologic and biochemical abnormalities (normocytic normochromic nonregenerative anemia, hypercholesterolemia) and thyroid function testing (total T_4, free T_4, TSH)
• Hyperadrenocorticism—clinical signs usually include polyuria, polydipsia, and exercise intolerance; CBC may reveal leukocytosis and erythrocytosis; serum biochemistry abnormalities include elevated ALP, ALT, and cholesterol, and decreased BUN; additional testing includes ACTH stimulation, LDDS test, endogenous ACTH, abdominal ultrasonography, and abdominal radiography
• GH-responsive dermatosis—see Hyperandrogenism
• Adrenal sex hormone dermatosis—see Hyperandrogenism

Attractive to Male Dogs
• Vaginitis—may be differentiated from hyperestrogenism via examination of vaginal cytology (lack of vaginal epithelial cell cornification), lack of evidence of ovarian abnormalities, or history of ovariohysterectomy • Behavioral abnormality—diagnosis of exclusion • Urinary tract infection—uncommon cause

Infertility
• Testicular degeneration/atrophy/immune-mediated orchitis—diagnosis based on physical examination, lack of testicular or intra-abdominal masses, semen evaluation (azoospermia), and testicular biopsy
• Intersex abnormalities—uncommon; diagnosis supported by physical examination findings (abnormal external genitalia), abnormal karyotype, and histologic examination of the reproductive tract, where available

CBC/BIOCHEMISTRY/URINALYSIS
CBC—changes are extremely variable; if present, initial 2–3 weeks characterized by thrombocytopenia or thrombocytosis, progressive anemia, and leukocytosis (white cell counts may exceed 100,000 WBC/μL); after 3 weeks, pancytopenia and aplastic anemia may be noted; hematuria (secondary to thrombocytopenia)

OTHER LABORATORY TESTS
• Serum estrogen (estradiol) concentrations—may be evaluated via radioimmunoassay; however, physiologic serum concentrations may be within normal limits due to accuracy of assay
• Vaginal/preputial cytology—extremely reliable as a bioassay for estrogen; under the influence of estrogen, will reveal a predominance of cornified epithelial cells that are anuclear or have pyknotic nuclei
• GnRH—may be administered to induce luteinization for cases of ovarian remnant syndrome or follicular cysts; 50 μg HCG is administered intramuscularly and serum progesterone assessed 7–10 days later for verification of luteinization; results are variable

IMAGING
• Ultrasonography of the abdomen and testes—to assess for testicular masses, cystic or enlarged ovarian structures, intra-abdominal masses, and local lymph node size and echogenicity
• Vaginoscopy—may be completed to evaluate the vaginal mucosa; under the influence of estrogen, the vaginal mucosa should appear either edematous and pink or crenulated

DIAGNOSTIC PROCEDURES
• Fine-needle aspiration cytology of testicular masses—may provide a cytologic diagnosis prior to pursuing surgery
• Three-view metastatic radiographic evaluation of the thoracic cavity—complete prior to any surgical intervention
• Complete hemogram and serum chemistries—always perform preoperatively
• Examination and biopsy of local lymph nodes—for evaluation of metastatic disease; may be completed, if indicated, at time of surgical exploration or ultrasonography
• Bone marrow core biopsy—may be used to confirm the presence of aplastic anemia
• Laparoscopy or laparotomy—may be used to identify and remove intra-abdominal masses, ovarian tissue, or testicular tissue
• Skin biopsy—may reveal nonspecific changes associated with endocrine alopecia such as orthokeratotic hyperkeratosis, epidermal atrophy and melanosis, follicular keratosis, telogen hair follicles, and sebaceous gland atrophy

TREATMENT
• Treatment of choice for endogenous hyperestrogenism in the intact female and male is surgical neutering.
• Unilateral orchiectomy or ovariectomy of the affected neoplastic testicle or ovary may be considered in valuable breeding animals. Use of testicular prosthetic devices is not advised.
• Discontinue exogenous estrogen administration in cases of exogenous hyperestrogenism.

MEDICATIONS

DRUG(S)
• Supportive care—including administration of appropriate antimicrobial therapy and blood products
• Synthetic erythropoietin, G-CSF, GM-CSF—may be considered to stimulate erythroid and granulocytic production at the level of the bone marrow
• GnRH—may induce ovulation in cases of follicular cysts; however, results are unreliable

CONTRAINDICATIONS/POSSIBLE INTERACTIONS
Administration of chemotherapeutic agents for treatment of metastatic testicular or ovarian neoplasia should be pursued with caution due to increased risk of bone marrow suppression secondary to hyperestrogenism.

FOLLOW-UP
• Repeat serial CBC analysis—to evaluate response to therapy and progression of disease
• Repeat serial bone marrow aspiration cytology—to evaluate bone marrow response and erythroid, myeloid, and megakaryocytic regeneration when myelosuppression is present. Peripheral signs of regeneration may not occur for weeks to months after initial insult.
• Concurrent administration of iron dextran intramuscularly or multiple daily doses of oral iron—paramount to support erythrocyte regeneration
• Use of erythropoietin, G-CSF, GM-CSF—closely monitor erythrocyte and leukocyte regeneration
• Evaluation of serum progesterone concentration—may be used to evaluate ovulation; serum progesterone concentration > 2 ng/dL (usually > 5) supports that ovulation has occurred

• Clinical signs of male feminization syndrome should resolve within 2–6 weeks after testicular tumor removal.
• Lack of resolving pancytopenia and continued bone marrow hypoplasia 3 weeks after surgical removal of ovarian or testicular neoplasia or removal of follicular cysts—associated with a grave prognosis

MISCELLANEOUS

ASSOCIATED CONDITIONS
• Prostatomegaly
• Cystic-endometrial hyperplasia
• Hepatotoxicity (secondary to exogenous estrogen administration)
• Infertility
• Bone marrow aplasia, pancytopenia
• Sepsis

ABBREVIATIONS
• ACTH = adrenocorticotropic hormone
• ALP = alanine phosphatase
• ALT = alanine aminotransferase
• BUN = blood urea nitrogen
• G-CSF = granulocyte colony-stimulating factor
• GH = growth hormone
• GM-CSF = granulocyte-macrophage colony-stimulating factor
• GnRH = gonadotropin-releasing hormone
• HCG = human chorionic gonadotropin
• LDDS = low-dose dexamethasone suppression
• T_4 = thyroxine
• TSH = thyroid-stimulating hormone

Suggested Reading
Disorders of the canine ovary. In: Johnston SD, Root Kustritz MV, Olson PNS, eds. Canine and feline theriogenology. Philadelphia: Saunders, 2001:193–205.
Disorders of the canine testes and epididymis. In: Johnston SD, Root Kustritz MV, Olson PNS, eds. Canine and feline theriogenology. Philadelphia: Saunders, 2001:312–332.
Authors Sophie A. Grundy and Autumn P. Davidson
Consulting Editor Deborah S. Greco

HYPERGLYCEMIA

 BASICS

DEFINITION
High concentration of glucose in whole blood, plasma, or serum

PATHOPHYSIOLOGY
• May result from absolute or relative insulin deficiency, reduced use of glucose in peripheral tissue, increased gluconeogenesis in the liver, and increased glycogenolysis
• Insulin antagonists or counterregulatory hormones (e.g., cortisol, adrenocorticotropic hormone [ACTH], growth hormone, epinephrine, and glucagon) also contribute to hyperglycemia.

SYSTEMS AFFECTED
• Endocrine/Metabolic—primarily because of regulating carbohydrate metabolism
• Renal/Urologic—osmotic diuresis caused by hyperglycemia causes polyuria with secondary polydipsia.
• Nervous—severe hyperglycemia may cause CNS dysfunction by increasing serum osmolality.
• Ophthalmic—persistent hyperglycemia (e.g., diabetes mellitus) can cause cataracts in dogs.

SIGNALMENT
Dog and cat

SIGNS

General Comments
• Clinical signs vary and often reflect underlying disease.
• Some patients are asymptomatic, especially those with transient, stress-induced, and postprandial hyperglycemia.

Historical Findings
• Variable
• Polydipsia, polyuria, depression, weight loss, obesity, polyphagia
• CNS depression—severe hyperglycemia

Physical Examination Findings
Often normal, but can include nonhealing wounds, abscesses, obesity, cataracts, and hepatomegaly

CAUSES
• Low glucose use—diabetes mellitus, acute pancreatitis, acromegaly (increased growth hormone) in cats, high progesterone during diestrus (dogs), renal insufficiency, and pancreatectomy to treat insulinoma
• High glucose production—hyperadrenocorticism, pheochromocytoma, glucagonoma, exocrine pancreatic neoplasia
• Physiologic—postprandial fluctuation, exertion or excitement, and stress (epinephrine induced), especially in cats
• Drugs—thiazide diuretics, morphine, dextrose-containing fluids, progestins (e.g., megestrol acetate [Ovaban]), growth hormone, glucocorticoids, and ACTH
• Insulin administration problems in confirmed diabetics—Somogyi phenomenon, antiinsulin antibodies, and poor insulin absorption
• Parenteral administration of nutritional solutions
• Laboratory error

RISK FACTORS
• Concurrent disease—hyperadrenocorticism, acromegaly, and acute pancreatitis
• Diabetogenic drugs
• Dextrose-containing fluids

 DIAGNOSIS

DIFFERENTIAL DIAGNOSIS
• Mild, transiently high blood glucose can be associated with stress and epinephrine-induced excitement or normal postprandial fluctuation.
• In patients with mild hyperglycemia and no history of polydipsia/polyuria, repeat blood glucose determination after 12-hour fast and eliminate or minimize stress (i.e., allow time for acclimation to hospital environment).

LABORATORY FINDINGS

Drugs That May Alter Laboratory Results
• High blood glucose concentration—glucocorticoids, ACTH, dextrose-containing fluids, epinephrine, asparaginase, β-adrenergic agonists, and diazoxide
• Low blood glucose concentration determined enzymatically—aspirin, ascorbic acid, and acetaminophen

Disorders That May Alter Laboratory Results
• Lipemia, hemolysis, and icterus may interfere with spectrophotometric assays.
• Delayed serum separation artificially lowers glucose concentration; must separate serum within 1 hour of collection to prevent cellular glucose use
• Refrigerate or freeze serum sample not analyzed within 12 hours.
• Blood glucose reagent strips require whole blood.
• Measure glucose concentration in whole blood within 30 min of collection.
• Sodium fluoride collection tubes allow more-stable readings and can prevent artificially low readings by spectrophotometry; do not use for enzymatic assays.

Valid If Run in Human Laboratory?
Yes

CBC/BIOCHEMISTRY/URINALYSIS
• Hyperglycemia may be the only abnormal finding.
• CBC—may be normal; possible inflammatory leukogram in patients with infection
• Urinalysis—may be normal; possible abnormalities include glucosuria, pyuria, bacteruria, and ketonuria.
• Fasting hyperglycemia plus glucosuria suggests diabetes mellitus, although mild hyperglycemia and glucosuria can be physiologic in cats.

• Lipemia is associated with low lipoprotein lipase, hyperadrenocorticism, acute pancreatitis, and postprandial blood sampling.
• High amylase and lipase activity suggests acute pancreatitis, especially in nonazotemic patients.
• High liver enzyme activity may accompany fatty infiltration.

OTHER LABORATORY TESTS
• ACTH stimulation or low-dose dexamethasone suppression test to rule out hyperadrenocorticism
• Serum insulin concentration—hyperglycemia is usually accompanied by hyperinsulinemia.
• Hyperglycemia with low serum insulin suggests diabetes mellitus.
• Although rarely indicated, IV glucose and a glucagon tolerance test may help demonstrate carbohydrate intolerance; blood glucose should return to normal within 60 min and serum insulin should increase after IV glucose or glucagon administration.
• Determine serum osmolarity in patients with moderate-to-severe hyperglycemia.

IMAGING
Abdominal radiography and ultrasonography may provide valuable information regarding underlying causes.

DIAGNOSTIC PROCEDURES
N/A

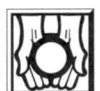

TREATMENT
• Minimize or eliminate stress.
• Avoid abrupt decreases in blood glucose.
• Discontinue diabetogenic drugs or adjust their dosage to normalize blood glucose while maintaining therapeutic concentration.
• Dextrose-free fluids
• Avoid semimoist commercial foods because of the higher content of simple sugars.
• Offer a high-protein, low-carbohydrate, low-fat, high-fiber diet.

MEDICATIONS
DRUG(S) OF CHOICE
Insulin—regular (crystalline) insulin has a more rapid onset of effect but a shorter duration of action than other types of insulin.

CONTRAINDICATIONS
• Diabetogenic drugs (e.g., glucocorticoids)
• Dextrose-containing fluids

PRECAUTIONS
Avoid lowering blood glucose abruptly and causing hypoglycemia.

POSSIBLE INTERACTIONS
N/A

ALTERNATIVE DRUG(S)
Oral administration of hypoglycemic agents—sulfonylureas (e.g., glipizide [Glucotrol]) and biguanides are most useful in cats with type II (non-insulin-dependent) diabetes mellitus.

FOLLOW-UP
PATIENT MONITORING
• Blood glucose after initiating treatment and discontinuing diabetogenic drugs
• Glucose curves by measuring blood glucose hourly or every 2 h for 12–24 h after insulin administration
• Glycosylated hemoglobin and fructosamine on an outpatient basis to monitor long-term glucose control
• Insulin concentrations after treatment
• For return of clinical signs such as polyuria, polydipsia, and polyphagia

POSSIBLE COMPLICATIONS
• High incidence of sepsis (and infection)
• Severe hyperglycemia may be associated with CNS depression and coma because of hyperosmolarity

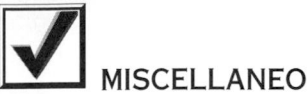

MISCELLANEOUS
ASSOCIATED CONDITIONS
• Severe hyperglycemia associated with hyperosmolarity
• Uremia may be associated with hyperglycemia.
• Hyperglycemia associated with acidosis, hyponatremia, hypokalemia, and hypophosphatemia; although total body concentrations of these electrolytes are low, serum chemistry measurements may be normal, high, or low.

AGE-RELATED FACTORS
N/A

ZOONOTIC POTENTIAL
N/A

PREGNANCY
Pregnancy-induced diabetes mellitus caused by high progesterone concentration is reported in humans.

SYNONYMS
"High blood sugar"

SEE ALSO
• Diabetes Mellitus
• Hyperosmolarity

ABBREVIATION
ACTH = adrenocorticotropic hormone

Suggested Reading
Kaneko JJ, ed. Carbohydrate metabolism and its diseases. In: Kaneko JJ, ed. Clinical biochemistry of domestic animals. 4th ed. San Diego: Academic Press, 1989:44–85.
Rich LJ, Coles EH. Tables of abnormal blood values as a guide to disease syndromes. In: Ettinger SJ, Feldman EC, eds. Textbook of veterinary internal medicine. 4th ed. Philadelphia: Saunders, 1995:11–17.
Willard MD, Tvedten H, Turnwald GH. Small animal clinical diagnosis by laboratory methods. 2nd ed. Philadelphia: Saunders, 1994:154–160.
Author Margaret R. Kern
Consulting Editor Deborah S. Greco

HYPERKALEMIA

 BASICS

DEFINITION
Serum potassium concentration higher than the testing laboratory's upper limit of normal, generally > 5.7 mEq/L (mmol/L)

PATHOPHYSIOLOGY
• Potassium is primarily intracellular; serum concentrations do not accurately reflect tissue concentrations. • Hyperkalemia is often associated with cellular injury (e.g., trauma and ischemia) and other causes of translocation of potassium out of the intracellular space (e.g., acidosis). • Potassium is eliminated in the kidneys and elimination is enhanced by aldosterone; conditions that inhibit renal elimination of potassium will cause hyperkalemia.

SYSTEMS AFFECTED
• Cardiovascular—potassium affects cardiac conduction, and changes are reflected on the ECG; as potassium rises, the T waves become tall and spiked with a narrow base, the QRS complexes widen, and the P-R intervals lengthen; the P waves become smaller and wider and, in animals with severe hyperkalemia, disappear (atrial standstill); higher concentrations of potassium cause fusion of the QRS-T, which causes a wide, complex idioventricular rhythm followed by ventricular fibrillation or asystole; ECG changes in animals with hyperkalemia vary and are diminished by hypernatremia, hypercalcemia, and alkalosis.
• Nervous—neuromuscular function affected

SIGNALMENT
• Dogs and cats
• Pseudohyperkalemia in Akita

SIGNS

Historical Findings
• Weakness • Collapse • Flaccid paralysis
• Death

Physical Examination Findings
In addition to historical findings, arrhythmias, especially bradyarrhythmias, in some animals

CAUSES
• Pseudohyperkalemia—some blood cells (i.e., platelets, WBCs, and RBCs in Akita), contain high concentrations of potassium; if the blood sample is not analyzed or separated promptly, this intracellular potassium is released into the serum, causing the potassium concentration to be artificially high (pseudohyperkalemia).
• Low potassium elimination—anuric or oliguric renal failure; urinary tract rupture or urethral obstruction; administration of potassium-sparing diuretics, ACE inhibitors, trimethoprim, nonsteroidal antiinflammatory drugs, or heparin (causing hypoaldosteronism); some gastrointestinal diseases (e.g.,

salmonellosis, trichuriasis, duodenal perforation) • Translocation of potassium—acidosis, reperfusion syndrome, tumor lysis syndrome, muscle trauma, severe digitalis overdose, infusion of mannitol, and hyperglycemia causing hyperosmolality
• High potassium intake—oral or parenteral potassium supplements • Miscellaneous—pleural effusion and ascites

RISK FACTORS
• Akita breed—pseudohyperkalemia • Fluid therapy with potassium supplementation
• Administration of potassium-sparing diuretics and ACE inhibitors • Conditions associated with acidosis • Trauma • Renal disease • Lower urinary tract disease in male cats • Cystic calculi in male dogs
• Thrombocytosis and leukemia

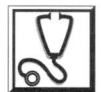 **DIAGNOSIS**

DIFFERENTIAL DIAGNOSIS
• Waxing and waning history of gastrointestinal complaints, weakness, collapse—consider hypoadrenocorticism.
• Straining to urinate or low urine output—consider urinary obstruction or oliguric/anuric renal failure.

LABORATORY FINDINGS

Drugs That May Alter Laboratory Results
None

Disorders That May Alter Laboratory Results
Thrombocytosis (>1,000,000 cells/mm³), leukocytosis (>200,000 cells /mm³), and abnormal (leukemic) leukocytes can cause release of large amounts of potassium into the serum if not separated quickly.

Valid If Run in Human Laboratory?
Yes

CBC/BIOCHEMISTRY/URINALYSIS
• In patients with Na:K ratio < 27, consider hypoadrenocorticism; some patients with diarrhea and metabolic acidosis, ascites, chylothorax, or pregnancy may also have a low Na:K ratio. • In patients with azotemia, consider hypoadrenocorticism, anuric or oliguric renal failure, and ruptured or obstructed urinary tract. • In patients with high creatine kinase, aspartate aminotransferase, and lactic dehydrogenase, consider muscle injury. • In patients with severe thrombocytosis or leukocytosis or if the patient is an Akita, consider pseudohyperkalemia.

OTHER LABORATORY TESTS
ACTH response test to rule out hypoadrenocorticism

IMAGING
Radiographic contrast studies or ultrasound to rule out urinary tract rupture or obstruction.

DIAGNOSTIC PROCEDURES
None

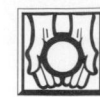 **TREATMENT**

• Varies, depending on the underlying cause of hyperkalemia
• Aggressiveness is dictated by patient's appearance and severity of ECG abnormalities.
• Initiate supportive measures to lower potassium while pursuing definitive diagnosis.
• Saline (0.9%) is the fluid of choice for lowering potassium concentrations and blunting the effects of hyperkalemia on cardiac conduction; if the patient is dehydrated or hypotensive, fluids can be administered rapidly (dogs, up to 90 mL/kg/h; cats, 60 mL/kg/h or faster with monitoring of central venous pressure).

 MEDICATIONS

DRUG(S) OF CHOICE
• Can administer sodium bicarbonate to patients with severe hyperkalemia to induce translocation of potassium into cells; if blood pH and base deficit cannot be determined, administer 1–2 mEq/kg slowly IV; to calculate bicarbonate dose more accurately:

$$\text{dogs, } 0.3 \times \text{body weight (kg)} \times (21 - \text{patient } HCO_3^-)$$

$$\text{cats, } 0.3 \times \text{body weight (kg)} \times (19 - \text{patient } HCO_3^-)$$

Administer half of dose and reevaluate.
• Can administer dextrose and regular insulin to patients with severe hyperkalemia to induce translocation of potassium into cells (regular insulin, 0.5 U/kg IV with 50% dextrose, 1 g/kg IV); dextrose can also be used without insulin.
• For patients with life-threatening hyperkalemia, administer calcium gluconate 10% (0.5–1 mL/kg slowly IV over 10 min) while monitoring the ECG; calcium antagonizes the effect of potassium on the conduction system without lowering the potassium concentration.

CONTRAINDICATIONS
• Avoid potassium-containing fluids and fluids that cause hyponatremia, acidosis, or hypocalcemia.
• Avoid drugs that contain potassium or interfere with potassium elimination (e.g., ACE inhibitors, trimethoprim antibiotics, and potassium-sparing diuretics).

PRECAUTIONS
• Kayexalate and sodium bicarbonate cause a sodium load that may lead to fluid retention in patients with cardiac or renal failure.
• Sodium bicarbonate lowers ionized calcium levels. Use cautiously in hypocalcemic

patients.

POSSIBLE INTERACTIONS
N/A

ALTERNATIVE DRUG(S)
Sodium polystyrene sulfonate (Kayexalate) per os or per rectum binds potassium within the intestinal tract, limiting absorption and reabsorption; rarely used in veterinary practice

FOLLOW-UP

PATIENT MONITORING
• Recheck potassium at frequency dictated by the underlying disease. • Check ECG frequently until rhythm disturbances resolve.

PREVENTION/AVOIDANCE
• Monitor potassium in patients receiving drugs that alter potassium elimination.

• Administer IV potassium at a rate less than 0.5 mEq/kg/h.

POSSIBLE COMPLICATIONS
Death of animals with severe hyperkalemia

EXPECTED COURSE AND PROGNOSIS
Vary with severity of hyperkalemia and underlying cause

MISCELLANEOUS

ASSOCIATED CONDITIONS
N/A

AGE-RELATED FACTORS
N/A

ZOONOTIC POTENTIAL
N/A

PREGNANCY
Combined hyperkalemia and hyponatremia reported in several pregnant dogs

SYNONYMS
N/A

SEE ALSO
• Acidosis, Metabolic • Atrial Standstill
• Hypoadrenocorticism • Renal Failure, Acute
• Urinary Tract Obstruction

ABBREVIATION
ACE = angiotensin-converting enzyme

Suggested Reading
Di Bartola SP. Management of hypokalaemia and hyperkalaemic. J Feline Med Surg 2001;3:181–183.
Philips SL, Polzin DJ. Clinical disorders of potassium homeostasis. Hyperkalemic and hypokalemia. Vet Clin North Am Small Anim Pract 1998;28:545–564.
Author Francis W. K. Smith, Jr.
Consulting Editor Deborah S. Greco

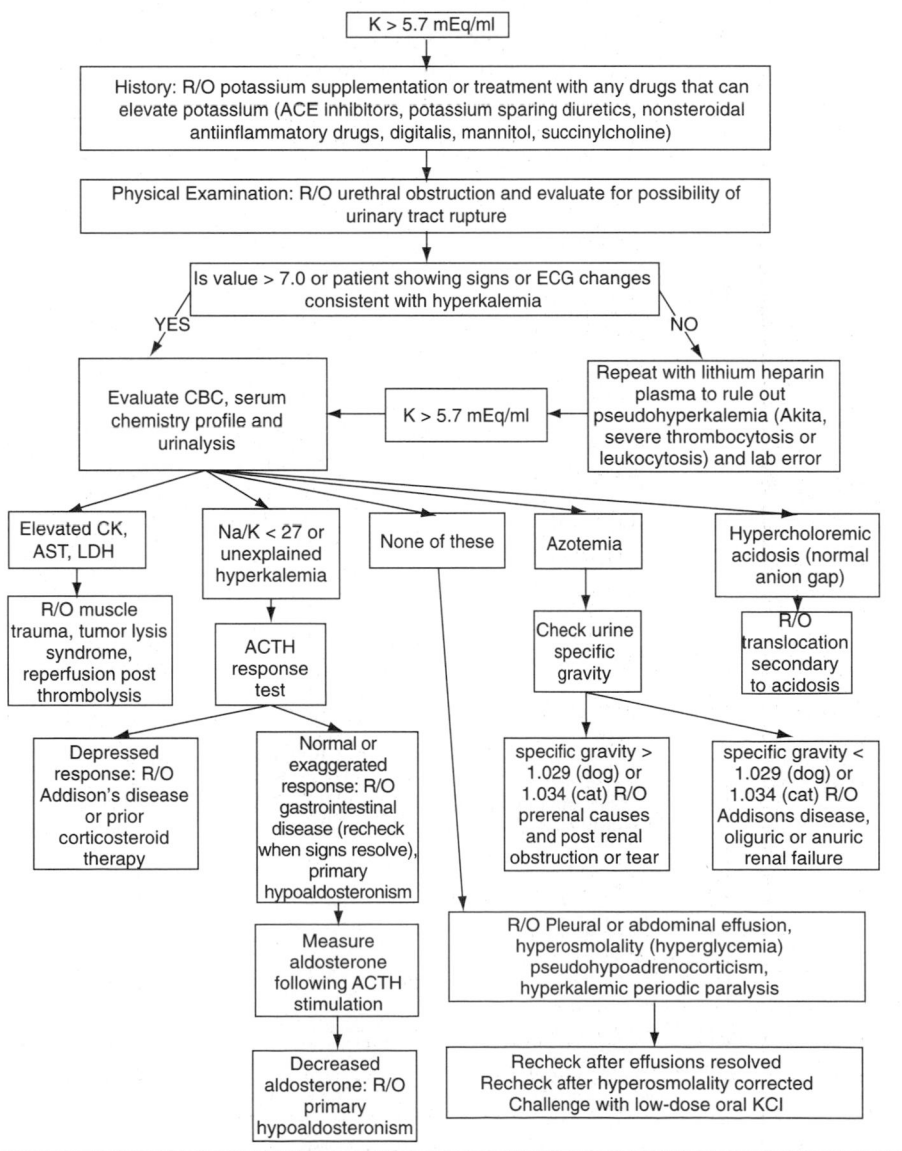

HYPERLIPIDEMIA

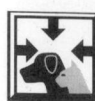 BASICS

DEFINITIONS
• Concentration of lipid in the blood of a fasted (>12 h) patient that exceeds the upper range of normal for that species; includes both hypercholesterolemia and hypertriglyceridemia
• Lipemic—serum or plasma separated from blood that contains an excess concentration of triglycerides (>200 mg/dL)
• Lactescence—opaque, milklike appearance of serum or plasma that contains an even higher concentration of triglycerides (>1000 mg/dL) than lipemic serum

PATHOPHYSIOLOGY
Primary Hyperlipidemia
• Idiopathic hyperchylomicronemia—defect in lipid metabolism causing hypertriglyceridemia and hyperchylomicronemia; possibly caused by a defect in lipoprotein lipase activity or the absence of the surface apoprotein CII; familial disorder in the miniature schnauzer
• Hyperchylomicronemia in cats—familial, autosomal recessive defect in lipoprotein lipase activity
• Idiopathic hypercholesterolemia—occurs in some families of Doberman pinschers and rottweilers; LDL cholesterol is high.

Secondary Hyperlipidemia
• Postprandial—absorption of chylomicrons from the gastrointestinal tract occurs 30–60 min after ingestion of a meal containing fat; may increase serum triglycerides for 3–10 hours
• Diabetes mellitus—low lipoprotein lipase (LPL) activity; high synthesis of very-low-density lipoprotein (VLDL) by the liver
• Hypothyroidism—low LPL activity and lipolytic activity by other hormones (e.g., catecholamines); reduced hepatic degradation of cholesterol to bile acids
• Hyperadrenocorticism—increased synthesis of VLDL by the liver and low LPL activity causes both hypercholesterolemia and hyper-triglyceridemia.
• Liver disease—hypercholesterolemia caused by reduced excretion of cholesterol in the bile
• Nephrotic syndrome—common synthetic pathway for albumin and cholesterol and possibly low oncotic pressure lead to increased cholesterol synthesis.
• Obesity— excessive hepatic synthesis of VLDL

SYSTEMS AFFECTED
• Ophthalmic
• Nervous
• Endocrine/Metabolism
• Gastrointestinal
• Hepatobiliary

SIGNALMENT
• Dog and cat
• Variable, depending on the cause
• Hereditary hyperlipidemias—age of onset is >8 months in cats and >4 years in predisposed breeds of dog such as the miniature schnauzer.

SIGNS
Historical Findings
• Recent ingestion of a meal
• Seizures
• Abdominal pain and distress
• Neuropathies

Physical Examination Findings
• Lipemia retinalis
• Lipemic aqueous
• Neuropathy
• Cutaneous xanthomata
• Lipid granulomas in abdominal organs

CAUSES
Increased Absorption of Triglycerides or Cholesterol
Postprandial

Increased Production of Triglycerides or Cholesterol
• Nephrotic syndrome
• Pregnancy
• Defects in lipid clearance enzymes or lipid carrier proteins
• Idiopathic hyperchylomicronemia
• Hyperchylomicronemia in cats
• Idiopathic hypercholesterolemia

Decreased Clearance of Triglycerides or Cholesterol
• Hypothyroidism
• Hyperadrenocorticism
• Diabetes mellitus
• Pancreatitis
• Cholestasis

RISK FACTORS
• Obesity
• High dietary intake of fats
• Genetic predisposition in miniature schnauzer and Himalayan cat
• Idiopathic hypercholesterolemia observed in families of Doberman pinschers and rottweilers

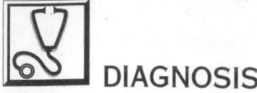 DIAGNOSIS

DIFFERENTIAL DIAGNOSIS
Fasting Hyperlipidemia
Rule out postprandial lipemia with a 12-hour fast.

Primary Hyperlipoproteinemia
• Idiopathic hyperchylomicronemia is observed most commonly in the miniature schnauzer breed.
• Hyperchylomicronemia in cats often manifests as polyneuropathies and lipogranulomas.
• Idiopathic hypercholesterolemia is observed most frequently in the Doberman pinscher and rottweiler breeds; animals are often asymptomatic.

Secondary Hyperlipidemia
• Diabetes mellitus—signs include polyphagia, weight loss, polydypsia, and polyuria; glycosuria and fasting hyperglycemia confirm the diagnosis.
• Hypothyroidism—signs include lethargy, hypothermia, heat seeking, and dermatologic changes (e.g., alopecia and hyperpigmentation).
• Pancreatitis—signs include abdominal pain, vomiting, diarrhea, and anorexia; often hyperlipidemia is accompanied by high liver enzyme activities and high lipase and amylase.
• Hyperadrenocorticism—signs include polydypsia, polyuria, polyphagia, dermatologic changes (e.g., alopecia and thin skin), and hepatomegaly; hypercholesterolemia often is attended by high ALP isoenzyme.
• Hepatic disease and cholestatic disorders—signs include anorexia, weight loss, and icterus.
• Nephrotic syndrome—signs include ascites and peripheral edema; hypercholesterolemia is observed in conjunction with hypoproteinemia and proteinuria.

LABORATORY FINDINGS
Sample Handling
• Submit serum.
• Lipemia causes hemolysis if serum remains on RBC for a long time; inquire about the laboratory method of clearing lipemic samples before submission.
• Two samples may be submitted: one for biochemical analysis, which may be cleared, and one for triglycerides and cholesterol concentrations.

Drugs That May Alter Laboratory Results
- Corticosteroids
- Phenytoin
- Prochlorperazine
- Thiazides
- Phenothiazines

Disorders That May Alter Laboratory Results
- Falsely high cholesterol
- Nonfasted samples (<12 hours)
- Icterus—spectrophotometric techniques
- Fluoride and oxalate anticoagulants—enzymatic techniques
- Lipemia

Valid If Run in Human Laboratory?
Yes

CBC/BIOCHEMISTRY/URINALYSIS
- Results of hemogram usually normal
- Hyperadrenocorticism—polycythemia and nucleated RBCs
- Hypothyroidism—mild normocytic, normochromic anemia
- High triglycerides—dogs, >150 mg/dL; cats, >100 mg/dL
- High cholesterol—dogs, >300 mg/dL; cats, >200 mg/dL
- Nephrotic syndrome—low albumin
- Diabetes mellitus—high serum glucose
- Hyperadrenocorticism— high ALP activity
- Pancreatitis—high serum lipase
- Results of urinalysis often normal
- Nephrotic syndrome—proteinuria

OTHER LABORATORY TESTS
- HDL and LDL determinations—used in human medicine; values reported for HDL and LDL in dogs and cats cannot be assumed to be reliable.
- Chylomicron test—obtain serum sample after a 12-hour fast and refrigerate for 12–14 hours; do not freeze; chylomicrons rise to the surface and form a creamy layer.
- Lipoprotein electrophoresis—separates LDL, VLDL, HDL1, and HDL2
- LPL activity—collect serum for triglycerides and cholesterol concentrations and lipoprotein electrophoresis before and 15 min after IV administration of heparin (90 IU/kg); if there is no change in values before and after heparin administration, a defective LPL enzyme system should be suspected.

- T_4 and T_3 determinations indicated if hypothyroidism is suspected
- Adrenocorticotropic hormone (ACTH) stimulation test indicated if hyperadrenocorticism is suspected

IMAGING
N/A

DIAGNOSTIC PROCEDURES
N/A

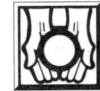 TREATMENT
Diet should contain <10% fat (e.g., Hill's r/d, Iams restricted calorie).

 MEDICATIONS

DRUG(S) OF CHOICE
- Initial management is dietary.
- See Alternative Drugs if diet fails to control hyperlipidemia.

CONTRAINDICATIONS
N/A

PRECAUTIONS
N/A

POSSIBLE INTERACTIONS
N/A

ALTERNATIVE DRUG(S)
- Gemfibrozil—7.5 mg/kg PO q12h
- Fish oils—linolenic acid (omega-3 polyunsaturated fat), 10–30 mg/kg PO q24h
- Clofibrate and niacin—not currently recommended in cats or dogs

 FOLLOW-UP

PATIENT MONITORING
- Keep triglyceride concentrations < 500 mg/dL to avoid possibly fatal episodes of acute pancreatitis.
- Checking cholesterol often is not necessary because hypercholesterolemia is not associated with clinical signs.

POSSIBLE COMPLICATIONS
- Pancreatitis and seizures are common complications of hyperlipidemia in the miniature schnauzer.

- In cats with hereditary chylomicronemia, xanthoma formation, lipemia retinalis, and neuropathies have been reported; peripheral neuropathies usually resolve 2–3 months after institution of a low-fat diet.

 MISCELLANEOUS

ASSOCIATED CONDITIONS
- Pancreatitis
- Seizures
- Neuropathies

AGE-RELATED FACTORS
N/A

ZOONOTIC POTENTIAL
N/A

PREGNANCY
Potential cause of high cholesterol

SYNONYMS
- Lipemia
- Hyperlipoproteinemia

SEE ALSO
See Causes.

ABBREVIATIONS
- ALP = alkaline phosphatase
- HDL = high-density lipoprotein
- LDL = low-density lipoprotein
- LPL = lipoprotein lipase
- T_4 = thyroxine
- T_3 = triiodothyronine
- VLDL = very-low-density lipoprotein

Suggested Reading

Barrie J, Watson TOG. Hyperlipidemia. In: Bonagura JD, ed. Kirk's Current veterinary therapy XII. Philadelphia: Saunders, 1995:430–434.

Ford R. Canine hyperlipidemias. In: Ettinger ST, Feldman EC, eds. Textbook of veterinary internal medicine. 4th ed. Philadelphia: Saunders, 1994:1414–1418.

Jones B. Feline hyperlipidemias. In: Ettinger ST, Feldman EC, eds. Textbook of veterinary internal medicine. 4th ed. Philadelphia: Saunders, 1994:1410–1413.

Author Deborah S. Greco
Consulting Editor Deborah S. Greco

HYPERMAGNESEMIA

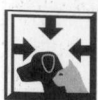 ## BASICS

DEFINITION
• Dogs—serum magnesium > 2.51 mg/dL
• Cats—serum magnesium > 2.3 mg/dL

PATHOPHYSIOLOGY
• Magnesium—second only to potassium as the most abundant intracellular cation; most is found in bone and muscle; required for many metabolic functions
• Magnesium is an important cofactor in the sodium-potassium ATPase pump that maintains an electrical gradient across membranes and thus plays an important role in the activity of electrically excitable tissues.
• Interference with the electrical gradient can change resting membrane potentials; repolarization disturbances result in neuromuscular and cardiac abnormalities.
• Magnesium homeostasis is largely controlled by renal elimination; any condition that severely lowers the glomerular filtration rate can elicit hypermagnesemia.
• High magnesium concentration impairs transmission of nerve impulses and decreases the postsynaptic response at the neuromuscular junction.
• Magnesium has been called nature's calcium blocker; the most serious complications of hypermagnesemia result from calcium antagonism in the cardiac conduction system.

SYSTEMS AFFECTED
• Cardiovascular
• Musculoskeletal
• Nervous

SIGNALMENT
Dog and cat

SIGNS

General Comments
• Usually caused by renal failure; clinical signs may be referable to azotemia and renal insufficiency.
• Characterized by progressive loss of neuromuscular, respiratory, and cardiovascular function

Historical and Physical Examination Findings
• Earliest symptoms—nausea, vomiting, weakness, and hyporeflexia
• Hypotension and ECG changes, including delayed intraventricular conduction and prolonged QT interval, are noted as serum magnesium levels climb.
• Atrioventricular block, respiratory depression, coma, and cardiac arrest have been seen in people with serum magnesium concentrations > 16 mg/dL.

CAUSES
• Renal failure
• Intestinal hypomotility disorders and constipation
• Endocrine disorders including hypoadrenocorticism, hypothyroidism, and hyperparathyroidism
• Excessive magnesium administration from magnesium-containing cathartic solutions given in conjunction with activated charcoal, magnesium-containing laxatives, and excess magnesium in peritoneal dialysis solutions

RISK FACTORS
• Renal disease
• Massive hemolysis
• Hypoadrenocorticism
• Hyperparathyroidism
• Excessive use of magnesium-containing cathartic solutions, especially in patients with renal insufficiency
• Intestinal hypomotility

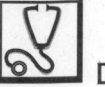 ## DIAGNOSIS

DIFFERENTIAL DIAGNOSIS
• Signs are most similar to those of hypocalcemia, which often occurs simultaneously.
• Bradycardia can be caused by neurologic disease, hyperkalemia, hypertension, hypothyroidism, sick sinus syndrome, and various drugs.

Laboratory Findings
Note: 12 mg of magnesium = 1 mEq of magnesium; to convert from mg/dL to mEq/L, divide by 1.2

Drugs That May Alter Laboratory Results
• Serum is favored over plasma because the anticoagulant used for plasma samples can contain citrate or other ions that may bind magnesium.
• EDTA, sodium fluoride-oxalate, sodium citrate, and intravenous calcium gluconate can cause falsely low serum magnesium values.

Disorders That May Alter Laboratory Results
• Hemolysis may cause false increases in serum magnesium; the magnesium concentration in erythrocytes is approximately three times that in serum.
• Holding serum or urine in metal containers can falsely elevate magnesium values.
• Hyperbilirubinemia can cause false decreases in serum magnesium.

Valid if Run in Human Laboratory?
Yes

CBC/BIOCHEMISTRY/URINALYSIS
• Serum magnesium—dogs, > 2.51 mg/dL; cats, > 2.3 mg/dL
• Hypocalcemia is common.
• Azotemia in some patients

OTHER LABORATORY TESTS
N/A

IMAGING
N/A

DIAGNOSTIC PROCEDURES
Electrodiagnostics (e.g. electromyelography and ECG) reveal effects of hypermagnesemia but do not help differentiate the cause.

TREATMENT
• Management involves enhancing elimination from the body and symptomatic therapy.
• Discontinue all magnesium-containing medications and nutritional supplements.
• Saline diuresis enhances renal clearance of magnesium and provides fluid volume.
• Patients with oliguria may require peritoneal dialysis to treat severe hypermagnesemia.
• Parenteral calcium directly antagonizes the effect of magnesium, reversing respiratory depression, cardiac arrhythmias, and hypotension; calcium also enhances magnesium excretion.
• Fluid therapy with 0.9% NaCl provides fluid volume to address hypotension and azotemia.

MEDICATIONS

DRUG(S) OF CHOICE
• Furosemide promotes renal excretion of magnesium by decreasing absorption of magnesium in the loop of Henle.
• Enteral and parenteral calcium administration helps reverse clinical manifestations of hypermagnesemia and correct concurrent hypocalcemia; oral supplementation with any preparation can be given at a dosage of 25–50 mg/kg/ day; severe hypermagnesemia can be treated with 10% calcium gluconate: 1–2 mL/kg (diluted 1:1 with saline) IV or SC q8h, administered very slowly.

CONTRAINDICATIONS
Magnesium-containing compounds

PRECAUTIONS
Monitor ECG during calcium infusions.

POSSIBLE INTERACTIONS
N/A

ALTERNATIVE DRUG(S)
N/A

FOLLOW-UP

PATIENT MONITORING
• Serum magnesium and calcium concentrations
• Renal function—azotemia and urine output
• Continuous electrocardiogram if possible

POSSIBLE COMPLICATIONS
• Severe hypermagnesemia and hypocalcemia can be fatal.
• Hypermagnesemic dogs were 2.6 times more likely not to survive their illness than patients with normal serum magnesium levels.

MISCELLANEOUS

ASSOCIATED CONDITIONS
• Hypocalcemia
• Hyperphosphatemia
• Azotemia

AGE-RELATED FACTORS
N/A

ZOONOTIC POTENTIAL
N/A

PREGNANCY
Effects on the fetus identical to the effects on the dam

SYNONYMS
None

SEE ALSO
Hypocalcemia

ABBREVIATIONS
N/A

Suggested Reading
Macintire DK. Disorders of potassium, phosphorus, and magnesium in critical illness. Compend Cont Educ 1997;19:41–48.
Marino PL. Magnesium. In: Marino PL, ed. The ICU book. Baltimore: Williams & Wilkins, 1998:660–672.
Martin LG. Hypercalcemia and hypermagnesemia. Vet Clin North Am Small Anim Pract 1998;28(3):565–585.
McClean RM. Magnesium and its therapeutic uses: a review. Am J Med 1994; 96:63–76.
Author Tim Hackett
Consulting Editor Deborah S. Greco

HYPERMETRIA AND DYSMETRIA

 BASICS

DEFINITION
• Dysmetria describes incoordination of the limbs during voluntary movement characterized by an inability to judge the rate, range, and force of movements.
• Hypermetria specifically describes overreaching limb movements giving a characteristic goose-stepping gait. Dysmetria includes both hypo- and hypermetria.

PATHOPHYSIOLOGY
• The cerebellum plays a central role in generating skilled movements and maintaining muscle tone and body posture. It does not initiate but coordinates and smooths movements. • Damage to the cerebellum results in inaccurate gauging of voluntary movements and hence a dysmetric or hypermetric gait. Motor strength is preserved; conscious proprioception is unaffected.
• Rarely, spinal cord compression can produce dysmetria or hypermetria, rather than the more typical sensory ataxia, as a result of compression of the spinocerebellar tracts. This is more likely to occur with dorsally located lesions (e.g., subarachnoid cysts).

SYSTEMS AFFECTED
Nervous—specifically the cerebellum and the spinocerebellar tracts

SIGNALMENT
Dogs and cats of any age, breed, or sex

SIGNS
Other signs of cerebellar disease that may be present include a truncal sway, intention tremor, wide-based stance, head tilt, loss of the menace response, and anisocoria.

CAUSES
Cerebellar
• Dogs—hypoplasia (inherited or secondary to infection with canine herpesvirus in the perinatal period); abiotrophy; Chiari malformations; lysosomal storage diseases; canine distemper virus; protozoal infections (*Toxoplasma gondii* and *Neospora caninum*); rickettsial infections (*Ehrlichia canis* and Rocky Mountain spotted fever); *Cryptococcus* and other fungal infections; granulomatous meningoencephalitis; steroid-responsive tremor syndrome (idiopathic tremor or "white shaker" syndrome); neoplasia; trauma; hemorrhage; and metronidazole toxicity
• Cats—hypoplasia most commonly secondary to in utero infection with feline panleukopenia virus; lysosomal storage diseases; Chiari malformations; feline infectious peritonitis; feline leukemia virus and feline immunodeficiency virus (associated immunosuppression predisposes to other encephalitides and to neoplasia); toxoplasmosis; *Cryptococcus* and other fungal infections; neoplasia; hemorrhage; and trauma

Spinal
Dogs—subarachnoid cysts; neoplasia; vertebral malformation; and calcinosis circumscripta

RISK FACTORS
Cerebellar
• Cerebellar abiotrophy has been reported in Gordon and Irish setters, Kerry blue terriers, Airedale terriers, Finnish harriers, Samoyeds, Bern running dogs, cocker spaniels, cairn terriers, Australian kelpies, bullmastiffs, Old English sheepdogs, Rhodesian Ridgebacks, Border and rough-coated collies, American Staffordshire terriers, and Brittany spaniels.

• Cerebellar hypoplasia has been reported in chow chows, Irish setters, and wire fox terriers. • Lysosomal storage diseases causing dysmetria and hypermetria have been reported in Siamese, Balinese, Persian, and domestic shorthair cats, and in English springer spaniels, Portuguese water dogs, German shorthaired pointers, Australian silky terriers, schipperkes, English setters, Border collies, salukis, Chihuahuas, Queensland blue heelers, dachshunds, Yugoslavian shepherds, and Tibetan terriers. • Cavalier King Charles spaniels are predisposed to Chiari malformations.
• Small-breed white dogs, such as Maltese and West Highland white terriers, are predisposed to steroid-responsive (idiopathic) tremor syndrome. • Metronidazole at dosages > 60 mg/kg/day can induce cerebellar signs in dogs.

Spinal
• Giant-breed dogs are predisposed to vertebral malformation and instability.
• Young large-breed dogs are predisposed to subarachnoid cysts and calcinosis circumscripta.

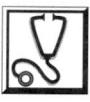 DIAGNOSIS

DIFFERENTIAL DIAGNOSIS
• Some dogs, especially small breeds, have a high-stepping gait in their thoracic limbs as a normal finding. If there are no other signs of cerebellar disease, it is important to establish from the owner whether a high-stepping thoracic limb gait is normal for his or her dog. • For differential diagnosis, see Causes.

CBC/BIOCHEMISTRY/URINALYSIS
• CBC may reflect infectious/inflammatory disease. • Storage products may be present in leukocytes in some lysosomal storage diseases.

OTHER LABORATORY TESTS
• Acute and convalescent serologic titers—to diagnose rickettsial, protozoal, fungal, and viral diseases • CSF antibody or antigen (*Cryptococcus*) titers—for some infections (e.g., canine distemper virus, *Toxoplasma*, *Cryptococcus*), measure in addition to serologic titers.

IMAGING
• Thoracic radiography—recommended in older patients to identify metastatic disease • Abdominal ultrasonography—recommended in older patients if intra-abdominal neoplasia is suspected • Brain CT or MRI—recommended to diagnose neoplasia, cerebellar hypoplasia, and Chiari malformations; MRI is the preferred modality for evaluating the caudal fossa as significant artifacts occur on CT images as a consequence of the thickness of the bones in this region of the skull • Survey spinal radiography—if spinal cord disease is suspected; may be helpful in identifying vertebral malformations and calcinosis circumscripta • Myelography—if spinal cord disease is suspected

DIAGNOSTIC PROCEDURES
• Fundic examination—to identify chorioretinitis (evidence of infectious/inflammatory disease) and vascular lesions • CSF analysis—to diagnose encephalitis; storage products may be present in CSF leukocytes in some lysosomal storage diseases • Liver biopsy—may be helpful in diagnosing certain lysosomal storage diseases in animals with hepatomegaly

TREATMENT
• Severe and/or rapidly progressive clinical signs—hospitalization for immediate diagnostic work-up and treatment • Mild and slowly progressive clinical signs—outpatient management, but diagnostic tests requiring anesthesia necessitate hospitalization • Patients should be restricted to areas and activities where they are unlikely to fall and injure themselves.

MEDICATIONS
DRUG(S) OF CHOICE
• Do not initiate therapy until a diagnosis has been established. • Discontinue metronidazole, regardless of the dose rate, to see if there is an improvement in signs.

ALTERNATIVE DRUG(S)
N/A

FOLLOW-UP
PATIENT MONITORING
• Periodic repeat neurologic examinations to monitor progress • See specific diseases for specific instructions.

MISCELLANEOUS
ZOONOTIC POTENTIAL
Fungal infections can be zoonotic if spores are released. This is most likely to occur if exudative skin lesions are present.

SEE ALSO
• Brain Injury • Cerebellar Degeneration • Encephalitis

ABBREVIATIONS
• CSF = cerebrospinal fluid
• CT = computed tomography
• MRI = magnetic resonance imaging

Suggested Reading
Bagley RS. Intracranial disease. Vet Clin North Am Small Anim Pract 1996; 26:857–874, 945–972.
Braund KG. Clinical syndromes in veterinary neurology, 2nd ed. Baltimore: Mosby, 1994.
Author Natasha J. Olby
Consulting Editor Joane M. Parent

HYPERNATREMIA

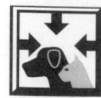BASICS

DEFINITION
Serum sodium concentration >158 mEq/L in dogs or >165 mEq/L in cats

PATHOPHYSIOLOGY
• Sodium is the most abundant cation in the extracellular fluid, so hypernatremia usually reflects hyperosmolality.
• Common causes of hypernatremia include renal or gastrointestinal loss of water in excess of sodium loss and low water intake.

SYSTEMS AFFECTED
• Endocrine/Metabolic
• Nervous

SIGNALMENT
Dogs and cats

SIGNS
• Polydypsia
• Disorientation
• Coma
• Seizures
• Other findings depend on underlying cause
• Severity of signs usually correlates to the degree of hypernatremia

CAUSES
• Total body sodium high—oral ingestion (rare); IV administration of NaCl during cardiovascular resuscitation; hyperaldosteronism (rare)
• Total body sodium normal plus water deficit—low water intake (e.g., no access to water and adipsia or hypodipsia); high urinary water loss (e.g., diabetes insipidus); high insensible water loss (e.g., panting and hyperthermia)
• Total body sodium low and hypotonic fluid loss (i.e., loss of fluid containing sodium without adequate water replacement)—urinary loss (e.g., diabetes mellitus, osmotic diuresis, and diuresis after acute urinary obstruction); gastrointestinal sodium loss (e.g., administration of osmotic cathartic, vomiting, and diarrhea)

RISK FACTORS
N/A

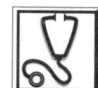DIAGNOSIS

DIFFERENTIAL DIAGNOSIS
• Diabetes insipidus
• Hyperosmolar nonketotic syndrome
• Hypertonic dehydration
• Salt ingestion—rare

LABORATORY FINDINGS

Drugs That May Alter Laboratory Results
A wide variety of drugs interfere with renal capacity to concentrate urine, leading to water loss in excess of sodium and high serum sodium concentration; these drugs include lithium, demeclocycline, and amphotericin.

Disorders That May Alter Laboratory Results
Lipemia or hyperproteinemia (>11 g/dL) can artifactually raise sodium concentration when the flame photometry method is used.

Valid If Run in a Human Laboratory?
Yes

CBC/BIOCHEMISTRY/URINALYSIS
• High serum sodium concentration
• Diabetes insipidus—polyuria, low urinary specific gravity, and low urinary sodium concentration
• Hyperosmolar nonketotic syndrome—high blood glucose, low urine output, and high urinary specific gravity (usually >1.025)
• Hypertonic dehydration—low urinary sodium concentration and high urinary specific gravity (usually >1.030)

OTHER LABORATORY TESTS
• Modified water deprivation test (see Appendix for test protocol) to differentiate diabetes insipidus from other causes of polyuria and polydipsia; performed after results of CBC, biochemical analysis, urinalysis, and endocrine testing are evaluated to rule out hyperadrenocorticism
• After water restriction, patients with diabetes insipidus have little or no increase in urinary specific gravity or osmolality.
• After ADH or DDAVP administration, patients with nephrogenic diabetes insipidus have <10% increase in urinary specific gravity; those with central diabetes insipidus have a 10–800% increase.

IMAGING
CT scan or MRI in patients with diabetes insipidus to rule out pituitary tumor

DIAGNOSTIC PROCEDURES
N/A

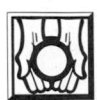 TREATMENT

• After resolution of the hypernatremia, consider a sodium-restricted diet (especially in patients with nephrogenic diabetes insipidus).
• Water must be available at all times for patients with diabetes insipidus.

 MEDICATIONS

DRUG(S) OF CHOICE
• If hypovolemia is severe—replace volume with isotonic saline (i.e., lactated Ringer or normal saline) or isotonic fluids (i.e., 5% dextrose with half-normal saline)
• Hypernatremia—administer hypotonic fluids (e.g., 5% dextrose in water) to reduce serum sodium by 0.5 mEq/h or by no more than 20 mEq/L/day; supplement with potassium and phosphate if needed.

• Central diabetes insipidus—DDAVP (1–2 drops in subconjunctival sac q12–24h)
• Nephrogenic diabetes insipidus—chlorothiazide (10–40 mg/kg PO q12h)

CONTRAINDICATIONS
Refer to manufacturer's literature.

PRECAUTIONS
• Rapid correction of hypernatremia can cause pulmonary edema.
• Hypocalcemia may develop during correction of hypernatremia.

POSSIBLE INTERACTIONS
N/A

ALTERNATIVE DRUG(S)
N/A

FOLLOW-UP

PATIENT MONITORING
• Acute setting—electrolytes, urine output, and body weight
• Diabetes insipidus—water intake

POSSIBLE COMPLICATIONS
• CNS thrombosis or hemorrhage
• Hyperactivity
• Seizures
• Serum sodium >180 mEq/L often associated with residual CNS damage
• Many patients recover, but possibility of neurologic damage is high.

MISCELLANEOUS

ASSOCIATED CONDITIONS
N/A

AGE-RELATED FACTORS
N/A

ZOONOTIC POTENTIAL
N/A

PREGNANCY
N/A

SYNONYMS
None

SEE ALSO
• Diabetes Insipidus
• Hyposthenuria

ABBREVIATIONS
• ADH = antidiuretic hormone
• DDAVP = brand name of desmopressin, a synthetic ADH preparation

Suggested Reading
DiBartola SP. Fluid therapy in small animal practice. Philadelphia: Saunders, 1992.
Marks SL, Taboada J. Hypernatremia and hypertonic syndromes. Vet Clin North Am Small Anim Pract 1998;28(3):533–543.
Ross DB. Clinical physiology of acid-base and electrolyte disorders. 3rd ed. New York: McGraw-Hill, 1989.
Author Rhett Nichols
Consulting Editor Deborah S. Greco

HYPEROSMOLARITY

 **BASICS**

DEFINITION
• Osmolarity—expressed in mOsm/L; represents the number of solute particles per liter of solution
• Osmolality—expressed in mOsm/kg; represents the number of solute particles per kilogram of solution
• Hyperosmolarity—a high concentration of solute particles per liter of solution
• Serum concentrations > 310 mOsm/L in dogs and > 330 mOsm/L in cats are usually considered hyperosmolar.

PATHOPHYSIOLOGY
• Serum sodium is responsible for most of the osmotically active particles that contribute to serum osmolarity; serum glucose and urea also contribute to serum osmolarity.
• Anything that causes water loss increases concentrations of solutes in plasma or serum, thereby increasing serum osmolarity.
• Blood volume, hydration status, and ADH are intimately involved in controlling extracellular fluid volume.
• Low circulating blood volume stimulates carotid and aortic baroreceptors to respond to changes in blood pressure, causing ADH secretion.
• Hyperosmolarity affects the osmoreceptors in the hypothalamus and stimulates ADH secretion from the neurohypophysis; the hypothalamic thirst center is also stimulated and causes an increase in water consumption to counteract serum hyperosmolarity by solute dilution.
• Rapid increases in serum osmolarity cause water movement along its concentration gradient from intracellular to extracellular spaces, resulting in neuronal dehydration, cell shrinkage, and cell death; cerebral vessels may weaken and hemorrhage.

SYSTEMS AFFECTED
• Nervous—excessive thirst may be the first sign of hyperosmolarity. Central nervous system depression may lead to coma.
• Cardiovascular—hypotension and decreased ventricular contractility
• Renal/Urologic—low urine output

SIGNALMENT
• Dogs and cats
• Hypodipsia and hyperosmolarity have been reported in young female miniature schnauzers.

SIGNS

General Comments
• Primarily neurologic or behavioral
• Severity is related more to how quickly hyperosmolarity occurs than to the absolute magnitude of change.
• Most likely to occur if serum osmolarity is >350 mOsm/L and usually severe if >375 mOsm/L

Historical Findings
Anorexia, lethargy, vomiting, weakness, disorientation, ataxia, seizures, and coma; polydipsia followed by hypodipsia

Physical Examination Findings
• Normal, or abnormalities may reflect underlying disease
• In addition to historical findings, dehydration, tachycardia, hypotension, weak pulses, and fever may be detected.

CAUSES

Increased Solutes
Hypernatremia, hyperglycemia, severe azotemia, ethylene glycol toxicosis, salt poisoning, sodium phosphate enemas in cats and small dogs, mannitol, radiographic contrast solution, administration of ethanol, aspirin toxicosis, shock, lactate in patients with lactic acidosis, acetoacetate and β-hydroxybutyrate in patients with ketoacidosis, liquid enteral nutrition, and parenteral nutrition solutions

Decreased Extracellular Fluid Volume
Dehydration—gastrointestinal loss, cutaneous loss, third space loss, low water consumption, and polyuria without adequate compensatory polydipsia

RISK FACTORS
• Medical conditions that predispose—renal failure, diabetes insipidus, diabetes mellitus, hyperadrenocorticism, hyperaldosteronism, and heat stroke
• Therapeutic hyperosmolar solutions—hypertonic saline, sodium bicarbonate, sodium phosphate enemas in cats and small dogs, mannitol, and parenteral nutrition solutions
• High environmental temperatures
• Fever

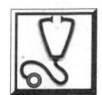 **DIAGNOSIS**

DIFFERENTIAL DIAGNOSIS
• Primary CNS disease and neoplasia may be characterized by altered mentation, but serum osmolarity is usually normal.
• Physical evidence or history of injury usually helps to rule out CNS depression caused by cranial trauma.
• Perform a thorough physical examination to assess hydration status and obtain information regarding previous therapy that may have included sodium-containing fluids or hyperosmolar solutions.

LABORATORY FINDINGS

Drugs That May Alter Laboratory Results
Excessive administration of sodium-containing fluids or hyperosmolar solutions increase serum osmolarity.

Disorders That May Alter Laboratory Results
N/A

Valid If Run in Human Laboratory?
Yes

CBC/BIOCHEMISTRY/URINALYSIS
• High PCV, hemoglobin, and plasma proteins in dehydrated patients; serum electrolytes may also be increased.
• Hyperosmolarity is an indication to evaluate serum sodium and glucose concentrations.
• Without the presence of excessive unmeasured osmoles, estimated serum osmolarity may be calculated from serum chemistries as follows:

$$\frac{1.86(\text{Na} + \text{K}) + \text{BUN} + \text{glucose}}{2.8 \times 18}$$

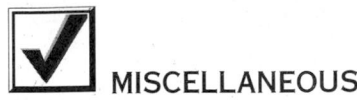
• Normally, calculated osmolarity should not exceed measured osmolarity; if it is, consider laboratory error.
• If measured osmolarity exceeds the calculated osmolarity, determine the osmolar gap.
• Osmolar gap = measured osmolarity − calculated osmolarity.
• High measured osmolarity and normal calculated osmolarity with a high osmolar gap indicate the presence of unmeasured solutes (not Na, K, glucose, BUN).
• High measured osmolarity and high calculated osmolarity with a normal osmolar gap usually indicate that the hyperosmolarity is caused by hyperglycemia or hypernatremia.
• Serum sodium concentration may be artificially low in patients with severe hyperglycemia and hyperosmolarity.
• Fasting hyperglycemia and glucosuria support a diagnosis of diabetes mellitus.
• Numerous calcium oxalate crystals in the urine suggest ethylene glycol toxicosis.
• High urinary specific gravity rules out diabetes insipidus.
• Low urinary specific gravity, especially hyposthenuria, suggests diabetes insipidus.

OTHER LABORATORY TESTS
Urinary osmolarity lower than serum osmolarity suggests diabetes insipidus; concentrated urine rules out diabetes insipidus.

IMAGING
Renal ultrasonography may reveal bright, hyperechoic kidneys in patients with ethylene glycol toxicosis.

DIAGNOSTIC PROCEDURES
N/A

 TREATMENT
• Mild hyperosmolarity without clinical signs may not warrant specific treatment, but diagnose and treat underlying diseases.
• Hospitalize patients with moderate-to-high osmolarity (>350 mOsm/L) and patients exhibiting clinical signs and gradually lower serum osmolarity with intravenous fluids while a definitive diagnosis is pursued.
• Administer D_5W or 0.45% saline slowly IV.

• Free water deficit can be calculated by the following formula:

Free water deficit = 0.4 × lean body weight in kg × [(Plasma Na/140) − 1].

The goal is to not drop sodium more than 15 mEq/L in an 8 hour period; that is, the ultimate goal is to not drop the sodium by more than 2 mEq/L per hour.
• Initially, 0.9% saline may be used to restore normal hemodynamics and replace dehydration deficits; replace one-half of dehydration deficits over 12 hours and the remainder over 24 hours; then switch to D_5W or 0.45% saline.

 MEDICATIONS

DRUG(S) OF CHOICE
Seizures can be controlled with diazepam, phenobarbital, or pentobarbital.

CONTRAINDICATIONS
Hypertonic saline and hyperosmolar solutions

PRECAUTIONS
• May use normal saline initially, but rapid administration may worsen neurologic signs.
• Rapid administration of hypotonic fluids (e.g., D_5W and 0.45% saline) may also cause cerebral edema and worsen neurologic signs.

POSSIBLE INTERACTIONS
N/A

ALTERNATIVE DRUG(S)
Regular insulin 0.1 unit/kg IM or IV can be administered if a hyperglycemic crisis occurs secondary to parenteral nutrition administration.

 FOLLOW-UP

PATIENT MONITORING
• Hydration status; avoid overhydration.
• Bladder size, urine output, and breathing patterns during IV fluid administration
• Anuria, irregular breathing patterns, worsening depression, coma, or seizures may be signs of deterioration.

POSSIBLE COMPLICATIONS
Altered consciousness and abnormal behavior

✓ MISCELLANEOUS

ASSOCIATED CONDITIONS
Hypernatremia and hyperglycemia

AGE-RELATED FACTORS
N/A

ZOONOTIC POTENTIAL
N/A

PREGNANCY
N/A

SYNONYMS
N/A

SEE ALSO
• Diabetes with Hyperosmolar Coma
• Hyperglycemia
• Hypernatremia

ABBREVIATION
ADH = antidiuretic hormone

Suggested Reading
DiBartola SP, ed. Fluid therapy in small animal practice. Philadelphia: Saunders, 1992.
DiBartola SP, Green RA, Autran de Morais HS. Osmolality and osmolal gap. In: Willard MD, Tvedten H, Turnwald GH, eds. Small animal clinical diagnosis by laboratory methods. 2nd ed. Philadelphia: Saunders, 1994:106–107.
Moens NMM, Remedios AM. Hyperosmolar hyperglycemic syndrome in a dog resulting from parenteral nutrition overload. J Sm Anim Pract 1997;38:417–420.
Riley JH, Cornelius LM. Osmolality. In: Loeb WF, Quimby FW, eds. The clinical chemistry of laboratory animals. New York: Pergamon Press, 1989:395–397.

Acknowledgment
The author/editors acknowledge the contributions of Margaret R. Kern, who authored this topic in the previous edition.

Author Elisa M. Mazzaferro
Consulting Editor Deborah S. Greco

HYPERPARATHYROIDISM

 **BASICS**

DEFINITION
A pathologic, sustained, high, circulating concentration of PTH

PATHOPHYSIOLOGY
• PTH—secreted by the parathyroid glands in response to changes in the concentration of ionized calcium in the serum; raises the serum calcium concentration through its effects on bone and renal tubular calcium resorption and vitamin D–dependent intestinal calcium absorption
• Can develop as a primary condition or be secondary to a disorder of calcium homeostasis; primary hyperparathyroidism is associated with benign (usually) adenoma of the parathyroid gland(s); secondary hyperparathyroidism can be caused by a deficiency of calcium and vitamin D associated with malnutrition or chronic renal disease

SYSTEMS AFFECTED
• Renal/urologic
• Gastrointestinal
• Neuromuscular
• Cardiovascular

GENETICS
• None known for primary hyperparathyroidism, but its association with certain breeds suggests a possible hereditary basis in some cases.
• Secondary hyperparathyroidism can develop in association with hereditary nephropathy, but is not inherited per se.

INCIDENCE/PREVALENCE
• Prevalence of primary form is unknown.
• More commonly diagnosed in dogs than in cats.
• Fairly common among causes of hypercalcemia, but much less common than hypercalcemia of malignancy (at least in dogs)
• Nutritional secondary hyperparathyroidism is decreasing in prevalence as the public becomes more educated in pet nutrition.
• Chronic renal failure with secondary hyperparathyroidism is extremely common, more so in cats than in dogs.

GEOGRAPHIC DISTRIBUTION
N/A

SIGNALMENT

Species
Cats and dogs

Breed Predilections
• Keeshond
• Siamese cat

Mean Age and Range
• Cats—mean age, 13 years; range 8–15 years
• Dogs—mean age, 10 years; range 5–15 years

Predominant Sex
None

SIGNS

General Comments
• Most dogs and cats with primary hyperparathyroidism do not appear ill.
• Signs are usually mild and are due solely to the effects of hypercalcemia.
• Signs become apparent when hypercalcemia is severe and chronic.

Historical Findings
• Polyuria
• Polydipsia
• Anorexia
• Lethargy
• Vomiting
• Weakness
• Urolithiasis
• Stupor and coma

Physical Examination Findings
• Often unremarkable
• Parathyroid adenoma is not palpable in dogs but often is in cats.
• Nutritional secondary disease is sometimes associated with pathologic bone fractures and general poor body condition.

CAUSES
• Primary hyperparathyroidism—PTH-secreting adenoma of the parathyroid gland
• Renal secondary hyperparathyroidism—renal calcium loss and reduced gut absorption of calcium due to deficiency in calcitriol production by the renal tubular cells
• Nutritional secondary hyperparathyroidism—a nutritional deficiency of calcium and vitamin D

RISK FACTORS
• Primary hyperparathyroidism—unknown
• Secondary hyperparathyroidism—coexisting renal tubular disease or calcium/vitamin D malnutrition

 DIAGNOSIS

DIFFERENTIAL DIAGNOSIS
The differential list includes causes of hypercalcemia.
• Lymphosarcoma—common in dogs, rare in cats
• Anal sac apocrine gland adenocarcinoma—dogs
• Other miscellaneous carcinomas—dogs and cats
• Myeloproliferative disease—cats
• Fibrosarcoma—cats
• Chronic renal failure
• Hypoadrenocorticism
• Vitamin D rodenticide intoxication—no such products are currently marketed in the U.S.

CBC/BIOCHEMISTRY/URINALYSIS
• High serum calcium concentration
• Low or low-normal serum phosphorus concentration in primary hyperparathyroidism
• Hyperphosphatemia in secondary hyperparathyroidism or hypervitaminosis D
• BUN and creatinine concentrations are usually normal in patients with primary hyperparathyroidism, except those with hypercalcemia-induced renal failure.

OTHER LABORATORY TESTS
• Serum ionized calcium determination is often normal in patients with chronic renal failure and high in patients with primary hyperparathyroidism or hypercalcemia associated with malignancy.
• High serum PTH concentration is diagnostic for primary hyperparathyroidism in the absence of azotemia; assays that measure the intact PTH molecule are most useful.

IMAGING
• Radiography can be useful to assess urolithiasis, renal morphology, and bone density and to identify occult neoplasia.
• Ultrasonography of the ventral cervical area sometimes reveals a parathyroid gland adenoma.
• Ultrasound of the abdomen can reveal lymphadenopathy, urolithiasis, or renal morphologic abnormalities.

DIAGNOSTIC PROCEDURES
Surgical exploration of the ventral cervical area

PATHOLOGIC FINDINGS
• Parathyroid adenoma is usually a solitary, small (=1 cm), round, light brown or reddish mass located in the proximity of the thyroid gland.
• Occasionally multiple adenomas are found.
• The histologic distinctions between adenomas, hyperplasia, and carcinomas of the parathyroid gland are often unclear.

 TREATMENT

APPROPRIATE HEALTH CARE
• Primary hyperparathyroidism generally requires inpatient care and surgery.
• Nutritional or renal secondary hyperparathyroidism in noncritical patients can be managed on an outpatient basis.

NURSING CARE
N/A

ACTIVITY
No alterations recommended

DIET
Calcium supplementation for secondary forms

CLIENT EDUCATION
Explain signs referable to changes in calcium status, since hypocalcemia is a potential complication of parathyroidectomy.

SURGICAL CONSIDERATIONS
Surgery is the treatment of choice for primary hyperparathyroidism and is often important in establishing the diagnosis.

 MEDICATIONS

DRUG(S) OF CHOICE
• Normal saline is the fluid of choice for treatment of hypercalcemia
• Diuretics (furosemide) and corticosteroids can be useful in treating hypercalcemia.
• No medical treatment exists for primary hyperparathyroidism per se.

CONTRAINDICATIONS
• Do not use glucocorticoids until the diagnosis of lymphoma has been excluded; they can obfuscate the diagnosis.
• Avoid calcium-containing fluids.

PRECAUTIONS
Use furosemide only in patients with adequate hydration.

POSSIBLE INTERACTIONS
N/A

ALTERNATIVE DRUG(S)
Mithramycin has been used in patients with severe hypercalcemic crises; avoid if possible, because of associated nephrotoxicity and hepatotoxicity.

 FOLLOW-UP

PATIENT MONITORING
• Postoperative hypocalcemia is relatively common after treatment of primary hyperparathyroidism in patients with a presurgery serum calcium concentration >14 mg/dL; check serum calcium once or twice daily for 1 week after surgery.
• In patients with renal impairment, check serum concentrations of urea nitrogen and creatinine.

PREVENTION/AVOIDANCE
• No strategies exist for prevention of primary hyperparathyroidism.
• Nutritional secondary hyperparathyroidism is prevented by proper nutrition.

POSSIBLE COMPLICATIONS
Irreversible renal failure secondary to hypercalcemia

EXPECTED COURSE AND PROGNOSIS
• Untreated disease usually progresses to end-stage kidney or neurologic disease.
• Prognosis for treatment of parathyroid adenoma is excellent.
• Recurrence is seen in a small percentage of cases.

 MISCELLANEOUS

ASSOCIATED CONDITIONS
Calcium-containing urolithiasis

AGE-RELATED FACTORS
N/A

ZOONOTIC POTENTIAL
N/A

PREGNANCY
N/A

SYNONYMS
None

SEE ALSO
• Hypercalcemia
• Hyperparathyroidism, Renal Secondary
• Renal Failure, Chronic

ABBREVIATIONS
BUN = blood urea nitrogen
PTH = parathyroid hormone

Suggested Reading

Chew DJ, Nagode LA, Carothers M. Disorders of calcium: hypercalcemia and hypocalcemia. In: DiBartola SP. Fluid therapy in small animal practice. Philadelphia: Saunders, 1992:116–176.

Feldman EC, Nelson RW. Hypercalcemia and primary hyperparathyroidism. In: Canine and feline endocrinology and reproduction. 2nd ed. Philadelphia: Saunders, 1996: 455–495.

Richter KP, Kallet AJ, Feldman EC. Primary hyperparathyroidism in the cat. In: Kirk RW, Bonagura JD, eds. Current veterinary therapy XI. Philadelphia: Saunders, 1992.

Author Thomas K. Graves
Consulting Editor Deborah S. Greco

HYPERPARATHYROIDISM, RENAL SECONDARY

BASICS

OVERVIEW
• Clinical syndrome characterized by a high concentration of biologically active PTH secondary to chronic renal failure; major cause is the absolute or relative lack of calcitriol synthesis, though low concentrations of ionized calcium also contribute.
• Hyperphosphatemia secondary to declining renal function reduces the activity of 1-α-hydroxylase in the kidney, which in turn reduces production of calcitriol (1,25-dihydroxycholecalciferol). Reduced renal tubular mass also contributes to reduced calcitriol synthesis. Normal calcitriol concentrations exert a negative effect on PTH synthesis within the parathyroid gland nucleus. Low calcitriol and serum ionized calcium concentrations result in increased PTH production and parathyroid gland hyperplasia. High PTH production increases serum calcitriol and calcium concentrations at the expense of chronically high PTH concentration.
• Calcitrol synthesis is impaired in patients with severe chronic renal failure and low numbers of renal tubules regardless of the level of PTH compensation. PTH may act as a uremic toxin and may promote nephrocalcinosis and progression of chronic renal failure.

SIGNALMENT
Dogs and cats; see Chronic Renal Failure for age and breed predilections.

SIGNS
• Those associated with underlying chronic renal failure are the usual reason for examination.
• Severe renal osteodystrophy or "rubber jaw" occurs in some patients, most commonly young dogs with severe renal secondary hyperparathyroidism.

CAUSES & RISK FACTORS
Any disease that causes chronic renal failure

DIAGNOSIS

DIFFERENTIAL DIAGNOSIS
• Hypercalcemic nephropathy—renal disease (or failure) caused by ionized hypercalcemia; can be difficult to differentiate from long-standing renal secondary hyperparathyroidism in which the parathyroid glands lose their negative feedback responsiveness to high levels of ionized calcium (tertiary hyperparathyroidism)
• The total serum calcium concentration is usually higher in patients with hypercalcemic nephropathy than in those with renal secondary hyperparathyroidism; the ionized serum calcium concentration is usually low or normal with renal secondary hyperparathyroidism and high with hypercalcemic nephropathy.
• Serum PTH concentration is low in animals with hypercalcemia of malignancy; may detect underlying causes of hypercalcemia such as lymphoma or apocrine gland adenocarcinoma of the anal sac
• Primary hyperparathyroidism—initially characterized by hypercalcemia (ionized and total), normal or low serum phosphorus concentration, and high PTH concentration; renal function is initially normal but may become compromised later in the course of disease.

CBC/BIOCHEMISTRY/URINALYSIS
• Azotemia
• Hyperphosphatemia
• Urine specific gravity < 1.030 in dogs and < 1.035 in cats
• Possible hypocalcemia (ionized calcium); the total serum calcium concentration may be low, normal, or slightly high; see Chronic Renal Failure.

OTHER LABORATORY TESTS
• Definitive diagnosis and therapeutic monitoring of renal secondary hyperparathroidism require measurement of high serum PTH concentration; an immunoassay for PTH directed against the amino-terminal or intact PTH molecule and validated for dogs or cats is necessary for interpretation of meaningful results.
• A low to normal ionized serum calcium concentration is useful to differentiate renal secondary hyperparathyroidism from other causes of hypercalcemia.

IMAGING
Radiographs may reveal low bone density, loss of the lamina dura around the teeth, and soft-tissue mineralization of the gastric mucosa or other tissues.

DIAGNOSTIC PROCEDURES
N/A

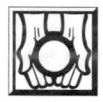

TREATMENT
• See Chronic Renal Failure for general treatment principles.
• Patients with renal secondary hyperparathyroidism—feed a diet low in phosphorus content and give free access to fresh water.

MEDICATIONS

DRUG(S)

Intestinal Phosphate Binders
• Prescribe if dietary management does not return phosphorous concentration to normal.
• Aluminum hydroxide (30–90 mg/kg/day PO with meals), calcium carbonate (90–150

mg/kg/day PO with meals), or calcium acetate (60–90 mg/kg/day PO with meals)
• Hypercalcemia may uncommonly develop when a calcium-containing phosphate binder is combined with calcitriol. Aluminum- and calcium-containing phosphate binders can be used in combination to reduce the dosage of each and minimize the risk of hypercalcemia.

Calcitriol
• Low-dose calcitriol (2.5–3.5 ng/kg PO q24h)—may use after initiation of dietary phosphorus restriction and oral phosphate binders; note that this dose is in ng/kg rather than mg/kg; a pharmacy that specializes in reformulation into low doses is needed to provide this prescription.
• Maintain serum phosphorus concentration within the normal range before and during calcitriol therapy.

CONTRAINDICATIONS/POSSIBLE INTERACTIONS
• Calcitriol administration may result in hypercalcemia, especially if combined with a calcium-containing intestinal phosphate binder. Hypercalcemia sometimes develops in patients with longstanding chronic renal failure but is not related to calcitriol treatment. In these instances, ionized calcium concentration is normal or low, and hypercalcemia does not resolve when calcitriol treatment is discontinued.
• Do not use calcium-containing intestinal phosphate binders in patients with hyperphosphatemia or with a calcium × phosphorus product > 70. Use aluminum-containing intestinal phosphate binders initially to correct hyperphosphatemia, followed by calcium-containing intestinal phosphate binders once the serum phosphorus concentration is normal.

FOLLOW-UP

PATIENT MONITORING
• Serum concentrations of calcium, phosphorus, creatinine, and urea nitrogen—weekly to monthly depending on therapy and the severity of chronic renal failure
• Patients receiving calcitriol should be monitored for hypercalcemia and/or hyperphosphatemia weekly for 4 weeks, then monthly if the patient is stable, and then every 3–4 months.
• Serial evaluations of PTH concentration—most dogs and cats treated with low doses of calcitriol achieve near-normal levels of PTH within 3 months; it may be necessary to increase the dose in those with severe parathyroid gland hyperplasia.
• If hypercalcemia develops, discontinue use of calcitriol. Measurement of ionized calcium is recommended since some animals with chronic renal failure develop nonionized hypercalcemia that is unrelated to calcitriol treatment. If hypercalcemia is due to calcitriol treatment (high-ionized calcium), it should abate within 5 days. Intermittent-dose calcitriol treatment at twice the dose every other day may alleviate a mild degree of hypercalcemia. Patients with more severe hypercalcemia may benefit from 3.5 times the normal dose given every 3.5 days. These effects on reduction in calcemia are due to decreased programming of intestinal epithelial cells for calcium absorption.

PREVENTION/AVOIDANCE
Dietary phosphorus restriction in patients with chronic renal failure may delay the onset of renal secondary hyperparathyroidism.

POSSIBLE COMPLICATIONS
Renal osteodystrophy and pathologic fractures (rare)

EXPECTED COURSE AND PROGNOSIS
• Progression of the underlying chronic renal failure may be slowed by treatment of renal secondary hyperparathyroidism.
• Long-term prognosis is guarded to poor for patients with chronic renal failure and renal secondary hyperparathyroidism.
• Short-term prognosis depends on severity of chronic renal failure.

MISCELLANEOUS

AGE-RELATED FACTORS
Young animals can develop severe renal osteodystrophy and may benefit from treatment with calcitriol and calcium carbonate.

ABBREVIATION
PTH = parathyroid hormone

Suggested Reading
Chew DJ, Nagode LA. Calcitriol in the treatment of chronic renal failure. In: Kirk RW, Bonagura JD, eds. Current veterinary therapy XI. Philadelphia: Saunders, 1992: 857–860.
Nagode LA, Chew DJ, Podell M. Benefits of calcitriol therapy and serum phosphorus control in dogs and cats with chronic renal failure. Vet Clin North Am 1996;26:1293–1330.
Authors Larry G. Adams and Dennis J. Chew
Consulting Editors Larry G. Adams and Carl A. Osborne

HYPERPHOSPHATEMIA

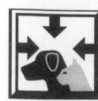 BASICS

DEFINITION
• Serum total phosphorus > 5.5 mg/dL (dogs)
• Serum total phosphorus > 6.0 mg/dL (cats)

PATHOPHYSIOLOGY
• Control of phosphorus is complex and is influenced by the actions of PTH and vitamin D and the interaction of these hormones with the gut, bone, kidneys, and parathyroid glands.
• High serum phosphorus results from excessive gastrointestinal absorption of phosphorus, excessive bone resorption of phosphorus, and reduced renal excretion of phosphorus.

SYSTEMS AFFECTED
• Renal
• Endocrine
• Metabolic

SIGNALMENT
• Dog and cat
• Any age, but commonly young, growing animals or old animals with renal insufficiency

SIGNS

Historical Findings
• Depend on the underlying cause of hyperphosphatemia
• No specific signs directly attributable to hyperphosphatemia
• Acute hyperphosphatemia causes hypocalcemic tetany and/or vascular collapse.

Physical Examination Findings
Chronic hyperphosphatemia causes calcification of soft tissues, resulting in chronic renal failure and tumoral calcinosis.

CAUSES
• Reduced glomerular filtration rate
• Prerenal azotemia
• Renal azotemia
• Postrenal azotemia
• Hyperphosphatemia secondary to excessive bone resorption or muscle breakdown
• Young growing dogs
• Hypoparathyroidism
• Hypersomatotropism
• Hyperphosphatemia caused by excessive gastrointestinal absorption of phosphorus
• Osteolysis
• Disuse osteoporosis
• Osseous neoplasia
• Hyperthyroidism
• Phosphorus-containing enemas
• Vitamin D toxicosis
• Phosphorus dietary supplementation
• Nutritional secondary hyperparathyroidism

RISK FACTORS
Use of phosphorus-containing enemas to small animals such as cats

 DIAGNOSIS

DIFFERENTIAL DIAGNOSIS
• Hypoparathyroidism—also characterized by clinical signs of hypocalcemia such as seizures and tetany
• Prerenal azotemia as a cause of hyperphosphatemia—associated with disease states that result in low cardiac output such as congestive heart failure, dehydration, hypoadrenocorticism and shock
• Renal insufficiency, either acute or chronic renal failure—attended by azotemia and abnormal findings on urinalysis (low urinary specific gravity)
• Young, growing animals—can have serum phosphorus concentrations twice those of adults
• Vitamin D intoxication—history of vitamin D supplementation or ingestion of rodenticides (e.g., Rampage)
• Nutritional secondary hyperparathyroidism—history of dietary calcium–phosphorus imbalance
• Hyperthyroidism in cats—clinical signs of weight loss, polyphagia, and polydipsia and polyuria
• Hypersomatotropism—attended by a history of progesterone administration in dogs and insulin-resistant diabetes mellitus in cats
• Nonazotemia tumoral calcinosis—observed in human beings as an autosomal dominant disorder; rare cause of hyperphosphatemia associated with large bone lesions
• Jasmine toxicity—history of plant ingestion
• Factitious

LABORATORY FINDINGS

Drugs That May Alter Laboratory Results
• Phosphorus-containing enemas
• Intravenous KPO_4
• Anabolic steroids
• Furosemide
• Hydrochlorothiazide
• Minocycline

Disorders That May Alter Laboratory Results
• Hemolysis and lipemia can falsely raise phosphorus concentrations.
• Collection in citrate, oxalate, or EDTA

Valid If Run in Human Laboratory?
Valid

CBC/BIOCHEMISTRY/URINALYSIS
• Serum phosphorus > 6.0 mg/dL
• Low serum calcium in patients with primary hypoparathyroidism
• High serum calcium in patients with vitamin D intoxication
• Azotemia and isosthenuria help define degree of renal impairment.
• Hyperkalemia and hyponatremia suggest hypoadrenocorticism.

OTHER LABORATORY TESTS
• Serum PTH measurement—intact molecule and two-site assay methods have the greatest specificity; high-normal or high concentrations suggest primary hyperparathyroidism; low concentrations suggest neoplasia.
• Thyroxine concentrations—indicated in cats with hyperphosphatemia and clinical signs consistent with hyperthyroidism
• Insulin-like growth factor I (IGF-1) concentrations—indicated in dogs or cats with unexplained hyperphosphatemia and clinical signs consistent with acromegaly; IGF-1 concentrations are elevated in animals with hypersomatotropism.
• Vitamin D assays are not readily available.
• ACTH stimulation testing to confirm hypo-adrenocorticism

IMAGING
• Abdominal radiography to assess renal size and symmetry
• Renal ultrasonography to detect soft-tissue mineralization
• Thyroid scan to rule out hyperthyroidism
• Radiography of long bones to detect osteo-porosis or neoplasia

DIAGNOSTIC PROCEDURES
Renal biopsy

TREATMENT
• Inpatient, because of the deleterious effects of hyperphosphatemia and the need for fluid therapy; consider severe hyperphosphatemia a medical emergency.
• Restrict dietary phosphorus.
• Normal saline is the fluid of choice.

MEDICATIONS

DRUG(S) OF CHOICE
Acute Hyperphosphatemia
• Dextrose (1g/kg IV) and insulin (0.5 U/kg IV)
• Avoid phosphorus-containing fluids.

Chronic Hyperphosphatemia
Oral administration of phosphorus binders (e.g., Amphojel)

CONTRAINDICATIONS
N/A

PRECAUTIONS
N/A

POSSIBLE INTERACTIONS
N/A

ALTERNATIVE DRUG(S)
N/A

FOLLOW-UP

PATIENT MONITORING
• Serum calcium every 12 h
• Renal function tests—urine output must be monitored, particularly if oliguric renal failure is suspected, in which case urine output should be measured carefully; oliguria cannot be determined unless the patient is fully hydrated.
• Hydration status—indicators of overhydration include increased body weight, increased central venous pressure, and edema (pulmonary or subcutaneous).

POSSIBLE COMPLICATIONS
• Hypophosphatemia resulting in hemolysis
• Soft-tissue mineralization

MISCELLANEOUS

ASSOCIATED CONDITIONS
Hypocalcemia

AGE-RELATED FACTORS
Mild elevations in phosphorus may be normal in growing animals.

ZOONOTIC POTENTIAL
N/A

PREGNANCY
N/A

SYNONYMS
None

SEE ALSO
• Hypoparathyroidism
• Renal Failure, Acute
• Renal Failure, Chronic

ABBREVIATIONS
• ACTH = adrenocorticotropin
• IGF-1 = insulin-like growth factor I
• PTH = parathyroid hormone

Suggested Reading
Aurbach GD, Marx SJ, Spiegel AM. Parathyroid hormone, calcitonin, and the calciferols. In: Wilson JD, Foster DW, eds. Williams textbook of endocrinology. 7th ed. Philadelphia: Saunders, 1985:1208–1209.
Willard MD, Tvedten H, Turnwald GH. Clinical diagnosis by laboratory methods. Philadelphia: Saunders, 1989.
Author Deborah S. Greco
Consulting Editor Deborah S. Greco

HYPERTENSION, PORTAL

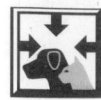

BASICS

DEFINITION
Portal pressure > 13 cm H_2O

PATHOPHYSIOLOGY
• Caused by an increase in portal blood flow, an increase in resistance to portal blood flow, or a combination • Increased resistance—most commonly as a consequence of acquired disease; anatomic site used to classify mechanisms: prehepatic (abdominal portion of the portal vein), hepatic (within the liver), or posthepatic (hepatic veins, caudal vena cava, and heart) • Consequences—development of multiple APSS with subsequent hepatic encephalopathy from prehepatic and hepatic causes; results in increased abdominal lymph production • APSS—typically connect the abdominal portal system and the caudal vena cava; become apparent within 1–2 months of onset of hypertension • Ascites associated with hepatic causes—pure transudate; most likely to develop when portal hypertension and hypoalbuminemia coexist (albumin < 1.5 g/dL) • Ascites secondary to posthepatic disorders—modified transudate (protein > 2.5 g/dL and hypocellular) • Ascites from prehepatic causes—often short lived; low protein content, reflects splanchnic lymph

SYSTEMS AFFECTED
• Hepatobiliary—obstruction of blood flow causes distention of the venous bed behind the obstruction; passive congestion of the spleen causes splenomegaly; passive congestion of the liver caused by posthepatic disorders usually results in only hepatomegaly • Nervous—hepatic encephalopathy • Cardiovascular—multiple portosystemic shunts and ascites with vena caval obstruction, not with congestive heart failure or pericardial tamponade as these cause increased hydrostatic pressure in both hepatic and vena caval systems • Gastrointestinal—splanchnic hypertension associated with tissue edema; increased gut wall permeability; predisposition to ulceration, endotoxemia, and malnutrition owing to reduced nutrient assimilation

GENETICS
Increased occurrence in some breeds and kindreds—certain hepatic vascular anomalies; idiopathic hepatic fibrosis; copper hepatopathy

SIGNALMENT

Species
Dogs and rarely cats

Breed Predilections
Familial hepatic vascular disorders reported—Doberman pinschers (noncirrhotic portal hypertension); Saint Bernards (arteriovenous fistula); black standard poodles; and German shepherd dogs (idiopathic or juvenile hepatic fibrosis)

Mean Age and Range
• Juveniles—inherited or congenital disorders; vena caval and cardiac malformations • Young dogs (< 2 years of age)—idiopathic juvenile hepatic fibrosis • Young dogs with onset of signs < 1.5 years of age—congenital hepatic vascular malformations • Middle-aged and older animals—acquired hepatic and biliary disorders

Predominant Sex N/A

SIGNS

General Comments
• Depend on site, degree, and rate of development of hypertension and the underlying cause • Most underlying disorders are chronic.

Historical Findings
• Abdominal distention • Ascites and hepatomegaly • Hepatic encephalopathy—may be secondary to APSS • Cardiac disorders—cough; exercise intolerance; dyspnea • Portal thromboembolism—bloody diarrhea; ileus; abdominal pain

Physical Examination Findings
• Abdominal effusion • Splenomegaly • Hepatomegaly—posthepatic causes only • Jugular vein distention—cardiopulmonary causes • Muffled heart sounds—pericardial or pleural effusion • Cardiac arrhythmias or murmur—cardiac disease • Pulmonary "crackles" (edema)—cardiogenic causes • Hepatic encephalopathy • Jaundice • Hepatic bruit (AV fistula)—see Arteriovenous Malformation of Liver) • Consequent to surgical ligation of PSVA (see Portosystemic Vascular Anomaly, Congenital)

CAUSES

Prehepatic
• Portal vein thrombosis, stenosis, or neoplasia • Portal vein compression—large lymph nodes; neoplasia, granuloma; abscess • Postoperative complication of PSVA shunt ligation • Congenital portal vein atresia

Intrahepatic
• Hepatic fibrosis/cirrhosis • Chronic inflammatory liver disease • Chronic extrahepatic bile duct obstruction (> 6 weeks) • Idiopathic juvenile hepatic fibrosis • Hepatic neoplasia—porta hepatis location • Liver entrapment—in diaphragmatic hernia • Veno-occlusive disease • Noncirrhotic portal hypertension • Portal vein atresia/hypoplasia • Hepatic AV fistula

Posthepatic
• Right-sided congestive heart failure • Heartworm disease • Pericardial tamponade • Severe pulmonary thromboembolism • Pericarditis—restrictive or constrictive • Cardiac neoplasia • Cor triatriatum dexter • Disorders affecting the supradiaphragmatic caudal vena cava—thrombosis; congenital kink or web; heartworm vena cava syndrome; occlusion by neoplasia; entrapment in diaphragmatic hernia

RISK FACTORS
Depend on underlying cause

DIAGNOSIS

DIFFERENTIAL DIAGNOSIS
• Physicochemical analysis of abdominal effusion—helps narrow diagnosis • Pure transudate—hypoalbuminemia secondary to PLE; PLN; liver failure • Modified transudate with normal or low albumin—PLE; PLN; liver failure (chronic effusion); neoplasia; abdominal thromboembolism; visceral entrapment in diaphragmatic hernia • Modified transudate with large liver and jugular distention—cardiac or pericardial abnormalities; heartworm; right atrial tumor • Modified transudate with large liver, without jugular distention, muffled heart, or pulmonary edema—kinked vena cava; Budd-Chiari like syndrome • Hepatic encephalopathy—liver fibrosis; cirrhosis; juvenile fibrosing liver disease; hepatic AV fistula • Jaundice—chronic hepatitis or cholangitis; chronic bile duct obstruction; infiltrative hepatic neoplasm • Bloody diarrhea, abdominal pain, ileus, signs of endotoxemia—acute extrahepatic portal thromboembolism

CBC/BIOCHEMISTRY/URINALYSIS
• CBC—schistocytes with thromboembolism; RBC microcytosis with PSVA or APSS; icteric plasma with liver disease • Biochemistry—liver disease associated variably with high liver enzymes, low concentration of BUN, creatinine, cholesterol, and glucose, hyperbilirubinemia, and coagulation abnormalities; posthepatic disorders associated with high liver enzymes, sometimes azotemia, and normal plasma color. • Urinalysis—ammonium biurate crystalluria with hepatobiliary diseases causing APSS; may note granular casts with thromboembolism; may note proteinuria with heartworm disease

OTHER LABORATORY TESTS
• Total serum bile acids—normal to high fasting and high 2-hr postprandial concentrations with hepatobiliary disease; shunting pattern typified by normal fasting and markedly high postprandial values • Blood ammonia—hyperammonemia associated with underlying liver disease and APSS • Physicochemical characterization of abdominal effusion—high serum albumin:effusion albumin ratio (> 1.1) consistent with portal hypertension; high ratio may predict positive response to diuretic therapy

IMAGING

Radiography
• Thoracic radiography—reveals abnormalities causing posthepatic portal hypertension (e.g., kinked vena cava, pericardial effusion, pulmonary disease, pleural effusion, diaphragmatic hernia) • Abdominal radiography—may reveal effusion, splenomegaly, or large liver (e.g., with congestion, diffuse neoplasia, or hepatic AV fistula); liver small in most disorders causing APSS and in PSVA

Abdominal Ultrasonography
• Inspect portal perfusion dynamics and vessel distention; use Doppler color flow interrogation to demonstrate hepatofugal perfusion (blood flow around the liver as in portosystemic shunting) • Identify lobe(s) containing AV fistula(e) • Detect APSS and PSVA • Appraise visceral parenchyma and lymph nodes (neoplasia, other disorders) • Identify portal hypoplasia, stricture, and occlusion in porta hepatis • Estimate hepatic venous distention—intrahepatic and supradiaphragmatic segments

Echocardiography
To detect congenital and acquired cardiac and pericardial disorders, neoplasia, thrombi, heartworms, pleural effusion, malformed or thrombosed vena cava, and diaphragmatic hernia

Angiography and Nuclear Imaging
• Colorectal scintigraphy—confirms portosystemic shunting • Angiography—demonstrates celiac trunk or proper hepatic artery for diagnosis of hepatic AV fistula • Nonselective or selective studies—congenital cardiac disease; thromboembolic disorders; hepatic vein disorders • Portovenography—portal vein and hepatic vein disorders

DIAGNOSTIC PROCEDURES
• Electrocardiography and central venous pressure—with cardiac disease • Liver biopsy—required with hepatic or hepatic vascular disorders • Portal pressure—may be measured during laparotomy; unreliable in deducing underlying causes (high pressure blunted by APSS); portal hypertension deduced with ultrasound interrogation with Doppler color flow

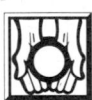

TREATMENT

APPROPRIATE HEALTH CARE
Inpatient—for signs of hepatic encephalopathy; amelioration of tense ascites by therapeutic abdominocentesis

NURSING CARE
• Fluid therapy—with all causes, restrict sodium concentration (avoid 0.9% NaCl) because of the high likelihood of total-body sodium loading • Monitor body weight and condition, girth circumference, plasma proteins, and PCV—assess hydration status and tolerance of fluid infusion • Low oncotic pressure—colloid or albumin indicated; avoid dextran with hepatic dysfunction; plasma preferred for liver patients (or use hetastarch at 20 mL/kg/day given by CRI) • Glucose supplementation—with hepatic dysfunction and hypoglycemia; 2.5%–5.0% dextrose with half-strength polyionic fluids initially; titrate dextrose concentration to achieve euglycemia and yet avoid hyperglycemia • Therapeutic abdominocentesis—only if abdominal distention is causing discomfort, impairing breathing or sleeping, or reducing food ingestion, or when medical efforts at ascites mobilization fail; repeated large-volume procedure

may cause dehydration, hypoproteinemia, and electrolyte depletion and introduce infection; use aseptic technique and concurrently provide polyionic fluids in moderation with colloid

ACTIVITY
Depends on cause

DIET
• Ascites—restricted sodium • Hepatic encephalopathy—restricted protein (see Hepatic Encephalopathy); **Caution:** restrict protein only if protein intolerance is detected

CLIENT EDUCATION
Inform client that definitive diagnosis requires a progressive logical diagnostic strategy and that there can be no prediction for cure or chronic amelioration until a definitive diagnosis is ascertained.

SURGICAL CONSIDERATIONS
• Ligation of APSS strongly contraindicated • If acute symptomatic portal hypertension develops after surgical ligation of PSVA—ligature removal imperative (see Portosystemic Vascular Anomaly, Congenital) • Embolectomy of thrombi not recommended; rather, use streptokinase or TPA and LMW heparin (see Coagulopathy of Liver Disease), definitive treatments remain controversial: streptokinase and TPA have severe side effects and are expensive • Correction of chronic diaphragmatic hernia—high risk • Surgical correction and cure of cor triatriatum and kinked vena cava possible • Pericardectomy—pericardial restriction or tamponade; thoracoscopic procedure is least invasive, with lowest mortality and best outcome • Removal of tumor or fibrous adhesions causing veno-occlusion • Removal of liver lobe(s) containing AV fistula(e)

MEDICATIONS

DRUG(S) OF CHOICE
• Diuretics—spironolactone (1–4 mg/kg PO q12h) combined with furosemide (1–4 mg/kg PO q12h) with liver disease; spironolactone requires a doubled loading dose one time; start low, then titrate diuretic dose higher after observing response for 4 days (body weight, girth, hydration, electrolytes); furosemide and enalapril with cardiac dysfunction (some clinicians also use low-dose spironolactone) • See also Hepatic Encephalopathy

CONTRAINDICATIONS N/A

PRECAUTIONS N/A

POSSIBLE INTERACTIONS
• Avoid drugs that rely on first-pass hepatic extraction, biotransformation, or hepatic elimination, if possible; if not possible, reduce drug dosage appropriately.
• Reduce dose of highly protein-bound drugs with hypoalbuminemia

ALTERNATIVE DRUG(S) N/A

FOLLOW-UP

PATIENT MONITORING
• Body weight, body condition, and girth—sequentially • Hydration • Electrolytes • Acid–base status • Central venous pressure (take care if coagulopathy or high risk for thrombosis; avoid catheters in vena cava or other large central vessels) • Blood pressure • Albumin—with hypoalbuminemia • Glucose—with liver disease • Lung sounds, pulse oximetry, ventilatory effort, and central venous pressure—with cardiovascular and/or pulmonary disorder; avoid iatrogenic pulmonary edema during fluid therapy (especially with hypoalbuminemia)

PREVENTION/AVOIDANCE N/A

POSSIBLE COMPLICATIONS
• Thrombosis • Endotoxemia • Hypotension • Hepatic encephalopathy

EXPECTED COURSE AND PROGNOSIS
Depends on cause

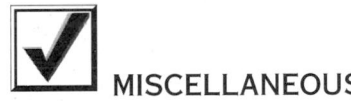

MISCELLANEOUS

ASSOCIATED CONDITIONS
• Chronic liver disease • Numerous disorders causing prehepatic or posthepatic venous occlusion

PREGNANCY
Affects uterine perfusion and likely leads to abortion or stillbirths

SEE ALSO
• Ascites • Cirrhosis and Fibrosis of the Liver • Congestive Heart Failure, Right-sided • Hepatic Encephalopathy • Pericarditis • Portosystemic Shunt, Acquired • Portosystemic Vascular Anomaly, Congenital

ABBREVIATIONS
• APSS = acquired portosystemic shunt(s) • AV = arteriovenous • CRI = constant rate infusion • LMW = low molecular weight • PLE = protein-losing enteropathy • PLN = protein-losing nephropathy • PSVA = portosystemic venous anomaly • TPA = tissue plasminogen activator

Suggested Reading
Center SA. Pathophysiology of liver disease: normal and abnormal function. In: Guilford WG, Center SA, Strombeck DR, et al., eds. Strombeck's small animal gastroenterology. 3rd ed. Philadelphia: Saunders, 1996:553–632.
Authors Susan E. Bunch and Susan E. Johnson
Consulting Editor Sharon A. Center

HYPERTENSION, PULMONARY

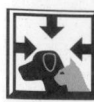

BASICS

DEFINITION
Elevation in systolic pulmonary artery pressure > 30 mm Hg or mean pulmonary arterial pressure > 20 mm Hg

PATHOPHYSIOLOGY
• Several events can lead to elevations in pulmonary artery pressure. Primary pulmonary hypertension, a congenital abnormality in the pulmonary vasculature, has not been identified in cats or dogs. Secondary pulmonary hypertension can be caused by pulmonary artery or capillary vasoconstriction, pulmonary artery obstruction, high left atrial pressure with resultant pulmonary capillary pressure elevation, or excessive pulmonary arterial blood flow. Hypoxia and associated acidemia associated with pulmonary disease or other abnormalities commonly result in pulmonary vasoconstriction. • As pressures in the pulmonary capillaries and pulmonary artery rise, the right ventricle hypertrophies to maintain pulmonary blood flow. Pulmonary hypertension leads to abnormalities in pulmonary blood flow and filling of the left ventricle, which can cause dyspnea, weakness, exercise intolerance, and cyanosis. High right heart pressures can cause venous congestion, tricuspid regurgitation, and right-sided congestive heart failure (R-CHF). • Secondary causes of pulmonary hypertension include severe pulmonary disease (vasoconstriction and obstruction), heartworm disease (vasoconstriction and obstruction), severe left heart disease (high left atrial pressure), pulmonary thromboembolism (obstruction and vasoconstriction), and congenital heart disease with left-to-right shunting (excessive pulmonary blood flow). Extrapulmonary causes of chronic hypoxia such as hypoventilation and high altitude disease can also lead to pulmonary hypertension.

SYSTEMS AFFECTED
• Cardiovascular—pulmonary artery hypertrophy and dilation, right ventricular hypertrophy and dilation (cor pulmonale), right atrial dilation, possible R-CHF (especially if significant tricuspid value disease is present) • Respiratory— pulmonary abnormalities may cause pulmonary hypertension

GENETICS
No genetic basis found; pulmonary hypertension can be secondary to several congenital heart defects that may have a genetic basis.

INCIDENCE/PREVALENCE
• Unknown • No cases of idiopathic primary pulmonary hypertension documented in the veterinary literature.

GEOGRAPHIC DISTRIBUTION
Unknown; may be a relatively higher prevalence in heartworm endemic areas and at high altitudes

SIGNALMENT

Species
Dogs and cats

Breed Predilections
May be based on underlying cause of pulmonary hypertension (e.g. congenital heart disease)

SIGNS

General Comments
May be due to pulmonary hypertension or the underlying primary disease

Historical Findings
• Exercise intolerance • Dyspnea • Coughing/hemoptysis • Syncope • Abdominal distention • Weight loss

Physical Examination Findings
• Dyspnea • Coughing • Hemoptysis • Loud or split second heart sound • Abnormal lung sounds • Cyanosis • Heart murmur • Abdominal distention • Jugular distention • Weight loss

CAUSES

Pulmonary Parenchymal Disease (Vasoconstriction from Chronic Hypoxia and Acidemia)
• Vascular obstruction from pulmonary fibrosis, vascular hypertrophy, and infiltrative disease • Chronic bronchitis • Eosinophilic bronchitis • Disseminated neoplasia • Adult respiratory distress syndrome

Pulmonary Thromboembolism (Vascular Obstruction and Secondary Vasoconstriction)
• Hyperadrenocorticism • Protein-losing nephropathy • Sepsis • Heartworm disease • Immune-mediated hemolytic anemia • Neoplasia • Pancreatitis • Endocarditis • Disseminated intravascular coagulation • Cardiac disease

Congenital Heart Disease with Left-to-Right Shunting (Excessive Pulmonary Blood Flow and Reactive Vasoconstriction)
• Patent ductus arteriosus • Ventricular septal defect • Atrial septal defect • Probably a rare cause of pulmonary hypertension

Vascular Obstruction Secondary to Vascular Hypertrophy and Thromboembolism—Reactive Vasoconstriction
• Heartworm disease

Left Heart Disease (High Left Atrial Pressure)
• Mitral regurgitation • Dilated cardiomyopathy • Hypertrophic cardiomyopathy • Restrictive cardiomyopathy • Mitral stenosis

• Congenital pulmonary venous obstruction (cor triatriatum sinister) • Left atrial tumors

Extrapulmonary Causes of Chronic Hypoxia (Vasoconstriction from Hypoxia and Acidemia)
• Hypoventilation (Pickwickian syndrome, neuromuscular disorders) • High altitude disease • Idiopathic primary pulmonary hypertension (not documented in dogs or cats)

RISK FACTORS
• Cardiac and pulmonary disease • Heartworm disease • Diseases associated with pulmonary thromboembolism • Obesity • High altitude

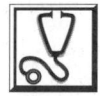

DIAGNOSIS

DIFFERENTIAL DIAGNOSIS
• L-CHF without pulmonary hypertension • Collapsing trachea • Primary right-sided heart disease • Significant pulmonary disease without pulmonary hypertension • Heartworm disease • Pneumothorax • Pyothorax • Hemothorax • Laryngeal paralysis

CBC/BIOCHEMISTRY/URINALYSIS
• Findings vary with underlying cause. • No consistent findings associated with pulmonary hypertension • Polycythemia can be seen if marked hypoxia

OTHER LABORATORY TESTS
• Arterial blood gases (hypoxemia) • Occult heartworm test • Workup for causes of pulmonary thromboembolism (urine protein: creatinine ratio, antithrombin III level, coagulation profile, ACTH stimulation test, low-dose dexamethasone suppression test) • Fluid analysis of pleural or abdominal effusions

IMAGING

Radiography
• Large pulmonary artery • Large right ventricle • Dilated caudal vena cava • Pleural effusion • Hepatomegaly • Ascites • Other findings vary with cause, but might include evidence of primary pulmonary disease, pulmonary embolism, and heartworm disease.

Echocardiography
• Right ventricular hypertrophy • Right ventricular dilation • Right atrial dilation • Pulmonary artery dilation • Pleural effusion • Pericardial effusion • If tricuspid valve insufficiency, systolic pressure gradients can be estimated with Doppler (>30 mm Hg is abnormal) • Evidence of left heart disease, heartworm disease, congenital heart disease, or pulmonary thromboembolism, depending on cause of pulmonary hypertension

DIAGNOSTIC PROCEDURES
Transtracheal wash or bronchoalveolar lavage

Electrocardiography
• Right mean electrical axis deviation • Deep S waves in leads I, II, III, and aVF • Widening of QRS complex • Tall P waves (i.e., P pulmonale) • ST segment depression may occur with significant hypoxia. Hypoxia could induce arrhythmias such as ventricular premature complexes.

Cardiac Catheterization and Pulmonary Angiography
• May be required to confirm pulmonary hypertension • May demonstrate abnormalities such as heartworms, pulmonary thromboembolism, vascular changes, or congenital heart disease supporting the underlying cause of pulmonary hypertension

PATHOLOGIC FINDINGS
• Consistent with underlying disease • Pulmonary artery thrombus • Dilated pulmonary artery • Right heart enlargement • Heartworms • Pleural effusion • Ascites • Medial hypertrophy of pulmonary vasculature • Intimal proliferation and sclerosis of pulmonary vasculature • Necrotizing arteritis

 TREATMENT

APPROPRIATE HEALTH CARE
• Hospitalize patients in severe respiratory distress until stable. • Administer oxygen therapy, bronchodilators, diuretics, and antibiotics on an emergency basis in accordance with underlying disease.

NURSING CARE
• Monitor hydration and body temperature closely. • Administer fluid therapy judiciously on basis of hydration status and severity of right-sided cardiac disease; right-sided cardiac disease may contraindicate fluid therapy. • Maintain low-stress environment.

ACTIVITY
Restricted

DIET
Specific guidelines based on underlying disease; if heart failure, restricted sodium diet may have benefit

CLIENT EDUCATION
• Diagnosis often presumptive without catheterization or Doppler echocardiography • Prognosis varies with reversibility of the underlying disease, but is very guarded in most cases. • Avoid environments that may predispose to respiratory distress—excessively cold or dry air, excessive heat, second-hand smoke, high altitudes

SURGICAL CONSIDERATIONS
N/A

 MEDICATIONS

DRUG(S) OF CHOICE
• Medical management is controversial; direct treatment at the primary underlying disease process. • The ideal therapeutic agent should reduce pulmonary vascular resistance and hypertension without affecting the systemic circulation; oxygen can accomplish this, but long-term oxygen administration is not feasible in these patients; short-term or intermittent use of oxygen may be beneficial.

Vasodilators
• Ideally, base selection on pulmonary and systemic blood pressure response during cardiac catheterization. • Choices include ACE inhibitors (e.g., enalapril, benazepril), hydralazine, and calcium channel blockers. • Often not useful due to development of systemic hypotension.

Bronchodilators
• May benefit treatment of hypoxia-mediated pulmonary hypertension (i.e. pulmonary disease) • Choices include sympathomimetics (e.g., terbutaline) and methylxanthines (e.g., theophylline, aminophylline). • Bronchodilators may have additional positive inotropic effects.

Positive Inotropes (Digoxin, Dobutamine)
• Not a primary treatment of pulmonary hypertension • May improve right heart function and resolve CHF • Monitor closely for digoxin-related arrhythmias.

Anticoagulant Therapy
• Indicated if thromboembolic disease diagnosed • Questionable efficacy • Choices include heparin, warfarin, and aspirin

CONTRAINDICATIONS
• Drugs or situations that worsen pulmonary hypoxia (e.g., respiratory depressants) • Drugs that depress cardiac function (e.g., β-blockers) • Drugs that cause vasoconstriction

PRECAUTIONS
• Excessive administration of vasodilators can cause systemic hypotension. • Excessive use of bronchodilators can lead to detrimental tachycardia and hyperexcitability. • Monitor coagulation profiles closely during anticoagulation.

ALTERNATIVE DRUG(S) N/A

 FOLLOW-UP

PATIENT MONITORING
• Physical examination with careful cardiac and pulmonary auscultation • Monitor for worsening in clinical signs • Thoracic radiography • Arterial blood gases • Echocardiography • Electrocardiography

PREVENTION/AVOIDANCE
Early evaluation and prevention of conditions that predispose to pulmonary hypertension

POSSIBLE COMPLICATIONS
• Right-sided heart failure • Syncope • Cardiac arrhythmias • Sudden death

EXPECTED COURSE AND PROGNOSIS
• Based on ability to reverse underlying disease • When changes are irreversible, treatment is palliative. • In general very guarded

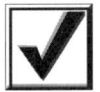 MISCELLANEOUS

ASSOCIATED CONDITIONS
See causes

AGE-RELATED FACTORS
N/A

PREGNANCY
High risk

SEE ALSO
Diseases causing pulmonary hypertension

ABBREVIATIONS
ACE = angiotensin-converting enzyme
ACTH = adrenocorticotropic hormone
L-CHF = left-sided congestive heart failure
R-CHF = right-sided congestive heart failure

Suggested Reading
Johnson LR, Hamlin RL. Recognition and treatment of pulmonary hypertension. In: Bonagura, JD, ed. Current veterinary therapy XII. Philadelphia: Saunders, 1995: 887–892.
Rich S, Braunwald E, Grossman W. Pulmonary hypertension. In: Braunwald E, ed. Heart disease. 5th ed. Philadelphia: Saunders, 1997:780–807.
Author Donald P. Schrope
Consulting Editors Larry P. Tilley and Francis W. K. Smith, Jr.

HYPERTENSION, SYSTEMIC

BASICS

DEFINITION
Sustained elevation in systolic or diastolic (or both) arterial blood pressure

PATHOPHYSIOLOGY
• Blood pressure is determined by cardiac output and systemic vascular resistance; cardiac output is determined by heart rate and stroke volume; systemic arterial blood pressure regulation depends on integration of complex mechanisms within the central and peripheral nervous systems, renal and cardiac tissues, and humoral factors, which synergistically affect cardiac output and peripheral vascular resistance.
• Baroreceptors in the carotid sinus and aortic arch respond to changes in blood pressure; a fall in blood pressure increases sympathetic discharge, causing vasoconstriction and increased cardiac contractility and heart rate to return blood pressure to normal; humoral substances that modulate blood pressure include catecholamines, vasopressin, kinins, renin, angiotensin, aldosterone, prostaglandins, and atrial natriuretic peptide; the renin-angiotensin-aldosterone system is probably the most important component.
• Hypertension—primary (e.g., essential or idiopathic) or secondary to an underlying disease process; secondary hypertension is more common in veterinary medicine; cause of primary hypertension is not fully understood but some cases have a hereditary component.

SYSTEMS AFFECTED
• Cardiovascular • Renal/Urologic • Ocular • Nervous

GENETICS
Colonies of hypertensive dogs have been produced by mating dogs with essential hypertension; mode of inheritance not known

INCIDENCE/PREVALENCE
Unknown; diagnosed more frequently now that more veterinarians are monitoring blood pressure. One study found that 65% of cats with chronic renal failure and 87% of cats with hyperthyroidism had mild hypertension. A study of clinically normal dogs documented hypertension in 10% (blood pressure more than 2 standard deviations above the mean).

SIGNALMENT

Species
Dogs and cats

Breed Predilection
None

Mean Age and Range
• Dogs—mean age 8.9 ± 3.6 years; range 2–14 years • Cats—mean age 15.1 ± 3.8 years; range 4–20 years

SIGNS
• Acute blindness • Ocular hemorrhage • Dilated pupils • Retinal detachment • Swollen or shrunken kidneys • Hematuria • Epistaxis • Seizures, disorientation, ataxia, circling, hemiparesis, paraparesis, nystagmus • Cardiac murmurs and gallops; less commonly, CHF • Palpable thyroid gland (when hyperthyroid)

CAUSES

Primary or Essential
Not known

Secondary
• Renal disease—end-stage renal disease, glomerulonephritis, amyloidosis, renal artery stenosis • Hyperadrenocorticism • Hyperthyroidism • Diabetes mellitus—uncommon • Pheochromocytoma—rare condition • Hyperaldosteronism—rare condition • Central nervous system disease—rare cause

DIAGNOSIS

DIFFERENTIAL DIAGNOSIS
• Cardiovascular—hypertrophic cardiomyopathy, hyperthyroid heart disease, aortic stenosis, arterial thromboembolic disease • Ophthalmic—ocular trauma, systemic infections (bacterial, fungal, viral), coagulopathies, vasculopathy • Neurologic—primary brain, spinal cord, or peripheral nerve disease • Physical examination and results of biochemistry tests and urinalysis important for establishing the underlying cause for secondary hypertension

CBC/BIOCHEMISTRY/URINALYSIS
• CBC usually normal • Biochemistry may reveal azotemia and hyperphosphatemia (renal insufficiency), hyperglycemia (diabetes mellitus), or high serum alkaline phosphatase (hyperadrenocorticism).
• Urinalysis may reveal proteinuria (glomerulonephritis and amyloidosis), hematuria, poor concentration ability (renal insufficiency, hyperadrenocorticism), or glucosuria (diabetes mellitus).

OTHER LABORATORY TESTS
• Glomerulonephropathy—high urine protein:urine creatinine ratio, low creatinine clearance • Renal dysfunction—low creatinine clearance • Hyperadrenocorticism—exaggerated ACTH response test, failure to suppress with dexamethasone, high urine cortisol:creatinine ratio • Hyperthyroidism (cats)—high T_4, inadequate suppression with a T_3 suppression test • Hypothyroidism (dogs)—low T_3, T_4, free T_3, free T_4; possibly high T_3 and T_4 autoantibodies, high endogenous TSH • Pheochromocytoma—high urinary vanillylmandelic acid • Hyperaldosteronism—24-hour urine aldosterone and plasma aldosterone concentrations high

IMAGING
• Thoracic radiograph to evaluate secondary cardiac changes (mild cardiomegaly) • Abdominal radiographs to evaluate liver, adrenals, and kidneys • Echocardiogram to evaluate hypertensive heart disease (left ventricular free wall and/or interventricular septal hypertrophy and mild left atrial dilation) • Abdominal ultrasound to evaluate kidneys and adrenal glands • CT or MRI scan if brain tumor or hyperadrenocorticism suspected • CT, MRI, or myelogram to determine cause for paresis • Thyroid scintigraphy to evaluate hyperthyroidism

DIAGNOSTIC PROCEDURES
Definitive diagnosis of hypertension requires documentation of high arterial blood pressure via direct or indirect methods.

Direct (Invasive)
Measurement using arterial catheterization or puncture and pressure transducer (PDS Monitor, Baxter) is considered the gold standard; equipment is expensive and the technique can cause animal discomfort and is seldom performed in clinical practice.

Indirect (Noninvasive)
Performed correctly, indirect blood pressure measurements correlate well with direct blood pressure measurements. Indirect blood pressure measurements obtained with oscillometric or Doppler techniques—require an inflatable cuff (width of the cuff should be approximately 40% of the circumference of the limb at the site of placement) wrapped around a distal limb or tail; hold limb at or near level of heart when measuring blood pressure.

Oscillometric Technique
• Oscillometric technique (Cardell, Memoprint) detects pulse pressure oscillations beneath the cuff bladder that result from changes in arterial diameter; proper cuff size critical for accurate measurement
• Place animal in lateral or sternal recumbency or allow to stand in a calm environment. Place artery arrow marker on the cuff on the palmar aspect of the metacarpal region (or proximal to the carpus with arrow pointed medially), over the craniomedial metatarsal region (or proximal to the tarsus) or on the ventral aspect of the tail in a snug position. Cuff inflates and deflates automatically with blood pressure (systolic, diastolic, and mean); heart rate is automatically calculated and digitally displayed.

Doppler Technique
• Ultrasonic Doppler flow detector (Parks Medical Electronics; Silogic; SDI; Thames Medical) • Uses ultrasound waves to detect and audibilize blood flow in an artery distal to the blood pressure cuff • Apply pneumatic cuff in snug position. Distal to the cuff, place the transducer probe crystal over moistened skin, just proximal to the large carpal pad (common digital branch of the radial artery),

in a bed of ultrasound gel, and tape or hold in place. Inflate cuff bladder to suprasystemic pressure until the audible signal is cut off. Deflate cuff at approximately 3 mm Hg/sec. Return of the Doppler signal determines systolic blood pressure. Mark diastolic pressure (not as easy to detect) when Doppler signal pitch changes abruptly or disappears. Doppler technique also detects blood pressure on the ventral aspect of the proximal tail and over the craniomedial aspect of the tarsus.

Blood Pressure Guidelines for Dogs and Cats
Hypertension is currently defined by most investigators as the following:
• Dog: systolic > 180 mm Hg; diastolic > 100 mm Hg • Cat: systolic > 170–180 mm Hg; diastolic > 120 mm Hg
• Average a series of 3–5 measurements for the most reliable measurement. Interpret all results in light of the animal's excitement level during the procedure and repeat if results are questionable.

PATHOLOGIC FINDINGS
• Arteriolar hypertrophy, tunica media vasorum hyperplasia, and destruction of the internal elastic lamina layer; vascular damage in the eye, kidney, and cardiovascular and nervous system tissues leads to hemorrhage, thrombosis, edema, and necrosis.
• Ventricular hypertrophy develops in response to an increased workload.

TREATMENT

APPROPRIATE HEALTH CARE
Hospitalization may be stressful to the patient; make every attempt to manage them as outpatients. Inpatient care may be necessary depending upon the underlying condition (e.g., fluid therapy in a cat with renal failure) or serious complications related to hypertension (e.g., neurologic signs).

DIET
Influenced by underlying cause; sodium restriction generally advised, although unlikely to lower blood pressure when used alone

CLIENT EDUCATION
• Unless underlying cause is curable (e.g., hyperthyroidism) or controllable (e.g., hyperadrenocorticism), patient is likely to be on antihypertensive medication indefinitely.
• Alert owners to end-organ effects of uncontrolled hypertension (e.g., retinal hemorrhage, retinal detachment, progressive renal impairment, cardiac disease, neurologic signs).

SURGICAL CONSIDERATIONS
Dictated by underlying cause; may be indicated for hyperthyroidism, pheochromocytoma, some forms of hyperadrenocorticism

MEDICATIONS

DRUG(S) OF CHOICE
Preferred Therapy
• Treat underlying cause. • Cats—calcium channel blocker (i.e., amlodipine) or ACE inhibitor (i.e., benazepril) and sodium-restricted diet • Dogs—calcium channel blocker (i.e., amlodipine) or ACE inhibitor (e.g., enalapril or benazepril) and sodium-restricted diet • β-Blocker or α-adrenergic blocker if no response to ACE inhibitor or calcium channel blocker

ACE Inhibitors
• Lower peripheral vascular resistance and stroke volume by blocking the conversion of angiotensin I to angiotensin II • Enalapril—dogs, 0.5 mg/kg PO q12–24h; cats, 0.25–0.5 mg/kg PO q12–48h • Benazepril—dogs and cats, 0.25–1.0 mg/kg PO q24h

Calcium Channel Blockers
• Lower peripheral vascular resistance by vasodilation; some lower cardiac output through negative chronotropic and inotropic effects. • Amlodipine—dogs, 0.2–0.4 mg/kg q24h (anecdotal); cats, 0.18–0.3 mg/kg PO q24h • Diltiazem: dogs, 0.5–1.5 mg/kg PO q8h; cats, 1.5–2.5 mg/kg PO q8h; diltiazem-CD: cats, 10 mg/kg PO q24h

CONTRAINDICATIONS
• β-Blockers might worsen bronchiolar disease, CHF; do not use in patients with second- and third-degree AV blocks.
• Diltiazem—use with caution in patients with CHF and do not use in patients with second- or third-degree AV block.

PRECAUTIONS
Diuretics might induce hypokalemia and metabolic alkalosis; arterial vasodilators can cause reflex tachycardia; any treatment can cause hypotension.

POSSIBLE INTERACTIONS
Combinations of drugs may increase risk of hypotension.

ALTERNATIVE DRUG(S)
β-Adrenergic Blockers
• Lower heart rate and cardiac output and suppress renin secretion • Propranolol—dogs, 0.2–1.0 mg/kg PO q8h; cats, 2.5–5 mg/cat PO q8–12h • Atenolol—dogs, 0.25–1 mg/kg PO q12–24h PO; cats, 6.25–12.5 mg/cat PO q12–24h

Vasodilators
• Lower peripheral vascular resistance by direct action on arteriole smooth muscle
• Hydralazine HCl—dogs, 0.5–3 mg/kg PO q12h; cats, 0.5–0.8 mg/kg PO q12h
• Phenoxybenzamine—cats, 2.5–7.5 mg/cat q8–12h

FOLLOW-UP

PATIENT MONITORING
• Blood pressure and hypertensive complications (especially retinopathy) checked weekly until blood pressure is controlled • Laboratory tests to measure side effects of medications and clinical disease response (e.g., proteinuria, hematuria, anemia, thrombocytopenia, potassium balance, sodium balance, azotemia, albumin)

POSSIBLE COMPLICATIONS
• CHF • Glomerulonephropathy (proteinuria, hematuria) • Renal failure
• Retinopathy (hemorrhage, detached retina)
• Cerebral vascular accident (various central nervous system signs)

EXPECTED COURSE AND PROGNOSIS
Dictated by underlying cause; in most patients can be controlled with appropriate therapy

MISCELLANEOUS

AGE-RELATED FACTORS
Renal failure and hyperthyroidism—more common in older animals

SYNONYMS
High blood pressure

SEE ALSO
• Diabetes Mellitus, Uncomplicated
• Glomerulonephritis • Hyperadrenocorticism
• Hyperthyroidism • Pheochromocytoma
• Renal Failure, Acute • Renal Failure, Chronic

ABBREVIATIONS
• ACE = angiotensin-converting enzyme
• CHF = congestive heart failure

Suggested Reading
Kobayashi DL, Peterson ME, Graves TK, et al. Hypertension in cats with chronic renal failure or hyperthyroidism. J Vet Intern Med 1990;4:58–62.
Littman MP. Spontaneous systemic hypertension in 24 cats. J Vet Intern Med 1994;8:79–86.
Maggio F, DeFrancesco T, Atkins C, et al. Ocular lesions associated with systemic hypertension in cats: 69 cases (1985–1998). J Am Med Assoc 2000;695–702.
Snyder PS. Amlodipine: a randomized, blinded clinical trial in 9 cats with systemic hypertension. J Vet Intern Med 1998;12(3):157–162.
Snyder PS. Canine hypertensive disease. Compend Cont Ed Pract Vet 1991;13:1785–1793.
Author Patti S. Snyder
Consulting Editors Larry P. Tilley and Francis W. K. Smith, Jr.

HYPERTHYROIDISM

 BASICS

DEFINITION
A pathologic, sustained, high overall metabolism caused by high circulating concentrations of thyroid hormones

PATHOPHYSIOLOGY
• Hyperthyroidism in cats is most often caused by autonomously hyperfunctioning nodules of the thyroid gland that secrete T_4 and T_3, uncontrolled by normal physiologic influences (e.g., TSH secretion); one or both lobes of the thyroid gland can be affected.
• Rare cases of feline hyperthyroidism (1–2%) are caused by hyperfunctioning thyroid carcinoma.
• Extremely uncommon in dogs, it has been seen in some dogs with thyroid carcinoma (most dogs with thyroid gland neoplasia are euthyroid) and in dogs with oversupplementation of exogenous thyroid hormone.

SYSTEMS AFFECTED
• Musculoskeletal—cachexia
• Cardiovascular—myocardial hypertrophy and hypertension
• Gastrointestinal—chronic cellular malnutrition, decreased gastrointestinal transit time, malabsorption, and hepatocellular damage
• Renal/urologic—high GFR may mask underlying chronic renal failure, possible hyperfiltration injury, and decreased urine-concentrating ability
• Nervous
• Behavioral

GENETICS
No known genetic predisposition

INCIDENCE/PREVALENCE
• Most common endocrine disease of cats; one of the most common diseases in late middle-aged and old cats; true incidence is unknown, but diagnosis of the disease is increasing.
• Rare in dogs

GEOGRAPHIC DISTRIBUTION
N/A

SIGNALMENT

Species
Cats and (rarely) dogs

Breed Predilections
None

Mean Age and Range
Mean age in cats, approximately 13 years; range 4–22 years

Predominant Sex
None

SIGNS

General Comments
• Multisystemic; reflect the overall increase in metabolism
• Less than 10% of patients are referred to as "apathetic"; these patients exhibit atypical signs (e.g. poor appetite, anorexia, depression, and weakness).

Historical Findings
• Weight loss
• Polyphagia
• Vomiting
• Diarrhea
• Polydipsia
• Tachypnea
• Hyperactivity
• Dyspnea
• Aggression

Physical Examination Findings
• Large thyroid gland—70% of patients are affected bilaterally
• Poor body condition
• Heart murmur
• Tachycardia
• Gallop rhythm
• Unkempt appearance
• Thickened nails

CAUSES
• Cats—Autonomously hyperfunctioning nodules; rarely, thyroid carcinoma
• Dogs—T_4 or T_3 secretion by a thyroid carcinoma

RISK FACTORS
Unknown

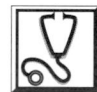 DIAGNOSIS

DIFFERENTIAL DIAGNOSIS
The clinical signs of feline hyperthyroidism can overlap with those of chronic renal failure, chronic hepatic disease, and neoplasia (especially intestinal lymphoma); they can be excluded on the basis of routine laboratory findings and thyroid function tests.

CBC/BIOCHEMISTRY/URINALYSIS
• Erythrocytosis (mild) and, less commonly, leukocytosis, lymphopenia, and eosinopenia—stress response associated with high T_3 and T_4
• High ALT activity—common
• High ALP, LDH, AST, BUN, creatinine, glucose, phosphorus, and bilirubin—less common; caused by more severe complications of hyperthyroidism

OTHER LABORATORY TESTS
• Serum total T_4 concentration (TT_4)—measures for protein-bound and free (unbound) T_4; high resting concentration confirms the diagnosis of hyperthyroidism
• Serum total T_3 concentration—high concentration less reliable than serum TT_4
• Free T_4 (FT_4) by equilibrium dialysis—useful to diagnose mild or early hyperthyroidism in cats, which may have normal resting serum TT_4 concentrations
• In theory, FT_4 more accurately reflects true thyroid gland secretory status, but some cats with nonthyroidal illness exhibit unexplained elevations in FT_4; do not use FT_4 alone as a first-line screening test.
• T_3 suppression test—useful to diagnose mild hyperthyroidism (see Appendix for protocol and interpretation)
• TRH stimulation test—useful to diagnose mild hyperthyroidism (see Appendix for protocol and interpretation)

IMAGING
• Thoracic radiography and echocardiography may be useful in assessing the severity of myocardial disease.
• Dogs—do thoracic radiography to detect pulmonary metastasis.
• Cats—abdominal ultrasound may be useful to explore underlying renal disease.

DIAGNOSTIC PROCEDURES
• Treatment of hyperthyroidism can significantly decrease renal function; pursue any abnormal value revealed by CBC, serum biochemical testing, or urinalysis by bacterial culture of the urine, abdominal radiography, and ultrasonography of the urinary tract.
• Can measure GFR by plasma disappearance of iohexol or appropriate radiopharmaceuticals (if available) in cats with suspected underlying renal disease
• Noninvasive blood pressure measurement may be useful in complete pretreatment assessment and monitoring or therapy.

PATHOLOGIC FINDINGS
• Adenomatous hyperplasia of one or both lobes of the thyroid gland
• Carcinoma in dogs and 1–2% of cats

 TREATMENT

APPROPRIATE HEALTH CARE
• Outpatient management usually suffices for cats, if antithyroid drugs are used.
• Radioiodine treatment and surgical thyroidectomy require inpatient treatment and monitoring.
• Rare cases of overt congestive heart failure require emergency inpatient intensive care.

NURSING CARE
N/A

ACTIVITY
No alterations recommended

DIET
• Resolution of thyrotoxicosis obviates the need for modifications.
• Poor absorption of many nutrients and high metabolism suggest the need for a highly digestible diet with high bioavailability of protein in untreated hyperthyroidism.

CLIENT EDUCATION
• Inform clients of adverse effects of antithyroid drugs (see below) and surgical complications.
• Clients should be aware of possible (rare) recurrence after treatment.

SURGICAL CONSIDERATIONS
• Surgical thyroidectomy is one recommended treatment for hyperthyroidism in cats.
• Surgical treatment of thyroid carcinoma (dogs and cats) is usually not curative, but can be palliative.

 MEDICATIONS

DRUG(S) OF CHOICE
• Methimazole (Tapazole) is most often recommended (10–15 mg/day divided q8–12h).
• β-Adrenergic blocking drugs—sometimes used to treat some of the cardiovascular and neurologic effects of excess thyroid hormone; can be used in combination with methimazole; mainly used to prepare the patient for surgical thyroidectomy or radioiodine therapy
• Radioiodine is a safe and effective treatment; availability of veterinary facilities offering this treatment is limited but increasing.

CONTRAINDICATIONS
N/A

PRECAUTIONS
• Antithyroid drugs have several side effects.
• Anorexia and vomiting are common side effects of methimazole; rare side effects include self-induced excoriation of the face, thrombocytopenia, bleeding diathesis, agranulocytosis, serum antinuclear antibodies, and hepatopathy.
• Side effects usually develop within the first 3 months of treatment and may or may not necessitate drug cessation and alternative treatment (depending on severity).
• Bleeding, jaundice, and agranulocytosis necessitate immediate withdrawal of the drug.

POSSIBLE INTERACTIONS
N/A

ALTERNATIVE DRUG(S)
• Carbimazole—another useful antithyroid drug; not available in the United States
• Propylthiouracil—can be useful if methimazole is unavailable; adverse effects may be more common and more severe than with methimazole.
• Ipodate—a radiographic contrast agent; can be used to treat some cases of mild hyperthyroidism, but not effective in most hyperthyroid patients; long-term effectiveness has not been established.

 FOLLOW-UP

PATIENT MONITORING
• Methimazole—physical examination, CBC (with platelet count), serum biochemical analysis, and serum T_4 determination every 2–3 weeks for the initial 3 months of treatment; adjust the dosage to maintain serum T_4 concentration in the low-normal range
• Surgical thyroidectomy—watch for development of hypocalcemia and/or laryngeal paralysis during the initial postoperative period; measure serum T_4 concentrations in the first week of surgery and every 3–6 months thereafter to check for recurrence
• Radioiodine—measure serum T_4 concentrations 2 weeks after treatment and every 3–6 months subsequently.
• Renal function—GFR declines following treatment in most patients; therefore, perform a physical examination, serum biochemistry, and urinalysis 1 month after treatment and then as indicated by the clinical history.

PREVENTION/AVOIDANCE
N/A

POSSIBLE COMPLICATIONS
• Untreated disease can lead to congestive heart failure, intractable diarrhea, renal damage, retinal detachment (as a result of hypertension), and death.
• Complications of surgical treatment include hypoparathyroidism, hypothyroidism, and laryngeal paralysis.
• Hypothyroidism is rare following radioiodine therapy

EXPECTED COURSE AND PROGNOSIS
• Uncomplicated disease—prognosis is excellent; recurrence is possible and is most commonly associated with poor owner compliance with medical management; regrowth of hyperthyroid tissue is possible but uncommon after surgical thyroidectomy or radioiodine treatment.
• Dogs or cats with thyroid carcinoma—prognosis is poor; treatment with radioiodine, surgery, or both is usually followed by recurrence of disease; adjuvant chemotherapy is of questionable benefit.

 MISCELLANEOUS

ASSOCIATED CONDITIONS
• In cats with underlying renal disease (either secondary to chronic hypertension or unrelated to thyroid disease), the prognosis is less favorable.
• Renal insufficiency may not become apparent until euthyroidism has been established; for this reason, a reversible form of treatment (i.e., antithyroid drugs) is recommended if renal disease is suspected in a cat with hyperthyroidism.
• In some patients, hyperthyroidism might be best left untreated.

AGE-RELATED FACTORS
N/A

ZOONOTIC POTENTIAL
N/A

PREGNANCY
N/A

SYNONYMS
• Thyrotoxicosis
• Multinodular toxic goiter
• Plummer's disease

SEE ALSO
• Cardiomyopathy, Hypertrophic—Cats
• Congestive Heart Failure, Left-sided
• Hypertension, Systemic
• Hypoparathyroidism

ABBREVIATIONS
• ALP = alkaline phosphatase
• AST = aspartate transaminase
• BUN = blood urea nitrogen
• CBC = complete blood count
• FT_4 = free thyroxine
• GFR = glomerular filtration rate
• LDH = lactate dehydrogenase
• T_3 = triiodothyronine
• T_4 = thyroxine
• TRH = thyrotropin-releasing hormone
• TSH = thyrotropin
• TT_4 = total thyroxine

Suggested Reading

Graves TK, Peterson ME. Occult hyperthyroidism in cats. In: Kirk RW, Bonagura JD, eds. Current veterinary therapy XI. Philadelphia: Saunders, 1992:334–337

Graves TK. Complications of treatment and concurrent illness associated with feline hyperthyroidism. In: Kirk RW, Bonagura JD, eds. Current veterinary therapy XII. Philadelphia: Saunders, 1995:

Graves TK. Hyperthyroidism and the kidney. In August JR, ed. Consultations in feline internal medicine 3, Philadelphia: Saunders, 1997:

Author Thomas K. Graves
Consulting Editor Deborah S. Greco

HYPERTROPHIC OSTEODYSTROPHY

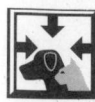 BASICS

DEFINITION
An inflammatory disease of bone that affects rapidly growing puppies

PATHOPHYSIOLOGY
• Characterized by nonseptic suppurative inflammation within metaphyseal trabeculae of long bones
• Rapidly growing bones more severely affected
• Metaphyses—widened owing to perimetaphyseal swelling and bone deposition
• Trabecular microfracture and metaphyseal separation—occur adjacent and parallel to the physis
• Bone formation defective
• Ossifying periostitis—may be extensive

SYSTEMS AFFECTED
• Musculoskeletal—symmetrical distribution; distal forelimbs most severely affected; may note soft tissue mineralization in other organs; widened costochondral junctions
• Respiratory—interstitial pneumonia
• Gastrointestinal—diarrhea

GENETICS
No basis

INCIDENCE/PREVALENCE
Low

GEOGRAPHIC DISTRIBUTION
N/A

SIGNALMENT

Species
Dogs

Breed Predilections
• Large, rapidly growing breeds
• Great Danes—most common
• Reported—Irish wolfhounds; St. Bernards; Kuvasz; Irish setters; Weimaraners; Doberman pinschers; German shepherds; Labrador retrievers; many others

Mean Age and Range
• Affects only growing puppies
• Mean—3–4 months
• Range of onset—2–8 months

Predominant Sex
Males more than females

SIGNS

General Comments
Lameness—may be episodic; degree varies from mild to non–weight-bearing; initial episode may resolve without relapse.

Historical Findings
• Depend on severity of the episode
• Owners often describe a depressed puppy that is reluctant to move.
• Inappetence—common

Physical Examination Findings
• Lameness—symmetrical, more severe in forelimbs
• Metaphyses—painful; warm; swollen
• Pyrexia—as high as 41.1°C (106°F)
• Inappetence
• Depression
• Weight loss
• Dehydration
• Diarrhea
• Cachexia
• Debilitation
• Manifestations of systemic illness—respiratory or gastrointestinal

CAUSES
Unknown; the following hypotheses have been proposed.

Metabolic
• Hypovitaminosis C—discounted; many patients have normal ascorbic acid values; supplementation does not resolve disease or prevent relapses; dogs synthesize their own vitamin C; histologic changes differ from those of disease.
• Hypocuprosis—produces histologic changes in rats similar to those seen in affected puppies; does not cause similar changes in dogs

Nutritional
• Overnutrition and oversupplementation—association inconsistent at best
• Only one or two affected puppies within a litter; however, all receive the same diet and supplementation.
• Has occurred in puppies that were not over-fed or oversupplemented
• Correcting diet does not alter the course of the disease or eliminate relapses.

Infectious
• Bacterial or fungal organisms—not identified histopathologically in tissues from affected puppies
• Unable to transmit the disease hematogenously from affected to unaffected puppies
• Canine distemper virus RNA—detected in bone cells of patients; unaffected dogs injected with blood from patients developed distemper (3 of 7 dogs) but not hypertrophic osteodystrophy.
• Secondary development may depend on the timing of the neonate's exposure.

RISK FACTORS
None proven

 DIAGNOSIS

DIFFERENTIAL DIAGNOSIS
• Juvenile bone and joint disorders
• Panosteitis—no metaphyseal swelling; cottony intramedullary densities in long bones on radiographs

• Elbow dysplasia—no metaphyseal swelling; no fever; pain localized to the elbow(s); typical radiographic signs
• Osteochondritis dissecans—no metaphyseal swelling or fever; pain localized to shoulder or elbow; subchondral defects on radiographs
• Septic polyarthritis—swelling more localized to joint capsule; soft tissue swelling localized to the joint on radiographs; septic suppurative inflammation on arthrocentesis; culture
• Nonseptic polyarthritis—nonseptic suppurative inflammation on arthrocentesis; direct diagnostics toward other causes (e.g., *Ehrlichia canis*)
• Septic metaphysitis—radiographs of the extremities not typical of hypertrophic osteodystrophy; asymmetrical; may note septic suppurative inflammation on needle aspiration of metaphyseal lesions; hematologic findings implicate bacterial infection (neutrophilia with accompanying left shift).
• Retained cartilage cores—young large and giant breeds; valgus deformity of the distal forelimbs caused by retained cartilage core in the distal ulnar physes; retained cartilage on radiographs; afebrile; less perimetaphyseal swelling; less or no pain with manipulation
• Canine osteochondrodysplasias—developmental disorders; various breeds; cartilage abnormalities and abnormal bone growth result in limb shortening and bowing deformities of the distal limbs; afebrile; nonpainful; heritable

CBC/BIOCHEMISTRY/URINALYSIS
• Do not contribute to diagnosis
• Stress leukogram
• Normal serum parameters
• Hypocalcemia uncommon

OTHER LABORATORY TESTS
N/A

IMAGING
• Distal extremity radiographs—irregular radiolucent zones within metaphyses, parallel and adjacent to physes; flared metaphyses; extraperiosteal new bone extending up the diaphyses; mineralization of perimetaphyseal soft tissues; asynchronous growth in paired bones; cranial bowing; valgus deformity
• Vertebrae and mandible—rarely affected
• Thoracic radiographs—may reveal interstitial infiltrates

DIAGNOSTIC PROCEDURES
N/A

PATHOLOGIC FINDINGS
• Distal metaphyses of the radius and ulna—most severe changes; similar abnormalities in all long bones
• Gross—wide metaphyses; peripheral mineralization; soft tissue swelling

Histologic
• Nonseptic suppurative inflammation of the metaphysis (osteochondritis), especially adjacent to growth plates
• Necrosis and probable secondary failure of osseous tissue deposition onto the calcified cartilage lattice of the primary spongiosa
• Trabecular microfractures and impaction
• Defective bone formation—thought to be secondary to osteochondral complex inflammation
• Mineralization of perimetaphyseal soft tissues and soft tissues in other regions of the body
• Interstitial pneumonia

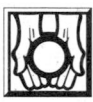 TREATMENT

APPROPRIATE HEALTH CARE
• None specific
• Supportive—from none to intensive care for severely affected puppies
• Depends on the severity of the episode, pyrexia, and the patient's ability to maintain normal hydration and willingness to eat

NURSING CARE
• Some patients will not stand or move—prone to develop pressure sores; turn every 2–4 hr to prevent sores and hypostatic congestion of the dependent lung
• Intravenous fluid therapy—for dehydration; maintenance fluid thereafter

ACTIVITY
• Restricted—running and jumping may exacerbate metaphyseal injury and result in further inflammation.
• Confine to a small well-padded area—recommended
• Leash walking only

DIET
• Normal commercial puppy ration
• Avoid supplements

CLIENT EDUCATION
• Warn the client of the disease's relapsing nature.
• Inform client that bony deformities will remodel to some degree with time but that bowing and valgus deformations are permanent.
• Warn client that the more severe the disease, the more severe the bowing deformity.

SURGICAL CONSIDERATIONS
• Generally none
• Consider surgical methods of alimentation (pharyngostomy tube, esophagostomy tube,

gastrostomy tube)—debilitated puppies that will not eat or drink and have frequently relapsing episodes of acute clinical signs

 MEDICATIONS

DRUG(S) OF CHOICE
• Antiinflammatory drugs—for pain and antipyretic effects; may try aspirin (10 mg/kg PO q12h), carprofen (1–2 mg/kg IM or PO q12h), or etodalac (10–15 mg/kg PO q24h)
• Prednisone—0.5–1.0 mg/kg PO q24h); only when there is no response to NSAIDs

CONTRAINDICATIONS
Vitamin C—may be contraindicated; may accelerate dystrophic calcification and decrease bone remodeling

PRECAUTIONS
• Avoid immunosuppressive drugs if an infectious cause is proven or if secondary infection is seen.
• NSAIDs—may cause gastric ulceration; watch for hematemesis or melena.

POSSIBLE INTERACTIONS
None

ALTERNATIVE DRUG(S)
None

 FOLLOW-UP

PATIENT MONITORING
Signs of improvement—less metaphyseal sensitivity; patient gets up; appetite improves; pyrexia resolves.

PREVENTION/AVOIDANCE
N/A

POSSIBLE COMPLICATIONS
• Cachexia
• Permanent bowing deformities
• Secondary bacterial infection
• Pressure sores
• Muscle fasciculations, seizure—with hypocalcemia
• May see secondary septicemia

EXPECTED COURSE AND PROGNOSIS
• Course—days to weeks
• Most patients—one or two episodes and recover
• Some patients—seem to have intractable relapsing episodes of pain and pyrexia; rarely die or are euthanized

• Prognosis—usually good; guarded with multiple relapses or complicating secondary problems
• Persistent bowing deformity—eliminates many purebred puppies from the show ring

 MISCELLANEOUS

ASSOCIATED CONDITIONS
Craniomandibular osteopathy—may be associated with mineralization of soft tissues (ossifying periostitis) around long bones; similar to hypertrophic osteodystrophy; may result in lameness

AGE-RELATED FACTORS
None

ZOONOTIC POTENTIAL
None

PREGNANCY
Occurs only in juveniles

SYNONYMS
Metaphyseal osteopathy

SEE ALSO
• Elbow Dysplasia
• Osteochondrosis
• Panosteitis

Suggested Reading
Abeles V, Harrus S, Amgles JM. Hypertrophic osteodystrophy in six Weimaraner puppies associated with systemic signs. Vet Rec 1999;145(5):130–134.
Bellah JR. Hypertrophic osteodystrophy. In: Bojrab MJ, ed. Disease mechanisms in small animal surgery. 2nd ed. Philadelphia: Lea & Febiger, 1993:858–864.
Lenehan TM, Fetter AW. Hypertrophic osteodystrophy. In: Newton CD, Nunamaker DM, eds. Textbook of small animal orthopedics. Philadelphia: Lippincott, 1985:597–601.
Mee AP, Gordon MT, May C, et al. Canine virus transcripts detected in the bone cells of dogs with metaphyseal osteopathy. Bone 1993;14:59–67.
Schulz KS, Payne JT, Aronson E. *Escherichia coli* bacteremia associated with hypertrophic osteodystrophy in a dog. JAVMA 1991;199:1170–1173.
Author Jamie R. Bellah
Consulting Editor Peter K. Shires

HYPERTROPHIC OSTEOPATHY

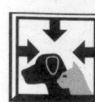

BASICS

OVERVIEW
• Results in increased peripheral blood flow and periosteal new bone proliferation along the diaphyseal region of long bones, often beginning in the distal phalanges, meta-carpals, and metatarsals
• Pathogenesis—speculative; theories: chronic anoxia, obscure toxins, hyperestrogenism, and autonomic neurovascular reflex mechanisms mediated by afferent branches of the vagus or intercostal nerves
• Considered a manifestation of a primary disease process
• Affects the musculoskeletal system

SIGNALMENT
• More common in dogs than cats
• Age of highest frequency—8 years; coincides with the peak incidence of pulmonary neo-plasms
• Mean age—5.6 years for dogs with nonneo-plastic lung lesions
• Large-breed dogs—12 years of age with embryonal rhabdomyosarcoma

SIGNS

Historical Findings
• Listlessness
• Reluctance to move
• Enlargement of the distal portion of the extremities

Physical Examination Findings
• Lame, sore, and painful limbs
• Extremities—enlarged and firm to the touch; not edematous
• Swelling—predominantly below level of elbow and stifle joints, extending distally to toes

CAUSES & RISK FACTORS
• Primary and metastatic lung tumors
• Nonneoplastic thoracic conditions—pneumonia; heartworm disease; congenital or acquired heart disease; bronchial foreign bodies; *Spirocerca lupi* infestation of esophagus; focal lung atelectasis
• Esophageal sarcoma
• Embryonal rhabdomyosarcoma of the urinary bladder
• Adenocarcinoma of the liver or prostate gland
• Thoracic and abdominal mesotheliomas

DIAGNOSIS

DIFFERENTIAL DIAGNOSIS
• Osteomyelitis—not symmetrical and generally edematous; lysis; history of penetrating trauma or systemic infection
• Metastatic neoplasia—not symmetrical

CBC/BIOCHEMISTRY/URINALYSIS
• Depend on the underlying cause
• Serum ALP—may be elevated

OTHER LABORATORY TESTS
Ultrasound—help identify and differentiate primary lesions

IMAGING
• Radiographs of affected long bones—bilaterally symmetric extensive, rough, periosteal new bone formation on diaphyseal regions; buds project outward from the cortex and perpendicular to the long axis; periosteal new bone forms around the entire circumference of the bone; joints not affected
• Radiographs of the thoracic and abdominal cavities—indicated; identify underlying cause

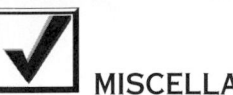
DIAGNOSTIC PROCEDURES
Bone biopsy and culture (bacterial and fungal)—necessary only in atypical cases; rule out neoplasia and osteomyelitis

TREATMENT
• Directed at underlying primary cause
• Options in selected cases—unilateral vagotomy on the side of a lung lesion; incising through parietal pleura; subperiosteal rib resection; bilateral cervical vagotomy

MEDICATIONS

DRUG(S)
• Depend on underlying cause
• Glucocorticoids (e.g., prednisone)—may be used to improve clinical signs and reduce the extent of swelling
• Analgesics—as needed

CONTRAINDICATIONS/POSSIBLE INTERACTIONS
N/A

FOLLOW-UP

PATIENT MONITORING
• Condition indicates other disease processes—important to recognize need for further diagnostic tests to identify the primary cause
• Removal of the inciting cause—may bring about regression of clinical signs

EXPECTED COURSE AND PROGNOSIS
• Bony changes—may take several months to regress
• Prognosis—guarded to poor owing to the common occurrence of neoplastic causes

MISCELLANEOUS

SYNONYMS
• Hypertrophic pulmonary osteopathy (HPO)
• Hypertrophic pulmonary osteoarthropathy (HPOA)
• Hypertrophic osteoarthropathy (HOA)

ABBREVIATION
ALP = alkaline phosphatase

Suggested Reading
Halliwell WH. Tumorlike lesions of bone. In: Bojrab MJ, ed. Disease mechanisms in small animal surgery. Philadelphia: Lea & Febiger, 1993:933–934.
Author Peter D. Schwarz
Consulting Editor Peter K. Shires

HYPERTROPHIC PYLORIC GASTROPATHY, CHRONIC

 BASICS

DEFINITION
Pyloric stenosis or chronic hypertrophic pyloric gastropathy is an obstructive narrowing of the pyloric canal resulting from varying degrees of muscular hypertrophy or mucosal hyperplasia.

PATHOPHYSIOLOGY
• Can result from a congenital lesion composed primarily of hypertrophy of the smooth muscle or be one of three types of acquired form—primarily circular muscle hypertrophy (type 1), a combination of muscular hypertrophy and mucosal hyperplasia (type 2), or primarily mucosal hyperplasia (type 3)
• The cause is unknown; proposed factors include increased gastrin levels (which have a trophic effect on the muscle and mucosa) or changes in the myenteric plexus that lead to chronic antral distension and its associated effects.

SYSTEMS AFFECTED
• Gastrointestinal—chronic intermittent vomiting
• Musculoskeletal—weight loss
• Respiratory—possible aspiration pneumonia

GENETICS
Inheritance pattern unknown

INCIDENCE/PREVALENCE
Uncommon

GEOGRAPHIC DISTRIBUTION
N/A

SIGNALMENT
Species
• More common in dogs
• Rare in cats

Breed Predilections
• Congenital—brachycephalic breeds (boxer, Boston terrier, bulldog); Siamese cats
• Acquired—Lhasa apso, shih tzu, Pekingese, poodle

Mean Age and Range
• Congenital—shortly after weaning and up to 1 year of age
• Acquired—9.8 years of age

Predominant Sex
Twice as many males as females

SIGNS
General Comments
• Clinical signs are related to the degree of pyloric narrowing.
• Projectile vomiting is generally not a presenting complaint. Animals are well fleshed.

Historical Findings
• Chronic intermittent vomiting of undigested or partially digested food (rarely containing bile) often several hours after eating
• Congenital lesions begin to produce clinical signs shortly after weaning.
• Frequency of vomiting increases with time.
• Lack of response to antiemetics or motility agents
• Occasional anorexia with weight loss

Physical Examination Findings
Most dogs are generally in good physical condition.

CAUSES
• Congenital or acquired
• May be influenced by infiltrative mural diseases
• Chronic elevations in gastrin levels
• Neuroendocrine factors may play a role.

RISK FACTORS
Chronic stress, inflammatory disorders, chronic gastritis, gastric ulcers, and genetic predispositions influence the disease process in humans and may play a role in small animals.

 DIAGNOSIS

DIFFERENTIAL DIAGNOSIS
• Gastric neoplasia
• Gastric foreign body
• Granulomatous fungal disease (e.g., pythiosis)
• Eosinophilic granuloma
• Motility disorders
• Cranial abdominal mass—pancreatic or duodenal

CBC/BIOCHEMISTRY/URINALYSIS
• Findings vary, depending on the degree and chronicity of obstruction.
• Hypochloremic metabolic alkalosis (characteristic of pyloric outflow obstruction) or metabolic acidosis (or mixed acid–base imbalance)
• Hypokalemia
• Anemia—if concurrent gastrointestinal (GI) ulceration
• Prerenal azotemia—if dehydration present

OTHER LABORATORY TESTS
N/A

IMAGING
Abdominal Radiographs
Normal to markedly distended stomach

Upper GI Barium Contrast Study
• May display a "beak" sign created by pyloric narrowing, allowing minimal barium to pass into the pyloric antrum
• Retention of most of the barium in the stomach after 6 h indicates delayed gastric emptying.
• Intraluminal filling defects or pyloric wall thickening

Fluoroscopy
• Normal gastric contractility
• Delayed passage of barium through the pylorus

Abdominal Ultrasound
Measurable thickening of the wall of the pylorus and antrum

HYPERTROPHIC PYLORIC GASTROPATHY, CHRONIC

DIAGNOSTIC PROCEDURES

Endoscopy—allows evaluation of the mucosa for ulceration, hyperplasia, and mass lesions; specimens can be obtained for histopathologic evaluation.

PATHOLOGIC FINDINGS

• Include focal to multifocal mucosal polyps, diffuse mucosal thickening, and pyloric wall-thickening, with variable degree of pyloric narrowing
• Changes range from hypertrophy of the circular smooth muscle to hyperplasia of the mucosa and associated glandular structures; a wide spectrum of inflammatory cell infiltration exists.

 TREATMENT

APPROPRIATE HEALTH CARE

• Depends on severity of clinical signs
• Patients should be evaluated and surgery scheduled at the earliest convenience.

NURSING CARE

• Appropriate parenteral fluids to correct any electrolyte imbalances and metabolic alkalosis or acidosis
• Isotonic saline (with potassium supplementation) is the fluid of choice for hypochloremic metabolic alkalosis.
• Consideration of postoperative nutritional support is important.
• In severe cases treated with gastroduodenostomy or gastrojejunostomy, surgical placement of a jejunostomy tube for enteral nutrition may be advantageous.

ACTIVITY

Restrict

DIET

Highly digestible, low-fat—until surgical intervention is feasible

CLIENT EDUCATION

• Surgical treatment is highly successful.
• If clinical signs recur postoperatively, more-aggressive surgical procedures may be indicated.

SURGICAL CONSIDERATIONS

• Surgical intervention is the treatment of choice.
• Goals involve establishing a diagnosis with histopathologic samples, excising abnormal tissue, and restoring GI function with the least-invasive procedure.
• Surgical procedures depend on the extent of obstruction—pyloromyotomy (Fredet-Ramstedt), pyloroplasty (Heineke-Mikulicz or antral advancement flap), gastroduodenostomy (Billroth 1), gastrojejunostomy (Billroth 2)

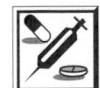 **MEDICATIONS**

DRUG(S) OF CHOICE

Antiemetics and motility modifiers are generally ineffective.

CONTRAINDICATIONS

• Evidence of complete pyloric obstruction precludes promotility drugs.
• Avoid anticholinergic agents because of their inhibitory effects on GI motility.

PRECAUTIONS

N/A

POSSIBLE INTERACTIONS

N/A

ALTERNATIVE DRUG(S)

N/A

 FOLLOW-UP

PATIENT MONITORING

Postoperatively for recurrence of clinical signs because of poor choice of surgical procedure

PREVENTION/AVOIDANCE

N/A

POSSIBLE COMPLICATIONS

Postoperative surgical complications include recurrence of clinical signs, gastric ulceration, pancreatitis, bile duct obstruction, and incisional dehiscence with peritonitis.

EXPECTED COURSE AND PROGNOSIS

• 85% of dogs show good-to-excellent results with resolution of clinical signs upon proper surgical intervention.
• Poor prognosis if gastric neoplasia (especially adenocarcinoma) is an underlying cause

 MISCELLANEOUS

ASSOCIATED CONDITIONS

Gastric ulceration

AGE-RELATED FACTORS

• Intermittent vomiting in young brachycephalic breeds upon weaning indicates congenital stenosis.
• Chronic intermittent vomiting in adult (8–10 years old) small breed dogs supports a diagnosis of an acquired pyloric hypertrophy.

ZOONOTIC POTENTIAL

None

PREGNANCY

High gastrin levels in pregnant females may predispose to development of the syndrome.

SYNONYMS

• Chronic hypertrophic antral gastropathy
• Hypertrophic gastritis
• Acquired antral pyloric hypertrophy
• Congenital pyloric stenosis

SEE ALSO

N/A

Suggested Reading

Matthiesen D. Chronic gastric outflow obstruction. In: Slatter D, ed. Textbook of small animal surgery. 2nd ed. Philadelphia: Saunders, 1993:561–571.

Stanton M. Gastric outlet obstruction. In: Bojrab MJ, ed. Disease mechanisms in small animal surgery. 2nd ed. Philadelphia: Lea & Febiger, 1993:235–236.

Authors Albert E. Jergens and James E. Williams, Jr.
Consulting Editor Albert E. Jergens

HYPERVISCOSITY SYNDROME

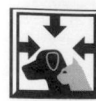 BASICS

OVERVIEW
• An assortment of clinical signs caused by high blood viscosity
• Typically results from markedly high concentration of plasma proteins, although can result (rarely) from extremely high erythrocyte count
• Most frequently seen as a paraneoplastic syndrome, often associated with multiple myeloma and other lymphoid tumors or leukemia
• Total plasma protein may exceed 10 g/dL, with serum protein electrophoresis showing monoclonal gammopathy.
• Clinical signs caused by reduced blood flow through smaller vessels, high plasma volume, and associated coagulopathy
• Systems affected include hemic/lymphatic/immune, ophthalmic, and nervous.

SIGNALMENT
• Dogs more frequently affected than cats
• No sex or breed predilections
• More common in older animals

SIGNS

Historical Findings
• No consistent signs
• Anorexia
• Lethargy
• Depression
• Polyuria and polydipsia
• Blindness, ataxia, and seizures
• Bleeding tendencies

Physical Examination Findings
• Neurologic deficits, including seizures and disorientation
• Tachycardia and tachypnea if congestive heart failure present owing to volume overload
• Epistaxis or other mucosal bleeding
• Hepatomegaly/splenomegaly/lymphadenopathy
• Visual deficits associated with engorged retinal vessels, retinal hemorrhage or detachment, and papilledema

CAUSES & RISK FACTORS
• Multiple myeloma and plasma cell tumors (IgM > IgA > IgG)
• Lymphocytic leukemia or lymphoma
• Marked polycythemia (PCV > 65%)
• Chronic atypical inflammation with monoclonal gammopathy (e.g., ehrlichiosis in dogs)
• Chronic autoimmune disease (e.g., systemic lupus erythematosus and rheumatoid arthritis)

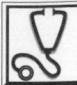 DIAGNOSIS

DIFFERENTIAL DIAGNOSIS
• Other unexplained neurologic disease or bleeding disorders
• Appropriate polycythemia (e.g., right to left cardiac shunt)
• Hyperviscosity is a syndrome, not a final diagnosis.

CBC/BIOCHEMISTRY/URINALYSIS
• Nonregenerative anemia (in patients without polycythemia as a cause of hyperviscosity), thrombocytopenia, or leukopenia
• Hyperproteinemia (total plasma protein > 9.0 g/dL) and hyperglobulinemia (> 5.0 g/dL)
• Azotemia and hypercalcemia if hyperviscosity caused by a paraneoplastic syndrome
• Isosthenuria and marked proteinuria

OTHER LABORATORY TESTS
• High concentration of IgG, IgA, or IgM, as detected by radial immunodiffusion
• High plasma or serum viscosity (> 3 relative to water)
• Prolonged prothrombin time or activated partial thromboplastin time

IMAGING
Hepatosplenomegaly, cardiomegaly, and osteolytic lesions (in association with multiple myeloma) are possible.

DIAGNOSTIC PROCEDURES
• Plasma cell or lymphoid infiltrate revealed by bone marrow biopsy
• Bence-Jones proteinuria in patients with multiple myeloma

 TREATMENT

APPROPRIATE HEALTH CARE
• Generally treat as inpatient
• Treat underlying disease
• Phlebotomy (15–20 mL/kg) with crystalloid fluid volume replacement
• Plasmapheresis (10–15 mL/kg), if available

NURSING CARE
As dictated by underlying disease

 MEDICATIONS

DRUG(S)
• Provide treatment for underlying neoplastic or inflammatory condition.
• See other topics for drug therapy for the underlying cause (e.g., plasma cell tumor, lymphocytic leukemia, lymphoma, ehrlichiosis, and polycythemia).

CONTRAINDICATIONS/POSSIBLE INTERACTIONS
• Avoid use of medications that might increase vascular volume, including synthetic colloids (e.g., hetastarch and dextran).
• Avoid medications that alter platelet function (e.g., NSAIDs).

 FOLLOW-UP
• Monitor serum or plasma proteins frequently as a marker of treatment efficacy.
• CBC, biochemistry panel, and urinalysis to monitor other laboratory abnormalities

 MISCELLANEOUS

SEE ALSO
• Ehrlichiosis
• Leukemia, Chronic Lymphocytic
• Lymphosarcoma (Lymphoma)—Cats
• Lymphosarcoma (Lymphoma)—Dogs
• Multiple Myeloma
• Plasmacytoma, Mucocutaneous
• Polycythemia

ABBREVIATION
PCV = packed cell volume

Suggested Reading
Hohenhaus AE. Syndromes of hyperglobulinemia: diagnosis and therapy. In: Kirk RW, ed. Current veterinary therapy XII. Philadelphia: Saunders, 1995:523–530.
Author Elizabeth A. Rozanski
Consulting Editor Stephen A. Kruth

HYPHEMA

BASICS

DEFINITION
Blood in the anterior chamber

PATHOPHYSIOLOGY
• Results from any condition that causes intraocular vessel damage sufficient to allow egress of erythrocytes
• Bleeding vessels—resident or acquired vessels (neovascularization); may be in the retina, vitreous (hyaloid artery or primary vitreous), choroid, ciliary body, or iris; resident: bleed as a result of trauma, inflammation, defects in hemostasis, or neoplastic infiltration; new: inherently leaky and prone to bleed spontaneously
• Most common causes of iris neovascularization—chronic retinal detachment, chronic uveitis, and intraocular neoplasia, especially lymphosarcoma
• May be the presenting sign of systemic hypertension, especially in old cats—occurs as a result of precapillary, arteriole ischemia secondary to the eye's attempt to autoregulate blood flow to maintain normal perfusion of ocular tissue
• Usually does not in itself cause any adverse secondary effects
• Secondary glaucoma—persistent bleeding; referred to as ghost cell glaucoma; occurs because the plasma membranes of aged erythrocytes lose their plasticity, predisposing the patient to plugging of the trabecular spaces

SYSTEMS AFFECTED
Ophthalmic

GENETICS
N/A

INCIDENCE/PREVALENCE
May be a presenting sign of many ocular and systemic diseases

GEOGRAPHIC DISTRIBUTION
N/A

SIGNALMENT

Species
Dogs and cats

Breed Predilections
N/A

Mean Age and Range
Any

Predominant Sex
N/A

SIGNS

General Comments
Depend on how much bleeding has occurred, whether vision is impaired, and whether there is an associated systemic disease

Historical Findings
• Extremely diverse, reflecting the multitude of causes
• History of vision loss uncommon
• Rarely bilateral and complete

Physical Examination Findings
• Blood seen within the anterior chamber of the eye; if severe, cannot see other intraocular structures
• Corneal edema—common
• Lymphosarcoma—blood often mixed with WBCs
• Secondary to trauma—often see eyelid, conjunctival, or corneal lesions
• IOP—may be elevated with long-standing duration of condition

CAUSES
• Trauma
• Chronic retinal detachment
• Uveal neoplasia—especially lymphosarcoma, hemangiosarcoma, and primary uveal melanoma
• Uveitis—especially if caused by FIP (cats) and rickettsial disease (dogs)
• Coagulopathies
• Vasculitis—immune-mediated or secondary to rickettsial diseases (e.g., Rocky mountain spotted fever, ehrlichiosis)
• Systemic hypertension—primary or secondary to renal disease; hyperthyroidism
• Parasite migration—ophthalmomyiasis interna
• Secondary to congenital ocular defects—collie eye anomaly; persistent primary vitreous; severe retinal dysplasia

RISK FACTORS
• Uveitis
• Metastatic neoplasia
• Chronic retinal detachment
• Any disease causing vasculitis or vascular fragility
• Chronic renal disease
• Coagulopathies
• Congenital ocular defects

DIAGNOSIS

DIFFERENTIAL DIAGNOSIS
• Bilateral condition—indicates systemic disease
• Unilateral condition in old dogs—suspect retinal detachment
• No conjunctival or episcleral vascular injection—suspect coagulopathy
• With retinal hemorrhage or detachment in old cats—strongly suspect systemic hypertension
• With chronic uveitis or recurrent condition—rule out intraocular neoplasia

CBC/BIOCHEMISTRY/URINALYSIS
• Usually normal with localized ocular disease
• Anemia or thrombocytopenia—may be noted with a systemic bleeding disorder

OTHER LABORATORY TESTS
• Suspected coagulopathy—special laboratory tests to assess hemostasis indicated; intrinsic coagulation (ACT and PTT); extrinsic coagulation (one-stage PT); thrombocyte and reticulocyte counts; thrombin time; fibrinogen levels; fibrinogen degradation products
• Secondary to chronic uveitis—uveitis workup indicated (see Anterior Uveitis—Dogs and Anterior Uveitis—Cats)

IMAGING
• Ocular ultrasonography—indicated when condition is severe enough to obstruct view of the intraocular structures; easily identify retinal detachment and intraocular tumors
• Thoracic radiographs and possibly abdominal ultrasound—may help rule out disseminated neoplasia

DIAGNOSTIC PROCEDURES
• Suspected bleeding disorders—bone marrow examination; buccal bleeding time
• Blood pressure measurement—indicated when condition cannot be attributed to ocular disease
• Lymph node aspiration and biopsy—indicated for suspected lymphosarcoma

PATHOLOGIC FINDINGS
Gross—anterior chamber partially or completely filled with blood

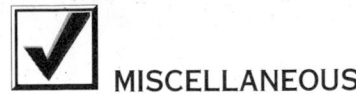
Histologic
• Erythrocytes—in a matrix of proteinaceous fluid
• RBCs—in the iridocorneal angle and trabecular spaces
• Vitreal hemorrhage
• Posterior synechiae and inflammatory cells in the anterior uvea—common with primary uveitis
• Pre-iridal fibrovascular membranes—common with primary retinal detachment or chronic uveitis

 TREATMENT

APPROPRIATE HEALTH CARE
Usually outpatient

NURSING CARE
N/A

ACTIVITY
Restricted only if caused by a clotting disorder

DIET
N/A

CLIENT EDUCATION
• Explain that hyphema is a clinical sign and not a specific disease.
• Inform client that no specific treatments for hyphema exist and that treatment is directed at eliminating the underlying cause.

SURGICAL CONSIDERATIONS
• Trauma—surgical intervention indicated to repair accompanying adnexal or corneal defects
• Secondary glaucoma caused by chronic condition—surgical procedure indicated to remove (e.g., enucleation) or possibly salvage the globe (e.g., evisceration and intrascleral prosthesis; gentamicin injection)
• Irreversibly lost vision—consider enucleation or possibly a globe salvage procedure.
• Surgical evacuation of blood from the anterior chamber—rarely indicated

 MEDICATIONS

DRUG(S) OF CHOICE
• None specific
• Topical antibiotics—not indicated unless associated with conjunctival or corneal epithelial defects (trauma)
• Topical corticosteroids—q6h; 1% prednisolone acetate or 0.1% dexamethasone; often empirically used to control uveal inflammation

• Systemic corticosteroids—usually indicated only when caused by a corticosteroid-responsive systemic disease (e.g., lymphosarcoma) or posterior segment inflammation
• Systemic hypotensive therapy—indicated if caused by hypertension
• Topical 1% atropine solution—given to effect; indicated to prevent synechia formation unless secondary glaucoma has occurred
• Dichlorphenamide—2–4 mg/kg PO q8–12h; for secondary glaucoma; may help lower IOP
• Topical 0.5% timolol (q12 h) or dipivefrin HCl (q8–12h)—may be used in place of epinephrine
• Formed clots—may be dissolved if tissue-plasminogen activator (0.1–0.2 mL, 250 μg/mL) is injected into the anterior chamber within 5–7 days of hemorrhage

CONTRAINDICATIONS
Do not treat with tissue plasminogen activator if a clot has not formed and if the cause of the bleeding has not been eliminated, because rebleeding is likely.

PRECAUTIONS
Pilocarpine—may exacerbate breakdown of the blood–aqueous barrier; may cause further bleeding

POSSIBLE INTERACTIONS
N/A

ALTERNATIVE DRUG(S)
N/A

 FOLLOW-UP

PATIENT MONITORING
• Severe disease—IOP monitored daily
• Less severe disease—examined every 2–3 days until resolution

PREVENTION/AVOIDANCE
Restricted activity if caused by a clotting disorder

POSSIBLE COMPLICATIONS
• Glaucoma
• Vision loss

EXPECTED COURSE AND PROGNOSIS
• Trauma—prognosis generally good unless irrevocable damage has occurred to the lens, ciliary body, or retina
• Secondary to retinal detachment and anterior segment neovascularization—typically will not resolve; secondary glaucoma eventually results, necessitating some type of surgical intervention to relieve pain (e.g., enucleation; evisceration with prosthesis)

MISCELLANEOUS

ASSOCIATED CONDITIONS
• Clotting disorders
• Systemic hypertension
• Uveitis
• Metastatic neoplasia—lymphosarcoma; hemangiosarcoma
• Retinal detachment
• Von Willebrand disease

AGE-RELATED FACTORS
Systemic hypertension—more common in elderly patients

ZOONOTIC POTENTIAL
N/A

PREGNANCY
N/A

SEE ALSO
• Anterior Uveitis—Cats
• Anterior Uveitis—Dogs
• Coagulation Factor Deficiency
• Hypertension, Systemic
• Red Eye

ABBREVIATIONS
• ACT = activated clotting time
• FIP = feline infectious peritonitis
• IOP = intraocular pressure
• PT = prothrombin time
• PTT = partial thromboplastin time

Suggested Reading
Collins BK, Moore CP. Diseases and surgery of the canine anterior uvea. In: Gelatt KN, ed., Veterinary ophthalmology. 3rd ed. Philadelphia: Lippincott Williams & Wilkins, 1999:755–795.
Littman MP. Spontaneous systemic hypertension in 24 cats. J Vet Intern Med 1994; 8:79–86.
Nelms S, Nasisse MP, Davidson MG, Kirschner S. Hyphema associated with retinal disease in dogs: 17 cases. J Am Vet Med Assoc 1993;202:1289–1292.
Author Mark P. Nasisse
Consulting Editor Paul E. Miller

HYPOADRENOCORTICISM (ADDISON'S DISEASE)

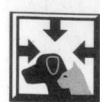 **BASICS**

DEFINITION
An endocrine disorder resulting from deficient production of glucocorticoids and/or mineralocorticoids

PATHOPHYSIOLOGY
• Mineralocorticoid (aldosterone) deficiency results in an inability to excrete potassium and retain sodium; sodium deficiency leads to diminished effective circulating volume that in turn contributes to prerenal azotemia, hypotension, dehydration, weakness, and depression.
• Hyperkalemia (along with other metabolic derangements) may result in myocardial toxicity.
• Glucocorticoid (cortisol) deficiency contributes to anorexia, vomiting, melena, lethargy, and weight loss; predisposes to hypoglycemia and results in impaired excretion of water.

SYSTEMS AFFECTED
Multiple organ systems involved; extent of involvement varies from case to case.

GENETICS
N/A

INCIDENCE/PREVALENCE
No exact figures available; considered uncommon to rare in dogs and very rare in cats

GEOGRAPHIC DISTRIBUTION
N/A

SIGNALMENT
Species
Dogs and cats

Breed Predilections
• Great Danes, rottweilers, Portuguese water dogs, standard poodles, West Highland white terriers, and wheaten terriers have increased relative risk.
• No predilection in cats

Mean Age and Range
• Dogs—range, < 1 to > 12 years; median, 4 years
• Cats—range, 1–9 years; most are middle-aged

Predominant Sex
Female dogs are at an increased relative risk; no predilection in cats.

SIGNS
General Comments
Vary from mild and few in some patients with chronic hypoadrenocorticism to severe and life-threatening in an acute addisonian crisis

Historical Findings
• Dogs—lethargy, anorexia, vomiting, weight loss, waxing/waning course, diarrhea, previous response to therapy, shaking, PU/PD
• Cats—lethargy, anorexia, vomiting, PU/PD, weight loss

Physical Examination Findings
• Dogs—depression, weakness, dehydration, collapse, hypothermia, slow CRT, melena, weak pulse, bradycardia, painful abdomen, hair loss
• Cats—dehydration, weakness, slow CRT, weak pulse, bradycardia

CAUSES
• Primary hypoadrenocorticism—idiopathic (immune-mediated), mitotane overdose, granulomatous disease, metastatic tumors
• Secondary hypoadrenocorticism—iatrogenic following withdrawal of long-term glucocorticoid administration, isolated ACTH deficiency, panhypopituitarism, nonfunctional pituitary tumor

RISK FACTORS
N/A

 DIAGNOSIS

DIFFERENTIAL DIAGNOSIS
• Signs are nonspecific and are seen in other, more common medical disorders, particularly gastrointestinal and renal diseases.
• Although no signs are pathognomonic, a waxing and waning course and previous response to nonspecific medical intervention ("fluids and steroids") should alert the clinician to consider the diagnosis.

CBC/BIOCHEMISTRY/URINALYSIS
• Hematologic abnormalities may include anemia, eosinophilia, and lymphocytosis.
• Serum biochemical findings may include hyperkalemia, azotemia, hyponatremia, hypochloremia, decreased total CO_2, hypercalcemia, increased liver enzymes, increased serum alkaline phosphatase, and hypoglycemia.
• Urinalysis often reveals impaired urine-concentrating ability.
• Some patients with hypoadrenocorticism exhibit normal electrolyte levels.

OTHER LABORATORY TESTS
• Definitive diagnosis is by demonstration of undetectable-to-low serum cortisol concentrations that fail to increase after administration of either ACTH gel IM (20 U in dogs, 10 U in cats) or synthetic ACTH IV (5 μg in dogs, 0.125 mg in cats).
• In hypovolemic dehydrated animals, use synthetic ACTH IV or delay testing until after initial fluid administration is completed.
• Determine the plasma ACTH concentration in patients with normal electrolyte levels, to differentiate primary from secondary hypoadrenocorticism; must collect sample before administering glucocorticoids.

IMAGING
Radiographs may reveal microcardia, narrowed vena cava or descending aorta, hypoperfused lung fields, and very rarely megaesophagus.

DIAGNOSTIC PROCEDURES
N/A

PATHOLOGIC FINDINGS
• Gross examination—atrophy of the adrenal glands
• Microscopically—lymphocytic-plasmacytic adrenalitis and/or adrenocortical atrophy

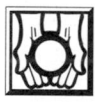 **TREATMENT**

APPROPRIATE HEALTH CARE
• An acute addisonian crisis is a medical emergency requiring intensive therapy.
• Treatment of chronic hypoadrenocorticism depends on severity of clinical signs; usually initial stabilization and therapy are conducted on an inpatient basis.

NURSING CARE
Treat acute addisonian crisis with rapid correction of hypovolemia using isotonic fluids (preferably 0.9% NaCl).

ACTIVITY
No alteration necessary

DIET
No need to alter

CLIENT EDUCATION
• Lifelong glucocorticoid and/or mineralo-corticoid replacement therapy is required.
• Increased dosages of replacement glucocorticoid are required during periods of stress such as travel, hospitalization, and surgery.

SURGICAL CONSIDERATIONS
N/A

 MEDICATIONS

DRUG(S) OF CHOICE
• Chronic primary hypoadrenocorticism—treat with glucocorticoid replacement (prednisone, 0.2 mg/kg/day) and mineralocorticoid replacement (fludrocortisone acetate, 10–20 μg/kg/day divided, adjusted by 0.05- to 0.1-mg increments on the basis of serial serum electrolyte determinations or DOCP, 2 mg/kg IM or SC every 21–30 days adjusted if needed on the basis of serum electrolyte determinations)
• Parenteral administration of a rapidly acting glucocorticoid such as dexamethasone sodium phosphate or prednisolone sodium succinate; dexamethasone sodium phosphate is preferred because prednisolone cross-reacts with cortisol assays
• Patients with confirmed secondary hypoadrenocorticism require only glucocorticoid supplementation (prednisone, 0.2 mg/kg/day).

CONTRAINDICATIONS
N/A

PRECAUTIONS
N/A

POSSIBLE INTERACTIONS
N/A

ALTERNATIVE DRUG(S)
N/A

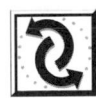 FOLLOW-UP

PATIENT MONITORING
• Adjust the daily dose of fludrocortisone by 0.05- to 0.1-mg increments as needed, based on serial serum electrolyte determinations;

following initiation of therapy, check serum electrolyte levels weekly until they stabilize in the normal range; thereafter, check serum electrolyte concentrations and BUN or creatinine monthly for the first 3–6 months and then every 3–12 months.
• In many dogs given fludrocortisone, the daily dose required to control the disorder increases incrementally, usually during the first 6–24 months of therapy; in most dogs, the final fludrocortisone dosage needed is 20–30 μg/kg/day; very few can be controlled on 10 μg/kg/day or less.
• After the first 2 injections of DOCP, ideally measure serum electrolyte levels at 2, 3, and 4 weeks to determine the duration of effect; thereafter, check electrolyte levels at the time of injection for the next 6 months (and adjust the dosage of DOCP if necessary) and then every 6–12 months.
• DOCP is usually required at 3- to 4-week intervals, but a few patients need injections every 2 weeks; alternatively, to maintain monthly injections, the dosage of DOCP can be incrementally increased; almost all hypoadrenocorticism will be well controlled on a maintenance DOCP dose of 2 mg/kg/injection.

PREVENTION/AVOIDANCE
• Continue hormonal replacement therapy for the lifetime of the patient.
• Increase the dosage of replacement glucocorticoid during periods of stress such as travel, hospitalization, and surgery.

POSSIBLE COMPLICATIONS
• PU/PD may occur from prednisone administration, necessitating decreasing or discontinuing the drug.
• PU/PD may occur from fludrocortisone administration, necessitating a change to DOCP therapy.

EXPECTED COURSE AND PROGNOSIS
Except for patients with primary hypoadrenocorticism caused by granulomatous or metastatic disease and secondary hypoadrenocorticism caused by a pituitary mass, the vast majority of patients carry a good to excellent prognosis following proper stabilization and treatment.

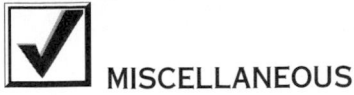 MISCELLANEOUS

ASSOCIATED CONDITIONS
Concurrent endocrine gland failure occurs in up to 5% of dogs—hypothyroidism, diabetes mellitus, and/or hypoparathyroidism

AGE-RELATED FACTORS
N/A

ZOONOTIC POTENTIAL
N/A

PREGNANCY
N/A

SYNONYMS
Addison's disease (primary hypoadrenocorticism)

SEE ALSO
• Hyperkalemia
• Hyponatremia

ABBREVIATION
PD/PU = polydipsia, polyuria

Suggested Reading

Greco DS, Peterson ME. Feline hypoadrenocorticism. In: Kirk RW, ed. Current veterinary therapy X. Philadelphia: Saunders, 1989:1042–1045.

Kintzer PP, Peterson ME. Canine hypoadrenocorticism. In: Kirk RW, Bonagura JD, eds. Current veterinary therapy XII. Philadelphia: Saunders, 1995:425–429.

Kintzer PP, Peterson ME. Primary and secondary hypoadrenocorticism. Vet Clin N Am 1997;27(2):349–358.

Peterson ME, Kintzer PP, Kass PH. Pretreatment clinical and laboratory findings in dogs with hypoadrenocorticism: 225 cases (1979–1993). J Am Vet Med Assoc 1996;208:85–91.

Author Peter P. Kintzer
Consulting Editor Deborah S. Greco

HYPOALBUMINEMIA

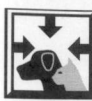 BASICS

DEFINITION
Low serum albumin concentration exists for most assays if < 2.0 g/dL

Pathophysiology
• Albumin—produced exclusively in the liver.
• Provides 75%–80% of plasma colloid oncotic pressure; important for retaining fluid within the vascular compartment • Low oncotic pressure permits loss of fluid into the interstitial space and potential third-space compartments, causing edema and body cavity effusion. • Serum albumin < 1.5 g/dL causes edema and effusion. • Serum albumin 1.5–2.5 gm/dL is not associated with edema or effusion unless other factors provoke fluid extravasation (e.g., increased hydrostatic pressure [venous occlusion, vascular bed hypertension], renal sodium retention, fluid overload, increased vascular permeability).
• Symptomatic hypoalbuminemia develops as a result of chronic liver disease, extracorporeal loss in the gut (PLE), loss through the glomeruli (PLN), cutaneous loss (severe exudative dermatitis, third-degree burns), or malnutrition/starvation. • Albumin and globulin concentrations—may help differentiate cause; equivalent losses occur in PLE and blood loss

SYSTEMS AFFECTED
• Cardiovascular and respiratory—transudative body cavity effusion (e.g., pleural effusion, ascites); peripheral edema; pulmonary edema
• Endocrine and metabolic—altered protein binding permits increased unbound-free drug and adverse drug effects • Cutaneous and musculoskeletal—delayed wound healing (controversial); altered skin turgor (e.g., overestimation of hydration status)

SIGNALMENT
Species Dogs and cats
Breed Predilections N/A
Mean Age and Range N/A
Predominant Sex N/A

SIGNS
Historical Findings
• Abdominal distention: ascites • Diarrhea and/or vomiting: PLE • Dyspnea—owing to pulmonary edema or pleural effusion
• Swollen limbs—with edema

Physical Examination Findings
• Ascites • Muffled heart sounds—pleural effusion • Pulmonary crackles—edema
• Peripheral edema • Dyspnea • Thickened bowel loops—PLE

CAUSES
Decreased Albumin Production
• Chronic liver disease—chronic hepatitis; cirrhosis; idiopathic hepatic fibrosis; variable in congenital portosystemic shunt (dogs) • Inadequate intake—malnutrition/malassimilation

Extracorporeal Albumin Loss
• PLN—amyloidosis; glomerulonephritis
• PLE—lymphangiectasia; lymphoma; severe inflammatory bowel disease; histoplasmosis
• Extensive exudative cutaneous lesions
• Chronic severe blood loss
• Repeated large volume paracentesis—abdominal or pleural effusion

Sequestration: Body Cavities and Tissues
• Inflammatory effusions—pancreatitis; peritonitis; chylous effusions; pyothorax
• Vasculopathy, vasculitis—immune mediated; infectious (*Ehrlichia*, Rocky Mountain spotted fever); sepsis syndrome; infectious canine hepatitis

Miscellaneous
• Hyperglobulinemia • Negative acute-phase response • Catabolism • Dilution—iatrogenic vascular expansion; syndrome of inappropriate ADH release • Hypoadrenocorticism

RISK FACTORS
• Diseases of the liver, kidney, intestines, and blood vessels • Negative nitrogen balance

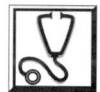 DIAGNOSIS

DIFFERENTIAL DIAGNOSIS
• Severe liver disease—patient may or may not be jaundiced; may develop hepatic encephalopathy or polyuria and polydipsia; predisposed to ascites • PLE—diarrhea common; usually thickened bowel segments
• Cutaneous lesions—must be severe and exudative • External blood loss—associated with pallor; vital signs indicate anemia; extracorporeal evidence of blood loss (enteric, urinary, respiratory tract) • Malnutrition—mild hypoalbuminemia • Aggressive fluid therapy—may exacerbate hypoalbuminemia or create spurious findings

LABORATORY FINDINGS
Drugs That May Alter Laboratory Results
Ampicillin may cause falsely high values (depending on assay system).

Disorders That May Alter Laboratory Results
Extreme lipemia or excessive hemolysis—artificially high values with bromocresol green method

Valid if Run in Human Laboratory?
Yes

CBC/BIOCHEMISTRY/URINALYSIS
CBC
• Depends on underlying cause • Severe liver disease—RBC microcytosis (common)
• Severe blood loss—regenerative anemia
• PLE—lymphopenia in lymphangiectasia

Biochemistry
• Fractionation of total protein—may disclose clues to underlying disorder; patterns influenced by acute-phase response, which increases globulins and provides a negative feedback on albumin synthesis • Chronic liver disease—low albumin; normal to high globulin • PLE—low albumin; low globulin
• PLN—low albumin; globulin usually normal but may be variable • Exudative losses—low albumin; variable globulin
• Malnutrition—low albumin; normal globulin • Severe blood loss—low albumin; low to normal globulin • Cholesterol—low with chronic liver disease, severe PLE, Addison's disease, and severe malnutrition; high with PLN and pancreatitis • Liver enzymes—may be high with chronic hepatitis, inflammatory bowel disease causing PLE, and a general systemic response to inflammation. • Bilirubin—may be high with chronic liver disease • BUN—may be low in chronic liver disease or patients undergoing diuresis; high with reduced renal function or dehydration • Hyperkalemia and hyponatremia—indicate Addison's disease or gut-associated pseudohypoadrenocorticism
• Spurious hypocalcemia—calculate: corrected calcium = measured calcium − measured albumin + albumin midrange for laboratory used (primarily dogs)

Urinalysis
• Complete urine examination—essential; rules out PLN • Obtain urine by cystocentesis to avoid lower-tract contamination; **Caution:** avoid cystocentesis-induced hematuria
• Proteinuria—substantiate dipstick detection with chemical determination • Urine protein:creatinine ratio—essential; > 3.0 compatible with nephrotic range proteinuria; must interpret along with urine sediment; spurious positive values with active sediment (WBCs, RBCs) and macroscopic hematuria; many dogs with glomerulonephritis have hyaline, waxy, or granular casts in their urine

OTHER LABORATORY TESTS
• TSBA—high with severe liver disease; may note spurious low values with PLE (fat malabsorption) • Physicochemical evaluation of effusion—transudate (pure or modified) if hypoalbuminemia is a leading cause; exudate (septic, nonseptic) in other disorders

IMAGING
• Thoracic radiography—pleural effusion; pulmonary edema • Barium contrast studies—limited utility for differential diagnosis • Abdominal radiographs—effusion; altered liver size; mass lesions; quadrant signs of pancreatic disease
• Abdominal ultrasonography—helps differentiate visceral abnormalities (e.g., small liver, thickened gut wall), mass lesions, fluid pockets, altered portal blood flow, mesenteric lymphadenopathy, and biliary tree abnormalities

OTHER DIAGNOSTIC PROCEDURES
• Antithrombin III—Molecular weight similar to albumin; may be low with PLE, PLN, and other conditions associated with albumin loss; low with hepatic synthetic failure • Liver biopsy—after evaluating coagulation (mucosal bleeding time, PIVKA, PT, APTT, platelet count) • Renal biopsy—differentiates amyloidosis from glomerulonephritis; limited use owing to few treatment options for these disorders • Intestinal biopsy—via endoscopy (pinch) or surgery (full-thickness); delayed healing of surgical wounds and seroma formation may occur with laparotomy in patient with severe hypoalbuminemia

 TREATMENT

APPROPRIATE HEALTH CARE
• Depends on definitive cause
• Pleural effusion restricting ventilation—perform thoracentesis with or without chest tube.

NURSING CARE
Provide physical therapy and walk patient to improve drainage of peripheral edema.

Fluid Therapy
• Avoid excessive sodium loading
• Colloids—use to increase oncotic pressure and reduce quantity of crystalloids required for volume expansion; anticipate continued intravenous administration by CRI; not retained by patients with extracorporeal losses (PLE, PLN, surface exudation), administer for acute needs or volume expansion
• Plasma—best colloid, especially with coagulopathy or high risk of thrombosis; also provides antithrombin III; longer oncotic effect compared with synthetic colloids
• Hetastarch—synthetic polymer; increases oncotic pressure; 6% solution in 0.9% NaCl (10–20 mL/kg IV over 6–8 hr or dripped slowly for 24 hr); multiple doses usually given; may exacerbate or create bleeding tendencies; does not negate loss of protein binding • Dextran 70—polysaccharide; increases oncotic pressure; considered last-resort alternative colloid; 6% solution in 0.9% NaCl (1 mL/kg/hr IV); may exacerbate or create bleeding tendencies by interfering with platelet function; does not negate loss of protein binding; avoid use in liver patients as it may provoke bleeding • Human albumin—12.5 g/20 g lean body weight IV over 24 hr (use is controversial)

DIET
• Achieve positive energy and nitrogen balance • Hepatic encephalopathy—restrict protein intake (see Hepatic Encephalopathy) • Effusions or edema due to hypoalbuminemia—restrict sodium • PLE associated with lymphangectasia—medium-chain triglycerides (dogs only; controversial) combined with fat-restricted diet

 MEDICATIONS

DRUG(S)
• Glucocorticoids—used for some types of chronic hepatitis and inflammatory bowel disease; select agent with minimal mineralocorticoid effects (e.g., dexamethasone) to avoid sodium and water retention • Diuretics—assist in mobilization and excretion of excess body water and sodium; furosemide (1–4 mg/kg IV, IM, or PO q4–12h): use judiciously to avoid intravascular volume contraction and in combination with spironolactone (1–4 mg/kg q12h) with liver or heart disease • Antithrombotic treatment—aspirin (0.5 mg/kg PO or rectally q12h) with low antithrombin III, especially in cases of PLN • Enalapril (0.5 mg/kg PO q12–24h)–for dogs with PLN; alternative is benazepril

CONTRAINDICATIONS
Synthetic colloids—avoid with anuria, renal failure, congestive heart failure, severe coagulopathy, or von Willebrand's disease

PRECAUTIONS
• Fluid therapy—large doses of synthetic colloids may cause volume overload and coagulopathy (especially dextrans); do not overload with crystalloid fluids (e.g., lactated Ringer's solution, Plasma-Lyte), which are rapidly distributed into the interstitial space (70% volume within 1 hr), worsening pulmonary edema, limb edema, and body cavity effusions; restrict maintenance fluid volume with crystalloids to one-third to one-half normal, depending on contemporary losses, if used with colloids • Plasma or human albumin transfusion—may be complicated by transfusion or allergic reaction • Diuretic therapy—may cause serious volume contraction, predisposing patients to azotemia and hypotension, and electrolyte and acid–base derangements • Unanticipated drug side effects—owing to reduced albumin concentration for drug binding • Use of DDAVP for bleeding—may aggravate fluid retention and complications

POSSIBLE INTERACTIONS N/A
ALTERNATIVE DRUG(S) N/A

 FOLLOW-UP

PATIENT MONITORING
• Body weight—especially during fluid therapy; monitor fluid retention • Vital signs, thoracic auscultation for crackles—monitor for pulmonary edema • Serum albumin concentration • Blood pressure—monitor for vascular expansion • Abdominal girth—monitor for severity of ascites • Pulse oximetry—to detect hypoxemia secondary to pulmonary edema

POSSIBLE COMPLICATIONS
• PLN—may be complicated by thromboembolism; minimize intravenous catheterization and iatrogenic trauma
• Hypovolemia—in dehydrated animals, animals with Addison's disease or blood loss, or animals overtreated with diuretics; predisposes to acute renal failure and DIC

EXPECTED COURSE AND PROGNOSIS
Depend on underlying cause

 MISCELLANEOUS

PREGNANCY
Condition complicates pregnancy.

SEE ALSO
• Amyloidosis • Cirrhosis and Fibrosis of the Liver • Glomerulonephritis • Juvenile Fibrosing Liver Disease • Portosystemic Shunt, Acquired • Portosystemic Vascular Anomaly, Congenital • Protein-losing Enteropathy

ABBREVIATIONS
• ADH = antidiuretic hormone • APTT = activated partial thromboplastin time
• BUN = blood urea nitrogen • CRI = constant rate infusion • DDAVP = 1 deamino-8-D-arginine vasopressin • DIC = disseminated intravascular coagulation
• PIVKA = proteins invoked by vitamin K absence or antagonism • PLE = protein-losing enteropathy • PLN = protein-losing nephropathy • PT = prothrombin time
• TSBA = total serum bile acids

Suggested Reading
Center SA. Effusions. In: Willard MD, Tvedten H, Turnwald GH, eds. Small animal clinical diagnosis by laboratory methods. Philadelphia: Saunders, 2002.
Rudloff E, Kirby R. Colloids: current recommendations. In: Bonagura JD, ed. Kirk's current veterinary therapy XIII. Phladelphia: Saunders, 2000:131–136.
Smiley LE, Garvey MS. The uses of hetastarch as adjunct therapy in 26 dogs with hypoalbuminemia: a phase two clinical trial. J Vet Intern Med 1994;8:195–202.
Turnwald GH, Barta O. Immunologic and plasma protein disorders. In: Willard MD, Tvedten H, Turnwald GH, eds. Small animal clinical diagnosis by laboratory methods. Philadelphia: Saunders, 2002.
Authors Susan E. Bunch and Susan E Johnson
Consulting Editor Sharon A. Center

HYPOANDROGENISM

 BASICS

OVERVIEW
• Hypoandrogenism refers to the relative or absolute deficiency of masculinizing sex hormones, such as testosterone and its derivatives. Androgens are produced by the adrenal cortex, the ovary in the female, and the interstitial (Leydig) cells of the testes in the male.
• Males—Primary hypoandrogenism in the male is a rare condition associated with bilaterally symmetric alopecia (endocrine alopecia) in old castrated male dogs. It may also be seen in association with testicular destruction in association with inflammatory testicular disease; however, the latter is not usually associated with clinical signs other than a lack of libido and spermatogenesis.
• Females—Primary hypoandrogenism is documented in the bitch, but secondary hypoandrogenism due to such conditions as hyperadrenocorticism and hypothyroidism is far more common.

SIGNALMENT
• Dogs and cats
• More common in older animals, although congenital forms exist.
• Primary hypoandrogenism rare in females, most common in castrated male dogs (especially the Afghan hound)

SIGNS

Historical Findings
• Failure to cycle
• Low libido

Physical Examination Findings
• Dry, dull hair coat
• Coat color change
• Small, underdeveloped testes
• Poor semen quality
• Absence of penile spines in toms

CAUSES & RISK FACTORS
• Boston terriers—low fetal androgen production is thought to be associated with the occurrence of hypospadias
• Calico and tortoiseshell male cats—in association with Klinefelter's (39 XXY) syndrome
• Antiandrogenic drug administration—mitotane, ketoconazole, megestrol acetate
• Testicular degeneration
• Castration

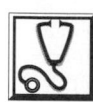 **DIAGNOSIS**

DIFFERENTIAL DIAGNOSIS
• Hypothyroidism—diagnosis based on appropriate clinical signs, in conjunction with typical hematologic and biochemical abnormalities (normocytic normochromic nonregenerative anemia, hypercholesterolemia) and thyroid function testing (total T_4, free T_4, TSH)
• Hyperadrenocorticism—clinical signs usually include polyuria/polydipsia and exercise intolerance; CBC may reveal leukocytosis, erythrocytosis; serum biochemistry abnormalities include high ALP, ALT, and cholesterol, and low BUN; additional testing includes ACTH stimulation, LDDS test, endogenous ACTH, abdominal ultrasonography, abdominal radiography
• Hyposomatotropism—also known as GH-responsive dermatosis. This syndrome is thought to be a secondary problem that occurs in association with alopecia-X (see Hyperandrogenism). Definitive diagnosis is made with careful consideration to breed; history; physical examination; laboratory results, excluding other endocrine causes of alopecia; skin biopsy; and response to therapy.

CBC/BIOCHEMISTRY/URINALYSIS
Usually unremarkable

OTHER LABORATORY TESTS
• Skin biopsy may reveal nonspecific changes associated with endocrine alopecia, such as orthokeratotic hyperkeratosis, epidermal atrophy and melanosis, follicular keratosis, telogen hair follicles, and sebaceous gland atrophy.
• Karyotype—to detect intersex abnormalities
• Serum testosterone concentrations—single values of little clinical significance due to daily fluctuation in serum concentration in the normal animal
• Testicular biopsy—to document inflammatory testicular disease
• Semen analysis
• Serum LH concentration—to assess Leydig cell function

IMAGING
N/A

DIAGNOSTIC PROCEDURES
Diagnosis is based on evaluation of history, physical examination, laboratory testing to rule out other differential diagnoses, and response to therapy.

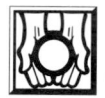 **TREATMENT**

May attempt hormone replacement therapy

MEDICATIONS

DRUG(S) OF CHOICE
Methyltestosterone
Dog: 5–25 mg/dog PO q24–48h
Cat: 1–2.5 mg/cat PO q48h

CONTRAINDICATIONS/POSSIBLE INTERACTIONS
• Use of methyltestosterone may result in cholestatic liver disease and behavioral changes, such as aggression.
• Drugs that interfere with steroid synthesis should be avoided.

 FOLLOW-UP

PATIENT MONITORING
Response to therapy

PREVENTION/AVOIDANCE
Avoid drugs known to cause hypoandrogenism in breeding animals.

POSSIBLE COMPLICATIONS
Permanent hypogonadism and infertility are possible.

EXPECTED COURSE AND PROGNOSIS
Varies with cause; may be permanent, temporary, or intermittent

 **MISCELLANEOUS**

ASSOCIATED CONDITIONS
• Testosterone-responsive dermatosis of male animals
• Hypogonadism
• Intersex abnormalities

ABBREVIATIONS
• ACTH = adrenocorticotropic hormone
• ALP = alkaline phosphatase
• ALT = alanine aminotransferase
• BUN = blood urea nitrogen
• GH = growth hormone
• LDDS = low-dose dexamethasone suppression test
• LH = luteinizing hormone
• T_4 = thyroxine
• TSH = thyroid-stimulating hormone

Suggested Reading
Griffin CE, Scott DW, Miller WH. Endocrine and metabolic diseases. In: Scott DW, Miller WH, Griffin CE, eds. Muller and Kirk's small animal dermatology. Philadelphia: Saunders, 2001:780–885.
Authors Sophie A. Grundy and Autumn P. Davidson
Consulting Editor Deborah S. Greco

HYPOCALCEMIA

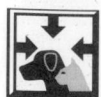 BASICS

DEFINITION

Low total serum calcium concentration

PATHOPHYSIOLOGY

Of the total circulating serum calcium, 50% is protein bound, 40% is ionized, and 10% is complexed with other substances. Protein-bound calcium cannot diffuse through membranes and thus is unusable by the tissues. Complexed calcium can diffuse through membranes but is unavailable for use by tissues. Only the ionized form is available to tissues, so only changes in this fraction of total serum calcium are responsible for clinical problems (hypo- and hypercalcemia). Measurement of ionized calcium is difficult for routine performance, and biochemical profiles record only total serum calcium. Mechanisms involved in hypocalcemia include:
• Low concentrations of binding proteins—hypoalbuminemia
• Reduced intestinal absorption—deficient vitamin D (renal disease, severe intestinal disease)
• Reduced renal and bone resorption—hypoparathyroidism
• Inadequate dietary intake
• Excessive loss—lactation
• Sequestration—saponification (acute pancreatitis)
• Binding/complexing with administered or ingested chemicals—phosphate-containing enemas, citrate toxicity, ethylene glycol toxicity, low calcium/high phosphorus diet (nutritional secondary hyperparathyroidism)
• Impaired synthesis or refractoriness to PTH—hypomagnesemia

SYSTEMS AFFECTED

• Nervous/Neuromuscular—seizures, tetany, ataxia, and weakness
• Cardiovascular—ECG changes and bradycardia
• Gastrointestinal—anorexia and vomiting (especially cats)
• Ophthalmic—posterior lenticular cataracts
• Respiratory—panting

SIGNALMENT

• Dog and cat
• Varies depending on the underlying cause

SIGNS

General Comments

Signs of the underlying disease may be seen without clinical signs of hypocalcemia, because the latter do not occur until total serum calcium falls below 6.7 mg/dL.

Historical Findings

• Seizures
• Muscle trembling, twitching, or fasciculations
• Ataxia or stiff gait
• Weakness
• Panting
• Facial rubbing
• Vomiting
• Anorexia

Physical Examination Findings

• Fever
• Posterior lenticular cataracts in patients with primary hypoparathyroidism

CAUSES

Nonpathologic Hypocalcemia

• Laboratory error—occurs up to 13% of the time; repeat serum calcium determinations recommended to confirm true hypocalcemia, especially if results indicate significant hypocalcemia despite absence of clinical signs.
• Hypoalbuminemia—most common cause; accounts for over 50% of patients; leads to reduction of protein-bound calcium without affecting ionized calcium; not associated with clinical signs
• Correct for hypoalbuminemia by use of one of the following formulas:

$$\text{Corrected Ca} = \text{Ca (mg/dL)} - \text{albumin (g/dL)} + 3.5$$

or

$$\text{Corrected Ca} = \text{Ca (mg/dL)} - [0.4 \times \text{total protein (g/dL)}] + 3.3$$

Note: In cats, hypoalbuminemia causes a drop in the calcium concentration; these formulas were developed in dogs and cannot be applied to cats.
• Alkalosis—causes a shift from protein-bound calcium to ionized calcium as well as a reduction in measured calcium; not associated with clinical signs

Pathologic Hypocalcemia

• Primary hypoparathyroidism
• Hypoparathyroidism secondary to thyroidectomy and parathyroid damage
• Renal failure—acute or chronic
• Ethylene glycol toxicity
• Acute pancreatitis
• Puerperal tetany—eclampsia
• Phosphate-containing enemas
• Nutritional secondary hyperparathyroidism
• Hypomagnesemia
• Intestinal malabsorption

• Citrate toxicity—multiple blood transfusions or improper citrate–blood ratio

RISK FACTORS

Puerperal tetany (eclampsia)—usually seen in small-breed bitches during the first 21 days of nursing a litter

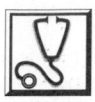 DIAGNOSIS

DIFFERENTIAL DIAGNOSIS

• Clinical signs of hypocalcemia—rule out primary hypoparathyroidism, hypoparathyroidism secondary to thyroidectomy and parathyroid damage, and puerperal tetany (eclampsia); other causes rarely lower the serum calcium enough to cause clinical signs.
• Polyuria and polydipsia—rule out renal failure.
• Neurologic signs—rule out ethylene glycol toxicity.
• Vomiting and diarrhea—rule out acute pancreatitis, intestinal malabsorption, renal failure, and ethylene glycol toxicity.
• Bone pain or fractures—rule out nutritional secondary hyperparathyroidism.

LABORATORY FINDINGS

Drugs That May Alter Laboratory Results

• Sodium bicarbonate may cause alkalosis and lower the serum calcium concentration.
• Samples collected in EDTA tubes may have a falsely low serum calcium concentration because of calcium chelation.

Disorders That May Alter Laboratory Results

• Lipemia can raise the serum calcium significantly.
• Any cause of hypoalbumenia can falsely lower the serum calcium (see causes of nonpathogenic hypocalcemia).

Valid If Run in Human Laboratory?

Yes

CBC/BIOCHEMISTRY/URINALYSIS

• Low calcium
• Mild-to-moderate anemia possible in patients with chronic renal failure, nutritional secondary hyperparathyroidism, and intestinal malabsorption
• Leukocytosis possible in patients with acute pancreatitis
• Hypoalbuminemia in patients with hypoproteinemia-induced hypocalcemia—intestinal malabsorption, protein-losing nephropathy, other causes
• High total CO_2 in patients with alkalosis-induced hypocalcemia

• High BUN and creatinine in patients with acute and chronic renal failure and ethylene glycol toxicity
• High phosphorus in patients with acute and chronic renal failure, ethylene glycol toxicity, primary hypoparathyroidism, hypoparathyroidism secondary to thyroidectomy and parathyroid damage, and in patients receiving phosphate-containing enemas
• High amylase and lipase in many, but not all, patients with acute pancreatitis
• Isosthenuria in patients with chronic renal failure, moderate-to-advanced acute renal failure, and ethylene glycol toxicity
• Glucosuria in patients with acute renal failure and ethylene glycol toxicity

OTHER LABORATORY TESTS
• Ethylene glycol test—indicated in patients suspected of ingesting ethylene glycol within the previous 12–16 hours
• PTH assay—indicated when primary hypoparathyroidism is suspected
• Serum magnesium concentration—hypomagnesemia is a rare cause of hypocalcemia; indicated when all other causes of hypocalcemia have been ruled out

IMAGING
• Radiography usually normal
• Possibly, small kidneys in patients with chronic renal failure and large kidneys in patients with acute renal failure and ethylene glycol toxicity
• Possibly, decreased bone density in patients with nutritional secondary hyperparathyroidism
• Possibly, mild pleural effusion and decreased abdominal detail from effusion with pancreatitis

DIAGNOSTIC PROCEDURES
ECG changes include prolongation of the ST and QT segments; sinus bradycardia and wide T waves or T wave alternans in some patients

 TREATMENT

• Inpatient treatment for patients with clinical hypocalcemia whose underlying disease requires support
• Emergency treatment is usually only needed for patients with primary hypoparathyroidism, hypoparathyroidism secondary to thyroidectomy and parathyroid damage, puerperal tetany (eclampsia), recent phosphate-containing enema administration, and citrate toxicity (rare).

• Short-term and long-term treatment is usually needed only to treat primary hypoparathyroidism and puerperal tetany (eclampsia).
• Diet change recommended in patients with nutritional secondary hyperparathyroidism (to a balanced diet) and renal failure (see Renal Failure, Chronic).

 MEDICATIONS

DRUG(S) AND FLUIDS
Emergency Treatment
• Calcium gluconate 10% solution—5–15 mg/kg (0.5–1.5 mL/kg) slowly to effect over a 10-min period; monitor heart rate and stop administration temporarily if bradycardia occurs; if ECG monitoring is possible, QT interval shortening is an indication to temporarily stop administration.
• Calcium chloride 10% solution—also effective; extremely caustic if administered extravascularly, and three times more potent than calcium gluconate; the mg/kg dosage is the same as for calcium gluconate (5–15 mg/kg), but only one third the volume is needed (0.15–0.5 mL/kg).
• If the patient has puerperal tetany (eclampsia), remove the puppies from the mother and hand-nurse until weaned.

Short-term Treatment Immediately After Correction of Tetany
With calcium gluconate 10% solution, relapse of clinical signs after emergency treatment can be prevented by use of one of the following:
• Constant-rate IV infusion of 60–90 mg/kg/day (6.5–9.75 mL/kg/day) added to the fluids
• Subcutaneous administration 3–4 times daily of the dosage determined necessary for initial control of tetany; dilute this dose in an equal volume of saline.

Long-term Treatment
See Hypoparathyroidism.

CONTRAINDICATIONS
N/A

PRECAUTIONS
See Hypoparathyroidism.

POSSIBLE INTERACTIONS
See Hypoparathyroidism.

ALTERNATIVE DRUG(S)
N/A

 FOLLOW-UP

PATIENT MONITORING
• Serum calcium concentration monthly for the first 6 months, then every 2–4 months
• Goal is to maintain serum calcium concentration between 8 and 10 mg/dL.

POSSIBLE COMPLICATIONS
Hypocalcemia and hypercalcemia (which can lead to renal failure) are both concerns in patients on long-term therapy.

 MISCELLANEOUS

ASSOCIATED CONDITIONS
N/A

AGE-RELATED FACTORS
N/A

ZOONOTIC POTENTIAL
N/A

PREGNANCY
• Hypocalcemia can lead to weakness and dystocia.
• Clinical hypocalcemia caused by puerperal tetany (eclampsia) usually is seen in small-breed bitches during the first 21 days of nursing a litter.

SYNONYMS
N/A

SEE ALSO
• See Causes.
• Hypoparathyroidism

ABBREVIATIONS
• Ca = calcium
• EDTA = ethylene diamine tetraacetic acid
• PTH = parathyroid hormone

Suggested Reading
Feldman EC, Nelson RW. Hypocalcemia and primary hypoparathyroidism. In: Feldman EC, Nelson RW, eds. Canine and feline endocrinology and reproduction. Philadelphia: Saunders, 1996:497–516.
Meuten DJ, Armstrong PJ. Parathyroid disease and calcium metabolism. In: Ettinger SJ, ed. Textbook of veterinary internal medicine. Philadelphia: Saunders, 1989:1610–1631.
Waters CB, Scott-Moncrieff JCR. Hypocalcemia in cats. Compend Contin Educ Pract Vet 1992;14:497–507.
Author Mitchell A. Crystal
Consulting Editor Deborah Greco

HYPOCHLOREMIA

 BASICS

DEFINITION
Serum chloride concentration below the lower limit of normal—dogs, < 105 mEq/L; cats, < 117 mEq/L

PATHOPHYSIOLOGY
• Chloride is the most abundant anion in the extracellular fluid.
• Chloride concentration is controlled by electrochemical gradients resulting from the active transport of sodium.
• In general, chloride concentration varies directly with sodium concentration and inversely with bicarbonate concentration.

SYSTEMS AFFECTED
Depend on underlying disorder

SIGNALMENT
Dog and cat

CAUSES
• Gastric vomiting
• Hypoadrenocorticism
• Metabolic alkalosis
• Salt-losing nephropathy
• Diuretic therapy

RISK FACTORS
N/A

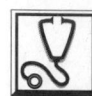 DIAGNOSIS

DIFFERENTIAL DIAGNOSIS
If the degree of hypochloremia exceeds that of hyponatremia, it suggests selective chloride loss as seen in patients with gastric vomiting.

LABORATORY FINDINGS
Drugs That May Alter Laboratory Results
Furosemide, thiazides, bicarbonate, and laxatives lower the serum concentration.

Disorders That May Alter Laboratory Results
Lipemia and hyperproteinemia can falsely lower chloride concentration if ion-specific electrodes are not used.

Valid if Run in Human Laboratory?
Yes

CBC/BIOCHEMISTRY/URINALYSIS
• Low chloride
• Other abnormalities depend on underlying disorder; possibly, hyponatremia, hyperkalemia, and high bicarbonate concentration

OTHER LABORATORY TESTS
• Measurement of urine fractional excretion of chloride may demonstrate high excretion.
• Blood gas measurement may reveal metabolic alkalosis.

IMAGING
N/A

DIAGNOSTIC PROCEDURES
N/A

 TREATMENT

• Depends on underlying disorder
• Use 0.9% NaCl if fluid administration is indicated.

DIET
No need to alter

CLIENT EDUCATION
Depends on underlying disorder

SURGICAL CONSIDERATIONS
N/A

 MEDICATIONS

DRUG(S) OF CHOICE
Other fluid therapy and medication as dictated by underlying cause

CONTRAINDICATIONS
N/A

PRECAUTIONS
N/A

POSSIBLE INTERACTIONS
N/A

ALTERNATIVE DRUG(S)
N/A

 FOLLOW-UP

PATIENT MONITORING
Serum electrolyte concentrations as needed to ensure appropriate response

POSSIBLE COMPLICATIONS
Depend on underlying disorder

PREVENTION/AVOIDANCE
Depends on underlying disorder

EXPECTED COURSE AND PROGNOSIS
Depends on underlying cause

✔ MISCELLANEOUS

ASSOCIATED CONDITIONS
Often accompanied by hyponatremia

AGE-RELATED FACTORS
N/A

ZOONOTIC POTENTIAL
N/A

PREGNANCY
N/A

SYNONYMS
N/A

SEE ALSO
N/A

ABBREVIATIONS
N/A

Suggested Reading
DiBartola SP. Fluid therapy in small animal practice. Philadelphia: Saunders, 1992.
Rose DB. Clinical physiology of acid-base and electrolyte disorders. 3rd ed. New York: McGraw-Hill, 1989.
Author Peter P. Kintzer
Consulting Editor Deborah S. Greco

HYPOGLYCEMIA

 BASICS

DEFINITION
Abnormally low blood glucose concentration

PATHOPHYSIOLOGY
Mechanisms responsible for hypoglycemia:
• Excess insulin or insulin-like factors (e.g., insulinoma, extrapancreatic paraneoplasia, and iatrogenic insulin overdose)
• Reduction of hormones needed to maintain normal serum glucose (e.g., hypoadrenocorticism)
• Reduced hepatic gluconeogenesis (e.g., hepatic disease, glycogen storage diseases, and sepsis)
• Excessive metabolic use of glucose (e.g., in hunting dogs, pregnancy, neoplasia, polycythemia, and sepsis)
• Reduced intake or underproduction of glucose (e.g., in puppies and kittens, toy breeds, and severe malnutrition or starvation)

SYSTEMS AFFECTED
• Nervous
• Musculoskeletal

SIGNALMENT
• Dog and cat
• Variable, depending on the underlying cause

SIGNS
• Seizures
• Posterior paresis
• Weakness
• Collapse
• Muscle fasciculations
• Abnormal behavior
• Lethargy and depression
• Ataxia
• Polyphagia
• Weight gain
• PU/PD
• Exercise intolerance
• Some animals appear normal aside from findings associated with underlying disease.
• Many animals have episodic signs.

CAUSES

Endocrine
• Insulinoma
• Extrapancreatic paraneoplasia
• Iatrogenic insulin overdose
• Hypoadrenocorticism

Hepatic Disease
• Portosystemic shunt
• Cirrhosis
• Severe hepatitis (e.g., toxic and inflammatory)
• Glycogen storage diseases

Overuse
• Hunting dog hypoglycemia
• Pregnancy
• Polycythemia
• Neoplasia
• Sepsis

Reduced Intake/Underproduction
• Young puppies and kittens
• Toy-breed dogs
• Severe malnutrition or starvation

RISK FACTORS
• Low energy intake predisposes to hypoglycemia in patients with conditions causing overuse and underproduction.
• Fasting, excitement, exercise, and eating may or may not increase the risk of hypoglycemic episodes in patients with insulinoma.

 DIAGNOSIS

DIFFERENTIAL DIAGNOSIS
• Patients with hyperinsulinism—signs of hypoglycemia or a normal physical examination
• Patients with hypoadrenocorticism—waxing, waning, nonspecific signs (e.g., vomiting, diarrhea, melena, and weakness); addisonian patients that present in a crisis usually display hypovolemia and hyperkalemia rather than hypoglycemia (e.g., shock, bradycardia, and dehydration).
• Patients with portosystemic shunts—usually young to middle-aged; often thin or appear to have stunted growth; rarely, they have ascites or edema.
• Patients with cirrhosis and severe hepatitis usually have other signs of their disease (e.g., gastrointestinal signs, icterus, and ascites or edema).
• Patients with sepsis—critical; usually in shock; pyrexia or hypothermia revealed by examination; may have gastrointestinal signs
• Glycogen storage diseases—rare; usually seen in animals <1 year old
• Extrapancreatic paraneoplasia and large neoplastic processes that cause hypoglycemia can often be detected by physical examination.

LABORATORY FINDINGS

Drugs That May Alter Laboratory Results
None

Disorders That May Alter Laboratory Results
Delayed separation of serum causes falsely low serum glucose values; if blood cannot be centrifuged and the serum separated within 30 min of collection, it should be collected in a sodium fluoride tube.

Valid If Run in Human Laboratory?
Yes

CBC/BIOCHEMISTRY/URINALYSIS
• Patients with hyperinsulinism may have normal results.
• Patients with hypoadrenocorticism may have lymphocytosis, eosinophilia, hyperkalemia, hyponatremia, azotemia, or hypercalcemia.
• Patients with portosystemic shunts may have microcytosis, hypoalbuminemia, low BUN, mildly high liver enzyme activities, urate crystals, and low urinary specific gravity.
• Patients with cirrhosis, severe hepatitis, and hepatic neoplasia may have anemia associated with chronic disease, high liver enzyme activities, hyperbilirubinemia, hypoalbuminemia, bilirubinuria, and low urinary specific gravity.
• Patients with polycythemia have a PCV >65.

OTHER LABORATORY TESTS
• Simultaneous fasting glucose/insulin determination—indicated when insulinoma is suspected; high plasma insulin in the face of hypoglycemia suggests insulinoma.
• AIGR—indicated when insulinoma is suspected:

$$AIGR = \frac{plasma\ insulin\ [\mu U/mL] \times 100}{plasma\ glucose\ [mg/dL] - 30}$$

Use 1 as denominator if glucose is <30; AIGR > 30 suggests an insulinoma; AIGR = 19–30 is a gray zone—repeat test; AIGR < 19 indicates insulinoma is unlikely. (**Note:** False-positive results are possible, especially when the blood glucose concentration is <40 mg/dL.)
• ACTH stimulation test—indicated when hypoadrenocorticism is suspected
• Fasting and postprandial serum bile acids—indicated when a portosystemic shunt or functional hepatic disease is suspected
• Bacterial culture of blood—indicated when sepsis is suspected

IMAGING
• Abdominal radiography and ultrasonography—useful in patients with extrapancreatic paraneoplasia and large neoplastic processes (may see organomegaly or masses), as well as portosystemic shunt (microhepatica), cirrhosis (microhepatica, hyperechogenicity), and severe hepatitis (hepatomegaly)
• Thoracic radiography—to detect metastasis if neoplasia is suspected

• Technetium-99m per rectal quantitative hepatic scintigraphy—useful to detect portosystemic shunt
• Mesenteric portography—useful to detect portosystemic shunt (requires surgery)

DIAGNOSTIC PROCEDURES
• ECG—useful to evaluate bradycardia in patients with hypoadrenocorticism
• Ultrasound-guided or surgical hepatic biopsy—useful to evaluate for cirrhosis, hepatitis, and glycogen storage diseases

TREATMENT
• Treat animals with clinical hypoglycemia whose underlying disease needs support as inpatients.
• If able to eat (i.e., responsive, no vomiting), feeding should be part or all of initial treatment.
• If unable to eat, start continuous fluid therapy with 2.5% dextrose; if clinical signs persist, use a 5% dextrose solution.
• Surgery is indicated if a portosystemic shunt or insulinoma is the cause of hypoglycemia.

MEDICATIONS

DRUG(S) OF CHOICE

Emergency/Acute Treatment
• In hospital—administer 50% dextrose, 1 mL/kg IV slow bolus (1–3 min).
• At home—do not attempt to have the owner administer medication orally during a seizure; hypoglycemic seizures usually abate within 1–2 min; if a seizure is prolonged, recommend transportation to hospital; if a short seizure has ended or other signs of a hypoglycemic crisis exist, recommend rubbing corn syrup or 50% dextrose on the buccal mucosa, followed by 2 mL/kg of the same solution orally once the patient can swallow; then seek immediate attention.
• Initiate frequent feeding of a diet low in simple sugars or, if patient is unable to eat, continuous fluid therapy with 2.5% dextrose.

Long-term Treatment
• See Insulinoma for treatment of insulinoma and extrapancreatic paraneoplasia.
• Hunting dog hypoglycemia—feed moderate meal of fat, protein, and complex carbohydrates a few hours before hunting; can feed snacks (e.g., dog biscuits) every 3–5 hours during the hunt
• Toy-breed hypoglycemia—increase the frequency of feeding.
• Puppy and kitten hypoglycemia—increase the frequency of feeding (nursing or hand feeding).
• Other causes of hypoglycemia require treating the underlying disease and do not usually need long-term treatment.

CONTRAINDICATIONS
• Insulin
• Barbiturates and diazepam in patients with hypoglycemic seizures—they do not treat the cause of the seizure and they may worsen hepatoencephalopathy in patients with portosystemic shunt and cirrhosis.

PRECAUTIONS
• 50% dextrose causes tissue necrosis and sloughing if given extravascularly; never give dextrose in concentrations over 5% without confirmed vascular access.
• Administering a dextrose bolus without following with frequent feedings or continuous IV fluids with dextrose can predispose to subsequent hypoglycemic episodes.

POSSIBLE INTERACTIONS
N/A

ALTERNATIVE DRUG(S)
N/A

FOLLOW-UP

PATIENT MONITORING
• At home—for return or progression of clinical signs of hypoglycemia; assess serum glucose if signs recur.
• Single, intermittent serum glucose determinations may not truly reflect the glycemic status of the patient because of normal production of counterregulatory hormones.
• Other monitoring is based on the underlying disease.

POSSIBLE COMPLICATIONS
Recurrent, progressive episodes of hypoglycemia

MISCELLANEOUS

ASSOCIATED CONDITIONS
Prolonged hypoglycemia can cause transient (hours to days) to permanent blindness from laminar necrosis of the occipital cerebral cortex.

AGE-RELATED FACTORS
Neonatal animals have poor glycogen storage capacity and a reduced ability to perform gluconeogenesis; thus, short periods of fasting (6–12 hours) can cause hypoglycemia.

ZOONOTIC POTENTIAL
None

PREGNANCY
• Hypoglycemia can lead to weakness and dystocia.
• Pregnancy coupled with fasting causes hypoglycemia in rare instances.

SYNONYMS
N/A

SEE ALSO
• See Causes.
• Insulinoma

ABBREVIATIONS
• AIGR = amended insulin:glucose ratio
• PCV = packed cell volume
• PU/PD = polyuria and polydipsia

Suggested Reading
Leifer CE. Hypoglycemia. In: Kirk RW, ed. Current veterinary therapy IX. Philadelphia: Saunders, 1986:982–987.
Nelson RW. Disorders of the endocrine pancreas. In: Ettinger SJ, ed. Textbook of veterinary internal medicine. Philadelphia: Saunders, 1989:1676–1720.
Author Mitchell A. Crystal
Consulting Editor Deborah S. Greco

HYPOKALEMIA

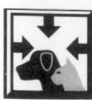 BASICS

DEFINITION
Serum potassium concentration < 3.5 mEq/L

PATHOPHYSIOLOGY
• Potassium is the major intracellular cation and thereby largely responsible for maintenance of intracellular volume.
• The ratio of intracellular to extracellular potassium concentration is important in determining the cellular membrane potential. Rapid alterations in extracellular potassium concentration alter this ratio and predispose an animal to arrhythmias and conduction disturbances in excitable tissues (e.g., heart, nerve, and muscle).
• Hypokalemia can be caused by excessive potassium loss via the gastrointestinal tract or kidneys or movement of potassium from the extracellular fluid compartment into cells (i.e., translocation).

SYSTEMS AFFECTED
• Endocrine/Metabolic—carbohydrate intolerance
• Neuromuscular—skeletal muscle weakness and intestinal ileus
• Cardiovascular—arrhythmias
• Renal/Urologic—hyposthenuria and renal failure

SIGNALMENT
Burmese cats 4–12 months old; recurrent episodes of hypokalemic periodic paralysis

SIGNS
• Historical complaints are often referable to the disease or factors contributing to the hypokalemia
• Weakness
• Lethargy
• Anorexia
• Polyuria
• Polydipsia
• Vomiting
• Ventroflexion of the neck (cats)
• Stilted gait in the forelimbs (cats)

CAUSES

Urinary Potassium Loss
• Chronic renal failure
• Renal tubular acidosis
• Diuretic administration (other than potassium-sparing diuretics)
• Postobstructive diuresis
• Dialysis
• Intravenous fluid diuresis
• Mineralocorticoid excess
• Administration of penicillins
• Administration of amphotericin B

Gastrointestinal Potassium Loss
• Vomiting
• Diarrhea

Insufficient Potassium Intake
• Anorexia
• Potassium-deficient diet
• Potassium-free fluids

Translocation (Extracellular Fluid to Intracellular Fluid)
• Insulin and glucose administration
• Sodium bicarbonate administration
• Catecholamine administration
• Alkalemia
• Hypokalemic periodic paralysis

RISK FACTORS
Feeding cats acidifying diet that is marginal in potassium

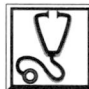 DIAGNOSIS

DIFFERENTIAL DIAGNOSIS
• Azotemia, isosthenuria, and historical PU/PD—rule out chronic renal failure and hypokalemic nephropathy.
• Glucosuria, hyperglycemia, and historical PU/PD—rule out diabetes mellitus
• Metabolic acidosis and urine pH > 6.5—rule out renal tubular acidosis
• Metabolic alkalosis and hypochloremia—rule out upper gastrointestinal obstruction and severe vomiting.
• Young Burmese cat with episodes of severe muscle weakness—rule out hypokalemic periodic paralysis
• Historical urethral obstruction—rule out postobstructive diuresis

LABORATORY FINDINGS

Drugs That May Alter Laboratory Results
Excessive volume of K_3EDTA raises plasma potassium concentration.

Disorders That May Alter Laboratory Results
• Hemolysis in dogs with high RBC potassium (e.g., Akitas) and phosphofructo-kinase deficiency in the English springer spaniel can cause falsely high potassium concentration.
• Thrombocytosis increases serum potassium due to release from platelets during clot formation.

Valid if Run in Human Laboratory?
Yes

CBC/BIOCHEMISTRY/URINALYSIS
• Results may reveal normocytic normochromic nonregenerative anemia in patients with chronic renal failure.
• High BUN and creatinine (with or without phosphate) in patients with chronic renal failure or hypokalemic nephropathy
• Low total CO_2 in patients with renal tubular acidosis or renal failure
• High total CO_2 in patients with metabolic alkalosis
• High glucose in patients with diabetes mellitus
• Glucosuria in patients with diabetes mellitus
• pH > 6.5 in patients with renal tubular acidosis
• Isosthenuria in patients with chronic renal failure or hypokalemic nephropathy

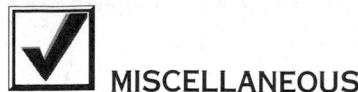
OTHER LABORATORY TESTS
• Aldosterone measurement to diagnose primary hyperaldosteronism
• ACTH stimulation or low-dose dexamethasone suppression test to diagnose hyperadrenocorticism (cause of mineralocorticoid excess)
• Urinary fractional excretion of potassium is elevated in chronic renal failure and hypokalemic nephropathy.

IMAGING
• Ultrasonography may reveal an adrenal tumor—rule out hyperaldosteronism or hyperadrenocorticism.
• Radiographs and ultrasonography—useful in chronic renal failure work-up
• Upper G.I. barium studies—to diagnose upper G.I. disorders (anatomic or functional) causing metabolic alkalosis

OTHER DIAGNOSTIC PROCEDURES
Gastroscopy is useful in diagnosis of upper gastrointestinal disorders resulting in metabolic alkalosis, such as pyloric hypertrophy or gastric neoplasia.

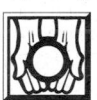

TREATMENT
• Animals with mild hypokalemia (potassium 3.0–3.5) can be treated as outpatients by oral supplementation.
• Severely affected patients should be hospitalized; these animals are at risk of respiratory muscle paralysis and cardiac arrhythmias and should be handled with minimal stress.

MEDICATIONS

DRUG(S) OF CHOICE
• Oral supplementation—potassium gluconate (Tumil-K, Kaon) is an effective treatment, and is the only treatment required in mildly affected animals (initial dosage, 1–3 mEq/kg/day divided q8h).
• Once serum potassium has normalized, administer a maintenance dosage (1.0 mEq/kg/day divided q12h).
• Parenteral supplementation—in patients with anorexia or vomiting, parenteral supplementation is required. Potassium chloride is added to maintenance fluid therapy according to the schedule below and is adjusted according to the patient's response. *Do not exceed an intravenous rate of 0.5 mEq/kg/hr.* At high rates of supplementation, an infusion pump is required to avoid overdosage.

SERUM K^+ SUPPLEMENT (MEQ/L)
3.5–4.5	20
3.0–3.5	30
2.5–3.0	40
2.0–2.5	60
< 2.0	80

CONTRAINDICATIONS
Avoid sodium bicarbonate, insulin, and glucose (if possible) in patients with severe hypokalemia.

PRECAUTIONS
See above

POSSIBLE INTERACTIONS
Potassium supplementation in conjunction with ACE inhibitor, potassium-sparing diuretic, prostaglandin inhibitor, or beta blocker may cause hyperkalemia.

ALTERNATIVE DRUG(S)
Potassium phosphate is used in patients with concurrent hypophosphatemia. Dosage is based on phosphate content (see Phosphorus, Hypophosphatemia).

FOLLOW-UP

PATIENT MONITORING
Serum potassium with the frequency dictated by the degree of hypokalemia and the severity of clinical signs

POSSIBLE COMPLICATIONS
Arrhythmias

✔ MISCELLANEOUS

ASSOCIATED CONDITIONS
• Hypomagnesemia
• Hypophosphatemia

AGE-RELATED FACTORS
N/A

ZOONOTIC POTENTIAL
N/A

PREGNANCY
N/A

SYNONYMS
N/A

SEE ALSO
See Causes

ABBREVIATIONS
• ACE = angiotensin converting enzyme
• CO_2 = carbon dioxide
• ECF = extracellular fluid
• ICF = intracellular fluid
• K^+ = potassium
• PU/PD = polyuria/polydipsia

Suggested Reading
DiBartola SP, Autran de Morais HS. Disorders of potassium: hypokalemia and hyperkalemia. In: DiBartola SP, ed. Fluid therapy in small animal practice. Philadelphia: Saunders, 1992:89–115.
DiBartola SP, Green RA, Autran de Morais HS. Electrolytes and acid-base. In: Willard MD, Tvedten H, Turnwald GH, eds. Small animal clinical diagnosis by laboratory methods. 2nd ed. Philadelphia: Saunders, 1994:97–113.
Willard MD. Disorders of potassium homeostasis. Vet Clin North Am Small Anim Pract 1989;19:241–263.
Author Melissa S. Wallace
Consulting Editor Deborah S. Greco

HYPOMAGNESEMIA

 BASICS

DEFINITION
- Dogs—serum magnesium < 1.89 mg/dL
- Cats—serum magnesium < 1.8 mg/dL

PATHOPHYSIOLOGY
- Magnesium—second only to potassium as the most abundant intracellular cation; most is found in bone (60%) and soft tissue (38%); most of the soft tissue magnesium resides in skeletal muscle and liver; required for many metabolic functions; an activator or catalyst for over 300 enzyme systems including phosphatases and enzymes that involve ATP
- Because only 1–2% of total magnesium resides in the extracellular compartment, serum magnesium concentration does not always reflect the whole-body magnesium status.
- Hypomagnesemia—many causes; incidence rates > 50% have been reported in critically ill human patients, but it has often been ignored in veterinary practice.
- Magnesium is an important cofactor in the sodium–potassium ATPase pump that maintains an electrical gradient across membranes; as a result, it plays an important role in the activity of electrically excitable tissues.
- Magnesium is also important in the production and elimination of acetylcholine; a low concentration of magnesium in the extracellular fluid can increase concentrations of acetylcholine at motor endplates and cause tetany.
- Interference with the electrical gradient can change resting membrane potentials and repolarization disturbances, resulting in neuromuscular and cardiac abnormalities.
- Magnesium regulates calcium movement into smooth muscle cells important to contractile strength and peripheral vascular tone.
- Hypomagnesemia can alter the functions of the skeletal muscles, resulting in tetany and a variety of myopathies seen in patients receiving cisplatin and other nephrotoxic drugs.
- Magnesium depletion can affect the membrane pump on cardiac cell membranes, resulting in the depolarization of cardiac cells and tachyarrhythmias; cardiac arrhythmias associated with hypomagnesemia include ventricular arrhythmias, torsades de pointes, QT prolongation, ST segment shortening, and widening of T waves; hypomagnesemia increases the risk of digoxin toxicity because both inhibit the membrane pump.
- Hypomagnesemia causes resistance to the effects of PTH and can increase the uptake of calcium into bone.

SYSTEMS AFFECTED
- Multiple organ systems
- Gastrointestinal
- Renal
- Endocrine

SIGNALMENT
Dog and cat

SIGNS
- Hypomagnesemia occurs with a variety of diseases with diverse signs:
- Weakness
- Muscle fibrillation
- Ataxia and depression
- Hyperreflexia
- Tetany
- Behavior changes
- Arrhythmias

CAUSES
- Four general categories—gastrointestinal, renal, endocrine, and miscellaneous
- Severe malnutrition or significant malabsorptive intestinal diseases can lead to hypomagnesemia; hypomagnesemia can occur after excessive loss of body fluids (e.g., severe, prolonged diarrhea); magnesium is found in high concentration in the lower gastrointestinal tract, so secretory diarrhea in humans has been associated with profound hypomagnesemia; this is not well documented in veterinary patients.
- Magnesium homeostasis is regulated by the kidney; renal control of tubular reabsorption takes place primarily in the ascending limb of the loop of Henle; renal magnesium loss can be due to nephrotoxic drugs, including cisplatin, aminoglycosides, and amphotericin B; magnesium reabsorption can also be impaired with osmotic diuresis (diabetes mellitus), loop diuretics, hypercalciuria, and tubular acidosis.
- Hypomagnesemia associated with diuretic administration is a significant problem in human heart failure patients but has not been noted in animals.
- Endocrine problems associated with hypomagnesemia include hypercalcemia, hyperthyroidism, and hyperparathyroidism.
- Magnesium can be redistributed by refeeding after starvation, insulin therapy in diabetic ketoacidotic patients, parathyroidectomy, use of a total parenteral nutrition formulation with inadequate magnesium content, and in patients with acute pancreatitis.
- Causes of hypomagnesemia in the critically ill include decreased intake, lack of magnesium in parenteral fluids in patients receiving long-term fluid therapy or dialysis, excessive gastrointestinal loss, redistribution, and sequestration.

- Hypomagnesemia is associated with diabetes mellitus, especially following aggressive insulin therapy for diabetic ketoacidosis; nearly 25% of human diabetic outpatients were found to have low serum magnesium.

RISK FACTORS
- Total parenteral nutrition
- Diuretic administration
- Peritoneal dialysis
- Intestinal lymphangiectasia
- Diabetes mellitus

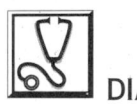 **DIAGNOSIS**

DIFFERENTIAL DIAGNOSIS
- Signs of hypomagnesemia are vague and multisystemic, and other causes of neuromuscular abnormalities, especially other electrolyte abnormalities, must be investigated.
- Consider cardiac abnormalities, intoxications, and renal diseases.

LABORATORY FINDINGS
Note: 12 mg of magnesium = 1 mEq of magnesium; to convert from mg/dL to mEq/L, divide by 1.2.

Drugs That May Alter Laboratory Results
- Serum is favored over plasma because the anticoagulant used for plasma samples can contain citrate or other ions that bind magnesium.
- EDTA, sodium fluoride–oxalate, sodium citrate, and intravenous calcium gluconate can cause falsely decreased serum magnesium values.

Disorders That May Alter Laboratory Results
- Hemolysis can falsely elevate serum magnesium.
- Hypercalcemia (> 16 mg/dL) and hyperproteinemia (> 10.0 g/dL) can also falsely elevate serum magnesium.
- Hyperbilirubinemia and lipemia can cause false decreases in serum magnesium.

Valid if Run in Human Laboratory?
Yes

CBC/BIOCHEMISTRY/URINALYSIS
- Serum magnesium < 1.89 mg/dL
- If patient is azotemic, consider renal causes.
- Tubular casts in urinary sediment may indicate nephrotoxicity.
- Hypokalemia, hyponatremia, and hypocalcemia are common findings, regardless of the cause of hypomagnesemia; because serum magnesium is not routinely measured, hypokalemia or hyponatremia should alert the clinician to the possibility of hypomagnesemia.

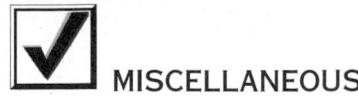
OTHER LABORATORY TESTS

- The diagnosis of magnesium depletion can be difficult since < 1% of total body magnesium is located in serum; only 55% of the magnesium in plasma is in the active (ionized) form; 33% is bound to plasma proteins and 12% is chelated with divalent anions such as phosphate and sulfate; magnesium assays (spectrophotometry) measure all three fractions.
- Ionized magnesium can be measured with an ion-specific electrode or by ultrafiltration of plasma; alternative methods of evaluating magnesium status include mononuclear blood cell magnesium levels or quantifying retention from a loading dose.
- Urinary magnesium determination may help differentiate conditions associated with high urinary magnesium loss from conditions of low intake or absorption.
- Human studies suggest that retention of > 40–50% of an administered magnesium load indicates magnesium depletion, while retention of < 20% indicates adequate magnesium stores.

IMAGING
N/A

DIAGNOSTIC PROCEDURES
Electrodiagnostics (e.g., electromyelography and electrocardiography) may reveal effects of hypomagnesemia but will not help differentiate the cause.

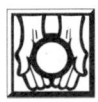

TREATMENT

- Treatment depends on the underlying cause of the abnormality and the severity of hypomagnesemia.
- Since experience in treating veterinary patients with hypomagnesemia is extremely limited, recommendations are difficult.
- Mild hypomagnesemia may resolve with treatment of the underlying disorder; however, if hypomagnesemia is severe, intensive care is needed.

MEDICATIONS

DRUG(S) OF CHOICE
Can dilute magnesium sulfate in 5% dextrose in water and administer 0.75–1 mEq/kg/day as a constant-rate intravenous infusion; the solution of magnesium sulfate should be less than 20%; the magnesium infusion should use a separate intravenous line to minimize interactions with other minerals.

CONTRAINDICATIONS
- Do not use aminoglycosides; hypomagnesemia potentiates their nephrotoxicity.
- Do not use cisplatin chemotherapy.

PRECAUTIONS
- Discontinue digoxin if possible.
- Use diuretics with caution.
- Hypermagnesemia is possible with overzealous treatment.
- Azotemic patients requiring magnesium therapy should receive a lower dose and more frequent monitoring than patients with normal kidney function, to prevent iatrogenic hypermagnesemia.

POSSIBLE INTERACTIONS
- Magnesium sulfate is incompatible with sodium bicarbonate, hydrocortisone, and dobutamine HCl; avoid mixing other drugs with magnesium sulfate solution.
- Avoid calcium-containing compounds; they lower the serum magnesium concentration.
- Additive CNS depression can occur when parenteral magnesium sulfate is used with CNS depressant sedatives, neuromuscular blocking agents, and anesthetics.
- Parenteral magnesium sulfate used with nondepolarizing neuromuscular blocking agents has caused excessive neuromuscular blockade.
- Use magnesium supplementation cautiously with digitalis compounds to avoid serious conduction disturbances.
- Calcium supplements may negate the effects of parenteral magnesium.

ALTERNATIVE DRUG(S)
N/A

FOLLOW-UP

PATIENT MONITORING
- Serum magnesium and calcium concentrations daily
- ECG continuously, especially during magnesium infusion

POSSIBLE COMPLICATIONS
Severe hypomagnesemia can be fatal.

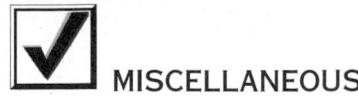

MISCELLANEOUS

ASSOCIATED CONDITIONS
- Hypokalemia
- Hyponatremia
- Hypocalcemia
- Hypophosphatemia

AGE-RELATED FACTORS
N/A

ZOONOTIC POTENTIAL
N/A

PREGNANCY
Effects on the fetus are identical to the effects on the dam.

SYNONYMS
None

SEE ALSO
See Causes.

ABBREVIATIONS
- ATP = adenosine triphosphate
- CNS = central nervous system
- EDTA = ethylene diamine tetraacetic acid
- PTH = parathyroid hormone

Suggested Reading

Dhupa N. Magnesium therapy. In: Bonagura JD, ed. Kirk's current veterinary therapy XII. Philadelphia: Saunders, 1995:132–133.

Flanders JA, Neth S, Erb HN, et al. Functional analysis of ectopic parathyroid activity in cats. Am J Vet Res 1991; 52:1336–1340.

Hebert P, Mehta N, Wang J, et al. Functional magnesium deficiency in critically ill patients identified using a magnesium-loading test. Crit Care Med 1997;25:749–755.

Macintire DK. Disorders of potassium, phosphorus, and magnesium in critical illness. Compend Cont Educ 1997; 19:41–48.

Marino PL. Magnesium. In: Marino PL, ed. The ICU book. Baltimore: Williams & Wilkins, 1998:660–672.

Martin LG, Wingfield WE, Van Pelt DR, et. al. Magnesium in the 1990's: Implications for veterinary critical care. J Vet Emerg Crit Care 1993;3:105–114.

Martin LG, Matteson VL, Wingfield WE, et al. Abnormalities of serum magnesium in critically ill dogs: incidence and implications. J Vet Emerg Crit Care 1994;4:15–20.

Rosol TJ, Capen CC. Calcium-regulating hormones and diseases of abnormal mineral metabolism. In: Kaneko JJ, Harvey JW, Bruss MJ, eds. Clinical biochemistry of domestic animals. 5th ed. San Diego: Academic Press, 1997:674–687.

Author Tim Hackett
Consulting Editor Deborah S. Greco

HYPOMYELINATION

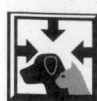

BASICS

DEFINITION
• Congenital condition caused by insufficient myelin production
• All axons > 1–2 mm in diameter are invested with a covering of myelin that arises from oligodendrocytes in the CNS and Schwann cells in the PNS.
• Myelin insulates axons and facilitates propagation of action potentials.

SIGNALMENT

CNS
• Dogs & cats
• Welsh springer spaniels, Samoyeds, chow chows, Weimaraners, Bernese mountain dogs, Dalmatians, and lurchers (an English cross-breed)—reported in dogs
• Siamese cats
• Predominant sex—springer spaniels and Samoyed male puppies clinically affected, whereas females remain largely asymptomatic carriers; no sex differences reported in other breeds

PNS
• Dogs
• Golden retrievers—reported in both sexes

SIGNS

CNS
• Clinical signs appear within days of birth.
• Generalized body tremors that worsen with exercise and subside during rest
• Improve by 1 year of age, except for springer spaniels and Samoyeds, which are affected for life

PNS
• Clinical signs appear at 5–7 weeks of age.
• Generalized weakness, pelvic limb ataxia, muscle wasting, and hyporeflexia
• Improve with age

CAUSES & RISK FACTORS
• Genetic—sex-linked recessive condition proven for CNS disease in springer spaniels; speculative for other breeds
• Viral or toxic—possible in chow chows, Weimaraners, Bernese mountain dogs, Dalmatians, and lurchers because clinical signs of CNS disease improve or resolve
• PNS—undetermined; possibly genetic

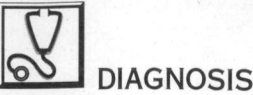

DIAGNOSIS

DIFFERENTIAL DIAGNOSIS

CNS
• Cerebellar hypoplasia or abiotrophy—tremors in neonates; but ataxia and intention tremors more prominent
• Storage diseases—associated with tremors; neonates are normal.
• Idiopathic tremors in white dogs do not develop before 8 months of age.

PNS
• Muscular dystrophy
• Congenital myasthenia gravis
• Other polyneuropathies or myopathies

CBC/BIOCHEMISTRY/URINALYSIS
Usually normal

OTHER LABORATORY TESTS
N/A

IMAGING
MRI—detect CNS form

DIAGNOSTIC PROCEDURES

CNS
- Diagnosis based on clinical signs
- Brain biopsy
- Necropsy

PNS
- Electromyography—usually normal to mild diffuse spontaneous activity
- Motor nerve conduction velocity—small or no evoked potentials and slowed conduction
- Nerve biopsy—insufficient myelin surrounding peripheral axons

 TREATMENT
- None effective for either form

 MEDICATIONS

DRUG(S)
N/A

CONTRAINDICATIONS/POSSIBLE INTERACTIONS
N/A

 FOLLOW-UP

PREVENTION/AVOIDANCE
Avoid breeding animals in which a genetic cause is suspected.

EXPECTED COURSE AND PROGNOSIS
- CNS—springer spaniels and Samoyeds affected for life; other breeds improve by 1 year of age
- PNS—dogs have normal lifespan

 MISCELLANEOUS

ABBREVIATIONS
CNS = central nervous system
MRI = magnetic resonance imaging
PNS = peripheral nervous system

Suggested Reading

Braund KG, Mehta JR, Toivio-Kinnucan M, Amling KA, Shell LG, Matz ME. Congenital hypomyelinating polyneuropathy in two golden retriever littermates. Vet Pathol 1989;26:202–208.

Duncan ID. Abnormalities of myelination of the central nervous system associated with congenital tremor. J Vet Intern Med 1987;1:10–23.

Matz ME, Shell L, Braund K. Peripheral hypomyelinization in two golden retriever litter mates. J Am Vet Med Assoc 1990; 197:228–230.

Stoffregen DA, Huxtable CR, Cummings JF, et al. Hypomyelination of the central nervous system of two Siamese kitten littermates. Vet Pathol 1993;30:388–391.

Author Karen Dyer Inzana
Consulting Editor Joane M. Parent

HYPONATREMIA

 BASICS

DEFINITION
Serum sodium concentration below the lower limit of normal. Usually associated with low total body sodium

PATHOPHYSIOLOGY
Sodium is the most abundant cation in the extracellular fluid and, therefore, hyponatremia usually reflects hypoosmolality. Either solute loss or water retention can theoretically cause hyponatremia. Most solute loss occurs in isoosmotic solutions (e.g., vomit and diarrhea) and, as a result, water retention in relation to solute is the underlying cause in almost all patients with hyponatremia. In general, hyponatremia occurs only when a defect in renal water excretion is present.

SYSTEMS AFFECTED
Nervous—severe neurologic dysfunction is not usually seen until serum sodium concentration falls below 110–115 mEq/L. Overly rapid correction of hyponatremia can also cause neurologic damage.

SIGNALMENT
Dogs and cats.

SIGNS
• Lethargy
• Seizures
• Obtundation
• Coma
• Other findings depend on the underlying cause.

CAUSES
Disorders Associated with Normal Renal Water Excretion
• Primary polydipsia
• Reset osmostat

Disorders Associated with Reduced Renal Water Excretion
• Low effective circulating volume—gastrointestinal losses, renal losses (including mineralocorticoid deficiency), skin losses, and edematous states (e.g., heart failure, end stage liver disease, and nephrotic syndrome)
• Diuretic administration
• Renal failure
• ADH excess with normovolemia—syndrome of inappropriate ADH secretion, hypocortisolemia, and hypothyroidism
• Low solute intake

RISK FACTORS
N/A

 DIAGNOSIS

DIFFERENTIAL DIAGNOSIS
N/A

LABORATORY FINDINGS
Drugs That May Alter Lab Results
Mannitol can cause pseudohyponatremia.

Disorders That May Alter Lab Results
Hyperlipidemia, hyperglycemia, and hyperproteinemia can cause pseudohyponatremia.

Valid if Run in a Human Laboratory?
Yes

CBC/BIOCHEMISTRY/URINALYSIS
• Low serum sodium concentration.
• Other abnormalities may point to the underlying cause.

OTHER LABORATORY TESTS
• Plasma osmolality is low; if plasma osmolality is normal or high, exclude renal failure or causes of pseudohyponatremia (e.g., hyperlipidemia, hyperglycemia, hyperproteinemia, and mannitol administration).
• Urine osmolality < 100–150 mosmol/kg indicates primary polydipsia or reset osmostat. Urine osmolality > 150–200 mosmol/kg indicates impaired renal water excretion.
• Urine sodium concentration < 15–20 mEq/L indicates low effective circulating volume, pure cortisol deficiency, primary polydipsia with high urine output. Urine sodium concentration > 20 to 25 mEq/L indicates syndrome of inappropriate ADH secretion, adrenal insufficiency, renal failure, reset osmostat, diuretic administration, or vomiting with marked bicarbonate loss.

IMAGING
N/A

DIAGNOSTIC PROCEDURES
N/A

PATHOLOGIC FINDINGS
N/A

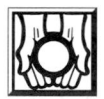 **TREATMENT**

INPATIENT VERSUS OUTPATIENT
Depends on severity of hyponatremia, associated neurologic dysfunction, and the underlying disorder

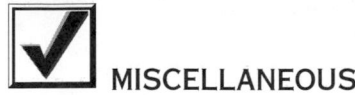
DIET
N/A

CLIENT EDUCATION
Depends on the underlying disorder

SURGICAL CONSIDERATIONS
N/A

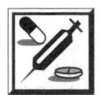 **MEDICATIONS**

DRUG(S)
Treatment consists of increasing the serum sodium concentration and treating the underlying cause. Hyponatremia is corrected by administering NaCl if the patient has hypovolemia (e.g., volume depletion, adrenal insufficiency, and diuretic administration) and by restricting water if the patient has normovolemia or edema (e.g., renal failure, SIADH, primary polydipsia, and edematous states). Hypertonic saline administration is usually indicated if the patient has clinical signs or serum sodium concentration < 105–110 mEq/L. The sodium deficit is estimated by 0.5 × lean BW (kg) × (120 − serum sodium concentration). If the patient has no to mild clinical signs, increase sodium concentration at a rate of 0.5 mEq/L per hour until sodium concentration is 120–125 mEq/L, then discontinue hypertonic saline and normalize serum sodium concentration over several days with isotonic saline or water restriction as dictated by the cause of hyponatremia. If the patient has seizures or coma, a rate of 1–1.5 mEq/L per hour for the first 10 mEq/L may be indicated. True volume depletion must also be corrected. In edematous patients with symptomatic hyponatremia, administration of a loop diuretic in addition to hypertonic saline may be necessary. Other medications are dictated by the underlying cause.

CONTRAINDICATIONS
N/A

PRECAUTIONS
Overly rapid correction of hyponatremia can result in neurologic damage (demyelination); avoid increasing serum sodium concentration by more than 25 mEq/L in the first 48 hours.

POSSIBLE INTERACTIONS
N/A

 FOLLOW-UP

PATIENT MONITORING
Serum electrolyte concentrations as needed to assure appropriate response to NaCl and other indicated therapies

PREVENTION/AVOIDANCE
Depends on the underlying disorder

POSSIBLE COMPLICATIONS
Depends on the underlying disorder

EXPECTED COURSE AND PROGNOSIS
Depends on the underlying disorder

✓ **MISCELLANEOUS**

ASSOCIATED CONDITIONS
Other electrolyte and acid–base abnormalities are often associated with the clinical disorders that cause hyponatremia.

AGE-RELATED FACTORS
Depends on the underlying cause

ZOONOTIC POTENTIAL
N/A

PREGNANCY
N/A

SYNONYMS
N/A

SEE ALSO
N/A

ABBREVIATIONS
ADH = antidiuretic hormone
SIADH = syndrome of inappropriate ADH secretion

Suggested Reading
DiBartola SP. Fluid therapy in small animal practice. Philadelphia: Saunders, 1992.
Rose DB. Clinical physiology of acid–base and electrolyte disorders. 3rd ed. New York: McGraw-Hill, 1989.
Author Peter P. Kintzer
Consulting Editor Deborah S. Greco

HYPOPARATHYROIDISM

 **BASICS**

DEFINITION
Absolute or relative deficiency of parathyroid hormone secretion leading to hypocalcemia

PATHOPHYSIOLOGY
• Dogs—most commonly idiopathic immune-mediated parathyroiditis • Cats—most commonly iatrogenic secondary to damaged or removed parathyroid glands during thyroidectomy for hyperthyroidism; idiopathic atrophy and immune-mediated parathyroiditis also seen (uncommon)

SYSTEMS AFFECTED
• Nervous/neuromuscular—seizures, tetany, ataxia, and weakness caused by increased neuromuscular activity resulting from diminished neuronal membrane stability
• Cardiovascular—ECG changes and bradycardia caused by altered neuromuscular activity
• Gastrointestinal—anorexia and vomiting (especially cats) of unknown cause, possibly changes in gastrointestinal muscular activity
• Ophthalmic—posterior lenticular cataracts of unknown cause • Respiratory—panting caused by neuromuscular weakness and anxiety associated with neurologic and neuromuscular changes • Renal/urologic—polyuria and polydipsia (PU/PD) of unknown cause

INCIDENCE/PREVALENCE
• Dogs—uncommon; exact prevalence not reported • Cats—common in thyroidectomized cats (10–82% of patients, depending on surgical technique and surgical skill); spontaneous occurrence rare (6 cases reported)

SIGNALMENT

Species
Dogs and cats

Breed Predilections
Toy poodle, miniature schnauzer, German shepherd, Labrador retriever, and Scottish terrier; mixed-breed cats

Mean Age and Range
• Dogs—mean age, 6 years; range, 6 weeks to 12 years • Cats—secondary to thyroidectomy: mean age 12–13 years, range 4–22 years; spontaneous: mean age 2.25 years, range 6 months to 6.7 years

Predominant Sex
• Dogs—female • Cats—none

SIGNS

Dogs
• Seizures (54–73%) • Muscle trembling, twitching, and fasciculations (54%) • Tense, splinted abdomen (50%) • Ataxia/stiff gait (43%) • Fever (30–40%) • Panting (35%)
• Posterior lenticular cataracts (15–20%)
• Weakness • PU/PD • Facial rubbing
• Vomiting • Anorexia • Up to 20% may have normal physical examination results

Cats (based on 6 reported cases)
• Lethargy, anorexia, and depression (100%)
• Seizures (50%) • Muscle trembling, twitching, and fasciculations (83%) • Panting (33%)
• Posterior lenticular cataracts (33%)
• Bradycardia (17%) • Fever (17%)
• Hypothermia (17%)

RISK FACTORS
• Dogs—N/A • Cats—thyroidectomy for hyperthyroidism

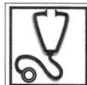 **DIAGNOSIS**

DIFFERENTIAL DIAGNOSIS
The main problems associated with hypoparathyroidism, which must be differentiated from other disease processes, are seizures, weakness, and muscle trembling, twitching, and fasciculations.

Seizures
• Cardiovascular—syncope • Metabolic—hepatoencephalopathy and hypoglycemia
• Neurologic—epilepsy, neoplasia, toxin, and inflammatory disease

Weakness
• Cardiovascular—congenital anatomic defects, arrhythmias, heart failure, and pericardial effusion • Metabolic—hypoadrenocorticism, hypoglycemia, anemia, hypokalemia (especially cats), and hypothyroidism
• Neurologic/neuromuscular—myasthenia gravis, polymyositis, polyradiculoneuropathy, and spinal cord disease • Toxic—tick paralysis, botulism, chronic organophosphate exposure, and lead poisoning

Muscle Trembling, Twitching, and Fasciculations
• Metabolic—hypercalcemia, hyperadrenocorticism, and puerperal tetany (i.e., eclampsia) • Toxic—tetanus and strychnine poisoning

CBC/BIOCHEMISTRY/URINALYSIS
• Results of hemogram and urinalysis usually normal; these tests are performed to rule out other differential diagnoses • Hypocalcemia (usually <6.5 mg/dL) and normal or mild to moderate hyperphosphatemia • Evaluate serum albumin carefully in all patients with hypocalcemia; hypoalbuminemia is the most common cause of hypocalcemia; in dogs with hypoalbuminemia, one of the following formulas should be used to correct the serum calcium:

$$\text{Corrected Ca} = \text{Ca (mg/dL)} - \text{albumin (g/dL)} + 3.5$$

or

$$\text{Corrected Ca} = \text{Ca (mg/dL)} - [0.4 \times \text{total protein (g/dL)}] + 3.3$$

• Hypocalcemia caused by hypoalbuminemia in cats cannot be corrected by these formulas, although hypoalbuminemia causes reduced serum calcium in cats. • The only other disease process that reduces serum calcium and raises serum phosphorus is renal failure, which is easily distinguished from hypoparathyroidism by the presence of azotemia.

OTHER LABORATORY TESTS
Serum PTH determination—demonstrates undetectable or very low concentration of PTH; patients with other processes causing hypocalcemia (e.g., renal failure) have a normal-to-high concentration of PTH.

IMAGING
Radiography and ultrasonography are normal

DIAGNOSTIC PROCEDURES
• ECG changes seen in patients with hypocalcemia include prolongation of the ST and QT segments; sinus bradycardia and wide T waves or T wave alternans is occasionally seen.
• Cervical exploration reveals absence or atrophy of the parathyroid glands.

PATHOLOGIC FINDINGS
• Dogs—normal tissue with mature lymphocytes, plasma cells, and fibrous connective tissue along with chief cell degeneration
• Cats—parathyroid gland atrophy is more common, although histopathologic findings similar to those in dogs were found in one cat

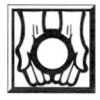 **TREATMENT**

APPROPRIATE HEALTH CARE
• Hospitalize for medical management of hypocalcemia until clinical signs of hypocalcemia are controlled and serum calcium concentration is >7.0 mg/dL. • See Hypocalcemia for emergency inpatient management and appropriate fluid therapy.

 MEDICATIONS

DRUG(S)

Emergency/Acute Therapy
See Hypocalcemia.

Short-term Post-tetany Therapy
See Hypocalcemia.

Long-term Therapy
• Vitamin D administration is needed indefinitely; The dosage should be increased or tapered on the basis of serum calcium concentration. • Shorter-acting preparations of vitamin D are preferred so that overdosage (hypercalcemia) can be quickly corrected (see Table 1). • A more economical approach to treatment is to maximize oral administration of calcium and reduce oral administration of vitamin D; calcium is usually less expensive than vitamin D (see Table 2).

PRECAUTIONS

All calcium preparations given orally can cause gastrointestinal disturbances; calcium carbonate may be less irritating because of its high calcium availability and lower dosage requirement.

POSSIBLE INTERACTIONS

• Injectable calcium solutions are reportedly incompatible with tetracycline drugs, cephalothin, methylprednisolone sodium succinate, dobutamine, metoclopramide, and amphotericin B. • Thiazide diuretics used in conjunction with large doses of calcium may cause hypercalcemia. • Patients on digitalis are more likely to develop arrhythmias if calcium is administered intravenously. • Calcium administration may antagonize effects of calcium channel blocking agents (e.g., diltiazem, verapamil, nifedipine, and amlodipine).

 FOLLOW-UP

PATIENT MONITORING

• Hypocalcemia and hypercalcemia are both concerns with long-term management.
• Serum calcium concentration monthly for the first 6 months then every 2–4 months; goal is to maintain serum calcium between 8 and 10 mg/dL.

• Inform clients about clinical signs of hypo- and hypercalcemia.

POSSIBLE COMPLICATIONS
• Hypocalcemia
• Hypercalcemia, which can lead to renal failure (see Hypercalcemia)

EXPECTED COURSE AND PROGNOSIS
• With close monitoring of serum calcium and client dedication, the prognosis for long-term survival is excellent.
• Adjustments in vitamin D and oral calcium administration can be expected during the course of management, especially during the initial 2–6 months.
• Cats with hypoparathyroidism secondary to thyroidectomy usually require only transient treatment because they typically regain normal parathyroid function within 4–6 months, often within 2–3 weeks.

 MISCELLANEOUS

ASSOCIATED CONDITIONS
Excess muscular activity can lead to hyperthermia, which may necessitate treatment.

PREGNANCY
Hypocalcemia can lead to weakness and dystocia.

SEE ALSO
• Hypercalcemia • Hyperthyroidism
• Hypocalcemia

ABBREVIATIONS
• Ca = calcium
• ECG = electrocardiography
• PTH = parathyroid hormone
• PU/PD = polyuria and polydipsia

Suggested Reading

Bruyette DS, Feldman EC. Primary hypoparathyroidism in the dog. Report of 15 cases and review of 13 previously reported cases. J Vet Intern Med 1988;2:7–14.

Feldman EC, Nelson RW. Hypocalcemia and primary hypoparathyroidism. In: Feldman EC, Nelson RW, eds. Canine and feline endocrinology and reproduction. Philadelphia: WB Saunders, 1996:497–516.

Peterson ME, James KM, Wallace M, et al. Idiopathic hypoparathyroidism in five cats. J Vet Intern Med 1991;5:47–51.

Waters CB, Scott-Moncrieff JCR. Hypocalcemia in cats. Compend Contin Educ Pract Vet 1992;14:497–507.

Author Mitchell A. Crystal
Consulting Editor Deborah S. Greco

Table 1

Vitamin D Preparations			
Preparation	*Dose*	*Maximal Effect*	*Size*
1,25 Dihydroxycholecalciferol (active vitamin D_3, calcitriol)	0.005–0.015 µg/kg/day	1–4 days	0.25 and 0.5 µg capsules and 1.0 µg/ml oral solution
Dihydrotachysterol	Initial: 0.02–0.03 mg/kg/day Maint: 0.01–0.02 mg/kg/24–48 h	1–7 days	0.125, 0.2, 0.4 mg capsules and 0.2 mg/mL syrup
Ergocalciferol (vitamin D_2)	Initial: 4000–6000 U/kg/day Maint: 1000–2000 U/kg/day-week	5–21 days	25,000 and 50,000 U capsules and 8,000 U/mL syrup

Table 2

Calcium Preparations			
Preparation	*Dose*	*Available Calcium*	*Size Available*
Calcium carbonate	Canine: 1–4 g/day Feline: 0.5–1 g/day	40%	250–1500 mg tablets and 125 mg capsules
Calcium gluconate	Canine: 1–4 g/day Feline: 0.5–1 g/day	10%	500–1000 mg tablets
Calcium lactate	Canine: 1–4 g/day Feline: 0.5–1 g/day	13%	325, 650 mg tablets and 500 mg capsules
Calcium acetate	Canine: 1–4 g/day Feline: 0.5–1 g/day	25%	667 mg tablets
Calcium citrate	Canine: 1–4 g/day Feline: 0.5–1 g/day	21%	250, 950 mg tablets

HYPOPHOSPHATEMIA

 **BASICS**

DEFINITION
Serum phosphorus concentration < 2.5 mg/dL

PATHOPHYSIOLOGY
• A low phosphorus concentration can be caused by shifts of phosphorus from the extracellular fluid into body cells, reduced intestinal absorption of phosphorus, or reduced renal phosphorus reabsorption.
• Because phosphorus is an important component of ATP, low serum phosphorus concentration can cause ATP depletion and affect cells that are high energy users, including RBCs, skeletal muscle cells, and brain cells.

SYSTEMS AFFECTED
• Hemic/Lymphatic/Immune—hemolysis
• Musculoskeletal—weakness and respiratory paralysis
• Nervous—seizures

SIGNALMENT
Dog and cat

SIGNS

Historical Findings
Consistent with the primary disease responsible for the hypophosphatemia rather than relating to the phosphate concentration itself

Physical Examination Findings
• Pallor from hemolytic anemia (severe hypophosphatemia)
• Red or dark-colored urine due to hemoglobinuria—severe hypophosphatemia
• Tachypnea, dyspnea, and anxiety secondary to hypoxia
• Muscle weakness
• Mental depression
• Rapid, shallow respirations because of poor respiratory muscle function

CAUSES
• Laboratory error
• Mannitol administration
• Transcellular shift (maldistribution)—enteral nutrition and total parenteral nutrition; diabetes mellitus; carbohydrate loading with insulin administration; respiratory alkalosis
• Reduced intestinal absorption of phosphorus—phosphorus-poor diet; vitamin D deficiency; phosphate-binding agent; malabsorption syndrome
• Reduced renal phosphate reabsorption—primary hyperparathyroidism; renal tubular defects (e.g., Fanconi's syndrome); hyperadrenocorticism; proximal tubular diuretics (e.g., carbonic anhydrase inhibitors); hypocalcemic tetany (eclampsia); sodium bicarbonate administration

RISK FACTORS
• Undiagnosed or poorly regulated diabetes mellitus
• Prolonged anorexia, starvation, or malnutrition

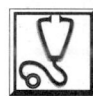 **DIAGNOSIS**

DIFFERENTIAL DIAGNOSIS
• Severe hypophosphatemia (< 1.0 mg/dL) is seen most often as a complication of diabetic ketoacidosis; monitor severely ill diabetics closely during the first few days of treatment for the development of hypophosphatemia.
• Patients with prolonged anorexia, starvation, or severe intestinal malabsorption may develop hypophosphatemia if given hyperalimentation, especially if the formulas have marginal phosphorus content.

LABORATORY FINDINGS

Drugs That May Alter Laboratory Results
Mannitol interferes with analysis, falsely lowering serum phosphorus concentration.

Disorders That May Alter Laboratory Results
Hemolysis, hyperlipidemia, and hyperproteinemia may falsely elevate serum phosphorus.

Valid if Run in Human Laboratory?
Yes

CBC/BIOCHEMISTRY/URINALYSIS
• Concurrent findings of hyperglycemia, glucosuria, ketonuria, and a high anion gap metabolic acidosis confirm that the hypophosphatemia is a complication of diabetic ketoacidosis.
• Hypercalcemia in association with hypophosphatemia suggests primary hyperparathyroidism.
• Hypocalcemia with hypophosphatemia is reported in patients with eclampsia.
• Moderate hypophosphatemia with high serum alkaline phosphatase activity suggests hyperadrenocorticism.
• Panhypoproteinemia suggests an intestinal malabsorption disorder.
• Hypophosphatemia in association with glucosuria, normoglycemia, isosthenuria, or azotemia suggests a renal tubular defect such as Fanconi's syndrome.

OTHER LABORATORY TESTS
• PTH assay—useful to diagnose primary hyperparathyroidism
• Measurement of vitamin D metabolites, particularly cholecalciferol—useful to diagnose vitamin D deficiency

IMAGING
Radiology may reveal poor bone quality or pathologic fractures in patients with disorders of calcium, phosphorus, and vitamin D.

DIAGNOSTIC PROCEDURES
Exploratory surgery of the cervical region confirms hyperparathyroidism.

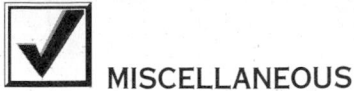

TREATMENT

• Hospitalize patients with severe hypophosphatemia (phosphorus concentration < 1.5 mg/dL) to observe for hemolysis and provide treatment as needed.
• If the condition is caused by initiation of insulin therapy or hyperalimentation, suspend these treatments until phosphate has been administered for a few hours.
• Obtain fresh whole blood in case a transfusion is required.
• Can evaluate patients with moderate hypophosphatemia (1.5–2.5) as outpatients if other conditions are stable
• If the serum phosphorus is < 1.5 mg/dL, administer a balanced electrolyte solution IV (e.g., 0.9% saline, lactated Ringer's solution, Normosol-R, or Plasma-Lyte), supplemented with either sodium or potassium phosphate.

MEDICATIONS

DRUG(S) OF CHOICE

• Potassium phosphate for injection has 3 mmol of phosphate and 4.4 mEq of potassium per milliliter; the dose of phosphate is 0.01–0.03 mmol/kg/h for 6 hours; however, many cats with diabetic ketoacidosis who develop hypophosphatemia require higher dosages and a longer duration of therapy; a rate of 0.06–0.12 mmol/kg/h for 6–24 hours is typical.
• Oral supplementation of phosphate may benefit animals with moderate hypophosphatemia; sodium and potassium phosphate powders and tablets are commercially available, but current dosing in veterinary medicine is empirical.

CONTRAINDICATIONS

• Avoid diuretics, especially carbonic anhydrase inhibitors.
• Avoid phosphate-poor enteral feeding formulas and total parenteral nutrition solutions in patients with hypophosphatemia and patients with predisposing disorders.

• Avoid intravenous supplementation of phosphate in hypercalcemic patients; precipitation of calcium and phosphate causes soft tissue mineralization and renal damage.

PRECAUTIONS

Oversupplementation, especially in patients with renal impairment or inadequate hydration, can cause hyperphosphatemia; acute hyperphosphatemia can result in hypocalcemia.

ALTERNATIVE DRUG(S)

If an oral or parenteral phosphate supplement is unavailable, skim or low-fat milk may be administered; this will be insufficient in severely affected patients.

FOLLOW-UP

PATIENT MONITORING

• Measure serum phosphorus every 12–24 hours until the concentration is stable within the normal range.
• If hyperphosphatemia develops, stop all supplementation and provide intravenous fluid diuresis until the phosphorus returns to normal.
• Administer calcium gluconate intravenously *only* if tetany from hypocalcemia develops.
• Monitor hyperphosphatemic animals for acute renal failure.
• Check the serum potassium concentration daily until stable.

POSSIBLE COMPLICATIONS

• Hemolysis from hypophosphatemia may be acute and severe, requiring transfusion; fresh blood is preferred over stored blood products because stored RBCs may use serum phosphate and exacerbate the condition.
• Cardiac arrest and respiratory failure are life-threatening complications of severe hypophosphatemia.
• Respiratory support with positive pressure ventilation is an option.
• See Patient Monitoring for other complications.

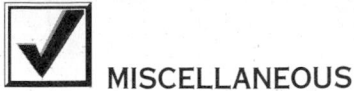

MISCELLANEOUS

ASSOCIATED CONDITIONS

Hypokalemia is often concurrent, especially in patients with diabetic ketoacidosis.

AGE-RELATED FACTORS

N/A

ZOONOTIC POTENTIAL

N/A

PREGNANCY

• Hypophosphatemia in the periparturient animal may be associated with hypocalcemia caused by secretion of PTH to mobilize calcium for neonatal bone growth and lactation.
• PTH promotes phosphaturia and hypophosphatemia.

SYNONYMS

N/A

SEE ALSO

• Diabetes with ketoacidosis
• Hyperparathyroidism

ABBREVIATIONS

• ALP = alkaline phosphatase
• ATP = adenosine triphosphate
• PTH = parathyroid hormone
• RBC = red blood cells

Suggested Reading

DiBartola SP. Disorders of phosphorus: hypophosphatemia and hyperphosphatemia. In: DiBartola SP, ed. Fluid therapy in small animal practice. Philadelphia: Saunders, 1992:177–191.
Forrester SD, Moreland RJ. Hypophosphatemia: causes and clinical consequences. J Vet Intern Med 1989;3:149–159.
Willard MD, Zerbe CA, Schall WD, et al. Severe hypophosphatemia associated with diabetes mellitus in six dogs and one cat. J Am Vet Med Assoc 1987;190:1007–1010.
Author Melissa S. Wallace
Consulting Editor Deborah S. Greco

HYPOPITUITARISM

 BASICS

OVERVIEW
• A condition resulting from destruction of the pituitary gland by a neoplastic, degenerative, or anomalous process
• Associated with low production of pituitary hormones including thyroid-stimulating hormone (TSH), adrenocorticotropin hormone (ACTH), luteinizing hormone, follicle-stimulating hormone, and growth hormone (GH)

SIGNALMENT
• Age: 2–6 months
• Breeds—German shepherd dog, Carnelian bear dog, spitz, toy pinscher, and Weimaraner
• Simple autosomal recessive in German shepherd dog and Carnelian bear dog

SIGNS

Historical Findings
• Mental retardation manifested as difficulty in house-breaking
• Slow growth noticed in first 2–3 months of life
• Proportionate dwarfism

Physical Examination Findings
• Retained puppy haircoat
• Thin, hypotonic skin
• Shrill bark
• Truncal alopecia
• Cutaneous hyperpigmentation
• Infantile genitalia
• Delayed dental eruption

CAUSES & RISK FACTORS

Congenital
• Cystic Rathke's pouch
• Isolated GH deficiency

Acquired
• Pituitary tumor
• Trauma
• Radiotherapy

 DIAGNOSIS

DIFFERENTIAL DIAGNOSIS
• Hypothyroid dwarfism; breed predilection and disproportionate dwarfism observed in patients with hypothyroidism.
• Other causes of stunted growth—portosystemic shunt, diabetes mellitus, hyperadrenocorticism, malnutrition, parasitism

CBC/BIOCHEMISTRY/URINALYSIS
• Eosinophilia
• Lymphocytosis
• Hypophosphatemia
• Hypoglycemia

OTHER LABORATORY TESTS
• Corticotropin and TSH response tests
• Subnormal response to TSH and ACTH
• Growth hormone and insulin-like growth factor assays
• Growth hormone assay not currently available in the U.S.; recommend measurement of IGF-1, which is low.

IMAGING
Radiography may reveal epiphyseal dysgenesis and abnormal retention of physeal growth plates.

DIAGNOSIS
N/A

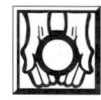 TREATMENT

Manage medically on an outpatient basis

 MEDICATIONS

DRUG(S)
• Growth hormone—human, porcine, or bovine, if available; 0.1 IU/kg SC 3 times weekly for 4–6 weeks; repeat if necessary.
• Treat hypothyroidism with levothyroxine (22 µg/kg PO q24h).
• Glucocorticoids (e.g., prednisone, 0.2 mg/kg PO q24h) if ACTH response test

results are subnormal; higher dosage of steroids is needed during periods of stress.

CONTRAINDICATIONS/POSSIBLE INTERACTIONS
Hypersensitivity reactions and carbohydrate intolerance may develop with growth hormone supplementation.

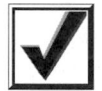 FOLLOW-UP

PATIENT MONITORING
• Blood and urinary glucose concentration
• Stop growth hormone supplementation if glucosuria develops or blood glucose is >150 mg/dL.

POSSIBLE COMPLICATIONS
Neurologic complications of expansion of Rathke's pouch

EXPECTED COURSE AND PROGNOSIS
• Skin and haircoat improve within 6–8 weeks of initiating growth hormone and thyroid supplementation.
• Generally no increase in stature because growth plates have usually closed by the time of diagnosis
• Dogs often die at a young age (3–4 years) because of neurologic complications.
• Poor long-term prognosis

✓ MISCELLANEOUS

SEE ALSO
• Hypothyroidism
• Hypoadrenocorticism (Addison's Disease)

ABBREVIATIONS
• ACTH = adrenocorticotropin
• GH = growth hormone
• TSH = thyroid-stimulating hormone

Suggested Reading
Campbell KL. Growth hormone-related disorders in dogs. Compend Cont Educ Pract Vet 1988;10:477–482.
Author Deborah S. Greco
Consulting Editor Deborah S. Greco

BASICS

OVERVIEW
• **Hypopyon**—accumulation of white blood cells in anterior chamber of eye. Inflammatory breakdown of blood-aqueous barrier allows entry of blood cells into anterior chamber. Cells often settle because of gravity, forming a fluid line in ventral anterior chamber. • **Lipid flare**—turbidity of anterior chamber caused by a high concentration of lipids in aqueous humor. Requires breakdown of blood–aqueous barrier and concurrent hyperlipidemia to occur

SIGNALMENT
Affects both dogs and cats; no age or sex predilection

SIGNS
Hypopyon—white to yellow opacity within anterior chamber; may be a ventral accumulation of cells or may completely fill anterior chamber. Concurrent ophthalmic signs include blepharospasm, epiphora, diffuse corneal edema, aqueous flare, miosis, iridal swelling, and vision loss.
Lipid flare—diffuse milky appearance to anterior chamber; usually obscures visualization of intraocular structures. Concurrent ophthalmic signs may include vision loss, mild blepharospasm, and mild to moderate diffuse corneal edema.

CAUSES & RISK FACTORS
Hypopyon
Any cause of uveitis can result in hypopyon. Most commonly, hypopyon is associated with severe uveitis. Hypopyon can also result from neoplastic cell accumulation in ocular lymphoma.

Lipid Flare
Lipid flare results from hyperlipidemia and concurrent breakdown of blood–aqueous barrier (due to uveitis). Hyperlipidemia may also destabilize blood–aqueous barrier directly. Postprandial lipemia may occasionally result in lipemic aqueous if uveitis is present.

DIAGNOSIS

DIFFERENTIAL DIAGNOSIS
Hypopyon
Fibrin in anterior chamber—generally forms an irregular clot, not a ventrally located horizontal line

Lipid Flare
• Severe aqueous flare—does not appear as milky/white as lipid flare. Animals with severe aqueous flare generally exhibit much more ocular pain than animals with lipid flare.
• Diffuse corneal edema—severe corneal edema may be confused with anterior chamber opacity, but corneal stromal thickening, keratoconus, and corneal bullae are noted with the former

CBC/BIOCHEMISTRY/URINALYSIS
Hypopyon
Often normal; abnormalities related to underlying cause of uveitis may be present

Lipid Flare
Elevated serum triglycerides and cholesterol; other abnormalities may be present related to underlying metabolic disorder(s)

OTHER LABORATORY TESTS
Hypopyon
None if hypopyon is related to obvious corneal disease; if related to uveitis, look for underlying cause of uveitis (see Anterior Uveitis—Dogs; Anterior Uveitis—Cats)

Lipid Flare
See Lipids/Hyperlipidemia.

DIAGNOSTIC PROCEDURES
Anterior chamber centesis indicated with suspicion of neoplastic origin of hypopyon (e.g., lymphoma); unrewarding under other circumstances

TREATMENT

• Hypopyon requires aggressive treatment for uveitis and underlying cause. Outpatient treatment is generally adequate. • Lipid flare requires treatment for uveitis (which is usually mild) and underlying metabolic disorder. Outpatient treatment is adequate.

MEDICATIONS

DRUG(S)
Hypopyon
Corticosteroids
Topical
• Prednisolone acetate 1%—apply 2–6 times daily, depending on severity of disease.
• Dexamethasone 0.1%—apply 2–6 times daily, depending on severity of disease. • Taper medication frequency as condition resolves.
Subconjunctival
• Triamcinolone acetonide—4–6 mg (dog); 4 mg (cat) by subconjunctival injection
• Methylprednisolone—3–10 mg (dog); 4 mg (cat) by subconjunctival injection
Indicated as one-time injection followed by topical and/or systemic antiinflammatories
Systemic
• Prednisone—0.5–2.2 mg/kg/day (dog); 1–3 mg/kg/day (cat); taper dose after 7–10 days. Only use if systemic infectious causes of uveitis have been ruled out.
Nonsteroidal Antiinflammatory Drugs
Topical
• Flurbiprofen—apply 2–4 times daily, depending on severity of disease.
• Diclofenac—apply 2–4 times daily, depending on severity of disease.
Systemic
• Carprofen–2.2 mg/kg PO BID (dog)
• Etodolac—10–15 mg/kg PO QD (dog)
• Aspirin—10–25 mg/kg PO BID (dog); 10 mg/kg PO q48hr (cat).
Do not use concurrently with systemic corticosteroids.
Topical mydriatic/cycloplegic
Atropine sulfate 1%—apply 1–4 times daily, depending on severity of disease. Use lowest frequency adequate to maintain dilated pupil and ocular comfort. Use ointment instead of solution in cats to minimize salivation.

Lipid Flare
Topical Corticosteroids
• Prednisolone acetate 1%—apply 2–4 times daily, depending on severity of disease.
• Dexamethasone 0.1%—apply 2–4 times daily, depending on severity of disease. • Taper medication frequency as condition resolves.
Topical Mydriatic/Cycloplegic
Atropine sulfate 1%—apply 1–2 times daily, if necessary for perceived ocular discomfort.

CONTRAINDICATIONS/POSSIBLE INTERACTIONS
• Avoid the use of miotic medications (e.g., pilocarpine, demecarium bromide, latanoprost) in presence of hypopyon or lipid flare. • Topical and subconjunctival corticosteroids contraindicated if ulcerative keratitis is the cause of hypopyon • Out of concern for secondary glaucoma, topical atropine should be used judiciously and IOP should be monitored periodically.

FOLLOW-UP

PATIENT MONITORING
Recheck in 2–3 days. Intraocular pressure should be monitored to detect secondary glaucoma. Frequency of subsequent rechecks dictated by severity of disease and response to treatment

EXPECTED COURSE AND PROGNOSIS
• Hypopyon—prognosis guarded; depends on underlying disease and response to treatment
• Lipid flare—prognosis good; generally responds quickly (within 24–72 hours) to moderate anti-inflammatory therapy; recurrence possible

MISCELLANEOUS

Suggested Reading
Slatter D. Uvea. In: Slatter D, ed. Fundamentals of veterinary ophthalmology, 3rd ed. Philadelphia: Saunders, 2001:314–349.
Author Ian P. Herring
Consulting Editor Paul E. Miller

HYPOSTHENURIA

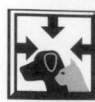 **BASICS**

DEFINITION
Urinary specific gravity between 1.000 and 1.006

PATHOPHYSIOLOGY
The ability to concentrate urine normally (dogs, >1.030; cats, >1.035) depends on a complex interaction between ADH, the protein receptor for ADH on the renal tubule, and a hypertonic renal medullary interstitium; interference with the synthesis, release, or actions of ADH, damage to the renal tubule, and altered tonicity of the medullary interstitium (medullary washout) can cause hyposthenuria.

SYSTEMS AFFECTED
Depends on the underlying disorder

GENETICS
N/A

INCIDENCE
N/A

GEOGRAPHIC DISTRIBUTION
N/A

SIGNALMENT

Species
Dogs and cats

Breed Predilection
None

Predominant Sex
None

Mean Age and Range
None

SIGNS
• Polyuria and polydipsia
• Urinary incontinence—occasional
• Other signs depend on the underlying disorder.

CAUSES
Any disorder or drug that interferes with the release or action of ADH, damages the renal tubule, causes medullary washout, or causes a primary thirst disorder (see Differential Diagnosis)

RISK FACTORS
N/A

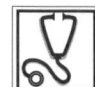 **DIAGNOSIS**

DIFFERENTIAL DIAGNOSIS
• Pyometra
• Cushing's disease
• Diabetes insipidus
• Pyelonephritis
• Hypercalcemia
• Early renal failure
• Primary liver disease
• Hypokalemia
• Hypoadrenocorticism
• Primary polydipsia—compulsive water drinking

LABORATORY FINDINGS

Drugs That May Alter Laboratory Results
Cortisone, lithium, demeclocycline, methoxyflurane, thiazide diuretics, and intravenous administration of fluids can all lower urine specific gravity into the hyposthenuric range.

Disorders That May Alter Laboratory Results
N/A

Valid If Run in a Human Laboratory?
Yes

CBC/BIOCHEMISTRY/URINALYSIS
• Low urinary specific gravity (1.000 to 1.006), other abnormalities may point to the underlying cause.
• High serum ALP activity suggests hyperadrenocorticism or primary liver disease.
• High cholesterol common in patients with hyperadrenocorticism
• Leukocytosis with a left shift in some patients with pyometra or pyelonephritis
• Hyperkalemia and hyponatremia suggest hypoadrenocorticism.
• Low serum potassium confirms hypokalemia.
• Inflammatory sediment or bacteriuria consistent with pyelonephritis
• Proteinuria common in patients with pyelonephritis, pyometra, and hyperadrenocorticism

OTHER LABORATORY TESTS
ACTH levels to determine the cause of hyperadrenocorticism (i.e., pituitary dependent versus adrenal tumor)

IMAGING
• Radiography to assess renal size and shape and to detect calcified adrenal tumor or large uterus

- Intravenous pyelogram to help diagnose pyelonephritis
- Ultrasonography to assess adrenal size, renal and hepatic size and architecture, and uterine size
- MRI or CT scan to assess a pituitary or hypothalamic mass that may be the cause of central diabetes insipidus or hyperadreno-corticism

DIAGNOSTIC PROCEDURES
- ACTH stimulation test to screen for hyperadrenocorticism and hypoadreno-corticism
- Low-dose dexamethasone suppression test and urine/cortisol creatinine test to screen for hyperadrenocorticism
- Serum bile acids to evaluate liver function
- **Note:** dogs with hyperadrenocorticism often have mildly high bile acids.
- Modified water deprivation test to differentiate diabetes insipidus from psychogenic polydipsia; see Appendix for test protocol.

PATHOLOGIC FINDINGS
N/A

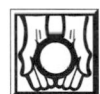

TREATMENT
- Depends on the underlying disorder
- Do not restrict patient's water intake unless appropriate to the definitive diagnosis.
- Depends on the underlying disorder

MEDICATIONS

DRUG(S) OF CHOICE
Depends on the underlying disorder

CONTRAINDICATIONS
N/A

PRECAUTIONS
N/A

POSSIBLE INTERACTIONS
N/A

ALTERNATIVE DRUG(S)
N/A

FOLLOW-UP

PATIENT MONITORING
Urine specific gravity, hydration status, renal function, and electrolytes

POSSIBLE COMPLICATIONS
Dehydration

MISCELLANEOUS

ASSOCIATED CONDITIONS
See Differential Diagnosis

AGE-RELATED FACTORS
N/A

ZOONOTIC POTENTIAL
N/A

PREGNANCY
N/A

SYNONYMS
N/A

SEE ALSO
- Diabetes Insipidus • Hyperadrenocorticism (Cushing's Disease)

ABBREVIATIONS
- ACTH = adrenocorticotrophic hormone
- ADH = antidiuretic hormone
- ALP = alkaline phosphatase
- CT = computed tomography
- MRI = magnetic resonance imaging

Suggested Reading

DiBartola SP. Fluid therapy in small animal practice. Philadelphia: Saunders, 1992.

Rose DB. Clinical physiology of acid-base and electrolyte disorders. 3rd ed. New York: McGraw-Hill, 1989.

Author Rhett Nichols

Consulting Editor Deborah S. Greco

HYPOTHERMIA

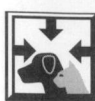 BASICS

DEFINITION
• Body temperature below normal in a homothermic organism
• Mild hypothermia—90–99°F (32–35°C)
• Moderate hypothermia—82–90°F (28–32°C)
• Severe hypothermia—any temperature < 82°F (28°C)

PATHOPHYSIOLOGY
• The hypothalamus regulates body temperature in response to changes in blood and skin temperature. Animals conserve heat by behavioral responses and physiologic responses (e.g., peripheral vasoconstriction to reduce heat loss to the environment, and piloerection to trap a layer of air next to the skin to provide thermal insulation. Active heat production—increased cardiac output, metabolic rate, and muscle activity (i.e., shivering)
• Thermoregulatory responses may be inadequate in neonates, geriatric animals, and hypothyroid or anesthetized animals. During prolonged exposure to cold, thermal homeostasis may fail, even in healthy animals.
• Hypothermia causes CNS depression. Peripheral vasoconstriction and fluid shifts increase blood viscosity and reduce cardiac output. Severe hypothermia is associated with hypotension. Reduced respiratory rate and depth leads to hypercapnia and respiratory acidosis. Fluid shifts into the alveoli affect alveolar gas exchange, resulting in hypoxemia. Increased hemoglobin affinity for oxygen causes reduced oxyhemoglobin unloading at the tissue level. Reduction of cellular metabolism may have a protective effect in animals with severe hypothermia.

SYSTEMS AFFECTED
• Nervous—impaired consciousness ranging from obtundation to coma
• Cardiovascular—arrhythmias, conduction disturbances, changes in vasomotor tone, hypotension, and low cardiac output
• Respiratory—respiratory depression, respiratory acidosis, and hypoxemia
• Hemic/Lymph/Immune—reversible platelet and coagulation factor dysfunction and disseminated intravascular coagulation (DIC)

GENETICS
N/A

INCIDENCE/PREVALENCE
Varies with geographic location

GEOGRAPHIC DISTRIBUTION
Most common in cold climates

SIGNALMENT

Species
Dog and cat

Breed Predilection
More common in small breeds with a predisposition to surface heat loss

Mean Age and Range
More common in neonates and geriatrics

Predominant Sex
None

SIGNS

Historical Findings
• Known prolonged exposure to cold ambient temperatures
• Possibly, disappearance from home or a history of trauma
• Cold, unresponsive animal

Physical Examination Findings
Mild hypothermia (90–99°F)
• Mental depression
• Lethargy
• Weakness
• Shivering
Moderate hypothermia (82–90°F)
• Muscle stiffness
• Bradycardia
• Hypotension
• Reduced respiratory rate and depth
• Stupor/obtundation
Severe hypothermia (< 82°F)
• Inaudible heart sounds
• Difficulty breathing
• Coma
• Fixed and dilated pupils

CAUSES
• Cold ambient temperature
• Impaired thermoregulation (e.g., neonates, geriatrics, animals with hypothyroidism or hypothalamic disease)
• Impaired behavioral responses—as seen in neonates, sick, debilitated, or injured animals)
• Predisposition to surface heat loss—as in neonates and small animals
• Inadequate heat generation—as in neonates and cachectic and hypothyroid animals

RISK FACTORS
• Hypothyroidism
• Hypothalamic disease
• Very young or old age
• Low body fat and glycogen stores
• Anesthesia and surgery

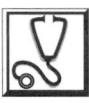 DIAGNOSIS

DIFFERENTIAL DIAGNOSIS

Differentiating Similar Signs
Must differentiate from death in animals with severe hypothermia

Differentiating Causes
• Must differentiate from other causes of CNS depression, including primary CNS disease, metabolic disorders, such as hypoglycemia and hepatic encephalopathy, electrolyte disturbances, systemic infection, and neoplasia
• Must differentiate from other causes of bradycardia and cardiac arrhythmias, such as primary cardiac disease, hyperthyroidism in cats, and anesthetic or sedative agents

CBC/BIOCHEMISTRY/URINALYSIS
• Usually normal
• Mild hemoconcentration and hyperglycemia in some animals

OTHER LABORATORY TESTS
• Platelet count and coagulation panel may reveal thrombocytopenia and prolongation of activated partial thromboplastin and prothrombin times.
• Thyroid hormone evaluation may confirm underlying hypothyroidism.

IMAGING
N/A

DIAGNOSTIC PROCEDURES
Rectal or esophageal probes or low recording thermometers may be useful for monitoring body temperatures below 93°F in patients with severe hypothermia.

Electrocardiography
• Sinus bradycardia with lengthening of PR, QRS, and QT intervals
• Atrial arrhythmias initially in some patients
• Ventricular arrhythmias (e.g., ventricular premature complex and ventricular tachycardia) occur as body temperature decreases further.
• Ventricular fibrillation likely at body temperatures < 82°F

TREATMENT
• Treat most as inpatients until normothermia is reached.
• Minimize movement to prevent lethal cardiac arrhythmias, especially in patients with severe hypothermia.
• Anticipate further decline in body temperature during initial rewarming, because of contact of warmer "core" blood with the colder surface of the body.
• Aim to support vital organ systems, rewarm the patient, and prevent further heat loss.
• Airway management and oxygen supplementation are essential; ventilatory support may be required in animals with severe hypothermia.
• Mild hypothermia—use passive rewarming techniques, including thermal insulation with blankets
• Mild hypothermia—use active external rewarming with heat sources such as heating pads and radiant heat; apply heat to the trunk to rewarm the body's "core" without causing peripheral vasodilation in the limbs; provide a protective layer between the heat source and the patient's skin.
• Severe hypothermia—use core rewarming techniques, including warm water gastric and peritoneal lavage, warm water enemas, warm IV fluid administration, and airway rewarming (using warmed air).

MEDICATIONS

DRUG(S) OF CHOICE
• Oxygen supplementation may be provided via a face mask or endotracheal tube.
• Blood volume support—essential; most isotonic, balanced electrolyte solutions can be used
• Fluid solutions should be warm to prevent additional heat loss.
• Fluid supplementation with dextrose may be helpful.

CONTRAINDICATIONS
• Severe hypothermia—avoid lactated Ringer's solution because of impaired hepatic metabolism of lactate.
• At temperatures < 82°F the heart is refractory to atropine and antiarrhythmic agents.

PRECAUTIONS
N/A

POSSIBLE INTERACTIONS
N/A

ALTERNATIVE DRUG(S)
N/A

FOLLOW-UP

PATIENT MONITORING
• Core body temperature during rewarming
• ECG and blood pressure to assess cardiovascular status during rewarming
• Observe for development of frostbite

PREVENTION/AVOIDANCE
• Avoid prolonged exposure to cold, especially with at-risk animals.
• Warm patient and monitor body temperature in anesthetized animals.

POSSIBLE COMPLICATIONS
• Peripheral vasodilation during rewarming may further drop body temperature.
• Return of cool peripheral blood to the heart may precipitate cardiac arrhythmias.
• Severe hypothermia may cause cardiac arrest.

EXPECTED CAUSE AND PROGNOSIS
Varies with severity of hypothermia, underlying cause, and patient health status prior to hypothermic episode

MISCELLANEOUS

ASSOCIATED CONDITIONS
N/A

AGE-RELATED FACTORS
Sick or hypoglycemic neonates can become markedly hypothermic in normal environments; treatment may extend to long-term management of ambient temperature of environment.

ZOONOTIC POTENTIAL
N/A

PREGNANCY
N/A

SYNONYMS
None

SEE ALSO
Shock, Cardiogenic

ABBREVIATIONS
DIC = disseminated intravascular coagulation

Suggested Reading
Ahn AH. Approach to the hypothermic patient. In: Bonagura JD, ed. Current veterinary therapy XII. Philadelphia: Saunders, 1995:157–161.
Dhupa N. Hypothermia in dogs and cats. Compend Contin Educ Pract Vet 1995;17:61–69.
Author Nishi Dhupa
Consulting Editors Larry P. Tilley and Francis W. K. Smith, Jr.

HYPOTHYROIDISM

 **BASICS**

DEFINITION
• Clinical condition that results from inadequate production and release of tetraiodothyronine (levothyroxine, T_4) and triiodothyronine (liothyronine, T_3) by the thyroid gland
• Characterized by a generalized decrease in cellular metabolic activity

PATHOPHYSIOLOGY

Acquired Hypothyroidism
• In dogs, primary acquired hypothyroidism is the most common type (>95% of cases).
• Caused by lymphocytic thyroiditis (50%) or idiopathic thyroid atrophy (50%)
• Lymphocytic thyroiditis is thought to be immune mediated (cellular and humoral).
• Circulating autoantibodies to thyroglobulin are often present, but these autoantibodies can also be found in a variable percentage (15%–40%) of normal, euthyroid dogs.
• Rarely, primary hypothyroidism is caused by neoplastic (primary or metastatic) destruction of the thyroid gland or dietary iodine deficiency.
• Rare in cats and is most commonly seen following bilateral thyroidectomy or radioactive iodine therapy; it is often transitory and frequently does not require therapy.
• Accessory thyroid tissue in the neck or thoracic cavity usually undergoes hyperplasia and produces physiologic amounts of thyroid hormones.
• Acquired secondary hypothyroidism is uncommon in dogs and cats; it is caused by pituitary dysfunction or destruction leading to decreased thyrotropin (thyroid-stimulating hormone, TSH) production.
• Thyrotropin is the pituitary hormone responsible for stimulating thyroid hormone synthesis and secretion.
• Increased circulating levels of glucocorticoids (endogenous or exogenous) can transitorily suppress TSH secretion by anterior pituitary thyrotropes; this leads to decreased blood levels of T_4 and free T_4. Thyrotrope secretion of TSH normalizes when blood glucocorticosteroid levels return to normal.
• Tertiary hypo-thyroidism caused by decreased thyrotropin-releasing hormone (TRH) production by the hypothalamus has not been documented in dogs or cats.

Congenital Hypothyroidism
• Congenital hypothyroidism is very rare in both dogs and cats.
• Reported causes of primary congenital hypothyroidism in dogs and cats include thyroid agenesis or dysgenesis, dyshormonogenesis, and iodine deficiency.
• Secondary congenital hypothyroidism is most commonly observed in German shepherd dogs with a panhypopituitarism caused by a cystic Rathke's pouch.
• A congenital deficiency in pituitary TSH production was reported in a family of giant schnauzers.

SYSTEMS AFFECTED
• Endocrine/Metabolic
• Skin/Exocrine
• Behavioral
• Neuromuscular
• Reproductive
• Gastrointestinal
• Ophthalmic
• Cardiovascular
• Nervous

GENETICS
• No known genetic basis for the inheritance of primary hypothyroidism in canines
• Familial lymphocytic thyroiditis has been reported in individual colonies of borzois, beagles, and great Danes.

INCIDENCE/PREVALENCE
• Primary hypothyroidism is a common endocrinopathy in dogs; the reported prevalence of hypothyroidism in dogs ranges from 1:500 to 3:500.
• Hypothyroidism is rare in cats.

GEOGRAPHIC DISTRIBUTION
N/A

SIGNALMENT

Species
Dogs and rarely cats

Breed Predilection
• Primary acquired hypothyroidism is more common in medium to large-sized dogs.
• Breeds reported to be predisposed to developing primary acquired hypothyroidism include the golden retriever, Doberman pinscher, Irish setter, great Dane, airedale terrier, Old English sheepdog, dachshund, miniature schnauzer, cocker spaniel, poodle, and boxer.

Mean Age and Range
Most common in middle-aged dogs (4–10 years)

Predominant Sex
No definitive sex predilection has been identified; however, castrated male dogs and spayed female dogs appear to be at increased risk.

SIGNS

Historical Findings
• Most common—lethargy, inactivity, mental dullness, weight gain, hair loss or excessive shedding, lack of hair regrowth following clipping, dry or lusterless haircoat, excessive scaling, hyperpigmentation, recurrent skin infections, and cold intolerance
• Uncommon—generalized weakness, incoordination, head tilt, facial paralysis, seizures, and infertility
• Clinical signs develop slowly and are progressive.

Physical Examination Findings
Dermatologic Abnormalities—Very Common
• Bilaterally symmetric truncal alopecia that spares the head and extremities—common
• Alopecia is usually nonpruritic unless a secondary pyoderma or other pruritic dermatitis is also present.
• Hairs epilate easily; the haircoat is often dry and lusterless. Hair loss occurs in areas of friction.
• Alopecia often initially involves the flank area, base of the ears, tail (rat tail) and friction areas (axillae, ventrum of thorax, abdomen and neck, and under the collar).
• Early in the disease course, alopecia may be multifocal and asymmetric; alopecic lesions may have irregular margins.
• Hyperpigmentation and increased thickness of the epidermis are common, particularly in friction areas.
• Seborrhea—common; can be generalized, multifocal, or localized. Dull, dry coat.
• A secondary superficial pyoderma occurs occasionally; deep pyoderma is less common.
• Dermal accumulation of mucopolysaccharides can lead to nonpitting edema (myxedema), particularly in the facial area; this produces the classic "tragic" expression associated with hypothyroidism.
• Ceruminous otitis externa may be seen.

General/Metabolic—Very Common
• Lethargy, mental dullness
• Weight gain
• Mild hypothermia
Reproductive
• Infertility and prolonged anestrus in females
• Inappropriate galactorrhea in sexually intact bitches
Neuromuscular—Uncommon
• A peripheral neuropathy (localized or generalized) involving lower motor neurons occasionally occurs in hypothyroid dogs.
• Generalized weakness is the most common clinical sign; dogs may have a stiff, stilted gait.
• Other neurologic findings may include proprioceptive deficits, hyporeflexia, head tilt, facial paralysis/paresis, and ataxia.
• A secondary myopathy characterized by denervation atrophy is usually present in dogs with hypothyroid polyneuropathy.
• Some hypothyroid dogs develop a generalized myopathy without concurrent neurologic involvement; these dogs present for generalized weakness.
• Seizures secondary to marked cerebral atherosclerosis have been rarely reported in hypothyroid dogs with marked hyperlipidemia.
• Laryngeal paralysis, megaesophagus, and Horner's syndrome have been suggested with hypothyroidism, but definitive proof of a causal relationship is lacking.
Ophthalmic
• Corneal lipid deposits
• Lipemia retinalis
Felines—Rare
• Unkempt appearance, matting of hair, nonpruritic seborrhea sicca, pinnal alopecia
• Lethargy
• Obesity
Congenital Hypothyroidism—Cretinism
• Mental dullness/retardation, lethargy, inactivity
• Disproportionate dwarfism (large, broad head with short neck and limbs), shortened mandible, protruding tongue, delayed dental eruption
• Constipation/obstipation—particularly in cats
• Hypothermia
• Retention of puppy coat, progressive truncal alopecia (dogs)

CAUSES
Lymphocytic thyroiditis, idiopathic thyroid atrophy, congenital disease, pituitary disease, dietary iodine deficiency, neoplasia, and iatrogenic

RISK FACTORS
• Neutering may slightly increase risk of developing primary hypothyroidism.
• Bilateral thyroidectomy may result in hypothyroidism.

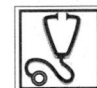 **DIAGNOSIS**

DIFFERENTIAL DIAGNOSIS
• Dermatologic abnormalities are frequently the predominant clinical abnormality in dogs with hypothyroidism.
• Consider endocrine causes of alopecia (e.g., hyperadrenocorticism, sex hormone–related dermatopathies, growth hormone–responsive dermatosis, and adrenal sex hormone abnormalities).
• If fasting hyperlipidemia detected (most common laboratory abnormality in hypothyroid dogs), must rule out diabetes mellitus, hyperadrenocorticism, nephrotic syndrome, acute pancreatitis, biliary obstruction, and primary lipid metabolism abnormalities

CBC/BIOCHEMISTRY/URINALYSIS
• Hypercholesterolemia—observed in up to 80% of hypothyroid dogs
• Hypertriglyceridemia and gross lipemia—less common
• Mild, normochromic, normocytic, nonregenerative anemia—up to 50% of hypothyroid dogs
• Mildly elevated serum creatine kinase levels are intermittently identified.

OTHER LABORATORY TESTS
• Do endocrine testing in dogs with clinical signs or laboratory abnormalities suggesting hypothyroidism.
• Routine endocrine testing of sick dogs for hypothyroidism is unnecessary if they do not show signs consistent with hypothyroidism.
• Please see Appendix for table of endocrine test protocols.

Basal Serum Thyroid Hormone Concentrations
• Basal serum T_4 levels in the mid-normal to high-normal range rule out a diagnosis of hypothyroidism; further endocrine testing is not indicated.
• A subnormal T_4 concentration is compatible with, but not diagnostic for, hypothyroidism.
• Subnormal T_4 levels can be seen in healthy, euthyroid dogs.
• Serum T_4 levels often drop below normal in dogs with nonthyroidal illness (sick euthyroid syndrome); these animals are not hypothyroid and do not require thyroid hormone supplementation.
• Basal serum T_3 levels are not an accurate means for evaluating thyroid function; one study found normal serum T_3 levels in 74% of hypothyroid dogs; serum T_3 levels can be subnormal in healthy, euthyroid dogs and in euthyroid dogs with nonthyroidal illness.
• Markedly elevated T_4 or T_3 levels in dogs may indicate the presence of thyroid hormone autoantibodies; these autoantibodies can cause false elevations or, less commonly, false decreases in T_4 or T_3 concentrations determined by radioimmunoassay.
• Determination of serum free T_4 (FT_4) levels by equilibrium or direct dialysis is a sensitive and specific way to evaluate a patient for hypothyroidism.
• Low FT_4 concentrations in a patient with compatible clinical signs and low total T_4 levels strongly indicate hypothyroidism; however, FT_4 levels are low in up to 25% of euthyroid dogs with hyperadrenocorticism.
• Dogs with hyperadrenocorticism and low T_4 or low FT_4 levels should receive treatment for hyperadrenocorticism followed by retesting of thyroid levels; often T_4 and FT_4 levels will increase into normal range
• Severe nonthyroidal illness may suppress FT_4 levels in some euthyroid dogs.
• Determination of serum FT_3 levels is noncontributory to diagnosing hypothyroidism.

Endogenous Thyrotropin (TSH) Concentrations
• Thyrotropin concentrations are increased in most dogs with primary hypothyroidism, but 25–40% of dogs with confirmed hypothyroidism have normal serum TSH levels (false-negatives).

HYPOTHYROIDISM

• Elevated TSH levels have been reported in 10%–20% of euthyroid dogs with nonthyroidal illness (false-positives).
• High TSH levels in conjunction with low T_4 or low FT_4 concentrations strongly indicate hypothyroidism.
• Measurement of TSH is best used in conjunction with other thyroid tests.

Autoantibodies to Thyroid Hormones and Thyroglobulin (Tg)
• Autoantibodies to Tg and, to a much lesser extent, T_3 and T_4 occur in 30%–50% of dogs with hypothyroidism and are consistent with a diagnosis of lymphocytic thyroiditis; these autoantibodies can also occur in healthy, euthyroid dogs.
• Healthy dogs with normal T_4 concentrations and autoantibodies to Tg, T_3, or T_4 may be at increased risk for developing hypothyroidism, but this is not proven.

TSH Stimulation Test
• In past years, was considered the gold standard for the diagnosis of canine hypothyroidism
• Recombinant human TSH is available but expensive; its high cost precludes routine use.
• Dogs with primary hypothyroidism show little or no increase in serum T_4 in response to TSH; normal dogs show a robust increase.
• Borderline or equivocal responses occur; retesting at a later time or use of other thyroid function tests may be best in such circumstances.

TRH Stimulation Testing
• TRH results in a small and variable increase in serum T_4 levels.
• This test is unreliable for the diagnosis of canine hypothyroidism.
• Measurement of TSH in response to TRH could potentially be used to differentiate primary from secondary hypothyroidism.

IMAGING

Radiography
• Epiphyseal dysgenesis, delayed epiphyseal ossification, and shortened vertebral bodies are present in patients with congenital hypothyroidism; these patients frequently develop radiographic signs of degenerative joint disease as adults.

• Megacolon is a common radiographic finding in cats with congenital hypothyroidism.

Echocardiography
Indices of left ventricular systolic function are commonly abnormal; these changes are usually not clinically significant unless the dog has concurrent primary heart disease.

DIAGNOSTIC PROCEDURES
Electrocardiography—low-amplitude R-waves commonly observed; bradycardia less frequently

PATHOLOGIC FINDINGS
• Lymphocytic thyroiditis is characterized by a diffuse infiltration of lymphocytes and plasma cells into the thyroid parenchyma with eventual destruction of the gland.
• Idiopathic thyroid atrophy is characterized by parenchymal atrophy and replacement with adipose and connective tissue.
• Epidermal and dermal abnormalities are common.
• Dermatohistopathologic abnormalities commonly seen with hypothyroidism include orthokeratotic hyperkeratosis, sebaceous gland atrophy, epidermal hyperplasia, follicular atrophy, myxedema, and vacuolation of the arrector pili muscles.

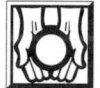

TREATMENT

APPROPRIATE HEALTH CARE
Outpatient

NURSING CARE
N/A

ACTIVITY
N/A

DIET
Reduced-fat diet until body weight is satisfactory and T_4 concentrations are normal

CLIENT EDUCATION
• Dogs with primary hypothyroidism respond well to treatment with oral synthetic levothyroxine (L-thyroxine).

• The appropriate dosage for L-thyroxine varies between individuals because of differences in gastrointestinal (GI) absorption and hormone metabolism.
• Treatment is lifelong.
• Most clinical and laboratory abnormalities resolve over a few weeks to a few months.
• Occasionally, dermatologic abnormalities worsen transiently during the first month of therapy.

SURGICAL CONSIDERATIONS
N/A

MEDICATIONS

DRUG(S) OF CHOICE
• Levothyroxine is the treatment of choice.
• The starting dosage is 0.02–0.04 mg/kg/day or 0.5 mg/m²/day divided q12h.
• Adjust dosage on the basis of post-pill serum T_4 concentration and clinical response to therapy; initially, use a veterinary name brand product.
• If the patient responds to therapy, once-daily therapy can be tried; however, some patients require continued q12h therapy.
• Different brands of L-thyroxine frequently have different GI absorption kinetics; the dosage may change if the brand is changed.

CONTRAINDICATIONS
None

PRECAUTIONS
• The initial dosage of L-thyroxine may need to be decreased in animals with concurrent heart failure, diabetes mellitus, renal failure, liver disease, or hypoadrenocorticism.
• The initial dosage of L-thyroxine is 25% of the standard daily dosage in these patients.
• Slowly increase the dosage over 2–4 months until the appropriate dosage is obtained; this allows the patient to adjust slowly to the increased basal metabolic rate.
• Start glucocorticoid replacement therapy prior to L-thyroxine therapy in hypothyroid animals with concurrent hypoadrenocorticism.

POSSIBLE INTERACTIONS
• Glucocorticoids, phenytoin, salicylates, androgens, and furosemide may enhance the metabolism of L-thyroxine by inhibiting serum protein binding.
• Sucralfate and aluminum hydroxide can inhibit GI absorption.

ALTERNATIVE DRUG(S)
• Therapy with synthetic liothyronine (T_3) is not indicated or recommended in the vast majority of hypothyroid dogs.
• Liothyronine therapy is indicated only if a dog fails to achieve a normal serum T_4 concentration following appropriate therapy with at least two different brands of L-thyroxine. This probably indicates a lack of intestinal absorption; liothyronine is almost completely absorbed from the gut.
• The initial dosage is 4–6 μg/kg PO q8h; final dosage is based on clinical response and on serum T_3 levels in the normal range; some patients can be maintained on q12h therapy.

 FOLLOW-UP

PATIENT MONITORING
• Mental alertness and activity levels usually increase within 1–2 weeks after initiation of therapy.
• Dermatologic abnormalities slowly resolve over 1–4 months, as do neurologic deficits that are secondary to hypothyroidism.
• Reproductive abnormalities resolve more slowly.
• If significant clinical improvement does not occur within 3 months of initiation of therapy, with serum T_4 levels in the normal range, the diagnosis of hypothyroidism may be incorrect.
• Check serum T_4 levels after 1 month of therapy.
• Determine peak serum T_4 concentrations 4–8 hours after L-thyroxine administration.

• Serum T_4 concentrations should be in the normal range or mildly increased. Patients on once-daily therapy that do not respond to therapy and have a normal or high peak T_4 concentration should have their pre-pill T_4 concentration (trough T_4) assessed; if the trough T_4 concentration is low, twice-daily therapy is indicated.
• Following initial normalization of serum T_4 values, check them yearly, or sooner if clinical signs of hypothyroidism or thyrotoxicosis develop.
• Recheck serum T_4 concentrations 1 month after any change in dosage or brand of L-thyroxine being administered.

PREVENTION/AVOIDANCE
Proper treatment prevents disease recurrence.

POSSIBLE COMPLICATIONS
• Prolonged administration of an inappropriately high dosage of L-thyroxine can cause iatrogenic hyperthyroidism.
• Clinical signs of thyrotoxicosis include panting, polyphagia, weight loss, polyuria/polydipsia, anxiety, and diarrhea.
• Keep peak serum T_4 concentrations at or below 5μg/dL (64 nmol/L).

EXPECTED COURSE AND PROGNOSIS
• Dogs treated for acquired primary hypothyroidism have an excellent prognosis; life expectancy is normal.
• Patients with acquired central hypothyroidism may have a poor prognosis if condition is secondary to a tumor or destructive process affecting the pituitary or hypothalamus.

 MISCELLANEOUS

ASSOCIATED CONDITIONS
Primary hypothyroidism has been reported to occur concurrently with primary hypoadrenocorticism and/or insulin-dependent diabetes mellitus in a small number of animals.

AGE-RELATED FACTORS
None

ZOONOTIC POTENTIAL
None

PREGNANCY
N/A

SYNONYMS
None

SEE ALSO
Myxedema and Myxedema Coma

ABBREVIATIONS
• FT_3 = free T_3
• FT_4 = free T_4
• T_3 = liothyronine, triiodothyronine
• T_4 = L-thyroxine, tetraiodothyronine
• TRH = thyrotropin-releasing hormone
• TSH = thyroid-stimulating hormone, thyrotropin

Suggested Readings

Kantrowitz LB, Peterson ME, Melian C, Nichols R. Serum total thyroxine, total triiodothyronine, free thyroxine, and thyrotropin concentrations in dogs with non-thyroidal disease. J Am Vet Med Assoc 2001;219:765–769.

Kemppainen RJ, Behrend EN. Diagnosis of canine hypothyroidism: perspective from a testing laboratory. Vet Clin N Amer Small Anim Pract 2001;31:951–962.

Panciera DL. Canine hypothyroidism. In: Torrance AG, Mooney CT, eds. BSAVA manual of small animal endocrinology. 2nd ed. Cheltenham, UK: British Small Animal Veterinary Association, 1998:103–113.

Panciera DL. Conditions associated with canine hypothyroidism. Vet Clin N Amer Small Anim Pract 2001;31:935–950.

Author Robert J. Kemppainen, John W. Tyler
Consulting Editor Deborah S. Greco

HYPOXEMIA

 BASICS

DEFINITION
• A decrease in PaO_2, resulting in marked desaturation of hemoglobin
• Clinically significant desaturation of hemoglobin begins at a $PaO_2 < 60$ mm Hg.

PATHOPHYSIOLOGY
Six physiologic causes—(1) low P_1O_2; (2) hypoventilation (increase in $PaCO_2$); (3) mismatching of alveolar ventilation and perfusion so that areas of the lung that are not ventilated properly are still perfused adequately; (4) alveolar–capillary membrane diffusion defect; (5) right-to-left cardiac or pulmonary shunting; (6) low cardiac output

SYSTEMS AFFECTED
• All organs—oxygen essential for normal cellular function; individual tissue oxygen requirements vary by organ.
• Nervous—brain and CNS most important; may result in irreversible brain damage; there are no large oxygen stores in brain tissue.
• Cardiovascular—may result in focal or global ischemia; if prolonged, may develop arrhythmias and cardiac failure

SIGNALMENT
Any breed, age, and sex of dogs and cats

SIGNS

Historical Findings
• Episodes of coughing
• Breathing problems—especially open-mouth breathing
• Trauma
• Gagging
• Exercise intolerance
• Cyanosis
• Collapse

Physical Examination Findings
• Tachypnea
• Dyspnea
• Orthopnea
• Pale mucous membranes
• Cyanosis
• Coughing
• Open-mouth breathing
• Tachycardia
• Poor peripheral pulse
• Abnormal thoracic auscultation

CAUSES
• Low P_1O_2—high altitude (the higher the elevation, the lower the barometric pressure, which results in a decrease in P_1O_2; F_1O_2 is fixed at 0.21); suffocation; enclosure in small areas with improper ventilation
• Hypoventilation—result of inadequate alveolar ventilation; muscular paralysis; upper airway obstruction; air or fluid in the pleural space; restriction of the thoracic cage, diaphragmatic hernia; CNS disease
• Mismatching of alveolar ventilation and perfusion—usually during anesthesia or prolonged recumbency in which a large area of lung becomes atelectatic; pulmonary edema; pulmonary thromboembolism; pulmonary parenchymal disease (infectious or neoplastic); lower airway disease; pneumonia; pulmonary contusions
• Alveolar–capillary membrane diffusion defect—rarely clinically important
• Right-to-left cardiac or pulmonary shunting—tetralogy of Fallot; ventricular septal defect; reversed patent ductus arteriosus; intrapulmonary arteriovenous shunt
• Low cardiac output—cardiac failure from any cause; shock from any cause

RISK FACTORS
• Sudden move to higher elevations
• Trauma
• Bronchopneumonia
• Pleural disease
• Anesthesia
• Cardiac disease
• Bronchial disease—chronic obstructive pulmonary disease; feline asthma
• Geriatric pulmonary or cardiac changes

 DIAGNOSIS

DIFFERENTIAL DIAGNOSIS
• Signs of tachypnea and/or dyspnea
• Excitement or anxiety
• Hyperthermia
• Pyrexia
• Head trauma
• Pain

LABORATORY FINDINGS

Drugs That May Alter Laboratory Results
N/A

Disorders That May Alter Laboratory Results
• Air bubbles in the arterial blood sample—falsely high PaO_2 values
• Improper packaging of the arterial blood sample—falsely high PaO_2 values after approximately 30 min at room temperature

Valid If Run in Human Laboratory?
Yes

CBC/BIOCHEMISTRY/URINALYSIS
PCV—may be high with chronic condition; may be low if inflammatory cause

OTHER LABORATORY TESTS

Arterial Blood Gases
Collect arterial blood sample in an anaerobic manner, as follows:
• Use enough heparin to coat the needle and the inside of the syringe.
• Place a rubber stopper on the needle or covering the hub of the syringe, to prevent room air from entering the sample.
• Analyze sample within 15 min if left at room temperature; place sample on ice to extend safe time for analysis to 24 hours.
• Bedside or portable blood gas analyzers—several models available; make analysis more convenient

IMAGING
Thoracic radiographs and echocardiography—evaluate intrathoracic disease; differentiate pulmonary and cardiac disease.

DIAGNOSTIC PROCEDURES

Pulse Oximetry
• Indirectly determines SaO_2; relation between PaO_2 and SaO_2 based on the oxyhemoglobin dissociation curve: $SaO_2 > 90\%$ when $PaO_2 > 60$ mm Hg
• $SaO_2 < 95\%$—considered abnormal
• Best results when probe used on the tongue of animals; thus may be limited to anesthetized, heavily sedated, or seriously ill patients with a low level of consciousness; keep tongue moistened for most accurate readings.
• Other successful probe sites—ear; vulva (female), and prepuce (male); skin between toes; thin skin in the flank area
• Poor results—least accurate in low-flow states such as hypotension (global low flow)

or hypothermia (low flow to skin); falsely low values (usually < 85%) during carboxyhemo-globinemia (smoke inhalation)
• Rectal probes—should become available; will allow readings in awake patients

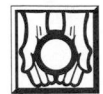

TREATMENT
Must identify and correct the primary cause

Oxygen Therapy
• Most common supportive treatment
• Corrects low-inspired oxygen, hypoventil-ation, and alveolar–capillary membrane diffusion defects; may not always correct mismatching of ventilation and perfusion; often does not correct right-to-left cardiac or pulmonary shunts and low cardiac output
• May not be completely beneficial until adequate blood volume is established
• Delivery—directly from an oxygen source from the anesthetic machine via a face mask placed securely around the muzzle or from an E-tank fitted with an oxygen regulator through a face mask, intranasal catheter, or oxygen cage
• Increase in F_IO_2—determined by the oxygen flow rate and the amount of oxygen mixed with room air
• PPV—may be needed for ARDS or severe hypoventilation

Fluid Therapy
• Low cardiac output—fluid administration and inotropic support (e.g., dobutamine or dopamine) important
• Cardiac failure—requires aggressive medical treatment; diuretics; afterload and preload reduction; inotropic support; oxygen administration; fluids indicated after institu-tion of primary treatment; use caution with type and rate of fluids after initial stabiliza-tion.
• Hypovolemic, hemorrhagic, traumatic, or septic shock—requires aggressive fluid administration; crystalloids (90 mL/kg as fast as possible), hypertonic solutions (7% NaCl, 4 mL/kg), colloids (hetastarch, 20 mL/kg), hemoglobin-based oxygen-carrying solutions, or combination

• Severe pulmonary contusion—hypertonic fluids or colloids, or combination preferred

MEDICATIONS

DRUG(S) OF CHOICE
Bronchospasm—bronchodilators; terbutaline (0.01 mg/kg SC, IM, or IV q8h) or extended release theophylline 10 mg/kg PO q12h (dog), q24h (cat)

CONTRAINDICATIONS
• Aggressive fluid administration—not indicated for cardiac failure and pulmonary edema
• Diuretics—not indicated for shock, low P_IO_2, alveolar–capillary membrane diffusion defects, mismatching of alveolar ventilation and perfusion, and right-to-left shunts

PRECAUTIONS
• Inotropic drugs—arrhythmias may develop.
• Oxygen toxicity—from prolonged (> 12 hr) exposure to high-concentration (> 70%) oxygen; pulmonary edema, seizures, and death

POSSIBLE INTERACTIONS
N/A

ALTERNATIVE DRUG(S)
N/A

FOLLOW-UP

PATIENT MONITORING
• Decrease in respiratory effort and a decrease in cyanosis (if initially noted)—check efficacy of treatment and support.
• Arterial blood gas—determine resolution
• Pulse oximetry—alternative; interpret results cautiously with hypotension, hypo-thermia, smoke inhalation, and non-tongue probe site.

POSSIBLE COMPLICATIONS
• Brain damage—depends on severity and duration of hypoxemia; partial or complete loss of neuronal function; dementia; seizures; loss of consciousness

• Arrhythmias—may develop secondary to myocardial hypoxia; may be very difficult to treat effectively

MISCELLANEOUS

ASSOCIATED CONDITIONS
N/A

AGE-RELATED FACTORS
N/A

ZOONOTIC POTENTIAL
N/A

PREGNANCY
May adversely affect fetuses, especially during the first trimester of pregnancy

SEE ALSO
• Cyanosis
• Dyspnea, Tachypnea, and Panting
• See also Causes.

ABBREVIATIONS
• ARDS = acute respiratory distress syndrome
• F_IO_2 = fraction of oxygen in inspired air
• PaO_2 = partial pressure of arterial oxygen
• $PaCO_2$ = partial pressure of arterial carbon dioxide
• PCV = packed cell volume
• P_IO_2 = partial pressure of inspired oxygen
• PPV = positive-pressure ventilation
• SaO_2 = saturation of arterial blood with oxygen

Suggested Reading
Martin L. All you really need to know to in-terpret arterial blood gases. Philadelphia: Lippincott Williams & Wilkins, 1999, 48–106.
West JB. Pulmonary physiology and patho-physiology. Philadelphia: Lippincott Williams & Wilkins, 1999:16–32, 100–111, 125–144.
West JB. Respiratory physiology: the essen-tials. 6th ed. Philadelphia: Lippincott Williams & Wilkins, 2000:21–78, 45–62.
Author Thomas Kevin Day
Consulting Editor Lynelle R. Johnson

IDIOVENTRICULAR RHYTHM

 BASICS

DEFINITION

If conduction of sinus node pacemaker impulses to the ventricles is blocked or the impulses decrease in frequency, the lower regions of the heart automatically take over the role of pacemaker for the ventricles, which results in ventricular escape complexes (Figure 1) or an idioventricular rhythm (Figure 2).

ECG Features

• A series of ventricular escape beats with a heart rate < 65 bpm in dogs and < 100 bpm in cats; heart rates of 65–100 bpm in dogs and 100–160 bpm in cats are often termed *accelerated idioventricular rhythms*
• P waves may be absent or may precede, be hidden within, or follow the ectopic QRS complex.
• P waves are unrelated to the QRS complexes • QRS configuration—wide and bizarre; similar to that of a ventricular premature complex

PATHOPHYSIOLOGY

• May be hemodynamically important with slow ventricular rates
• Does not occur in healthy animals
• Subsidiary pacemakers seem to discharge more rapidly in cats than in dogs.

SYSTEMS AFFECTED

Cardiovascular

GENETICS

N/A

INCIDENCE/PREVALENCE

Unknown

GEOGRAPHIC DISTRIBUTION

N/A

SIGNALMENT

Species

Dogs and cats

Breed Predilections

• Atrial standstill in English springer spaniels and Siamese cats
• Pugs, miniature schnauzers, and dalmatians prone to conduction abnormalities

Mean Age and Range

N/A

Predominant Sex

N/A

SIGNS

Historical Findings

• Some animals asymptomatic
• Weakness
• Lethargy
• Exercise intolerance
• Syncope
• Heart failure

PHYSICAL EXAMINATION FINDINGS

• Irregular rhythm associated with pulse deficits
• Variation in heart sounds
• Possible intermittent "cannon" waves in the jugular venous pulses (with atrioventricular [AV] block)

CAUSES

• Not a primary disease—a secondary result of a primary disease
• The escape rhythm is a safety mechanism to maintain cardiac output.

Causes of Sinus Bradycardia and Sinus Arrest

• Increased vagal tone (high intracranial pressure, high ocular pressure)
• Drugs—digoxin, tranquilizers, propranolol, quinidine, and anesthetics
• Addison's disease
• Hypoglycemia
• Renal failure

• Hypothermia
• Hyperkalemia
• Hypothyroidism

Causes of AV Block

• Congenital
• Neoplasia
• Fibrosis
• Lyme disease

RISK FACTORS

N/A

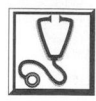 DIAGNOSIS

DIFFERENTIAL DIAGNOSIS

• Ventricular tachycardia—dogs have a cardiac rate > 100 bpm; cats > 150 bpm
• Slow heart rate in animals with right bundle branch block, left bundle branch block, or left anterior fascicular block; animals with these disturbances have the P waves associated with the QRS complexes.

CBC/BIOCHEMISTRY/URINALYSIS

• No specific findings
• Complete blood testing may suggest a metabolic abnormality.

OTHER LABORATORY TESTS

• Drug toxicity
• Lyme's titer in animals with complete AV block

IMAGING

Echocardiogram may show structural heart disease.

DIAGNOSTIC PROCEDURES

Electrocardiography

PATHOLOGIC FINDINGS

Depend on underlying cause

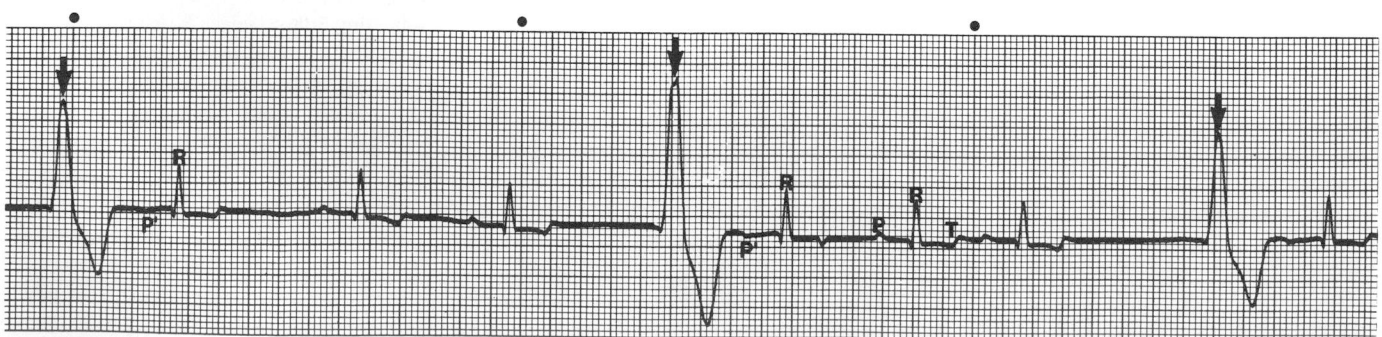

Figure 1.

Ventricular escape complexes (arrows) during various phases in the dominant sinus rhythm in a dog during anesthesia. The sinus rate increased (not shown) after anesthesia was stopped; ¹/₂ cm = 1 mv. (From: Tilley LP: Essentials of canine and feline electrocardiography. 3rd ed. Baltimore: Lippincott Williams & Wilkins, 1992, with permission.)

IDIOVENTRICULAR RHYTHM

TREATMENT

APPROPRIATE HEALTH CARE
• Rhythm is an escape or safety mechanism for maintaining cardiac output; do *not* direct treatment toward suppressing this escape rhythm, but toward the primary disease process that allows the escape rhythm to assume pacemaker control of the heart.
• Symptomatic treatment is directed toward increasing the heart rate.

NURSING CARE
May be required for underlying disease

ACTIVITY
Symptomatic animals may require cage rest.

DIET
No modifications or restrictions unless required for management of the underlying condition

CLIENT EDUCATION
Inform of the need to seek and specifically treat an underlying cause.

SURGICAL CONSIDERATIONS
Pacemaker implantation may be necessary.

MEDICATIONS

DRUG(S) OF CHOICE
• Atropine or glycopyrrolate usually indicated to block vagal tone or increase the heart rate
• If those drugs are ineffective, isoproterenol, dopamine, dobutamine, or artificial pacing may be needed.

CONTRAINDICATIONS
Lidocaine, procainamide, quinidine, propranolol, diltiazem, or any other drug that slows the cardiac rate or reduces contractility

PRECAUTIONS
Atropine is briefly vagotonic immediately postinjection and can temporarily exacerbate the condition.

POSSIBLE INTERACTIONS
N/A

ALTERNATIVE DRUG(S)
N/A

FOLLOW-UP

PATIENT MONITORING
• Serial ECG may show clearing of the lesion or progression to complete heart block.
• Serial blood profiles may be needed to monitor progress of the primary disease process.
• Serial echocardiograms may show improvement or progressive changes in cardiac structure

PREVENTION/AVOIDANCE
N/A

POSSIBLE COMPLICATIONS
Prolonged bradycardia may cause secondary congestive heart failure or inadequate renal perfusion.

EXPECTED COURSE AND PROGNOSIS
• Arrhythmia may abate when the primary disorder is corrected.
• Guarded if condition is associated with cardiac or metabolic disorder; poor if the rate

is not increased pharmacologically or if underlying cause cannot be identified and treated

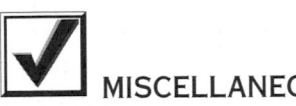

MISCELLANEOUS

ASSOCIATED CONDITIONS
N/A

AGE-RELATED FACTORS
N/A

ZOONOTIC POTENTIAL
N/A

PREGNANCY
N/A

SYNONYMS
None

SEE ALSO
• Atrial Standstill
• Atrioventricular Block, Complete
• Atrioventricular Dissociation

ABBREVIATION
• AV = atrioventricular
• bpm = beats per minute

Suggested Reading
Tilley LP. Essentials of canine and feline electrocardiography. 3rd ed. Baltimore: Williams & Wilkins, 1992:152, 222.
Authors Larry P. Tilley and Naomi L. Burtnick
Consulting Editors Larry P. Tilley and Francis W. K. Smith, Jr.

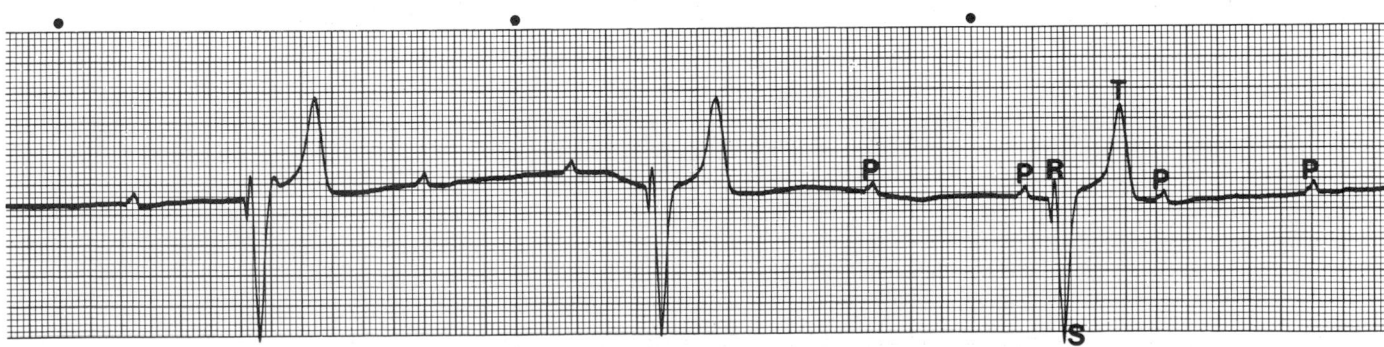

Figure 2.

Complete heart block. The P waves occur at a rate of 120, independent of the ventricular rate of 50. The QRS configuration is a right bundle branch block pattern. The regular rate and stable QRS indicate that the rescuing focus is probably near the AV junction. (From: Tilley LP: Essentials of canine and feline electrocardiography. 3rd ed. Baltimore: Lippincott Williams & Wilkins, 1992, with permission.)

ILEUS

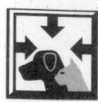 **BASICS**

OVERVIEW

• Adynamic (paralytic, functional) ileus is defined as a transient and reversible intestinal obstruction resulting from inhibition of bowel motility.

• Lack of peristalsis of stomach, small bowel, or large bowel causes functional obstruction, as intestinal contents accumulate in the dependent areas of the gastrointestinal tract instead of being propelled in an aborad direction.

• Ileus is not a primary disease but a secondary complication of a number of disorders.

• Adynamic ileus is thought to occur secondary to electromechanical dissociation of the intestinal musculature due to increased sympathetic tone, release of humoral inhibitory factors (catecholamines, vasopressin, endogenous opiates), impaired release of prokinetic hormones (neurotensin, motilin), or hypokalemia.

SYSTEMS AFFECTED

Gastrointestinal

SIGNALMENT

Cats and dogs

SIGNS

• Anorexia
• Vomiting
• Depression
• Mild abdominal distention or discomfort secondary to accumulation of gas in the hypomotile bowel.

• Failure to auscultate gut sounds after two to three minutes is suggestive of ileus.
• During the initial state (partial loss of motility), the gut sounds can be increased.

CAUSES & RISK FACTORS

• Surgical operations (especially gastrointestinal surgery)
• Electrolyte imbalance (hypokalemia, hypomagnesemia, hypocalcemia)
• Acute inflammatory lesions of the bowel, peritoneal cavity, or other abdominal organs (particularly associated with canine parvoviral enteritis, acute pancreatitis)
• Unrelieved mechanical obstruction
• Intestinal ischemia
• Gram-negative sepsis
• Endotoxemia
• Shock
• Retroperitoneal injury
• Uremia
• Autonomous neuropathies (dysautonomia, spinal cord injury)
• Visceral myopathies
• Use of anticholinergic drugs
• Intestinal overdistention (aerophagia)
• Lead poisoning

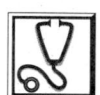 **DIAGNOSIS**

DIFFERENTIAL DIAGNOSIS

Adynamic ileus must be differentiated from mechanical obstructions by:
• Intestinal foreign bodies
• Intussusception
• Intramural abscess
• Incarcerated or strangulated hernia
• Volvulus

• Mesenteric infarction
• Parasites
• Adhesions
• Postoperative stricture
• Impaction
• Congenital malformation
• Inflammatory or traumatic lesions
• Neoplasia

CBC/BIOCHEMISTRY/URINALYSIS

• Hemogram changes depend on primary cause of ileus.
• Serum chemistry profiles and urinalysis help assess electrolyte disturbances (especially hypokalemia) and presence of azotemia.

OTHER LABORATORY TESTS

• TLI and pancreatic lipase tests to identify pancreatitis
• Fecal parvovirus ELISA test in puppies with ileus and diarrhea

IMAGING

Abdominal Radiographic Findings

• Bowel loops are distended with gas and fluid. Common radiographic patterns include:
• Generalized gas ileus—consider aerophagia, smooth muscle paralyzing drugs, generalized peritonitis, or enteritis.
• Generalized fluid ileus—consider enteritis, diffuse intestinal neoplasia.
• Localized gas ileus—consider localized peritonitis (pancreatitis), early stage bowel obstruction, disruption of the arterial supply.
• Localized fluid ileus—consider foreign body, neoplastic obstruction, intussusception.

Ultrasonography
• Differentiate adynamic ileus from mechanical intestinal obstructions.
• Identify pancreatitis or peritonitis.

DIAGNOSTIC PROCEDURES

BIPS (Barium-Impregnated Polyethylene Spheres)
• Confirm adynamic ileus.
• Delayed gastrointestinal transit along with retention of BIPS in the stomach
• Scattering of BIPS throughout the entire upper gastrointestinal tract

Other Procedures to Consider
• Abdominocentesis with peritoneal effusion to confirm peritonitis
• Gastrointestinal endoscopy or exploratory laparotomy to rule out mechanical obstruction
• Spinal radiographs, myelogram, spinal MRI, CT, CSF analysis to identify spinal cord injury
• Ocular response test with 0.1% pilocarpine and 0.25% physostigmine for dysautonomia

TREATMENT
• Identify and treat the primary underlying cause.
• Correct electrolyte abnormalities (especially hypokalemia) if present.
• Use of prokinetic drugs is thought to be helpful.
• Gastrointestinal decompression via nasogastric tube is rarely necessary.

MEDICATIONS

DRUG(S)
Metoclopramide (0.4 mg/kg IV q6h)

CONTRAINDICATIONS/POSSIBLE INTERACTIONS
• Anticholinergic drugs (e.g., atropine, glycopyrrolate)
• Opiates (e.g., morphine, hydromorphone, oxymorphone, butorphanol)
• Opiate antidiarrheals (e.g., paregoric, diphenoxylate hydrochloride/atropine sulfate, loperamide hydrochloride)

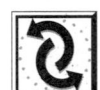

FOLLOW-UP

PATIENT MONITORING
• Monitor correction of electrolyte imbalance if present.
• Abdominal auscultation to evaluate gastrointestinal motility

PREVENTION/AVOIDANCE
Avoid anticholinergic drugs and opiates if not indicated.

POSSIBLE COMPLICATIONS
Animals with adynamic ileus are predisposed to the development of small intestinal bacterial overgrowth, bacterial translocation, and sepsis.

EXPECTED COURSE AND PROGNOSIS
Prognosis depends on successful resolution of primary disease process.

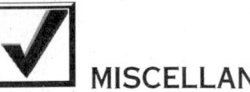

MISCELLANEOUS

ASSOCIATED CONDITIONS
See under Causes & Risk Factors.

AGE-RELATED FACTORS
N/A

ZOONOTIC POTENTIAL
N/A

PREGNANCY
Ileus has been reported in a lactating bitch with hypomagnesemia and hypocalcemia.

SYNONYMS
• Adynamic ileus—functional ileus, paralytic ileus
• Pseudo-obstruction—chronic, more segmental adynamic ileus
• Mechanical ileus—generally addressed in current literature as mechanical obstruction

ABBREVIATIONS
• ELISA = enzyme-linked immunosorbent assay
• TLI = trypsin-like immunoreactivity

Suggested Reading
Guilford WG. Motility disorders of the bowel. In: Guilford WG, Center SA, Strombeck DR, Williams DA, Meyer DJ. Strombeck's small animal gastroenterology. 3rd ed. Philadelphia: Saunders, 1996:335–336.
Author Susanne K Lauer
Consulting Editor Albert E. Jergens

IMMUNODEFICIENCY DISORDERS, PRIMARY

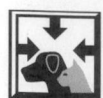

BASICS

DEFINITION
• Diminished ability to mount an effective immune response
• Caused by heritable defects in the immune system (secondary disease—diminished immune response acquired as a consequence of some other primary disease)

PATHOPHYSIOLOGY
• The identification of a specific defect in the immune response requires an adequate understanding of the cellular and genetic basis of the immune system.
• The types and causes are diverse; defects in the cell-mediated, humoral, complement, and phagocytic systems have all been described in the veterinary literature.
• Defects involving the humoral immune response—associated with a high susceptibility to bacterial infection
• Defects involving the cell-mediated immune response—associated with a high susceptibility to viral, fungal, and protozoal infections
• Defects in the phagocytic or complement system—associated with disseminated infection

SYSTEMS AFFECTED
• Hemic/Lymph/Immune—defect in a specific cell population in lymphoid tissue
• Skin/Exocrine, Respiratory, Gastrointestinal—chronic or recurrent infections
• Other organ systems—dissemination of infection, failure to thrive

GENETICS
Typically breed-specific with variable modes of inheritance

INCIDENCE/PREVALENCE
Rare

GEOGRAPHIC DISTRIBUTION
None

SIGNALMENT

Species
Dogs and cats

Breed Predilections
• X-linked severe combined immunodeficiency—Basset hounds, Cardigan Welsh Corgis
• Severe combined immunodeficiency disease (SCID)—Jack Russell terriers
• IgA deficiency—beagles, German shepherds, and Chinese shar-peis
• IgM deficiency—Doberman pinschers
• Thymic hypoplasia—dwarfed Weimaraners
• Cyclic hematopoiesis—gray collies
• Chediak-Higashi syndrome—Persian cats
• Leukocyte adhesion deficiency—Irish setters
• Complement deficiency—Brittany spaniels
• Bactericidal defect—Doberman pinschers
• Transient hypogammaglobulinemia—Samoyeds

Mean Age and Range
Primary immunodeficiency diseases typically expressed in the first year of life

Predominant Sex
X-linked recessive severe combined immunodeficiency disease of Basset hounds—males affected and females carriers for the defect

SIGNS

General Comments
Depend on the level at which the immune response is defective; range from chronic respiratory and gastrointestinal signs and skin infections to life-threatening conditions

Historical Findings
• High susceptibility to infection and failure to respond to appropriate, conventional antibiotic therapy
• Lethargy
• Anorexia
• Skin infection
• Failure to thrive
• Signs often appear when maternal antibody concentrations decline.
• Vaccine-induced disease by modified live virus preparation

Physical Examination Findings
• Hallmark—failure to thrive
• Clinical signs attributable to infections

CAUSES
Congenital

RISK FACTORS
None

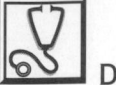

DIAGNOSIS

DIFFERENTIAL DIAGNOSIS
• Patients must be rigorously evaluated for underlying disease process that may cause secondary (acquired) immunodeficient state (e.g., hyperadrenocorticism, FeLV, and FIV).
• Patients are typically young with recurrent infection that fails to respond to conventional treatment

CBC/BIOCHEMISTRY/URINALYSIS
CBC may indicate deficiencies in specifically affected cell lines or a chronic inflammatory process.

OTHER LABORATORY TESTS
• Serum protein electrophoresis—demonstrate gross deficiency in immunoglobulin concentration
• Serum immunoglobulin quantitation—evaluate humoral immune system, identify selective immunoglobulin deficiency, support diagnosis of agammaglobulinemia
• The lymphocyte transformation test—evaluate the cell-mediated immune system and identify animals with T lymphocyte deficiency.
• Bactericidal assays—evaluate neutrophil function.
• Serum concentration of complement components—diagnose complement deficiency.
• Enumeration of lymphocyte subsets by immunofluorescence with monoclonal antibodies—identify deficiency of specific cell lines.
• Other more specific tests to evaluate immune function in veterinary species are available, but to get reliable results generally requires access to research laboratories that perform these tests.

IMAGING
N/A

DIAGNOSTIC PROCEDURES
In some patients, bone marrow and lymph node biopsy aids in classifying the type of immune deficiency.

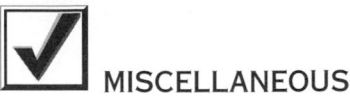

PATHOLOGIC FINDINGS
• Lesions vary; depend on the specific defect; most the result of recurrent or opportunistic infection involving the skin, ear canal, and respiratory and gastrointestinal systems
• Lesions of septicemia common in animals with severe defects
• T lymphocyte defects—hypoplastic or dysplastic lesions of the thymus and T lymphocyte–dependent areas of secondary lymphoid tissues
• B lymphocyte defects—hypoplastic or dysplastic lesions of the bone marrow or B lymphocyte–dependent areas of secondary lymphoid tissues
• Lymphoid hypoplasia or hyperplasia may be seen, depending on the overall defect and the occurrence of infection.

TREATMENT

APPROPRIATE HEALTH CARE
• Hospitalization may be necessary to control life-threatening infection.
• Outpatient management possible for some patients

NURSING CARE
Supportive care appropriate to the nature of the infection

ACTIVITY
Determined largely by the severity of the defect and the occurrence of infection

DIET
• Dietary management may be required to ensure that the patient is maintained at an adequate level of nutrition.
• Potential sources of infectious agents such as raw meat must be avoided.

CLIENT EDUCATION
• Inform client that the animal cannot be cured.
• Discuss why the patient has high susceptibility to infection.
• Discuss and advise as to the heritability of the disease.
• Discuss the possibility of other litter mates being affected.
• Avoid exposure to ill animals.

SURGICAL CONSIDERATIONS
N/A

MEDICATIONS

DRUG(S) OF CHOICE
• Antibiotics to control infections
• γ-Globulin or plasma preparations can be used in conjunction with antibiotics to control infection in patients with humoral defect.
• Symptomatic treatment for secondary disease states

CONTRAINDICATIONS
γ-Globulin or plasma preparations should not be administered to patients with selective IgA deficiency, because many affected patients have high concentrations of anti-IgA antibodies and may develop an anaphylactic reaction.

PRECAUTIONS
Modified live virus vaccines should not be administered to patients with suspected T lymphocyte deficiencies, because they may induce disease in these patients.

POSSIBLE INTERACTIONS
None

ALTERNATIVE DRUG(S)
None

FOLLOW-UP

PATIENT MONITORING
• For clinical signs of secondary infection
• Routine physical examination to assess efficacy of antibiotic therapy in control of secondary infection

PREVENTION/AVOIDANCE
• Affected animals should not be bred.
• Pedigree analysis to determine the mode of inheritance and prevent propagating the defect

POSSIBLE COMPLICATIONS
Infection

EXPECTED COURSE AND PROGNOSIS
• The severity of the defect determines the course of disease and prognosis.
• Patients with minor defects can be successfully managed.

MISCELLANEOUS

ASSOCIATED CONDITIONS
None

AGE-RELATED FACTORS
Usually expressed early in life

ZOONOTIC POTENTIAL
None

PREGNANCY
N/A

SYNONYMS
None

SEE ALSO
Neutropenia

ABBREVIATIONS
• FeLV = feline leukemia virus
• FIV = feline immunodeficiency virus

Suggested Reading
Guilford WG. Primary immunodeficiency diseases of dogs and cats. Compend Cont Ed Pract Vet 1987;9:641–648.
Lewis RM, Picut CA. Veterinary clinical immunology. Philadelphia: Lea & Febiger, 1989.
Author Paul W. Snyder
Consulting Editor Stephen A. Kruth

IMMUNOPROLIFERATIVE ENTEROPATHY OF BASENJIS

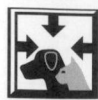 BASICS

OVERVIEW
• An immunologically mediated disease characterized by chronic intermittent diarrhea, anorexia, and weight loss associated with lymphoplasmacytic enteritis, protein-losing enteropathy, malabsorption, maldigestion, and hypergammaglobulinemia due to increased concentrations of serum IgA
• Pathogenesis unclear but related to abnormal immune responses
• Systems affected include gastrointestinal, immune, skin, renal, endocrine, and hepatobiliary

SIGNALMENT
• Young to middle-aged basenjis—usually <3 years of age
• Related dogs often affected

SIGNS
• Chronic intermittent diarrhea
• Severe progressive weight loss
• Anorexia often preceding diarrhea
• Bilaterally symmetric alopecia
• Scaling and ulceration of ear margins
• Attitude—usually bright and alert
• Vomiting occasionally noted

CAUSES & RISK FACTORS
• Cause unknown
• Immune, genetic, and environmental factors are likely.
• Episodes of diarrhea are associated with stressful events—boarding, estrus, transport, vaccination, etc.

 DIAGNOSIS

DIFFERENTIAL DIAGNOSIS
• Lymphangiectasia, lymphoplasmacytic enteritis, eosinophilic enteritis, histoplasmosis, exocrine pancreatic insufficiency, intestinal lymphoma, metabolic disorders, intestinal parasitism
• Signalment, age of onset, fecal, CBC, chemistry profile, urinalysis, serum trypsin-like immunoreactivity (TLI)/ B_{12}/folate, serum IgA levels, and gastrointestinal histology are used to differentiate.

CBC/BIOCHEMISTRY/URINALYSIS
• Hypoproteinemia
• Severe hypoalbuminemia
• Hyperglobulinemia
• Mature neutrophilia often present
• Poorly regenerative anemia—advanced disease
• Moderately increased hepatic enzymes—advanced disease

OTHER LABORATORY TESTS
• Hypergammaglobulinemia due to increased serum IgA
• Depression of xylose absorption curve correlates with severity of clinical disease.
• Small intestinal bacterial overgrowth may cause functional exocrine pancreatic insufficiency, but TLI is normal.
• May be hypergastrinemia and hyperchlorhydria

IMAGING
Abdominal ultrasound may demonstrate diffuse small bowel thickening, normal gastrointestinal wall layering, and lack of other visceral abnormalities.

OTHER DIAGNOSTIC PROCEDURES
Endoscopic appearance of the small bowel typically is abnormal.

PATHOLOGIC FINDINGS
• Consistent pathologic lesions include uniform thickening of the small bowel,

generalized infiltration of the intestinal lamina propria with lymphocytes and plasma cells, and blunting and fusion of villous tips.
• May be gastric mucosal hypertrophy, lymphocytic gastritis, parietal and chief cell hyperplasia, and gastric ulceration
• Presence and severity of gastric lesions do not correlate with severity of intestinal lesions.
• Other associated lesions include thyroid parafollicular cell atrophy, gastric acinar atrophy, and glomerulonephritis.

 ## TREATMENT

• Outpatient medical management unless dehydration or other severe complications exist
• Advise owners not to breed affected dogs or their littermates.
• Minimize stressful episodes.
• Use dietary trials to determine what diet is best tolerated.

 ## MEDICATIONS

DRUG(S)

Antibiotics
• Used for small intestinal bacterial overgrowth
• Metronidazole (10–20 mg/kg PO q12–24h)
• Tylosin (10 mg/kg PO q12h)
• Oxytetracycline (10–20 mg/kg PO q8h)

Corticosteroids
• Used for immunosuppression and anti-inflammation
• Prednisone (1 mg/kg PO q12h for 2–4 weeks, then slowly taper over 4–6 months to achieve 0.5–1 mg/kg PO q48h)

CONTRAINDICATIONS/POSSIBLE INTERACTIONS
Anticholinergics contraindicated

 ## FOLLOW-UP

• Diarrhea and weight loss usually show initial improvement with antibiotic or corticosteroid therapy.
• Recurrence of signs is common.
• Long-term prognosis poor

 ## MISCELLANEOUS

ABBREVIATIONS
TLI = trypsin-like immunoreactivity

Suggested Reading
Breitschwerdt EB. Immuno-proliferative enteropathy of Basenjis. Semin Vet Med Surg (Sm Anim) 1992;7:153–161.
Author Amy M. Grooters
Consulting Editor Albert E. Jergens

INCONTINENCE, FECAL

BASICS

DEFINITION
Inability to retain feces, resulting in involuntary passage of fecal material

PATHOPHYSIOLOGY
• Reservoir fecal incontinence develops when disease processes reduce the capacity or compliance of the rectum.
• Sphincter incontinence develops when the external anal sphincter is anatomically disrupted (i.e. nonneurogenic sphincter incontinence) or denervated (i.e. neurogenic sphincter incontinence).
• Neurogenic sphincter incontinence can be caused by pudendal nerve damage, sacral spinal cord disease, autonomic dysfunction, and generalized peripheral neuropathy or myopathy.
• Damage to, or degeneration of, the levator ani and coccygeus muscles may also contribute.

SYSTEMS AFFECTED
• Nervous
• Gastrointestinal

SIGNALMENT
• Dogs and cats
• Although any age animal may be affected, incidence increases in older patients.

SIGNS

Historical Findings
• Reservoir incontinence—promotes an urge to defecate; signs include frequent, conscious defecation without dribbling of feces; defecation may be associated with tenesmus, dyschezia, or hematochezia.
• Sphincter incontinence—associated with involuntary expulsion or dribbling of fecal material, especially during excitement or barking and coughing
• Question clients about previous neurologic disease, anorectal surgery and/or trauma, house training, deworming, and whether the pet seems to defecate voluntarily or involuntarily; also obtain information regarding the pet's diet, current medications, and concurrent systemic clinical signs, especially neurologic signs.
• Concurrent urinary incontinence suggests neurogenic sphincter incontinence.

Physical Examination Findings
• Reservoir incontinence—may include anorectal sensitivity or pain on digital palpation, a rectal mass or thickening of the rectal mucosa; external anal sphincter tone and nonneurogenic sphincter incontinence anal reflex are normal.

• Nonneurogenic sphincter incontinence—may include evidence of perineal trauma or perianal fistulas; the anal reflex is present, but the external anal sphincter may not completely close if the sphincter has been anatomically disrupted.
• Neurogenic sphincter incontinence—may include loss of tone to the external anal sphincter, but anal tone is a poor indicator of anal sphincter function; the anal reflex is absent or diminished.
• Do a complete neurologic examination on all animals with sphincter incontinence; additional findings suggesting lumbosacral spinal cord disease include loss of voluntary movement and tone to the tail, lumbosacral pain, flaccid posterior paresis or paralysis, and hyporeflexic myotatic reflexes to the pelvic limbs.
• Diffuse lower motor neuron signs suggest generalized peripheral neuropathy or myopathy; upper motor neuron signs to the pelvic limbs suggest CNS disease cranial to the lumbosacral plexus.

CAUSES

Reservoir Incontinence
• Colorectal disease—colitis and neoplasia
• Diarrhea—large volumes of feces from any cause can overwhelm the absorptive and storage capacity of the colon.

Nonneurogenic Sphincter Incontinence
• Traumatic anal injuries—bite wounds, laceration, or gunshot
• Iatrogenic—the external anal sphincter and levator ani muscles can be anatomically disrupted during anorectal surgery.
• Perianal fistulas

Neurogenic Sphincter Incontinence
• CNS—degenerative myelopathy, spinal dysraphism, spina bifida, trauma, intervertebral disk extrusion, neoplasia, meningomyelitis (various causes), fibrocartilaginous embolism, other vascular compromises
• Cauda equina syndrome—L6-L7 or L7-S1 intervertebral disk extrusion, spondylosis deformans, congenital spinal canal stenosis, lumbosacral instability, diskospondylitis, and neoplasia
• Peripheral neuropathy—infectious, immune-mediated, drug-induced (e.g., vincristine sulfate), dysautonomia, and idiopathic
• Myopathy/neuromuscular disorder
• Degeneration (aging)—multiple factors are likely involved, including atrophy of the muscles involved in fecal continence, weakness, degenerative neuropathy, and senility.

RISK FACTORS
• Anorectal disease and surgery
• CNS disease and peripheral neuropathy

DIAGNOSIS

DIFFERENTIAL DIAGNOSIS
• Gastrointestinal disease from any cause can increase the urge to defecate without directly altering the reservoir capacity of the colon.
• Unlike sphincter incontinence, gastrointestinal disease is often associated with weight loss, vomiting, tenesmus, dyschezia, and hematochezia.
• Behavior disorders (e.g., separation anxiety), unlike fecal incontinence, are often associated with destructive activities or excessive vocalization.
• Inadequate house training usually occurs in young dogs or dogs recently introduced to an indoor environment.

CBC/BIOCHEMISTRY/URINALYSIS
• Results usually normal
• Urinalysis may show evidence of lower urinary tract infection (e.g., pyuria, hematuria), especially with concurrent urinary incontinence.

OTHER LABORATORY TESTS
Perform fecal flotation to help rule out parasitism as a cause of diarrhea.

IMAGING
• Lateral and ventrodorsal survey radiography of the lumbosacral spine may show evidence of intervertebral disk extrusion, diskospondylitis, vertebral neoplasia, spina bifida, lumbosacral trauma, or vertebral malformation.
• Myelography and epidurography are also useful in demonstrating compressive lesions within the spinal canal.
• CT and MRI may be necessary to demonstrate some compressive lesions and intraparenchymal spinal cord lesions.

OTHER DIAGNOSTIC PROCEDURES
• Electromyography (EMG) to evaluate external anal sphincter, levator ani, and coccygeus muscles for evidence of denervation or myopathy
• Evaluation of other muscles recommended to help localize the neurologic lesion—diffuse denervation versus focal spinal cord lesion
• Can evaluate the pudendal-anal reflex electrophysiologically
• Muscle and nerve biopsy for myopathy and peripheral neuropathy
• Analysis of cerebrospinal fluid (CSF) collected by lumbar puncture may reveal evidence of a CNS infectious or inflammatory process, neoplasia, or trauma.
• Perform colonoscopy and colorectal mucosal biopsy if reservoir incontinence is suspected.

TREATMENT

- If possible, identify the underlying cause; fecal incontinence may resolve if the underlying cause is successfully treated (e.g., spinal cord decompression).
- Dietary—fecal volume can be reduced by feeding low-residue diets such as cottage cheese and rice and/or tofu
- Frequent warm water enemas will diminish the volume of feces in the colon and thus decrease the incidence of inappropriate defecation.
- Environmental changes (e.g., making the pet an outside pet) may increase client satisfaction and thus avoid euthanasia of an otherwise healthy animal.
- Reflex defecation can sometimes be induced in animals with posterior paralysis (e.g., a mild pinch of the toe on a pelvic limb or tail); similarly, applying a warm washcloth to the anus or perineum may stimulate defecation.
- Surgical reconstruction of anorectal lesions may markedly improve fecal continence in patients with nonneurogenic sphincter incontinence.
- Fascial slings and silicone elastomer slings have met with variable success in treating neurogenic sphincter incontinence in dogs.
- Prognosis is poor if the underlying cause cannot be identified and successfully corrected; discuss the prognosis with the client early in the evaluation, to avoid unrealistic expectations.

MEDICATIONS

DRUG(S) OF CHOICE

- Opiate motility-modifying drugs (e.g., diphenoxylate hydrochloride and loperamide hydrochloride) increase segmental contraction of the bowel and slow passage of fecal material, thus increasing the amount of water absorbed from the feces.

- Antiinflammatory agents, such as glucocorticoids and sulfasalazine, may benefit patients with suspected reservoir incontinence due to inflammatory bowel disease.

CONTRAINDICATIONS

- Do not use motility modifying drugs in patients with diarrhea if an infectious or toxic cause is suspected.
- Do not use opiate motility modifiers in patients with respiratory disease; use cautiously in patients with liver disease.
- Use of opiates in cats is generally not recommended.

PRECAUTIONS

- Motility-modifying drugs may cause constipation and bloat.
- Opiate motility-modifying drugs may cause sedation.

POSSIBLE INTERACTIONS

Increased sedation and respiratory depression are possible when opiates are used concurrently with other CNS depressants (e.g., barbiturates, general anesthetics, and tranquilizers).

ALTERNATIVE DRUG(S)

N/A

FOLLOW-UP

PATIENT MONITORING

- If fecal incontinence is due to an underlying neurologic cause, use serial neurologic examinations to monitor patient progress.
- Radiographic procedures, EMG, CSF analysis, and electrodiagnostic studies can also be used to follow progress.
- Check fecal consistency and volume.
- Adjust diet and motility-modifying drug dosages to find the appropriate therapy for each individual patient.

POSSIBLE COMPLICATIONS

- Neurogenic sphincter incontinence is often unresponsive despite appropriate dietary, medical, and surgical treatment.
- Fifty percent of pets with fecal incontinence were euthanized in one recent study.

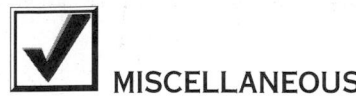

MISCELLANEOUS

ASSOCIATED CONDITIONS

N/A

AGE-RELATED FACTORS

N/A

ZOONOTIC POTENTIAL

- Exposure to animal feces increases the risk of exposure to zoonotic parasites.
- Advise clients about zoonotic diseases (e.g., cutaneous and visceral larval migrans and toxoplasmosis).

PREGNANCY

N/A

SYNONYMS

N/A

SEE ALSO

- Incontinence, Urinary
- Intervertebral Disk Disease, Thoracolumbar

ABBREVIATIONS

CSF = cerebrospinal fluid
CT = computed tomography
EMG = electromyography
MRI = magnetic resonance imaging

Suggested Reading

Guilford WG. Fecal incontinence in dogs and cats. Compend Contin Educ Pract Vet 1990;12:313–326.

Richter KP. Diseases of the rectum and anus. In: Kirk's current veterinary therapy XI. Philadelphia: Saunders, 1992:615–616.

Washabau RJ, Brockman DJ. Recto-anal disease. In: Ettinger SJ, Feldman EC, eds. Textbook of veterinary internal medicine. 4th ed. Philadelphia: Saunders, 1995: 1408–1409.

Author Randall C. Longshore
Consulting Editor Albert E. Jergens

INCONTINENCE, URINARY

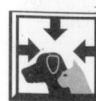

BASICS

DEFINITION
Loss of voluntary control of micturition, usually observed as involuntary urine leakage

PATHOPHYSIOLOGY
Usually a disorder of the storage phase of micturition. Urine storage failure is caused by failure of urinary bladder accommodation, failure of urethral continence mechanisms, or anatomic bypass of urinary storage structures. Partial outlet obstruction and other causes of urinary bladder overdistension may result in paradoxical, or overflow, urinary incontinence.

SYSTEMS AFFECTED
• Renal/Urologic
• Nervous
• Skin/Exocrine—urine scald and perineal and ventral dermatitis, recessed vulva

INCIDENCE/PREVALENCE
Urinary incontinence may affect more than 20% of spayed female dogs, especially large-breed dogs.

SIGNALMENT
• Dogs and (rarely) cats
• Most common in middle-aged to old neutered female dogs; also observed in juvenile females and (rarely) neutered males
• Medium to large-breed dogs most often affected

SIGNS
N/A

CAUSES

Neurologic
• Disruption of local neuroreceptors, peripheral nerves, spinal pathways, or higher centers involved in the control of micturition can disrupt urine storage.
• Lesions of the sacral spinal cord, such as a congenital malformation, cauda equina compression, lumbosacral disk disease, or traumatic fractures or dislocation, can result in a flaccid, overdistended urinary bladder with weak outlet resistance. Urine retention and overflow incontinence develop.
• Lesions of the cerebellum or cerebral micturition center affect inhibition and voluntary control of voiding, usually resulting in frequent, involuntary urination or leakage of small volumes of urine.

Urinary Bladder Storage Dysfunction
• Poor accommodation of urine during storage or urinary bladder hypercontractility leads to frequent leakage of small amounts of urine.
• Urinary tract infection, chronic inflammatory disorder, infiltrative neoplastic lesions, external compression, and chronic partial outlet obstruction are potential causes.

• Congenital urinary bladder hypoplasia may accompany ectopic ureters or other developmental disorders of the urogenital tract.
• Idiopathic detrusor instability has been associated with FeLV infection in cats and unknown causes in dogs.

Urethral Disorders
• If urethral closure provided by urethral smooth muscle, striated muscle, and connective tissue does not prevent leakage of urine during storage, intermittent urinary incontinence is observed.
• Examples—congenital urethral hypoplasia or incompetence, acquired urethral incompetence (i.e., reproductive hormone–responsive urinary incontinence), urinary tract infection or inflammation, prostatic disease or prostatic surgery (males), and vestibulovaginal anomaly (females)

Anatomic
• Developmental or acquired anatomic abnormalities that divert urine from normal storage mechanisms or interfere with urinary bladder or urethral function
• Ectopic ureters can terminate in the distal urethra, uterus, or vagina.
• Patent urachal remnants divert urine outflow to the umbilicus.
• Vestibulovaginal anomalies, congenital urocystic hypoplasia, or urethral hypoplasia
• Intrapelvic bladder neck location may contribute to urine leakage due to urethral incompetence.
• Vulvar and perivulvar conformation abnormalities may contribute.

Urine Retention
Overflow observed when intravesicular pressure exceeds outlet resistance

Mixed Urinary Incontinence
Mixed or multiple causes are observed in humans and probably occur in dogs and cats. Combinations of urethral and bladder storage dysfunction and combinations of anatomic and functional disorders are most likely.

RISK FACTORS
• Neutering increases the risk of development of urethral incompetence.
• Early neutering has not been shown to significantly increase the risk of urinary incontinence in dogs.
• Conformational characteristics such as bladder neck position, urethral length, and concurrent vaginal anomalies may increase the risk of urinary incontinence in female dogs.
• Obesity may increase the risk of urinary incontinence in neutered female dogs.
• Other possible risk factors for urethral incompetence include breed, large body size, and early tail docking.

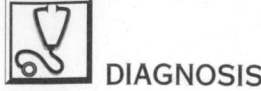

DIAGNOSIS

DIFFERENTIAL DIAGNOSIS

Differentiating Similar Signs
• Voluntary but inappropriate urination (usually behavioral)
• Urethral discharges, often associated with prostatic disease in male dogs and vaginal disorders in female dogs
• Urine spraying or inappropriate urination in cats can be confused with urinary incontinence; spraying is more likely to be done by cats in an upright position, with urine soiling found on vertical surfaces of furniture, walls, and drapes.
• Polyuria—may precipitate or exacerbate urinary incontinence or lead to nocturia and inappropriate urination; measure urine specific gravity in a random urine sample to rule in or out clinically important polyuria.

Differentiating Causes
• Neurogenic causes of urinary incontinence—usually cause a large, distended urinary bladder and other neurologic deficits such as weak anal or tail tone, depressed perineal sensation, and proprioceptive deficits
• Dogs with urethral incompetence typically exhibit intermittent occurrences of urinary incontinence, observed most often at night or while the animal is sleeping. Physical examination reveals a small urinary bladder and no other defects.
• Historical and physical findings in patients with urinary bladder storage dysfunction resemble those observed in patients with urethral incompetence, although increased frequency of urination or apparent urgency may be additional clinical signs.
• Anisocoria is found frequently in cats with urinary incontinence associated with FeLV infection.
• Historical signs in male dogs with prostatic disease include tenesmus, hind limb weakness, dysuria, and pollakiuria. Physical findings include prostatomegaly, lumbosacral pain, pain on prostatic palpation, and hind limb trembling or weakness.

CBC/BIOCHEMISTRY/URINALYSIS
• Hematologic and biochemical analyses may be indicated in patients with polyuric disorders (see Polyuria and Polydipsia).
• Urinalysis is always recommended and may reveal evidence of urinary tract infection (e.g., pyuria, hematuria, and bacteria) or polyuria (e.g., low urine specific gravity).

OTHER LABORATORY TESTS
Test cats for FeLV infection.

IMAGING

Radiographic Findings
• Contrast radiography is indicated in juvenile animals and animals exhibiting urinary incontinence shortly after surgical procedures or traumatic incidents
• Excretory urography allows visualization of the kidneys, ureteral terminations, and urinary bladder.
• Retrograde vaginourethrography allows visualization of the vaginal vault, urethra, and urinary bladder. Ectopic ureters usually fill with contrast media in these retrograde studies as well.
• Double-contrast cystography may be required for full visualization of urinary bladder structure and identification of urinary bladder lesions.

Ultrasonographic Findings
Can use for evaluation of the kidneys, ureters, and urinary bladder to identify uroliths, masses, hydronephrosis or hydroureter, or evidence of pyelonephritis

DIAGNOSTIC PROCEDURES
• Neurologic examination—examination of anal tone, tail tone, perineal sensation, and bulbospongiosus reflexes provides a brief assessment of caudal spinal and peripheral nerve function
• Urethral catheterization—may be required to assess patency of the urethra if urine retention is observed
• Urodynamic procedures—consider cystometrography, urethral pressure profilometry, and electromyography to evaluate urinary bladder, urethral, and neurologic function more objectively.
• Cystoscopy—may visualize bladder, urethra, and ectopic ureteral terminations

 TREATMENT

APPROPRIATE HEALTH CARE
• Usually as outpatient
• Address partial obstructive disorders and primary neurologic disorders specifically if possible.
• Identify urinary tract infection and treat appropriately.
• Ectopic ureters and congenital urethral hypoplasia can be surgically corrected; functional abnormalities of urethral competence or urinary bladder storage function may accompany the anatomic disorder and require ancillary medical treatment.
• Surgical procedures such as colposuspension, cystourethropexy, Teflon or collagen implants, and prosthetic sphincter implantation have been described for the treatment of refractory incontinence.

 MEDICATIONS

DRUG(S) OF CHOICE

Urethral Incompetence
• Manage with reproductive hormones (e.g., stilbestrol, diethylstilbestrol [0.1–1.0 mg/dog PO q24h for 5–7 days followed by 0.1–1.0 mg/dog PO q4–7 days prn], conjugated estrogens, estriol, and testosterone) or α-adrenergic agonists (e.g., phenylpropanolamine [1.5 mg/kg PO q8–12h], phenylephrine, pseudoephedrine [1.1 mg/kg PO q12h]).
• α-Adrenergic agents and reproductive hormones can be administered in combination for a synergistic therapeutic effect.
• Availability of diethylstilbestrol and phenylpropanolamine may be limited to veterinary compounding pharmacies.
• Imipramine (5–15 mg/dog PO q12h), a tricyclic antidepressant with anticholinergic and α-agonist actions, provides an alternative method of treatment.

Detrusor Instability
Manage with anticholinergic or antispasmodic agents (e.g., oxybutynin [approximately 0.2 mg/kg PO q8–12h, up to 5 mg total dose], propantheline, imipramine, flavoxate, and dicyclomine).

Prostatic Disease
See Prostatomegaly; Prostatitis and Prostatic Abscesses.

CONTRAINDICATIONS
• Adrenergic agonists in patients with cardiac disease, renal disease, and hypertensive disorders
• Anticholinergic agents in patients with glaucoma or cardiac disease

PRECAUTIONS
• Estrogen compounds (rarely) cause signs of estrus, bone marrow suppression, and exacerbate immune-mediated disease.
• Testosterone administration can cause signs of aggression or libido, exacerbate prostatic disease, and contribute to the development of perineal hernia or perianal adenoma.
• Adrenergic agonists can cause restlessness, tachycardia, and hypertension.
• Anticholinergic agents can cause nausea, vomiting, and constipation.

POSSIBLE INTERACTIONS
• Tricyclic antidepressants should not be administered concurrently with monoamine-oxidase inhibitors (e.g., Anipryl).
• The risk of hypertension increases if α-adrenergic agonists are administered concurrently with tricyclic antidepressants.

ALTERNATIVE DRUG(S)
N/A

 FOLLOW-UP

PATIENT MONITORING
• Patients receiving α-adrenergic agents—observe during the initial treatment period for adverse effects of the drug including tachycardia, anxiety, and hypertension. • Patients receiving estrogen—initial, 1-month, and periodic hemograms • Periodic urinalysis and urine culture • Expect excellent response to medical treatment in 60–90% of treated patients. • Once a therapeutic effect has been observed, slowly reduce the dosage and frequency of administration of pharmacologic agents to the minimum required. • Consider combination treatment (α-adrenergic agonist with reproductive hormones or anticholinergic agents) or surgical options if poor response to single-agent medication

POSSIBLE COMPLICATIONS
• Recurrent and ascending urinary tract infection • Urine scald and perineal and ventral dermatitis • Refractory and unmanageable incontinence

 MISCELLANEOUS

ASSOCIATED CONDITIONS
Urinary tract infection

PREGNANCY
Although urinary incontinence is rare in pregnant animals, the use of estrogens or anticholinergic agents is not advised.

SYNONYMS
Enuresis

SEE ALSO
• Polyuria and Polydipsia • Prostatitis and Prostatic Abscess • Urinary Tract Obstruction • Urinary Retention, Functional

ABBREVIATION
FeLV = feline leukemia virus

Suggested Reading
Holt PE. Pathophysiology and treatment of urethral sphincter mechanism incompetence in the incontinent bitch. Vet Intern 1992;3:15.
Lane IF. Treating urinary incontinence. Vet Med 2003;98:58–65.
Lane IF, Barsanti JA. Urinary incontinence. In: August J. ed. Consultations in feline internal medicine. 2nd ed. Philadelphia: Saunders, 1994:373–382.
Rawlings C, Barsanti JA, Mahaffey MB, Bement S. Evaluation of colposuspension for treatment of incontinence in spayed female dogs. J Am Vet Med Assoc 2001;219:770–775.
Author India F. Lane
Consulting Editors Larry G. Adams and Carl A. Osborne

INFECTIOUS CANINE TRACHEOBRONCHITIS (KENNEL COUGH)

 BASICS

DEFINITION
Any contagious respiratory disease of dogs that is manifested by coughing and seemingly not caused by canine distemper virus

PATHOPHYSIOLOGY
Pathogenesis usually involves an injury to the respiratory epithelium, viral infection, or both, followed by invasion of the damaged tissue by bacterial, fungal, mycoplasmal, parasitic, or other virulent organisms, resulting in further damage and clinical signs.

SYSTEMS AFFECTED
Respiratory—primarily affected unless associated with sepsis or congenital anomaly

GENETICS
N/A

INCIDENCE/PREVALENCE
Occurs most commonly in places where dogs of varying ages and susceptibility congregate, often under less than ideal hygienic conditions

GEOGRAPHIC DISTRIBUTION
Worldwide

SIGNALMENT

Species
Dogs

Breed Predilection
None

Mean Age and Range
• Most severe in puppies 6 weeks to 6 months old
• May develop in dogs of all ages and often with pre-existing subclinical airway disease (e.g., congenital anomaly, chronic bronchitis, and bronchiectasis)

Predominant Sex
None

SIGNS

General Comments
• Related to the degree of respiratory tract damage and age of the affected dog
• May be nonexistent, mild, or severe with pneumonia
• Most viral, bacterial, and mycoplasmal agents spread rapidly from seemingly healthy dogs to others in the same environment; signs usually begin about 4 days after exposure to the infecting agent(s).

Historical Findings
• Uncomplicated—cough in an otherwise healthy animal is characteristic; may be dry and hacking, soft and dry, moist and hacking, or paroxysmal, followed by gagging or expectoration of mucus; excitement, exercise, changes in temperature or humidity of the inspired air, and gentle pressure (e.g., from collar) on the trachea induce a paroxysm of coughing.
• Severe—affect on appetite severe; cough (when noted) is moist and productive; may see lethargy, anorexia, dyspnea, and exercise intolerance

Physical Examination Findings
• Uncomplicated—cough readily induced with tracheal pressure; lung sounds often normal; otherwise healthy
• Severe—may detect constant, low-grade, or fluctuating fever (39.4–40.0°C; 103–104°F); may detect increased intensity of normal lung sounds, crackles, or (less frequently) wheezes

CAUSES
• Viral—canine distemper virus; CAV-2; CPI; CAV-1; canine reovirus type 1, 2, or 3; canine herpesvirus
• CAV-2 and CPI—may damage respiratory epithelium to such an extent that invasion by various bacteria and mycoplasmas causes severe airway disease
• Bacterial—*Bordetella bronchiseptica*, with no other respiratory pathogens, produces clinical signs indistinguishable from those of other bacterial causes; *Pseudomonas, Escherichia coli, Klebsiella, Pasteurella, Streptococcus, Mycoplasma,* and other species equally likely

RISK FACTORS
• Less than ideal hygienic conditions—seen in some pet shops, humane society shelters, research facilities, and boarding and training kennels
• Coexisting subclinical airway disease—congenital anomalies; chronic bronchitis; bronchiectasis

 DIAGNOSIS

DIFFERENTIAL DIAGNOSIS
• The diagnosis is usually provisionally established by eliminating noninfectious causes of coughing.
• Numerous organisms that infect the lungs
• History that reveals a source of exposure
• Patient's vaccination status
• See Cough.

CBC/BIOCHEMISTRY/URINALYSIS
• Early mild leukopenia (5000–6000 cells/dL)—may be detected; suggests viral cause
• Neutrophilic leukocytosis with a left shift—frequently found with severe pneumonia
• Serum chemistry profile and urinalysis—usually normal

OTHER LABORATORY TESTS
Arterial blood gas analysis—may be useful with pneumonia

IMAGING
• Radiographs—unremarkable with uncomplicated disease; of value primarily to rule out noninfectious causes of a cough
• Thoracic radiographs—severe cases: may demonstrate an interstitial and alveolar lung pattern with a cranioventral distribution typical of bacterial pneumonia; may see a diffuse interstitial lung pattern typical of viral pneumonia; may note a mixed lung pattern (e.g., combination of alveolar, interstitial, and peribronchial lung patterns)

DIAGNOSTIC PROCEDURES
• With suspected severe disease—perform transtracheal washing or tracheobronchial lavage via bronchoscopy.
• Antimicrobial sensitivity pattern of cultured bacteria—identification aids markedly in providing an effective treatment plan

PATHOLOGIC FINDINGS
• CPI—causes few to no clinical signs; lungs of infected dogs 6–10 days after exposure may contain petechial hemorrhages that are evenly distributed over the surfaces; detected by immunofluorescence in columnar epithelial cells of the bronchi and bronchioles 6–10 days after aerosol exposure
• CAV-2—lesions confined to the respiratory system; large intranuclear inclusion bodies found in bronchial epithelial cells and alveolar septal cells; clinical signs tend to be mild and short-lasting; lesions persist for at least a month after infection
• Bordetellosis and severe bacterial infection—evidence of purulent bronchitis, tracheitis, and rhinitis with hyperemia and enlargement of the bronchial, mediastinal, and retropharyngeal lymph nodes; may see large numbers of gram-positive or -negative organisms in the mucus of the tracheal and bronchial epithelium

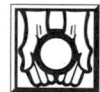 **TREATMENT**

APPROPRIATE HEALTH CARE
• Outpatient—strongly recommended for uncomplicated disease
• Inpatient—strongly recommended for complicated disease and/or pneumonia

NURSING CARE
Fluid administration—indicated for complicated disease and/or pneumonia

INFECTIOUS CANINE TRACHEOBRONCHITIS (KENNEL COUGH)

ACTIVITY
Enforce rest—for at least 14–21 days with uncomplicated disease; for at least the duration of radiographic evidence of pneumonia

DIET
Good-quality canned or dry commercial food

CLIENT EDUCATION
• Encourage client to isolate patient from other animals; infected dogs can transmit the agent(s) before onset of clinical signs and afterward until immunity develops.
• Inform client that patients with uncomplicated disease should respond to treatment in 10–14 days.
• Inform client that once infection spreads in a kennel, it can be controlled by evacuation for 1–2 weeks and disinfecting with commonly used chemicals, such as sodium hypochlorite (1:30 dilution), chlorhexidine, and benzalkonium.

SURGICAL CONSIDERATIONS
N/A

MEDICATIONS

DRUG(S) OF CHOICE
• Amoxicillin/clavulanic acid (12.5–25 mg/kg PO q12h) or doxycycline (5 mg/kg PO q12h)—initial treatment of uncomplicated disease
• Gentamicin (2–4 mg/kg IV, IM, SC q6–8h) or amikacin (6.5 mg/kg IV, IM, SC q8h) and a first-generation cephalosporin (cefazolin, 20–35 mg/kg IV, IM q8h) or enrofloxacin (2.5–5 mg/kg PO, IM, IV q12h)—usually effective for severe disease
• Antimicrobial therapy—continue for at least 10 days beyond radiographic resolution.
• *B. bronchiseptica* and other resistant species—some antimicrobials may not reach adequate therapeutic concentrations in the lumen of the lower respiratory tract, so oral or parenteral administration may have limited effectiveness; nebulization with kanamycin (250 mg), gentamicin (50 mg), or polymyxin B (333,000 IU) may eliminate species when administered daily for 3–5 days.
• Butorphanol (0.55 mg/kg PO q8–12h) or hydrocodone bitartrate (0.22 mg/kg PO q6–8h)—effective suppression of dry, nonproductive cough

• Bronchodilators (e.g., Theo-Dur, 10–20 mg/kg PO q12h)—may use to control bronchospasm; made clinically apparent by wheezing

CONTRAINDICATIONS
Do not use cough suppressants in patients with pneumonia.

PRECAUTIONS
None

POSSIBLE INTERACTIONS
Fluoroquinolones and theophylline derivatives—concurrent use causes high and possibly toxic plasma theophylline concentration.

ALTERNATIVE DRUG(S)
None

FOLLOW-UP

PATIENT MONITORING
• Uncomplicated disease—should respond to treatment in 10–14 days; if patient continues to cough 14 days or more after establishment of an adequate treatment plan, question the diagnosis of uncomplicated disease.
• Severe disease—repeat thoracic radiography until at least 14 days beyond resolution of all clinical signs.

PREVENTION/AVOIDANCE
Shedding of the causative agent(s) of infectious tracheobronchitis in respiratory secretions of dogs undoubtedly accounts for the persistence of this problem in kennels, animal shelters, boarding facilities, and veterinary hospitals.

Viral and Bacterial Vaccines
• Available to control the principal agents involved
• *B. bronchiseptica* and CPI vaccine—may vaccinate puppies intranasally as early as 2–4 weeks of age without interference from maternal antibody and follow with annual revaccination; may vaccinate mature dogs with a one-dose intranasal vaccination (at the same time as their puppies or when they receive their annual vaccinations)
• Inactivated *B. bronchiseptica* parenteral vaccine—administered as two doses, 2–4 weeks apart; initial vaccination of puppies is recommended at or about 6–8 weeks of age; revaccinate at 4 months of age.

POSSIBLE COMPLICATIONS
N/A

EXPECTED COURSE AND PROGNOSIS
• Natural course of uncomplicated disease, if untreated—10–14 days; simple restriction of exercise and prevention of excitement shortens the course.
• Typical course of severe disease—2–6 weeks; patients that die often developed severe pneumonia that affected multiple lung lobes.

MISCELLANEOUS

ASSOCIATED CONDITIONS
May accompany other respiratory tract anomalies

AGE-RELATED FACTORS
Most severe in puppies 6 weeks to 6 months old and in puppies from commercial pet shops and humane society shelters

ZOONOTIC POTENTIAL
None

PREGNANCY
High risk in dogs on extensive medical treatment; especially risky for developing puppies

SYNONYMS
Kennel cough—uncomplicated disease

ABBREVIATIONS
• CAV = canine adenovirus
• CPI = canine parainfluenza

Suggested Reading
Bemis DA. Bordetella and mycoplasma respiratory infection in dogs. Vet Clin North Am Small Anim Pract 1992;22:1173–1186.
Ford RB, Vaden SL. Canine infectious tracheobronchitis. In: Greene CE, ed. Infectious diseases of the dog and cat. Philadelphia: Saunders, 1990:259–265.
Hoskins JD, Taboada J. Specific treatment of infectious causes of respiratory disease in dogs and cats. Vet Med 1994;89:443–452.
Padrid P. Chronic lower airway disease in the dog and cat. Probl Vet Med 1992; 4:320–344.
Author Johnny D. Hoskins
Consulting Editor Lynelle R. Johnson

INFERTILITY, FEMALE

 BASICS

DEFINITION
Historical complaint that occurs in bitches showing abnormal cycling, copulation failure, conception failure, or pregnancy loss

PATHOPHYSIOLOGY
• Normal fertility—requires normal estrus cycling with ovulation of normal ova into a patent, healthy reproductive tract; fertilization by normal spermatozoa; implantation of the conceptus into the endometrium; formation of the normal zonary placenta; and maintenance of pregnancy in the presence of high progesterone concentration throughout the approximately 2-month gestation
• Breakdown in any of the processes causes infertility.

SYSTEMS AFFECTED
Reproductive

SIGNALMENT
• Animals of all ages; may be more common in old animals
• Dogs > 6 years old—more likely to have underlying cystic endometrial hyperplasia; may be predisposed to uterine infection and failure of conception or implantation
• Dog breeds predisposed to thyroid insufficiency—may have a higher prevalence; include golden retrievers, Doberman pinschers, dachshunds, Irish setters, miniature schnauzers, Great Danes, poodles, and boxers

SIGNS

Historical Findings
• Failure to cycle
• Failure to copulate
• Normal copulation with no subsequent pregnancy or parturition

Physical Examination Findings
Positive pregnancy with no subsequent parturition

CAUSES
Animals acquired when already mature—possibility of previous ovariohysterectomy

Dogs
• Insemination at the improper time in the estrus cycle—most common
• Subclinical uterine infection
• Male infertility factors
• Thyroid insufficiency
• Hypercortisolism
• Anatomic abnormality
• Chromosomal abnormality
• Abnormal ovarian function
• *Brucella canis*—always a possibility

Cats
• Similar causes to those of dogs
• Lack of sufficient copulatory stimulus to induce ovulation
• Systemic viral or protozoal infection

RISK FACTORS
• *B. canis* (dogs)
• Thyroid insufficiency (dogs)
• Hypercortisolism (dogs and cats)—endogenous or exogenous
• Systemic viral infection (dogs and cats)—canine herpesvirus; FeLV; FIV
• Systemic protozoal infection (dogs and cats)—e.g., toxoplasmosis
• Any chronic, debilitating disease condition (dogs and cats)
• Congenital vaginal anomaly (dogs and cats)

 DIAGNOSIS

DIFFERENTIAL DIAGNOSIS

Historical Information
• Extremely useful in distinguishing causes
• Is the patient cycling? Primary anestrus = no overt estrus cycle by 2 years of age; secondary anestrus = no overt estrus cycle within 1 year of a normal cycle
• Has the patient conceived or given birth in the past? If so, how recently? What was the litter size? What percentage of the litter was weaned?
• Is the patient free of systemic viral or protozoal infection?
• Is the patient capable of normal copulation?
• Was the patient bred to a male of proven fertility at the proper time of the estrus cycle?
• Did the patient ovulate during the estrus cycle and maintain progesterone concentration consistent with pregnancy during the entire gestation?
• Is the bitch euthyroid?

CBC/BIOCHEMISTRY/URINALYSIS
Usually normal

OTHER LABORATORY TESTS

Serologic Test for *B. canis* (Dogs)
• Rapid slide agglutination test—used as a screen; sensitive but not specific
• If positive results—recommend recheck by an agar gel immunodiffusion test (Cornell University Diagnostic Laboratory, 607-253-3900) or bacterial culture of whole blood lymph node aspirate.

Serum Progesterone Measurement
• Should remain high throughout gestation
• May measure at the time of examination
• If concentration < 2 ng/mL in midgestation and pregnancy loss occurs, insufficient luteal function indicated (Hypoluteodism) (See Abortion, Spontaneous, and Pregnancy Loss—Dogs)
• Concentration > 2 ng/mL—may indicate silent heat; estrus with no overt behavioral or physical changes; or pathologic production of progesterone from a luteal ovarian structure, functional ovarian neoplasm, or the adrenal gland

Dogs
• May be measured during proestrus and estrus to predict ovulation time and optimize breeding management
• Concentration and ovulation—1.0–1.9 ng/mL, ovulation in 3 days; 2.0–2.9 ng/mL, ovulation in 2 days; 3.0–3.9 ng/mL, ovulation in 1 day; 4.0–10.0 ng/mL, ovulation that day
• Optimal breeding day for maximum litter size—2 days after ovulation
• Day of ovulation—extremely variable; not well correlated with standing behavior (see Breeding, Timing)

Cats
• May be measured after breeding to assess induction of ovulation
• Concentration > 2 ng/mL—indicates functional luteal tissue

Other Tests
• Bacterial culture for uterine organisms (dogs and cats)—vaginal discharge originating in the uterus during proestrus or estrus is collected directly by hysterotomy or indirectly from the anterior vagina by a guarded swab.
• Thyroid hormone testing (dogs)—may measure resting serum concentration of T_3 or T_4; may measure T_4 after challenge with TSH to assess insufficiency
• Serologic testing—canine herpesvirus and toxoplasmosis (see Abortion, Spontaneous, and Pregnancy Loss—Dogs); FeLV, FIV, and toxoplasmosis (see Abortion, Spontaneous, and Pregnancy Loss—Cats)
• Karyotype (dogs and cats)—performed on heparinized blood samples of patients with primary or persistent anestrus; look for chromosomal abnormalities that can cause abnormal sexual differentiation (testing done by University of Minnesota Cytogenetics Laboratory, 612-624-4767; see Sexual Development Disorders).
• Serum cortisol assay (dogs and cats)—if the resting serum concentration is high, investigate the underlying cause.

• Semen evaluation (dogs and cats)—direct evaluation to rule out oligospermia or azoospermia recommmended; alternatively, may test-breed the male to another female to prove fertility; rule out azoospermia in tom-cat by finding spermatozoa in a vaginal flush or swab specimens from the queen or in urine collected by cystocentesis from the tom. (See also Infertility, Male—Dogs.)

IMAGING
• Radiography and ultrasonography—normal ovaries and a nongravid uterus usually not visible; large ovaries may indicate cystic ovarian disease or neoplasia; visible uterus may indicate cystic endometrial hyperplasia.
• Positive-contrast procedures—vaginography in dogs; hysterography in dogs and cats; performed prepuberally or when the patient is in estrus; may reveal anatomic abnormality (e.g., abnormal structure and impatency)
• Ultrasound—may diagnose pregnancy as early as 20–24 days after ovulation; useful for documenting pregnancy loss

DIAGNOSTIC PROCEDURES
• Laparotomy (dogs and cats)—assess anatomy of the tubular tract and gonads.
• Hysterotomy—to obtain a direct uterine culture specimen; biopsy of the uterus or ovaries

 TREATMENT
• Cats—seasonal breeders; depend on photoperiod; cycle when exposed to long day length, normally from late January to mid-October; induce year-round cycling by a daily light exposure of ≥ 12 hours; for a noncycling cat during the physiologic breeding season, ask client about the queen's housing and exposure to light
• Heritable cause (e.g., thyroid insuffi-ciency)—counsel owner regarding the advisability of retaining the patient in the breeding program.
• Surgical resection of vaginal anomalies (dogs)—may ease natural service and vaginal delivery of pups
• Surgical repair of impatent tubular tract (dogs and cats)—difficult procedure; prognosis for future fertility guarded
• Surgical drainage of ovarian cysts (dogs and cats)—efficacy unknown
• Unilateral ovariectomy of neoplastic ovary (dogs and cats)—future fertility depends on resumption of normal function of the remaining ovary and lack of metastasis

• Prognosis for future fertility—initially good, because the most common cause is improper breeding management; worsens with other causes

 MEDICATIONS

DRUG(S) OF CHOICE
• Antibiotics (dogs and cats)—for uterine infection; choice depends on bacterial culture and sensitivity test of the uterus or of vaginal discharge during proestrus or estrus
• L-Thyroxine—for thyroid insufficiency; dogs: 0.01 mg/kg PO q12h; prognosis for future fertility with return to euthyroid state guarded

Gonadotropin Therapy
• For induction of ovulation
• GnRH, which causes release of endogenous LH from the pituitary, or hCG, which has LH-like activity
• Cats not adequately stimulated to ovulate at the time of copulation—GnRH (25 µg/cat IM or hCG 250 IU/cat IM) at time of breeding
• Ovarian cystic disease—cats: GnRH (25 µg/cat IM) or hCG (250 IU/cat IM); dogs: GnRH (50 µg/dog IM) or hCG (1000 IU/dog half IV, half IM); causes ovulation or luteinization of cystic ovarian tissue
• Estrus induction (dogs)—diethylstilbestrol (5 mg q24h PO until signs of proestrus induced); bromocriptine (20 mcg/kg q12h PO for 21 days); cabergoline (5 mcg/kg q24h PO for 7–10 days or until signs of proestrus induced)

CONTRAINDICATIONS
N/A

PRECAUTIONS
N/A

POSSIBLE INTERACTIONS
N/A

ALTERNATIVE DRUG(S)
N/A

 FOLLOW-UP

PATIENT MONITORING
• L-Thyroxine (dogs)—blood concentrations of T_3 and T_4 rechecked after 1 month of supplementation to ensure adequate absorption of medication and resumption of a euthyroid state

• Ultrasonography (dogs and cats)—to definitively diagnose pregnancy; monitor gestation
• Progesterone assay (dogs and cats)

POSSIBLE COMPLICATIONS
N/A

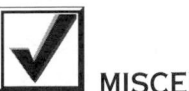 MISCELLANEOUS

ASSOCIATED CONDITIONS
• Infertility caused by endocrinopathy—signs of dermatologic abnormality (e.g., alopecia with thyroid insufficiency or hypercortisolism); systemic signs of disease (e.g., polydipsia and polyuria with hypercortisolism)
• Bitches with a vaginal anatomic abnormality—persistent or recurrent urinary tract disease or vaginitis

AGE-RELATED FACTORS
N/A

ZOONOTIC POTENTIAL
B. canis infection—organism is less readily shed if affected animals are gonadectomized; stress good hygiene.

PREGNANCY
N/A

SEE ALSO
• See Causes.

ABBREVIATIONS
FeLV = feline leukemia virus
FIV = feline immunodeficiency virus
GnRH = gonadotropin-releasing hormone
hCG = human chorionic gonadotropin
LH = luteinizing hormone
T_3 = triiodothyronine
T_4 = thyroxine
TSH = thyroid-stimulating hormone

Suggested Reading
Freshman JL. Clinical approach to infertility in the cycling bitch. Vet Clin North Am Small Anim Pract 1991;21:427–436.
Johnston SD, Olson PNS, Root MV. Clinical approach to infertility in the bitch. Semin Vet Med Surg Small Anim 1994;9:2–6.
Authors Margaret V. Root Kustritz and Shirley D. Johnston
Consulting Editor Sara K. Lyle

INFERTILITY, MALE—DOGS

BASICS

DEFINITION
• Diminished or absent fertility; does not imply sterility • Results from a wide range of problems that prevent the delivery of sufficient numbers of spermatozoa to fertilize ovulated, mature oocytes in the bitch

PATHOPHYSIOLOGY
• Spermatogenesis—encompasses the formation and development of spermatozoa from primordial germ cells; a coordinated, hormonally controlled, cyclic process; approximately 60 days required for a complete phase (46 days for the testicular phase; remainder for the epididymal phase); thus, testicular problems require at least 60 days for recovery, and epididymal problems require at least 2 weeks. • Azoospermia—ejaculate completely devoid of spermatozoa • Oligozoospermia—ejaculate with low numbers of spermatozoa • Primary causes—impaired or arrested spermatogenesis; blockage of the excurrent ducts; genitourinary inflammation; testicular neoplasia; environmental stress; congenital abnormality; endocrine abnormality

SYSTEMS AFFECTED
• Reproductive • Endocrine/Metabolic • Musculoskeletal • Nervous

GENETICS
• There are very few substantiated heritable causes of infertility in the stud dog.
• Alpha-L-fucosidase deficiency—in male dogs a heritable lysosomal storage disorder has been reported; causes a specific deleterious effect on acrosomal dysgenesis and impaired sperm maturation • Primary ciliary dyskinesia (PCD)—congenital abnormality of ciliary ultrastructure; absent, irregular, or asynchronous motility patterns of all ciliated cells; diagnosed by electron microscopy of spermatozoa • Hypothyroidism—in females some thyroid disorders appear to be heritable and have specific effects on cyclicity; the effect of hypothyroidism on male fertility is less clearly defined and probably is minimal.

INCIDENCE/PREVALENCE
True incidence unknown

GEOGRAPHIC DISTRIBUTION
N/A

SIGNALMENT

Species
Dogs

Breed Predilections
Relatively higher prevalence of specific problems seen in certain breeds

Mean Age and Range
Prevalence increases with age.

Predominant Sex
Males

SIGNS

General Comments
General complaint—no puppies produced; whelping rate < 75% when bred with correct timing to fertile bitches; owner suspects male dog infertility.

Historical Findings
• Age of testicular descent • Age at first attempted mating • Libido and breeding behavior • Frequency and number of matings • Method used to time breedings • Type of semen used for breeding (fresh, fresh-extended, chilled-extended, or frozen) • Handling of semen and route of insemination • Litter size(s) • Familial history of infertility • Degree of inbreeding • Fertility status of bitches bred • *Brucella canis* status of all breeding partners • Current and previous drug and dietary therapies • Previous medical or surgical illnesses

Physical Examination Findings
• Sheath and penis—palpated to identify masses or adhesions • Non-erect penis exteriorized to determine if the superficial mucosa contains any clinically important lesions and if the os penis is undamaged • Testes and epididymis—palpated and examined, size and symmetry of the epididymis relative to the testes noted • Internal urethra and prostate—digital rectal palpation to determine location, size, and symmetry

CAUSES
Incorrect timing of breeding—most common cause

Congenital
• Chromosomal abnormalities (XXY syndrome) and XX sex reversal (XX male syndrome)—phenotypic males with hypoplastic testes and no spermatogenesis; see Sexual Development Disorders • Germinal cell aplasia—biopsy reveals "Sertoli cell only" syndrome • Unilateral or bilateral segmental aplasia of the epididymis or vas deferens—causes either oligospermia or azoospermia

Acquired
• Incomplete ejaculation—unfamiliar surroundings; slippery flooring; no estrous bitch; dominant owner or bitch present • Obstruction of the efferent ducts, epididymides, or ductus deferens—leads to azoospermia if bilateral; sperm granuloma, spermatocele, acute inflammation, chronic inflammatory stenosis, segmental aplasia, neoplasia, previous vasectomy, and attempts to tack testes into a scrotal location • Inflammation or infection of the testes—especially *B. canis* and *Escherichia coli*; requires prompt and aggressive treatment to prevent infertility • Hypothyroidism—role unclear; evaluate thyroid function with poor semen quality; may be associated with decreased libido • Hyperprolactinemia—role unclear; evaluate prolactin levels with azoospermia • Hyperadrenocorticism—causes testicular atrophy; probably reversible • Drugs—parasiticides, corticosteroids, anabolic steroids, estrogens, androgens, progestogens, GnRH agonists/antagonists, ketoconazole, amphotericin B, agents, may interfere with or interrupt spermatogenesis; assess all topical and systemic therapies • Environmental toxins—endocrine-disrupting contaminants can affect the hypothalamic-pituitary axis and gonadal steroidogenesis; effects in the dog unknown • Trauma, environmental damage, testicular neoplasia, systemic disease, ischemia, and heat stress—may cause transient infertility or sterility • Prostatic disease—appears to markedly reduce semen quality and libido • Inbreeding—initially reduces fertility; eventually a rebound effect and fertility starts to return to near normal if the breeder selects for fertile individuals • Lymphocytic orchitis—familial in some breeds (e.g., beagles and borzois); affected animals may be fertile when young; fertility declines at an accelerated rate with age • Retrograde ejaculation—some retrograde flow into the bladder normal; complete retrograde ejaculation (aspermia) rare; diagnosis aided by urinalysis (cystocentesis) after ejaculation

RISK FACTORS
• Congenital disorders affecting reproductive function—not uncommon; tend to occur in selected breeds
• Teaser bitches and stud dogs not tested for infectious disease (e.g., *B. canis* and bacterial culture of genital tract) before breeding

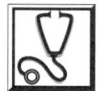

DIAGNOSIS

DIFFERENTIAL DIAGNOSIS
Before extensive diagnostic work on the male, determine that the bitches are fertile (previous litters) and that the breedings were optimally timed (see Infertility, Female; and Breeding, Timing)

CBC/BIOCHEMISTRY/URINALYSIS
• Usually normal • Brucellosis or prostatitis—variable changes in the leukogram (normal or leukocytosis) and urinalysis (high numbers of leukocytes); depends on the time-course of the infection • Systemic illness—may impair reproductive function, but infertility is usually not the primary complaint on examination

OTHER LABORATORY TESTS

Endocrine Profile

• Resting testosterone—normal, intact dogs, 0.4–10 ng/mL; most common range, 1–4 ng/mL • Androgenic tissue—confirmed if serum concentration of testosterone increases 100% over the resting value 2–3 hr after injection with either 1–2 μg/kg GnRH or 40 lU/kg hCG; useful to detect bilaterally cryptorchid condition • Serum FSH concentration—rises with marked reduction in spermatogenesis because of loss of inhibin secretion • Serum LH concentration—difficult to interpret because of its episodic secretion • Thyroid function—evaluated by baseline T_3 and T_4, TSH values, and stimulation testing (see Hypothyroidism)

IMAGING

Ultrasonography—helps identify lesions that alter the testicular and epididymal architecture (e.g., neoplasia and spermatocele); evaluates the prostate gland for hyperplasia, chronic prostatitis, cyst, abscess, or neoplasia (see Benign Prostatic Hyperplasia; Prostatic Cysts; Prostatitis and Prostatic Abscess; Prostatomegaly)

DIAGNOSTIC PROCEDURES

Breeding Soundness Examination

• Pivotal to ensure that all appropriate information is collected • Sperm-rich and prostatic portions of the ejaculate—collected as separate fractions by use of a sterile artificial vagina and sterile, graduated, nontoxic plastic tubes in the presence of an estrous bitch; use 4 × 4 gauze pads or swabs containing estrual vaginal discharge (can be frozen and stored) if estrous bitch unavailable • Sperm-rich fraction—volume; concentration, motility, and morphologic characteristics of sperm cells; cytologic examination; qualitative and quantitative cultures • Prostatic fraction and urine (collected by cystocentesis)—cytologic examination; qualitative and quantitative cultures • Culture results—must be correlated with clinical and cytologic evidence of an active infection; evidence of inflammation if greater than 1–3 WBC/hpf observed (especially sperm-rich fraction) • Prostatic fraction that indicates a clinically important infection—re-evaluate by other sampling techniques that avoid contamination from the penile mucosa and prepuce • Azoospermic or oligospermic ejaculate—re-collect 1 hour later and again on several occasions before confirming infertility

Epididymal Markers

ALP concentration in seminal fluid—normal 8,000–40,000 U/mL; epididymal in origin; may indicate obstruction if < 5,000 U/mL and a complete ejaculate was obtained; pathologic effects of obstruction are more easily seen if ALP is performed on two ejaculates collected 60 minutes apart.

PATHOLOGIC FINDINGS

• Testicular biopsy—determines the degree of spermatogenesis and the integrity of the blood-testis barrier; differentiates obstruction of efferent ducts from testicular hypoplasia and degeneration; allows an informed prognosis • Incisional biopsy—superior to aspiration or needle biopsy for obtaining a diagnostic sample; Bouin's fixative required for processing the tissue

TREATMENT

APPROPRIATE HEALTH CARE

Supportive regimens—reducing environmental heat or other stress

ACTIVITY

• Restrict if activity or use is thought to be producing hyperthermia (see Heat Stroke and Hyperthermia). • No restriction for other causes of infertility

DIET

Ensure adequate diet and mineral supplementation.

CLIENT EDUCATION

• Inform client that the testis will require at least 60 days from correction of identified causes to return to function. • Stress patience while the patient is regularly checked to ensure there is no worsening of the condition.

SURGICAL CONSIDERATIONS

Re-anastomosis of blocked excurrent ducts is successful for sperm production in several cases.

MEDICATIONS

DRUG(S) OF CHOICE

• Specific medications must be administered long enough and at a dosage that will ensure tissue penetration. Antibiotics (for penetration and spectrum)—chloramphenicol, trimethoprim-sulfa, erythromycin, and enrofloxacin; usually recommended for a minimum of 3–4 weeks to allow adequate and sustained levels within the reproductive tract • Pseudoephedrine—used with limited success in humans with retrograde ejaculation; 4–5 mg/kg PO q8h, or 1 and 3 hr before collection

CONTRAINDICATIONS

• Trimethoprim-sulfas—contraindicated if predisposed to keratitis sicca • Chloramphenicol and trimethoprim-sulfas—reportedly induce blood dyscrasias

PRECAUTIONS N/A

POSSIBLE INTERACTIONS N/A

ALTERNATIVE DRUG(S) N/A

FOLLOW-UP

PATIENT MONITORING

Recheck at intervals that take into account the length of the spermatogenic cycle (60 days) but are frequent enough to allow detection of deteriorating condition.

PREVENTION/AVOIDANCE

Avoid exposure to environmental temperature extremes (heat or cold).

POSSIBLE COMPLICATIONS N/A

EXPECTED COURSE AND PROGNOSIS

• Fair to good—cases of mistimed breeding; appropriately breed to fertile bitch. • Guarded—cases of confirmed infertility; < 10% return to fertility after diagnosis and appropriate treatment.

MISCELLANEOUS

ASSOCIATED CONDITIONS

• Brucellosis infection—diskospondylitis, polyarthritis, posterior paresis, fever, and uveitis • Prostatic disease—obstipation, locomotor difficulties, fever, hematuria, pollakiuria, and dysuria • Lymphocytic orchitis—lymphocytic thyroiditis

AGE-RELATED FACTORS

• Reduction in daily sperm output and morphologically normal sperm cells—with age • Difficult to assess the effect of age alone on fertility • Most old, infertile dogs have concurrent diseases (e.g., systemic or prostatic disease and testicular neoplasia) that have documented effects on fertility.

ZOONOTIC POTENTIAL N/A

SEE ALSO

See Causes

ABBREVIATIONS

• ALP = alkaline phosphatase
• FSH = follicle-stimulating hormone
• GnRH = gonadotropin-releasing hormone
• hCG = human chorionic gonadotropin
• hpf = high-power field
• LH = luteinizing hormone
• TSH = thyroid-stimulating hormone
• WBC = white blood cell

Suggested Reading

Johnston SD, Root Kustritz MV, Olson PNS. Clinical approach to infertility in the male dog. In: Johnston SD, Root Kustritz MV, Olson PNS. Canine and feline theriogenology. Philadelphia: Saunders, 2001:370–387.

Wallace MS. Infertility in the male dog. Prob Vet Med 1992;4(3):531–544.

Author Richard A. Fayrer-Hosken
Consulting Editor Sara K. Lyle

INFLAMMATORY BOWEL DISEASE

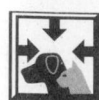 **BASICS**

DEFINITION
A group of gastrointestinal diseases characterized by inflammatory cellular infiltrates in the lamina propria of the small or large intestine, with associated clinical signs

PATHOPHYSIOLOGY
• An abnormal mucosal immune response to certain causative factors that results in the recruitment of inflammatory cells to the intestine
• Damage results from the elaboration of cytokines, release of proteolytic and lysosomal enzymes, complement activation secondary to immune complex deposition, and generation of oxygen free radicals.
• Certain environmental agents and hereditary factors may also influence the development of IBD.

SYSTEMS AFFECTED
• Gastrointestinal
• Hepatobiliary
• Hemic/Lymphatic/Immune—rarely
• Musculoskeletal—rarely
• Ophthalmic—rarely
• Respiratory—rarely
• Skin/Exocrine—rarely

GENETICS
N/A

INCIDENCE/PREVALENCE
Common

GEOGRAPHIC DISTRIBUTION
N/A

SIGNALMENT

Species
Dogs and cats

Breed Predilection
Breed predisposition with some forms of the disease (e.g., immunoproliferative enteropathy of basenjis and lundehunds, histiocytic colitis of French bulldogs and boxers, and gluten-sensitive enteropathy in Irish setters)

Mean Age and Range
More common in animals >2 years of age, although younger animals can be affected

Predominant Sex
N/A

SIGNS

Historical Findings
• Dogs—chronic intermittent vomiting, diarrhea, and weight loss are common.
• Cats—vomiting is most common, followed by diarrhea.
• Borborygmus, flatulence, anorexia or ravenous appetite, hematochezia, abdominal pain, and mucoid stools are less commonly reported.

Physical Examination Findings
• Vary from an apparently healthy animal to a thin, depressed animal
• Poor haircoat is frequently noted.
• Abdominal palpation may reveal pain, thickened bowel loops, and mesenteric lymphadenopathy (especially in cats).

CAUSES
• Pathogenesis is most likely multifactorial.
• Several causative factors have been identified.

Infectious Agents
• No convincing link definitively established between one specific microbial agent and IBD
• *Giardia, Salmonella, Campylobacter,* and normal resident gastrointestinal flora have been implicated.

Dietary Agents
Meat proteins, food additives, artificial coloring, preservatives, milk proteins, and gluten (wheat) are all proposed causative agents.

Genetic Factors
• Certain forms of IBD are more common in some breeds of dogs (see above).
• Association of inherited chromosome fragility with IBD suggested in humans
• Certain major histocompatibility genes, which are important components of normal immune responses, may render an individual susceptible to the development of IBD.

RISK FACTORS
See Causes.

 DIAGNOSIS

DIFFERENTIAL DIAGNOSIS
• Cats—hyperthyroidism, intestinal neoplasia (especially infiltrative lymphosarcoma or mast cell tumor), dietary intolerance/hypersensitivity, granulomatous FIP, other viral infections (e.g., FeLV and FIV), exocrine pancreatic insufficiency, intestinal parasitism, and bacterial overgrowth are primary differentials.
• Dogs—intestinal neoplasia, motility disorders, dietary intolerance/hypersensitivity, lymphangiectasia, exocrine pancreatic insufficiency, intestinal parasitism, and bacterial overgrowth are primary differentials.

CBC/BIOCHEMISTRY/URINALYSIS
• Results often normal; these tests help rule in or out some other differential diagnoses.
• Occasionally a mild, nonregenerative anemia and mild leukocytosis without a left shift occur in cats.
• Dogs with IBD frequently have a neutrophilic leukocytosis with a left shift.
• Hypoproteinemia tends to be more common in dogs with IBD than in cats.
• Cobalamin deficiency reported in cats

OTHER LABORATORY TESTS
• Useful to eliminate other differentials
• Dogs—tests include fasting serum TLI to evaluate exocrine pancreatic function and fasting serum cobalamin and folate assays to evaluate small intestinal function and bacterial overgrowth
• Cats—T_4 and FeLV/FIV serology are recommended; fasting serum TLI (if exocrine pancreatic insufficiency is suspected); serum cobalamin and folate assays to evaluate small intestinal function and bacterial overgrowth

IMAGING
• Survey abdominal radiographs—usually normal
• Barium contrast studies—occasionally reveal mucosal abnormalities and thickened bowel loops, but are generally not helpful in establishing a definitive diagnosis; can be normal in animals with even severe disease
• Ultrasonography—may use to measure stomach and intestinal wall thickness and to rule out other diseases

DIAGNOSTIC PROCEDURES
• May initiate a hypoallergenic diet trial first to rule in or rule out dietary allergy or intolerance
• Occasionally, certain forms of IBD respond to dietary manipulations alone; if signs resolve completely, a diagnosis of dietary allergy or intolerance is likely and no further workup is necessary.

- Always perform fecal examination for parasites.
- Definitive diagnosis requires biopsy and histopathology, usually obtained via endoscopy.
- May collect duodenal aspirates for *Giardia* spp. detection during endoscopy
- Intestinal fluid obtained during endoscopy can also be submitted for quantitative culture if bacterial overgrowth is suspected.
- Exploratory laparotomy may be indicated if involved portions of the gastrointestinal tract are unapproachable by endoscopy or if abdominal organomegaly is present.

PATHOLOGIC FINDINGS

Infiltration of intestines with inflammatory cells

 TREATMENT

APPROPRIATE HEALTH CARE

Outpatient, unless the patient is debilitated from dehydration, hypoproteinemia, or cachexia

NURSING CARE

- If the patient is dehydrated or must be NPO because of vomiting, any balanced fluid such as lactated Ringer's solution is adequate (for a patient without other concurrent disease); otherwise, select fluids on the basis of secondary diseases.
- If there is severe hypoalbuminemia from protein-losing enteropathy, consider colloids such as dextrans or hetastarch.

ACTIVITY

No restrictions

DIET

- Manipulation is important.
- For detailed description of possible regimens, see specific diseases.

CLIENT EDUCATION

- Emphasize to the client that IBD is not necessarily cured as much as controlled.
- Relapses are common; the client must be prepared to be patient during the various

food and medication trials that are often necessary to get the disease under control.
- A severely debilitated patient may need hospitalization and parenteral nutrition.

SURGICAL CONSIDERATIONS

Unlike the situation with human beings, no surgical procedures are available for relief of IBD in veterinary patients.

 MEDICATIONS

DRUG(S) OF CHOICE

See discussion under specific diseases.

CONTRAINDICATIONS

If secondary problems are present, avoid therapeutic agents that might be contraindicated for those conditions.

PRECAUTIONS

See discussion under specific diseases.

POSSIBLE INTERACTIONS

See discussion under specific diseases.

ALTERNATIVE DRUG(S)

See discussion under specific diseases.

 FOLLOW-UP

PATIENT MONITORING

- Periodic reevaluation may be necessary until the patient's condition stabilizes.
- No other follow-up may be required except yearly physical examinations and assessment during relapse.

PREVENTION/AVOIDANCE

N/A

POSSIBLE COMPLICATIONS

Dehydration, malnutrition, adverse drug reactions, hypoproteinemia, anemia, and diseases secondary to therapy or resulting from the above-mentioned problems

EXPECTED COURSE AND PROGNOSIS

- Vary with specific type of IBD
- See discussion under specific diseases.

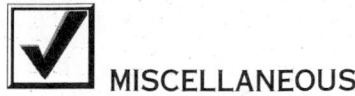 MISCELLANEOUS

ASSOCIATED CONDITIONS

See discussion under specific diseases.

AGE-RELATED FACTORS

- See discussion under specific diseases.
- The workup and differentials are essentially the same, regardless of age.
- Some differentials are more likely in younger individuals (i.e., intestinal parasitism versus neoplasia).
- Younger individuals with confirmed IBD may have other immune system defects.
- Counsel clients about breeding and monitoring for the appearance of other diseases.

ZOONOTIC POTENTIAL

N/A

PREGNANCY

See discussion under specific diseases.

SYNONYMS

N/A

SEE ALSO

- Gastroenteritis, Lymphocytic-Plasmacytic
- Gastroenteritis, Eosinophilic
- Colitis and Proctitis

ABBREVIATIONS

- FeLV = feline leukemia virus
- FIP = feline infectious peritonitis
- FIV = feline immunodeficiency virus
- IBD = inflammatory bowel disease
- TLI = trypsin-like immunoreactivity
- T_4 = thyroxine

Suggested Reading

Strombeck DR, Guilford WG. Idiopathic inflammatory bowel diseases. In: Guilford WG, Center SA, Strombeck DR, et al., eds. Strombeck's small animal gastroenterology. 3rd ed. Philadelphia: Saunders, 1996: 451–486.

Tams TR. Feline inflammatory bowel disease. Vet Clin North Am 1993;23.

Author Kelly J. Diehl

Consulting Editor Albert E. Jergens

INSULINOMA

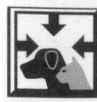 **BASICS**

DEFINITION
Pancreatic islet β-cell neoplasm that secretes an excess quantity of insulin

PATHOPHYSIOLOGY
Excessive insulin secretion leads to excessive glucose uptake and use by insulin-sensitive tissues and reduced hepatic production of glucose; this causes hypoglycemia and its associated clinical signs.

SYSTEMS AFFECTED
• Nervous—seizures, disorientation, abnormal behavior, collapse, posterior paresis, and ataxia
• Musculoskeletal—weakness and muscle fasciculations
• Gastrointestinal—polyphagia and weight gain

GENETICS
N/A

INCIDENCE/PREVALENCE
• Dogs—uncommon
• Cats—rare (4 reports)

GEOGRAPHIC DISTRIBUTION
N/A

SIGNALMENT

Species
Dogs and cats

Breed Predilections
• Dogs—standard poodle, boxer, fox terrier, Irish setter, German shepherd, golden retriever, and collie
• Cats—none; possibly Siamese

Mean Age and Range
• Dogs—middle-aged to old; mean, 10.5 years; range, 3–14 years (rare in dogs < 6 years old)
• Cats—(4 cases) mean, 14.75 years; range, 12–17 years

Predominant Sex
None

SIGNS

General Comments
• Episodic
• May or may not be related to fasting, excitement, exercise, and eating
• Dogs usually demonstrate more than one clinical sign, and they progress with time.

Historical Findings
• Dogs—seizures (generalized and focal) most common; also, posterior paresis, weakness, collapse, muscle fasciculations, abnormal behavior, lethargy and depression, ataxia, polyphagia, weight gain, polyuria and polydipsia, and exercise intolerance
• Cats—seizures, ataxia, muscle fasciculations, weakness, lethargy and depression, anorexia, weight loss, and polydipsia

Physical Examination Findings
• Usually within normal limits
• Obesity in some dogs
• Rarely, polyneuropathy in dogs

CAUSES
Most patients have malignant, insulin-producing carcinoma or adenocarcinoma of the pancreas; tumors considered benign according to histopathologic findings usually metastasize later.

RISK FACTORS
Fasting, excitement, exercise, and eating may increase the risk of hypoglycemic episodes.

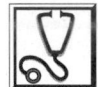 **DIAGNOSIS**

DIFFERENTIAL DIAGNOSIS
• Extrapancreatic tumor hypoglycemia—paraneoplastic hypoglycemia has been documented in dogs with hepatocellular carcinoma, metastatic mammary carcinoma, primary pulmonary carcinoma, and others; these tumors secrete insulin or insulin-like factors.
• Differentiate from beta-cell pancreatic tumor by a complete hypoglycemic workup, including imaging.
• Seizures and collapse—must consider cardiovascular (e.g., syncope), metabolic (e.g., hepatoencephalopathy, hypocalcemia, anemia, and hypoadrenocorticism), and neurologic (e.g., epilepsy, neoplasia, toxin, and inflammatory disease) causes
• Posterior paresis and weakness—consider cardiovascular (e.g., congenital anatomic defect, arrhythmias, heart failure, and pericardial effusion), metabolic (e.g., hypoadrenocorticism, hypocalcemia, anemia, hypokalemia, and hypothyroidism), neurologic and neuromuscular (e.g., spinal cord disease, myasthenia gravis, polymyositis, and polyradiculoneuropathy), and toxic (e.g., tick paralysis, botulism, chronic organophosphate exposure, and lead poisoning) causes

• Muscle fasciculations—consider metabolic (e.g., hypercalcemia, hypocalcemia, and hyperadrenocorticism) and toxic (e.g., tetanus and strychnine poisoning) causes

CBC/BIOCHEMISTRY/URINALYSIS
• Results usually normal, except hypoglycemia (< 70 mg/dL in > 90% of patients)
• Normoglycemia in some patients, due to counterregulatory hormone production (epinephrine, glucocorticoids, etc.)

OTHER LABORATORY TESTS
• Simultaneous fasting glucose and insulin determination—on initiating fasting, collect blood samples hourly or bihourly for serum glucose determination and serum storage; when the serum glucose drops below 60 mg/dL (usually within 8–10 hr in dogs, at presentation in cats), submit that sample for serum insulin determination; interpretation: high insulin, insulinoma likely; normal insulin, insulinoma possible; low insulin, insulinoma unlikely
• Amended insulin:glucose ratio (AIGR)—this test is intended to diagnose insulinoma when the insulin concentration is within the normal range but inappropriately high for the degree of hypoglycemia.

$$AIGR = \frac{[\text{plasma insulin } (\mu U/mL) \times 100]}{[\text{plasma glucose } (mg/dL) - 30]}$$

use 1 as denominator if glucose is < 30; AIGR > 30 suggests insulinoma, AIGR = 19–30, gray zone, repeat test; AIGR < 19, insulinoma unlikely
• **Note:** False-positive results are possible, especially when serum glucose is < 40 mg/dL.

IMAGING
Thoracic and abdominal radiography and abdominal ultrasonography are usually normal but help evaluate for extrapancreatic tumor–induced hypoglycemia as well as some other differential diagnoses.

DIAGNOSTIC PROCEDURES
N/A

PATHOLOGIC FINDINGS
• Insulinoma is usually a small, solitary nodule, but multiple nodules or diffuse infiltration can be seen.
• Most insulinomas can be identified grossly at surgery, occasionally gentle palpation is required for detection, and very rarely no tumor can be identified.
• Metastasis is seen in 40% of patients at surgery; common areas include the regional lymph nodes and liver; other areas include the duodenum, mesentery, omentum, and spleen.
• Histopathologically they appear as either carcinoma or adenoma, but both behave malignantly.

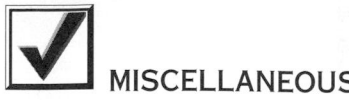

TREATMENT

APPROPRIATE HEALTH CARE
• Hospitalize for workup, surgery, and (if clinically hypoglycemic) treatment.
• Treat as outpatient if the owner declines surgery and the patient is not clinically hypoglycemic.

NURSING CARE
• Administer 50% dextrose, 1 mL/kg IV slow bolus (1–3 min) to control seizures/severe hypoglycemic signs.
• Fluid therapy with 2.5% dextrose (increase to 5% if needed to control clinical signs) should follow dextrose bolus; alternatively, if the patient can eat, frequent feedings of an appropriate diet (see Diet) may replace dextrose-containing fluids in many patients.

ACTIVITY
Restricted

DIET
• The first and most important aspect of management (with or without surgery)
• Feed 4–6 small meals a day.
• Should be high in protein, fat, and complex carbohydrates and low in simple sugars; avoid semimoist food

CLIENT EDUCATION
Owner should be aware of signs of hypoglycemia and seek immediate attention if they occur.

SURGICAL CONSIDERATIONS
Confirms diagnosis, improves survival time, can potentially provide prolonged remission, and improves response to medical treatment

MEDICATIONS

DRUG(S) OF CHOICE

Emergency/Acute Therapy
See Nursing Care above.

Long-term Therapy
• Glucocorticoids (prednisone at an initial dosage of 0.25 mg/kg PO q12h; increased to 2–3 mg/kg PO q12h if needed)—initial medical treatment if diet alone is ineffective; begin with the low dosage and gradually increase as signs of hypoglycemia recur.
• Diazoxide (Proglycem, 5 mg/kg PO q12h; gradually increased to 30 mg/kg PO q12h if needed)—added after diet and glucocorticoids have proven ineffective

• Sandostatin (ocreotide, 10–20 μg SC q8–12h)—a synthetic somatostatin analogue; prevents hypoglycemia in some dogs refractory to conventional treatment; can be used with diet, steroids, and diazoxide; expensive

CONTRAINDICATIONS
Insulin

PRECAUTIONS
• Dextrose bolus—suitable for acute hypoglycemic crisis if followed by continuous dextrose-containing fluids or appropriate feeding; may precipitate further hypoglycemic crises if given alone
• Glucocorticoids used at high dosages for prolonged periods can cause iatrogenic hyperadrenocorticism.
• Diazoxide—can cause gastrointestinal irritation; causes bone marrow suppression, cataract formation, aplastic anemia, tachycardia, and thrombocytopenia in humans

POSSIBLE INTERACTIONS
N/A

ALTERNATIVE DRUG(S)
One case report has published the use of continuous-rate infusion of glucagon to control seizures and glycemic regulation without inducing a rebound effect.

FOLLOW-UP

PATIENT MONITORING
• At home for return or progression of clinical signs of hypoglycemia
• In-hospital serum glucose determinations—single, intermittent serum glucose determinations may not truly reflect the glycemic status of the patient because insulinomas occasionally respond to normal feedback mechanisms and because of production of counterregulatory hormones.
• Adjust medication on the basis of clinical signs and serum glucose levels.

PREVENTION/AVOIDANCE
N/A

POSSIBLE COMPLICATIONS
Recurrent or progressive episodes of hypoglycemia

EXPECTED COURSE AND PROGNOSIS
• Likelihood of malignancy is high; metastasis is seen in 40% of patients at the time of surgery.
• Dogs—mean survival time, about 16–19 months; range, 2–60 months; surgery improves survival time.
• Cats—mean survival time, about 6.5 months; range, 0–18 months

MISCELLANEOUS

ASSOCIATED CONDITIONS
Obesity

AGE-RELATED FACTORS
Younger dogs have shorter survival times.

ZOONOTIC POTENTIAL
N/A

PREGNANCY
N/A

SYNONYMS
• Insulin-secreting tumor
• B-cell tumor
• Hyperinsulinism
• Islet cell tumor
• Islet cell adenocarcinoma
• Insulin-producing pancreatic tumor

SEE ALSO
Glucose, Hypoglycemia

ABBREVIATION
AIGR = amended insulin:glucose ratio

Suggested Reading

Cox D. Pancreatic insulin-secreting neoplasm (insulinoma) in a West Highland white terrier. Can Vet J 1999;40:343–345.
Fischer JR, Smith SA, Harkin KR. Glucagon constant-rate infusion: a novel strategy for the management of hyperinsulinemic-hypoglycemic crisis in the dog. J Am Vet Med Assoc 2000;36:27–32.
Greco D. APUDomas: pheochromocytoma, insulinoma and gastrinoma. In: August JR, ed. Consultations in feline internal medicine, 4th ed. Philadelphia: Saunders, 2000:181–185.
Lester NV, Newell SM, Hill RC, Lanz OI. Scintigraphic diagnosis of insulinoma in a dog. Vet Rad Ultrasound 1999; 40:174–178.
McDermott L, Swainson S, Howard M. Canine insulinoma: a case report and review of the current literature. Iowa State University Veterinarian 1999;61:60–66.

Acknowledgment

The author and editors acknowledge the prior contributions of Dr. Mitchell A. Crystal, who authored this topic in the previous edition.
Author Nicole Bennett
Consulting Editor Deborah S. Greco

INTERDIGITAL DERMATITIS

 BASICS

OVERVIEW
• Disease of the feet of dogs
• Also known as pododermatitis, interdigital pyoderma, pedal folliculitis, and furunculosis

SIGNALMENT
• Dogs of any age, sex, or breed
• Short-coated male dogs (e.g., English bull dogs, Great Danes, basset hounds, mastiffs, bull terriers, boxers, dachshunds, Dalmatians, German short-haired pointers, and Weimaraners) may be predisposed.
• Some long-coated breeds (e.g., German shepherds, Labrador retrievers, golden retrievers, Irish setters, and Pekingese) are possibly predisposed.

SIGNS
• May affect one foot and one interdigital space or multiple interdigital spaces and feet
• Diseased tissue—usually erythematous and swollen; has either intact bullae, ruptured draining tracts, or both
• Sometimes mild to severe swelling of the affected feet
• Mild to severe lameness may be seen.

CAUSES & RISK FACTORS
One Affected Foot
• Foreign bodies (e.g., grass awns, wood slivers, suture material)
• Osteomyelitis
• Neoplasia
• Infection

More Than One Affected Foot
• Hypersensitivity reaction—food, atopy, contact dermatitis
• Infection—bacterial, fungal, yeast
• Trauma—clipper burns, cuts
• Chemical—contact irritant dermatitis
• Metabolic—hypothyroidism, hyperadrenocorticism
• Parasitic—demodicosis often complicated by the presence of furunculosis and draining tracts; heartworm, hookworm, and pelodera result in erythema, pruritus, and patchy alopecia of the feet; pelodera affects the limbs and the ventral abdomen.
• Idiopathic
• Recurrent pododermatitis—clinically important footpad involvement with the interdigital dermatitis
• Immune-mediated—pemphigus, pemphigoid, systemic lupus erythematosus
• Zinc deficiency or zinc responsive
• Superficial necrolytic dermatitis
• Follicular cysts

 DIAGNOSIS

DIFFERENTIAL DIAGNOSIS
Adult onset demodicosis—underlying hypothyroidism, hyperadrenocorticism, allergic disease, neoplasia, or idiopathic

CBC/BIOCHEMISTRY/URINALYSIS
• Usually normal
• Superficial necrolytic dermatitis—may have high liver and pancreatic enzyme activities

OTHER LABORATORY TESTS
• Blood tests—heartworm microfilaria
• Thyroid hormone tests—hypothyroidism
• Adrenal response tests (low-dose dexamethasone-suppression test, urine cortisol: creatinine ratio, ACTH stimulation)—hyperadrenocorticism

IMAGING
Radiographs—underlying osteomyelitis

DIAGNOSTIC PROCEDURES
• Biopsies—foreign bodies, demodicosis, neoplasia, infectious agents (fungi, bacteria) or other parasites (heartworm and, rarely, hookworm)
• Skin scrapings—identify parasites (demodicosis), pelodera, or fungi (dermatophytosis)
• Fecal flotation—identify hookworm ova
• Cytologic examination of the exudate with Wright-Giemsa stain—identify yeast, bacteria, and (rarely) parasites; evaluate the type of inflammatory response (e.g., eosinophils may suggest parasites or hypersensitivity)

PATHOLOGIC FINDINGS
Other than causal findings listed above (e.g., parasites and bacteria), the reaction pattern is a folliculitis, perifolliculitis, and pyogranulomatous dermatitis if the follicles or follicular cysts have ruptured.

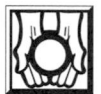 TREATMENT

• Treatments directed at underlying cause, if known
• Antibiotics—if bacteria are present; must be used until the deep tissues have healed; selection of appropriate drug depends on culture and sensitivity; begin as soon as possible with the correct drug, because treatment usually lasts several months.
• Draining lesions—twice-daily foot soaks (10 min each) until draining stops
• May be beneficial to restrict activity or protect feet
• Severe refractory cases—surgical débridement and removal of the affected interdigital tissue
• Follicular cysts may be ablated with CO_2 laser treatment.

 MEDICATIONS

DRUG(S)
• Broad-spectrum antibiotic—for the deep bacterial infection (furunculosis); use one that is effective against the staphylococcal organisms based on culture and sensitivity; try amoxicillin with clavulanate, fluoroquinolones, or cephalosporin; 6–8 weeks of therapy needed
• Rifampin—use with caution for short periods (30–60 days) at 5–10 mg/kg q24h; penetrates deep lesions well, owing to its lipid solubility; must be accompanied by a good antibiotic, because bacteria rapidly develop resistance

CONTRAINDICATIONS/POSSIBLE INTERACTIONS
Rifampin
• Monitor liver enzymes and CBC every 2 weeks.
• Do not use with liver disease.
• Stimulates liver enzymes involved in drug metabolism and thus can influence the metabolism of concurrently administered drugs; concentrations of anticoagulants, digitoxin, corticosteroids, and other drugs become subtherapeutic.
• When rifampin and ketoconazole are administered concurrently, both drugs are subtherapeutic.
• Use caution when concurrently administering other drugs.

 FOLLOW-UP

• Monitor closely to detect the underlying cause, if not previously determined; determining the cause can be tedious and frustrating but is essential for complete resolution and healing.
• Continue medication for bacterial infection for 2 weeks after all palpable dermal lesions are resolved.

 MISCELLANEOUS

ABBREVIATION
ACTH = adrenocorticotropic hormone

Suggested Reading
Scott DW. Canine pododermatitis. In: Kirk RW, ed. Current veterinary therapy, small animal practice VII. Philadelphia: Saunders, 1980:467–469
Author David Duclos
Consulting Editor Karen Helton Rhodes

INTERSTITIAL CELL TUMOR, TESTICLE

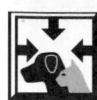

BASICS

OVERVIEW
Benign tumor of the testicle that arises from interstitial (e.g., Leydig) cells

SIGNALMENT
• Common in dogs and rare in cats
• Usually old male dogs

SIGNS
• Usually none unless associated with estrogen secretion, causing feminization and bone marrow hypoplasia (see Sertoli Cell Tumor)
• Single or multiple discrete tumor masses (usually 1 to 2 cm) within a single testis

CAUSES & RISK FACTORS
• Generally unknown
• Cryptorchidism—may predispose

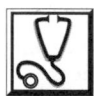

DIAGNOSIS

DIFFERENTIAL DIAGNOSIS
• Sertoli cell tumor
• Seminoma
• Hyperadrenocorticism—with feminization
• Hypothyroidism—with feminization

CBC/BIOCHEMISTRY/URINALYSIS
• Usually normal, unless estrogen excess causes bone marrow hypoplasia
• Various cytopenias—with estrogen excess

OTHER LABORATORY TESTS
• High serum estradiol concentration
• Low serum testosterone concentration

IMAGING
Ultrasonography—tumors < 3 cm in diameter tend to be hypoechoic; tumors > 5 cm tend to have mixed echogenic patterns.

DIAGNOSTIC PROCEDURES
N/A

TREATMENT
Castration and histopathologic examination of appropriate tissue

MEDICATIONS

DRUG(S)
• None, unless bone marrow hypoplasia
• Recombinant hematopoietic colony-stimulating factors—may be useful in treating bone marrow hypoplasia

CONTRAINDICATIONS/POSSIBLE INTERACTIONS
N/A

FOLLOW-UP

PATIENT MONITORING
None required, unless bone marrow hypoplasia

POSSIBLE COMPLICATIONS
Cytopenias caused by estrogen excess

EXPECTED COURSE AND PROGNOSIS
Usually excellent

MISCELLANEOUS

ASSOCIATED CONDITIONS
• Prostate disease—with testicular tumor
• Reported as a functional ectopic tumor in one cat

Suggested Reading
Morrison WB. Cancers of the reproductive tract. In: Morrison WB, ed., Cancer in dogs and cats: medical and surgical management. Baltimore: Williams & Wilkins, 1998.
Suess RP, Barr SC, Sacre BJ, et al. Bone marrow hypoplasia in a feminized dog with an interstitial cell tumor. J Am Vet Med Assoc 1992;200:1346–1348.

Author Wallace B. Morrison
Consulting Editor Wallace B. Morrison

INTERVERTEBRAL DISC DISEASE, CERVICAL

 BASICS

DEFINITION
A degeneration of the cervical intervertebral discs that causes protrusion or extrusion of disc material into the spinal canal. The protruded or extruded disc material causes spinal cord compression (myelopathy) and/or nerve root entrapment (radiculopathy).

PATHOPHYSIOLOGY
• Classified as acute disc herniation (Hansen type I disc) or chronic disc protrusion (Hansen type II disc). • Hansen type I disc degeneration is characterized by chondroid degeneration of the nucleus pulposus and acute rupture of the anulus fibrosus with extrusion of the nucleus pulposus into the spinal canal. • Hansen type II disc degeneration is characterized by fibrinoid degeneration of the nucleus pulposus. This causes bulging and protrusion of the dorsal anulus fibrosus into the vertebral canal.
• Disc extrusion or protrusion into the spinal canal causes focal compression of the spinal cord (myelopathy) and/or focal compression of a nerve root (radiculopathy).
• Consequences of spinal cord compression are ischemia and demyelination. • Dorsal disc extrusion or protrusion is more common than lateral disc extrusion or protrusion. • Disc extrusion may be secondary to trauma.
• Surgical fusion of cervical vertebrae may alter the biomechanics on adjacent vertebral bodies and therefore predispose discs to protrusion or extrusion.

SYSTEM AFFECTED
• Nervous system—either focal myelopathy or focal radiculopathy

GENETICS
• Not known • Chondrodystrophoid breeds (e.g., dachshunds, beagles, cocker spaniels) are most commonly affected with Hansen type I disc extrusion. • Large breed dogs (e.g., Doberman pinschers) are most commonly affected with Hansen type II disc extrusion.

INCIDENCE/PREVALENCE
• Cervical disc disease accounts for roughly 15% of all canine intervertebral disc disease.
• Eighty percent of disc extrusion occurs in dachshunds, beagles, and poodles.
• C3–C4 is the reported to be the most common site of disc extrusion.

SIGNALMENT

Species
Dogs

Breed Predisposition
• Hansen type I—dachshunds, poodles. Beagles, cocker spaniels
• Hansen type II—Doberman pinschers

Mean Age and Range
• Hansen type I—3–6 years of age
• Hansen type II—8–10 years of age

Predominant Sex
None recognized

SIGNS
Severity of clinical signs and spinal cord injury is dependent on several factors, including the rate and volume of disc extrusion or protrusion, spinal cord diameter relative to vertebral canal diameter, and the velocity of disc material that was extruded.

Historical Findings
• Neck pain—most common owner complaint • Stiff, stilted gait, reluctance to move the head and neck • Lowered head stance and muscle spasms of the head and neck • It has been reported that 10% of affected patients are tetraparetic. • Muscle atrophy over the scapula • Patients may have neck pain and front leg lameness secondary to dorsolateral disc extrusion.

Physical Examination Findings
• Neck pain—elicited upon flexion and extension of the neck or by turning the neck from side to side. Pain can also be elicited by deep palpation of the cervical muscles.
• Occasionally patients have neck pain and apparent forelimb lameness as a result of dorsolateral disc herniation (root signature/radiculopathy). This helps localize the lesion to C4–C7. • Paresis with postural reaction deficits involving both thoracic and pelvic limbs may be present. The deficits can also be ipsilateral in nature. • Pelvic limb paresis may be more severe than thoracic limb paresis. • Pelvic limb spinal reflexes may be normal to exaggerated. • Thoracic limb spinal reflexes may be normal to exaggerated when lesions are located in the C1–C6 spinal cord segments and may be normal to decreased when the C6–T2 spinal cord segment is affected. • Bladder function may be upper motor neuron in nature or normal.

CAUSES
• Hansen type I—early chondroid degeneration of the cervical intervertebral disc and subsequent disc mineralization
• Hansen type II—gradual fibroid degeneration of the cervical intervertebral disc

RISK FACTORS
Obesity and repeated traumatic events

 DIAGNOSIS

DIFFERENTIAL DIAGNOSIS
• Hansen type I disc disease • Hansen type II disc disease • Neoplasia • Atlantoaxial instability • Discospondylitis • Meningitis • Fibrocartilaginous embolism • Cervical vertebral instability • Spinal fracture/luxation • Endocrine—hypothyroidism

CBC/BIOCHEMISTRY/URINALYSIS
Should be performed in older animals in anticipation of general anesthesia and surgery

OTHER LABORATORY TESTS
• Cerebrospinal fluid (CSF) analysis— performed under general anesthesia prior to myelography. CSF should be collected from a cisternal tap since this site is closer to the lesion than a lumbar tap. • CSF analysis reveals mild to moderate elevation in protein levels and mild to moderate pleocytosis.
• Hansen type I disc herniation is usually associated with more severe CSF changes than in Hansen type II disc disease.

IMAGING

Cervical Spinal Radiography
• Well-positioned lateral and ventrodorsal survey radiographs of the cervical spine are always indicated. • Animals should be anesthetized for this procedure.
• Classic findings include narrowed intervertebral disc space, collapse of the articular facets, calcified disc material present in the intervertebral foramen or in the spinal canal • Hansen type II disc disease may be associated with spondylosis deformans.
• May reveal evidence of discospondylitis, fracture/luxation, atlantoaxial instability, or lytic vertebrae suggestive of a bone tumor

Myelography
• Myelography is indicated in 90% to 95% of cervical disc patients. • Survey cervical radiographs may be misleading. • Either a cisternal or lumbar injection between L5 and L6 or L4 and L5 can be used. • Lateral radiographs—reveal dorsal deviation of the ventral contrast column over the inter-vertebral disc space consistent with an extradural mass
• An intraforaminal or dorsolateral disc herniation is best seen on an oblique cervical radiograph, with the entire cervical spine positioned at a 45- to 60-degree angle to the table.

Enhanced Diagnostic Imaging
Magnetic resonance imaging (MRI) and computed tomography have also been used for diagnosis of cervical intervertebral disc disease.

DIAGNOSTIC PROCEDURES
Cerebral spinal fluid analysis

PATHOLOGIC FINDINGS

Gross Findings
• Hansen type I disc—white extruded disc material that has a granular consistency and is usually easily removed from the spinal canal
• Hansen type II disc—firm protrusion of the dorsal anulus fibrosus that is adherent to the floor of the spinal canal and to the dura of the spinal cord. Type II discs are much more difficult to remove from the spinal canal.
• Spinal cord—in acute disc extrusion the spinal cord may appear bruised and swollen;

in chronic disc protrusion the spinal cord may appear to be atrophied but is often normal in appearance.

Histopathologic Findings
• Hansen type I disc—shifting concentration of glycosaminoglycans, loss of water and proteoglycan content, and increased collagen content. The disc becomes more cartilaginous and undergoes dystrophic calcification.
• Hansen type II disc—a gradual fibroid metaplasia leaves the disc with increased glycosaminoglycan level and lower collagen content. The nucleus does not undergo cartilaginous metaplasia.
• Spinal cord—dependent on the severity of the disease and type of disc disease. Hansen type II—demyelination and gliosis are seen. Hansen type I—hemorrhage and edema can be seen and with severe disease myelomalacia can be observed

TREATMENT

APPROPRIATE HEALTH CARE
• Conservative management—dependent on patient's history and presenting neurologic status • Surgical management—patients with repeated episodes of neck pain, patients presented with severe neck pain and neurologic deficits, or patients that have not responded to conservative management

NURSING CARE
• Handling—minimal manipulation of the cervical spine and avoidance of jugular venipuncture if at all possible
• Urination—monitor patients for complete emptying of the bladder; patients may need to have bladder manually expressed or intermittent bladder catheterization. In some cases indwelling urinary catheter may need to be placed. Urinalysis, including culture and sensitivity, should be performed after removal of an indwelling catheter to make sure the patient did not obtain a nosocomial bacterial cystitis. • Defecation—patients may need enemas and can be switched to a low-residue diet to decrease the volume of feces
• Recumbent patients—should be kept on a well-padded mat and turned every 4 hours. Patients should be checked for pressure sores over bony prominences, which can lead to prolonged hospital stays and more surgeries.
• Physical therapy—hydrotherapy and passive range of motion of all joints should be performed as often as possible to prevent severe muscle atrophy

ACTIVITY
• Minimal, no running or jumping. When patients are being leash-walked, a harness should be used instead of a collar.
• With conservative management patients should be strictly confined to cage rest for 3 to 4 weeks.

• Following surgery patients should have minimal activity and be leash-walked only for 4 to 6 weeks, then slowly re-introduced to full activity.

DIET
For obese patients, a reducing diet should be instituted.

CLIENT EDUCATION
• For conservative management, strict cage confinement should be emphasized.
• Weight loss if the animal is obese
• Common clinical signs of animals with cervical disc disease

SURGICAL CONSIDERATIONS
• When indicated the goal of surgery is to remove disc material from the spinal canal and therefore decompress the spinal cord and/or nerve root. • Surgery usually provides immediate pain relief and eventual normal motor function. • A ventral cervical slot is the most common surgical approach for the removal of disc material from the spinal canal. • Disc material that has extruded dorsolaterally into the intervertebral foramen is removed via a lateral approach to the cervical spine or through a dorsal laminectomy, with or without a facetectomy.
• Fenestration alone for dogs with neck pain only usually does not resolve clinical signs.

MEDICATIONS

DRUG(S)
• Low-dose glucocorticoid therapy may be beneficial in order to decrease the pain in animals that are being treated conservatively.
• Glucocorticoids given to animals without simultaneous strict cage confinement could exacerbate disc extrusion by encouraging exercise. • Methylprednisolone sodium succinate—30 mg/kg intravenously within the first 8 hr of clinical onset can be given in acute cases. This can be followed by a dose of 15 mg/kg 2 hr after the initial dose, then every 6 hr for 24 hr. • If high-dose steroid therapy is initiated, gastrointestinal protectants should also be given. Common drugs used are cimetidine, ranitidine, misoprostol, and sucralfate.
• Nonsteroidal antiinflammatory drugs (NSAIDs) should be avoided, since they may cause severe gastric irritation and ulceration.
• Muscle relaxants can be used, but are generally unsuccessful when used alone.

CONTRAINDICATIONS
Never use glucocorticoids simultaneously with NSAIDs—this can cause severe gastrointestinal irritation and possibly intestinal perforation.

PRECAUTIONS
When using high-dose corticosteroids for cervical disc disease, patients should be placed on gastro-protectants to prevent the gastrointestinal side effects associated with corticosteroids.

POSSIBLE INTERACTIONS
NSAIDs in combination with glucocorticoids can cause gastrointestinal perforation or severe gastrointestinal bleeding, both situations leading to death.

FOLLOW-UP

PATIENT MONITORING
• Weekly evaluations should be performed until the resolution of clinical signs.
• All patients should be fitted with a harness, and neck collars should be avoided.

PREVENTION/AVOIDANCE
• Inherent in particular breeds • Keeping patients at an ideal weight may help.

POSSIBLE COMPLICATIONS
• Complications are uncommon.
• Continued neck pain • Deteriorating motor status • Subluxation/luxation of vertebral bodies

EXPECTED COURSE AND PROGNOSIS
• Prognosis for patients treated surgically or conservatively depends on neurologic signs at the time of presentation. • Prognosis is generally favorable for most patients.
• Most patients treated conservatively have recurrence of disease and may require surgical intervention.

MISCELLANEOUS

ASSOCIATED CONDITIONS
Animals predisposed to cervical disc disease are also the same breeds that are predisposed to thoracolumbar disc disease.

SEE ALSO
Intervertebral Disc Disease, Thoracolumbar

Suggested Reading
Oliver JE, Lorenz MD, Kornegay JN. Handbook of veterinary neurology. 3rd ed. Philadelphia: Saunders, 1997:174–187.
Seim HB. Surgery of the cervical spine. In: Small animal surgery. 2nd ed. St. Louis: Mosby, 2002:1213–1268.
Toombs JP: Cervical intervertebral disc disease in dogs, Compend Contin Educ Pract Vet 1992;14:1477.

Acknowledgment
The author and editors acknowledge the prior contributions of Mary O. Smith, who authored this topic in the previous edition.
Author Otto L. Lanz
Consulting Editor Peter K. Shires

INTERVERTEBRAL DISC DISEASE, THORACOLUMBAR

 BASICS

DEFINITION
Degenerative changes within the intervertebral discs characterized by loss of water, cellular necrosis, and calcification. Biomechanical properties of the disc deteriorate, resulting in extrusion or protrusion of disc material.

PATHOPHYSIOLOGY
• Accelerated degeneration of discs in chondrodystrophic breeds has been termed chondroid metaplasia. • Hansen Type I refers to acute extrusion of nucleus pulposus through the anulus into the vertebral canal; typically occurs in small chondrodystrophic breeds but may occur in larger non-chondrodystrophic dogs as well. • Hansen Type II lesions involve gradual protrusion (bulging) of the dorsal anular fibers into the vertebral canal; this is associated with fibroid metaplasia of the disc. • Acute disc extrusion results in disc material causing direct spinal cord injury and disc mass causing spinal cord compression. Disc mass (spinal cord compression) results in ischemia and spinal cord changes that vary from mild demyelination to necrosis of both gray and white matter; events at the cellular level include release of vasoactive substances, increased intracellular calcium, and increased free radical formation and lipid peroxides. • Pain due to dural irritation, nerve root impingement, or possibly discogenic in origin • Disc herniation rare between T3 and T10 owing to presence of intercapital ligament

SYSTEM AFFECTED
Nervous

GENETICS
Chondrodystrophic breeds (e.g., dachshunds; shih tzu, Pekingese) are predisposed to Hansen type I disease; larger breeds more commonly have Hansen type II disease.

INCIDENCE/PREVALENCE
• Most common neurologic dysfunction in small animals; affects 2% of the canine population • Rarely occurs in felines • Thoracolumbar disc disease comprises 85% of all disc herniations.

SIGNALMENT

Species
Dogs and occasionally cats

Breed Predilections
• Type I—Dachshunds; shih tzus, Lhaso apso; Pekingese, cocker spaniels, Welsh corgis; toy and miniature poodles • Type II—large breeds but may occur in any breed

Mean Age and Range
• Type I—3–7 years of age • Type II—8–10 years of age; cats mean age of 10 years

SIGNS

General Comments
Signs depend on the type of herniation, the velocity of disc contact with the spinal cord, the amount and duration of cord compression, the location (UMN or LMN), and the spinal canal/spinal cord diameter ratio (cervical vs thoracolumbar).

Historical Findings
• Onset may be peracute or acute in chondrodystrophoid dogs (type I disease), and may occur during vigorous activity. • Larger dogs or smaller dogs with type II disease have a more insidious onset, and tend to worsen with time.

Physical Examination Findings
• Varies considerably depending on type of herniation and anatomic location of lesion • Thoracolumbar pain common in dogs; reluctant to ambulate and hunched posture; careful palpation of spinous processes and epaxial musculature produces distinct localized pain; often some degree of paraparesis with decreased or absent proprioception in the rear limbs • Spinal reflexes in the rear limbs are usually exaggerated (hyper) when lesion is between T3 and L3; reflexes are decreased (hypo) when lesion is caudal to L3. • 75% of thoracolumbar herniations occur between T11 and L3. • Superficial and deep pain perception may be decreased or absent in the rear limbs; presence of deep pain sensation is the single most reliable prognostic factor for return to acceptable function; pain perception should be cerebral in nature and not confused with a withdrawal reflex (local spinal reflex). • Forelimb function is normal; occasionally Schiff-Sherrington phenomena may cause increased muscle tone in the forelimbs. • Urinary incontinence or retention is common when the lesion affects motor function. • Pain is less obvious in cats; the site of herniation is often lumbar.

CAUSES
• Chondroid or fibroid degeneration of the thoracolumbar intervertebral discs • 15% of animals with spinal fractures have been reported to have disc extrusions in addition to the fracture/luxation.

RISK FACTORS
Type I disease most often affects chondrodystrophic breeds.

 DIAGNOSIS

DIFFERENTIAL DIAGNOSIS
• Type I—Trauma causing fracture/luxation, neoplasia, discospondylitis, fibrocartilaginous embolism; differentiated by history, survey radiography, and myelography • Type II—degenerative myelopathy, neoplasia, discospondylitis, orthopedic disease; differentiated by history, radiography, and careful orthopedic and neurologic examination

CBC/BIOCHEMISTRY/URINALYSIS
• Elevation of liver enzymes common if patient has received corticosteroids for pain or neurologic disease • Urine retention/incontinence increases risk of urinary tract infection characterized by leukocytes, protein, and bacteruria on urinalysis.

OTHER LABORATORY TESTS
CSF analysis performed routinely in conjunction with myelography and if there is high suspicion of another disease process; may be normal but more typically shows mild to moderate increase in protein with or without pleocytosis

IMAGING
• Thoracolumbar spinal radiography • Survey radiographs rule out some other disease processes. • Diagnostic radiographs taken under general anesthesia may reveal a narrowed or wedged disc space, collapsed articular facet space, and small intervertebral foramen with increased or mineralized density within the spinal canal.

DIAGNOSTIC PROCEDURES
• Myelography performed with iohexol recommended in all patients when surgery is indicated; contrast usually introduced at L5–L6; usually shows an extradural mass lesion causing spinal cord compression adjacent to the affected disc; spinal cord swelling may be evidenced by thinning of contrast columns over several intervertebral space • CT, MRI, or repeat myelography may be indicated when results are not definitive. • CSF analysis

PATHOLOGIC FINDINGS

Gross
• Extruded disc material (type I disease)—white to yellow and "toothpaste" consistency; if chronic, may be hardened and adhered to surrounding structures. • Protruded disc material (type II disease)—usually firm, grayish white and may be adherent to surrounding structures • Spinal cord may appear normal or be swollen and discolored in acute severe disease.

Histopathologic
• Degenerated discs have decreased amounts of proteoglycans, glycosaminoglycans, and water; discs may become mineralized or cartilaginous. • Spinal cord lesion depends upon type and severity of disc extrusion or protrusion; acute, severe disease may cause hemorrhage, edema, tissue necrosis; chronic disease demyelination of white and in some cases gray matter

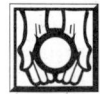 TREATMENT

APPROPRIATE HEALTH CARE
• Guidelines for therapy based on classification of clinical condition
Class 1—back-pain only
Class 2—back pain, ataxia, mild paraparesis, motor ability good
Class 3—proprioceptive deficits, motor ability affected but still present
Class 4—complete paraparesis (no motor ability) with deep pain perception present
Class 5—complete paraparesis, no deep pain present

INTERVERTEBRAL DISC DISEASE, THORACOLUMBAR

• Class 1 patients treated medically • Class 2 patients treated medically initially with serial neurologic exam, surgery if patient remains static or condition declines • Classes 3 and 4 surgical therapy • Class 5 surgical therapy if within the first 12–24 hours of occurrence • Serial neurologic examination important for all affected animals

NURSING CARE

• Absolute restricted confinement for 2–4 weeks • Minimize spinal manipulation and support spine when handling patient. • Ensure ability to urinate or consider bladder expression, intermittent catheterization, or indwelling urinary catheter for patients in classes 3–5 • Recumbent patients should be kept clean on padded bedding placed on elevated cage racks and turned frequently to prevent formation of decubital ulcers.
• Manual evacuation of the bowel or enemas may be necessary to promote defecation.
• Physical therapy with passive manipulation of rear limbs begun early followed by more intense therapy (hydrotherapy) for animals with neurologic deficits • Carts useful in many patients in promoting return to function; patient tolerance is limiting factor.

ACTIVITY

• Restricted movement most important part of medical management • Cage rest in hospital or enforced cage rest as an outpatient for 2–4 weeks for class 1 patients or postoperative animals

DIET

Weight reduction if patient is obese

CLIENT EDUCATION

• Describe signs of spinal cord compression and advise client of need for reevaluation in the case of worsening clinical signs.
• Emphasize the importance of restricted activity and how that may be accomplished when treating the patient medically or following surgery. • Some degree of restricted activity may be important for the remainder of the animal's life since it has disc disease.
• Most animals in classes 1–4 have a good to excellent prognosis for return to function, i.e., ambulation with bowel and bladder continence; patients in class 5 have a poorer but not hopeless prognosis; percentages vary but up to approximately 50% may regain deep pain and some function.

SURGICAL CONSIDERATIONS

• Strongly indicated for animals in classes 3 and 4, also within the first 12–24 hours for class 5 dogs; also indicated for static or worsening class 1 and 2 dogs • Primary surgical goal is to relieve spinal cord compression by disc mass removal via hemilaminectomy, dorsal laminectomy, or pediculectomy; disk fenestration alone rarely indicated • Recurrence of clinical signs in animals who have been operated on may be due to further extrusion of disc from the original site in many cases. • Surgical controversies remain over the issues of

prophylactic disc fenestration performed concurrently with decompressive surgery and the prognosis for return to function after surgery in negative deep pain patients.

MEDICATIONS

DRUG(S) OF CHOICE

• Methylprednisolone sodium succinate—30 mg/kg IV, within 8 hours of onset or presurgically in classes 2–5; some clinicians recommend repeat administration 12 hours later of 30 mg/kg or at 15 mg/kg 2 and 6 hours after first dose for severe acute disease (classes 4 and 5) • Prednisone or prednisolone—0.25–0.50 mg/kg PO twice daily for 2–4 days, then taper dose over 10 days for animals not having surgery; important that therapy be combined with strict cage rest and repeated neurologic examinations
• NSAIDs may be used as an analgesic in class 1 cases rather than prednisone or prednisolone.
• Narcotic analgesics may be necessary postoperatively; oxymorphone (0.05–0.1 mg/kg IV or IM q4h), butorphanol (0.2–0.4 mg/kg IV, IM, or SC every 2–4 hours), or buprenorphine (5–15 µg/kg IV or IM q6h)
• Methocarbamol (25–45 mg/kg q8h) may be useful in cases where muscle spasm is contributing to pain; more applicable with cervical disease • Bethanechol (5–15 mg/dog PO) and phenoxybenzamine (0.25 mg/kg PO q8–12h) variably helpful in managing bladder dysfunction associated with spinal cord lesion.

CONTRAINDICATIONS

Avoid concomitant use of glucocorticoids and NSAIDs because of combined negative effects on the gastrointestinal tract.

PRECAUTIONS

• Use of glucocorticoids without cage confinement may decrease pain, thereby encouraging excessive activity and leading to further disc herniation and deterioration of clinical condition. • High doses of glucocorticoids such as dexamethasone especially in combination with surgical therapy may result in extensive gastrointestinal hemorrhage and intestinal perforation; less common with other glucocorticoids

ALTERNATIVE DRUG(S) & THERAPIES

• Acupuncture may be effective for animals with chronic pain where no compressive lesion can be demonstrated by myelography. • Discolysis by enzymatic injection or laser ablation described but not proven therapy in dogs

FOLLOW-UP

PATIENT MONITORING

• Patients treated medically should be reevaluated 2–3 times daily for worsening neurologic signs for the first 48 hours after onset • If stable, re-evaluate daily, then weekly, until clinical signs have resolved. • Patients

treated surgically are evaluated twice daily until improvement is noted; urinary bladder function or awaiting development of an autonomic bladder are the limiting factors for hospitalization.

PREVENTION/AVOIDANCE

Prevention of obesity and avoiding strenuous exercise or jumping may or may not avoid exacerbation of clinical signs.

POSSIBLE COMPLICATIONS

• Recurrence of signs associated with disc herniation at original or at new site
• Deterioration of clinical signs with or without surgery; hard-to-predict clinical course in some cases, especially those with severe type 1 lesions • Rarely, development of ascending or descending myelomalacia; occurs in class 4 or 5 dogs 3–5 days following injury and characterized by variable and changing neurologic findings, possible fever, possible dyspnea; euthanasia event when diagnosed

EXPECTED COURSE AND PROGNOSIS

• Overall prognosis for dogs in class 1–4 good; those treated conservatively may experience recurrence of clinical signs. • Recurrence rates of dogs without fenestration at the time of laminectomy range from 5–30%. • Dogs in class 5 have a variable (10–75%) chance of recovery; overall a guarded prognosis

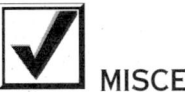

MISCELLANEOUS

ASSOCIATED CONDITIONS

Predisposed patients and breeds may have concurrent cervical disk disease

SEE ALSO

Intervertebral Disc Disease, Cervical

ABBREVIATIONS

• CSF = cerebrospinal fluid • NSAID = nonsteroidal antiinflammatory drug

Suggested Reading

Fingeroth JM. Treatment of canine intervertebral disk disease: recommendations and controversies. In Bonagura JD, ed. Current veterinary therapy XII. Philadelphia: Saunders, 1995:1146–1152.

Munana KR, Olby N, Sharp NJH, et al. Intervertebral disc disease in 10 cats. J Am Anim Hosp Assoc 2001; 37:384–389.

Seim HB. Conditions of the thoracolumbar spine. Semin Vet Med Surg 1996; 11:235–253.

Seim HB. Surgery of the thoracolumbar spine. In: Fossum TW, ed. Small Animal Surgery, 2nd ed. St. Louis: Mosby, 2002: 1269–1287.

Acknowledgment

The author/editors acknowledge the prior contributions of Dr. Mary Smith, who authored this topic in the previous edition.

Author Don R. Waldron
Consulting Editor Peter K. Shires

INTUSSUSCEPTION

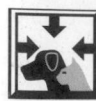

BASICS

DEFINITION
• Prolapse or invagination of one portion of the GI tract into the lumen of an adjoining segment
• The invaginated segment is the *intussusceptum* and the ensheathing segment is the *intussuscipiens.*
• Classified according to location within the alimentary tract—enterocolic (ileocolic; most common location), cecocolic, enteroenteric, duodenogastric, gastroesophageal
• High intussusceptions may be defined as those proximal to the jejunum; low intussusceptions are those distal to the duodenum.

PATHOPHYSIOLOGY
• Exact physical and mechanical events that lead to intussusception are unknown.
• Uncoordinated peristalsis is probably involved; vigorous contraction of a bowel segment causes invagination of that segment into an adjacent flaccid segment.
• Regions of the GI tract that undergo abrupt change in anatomic diameter (e.g., ileocolic, or gastroesophageal junctions) are at high risk.
• Results in partial or complete GI obstruction leading to hypovolemia and dehydration
• Vascular compromise is common, especially to the intussusceptum, ranging from venous and lymphatic obstruction to arterial obstruction with full-thickness necrosis.
• Disruption of the mucosal barrier may allow absorption of bacteria and/or endotoxin and resultant shock.

SYSTEMS AFFECTED
• Gastrointestinal
• Cardiovascular—hypovolemic or septic shock
• May be multiple organ failure in severe, untreated cases

GENETICS
Heritability unproven, although gastroesophageal intussusception (GEI) has been reported in multiple littermates.

INCIDENCE/PREVALENCE
Unknown

GEOGRAPHIC DISTRIBUTION
N/A

SIGNALMENT

Species
• Dogs and cats
• GEI reported only in dogs.

Breed Predilection
• German shepherd dogs and Siamese cats
• German shepherd dogs have an especially high prevalence of GEI (64%).

Mean Age and Range
• Higher incidence in puppies and kittens: ~ 80% are <1 year of age; for GEI, 80% of dogs are >3 months of age).
• Reported range—5 days to 9 years

Predominant Sex
• None for intussusception in general
• Male:female ratio approximately 2:1 for GEI

SIGNS

General Comments
• Clinical signs and disease progression vary markedly depending upon location, degree of vascular compromise, and completeness of obstruction.
• In general, high intussusceptions have a more acute onset of signs and a more rapid clinical deterioration with higher mortality than do low intussusceptions.

Historical Findings
• High intussusceptions—frequent vomiting, regurgitation, hematemesis, dyspnea, abdominal discomfort, and collapse
• Low intussusceptions—may include bloody mucoid diarrhea, tenesmus, intermittent vomiting, and weight loss

Physical Examination Findings
• Intermittent vomiting, bloody mucoid stools, and/or palpation of a sausage-shaped abdominal mass—mass is often caudal since ileocolic intussusception is most common.
• Most patients are mildly to severely dehydrated.
• May be signs of shock
• Abdominal pain—variable; may make palpation of the mass more difficult
• Ileocolic intussusception may present with the intussusceptum protruding through the anus.

CAUSES
• Idiopathic
• Enteritis—viral, bacterial
• Intestinal parasites
• Foreign bodies
• Previous abdominal surgery
• Intestinal mass
• Megaesophagus associated with GEI

RISK FACTORS
Any condition leading to altered GI motility

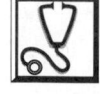

DIAGNOSIS

DIFFERENTIAL DIAGNOSIS
• Many of the disease conditions that may mimic intussusception are also predisposing factors for development of intussusception; thorough examination and close patient monitoring are of utmost importance.

• Viral enteritis—usually can diagnose on the basis of typical changes in CBC (leukopenia/neutropenia) and commercial fecal antigen test kits
• Foreign bodies—may be radiopaque or may cause plication of intestinal loops (linear foreign bodies); contrast studies can usually differentiate a foreign body from an intussusception, although the distinction is often made at the time of exploratory celiotomy.
• Mesenteric volvulus—can exhibit signs similar to those of intussusception; plain radiographic distinction may be difficult; mesenteric volvulus tends to have a more rapidly fatal course, and emergency celiotomy is indicated to differentiate the two conditions.
• Intestinal parasites—diagnosed by fecal examination and response to an anthelmintic
• HGE can be differentiated by a lack of radiographic signs of obstruction.
• Ileocolic intussusception with the intussusceptum protruding through the anus is differentiated from rectal prolapse by passing a blunt probe between the prolapsed segment and the anus; if the probe passes into the pelvic canal, the protrusion is due to an intussusception.
• GEI has inappropriately been confused with hiatal hernia.

CBC/BIOCHEMISTRY/URINALYSIS
• Leukogram—variable; ranges from leukopenia (underlying viral enteritis) to leukocytosis (with bowel necrosis or peritonitis)
• Hematocrit—may be low if significant GI hemorrhage; high with dehydration
• Electrolyte abnormalities—hyponatremia, hypochloremia, and hypokalemia tend to be more profound with high intussusceptions.
• Prerenal azotemia with dehydration
• Urinalysis—usually normal or nonspecific

OTHER LABORATORY TESTS
• Blood gas evaluation usually reveals a metabolic acidosis.
• High intussusception—metabolic alkalosis may prevail from loss of gastric acid in the vomitus (hypochloremia with metabolic alkalosis strongly supports pyloric outflow obstruction).

IMAGING
• Definitive diagnosis from plain films may be difficult.
• Usually radiographic signs of obstruction—bowel loops distended with gas and fluid; more pronounced with complete obstruction
• A tissue-dense tubular mass strongly supports a diagnosis of intussusception.
• In GEI, thoracic radiographs show dilation of the esophagus with a tissue-dense mass in the caudal esophagus; the normal gastric air bubble may be absent in the cranial abdomen.

- Abdominal ultrasound—can be used to identify the intussusception; a cylindrical intestinal mass with excessive wall layering is highly specific for intussusception.
- Contrast studies (upper GI, barium enema)—can be used to outline an intussusception, but often result in unnecessary delays in definitive treatment

DIAGNOSTIC PROCEDURES
- Esophagoscopy can identify a soft tissue mass (stomach) within the lumen of the esophagus in patients with GEI.
- Colonoscopy may help identify enterocolic or cecocolic intussusceptions.

PATHOLOGIC FINDINGS
- The basic lesion is grossly obvious.
- Histopathologic changes in the affected bowel range from areas of mucosal erosion and hemorrhages to full-thickness mural necrosis.

TREATMENT

APPROPRIATE HEALTH CARE
- Inpatient medical and surgical management; surgical emergency once patient is stabilized
- Life-threatening condition

NURSING CARE
- Aggressive intravenous fluid support to correct dehydration and replace ongoing GI losses—use a balanced electrolyte solution (e.g., lactated Ringer's solution); use NaCl if dehydration is profound.
- Profound hyponatremia and hypochloremia indicates 0.9% NaCl.
- Potassium supplementation—based on measured serum levels, but usually required; use 20 mEq of KCl/L of IV fluid if serum potassium concentration is unknown; do not exceed an administration rate of 0.5 mEq/kg/h.

ACTIVITY
Restrict during treatment and postoperative periods (~ 7–10 days).

DIET
- Maintain vomiting patients NPO.
- Can usually initiate oral intake of fluid and food 12–24 hours following surgical correction
- Early oral alimentation with small, frequent meals promotes normal peristalsis and avoids further ileus.

CLIENT EDUCATION
- A poor-to-grave prognosis is associated with nonoperative treatment of intussusception.
- GEI is associated with a high mortality in all cases.
- Correction of the intussusception may not address the underlying GI disorder.

SURGICAL CONSIDERATIONS
- A surgical emergency
- Celiotomy and correction should follow initial patient stabilization.
- Attempt manual reduction of the intussusception by gently "milking" the invaginated segment.
- Assess bowel viability by color, pulsation, intestinal contraction, and Wood's lamp fluorescence following IV fluorescein injection.
- If the intussusception is nonreducible or nonviable, resection and anastomosis are indicated.
- Can minimize risk of postoperative recurrence by enteroplication of the small intestine
- GEI recurrence is prevented by a left-sided gastropexy of the fundus.

MEDICATIONS

DRUG(S) OF CHOICE
- Administer broad-spectrum antibiotics or combinations with efficacy against coliforms and anaerobes, intravenously prior to surgery.
- Histamine blockers (e.g., famotidine, ranitidine) and/or protectants (e.g., sucralfate) may be indicated if GI ulceration is suspected.

CONTRAINDICATIONS
- Motility-enhancing antiemetics (e.g., metoclopramide, cisapride)
- Antiemetics mask signs of GI obstruction.

PRECAUTIONS
Anticholinergics exacerbate postoperative ileus and are not recommended.

POSSIBLE INTERACTIONS
N/A

ALTERNATIVE DRUG(S)
N/A

FOLLOW-UP

PATIENT MONITORING
- Watch closely for recurrence or worsening of signs for the first 3–5 days following surgery, when serious complications are most likely to occur.
- Recurrence is common (20–30%) in patients that do not receive enteroplication and usually occurs within 3 days.
- Suspect anastomotic dehiscence or leakage with a deterioration of clinical signs; diagnostic peritoneal lavage is the most sensitive method for detecting dehiscence.

PREVENTION/AVOIDANCE
Routine veterinary care of puppies and kittens (e.g., vaccinations and treatment of intestinal parasites) will eliminate many predisposing factors.

POSSIBLE COMPLICATIONS
- Recurrence
- Persistence of underlying GI problem if undiagnosed or untreated
- Peritonitis
- Short bowel syndrome may occur with resection of large segments of intestine.

EXPECTED COURSE AND PROGNOSIS
- Presence and severity of underlying condition will affect prognosis.
- Low intussusceptions: <20% mortality with proper treatment
- GEI: ~ 95% mortality

MISCELLANEOUS

ASSOCIATED CONDITIONS
May accompany other GI abnormalities

AGE-RELATED FACTORS
In old animals may be more commonly associated with mural mass lesions; routinely submit resected bowel segments in old patients for histopathology.

ZOONOTIC POTENTIAL
N/A

PREGNANCY
The stress of the metabolic and hemodynamic derangements, coupled with anesthesia and surgery, may result in pregnancy termination.

SYNONYMS
Cecocolic intussusception is commonly termed *cecal inversion.*

SEE ALSO
- Shock • Peritonitis
- Gastrointestinal Obstruction

ABBREVIATIONS
- GEI = gastroesophageal intussusception
- GI = gastrointestinal
- HGE = hemorrhagic gastroenteritis

Suggested Reading
Leib MS, Blass CE. Gastroesophageal intussusception in the dog: a review of the literature and a case report. J Am Anim Hosp Assoc 984;20:783–790.
Lewis DD. Intussusception in dogs and cats. Compend Contin Educ Pract Vet 1987;9:523–533.
Oaks MG, Lewis DD, Hosgood G, et al. Enteroplication for the prevention of intussusception recurrence in dogs: 31 cases. J Am Vet Med Assoc 1994;205:72–75.
Orsher RJ, Rosin E. Small intestine. In: Slatter D, ed. Textbook of small animal surgery. 2nd ed. Philadelphia: Saunders, 1993:593–612.

Author Bradford C. Dixon
Consulting Editor Albert E. Jergens

IRIS ATROPHY

 BASICS

OVERVIEW
• Degeneration of the pupillary margin or stroma (or both portions) of the iris, resulting in an iris that is thin or has areas of full-thickness tissue loss
• May be a senile or secondary change
• Secondary—may be a potential sequela of chronic inflammation (uveitis)
• Iris sphincter muscle—frequently affected, resulting in incomplete pupillary constriction
• Margin may remain unaffected; loss of stroma and iris dilator muscle causes large holes in the iris that resemble multiple pupillary openings
• Vision unaffected
• May cause discomfort in bright-light settings

SIGNALMENT
• Dogs—common aging change; all breeds, but affects small breeds (e.g., miniature and toy poodles, miniature schnauzers, and Chihuahuas) more commonly
• Cats—uncommon; most common with blue irides
• Secondary—any breed of dog or cat

SIGNS
Historical Findings
• Photophobia
• Previous episodes of uveitis

PHYSICAL EXAMINATION FINDINGS
• Incomplete pupillary light reflex, accompanied by a normal menace response
• Unilateral—may note anisocoria
• Irregular, scalloped edge to the pupillary margin
• Thin or absent areas of the iris on transillumination
• Strands of iris occasionally remain, spanning across portions of the pupil.
• Holes within the iris stroma—may resemble additional pupils
• Secondary—may be accompanied by any sign associated with chronic uveitis

CAUSES & RISK FACTORS
• Normal aging
• Uveitis
• Glaucoma

 DIAGNOSIS

DIFFERENTIAL DIAGNOSIS
• Must differentiate from congenital iris anomalies
• Iris aplasia—rare in dog and cats
• Iris hypoplasia
• Iris coloboma—a complete, full-thickness area of lack of development of all layers of the iris; frequently associated with the merle condition; may also see associated lack of lens zonules and an indentation of the lens deep to the colobomatous area
• Polycoria—more than one pupil, each with the ability to constrict
• Persistent pupillary membranes—arise from the collarette (midportion) of the iris, not from the free pupillary margin
• Pupil dilation due to glaucoma will also have an elevated IOP, will usually have corneal edema, conjunctival +/− scleral infection, may also be blind

CBC/BIOCHEMISTRY/URINALYSIS
N/A

OTHER LABORATORY TESTS
N/A

IMAGING
N/A

DIAGNOSTIC PROCEDURES
Tonometry—possibly low IOP if secondary to uveitis; high IOP if the uveitis has advanced to a secondary glaucoma

 TREATMENT

• Nonreversible
• Secondary—aimed at controlling the underlying disease. May halt progression of the condition
• Patient may exhibit photophobia because of inability to constrict the pupil; provide adequate shade.

 MEDICATIONS

DRUG(S)
• Senile—none
• Secondary—depend on underlying disease

CONTRAINDICATIONS/POSSIBLE INTERACTIONS
Topical atropine—exacerbates photophobia and pupillary dilation

 FOLLOW-UP

• Senile—may continue to progress with age
• Secondary—usually does not progress once the primary disease is controlled

 MISCELLANEOUS

SEE ALSO
• Anterior Uveitis—Cats
• Anterior Uveitis—Dogs
• Glaucoma

ABBREVIATION
• IOP = intraocular pressure

Suggested Reading
Collins BK, Moore CP. Diseases and surgery of canine anterior uvea. In: Gelatt KN, ed., Veterinary ophthalmology. 3rd ed. Philadelphia: Lippincott Williams & Wilkins, 1999: 755–795.
Author Stephanie L. Smedes
Consulting Editor Paul E. Miller

BASICS

OVERVIEW
• Iron—essential element for living organisms; may be lethal when ingested in large quantities
• Sources of large concentrations of readily ionizable iron—multivitamins; dietary mineral supplements; human pregnancy supplements
• Overdose—loss of the normal mucosal limitations of iron absorption; corrosive to the gastrointestinal mucosa • Circulating iron in excess of the TIBC—very reactive; causes oxidative damage to any cell type • Damage to mitochondria—loss of oxidative metabolism
• Affected primary systems—gastrointestinal; hepatic; cardiovascular; nervous

SIGNALMENT
Dogs; possible in other species

SIGNS

General Comments
• History—generally indicates pill ingestion
• Unlikely to develop in patients that remain asymptomatic for 6–8 hr • Occur in four stages

Stage I (0–6 hr)
• Vomiting • Diarrhea • Depression
• Gastrointestinal hemorrhage • Abdominal pain

Stage II (6–24 hr)
Apparent recovery

Stage III (12–96 hr)
• Vomiting • Diarrhea • Depression
• Gastrointestinal hemorrhage • Shock
• Tremors • Abdominal pain

Stage IV (2–6 weeks)
Gastrointestinal obstruction

CAUSES & RISK FACTORS
• Generally associated with ingestion of iron-fortified pills • Dogs—likely to ingest a large number of pills, owing to relatively indiscriminate eating behavior • Toxic dose (dogs)—> 20 mg/kg of elemental iron
• Metallic iron and iron oxide (rust)—not readily ionizable; not associated with toxicoses • Take care when calculating iron ingestion; iron salts in supplements and medications vary in elemental iron content (between 12% and 63%).

ELEMENTAL IRON IN IRON SALTS

Salt Form	Elemental Iron (%)
Ferric ammonium citrate	15%
Ferric chloride	34%
Ferric hydroxide	63%
Ferric phosphate	37%
Ferrous fumarate	33%
Ferrous carbonate	48%
Ferrous gluconate	12%
Ferrous lactate	24%
Ferrous sulfate	20%
Peptonized iron	16%

DIAGNOSIS

DIFFERENTIAL DIAGNOSIS
Other causes of gastroenteritis

CBC/BIOCHEMISTRY/URINALYSIS
• Leukocytosis
• Hyperglycemia
• Normal to high AST, ALT, ALP, and serum bilirubin

OTHER LABORATORY TESTS
Metabolic acidosis

Serum Analysis for Total Iron and TIBC
• Normal binding capacity—3–4 times the serum iron
• Serum iron in excess of TIBC—indicates poisoning; treatment required; monitor at 2–3 hr and at 5–6 hr postingestion and in asymptomatic patients (absorption rates vary with tablet dissolution and serum iron concentrations change rapidly).

IMAGING
Radiography—intact iron-containing pills are radiodense; able to visualize pill bezoars or pills adhered to the esophageal mucosa

DIAGNOSTIC PROCEDURES
• Postmortem analysis for iron in tissues—often ineffective, because of the reactive nature of free iron and the systemic distribution of reactive binding
• Analysis of gastrointestinal or stomach contents—may aid in documenting high iron exposures

PATHOLOGIC FINDINGS
Primary gross lesions—hemorrhage in the gastrointestinal tract and liver; hepatomegaly

TREATMENT
• Correct hypovolemic shock—intravenous fluids
• Correct acidosis—bicarbonate added to intravenous fluids

DECONTAMINATION AND PROTECTION
• Prevent further gastrointestinal and systemic damage—removal of unabsorbed iron from the stomach; lessens duration and severity of signs
• Treat gastrointestinal damage—gastric demulcents or sucralfate for severe gastrointestinal damage
• Emesis—induced for asymptomatic patient

• Gastric or enterogastric lavage—lessens absorption; performed when emesis is contraindicated or when pill bezoars are identified
• Emergency gastrotomy—indicated if lavage fails to remove adherent pills or bezoars

CHELATION
• Chelate excess systemic iron.
• Deferoxamine mesylate—iron chelator
• Duration of therapy—until TIBC is greater than serum iron

MEDICATIONS

DRUG(S)
• Deferoxamine mesylate—15 mg/kg/hr IV infusion or 40 mg/kg IM q4–6h or 40 mg/kg slow IV q4–6h; for chelation; indicated when serum iron exceeds TIBC
• Sucralfate—0.5–1 g PO q8–12h; for gastrointestinal protection

CONTRAINDICATIONS/POSSIBLE INTERACTIONS
• Activated charcoal—does not bind iron
• Gastric lavage—contraindicated with hematemesis, owing to increased risk of perforation
• Intravenous deferoxamine—must be given slowly or may precipitate cardiac arrhythmias
• Deferoxamine—teratogenic; use in pregnant patients only if the benefits outweighs the risks.

FOLLOW-UP
• Liver enzymes—monitored up to 24 hr after excess circulating iron is controlled
• Instruct client to watch for evidence of gastrointestinal obstruction for 4–6 weeks after poisoning.

MISCELLANEOUS

SEE ALSO
Poisoning (Intoxication)

ABBREVIATIONS
• ALP = alkaline phosphatase • ALT = alanine aminotransferase • AST = aspartate aminotransferase • TIBC = total iron binding capacity

Suggested Reading
Greentree WF, Hall JO. Iron toxicosis. In: Bonagura JD, ed. Kirk's current veterinary therapy XII. Philadelphia: Saunders, 1983:240–242.
Author Jeffery O. Hall
Consulting Editor Gary D. Osweiller

IRRITABLE BOWEL SYNDROME

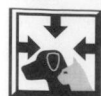 BASICS

DEFINITION
A condition characterized by chronic intermittent signs of colonic dysfunction in the absence of structural gastrointestinal pathology

PATHOPHYSIOLOGY
• Unknown causes
• Potential causes include abnormal colonic myoelectrical activity and motility, dietary fiber deficiency, dietary intolerances, stress, and changes in neural or neurochemical regulation of colonic function.

SYSTEMS AFFECTED
Gastrointestinal

GENETICS
N/A

INCIDENCE/PREVALENCE
• An estimated 10–15% of dogs with chronic large bowel diarrhea have IBS.
• This disorder is poorly characterized and the diagnosis is based on exclusion of other causes, so accurate assessment of its prevalence is difficult.

GEOGRAPHIC DISTRIBUTION
N/A

SIGNALMENT
Species
Dogs

Breed Predilections
Any breed; especially working dogs

Mean Age and Range
N/A

Predominant Sex
N/A

SIGNS
Historical Findings
• Chronic, intermittent signs of large bowel diarrhea, including frequent passage of small amounts of feces and mucus, and dyschezia
• Hematochezia is uncommon.
• Abdominal pain, bloating, vomiting, and nausea may also occur.

Physical Examination Findings
• Often unremarkable
• May be evident abdominal pain
• Rectal examination is normal aside from large bowel diarrhea.

CAUSES
Unknown

RISK FACTORS
• Stress (e.g., changes in the household or being left alone for extended periods) may be associated with episodes of diarrhea.
• In many dogs, stress appears to play no role.

 DIAGNOSIS

• Based on the exclusion of all other potential causes of large bowel diarrhea
• Reserve for patients that have undergone a thorough diagnostic evaluation, therapeutic deworming, and bland diet trials without resolution of signs.

DIFFERENTIAL DIAGNOSIS
Causes of Large Bowel Diarrhea
• Whipworms
• Inflammatory colitis
• *Clostridium perfringens*
• Fiber-responsive large bowel diarrhea
• Dietary indiscretion or intolerance
• *Giardia*
• Histoplasmosis
• Pythiosis
• Colonic neoplasia
• Cecal inversion

Diseases with Similar Signs
• Dysuria/stranguria—exclude with observation, urinalysis, and imaging.
• Prostatic disease—exclude with rectal examination and imaging.

CBC/BIOCHEMISTRY/URINALYSIS
Normal

OTHER LABORATORY TESTS
Direct fecal examination, fecal flotation, and fecal/rectal scraping cytology—normal

IMAGING
• Survey and contrast radiographic studies of the abdomen—normal
• Abdominal ultrasonography—normal

DIAGNOSTIC PROCEDURES
• Colonoscopy generally normal; colonic spasm, excessive intraluminal mucus, and hypermotility are occasionally present.
• Mucosal biopsy specimens from multiple areas in the colon are histologically normal.

PATHOLOGIC FINDINGS
Normal

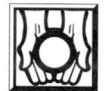 TREATMENT

APPROPRIATE HEALTH CARE
Outpatient medical management

ACTIVITY
N/A

IRRITABLE BOWEL SYNDROME

DIET
A highly digestible diet with added soluble fiber (Metamucil, 1–3 tbs per day) often improves the diarrhea, but rarely completely resolves clinical signs.

CLIENT EDUCATION
• Inform clients that response to treatment varies and affected dogs may have long-term intermittent clinical signs.
• Eliminate any stressful factors in the dog's environment if possible.

SURGICAL CONSIDERATIONS
N/A

MEDICATIONS

DRUGS OF CHOICE
Drug therapy for several days up to 1 to 2 weeks during episodes

Motility Modifiers
• Opiate antidiarrheals improve signs by increasing rhythmic segmentation.
• Loperamide (Imodium), 0.1–0.2 mg/kg PO q8–12h
• Diphenoxylate (Lomotil), 0.05–0.2 mg/kg PO q8–12h

Antispasmodic–Tranquilizer Combinations
• Used to relieve abdominal cramping, bloating, and distress
• Chlordiazepoxide and clidinium bromide (Librax), 0.1–0.25 mg of clidinium/kg PO q8–12h
• Isopropamide and prochlorperazine (Darbazine), 0.14–0.22 mg/kg SC q12h; oral: see package insert.

Parenteral Antiemetics
• If nausea and vomiting preclude the use of oral medication, administer antiemetics parenterally for 1–2 days.

• Chlorpromazine (Thorazine), 0.2–0.5 mg/kg q6–24h SC or IM

CONTRAINDICATIONS
• Opiates—respiratory dysfunction, hepatic encephalopathy, and/or severe debilitation
• Anticholinergics—cardiac disease, hepatobiliary disease, renal disease, hypertension, and/or hyperthyroidism

PRECAUTIONS
N/A

POSSIBLE INTERACTIONS
N/A

ALTERNATIVE DRUGS
Sulfasalazine (Azulfidine), 22–30 mg/kg PO q8h—reported to improve signs in some dogs with significant dyschezia

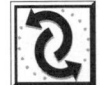
FOLLOW-UP

PATIENT MONITORING
Have owner monitor stool consistency and watch for signs of dyschezia and abdominal discomfort.

PREVENTION/AVOIDANCE
Minimize any stressful factors in the patient's environment that might precipitate an episode.

POSSIBLE COMPLICATIONS
N/A

EXPECTED COURSE AND PROGNOSIS
• Should see improved stools, decreased mucus, and relief of dyschezia and abdominal distress within 1–2 days of starting medication
• In some dogs, signs completely resolve following treatment and dietary alterations; others have long-term episodic signs.

✓
MISCELLANEOUS

ASSOCIATED CONDITIONS
None

AGE-RELATED FACTORS
None

ZOONOTIC POTENTIAL
None

PREGNANCY
N/A

SYNONYMS
• Spastic colon
• Nervous colon
• Spastic colitis
• Mucous colitis

SEE ALSO
• Diarrhea, Chronic—Dogs
• Colitis and Proctitis
• Dyschezia and Hematochezia

ABBREVIATION
IBS = irritable bowel syndrome

Suggested Reading

Leib MS, Monroe WE, Codner EC. Management of chronic large bowel diarrhea in dogs. Vet Med 1991;86:922–929.

Strombeck DR, Guilford WG. Strombeck's small animal gastroenterology. 3rd ed. Philadelphia: Saunders, 1996.

Tams TR. Irritable bowel syndrome. In: Kirk RW, Bonagura JD, eds. Current veterinary therapy XI. Philadelphia: Saunders, 1992:604–608.

Author Amy M. Grooters

Consulting Editor Albert E. Jergens

IVERMECTIN TOXICITY

 BASICS

OVERVIEW
• Toxicity—dogs given large extra-label dosages (≥ 10–15 times recommended dosage)
• Ivermectin—potentiates the release and binding of the neuroinhibitory substance GABA at certain synapses in the CNS; metabolized and excreted by the liver
• Sensitivity—some dogs unusually sensitive; differences may relate to a defect in the blood–brain barrier, higher than normal amounts of unbound ivermectin in the plasma, or an ivermectin-specific blood–brain transport mechanism

SIGNALMENT
• Collies—most commonly affected; not all are sensitive
• Australian shepherds—common
• May be a genetic component in sensitive animals
• No age or sex predilections

SIGNS
• Mydriasis
• Depression
• Drooling
• Vomiting
• Ataxia
• Tremors
• Disorientation
• Weakness, recumbency
• Nonresponsiveness
• Blindness
• Bradycardia
• Hypoventilation
• Coma
• Death

CAUSES & RISK FACTORS
• Extra-label use at high dosage
• Breed sensitivity—collies; Australian shepherds

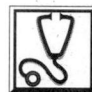 **DIAGNOSIS**

• Based on history and clinical signs
• No specific tests useful in confirming the diagnosis

DIFFERENTIAL DIAGNOSIS
• Overdoses of other ivermectin compounds—milbemycin oxime
• Other toxicants or diseases affecting CNS

CBC/BIOCHEMISTRY/URINALYSIS
N/A

OTHER LABORATORY TESTS
Arterial blood gases—may reveal high $PaCO_2$ and low PaO_2 caused by respiratory depression and hypoventilation

IMAGING
N/A

DIAGNOSTIC PROCEDURES
Physostigmine—1 mg IV; temporary (30–40-min) return to consciousness or resumed alertness and muscle activity after the administration supports but does not confirm diagnosis; does not speed recovery; not indicated for treatment; glycopyrrolate administered first may prevent severe bradycardia

TREATMENT

• Mainstay—supportive and symptomatic care
• Proper fluid therapy, maintenance of electrolyte balance, nutritional support, and prevention of secondary complications—important goals
• Nutritional support—institute early, preferably within 2–3 days of exposure; severe CNS depression or coma may last for weeks
• Frequent turning of patient, appropriate bedding, physical therapy, attentive nursing care, and other standard treatment measures for a recumbent patient important
• Apply ocular lubricants.
• Mechanical ventilation—may be required with respiratory depression

MEDICATIONS

DRUG(S)
• No known reversal agent
• Atropine or glycopyrrolate—may be administered as needed to treat bradycardia

CONTRAINDICATIONS/POSSIBLE INTERACTIONS
Avoid other drugs that stimulate the GABA receptor—benzodiazepine tranquilizers

FOLLOW-UP

• Prognosis and eventual outcome—depend on individual and breed sensitivity, amount of drug ingested or injected, how rapidly clinical signs develop, response to supportive treatment, and overall health of patient

• Convalescence may be prolonged (several weeks); good supportive care in many seemingly hopeless cases has resulted in complete recovery.

MISCELLANEOUS

SEE ALSO
• Heartworm Disease—Dogs
• Poisoning (Intoxication)

ABBREVIATIONS
CNS = central nervous system
GABA = γ-aminobutyric acid

Suggested Reading
Paul AJ, Tranquilli WJ. Ivermectin. In: Kirk RW, ed. Current veterinary therapy X. Philadelphia: Saunders, 1989:140–142.
Author Allan J. Paul
Consulting Editor Gary D. Osweiler

JUVENILE FIBROSING LIVER DISEASE

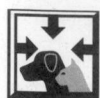

BASICS

DEFINITION
• Noninflammatory hepatopathy of young adult dogs, characterized by mild to moderate hepatic fibrosis • Usually associated with portal hypertension, ascites, and hepatic encephalopathy

PATHOPHYSIOLOGY
• Hepatic fibrosis—variable; basis unknown; may be related to intrahepatic hypoplasia of hepatic portal vein venules, long-standing portosystemic shunting, and/or exposure to toxic bile acids and toxin absorption; lesion may also represent a juvenile response to hepatic injury; fibrosis is more severe in long-standing cases • Speculation of portal hypoplasia confused by physiologic response of hepatic artery to deprivation of portal blood flow • Microhepatia—due to deviated portal blood flow (lack of hepatotrophic factors)

SYSTEMS AFFECTED
• Gastrointestinal—ascites; anorexia; intermittent vomiting or diarrhea; enteric hypertensive vasculopathy causing ulceration • Nervous—episodic hepatic encephalopathy • Musculoskeletal—stunted growth in some dogs; weight loss • Urogenital—polyuria and polydipsia; ammonium biurate urolithiasis • Hemic/lymphatic/immune—RBC microcytosis

SIGNALMENT
• Dogs only • Breeds—Doberman pinschers, cocker spaniels, and German shepherds, but may occur in any breed • No sex predilection • Young adult dogs; mean age 2 years, range 0.2–8 years • Genetic basis—unknown; may affect littermates

SIGNS
• Episodic CNS signs (hepatic encephalopathy) • Ascites • Stunted growth (very young dogs) • Weight loss • Inappetence • Intermittent vomiting or diarrhea • Enteric hemorrhage • Polyuria and polydipsia • Obstructive urolithiasis (ammonium urates)

CAUSES & RISK FACTORS
• Purebred, large-breed dogs • Chronic exposure to gastrointestinally absorbed toxins—possible risk factor • Congenital malformation (portal hypoplasia)—speculated risk factor

DIAGNOSIS

DIFFERENTIAL DIAGNOSIS
• CNS signs—infectious disorders (e.g., distemper); toxicities (e.g., lead); hydrocephalus; idiopathic epilepsy; metabolic disorders (e.g., hypoglycemia, hypokalemia, hyperkalemia) • Hepatic encephalopathy—severe liver disease (e.g., cirrhosis); PSVA; symptomatic MVD; urea cycle enzyme deficiencies • Ascites—pure transudate (protein-losing nephropathy, protein-losing enteropathy, liver disease, hepatic arteriovenous portal fistula[e]); modified transudate (right-sided heart failure, supradiaphragmatic vena caval obstruction, liver disease, neoplasia, portal vein thrombosis); hemorrhage • Portal hypertension—chronic hepatic disease; portal venous thromboembolism; hepatic AV fistula(e)

CBC/BIOCHEMISTRY/URINALYSIS
• CBC—erythrocyte microcytosis; target cells • Biochemistry—hypoalbuminemia; normal or low serum globulin; moderately increased ALP and ALT activity; variable low BUN and hypocholesterolemia • Urinalysis—hyposthenuria or isosthenuria; occasionally ammonium biurate crystalluria

OTHER LABORATORY TESTS
• Coagulation tests—variable coagulation abnormalities, including prolonged PT, APTT, ACT, and PIVKA, low fibrinogen, and marginal thrombocytopenia; prolonged buccal mucosal bleeding times indicate high risk for bleeding during liver biopsy • Peritoneal fluid analysis—pure transudate (total protein < 2.5 g/dL) • TSBA—fasting values increased in most; postprandial values always increased • Plasma ammonia concentration—usually abnormal; inconsistent in reliability

IMAGING

Radiography
• Abdominal effusion • Microhepatia • Thoracic radiography—normal (rules out right-sided heart disease)

Abdominal Ultrasonography
• Abdominal effusion • Subjectively small liver; variable liver texture; nonremarkable intrahepatic vasculature • Multiple APSS • Color-flow Doppler—hepatofugal circulation; rules out portal thrombosis; hepatic AV fistula(e)

Contrast Angiography
• Venous portography—if ultrasonography is inconclusive; demonstrates APSS; intrahepatic perfusion may be normal or attenuated; may see reduced size of extrahepatic portal vein/portal atresia • Hepatic arteriography—rarely done; rules out hepatic AV fistula(e); discloses coiled hepatic arteries (physiologic compensatory response to diminished portal blood flow)

Echocardiography
Rules out right-sided heart disease and vena caval occlusion

DIAGNOSTIC PROCEDURES
• Liver biopsy • High portal pressure—at mesenteric venous portography; >13 cm H_2O; attenuated by APSS; portal pressure determination not clinically indicated or needed

PATHOLOGIC FINDINGS
• Gross—small liver; fine nodular appearance • Microscopic—very mild to severe changes; small portal venules reflect underperfusion due to portosystemic shunts; very small or absent portal venules may suggest developmental anomaly; multiple cross-sections of portal arterioles reflect "coiled" arterioles • Fibrosis may involve different portions of the hepatic architecture: surrounding portal triad (zone 1); perisinusoidal (zone 2); around hepatic venules (zone 3) • Variable size of hepatic lobules—reflects portosystemic shunting

TREATMENT

APPROPRIATE HEALTH CARE
• Inpatient—for severe hepatic encephalopathy (see Hepatic Encephalopathy) • Outpatient—adjust nutritional support; avoid endoparasitism; avoid NSAIDs (augment sodium and water retention and gastrointestinal ulceration); treat infections promptly (predisposed to septicemia); remain vigilant for ammonium urate obstructive uropathies (all levels of urinary system)

NURSING CARE

Hepatic Encephalopathy
• Eliminate causal factors—dehydration, hypokalemia, gastrointestinal bleeding, infections, catabolism, hypoglycemia, and metabolic alkalosis • Diet—modified quality and quantity of protein; dairy and soy protein are optimal sources • Optimize nitrogen tolerance by concurrent treatment with

lactulose, metronidazole, or neomycin (see Hepatic Encephalopathy) • Maintain body condition—adjust nutritional management accordingly; muscle mass attenuates ammonia toxicity • Multiple small feedings daily • Medical treatment to alter enteric uptake and formation of hepatic encephalopathy toxins

Ascites
• Restricted activity—improves hepatic perfusion; assists in ascites mobilization • Dietary sodium restriction • Diuretics—combined use of spironolactone and furosemide, titrated to optimal response • Therapeutic abdominocentesis—for tense ascites and respiratory compromise • Parenteral vitamin K_1 and additional blood component therapy—initial treatment for all patients with bleeding tendencies as indicated (see Coagulopathy of Liver Disease)

MEDICATIONS

DRUG(S) OF CHOICE

Hepatic Encephalopathy
• Lactulose (0.5–1.0 mL/kg PO q8–12h)—tailor dose to maintain soft stool; early management and later as necessary • Oral antibiotics—first choice is metronidazole (7.5 mg/kg PO q12h); neomycin (22 mg/kg PO q8–12h PO): beware of increased enteric absorption with inflammatory bowel disease and possible nephrotoxicity and ototoxicity; chronic neomycin (3% absorbed per dose) may lead to toxicity; amoxicillin (22 mg/kg PO q12h)

Ascites
• Furosemide (1–4 mg/kg PO, IM, or IV q12–24h)—potassium wasting; best used in combination with spironolactone • Spironolactone (1–4 mg/kg PO q12h, initiated with loading dose of at least 2–4 mg/kg)—potassium sparing; less potent than furosemide • Taper diuretic dose once response is achieved; individualize chronic treatment to response; diuretics may be used intermittently to mobilize recurring ascitic effusion

Antifibrotic Medications
• Ursodiol (10–15 mg/kg/day PO q24h)—use indefinitely; also provides important hepatoprotectant, choleretic, antioxidant, and other beneficial influences • Polyunsaturated phosphatidylcholine (50–100 mg/kg, not to exceed 3 g PO q24h)—mix with food • Colchicine (0.03 mg/kg PO q24h)—efficacy unproven

• Bleeding tendencies—initial treatment with vitamin K_1 (0.5–1.5 mg/kg IM or SC, up to three doses at 12-hr intervals); blood component therapy as necessary to rescue from spontaneous or iatrogenic induced bleeding; DDAVP (0.5–1.0 μg/kg IV in saline) may increase coagulation factors, shorten mucosal bleeding time, and reduce bleeding tendencies (mechanism not fully explained but effective clinically and reported beneficial in humans with liver disease–associated coagulopathies and active bleeding from biopsy sites)

Gastrointestinal Hemorrhage
• H_2-receptor antagonists—famotidine (0.5 mg/kg PO, IM, or SC q12–24h); avoid cimetidine because of danger of induced drug interactions • Gastroprotectant—sucralfate 0.25 g/10 kg PO q8–12h • Give hepatoprotectants or antacids indefinitely to suppress symptomatic gastrointestinal bleeding and ulceration, common long-term problems in serious hepatic disorders associated with APSS • Eliminate endoparasitism

CONTRAINDICATIONS/POSSIBLE INTERACTIONS
• Avoid drugs that rely on hepatic biotransformation • Avoid drugs that react with GABA-benzodiazepine receptors • Avoid drugs that inhibit biotransformation and metabolism of other drugs (e.g., cimetidine, chloramphenicol, quinidine, certain calcium channel blockers)

FOLLOW-UP

PATIENT MONITORING
• Biochemistry—initially, monitor biweekly to monthly until stabilized, then every 4–6 months; monitor for iatrogenic drug toxicity and decompensation and progressive or active liver injury • Follow-up liver biopsy (after 12 months of therapy)—monitor progression and need for further therapy.

POSSIBLE COMPLICATIONS
• Hepatic encephalopathy—requires indefinite nutritional and medical management • Gastrointestinal bleeding and ulceration—may need chronic H_2-receptor antagonists and sucralfate • Ascites—sodium restriction and diuretics titrated to response

EXPECTED COURSE AND PROGNOSIS
• Prognosis fair to favorable—if patient survives initial stages and is stabilized and diagnosis is confirmed • Life-long treatment—for hepatic encephalopathy, hypertensive portal vasculopathy, and enteric hemorrhage; occasional flare-ups of hepatic encephalopathy and ascites may require hospitalizations and adjustment of medical interventions • No large database substantiates that treatment improves survival.

MISCELLANEOUS

ASSOCIATED CONDITIONS
• Hepatic encephalopathy • Ascites • Gastrointestinal ulceration • APSS

AGE-RELATED FACTORS
• Prognosis depends on degree of fibrosis and hepatic insufficiency at initial diagnosis. • Fibrosis may progress with age; poorly substantiated due to paucity of follow-up liver biopsies

ZOONOTIC POTENTIAL
N/A

SEE ALSO
• Hepatic Encephalopathy • Portosystemic Shunting, Acquired • Ascites • Hypertension, Portal

ABBREVIATIONS
• ACT = activated clotting time • APSS = acquired portosystemic shunts • APTT = activated partial thromboplastin time • ALP = alkaline phosphatase • ALT = alanine aminotransferase • AV = arteriovenous • BUN = blood urea nitrogen • CNS = central nervous system • DDAVP = 1 deamino-8-D-arginine vasopressin • MVD = hepatoportal microvascular dysplasia • NSAID = nonsteroidal anti-inflammatory drug • PIVKA = proteins invoked by vitamin K absence or antagonism • PSVA = portosystemic vascular anomaly • PT = prothrombin time • TSBA = total serum bile acids

Suggested Reading
Bunch SE, Johnson SE, Cullen JM. Idiopathic noncirrhotic portal hypertension in dogs: 33 cases (1982–1998). J Am Vet Med Assoc 2000;218:392–399.
Rutgers HC, Haywood S, Kelly DF. Idiopathic hepatic fibrosis in 15 dogs. Vet Rec 1993;133:115–118.
Author H. Carolien Rutgers
Consulting Editor Sharon A. Center

JUVENILE POLYARTERITIS (BEAGLE PAIN SYNDROME)

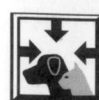

BASICS

OVERVIEW
A systemic necrotizing vasculitis most commonly reported in young beagles; a similar syndrome has been reported in a number of other breeds, including Bernese mountain dogs and boxers; also termed steroid-responsive meningitis-arteritis

SIGNALMENT
• Age at onset—4–10 months (beagles); other breeds may present at older ages
• Males and females equally affected
• Most reported cases from colonies of beagles bred for research; pet beagles also are affected

SIGNS
• Cervical pain
• Fever—40°–41.5° C (104°–107° F)
• Lethargy
• Anorexia
• Weight loss
• Hunched stance
• Unwillingness to move the head and neck
• General hyperesthesia

CAUSES & RISK FACTORS
• Hereditary predisposition in some colonies of beagles
• Suspected to be immune mediated

DIAGNOSIS

DIFFERENTIAL DIAGNOSIS
• Bacterial meningitis—cervical pain and fever; signs are persistent and progressive rather than relapsing and remitting; ruled out by CSF analysis and culture
• Cervical disk disease—cervical pain; affected dogs usually older; no fever, leukocytosis, or CSF pleocytosis
• Diskospondylitis—cervical pain and fever; CSF usually normal
• Granulomatous and infectious meningo-encephalomyelitis—differentiated by signalment, CSF analysis, and appropriate serologic testing and culture; other neurologic deficits are usually present
• Polyarthritis—cervical pain and fever; other joints usually affected; CSF normal; some beagles may have concurrent polyarthritis
• Protozoal infection—toxoplasmosis, *Neospora caninum*, leishmaniasis, or hepatozoonosis; may cause fever and muscle pain; differentiated by serology and muscle biopsy

CBC/BIOCHEMISTRY/URINALYSIS
• Moderate to marked leukocytosis with neutrophilia
• Mild to moderate nonregenerative anemia
• Mild to moderate hypoalbuminemia
• Urinalysis—usually normal; occasionally, mild increase in protein:creatinine ratio

OTHER LABORATORY TESTS
• Serum electrophoresis—hypoalbuminemia with high α_2-globulin fraction
• Antinuclear antibody test, lupus erythematosus preparation, and rheumatoid factor test—negative in beagles; positive results reported for some other breeds
• Serum IgA—increased

IMAGING
• Thoracic, abdominal, and cervical radiography—normal

DIAGNOSTIC PROCEDURES
• CSF analysis—neutrophilic pleocytosis with mild to moderate increase in microprotein; normal results do not rule out the diagnosis
• Synovial fluid analysis—may show neutrophilic inflammation
• Bacterial cultures (CSF, blood, and urine)—negative
• Serology for other infectious diseases—negative

JUVENILE POLYARTERITIS (BEAGLE PAIN SYNDROME)

PATHOLOGIC FINDINGS
• Severe necrotizing vasculitis, perivasculitis, and thrombosis of small to medium vessels in the leptomeninges of the cervical spinal cord
• Other affected organs—cranial mediastinum, coronary arteries, thyroid, thymus, lymph nodes, testes, small intestine, diaphragm, esophagus, and urinary bladder; lesions outside the CNS are common in beagles but rare in other breeds
• Clinically asymptomatic dogs—minimal vascular lesions
• Amyloidosis—identified occasionally in severely affected patients

TREATMENT
• Restrict activity
• Fluid therapy—may be necessary in severely affected patients that are unwilling to eat or drink

MEDICATIONS

DRUG(S)
Prednisone—1 mg/kg q12h; clinical signs should resolve in 12–48 hr; taper to minimum dose that will control signs (usually 0.25–0.5 mg/kg q48h); usually can be discontinued after 2–6 months of treatment

CONTRAINDICATIONS/POSSIBLE INTERACTIONS
N/A

FOLLOW-UP

PATIENT MONITORING
• Monitor for neck pain and gastrointestinal hemorrhage.
• Monitor CBC and biochemical panel for inflammation or organ dysfunction.
• Some patients may relapse despite treatment.

PREVENTION/AVOIDANCE
N/A

POSSIBLE COMPLICATIONS
N/A

EXPECTED COURSE AND PROGNOSIS
• Episodic—signs usually persist 2–7 days and then resolve; most patients experience multiple episodes, but some have only 1–2 episodes before apparently becoming normal
• Some patients may have persistent clinical signs.
• Clinical signs appear to resolve in all but the most severely affected patients by 12–18 months of age.

MISCELLANEOUS

ASSOCIATED CONDITIONS
Polyarthritis

AGE-RELATED FACTORS
N/A

ZOONOTIC POTENTIAL
N/A

PREGNANCY
N/A

SEE ALSO
• Neck and Back Pain • Steroid-responsive Meningitis-Arteritis—Dogs

ABBREVIATIONS
• CNS = central nervous system
• CSF = cerebrospinal fluid

Suggested Reading
Scott-Moncrieff JCR, Snyder PW, Glickman LT, et al. Systemic necrotizing vasculitis in nine young beagles. J Am Vet Med Assoc 1992;201:1553–1558.
Tipold A, Jaggy A. Steroid responsive menigitis-arteritis in dogs: long term study of 32 cases. J Small Anim Pract 1994; 35:311–316.
Author J. Catharine Scott-Moncrieff
Consulting Editor Joane M. Parent

BASICS

DEFINITION
Any inflammation of the cornea that does not retain fluorescein stain

PATHOPHYSIOLOGY
• A pathologic response that decreases the clarity of the cornea; associated with edema, inflammatory cell infiltration, neovascularization, pigmentation, lipid or calcium deposition, scarring
• Neovascularization—superficial corneal vessels are usually dendritic or tree-branching and indicate superficial or external eye disease; deep corneal vessels are shorter and straighter, indicating deep corneal or intraocular disease

GENETICS
• No proven genetic basis in dogs or cats
• Chronic superficial keratitis (pannus)—inherited predisposition considered in the German shepherd

INCIDENCE/PREVALENCE
Common cause of eye disease in dogs and cats

GEOGRAPHIC DISTRIBUTION
Chronic superficial keratitis more common in high-altitude, intense-sunlight climates

SIGNALMENT
Species
• Common cause of eye disease in dogs and cats • Dogs—chronic superficial keratitis (pannus); pigmentary keratitis; nodular granulomatous episcleritis; KCS (see Keratoconjunctivitis Sicca) • Cats—eosinophilic keratitis, herpesvirus (stromal form); corneal sequestration; KCS uncommon and usually secondary to chronic herpesvirus infection

Breed Predilections
Dogs
• Chronic superficial keratitis (pannus)—may occur in any breed; high prevalence in German shepherds and Belgian Tervurens
• Pigmentary keratitis—brachycephalic breeds with exposure keratopathy from lagophthalmia and tear film deficiencies, nasal folds, and nasal trichiasis; notably pugs, Lhasa apsos, shih tzus, Pekingese • Nodular granulomatous episcleritis—may occur in any breed; prevalent in cocker spaniels, greyhounds; collies and Shetland sheepdogs have predisposition for nictitating membrane involvement as well • KCS—brachycephalic breeds; notably cocker spaniels, English bulldogs, Lhasa apsos, shih tzus, pugs, West Highland white terriers, Pekingese, cavalier King Charles spaniels
Cats
• Eosinophilic keratitis and herpesvirus—none known • Corneal sequestration—most

prevalent in Persians, Siamese, Burmese, and Himalayans
Mean Age and Range
• Dogs: Chronic superficial keratitis—may occur at any age; higher risk at 4–7 years of age; pigmentary keratitis—may occur at any age; nodular granulomatous episcleritis—may occur at any age; in collies—young to middle-aged (mean 3.8 years); KCS—usually middle-aged or old • Cats: Herpesvirus—all ages; eosinophilic keratitis and corneal sequestrum—all ages except neonates

SIGNS
Historical Findings
May cause variable corneal discoloration and ocular discomfort

Physical Examination Findings
Dogs
• Chronic superficial keratitis—usually bilateral, often symmetrical pinkish white lesions (i.e., granulation tissue) with variable pigmentation; usually lateral or ventrolateral cornea with medial, ventral, and dorsal quadrants affected in that order; third eyelids may be affected and appear thickened or depigmented; white lipid deposits may be present at adjacent corneal edge; may lead to blindness in advanced disease • Pigmentary keratitis—appears as focal to diffuse brown to black discoloration of the cornea; often associated with corneal vascularization or scarring • Nodular granulomatous episcleritis—usually bilateral, raised pink to tan lesions of the lateral cornea; may be slowly to rapidly progressive; white deposits and neovascularization may occur in adjacent corneal stroma; third eyelids may appear thickened • KCS—variable findings; may be unilateral or bilateral; mucoid to mucopurulent ocular discharge, conjunctival hyperemia, corneal neovascularization, pigmentation, and variable scarring
Cats
• Herpesvirus (nonulcerative; stromal)—may be unilateral or bilateral; often occurs with ulceration; stromal edema, infiltrates, neovascularization, scarring; may threaten vision if severe scarring • Eosinophilic keratitis—usually unilateral; usually affects the lateral or medial cornea but may affect any quadrant; appears as raised white, pink, or gray corneal plaque with roughened surface; may retain fluorescein stain at the periphery of the lesion • Corneal sequestrum—usually unilateral but can be bilateral; appears as amber, brown, or black oval to circular plaques of the central or paracentral cornea; can vary in size and corneal depth of the affected cornea; edges may appear raised because of corneal edema, thickened epithelium, or granulation tissue; corneal neovascularization is variable; may retain fluorescein at periphery of lesion

CAUSES
Dogs
• Chronic superficial keratitis—presumed to be immune-mediated; altitude and solar radiation increase the prevalence and severity of the disease. • Pigmentary keratitis—secondary to any chronic corneal irritation; evaluate for primary underlying ocular conditions; more frequently associated with exposure keratopathy and KCS • Nodular granulomatous episcleritis—presumed to be immune-mediated • KCS—usually caused by immune-mediated dacryoadenitis

Cats
• Herpesvirus—believed to be immune-mediated T-cell lymphocyte reaction to herpesvirus antigen rather than a cytopathic effect of the virus • Eosinophilic keratitis—unknown; some patients are concurrently affected with herpesvirus • Corneal sequestrum—unknown; likely due to chronic corneal irritation; some patients have history of previous trauma; suggested relationship with previous herpesvirus infection

RISK FACTORS
Dogs—chronic superficial keratitis more likely to occur at high altitudes with intense sunlight

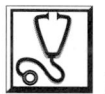
DIAGNOSIS

DIFFERENTIAL DIAGNOSIS
Dogs
• Infectious keratitis is usually ulcerative and painful; cytologic examination of cornea reveals white blood cells, organisms present.
• Neoplasia—rare involvement of sclera or cornea; distinguish based on color, age of animal, breed predilection, usually unilateral, response to topical antiinflammatory therapy

Cats
• Infectious keratitis—usually ulcerative and painful, stromal herpesvirus may be associated with secondary ulcerative keratitis; cytologic examination of cornea reveals white blood cells, organisms present • Neoplasia—very rare; usually involving limbal area

DIAGNOSTIC PROCEDURES
Dogs
Cytologic examination of corneal or conjunctival scrapings reveals a preponderance of lymphocytes and plasma cells in chronic superficial keratitis; biopsy of conjunctiva or cornea (superficial keratectomy) for confirmation of nodular granulomatous episcleritis, chronic superficial keratitis can be considered; Schirmer tear test for pigmentary keratitis, KCS, or any corneal disease of undetermined cause; normal values are > 15 mm/min; values consistent with KCS are < 10 mm/min; values between 10

and 15 mm/min suggest KCS but should be interpreted with consideration of the breed and concurrent ocular findings.

Cats

Conjunctival or corneal scrapings can be submitted for IFA, PCR, or viral culture for herpesvirus; interpretation can be difficult; obtain IFA samples before fluorescein stain is applied to eye; cytology of cornea usually reveals the presence of numerous eosinophils indicating eosinophilic keratitis; biopsy of the cornea (superficial keratectomy) can be considered for eosinophilic keratitis or sequestrum but diagnosis is usually possible by clinical signs (both) and cytology (eosinophils).

 TREATMENT

APPROPRIATE HEALTH CARE
• Outpatient—generally sufficient
• Inpatient—cases that warrant surgery due to inadequate response to medical therapy

CLIENT EDUCATION

Dogs
All patients require lifelong treatment; disease is controlled rather than cured; surgery may be needed for pigmentary keratitis or KCS.

Cats
• Herpesvirus—ocular discomfort and keratitis often recurrent • Eosinophilic keratitis—disease controlled rather than cured • Corneal sequestrum—sequestrum may slough spontaneously; may require months to years and clinical course may be prolonged without surgery; removal of sequestrum by superficial keratectomy may be incomplete and it may recur postoperatively.

SURGICAL CONSIDERATIONS

Dogs
• Chronic superficial keratitis—superficial keratectomy may be performed for severe disease; usually unnecessary; still requires indefinite medial treatment to prevent recurrence; β-irradiation with a strontium-90 probe is noninvasive and may be preferred since lymphocytes, plasma cells, and melanocytes are sensitive to effects of irradiation. • Pigmentary keratitis—superficial keratectomy may be performed only after initial underlying cause is corrected; only in severe cases that threaten vision; β-irradiation and cryotherapy have been used to resolve condition • Nodular granulomatous episcleritis—superficial keratectomy is diagnostic; usually unnecessary; only temporarily resolves clinical signs; medical treatment is still required • KCS—parotid duct transposition or permanent partial tarsorrhaphy may be indicated

Cats
• Eosinophilic keratitis—superficial keratectomy is diagnostic; usually unnecessary; only temporarily resolves clinical signs; medical treatment is preferred
• Corneal sequestrum—superficial keratectomy may be curative; recurrence is possible; ocular discomfort is primary indication for surgery

 MEDICATIONS

DRUG(S)

Dogs
• Chronic superficial keratitis—topical corticosteroids (1% prednisolone or 0.1% dexamethasone q6–12 hr; topical 1% or 2% cyclosporine in oil or 0.2% ointment q8–12h; either of the above can be used alone or in combination for more severe cases; subconjunctival corticosteroid injection can be used as an adjunct to topical therapy in severe cases (triamcinolone acetonide 4–8 mg). • Pigmentary keratitis—topical treatment directed at cause; topical corticosteroids if primary cause is inflammatory; lubricants or cyclosporine if primary condition is KCS; cyclosporin may be beneficial to reduce pigmentation in all cases. • Nodular granulomatous episcleritis—topical corticosteroids and/or cyclosporine as described above; systemic azathioprine (2mg/kg/day initially, then gradually reduce) may be effective when used alone or in combination with topical medications.
• KCS—topical 1% or 2% cyclosporine in oil or 0.2% ointment q8–12h (see Keratoconjunctivitis Sicca)

Cats
• Herpesvirus—topical antiviral agents (trifluridine—Viroptic) q4–6h; for stromal disease, topical corticosteroids can be used concurrent with antiviral agents but with extreme caution; oral lysine (250 mg BID to 500 mg SID) may be of benefit; oral antiviral agents should be used with extreme caution because of bone marrow suppression that could lead to death • Eosinophilic keratitis—topical corticosteroids (1/8 to1% prednisolone or 0.1% dexamethasone) q6–12h usually causes remission; corticosteroids should be used with caution and the patient monitored for ulceration or worsening of clinical signs; topical antivirals can be used in combination with corticosteroids if herpesvirus infection is suspected; for severe, refractory cases, megestrol acetate (Ovaban 5 mg PO q24h for 5 days, then 5 mg q48h for 1 week, then 5 mg weekly for maintenance) can be considered. • Corneal sequestrum—topical triple antibiotic BID to TID for associated corneal ulceration; artificial tear lubrication may be beneficial for relieving discomfort;

topical antivirals can be used if herpesvirus infection is suspected; topical 1% atropine ointment SID to q12h for pain associated with concurrent uveitis if clinical signs present

CONTRAINDICATIONS
Topical corticosteroids are contraindicated with corneal ulcers; topical atropine is contraindicated with KCS, glaucoma, or lens luxation.

PRECAUTIONS
• Azathioprine may cause gastrointestinal signs, hepatotoxicity, and myelosuppression.
• Megestrol acetate—not FDA-approved for use in cats; possible side effects include polyphagia, transient diabetes mellitus, mammary hyerplasia, mammary neoplasia, and pyometra

 FOLLOW-UP

PATIENT MONITORING
• Periodic ocular examination recommended to evaluate efficacy of topical and systemic medications; examine at 1–2 week intervals, gradually lengthening the interval with remission or resolution of clinical signs; evaluate response to therapy based on resolution of neovascularization and stabilization of pigmentation; complete resolution of pigmentation may not occur.

POSSIBLE COMPLICATIONS
All of the above may lead to continued ocular discomfort, visual defects, or blindness in severe cases.

 MISCELLANEOUS

SEE ALSO
• Keratitis, Ulcerative
• Keratoconjunctivitis Sicca

ABBREVIATIONS
• IFA = Immunofluorescent assay
• KCS = Keratoconjunctivitis sicca
• PCR = polymerase chain reaction

Suggested Reading
Chavkin MJ, Roberts SM, Salman MD, et al. Risk factors for development of chronic superficial keratitis in dogs. J Am Vet Med Assoc 1994;204:1630–1634.
Nassise MP, Feline herpesvirus ocular disease. Vet Clin North Am Small Anim Pract 1990;20:667–680.

Acknowledgment
The author wishes to acknowledge the contributions made by B. Keith Collins in preparing this chapter.
Author George A. Abrams
Consulting Editor Paul E. Miller

KERATITIS, ULCERATIVE

BASICS

DEFINITION
Inflammation of the cornea associated with loss of the corneal epithelium (corneal erosion) and possibly loss of variable amounts of the underlying corneal stroma (corneal ulcer)

PATHOPHYSIOLOGY
• May be caused by any condition (traumatic or nontraumatic) that disrupts the corneal epithelium or stroma • Ulcers—classified as superficial or deep, uncomplicated or complicated • Superficial—involves the epithelium and possibly the superficial stroma • Deep—involves a greater thickness of stroma and may extend to Descemet's membrane (descemetocele), possibly leading to rupture of the globe • Complicated—persistence of underlying/inciting cause, microbial infection, or production of degradative enzymes • Epithelial wound healing—adjacent corneal epithelial cells loosen and begin migration over the defect within a few hours; mitosis occurs within a few days to restore normal epithelial thickness; healing process complete in 5–7 days in uncomplicated, superficial ulcers • Stromal wound healing—slower, more complex; may occur in an avascular or vascular manner; in shallow wounds, epithelial migration and mitosis may be sufficient to fill the defect; epithelium may cover some deeper ulcers even when epithelium and stromal regeneration are insufficient to restore normal corneal thickness (nonulcerated divet defect is called a facet); stroma usually heals by fibrovascular infiltration, which may take several weeks and often results in loss of or decrease in corneal clarity. • Stromal ulcers—often complicated by microbial infection or enzymatic destruction initiated by microbial organisms, host inflammatory cells, or corneal epithelial or stromal cells; excessive enzymatic destruction may result in gelatinous appearance of the corneal stroma, called a melting or collagenase ulcer. • Spontaneous chronic corneal epithelial defects (SCCED)—delayed healing due to abnormalities of the anterior stroma and epithelial cells that prevent reassembly of normal epithelial adhesion complexes

GENETICS
• No proven basis, although breed predilections are seen • May occur secondary to other corneal diseases that have breed predispositions and presumably a genetic basis such as corneal epithelial dystrophy in Shetland sheepdogs and corneal endothelial dystrophy in Boston terriers

SIGNALMENT

Species
Dogs and cats

Breed Predilections
• Dogs—brachycephalic breeds predisposed • SCCED—occurs in any breed • Cats—Persian, Himalayans, Siamese, and Burmese predisposed to feline corneal sequestrums (see Keratitis, Nonulcerative)

Mean Age and Range
• Age of onset—variable; determined by cause • SCCED—middle-aged and older dogs

SIGNS

Historical Findings
• May be acute or chronic (SCCED) • Tearing, squinting, rubbing at eyes • Owners may report the appearance of a film over the eye (often corneal edema); prolapsed third eyelid • Sometimes history of trauma • Herpetic ulcers (cats)—may have history of respiratory disease

Physical Examination Findings
• Nonspecific—serous to mucopurulent ocular discharge; blepharospasm; photophobia; nictitans prolapse; conjunctival hyperemia • Superficial—may note one or more circumscribed, linear, or geographic defects in the cornea • Deep stromal ulcer or descemetocele—may appear as a crater-like defect • Depending on cause and duration—may see neovascularization, pigmentation, scarring, mineral or lipid deposition, inflammatory cell infiltrate (yellow to cream-colored opacity with indistinct margins, often surrounded by corneal edema), collagenolytic activity (melting) of the corneal stroma • SCCED—loose or redundant epithelial edges; may demonstrate fluorescein stain extending into areas with seemingly intact epithelium • Ulcerative corneal disease usually stimulates tear production; absence of obvious lacrimation suggests component of dry eye (KCS). • Reflex anterior uveitis—mild or severe, secondary to ulceration; severe may result in hypopyon; severe suggests concurrent bacterial infection

CAUSES
• Trauma—blunt; penetrating; perforating • Adnexal disease—ectopic cilia, entropion, ectropion, eyelid mass, distichiasis • Lagophthalmos (inability to close eyelids completely)—results in exposure keratitis; may be breed-related in brachycephalic dogs and cats; may be caused by exophthalmos, buphthalmos, or may be neuroparalytic from facial nerve paralysis • Tear-film abnormality—quantitative tear deficiency (KCS); qualitative tear film deficiency caused by mucin deficiency or some other unidentified tear abnormality • Infection—usually secondary in dogs; can be primary infection of herpesvirus in cats • Primary corneal disease—endothelial dystrophy; other endothelial disease • Miscellaneous—foreign body (corneal or conjunctival); chemical burns; neurotrophic keratitis (loss of trigeminal sensation); immune mediated disease

DIAGNOSIS

DIFFERENTIAL DIAGNOSIS
• Fluorescein dye retention—diagnostic • Other causes of a red and painful eye—conjunctivitis, uveitis, KCS, glaucoma (see Red Eye) • May develop concurrently with other causes of a red eye (e.g., secondary to KCS)

CBC/BIOCHEMISTRY/URINALYSIS
N/A

OTHER LABORATORY TESTS
• Corneal culture and sensitivity—aerobic bacteria; particularly for complicated, deep, or rapidly progressive corneal ulcers • Herpesvirus (cats)—PCR or IFA for herpesvirus available; negative test does not rule out herpesvirus infection.

DIAGNOSTIC PROCEDURES

Fluorescein Staining
• Homogeneous stain uptake—superficial or stromal ulcer; may be circular to geographic, linear, or combination; location and shape may help determine cause (e.g., linear may indicate foreign body or rubbing of ectopic cilia); interpretation of depth subjective • SCCED—may have leakage of stain under surrounding loose epithelium • Crater-like defect that retains stain at the periphery but is clear at center • Descemetocele—may see Descemet's membrane bulging forward if defect is large • Crater-like defect with pooling of stain transiently but can be easily rinsed–previous stromal ulcer that has epithelialized (facet); must be distinguished from a descemetocele

Other
• Rose Bengal corneal stain (cats) may delineate superficial, linear, epithelial ulcers (dendritic ulcers), which are considered pathognomonic for herpesvirus infection. • Schirmer tear test may identify ulceration associated with KCS; it is contraindicated in very deep ulcers or descemetoceles. • Cytologic evaluation of cornea and Gram, Giemsa, or Wright staining may reveal microbial or fungal organisms, and may help direct initial antimicrobial therapy.

TREATMENT

APPROPRIATE HEALTH CARE
Hospitalize deep or rapidly progressive ulcers; these may require surgery and/or frequent medical treatments.

NURSING CARE
Keep facial hair out of eyes and clean.

ACTIVITY
• Restrict with deep stromal ulcer or descemetocele to prevent rupture. • Prevent self-trauma with Elizabethan collar.

CLIENT EDUCATION
• Instruct client to wait at least 5 minutes between medications if more than one ophthalmic drug is prescribed; wait longer between ointments. • Advise client to contact veterinarian if patient appears more painful or the eye markedly changes in appearance. • SCCED—discuss protracted course with client; usually achieve healing within 2–6 weeks, but may require weekly rechecks and multiple procedures

SURGICAL CONSIDERATIONS
• Superficial ulcers do not usually require surgery if the inciting cause has been eliminated. • Ulcer that extends one-half or greater corneal thickness and particularly to Descemet's membrane may benefit from surgery. • Descemetocele and full thickness corneal laceration—considered a surgical emergency

Procedures
• SCCED—debridement of loose epithelium with a dry, sterile, cotton-tipped swab after application of topical anesthesia (50% success rate); punctate or grid keratotomy easily performed after epithelial debridement with topical anesthesia (80% success rate); superficial keratectomy is more invasive and may cause more scarring, but has 100% success rate; application of a contact lens or nictitans flap after any of these procedures will improve comfort and aid healing.
• Therapeutic contact lens placement—acts as a bandage to reduce both frictional irritation from the eyelids and pain; most useful in SCCED; easy application and can still see eye; most retained 1–2 weeks, then removed; plano lens (no correction, Bausch & Lomb) used most commonly; should monitor eye for increased pain and corneal edema, which indicate contact does not fit and is causing corneal hypoxia • Rotational pedicle conjunctival flap, corneoscleral transposition, corneal transplant—surgical procedures for ulcers greater than 50% thickness of the stroma and descemetoceles • Cyanoacrylate repair (corneal glue)—can be used for deep ulcers; promotes corneal vascularization and stabilizes cornea, but has somewhat lower success rate compared to other corneal surgeries

MEDICATIONS

DRUG(S) OF CHOICE

Antibiotics
• Topical agents—indicated for all patients
• Frequency of application—determined by severity and the preparation used; ointments have a relatively long contact time and are applied q6–12h; solutions are applied more frequently (4, 6, 8 or even 12 times daily) in the initial treatment of complicated ulcers; solutions probably more appropriate in deep ulcers • Commonly used agents—oxytetracycline/polymyxin B (cats); triple antibiotic, gentamicin, and tobramycin
• Uncomplicated ulcers or superficial erosions—combination of neomycin, polymyxin B, and bacitracin an excellent first choice; broad spectrum of antimicrobial activity; often used 2–3 times a day for prophylactic therapy • Complicated ulcers—often use combination therapy of cefazolin (use IV solution to make 33–50 mg solution in saline or artificial tears for topical use) with either an aminoglycoside (tobramycin, gentamicin) or fluoroquinolone (ciprofloxacin, ofloxacin); particularly in rapidly progressive, deep, or melting ulcers; frequency depends on severity but usually a minimum of q3–4h.

Atropine
• 1% ointment or solution • Indicated for reflex anterior uveitis; frequency—usually q8–24h to effect (mydriasis)

Antiviral Agents
• Indicated for herpetic ulcers in cats
• Trifluridine (Viroptic) solution—q4–6h until clinical response is observed; then reduce for 1–2 weeks after clinical signs have subsided

NSAIDs
• May be indicated for antiinflammatory and analgesic properties • Aspirin (dogs)—10–15 mg/kg PO q12h

CONTRAINDICATIONS
• Topical corticosteroids—contraindicated with any corneal erosion or ulcer • Topical NSAIDs—contraindicated with herpetic ulcers, melting ulcers • Topical atropine—contraindicated with glaucoma, KCS

PRECAUTIONS
• Topical NSAIDs (flurbiprofen, diclofenac)—may delay corneal healing, may potentiate corneal melting • Terramycin, trifluridine, neomycin—may be irritating
• Topical cyclosporine can be used safely in uncomplicated ulcer in KCS patients.

POSSIBLE INTERACTIONS
Combining antibiotics in solution may inactivate some antibiotics.

ALTERNATIVE DRUG(S)
• Acetylcystine—anticollagenolytic agent used for treatment of melting ulcers; efficacy is controversial; dilute 20% stock solution to 5%–10% with artificial tears; apply q2–4h.
• Autologous plasma (collected in EDTA)—anticollagenolytic agent; keep refrigerated; avoid contamination; discard after 48 hr.

FOLLOW-UP

PATIENT MONITORING
• Superficial ulcers—repeat fluorescein stain in 3–6 days; if it persists 7 days or longer, either inciting cause has not been eliminated or the patient has SCCED. • Deep stromal or rapidly progressive ulcers—assess every 24 hours initially if outpatient until improvement is seen; many of these patients are hospitalized or undergo surgery; decrease frequency of antibiotic therapy as condition improves.

PREVENTION/AVOIDANCE
• Brachycephalic dogs—lubricant ointment administration, permanent partial tarsorrhaphy surgery or both may help prevent recurrent ulceration • KCS-related ulcers—life-long treatment of KCS (cyclosporine) or parotid duct transposition surgery to prevent continued ulceration
• Herpesvirus (cats)–may try oral Lysine 250 mg PO BID to prevent viral replication; may decrease severity and/or frequency of outbreaks

POSSIBLE COMPLICATIONS
Progressive corneal ulceration—rupture of globe; endophthalmitis; secondary glaucoma; phthisis bulbi; blindness; blind and painful eye (may require enucleation)

EXPECTED COURSE AND PROGNOSIS
• Uncomplicated superficial ulcer—usually heals in 5–7 days • SCCED—may persist for weeks to months; may require multiple procedures • Deep corneal ulcer treated medically—may require several weeks for fibrovascular repair of defect; does not always granulate satisfactorily; continued deterioration of ulcer and globe rupture are possible. • Deep ulcer treated with conjunctival flap—frequently results in more comfort within a few days after surgery; blood supply to flap can be cut in 4–6 weeks if healed well to decrease scarring.

Suggested Reading
Kern TJ. Ulcerative keratitis. Vet Clin North Am Small Animal Pract 1990;20:643–666.
Murphy CJ. Disorders of the cornea and sclera. In: Kirk RW, Bonagura JD, eds. Current veterinary therapy XI. Philadelphia: Saunders, 1992:1101–1111.

Acknowledgment
The author would like to acknowledge the contributions of B. Keith Collins in preparing this chapter.
Author Ellison Bentley
Consulting Editor Paul E. Miller

KERATOCONJUNCTIVITIS SICCA

 BASICS

OVERVIEW
A deficiency of aqueous tear film, resulting in drying and inflammation of the cornea and conjunctiva

SIGNALMENT
• Very common in dogs; much rarer in cats
• Predisposed dog breeds—include cocker spaniels, bulldogs, West Highland white terriers, Lhasa apsos, and shih tzus
• Inheritance—undefined
• Age of onset—depends on inciting cause
• Some studies report females are predisposed.

SIGNS
• Cats tend to be less symptomatic than dogs.
• Blepharospasm
• Conjunctival hyperemia
• Chemosis
• Prominent nictitans
• Mucoid to mucopurulent ocular discharge
• Corneal changes (chronic disease)—superficial vascularization; pigmentation; ulceration
• Severe disease—impaired or loss of vision

CAUSES & RISK FACTORS
• Immunologic—immune-mediated adenitis most common and often associated with other immune-mediated diseases (e.g., atopy)
• Congenital—pugs; Yorkshire terriers; sporadically in other breeds
• Neurogenic—occasionally seen after traumatic proptosis or neurologic disease that interrupts innervation of the lacrimal gland, often has a dry nose on same side as dry eyes
• Drug-induced—general anesthesia and atropine cause transient keratoconjunctivitis sicca
• Drug toxicity—some sulfa-containing drugs (e.g., trimethoprim-sulfamethoxazole) or etodolac may cause transient or permanent condition
• Iatrogenic—removal of the nictitans gland may predispose, especially in at-risk breeds
• Radiotherapy— when periocular area is in or near the primary beam
• Systemic disease—canine distemper virus; any debilitating disease
• Chronic conjunctivitis (cats)—chronic herpes or chlamydia conjunctivitis
• Chronic blepharoconjunctivitis (dogs)
• Breed-related predisposition

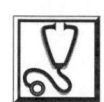 DIAGNOSIS

DIFFERENTIAL DIAGNOSIS
Often confused with bacterial conjunctivitis; most dogs with chronic KCS have secondary bacterial overgrowth; differentiated by use of the Schirmer tear test

CBC/BIOCHEMISTRY/URINALYSIS
N/A

DIAGNOSTIC PROCEDURES
• Schirmer tear test—decreased results diagnostic; normal value (dogs): at least 15 mm/min of wetting; symptomatic patients: usually < 10 mm/min of wetting
• Fluorescein staining—corneal ulcers
• Aerobic bacterial culture and sensitivity if initial treatment is unsuccessful; not routinely recommended because bacterial overgrowth common with chronic disease
• Conjunctival cytology—may indicate the nature and degree of bacterial overgrowth

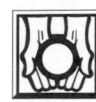 TREATMENT

• Outpatient—unless secondary disease (e.g., ulcerative keratitis) identified
• Clean eyes before instilling medication.
• Instruct owners to keep the eyes and adnexa clean and free of dried discharge.
• Advise owners to call at once if ocular pain increases because patients are predisposed to severe corneal ulceration.
• Parotid duct transposition—surgical procedure that reroutes the parotid duct to deliver saliva to the inferior cul-de-sac; performed much less frequently since cyclosporine was introduced; saliva can be irritating to the cornea; some patients are uncomfortable after surgery and require ongoing medical therapy.

MEDICATIONS

DRUG(S)
• Cyclosporine A (dogs)—may be used as a 0.2% ointment; most effective for immune-mediated disease; shown to be effective in promoting lacrimation in 80% of patients; for unresponsive disease, some ophthalmologists advocate use of a 1% or 2% solution in corn oil (q12h initially, then q12–24h thereafter, depending on response)
• Tacrolimus—0.02% tacrolimus in ointment or oil base was recently tested in a clinical trial and found to improve STT values in 92% of eyes. It is generally recommended for BID use. Currently the drug is available through compounding pharmacies. The method of action is proposed to be similar to cyclosporine; however, the receptors are distinct.
• Pilocarpine—0.25% topically q12h; alternatively may use 1 drop of 2% pilocarpine/10 kg body weight q12h on food and slowly increase by 1 drop increments until increased tearing or systemic side effects noted (anorexia, salivation, vomiting, diarrhea, bradycardia). Most effective in neurogenic KCS

• Artificial tears and lubricant ointments—help moisten the cornea; must be used frequently; only transiently relieve drying; preparations vary greatly in their composition; thicker agents (Hylashield) may be soothing for very dry eyes in patients that fail to respond to cyclosporine therapy.
• Broad-spectrum antibiotics—topical (solutions or ointments); frequently indicated for secondary bacterial overgrowth; rarely indicated once the bacterial overgrowth is controlled and tear production improves
• Corticosteroids—topical; frequently used before cyclosporine was introduced; minimize inflammation; effective in reducing corneal vascularization and pigmentation; now not commonly used
• Mucolytic agents (e.g., acetylcysteine)—occasionally used to help break up tenacious mucous discharge; add significantly to the cost of treatment; rarely indicated once tear production has improved

CONTRAINDICATIONS/POSSIBLE INTERACTIONS
• Topical cyclosporine—occasionally irritating
• Topical pilocarpine—initially irritating
• Topical corticosteroids—avoided with ulcerative keratitis

FOLLOW-UP
• Recheck at regular intervals—monitor response and progress.
• Schirmer tear test—performed 4–6 weeks after initiating cyclosporine; evaluate response (patient should have received the drug the day of the visit)
• Immune-mediated disease—usually requires life-long treatment
• Other types of disease—may be transient (e.g. atropine therapy); require treatment only until tear production returns

MISCELLANEOUS

ABBREVIATIONS
• KCS = keratoconjunctivitis sicca
• STT = Schirmer tear test

Suggested Reading
Moore CP. Diseases and surgery of the lacrimal system. In: Gelatt KN, ed. Philadelphia: Lippincott Williams & Wilkins 1999:583–607.
Author Erin S. Champagne
Consulting Editor Paul E. Miller

LACTIC ACIDOSIS

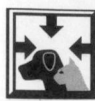

BASICS

DEFINITION

• Hyperlactatemia—serum lactate concentration > 1.5 mmol/L for dogs; no reported lactate kinetics for cats
• Lactic acidosis—hyperlactatemia with an arterial pH below the normal range

PATHOPHYSIOLOGY

• Lactic acid is the end product of both aerobic and anaerobic glucose metabolism; at physiologic pH, lactic acid immediately dissociates to lactate and hydrogen ion; small amounts of lactate are formed daily in healthy individuals, but clinically significant lactate accumulation is from anaerobic glycolysis. Lactic acid is produced during normal physiologic processes (e.g., exercise) and during pathologic processes (e.g., shock).
• Cori cycle—the preferred route of lactate use by the liver and kidneys; helps maintain the balance between lactate production and clearance, while providing a consistent source of glucose to critical tissues such as the brain and red blood cells, which preferentially use glucose; important in maintaining acid–base balance because the hydrogen ion produced during lactic acid dissociation is used during gluconeogenesis
• In most critically ill patients, hyperlactatemia and lactic acidosis are due to conditions that induce tissue hypoxia, with the shift to anaerobic glycolysis.
• Inadequate perfusion, severe hypoxemia, increased oxygen demands, decreased hemoglobin concentration, or combinations of these factors cause tissue hypoxia.
• Depending on the duration and severity of hypoxia, hyperlactatemia and possibly lactic acidosis may develop.
• Hyperlactatemia generally develops when tissue perfusion is adequate and acid–base buffering systems are intact.
• Clinically evident tissue hypoperfusion does not usually occur in patients with hyperlactatemia alone, but "occult" hypoperfusion may be present that is not detectable by routine monitoring and may represent a precursor phase to overt hypoperfusion.
• Lactic acidosis is usually present in association with abnormal metabolic regulation secondary to marked tissue hypoxia and hypoperfusion, certain drugs or toxins, or congenital defects in carbohydrate metabolism;

buffering systems usually cannot cope with the developing acidosis.
• The severity of hyperlactatemia and acidosis that develops in critically ill patients with inadequate tissue perfusion and oxygen delivery or inadequate oxygen uptake reflects the severity of tissue hypoxia; thus evaluation of lactate levels in these patients helps in assessing the degree of tissue hypoperfusion and hypoxia.
• Studies in human trauma and shock patients demonstrate that lactate predicts outcome and that mortality is correlated with the severity of the lactic acidosis: the higher the lactate level, the greater the mortality.
• Lactate measurement allows reliable assessment of the response by critically ill or injured people to initial and continuing resuscitative therapy.
• Lactate concentrations are increased in critically ill and injured dogs; and an apparent association exists between severity of increased lactate concentrations and outcome and differences in lactate concentrations between varying disease states and injury types (seizures, ethylene glycol and aspirin intoxication, and major trauma).
• Numerous clinical and experimental studies in critically ill human patients and recent results in critically ill and injured dogs clearly show blood lactate measurement to be a useful tool for assessing the severity of tissue hypoxia and the response to therapy and a prognostic tool for outcome.

SYSTEMS AFFECTED

• Persistent lactic acidosis directly affects myocardial function, reduces cardiac output, and increases organ hypoperfusion; these effects lead to deeper levels of tissue hypoxia.
• Hypoxia and acidosis eventually lead to such deleterious effects on cellular function, especially myocardial function, that multiple organ system failure ensues.

SIGNALMENT

Dog and cat

SIGNS

General Comments

Usually relate more to the underlying disorder causing the acidosis than to direct effects of the acidosis itself

Historical Findings

Disorders causing lactic acidosis are fairly common, and historical facts may prompt the clinician to suspect an underlying acidosis.

Physical Examination Findings

• Tachypnea is usually present in these patients as they attempt respiratory compensation.
• Most patients with acidosis are hypovolemic and thus demonstrate evidence of poor tissue perfusion or dehydration—dark mucous membranes, prolonged capillary refill time, and increased skin turgor.
• Severely acidotic patients may have cardiac dysrhythmias and poor contractility.

CAUSES

• Two types, A and B, based on the clinical presence or absence of hypoperfusion or tissue hypoxia
• Type A lactic acidosis—more common; due to decreased or inadequate oxygen delivery and oxygen consumption (i.e., poor tissue perfusion and tissue hypoxia)
• Causes of type A include shock, regional hypoperfusion, arterial obstruction, severe hypoxemia, severe anemia, carbon monoxide poisoning, severe asthma, and severe motor seizures.
• Type B lactic acidosis—includes all other causes of lactic acidosis; is subdivided into three subsets (B_1, B_2, B_3); is characterized by the absence of hypoxemia or poor tissue perfusion
• Many causes of type B lactic acidosis have recently been shown to be "occult" hypoperfusion not detectable by routine monitoring parameters or possibly combinations of types A and B lactic acidosis.
• The most common causes of type B lactic acidosis in veterinary medicine include neoplasia, alkalosis, sepsis, renal failure, liver disease, catecholamine use (norepinephrine, epinephrine), and intoxications (strychnine, cyanide, ethylene glycol, salicylates, acetaminophen, propylene glycol).

RISK FACTORS

• Risk factors for development of hyperlactatemia and lactic acidosis relate directly to risk factors for the specific disorders causing the underlying tissue hypoxia.
• In general, young animals are more at risk for traumatic shock and intoxications.
• Older animals are more likely to develop neoplasia, renal failure, heart failure, liver disease, severe anemias, and vascular disorders; consult Risk Factors for these specific disorders.

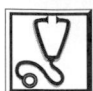

DIAGNOSIS

DIFFERENTIAL DIAGNOSIS
• Differential diagnoses for hyperlactatemia and lactic acidosis include those disorders described under Causes.
• Any severely ill animal is suspect for an underlying acidosis, and evaluating the lactate concentration can aid in diagnosis.

LABORATORY FINDINGS

Drugs That May Alter Laboratory Results
• Catecholamines, salicylates, acetaminophen, terbutaline, nitroprusside, halothane, bicarbonate, and propylene glycol all can cause mild-to-moderate increases in lactate concentrations in the absence of true tissue hypoperfusion and hypoxia.
• Lower lactate concentrations are found in samples with sodium citrate anticoagulant than in those with heparin and EDTA.
• Even small amounts of lactate-containing intravenous fluids (e.g., lactated Ringer's solution) may cause false increases in circulating lactate concentration in a blood sample if not properly cleared from the catheter or tubing through which the intravenous fluid was being given.

Disorders That May Alter Laboratory Results
• Several types of neoplasia increase lactate concentrations because the tumor cells preferentially use anaerobic glucose metabolism as part of the cancer cachexia syndrome.
• Alkalosis, sepsis, liver disease, and renal failure also can increase lactate concentrations by mechanisms other than poor tissue perfusion and hypoxia.
• Failure to detect elevated lactate concentrations does not ensure adequate perfusion to all organs; significant organ hypoperfusion may exist that may ultimately lead to multiple organ failure.
• Regional hypoperfusion, especially splanchnic, occurs in the absence of, or before, increases in systemic lactate and metabolic acidosis and often despite therapy that successfully maintains blood pressure, cardiac output, heart rate, DO_2, VO_2, and respiratory parameters.

Valid if Run in Human Laboratory?
• Yes; semiautomated and automated techniques are available for rapid measurement of lactate concentration in microliter samples of whole blood, serum, and plasma.
• Lactate concentration is ideally measured on an arterial sample; however, central venous and pulmonary artery samples are acceptable.
• Peripheral venous blood samples are not ideal, especially if the measurement will be used to assess global tissue perfusion.

CBC/BIOCHEMISTRY/URINALYSIS
• Few specific CBC findings would suggest causes for hyperlactatemia and lactic acidosis.
• Biochemical and urinalysis findings help determine the underlying cause; examples include renal azotemia and markedly increased serum osmolality seen with ethylene glycol intoxication; renal azotemia, hyperkalemia, and tubular casts seen with acute renal failure; and increased lactate concentration, increased total protein, and increased hematocrit with dehydration and poor tissue perfusion in a shock patient.

OTHER LABORATORY TESTS
• Arterial blood gas analysis may help define the extent of a concurrent respiratory disorder and a mixed acid–base disorder.
• Additional tests (e.g., ethylene glycol, serum and urine glucose, serum and urine ketones) may be helpful, depending on the suspected cause.

IMAGING
N/A

DIAGNOSTIC PROCEDURES
N/A

TREATMENT
• Hyperlactatemia alone is seldom significant enough to prompt specific therapy and is more important as a marker of possible severe or developing systemic problems.
• Lactic acidosis is often severe, and aggressive therapy to correct the underlying cause(s) and specifically treat the acidosis is usually indicated.
• Detection of hyperlactatemia, with or without acidosis, should drive the clinician to seek causes of hypoperfusion and should dictate early therapeutic interventions to improve tissue oxygen delivery to halt organ ischemia and avert progression to circulatory shock.

MEDICATIONS

DRUG(S) OF CHOICE
• Specific drug and fluid use depends on the underlying cause.
• Many causes of hyperlactatemia and lactic acidosis are characterized by fluid volume deficits; thus, aggressive fluid therapy is traditionally a hallmark initial step in treatment.

CONTRAINDICATIONS
N/A

PRECAUTIONS
N/A

POSSIBLE INTERACTIONS
N/A

ALTERNATIVE DRUG(S)
N/A

FOLLOW-UP

PATIENT MONITORING
• Serial lactate determinations are more valuable than single (admission, peak) lactate levels; monitor lactate over time in critical patients.
• The ability of a patient to clear lactate predicts response to therapy and survival.
• Continue checking other parameters that help gauge the response to therapy for the underlying cause.

POSSIBLE COMPLICATIONS
• Persons with lactic acidosis are at greater risk of developing multiple organ failure and have a higher mortality rate than patients without lactic acidosis.
• Dogs and horses with elevated lactate concentrations and lactic acidosis have poorer outcomes as well.

MISCELLANEOUS

ASSOCIATED CONDITIONS
N/A

AGE-RELATED FACTORS
N/A

ZOONOTIC POTENTIAL
N/A

PREGNANCY
N/A

SYNONYMS
N/A

SEE ALSO
Metabolic Acidosis

ABBREVIATIONS
N/A

Suggested Reading
Kruse JA. Lactic acidosis. In: Carlson RW, Geheb MA, eds. Principles and practice of medical intensive care. Philadelphia, Saunders, 1995:1231–1245.
Lagutchik MS, Ogilivie GK, Wingfield WE, Hackett TB. Lactate kinetics in veterinary critical care: a review. J Vet Emerg Crit Care 1996;6:81–95.
Mizock BA, Falk JL. Lactic acidosis in critical illness. Crit Care Med 1992;20:80–93.
Vail DM, Ogilive GK, Wheeler SL, et al. Alterations in carbohydrate metabolism in canine lymphoma. J Vet Intern Med 1990;4:8–11.
Author Michael S. Lagutchik
Consulting Editor Deborah S. Greco

LAMENESS

 BASICS

DEFINITION
A disturbance in gait and locomotion in response to pain or injury

PATHOPHYSIOLOGY
• Severe, sharp pain—when moving, patient carries or puts no weight on the affected limb.
• Milder, dull, or aching pain—when moving, patient limps or bears little weight on the affected limb; at rest, the patient bears less weight on the affected limb.
• Pain produced only during certain phases of movement—patient adjusts its motion and gait to minimize discomfort.

SYSTEMS AFFECTED
• Musculoskeletal
• Nervous

SIGNALMENT
• Any age or breed of dog
• Age, breed, and sex predilection—depend on specific disease

SIGNS

General Comments
• Unilateral forelimb—compensated for by moving the head and neck upward as the affected limb is placed on the ground and dropping the head and neck when the sound limb bears the weight
• Bilateral hindlimb—head and neck movement less pronounced; more weight shifted to the forelimbs by dropping the forequarters
• Unilateral hindlimb—may drop lower on the sound limb when it strikes the ground; elevated hindquarters when the affected limb is on the ground

• Always assess the patient's neurologic status, especially with a suspected proximal lesion.

Historical Findings
• Complete history—mandatory; signalment; identification of affected limb(s); known trauma; changes with weather, exercise, or rest; responsiveness to previous treatments
• Determine onset of lameness—acute or chronic
• Determine progression—static; slow; rapid
• Is the patient demonstrably painful?

Physical Examination Findings
• Perform a complete routine examination.
• Observe gait—walking; trotting; climbing stairs; doing figure-eights
• Palpate—asymmetry of muscle mass; bony prominences
• Manipulate bones and joints, beginning distally and working proximally.
• Assess—instability; incongruency; luxation or subluxation; pain; abnormal range of motion; abnormal sounds
• Examine suspected area of involvement last—by starting with normal limbs, patient may relax, allowing assessment of normal reaction to maneuvers.

CAUSES

Forelimb
Growing Dog (< 12 Months of Age)
• Osteochondrosis of the shoulder
• Shoulder luxation or subluxation—congential
• Osteochondrosis of the elbow
• Un-united anconeal process
• Fragmented medial coronoid process
• Elbow incongruity
• Avulsion or calcification of the flexor muscles—elbow
• Asymmetric growth of the radius and ulna
• Panosteitis

• Hypertrophic osteodystrophy
• Trauma—soft tissue; bone; joint
• Infection—local; systemic
• Nutritional imbalances
• Congenital anomalies
Mature Dog (> 12 Months of Age)
• Degenerative joint disease
• Bicipital tenosynovitis
• Calcification or mineralization of supraspinatus or infraspinatus tendon
• Contracture of supraspinatus or infraspinatus muscle
• Soft tissue or bone neoplasia—primary; metastatic
• Trauma—soft tissue; bone; joint
• Panosteitis
• Polyarthropathies
• Polymyositis
• Polyneuritis

Hindlimb
Growing Dog (< 12 Months of Age)
• Hip dysplasia
• Avascular necrosis of femoral head—Legg-Calvé-Perthes disease
• Osteochondrosis of stifle
• Patella luxation—medial or lateral condyle
• Osteochondrosis of hock
• Panosteitis
• Hypertrophic osteodystrophy
• Trauma—soft tissue; bone; joint
• Infection—local; systemic
• Nutritional imbalances
• Congenital anomalies
Mature Dog (> 12 Months of age)
• Degenerative joint disease
• Cruciate ligament disease
• Avulsion of long digital extensor tendon—stifle
• Soft tissue or bone neoplasia—primary; metastatic
• Trauma—soft tissue; bone; joint

- Panosteitis
- Polyarthropathies
- Polymyositis
- Polyneuritis

RISK FACTORS
N/A

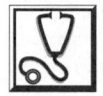

DIAGNOSIS

DIFFERENTIAL DIAGNOSIS
Must differentiate musculoskeletal from neurogenic causes

CBC/BIOCHEMISTRY/URINALYSIS
Usually normal

OTHER LABORATORY TESTS
Depend on suspected cause

IMAGING
- Radiographs recommended for all suspected musculoskeletal causes
- CT, MRI, and bone scans with radio-isotopes—help identify and delineate causative lesions

DIAGNOSTIC PROCEDURES
- Cytologic examination of joint fluid—identify and differentiate intraarticular disease
- EMG—differentiate neuromuscular from musculoskeletal disease
- Muscle and/or nerve biopsy—reveal and identify neuromuscular disease

TREATMENT
Depends on underlying cause

MEDICATIONS

DRUG(S) OF CHOICE
- Analgesics and NSAIDs—often indicated for symptomatic treatment; try buffered or enteric-coated aspirin (10–25 mg/kg PO q8–12h), carprofen (2.2 mg/kg PO q12h), etodolac (10–15 mg/kg PO q24h), phenyl-butazone (3–7 mg/kg PO q8h, total dose < 800 mg/day), meclofenamic acid (0.5 mg/kg PO q12h), or piroxicam (0.3 mg/kg PO q24h for 3 days, then q48h)
- Corticosteroids—use judiciously, unless specifically indicated (potential side effects; articular cartilage damage associated with long-term use)

CONTRAINDICATIONS
N/A

PRECAUTIONS
NSAIDs—gastrointestinal irritation may preclude use in some patients

POSSIBLE INTERACTIONS
N/A

ALTERNATIVE DRUG(S)
Chondroprotective drugs (e.g., polysulfated glycosaminoglycans, glucosamine, and chondroitin sulfate)—for degenerative joint disease; may be of benefit in limiting cartilage damage and degeneration; may help alleviate pain and inflammation

FOLLOW-UP

PATIENT MONITORING
Depends on underlying cause

POSSIBLE COMPLICATIONS
N/A

MISCELLANEOUS

ASSOCIATED CONDITIONS
N/A

AGE-RELATED FACTORS
N/A

ZOONOTIC POTENTIAL
N/A

PREGNANCY
N/A

SEE ALSO
Chapters covering musculoskeletal and neuromuscular disorders

ABBREVIATIONS
- CT = computed tomography
- EMG = electromyogram
- MRI = magnetic resonance imaging
- NSAIDs = nonsteroidal antiinflammatory drugs

Suggested Reading
Brinker WO, Piermattei DL, Flo GL. Physical examination for lameness. In: Handbook of small animal orthopedics and fracture repair. 3rd ed. Philadelphia: Saunders, 1997:228–230.
Author Peter D. Schwarz
Consulting Editor Peter K. Shires

LARYNGEAL DISEASE

 BASICS

DEFINITION

Suggests a disease process that alters normal structure and, usually, function of the larynx

PATHOPHYSIOLOGY

• Signs depend on the cause and severity of the resulting dysfunction. • With severe obstruction to laryngeal airflow—hyperpyrexia and heat prostration possible
• Air hunger syndrome (e.g., hypoventilation, hypoxemia)—may note retching, vomiting, aspiration pneumonia, and even respiratory or cardiac arrest. Signs most commonly observed in association with physical activity or in a stressful environment.

SYSTEMS AFFECTED

• Respiratory—interference with air–oxygen delivery to the alveoli (hypoventilation); aspiration pneumonia; pulmonary edema possible in dogs • Gastrointestinal—retching and vomiting secondary to severe hypoxemia; esophageal motor dysfunction secondary to a generalized polyneuropathy–like disorder may play a significant role in the occurrence of upper gastrointestinal clinical signs.
• Cardiovascular and nervous—hyperpyrexia and heat prostration • Endocrine—hypothyroidism is recognized in association with neuromuscular disorders, including esophageal motor dysfunction and laryngeal paralysis.

GENETICS

• Paralysis (dogs)—Bouvier des Flandres (autosomal dominant trait); Siberian huskies and husky mixed breeds (mode of inheritance under study); laryngeal paralysis–polyneuropathy complex in young Dalmatians and Rottweilers (these conditions are considered to be inherited, but this is presently unproven) • Cats—no studies reported

INCIDENCE/PREVALENCE

• Paralysis—hereditary forms: high incidence; acquired (idiopathic) form: fairly high prevalence, undefined incidence; rare in cats
• Trauma—rare in dogs and cats • Tumors (primary and as part of a generalized neoplastic process)—rare in dogs; more common in domestic cats but incidence poorly defined

SIGNALMENT

Species
Dogs and cats

Breed Predilections
Paralysis (Dogs)
• Hereditary—Bouvier des Flandres, Siberian huskies, and husky mixed breeds • Part of a generalized polyneuropathy syndrome—Dalmatians, and probably Rottweilers
• Acquired—overrepresented in giant breeds (St. Bernards, Newfoundlands) and large

breeds (Irish setters, Labradors, golden retrievers)

Mean Age and Range
Paralysis
• Hereditary—onset of signs varies in the different breeds: Rottweilers—11 to 13 weeks of age; Dalmatians—4 to 8 months of age; Bouviers—4 to 6 months of age; white-coated German shepherds—4 to 6 months of age. • Acquired—1–12 years of age; reported mean, 9–12 years • Cats—usually older, but seen occasionally in younger cats secondary to trauma or surgical procedures
Neoplasia
• Middle-aged to old dogs and cats

Predominant Sex
Paralysis—hereditary: reported incidence varies from 3:1 male predominance to a 1:1 M:F incidence; acquired: reported 2:1 male predominance

SIGNS

General Comments
Directly related to the degree of impairment of laryngeal airflow

Historical Findings
• Change in character of the bark or meow
• Occasional coughing • Reduced activity
• Exercise intolerance • Abnormal breathing sounds with exertion or stress • Associated with exertion, stress, or heat—severely difficult breathing; gagging and retching; vomiting; weakness and lethargy; collapse; even sudden death

Physical Examination Findings
• Noisy respiration and a high-pitched inspiratory sound (stridor)—most common
• Cats—inspiratory stridor less characteristic than in dogs • Upper airway sounds—referred over the trachea and to hilar lung fields, bilaterally • With aspiration—focal or bilateral rales may be ausculted • Rectal temperature—usually elevated above normal, especially in warm weather

CAUSES

Paralysis
• Congenital • Acquired—suggested hormonal deficiencies (e.g., hypothyroidism), central or peripheral vagal nerve abnormality, cervical trauma, abnormality involving the recurrent laryngeal nerves, disease in the anterior thorax, generalized peripheral neuropathy, myopathy, and other immune-mediated disorders; the high incidence of laryngeal paralysis in large-breed dogs and certain specific breeds (i.e., Labrador retrievers) strongly suggests genetic predisposition. • Thyroid adenocarcinoma—may impinge or invade recurrent laryngeal nerves

Trauma
• Penetrating (e.g., bite wounds) or blunt neck • Injury secondary to ingested foreign materials—bones; sticks; needles; pins

Neoplasia
• May be seen as a primary tumor arising within the larynx, or as part of a systemic neoplastic process. • Dogs—a variety of neoplasms have been reported; including squamous cell carcinoma, rhabdomyosarcoma, undifferentiated carcinoma, oncocytoma, lipoma, thyroid carcinoma, mast cell tumor, osteosarcoma, fibrosarcoma, and melanoma. • Cats—the predominant neoplasm is lymphosarcoma, with squamous cell carcinoma and primary adenocarcinoma also being reported.

RISK FACTORS
• Systemic disorders—See Causes
• Concomitant pulmonary abnormalities

 DIAGNOSIS

DIFFERENTIAL DIAGNOSIS

• Laryngeal collapse—potential complication of long-standing brachycephalic airway syndrome and (rarely) laryngeal paralysis; noisy, obstructed breathing pattern with no inspiratory stridor; more likely than paralysis in brachycephalic dog; complete laryngeal examination under heavy sedation needed to confirm the diagnosis. • Chronic proliferative, pyogranulomatous laryngitis—may cause a mass lesion requiring surgical removal; histopathologic examination; tapered administration of corticosteroids
• Obstructing processes involving the trachea and the tracheobronchial junction—may mimic laryngeal disease on physical examination; causes include tracheal collapse (e.g., tracheomalacia) and intraluminal and peritracheal masses (osteochondroma being the most commonly reported intratracheal tumor in the dog; whereas epithelial malignancies are most common in the domestic cat. Both are quite rare.)

CBC/BIOCHEMISTRY/URINALYSIS
• Usually normal • With aspiration pneumonia—high WBC count with a left shift possible

OTHER LABORATORY TESTS
• Arterial blood gas analysis—detect hypoxemia and respiratory acidosis
• Thyroid testing—routinely performed because hypothyroidism is a suggested cause for idiopathic paralysis; < 10% of affected dogs test positive; hormone replacement in a few dogs did not result in improved laryngeal function.

IMAGING
• Routine imaging procedures—little benefit as primary diagnostic procedures
• Radiography, fluoroscopy, and bronchoscopy—help rule out the differential diagnoses; detect aspiration pneumonia
• Ultrasonography has recently been demonstrated as a useful diagnostic tool in

the non-invasive diagnosis of laryngeal masses. • Barium swallow with or without fluoroscopy (dogs)—perform in every patient in which occasional vomiting is reported; a low incidence (< 10%) of esophageal motor dysfunction found with idiopathic paralysis

DIAGNOSTIC PROCEDURES
Electromyography—define partial or complete denervation potentials (e.g., fibrillation and/or positive waves) with or without pseudomyotonia

Laryngoscope
• Visual inspection with the patient under heavy sedation or anesthesia required for proper evaluation • Paralysis—dogs: even light barbiturate anesthesia makes evaluation difficult; recommend acepromazine (0.033 mg/kg IM, SC); cats: ketamine HCl (6–10 mg/kg IV) alone or ketamine HCl (3–5 mg/kg) with diazepam (0.1–0.2 mg/kg), or Telazol (9–12 mg/kg IM, SC) provides sedation without interfering with laryngeal function • Stimulating respiratory effort with doxapram administration can facilitate the diagnosis. • Abduction of laryngeal cartilages—normally observed during deep inspiration; with paralysis may note passive opening of the larynx during expiration

PATHOLOGIC FINDINGS
• Gross—redness and swelling of the mucosa over the arytenoid cartilages and the vocal folds • Histopathologic—inflammation and edema of the perilaryngeal mucous membranes; denervation atrophy of the laryngeal muscles

 TREATMENT

APPROPRIATE HEALTH CARE
• Outpatient—while awaiting surgery if stable • Emergency—marked respiratory distress; oxygen therapy combined with sedation and corticosteroids (dexamethasone sodium phosphate at 1–2 mg/kg IV; then 0.5–1.0 mg/kg SC q12h for 24 hr; then 0.2 mg/kg SC q12h in tapering doses) or emergency tracheotomy

NURSING CARE
• Avoid warm poorly ventilated environments, as these further compromise normal cooling mechanisms, as well as proper air exchange. • Avoid cervical collars and choke chains, as they will also interfere with normal air exchange, especially if there is associated tracheal collapse.

ACTIVITY
Severe restriction—patients pending surgery; when owner refuses surgery

CLIENT EDUCATION
Paralysis
• Discuss potential complications of heat prostration and asphyxia if surgery is not pursued. • Discuss the improved quality of life and normal life expectancy with successful surgery. • Discuss the heritability of the congenital forms of laryngeal paralysis. • Discuss the increased risk for aspiration pneumonia after surgery.

SURGICAL CONSIDERATIONS
• Paralysis—surgical management treatment of choice; variety of procedures reported; efficacy of any one procedure depends on the surgeon's experience and expertise and perhaps other minor factors. • Trauma—temporary tracheotomy may be life-saving and curative. • Neoplasia—tumor excision with or without modified surgery to enlarge the laryngeal airway may be curative in dogs; for squamous cell adenocarcinoma, surgical excision coupled with radiotherapy management of choice; permanent tracheostomy may improve quality of life.

 MEDICATIONS

DRUG(S)
• Acquired paralysis (dogs) when surgery is declined—may benefit from mild sedatives (acepromazine, promazine, or diazepam) and corticosteroids (prednisone at 2.2 mg/kg divided q12h initially; then gradually reduce to alternate-day administration)
• Lymphosarcoma involving the larynx or tonsils is potentially responsive to chemotherapy in affected cats and dogs; a temporary tracheostomy may be beneficial at the initiation of therapy.

PRECAUTIONS
• Heavy sedation without a tracheotomy in a hot environment may predispose the patient to heat prostration.
• Corticosteroids—chronic use may predispose the patient to gastric ulcerations and, if susceptible, to diabetes mellitus and systemic or focal infections

 FOLLOW-UP

PATIENT MONITORING
• Reexamination of larynx—recommended 3–4 weeks after surgery • Arterial blood gases—should normalize after surgery
• Improvement in activity and exercise tolerance—reported by owners after surgery

PREVENTION/AVOIDANCE
Dogs with inheritable laryngeal paralysis should not be used for breeding.

POSSIBLE COMPLICATIONS
• Recurrence of clinical signs—with tumor regrowth; with inadequate surgery to treat paralysis • Laryngeal web formation (dogs)—after bilateral vocal cord resection; transect and treat with tapered corticosteroids

• Increased risk of aspiration pneumonia—after any laryngeal surgical protocol, as surgery places the larynx in a fixed open position • Risk of aspiration—particularly high if evidence of aspiration noted before surgical treatment of paralysis

EXPECTED COURSE AND PROGNOSIS
• Paralysis—long-term prognosis good to excellent with successful surgery; with unsatisfactory initial surgery, additional surgery may improve prognosis. • Trauma—progress usually satisfactory with conservative management, even after emergency tracheotomy • Neoplasia—squamous cell adenocarcinoma (dogs and cats): prognosis poor, even with radiotherapy; lymphosarcoma (cats): prognosis depends on chemotherapy used and patient response.

 MISCELLANEOUS

ASSOCIATED CONDITIONS
• Cervical masses, notably thyroid adenocarcinoma, occasionally • Generalized esophageal motor dysfunction—low incidence in dogs with acquired paralysis, suggesting polyneuropathy

AGE-RELATED FACTORS
Hereditary paralysis—onset of clinical signs within the first year of life

PREGNANCY
Increased risk in patients with clinical signs of laryngeal dysfunction

SEE ALSO
• Brachycephalic Airway Syndrome • Lymphosarcoma—Cats • Stertor and Stridor • Tracheal Collapse—Dogs

Suggested Reading
Braund KG, et al: Laryngeal paralysis–polyneuropathy complex in young Dalmatians. Am J Vet Res 1994; 55:534–542.
Jaggy A, Oliver JE, Ferguson DC, et al. Neurological manifestations of hypothyroidism: a retrospective study of 29 dogs. J Vet Intern Med 1994;8:328–336.
Mahony OM, Knowles KE, Kyle G, et al. Laryngeal paralysis–polyneuropathy complex in young Rottweilers. J Vet Intern Med 1998;12:330–337.
Ridyard AE, et al. Spontaneous laryngeal paralysis in four white-coated German shepherd dogs. J Sm Anim Pract 2000; 41:558–561.
Rudorf H, Brown P. Ultrasonography of laryngeal masses in six cats and one dog. Vet Radiol Ultras 1998;37:442–446.
White RN. Unilateral arytenoid lateralization for the treatment of laryngeal paralysis in four cats. J Sm Anim Pract 1994;35: 455–458.
Author Neil K. Harpster
Consulting Editor Lynelle R. Johnson

LEAD POISONING

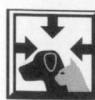 **BASICS**

DEFINITION
Intoxication (blood lead > 0.4 ppm) owing to acute or chronic exposure to some form of lead

PATHOPHYSIOLOGY
• Lead—interacts with sulfhydryl groups; interferes with numerous enzymes, including those involved in heme synthesis; causes fragility and decreased survival of RBCs
• Release of reticulocytes and nucleated RBCs from bone marrow
• Inhibition of 5'-pyrimidine nucleotidase—retention of RNA degradation products; aggregation of ribosomes (e.g., basophilic stippling)
• Damage to CNS capillaries—may account for brain lesions
• Young patients—weaker blood–brain barrier may permit more lead to reach the brain.

SYSTEMS AFFECTED
• Hemic/Lymph/Immune—interference with hemoglobin synthesis
• Gastrointestinal—unknown mechanism
• Nervous—capillary damage; possible direct toxic affect
• Renal/Urologic—damage to proximal tubule cells

GENETICS
N/A

INCIDENCE/PREVALENCE
• Incidence unknown
• Decreasing prevalence in dogs—owing to elimination of sources
• Increasing prevalence in cats—increased awareness and diagnosis
• Higher number of cases during warmer months

GEOGRAPHIC DISTRIBUTION
Low socioeconomic status of pet-owning family associated with high blood lead concentration in pets

SIGNALMENT
Species
Dogs more commonly than cats
Breed Predilections
N/A

Mean Age and Range
Mainly dogs < 1 year of age
Predominant Sex
N/A

SIGNS
General Comments
• Primarily gastrointestinal and neurologic
• Gastrointestinal—often precede CNS signs; predominant with chronic, low-level exposure
• CNS—occur more often with acute exposure
• History of renovation of older house or ingestion of lead objects

Physical Examination Findings
• Vomiting
• Diarrhea
• Anorexia
• Abdominal pain
• Lethargy
• Hysteria
• Seizures
• Blindness
• Cats—central vestibular abnormalities such as vertical nystagmus and ataxia reported

CAUSES
• Ingestion of some form of lead—paint and paint residues or dust from sanding; car batteries; linoleum; solder; plumbing materials and supplies; lubricating compounds; putty; tar paper; lead foil; golf balls; lead object (e.g., shot, fishing sinkers, drapery weights)
• Use of improperly glazed ceramic food or water bowl

RISK FACTORS
• Age < 1 year
• Living in economically depressed areas
• Living in old house or building that is being renovated

 DIAGNOSIS

DIFFERENTIAL DIAGNOSIS
Dogs
• Canine distemper
• Infectious encephalitides
• Bromethalin or methylxanthine toxicosis
• NSAID toxicosis
• Heat stroke
• Intestinal parasitism
• Intussusception

• Pancreatitis
• Infectious canine hepatitis
Cats
• Degenerative or storage diseases
• Hepatic encephalopathy
• Infectious encephalitides
• Organophosphate toxicosis

CBC/BIOCHEMISTRY/URINALYSIS
• Between 5 and 40 nucleated RBCs/100 WBCs without anemia
• Absence of nucleated RBC changes does not rule out the diagnosis.
• Anisocytosis, polychromasia, poikilocytosis, target cells, hypochromasia
• Basophilic stippling of RBCs
• Neutrophilic leukocytosis
• Cats—elevated AST and ALP reported
• Urinalysis—mild non-specific renal damage; glucosuria; hemoglobinuria

OTHER LABORATORY TESTS
Lead Concentration
• Toxic—antemortem whole blood: > 0.4 ppm (40 µg/dL); postmortem liver and/or kidney: > 5 ppm (wet weight)
• Lower values—must be interpreted in conjunction with history and clinical signs
• Blood levels—do not correlate with occurrence or severity of clinical signs
• $CaNa_2EDTA$ mobilization test—collect one 24-hr urine sample; administer $CaNa_2EDTA$ (75 mg/kg IM); collect a second 24-hr urine sample; with toxicosis, urine lead increases 10–60-fold post-EDTA.

IMAGING
May note radiopaque material in gastro-intestinal tract; not diagnostic

DIAGNOSTIC PROCEDURES
N/A

PATHOLOGIC FINDINGS
• Gross—may note paint chips or lead objects in gastrointestinal tract
• Intranuclear inclusion bodies—may note in hepatocytes or renal tubule epithelial cells; intracellular storage form of lead; considered pathognomonic

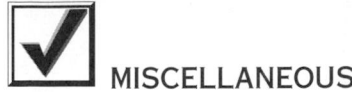

TREATMENT

APPROPRIATE HEALTH CARE
• Inpatient—first course of chelation, depending on severity of clinical signs
• Outpatient—orally administered chelators

NURSING CARE
• Balanced electrolyte fluids—Ringer's solution; replacement of hydration deficit
• Gastric or enterogastric lavage—may be indicated

ACTIVITY
N/A

DIET
N/A

CLIENT EDUCATION
• Inform client of the potential of adverse human health effects of lead.
• Notify public health officials.
• Determine the source of the lead.

SURGICAL CONSIDERATIONS
Removal of lead objects from the gastrointestinal tract

MEDICATIONS

DRUG(S) OF CHOICE
• Evacuation of gastrointestinal tract—saline cathartics; sodium or magnesium sulfate (dogs, 2–25 g; cats 2–5 g PO as 20% solution or less)
• Control of seizures—diazepam (given to effect; dogs, 5 to 20 mg; cats, 5 to 10 mg IV) or phenobarbital sodium (IV to effect)
• Alleviation of CNS signs—mannitol (0.25–2 g/kg IV, slow infusion over 30 to 60 minutes) and dexamethasone (2.2–4.4 mg/kg IV)
• Reduction of lead body burden-chelation therapy—$CaNa_2EDTA$ (dogs and cats, 25 mg/kg SC, IM, IV q6h for 2–5 days); dilute to a 1% solution with D_5W before administration; may need multiple treatment courses if blood lead concentration is high; allow 5-day rest period between treatment courses. Succimer–alternative to $CaNa_2EDTA$; orally administered chelating agent; 10 mg/kg PO q8h for 5 days followed by 10 mg PO q12h for 2 weeks; allow 2-week rest period between treatments; may

administer per rectum if clinical signs such as emesis preclude oral administration; cats successfully treated with 10 mg/kg PO q8h for 17 days; advantages over other chelators: can be given PO allowing for outpatient treatment; does not increase lead absorption from the gastrointestinal tract; not reported to be nephrotoxic; will not chelate essential elements such as zinc

CONTRAINDICATIONS
• $CaNa_2EDTA$—do not administer to patients with renal impairment or anuria; establish urine flow before administration; do not administer orally.
• D-Penicillamine—do not give if there is lead in the gastrointestinal tract (increases absorption)
• Succimer—does not increase gastrointestinal absorption

PRECAUTIONS
$CaNa_2EDTA$—safety in pregnancy not established.

POSSIBLE INTERACTIONS
• $CaNa_2EDTA$—depletion of zinc, iron and manganese with long-term therapy

ALTERNATIVE DRUG(S)
• D-Penicillamine—10–15 mg/kg PO q12h for 7 to 14 days; allow a 7-day rest period between treatments; do not give if there is lead in the gastrointestinal tract (increases absorption)

FOLLOW-UP

PATIENT MONITORING
Blood lead—should be < 0.4 ppm; assess 10–14 days after cessation of chelation therapy.

PREVENTION/AVOIDANCE
Determine source of lead and remove it from the patient's environment.

POSSIBLE COMPLICATIONS
Permanent neurologic signs (e.g., blindness) occasionally

EXPECTED COURSE AND PROGNOSIS
• Signs should dramatically improve within 24–48 hr after initiating chelation therapy.
• Prognosis—favorable with treatment
• Uncontrolled seizures—guarded prognosis

MISCELLANEOUS

ASSOCIATED CONDITIONS
N/A

AGE-RELATED FACTORS
Dogs < 1 year of age—more likely to be affected

ZOONOTIC POTENTIAL
None; however, humans in the same environment may be at risk for exposure.

PREGNANCY
• Transplacental passage—may cause neonatal poisoning
• Lactation—lead mobilized from bones unlikely to poison nursing animals

SYNONYMS
Plumbism

SEE ALSO
Poisoning (Intoxication)

Suggested Reading

Braton R, Kowalczyk D. Lead poisoning. In: Kirk R, ed. Current veterinary therapy X. Philadelphia: Saunders, 1989:152–159.

Knight TE, Kent M, Junk JE. Succimer for treatment of lead toxicosis in two cats. J Am Vet Med Assoc 2001;218:1946–1948.

Morgan RV, Moore FM, Pearce LK, et al. Clinical and laboratory findings in small companion animals with lead poisoning: 347 cases (1977–1986). J Am Vet Med Assoc 1991;199:93–97.

Morgan RV, Pearce LK, Moore FM, et al. Demographic data and treatment of small companion animals with lead poisoning: 347 cases (1977–1986). J Am Vet Med Assoc 1991;199:98–102.

Morgan RV. Lead poisoning in small companion animals: an update (1987–1992). Vet Hum Toxicol 1994;36:18–22.

Ramsey DT, Casteel SW, Fagella AM, et al. Use of orally administered succimer (meso-2,3-dimercaptosuccinic acid) for treatment of lead poisoning in dogs. J Am Vet Med Assoc 1996;208:371–375.

VanAlstine WG, Wickliffe LW, Everson RJ, et al. Acute lead toxicosis in a household of cats. J Vet Diagn Invest 1993;5:496–498.

Author Robert H. Poppenga
Consulting Editor Gary D. Osweiler

LEFT ANTERIOR FASCICULAR BLOCK

BASICS

DEFINITION
• Conduction delay or block in the anterior fascicle of the left bundle branch (Figures 1 and 2)
• Left ventricle activation then altered or delayed toward the blocked fascicle and corresponding papillary muscle

ECG Features
• QRS complex—normal duration
• Left axis deviation—dogs, < +40°; cats, < 0°
• Small q waves and tall R waves in leads I and aVL—small q not essential
• Deep S waves (exceeding the R waves) in leads II, III, and aVF

PATHOPHYSIOLOGY
• Anatomic basis still speculative—anterior fascicle vulnerable because it has a single blood supply, is long and thin, and is located in the turbulent outflow tract of the left ventricle
• No hemodynamic compromise

SYSTEMS AFFECTED
Cardiovascular

GENETICS
N/A

INCIDENCE/PREVALENCE
• Most commonly described form of bundle branch block in cats
• Uncommon in dogs

GEOGRAPHIC DISTRIBUTION
N/A

SIGNALMENT

Species
Dogs and cats

Breed Predilections
N/A

Mean Age and Range
N/A

Predominant Sex
N/A

SIGNS

Historical Findings
• Signs usually associated with the underlying cause
• Usually an incidental ECG finding

Physical Examination Findings
No associated signs or hemodynamic compromise

CAUSES
• Hypertrophic cardiomyopathy (cats)
• Left ventricular hypertrophy (e.g., mitral insufficiency, aortic stenosis, aortic body tumor, hypertension, and hyperthyroidism)
• Hyperkalemia (e.g., urethral obstruction, acute renal insufficiency, and Addison's disease)
• Ischemic cardiomyopathy (e.g., arteriosclerosis of the coronary arteries, myocardial infarction, and myocardial hypertrophy that obstructs coronary arteries)
• Surgical repair of a cardiac defect (e.g., ventricular septal defect or aortic valvular disease)
• Restrictive cardiomyopathy (cats)
• Fibrosis

RISK FACTORS
N/A

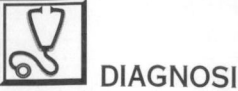

DIAGNOSIS

DIFFERENTIAL DIAGNOSIS
• Left ventricular enlargement—absence of left ventricular enlargement on thoracic radiograph or cardiac ultrasound supports a diagnosis of left anterior fascicular block.
• Right bundle branch block—deep, wide S waves in leads I, II, III and aVF causing a right axis deviation; in patients with left anterior fascicular block, leads I and aVL are positive and leads II, III, and aVF have deep S waves resulting in a left axis deviation.
• Altered position of the heart within the thorax—thoracic radiographs help identify mass or foreign body that may be displacing the heart.
• Suspect hyperkalemia if signs of urethral obstruction, renal insufficiency, or hypoadrenocorticism (Addison's disease); determine serum potassium concentration.

CBC/BIOCHEMISTRY/URINALYSIS
Hyperkalemia possible

OTHER LABORATORY TESTS
N/A

IMAGING
• Echocardiogram may show structural heart disease.
• Thoracic and abdominal radiographs may show mass, pulmonary metastatic lesion, foreign body, or abnormal cardiac position.

DIAGNOSTIC PROCEDURES
• Electrocardiography
• Long-term ambulatory monitoring (Holter) may reveal intermittent bundle branch block.

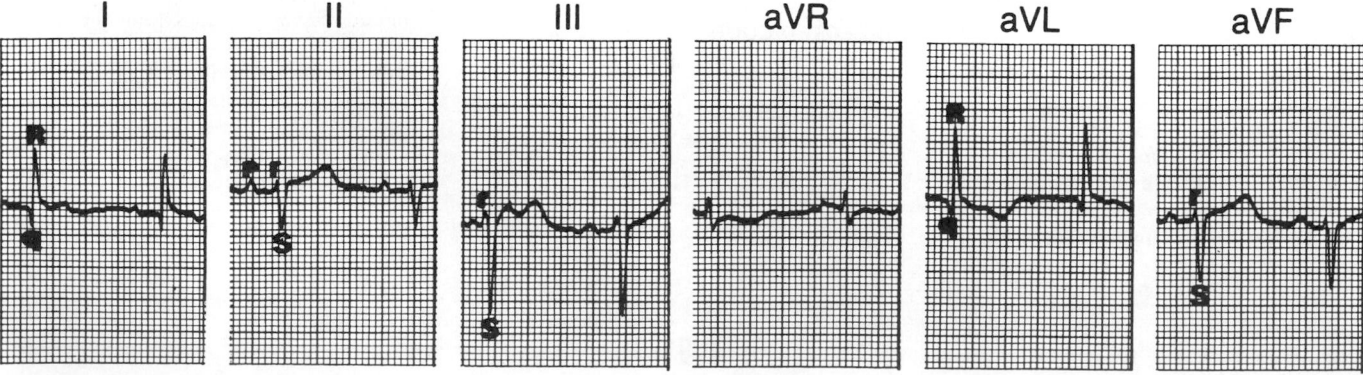

I   II   III   aVR   aVL   aVF

Figure 1.

Left anterior fascicular block in a cat with hypertrophic cardiomyopathy. Severe left axis deviation (260°) with a qR pattern in leads I and aVL and an rS pattern in leads II, III, and aVF. The QRS complexes are of normal duration. (From: Tilley LP: Essentials of canine and feline electrocardiography. 3rd ed. Baltimore: Lippincott Williams & Wilkins, 1992, with permission.)

PATHOLOGIC FINDINGS

Possible lesions or scarring on endocardial surface in the path of the bundle branches; applying Lugol's iodine to the endocardial surface within 2 hr postmortem enables clear visualization of the conduction system.

 TREATMENT

APPROPRIATE HEALTH CARE

• Treatment unnecessary
• Treat underlying cause.

NURSING CARE

Unnecessary

ACTIVITY

Unrestricted unless indicated by underlying condition

DIET

No modifications unless indicated by underlying condition

CLIENT EDUCATION

Fascicular block per se does not cause hemodynamic compromise; combined with right bundle branch block it may develop into second- or third-degree AV block, making treatment essential; need to treat underlying cause

SURGICAL CONSIDERATIONS

N/A

 MEDICATIONS

DRUG(S) OF CHOICE

Treatment directed toward the underlying primary disease (e.g., drugs to lower the serum potassium in hyperkalemia)

CONTRAINDICATIONS

N/A

PRECAUTIONS

N/A

POSSIBLE INTERACTIONS

N/A

ALTERNATIVE DRUG(S)

N/A

 FOLLOW-UP

PATIENT MONITORING

ECG regularly.

PREVENTION/AVOIDANCE

N/A

POSSIBLE COMPLICATIONS

Causative lesion could progress and lead to a more serious arrhythmia or complete heart block

EXPECTED COURSE AND PROGNOSIS

No hemodynamic compromise

 **MISCELLANEOUS**

ASSOCIATED CONDITIONS

N/A

AGE-RELATED FACTORS

N/A

ZOONOTIC POTENTIAL

N/A

PREGNANCY

N/A

SYNONYMS

None

SEE ALSO

• Atrioventricular Block, Complete
• Atrioventricular Block, First-degree
• Atrioventricular Block, Second-degree
• Left Bundle Branch Block
• Right Bundle Branch Block

ABBREVIATION

AV = atrioventricular

Suggested Reading

Tilley LP. Essentials of canine and feline electrocardiography. 3rd ed. Baltimore: Williams & Wilkins, 1992

Authors Larry P. Tilley and Naomi L. Burtnick

Consulting Editors Larry P. Tilley and Francis W. K. Smith, Jr.

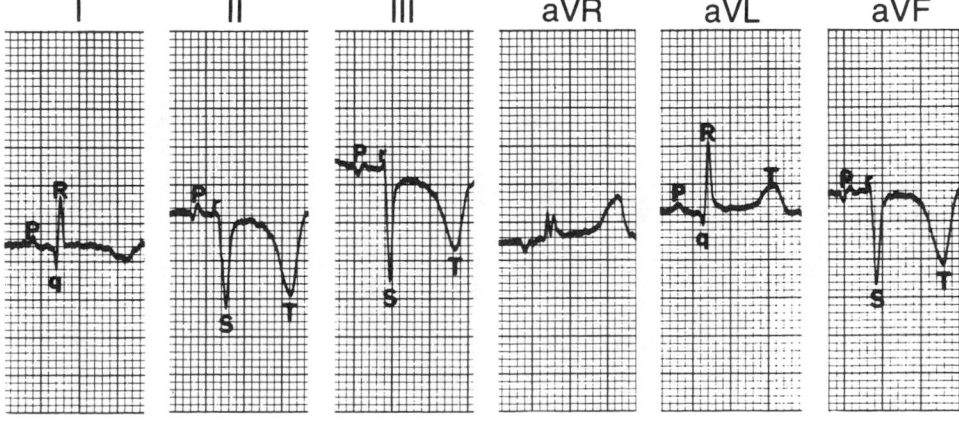

Figure 2.

Left anterior fascicular block in a dog with hyperkalemia (serum potassium, 5.3 mEq/L). There is abnormal left axis deviation ($-60°$) with a qR pattern in leads I and aVL and an rS pattern in leads II, III, and aVF. The large T waves are compatible with hyperkalemia. (From: Tilley LP: Essentials of canine and feline electrocardiography, 3rd ed. Baltimore: Lippincott Williams & Wilkins, 1992, with permission.)

LEFT BUNDLE BRANCH BLOCK

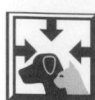 BASICS

DEFINITION
Conduction delay or block in both the left posterior and left anterior fascicles of the left bundle (Figures 1 and 2); a supraventricular impulse activates the right ventricle first through the right bundle branch; the left ventricle is activated late, causing the QRS to become wide and bizarre.

ECG Features
• QRS prolonged—dogs, > 0.08 sec, cats, > 0.06 sec
• QRS wide and positive in leads I, II, III, and aVF
• Block can be intermittent or constant.

PATHOPHYSIOLOGY
• Because the left bundle branch is thick and extensive, the lesion causing the block must be large.
• Usually an incidental ECG finding—does not cause hemodynamic abnormalities

SYSTEMS AFFECTED
Cardiovascular

GENETICS
N/A

INCIDENCE/PREVALENCE
Uncommon in cats and dogs. In cats with hypertrophic cardiomyopathy, left bundle branch block is not as commonly seen as left anterior fascicular block.

GEOGRAPHIC DISTRIBUTION
N/A

SIGNALMENT
Species
Cats and dogs
Breed Predilections
N/A
Mean Age and Range
N/A
Predominant Sex
N/A

SIGNS
Historical Findings
• Usually an incidental ECG finding—does not cause hemodynamic abnormalities
• Signs usually associated with the underlying condition
Physical Examination Findings
Does not cause signs or hemodynamic compromise

CAUSES
• Cardiomyopathy
• Direct or indirect cardiac trauma (e.g., hit by car and cardiac needle puncture)
• Neoplasia
• Subvalvular aortic stenosis
• Fibrosis • Ischemic cardiomyopathy (e.g., arteriosclerosis of the coronary arteries, myocardial infarction, and myocardial hypertrophy that obstructs coronary arteries)

RISK FACTORS
N/A

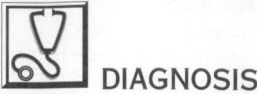 DIAGNOSIS

DIFFERENTIAL DIAGNOSIS
• Left ventricular enlargement
• No left ventricular enlargement on thoracic radiograph or cardiac ultrasound studies supports diagnosis of isolated left bundle branch block.
• Can also be confused with ventricular ectopic beats, but the PR interval is usually constant and left bundle branch block has no pulse deficits

CBC/BIOCHEMISTRY/URINALYSIS
N/A

OTHER LABORATORY TESTS
N/A

IMAGING
• Echocardiography may reveal structural heart disease; absence of left heart enlargement supports a diagnosis of left bundle branch block.
• Thoracic and abdominal radiographs may show masses or pulmonary metastatic lesions; traumatic injuries could result in localized or diffuse pulmonary densities.

DIAGNOSTIC PROCEDURES
• Electrocardiography
• Long-term ambulatory monitoring (Holter) may reveal intermittent left bundle branch block.

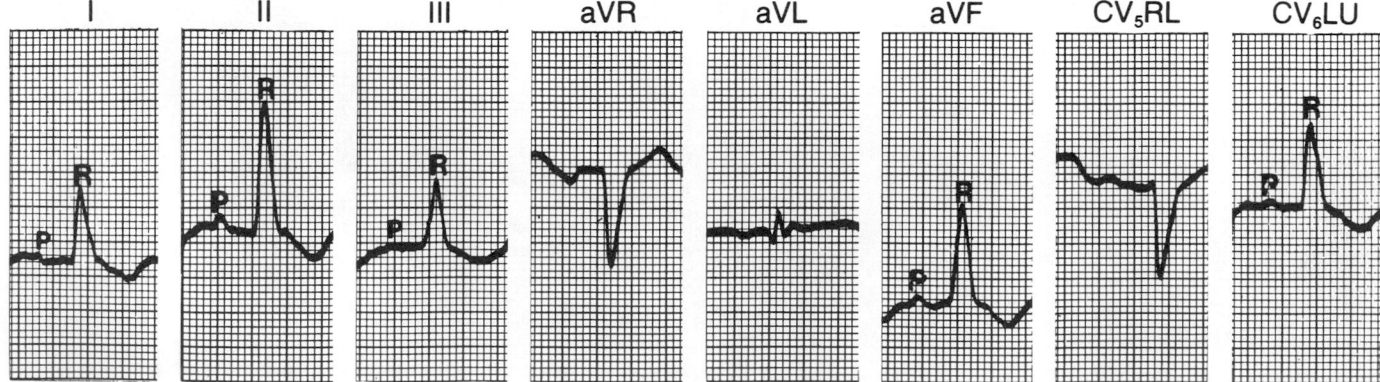

Figure 1.

Left bundle branch block in a cat with hypertrophic cardiomyopathy. The QRS complex is of 0.07-sec duration and is positive in leads I, II, III, aVF. Neither a Q wave nor an S wave occurs in these leads. The QRS complex is inverted in leads aVR. (From: Tilley LP. Essentials of canine and feline electrocardiography. 3rd ed. Baltimore: Lippincott Williams & Wilkins, 1992, with permission.)

PATHOLOGIC FINDINGS

Possible lesions or scarring on endocardial surface in the path of the bundle branches; applying Lugol's iodine to the endocardial surface within 2 h postmortem enables clear visualization of the conduction system.

 TREATMENT

APPROPRIATE HEALTH CARE

Directed toward the underlying cause

NURSING CARE

Generally not necessary

ACTIVITY

Unrestricted unless required for management of underlying condition

DIET

No modifications unless required for management of underlying condition

CLIENT EDUCATION

• Left bundle branch block per se does not cause hemodynamic abnormalities.
• Lesion causing the block could progress, leading to more serious arrhythmias or complete heart block.

SURGICAL CONSIDERATIONS

N/A

 MEDICATIONS

DRUG(S) OF CHOICE

N/A (unless required for management of underlying condition)

CONTRAINDICATIONS

N/A

PRECAUTIONS

N/A

POSSIBLE INTERACTIONS

N/A

ALTERNATIVE DRUG(S)

N/A

 FOLLOW-UP

PATIENT MONITORING

Serial ECG may show clearing or progression to complete heart block.

PREVENTION/ AVOIDANCE

N/A

POSSIBLE COMPLICATIONS

• Causative lesion could progress, leading to a more serious arrhythmia or complete heart block.
• First- or second-degree AV block may indicate involvement of the right bundle branch.

EXPECTED COURSE AND PROGNOSIS

No hemodynamic compromise

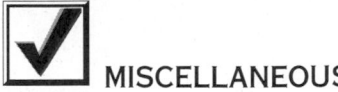 MISCELLANEOUS

ASSOCIATED CONDITIONS

N/A

AGE-RELATED FACTORS

N/A

ZOONOTIC POTENTIAL

N/A

PREGNANCY

N/A

SYNONYMS

N/A

SEE ALSO

• Atrioventricular Block, Complete
• Atrioventricular Block, First-degree
• Atrioventricular Block, Second-degree
• Left Anterior Fascicular Block
• Right Bundle Branch Block

ABBREVIATION

AV = atrioventricular

Suggested Readings

Tilley LP. Essentials of canine and feline electrocardiography. 3rd ed. Baltimore: Williams & Wilkins, 1992.
Authors Larry P. Tilley and Naomi L. Burtnick
Consulting Editors Larry P. Tilley and Francis W. K. Smith, Jr.

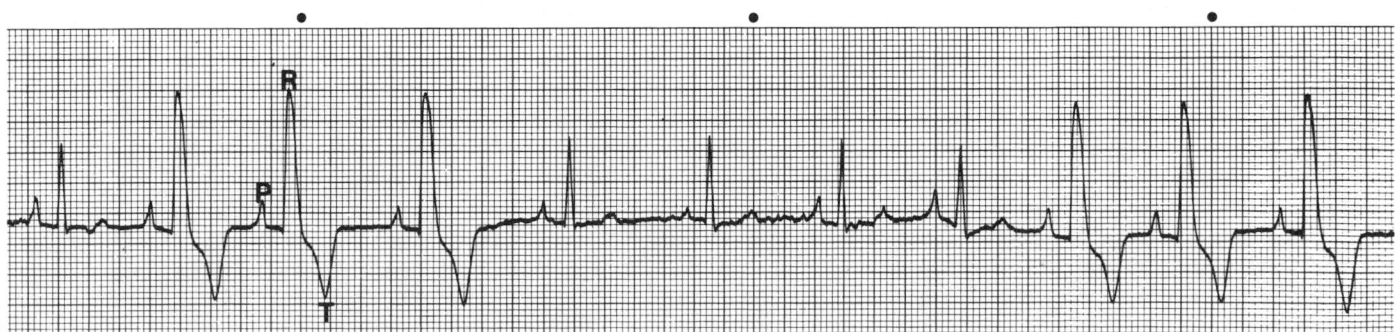

Figure 2.

Intermittent left bundle branch block in a Chihuahua. QRS complexes are wider (0.07–0.08 sec) in the second, third, and fourth complexes and in the last three complexes. Consistent P-R interval confirms a sinus origin for the abnormal-appearing QRS complexes (lead II, 50 mm/sec, 1 cm = 1 mV). (From: Tilley LP. Essentials of canine and feline electrocardiography 3rd ed. Baltimore: Lippincott Williams & Wilkins, 1992, with permission.)

LEGG-CALVÉ-PERTHES DISEASE

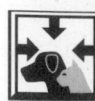

BASICS

DEFINITION
A spontaneous degeneration of the femoral head and neck leading to collapse of the coxofemoral joint and osteoarthritis

PATHOPHYSIOLOGY
• Precise cause unknown; a specific vascular lesion not identified
• Histologic evidence—points to infarction of vessels serving the proximal femur
• Necrosis of subchondral bone—leading to collapse and deformation of the femoral head during normal loading
• Articular cartilage—becomes thickened; cleft development; fraying of superficial layers
• Simultaneous osseous degeneration and repair—characteristic of ischemia and revascularization of bone
• No evidence of hypercoagulability or other blood clotting abnormalities

SYSTEMS AFFECTED
Musculoskeletal—causes a hind leg lameness; insidious in onset

GENETICS
• Manchester terriers—multifactorial inheritance pattern with a high degree of heritability
• Hereditary predisposition likely

INCIDENCE/PREVALENCE
• Common among miniature, toy, and small dog breeds
• No accurate estimates available

GEOGRAPHIC DISTRIBUTION
N/A

SIGNALMENT

Species
Dogs

Breed Predilections
• Toy breeds and terriers—most susceptible
• Manchester terriers, miniature pinschers, toy poodles, Lakeland terriers, west Highland white terriers, and cairn terriers—higher than expected incidence

Mean Age and Range
• Most patients are 5–8 months of age.
• Range—3–13 months

Predominant Sex
None

SIGNS

General Comments
Usually unilateral; only 12%–16% of cases are bilateral.

Historical Findings
Lameness—usually gradual onset over 2–3 months; weight-bearing; occasionally leg is carried.

Physical Examination Findings
• Pain on manipulation of the hip—most common
• Crepitation of the joint—inconsistent
• Atrophy of the thigh muscles—nearly always noted
• Patient otherwise normal

CAUSES
• Unknown
• Tamponade of the intracapsular subsynovial vessels serving the femoral head—suggested cause of ischemia leading to the pathologic changes

RISK FACTORS
• Small, toy, and miniature breeds—increased risk
• Trauma to the hip region

DIAGNOSIS

DIFFERENTIAL DIAGNOSIS
• Medial patellar luxation—may occur independently; primary differential in young dogs
• Rupture of the cranial cruciate ligament—primary differential in old dogs

CBC/BIOCHEMISTRY/URINALYSIS
N/A

OTHER LABORATORY TESTS
N/A

IMAGING
• Early radiographic changes—widening of the joint space; decreased bone density of the epiphysis; sclerosis and thickening of the femoral neck
• Later radiographic changes—lucent areas within the femoral head
• End-stage radiographic changes—flattening and extreme deformation of the femoral head; severe osteoarthrosis

DIAGNOSTIC PROCEDURES
N/A

PATHOLOGIC FINDINGS
• Femoral head—removed during FHNE; usually deformed with a thickened irregular articular surface
• Early disease—histologically characterized by loss of lacunar osteocytes and necrosis of marrow elements; trabeculae surrounded by granulation tissue
• Later disease—thickened metaphyseal trabeculae; mixture of necrosis and repair tissue typical of revascularization of bone
• Advanced disease—osteoclastic activity; new bone formation

TREATMENT

APPROPRIATE HEALTH CARE
• Rest and analgesics—reportedly successful in alleviating lameness in a minority of patients
• Ehmer sling—successful in one patient; maintained for 10 weeks
• Insidious onset often prevents early recognition and possibility of conservative treatment.
• FHNE with early and vigorous exercise after surgery—treatment of choice

NURSING CARE

Postsurgery
• Physical therapy—extremely important for rehabilitating the affected limb
• Analgesics, anti-inflammatory drugs, and cold packing—3–5 days; important
• Range-of-motion exercises—extension and flexion; initiated immediately
• Small lead weights—attached as ankle bracelets above the hock joint; encourage early use of the treated limb

ACTIVITY
• Postsurgery—early activity encouraged to improve leg use
• Conservative therapy—restricted activity recommended

DIET
Avoid obesity.

CLIENT EDUCATION
• Warn owners of Manchester terriers of the genetic basis of the disease; discourage breeding affected dogs.
• Warn client that recovery after FHNE may take 3–6 months.

SURGICAL CONSIDERATIONS
FHNE—treatment of choice

MEDICATIONS

DRUG(S) OF CHOICE
NSAIDs—preoperative or postoperatively; minimize joint pain; reduce synovitis; may try buffered or enteric-coated aspirin (10–25 mg/kg PO q8h or q12h), carprofen (2.2 mg/kg PO q12h), etodolac (10–15 mg/kg PO q24h), phenylbutazone (3–7 mg/kg PO q8h, total dose < 800 mg/day), meclofenemic acid (0.5 mg/kg PO q12h), or piroxicam (0.3 mg/kg PO q24h for 3 days, then q48h)

CONTRAINDICATIONS
NSAIDs—gastrointestinal upset may preclude use in some patients.

PRECAUTIONS
• NSAIDs—inhibition of platelet activity may increase hemorrhage at surgery; discontinue aspirin for at least 1 week before surgery, if possible; usually cause some degree of gastric ulceration
• Acetaminophen—unsuitable; potential for toxicity

POSSIBLE INTERACTIONS
NSAIDs—do not use in conjunction with glucocorticoids; risk of gastrointestinal tract ulceration

ALTERNATIVE DRUG(S)
Chondroprotective drugs (e.g., polysulfated glycosaminoglycans, glucosamine, and chondroitin sulfate)—little help in advanced disease; no evidence to suggest that these drugs prevent or reverse the disease process

FOLLOW-UP

PATIENT MONITORING
• Postsurgical progress checks—2-week intervals; necessary to ensure compliance with exercise recommendations
• Conservative therapy—re-evaluated (physical examination, radiographs) to determine if surgery is needed

PREVENTION/AVOIDANCE
• Discourage breeding of affected animals.
• Do not repeat dam–sire breedings that result in affected offspring.

POSSIBLE COMPLICATIONS
Limiting postoperative exercise may result in less than optimal limb function.

EXPECTED COURSE AND PROGNOSIS
• FHNE—good to excellent prognosis for full recovery (84%–100% success rate)
• Conservative therapy—reported to alleviate lameness after 2–3 months in about 25% of patients

MISCELLANEOUS

ASSOCIATED CONDITIONS
N/A

AGE-RELATED FACTORS
Usually affects juvenile small-breed dogs, but maturer dogs may be affected by chronic disease.

ZOONOTIC POTENTIAL
N/A

PREGNANCY
N/A

SYNONYMS
• Perthes disease
• Coxa plana

• Coxa magna
• Avascular necrosis of the femoral head
• Aseptic necrosis of the femoral head
• Osteochondritis juvenilis

SEE ALSO
• Cruciate Disease, Cranial
• Hip Dysplasia—Dogs
• Patella Luxation

ABBREVIATIONS
• FHNE = femoral head and neck excision
• NSAID = nonsteroidal antiinflammatory drug

Suggested Reading
Brenig B, Leeb T, Jansen S, Kopp T. Analysis of blood clotting factor activities in canine Legg-Calvé-Perthes' disease. J Vet Intern Med 1999;13:570–573.
Brinker WO, Piermattei DL, Flo GL, eds. Diagnosis and treatment of orthopedic conditions of the hindlimb. In: Handbook of small animal orthopedics and fracture treatment. 3rd ed. Philadelphia: Saunders 1997:465–466.
Gambardella PC. Legg-Calvé-Perthes disease in dogs. In: Bojrab MJ, ed. Disease mechanisms in small animal surgery. 2nd ed. Philadelphia: Saunders, 1993:804–807.
Gibson KL, Lewis DD, Perchman RD. Use of external coaptation for the treatment of avascular necrosis of the femoral head in a dog. J Am Vet Med Assoc 1990; 197:868–869.
Piek, CJ, Hazewinkel HAW, Wolvekamp WTC, et al. Long term follow-up of avascular necrosis of the femoral head in the dog. J Small Anim Pract 1996;37:12–18.
Author Larry Carpenter
Consulting Editor Peter K. Shires

LEIOMYOMA, STOMACH, SMALL AND LARGE INTESTINE

BASICS

OVERVIEW
Uncommon benign tumor arising from the smooth muscle of the stomach and intestinal tract

SIGNALMENT
• Middle-aged to older (> 6 years) dogs and cats
• Dogs more commonly affected than cats
• No breed predisposition

SIGNS

Historical Findings
• Related to gastrointestinal tract
• Stomach—vomiting
• Small intestine—vomiting; weight loss; borborygmus; flatulence
• Large intestine and rectum—tenesmus; hematochezia; sometimes rectal prolapse

Physical Examination Findings
• Stomach—no specific abnormalities
• Small intestine—often no abnormal findings; may feel midabdominal mass; occasionally distended, painful loops of small bowel
• Large intestine and rectum—may feel palpable mass per rectum

CAUSES & RISK FACTORS
Unknown

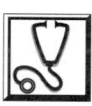

DIAGNOSIS

DIFFERENTIAL DIAGNOSIS
• Foreign body
• Inflammatory bowel disease
• Parasites
• Adenocarcinoma
• Leiomyosarcoma
• Lymphoma
• Pancreatitis

CBC/BIOCHEMISTRY/URINALYSIS
• Usually normal
• Hypoglycemia—occasionally
• Stomach and small intestine—may see microcytic hypochromic anemia

OTHER LABORATORY TESTS
N/A

IMAGING
• Abdominal ultrasound—may reveal a thickened wall of stomach or bowel; gastric leiomyoma most common at esophageal–gastric junction
• Contrast radiography (stomach and small intestine)—may reveal a space-occupying mass
• Double-contrast radiography (large intestine and rectum)—reveals a space-occupying mass

DIAGNOSTIC PROCEDURES

Upper Gastrointestinal Tract
Perform upper gastrointestinal tract endoscopy and mucosal biopsy. Frequently nondiagnostic because tumors are deep to the mucosal surface or distal to scope length; surgical biopsy often required to confirm the diagnosis

Large Intestine and Rectum
Colonoscopy may reveal a mass; mucosal biopsy may be nondiagnostic because of normal mucosal covering of the tumor; surgical biopsy often required

TREATMENT
• Surgical resection—treatment of choice; curative if tumor is resectable
• Even large leiomyomas often can be removed successfully with narrow margins.

MEDICATIONS

DRUG(S)
N/A

CONTRAINDICATIONS/POSSIBLE INTERACTIONS
N/A

FOLLOW-UP
• Complete resection—normal postoperative care; no additional follow-up necessary
• Monitor blood glucose postoperatively if hypoglycemic prior to surgery.

MISCELLANEOUS

ASSOCIATED CONDITIONS
Hypoglycemia—recognized as an associated paraneoplastic syndrome

Suggested Reading
McPherron MA, Withrow SJ, Seim HB, Powers BE: Colorectal leiomyoma in seven dogs. J Am Anim Hosp Assoc 1992;28:43–46.
Morrison WB. Nonlymphomatous cancers of the esophagus, stomach, and intestines. In: Morrison WB, ed., Cancer in dogs and cats: medical and surgical management. Baltimore: Williams & Wilkins, 1998:551–558.

Acknowledgment
The author and editors acknowledge the prior contribution of Dr. Ralph C. Richardson, who authored this topic in the previous edition.
Author Laura D. Garrett
Consulting Editor Wallace B. Morrison

LEIOMYOSARCOMA, STOMACH, SMALL AND LARGE INTESTINE

BASICS

OVERVIEW
• Uncommon malignant tumor arising from the smooth muscle of the stomach and intestinal tract
• Tends to be locally invasive; metastatic rate up to 50%, usually intra-abdominal sites
• Prognosis fair to guarded

SIGNALMENT
• Mostly middle-aged to older (> 6 years) dogs and cats
• Dogs more commonly affected than cats
• No breed predisposition

SIGNS

Historical Findings
• Related to gastrointestinal tract
• Stomach—vomiting; weight loss
• Small intestine—vomiting; weight loss; diarrhea; borborygmus; flatulence
• Large intestine and rectum—tenesmus, may lead to rectal prolapse; hematochezia

Physical Examination Findings
• Stomach—nonspecific
• Small intestine—may feel midabdominal mass; sometimes distended, painful loops of small bowel on abdominal palpation
• Large intestine and rectum—may feel palpable mass per rectum

CAUSES & RISK FACTORS
Unknown

DIAGNOSIS

DIFFERENTIAL DIAGNOSIS
• Foreign body
• Inflammatory bowel disease
• Parasites
• Adenocarcinoma
• Leiomyoma
• Lymphoma
• Pancreatitis

CBC/BIOCHEMISTRY/URINALYSIS
• Usually normal
• Anemia—may be hypochromic, microcytic
• Leukocytosis
• Hypoglycemia—reported as a paraneoplastic syndrome

OTHER LABORATORY TESTS
N/A

IMAGING
• Abdominal ultrasonography—may reveal a thickened wall of the stomach or bowel
• Positive contrast radiography (stomach and small intestine)—reveals a space-occupying mass
• Double-contrast radiography (large intestine and rectum)—reveals a space-occupying mass

DIAGNOSTIC PROCEDURES

Upper Gastrointestinal Tract
• Endoscopy and mucosal biopsy—perform, but results are frequently nondiagnostic because in some tumors deep to the mucosal surface, mass may be beyond reach of endoscope.
• Surgical biopsy—often required to confirm diagnosis

Large Intestine and Rectum
• Colonoscopy—may allow a mass to be seen; mucosal biopsy may be nondiagnostic because of the normal mucosal covering of the tumor
• Deep biopsy—perform if possible

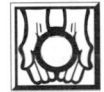

TREATMENT
• Surgical resection—treatment of choice
• Cecal leiomyosarcoma least likely to have metastases
• Surgery can provide prolonged survival for small intestinal masses
• Carefully evaluate for metastasis before extensive surgery (e.g., mesenteric lymph nodes, liver, and lungs)

MEDICATIONS

DRUG(S)
Chemotherapy not evaluated.

CONTRAINDICATIONS/POSSIBLE INTERACTIONS
N/A

FOLLOW-UP

EXPECTED COURSE AND PROGNOSIS
• Leiomyosarcomas often metastasize to the liver; local lymph nodes next frequently
• Small intestinal cases had median survival of 12 months.
• Cecal cases had median survival of 7.5 months, but most died of other diseases.
• Gastric cases most rare, but the few reported had high rate of metastasis and short survival times
• Complete resection—routine physical examination, thoracic radiography, and abdominal ultrasonography at 1, 3, 6, 9, and 12 months after surgery
• Incomplete resection—symptomatic support to relieve clinical signs

MISCELLANEOUS

ASSOCIATED CONDITIONS
• Hypoglycemia—reported as a paraneoplastic syndrome
• Erythrocytosis—recent report as a paraneoplastic syndrome

Suggested Reading
Crawshaw J, Berg J, Sardinas JC, et al. Prognosis for dogs with nonlymphomatous, small intestinal tumors treated by surgical excisions. J Am Anim Hosp Assoc 1998;34:451–456.
Kapatkin AS, Mullen HS, Matthiesen DT, Patnaik AK. Leiomyosarcoma in dogs: 44 cases (1983–1988). J Am Vet Med Assoc 1992;201:107.
Morrison WB. Nonlymphomatous cancers of the esophagus, stomach, and intestines. In: Morrison WB, ed. Cancer in dogs and cats: medical and surgical management. Baltimore: Williams & Wilkins, 1998:551–558.
Swann HM, Holt DE. Canine gastric adenocarcinoma and leiomyosarcoma: a retrospective study of 21 cases (1986–1999) and literature review. J Am Anim Hosp Assoc 2002;38:157–164.

Acknowledgment
The author acknowledges the prior contributions of Dr. Ralph C. Richardson, who authored this topic in the previous edition.
Author Laura D. Garrett
Consulting Editor Wallace B. Morrison

LEISHMANIASIS

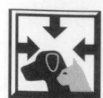

BASICS

OVERVIEW
- Protozoan—genus *Leishmania;* causes two types of disease: cutaneous and visceral
- Organ systems affected—cutaneous: skin, hepatobiliary, spleen, kidneys, eyes, and joints; visceral: hemorrhagic diathesis
- Affected dogs in the U.S. invariably acquired infection in another country.
- *L. donovani infantum*—Mediterranean basin, Portugal, and Spain; sporadic cases in Switzerland, northern France, and the Netherlands
- *L. donovani* complex or *L. braziliensis*—endemic areas of South and Central America and southern Mexico
- Endemic cases in dogs (Oklahoma and Ohio) and cats (Texas) have been reported in the U.S. Considered endemic in foxhounds in the U.S.
- Sandfly vectors—transmit flagellated parasites into the skin of a host. Vector unknown in U.S.
- Cats—often localizes in skin
- Dogs—invariably spreads throughout the body to most organs; renal failure is the most common cause of death.
- Incubation period—1 month to several years

SIGNALMENT
- Dogs—virtually all develop visceral, or systemic, disease; 90% also have cutaneous involvement; no sex or breed predilection
- Cats—cutaneous disease (rare); no sex or breed predilection

SIGNS

Visceral
- Exercise intolerance
- Severe weight loss and anorexia
- Diarrhea, vomiting, epistaxis, and melena—less common
- Dogs—lymphadenopathy; cutaneous lesions; emaciation; signs of renal failure (polyuria, polydipsia, vomiting) possible; neuralgia, polyarthritis, polymyositis, osteolytic lesions, and proliferative periostitis rare; about one-third of patients have fever and splenomegaly.

Cutaneous
- Hyperkeratosis—most prominent finding; excessive epidermal scale with thickening, depigmentation, and chapping of the muzzle and footpads
- Hair coat—dry; brittle; hair loss
- Dogs—intradermal nodules and ulcers may be seen; abnormally long or brittle nails are a specific finding in some patients.
- Cats—cutaneous nodules usually develop.

CAUSES & RISK FACTORS
- Travel to endemic regions (usually the Mediterranean), where dogs are exposed to infected sandflies
- Transfusion from infected animals can occur.
- Dog-to-dog transmission by direct contact can occur.

DIAGNOSIS

DIFFERENTIAL DIAGNOSIS
- Visceral—mycoses (blastomycosis, histoplasmosis); systemic lupus erythematosus; metastatic neoplasia; distemper; vasculitis
- Cutaneous—other causes of hyperkeratosis: primary idiopathic seborrhea and nutritional dermatoses (vitamin A responsive, zinc responsive); idiopathic nasodigital hyperkeratosis, lichenoid-psoriasiform dermatosis, epidermal dysplasia, and Schnauzer comedo syndrome are rare and breed-specific
- Skin biopsy—hyperkeratotic and nodular lesions; existence of organisms confirms diagnosis
- Hyperglobulinemia—differentiate from chronic ehrlichiosis and multiple myeloma

CBC/BIOCHEMISTRY/URINALYSIS
- Hyperproteinemia with hyperglobulinemia—100% of cases
- Hypoalbuminemia—95% of cases
- Proteinuria—85% of cases
- High liver enzyme activity—55% of cases
- Thrombocytopenia—50% of cases
- Azotemia—45% of cases
- Leukopenia with lymphopenia—20% of cases

OTHER LABORATORY TESTS
- Coombs, antinuclear antibody, and lupus erythematosus cell tests—sometimes positive
- Serologic diagnosis available

IMAGING
N/A

DIAGNOSTIC PROCEDURES
- Cultures—skin, spleen, bone marrow, or lymph node biopsies or aspirates; by the Center for Disease Control and Prevention
- Cytology and histopathology—identify intracellular organisms in biopsies or aspirate specimens (listed above)

PATHOLOGIC FINDINGS
- Cell infiltration (mainly histiocytes and macrophages) and characteristic intracellular amastigote forms—identified in many tissues: skin, lymph nodes, liver, spleen, and kidney
- Mucosal ulcerations—stomach, intestine, and colon, occasionally found

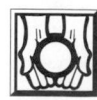

TREATMENT
- Outpatient
- Emaciated, chronically infected animals—consider euthanasia; prognosis very poor
- Diet—high-quality protein; special for renal insufficiency, if necessary
- Cats—single dermal nodule lesions are best surgically removed.
- Advise client of potential zoonotic transmission of organisms in lesions to humans.
- Inform client that organisms will never be eliminated, and relapse, requiring treatment, is inevitable.

MEDICATIONS

DRUG(S) OF CHOICE
- Sodium stibogluconate—available from the Center for Disease Control and Prevention; 30–50 mg/kg IV or SC q24h for 3–4 weeks
- Meglumine antimonate—100 mg/kg IV or SC q24h for 3–4 weeks
- Allopurinol—produces clinical cures but relapses occur. Best when used in combination with other drugs (meglumine or amphotericin B) as maintenance. Dose: 7 mg/kg PO q8h for 3 months, or 10 mg/kg/day PO for 2–24 months.
- Amphotericin B—0.5–0.8 mg/kg diluted in 50 mL dextrose 5% in water given IV over 1 min q48h for total dose of 8–15 mg/kg.

CONTRAINDICATIONS/POSSIBLE INTERACTIONS
- Seriously ill dogs—start antimonial drugs at lower doses
- Renal insufficiency—treat before giving antimonial drugs; prognosis depends on renal function at the onset of treatment

FOLLOW-UP
- Treatment efficacy—monitor by clinical improvement and identification of organisms in repeat biopsies
- Relapses—a few months to a year after therapy; recheck at least every 2 months after completion of treatment.
- Prognosis for a cure—very guarded

MISCELLANEOUS

Suggested Reading

Lindsay DS, Zajac AM, Barr SC. Canine leishmaniasis in American foxhounds: an emerging zoonosis? Comp Cont Ed Pract Vet 2002;24:304–312.

Author Stephen C. Barr

Consulting Editor Stephen C. Barr

BASICS

OVERVIEW
- Total dislocation of the lens from its normal location
- Anterior–forward through the pupil into the anterior chamber
- Posterior–into the posterior segment/vitreous chamber
- Occurs when the lens capsule separates 360° from the zonules that hold the lens in place
- Subluxation—partial separation of the lens from its zonular attachments; the lens remains in a normal or near-normal position in the pupil.
- Primary luxation—due to a pathologic alteration in the ciliary zonules including abnormal development or degeneration, usually inherited in dogs, often bilateral
- Congenital luxation—often associated with microphakia
- Secondary luxation–due to rupture or degeneration of the ciliary zonules as a result of chronic inflammation, buphthalmia, or intraocular neoplasia

SIGNALMENT
- Dogs–primary usually seen in adults (most 4–9 years), most commonly affected breeds: most Terrier breeds, Terrier mixed breeds, Tibetan terrier, Border collie, German shepherd dog, and some spaniels.
- Can also occur in older predisposed breeds presumably as a late-onset condition
- Dogs and cats—secondary; any age/breed

SIGNS
- Acute or chronically painful eye with episcleral injection and diffuse corneal edema, especially if glaucoma also present or anterior luxation
- Central corneal edema—may be caused by the lens touching the endothelium, resulting in mechanical disruption of endothelial cells
- Abnormally shallow or deep anterior chamber
- Iridodonesis (iris trembling); phacodonesis (lens trembling)
- Aphakic crescent (an area of pupil devoid of the lens)
- Malpositioned clear lens—sometimes observed in an otherwise asymptomatic eye

CAUSES & RISK FACTORS
- Primary—inheritance pattern uncertain
- Primary luxation and primary glaucoma—may occur simultaneously in some breeds (see under Signalment)
- Uveitis, especially chronic lens-induced uveitis
- Intraocular neoplasia—may physically luxate the lens or cause chronic inflammation leading to zonular degeneration
- Trauma—rarely causes a normal lens to luxate without signs of severe uveitis or hyphema

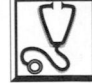

DIAGNOSIS

DIFFERENTIAL DIAGNOSIS
- Uveitis, glaucoma, and nodular granulomatous episclerokeratitis—also cause painful, red eyes with corneal edema and may be concurrent
- Buphthalmia may cause lens luxation; usually differentiated from primary lens luxation by history
- Corneal endothelial dystrophy or degeneration—may also cause corneal edema, making it difficult to see the intraocular structures; usually differentiated from primary lens luxation by history
- Diagnosis made by careful ophthalmic examination and history

CBC/BIOCHEMISTRY/URINALYSIS
Normal, unless sequela of a systemic disease that causes uveitis or dissemination of neoplasia

OTHER LABORATORY TESTS
N/A

IMAGING
- Thoracic radiographs and abdominal ultrasonography—may be indicated if secondary to intraocular neoplasia
- Ocular ultrasonography—useful if corneal edema or cloudy ocular media preclude examination and history
- Ultrasound biomicroscopy—in vivo examination of the anterior 4–5 mm of the globe, which includes microscopic resolution of the entire anterior segment, peripheral retina and some adnexa

DIAGNOSTIC PROCEDURES
Complete ophthalmic examination, including tonometry

TREATMENT
- Potentially visual eyes—best treated by removing the lens with or without sulcus intraocular lens prosthesis
- Occasionally topical miotic therapy can keep a posteriorly luxated lens behind the pupil and surgery can be prolonged
- Irreversibly blind eyes can be treated by enucleation or evisceration with intrascleral prosthesis; if secondary to neoplasia, enucleation is the best choice for therapeutic, and diagnostic purposes

MEDICATIONS

DRUG(S)
- Initiate the following medications, and if the eye has the potential for vision, refer the patient to a veterinary ophthalmologist immediately for intracapsular lens extraction.

- Topical miotic—prostaglandin analog (Xalatan, Lumigan, Travatan) q12h; indicated if the lens is primarily subluxated or posteriorly luxated; will lower IOP as well; lessens the chance of glaucoma and anterior luxation until intracapsular lens extraction can be performed
- If the pupil is blocked due to anterior lens luxation, tropicamide may allow the pupil to dilate, releasing the lens and relieving the pupillary block glaucoma; use with caution.
- Mannitol—1 g/kg IV over 20 min; indicated for high IOP (> 40 mm Hg)
- Carbonic anhydrase inhibitors— methazolamide (2–4 mg/kg PO q12h); initiated to reduce aqueous production
- Topical antiinflammatory—0.1% dexamethasone sodium phosphate (q6h)

CONTRAINDICATIONS/POSSIBLE INTERACTIONS
- Topical miotics—contraindicated if the lens is in the anterior chamber • Owner must verify location of lens prior to applying a miotic

FOLLOW-UP
- Medically treated primary posterior luxation—IOP rechecked 24 hr after starting treatment and frequently thereafter; once IOP is stable, reexamine patient at least quarterly; refer for evaluation as intracapsular lens extraction is also indicated for posterior luxations to decrease chance for retinal detachment and chronic uveitis
- Monitor for secondary glaucoma and retinal detachment
- If only one lens is involved at the time of examination, the other lens may eventually become involved.

MISCELLANEOUS

ABBREVIATION
IOP = intraocular pressure

Suggested Reading

Davidson MG, Nelms SR. Diseases of the lens and cataract formation. In: Gelatt KN, ed. Veterinary ophthalmology, 3rd ed. Philadelphia: Lippincott Williams & Wilkins, 1999:797–825.
Nasisse MP, Glover TL. Surgery for lens instability. Vet Clin North Am Small Anim Pract 1997;27:1175–1192.
Author Carmen Colitz
Consulting Editor Paul E. Miller

LEPTOSPIROSIS

 BASICS

DEFINITION

• Caused by pathogenic members of the genus *Leptospira* • Acute and chronic diseases of dogs (mainly nephritis and hepatitis) and other animals, including, although rarely, cats • Dogs—most disease caused by the serovars *L. grippotyphosa* and *L. pomona* • Vaccine (dogs)—contains the serovars *L. canicola* and *L. icterohaemorrhagiae;* promotes immunity to homologous serovars and protection from overt clinical disease; may not prevent colonization of the kidneys, resulting in a chronic carrier state; serovar specific; does not promote protection against other serovars present in nature

PATHOPHYSIOLOGY

• *Leptospira*—penetrate intact or cut skin or mucous membranes; rapidly invade bloodstream (4–7 days); spread to all parts of the body (2–4 days) • Invasion leads to fever, leukocytosis, transitory anemia (hemolysis), mild hemoglobinuria, and albuminuria. • Fever and bacteremia soon resolve. • Capillary and endothelial cell damage; occasionally results in petechial hemorrhages • Liver—hepatic necrosis and jaundice • Kidney—leptospiruria; *Leptospira* may localize in damaged renal tubules; organism replicates readily in tubular epithelial cell • Early serum antibodies appear • Death—usually a result of interstitial nephritis, vascular damage, and renal failure; may result from acute septicemia or DIC

SYSTEMS AFFECTED

Subacute to Acute/Severe Disease
• Renal/Urologic—focal interstitial nephritis; hemoglobinuric nephrosis; tubular damage/failure • Hepatobiliary—hepatitis; dysfunction; necrosis • Respiratory—vasculitis; interstitial pneumonia • Cardiovascular—endothelial cell damage; hemorrhage • Nervous—meningitis Chronic Disease • Renal/Urologic—chronic renal failure • Reproductive—abortion; weak puppies • Ophthalmic—anterior uveitis • Reproductive—*Salmonella typhimurium* and *Leptospira* linked to feline stillbirth

INCIDENCE/PREVALENCE

• Usually one or more serovars account for endemic disease in a geographic area. • *L. canicola* and *L. icterohaemorrhagiae*—usual serovars; clinical disease in dogs; *L. canicola* most common worldwide; *L. icterohaemorrhagiae* most common in Australia • *L. grippotyphosa* and *L. pomona* • *L. bratislava* becoming more prominent • Reported incidence (dogs)—falsely low; most infections are inapparent and remain undiagnosed • Prevalence (dogs)—city, 37.8%; suburban, 18.7%

GEOGRAPHIC DISTRIBUTION

• Worldwide, especially in warm, wet climates or seasons • Standing water and neutral or slightly alkaline soil promote presence in environment.

SIGNALMENT

Species
Dogs and rarely cats

Mean Age and Range
• Young dogs without passive maternal antibody—more likely to exhibit severe disease • Old dogs with adequate antibody titer levels—seldom exhibit clinical disease unless exposed to a serovar not in the vaccine

Predominant Sex
Traditionally, male dogs more commonly affected; disputed by recent reports

SIGNS

General Comments
• Vary with the age and immune status, environmental factors that affect leptospira survival, and virulence of the infecting serovar • Primary reservoir host—may spread particular serovar via urine shedding; may have no clinical signs or less severe disease (acute diffuse to chronic interstitial nephritis, e.g., *L. canicola* in dogs with relatively weak antibody response) • Incidental (accidental) host—acute severe disease (e.g., *L. icterohaemorrhagiae* in dogs with severe antibody response)

Historical Findings
Peracute to Subacute Disease
• Fever • Sore muscles • Stiffness • Shivering • Weakness • Anorexia • Depression • Vomiting • Rapid dehydration • Diarrhea—with or without blood • Icterus • Spontaneous cough • Difficulty breathing • PD-PU progressing to anuria • Bloody vaginal discharge • Death—without clinical signs
Chronic Disease
• No apparent illness • Fever of unknown origin • PD-PU—chronic renal failure

Physical Examination Findings
Peracute to Acute Disease
• Tachypnea • Rapid irregular pulse • Poor capillary perfusion • Hematemesis • Hematochezia • Melena • Epistaxis • Injected mucous membranes • Widespread petechial and ecchymotic hemorrhages • Reluctance to move, paraspinal hyperesthesia, stiff gait • Conjunctivitis • Rhinitis • Hematuria • Mild lymphadenopathy

CAUSES
• Dogs—*L. canicola, L. icterohaemorrhagiae, L. pomona, L. grippotyphosa, L. bratislava, L. copenhagenii, L. australis, L. autumnalis, L. ballum,* and *L. bataviae* • Cats—*L. canicola, L. grippotyphosa, L. pomona,* and *L. bataviae*

RISK FACTORS

Transmission
• Direct—host-to-host contact via infected urine, postabortion discharge, infected fetus/discharge, and sexual contact (semen) • Indirect—exposure (via urine) to a contaminated environment (vegetation, soil, food, water, bedding) under conditions in which *Leptospira* can survive • Disease agent—*Leptospira* serovar, each with its own virulence factors, infectious dose, and route of exposure

Host Factors
• Vaccine—protection is serovar-specific; prevents clinical disease as a result of homologous serovar; may not prevent kidney colonization and urine shedding; nonvaccine serovars may infect and cause disease in vaccinated host • Outdoor animals or hunting dogs—exposure of mucous membranes to water; exposure of abraded or water-softened skin increases risk of infection

Environmental Factors
• Warm and moist environment; wet season (high rainfall areas) of temperate regions; low-lying areas (marshy, muddy, irrigated); warm humid climates of tropical and subtropical regions • Temperature range—7–10°C (44.6–50°F) to 34–36°C (93–96°F) • Water—organism survives better in stagnant than in flowing water; neutral or slightly alkaline pH • Organism survives 180 days in wet soil and longer in standing water • Dense animal population—kennels and urban settings; increases chances of urine exposure • Exposure to rodents and other wildlife

 DIAGNOSIS

DIFFERENTIAL DIAGNOSIS
Subclinical infections and chronic carrier states generally go undetected.

Subacute to Acute Disease
• Dogs—heartworm disease; immune-mediated hemolytic anemia; bacteremia/septicemia (bite wound, prostatitis, endocarditis, dental disease); infectious canine hepatitis virus; canine herpesvirus; hepatic neoplasia; trauma; lupus; Rocky Mountain spotted fever; ehrlichiosis; toxoplasmosis; renal neoplasia; renal calculi • Cats—haemobartonellosis; drugs (acetaminophen); bacteremia/septicemia; FIV- and FeLV-associated diseases; cholangitis; toxoplasmosis; FIP; hepatic neoplasia; autoimmune disease (e.g., systemic lupus erythematosus); trauma; renal calculi; renal neoplasia

Reproductive/Neonatal Disease
• Dogs—brucellosis; distemper; herpes • Cats—FIP; FeLV; panleukopenia; herpesvirus; toxoplasmosis; salmonellosis

CBC/BIOCHEMISTRY/URINALYSIS
• PCV and total plasma solids—high owing to dehydration; rarely PCV low (hemolysis) • Leukocytosis with left shift—leukopenia initially during leptospiremic phase • Thrombocytopenia • Increased fibrin degradation products • BUN—high • Creatinine—high; mainly renal; depends on degree of renal failure • Electrolyte alterations—depend on degree of renal and gastrointestinal dysfunction • Hyponatremia • Hypochloremia • Hypokalemia—hyperkalemia with kidney failure • Hyperphosphatemia • Hypoalbuminemia • Acidosis—serum bicarbonate low • Alanine aminotransferase, aspartate aminotransferase, lactate dehydrogenase, and

alkaline phosphatase—high • Proteinuria
• Isosthenuria—acute renal failure

OTHER LABORATORY TESTS

Serology (Microscopic Agglutination Test)
• Test in acute stage and 3–4 weeks later (convalescent serum) • Unvaccinated patients—titers may be low initially (1:100–1:200); may be higher in the convalescent serum (1:800– 1:1600 or higher) if a homologous *Leptospira* serovar is tested • Vaccinated patients, older whole cell bacteria—expect high titers (up to 12–16 WBC post vaccination), then drop off to < 1:400; new subunit vaccine (*L. grippotyphosa, L. pomona*) titers rise to < 1:600 for less than 6 wk for serovars *L. canicola* and *L. icterohaemorrhagiae*; titers for other serovars are the same as for unvaccinated patients; run all serum samples at the same time, if possible

Darkfield Microscopy of Urine
• Often inconclusive • Difficult to read
• Requires fresh urine

Fluorescent Antibody Test of Urine
• More conclusive • *Leptospira* does not need to be viable; submit urine to laboratory on ice by overnight courier • Pretreat with furosemide 15 min before urine collection to increase success rate. • Correlate results with clinical history. • PCR—Promising but still experimental

Immunohistochemistry
• On fixed tissue

DIAGNOSTIC PROCEDURES
• Culture of body fluids antemortem (urine, blood, aqueous humor) and tissues postmortem (kidney, liver, fetus, placenta)—usually not practical because of the fastidiousness of *Leptospiras;* contact laboratory for the proper transport medium • Fluorescent antibody test—done on all tissues submitted for post-mortem workup, especially kidney and liver
• Special stains (Warthin-Starry silver stain)—attempt immunohistochemistry with monoclonal antibodies on formalin-fixed sections of kidney, liver, and fetal/placental tissue
• Polymerase chain reaction—some laboratories have developed protocols for both urine and tissue specimens

PATHOLOGIC FINDINGS
• Degree of kidney and liver disease depends on the serovar and the host's immunity • Cats—generally less severe lesions • Dogs (acute disease)—lungs may be edematous; kidneys pale and enlarged; liver enlarged and may be friable with multifocal necrosis and hemorrhage; gastrointestinal tract may hemorrhage

TREATMENT

APPROPRIATE HEALTH CARE
Acute severe disease—inpatient; extent of supportive therapy depends on severity; renal failure requires closely monitored diuresis.

NURSING CARE
• Depends on severity • Dehydration and shock—parenteral, balanced, polyionic, isotonic intravenous solution (lactated Ringer's)
• Severe hemorrhage—blood transfusion may be needed in association with treatment for DIC • Oliguria or anuria—initially rehydrate; then give intravenous osmotic diuretics or tubular diuretics; peritoneal dialysis may be necessary

ACTIVITY
Acutely ill and bacteremic/septicemic patients—restricted activity; cage rest; monitoring; and warmth

DIET
Severely ill patients—often anorexic, in shock, and lethargic; parenteral nutrition for prolonged anorexia

CLIENT EDUCATION
Inform client of zoonotic potential from contaminated urine of affected dogs and their environment.

MEDICATIONS

DRUG(S) OF CHOICE
• Procaine penicillin G—40,000–80,000 U/kg IM q24h or divided q12h until kidney function returns to normal • Dihydro-streptomycin—10–15 mg/kg IM q12h for 2 weeks to eliminate organism from kidney interstitial tissues; try streptomycin if no renal failure • Doxycycline—5 mg/kg PO or IV q12h for 2 weeks; use alone to clear both leptospiremia and leptospiruria

PRECAUTIONS
• Aminoglycoside—monitor patients with renal insufficiency carefully • Penicillins (dogs)—adjust doses with renal insufficiency

ALTERNATIVE DRUG(S)
• Ampicillin or amoxicillin—instead of penicillin • Erythromycin

FOLLOW-UP

PATIENT MONITORING
• Monitor kidney function, liver function, and electrolytes. • Monitor BUN, serum creatinine, and urine specific gravity in dogs with renal failure for indication of prognosis.

PREVENTION/AVOIDANCE
• Vaccines—vaccinate dogs per current label recommendations; bacteria-induced immunity lasts only 6–8 months and is serovar specific (no cross-protection outside of the serogroup); revaccination at least yearly; vaccinate dogs at risk (hunter, show dogs, dogs with access to water/ponds) every 4–6 months, especially in endemic areas • Kennels—strict sanitation to avoid contact with infected urine; control rodents; monitor and remove carrier dogs

until treated; isolate affected animals during treatment • Activity—limit access to marshy/muddy areas, ponds, low-lying areas with stagnant surface water, heavily irrigated pastures, and access to wildlife

POSSIBLE COMPLICATIONS
• DIC • Liver and kidney dysfunction may be permanent. • Uveitis and abortion sequelae

EXPECTED COURSE AND PROGNOSIS
• Most infections subclinical or chronic
• Prognosis guarded for acute severe disease

MISCELLANEOUS

AGE-RELATED FACTORS
Severe clinical disease in young dogs (nonvaccinated or lacking maternal antibody)

ZOONOTIC POTENTIAL
• High; organisms spread in urine of infected animals • Strict kennel hygiene and disinfection of premises (iodine-based disinfectant or stabilized bleach solutions) • Acutely infected and carrier animals must be treated.

PREGNANCY
• Possible abortion sequelae • Antimicrobial therapy—consider effect of drug on developing fetus.

SYNONYMS
In humans—Weil disease; swineherd disease; rice field disease; water-fever disease; cane-fever disease

ABBREVIATIONS
• BUN = blood urea nitrogen • DIC = disseminated intravascular coagulation
• FeLV = feline leukemia virus • FIP = feline infectious peritonitis • FIV = feline immunodeficiency virus • PCR = polymerase chain reaction • PCV = packed cell volume
• PD-PU = polydipsia and polyuria
• WBC = white blood cell

Suggested Reading
Baldwin CJ, Atkins CE. Leptospirosis in dogs. Compend Contin Educ Pract Vet 1987; 9:499–508.
Birnbaum N, Barr SC, Center SA, et al. Naturally acquired leptospirosis in 36 dogs: serological and clinicopathological features. J Small Anim Pract 1998;39:231–236.
Greene CE, Miller MA, Brown CA. Leptospirosis. In: Greene CE, ed. Infectious diseases of the dog and cat. Philadelphia: Saunders, 1998:273–281.
Heath SE, Johnson R. Leptospirosis. J Am Vet Med Assoc 1994;205:1518–1523.
Author Patrick L. McDonough
Consulting Editor Stephen C. Barr

LEUKEMIA, ACUTE LYMPHOBLASTIC

BASICS

OVERVIEW
• Lymphoproliferative disorder defined as the presence of circulating neoplastic prolymphocytes and lymphoblasts in the blood
• Patients have impaired humoral and cellular immunity.
• Characterized by bone marrow infiltration (and extramedullary sites) and displacement of normal hematopoietic stem cells
• May infiltrate other organs

SIGNALMENT
• Dogs—male to female ratio, 3:2; mean age, 6.2 years (range, 1–12 years)
• Rare in cats

SIGNS
• Often nonspecific
• Large liver and spleen
• Lymphadenomegaly
• Petechial or ecchymotic hemorrhages
• Other—reflect specific organ infiltration; any organ may be involved

CAUSES & RISK FACTORS
• Dogs—ionizing radiation; oncogenic viruses; chemical agents suspected but unproved
• Cats—FeLV infection

DIAGNOSIS

DIFFERENTIAL DIAGNOSIS
• Acute or chronic infection—toxoplasmosis; canine distemper; ehrlichiosis
• Aplastic anemia
• Metastatic neoplasia
• Multicentric lymphosarcoma—with acute lymphoblastic leukemia, only moderately large peripheral lymph nodes, marked splenomegaly, and signs of systemic illness with relatively acute onset. Note: may be difficult to differentiate.
• Other leukemias and myeloproliferative disorders

CBC/BIOCHEMISTRY/URINALYSIS
• CBC—normocytic, normochromic, nonregenerative anemia; thrombocytopenia; lymphoblastosis; leukocytosis or leukopenia
• Serum chemistry profile—high liver enzyme activities

OTHER LABORATORY TESTS
• Cytologic examination (bone marrow or core biopsies)—lymphoblastic infiltration with low numbers of myeloid and erythroid precursors and low numbers of megakaryocytes
• Immunohistochemical or enzymatic biochemical studies—may be needed to differentiate from other types of leukemia

IMAGING
Plain film radiography and ultrasound—often reveal hepatomegaly and splenomegaly

DIAGNOSTIC PROCEDURES
Bone marrow biopsy

TREATMENT
• Usually outpatient, unless supportive care required
• Patients are immunocompromised and should not be exposed to infectious disease.
• Transfusions—as indicated, to restore RBCs, platelets, or coagulation factors

MEDICATIONS

DRUG(S)
• Combination chemotherapy—prednisone (20 mg/m^2 PO q12h) and vincristine (0.7 mg/m^2 IV weekly); may result in partial or short-lived complete remission
• Cytosine arabinoside (400 mg/m^2 weekly); administer as constant rate infusion over 6–8 hours

CONTRAINDICATIONS/POSSIBLE INTERACTIONS
Chemotherapy may have toxic side effects; seek advice before starting treatment if you are unfamiliar with cytotoxic drugs.

FOLLOW-UP
• Monitor peripheral blood count and bone marrow—judge success and toxicity of treatment
• Hemorrhage from thrombocytopenia—major cause of death in dogs
• Prognosis grave

MISCELLANEOUS

PREGNANCY
Chemotherapy—contraindicated in pregnant animals

ABBREVIATION
FeLV = feline leukemia virus

Suggested Reading
Hamilton TA. The leukemias. In: Morrison WB, ed. Cancer in dogs and cats: medical and surgical management. Baltimore: Williams & Wilkins, 1998:721–729.
Reagan WJ, DeNicola DB. Myeloproliferative and lymphoproliferative disorders. In: Morrison WB, ed. Cancer in dogs and cats: medical and surgical management. Baltimore: Williams & Wilkins, 1998:95–122.
Author Linda S. Fineman
Consulting Editor Wallace B. Morrison

BASICS

OVERVIEW
• Rare, lymphoproliferative disorder
• Circulating neoplastic lymphocytes that are mature and well differentiated
• May note impaired humoral and cellular immunity
• Systems affected—hematopoietic, lymphatic, and integument

SIGNALMENT
• Dogs and cats
• Dogs—mean age, 9.4 years (range, 3–15 years); male to female ratio, 2:1

SIGNS
• Nonspecific
• Polydipsia and polyuria
• Lymphadenomegaly
• Lameness
• Fever
• Bruising

CAUSES & RISK FACTORS
Ionizing radiation, oncogenic viruses, and chemical agents—suspected but unproved

DIAGNOSIS

DIFFERENTIAL DIAGNOSIS
• Lymphosarcoma—may have a leukemic phase
• Immune-mediated hematologic diseases
• Ehrlichiosis

CBC/BIOCHEMISTRY/URINALYSIS
• Mild to moderate normocytic, normochromic anemia
• Normal to low platelet count
• Lymphocytosis—range, 5,000>100,000 cells/μL
• Normal to mildly high serum globulins
• May see high ALP

OTHER LABORATORY TESTS
• Cytologic examination (bone marrow aspirate or core biopsy)—shows high numbers of mature lymphocytes; crowding out of normal cell lines in advanced stages
• Serum protein electrophoresis—detects monoclonal spikes (usually IgM) in about 50% of patients
• Bence Jones proteinuria—about 50% of patients
• Direct Coombs test—may be positive with secondary immune-mediated hemolytic anemia

IMAGING
Radiography and ultrasonography—may reveal cranial organomegaly or internal lymphadenomegaly

DIAGNOSTIC PROCEDURES
Bone marrow biopsy

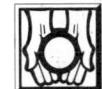

TREATMENT
• Usually outpatients
• Splenectomy—rarely indicated with secondary, immune-mediated hemolytic anemia or thrombocytopenia or if hypersplenism cannot be controlled medically
• Treatment advised only when patient is symptomatic.

MEDICATIONS

DRUG(S)
• Chlorambucil—0.2 mg/kg PO q24h for 7 days; then 0.1 mg/kg q24h to effect or 6 mg/m^2 PO eod (dogs); 2 mg q3–4 days (cats)
• Prednisone—20 mg/m^2 PO q12h; in combination with chlorambucil

CONTRAINDICATIONS/POSSIBLE INTERACTIONS
Chemotherapy—myelosuppression; may need to alter dosage, depending on neutrophil and platelet counts

FOLLOW-UP
• Periodic cytologic examination of bone marrow—response to treatment and disease progression
• Biweekly examination of CBC—response to treatment and disease progression
• Variable course, but progressive
• Severe hemolytic anemia and pneumonia may cause death.

MISCELLANEOUS

PREGNANCY
Chemotherapy contraindicated in pregnant animals.

ABBREVIATION
ALP = alkaline phosphatase

Suggested Reading
Hamilton TA. The leukemias. In: Morrison WB, ed. Cancer in dogs and cats: medical and surgical management. Baltimore: Williams & Wilkins, 1998:721–729.
Reagan WJ, DeNicola DB. Myeloproliferative and lymphoproliferative disorders. In: Morrison WB, ed. Cancer in dogs and cats: medical and surgical management. Baltimore: Williams & Wilkins, 1998:95–122.
Author Linda S. Fineman
Consulting Editor Wallace B. Morrison

LEUKOENCEPHALOMYELOPATHY IN ROTTWEILERS

BASICS

OVERVIEW
• A progressive, degenerative, demyelinating disease primarily affecting the cervical spinal cord in rottweilers
• Occurs worldwide
• Probably inherited

SIGNALMENT
• Dogs
• Rottweilers—either sex; 1.5–3.5 years old at onset

SIGNS
• No history of injury or illness
• Owners do not report discomfort.
• Insidious, progressive onset
• Proprioceptive ataxia and upper motor neuron weakness involving all four limbs; proprioceptive positioning postural reaction disappears as the disease progresses
• Spinal reflexes normal to exaggerated
• Crossed extensor reflexes in all four limbs in later stages

CAUSES & RISK FACTORS
Unknown; possibly a myelinolytic disease

DIAGNOSIS

DIFFERENTIAL DIAGNOSIS
• Neuroaxonal dystrophy and distal sensorimotor polyneuropathy—neurologic disorders in rottweilers; differentiated on the basis of neurologic deficits; neuroaxonal dystrophy: deficits relate to the cerebellum; distal sensorimotor polyneuropathy: tetraparesis associated with lower motor neuron signs

• Diskospondylitis, fracture or luxation, and intervertebral disk disease—neck pain; disk disease rarely seen in large-breed dogs at a young age
• Cervical vertebral instability (wobbler)—differentiate on the basis of spinal survey and myelographic studies; stenosis of the vertebral canal
• Canine distemper virus or other inflammatory cause of myelitis—progresses faster; CSF analysis abnormal
• Spinal cord tumors—old dogs; myelography reveals spinal cord compression

CBC/BIOCHEMISTRY/URINALYSIS
Normal

OTHER LABORATORY TESTS
N/A

IMAGING
Spinal cervical survey radiographs normal

DIAGNOSTIC PROCEDURES
• CSF analysis normal
• Myelography normal

PATHOLOGIC FINDINGS
• Widespread demyelination in brain stem, caudal cerebellar peduncles, pyramids, optic nerves, optic tracts, and extending into the thoracic spinal cord; most severe lesion in midcervical spinal cord
• Lesions bilateral with some asymmetry

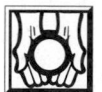

TREATMENT
• Outpatient, unless the severity of neurologic deficits precludes nursing care at home
• Activity—whatever can be tolerated
• Diet—ensure proper intake of food; patient may have difficulty reaching the feeding area.
• Neurologic status—slowly and progressively deteriorates; eventually, the patient is unable to walk or get up

MEDICATIONS

DRUG(S)
None available

CONTRAINDICATIONS/POSSIBLE INTERACTIONS
N/A

FOLLOW-UP
• Neurologic examination—monitor monthly to assess progression
• Avoid bed sores and urine and fecal scalding by keeping the patient on a clean, dry, and cushioned pad (e.g., synthetic sheepskin).
• Severe tetraparesis—within 6–12 months after onset of clinical signs
• Euthanasia—because of severe debility

MISCELLANEOUS

ABBREVIATION
CSF = cerebrospinal fluid

Suggested Reading
Wouda W, van Nes JJ. Progressive ataxia due to central demyelination in rottweiler dogs. Vet Q 1986;8:89–97.
Author Joane M. Parent
Consulting Editor Joane M. Parent

L-FORM BACTERIAL INFECTIONS

 BASICS

OVERVIEW
Caused by bacterial variants with defective or absent cell walls

L-Form Bacteria
• Isolated from humans, animals, and plants
• Named for Lister Institute (London), where discovered in 1935
• Differ from the mycoplasma by lack of sterols in their membranes (similar to bacteria)
• Soft, fragile, pleomorphic, spherical, and osmotically fragile; structurally equivalent to protoplasts and spheroplasts, which cannot divide
• Can grow and replicate by cell fission in an irregular manner, yielding daughter cells that differ in size, nucleic acid content, and amount of cytoplasm
• Formed as spontaneous variant of bacteria or when cell wall synthesis is inhibited or impaired by antibiotics (e.g., penicillin), specific immunoglobulins, or lysosomal enzymes that degrade cell walls
• Can be induced from virtually all gram-positive and -negative bacteria under suitable conditions
• May revert to normal cell wall strain in a suitable host or favorable medium
• Usually no pathogenicity

SIGNALMENT
• Sporadic in cats and dogs
• Most common in free-roaming cats of all ages

SIGNS
• Dogs—arthritis
• Cats—penetrating wound (usually cat bite); infected surgical site; cellulitis; fever; arthritis; synovitis

CAUSES & RISK FACTORS
• Bites, scratches, or trauma may allow organism to enter skin and subcutaneous tissue.
• Environmental reservoir unknown
• Formation encouraged by antibiotic treatment of host, resistance of host, suitability of in vivo site for establishment of infective locus, and relatively low to moderate virulence of the infecting bacterium
• Greatly reduced infectivity but may revert and display the pathogenic properties of the original bacterium

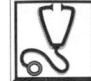 DIAGNOSIS

DIFFERENTIAL DIAGNOSIS
• Mycoplasma—differentiate by phase microscopy, by electron microscopy, or by measuring penicillin-binding proteins
• Suppurative skin infections caused by mycobacteria, yeast, or fungi
• Arthritis caused by immune-mediated disease, bacteria, spirochetes, mycoplasma, rickettsia, chlamydia, viruses, or fungus

CBC/BIOCHEMISTRY/URINALYSIS
• Neutrophilia with left shift
• Monocytosis
• Lymphocytosis
• Eosinophilia
• Mild normochromic, normocytic anemia
• High serum total protein

OTHER LABORATORY TESTS
• Cytology—exudate from draining lesions contains macrophages and neutrophils.
• Joint fluid—high neutrophil count
• Culture—difficult; requires special media (Hayflick); "fried-egg" appearance of colonies on solid agar (center portion embedded in agar; thin vacuolated growth on agar surface)
• Light microscopy—difficult to demonstrate
• Electron microscopy—may show characteristic pleomorphic, cell wall–deficient organisms in phagocytes
• Precise characterization and speciation—the organism must revert to the parental cell-walled state (may take years).

IMAGING
Radiographs—periarticular soft tissue swelling; periosteal proliferation

DIAGNOSTIC PROCEDURES
N/A

PATHOLOGIC FINDINGS
• Biopsy—pyogenic cellulitis; panniculitis; chronic pyogranulomatous arthritis; tenosynovitis
• Stains—neither conventional (H&E) nor specialized (gram, acid-fast, silver, PAS) reveal organisms

 TREATMENT

• Gentle cleaning degrades fragile organisms.
• Allow open wounds to heal by secondary intention.

 MEDICATIONS

DRUG(S)
• Variable antibiotic sensitivity
• Tetracycline—22 mg/kg PO q8h for at least 1 week after signs disappear
• Fever usually breaks within 24–48 hr.
• β-lactam antibiotics—inhibit cell wall synthesis; not effective

CONTRAINDICATIONS/POSSIBLE INTERACTIONS
N/A

 FOLLOW-UP

Arthritic changes persistent

 MISCELLANEOUS

• Public health significance unknown
• Ubiquitous; therefore, role in disease questioned

ABBREVIATIONS
• H&E = hematoxylin and eosin
• PAS = periodic acid–Schiff

Suggested Reading
Carro T. L-forms and mycoplasmal infections. In: August JR, ed. Consultations in feline internal medicine. 2nd ed. Philadelphia: Saunders, 1994:13–20.
Author J. Paul Woods
Consulting Editor Stephen C. Barr

LILY POISONING

 BASICS

OVERVIEW
• Plants in the *Lilium* and *Hemerocallis* genera—widely used ornamental plants; very toxic to cats; Easter lilies, tiger lilies, Japanese show lilies, rubrum lilies, numerous *Lilium* hybrids, and day lilies
• Ingestion of leaves or flowers—results in a severe nephrotoxic syndrome; as little as 2–3 leaves reported to be lethal
• Toxic principle(s) not elucidated

SIGNALMENT
• Cats—systemic poisoning
• Dogs—only mild gastrointestinal upset, even after ingestion of large quantities of plant material
• No age or breed predilections noted

SIGNS
• Sudden onset of vomiting—gradually subsides within 2–4 hr
• Depression and anorexia—onset about the same time as vomiting; persist throughout the syndrome
• Polyuria and dehydration—by 12–24 hr; lead to anuric renal failure
• Vomiting—recurs by 36 hr; accompanied by progressive weakness
• Recumbency—by 3–4 days
• Death—by 4–7 days postingestion

CAUSES & RISK FACTORS
• Plants—Easter lilies; tiger lilies; Asiatic hybrid lilies; Japanese show lilies; *Lilium* hybrids; day lilies; primarily when used in cut-flower arrangement or as household potted plants
• All ingestions by cats of plant material from the *Lilium* and *Hemerocallis* genera should be considered potentially toxic.
• Indoor cats—exclusively predisposed to ingestion of newly introduced plants

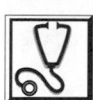 DIAGNOSIS

DIFFERENTIAL DIAGNOSIS
Nephrotoxins
• Aspirin and other NSAIDs
• Zinc
• Boric acid
• Ethylene glycol
• Mercury
• Nephrotoxic antibacterials—aminoglycosides

Systemic Diseases
• Acute chronic renal failure
• Urinary obstruction
• Immune-mediated renal disease
• Leptospirosis
• Pyelonephritis
• Lymphosarcoma

CBC/BIOCHEMISTRY/URINALYSIS
• Stress leukogram
• Moderate to severely high BUN, phosphate, and potassium
• Creatinine—severe increase common; usually 15–29 mg/dl; may be into the 40s
• Increased AST, ALT, and ALP late in disease
• Severe proteinuria, glucosuria, low specific gravity, and numerous tubular epithelial casts
• Crystalluria—not caused by ingestion of these plants

OTHER LABORATORY TESTS
N/A

IMAGING
N/A

DIAGNOSTIC PROCEDURES
If possible, examine plant to verify that it has been chewed

PATHOLOGIC FINDINGS
• Gross—swollen kidneys; empty gastrointestinal tract; moderate to severe perirenal edema
• Histologic—severe acute renal tubular necrosis with intact basement membranes; mild to severe interstitial edema; severe cast formation in the collecting ducts; may note evidence of mitotic figures in the remaining tubular epithelium

 TREATMENT

• Early decontamination—lessens duration and severity of signs
• Fluid therapy—initiation within 24 hr of ingestion prevents anuric renal failure; intravenous normal saline at two to three times maintenance for 24 hr
• Anuric renal failure—peritoneal dialysis only treatment; 7 days of therapy has returned renal function

 MEDICATIONS

DRUG(S)
• Decontamination—activated charcoal (2 g/kg)
• Cathartic—sorbitol (2.1 g/kg) or magnesium sulfate (0.5 g/kg)

CONTRAINDICATIONS/POSSIBLE INTERACTIONS
• Avoid fluids containing potassium.
• Avoid drugs eliminated by renal clearance.
• Diuretics (mannitol, hypertonic fluids, furosemide, thiazides)—not effective at initiating urine production

 FOLLOW-UP

• Successful prevention of anuric renal failure or after peritoneal dialysis—periodically follow serum chemistries to ensure normal renal function

EXPECTED COURSE AND PROGNOSIS
• Dehydration—from polyuric renal failure; required for the disease to progress to anuria

 MISCELLANEOUS

SEE ALSO
• Poisoning (Intoxication)
• Renal Failure, Acute

ABBREVIATIONS
• ALP = alkaline phosphatase
• ALT = alanine aminotransferase
• AST = aspartate aminotransferase
• BUN = blood urea nitrogen

Suggested Reading
Groff RM, Miller JM, Stair EL, et al. Toxicoses and toxins. In: Norsworthy GD, ed. Feline practice. Philadelphia: Lippincott, 1993:551–569.
Author Jeffery O. Hall
Consulting Editor Gary D. Osweiller

BASICS

OVERVIEW
Lipomas are benign tumors of adipocytes (fat cells). They are reported to occur in about 16% of dogs and 12% of cats; however, their true incidence is probably higher, since many lipomas are diagnosed by clinical appearance without histology. This tumor may occur anywhere on the body, although the subcutaneous areas of the chest, abdomen, limbs, and axillae may be most commonly affected. Lipomas have also been reported within the chest and abdominal cavities, uterus, vagina, and vulva.

SIGNALMENT
• Most common in middle-aged to older dogs; rarely seen in cats
• There is no breed predisposition, although Labrador retrievers, Doberman pinschers, miniature schnauzers, cocker spaniels, dachshunds, and Weimaraners have been reported to be at increased risk.
• Obese animals may be more susceptible.
• Female dogs are predisposed.
• Lipomas in cats may occur more frequently in neutered males.

SIGNS
• Usually solitary, but multiple lipomas may occur in the same individual
• Variable size, shape (often round), and growth rate (usually slow)
• Animals are often not symptomatic unless the mass becomes large enough to cause functional difficulties. Lipomas enlarge by expansion and not invasion. They may compress adjacent organs when they occur in the thoracic or abdominal cavity.
• Lipomas usually feel soft, but those that develop between muscle planes may feel firm and may be mistaken for infiltrative lipomas or soft tissue sarcomas. The caudal thigh region is a common place for intermuscular lipomas (between the semimembranosus and semitendinosus muscles).
• In many cases, the tumor is present for a long period of time (one year or more) before presentation to a veterinarian.

CAUSES & RISK FACTORS
Unknown

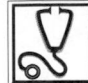

DIAGNOSIS

DIFFERENTIAL DIAGNOSIS
• Hemangiopericytoma
• Infiltrative lipoma
• Liposarcoma or other soft tissue sarcomas (e.g., myxosarcoma, fibrosarcoma)
• Mast cell tumor

CBC/BIOCHEMISTRY/URINALYSIS
Normal

OTHER LABORATORY TESTS
N/A

IMAGING
Radiography—reveals fat density tissue/mass surrounded by soft tissue density structures

DIAGNOSTIC PROCEDURES
Fine-needle aspiration cytology—reveals normal, mature adipocytes; fat tends to coalesce into droplets that wash off the slide during staining, leaving a fairly acellular specimen

PATHOLOGIC FINDINGS
Histologically consistent with normal adipose tissue, which may be subclassified if other tissue elements are present, e.g., cartilage (chondrolipoma), blood vessels (angiolipoma), or collagen (fibrolipoma); no tumor infiltration into surrounding structures (e.g., muscle)

TREATMENT
• Surgical excision is curative as these tumors are well encapsulated.
• Intermuscular lipomas of the caudal thigh region extend deep between muscle planes but do not invade adjacent structures; successful outcome with surgical removal
• Intralesional injection of 10% calcium chloride has been reported but is not recommended due to local irritation and tissue necrosis.

MEDICATIONS

DRUG(S)
Medical therapy is unnecessary and unlikely to be effective.

CONTRAINDICATIONS/POSSIBLE INTERACTIONS
N/A

FOLLOW-UP

PATIENT MONITORING
Have owner monitor for recurrence, which is rare and may be addressed successfully with a second surgery. If tumor recurs, consider the possibility of an infiltrative lipoma or soft tissue sarcoma.

PREVENTION/AVOIDANCE
No specific preventive measures, except possibly avoidance of obesity. Obesity may exacerbate the condition rather than promote lipoma development.

POSSIBLE COMPLICATIONS
N/A

EXPECTED COURSE AND PROGNOSIS
Cure with surgical excision is expected. Surgery is best performed before the tumor interferes with function or mobility. Development of other primary lipomas in other locations may occur.

MISCELLANEOUS

ASSOCIATED CONDITIONS
Possibly obesity

AGE-RELATED FACTORS
No specific factors, except age-related predisposition to tumor development

PREGNANCY
Surgery can likely be delayed until after whelping.

SEE ALSO
Lipoma, Infiltrative

ABBREVIATIONS
N/A

Suggested Reading
Thomas RC, Fox LE. Tumors of the skin and subcutis. In: Morrison WB, ed. Cancer in dogs and cats: medical and surgical management. Baltimore: Williams & Wilkins, 1998:500.
Author Anthony J. Mutsaers
Consulting Editor Wallace B. Morrison

LIPOMA, INFILTRATIVE

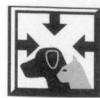

BASICS

OVERVIEW
• Invasive, nonencapsulated, lipoma variant that does not metastasize
• A benign neoplasm that infiltrates soft tissues, particularly muscles, and including fasciae, tendons, nerves, blood vessels, salivary glands, lymph nodes, and joint capsules, and occasionally bones
• Muscle infiltration typically extensive
• Surgical cures difficult to obtain
• Occurs much less frequently than does lipoma

SIGNALMENT
• Usually middle-aged dogs
• Cats—one report; extremely rare
• Labrador retrievers—possibly over-represented
• No breed predilection definitively demonstrated
• May be more common in females than in males

SIGNS
• Large, diffuse, soft tissue mass
• Clinically appears as localized muscle swelling
• Infiltration of pelvic, thigh, shoulder, sternal, and lateral cervical musculature—most common; recent evidence suggests no clear site prediction.

CAUSES & RISK FACTORS
Unknown

DIAGNOSIS

DIFFERENTIAL DIAGNOSIS
• Soft tissue sarcoma, particularly liposarcoma, hemangiopericytoma, myxosarcoma, rhabdomyosarcoma, and fibrosarcoma
• Lipoma
• Intermuscular lipoma
• Mast cell neoplasia

CBC/BIOCHEMISTRY/URINALYSIS
Normal

OTHER LABORATORY TESTS
N/A

IMAGING
• Radiography—reveals fat dense tissue between soft tissue dense structures
• CT imaging—allows adequate discrimination of tumor for radiation treatment planning; however, differentiation of normal fat from infiltrative lipoma can be problematic.

DIAGNOSTIC PROCEDURES
Cytologic examination of aspirate—reveals mature adipocytes

PATHOLOGIC FINDINGS
• Histologic examination—well-differentiated adipocytes; may be indistinguishable from normal adipose tissue
• Distinctive feature—tumor infiltration into and between muscle bundles

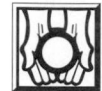

TREATMENT

Surgery
• Characteristic invasiveness makes excision extremely difficult; difficult to distinguish between tumor and normal adipose tissue
• Poorly defined tumor margins—may contribute to the observed high recurrence rate after surgical excision
• 36–50% of patients have recurrence within 3–16 months, except with limb amputation for appendicular tumor.
• Amputation of an affected limb—recommended only when quality of life is affected; tumor causes little inconvenience unless it interferes with movement, causes pressure-related pain, or develops in a vitally important anatomic site. Amputation also recommended before growth of proximal extent of tumor crosses attainable surgical margin

External Beam Radiotherapy
• Beneficial for long-term tumor control—median survival 40 months in a retrospective study of 13 dogs, with only 1 dog (7.7%) euthanized owing to tumor-related signs (vs. 26.7% with surgery alone)
• Dogs with measurable disease may only have stabilization of the tumor.
• Cytoreductive surgery for microscopic disease prior to radiation may result in long-term disease control.
• Unlikely to kill mitotically inactive mature adipocytes but may inhibit progressive infiltration by damaging tumor microcirculation

MEDICATIONS

DRUG(S)
Chemotherapy—partial response observed after doxorubicin administration in one dog

CONTRAINDICATIONS/POSSIBLE INTERACTIONS
N/A

FOLLOW-UP
• Focus—whether and when to recommend surgery and adjunctive radiation therapy for incomplete surgical margins
• Re-evaluations—schedule as dictated by tumor growth and choice of therapy

POSSIBLE COMPLICATIONS
Temporary acute side effects (e.g., moist dermatitis and alopecia) expected with radiation therapy

MISCELLANEOUS

SYNONYMS
• Lipomatosis
• Well-differentiated liposarcoma

SEE ALSO
Lipoma

Suggested Reading
McEntee MC, Page RL, Mauldin GN, et al. Results of irradiation of infiltrative lipoma in 13 dogs. Vet Radiol Ultrasound 2000; 41:554–556.

Acknowledgment
The author and editors acknowledge the prior contributions of Dr. James Thompson, who authored this topic in the previous edition.
Author Anthony J. Mutsaers
Consulting Editor Wallace B. Morrison

BASICS

OVERVIEW
• *Platynosomum concinnum* infection occurs in cats in Florida, Hawaii, and many other tropical areas • Infestation acquired from ingestion of an infected intermediate host, usually a lizard or frog • In endemic areas, 15%–85% of cats are infected.

SIGNALMENT
The typical patient is a young (6–24 months) feral cat with access to local fauna.

SIGNS
• Depend on severity of infection • Most affected cats have no clinical signs • Jaundice • Emaciation • Anorexia • Mucoid diarrhea • Hepatomegaly • Abdominal distention • Vomiting • Malaise

CAUSES & RISK FACTORS
• *P. concinnum*—adults normally reside in the bile ducts and gallbladder; life cycle requires two intermediate hosts and tropical or semitropical climate • Embryonated eggs—passed in the cat's feces, ingested by first intermediate host: a land snail • Miracidia—hatch from eggs in the snail; penetrate host tissues; change into sporocysts • Mature daughter sporocysts—emerge from the snail; ingested by the second intermediate host: usually an anole lizard (but also ingested by skinks, geckos, frogs, and toads); enter bile ducts and reside there until host is ingested by the cat • Cercariae—released in the upper digestive tract of cat; migrate to the bile ducts; mature and shed eggs in about 8 weeks • Risk factors for infection—tropical or subtropical climate; existence of intermediate hosts; an outdoor or indoor/outdoor environment; successful hunting skills; consumption of infected intermediate host

 DIAGNOSIS

DIFFERENTIAL DIAGNOSIS
• Cholangiohepatitis; hepatic lipidosis; bile duct carcinoma; hepatic lymphoma and any disorder causing major bile duct occlusion • Differentiated by examination of cytologic specimens from hepatic or bile aspirates; most definitively from histopathology of biopsied liver tissue; diagnoses also made by examining feces and finding trematode eggs

CBC/BIOCHEMISTRY/URINALYSIS
• CBC—various; usually circulating eosinophilia beginning 3 weeks after infection; persists for months • Biochemistry—High liver enzyme activities, especially ALT and AST; ALP may be normal or only slightly high • Bilirubin—increased; markedly high in advanced severe disease • Urinalysis—bilirubinuria

OTHER LABORATORY TESTS
• Fasting/postprandial bile acid—increased • Fecal examination—definitive diagnostic test; identification of *P. concinnum* eggs • Technique—sedimentation most successful; formalin-ether or sodium acetate most reliable (demonstrates eight times more eggs than direct fecal examination); fecal eggs detected in only 25% of cats • Patients with few parasites (one to five flukes)—may shed only 2–10 eggs/g of feces; may not discover eggs by fecal testing • Serial examinations—may be necessary

IMAGING
• Abdominal radiography—not helpful for diagnosis; may show mild hepatomegaly • Abdominal ultrasonography—differentiates biliary obstruction from hepatocellular disease; shows one or more of the following: (1) biliary obstruction: dilated gallbladder, common bile duct (> 2 mm), and intrahepatic ducts; (2) gallbladder sediment with flukes (oval hypoechoic structures with an echoic center), mildly thick gallbladder wall with a double-layered appearance (cholecystitis); (3) overall hypoechoic hepatic parenchyma with prominent hyperechoic portal areas (ducts) associated with cholangiohepatitis

DIAGNOSTIC PROCEDURES
• Liver biopsy—reveals signs of infection • Cholecystocentesis—reveals fluke eggs

PATHOLOGIC FINDINGS
• Gross—liver may appear large, yellow-green discolored, with dilated bile ducts; may see flukes in bile ducts or gallbladder; increased size and tortuosity of bile ducts on cut section • Histopathologic—depends on the number of flukes and duration of infestation; early (4–6 weeks): enlarged bile ducts and periductal areas infiltrated with inflammatory cells, especially eosinophils; middle (by 4 months): severe adenomatous hyperplasia of bile duct epithelium and coincident periductal inflammation; late (by 6 months): extensive peribiliary fibrous connective tissue that may cause bile duct stenosis

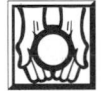 TREATMENT

Outpatient versus inpatient—depends on severity of illness

Inpatient
• Balanced polyionic solution with supplemental potassium chloride—20–40 mEq/L; as appropriate; based on serum electrolytes • Nutritional support—important to avoid development of hepatic lipidosis; feed high-protein canned food; ensure food intake; if cat is anorectic, use feeding tube (nasogastric initially, place esophageal or gastrostomy once condition stable); in cats with severe clinical signs, partial parenteral nutrition (not > 5 days) or total parenteral nutrition may be necessary; rarely, hepatic encephalopathy develops, necessitating protein restriction • B vitamin supplementation—important for anorectic and ill cats on fluid therapy; 2 mL B-soluble vitamins/L fluids

 MEDICATIONS

DRUG(S)
• Praziquantel—20 mg/kg SC q24h for 3–5 days; treatment of choice; eggs may pass in feces for up to 2 months after treatment • Prednisolone—initial dose for cats showing eosinophilia: 2.0 mg/kg/day for 2–4 weeks; then taper in 50% decrements every 2 weeks • Ursodeoxycholic acid—10–15 mg/kg PO • Broad-spectrum antibiotic coverage to protect from retrograde biliary tree infection with enteric organisms introduced by parasite; growth permissively encouraged by parasite death in tissues • Antioxidant therapy—suggested by necroinflammatory tissue injury; vitamin E (10 IU/kg daily) and S-adenosylmethionine (20 mg/kg PO daily, enteric coated tablets), until liver enzymes normalize • Antiemetics—for vomiting; e.g., metoclopramide (0.2–0.5 mg/kg PO or SC q6–8h or by CRI)

CONTRAINDICATIONS
Pregnancy—use caution with drug use.

 FOLLOW-UP

PATIENT MONITORING
• Monitor clinical signs, appetite, body condition and weight, liver enzymes, bilirubin, and fecal sedimentation. • Watch for signs of biliary tree occlusion after administration of praziquantel.

PREVENTION/AVOIDANCE
• Restrict outdoor access. • Praziquantel prophylaxis—every 3 months; may be required for outdoor cats in endemic, tropical climates

POSSIBLE COMPLICATIONS
• Death from liver failure; untreated symptomatic disease • Biliary tree obstruction • Pancreatitis (rare) • Pancreatic exocrine insufficiency—with chronic infection • Cholangitis/cholangiohepatitis (suppurative or nonsuppurative)

EXPECTED COURSE AND PROGNOSIS
Uncomplicated recovery in most patients treated

 MISCELLANEOUS

ZOONOTIC POTENTIAL N/A

SEE ALSO
• Bile Duct Obstruction • Cholangitis/Cholangiohepatitis Syndrome

Suggested Reading
Tams TR. Hepatobiliary parasites. In: Sherding RG, ed. The cat: disease and management. Philadelphia: Saunders, 1994: 607–611.

Authors Colin F. Burrows & Julie Corbet Pembleton

Consulting Editor Sharon A. Center

LIZARD VENOM TOXICITY

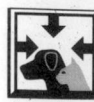

BASICS

OVERVIEW
• Poisonous lizards—found only in the U.S. Southwest and Mexico; *Heloderma suspectum* (Gila monster) and *H. horridum* (Mexican beaded lizard); tenacious bite; deliver venom from glands on the lower jaw by aggressive chewing action over grooved teeth; non-aggressive; animal envenomations rare
• Venom components—less well-characterized than other venoms; no evidence of altered coagulation in the victim

SIGNALMENT
Dogs and cats

SIGNS

Historical Findings
• Sudden onset of pain
• Bite—usually on the face, especially the lower lip; lizard may still be attached to patient (pathognomonic).

Physical Examination Findings
• Bleeding from bite site
• May note hypotension
• Extremely painful bite site
• Localized swelling
• Ptyalism—excessive salivation
• Excessive lacrimation
• Frequent urination and defecation
• May note aphonia in cats

CAUSES & RISK FACTORS
Outdoor activities

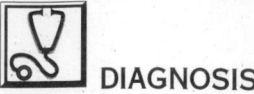

DIAGNOSIS

DIFFERENTIAL DIAGNOSIS
• Trauma
• Venomous snake bite—usually fewer punctures; depression and clotting abnormalities more prominent

CBC/BIOCHEMISTRY/URINALYSIS
N/A

OTHER LABORATORY TESTS
N/A

IMAGING
N/A

DIAGNOSTIC PROCEDURES
Electrocardiography—may detect arrhythmias

TREATMENT

• Remove lizard—place a prying instrument between the jaws; push into the back of the mouth; a flame held underneath the jaw often releases grip.
• Inpatient—monitor and treat hypotension, as necessary, with crystalloid fluid therapy
• Bite site—flush with lidocaine; probe to identify and remove fragments of lizard teeth (if not removed, they will become sequestra and abscess); soak with Burow solution or similar solution every 8 hr.

MEDICATIONS

DRUG(S)
• Control pain—can use narcotics (if severe)
• Broad-spectrum antibiotics indicated

CONTRAINDICATIONS/POSSIBLE INTERACTIONS
• Corticosteroids—not generally used by the author; authorities differ on the value of corticosteroids
• Antihistamines—not useful

FOLLOW-UP

• ECG—monitor for arrhythmias.
• Bite site—monitor for infection.

MISCELLANEOUS

Suggested Reading
Peterson ME, Meerdink G. Bites and stings of venomous animals. In: Kirk RW, ed. Current veterinary therapy X. Philadelphia: Saunders, 1989:177–186.
Author Michael E. Peterson
Consulting Editor Gary D. Osweiler

LOWER URINARY TRACT INFECTION

 BASICS

DEFINITION
Result of microbial colonization of the urinary bladder and/or proximal portion of the urethra

PATHOPHYSIOLOGY
Microbes, usually aerobic bacteria, ascend the urinary tract under conditions that permit them to persist in the urine or adhere to the epithelium and subsequently multiply. Urinary tract colonization requires at least transient impairment of the mechanisms that normally defend against infection. Inflammation of infected tissues results in the clinical signs and laboratory test abnormalities exhibited by patients.

SYSTEMS AFFECTED
Renal/Urologic—lower urinary tract

GENETICS
N/A

INCIDENCE/PREVALENCE
Common in female dogs; less common in male dogs; uncommon in cats

GEOGRAPHIC DISTRIBUTION
N/A

SIGNALMENT
Species
More common in dogs than in cats

Breed Predilection
None

Mean Age and Range
All ages affected, but occurrence increases with age because of a greater frequency of other urinary lesions (e.g., uroliths, prostate disease, and tumors) that predispose to secondary urinary tract infection.

Predominant Sex
More common in female than in male dogs; occurrence in male and female cats is similar.

SIGNS
Historical Findings
• None in some patients
• Pollakiuria—frequent voiding of small volumes
• Dysuria
• Urgency (or an apparent loss of ability to control urination during periods of confinement)
• Urinating in places that are not customary
• Hematuria and cloudy or malodorous urine in some patients

Physical Examination Findings
• No abnormalities in some animals
• Acute infection—bladder or urethra may seem tender on palpation.

• Palpation of the bladder may stimulate urination.
• Chronic infection—wall of the bladder or urethra may be palpably thickened or abnormally firm.
• Secondary infection—findings referable to the underlying problem

CAUSES
• Aerobic bacteria—most common
• Most common—*Escherichia, Staphylococcus,* and *Proteus* spp. (more than half of all cases)
• Common—*Streptococcus, Klebsiella, Enterobacter, Pseudomonas,* and *Corynebacterium* spp.
• Rare—a few other bacterial and fungal agents

RISK FACTORS
• Conditions that cause urine stasis or incomplete emptying of the bladder
• Conditions that disrupt mucosal defense properties
• Conditions that reduce or bypass anatomic and functional barriers to microbial ascent of the urinary tract (e.g., loss of muscle tone or length of the urethra and the vesicoureteral junctions)
• Conditions that compromise the antibacterial properties of urine (e.g., changes in urine pH or osmolality and low concentrations of urea and certain organic acids)

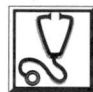 **DIAGNOSIS**

DIFFERENTIAL DIAGNOSIS
• Any other disease of the bladder or urethra
• Conditions commonly confused with, or complicated by, urinary tract infection include urolithiasis and neoplasia. In cats, idiopathic hemorrhagic cystitis is also a common problem that must be distinguished.
• Lower urinary tract disease can become complicated by secondary urinary tract infection; this is termed *complicated urinary tract infection* and requires different therapeutic strategies than are used for uncomplicated (i.e., simple) episodes of urinary tract infection.
• Frequent reinfection (more than one episode of newly acquired urinary tract infection within a year) usually indicates impaired host defense mechanisms. Seek an underlying cause. If no underlying cause can be identified and corrected, consider prophylactic antibacterial drug therapy.

CBC/BIOCHEMISTRY/URINALYSIS
• Results of CBC and serum biochemistry normal
• Pyuria is most commonly associated with urinary tract infection, but noninfectious

urinary lesions can also cause pyuria. Hematuria and proteinuria are also common. Bacteria may or may not be detected by microscopic examination of urinary sediment. Bacteriuria is sometimes reported in animals that do not have urinary tract infection.

OTHER LABORATORY TESTS
Urine Culture and Sensitivity Testing
• Urine culture is necessary for definitive diagnosis.
• Correct interpretation of urine culture results requires obtaining the specimen in a manner that minimizes contamination, handling and storing the specimen so that numbers of viable bacteria do not change in vitro, and using a quantitative culture method. Keep the specimen in a sealed sterile container; if the culture is not started right away, the urine can be refrigerated up to 8 hours without important changes in the results.
• Cystocentesis is the preferred technique for obtaining urine for culture.
• Cutoff values for significant bacteriuria in urine of dogs—obtained by cystocentesis, >1,000/mL; obtained by catheterization, >10,000/mL; obtained by voided urine specimen, >100,000/mL
• Cutoff values for significant bacteriuria in urine of cats—obtained by cystocentesis or catheterization, >1,000/mL; obtained by voided urine specimen, >10,000/mL
• Values that approach but do not exceed these cutoffs (i.e., less than one order of magnitude below) are suspicious, and retesting is indicated. Urine cultures that produce values more than one order of magnitude below these cutoffs are negative.
• In vitro susceptibility testing that determines the minimum inhibitory concentration (MIC) of each drug against the isolated organism is preferred for urinary pathogens. Drugs commonly used to treat urinary tract infection are highly concentrated in the urine, and any drug with an MIC value of one fourth or less of the average urine concentration of the drug during treatment is likely to be effective.

IMAGING
Survey and contrast radiographic studies as well as ultrasound of the bladder or urethra may detect an underlying urinary tract lesion (i.e., complicated urinary tract infection).

 TREATMENT

APPROPRIATE HEALTH CARE
Treat as outpatient unless another urinary abnormality (e.g., obstruction) requires inpatient treatment

LOWER URINARY TRACT INFECTION

ACTIVITY
• Unrestricted
• Regulating the patient's urination to coordinate with antibacterial drug treatments may improve therapeutic efficacy.

DIET
Restrictions not necessary but may be indicated for other concurrent urinary diseases (e.g., urolithiasis)

CLIENT EDUCATION
Prognosis for cure of simple urinary tract infection is excellent; prognosis for complicated urinary tract infection depends on the underlying abnormality. Compliance with recommendations for treatment and follow-up evaluations is crucial for optimum results.

SURGICAL CONSIDERATIONS
Except when a concomitant disorder requires surgical intervention, management does not involve surgery.

 MEDICATIONS

DRUG(S) OF CHOICE
• An appropriate antibiotic can be selected on the basis of the genus of the infecting bacteria—penicillin (e.g., ampicillin, 25 mg/kg PO q8h) for *Staphylococcus, Streptococcus,* or *Proteus* spp; trimethoprim-sulfadiazine (15 mg/kg combined PO q12h) for *Escherichia coli*; cephalexin (30 mg/kg PO q8h) for *Klebsiella* spp.; tetracycline (20 mg/kg PO q8h) for *Pseudomonas* spp.
• For an organism whose predictable susceptibility to a specific drug is not known or that does not respond as expected to the first drug, base choice of drug on results of sensitivity test.
• Antibacterial drugs are usually most effective when given q8h; however, fluoroquinolones and trimethoprim-sulfa products are effective when given q12h.
• For acute, uncomplicated infection, treat with antimicrobial drugs for 7–10 days. Chronic bacterial cystitis may need treatment for up to 4–6 weeks. Appropriate duration of treatment for complicated lower urinary tract infection depends on the underlying problem.
• Low-dose, bedtime antibacterial therapy can be used to prevent infections in animals that have frequent reinfections. Start such prophylactic treatment immediately after cure of the most recent episode of urinary tract infection by conventional treatment. Administer an appropriate antibacterial drug, usually ampicillin or nitrofurantoin, once daily for 4–6 months or longer. Dosage should be about one third of the conventional daily dose for the chosen drug, and the drug should be given after the animal has urinated for the last time each evening.

CONTRAINDICATIONS
Allergic reaction to a drug

PRECAUTIONS
• Long-term or repeated use of antimicrobial drugs is associated with adverse effects (e.g., allergic reaction) in some animals.
• Keratoconjunctivitis sicca is associated with administration of trimethoprim-sulfa products.
• Because of potential nephrotoxicity with long-term administration, use aminoglycosides only when there are no alternatives.

POSSIBLE INTERACTIONS
Patients with impaired renal function may have reduced urinary excretion of drugs used to treat urinary tract infection. Besides leading to unintended drug accumulation in such patients, impaired urinary excretion might reduce the drug's effectiveness.

ALTERNATIVE DRUG(S)
• Enrofloxacin and nitrofurantoin
• Ceftiofur, gentamicin, or amikacin, which must be given by injection

 FOLLOW-UP

PATIENT MONITORING
• When antibacterial drug efficacy is in doubt, culture the urine 2–3 days after starting treatment. If the drug is effective, the culture will be negative. • Continue treating at least 1 week after resolution of hematuria, pyuria, and proteinuria. Failure of urinalysis findings to return to normal while an episode of urinary tract infection is being treated with an effective antibiotic (i.e., as indicated by negative urine culture) generally indicates some other urinary tract abnormality (e.g., urolith, tumor). Rapid recrudescence of signs when treatment is stopped generally indicates either a concurrent urinary tract abnormality or that the infection extends into some deep-seated site (e.g., prostatic or renal parenchyma). • Successful cure of an episode of urinary tract infection is best demonstrated by performing a urine culture 7–10 days after completing antimicrobial therapy. • Animals being given low-dose bedtime antibacterial prophylactic treatment for frequent reinfection should have a urine culture performed via cystocentesis every 1–2 months.

PREVENTION/AVOIDANCE
• Avoid indiscriminate use of urinary catheters • Animals with frequent reinfection can be given bedtime therapy to augment host defenses and prevent reinfection.

POSSIBLE COMPLICATIONS
Failure to detect or treat effectively may lead to pyelonephritis or formation of struvite uroliths.

EXPECTED COURSE AND PROGNOSIS
• If not treated, expect infection to persist indefinitely. Associated health risks include development of urolithiasis and extension of infection to other portions of the urinary tract (e.g., the kidneys) or beyond (e.g., septicemia, diskospondylitis, and bacterial endocarditis). • Generally, the prognosis for animals with uncomplicated lower urinary tract infection is good-to-excellent. Patients that have frequent reinfection are candidates for low-dose bedtime prophylactic therapy, as described, but even these patients usually do well. The prognosis for animals with complicated infection is determined by the prognosis for the other urinary abnormality.

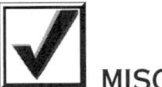 **MISCELLANEOUS**

ASSOCIATED CONDITIONS
• Struvite urolithiasis • Diabetes mellitus or hyperadrenocorticism

AGE-RELATED FACTORS
Complicated infection is more common in middle-aged to old than in young animals.

PREGNANCY
Depending on the stage of pregnancy, intensity of signs, and presence or absence of concomitant abnormalities, consider deferring treatment. Avoid using tetracycline, nitrofurantoin, or enrofloxacin.

SYNONYMS
• Bacterial cystitis • Urethrocystitis
• Urethritis

SEE ALSO
• Pyelonephritis • Urolithiasis, Struvite—Cats
• Urolithiasis, Struvite—Dogs

ABBREVIATION
MIC = minimum inhibitory concentration

Suggested Reading
Bartges JW, Barsanti JA. Bacterial urinary tract infections in cats. In: Bonagura JD, ed. Kirk's current veterinary therapy XIII. 13th ed. Philadelphia: Saunders, 2000:880–882.
Ling GV. Bacterial infections of the urinary tract. In: Ettinger SJ, Feldman EC, eds. Textbook of veterinary internal medicine. 5th ed. Philadelphia: Saunders, 2000:1678–1686.
Senior DF. Management of difficult urinary tract infections. In: Bonagura JD, ed. Kirk's current veterinary therapy XIII. 13th ed. Philadelphia: Saunders, 2000:883–886.
Author George E. Lees
Consulting Editors Larry G. Adams and Carl A. Osborne

LUMBOSACRAL STENOSIS AND CAUDA EQUINA SYNDROME

 BASICS

DEFINITION
• Caused by dorsoventral narrowing of the lumbosacral vertebral canal with compression of the L7, sacral, or caudal nerve roots
• Syndrome refers to the clinical signs related to injury of these nerve roots.

PATHOPHYSIOLOGY
• Congenital—abnormal development of the dorsal arch of the L7-S1 vertebrae causes narrowing of the lumbosacral spinal canal; chronic biomechanical stress may contribute to degenerative changes that reduce the canal diameter and cause compression of the spinal nerve roots; the smaller the canal, the less stenosis required before clinical signs appear
• Acquired—caused by bony and soft tissue degenerative changes that lead to a gradual reduction in the lumbosacral spinal canal

SYSTEMS AFFECTED
Nervous—specifically nerve roots, from L7 caudally

GENETICS
No known genetic basis

INCIDENCE/PREVALENCE
Unknown

GEOGRAPHIC DISTRIBUTION
N/A

SIGNALMENT
Species
• Common in dogs
• Rare in cats

Breed Predilections
• Congenital—small to medium dogs; border collies
• Acquired—large-breed dogs; German shepherds, boxers, rottweilers

Mean Age and Range
• Congenital—3–8 years
• Acquired—average age at onset 6–7 years

Predominant Sex
• Congenital—none
• Acquired—male

SIGNS
• Relate to varying degrees of compression of the L7, sacral, and caudal nerve roots
• Lumbosacral pain—salient clinical feature; may be the only sign
• Sciatic nerve dysfunction—may initially manifest as a lameness; may progress to pelvic limb weakness, muscle wasting, and postural reaction deficits
• Pudendal nerve root involvement—urinary and/or fecal incontinence
• Caudal nerve root involvement—weakness to paralysis of the tail
• Both meninges and nerve root compression—sensory disturbances that vary from unpleasant sensations to obvious low lumbar pain
• Congenital—self-inflicted lesions common
• Patients with both forms—extension of the pelvic limbs or dorsiflexion of the tail over the back reduces the lumbosacral canal diameter and usually elicits a painful response.

CAUSES
• Congenital vertebral malformation including transitional vertebral
• Type II disk protrusion
• Hypertrophy or hyperplasia of the inter-arcuate ligament
• Proliferation of the articular facets
• Subluxation or instability of the lumbosacral junction

RISK FACTORS
N/A

 DIAGNOSIS

DIFFERENTIAL DIAGNOSIS
• Hip dysplasia or other orthopedic injury—low lumbar pain; distinguish via thorough orthopedic examination
• Chronic diskospondylitis, osteomyelitis, and primary or metastatic vertebral tumors—cannot be differentiated by clinical signs alone
• Vertebral fractures and subluxations—acute; characterized by more bilateral signs
• Localized myelitis or radiculoneuritis—usually more diffuse pain

CBC/BIOCHEMISTRY/URINALYSIS
• Usually normal
• Urinalysis—may reveal lower urinary tract infection secondary to urinary incontinence

OTHER LABORATORY TESTS
N/A

IMAGING
• Radiology—spondylosis at the lumbosacral junction; narrowing of the L7-S1 disk space; ventral displacement of the sacrum relative to the lumbar vertebrae; interpret with caution because all can be seen in clinically normal animals.
• Myelography—rarely of benefit because the subarachnoid space rarely extends beyond vertebra L6 in large-breed dogs; indicated to rule out lesions rostral to the lumbosacral junction
• Epidurography—may outline a space-occupying mass over the lumbosacral disk space
• Discography of the L7-S1 space—may help highlight elevation of the dorsal annulus fibrosis
• CT and MRI—enhance the ability to recognize the condition

DIAGNOSTIC PROCEDURES
Electromyography—diagnostic and prognostic; denervation may be detected in the muscles innervated by the nerve roots L7 to caudal; denervation confirms the localization of the lesion and implies permanent deficits.

PATHOLOGIC FINDINGS
• May see one or more of the following features
• Type II disk disease with bulging of dorsal amnulus
• Hypertrophy of the interarcuate ligament
• Spondylosis causing stenosis of the intervertebral foramen with ensuing compression of nerve roots
• Ventral displacement of the sacrum in relation to lumbar vertebrae
• Proliferation of articular facets and hypertrophy of joint capsule
• Congenital malformation consisting of shortened pedicles
• Thickened and sclerotic lamina and articular processes

LUMBOSACRAL STENOSIS AND CAUDA EQUINA SYNDROME

TREATMENT

APPROPRIATE HEALTH CARE
• Urinary continence—outpatient pending surgery
• Urinary incontinence—inpatient for initial medical management

NURSING CARE
Urinary incontinence—catheterize the bladder until adequate voluntary control returns; monitor closely for urinary tract infection and administer appropriate antibiotics if necessary.

ACTIVITY
• After surgical decompression—restrict for 4 weeks; then gradually return to athletic function
• Nonsurgical treatment—confinement and restricted leash walks, alone or combined with corticosteroids, frequently alleviate pain; clinical signs often return with increasing levels of exercise.

DIET
Avoid obesity; excess weight increases biomechanical stress on the spine.

CLIENT EDUCATION
• Inform client that without treatment there will be progressive neurologic impairment of the pelvic limbs, urinary and fecal incontinence, and paralysis of the tail.
• Inform client that pelvic limb lameness and self-inflicted lesions result from pain associated with nerve root irritation and compression.
• Discuss surgical treatment, noting that it stops the progression and removes the source of pain, that some neurologic deficits may remain, and that medical management alone is usually unsatisfactory.

SURGICAL CONSIDERATIONS
• Surgical decompression—preferred treatment
• Dorsal laminectomy of the L7-S1 vertebrae—effectively relieves compression in most patients; may combine with facetectomy or foraminotomy if nerve roots are compressed
• Distraction fusion with or without laminectomy should be considered if the lumbosacral junction appears unstable (on radiographs or during surgery)

MEDICATIONS

DRUG(S) OF CHOICE
NSAIDs or corticosteroids—usually unsatisfactory

CONTRAINDICATIONS
N/A

PRECAUTIONS
N/A

POSSIBLE INTERACTIONS
N/A

ALTERNATIVE DRUG(S)
N/A

FOLLOW-UP

PATIENT MONITORING
N/A

PREVENTION/AVOIDANCE
N/A

POSSIBLE COMPLICATIONS
• Seroma formation—frequent sequela to surgery; can be effectively managed by cage rest and surgical drainage
• Excessive fibrous tissue formation (laminectomy membrane) in the surgical area—infrequent cause of recurrence of clinical signs; minimize by proper surgical technique; surgical removal is difficult and has a lower success rate than the initial dorsal laminectomy.
• Recurrence of signs > 6 months after surgery

EXPECTED COURSE AND PROGNOSIS
• Vary with the degree of neurologic injury
• Low lumbar pain and mild neurologic deficits (dogs)—good prognosis after surgery
• 80–90% have an excellent or good outcome
• Fecal and urinary incontinence (dogs)—guarded prognosis

MISCELLANEOUS

ASSOCIATED CONDITIONS
Lower urinary tract infections frequently accompany urinary incontinence.

AGE-RELATED FACTORS
German shepherds—concurrent coxofemoral osteoarthritis and/or degenerative myelopathy

ZOONOTIC POTENTIAL
N/A

PREGNANCY
N/A

SYNONYMS
• Lumbosacral malarticulation or malformation
• Lumbosacral instability
• Lumbosacral spondylopathy
• Lumbosacral spondylolisthesis

SEE ALSO
• Diskospondylitis
• Intervertebral Disk Disease—Thoracolumbar

ABBREVIATIONS
CT = computed tomography
MRI = magnetic resonance imaging
NSAIDs = nonsteroidal antiinflammatory drugs

Suggested Reading
Danielsson F, Sjostrom L. Surgical treatment of degenerative lumbosacral stenosis in dogs. Vet Surg 1999;28:91–98.
De Risio L, Thomas WB, Sharp NJH. Degenerative lumbosacral stenosis. Vet Clin North Am Small Anim Pract 2000; 30(1):111–132.
De Risio L, Sharp NJ, Olby NJ, Munana KR, Thomas WB. Predictors of outcome after dorsal decompressive laminectomy for degenerative lumbosacral stenosis in dogs: 69 cases (1987–1997). J Am Vet Med Assoc 2001;219(5):624–628.
Jones JC, Banfield CM, Ward DL. Association between postoperative outcome and results of magnetic resonance imaging and computed tomography in working dogs with degenerative lumbosacral stenosis. J Am Vet Med Assoc 2000; 216(11):1769–1774.
Jones JC, Shires PK, Inzana KD, Sponenberg DP, Massicotte C, Renberg W, Giroux A. Evaluation of canine lumbosacral stenosis using intravenous contrast-enhanced computed tomography. Vet Radiol Ultrasound 1999;40(2):108–114
Ramirez O, Thrall DE. A review of imaging techniques for canine cauda equina syndrome. Vet Radiol Ultrasound 1998; 39:283–296.
Author Karen Dyer Inzana, Brett C. Wood
Consulting Editor Joane M. Parent

LUNG LOBE TORSION

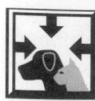 BASICS

OVERVIEW
- Twisting of lung lobe(s) at the hilus with occlusion of the bronchus, lymphatics, vein, and (finally) arteries
- Affected lobes—right middle lobe most commonly affected; other lobes may twist singly or in pairs.
- Initially, the lobe becomes engorged with blood, which causes it to enlarge; infarction and necrosis may follow; hemorrhagic pleural effusion typically develops.
- Chronic survivors—may note shrinkage and fibrosis of the lobe

SIGNALMENT
- Most common in large, deep-chested dogs
- Afghans (chylothorax)
- Spontaneous syndrome in pugs
- Less common in cats

SIGNS
- Fever
- Weakness
- Collapse
- Acute respiratory distress and shortness of breath
- Orthopnea
- Cough
- Retching
- Hemoptysis
- Ventral thoracic dullness
- Tachycardia
- Cyanosis
- Shock

CAUSES & RISK FACTORS
- Lobar torsion—usually associated with pre-existing condition that causes pleural effusion (e.g., trauma, neoplasia, and chylothorax)
- Thoracic or diaphragmatic surgery
- Spontaneous or idiopathic

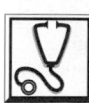 DIAGNOSIS

DIFFERENTIAL DIAGNOSIS
- Pulmonary contusion
- Diaphragmatic hernia
- Pulmonary abscess or infarction
- Neoplasia—lymphomatoid granulomatosis
- Coagulopathy
- Pneumonia, embolization, or thrombosis
- Uncomplicated pleural effusion and compression atelectasis
- Fungal or foreign body granuloma
- Lobar consolidation or bronchial obstruction from a foreign body

CBC/BIOCHEMISTRY/URINALYSIS
N/A

OTHER LABORATORY TESTS
N/A

IMAGING

Radiography
- Initially may reveal air bronchograms with disorientation of the torsed bronchus
- Pleural effusion—suggested by ventral leafing and interlobar fissures
- Consolidation and swelling of the torsed lobe with possible displacement of the heart and mediastinum
- May see lack of expansion of other lobes
- Thoracentesis may improve visualization and provide therapeutic benefits; ultrasound may be more successful before fluid is removed.

Ultrasound
- May allow further characterization
- Fine-needle aspiration contraindicated

DIAGNOSTIC PROCEDURES
- Pleural effusion—typically hemorrhagic or a modified transudate; PCV and WBC count similar to that of the peripheral blood; no platelets; chronicity or pre-existing effusions (e.g., chyle) may alter observations.
- Bronchoscopy—may reveal occlusion of the associated bronchus
- Surgical exploration—for definitive diagnosis and treatment

 TREATMENT

- Thoracentesis or chest tube placement
- Re-expansion pulmonary edema—may be a serious problem (especially in cats) if large volumes of pleural fluid are withdrawn quickly or if chronically compressed lungs are acutely inflated at surgery.
- Intravenous fluid administration; antibiotics
- Administer oxygen and treat for shock—when indicated
- Anesthesia—requires adequate ventilatory support; carefully monitor patient.
- Surgical removal of the involved lobe(s)—only effective treatment; do not untwist lobe and salvage (may lead to recurrence or necrosis); in situ ligation of the vessels or clamping with noncrushing forceps has been advocated; closely inspect remaining thoracic structures for any abnormalities; perform culture and pathologic examination of excised specimen.
- Postsurgery—monitoring; supportive care; tube drainage

 MEDICATIONS

DRUG(S)
- Antibiotics—perioperatively
- Treatment for shock—when indicated

CONTRAINDICATIONS/POSSIBLE INTERACTIONS
N/A

 FOLLOW-UP

- Observe for recurrence of pleural effusion.
- Thoracic radiographs—before discharge; as needed thereafter
- Prognosis—good if no underlying abnormality remains

 MISCELLANEOUS

ABBREVIATION
PCV = packed cell volume

Suggested Reading
Dye TL, Teague HD, Poundstone ML. Lung lobe torsion in a cat with chronic feline asthma. J Am Anim Hosp Assoc 1998;34:493–495.

Fossum TW. Small animal surgery. St. Louis: Mosby, 1997:665–667.

Neath PJ, Brockman DJ, King LG. Lung lobe torsion in dogs: 22 cases (1981–1999). J Am Vet Med Assoc 2000;217:1041–1044.

Rooney MB, Lanz O, Monnet E. Spontaneous lung lobe torsion in two pugs. J Am Anim Hosp Assoc 2001;37:128–130.

Author Bradley L. Moses
Consulting Editor Lynelle R. Johnson

LUPUS ERYTHEMATOSUS, CUTANEOUS (DISCOID)

BASICS

OVERVIEW
• Considered to be a benign variant of SLE
• Its comparative nature to the human form is controversial.
• One of the most common immune-mediated skin diseases
• Predominantly involves the planum nasale, face, ears, and mucous membranes; rarely other areas

SIGNALMENT
• Predominantly in dogs; rarely in cats
• Predominant breeds—collies, German shepherds, Siberian huskies, Shetland sheepdogs, Alaskan malamutes, chow chows, and their crosses
• No age predilection

SIGNS
• Usually starts with depigmentation of planum nasale and/or lips
• Depigmentation progresses to erosions and ulcerations.
• Tissue loss and scarring can occur.
• May also involve pinnae and periocular region; rarely feet and genitalia

CAUSES & RISK FACTORS
• Exact mechanism undetermined
• Genetic predisposition likely
• Suspected causes—drug reactions, viral initiation, and UV light exposure
• Seasonal exacerbations—associated with increased photoperiod and UV radiation
• UV exposure is a major concern.

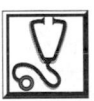

DIAGNOSIS

DIFFERENTIAL DIAGNOSIS

Major Considerations
• Other immune-mediated diseases—pemphigus foliaceus, pemphigus erythematosus, SLE, and uveodermatologic syndrome
• Drug reactions, erythema multiforme, and toxic epidermal necrolysis—nasal and facial lesions
• Dermatomyositis—affects some of the same predisposed breeds (collies and Shetland sheepdogs)
• Nasal pyoderma and nasal dermatophytosis—infectious conditions; can mimic discoid lupus erythematosus
• Insect hypersensitivity—one form creates a nasal inflammatory disease.

Other (Rare) Considerations
• Contact allergy
• Zinc-responsive dermatosis
• Metabolic epidermal necrosis
• T cell epidermotropic lymphoma—may start on the planum and rostral aspect of the muzzle and lips
• Squamous cell carcinoma—may affect the planum; may occur at a slightly higher incidence in chronic discoid lupus lesions
• Idiopathic leukoderma leukotrichia (vitiligo)—may cause depigmentation of the tissue and hair without concurrent inflammation

CBC/BIOCHEMISTRY/URINALYSIS
Usually normal

OTHER LABORATORY TESTS
ANA, LE preparation, and Coombs tests—usually normal or negative

IMAGING
N/A

OTHER DIAGNOSTIC PROCEDURES
Biopsies of nonulcerated, slate gray depigmented lesions—often characterized by interface lichenoid dermatitis with pigment incontinence and variable degrees of dermal mucin

PATHOLOGIC FINDINGS
Immunopathologic examination of nonulcerated samples preserved in Michel's solution—may reveal positive basal laminal fluorescence

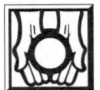

TREATMENT
• Not life-threatening
• May be disfiguring
• May create a source of trauma-induced bleeding
• Avoid direct solar exposure and use waterproof sunblocks with an SPF > 15.

MEDICATIONS

DRUG(S)
• Tetracycline and niacinamide—250 mg each PO q8h for dogs < 10 kg; 500 mg PO q8h for larger dogs
• Vitamin E—10–20 IU/kg PO q12h; may help reduce inflammation
• Topical corticosteroids—initially, a potent fluorinated product (e.g., 0.1% amcinonide) q24h for 14 days; then q48–72h for 28 days; if in remission switch to less-potent product (e.g., 0.5% or 2.5% hydrocortisone)
• Topical tacrolimus—0.1% tacrolimus (Protopic) q12h initially then taper to q24h when response seen
• Prednisone—consider for severe or nonresponsive cases; 2–3 mg/kg daily either solely or in combination with azathioprine 2 mg/kg PO on alternate days; taper prednisone to 0.5–1 mg/kg PO q48h for long-term maintenance

CONTRAINDICATIONS/POSSIBLE INTERACTIONS
N/A

FOLLOW-UP

PATIENT MONITORING
• Recheck 14 days after initiating treatment for clinical response.
• CBC and biochemistry—every 3–6 months if using topical tacrolimus and topical or oral corticosteroids for control
• CBC and platelet counts—every 2 weeks for the first 3–4 months; then every 3–6 months while on azathioprine

PREVENTION/AVOIDANCE
• Avoid using affected animals for breeding.
• Prone animals should avoid sunlight.

POSSIBLE COMPLICATIONS
• Scarring
• Secondary pyoderma
• Bleeding
• Disfigurement

EXPECTED COURSE AND PROGNOSIS
• Progressive but not usually life-threatening if left untreated
• With proper treatment, expect remission in majority of cases.
• The need for chronic immunosuppressive therapy suggests a more guarded prognosis, but remissions are common with more aggressive therapy.

MISCELLANEOUS

ABBREVIATIONS
• ANA = antinuclear antibody
• LE = lupus erythematosus
• SLE = systemic lupus erythematosus

Suggested Reading
Rosenkrantz WS. Discoid lupus erythematosus: current veterinary dermatology. St. Loius: Mosby, 1993.
Author Wayne S. Rosenkrantz
Consulting Editor Karen Helton Rhodes

LUPUS ERYTHEMATOSUS, SYSTEMIC (SLE)

BASICS

DEFINITION
A multisystem autoimmune disease characterized by the formation of antibodies against a wide array of self-antigens and circulating immune complexes

PATHOPHYSIOLOGY
• Cause unknown • High levels of circulating antigen-antibody complexes (type III hypersensitivity) are formed and deposited in the glomerular basement membrane, synovial membrane, skin, blood vessels, and other sites. • Antibodies directed toward self-antigen on cells such as erythrocytes, leukocytes, and platelets (type II hypersensitivity) may also be produced, and to a lesser degree, type IV hypersensitivity may be involved when cell-mediated immunity is directed against self-antigen. • Tissue injury—caused by activation of complement by circulating immune complexes and infiltration of inflammatory cells and by a direct cytotoxic effect of autoantibodies against membrane-bound antigens • Clinical manifestations depend on the localization of the immune complexes and the specificity of the autoantibodies. • Genetic, environmental, pharmacologic, and infectious factors may play a role in the production of clinical signs.

SYSTEMS AFFECTED
• Musculoskeletal—deposition of immune complexes in the synovial membranes • Skin/exocrine—deposition of immune complexes in the skin • Renal/urologic—deposition of immune complexes in the glomeruli • Hemic/lymph/immune—autoantibodies against RBCs, leukocytes, or platelets • Other organ systems—if there is deposition of immune complexes or antibodies

GENETICS
Hereditary in a colony of German shepherds; linked to the major histocompatibility complex allele DLA-A7

INCIDENCE/PREVALENCE
Rare, but probably underdiagnosed

GEOGRAPHIC DISTRIBUTION
N/A

SIGNALMENT
Species
Dogs and cats

Breed Predilections
• Shetland sheepdogs, collies, German shepherds, Old English sheepdogs, Afghan hounds, beagles, Irish setters, and poodles—overrepresented • Persian, Siamese, and Himalayan cats—may be predisposed

Mean Age and Range
The mean age is 6 years, but SLE can occur at any age.

Predominant Sex
None

SIGNS
Historical Findings
• Onset of signs can be acute or insidious. • Depend on the site of immune complexes and specificity of the autoantibodies • Waxing and waning course with clinical manifestations often sequential rather than concurrent • Lethargy • Anorexia • Shifting-leg lameness • Skin lesions

Physical Examination Findings
• Swollen and/or painful joints—major presenting sign in most patients • Symmetric or focal cutaneous lesions—characterized by erythema, scaling, ulceration, and alopecia • Fever—especially in the acute phase • Lymphadenopathy and hepatosplenomegaly • Ulceration of mucocutaneous junctions and oral mucosa may develop. • Arrhythmias, heart murmurs, and pleural friction rubs (i.e., associated with myocarditis, pericarditis, or pleuritis) • Muscle wasting

CAUSES
• Definitive causes unidentified • Exposure to drugs and viral infection suspected

RISK FACTORS
Exposure to ultraviolet light may exacerbate the disease.

DIAGNOSIS
• Definitive diagnosis—positive ANA or LE test (or both), and two major signs or one major *and* two minor signs • Probable diagnosis—positive ANA or LE cell test (or both) and one major *or* two minor signs • Major signs—polyarthritis, glomerulonephritis, skin lesions, hemolytic anemia, thrombocytopenia, and polymyositis • Minor signs—fever of unknown origin, oral ulcers, peripheral lymphadenopathy, pleuritis, pericarditis, myocarditis, depression, and seizures

DIFFERENTIAL DIAGNOSIS
• Neoplastic disease—may be associated with circulating immune complexes; patient may have signs similar to those of SLE • Important to exclude infectious disease because SLE is treated with immuno-suppressive drugs.

CBC/BIOCHEMISTRY/URINALYSIS
• CBC—may reveal anemia, leukopenia or leukocytosis, and thrombocytopenia; anemia may be moderate and nonregenerative (e.g., anemia of chronic disease) or severe and regenerative (e.g., hemolytic); leukogram: leukopenia and neutrophilia with or without monocytosis (inflammation) • Biochemistry—results vary widely, depending on the organ(s) affected • Urinalysis—high protein:creatinine ratio (> 1) with benign sediment indicates true proteinuria that may be caused by glomerulonephritis

OTHER LABORATORY TESTS
• Serum electrophoresis—usually shows high concentration of β- and γ-globulins (polyclonal gammopathy) • ANA test—a sensitive assay; positive results support a diagnosis of SLE; may also see positives in normal dogs and cats and in those with infectious diseases or being treated with certain drugs (e.g., penicillins, sulfonamides, tetracyclines) • LE test—identifies opsonized nuclear material within neutrophils and macrophages; positive result supports diagnosis of SLE; cumbersome to perform • Direct antiglobulin (Coombs) test—identifies complement or antibody on the surface of RBCs; not specific for SLE

IMAGING
Radiography of affected joints—reveals nonerosive arthritis, which is in contrast to the erosive lesions of rheumatoid arthritis

DIAGNOSTIC PROCEDURES
• Arthrocentesis—high cell count with nondegenerate neutrophils and monocytes and low viscosity is a characteristic finding • Synovial biopsy—may also help confirm a diagnosis of SLE • Bacterial culture of synovial fluid—negative • Skin biopsy—in patients with skin lesions; save specimen in 10% buffered formalin (for histopathologic examination) or Michel's solution (for immunofluorescence testing)

PATHOLOGIC FINDINGS
• Nonerosive polyarthritis with infiltration of synovial membranes with neutrophils and lymphocytes; no pannus formation
• Membranous or membranoproliferative glomerulonephritis • Mononuclear interface dermatitis with hydropic degeneration of keratinocytes and eosinophilic round bodies representing apoptotic basal keratinocytes
• Vasculitis and panniculitis in some patients
• Immunofluorescence—deposition of immune complexes along the basement membrane of the dermal-epidermal junction
• Vasculitis may be seen in any organ, especially myocardium, pericardium, and meninges.
• Reactive lymphoid hyperplasia in the lymph nodes and spleen

TREATMENT

APPROPRIATE HEALTH CARE
• Hospitalization—may be necessary for initial management (e.g., in a patient with hemolytic crisis)
• Outpatient management—usually possible

NURSING CARE
Supportive care varies with systems affected.

ACTIVITY
Enforced rest—during episodes of acute polyarthritis

DIET
Protein restriction—recommended in animals with glomerulonephritis

CLIENT EDUCATION
• Discuss the progressive and unpredictable course of the disease.
• Discuss the need for long-term, immunosuppressive therapy and its side effects.
• Discuss heritability of the disease.

SURGICAL CONSIDERATIONS
None

MEDICATIONS

DRUG(S) OF CHOICE
• Corticosteroids—target both objectives (i.e., to control the abnormal immune response and reduce inflammation) and form the basis of treatment; prednisone (1–2 mg/kg PO q12h)

• Cytotoxic immunosuppressive drugs—add when prednisone fails to improve the condition after 7–10 days or when the patient is steroid intolerant; reduce prednisone to 0.5–1 mg/kg PO q12h; use azathioprine (dogs: 2 mg/kg PO q24h), cyclophosphamide (dogs: 50 mg/m² PO for 4 consecutive days then 3 days off, repeat weekly), or chlorambucil (dogs: 2–3 mg/m² PO, cats: 1.5 mg/m² PO)
• Levamisole (dogs: 3–7 mg/kg PO every other day for 4 months)—may also be useful in achieving remission
• Gradually taper doses (no more often than every 2–3 weeks) once remission is achieved.

PRECAUTIONS
• Cats are susceptible to azathioprine toxicity; this drug should be used with caution, if at all (dosage: 0.3 mg/kg PO q48h).
• Cyclophosphamide can induce hemorrhagic cystitis.
• Cyclophosphamide, azathioprine, and chlorambucil may cause bone marrow suppression.
• Treatment with immunosuppressive drugs can increase the risk of severe infection.

POSSIBLE INTERACTIONS
Concurrent use of aspirin and prednisone increases the risk of gastrointestinal ulceration.

ALTERNATIVE DRUG(S)
Cyclosporin A (5–10 mg/kg PO q12h)—may be tried in refractory patients; use with caution, and withdraw if side effects occur (e.g., gastritis, lymphocytoid dermatitis, papillomatosis, gingival hyperplasia). Requires measurement of blood cyclosporine concentration at regular intervals.

FOLLOW-UP

PATIENT MONITORING
• Physical examination—weekly • CBC and biochemical analysis—to monitor the side effects of immunosuppressive drugs; initially, weekly • ANA—remains high during remission, so is not useful for monitoring the disease

PREVENTION/AVOIDANCE
Do not breed affected animals.

POSSIBLE COMPLICATIONS
• Renal failure and nephrotic syndrome secondary to glomerulonephritis

• Bronchopneumonia or sepsis secondary to immunosuppression

EXPECTED COURSE AND PROGNOSIS
Prognosis is guarded. The presence of hemolytic anemia and glomerulonephritis and the development of bacterial infection warrant a poor prognosis.

MISCELLANEOUS

ASSOCIATED CONDITIONS
N/A

ZOONOTIC POTENTIAL
N/A

PREGNANCY
The use of cytotoxic immunosuppressive drugs in pregnant animals is contraindicated.

SYNONYMS
N/A

SEE ALSO
• Anemia, Immune-mediated
• Glomerulonephritis • Polyarthritis, Nonerosive Immune-mediated
• Thrombocytopenia, Primary Immune-mediated

ABBREVIATIONS
• ANA = antinuclear antibody
• LE = lupus erythematosus
• RBC = red blood cell

Suggested Reading
Chabanne L, Fournel C, Monier JC, Rigal D. Canine systemic lupus erythematosus: part 1: clinical and biologic aspects. Compendium 1999;21:135–141.
Chabanne L, Fournel C, Rigal D, Monier JC. Canine systemic lupus erythematosus: part 2: diagnosis and treatment. Compendium 1999;21:402–421.
Tizard IR. Veterinary immunology: an introduction. Philadelphia: Saunders, 2000.
Author Mary F. Thompson
Consulting Editor Stephen Kruth

LYME DISEASE

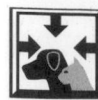

BASICS

DEFINITION
• One of the most common tick-transmitted zoonotic diseases in the world
• Caused by the spirochete *Borrelia burgdorferi*
• Dominant clinical feature (dogs)—recurrent acute arthritis with lameness, sometimes with anorexia and depression; may develop cardiac, neurologic, or renal diseases
• Reported in horses, cattle, and cats

PATHOPHYSIOLOGY
• Arthritis—pathogenesis unclear; caused directly by migrating spirochetes
• Local skin infestation after a tick bite is followed by a generalized infection of predominantly connective tissues, joint capsules, muscle, and lymph nodes.
• The incubation period in experimental dogs is 2–5 months.

SYSTEMS AFFECTED
• Persistent *B. burgdorferi*—found in skin, muscle, connective tissues, joints, and lymph nodes; rarely in body fluids (blood, CSF, and synovial fluid)
• Pathologic changes—with few exceptions restricted to joints, local lymph nodes, skin at the tick bite site; in specific cases, glomeruli of the kidney

GENETICS
Genetic basis known for mice; not established for dogs

INCIDENCE/PREVALENCE
• Percentage of seropositive dogs within a population varies greatly with exposure to infected ticks in endemic areas; reported range 5%–80%.
• About 5% of seropositive dogs in endemic areas develop Lyme disease.

GEOGRAPHIC DISTRIBUTION
• Worldwide distribution
• Variation in distribution of endemic areas
• U.S.—northeast > 90% of cases; also upper Mississippi region, California, and some southern states

SIGNALMENT

Species
Dogs and rarely cats

Breed Predilections
None

Mean Age and Range
Young dogs appear to be more susceptible than old dogs.

Sex Predispositions
None

SIGNS
• Recurrent acute arthritis with lameness—characteristic
• Lameness—lasts for only 3–4 days; responds well to antibiotic treatment; when acute, one or more joints may be swollen and warm; a pain response is elicited by palpation.
• Affected dogs may walk stiffly with an arched back and may be sensitive to touch.
• Fever, anorexia, and depression may accompany arthritis.
• Superficial cervical and/or popliteal lymph nodes may be swollen.
• Cardiac—reported but rare; include complete heart block
• Neurologic complications—rare
• Kidneys—reported glomerulonephritis with immune complex deposition in the glomeruli leading to fatal renal disease; patients may present with renal failure (vomiting, diarrhea, anorexia, weight loss, polyuria/polydipsia, peripheral edema or ascites).

CAUSES
• *B. burgdorferi* or related *Borrelia* sp.—transmitted by the small, hard-shell deer tick *Ixodes scapularis* or related *Ixodes* tick
• Infection—only after tick (nymphal stage in spring or adult female in fall) is partially engorged; 24–48 hr after the initial infestation

Ixodes ticks
• Have a 2-year life cycle
• Larvae—hatch in spring; become infected by feeding on white-footed mice (*Peromyscus leucopus*), which are persistently infected
• Nymphs—larvae molt into nymphs in the spring of the following year; stay infected or become infected by feeding on mice
• Adults—nymphs molt into adults in late fall of the second year; females engorge after mating on deer or other mammals, fall off, and hide under leaves until the following spring, when they each lay about 2000 eggs; males tend to stay on the deer.

RISK FACTORS
• Roaming tick-infested environment in Lyme-endemic area
• Speculated that urine from infected dogs and vectors other than ticks may be sources of infection; little supporting evidence

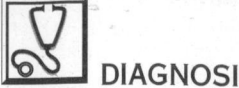

DIAGNOSIS

DIFFERENTIAL DIAGNOSIS
• Lyme arthritis—differentiate from other inflammatory arthritides
• Infectious agents—Rocky Mountain spotted fever; ehrlichiosis
• Fungal agents—histoplasma; cryptococcus; blastomycosis
• Protozoa—leishmania
• Bacteria—streptococcus; staphylococcus; others
• Immune-mediated diseases—idiopathic, lupus erythematosus, rheumatoid arthritis
• Specific breed diseases—akita arthritis, sharpei fever
• Culture of the joint fluid, serological assays, and immune testing (antinuclear antibodies; lupus erythematosus preparations)—rule out other disorders

CBC/BIOCHEMISTRY/URINALYSIS
• Arthritis only—unremarkable
• With protein-losing glomerulopathy—uremia, proteinuria, hypercholesterolemia, hyperphosphatemia, and hypoalbuminemia usually occur.

OTHER LABORATORY TESTS
• Fluid from affected joints—high WBC counts
• Positive serology by ELISA and Western blot—indicates previous exposure to *B. burgdorferi;* may indicate disease; ELISA cannot differentiate between sera from vaccinated and from naturally infected dogs but Western blot can; cross-reactions with antibody responses to *Leptospira* spp. minimal
• The 3Dx membrane ELISA bench test (IDEXX Laboratories, Westbrook, ME) measures antibody to the C6 *B. burgdorferi* protein. It is a convenient test and eliminates antibody responses to Lyme vaccines. However, 10% false positive reactions were recently found with this test in field samples.

IMAGING
Radiographs—help identify effusions in the joint; may help distinguish erosive from nonerosive joint disease

DIAGNOSTIC PROCEDURES
PCR from skin biopsy specimens—*B. burgdorferi* frequently isolated or demonstrated; time-consuming and expensive (not practical)

PATHOLOGIC FINDINGS

Gross
- Swollen joints with excess synovial fluid
- Sometimes enlarged lymph nodes

Histopathology
- Acute arthritis—fibrinopurulent synovitis
- Other joints—may have mild synovitis with infiltration of lymphocytes and plasma cells
- Lymph nodes—may show cortical hyperplasia with multiple enlarged follicles and expanded parafollicular areas
- Skin near tick bite site—may be perivascular infiltrates of plasma cells, lymphocytes, and some mast cells in the superficial dermis
- Renal lesions—glomerulonephritis, diffuse tubular necrosis with regeneration, and interstitial inflammation

TREATMENT

APPROPRIATE HEALTH CARE
Outpatient

NURSING CARE
Keep patient warm and dry.

ACTIVITY
Reduced activity advisable until clinical signs improve

DIET
No change needed

CLIENT EDUCATION
Inform client of importance of regular application of antibiotics as prescribed.

SURGICAL CONSIDERATIONS
Aspiration of synovial fluid—consider for diagnostic purposes

MEDICATIONS

DRUG(S) OF CHOICE
- Most commonly used antibiotics—doxycycline (10 mg/kg PO q12h) or amoxicillin (20 mg/kg PO q8–12h)
- Antibiotics—do not eliminate persistent infection; significantly improve clinical signs and pathology
- Recommended treatment period—4 weeks

CONTRAINDICATIONS
N/A

PRECAUTIONS
Do not treat young and growing animals with tetracyclines (doxycycline).

POSSIBLE INTERACTIONS
Jarisch-Herxheimer reaction—rare occurrence within the first 3 days of antibiotic treatment

reported in humans; not known in animals; toxic byproducts from killed spirochetes may intensify symptoms.

ALTERNATIVE DRUG(S)
- Corticosteroids—may initially ameliorate signs; mask effects of antibiotics for diagnostic purposes; enhance clinical signs later by immunosuppression
- Pain medications (nonsteroidal)—use judiciously to avoid masking signs

FOLLOW-UP

PATIENT MONITORING
- Improvement—seen within 3 days of antibiotic treatment
- If no improvement—consider a differential diagnosis.

PREVENTION/AVOIDANCE
- Prevent tick engorgement—repellents containing DEET or permethrin; tick collars; groom dogs daily
- Controlling tick population in the environment—restricted to small areas; limited results from reducing deer and/or rodent population
- Vaccine—two commercially available bacterins consisting of killed *B. burgdorferi* in adjuvant; one was shown to reduce the incidence of disease from 4.7% of seropositive dogs to about 1%; value still debated; single protein vaccine (OspA) protects dogs from infection and disease.

POSSIBLE COMPLICATIONS
- Heart block
- CNS disorders
- Fatal renal failure

EXPECTED COURSE AND PROGNOSIS
- Recovery from initial lameness expected 2–3 days after initiation of antibiotic treatment
- Disease may be recurrent with intervals of weeks to months; responds again to antibiotic treatment
- The nonresponsive chronic arthritis seen in humans is not known in dogs.

MISCELLANEOUS

ASSOCIATED CONDITIONS
N/A

AGE-RELATED FACTORS
- Young pups appear to be more susceptible than old dogs.
- Disease can occur in dogs of all ages; there is no difference in treatment.

ZOONOTIC POTENTIAL
- Occurs in humans; source of infection is ticks.
- Speculated that *B. burgdorferi* in the saliva or urine of affected dogs might be transmissible to humans—experiments have failed to prove this.
- Speculated that dogs can transport ticks home that then become attached to humans—*Ixodid* are not intermittent feeders and attach quickly; once tick starts feeding on a dog, it feeds to repletion and does not change hosts.

PREGNANCY
- Although possible, there is no convincing evidence that *B. burgdorferi* infection is transmitted in utero in dogs.
- Pregnant animals tolerate antibiotic treatment; do not use tetracyclines.

SYNONYMS
- Lyme borreliosis
- Lyme arthritis

ABBREVIATIONS
- CSF = cerebrospinal fluid
- ELISA = enzyme-linked immunosorbent assay
- PCR = polymerase chain reaction

Suggested Reading
Appel MJG, Allan S, Jacobson RH, et al. Experimental Lyme disease in dogs produces arthritis and persistent infection. J Infect Dis 1993;167:651–664.

Dambach DM, Smith CA, Lewis RM, et al. Morphological, immunohistochemical, and ultrastructural characterization of a distinctive renal lesion in dogs putatively associated with *Borrelia burgdorferi* infection: 49 cases (1987–1992). Vet Pathol 1997;34:85–170.

Greene CE, Appel MJG, Straubinger RK. Lyme borreliosis. In: Greene CE, ed. Infectious diseases of the dog and cat. Philadelphia: Saunders, 1998:282–293.

Levy SA, Barthold SW, Daubach DM, et al. Canine Lyme borreliosis. Compend Contin Educ Pract Vet 1993;15:833–848.

Liang ET, Jacobson RH, Straubinger RK, et al. Characterization of *Borrelia burgdorferi* VlsE invariable region useful in canine Lyme disease serodiagnosis by enzyme-linked immunosorbent assay. J Clin Microbiol 2000;38:4160–4166.

Straubinger RK, Summers BA, Chang Y-F, et al. Persistence of *Borrelia burgdorferi* in experimentally infected dogs after antibiotic treatment. J Clin Microbiol 1997;35:111–116.

Author Max J. G. Appel
Consulting Editor Stephen C. Barr

LYMPHADENITIS

 BASICS

DEFINITION
• Inflammation of one or more lymph nodes characterized by active migration of neutrophils, macrophages, or eosinophils into the node
• Lymphoid hyperplasia is not a form of lymphadenitis.

PATHOPHYSIOLOGY
• Usually the result of an infectious agent gaining access to a lymph node and establishing infection; because of the filtration functions of lymph nodes, they are likely to be exposed to infectious agents.
• Many organisms can cause inflammation; but agents such as fungi and mycobacteria that reside within macrophages and elicit a granulomatous inflammatory response are especially prone to establish infection within lymph nodes.
• Noninfectious—occurs infrequently; an example is eosinophilic lymphadenitis that occurs as an occasional component of eosinophilic inflammatory diseases.

SYSTEMS AFFECTED
• Hemic/Lymphatic/Immune
• May be a component of a more widespread infectious disease

GENETICS
• No known genetic basis
• Exception—rare cases of immunodeficiency; e.g., the familial susceptibility of certain basset hounds to mycobacteriosis, of which lymphadenitis is a frequent manifestation, Rottweilers may be predisposed to idiopathic hypereosinophilic syndromes causing eosinophilic lymphadenitis.

INCIDENCE/PREVALENCE
• Frequent manifestation of a number of infectious diseases
• Precise incidence is unknown.

GEOGRAPHIC DISTRIBUTION
Same as for systemic fungal infections such as histoplasmosis (central U.S.) and blastomycosis (central and eastern U.S.) and, less commonly, leishmaniasis (southern and southwestern U.S.)

SIGNALMENT
Species
Dogs and cats
Breed Predilection
None

Mean Age and Range
Because of their susceptibility to infection, neonates may have a higher rate of occurrence than older animals.
Predominant Sex
None

SIGNS
General Comments
• Complications of infection in another organ—usually relate to that organ rather than to the inflamed lymph node
• Component of systemic infection—associated with systemic inflammatory disease: fever, malaise, and anorexia

Historical Findings
• Seldom causes lymph node enlargement that is severe enough to be observed by owners
• Systemic signs of inflammatory disease or organ dysfunction

Physical Examination Findings
• Inflamed lymph nodes are typically large and firm and may be painful.
• Bacterial—animal may develop abscesses within the nodes that may open to the exterior and present as draining tracts.
• Animals may also have fever and other systemic signs of infection.

CAUSES
Bacteria
• Most pathogenic aerobic and anaerobic species have occasionally been reported.
• More likely agents—*Pasteurella, Bacteroides,* and *Fusobacterium* spp.
• A few, such as *Yersinia pestis* (bubonic plague) and *Francisella tularensis* (tularemia), have a particular affinity for lymph nodes and are especially likely to be manifest as lymphadenitis, especially in cats.
• *Bartonella vinsonii* infection may cause granulomatous lymphadenitis in dogs. *Bartonella* spp. can cause lymphoid hyperplasia in cats; however, organisms are not detected with routine stains.

Fungi
• Infections commonly include lymphadenitis as one manifestation of systemic disease.
• Likely organisms include *Blastomyces, Cryptococcus, Histoplasma, Coccidiodes,* and *Sporothrix.*
• Many other mycotic agents have occasionally been reported.

Viruses
• Many viral infections implicated because of lymphoid hyperplasia
• Coronavirus FIP
• Mesenteric lymph nodes are most commonly affected.

Other
• Protozoa—animals with toxoplasmosis and leishmaniasis frequently have lymphadenitis, although it is unlikely to be the most obvious clinical finding.
• Algae—lymphadenitis is often one manifestation of canine prototothecosis.
• Noninfectious (e.g., associated with pulmonary or systemic eosinophilic disease)—usually unknown

RISK FACTORS
• Animals with compromised immune function are susceptible to infection and, therefore, to lymphadenitis.
• FeLV and FIV are among the more common causes of immune compromise in veterinary patients.

 DIAGNOSIS

DIFFERENTIAL DIAGNOSIS
• Must ascertain that a palpable or visible mass is actually a lymph node and not a neoplastic mass or inflammatory process such as sialoadenitis
• Frequently cannot be distinguished on the basis of clinical findings from other causes of lymphadenomegaly, such as lymphoid hyperplasia, lymphoma, and metastatic neoplasia
• Fever and painful lymph nodes are likely to be associated with lymphadenitis.
• Lymphoma and lymphoid hyperplasia are more common causes of generalized lymph node enlargement than is lymphadenitis.

CBC/BIOCHEMISTRY/URINALYSIS
• Although affected animals may have an inflammatory leukogram, the absence of such changes does not exclude the diagnosis.
• Some animals with systemic causes of lymphadenitis (e.g., fungal infections, leishmaniasis) may have marked hyperglobulinemia.
• Circulating eosinophilia, often severe, is a relatively consistent finding in animals with eosinophilic diseases that are extensive and severe enough to cause lymphadenitis.
• Biochemistry results may reflect the degree of organ involvement from the underlying disease process.

OTHER LABORATORY TESTS
Serologic tests for the various systemic fungal diseases and possibly *Bartonella* spp. can be useful for identification, although these tests are best used only when attempts to demonstrate the organisms fail.

IMAGING

Radiography and ultrasonography—involvement of internal nodes, such as those in the thoracic and abdominal cavities, in patients with systemic inflammatory disease; valuable in assessing involvement of other organs, e.g., pneumonia in a patient with blastomycosis or histoplasmosis

DIAGNOSTIC PROCEDURES

• Fine-needle aspiration cytology is sufficient to diagnose most cases; a simple differential stain (e.g., Diff-Quik) is usually suitable.
• Gram staining can be performed in patients suspected of bacterial infection.
• Cytologic findings—high proportion of neutrophils, macrophages, eosinophils, or some combination of those cell types, which are only rarely seen in normal lymph nodes
• Bacteria, fungal agents, protozoa, and algae—often present in fine-needle aspirates of lymph nodes from animals with those infections; cytologic examination frequently is the most efficient means of detecting and identifying specific infectious agents in animals with either lymphadenitis of an isolated node or systemic infection.
• Eosinophilic lymphadenitis should not be diagnosed by cytologic examination of specimens, unless the proportion of eosinophils is markedly high, because mild eosinophilic infiltrates occur commonly in peripheral nodes of animals with allergic or parasitic skin disease.
• When a diagnosis is not made by cytologic examination, a lymph node biopsy may be indicated; specimens can be used for both histopathologic evaluation and culture.

PATHOLOGIC FINDINGS

• Although affected lymph nodes may be grossly normal, they are more frequently large and firm; the extent of enlargement varies widely and often distorts the shape of the node.
• Severe lymphadenitis may extend through the capsule of the node into adjacent tissues.
• On cut surface, affected nodes are often hyperemic and may have poorly defined nodules; in extreme examples of purulent lymphadenitis, abscesses may develop.
• Histologic lesions of purulent lymphadenitis include diffuse or multifocal infiltration of the affected node by neutrophils; the normal cortical-medullary architecture of the node may be disrupted.

• Granulomatous lymphadenitis—accumulations of activated macrophages involving the parenchyma of the node
• Eosinophilic lymphadenitis—large numbers of eosinophils both within sinuses and in the cortical parenchyma
• Necrosis common in all forms

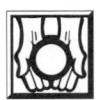 **TREATMENT**

APPROPRIATE HEALTH CARE

• Because lymphadenitis is a lesion rather than a specific disease, no single set of therapeutic recommendations is appropriate.
• The characteristics of the inflammation and the causative agent dictate appropriate treatment.

NURSING CARE
N/A

ACTIVITY
N/A

DIET
N/A

CLIENT EDUCATION
N/A

SURGICAL CONSIDERATIONS
N/A

 MEDICATIONS

DRUG(S) OF CHOICE

• Effective drug therapy requires identification of the causative agent.
• Purulent lymphadenitis of a single lymph node is likely to be of bacterial cause and can be treated with broad-spectrum systemic antibiotics if no organism is detected on initial cytologic evaluation.

CONTRAINDICATIONS
N/A

PRECAUTIONS
N/A

POSSIBLE INTERACTIONS
N/A

ALTERNATIVE DRUG(S)
N/A

 FOLLOW-UP

PATIENT MONITORING
N/A

PREVENTION/AVOIDANCE
N/A

POSSIBLE COMPLICATIONS
N/A

EXPECTED COURSE AND PROGNOSIS
N/A

 **MISCELLANEOUS**

ASSOCIATED CONDITIONS

• Multiple affected lymph nodes—frequently a manifestation of systemic infection that also affects many other organs
• Detection of fungi, protozoa, or algae in any inflamed node should alert one to the possibility of systemic infection by that agent.

AGE-RELATED FACTORS
None

ZOONOTIC POTENTIAL

• Bubonic plague, tularemia, and mycotic organisms present some risk of human infection.
• Specimens from affected animals should be handled cautiously.

PREGNANCY
N/A

SYNONYMS
None

SEE ALSO
See Causes.

ABBREVIATIONS

• FeLV = feline leukemia virus
• FIP = feline infectious peritonitis
• FIV = feline immunodeficiency virus

Suggested Reading

Duncan JR. The lymph nodes. In: RL Cowell, RD Tyler, eds. Diagnostic cytology of the dog and cat. Goleta, CA: American Veterinary, 1989:93–98.

Rogers KS, Barton CL, Landis M. Canine and feline lymph nodes. II. Diagnostic evaluation of lymphadenopathy. Compend Contin Ed Pract Vet 15:1493–1503.

Author Kenneth M. Rassnick

Consulting Editor Stephen A. Kruth

LYMPHADENOMEGALY

 BASICS

DEFINITION
Abnormally large lymph nodes, generalized or localized to a single node or group of regional nodes

PATHOPHYSIOLOGY
• Can result from hyperplasia of lymphoid elements, inflammatory infiltration, or neoplastic proliferation within the lymph node
• Because of their filtration function, lymph nodes often act as sentinels of disease in the tissues they drain; inflammation of any tissue is often accompanied by enlargement of the draining nodes, which most likely results from reactive lymphoid hyperplasia but may also be caused by extension of the inflammatory process into the nodes (lymphadenitis).
• Reactive hyperplasia involves proliferation of lymphocytes and plasma cells in response to antigenic stimulation.
• Lymphadenitis—implies active migration of neutrophils, activated macrophages, or eosinophils into the lymph node
• Infectious agents may be involved.
• Neoplastic proliferation may be either primary (malignant lymphoma) or metastatic.

SYSTEMS AFFECTED
Hemic/Lymph/Immune

SIGNALMENT
• Dogs and cats
• No breed, sex, or age predilection

SIGNS
• Typically does not cause clinical signs
• Severe—may cause mechanical obstruction and interference with the function of adjacent organs, signs of which depend on the affected lymph node and may include dysphagia, regurgitation, respiratory distress, dyschezia, and limb swelling
• Dogs and cats may be systemically ill from the underlying disease process.

CAUSES

Lymphoid Hyperplasia
• Localized or systemic infection caused by infectious agents of all categories (i.e., bacteria, viruses, fungi, protozoa, and algae) when infection does not directly involve the node
• Some infectious agents may produce lymphadenitis of certain lymph nodes with concurrent hyperplasia of other nodes that are not directly infected.

• Other infectious agents (e.g., rickettsia, *Bartonella* spp., and *Brucella canis*)—hyperplasia without overt lymphadenitis
• FIV and FeLV infection—generalized hyperplasia, although lymphoid depletion may occur late in the course of the disease; lymphadenitis can develop with a secondary infection.
• Antigenic stimulation by factors other than infectious agents (e.g., allergens)
• May develop in animals with immune-mediated disease (e.g, SLE and rheumatoid arthritis)

Lymphadenitis
• Bacteria—capable of causing purulent lymphadenitis, which may progress to abscessation; a few (e.g., *Mycobacterium* spp., *Bartonella* spp.) induce granulomatous lymphadenitis; other agents include aerobic and anaerobic organisms, *Pasteurella, Bacteroides,* fusobacterium, *Yersinia pestis,* and *Francisella tularensis.*
• Fungi—systemic infections from histoplasmosis, blastomycosis, cryptococcosis, and sporotrichosis
• Uncommon—protozoa, algae, and metazoan parasites
• Several involved lymph nodes—frequently a manifestation of systemic infection, such as histoplasmosis or blastomycosis
• Although primary infection of the lymph nodes does occur, lymphadenitis is usually accompanied by (and often results from) infection of other tissues being drained by the affected node.
• Eosinophilic—may be associated with allergic inflammation of the organ being drained by the affected lymph node (e.g., skin affected with flea allergy dermatitis); may be encountered in a patient with multisystemic idiopathic eosinophilic disease, such as feline and canine hypereosinophilic syndromes or in a lymph node draining a mast cell tumor

Neoplasia
• Cats—neoplastic transformation of lymphocytes by FeLV
• Dogs—lymphoma, cause unknown
• Most tumors that metastasize to the lymph nodes—unknown

RISK FACTORS
• Impaired immune function predisposes to infection and, therefore, to lymphadenitis.
• Animals with allergic diseases are likely to develop lymph node hyperplasia or eosinophilic lymphadenitis.
• Malignant lymphoma (cats)—infection with FeLV, FIV.
• Lymphadenomegaly caused by metastatic neoplasms—vary with the type of primary neoplasm

 DIAGNOSIS

DIFFERENTIAL DIAGNOSIS
• A mass in a location characteristic of a lymph node usually can be assumed to be one; cytologic evaluation of a fine-needle aspirate usually resolves any doubt.
• Palpable lymph nodes in normal dogs—mandibular, prescapular, axillary, superficial inguinal, and popliteal nodes; facial, retropharyngeal, and iliac nodes are palpable when larger than normal
• Severe lymph node enlargement (> 5 times normal size)—most likely to develop in patients with abscessation (lymphadenitis) and lymphoma
• Lesser degrees of enlargement—attributable to reactive hyperplasia, lymphadenitis, or neoplasia
• Extent of enlargement in patients with metastatic disease varies widely.
• Multiple lymph nodes affected throughout the body—likely the result of lymphoma or systemic infection that causes either lymphadenitis or lymphoid hyperplasia
• Abscessation and metastatic neoplasms usually affect a single lymph node.

CBC/BIOCHEMISTRY/URINALYSIS
• Cytopenias—seen with lymphoma, anemia of chronic disease, stress, splenic disease, or neoplastic infiltration of the bone marrow; also seen with rickettsial or viral disease
• Lymphocytosis—suggests rickettsial disease (dogs) and lymphoid neoplasia (dogs and cats); atypical lymphocytes in the blood help establish a diagnosis of lymphoid neoplasia
• Eosinophilia—may occur in animals with lymphadenopathy due to allergic or parasitic skin disease
• Neutrophilia, with or without a left shift—may develop in patients with lymphadenitis, lymphoid hyperplasia, or neoplasia
• Hypercalcemia—relatively common in dogs and rare in cats with lymphoma
• Hyperglobulinemia—may develop in patients with chronic inflammatory disease or lymphoid neoplasia

OTHER LABORATORY TESTS
• Cats—test for FeLV antigen and FIV in animals with large lymph nodes; infected animals may have lymphoma, lymphoid hyperplasia, or even lymphadenitis caused by immunosuppression.
• Serologic tests for antibodies against systemic fungal agents such as *Blastomyces* and *Cryptococcus* or bacteria such as *Bartonella* spp. may help establish those diagnoses.

IMAGING
- Radiography and ultrasonography—involvement of lymph nodes within the body cavity
- Lesions associated with lymph node enlargement may be detected in other organs, e.g., diffuse pneumonia in dogs with blastomycosis, and primary tumor in animals with lymphadenomegaly caused by metastatic neoplasia.

DIAGNOSTIC PROCEDURES

Cytologic Examination
- Aspirates from affected lymph nodes help determine the major category of lymphadenomegaly (i.e., hyperplasia, inflammation, or neoplasia) and may provide a specific diagnosis in patients with certain infectious diseases or neoplasms; a differential stain (e.g., Diff-Quik) is suitable in most cases.
- Gram staining can be performed in animals suspected of bacterial lymphadenitis.
- Aspirates from hyperplastic lymph nodes contain a mixed cell population in which small lymphocytes predominate along with large lymphocytes, plasma cells, occasional neutrophils and (perhaps) a few eosinophils and mast cells.
- Hyperplastic and normal lymph nodes are cytologically indistinguishable.
- Aspirates from lymph nodes affected by lymphadenitis contain high proportions of neutrophils, macrophages, and/or eosinophils, depending on the cause of the inflammation; specific infectious agents, such as bacteria and systemic fungi, may be evident.
- Frequently the means of diagnosis in animals with systemic fungal infection, such as blastomycosis and cryptococcosis
- Aspirates from lymph nodes affected by lymphoma typically contain a high proportion of (usually > 50%) large lymphocytes.
- Aspirates from lymph nodes containing metastatic neoplasia contain populations of cells that are not seen in normal nodes; the appearance of such cells varies widely, depending on the type of neoplasm.

Other
- In cats, severe lymphoid hyperplasia has been misdiagnosed as lymphoma; thus a biopsy is essential for animals with lymphadenomegaly.
- When a diagnosis cannot be made by cytologic examination, a surgical biopsy may be needed; excisional biopsy is preferable to needle biopsy.

- The cytologic diagnosis of lymphoma should be confirmed by histopathologic examination of an excised lymph node for accurate grading and to obtain potential prognostic information.

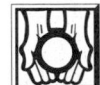

TREATMENT
- Because of the many disease processes and specific agents that can cause lymphadenomegaly, treatment depends on establishing the underlying cause.
- In animals suspected of lymphoma, corticosteroids should not be administered before completing staging tests if chemotherapy may be instituted.

MEDICATIONS

DRUG(S) OF CHOICE
Appropriate medications vary with the cause of lymph node enlargement.

CONTRAINDICATIONS
N/A

PRECAUTIONS
N/A

POSSIBLE INTERACTIONS
N/A

ALTERNATIVE DRUG(S)
N/A

FOLLOW-UP

PATIENT MONITORING
Lymph node size to assess efficacy of treatment

POSSIBLE COMPLICATIONS
N/A

MISCELLANEOUS

ASSOCIATED CONDITIONS
- Lymph node hyperplasia and lymphadenitis are often components or manifestations of systemic disease.
- Lymphoma may involve other organs (e.g., liver, spleen, intestines, kidneys, and meninges) with a variety of clinical consequences.

- Clinical disease in animals with metastatic neoplasms in the lymph nodes is usually attributable to the primary tumor rather than to the metastasis; however, exceptions are dogs with tonsillar carcinoma, who may have massively large mandibular lymph nodes, and dogs with adenocarcinoma of the anal sac, who often have dramatically large sublumbar lymph nodes.

AGE-RELATED FACTORS
None

ZOONOTIC POTENTIAL
- Direct transmission of diseases that cause lymphadenitis to humans is unlikely, with the exception of systemic mycotic disease, sporotrichosis, tularemia, plague, and *Bartonella* spp.
- Caution should be exercised when performing fine-needle aspiration in animals that may have systemic fungal disease.

PREGNANCY
N/A

SEE ALSO
- Lymphadenitis
- Lymphosarcoma (lymphoma)—Cats
- Lymphosarcoma (lymphoma)—Dogs

ABBREVIATIONS
FeLV = feline leukemia virus
FIV = feline immunodeficiency virus
SLE = systemic lupus erythematosus

Suggested Reading
Day MJ, Whitbread TJ. Pathological diagnoses in dogs with lymph node enlargement. Vet Rec 1988;136:72–73.
Duncan JR. The lymph nodes. In: Cowell RL, Tyler RD, eds. Diagnostic cytology of the dog and cat. Goleta, CA: American Veterinary, 1989:93–98.
Rogers KS, Barton CL, Landis M. Canine and feline lymph nodes. II. Diagnostic evaluation of lymphadenopathy. Compend Contin Ed Pract Vet 1993;15:1493–1503.

Author Kenneth M. Rassnick
Consulting Editor Stephen A. Kruth

LYMPHANGIECTASIA

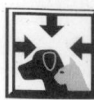 **BASICS**

DEFINITION
An obstructive disorder involving the lymphatic system of the gastrointestinal tract resulting in protein-losing enteropathy

PATHOPHYSIOLOGY
• Lymphatic obstruction results in dilation and rupture of intestinal lacteals with subsequent loss of lymphatic contents (plasma proteins, lymphocytes, and chylomicrons) into the intestinal lumen.
• Although some of the proteins may be digested and reabsorbed, excessive enteric loss results in hypoproteinemia.
• Hypoproteinemia causes a decrease in plasma oncotic pressure, leading to edema, ascites, and/or pleural effusion.

SYSTEMS AFFECTED
• Gastrointestinal—diarrhea, ascites
• Respiratory—pleural effusion
• Skin—subcutaneous edema

GENETICS
• Familial tendency for protein-losing enteropathy reported in soft-coated Wheaten terriers, basenjis, and Norwegian Lundehunds would suggest inheritance.
• Mode of inheritance unknown

INCIDENCE/PREVALENCE
Uncommon

GEOGRAPHIC DISTRIBUTION
N/A

SIGNALMENT
Species
Dogs

Breed Predilections
Increased prevalence in soft-coated Wheaten terriers, basenjis, Norwegian Lundehunds, and Yorkshire terriers.

Mean Age and Range
Mean ± SD age, 4.9 ± 1.9 years; age range, 2–9 years

Predominant Sex
Increased prevalence seen in female soft-coated Wheaten terriers; no sex predilection reported in other breeds

SIGNS
• Clinical signs are variable
• Diarrhea—chronic, intermittent or continuous, watery to semisolid consistency; however, not all patients have diarrhea
• Ascites
• Subcutaneous edema
• Dyspnea from pleural effusion
• Weight loss
• Flatulence
• Vomiting

CAUSES
Primary or Congenital Lymphangiectasia
• Focal—intestinal lymphatics only
• Diffuse lymphatic abnormalities (e.g., chylothorax, lymphedema, chyloabdomen, thoracic duct obstruction)

Secondary Lymphangiectasia
• Right-sided congestive heart failure
• Constrictive pericarditis
• Budd-Chiari syndrome
• Neoplasia (lymphosarcoma)

RISK FACTORS
N/A

 DIAGNOSIS

DIFFERENTIAL DIAGNOSIS
• Lymphangiectasia must be differentiated from other causes of protein-losing enteropathy (PLE).
• PLE must be differentiated from other causes of hypoalbuminemia.

CBC/BIOCHEMISTRY/URINALYSIS
• Hypoalbuminemia and hypoglobulinemia (panhypoproteinemia)
• Hypocholesterolemia
• Hypocalcemia
• Lymphopenia

OTHER LABORATORY TESTS
Tests to Differentiate PLE from Other Causes of Hypoalbuminemia
• Serum bile acid concentrations (pre- and post-prandial)—to rule out hepatic disease
• Urine protein/creatinine ratio—to rule out protein-losing nephropathy
• Occult fecal blood test—to rule out gastrointestinal blood loss
• Fecal α_1-proteinase inhibitor concentration—to confirm PLE

Tests to Differentiate Other Causes of PLE
• Fecal smear and flotation—to rule out parasites
• Serum cobalamin and folate concentrations—to rule out SIBO and cobalamin deficiency (while cobalamin deficiency does not cause PLE it is an indicator of long-standing and severe distal small intestinal disease)
• Fecal culture for specific enteric pathogens (i.e., *Salmonella* spp., *Campylobacter* spp., *Yersinia* spp.)—if infectious gastroenteritis is suspected
• *Clostridium* enterotoxin test—if infectious enteritis is suspected
• Other non-laboratory diagnostic procedures (discussed below)—important to aid these tests
• Fluid analysis of body cavity effusions—the effusion associated with lymphangiectasia is usually a transudate, but chyloabdomen and chylothorax are occasionally present.

IMAGING
• Survey thoracic and abdominal radiographs—to rule out cardiac disease and neoplasia
• Abdominal radiographs—to rule out mechanical intestinal disease and other causes of PLE
• Abdominal ultrasound—to rule out mechanical intestinal disease and other causes of PLE
• Cardiac ultrasound—to rule out right-sided congestive heart failure

DIAGNOSTIC PROCEDURES
• Endoscopy allows mucosal visualization and biopsy.
• Laparotomy allows visualization of dilated intestinal lymphatics and biopsies of intestines (full-thickness) and lymph nodes.
• An ECG can aid in evaluating the heart and ruling out right-sided congestive heart failure.

PATHOLOGIC FINDINGS
• Gross findings at laparotomy may include dilated lymphatics that are visible as a web-like network throughout the mesentery and serosal surface.

- May see small yellow-white nodules and foamy granular deposits adjacent to lymphatics
- Histopathology findings include ballooning distortion of villi, caused by markedly dilated lacteals.
- Villi can be edematous; some have a blunted appearance.
- Usually mucosal edema; diffuse or multifocal accumulations of lymphocytes and plasma cells can be identified in the lamina propria.

 TREATMENT

APPROPRIATE HEALTH CARE
- Mostly treated as outpatients
- May need hospitalization if complications due to hypoalbuminemia occur

NURSING CARE
N/A

ACTIVITY
Normal

DIET
- Low-fat diet with ample high-quality protein
- Long-chain triglycerides stimulate intestinal lymph flow and may lead to increased intestinal protein loss.
- Diets fortified with medium-chain triglycerides (MCTs) may be beneficial
- May feed MCTs to supplement fat and increase the calorie intake.
- Commercial sources of MCTs—MCT oil or Portagen (Mead Johnson, Evansville, IN)
- Supplement with fat-soluble vitamins—A, D, E, and K

CLIENT EDUCATION
Discuss unpredictable disease progression and response to therapy.

SURGICAL CONSIDERATIONS
- When intestinal lymphangiectasia is secondary to an identifiable lymphatic obstruction, consider surgery to relieve the obstruction.
- Pericardiectomy is indicated in cases of constrictive pericarditis.
- Cases that benefit from surgical intervention are rare.

 MEDICATIONS

DRUG(S) OF CHOICE
- Try corticosteroids if dietary therapy alone is unsuccessful (however, such therapy is not intended to treat lymphangiectasia but rather concurrent gastrointestinal inflammation).
- Oral prednisone at a dose of 2 mg/kg q12h for 5–7 days, followed by 1 mg/kg q12h for at least 6 weeks; after remission of the disease, dosage can be slowly decreased to the lowest dose effective at controlling the disease.

CONTRAINDICATIONS
N/A

PRECAUTIONS
N/A

POSSIBLE INTERACTIONS
N/A

ALTERNATIVE DRUGS
N/A

 FOLLOW-UP

PATIENT MONITORING
Body weight, serum protein concentration, and evidence of recurrent clinical signs (pleural effusion, ascites, and/or edema) need to be re-evaluated dependant on severity of the disease process.

PREVENTION/AVOIDANCE
N/A

POSSIBLE COMPLICATIONS
- Respiratory difficulty from pleural effusion
- Severe protein-calorie depletion
- Intractable diarrhea

EXPECTED COURSE AND PROGNOSIS
- Prognosis guarded
- Some animals fail to respond to treatment.
- Remissions of several months to more than 2 years can be maintained in some patients.

MISCELLANEOUS

ASSOCIATED CONDITIONS
Soft-coated Wheaten terriers may have concurrent protein-losing nephropathy (PLN).

AGE-RELATED FACTORS
N/A

ZOONOTIC POTENTIAL
N/A

PREGNANCY
N/A

SYNONYMS
N/A

SEE ALSO
Protein-losing Enteropathy

ABBREVIATIONS
- MCTs = medium-chain triglycerides
- PLE = protein-losing enteropathy
- SIBO = small intestinal bacterial overgrowth

Suggested Readings
Fossum TW, Sherding RG, Zack PM, et al. Intestinal lymphangiectasia associated with chylothorax in two dogs. J Am Vet Med Assoc 1987;190:61–64.
Kull PA, Hess RS, Craig LE, et al. Clinical, clinicopathologic, radiographic, and ultra-sonographic characteristics of intestinal lymphangiectasia in dogs: 17 cases (1996–1998). J Am Vet Med Assoc 2001;219:197–202.
Littman MP, Dambach DM, Vaden SL, et al. Familial protein-losing enteropathy and protein-losing nephropathy in soft coated Wheaten terriers: 222 cases (1983–1997). J Vet Int Med 2000;14:68–80.
Suter MM, Palmer DG, Schenk H. Primary intestinal lymphangiectasia in three dogs: a morphological and immunopathological investigation. Vet Pathol 1985;22:123–130.

Acknowledgment
The author and editors acknowledge the prior contributions of Dr. Mollyann Holland, who authored this topic in the previous edition.
Author Jörg M. Steiner
Consulting Editor Albert E. Jergens

LYMPHEDEMA

 BASICS

OVERVIEW
• Abnormal accumulation of protein-rich lymph fluid into interstitial spaces, especially subcutaneous fat
• Chronic lymphedema causes tissue fibrosis.
• May be congenital or acquired

SIGNALMENT
• More common in dogs than in cats
• Congenital in bulldogs and reported to be hereditary/congenital in a family of poodles; possible breed predilection in Labrador retrievers and Old English sheepdogs

SIGNS

Historical Findings
• Primary/congenital—usually peripheral limb swelling at birth or develops in first several months
• Typically starts at distal extremity and slowly advances proximally

Physical Examination Findings
• Most common in limbs, especially pelvic limbs; may be unilateral or bilateral
• Less common in ventral thorax, abdomen, ears, and tail
• Pitting, nonpainful; temperature of affected area is normal.
• Pitting quality lost with chronicity as fibrosis occurs
• Lameness and pain uncommon unless cellulitis develops

CAUSES & RISK FACTORS
• Hereditary/congenital malformation of the lymphatic system—aplasia, valvular incompetence, and lymph node fibrosis
• Excessive interstitial fluid production secondary to venous hypertension (associated with congestive heart failure and obstruction of venous drainage) or increased vascular permeability (associated with infection, trauma, heat, and irradiation)
• Secondary damage to lymphatic vessels or lymph nodes—associated with trauma, infection, and neoplasia

 DIAGNOSIS

DIFFERENTIAL DIAGNOSIS
• Edema caused by venous stasis (e.g., congestive heart failure and cirrhosis); look for varices, hyperpigmentation, and ulceration.
• Arteriovenous fistulae—listen for machinery murmur; feel for pulsatile vessels; confirm with angiogram.
• Edema caused by hypoproteinemia—protein-losing nephropathy or enteropathy, hepatic failure, serum loss from burns or hemorrhage; check serum protein concentration.
• Trauma—review history; look for bruising and lacerations.
• Neoplasia—if swelling is firm, obtain aspirate for cytologic examination.
• Cellulitis—look for fever, pain, and warm swelling.

CBC/BIOCHEMSITRY/URINALYSIS
Results normal

OTHER LABORATORY TESTS
N/A

IMAGING
Lymphography useful in documenting abnormalities within the lymphatic system; best results obtained with an injection of water-based contrast media directly into a lymphatic vessel. See references for detailed description of the technique.

DIAGNOSTIC PROCEDURES
N/A

TREATMENT

• No curative therapy—a number of surgical and medical treatments may be tried.
• Rest and massage of the affected limbs does not help.
• Conservative care—long-term use of pressure wraps, coupled with skin care and use of antibiotics to treat cellulitis and lymphangitis; may be successful in some patients
• Surgical procedures—can be attempted when conservative care and medications fail; lymph-angioplasty, bridging techniques, lymphatico-venous shunts, superficial and deep lymphatic anastomosis, and excisional procedures; none is consistently beneficial, and excisional procedures have been reported only in dogs.
• In humans—microwave heating of affected areas appears beneficial and adds to the effect of benzopyrones (see Drugs[s])
• Diets severely restricted in long-chain triglycerides are being investigated in humans.

MEDICATIONS

DRUG(S)

• Benzopyrones reduce high-protein edema by stimulating macrophages to release proteases; beneficial effects have been recorded in experimental studies in dogs. Rutin, 50 mg/kg PO q8h, may benefit. A study in humans showed combined usage of oral and topical benzopyrones to be more effective than either alone.
• Diuretics, steroids, anticoagulants, and fibrinolytic agents have been used, but no confirmed benefit.

CONTRAINDICATIONS/POSSIBLE INTERACTIONS

Diuretics—initially reduce swelling but increase protein content of interstitial fluid, resulting in further tissue damage and fibrosis.

FOLLOW-UP

• Puppies with severe lymphedema may die.
• Resolution seen in some puppies with pelvic limb involvement only

MISCELLANEOUS

Suggested Reading
Fossum TW, King LA, Miller MW, et al. Lymphedema: clinical signs, diagnosis, and treatment. J Vet Intern Med 1992;6:312–319.
Fossum TW, Miller MW. Lymphedema: etiopathogenesis. J Vet Intern Med 1992;6:283–293.
Author Francis W. K. Smith, Jr.
Consulting Editors Larry P. Tilley and Francis W. K. Smith, Jr.

LYMPHOCYTOSIS

 BASICS

DEFINITION
• Absolute number of circulating lymphocytes greater than the reference range: dogs, $> 5 \times 10^9$/L or > 5000/μL or mm³; cats, $> 7 \times 10^9$/L or > 7000/μL or mm³
• Absolute lymphocyte counts are greater in juveniles than in adults.

PATHOPHYSIOLOGY
• Lymphocytes are imperative for humoral- (B lymphocytes) and cell-mediated immunity (T lymphocytes). • B lymphocytes—derived from lymphoid stem cells in the bone marrow; responsible for the production of antibodies; differentiation of pre-B cells in the bone marrow is antibody independent; these undergo transformation into antibody-producing plasma cells. • T lymphocytes—derived from lymphoid stem cells in the bone marrow; differentiation in the thymus is influenced by interleukins and other substances produced by macrophages and cells in the thymic medulla and is antibody independent; responsible for cytotoxicity (a delayed-type hypersensitivity reaction), graft rejection, and regulation of the immune system through production of lymphokines
• Lymphoid cells produced in the bone marrow and thymus migrate to secondary lymphoid organs (e.g., lymph nodes, spleen, and gut-associated lymphoid tissue) where they give rise to immunocompetent cells in response to antigenic stimulation. • Under the proper stimulus, lymphocytes transform into lymphoblasts and then proliferate to make a clonal population of cells; the process is promoted by γ-interferon; some of the progeny become memory cells, but most express the appropriate immune response (humoral or cellular). • Lymphocyte generation time is 6–8 hr; stimulated by antigens; suppressed by corticosteroids, sex hormones, and malnutrition • Most B lymphocytes are short lived, with a survival time of several hours to about 5 days; most T lymphocytes and memory B lymphocytes are long lived, with an average lifespan of about 4 years; some memory cells can persist for decades. • B and T lymphocytes are responsible for approximately 95% of all lymphocytes; the remainder are "null" lymphocytes (i.e., large, granular lymphocytes), which serve as natural killer cells and other diverse functions. • Generally, the different types of lymphocytes cannot be identified on a blood film; occasionally, activated B lymphocytes (reactive lymphocytes) can be recognized by their large size, deep blue cytoplasm, and perinuclear clear zone; large, granular lymphocytes can be recognized by the presence of small, red cytoplasmic granules. • Reactive cells that have undergone blast transformation are known as immunoblasts.

RECIRCULATION
• Unlike granulocytes, about 70% of the lymphocytes that enter tissues return to the vasculature and recirculate. • Most recirculating lymphocytes are T cells along with small numbers of B memory cells. • Nonactivated lymphocytes circulate randomly in the blood. Once stimulated by antigen, further migration is altered. Lymphocytes stimulated in MALT undergo clonal expansion locally or complete the process in a local lymph node. Newly activated B cells migrate to MALT anywhere in the body, whereas T cells migrate to peripheral lymph nodes. Thus the immune response is dispersed throughout the entire body. • Lymphocyte migration is regulated by expression of specific adhesion molecules by HEV in the paracortical areas. Antigenic stimulation results in an increase in prominence and number of high endothelial venules. • Cytokines secreted at sites of inflammation increase expression of homing molecules and facilitate lymphocyte adhesion to HEV and migration into tissues.

SYSTEMS AFFECTED
• Hemic/Lymph/Immune—spleen, liver, and bone marrow owing to hyperplasia or neoplasia • Lymphoma can involve all systems and produce specific problems, including ocular, CNS, gastrointestinal, and renal.

SIGNALMENT
Dogs and cats

SIGNS
• Physiologic lymphocytosis—excited, vicious, or scared cat
• Lymphoma—large lymph nodes and, possibly, splenomegaly and hepatomegaly

CAUSES

Physiologic
• Epinephrine surge, especially common in excited cats • The change occurs in minutes and lasts about 30 min. • Can be produced by exogenous epinephrine injection, excitement, and fear; usually seen in young, healthy animals • Can be induced by difficulty collecting a blood sample • The change is much less common in cats that are sick. • The absolute lymphocyte count can occasionally rise to $> 20,000$/μL and is much greater than the relatively mild increase in mature neutrophils that accompanies this type of lymphocytosis.

Antigenic Stimulation
• Chronic inflammation, often with a suppurative component, such as pyometra and pyoderma • Immune-mediated diseases, acquired and autoimmune • Canine ehrlichiosis • Occasional cats with FeLV or FIV, although lymphopenia is more common • Vaccination • The increase in lymphocyte numbers associated with these problems is relatively mild and can range from the higher end of the reference range to approximately 10,000/μL. • Lymphocytosis in the face of an obvious clinical disease is particularly important because lymphopenia is a common response to the stress of disease.
• Immunocytes and immunoblasts (activated B lymphocytes) in the circulation generally indicate antigenic stimulation; however, morphologically, reactive lymphocytes cannot be readily distinguished from neoplastic lymphocytes.

Lymphoma
• Peripheral blood lymphocyte count can range from lymphopenia to counts $> 100,000$/μL. • Found in approximately 20% of dogs with lymphoma; usually mild to moderate (i.e., 5,000–15,000/μL); markedly high counts (i.e., $> 30,000$/μL) are uncommon. • Lymphopenia occurs in $> 50\%$ of dogs and cats with lymphoma and is more common than lymphocytosis in dogs with lymphoma because of the release of endogenous corticosteroids caused by the stress of the disease. • Immature and atypical-appearing lymphocytes should be searched for in a blood film; be sure to examine carefully the feathered edge or lateral margins of the blood smear.

Acute Lymphoblastic Leukemia
• Lymphoid neoplasia arises from and primarily involves the bone marrow and is unassociated with solid tumor masses.
• Counts of $> 20,000$/μL are usually seen owing to circulating lymphoblasts (usually T cells in cats and B cells in dogs).
• Occasionally, leukemia involves large granular lymphocytes characterized by large, pink, cytoplasmic granules. • Some animals are "aleukemic" (leukopenia with no circulating blasts) or subleukemic (normal leukocyte count with few circulating blasts). • Pancytopenia may result from myelophthisis, with lymphoblasts composing $> 30\%$ of the nucleated cells in the bone marrow.

Chronic Lymphocytic Leukemia
• Lymphoid neoplasm characterized by excessive numbers of small mature lymphocytes in the blood and bone marrow
• Lymphocyte counts range from 10,000–100,000/μL. • Lymphocytes appear normal or may have slightly more cytoplasm than normal. • Although the bone marrow usually contains high numbers of small lymphocytes, the level of infiltration is less than in patients with acute lymphoblastic leukemia. • Pancytopenia is uncommon.
• Clinical signs caused by tissue infiltration

Hypoadrenocorticism
• Occurs in 25–33% of dogs with hypoadrenocorticism due to the absence of glucocorticoids • Classically, accompanied by mild eosinophilia and the absence of neutrophilia or monocytosis in a sick and stressed animal

• A normal lymphocyte count in a sick and stressed animal suggests low glucocorticoids and, therefore, the possibility of hypoadrenocorticism.

Hyperthyroidism
• Approximately 10% of cats with hyperthyroidism have lymphocytosis.
• Lymphocyte count 4,000–14,000/μL

Drugs
• Methimazole associated with lymphocytosis in 7% of cats treated for hyperthyroidism
• Epinephrine and other β-adrenergic agonists can cause marked, transient lymphocytosis owing to recruitment from a noncirculating pool of lymphocytes.

RISK FACTORS
• FeLV infection—about 10–20% of feline lymphomas are positive for either FeLV antigen or DNA; insertion of viral DNA is thought to alter normal gene function and play a role in development of feline lymphoma. • FIV infection—lymphoma reported in a small percentage of affected cats, although the role of this virus in tumorigenesis appears to be indirect; recurrent infections and subsequent polyclonal B cell activation may set up the potential for malignant transformation.

DIAGNOSIS

DIFFERENTIAL DIAGNOSIS
• Ill, lethargic dog—consider hypoadrenocorticism, lymphoma, and acute lymphoblastic leukemia • Lymphadenopathy—consider lymphoma or ehrlichiosis • Thin, hyperactive, polyphagic cat—consider hyperthyroidism • Thin, lethargic cat—consider lymphoma

LABORATORY FINDINGS

Drugs That May Alter Laboratory Results
Corticosteroids cause lymphopenia.

Disorders That May Alter Laboratory Results
Incorrect identification of nucleated RBCs or monocytes as lymphocytes

Valid if Run in Human Laboratory?
Yes

CBC/BIOCHEMISTRY/URINALYSIS
• Severe lymphocytosis (> 15,000/μL)—consider acute lymphoblastic lymphoma or chronic lymphocytic leukemia
• Immature, bizarre, and abnormal lymphocytes in circulation—consider lymphoma or acute lymphoblastic leukemia
• Mature neutrophilia—consider physiologic epinephrine response and chronic inflammation

• Nonregenerative anemia, leukopenia, and/or thrombocytopenia—consider intramarrow disease, such as lymphoma and lymphocytic leukemia
• Eosinophilia—consider hypoadrenocorticism
• Polycythemia—consider hyperthyroidism
• Hypercalcemia—consider lymphoma

OTHER LABORATORY TESTS
• Serum protein electrophoresis monoclonal gammopathy suggests lymphoma and ehrlichiosis.
• Thyroid testing—high resting T_3, T_4 diagnoses hyperthyroidism
• Immunophenotyping—morphologic features may be insufficient to distinguish lymphoblasts from other hematopoietic progenitor cells (e.g., rubriblasts or myeloblasts). Immunophenotyping utilizes antibodies against cell surface molecules (cluster of differentiation antigens; CD antigens) to determine the specific cell type. Technique can be performed on formalin-fixed tissue sections, cytology smears, or cells in suspension (flow cytometry). ALL can be distinguished from AML by the presence of CD3 (T cells) or CD79a (B cells). The presence of CD34, an antigen expressed on early lymphohematopoietic progenitor cells, can be used to distinguish ALL that has infiltrated solid organs from stage V lymphoma. ALL tends to be CD34 positive. This antigen is not expressed by lymphoma, chronic lymphocytic leukemia, or myeloma, all of which involve less primitive cells.

IMAGING
Hepatosplenomegaly—consider lymphoma

DIAGNOSTIC PROCEDURES
• Biopsy helps confirm lymphoma.
• Examination of bone marrow aspirate used to diagnose acute lymphoblastic leukemia or stage lymphoma

TREATMENT
Treatment must be directed at the primary disease.

MEDICATIONS

DRUG(S)
Lymphoma—chemotherapy (see appropriate topics)

POSSIBLE INTERACTIONS
Complex interactions between levamisole, an immunomodulator that restores depressed immune function, and B and T lymphocytes.

FOLLOW-UP

PATIENT MONITORING
N/A

POSSIBLE COMPLICATIONS
N/A

MISCELLANEOUS

ASSOCIATED CONDITIONS
None

AGE-RELATED FACTORS
• Young puppies—lymphocyte count increases from birth to a maximum of 6,000/μL at approximately 6 weeks of age; value is within adult reference range for adults by 8 weeks of age. • Young kittens—absolute lymphocyte count increases from birth to a maximum of 10,500/μL at 12–14 weeks of age; value is within reference range for adults by 16–20 weeks of age.

SEE ALSO
• Ehrlichiosis • Hypoadrenocorticism (Addison's Disease) • Leukemia, Acute Lymphoblastic • Leukemia, Chronic Lymphocytic • Lymphoma—Cats • Lymphoma—Dogs

ABBREVIATIONS
• AML = acute myelogenous leukemia
• ALL = acute lymphoblastic leukemia
• FeLV = feline leukemia virus
• FIV = feline immunodeficiency virus
• HEV = high endothelial venules
• MALT = mucosa-associated lymphatic tissue

Suggested Reading
Dean GA. CD antigens and immunophenotyping. In: Feldman BF, Zinkl JG, Jain NC, eds. Schalm's veterinary hematology. 5th ed. Philadelphia: Lippincott Williams & Wilkins, 2000:689–695.
Tompkins M, Nelson PD, English RV, et al. Early events in the immunopathogenesis of feline retrovirus infections. J Am Vet Med Assoc 1991;199:1311–1316.
Wellman ML, Couto CG, Starkey RJ, Rajok JL. Lymphocytosis of large granular lymphocytes in three dogs. Vet Pathol 1989; 26:158–163.

Acknowledgment
The author and editors acknowledge the prior contributions of Dr. Donald Meuten, who authored this topic in a previous edition.

Author Joyce S. Knoll
Consulting Editor Stephen A. Kruth

LYMPHOMATOID GRANULOMATOSIS

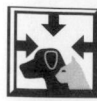 **BASICS**

OVERVIEW
• Rare pulmonary disease of dogs characterized by angiocentric and angiodestructive infiltration by atypical lymphoid cells
• Not a granulomatous disease as previously reported

SIGNALMENT
• Dogs
• Median age—5.75 years (range, 1.5–14 years)
• No breed predilection, but more common in large breeds and pure breeds

SIGNS
• Progressive respiratory signs including cough and dyspnea
• Exercise intolerance
• Weight loss
• Anorexia
• Fever in 50% of patients
• Duration—days to weeks

CAUSES & RISK FACTORS
Unknown

 DIAGNOSIS

DIFFERENTIAL DIAGNOSIS
• Mycotic, bacterial, or aspiration pneumonia
• Primary or metastatic pulmonary neoplasia

CBC/BIOCHEMISTRY/URINALYSIS
• Neutrophilic leukocytosis common
• Eosinophilia common
• Basophilia common

OTHER LABORATORY TESTS
N/A

IMAGING
• Radiography—reveals lobar pulmonary consolidation (e.g., mass lesions), hilar lymphadenomegaly, and pleural effusion
• Lesions—unilateral or bilateral

DIAGNOSTIC PROCEDURES
Biopsy—for definitive diagnosis

PATHOLOGIC FINDINGS
• Histologic—characterized by pleomorphic, angioinvasive mononuclear cells that often cause vascular obliteration
• Cytologic—may appear as sterile eosinophilic and neutrophilic inflammation with reactive macrophages

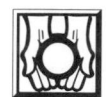 **TREATMENT**

Cytotoxic drugs combined with surgical excision when appropriate

MEDICATIONS

DRUG(S)
Combination protocol—COP suitable for lymphosarcoma

CONTRAINDICATIONS/POSSIBLE INTERACTIONS
• Myelosuppression—caused by cytotoxic drugs
• Hemorrhagic cystitis—caused by cyclophosphamide

 FOLLOW-UP

PATIENT MONITORING
Same as for lymphosarcoma treated by chemotherapy

POSSIBLE COMPLICATIONS
• Dyspnea as disease progresses
• Depression
• Anorexia
• Myelosuppression caused by chemotherapy

EXPECTED COURSE AND PROGNOSIS
Median survival with COP chemotherapy—12.5 months (range, days to 4 years)

 **MISCELLANEOUS**

ASSOCIATED CONDITIONS
May progress to lymphosarcoma

SYNONYMS
• Eosinophilic pulmonary granulomatosis
• Lymphoid granulomatosis
• Lymphoproliferative angiitis
• Granulomatosis

ABBREVIATION
COP = cyclophosphamide, vincristine (Oncovin), and prednisone

Suggested Reading
Berry CR, Moore PF, Thomas WP, et al. Pulmonary lymphomatoid granulomatosis in seven dogs (1976–1987). J Vet Intern Med 1990;4:157–166.
Morrison WB. Tumors of uncertain origin. In: Morrison WB, ed. Cancer in dogs and cats: medical and surgical management. Baltimore: Williams & Wilkins, 1998: 779–784.
Author Wallace B. Morrison
Consulting Editor Wallace B. Morrison

LYMPHOPENIA

 BASICS

DEFINITION
Absolute number of circulating lymphocytes less than reference range: dogs, $< 1 \times 10^9$/L or $< 1000/\mu$L or mm^3; cats, $< 1.5 \times 10^9$/L or $< 1,500/\mu$L or mm^3

PATHOPHYSIOLOGY
• B lymphocytes—derived from lymphoid stem cells in the bone marrow; responsible for the production of antibodies (humoral immunity)
• T lymphocytes—derived from lymphoid stem cells in the bone marrow; undergo further differentiation in the thymus; responsible for cytotoxicity (a delayed-type hypersensitivity reaction), graft rejection, and regulation of the immune system through production of lymphokines.
• Lymphoid cells produced in the bone marrow and thymus migrate to secondary lymphoid organs (e.g., lymph nodes, spleen, and gut-associated lymphoid tissue) where they give rise to immunocompetent cells in response to antigenic stimulation.
• Most antibody production takes place in the lymph nodes and involves participation of macrophages, B lymphocytes, and T lymphocytes; the interaction of these cells stimulates a clonal expansion of B and T cells; some of the progeny become memory cells, but most express the appropriate immune response (humoral or cellular).
• Lymphopoiesis is suppressed by corticosteroids, sex hormones, and malnutrition
• The number of lymphocytes in the blood depends on rates of production, recirculation, use, and destruction and does not necessarily reflect the level of lymphopoiesis.
• B and T lymphocytes are responsible for approximately 95% of all lymphocytes; the remainder are "null" lymphocytes (i.e., large, granular lymphocytes), which serve as natural killer cells and other diverse functions.
• Generally, the different types of lymphocytes cannot be identified on a blood film.
Recirculation
• Unlike granulocytes, about 70% of the lymphocytes that enter tissues return to the vasculature and recirculate.

• Most recirculating lymphocytes are T cells along with small numbers of B memory cells.
• Circulating T cells exercise immunologic surveillance.
• Most lymphocytes enter lymph nodes from the blood via HEV in the paracortical areas, but some enter from lymph.
• Nonactivated lymphocytes circulate randomly in the blood. Once stimulated by antigen, further migration is altered. Lymphocytes stimulated in MALT may undergo clonal expansion locally or travel to a local lymph node, where they complete the process. Newly activated B cells migrate to MALT anywhere in the body, whereas T cells migrate to peripheral lymph nodes. Thus the immune response is dispersed throughout the entire body.
• Lymphocyte migration is regulated by expression of specific adhesion molecules by HEV. Antigenic stimulation results in an increase in prominence and number of high endothelial or postcapillary venules.
• Cytokines secreted at sites of inflammation increase expression of homing molecules and facilitate lymphocyte adhesion to HEV and migration into tissues.

SYSTEMS AFFECTED
Hemic/Lymph/Immune—atrophy of lymph nodes and lymphoid tissue in spleen can be caused by some infectious agents.

SIGNALMENT
Dogs and cats

SIGNS
Relate to primary cause

CAUSES
Corticosteroid-induced
• Stress of systemic illness
• Hyperadrenocorticism—lymphopenia occurs in approximately 88% of affected dogs because of excess glucocorticoids
• Corticosteroid administration
• Corticosteroid-induced lympholysis and an increased shift of lymphocytes into tissue compartments
• Glucocorticoids inhibit interleukin synthesis by activated T lymphocytes and macrophages, resulting in immunosuppression.
• Classically accompanied by neutrophilia, monocytosis, and eosinopenia, but these are not consistent findings.

Acute Viral Infection
• FeLV—loss of both CD4$^+$ helper T lymphocytes and CD8$^+$ suppressor T lymphocytes; the CD4$^+$:CD8$^+$ ratio remains normal.
• FIV—selective loss of CD4$^+$ helper T cells and a relative lymphocytosis of CD8$^+$ suppressor T cells; an inverted CD4$^+$:CD8$^+$ ratio is seen
• Canine distemper virus—widespread atrophy and necrosis of lymphoid tissue results in depletion of both B and T lymphocytes; viral inclusions are occasionally seen in leukocytes (especially lymphocytes) or erythrocytes during the early stage of disease. Inclusions are large (up to 3 μm), homogeneous structures that stain from pale blue to reddish purple with Romanowsky stains
• Canine and feline parvovirus (feline panleukopenia virus)—destruction of rapidly dividing cells in both lymph nodes and bone marrow causes lymphopenia and neutropenia
• Infectious canine hepatitis

Loss of Lymphocytes
Loss of lymphocyte-rich lymph in patients with chylothorax, intestinal lymphangiectasia, or other protein-losing enteropathy

RISK FACTORS
None

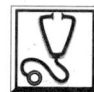 DIAGNOSIS

DIFFERENTIAL DIAGNOSIS
• Acute diarrhea—consider parvovirus or distemper infection
• Chronic diarrhea—consider protein-losing enteropathy
• Ill, lethargic cat—consider FeLV or FIV infection
• Cat with recurrent infection—consider FIV infection
• Thin-skinned, polyphagic, polyuric dog—consider hyperadrenocorticism
• Dyspnea—consider chylothorax
• Nasal discharge, cough—consider canine distemper infection
• Seizures—consider canine distemper infection

LABORATORY FINDINGS

Drugs That May Alter Laboratory Results
None

Disorders That May Alter Laboratory Results
Incorrect identification of nucleated RBCs or monocytes as lymphocytes

Valid if Run in Human Laboratory?
Yes

CBC/BIOCHEMISTRY/URINALYSIS
• Severe neutropenia—consider parvovirus
• Mature neutrophilia, monocytosis, and eosinopenia—consider glucocorticoid response to stress, exogenous glucocorticoid administration, and hyperadrenocorticism
• Marked elevation in alkaline phosphatase—consider canine hyperadrenocorticism
• Low serum total protein—consider protein-losing enteropathy and lymphangiectasia
• Nonregenerative anemia—consider FeLV

OTHER LABORATORY TESTS
• Serology—detect FeLV antigen in serum, canine parvovirus antigen in feces, and serum antibody titers to FIV and canine distemper
• Adrenal function testing—ACTH stimulation and low-dose dexamethasone suppression tests to diagnose hyperadrenocorticism; urine cortisol:creatinine ratio is a quick screen to rule out hyperadrenocorticism.

IMAGING
Large adrenal gland(s)—consider hyperadrenocorticism

DIAGNOSTIC PROCEDURES
Intestinal biopsy if lymphangiectasia suspected

 TREATMENT

Must be directed at the primary disease

 MEDICATIONS

DRUG(S) OF CHOICE
Hyperadrenocorticism—(see appropriate topics)

CONTRAINDICATIONS
None

PRECAUTIONS
None

POSSIBLE INTERACTIONS
Levamisole—an immunomodulator that restores depressed immune function; complex interactions with B and T lymphocytes affect their function

ALTERNATIVE DRUG(S)
None

 FOLLOW-UP

PATIENT MONITORING
N/A

POSSIBLE COMPLICATIONS
N/A

 MISCELLANEOUS

ASSOCIATED CONDITIONS
None

AGE-RELATED FACTORS
• Young puppies—lymphocyte count increases from birth to a maximum of 6000/μL at approximately 6 weeks of age; value is within adult reference range for adults by 8 weeks of age
• Young kittens—absolute lymphocyte count increases from birth to a maximum of 10,500/μL at 12–14 weeks of age; value is within reference range for adults by 16–20 weeks of age

ZOONOTIC POTENTIAL
None

PREGNANCY
N/A

SYNONYMS
None

SEE ALSO
• Distemper—Dogs
• Feline Immunodeficiency Virus
• Feline Panleukopenia
• Hyperadrenocorticism (Cushing disease)
• Protein-Losing Enteropathy

ABBREVIATIONS
• FeLV = feline leukemia virus
• FIV = feline immunodeficiency virus
• HEV = high endothelial venules
• MALT = mucosa-associated lymphatic tissue

Suggested Reading

Feldman BF, Zinkl JE, Jain NC, eds. Schalm's veterinary hematology. 5th ed. Philadelphia: Lippincott Williams & Wilkins, 2000.
Grindem CB. Blood cell markers. Vet Clin North Am Small Anim Pract 1996; 26:1043–1064.
Shelton GH, Linenberger MD, Abkowitz JL. Hematologic abnormalities in cats seropositive for feline immunodeficiency virus. J Am Vet Med Assoc 1991;199:1353–1357.
Tompkins M, Nelson PD, English RV, Novotney C, et al. Early events in the immunopathogenesis of feline retrovirus infections. J Am Vet Med Assoc 1991; 199:1311–1316.

Acknowledgment

The author and editors acknowledge the prior contributions of Dr. Kenneth S. Latimer, who authored this topic in a previous edition.
Author Joyce S. Knoll
Consulting Editor Stephen A. Kruth

LYMPHOSARCOMA—CATS

BASICS

DEFINITION
Malignant transformation of lymphocytes that reside mainly in lymphoid tissues

PATHOPHYSIOLOGY
Depends on the organs involved

SYSTEMS AFFECTED
• Hemic/Lymphatic/Immune
• Gastrointestinal
• Renal/Urologic
• Ophthalmic
• Nervous
• Skin/Exocrine
• Nasal

GENETICS
N/A

INCIDENCE/PREVALENCE
• About 90% of hematopoietic tumors and 33% of all tumors in cats
• Prevalence—41.6–200 per 100,000 cats

GEOGRAPHIC DISTRIBUTION
• On the East Coast (U.S.)—mediastinal lymphosarcoma most common (40%–52% of all patients)
• On the West Coast (U.S.)—alimentary lymphosarcoma most common (36% of all patients)

SIGNALMENT

Species
Cats

Breed Predilections
None

Mean Age and Range
• Mean age of FeLV-positive cats—3 years
• Mean age of FeLV-negative cats—7 years
• Median age of cats with localized extranodal lymphosarcoma—13 years

Predominant Sex
None

SIGNS

General Comments
• Depend on anatomic form

Historical Findings
• Mediastinal form—open-mouthed breathing; coughing; regurgitation; anorexia; weight loss
• Alimentary form—anorexia; weight loss; lethargy; vomiting; constipation; diarrhea; melena; frank blood in the stool
• Renal form—consistent with renal failure (e.g., vomiting, anorexia, polydipsia, polyuria, and lethargy)
• Multicentric form—possibly none in early stages; anorexia, weight loss, and depression with progression of disease
• Solitary form—depends on location; nasal lymphosarcoma: usually sneezing, nasal discharge, and occasionally facial deformity; spinal cord lymphosarcoma: quickly progressing posterior paresis may be seen; cutaneous lymphosarcoma: pruritic, hemorrhagic, or alopecic dermal masses may be seen

Physical Examination Findings
• Mediastinal form—noncompressible cranial thorax
• Alimentary form—thickened intestines or abdominal masses
• Renal form—large, irregular kidneys
• Multicentric form—generalized lymphadenomegaly
• All forms—fever; dehydration; depression; cachexia in some patients

CAUSES
FeLV—patients inconsistently test positive during illness (e.g., 85% with mediastinal, 45% with renal, 20% with multicentric, and 15% with alimentary)

RISK FACTORS
FeLV exposure

DIAGNOSIS

DIFFERENTIAL DIAGNOSIS
• Mediastinal form—congestive heart failure; cardiomyopathy; chylothorax; pyothorax; hemothorax; pneumothorax; diaphragmatic hernia; allergic lung disease; thymoma; ectopic thyroid carcinoma; pleural carcinomatosis; acetaminophen toxicity
• Alimentary form—foreign body ingestion; intestinal ulceration; intestinal fungal infection; inflammatory bowel disease; intussusception; lymphangiectasia; other gastrointestinal tumor
• Renal form—pyelonephritis; amyloidosis; glomerulonephritis; chronic renal failure
• Multicentric form—systemic mycotic infection; immune-mediated disease; toxoplasmosis; lymphoid hyperplasia; hypersensitivity reaction

CBC/BIOCHEMISTRY/URINALYSIS
• May see anemia, leukocytosis, and lymphoblastosis
• May find high creatinine, high serum urea nitrogen, high hepatic enzyme activity, hypercalcemia (rare), and monoclonal gammopathy
• May see isosthenuria, bilirubinuria, and proteinuria

OTHER LABORATORY TESTS
FeLV testing

IMAGING
• Thoracic radiography—evaluate for a mediastinal mass, pleural effusion, abnormal pulmonary parenchymal patterns (rare), and perihilar or retrosternal lymphadenomegaly
• Abdominal radiography—detect masses, hepatomegaly, splenomegaly, mesenteric or ileac (sublumbar) lymphadenomegaly, and unilateral or bilateral renomegaly
• Abdominal ultrasonography—reveal diffuse echotexture changes in the liver, spleen, and kidneys and focal thickening of the intestines

DIAGNOSTIC PROCEDURES
• Examination of bone marrow aspirate or core biopsy—evaluate bone marrow reserves
• Cytologic examination of a mass or lymph node
• Biopsy of a mass or lymph node

PATHOLOGIC FINDINGS
• Gross—likely to be white to gray in color with areas of hemorrhage and necrosis
• Cytologic—monomorphic population of pleomorphic lymphoid cells, sometimes with prominent, multiple nucleoli and coarse nuclear chromatin
• Histopathologic—vary; several morphologic classification schemes in use

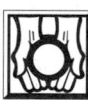

TREATMENT

APPROPRIATE HEALTH CARE
Outpatient whenever possible

NURSING CARE
N/A

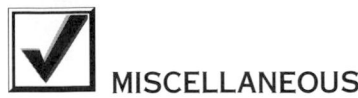
ACTIVITY
Normal

DIET
No change

CLIENT EDUCATION
• Warn client that a cure is possible but not likely.
• Inform client that the goal is to induce remission and achieve a good quality of life for patients for as long as possible.

SURGICAL CONSIDERATIONS
• To relieve intestinal obstructions and remove solitary masses
• To obtain specimens for histopathologic examination

MEDICATIONS

DRUG(S) OF CHOICE
• Chemotherapy—used in a combination or sequential protocol; some protocols have induction and maintenance periods
• Induction for combination chemotherapy—vincristine (0.5 mg/m² IV once weekly), cyclophosphamide (50 mg/m² PO q48h), cytosine arabinoside (100 mg/m² SC days 1 and 2), and prednisone (40 mg/m² q24h for 1 week; then 20 mg/m² PO q48h); use for 6 weeks.
• Maintenance for combination chemotherapy—methotrexate (2.5 mg/m² PO 3 times a week), chlorambucil (20 mg/m² PO every 2 weeks), prednisone (20 mg/m² PO q48h), and vincristine (0.5 mg/m² IV every 4 weeks)
• Relapsing lymphoma—doxorubicin, vinblastine, actinomycin-D, mitoxantrone, nitrogen mustard, procarbazine, and lomustine.
• Low-grade intestinal lymphoma has responded to Leukeran and prednisone.
• Radiotherapy—may be used for localized lymphoma; relapses outside the radiation field are not uncommon.

CONTRAINDICATIONS
None

PRECAUTIONS
• Myelosuppression secondary to chemotherapy—more common than average in FeLV-positive cats
• Seek advice before initiating treatment if you are unfamiliar with cytotoxic drugs.

POSSIBLE INTERACTIONS
None

ALTERNATIVE DRUG(S)
• Sequential chemotherapy—week 1: vincristine (0.025 mg/kg IV), L-asparaginase (400 IU/kg IM), and prednisone (2 mg/kg PO divided twice a day); week 2: cyclophosphamide (10 mg/kg IV); week 3: vincristine (0.025 mg/kg IV); week 4: methotrexate (0.8 mg/kg IV); then repeat the cycle; maintenance: lengthen the time between each treatment.
• Prednisone alone—temporary palliation

FOLLOW-UP

PATIENT MONITORING
• Physical examination, CBC, and platelet count—before each weekly cycle
• Radiography—as necessary

PREVENTION/AVOIDANCE
Avoid exposure to or breeding FeLV-positive cats.

POSSIBLE COMPLICATIONS
• Leukopenia
• Sepsis

EXPECTED COURSE AND PROGNOSIS
• Depends on initial response to chemotherapy, anatomic type, FeLV status, and tumor burden
• Mean survival with complete remission—7 months
• Median survival with partial remission—2.5 months
• Median survival with no response to treatment—1.5 months
• Mediastinal—about 10% of patients with live > 2 years
• Median survival with alimentary form—8 months
• Median survival with peripheral multicentric form—23.5 months
• Median survival with renal form—FeLV-negative, 11.5 months; FeLV-positive, 6.5 months
• Median survival with lymphosarcoma—FeLV-negative, 7 months; FeLV-positive, 3.5 months
• Median survival with a low tumor burden—FeLV-negative, 17.5 months; FeLV-positive, 4 months
• Treated with prednisone alone—patients live 1.5–2 months.
• Median duration of complete remission from localized lymphosarcoma—114 weeks

MISCELLANEOUS

ASSOCIATED CONDITIONS
• Hypoglycemia (rare)
• Monoclonal gammopathy (rare)
• Hypercalcemia (rare)

AGE-RELATED FACTORS
• Young cats with lymphosarcoma are generally FeLV-positive.

ZOONOTIC POTENTIAL
None

PREGNANCY
Do not use chemotherapy in pregnant animals.

SYNONYMS
• Lymphoma
• Malignant lymphoma

ABBREVIATION
FeLV = feline leukemia virus

Suggested Reading

Elmslie RE, Ogilive GK, Gillette EL, et al. Radiotherapy with and without chemotherapy for localized lymphoma in 10 cats. Vet Radiol 1991;32:277–280.

Jeglum KA, Whereat A, Young KA. Chemotherapy of lymphoma in 75 cats. J Am Vet Med Assoc 1987;190:174–178.

Mooney SC, Hayes AA, MacEwen EG, et al. Treatment and prognostic factors in lymphoma in cats: 103 cases (1977–1981). J Am Vet Med Assoc 1989;194:696–699.

Mooney SC, Hayes AA, Matus RE, et al. Renal lymphoma in cats: 28 cases (1977–1984). J Am Vet Med Assoc 1987;191:1473–1477.

Vonderhaar MA, Morrison WB. Lymphosarcoma. In: Morrison WB, ed. Cancer in dogs and cats: medical and surgical management. Jackson, Wyoming; Teton NewMedia, 2002;641–670.

Author Terrance A. Hamilton
Consulting Editor Wallace B. Morrison

LYMPHOSARCOMA—DOGS

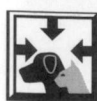 **BASICS**

DEFINITION
Clonal proliferation of neoplastic lymphocytes in solid tissues, primarily in lymph nodes, bone marrow, and visceral organs

PATHOPHYSIOLOGY
• Usually unifocal in origin with follicle-associated B lymphocytes that retain growth characteristics and the ability to migrate
• Ease of migration may account for spread of clinical disease.
• T lymphocyte lymphosarcoma—usually epitheliotropic (cutaneous) or mediastinal
• Clonal proliferation and high growth fraction may account for sudden onset of clinical signs.

SYSTEMS AFFECTED
• Hemic/Lymphatic/Immune—generalized, often peripheral, lymphadenomegaly with or without splenic, hepatic, and or bone marrow involvement and circulating malignant lymphocytes
• Gastrointestinal—infiltration of stomach, intestines, and associated lymph nodes
• Respiratory—proliferation of neoplastic lymphocytes in mediastinal lymph nodes, thymus, or lung parenchyma
• Miscellaneous (extranodal)—proliferation of or invasion by neoplastic lymphocytes in the bone marrow and ocular, cutaneous, mucocutaneous, neural, renal, cardiac, and other tissues

GENETICS
No consistent documentation of genetic basis

INCIDENCE/PREVALENCE
Reported as 6–30 per 100,000 dogs per year

SIGNALMENT

Species
Dogs

Breed Predilections
• Boxers, basset hounds, golden retrievers, Saint Bernards, Scottish terriers, Airedale terriers, and bulldogs—reported high-risk breeds
• Dachshunds and Pomeranians—reported low-risk breeds

Mean Age and Range
Patients usually 5–10 years old

Predominant Sex
None

SIGNS

General Comments
Depend on anatomic form and stage of disease

Historical Findings
• All forms of malignant lymphoma—nonspecific; anorexia; lethargy; weight loss
• Multicentric—generalized, painless lymphadenomegaly most common; may note distended abdomen secondary to hepatomegaly, splenomegaly, or ascites
• Gastrointestinal—vomiting; diarrhea; anorexia; abdominal discomfort
• Mediastinal—coughing; difficulty swallowing; anorexia; drooling; labored breathing; exercise intolerance secondary to mass(es) and/or effusion
• Extranodal—vary with the anatomic site; ocular: photophobia and conjunctivitis; CNS: seizures; cutaneous: plaque-like lesion; renal: lumbar pain; cardiac: exercise intolerance or syncope

Physical Examination Findings
• Multicentric—generalized, painless, irregular, movable, large lymph node(s) with or without hepatosplenomegaly
• Gastrointestinal—marked weight loss or palpable abdominal mass; thickened gut loops; rectal mucosal irregularities
• Mediastinal—dyspnea; tachypnea; muffled heart sounds secondary to pleural effusion
• Extranodal—ocular: anterior uveitis, retinal hemorrhages, and hyphema; cutaneous: raised plaque; neural: dementia, seizures, and paralysis; renal: renomegaly and renal failure; cardiac: arrhythmias

CAUSES
No specific cause proven

 DIAGNOSIS

DIFFERENTIAL DIAGNOSIS
• Infectious, neoplastic, immune-mediated, and inflammatory disease
• Cytologic and histologic evaluation and complete staging—differentiate from other diseases

CBC/BIOCHEMISTRY/URINALYSIS
• Anemia, lymphocytosis, lymphopenia, neutrophilia, monocytosis, circulating blasts, and thrombocytopenia common
• High ALT or ALP activity and hypercalcemia common
• Urinalysis usually normal

OTHER LABORATORY TESTS
Immunophenotyping to determine T or B cell characteristics

IMAGING
• Thoracic radiography—may reveal sternal or tracheobronchial lymphadenomegaly, widened mediastinum, pulmonary densities, and pleural effusion
• Abdominal radiography—may reveal sublumbar or mesenteric lymphadenomegaly, intestinal mass, abdominal effusions, and hepato(spleno)megaly
• Ultrasonography—lymphadenomegaly (obscured by effusion on radiographs) or nodules in visceral organs
• ECHO—evaluate cardiac contractility before doxorubicin administration

DIAGNOSTIC PROCEDURES
• Examine bone marrow aspirate and core biopsy—identify the extent of disease, which affects the chemotherapy choices
• CSF tap—if patient has CNS signs
• ECG—identify arrhythmias before doxorubicin administration

PATHOLOGIC FINDINGS
• Cut section—homogenous, white masses with areas of necrosis
• Monomorphic population of discrete round neoplastic cells that efface and replace parenchyma of lymph nodes and visceral organs or bone marrow

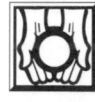 **TREATMENT**

APPROPRIATE HEALTH CARE
• Inpatient—intravenous chemotherapy
• Outpatient—after remission, some protocols allow owner to administer drugs orally at home; instruct owner to wear latex gloves when administering these drugs.
• Radiotherapy—may be used to treat refractory lymph nodes, large mediastinal involvement, and solitary cutaneous areas. Radiation therapy is also being used as an adjunct to chemotherapy in some oncology centers.

NURSING CARE
• Fluid therapy—may benefit patients with advanced disease; may benefit clinically ill and dehydrated patients
• Thoracocentesis or abdominocentesis—recommended with marked pleural or abdominal effusion

ACTIVITY
Restrict in patients with low WBC or platelet count

CLIENT EDUCATION
• Warn client that chemotherapy is rarely curative and relapse usually occurs.
• Inform client that the side effects of chemotherapy drugs depend on the type used but are usually associated with the gastrointestinal tract and bone marrow.
• Advise client that most dogs have leukopenia by day 7–10.
• Inform client that there is a 70%–80% response rate to most chemotherapy protocols.
• Note that the quality of life is good while the patient is receiving chemotherapy and while it is in remission; add that some protocols are associated with serious morbidity, whereas others have little morbidity.

SURGICAL CONSIDERATIONS
Rarely successful unless limited to one accessible site

MEDICATIONS

DRUG(S) OF CHOICE
• Combination chemotherapy—many protocols exist with similar remission and survival times
• Single-agent therapy (doxorubicin)—associated with remission and survival times that are similar to those for combination chemotherapy
• Corticosteroids alone—effective in the short term (1–2 months)
• Retinoids—may be used for cutaneous lymphosarcoma (3–4 mg/kg isotretinoin PO q24h)

Doxorubicin Protocol
Administer 30 mg/m² IV every 21 days (1 mg/kg for dog < 10 kg) for 3–5 treatments past complete remission (4–6 total treatments)

Combination Chemotherapy Protocol I
Induction
• Vincristine—0.5 mg/m² IV; day 1
• Cyclophosphamide—50 mg/m² PO; days 4–7
• Prednisone—20 mg/m² PO q12h
• Repeat weekly for 6 weeks; then begin maintenance
Maintenance
• Methotrexate—5.0 mg/m² PO; days 1 and 5
• Cyclophosphamide—100 mg/m² PO; day 3
• Prednisone—20 mg/m² q48h
• Continue for 6 weeks; then administer 1 week of induction; then 6 weeks of maintenance
• Continue for 1 year or until relapse

Combination Chemotherapy Protocol II (COPLA)
Induction
• L-asparaginase—10,000 units/m² SC; day 1 of weeks 1 and 2
• Vincristine—0.5–0.7 mg/m² IV; day 1 of weeks 1–8
• Cyclophosphamide—50 mg/m² PO q48h
• Prednisone—20 mg/m² PO q24h for 7 days; then q48h for 2–5 weeks; then 10 mg/m² PO q48h for 6 weeks; then stop
• Doxorubicin—30 mg/m² IV (1 mg/kg for dog < 10 kg); day 1 of weeks 6, 9, and 12
Maintenance
• Vincristine—0.5–0.7 mg/m² IV; day 1 every other week for 2 times; then day 1 every third week for 3 times; then day 1 every fourth week for 4 times; then day 1 every sixth week for 1 year
• Chlorambucil—4 mg/m² PO q48h for up to 2 years, starting on day 1 of week 1 and continuing for up to 2 years if remission is maintained

CONTRAINDICATIONS
N/A

PRECAUTIONS
• Doxorubicin—use cautiously or not at all with poor cardiac contractility or arrhythmias; use cautiously in patients with > 80% of bone marrow replaced by cancer cells
• L-asparaginase or doxorubicin—pretreat with diphenhydramine (1 mg/kg SC) 20 min before administration
• Always use a catheter when administering intravenous drugs.

POSSIBLE INTERACTIONS
All chemotherapy drugs must be given according to published protocols, because many have overlapping side effects.

ALTERNATIVE DRUG(S)
• Many alternative treatment protocols exist
• Lomustine (CCNU) or dacarbazine (DTIC)—may use for refractory cases

 FOLLOW-UP

PATIENT MONITORING
• Physical examination and cytologic or histologic evaluation—all nonresponsive lymph nodes
• CBC and platelet count—(1) on day 10 after first treatment; if severe leukopenia or neutropenia (WBC < 2000 cells/mm³; neutrophils < 1000 cells/mm³) is noted, reduce dosage (15%–25%) or add colony-stimulating factors to the protocol; (2) before each anthracycline chemotherapy or weekly (on day 1) with combination chemotherapy; if moderate or severe leukopenia (WBC < 4000 cells/mm³) is noted, delay treatment until cell counts return to normal (usually 1 week)
• After 2–3 courses of chemotherapy treatments, repeat tests with abnormal results before administering next treatment to confirm response.
• Echocardiography and ECG—periodically during and after doxorubicin administration to identify development of cardiotoxicity

POSSIBLE COMPLICATIONS
• Leukopenia and neutropenia
• Vomiting and diarrhea
• Anorexia
• Cardiotoxicity—due to doxorubicin; usually after total cumulative dose of 180–240 mg/m²
• Alopecia
• Pancreatitis
• Sepsis
• Tissue sloughing—with extravasated dose

EXPECTED COURSE AND PROGNOSIS
• Median duration of first remission with combination chemotherapy or doxorubicin—6 months (range, 45–334 days); 58%–90% of patients achieve complete remission.
• Median survival time with combination chemotherapy or doxorubicin—6–12 months (range, 112–365 days)
• Mediastinal form and/or hypercalcemia—poorer prognosis
• Primary CNS, diffuse gastrointestinal, and multisite cutaneous forms—associated with poor response to treatment

 MISCELLANEOUS

PREGNANCY
Treatment of pregnant dogs is contraindicated.

SYNONYMS
• Lymphoma • Malignant lymphoma

SEE ALSO
• Hypercalcemia
• Leukemia, Acute Lymphoblastic
• Leukemia, Chronic Lymphocytic

ABBREVIATIONS
• ALP = alkaline phosphatase • ALT = alanine aminotransferase • CCNU = chloroethylcyclohexylnitrosourea • CNS = central nervous system • COPLA = cyclophosphamide, vincristine (Oncovin), prednisone, and L-asparaginase • CSF = cerebrospinal fluid • DTIC = (dimethyltriazeno)imidazole carboxamide • ECG = electrocardiogram • ECHO = echocardiogram • WBC = white blood cell

Suggested Reading
Keller E, MacEwen E, Rosenthal R, et al. Evaluation of prognostic factors and sequential combination chemotherapy for canine lymphoma. J Vet Intern Med 1993:7;289–295.
Teske E. Canine malignant lymphosarcoma: a review and comparison with human non-Hodgkin's lymphosarcoma. Vet Q 1994;4:209–219.
Vonderhaar MA, Morrison WB. Lymphosarcoma. In: Morrison WB, ed. Cancer in dogs and cats: medical and surgical management. 2nd ed. Jackson, WY: Teton NewMedia, 2002:641–670.
Author Mary Ann Vonderhaar
Consulting Editor Wallace B. Morrison

LYMPHOSARCOMA, EPIDERMOTROPIC

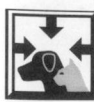 BASICS

OVERVIEW
• A subset of cutaneous T cell lymphosarcoma
• An uncommon malignant neoplasia affecting many species, including dogs and cats
• Mycosis fungoides and Sézary syndrome (mycosis fungoides with associated leukemia)—most common forms of cutaneous T cell lymphosarcoma
• Pagetoid reticulosis—rare; the lymphoid infiltrate is generally confined to the epidermis in the early stages of the disease.

SIGNALMENT
• More common in dogs than in cats
• Affects old dogs and cats; mean age 9–12 years
• No apparent breed or sex predilection

SIGNS
Historical Findings
• Chronic skin disease—months to years before diagnosis
• Erythema
• Depigmentation
• Scaling
• Alopecia
• Sometimes pruritus

Physical Examination Findings
• Erythema
• Scaling
• Depigmentation
• Alopecia
• Infiltrative plaques
• Ulceration
• Crusting
• Multiple nodules or mass formation
• Pruritus
• Lesions—throughout the skin; marked tendency for involvement of mucocutaneous junctions (lip, eyelids, nasal planum, anorectal junction, or vulva) or the oral cavity (gingiva, palate, or tongue)
• Usually three principal phases—patch, plaque, and tumor; progression to the tumor stage is very rapid in dogs (compared to humans); may also occur in tumor stage from the onset (tumor d'emblee form)

CAUSES & RISK FACTORS
None identified

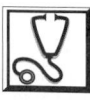 DIAGNOSIS

DIFFERENTIAL DIAGNOSIS
• Dermatophytosis, demodicosis—alopecia, erythema, scaling
• Allergies, scabies—generalized pruritus, erythema, scaling
• Cutaneous lupus erythematosus, erythema multiforme, other immune-mediated diseases—mucocutaneous depigmentation/ulceration
• Nonneoplastic chronic stomatitis—infiltrative and ulcerative oral mucosal disease
• Histiocytoma, cutaneous histiocytosis, mast cell tumor, or any other cutaneous neoplasia—nodule or mass formation

CBC/BIOCHEMISTRY/URINALYSIS
• Laboratory abnormalities—vary, depending on the stage and form of cutaneous T cell lymphosarcoma (mycosis fungoides vs. Sézary syndrome)
• Generally not helpful in the early stages

OTHER LABORATORY TESTS
N/A

IMAGING
Radiographs and ultrasound—not commonly used in the early stages; imaging is eventually necessary to confirm systemic disease and/or for tumor staging.

DIAGNOSTIC PROCEDURES
• Skin scrapings and fungal culture—rule out demodicosis and dermatophytosis, if applicable.
• Skin biopsy—definitive diagnosis

PATHOLOGIC FINDINGS
• Lymphoid infiltrate—into epidermis and epithelium of hair follicles and adnexal structures; distributed diffusely or as discrete Pautrier microaggregates within the epithelium
• Dermal infiltrate—polymorphous; also consists of malignant lymphocytes that obscure the dermoepidermal junction; in the patch and plaque stages, limited to the superficial dermis; in the tumor stage, extends to the deep dermis and subcutis
• Lymphocyte epitheliotropism—usually remains prominent throughout all stages

 TREATMENT

• Inform the client that a cure is extremely unlikely.
• The goal is to maintain a good quality of life for as long as possible.
• Therapy is usually of little benefit; rarely, solitary nodules can be surgically excised, resulting in long-term remissions or "cures."

 MEDICATIONS

DRUG(S)
• Chemotherapy—several protocols used with limited to no success, including various combinations of prednisolone, chlorambucil, vincristine, cyclophosphamide, doxorubicin, and methotrexate
• Topical chemotherapy—mechlorethamine (nitrogen mustard) has resulted in some success in managing early lesions; it has not been shown to alter the fatal course of the disease.
• α-Interferon, retinoids, extracorporeal photophoresis, and anti–T cell monoclonal antibodies—recently investigated in therapeutic trials with variable results
• Recent medication trials: lomustine 30 to 90 mg/m² every 4 weeks for 4–5 treatments; carmustine, topical; bexarotene (expensive retinoid); cyclosporine 5–10 mg/kg/day; doxorubicin 30 mg/m² every 3 weeks; tacrolimus, topical (especially nasal lesions); safflower oil (Hollywood brand) 3 mL/kg twice weekly

CONTRAINDICATIONS/POSSIBLE INTERACTIONS
• Depend on the chemotherapeutic or treatment protocol
• Seek advice from a veterinary oncologist or dermatologist before initiating therapy if you are unfamiliar with cytotoxic drugs and/or to learn about the most recent treatment protocols.

 FOLLOW-UP

• Prognosis grave
• Average survival time for dogs, from the onset of skin lesions to death, is 5–10 months.
• Death is usually the result of euthanasia.
• Rarely, dogs and cats may live for longer than 2 years after the diagnosis is made.

 MISCELLANEOUS

Suggested Reading
Moore PF, Olivry T. Cutaneous lymphomas in companion animals. Clin Dermatol 1994;12:499–505.
Scott DW, Miller WH, Griffin CE. Muller & Kirk's small animal dermatology. 5th ed. Philadelphia: Saunders, 1995.
Authors K. Marcia Murphy and Karen Helton Rhodes
Consulting Editor Karen Helton Rhodes

BASICS

OVERVIEW
• Rare inherited disorders caused by partial or complete deficiency of a lysosomal enzyme or an enzyme-activator protein, which leads to intracytoplasmic accumulation (storage) of the substrate of that enzyme
• Storage products—proteins, carbohydrates, lipids, or a combination
• Major classes of disease—proteinoses, glycoproteinoses, oligosaccharidoses, sphingolipidoses, mucopolysaccharidoses
• Many different types are reported in both dogs and cats.
• Inheritance is autosomal recessive

SIGNALMENT
• Dogs—German short-haired pointer, English setter, beagle, cairn terrier, bluetick hound, West Highland terrier, Sidney silky terrier, English springer spaniel, Portuguese water dog, Japanese spaniel, Labrador retriever, mixed breed dogs, many others.
• Cats—Persian, Siamese, Korat, Balinese, domestic shorthaired.
• Most affected animals are < 1 year old, but a few adult-onset diseases have been described.

SIGNS
General Comments
• Vary with the severity of the enzyme deficiency
• Carrier animals can be affected with a milder form of the disease.
• Many organ systems are affected, but neurologic signs tend to predominate.

Historical Findings
• Affected animals usually normal at birth
• Fail to thrive and may manifest skeletal malformations, particularly in the mucopolysaccharidoses
• Manifest a variety of neurologic signs within the first few months of life that suggest multifocal neurologic disease

Physical Examination Findings
• Cerebellar dysfunction common—intention tremor, nystagmus, dysmetria
• Peripheral neuropathy occurs in some diseases—weakness, hyporeflexia or areflexia, wasting
• Other neurologic—ataxia; exercise intolerance; seizures; behavioral changes; visual deficits, deafness, stereotypical behaviors, proprioceptive deficits
• Non-neurologic—may see organomegaly or skeletal malformations
• Ocular pathology present in some diseases—corneal opacification, cataract formation

CAUSES & RISK FACTORS
• Genetic—deletion or mutation involving a single gene that causes an absolute or partial deficiency of a lysosomal enzyme or activator protein; deficient production of enzymes that do not have normal biologic activity
• Susceptible breed

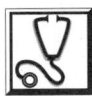

DIAGNOSIS

DIFFERENTIAL DIAGNOSIS
• Metabolic encephalopathy—usually episodic clinical signs; results of hemogram, biochemistry analysis, and urinalysis are often diagnostic
• Toxicities—acute onset of clinical signs; history of exposure
• Cerebellar hypoplasia—onset at 3–6 weeks of age; nonprogressive
• Cerebellar abiotrophy—deficits limited to the cerebellum; may be difficult to differentiate in the early stages without specific tests
• Prenatal or neonatal infections (especially viral) resulting in meningoencephalomyelitis—differentiated by CSF analysis; may be other signs, such as chorioretinitis
• Metabolic diseases—especially organic and amino acidurias

CBC/BIOCHEMISTRY/URINALYSIS
• Regular blood smears and CSF analysis—cytoplasmic vacuolation of leukocytes caused by accumulation of storage products is present in some cases.
• Urine—may find abnormal accumulation of substances (e.g., oligosaccharide in α-mannosidosis)

OTHER LABORATORY TESTS
N/A

IMAGING
• Radiographic evidence of bony malformation may be present in those diseases where skeletal pathology is a feature, e.g., the mucopolysaccharidoses
• Magnetic resonance imaging was used in one case to reveal diffuse white matter pathology in the brain of a dog with globoid cell leukodystrophy, and may be abnormal in some other diseases.

DIAGNOSTIC PROCEDURES
• Aspirates or biopsies of parenchymal organs, particularly the liver and spleen, may reveal intracellular storage material.
• Electromyography and nerve conduction studies frequently are abnormal in those diseases where peripheral neuropathy or myopathy is a feature.
• Biopsy of peripheral nerve or skeletal muscle may demonstrate specific pathology.
• Specific diagnosis is made by demonstrating low enzyme activity in preparations of serum, brain, viscera, leukocytes, or skin fibroblasts.
• Molecular genetic testing—now available for the specific diagnosis of a small number of lysosomal storage diseases; may be used to identify potential carriers of these diseases

TREATMENT
• Outpatient—unless severe deficits preclude nursing care at home
• Activity—restrict to safe areas; avoid stairs.
• Diet and fluids—ensure proper intake (patients are often debilitated); parenteral fluid therapy and enteral or parenteral nutritional support may be needed with severe disease
• Bone marrow transplantation—used experimentally with some success
• Gene therapy—may offer hope for specific treatment
• Primary treatment—preventive; control of breeding; genetic counseling
• Patients may be at high risk of developing secondary infection; monitor closely; initiate appropriate treatment if infection develops.

MEDICATIONS

DRUG(S)
N/A

CONTRAINDICATIONS/POSSIBLE INTERACTIONS
N/A

FOLLOW-UP
• Progressive and ultimately fatal
• Pedigree analysis—may be useful in diagnosis; important for identification of potential carrier animals

MISCELLANEOUS

ABBREVIATION
• CSF = cerebrospinal fluid

Suggested Reading
Jolly RD, Walkley SU. Lysosomal storage diseases of animals: an essay in comparative pathology. Vet Pathol 1997;34:527–548.
Skelly BJ, Franklin RJM. Recognition and diagnosis of lysosomal storage diseases in the cat and dog. J Vet Intern Med 2002; 16:133–141.
Author Mary O. Smith
Consulting Editor Joane M. Parent

MALASSEZIA DERMATITIS

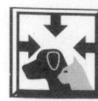

BASICS

OVERVIEW
• *Malassezia pachydermatis* (syn. *Pityrosporum canis*)—yeast; normal commensal of the skin, ears, and mucocutaneous areas; can overgrow and cause dermatitis, cheilitis, and otitis in dogs and cats • *M. pachydermatis* is lipid loving, but several species isolated from the cat are lipid dependent. • Yeast numbers in diseased areas are usually excessive, although this is a variable finding. • The causes of the transformation from harmless commensal to pathogen are poorly understood but seem related to allergy, seborrheic conditions, and possibly congenital and hormonal factors. • Canine *Malassezia dermatitis* and *Malassezia*-associated seborrheic dermatitis—common in all geographic regions of the world

SIGNALMENT
• Dogs—any dog breed; however, West Highland white terriers, poodles, basset hounds, cocker spaniels, and dachshunds are predisposed • Cats—less common than in dogs; disease and predisposing causes are speculated to be similar to those in the dog in young to middle-aged cats; aged cats may have *Malassezia dermatitis* associated with internal neoplasia; any breed may be affected; however, young rex cats are predisposed • No gender predilection

SIGNS
• Pruritus—with varying degrees of erythema, alopecia, scale, and greasy, malodorous exudation; affects lips, ears, feet, axillae, inguinal area, and ventral neck • Hyperpigmentation and lichenification—chronic cases • Concurrent black waxy to seborrheic otitis—frequent • Frenzied facial pruritus—uncommon but characteristic • Often a history of suspected allergy that worsens and seems to develop resistance or is resistant to glucocorticoid treatment • Concurrent pyoderma, hypersensitivities, and endocrine and keratinization disorders

CAUSES & RISK FACTORS
• High humidity and temperature—may increase the frequency • Concurrent hypersensitivity disease (particularly atopy, flea allergy, and some food allergy/intolerances)—may be a predisposing factor • Defects of cornification and seborrheas (especially in young dogs)—in predisposed breeds • Endocrinopathies (especially in old dogs)—suspected to be associated predisposing factors • Genetic factors—suspected for young onset in predisposed dog breeds and rex cats • Concurrent increase in cutaneous *Staphylococcus intermedius* population and resultant pyoderma—confirmed finding; canine seborrheic dermatitis is proposed, in selected cases, to be a result of this combination pathogen overgrowth; treatment of one alone does not result in resolution of all signs, but just unmasks the other; antiyeast treatment alone resolves all signs of *Malassezia dermatitis*

• Cats have both a young- and adult-age disease, which can be allergy associated. In rex cats, genetic features related to their unique coat or skin features or their predisposition to a mast cell abnormality called urticaria pigmentosa may be factors. Aged cats may have *Malassezia dermatitis* associated with thymomas and carcinomas of the pancreas and liver.

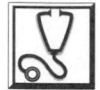

DIAGNOSIS

Diagnosis is made by demonstrating the organism on diseased skin usually associated with signs of scale and inflammation and a variable degree of seborrhea (as in abnormality of sebum) and pruritus; confirmed by finding a significant improvement in clinical signs on removal of the yeast

DIFFERENTIAL DIAGNOSIS
• Allergic dermatitis—including flea allergy, atopy, and food allergy • Superficial pyoderma • Primary and secondary seborrheas

CBC/BIOCHEMISTRY/URINALYSIS
Changes reflect predisposing conditions (e.g., hypothyroidism, hyperadrenocorticism) rather than yeast infection.

OTHER LABORATORY TESTS
• Fungal culture—use contact plates (small agar plates made from bottle lids and filled with Sabouraud agar or, preferably, modified Dixon agar, especially in the cat); press plates onto the affected skin surface; incubate at 32°–37°C for 3–7 days; count the distinctive yellow or buff, round, domed colonies (1–1.5 mm); provides semiqualitative data • Nonquantitative culture methods—no value because *Malassezia* is a normal commensal

IMAGING
• Dog—not appropriate • Aged cat—ultrasonography and radiography to investigate possible internal malignancy

DIAGNOSTIC PROCEDURES
Skin cytology—touch, cotton swab, or cellophane tape preparation stained with Diff-Quik; apply stain as a drop directly onto the slide (yeast may wash off during staining); pass a flame under the slide to improve stain penetration and visualization

TREATMENT

• Goals—confirm diagnosis by associating elimination of signs with reduction in yeast and bacterial numbers • Identify and treat any predisposing factors or diseases. • Topical therapy—yeast is principally located in the stratum corneum • Shampoo treatment—to remove scale, exudation, and malodor • Topical therapies (based on trial data)—Malaseb (DVM Pharmaceuticals, Miami, FL), a miconazole and chlorhexidine shampoo; less effective but useful is selenium sulfide shampoo; twice-weekly treat-

ments effective • Other topical antifungal and antibacterial shampoo treatments may also be of value if given with suitable systemic drugs. • Alternative combinations—topical keratolytic shampoo treatment with systemic antiyeast and antibacterial drugs

MEDICATIONS

DRUG(S)
• Localized cases—may respond to creams and lotions containing imidazole compounds • Ketoconazole—10 mg/kg q24h for 2–4 weeks in widespread or chronic lichenified cases • Chronic lichenified cases—ketoconazole (7–10 mg/kg q24h) as a short diagnostic for 7–10 days with effective topical antimycotic shampoo (miconazole and chlorhexidine combination) treatment; a good response confirms the diagnosis; response may be slow in chronic cases in which yeasts are buried deep in epidermal folds • Topical antimicrobial antibacterial (Malaseb) shampoo—to maintain remission in chronic cases

CONTRAINDICATIONS/POSSIBLE INTERACTIONS
• Ketoconazole—rarely may cause hepatic reaction; masks signs of hyperadrenocorticism and interferes with adrenal function tests due to blocking of cortisol production (via inhibition of P-450) in the adrenal gland; contraindicated in cats with hepatic and severe debilitating internal malignancy as they may not be able to metabolize the drug

FOLLOW-UP

• Physical examination and skin cytology—after 2–4 weeks, to monitor therapy • Treat until only rare organisms can be demonstrated or 7 days after a complete response is achieved. • Pruritus and odor—usually noticeably improved within 1 week • Recurrences—common when underlying dermatoses are not well controlled; regular bathing with antifungal antibacterial shampoo combinations (miconazole plus chlorhexidine) helps decrease recurrence

MISCELLANEOUS

PREGNANCY
Ketoconazole contraindicated

Suggested Reading
Scott DW, Miller WH, Griffin CE. Muller & Kirk's small animal dermatology. 5th ed. Philadelphia: Saunders, 1995.
Author K. V. Mason
Consulting Editor Karen Helton Rhodes

MALIGNANT FIBROUS HISTIOCYTOMA (GIANT CELL TUMOR)

BASICS

OVERVIEW
• Name based on histologic features of fibroblast- and histiocyte-like cells
• Mesenchymal neoplasm, but definitive cellular origin unknown; likely possibilities include fibroblasts, histiocytes, and undifferentiated mesenchymal cells
• Several histologic variants
• Storiform-pleomorphic and giant-cell—two major variants; both locally invasive; firm, subcutaneous or visceral masses on examination
• Despite previous reports to the contrary, metastatic potential in dogs appears to be moderate to high.
• Have been reported as injection site–related sarcomas of cats

SIGNALMENT
• More commonly reported in cats than in dogs
• Similar biologic behavior in both species
• Mean age—cats: 9 years (range, 2–12 years); dogs: 8 years (range, < 1–10 years); reported in a 4-month-old, mixed-breed, male puppy
• No breed or sex predilection

SIGNS
Historical Findings
• Anorexia, weight loss, and lethargy may occur.
• Depend on site of involvement
Physical Examination Findings
• Firm, invasive tumor arising in subcutaneous tissue
• May exhibit deep extension into underlying skeletal muscle
• May develop adjacent to bone and induce bone destruction and proliferation
• Most common sites—dorsal thoracic and scapular area, limbs, and pelvic region
• May also be a primary splenic tumor; palpable splenomegaly may be found
• Distant metastasis—common

CAUSES & RISK FACTORS
• Unknown
• Can be induced with carcinogens in laboratory animal species
• Injection sites in cats

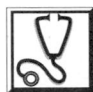

DIAGNOSIS

DIFFERENTIAL DIAGNOSIS
• Fibrosarcoma
• Chondrosarcoma
• Osteosarcoma (extraskeletal)
• Mast cell neoplasia
• Rhabdomyoma or rhabdomyosarcoma
• Liposarcoma
• Peripheral nerve sheath tumors
• Histiocytic diseases, like malignant or systemic histiocytosis
• Histiocytes sarcoma

CBC/BIOCHEMISTRY/URINALYSIS
• CBC—may vary; may be normal; may see regenerative or nonregenerative anemia
• Biochemistry—variably abnormal
• Urinalysis—usually normal

OTHER LABORATORY TESTS
Cytologic examination of aspirate—may reveal histiocyte- and fibroblast-like cells

IMAGING
• Radiography—reveals soft tissue dense mass; may note bone proliferation or destruction
• Ultrasonography—may detect abnormalities consistent with abdominal metastasis (most common in lymph nodes and liver)
• Metastasis potential would suggest physical examination and possible imaging—monthly for three months, then every 3–6 months

DIAGNOSTIC PROCEDURES
Histologic examination of biopsy specimen—necessary for definitive diagnosis

PATHOLOGIC FINDINGS
• Classification—considerable debate exists among pathologists, which may account for the apparent differences in behavior reported in the literature
• Many are histologically high grade
• Recent report of considerable overlapping histopathologic characteristics with histiocytic diseases in the splenic form.

TREATMENT
• Surgical excision—difficult owing to local invasive nature; recurrence rate is high.
• Amputation of an affected limb—may be appropriate; thoracic and abdominal radiographs and abdominal ultrasound critical for evaluating for detectable metastasis before amputation
• Radiotherapy—may be helpful as adjuvant treatment for localized tumor not amenable to surgical resection

MEDICATIONS

DRUG(S)
Chemotherapy—may be helpful in residual, high grade tumor or metastatic disease setting; doxorubicin (patient > 10 kg, 30 mg/m^2 IV every 3 weeks; patients < 10 kg, 1 mg/kg IV every 3 weeks).

CONTRAINDICATIONS/POSSIBLE INTERACTIONS
N/A

FOLLOW-UP
Reexamination—according to growth of tumor

MISCELLANEOUS

Suggested Reading
MacEwen EG, Powers BE, Macy D, et al. Soft tissue sarcomas. In: Withrow SJ, MacEwen EG, eds. Small animal clinical oncology. 3rd ed. Philadelphia: Saunders, 2001:287.

Acknowledgment
The author and editors acknowledge the prior contributions of James P. Thompson, who authored this topic in a previous edition.
Author Anthony J. Mutsaers
Consulting Editor Wallace B. Morrison

MALOCCLUSION OF TEETH

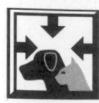

BASICS

OVERVIEW

The accurate assessment of abnormalities of occlusion will help determine if treatment is warranted and what treatment is appropriate.

Modified Angle Classification System of Malocclusion

• Class 0—normal occlusion: evaluate alignment of incisors (scissor bite), premolars (pinking shear effect), and carnassial teeth (close alignment of the developmental grooves: upper fourth premolar to lower first molar)
• Class 0, type 3—normal in brachycephalic breeds (e.g., boxers, bulldogs); some breeds allow "level" bite
• Class 1—jaws correct length, but specific teeth malpositioned (dental malocclusion); anterior crossbite; lance tooth; base-narrow canine teeth; and posterior crossbite
• Class 2—lower jaw (mandible) short in relation to upper jaw (maxilla) (skeletal malocclusion); tooth inclination or location may be improper (overshot)
• Class 3—lower jaw (mandible) long in relation to upper jaw (maxilla) (skeletal malocclusion); tooth inclination or location may be improper (undershot)
• Class 4—type of "wry bite" in which one quadrant is elongated and one quadrant is shortened (skeletal malocclusion); simple unilateral-type wry bites come within classes 1, 2, and 3, respectively

SIGNALMENT

• No sex or age predilection, though malocclusion usually apparent after eruption of teeth (permanent or deciduous)
• Breed predilection for certain malocclusions (e.g., lance teeth in Shetland sheepdogs)

SIGNS

• Vary greatly according to type, extent, and consequent injuries caused by the malocclusion
• May be associated with open or closed bites or overcrowding of the teeth
• Periodontal disease—may result from crowding or misalignment of teeth
• Soft tissue defects—from traumatic tooth contact; may be seen in the floor of the mouth and palate; palatal trauma may eventually result in oronasal fistula formation

• Fractures or attrition (wear) of teeth—may result from improper tooth contact

Class 1 Malocclusions

• Anterior crossbite (AXB)—palatally displaced maxillary incisors or labially displaced mandibular incisors
• Base-narrow canines—tips of mandibular canines touch palate lingual to normal contact point, just labial to the diastema between corner incisor and maxillary canine
• Lance teeth—mesioversion or rostroversion of maxillary canine(s); the diastema between the corner incisor and this canine is often diminished and may force the mandibular canine into an abnormal position
• Posterior crossbite (PXB)—most are due to reversal of the relationship (labial/lingual) between the upper and lower carnassial teeth; more common in dolichocephalic breeds (e.g., collies, shelties, some sight hounds)

CAUSES & RISK FACTORS

• Congenital or hereditary factors—skeletal malocclusions (classes 2, 3, and 4) and breed predilection
• Impediment to tooth eruption—operculum; retention of soft tissue covering
• Delayed eruption of deciduous or permanent teeth
• Retention or delayed loss of deciduous teeth
• Traumatic injury affecting the jaws or teeth

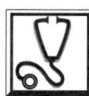

DIAGNOSIS

Based on visual and radiographic findings and the Modified Angle Classification System of Malocclusion (see Overview)

DIFFERENTIAL DIAGNOSIS

• Tooth displacement—due to trauma, oral masses, or other causes
• Mechanical block—due to jaw fractures, luxated or subluxated teeth, or foreign bodies causing open bite

IMAGING

• Oral photography—pre-, peri-, and post-therapy
• Intraoral radiography—to evaluate roots and abnormalities

DIAGNOSTIC PROCEDURES

Impressions and models—for evaluation and appliance manufacture

PATHOLOGIC FINDINGS

N/A

TREATMENT

Not every malocclusion needs orthodontic correction. If the bite is functional and nontraumatic to the animal, treatment may not be necessary. Additionally, extraction (or crown reduction with pulp capping) of offending teeth often can be an effective alternative to more classic orthodontic treatments. Orthodontic treatment is usually based on prevention of improper contact trauma, wear, or injury to hard or soft tissues.

Permanent Tooth Class 1 Malocclusion

Treatment primarily involves tipping movements of the teeth, although extrusion may be required to provide proper retention.
• Anterior crossbite—crowding: odontoplasty to thin teeth (use caution); labial maxillary arch bar with button brackets and elastic ligatures or chains (to move maxillary incisors forward or to extrude) is one of the best treatment methods; lingual maxillary arch bar with finger spring, mandibular or maxillary incline plane, maxillary expansion screw appliance, or mandibular brackets and elastic chains are all possible treatment modalities
• Base-narrow canine teeth—prevention of contact trauma, pain and discomfort, and oronasal fistula formation; if very mild, a gingivoplasty or gingivectomy in the diastema may release the contact; an orthodontic appliance may be needed to help guide a more significant deviation, tipping the tooth to a functional location or proper occlusion; orthodontic tipping movements can be provided by a number of different appliances, e.g., acrylic or composite inclined plane, expansion screws, W springs, cast-metal incline planes, and composite auto-incline planes (build-up on tooth)
• Lance tooth—button or brackets applied toward the tip of the canine tooth to be moved (target tooth) and near the gingiva of the anchor teeth (upper fourth premolar and first molar), with an elastic power chain applied between the two; careful monitoring to avoid anchor tooth movement (root surface area should exceed that of target tooth)
• Posterior crossbite—in most cases, no treatment is necessary as the bite is typically functional; in traumatic situations, extract of one of the offending teeth; orthodontic

correction is long and tedious and requires more advanced orthodontic appliances and blocking the bite open

Permanent Tooth Class 2, 3, and 4 Malocclusion
• Based on providing a functional, nontraumatic occlusion for the animal's medical health; if one is already present, treatment may not be necessary
• May require advanced orthodontic and surgical procedure and is generally best handled by a specialist

Deciduous Tooth Class 1 Malocclusion
Careful and gentle extraction of the maloccluded deciduous tooth to remove inappropriate physical impediment (interceptive orthodontics) in hopes that the permanent tooth will erupt in the appropriate position; when performed at least 4 weeks prior to permanent tooth eruption, success rate > 80% is not uncommon

Deciduous Tooth Class 2, 3, and 4 Malocclusion
Careful and gentle extraction of the maloccluded deciduous tooth in hopes that the short jaws will be released from the bite interlock, allowing it to grow (if the genetic potential is present), prior to eruption of permanent teeth and reestablishment of bite interlock; performed at least 6 weeks prior to permanent tooth eruption, success rate < 20% is common

MEDICATIONS

DRUG(S)
N/A

FOLLOW-UP

HOME CARE WITH APPLIANCE
• Examine the appliance twice daily.
• Flush the mouth with an oral hygiene solution or gel.
• Prevent chewing of items and provide a soft diet until the appliance is removed.

PATIENT MONITORING
• For the corrected occlusion to be stable, it needs to be self-retaining or it may tend to revert to malocclusion; examine at 2 weeks, 2 months, and 6 months after the treatment is complete to see if desired outcome is stable
• It is advisable at around 6 months post-therapy for radiographs to be taken and compared to the pretreatment films to determine if all teeth still appear vital (alive) and to evaluate any root changes that may have occurred due to the pressures of tooth and root movement during orthodontics.

EXPECTED COURSE AND PROGNOSIS
• Course of treatment may vary with the type of malocclusion and the animal's nature and habits (e.g., inappropriate chewing).
• Generally, most cases take 1–7 months for movement and retention phase, depending on severity and if extrusion of tooth/teeth is required for stabilization of the bite. Prognosis is good to excellent in most treated patients.
• Prognosis is fair to good in most untreated malocclusions.
• Complications in untreated cases—periodontal disease; attrition or fractures of teeth; trauma to soft tissues; oronasal fistula formation; drying or desiccation of exposed tooth surfaces, resulting in beige to brown discoloration
• Some cases DO NOT need or require orthodontic intervention; only routine observation for early detection and treatment of any secondary complications (e.g., periodontal disease, worn or chipped teeth) are advised

PREVENTION/AVOIDANCE
• Careful selection of puppies, with oral and general examination, as well as examination and history of sire and dame, prior to purchase
• Selective breeding based on preferred breed characteristics
• Careful monitoring of deciduous and permanent tooth eruption for early detection and treatment, if required

POSSIBLE COMPLICATIONS
• Selective extraction of deciduous tooth prior to permanent tooth eruption—potential for injury to underlying permanent tooth buds either by direct injury with extraction

instruments or subsequent traumatic inflammation affecting tooth growth and maturity; injuries may result in tooth buds dying, teeth becoming nonvital as they erupt, root dysplasia or dilaceration, crown hypoplasia, or hypomineralization
• Orthodontic movement of permanent teeth—several conditions may result from root resorption, root ankylosis, or nonvitality of the tooth; these conditions are uncommon in properly managed orthodontic procedures

MISCELLANEOUS

ASSOCIATED CONDITIONS
• Lack of head symmetry
• Oral soft tissue trauma
• Chipped teeth
• Desiccation of exposed tooth surfaces
• Periodontal disease

AGE-RELATED FACTORS
Typically, the condition is initially observed at < 14 months of age, usually shortly following tooth eruption.

ETHICAL CONSIDERATIONS
Although animals have the medical right to as functional and correct an occlusion as can be reasonably provided by therapy, animal club rules, professional association principles, and state and national laws may conflict with an animal's right to proper medical therapy. Some kennel club rules disqualify animals with modification to natural appearance (with certain exceptions), and owners should be made aware of this. If hereditary involvement is suspected, inform the owner. If treatment is being considered, the owner or agent should acknowledge his or her responsibility to inform anyone who has the right to know of such alterations. Additionally, the possibility of removing the animal from the genetic pool by appropriate methods should be discussed.

Suggested Reading
Wiggs BW, Lobprise HB. Veterinary dentistry—principles and practice. Philadelphia: Lippincott-Raven, 1997:457–463.
Authors Bob Wiggs and Stephen Coles
Consulting Editor Heidi B. Lobprise

MAMMARY GLAND HYPERPLASIA—CATS

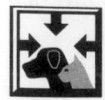

BASICS

OVERVIEW
A progesterone-dependent enlargement of one or more mammary glands

SIGNALMENT
• Young, intact, cycling, or pregnant queens
• Cats of either gender that are receiving exogenous progestogen (e.g., megestrol acetate)

SIGNS
• Localized or diffuse enlargement of one or more mammary glands
• Firm and nonpainful masses
• No concurrent signs of systemic illness

CAUSES & RISK FACTORS
• Secondary to a progesterone influence
• High progesterone—false pregnancy in queen induced to ovulate but nonpregnant

for 40–50 days after ovulation induction; throughout gestation; with exogenous progestogens

DIAGNOSIS

DIFFERENTIAL DIAGNOSIS
• Mastitis—lactating queen; mammary glands erythematous and painful; systemic illness with fever and immature neutrophilia; inflammatory cells and bacteria in fluid expressed from the affected gland(s)
• Mammary neoplasia—old queens (> 6 years of age); gross appearance may be indistinguishable; differentiated by biopsy of affected tissue

CBC/BIOCHEMISTRY/URINALYSIS
Normal

OTHER LABORATORY TESTS
N/A

IMAGING
N/A

DIAGNOSTIC PROCEDURES
• Cytologic examination of fluid expressed from affected glands—noninflammatory
• Excision biopsy—benign fibroglandular proliferation with no inflammation or necrosis

TREATMENT
• Hypertrophy owing to high endogenous progesterone—regresses when progesterone falls at the end of false pregnancy or gestation; consider ovariohysterectomy if fertility is not an issue.
• Hypertrophy owing to exogenous progestogens—regresses when medication is withdrawn

MEDICATIONS

DRUG(S)
• Bromocriptine mesylate—0.25 mg PO q24h for 5–7 days; not approved for use in cats; may cause nausea
• Nausea—metoclopramide (0.2 mg/kg PO q6–8h) or divided bromocriptine dose (give twice daily)
• Megestrol acetate (Ovaban)—reported success equivocal

CONTRAINDICATIONS/POSSIBLE INTERACTIONS
N/A

FOLLOW-UP
• Likelihood of recurrence in cats left intact—unknown
• Correlation with other abnormal conditions of the reproductive tract—unknown

MISCELLANEOUS

SYNONYMS
• Benign mammary hypertrophy
• Mammary fibroadenomatosis
• Fibroglandular mammary hypertrophy

Suggested Reading
Hayden DW, Johnston SD, Krang DT, et al. Feline mammary hypertrophy/fibroadenoma complex: clinical and hormonal aspects. Am J Vet Res 1981;42:1699–1703.
Author Margaret V. Root Kustritz
Consulting Editor Sara K. Lyle

MAMMARY GLAND TUMORS—CATS

 BASICS

DEFINITION
Malignant and benign tumors of the mammary glands in cats

PATHOPHYSIOLOGY
• Hormonal influences—may be involved
• Between 80% and 90% are malignant.

SYSTEMS AFFECTED
• Reproductive—mammary glands and metastatic sites
• Metastases at the time of euthanasia—> 80% of patients; one or more of the following sites: lymph nodes, lungs, pleura, liver, diaphragm, adrenal gland, and kidneys

GENETICS
• Unknown
• Siamese cats—may have twice the risk of other breeds

INCIDENCE/PREVALENCE
• Third most common neoplasia in cats (after hematopoietic and skin tumors)
• Accounts for 17% of neoplasms in female cats

GEOGRAPHIC DISTRIBUTION
N/A

SIGNALMENT
Species
Cats

Breed Predilections
Domestic shorthair and Siamese cats—higher reported incidence rates than other breeds

Mean Age and Range
• Mean—10–12 years
• Range—9 months to 23 years

Predominant Sex
Most (99%) develop in intact females

SIGNS
Historical Findings
Many patients have advanced disease on examination—average of 5 months after the tumors are first noticed

Physical Examination Findings
• Firm, nodular mass which may adhere to the skin but not to underlying abdominal wall
• Approximately 60% of patients have multiple gland involvement; one third have simultaneous involvement of both right and left mammary gland chains
• Any or all glands may be involved; slightly higher incidence observed for the two cranial glands
• Nipples—often red and swollen; may exude tan or yellow fluid
• Ulceration—noted in one quarter of patients
• Infiltrated lymphatic vessels—may appear as subcutaneous, linear, beaded chains
• Pelvic limbs—may be edematous and uncomfortable; temperature may be abnormal owing to tumor thrombi or impaired vascular return

CAUSES
• Unknown
• Strong association with prior use of progesterone-like drugs
• Only 10% of tumors are positive for estrogen receptors.

RISK FACTORS
• Intact females have a sevenfold higher risk than do spayed females.
• Genetic—Siamese breed
• Administration of progesterone-like drugs (e.g., megestrol acetate)—associated with development of benign and malignant masses
• Early ovariohysterectomy—protective effect not as clearly defined as in dogs

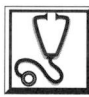 **DIAGNOSIS**

DIFFERENTIAL DIAGNOSIS
• Lobular hyperplasia
• Fibroepithelial hyperplasia
• Papillary cystic hyperplasia
• Mastitis
• Cysts

CBC/BIOCHEMISTRY/URINALYSIS
Anemia and leukocytosis—may occur

OTHER LABORATORY TESTS
Coagulation profile—with large, ulcerated tumors; rule out DIC

IMAGING
• Thoracic radiographs—detect lung metastases or pleural effusion; metastatic patterns may vary from discreet nodules to a diffuse interstitial pattern.
• Abdominal radiographs or ultrasound of sublumbar lymph nodes or ascites

DIAGNOSTIC PROCEDURES
• Preliminary biopsy—not recommended because of the high frequency of malignancy, unless results will change owner's willingness to treat; tissue for histopathologic examination obtained at the time of mastectomy
• Cytologic examination—mass(es): may rule out nonmammary malignancies; lymph nodes: with suspected metastasis; pleural fluid (if noted)

PATHOLOGIC FINDINGS
• Gross—adherence to overlying skin and ulceration common
• Histopathology—> 80% of tumors are adenocarcinomas: tubular, papillary, and solid most common; most are a combination of tumor types; often contain extensive areas of necrosis with lymphocytic and plasma-cell infiltration
• Metastasis to regional lymph nodes—50% of patients

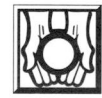 **TREATMENT**

APPROPRIATE HEALTH CARE
Discharge after surgery if stable.

NURSING CARE
Provide supportive fluids and appropriate antibiotics as needed.

ACTIVITY
N/A

DIET
N/A

CLIENT EDUCATION
• Stress the importance of early detection and removal.
• Stress the potential benefits of early ovariohysterectomy.

SURGICAL CONSIDERATIONS
• Radical mastectomy—patients without radiographic evidence of metastasis regardless of tumor size; removal of all four glands of the affected chain significantly reduces the chance of local recurrence; include the ipsilateral axillary (if large or cytologically suspect) and inguinal lymph nodes.
• Tumors in both mammary chains—perform two radical mastectomies, usually 2–4 weeks apart.
• Concurrent ovariohysterectomy—may address coexisting ovarian and uterine disease

MEDICATIONS

DRUG(S) OF CHOICE
• Combination chemotherapy—doxorubicin (1 mg/kg IV q 3 weeks) and cyclophosphamide (50 mg/m^2 PO on days 3, 4, 5, and 6); repeat every 3–4 weeks; shown to induce short-term partial and complete responses in about half of patients with metastatic or nonresectable local disease
• Other agents (carboplatin, mitoxantrone) may have activity.

CONTRAINDICATIONS
• Doxorubicin—renal disease
• Doxorubicin—compromised myocardial function
• Severe myelosuppression

PRECAUTIONS
• Doxorubicin—do not exceed a cumulative dose of 200 mg/m^2.

• Chemotherapy may be toxic; seek advice before initiating treatment if you are unfamiliar with cytotoxic drugs.
• Hepatic disease
• Renal disease

POSSIBLE INTERACTIONS
Verapamil—may potentiate doxorubicin-induced cardiomyopathy; avoid concurrent use.

ALTERNATIVE DRUG(S)
• Mitoxantrone—may substitute for doxorubicin
• No available biological response modifier has shown efficacy.

FOLLOW-UP

PATIENT MONITORING
• Complete physical examination—bimonthly; emphasis on palpation of previous incision line(s), remaining mammary glands, and axillary and inguinal lymph node regions
• Thoracic radiographs—every 1–3 months

PREVENTION/AVOIDANCE
Ovariohysterectomy—reduces the risk considerably; age for procedure to be done that will provide optimum effectiveness is unknown.

POSSIBLE COMPLICATIONS
• Tumor—anemia; osteoporosis; hypercalcemia; DIC; ascites; pleural effusion
• Chemotherapy—dilated cardiomyopathy; myelosuppression; anorexia; gastrointestinal toxicity; renal insufficiency; hepatopathy; agents may be carcinogenic and mutagenic.

EXPECTED COURSE AND PROGNOSIS
• High incidence of recurrence (66% with conservative surgery) and metastasis
• Time to recurrence—related to the type of surgery; radical mastectomy disease-free interval, 575 days (survival, 800 days); conservative surgery disease-free interval, 325 days (survival, 500 days)

• Single most important prognostic factor—tumor size; median survival with diameter > 3 cm, 6 months after surgery; median survival with diameter < 2 cm, approximately 3 years

MISCELLANEOUS

ASSOCIATED CONDITIONS
• Cystic ovaries
• Mastitis
• Uterine disease
• Other unrelated tumors

AGE-RELATED FACTORS
• Middle-aged cats most commonly affected
• Siamese cats—develop tumors at a younger age; incidence reaches a plateau at approximately 9 years.

ZOONOTIC POTENTIAL
None

PREGNANCY
Do not use chemotherapy in pregnant animals.

ABBREVIATION
DIC = disseminated intravascular coagulation

Suggested Reading
Jeglum KA, DeGuzman E, Young KM. Chemotherapy of advanced mammary adenocarcinoma in 14 cats. J Am Vet Med Assoc 1985;187:157–160.
MacEwen EG, Withrow SJ. Tumors of the mammary gland. In: Withrow SJ, MacEwen EG, eds. Small animal clinical oncology. 2nd ed. Philadelphia: Saunders, 1996:365–372.
Morrison WB. Canine and feline mammary gland tumors. In: Morrison WB, ed. Cancer in dogs and cats: medical and surgical management. Baltimore: Williams & Wilkins, 1998:591–598.
Author Sue Downing
Consulting Editor Wallace B. Morrison

MAMMARY GLAND TUMORS—DOGS

 BASICS

DEFINITION
Benign or malignant tumors of the mammary glands in dogs

PATHOPHYSIOLOGY
• Malignancy—about 50%
• About 50% of patients have multiple tumors.
• Lymphatic connections—exist between right and left series of glands; generally, cranial glands drain to axillary lymph nodes, caudal glands drain to inguinal lymph nodes, and in-between glands drain variably to either or both types of nodes; plexiform connections help explain occurrence of lymphatic metastasis against predicted lymph flow.
• Hormonal influence—suggested by lower incidence in dogs spayed at an early age (see Prevention/Avoidance)

SYSTEMS AFFECTED
• Reproductive
• Metastasis—respiratory, nervous, and other systems

GENETICS
N/A

INCIDENCE/PREVALENCE
Females—198.8 per 100,000

GEOGRAPHIC DISTRIBUTION
Similar worldwide

SIGNALMENT

Species
Dogs

Breed Predilection
None

Mean Age and Range
• Median age—about 10.5 years (range, 1–15 years)
• Uncommon in dogs < 5 years

Predominant Sex
Female; extremely rare in males

SIGNS

Historical Findings
Usually slow-growing single or multiple masses

Physical Examination Findings
• Single or multiple masses—about 50% of patients have multiple tumors.
• May be ulcerated
• May be freely movable—implies benign behavior
• May be fixed to skin or body wall—implies malignant behavior

CAUSES
Unknown; likely hormonal

RISK FACTORS
Circumstantial evidence—incriminates treatment with progestins and estrogen in combination, prolactin, and growth hormone

 DIAGNOSIS

DIFFERENTIAL DIAGNOSIS
• Lipoma
• Mast cell tumor
• Mammary hyperplasia
• Mastitis

CBC/BIOCHEMISTRY/URINALYSIS
• Usually normal
• Hypercalcemia and hypoglycemia—occasionally reported

OTHER LABORATORY TESTS
N/A

IMAGING
• Thoracic radiography—may detect metastasis
• Abdominal radiography—may detect metastasis to iliac (sublumbar) lymph nodes
• Radionuclide bone scanning—rarely positive in dogs

DIAGNOSTIC PROCEDURES
• Examination of cytologic preparations—often misleading; inflammation may mimic criteria of malignancy.
• Excisional biopsy—definitive diagnosis

PATHOLOGIC FINDINGS
• Gross—associated with considerable inflammation; may find ulceration
• Histopathologic—50% benign; 42% adenocarcinoma; 4% inflammatory carcinoma; 4% sarcoma

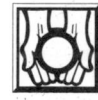 TREATMENT

APPROPRIATE HEALTH CARE
• Surgery—primary mode of treatment
• Chemotherapy—may be effective; infrequently reported

NURSING CARE
N/A

ACTIVITY
N/A

DIET
N/A

CLIENT EDUCATION
• Advise client that a mammary lump should never be left in place and observed.
• Inform client that early surgical intervention is best.
• Advise spaying before first estrus.

SURGICAL CONSIDERATIONS
Local excision (e.g., simple, regional, or unilateral mastectomy) with wide and deep margins (at least 2 cm in all directions)—may be as effective in terms of disease-free interval as radical bilateral mastectomy

MEDICATIONS

DRUG(S) OF CHOICE
Doxorubicin—30 mg/m² IV every 21days; reported to have induced partial remission in two dogs for 12 and 16 months, respectively

CONTRAINDICATIONS
Myocardial failure

PRECAUTIONS
Chemotherapy may be toxic; seek advice before treatment if you are unfamiliar with cytotoxic drugs.

POSSIBLE INTERACTIONS
Doxorubicin—side effects include myelotoxicity, vomiting and diarrhea, pancreatitis, and cardiac damage.

ALTERNATIVE DRUG(S)
Tamoxifen—helpful in some humans with breast cancer; ineffective in dogs and has serious side effects; do not use in dogs and cats.

FOLLOW-UP

PATIENT MONITORING
Physical examination and thoracic radiographs—1, 3, 6, 9, and 12 months after treatment

PREVENTION/AVOIDANCE
• Spayed before first estrous cycle—0.5% risk compared to intact bitch
• Spayed before second estrous cycle—8.0% risk compared to intact bitch
• Spayed after second estrus—26% risk compared to intact bitch
• Spayed after 2.5 years of age—no sparing effect on risk

POSSIBLE COMPLICATIONS
N/A

EXPECTED COURSE AND PROGNOSIS
• Median survival after mastectomy with tubular adenocarcinoma—24.6 months
• Median survival after mastectomy with solid carcinoma—6.5 months
• Benign tumor—excellent prognosis after mastectomy
• Carcinoma < 5 cm in diameter—usually a good prognosis if excision is complete

MISCELLANEOUS

Inflammatory carcinoma—very aggressive subtype; characterized by rapid growth, firmness, diffuse involvement, erythema, limb edema, color change, and pain; patient may be anemic, have leukocytosis, and develop DIC; tumor may be mistaken for mastitis, abscess, or dermatitis; prognosis poor

ASSOCIATED CONDITIONS
• Hypertrophic osteopathy
• Metastasis to lungs and CNS

AGE-RELATED FACTORS
N/A

ZOONOTIC POTENTIAL
N/A

PREGNANCY
N/A

ABBREVIATIONS
• CNS = central nervous system
• DIC = disseminated intravascular coagulation

Suggested Reading

Allen SW, Mahaffey EA. Canine mammary neoplasia: prognostic indicators and response to surgical therapy. J Am Anim Hosp Assoc 1989;25:540–546.

Hahn KA, Richardson RC, Knapp DW. Canine malignant mammary neoplasia: biological behavior, diagnosis, and treatment alternatives. J Am Anim Hosp Assoc 1992;28:251–256.

Morris JS, Dobson JM, Bostock DE. Use of tamoxifen in control of canine mammary neoplasia. Vet Rec 1993;133:539–542.

Morrison WB. Canine and feline mammary tumors. In: Morrison WB, ed. Cancer in dogs and cats: medical and surgical management. Baltimore: Williams & Wilkins, 1998:591–598.

Authors Wallace B. Morrison and Kevin A. Hahn

Consulting Editor Wallace B. Morrison

MARKING AND ROAMING BEHAVIOR

BASICS

OVERVIEW
• Marking—leaving scent (urine, feces, anal sacs, or sebaceous glands) on an object or to define territory; occurs on vertical and horizontal surfaces
• Middening—marking with feces
• Bunting—facial marking in cats
• Spraying—urine marking in cats
• Roaming—free wandering of an animal to locate, explore, or define an area, object, or individual.
• Normal behaviors with multiple causes—may be maladaptive owing to stimuli in the animal's environment

SIGNALMENT
• Dogs and cats, any sex or breed
• Age at onset—puberty in male dogs, first estrus cycle in females
• Most common in intact males, or intact females in estrus
• Exhibited by castrated males and spayed females

SIGNS
• Marking—deposition of urine and/or fecal matter, often in locations unacceptable to owners; occurs inside and outside of the home
• Roaming—wandering behavior that takes the animal away from its home; may occur secondary to other behavior problems
• Physical examination findings unremarkable unless a medical etiology for marking behavior

CAUSES
• Normal dog and cat behaviors
• Hormonally regulated; intact males likely to roam and mark
• Learned components possible; reproductive status not sole variable

Roaming
• Hunger
• Anxiety
• Curiosity

• Reproduction
• Social contact and play

Marking
• Medical condition
• Communication with conspecifics; communicates social rank, dominance, sexual status, territorial boundaries, general information about the animal itself and others
• Anxiety

RISK FACTORS
• Intact males more likely to roam and mark.
• Marking on walks; learned behavior
• Intact bitches, queens, or females spayed after first heat
• Cats with history of urinary tract disease
• Poor litterbox hygiene, multiple cats in home, cats roaming into yard

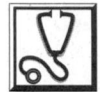

DIAGNOSIS

DIFFERENTIAL DIAGNOSIS
Define the cause of the behavior as either normal or a sign of another diagnosis.

Roaming
• Sexually motivated behavior
• Hunger/searching for food
• Separation anxiety
• Noise phobias
• Territorial behavior
• Social facilitation
• Predatory behavior
• Play/investigative behavior

Marking
• Sexually motivated behavior
• Territorial behavior
• Social dominance behavior
• Conflict behavior
• Anxiety
• Housesoiling
• Urinary tract disease
• Constipation or diarrhea
• Anal sac disease

CBC/BIOCHEMISTRY/URINALYSIS
Normal without urinary tract disease

OTHER LABORATORY TESTS
As indicated:
• Thyroid testing if roaming due to hunger
• Urine culture and sensitivity
• Vaginal cytology to determine estrus status

IMAGING
Radiographs or ultrasound if urinary tract disease

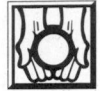

TREATMENT

Roaming
• Neuter intact males.
• Secure enclosure to prevent escape.
• Leash walk.
• Adequate exercise, attention, supervision, stimulation
• Doggie day care
• Ad libitum feeding—decrease need to search for food
• Treat separation anxiety—gradual desensitization, counterconditioning
• Treat other phobias and anxiety.

Marking
• Neuter intact males.
• Spay females early—before first estrus to prevent hormone effects.
• Treat urinary tract disease if present.
• Appropriate environmental changes as necessary (litterbox hygiene, litter preference testing, increasing available boxes in home)
• Deter other outdoor animals from interacting with pet.
• Remove stimuli or triggers.
• Express anal sacs if necessary.
• Treat constipation if necessary.
• Clean marked areas with effective enzymatic cleaners.
• Decrease motivation to urine mark—use synthetic pheromone to encourage bunting.

MEDICATIONS

DRUG(S)
• Medication is not necessary for roaming unless the primary problem (separation anxiety or noise phobias) warrants its use. Spraying due to medical etiologies should be treated accordingly.
• No drugs approved for the treatment of spraying in cats; informed owner consent is appropriate.
• Antianxiety medications—used for spraying due to anxiety or social conflict

Tricyclic Antidepressants
• Amitriptyline—dog: 2.2–4.4 mg/kg PO q24h; cat: 2.5–5.0 mg/cat/day
• Clomipramine—dog: 1–3 mg/kg PO q12h; cat: 0.5–1.0 mg/kg PO q12–24h
• Side effects include sedation, anticholinergic effects, cardiac conduction disturbances, and GI signs.

Selective Serotonin Reuptake Inhibitors
• Fluoxetine—dog: 0.5–2 mg/kg PO q24h; cat: 0.5–1.0 mg/kg PO q24h
• Paroxetine—dog: 1–2 mg/kg PO q24h; cat: 0.5–1.0 mg/kg PO q24h
• Side effects include sedation, inappetence, lethargy; irritability, urine retention, constipation.

Azaperone
• Buspirone—dog: 0.5–2.0 mg/kg PO q8–12h; cat: 2.5–10 mg/cat/day PO
• Side effects—GI signs, increased social conflict possible in cats

Benzodiazepines
• In dogs with concurrent anxiety diagnoses—alprazolam, 1 mg/15 kg PO q8h as needed
• Diazepam for spraying cats—0.2–0.4 mg/kg PO q12–24h. Use with extreme caution, as cases of fatality due to hepatotoxicity have been reported.

Megestrol Acetate
• Outdated treatment—use only as last resort.
• Side effects—obesity, pyometra, polyuria/polydipsia, diabetes mellitus, mammary hyperplasia, and carcinoma

CONTRAINDICATIONS/POSSIBLE INTERACTIONS
• Tricyclic antidepressants are contraindicated in animals with cardiac conduction disturbances or glaucoma.
• Clomipramine should not be used in aggressive dogs.
• Use caution with all drugs if animals have hepatic or renal compromise.
• Use benzodiazepines with caution in aggressive dogs because of disinhibition.
• Do not use tricyclic antidepressants or selective serotonin reuptake inhibitors with monoamine oxidase inhibitors, including amitraz products and selegiline.

FOLLOW-UP

PATIENT MONITORING
Follow up is variable depending on the severity of the problem, the diagnosis, and whether medication is prescribed. Help may be needed implementing changes to the environment and behavior modification.

PREVENTION/AVOIDANCE
• Neutering males and spaying females reduces likelihood of marking behaviors.
• Client education via proper husbandry techniques helpful

POSSIBLE COMPLICATIONS
• Roaming—possible injury from being hit by car, fighting with other animals
• Marking—property damage when it occurs inside the home
• Pet relinquishment

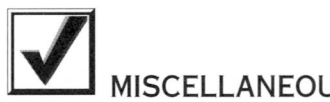

MISCELLANEOUS

AGE-RELATED FACTORS
Intact animals at or older than sexual maturity

ZOONOTIC POTENTIAL
Roaming exposes pet to other animals, including wildlife—rabies exposure possible

PREGNANCY
Listed medications should be avoided in pregnant animal.

Suggested Reading
Borchelt PL. Cat elimination behavior problems. Vet Clin N Am Sm Anim Pract 1991;21:257–264.
Hopkins SG, Schubert TA, Hart BL. Castration of adult male dogs: Effects on roaming, aggression, urine marking, and mounting. J Am Vet Med Assoc 1976;168:1108–1110.
Author Tracy L. Kroll
Consulting Editor Debra F. Horwitz

MAST CELL TUMORS

BASICS

DEFINITION
Neoplasia arising from mast cells

PATHOPHYSIOLOGY
• Histamine and other vasoactive substances released from mast cell tumors—may cause erythema and edema; histamine may cause gastric and duodenal ulcers. • Heparin release—increases likelihood of bleeding

SYSTEMS AFFECTED
• Skin/Exocrine—skin and subcutaneous tissue most common tumor sites in dogs and cats • Hemic/Lymphatic/Immune—spleen: common primary location in cats and uncommon primary location in dogs; common location for metastasis from the skin or subcutaneous sites • Gastrointestinal—intestinal mast cell tumor uncommon in cats and rare in dogs; gastric and duodenal ulcers possible

INCIDENCE/PREVALENCE
• Compose 20–25% of all skin and subcutaneous tumors in dogs • Fourth most common skin tumor in cats

SIGNALMENT

Species
Dogs and cats

Breed Predilections
• Boxers and Boston terriers • Siamese cats—predisposed to histiocytic cutaneous mast cell tumors

Mean Age and Range
• Dogs—mean age, 8 years • Cats—mean age, 10 years • Reported in animals < 1 year old and in cats as old as 18 years

Predominant Sex
None

SIGNS

General Comments
Depend on the location and grade of the tumor

Historical Findings
Dogs
• Patient may have had skin or subcutaneous tumor for days to months at the time of examination. • May have appeared to fluctuate in size • Recent rapid growth after months of quiescence common • Recent onset of erythema and edema most common with high-grade skin and subcutaneous tumors
Cats
• Anorexia—most common complaint with splenic tumor • Vomiting—may occur secondary to both splenic and gastrointestinal tumors

Physical Examination Findings
Dogs
• Extremely variable; may resemble any other type of skin or subcutaneous tumor (benign and malignant); may resemble an insect bite or allergic reaction • Primarily a solitary skin or subcutaneous mass; but may be multifocal • Approximately 50% located on the trunk and perineum; 40% on extremities; 10% on the head and neck region • Regional lymphadenopathy—may develop when a high-grade tumor metastasizes to draining lymph nodes • Hepatomegaly and spleno-megaly—features of disseminated mast cell neoplasia
Cats
• Cutaneous—primarily found in the subcutaneous tissue or dermis; may be papular or nodular, solitary or multiple, and hairy or alopecic or have an ulcerated surface; slight predilection for the head and neck regions • Splenic—splenomegaly is only consistent finding • Intestinal—firm, segmental thickenings of the small intestinal wall; measure 1–7 cm in diameter; metastases to the mesenteric lymph nodes, spleen, liver, and (rarely) lungs

CAUSES
Unknown

RISK FACTORS
• Hereditary • Previous inflammation

DIAGNOSIS

DIFFERENTIAL DIAGNOSIS
• Any other skin or subcutaneous tumor, be-nign or malignant, including lipoma • Insect bite or allergic reaction • Splenic—most common cause of splenomegaly in cats; must differentiate from lymphoma • Intestinal (cats)—may resemble any primary gastro-intestinal disorder (e.g., inflammatory and neoplasia)

CBC/BIOCHEMISTRY/URINALYSIS
Anemia and mastocythemia—may find in cats with splenic tumor and dogs with systemic mastocytosis

OTHER LABORATORY TESTS
N/A

IMAGING
• Abdominal radiography—may reveal splenomegaly in cats with splenic tumor and dogs with systemic mastocytosis
• Ultrasonography—helpful for evaluating visceral (liver, spleen) metastasis in dogs with high-grade tumors

DIAGNOSTIC PROCEDURES
• Cytologic examination of fine-needle aspirate—most important preliminary diagnostic test; reveals round cells with basophilic cytoplasmic granules that do not form sheets or clumps; if malignant mast cells are agranular, occurrence of large eosinophilic infiltrate may suggest mast cell tumor
• Tissue biopsy—necessary for definitive diagnosis and grading • Staging—to determine the extent of disease and appropriate treatment • Additional tests to achieve complete staging—cytologic examination or biopsy of local draining lymph node; cytologic examination of bone marrow aspirate; and thoracic radiography and abdominal ultrasonography with cytologic evaluation of hepatic and splenic aspirates

PATHOLOGIC FINDINGS
• Histopathologic examination (dogs)—grad-ing of tumor to predict biologic behavior; graded I–III (III is the most aggressive type)
• Cats—grading system; no correlation between histopathologic appearance of cutaneous tumor and prognosis

TREATMENT

APPROPRIATE HEALTH CARE
Dogs
• Aggressive surgical excision—treatment of choice • Histopathologic evaluation of the entire surgically excised tissue—essential to determine completeness of excision and predict the biologic behavior; if tumor cells extend close to the surgical margins, perform a second aggressive surgery as soon as possible • Lymph node involvement but no systemic involvement—aggressive excision of the affected lymph node(s) and the primary tumor required; follow-up chemotherapy useful to prevent further metastasis • Primary tumor and/or affected lymph nodes cannot be excised for microscopic disease—chemother-apy will have short-term palliative benefit (1–4 months) • Systemic metastasis—excision of primary tumor and affected lymph nodes of minimal benefit but chemotherapy may have short-term palliative benefit (< 2 months) • Radiotherapy—good treatment option for cutaneous tumor in a location that does not allow aggressive surgical excision; if possible, perform surgery before radiotherapy to reduce the tumor to a microscopic volume; tumors on an extremity respond better than do tumors located on the trunk

Cats
• Surgery—treatment of choice for cutaneous tumors • Splenectomy—treatment of choice for splenic tumor • Splenectomy and chemotherapy—recommended when mastocythemia accompanies splenic tumor

CLIENT EDUCATION
• Twenty percent of dogs diagnosed with a mast cell tumor will have two or more unrelated mast cell tumors in their lifetime. Each of these has the potential for being cured with appropriate surgical intervention. • Advise client that fine-needle aspiration and cytologic examination should be performed as soon as possible on any new mass. • Inform client that appropriate surgical excision should be done as soon as possible.

SURGICAL CONSIDERATIONS
• Excisional biopsy rather than incisional biopsy—necessary • Biopsy of lymph nodes and other suspicious visceral organs—appropriate • Complete surgical excision with 3-cm margins in all planes recommended for all moderate grade 2, high grade 2, and grade 3 tumors. Margins of 2 cm or less may be adequate for grade 1 and low grade 2 tumors. Resection of draining lymph nodes recommended for all high grade 2 and grade 3 tumors. Excisional biopsy with wide margins reasonable for very small tumors. Incisional biopsy of large mast cell tumors is recommended to obtain a tumor grade, predict prognosis, and establish a treatment plan.

MEDICATIONS

DRUG(S) OF CHOICE
• Prednisone—1 mg/kg PO q24h. Short-term remission only when used alone (although occasional exceptions do occur). Is beneficial in some cases to achieve cytoreduction before surgery • Other drugs (e.g., lomustine, vinblastine, cyclophosphamide)—add to length of remission of prednisone-sensitive tumors • Cutaneous tumor not controlled by surgery or radiotherapy—medical treatment appropriate; in author's experience, prednisone and chemotherapy not beneficial for aggressive tumors in cats • Prednisone-resistant tumor—chemotherapy does not appear to be beneficial • Intestinal tumor and systemic mastocytosis after splenectomy (cats)—prednisone and chemotherapy indicated • Measurable tumor (dogs)—vincristine alone induced partial remission in 21% of patients

Combination Chemotherapy
• Author's preferred treatment • Prednisone—1 mg/kg PO q24h; taper slowly after 4 months; discontinue after 7 months • Vinblastine—2–3 mg/m² IV; administer on day 1 of each 21-day cycle; initiate at a dosage of 2 mg/m²; increase by 10%–30% with each subsequent cycle, depending on tolerance and response (e.g., check CBC 1 week after administration); perform CBC before each administration; continue for 6 months

• Cyclophosphamide—250–300 mg/m² PO divided over 4 days; administer on days 8, 9, 10, and 11 of each 21-day cycle; initiate at 250 mg/m² for two cycles; increase to 300 mg/m² for cycle three if well tolerated; continue for 6 months • Recent information suggests that lomustine 60–90 mg/m² PO may be more effective than cyclophosphamide. When used with vinblastine, give lomustine on day 8 of cycle, but lengthen cycle from 21 to 28 days. Verify CBC at 7 and 14 days after first dose of lomustine to assess degree of neutropenia. Severe, prolonged myelosuppression can occur in some patients from a single dose. When used alone, lomustine can be given at 3-week intervals.

ALTERNATIVE DRUG(S)
Histamine-blocking agents (e.g., cimetidine)—helpful, particularly for systemic mastocytosis or when massive histamine release is a concern

FOLLOW-UP

PATIENT MONITORING
• Evaluate any new masses cytologically or histologically. • Evaluate regional lymph nodes at regular intervals to detect metastasis of grade II to III tumor.

POSSIBLE COMPLICATIONS
• Bleeding • Hemorrhagic gastroenteritis

EXPECTED COURSE AND PROGNOSIS

Dogs
• Tumors of the inguinal and perineal regions tend to be more aggressive than their histologic grade might suggest. These tumors should always be considered to have the potential for metastasis. • Historical survival data (Bostock) after surgery only indicates the following survival times—grade I, 77% alive; grade II, 45% alive; grade III, 13% alive • The relevance of these historical statistics is questionable as patients with mast cell tumor currently undergo aggressive staging and are treated more aggressively with surgery (i.e., resection of draining lymph nodes). • Lymph node metastasis—degree of lymph node involvement does affect prognosis (i.e., lymph node enlargement and cytologic effacement by mast cell tumor metastasis). Patients with grade 2 mast cell tumors with cytologic confirmation of lymph node metastasis without evidence of lymph node enlargement have a very good long-term prognosis when complete surgical resection of the primary tumor and lymph node is performed, followed by a 6-month chemotherapy regimen. Survival time for patients with grade 3 tumors is also improved

compared to less-aggressive surgery or no follow-up chemotherapy, but most do not survive beyond 1 year. When the lymph nodes are grossly enlarged, prognosis remains guarded even when aggressive resection and chemotherapy are administered. • Prednisone alone—effectively induced remission and prolonged survival time in 20% of patients with grade 2 or 3 tumors; only one of the five responding patients had documented lymph node metastasis when prednisone was initiated.

Cats
• Solitary cutaneous tumor—prognosis excellent; rate of recurrence low (16%–36%) despite incomplete excision; < 20% of patients develop metastasis • Survival after splenectomy for splenic tumor—reports of > 1 year • Concurrent development of mastocythemia—prognosis poor; prednisone and chemotherapy may achieve short-term remission • Intestinal tumor—prognosis poor; survival times rarely > 4 months after surgery

MISCELLANEOUS

Suggested Reading
LaDue T, Price GS, Dodge R, et al. Radiation therapy for incompletely resected canine mast cell tumors. Vet Radiol Ultrasound 1998;39:57–62.
McManus PM. Frequency and severity of mastocytemia in dogs with and without mast cell tumors: 120 cases (1995–1997). J Am Vet Med Assoc 1999;215:355–357
Rassnick KM, Moore AS, Williams LE, et al. Treatment of canine mast cell tumors with CCNU (lomustine). J Vet Intern Med 1999;13:601–605.
Seguin B, Leibman NF, Bregazzi VS, et al. Clinical outcome of dogs with grade-II mast cell tumors treated with surgery alone: 55 cases (1996–1999). J Am Vet Med Assoc 2001;218:1120–1123.
Takahashi T, Kadosawa T, Nagase M, et al. Visceral mast cell tumors in dogs: 10 cases (1982–1997). J Am Vet Med Assoc 2000; 216:222–226.
Thamm DH, Mauldin EA, Vail DM. Prednisone and vinblastine chemotherapy for canine mast cell tumor—41 cases (1992–1997). J Vet Intern Med 1999;13:491–497.
Weisse C, Shofer FS, Sorenmo K. Recurrence rates and sites for grade II canine cutaneous mast cell tumors following complete surgical excision. J Am Anim Hosp Assoc 2002; 38:71–73.

Author Robyn Elmslie
Consulting Editor Wallace B. Morrison

MASTITIS

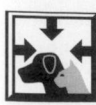

BASICS

OVERVIEW
• Bacterial infection of one or more lactating glands
• Result of ascending infection, trauma to the gland, or hematogenous spread
• *Escherichia coli, Staphylococci,* and B-hemolytic *Streptococci*—most commonly involved
• Potentially life-threatening infection; may lead to septic shock
• Sepsis—direct effect of mammary glands with systemic involvement

SIGNALMENT
• Postpartum bitch and queen
• Pseudopregnant lactating bitch or queen (rare)

SIGNS

Historical Findings
• Anorexia
• Lethargy
• Neglect of puppies or kittens
• Failure of puppies or kittens to thrive

Physical Examination Findings
• Firm, swollen, warm, and painful mammary gland(s) from which purulent or hemorrhagic fluid can be expressed
• Fever, dehydration, and septic shock—with systemic involvement
• Abscessation or gangrene of gland(s) can result

CAUSES & RISK FACTORS
• Trauma inflicted by puppy or kitten toenails and teeth
• Poor hygiene
• Systemic infection originating elsewhere (e.g., metritis)

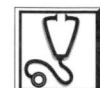

DIAGNOSIS

DIFFERENTIAL DIAGNOSIS
• Galactostasis—no systemic illness; cytologic examination and culture of milk help with differentiation
• Inflammatory mammary adenocarcinoma—affected gland does not produce milk; differentiated by biopsy

CBC/BIOCHEMISTRY/URINALYSIS
• Leukocytosis with left shift
• Leukopenia—with sepsis
• Mildly high PCV, total protein, and BUN—with dehydration

IMAGING
N/A

OTHER LABORATORY TESTS
N/A

DIAGNOSTIC PROCEDURES
Milk—normally slightly more acidic than serum; may become alkaline with infection; neutrophils, macrophages, and other mononuclear cells can be observed in high numbers in normal milk; the presence of large numbers of free and phagocytosed bacteria and degenerative neutrophils are noted with septic disease; bacterial culture to identify the organism

TREATMENT
• Inpatient until stable
• Puppies and kittens—hand-raised or placed on healthy surrogate dam; for selected

patients, neonates may be allowed to continue nursing (pay special attention to antibiotics used and weight gain of neonates)
• Dehydration or sepsis—intravenous fluid therapy
• Correct electrolyte imbalances and hypoglycemia.
• Treat shock, if indicated.
• Apply warm compress and milk out affected gland(s) several times daily.
• Abscessed or gangrenous glands—require surgical débridement

MEDICATIONS

DRUG(S)
• Acidic milk—weak bases; erythromycin (10 mg/kg PO q8h, dogs and cats) or lincomycin (15 mg/kg PO q8h, dogs and cats)
• Alkaline milk—weak acids; amoxicillin or cephalosporin (20 mg/kg q8h, dogs and cats)
• Either alkaline or acidic milk—chloramphenicol and enrofloxacin (2.5 mg/kg q12h)

• May infuse affected gland(s) with 1% Betadine solution by lacrimal cannula

CONTRAINDICATIONS/POSSIBLE INTERACTIONS
Patient allowed to nurse—avoid tetracycline, enrofloxacin, and chloramphenicol; may use cephalosporins, amoxicillin, and amoxicillin with clavulanic acid

FOLLOW-UP

PATIENT MONITORING
Physical examination and CBC

PREVENTION/AVOIDANCE
• Clean environment
• Hair shaved from around mammary glands
• Toenails of puppies and kittens clipped

POSSIBLE COMPLICATIONS
• Abscessation or gangrene—may cause loss of gland(s)
• Hand-raising puppies and kittens—requires considerable commitment by the owner

EXPECTED COURSE AND PROGNOSIS
Prognosis—good with treatment

MISCELLANEOUS

ABBREVIATION
PCV = packed cell volume

Suggested Reading
Johnston SD, Root Kustritz MV, Olson PNS. Periparturient disorders in the bitch. In: Johnston SD, Root Kustritz MV, Olson PNS, eds., Canine and feline theriogenology. Philadelphia: Saunders, 2001:131–134.
Olson JD, Olson PN. Disorders of the canine mammary gland. In: Morrow DA, ed., Current therapy in theriogenology 2. Philadelphia: Saunders, 1986:506–509.
Author Joni L. Freshman
Consulting Editor Sara K. Lyle

MATERNAL BEHAVIOR PROBLEMS

 **BASICS**

DEFINITION
Abnormal maternal behavior is either excessive maternal behavior in the absence of neonates or deficient maternal behavior in the presence of the dam's own neonates.

PATHOPHYSIOLOGY
The pathophysiology of one type of excessive maternal behavior, pseudocyesis, appears to be elevated progesterone levels following estrus in unbred bitches followed by an abrupt drop in levels. The pathophysiology of refusal to accept puppies by females after caesarean section is the waning of factors including oxytocin needed during the sensitive period for acceptance of the neonate. The pathophysiology of other types of deficient maternal behavior is unknown.

SYSTEM AFFECTED
Behavioral

GENETICS
There is no identified genetic predisposition, but a breed disposition in Jack Russell terriers indicates that there may be a genetic component. There are genetic models of deficient maternal behavior in mice. The genetic basis should be investigated in dogs and cats.

INCIDENCE/PREVALENCE
The incidence of deficient maternal behavior has not been determined, but seems to be low. Maternal behavior in cats and dogs that do not have offspring is more common.

GEOGRAPHIC DISTRIBUTION
N/A

SIGNALMENT

Species
Dogs and cats

Breed Predilections
Poor maternal behavior may be more common in Jack Russell terriers, but there has been no quantitative study.

Mean Age and Range
N/A

Predominant Sex
Female only

SIGNS

Deficient Maternal Behavior
Absent maternal behavior; the mother simply abandons her offspring. This is most apt to occur after caesarean section.

Poor Maternal Behavior
• The mother stays with her offspring, but will not allow them to nurse.
• In other cases the mother may show inadequate retrieval of young, insufficient cleaning of the young, or failure to stimulate elimination.
• In another form of poor maternal behavior the bitch carries the puppies from place to place without settling down or, in the most extreme form, kills some or all of her litter.

Abnormal Maternal Behavior
• The bitch or queen may allow her offspring to suckle, but kills her offspring either at birth or over a period of days. Occasionally the bitch, or more rarely the queen, will abandon or attack her offspring if it has changed in odor or appearance. A female may be disturbed by another animal or by people and can redirect her aggression to her offspring.
• A bitch may accidentally disembowel or even consume offspring completely while eating the fetal membranes and umbilical cord. This should be distinguished from normal licking, which can be quite vigorous, even dislodging the pup from a teat.

Maternal Aggression
Cats with kittens may be aggressive to other animals in the same household.

Excessive Maternal Behavior
• The pseudopregnant bitch or bitch spayed during the late luteal phase of the estrous cycle adopts, attempts to nurse, and guards inanimate objects (stuffed animals or even leashes). The pseudopregnant bitch may have mammary development and may be lactating.
• The newly spayed queen may steal kittens from a lactating queen. Queens post-spaying may also lactate if suckled.

CAUSES AND RISK FACTORS
• The presence of kittens in the environment of the recently spayed cat is a risk factor for excessive maternal behavior and kitten stealing.
• The risk of excessive carrying of pups, redirected aggression, or even cannibalism is increased if there are other dogs or too many people present in the nest area.

 DIAGNOSIS

DIFFERENTIAL DIAGNOSIS
• The most important differential is between primary abnormal maternal behavior and poor maternal behavior secondary to mastitis or metritis.
• Lactation tetany can result in aggressive behavior, although this behavior is rarely directed at the puppies and occurs later in lactation, not at parturition.

CBC/BIOCHEMISTRY/URINALYSIS
Usually normal unless other medical conditions are present

OTHER LABORATORY TESTS
Only as indicated by metabolic conditions of the bitch or queen

IMAGING
Only as indicated by other problems

DIAGNOSTIC PROCEDURES
N/A

PATHOLOGIC FINDINGS
Presence of milk in the mammary glands of females with excessive maternal behavior

 TREATMENT

APPROPRIATE HEALTH CARE
Normal health care

NURSING CARE
N/A

ACTIVITY
N/A

DIET
• Adequate diet for nursing bitches and queens to meet energy demands
• Restricted diets for pseudocyesis to discourage lactation
• In the case of deficient maternal behavior, the bitch or queen should be fed ad libitum to encourage lactation.

CLIENT EDUCATION

Abnormal or Poor Maternal Behavior
• The bitch that is carrying her pups or exhibiting redirected aggression to them should be isolated in a quiet, dark area. The bitch that bites her pups should be muzzled. The owner must stimulate elimination of the

puppies or kittens because the muzzled female cannot. An Elizabethan collar inhibits cannibalism in queens.

• The bitch should be attended at parturition and the pups removed temporarily if she is biting the pups themselves in addition to the umbilical cord.

• Bitches and queens with poor maternal behavior may exhibit the same behavior with subsequent litters.

Excessive Maternal Behavior

• Cats that have stolen kittens should be separated from the natural mother and kittens.

• The mothered objects should be removed from the pseudopregnant bitch.

• Food intake should be restricted to inhibit lactation.

Maternal Aggression

The best treatment for excessive maternal aggression is to separate the kittens; weaning alone may not suffice because the presence of the kittens alone may sustain or even reinstate maternal aggression in a queen separated from her kittens for several weeks.

SURGICAL CONSIDERATIONS

• Delay spaying for four months post-estrus to avoid post-spaying maternal behavior and its accompanying aggression.

• Spaying avoids future excessive maternal behavior in the absence of young.

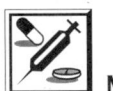

MEDICATIONS

DRUG(S) OF CHOICE

Excessive Maternal Behavior

Milbolerone (Cheque drops) is the drug of choice for pseudopregnant bitches or those exhibiting maternal behavior and lactation following spaying. The dose is 16 μg/kg PO once daily for 5 days. Milbolerone inhibits prolactin and thereby inhibits lactation.

CONTRAINDICATIONS

Do not use milbolerone in cats because it has a narrow margin of safety in that species. It should not be administered to Bedlington terriers.

PRECAUTIONS

Milbolerone can cause masculinization in females that may include male sexual behavior, clitoral hypertrophy, vulvovaginitis, and urinary incontinence.

POSSIBLE INTERACTIONS

• If tranquilizers are administered, care must be taken that the puppies or kittens are not sedated.

• Do not use estrogen or progesterones at the same time as milbolerone.

ALTERNATIVE DRUG(S)

Drugs are usually not needed.

FOLLOW-UP

PATIENT MONITORING

The puppies or kittens of females with deficient or poor maternal behavior should be monitored daily to be sure that they are gaining weight.

PREVENTION/AVOIDANCE

• Placing a nursing female in quiet, comfortable quarters away from noise and disturbances by other animals or people

• Do not re-breed females with poor maternal behavior. Determine whether any other female offspring of the female with abnormal behavior have also exhibited poor maternal behavior. In other species, poor maternal behavior is a paternally imprinted gene; the father must contribute the gene for poor maternal behavior. The daughters of rejecting mothers will not reject, but the daughters of their sons may.

• Deficient maternal behavior can occur with each litter; do not re-breed.

POSSIBLE COMPLICATIONS

Loss of offspring

EXPECTED COURSE AND PROGNOSIS

• Excessive maternal behavior usually wanes around the time of normal weaning (6–8 weeks).

• Poor and deficient maternal behavior can occur with each litter.

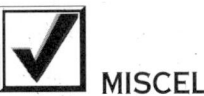

MISCELLANEOUS

ASSOCIATED CONDITIONS

N/A

AGE-RELATED FACTORS

N/A

ZOONOTIC POTENTIAL

N/A

PREGNANCY

• Consider especially drug use and effect of disease on the fetus.

• Do not breed dogs with history of poor maternal behavior.

SYNONYM

Mismothering

Suggested Reading

Connolly PB. Reproductive behaviour problems. In: Horwitz, Mills, Health, Eds. BSAVA manual of canine and feline behavioural medicine. 128–143, 2002.

Houpt, KA and Concannon, P.W. 1996. Sexual and maternal behavior in cats. In: L. Ackerman, ed. Cat Behavior and Training. Neptune City, NJ: T.F.H. Publications.

Houpt, KA. 2000. Maternal behavior and its aberrations. In: Recent advances in companion animal behavior problems. K.A. Houpt, Ed. International Veterinary Information Services (www.ivis.org).

Misner, TL and Houpt, KA 1998. Animal behavior case of the month. J Am Vet Med Assoc 213:1260–1262.

Author Katherine A. Houpt
Consulting Editor Debra F. Horwitz

MAXILLARY AND MANDIBULAR FRACTURES

BASICS

OVERVIEW
Fractures of the mandible, maxilla, and associated structures are classified as to location, severity (i.e., tooth involvement, soft tissue tears, and type of bone fracture), and effects of the muscles of mastication on reduction.

Effects of the Muscles of Mastication
• The muscles opening the mouth (e.g., digastric muscle) may help reduce or displace a fracture. • Favorable—fracture reduced by muscles of mastication • Nonfavorable—fracture displaced by muscles of mastication

Classification of Jaw Injury
• Type I—separation; no break in soft tissue
• Type II—separation; break in soft tissue
• Type III—separation; break in soft tissue and comminution of bone; broken teeth not unusual • Teeth involved may be maintained during osseous process (i.e., with endodontics or restoration). If required, they can be extracted following bone healing.

Classification of Jaw Fracture by Location
• A—central incisors (mesial midline) to canine teeth (A–symphysis is a common jaw fracture site in the cat)
• B—from canine to secnd premolar
• C—secnd premolar to first molar (carnassial tooth)
• D—from first molar to the angle of the mandible
• E—angle of the mandible
• F—coronoid process
• G—condylar process
• H—midline palate
• I—non-midline palate
• J—massive or combination of fractures

SIGNALMENT
• Dogs and cats
• No sex, age, or breed predilections

SIGNS
• Vary greatly according to the location, type, extent, cause, and underlying risk factors resulting in the injury • Facial deformity, malocclusion, fractured teeth, oral or nasal bleeding, and inability to properly close the jaw are not uncommon signs.

CAUSES
Injury, trauma, and predisposing factors

RISK FACTORS
• High-risk environment or temperament
• Oral infections (e.g., periodontal disease, osteomyelitis), neoplasia, or certain metabolic diseases—may result in weaker jaws that are more prone to injury.
• Traumatic injury affecting the jaws or teeth
• Congenital or hereditary factors resulting in weakened or deformed jaw bone

DIAGNOSIS

Based on visualization, palpation, and radiographic findings

DIFFERENTIAL DIAGNOSIS
• TMJ conditions—see Temporomandibular Joint—Dislocation/Luxation/Intermittent
• Tooth subluxation or luxation (i.e., interference with jaw closure)
• Endodontic disease (e.g., tooth abscess)
• Foreign body lodged in or near the oral cavity
• Maxillary or mandibular nerve injury or disease
• Eosinophilic myositis
• CMO
• Neoplasia

CBC/BIOCHEMISTRY/URINALYSIS/OTHER LABORATORY TESTS
As required—to assess and treat shock from initial injury; to assess animal prior to surgery

DIAGNOSTIC PROCEDURES
• Oral examination
• Radiography—intraoral and extraoral
• Neurologic examination
• Histopathology, if indicated

PATHOLOGIC FINDINGS
• Nonunions
• Neoplasia
• Osteomyelitis
• Periodontal or endodontic disease

TREATMENT

• Based on type of fracture, available equipment, supplies, and the doctor's knowledge, experience, and comfort level
• Treatment selection is based on four major points: (1) reduction of fracture and reasonable contact of fracture ends, if possible; (2) re-establishment of natural occlusion, if possible; (3) stabilization sufficient for proper healing; (4) salvage condition (nonrepairable or nonstabilizable condition)

TYPICAL TYPES OF TREATMENTS FOR CLASSES OF FRACTURES

Interarch Stabilization (typically for classes D, E, F, G, and J)
• Tape muzzle
• Cross-arch wiring (maxilla to mandible)
• Composite fixation of cross-arch teeth; sometimes used in combination with dental pins (i.e., TMS; Whaledent, New York, NY)

Intra-arch Stabilization (typically for classes H and I)
• Pin and wire combination
• Dental wiring
• Acrylic or composite splint

Intraoral Stabilization with Splint
Composite or acrylic splint (typically for classes A, B, C, H, I and J)

Intraoral Stabilization with Wire (typically for classes A, B, C, H, I, and J)
• Interdental wiring—ivy loop, Stout's multiple loop, Essig, and Risdon wiring techniques
• Dental wiring—circumdental used for anchorage for composite and acrylic splints (pig tails, cerclage, or twists)
• Osseous wiring—circumferential; transosseous; transcircumferential

Internal Fixation (for most classes of fractures, but must be used selectively with consideration of teeth and roots)
Orthopedic wire; IM pins; plates; screws

External Fixation (for most classes of fractures, but must be used selectively with consideration of teeth and roots)
IM pins with bars (stainless steel or carbon) or tubing (e.g., Penrose) reinforced with composite or acrylic

Salvage Surgery (typically for class J fractures)
• Condylectomy—nonrepairable fractures of the TMJ
• Cheiloplasty—salvage procedure to maintain reasonable mandibular support in certain nonunion conditions
• Rostral (or other) mandibulectomy—used in certain nonunion cases or with massive injury

TECHNIQUES
Below are more commonly used techniques; more advanced options are beyond the scope of this chapter (see Suggested Reading).
• Disinfect with chlorhexidine and clean and polish teeth.
• Objectives of fracture reduction—to re-establish occlusion and use appropriate stabilization
• Acrylic or composite splint—acrylics are reasonably priced and simple to use, but require adequate ventilation due to hazardous vapors; composites are easy to use, but are more expensive and require some specialized equipment.
• Reduce fracture in proper occlusion.
• Coat adjacent teeth and soft tissue with petroleum jelly.
• Apply dental wiring (e.g., cerclage around teeth) as needed for anchorage of acrylic, if needed.
• Acid etch the teeth with a 37% phosphoric acid gel; leave on for 30–60 seconds; rinse off thoroughly and air dry the teeth.
• The powder and liquid can now be placed in a simple salt-and-pepper fashion, adding one and then the other in small increments to begin the polymerizing action to harden the acrylic.
• Add acrylic until the desired shape and density of splint are obtained.

MAXILLARY AND MANDIBULAR FRACTURES

• Overbuilt areas may be reduced using acrylic burs on dental handpieces or with hand files to allow for a functional occlusion.

Circumferential Osseous Wiring or Suturing
• Wiring around the bone—used most commonly for symphysis separations
• 20- or 18-gauge needle—to pass wire
• 24- to 28-gauge wire—in small dogs or cats, absorbable (long-acting) or nonabsorbable 1- to 2-0 suture material can sometimes be substituted for wire
• Run wire from stab incision (ventral intermandibular space) to vestibule; pass behind canines, down through vestibule on opposite side, and back down through the ventral incision.
• Tighten wire to reduce fracture, but do not overtighten the wire ends or the teeth may be pulled too far medially (base narrow) and hit the palate.
• If teeth go base narrow, either loosen the wire ends or place a second figure-8 wire looped around the canine teeth and under the jaw.

Additional Treatment Considerations
• Bone graft—use in any class of fracture for areas of bone loss to reestablish structural stability; autograft: bone graft from same individual; allograft: bone graft from same species; alloplast: artificial graft material (Consil, Nutramax Labs Inc., Edgewood, MD); xenograft: graft material from another species
• Teeth in the fracture line should be maintained by appropriate treatment until the fracture heals, if possible, as removal may result in instability.
• Awareness of occlusion, tooth roots, and anatomy during treatment is critical.
• Treatment with composite/acrylic splints in association with wiring is generally very effective; may allow for improved occlusal reestablishment and less dental trauma.
• Pharyngostomy tube aids in occlusal checks intraoperatively.

HOME CARE
• Orthodontic wax—soft, pliable wax sent with owner to periodically cover irritating wires
• Oral irrigants—use twice daily for oral hygiene and to reduce bacteria; chlorhexidine solutions help reduce bacteria; zinc and ascorbic acid solutions help reduce bacteria and stimulate soft tissue healing
• Diet—soft food or gruel may be required during healing
• Nutritional and fluid maintenance required
• Chewing exercise—avoid hard chew items during healing process

MEDICATIONS

DRUG(S)

Pain Management
• Local anesthesia—intraoral local blocks; regional nerve blocks: mental n., mandibular n., infraorbital n., and maxillary n.
• Injectables—butorphanol tartrate (Torbugesic; Fort Dodge AH, Fort Dodge, IA); buprenorphine; nalbuphine
• Patches—fentanyl (Duragesic; Janssen, Titusville, NJ)
• Oral—carprofen (Rimadyl; Pfizer AH, Exton, PA); butorphanol tartrate (Torbugesic); hydrocodone

Antibiotics
Broad spectrum based on history, health, and chemical profile

FOLLOW-UP

PATIENT MONITORING
• Physical—recheck 2 weeks postoperative
• Radiographic—recheck 4–6 weeks postoperative, then every 2 weeks until fracture is healed and/or appliance is removed
• Fracture site may temporarily (1–2 weeks) be more at risk to refracture after the support of the appliance is removed. • Once the fracture line is stable, compromised teeth may need additional endodontic treatment (e.g., root canal) or careful extraction. • If the healing process results in a malocclusion—orthodontics or endodontic or selective exodontia (extraction) may be required
• Other considerations—stability of fracture and appliance; oral hygiene; oral intake of food and water; maintenence of weight; appropriate urination and defecation; indications of pain or swelling

POSSIBLE COMPLICATIONS
• Malocclusion • Endodontic disease
• Osteomyelitis • Nonunion • Sequestrum
• Dehiscence • Neurologic defects • Facial pain syndrome • Impaired mastication
• Temporary weight loss • Soft tissue trauma due to appliance or wires

POSSIBLE SEQUELAE

Impaired Mastication
• TMJ arthritis—chronic or intermittent TMJ pain; may require condylectomy
• Malocclusion—dental attrition; may require extractions

• Nonunion—may require partial or complete mandibulectomy or maxillectomy
• Ankylosis of mandible at the TMJ or zygomatic arch area

Facial Pain Syndrome
• Acute or chronic
• Due to nerve trauma from injury or as a complication of surgery

Nerve Damage
Affecting motor function

EXPECTED COURSE AND PROGNOSIS
• Generally good; however, predisposing factors, initiating force, location, type of fracture, quality of home care, and selection of treatment modality all affect the healing outcome.
• 4–12 weeks to bony union

MISCELLANEOUS

ASSOCIATED CONDITIONS
• Malocclusion
• Mastication difficulty
• Lack of head symmetry
• Soft tissue trauma
• Periodontal disease
• Chipped, broken, luxated, or avulsed teeth

AGE-RELATED FACTORS
Typically, condition initially is observed at < 14 months of age, usually shortly following tooth eruption

ABBREVIATIONS
• CMO = craniomandibular osteopathy
• IM = intramedullary
• TMJ = temporomandibular joint

Suggested Reading
Fossum TW. Small animal surgery. 2nd ed. St. Louis: Mosby, 2002:901–913.
Lobprise HB, Wiggs RB. The veterinarian's companion for common dental procedures. Lakewood, CO: AAHA Press, 2000: 115–136.
Marretta SM. Maxillofacial surgery. Vet Clin North Am Small Anim Pract 1998:1285–1296.
Wiggs RB, Lobprise HB. Veterinary dentistry principles and practice. Philadelphia: Lippincott-Raven, 1997:259–279.
Wiggs RB, Lobprise H, Mitchell PQ. Oral and periodontal tissue maintenance, augmentation, rejuvenation and regeneration. Vet Clin North Am Small Anim Pract 1998;28(5):1165–1188.
Authors R. B. Wiggs and B. P. Hall
Consulting Editor Heidi B. Lobprise

MEDIASTINITIS

 BASICS

OVERVIEW
• The mediastinum occupies the central portion of the chest, and is defined anatomically by the thoracic inlet cranially, the diaphragm caudally, the mediastinal pleura laterally, the paravertebral gutter and ribs dorsally, and the sternum ventrally.
• An inflammatory process involving the mediastinal space, usually the result of an infectious process
• Acute disease—severe infection may be life-threatening and may spread to the pleural space; sepsis may develop
• Chronic—mediastinal granuloma or abscess may develop and may result in cranial vena cava syndrome.
• Systems affected—primarily cardiovascular system because of interference with venous return or respiratory system secondary to intrathoracic mass effect or pleural effusion; may also interfere with esophageal function

SIGNALMENT
Rare in dogs and cats

SIGNS
• Lethargy and weakness
• Dysphagia and regurgitation
• Edema of head, neck, and forelimbs
• Polypnea and dyspnea

CAUSES & RISK FACTORS
• Acute disease—usually result of esophageal perforation or tracheal tear; may be secondary to neck wounds (e.g., bite or gunshot), sepsis, pneumonia, pericarditis, or pyothorax; mediastinal abscesses may develop subsequent to infections or neoplastic disorders arising in the mediastinum or adjacent tissues; may be complicated by gram-negative bacteria
• Chronic disease—usually result of a bacterial (e.g., *Actinomyces* and *Nocardia* spp.) or fungal (e.g., *Coccidioides, Cryptococcus, Blastomyces,* and *Histoplasma* spp.) infection
• Predisposing factors—esophageal foreign body; cervical or thoracic trauma; immuno-suppressed state
• Common occurrence in man following median sternotomy for cardiac surgery

 DIAGNOSIS

DIFFERENTIAL DIAGNOSIS
• Isolated pericarditis, pyothorax, and pneumonia
• Cranial mediastinal mass—lymphosarcoma; thymoma, thyroid, or parathyroid tumor; neurogenic tumor; mesenchymal tumor (usually lipoma or other fat accumulation); mediastinal cyst
• Esophageal motor dysfunction or other esophageal abnormality
• Gastroesophageal disorder

CBC/BIOCHEMISTRY/URINALYSIS
• High WBC count with left shift
• PCV and total protein—may be high owing to volume depletion

OTHER LABORATORY TESTS
N/A

IMAGING
• Thoracic radiographs—reveal a wide mediastinum; may see pneumothorax or bilateral pleural effusion
• Esophageal contrast study—evaluate esophageal perforation or other abnormality; use a water-soluble contrast medium with suspected perforation
• Thoracic ultrasound—differentiate between mediastinal fluid accumulation (e.g., cyst and abscess), inflammatory reaction, and tumor
• Computed tomography and MRI—more definitive than ultrasound

DIAGNOSTIC PROCEDURES
• Cytology—thoracentesis of any pleural effusion; transthoracic fine-needle aspirate; cutting-needle biopsy of the mediastinal enlargement
• Ultrasound-guided aspirate or biopsy may be very helpful in accurate sampling of tissues.
• Submit all samples (collected) for bacterial culture and sensitivity testing.

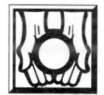 TREATMENT

• Inpatient with restricted activity until infection is controlled and condition is stable
• Pleural effusion of marked quantity or pyothorax of any degree—managed by tube thoracostomy
• Physiologically balanced electrolyte solutions, or parenteral alimenation—administer parenterally until oral alimentation is possible and water and food intake returns to normal or near normal

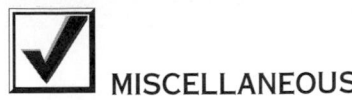
• Esophageal perforation—surgical emergency; after surgical repair, enforce either parenteral alimentation or gastric tube feeding for 3–5 days.
• Chronic disease—best treated by surgical exploration when associated with an abscess or a granuloma
• Tube thoracostomy—maintain postsurgery by continuous water seal suction for 5–7 days or until negligible fluid is removed; follow a similar course with or without pleural cavity lavage when surgery is not performed.
• Warn client that this is a serious disease with a guarded prognosis.

MEDICATIONS

DRUG(S)
• Broad-spectrum bactericidal antibiotic—choose on the basis of bacterial culture and sensitivity testing; parenterally for at least the first week of treatment, then orally
• Antifungal treatment is indicated when mycotic organisms are isolated.

CONTRAINDICATIONS/POSSIBLE INTERACTIONS
• Aminoglycoside antibiotics—avoid or accurately base dosage on creatinine clearance with azotemia
• Avoid excess fluid administration following removal of chest tube, as this may contribute to mediastinal and pleural fluid accumulation.

FOLLOW-UP

PATIENT MONITORING
• Daily temperature recording
• Hemogram—every 2–3 days during hospitalization (usually 7–10 days)
• Thoracic radiographs—at 7–10-day intervals (more often if drainage is needed)
• Antibiotics—generally continue for 1 week after hemogram and radiographs return to normal; with abscessation, continue an additional 4–6 weeks.

POSSIBLE COMPLICATIONS
• Pyothorax
• Sepsis
• Mediastinal fibrosis

EXPECTED COURSE AND PROGNOSIS
• With early diagnosis and aggressive treatment—prognosis fair to good
• With mediastinal fibrosis—long-term prognosis guarded to poor

MISCELLANEOUS

ABBREVIATIONS
MRI = magnetic resonance imaging
PCV = packed cell volume

Suggested Reading
Biller DS: Mediastinal disease. In: Ettinger ST, Feldman EC, eds. Textbook of veterinary internal medicine. 5th ed. Philadelphia: Saunders, 2000:1094–1096.
Hoffman OA, et al.: Primary mediastinal neoplasms (other than thymoma). Mayo Clin Proc 1993;68:880–1091.
Kneller SK: Thoracic radiography. In: Kirk RW, ed. Current veterinary therapy IX. Philadelphia: Saunders, 1986:250–261.
Light RM: Disorders of the pleura, mediastinum, and diaphragm. In: Harrison's principles of internal medicine. 14th ed. New York: McGraw-Hill, 1998:1472–1476.
Moon ML: Thoracic radiology. In: August JR, ed. Consultations in feline internal medicine. 3rd ed. Philadelphia: Saunders, 1997:251–253.
Author Neil K. Harpster
Consulting Editor Lynell R. Johnson

MEGACOLON

 BASICS

DEFINITION
A condition of persistent increased large bowel diameter associated with chronic constipation/obstipation and low-to-absent colonic motility

PATHOPHYSIOLOGY
• Acquired megacolon results from chronic retention of fecal material that leads to colonic absorption of fecal water and solidified fecal concretions.
• Prolonged distension of the colon results in irreversible changes in colonic motility that leads to colonic inertia.
• Congenital absence of colonic ganglionic cells (Hirschsprung's disease) is not clearly documented in small animals.
• Recent work strongly suggests that the pathogenesis of idiopathic megacolon in cats involves a disturbance of colonic smooth muscle function.

SYSTEMS AFFECTED
Gastrointestinal

GENETICS
N/A

INCIDENCE/PREVALENCE
Unknown

GEOGRAPHIC DISTRIBUTION
N/A

SIGNALMENT
Species
• Idiopathic megacolon—cats
• Acquired megacolon—cats and dogs

Breed Predilections
Some evidence for increased risk in Manx cats

Mean Age and Range
• Idiopathic megacolon—middle-aged to old cats (mean age, 4.9 years; range, 1–15 years)
• Acquired megacolon—none

Predominant Sex
None

SIGNS
Historical Findings
• Idiopathic megacolon—typically a chronic/recurrent problem; signs often present for months to years.
• Acquired megacolon—signs may be acute or chronic.
• Constipation/obstipation
• Tenesmus with small or no fecal volume
• Hard, dry feces

• Infrequent defecation
• Small amount of diarrhea (often mucoid) may occur after prolonged tenesmus.
• Occasional vomiting, anorexia, and/or depression
• Weight loss

Physical Examination Findings
• Abdominal palpation reveals an enlarged colon with a hard fecal mass.
• Digital rectal examination may indicate an underlying (obstructive) cause and confirms fecal impaction.
• Dehydration
• Scruffy, unkempt haircoat

CAUSES
• Idiopathic—cats
• Mechanical obstruction—pelvic fracture malunion, foreign body or improper diet (especially bones), stricture, pseudocoprostasis, prostatic disease, perineal hernia, neoplasia, anal or rectal atresia
• Causes of dyschezia—anorectal disease (anal sacculitis, anal sac abscess, perianal fistula, proctitis), trauma (fractured pelvis, fractured limb, dislocated hip, perianal bite wound or laceration, perineal abscess)
• Metabolic disorders—hypokalemia, severe dehydration
• Drugs—vincristine, barium, antacids, sucralfate, anticholinergics
• Neurologic/neuromuscular disease—congenital abnormalities of the caudal spine (especially Manx cats), paraplegia, spinal cord disease, intervertebral disk disease, dysautonomia, sacral nerve disease, sacral nerve trauma (e.g., tail fracture/pull injury), trauma to colonic innervation

RISK FACTORS
• Conditions leading to inability to posture (limb and pelvic fractures, neuromuscular disease, etc.) or rectoanal pain
• Prior pelvic fractures
• Possible association with low physical activity and obesity
• Perineal hernias

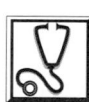 **DIAGNOSIS**

DIFFERENTIAL DIAGNOSIS
• Other causes of palpable colonic masses (e.g., lymphoma, carcinoma, intussusception)—distinguish on the basis of texture, rectal examination, and imaging.
• Dysuria/stranguria—exclude by palpation of the bladder and colon, and by urinalysis.

• Tenesmus due to inflammation of the lower bowel (colitis)—exclude by palpation, rectal examination, and imaging.

CBC/BIOCHEMISTRY/URINALYSIS
• May show evidence of dehydration (elevated packed cell volume, total protein) and stress leukogram
• Electrolyte abnormalities may develop depending on duration of obstipation; may be prerenal azotemia with dehydration
• Urinalysis—no consistent changes; important to confirm normal renal function in dehydrated animals and to rule out lower urinary tract disease as a differential diagnosis

OTHER LABORATORY TESTS
N/A

IMAGING
• Abdominal/pelvic radiographs to identify any underlying causes
• Can easily see the enlarged, fecal-filled colon on plain abdominal radiographs
• Abdominal ultrasound may help to identify mural or obstructive masses.

DIAGNOSTIC PROCEDURES
May need colonoscopy to rule out mural or intraluminal obstructive lesions

PATHOLOGIC FINDINGS
• The most severe dilation typically occurs in the transverse and descending colon, although the entire length of the colon can be involved.
• The colon is usually histologically normal.

 TREATMENT

APPROPRIATE HEALTH CARE
• Inpatient medical management; surgery may be indicated if recurrent/severe problem
• Medical therapy—restore normal hydration, followed by anesthesia and manual evacuation of the colon using warm water enemas, water-soluble jelly, and gentle extraction of feces with a gloved finger or sponge forceps; do not traumatize the colonic mucosa excessively.
• Continue long-term therapy at home.

NURSING CARE
• Most patients require parenteral fluid support to correct dehydration.
• Intravenous administration of balanced electrolyte solutions is the preferred route.

ACTIVITY
• Encourage activity and exercise.
• Restriction indicated in the postoperative period if surgery is performed.

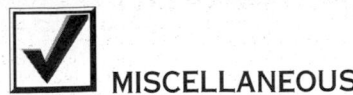

DIET
• Many patients require a low-residue-producing diet; bulk-forming fiber diets can worsen or lead to recurrence of colonic fecal distension.
• A high-fiber diet is occassionally helpful.
• A more palatable, maintenance-type diet can be supplemented with products such as Metamucil or pumpkin pie filler.

CLIENT EDUCATION
• In idiopathic disease or with severe colonic injury, medical therapy is often lifelong and can be frustrating.
• Recurrence is common.
• Surgery (subtotal colectomy) is indicated if medical therapy fails.

SURGICAL CONSIDERATIONS
• An underlying obstructive cause requires surgical correction.
• Avoid enema administration/colonic evacuation prior to subtotal colectomy.
• Subtotal colectomy with ileorectal or colorectal anastomosis—treatment of choice for idiopathic megacolon refractory to medical management
• Colectomy may also be required with obstructive megacolon caused by irreversible changes in colonic motility.

MEDICATIONS

DRUG(S) OF CHOICE
• Can improve colonic motility in less severe cases with cisapride, a prokinetic GI drug (dogs, 0.1–0.5 mg/kg PO q8–12h; cats, 2.5–10.0 mg/cat q8–12h)
• Stool softeners (e.g., lactulose, 1 mL/4.5 kg PO q8–12h to effect) are recommended in conjunction with cisapride and diet.
• Broad-spectrum prophylactic antibiotics are recommended prior to colon evacuation and during the perioperative period if surgery is elected.

CONTRAINDICATIONS
• Sodium phosphate retention enemas (e.g., Fleet; C.B. Fleet Co., Inc.)—because of their association with severe hypocalcemia
• Mineral oil and white petrolatum—because of danger of fatal lipoid aspiration pneumonia due to lack of taste

PRECAUTIONS
Common hairball laxatives (e.g., Laxatone, Cat-a-Lax) are typically ineffective.

POSSIBLE INTERACTIONS
N/A

ALTERNATIVE DRUG(S)
Docusate sodium can be used as a stool softener in place of lactulose.

FOLLOW-UP

PATIENT MONITORING
• Following colonic resection and anastomosis—for 3–5 days check for signs of dehiscence and peritonitis.
• Clinical deterioration warrants abdominocentesis and/or peritoneal lavage to detect anastomotic leakage.
• Continue fluid support until the patient is willing to eat and drink.

PREVENTION/AVOIDANCE
• Repair pelvic fractures that narrow the pelvic canal.
• Avoid exposure to foreign bodies and feeding bones.

POSSIBLE COMPLICATIONS
• Recurrence or persistence—most common
• Potential surgical complications include peritonitis, persistent diarrhea, stricture formation, and recurrence of obstipation.
• Traumatic perforation of the colon is a serious complication of overzealous fecal evacuation.

EXPECTED COURSE AND PROGNOSIS
• Historically, medical management has been unrewarding.
• Cisapride appears to improve the prognosis with medical management in some patients, but may not suffice in severe or long-standing cases.
• Postoperative diarrhea—expected; typically resolves within 6 weeks (80% of cats with idiopathic megacolon undergoing subtotal colectomy) but can persist for several months; stools become more formed as the ileum adapts by increasing reservoir capacity and water absorption.
• Subtotal colectomy is well tolerated by cats; constipation recurrence rates are typically low.

MISCELLANEOUS

ASSOCIATED CONDITIONS
Perineal hernia

AGE-RELATED FACTORS
Concurrent medical conditions (e.g., chronic renal insufficiency, hyperthyroidism) may occur with idiopathic megacolon, since many cats are old.

ZOONOTIC POTENTIAL
N/A

PREGNANCY
• The effect of cisapride on the fetus is unknown.
• Patients would be at increased risk for dystocia if they carried a pregnancy to term.

SYNONYMS
N/A

SEE ALSO
• Constipation and Obstipation
• Dyschezia and Hematochezia
• Perineal Hernia

ABBREVIATIONS
N/A

Suggested Reading
Bertoy RW. Megacolon. In: Bojrab MJ, ed. Disease mechanisms in small animal surgery. 2nd ed. Philadelphia: Lea & Febiger, 1993:262–265.
Holt D, Johnston DE. Idiopathic megacolon in cats. Compend Contin Educ Pract Vet 1991;13:1411–1416.
Rosin E. Megacolon in cats: the role of colectomy. In: Lieb MS, ed. Small animal practice. Philadelphia: Saunders, Vet Clin North Am 1993;23(3):587–594.
Tams TR. Cisapride: clinical experience with the newest GI prokinetic drug. (Abstract) Proceedings of the 12th Annual Veterinary Medical Forum-ACVIM. 1994:100–101.

Author Bradford C. Dixon
Consulting Editor Albert E. Jergens

MEGAESOPHAGUS

 BASICS

DEFINITION
Rather than a single disease entity, mega-esophagus refers to esophageal dilation and hypomotility, which may be a primary disorder or secondary to esophageal obstruction or neuromuscular dysfunction.

PATHOPHYSIOLOGY
• Esophageal motility is decreased or absent, resulting in accumulation and retention of food and liquid in the esophagus. • Reflex esophageal motility begins when food stimulates sensory afferents in the esophageal mucosa, which then sends afferent messages to the brain stem swallowing center via the vagus nerve. • Efferent messages from lower motor neurons in the nucleus ambiguus travel via the vagus to stimulate contraction of esophageal striated and smooth muscle. • Lesions anywhere along this pathway, including the myoneural junction, may result in esophageal hypomotility and distention. • Afferent nerve dysfunction appears to be more important than efferent dysfunction, as upper and lower esophageal sphincter function is normal after swallowing. • Increased lower esophageal sphincter tone is not an important cause of megaesophagus in veterinary patients.

SYSTEMS AFFECTED
• Gastrointestinal—regurgitation, weight loss/cachexia • Neuromuscular—may be manifestation of neuromuscular disease • Respiratory—if aspiration pneumonia occurs

GENETICS
Congenital idiopathic megaesophagus is heritable in wire-haired fox terriers (simple autosomal recessive) and miniature schnauzers (simple autosomal dominant or 60% penetrance autosomal recessive).

INCIDENCE/PREVALENCE
Most common cause of regurgitation in dogs and cats

GEOGRAPHIC DISTRIBUTION
N/A

SIGNALMENT

Species
More common in dogs than cats

Breed Predilections
• Hereditary in wire-haired fox terriers and miniature schnauzers • Familial predispositions reported in the German shepherd, Newfoundland, Great Dane, Irish setter, sharpei, pug, greyhound, Labrador retriever, and Siamese cats.

Mean Age and Range
• Congenital megaesophagus—signs of regurgitation first appear at weaning • Acquired forms—reported most often in young adults to middle-aged animals

Predominant Sex
N/A

SIGNS

Historical Findings
• May include regurgitation of food and water, weight loss or poor growth, hypersalivation, and a gurgling sound with swallowing • History relating to the underlying cause of megaesophagus may include weakness, paresis or paralysis, ataxia, gagging, dysphagia, pain, or depression. • May see coughing, mucopurulent nasal discharge, and dyspnea with concurrent aspiration pneumonia

Physical Examination Findings
• Occasionally normal • Related to mega-esophagus—regurgitation, weight loss, auscultation of retained fluid and food in the esophagus, halitosis, ptyalism, bulging of the esophagus at the thoracic inlet, and pain associated with palpation of the cervical esophagus • Related to the cause or sequelae of mega-esophagus—respiratory crackles, tachypnea, pyrexia, myalgia, muscle weakness, muscle atrophy, hyporeflexia, proprioceptive and postural deficits, autonomic disorders (mydriasis with loss of pupillary light reflex, dry nasal and ocular mucous membranes, diarrhea, bradycardia), cranial nerve deficits (especially cranial nerves VI, IX, and X), paresis or paralysis, and mentation changes

CAUSES
• Congenital idiopathic megaesophagus • Primary acquired—idiopathic adult onset megaesophagus • Secondary acquired— 1. Peripheral neuropathy and neuromuscular junction—myasthenia gravis (focal and generalized); polymyositis (including systemic lupus erythematosus); polyneuritis; polyradiculoneuritis; botulism; dysautonomia; tetanus; bilateral vagal damage. 2. Central nervous system—degenerative, infectious/inflammatory, neoplastic, trauma to the brain stem and cervical spinal cord. 3. Esophageal obstruction—esophageal foreign body, stricture, neoplasia, granuloma, vascular ring anomalies (e.g., persistent right aortic arch), periesophageal compression. 4. Miscellaneous—esophagitis, hypothyroidism, hypoadrenocorticism, thymoma (with secondarily acquired myasthenia gravis), toxicosis (lead, thallium, acetylcholinesterase inhibitors)

RISK FACTORS
N/A

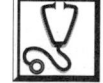 DIAGNOSIS

DIFFERENTIAL DIAGNOSIS
• Other disorders causing regurgitation. • Obstructive pharyngeal disease (foreign bodies, inflammation, neoplasia, cricopharyngeal achalasia) and palate disorders may produce regurgitation with normal esophageal motility. • Pharyngeal pain and dysphagia often occur with obstructive pharyngeal disease. • Distinguish regurgitation from dysphagia and vomition. • Regurgitation is a passive process with no forceful abdominal contraction, anticipatory salivation, nausea, or retching. • Bile-stained ingesta suggests vomition. • The time relationship between eating and expulsion of food does not help to distinguish regurgitation and vomiting.

CBC/BIOCHEMISTRY/URINALYSIS
• No characteristic findings, but may aid in identifying the underlying cause • Hyponatremia and hyperkalemia suggest hypoadrenocorticism. • Hypercholesterolemia is usually present with hypothyroidism. • Elevated creatine kinase (CK) suggests a primary muscle disorder.

OTHER LABORATORY TESTS
• Acetylcholine receptor antibody titers to screen for acquired myasthenia gravis should be performed in all patients with mega-esophagus. • Antinuclear antibody titers to evaluate for SLE • ACTH stimulation to evaluate adrenal function • Free T_4/TSH level to evaluate thyroid function • Blood lead and cholinesterase levels to evaluate for toxicity

IMAGING

Survey Thoracic Radiographs
• Esophagus dilated with gas, fluid, or ingesta • The trachea is often displaced ventrally by the distended esophagus.

Contrast Esophagram and Fluoroscopy
• An esophagram using either barium liquid or paste may demonstrate contrast pooling, abnormal esophageal motility, or stricture. • Abnormal primary and secondary esophageal peristalsis can be visualized with fluoroscopy. • Contrast studies—not necessary for diagnosing most cases of megaesophagus; use with caution in patients with known mega-esophagus, because of the risk of aspiration.

Nuclear Scintigraphy
Measures the rate of transport of radiolabeled food through the esophagus

DIAGNOSTIC PROCEDURES
• Endoscopy—can use to visualize a dilated esophagus, foreign bodies, neoplasia, and esophagitis; mucosal biopsy specimens and cytology samples may be obtained; esophageal foreign bodies may be removed • EMG and NCV—fibrillation potentials, positive sharp waves, and complex repetitive discharges suggest neuromuscular disease; prolonged NCV suggests peripheral neuropathy • Esophageal manometry—measures esophageal pressure and transit time during swallowing • Muscle and nerve biopsies/histopathology—useful to confirm diagnosis of inflammatory and degenerative disorders of muscles and nerves

• Cerebrospinal fluid analysis—pleocytosis and/or protein elevations suggest central nervous system disease • Autonomic nervous system testing—ocular pharmacologic testing (e.g. 0.05–0.1% pilocarpine eyedrops to demonstrate postganglionic denervation of the iris constrictor muscle) and measurement of blood pressure (hypotension) support autonomic dysfunction • Fecal examination for *Spirocerca lupi* ova

PATHOLOGIC FINDINGS
Gross and histopathologic findings vary, depending on the underlying disease.

TREATMENT

APPROPRIATE HEALTH CARE
• Many can be diagnosed and treated as outpatients. • Hospitalize patients with aspiration pneumonia, obstructive megaesophagus, severe debilitation, or advanced neurologic disease.

NURSING CARE
Aspiration pneumonia and/or dehydration warrant appropriate antibiotic and fluid therapy.

ACTIVITY
No change necessary for megaesophagus alone; restriction may be necessary for associated neuromuscular disorders.

DIET
• A high-calorie food should be chosen. • Feed in upright position (45–90° angle to floor) and maintain position for 10–15 minutes following feeding. • Dietary consistency must be tailored to the individual patient. Feeding a gruel may produce less regurgitation, but meat balls have less risk of aspiration and may stimulate more peristalsis. • Patients with severe regurgitation may need parenteral feeding via gastrotomy tube.

CLIENT EDUCATION
Emphasize the danger of aspiration pneumonia and the importance of the special feeding requirements.

SURGICAL CONSIDERATIONS
• Surgery may be necessary to remove esophageal foreign bodies or neoplasia or correct vascular ring anomalies. • No surgical procedures improve esophageal motility. • The modified Heller cardiomyotomy reduces lower esophageal tone and may improve gravity-facilitated movement of ingesta into the stomach. • Surgical treatment of megaesophagus has not been critically evaluated in dogs and cats and is not currently recommended.

MEDICATIONS

DRUG(S)
• No drugs are commonly used to treat megaesophagus alone; direct treatment at the underlying disease or associated conditions (e.g., aspiration pneumonia). • Sucralfate (0.5–1.0 g/dog PO q8h), H$_2$ blockers (e.g., famotidine 0.5 mg/kg PO q12–24h in dogs), or omeprazole (0.7 mg/kg PO q24h in dogs) can be used if reflux esophagitis is present. • Metoclopramide (0.2–0.5 mg/kg PO q6–8h in dogs) speeds gastric emptying, increases gastroesophageal sphincter tone, and is most useful when reflux esophagitis is a contributing or the primary cause; use of metoclopramide for other causes has had limited success. • Broad-spectrum antibiotics—necessary for patients with aspiration pneumonia; parenteral antibiotics or enteral administration via a gastrotomy tube may be required for patients with severe regurgitation • Immunosuppressive agents (e.g., prednisone, cyclophosphamide, azathioprine) are required for immune-mediated diseases. • Prednisone and acetylcholinesterase inhibitors (pyridostigmine) are used to treat myasthenia gravis.

PRECAUTIONS
• Corticosteroids may be necessary to treat conditions causing megaesophagus; use with caution in patients with aspiration pneumonia. • Cisapride (0.1–0.5 mg/kg PO q8–12h in dogs) has been used to treat megaesophagus, but its use is controversial; it decreases esophageal transit time and increases lower esophageal tone in normal dogs; both of these effects are undesirable when treating megaesophagus; despite this, regurgitation decreases in some patients receiving cisapride; if symptoms of megaesophagus worsen, discontinue cisapride.

FOLLOW-UP

PATIENT MONITORING
• Reexamine patients if signs of aspiration pneumonia develop—fever, cough, mucopurulent nasal discharge. • May use repeat thoracic radiographs, esophagrams, and fluoroscopic and neurologic examinations to follow progression or resolution of megaesophagus

PREVENTION/AVOIDANCE
Esophageal obstruction may be prevented if pets are not allowed access to bones, garbage, or other tempting items.

POSSIBLE COMPLICATIONS
Aspiration pneumonia

EXPECTED COURSE AND PROGNOSIS
• Poor, with or without treatment • Aspiration pneumonia, owner noncompliance, and malnutrition are leading causes of death. • Additional neurologic abnormalities may develop if the megaesophagus is caused by neuromuscular disease. • Megaesophagus caused by myasthenia gravis may improve with treatment. • Occasionally, congenital idiopathic megaesophagus may resolve with age. • Treatment of underlying conditions may also result in improved esophageal function.

MISCELLANEOUS

ASSOCIATED CONDITIONS
Aspiration pneumonia

AGE-RELATED FACTORS
Regurgitation at weaning suggests congenital or obstructive megaesophagus.

ZOONOTIC POTENTIAL
Determine rabies vaccination status for all patients.

PREGNANCY
N/A

SYNONYMS
Do not use the term *achalasia,* which describes esophageal hypomotility and lower esophageal sphincter hypertonicity in humans, because megaesophagus in animals is rarely associated with lower esophageal sphincter hypertonicity.

SEE ALSO
• Dysphagia • Esophageal Foreign Bodies • Myasthenia Gravis • Pneumonia, Bacterial • Regurgitation

ABBREVIATIONS
• ACTH = adenocorticotropic hormone
• EMG = electromyography
• NCV = nerve conduction velocity
• SLE = systemic lupus erythematosus
• T$_4$ = thyroxine
• TSH = thyroid stimulating hormone

Suggested Reading
Boudrieau RJ. Megaesophagus in the dog: a review of 50 cases. JAAHA 1985;21:33–40.
Guilford WG. Megaesophagus in the dog and cat. Semin Vet Med Surg (Small Anim) 1990;5:37–45.
Leib MS. Megaesophagus. In: Bojrab MJ, ed. Disease mechanisms in small animal surgery. 2nd ed. Philadelphia: Lea & Febiger, 1993:205–209.
Mears EA, DeNovo RC. Canine megaesophagus. In: Bonagura JD, ed. Kirk's current veterinary therapy XIII small animal practice. Philadelphia: Saunders, 2000; 602–607.
Washabau RJ, Hall JA. Diagnosis and management of gastrointestinal motility disorders in dogs and cats. Compend Cont Educ Pract Vet 1997;19:721–736.

Author Randall C. Longshore
Consulting Editor Albert E. Jergens

MELANOCYTIC TUMORS, ORAL

 BASICS

OVERVIEW
• Tumors characterized by progressive local invasion of neoplastic melanocytic cells within the oral cavity of dogs or cats
• Arise from the gingival surface and grow rapidly
• Generally characterized by a nonencapsulated, raised, irregular, ulcerated, and/or necrotic surface; highly invasive to bone
• Melanoma—most common oral malignancy in dogs; third most common in cats
• Metastatic—common (80% metastatic rate in dogs); spread to the lymph nodes more common than to the lungs
• Cause of death—secondary to local recurrence, dysphagia, and subsequent cachexia or metastatic disease

SIGNALMENT
• Occurs more commonly in dogs and cats > 10 years in age
• No sex or breed predilection

SIGNS

Historical Findings
• Excessive salivation
• Halitosis
• Dysphagia
• Bloody oral discharge
• Weight loss

Physical Examination Findings
• Oral mass
• Loose teeth
• Facial deformity
• Occasionally, cervical lymphadenomegaly

CAUSES & RISK FACTORS
None identified

 DIAGNOSIS

DIFFERENTIAL DIAGNOSIS
• Other oral malignancy
• Epulis
• Abscess
• Benign polyp

CBC/BIOCHEMISTRY/URINALYSIS
Usually normal

OTHER LABORATORY TESTS
Cytologic evaluation of an impression smear—obtain from an incisional biopsy specimen (wedge); may yield a diagnosis

IMAGING
• Skull radiography—evaluate for bone involvement deep to the mass.
• Thoracic radiographs—evaluate lungs for metastasis.

DIAGNOSTIC PROCEDURES
• Large, deep tissue biopsy (down to bone)—required to sufficiently differentiate from other oral malignancies

• Carefully palpate regional lymph nodes (mandibular and retropharyngeal).

IMMUNOHISTOCHEMISTRY
• May help confirm a diagnosis, especially if amelanotic

 TREATMENT

SURGERY
• Radical surgical excision—required (e.g., hemimaxillectomy); well tolerated by most patients; must have margins of at least 2 cm; improved survival when excisional margins are free of neoplastic cells
• Cryosurgery—not indicated because of extensive bony invasion
• Soft foods—may be recommended to prevent tumor ulceration or after radical oral excision

RADIATION
• Course of fraction external beam radiotherapy (teletherapy)—may offer considerable long-term control if tumor is deemed inoperable
• Current radiotherapy plans—attempt 24 Gy given in three fractions at 0, 7, and 21 days; 36 Gy given in 6 weekly fractions
• Response in cats not reported
• Complications—depends on protocol; include mucositis, anorexia, and dehydration requiring aggressive supportive care

• Combined with low-dose cisplatin or carboplatin—may improve overall survival
• Combined with hyperthermia—does not improve overall survival

OTHER
• Piroxicam—may play a role in pain control and tumor control

MEDICATIONS

DRUG(S)
• Carboplatin has been described for local or systemic control of oral melanoma in dogs.
• No effective chemotherapy has been described in cats.
• Local control (palliation) with intralesionally administered cisplatin reported

CONTRAINDICATIONS/POSSIBLE INTERACTIONS
• Chemotherapy can be toxic; seek advice before initiating treatment if you are unfamiliar with cytotoxic drugs.
• Cisplatin should not be used in cats.

FOLLOW-UP

EXPECTED COURSE AND PROGNOSIS
• Depends on staging of disease
• Radical excision involving normal bone—best long-term control and survival
• Survival after complete surgical excision (dogs)—median, 340 days; mean, 567 days
• Survival after incomplete surgical excision (dogs)—median, 260 days; mean, 210 days
• Survival after any form of surgical excision (cats)—< 60 days
• Survival with radiotherapy treatment (dogs)—5–8 mos
• Positive prognostic features at the time of diagnosis—location (e.g., rostral mandible and caudal maxilla), small tumor size, and low mitotic index
• Distant metastasis at examination—low (< 10%); but is most often the cause of death late in the course of the disease
• Overall prognosis in cats—poor; most tumors are locally invasive and diagnosed late in the course of the disease; cause of death is secondary to local recurrence, dysphagia, and subsequent cachexia

MISCELLANEOUS

Suggested Reading

Freeman KP, Hahn KA, King GK, Harris DF. Treatment of dogs with oral melanoma by hypofractionated radiation therapy and platinum-based chemotherapy (1987–1997). J Vet Intern Med 2003; Jan-Feb; 17(1):96–101.

Hahn KA, DeNicola DB, Richardson RC, Hahn EA. Canine oral malignant melanoma: prognostic utility of an alternative staging system. J Small Anim Pract 1994;35:251–256.

Patnaik AK, Mooney S. Feline melanoma: a comparative study of ocular, oral, and dermal neoplasms. Vet Pathol 1988; 25:105–112.

Rassnick KM, Ruslander DM, Cotter SM, et al. Use of carboplatin for treatment of dogs with malignant melanoma: 27 cases (1989–2000). J Am Vet Med Assoc 2001;218:1444–1448.

Authors Kevin A. Hahn and Kimberly P. Freeman

Consulting Editor Wallace B. Morrison

MELANOCYTIC TUMORS, SKIN AND DIGIT

 BASICS

DEFINITION
Benign or malignant neoplasm arising from melanocytes and melanoblasts (melanin-producing cells)

PATHOPHYSIOLOGY
• Locally invasive
• Malignant—may invade bone and metastasize to regional lymph nodes

SYSTEMS AFFECTED
• Skin/Exocrine
• Metastatic sites—bone, lymph nodes, lung, and viscera

GENETICS
Unknown

INCIDENCE/PREVALENCE
• Dogs—4%–20% of all skin tumors
• Cats—0.8%–7% of all skin tumors

GEOGRAPHIC DISTRIBUTION
N/A

SIGNALMENT

Species
Dogs and cats

Breed Predilections
• Dogs—Scottish terriers, Boston terriers, Airedale terriers, cocker spaniels, boxers, springer spaniels, Irish setters, Irish terriers, chow chows, Chihuahuas, and Doberman pinschers
• Cats—none

Mean Age and Range
• Dogs—9 years
• Cats—8–14 years

Predominant Sex
• Dogs—males may be predisposed.
• Cats—none

SIGNS

Historical Findings
• Slow or rapidly growing mass
• Lameness if digit is involved

Physical Examination Findings
• Pigmented or nonpigmented (amelanotic) mass, usually solitary
• Develops anywhere but may be more common on face, trunk, feet, and scrotum in dogs and head, digit, pinna, and nose in cats
• Regional lymph nodes—may be large
• Advanced disease—may have dyspnea or harsh lung sounds because of pulmonary metastasis

CAUSES
Unknown

RISK FACTORS
Unknown

 DIAGNOSIS

DIFFERENTIAL DIAGNOSIS
Histopathologic examination and special stains—may distinguish amelanotic melanoma from poorly differentiated mast cell tumors, lymphosarcoma, and carcinoma

CBC/BIOCHEMISTRY/URINALYSIS
Usually normal

OTHER LABORATORY TESTS
Immunohistochemical stains—may help differentiate melanoma (especially amelanotic) from other tumors; melanoma stains positive with vimentin, S-100, neuron-specific enolase, and human melanosome–specific antigen.

IMAGING
• Thoracic radiography—detect metastasis
• Area radiography—determine if underlying bone is involved, especially with melanoma of the digit.

DIAGNOSTIC PROCEDURES
Cytologic examination of fine-needle aspirate—reveals brown, rod-like intracellular granules (melanin) in cells of various sizes and shapes; pigment may be absent in the case of amelanotic melanoma; may see macrophages (melanophages) containing phagocytosed melanin

PATHOLOGIC FINDINGS

Gross
• Masses—vary in color and appearance; may be ulcerated
• Benign—generally slow-growing; brown to black; varies from macules and plaques to firm, dome-shaped nodules, 0.5–2 cm in diameter
• Malignant—generally rapidly growing; amelanotic to dark brown, gray, or black
• Melanomas of the digit (dog and cat) and eyelid (cat) tend to be malignant.

Histopathologic Findings
• Often difficult to distinguish benign from malignant lesions because both may have cells that vary in shape (e.g., epithelioid, fusiform, dendritic, and mixed), degree of pigmentation, and cytoplasmic morphology
• Malignant—generally high mitotic index; nuclear and nucleolar pleomorphism; invasive into surrounding tissues; amelanotic may pose a diagnostic challenge; special stains may be particularly useful.
• Benign and malignant—may note associated inflammation, predominantly lymphoplasmacytic

 TREATMENT

APPROPRIATE HEALTH CARE
Inpatient if undergoing surgery

NURSING CARE
• Fluid administration—indicated during surgery
• Melanoma of the digit—may require bandaging of the distal limb after surgery

ACTIVITY
• Depends on location of tumor
• Generally, restrict until sutures are removed.

DIET
Normal

CLIENT EDUCATION
• Discuss the need for early surgical removal.
• Do not advise a wait-and-see approach.

• Warn client that malignant melanoma may metastasize early in the course of the disease; thus prognosis is guarded.

SURGICAL CONSIDERATIONS
• Wide surgical excision—treatment of choice
• Amputation of digit—nail bed or digit affected

 MEDICATIONS

DRUG(S) OF CHOICE
• Adjunctive chemotherapy—recommended if surgical excision is incomplete or the mass is nonresectable
• Dacarbazine (DTIC) (dogs), doxorubicin, and carboplatin—reported to induce partial and complete remission in a small number of animals; may be the drugs of choice

CONTRAINDICATIONS
Doxorubicin—cardiotoxic; contraindicated with heart disease

PRECAUTIONS
Veterinarians administering chemotherapeutics should follow published guidelines on the safe use of these drugs and should be familiar with potential side effects.

POSSIBLE INTERACTIONS
None reported

ALTERNATIVE DRUG(S)
Cimetidine—shown to be of some benefit in horses and humans with malignant melanoma; believed to act as a biologic response modifier by reversing suppressor T-cell–mediated immune suppression; has not been evaluated for this purpose in dogs and cats

 FOLLOW-UP

PATIENT MONITORING
• Evaluate for evidence of recurrence and metastasis—1, 3, 6, 9, 12, 18, and 24 months after surgery; if the owner believes the mass is returning; if the patient is otherwise not normal
• Thoracic radiography—at the time of rechecks and periodically thereafter

PREVENTION/AVOIDANCE
N/A

POSSIBLE COMPLICATIONS
None

EXPECTED COURSE AND PROGNOSIS
• Dogs—25%–50% of melanomas reported to be malignant; melanomas on the digit and scrotum have a greater likelihood of being malignant.
• Survival with benign melanomas (dogs)—mean: skin, > 24 months; digit, 19.3 months; 2-year: skin, 94.3%; digit: 38%
• Survival with malignant melanoma (dogs)—skin: 8–13.5 months; digit: 16.9 months; 2-year: skin, 34.1%; digit: 22%–36%
• Cats—35%–50% of melanomas reported to be malignant
• Mean survival with melanoma of the skin or digit (cats)—not frequently reported; 4.5 months after surgery in one study of 57 cats

 MISCELLANEOUS

ASSOCIATED CONDITIONS
None

AGE-RELATED FACTORS
None

ZOONOTIC POTENTIAL
None

PREGNANCY
N/A

SYNONYMS
• Benign—melanocytic nevus; melanocytoma
• Malignant—melanosarcoma (rarely used)

ABBREVIATION
DTIC = (dimethyltriazeno)imidazole carboxamide

Suggested Reading

Aronsohn MG, Carpenter JL. Distal extremity melanocytic nevi and malignant melanomas in dogs. J Am Anim Hosp Assoc 1990;26:605–612.

Luna LD, Higginbotham ML, Henry CJ. Feline non-ocular melanoma: a retrospective study of 23 cases (1991–1999). J Feline Med Surg 2000;2:173–181.

Miller WH, Scott DW, Anderson WI. Feline cutaneous melanocytic neoplasms: a retrospective analysis of 43 cases (1979–1991). Vet Dermatol 1993;4:19–26.

Pulley LT, Stannard AA. Tumors of the skin and soft tissues. In: Moulton JE, ed. Tumors in domestic animals. 3rd ed. Berkeley: University of California Press, 1990:75–82.

Thomas RC, Fox LE. Tumors of the skin and subcutis. In: Morrison WB, ed. Cancer in dogs and cats: medical and surgical management. Baltimore: Williams & Wilkins, 1998:489–510.

Author Joanne C. Graham
Consulting Editor Wallace B. Morrison

MELENA

BASICS

DEFINITION
Presence of digested blood in the feces, which gives a black, tarry appearance

PATHOPHYSIOLOGY
Usually results from upper GI bleeding, but can be associated with ingested blood from the oral cavity or respiratory tract

SYSTEMS AFFECTED
• Gastrointestinal
• Respiratory
• Coagulation

SIGNALMENT
• More common in dogs than cats
• No breed or sex predilection

SIGNS

Historical Findings
• Patients with upper GI tract hemorrhage may demonstrate vomiting, inappetance, weight loss, weakness, and/or mucous membrane pallor.
• Patients with respiratory tract hemorrhage may demonstrate epistaxis, sneezing, hemoptysis, mucous membrane pallor, weakness, and/or dyspnea.
• Patients with abnormal coagulation may demonstrate petechia, ecchymosis, mucous membrane pallor, epistaxis, hematuria, hyphema, and/or weakness.

Physical Examination Findings
Depends on the underlying cause

CAUSES

Primary GI Ulceration/Erosion
• Neoplasia—lymphoma, adenocarcinoma
• Infectious—pythiosis, fungal, parasitic, *Helicobacter* spp.
• Mechanical—foreign body
• Inflammatory—acute gastritis; hemorrhagic gastropathy, lymphoplasmacytic, eosinophilic, granulomatous, and/or histiocytic enteritis
• Drugs—NSAIDs, corticosteroids

Metabolic/Other Diseases That Cause GI Ulceration
• Renal failure
• Hepatic disease
• Pancreatitis
• Hypoadrenocorticism
• Neoplasia—gastrinoma, mast cell tumor
• Shock, poor perfusion

Ingestion of Blood
• Diet
• Esophageal lesion—neoplasia, esophagitis
• Oral or pharyngeal lesion—neoplasia, abscess
• Nasal lesion—neoplasia, fungal rhinitis
• Respiratory lesion—lung lobe torsion, neoplasia, pneumonia, trauma

Coagulopathy
• Thrombocytopenia
• Platelet dysfunction—von Willebrand's disease, thrombasthenia, thrombopathia, NSAIDs
• Clotting factor abnormalities—anti-coagulant rodenticide ingestion, clotting factor deficiency
• DIC

RISK FACTORS
Arthritis or other conditions requiring use of NSAIDs or corticosteroids

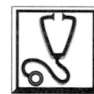

DIAGNOSIS

DIFFERENTIAL DIAGNOSIS
• Medications that cause dark stool—bismuth subsalicylate, oral iron therapy
• Must distinguish intestinal from extra-intestinal disease

CBC/BIOCHEMISTRY/URINALYSIS
• Microcytic, hypochromic, poorly regenerative anemia if chronic blood loss
• Regenerative anemia in early blood loss—may be poorly regenerative if <3 days
• Panhypoproteinemia if significant blood loss
• Thrombocytopenia, neutrophilia in some patients; pancytopenia in some
• Biochemistry analysis may reveal extra-intestinal cause of melena—renal failure, hepatic disease, hypoadrenocorticism
• Urinalysis may demonstrate hematuria in patients with coagulation defects.

OTHER LABORATORY TESTS
• Coagulation profile may reveal clotting abnormality.
• Bleeding time may be prolonged.
• Fecal examination may reveal infectious cause—parasites
• ACTH stimulation test abnormally low with hypoadrenocorticism
• Urease testing for *Helicobacter* spp.

IMAGING
• Abdominal radiography may reveal a mass, foreign body, or abnormalities in renal or hepatic size/shape.
• Thoracic radiographs may identify intra-thoracic lesions.
• Nasal radiographs or nasal CT may indicate intranasal lesions.
• Ultrasonography may reveal a mass, hepatic disease, pancreatitis, or renal disease.
• Upper GI barium series may delineate gastric or upper small intestinal mass, ulceration, or filling defect.

DIAGNOSTIC PROCEDURES
• Endoscopy allows visualization of masses and/or ulcers (esophageal, gastric, and/or

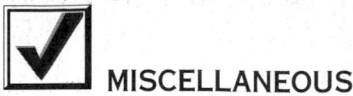
duodenal), retrieval of GI foreign bodies, and biopsy.
• Rhinoscopy occasionally allows visualization of nasal lesions (endoscope or bronchoscope retroflexion and choanal evaluation is often helpful).
• Bronchoscopy allows visualization of airway lesions.
• Bone marrow aspiration and cytology indicated if pancytopenia is present

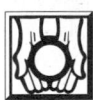
TREATMENT

• Inpatient—exception may be animal with intestinal parasites
• Treat underlying disease—renal failure, hepatic disease, hypoadrenocorticism, respiratory disease, etc.
• Fluid replacement with balanced electrolyte solutions and potassium supplementation
• Whole blood or packed red cell transfusions if anemia is severe
• Whole blood or plasma transfusion if the patient has a coagulopathy
• Temporarily discontinue oral intake if vomiting
• Surgery may be required for severe gastroduodenal ulceration or neoplasia

MEDICATIONS

DRUG(S) OF CHOICE
• Mucosal protectants for gastroduodenal ulceration/erosion—H_2-receptor antagonists

(e.g., ranitidine 2 mg/kg IV or PO q12h or famotidine 0.5 mg/kg IV or PO q12–24h); sucralfate 0.5–1g PO q6–8h); misoprostol 3–5 mcg/kg PO q8h.
• Triple therapy if *Helicobacter* suspected or confirmed (see *Helicobacter*)

CONTRAINDICATIONS
Avoid corticosteroids and NSAIDs in patients with gastroduodenal ulceration/erosion

PRECAUTIONS
N/A

POSSIBLE INTERACTIONS
N/A

ALTERNATIVE DRUG(S)
Na/K-ATPase pump blocker (omeprazole 0.7 mg/kg PO q24h) can be used if H_2-receptor antagonists are unsuccessful or initially in severe gastroduodenal ulcer disease.

FOLLOW-UP

PATIENT MONITORING
• PCV daily until anemia stabilized, then weekly
• Hydration daily if patient vomiting
• Daily for respiratory distress if respiratory tract involved

POSSIBLE COMPLICATIONS
• Gastric or duodenal perforation and peritonitis
• Hypovolemic shock and death if severe, acute blood loss

MISCELLANEOUS

ASSOCIATED CONDITIONS
N/A

AGE-RELATED FACTORS
N/A

ZOONOTIC POTENTIAL
Helicobacter spp. have unknown zoonotic potential.

PREGNANCY
N/A

SYNONYMS
N/A

SEE ALSO
Individual causative diseases—Hypoadrenocorticism, *Helicobacter*, etc.

ABBREVIATIONS
• CT = computed tomography
• DIC = disseminated intravascular coagulation
• GI = gastrointestinal
• NSAIDs = nonsteroidal antiinflammatory drugs

Suggested Reading
Willard MD. Diseases of the stomach. In: Ettinger SJ, Feldman EC, eds. Textbook of veterinary internal medicine. Philadelphia: Saunders, 1995:1143–1168.
Authors Lisa E. Moore and Colin F. Burrows
Consulting Editor Albert E. Jergens

MENINGIOMA

 BASICS

OVERVIEW
• Tumors of the meninges most commonly found intracranially over the cerebrum
• Usually solitary masses; occasionally multiple (cats)
• May occur as plaque-like masses on the floor of the calvaria, paranasally, or (rarely) in a retrobulbar location in dogs more than cats; also develop along the spinal cord but less frequently and with an intradural, extramedullary predilection site
• Compress the adjacent tissue, causing vasogenic edema
• Dogs—tends to be more invasive into brain parenchyma or surrounding vasculature

SIGNALMENT
• Dogs and cats
• Dogs—no breed predilection; mesocephalic breeds may have a higher incidence of paranasal meningiomas; most > 7 years of age; range 11 weeks to 14 years; a spinal meningeal sarcoma was diagnosed in an 11-week-old rottweiler; slight predominance for females
• Cats—most > 9 years of age; range 1–24 years; slight predominance for males

SIGNS
• Vary with tumor location
• Typically chronic and insidiously progressive over weeks to months
• May be acute if vascular invasion results in focal ischemia or if edema develops rapidly
• Lateralizing deficits predominate.

Intracranial
• Cerebral disease—predominates; abnormal behavior and mentation; contralateral visual and proprioceptive deficits; seizures
• Dogs—late-onset seizures common presenting sign without evidence of neurologic examination deficits (silent area disease)
• Cats—seizures less common than in dogs

Intraspinal
• Ataxia and motor dysfunction—vary with location of the tumor along the spinal column
• Neck or back pain

CAUSE & RISK FACTORS
• Uncertain
• Documentation in young cats with mucopolysaccharidosis type I suggests a causal relationship.

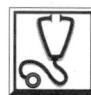 **DIAGNOSIS**

DIFFERENTIAL DIAGNOSIS
• Other primary CNS (e.g., glioma) or secondary (e.g., extensional or metastatic) tumors—more rapid onset and progression of signs; differentiate by brain imaging
• Cryptococcus granuloma—reported to have same appearance on CT as a meningioma in a cat
• Granulomatous meningoencephalitis—may cause progressive focal deficits in dogs
• Silent area meningiomas—may mimic a metabolic encephalopathy
• Nerve sheath tumors, gliomas, and type II intervertebral disk disease—differentiate from a spinal cord syndrome

CBC/BIOCHEMISTRY/URINALYSIS
Usually normal

OTHER LABORATORY TESTS
CSF analysis—infrequently performed because of the characteristic results of diagnostic imaging; results normal or reveal high protein, sometimes with a neutrophilic pleocytosis

IMAGING
• CT and MRI scans of the head—preferred diagnostic techniques for intracranial disease
• MRI—often appear as hyperintense on T_2WI, isointense on T_1WI and homogeneously enhancing post-contrast mass lesion of the brain or spinal cord.
• CT—commonly reveals homogeneous enhancement of well circumscribed lesion
• Skull radiography and CT—may reveal hyperostosis of the calvaria adjacent to the meningioma and increased tissue density if the tumor is calcified
• Myelography—typically reveals an intradural–extramedullary mass with spinal disease; golf tee appearance makes differentiation from a nerve sheath tumor difficult without biopsy.
• Tissue biopsy remains necessary for definitive diagnosis

DIAGNOSTIC PROCEDURES
Electroencephalography—reveals slow-wave, medium- to high-voltage activity indicating cortical depression; may show paroxysmal waveforms characteristic of seizure activity

TREATMENT

- Outpatient, if treated medically
- Inpatient—dehydration; anorexia; frequent seizures
- Surgical excision—necessary for definitive management; usually successful if the tumor is accessible; incomplete excision more common in dogs because of invasiveness
- Radiation therapy—after excision; may be associated with prolonged survival time
- Medical management—palliative only; expect patient to deteriorate
- Fluids—avoid overzealous administration; may exacerbate cerebral edema and neurologic deficits

MEDICATIONS

DRUG(S)

Cerebral Edema
- Corticosteroids—improve neurologic deficits associated with vasogenic edema
- Stuporous, severely ataxic, or showing signs of herniation—methylprednisolone sodium succinate (30 mg/kg IV) or dexamethasone sodium phosphate (0.25 mg/kg IV)
- Continued deterioration or no improvement—20% mannitol solution (0.5–2.0 g/kg CRI over 20 min)

- Once stable—prednisone (0.5 mg/kg q12h) or dexamethasone (0.02–0.05 mg/kg PO q8h; then taper as needed)

Seizures
- Anticonvulsants—if seizures occur more frequently than one per 6–8 weeks
- Phenobarbital (first choice)—2–3 mg/kg IV or PO q12h or KBr 250 mg/ml—100 mg/kg divided q12hr × 4 day (loading dose) then 40 mg/kg divided q12h (maintenance dose)
- Cluster seizures—consider a loading dose of phenobarbital (12–16 mg/kg IV) or diazepam (0.5 mg/kg/hr CRI)

CONTRAINDICATIONS/POSSIBLE INTERACTIONS

Chloramphenicol and cimetidine—avoid with phenobarbital because they delay its metabolism

FOLLOW-UP

- Serial neurologic examinations—detect marked improvement in deficits within 24–48 hr after initiation of corticosteroids

Cats
- Surgical excision—prognosis good; 75% of patients that undergo surgical excision are cured; seizure activity may persist despite successful excision

- Medical management—neurologic deficits become more severe, but may take many months because meningiomas tend to be slow growing; thoracolumbar disease progresses to paralysis and inability to control urination; causes urinary retention and (possibly) bladder atony and cystitis.

MISCELLANEOUS

ABBREVIATIONS
- CNS = central nervous system
- CRI = constant rate infusion
- CSF = cerebrospinal fluid
- CT = computed tomography
- MRI = magnetic resonance imaging

Suggested Reading

Braund KG, Ribas JL. Central nervous system meningiomas. Compend Contin Educ Pract Vet 1986;8:241–248.

Gallagher JG, Berg J, Knowles KE, Williams LL, Bronson RT. Prognosis after surgical excision of cerebral meningiomas in cats: 17 cases (1986–1992). J Am Vet Med Assoc 1993;15:10:1437–1440.

Author Richard J. Joseph
Consulting Editor Joane M. Parent

MENINGITIS/MENINGOENCEPHALITIS/MENINGOMYELITIS, BACTERIAL

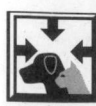 BASICS

DEFINITION
• Meningitis—inflammation of the meninges
• Meningoencephalitis—inflammation of the meninges and brain
• Meningomyelitis—inflammation of the meninges and spinal cord

PATHOPHYSIOLOGY
• Bacterial infection of the CNS by extension of an infected extraneural site by direct inoculation or by hematogenous route
• Inflammation of the meninges can lead to secondary inflammation of the brain or spinal cord, resulting in neurologic deficits.
• Inflammatory debris and scarring can obstruct CSF flow, leading to secondary hydrocephalus.

SYSTEMS AFFECTED
• Nervous—meninges, brain, or spinal cord
• Multisystemic signs—may be present because the infection usually originates in an extraneural site

GENETICS
N/A

INCIDENCE/PREVALENCE
Rare

GEOGRAPHIC DISTRIBUTION
N/A

SIGNALMENT

Species
Dogs and cats

Breed Predilections
N/A

Mean Age and Range
• Any age
• Neonates may have a relatively higher risk because of omphalophlebitis.

Predominant Sex
N/A

SIGNS

General Comments
• Patients are nearly always systemically ill.
• Depression, shock, hypotension, and DIC may be found.
• CNS signs may be profound and rapidly progressive.

Physical Examination Findings
• May find site of underlying infection
• Cervical rigidity
• Hyperesthesia
• Pyrexia

• Vomiting and bradycardia—may occur
• Neurologic deficits—reflect the location of the involved parenchyma (e.g., altered mentation, cranial nerve deficits, postural reaction deficits, paresis, seizures); increased intracranial pressure may be present

CAUSES
• Meningoencephalitis—usually secondary to local extension from infection of the ears, eyes, sinuses, nasal passages
• Meningomyelitis—secondary from diskospondylitis or osteomyelitis
• Hematogenous spread of bacterial infection less often occurs from extracranial foci in dogs with bacterial endocarditis, prostatitis, diskospondylitis, pneumonia, or gastroenteritis.
• The point of origin is not always found.

RISK FACTORS
• Untreated bacterial infection
• Immunocompromised state
• Injury involving the CNS or adjacent structures

 DIAGNOSIS

DIFFERENTIAL DIAGNOSIS

Fungal Meningitis
• Affected extraneural sites (dogs)—common with CNS cryptococcus (e.g., nasal, skin, and bone), blastomycosis (e.g., lung, lymph nodes, eyes, skin, and bone), and coccidioidomycosis (e.g., lung, bones, and joints)
• Diagnosis often made by biopsy or cytologic examination of affected tissues
• Serologic testing available
• Organisms—sometimes observed in the CSF; may be cultured

Distemper Virus Meningoencephalitis
• Patients usually young and unvaccinated
• CNS signs may be preceded by mild gastrointestinal and respiratory signs.
• Chorioretinitis common
• Inclusion bodies—may be observed on cytologic examination of blood smears
• Virus—may be detected in a conjunctival scraping or tracheal wash specimen by fluorescent antibody technique
• Biopsy of the haired skin of the dorsal neck can be used for immunohistochemical diagnosis.
• CSF analysis—typically reveals a high number of small lymphocytes and high protein concentration. Antibody against CDV may be increased in CSF. Viral antigen may also be detected.

FIP Virus Meningoencephalitis
• Often accompanied by fever, anorexia, uveitis, and chorioretinitis • CSF analysis—nonseptic mixed inflammation with neutrophils, lymphocytes, monocytes macrophages • CSF protein, increased; coronavirus antibody present

Toxoplasma/Neospora Meningoencephalitis
• Toxoplasma may accompanied by pneumonia, hepatitis, myositis, and uveitis, especially in cats. • In young dogs, nerve roots and muscles involved • Serum titer—may rise with active infection • CSF titer may be increased with active CNS infection. • Biopsy of affected tissues—may reveal the organism

Aseptic (Immune-mediated) Meningitis
• Observed mainly in young large-breed dogs that have cervical pain alone and are not systemically ill
• Cervical pain/fever common
• Neurologic deficits may occur chronically.
• CSF analysis—neutrophilic pleocytosis in acute cases—culture negative
• Serum and CSF IgA increased

Primary Neoplasia of the CNS
• Signs—limited to the CNS
• Standard laboratory tests—normal
• The diagnosis is made by CT or MRI and CSF analysis.

Granulomatous Meningoencephalomyelitis
• Clinical signs—usually not systemic
• CSF analysis—lymphocytes, monocytes, occasional plasma cells, and anaplastic mono-nuclear cells; sometimes mature nontoxic neutrophils
• CSF culture—negative

CBC/BIOCHEMISTRY/URINALYSIS
• Leukocytosis is common; left shift or toxicity may be seen.
• Evidence of other organ involvement (e.g., liver and kidney) and hyperglobulinemia in response to chronic infection
• Pyuria and bacteriuria—with underlying urinary tract or prostatic infection; with hematogenous spread of bacteria

OTHER LABORATORY TESTS
• Positive serologic tests—differentiate fungal, protozoal, rickettsial, and viral from bacterial disease; cats: toxoplasma titer may be positive without clinical disease.
• Cytologic examination of infected tissues—skin, eyes, nasal discharge, and sputum; helps identify the organism, especially in patients with fungal disease
• Blood and urine culture—may be positive

MENINGITIS/MENINGOENCEPHALITIS/MENINGOMYELITIS, BACTERIAL

IMAGING
- Thorax/abdominal radiography—identifies underlying infection or other significant disease
- Spinal radiography—diskospondylitis as a focus of infection
- Skull radiography—sinus, nasal cavity, or ear as initiating site (insensitive)
- Echocardiography—valvular endocarditis suspected based on murmur/arrhythmia
- MRI/CT to rule out other disease or identify site of infection (sinus, nasal, ear)

DIAGNOSTIC PROCEDURES
Biopsy—infected tissue; may help identify the organism

CSF Analysis
- Collection—contraindicated with signs that suggest high intracranial pressure, because it may precipitate brain herniation—pretreat with mannitol
- Analysis—neutrophilic pleocytosis with high protein concentration; sometimes the neutrophils appear toxic or degenerated and bacteria are seen; difficult to differentiate aseptic from bacterial meningitis by this alone
- Culture—aerobic or anaerobic; may be positive (< 40%)

PATHOLOGIC FINDINGS
- May note subdural empyema, herniation, or purulent material on the surface of the brain
- Diffuse suppurative leptomeningeal infiltration common

TREATMENT

APPROPRIATE HEALTH CARE
Inpatient—treat aggressively; intensive care monitoring often necessary

NURSING CARE
Fluid therapy and supportive care—as indicated for shock

ACTIVITY
Restricted

DIET
N/A

CLIENT EDUCATION
Inform client that rapid and aggressive treatment is important.

SURGICAL CONSIDERATIONS
N/A

MEDICATIONS

DRUG(S) OF CHOICE

Antibiotics
- Agents that penetrate the blood–brain barrier—chloramphenicol, trimethoprim, sulfonamides, metronidazole, quinolines, and cefotaxime
- Cultures—CSF, blood, urine, primary site; determine drug sensitivity; if cultures cannot be obtained, choose a broad-spectrum agent that is effective against aerobes and anaerobes
- Inflammation and suspected staphylococcal infection—use penicillin or ampicillin, which enter the CNS with inflammation; use in combination with another antibiotic that enters the CNS.

Anticonvulsants
- Indicated for seizures
- Diazepam initially and then phenobarbital

CONTRAINDICATIONS
Aminoglycosides and first-generation cephalosporins—do not penetrate the blood–brain barrier even in the presence of inflamed meninges; do not use.

PRECAUTIONS
N/A

POSSIBLE INTERACTIONS
Chloramphenicol—do not use in combination with phenobarbital; inhibits the hepatic metabolism of phenobarbital, leading to a toxic concentration

ALTERNATIVE DRUG(S)
N/A

FOLLOW-UP

PATIENT MONITORING
Nervous system signs, fever, leukocytosis, and systemic signs

PREVENTION/AVOIDANCE
Treat local infections adjacent to the CNS (e.g., infections of the eyes, ears, sinuses, nose, and spine) early and aggressively to prevent extension to the CNS.

POSSIBLE COMPLICATIONS
Damage caused by inflammation of the brain and spinal cord or associated thrombosis may be irreversible.

EXPECTED COURSE AND PROGNOSIS
- Response to antibiotics—variable; prognosis guarded
- Many patients die despite treatment.
- Some patients recover completely.
- Treatment for at least 4 weeks after resolution of all signs is recommended.

MISCELLANEOUS

ASSOCIATED CONDITIONS
N/A

AGE-RELATED FACTORS
N/A

ZOONOTIC POTENTIAL
N/A

PREGNANCY
N/A

SYNONYMS
N/A

SEE ALSO
- Encephalitis
- Meningoencephalomyelitis, Granulomatous

ABBREVIATIONS
- CDV = canine distemper virus
- CNS = central nervous system
- CSF = cerebrospinal fluid
- CT = computed tomography
- DIC = disseminated intravascular coagulation
- FIP = feline infectious peritonitis
- MRI = magnetic resonance imaging

Suggested Reading
Fenner WR. Central nervous system infections. In: Greene CE, ed. Infectious diseases of the dog and cat. Philadelphia: Saunders, 1998:647–657.
Meric SM. Canine meningitis: A changing emphasis. J Vet Intern Med 1998;2:26–35.
Radaelli ST, Platt SR. Bacterial menigoencephalomyelitis in dogs: a retrospective study in 23 cases (1990–1999). J Vet Intern Med 2002;16:159–163.
Sarfaty D, Carillo JM, Greenlee PG. Differential diagnosis of granulomatous meningoencephalomyelitis, distemper and suppurative meningoencephalitis in the dog. J Am Vet Med Assoc 1986;4:387–392.
Tipold A. Diagnosis of inflammatory and infectious diseases of the central nervous system in dogs. A retrospective study. J Vet Intern Med 1995;5:304–314.

Author Susan M. Taylor
Consulting Editor Joane M. Parent

MENINGOENCEPHALOMYELITIS, EOSINOPHILIC

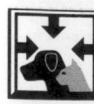 BASICS

OVERVIEW
• Diffuse or multifocal meningoencephalo-myelitis
• CSF analysis reveals eosinophilic pleocytosis.
• Eosinophils—in response to a parasite or an allergic reaction
• Underlying cause of the idiopathic syndrome unknown
• Meningeal involvement can be marked.

SIGNALMENT
• Dogs, and rarely cats
• Golden retrievers may be predisposed.
• Any age

SIGNS
• Vary in location and severity
• Neurologic abnormalities—often relate to the cerebrum; dementia, seizures, circling, and cortical blindness

CAUSES & RISK FACTORS
• Idiopathic or allergic—more common than other causes
• Neoplasia—reaction to foreign material

• Parasitic—cerebral cysticerci, *Dirofilaria immitis*
• Protozoal—*Neospora caninum, Toxoplasma gondii*
• Fungal—*Cryptococcus neoformans*
• Vaccination

 DIAGNOSIS

DIFFERENTIAL DIAGNOSIS
• Cannot be differentiated from the other encephalitides on the basis of clinical signs alone; CSF analysis must be done.
• After eosinophils are identified in the CSF—consider parasitic disease, allergic response, tumor, fungal disease.
• Parasitic disease—differentiate on the basis of systemic signs, laboratory data, and serologic test results
• Allergic and idiopathic disease—predominance of cerebral signs; negative serologic test results; marked eosinophilic pleocytosis
• Brain tumor—old patient; relatively long history; clinical signs relate to a focal lesion; eosinophils may be found, but usually in low numbers; confirm by brain imaging and biopsy.

CBC/BIOCHEMISTRY/URINALYSIS
• Peripheral eosinophilia—not always a reliable indicator of brain disease; degree does not correlate with the number of eosinophils in the CSF.
• Biochemical analysis and urinalysis—usually normal with idiopathic and allergic disease; liver enzyme activity and creatine kinase may be high with parasitic disease.

OTHER LABORATORY TESTS
N/A

IMAGING
• MRI—diffuse meningeal enhancement following contrast injection in diffuse meningocephalitis; space-occupying lesion if tumor present; hyperintense patchy lesions focally after contrast with larval migration

DIAGNOSTIC PROCEDURES

CSF Analysis
• Idiopathic and allergic disease—marked eosinophilic pleocytosis
• Parasitic and protozoal disease—less pleocytosis; may see neutrophils
• Neoplasia—low WBC; small numbers of eosinophils
• Fungal—marked eosinophilic pleocytosis may be present with *Cryptococcus;* organisms usually present as well

Serologic Testing
• If CSF analysis confirms existence of eosinophils, look thoroughly for parasitic and fungal disease.
• Always test for heartworm, *N. caninum, T. gondii,* and *C. neoformans*

TREATMENT
• Usually inpatient, because of severity of clinical signs
• Activity—as tolerated
• Regular diet

MEDICATIONS
DRUG(S)
• Idiopathic disease—steroid administration; dexamethasone (0.25 mg/kg q24hr for 1 day; then 0.1 mg/kg q24h for 6 days); follow with prednisone (0.5 mg/kg q24h for 2 weeks); then slowly wean patient over 6 weeks
• Protozoal disease—clindamycin, sulfonamides, and pyrimethamine

• Heartworm—microfilarial migration to the CNS is rare; no available treatment other than supportive
• Parasitic vs. parasite

CONTRAINDICATIONS/POSSIBLE INTERACTIONS
Steroids—contraindicated with protozoal disease

FOLLOW-UP
PATIENT MONITORING
Repeat neurologic examination every 6 hr to monitor progress if inpatient

EXPECTED COURSE AND PROGNOSIS
• Idiopathic disease—good prognosis with early and aggressive treatment; improvement usually seen in the first 72 hr; full recovery in 6–8 weeks; may repeat CSF analysis to determine if treatment can be stopped
• Protozoal disease—poor to grave prognosis
• Larval migration prognosis guarded to poor and depends on location of the lesion; signs may resolve, but larvae often continue to migrate and death may ensue.

• Degradation of eosinophils is toxic to nervous tissue; patient may have permanent deficits from not only the primary disease but also the eosinophils.

MISCELLANEOUS
ABBREVIATIONS
• CNS = central nervous system
• CSF = cerebrospinal fluid
• MRI = magnetic resonance imaging
• WBC = white blood cell

Suggested Reading
Smith-Maxie LL, Parent JM, Rand J, et al. Cerebrospinal fluid analysis and clinical outcome of eight dogs with eosinophilic meningoencephalomyelitis. J Vet Intern Med 1989;3:167–174.

Author Joane M. Parent
Consulting Editor Joane M. Parent

MENINGOENCEPHALOMYELITIS, GRANULOMATOUS

 BASICS

DEFINITION
Progressive, idiopathic, inflammatory disease that can affect the brain, spinal cord, and meninges in dogs

PATHOPHYSIOLOGY
• Host response to an infectious agent suggested by similarities to viral encephalomyelitis
• No infectious agents have been identified.
• Three forms—focal, disseminated, and ocular
• Focal—usually affects the brain stem, cerebral cortex, cerebellum, or cervical spinal cord
• Disseminated—usually affects the caudal brain stem (vestibular system), cervical cord, and meninges
• Ocular—primarily affects the optic nerves and optic chiasm; may occur alone or in combination with the CNS form, focal or disseminated

SYSTEMS AFFECTED
• Nervous
• Ophthalmic

GENETICS
No heritability demonstrated

INCIDENCE/PREVALENCE
The literature indicates sporadic occurrence, but field evidence suggests it may be one of the most common causes of progressive CNS dysfunction in adult dogs.

GEOGRAPHIC DISTRIBUTION
N/A

SIGNALMENT

Species
• Dogs
• Inflammatory CNS lesions without recognized infectious agents can occur in any species, including cats.

Breed Predilections
• Poodles and terriers—may be predisposed
• Other small breeds—commonly affected
• Large-breed dogs—may be affected, particularly with disseminated disease

MEAN AGE AND RANGE
• Mean—5 years
• Range—6 months to 10 years
• Approximately 30% of affected dogs < 2 years old; most are 1–3 years of age

Predominant Sex
Both sexes affected with a slightly higher prevalence in females

SIGNS

Historical Findings
• Focal—acts as a slowly enlarging, space-occupying mass; signs progressing over 3–6 months
• Disseminated—acute onset; rapid progression over 1–8 weeks; 25% die within 1 week.
• Ocular—acute blindness; often remains static; progression usually occurs when other forms coexist

Physical Examination Findings
• Fever—in some patients with the disseminated form
• Neurologic abnormalities—reflect location of the lesion(s)
• Cerebral involvement—seizures, circling, head pressing, and central blindness
• Brain stem involvement—head tilt, nystagmus, and trigeminal or facial nerve involvement
• Ocular form—acute blindness; bilaterally dilated, nonresponsive pupils
• Meningeal and cervical spinal cord involvement—cervical pain with ataxia and tetraparesis common

CAUSES
Unknown

RISK FACTORS
Unknown

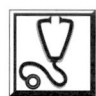 **DIAGNOSIS**

DIFFERENTIAL DIAGNOSIS
• Cannot be differentiated from other causes of meningoencephalomyelitis by clinical signs alone
• Infectious causes—viral, fungal, rickettsial, and protozoal diseases; differentiate by signalment (e.g., rarely occurs in dogs < 2 years old, whereas canine distemper, toxoplasmosis, and *Neosporum* meningoencephalomyelitis are most common in young dogs), systemic signs, and results of serologic testing and CSF analysis and culture
• CSF analysis—typically not pathognomonic for a specific cause; the following generalizations have been reported; bacterial infections: severe polymorphonuclear pleocytosis and very high protein levels; distemper: mild mononuclear pleocytosis and mildly elevated protein levels; protozoal and fungal infections: mixed mononuclear and polymorphonuclear pleocytosis and fungal organisms (especially cryptococcosis) may be noted; rickettsial infections: mild mononuclear pleocytosis with mildly high protein levels

• Aseptic meningitis—cervical pain without neurologic deficits; CSF analysis usually reveals neutrophilic pleocytosis.
• Brain tumors—differentiate from focal by CSF analysis combined with diagnostic imaging
• Cervical intervertebral disk disease—dogs have neck pain but usually have no accompanying systemic signs or brain stem involvement.
• Atlanto-axial luxation: young toy breeds. No systemic or brain stem signs

CBC/BIOCHEMISTRY/URINALYSIS
• Usually normal
• Occasional leukocytosis may be seen

OTHER LABORATORY TESTS
• None required
• Serum titers help rule out infectious disease.

IMAGING
• CT (brain)—variably dense, nonenhancing intra-axial mass most common finding
• MRI (brain)—nonenhancing intra-axial mass with attendant edema

DIAGNOSTIC PROCEDURES

CSF Analysis
• Total WBC—varies widely; mean = 800 cells/mm^3; range = 9–5400 cells/mm^3
• Mixed mononuclear pleocytosis with a high number of lymphocytes and monocytes and occasional plasma cells common
• Large, foamy mononuclear cells frequently seen
• Neutrophil population—1–20% in most patients
• Total protein—varies widely; range = 40–250 mg/dL
• Occasionally, proteins are high without pleocytosis or results are normal.

PATHOLOGIC FINDINGS
• Meninges may be thickened and cloudy.
• Brain sections—may have circumscribed areas that are soft and grayish
• Optic nerves—large with ocular form
• Lesions predominate in white matter.
• Dense perivascular aggregations of mononuclear cells (lymphocytes, monocytes, and plasma cells) arranged in a whirling pattern—characteristic

 TREATMENT

APPROPRIATE HEALTH CARE
• Inpatient—initial treatment for severe or progressive disease
• Antiepileptics—patients with seizures

• Diuretics—Lasix (1 mg/kg IV q6–8h) and/or mannitol (1 g/kg IV q6h); for patients with marked neurologic disabilities and/or evidence of edema on imaging
• Outpatient—stable patients can be discharged after the diagnosis has been made.

NURSING CARE
• Intravenous fluids—patients that are not drinking; maintenance fluid therapy indicated, unless the patient is dehydrated; avoid overhydration, which leads to cerebral edema.
• Seizures—monitor patient continuously; treat as needed.
• Patients unable to ambulate should be maintained on soft bedding, turned frequently, and checked for appropriate urinary and fecal function.

ACTIVITY
Restricted

DIET
• Adequate caloric intake is indicated.
• Special diet and caloric considerations—for patients undergoing stress, anorexia, or accelerated metabolism because of illness

CLIENT EDUCATION
• Inform client that this condition has an inexorable course, although some dogs respond to treatment for a short time (weeks to a few months).
• Discuss the importance of the initial diagnostic evaluation for differentiating the disease from more treatable disorders.

SURGICAL CONSIDERATIONS
• Histologic evaluation of affected CNS tissue—diagnostic gold standard
• Low-morbidity brain biopsy—for a confirmed focal mass to differentiate from other focal diseases

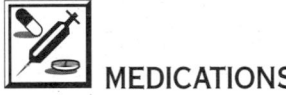

MEDICATIONS

DRUG(S) OF CHOICE
Corticosteroids
• Primary treatment
• Relatively benign clinical conditions—prednisolone (1 mg/kg PO q12h); continue treatment until the patient achieves a response zenith; then slowly decrease dose; recrudescence of signs prompts re-establishment of the lowest dose that maintains a clinically acceptable pet.

• Severe clinical conditions—high-dose (prednisone 2–4 mg/kg IV) for the first 48–72 hr; after signs improve, initiate oral corticosteroids.
• Some patients do not respond to corticosteroid treatment.
• Most patients require continued treatment to prevent recrudescence of clinical signs.
• To prevent steroid-induced gastric ulceration—cimetidine (10 mg/kg PO q8h) and/or sucralfate (0.5–1.0 g PO q8–12h)

CONTRAINDICATIONS
It is important to eliminate infectious differentials before treating with corticosteroids.

PRECAUTIONS
Rapid reduction in corticosteroid dosage may precipitate a refractory recrudescence of clinical signs.

POSSIBLE INTERACTIONS
N/A

ALTERNATIVE DRUG(S)
• Azathioprine—2 mg/kg PO daily; add to the regimen when the side effects of prednisolone (e.g., polyuria and polyphagia) are too pronounced or when prednisolone has failed.
• Cyclophosphamide—50 mg/m² PO q48h; try when prednisolone is ineffective.
• Radiotherapy—may be beneficial

FOLLOW-UP

PATIENT MONITORING
• Perform weekly neurologic reevaluation in the first 2–4 weeks of treatment
• Perform CBC and biochemical analysis regularly to monitor steroid side effects and for toxicity if azathioprine or cyclophosphamide is administered.

PREVENTION/AVOIDANCE
N/A

POSSIBLE COMPLICATIONS
Disease may progress despite appropriate treatment.

EXPECTED COURSE AND PROGNOSIS
• Corticosteroids—may slow or reverse signs; must be continued for life
• Disease progresses in most patients despite treatment.

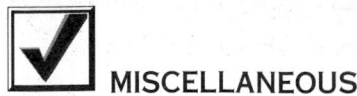

MISCELLANEOUS

ASSOCIATED CONDITIONS
N/A

AGE-RELATED FACTORS
N/A

ZOONOTIC POTENTIAL
N/A

PREGNANCY
Corticosteroid administration and the short life expectancy of affected dogs make successful gestation unlikely.

SYNONYMS
Inflammatory reticulosis

SEE ALSO
• Encephalitis
• Meningitis/Meningoencephalitis/Meningomyelitis, Bacterial
• Meningoencephalomyelitis, Eosinophilic

ABBREVIATIONS
• CNS = central nervous system
• CSF = cerebrospinal fluid
• CT = computed tomography
• MRI = magnetic resonance imaging

Suggested Reading
Bailey CS, Higgins RJ. Characteristics of cerebrospinal fluid associated with canine granulomatous meningoencephalomyelitis: a retrospective study. J Am Vet Med Assoc 1986;188:418–421.
Oliver JE, Lorenz MO, Kornegay JN. Handbook of veterinary neurology. 3rd ed. Philadelphia: Saunders, 1997.
Sorjonen DC. Clinical and histopathological features of granulomatous meningoencephalomyelitis in dogs. J Am Anim Hosp Assoc 1990;26:141–147.
Summers BA, Cummings JF, de Lahunta A. Veterinary neuropathology. St. Louis: Mosby, 1995:110–111.
Thomas JB, Eger C. Granulomatous meningoencephalomyelitis in 21 dogs. J Small Anim Pract 1989;30:287–293.
Author D. C. Sorjonen
Consulting Editor Joane M. Parent

MESOTHELIOMA

 BASICS

OVERVIEW
• Rare tumor of the epithelial lining of body cavities
• Dogs—thoracic cavity, pericardial sac, abdominal cavity, and vaginal tunic of the scrotum
• Cats—thoracic cavity, pericardial sac, and abdominal cavity
• Highly effusive

SIGNALMENT
• Dogs and cats
• Sclerosing mesothelioma—primarily in male dogs
• German shepherds—most commonly affected breed

SIGNS
• Displacement of viscera
• Dyspnea
• Exercise intolerance
• Muffled heart and ventral lung sounds
• Vomiting
• Large scrotum
• Abdominal distension with ascites
• Low chest compliance owing to mediastinal mass and pleural effusion

CAUSES & RISK FACTORS
Exposure to asbestos

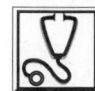 DIAGNOSIS

DIFFERENTIAL DIAGNOSIS
• Other causes of effusion—congestive heart failure; liver disease; hypoalbuminemia; pyothorax; lymphosarcoma; idiopathic pericardial effusion
• Other mediastinal masses—lymphosarcoma; thymoma; thyroid carcinoma; chemodectoma

CBC/BIOCHEMISTRY/URINALYSIS
No specific abnormalities

OTHER LABORATORY TESTS
N/A

IMAGING
• Radiography—shows body cavity effusion and/or masses
• Ultrasound—detects pericardial sac thickening and effusion

DIAGNOSTIC PROCEDURES
• Cytologic examination of fluid—interpret results cautiously because it can be difficult to distinguish mesothelioma from physiologic mesothelial proliferation.
• Exploratory surgery or laparoscopy—reveals nodules, plaques, or thickenings of the mesothelial lining of the body cavity
• Histologic evaluation—reveals morphologic characteristics of epithelial neoplasms and mesenchymal proliferation

 TREATMENT

• Outpatient
• Activity—restrict with dyspnea
• Partial pericardectomy—relieve pericardial effusion
• Centesis or pleurodesis—palliative therapy for pleural effusion

MEDICATIONS

DRUG(S)
• Cisplatin—has been successful; may be given intracavitary but penetrates the tumor only a few cells deep and is effective only when the mass is not large; administer according to established protocols that include adequate diuresis.
• Mitoxantrone and doxorubicin have also been used.

CONTRAINDICATIONS/POSSIBLE INTERACTIONS
Cisplatin—do not use in cats; do not use in dogs with renal disease.

 FOLLOW-UP
• Thoracic radiography—every treatment and every 3 months after treatment
• Laboratory tests—assess renal status after cisplatin administration.
• Avoid exposure to asbestos.
• Survival after intracavitary cisplatin—3 dogs: 410 days, > 129 days, and 306 days

 MISCELLANEOUS

Suggested Reading
Moore AS, Kirk C, Cardona A. Intracavitary cisplatin chemotherapy experience with six dogs. J Vet Intern Med 1991;5:227–231.
Morrison WB. Nonpulmonary intrathoracic cancer. In: Morrison WB, ed. Cancer in dogs and cats: medical and surgical management. Jackson, Wyoming: Teton NewMedia, 2002:513–526.
Author Terrance A. Hamilton
Consulting Editor Wallace B. Morrison

METALDEHYDE POISONING

BASICS

DEFINITION
• Metaldehyde—polycyclic polymer of acetaldehyde; primarily affects the nervous system; an ingredient of slug and snail baits; used as solid fuel for some camp stoves
• Baits—liquid or dry; usually pellets mixed with feed material (e.g., soybeans, rice, oats, sorghum, and apples); may contain other toxicants (e.g., arsenate and insecticides)

PATHOPHYSIOLOGY
• Exact mechanism unknown
• May increase excitatory neurotransmitters or decrease inhibitory neurotransmitters

SYSTEMS AFFECTED
• Nervous
• Respiratory—death usually as a result of respiratory failure
• Hepatobiliary—even if patient survives the initial convulsive period, it may develop liver disease 2–3 days later.

GENETICS
N/A

INCIDENCE/PREVALENCE
Depends on geographic location

GEOGRAPHIC DISTRIBUTION
More commonly found in coastal and low-lying areas, which have a higher prevalence of snails and slugs than other areas

SIGNALMENT
Species
Dogs and cats

Breed Predilections
N/A

Mean Age and Range
Any

Predominant Sex
N/A

SIGNS

General Comments
May occur immediately after ingestion or may be delayed for up to 3 hr

Historical Findings
• Bizarre behavior
• Ataxia
• Muscle tremors
• Convulsions

.Physical Examination Findings
• Convulsions—continuous or intermittent; not necessarily evoked by external stimuli
• Between convulsions—may note muscle tremors and anxiety; may be hyperesthetic
• Hyperthermia—temperature up to 42.2°C (108°F) common; probably caused by excessive muscle activity
• Tachycardia
• Nystagmus
• Mydriasis
• Hyperpnea
• Hypersalivation
• Ataxia
• Vomiting
• Cyanosis
• Diarrhea
• Dehydration
• Depression or narcosis—may occur late in the course
• Death—usually owing to respiratory failure, which occurs 4–24 hr after exposure; owing to liver disease, delayed after exposure if patient survives initial convulsive period

CAUSES
Ingestion of metaldehyde

RISK FACTORS
Living in area with high prevalence of snails and slugs

DIAGNOSIS

DIFFERENTIAL DIAGNOSIS
• Strychnine toxicosis—causes intermittent seizures that can be evoked by external stimuli
• Penitrem A—mycotoxin usually found in moldy English walnuts or cream cheese; has been reported in other foodstuffs; causes a tremorgenic syndrome
• Roquefortine—mycotoxin found in moldy bleu cheese and other foodstuffs; causes a tremorgenic syndrome
• Lead toxicosis—may cause seizures, behavior changes, blindness, and gastrointestinal upset
• Zinc phosphide
• Bromethalin
• Organochlorine insecticides—cause seizures in most mammals
• Anticholinesterase insecticides—organophosphates and carbamates; may cause seizures; often accompanied by excessive salivation, lacrimation, urination, and defecation
• Seizures—may be the result of a host of nontoxic conditions (e.g., neoplasia, trauma, infection, metabolic disorder, and congenital disorder)

CBC/BIOCHEMISTRY/URINALYSIS
• Not diagnostic
• Severe metabolic acidosis can occur

OTHER LABORATORY TESTS
Metaldehyde testing—vomitus, stomach contents, serum, urine, or liver

IMAGING
N/A

DIAGNOSTIC PROCEDURES
N/A

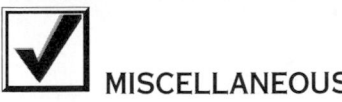

PATHOLOGIC FINDINGS
- Hepatic, renal, and pulmonary congestion
- Petechial and ecchymotic hemorrhages
- Subendocardial and subepicardial hemorrhages
- Stomach contents may have odor of formaldehyde

TREATMENT

APPROPRIATE HEALTH CARE
Emergency inpatient intensive care management until convulsions cease

NURSING CARE
Fluids—often necessary for dehydration or acidosis

ACTIVITY
Restricted

DIET
Do not feed patients that are vomiting, convulsing, or heavily sedated.

CLIENT EDUCATION
N/A

SURGICAL CONSIDERATIONS
N/A

MEDICATIONS

DRUG(S) OF CHOICE
- No antidote available
- Prevent further absorption—emetics or gastric lavage followed by administration of activated charcoal
- Convulsions—tranquilize with diazepam, barbiturates, or methocarbamol

CONTRAINDICATIONS
Never induce vomiting in a convulsing patient.

PRECAUTIONS
- Do not use depressants in an already depressed patient
- Barbiturates—may lead to cardiac arrest

POSSIBLE INTERACTIONS
N/A

ALTERNATIVE DRUG(S)
N/A

FOLLOW-UP

PATIENT MONITORING
Periodically allow tranquilizers to wear off to re-evaluate convulsive condition.

PREVENTION/AVOIDANCE
Do not apply metaldehyde in areas accessible to pets.

POSSIBLE COMPLICATIONS
Liver disease—if patient survives the initial convulsive phase

EXPECTED COURSE AND PROGNOSIS
- Reported sequelae—diarrhea; memory loss; temporary blindness
- Liver disease—may be a secondary problem
- Prognosis—principally depends on the amount ingested
- Without successful treatment—death 4–12 hr after exposure

MISCELLANEOUS

ASSOCIATED CONDITIONS
Concurrent toxicoses from additional ingredients (arsenate and insecticides) in the molluscicide

AGE-RELATED FACTORS
N/A

ZOONOTIC POTENTIAL
N/A

PREGNANCY
Not known to be mutagenic, genotoxic, or immunotoxic

SYNONYMS
- Polyacetaldehyde
- Limovet
- Limax
- Antimilace
- Snail bait

SEE ALSO
Poisoning (Intoxication)

Suggested Reading

Andreasen JR. Metaldehyde toxicosis in ducklings. J Vet Diagn Invest 1993; 5:500–501.
Booze TF, Oehme FW. Metaldehyde toxicity: a review. Vet Hum Toxicol 1985;27:11–19.
Von Burg R, Stout T. Metaldehyde. J Appl Toxicol 1991;11:377–378.

Author Konstanze H. Plumlee
Consulting Editor Gary D. Osweiler

METHEMOGLOBINEMIA

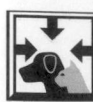 **BASICS**

DEFINITION
• Methemoglobin content in blood > 1.5% of total hemoglobin
• Methemoglobin differs from hemoglobin in that the iron moiety of heme groups has been oxidized from the ferrous (+2) to the ferric (+3) state

PATHOPHYSIOLOGY
• About 3% of hemoglobin is oxidized to methemoglobin each day in normal animals as a result of autoxidation of hemoglobin or secondary to oxidants produced in normal metabolic reactions.
• Methemoglobin usually accounts for < 1% of total hemoglobin, because it is constantly reduced back to hemoglobin by an NADH-dependent methemoglobin reductase (cytochrome b_5 reductase) enzyme reaction within RBCs.
• Caused by either increased production of methemoglobin by oxidants or decreased reduction of methemoglobin associated with a deficiency of the RBC methemoglobin reductase enzyme

SYSTEMS AFFECTED
• Hemic/Lymph/Immune—reduced oxygen-carrying capacity of blood, because methemoglobin cannot bind oxygen; if methemoglobin content reaches high values (e.g., > 50% of total hemoglobin), various organs may suffer hypoxic injury.
• Hepatobiliary—in addition to hypoxic injury, the liver may be damaged directly by oxidant drugs that it metabolizes.
• Renal/Urologic—in addition to hypoxic injury, the kidneys may be damaged if intravascular hemolysis occurs.

SIGNALMENT
• Dogs and cats
• Deficiency in RBC methemoglobin reductase has been recognized in Chihuahuas, borzois, English setters, terrier mixes, cockapoos, coonhounds, poodles, corgis, Pomeranians, and toy Eskimo dogs and in domestic short-haired cats.

SIGNS
Caused Directly
• Possibly none in animals with mild to moderate methemoglobinemia
• Cyanotic-appearing mucous membranes—may be difficult to recognize in heavily pigmented animals
• Lethargy, tachycardia, tachypnea, ataxia, and stupor caused by hypoxia when methemoglobin content exceeds 50%
• Coma-like state and death when methemoglobin content reaches 80%

Caused by Associated Diseases
• Vomiting, anorexia, and diarrhea possible in patients with drug toxicity
• Hemoglobinuria secondary to severe intravascular hemolysis in some patients with concomitant Heinz body hemolytic anemia
• Subcutaneous edema, especially involving the face, and salivation in cats with acetaminophen toxicity

CAUSES
• Toxicity—acetaminophen, benzocaine, and phenazopyridine in cats and dogs; these drugs can also cause Heinz body hemolytic anemia.
• Deficiency in RBC methemoglobin reductase

RISK FACTORS
• Application of benzocaine to traumatized skin or mucous membranes increases the likelihood of systemic absorption and methemoglobinemia.
• Cats are much more likely to develop clinically significant methemoglobinemia than are dogs after acetaminophen administration; this drug is not recommended for use in cats.
• Methemoglobinemia secondary to methemoglobin reductase deficiency is an inherited disorder.

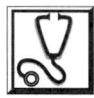 **DIAGNOSIS**

DIFFERENTIAL DIAGNOSIS
• Both low blood oxygen tension and methemoglobinemia can cause cyanotic-appearing mucous membranes and dark-colored blood samples.
• Hypoxemia is documented by measuring low PO_2 in an arterial blood sample.
• Methemoglobinemia is suspected when arterial blood with normal or high PO_2 is dark colored.

LABORATORY FINDINGS
Drugs That Alter Laboratory Results
None

Disorders That May Alter Laboratory Results
Hemolysis in the sample may raise the methemoglobin value, especially if the methemoglobin assay is not conducted soon after sample collection.

Valid if Run in Human Laboratory?
• Valid, as long as the method to lyse RBCs does not cause methemoglobin formation in the animal being tested
• Saponin should not be used to lyse RBCs, because it raises the methemoglobin value in some species.

CBC/BIOCHEMISTRY/URINALYSIS
• Chronic methemoglobinemia secondary to methemoglobin reductase deficiency can result in a slightly high PCV; in contrast, anemia may accompany methemoglobinemia caused by oxidant drugs.
• If severe or induced by oxidant drugs, evidence of injury to various organs (e.g., high BUN and ALT) may be seen.

OTHER LABORATORY TESTS
• Spot test—determine if the patient's methemoglobin content is clinically important: one drop of blood from the patient is placed on a piece of absorbent white paper and a drop of normal control blood is placed next to it. If the methemoglobin content is ≥ 10%, the patient's blood will be noticeably browner than the bright red of the control blood.
• Accurate determination of methemoglobin content requires that blood be rapidly submitted to a laboratory.
• Methemoglobin content in dogs with methemoglobin reductase deficiency varies from 13 to 41%; the methemoglobin content in five deficient cats was 44–52%.
• A definitive diagnosis of methemoglobin reductase deficiency is made by measuring

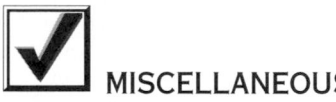

enzyme activity in RBCs; this assay is done in a few research laboratories and requires that arrangements be made before blood samples are submitted.

IMAGING
N/A

DIAGNOSTIC PROCEDURES
• Blood should be stained for Heinz bodies if evidence of toxicity is present.
• The presence of Heinz bodies indicates exposure to an oxidant drug that may also cause hemolytic anemia.

TREATMENT

• Mild to moderate—does not require specific treatment to reduce the methemoglobin content
• Drug-induced—the use of the drug should be discontinued; RBCs can convert much of the methemoglobin back to hemoglobin within 24 hr after elimination of drug exposure.
• Inherited methemoglobin reductase deficiency—animals have normal life expectancy and generally do not require treatment, although veterinarians may wish to give a single IV injection of methylene blue (see below) 1 hr before a deficient animal is anesthetized for surgery to maximize the amount of hemoglobin that is capable of binding oxygen.
• Whole blood transfusions should be given to patients with severe anemia and those with rapidly decreasing PCV and clinical signs suggesting a deteriorating condition.
• Severe intravascular hemolysis—IV fluid administration recommended
• Treatment of electrolyte or acid–base imbalances may also be indicated in patients with severe vomiting or diarrhea, concomitant renal injury, or impending shock.
• Administration of oxygen is of limited value because methemoglobin cannot bind oxygen, and an increase in dissolved oxygen results in only a small increase in blood oxygen content.

MEDICATIONS

DRUG(S) OF CHOICE
• Methylene blue—given slowly over several minutes as a 1% solution (1 mg/kg IV), may be administered in patients with severe methemoglobinemia; a dramatic response should occur during the first 30 min of treatment; CAUTION: Although this dose can be repeated if necessary, methylene blue can cause Heinz body hemolytic anemia in cats and dogs.
• N-acetylcysteine is efficacious in the treatment of acetaminophen toxicity in cats if given within a few hours after exposure; recommended dosage is 140 mg/kg PO followed by 70 mg/kg q6h for 7 treatments.

CONTRAINDICATIONS
None

PRECAUTIONS
In patients that have been given drugs that cause substantial Heinz body formation and methemoglobinemia, methylene blue treatment can potentiate the formation of Heinz bodies and anemia; consequently, it is prudent to measure the PCV for 3 days after methylene blue treatment to ensure that clinically important anemia does not develop.

POSSIBLE INTERACTIONS
None

ALTERNATIVE DRUG(S)
None

FOLLOW-UP

PATIENT MONITORING
• The cyanotic appearance of skin and mucous membranes should disappear after reduction of methemoglobin to an amount that does not produce clinical signs.
• Blood on the spot test should appear bright red after reduction of methemoglobin to values < 10% of total hemoglobin.

• If methylene blue treatment is given or Heinz bodies are present within RBCs, the PCV should be monitored closely, because it usually does not reach its lowest point until approximately 3 days after initial oxidant exposure.

POSSIBLE COMPLICATIONS
Coma and death can occur if methemoglobin content reaches 80% of total hemoglobin.

MISCELLANEOUS

ASSOCIATED CONDITIONS
Heinz body anemia

AGE-RELATED FACTORS
None

ZOONOTIC POTENTIAL
None

PREGNANCY
N/A

SYNONYMS
None

SEE ALSO
• Acetaminophen Toxicity
• Anemia, Heinz Body

ABBREVIATIONS
• ALT = alanine aminotransferase
• PCV = packed cell volume

Suggested Reading

Cullison RF. Acetaminophen toxicosis in small animals: clinical signs, mode of action, and treatment. Comp Cont Ed Pract Vet 1984;6:315–321.
Harvey JW. Hereditary methemoglobinemia. In: Feldman BF, Zinkl JG, Jain NC, eds. Schalm's veterinary hematology. 5th ed. Philadelphia: Lippincott Williams & Wilkins, 2000;1008–1011.
Harvey JW. Methemoglobinemia and Heinz body hemolytic anemia. In: Kirk RW, Bonagura J, eds. Current veterinary therapy XII, Philadelphia: Saunders, 1995:443–446.

Author John W. Harvey
Consulting Editor Stephen A. Kruth

METRITIS

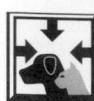 **BASICS**

OVERVIEW
• Bacterial uterine infection that develops in the immediate postpartum period (usually within the first week); occasionally develops after an abortion or non-sterile artificial insemination—rarely after breeding
• Bacteria—ascend through the open cervix to the uterus; a large, flaccid, postpartum uterus provides an ideal environment for growth; gram-negative bacteria (e.g., *Escherichia coli*) commonly isolated
• Potentially life-threatening infection; may lead to septic shock
• Directly affects uterus; systemic involvement as sepsis develops
• Can become chronic and lead to infertility

SIGNALMENT
• Postpartum bitch and queen
• No age or breed predilection

SIGNS

Historical Findings
• Malodorous, purulent, sanguinopurulent, or dark green vulvar discharge
• Depression
• Anorexia
• Neglect of puppies and kittens
• Reduced milk production

Physical Examination Findings
• Fever
• Large uterus on abdominal palpation
• Dehydration
• Injected mucous membranes
• Tachycardia—with sepsis

CAUSES & RISK FACTORS
• Dystocia
• Obstetric manipulation
• Retained fetuses or placentas
• Prolonged delivery (large litter)
• Postabortion, and postnatural or artificial insemination (rare)

 DIAGNOSIS

DIFFERENTIAL DIAGNOSIS
• Subinvolution of placental sites—no sign of infection on cytologic examination of vagina
• Eclampsia—differentiated by serum calcium concentration
• Mastitis—differentiated by physical examination findings

CBC/BIOCHEMISTRY/URINALYSIS
• Neutrophilia with left shift
• Leukopenia—occasionally with endotoxic shock
• High PCV, total protein, creatinine, BUN, and urine specific gravity—secondary to dehydration
• High liver enzyme—with endotoxemia
• Low urine specific gravity—may see with endotoxemia

OTHER LABORATORY TESTS
N/A

IMAGING
• Radiography—reveals a large uterus and possibly retained fetuses.
• Ultrasonography—reveals intrauterine fluid accumulation, retained placentas, and retained fetuses; shows abdominal effusion secondary to uterine rupture

DIAGNOSTIC PROCEDURES
• Vaginal cytologic examination—detect degenerative neutrophils with intracellular and extracellular bacteria
• Guarded anterior vaginal or transcervical culture—aerobes and anaerobes; identify organism and its antibiotic sensitivity pattern

 TREATMENT

• Inpatient until systemic signs resolve
• Dehydration—intravenous balanced electrolyte solution
• Treat shock
• Electrolyte imbalances and hypoglycemia—correct; identified by serum chemistry profile
• Ovariohysterectomy—treatment of choice for retained fetus or placenta, uterine rupture,

or severe infection and if future breeding is not desired
• Chronically affected patient that does not respond to medical treatment—may perform hysterotomy and lavage as long as the uterus has no friable areas
• Friable uterus—pack off and handle gently at surgery.

MEDICATIONS

DRUG(S)
• Antibiotics—start with broad-spectrum agents (oral if patient is stable; intravenous if patient is in shock); choice confirmed by bacterial culture and sensitivity; continued at least 14 days
• Nursing planned—amoxicillin-clavulanic acid (dogs, 12.5–25 mg/kg PO q12h; cats, 62.5 mg/cat PO q12h); can administer q8h with gram-negative infections; or oxacillin to start
• Nursing not planned—enrofloxacin (2.5–10 mg/kg PO q12h) to start
• Oxytocin—0.5–1.0 U/kg IM; then repeat in 1–2 hr; may note inadequate response if > 48 hr since parturition

• $PGF_{2\alpha}$—100–250 μg/kg SC q12h for 5–8 days; to evacuate uterus; safety and efficacy not established

CONTRAINDICATIONS/POSSIBLE INTERACTIONS
• Prostaglandin—may induce uterine rupture if the tissue is devitalized
• Oxytocin—may not be effective beyond 48 hr postpartum
• Uterine flushing—may cause rupture of devitalized wall

FOLLOW-UP

PATIENT MONITORING
• CBC, temperature, vaginal cytologic examination, and clinical signs
• Ultrasonography—monitor evacuation of uterine fluid

POSSIBLE COMPLICATIONS
• Ovariohysterectomy—necessary when medical treatment is ineffective
• Uterine rupture and peritonitis—may occur with medical treatment

• Owners may need to handraise puppies and kittens

EXPECTED COURSE AND PROGNOSIS
• Ovariohysterectomy—prognosis for recovery good; recommended for old patients
• Medical treatment—prognosis for recovery fair; may adversely affect future reproduction

MISCELLANEOUS

ABBREVIATION
PCV = packed cell volume

Suggested Reading
Johnston SD, Root Kustritz MV, Olson PNS. Periparturient disorders in the bitch. In: Johnston SD, Root Kustritz MV, Olson PNS, eds. Canine and feline theriogenology. Philadelphia: Saunders, 2001:129–145.
Magne ML. Acute metritis in the bitch. In: Morrow DA, ed. Current therapy in theriogenology 2. Philadelphia: Saunders, 1986:505–506.
Author Joni L. Freshman
Consulting Editor Sara K. Lyle

MONOCYTOSIS

 BASICS

DEFINITION
Absolute number of circulating monocytes greater than the reference range: dogs, $> 1.3 \times 10^9$/L or $> 1300/\mu$L or mm³; cats, $> 0.9 \times 10^9$/L or $900/\mu$L or mm³

PATHOPHYSIOLOGY
• Monocytes are derived from hematopoietic stem cells named CFU-GM, which (with the appropriate stimulus) differentiate into monoblasts (or myeloblasts) and then into monocytes.
• The production, differentiation, and release of monocytes are regulated by a variety of substances derived from macrophages, T lymphocytes, endothelial cells, and fibroblasts.
• Monocytopoiesis is stimulated by substances such as IL-3, IL-11, GM-CSF, monocyto-poietin, an MS-CSF, and a macrophage-derived factor that increases the mitotic activity of monocyte precursors in the bone marrow.
• Monocyte production is inhibited by PGE_1, PGE_2, and corticosteroids.
• Production to release of monocytes normally takes 36–60 hr, although with disease, production time can be shortened to a minimum emergence time of about 6 hr.
• The bone marrow lacks a reserve of monocytes because newly formed monocytes are released immediately to the circulation.
• Monocytes have a circulating half-life of about 20 hr before exiting the circulation to reside in various tissues; this process triggers another stage of differentiation, involving changes in ultrastructure, cell receptors, and metabolism; these transformed cells are referred to as macrophages, or histiocytes, and are part of the mononuclear phagocyte system.
• Fixed macrophages can be found in most tissues, including lymph nodes, bone marrow, spleen, liver (Kupffer cells), bone (osteo-clasts), lamina propria of the intestinal tract, and the CNS (microglial cells).
• Free macrophages—found primarily in the pleural, peritoneal, and synovial cavities; lungs (alveolar macrophages); and inflammatory sites; can migrate through the lymphatic system into another tissue
• Several macrophages may fuse to form multinucleated giant cells, a common response to fungi, mycobacteria, syncytial virus, and foreign material.

• There are far more tissue macrophages than circulating monocytes, perhaps owing to their long life span of several months to more than a year.
• Most macrophages in a region originate from circulating monocytes; but under specific microenvironmental stimuli, they can be derived from local production; accumulation of monocytes in an area of acute or chronic inflammation is caused by chemotactic factors that attract monocytes to these specific foci.

FUNCTIONS OF THE MONONUCLEAR PHAGOCYTE SYSTEM
• Phagocytic removal of damaged or aged cells or debris, tumor cytolysis, and micro-bicidal activity
• Regulation of the immune system via antigen processing and presentation and by secretion of interleukins responsible for promoting granulopoiesis, lymphocyte proliferation, and lymphokine production
• Vital in controlling certain pathogens, including intracellular bacteria (e.g., *Mycobacterium, Listeria,* and *Brucella*), mycotic agents, protozoa, and viruses
• Involved in regulation of coagulation, fibrinolysis, healing, and bone repair
• Exerts cytotoxicity against tumor or foreign cells

SYSTEMS AFFECTED
• Respiratory—alveolar macrophages
• Hemic/Lymph/Immune—lymph nodes (histiocytic proliferation), spleen (mono-nuclear phagocyte system proliferation), and bone marrow
• Hepatobiliary—Kupffer cells
• Musculoskeletal—osteoclasts
• Nervous system—microglial cells
• Thoracic and abdominal cavities—macrophage proliferation

SIGNALMENT
Dogs and cats

SIGNS
Related to primary cause

CAUSES
General
Any process that stimulates neutrophilia, because monocytes and neutrophils share the same stem-cell precursor CFU-GM

Glucocorticoids
• Corticosteroids stimulate absolute mono-cytosis in dogs and less frequently in cats.
• Monocytosis develops within hours of steroid exposure and resolves within 24 hr after removing the corticosteroid stimulus.

• Glucocorticoid treatment, stress of disease, and hyperadrenocorticism

Inflammation
• Infectious—mycotic (e.g., *Aspergillus* and *Blastomycosis*), protozoal (e.g., *Toxoplasma*), viral (e.g., FIP and FIV), bacterial (e.g., *Mycobacterium* and *Brucella*); unlike most infectious diseases in which monocytosis is accompanied by neutrophilia, in some animals with bacterial endocarditis monocytosis is the only leukogram abnormality.
• Noninfectious—foreign material, necrotic tissue, malignant tumor, hemolytic anemia, trauma, immune-mediated disease, and hemorrhage

Bone Marrow Disease
• Marrow recovery from leukopenia—because of the rapid induction of monocytes and their uniquely short marrow transit time, mono-cytosis is often the earliest sign of marrow recovery and can exceed $20,000/\mu$L.
• Monocytic or myelomonocytic leukemia—neoplastic proliferation of the monocyte cell line or a combined myeloid and monocyte cell line produces monocytosis; immature, bizarre cells are present in the circulation.
• Canine cyclic hematopoiesis (silver-gray collies)—cyclic neutropenia occurs at 10–14-day intervals, lasts 2–4 days, and is soon followed by a monocytosis; a "rebound" neutrophilia appears 2–4 days later.
• Canine granulocytopathy syndrome (Irish setters)—a defect in neutrophil intracellular bactericidal activity resulting in recurrent bacterial infection, marked neutrophilia, and variable monocytosis
• Leukocyte surface glycoprotein deficiency—abnormality reported in one Irish setter cross-bred dog with a history of recurrent bacterial infection associated with marked neutrophilia and variable monocytosis; this deficiency in adhesion molecules resulted in impaired granulocyte aggregation and adhesion.

RISK FACTORS
N/A

 DIAGNOSIS

DIFFERENTIAL DIAGNOSIS
• Severely stressed or ill dogs—consider endogenous glucocorticoids.
• Concurrent alopecia, potbelly, thin skin, and muscle atrophy—consider hyper-adrenocorticism.

- Fever of undetermined origin—consider endocarditis and immune-mediated disease.
- Draining cutaneous wound—consider mycotic infection and foreign body.
- Splenomegaly, hepatomegaly, or lymphadenopathy—consider leukemia, mycotic infection, and malignant histiocytosis.

LABORATORY FINDINGS

Drugs That May Alter Laboratory Results
None

Disorders That May Alter Laboratory Results
None

Valid if Run in Human Laboratory?
- Yes, but certain automated techniques for counting monocytes can yield errors
- Mechanical blood-spreading devices shift larger cells, such as monocytes, into the "counting area," with absolute, artifactual monocytosis reported.
- Incorrect identification of metamyelocytes, other immature neutrophils, or toxic neutrophils can result in erroneous monocytosis.

CBC/BIOCHEMISTRY/URINALYSIS
- Severe monocytosis (e.g., > 20,000/μL)—consider leukemia or rebound phase of cyclic hematopoiesis
- Immature, bizarre, and abnormal cells in circulation—consider monocytic leukemia and myelomonocytic leukemia
- Mature neutrophilia, lymphopenia, and eosinopenia—consider stress and hyperadrenocorticism
- Neutrophilia—consider chronic inflammation or inherited neutrophil dysfunction
- Anemia—consider immune-mediated hemolytic anemia

OTHER LABORATORY TESTS
- Serology—serum antibody titer to FIV, *Brucella,* and *Toxoplasma*; antibody titers to feline coronavirus can be difficult to interpret, but PCR on effusion or a biopsied lesion can provide a diagnosis of FIP
- Adrenal function testing—ACTH stimulation and low-dose dexamethasone suppression tests to diagnose hyperadrenocorticism; urine cortisol: creatinine ratio is a quick screen to rule out hyperadrenocorticism
- ANA to rule out systemic lupus erythematosus
- Coombs test for immune-mediated hemolytic anemia

- Acid fast stain to rule out *Mycobacterium* spp.
- Fungal culture of lesion to rule out mycotic infection

IMAGING
Echocardiogram for bacterial endocarditis

DIAGNOSTIC PROCEDURES
- Blood cultures for bacterial endocarditis
- Fine-needle aspiration or biopsy of solid mass to rule out malignant histiocytosis
- Fine-needle aspiration or biopsy of lesion to rule out mycotic infection

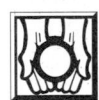 TREATMENT
Treatment directed at the underlying cause of monocytosis

 MEDICATIONS

DRUG(S) OF CHOICE
N/A

CONTRAINDICATIONS
N/A

PRECAUTIONS
N/A

POSSIBLE INTERACTIONS
N/A

ALTERNATIVE DRUG(S)
N/A

 FOLLOW-UP

PATIENT MONITORING
N/A

POSSIBLE COMPLICATIONS
N/A

 MISCELLANEOUS

ASSOCIATED CONDITIONS
- Other diseases that affect the mononuclear phagocyte system but do not cause consistent monocytosis

- Malignant and systemic histiocytosis—although Bernese mountain dogs have a predilection for this solid histiocytic neoplasm, it has been reported in other breeds as well as in a few cats; occasionally, abnormal macrophages can be found in the circulation.
- Lysosomal storage diseases

AGE-RELATED FACTORS
None

ZOONOTIC POTENTIAL
None

PREGNANCY
N/A

SYNONYMS
N/A

SEE ALSO
None

ABBREVIATIONS
- ACTH = adrenocorticotropic hormone
- CFU-GM = colony-forming unit–granulocyte, monocyte
- FIP = feline infectious peritonitis
- FIV = feline immunodeficiency virus
- GM-CSF = granulocyte-monocyte colony-stimulating factor
- IL-3, IL-11 = interleukin 3, interleukin 11
- MS-CSF = monocyte-specific colony-stimulating factor
- PCR = polymerase chain reaction
- PGE_1, PGE_2 = prostaglandin E_1, prostaglandin E_2

Suggested Reading
Bienzle D. Monocytes and macrophages. In: Feldman BF, Zinkl JG, Jain NC, eds. Schalm's veterinary hematology. 5th ed. Philadelphia: Lippincott William & Wilkins, 2000:318–325.

Giger U, Boxer LA, Simpson PJ, et al. Deficiency of leukocyte surface glycoproteins Mo1, LFA-1 and Leu M5 in a dog with recurrent bacterial infections. Blood 1987; 69:1622–1630.

Renshaw HW, Davis WC. Canine granulocytopathy syndrome. Am J Pathol 1979; 95:731–744.

Acknowledgment
The author and editors acknowledge the prior contributions of Dr. Donald Meuten, who authored this topic in a previous edition.
Author Joyce S. Knoll
Consulting Editor Stephen A. Kruth

MUCOPOLYSACCHARIDOSIS

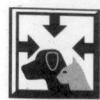 BASICS

OVERVIEW
- A group of heritable lysosomal storage disorders caused by deficiency of lysosomal enzymes needed for the stepwise degradation of GAGs (mucopolysaccharides)
- Undegraded GAGs are stored in lysosomes, resulting in progressive tissue and organ dysfunction.
- Features depend on the specific lysosomal enzyme deficiency, type of GAG stored, and the tissues in which storage occurs.

Types of MPSs Reported in Dogs and Cats
- MPS I—α-L-iduronidase deficiency; dermatan and heparan sulfate stored
- MPS II—iduronate sulfatase deficiency; dermatan and heparan sulfate stored
- MPS IIIA—heparan N-sulfatase deficiency; heparan sulfate stored
- MPS VI—arylsulfatase B deficiency; dermatan sulfate stored
- MPS VII—β-glucuronidase deficiency; dermatan, heparan, and chondroitin sulfate stored

SIGNALMENT
- Cats—MPS I and VII, domestic shorthair; MPS VI, Siamese and domestic shorthair
- Dogs—MPS I, Plott hounds; MPS II, Labrador retrievers; MPS IIIA, wire-haired dachshunds and Huntaway (Sheep) dogs; MPS VI, miniature pinschers, miniature schnauzers, and Welsh corgis; MPS VII, mixed breeds and German shepherds

- Both sexes equally affected by MPS I, III, VI, and VII; primarily males affected by MPS II

SIGNS
- Dwarfism (except cats with MPS I)
- Severe bone disease (dysostosis multiplex)
- Degenerative joint disease, including hip subluxation
- Facial dysmorphia—more evident in Siamese cats, which normally have an elongated face, than in other cats
- Hepatomegaly (except cats with MPS VI)
- Corneal clouding—a result of fine granular opacities in the corneal stroma, first apparent at approximately 8 weeks of age
- Large tongue (dogs)
- Thickening of the heart valves
- Excess urinary excretion of GAG
- Metachromatic granules (Alder-Reilly bodies) in blood leukocytes
- Disease progresses; clinical signs apparent at 2–4 months of age
- Affected animals may live several years, but locomotor difficulty is progressive.
- Skeletal abnormalities more severe in cats with MPS VI than in those with MPS I; some MPS VI cats develop posterior paresis owing to spinal cord compression.
- Manipulation of the head or neck usually painful
- CNS disease not clinically apparent in dogs or cats with any type of MPS, although there is microscopic evidence of neuronal storage.

CAUSES & RISK FACTORS
- MPS transmission is autosomal recessive, except MPS II, which is X-linked recessive.
- In-breeding increases risk if the defective gene is present in the family.

 DIAGNOSIS

DIFFERENTIAL DIAGNOSIS
- Metachromatic granules within neutrophils and lymphocytes—suggest MPS; also observed with GM_2 gangliosidosis, a lysosomal storage disease that, unlike MPS, is characterized by progressive neurologic disease and early death; granules may also be observed in neutrophils of some Burmese cats that have normal lymphocytes and have no clinical abnormalities; very rarely, toxic granulation of neutrophils can have a similar appearance.
- Corneal clouding—also observed with numerous other lysosomal storage diseases, including acid lipase deficiency, GM_1 and GM_2 gangliosidosis, and mannosidosis; lysosomal enzyme panels can be performed to definitively diagnose the type of storage disorder; corneal edema and corneal dystrophy may have a similar appearance.
- Whereas the radiographic appearance of MPS is characteristic, other disorders with similarities include congenital hypothyroidism, epiphyseal dysplasia, and hypervitaminosis A.

CBC/BIOCHEMISTRY/URINALYSIS
- Examination of Wright's-stained blood films reveals neutrophils and monocytes containing numerous distinctive metachromatic granules.
- Granules quite indistinct in animals with MPS I
- Granules usually not apparent when stained with Diff-Quik

• Occasional lymphocytes have vacuoles that contain metachromatic granules, particularly in animals with MPS VII.

OTHER LABORATORY TESTS
• Wright's-stained cytologic preparations of lymph node, liver, bone marrow, and joint fluid specimens reveal characteristic metachromatic granules within cells.
• Presence of excess GAG in urine usually indicates MPS.
• Definitive diagnosis made by measuring lysosomal enzyme activity in serum, leukocyte pellets, or frozen liver.

IMAGING
• Radiography—low bone density with thin cortices
• Epiphyseal abnormalities—vary from slight irregularities to large scalloped defects in subchondral bone
• Joint changes—acetabular flattening and periarticular osteophyte formation
• In some cats, proliferative bone is present around all articular facets of vertebrae, causing fusion of cervical vertebrae.

DIAGNOSTIC PROCEDURES
None

PATHOLOGIC FINDINGS
Distended lysosomes seen in cells of many tissues examined by light and electron microscopy

TREATMENT

DEFINITIVE TREATMENT
• BMT—the most successful treatment to date; after engraftment, donor-derived normal leukocytes provide missing enzyme to various tissues; when performed at a very early age, affected animals lead near-normal lives; not as helpful when performed after skeletal maturity; expensive, life-threatening, and a normal sibling is needed as a donor
• Enzyme-replacement therapy, using recombinant enzyme at birth, followed by BMT, has been quite effective in animal models of MPS.
• Both BMT and enzyme replacement are expensive and have been employed primarily in animal models to determine the potential success in children; very few privately owned animals have been treated.
• Gene therapy is effective in some animal models.

NURSING CARE
• Fluid administration is often required to correct dehydration.
• With increasing age, difficulty eating progresses; a diet of soft food may be helpful.

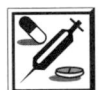

MEDICATIONS

DRUG(S)
Affected animals are susceptible to viral and bacterial respiratory infection; antibiotics may be indicated.

CONTRAINDICATIONS/POSSIBLE INTERACTIONS
None

FOLLOW-UP

PREVENTION/AVOIDANCE
• Avoid inbreeding in family with history of disease
• Enzyme assays should be performed to diagnose heterozygotes.

EXPECTED COURSE AND PROGNOSIS
• Prognosis reasonably good in animals treated with BMT
• Untreated animals usually develop severe skeletal and joint disease and may become nonambulatory at 3 to 5 years of age.

MISCELLANEOUS

ABBREVIATIONS
• BMT = bone marrow transplant
• GAG = glycosaminoglycan

Suggested Reading
Haskins M, Giger U. Lysosomal storage diseases. In: Kaneko JJ, Harvey JW, Bruss ML, eds. Clinical biochemistry of domestic animals. 5th ed. San Diego: Academic Press, 1997:741–760.
Author Mary Anna Thrall
Consulting Editor Stephen A. Kruth

MULTIPLE MYELOMA

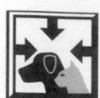 BASICS

DEFINITION
• Uncommon malignant neoplasm of hematopoietic tissue derived from a clonal population of plasma cells in the bone marrow
• Three of four defining features must be present for diagnosis: monoclonal gammopathy; neoplastic plasma cells or bone marrow plasmacytosis; lytic bone lesions; and Bence Jones (light-chain) proteinuria

PATHOPHYSIOLOGY
• Proliferation of a single clone of plasma cells that produces immunoglobulins (IgA or IgG) or subunits (heavy or light chains)
• Overproduction of IgM—Waldenstrom's macroglobulinemia
• Polymerized IgA or IgG—may increase serum viscosity (8–10 times normal)
• Bleeding diathesis—caused by effect of paraprotein coating of platelets, thrombocytopenia, increased viscosity of blood, and interference with normal coagulation factors
• Nephrotoxicity—secondary to protein deposition of amyloid or direct effect of the protein on renal tubular epithelial cells

SYSTEMS AFFECTED
• Musculoskeletal—multiple areas of active bone lysis in the skeleton including vertebral column (especially lumbar), pelvis, skull, and, occasionally, appendicular bones
• Soft tissues—neoplastic plasma cells may be present in extraskeletal sites (e.g., liver, spleen, lymph nodes, kidney, pharynx, lung, muscle, and gastrointestinal tract)
• Nervous, cardiovascular, and respiratory—possible abnormalities secondary to hyperviscosity

GENETICS
N/A

INCIDENCE/PREVALENCE
• Dogs—reported prevalence < 1% of all malignant tumors; < 8% of hematopoietic malignant tumors; 3.6% of all bone tumors
• Cats—reported prevalence < 1% of hematopoietic tumors

GEOGRAPHIC DISTRIBUTION
N/A

SIGNALMENT

Species
Dogs and cats

Breed Predilections
German shepherds and other purebred dogs

Mean Age and Range
Primarily middle-aged or old dogs and cats (6–13 years)

Predominant Sex
None

SIGNS

General Comments
Attributed to bone infiltration and lysis, effects of proteins produced by the tumor (e.g., hyperviscosity and nephrotoxicity), and infiltration of organ(s) by neoplastic cells

Historical Findings
• Depend on location and extent of disease
• Weakness
• Lameness
• Pain
• Paresis
• Urinary incontinence
• Epistaxis—unilateral or bilateral
• Blindness
• Dementia
• Malaise
• Labored breathing
• Polyuria
• Polydipsia
• Gastrointestinal bleeding

Physical Examination Findings
Dogs
• Bleeding—especially from the nose or mucous membranes (36%)
• Blindness, retinal hemorrhage, or dilated retinal vessels (35%); detached retina; glaucoma; anterior uveitis
• Lameness (47%), bone pain and weakness (60%)—with lytic bone lesions
• Dementia, malaise (11%), and coma (rare)
• Polydipsia and polyuria (25%)—with hypercalcemia or renal dysfunction
• Pale mucous membranes
• Fever
• Lethargy
• Hepatosplenomegaly
Cats
• Anorexia
• Weight loss
• Malaise
• Polydipsia
• Polyuria
• Fever

CAUSES
Unknown

RISK FACTORS
N/A

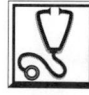 DIAGNOSIS

DIFFERENTIAL DIAGNOSIS
• Infectious—bacterial, fungal, and parasitic disorders
• Monoclonal gammopathy can occur in ehrlichiosis.
• Neoplastic—metastatic (e.g., carcinoma, sarcoma, mast cell tumor, lymphosarcoma, and lymphoid leukemia)
• Immune-mediated—benign hypergammaglobulinemia; rheumatoid arthritis; plasmacytic gastroenterocolitis

CBC/BIOCHEMISTRY/URINALYSIS
• Hemogram—anemia (70% of dogs); neutropenia (25% of dogs); thrombocytopenia (30% of dogs); eosinophilia; plasma cell leukemia (very rare)
• High RBC rouleaux formation, high serum viscosity, or high serum total protein with hypoalbuminemia (65% of dogs) and hyperglobulinemia
• Hypercalcemia (17% of dogs; very rare in cats)
• High BUN, creatinine, ALP, or ALT
• Bence Jones proteins—undetectable on routine urinalysis (dip stick)
• Urine proteinuria, isosthenuria, cylindruria, pyuria, hematuria, or bacteruria

OTHER LABORATORY TESTS
• Serum protein electrophoresis—identify monoclonal gammopathy (i.e., protein spike), even if globulin concentration is normal
• Serum immunoglobulin quantification
• Urine protein electrophoresis—identify Bence Jones proteins (immunoglobulin light chain); positive in 30%–40% of dogs
• Protein:creatinine ratio—assess the extent of urine protein loss
• Coagulation profile
• Serum viscosity—high
• Bleeding time or platelet function tests

IMAGING
• Radiography (dogs)—axial and appendicular skeleton; show multifocal, lytic (punched-out) lesions in 50%
• Radiography (cats)—bony lesions rare
• Extraskeletal sites may be identified by organomegaly.
• Ultrasonography—detect changes in echotexture of visceral organs (e.g., infiltration)

DIAGNOSTIC PROCEDURES
Cytologic examination of bone marrow and skeletal and extraskeletal lesions—determine if > 20%–25% of normal cell population are plasma cells

PATHOLOGIC FINDINGS
• Color—greenish in soft tissue; red-grey within bone marrow
• Sheets or isolated discrete round cells with eosinophilic cytoplasm, eccentric nuclei, perinuclear clear zone, and cartwheel appearance of the nuclear chromatin
• Neoplastic cells may grow between osseous trabeculae or cause erosion and lysis of bony trabeculae and cortex.

TREATMENT

APPROPRIATE HEALTH CARE
• Inpatient—azotemia, hypercalcemia, or clinically important bacterial infection
• Plasmapheresis—lowers protein burden; for symptomatic patient, withdraw a volume of venous blood, centrifuge it, discard the plasma, and return the RBCs in intravenous fluids (crystalloid) to the patient; with signs of hyperviscosity, perform phlebotomy and replace intravenously with an equal volume of isotonic fluids
• Radiotherapy—may be used on isolated areas with curative or palliative intent

NURSING CARE
• Venipuncture—use aseptic technique
• Bacterial infection—treat aggressively with appropriate antibiotics
• Hypercalcemia and renal failure—treat appropriately

ACTIVITY
Multiple myeloma—treat as immune compromised; take care to prevent bacterial infection (e.g., caused by puncture wounds from dog or cat fights)

DIET
N/A

CLIENT EDUCATION
• Inform client that chemotherapy is palliative but long remissions are possible.
• Warn client that relapse will occur.
• Discuss side effects, which depend on the drugs used.
• Inform client that most patients develop mild leukopenia with chemotherapy.

SURGICAL CONSIDERATIONS
Areas nonresponsive to chemotherapy or solitary lesions can be removed surgically.

MEDICATIONS

DRUG(S) OF CHOICE
• Dogs—melphalan (0.1 mg/kg PO q24h for 10 days; then 0.05 mg/kg PO q24h) and prednisone (0.5 mg/kg PO q24h for 10 days; then 0.5 mg/kg q48h for 60 days, then stop); cyclophosphamide can be used in addition to or in place of melphalan (200–300 mg/m² IV once weekly or 50 mg/m² PO q24h for 4 days/week).
• Liposome-encapsulated doxorubicin was reported to be effective in one dog.
• Cats—melphalan (0.5 mg PO q24h for 10 days; then 0.5 mg PO q48h) and prednisone (2.5 mg PO q24h)

CONTRAINDICATIONS
N/A

PRECAUTIONS
• Melphalan—very bone marrow suppressive, especially to platelets
• Cyclophosphamide—may be beneficial to substitute for melphalan with thrombocytopenia
• Affected animals may have low numbers of neutrophils or nonfunctional lymphocytes; take care to minimize exposure to infectious agents (e.g., viral, bacterial, and fungal).
• Use septic or very clean technique when performing any invasive techniques, even drawing blood.
• Chemotherapy may be toxic; seek advice before initiating any treatment if you are not familiar with cytotoxic drugs.

ALTERNATIVE DRUG(S)
Dogs—more aggressive combination chemotherapy protocol; cyclophosphamide (200 mg/m² IV every 14 days), vincristine (0.7 mg/m² IV every 14 days), melphalan (0.10 mg/kg PO q24h for 10 days; then 0.05 mg/kg PO q24h), and prednisone (0.5 mg/kg PO q24h)

FOLLOW-UP

PATIENT MONITORING
• CBC and platelet counts—weekly for at least 4 weeks; assess bone marrow response
• Tests with abnormal results—monthly 2 times; evaluate response to treatment
• Protein electrophoresis; monthly for several months, until normal levels obtained; monitor periodically for relapse
• Abnormal skeletal radiographs—monthly 2 times; then every other month until normal; evaluate response to treatment

PREVENTION/AVOIDANCE
N/A

POSSIBLE COMPLICATIONS
• Bleeding
• Secondary infections
• Pathologic fractures
• Even with treatment, it may be several months before clinical signs resolve.
• Chemotherapy—may cause leukopenia or thrombocytopenia, anorexia, alopecia, hemorrhagic cystitis, or pancreatitis

EXPECTED COURSE AND PROGNOSIS
Continuous care must be taken to protect patients from secondary infection.

Dogs
• Median survival with alkylating agents and prednisone—18 months
• Median survival with prednisone—7 months
• Complete response in 43%; partial response in 49%

• Hypercalcemia, extensive bone lysis, or Bence Jones proteinuria—shorter survival times

Cats
Survival with alkylating agents and prednisone—2–9 months

MISCELLANEOUS

ASSOCIATED CONDITIONS
None

AGE-RELATED FACTORS
None

PREGNANCY
Chemotherapy is contraindicated in pregnant animals.

SYNONYMS
• Plasma cell myeloma
• Plasmacytoma
• Myelocytoma
• Myelosarcoma
• Plasma cell leukemia
• Erythrocytoma
• Lymphocytoma

SEE ALSO
• Hypercalcemia
• Renal Failure, Chronic

ABBREVIATIONS
• ALP = alkaline phosphatase
• ALT = alanine aminotransferase
• BUN = blood urea nitrogen
• RBC = red blood cell

Suggested Reading
Couto CG. Oncology. In: Sherding RD, ed. The cat: diseases and clinical management. New York: Churchill Livingstone, 1989:589–647.
Hammer AS, Couto CG. Complications of multiple myeloma. J Am Anim Hosp Assoc 1994;30:9–14.
Kisselberth WC, MacEwan EG, Helfand SC, et al. Response to liposome-encapsulated doxorubicin (TLC D-99) in a dog with myeloma. J Vet Intern Med 1998;9:425–428.
Matus RE, Leifer CE, MacEwan EG, Hurvitz AI. Prognostic factors for multiple myeloma in the dog. J Am Vet Med Assoc 1986;11:1288–1292.
Morrison WB. Plasma cell neoplasms. In: Morrison WB, ed. Cancer in dogs and cats: medical and surgical management. Baltimore: Williams & Wilkins, 1998:697–704.
Vail DM. Hematopoietic tumors: plasma cell neoplasms. In: Withrow SJ, MacEwan EG, eds., Clinical veterinary oncology. Philadelphia: Lippincott, 1996:509–520.
Authors Mary Ann Vonderhaar and Wallace B. Morrison
Consulting Editor Wallace B. Morrison

MUMPS

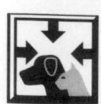

BASICS

OVERVIEW
• Common illness in humans
• Dogs contract the disease from infected children.
• Incidence (dogs)—low

SIGNALMENT
• Dogs of all ages
• No sex or breed predilections

SIGNS
• Enlarged parotid salivary glands
• Fever
• Anorexia

CAUSES & RISK FACTORS
Mumps virus—family Paramyxoviridae; genus *Paramyxovirus*

DIAGNOSIS

DIFFERENTIAL DIAGNOSIS
• Benign parotid salivary gland enlargement
• Neoplasia

CBC/BIOCHEMISTRY/URINALYSIS
No specific findings

OTHER LABORATORY TESTS
N/A

IMAGING
N/A

DIAGNOSTIC PROCEDURES
Serologic—mumps viral antibodies

TREATMENT
Usually not required

MEDICATIONS

DRUG(S)
None

CONTRAINDICATIONS/POSSIBLE INTERACTIONS
None

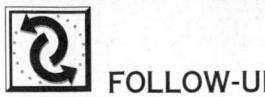
FOLLOW-UP

PATIENT MONITORING
Monitor hydration, electrolytes, acid–base balance, and body temperature.

EXPECTED COURSE AND PROGNOSIS
Patients usually recover within 5–10 days of infection.

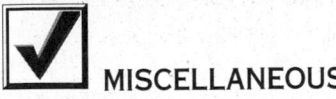
MISCELLANEOUS

ZOONOTIC POTENTIAL
Mumps virus spreads only from acutely infected humans to susceptible dogs.

Suggested Reading
Greene CE. Mumps and influenza virus infections. In: Greene CE, ed. Infectious diseases of the dog and cat. 2nd ed. Philadelphia: Saunders, 1998:130.

Author Johnny D. Hoskins
Consulting Editor Stephen C. Barr

MURMURS, HEART

BASICS

DEFINITION
Vibrations caused by disturbed blood flow

Timing of Murmurs
• Systolic murmurs occur between S1 and S2 (systole).
• Diastolic murmurs occur between S2 and S1 (diastole).
• Continuous and to-and-fro murmurs occur throughout all or most of the cardiac cycle.
• Continuous murmurs are usually accentuated near S2 and to-and-fro murmurs are usually absent near S2.

Grading Scale for Murmurs
• Grade I—barely audible
• Grade II—soft, but easily auscultated
• Grade III—intermediate loudness; most hemodynamically important murmurs are at least grade III.
• Grade IV—loud with palpable thrill
• Grade V—very loud, audible with stethoscope barely touching the chest; palpable thrill
• Grade VI—very loud, audible without the stethoscope touching the chest; palpable thrill

Configuration
• Plateau murmurs have uniform loudness and are typical of regurgitant murmurs such as mitral and tricuspid insufficiency and ventricular septal defect.
• Crescendo-decrescendo murmurs get louder and then softer and are typical of ejection murmurs such as pulmonic and aortic stenosis and atrial septal defect.
• Decrescendo murmurs start loud and then get softer and are typical of diastolic murmurs such as aortic or pulmonic insufficiency and mitral or tricuspid stenosis.

Location
Dogs
• Mitral area—left fifth intercostal space at costochondral junction
• Aortic area—left fourth intercostal space above costochondral junction
• Pulmonic area—left second to fourth intercostal space at sternal border
• Tricuspid area—right third to fifth intercostal space near costochondral junction

Cats
• Mitral area—left fifth to sixth intercostal space 1/4 ventrodorsal distance from sternum
• Aortic area—left second to third intercostal space just above the pulmonic area
• Pulmonic area—left second to third intercostal space 1/3–1/2 ventrodorsal distance from sternum
• Tricuspid area—right fourth to fifth intercostal space 1/4 ventrodorsal distance from sternum

PATHOPHYSIOLOGY
• Disturbed blood flow associated with high flow through normal or abnormal valves or with structures vibrating in the blood flow
• Flow disturbances associated with outflow obstruction or forward flow through stenosed valves or into a dilated great vessel
• Flow disturbances associated with regurgitant flow through an incompetent valve, septal defect, or patent ductus arteriosus

SYSTEMS AFFECTED
Cardiovascular

SIGNALMENT
Dogs and cats

SIGNS
Relate to cause of the murmur

CAUSES
Systolic Murmurs
• Mitral and tricuspid valve endocardiosis
• Cardiomyopathy and AV valve insufficiency
• Physiologic flow murmurs
• Anemia
• Mitral and tricuspid valve dysplasia
• Systolic anterior mitral motion (SAM)
• Dynamic right ventricular outflow obstruction
• Dynamic subaortic stenosis
• Atrial septal defect
• Ventricular septal defect
• Pulmonic stenosis
• Aortic stenosis
• Tetralogy of Fallot
• Mitral and tricuspid valve endocarditis
• Hyperthyroidism
• Heartworm disease

Continuous or To-and-Fro Murmurs
• Patent ductus arteriosus
• Ventricular septal defect with aortic regurgitation
• Aortic stenosis with aortic regurgitation

Diastolic Murmurs
• Mitral and tricuspid valve stenosis
• Aortic and pulmonic valve endocarditis

RISK FACTORS
Cardiac disease

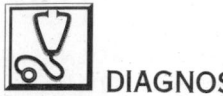

DIAGNOSIS

DIFFERENTIAL DIAGNOSIS
Differential Signs
• Must differentiate from other abnormal heart sounds—split sounds, ejection sounds, gallop rhythms, and clicks
• Must differentiate from abnormal lung sounds and pleural rubs; listen to see if timing of abnormal sound is correlated with respiration or heartbeat.

Differential Causes
• Pale mucous membranes support diagnosis of anemic murmur.
• Location and radiation of murmur and timing during cardiac cycle can help determine cause; see algorithm.

CBC/BIOCHEMISTRY/URINALYSIS
• Anemia in animals with anemic murmurs
• Polycythemia in animals with right-to-left shunting congenital defects
• Leukocytosis with left shift in animals with endocarditis

OTHER LABORATORY TESTS
N/A

IMAGING
• Thoracic radiography—useful for evaluating heart size and pulmonary vasculature in hopes of determining cause and significance of murmur
• Echocardiography—recommended when a cardiac cause is suspected and the nature of the defect is unknown
• Doppler studies sometimes required to confirm cause of murmur

Diagnostic Procedures
Electrocardiography may be useful in assessing heart enlargement patterns in animals with murmurs.

TREATMENT
• Outpatient unless heart failure is evident
• Base decisions on the cause of the murmur and associated clinical signs.
• None indicated for murmur alone

MEDICATIONS

DRUG(S)
N/A

CONTRAINDICATIONS
N/A

PRECAUTIONS
N/A

POSSIBLE INTERACTIONS
N/A

FOLLOW-UP

PATIENT MONITORING
Low-grade systolic ejection murmurs in puppies may be physiologic; most resolve by 6 months of age. If murmur still present after 6 months, include diagnostic imaging.

POSSIBLE COMPLICATIONS
If murmur is associated with structural heart disease, may see signs of congestive heart failure (e.g., coughing, dyspnea, and ascites) or exercise intolerance

MISCELLANEOUS

ASSOCIATED CONDITIONS
N/A

AGE-RELATED FACTORS
• Murmurs present since birth generally associated with a congenital defect or physiologic flow murmur
• Acquired murmurs in geriatric, small-breed dogs usually associated with degenerative valve disease
• Acquired murmurs in large-breed dogs usually associated with dilated cardiomyopathy
• Acquired murmurs in geriatric cats usually associated with cardiomyopathy or hyperthyroidism

ZOONOTIC POTENTIAL
N/A

PREGNANCY
N/A

SYNONYMS
N/A

SEE ALSO
See Causes.

ABBREVIATIONS
• AV = atrioventricular
• S1 = first heart sound
• S2 = second heart sound

Suggested Reading
Smith FWK Jr., Tilley LP. Rapid interpretation of heart sounds, murmurs, and arrhythmias. Philadelphia: Lea & Febiger, 1992.
Authors Francis W. K. Smith, Jr., and Robert L. Hamlin
Consulting Editors Larry P. Tilley and Francis W. K. Smith, Jr.

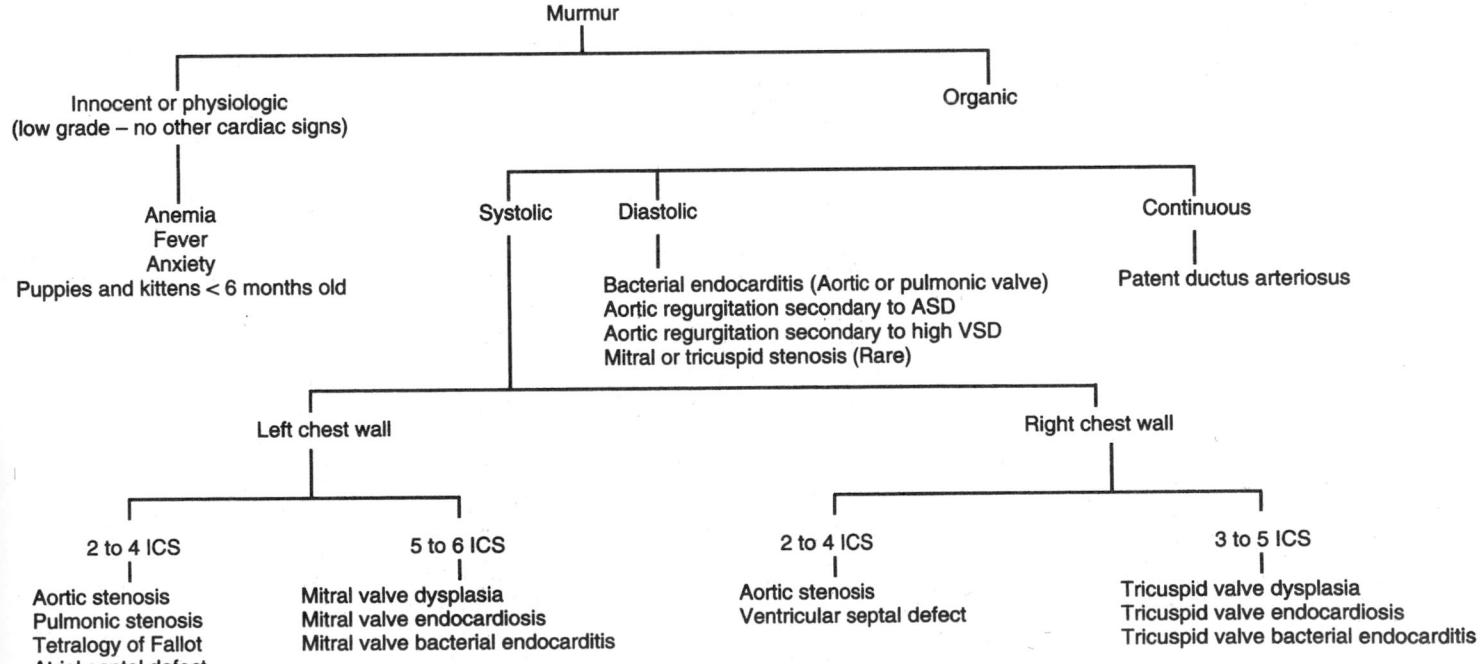

Figure 1.

Differential diagnosis of cardiac disease based on the timing and location of murmurs. ASD = atrial septal defect; VSD = ventricular septal defect; ICS = intercostal space. Adapted from Allen DG. Murmurs and abnormal heart sounds. By permission of Mosby-Year Book, Inc. In: Allen DG, Kruth SA, eds. Small animal cardiopulmonary medicine. Philadelphia: BC Decker, 1988:13.

MUSCLE RUPTURE (MUSCLE TEAR)

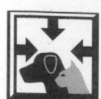

BASICS

OVERVIEW
A normal muscle may be stretched, pinched, or injured directly, resulting in fiber disruption, weakening, and immediate or delayed separation of the uninjured portions. Alternatively the muscle structure may be compromised by systemic or iatrogenic conditions, and normal activity may cause muscle disruption. The rupture may be complete or incomplete, and may be mid-substance or at the muscle-tendon junction. The acute stage is characterized by a typical inflammatory reaction that becomes chronic with collagen maturation, cross-linking, and adhesion development over time. Frequently the acute phase is overlooked as the signs may be temporary and respond well to rest. The chronic effects are often progressive and unresponsive to support therapies.

SIGNALMENT
Limb and masticatory muscles are the primary structures affected. Traumatic injury is indiscriminate, although certain activities may predispose because of exposure. The ruptures that are apparently unrelated to trauma seem to affect middle-aged to older working dogs, with no reported sex predilection. Cats affected less frequently than dogs

SIGNS

Acute Injury
• Immediate lameness that is characterized by the specific muscle affected • Localized swelling, heat, and pain • Generally present for a few days to a week

Chronic Phase (if it develops)
• Progressive • Painless • Usually associated with scar tissue that impedes normal function of an extremity

Causes & Risk Factors
• Trauma • Over-extension • Myositis • Degenerative (unknown etiology) • Myopathy secondary to medical conditions like Cushing's disease • Apparent risk factor for dogs is involvement in hunting, tracking, or similar activities in the outdoors.

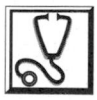

DIAGNOSIS

DIFFERENTIAL DIAGNOSIS
• Neurologic dysfunction—recognized by neurologic abnormalities • Tendon rupture—visible or palpable disruption in the tendon • Origin/insertion avulsion fracture—radiographic evidence of bone fragment defect and translocation • Luxation/subluxation—palpable or radiographic evidence of joint instability or malalignment

CBC/BIOCHEMISTRY/URINANALYSIS
No injury-specific findings

OTHER LABORATORY TESTS
• CPK may be elevated in acute cases.

• No known specific tests available

IMAGING

Radiographic Findings
Soft tissue swelling may be evident in the early stages. Calcification of muscle can occur in the traumatized area in chronic situations.

Ultrasonographic Findings
• Local swelling and disorientation of the normal muscle fiber orientation may be seen at the site of injury in acute cases. • Scar tissue and contracted areas of fibrous tissue can be seen in the muscle in chronic cases. • Measurable differences between normal and abnormal sides may be useful in documenting the affected muscle site.

CT Findings
Produces better tissue contrast than the above but still constrained to an axial plane of view.

MRI Findings
Edema and hemorrhage cause a change in the signal that can be differentiated from changes due to fibrous tissue replacement of muscle. This allows localization of the problem and helps to identify the type of problem.

DIAGNOSTIC PROCEDURES

Muscle Biopsy
The presence of fibrous tissue and the loss of muscle cells may be documented. Differentiating disuse atrophy from neurologic atrophy and from injury-induced scarring may be impossible without corroborating evidence.

TREATMENT
• There is no documented evidence to support a single "best" way to treat acute muscle injuries in order to prevent fibrous contracture and adhesions. It is generally believed that immediate postinjury care should involve rest, local cold application followed within hours by heat, and passive physical therapy (movement). It would be inappropriate to hospitalize or cage a recently injured animal for muscle problems unless surgical repair is planned. Light or non–weight bearing activity would be appropriate for an extended period of time (4–6 weeks). Analgesics and antiinflammatory drugs would be recommended for several days to a week. Surgery may be performed within a few days of the injury to repair obvious, acute muscle rupture that results in a separation of the uninjured muscle segments. An essential part of muscle repair is effective tension relief for the injured muscle so that healing can occur without disruption as function returns. Internal or external orthopedic devices may be necessary to provide effective tension relief. Owners should be made aware of the possibility of scar-related problems affecting the patient's gait in the long term. • Once the muscle injury becomes chronic and associated with contracture or adhesions, treatment is aimed at function salvage. Surgical release of the adhesions or fibrous tissue bands is often accompanied by instantaneous symptomatic relief. The prevention of re-adhesion and progressive contracture is much less rewarding. • Specific

muscle injuries have widely disparate prognoses. Infraspinatus contracture responds well to surgical excision of the tendon of insertion. Gracilis contracture has a 100% recurrence rate after surgical resection. Quadriceps contracture has a similarly dismal failure rate after surgery. • Muscle injuries that have healed in an elongated state have a better prognosis for surgical improvement of function than contracted muscles. The most common elongation injury affects the muscles of the Achilles group. Hock hyperflexion can be surgically reconstructed to return these animals to relatively normal function. This is usually accomplished by shortening the Achilles tendon rather than the injured muscle or musculotendinous junction.

MEDICATIONS

DRUG(S)
None are specific. Antiinflammatory drugs may be indicated in acute situations.

CONTRAINDICATIONS/POSSIBLE INTERACTIONS
Immobilization of the injured muscle in a position that allows adhesions to develop to nearby bone will often result in "tie down" contractures.

FOLLOW-UP

PATIENT MONITORING
Repetitive range of motion monitoring

PREVENTION/AVOIDANCE
Early inflammation control and non–weight bearing passive physical therapy may be beneficial.

POSSIBLE COMPLICATIONS
Contracture of the muscle and fibrous replacement of muscle tissue

EXPECTED COURSE AND PROGNOSIS
Specific to the muscle and the type of injury.

MISCELLANEOUS

ASSOCIATED CONDITIONS
Joint hypermobility, angular limb deformities, flexion/extension joint abnormalities

AGE-RELATED FACTORS
Growth plate fractures in young dogs are associated with quadriceps contracture.

ABBREVIATIONS
• CT = computed tomography • MRI = magnetic resonance imaging

Suggested Reading
Vaughan LC. Muscle and tendon injuries in dogs. J Small Anim Pract 20:711–736, 1979.

Author Peter K. Shires
Consulting Editor Peter K. Shires

BASICS

OVERVIEW
• Toxic mushrooms—classified into four categories on the basis of clinical signs and their time of onset and into seven groups on the basis of the toxin; *Amanita* most important genus
• Onset of signs after ingestion of category B, C, or D mushrooms—20 min to 3 hr
• Systems affected—hepatobiliary (hepatic necrosis); renal/urologic (renal tubular necrosis); nervous (autonomic and central)

Category A
• Most toxic
• Cause of cellular destruction, most often of liver and kidneys
• Group I toxin—cyclopeptides; found in *Amanita* spp. and *Galerina* spp.
• Group II toxin—monomethylhydrazine; found in *Gyromitra* spp.; onset of signs > 6 hr after ingestion

Category B
• Affect the autonomic nervous system
• Group III toxin—coprine; found in *Coprinus* spp.
• Group IV toxin—muscarinic effects; found in *Clitocybe* spp. and *Inocybe* spp.

Category C
• Affect the CNS; cause delirium
• Group V toxin—ibotenic acid-muscimol; found in *Amanita* spp.
• Group VI toxin—hallucinogens; *Psilocybe* spp. and *Panceobus* spp.

Category D
• Cause gastrointestinal irritation
• Group VII toxin—found in a variety of genera

SIGNALMENT
Primarily dogs; mostly puppies

SIGNS

General Comments
• Depend on the type of mushroom ingested
• Toxicity of a particular species—not consistent; depends on the local environment

Physical Examination Findings
• Vomiting
• Diarrhea
• Abdominal pain
• Lethargy
• Icterus
• Ataxia
• Seizures
• Coma

Group IV Toxins
• Ptyalism (excess salivation)
• Lacrimation
• Diarrhea

CAUSES & RISK FACTORS
Exposure to and ingestion of toxic mushroom

DIAGNOSIS

DIFFERENTIAL DIAGNOSIS
• Diagnosis usually relies on owner observation.
• Seasonal occurrence; primarily summer and fall

CBC/BIOCHEMISTRY/URINALYSIS
• High ALT, AST, total bilirubin, BUN, and creatinine; may be delayed 24–48 hr after ingestion
• Hypoglycemia
• Hypokalemia

OTHER LABORATORY TESTS
• Identification of mushroom (refrigerate) or spores in vomitus or stomach contents—submit to an experienced mycologist

IMAGING
N/A

DIAGNOSTIC PROCEDURES
N/A

PATHOLOGIC FINDINGS
Hepatocellular and renal tubular necrosis

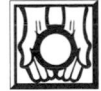

TREATMENT
• Inpatient—monitor vital signs; supportive and symptomatic care
• NPO if vomiting
• Parenteral fluids—maintain hydration and induce diuresis
• Warn client that temporary improvement in gastrointestinal signs with group I toxicity is often followed by delayed onset of hepatic and renal failure.

MEDICATIONS

DRUG(S)
• Induce emesis—ipecac syrup (1–2 mL/kg PO up to 15 mL) or apomorphine (0.04 mg/kg IV)
• Activated charcoal—1–4 g/kg q3–6h for 24–36 hr; mix in water (1 g/5–10 mL water)
• Furosemide—2–4 mg/kg IV q8–12h; for oliguric or anuric renal failure in patents with normal hydration status
• Atropine—0.02–0.04 mg/kg half-dose IV, half-dose IM; block muscarinic signs; group IV toxins only
• Penicillin G—20,000 U/kg IM q12–24h
• Diazepam—0.25–0.5 mg/kg IV or IM; for seizures

CONTRAINDICATIONS/POSSIBLE INTERACTIONS
Atropine—contraindicated with group IV toxicosis

FOLLOW-UP
• Monitor hepatic and renal function for at least 48 hr.
• Group I toxicosis—temporary improvement in gastrointestinal signs often followed by delayed onset of hepatic and renal failure
• Prognosis—good, except for group I toxicosis

MISCELLANEOUS

SEE ALSO
Poisoning (Intoxication)

ABBREVIATIONS
• ALT = alanine aminotransferase
• AST = aspartate aminotransferase

Suggested Reading
Lincoft G, Mitchel DH. Toxic and hallucinogenic mushroom poisoning. New York: Van Nostrand Reinhold, 1977.
Author Ronald B. Wilson
Consulting Editor Gary D. Osweiler

MYASTHENIA GRAVIS

 BASICS

DEFINITION
A disorder of neuromuscular transmission characterized by muscular weakness and excessive fatigability

PATHOPHYSIOLOGY
Transmission failure at the neuromuscular junction—results from structural or functional abnormalities of the nicotinic AChRs (congenital form) and from autoantibody-mediated destruction of AChRs and post-synaptic membranes (acquired form)

SYSTEMS AFFECTED
• Neuromuscular—result of abnormalities or destruction of AChRs
• Respiratory—may find aspiration pneumonia secondary to megaesophagus

GENETICS
• Congenital familial forms—Jack Russell terriers, springer spaniels, smooth fox terriers; autosomal recessive mode of inheritance
• Acquired—as with other autoimmune diseases, requires appropriate genetic background for disease to occur; multifactorial, involving environmental, infectious, and hormonal influences

INCIDENCE/PREVALENCE
• Congenital—rare
• Acquired—not uncommon in dogs; rare in cats

GEOGRAPHIC DISTRIBUTION
Worldwide

SIGNALMENT
Species
Dogs and cats

Breed Predilections
• Congenital—Jack Russell terriers; springer spaniels; smooth fox terriers
• Acquired—several breeds: golden retrievers; German shepherds; Labrador retrievers; dachshunds; Scottish terriers; Akitas

Mean Age and Range
• Congenital—6–8 weeks of age
• Acquired—bimodal age of onset; dogs: 1–4 years of age and 9–13 years of age

Predominant Sex
• Congenital—none
• Acquired—may be a slight predilection for females in the young age group; none in the old age group

SIGNS
General Comments
• Acquired—may have several clinical presentations ranging from focal involvement of the esophageal, pharyngeal, and extraocular muscles to acute generalized collapse
• Should be on the differential diagnosis of any dog with acquired megaesophagus or lower motor neuron weakness

Historical Findings
• Regurgitation—common; important to differentiate between vomiting and regurgitation
• Voice change
• Exercise-related weakness
• Acute collapse
• Progressive weakness

Physical Examination Findings
• Patient may look normal at rest.
• Excessive drooling, regurgitation, and repeated attempts at swallowing
• Muscle atrophy—usually not found
• Dyspnea—with aspiration pneumonia
• Fatigue or cramping—with mild exercise
• Careful neurologic examination—subtle findings: decreased or absent palpebral reflex (may be fatigable); may note a poor or absent gag reflex; spinal reflexes usually normal but fatigable (rarely absent and dog unable to support its weight)

CAUSES
• Congenital
• Immune-mediated
• Paraneoplastic

RISK FACTORS
• Appropriate genetic background
• Neoplasia—particularly thymoma
• Methimazole treatment (cats)—may result in reversible disease

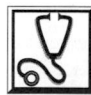 DIAGNOSIS

DIFFERENTIAL DIAGNOSIS
• Other disorders of neuromuscular transmission—tick paralysis; botulism; cholinesterase toxicity
• Acute or chronic polyneuropathies
• Polymyopathies—including polymyositis
• Diagnosis depends upon a careful history, thorough physical and neurologic examinations, and specialized laboratory testing.

CBC/BIOCHEMISTRY/URINALYSIS
• Normal
• Serum creatine kinase—usually normal; may be elevated with polymyositis associated with concurrent thymoma

OTHER LABORATORY TESTS
• Serum AChR antibody titer—diagnostic for acquired form
• Thyroid and adrenal function—may see abnormalities associated with acquired form

IMAGING
Thoracic radiographs—megaesophagus; cranial mediastinal mass

DIAGNOSTIC PROCEDURES
• Ultrasound-guided biopsy of cranial mediastinal mass—may support diagnosis of thymoma
• Dramatic increase in muscle strength after administration of edrophonium chloride (0.1 mg/kg IV)—may see false-negative and false-positive responses
• Decreased or absent palpebral reflex—may return after edrophonium chloride administration
• Electrophysiologic evaluation—necessity questionable with increased availability of AChR antibody testing; many patients with acquired form are poor anesthetic risks.
• Electrocardiogram—with bradycardia; third-degree heart block was recently documented in some patients with acquired disease.

PATHOLOGIC FINDINGS
Biopsy of a cranial mediastinal mass may reveal thymoma, thymic hyperplasia, or thymic atrophy.

 TREATMENT

APPROPRIATE HEALTH CARE
• Inpatient—until adequate dosages of anticholinesterase drugs are achieved
• Aspiration pneumonia—may require intensive care
• Gastrostomy tube—may be required if patient is unable to eat or drink without significant regurgitation

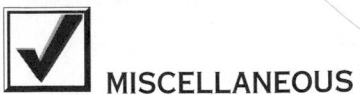
NURSING CARE
• Oxygen therapy, intensive antibiotic therapy, intravenous fluid therapy, and supportive care—generally required for aspiration pneumonia
• Nutritional maintenance with a gastrostomy tube—multiple feedings of a high-caloric diet; good hygiene care

ACTIVITY
Self-limited owing to the severity of muscle weakness and extent of aspiration pneumonia

DIET
May try different consistencies of food—gruel; hard food; soft food; evaluate what is best tolerated

CLIENT EDUCATION
• Warn client that, although the disease is treatable, most patients require months of special feeding and medication.
• Inform client that a dedicated owner is important to a favorable outcome for acquired myasthenia.

SURGICAL CONSIDERATIONS
• Cranial mediastinal mass—thymoma
• Before attempting surgical removal, stabilize patient with anticholinesterase drugs and treat aspiration pneumonia.
• Weakness may not be seen initially.
• Suspected thymoma—test all patients for acquired disease before surgery.

 MEDICATIONS

DRUG(S) OF CHOICE
• Anticholinesterase drugs—prolong the action of acetylcholine at the neuromuscular junction; pyridostigmine bromide syrup (Mestinon syrup) at 1–3 mg/kg PO q8–12h diluted half and half in water
• Corticosteroids—0.5 mg/kg q24h; initiated if there is a poor response to pyridostigmine or if there is no response to the edrophonium chloride challenge

CONTRAINDICATIONS
Avoid drugs that may reduce the safety margin of neuromuscular transmission—aminoglycoside antibiotics; antiarrhythmic agents; phenothiazines; anesthetics; narcotics; muscle relaxants; magnesium

PRECAUTIONS
• Avoid large volumes of barium for evaluating megaesophagus.
• Large air-filled esophagus seen on survey radiographs—barium study not indicated
• Avoid immunosuppressive dosages of prednisone—may worsen muscle weakness
• Avoid unnecessary vaccinations.

POSSIBLE INTERACTIONS
N/A

ALTERNATIVE DRUG(S)
Azathroprine—2.0 mg/kg PO through gastrostomy tube q24h. Taper to q48h when clinical remission of the disease.

 FOLLOW-UP

PATIENT MONITORING
• Return of muscle strength should be evident.
• Thoracic radiographs—evaluated every 4–6 weeks for resolution of megaesophagus
• AChR antibody titers—evaluated every 6–8 weeks; decrease to the normal range with clinical remission

PREVENTION/AVOIDANCE
N/A

POSSIBLE COMPLICATIONS
• Aspiration pneumonia
• Respiratory arrest

EXPECTED COURSE AND PROGNOSIS
• No severe aspiration pneumonia or pharyngeal weakness—good prognosis for complete recovery; resolution usually within 4–6 months
• Thymoma present—guarded prognosis unless complete surgical removal and control of myasthenic symptoms are achieved

✓ MISCELLANEOUS

ASSOCIATED CONDITIONS
• Other autoimmune disorders—thyroiditis; skin disorders; hypoadrenocorticism
• Disorders of the thymus—thymoma; thymic hyperplasia
• Other neoplasias

AGE-RELATED FACTORS
Bimodal age of onset—1–4 years of age and 9–13 years of age

ZOONOTIC POTENTIAL
N/A

PREGNANCY
• Humans—weakness may improve during pregnancy but worsens after delivery; some neonates of affected mothers have a temporary myasthenia gravis–like weakness that lasts several days to weeks that is due to in utero transfer of autoantibodies from the mother.
• Documented in dogs after whelping

SEE ALSO
• Chapters covering autoimmune diseases
• Megaesophagus

ABBREVIATION
AChR = acetylcholine receptor

Suggested Reading
Drachman DB. Myasthenia gravis. N Eng J Med 1994;330:1797–1810.
Shelton GD. Canine myasthenia gravis. In: Kirk WR, Bangor JD, eds. Current veterinary Therapy XI. Philadelphia: Saunders, 1992:1039–1040.
Shelton GD. Megaesophagus secondary to myasthenia gravis. In: Kirk WR, Bonagura JD, eds. Current veterinary therapy XI. Philadelphia: Saunders, 1992:580–583.
Shelton GD, Lendstrom JM. Spontaneous remission in canine myasthenia gravis: Implications for assessing human MG therapies. Neurology 2001;57:2139–2141.
Shelton GD. Myasthenia gravis and disorders of neuromuscular transmission. Vet Clin North Am 2002;31:189–200.
Author G. Diane Shelton
Consulting Editor Peter K. Shires

MYCOBACTERIAL INFECTIONS

 BASICS

OVERVIEW
• Mycobacteria—Gram-positive, acid-fast higher bacteria (genus *Mycobacterium*); obligate or sporadic pathogens in humans and animals • Tuberculosis—caused by *Mycobacterium tuberculosis* (humans), *M. bovis* (cattle and some wild mammals), and *M. microti* (voles); dogs and cats exposed to infected primary hosts sporadically infected; disseminated or multi-organ disease caused by obligately parasitic organism; rare in dogs and cats in developed countries. • Leprosy—*M. lepraemurium* (from rodents) and 2 unnamed leprosy organisms • Cats: two syndromes—Syndrome 1 affecting young cats with localized nodular disease affecting limbs with sparse to moderate numbers of acid-fast bacilli present in lesions (*M. lepraemurium*); syndrome 2 affecting old cats with generalized skin lesions with large numbers of acid-fast bacilli in lesions (unnamed species with affinity to *M. malmoense*) • Dogs: canine leproid granuloma syndrome caused by unnamed and uncultured *Mycobacterium* spp. identified by DNA sequencing. • Systemic or non-cutaneous infection with non-tuberculosis mycobacteria—*M. chelonae-abscessus, M. avium* complex, *M. fortuitum, M. genavense, M. kansasii, M. smegmatis, M. thermoresistibile, M. xenopi*; sporadic infections in dogs and cats; some patients with concurrent or immunosupressing disease or the result of traumatic tissue introduction of saprophytic organism; syndromes include pleuritis, localized or disseminated granulomas, disseminated disease, neuritis, bronchopneumonia. • Cutaneous/subcutaneous infections due to rapidly growing mycobacteria—also known as mycobacterial panniculitis. • Dogs and cats: caused by saprophytic mycobacteria *M. fortuitum, M. chelonae-abscessus, M. smegmatis, M. phlei, M. thermoresistibile*.

SIGNALMENT
Tuberculosis
• Cats and dogs of any age • Basset hounds and Siamese cats reported as most susceptible; evidence unclear (possible statistical aberration)

Feline Leprosy
Adult free-roaming cats and kittens; kittens and young adult cats in syndrome 1; older cats (avg 9 years) in syndrome 2.

Canine Leproid Granuloma
Reported cases have been in mostly short-haired outdoor-housed large-breed dogs, especially boxers and German Shepherd dogs.

Systemic Non-tuberculous Mycobacteriosis
A sporadic disease that can affect dogs and cats of any age

Mycobacterial Panniculitis
Adult cats and dogs

SIGNS
Tuberculosis
• Correlated with the route of exposure. Major sites of involvement–oropharyngeal lymph nodes, cutaneous and subcutaneous tissues of the head and extremities; pulmonary system; gastrointestinal system • Dogs—respiratory, especially coughing; dyspnea uncommon • Cats—from contaminated milk: weight loss, chronic diarrhea and thickened intestines; from predation: cutaneous nodules, ulcers and draining tracts • Virtually all dogs and many cats—pharyngeal and cervical lymph-adenopathy; retching, ptyalism, or tonsillar abscess; lymph nodes are visible or palpably firm, fixed, tender; may ulcerate and drain • Fever • Depression • Partial anorexia and weight loss • Hypertrophic osteopathy may occur. • Disseminated disease—body cavity effusion; visceral masses; bone or joint lesions; dermal and subcutaneous masses and ulcers; lymphadenopathy and/or abscesses; CNS signs; sudden death

Feline Leprosy
• Syndrome 1—initial localized nodules on limbs; progress rapidly, may ulcerate; aggressive clinical course; recurrence after surgical excision; widespread lesions develop in several weeks. • Syndrome 2—initial localized or generalized skin nodules that do not ulcerate, slowly progressive over months to years

Canine Leproid Granuloma
• One or more well-circumscribed painless nodules (2 mm–5 cm) in dermis or subcutis; often on head or ear, but may be anywhere on the body; only very large lesions ulcerate. • No systemic signs of illness

Systemic Non-tuberculous Mycobacteriosis
• Pulmonary and systemic infections with AM are reported rarely in dogs, in which case the signs are as for TB. • With *M. avium* infection, disease is most often disseminated.

Mycobacterial Panniculitis
• Cutaneous–traumatic lesion that fails to heal with appropriate therapy; spreads locally in the subcutaneous tissue (panniculitis); original lesion enlarges, forming a deep ulcer that drains greasy hemorrhagic exudate; surrounding tissue becomes firm; satellite pinpoint ulcerations open and drain. • Wound dehiscence at surgery sites • Systemic signs uncommon

CAUSES AND RISK FACTORS
Tuberculosis
• Source of exposure–always an infected typical host • Dogs—usually exposed from an infected person in the household (*M. tuberculosis*); route is ingestion of expectorated infectious material; aerosol exposure possible; patients most often found in urban areas with immigrants from the developing world • Cats—classically exposed by drinking unpasteurized milk of infected cattle (*M. bovis*); much less common now than in the past; may be exposed by predation on infected small mammals (*M. bovis*, undefined tuberculosis species)

Feline Leprosy
In Syndrome 1, cases have been reported from temperate coastal areas and port cities; cool climate may facilitate growth of the organism in extremities. In Syndrome 2, cases are from rural or semi-rural environments; old age or immunoincompetence may be a risk factor. The exact risk factors remain undefined; exposure to rodents is postulated.

Canine Leproid Granuloma
Cases have been associated with fly bites; short coat may predispose. The disease is likely to be found world-wide but most cases have been reported from Australasia and Brazil. In the United States, cases have come from California, Hawaii, and Florida.

Systemic Non-tuberculous Mycobacteriosis
• Most reported patients are immuno-suppressed or have concurrent systemic diseases. • Exposure—routes of exposure in pulmonary and systemic disease are unknown.

Mycobacterial Panniculitis
• Most infections have had antecedent trauma or surgical wound. Most patients are immunocompetent. • Trauma and accidental inoculation of the subcutaneous fat may result in infection; history of bite wound possible (subcutaneous disease) • Fat animals may be more at risk than lean ones.

 DIAGNOSIS

DIFFERENTIAL DIAGNOSIS
The mycobacterial infections have different prognoses, treatment recommendations, and public health consequences but may initially have similar signs, especially cutaneous lesions.

OTHER LABORATORY TESTS
Tuberculosis
Tuberculosis (dogs)—intradermal skin testing with BCG may produce false-positive results.

IMAGING

Radiography

• Thoracic, abdominal, or skeletal lesions—suggest granulomatous infectious disease
• No specific lesions for the mycobacterioses
• Pulmonary tuberculosis lesions—may become calcified or cavitated

DIAGNOSTIC PROCEDURES

• Based on histopathologic and microbiologic evaluation of biopsy material from affected tissue • Biopsy specimens—should be uncontaminated by surface bacteria; must incorporate the center of a granulomatous focus • Smears from infected tissues—for detection with acid-fast stains. On routine staining, organisms are negatively stained, showing "ghosts" of bacilli within macrophages; swabs or aspirations of draining cutaneous lesions or lymph nodes, transtracheal wash; endoscopic brushings; rectal cytology; impressions taken at surgical biopsy. Heat-fixed smears should be submitted along with tissue for culture. • Culture—special media and techniques required; identification of isolates may take several weeks.
• PCR methodologies—may be useful for any of the mycobacterial infections; for canine leproid granuloma and the two feline leprosy syndromes the primers are not commercially available, but can be used to identify the suspect organisms

TREATMENT

Tuberculosis

Permission of local health authorities should be obtained in cases of *Mycobacterium tuberculosis* infection.

Feline Leprosy

There is no known treatment. In syndrome 2, individual lesions may be excised, which may be curative.

Canine Leproid Granuloma

Excision is curative. In systemic and subcutaneous infections with rapid- or slow-growing mycobacteriosis, treatment should be based on organism identification and antibiotic sensitivity testing. Multiple drug therapy is often warranted. Surgical debulking may aid resolution.

 MEDICATIONS

DRUG(S)

Tuberculosis

• Always use double- or triple-drug oral therapy; never attempt single-drug therapy for any organism.
• Current recommendation—fluoroquinolone (e.g., enrofloxacin), clarithromycin, and rifampin for 6–9 months

• Enrofloxacin, orbifloxacin, and ciprofloxacin—5–15 mg/kg PO q24h
• Rifampin—10–20 mg/kg PO q24h or divided q12h (maximum, 600 mg/day)
• Clarithromycin—5–10 mg/kg PO q24h
Alternatives
• Isoniazid and rifampin—combinations have been used; little is known about their use in cats; one recent report of treatment (cat) with isoniazid, rifampin, and dihydrostreptomycin for 3 months noted weight loss but eventual successful outcome
• Isoniazid—10–20 mg/kg (up to 300 mg total) PO q24h
• Ethambutol—15 mg/kg PO q24h
• Pyrazinamide—instead of ethambutol; 15–40 mg/kg PO q24h
• Dihydrostreptomycin—15 mg/kg IM q24h

Feline Leprosy

• Clofazimine 2–8 mg/kg PO q 24hr × 6 weeks, then q 3–4 days for 1–2 months
• Rifampin 10–20 mg/kg q24h or divided q12h.

Subcutaneous and Systemic Non-tuberculous infections

• In vitro sensitivity testing may be used to choose chemotherapy for these cases. Among antibiotics reported to be effective against various AM isolates are macrolides, sulfonamides, tetracyclines, aminoglycosides, and fluoroquinolones. • Anti-TB drugs are not generally effective. • Typically, single-agent therapy has been recommended, but owing to poor response over the long term, double agent therapy may be warranted.
• Fluoroquinolone antibiotics and/or clarithromycin would be good empirical treatment. Use dosages as recommended above for TB. • Clofazimine may be useful for *M. avium* infections. Dosage is 2–8 mg/kg PO q 24 hr × 6 weeks, then q 3–4 days for 1–2 months • Treatment should be continued for 2–6 months. Relapses upon cessation of treatment or during the course of treatment are common.

CONTRAINDICATIONS/POSSIBLE INTERACTIONS

• Traditional antituberculosis drugs—be alert for any adverse reactions; experience limited, especially in cats

 FOLLOW-UP

PATIENT MONITORING

• Antituberculosis and antileprosy drugs—examine at least monthly; monitor for anorexia and weight loss.

• Monitor liver enzymes monthly.
• Instruct owners to report cutaneous lesions immediately.

PREVENTION/AVOIDANCE

Clinicians aware of a human tuberculosis case in a household with dogs or cats should counsel owners about the risk of reverse zoonosis.

EXPECTED COURSE AND PROGNOSIS

Tuberculosis

Guarded, but in reality, currently undefined as experience with modern drugs that are better tolerated for long courses is limited.

Feline Leprosy

Fair for syndrome 2, especially if lesions are amenable to surgical excision. For syndrome 1, prognosis is guarded to poor.

Canine Leproid Granuloma

Prognosis is good with surgical excision.

 MISCELLANEOUS

ZOONOTIC POTENTIAL

• Tuberculosis—affected domestic pets are possible serious zoonotic threats to owners; public health authorities should be notified of any antemortem or postmortem diagnosis (may be required by law); do not attempt treatment without concurrence of public health authorities.
• *M. tuberculosis*—greatest potential for zoonosis, especially with draining cutaneous lesions
• Disease transmission from dogs and cats to humans—very rarely recorded; in recent outbreaks of tuberculosis in cats, no such case was documented.

ABBREVIATIONS

• AM = Atypical mycobacteriosis
• DMSO = dimethyl sulfoxide
• DNA = deoxyribonucleic acid
• FL = feline leprosy
• PCR = polymerase chain reaction
• TB = tuberculosis
• ZN = Ziehl-Neelsen acid-fast stain

Suggested Reading

Greene CE. Mycobacterial Infections. In: Greene CE, ed. Infectious diseases of the dog and cat. Philadelphia: Saunders, 1998: 313–325.
Malik R, Hughes MS, James G et al. Feline leprosy: Two different clinical syndromes. J Fel Med Surg 2002;4:43–59.
Author Carol Foil
Consulting Editor Stephen C. Barr

MYCOPLASMOSIS

 **BASICS**

DEFINITION
• Class Mollicutes (Latin, *mollis,* "soft"; *cutis,* "skin"); > 80 genera; three families: myco-plasmas, T-mycoplasmas or ureaplasmas, and acholeplasmas
• Smallest (0.2–0.3 μm) and simplest procaryotic cells capable of self-replication
• Fastidious, facultative anaerobic, gram-negative rods
• Lack a cell wall; thus plastic, highly pleo-morphic, and sensitive to lysis by osmotic shock, detergents, alcohols, and specific anti-body plus complement; enclosed by a trilayered cell membrane built of amphipathic lipids (phospholipids, glycolipids, lipoglycans, sterols) and proteins; most require sterols for growth.
• Different from wall-defective or wall-less L-form bacteria, which can revert to the normal cell wall strain
• Reproduce by binary fission; genome replication not necessarily synchronized with cell division, resulting in budding forms and chains of beads
• Ubiquitous in nature as parasites, commensals, or saprophytes in animals, plants, and insects; many are pathogens of humans, animals, plants, and insects.

PATHOPHYSIOLOGY
• Often part of the resident flora as commensals on mucous membranes of the upper respiratory, digestive, and genital tracts; pathogenicity and role in disease often controversial
• Species show considerable host specificity
• Mechanisms by which disease is caused are poorly understood.
• Some species attach to cells by specific receptors; small size and plastic nature enable them to adapt to the shape and contours of host cell surfaces.
• Intimate contact with host cells—necessary for assimilation of vital nutrients and growth factors (e.g., nucleic acid precursors), which organism cannot synthesize; along with the tendency of exogenous proteins to bind to mycoplasmal membrane may allow organism to evade the host's immune response; may incorporate host cell antigen onto myco-plasma membrane (capping) because lack of cell wall; conversely, mycoplasmal protein antigen may become incorporated onto surface of host cell, thereby involving host cell in deleterious immunologic reactions intended against the organism.
• Products produced during growth—capsular carbohydrate, hemolysins, proteolytic enzymes, ammonia, and endonucleases; accumulation of mycoplasma metabolites (i.e., H_2O_2, NH_3) may contribute to cytopathic effects and tissue damage; cytotoxic glycoproteins and proteins have been isolated from the membranes of several species.
• Immune response—predominantly humoral; as with bacterial infections, IgM and IgA are first antibodies to appear, followed by IgG.
• Fibrinous exudate accompanying infections—protects organism from antibodies and anti-microbial drugs; contributes to chronicity
• Secondary bacterial invaders—common (e.g., attachment to respiratory tract cells results in destruction of cilia, which predisposes patient to secondary bacterial infection)

SYSTEMS AFFECTED
Dogs
• Respiratory—pneumonia and upper respiratory infections; caused by *M. cynos;* associated with *M. canis, M. spumans, M. edwardii, M. feliminutum, M. gateae,* and *M. bovigenitalium*
• Renal/Urologic—urinary and genital tract infections (e.g., balanoposthitis, urethritis, prostatitis, cystitis, nephritis, vaginitis, endometritis); caused by *M. canis* and *M. spumans*
• Reproductive—mycoplasma and ureaplasma; associated with infertility, early embryonic death, abortion, stillbirths or weak newborns, and neonatal mortality
• Musculoskeletal—arthritis; from *M. spumans*
• Gastrointestinal—associated with colitis
Cats
• Ophthalmic—conjunctivitis; associated with *M. felis* (5%–25%)
• Respiratory—pneumonia, associated with *M. gateae, M. feliminutum,* and *M. felis;* upper respiratory infections, associated with *M. felis*
• Musculoskeletal—chronic fibrinopurulent polyarthritis and tenosynovitis; associated with *M. gateae* and unspecified mycoplasmal organisms
• Renal/Urologic—urinary tract infections
• Reproductive—abortions and fetal deaths; associated with *M. gateae* and ureaplasmas
• Skin/Exocrine—chronic cutaneous abscesses

GENETICS
N/A

INCIDENCE/PREVALENCE
• Frequent inhabitants of mucosal membranes; *M. gateae* and/or *M. felis* found in oral cavity or urogenital tract of 70%–80% of healthy cats
• Rate of isolation in diseased dogs much higher than in normal dogs (e.g., lung, uterus, prepuce)

GEOGRAPHIC DISTRIBUTION
Ubiquitous

SIGNALMENT

Species
Dogs and cats

Breed Predilections
None

Mean Age and Range
All ages

Predominant Sex
None

SIGNS

General Comments
Pathogenic role controversial

Historical Findings
• Polyarthritis—chronic intermittent lameness; reluctance to move; joint pain
• Fever
• Malaise
• Conjunctivitis—unilateral or bilateral

Physical Examination Findings
• Polyarthritis—diffuse limb edema; joint swelling; pain
• Conjunctivitis—blepharospasm; chemosis; conjunctival hyperemia; epiphora; and serous or purulent ocular discharge
• Mild rhinitis—sneezing

CAUSES
• Mycoplasma flora of dogs—*M. canis, M. spumans, M. maculosum, M. edwardii, M. cynos, M. molare, M. opalescens, M. feliminutum, M. gateae, M. arginini, M. bovigenitalium, Acholeplasma laidlawii,* and ureaplasmas
• Mycoplasma flora of cats—*M. felis, M. gateae, M. feliminutum, M. arginini, M. pulmonis, M. arthritidis, M. gallisepticum, Acholeplasma laidlawi,* and ureaplasmas

RISK FACTORS
• Commensals—occasionally cause systemic infection associated with immunodeficiency, immunosuppression, or cancer
• Impaired resistance of the host—may allow organism to cross the mucosal barrier and disseminate
• Organism may be opportunistic—one factor in a multifactorial causal complex (e.g., impaired pulmonary clearance from viral infection may allow organism to establish infection in lungs as secondary opportunistic pathogen)
• Predisposing factors—stresses (e.g., reproductive problems associated with overcrowded operations) and other factors (e.g., urinary tumors and urinary calculi)
• Rate of isolation of organism in diseased dogs much higher than in normal dogs

DIAGNOSIS

DIFFERENTIAL DIAGNOSIS
• Upper respiratory infection (dogs and cats)—viruses (parainfluenza virus, canine distemper, herpesvirus, feline calcivirus, reovirus); *Chlamydia psittaci;* bacteria (*Bordetella bronchiseptica,* staphylococci, streptococci, coliforms)
• Urinary tract infection (dogs and cats)—bacteria (staphylococci, streptococci, coliforms); fungus (*Candida*); parasites
• Infertility, early embryonic death, abortion, stillbirths or weak newborns, and neonatal mortality (dogs)—bacteria (*Brucella, Salmonella, Campylobacter, E. coli,* streptococcus); viruses (canine herpesvirus, canine distemper, canine adenovirus); *Toxoplasma gondii,* endocrinopathies (progesterone deficiency, hypothyroidism)
• Prostatitis (dogs)—bacteria (*E. coli, Brucella canis*); fungi (*Blastomyces, Cryptococcus*)
• Arthritis (dogs and cats)—immune-mediated, bacteria (staphylococci, streptococci, coliforms, anaerobes); L-form bacteria; rickettsia (*Ehrlichia*); *Borrelia burgdorferi;* fungi (*Coccidioides, Cryptococcus, Blastomyces*); protozoa (*Leishmania*); viruses (feline calicivirus)
• Conjunctivitis (cats)—feline herpesvirus; feline calicivirus; feline reovirus; *Chlamydia psittaci;* bacteria

CBC/BIOCHEMISTRY/URINALYSIS

With Polyarthritis
• Mild anemia
• Neutrophilic leukocytosis
• Hypoalbuminemia
• Hypoglobulinemia
• Proteinuria, resulting from immune-complex glomerulonephritis

OTHER LABORATORY TESTS
• Serologic tests—complement fixation, agar gel immunodiffusion, ELISA; detect organism
• Difficult to demonstrate in and from tissues
• Extremely pleomorphic—in smears (e.g., conjunctival scrapings) seen as coccobacilli, coccal forms, ring forms, spirals, and filaments
• Stains—stain poorly (gram-negative); preferred: Giemsa or other Romanowsky stain
• Fluorescent antibody test—definitive diagnosis; isolate and identify or detect the organism in tissues; can submit cotton swabs placed in Hayflick broth medium or commercially available swabs; organisms fragile; refrigerate specimens and deliver to the laboratory within 48 hr; freeze to preserve longer.

IMAGING
Polyarthritis—no radiographic changes

DIAGNOSTIC PROCEDURES
• Polyarthritis—high numbers of nondegenerative neutrophils in synovial fluid
• Prostatic fluid—inflammatory cells with negative bacterial culture

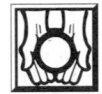

TREATMENT

APPROPRIATE HEALTH CARE
Outpatient

NURSING CARE
N/A

ACTIVITY
N/A

DIET
N/A

CLIENT EDUCATION
N/A

SURGICAL CONSIDERATIONS
N/A

MEDICATIONS

DRUG(S) OF CHOICE
• Sensitive to antibiotics that specifically inhibit synthesis in procaryotes
• Tetracyclines—22 mg/kg PO q8h
• Doxycycline—5mg/kg PO q12h
• Chloramphenicol—40–50 mg/kg IV, IM, SC, PO q8–12h
• No standardized procedure for in vitro antimicrobial susceptibility tests
• Topical antibiotic—conjunctivitis

CONTRAINDICATIONS
• Topical steroid ointments—improper use for conjunctivitis may prolong infection and predispose patient to corneal ulceration.
• Tetracyclines—avoid use in animals < 6 months of age.
• Tetracycline and chloramphenicol—avoid use in pregnant animals.

PRECAUTIONS
Sulfonamides and β-lactams—inhibit peptidoglycan synthesis; organism resistant because of lack of cell walls

POSSIBLE INTERACTIONS
N/A

ALTERNATIVE DRUG(S)
• Gentamicin
• Kanamycin
• Spectinomycin
• Spiramycin
• Tylosin
• Erythromycin
• Nitrofurans
• Fluoroquinolones

CONTRAINDICATIONS/POSSIBLE INTERACTIONS
N/A

FOLLOW-UP

PATIENT MONITORING
Treat for an extended period of time.

PREVENTION/AVOIDANCE
• No vaccines are available.
• Organism readily killed by drying, sunshine, and chemical disinfection

POSSIBLE COMPLICATIONS
N/A

EXPECTED COURSE AND PROGNOSIS
Prognosis good in animals with competent immune systems and given appropriate antibiotic therapy

MISCELLANEOUS

ASSOCIATED CONDITIONS
M. pneumoniae—infects respiratory tracts in humans worldwide; causes mycoplasmal pneumonia, bronchitis, or upper respiratory infection; usually self-limited; rarely fatal

AGE-RELATED FACTORS
Tetracyclines—avoid in animals < 6 months of age.

ZOONOTIC POTENTIAL
• Not generally considered zoonotic
• Reported development of suppurative mycoplasmal tenosynovitis in a veterinarian who was scratched by a cat being treated for colitis

PREGNANCY
Tetracycline and chloramphenicol—do not use in pregnant animals.

SYNONYMS
Pleuropneumonia-like organisms

ABBREVIATION
ELISA = enzyme-linked immunosorbent assay

Suggested Reading
Greene CE. Mycoplasmal, ureaplasmal, and L-form infections. In: Greene CE, ed. Infectious diseases of the dog and cat. Philadelphia: Saunders, 1998:174–178.
Author J. Paul Woods
Consulting Editor Stephen C. Barr

MYCOTOXICOSIS—AFLATOXIN

BASICS

OVERVIEW
- Result of a fungal toxin that affects the liver of dogs
- Rarely reported; possible in hot, humid climates where grain-based foods are exposed to moisture or if contaminated grains are used in production of feeds
- Clinical signs and lesions—dose and time dependent

SIGNALMENT
- Dogs
- Not reported in cats
- Young males and pregnant females—probably more susceptible

SIGNS
- Sudden death
- Anorexia
- Weight loss
- Icterus
- Ascites
- Hemorrhage

CAUSES & RISK FACTORS
- Grain-based feeds contaminated with *Aspergillus flavus, A. parasiticus,* or *Penicillium puberulum*
- Feeds exposed to elements with obvious mold spoilage
- Outside dogs at more risk

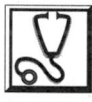

DIAGNOSIS

DIFFERENTIAL DIAGNOSIS
- Other causes of subacute to chronic liver disease and associated DIC
- No differentiating tests

CBC/BIOCHEMISTRY/URINALYSIS
- Thrombocytopenia
- High ALT and SAP
- Hypoalbuminemia
- High blood ammonia
- Hyperbilirubinemia

OTHER LABORATORY TESTS
- PT and APTT—prolonged; reduction in absolute concentrations and/or reduction in activated liver–produced clotting factors
- High FDP
- Hypofibrinogenemia

IMAGING
N/A

DIAGNOSTIC PROCEDURES
- Liver biopsy—not definitive

PATHOLOGIC FINDINGS
- Fatty change
- Icterus
- Ascites
- Mottled liver
- Biliary proliferation
- Hepatocellular necrosis
- Cholestasis
- Cholecystic edema

TREATMENT
- Aimed at reducing liver stress
- Diet—high-quality protein; dietary glucose source (e.g., corn syrup)
- Intravenous fluid therapy
- Possibly heparin and antithrombin III—with DIC

MEDICATIONS

DRUG(S)
No specific therapy

CONTRAINDICATIONS/ POSSIBLE INTERACTIONS
- Avoid drugs metabolized by the liver for activation.
- Do not expose patient to organophosphates or strong pyrethroid insecticides.

FOLLOW-UP

PREVENTION/AVOIDANCE
- Avoid using feedstuff that is obviously moldy.
- Store feed in clean dry area.
- Clean feed dispensers and feed bowls regularly.

POSSIBLE COMPLICATIONS
- With significant liver damage—persistent liver dysfunction
- Nephropathy—liver induced

EXPECTED COURSE AND PROGNOSIS
Prognosis—poor, even with treatment

MISCELLANEOUS

PREGNANCY
- Indirect effects on uterus
- Potentially teratogenic
- Pregnant animals may be more susceptible to toxicosis.

ABBREVIATIONS
- ALT = alanine aminotransferase
- APTT = activated partial thromboplastin time
- DIC = disseminated intravascular coagulation
- FDP = fibrin degradation products
- PT = prothrombin time
- SAP = serum alkaline phosphatase

Suggested Reading
Nicholson SS. Mycotoxicosis. In: Kirk RW, ed. Current veterinary therapy IX. Small animal practice. Philadelphia: Saunders, 1986:225–226.
Author George H. D'Andrea
Consulting Editor Gary D. Osweiler

BASICS

OVERVIEW

• DON (vomitoxin) is a toxin that can be produced by *Fusarium* fungi in grains such as wheat, oats, barley, and corn.
• The main source of exposure for dogs and cats is through the ingestion of pet food made with DON-contaminated grain.
• Although the exact mechanism is not well defined, ingestion of DON can cause feed refusal; it may have a central emetic effect that results in vomiting.

SIGNALMENT

• Experimental and anecdotal reports have shown evidence that dogs experience a sudden onset of feed refusal and/or vomiting following ingestion of food containing DON.
• Experimental studies indicate that cats have similar signs.

SIGNS

• Dogs and cats experience sudden onset of feed refusal and vomiting, which may result in weight loss.
• Onset of clinical signs can occur within minutes of exposure.
• The abnormal clinical signs may also resolve rapidly following removal of contaminated food.

CAUSES & RISK FACTORS

• Animals are exposed to DON when grain containing DON is mixed into their complete feed.
• Experimentally, food intake of beagles and Brittany dogs is reduced when DON concentrations in their food are $> 4.5 \pm 1.7$ mg DON/kg of food.
• Food intake in cats is reduced with DON concentrations $> 7.7 \pm 1.1$ mg/kg.
• Vomiting in dogs and cats is common when DON concentration in their food is > 8 mg/kg.

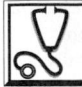 **DIAGNOSIS**

DIFFERENTIAL DIAGNOSIS

Numerous other causes of inappetence and vomiting—viral, bacterial, or parasitic infections; other toxicoses (e.g., exposure to organophosphates/carbamates or ethylene glycol); ingestion of poisonous plants causing irritation to the gastrointestinal tract; ingestion of lilies by cats, resulting in severe kidney failure; other medical conditions, such as pancreatitis, neoplasia, and inflammation of the gastrointestianl tract

CBC/BIOCHEMISTRY/URINALYSIS

These may be used to rule out other causes of inappetence and vomiting.

OTHER LABORATORY TESTS

N/A

IMAGING

May be used to rule out other causes of inappetence and vomiting

DIAGNOSTIC PROCEDURES

Analysis of pet food for DON by thin-layer chromatography or high-pressure liquid chromatography

PATHOLOGIC FINDINGS

There are no pathognomonic gross or microscopic lesions.

 TREATMENT

Removal of contaminated pet food should result in rapid cessation of vomiting and return to normal food intake.

 MEDICATIONS

DRUG(S)

N/A

 FOLLOW-UP

PATIENT MONITORING

• Monitor hydration and electrolytes if vomiting has been severe.
• Ensure animal returns to normal weight following removal of pet food containing DON.

PREVENTION/AVOIDANCE

Provide high-quality pet food free of DON.

EXPECTED COURSE AND PROGNOSIS

The prognosis is excellent following removal of feed containing DON.

 MISCELLANEOUS

AGE-RELATED FACTORS

In other, more well-studied species (e.g., swine), young animals are more severely affected and at lower concentrations of DON in the feed than are adults.

ABBREVIATION

DON = deoxynivalenol

Suggested Reading

Hughes DM, Gahl MJ, Graham CH, Grieb SL. Overt signs of toxicity to dogs and cats of dietary deoxynivalenol. J Anim Sci 1999;77:693–700.

Author Stephen B. Hooser
Consulting Editor Gary Osweiler

MYCOTOXICOSIS—TREMORGENIC TOXINS

BASICS

OVERVIEW
• Penitrem A—produced by the fungus *Penicillium crustosum* (and perhaps other *Penicillium* spp.); poisoning by this toxin has been reported in dogs ingesting moldy bread, cheese, and English walnuts
• Roquefortine—produced by *Penicillium roquefortii* (and perhaps other *Penicillium* spp.); has been reported to cause poisoning in dogs through ingestion of moldy cheese or decaying organic material (compost)

SIGNALMENT
Poisoning by penitrem A and roquefortine has been reported in dogs of various ages and breeds soon after the ingestion of moldy foods or compost.

SIGNS
• Moderate to severe muscle tremors and seizures—begin minutes to hours (2–4 hr in case reports) after ingestion of moldy food or compost
• Affected dogs may be hyperresponsive to external stimuli.
• Early signs—may include panting, hyperactivity, vomiting, ataxia, incoordination, weakness, and/or rigidity
• Prolonged muscle tremors or seizures—may lead to hyperthermia, hypoglycemia, dehydration, and anorexia
• Severe cases—may result in death
• Liver necrosis—has been reported experimentally

CAUSES & RISK FACTORS
Dogs (and potentially cats) are exposed to penitrem A and roquefortine when they ingest moldy food or decomposing organic matter (compost). Experimentally, doses of 0.125 mg/kg penitrem A produced tremors within 30 minutes. Doses of 0.5 mg/kg of penitrem A resulted in acute onset of tremors, severe liver necrosis, and death.

DIAGNOSIS

DIFFERENTIAL DIAGNOSIS
• Toxic causes of seizures—strychnine; insecticides (e.g., organophosphate, carbamate, organochlorine, nicotine, pyrethroid); metaldehyde; zinc phosphide; bromethaline; methylxanthines (theobromine and caffeine)
• Nontoxic causes of seizures—inflammation; congenital abnormal myelin formation; metabolic conditions (e.g., hepatic or uremic encephalopathy)

CBC/BIOCHEMISTRY/URINALYSIS
Perform CBC, biochemistry, and urinalysis to assess the patient's status and to help rule out other causes of tremors and seizures.

OTHER LABORATORY TESTS
N/A

IMAGING
N/A

DIAGNOSTIC PROCEDURES
• Thin-layer chromatography or high-pressure liquid chromatography—analysis of vomitus, stomach contents, and gastric lavage washings for penitrem A or roquefortine
• Bile analysis—reported to be of value

PATHOLOGIC FINDINGS
• There are no pathognomonic lesions associated with penitrem A or roquefortine toxicosis.
• High doses of penitrem A have been reported to cause severe liver damage experimentally.

TREATMENT
• Remove contaminated food or organic material.
• Induce vomiting (if patient is not at risk of aspirating vomitus) or institute gastric lavage followed by administration of activated charcoal.

MEDICATIONS

DRUG(S)
• Diazepam—to control seizures
• Barbiturates—if tremors and seizures cannot be controlled with diazepam
• Sodium bicarbonate—may be required if an acid–base imbalance exists
• Other symptomatic and supportive therapy—as indicated

CONTRAINDICATIONS/POSSIBLE INTERACTIONS
N/A

FOLLOW-UP

PATIENT MONITORING
Patients should be monitored for occurrence of tremors or seizures, hyperthermia, dehydration, acid–base imbalances, liver damage, and rhabdomyolysis.

PREVENTION/AVOIDANCE
Prevent animals from eating moldy food items, garbage, or compost.

POSSIBLE COMPLICATIONS
• Seizures—may not be controlled with diazepam
• Acid–base imbalances—may develop
• Hepatic damage and rhabdomyolysis—may occur
• Exposure can be fatal if lethal doses are consumed and are absorbed before gastro-intestinal decontamination and therapy are instituted.

EXPECTED COURSE AND PROGNOSIS
• Very good if aggressive therapy is instituted, the toxin is removed from the gastrointestinal tract, and the seizures are controlled with diazepam or barbiturates
• Recovery in most clinical cases is reported to be complete within 24–48 hr.
• In a few reported cases, signs of weakness, muscle rigidity, and incoordination were persistent and slowly resolved over 1–2 weeks.
• A few severe cases have been reported to be fatal.

MISCELLANEOUS

Suggested Reading
Puschner B. Mycotoxins. Vet Clin North Am Small Anim Pract 2002;32:409–419.
Author Stephen B. Hooser
Consulting Editor Gary Osweiler

BASICS

OVERVIEW
Characterized by alterations in the normal development and maturation of hematopoietic stem cells

SIGNALMENT
More common in cats than in dogs

SIGNS
• Pale mucous membranes
• Lethargy
• Weight loss
• Hepatosplenomegaly
• Peripheral lymphadenomegaly varies

CAUSES & RISK FACTORS
• Associated with FeLV infection in cats
• Bone marrow dysplasia—may be caused by ehrlichiosis and Rocky Mountain spotted fever
• Drugs (e.g., trimethoprim and sulfa combination, estrogen, Butazolidin, and cytotoxic anticancer agents)—may cause myelodysplasia

DIAGNOSIS

DIFFERENTIAL DIAGNOSIS
Differentiate from infectious causes and drug toxicity (see Causes & Risk Factors)

CBC/BIOCHEMISTRY/URINALYSIS
• Cytopenias
• Megaloblastic anemia
• Circulating, nucleated RBC
• Large, bizarre platelets
• Immature granulocytes with abnormal morphologic characteristics
• Monocytosis

OTHER LABORATORY TESTS
Examination of bone marrow aspirate and core biopsy—reveals ineffective erythropoiesis and granulopoiesis within a specimen with normal cellularity

IMAGING
N/A

DIAGNOSTIC PROCEDURES
Bone marrow biopsy

TREATMENT

• Nonspecific, unless a treatable cause is identified
• Intensive nursing care often necessary
• Supportive care—may require multiple blood transfusions and nutritional support

MEDICATIONS

DRUG(S)
Antibiotics—for secondary bacterial infection, if necessary

CONTRAINDICATIONS/POSSIBLE INTERACTIONS
N/A

FOLLOW-UP

• CBC and cytologic examination of bone marrow aspirate or biopsy—repeat to monitor progression of disease
• Transfuse as necessary.
• Possible complications—sepsis; hemorrhage; profound anemia
• Prognosis—guarded to poor

MISCELLANEOUS

ABBREVIATON
• FeLV = feline leukemia virus

Suggested Reading
Harvey JW. Myeloproliferative disorders in dogs and cats. Vet Clin North Am Small Anim Pract 1981;11:349–381.
Reagan WJ, DeNicola DB. Myeloproliferative and lymphoproliferative disorders. In: Morrison WB, ed. Cancer in dogs and cats: medical and surgical management. Baltimore: Williams & Wilkins, 1998:95–122.
Author Linda S. Fineman
Consulting Editor Wallace B. Morrison

MYELOMALACIA AND HEMATOMYELIA

 BASICS

OVERVIEW
• Acute, progressive, ischemic necrosis of the spinal cord after acute spinal cord trauma
• First appears at the site of injury; then progresses both cranially and caudally
• Death may be caused by respiratory paralysis if the intercostal and phrenic nerves are affected.

SIGNALMENT
• Any age or breed
• Because of the close association between acute type I disk herniation and myelomalacia, breeds predisposed to the former are more commonly affected.

SIGNS
• Acute paralysis from spinal injury—initial clinical sign
• Thoracolumbar injury—paralysis with exaggerated spinal reflexes in the pelvic limbs
• Pain perception—usually absent caudal to the lesion
• Spinal cord malacia—progresses to involve the lumbosacral spinal segments within 72 hr, causing pelvic limb areflexia and atonia, dilated anus, and flaccid, easily expressed urinary bladder; thoracic and cervical spinal cord segments may be involved 7–10 days after the initial insult.
• Subarachnoid hemorrhage secondary to necrosis of the microvasculature in the spinal cord—may cause hyperthermia and extreme meningeal pain

CAUSES & RISK FACTORS
• Type I disk disease
• Vertebral or spinal cord trauma

 DIAGNOSIS

DIFFERENTIAL DIAGNOSIS
• Cannot be differentiated from spinal trauma
• Diagnosis based on hind limb upper motor neuron paralysis that progresses to a lower motor neuron paralysis and a rostrally advancing line of analgesia

CBC/BIOCHEMISTRY/URINALYSIS
• Usually normal, initially
• Road accident—nonspecific abnormalities related to other organ injury
• After condition has developed, degenerative left shift caused by massive spinal cord necrosis may occur.

OTHER LABORATORY TESTS
N/A

IMAGING
• Spinal survey radiography—evidence of herniated disk; vertebral fracture or luxation
• Myelogram—cord compression; edema

DIAGNOSTIC PROCEDURES
Cerebellomedullary cistern CSF—results unspecific; relate to stage of development of clinical ascending/descending myelomalacia; neutrophilic pleocytosis is often present.

 TREATMENT

• None to reverse spinal cord damage
• Agents useful for treating the secondary effects of spinal cord trauma (e.g., methylprednisolone sodium succinate and 21-aminosteroid compounds)—not evaluated for myelomalacia; may be useful in halting progression

 MEDICATIONS

DRUG(S)
• If treatment initiated within 8 hr of trauma, methylprednisolone sodium succinate—30 mg/kg IV initially; follow with 15 mg/kg IV 2 and 6 hr after the initial dose; follow with 2.4 mg/kg/hr for 42 hr
• Histamine H_2-blocker (e.g., cimetidine), sucralfate, or misoprostol—protect against gastrointestinal ulcers in patients receiving corticosteroids

CONTRAINDICATIONS/POSSIBLE INTERACTIONS
• Methylprednisolone therapy maybe harmful if administered 8 hr or longer after trauma;
• Rise in incidence of infection associated with methylprednisolone administration in humans

 FOLLOW-UP

• In a few patients, condition progresses only caudally; paralysis is permanent, but respiratory compromise does not occur.
• Reported after decompressive laminectomy, suggesting that surgery does not prevent its occurrence

 MISCELLANEOUS

ABBREVIATION
CSF = cerebrospinal fluid

Suggested Reading
Olby N. Current concepts in the management of acute spinal cord injury. J Vet Intern Med 1999;13:399–407.
Author Karen Dyer Inzana
Consulting editor Joane M. Parent

BASICS

OVERVIEW
• Neoplastic proliferation of nonlymphoid cell lines of bone marrow origin
• Believed to represent a spectrum of disorders in which the stem cell involved is a hematopoietic precursor capable of differentiating into all blood cell types except lymphocytes
• Leukemia (acute and chronic)—may develop from granulocytic, monocytic, erythrocytic, and megakaryocytic cell lines

SIGNALMENT
Dogs and cats

SIGNS
• Pale mucous membranes
• Lethargy
• Weight loss
• Hepatosplenomegaly
• Peripheral lymphadenomegaly—occasionally

CAUSES & RISK FACTORS
• Cats—most commonly associated with FeLV infection; when recovering from panleukopenia or hemobartonellosis, may be a relatively higher risk of developing a mutant cell line induced by FeLV
• Dogs—unknown

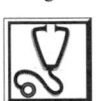

DIAGNOSIS

DIFFERENTIAL DIAGNOSIS
• Acute lymphocytic leukemia—usually differentiated by special staining techniques
• Leukemoid response
• Other causes of eosinophilia—parasitism; allergic disease; eosinophilic gastroenteritis; mast cell neoplasia; differentiate from eosinophilic leukemia

• Severe hemolytic anemia must be differentiated from acute erythroleukemia.

CBC/BIOCHEMISTRY/URINALYSIS
• Severe, nonregenerative anemia
• Circulating nucleated RBCs
• Megaloblastic erythrocytes
• Leukocytosis or leukopenia
• Thrombocytopenia with abnormal platelet morphology

OTHER LABORATORY TESTS
• Examination of bone marrow aspirate or core biopsy—reveals hypercellular bone marrow with abnormal morphology in all cell lines; neoplastic proliferation or absence of one cell line
• Immunohistochemical or other special stain—may be necessary to determine cell type

IMAGING
Plain radiographs and ultrasound—hepatomegaly and splenomegaly common

DIAGNOSTIC PROCEDURES
Examination of bone marrow aspirate or core biopsy

TREATMENT
• Outpatient or inpatient
• Supportive care—blood transfusions and fluid administration to correct dehydration

MEDICATIONS

DRUG(S)
• Little information available in the literature regarding treatment
• Cytosine arabinoside—may be used; 100 mg/m^2 SC divided q12h 4 days per week

• Hydroxyurea—30–45 mg/kg q24h for 7–10 days; then 30–45 mg/kg q48h; essentially, titrate dosage to patient response
• Antibiotics—may be indicated to combat secondary infection

CONTRAINDICATIONS/POSSIBLE INTERACTIONS
Chemotherapy can be toxic; seek advice before treatment if unfamiliar with cytotoxic drugs.

FOLLOW-UP
• CBC and examination of bone marrow aspirate—determine response to treatment and progression of disease.
• Prognosis—grave; usually rapid and fatal clinical course

MISCELLANEOUS

PREGNANCY
Chemotherapy drugs are contraindicated in pregnant animals

ABBREVIATION
FeLV = feline leukemia virus

Suggested Reading
Hamilton TA. The leukemias. In: Morrison WB, ed. Cancer in dogs and cats: medical and surgical management. Baltimore: Williams & Wilkins, 1998:721–729.
Reagan WJ, DeNicola DB. Myeloproliferative and lymphoproliferative disorders. In: Morrison WB, ed. Cancer in dogs and cats: medical and surgical management. Baltimore: Williams & Wilkins, 1998:95–122.
Author Linda S. Fineman
Consulting Editor Wallace B. Morrison

MYOCARDIAL INFARCTION

BASICS

OVERVIEW
• Rapid development of myocardial necrosis resulting from sustained, complete reduction of blood flow to a portion of the myocardium, caused by thrombus formation • Uncommon as a naturally occurring disease in dogs • Microscopic intramural myocardial infarctions and focal areas of myocardial fibrosis are common in dogs with acquired cardiovascular disease. • Consistent ECG characteristics of spontaneous myocardial infarction are not well characterized in dogs and cats.

SIGNALMENT
Rare in dogs and cats

SIGNS

Historical Findings
• Lethargy • Anorexia • Weakness • Dyspnea • Collapse • Vomiting • Obesity • Unexpected death

Physical Examination Findings
• Lameness • Tachycardia • Heart murmur • Cardiac rhythm disturbances • Low-grade fever

CAUSES AND RISK FACTORS
• Atherosclerosis and coronary artery disease • Nephrotic syndrome • Vasculitis • Hypothyroidism • Bacterial endocarditis • Neoplasia • Septicemia • Intramural coronary arteriosclerosis in old dogs • Subvalvular aortic stenosis

Cats
• Cardiomyopathy • Thromboembolism

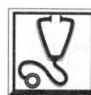

DIAGNOSIS
Generally presumptive, based on acute onset of signs in a patient with predisposing factors and consistent ECG changes

DIFFERENTIAL DIAGNOSIS

Other Causes of S-T Segment Changes
• Normal variation • Myocardial ischemia/hypoxia • Hyper-, hypokalemia • Digitalis toxicity • Trauma to the heart • Pericarditis • Artifact—wandering baseline

Other Causes of Weakness and Collapse
• Trauma • Neurologic disease • Thromboembolism • Pericardial effusion • Arrhythmia

CBC/BIOCHEMISTRY/URINALYSIS
• Mild leukocytosis • High liver enzymes • Hyperlipidemia—if animal is hypothyroid • High amylase • High creatine kinase and cardiac isoenzymes

OTHER LABORATORY TESTS
Low T_4 and T_3

IMAGING
• Echocardiography—2-D and M-mode echocardiography useful in evaluating wall motion abnormalities and overall left ventricular function • Angiocardiography—rarely, if ever, used in clinical veterinary cardiology

DIAGNOSTIC PROCEDURES

Electrocardiographic Findings
• Sudden deviation of the ST segment • Tall peaked T waves—first few hours • Sudden development of Q waves or a change in direction of the T wave • Axis shift of the frontal plane • Low-voltage QRS complexes • Sudden development of bundle branch block or heart block • Sudden onset of ventricular arrhythmias because of myocardial ischemia • Sloppy "R" wave descent may be associated with intramural myocardial infarction.

TREATMENT
• Direct at the underlying disorder; likewise the symptomatic therapy (e.g., congestive heart failure [CHF]) • Must identify and immediately treat life-threatening arrhythmias • Restrict activity

MEDICATIONS

DRUG(S)
• Thrombolytic agents, IV—(e.g., streptokinase); cost prohibitive and lack of experience in veterinary medicine with dosage and use • Lidocaine for ventricular arrhythmias • β-Blockers—use cautiously with dilated cardiomyopathy because of possible development of low-output CHF. • Propranolol—dogs, 0.2–1.0 mg/kg PO q8h; cats, 2.5–5 mg/cat PO q8–12h • Atenolol—dogs, 0.25–1.0 mg/kg PO q12–24h; cats, 6.25–12.5 mg PO q24h • Antithrombotic agents (e.g., warfarin, heparin, and aspirin)

FOLLOW-UP
• Determined by clinical status and diagnosis of underlying disorder • Monitor anticoagulated patient; CBC and bleeding profiles, including fibrinogen

MISCELLANEOUS

ABBREVIATON
ECG = electrocardiogram

Suggested Reading
Driehuys E, Van Winkle TJ, Sammarco CD, Drobatz KJ. Myocardial infarction in dogs and cats: 37 cases (1985–1994). JAVMA 1998;213:1444–1448.

Kidd L, Stepien RL, Amoheim DP. Clinical findings and coronary artery disease in dogs and cats with acute & subacute myocardial necrosis: 28 cases. J Am Anim Hosp Assoc 2000;36:199–208.

Liu SK, Fox PR. Cardiovascular pathology. In: Fox PR, Sisson D, Moise NS, eds. Canine and feline cardiology. 2nd ed. Philadelphia: Saunders, 1999:837–838.

Author Larry P. Tilley

Consulting Editors Larry P. Tilley and Francis W. K. Smith, Jr.

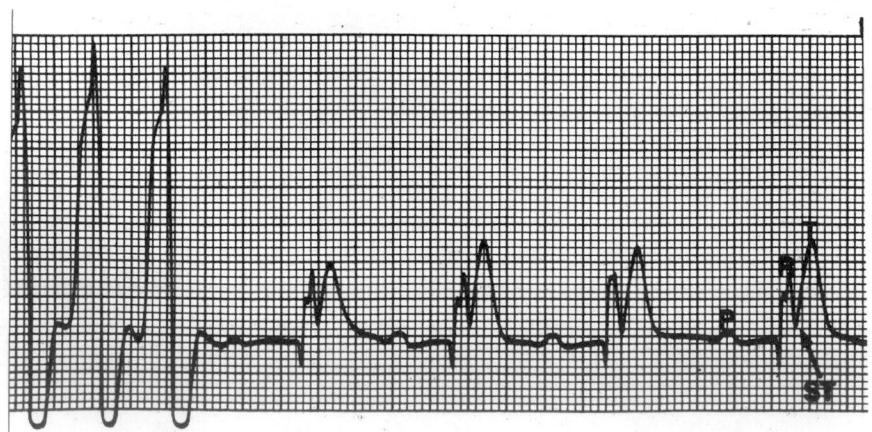

Transmural infarction of the left ventricle in a dog with arteriosclerosis and hypothyroidism. The first three rapid successive complexes represent ventricular tachycardia. The sinus rhythm that follows illustrates small complexes, marked elevation of the S-T segment, and first degree AV block (prolonged P-R interval). (From: Tilley LP. Essentials of canine and feline electrocardiography. 3rd ed. Baltimore: Lippincott Williams & Wilkins, 1992, with permission).

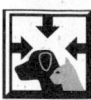

BASICS

OVERVIEW
• Rare—0.19% incidence
• Reported types—hemangiosarcoma, hemangioma, fibrosarcoma, fibroma, lymphosarcoma, myxosarcoma, myxoma, rhabdomyosarcoma, neurofibroma, granular cell tumor, and osteosarcoma

SIGNALMENT
• Dogs and cats
• More common in old animals

SIGNS
• Depend on location and infiltration
• May include—sudden collapse caused by cardiac arrhythmia or signs of heart failure caused by pericardial effusion, venous obstruction, myodynamic failure, or valvular obstruction

CAUSES & RISK FACTORS
Unknown

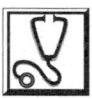

DIAGNOSIS

DIFFERENTIAL DIAGNOSIS
• Idiopathic pericardial effusion
• Pericarditis
• Cardiomyopathy
• Congestive heart failure
• Valvular insufficiency
• Heart base tumor

CBC/BIOCHEMISTRY/URINALYSIS
Anemia in a few patients

OTHER LABORATORY TESTS
N/A

IMAGING
• Thoracic radiography—evaluate heart size and shape.
• Echocardiography—assess myocardial texture and see mass.

DIAGNOSTIC PROCEDURES
• Electrocardiography—determine presence of arrhythmia
• Surgical biopsy

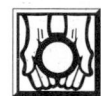

TREATMENT
• Inpatient—restrict activity until recovered from surgery
• Surgical excision—may be curative for benign tumors
• Pericardiectomy—may provide relief from cardiac tamponade
• Chemotherapy—probably most effective after surgical excision
• Alert the client to the potential for sudden death.

MEDICATIONS

DRUG(S)
• Lidocaine infusion (25–75 μg/kg/min) or procainamide (8–20 mg/kg PO q8h)—treat symptomatic ventricular premature contractions and ventricular tachycardia
• Atenolol (cats: 6.25–12.5 mg/cat PO q12h; dogs: 0.25–1.0 mg/kg PO q12–24h) or propranolol (dogs: 0.2–1.0 mg/kg PO q8h) or diltiazem (1–1.5 mg/kg PO q8h)—treat paroxysmal supraventricular tachycardia
• Combination chemotherapy—doxorubicin (30 mg/m² every 3 weeks), cyclophosphamide (100–150 mg/m² every 3 weeks), and

vincristine (0.7 mg/m² weeks 2 and 3); used successfully to treat cardiac hemangiosarcoma

CONTRAINDICATIONS/POSSIBLE INTERACTIONS
Chemotherapy may have gastrointestinal, bone marrow, cardiac, and other toxicities; seek advice before treatment if you are unfamiliar with cytotoxic drugs.

FOLLOW-UP
• Serial cardiac ultrasonography—monitor response to treatment and doxorubicin toxicity
• Thoracic radiography—monitor effusion and metastasis
• CBC and platelet count—monitor myelosuppression caused by chemotherapy
• Prognosis—guarded to poor

MISCELLANEOUS

PREGNANCY
Chemotherapy should not be used in pregnant animals.

Suggested Reading
deMadron NE, Helfand SC, Stebbins KE. Use of chemotherapy for treatment of cardiac hemangiosarcoma in a dog. J Am Vet Med Assoc 1987;190:887–891.
Morrison WB. Nonpulmonary intrathoracic cancer. In: Morrison WB, ed. Cancer in dogs and cats: medical and surgical management. Jackson, Wyoming: Teton NewMedia, 2002:513–526.
Author Terrance A. Hamilton
Consulting Editor Wallace B. Morrison

MYOCARDITIS

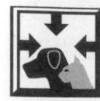 BASICS

DEFINITION
• Inflammation of the heart muscle, often caused by infectious agents affecting the myocytes, interstitium, vascular elements, or pericardium.
• Viral, bacterial, rickettsial, fungal, and protozoal diseases are all associated with myocardial inflammation (i.e., myocarditis).
• Pharmacologic agents (e.g., doxorubicin) can also be causative.

PATHOPHYSIOLOGY
• Mechanisms—toxin production, direct invasion of myocardial tissue, and immune-mediated myocardial damage; vasculitis associated with systemic disease; allergic reactions and direct myocyte damage caused by pharmacologic agents. Protozoa (e.g., *Trypanosoma cruzi*) lead to granulomatous myocarditis; viral myocarditis is associated with cell-mediated immunologic reactions.
• Myocardial involvement may be focal or diffuse. Clinical manifestations depend on the extent of the lesions. Diffuse, severe involvement may lead to global myocardial damage and CHF; discrete lesions involving the conduction system may cause profound arrhythmias.

SYSTEMS AFFECTED
• Systemic organ involvement depends on the causative agent.
• Cardiovascular—myocardial failure or arrhythmias
• Respiratory—if pulmonary edema develops

GENETICS
N/A

INCIDENCE/PREVALENCE
• Viral myocarditis (e.g., parvovirus, distemper virus, and herpesvirus)—rare; very young puppies in their first months of life may be profoundly affected; in a second form (parvoviral), dilated cardiomyopathy develops in dogs 5–6 months of age that were infected during their first weeks of life.
• Protozoal myocarditis associated with *T. cruzi* (i.e., Chagas' disease) reported in dogs < 2 years old from the southeastern United States. Males are more commonly affected than females. *Toxoplasma gondii* occasionally causes myocarditis. Immunosuppressed animals (e.g., cats with feline leukemia virus) are at high risk. *Hepatozoon canis* reported in dogs living in the Texas Gulf.
• Fungal myocarditis—primarily seen in association with systemic fungal infection; myocardial involvement varies with regional prevalence and prevalence of the systemic manifestation.

• Bacterial myocarditis—can be caused by generalized sepsis and bacteremia
• Doxorubicin cardiotoxicity—reported in dogs receiving cumulative doses = 150–240 mg/m^2
• Spirochetal myocarditis associated with *Borrelia burgdorferi*—documented in 10% of humans with Lyme disease; incidence and prevalence in dogs not well documented

GEOGRAPHIC DISTRIBUTION
Suspect myocarditis associated with infectious agents wherever these diseases are endemic (see above).

SIGNALMENT
Species
Dogs and cats

Breed Predilections
N/A

Mean Age and Range
Viral myocarditis—seen primarily in animals < 1 year of age

Predominant Sex
N/A

SIGNS
General Comments
• Related to the degree and location of myocardial involvement
• Range from those of arrhythmias to those of CHF
• Onset of cardiac dysfunction in association with systemic illness or the use of specific pharmacologic agents is often the hallmark of myocarditis.

Historical Findings
• Coughing, exercise intolerance, dyspnea—associated with CHF
• Syncope and weakness—associated with arrhythmias
• Concurrent systemic manifestations—often seen with infective myocarditis
• Use of antineoplastic or other pharmacologic agents—associated with the onset of cardiac dysfunction

Physical Examination Findings
• Gallop rhythm or murmur may be found—depends on the nature of the myocardial damage
• Arrhythmias—may be auscultated.
• Fever—common in patients with active infection associated with myocarditis

CAUSES
• Virus (e.g., parvovirus, distemper virus, herpesvirus)
• Protozoa (e.g., *T. cruzi, T. gondii,* and *H. canis*)
• Bacteria
• Fungus (e.g., *Cryptococcus neoformans, Coccidioides immitis,* and *Aspergillus terreus*)
• Algae (e.g., *Prototheca* spp.)
• Doxorubicin

RISK FACTORS
• Exposure to infectious agents
• Use of myocardiotoxic compounds
• Immunosuppression
• Debilitating diseases

 DIAGNOSIS

DIFFERENTIAL DIAGNOSIS
• Always consider preexisting heart disease, including congenital defects, cardiomyopathy, and acquired valvular disease.
• History of a heart murmur or the presence of arrhythmias before onset of systemic illness helps differentiate from other diseases.
• Extracardiac organ involvement and identification of infectious agents may aid in the diagnosis.

CBC/BIOCHEMISTRY/URINALYSIS
Abnormalities—vary, depending on organ involvement

OTHER LABORATORY TESTS
Serologic Tests to Help Identify an Infectious Agent
• Cytologic examination of pericardial, pleural, and peritoneal effusions to identify the infectious organism
• Blood culture to diagnose bacteremia

IMAGING
Thoracic Radiographic Findings
• Cardiac silhouette may appear large or normal depending on the extent of involvement.
• Pulmonary edema, congestion, or pleural effusion in patients with CHF
• Globoid heart in some animals with pericardial effusion
• Pulmonary granuloma may be found in animals with granulomatous myocardial infection.

Echocardiographic Findings
• Reflect the extent of myocardial damage; may be normal if lesions are small or primarily affect the conduction system
• Pericardial effusion in some patients; pericardium may appear thickened and hyperechoic, depending on the extent of pericardial involvement.
• Myocardium may appear mottled with patchy areas of hyperechogenicity caused by myocardial inflammation, fibrosis, or granulomas.
• Regional dyskinesis caused by focal involvement may be appreciated on 2-D echocardiography.

Angiography
• Because of the quality and noninvasive nature of echocardiography, cardiac catheterization is rarely indicated for the diagnosis.

• May use angiography to detect specific chamber involvement or pericardial effusion, if echocardiography is not available

DIAGNOSTIC PROCEDURES

Electrocardiographic Findings
• LV, LA, RV, or RA enlargement patterns in some patients—depending on the extent of chamber involvement
• Arrhythmias—include both atrial and ventricular tachyarrhythmias
• Differentiate right and left bundle branch blocks and hemiblocks from ventricular enlargement patterns.
• Atrioventricular nodal conduction disturbances in some patients

Endomyocardial Biopsy
Useful for detection of infectious agents (e.g., protozoa, fungal elements) or inflammatory cell infiltrates

Pericardiocentesis
• Alleviates pericardial effusion
• Submit fluid for cytologic examination and possible bacterial culture.

Holter Monitor Study
• To detect arrhythmias, frequency and severity
• To monitor antiarrhythmic therapy

Pathologic Findings
• Dilated cardiac chambers with patchy areas of hyperemia, necrosis, or fibrosis
• Granulomas seen grossly in some patients
• Microscopic examination of the myocardium or pericardium may reveal inflammatory cells (e.g., lymphocytes, plasma cells, and macrophages), patchy fibrosis, or the infectious agents themselves.
• Myofiber dropout—seen in patients with doxorubicin toxicity

TREATMENT

APPROPRIATE HEALTH CARE
• Hospitalize patients with CHF for initial medical management.
• Hospitalize patients with severe ventricular arrhythmias for initial antiarrhythmic therapy.
• Hospitalize patients with severe systemic manifestations for aggressive medical therapy.

NURSING CARE
N/A

ACTIVITY
Restricted

DIET
Sodium restriction if CHF

CLIENT EDUCATION
• Cardiac manifestations may persist even with resolution of systemic illness.
• Certain arrhythmias (i.e., ventricular tachyarrhythmias) may predispose to sudden death.
• Antemortem diagnosis may be difficult.
• Some infectious agents may pose a public health risk.

SURGICAL CONSIDERATIONS
Complete atrioventricular block may require pacemaker implantation.

MEDICATIONS

DRUG(S) OF CHOICE
• If a specific etiologic agent is identified, direct treatment against it.
• Tailor antiarrhythmic therapy to the predominant arrhythmia.
• Treat CHF with furosemide (1–2 mg/kg PO q6–12h), enalapril (0.25–0.5 mg/kg PO q12–24h), and digoxin (0.22 mg/m^2 PO q12h)

CONTRAINDICATIONS
Public health considerations may preclude treatment of some infectious diseases (i.e., *T. cruzi*).

PRECAUTIONS
• All antiarrhythmic drugs have proarrhythmic properties and should be monitored closely.
• Systemic organ involvement (e.g., renal involvement) may necessitate modifying drug dosages or use of various cardiac drugs; monitor systemic function carefully.

POSSIBLE INTERACTIONS
N/A

ALTERNATIVE DRUG(S)
N/A

FOLLOW-UP

PATIENT MONITORING
• Antiarrhythmic therapy—frequent auscultation and ECG
• Serologic titers when appropriate
• Auscultation and follow-up radiographs—treatment of CHF
• Hemograms and serum biochemical analysis—systemic effects

PREVENTION/AVOIDANCE
• Avoid breeding animals with a poor vaccination history.
• Avoid endemic areas if possible.
• Monitor ECG and echocardiogram when using doxorubicin.

EXPECTED COURSE AND PROGNOSIS
• Depend on the extent and severity of myocardial involvement
• Many systemic fungal and protozoal diseases do not respond well to medical management.
• Patients with extensive myocardial inflammation, degeneration, and signs of CHF—very poor prognosis
• Patients with isolated, controllable arrhythmias—good prognosis if the underlying cause can be treated successfully

MISCELLANEOUS

ASSOCIATED CONDITIONS
Often accompanies systemic illness

AGE-RELATED FACTORS
Viral myocarditis—most often seen in animals < 1 year old

ZOONOTIC POTENTIAL
• Varies with infectious agent involved
• May be high with protozoal and mycotic infections

PREGNANCY
Some viral diseases (e.g., canine herpesvirus and parvovirus) have been passed to the fetus during pregnancy.

SYNONYMS
N/A

SEE ALSO
• Infectious diseases listed under causes
• Ventricular premature complexes
• Ventricular tachycardia

ABBREVIATIONS
• CHF = congestive heart failure
• ECG = electrocardiogram
• LA = left atrium
• LV = left ventricle
• RA = right atrium
• RV = right ventricle

Suggested Reading
Liu SK, Fox PR. Cardiovascular pathology. In: Fox PR, Sisson D, Moise NS, eds. Textbook of canine and feline cardiology. 2nd ed. Philadelphia: Saunders, 1999: 817–844.
Wynne J, Braunwald E. The cardiomyopathies and myocarditides In: Braunwald E, ed. Heart disease: a textbook of cardiovascular medicine. 5th ed. Philadelphia: Saunders, 1997:1404–1463.
Author Michael B. Lesser
Consulting Editors Larry P. Tilley and Francis W. K. Smith, Jr.

MYOCLONUS

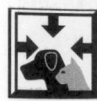 **BASICS**

OVERVIEW
• A coarse, repetitive, involuntary, and rhythmic contraction of a portion of a muscle, entire muscle, or group of muscles
• May affect one or several muscle groups
• May occur synchronously or asynchronously in several areas
• A CNS dysfunction involving the lower motor neurons and interneurons at the segmental level of the spinal cord or the brain stem
• A clinical sign; although reported most commonly with canine distemper virus infection, may be caused by other encephalitides and degenerative processes affecting motor neurons

SIGNALMENT

Acquired
• Dogs and rarely cats
• No breed, sex, or age predispositions

Congenital
• Dogs
• Reflex myoclonus—Labrador retrievers and Dalmatians; develops in the first few weeks of life
• Neonatal myoclonus of the paravertebral muscles—silky terriers; caused by spongy degeneration

SIGNS

Historical Findings
• With distemper—observed after a bout of gastrointestinal signs, cough, and/or ocular or nasal purulent discharge; persists at rest and even during sleep or light anesthesia; consistent frequency within a given patient; distemper diagnosis may precede the myoclonus by months to years; occurs more frequently in chronic phase of distemper
• With familial reflex—observed when the patient starts to walk; intermittent muscle contractions induced by auditory or tactile stimulus and by exercise; involves all limbs, neck, and head (e.g., the facial and masticatory muscles); patient unable to rise without assistance

Physical Examination Findings
• Masticatory and appendicular muscles—most frequently affected with distemper-induced disease; may be paresis of the affected limb
• May see other signs suggesting distemper (e.g., hard pads, ocular and nasal purulent discharge, and chorioretinitis)
• Neurologic deficits suggesting multifocal lesions in some patients
• The patient may be otherwise healthy.

CAUSES & RISK FACTORS

Congenital
• Familial in Labrador retrievers
• Spongy degeneration in silky terriers
• Other congenital anomalies of unknown cause

Acquired
• Canine distemper virus—most frequent cause; the only CNS disease repeatedly associated with myoclonus in dogs; unvaccinated dogs are at risk.
• Encephalitis of any cause—dogs and cats
• Degenerative disease—especially spongy degeneration
• Described in a dog with lead poisoning

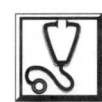 **DIAGNOSIS**

DIFFERENTIAL DIAGNOSIS
• Canine distemper virus—systemic signs (e.g., gastroenteritis, pneumonia, and ocular or nasal purulent discharge)
• Other disorders that are limited to parts of the body—differentiate from acquired form
• Partial seizures—Dobermans, Labrador retrievers, and English bulldogs; occasional head nods in a yes or no direction; occur

infrequently and intermittently; limited to the head; last from few seconds to minutes; affected dog continues its activity and is otherwise normal.
• Dancing Doberman disease—differentiated on the basis of breed and the movements observed (e.g., the dog holds one pelvic limb flexed while standing; both limbs usually become affected, giving a dancing aspect to the standing position)

CBC/BIOCHEMISTRY/URINALYSIS
• Congenital or secondary to a past canine distemper virus infection—normal
• Other acquired forms—may suggest a specific cause if the patient has infectious encephalomyelitis; otherwise, normal

OTHER LABORATORY TESTS
N/A

IMAGING
MRI—may help determine diagnosis in acute disease

DIAGNOSTIC PROCEDURES
Acute development—CSF analysis, serologic testing may help determine the diagnosis.

TREATMENT
• Active encephalomyelitis—inpatient; establish a diagnosis and initiate treatment
• Exercise—as tolerated
• Diet—ensure proper nutrition with active CNS disease; modify, if necessary, with vomiting or diarrhea
• Usually persists for years but spontaneous remission can occur
• Familial—clinical signs in Labrador retrievers and Dalmatians are severe and usually not compatible with quality of life.

MEDICATIONS

DRUG(S)
• With chronic, inactive canine distemper—treatment often unnecessary; alleviation may be obtained with procainamide (125–250 mg/dog PO q6–12h).
• Chlorazepate or acetylpromazine—reflex disease; may see improvement
• Active encephalomyelitis—treat accordingly

CONTRAINDICATIONS/POSSIBLE INTERACTIONS
N/A

FOLLOW-UP
• Monitor CNS disease.
• Usually persists indefinitely; remission occasionally seen
• Active distemper virus infection—poor to grave prognosis

MISCELLANEOUS

SYNONYMS
• Flexor spasm
• Canine chorea

ABBREVIATIONS
CNS = central nervous system
CSF = cerebrospinal fluid
MRI = magnetic resonance imaging

Suggested Reading
Oliver JE, Lorenz MD, Kornegay JN. Handbook of veterinary neurology. 3rd ed. Philadelphia: Saunders, 1997.
Author Joane M. Parent
Consulting Editor Joane M. Parent

MYOPATHY, FOCAL INFLAMMATORY—MASTICATORY MUSCLE MYOSITIS AND EXTRAOCULAR MYOSITIS

 BASICS

DEFINITION
• Masticatory—focal inflammatory myopathy affecting the muscles of mastication (temporalis and masseter muscles) and sparing the limb muscles
• Extraocular—selectively affects the extraocular muscles, sparing limb and masticatory muscles

PATHOPHYSIOLOGY
• Masticatory—suspected immune-mediated cause owing to autoantibodies against type 2M fibers and a positive clinical response to immunosuppressive doses of corticosteroids
• Extraocular—suspected immune-mediated cause owing to positive clinical response to corticosteroids

SYSTEMS AFFECTED
Neuromuscular—muscles of mastication; extraocular muscles

GENETICS
• Unknown
• As with autoimmune diseases in general, the appropriate genetic background must exist.
• Extraocular—golden retrievers may have a genetic predisposition.

INCIDENCE/PREVALENCE
• Unknown
• Masticatory—not rare

GEOGRAPHIC DISTRIBUTION
Probably worldwide

SIGNALMENT

Species
Dogs

Breed Predilections
• Various
• Extraocular—golden retrievers

Mean Age and Range
• No obvious age predisposition

Predominant Sex
• None obvious

SIGNS

General Comments
Masticatory—usually related to abnormalities of jaw movement and jaw pain; not a "table-top" diagnosis; usually requires laboratory testing to confirm diagnosis

Historical Findings
• Masticatory—acute or chronic pain when opening the jaw; inability to pick up a ball or get food into the mouth; acutely swollen muscles; progressive muscle atrophy
• Extraocular—bilateral exophthalmos

Physical Examination Findings
• Masticatory—marked jaw pain with manipulation and/or trismus; acute muscle swelling with exophthalmos; muscle atrophy with enophthalmos; inability to open the jaw under anesthesia
• Extraocular—bilateral exophthalmos; impaired vision

CAUSES
Immune mediated

RISK FACTORS
• Appropriate genetic background
• Possible previous bacterial or viral infection

 DIAGNOSIS

DIFFERENTIAL DIAGNOSIS
• Retro-orbital abscess—probe behind last upper molar
• Temporomandibular joint disease—radiographically abnormal joint
• Polymyositis—high serum creatine kinase; generalized EMG abnormalities; diagnostic muscle biopsies
• Neurogenic atrophy of temporalis muscles—determined by EMG and muscle biopsy
• Atrophy of masticatory muscles from corticosteroids—history of corticosteroid use; characteristic changes on muscle biopsy

CBC/BIOCHEMISTRY/URINALYSIS
Serum creatine kinase—normal or mildly elevated

OTHER LABORATORY TESTS
• Muscle biopsy—diagnostic test of choice for masticatory disease
• Immunocytochemical assay—demonstrate autoantibodies against masticatory muscle type 2M fibers; negative in polymyositis and extraocular disease

IMAGING
• Radiography of the temporomandibular joints
• Orbital sonogram—for extraorbital disease; demonstrate swollen extraocular muscles
• MRI—for demonstration of inflammation in muscles

DIAGNOSTIC PROCEDURES
EMG—differentiate between extraocular disease and polymyositis; abnormal masticatory muscles in masticatory myositis only; generalized abnormalities in polymyositis

PATHOLOGIC FINDINGS

Masticatory
• Swelling or atrophy of the masticatory muscles
• Biopsy specimen—may see myofiber necrosis, phagocytosis, mononuclear cell infiltration with a multifocal and perivascular distribution; may see myofiber atrophy and fibrosis with chronic condition; eosinophils rare

Extraocular
Mononuclear cell infiltration—restricted to extraocular muscles

 TREATMENT

APPROPRIATE HEALTH CARE
Outpatient

NURSING CARE
Gastrostomy tube—may be required with severe restrictions in jaw mobility; requires good hygiene and supportive care

ACTIVITY
N/A

MYOPATHY, FOCAL INFLAMMATORY—MASTICATORY MUSCLE MYOSITIS AND EXTRAOCULAR MYOSITIS

DIET
Masticatory—may require liquid food or gruel until jaw mobility is regained; may need a gastric feeding tube to facilitate fluid and caloric intake

CLIENT EDUCATION
• Warn client that long-term corticosteroid therapy may be required.
• Inform client that residual muscle atrophy and restricted jaw movement may occur with chronic masticatory disease.

SURGICAL CONSIDERATIONS
Not indicated

 MEDICATIONS

DRUG(S) OF CHOICE
Coricosteroids—immunosuppressive dosages, tapered as jaw mobility, swelling, and serum creatine kinase return to normal; maintained at lowest alternate-day dosage that prevents restricted jaw mobility; treated for a minimum of 6 months

CONTRAINDICATIONS
N/A

PRECAUTIONS
• Corticosteroids—watch for infection and undesirable side effects.
• Clinical signs may recur if treatment is stopped too soon.

POSSIBLE INTERACTIONS
N/A

ALTERNATIVE DRUG(S)
Intolerable side effects of corticosteroids—institute a lower dose of corticosteroids and combine with another drug (e.g., azathioprine).

 FOLLOW-UP

PATIENT MONITORING
• Masticatory—return of jaw mobility and decreased serum creatine kinase
• Extraocular—decreased swelling of extraocular muscles

PREVENTION/AVOIDANCE
N/A

POSSIBLE COMPLICATIONS
• Corticosteroids—undesirable side effects
• Recurrence of clinical signs—treatment stopped too early
• Poor clinical response—inadequate dosages of corticosteroids
• Restrictive strabismus (extraocular myositis)

EXPECTED COURSE AND PROGNOSIS
• Masticatory—jaw mobility should return to normal unless the condition is chronic and severe fibrosis develops; good prognosis if treated early with adequate dosages of corticosteroids
• Extraocular—good response to corticosteroids; good prognosis

 MISCELLANEOUS

ASSOCIATED CONDITIONS
Other concurrent autoimmune disorders

AGE-RELATED FACTORS
N/A

ZOONOTIC POTENTIAL
N/A

PREGNANCY
Unknown

SYNONYMS
• Eosinophilic myositis
• Atrophic myositis

SEE ALSO
• Myopathy, Generalized Inflammatory–Polymyositis and Dermatomyositis
• Myopathy, Noninflammatory–Endocrine

ABBREVIATIONS
• EMG = electromyogram
• MRI = magnetic resonance imaging

Suggested Reading
Allgoewer I, Blair M, Basher T, Davidson M et al. Extraocular myositis and restrictive strabismus in 10 dogs. Vet Ophth 2003;21–26.
Carpenter JL, Schmidt GM, Moore FM, et al. Canine bilateral extraocular polymyositis. Vet Pathol 1989;26:510–512.
Orvis JS, Cardinet GH III. Canine muscle fiber types and susceptibility of masticatory muscles to myositis. Muscle Nerve 1981; 4:354–359.
Podell M. Inflammatory myopathies. Vet Clin North Am 2002;31:147–167.
Shelton GD, Cardinet GH III, Bandman E. Canine masticatory muscle disorders: a clinicopathological and immunochemical study of 29 cases. Muscle Nerve 1987; 10:753–766.
Shelton GD. Canine masticatory muscle disorders. In Kirk RW, ed. Current veterinary therapy X. Philadelphia: Saunders, 1989; 816–819.

Author G. Diane Shelton
Consulting Editor Peter K. Shires

MYOPATHY, GENERALIZED INFLAMMATORY—POLYMYOSITIS AND DERMATOMYOSITIS

 **BASICS**

DEFINITION

• Polymyositis—a condition in which skeletal muscles are damaged by a nonsuppurative inflammatory process dominated by lymphocytic infiltration
• Dermatomyositis—polymyositis is associated with characteristic skin lesions

PATHOPHYSIOLOGY

• Inflammation of skeletal muscles—results in muscle weakness, myalgia, and atrophy
• Muscle inflammation—may be a result of immune-mediated, infectious, or paraneoplastic disorders; may be a sequela to certain drug therapies

SYSTEMS AFFECTED

• Neuromuscular—generalized muscle involvement including masticatory and limb muscles
• Gastrointestinal—particularly the pharyngeal and esophageal muscles, because they are composed predominantly of skeletal muscle in dogs
• Skin/Exocrine—particularly if related to a generalized immune-mediated connective tissue disorder

GENETICS

• Unknown
• As for autoimmune diseases in general, the appropriate genetic background must exist.
• Dermatomyositis—reported to have an autosomal dominant inheritance pattern in rough-coated collies and Shetland sheepdogs

INCIDENCE/PREVALENCE

• Unknown
• Generalized inflammatory myopathies—not common

GEOGRAPHIC DISTRIBUTION

Probably worldwide

SIGNALMENT

Species

Dogs and rarely cats

Breed Predilections

• Polymyositis—various breeds of dogs and cats may be affected; breed-associated in Newfoundland and boxer
• Dermatomyositis—reported in rough-coated collies, Shetland sheepdogs, and Australian cattle dogs

Mean Age and Range

• Polymyositis—none obvious
• Dermatomyositis—3–5 months of age

Predominant Sex

None obvious

SIGNS

General Comments

• Polymyositis—usually associated with a stiff-stilted gait, muscle pain, and/or muscle weakness. May see regurgitation and megaesophagus
• Elevated serum creatine kinase—supports but does not make the diagnosis of myositis
• Muscle biopsy—needed to confirm the diagnosis

Historical Findings

• Stiff-stilted gait—acute or chronic
• Muscle swelling and/or atrophy
• Generalized muscle pain
• Generalized muscle weakness and exercise intolerance
• Regurgitation of food or difficulty swallowing

Physical Examination Findings

• Pain upon palpation of muscle groups
• Generalized muscle atrophy, including the muscles of mastication
• Gait abnormalities, including a stiff-stilted gait
• Neurologic examination—not abnormal; may be a decreased gag reflex if the pharyngeal muscles are affected
• Dermatomyositis (dogs)—typical skin lesions

CAUSES

• Immune-mediated
• Infectious—*Toxoplasma gondii; Neospora canis; Hepatozoon canis; Ehrlichia canis;* bacterial infection uncommon
• Drug-induced
• Paraneoplastic syndrome

RISK FACTORS

• Appropriate genetic background
• Possibly previous bacterial or viral infection
• Neoplasia, possibly occult

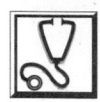 **DIAGNOSIS**

DIFFERENTIAL DIAGNOSIS

• Polyarthritis—differentiated by physical examination and evaluation of joint fluid
• Noninflammatory muscle disorders—differentiated by muscle biopsy
• Polyneuropathy—differentiated by neurologic examination, electrophysiology, and muscle biopsy
• Chronic intervertebral disk disease—differentiated by physical examination and serum creatine kinase

CBC/BIOCHEMISTRY/URINALYSIS

Serum creatine kinase—variably elevated

OTHER LABORATORY TESTS

• Serum antinuclear antibody titer—may be positive in connective tissue disorders
• May see concurrent hypothyroidism

IMAGING

• Regurgitation—evaluate thoracic radiography for esophageal dilatation.
• Pharyngeal weakness—perform a dynamic study for the evaluation of the swallowing process.

DIAGNOSTIC PROCEDURES

• Muscle biopsy—single most important test for diagnosing polymyositis; sample multiple muscles, because condition may be missed if distribution is patchy

MYOPATHY, GENERALIZED INFLAMMATORY—POLYMYOSITIS AND DERMATOMYOSITIS

• Electromyographic evaluation—performed to determine the distribution of muscle involvement and the muscles to be biopsied; should help differentiate myopathic from neuropathic causes of muscle weakness

PATHOLOGIC FINDINGS
• Muscle swelling or atrophy
• Biopsy specimens—usually contain mononuclear cell infiltrates
• Rare neutrophils or eosinophils—may be noted
• Regenerating myofibers—may be observed
• Intramyofiber parasite cyst—rare
• Chronic condition—may see extensive myofiber atrophy and fibrosis

TREATMENT

APPROPRIATE HEALTH CARE
Outpatient

NURSING CARE
Supportive care—may be required to prevent skin wounds and decubital ulcers in non-ambulatory severely affected patients

ACTIVITY
Should increase, along with muscle strength, as muscle inflammation decreases

DIET
• Megaesophagus—may require feeding from an elevation; try foods of different consistencies.
• Severe regurgitation—may need to place a gastric feeding tube to maintain hydration and nutrition

CLIENT EDUCATION
• Warn client that long-term immunosuppressive therapy may be required for an immune-mediated condition.
• Inform client that residual muscle atrophy may occur with chronic disease and extensive fibrosis.

• Suggest genetic counseling for familial disorders.

SURGICAL CONSIDERATIONS
Only for concurrent neoplasia.

MEDICATIONS

DRUG(S) OF CHOICE
• Corticosteroids—immunosuppressive dosages usually result in clinical improvement of immune-mediated condition; decrease to the lowest alternate-day dosage that maintains normal creatine kinase and improved muscle strength and mobility; may require long-term therapy
• Identified infectious agent—initiate specific therapy.

CONTRAINDICATIONS
N/A

PRECAUTIONS
Corticosteroids—observe for infection and undesirable side effects; remember that chronic therapy may lead to muscle atrophy

POSSIBLE INTERACTIONS
N/A

ALTERNATIVE DRUG(S)
Intolerable side effects of corticosteroids—institute a lower dose of corticosteroids combined with another drug (e.g., azathioprine)

FOLLOW-UP

PATIENT MONITORING
• Serum creatine kinase—periodic evaluation; if elevated, should decrease into the normal range
• Corticosteroids—side effects

PREVENTION/AVOIDANCE
N/A

POSSIBLE COMPLICATIONS
• Corticosteroids—undesirable side effects
• Recurrence of clinical signs—treatment stopped too early
• Poor clinical response—inadequate dosages of corticosteroids

EXPECTED COURSE AND PROGNOSIS
• Immune-mediated condition—good to fair prognosis
• Paraneoplastic disorder associated with occult neoplasia—guarded prognosis

MISCELLANEOUS

ASSOCIATED CONDITIONS
• Other concurrent autoimmune disorders
• Neoplasia

AGE-RELATED FACTORS
N/A

ZOONOTIC POTENTIAL
N/A

PREGNANCY
Unknown

SEE ALSO
Myopathy, Noninflammatory—Endocrine

Suggested Reading

Hargis AM, Haupt KH, Prieur DJ, Moore MP. A skin disorder in three Shetland sheepdogs: comparison with familial canine dermatomyositis of collies. Compend Contin Educ Pract Vet 1985;7:306–318.

Kornegay JN, Gorgacz EJ, Dawe DL, et al. Polymyositis in dogs. J Am Vet Med Assoc 1980;176:431–438.

Podell M. Inflammatory myopathies. Vet Clin North Am 2002;31:147–167.

Shelton GD, Cardinet GH III. Pathophysiologic basis of canine muscle disorders. J Vet Intern Med 1987;1:36–44.

Author G. Diane Shelton

Consulting Editor Peter K. Shires

MYOPATHY, NONINFLAMMATORY—ENDOCRINE

 BASICS

DEFINITION
Myopathies associated with various endocrinopathies (including hypothyroidism, hyperthyroidism, hypoadrenocorticism, hyperadrenocorticism) and associated with exogenous corticosteroid use (steroid myopathy)

PATHOPHYSIOLOGY

With Adrenal Dysfunction
• Glucocorticoid excess—impaired muscle protein metabolism; may accelerate degradation of myofibrillar and soluble protein in skeletal muscle; impairment of carbohydrate metabolism owing to induction of an insulin-resistant state; may note elevated ACTH levels
• Adrenal insufficiency—circulatory insufficiency; fluid and electrolyte imbalance; impaired carbohydrate metabolism

With Thyroid Disease
• Hyperthyroidism—increased mitochondrial respiration; accelerated protein degradation and lipid oxidation; glycogen depletion; impaired glucose uptake
• Hypothyroidism—impaired muscle energy metabolism by reduced glycogen breakdown, gluconeogenesis, and oxidative and glycolytic capacity; impaired insulin-stimulated carbohydrate metabolism

SYSTEMS AFFECTED
• Neuromuscular—impaired energy metabolism
• Cardiovascular—impaired energy metabolism; circulatory disorders

GENETICS
N/A

INCIDENCE/PREVALENCE
• Exact incidence unknown
• Myopathies related to exogenous corticosteroids—common
• Myopathies associated with Cushing syndrome and hypothyroidism—not uncommon

GEOGRAPHIC DISTRIBUTION
Probably worldwide

SIGNALMENT

Species
• Dogs—steroid myopathy; weakness associated with hyperadrenocorticism and hypoadrenocorticism; hypothyroidism
• Cats—weakness associated with hyperthyroidism

Breed Predilections
Affects several breeds

MEAN AGE AND RANGE
• Steroid myopathy—dogs of any age
• Other disorders—see specific disease

Predominant Sex
None found

SIGNS

General Comments
Corticosteroid use in dogs—muscles very susceptible; muscle atrophy (particularly the masticatory muscles) is not uncommon with prolonged corticosteroid use

Historical Findings
• Muscle weakness, atrophy, and stiffness
• Regurgitation
• Dysphagia
• Dysphonia

Physical Examination Findings
• Muscle weakness, stiffness, cramping, and myalgia
• Muscle hypertrophy or atrophy
• May not note other clinical signs of an endocrine disorder

CAUSES
• Endocrine dysfunction
• Autoimmune
• Neoplastic

RISK FACTORS
N/A

 DIAGNOSIS

DIFFERENTIAL DIAGNOSIS
• Inflammatory myopathies—distinguished by muscle biopsy
• Noninflammatory myopathies—distinguished by muscle biopsy

CBC/BIOCHEMISTRY/URINALYSIS
• Baseline testing—abnormalities consistent with endocrine disorder
• Serum creatine kinase—usually normal

OTHER LABORATORY TESTS
Thyroid and adrenal function tests—should be diagnostic

IMAGING
• Dynamic studies—evaluate pharyngeal and esophageal function; with regurgitation and dysphagia
• Cardiac evaluation—for cats with hyperthyroidism

DIAGNOSTIC PROCEDURES
• Muscle biopsy—fresh frozen sections
• Electromyography

PATHOLOGIC FINDINGS
• Hyperadrenocorticism and steroid myopathies—selective atrophy of type 2 muscle fibers; may see lobulated or ragged-red fibers with associated myotonia
• Hypoadrenocorticism—normal
• Hyperthyroidism (cats)—unknown if pathologic abnormalities occur within muscle
• Hypothyroidism—atrophy of type 2 fibers; may see an increase in type 1 fibers; may see PAS-positive deposits and nemaline rods in type 2 fibers

MYOPATHY, NONINFLAMMATORY—ENDOCRINE

TREATMENT

APPROPRIATE HEALTH CARE
Depends on specific endocrine disorder

NURSING CARE
Support bandaging, wound management (decubital ulcers), and physical therapy—with musculoskeletal manifestations

ACTIVITY
• Clinical corticosteroid myopathy (humans)—inactivity worsens condition; increased muscle activity may partially prevent atrophy.
• Physical therapy—may help prevent and treat muscle weakness and wasting in dogs receiving glucocorticoids

DIET
• Regurgitation and megaesophagus—feed from an elevation.
• Dysphagia and esophageal dilation—give food with the best-tolerated consistency.
• Gastric feeding tube—if oral feeding is not tolerated

CLIENT EDUCATION
Depends on specific endocrine disorder

SURGICAL CONSIDERATIONS
Removal of neoplasia

MEDICATIONS

DRUG(S) OF CHOICE
• Depend on specific endocrine disorder
• Corticosteroid myopathy—decrease corticosteroid dosage to the lowest possible level; use a nonfluorinated corticosteroid and alternate-day dosing.

• Intramyofiber lipid storage with steroid myopathy—L-carnitine (50 mg/kg q12h) may improve muscle strength.

CONTRAINDICATIONS
N/A

PRECAUTIONS
Depend on specific endocrine disorder

POSSIBLE INTERACTIONS
N/A

ALTERNATIVE DRUG(S)
Fluorinated corticosteroids, triamcinolone, betamethasone, and dexamethasone—most likely to produce muscle weakness; use an equivalent dose of another corticosteroid.

FOLLOW-UP

PATIENT MONITORING
• Depends on specific endocrine disorder
• Steroid myopathy—should note return of muscle strength and mass with decreased steroid use

PREVENTION/AVOIDANCE
N/A

POSSIBLE COMPLICATIONS
Depend on specific endocrine disorders

EXPECTED COURSE AND PROGNOSIS
• Myotonia associated with hyperadrenocorticism—poor prognosis for resolution
• Steroid myopathy—good prognosis for return of muscle strength and mass; recovery may take weeks
• Hypothyroid myopathy—improvement in muscle pain and stiffness common
• Hyperthyroidism (cats)—good prognosis for return of muscle strength following return to euthyroid state

• Hypoadrenocorticism—good prognosis for return of muscle strength
• Dysphagia and regurgitation—may resolve with adequate treatment

MISCELLANEOUS

ASSOCIATED CONDITIONS
• May note multiple endocrinopathies
• Hypothyroidism (dogs)—concurrent myasthenia gravis

AGE-RELATED FACTORS
N/A

ZOONOTIC POTENTIAL
N/A

PREGNANCY
Unknown

ABBREVIATIONS
• ACTH = adrenocorticotropic hormone
• PAS = periodic acid–Schiff

Suggested Reading
Jaggy A, Oliver JE, Ferguson DC, et al. Neurological manifestations of hypothyroidism: a retrospective study of 29 cases. J Vet Intern Med 1994;8:328–330.
LeCouteur RA, Dow SW, Sisson AF. Metabolic and endocrine myopathies of dogs and cats. Semin Vet Med Surg Small Anim 1989;4:146–155.
Platt SR. Neuromuscular complications in endocrine and metabolic disorders. Vet Clin North Am 2002;31:125–146.
Shelton GD, Cardinet GH III. Pathophysiologic basis of canine muscle disorders. J Vet Intern Med 1987;1:36–44.

Author G. Diane Shelton
Consulting Editor Peter K. Shires

MYOPATHY, NONINFLAMMATORY—HEREDITARY LABRADOR RETRIEVER

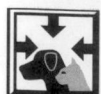 BASICS

OVERVIEW
- An inherited progressive and degenerative generalized myopathy of Labrador retrievers
- Simple autosomal recessive mode of inheritance
- Pathophysiologic mechanism(s) unknown
- Histologic examination of muscle—more typical of a neurogenic than a myopathic cause; no morphologic changes in the CNS or peripheral nerves identified

SIGNALMENT
- Occurs in black and yellow Labrador retrievers
- Age of onset—variable (6 weeks to 7 months); most common at 3–4 months
- Affects males and females

SIGNS
- Severity ranges from stilted gait to muscle weakness, bunny hopping pelvic limb gait, ventroflexion of the neck, arched back, and abnormal joint posture (cow-hocked stance, hyperextended carpi)
- Worsen with exercise, excitement, and cold weather
- Patient may collapse with forced exercise.
- Some improvement with rest
- Generalized muscle atrophy—mild to severe
- Atrophy of proximal limb and masticatory muscles often most prominent
- Tendon reflexes—normal, hypoactive, or absent
- Occasionally, patients become recumbent or develop megaesophagus.

CAUSE & RISK FACTORS
Autosomal recessive mode of inheritance

 DIAGNOSIS

DIFFERENTIAL DIAGNOSIS
- With little muscle atrophy—exercise intolerance may mimic signs of myasthenia gravis or cardiac or orthopedic disease.
- With marked muscle atrophy—consider other myopathies (infectious, immune-mediated, metabolic, congenital) and generalized lower motor neuron disorders.

CBC/BIOCHEMISTRY/URINALYSIS
Creatine kinase—normal or mildly or moderately elevated

OTHER LABORATORY TESTS
N/A

IMAGING
N/A

DIAGNOSTIC PROCEDURES
- EMG—spontaneous activity, including complex repetitive discharges, especially in proximal limb and masticatory muscles; may reveal no abnormalities with mild disease
- Muscle histology—reveals variation in fiber size, angular atrophy of both type 1 and 2 myofibers, grouped atrophy, increase in central nuclei, muscle degeneration and regeneration, and fibrosis; may note deficiency or increase in type 2 myofibers

 TREATMENT

- None specific
- Avoid cold, because it exacerbates clinical signs.
- Discourage breeding of affected animals.
- Do not repeat dam–sire breedings that result in affected offspring.

 MEDICATIONS

DRUG(S)
Diazepam may be beneficial.

CONTRAINDICATIONS/POSSIBLE INTERACTIONS
None known

 FOLLOW-UP

- Clinical signs generally stabilize.
- Mild disease—may be an acceptable pet; may show some improvement in exercise tolerance
- Aspiration pneumonia—a risk with megaesophagus

 MISCELLANEOUS

ASSOCIATED CONDITIONS
N/A

AGE-RELATED FACTORS
N/A

ZOONOTIC POTENTIAL
N/A

PREGNANCY
N/A

ABBREVIATION
EMG = electromyography

Suggested Reading
McKerrell RE, Braud KG. Hereditary myopathy of Labrador retrievers. In: Kirk RW, Bonagura JD, eds. Current veterinary therapy X. Philadelphia: Saunders, 1989:820–821.

Author Georgina Child
Consulting Editor Peter K. Shires

MYOPATHY, NONINFLAMMATORY—HEREDITARY MYOTONIA

BASICS

OVERVIEW
• Myopathy characterized by persistent contraction of muscle fibers on initiation of movement or when stimulated to contract
• May affect all skeletal muscles
• Congenital or acquired
• Congenital—may be associated with abnormal chloride conductance of muscle membrane

SIGNALMENT
• Congenital—described in young chow chows; rarely seen in other dog breeds
• Acquired—all breeds potentially susceptible
• Reported in cats

SIGNS
Historical Findings
• Difficulty rising
• Stiffness after rest
• May note dyspnea, dysphagia, and/or regurgitation
• May improve with exercise
• Exacerbated by cold

PHYSICAL EXAMINATION FINDINGS
• Hypertrophy of proximal limb muscles, neck muscles, and tongue
• Abduction of thoracic limbs
• Bunny-hopping pelvic limb gait
• Patient may fall and remain rigid in lateral recumbency for short periods.

CAUSES & RISK FACTORS
Chow chows—suspected autosomal recessive mode of inheritance

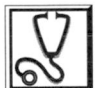

DIAGNOSIS

DIFFERENTIAL DIAGNOSIS
Other myopathies—distinguished by signalment and clinical and electromyographic findings

CBC/BIOCHEMISTRY/URINALYSIS
Creatine kinase—may be slightly elevated

OTHER LABORATORY TESTS
N/A

IMAGING
N/A

DIAGNOSTIC PROCEDURES
• Percussion of muscles and tongue in conscious and anesthetized dogs—causes sustained dimpling
• Electromyography—reveals multifocal or generalized high-frequency discharges that wax and wane in amplitude and frequency (dive bomber–sounding potentials) and that are increased after muscle percussion

PATHOLOGIC FINDINGS
• Muscle histology—shows mild changes (e.g., some angular atrophy, central nuclei, variation in fiber size)

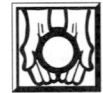

TREATMENT
• None specific
• Discourage activities that result in hyperventilation.
• Avoid cold.
• Anesthesia (induction and recovery)—possible risk of respiratory obstruction owing to adduction of vocal cords or regurgitation

MEDICATIONS

DRUG(S)
Membrane-stabilizing drugs—procainamide and quinidine; may decrease severity of clinical signs

CONTRAINDICATIONS/POSSIBLE INTERACTIONS
None

FOLLOW-UP

PREVENTION/AVOIDANCE
• Chow chows—inherited condition; advise owner regarding breeding.
• Discourage breeding of affected animals.
• Do not repeat dam–sire breedings that resulted in affected offspring.

POSSIBLE COMPLICATIONS
Respiratory obstruction and/or aspiration of regurgitated food—may be life-threatening; advise owners of the clinical symptoms and treatment.

EXPECTED COURSE AND PROGNOSIS
Prognosis guarded

MISCELLANEOUS

ASSOCIATED CONDITIONS
N/A

AGE-RELATED FACTORS
Aging—signs may stabilize or worsen.

ZOONOTIC POTENTIAL
N/A

PREGNANCY
N/A

Suggested Reading
Amann JF, Tomlinson J, Hankison JK. Myotonia in a chow chow. J Am Vet Med Assoc 1985;187:415–417.
Duncan ID, Griffiths IR. Myotonia in the dog. In: Kirk RW, ed. Current veterinary therapy VlII. Philadelphia: Saunders, 1983:686–689.
Hill SL, Shelton GD, Lemehan TM. Myotonia in a cocker spaniel. J Am Anim Hosp Assoc 1995;31:506–509.
Honhold N, Smith DA. Myotonia in the Great Dane, Vet Rec 1986;119:162.
Shires PK, Nafe LA, Hulsie DA. Myotonia in a Staffordshire terrier J Am Vet Med Assoc 1983;183(2):229–232.
Toll J, Copper B, Altschul M. Congenital myotonia in 2 domestic cats. J Vet Intern Med 1998;12:116–119.
Vite CH, Melniczel J, Patterson D. Congenital myotonic myopathy in the miniature schnauzer: an autosomal recessive trait. J Hered. 1999;90(5):578–80.

Author Georgina Child
Consulting Editor Peter K. Shires

MYOPATHY, NONINFLAMMATORY—HEREDITARY SCOTTY CRAMP

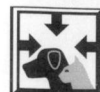

BASICS

OVERVIEW
• Inherited neurologic disorder in Scottish terriers characterized by episodic muscle hypertonicity or cramping
• Not associated with any morphologic changes in muscle, peripheral nerve, or the CNS
• Thought to be the result of a disorder in serotonin metabolism within the CNS
• Similar condition reported in young Dalmatians and Labrador retrievers—may be result of low numbers of neurotransmitter glycine receptors in the CNS

SIGNALMENT
• Young Scottish terriers, typically < 1 year of age
• No known sex predilection

SIGNS
• Normal at rest and on initial exercise
• Further exercise or excitement—abduction of the thoracic limbs; arching of the lumbar spine; stiffening or overflexion of the pelvic limbs (goose-stepping gait)
• Patient may fall, with tail and pelvic limbs flexed tightly against the body
• Respiration—may cease for a short time
• Facial muscles—may be contracted
• No loss of consciousness
• Severity varies
• Episodes—may last up to 30 min

CAUSES & RISK FACTORS
Inherited condition with probable recessive mode of transmission

DIAGNOSIS

DIFFERENTIAL DIAGNOSIS
Seizure disorder—distinguished on basis of family history, typical clinical signs with no loss of consciousness, and induction of signs with serotonin antagonists

CBC/BIOCHEMISTRY/URINALYSIS
Normal

OTHER LABORATORY TESTS
N/A

IMAGING
N/A

DIAGNOSTIC PROCEDURES
Clinical signs may be induced by giving the serotonin antagonist, methysergide.

TREATMENT
Behavioral modification and/or environmental changes—eliminating triggering situations (excitement, stress); may be adequate

MEDICATIONS

DRUG(S)
Acepromazine, diazepam, or vitamin E—may reduce the incidence and severity of episodes

CONTRAINDICATIONS/POSSIBLE INTERACTIONS
• Serotonin antagonists—increase severity of clinical signs
• Aspirin, indomethacin, phenylbutazone, Banamine (flunixin meglumine), and penicillin—may exacerbate clinical signs

FOLLOW-UP

PATIENT MONITORING
Nonprogressive

PREVENTION/AVOIDANCE
• Discourage breeding affected animals.
• Do not repeat dam–sire breedings that result in affected offspring.

EXPECTED COURSE AND PROGNOSIS
• Mild to moderate—fair to good long-term prognosis; usually acceptable disability to owners; nonprogressive
• Severe—guarded to poor prognosis

MISCELLANEOUS

ASSOCIATED CONDITIONS
N/A

AGE-RELATED FACTORS
N/A

ZOONOTIC POTENTIAL
N/A

PREGNANCY
N/A

Suggested Reading
Meyers KM, Clemmons RM. Scotty cramp. In: Kirk RW, ed. Current veterinary therapy VIII. Philadelphia: Saunders, 1983:702–704.

Author Georgina Child
Consulting Editor Peter K. Shires

BASICS

OVERVIEW
• Inherited, progressive, and degenerative generalized myopathy with X-linked mode of inheritance
• Patients lack muscle membrane–associated protein dystrophin
• RNA processing defect—identified in golden retrievers, Irish terriers, Samoyeds, rottweilers, Belgian shepherds, and one miniature schnauzer

SIGNALMENT
• Seen primarily in neonate and young dogs
• Described in cats
• Primarily affects males
• Females—usually carriers of gene defect; homozygotes may be affected.

SIGNS

Dogs
• Golden retrievers—exercise intolerance; stilted gait; bunny-hopping pelvic limb gait; plantigrade stance; partial trismus; muscle atrophy (especially the truncal and temporalis muscles); hypertrophy of some muscles (especially the tongue); kyphosis; lordosis; drooling; dysphagia; aspiration pneumonia (due to pharyngeal and/or esophageal involvement)
• Other breeds—similar; include vomiting and megaesophagus
• Vary in severity, onset, and progression; may be seen as early as 6 weeks; tend to stabilize by 6 months
• Stunting and ineffective suckling—may be evident in younger pups
• Cardiac failure—may occur owing to cardiomyopathy
• Severe muscle contractures
• Spinal reflexes—normal initially; may become hypoactive

Cats
• Dystrophin deficient—muscle hypertrophy; stiff gait; cervical rigidity; exercise intolerance; vomiting

• Not apparent in one cat until 21 months of age

CAUSES & RISK FACTORS
Inherited defect of the X chromosome

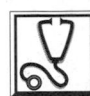

DIAGNOSIS

DIFFERENTIAL DIAGNOSIS
Other inherited, infectious (protozoal), immune-mediated, or metabolic myopathies; distinguished by muscle histology and demonstration of dystrophin deficiency

CBC/BIOCHEMISTRY/URINALYSIS
Normal except for marked elevation in serum creatine kinase (may be > 10,000 U/L; further increased after exercise)

OTHER LABORATORY TESTS
• Dystrophin deficiency—demonstrated immunocytochemically or by Western blot analysis; diagnostic
• Serologic testing—may be warranted to rule out infectious and immune-mediated causes

IMAGING
N/A

DIAGNOSTIC PROCEDURES
Electromyography—shows complex repetitive discharges

PATHOLOGIC FINDINGS
Histologic examination of muscle—muscle fiber necrosis and regeneration; myofiber mineralization (may be dramatic); myofiber hypertrophy (may be variation in myofiber size or fibrosis)

TREATMENT
None proven effective

MEDICATIONS

DRUG(S)
Glucocorticosteriods—may provide some improvement; reason unknown

CONTRAINDICATIONS/POSSIBLE INTERACTIONS
None

FOLLOW-UP

PATIENT MONITORING
Monitor periodically for aspiration pneumonia or cardiomyopathy.

PREVENTION/AVOIDANCE
• Discourage breeding of affected animals.
• Do not repeat dam–sire breedings that result in affected offspring.

POSSIBLE COMPLICATIONS
Aspiration pneumonia or cardiomyopathy may be life threatening.

EXPECTED COURSE AND PROGNOSIS
• Overall prognosis—guarded to poor as no effective palliative treatment
• Golden retrievers—signs tend to stabilize at 6 months.
• Other dog breeds and cats—progression variable

MISCELLANEOUS

ASSOCIATED CONDITIONS
N/A

AGE-RELATED FACTORS
N/A

ZOONOTIC POTENTIAL
N/A

PREGNANCY
N/A

Suggested Reading
Kornegay JN. The X-linked muscular dystrophies. In: Kirk RW, Bonagura JD, eds. Current veterinary therapy XI. Philadelphia: Saunders, 1992:1042–1047.
Author Georgina Child
Consulting Editor Peter K. Shires

MYOPATHY, NONINFLAMMATORY—METABOLIC

 BASICS

DEFINITION
• Myopathy associated with disorders of glycogen metabolism, lipid metabolism, or oxidative phosphorylation and mitochondrial metabolism
• Currently poorly characterized in veterinary medicine

PATHOPHYSIOLOGY
• Usually associated with inherited or acquired enzyme defects involving major metabolic pathways
• May result in storage of the abnormal metabolic byproduct or morphologic abnormalities of mitochondria

SYSTEMS AFFECTED
• Neuromuscular—dependence on oxidative metabolism for energy
• Nervous—dependence on glycolytic and oxidative metabolism for energy
• Cardiovascular—dependence on oxidative metabolism for energy
• Hemic/Lymphatic/Immune—RBCs depend on glycolytic metabolism.
• Storage products in other organs—liver; spleen

GENETICS
Undetermined

INCIDENCE/PREVALENCE
Rare, except lipid-storage myopathies

GEOGRAPHIC DISTRIBUTION
Unknown; probably worldwide

SIGNALMENT
Species
Dogs and cats

Breed Predilections
• Inherited muscle phosphofructokinase deficiency—English springer spaniels, American cocker spaniels
• Acid maltase deficiency—Laplands
• Debranching enzyme deficiency—German shepherds
• Mitochondrial myopathy—clumber spaniels, Sussex spaniels, Old English sheepdogs

Mean Age and Range
• Inherited metabolic defects—2–3 months
• Acquired metabolic defects—adults

Predominant Sex
None found

SIGNS
General Comments
Very few of these conditions have been adequately described.

Historical Findings
• Muscular weakness
• Exercise intolerance
• Cramping
• Collapse
• Regurgitation and/or dysphagia
• Esophageal and/or pharyngeal abnormalities
• Dark urine; myoglobinuria; hemoglobinuria
• Encephalopathy
• Vomiting

Physical Examination Findings
• Exercise-related weakness, stiffness, and/or cramping
• Abnormal neurologic examination—disorientation; stupor; coma
• Abdominal distention—storage product accumulation in liver
• May appear normal, with fluctuating clinical signs

CAUSES
• Inborn error of metabolism
• Acquired metabolic defect
• Viral infections
• Drug induced
• Environmental factors

RISK FACTORS
• Inherited disorders
• Appropriate genetic background
• Others unknown

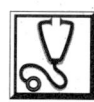 **DIAGNOSIS**

DIFFERENTIAL DIAGNOSIS
• Inflammatory myopathies—differentiated by muscle biopsy
• Other noninflammatory myopathies—differentiated by muscle biopsy
• Other metabolic encephalopathies—differentiated by laboratory evaluation

CBC/BIOCHEMISTRY/URINALYSIS
• Plasma lactate levels—elevated resting or postexcercise with disorders of fatty acid oxidation or oxidative phosphorylation; no elevation with glycolytic disorders
• Serum creatine kinase levels—may be elevated with exercise and normal at rest; may be persistently elevated
• Hypoglycemia—may occur with some glycolytic and oxidative disorders
• Hyperammonemia—may occur with urea cycle defects

OTHER LABORATORY TESTS
• Quantitation of plasma amino acids—abnormal accumulations
• Quantitation of urine organic acids—demonstrate abnormal organic acid production
• Quantitation of plasma, urine, and muscle carnitine—may be low with primary or secondary disorders of carnitine; low with primary organic acidurias
• Specific enzyme assays—depend on suspected metabolic defect
• Fibroblast cultures—study metabolic defect

IMAGING
MRI—evaluate the CNS; reveals abnormalities in humans

DIAGNOSTIC PROCEDURES
• Light microscopy—fresh frozen muscle sections; demonstrates storage products (glycogen, lipid) or abnormal mitochondria
• Electron microscopy of muscle reveals abnormal mitochondria, paracrystalline inclusions, and glycogen or lipid accumulation.
• Cardiovascular system evaluation—may have concurrent cardiomyopathy
• Other organ biopsies—with organomegaly

PATHOLOGIC FINDINGS
• Triglyceride droplets in muscle—lipid storage myopathy
• Ragged-red fibers in muscle—mitochondrial myopathy
• Glycogen deposition in muscle—glycogen storage disorder

MYOPATHY, NONINFLAMMATORY—METABOLIC

 TREATMENT

APPROPRIATE HEALTH CARE
• Inpatient—may required intensive care for severe encephalopathy, seizures, lactic acidemia, hypoglycemia, or hyperammonemia
• Outpatient—clinical signs related only to neuromuscular system

NURSING CARE
Depends on type and severity of disorder

ACTIVITY
Exercise restriction—with muscle weakness, stiffness, or exercise-induced collapse

DIET
• Avoid prolonged periods of fasting.
• Restrictions—depend on underlying defect
• Vitamin and co-factor therapy—determined by underlying defect

CLIENT EDUCATION
• Warn client that most inherited metabolic defects cannot be cured, although some can be treated.
• Advise against breeding affected individuals.

SURGICAL CONSIDERATIONS
N/A

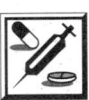 MEDICATIONS

DRUG(S) OF CHOICE
• Depend on the abnormality and clinical signs
• Lipid storage myopathies—L-carnitine (50 mg/kg PO q12h); riboflavin (50–100 mg PO q24h); coenzyme Q_{10} (1 mg/kg PO q24h)
• Mitochondrial myopathies—may benefit from therapy similar to that listed for lipid storage myopathies

CONTRAINDICATIONS
None known

PRECAUTIONS
Avoid fasting and strenuous exercise if they precipitate clinical signs.

POSSIBLE INTERACTIONS
N/A

ALTERNATIVE DRUG(S)
N/A

 FOLLOW-UP

PATIENT MONITORING
• Lipid storage myopathies—return of muscle strength; elimination of muscle pain
• Elevated serum creatine kinase—should return to normal

PREVENTION/AVOIDANCE
N/A

POSSIBLE COMPLICATIONS
Severe neurologic impairment

EXPECTED COURSE AND PROGNOSIS
• Untreatable disorder—poor prognosis
• Lipid storage myopathies—good prognosis if no underlying organic acidemia

 MISCELLANEOUS

ASSOCIATED CONDITIONS
• Iatrogenic and naturally occurring Cushing syndrome
• Lipid storage myopathies—found in some dogs
• Hemolytic anemia—due to underlying metabolic defect

AGE-RELATED FACTORS
• Inborn errors—usually found in young dogs
• Acquired defects—found in adult dogs

ZOONOTIC POTENTIAL
N/A

PREGNANCY
Unknown

SYNONYMS
• Lipid storage myopathies
• Mitochondrial myopathies
• Glycogen storage disorders
• Cori disease—glycogenosis type III
• Phosphofructokinase deficiency—glycogenosis type VII
• Acid maltase deficiency—glycogenosis type II)

ABBREVIATIONS
• CNS = central nervous system
• MRI = magnetic resonance imaging
• RBC = red blood cell

Suggested Reading
Fyfe JC. Molecular diagnosis of inherited neuromuscular disease. Vet Clin North Am 2002;31:287–300.
LeCouteur RA, Dow SW, Sisson AF. Metabolic and endocrine myopathies of dogs and cats. Semin Vet Med Surg Small Anim 1989;4:146–155.
Platt SR. Neuromuscular complications in endocrine and metabolic disorders. Vet Clin North Am 2002;31:125–146.
Shelton GD, Gardinet GH III. Pathophysiologic basis of canine muscle disorders. J Vet Intern Med 1987;1:36–44.
Shelton GD. Canine lipid storage myopathies. In: Bonagura JD, Kirk RW, eds. Current veterinary therapy XII. Philadelphia: Saunders, 1995;1161–1163.
Shelton GD, Engvall E. Muscular dystrophies and other inherited myopathies. Vet Clin North Am 2002;31:103–124.
Author G. Diane Shelton
Consulting Editor Peter K. Shires

MYXEDEMA AND MYXEDEMA COMA

BASICS

OVERVIEW
• Myxedema coma is a rare complication that can develop in dogs with severe hypothyroidism; in addition to the clinical signs usually seen with hypothyroidism, patients also develop hypothermia, extreme weakness, lethargy, and profound mental obtundation that can progress from marked depression to coma and death.
• Clinical signs develop secondary to a marked decrease in cellular oxidative metabolism, calorigenesis, and an overall decreased basal metabolic rate; myxedema refers to the nonpitting edema that frequently occurs in patients, most prominently in the skin of the facial region, particularly above the eyes and in the jowls; myxedema develops because of increased dermal ground substance (mucopolysaccharides, hyaluronic acid, and water).
• Myxedema coma has a high mortality rate; successful treatment depends on appropriate and timely therapy, based on clinical recognition of the syndrome.

SIGNALMENT
• Dogs
• Myxedema coma is a rare syndrome; the great majority of reported cases have been in Doberman pinschers.
• Age range was 2.5–5 years.
• No apparent sex predilection
• Myxedema coma not reported in felines

SIGNS

Historical Findings
• Dogs are usually presented for profound weakness, collapse, lethargy, and mental obtundation; these signs may develop acutely over a day or may exist for a few weeks before presentation.
• Rapid development of clinical signs has been most commonly observed in animals that were being boarded or were hospitalized.
• In addition, affected animals commonly have a history of alopecic skin disease or a poor haircoat; the owner may report other clinical signs of hypothyroidism.

Physical Examination
• Extreme weakness, depressed level of consciousness, and hypothermia without shivering have been present in all reported cases of myxedema coma.
• Other common abnormalities are bradycardia, bradypnea, alopecia, dry haircoat, and myxedema of the face and jowls.
• Mucous membranes may be slightly cyanotic secondary to poor peripheral perfusion and hypoxia; hypoxia can be caused by hypoventilation and/or pulmonary edema; 50% of reported patients have had hilar pulmonary edema and pleural effusion; heart and lung sounds may be diminished or crackles may be heard if pulmonary edema exists.
• A small percentage of patients have abdominal fluid detected by abdominal palpation.

CAUSES & RISK FACTORS
• Myxedema coma develops in canines secondary to severe primary hypothyroidism.
• Both lymphocytic thyroiditis and thyroid atrophy have been reported in affected dogs.
• Risk factors for development of myxedema coma include infectious diseases, respiratory disease, central nervous system or respiratory system depressants (anesthetics and tranquilizers), heart failure, and hypovolemia.
• Exposure to cold environmental temperatures can also precipitate myxedema coma.

DIAGNOSIS

DIFFERENTIAL DIAGNOSIS
• Consider diseases that cause cardiovascular, metabolic/endocrine, respiratory, neuromuscular, or central nervous system abnormalities when patients present with a primary complaint of weakness; however, metabolic/endocrine and central nervous system diseases are more likely to be associated with marked mental dullness.
• Hypothermia may be seen with shock, fulminant heart failure, hypothalamic and metabolic/endocrine disorders, or with exposure to cold temperatures.
• Dilated cardiomyopathy is a primary differential in Doberman pinschers.
• Specific metabolic/ endocrine diseases that should be ruled out include hypoadrenocorticism, hypoglycemia, diabetic ketoacidosis, and hepatoencephalopathy.
• Clinical abnormalities that help differentiate myxedema coma include hypothermia without shivering, myxedema, bradycardia, and epidermal abnormalities (nonpruritic alopecia and poor haircoat).

CBC/BIOCHEMISTRY/URINALYSIS
• Mild, nonregenerative anemia
• Inappropriately normal lymphocyte count
• Inflammatory leukogram—increased bands
• Hypercholesterolemia
• Hyponatremia
• Hypertriglyceridemia
• Hypoxemia
• Hypercarbia
• Hypoglycemia

OTHER LABORATORY TESTS

Endocrine Testing
• A definitive diagnosis is made when subnormal baseline serum T_4 levels and either

subnormal free T_4 or increased endogenous TSH levels are documented in a dog with compatible clinical signs.
• A TSH stimulation test is not recommended because it would delay definitive treatment for 6 hours.

Cytology and Fluid Analysis
Pleural and peritoneal effusions are usually identified as high-protein transudates.

IMAGING
• Thoracic radiographs—50% of reported patients have had hilar pulmonary edema; pleural effusion also observed
• Abdominal radiographs—may be loss of abdominal serosal detail secondary to intraabdominal fluid
• Echocardiography—method of choice for ruling out dilated cardiomyopathy; dogs with hypothyroidism can have echocardiographic evidence of abnormal left ventricular systolic function (decreased fractional shortening, increased end-systolic diameter, increased preejection period, and decreased left ventricular free wall and interventricular septal wall thickness); these abnormalities are usually mild and not as severe as those seen in patients with dilated cardiomyopathy.

DIAGNOSTIC PROCEDURES
ECG—bradycardia, decreased P- and R-wave amplitude, and a prolonged PR interval may be seen.

PATHOLOGIC FINDINGS
• Thyroid gland—lymphocytic thyroiditis and/or atrophy
• Skin—may see increased dermal thickness, myxedema, orthokeratotic hyperkeratosis, follicular atrophy, and vacuolation of the arrector pili muscles

TREATMENT
• Myxedema coma is a medical emergency.
• Successful treatment depends on early clinical recognition of the characteristic clinical signs and laboratory abnormalities.
• Treatment is initiated on the basis of a presumptive clinical diagnosis.

NURSING CARE
• Rewarm patients passively with blankets and place them in a warm environment.
• Avoid active attempts (e.g., warm fluids or heating pads) to warm patients; they could cause a precipitous increase in peripheral tissue perfusion and oxygen use.
• Cautious intravenous administration of sodium-containing isotonic fluids at maintenance rates (44 mL/kg/day) is indicated; can add dextrose to the fluids if hypoglycemia is present
• Patients with marked hypoxia should receive oxygen therapy (oxygen cage, oxygen face mask, or oxygen nasal catheter); however, the profound hypoventilation that is causing the hypoxia may necessitate mechanical respiratory support in patients with severe hypoxia and hypercarbia.

MEDICATIONS

DRUG(S)
• Intravenous levothyroxine (0.02 mg/kg q12h for 1–2 doses as needed) is the definitive treatment.
• Can switch patients to oral levothyroxine therapy (0.01 mg/kg q12h) after their condition has stabilized

• Treatment with glucocorticosteroids and broad-spectrum antibiotics is recommended.

CONTRAINDICATIONS/POSSIBLE INTERACTIONS
• Avoid active rewarming.
• Inappropriate intravenous fluid therapy can precipitate or aggravate pulmonary edema.
• Avoid the use of narcotics, tranquilizers, or anesthetics in most instances.

FOLLOW-UP
• The patient's mental alertness, temperature, pulse, and respiration should improve significantly within 6–8 hours.
• Most reported patients have died within 12–24 hours following initiation of therapy, even though their vital signs have improved.
• Myxedema coma has a grave prognosis.

MISCELLANEOUS

SEE ALSO
Hypothyroidism

ABBREVIATIONS
• T_4 = levothyroxine
• TSH = thyroid-stimulating hormone

Suggested Readings
Chastain CB, Graham CL, Riley MG. Myxedema coma in two dogs. Canine Pract 1982;9:20–34.
Kelly MJ, Hill JR. Canine myxedema stupor and coma. Compend Contin Ed Pract Vet 1984;6:1049–1055.
Author John W. Tyler
Consulting Editor: Deborah S. Greco

NAIL AND NAILBED DISORDERS

BASICS

DEFINITION
• Paronychia—inflammation of soft tissue around the nail
• Onychomycosis—fungal infection of the nail
• Onychorrhexis—brittle nails that tend to split or break
• Onychomadesis—sloughing of the nail
• Nail dystrophy—deformity caused by abnormal growth

PATHOPHYSIOLOGY
• Nails and nailfolds—subject to trauma, infection, vascular insufficiency, immune-mediated disease, neoplasia, defects in keratinization, and congenital abnormalities
• A particular nail deformity may be caused by a variety of diseases.
• A single disease can present with various nail lesions.
• Sometimes the cause is unknown and there is no response to treatment.

SYSTEMS AFFECTED
Skin/Exocrine

SIGNALMENT
• Dogs and cats
• Dachshund—predisposed to onychorrhexis

SIGNS
• Licking
• Lameness
• Pain
• Swelling, erythema, and exudate of nailfold
• Deformity or sloughing of nail

CAUSES

Paronychia
• Infection—bacteria, dermatophyte, yeast (*Candida*), demodicosis, leishmaniasis

• Immune-mediated—pemphigus, bullous pemphigoid, SLE, drug eruption, lupoid onychodystrophy
• Neoplasia—squamous cell carcinoma, melanoma, eccrine carcinoma, osteosarcoma, subungual keratoacanthoma, inverted squamous papilloma
• Arteriovenous fistula

Onychomycosis
• Dogs—*Trichophyton mentagrophytes*—usually generalized
• Cats—*Microsporum canis*

Onychorrhexis
• Idiopathic—especially in dachshunds; multiple nails
• Trauma
• Infection—dermatophytosis, leishmaniasis

Onychomadesis
• Trauma
• Infection
• Immune-mediated—pemphigus, bullous pemphigoid, SLE, drug eruption, lupoid onychodystrophy
• Vascular insufficiency—vasculitis, cold agglutinin disease
• Neoplasia—see above
• Idiopathic

Nail Dystrophy
• Acromegaly
• Feline hyperthyroidism
• Zinc-responsive dermatosis
• Congenital malformations

RISK FACTORS
• Paronychia (infectious)—immunosuppression (endogenous or exogenous), FeLV infection, trauma, and diabetes mellitus
• Bacterial onychomadesis—excessively short nail trimming (into the quick) postulated to predispose animal

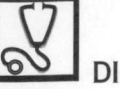

DIAGNOSIS

DIFFERENTIAL DIAGNOSIS
• Trauma or neoplasia often affects a single nail.
• Involvement of multiple nails suggests a systemic disease.
• Immune-mediated diseases (except lupoid onychodystrophy) usually have other skin lesions in addition to nail/nailfold lesions.

CBC/BIOCHEMISTRY/URINALYSIS
May show evidence of SLE, diabetes mellitus, hyperthyroidism, or other systemic illness

OTHER LABORATORY TESTS
• FeLV
• T_4
• ANA titer

IMAGING
Radiographs—osteomyelitis of third phalanx

OTHER DIAGNOSTIC PROCEDURES
• Biopsy—histopathology and direct immunofluorescence; often involves a third phalanx amputation
• Cytology of exudate
• Skin scraping
• Bacterial and fungal culture

TREATMENT

PARONYCHIA
• Surgical removal of nail plate (shell)—provide adequate drainage; grasp nail firmly with hemostat and strip it from its attachments with one swift downward motion; bandage foot following procedure.
• Antimicrobial soaks
• Identify underlying condition and treat specifically.

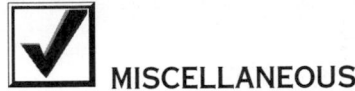

ONYCHOMYCOSIS
• Antifungal soaks—chlorhexidine, povidone iodine, lime sulfur
• Surgical removal of nail plate—may improve response to systemic medication
• Amputation of third phalanx

ONYCHORRHEXIS
• Repair with fingernail glue (type used to attach false nails in humans).
• Remove splintered pieces.
• Amputation of third phalanx
• Treat underlying cause.

ONYCHOMADESIS
• Antimicrobial soaks
• Treat underlying cause.

NEOPLASIA
• Depends on biologic behavior of specific tumor
• Surgical excision
• Amputation of digit
• Amputation of leg
• Chemotherapy
• Radiation therapy

NAIL DYSTROPHY
Treat underlying cause.

MEDICATIONS

DRUG(S) OF CHOICE
• Bacterial paronychia—systemic antibiotics based on culture and sensitivity; cephalosporins pending culture result
• *Candida paronychia*—ketoconazole (10 mg/kg PO q12h); topical nystatin or miconazole
• Onychomycosis—griseofulvin (50–150 mg/kg PO per day) or ketoconazole (10 mg/kg PO q12h) for 6–12 months until negative cultures; itraconazole (10 mg/kg PO daily) for 3 weeks and then pulse therapy twice a week until resolved
• Onychomadesis—depends on cause; immunosuppressive therapy for immune-mediated diseases
• Often-used medications include cyclosporine, tetracycline with niacinamide, pentoxifylline, vitamin E, essential fatty acid supplementations, and chemotherapeutic agents (azathioprine, chlorambucil, etc).

CONTRAINDICATIONS
Griseofulvin—do not use in pregnant animals

PRECAUTIONS
• Griseofulvin—may cause bone marrow suppression, anorexia, vomiting, and diarrhea; absorption enhanced if given with a high-fat meal
• Ketoconazole—may cause anorexia, gastric irritation, hepatic toxicity, and lightening of the hair coat

POSSIBLE INTERACTIONS
N/A

ALTERNATIVE DRUG(S)
N/A

FOLLOW-UP

PATIENT MONITORING
Depends on underlying cause

POSSIBLE COMPLICATIONS
N/A

EXPECTED COURSE AND PROGNOSIS
• Bacterial or fungal paronychia and onychomycosis—treatment may be prolonged and response may be influenced by underlying immunosuppressive factors.
• Onychomycosis and onychorrhexis—may require amputation of the third phalanx for resolution
• Nail dystrophy—prognosis is good when underlying cause can be effectively treated (e.g., hyperthyroidism, zinc-responsive dermatosis).
• Onychomadesis—prognosis depends on underlying cause; immune-mediated diseases and vascular problems carry a more guarded prognosis than do trauma or infectious causes
• Neoplasia—some can be totally excised or removed by amputation of the digit; others are highly malignant and may have already spread by the time of diagnosis

MISCELLANEOUS

ASSOCIATED CONDITIONS
N/A

AGE-RELATED FACTORS
N/A

ZOONOTIC POTENTIAL
Dermatophyte infections

PREGNANCY
N/A

SYNONYMS
Nailfold = nail bed

SEE ALSO
• Demodicosis
• Dermatophytosis
• Pemphigoid, Bullous
• Pemphigus
• Pododermatitis
• Pyoderma
• Vasculitis, Cutaneous

ABBREVIATIONS
• ANA = antinuclear antibody
• FeLV = feline leukemia virus
• SLE = systemic lupus erythematosus
• T_4 = thyroxine

Suggested Reading
Muller GH, Kirk RW, Scott DW. Small animal dermatology. 4th ed. Philadelphia: Saunders, 1989.
Authors Ellen C. Codner and Karen Helton Rhodes
Consulting Editor Karen Helton Rhodes

NARCOLEPSY AND CATAPLEXY

BASICS

OVERVIEW
Sleep disorders

Narcolepsy
Excessive daytime sleepiness, lethargy, or brief periods of collapse and unconsciousness that resolve spontaneously

Cataplexy
• Brief episodes of muscle paralysis with loss of tendon reflexes that are completely and spontaneously reversible
• Patient stays alert and will follow with its eyes.

SIGNALMENT
• Dogs and rarely cats
• Multiple breeds of dogs
• Proven hereditary—Labrador retrievers, poodles, dachshunds, and Doberman pinschers
• Recessive inheritance with complete penetrance—Labradors and Dobermans
• Clinical signs usually appear < 6 months of age.

SIGNS
• Physical and neurologic examinations—normal except during an attack
• Onset—rapid (peracute) in both conditions
• Episodes—usually last only a few seconds to minutes, but can last up to 30 min; usually characterized by collapse into lateral or sternal recumbency with no movements and atonic muscles; commonly elicited during eating, excitement, playing, and sexual activity; may see multiple episodes in one day
• Eye movements, muscular twitching, and whining (as in REM sleep)—frequently observed during episodes
• Patients are usually aroused by loud noises, petting, or other external stimuli.

CAUSES & RISK FACTORS
• Unknown
• Neurotransmitter disturbance
• Possible immune system involvement

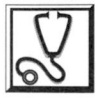

DIAGNOSIS

DIFFERENTIAL DIAGNOSIS
• Seizure activity—urinary or fecal incontinence, excessive salivation, and muscle rigidity are not characteristic of sleep disorders.

• Cataplexy—myasthenia gravis; hypoglycemia; hypocalcemia; hypokalemia; adrenal insufficiency; polymyositis; syncope; nonconvulsive seizure (drop attacks)
• Narcolepsy—hypothyroidism; chronic hypoxia; obesity (Pickwickian syndrome); other metabolic illnesses

CBC/BIOCHEMISTRY/URINALYSIS
• Normal
• Perform to rule out differentials.

OTHER LABORATORY TESTS
N/A

IMAGING
N/A

DIAGNOSTIC PROCEDURES
• Observe an episode—if a consistent activity elicits attacks, attempt to simulate the activity; probably helpful only for severely affected animals
• Food-elicited cataplexy test—place 10 pieces of food in a row 12–24 in. apart; record the time required for the patient to eat all the pieces and the number, type, and duration of any attacks that occur; normal dogs eat all food in < 45 sec and have no attacks; affected dogs take > 2 min to eat the food and can have 2–20 attacks.
• Yohimbine challenge (cataplexy)—administer 25–50 µg/kg IV bolus; positive: 90% reduction in the number or severity of episodes; response should occur within 20–30 min after administration and last for about 4 hr
• Physostigmine challenge (cataplexy)—administer 0.025 mg/kg IV; repeat the food-elicited test 5–15 min after the injection; increase dosage if necessary (0.05 mg/kg; 0.075 mg/kg; 0.10 mg/kg); produces signs in affected patients, causing up to a 300% increase in the number and duration of episodes; effects of each dose last 15–45 min.

TREATMENT
• Primary goal—reduce the severity and frequency of cataplectic attacks
• Inform client that cataplexy is not a fatal disease, choking on food and airway obstruction do not occur, and the pet is not suffering.

• Inform client that activities such as hunting, swimming, and unleashed exercise put the patient at risk.

MEDICATIONS

DRUG(S)
• Yohimbine—drug of choice; 50–100 µg/kg SC or PO q8–12h
• Imipramine—Tofranil; 0.5–1.0 mg/kg PO q8h
• Methylphenidate—Ritalin—5–10 mg PO q24h
• Dextroamphetamine—5–10 mg PO q24h

CONTRAINDICATIONS/POSSIBLE INTERACTIONS
• Many patients develop drug tolerance; change of drug may become necessary.
• Monamine oxidase inhibitors—contraindicated in dogs because of possible toxic cardiovascular side effects

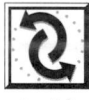

FOLLOW-UP
• Avoiding inciting activities may reduce episodes so that medication is not needed.
• Patients with the inherited form may improve with age.
• Prognosis—varies even with treatment; some patients remain symptomatic.

MISCELLANEOUS

ABBREVIATION
REM = rapid eye movement

Suggested Reading
Fenner WR. Seizures, narcolepsy, and cataplexy. In: Birchard SJ, Sherding RG, eds. Saunders manual of small animal practice. Philadelphia: Saunders, 1994:1147–1156.
Author T. Mark Neer
Consulting Editor Joane M. Parent

NASAL AND NASOPHARYNGEAL POLYPS

BASICS

OVERVIEW
• Protruding pink, polypoid growths (benign) arising from the mucous membranes after arising from a stalk.
• Nasal—originate from the nasal mucosa in dogs and cats.
• Nasopharyngeal—originate from the base of the eustachian tube in cats; may extend into the external or middle ear canal, pharynx, and nasal cavity

SIGNALMENT
• Nasopharyngeal polyps—kittens and young adult cats
• Nasal polyps—dogs and cats

SIGNS

Nasal Polyps
• Chronic mucopurulent nasal discharge
• Noisy breathing—stertor
• Nasal congestion
• Sneezing or epistaxis
• Decreased nasal airflow, generally unilateral
• Nonresponsive to antibiotics or recurrent

Nasopharyngeal Polyps
• Same as for nasal polyps; may be unilateral or bilateral
• Inspiratory dyspnea and choking or gagging
• Dysphagia
• Chronic, nonresponsive otitis
• Head tilt and/or nystagmus
• Horner's syndrome

Causes & Risk Factors
Unknown

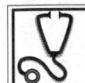

DIAGNOSIS

DIFFERENTIAL DIAGNOSIS
• Feline upper respiratory disease complex
• Upper airway obstruction
• Chronic otitis
• Neurologic disease
• Nasopharyngeal stenosis
• Foreign body
• Neoplasia

CBC/BIOCHEMISTRY/URINALYSIS
N/A

OTHER LABORATORY TESTS
N/A

IMAGING
• Radiographs of nasal cavity—may show a soft tissue structure within the nasal passages
• Radiographs of nasopharynx—may show a soft tissue mass
• Closely evaluate radiographs for involvement of the tympanic bullae (osseous bullae).
• Ultrasonography may reveal cysts or masses in the nasopharynx. Guided needle aspiration or biopsy can be performed.
• MRI and CT can be helpful in detecting lesions better, determining anatomic relationships, and determining involvement in adjacent structures, i.e., bullae.

DIAGNOSTIC PROCEDURES
• While animal is under anesthesia, palpation and visual examination often reveal polyp.
• Caudal rhinoscopy—a spay hook and dental mirror or flexible endoscope are used to visualize the caudal nasopharynx.
• Rostral rhinoscopy (rigid or flexible cystoscope or arthroscope)—allows visualization and biopsy of the mass
• Deep otoscopic cytology examination
• Histopathology

TREATMENT
• Surgery—treatment of choice: excision via the oral cavity for nasopharyngeal polyps, or rhinotomy for nasal polyps; complete excision of root and base of polyp is mandatory to prevent recurrence.
• Concurrent bulla osteotomy—may prevent recurrence of nasopharyngeal polyps

MEDICATIONS

DRUG(S)
Postsurgery—use an appropriate agent for secondary bacterial or yeast infection of the nasal or otic cavity; choose on the basis of culture and sensitivity testing.

CONTRAINDICATIONS/POSSIBLE INTERACTIONS
N/A

FOLLOW-UP
• Incomplete removal of polyp and stalk may result in recurrence.
• Horner's syndrome or facial paralysis may develop after bulla osteotomy, but is generally transient.
• Prognosis excellent with complete removal

MISCELLANEOUS

Suggested Reading
Hendricks JC. Brachycephalic airway syndrome. Update on respiratory disease. Vet Clin North Am Small Anim Pract 1989; 19:1167–1188.
Author James C. Prueter
Consulting Editor Lynelle R. Johnson

NASAL DERMATOSES

 BASICS

DEFINITION
Pathologic condition of the nasal skin involving either the haired portion (bridge of the nose) or nonhaired portion (nasal planum)

PATHOPHYSIOLOGY
N/A

SYSTEMS AFFECTED
- Skin/exocrine
- Multisystemic—SLE

SIGNALMENT
- Dermatophytosis, zinc-responsive dermatosis, dermatomyositis, and demodicosis—more likely in dogs < 1 year of age
- Zinc-responsive dermatosis—Siberian huskies, Alaskan malamutes
- Dermatomyositis—collies, Shetland sheepdogs
- Uveodermatologic syndrome—akitas, Samoyeds, Siberian huskies
- SLE and DLE—collies, Shetland sheepdogs, German shepherds; DLE may occur more often in females
- Epidermotropic lymphoma—old dogs

SIGNS
- Depigmentation
- Hyperpigmentation
- Erythema
- Erosion/ulceration
- Vesicles/pustules
- Crusts
- Scarring
- Alopecia
- Nodules/plaques

CAUSES
- Nasal pyoderma
- Demodicosis
- Dermatophytosis
- Other fungal infections—cryptococcosis, sporotrichosis, aspergillosis
- DLE and SLE
- Pemphigus foliaceus
- Pemphigus erythematosus
- Nasal solar dermatitis
- Dermatomyositis
- Zinc-responsive dermatosis
- Uveodermatologic syndrome
- Vitiligo
- Nasal depigmentation
- Contact hypersensitivity—plastic dish dermatitis, topical drug hypersensitivity (neomycin)
- Tumors—squamous cell carcinoma, basal cell carcinoma, mycosis fungoides, fibrosarcoma
- Trauma

- Idiopathic sterile granuloma
- Idiopathic nasal hyperkeratosis

RISK FACTORS
- Adult cats—may be inapparent carriers of dermatophytes
- Rooting behavior—pyoderma, dermatophytosis
- Sun exposure—nasal solar dermatitis, DLE, SLE, pemphigus erythematosus
- Poorly pigmented nose—nasal solar dermatitis, squamous cell carcinoma
- Large, rapidly growing breeds over-supplemented with calcium or fed high-cereal diet—zinc-responsive dermatosis
- Immunosuppression—demodicosis, pyoderma, dermatophytosis

 DIAGNOSIS

DIFFERENTIAL DIAGNOSIS

Nasal Solar Dermatitis
- Lesions—confined to nose; precipitated by heavy sunlight exposure
- Begins in poorly pigmented skin at junction of nasal planum and bridge of nose
- Negative DIF

DLE
- Primarily affects nasal area
- Exacerbated by sunlight
- Positive DIF at basement membrane zone
- Biopsy—interface dermatitis

SLE
- Multisystemic disease
- Skin lesions—often involve nose, face, mucocutaneous junctions; multifocal or generalized
- ANA positive
- Positive DIF at basement membrane zone

Pemphigus Foliaceus
- Lesions—usually start on face and ears; commonly involve footpads; eventually generalize
- Biopsy—subcorneal pustules with acantholysis
- Positive DIF in intercellular spaces of epidermis

Pemphigus Erythematosus
- Lesions—primarily confined to face and ears
- Biopsy—intraepidermal pustules with acantholysis
- Positive DIF at basement membrane zone and intercellular spaces

Demodicosis
- Often starts on face or forelimbs
- May generalize
- Diagnose with skin scrapings

Plastic (or Rubber) Dish Dermatitis
- Depigmentation and erythema of anterior nasal planum and anterior lips
- No ulceration or crusting
- History of exposure

Dermatomyositis
- Typical breed
- Nasal, facial, and extremity lesions—characterized by erosion, alopecia, scarring, and hyperpigmentation
- Polymyositis or megaesophagus may be seen.
- Biopsy—interface dermatitis with follicular atrophy
- Negative DIF

Uveodermatologic Syndrome
- Typical breed
- Uveitis and cutaneous macular depigmentation without inflammation—nose, lips, and eyelids
- Biopsy of early lesions—interface dermatitis, pigmentary incontinence

Zinc-responsive Dermatosis
- Typical signalment or diet (i.e., high-fiber or calcium supplementation)
- Crusted lesions—face, mucocutaneous junctions, pressure points, footpads
- Biopsy—parakeratotic hyperkeratosis

Other
- Nasal pyoderma—acute onset of folliculitis on haired portion of nose
- Dermatophytosis—haired portion of the nose; diagnose with culture or biopsy
- Vitiligo—cutaneous macular depigmentation without inflammation on nose, lips, eyelids, footpads, and nails; leukotrichia with leukoderma may be seen.
- Nasal hypopigmentation—normal black coloration of nasal planum fades to light brown or whitish color; may be seasonal or wax and wane
- Idiopathic nasal hyperkeratosis—dry, horny growths of keratin localized to nasal planum
- Other diseases—differentiate with history or biopsy

CBC/BIOCHEMISTRY/URINALYSIS
- Usually normal
- SLE—may see hemolytic anemia, thrombocytopenia, or evidence of glomerulonephritis (high BUN, proteinuria)

OTHER LABORATORY TESTS
N/A

IMAGING
N/A

DIAGNOSTIC PROCEDURES
- Skin scrapings—*Demodex*
- Cytology—fungal organisms, bacteria, or acantholytic cells (pemphigus)

- Dermatophyte test medium—dermatophytosis
- Culture on Sabouraud agar—other fungal infections
- Bacterial culture and sensitivity or cytologic evaluation—pyoderma
- Joint tap—evidence of polyarthritis in SLE
- ANA—positive in most cases of SLE
- Ocular examination—uveitis in uveodermatologic syndrome
- ECG—evidence of myocarditis in SLE
- EMG—evidence of polymyositis in SLE and dermatomyositis
- DIF—deposition of immunoglobulin at the basement membrane zone in DLE, SLE, and pemphigus erythematosus and intercellular spaces of epidermis in pemphigus foliaceus and pemphigus erythematosus
- Skin biopsy

IMAGING
N/A

PATHOLOGIC FINDINGS
- Folliculitis/furunculosis (± mites, bacteria, or fungal elements)—demodicosis, dermatophytosis, nasal pyoderma
- Follicular atrophy and perifollicular fibrosis—dermatomyositis
- Interface dermatitis—DLE, SLE, dermatomyositis, uveodermatologic syndrome
- Intraepidermal pustules with acantholysis—pemphigus foliaceus and pemphigus erythematosus
- Parakeratotic hyperkeratosis—zinc-responsive dermatosis
- Hypomelanosis—vitiligo, uveodermatologic syndrome
- Granulomatous/pyogranulomatous dermatitis—pyoderma, fungal, foreign body, idiopathic sterile granuloma

TREATMENT
- Outpatient, except SLE with severe multiorgan dysfunction or tumors requiring surgical excision or radiation therapy
- Reduce exposure to sunlight—DLE, SLE, pemphigus erythematosus, nasal solar dermatitis, squamous cell carcinoma
- Discourage rooting behavior—pyoderma, dermatophytosis

- Warm soaks—aid removal of exudate and crusts
- Replace plastic or rubber dish and avoid contact with topical drug or other agent causing hypersensitivity reaction.

MEDICATIONS

DRUG(S) OF CHOICE
- Fungal infections—systemic antifungals: griseofulvin, ketoconazole, itraconazole (drug of choice in the cat); topical enilconazole for aspergillosis; surgical excision of early discrete lesions
- Nasal solar dermatitis—topical corticosteroids; antibiotics for secondary infection; sunscreens; tattoo hypopigmented skin (not currently used)
- Idiopathic sterile granuloma—surgical excision when feasible; immunosuppressive therapy with glucocorticoids ± azathioprine, cyclosporine, tetracycline, and niacinamide
- SLE—immunosuppressive therapy with prednisolone ± azathioprine (dogs), chlorambucil, or gold salts (cats)
- Vitiligo/nasal depigmentation—no treatment
- Tumors—surgical excision; chemotherapy; radiation therapy
- Idiopathic nasal hyperkeratosis—antibiotic-corticosteroid cream for fissures, topical humectant (Kerasolv from DVM Pharmaceuticals), topical tacrolimus (Protopic)
- Other diseases—see specific disease

CONTRAINDICATIONS
- Avoid chrysotherapy in patients with renal disease.
- Azathioprine—use cautiously in cats; may cause fatal leukopenia or thrombocytopenia

PRECAUTIONS
- Griseofulvin—can cause anorexia, vomiting, diarrhea, and bone marrow suppression; feed with high-fat diet
- Ketoconazole—may cause anorexia, gastric irritation, hepatotoxicity, and lightening of hair coat

POSSIBLE INTERACTIONS
N/A

ALTERNATIVE DRUG(S)
N/A

FOLLOW-UP

PATIENT MONITORING
Varies with specific disease and treatment prescribed

POSSIBLE COMPLICATIONS
Scarring with deep infections or overly vigorous cleaning

MISCELLANEOUS

ASSOCIATED CONDITIONS
N/A

AGE-RELATED FACTORS
N/A

ZOONOTIC POTENTIAL
Dermatophytosis

PREGNANCY
Griseofulvin is teratogenic.

SYNONYMS
Uveodermatologic = Vogt-Koyanagi-Harada syndrome

ABBREVIATIONS
- ANA = antinuclear antibody
- BUN = blood urea nitrogen
- DIF = direct immunofluorescence
- DLE = discoid lupus erythematosus
- ECG = electrocardiogram
- EMG = electromyography
- SLE = systemic lupus erythematosus

Suggested Reading
Muller GH, Kirk RW, Scott DW. Small animal dermatology. 4th ed. Philadelphia: Saunders, 1989.
Authors Ellen C. Codner and Karen Helton Rhodes
Consulting Editor Karen Helton Rhodes

NASAL DISCHARGE (SNEEZING, REVERSE SNEEZING)

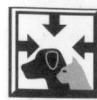

BASICS

DEFINITION
• May be serous, mucoid, mucopurulent, purulent, blood tinged, frank blood (epistaxis), or contain food debris
• Sneezing—reflexive expulsion of air through the nasal cavity; commonly associated with nasal discharge
• Reverse sneezing—repetitive, forceful inspiratory efforts elicited after irritation of the mucosa in the caudal-dorsal nasopharynx

PATHOPHYSIOLOGY
• Secretions—produced by mucous cells of the epithelium and submucosal glands; increased production owing to irritation of the nasal mucosa by mechanical, chemical, or inflammatory stimuli
• Mucosal irritation and accumulated secretions—potent stimulus of the sneeze reflex
• Sneezing—frequency often diminishes with chronic disease
• Reverse sneezing—caused by irritation of the mucosa of the caudo-dorsal nasopharynx
• Gagging protective reflex elicited by oropharyngeal stimulation; usually functions to clear material from the oropharynx; often follows a coughing episode as secretions are brought through the larynx into the oropharynx

SYSTEMS AFFECTED
• Respiratory—mucosa of the upper tract, including the nasal cavities, sinuses, and naso-pharynx; lower tract disease often produces secretions that affect the upper airways.
• Cardiovascular—systemic hypertension
• Gastrointestinal—signs may be observed with extranasal diseases (e.g., swallowing disorders and esophageal or gastrointestinal diseases) • Hemic/Lymphatic/Immune—blood-tinged discharge or epistaxis owing to platelet or hemostatic defects

SIGNALMENT
• Dogs and cats • Young animals—cleft palate; ciliary dyskinesia; immunoglobulin deficiency; nasal polyps • Older animals—nasal tumors; primary dental disease
• Hunting dogs—foreign body
• Dolichocephalic dogs—aspergillosis
• Male dogs may have a higher incidence of nasal fungal infection than do females.

SIGNS

Historical Findings
• Sneezing—commonly reported as a concurrent problem • Important to know both the initial and current character of the discharge as well as whether it was originally unilateral or bilateral
• Stertor—owners frequently report noisy breathing especially when animal is sleeping
• Response to previous antibiotic therapy—may help determine secondary bacterial involvement; foreign body, dental-related disease, and pneumonia usually respond initially to antibiotic treatment but commonly relapse; nasal tumors and fungal rhinitis typically show little response.

Physical Examination Findings
• Secretions or dried discharge on the hair of the muzzle or forelimbs • May note reduction in nasal air flow • Concurrent dental disease
• Bony involvement—with a tumor or fourth premolar abscess; may be detected as facial or hard palate swelling or as pain secondary to osteomyelitis due to fungal or bacterial infection or to tumor invasion • Mucosal de-pigmentation of the nasal alar cartilage—often observed with chronic nasal discharge, especially dogs with nasal aspergillosis
• Mandibular lymphadenomegaly—neoplasia, fungal infection, dental disease
• Polyp—may be visible on otoscopic exam
• Chorioretinitis—may be seen with canine distemper or feline cryptococcosis

CAUSES
• Unilateral—often associated with non-systemic processes; foreign body; dental-related disease (e.g., abscess and oronasal fistula); fungal infections (e.g., aspergillosis, penicilliosis, cryptococcosis, and *Sporothrix*); nasal tumor (e.g., adenocarcinoma, squamous cell carcinoma, and fibrosarcoma)
• Bilateral—infectious agent (e.g., feline viral rhinotracheitis, feline calicivirus, canine distemper, and secondary bacterial infection); airborne irritant; allergy; ciliary dyskinesia; IgA deficiency; lymphoplasmacytic or hyperplastic rhinitis • Unilateral progressing to bilateral—*Aspergillus;* nasal tumor • Either unilateral or bilateral—epistaxis (e.g., coagulopathy and systemic hypertension); foreign body; nasal parasites (dogs, *Pneumonyssoides;* dogs and cats, *Cuterebra* and *Capillaria;* cats, *Linguatula*) • Extranasal diseases—pneumonia, megaesophagus, chronic vomiting, cricopharyngeal achalasia; secretions may be forced up into the nasopharynx, resulting in nasal discharge

RISK FACTORS
• Exposure to other animals • Dental disease
• Foreign bodies—more common in outdoor animals • Infectious—poorly vaccinated animal; kennel situations • Nasal asper-gillosis—dogs bedded on straw • Nasal mites—kennel-raised dogs
• Immunosuppression, chronic corticosteroid use, and FeLV or FIV infection • Chronic, low grade pneumonia • Chronic vomiting

DIAGNOSIS

DIFFERENTIAL DIAGNOSIS

Similar Signs
Differentiate regular sneezing (occurs on expiration) from reverse sneezing (occurs on inspiration and localizes the site of irritation to the caudal-dorsal nasopharynx).

Causes
• Serous—mild irritation; viral and parasitic (e.g., nasal mites) disorders
• Mucoid—allergy; nonspecific airborne irritants early neoplastic condition
• Purulent (or mucopurulent)—secondary bacterial or fungal infection
• Serosanguinous to epistaxis—destructive process (e.g., primary nasal tumor and aspergillosis in dogs); after violent or paroxysmal sneezing episodes (e.g., traumatic capillary rupture); associated with selected systemic disease (e.g., coagulopathy, platelet disorder, and systemic hypertension)

CBC/BIOCHEMISTRY/URINALYSIS
• Results not specific for any particular cause
• Valuable—detect concurrent problems; part of a thorough evaluation before general anesthesia for diagnostic procedures

OTHER LABORATORY TESTS
• Serologic tests—help to diagnose fungal (e.g., aspergillosis and cryptococcosis) and rickettsial (e.g., ehrlichiosis and Rocky Mountain spotted fever) diseases
• Coagulation studies—determine platelet numbers and function
• Immunoglobulin quantification—diagnose IgA deficiency

IMAGING

Skull Radiography
• Anesthetize and carefully position patient
• Perform before rhinoscopy and periodontal probing, which may cause nasal bleeding and alter radiographic density
• Lateral view—detect any periosteal reaction over the nasal bone; note gross changes in the maxillary teeth, nasal cavity, and frontal sinuses (without identifying which side is involved); evaluate air column outlining the nasopharynx for filling defects
• Open-mouth ventrodorsal and intraoral views (using sheet film)—excellent for evaluating nasal cavities and turbinates
• Rostrocaudal view—evaluate each frontal sinus (periosteal reaction and filling)
• CT and MRI—help detect the extent of bony changes associated with nasal tumors and fungal rhinitis

NASAL DISCHARGE (SNEEZING, REVERSE SNEEZING)

Dental Radiography
• Lateral oblique views (use high-speed screen film)—best for detecting maxillary tooth abnormalities • Ultraspeed, nonscreen, intraoral dental film—provides excellent detail of nasal and dental disorders

Thoracic Radiography
May reveal areas of alveolar infiltrates—secretions coughed-up in a patient with chronic pneumonia may cause nasopharyngeal irritation and clinical nasal discharge.

DIAGNOSTIC PROCEDURES
• Rhinoscopy—indicated with chronic or recurrent nasal discharge; may be indicated with reverse sneezing and acute epistaxis; evaluate both anterior and posterior; may be contraindicated with bleeding disorders
• Nasal cytologic examination—nonspecific inflammation (nondegenerative poly-morphonuclear cells) most commonly found; large numbers of eosinophils suggest hypersensitivity or allergic rhinitis; hyphae or microconidia diagnostic for *Aspergillus;* yeast bodies diagnostic for *Cryptococcus;* may note neoplastic cells • Fungal culture—difficult to interpret; up to 40% of normal dogs may have positive fungal cultures • Bacterial cultures are suspect as most infections are secondary; useful when resistant organisms suspected • Biopsy of the nasal cavity—indicated with chronic nasal discharge and with suspected tissue growth (tumor or granuloma); various techniques may be used (directed endoscopic biopsy best, rigid catheter or the blind coring technique, and rhinotomy); multiple samples required to ensure adequate representation because necrosis of the leading tissue edge is common; perform electron microscopy for suspected ciliary dyskinesia. • Bronchoscopy—indicated when rhinoscopy reveals only minimal changes; exudate often observed in the middle lung lobes of dogs that do not show typical lower respiratory signs and serves as an extranasal source of secretions • Periodontal probing of all upper teeth—part of every evaluation of sneezing and nasal discharge; perform after rhinoscopy; the normal gingival sulcus: dogs, < 4.0 mm; cats, < 1.0 mm
• Blood pressure, platelets, and coagulation profile for epistaxis

TREATMENT
• Outpatient—acceptable except when surgery is required
• Adequate hydration, nutrition, warmth, and hygiene (keeping nares clean)—important with chronic sneezing and nasal discharge
• Surgery—for exploratory rhinotomy; to treat *Rhinosporidium* or foreign body; to place tubes to deliver antifungal medications

MEDICATIONS
DRUG(S)
• Secondary bacterial infection—antibiotics; choose a good gram-positive spectrum of activity (e.g., amoxicillin, clavamox, clindamycin, Zithromax, and one of the cephalosporins); tetracyclines are actively secreted into the gingival sulcus and may be used with chronic rhinitis secondary to dental disease.
• Attempt to dry up nasal secretions—decongestants (ephedrine at 10–50 mg total PO q8–12h, to a maximum of 4 mg/kg, dogs; 2–4 mg/kg q8–12h, cats); topical vasoconstrictors (neosynephrine at 0.25%–0.5% q8–24h or oxymetazoline at 0.25% q24h)
• Dental-associated rhinitis—antibiotics; dental work (e.g., extractions, gingivectomy, and flap closure to treat fistula)
• Foreign body removal—antibiotics
• Nasal parasites—ivermectin (300 µg/kg PO weekly for 2–3 weeks) to treat *Pneumonyssoides;* fenbendazole (50 mg/kg q6h for 10 days) to treat *Capillaria*
• Nonspecific inflammation—prednisolone (1–2 mg/kg PO q12–24h) or piroxicam (0.3 mg/kg PO q24–48h)
• Canine nasal aspergillosis—topical treatment with an antifungal agent delivered through surgically or endoscopically placed frontal sinus tubes (e.g., enilconazole or clotrimazole); curettage (surgical or endoscopic) is critical to successful treatment
• Feline cryptococcosis or sporothricosis—itraconazole (5–10 mg/kg PO q24h) or fluconazole (50 mg/cat q12h)
• Neoplasia—radiotherapy and chemotherapy

CONTRAINDICATIONS
• Ephedrine—in cardiac patients
• Ivermectin—in collies and similar breeds

PRECAUTIONS
• Itraconazole—anorexia, nausea, vomiting, and high liver enzymes (e.g., ALT) reverse when the drug is discontinued
• Rebound phenomenon—reported with overuse of topical nasal vasoconstrictors

FOLLOW-UP
PATIENT MONITORING
• Nasal discharge and sneezing—note changes in frequency, volume, and character.
• Surgically placed nasal tubes—inpatient monitoring; watch for subcutaneous emphysema and local cellulitis.
• Repeat rhinoscopy—indicated to ensure adequate response to treatment for fungal rhinitis

• Recheck thoracic radiographs or bronchoscopy—monitor response to treatment for chronic pneumonia

POSSIBLE COMPLICATIONS
• Loss of appetite—especially in cats
• Extension of primary disease (e.g., fungal infection and tumor) into the mouth, eye, or brain • Respiratory distress—caused by nasal obstruction • Involvement of the cribriform plate in dogs with aspergillosis—CNS damage during topical drug therapy and tube placement is a risk

MISCELLANEOUS
ASSOCIATED CONDITIONS
• Sinusitis • Dental disease • Secondary causes—coagulopathy, pneumonia, crico-pharyngeal disease, megaesophagus • Cats—immunosuppression caused by FeLV or FIV; fungal disease (e.g., cryptococcosis and *Sporothrix*); upper respiratory viral infection

AGE-RELATED FACTORS
Middle-aged to old patients—often associated with dental or neoplastic conditions

ZOONOTIC POTENTIAL
Sporothrix infection may represent a zoonotic health concern.

PREGNANCY
The safety of most recommended drugs has not been established in pregnant animals.

SEE ALSO
• Aspergillosis • Ciliary Dyskinesia, Primary • Cryptococcosis • Epistaxis • Nasal and Nasopharyngeal Polyps • Nasopharyngeal Stenosis • Rhinitis and Sinusitis • Nasal Tumors

ABBREVIATIONS
• ALT = alanine aminotransferase
• CNS = central nervous system • CT = computed tomography • FeLV = feline leukemia virus • FIV = feline immunodeficiency virus • MRI = magnetic resonance imaging

Suggested Reading
McKiernan BC. Sneezing and nasal discharge. In: Ettinger SJ, Feldman EC, eds. Textbook of veterinary internal medicine. 4th ed. Philadelphia: Saunders, 1994:79–85.

Ogilvie GK, LaRue SM. Canine and feline nasal and paranasal sinus tumors. Vet Clin North Am 1992;22:1133–1144.

Van Pelt DR, Lappin MR. Pathogenesis and treatment of feline rhinitis. Vet Clin North Am 1994;24:807–823.

Van Pelt DR, McKiernan BC. Pathogenesis and treatment of canine rhinitis. Vet Clin North Am Small Anim Pract 1994;24:789–806.

Author Brendan C. McKiernan
Consulting Editor Lynelle R. Johnson

NASOPHARYNGEAL STENOSIS

BASICS

OVERVIEW
• Formation of a thin but tough membrane at the internal nasal meatus, resulting in the narrowing of the orifice from a 5–6-mm oval opening to a 1–2-mm opening
• Chronic inflammation and fibrosis on histologic examination suggest an infectious or allergic cause.

SIGNALMENT
• Cats of any breed or sex
• Age—range, usually 8 months to 10 years; any age as long as ample time has passed since exposure to the inciting cause

SIGNS
• Evidence of upper respiratory obstruction
• Whistling or snoring noise
• Minimal nasal discharge
• Duration of signs for at least several months
• Aggravation of signs during eating
• Failure to respond to antibiotics or corticosteroids

CAUSES & RISK FACTORS
• Viral upper respiratory or chlamydial infection
• Foreign body or irritant contacting affected area

DIAGNOSIS

DIFFERENTIAL DIAGNOSIS
• Nasopharyngeal polyps—seen during oral examination or by radiography or endoscopy
• Chronic rhinitis or sinusitis—moderate to severe nasal discharge and sneezing; obvious radiographic changes commonly seen
• Foreign body—unilateral mucopurulent nasal discharge; radiographic abnormalities
• Intranasal neoplasia—unilateral obstruction; nasal discharge often bloody; radiographic changes
• Mycotic rhinitis—moderate to severe nasal discharge, often hemorrhagic; radiographic changes

• Laryngeal disease—no improvement with open-mouth breathing; lack of snorting and nasal discharge; abnormalities on oral examination

CBC/BIOCHEMISTRY/URINALYSIS
N/A

OTHER LABORATORY TESTS
N/A

IMAGING
Near-normal radiographic findings

DIAGNOSTIC PROCEDURES
• Inability to pass a 3.5 French catheter through the ventral meatus into the pharynx
• Visualization of the membrane by use of a retroflexed pediatric bronchoscope or a dental mirror

TREATMENT
Surgery—under general anesthesia; patient in dorsal recumbency with the mouth wide open; incise soft palate; resect membrane; suture soft palate.

MEDICATIONS

DRUG(S)
Antibiotics after surgery

CONTRAINDICATIONS/POSSIBLE INTERACTIONS
N/A

FOLLOW-UP
• Warn client that recurrence is possible.
• Consider high levels of corticosteroids if a second surgery is necessary.

MISCELLANEOUS

Suggested Reading

Mitten RW. Acquired nasopharyngeal stenosis in cats. In: Kirk RW, Bonagura JD, eds. Current veterinary therapy XI. Philadelphia: Saunders, 1992:801–803.

Author Justin H. Straus
Consulting Editor Lynelle R. Johnson

NECK AND BACK PAIN

 **BASICS**

DEFINITION
Discomfort along the spinal column

PATHOPHYSIOLOGY
Pain may originate in the epaxial muscle, vertebrae and associated structures, spinal nerves, nerve roots or dorsal root ganglia, and meninges.

SYSTEMS AFFECTED
• Nervous
• Musculoskeletal

SIGNALMENT
• Dogs and cats
• Disk disease—dogs: usually develops at 3–8 years old, occasionally outside this range; rare in cats
• Wobbler syndrome—large-breed dogs; more often in middle-aged to old Doberman pinschers and young Great Danes
• Atlantoaxial luxation and subluxation—occurs in young to middle-aged miniature breeds
• Steroid-responsive meningitis-arteritis—dogs < 2 years; Bernese mountain dog, boxer, beagle, toller retriever

SIGNS

Historical Findings
Complaints—relate to perceived discomfort; reluctance in going up or down stairs most common

Physical Examination Findings
• Head down posture—neck
• Arched back—neck or back
• Pain on epaxial palpation
• Guarded posture
• Reluctance to walk
• Epaxial muscle rigidity
• Palpable heat in the epaxial musculature
• Low grade fever—primarily in patients with meningeal involvement

CAUSES

Epaxial Muscle
• Traumatic myositis
• Exertional rhabdomyolysis
• Muscle neoplasia—rhabdomyosarcoma
• Inflammatory myositis—parasitic, bacterial, protozoal, or immune mediated
• Foreign body myositis—grass awn migration

Vertebrae and Associated Structures
• Disk disease
• Diskospondylitis
• Osteoarthritis of facets

• Unstable vertebral anomalies—hemivertebrae and atlantoaxial luxation or subluxation
• Vertebral neoplasia—osteosarcoma, chondrosarcoma, multiple myeloma, and metastatic tumors
• Vertebral osteomyelitis
• Fracture
• Luxation and subluxation
• Malformation and malarticulation

Spinal Nerves
• Entrapment by disk herniation
• Neoplasia—neurofibroma and neurofibrosarcoma
• Traumatic entrapment, tearing, or laceration
• Neuritis—viral, bacterial, and parasitic
• Compression or inflammation of dorsal root ganglion

Meninges
• Meningioma and metastatic neoplasia
• Meningitis—bacterial, viral, parasitic, protozoal, rickettsial, immune mediated, or idiopathic

RISK FACTORS
• Trauma
• Very active animal
• Previous diagnosis of cancer

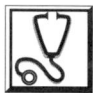 **DIAGNOSIS**

DIFFERENTIAL DIAGNOSIS
• Diseases involving thoracic structures—pleura, cardiovascular system, and lungs
• Diseases involving abdominal structures—kidneys, prostate gland, pancreas, and intestines
• Rule out limb musculoskeletal pain.
• Degenerative radiculomyelopathy and fibrocartilaginous myelopathy—nonpainful diseases of the spinal cord
• Often associated with neoplasia in cats

CBC/BIOCHEMISTRY/URINALYSIS

Epaxial Muscle
• Creatine kinase—can be high with any diseases affecting the muscle
• High WBC count—may indicate an abscess
• Myoglobinuria—may reflect the extent of damage

Vertebrae and Associated Structures
• Usually normal with degenerative, anomalous, and neoplastic disease
• Hemogram—may be abnormal with inflammatory diseases (e.g., acute diskospondylitis and multisystemic involvement)

Spinal Nerves
Usually normal

Meninges
• Usually normal, even with severe meningitis
• Leucocytosis—some patients with aseptic meningitis

OTHER LABORATORY TESTS

Vertebrae and Associated Structures
Multiple myeloma—may note Bence Jones protein in the urine; bone marrow examination may reveal neoplastic cells.

Meninges
• Specific serologic tests—depend on suspected cause; canine distemper, ehrlichiosis, Rocky Mountain spotted fever, neosporosis, toxoplasmosis
• Serum IgA—often high with aseptic meningitis

IMAGING

Epaxial Muscle
• Applicable only in patients with suspected neoplasia or foreign body
• Thoracic radiography—detect metastasis

Vertebrae and Associated Structures
• Survey radiography—thoracic: detect metastasis; spinal: detect obvious bony abnormalities (e.g., fracture or luxation, diskospondylitis, neoplasia, osteoarthritis, and extruded calcified disk)
• Myelography—delineate extradural (e.g., disk herniation), intradural-extramedullary (e.g., meningioma), and intramedullary (e.g., spinal neoplasia) lesions
• CT—cross-sectional and other special views; more clearly defines bony lesions
• MRI—cross-sectional and other special views; more clearly defines soft tissue lesions

Spinal Nerves
• Survey radiograph—seldom of benefit
• Myelography—seldom of benefit unless the lesion is pressing on or invading the meninges
• MRI—most rewarding imaging technique for identifying the location and extent of the lesion

Meninges
• Myelography—can identify neoplastic involvement (e.g., meningioma)
• MRI—more clearly defines soft tissue lesions

DIAGNOSTIC PROCEDURES

Epaxial Muscle
• Muscle biopsy—may reveal neoplastic or inflammatory cells
• EMG—may identify an irritating or denervating process affecting the muscles

Vertebrae and Associated Structures
• Bone biopsy—helps confirm vertebral neoplasia and infection
• Cytology and culture (diskospondylitis)—obtain aspirate from the affected intervertebral space; may help identify cause

Spinal Nerves
• Electrodiagnostic testing—EMG, nerve conduction velocity, and F waves; helps differentiate and confirm muscle versus nerve disease and location of the lesion

Meninges
CSF analysis—diagnostic test of choice; include measurement of immunoglobulins, serologic testing, and bacterial culture.

TREATMENT
• Varies widely according to the nature and extent of the tissues involved
• **CAUTION:** symptomatic treatment without first establishing a diagnosis can be dangerous.
• Inpatient vs. outpatient—depends on severity of disease
• Surgical intervention—inpatient; indicated for disk herniation, trauma, congenital anomalies, and neoplasia; foreign body may require removal or drainage to treat an associated abscess
• Acupuncture—may alleviate neck/back pain

MEDICATIONS

DRUG(S) OF CHOICE

Epaxial Muscle
• Antimicrobial therapy—for infection; depends on the causative agent
• Glucocorticosteroids—may be required; depends on the diagnosis
• Chemotherapy or radiotherapy—for neoplasia; depends on tumor type

Vertebrae and Associated Structures
• Glucocorticosteroids—indicated in some patients and contraindicated in others; establish a diagnosis, if at all possible, before initiating
• Antimicrobials—indicated when a specific organism can be identified or is suspected (e.g., with diskospondylitis)
• Chemotherapy and radiotherapy—depends on tumor type

Spinal Nerves
Corticosteroids—useful for trauma, inflammation, and nerve compression; may help some patients with neoplasia

Meninges
• Antimicrobials that cross the blood–brain barrier—when delivery to the CNS is desired
• Corticosteroids—may be indicated; establish a diagnosis, if at all possible, before initiating.

CONTRAINDICATIONS
Glucocorticosteroids—may be detrimental for patients with infectious conditions and with gastroenteritis or cystitis

PRECAUTIONS
• Glucocorticosteroids—watch for signs of gastroenteritis or cystitis before initiating and while administering.
• With instability or possible disk disease—cage rest indicated for patients using drugs with analgesic effects to prevent exacerbation of the primary problem and further neurologic damage
• Steroids and NSAIDs—do not use in combination; life-threatening gastroenteritis may result.

POSSIBLE INTERACTIONS
N/A

ALTERNATIVE DRUG(S)
• NSAIDs
• Polysulfated glycosaminoglycan
• Methocarbamol—muscle relaxation
• Benzodiazepines (e.g., diazepam)—muscle relaxation and antianxiety effects
• Phenylbutazone—may alleviate musculoskeletal pain; ineffective against neurologic pain
• Fentanyl patches

FOLLOW-UP

PATIENT MONITORING
• Monitor response to treatment closely and make adjustments as necessary.
• Instruct client to watch for signs of gastroenteritis and cystitis.

POSSIBLE COMPLICATIONS

Epaxial Muscle
• Abscess
• Chronic pain
• Fibrous replacement of muscle fibers, causing chronic pain and immobility

Vertebrae and Associated Structures
• Frequent recurrence in patients with disk disease that receive medical management only
• Permanent paralysis or dysfunction
• Urinary and fecal incontinence

• Chronic pain
• Spread to adjacent tissues

Spinal Nerves
• Permanent paralysis or dysfunction
• Chronic pain

Meninges
• Involvement of surrounding spinal cord and brain tissue

MISCELLANEOUS

ASSOCIATED CONDITIONS
• Cardiac muscle disease in patients with myositis
• Sites of infection in other tissues as a source of CNS or vertebral involvement (e.g., bacterial endocarditis or cystitis as a cause of diskospondylitis)
• Metastatic disease from a primary tumor in another organ system
• Immunologic incompetence

AGE-RELATED FACTORS
• Anomalous conditions—usually seen in younger animals
• Disk disease—most frequently seen in active, middle-aged dogs
• Neoplastic conditions—more often seen in middle-aged to old animals

ZOONOTIC POTENTIAL
N/A

PREGNANCY
Use of glucocorticosteroids is contraindicated.

SEE ALSO
See causes

ABBREVIATIONS
• CT = computed tomography
• EMG = electromyography
• MRI = magnetic resonance imaging
• NSAIDS = nonsteroidal antiinflammatory drugs

Suggested Reading
Aron DM. Pain. In: Lorenz MD, Cornelius LM, eds. Small animal medical diagnosis. Philadelphia: Lippincott, 1987:411–424.
Oliver JE, Lorenz MD, Kornegay JN. Pain. In: Handbook of veterinary neurology. Philadelphia: Saunders, 1997:333–340.
Author Patricia J. Luttgen
Consulting Editor Joane M. Parent

NECROTIZING ENCEPHALITIS IN YORKSHIRE TERRIERS

BASICS

OVERVIEW
• One of the breed-restricted encephalitides defined by highly characteristic morphologic features
• First described in 1993 in Switzerland; occurs in several other European countries and in North America
• CNS only organ system affected
• A genetic basis probable

SIGNALMENT
• Dogs
• Yorkshire terriers
• Occasionally in other small breeds—Chihuahuas; Shi-Tzus
• Usually affects young adults (1–5 years of age); may affect older animals

SIGNS
• Initially variable
• Acute in onset; uniformly progressive
• Seizures—may occur; not always observed (unlike the breed-specific encephalitides of Maltese and pug dogs)
• Brain stem symptoms with central vestibular signs—predominate
• Rarely, cortical involvement

CAUSES & RISK FACTORS
• Unknown
• An infectious agent might be suspected.

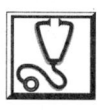

DIAGNOSIS

DIFFERENTIAL DIAGNOSIS
• Rule out other inflammatory or infectious diseases of the CNS.
• Neoplasia

CBC/BIOCHEMISTRY/URINALYSIS
Usually normal

OTHER LABORATORY TESTS
N/A

IMAGING
• CT and MRI (brain)—nonspecific changes; decreased opacity in CT scans; may support the clinical diagnosis considering breed, age, multifocal lesions, and course of the disease
• Neurosonography, CT, and MRI (brain)—nonspecific moderate hydrocephalus

DIAGNOSTIC PROCEDURES
CSF analysis—moderate mononuclear pleocytosis (12–76 leukocytes/mm^3); mild to marked elevation of protein

PATHOLOGIC FINDINGS
Lesions
• In the CNS—multifocal; predominantly in the brain stem and cerebral white matter
• Active—large malacic gliotic center surrounded by a wall of extremely severe mononuclear inflammation
• Old—rarefied or cystic areas surrounded by intense astroglial sclerosis

TREATMENT
• Outpatient
• No specific treatment known
• Supportive only—prevent seizures

MEDICATIONS

DRUG(S)
• None specific
• Steroids—may suppress the clinical signs to a considerable degree; prednisolone or prednisone (1–2 mg/kg PO q24h for the first 1–2 weeks; then taper dosage slowly).
• Phenobarbital—to reduce seizures; 2–8 mg/kg PO q12h; monitor serum concentration

CONTRAINDICATIONS/POSSIBLE INTERACTIONS
N/A

FOLLOW-UP

PATIENT MONITORING
• Monitor serum concentration of phenobarbital.
• Perform regular clinical and neurologic examinations.

PREVENTION/AVOIDANCE
N/A

POSSIBLE COMPLICATIONS
N/A

EXPECTED COURSE AND PROGNOSIS
• Chronic for months or even years
• In every described case, the neurologic signs were progressive.
• Prognosis—guarded

MISCELLANEOUS

SEE ALSO
• Necrotizing Meningoencephalitis of Maltese Dogs
• Pug Encephalitis (Meningoencephalitis)
• Seizures (Convulsions, Status Epilepticus)—Dogs

ABBREVIATIONS
• CNS = central nervous system
• CSF = cerebrospinal fluid
• CT = computed tomography
• MRI = magnetic resonance imaging

Suggested Reading
Ducote JM, Johnson KE, Dewey CW, Walker MA, Coates JR, Berridge BR. Computed tomography of necrotizing meningoencephalomyelitis in 3 Yorkshire Terriers. Vet Radiol Ultrasound 1999;40: 617–621.
Tipold A, Fatzer R, Jaggy A, et al. Necrotizing encephalitis in Yorkshire terriers. J Small Anim Pract 1993;34:623–628.
Author Andrea Tipold
Consulting Editor Joane M. Parent

NECROTIZING MENINGOENCEPHALITIS OF MALTESE DOGS

 BASICS

OVERVIEW
• One of the breed-restricted encephalitides that are defined by highly characteristic morphologic features
• Rare; found in North America and Europe
• CNS only organ system affected

SIGNALMENT
• Maltese dogs between 9 months and 4 years of age
• A genetic basis probable

SIGNS
• Acute and progressive
• Mostly mild to severe symptoms consistent with a forebrain lesion
• Seizures—observed in all described patients

CAUSES & RISK FACTORS
• Unknown
• An infectious agent might be suspected.

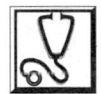 DIAGNOSIS

DIFFERENTIAL DIAGNOSIS
Rule out neoplasia and other inflammatory or infectious CNS diseases.

CBC/BIOCHEMISTRY/URINALYSIS
Usually normal

OTHER LABORATORY TESTS
N/A

IMAGING
CT and MRI (brain)—nonspecific changes

DIAGNOSTIC PROCEDURES
• CSF analysis—moderate mononuclear or mixed-cell pleocytosis; (50–247 leucocytes/mm^3); mild protein elevation
• Brain biopsy—helps the diagnosis in vivo

PATHOLOGIC FINDINGS
Necrosis and nonsuppurative inflammation of the cerebral gray and white matter

 TREATMENT

• Inpatient or outpatient
• No specific treatment known
• Supportive only—prevent seizures

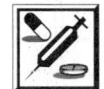 MEDICATIONS

DRUG(S)
• None specific
• Seizures—phenobarbital (2–8 mg/kg PO q12h); monitor serum concentrations
• Inflammatory response—corticosteroids; prednisolone or prednisone (1–2 mg/kg PO q24h for the first 1–2 weeks; then taper dosage slowly)

CONTRAINDICATIONS/POSSIBLE INTERACTIONS
N/A

 FOLLOW-UP

PATIENT MONITORING
• Monitor serum concentration of phenobarbital.
• Perform regular clinical and neurologic examinations.

EXPECTED COURSE AND PROGNOSIS
• Outcome not known exactly because only a few cases have been described
• Prognosis—regarded as poor; because pug dogs with a similar disease may survive a few years, a prolonged course of the disease may be expected in Maltese dogs too.

 MISCELLANEOUS

SEE ALSO
• Necrotizing Encephalitis in Yorkshire Terriers
• Pug Encephalitis (Meningoencephalitis)
• Seizures (Convulsions, Status Epilepticus)—Dogs

ABBREVIATIONS
• CNS = central nervous system
• CSF = cerebrospinal fluid
• CT = computed tomography
• MRI = magnetic resonance imaging

Suggested Reading
Stalis IH, Chadwick B, Dayrell-Hart B, et al. Necrotizing meningoencephalitis of Maltese dogs. Vet Pathol 1995;32:230–235.
Author Andrea Tipold
Consulting Editor Joane M. Parent

NEONATAL MORTALITY (FADING SYNDROME)

 **BASICS**

DEFINITION
Death occuring from birth to 2 weeks of age

PATHOPHYSIOLOGY
• Inadequate thermoregulatory activity, immunologic responses, and glucose control allow greater susceptibility to a number of insults, usually combination of environmental, infectious, nutritional, and metabolic factors.
• Hypothermia, hypoglycemia, dehydration, and hypoxia—common preludes

SYSTEMS AFFECTED
• Respiratory
• Endocrine/Metabolic
• Cardiovascular
• Nervous
• Hepatobiliary
• Renal/Urologic

SIGNALMENT
• Dogs and cats
• Pedigree puppies and kittens—more prone to congenital (and hereditary) defects

SIGNS
General Comments
• Preweaning losses—typically 10%–30%; about 65% occur during the first week; greater losses in a cattery or kennel should be considered abnormal.
• Historical and physical examination findings rarely narrow the differential diagnosis, because of the limited number of ways neonates can respond to illness.

Historical Findings
• Low birth weight, loss of weight, and/or failure to gain weight
• Decreased activity and appetite
• Weakness
• Constantly vocal or restless early, quiet and inactive later
• Tendency to remain separate from the dam and the rest of the litter

Physical Examination Findings
• Nonspecific
• Weakness, hypothermia (newborn temperature is about 35.5°C [96°F], rising to 37–37.8°C [99°–100°F] during the fourth week of life), hypoglycemia, dehydration—common and inter-related
• Respiratory distress, diarrhea, or hemoglobinuria—may be seen
• Gross anatomic defects—may be detectable

CAUSES
Noninfectious
• Dam-related—dystocia or prolonged labor; cannibalism; lactation failure; trauma; inattention or overattention; inadequate nutrition, including taurine deficiency in kittens
• Environmental—any factor that discourages nursing and allows hypothermia, including temperature extremes, humidity extremes, inadequate sanitation, overcrowding, and stress
• Nutritional—inadequate or ineffective nursing; hypoglycemia; hypothermia-induced digestive malfunction
• Neonatal isoerythrolysis—queen with blood type B; kitten with blood type A
Birth Defects
• Gross anatomic defects—more frequently in kittens (about 10% of nonsurviving neonates) than in puppies
• Gastrointestinal abnormalities—cleft palate; segmental intestinal agenesis or atresia
• Craniofacial abnormalities—failure of midline closure, causing herniation
• Cardiac defects—valvular dysplasia; VSD; atrioventricular fistula
• Respiratory defects—thoracic wall abnormalities; pectus excavatum; primary ciliary dyskinesia; surfactant deficiency
• Inborn errors of metabolism—usually autosomal recessive traits

Infectious
• Viral (kittens)—feline calicivirus; FeLV; FIV; feline herpesvirus type 1, feline panleukopenia virus
• Viral (puppies)—canine adenovirus type 1; canine distemper virus; canine herpesvirus; canine parvovirus type 1
• Bacterial—acquired mainly across the placenta, in the birth canal, via the umbilicus, gastrointestinal tract, respiratory tract, urinary tract, or skin wounds
• Neonatal sepsis—primarily from *E. coli*, β-hemolytic streptococcus, coagulase-positive staphylococcus, and gram-negative enteric organisms
• Respiratory—*Bordetella bronchiseptica; Pasteurella multocida*
• Enteric—*E. coli; Salmonella* spp.; *Campylobacter* spp.
• *Brucella canis*—puppies
• Parasitic—heavy infection with helminths *Toxocara canis, Toxocara cati, Toxascaris leonina, Ancylostoma caninum,* or *Ancylostoma tubaeforme;* coccidian parasites such as *Toxoplasma, Neospora, Isospora, Cryptosporidium,* or *Giardia*

RISK FACTORS
• Subnormal birth weight or failure to grow normally—kittens: minimum daily gain of 7–10 g; puppies: should double in weight by 10–12 days; both: 5%–10% gain per day generally acceptable
• Dystocia or prolonged labor
• Inbreeding—higher incidence of homozygous recessive genotype
• Sire with blood type A and queen with blood type B

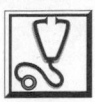 **DIAGNOSIS**

DIFFERENTIAL DIAGNOSIS
Excessive losses often due to a combination of environmental, immunologic, nutritional, infectious, and metabolic factors; detection and correction of problems in each area necessary to prevent ongoing losses

CBC/BIOCHEMISTRY/URINALYSIS
Premortem blood samples from affected individuals usually not obtainable and not pathognomonic
CBC
• Hydration status and age influence results.
• Mild normocytic, normochromic anemia
• White cell counts variable; may note thrombocytopenia and mild to moderate neutrophilia (with left shift) if septic
Biochemistry
• Hypoglycemia
• Other changes depend on organ system involved.
Urinalysis
• Hemoglobinuria—with neonatal isoerythrolysis
• Bacteria—with infection
• Urine specific gravity—> 1.017 suggests inadequate hydration

OTHER LABORATORY TESTS
• FeLV antigen test
• FIV antibody test
• Serology—*Brucella canis;* canine herpesvirus; *Toxoplasma; Neospora*

IMAGING
N/A

DIAGNOSTIC PROCEDURES
• Histopathologic—examination of multiple tissues collected at necropsy
• Metabolic screening of urine sample—rule out inborn errors of metabolism
• Virus isolation
• Bacterial culture
• Blood typing in pedigree cats
• Fecal examination—parasites

PATHOLOGIC FINDINGS
• Postmortem—extremely important; examine as soon after death as possible advisable to minimize autolysis; give special notice to the following items
• Stomach—devoid of contents: lack of nursing; consider dam-related causes (e.g., inappropriate behavior or lactation) or neonatal problems (e.g., weakness, trauma, or physiologic abnormality); filled with milk: suggests sudden death (e.g., trauma, peracute illness) or gastrointestinal dysfunction (body temperature < 35°C [95°F])
• Thymus subnormal size—not pathognomonic; can be a result of multiple causes (e.g., viral infection, nutrition, and defective immune system)
• Petechiation—common; accompanied by hemorrhage in other organ systems suggests coagulopathy or septicemia
• Urine in the urinary bladder—implies a degree of renal dysfunction or inadequate care by the dam
• Lungs—should appear the same as an adult's; homogeneous dark red color typical of a stillborn animal that has not taken a breath; hemorrhage, edema, congestion, and mottled color abnormal but nonspecific
• Note malformations.
• Multiple tissue samples—submit to a diagnostic laboratory; virus isolation, bacterial culture and sensitivity, and histopathology; check with laboratory for proper submission

 TREATMENT
• Correct any underlying deficiencies in husbandry or breeding selection.
• Warmth—slowly warm neonate to 36–36.7°C (97°–98°F) over several hours, if necessary; provide ambient temperature of 29–35°C (85°–95°F) and relative humidity of 55%–65%.
• Oxygen—supplement at 30%–40%, if necessary
• Intravenous fluids—consider administration of warmed D_5W solution if hypoglycemic; administer warm lactated Ringer's solution or half-strength lactated Ringer's and $D_{2.5}W$ (intravenously, intraosseously, or subcutaneously) at 1.0 mL/30 g body weight

• Do not attempt to feed if body temperature < 35°C (95°F) and no sucking reflex; once warmed, encourage nursing
• Neonatal isoerythrolysis—disallow nursing for first 24 hr after birth

 MEDICATIONS
DRUG(S) OF CHOICE
• Antibiotics—commonly used are penicillins (penicillin G, ampicillin, amoxicillin, amoxicillin with clavulanic acid) and first-generation cephalosporins; reduce adult dose by one-half and use same dosage interval
• Supplement—milk replacer formula
• Vitamin K_1—0.01–0.1 mg SC or IM once

CONTRAINDICATIONS
Aminoglycosides, tetracyclines, fluoroquinolones, trimethoprim/sulfonamide, and chloramphenicol—avoid during the neonatal period

PRECAUTIONS
Drug absorption, distribution, metabolism, and excretion for dogs and cats differ significantly during the first 5 weeks of life from those of adults.

POSSIBLE INTERACTIONS
N/A

ALTERNATIVE DRUG(S)
N/A

 FOLLOW-UP
PATIENT MONITORING
• Hydration status—check daily; dryness of mouth and yellow golden urine indicate dehydration
• Body weight—monitor daily or every other day in growing neonates
• Dam—check that nursing and care are adequate; supplement with milk replacer formula, if necessary

POSSIBLE COMPLICATIONS
N/A

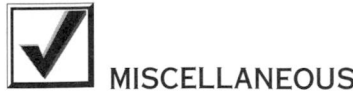 MISCELLANEOUS
ASSOCIATED CONDITIONS
N/A

AGE-RELATED FACTORS
N/A

ZOONOTIC POTENTIAL
N/A

PREGNANCY
N/A

SYNONYMS
• Wasting syndrome
• Fading puppy or kitten syndrome

SEE ALSO
See Causes

ABBREVIATIONS
• FeLV = feline leukemia virus
• FIV = feline immunodeficiency virus
• VSD = ventricular septal defect

Suggested Reading

Hoskins JD. Clinical evaluation of the kitten: from birth to eight weeks of age. Compend Contin Educ Pract Vet 1990; 12:1215–1225.
Hoskins JD. Fading puppy and kitten syndromes. Feline Pract 1993;21:19–22.
Jones RL. Special considerations for appropriate antimicrobial therapy in neonates. Vet Clin North Am Small Anim Pract 1987;17:577–602.
Lawler DF. Care and diseases of neonatal puppies and kittens. In: Kirk RW, Bonagura JD, eds. Current veterinary therapy X. Philadelphia: Saunders, 1989:1325–1333.
Lawler DF. Investigating kitten deaths in catteries. In: August JR, ed. Consultations in feline internal medicine. Philadelphia: Saunders, 1991:47–54.
Author Johnny D. Hoskins
Consulting Editor Stephen C. Barr

NEOSPOROSIS

 BASICS

OVERVIEW
• *Neospora caninum*—recently recognized coccidian protozoon previously confused with *Toxoplasma gondii;* tachyzoites and tissue cysts resemble *T. gondii* under light microscopy.
• Complete life cycle unknown.
• Dogs—definitive hosts. Oocysts excreted in feces are infective to other dogs and cattle by contaminating feed. Neosporosis is a major cause of abortion in cattle (intermediate host). Also infects red foxes and coyotes.
• Disease caused by necrosis associated with tissue damage from cyst rupture and tachyzoite invasion
• Transmission—transplacental, resulting in congenital infection. Ingestion of sporulated oocysts passed in feces of dog, or tissue cysts in tissues from intermediate hosts.

SIGNALMENT
• Dogs—natural infections (mainly puppies); hunting dogs overrepresented
• Cats—experimentally infected

SIGNS
• Similar to those of toxoplasmosis, except neurologic and muscular abnormalities predominate and are often more severe
• Young dogs (< 6 months)—ascending paralysis more common; distinguished from other forms of paralysis by gradual muscle atrophy; stiffness of pelvic limbs more affected than thoracic limbs; progresses to rigid contracture of limbs
• Cervical weakness and dysphagia—gradually develop, eventually leading to death
• Ataxia secondary to atrophy of the cerebellum
• Old dogs—usually CNS involvement (seizures, tremors), polymyositis, myocarditis, and dermatitis; as in toxoplasmosis, virtually any organ may be affected; head tremor; postural deficits from cerebellar disease; Horner's syndrome
• Generalized ulcerative and pyogranulomatous dermatitis seen in dogs on immunosuppressive treatment for SLE and lymphosarcoma

CAUSES & RISK FACTORS
N. caninum

 DIAGNOSIS

DIFFERENTIAL DIAGNOSIS
• Young dogs—other causes of peripheral multifocal neurologic signs, mainly including infectious diseases (toxoplasmosis, distemper); progressive polyradiculomyositis; other causes of diffuse lower motor neuron muscular diseases rare
• Old dogs with CNS disease—other infectious diseases (fungal, rabies, pseudo-rabies); toxicity (lead, organophosphorus, carbamate, chlorinated hydrocarbon, strychnine); nonsuppurative encephalitis; meningitis; granulomatous meningo-encephalitis; metabolic disease (hypo-glycemia, hepatic encephalopathy)

CBC/BIOCHEMISTRY/URINALYSIS
• Depending on the organ system involved
• Muscle involvement—creatine phosphokinase and AST activities may be high.

OTHER LABORATORY TESTS
• Serologic testing (IFA)—CSF or serum
• Antibodies do not cross-react with *T. gondii.*

IMAGING
N/A

DIAGNOSTIC PROCEDURES
CSF—slight increase in protein and nucleated cell number; cells mainly mononuclear; neutrophils may be seen

PATHOLOGIC FINDINGS
• Nonsuppurative encephalomyelitis
• Severe nonsuppurative inflammation of cerebella leptomeninges and cerebella cortex
• Myositis
• Myofibrosis
• Polyradiculoneuritis
• Pneumonia, cerebella atrophy, multifocal necrotizing myocarditis, and nodular dermatitis—described
• Ulcerative and pyogranulomatous dermatitis
• *N. caninum* seems to induce more inflammation than does *T. gondii*.
• Histology—differentiation by location in host cell cytoplasm (not within a parasitophorous vacuole as *T. gondii*)
• Tissue cysts—those of *N. caninum* have thicker walls; differentiated from *T. gondii* by immunohistochemical staining
• Electronmicroscopy—rhoptries of *N. caninum* tachyzoites electron dense; those of *T. gondii* honeycomb

TREATMENT
• Once muscle contracture or ascending paralysis has occurred, the prognosis for clinical improvement is poor.
• Progression of clinical disease might be arrested by treatment.

MEDICATIONS

DRUG(S)
• See Toxoplasmosis
• Clindamycin—25–50 mg/kg PO or IM per day, divided into 2 doses; continue for at least 2 weeks after clinical signs cleared

CONTRAINDICATIONS/POSSIBLE INTERACTIONS
N/A

FOLLOW-UP
• Treat for an extended period of time.
• Serologically test dam or other in-contact dogs and cattle.

MISCELLANEOUS

ZOONOTIC POTENTIAL
None identified (unlike *T. gondii*)

SEE ALSO
Toxoplasmosis

ABBREVIATIONS
• AST = aspartate aminotransferase
• CSF = cerebrospinal fluid
• IFA = immunofluorescent antibody
• SLE = systemic lupus erythematosus

Suggested Reading
Basso W, Venturini L, Venturini MC, et al. First isolation of *Neospora caninum* from the feces of a naturally infected dog. J Parasitol 2001;87:612–618.
Author Stephen C. Barr
Consulting Editor Stephen C. Barr

NEPHROLITHIASIS

BASICS

DEFINITION
• Nephroliths—uroliths (i.e., polycrystalline concretions or calculi) located in the renal pelvis or collecting diverticula of the kidney • Nephroliths or nephrolith fragments may pass into the ureters (ureteroliths). • Nephroliths that are not infected, not causing obstruction or clinical signs, and not progressively enlarging are termed *inactive*.

PATHOPHYSIOLOGY
Nephroliths can obstruct the renal pelvis or ureter, predispose to pyelonephritis, and result in compressive injury of the renal parenchyma leading to renal failure; see chapters on the different urolith types for pathophysiology of urolithiasis; in cats, nephroliths composed of blood clots mineralized with calcium phosphate can form secondarily to chronic renal hematuria.

SYSTEMS AFFECTED
• Renal/Urologic—affects the urinary tract, with potential for obstruction, recurrent urinary tract infections, or renal failure • Obstruction of the renal pelvis or ureter in an animal with pyelonephritis may result in septicemia (urosepsis) and thus affect any body system.

GENETICS
N/A

INCIDENCE/PREVALENCE
• Nephroliths compose ~1.3–2.8% of uroliths in dogs and cats submitted to stone centers for analysis; the true incidence of nephroliths is likely much higher because many animals with nephroliths are asymptomatic. • Most common mineral compositions of canine nephroliths submitted for analysis, in descending frequency—calcium oxalate, struvite, ammonium urate, mixed, calcium phosphate, and cystine • Most common mineral compositions of nephroliths in cats submitted for analysis, in descending frequency—calcium oxalate, matrix, calcium phosphate, mixed, and struvite

SIGNALMENT

Species
Dogs and cats

Breed Predilections
Canine
• Calcium oxalate nephroliths—miniature schnauzer, Lhasa apso, Yorkshire terrier, miniature poodle, and shih tzu
• Struvite nephroliths—miniature schnauzer, bichon frise, shih tzu, Yorkshire terrier, Lhasa apso, cocker spaniel, and miniature poodle
• Urate nephroliths—dalmatian, Yorkshire terrier, and English bulldog
• Cystine—Newfoundland

Feline
Domestic shorthair (33%), domestic longhair (17%), Persian (8%), Siamese (6%), unknown breed (19%)

Mean Age and Range
• Dogs—mean age of affected animals, 9 years (range, 4 months to 14 years)
• Cats—mean age of affected animals, 8 years (range, 2 months to 18 years)

Predominant Sex
• Overall, nephroliths in dogs are slightly more common in females (55%) than males (41%), with 4% unspecified; for struvite nephroliths, females > males; for calcium oxalate, cystine, and urate nephroliths males > females
• In cats, nephroliths are slightly more common in females (55%) than males (45%).

SIGNS

General Comments
Many patients are asymptomatic, and the nephroliths are diagnosed during workup of other problems.

Historical Findings
• None or hematuria, vomiting, and recurrent urinary tract infection; dysuria and pollakiuria in animals with urinary tract infection • Signs attributable to uremia in animals with bilateral obstruction or renal failure • Signs referable to lower urinary tract urolithiasis if uroliths are present in the upper and lower urinary tract
• So-called renal colic with acute abdominal/lumbar pain and vomiting is uncommon.

Physical Examination Findings
Abdominal or lumbar pain upon palpation or no significant findings

CAUSES
• For an extensive listing of causes, see chapters on each urolith type. Oversaturation of the urine with calculogenic minerals may contribute to urolithiasis. • Calcium oxalate urolithiasis—hypercalciuria, hypercalcemia, hypocitraturia, hyperoxaluria, primary hyperparathyroidism, excessive dietary calcium intake • Calcium phosphate urolithiasis—chronic renal bleeding (cats), hypercalcemia, hyperparathyroidism, excessive dietary calcium and phosphorus, renal tubular acidosis
• Cystine urolithiasis—cystinuria • Struvite urolithiasis—urinary tract infection with urease-producing microbes, diets that produce alkaline urine pH • Urate urolithiasis—genetic defect in conversion of uric acid to allantoin (dalmatians), portosystemic shunt
• Xanthine urolithiasis—allopurinol administration and high dietary purine intake in dogs predisposed to urate urolithiasis

RISK FACTORS
• Alkaline urine—struvite and calcium phosphate uroliths • Acid urine—calcium oxalate, cystine, urate, and xanthine uroliths
• Urine retention and formation of highly concentrated urine • Lower urinary tract infection—ascending infection and pyelonephritis • Conditions that predispose to urinary tract infection (e.g., perineal urethrostomy, ectopic ureters, hyperadrenocorticism), vesicoureteral reflux, and exogenous steroid administration or hyperadrenocorticism (calcium oxalate uroliths)

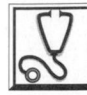

DIAGNOSIS

DIFFERENTIAL DIAGNOSIS
Consider nephroliths in any patient with renal failure, recurrent urinary tract infection, acute vomiting (acute pancreatitis, acute gastroenteritis, intestinal or gastric obstruction, etc.), or abdominal or lumbar pain (e.g., intervertebral disk protrusion, peritonitis); nephroliths are usually confirmed by radiographs or ultrasonography; differentiate mineralization of the renal pelvis or collecting diverticula from true nephrolithiasis.

CBC/BIOCHEMISTRY/URINALYSIS
• CBC results—usually normal unless the patient has pyelonephritis; patients with pyelonephritis may have leukocytosis and neutrophilia with a left shift.
• Serum biochemistry analysis—usually normal unless bilateral obstruction, pyelonephritis, or compressive renal injury leads to renal failure (azotemia with an inappropriate urine specific gravity, hyperphosphatemia); hypercalcemia may contribute to formation of calcium oxalate or calcium phosphate nephroliths.
• Urinalysis—may reveal hematuria and crystalluria; crystal type may indicate mineral composition; pyuria, proteinuria, and bacteriuria may also be seen in animals with urinary tract infection.

OTHER LABORATORY TESTS
• Submit all retrieved nephroliths or nephrolith fragments for quantitative analysis to allow implementation of appropriate preventive strategies. Although definitive identification of nephrolith type requires quantitative analysis, composition can frequently be predicted on the basis of signalment, radiographic appearance, and urinalysis findings.
• Results of bacterial culture of urine may confirm urinary tract infection in animals with concurrent pyelonephritis.

IMAGING
• Can detect radiopaque nephroliths (e.g., calcium phosphate, calcium oxalate, struvite) by survey radiography; cystine, urate, and xanthine are radiolucent to slightly radiopaque.
• May use ultrasonography or excretory urography to confirm the presence, size, and number of nephroliths or ureteroliths regardless of radiographic density

DIAGNOSTIC PROCEDURES

After ESWL, nephrolith fragments can be retrieved for quantitative analysis by voiding, cystoscopy, catheter-assisted retrieval, or voiding urohydropropulsion.

PATHOLOGIC FINDINGS

Histopathology required only to confirm the presence of secondary renal lesions.

 TREATMENT

APPROPRIATE HEALTH CARE

Manage patients with inactive nephroliths as outpatients. Medical dissolution protocols can be administered to outpatients. Removal of nephroliths by surgery or ESWL requires hospitalization.

ACTIVITY

Unlimited

DIET

Medical dissolution of nephroliths requires a diet appropriate to the specific nephrolith type. See Medications section.

CLIENT EDUCATION

• Inactive nephroliths—may not require removal but should be monitored periodically by urinalysis, urine culture, and radiography; can potentially cause obstruction at any time, which can result in hydronephrosis without clinical signs, so conservative management and monitoring carries a slight risk of undetected and potentially irreversible renal damage, which must be weighed against the potential renal damage from nephrotomy
• Nephroliths (especially metabolic uroliths) tend to recur after removal; monitor the patient every 3 to 6 months.

SURGICAL CONSIDERATIONS

• Indications for removal of nephroliths—obstruction, recurrent infection, symptomatic nephroliths, progressive nephrolith enlargement, and a nonfunctional contralateral kidney
• Treatment options for nephroliths—medical dissolution, surgery, and ESWL. Calcium oxalate nephroliths, the most common mineral composition in dogs and cats, are not amenable to medical dissolution. Ureteroliths or nephroliths causing complete obstruction are also not amenable to medical dissolution. • Surgical options—nephrotomy or pyelolithotomy. Because the nephroliths are surrounded by renal tissue, nephrotomy is required in most dogs and cats. Nephrolith removal by percutaneous nephrolithotomy has been reported in dogs.
• ESWL—safe and effective method of treating canine nephroliths and ureteroliths; nephrolith fragments pass down the ureter into the bladder and are voided in the urine. • ESWL—not as effective for treatment of nephroliths and ureteroliths in cats compared with dogs.

 MEDICATIONS

DRUG(S) OF CHOICE

• Antibiotics selected on the basis of urine culture and sensitivity testing as needed; periprocedural antibiotics are recommended when infected nephroliths are treated by ESWL or surgically removed.
• Medical dissolution protocols are limited to struvite, urate, and cystine uroliths.
• Medical dissolution protocols for *struvite* nephroliths include a calculolytic diet (Prescription Diet s/d, Hill's) and appropriate antibiotic therapy (i.e., if patient has a urinary tract infection) for the duration of treatment.
• Medical dissolution of canine *urate* nephrolithiasis can be attempted by a protein- and purine-restricted, alkalinizing diet (Prescription diet Canine u/d, Hill's), allopurinol (15 mg/kg PO q12h), and supplemental potassium citrate as needed to maintain urine pH ~7.0.
• Medical dissolution of canine *cystine* nephrolithiasis can be attempted using a protein-restricted, alkalinizing diet (Prescription diet Canine u/d, Hill's), 2-MPG (Thiola, 15 mg/kg PO q12h), and supplemental potassium citrate as needed to maintain urine pH ~7.5.

CONTRAINDICATIONS

• Do not use allopurinol without dietary purine restriction—it may cause xanthine nephrolithiasis in dogs predisposed to urate urolithiasis. • Do not give acidifying diets to azotemic patients unless blood pH and total CO_2 are monitored for development of metabolic acidosis.

POSSIBLE INTERACTIONS N/A

PRECAUTIONS N/A

ALTERNATIVE DRUG(S) N/A

 FOLLOW-UP

PATIENT MONITORING

Abdominal radiographs (ultrasonography for radiolucent uroliths), urinalysis, and urine culture every 3 to 6 months to detect nephrolith recurrence. Dogs treated with ESWL—check every 2 to 4 weeks by radiographs and ultrasonography until nephrolith fragments have passed through the excretory system.

PREVENTION/AVOIDANCE

Eliminate factors predisposing to individual urolith type, augment urine volume, and correct factors contributing to urine retention.

POSSIBLE COMPLICATIONS

Hydronephrosis, renal failure, recurrent urinary tract infection, and pyelonephritis

EXPECTED COURSE AND PROGNOSIS

• Highly variable; depends on nephrolith type, location, and size, and the presence of secondary complications (e.g., obstruction, infection, renal failure) • Inactive nephroliths may remain inactive for years, resulting in an excellent prognosis. • We have had excellent results using ESWL to treat dogs with nephroliths—return to normal health and an excellent prognosis. • The prognosis for patients with renal failure caused by nephrolithiasis depends on the severity and rate of progression of renal failure.

 MISCELLANEOUS

ASSOCIATED CONDITIONS

Hyperadrenocorticism and chronic glucocorticoid administration are associated with calcium oxalate uroliths and with urinary tract infection resulting in struvite urolithiasis.

AGE-RELATED FACTORS

Geriatric dogs that are poor surgical candidates may be treated with ESWL.

PREGNANCY

Contraindication to ESWL

SYNONYMS

Kidney stones, renal calculi, renoliths, kidney calculi

SEE ALSO

• Hydronephrosis • Pyelonephritis • Renal Failure, Chronic • Urinary Tract Obstruction • Urolithiasis, Calcium Oxalate • Urolithiasis, Calcium Phosphate • Urolithiasis, Cystine • Urolithiasis, Struvite—Cats • Urolithiasis, Struvite—Dogs • Urolithiasis, Urate • Urolithiasis, Xanthine

ABBREVIATION

ESWL = extracorporeal shock wave lithotripsy

Suggested Reading

Block G, Adams LG, Widmer WR, et al. The use of extracorporeal shock wave lithotripsy for treatment of spontaneous nephrolithiasis and ureterolithiasis in dogs. J Am Vet Med Assoc 1996;208:531–536.

Ling GV. Nephrolithiasis: prevalence of mineral type. In: Kirk RW, Bonagura JD, eds. Current veterinary therapy. XII. Philadelphia: Saunders, 1995:980.

Osborne CA, Unger LK, Lulich JP. Canine and feline nephroliths. In: Kirk RW, Bonagura JD, eds. Current veterinary therapy. XII. Philadelphia: Saunders, 1995: 981–985.

Stone EA. Canine nephrotomy. Compend Contin Educ Pract Vet 1987;9:883–888.

Author Larry G. Adams
Consulting Editors Larry G. Adams and Carl A. Osborne

NEPHROTIC SYNDROME

 BASICS

DEFINITION

The combination of significant proteinuria, hypoalbuminemia, ascites or edema, and hypercholesterolemia; in addition, systemic hypertension and hypercoagulability are commonly associated; usually occurs secondary to either glomerulonephritis or renal amyloidosis

PATHOPHYSIOLOGY

• Persistent protein loss exceeding 3.5 g/day often leads to clinical signs; consequences of severe proteinuria include sodium retention and edema, hypercholesterolemia, hypertension, hypercoagulability, muscle wasting, and weight loss. • A combination of low plasma oncotic pressure and hyperaldosteronism causing sodium retention often causes ascites and edema, but it has been hypothesized that intrarenal mechanisms, independent of aldosterone, may also contribute to sodium retention. The hypercholesterolemia probably results from a combination of decreased catabolism and increased hepatic synthesis of proteins and lipoproteins, which results in accumulation of large-molecular-weight, cholesterol-rich lipoproteins that are not lost through the damaged capillary wall as are the smaller-molecular-weight proteins such as albumin.
• Systemic hypertension is a frequent complication in dogs. It probably results from a combination of sodium retention, glomerular capillary and arteriolar scarring, decreased renal production of vasodilators, increased responsiveness to normal pressor mechanisms, and activation of the renin-angiotensin system. In one study, 84% of dogs with glomerular disease (e.g., glomerulonephritis, glomerulosclerosis, and amyloidosis) had systemic hypertension.
• Hypercoagulability and thromboembolism occur secondary to several abnormalities in the clotting system. In addition to a mild thrombocytosis, hypoalbuminemia-related platelet hypersensitivity increases platelet adhesion and aggregation inversely proportional to the magnitude of hypoalbuminemia. Loss of antithrombin III in urine also contributes to hypercoagulability. Antithrombin III works in concert with heparin to inhibit serine proteases (clotting factors II, IX, X, XI, and XII) and normally plays a vital role in modulating thrombin and fibrin production. • Finally, altered fibrinolysis and an increased concentration of large-molecular-weight clotting factors (fibrinogen, and clotting factors V, VII, VIII, and X) may lead to a relative increase in clotting factors compared with regulatory proteins.

SYSTEMS AFFECTED

• Renal/Urologic—proteinuria initially; often the underlying disease is progressive, resulting in irreversible glomerular damage, loss of nephrons, azotemia, and chronic renal failure. • Proteinuria itself can be harmful to the glomeruli and tubules. • Cardiovascular—edema, ascites, hypercholesterolemia/hyperlipidemia, hypertension, hypercoagulability, and thromboembolic disease

GENETICS

• Familial glomerular lesions have been reported in Bernese mountain dogs, samoyeds, dobermans, English cocker spaniels, rottweilers, greyhounds, and soft-coated wheaten terriers, as well as cats. • Familial amyloidosis has been reported in Abyssinian, Oriental shorthair, and Siamese cats and in Chinese shar pei dogs. Renal deposition of amyloid in these breeds with familial disease often occurs in the renal medulla, and therefore proteinuria may not be present.

INCIDENCE/PREVALENCE

More common in dogs than in cats

SIGNALMENT

Species
Dogs and cats

Breed Predilection
In some glomerulonephritis studies, golden retrievers, miniature schnauzers, and long-haired dachshunds appear to be overrepresented. Beagles, collies, and Walker hounds are reportedly at increased risk for renal amyloidosis.

Mean Age and Range
• Mean age of dogs with glomerulonephritis—6.5–7.0 years; range, 0.8–17 years • Cats with glomerulonephritis—mean age at presentation is 4.0 years • Most dogs and cats with renal amyloidosis are over 5 years of age.

Predominant Sex
None

SIGNS

Historical Findings
• Edema and/or ascites are the most common presenting complaint. • Occasionally, signs associated with an underlying infectious, inflammatory, or neoplastic disease may be why owners seek veterinary care. • Rarely, dogs may exhibit acute dyspnea or severe panting due to a pulmonary thromboembolism, or acute blindness due to retinal hemorrhage or detachment.

Physical Examination Findings
• Edema and ascites • Retinal hemorrhage, detachment, and papilledema can indicate systemic hypertension. • Arrhythmias and/or murmurs secondary to left ventricular hypertrophy caused by systemic hypertension • Dyspnea and cyanosis in dogs with pulmonary thromboembolism

CAUSES
Glomerulonephritis and amyloidosis occur secondary to chronic inflammatory conditions (e.g., infection, neoplasia, and immune-mediated disease).

RISK FACTORS
See Causes above.

 DIAGNOSIS

DIFFERENTIAL DIAGNOSIS

Proteinuria
• Most common cause is inflammatory urinary tract disease (e.g., bacterial cystitis/pyelonephritis, urolithiasis, and neoplasia); inflammation of the urinary tract is usually associated with active urine sediment—increased numbers of RBCs, WBCs, epithelial cells, and bacteria are observed in the urine sediment. • Glomerulonephritis and renal amyloidosis often cause severe proteinuria with inactive urine sediment (hyaline casts may be present); renal biopsy is the only accurate way to distinguish amyloidosis from glomerulonephritis.

Hypoalbuminemia
Can be associated with decreased albumin production (severe liver disease) and increased albumin loss (protein-losing enteropathies and protein-losing nephropathies)

CBC/BIOCHEMISTRY/URINALYSIS

• Persistent, significant proteinuria with inactive urine sediment (hyaline casts may be observed) is the hallmark laboratory abnormality associated with protein-losing nephropathies. • Hypoalbuminemia and hypercholesterolemia are common.
• Microalbuminuria often precedes overt proteinuria and may become an important early diagnostic tool.

OTHER LABORATORY TESTS

Urine Protein:Creatinine Ratio
Used to confirm and quantify abnormal proteinuria; the magnitude of proteinuria roughly correlates with the severity of glomerular lesions, making this ratio a useful parameter for assessing response to therapy or progression of disease.

Protein Electrophoresis
• Of urine and serum—may help identify the source of the proteinuria and establish a prognosis • Proteinuria associated with hemorrhage into the urinary tract may have an electrophoretic pattern similar to that of the serum. • Light chain immunoglobulins (Bence Jones proteins) may be present in the urine in cases of lymphoid malignancy.
• Early glomerular damage usually results principally in albuminuria; with progression of the glomerular disease, an increasing amount of globulin may be lost as well.
• Marked decreases in serum albumin and increased concentrations of larger-molecular-weight proteins, such as IgM, in the serum suggest severe proteinuria and the nephrotic syndrome. As the glomerular disease progresses and causes loss of at least three-

quarters of the nephrons, the resultant decreased glomerular filtration usually results in decreased proteinuria.

IMAGING
Protein-losing nephropathies do not cause specific changes on abdominal radiographs or renal ultrasound (with severe renal cortical amyloidosis there may be increased renal cortical echogenicity and the cortex may be thickened); however, these tests are useful in ruling out other concurrent conditions. Ultrasound can be used to guide percutaneous renal biopsies.

DIAGNOSTIC PROCEDURES
Do a renal biopsy if significant and persistent proteinuria with inactive urine sediment exists. Histopathologic evaluation of renal tissue will establish a diagnosis (e.g., glomerulonephritis vs. amyloidosis) and help in formulating a prognosis. Consider renal biopsy only after less-invasive tests (CBC, serum biochemistry profile, urinalysis, quantitation of proteinuria) are completed and blood clotting ability has been assessed.

TREATMENT

APPROPRIATE HEALTH CARE
Most nephrotic syndrome patients can be treated as outpatients; exceptions include severely azotemic and/or hypertensive patients and patients with thromboembolic disease.

NURSING CARE
Paracentesis—reserved for patients with respiratory distress and abdominal discomfort caused by ascites

ACTIVITY
Restrict activity because of the possibility of thromboembolic disease.

DIET
Sodium-reduced, high-quality, low-quantity protein diets

CLIENT EDUCATION
• If the underlying cause cannot be identified and corrected, glomerulonephritis and amyloidosis are usually progressive, resulting in chronic renal failure. • Biopsy is required to differentiate between glomerulonephritis and amyloidosis.

SURGICAL CONSIDERATIONS
N/A

MEDICATIONS

DRUG(S)
Systemic Hypertension
• If hypertension is not controlled with dietary sodium reduction, consider vasodilator therapy. • Angiotensin-converting enzyme (ACE) inhibitors such as enalapril (0.5 mg/kg PO q24h) have decreased glomerular capillary pressure, proteinuria, and incidence of glomerulosclerosis in some studies in dogs. • Individual responses to ACE inhibitors vary, and acute renal decompensation associated with hypotension is a potential adverse side effect. • In some cases, calcium channel blockers (e.g., amlodipine) may be necessary, either alone or in combination with ACE inhibitors, to control hypertension.

Edema and Ascites
• Cage rest and dietary sodium reduction • Reserve paracentesis and diuretics for patients with respiratory distress and abdominal discomfort. Overzealous use of diuretics may cause dehydration and acute renal decompensation. • Plasma transfusions provide only temporary benefit. • Dietary protein supplementation was formerly recommended to offset the effects of proteinuria; however, normal or high dietary protein may contribute to the progression of renal disease by causing glomerular hyperfiltration, increased proteinuria, and, subsequently, glomerulosclerosis. Thus dietary therapy should include a reduced (not restricted) amount of high-quality protein such as Hill's Prescription Diets (canine and feline) k/d. • Dietary protein modulates the renin-angiotensin-aldosterone axis, and angiotensin II may be responsible for the increased glomerular permselectivity mediated by dietary protein. Enalapril and low dietary protein have an additive antiproteinuric effect in rats, and enalapril attenuates hypercholesterolemia and glomerular injury in hyperlipidemic rats. Thus, besides decreasing glomerular capillary hydraulic pressure, ACE inhibitors may attenuate proteinuria by another mechanism.

Antithrombotics
• Prophylactic anticoagulant treatment may benefit patients with significant proteinuria, and measurement of antithrombin III and fibrinogen concentrations may help identify patients at greatest risk of thromboembolism. Dogs with antithrombin III concentrations below 70% of normal and fibrinogen concentrations above 300 mg/dL have increased risk for thrombus formation and are candidates for anticoagulant treatment. • Warfarin is highly protein-bound. Individualize its dosage for each patient. An initial dosage of 0.22 mg/kg PO q24h is recommended for dogs. Monitor prothrombin time (with the goal of increasing the baseline prothrombin time by 150%). If new drugs (especially highly protein-bound drugs like aspirin, which may displace warfarin from protein-binding sites) are added to the treatment regimen or if marked changes occur in serum albumin concentrations, reevaluate the patient's prothrombin time. • Low-dose aspirin (0.5–5 mg/kg PO q12–24h) is easily administered on an outpatient basis and does not require the extensive monitoring of warfarin treatment.

CONTRAINDICATIONS
Do not use corticosteroids in azotemic patients.

PRECAUTIONS
• Dosages of highly protein-bound drugs (e.g., aspirin) may need adjustment; serum albumin concentrations change with treatment or progression of disease. • Use ACE inhibitors with more caution in azotemic patients.

POSSIBLE INTERACTIONS
See Precautions, above.

FOLLOW-UP

PATIENT MONITORING
Urinary protein:creatinine ratio; serum urea nitrogen, creatinine, albumin, and electrolyte concentrations; blood pressure; and body weight; ideally, recheck examinations should occur 1, 3, 6, 9, and 12 months after initiation of treatment.

POSSIBLE COMPLICATIONS
Chronic renal insufficiency or failure

MISCELLANEOUS

ASSOCIATED CONDITIONS
• Hypertension • Hypercoagulability

PREGNANCY
High risk in those patients with severe hypoalbuminemia and/or hypertension

SYNONYMS
• Glomerulopathy • Protein-losing nephropathy

SEE ALSO
• Glomerulonephritis • Amyloidosis • Proteinuria

ABBREVIATION
ACE = angiotensin-converting enzyme

Suggested Reading
Cook AK, Cowgill LD. Clinical and pathologic features of protein-losing glomerular disease in the dog. A review of 137 cases (1985–1992). J Am Anim Hosp Assoc 1996;32:313–322.
Grauer GF. Glomerulonephritis. Semin Vet Med Surg (Small Anim) 1992;7:187–197.
Grauer GF, Greco DS, Getzy DM, et al. Effects of enalapril versus placebo as a treatment for canine idiopathic glomerulonephritis. J Vet Intern Med 2000;14:562–533.
Author Gregory F. Grauer
Consulting Editors Larry G. Adams and Carl A. Osborne

NEPHROTOXICITY, DRUG-INDUCED

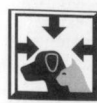 BASICS

DEFINITION
Renal injury caused by a pharmacologic agent used to diagnose or treat a medical disorder

PATHOPHYSIOLOGY
• Drugs can cause nephrotoxicosis by interfering with renal blood flow, glomerular function, or tubular function.
• Many drugs are nephrotoxic because they are excreted primarily by the kidneys.
• Most nephrotoxic drugs cause proximal renal tubular necrosis.
• If renal injury is severe, acute renal failure develops.

SYSTEMS AFFECTED
• Renal/Urologic
• Gastrointestinal—inappetence, vomiting, diarrhea, or melena due to gastrointestinal irritation or ulceration in patients with uremia
• Endocrine/Metabolic—metabolic acidosis due to decreased elimination of acid by kidneys and inability to resorb bicarbonate
• Hemic/Lymphatic/Immune—anemia due to blood loss or decreased red blood cell survival in patients with uremia; increased susceptibility to infections because of immune dysfunction in patients with uremia
• Nervous—depression, lethargy associated with effect of uremic toxins on central nervous system
• Respiratory—tachypnea or respiratory distress due to uremic pneumonitis or compensatory response for metabolic acidosis

GENETICS
N/A

INCIDENCE/PREVALENCE
N/A

GEOGRAPHIC DISTRIBUTION
N/A

SIGNALMENT

Species
More common in dogs than cats

Breed Predilection
N/A

Mean Age and Range
Any age; old patients are more susceptible.

Predominant Sex
N/A

SIGNS

Historical Findings
• Polyuria and polydipsia
• Inappetence
• Depression
• Vomiting
• Diarrhea

Physical Examination Findings
• Dehydration
• Oral ulcers
• Foul-smelling breath

CAUSES

Antimicrobial Drugs
• Aminoglycosides—all drugs in this class are potentially nephrotoxic, including neomycin, gentamicin, amikacin, kanamycin, and streptomycin. Nephrotoxicosis due to treatment with gentamicin occurs most often, probably because it is the most frequently used aminoglycoside.
• Tetracyclines—outdated products can cause acquired Fanconi-like syndrome characterized by glucosuria, proteinuria, and renal tubular acidosis; IV administration to dogs at high dosages (>30 mg/kg) can cause acute renal failure.
• Administration of sulfa drugs (e.g., trimethoprim-sulfadiazine) has been associated with acute renal failure in dogs, but no causal relationship has been proven.

Antifungal Drugs
Amphotericin B—only one that causes clinically important nephrotoxicosis

Antineoplastic Drugs
• Cisplatin—only antineoplastic agent that causes clinically important nephrotoxicosis in dogs
• Doxorubicin—may be associated with nephrotoxicosis in cats; rarely of clinical importance

NSAIDs
• Aspirin, ibuprofen, naproxen, piroxicam, and flunixin meglumine may cause nephrotoxicosis.
• Most likely to cause renal injury in patients with preexisting renal disease or those with concomitant dehydration or other causes of hypovolemia

ACE Inhibitors
• Include captopril, enalapril, and lisinopril
• Most likely to cause acute renal failure in patients with hyponatremia, dehydration, or congestive heart failure

Antiparasitic Drugs
Thiacestarsamide is the only antiparasitic drug that causes clinically important nephrotoxicosis.

Radiographic Contrast Agents
Intravenous administration of radiographic contrast agents can cause acute renal failure, especially in patients with dehydration, hypovolemia, or hypotension associated with inhalational anesthesia.

RISK FACTORS
• Dehydration
• Advanced age, probably because older patients have preexisting renal disease
• Renal disease, inactive or active
• Renal hypoperfusion; potential causes include any disorder associated with hypovolemia (e.g., vomiting, hemorrhage, hypoadrenocorticism), low cardiac output (e.g., congestive heart failure, pericardial disease, cardiac arrhythmias, inhalational anesthesia), or renal vasocontriction (e.g., NSAID administration)
• Electrolyte and acid–base abnormalities including hypokalemia, hyponatremia, hypocalcemia, and metabolic acidosis
• Concurrent drug therapy—administration of furosemide increases nephrotoxicosis of aminoglycosides; treatment with cytotoxic drugs (e.g., cyclophosphamide) may increase nephrotoxic potential of drugs.
• Fever
• Sepsis

 DIAGNOSIS

DIFFERENTIAL DIAGNOSIS
• Must differentiate from other causes of acute renal failure including causes of acute tubular necrosis such as ethylene glycol toxicosis and renal ischemia, and causes of nephritis such as leptospirosis and bacterial urinary tract infection
• Most patients have a history of recent treatment (i.e., within the previous 2 weeks) with a potentially nephrotoxic drug; acute renal failure may occur several days after discontinuation of an aminoglycoside.
• Determine all drugs that have been administered to the patient, including over-the-counter preparations (e.g., aspirin, ibuprofen, and naproxen) and medications prescribed for human use (e.g., NSAID or ACE inhibitor).

CBC/BIOCHEMISTRY/URINALYSIS
• Hemogram—usually normal unless concomitant problems exist (e.g., gastrointestinal hemorrhage associated with administration of NSAIDs)
• Biochemical analysis—normal in early stages of drug-induced nephrotoxicosis or reveals signs consistent with acute renal failure including azotemia, hyperphosphatemia, and metabolic acidosis
• Urinalysis—may reveal low urinary specific gravity (often < 1.025), proteinuria, glucosuria, or cylindruria

OTHER LABORATORY TESTS
Measuring serum aminoglycoside concentration may help prevent nephrotoxicosis in patients receiving these drugs, especially those with risk factors.

IMAGING
N/A

DIAGNOSTIC PROCEDURES

Renal biopsy may be indicated to determine cause of acute renal failure and potential for reversibility, especially in patients that do not respond to treatment as expected.

PATHOLOGIC FINDINGS

Most nephrotoxic drugs cause proximal renal tubular necrosis.

TREATMENT

APPROPRIATE HEALTH CARE

• Manage patients with acute renal failure as inpatients.
• Manage patients without azotemia that can eat and drink enough to maintain hydration as outpatients.

NURSING CARE

• Administer 0.9% saline intravenously in patients with renal failure; lactated Ringer's solution can be used but it contains a small amount of potassium, which may not be ideal in patients with acute renal failure and hyperkalemia.
• Correct hydration deficits rapidly (i.e., over 6–8 hours) to minimize further renal injury. Calculate volume of fluid to administer as follows: volume (mL) = body weight (kg) × % dehydration × 1000 mL.
• In addition to correcting hydration deficits, administer maintenance requirements (66 mL/kg/day) and replace any ongoing losses caused by vomiting and diarrhea. As a minimum, assume that patients with acute renal failure are losing 3–5% of their body weight because of ongoing losses.

ACTIVITY

Reduce

DIET

• Outpatients can be fed their regular diet.
• Modify diet for patients with acute renal failure; avoid oral feeding until vomiting is controlled.
• When oral feeding is initiated, a moderately protein-restricted diet such as canine k/d (Hill's Pet Products, Topeka) can help control signs of uremia.

CLIENT EDUCATION

• Avoid unnecessary stress (e.g., boarding or elective surgery); provide unlimited access to clean, fresh water at all times.
• If any signs of illness such as inappetence, vomiting, or diarrhea develop, return the patient immediately for veterinary care to minimize worsening of renal function.

SURGICAL CONSIDERATIONS

• Avoid elective surgery until renal disease is resolved.

• If surgery is necessary, administer fluids (5–20 mL/kg/h) during anesthesia to maintain adequate mean arterial blood pressure (>60 mm Hg) and renal perfusion. Monitor urine output and adjust rate of fluid administration to maintain urine production of 1–2 mL/kg/h.

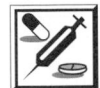

MEDICATIONS

DRUG(S)

None

CONTRAINDICATIONS

Do not use furosemide to promote diuresis in patients with aminoglycoside nephrotoxicosis.

PRECAUTIONS

Avoid drugs that may worsen renal injury in patients with nephrotoxicosis, including NSAIDs, vasodilators, and ACE inhibitors.

POSSIBLE INTERACTIONS

N/A

FOLLOW-UP

PATIENT MONITORING

• Weigh hospitalized patients several times daily to detect changes in fluid balance and adjust fluid therapy accordingly.
• Biochemical analysis and electrolytes every 1–2 days to evaluate severity of azotemia and detect electrolyte and acid/base abnormalities
• Patients receiving aminoglycosides—urinalysis every 1–2 days to detect early signs of nephrotoxicosis such as glucosuria, increased proteinuria, and cylindruria; discontinue aminoglycoside if any of these signs are observed.
• Urine output to determine if patient is polyuric or oliguric; adjust fluid therapy on the basis of these findings and determine need for additional treatment to stimulate urine production.

PREVENTION/AVOIDANCE

• Avoid or correct risk factors that predispose to development of drug-induced nephrotoxicosis.
• Administer saline diuresis to all dogs receiving cisplatin.
• Avoid using nephrotoxic drugs unless they are necessary (e.g., use aminoglycosides only if patient has overwhelming sepsis and culture results indicate aminoglycosides are the only effective antimicrobial).
• Monitor serum aminoglycoside concentration and perform frequent urinalyses while administering an aminoglycoside. Monitoring urinary GGT:creatinine ratio may detect

renal injury early in aminoglycoside toxicity.
• Do not administer furosemide with an aminoglycoside.

POSSIBLE COMPLICATIONS

• Acute renal failure
• Chronic renal failure

EXPECTED COURSE AND PROGNOSIS

• Patients without azotemia may develop acute renal failure within several days, especially with aminoglycosides.
• Renal injury caused by nephrotoxic drugs may lead to development of chronic renal failure months to years later.

MISCELLANEOUS

ASSOCIATED CONDITIONS

N/A

AGE-RELATED FACTORS

N/A

ZOONOTIC POTENTIAL

N/A

PREGNANCY

N/A

SYNONYMS

N/A

SEE ALSO

Renal failure, acute

ABBREVIATIONS

• ACE = angiotensin-converting enzyme
• GGT = γ-glutamyltransferase
• NSAID = nonsteroidal antiinflammatory drug

Suggested Reading

Behrend EN, Grauer GF, Mani I, et al. Hospital-acquired acute renal failure in dogs: 29 cases (1983–1992). J Am Vet Med Assoc 1996;208:537–541.

Brown SA, Barsanti JA. Gentamicin nephrotoxicosis in the dog. In: Kirk RW, ed. Current veterinary therapy IX. Philadelphia: Saunders, 1986:1146–1150.

Brown SA, Barsanti JA, Crowell WA. Gentamicin-associated acute renal failure in the dog. J Am Vet Med Assoc 1985;186:686–690.

Forrester SD, Troy GC. Renal effects of nonsteroidal antiinflammatory drugs. Compend Contin Educ Pract Vet 1999; 21:910–919.

Vaden SL, Levine J, Breitschwerdt EB. A retrospective case-control of acute renal failure in 99 dogs. J Vet Intern Med 1997;11:58–64.

Author S. Dru Forrester
Consulting Editors Larry G. Adams and Carl A. Osborne

NEUROAXONAL DYSTROPHY

 BASICS

OVERVIEW
• Inherited abiotrophies of neurons in diverse regions of the CNS, particularly the cerebellum and associated pathways
• Inheritance—usually thought to be autosomal recessive

SIGNALMENT
• Dogs and cats
• Dogs—rottweilers, collies, Chihuahuas, German shepherds, and boxers
• Age at onset—breed-specific, ranging from 5 weeks (cats) to 1–2 years (rottweilers)

SIGNS
• Cerebellar ataxia—progressive dysmetria and hypermetria of the limbs (rarely hypometria) with patellar hyperreflexia
• Strength and proprioception normal
• Loss of menace responses despite normal vision and facial nerve function
• Mild intention tremor or head and neck dysmetria in some patients

CAUSES & RISK FACTORS
• Specific cause unknown
• Believed to be neuronal abiotrophy with autosomal recessive inheritance
• Breed predisposition

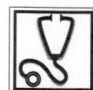 DIAGNOSIS

DIFFERENTIAL DIAGNOSIS
• Distemper encephalitis—differentiated on the basis of systemic signs preceding or accompanying the neurologic deficits and on results of CSF analysis (normal with neuroaxonal dystrophy)
• Cerebellar hypoplasia—apparent by 3–6 weeks of age; nonprogressive
• Infectious encephalitides—fungal, rickettsial, and protozoal; differentiated on the basis of multisystemic signs, serologic testing, and CSF analysis
• Cervical spinal cord disease—proprioceptive deficits and tetraparesis
• Diagnosis is by exclusion; it may not be possible to reach an antemortem diagnosis.

CBC/BIOCHEMISTRY/URINALYSIS
Normal

OTHER LABORATORY TESTS
N/A

IMAGING
N/A

DIAGNOSTIC PROCEDURES
All antemortem diagnostic tests are normal.

NEUROAXONAL DYSTROPHY

PATHOLOGIC FINDINGS
• Axonal spheroids—present throughout the CNS gray matter, except the cerebral cortex

 TREATMENT
• None available that will alter the course of the disease
• Outpatient, unless severe deficits preclude nursing care at home
• Activity—restrict activity to areas where a fall can be avoided (avoid stairs, swimming pools, etc.).

 MEDICATIONS

DRUG(S)
N/A

CONTRAINDICATIONS/POSSIBLE INTERACTIONS
N/A

 FOLLOW-UP
• Rottweilers—worsen over 1–5 years; develop clonic patellar reflexes and crossed extensor reflexes
• Not fatal but severely incapacitating

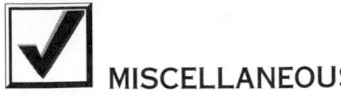 MISCELLANEOUS

ABBREVIATIONS
• CNS = central nervous system
• CSF = cerebrospinal fluid

Suggested Reading
De Lahunta A. Abiotrophy in domestic animals: a review. Can J Vet Res 1990; 54:65–76.
Author Mary O. Smith
Consulting Editor Joane M. Parent

NEUTROPENIA

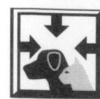 **BASICS**

DEFINITION
• Neutrophil count < 2900 neutrophils/μL in dogs and < 2500 neutrophils/μL in cats
• Can develop alone or as a component of pancytopenia
• Often accompanied by a left shift and toxic change (e.g., cytoplasmic basophilia, cytoplasmic vacuolation, Döhle bodies, and toxic granulation)

PATHOPHYSIOLOGY
• Results from one of three mechanisms—(1) deficient neutrophil production in the bone marrow, (2) cells shifting from the circulating neutrophil pool to the marginal neutrophil pool in the blood, and (3) reduced neutrophil survival because of excessive tissue demand or immune-mediated destruction of cells
• Most commonly associated with infection, because emigration of neutrophils from the blood into the tissues exceeds the rate at which the bone marrow can replace them

SYSTEMS AFFECTED
• Predisposes the patient to systemic infection by a variety of pathogens
• Many body systems can be affected in any combination, depending on the site(s) of infection.

SIGNALMENT
• Nothing specific for generalized infection
• Giant schnauzers with inherited vitamin B$_{12}$ malabsorption
• Gray collies and possibly border collies with cyclic neutropenia
• Belgian Tervuren dogs

SIGNS
• Signs of localized or systemic infection
• Pyrexia
• No clinical signs in Belgian Tervurens

CAUSES
Deficient Neutrophil Production
Stem Cell Death or Inhibition
• Infectious agents—dogs and cats, parvoviruses and bacteria-induced myelonecrosis; cats, FeLV and FIV; dogs, *Ehrlichia canis*
• Drugs, chemicals, and toxins—dogs and cats, chemotherapy agents and cephalosporins; cats, T-2 mycotoxin ingestion, chloramphenicol and benzene-ring compounds, and griseofulvin; dogs, estrogen, phenylbutazone, trimethoprim-sulfadiazine, Noxzema ingestion, thiacetarsamide administration (idiosyncratic)

• Lack of trophic factors—inherited malabsorption of vitamin B$_{12}$ (giant schnauzers); ionizing radiation

Reduced Hematopoietic Space Secondary to Myelophthisis
• Bone marrow necrosis
• Myelofibrosis
• Osteopetrosis
• Disseminated neoplasia, leukemia, and myelodysplastic syndrome
• Disseminated granulomatous disease (histoplasmosis)

Cyclic Stem Cell Proliferation
• Inherited cyclic hematopoiesis (gray collies)
• Cyclophosphamide treatment
• Idiopathic disease
• Immune-mediated suppression of granulopoiesis
• Poorly documented in dogs and cats

Neutrophil Migration
A shift in neutrophils from the circulating neutrophil pool (where they can be quantitated by the WBC count) to the marginal neutrophil pool (where they cannot be counted) occurs in patients with endotoxemia.

Reduced Survival
• Severe bacterial infection (most common cause)—pneumonia, peritonitis, and pyothorax
• Immune-mediated destruction
• Drug-induced destruction
• Hypersplenism (sequestration)
• Paraneoplastic syndrome (precise mechanism unknown)

Possible Benign Familial Neutropenia (Belgian Tervurens)
• Familial condition, inheritance pattern not determined
• Normal bone marrow
• Probable expansion of marginal neutrophil pool
• Treatment not necessary if healthy

RISK FACTORS
• Inherited disease—cyclic hematopoiesis in gray collies and possibly border collies; neutropenia in giant schnauzers
• Drug and chemical exposure—estrogen overdose in dogs (pancytopenia) and chloramphenicol and benzene-ring compounds in cats
• Exposure to various infectious agents—dogs and cats, overwhelming bacterial infection; dogs, acute *Ehrlichia canis* infection and parvovirus infection; cats, FeLV infection

• Middle-aged and old animals are less effective at repopulating the bone marrow after a severe toxic insult.

 DIAGNOSIS

DIFFERENTIAL DIAGNOSIS
• Breed of dog may promote suspicion of inherited disease (e.g., cyclic hematopoiesis in gray collies and neutropenia in giant schnauzers)
• History should include information concerning drugs, toxins, and radiation exposure.

LABORATORY FINDINGS
Drugs That May Alter Laboratory Results
None

Disorders That May Alter Laboratory Results
• Failure to properly mix the blood specimen before sampling for CBC (laboratory error)
• Obtaining blood specimen from an IV catheter used for fluid administration (diluted specimen)
• Partial clotting of the blood specimen with neutrophil entrapment or aggregation (poor anticoagulation)

Valid if Run in Human Laboratory?
Automated neutrophil counts are valid; however, technicians identify too many bands in animal blood (left shift).

CBC/BIOCHEMISTRY/URINALYSIS
• Diagnosis is verified by CBC and leukocyte differential counts.
• Multiple CBCs necessary to confirm or exclude a diagnosis of cyclic hematopoiesis

OTHER LABORATORY TESTS
• Serologic test—exclude ehrlichiosis in dogs and FeLV and FIV infections in cats
• Demonstration of antineutrophil antibodies—essential for diagnosing immune-mediated neutropenia
• Consider microbiologic culture of putative sites(s) of bacterial infection or empiric antibiotic administration if occult infection is suspected.

IMAGING
Survey radiography and ultrasonography may help locate occult sites of infection not apparent during physical examination.

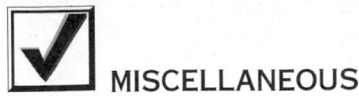
DIAGNOSTIC PROCEDURES

• Examination of a bone marrow aspirate and core biopsy—to evaluate neutrophil production and exclude myelophthisis, myelonecrosis, myelofibrosis, and osteopetrosis
• Provocative exposure to parenteral vitamin B_{12} should reverse anemia, neutropenia, and neutrophil hypersegmentation in affected giant schnauzers.
• Cytologic examination of preparations—to document excess tissue demand for neutrophils, verify sequestration of neutrophils in body cavities or between tissue planes, confirm bacterial infection, and identify sites of insensible or occult loss of neutrophils from mucous membranes or skin lesions
• Culture of infection site or blood culture in febrile animals

TREATMENT

• Primary concern is development of secondary infection
• In the absence of pyrexia, broad-spectrum antibiotics should be given prophylactically on an outpatient basis (especially if the count is < 1000 neutrophils/μL).
• Pyrexia—indicates current infection; treated more aggressively; inpatient treatment recommended for administration of parenteral antibiotics until the infection is contained
• Transfusion may be indicated in patients with severe anemia (PCV < 15%).

MEDICATIONS

DRUG(S)

• Nonfebrile (dogs and cats)—trimethoprim-sulfadiazine (15 mg/kg PO q12h) or cephalexin (30 mg/kg PO q12h) or a fluroquinolone (note potential for retinal toxicity in cats)
• Febrile (dogs and cats)—ampicillin (20 mg/kg IV q6–8h) or cephazolin (20–30 mg/kg IV q6–8h) or cephalothin (25–40 mg/kg IV q6–8h) *and* gentamicin sulfate (1–2 mg/kg IV q6–8h) or enrofloxicin (5 mg/kg IV q12h; note potential for retinal toxicity in cats)
• Severe sepsis (dogs and cats)—imipenem-cilastatin (5mg/kg IV q8h as 1-hour infusion

• rcG-CSF (dogs and cats)—5 μg/kg/day; may be of benefit in minimizing the duration; effective in dogs for prolonged periods and in cats for 42+ days; this drug not commercially available
• rhG-CSF—may be effective short term; however, development of antibodies to the protein takes place in 14–21 days
• Neutrophilia subsides within 5 days after G-CSF is discontinued.

CONTRAINDICATIONS

Adequately controlled safety studies of rcG-CSF and rhG-CSF have not been performed in dogs and cats (including pregnant animals); high-dose administration (80 μg/kg/day) of rhG-CSF in pregnant rabbits was associated with fetal resorption, abortion, and increased genitourinary tract hemorrhage.

Pregnant Animals

• Drugs listed should be used only if the benefits supersede the inherent risks.
• Sulfa drugs cross the placenta and can cause jaundice, hemolytic anemia, and kernicterus.
• Trimethoprim crosses the placenta; no harm accompanies drug administration in early pregnancy; however, this drug should not be used near term because of folic acid inhibition.
• Gentamicin sulfate crosses the placenta and may be associated with fetal ototoxicity.

PRECAUTIONS

• Maintain hydration when administering sulfa drugs to prevent renal crystallization.
• Gentamicin sulfate may be nephrotoxic and ototoxic.
• Risk of nephrotoxicity higher in dehydrated and overdosed animals

POSSIBLE INTERACTIONS

N/A

FOLLOW-UP

PATIENT MONITORING

• Periodic CBC; improvement denoted by a rising leukocyte or neutrophil count, resolution of left shift, and disappearance of toxic change
• Rebound neutrophilic leukocytosis expected during recovery from neutropenia

POSSIBLE COMPLICATIONS

Secondary infections

MISCELLANEOUS

ASSOCIATED CONDITIONS

Secondary infection

AGE-RELATED FACTORS

Repopulation of bone marrow with hematopoietic cells is more difficult in middle-aged and old animals because of age-related reduction in stem cell numbers.

ZOONOTIC POTENTIAL

None

PREGNANCY

N/A

SYNONYMS

None

SEE ALSO

• Ehrlichiosis
• Estrogen Toxicity
• Feline Immunodeficiency Virus
• Feline Leukemia Virus Infection
• Feline Panleukopenia
• Parvovirus Infection—Dogs

ABBREVIATIONS

• FeLV = feline leukemia virus
• FIV = feline immunodeficiency virus
• PCV = packed cell volume
• rcG-CSF = recombinant canine granulocyte colony-stimulating factor
• rhG-CSF = recombinant human granulocyte colony-stimulating factor

Suggested Reading

Abrams-Ogg ACG, Kruth SA. Antimicrobial therapy for the neutropenic dog and cat. In: Bonagura JD, ed Kirk's current veterinary therapy XIII. Philadelphia: Saunders, 2000.
August JR. Consultations in feline internal medicine. 2nd ed. Philadelphia: Saunders, 1994.
Greenfield CA, Messick JB, Solter PF, Schaeffer DJ. Results of hematologic analyses and prevalence of physiologic leukopenia in Belgian Tervurens. J Am Vet Med Assoc 2000;216:866–871.
Latimer KS, Mahaffey EA, Prasse KW. Duncan and Prasse's Veterinary Laboratory Medicine. 4th ed. Iowa State Press, 2003.
Sherding RG. Cat diseases and clinical management. New York: Churchill Livingstone, 1989.

Author Kenneth S. Latimer
Consulting Editor Stephen A. Kruth

NEUTROPHILIA

BASICS

DEFINITION
• Abnormally high absolute number of circulating neutrophils
• In adult dogs and cats, neutrophil counts > 12,000–13,000/μL
• The most common cause of leukocytosis

PATHOPHYSIOLOGY
• Neutrophils are produced in the bone marrow, released into the blood, circulate briefly, and migrate into tissue spaces and onto epithelial surfaces.
• CSFs govern the proliferation and maturation of immature neutrophils in the marrow.
• Injury or bacterial invasion of tissue results in the production and release of CSFs, which increase proliferation and maturation of neutrophilic progenitor cells in the bone marrow; other mediators of inflammation stimulate bone marrow release and promote margination and adhesion of neutrophils to vascular endothelium at the site of inflammation.
• Transit time for bone marrow granulopoiesis is 4–6 days.
• Neutrophils circulate for about 10 hr and are compartmentalized into a CNP and an MNP; neutrophils in the CNP circulate with other blood cells and are measured in the CBC; neutrophils in the MNP are intermittently adherent to endothelium, especially in small veins and capillaries.
• Migration of neutrophils into the tissues occurs randomly and is unidirectional.
• Neutrophils are also destroyed in spleen, liver, and bone marrow.
• Number of circulating neutrophils is affected by the rate of bone marrow production and release, the rate of exchange between the CNP and the MNP, and the rate of migration into tissue; changes in these rates can favor an increase in circulating neutrophils.
• Neutrophilia results when one or more of the following occurs: (1) rates of marrow production and release increase; (2) neutrophils demarginate from the MNP into the CNP; (3) tissue demand for neutrophils increases; and (4) granulocytic neoplasia develops.

SYSTEMS AFFECTED
Hemic/Lymph/Immune–a hematologic abnormality and is the result of a systemic response or disease rather than a cause thereof.

SIGNALMENT
Dogs and cats

SIGNS
• Vary with cause
• History and clinical findings evaluated for evidence of inflammation or sepsis as a cause; once eliminated, other causes explored

CAUSES

Physiologic Neutrophilia
• Fear, excitement, vigorous exercise, and seizure activity, which lead to epinephrine release
• Neutrophils demarginate from the MNP into the CNP, resulting in transient (1-hr), mature neutrophilia.
• In cats, marked lymphocytosis (6,000–15,000/μL) occurs concurrently.

Corticosteroid- or Stress-induced
• Endogenous release or exogenous administration of corticosteroids increases bone marrow release of mature neutrophils, demargination into the CNP, and diminished tissue migration.
• Leukocytosis (15,000–35,000/μL) and neutrophilia occur 4–8 hr after corticosteroid administration and return to normal 1–3 days after treatment.
• In dogs, lymphopenia, eosinopenia, and monocytosis occur concurrently.
• Associated with pain, traumatic injury, boarding, transport, or other stressful conditions

Acute Inflammation
• Inflammation, sepsis, necrosis, or immune-mediated disease cause an increase in tissue demand and bone marrow release of segmented and band neutrophils.
• Leukocytosis (15,000–35,000/μL), neutrophilia with left shift, toxic neutrophils, lymphopenia, eosinopenia, and variable monocytosis are usual responses.
• Surgical removal or drainage of septic focus may increase neutrophilia.

Chronic Inflammation
• Chronic suppuration (e.g., pyometra, abscesses, pyothorax, and pyoderma) and some neoplasms cause marrow granulocytic hyperplasia, resulting in severe leukocytosis (50,000–120,000/μL), neutrophilia with a left shift, variable numbers of toxic neutrophils, monocytosis, and hyperglobulinemia.
• Anemia of chronic disease may be noted.
• Leukemoid response—describes inflammatory neutrophilia with WBC counts > 100,000/μL. This response is similar to the CBC results in chronic granulocytic leukemia.

Hemolytic or Hemorrhagic Anemias
• Neutrophilia with a left shift can occur in dogs with immune-mediated hemolytic anemia.
• Mature neutrophilia occurs within 3 hr after acute hemorrhage.

Chronic Granulocytic Leukemia
• Hematologic response in dogs similar to neutrophilia of chronic inflammation
• Severe neutrophilic leukocytosis (> 80,000/μL), disordered left shift, and variable degrees of thrombocytopenia and anemia are observed.
• Splenomegaly and hepatomegaly may be pronounced.

Other Causes
• Granulocytopathy
• Cyclic hematopoiesis

RISK FACTORS
N/A

DIAGNOSIS

DIFFERENTIAL DIAGNOSIS
• Animals with inflammatory neutrophilia usually have historical or clinical evidence of septic or nonseptic inflammatory disease, such as pyrexia, weight loss, anorexia, and specific organ system involvement.
• Stress neutrophilia occurs frequently in dogs and cats examined because of noninflammatory disorders.
• Physiologic neutrophilia with concurrent lymphocytosis occurs in young healthy animals, especially apprehensive cats.

LABORATORY FINDINGS

Drugs That May Alter Laboratory Results
• Corticosteroid administration causes stress-induced neutrophil response.
• Neutrophilia subsides with long-term therapy but lymphopenia persists.

Disorders That May Alter Laboratory Results
• Falsely high electronic WBC counts—caused by large platelets, platelet clumps, and Heinz bodies
• Falsely low electronic WBC counts—caused by leukocyte clumping

Valid If Run in Human Laboratory?
• Yes, but some human laboratories overestimate the number of band cells at the expense of mature neutrophils.
• Normal animals will appear to have left shifts.

CBC/BIOCHEMISTRY/URINALYSIS
• Assessment of sequential leukograms—important because the number of segmented and band neutrophils can change dramatically in a few hours; trends important in diagnosis and prognosis
• Toxic neutrophils—observed in patients with neutrophilia caused by inflammation, especially those associated with toxemia; observed in blood and bone marrow characterized by diffuse cytoplasmic basophilia, foamy vacuolated cytoplasm, Döhle bodies, and giant forms with bizarre nuclear shapes
• Animals with acute sepsis and neutrophilia can become hypoglycemic.

OTHER LABORATORY TESTS
• Blood culture
• Bacterial or fungal culture of urine, tissue samples, and body fluids
• Serologic tests for fungi, protozoa, or rickettsia; organisms of special interest include *Blastomyces*, *Histoplasma*, *Coccidioides*, *Actinomyces*, *Nocardia*, *Toxoplasma*, *Hepatozoon*, and *Rickettsia*.
• Coombs' test, antinuclear antibody test, or rheumatoid factor test is indicated if immune-mediated disease suspected.

• Tests of neutrophil adhesion, chemotaxis, and bactericidal activity are indicated if granulocytopathy is suspected.

IMAGING
Radiography and ultrasonography of abdomen, thorax, soft tissue, or skeleton—inflammatory or neoplastic lesions (e.g., abscess, granulomatous lesion, effusions, foreign body, and organomegaly)

DIAGNOSTIC PROCEDURES
• Cytologic examination of suspect tissues or fluids for bacteria, fungi, protozoa, or neoplasia
• Aspiration of bone marrow and spleen if chronic granulocytic leukemia suspected

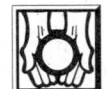 TREATMENT
• Varies with the identity and severity of underlying cause
• Animals with acute sepsis or hemolytic anemia require aggressive intervention.
• Animals with inflammatory neutrophilia caused by localized sites of suppuration may require surgical removal or drainage of affected tissues.
• Animals with chronic granulocytic leukemia require chemotherapy.

 MEDICATIONS

DRUG(S) OF CHOICE
Appropriate antimicrobial therapy for septic inflammation decided after identification of causative agent and sensitivity testing

CONTRAINDICATIONS
Corticosteroids should be avoided if bacterial, fungal, or protozoal infection is suspected.

PRECAUTIONS
N/A

POSSIBLE INTERACTIONS
N/A

ALTERNATIVE DRUG(S)
N/A

 FOLLOW-UP

PATIENT MONITORING
Animals with inflammatory neutrophilia, especially those of acute onset, may require daily or twice-daily hematologic assessment.

POSSIBLE COMPLICATIONS
• Animals with acute inflammatory neutrophilia may become neutropenic if neutrophil migration into the inflamed tissue exceeds the bone marrow production rate.
• If neutropenia develops with inflammation, prognosis is grave.

 MISCELLANEOUS

ASSOCIATED CONDITIONS
N/A

AGE-RELATED FACTORS
N/A

ZOONOTIC POTENTIAL
Some causes of neutrophilia

PREGNANCY
N/A

SYNONYMS
None

SEE ALSO
• Cyclic Hematopoiesis—Dogs
• Hyperadrenocorticism (Cushing's disease)
• Lymphocytosis
• Myeloproliferative Disorders

ABBREVIATIONS
• CBC = complete blood count
• CNP = circulating neutrophil pool
• CSF = colony-stimulating factor
• MNP = marginal neutrophil pool

Suggested Reading
Brady CA, Otto CM, VanWinkle TJ, King LG. Severe sepsis in cats: 29 cases (1986–1998). J Am Vet Med Assoc 2000;217:531–535.
Kociba G. Leukocyte changes in disease. In: Ettinger SJ, Feldman EC, eds. Textbook of veterinary internal medicine. Philadelphia: Saunders, 2000:1842–1860.
Author Peter S. MacWilliams
Consulting Editor Stephen A. Kruth

NOCARDIOSIS

BASICS

OVERVIEW
• An uncommon infection of dogs and cats
• Organism—soil saprophyte; enters body through contamination of wounds or by respiratory inhalation
• A compromised immune system enhances the likelihood of infection.
• Systems affected—respiratory, skin/exocrine, lymphatic, musculoskeletal, nervous

SIGNALMENT
Dogs and cats of any breed

SIGNS
• Depends on the site of infection
• Pleural—pyothorax, resulting in dyspnea, emaciation, and fever
• Cutaneous—chronic, nonhealing wounds; often accompanied by fistulous tracts; if extended, may result in lymphadenopathy, draining lymph nodes, and osteomyelitis
• Disseminated—most common in young dogs; usually begins in the respiratory tract; lethargy, fever, and weight loss; cyclic fever may be characteristic; CNS may be affected; pleural and/or abdominal effusion may occur.

CAUSES & RISK FACTORS
• *Nocardia asteroides* (dogs and cats)
• *N. brasiliensis* (cats only)
• *Proactinomyces* spp. (rare)

DIAGNOSIS

DIFFERENTIAL DIAGNOSES

Cutaneous
• Actinomycosis
• Atypical mycobacteriosis
• Leprosy
• Bite wound abscesses
• Draining tracts resulting from foreign bodies

Pleural
• Bacterial pyothorax
• Thoracic neoplasia
• Chronic diaphragmatic hernia

Disseminated
• Systemic fungal infections
• Feline infectious peritonitis

CBC/BIOCHEMISTRY/URINALYSIS
• Neutrophilic leukocytosis
• Nonregenerative anemia—with long-standing infections (anemia of chronic disease)
• Chemistries—usually normal; hypergamma-globulinemia may be seen with long-standing infections.

OTHER LABORATORY TESTS
N/A

IMAGING
Radiographs—may reveal pleural or peritoneal effusion, pleuropneumonia, or osteomyelitis

DIAGNOSTIC PROCEDURES
• Cytology—thoracentesis or abdomino-centesis for samples; stain these or other exudates with Romanowsky, gram, and modified acid-fast stains for rapid diagnosis; may reveal gram-positive branching fila-mentous rods and cocci; cannot be distin-guished from *Actinomyces* spp.
• Culture—diagnostic; aerobic culturing on Sabouraud medium

PATHOLOGIC FINDINGS
• *N. asteroides*—more suppurative pyogranulomatous reaction than with *Actinomyces* spp.
• *N. brasiliensis*—granulomatous reaction with extensive fibrosis
• Although the organism is usually present, it cannot be distinguished histopathologically from *Actinomyces* spp.

TREATMENT

- Pleural or peritoneal effusions and disseminated form—inpatient until clinically stable and effusion removed; fluid therapy for rehydration and maintenance often needed
- Long-term antibiotic therapy and draining fistulous tracts—outpatient
- Diet—encourage consumption by offering foods with appealing tastes and smells; forced enteral feeding for anorectic inpatients essential; orogastric tube feeding preferred
- Surgery—when feasible, surgical drainage should accompany medical therapy; important to place a thoracostomy tube for pleural effusion; attempt surgical drainage and débridement of draining tracts and lymph nodes; take care to identify foreign bodies.

MEDICATIONS

DRUG(S)

- Cultured organism—antibiotic sensitivity testing
- No culture or results pending—good first-choice drugs: sulfonamides (e.g., sulfadiazine at 100 mg/kg IV, PO as a loading dose followed by 50 mg/kg IV, PO q12h) and sulfonamide-trimethoprim combinations (30 mg/kg PO q24h)
- Aminoglycosides—gentamicin (3 mg/kg IV, IM, SC q8h); amikacin (6.5 mg/kg IV, IM, SC q8h)
- Tetracyclines—doxycycline (10 mg/kg PO q24h); tetracycline hydrochloride (15–20 mg/kg PO q8h); minocycline (5–12.5 mg/kg PO q12h)
- Erythromycin—10–20 mg/kg PO q8h; or combined with ampicillin (20–40 mg/kg PO q8h) or amoxicillin (6–20 mg/kg PO q8–12h)
- Amoxicillin plus an aminoglycoside—synergistic combination; consider in any serious infection when culturing is not possible or is pending
- Average treatment period is 6 weeks; however, medical treatment should extend several weeks past apparent remission of the disease.

CONTRAINDICATIONS/POSSIBLE INTERACTIONS

Tetracyclines (cats)—may cause fever up to 41.5°C (107°F); discontinue and replace if fever increases during therapy.

FOLLOW-UP

Monitor carefully for fever, weight loss, seizures, dyspnea, and lameness the first year after apparently successful therapy because of the potential for bone and CNS involvement.

MISCELLANEOUS

SEE ALSO

Actinomycosis

Suggested Reading

Edwards DF. Actinomycosis and nocardiosis. In: Greene CE, ed. Infectious diseases of the dog and cat. Philadelphia: Saunders, 1998:303–313.

Author Gary D. Norsworthy
Consulting Editor Stephen C. Barr

NONSTEROIDAL ANTIINFLAMMATORY DRUG TOXICITY

 **BASICS**

DEFINITION
• Toxicity secondary to the acute or chronic ingestion of an NSAID
• NSAIDs—classified as carboxylic acids (aspirin, indomethacin, and sulindac; ibuprofen, naproxen, and carprofen; meclofenamic acid and flunixin meglumine) or enolic acids (phenylbutazone, dipyrone, piroxicam); COX-2 inhibitors

PATHOPHYSIOLOGY
• Action—analgesic, antipyretic, and anti-inflammatory owing to the inhibition of cyclooxygenase; decreases production of prostaglandins that act as mediators of inflammation
• Well absorbed orally
• Clearance—varies greatly among species; eliminated slowly in dogs and cats
• Metabolized in the liver to active or inactive metabolites
• Excreted in the kidney via glomerular filtration and tubular secretion

SYSTEMS AFFECTED
• Gastrointestinal—erosions and ulcers
• Renal/Urologic—acute renal failure; acute interstitial nephritis
• Hemic/Lymphatic/Immune—may note bleeding disorders secondary to decreased platelet aggregation
• Hepatobiliary—idiosyncratic hepatocellular damage

GENETICS
Species differences in absorption, excretion, and metabolism of different agents are dramatic; avoid extrapolation of data from other species or dosages.

INCIDENCE/PREVALENCE
Among the 10 most common toxicoses reported to the National Animal Poison Control Center

GEOGRAPHIC DISTRIBUTION
N/A

SIGNALMENT
• Dogs and cats
• No breed, age or sex predilections

SIGNS
General Comments
• Gastrointestinal irritation—usually develops within a few hours
• Renal involvement or gastrointestinal ulceration—may be delayed several days

Historical Findings
• Evidence of accidental consumption of owner's medication
• Lethargy
• Anorexia
• Vomiting—with or without blood
• Diarrhea
• Icterus
• Melena
• Collapse and sudden death—may occur secondary to a perforated gastric ulcer
• Polyuria, polydipsia, and oliguria
• Ataxia, seizures, coma—may occur with large ingestions

Physical Examination Findings
• Depression
• Pale mucous membranes
• Painful abdomen
• Dehydration
• Fever
• Tachycardia
• Icterus

CAUSES
Accidental exposure or inappropriate administration

RISK FACTORS
Animals predisposed to renal disease—old age; pre-existing renal, hepatic, or cardiovascular disease; hypotension; other concurrent illness and/or medications; previous history of gastrointestinal ulcer or bleeding

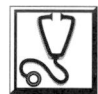 **DIAGNOSIS**

DIFFERENTIAL DIAGNOSIS
Other conditions (medical or toxicologic) that cause gastrointestinal and renal effects; diagnosis based on history of exposure and compatible clinical signs

CBC/BIOCHEMISTRY/URINALYSIS
• Anemia—regenerative or nonregenerative, depending on duration of bleeding
• Leukocytosis—associated with perforated gastric ulcer and accompanying peritonitis
• BUN and creatinine—may be high secondary to prerenal azotemia or primary renal insult
• High liver enzymes—occasionally
• May note hematuria, pyuria, proteinuria, and isosthenuria

OTHER LABORATORY TESTS
N/A

IMAGING
N/A

DIAGNOSTIC PROCEDURES
Endoscopy—verify gastrointestinal ulceration

PATHOLOGIC FINDINGS
• Gastrointestinal irritation, ulceration, or hemorrhage with possible gastric perforation and peritonitis
• Renal tubular or papillary necrosis or interstitial nephritis

 TREATMENT

APPROPRIATE HEALTH CARE
• Outpatient—mild clinical signs (with low ingested dose); managed at home with appropriate medication, dietary, and symptomatic measures
• Inpatient—high ingested dose; potential for renal toxicosis; relatively serious clinical signs (frequent vomiting, bloody vomitus, melena, anemia, or evidence of renal involvement); aggressive treatment to avoid life-threatening complications

NURSING CARE
• Fluid therapy—restore hydration when moderate to severe vomiting; administration of at least twice maintenance rates with known or potential renal involvement (see Renal Failure, Acute)
• If severely anemic, a blood transfusion may be indicated.

ACTIVITY
N/A

DIET
• Vomiting—NPO
• Vomiting resolved—begin with a bland, low-protein diet

NONSTEROIDAL ANTIINFLAMMATORY DRUG TOXICITY

CLIENT EDUCATION
• Stress the importance of contacting a veterinarian or the National Animal Poison Control Center whenever an animal is exposed to a nonprescribed NSAID.
• Inform client that dogs and particularly cats have a low tolerance to NSAIDs.
• With a prescribed NSAID, instruct client to look for adverse or idiosyncratic effects and to stop the drug and contact the clinic if they occur.

SURGICAL CONSIDERATIONS
Surgical intervention may be required for a perforated gastric ulcer.

 MEDICATIONS

DRUG(S) OF CHOICE

Recent Ingestion
• Ingestion within a few hours and no vomiting—induce emesis (apomorphine or hydrogen peroxide) unless patient has seizures or marked CNS depression.
• After emesis—activated charcoal (1–2 g/kg PO) and a cathartic (magnesium or sodium sulfate at 0.25 tsp/5 kg or 70% sorbitol at 3 mL/kg) if no diarrhea
• Repeat activated charcoal—one-half the original dose

H_2-Receptor Antagonists
• For gastrointestinal upset or ulceration
• Cimetidine—5–10 mg/kg PO, IV, IM q6–8h; primarily effective for treating ulcers from acute overdose or from chronic administration after the drug withdrawn
• Ranitidine—alternative; dogs, 2 mg/kg PO, IV q8h; cats, 2.5 mg/kg IV q12h or 3.5 mg/kg PO q12h; may be a better choice because cimetidine may inhibit liver microsomal enzymes

Other
• Sucralfate—dogs, 0.5–1 g PO q8–12h; cats, 0.25 g PO q8h; binds to proteins in the ulcer base; stimulates mucus and bicarbonate secretion
• Misoprostol—1–3 µg/kg PO q8h; PGE_2 analogue; prevents gastrointestinal bleeding and ulceration; promotes healing during chronic use in humans and dogs treated with aspirin

• Omeprazole—patients > 20 kg, 1 capsule (20 mg) daily; patients < 20 kg one-half capsule; patients < 5 kg, one-quarter capsule; potent inhibitor of gastric acid secretion; blocks the final step of hydrochloric acid production
• Dopamine—may be indicated for acute renal failure
• Standard anticonvulsant therapy—diazepam, pentobarbital, phenobarbital, if needed
• Duration of treatment—depends on the half-life of the particular agent ingested

CONTRAINDICATIONS
Avoid concomitant use of corticosteroids or multiple NSAIDs together; contraindicated in pregnancy (abortifacient effect)

PRECAUTIONS
Patients using other nephroactive or nephrotoxic drugs (e.g., aminoglycosides and ACE inhibitors)—at higher risk for developing NSAID nephropathy

POSSIBLE INTERACTIONS
NSAIDs—highly protein bound; may be affected by concurrent use of other highly protein bound drugs

ALTERNATIVE DRUG(S)
N/A

 **FOLLOW-UP**

PATIENT MONITORING
• Urine output—monitor carefully for oliguria; examine for casts, protein, and glucose
• Stool and vomitus—check for gastrointestinal bleeding (may not develop for several days)
• BUN and creatinine—twice daily for several days (full extent of renal damage may not be immediately evident)

PREVENTION/AVOIDANCE
• Store medications out of the reach of pets.
• Discourage owners from medicating pet without supervision of a veterinarian.
• Pretest high-risk patients with appropriate laboratory tests before beginning therapy.

POSSIBLE COMPLICATIONS
• Perforation of a gastric ulcer and peritonitis
• Irreversible acute and chronic renal failure

EXPECTED COURSE AND PROGNOSIS
• Gastric upset or ulceration—usually complete recovery with appropriate treatment
• Renal effects—generally reversible with early and aggressive treatment
• Acute hepatopathies—generally resolve after discontinuation of drug

 **MISCELLANEOUS**

ASSOCIATED CONDITIONS
N/A

ZOONOTIC POTENTIAL
N/A

PREGNANCY
• Exposure during pregnancy—risk for fetal cardiopulmonary and renal effects
• May prolong pregnancy, especially if administered during the third trimester and before the onset of labor

SEE ALSO
• Aspirin Toxicity
• Poisoning (Intoxication)
• Renal Failure, Acute

ABBREVIATIONS
• ACE = angiotensin-converting enzyme
• BUN = blood urea nitrogen
• CNS = central nervous system
• COX-2 = cyclooxygenase-2
• NPO = nothing by mouth
• NSAID = nonsteroidal antiinflammatory drug

Suggested Reading
Johnston SA, Budsburg SC. Nonsteroidal anti-inflammatory drugs and corticosteroids in the management of canine osteoarthritis. Vet Clin North Am Small Anim Pract 1997;27:841–862.
Kore AC. Toxicology of nonsteroidal anti-inflammatory drugs. Vet Clin North Am Small Anim Pract 1990;20:419–431.
Author Judy Holding
Consulting Editor Gary D. Osweiler

NYSTAGMUS

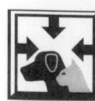

BASICS

DEFINITION
• Involuntary, rhythmic oscillation of the eyeballs
• Jerk nystagmus—most common; movements have a slow phase in one direction and a rapid recovery in the opposite direction
• Pendular nystagmus—seen less frequently; characterized by small oscillations of the eyes with no fast or slow component

PATHOPHYSIOLOGY
• Nystagmus at rest—abnormal; most commonly a reflection of vestibular dysfunction
• Projections from the vestibular nuclei in the brain stem influence the nuclei of cranial nerves III, IV, and VI, which innervate the extraocular muscles. This system controls normal physiologic nystagmus, which provides coordinated conjugate eye movements in association with changes in position of the head. When this system is disrupted, a jerk nystagmus develops independent of head movement (so-called spontaneous or pathologic nystagmus).
• Jerk nystagmus must be differentiated from pendular nystagmus, which is most often observed as an incidental finding in Siamese and Himalayan cats.
• Pendular nystagmus is the result of a congenital abnormality in which a larger-than-usual portion of the optic nerve fibers crosses in the chiasm; may also be seen with cerebellar disease and with visual deficits.

SYSTEMS AFFECTED
Nervous—central or peripheral

CAUSES & RISK FACTORS

Peripheral Vestibular Disease
• Metabolic—hypothyroidism; hyperadrenocorticism
• Neoplastic—nerve sheath tumor or tumor involving surrounding bone or soft tissues
• Inflammatory—otitis media-interna; inflammatory nasopharyngeal polyps (cats)
• Idiopathic—canine geriatric vestibular disease; feline idiopathic vestibular disease
• Toxic—e.g., aminoglycosides, topical iodophors, topical chlorhexidine
• Trauma

Central Vestibular Disease
• Degenerative—storage disorders; neuronal degeneration; demyelinating disease
• Neoplastic—primary or metastatic tumors
• Nutritional—thiamine deficiency
• Inflammatory/infectious—viral (canine distemper, feline infectious peritonitis); bacterial; protozoal (toxoplasmosis, neosporosis); fungal (cryptococcosis, blastomycosis, histoplasmosis, coccidioido-mycosis, aspergillosis); rickettsial (ehrlichiosis, Rocky Mountain spotted fever); inflammatory, noninfectious (granulomatous meningoencephalomyelitis)
• Toxic—lead; hexachlorophene; metronidazole
• Trauma
• Vascular—hemorrhage; infarction

DIAGNOSIS

DIFFERENTIAL DIAGNOSIS

Peripheral Vestibular Disease
• Nystagmus—either rotary or horizontal, with the fast phase directed away from the side of the lesion; does not change direction
• Other signs of vestibular disease—e.g., head tilt, circling, ataxia; often present and occur ipsilateral to the lesion
• Ipsilateral facial nerve paresis or paralysis and/or Horner's syndrome—may be seen because of the close association of CN VII and the sympathetic nerve to CN VIII as they course through the petrous temporal bone in the region of the middle ear

Central Vestibular Disease
• Nystagmus—may be horizontal, rotary, or vertical; may change direction with different head positions
• Other signs of vestibular disease—e.g., head tilt, circling, ataxia; often present
• Evidence of brain stem involvement—characteristically seen; includes alterations in level of consciousness, paresis, postural reaction deficits, and other CN deficits (V and VII are most commonly affected); deficits are typically ipsilateral to the lesion
• Paradoxical vestibular disease—may occur with certain lesions of the cerebellum; in these cases, postural reaction deficits occur ipsilateral to the lesion, whereas the head tilt and other vestibular signs are directed contralateral to the lesion

CBC/BIOCHEMISTRY/URINALYSIS
Results are usually normal.

OTHER LABORATORY TESTS
• Thyroid profile—if hypothyroidism is suspected
• Adrenal function testing—if hyperadrenocorticism is suspected
• Bacterial culture of sample obtained via myringotomy—if otitis media-interna is likely
• Serologic testing—for potential infectious agents

IMAGING
• Computed tomography of the tympanic bullae—more sensitive than survey radiography to assess for presence of otitis media-interna
• Computed tomography or magnetic resonance imaging of the brain—indicated for animals with central vestibular disease to identify any structural abnormalities in the brain stem

DIAGNOSTIC PROCEDURES
Analysis of cerebrospinal fluid collected from the cerebellomedullary cistern—to evaluate for inflammation

 TREATMENT
• The cause of the disease and the severity of signs determine whether the animal is best treated on an inpatient or an outpatient basis.
• Fluid therapy is indicated in the acute stages of disease for animals that experience anorexia and vomiting.

• As a rule, animals with central involvement require more intensive care than those with peripheral disease.
• Many animals show improvement over the first several days, as the nervous system is able to compensate for vestibular disturbances that remain static or are slowly progressive.

 **MEDICATIONS**

DRUG(S)
• Meclizine (dogs: 4 mg/kg PO q24h; cats: 2 mg/kg PO q24h)—an antihistamine used to treat motion sickness; may be helpful in alleviating nausea and vomiting associated with acute vestibular dysfunction
• Specific medical therapy is directed at the underlying cause, if one can be identified.

CONTRAINDICATIONS/POSSIBLE INTERACTIONS
• Avoid potential ototoxic drugs, such as aminoglycosides.
• Avoid instilling topical medications into the ear of an animal with suspected otitis media-interna, especially if the tympanic membrane cannot be visualized or is not intact. Such agents can exacerbate vestibular signs and cause deafness.
• Avoid the use of metronidazole at daily doses greater than 60 mg/kg, as this has been associated with vestibular dysfunction in dogs.

 FOLLOW-UP

PATIENT MONITORING
Repeat neurologic examination—perform at least 2 weeks after initial diagnosis to monitor for improvement or progression of disease

POSSIBLE COMPLICATIONS
• Dehydration and electrolyte imbalance associated with anorexia and vomiting
• Rare extension of otitis media-interna into the adjacent brain stem

EXPECTED COURSE AND PROGNOSIS
• Prognosis varies, depending on the cause of the vestibular disturbance.
• In general, animals with peripheral vestibular disease have a better prognosis than those with central involvement.

 **MISCELLANEOUS**

ABBREVIATION
CN = cranial nerve

Suggested Reading
Thomas WB. Vestibular dysfunction. Vet Clin North Am Small Anim Pract 2000; 30:227–249.
Author Karen R. Muñana
Consulting Editor Joane M. Parent

OBESITY

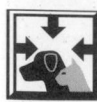 **BASICS**

DEFINITION
A pathologic increase in body fat resulting in an increase in body weight that may lead to a multitude of metabolic, musculoskeletal, and/or physiologic derangements

PATHOPHYSIOLOGY
• Animal factors—increased age, neutering, and inactivity are important risk factors for both dogs and cats.
• Feeding management—overfeeding or energy intake exceeding energy requirement is a common cause of obesity; Excessive food consumption may result from a lack of proper owner education, inappropriately generous feeding recommendations by pet food manufacturers, and emphasis on food palatability both by owners and manufacturers.
• Dietary factors—no specific diet other than an excessive amount of "table scraps" and "treats" has been shown to increase risk in dogs; in cats, consumption of "high-fat" diets reportedly increases risk
• Owner factors—many owners of overweight pets are overweight themselves and engage in feeding as a social activity; clients also may consider their pet to be "one of the family" and be unwilling to deprive a loved one of food; these factors may undermine simple-minded "eat less and exercise more!" approaches to management of obesity; they must be identified and acknowledged by both client and therapist for long-term resolution of obesity.

SYSTEMS AFFECTED
• Patients more than 40% above "optimum" (moderate) body weight are at increased risk.

Dogs
• Cardiovascular
• Musculoskeletal—articular and locomotor problems, including developmental orthopedic disease in growing dogs

Cats
• Endocrine/Metabolic—diabetes mellitus
• Musculoskeletal—lameness
• Dermatologic—nonallergic skin problems
• Hepatobiliary—hepatic lipidosis may occur if food intake ceases.

SIGNALMENT
• Dogs and cats
• Breeds predisposed include the Labrador retriever, Cairn terrier, cocker spaniel, dachshund, sheltie, basset hound, beagle, King Charles spaniel, collie, and, in our practice, Norwegian elkhounds
• Female dogs are at increased risk.
• In cats, apartment-dwelling, inactive, middle-aged neutered males of mixed-breed ancestry are at increased risk.

SIGNS
• Excess amounts of body fat for body size, often measured as body condition score of ≥ 4 on a 1–5 scale in which 1 = cachectic (> 20% underweight), 2 = lean (10–20% underweight), 3 = moderate, 4 = stout (20–40% overweight), 5 = obese (> 40% overweight)
• Sites of adipose tissue to evaluate during physical examination include the ribcage and abdomen; one should be able to feel the ribs easily and see an abdominal "waist" when viewing the animal either from above or from the side.
• Cats often exhibit excessive inguinal fat.

CAUSES
• Most commonly, excessive access to highly palatable food, often combined with insufficient activity; clinically, at least two types of owners may be distinguished: "mindless," for whom feeding the animal is an automatic chore, and "timeless," for whom feeding is a significant social, time-filling activity.
• Hypothyroidism
• Hyperadrenocorticism
• Insulinoma

RISK FACTORS
• Owner lifestyle
• Diet palatability and energy density
• Breed
• Activity level

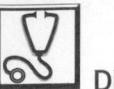 **DIAGNOSIS**

DIFFERENTIAL DIAGNOSIS
Differentiating Similar Signs
• Pregnancy
• Increased muscle mass
• Hypothyroidism
• Cushing's disease
• Insulinoma
• Organomegaly

Differentiating Causes
• Similar problems/diseases should be differentiated via history, physical examination, laboratory evaluation, and imaging.
• Document body condition score ≥ 4

CBC/BIOCHEMISTRY/URINALYSIS
Normal

OTHER LABORATORY TESTS
Normal

IMAGING
Demonstrates excess body fat

DIAGNOSTIC PROCEDURES
N/A

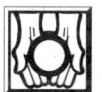 **TREATMENT**
Success is lifelong amelioration of the problem.

DIET
• Any of the many reduced-calorie diets currently available may be dispensed or prescribed.
• Changing the diet may help to reeducate the client about feeding, but diet per se does not cause obesity and is ancillary to its long-term treatment.
• In cats, it has been shown that an energy restriction to 60% of maintenance requirements at a target body weight over an 18-week period will result in the majority of weight loss being from body fat and thus minimize the loss of lean body tissue.
• Composition, type, and percentage of dietary fiber content have not conclusively

been determined to specifically aid in obesity management in dogs.

CLIENT EDUCATION

• Most important part of obesity therapy; must be tailored to each particular circumstance
• Mindless—demonstrate appropriate body condition score, explain that the pet should be fed the amount of food necessary to achieve this condition in this particular animal; reducing food availability to achieve the desired body condition often suffices
• Timeless—much more careful investigation of the circumstances and consideration of the necessity for maintaining a lower weight are necessary for this group; clients must come to want the animal to maintain a lower weight for demonstrable reasons and need the means and support to achieve this, while retaining the desired relationship with the pet. Therapeutic suggestions include reasonable, functional weight loss goals, rather than recommending achieving a poorly defined "optimal adult weight" for aesthetic reasons (e.g., sufficient weight loss to enhance glycemic control of a non–insulin-dependent diabetic or ability to walk for 20 min without exhaustion or lameness). Keeping a food record that identifies all food sources may help some clients appreciate how many the pet consumes. Suggest that "snacks" *replace* regular food rather than *supplement* it and that the snacks consist of a portion of the regularly allotted food.

MEDICATIONS

DRUG(S) OF CHOICE
N/A

CONTRAINDICATIONS
N/A

PRECAUTIONS
N/A

POSSIBLE INTERACTIONS
N/A

ALTERNATIVE DRUG(S)
N/A

FOLLOW-UP

PATIENT MONITORING
• As with any other chronic metabolic problem, lifelong follow-up, coaching, and support are essential to maintain the reduced weight.
• Frequent and regular body weight evaluations and veterinary examinations should be stressed upon initial examination.
• At the initial visit instruct clients to recognize moderate body condition score and to feed the quantity of food necessary to maintain this condition during the changing physiologic and environmental conditions of the pet's life; remind them at checkups.
• When clients express concern about how little food is needed to maintain moderate body condition, recommend increased activity and/or a reduced-calorie diet *before* the animal becomes obese.

POSSIBLE COMPLICATIONS
N/A

MISCELLANEOUS

ASSOCIATED CONDITIONS
• Orthopedic problems
• Dermatologic problems
• Respiratory problems
• Increased anesthetic risk
• Cardiovascular problems—dogs
• Diabetes mellitus—cats
• Hepatic lipidosis—cats

AGE-RELATED FACTORS
N/A

ZOONOTIC POTENTIAL
N/A

PREGNANCY
Obesity may increase risk of dystocia; but because of potential risk to the fetus, do not treat pregnant animals.

SYNONYMS
N/A

SEE ALSO
• Hyperadrenocorticism
• Hypothyroidism
• Insulinoma

Suggested Reading

Burkholder WJ, Bauer JE, Foods and techniques for managing obesity in companion animals. J Am Vet Med Assoc 1998; 212(5):858–862.
Butterwick RF, Markwell PJ. Body composition changes in cats during weight reduction by controlled calorie restriction. Vet Rec 1996;138:354–357.
Obesity in cats and dogs. Int J Obes Relat Metab Dis 1994;18(Suppl 1).
Scarlett JM, Donoghue S. Associations between body condition and disease in cats. J Am Vet Med Assoc 1998;212(11): 1725–1731.

Acknowledgment

The author and editors acknowledge the prior contributions of Dr. C.A. Tony Buffington, who authored this topic in the previous edition.

Author John Crandell
Consulting Editors Albert E. Jergens

ODONTOCLASTIC RESORPTIVE LESIONS—CATS

 BASICS

DEFINITION
Dental resorptions of unknown etiology affecting cats

PATHOPHYSIOLOGY
• Unlike cavities in humans, which result from bacterial enzymes and acids digesting the tooth substance, the cause of feline odontoclastic resorptive lesions (FORLs) is presently unknown; cells called odontoclasts, found in the defects, cause tooth structure to dissolve; odontoclasts originate from monocytes.
• In the acute phase, odontoclasts attach to the lacunar surface of intact dental tissue; resorption progresses and reparative bonelike or cementum-like tissue covers the excavated dentin; granulomatous tissue often occupies the excavated sites.
• Resorption also occurs in the periodontal ligament and alveolar bone; both external and internal resorption may take place; in time, remodeling replaces dentinal tissue with bonelike or cementum-like tissues, radiographically appearing as ankylosis.

SYSTEMS AFFECTED
Oral cavity

GENETICS
N/A

INCIDENCE/PREVALENCE
• A relatively newly recognized syndrome
• A large percentage of cats older than 1 year have at least one FORL.
• Most feline patients presented for diagnosis or treatment of oral or dental disease have their teeth affected with FORLs; presence consistently increases with age.

GEOGRAPHIC DISTRIBUTION
N/A

SIGNALMENT

Species
Cat

Breed Predilections
Asian short-haired, Siamese, Persian, and Abyssinian cats may show a breed predisposition.

Mean Age and Range
N/A

Predominant Sex
N/A

SIGNS

Historical Findings
• Most affected cats show no clinical signs; some show hypersalivation; others, oral bleeding or difficulty chewing; some cats pick up and drop food (especially hard food) when eating; others hiss while chewing.
• Some cats have behavior changes—reclusive or aggressive

Physical Examination Findings
• A cotton-tipped applicator applied to the suspected FORL (Stages 2–4) usually causes pain evidenced by jaw spasms.
• FORLs can occur above or below the free gingival margin; most occur at the labial or buccal surface near the cementoenamel junction where the free gingiva meets the tooth surface; calculus and hyperplastic gingival tissue may obscure the lesion.
• FORLs can be found on any tooth; most commonly affected are the mandibular third premolar and molar, followed by the maxillary third and fourth premolars.
• Under general anesthesia, the lesions are examined with an explorer; a fine Shepherd's hook type is preferred; the explorer helps identify subgingival lesions coronal to the alveolar bone; the furcation area is a frequent site, and the examiner must distinguish a resorptive lesion from disease limited to alveolar bone loss.
• Stage 1 FORL—enamel defect less than 0.5 mm deep; minimally sensitive because it has not entered the dentin
• Stage 2 FORL—penetrates the enamel and dentin, but does not enter the endodontic system; these teeth may be treated with glass ionomer restoratives, which release fluoride ions to desensitize the exposed dentin, strengthen the enamel, and chemically bind to tooth surfaces; only 20% success rate, long term (> 2 yr). The extent of root involvement (determined radiographically) helps to determine therapy; if root resorption is present, extraction is often the best choice.
• Stage 3 FORL—penetrates into the endodontic system; radiographs are needed to determine the full extent of penetration.
• Stage 4 FORL—the crown has been eroded or fractured; gingiva growing over the root fragments leaves a painful bleeding lesion upon probing.

• Stage 5 FORL—the tooth crown is gone; gingival swelling covers the retained root

CAUSES
• The etiology is unknown; likely a multitude of initiating factors exist.
• Affected cats may have calcium regulation problems; an improper ratio of dietary calcium, magnesium, and phosphorus; or parathyroid gland malfunction producing calcium imbalance.
• Hyperreactivity to inflammatory cells, dental plaque, and/or calculus; endotoxins; prostaglandins, cytokines, and proteinases are also under investigation.

RISK FACTORS
N/A

 DIAGNOSIS

DIFFERENTIAL DIAGNOSIS
• Lymphocytic plasmacytic stomatitis syndrome
• Another type of resorptive lesion may be seen where periodontal disease has resulted in gingival recession and root exposure. These exposed root surfaces may show extensive external resorption, but there will be no further root involvement (resorption).

CBC/BIOCHEMISTRY/URINALYSIS
N/A

IMAGING
• Intraoral radiology is essential in making definitive diagnosis and planning treatment.
• Radiographic appearance varies from minute radiolucent defects of the tooth primarily at the cementoenamel junction to internal resorption and ankylosis of the apex to the supporting bone.

PATHOLOGIC FINDINGS
• Odontoclasts are arranged regularly along the edge of resorptive lesions.
• No decalcification in the dentin, suggesting that the resorptive lesions are not derived from dental caries.
• Resorptive lesions appear to be induced by granulation tissue.

TREATMENT

APPROPRIATE HEALTH CARE
N/A

NURSING CARE
• Controversial; FORLs are considered to be progressive; treatment may be attempted if the lesion is shallow and does not involve the pulp chamber, and there is no indication of root resorption radiographically.
• Stage 1—an enamel defect is noted; the lesion is minimally sensitive because it has not entered dentin; therapy includes thorough cleaning and polishing; gingivectomy and odontoplasty have been adjunctive; pulse antibiotics (given the first 5 days of each month) may help control plaque accumulation in all stages; application of fluoride varnish and dental sealers has been advocated but not evaluated to determine effectiveness in halting or slowing lesion progression.
• Stage 2 lesions—penetrate the enamel and dentin, are painful and must be treated by extraction or glass ionomer restoration, which provides short-term results in most cases
• Glass ionomer restoratives release fluoride ions to desensitize the exposed dentin, strengthen enamel, and chemically bind to tooth surfaces; application does not automatically stop disease progression.
• Stage 2 FORL treatment procedure with self-cured glass ionomer—(1) clean the area to be treated, with a curette or scaler; use flower pumice and water as a polish (not prophy paste); (2) isolate the gingiva by packing with gingival retraction cord or perform a gingivectomy; (3) irrigate and dry the area (but not bone dry); (4) once mixed, glass ionomer cement is placed on top of the lesion; when set, a varnish or nonfilled, light-cured resin is place over the restoration; and (5) finish and shape the restoration with a finishing bur; place a second coat of varnish or resin over the restoration to maintain proper moisture levels while curing
• Stage 3 lesions—enter the endodontic system; require either endodontics to seal the canal from oral bacteria or extraction; restoration with glass ionomer restoratives as the sole treatment is not an option, and in most cases, extraction is necessary, especially with evidence of root resorption

ACTIVITY
N/A

DIET
Prewet diet to soften

CLIENT EDUCATION
Daily home brushing may help control plaque.

SURGICAL CONSIDERATIONS
• Stages 2 and 3 FORLs with root resorption—gingival flap for exposure, section multi-rooted teeth, elevate segments, close
• Stage 4 FORLs—the crown is eroded or fractured with part of the crown remaining; gingiva grows over the root fragments, yielding a sensitive bleeding lesion upon probing; treatment of choice is flap surgery and extraction of the root fragments
• Stage 5 FORLs—the crown is gone and roots remain; the decision to perform surgery to find and extract the retained root(s) is based on inflammation and/or pain; if the cat feels discomfort when the lesion is probed, then the root(s) is extracted via flap exposure
• When roots are resorbed or ankylosed, the remaining fragile crown will often snap off during attempts at elevation. With sufficient radiographic documentation, owner consent, as well as future monitoring, these sites can be smoothed and closed, and will often heal without complication.

MEDICATIONS

DRUG(S)
N/A

CONTRAINDICATIONS
N/A

PRECAUTIONS
N/A

POSSIBLE INTERACTIONS
N/A

FOLLOW-UP

PATIENT MONITORING
N/A

PREVENTION/AVOIDANCE
N/A

POSSIBLE COMPLICATIONS
N/A

EXPECTED COURSE AND PROGNOSIS
N/A

MISCELLANEOUS

ASSOCIATED CONDITIONS
N/A

AGE-RELATED FACTORS
N/A

ZOONOTIC POTENTIAL
N/A

PREGNANCY
N/A

SYNONYMS
• External osteodontoclastic resorptive lesions
• Neck lesions
• Idiopathic buccocervical erosion
• Chronic subgingival tooth erosion
• Cervical line erosion
• Subgingival resorptive lesions

SEE ALSO
See Causes

ABBREVIATIONS
FORL = feline odontoclastic resorptive lesions

Suggested Reading
Harvey CE, Emily PP. Small animal dentistry. Philadelphia: Mosby, 1993.
Wiggs RB, Lobprise HB. Veterinary dentistry: principles and practice. Philadelphia: Lippincott-Raven, 1997.
Author Jan Bellows
Consulting Editor Heidi B. Lobprise

OLIGURIA AND ANURIA

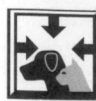

BASICS

DEFINITION
• Oliguria—the production of an abnormally small amount of urine (urine production rate < 0.25 mL/kg/h)
• Anuria—formation of essentially no urine (urine production rate < 0.08 mL/kg/h)

PATHOPHYSIOLOGY
• Physiologic oliguria occurs when the kidneys limit renal water loss during episodes of low renal perfusion to preserve body fluid and electrolyte balance. High plasma osmolality or low effective circulating fluid volume stimulate ADH synthesis and release. ADH acts on the kidneys to induce formation of small quantities of concentrated urine (the hallmark of physiologic oliguria).
• Pathologic oliguria results from severe renal parenchymal impairment. Factors include (1) high resistance in afferent glomerular vessels, (2) low glomerular permeability, (3) increased leakage ("back leak") of filtrate from damaged renal tubules, (4) renal intratubular obstruction, and (5) extensive loss of nephrons resulting in marked reduction in the quantity of glomerular filtrate produced.
• Anuria may be of renal or postrenal origin. Severe renal disease occasionally causes anuria. Mechanisms are the same as for pathologic oliguria (e.g., obstruction of urinary flow or rupture of the excretory pathway).

SYSTEMS AFFECTED
Renal/Urologic

SIGNALMENT
Dogs and cats

SIGNS
N/A

CAUSES
• Physiologic oliguria—renal hypoperfusion (caused by low blood volume or hypotension) or hypertonicity (usually caused by hypernatremia)
• Pathologic oliguria—acute oliguric renal failure or end-stage chronic renal failure
• Anuria—complete urinary tract obstruction, rupture of the urinary excretory pathway, or very severe, primary renal failure

RISK FACTORS
• Physiologic oliguria—dehydration, low cardiac output, hypotension
• Pathologic oliguria and anuria caused by primary renal failure (risk factors for acute renal failure)—preexisting renal disease, exposure to nephrotoxins, dehydration, low cardiac output, hypotension, electrolyte imbalance, acidosis, advanced age, fever, sepsis, liver disease, multiple organ failure, trauma, diabetes mellitus, hypoalbuminemia, hyperviscosity syndrome
• Anuria—urolithiasis, urinary tract neoplasia, idiopathic feline lower urinary tract disease (obstruction), micturition disorder, trauma

DIAGNOSIS

DIFFERENTIAL DIAGNOSIS
• Physiologic oliguria is suggested by physical signs of poor tissue perfusion (e.g., dehydration, prolonged capillary refill time, pale mucous membranes, weak pulse, rapid or irregular pulse, cool extremities); patient may have a history of recent fluid loss (vomiting, diarrhea, polyuria, hemorrhage); signs of uremia are typically absent and oliguria resolves rapidly when renal hypoperfusion is corrected
• Suspect pathologic oliguria and renal anuria with any of the risk factors given; the more risk factors, the more likely the patient has or will develop acute renal failure. Patients with pathologic oliguria caused by chronic renal failure typically have a history of progressive renal disease (including longstanding polyuria, polydipsia, poor appetite, and weight loss). Patients with chronic renal failure are at risk of developing acute renal failure. Signs of uremia are commonly observed, and fluid therapy and other measures designed to restore adequate renal perfusion often fail to increase urinary flow.
• Suspect anuria due to urinary obstruction or rupture of the excretory pathway in patients that repeatedly strain to void but cannot produce urinary flow. They may have a previous history of pollakiuria, dysuria, stranguria, hematuria, urolithiasis, trauma, or instrumentation of the urinary tract. In patients with urinary obstruction, physical examination may reveal an enlarged urinary bladder, painful posterior abdomen, and masses or uroliths in the urethra or bladder. Physical examination of patients with rupture of the urinary tract may reveal ascites, fluid infiltration in tissues around the urinary tract, painful caudal abdomen, masses or uroliths in the bladder or urethra, or evidence of trauma (e.g., pelvic fracture). Urinary obstruction caused by disorder of micturition may be suspected in patients with enlargement of the urinary bladder, increased resistance to manual expression of the bladder, and neurologic signs affecting the hind limbs and/or tail. Signs of uremia may develop. Restoration of urinary flow or correcting rents in the excretory pathway rapidly restores adequate urinary flow.

CBC/BIOCHEMISTRY/URINALYSIS
• Serum urea nitrogen and creatinine concentrations are typically high unless the onset of oliguria or anuria is very recent.
• Hyperkalemia is common with pathologic oliguria and anuria, less common and less severe in animals with physiologic oliguria (except in those with hypoadrenocorticism).
• Physiologic oliguria is characterized by urinary specific gravity values above 1.030 in dogs and 1.035 in cats. Oliguria associated with lower urinary specific gravity values suggests primary renal failure. Patients with urine-concentrating defects from other diseases or drugs are the exception to this rule.
• Renal anuria is often characterized by urinary specific gravity values above 1.030 (dogs) or 1.035 (cats). Urinary specific gravity in patients with postrenal anuria varies. Adequate urine-concentrating ability is often lost after urinary obstruction but may persist with rupture of the excretory pathway.

OTHER LABORATORY TESTS
N/A

IMAGING
• Abdominal radiographs and ultrasound are useful to rule out urinary obstruction and rupture of the excretory pathway. Distension of any portion of the excretory pathway or observation of uroliths within the ureters, bladder neck, or urethra suggests urinary obstruction.
• Detection of fluid within the peritoneal cavity or adjacent to the urinary tract supports a diagnosis of rupture of the excretory pathway.
• Excretory urography, retrograde urethrocystography, or vaginourethrocystography may provide definitive proof of urinary obstruction or rupture of the excretory pathway.

DIAGNOSTIC PROCEDURES
• Electrocardiography may quickly establish whether the patient has clinically important hyperkalemia. Hyperkalemic cardiotoxicity is characterized (in order of progressing hyperkalemia) by tall, peaked T waves with a narrow base; prolongation of the P-R interval and QRS complex; decreased amplitude and increased width of P waves; bradycardia; atrial standstill; QRS-T fusion causing a wide-complex, idioventricular rhythm; ventricular fibrillation or asystole.
• Urethrocystoscopy may provide evidence for obstruction or rupture of the urinary tract.
• Placing a urinary catheter may provide information about the integrity of the lower urinary tract, but this approach is not recommended as a diagnostic procedure because it may be misleading, it may cause additional trauma to the urinary tract, and it may introduce bacteria.

TREATMENT
• Oliguria and anuria are medical emergencies; left untreated, they may lead to death within hours to days. Death typically results from uremia, hyperkalemia, or sepsis (in patients with urinary tract infection).

• Correct persistent renal hypoperfusion rapidly; it may lead to acute ischemic renal injury.

• Correct renal hypoperfusion by intravenous administration of normal saline or lactated Ringer's solution. In selected animals, other fluids may be more appropriate (e.g., blood to correct hypoperfusion resulting from hemorrhage).

• Therapy for primary renal oliguria and anuria is usually limited to symptomatic and supportive care designed to allow the patient to survive long enough for some spontaneous recovery of renal function to occur. Elimination of causative factor may slow or stop further renal injury (e.g., terminating aminoglycoside administration, correcting hypercalcemia, or restoring adequate renal perfusion); however, once oliguria or anuria has developed, few if any renal diseases will be amenable to specific treatment

• Postrenal causes for anuria may be corrected by nonsurgical or surgical methods. Nonsurgical methods include hydropropulsion of uroliths or urethral plugs or placement of urinary catheters to restore low-pressure urinary flow. Surgical methods may include removal of uroliths, polyps, or neoplastic tissue or surgical correction of rents, strictures, or malposition of the excretory pathway.

 MEDICATIONS

DRUG(S)

• In patients with renal oliguria, diuretics are usually indicated after correcting renal hypoperfusion. Diuretic-induced increased urinary flow rate does not necessarily indicate improved renal function, but converting oliguria to nonoliguria facilitates managing the patient by fluid and electrolyte administration. Increased urinary flow after diuretic administration suggests a more favorable prognosis.

• Furosemide (2 mg/kg/IV q8h) is often used initially in patients with oliguric renal failure. Urinary flow should increase within 1 hr. If diuresis does not ensue within an hour, dosage may be increased to 4–6 mg/kg IV.

• Dopamine (0.5–3 μg/kg/min) has the potential to increase renal blood flow, glomerular filtration, and renal sodium excretion in dogs. Higher doses may cause renal vasoconstriction, tachycardia, and cardiac arrhythmias and are contraindicated in ARF. Dopamine is generally administered concurrently with furosemide. Diuresis should ensue within 1 to 2 hours. If diuresis ensues, dopamine should be continued until fluid and electrolyte balance can be maintained without further drug therapy. However, most recent data suggest that dopamine is usually ineffective in reversing established oliguria. If urine flow does not

increase within 2 hours, discontinue dopamine. Although limited data support use of dopamine with furosemide in dogs, recent data suggest that cats lack dopamine-specific receptor activity in their kidneys. Dopamine is not an appropriate therapy for oliguria in cats.

• Mannitol (0.5–1.0 g/kg IV) can be given as a 10 or 20% solution over 15–20 min. Urinary flow should increase within 1 hour. Do not repeat administration of mannitol if diuresis does not ensue; it may cause excessive volume expansion.

• A safer but possibly less effective alternative to mannitol is infusion of 10–20% dextrose solution (25–50 mL/kg/IV q8–12h) over 1–2 hours. Because dextrose is metabolized, the potential for volume expansion is minimized.

CONTRAINDICATIONS

Nephrotoxic drugs

PRECAUTIONS

• Administer fluids judiciously to patients that are persistently oliguric or anuric to avoid overhydration. In patients with unresponsive renal oliguria, peritoneal dialysis or hemodialysis may be the only means of correcting severe fluid-induced volume overexpansion.

• Correct fluid deficits before initiating diuretic administration. Otherwise renal hypoperfusion and ischemic renal injury may be exacerbated.

• Use drugs requiring renal excretion with caution. If resolution of oliguria or anuria can reasonably be expected within minutes to a few hours (e.g., physiologic oliguria and anuria due to urinary obstruction), normal dosages of drugs requiring renal excretion may be used.

• Avoid electrolyte solutions containing more than 4 mEq of potassium per liter in most animals.

• Dopamine can cause cardiac arrhythmias, particularly in animals with hyperkalemia. ECG monitoring is recommended when high dosages are used and in animals with hyperkalemia.

POSSIBLE INTERACTIONS

Furosemide may promote the nephrotoxicity associated with aminoglycoside antibiotics.

 FOLLOW-UP

PATIENT MONITORING

• Urinary flow rate—urinary catheterization may be necessary for accurate determination of urine volume, but it can induce bacterial urinary tract infection, an important cause of morbidity and mortality in patients with acute renal failure. Catheters must be placed using aseptic technique. Intermittent catheterization is less likely to cause urinary tract infection

than an indwelling catheter. The shorter the time that a catheter is indwelling, the lower the risk of urinary tract infection. Attach indwelling catheters to a closed, sterile, urinary drainage system.

• Creatinine, serum urea nitrogen, and potassium concentrations after 12–24 hr; patients with severe hyperkalemia may need more frequent monitoring of serum potassium concentrations

• ECG to assess cardiac effects of dopamine, hyperkalemia, and response to therapy

POSSIBLE COMPLICATIONS

• Hyperkalemia and associated cardiotoxicity

• Uremia leading to death

• Dehydration caused by vomiting, diarrhea, respiratory losses

• Overhydration caused by excessive fluid intake or administration leading to pulmonary edema

• Bacterial urinary tract infection and sepsis

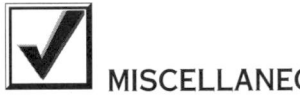 **MISCELLANEOUS**

ASSOCIATED CONDITIONS
N/A

AGE-RELATED FACTORS
N/A

ZOONOTIC POTENTIAL
N/A

PREGNANCY
N/A

SYNONYMS
N/A

SEE ALSO
• Azotemia and Uremia
• Hyperkalemia
• Nephrotoxicity, Drug-induced
• Renal Failure, Acute and Chronic
• Urinary Tract Obstruction

ABBREVIATIONS
• ADH = antidiuretic hormone
• ARF = acute renal failure
• ECG = electrocardiogram

Suggested Reading

Cowgill LD, Elliot DA: Acute renal failure. In: Ettinger SJ, Feldman EC, eds. Textbook of veterinary internal medicine. Philadelphia: Saunders, 2000:1615–1633.

Cowgill LD, Langston CE. Role of hemodialysis in the management of dogs and cats with renal failure. Vet Clin North Am Small Anim Pract 1996;26(6):1347–1348.

Labato MA: Strategies for management of acute renal failure. Vet Clin North Am Small Anim Pract 2001;31:1265–1287.

Author David J. Polzin
Consulting Editors Larry G. Adams and Carl A. Osborne

ONCOCYTOMA

 BASICS

OVERVIEW
• Rare benign neoplasm derived from oxyphil cells: atypical neuroendocrine cells that occur scattered throughout endocrine glands and epithelial tissues
• Most common location is the larynx
• Minimally invasive
• Nonmetastatic
• Special stains have shown most oncocytomas to actually be rhabdomyomas: benign striated muscle tumors
• Prognosis good to excellent

SIGNALMENT
• Young to middle-aged dogs; only one report in a cat
• No breed predisposition

SIGNS

Historical Findings
• Dependent on location of mass
• Dyspnea; voice change with laryngeal mass

Physical Examination Findings
• Inspiratory dyspnea
• Mass protruding into lumen of larynx on examination under sedation

CAUSES & RISK FACTORS
Unknown

 DIAGNOSIS

DIFFERENTIAL DIAGNOSIS
• Laryngeal paralysis
• Carcinoma
• Squamous cell carcinoma
• Mast cell tumor
• Lymphoma

CBC/BIOCHEMISTRY/URINALYSIS
Usually normal

OTHER LABORATORY TESTS
N/A

IMAGING
• Lateral cervical radiography—evaluation of laryngeal space
• Thoracic radiography—pulmonary metastasis evaluation in case of malignant tumor

DIAGNOSTIC PROCEDURES
• Laryngeal examination under sedation or general anesthesia
• Cytology of mass—may rule out other neoplasia, such as lymphoma and mast cell tumor
• Incisional biopsy for histopathology—required for definitive diagnosis

 TREATMENT

• Surgical resection—treatment of choice
• Despite a poor location, most oncocytomas (rhabdomyomas) can be removed ("peeled out") while preserving laryngeal function.

 MEDICATIONS

DRUG(S) OF CHOICE
N/A

 FOLLOW-UP

PATIENT MONITORING
• Complete resection—normal postoperative care; no additional follow-up necessary
• Incomplete resection—monitor for recurring clinical signs; may need to pursue more aggressive surgery (complete laryngectomy with permanent tracheostomy)

EXPECTED COURSE AND PROGNOSIS
Complete resection is curative.

 MISCELLANEOUS

Suggested Reading
Carlisle CH, Biery DN, Thrall DE. Tracheal and laryngeal tumors in the dog and cat: literature review and 13 additional patients. Vet Radiol 1991;32:229–235.
Author Laura D. Garrett
Consulting Editor Wallace B. Morrison

BASICS

OVERVIEW
• Infection of the conjunctiva or cornea before, or just after, the separation of the eyelids in the neonate
• Occurs in puppies and kittens
• Associated with *Staphylococcus* spp. or *Streptococcus* spp. in dogs and cats, and with Herpesvirus in cats
• Potentially vision-threatening
• Source of infection—believed to be from a vaginal infection of the dam at the time of birth or from a nonhygienic environment

SIGNALMENT
• Affects all breeds of cats and dogs
• Neonates before the time that they open their eyelids (10–14 days postpartum)

SIGNS
• Upper and lower eyelids are still adherent (physiologic ankyloblepharon) and bulge outward because of the accumulation of debris and discharge within the conjunctival fornices and between the cornea and lids
• May note a mucoid to mucopurulent discharge extruding through the medial canthus
• Cornea and conjunctiva—may be ulcerated
• May note adhesions (symblepharon) of the conjunctiva to the cornea or to other areas of the conjunctiva (including that of the nictitans)
• Perforation of the cornea with iris prolapse and collapse of the globe—occasionally seen

CAUSES & RISK FACTORS
• Vaginal infections in the dam near the time of birth
• Unclean environment for the neonates

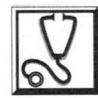
DIAGNOSIS

DIFFERENTIAL DIAGNOSIS
Neonates with entropion in which the eyelids have already separated—may have mucoid to mucopurulent discharge; view of the cornea may be obscured; may have appearance of ankyloblepharon; differentiated by age patients older than 10–14 days) and no ankyloblepharon when eyelids are everted

CBC/BIOCHEMISTRY/URINALYSIS
Normal unless there is a concurrent systemic infection

OTHER LABORATORY TESTS
• Cultures of neonate's ocular discharge and/or dam's vaginal discharge—may help diagnose bacterial infection
• Cytology of the affected tissues—may help determine presence of bacteria
• Immunofluorescent antibody or polymerase-chain reaction tests (cats)—feline herpesvirus

IMAGING
N/A

DIAGNOSTIC PROCEDURES
• Full physical examination of the dam and neonate
• Fluorescein staining—corneal or conjunctival ulceration

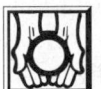
TREATMENT
• Separation of the eyelids—cornerstone of treatment; can be accomplished by manual traction beginning at the medial canthus or introduction into the medial canthus of a small blunt scissor blade or the blunt, butt end of a scalpel blade and gently separating (not cutting) the eyelids
• Conjunctival sacs and cornea—lavaged with warm saline to remove the discharge
• Warm compresses—may aid in separation of the eyelids and in preventing re-adherence
• Systemic support—as needed

MEDICATIONS

DRUG(S)
• Broad spectrum, topical antibiotics—neomycin, bacitracin, or polymyxin B; applied four times daily for at least 1 week; antibiotic chosen on basis of bacterial culture and sensitivity, if available

CONTRAINDICATIONS/POSSIBLE INTERACTIONS
• Tetracycline—do not use in neonates because of the risk of affecting bone or teeth; topical chloramphenicol or ciprofloxacin is drug of choice for *Chlamydia*.
• Topical corticosteroids—contraindicated

FOLLOW-UP

PATIENT MONITORING
• Warm compresses—may be necessary for a few days to keep the eyelids from re-adhering
• Topical antibiotics—continued for a minimum of 7 days
• Observe littermates that are not initially affected.
• Treat vaginal infections in the dam with appropriate medications.

PREVENTION/AVOIDANCE
• Keep the external environment and the dam's nipples clean.
• Treat vaginal infection in the dam before delivery, if possible.

POSSIBLE COMPLICATIONS
• Severe keratitis with scarring and symblepharon
• Rupture of the cornea with secondary phthisis; blindness may be irreversible

MISCELLANEOUS

Suggested Reading
Williams MM. Neonatal ophthalmic disorders. In: Kirk RW, ed. Current veterinary therapy X. Philadelphia: Saunders, 1989: 658–673.
Author Stephanie L. Smedes
Consulting Editor Paul E. Miller

OPTIC NEURITIS

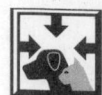

BASICS

OVERVIEW
• Inflammation of one or both optic nerves, resulting in reduction of visual function
• May be a primary disease or secondary to systemic CNS disease because the optic nerve communicates with the subarachnoid space
• Affects the ophthalmic and nervous systems

SIGNALMENT
• Dogs and cats
• Primary—uncommon; usually affects dogs > 3 years of age
• Secondary—N/A

SIGNS

Historical Findings
• Acute-onset blindness
• Partial visual deficits—often overlooked

Physical Examination Findings
• Blind or reduced vision in one or both eyes
• Pupils fixed and dilated—may have intact but diminished pupillary light reflex
• Funduscopic examination—optic disk swelling; focal hemorrhage; active or inactive chorioretinitis
• Often normal fundus with retrobulbar or intracranial optic nerve disease

CAUSES & RISK FACTORS
• Idiopathic
• Systemic mycoses
• Canine distemper
• FIP
• Neoplasm—primary or metastatic
• Toxoplasmosis
• Neosporum caninum
• Granulomatous meningoencephalomyelitis
• Toxicity—lead

DIAGNOSIS

DIFFERENTIAL DIAGNOSIS
• Cortical blindness—normal pupillary light reflex; normal fundus examination; possibly other neurologic deficits
• SARDS (dogs)—minimal to absent pupillary light reflex; normal fundus (early in course); flat electroretinogram

CBC/BIOCHEMISTRY/URINALYSIS
No specific abnormalities

OTHER LABORATORY TESTS
Specific viral, protozoal, or fungal serologic tests on serum

IMAGING
Neuroimaging—CT and/or MRI

DIAGNOSTIC PROCEDURES
• CSF analysis
• Electroretinogram—investigate retinal function; normal in optic neuritis, flat in SARDS
• Visual evoked potentials—investigate optic nerve function

TREATMENT
• Based on underlying disease

MEDICATIONS

DRUG(S)
• Depend on primary disease process when identifiable
• Idiopathic–Prednisone—2 mg/kg q12h for 14 days; then 1 mg/kg q12h for 14 days; then gradual reduction to maintenance dosage

CONTRAINDICATIONS/POSSIBLE INTERACTIONS
N/A

FOLLOW-UP
• Monitor clinical signs or visual evoked potentials, if available.
• Prognosis—depends on underlying disease
• Blindness may be permanent with idiopathic optic neuritis.
• Clinical course—unpredictable
• Flare ups—may occur if medication is inadequate

MISCELLANEOUS

ABBREVIATIONS
• CSF = cerebrospinal fluid
• FIP = feline infectious peritonitis
• SARDS= sudden acquired retinal degeneration syndrome

Suggested Reading
Braund KG. Clinical syndromes in veterinary neurology. 2nd ed. St. Louis: Mosby, 1994.
Author David Lipsitz
Consulting Editor Paul E. Miller

ORAL CAVITY TUMORS, UNDIFFERENTIATED MALIGNANT TUMORS

 BASICS

OVERVIEW
• Highly aggressive, rapidly growing masses in the area of the hard palate, upper molar teeth, or maxilla and orbit
• Most are highly invasive to the bone and are nonencapsulated with a smooth to slightly nodular surface (mistaken as benign); may become ulcerated
• Biopsy—reveals undifferentiated malignancy of undetermined histogenesis
• Highly metastatic
• Cervical lymphadenopathy common

SIGNALMENT
• All dogs < 2 years old; range, 6–22 months
• Primarily a disease of large breeds
• No sex predilection

SIGNS
Historical Findings
• Excessive salivation
• Halitosis
• Dysphagia
• Bloody oral discharge
• Weight loss
Physical Examination Findings
• Oral mass
• Loose teeth
• Facial deformity
• Cervical lymphadenopathy—occasionally

CAUSES & RISK FACTORS
None identified

 DIAGNOSIS

DIFFERENTIAL DIAGNOSIS
• Other oral malignancy
• Epulis
• Abscess
• Benign polyp

CBC/BIOCHEMISTRY/URINALYSIS
May be normal

OTHER LABORATORY TESTS
Cytologic evaluation of an impression smear obtained from an incisional biopsy specimen (wedge)—may yield diagnosis

IMAGING
• Skull radiography—detect bone invasion deep to the mass
• Thoracic radiography—detect lung metastasis

DIAGNOSTIC PROCEDURES
• Carefully palpate regional lymph nodes (mandibular and retropharyngeal).
• Large, deep tissue biopsy (down to bone)—required to differentiate from other oral malignancies

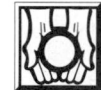 **TREATMENT**

SURGERY
Radical surgical excision—usually ineffective because of extensive local disease or metastasis on examination; if attempted, must have margins of at least 2 cm into normal bone and soft tissues

RADIATION
Efficacy unreported; most undifferentiated tumors are poorly responsive

OTHER
Soft foods—may be recommended to prevent tumor ulceration or after radical oral excision

 MEDICATIONS

DRUG(S)
• Chemotherapy—efficacy unreported; most undifferentiated tumors are poorly responsive.
• Local control (palliation) with intralesionally administered cisplatin—reported

CONTRAINDICATIONS/POSSIBLE INTERACTIONS
Chemotherapy can be toxic; seek advice before initiating treatment if you are unfamiliar with cytotoxic drugs.

 FOLLOW-UP

Dogs—most have lymph node metastasis on examination; usually euthanized within 30 days of diagnosis because tumor growth is progressive and uncontrolled, resulting in dysphagia and cachexia

 MISCELLANEOUS

Suggested Reading

Frazier DL, Hahn KA. Cancer chemotherapeutics. In: Hahn KA, Richardson RC, eds. Cancer chemotherapy, a veterinary handbook. Baltimore: Williams & Wilkins, 1995:77–150.

Patnaik AL, Lieberman PH, Erlandson RA, et al. A clinicopathologic and ultrastructural study of undifferentiated malignant tumors of the oral cavity in dogs. Vet Pathol 1986;23:170–175.

Author Kevin A. Hahn and Kimberly P. Freeman

Consulting Editor Wallace B. Morrison

ORAL MASSES

 BASICS

DEFINITION
Oral cavity growth

PATHOPHYSIOLOGY
N/A

SYSTEMS AFFECTED
N/A

GENETICS
N/A

INCIDENCE/PREVALENCE
• Males are more commonly affected with oral melanomas and fibrosarcomas than females.
• Breed predilection—golden retriever, German shorthaired pointer, Weimaraner, St. Bernard, and cocker spaniels more prone to oral tumors; dachshunds and beagles less prone to oral tumors; boxer, gingival hyperplasia

GEOGRAPHIC DISTRIBUTION
N/A

SIGNALMENT

Cat
• Squamous cell carcinoma—age range, 3–21 years (mean, 12.5); most common site, the sublingual area; two forms are tonsillar and nontonsillar; common presenting signs include excessive drooling and/or bleeding from the mouth; frequently invades bone, loosening teeth; morbidity and mortality result from local disease rather than distant metastasis.
• Fibrosarcomas—age range, 1–21 years (mean, 10.3); no particular predilection site; all associated with local tissue destruction; muscle and bone invasion are occasionally seen.

Dog
• Epulides are the most common benign oral tumor; three types occur.
　• Fibromatous epulis—common in dogs (and cats); age range 1–17 (mean, 7.5); both pedunculated and sessile forms; they usually have a smooth, pink surface
　• Peripheral odontogenic fibroma (ossifying epulis)—similar to fibromatous, but has an osteoid matrix
　• Peripheral ameloblastoma (acanthomatous epulis)—classified as benign but tends to invade adjacent bone

• Malignant melanoma—the most common oral malignant tumor in the dog; cocker spaniels, German shepherds, chow chows, and dogs with heavily pigmented mucous membranes are predisposed; males more frequently affected than females
• Melanoma—many places in the oral cavity (gingiva, buccal mucosa, hard or soft palate, and tongue); locally invasive and metastasize to lungs and regional lymph nodes; presenting complaint is commonly oral bleeding, ptyalism, or halitosis; tumor size on presentation is important to patient survival; in the dog, melanomas < 2 cm carry a better survival rate (median 511 days) than those > 2 cm (164 days); tumors located rostrally have better prognosis than those located distally.
• Squamous cell carcinoma—the next most common oral malignancy; originates from the gingival epithelium; red, ulcerated, and may have cauliflower projections; large-breed dogs are predisposed; prognosis depends on location in the oral cavity; those located rostrally carry a better prognosis than those at the base of the tongue or occurring in the tonsils, which tend to metastasize and are the most aggressive.
• Papillary squamous cell carcinoma—a rapidly growing tumor of young dogs (< 1 year); in the papillary gingiva; locally aggressive but does not metastasize; treatment of choice is excision.
• Fibrosarcomas—the third most common oral malignancy in dogs (and the second most common in the cat); fibrosarcomas have a predilection for the maxilla of large, male, older dogs; the gingiva is commonly affected, especially around the maxillary fourth premolar, followed by the hard palate and oral mucosa; invasive but rarely metastasize
• Tumors of dental laminar epithelium—originate from epithelial cells of the dental lamina; form from dental epithelium during development or may originate from nests of epithelial cells that maintain the ability to function as dental lamina
　• Ameloblastoma—the most common tumor of dental laminar epithelium in dogs; behave as slowly expansible tumors occurring deep within bone; may be cystic or solid
• Other tumor types include undifferentiated carcinomas, osteosarcomas, lymphosarcomas, mast cell tumors, giant cell tumors, neurofibromas, and myxofibrosarcomas.

SIGNS
May include halitosis, oral hemorrhage, and reluctance to chew; often are none

CAUSES
N/A

RISK FACTORS
• Tonsillar squamous cell carcinoma occurs ten times more commonly in dogs from urban settings than in rural dogs.
• Squamous cell carcinoma—more prevalent in white dogs in one study

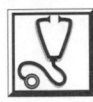 DIAGNOSIS

DIFFERENTIAL DIAGNOSIS
• Infection—viral/bacterial/fungal
• Odontoma • Dentigerous cyst

CBC/BIOCHEMISTRY/URINALYSIS
N/A

OTHER LABORATORY TESTS
N/A

IMAGING
Take radiographs of the affected jaw for bony invasion, lungs for metastases.

DIAGNOSTIC PROCEDURES
Aspirate enlarged regional lymph nodes for cytology or biopsy to evaluate metastasis.

PATHOLOGIC FINDINGS
• Must biopsy; sample deep tissue surrounding the mass; use excision, wedge, or needle-punch techniques.
• Cytology may also be helpful but is not as definitive as histopathology.

 TREATMENT

• Depends on the tumor type
• Benign tumors are treatable with long-term success via surgery.
• Malignant tumors are treated surgically with varying success depending on tumor type, location, and metastasis at presentation.
• In advanced circumstances, combined therapy (surgery, chemotherapy, and radiation) may provide the best care.
• Dogs with tumors caudal to the first premolar had a three times greater risk of dying from the disease than those with tumors rostral to the first premolar.

SURGICAL CONSIDERATIONS

- Fibromatous epulis—marginal excision is the treatment of choice; cryotherapy and radiation treatment also give long-term success.
- Peripheral odontogenic fibromas (ossifying epulis)—treat the same as fibromatous epulis.
- Acanthomatous epulis—excision with at least 1-cm margins is usually curative; radiation has also been used successfully; the combination of surgery and radiation may be most effective (requiring less aggressive surgery), but if radiation is not readily available, surgery may be the only option; surgery must be aggressive; the best chance to resolve the problem surgically is the first time; extract any teeth that may impede incisional healing.
- Multiple (10) injections of bleomycin (5 mg) injected at the tumor site have been effective in a small number of reported cases.
- Melanoma—prognosis improves if the tumor is small and located in the rostral mandible; if surgery is chosen for therapy, it should be aggressive; typically mandibulectomy or maxillectomy; median survival times average 8 months; combination of surgery, radiation, and chemotherapy (low-dose cisplatin) yielded a median survival of 14 months in one study; pigmentation does not affect the prognosis; relatively radioresistant; one study showed a median survival time of 14 months after radiation only; the problem with melanoma is not local disease management but metastasis.
- Squamous cell carcinoma—better long-term prognosis than malignant melanoma or fibrosarcoma in the dog; may be widely surgically excised or irradiated in the dog, especially if the lesion is rostral (better prognosis than those located caudally); perform a maxillectomy or mandibulectomy with a 2-cm clean surgical margin as a goal; in dogs, radiation alone delivers a median survival rate of 15–17 months; in dogs, prognosis for survival following treatment of lingual involvement is poor; dogs tolerate partial glossotomy involving 40–60% of the tongue; for tumors larger than 2 cm or those with incomplete resections surgery, radiation, and chemotherapy (mitoxantrone) may be the best options.
- Fibrosarcoma—surgical excision with at least 2-cm margins usually results in a 12-month median survival rate; usually require a maxillectomy or mandibulectomy; palatine fibrosarcomas carry the poorest prognosis because of the inability to surgically resect adequately

APPROPRIATE HEALTH CARE
N/A

NURSING CARE
N/A

ACTIVITY
N/A

DIET
N/A

CLIENT EDUCATION
N/A

 MEDICATIONS

DRUG(S) OF CHOICE
N/A

CONTRAINDICATIONS
N/A

PRECAUTIONS
N/A

POSSIBLE INTERACTIONS
N/A

ALTERNATIVE DRUG(S)
N/A

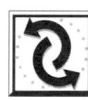 FOLLOW-UP

PATIENT MONITORING
N/A

PREVENTION/AVOIDANCE
N/A

POSSIBLE COMPLICATIONS
- Surgical removal of part of the tongue may result in avascular necrosis if the tongue is transected just caudal to the origin of dorsal branches of the lingual arteries.
- Postoperative complications of mandibulectomy include wound dehiscence, prehension dysfunction, tongue lag, medial drift, excessive drooling, palatal ulceration secondary to malocclusion, and pressure necrosis.

- Feline mandibulectomies can be performed, but they result in greater complications (tongue swelling, ranula formation) than in the canine patient.

EXPECTED COURSE AND PROGNOSIS
- Dogs with inadequate tumor-free surgical margins were two-and-a-half times more likely to die of the tumor than those with complete histologic excision; some surgical patients need gastrostomy tubes to facilitate nutritional supplementation during the treatment period.
- Dogs with tumors located caudal to the first premolar had three times greater risk of dying from the disease than those with tumors located rostral to the first premolar.

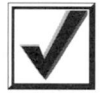 MISCELLANEOUS

ASSOCIATED CONDITIONS
N/A

AGE-RELATED FACTORS
N/A

ZOONOTIC POTENTIAL
N/A

PREGNANCY
N/A

SYNONYMS
N/A

SEE ALSO
N/A

ABBREVIATIONS
N/A

Suggested Reading

Harvey CE, Emily PP. Small animal dentistry. Philadelphia: Mosby, 1993.

Wiggs RB, Lobprise HB. Veterinary dentistry: principles and practice. Philadelphia: Lippincott-Raven, 1997.

Author James M-G. Anthony
Consulting Editor Heidi B. Lobprise

ORAL ULCERATION AND CHRONIC ULCERATIVE PERIODONTAL STOMATITIS

 BASICS

DEFINITION
Focal or multifocal loss of mucosal integrity of the superficial epithelial layers in specific areas of the oral cavity

SYSTEMS AFFECTED
Gastrointestinal—oral cavity

GENETICS
N/A

GEOGRAPHIC DISTRIBUTION
N/A

SIGNALMENT
• Dogs and cats of any age and either sex
• Breed predilection for ulcerative stomatitis (a.k.a. chronic ulcerative periodontal stomatitis [CUPS])—Maltese, Cavalier King Charles spaniels, cocker spaniels, Bouvier des Flandres.
• Feline LPS—may have predilection for Somali and Abyssinian cats (see Plasma Cell Gingivitis and Pharyngitis; Stomatitis)
• Idiopathic osteomyelitis—may have predilection for cocker spaniels; complication associated with CUPS

SIGNS
• Halitosis
• Gingivitis
• Faucitis
• Pharyngitis
• Buccitis/buccal mucosal ulceration
• Hypersalivation (thick, ropey saliva)
• Pain
• Anorexia
• Mucosal ulceration—"kissing ulcers" common in CUPS
• Plaque—with or without calculus
• Exposed, necrotic bone—with alveolar osteitis and idiopathic osteomyelitis
• Behavior changes secondary to oral sensitivity
• Scar formation on lateral margins of tongue—with CUPS
• Note: sometimes these signs will start following a routine dental cleaning on a previously "normal" patient; probably would have occurred eventually, just exacerbated by manipulation in the oral cavity

CAUSES

Metabolic
• Diabetes mellitus
• Hypoparathyroidism
• Hypothyroidism
• Renal disease—uremia

Nutritional
• Protein-calorie malnutrition
• Riboflavin deficiency

Neoplastic
• Dog—malignant melanoma; squamous cell carcinoma; fibrosarcoma
• Cat—squamous cell carcinoma; fibrosarcoma; malignant melanoma

Immune-mediated
• Pemphigus vulgaris—90% have oral involvement
• Bullous pemphigoid—80% have oral involvement
• Systemic lupus erythematosus—50% have oral involvement
• Discoid lupus erythematosus
• Drug-induced—toxic epidermal necrolysis

Infectious
• Retrovirus—FeLV/FIV
• Calicivirus—cat
• Herpesvirus—cat
• Leptospirosis—dog
• Periodontal disease—dog and cat

Traumatic
• Foreign body—bone or wood fragments
• Electric cord shock
• Malocclusion
• Gum-chewer's disease—chronic chewing of cheek

Chemical/Toxic
• Acids
• Thallium

Idiopathic
• Eosinophilic granuloma—cats, Siberian huskies, Samoyeds
• LPS—cats; see Plasma Cell Gingivitis and Pharyngitis, and Stomatitis
• CUPS—dogs; allergic, hypersensitivity reaction to plaque
• Idiopathic osteomyelitis—dogs

RISK FACTORS
N/A

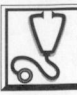 **DIAGNOSIS**

• History and oral examination—foreign bodies; malocclusions; chemical, toxic, and electrical burns
• Idiopathic conditions—clinical signs; history; breed predispositions; response to therapy

CBC/BIOCHEMISTRY/URINALYSIS
• CBC, biochemistry, urinalysis, and T_4—diabetes mellitus; hypoparathyroidism; renal disease; hypothyroidism; infections
• Chronic conditions may have elevated serum total protein and elevated globulin levels due to chronic antigen stimulation; T_4 may be decreased secondarily.

OTHER LABORATORY TESTS
• Serology—FeLV/FIV test; titers for specific infections
• Cultures—usually nonspecific; oral flora contaminants

DIAGNOSTIC PROCEDURES
Biopsy/cytology—neoplasia, immune-mediated disease, and chronic inflammation result in predominant lymphocytes and plasmocytes (CUPS and LPS)

IMAGING
Radiography—helps determine bony involvement and extent of idiopathic osteomyelitis

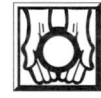 **TREATMENT**

APPROPRIATE HEALTH CARE
• Supportive therapy—soft diet; fluids; hospitalization in severe cases
• Nutritional support—via pharyngostomy or esophagostomy feeding tube
• CUPS—continuous, meticulous home care to prevent plaque accumulation; dental cleaning initially and frequently; periodontal therapy; extraction of diseased teeth
• Underlying metabolic or other disease—treat systemic illness appropriately.

ORAL ULCERATION AND CHRONIC ULCERATIVE PERIODONTAL STOMATITIS

CLIENT EDUCATION
• Warn client that prognosis is guarded, response to therapy depends on underlying cause, and prolonged treatment and/or further extractions may be necessary.
• In CUPS or LPS, any level of home care that can be provided is encouraged (brushing or topical antimicrobials).

SURGICAL CONSIDERATIONS
• Select extractions (partial, caudal, or full mouth)—may be indicated for chronic idiopathic conditions, e.g., CUPS and LPS, to remove the source of reaction (plaque/teeth)
• Removal of entire tooth structure—important in extraction treatment for LPS
• Removal of necrotic/avascular bone, gingival flap closure, and broad-spectrum antibiotics—indicated for idiopathic osteomyelitis; monitor for recurrence.

 MEDICATIONS

DRUG(S)
• Antimicrobials—treat primary and secondary bacterial infections, may be used intermittently between cleanings for therapeutic assistance, but the owner must be cautioned that chronic use could lead to antibiotic resistance; clindamycin (11 mg/kg PO q12h); amoxicillin-clavulanate (12.5–25 mg/kg PO q12h); tetracycline (10–22 mg/kg PO q8h)
• Antiinflammatory/immunosuppressive drugs—the comfort of the patient must be weighed against potential long-term side effects of corticosteroid usage; prednisone (0.5–1.0 mg/kg q12–24h PO, taper dosage)
• Mucosal protectants—for chemical insults; sucralfate (1g/25 kg q8h PO); cimetidine (5–10 mg/kg q8-12h PO)
• Analgesics—postextraction; carprofen (0.5 mg/kg PO q12–24h); hydrocodone (0.22 mg/kg q8–12h)

• Topical therapy—chlorhexidine solution or gel (antibacterial): CHX (VRx Products, Harbor City, CA) or CET Oral Hygiene Rinse (Virbac, Fort Worth, TX); zinc gluconate/ascorbic acid: MaxiGuard gel (Addison Biological Laboratory, Inc., Fayette, MO); stabilized chlorine dioxide for halitosis: Oxyfresh Pet Oral Hygiene Solution (Oxyfresh Worldwide, Inc., Spokane, WA)

CONTRAINDICATIONS
• Do not use these medications in patients with known hypersensitivities.
• Corticosteroids are contraindicated in patients with systemic fungal infections.

PRECAUTIONS
• Some antimicrobials may upset the gastrointestinal tract.
• Avoid corticosteroids in patients that may already be immunocompromised (i.e., those with FeLV or FIV).

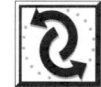 FOLLOW-UP

PATIENT MONITORING
Inflammation may take 4–6 weeks to subside after extractions due to plaque retention of sutures and tongue.

 MISCELLANEOUS

ASSOCIATED CONDITIONS
N/A

AGE-RELATED FACTORS
N/A

PREGNANCY
Avoid medications known to interact adversely with pregnant females or developing fetuses.

SYNONYMS
• Ulcerative stomatitis
• Vincent's stomatitis
• Necrotizing stomatitis

ABBREVIATIONS
• CUPS = chronic ulcerative periodontal stomatitis
• FeLV = feline leukemia virus
• FIV = feline immunodeficiency virus
• LPS = lymphocytic-plasmacytic stomatitis
• T_4 = thyroxine

Suggested Reading

Harvey CE. Veterinary dentistry. Philadelphia: Saunders, 1985.
Lobprise HB, Wiggs RB. The veterinarian's companion for common dental procedures. Lakewood, CO: AAHA Press, 2000.
Manfra Maretta S, Brine E, Smith CW, et al. Idiopathic mandibular and maxillary osteomyelitis and bone sequestra in cocker spaniels. In: Proceedings of the Veterinary Dental Forum, Denver, CO, 1997; sponsored by the American Veterinary Dental College, Academy of Veterinary Dentistry, and the American Veterinary Dental Society.
Smith MM. Oral and salivary gland disorders. In: Ettinger SJ, ed. Textbook of veterinary internal medicine. 5th ed. Philadelphia: Saunders, 2000:1114–1121.
Wiggs RB, Lobprise HB. Veterinary dentistry principles & practice. Philadelphia: Lippincott-Raven, 1997.

Acknowledgment

The author and editors acknowledge the prior contributions of Dr. Jan Bellaus, who authored this topic in the previous edition.
Author R. Michael Peak
Consulting Editor Heidi B. Lobprise

ORBITAL DISEASES (EXOPHTHALMOS, ENOPHTHALMOS, STRABISMUS)

BASICS

DEFINITION
- Abnormal position of the globe
- Exophthalmos—anterior displacement of the globe
- Enophthalmos—posterior displacement of the globe
- Strabismus—deviation of the globe from the correct position of fixation, which the patient cannot correct

PATHOPHYSIOLOGY
- Orbit cannot be examined directly; orbital disease manifested only by signs that alter the position, appearance, or function of the globe and adnexa
- Malpositioned globe—caused by changes in volume (loss or gain) of the orbital contents or abnormal extraocular muscle function
- Exophthalmos—caused by space-occupying lesions posterior to the equator of the globe
- Enophthalmos—caused by loss of orbital volume or space-occupying lesions anterior to the equator of the globe
- Strabismus—usually caused by an imbalance of extraocular muscle tone or lesions that restrict extraocular muscle mobility

SYSTEMS AFFECTED
- Ophthalmic
- Respiratory—because of the close proximity, the nasal cavity and frontal and maxillary sinuses are often involved

SIGNALMENT
- Dogs/Cats
- Orbital abscess or cellulitis and myositis— more common in young adult dogs
- Myositis—predisposed breeds: German shepherds, golden retrievers, Weimaraners
- Orbital neoplasia—more common in middle-aged to old dogs

SIGNS

Exophthalmos
- Secondary signs of space-occupying orbital disease
- Difficulty in retropulsing the globe
- Serous to mucopurulent ocular discharge
- Chemosis
- Eyelid swelling
- Lagophthalmos—inability to close the eyelids over the cornea adequately during blinking
- Exposure keratitis—with or without ulceration
- Pain on opening the mouth
- Third eyelid protrusion is due to extraconal mass or late in progression of intraconal mass.

- Visual impairment caused by optic neuropathy
- Fundic abnormalities, including retinal detachment
- Retinal vascular congestion
- Focal inward deviation of the posterior globe
- Optic disk swelling
- Neurotropic keratitis after damage to the ophthalmic branch of cranial nerve V
- Fever and malaise—with orbital abscess or cellulitis
- IOP—rarely high

Enophthalmos
- Ptosis
- Third eyelid protrusion
- Extraocular muscle atrophy
- Entropion—with severe disease

Strabismus
- Deviation of one or both eyes from the normal position
- May note exophthalmos or enophthalmos

CAUSES

Exophthalmos
- Neoplasm—primary or secondary
- Abscess or cellulitis—bacterial or fungal; fungal more likely in cats; look for foreign bodies
- Zygomatic mucocele—not described in cats
- Myositis—muscles of mastication or extraocular muscles
- Orbital hemorrhage secondary to trauma
- Arteriovenous fistula—rare

Enophthalmos
- Ocular pain
- Microphthalmia
- Phthisis bulbi
- Collapsed globe
- Horner syndrome
- Dehydration
- Loss of orbital fat or muscle
- Conformational enophthalmos in dolichocephalic breeds
- Neoplasia—especially those originating from rostral orbit

Strabimus
- Abnormal innervation of extraocular muscle
- Restriction of extraocular muscle mobility by scar tissue from previous trauma or inflammation
- Destruction of extraocular muscle attachments after proptosis
- Convergent strabismus—congenital; results from abnormal crossing of visual fibers in the CNS (Siamese cats)
- Shar-pei strabismus.

RISK FACTORS
Proptosis—more readily occurs in brachycephalic dogs with shallow orbits

DIAGNOSIS

DIFFERENTIAL DIAGNOSIS

Similar Signs
- Buphthalmic globe—may simulate a space-occupying mass and cause the eye to be displaced anteriorly owing to its size in relationship to the orbital volume; IOP usually high; corneal diameter is greater than normal, corneal edema, mydriatic pupil, ↓ vision (i.e., signs of glaucoma)
- Episcleritis—may cause severe diffuse or focal thickening of the fibrous tunic, often imitating a buphthalmic globe; corneal edema; low IOP; aqueous flare

Causes
- Acute onset of exophthalmos—often inflammatory orbital disease. Pain, especially on opening the mouth, is more likely due to inflammatory orbital disease than orbital neoplasia.
- Mucoceles—more variable in speed of onset and degree of patient discomfort
- Myositis—may be unilateral or bilateral
- Neoplasia—usually slowly progressive, not painful, unilateral exophthalmos

CBC/BIOCHEMISTRY/URINALYSIS
- Usually normal
- Leukogram—may show inflammation with abscess or cellulitis or myositis
- Peripheral eosinophilia—occasionally seen in dogs with masticatory muscle myositis

OTHER LABORATORY TESTS
N/A

IMAGING
- Skull radiographs (especially of the frontal sinuses and nasal cavity), orbital ultrasonography, and CT—are extremely helpful in defining the extent of the lesion
- Thoracic radiographs—may help identify metastatic disease

DIAGNOSTIC PROCEDURES
- Lack of globe retropulsion—confirms a space-occupying mass
- Oral examination, skull radiographs, and fine-needle aspiration of the orbit—may be completed after anesthetizing the patient
- Fine-needle aspiration (18–20-gauge)— submit samples for aerobic, anaerobic, and fungal cultures; gram staining; and cytologic examination
- Cytology—often diagnostic for abscess or cellulitis, zygomatic salivary gland mucocele, and neoplasia
- Biopsy—indicated if needle aspiration is undiagnostic. Biopsy of masseter, temporal, or extraocular muscle if myositis suspected

ORBITAL DISEASES (EXOPHTHALMOS, ENOPHTHALMOS, STRABISMUS)

• Forced duction of the globe (strabismus)—grasp the conjunctiva with a fine pair of forceps following topical anesthesia; differentiates neurologic disease (in which the globe moves freely) from restrictive condition (in which the globe cannot be moved manually)

 TREATMENT

PROPTOSIS
• See Proptosis.

ORBITAL ABSCESS OR CELLULITIS
• Inpatient—intravenous fluids to maintain hydration and replace fluid deficits until patient is able to eat
• Establish ventral orbital drainage while the patient is anesthetized.
• Incise the surgically prepared mucosa approximately 1 cm behind the last molar.
• Push a blunt-tipped forceps (e.g., Kelly or Carmalt) into the orbital space and open; in general, advance the forceps to the level of the box lock, or until movement of the eye occurs with forceps opening.
• Drainage is seen in less than half of patients.
• Take care to minimize retrobulbar trauma and optic nerve damage; use only blunt dissection; never cut or crush tissue.
• Collect samples for bacterial culture and cytologic examination through this port.
• Hot packing—q6h; helps decrease swelling and cleans discharge

ORBITAL NEOPLASMS
• Usually primary and malignant
• Early exenteration or orbital exploratory surgery and debulking of the mass via a lateral approach to the orbit to save the globe are rational therapeutic choices.
• Adjunctive chemotherapy or radiotherapy—depending on neoplasm type and extent of the lesion
• Without adjunct therapy—survival is weeks to months if malignant because the patient is usually examined late in the course of disease
• Consultation with an oncologist is recommended once the diagnosis is made.

ZYGOMATIC MUCOCELE
May resolve with antibiotic and corticosteroid administration; if not, surgical excision of the cyst and associated gland is usually curative.

STRABISMUS
• Neurologic—best treated by identifying the underlying cause and addressing that, if possible

• Restrictive or posttraumatic—may be treated surgically; repositioning or excising the attachments of the extraocular muscles; relieving excessive tension on those muscles; usually a very difficult procedure

 MEDICATIONS

DRUG(S) OF CHOICE
• Exophthalmos (all patients)—lubricate cornea (e.g., artificial tear ointment q6h) to prevent desiccation and ulceration
• Ulceration—topical antibiotic (e.g., bacitracin-neomycin-polymyxin, q8h) and cycloplegic (e.g., 1% atropine q12–24h), to prevent infection and reduce ciliary spasm, respectively

Orbital Abscess or Cellulitis
• Intravenous antibiotics—sodium ampicillin (20 mg/kg q6–8h) or chloramphenicol (25 mg/kg q8h); while awaiting results of bacterial culture and cytologic examination; if owners decline diagnostic testing
• Bacterial orbital infections—may be mixed; *Pasteurella multocida* and *Enterobacteriaceae* common
• Oral antibiotics—after patient begins to eat; based on culture and sensitivity
• Most patients recover within approximately 2 weeks of treatment.
• Itraconazole—2.5 mg/kg q12h; or fluconazole 2.5 mg/kg q12h or 5 mg/kg q24h may be considered for orbital aspergillosis
• Prednisone—1 mg/kg SC or IM q24h, once or twice; minimize optic neuritis and reduce orbital swelling and globe exposure

Acute Myositis
• Difficult prehension—systemic corticosteroids (prednisone, 2 mg/kg SC or IM); then oral corticosteroids for the following 4–6 weeks (prednisone, 2 mg/kg q24h) until the swelling subsides; then taper
• Azathioprine—1–2mg/kg PO q24h for 3–7 days; then q48h and taper; with or without corticosteroids, may be used chronically to manage recurrent disease

CONTRAINDICATIONS
N/A

PRECAUTIONS
• Systemic corticosteroids—use with extreme caution with deep fungal orbital disease
• Azathioprine—may be hepatotoxic and cause myelosuppression
• Follow CBC platelet count and liver enzymes every 1–2 weeks for 8 weeks, then periodically thereafter.

POSSIBLE INTERACTIONS

N/A

ALTERNATIVE DRUG(S)
N/A

 FOLLOW-UP

PATIENT MONITORING
• Inflammatory orbital disease—examine at least weekly until clinical signs abate.
• Advise client to watch for recurrence of signs, especially if an orbital foreign body is likely.
• Treat fungal infections for 60 days after signs cease.

POSSIBLE COMPLICATIONS
• Vision loss
• Loss of the eye
• Permanent malposition of the globe
• Death

 **MISCELLANEOUS**

ASSOCIATED CONDITIONS
N/A

AGE-RELATED FACTORS
N/A

ZOONOTIC POTENTIAL
N/A

PREGNANCY
Avoid systemic corticosteroids, antifungal medications, and azathioprine in pregnant animals.

SEE ALSO
• Proptosis
• Red Eye

ABBREVIATIONS
• CNS = central nervous system
• CT = computed tomography
• IOP = intraocular pressure

Suggested Reading
Lindley DM. Disorders of the orbit. In: Kirk RW, Bonagura JD, eds. Current veterinary therapy XI. Philadelphia: Saunders, 1992:1081–1085.
Speiss BM, Wallin-Hakenson N. Diseases of the canine orbit. In: Gelatt KN, ed. Veterinary Ophthalmology, 3rd ed. Philadelphia: Lippincott Williams & Wilkins, 1999:511–533.
Author Carmen M.H. Colitz
Consulting Editor Paul E. Miller

ORGANOPHOSPHATE AND CARBAMATE TOXICITY

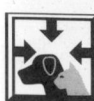 **BASICS**

DEFINITION
• Results from exposure to organophosphorous compounds or carbamates, which are common active ingredients in household and agricultural insecticide products
• Animal products—organophosphate: chlorpyrifos, coumaphos, cythioate, diazinon, famphur, fenthion, phosmet, and tetrachlorvinphos; carbamate: carbaryl and propoxur
• Agricultural, lawn, and garden products—organophosphate: acephate, chlorpyrifos, diazinon, disulfoton, fonofos, malathion, parathion, terbufos, and others; carbamate: carbofuran and methomyl

PATHOPHYSIOLOGY
• Cause nervous system effects by inhibiting cholinesterase, which includes acetylcholinesterase, pseudocholinesterase, and other esterases
• Acetylcholinesterase—normally hydrolyzes the neurotransmitter acetylcholine in nervous tissue, RBCs, and muscle, resulting in termination of nervous transmission
• Pseudocholinesterase—found in plasma, liver, pancreas, and nervous tissue, mainly in cats
• Cholinesterase inhibition—allows acetylcholine accumulation at the postsynaptic receptor; causes stimulation of effector organs; spontaneous reactivation after organophosphorous compound binding is very slow and once aging occurs is virtually nonexistent; reversible after carbamate binding

SYSTEMS AFFECTED
Nervous—result from overriding stimulation of parasympathetic pathways; may also result from sympathetic stimulation; acetylcholine stimulates nicotinic receptors of the somatic nervous system (skeletal muscle), parasympathetic preganglionic nicotinic and postganglionic muscarinic receptors (cardiac muscle, pupil, blood vessels, smooth muscles in lung and gastrointestinal tract, exocrine glands), and sympathetic preganglionic nicotinic receptors (adrenal and indirectly cardiac muscle, pupil, blood vessels, smooth muscles in lung and gastrointestinal tract, exocrine glands).

GENETICS
• Animals with inherently low cholinesterase activity—more susceptible to cholinesterase depression
• Cholinesterase activity—more easily inhibited in cats than in dogs

INCIDENCE/PREVALENCE
Common in small animals

GEOGRAPHIC DISTRIBUTION
• More common in areas of high flea prevalence and intense agricultural activity

SIGNALMENT

Species
Cats and small or exceptionally lean dogs—most susceptible

Breed Predilections
Lean dogs (e.g., sight hounds and racing breeds) and lean longhair cats—more susceptible to cholinesterase inhibition because of lack of fat; many organophosphorous compounds and metabolites are stored in fat and slowly released into circulation.
• Organophosphate-containing dips labeled for dogs only—inappropriately applied to cats

Mean Age and Range
Young animals—more likely intoxicated due to lower detoxification capability

Predominant Sex
Intact males more susceptible to some organophosphates

SIGNS

General Comments
• Parasympathetic stimulation—usually predominates
• Sympathetic stimulation—may result in lack of specific expected signs; may note opposite signs from those expected

Historical Findings
• Medical history—often discloses heavy or repeated applications of flea and tick insecticides; evidence of exposure to an agricultural or home and garden product
• Carbamate insecticides (methomyl and carbofuran)—may cause rapid onset of seizures and respiratory failure; treat aggressively without delay.
• Organophosphate insecticides (cats)—chronic anorexia, muscle weakness, and muscle twitching, with or without episodes of acute toxicosis, which may last for days to weeks

Physical Examination Findings
• Hypersalivation
• Vomiting
• Diarrhea
• Miosis
• Bradycardia
• Depression
• Ataxia
• Muscle tremors
• Seizures
• Hyperthermia

• Dyspnea
• Respiratory failure
• Death
• Patient may not exhibit all signs
• Sympathetic stimulation—signs reversed

CAUSES
• Overuse, misuse, or use of multiple cholinesterase-inhibiting insecticides
• Misuse of organophosphate insecticides in cats
• Intentional dermal application of house or yard insecticides

RISK FACTORS
• Concurrent exposure to multiple organophosphate- and/or carbamate-containing products
• Exposure to floors that are damp with organophosphorous premise products
• Incorrect dilution of insecticides

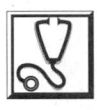 **DIAGNOSIS**

DIFFERENTIAL DIAGNOSIS
• History of exposure, amount of exposure, and clinical signs—should be consistent with toxicosis
• Exposure to other insecticidal products—pyrethrin/pyrethroids (flea and tick); D-limonene (citrus flea and tick); fipronil (flea and tick); imidacloprid (flea)
• Other pesticides—strychnine; fluoroacetate (1080); 4-aminopyridine (avicide); metaldehyde (snail bait); zinc/aluminum phosphide (rodenticide); bromethalin (rodenticide)
• Other toxicants—chocolate; caffeine; cocaine; amphetamine

CBC/BIOCHEMISTRY/URINALYSIS
N/A

OTHER LABORATORY TESTS

Cholinesterase Activity
• Reduced to < 25% of normal in whole blood, retina, or brain—suggests exposure to a cholinesterase-inhibiting compound
• Test results—must be interpreted in context of the amount of exposure and the clinical signs and the time of their onset
• Use laboratories experienced in handling animal samples.
• Chlorpyrifos—experimentally exposed animals may remain clinically normal with no detectable cholinesterase activity.
• Carbamate inhibition—reactivation can occur during sample transport and testing, giving false-negative results.

ORGANOPHOSPHATE AND CARBAMATE TOXICITY

IMAGING
N/A

DIAGNOSTIC PROCEDURES
• Detection of insecticides—tissue (e.g., brain, liver, kidney, and fat); stomach contents; gastrointestinal tract; fur or hair; negative results do not rule out toxicosis.
• May find pieces of chewed containers in the gastrointestinal tract

PATHOLOGIC FINDINGS
• Histopathologic lesions—rare
• Delayed neuropathy—not usually associated with commercially available organophosphorous compounds

 TREATMENT

APPROPRIATE HEALTH CARE
• Outpatient—mild signs from exposure to flea and tick collars and powders; treated by simply removing the collar or brushing excess powder from the coat
• Inpatient—continued salivation, tremors, or dyspnea

NURSING CARE
• Basis—stabilization; decontamination; antidotal treatment with atropine (and pralidoxime chloride for organophosphate toxicosis); supportive care
• Oxygen—if necessary, until respiration returns to normal
• Fluid therapy—may be needed in anorexic cats
• Bathing (dermal exposure)—use hand dishwashing detergent; rinse with copious amounts of water.

ACTIVITY
N/A

DIET
Chronically anorexic cats—maintain nutritional and fluid requirements.

CLIENT EDUCATION
• Stress the importance of following insecticide label directions.
• Caution client that cats with chronic anorexia and weakness may need days to weeks of supportive care for full recovery.

SURGICAL CONSIDERATIONS
N/A

 MEDICATIONS

DRUG(S) OF CHOICE
• Pentobarbital 5–15 mg/kg IV
• Diazepam (0.05–1.0 mg/kg IV) or phenobarbital (3.0–30 mg/kg IV to effect, low dosage in cats)—controls seizures
• Atropine sulfate—0.2 mg/kg one-quarter IV, remaining SC, as needed; administered immediately; repeated only as needed to control life-threatening clinical signs from muscarinic stimulation
• Pralidoxime chloride (Protopam)—10–15 mg/kg IM, SC q8–12h until recovery; discontinue after three doses if no response; reduces muscle fasciculations; most beneficial against organophosphorous insecticides when started within 24 hr of exposure; even several days after dermal exposure may stimulate anorexic cats (with or without tremors) to resume eating; if refrigerated and wrapped in foil, reconstituted bottles may be successfully used for up to 2 weeks
• Ingestion of liquid insecticidal solution—avoid inducing emesis; risk of aspiration because many solutions contain hydrocarbon solvents
• No clinical signs, liquid solvent not ingested, and very recent ingestion—3% hydrogen peroxide (2.2 mL/kg PO to a maximum of 45 mL) after feeding a moist meal
• Evacuation of the stomach for patient with clinical signs—gastric lavage with the patient intubated, under anesthesia, with a large-bore stomach tube; then administration of activated charcoal (2.0 g/kg PO) containing sorbitol as a cathartic in a water slurry
• Diarrhea—do not administer sorbitol-containing products

CONTRAINDICATIONS
Phenothiazine tranquilizers may potentiate organophosphate toxicosis.

PRECAUTIONS
Atropine—avoid overuse; may cause tachycardia, CNS stimulation, seizures, disorientation, drowsiness, and respiratory depression

POSSIBLE INTERACTIONS
N/A

ALTERNATIVE DRUG(S)
N/A

 FOLLOW-UP

PATIENT MONITORING
Monitor heart rate, respiration, and fluid and caloric intake.

PREVENTION/AVOIDANCE
• Closely follow directions on insecticidal labels.
• Avoid use on sick or debilitated animals.
• Avoid simultaneous use of organophosphate and carbamate products.

POSSIBLE COMPLICATIONS
N/A

EXPECTED COURSE AND PROGNOSIS
• Chronic organophosphate insecticide–induced weakness and anorexia (cats)—may last 2–4 weeks; most patients fully recover with aggressive nursing care.
• Acute toxicosis treated promptly—good prognosis

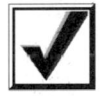 MISCELLANEOUS

ASSOCIATED CONDITIONS
N/A

AGE-RELATED FACTORS
N/A

ZOONOTIC POTENTIAL
N/A

PREGNANCY
N/A

SEE ALSO
Poisoning (Intoxication)

Suggested Reading

Fikes JD. Feline chlorpyrifos toxicosis. In: Kirk RW, Bonagura JD, eds. Current veterinary therapy XI. Philadelphia: Saunders, 1992:188–191.
Fikes JD. Organophosphate and carbamate insecticides. Vet Clin North Am Small Anim Pract 1990;20:353–367.
Authors Steven R. Hansen and Elizabeth A. Curry-Galvin
Consulting Editor Gary D. Osweiler

ORONASAL FISTULA

BASICS

OVERVIEW
- A hole between the oral and nasal cavity
- Communication between the mouth and nasal cavity can occur from pathology of any of the maxillary teeth; defects are vertical.

SIGNALMENT
Dog—dolichocephalic head types are affected most often, especially dachshunds.

SIGNS
- Chronic rhinitis—with or without blood
- Sneezing—also common, especially when the maxillary canines are digitally palpated

CAUSES & RISK FACTORS
- Can be caused by trauma, penetration of a foreign body, bite wounds, traumatic tooth extraction, electrical shock, or oral cancer
- Usually associated with end-stage periodontitis of the maxillary canine tooth leading to lysis of the bone separating the nasal and oral cavities
- Fistula width is related to the size of the dog; fistula depth to the chronicity of the periodontal infection.
- Dogs with uncorrected base-narrow canines and those with prognathic (overbite) mal-occlusions causing the mandibular canines to penetrate the hard palate are predisposed.

DIAGNOSIS

- Maxillary canines are most commonly affected.
- The palatal root of the maxillary fourth premolar is next most common.
- Inserting a periodontal probe into the pocket along the palatine surface of the maxillary canine tooth often causes hemorrhage from the ipsilateral nostril, confirming an oronasal fistula.

DIFFERENTIAL DIAGNOSIS
- Periodontal disease
- Oral cancer
- Trauma
- Foreign body penetration

CBC/BIOCHEMISTRY/URINALYSIS
N/A

IMAGING
- Radiographs rarely diagnose oronasal fistula because the lesions are generally isolated to the medial surface.
- Radiographs may show foreign body entrapment, or lysis consistent with neoplasia.

DIAGNOSTIC PROCEDURES
Periodontal probing—if probing leads to epistaxis, an oronasal fistula exists

TREATMENT

- Repair to prevent foreign material and infection from passing from the mouth into the nose causing rhinitis, sinusitis, and possibly pneumonia.
- Extract the tooth and close the defect; after extraction, the goal of surgical closure is to place an epithelial layer in both the oral and nasal cavities.
- Full-thickness flap—after tooth extraction, a mucoperiosteal pedical flap may be elevated from the dorsal aspect of the fistula, released, advanced to cover the defect, and sutured in place; a successful full-thickness flap requires some attached gingiva above the defect, sutures at the edge of the defect (not over the void), and no tension on the suture line.
- Double reposition flap—used for large fistulas or repair failures where no attached gingiva remains or where periosteal tissue cannot be included; after extraction, the first flap is harvested from the hard palate and inverted so that the oral epithelium is toward the nasal passage; the second flap is muco-buccal and harvested from the alveolar mucosa and underside of the lip rostral to the fistula; it is sutured over the first flap and donor site.
- Guided tissue regeneration of the maxillary canine—may be used for repair of a deep palatal pocket if not yet fistulated; a palatal flap is elevated to approach the infrabony defect; soft tissue and calculus are removed from the defect with a curette.

- Bone grafts such as PerioGlas, Consil (Nutramax Laboratories, Edgewood, MD), synthetic and natural hydroxyapatite, autogenous and heterologous bone, polylactic acid, and plaster of Paris have been used to exclude regrowth of gingival connective tissue and epithelium, promoting regeneration of bone and periodontal ligament.
- Can surgically repair oronasal fistulas located in the central portion of the hard palate with a transposition flap of the hard palate mucoperiosteum from tissue adjacent to the defect

MEDICATIONS

DRUG(S)
N/A

CONTRAINDICATIONS/POSSIBLE INTERACTIONS
N/A

FOLLOW-UP

Normal postoperative monitoring

MISCELLANEOUS

Suggested Reading
Harvey CE, Emily PP. Small animal dentistry. St. Louis: Mosby, 1993.
Wiggs RB, Lobprise HB. Veterinary dentistry: principles and practice. Philadelphia: Lippincott-Raven, 1997.
Author Jan Bellows
Consulting Editor Heidi B. Lobprise

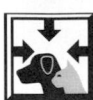

BASICS

OVERVIEW
• A growth and developmental abnormality of cartilage and bone; encompasses many disorders involving bone growth
• Results from delayed endochondral ossification
• Skeletal defects—usually involve the appendicular skeleton; specifically the metaphyseal growth plates
• Achondroplasia—failure of cartilage growth; characterized by a proportionate short-limbed dysplasia; evident soon after birth
• Hypochondrodysplasia—less severe form of achondrodysplasia
• Characteristic breeds—result of selection of certain desirable traits
• Affects musculoskeletal and ophthalmic systems

SIGNALMENT
• Achondroplastic breeds—bulldogs; Boston terriers; pugs; Pekingese; Japanese spaniels; shih tzus
• Hypochondroplastic breeds—dachshunds; basset hounds; beagles; Welsh corgis; dandie Dinmont terriers; Scottish terriers; Skye terriers
• Reported nonselected chondrodysplastic abnormalities—Alaskan malamutes; Samoyeds; Labrador retrievers; English pointers; Norwegian elkhounds; Great Pyrenees; cocker spaniels; Scottish terriers; Scottish deerhounds
• Ocular-skeletal dysplasia—diagnosed in Labrador retrievers and Samoyeds

SIGNS

Historical Findings
• Obvious skeletal deformities
• Retarded growth

Physical Examination Findings
• Usually affects the appendicular skeleton; may affect axial skeleton
• Long bones—appear shorter than normal; often bowed
• Major joints (elbow, stifle, carpus, tarsus)—appear enlarged
• Radius and ulna—often severely affected owing to asynchronous growth
• Lateral bowing of the forelimbs
• Enlarged carpal joints
• Valgus deformity of the paws

• Shortened maxilla—relative mandibular prognathism
• Spinal deviations—due to hemivertebrae
• Retina—dysplasia; partial to complete detachment

CAUSES & RISK FACTORS
• Achondrodysplastic and hypochondrodysplastic breeds—autosomal dominant trait
• Nonselected chondrodysplastic breeds—simple autosomal recessive or polygenic trait
• Littermates often affected

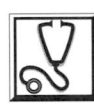

DIAGNOSIS

DIFFERENTIAL DIAGNOSIS
Premature closure of the ulnar or radial physes—history of trauma; no other bones affected; unilateral or bilateral abnormalities

CBC/BIOCHEMISTRY/URINALYSIS
N/A

OTHER LABORATORY TESTS   N/A

IMAGING
• Radiography of affected limbs—irregular flattening of the metaphysis; widening of the physeal line; retained endochondral cores; irregularities in ossification of the affected long bone; degenerative joint disease and joint laxity owing to abnormal stress and weight bearing on the limbs
• Radiography of the spine—hemivertebrae; wedge-shaped vertebrae

DIAGNOSTIC PROCEDURES
Bone biopsy of growth plate—definitive diagnosis

PATHOLOGIC FINDINGS
Histologic findings: disorganization of the proliferative zone, abnormalities within the hypertrophic zone, abnormal formation of the primary and secondary spongiosa

TREATMENT
• Achondrodysplasia—considered a normal abnormality in some (chondrodystrophic) breeds
• Surgery—usually of little benefit for nonselected chondrodysplasia
• Corrective osteotomy to realign limb(s) or joint(s)—may have limited benefit

MEDICATIONS

DRUG(S)
• Analgesics and antiinflammatory agents—palliative use warranted; may try buffered or enteric-coated aspirin (10–25 mg/kg PO q8h–12h), carprofen (2.2 mg/kg PO q12h), etodolac (10–15 mg/kg PO q24h), phenylbutazone (3–7 mg/kg PO q8h, total dose < 800 mg/day), meclofenamic acid (0.5 mg/kg PO q12h), or piroxicam (0.3 mg/kg PO q24h for 3 days; then every other day)
• Chondroprotective agents—polysulfated glycosaminoglycans, glucosamine, and chondroitin sulfate; may have limited benefit in preventing articular cartilage changes

CONTRAINDICATIONS/POSSIBLE INTERACTIONS
N/A

FOLLOW-UP

PREVENTION/AVOIDANCE
• Do not repeat dam–sire breedings that resulted in affected offspring.
• Discourage breeding affected animals.

POSSIBLE COMPLICATIONS
Intra-articular and periarticular joint structures—degenerate owing to abnormal conformation of the appendicular skeleton; leads to altered biomechanics; results in poor quality of life

EXPECTED COURSE AND PROGNOSIS
Depend on severity

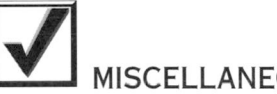

MISCELLANEOUS

SYNONYMS
Dwarfism

Suggested Reading
Sande RD, Bingel SA. Animal models of dwarfism. Vet Clin North Am Small Anim Pract 1982;13:71.
Author Peter D. Schwarz
Consulting Editor Peter K. Shires

OSTEOCHONDROSIS

BASICS

DEFINITION
A pathologic process in growing cartilage, primarily characterized by a disturbance of endochondral ossification that leads to excessive retention of cartilage

PATHOPHYSIOLOGY
• Cells of the immature articular joint cartilage and growth plates do not differentiate normally.
• The process of endochondral ossification is retarded, but the cartilage continues to grow, resulting in abnormally thick regions that are less resistant to mechanical stress.
• Bilateral disease common
• Most commonly affected joints—shoulder (caudocentral humeral head); elbow (medial aspect humeral condyle); stifle (femoral condyle: lateral more often than medial); hock (ridge of the talus: medial more common than lateral)
• Other reported locations—femoral head; dorsal rim of the acetabulum; glenoid cavity (scapula); patella; distal radius; medial malleolus; cranial end plate of the sacrum; vertebral articular facets; cervical vertebrae
Immature Joint Cartilage
• Nutrition maintained by diffusion of nutrients from the synovial fluid
• Thickened cartilage results in impaired metabolism, leading to degeneration and necrosis of the poorly supplied cells
• Fissure within the thickened cartilage—may result from mechanical stress; eventually leads to the formation of a cartilage flap, or OCD; may cause lameness
• Lameness (pain)—becomes evident once synovial fluid establishes contact with subchondral bone; affected by cartilage breakdown products released into the synovial fluid; inflammation
Retention of Cartilage in Growth Plates
• Usually does not lead to necrosis, probably owing to nutrition provided by vessels within the cartilage
• May lead to slippage and asymmetric growth; most marked in the distal ulnar physis

SYSTEMS AFFECTED
Musculoskeletal

GENETICS
• Polygenetic transmission—expression determined by an interaction of genetic and environmental factors
• Heritability index—depends on breed; 0.25–0.45

INCIDENCE/PREVALENCE
Frequent and serious problem in many dog breeds

GEOGRAPHIC DISTRIBUTION
N/A

SIGNALMENT

Species
• Dogs
• Demonstrated clinically—horses; pigs; broiler chickens; turkeys; humans

Breed Predilections
Large and giant breeds—great Danes, Labrador retrievers, Newfoundlands, rottweilers, Bernese mountain dogs, English setters, Old English sheepdogs

Mean Age and Range
• Onset of clinical signs—typically 4–8 months
• Diagnosis—generally 4–18 months
• Symptoms of secondary DJD—any age

Predominant Sex
• Shoulder—males (2:1)
• Elbow, stifle, and hock—none

SIGNS

General Comments
Depend on the affected joint(s) and concurrent DJD

Historical Findings
Lameness—most common; sudden or insidious in onset; one or more limbs; becomes worse after exercise; duration of several weeks to months; slight, moderate, or severe; patient may support little weight on the affected limb.

Physical Examination Findings
• Pain—usually elicited on palpation by flexing, extending, or rotating the involved joint
• Generally a weight-bearing lameness
• Joint effusion with capsular distention—common with OCD of elbow, stifle, and hock
• Muscle atrophy—consistent finding with chronic lameness
• Hock OCD—hyperextension of the tarsocrural joint

CAUSES
• Developmental
• Nutritional

RISK FACTORS
• Diet containing three times the recommended calcium levels
• Rapid growth and weight gain

DIAGNOSIS

DIFFERENTIAL DIAGNOSIS
• Intraarticular (osteochondral) fractures
• Elbow dysplasia
• Panosteitis

CBC/BIOCHEMISTRY/URINALYSIS
N/A

OTHER LABORATORY TESTS
N/A

IMAGING

Radiography
• Standard craniocaudal and mediolateral views—necessary for all involved joints
• Appears as flattening of the subchondral bone or as a subchondral lucency
• Cannot be differentiated from OCD
• Sclerosis of the underlying bone—common in chronic OCD lesions; may see flap if it is calcified
• Calcified bodies within the joint (joint mice)—indicate dislodged cartilage flap
• Contralateral joint—comparison; check for involvement
• Oblique views—may improve visualization, especially for hock, elbow, and shoulder lesions
• Skyline views of the talar ridges of the hock joint—help identify medial and lateral lesions

CT and MRI
• Useful for visualizing extent of subchondral lesions
• Not reliable for detecting a loose cartilage flap

Positive Contrast Arthrography
Useful for differentiating from OCD of the shoulder

DIAGNOSTIC PROCEDURES
• Joint tap and analysis of synovial fluid—confirms involvement; should note straw-colored fluid with normal to decreased viscosity; from cytology, should note

>10,000 nucleated cells/μL (> 90% should be mononuclear cells)
• Arthroscopy—minimally invasive; excellent method for differentiating from OCD and for corrective treatment

PATHOLOGIC FINDINGS
• Articular cartilage—initially may appear yellowish
• Retention of articular cartilage extending into subchondral bone surrounded by increased amount of trabecular bone
• Clefts between the underlying trabecular bone and the degenerated and necrotic deep layer of the overlying thickened (retained) cartilage

TREATMENT

APPROPRIATE HEALTH CARE
Not treatable

NURSING CARE
• Cryotherapy (ice packing) of affected joint—immediately postsurgery; 15–20 min three times a day for 3–5 days
• Range-of-motion exercises—initiated as soon as patient can tolerate

ACTIVITY
• Restricted
• Avoid hard concussive activities (e.g., running on concrete).

DIET
• Weight control—important for decreasing load and, therefore, the stress on the affected joint(s)

CLIENT EDUCATION
• Discuss the heritability of the disease.
• Warn client that DJD may develop.
• Discuss the influence of excessive intake of nutrients that promote rapid growth.

SURGICAL CONSIDERATIONS
• Nonsurgical condition
• May progress to OCD as the patient grows
• Arthrotomy or arthroscopy—indicated for most OCD patients
• Shoulder—indicated for all OCD lesions; exploratory procedure indicated for pain and lameness with radiographic evidence of osteochondrosis
• Elbow—indicated for all OCD lesions; indicated to assess for other conditions (see Elbow Dysplasia)

• Stifle—controversial; patients develop DJD even with procedure; arthroscopy may improve the recovery rate and long-term function
• Hock—remove osteochondral flap; controversial; all patients develop severe DJD even with procedure; attempt to reattach the flap to the underlying subchondral bone, if warranted.

MEDICATIONS

DRUG(S) OF CHOICE
Antiinflammatory drugs (NSAIDs) and analgesics—may be used to symptomatically treat associated DJD; do not promote healing of the cartilage flap (thus surgery is still indicated)

CONTRAINDICATIONS
Avoid corticosteroids owing to potential side effects and articular cartilage damage associated with long-term use.

PRECAUTIONS
NSAIDs—gastrointestinal irritation may preclude their use.

POSSIBLE INTERACTIONS
N/A

ALTERNATIVE DRUG(S)
Chondroprotective drugs (e.g., polysulfated glycosaminoglycans, glucosamine, and chondroitin sulfate)—may help limit cartilage damage and degeneration; may help alleviate pain and inflammation

FOLLOW-UP

PATIENT MONITORING
• Periodic monitoring until patient is skeletally mature—recommended to assess progression to an OCD lesion
• Postsurgery—limit activity for 4–6 weeks; encourage early, active movement of the affected joint(s).
• Yearly examinations—recommended to assess progression of DJD

PREVENTION/AVOIDANCE
• Discourage breeding of patients.
• Do not repeat dam–sire breedings that resulted in affected offspring.
• Restricted weight gain and growth in young dogs—may decrease incidence

POSSIBLE COMPLICATIONS
N/A

EXPECTED COURSE AND PROGNOSIS
• Shoulder—good to excellent prognosis for return to full function; minimal osteoarthritis development
• Elbow, stifle, and hock—fair to guarded prognosis; depends on size of lesion (most important), DJD, and age at diagnosis and treatment; progressive osteoarthritis development, even after surgery

MISCELLANEOUS

ASSOCIATED CONDITIONS
N/A

AGE-RELATED FACTORS
N/A

ZOONOTIC POTENTIAL
N/A

PREGNANCY
N/A

SEE ALSO
Elbow Dysplasia

ABBREVIATIONS
• CT = computed tomography
• DJD = degenerative joint disease
• MRI = magnetic resonance imaging
• NSAID = nonsteroidal antiinflammatory drug
• OCD = osteochondritis dissecans

Suggested Reading
Fox SM, Walker AM. The etiopathogenesis of osteochondrosis. Vet Med 1993;88:116–122.
Olsson SE. Lameness in the dog: a review of lesion causing osteoarthrosis of the shoulder, elbow, hip, stifle and hock joints. Proceedings of the American Animal Hospital Association, 1975;42:363–370.
Olsson SE. Osteochondritis dissecans in dogs: a study of pathogenesis, clinical signs, pathologic changes, natural course and sequelae [Abstract]. J Am Vet Radiol Soc 1973;14:4.
Author Peter D. Schwarz
Consulting Editor Peter K. Shires

OSTEOMYELITIS

BASICS

DEFINITION
An acute or chronic inflammation of bone and the associated soft tissue elements of marrow, endosteum, periosteum and vascular channels that is usually caused by bacteria and rarely by fungi and other microorganisms

PATHOPHYSIOLOGY
• Hematogenously disseminated micro-organisms—may localize in metaphyseal bone of young animals and vertebrae of adults; cause osteomyelitis when tissue defense mechanisms have been compromised • Direct inoculation of bone with pathogenic bacteria—may not initiate infection unless there is concurrent tissue injury, bone necrosis, sequestration, fracture instability, altered tissue defenses, foreign material, or surgical implants • Once bone infection is established, bacteria may persist by adhering to implants and sequestra.
• Biofilm—made up of slime produced by staphylococci and other bacteria together with host-derived proteins, cellular debris, and carbohydrate; enshrouds bacterial colonies; provides protection from antimicrobial drugs and host defenses; induces some bacteria to transform to more virulent strains that are more resistant to antimicrobial drugs • Fracture instability exacerbates infection; resorption of bone owing to infection and instability causes widening of the fracture gap and implant loosening, contributing to persistence of infection.

SYSTEMS AFFECTED
Musculoskeletal

GENETICS
Breeds with heritable immunodeficiency or hematogenous diseases

INCIDENCE/PREVALENCE
• Prevalence after open reduction and internal fixation of closed fractures not uncommon (probably similar incidence as diskospondylitis) • Prevalence after trauma and open fracture—unknown; relatively common • Hematogenous disease in young dogs—uncommon • Diskospondylitis in adult dogs and cats and fungal disease—not uncommon

GEOGRAPHIC DISTRIBUTION
• Actinomycosis—grass awns usually cause soft tissue infections, not osteomyelitis; with osteomyelitis, likely a soil contaminant: California, Florida, UK, and Australia
• Blastomycosis—central and eastern regions of the U.S: Great Lakes region and the Mississippi and Ohio River valleys
• Coccidioidomycosis—southwestern U.S., Mexico, and Central and South America

• Histoplasmosis—Ohio, Missouri, and Mississippi River valleys and tributaries

SIGNALMENT

Species
Dogs and cats

Breed Predilections
Breeds with immunodeficiency and hematogenous diseases

Mean Age and Range
Hematogenous metaphyseal infection—young dogs

Predominant Sex
Male dogs—for post-traumatic infection; blastomycosis

SIGNS

General Comments
• Acute postoperative wound infections after orthopedic surgery—may be indistinguishable from acute condition; may progress to chronic disease • Most patients have chronic disease at time of examination and diagnosis.

Historical Findings
• Episodes of lameness • Draining tracts
• Persistent ulcers • Previous trauma
• Fracture or surgery—post-traumatic disease
• Affected vertebrae or intervertebral disks (dogs)—may note hind limb weakness and difficulty in rising • Travel to regions endemic for mycotic infections—fungal infection

Physical Examination Findings
• Acute hematogenous disease (dogs)—sudden onset of systemic illness; pyrexia; lethargy; limb pain; local signs of acute inflammation
• Chronic condition—usually associated with chronic draining tracts, nonhealing ulcers, pain, secondary muscle atrophy, and joint stiffness • Unhealed fractures with concurrent infection—may note instability, crepitus, and limb deformity • Fungal infections—may see limb swelling, lameness, and intermittently draining tracts • Bone infections of the spine—may cause pain and neurologic deficits (e.g., paresis and paralysis)

CAUSES
• Open fracture • Traumatic injury • Open reduction and internal fixation of closed fracture • Elective orthopedic surgery
• Prosthetic joint implant • Gunshot wound
• Penetrating foreign body • Bite and claw wounds • Extension to bone of soft tissue infection—periodontitis; rhinitis; otitis media; paronychia • Hematogenous infection
• Staphylococci—cause approximately 50% of bone infections; often monomicrobial infections • Polymicrobial infection—common; may contain mixtures of aerobic gram-negative bacteria; anaerobic cultures should be submitted with potential isolates including: *Actinomyces, Clostridium, Peptostreptococcus, Bacteroides,* and *Fusobacterium*

• Fungal infection—*Coccidioides immitis; Blastomyces dermatitidis; Histoplasma capsulatum; Cryptococcus neoformans; Aspergillus*

RISK FACTORS
• Open fracture and bone contamination
• Soft tissue trauma • Bite and claw wounds
• Migrating foreign body • Orthopedic surgery • Prosthetic orthopedic implant
• Cortical bone allograft • Immunodeficiency

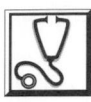

DIAGNOSIS

DIFFERENTIAL DIAGNOSIS
• Neoplasia • Bone cysts • Delayed fracture union as a result of instability • Hypertrophic osteodystrophy • Secondary hypertrophic osteopathy • Medullary bone infarction

CBC/BIOCHEMISTRY/URINALYSIS
Hemogram—inflammatory left shift usually evident only with acute disease

OTHER LABORATORY TESTS
Serology—confirms some fungal infections

IMAGING

Radiology
• Acute disease—bone architecture normal; see only soft tissue swelling • Chronic disease—sequestra (avascular segment of cortical bone); reactive periosteal new bone; involucrum formation (reactive tissue surrounding sequestrum); bone resorption
• Bone resorption—widening of fracture gaps; cortical thinning; generalized osteopenia; implant loosening • Contrast films—may help delineate sinuses and radiolucent foreign bodies; inject water-soluble contrast media through a Foley catheter into the sinuses.

Other
• Ultrasonography—localize large accumulations of fluid; guide fluid sampling by needle aspiration • Scintigraphy—^{99m}Tc-labeled methylene diphosphonate; highly sensitive for detecting increased vascularity of bone; not specific for osteomyelitis

DIAGNOSTIC PROCEDURES
• Fluid aspirates or Jamshidi-needle tissue biopsies—collected from focus of infection by sterile techniques; cultured aerobically and anaerobically; identify microorganisms; determine in vitro antimicrobial drug susceptibility • Open surgical biopsy—indicated when needle aspirates are negative or when débridement is necessary for treatment; culture samples of necrotic tissue, sequestra, implants, and foreign material; histopathologic examination for suspected fungal infection and to rule-out neoplasia • Fluid and tissue samples for anaerobic culture—immediately place into appropriate medium (e.g., reduced Cary-Blair anaerobic transport medium).

• Purulent fluid from draining tracts—culture may be misleading; tracts are colonized by skin organisms and gram-negative bacteria; cultures are often polymicrobic. • Blood cultures—may be positive with acute disease or chronic disease with septicemia.

PATHOLOGIC FINDINGS
• Bone sequestration—virtually diagnostic
• Inflammation and necrosis of bone and the adjacent tissues—pyogenic bacteria
• Cytologic or histopathologic examination of smears or sections—usually leads to diagnosis of fungal infection; special fungal stains (methenamine silver; PAS) for microorganism identification

 TREATMENT

APPROPRIATE HEALTH CARE
• Inpatient—surgical débridement, drainage, culturing, irrigation, and wound management until infection begins to resolve; infected fractures (surgical stabilization)
• Outpatient—long-term oral antimicrobial drug therapy

NURSING CARE
• Depends on severity, location, and degree of associated soft tissue injury • Take care to prevent nosocomial infections by pathogen contamination to other patients in the hospital.

ACTIVITY
Restricted—with any danger of a pathologic fracture developing; with an unhealed fracture

DIET
No restriction

CLIENT EDUCATION
• Warn the client about the expense of treatment, the likelihood of recurrence, the problems with sequestration, the need for repeated surgical intervention, and the long duration of therapy. • Discuss the prognosis.

SURGICAL CONSIDERATIONS
• Chronic disease—surgical débridement; removal of sequestrum; establishment of drainage • Infected stable fracture—leave pre-existing internal fixation implants in place during healing. • Infected unstable fracture—remove implants; stabilize with external or internal skeletal fixation. • Bone deficits—graft with autologous cancellous bone either acutely or after infection has abated and granulation tissue has formed in the wound.
• Large segmental deficits in long bones—bridge by Ilizarov technique or other bone segment transport. • Localized chronic infection—may be amenable to resolution by amputation (tail, digit, limb) or en bloc

resection (sternum, thoracic wall, mandible, maxilla) and primary wound closure
• Remove all implants after the fracture has healed; bacteria harbored by implant biofilm may lead to recurrence or be a pathogenic factor for fracture-associated sarcoma.

 MEDICATIONS

DRUG(S) OF CHOICE
• Antimicrobial drugs—depend on in vitro determination of susceptibility of microorganisms; also consider possible toxicity, frequency and route of administration, and expense; most penetrate normal and infected bone well; must be given for 4–8 weeks
• Staphylococci (dogs)—usually *S. intermedius,* which are resistant to penicillin because of β-lactamase production; highly susceptible to cloxacillin, amoxicillin-clavulanate, cefazolin, and clindamycin
• Anaerobes—more are sensitive to metronidazole and clindamycin.
• Aminoglycosides and quinolones (ciprofloxacin and enrofloxacin)   effective against gram-negative aerobic bacteria
• Quinolones—may give orally; not nephrotoxic; to protect against resistance, use only for infections caused by gram-negative organisms or *Pseudomonas* that are resistant to other oral antimicrobial drugs.
• Chronic disease—continuous local delivery of antimicrobial drugs by antibiotic-impregnated methylmethacrylate beads
• Itraconazole—5–10 mg/kg PO q24h; given continuously, may control disseminated aspergillosis for up to 2 years

CONTRAINDICATIONS
Quinolones—do not give to young patients; experimentally induce articular cartilage lesions in immature dogs

PRECAUTIONS
Aminoglycosides—may cause nephrotoxicity, especially in dehydrated patients and with electrolyte losses or pre-existing renal disease

POSSIBLE INTERACTIONS
N/A

ALTERNATIVE DRUG(S)
Identify other antimicrobial drugs by repeating cultures and susceptibility determination if the infection becomes unresponsive to the initial agent.

 FOLLOW-UP

PATIENT MONITORING
• Radiography—every 4–6 weeks; determine bone healing

• Reculture bone—suspected persistent infection

PREVENTION/AVOIDANCE
N/A

POSSIBLE COMPLICATIONS
• Recurrence
• Chronic disease—may result in limb deformity, impaired function, fracture disease, or neurologic deficits
• Malignant neoplasia—rare sequela to chronic infection of fractures repaired by internal fixation

EXPECTED COURSE AND PROGNOSIS
• Acute infection and chronic bacterial diskospondylitis—may be cured by 4–8 weeks of antimicrobial drug therapy if there is limited bone necrosis and no fracture
• Chronic disease—resolution with antimicrobial drug therapy alone unlikely; provide appropriate surgical treatment.
• Recurrence of chronic infection—evident by return of lameness or draining tracts; may occur weeks, months, or years after the last treatment; may require repeated sequestrectomy, débridement, microbiologic culturing, drainage, fracture stabilization, bone grafting, or implant removal

 MISCELLANEOUS

ASSOCIATED CONDITIONS N/A

AGE-RELATED FACTORS N/A

ZOONOTIC POTENTIAL N/A

PREGNANCY N/A

SYNONYMS
Bone infection

SEE ALSO
• Diskospondylitis • Fungal Infections

Suggested Reading
Doherty MA, Smith MM. Contamination and infection of fractures resulting from gunshot trauma in dogs: 20 cases (1987–1992). J Am Vet Med Assoc 1995;206(2):203–205.
Johnson KA. Osteomyelitis. In: Birchard SJ, Sherding RG, eds. Saunders manual of small animal practice. Philadelphia: Saunders, 1994:1091–1095.
Johnson KA. Osteomyelitis in dogs and cats. J Am Vet Med Assoc 1994;205:1882–1887.
Rochat MC. Preventing and treating osteomyelitis. Vet Med, 2001;96(a).
Authors Kenneth A. Johnson and Mark M. Smith
Consulting Editor Peter K. Shires

OSTEOSARCOMA

 BASICS

DEFINITION
• Most common primary bone tumor in dogs
• Typically affects the appendicular skeleton of large- to giant-breed dogs
• Malignant, with microscopic lung metastases in > 90% of dogs at the time of diagnosis
• Cats—less common; less aggressive biologic behavior than in dogs

Pathophysiology
Chronic low-grade bone trauma in large dogs—hypothesized as a cause

Systems Affected
• Musculoskeletal—appendicular skeleton (metaphyseal region of the distal radius, proximal humerus, distal femur, and proximal tibia) most commonly affected in dogs; may also occur in the axial skeleton
• Respiratory—most common metastatic site is the lungs
• Soft tissue sites such as spleen and mammary gland may also be primary sites.

Genetics
• Does not appear to be heritable; although breed predilections do occur
• Breed size and rate of maturity may be more important than breed or family line.

Incidence/Prevalence
• Dogs—accounts for up to 85% of all primary bone tumors
• Cats—most common primary bone tumor; accounts for < 7% of all reported malignancies

Geographic Distribution
N/A

SIGNALMENT

Species
Dogs and cats

Breed Predilections
• Dogs—large to giant breeds
• Cats—domestic shorthair

Mean Age and Range
• Dogs—bimodal peak at 2 years and 7 years; reported as young as 6 months
• Cats—mean age, 8.5 years; range, 4–18 years

Predominant Sex
• Dogs—males predominate (1.2:1) in most reports
• Cats—both males and females

SIGNS

Historical Findings
• Vary
• Lesions may be subtle—key features: localized swelling, a palpable mass, or pain
• Swelling, lameness, and pain common
• Other complaints—inappetence and lethargy

Physical Examination Findings
• Depend on site
• A firm, painful swelling of the affected site common
• Degree of lameness—varies from mild to non–weight bearing
• Pathologic fracture rare

CAUSES
Unknown in both species

RISK FACTORS
• Dogs—large to giant breeds; metallic implants at fracture repair sites; history of exposure to ionizing radiation
• Cats—unknown

 DIAGNOSIS

DIFFERENTIAL DIAGNOSIS
• Other primary or metastatic bone tumor
• Fungal or bacterial osteomyelitis

CBC/BIOCHEMISTRY/URINALYSIS
Alkaline phosphatase elevations are associated with a poorer prognosis.

OTHER LABORATORY TESTS
N/A

IMAGING

Radiographs—Primary Site
• Take at least two views.
• Typical findings—bony lysis; proliferation in the metaphyseal region of long bones
• Marked soft tissue swelling common
• Does not usually involve both sides of a joint cavity
• CT scan is more sensitive at detecting early bone lysis.

Radiographs—Thoracic
• Always take three views, although metastatic disease is seen in < 10% of patients at the time of examination.
• Metastatic lesions—typically discrete, round, soft-tissue density nodules

Nuclear Bone Scans
• May be useful for identifying bony or soft tissue metastatic disease earlier than via radiography
• Will not distinguish between sites of previous trauma or inflammation and metastatic neoplasia

DIAGNOSTIC PROCEDURES
• Cytologic examination of bone aspirate—may yield diagnosis
• Bone biopsy—gold standard for diagnosis

PATHOLOGIC FINDINGS
• Gross—mild to severe destruction of cortical bone with new bone proliferation
• Histologic—malignant population of mesenchymal cells that are plump and polygonal to spindyloid in shape; osteoid production is diagnostic.
• Parosteal (juxtacortical)—soft tissue variant; may be less aggressive than other forms

 TREATMENT

APPROPRIATE HEALTH CARE
• Diagnostic evaluation—outpatient
• Surgery and the first chemotherapy treatment—inpatient
• Subsequent chemotherapy—outpatient

NURSING CARE
Manage pain as needed (see Alternative Drugs).

ACTIVITY
Restricted after surgery until adequate healing has occurred

DIET
N/A

CLIENT EDUCATION
• Warn client that the long-term prognosis is poor; achievable goals should be to relieve discomfort and prolong a good quality of life.
• Prepare clients for possible chemotherapy-induced side effects.

SURGICAL CONSIDERATIONS

Dogs

Appendicular Sites
• Amputation of affected limb—forequarter or hip disarticulation
• Limb-salvage therapy—appropriate for distal radial lesions only; available at a limited number of referral hospitals
• Adjuvant chemotherapy—recommended after either surgical procedure
Axial Sites
• Aggressive surgical excision
• Chemotherapy—recommended after surgery
Soft Tissue Sites
• Aggressive surgical resection; chemotherapy recommended after surgery
Metastasectomy
• Pulmonary metastasectomy—has been described

Cats

Appendicular Sites
• Amputation of affected limb
• Adjuvant therapy may not be necessary.
Axial Sites
• Attempt aggressive surgical excision—depending on site of lesion
• Local recurrence—main reason for treatment failure

Both Species

Inoperable neoplasms—radiotherapy offers marked pain relief.

MEDICATIONS

DRUG(S) OF CHOICE

• Definitive treatment
• Postsurgical chemotherapy with a platinum-based protocol—current standard of care
• Cisplatin—70 mg/m^2 IV every 3 weeks for a minimum of 4 doses; must be given with saline-induced diuresis to prevent nephrotoxicity; begin diuresis (18.3 L/kg/hr) for 4 hr; administer chemotherapy over 20 min; then continue diuresis for another 2 hr; will cause vomiting within 2 hr of administration (give butorphanol at 0.4 mg/kg IM 20 min before cisplatin administration to minimize)
• Carboplatin—300 mg/m^2 IV every 3 weeks for a minimum of 4 doses; more expensive and less toxic than cisplatin; use in cats
• Doxorubicin—30 mg/m^2 IV every 2 weeks for 5 doses

CONTRAINDICATIONS

• Pre-existing renal dysfunction—do not treat with platinum-based drugs.
• Cisplatin—do not give to cats.

PRECAUTIONS

• Avoid aluminum or metal-containing catheters and needle hubs because aluminum interferes with the activity of platinum-containing drugs.
• Seek advice before initiating therapy if you are unfamiliar with cytotoxic drugs.

POSSIBLE INTERACTIONS

N/A

ALTERNATIVE DRUG(S)

Palliative treatment—pain management must be addressed for patients whose owners decline definitive treatment; in dogs, manage with aspirin (20 mg/kg PO q8h), piroxicam (0.3 mg/kg PO q24h with food), acetaminophen (15 mg/kg PO q8h) +/− codeine (1–2 mg/kg PO q8h), or consider fentanyl patches.

FOLLOW-UP

PATIENT MONITORING

• Monitor for myelosuppression 7–10 days after chemotherapy.
• Take thoracic radiographs every 2–3 months after surgery.
• Take radiographs of graft site every 2–3 months after surgery because local recurrence is possible after limb salvage.

PREVENTION/AVOIDANCE

N/A

POSSIBLE COMPLICATIONS

• Metastasis
• Hypertrophic osteopathy

EXPECTED COURSE AND PROGNOSIS

Dogs

• Median survival without treatment, with amputation alone, or with palliative radiotherapy alone—approximately 4 months
• Median survival with surgery and chemotherapy—10 months
• Mandibular osteosarcoma—less aggressive than other sites; 1-year survival with surgery alone—71% reported

Cats

• Appendicular—median survival with surgery: > 2 years
• Axial—median survival with surgery: 5.5 months

MISCELLANEOUS

ASSOCIATED CONDITIONS

N/A

AGE-RELATED FACTORS

N/A

ZOONOTIC POTENTIAL

None

PREGNANCY

Do not breed animals undergoing chemotherapy.

SYNONYM

Osteogenic sarcoma

SEE ALSO

• Chondrosarcoma, Bone
• Fibrosarcoma, Bone
• Hemangiosarcoma, Bone

Suggested Reading

Botettp WV, Patnaik AK, Schrader SC, et al. Osteosarcoma in cats: 22 cases (1974–1984). J Am Vet Med Assoc 1987;190:91–93.

Dernell WS, Straw RC, Withrow SJ. Tumors of the skeletal system. In: Withrow SJ, MacEwen EG, eds. Small animal clinical oncology. Philadelphia: Saunders, 2001:378–417.

Morrison WB. Cancer drug pharmacology and clinical experience. In: Morrison WB, ed. Cancer in dogs and cats: medical and surgical management. Baltimore: Williams & Wilkins, 1998:359–385.

Waters DJ, Cooley DM. Skeletal neoplasms. In: Morrison WB, ed. Cancer in dogs and cats: medical and surgical management. Baltimore: Williams & Wilkins, 1998:639–654.

Author Ruthanne Chun
Consulting Editor Wallace B. Morrison

OTITIS EXTERNA AND MEDIA

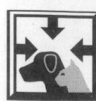

BASICS

DEFINITION
• Otis externa—inflammation of the external ear canal
• Otitis media—inflammation of the middle ear
• The terms are not diagnoses but descriptions of clinical signs.

PATHOPHYSIOLOGY
• Otis externa—chronic inflammation results in alterations in the normal environment of the canal; the external ear canal is lined with epithelium containing modified apocrine (cerumen) glands; the glands enlarge and produce excessive wax; the epidermis and dermis thicken and become fibrotic; thickened canal folds effectively reduce canal width; calcification of auricular cartilage is the end-stage result.
• Otitis media—often an extension of otitis externa through a ruptured tympanum; frequently occurs without rupture of tympanum; can occur from polyps or neoplasia within the middle ear

SYSTEMS AFFECTED
• Skin/Exocrine
• Nervous—inflammation of the vestibulo-cochlear nerve

GENETICS
N/A

INCIDENCE/PREVALENCE
N/A

GEOGRAPHIC DISTRIBUTION
N/A

SIGNALMENT

Species
Dogs and cats

Breed Predilections
• Pendulous-eared dogs, especially spaniels and retrievers
• Dogs with hirsute external canals—terriers and poodles
• Stenosis of the external ear canal is common in shar peis.

Mean Age And Range
N/A

Predominant Sex
None

SIGNS

General Comments
• Otitis externa—often a secondary symptom of an underlying disease
• Infection—purulent and malodorous exudate
• Inflammation—exudation, pain, pruritus, and erythema

• Chronic otitis externa (dogs)—results in tympanic membrane rupture (71%) and otitis media (82%)

Historical Findings
• Pain
• Head shaking
• Scratching at the pinnae
• Malodorous ears

Physical Examination Findings
• Redness and swelling of the external canal, leading to stenosis
• Scaling and exudation—may result in malodor and canal obstruction
• Cats—hold the pinna down or tilt the head
• Vestibular signs (with head tilt, nystagmus, anorexia, ataxia, and infrequent vomiting) indicate development of otitis media/interna.

CAUSES

Primary Causes
• Parasites (otitis externa)—*Otodectes cynotis, Demodex* spp., *Sarcoptes* and *Notoedres,* and *Otobius megnini*
• Hypersensitivities—atopy, food allergy, contact allergy, and systemic or local drug reaction
• Foreign bodies—plant awns
• Obstructions—neoplasia, polyps, cerumen gland hyperplasia, and accumulation of hair; may also be a secondary event
• Keratinization disorders and increased cerumen production—functional obstruction of the ear canal
• Autoimmune diseases—frequently affect the pinnae; sometimes affect the external ear canal

Perpetuating Factors
• Secondary bacterial infections—common; *Staphylococcus intermedius* most often cultured from the horizontal canal in otitis externa; *Pseudomonas* spp., *Proteus* spp., *Corynebacterium* spp., and *E. coli* frequently reported; *Pseudomonas* spp. most often cultured in otitis media
• Infections—often mixed with, or entirely the result of, *Malassezia pachydermatis;* other yeast (*Candida*) or fungal species rare
• Progressive changes—canal hypertrophy, cerumen gland hyperplasia and adenitis, fibrosis, and cartilage calcification; cause recalcitrant otitis externa; prevent return to a normal ear canal even with proper treatment
• Otitis media—can produce symptoms on its own; can act as a reservoir for organisms, causing recurrent condition

RISK FACTORS
• Abnormal or breed-related conformation of the external canal (e.g., stenosis, hirsutism, and pendulous pinnae) restricts proper air flow into the canal.

• Excessive moisture (e.g., from swimming or frequent cleanings with improper solutions) can lead to infection; overzealous client compliance with recommendations for ear cleanings common
• Topical drug reaction and irritation and trauma from abrasive cleaning techniques
• Underlying systemic diseases produce abnormalities in the environment and ear canal immune response.

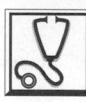

DIAGNOSIS

DIFFERENTIAL DIAGNOSIS
N/A

CBC/BIOCHEMISTRY/URINALYSIS
May indicate a primary underlying disease

OTHER LABORATORY TESTS
Allergy workup as indicated

IMAGING
Bullae radiographs—otitis media

DIAGNOSTIC PROCEDURES
• Skin scrapings from the pinna—parasites
• Skin biopsy—autoimmune disease, neoplasia, or cerumen gland hyperplasia
• Culture of exudate—rarely assists in devising a treatment plan; reserve for resistant infection
• Microscopic examination of aural exudate—single most important diagnostic tool after complete examination of the ear canal
• Appearance of the exudate—yeast infections commonly produce a yellow-tan thick exudate; bacterial infections commonly produce a brownish black thin exudate; however, appearance does not allow an accurate diagnosis of the type of infection; microscopic examination necessary
• Infections within the canal can change with prolonged or recurrent therapy; repeat examination of aural exudate is required in chronic cases.

Microscopic Examination
• Preparations—make from both canals (the contents of the canals may not be the same); spread samples thinly on a glass microscope slide; examine both unstained and modified Wright-stained samples.
• Mites—presumptive diagnosis
• Type(s) of bacteria or yeast—assist in the choice of therapy
• Findings (types of organisms; WBCs)—note in the record; rank the number of organisms and cell types on a scale of 0–4 to allow treatment monitoring
• WBCs within the exudate—active infection; systemic antibiotic therapy may be warranted.

PATHOLOGIC FINDINGS
N/A

TREATMENT

APPROPRIATE HEALTH CARE
Outpatient, unless severe vestibular signs are noted

NURSING CARE
N/A

ACTIVITY
No restrictions

DIET
No restrictions unless a food allergy is suspected

CLIENT EDUCATION
Teach clients, by demonstration, the proper method for cleaning ears.

SURGICAL CONSIDERATIONS
• Indicated when the canal is severely stenotic or obstructed or when neoplasia or a polyp is diagnosed
• Severe, unresponsive otitis media may require a bullae osteotomy.

MEDICATIONS

DRUG(S) OF CHOICE

Systemic
• Antibiotics—useful in severe cases of bacterial otitis externa; mandatory when the tympanum has ruptured; trimethoprim-potentiated sulfonamides (dosage varies by preparation), cephalexin (25 mg/kg q8–12h), enrofloxacin (2.5 mg/kg q12h), or clindamycin (10 mg/kg q12h)
• Antifungals—use with overwhelming yeast or fungal infection; ketoconazole (5–10 mg/kg q12h)
• Corticosteroids—reduce swelling and pain; reduce wax production; antiinflammatory dosages of prednisone (0.25–0.5 mg/kg q12h); use sparingly and for short durations only
• Selamectin—(Revolution®) applied topically every 2 weeks for 3 applications—FDA-labeled to treat *Otodectes cynotis*.

Topical
• Topical therapy paramount for resolution and control of otitis externa
• First, completely clean the external ear canal of debris; complete flushing under general anesthesia reserved for uncooperative patients or severe cases, including otitis media
• Second, thoroughly clean the ear daily during initial therapy; then every 3–7 days once signs resolve.

• Finally, apply appropriate topical medications frequently and in sufficient quantity to completely treat the entire canal.
• Not recommended—combination ointments (e.g., Otomax, Panalog, Liquachlor), which often accumulate and perpetuate the condition
• Recommended—antibacterial (e.g., gentocin) or antiyeast drops (miconazole), with or without corticosteroid; commercial ear cleansers with cerumenolytics, antiseptics, and astringents; Derma Pet® cleanser for routine cleaning or when the competence of the tympanic membrane is in question; chlorhexidine-containing solutions (e.g., Chlorhexiderm Flush®, Hexadene Flush®) for more severe cases when the tympanic membrane is intact (controversial)
• Cerumenolytics—dioctyl sodium sulfosuccinate or carbamide peroxide; emulsify waxes, facilitating removal
• Antiseptics—acetic acid or chlorhexidine gluconate; reduce or eliminate infectious organisms
• Astringents—isopropyl alcohol, boric acid, or salicylic acid; reduce moisture
• Antibiotics, antifungals, and/or parasiticides—use only when presence of organism(s) has been confirmed
• Ivermectin 0.01% (Acarexx) otic suspension—FDA-labeled to treat *Otodectes cynotis*
• Resistance to medications—perform a culture and sensitivity of the aural exudate; recently, suspensions of silver sulfadiazine and of enrofloxacin have been shown to be effective
• Generally, ingredients should be limited to those needed to treat a specific infection (i.e., antibiotics only for a bacterial infection).

CONTRAINDICATIONS
• Ruptured tympanum—use caution with topical cleansers and medications other than sterile saline or dilute acetic acid; potential for ototoxicity is a concern; controversial

PRECAUTIONS
• Use extreme caution when cleaning the external ear canals of all animals with severe and chronic otitis externa, because the tympanum can easily be ruptured.
• Postflushing vestibular complications are common in cats, although usually temporary; warn clients of possible complications and residual effects.

POSSIBLE INTERACTIONS
Several topical medications infrequently induce contact irritation or allergic response; reevaluate all worsening cases.

ALTERNATIVE DRUG(S)
N/A

FOLLOW-UP

PATIENT MONITORING
Repeat exudate examinations can assist in monitoring infection.

PREVENTION/AVOIDANCE
• Routine ear cleaning by the client
• Control of underlying diseases

POSSIBLE COMPLICATIONS
Uncontrolled otitis externa can lead to otitis media, deafness, vestibular disease, cellulitis, facial nerve paralysis, progression to otitis interna, and rarely meningoencephalitis.

EXPECTED COURSE AND PROGNOSIS
• Otitis externa—with proper therapy, most cases resolve in 3–4 weeks; failure to correct underlying primary cause results in recurrence.
• Perpetuating factors (e.g., stenosis of the ear canal and calcification of the auricular cartilage) will not resolve and may result in recurrence.
• Otitis media—may take 6+ weeks of systemic antibiotics until all signs have resolved and the tympanic membrane has healed

MISCELLANEOUS

ASSOCIATED CONDITIONS
N/A

AGE-RELATED FACTORS
N/A

ZOONOTIC POTENTIAL
Potenially *Sarcoptes* or *Notoedres* mite infestation and fungal infection

PREGNANCY
Do not use systemic glucocorticoids during pregnancy, if possible.

SYNONYMS
N/A

SEE ALSO
Causes

ABBREVIATION
WBC = white blood cell

Suggested Reading
Griffin CE. Otitis externa and otitis media. In: Griffin CE, Griffin CE, Kwochka KW, MacDonald JM, eds. Current veterinary dermatology: the science and art of therapy. St. Louis: 1993.
Author Alexander H. Werner
Consulting Editor Karen Helton Rhodes

OTITIS MEDIA AND INTERNA

BASICS

DEFINITION
Inflammation of the middle (otitis media) and inner (otitis interna) ears most commonly caused by bacterial infection

PATHOPHYSIOLOGY
• Most often arises from extension of infection of the external ear through the tympanic membrane; may extend from the oral and nasopharyngeal cavities via the eustachian tube • Interna—may also result from hematogenous spread of a systemic infection

SYSTEMS AFFECTED
• Nervous—vestibulocochlear receptors in the inner ear and the facial nerve and sympathetic chain in the middle ear (peripheral) with possible extension of infection intracranially (central) • Ophthalmic—cornea and conjunctiva; from exposure and/or lack of tear production after nerve damage
• Gastrointestinal—taste; from damage to the parasympathetic branch of the facial nerve (chordae tympani) supplying the ipsilateral rostral two thirds of the tongue

GENETICS
N/A

INCIDENCE/PREVALENCE
N/A

GEOGRAPHIC DISTRIBUTION
N/A

SIGNALMENT

Species
Dogs and cats

Breed Predilections
• Cocker spaniels and other long-eared breeds
• Poodles with chronic otitis or pharyngitis from dental disease

Mean Age and Range
Any age

Predominant Sex
N/A

SIGNS

General Comments
Depend on severity and extent of the infection; range from none to those related to bulla discomfort and nervous system involvement

Historical Findings
• Pain when opening the mouth; reluctance to chew; shaking the head; pawing at the affected ear • Head tilt • Patient may lean, veer, or roll toward the side affected with peripheral vestibulitis. • Vestibular deficits—transient and episodic • Bilateral involvement—wide head excursions, truncal ataxia, and deafness • Vomiting and nausea—may occur during the acute phase

• Facial nerve damage—saliva and food dropping from the corner of the mouth; an inability to blink; ocular discharge
• Anisocoria and/or protrusion of the third eyelid (Horner's syndrome)—may be noted

Physical Examination Findings
• Evidence of aural erythema, discharge, and thick and stenotic canals supports otitis externa. • Gray, dull, opaque, and bulging tympanic membrane on otoscopic examination indicates a middle ear exudate.
• Dental tartar, gingivitis, tonsillitis, or pharyngitis—may be associated
• Ipsilateral mandibular lymphadenopathy—may occur with severe infections • Pain upon opening the mouth or bulla palpation may be detected • Corneal ulcer—may be caused by inability to blink or a dry eye

Neurologic Examination Findings
• Damage to the associated neurologic structures depends on the severity and location. • Vestibular portion of cranial nerve VIII—when vestibular portion is affected, there is always an ipsilateral head tilt
• Bilateral damage of cranial nerve VIII—rare; patient is reluctant to move and may stay in a crouched posture with wide head excursions; physiologic nystagmus poor to absent • Nystagmus—resting or positional and rotatory or horizontal may be seen
• Vestibular strabismus—ipsilateral ventral deviation of eyeball with neck extension may be noted • Ipsilateral leaning, veering, falling, or rolling may occur. • Facial nerve damage—ipsilateral paresis/paralysis of the ear, eyelids, lips, and nares; may be reduced tear production (indicated by the Schirmer tear test); with chronic facial nerve paralysis, contracture of the affected side of the face caused by fibrosis of the denervated muscles; deficits can be bilateral.
• Affected sympathetic chain—Horner's syndrome; always miosis of the affected pupil; may note protrusion of the third eyelid, ptosis, and enophthalmos

CAUSES
• Bacteria—primary agents • Yeast (*Malassezia* spp., *Candida* spp.) and *Aspergillus*—agents to consider • Mites—predispose patient to secondary bacterial infections • Unilateral disease—foreign bodies, trauma, polyps, and tumors (e.g., fibromas, squamous cell carcinoma, ceruminous gland carcinoma, and primary bone tumors)

RISK FACTORS
• Nasopharyngeal polyps and inner, middle, or outer ear neoplasia—may predispose patient to bacterial infection
• Vigorous ear flush • Ear cleaning solutions (e.g., chlorhexidine)—may be irritating to the middle and inner ear; avoid if the tympanum is ruptured. • Inhalant anesthesia and traveling by airplane—change middle ear pressures

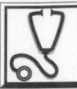

DIAGNOSIS

DIFFERENTIAL DIAGNOSIS
• Signs associated with congenital vestibular anomalies are present from birth.
• Hypothyroidism—may cause a polyneuropathy with a predilection for cranial nerves VII and VIII; abnormal thyroid profile (T_4, free T_4, TSH level) supports the diagnosis • Central vestibular diseases—differentiated by occurrence of lethargy, somnolence, stupor, and other brain stem signs • Neoplasia and nasopharyngeal polyps—common causes of refractory and relapsing otitis media and interna; diagnosed by imaging of the head • Thiamine deficiency (cats)—bilateral central vestibular signs; history of an all-fish diet or persistent anorexia helps the diagnosis • Metronidazole toxicity—bilateral cerebellar involvement (vestibular portion) signs after high dosage or prolonged use • Trauma—history and physical evidence of injury • Idiopathic vestibular disease (old dogs and young to middle-aged cats), idiopathic facial paralysis, and idiopathic Horner's syndrome—diagnoses made by exclusion • *Cryptococcus*—has been reported in association with peripheral vestibular disease in cats

CBC/BIOCHEMISTRY/URINALYSIS
• Leukocytosis with a left shift—may be noted • Globulins—may be high if infection is chronic • Urinalysis—usually normal; pyuria and bacteruria may be seen if the bacterial infection is hematogenous.

OTHER LABORATORY TESTS
• Blood and/or urine cultures—may be positive with a hematogenous source of infection • Low T_4, free T_4 with a high TSH level with hypothyroidism

IMAGING
• Video otoscopy—provides a detailed examination of the external ear canal and tympanic membrane; it also facilitates determining the integrity of the tympanic membrane, obtaining diagnostic samples for cytology and culture/sensitivity, and performing therapeutic lavages of the external ear canal and middle ear cavity • Bullae radiographs—tympanic bullae may appear cloudy if exudate is present; may see thickening of the bullae and petrous temporal bone with chronic disease; may see lysis of the bone with severe cases of osteomyelitis; may be normal; not a sensitive test • CT and MRI—detailed evidence of fluid and soft tissue density within the middle ear and the extent of involvement of the adjacent structures; CT better at revealing associated bony changes; MRI better for evaluating surrounding soft tissue structures including brain stem and cerebellum

DIAGNOSTIC PROCEDURES

• Myringotomy—insert a spinal needle (20 gauge; 2.5–3.5 in.) through the otoscope and tympanic membrane to aspirate middle ear fluid for cytologic examination and culture and sensitivity. • BAER—test the functional integrity of the peripheral and central auditory pathways; detect hearing loss • CSF analysis—if neutrophilic pleocytosis and increased protein with intracranial extension of the infection are noted, perform culture and sensitivity

PATHOLOGIC FINDINGS

Purulent exudate within the middle ear cavity surrounded by a thickened bullae and microscopic evidence of degenerative neutrophils with intracellular bacteria

TREATMENT

APPROPRIATE HEALTH CARE

• Inpatient—severe debilitating infection; neurologic signs • Discharge stable patients, pending further diagnostics and surgery, if indicated.

NURSING CARE

• Fluid therapy—if unable to eat or drink owing to vomiting and disorientation • Concurrent otitis externa—culture and clean the ear; use warm normal saline if the tympanum is ruptured; if a cleaning solution is used, follow with a thorough flush with normal saline; dry the ear canal with a cotton swab and low vacuum suction; astringents (e.g., Otic Domeboro or boric acid) can be effective

ACTIVITY

Restrict with substantial vestibular signs to avoid injury.

DIET

• Vomiting from vestibulitis—withhold food and water for 12–24 hr • Severe disorientation—hand feed and water small amounts frequently; elevate head to avoid aspiration pneumonia

CLIENT EDUCATION

• Inform client that most bacterial infections resolve with an early aggressive course of broad-spectrum antibiotics and do not recur. • Warn client that relapsing signs may occur and may require surgical drainage if bony structure changes and/or middle ear effusion are evident on imaging studies.

SURGICAL CONSIDERATIONS

• Reserve surgery for relapsing or nonresponsive patients. • Do not rely on severity of neurologic signs as an indication for surgical intervention; reserve surgery for patients with evidence of middle ear exudate, osteomyelitis refractory to medical management, and nasopharyngeal polyps or neoplasia. • Bullae osteotomy—allows drainage of the middle ear cavity • Ear ablation through the horizontal ear canal—indicated when otitis media is associated with recurrent otitis externa or neoplasia • Cytologic examination and culture and sensitivity of middle ear effusion and histopathologic evaluation of samples of abnormal tissue—perform at the time of surgery

MEDICATIONS

DRUG(S) OF CHOICE

• Topical water-based or ophthalmic antibiotic solutions—chloramphenicol or a triple antibiotic preparation; or ofloxacin (Floxin) otic solution bid—dogs and cats • Antibiotics—long-term (6–8 weeks); broad-spectrum systemic agents; select on basis of culture and sensitivity, if available • Amoxicillin/clavulanic acid (Clavamox)—12.5–22 mg/kg bid PO is a good first choice antibiotic • Fluoroquinolone or third generation cephalosporin antibiotics are good second choice alternatives, if culture and sensitivity unavailable and Clavamox ineffective; enrofloxacin (Baytril)—5 mg/kg q24h or Cefaclor (ceclor)—22 mg/kg bid to tid; metronidazole (Flagyl)—15–25 mg/kg bid for 2 weeks, if anaerobes are suspected.

CONTRAINDICATIONS

• Ruptured tympanum or associated neurologic deficits—avoid oil-based or irritating external ear preparations (e.g., chlorhexidine) and aminoglycosides, which are toxic to inner ear structures • Otitis media or interna—topical and systemic corticosteroids contraindicated; may exacerbate the signs associated with infection

PRECAUTIONS

Avoid rigorously flushing the external ear; may result in or exacerbate signs of otitis media or interna

POSSIBLE INTERACTIONS
N/A

ALTERNATIVE DRUG(S)
N/A

FOLLOW-UP

PATIENT MONITORING

Evaluate for resolution of signs after 10–14 days or sooner if the patient is deteriorating.

PREVENTION/AVOIDANCE

• Routine ear cleaning and dental prophyl-axis—may reduce chances of infection

POSSIBLE COMPLICATIONS

• Signs associated with vestibular and facial nerve damage or Horner's syndrome—may remain • Severe infections—may spread to the brain stem • Osteomyelitis of the petrous temporal bone and middle ear cavity effusion—common sequela to severe, chronic infections • Bulla osteotomy—postoperative complications include Horner's syndrome, facial paralysis, and onset or exacerbation of vestibular dysfunction • Cats—consider avoiding bilateral bullae osteotomies in patients with bilateral effusions; may be an increased incidence of death after surgery

EXPECTED COURSE AND PROGNOSIS

• Otitis media and interna—usually responsive to medical management • When medical management is ineffective, a surgical evaluation for lateral ear resection should be explored. • Vestibular signs—improvement in 2–6 weeks; more rapid in small dogs and in cats

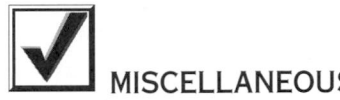

MISCELLANEOUS

ASSOCIATED CONDITIONS
N/A

AGE-RELATED FACTORS
Ear mites more common in kittens and puppies

ZOONOTIC POTENTIAL
N/A

PREGNANCY
N/A

SYNONYMS
Middle and inner ear infections

SEE ALSO

• Facial Nerve Paresis/Paralysis • Head Tilt (Vestibular Disease) • Horner's Syndrome • Otitis Externa and Media

ABBREVIATIONS

• BAER = brainstem auditory-evoked response • CSF = cerebrospinal fluid • CT = computed tomography • MRI = magnetic resonance imaging • TSH = thyroid-stimulating hormone

Suggested Reading

Angus JC, Campbell KL. Uses and indica-tions for video-otoscopy in small animal practice. Vet Clin North Am Small Anim Pract 2001;31(4):809–828.

Bruyette DS, Lorenz MD. Otitis externa and media: diagnostic and medical aspects. Semin Vet Med Surg Small Anim 1993;8:3–9.

Garosi LS, Dennis R, Penderis J, Lamb CR, Targett MP, Cappello R, Delauche AJ. Re-sults of magnetic resonance imaging in dogs with vestibular disorders: 85 cases (1996–1999). J Am Vet Med Assoc 2001; 218(3):385–391

Murphy KM. A review of techniques for the investigation of otitis externa and otitis media. Clin Tech Small Anim Pract 2001; 16:236–241.

Author Richard J. Joseph

Consulting Editor Joane M. Parent

OVARIAN REMNANT SYNDROME

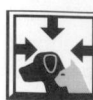

BASICS

OVERVIEW
• Ovarian remnant syndrome is the presence of behavioral and/or physical signs of estrus in a female dog or cat having previously undergone ovariohysterectomy (OHE). • Caused by to the presence of functional residual ovarian tissue • Ovarian remnant syndrome is reported to be responsible for 17% of all post-OHE complications.

SIGNALMENT
• Female dogs and cats; more common in cats • No breed predisposition or geographic distribution • Signs of estrus usually occur months to years after OHE, but can begin within days after surgery.

SIGNS

Bitches
• Attraction of male dogs • Swelling of the vulva • Mucoid to sanguineous vaginal discharge • Passive interaction with male dogs • Flagging • May allow copulation • Signs of proestrus last an average of 9 days, signs of estrus last an average of 9 days; average interval between signs of proestrus and estrus is 7 months.

Queens
• Vocalization • Lordosis • Restlessness • Head rubbing • Rolling • Tail deviation and treading the hind limbs • May allow copulation • Demonstrate typical behavioral signs of estrus in a cyclical (seasonally polyestrous) fashion • Estrus lasts 2–19 days, followed by postestrus (or interestrus), which lasts for 8–10 days.

CAUSES & RISK FACTORS
• Failure to remove both ovaries completely • No correlation with age at OHE, difficulty of surgery, obesity of patient, or experience of surgeon • Presence of anatomically abnormal ovarian tissue (fragmentation into the broad ligament) • Supernumerary ovary (rare) • Experimentally, functionality returns to ovarian tissue removed from its vascular supply and replaced into or onto the lateral abdominal wall.

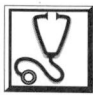

DIAGNOSIS

DIFFERENTIAL DIAGNOSIS
• Inflammation or infection of the genitourinary tract • Vaginal hemorrhage due to foreign body • Trauma • Uterine stump pyometra • Neoplasia • Vascular anomalies of the genitourinary tract • Coagulopathy • Exogenous estrogen administration • Endogenous extraovarian source of estrogen: adrenal pathology (rare)

CBC/BIOCHEMISTRY/URINALYSIS
• Usually normal • Anemia if vaginal hemorrhage is profound; uncommon unless concurrent ovarian neoplasia, follicular cysts, coagulopathy, or other systemic disease

OTHER LABORATORY TESTS
• Observation of behavioral and physical signs of estrus together with vaginal cytology and/or measurement of serum progesterone or estradiol concentrations confirming the presence of functional ovarian tissue • Vaginal cytology: vaginal mucosal cornification is a bioassay for elevated plasma estradiol concentrations (see Breeding, Timing). • Vaginal cytology (bitch): epithelial cell cornification is generally >90% during estrus (superficial and anuclear cells). • Vaginal cytology (queen): epithelial cell cornification ranges from 10%–40%; clearing (absence of debris and clumping of cells) occurs in 90% of smears during estrus. • Serum progesterone (bitch): serum progesterone concentrations >2 ng/ml (measured 1–3 weeks after behavioral estrus) is consistent with functional luteal tissue. GnRH (50 μg IM), hCG (400 IU IV), or hCG (1000 IU [1/2 IV, 1/2 IM]) can be used to induce ovulation or luteinization for diagnostic purposes; serum progesterone concentration is measured 2–3 weeks later. • Serum progesterone (queen): ovulation or luteinization is stimulated during behavioral estrus, and serum progesterone concentration is measured 2–3 weeks later; poststimulation serum progesterone concentrations >2 ng/mL are consistent with functional luteal tissue. GnRH (25 μg IM) can be used to induce ovulation or luteinization for diagnostic purposes; serum progesterone concentration is measured 2–3 weeks later. • Serum estradiol: peak levels triggering behavioral estrus range from 20 to >70 pg/mL; serum estradiol concentrations are less contributory to the diagnosis of ovarian remnant syndrome than is vaginal cytology.

IMAGING

Ultrasonography
• Can be used to support a diagnosis of ovarian remnant syndrome that is based on cytology and hormonal profiles; imaging should begin in a sagittal plane slightly caudomedial to the kidneys (where remnant ovarian tissue is expected). • Remnant ovarian tissue may be visible only during the follicular phase (anechoic and cystic) or the luteal phase (hypoechoic relative to renal tissue). • Ectopic ovarian tissue can be difficult to locate and image using ultrasonography. • Evaluate the adrenal glands for size and shape.

DIAGNOSTIC PROCEDURES
• Exploratory laparotomy—removal of residual ovarian tissue confirms and resolves the problem. • Identification of residual ovarian tissue is facilitated by the presence of corpora lutea or follicles; schedule procedure during times of elevated progesterone or during behavioral estrus. • Histopathology—submit visible functional ovarian tissue; if no visible ovarian tissue is identified, submit all scar tissue at the ovarian pedicles.

TREATMENT
Surgical removal of residual ovarian tissue

MEDICATIONS

DRUG(S)
• Progestational or androgenic compounds to suppress follicular ovarian activity—not recommended because of undesirable side effects (mammary neoplasia, diabetes, undesirable behavior) • Immunocontraception will offer a viable alternative to laparotomy when perfected and commercially available in the United States.

FOLLOW-UP

POSSIBLE COMPLICATIONS
Removal of functional luteal tissue may induce signs of pseudopregnancy in dogs postoperatively (see False Pregnancy).

EXPECTED COURSE AND PROGNOSIS
Successful removal of remnant ovarian tissue should result in cessation of clinical signs of estrus.

MISCELLANEOUS

SEE ALSO
• Breeding, Timing • False Pregnancy

ABBREVIATIONS
• FSH = follicle-stimulating hormone • GnRH = gonadotropin-releasing hormone • hCG = human chorionic gonadotropin • OHE = ovariohysterectomy

Suggested Reading
Johnston SD, Root-Kustritz MV, Olson PN. Disorders of the canine ovary. In: Canine and feline theriogenology. Philadelphia: Saunders, 2001:193–205.
Johnston SD, Root-Kustritz MV, Olson PN. Disorders of the feline ovaries. In: Canine and feline theriogenology. Philadelphia: Saunders, 2001:453–462.
Miller DM: Ovarian remnant syndrome in dogs and cats: 46 cases (1988–1992). J Vet Diagn Invest 1995;7:572–574.

Author Autumn P. Davidson
Consulting Editor Sara K. Lyle

BASICS

OVERVIEW
• Epithelial (carcinoma), germ cell (dysgerminoma and teratoma), and sex-cord stromal (granulosa cell tumor, Sertoli-Leydig cell tumor, thecoma, and luteoma) tumors
• Dogs—rare (0.5%–1.2% of tumors); 40% carcinomas, 10% germ cell, and 50% sex-cord
• Cats—extremely rare (0.7%–3.6% of tumors); 15% germ cell and 85% sex-cord
• Metastasis common
• Some tumors produce hormones.

SIGNALMENT
• Dogs and cats
• Middle-aged to old animals
• Teratoma develops in young patients.

SIGNS
• Tumors that produce steroid hormones—anestrus; persistent estrus; pyometra; gynecomastia; bilaterally symmetrical alopecia; pancytopenia; masculinization
• Ascites or pleural effusion—occasionally
• Other signs associated with mass effects of the tumor

CAUSES & RISK FACTORS
Intact sexual status

DIAGNOSIS

DIFFERENTIAL DIAGNOSIS
• Other causes of abdominal effusion
• Other midabdominal mass

CBC/BIOCHEMISTRY/URINALYSIS
No consistent abnormalities

OTHER LABORATORY TESTS
N/A

IMAGING
• Abdominal radiography—may reveal unilateral or bilateral midabdominal mass at the caudal pole of the kidney or effusion
• Abdominal ultrasound—confirm abdominal radiographic findings
• Thoracic radiography—may reveal metastasis

DIAGNOSTIC PROCEDURES
• Cytologic evaluation of pleural or abdominal fluid—may be diagnostic for malignant effusion
• Histopathologic examination—necessary for definitive diagnosis

TREATMENT
• Ovariohysterectomy—treatment of choice for a solitary mass
• Peritoneal transplantation during surgical removal is possible.

MEDICATIONS

DRUG(S)
• Chemotherapy—little information for dogs and cats
• Cyclophosphamide, chlorambucil, lomustine, and bleomycin—successful treatment in one patient (dog)
• Cisplatin—successful treatment in three dogs

CONTRAINDICATIONS/POSSIBLE INTERACTIONS
Cisplatin—do not use in cats; do not use in dogs with renal disease

FOLLOW-UP
• Abdominal and thoracic radiography—every 3 months; monitor for recurrence and metastasis
• Ovariohysterectomy—prevention
• Prognosis—guarded
• Chemotherapy—has potential to lengthen survival

MISCELLANEOUS

ASSOCIATED CONDITIONS
• Pyometra
• Ovarian cysts
• Cystic endometrial hyperplasia

Suggested Reading
Morrison WB. Cancer of the reproductive tract. In: Morrison WB, ed. Cancer in dogs and cats: medical and surgical management. Jackson, Wyoming: Teton NewMedia, 2002:555–564.
Patnaik AK, Greenlee PG. Canine ovarian neoplasms: a clinicopathologic study of 71 cases including histology of 12 granulosa cell tumors. Vet Pathol 1987;24:509–514.
Author Terrance A. Hamilton
Consulting Editor Wallace B. Morrison

PAIN (ACUTE, CHRONIC, AND POSTOPERATIVE)

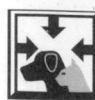 **BASICS**

DEFINITION
• Pain is an unpleasant sensory or emotional experience associated with actual or potential tissue damage, or described in terms of such damage.
• The inability to communicate in no way negates the possibility that an animal is experiencing pain and is in need of appropriate pain-relieving treatment.

PATHOPHYSIOLOGY
• Application of a noxious stimulus activates specialized nerve endings called nociceptors; nociceptors transduce noxious chemical, mechanical, or thermal stimuli into electrochemical potentials that are transmitted via sensory nerves, from the affected tissue to the spinal cord.
• In the dorsal horn of the spinal cord, the incoming first-order peripheral nerve synapses with ascending spinal neurons, which terminate in the brain stem. Incoming noxious information can be modulated at the level of the dorsal horn by other incoming information, descending inhibitory nerve impulses, or pharmacologic inhibition by several classes of drugs. The ascending neurons synapse in the brain stem to form ascending tracts that end in the cortex, where perception of the sensation of pain occurs. Neuroendocrine and physiologic responses (e.g., tachycardia, elevated cortisol) to noxious stimuli may originate from the level of the brain stem in response to ascending noxious information.

SYSTEMS AFFECTED
• Pain may originate from any tissue, including from within the nervous system itself. In humans, pain may be experienced in the absence of any observable injury and may be associated with fear, anxiety, or depression.

• The physiologic response to pain can include decreased immune function, increased catabolism, and elevated neuroendocrine markers of the stress response. Pain can result in a loss of function of affected tissues.

GENETICS
The influence of genetics on pain perception is poorly understood. However, there is evidence that age, sex, breeding strain, and species can alter responses to noxious stimuli. Recently, genes have been described that modify individual mouse behavioral responses to noxious stimuli.

INCIDENCE/PREVALENCE
Evolutionarily, aversion to noxious stimuli was protective to organisms, keeping them away from harm. In domestic species, this aversion is thought to be associated with the perception of pain. Similarities in anatomy and responses to noxious stimuli suggest that humans and nonhuman mammals may experience pain in similar ways. Less complex animals (e.g., fish, amphibians, insects) exhibit aversion to noxious stimuli, but it is unclear whether they experience the sensation of pain the way humans do.

GEOGRAPHIC DISTRIBUTION
N/A

SIGNALMENT
N/A

SIGNS
• Behavioral signs of pain and distress vary considerably among individuals.
• Experience, environment, age, species, and other factors can modify the intensity of the reaction to noxious stimuli.
• Most obvious clinical signs of distress in the dog and cat—vocalization; agitation; abnormal posture or gait; thrashing; hyperesthesia or hyperalgesia; and allodynia
• More subtle signs that are shared by many conditions include trembling; depression; reduced appetite; stupor; biting.

• Tachypnea, tachycardia, mydriasis, and hypertension—associated with the stress response; may accompany pain but are nonspecific signs that may be seen with many conditions
• Clinical signs associated with chronically painful conditions may be very subtle or difficult to evaluate since homeostatic mechanisms tend to help the animal compensate. Chronically painful conditions are often associated with decreased activity, lameness, or depression.

CAUSES
Pain can be caused by tissue disruption associated with trauma or surgery, but it also is caused by chronic degenerative changes such as osteoarthritis. Pain that outlives the initial tissue damage is pathologic and may indicate altered nervous system processing. In humans, just the thought of potential tissue damage may cause feelings of pain. Also, emotional states can trigger unpleasant or painful feelings. The contribution of emotion and expectation to veterinary patient pain is unknown.

RISK FACTORS
• All animals that experience surgical or traumatic tissue damage should be evaluated for the presence of pain. Pain intensity may not always correlate with the degree of tissue damage. However, more invasive soft tissue and orthopedic procedures are likely associated with a greater intensity of pain.
• Animals that exhibit nonspecific behavioral signs associated with pain should be evaluated for chronic or degenerative changes.
• Specific risk factors associated with the development of different pain syndromes have not been described well in veterinary patients.

PAIN (ACUTE, CHRONIC, AND POSTOPERATIVE)

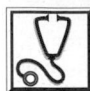

DIAGNOSIS

DIFFERENTIAL DIAGNOSIS

• Most human patients can indicate their personal feeling of pain, and their reports often become part of the medical record. Veterinary patients cannot indicate their personal feelings of pain; therefore, the veterinarian must use his/her diagnostic skills to gauge the intensity of pain and the need for therapy. Identifying pain in veterinary patients is a diagnosis, and the medical record should reflect the veterinarian's clinical diagnostic and treatment plan.

• Acute pain is almost always accompanied by tissue damage or disease, and diagnosis and treatment of the primary disorder should be done before or concomitantly with treatment of pain. The presence or absence of pain is sometimes used as a way of monitoring and diagnosing some conditions, and treatment should be in accordance with good medical practice. Pain should be differentiated from distress associated with other factors, such as restraint, restrictive bandaging, and separation from owners. Drugs used to treat pain, particularly opioids and dissociative anesthetics, may cause dysphoria, which often resembles signs of pain and distress. Tachycardia and other physiologic signs are also associated with shock, stress, or excessive sympathetic stimulation.

CBC/BIOCHEMISTRY/URINALYSIS

• There are few predictable changes in common laboratory tests that indicate pain.
• Cortisol increases associated with acute pain may appear as a stress leukogram.
• Hyperglycemia may also be observed in some patients.
• Normal laboratory tests should not be interpreted as lack of pain.

OTHER LABORATORY TESTS

• Serum cortisol—often increased in experimental studies of pain; however, use of this test is not common because of poor specificity and sensitivity for pain in the clinical setting
• Plasma norepinephrine and epinephrine concentrations—may also be increased with acute pain; these tests are expensive, difficult, and have poor sensitivity and specificity for pain.

IMAGING

Imaging of the nervous system with MRI, functional MRI, PET, and SPECT to detect pain is being investigated in humans and laboratory animals. The clinical application of these tests is questionable in veterinary patients at this time.

DIAGNOSTIC PROCEDURES

• Recognition of pain in animals is subjective. Many scoring systems have been reported, but clinical utility is better with some systems than with others.
• A routine for the evaluation process helps. The authors begin evaluation of pain with the signalment, history, and physical examination. Next, the animal's behavior is observed from a distance, and then behavior is noted during human interaction. Finally, gentle palpation of the body region of interest is performed, if necessary, to determine the animal response.
• When analgesics are administered, the process should be repeated periodically to assess effectiveness. Do not assume the administration of an analgesic will result in acceptable relief of pain.
• Complete abolishment of pain may not be possible or desirable if analgesic administration results in excessive adverse effects. Therapy should aim to make the pain tolerable.

PATHOLOGIC FINDINGS

Pain is not commonly associated with characteristic pathologic findings. Pain can be secondary to many diseases and pathologic conditions.

TREATMENT

APPROPRIATE HEALTH CARE

• Analgesic and anesthetic drug administration is common. Drug selection depends on species, pain intensity, and underlying cause.
• Treat the underlying cause at the same time if possible.
• If the patient's quality of life is not acceptable, euthanasia may be the most humane option.

NURSING CARE

• General good nursing practices
• Nonpharmacologic treatments, including bandaging and hydrotherapy, may be appropriate.

ACTIVITY

Cage rest, limited activity, or physical therapy may be useful for some types of conditions.

DIET

• Dietary changes to help treat the underlying condition (e.g., weight reduction for hip dysplasia) may be beneficial.
• No diet for the treatment of pain per se exists, although many supplements and nutraceuticals have been marketed.
• Evaluation of nutraceutical safety and efficacy is the responsibility of the veterinarian and owner since these compounds do not undergo FDA-Center for Veterinary Medicine review.

PAIN (ACUTE, CHRONIC, AND POSTOPERATIVE)

CLIENT EDUCATION
• Client communication is important for the successful treatment of pain.
• When pain medication is dispensed, educate the client on what to look for with effective treatment, as well as adverse effects.
• Inform the client that analgesic effectiveness varies and several drugs may need to be tried before an effective treatment is found.
• Clients should also participate in evaluation of pain, especially chronic pain. The use of simplified rating scales, such as the Oxford Pain Chart (see Appendix VIII [Figure VIII-A] can help document treatment effectiveness.)

SURGICAL CONSIDERATIONS
• Surgical treatment of the underlying condition causing pain may be the best treatment.
• Surgical disruption of nerves (neurectomy) to halt pain transmission—not always associated with positive results; may result in worsening of the painful condition

MEDICATIONS
DRUG(S) OF CHOICE
(SEE APPENDIX VIII)
• Opioids, alone or in combination with other classes of drugs, such as sedative/tranquilizers or NSAIDs, are widely used for the management of acute postoperative pain. Full μ-opioid receptor agonists, such as morphine, hydromorphone, and fentanyl, are usually effective for moderate to severe pain. Agonist-antagonist drugs, such as buprenorphine and butorphanol, are usually reserved for mild to moderate pain. Opioids generally have poor oral bioavailability, and oral doses should be adjusted accordingly. Full μ-opioid receptor agonists can be used safely in cats. However, doses are usually reduced relative to dog doses. Should dysphoria develop, tranquilization with an α2-agonist or acepromazine may be effective.
• NSAIDs are used most commonly for the chronic treatment of painful conditions in dogs. In general, newer NSAIDs have improved safety when administered chronically, but gastrointestinal and renal side effects are still possible. The safety and effectiveness of most NSAIDs have not been well demonstrated in cats, and their use in cats is limited. Carprofen and etodolac appear to be well tolerated in dogs, but some animals may experience gastrointestinal side effects. Appropriate owner education and follow-up are important.
• Treatment of neuropathic pain (pain originating from within the nervous system) is a subcategory of pathologic pain. Neuropathic pain may originate from brain or spinal masses, injury (such as with intervertebral disc disease), inflammation, or the repetitive stimulation of the pain transmission system by a chronic injury outside the nervous system. Classic signs that accompany neuropathic pain are allodynia and hyperalgesia. Neuropathic pain also does not always respond well to traditional analgesics, such as NSAIDs and opioids, although these drugs are usually tried initially (except for NSAIDs when neurosurgical intervention is imminent). Tricyclic antidepressants, anticonvulsants, NMDA receptor antagonists, and other alternative (complementary) therapies may be effective. Most of these treatments require extra- or off-label use of human medications, and the veterinarian assumes much of the liability for their use. Owner education and appropriate patient follow-up are important for successful therapy.

CONTRAINDICATIONS
• Opioids may be associated with severe respiratory depression in human patients, but most dogs and cats have only minimal respiratory depression. In patients with severe respiratory compromise or intracranial hypertension, opioids may be contra-indicated. Most μ-opioid receptor agonists may also alter gastrointestinal and urinary tract motility, resulting in constipation, urinary retention, and vomiting.
• NSAIDs can cause gastrointestinal ulceration, hepatopathies, and impaired renal function. Preexisting gastrointestinal, hepatic, or renal disease may be a contraindication to their use. Concomitant glucocorticoid therapy, severe stress, or anorexia may predispose many animals to side effects. NSAIDs that significantly inhibit COX-1 may also alter platelet function and may result in hemorrhage or prolonged bleeding times. Acetaminophen or acetaminophen-containing analgesics should not be used in cats.

PRECAUTIONS
Carefully monitor patients for adverse effects and clinical effectiveness following administration of analgesic drugs. Drugs should not be used, or be used on the advice of a specialist, when otherwise contraindicated.

POSSIBLE INTERACTIONS

Opioids can reduce the anesthetic requirements for most species, especially when combined with α_2-agonists or acepromazine as a premedication before anesthesia. Some opioids, such as meperidine, may also interact with MAO-B inhibitors, such as selegiline (L-deprenyl). Concurrent glucocorticoid therapy may enhance NSAID toxicity. Other drugs that predispose animals to gastrointestinal or renal impairment, such as aminoglycoside antimicrobials, should be used with caution when NSAIDs are also being administered.

ALTERNATIVE DRUG(S)

Nontraditional medical treatments are common, but should be evaluated for safety and effectiveness before recommendation and use.

 FOLLOW-UP

PATIENT MONITORING

• Because of concern for the humane care of animals, frequent evaluation of analgesic drug effectiveness should be performed.
• Patients receiving chronic analgesic medication, especially NSAIDs, should be evaluated periodically to monitor gastrointestinal, liver, and renal function.

PREVENTION/AVOIDANCE

Although some degree of pain is usually an unavoidable consequence of surgery or trauma, when possible, the preemptive administration of analgesic drugs may provide better control of the pain and reduce the potential for central nervous system wind-up. Use of proper anesthetic techniques incorporating analgesic premedications is an effective way of practicing preemptive analgesia.

POSSIBLE COMPLICATIONS

The complications associated with proper analgesic therapy are usually minimal. However, careful follow-up and monitoring are important, especially when treating animals in the immediate postoperative period and following trauma.

EXPECTED COURSE AND PROGNOSIS

Acute pain associated with surgery or trauma usually resolves with tissue healing. Opioids may be most effective for the 12–24 hr following surgery, whereas NSAIDs may be better after that period. Some NSAIDs are effective analgesics when given immediately after surgery. When pain signs persist beyond the normal course of a few days to weeks, suspect persistent disease, injury, or central nervous system changes and consult an anesthesiologist or a specialist trained in pain management for suggestions about appropriate therapy.

 MISCELLANEOUS

ASSOCIATED CONDITIONS

N/A

AGE-RELATED FACTORS

N/A

ZOONOTIC POTENTIAL

N/A

PREGNANCY

The effects of many of the analgesic drugs approved for use in dogs and cats on the fetus are not widely reported. Opioids may cause fetal respiratory depression following delivery. NSAIDs may alter maternal or fetal prostaglandin production, resulting in pregnancy complications.

ABBREVIATIONS

COX = cyclooxygenase
MAO = monoamine oxidase
MRI = magnetic resonance imaging
NMDA = N-methyl-D-aspartate
NSAIDs = nonsteroidal antiinflammatory drugs
PET = positron emission tomography
SPECT = single-photon emission computed tomography

Suggested Reading

Carroll GL. Small animal pain management. Lakewood, CO: AAHA Press, 1998.
Mathews KA, ed. Management of pain. Vet Clin North Am Small Anim Pract 2000;
Tranquilli WJ, Grimm KA, Lamont LA, eds. Pain management for the small animal practitioner. Jackson Hole, WY: Teton New Media, 2000.

Authors Kurt A. Grimm, Leigh A. Lamont, and William J. Tranquilli
Consulting Editor Joane Parent

PANCREATITIS

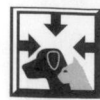 BASICS

DEFINITION
• Inflammation of the pancreas • Acute pancreatitis—inflammation of the pancreas that occurs abruptly with little or no permanent pathologic change
• Chronic pancreatitis—continuing inflammatory disease that is often accompanied by irreversible morphologic change

PATHOPHYSIOLOGY
• Host defense mechanisms normally prevent pancreatic autodigestion by pancreatic enzymes, but under select circumstances, these natural defenses fail; autodigestion occurs when these digestive enzymes are activated within acinar cells. • Local and systemic tissue injury is due to the activity of released pancreatic enzymes and a variety of inflammatory mediators such as kinins, free radicals, and complement factors.

SYSTEMS AFFECTED
• Gastrointestinal—altered GI motility (ileus) due to regional chemical peritonitis; local or generalized peritonitis due to enhanced vascular permeability; concurrent inflammatory bowel disease may be seen in cats.
• Hepatobiliary—lesions due to shock, pancreatic enzyme injury, inflammatory cellular infiltrates, and intra/extrahepatic cholestasis • Respiratory—pulmonary edema or pleural effusion; adult respiratory distress syndrome is an uncommon but potentially fatal sequela with systemic complications.
• Cardiovascular—cardiac arrhythmias may result from release of myocardial depressant factor. • Hematologic—activation of the coagulation cascade and systemic consumptive coagulopathy (DIC) occur.

INCIDENCE/PREVALENCE
• Unknown • Up to 1% of normal dogs have histologic evidence of pancreatitis. • Necropsy surveys suggest an increased prevalence in cats with cholangiohepatitis, hepatic lipidosis, and inflammatory bowel disease.

SIGNALMENT

Species
Dogs and cats

Breed Predilection
• Miniature schnauzer • Miniature poodle
• Cocker spaniel • Siamese cats

Mean Age and Range
• Acute pancreatitis is most common in middle-aged and old (>7 years) dogs; mean age at presentation is 6.5 years. • Mean age for acute pancreatitis in cats is 7.3 years.

Predominant Sex
Female—dogs

SIGNS
General Comments
• Dogs—GI tract signs • Cats—vague, non-specific, and nonlocalizing

Historical Findings
• Lethargy/depression/anorexia—common in dogs and cats • Vomiting—common in dogs, less common in cats • Weight loss—common in cats • Dogs may exhibit abdominal pain.
• Diarrhea—more frequently seen in dogs than in cats • Icterus—common in dogs and cats

Physical Examination Findings
• Severe lethargy—both species
• Dehydration—common; due to GI losses
• Abdominal pain • Mass lesions may be palpable in both dogs and cats. • Fever—common in dogs; both fever and hypothermia reported in cats • Icterus—more common in cats • Less common systemic abnormalities include respiratory distress, bleeding disorders, and cardiac arrhythmias.

CAUSES
Usually unknown; possibilities include:
• Nutritional factors (e.g., hyperlipoproteinemia) • Pancreatic trauma/ischemia
• Duodenal reflux • Drugs/toxins (see Contraindications) • Pancreatic duct obstruction • Hypercalcemia • Infectious agents—toxoplasmosis, feline infectious peritonitis (FIP) • Extension of feline hepatobiliary or intestinal inflammation.

RISK FACTORS
• Breed (see under Signalment) • Obesity in dogs • Concurrent disease in dogs (e.g., diabetes mellitus, hyperadrenocorticism, chronic renal failure, and neoplasia) • Recent drug administration (see Contraindications, under Medications) • Concurrent hepatic/gut inflammatory disease in cats • See also Causes.

 DIAGNOSIS

DIFFERENTIAL DIAGNOSIS
Other causes of acute abdomen:
• GI disease (obstruction, foreign body, perforation, gastroenteritis, ulcer disease)—exclude with CBC/biochemistry/urinalysis, imaging, paracentesis, and endoscopy with biopsy. • Splenic torsion—exclude with imaging. • Hypoadrenocorticism—exclude with CBC/biochemistry/urinalysis, ACTH stimulation test. • Urogenital disease (pyelonephritis, prostatitis or abscessation, pyometra, urinary tract rupture or obstruction, acute renal failure)—exclude with CBC/biochemistry/urinalysis, urine culture/sensitivity, and imaging. • Hepatobiliary disease (cholangiohepatitis)—exclude with CBC/biochemistry /urinalysis, bile acids, imaging, and biopsy. • Abdominal

neoplasia—exclude with imaging and cytology or biopsy.

CBC/BIOCHEMISTRY/URINALYSIS
• CBC—in dogs often reveals hemoconcentration, leukocytosis with a left shift, and toxic neutrophils; cats are more variable and may show neutrophilia (30%) and nonregenerative anemia (26%) • Serum biochemistries—often show prerenal azotemia; liver enzyme activities (ALT, ALP) are often high because of hepatic ischemia or exposure to pancreatic toxins; hyperbilirubinemia is more common in cats and is due to hepatocellular damage and intra/extrahepatic biliary obstruction; hyperglycemia is seen in dogs and cats with necrotizing pancreatitis due to hyperglucagonemia; may see mild hypoglycemia in dogs; cats with suppurative pancreatitis may be hypoglycemic; hypercholesterolemia and hypertriglyceridemia are common.
• Urinalysis—unremarkable

OTHER LABORATORY TESTS
• Serum amylase and lipase activities are unreliable serologic markers—may be elevated in dogs but are nonspecific; also increase with hepatic, renal, or neoplastic disease in the absence of pancreatitis; dexamethasone may increase serum lipase concentrations in dogs; lipase may be normal or high in cats.
• Pancreatic lipase immunoreactivity (cPLI) is a highly sensitive and specific serologic marker of pancreatic inflammation in the dog. • TLI assay—TLI is pancreatic specific, and serum concentrations may be increased with acute pancreatitis in cats; reduced glomerular filtration may also increase serum TLI. Serum TLI is the best serologic marker for feline pancreatitis with sensitivities and specificities ranging from 50–75%. Normal TLI assay results do not rule out feline pancreatitis.

IMAGING
• Abdominal radiographs—may include increased soft tissue opacity in the right cranial abdominal compartment; loss of visceral detail ("ground glass appearance") due to abdominal effusion; static gas pattern in the proximal duodenum; widened angle between pyloric antrum and proximal duodenum • Thoracic radiographs—may reveal mild pleural effusion or more severe pulmonary complications • Abdominal ultrasound—nonhomogeneous solid or cystic mass lesions suggest pancreatic abscess; may be a pancreatic mass or altered echogenicity (hypoechoic) in the area of the pancreas; may see peritoneal effusion and extrahepatic biliary obstruction

DIAGNOSTIC PROCEDURES
• Ultrasound-guided needle-aspiration biopsy may confirm inflammation, abscess, or cyst.
• Laparoscopy with pancreatic forceps biopsy for histologic diagnosis

PATHOLOGIC FINDINGS
• Gross findings (acute pancreatitis)—mild swelling with edematous pancreatitis; grayish yellow areas of pancreatic necrosis with varying amounts of hemorrhage with necrotizing pancreatitis • Gross findings (chronic pancreatitis)—pancreas is reduced in size, firm, gray, and irregular; may contain extensive adhesions to surrounding viscera • Microscopic changes (acute pancreatitis)—include edema, parenchymal necrosis, and neutrophilic cellular infiltrate with acute lesions • Microscopic changes (chronic pancreatitis)—pancreatic fibrosis around ducts, ductal epithelial hyperplasia, and mononuclear cellular infiltrate; inflammatory lesions may also be seen in the hepatic parenchyma and intestinal mucosa of cats

TREATMENT

APPROPRIATE HEALTH CARE
• Inpatient medical management • Aggressive IV fluid therapy • Fluid therapy goals—correct hypovolemia and maintain pancreatic microcirculation. • A balanced electrolyte solution such as lactated Ringer's solution (LRS) is the first-choice rehydration fluid. • Correct initial dehydration (mL = % dehydration × weight in kg × 1000) and give over 4–6 h. • May need colloids (oxyglobin, hetastarch) • Following replacement of deficits, give additional fluids to match maintenance requirements (2.5 × weight in kg) and on-going losses (estimated). • Potassium chloride (KCl) supplementation usually needed because of potassium loss in the vomitus; base potassium supplementation on measured serum levels (use 20 mEq of KCl/L of IV fluid if serum potassium levels are not known; do not administer faster than 0.5 mEq/kg/h).

ACTIVITY
Restrict

DIET
• Continue to feed orally unless vomiting is intractable; feeding maintains intestinal epithelial integrity and minimizes bacterial translocation. • Animals with intermittent vomiting should be treated with antiemetics—metoclopramide (continuous infusion) or phenothiazines (following correction of fluid deficits). • Jejunostomy catheter feeding is most ideal since it allows for enteral feeding while promoting pancreatic rest; percutaneous endoscopic jejunostomy (PEJ) catheter placement has recently been described. • NPO in animals with persistent vomiting; when there has been no vomiting for 24–48 hours, offer small volumes of water; if tolerated, begin small, frequent feedings of a carbohydrate (e.g., boiled rice); gradually introduce a protein source of high biologic value such as cottage cheese or lean meat.

• Avoid high-protein and high-fat diets • Patients needing extended NPO may require jejunostomy enteral feeding or total parenteral nutrition.

CLIENT EDUCATION
• Discuss the need for extended hospitalization. • Discuss the expense of diagnosis and treatment. • Discuss possible short-term and long-term complications (see Associated Conditions).

SURGICAL CONSIDERATIONS
• May need surgery to remove pseudocysts, abscesses, or devitalized tissue seen with necrotizing pancreatitis. • May need laparotomy and pancreatic biopsy to confirm pancreatitis and/or rule out other, nonpancreatic diseases • Extrahepatic biliary obstruction from pancreatitis requires surgical correction.

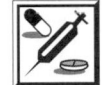

MEDICATIONS

DRUG(S)
• Corticosteroids only indicated in shock • Centrally acting antiemetics indicated with intractable vomiting—metoclopramide (1–2 mg/kg in 24h), chlorpromazine (0.5 mg/kg IM or SC q8h), or prochlorperazine (0.1 mg/kg q8h) • Antibiotics if evidence of sepsis—penicillin G (20,000 U/kg q6h), ampicillin sodium (20 mg/kg q8h), and enrofloxacin (5–20 mg/kg IV q12h in dogs) • Analgesics to relieve abdominal pain, e.g., buprenorphine (0.005–0.01 mg/kg IM, IV, or SC q6–12h)

CONTRAINDICATIONS
• Anticholinergics (e.g., atropine) • Azathioprine • Chlorothiazide • Estrogens • Furosemide • Tetracycline

PRECAUTIONS
• Only use phenothiazine antiemetics in well-hydrated patients; these drugs have hypotensive properties.

FOLLOW-UP

PATIENT MONITORING
• Evaluate hydration status closely during first 24 h of therapy; twice daily check physical examination, body weight, hematocrit, total plasma protein, BUN, and urine output. • Evaluate the effectiveness of fluid therapy after 24 h and adjust flow rates and fluid composition accordingly; repeat biochemistries to assess electrolyte/acid–base status • Repeat plasma enzyme concentrations (pancreatic lipase or TLI) after 48 h to evaluate the inflammatory process. • Watch closely for systemic complications involving a variety of organ systems; perform appropriate diagnostic tests as needed (see Associated Conditions).

• Gradually taper fluids down to maintenance requirements if possible. • Maintain oral alimentation or enteral nutrition as described above.

PREVENTION/AVOIDANCE
• Weight reduction if obese • Avoid high-fat diets. • Avoid drugs that may precipitate disease (see Contraindications).

POSSIBLE COMPLICATIONS
• Failed response to supportive therapy • Life-threatening associated conditions

EXPECTED COURSE AND PROGNOSIS
• Good for most patients with edematous pancreatitis; these patients usually respond to appropriate symptomatic therapy. • More guarded to poor for patients with necrotizing pancreatitis and systemic conditions

MISCELLANEOUS

ASSOCIATED CONDITIONS
Life-Threatening
• Pulmonary edema (e.g., adult respiratory distress syndrome) • Cardiac arrhythmias • Peritonitis • DIC • Feline hepatic lipidosis

Non–Life-Threatening
• Diabetes mellitus • EPI • Feline cholangiohepatitis • Feline inflammatory bowel disease

AGE-RELATED FACTORS
Most common in middle-aged animals

SEE ALSO
• Acute Abdomen • Exocrine Pancreatic Insufficiency

ABBREVIATIONS
• ALP = alkaline phosphatase • ALT = alanine aminotransferase • DIC = disseminated intravascular coagulation • EPI = exocrine pancreatic insufficiency • GI = gastrointestinal • NPO = nothing per os • TLI = trypsin-like immunoreactivity

Suggested Reading
Cook AK, Breitschwerdt EB, Levine JF, et al. Risk factors associated with acute pancreatitis in dogs: 101 cases (1985–1990). J Am Vet Med Assoc 1993;203:673–679.
Simpson KW. Acute pancreatitis. In: August JR, ed. Consultations in feline internal medicine. 3rd ed. Philadelphia: Saunders, 1997:91–98.
Simpson KW. The emergence of feline pancreatitis. J Vet Intern Med 2001;15:327–328.
Author Albert E. Jergens
Consulting Editor Albert E. Jergens

PANCYTOPENIA

 BASICS

DEFINITION
Simultaneous leukopenia, anemia, and thrombocytopenia; not a disease itself, rather a group of laboratory findings resulting from multiple causes

PATHOPHYSIOLOGY
• Mechanisms include decreased production of cells in the bone marrow or increased peripheral use, destruction, or sequestration; one or more of these mechanisms may occur together.
• Decreased production occurs when pluripotent, multipotent, or committed stem cells are destroyed, their proliferation or differentiation is suppressed, or the maturation of differentiated cells is delayed or arrested.
• If pluripotent stem cells are affected, pancytopenia develops; if committed stem cells are involved, cytopenia of the cell type develops.
• Use and destruction typically result in an increased production of cells in the bone marrow. At least 2 days are required before increased production begins to have an effect on peripheral blood counts, and peak output usually takes about a week; thus, the rate of destruction necessary to cause cytopenia is not as great during the first few days of disease as it is later.
• Sequestration of cells in the microcirculation, especially that of the spleen, intestine, and lungs, can cause cytopenia of the cell type involved.

SYSTEMS AFFECTED
Hemic/lymphatic/immune—bone marrow, spleen, lymph nodes, and other lymphoid tissues; depending on the cause, these organs can be affected by cellular depletion, degeneration, necrosis, hyperplasia, dysplasia, or dyscrasia; changes may occur alone or in combination

SIGNALMENT
• Dogs and cats
• No age or sex predilection

SIGNS

Historical Findings
• History reflects the underlying cause
• Lethargy or pallor from anemia
• Petechial hemorrhage or mucosal bleeding from thrombocytopenia
• Repeated febrile episodes or frequent or persistent infections from leukopenia

Physical Examination Findings
• Lethargy
• Pale mucous membranes
• Petechial hemorrhages
• Mucosal hemorrhage (e.g., hematuria, epistaxis, hemoptysis, melena)
• Fever

CAUSES

Infectious Diseases
• FeLV
• FIV
• Ehrlichiosis
• Feline infectious peritonitis
• Canine and feline parvovirus
• Infectious canine hepatitis virus
• Histoplasmosis
• Endotoxemia and septicemia (especially gram-negative organisms or tularemia)

Drugs, Chemicals, and Toxins
• Estrogen (exogenous administration, Sertoli cell tumor, interstitial cell tumor)
• Phenylbutazone
• Griseofulvin
• Methimazole (cats)
• Chloramphenicol
• Trimethoprim-sulfadiazine
• Albendazole
• Captopril
• Second-generation cephalosporins
• Chemotherapeutic drugs (azathioprine, doxorubicin, carboplatin, cyclophosphamide, cytosine arabinoside, vinblastine, hydroxyurea)
• Thallium
• *Fusarium* T-2 toxin
• Ionizing radiation

Proliferative and Infiltrative Diseases
• Hematopoietic neoplasia (e.g., leukemias, lymphoma, myelodysplasia)
• Myelofibrosis
• Myelophthisis

Immune-mediated Diseases
• Aplastic anemia (also known as aplastic pancytopenia)
• Immune-mediated hemolytic anemia and thrombocytopenia

RISK FACTORS
Vary with individual cause

 DIAGNOSIS

DIFFERENTIAL DIAGNOSIS
• Acute onset with severe clinical signs—more consistent with conditions that cause necrosis, destruction, or sequestration of cells
• Slow, insidious onset—more consistent with conditions that cause bone marrow suppression

LABORATORY FINDINGS

Drugs That May Alter Laboratory Results
Glucocorticoids often mildly to moderately increase the neutrophil count, which may then obscure the presence of neutropenia.

Disorders That May Alter Laboratory Results
Phlebotomy technique may result in platelet clumping and hemolysis, leading to spuriously low platelet count and PCV, respectively.

Valid if Run in Human Laboratory?
Varies with laboratory; ensure that instrumentation has been validated for dog and cat specimens and use appropriate reference intervals

CBC/BIOCHEMISTRY/URINALYSIS
• Leukopenia—characterized by neutropenia with or without lymphopenia
• Anemia—may be regenerative or nonregenerative, depending on underlying cause
• Thrombocytopenia
• Blood smear evaluation—may reveal infectious agents (e.g., *Ehrlichia* spp. *Histoplasma capsulatum*); may reveal abnormal cells of any lineage, suggesting myeloproliferative or lymphoproliferative diseases
• Toxic changes in leukocytes—may suggest bone marrow injury (e.g., from parvovirus or chemical agent), septicemia, or endotoxemia
• Biochemical alterations—depend on organ and degree of involvement (e.g., increased liver enzymes may be seen with certain infectious diseases, toxins, and infiltrative diseases)

OTHER LABORATORY TESTS
• Reticulocyte count—a regenerative response to anemia suggests destruction, use, or sequestration of RBCs; a nonregenerative response suggests bone marrow suppression and merits bone marrow examination
• Immunologic tests for infectious diseases (e.g., FeLV, FIV, *Ehrlichia* spp.)
• PCR for infectious diseases

IMAGING
N/A

OTHER DIAGNOSTIC PROCEDURES
• Bone marrow examination—indicated when cause of pancytopenia cannot be determined with other tests

• Hypercellular bone marrow associated with myelodysplasia, neoplasia, myelophthisis, or recovery from parvovirus
• Hypocellular bone marrow associated with necrosis, myelofibrosis, and suppression (e.g., drugs, estrogen, aplastic anemia)
• If a bone marrow aspirate cannot be obtained, myelofibrosis, necrosis, or marked hypocellularity should be suspected and a core biopsy should be evaluated.

PATHOLOGIC FINDINGS
Bone marrow core biopsy—may see replacement of normal hematopoietic tissue with necrotic, neoplastic, fibrous, or adipose tissue, depending on the underlying cause

TREATMENT
• Supportive treatment depends on the clinical situation and includes aggressive antibiotic therapy and blood component transfusions.
• Treatment of the underlying condition is paramount.

MEDICATIONS

DRUG(S) OF CHOICE
Treatment should be appropriate for the clinical situation (i.e., the degree to which each cell population is decreased, presence of fever or infection, and established or suspected specific diagnoses); see specific causes.

CONTRAINDICATIONS
• Drugs that may suppress hematopoiesis further (see Causes)
• Aspirin or other drugs that may interfere with platelet function

PRECAUTIONS
Because of the patient's compromised immune status, glucocorticoids and other immunosuppressive drugs should be used only when absolutely necessary and with extreme care.

POSSIBLE INTERACTIONS
N/A

ALTERNATIVE DRUG(S)

Recombinant Hematopoietic Growth Factors
• rhG-CSF—1–5 μg/kg/day SC; stimulates neutrophil production
• rhEPO—initial dosage: 100 U/kg SC three times/week; stimulates erythropoiesis

FOLLOW-UP

PATIENT MONITORING
• Daily physical examination, including frequent monitoring of body temperature
• Periodic CBC—frequency depends on severity of cytopenia, age, general physical condition of the patient, and underlying cause

PREVENTION/AVOIDANCE
• Castration of cryptorchid males
• Vaccination for infectious diseases
• Frequent monitoring of CBC in cancer patients receiving chemotherapy

POSSIBLE COMPLICATIONS
• Hemorrhage
• Sepsis

EXPECTED COURSE AND PROGNOSIS
• Depends on the underlying cause
• Often a guarded prognosis is warranted.

MISCELLANEOUS

ASSOCIATED CONDITIONS
Infections—in patients with neutropenia

AGE-RELATED FACTORS
N/A

ZOONOTIC POTENTIAL
• Tularemia
• An owner can contract histoplasmosis from the same source as the patient.

PREGNANCY
Stress of underlying disease may cause abortion; see respective topics for the effects of different causes on pregnancy.

SYNONYMS
N/A

SEE ALSO
• Anemia, Aplastic
• Anemia, Nonregenerative
• Anemia, Regenerative
• Neutropenia
• Specific causes of pancytopenia
• Thrombocytopenia

ABBREVIATIONS
• FeLV = feline leukemia virus
• FIV = feline immunodeficiency virus
• PCR = polymerase chain reaction
• PCV = packed cell volume
• rhEPO = recombinant human erythropoietin
• rhG-CSF = recombinant human granulocyte colony-stimulating factor

Suggested Reading
Tvedten H, Weiss DJ. Erythrocyte disorders. In: Willard MD, Tvedten H, Turnwald GH, eds. Small animal clinical diagnosis by laboratory methods. 3rd ed. Philadelphia: Saunders, 1999:31–51.
Weiss DJ. Detecting and diagnosing the cause of canine pancytopenia. Vet Med 2002; 97:21–32.
Weiss DJ, Evanson OA. A retrospective study of feline pancytopenia. Comp Haematol Int 2000;10:50–55.
Weiss DJ, Evanson OA, Sykes J. A retrospective study of canine pancytopenia. Vet Clin Pathol 1999;28:83–88.

Acknowledgment
The author and editors acknowledge the prior contributions of Gregory O. Freden, who authored this topic in the previous edition.
Author Darren Wood
Consulting Editor Stephen Kruth

PANNICULITIS

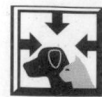 BASICS

OVERVIEW
• An inflammation of the subcutaneous fat tissue
• Uncommon in dogs and cats
• Multiple causes
• Single or multiple subcutaneous nodules or draining tracts
• Usually involves the trunk
• The lipocyte (fat cell) is susceptible to trauma, ischemic disease, and inflammation from adjacent tissues.
• Histology—divided into lobular (involves the fat lobules), septal (involves the interlobular connective tissue septa), and diffuse (involves both lobular and interlobular septa) types
• Diffuse most common in dogs
• Septal most common in cats

SIGNALMENT
• No age, sex, or breed predilection
• Sterile nodular panniculitis—dachshunds are predisposed; collies and miniature poodles are at risk; can occur in any breed

SIGNS
• Lesions—usually occur over the trunk; most dogs have a single nodular lesion over the ventral or lateral trunk; may become cystic and develop draining tracts; may be painful before and just after rupturing; ulcerations often heal with crusting and scarring
• Early cases of single or multifocal disease—nodules are freely movable underneath the skin; skin overlying the nodule is usually normal but may become erythematous or (less often) brown or yellow

• Nodules—vary from a few millimeters to several centimeters in diameter; may be firm and well circumscribed or soft and poorly defined; as they enlarge and develop, may fix to the deep dermis (thus the overlying skin is not freely movable)
• Involved fat may necrose.
• Exudate—usually a small amount of oily discharge; yellow-brown to bloody
• Multiple lesions (dogs and cats)—systemic signs common (e.g., anorexia, pyrexia, lethargy, and depression)

CAUSES & RISK FACTORS
• Infectious—bacterial, fungal, atypical mycobacteria, infectious embolism
• Immune-mediated—lupus panniculitis, erythema nodosum
• Idiopathic—sterile nodular panniculitis
• Trauma
• Neoplastic—multicentric mast cell tumors, cutaneous lymphosarcoma
• Foreign bodies
• Postinjection—corticosteroids, vaccines, other subcutaneous injections

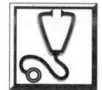 DIAGNOSIS

DIFFERENTIAL DIAGNOSIS

Deep Pyoderma
• More common than panniculitis
• More likely over pressure points
• May have associated lesions of superficial pyoderma (e.g., papules, pustules, and epidermal collarettes)
• Aspirates and impression smears—marked numbers of neutrophils with variable numbers of mononuclear cells and bacteria

• Culture/sensitivity and biopsies—confirm diagnosis

Cutaneous Cysts
• Usually nonpainful
• Well demarcated
• Usually no inflammation
• Aspirates—amorphous debris; no inflammatory cells
• Biopsies—confirm diagnosis

Cutaneous Neoplasia
• Lipomas—soft; usually well demarcated
• No inflammation or draining tracts
• Aspirates—lipocytes; no inflammatory cells
• Biopsies—confirm diagnosis

Mast Cell Tumors/Cutaneous Lymphosarcoma
• Multifocal
• May affect the head, legs, and mucous membranes
• Often erythematous
• Variable presentations
• Aspirates—often suggestive
• Biopsies—confirm diagnosis

Sterile Nodular Panniculitis
• A diagnosis made by ruling out other causes of panniculitis
• Biopsies, cultures, and other diagnostic tests—as indicated by the clinical presentation

CBC/BIOCHEMISTRY/URINALYSIS
• Most cases have no abnormalities.
• Occasional regenerative left shift or eosinophilia
• Mild leukocytosis
• Mild normochromic, normocytic nonregenerative anemia

OTHER LABORATORY TESTS

- Antinuclear antibody
- Direct immunofluorescence testing
- Serum protein electrophoresis
- Serum lipase/amylase levels

IMAGING

Ultrasound—pancreatitis may be a contributing factor (rare)

DIAGNOSTIC PROCEDURES

- Bacterial culture and sensitivity testing—necessary for identifying primary or secondary bacteria
- Fungal and atypical mycobacteria culture
- Biopsies—negative cultures help diagnose sterile nodular panniculitis
- Special stains of histologic samples—help identify causative agent

PATHOLOGIC FINDINGS

- Surgical excisional biopsies—much more accurate than punch biopsy specimens in most cases; punch biopsies do not provide a deep enough sample to make the diagnosis.
- Histologic lesions—required to make a diagnosis of panniculitis; determine septal, lobular, or diffuse inflammatory infiltrate by neutrophils, histiocytes, plasma cells, lymphocytes, eosinophils, or multinucleated giant cells; identify necrosis, fibrosis, or vasculitis.

TREATMENT

- Single lesions—cured with surgical excision
- Multiple lesions—require systemic medications

MEDICATIONS

DRUG(S)

- Positive culture results require appropriate antifungal, antibacterial, or antimycobacterial treatment.
- Sterile nodular panniculitis—systemic treatment with steroids; prednisone (2.2 mg/kg daily) until lesions completely regress (36 weeks); after remission, gradually taper dosage over 2 weeks; occasionally may need slower taper to minimize chance of recurrence; many patients cured; some patients need low-dose alternate-day treatment to maintain remission.
- Oral vitamin E—may control mild cases
- Oral potassium iodide or azathioprine (1 mg/kg daily)—alternatives when steroids are contraindicated

FOLLOW-UP

- Depends on type and duration of treatment
- Monitor CBC, platelet count, chemistry profile, and urinalysis if immune-suppressing agents or long-term glucocorticosteroids are used.

MISCELLANEOUS

Suggested Reading

Scott DW, Miller WH, Griffin CE. Muller and Kirk's Small animal dermatology. 5th ed. Philadelphia: Saunders, 1995.

Author Kevin Shanley

Consulting Editor Karen Helton Rhodes

PANOSTEITIS

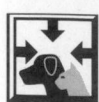

BASICS

DEFINITION

A self-limiting, painful condition affecting one or more of the long bones of young, medium- to large-breed dogs that is characterized clinically by lameness and radiographically by high density of the marrow cavity.

PATHOPHYSIOLOGY

- Cause unknown
- Attempts to isolate microorganisms have failed
- Metabolic, allergic, or endocrine aberrations—without support
- Pain—may be owing to disturbance of endosteal and periosteal elements, vascular congestion, or high intramedullary pressure

SYSTEMS AFFECTED

Musculoskeletal—lameness of variable intensity; may affect a single limb or become a shifting leg lameness

GENETICS

- No proven transmission
- Predominance of German shepherds in the affected population strongly suggests an inheritable basis.

INCIDENCE/PREVALENCE

No reliable estimates; common

GEOGRAPHIC DISTRIBUTION

N/A

SIGNALMENT

Species

Dogs

Breed Predilections

- German shepherds and German shepherd mixes—most commonly affected
- Medium to large breeds—most commonly affected

Mean Age and Range

- Usually 5–18 months of age
- As young as 2 months and as old as 5 years

Predominant Sex

Male

SIGNS

General Comments

Lameness—if no distinct abnormalities noted on physical examination or radiographs, repeat examinations 4-6 weeks later.

Historical Findings

- No associated trauma
- Lameness—varying intensity; usually involves the forelimbs initially; may affect the hind limbs; may see shifting leg lameness; may be non–weight bearing
- Severe disease—mild depression; inappetence; weight loss

Physical Examination Findings

- Pain—on deep palpation of the long bones (diaphysis) in an affected limb; distinguishing characteristic; palpate firmly along the entire shaft of each bone while carefully avoiding any pinching of nearby muscle.
- Bones—ulna most commonly affected; may affect radius, humerus, femur, and tibia (in decreasing order of frequency) either concurrently or subsequently
- May note low-grade fever
- May see muscle atrophy

CAUSES

Unknown

RISK FACTORS

Purebred German shepherd or German shepherd mix

DIAGNOSIS

DIFFERENTIAL DIAGNOSIS

- Always consider the diagnosis with lameness in a young German shepherd or German shepherd mix.
- May occur alone or with other juvenile orthopedic diseases
- Osteochondritis dissecans
- Fragmented medial coronoid process
- Un-united anconeal process

- Hip dysplasia
- Fractures and ligamentous injuries from unobserved trauma
- Shifting leg lameness—immune-mediated arthritides; Lyme disease; bacterial endocarditis
- Coccidioidomycosis
- Bacterial osteomyelitis

CBC/BIOCHEMISTRY/URINALYSIS

- Usually normal
- May note eosinophilia early in disease

OTHER LABORATORY TESTS

N/A

IMAGING

- Radiographic densities within the medulla of long bones—characteristic; confirm diagnosis
- Early, middle, and late radiographic lesions
- Early—trabecular pattern of the ends of the diaphysis becomes more prominent; may appear blurred; may see granular opacities
- Middle—patchy sclerotic opacities first around the nutrient foramen and later throughout the diaphysis; widened cortex; thickened periosteum with increased opacity
- Late—during resolution, diminished overall opacity of the medullary canal (toward normal); a coarse trabecular pattern and some granular opacity may remain; may be a period in which the medullary canal becomes more lucent than normal

DIAGNOSTIC PROCEDURES

Bone biopsy—occasionally indicated to rule out neoplasia and bacterial or fungal infections that have similar radiographic appearances

PATHOLOGIC FINDINGS

- Biopsy or necropsy—rarely performed because of excellent prognosis for recovery
- No gross pathologic lesions
- Degeneration of the marrow adipocytes surrounding the nutrient foramen followed by proliferation of vascular stromal cells within the marrow sinusoids
- Osteoid formation and endosteal new bone formation—progress proximally and distally

• Vascular congestion—may accompany the proliferation of new bone, secondarily stimulating endosteal and periosteal reaction
• Remodeling of the endosteum—occurs during resolution; reestablishes normal endosteal and marrow architecture

TREATMENT

APPROPRIATE HEALTH CARE
Outpatient

NURSING CARE
Maintenance and replacement fluid therapy—occasionally owing to prolonged periods of inappetence and pyrexia

ACTIVITY
• Limited—not shown to hasten recovery; lessens pain
• Moderate to severe disease—pain may cause self-limited movement leading to muscle atrophy.

DIET
N/A

CLIENT EDUCATION
• Warn client that patient may develop other juvenile orthopedic diseases.
• Inform client that signs of pain and lameness may last for several weeks.
• Warn client that recurrence of clinical signs is common up to 2 years of age.

SURGICAL CONSIDERATIONS
N/A

MEDICATIONS

DRUG(S) OF CHOICE
NSAIDs
• Minimize pain; decrease inflammation
• Symptomatic therapy has no bearing on the duration of the disease.
• May try buffered or enteric-coated aspirin (10–25 mg/kg PO q8h or q12h), carprofen

(2.2 mg/kg PO q12h), etodolac (10–15 mg/kg PO q24h), phenylbutazone (3–7 mg/kg PO q8h, total dose < 800 mg/day), meclofenamic acid (0.5 mg/kg PO q12h), or piroxicam (0.3 mg/kg PO q24h for 3 days, then q48h)

Glucocorticoids
• May give antiinflammatory dosage—prednisone (0.1–0.5 mg/kg PO)
• Potential side affects well documented
• Goal for chronic use—low-dose and alternate-day therapy

CONTRAINDICATIONS
NSAIDs—gastrointestinal upset may preclude use.

PRECAUTIONS
• NSAIDs—most cause some degree of gastric ulceration.
• Acetaminophen—unsuitable; potential for toxicity

POSSIBLE INTERACTIONS
NSAIDs—do not use in conjunction with glucocorticoids; risk of gastrointestinal tract ulceration

ALTERNATIVE DRUG(S)
N/A

FOLLOW-UP

PATIENT MONITORING
Recheck lameness every 2–4 weeks to detect more serious concurrent orthopedic problems.

PREVENTION/AVOIDANCE
N/A

POSSIBLE COMPLICATIONS
N/A

EXPECTED COURSE AND PROGNOSIS
• Self-limiting disease
• Treatment—symptomatic; appears to have no influence on duration of clinical signs.
• Multiple limb involvement—common
• Lameness—typically lasts from a few days to several weeks; may persist for months

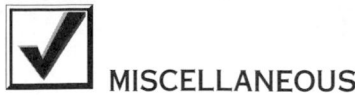

MISCELLANEOUS

ASSOCIATED CONDITIONS
N/A

AGE-RELATED FACTORS
Typically affects immature and young dogs

ZOONOTIC POTENTIAL
N/A

PREGNANCY
Females reported to be more susceptible to panosteitis during estrus; no proven relationship to reproductive hormones or pregnancy

SYNONYMS
• Enostosis
• Fibrous osteodystrophy
• Juvenile osteomyelitis
• Eosinophilic panosteitis

ABBREVIATION
NSAIDs = nonsteroidal antiinflammatory drugs

Suggested Reading
Piermattei DL, Flo GL. Disease conditions in small animals. In: Piermattei DL, Flo GL, eds. Handbook of small animal orthopedics and fracture treatment. 3rd ed. Philadelphia: Saunders 1997:715–718.
Halliwell WH. Tumorlike lesions of bone. In: Bojrab MJ, ed. Disease mechanisms in small animal surgery. 2nd ed. Philadelphia: Saunders 1993:932–933.
Manly PA, Romich JA. Miscellaneous orthopedic diseases. In: Slatter DH, ed. Textbook of small animal surgery. 2nd ed. Philadelphia: Saunders 1993:1984–1987.
Muir P, Dubielzig RR, Johnson KA. Panosteitis. Compend Contin Educ Pract Vet 1996;18:29–33.
Author Larry Carpenter
Consulting Editor Peter K. Shires

PAPILLEDEMA

BASICS

OVERVIEW
• Papilledema—swelling of optic disk secondary to increased intracranial pressure without discernible vision loss
• Optic disk edema
• Swelling of the optic disk reflecting other pathologies—including optic neuritis
• Affects the ophthalmic and nervous systems

SIGNALMENT
Dogs and cats

SIGNS

Historical Findings
• Cerebral signs
• Disk edema per se produces no visual deficits.

Physical Examination Findings
• CNS signs
• Elevation and hyperemia of optic nerve head
• Blurring of optic disk margin
• Filling in of physiologic cup
• Pupillary light reflexes are normal.

CAUSES & RISK FACTORS
• Hydrocephalus
• Hepatic encephalopathy
• Neoplasm—primary or metastatic
• Distemper (dogs)
• FIP (cats)
• Systemic mycoses
• Toxoplasmosis
• *Neosporum caninum*
• Granulomatous meningoencephalomyelitis
• Trauma

DIAGNOSIS

DIFFERENTIAL DIAGNOSIS
Diseases causing optic disk swelling—optic neuritis; congenital anomalies
• Optic neuritis—abnormal pupillary light reflexes

CBC/BIOCHEMISTRY/URINALYSIS
No specific abnormalities

OTHER LABORATORY TESTS
Specific viral, fungal or protozoal serologic testing

IMAGING
• Neuroimaging—CT or MRI
• Orbital ultrasound

DIAGNOSTIC PROCEDURES
CSF analysis—measure intracranial pressure

TREATMENT
• Resolve cause of increased intracranial pressure or orbital disease.
• Patients need critical monitoring.
• Maintain PaCO$_2$ at 30–35 mm Hg

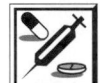

MEDICATIONS

DRUG(S)
• Mannitol—1 g/kg IV over 20 min; repeated as necessary
• Furosemide (Lasix)—1 mg/kg IV q8h

• Corticosteroids—prednisone (0.5 mg/kg PO q12h) or dexamethasone SP 0.25 mg/kg IV q8–12h); not indicated for head trauma

CONTRAINDICATIONS/POSSIBLE INTERACTIONS
• Beware of brain herniation.
• Systemic corticosteroids—do not use until infectious causes are ruled out.

FOLLOW-UP
Prognosis—depends on underlying disease

MISCELLANEOUS

ABBREVIATIONS
• CNS = central nervous system
• CSF = cerebrospinal fluid
• CT = computed tomography
• FIP = feline infectious peritonitis
• MRI = magnetic resonance imaging

Suggested Reading
Whiting AS, Johnson LN. Papilledema: clinical clues and differential diagnosis. Am Fam Physician 1994;5:1125–1134.
Author David Lipsitz
Consulting Editor Paul E. Miller

BASICS

OVERVIEW
• Papillomaviruses (PVs)—group of nonenveloped, double-stranded DNA viruses that induce proliferative cutaneous tumors in cats and dogs and mucosal tumors in dogs; each is host- and fairly site-specific, with characteristic clinical and microscopic changes in infected tissues. • Tumors—papillomas, warts, or verrucae; generally benign; spontaneously regress; rarely may undergo conversion to SCC • Lesions—often multiple, well demarcated, and exophytic; sometimes hyperkeratotic plaques or with papules; may be deeply pigmented (black or brown), pink, tan, or white • Infection—inoculation through breaks in the epidermis or mucosal epithelium; iatrogenic transmission through use of contaminated instruments possible

SIGNALMENT
Dogs
• At least five types of PV may infect dogs. • Oral and ocular papillomas—generally seen in young animals (6 months to 4 years); however, any age may be affected • Cutaneous papillomas—any age • Miniature schnauzers and pugs—pigmented sessile papillomas generally manifest before 5 years of age

Cats
• Feline papillomatosis and Bowen's disease—old animals (7 years and up) • PV-induced lesions have been identified in kittens. • No breed predisposition

SIGNS
Historical Findings
• Dysphagia • Ptyalism • Reluctance to eat • Halitosis—dogs with oral papillomas

Physical Examination Findings
Dogs
• True cutaneous papillomas—rare; lesion is an exophytic, often pedunculated, papilliferous growth consisting of multiple fronds of epithelium; may be found anywhere on the body; rarely exceed 1 cm in diameter • Venereal warts—affect the lower genital tract; probably caused by a novel PV • Cutaneous inverted papillomas—rare; caused by a unique PV; lesions: generally found on the ventral trunk and abdomen, 1–2 cm in diameter, raised and firm, small pore opening to the skin surface • Familial form—rare; pugs and miniature schnauzers; up to 80 scaly, black plaques scattered on the ventral neck, trunk, and medial aspects of limbs (pigmented epidermal nevi and lentiginosis profusa)
Oral
• Multiple tumors (as many as 100) on the mucocutaneous junctions around the mouth, lips, tongue, palate, epiglottis, and upper esophagus and on the mucosa of the oropharynx • Early papillomas—discrete, pale, smooth elevations of the mucosa; proceed to develop a filiform to cauliflower-like appearance • Lesions—may bleed and be ulcerated owing to trauma from teeth • Halitosis and discharge from the mouth—with secondary bacterial infection of traumatized lesions • Respiratory distress—rare; multiple tumors may obstruct the airway • The canine oral PV is believed to be the cause of some eyelid, corneal, and conjunctival papillomas.
Cats
• Exophytic papillomas—exceedingly rare • Cutaneous—multifocal to coalescing plaques of epidermal hyperplasia that may be pigmented or waxy and white • Lesions—persistent; may progress to SCC (Bowen's disease or multicentric SCC in situ) • SCC in situ lesions—well demarcated; deeply pigmented; erythematous; crusted; occasionally ulcerated; may progress to invasive SCC

CAUSES & RISK FACTORS
• Oral (dogs)—young and immunologically naive; recovered animals appear to be immune. • Cutaneous (dogs and cats)—immunosuppression (acquired, congenital, or iatrogenic from use of corticosteroids) facilitates all types of PV infection; defects in cell-mediated immunity thought to have a permissive effect on the persistence of PV-induced lesions

 DIAGNOSIS

DIFFERENTIAL DIAGNOSIS
Dogs
• Oral cavity and oropharynx—fibromatous epulis; transmissible venereal tumor; if ulcerated, SCC • Cutaneous—sebaceous hyperplasias; cutaneous tags • Pigmented—melanomas • Inverted—intracutaneous cornifying epitheliomas

Cats
Multiple sessile, hyperkeratotic lesions—eosinophilic granulomas or plaques; actinic keratosis; cutaneous lesions of FeLV; multicentric SCC in situ; SCC

DIAGNOSTIC PROCEDURES
• Oral papillomatosis—gross appearance and physical examination findings generally provide the diagnosis; biopsy of one or two lesions may be used for confirmation. • Histopathology—generally required for cutaneous, venereal, and some ocular papillomas • Immunohistochemistry—avidin–biotin complex method to detect PV group–related antigens; dogs: helps make the diagnosis; cats: recommended for confirmation of diagnosis

 TREATMENT
• Oral—self-limiting; lesions generally regress spontaneously. • Surgery to remove oral tumors (excision, cryosurgery, or electrosurgery)—airway is being occluded; patient is unable to eat comfortably; aesthetic reasons • Systemic corticosteroids—withdraw if severe or persistent oral or cutaneous disease recurs. • Persistent disease (dogs)—may treat with autovaccination; use heat-inactivated autogenous vaccine. • Cats—no efficacious therapy for chronic PV-induced skin lesions; SCC in situ lesions may respond to ^{90}Sr plesiotherapy.

 **MEDICATIONS** N/A

 FOLLOW-UP

PATIENT MONITORING
Monitor lesions carefully to detect signs (ulceration, purulent exudation, and rapid growth) of malignant transformation to SCC.

PREVENTION/AVOIDANCE
• Separate dogs with oral papillomatosis from susceptible animals. • Commercial kennels with outbreaks of oral papillomatosis—may use autogenous vaccines • Live canine oral PV vaccine—reported to induce hyperplastic epithelial tumors and SCC at vaccination sites; latency period 11–34 months

EXPECTED COURSE AND PROGNOSIS
• Dogs—prognosis usually good; incubation period 1–8 weeks; regression usually occurs at 1–5 months; lesions may persist for 24 months or more. • Cats—long-term prognosis for chronic papillomatosis and Bowen's disease uncertain

 **MISCELLANEOUS**

ZOONOTIC POTENTIAL
None

ABBREVIATIONS
• FeLV = feline leukemia virus • SCC = squamous cell carcinoma

Suggested Reading
Sundberg JP. Papillomaviruses. In: Castro AE, Heuscele WP, eds. Veterinary diagnostic virology. St. Louis: Mosby, 1992:148–150.
Authors Suzette M. LeClerc and Edward G. Clark
Consulting Editor Stephen C. Barr

PARALYSIS

 BASICS

DEFINITIONS
• Paresis—weakness of voluntary movement
• Paralysis—lack of voluntary movement
• Quadriparesis (tetraparesis)—weakness of voluntary movements in all limbs
• Quadriplegia (tetraplegia)—absence of all voluntary limb movement • Paraparesis—weakness of voluntary movements in pelvic limbs • Paraplegia—absence of all voluntary pelvic limb movement • Schiff-Sherrington syndrome—associated with severe spinal cord trauma, usually near the thoracolumbar spine; with the patient in lateral recumbency, front limbs and neck are in extension, with paralysis of pelvic limbs; front limbs normal; exaggerated pelvic limb spinal reflexes; prognosis is based on presence or absence of deep pain perception in pelvic limbs
• Spinal shock—associated with severe spinal cord trauma, usually located near the thoracolumbar spine; paralyzed pelvic limbs with initially areflexic pelvic limb reflexes that become exaggerated (and more indicative of a T3-L3 lesion localization) within minutes to a few hours after the trauma

PATHOPHYSIOLOGY
• Weakness—may be caused by lesions in the upper or lower motor neuron system
• Cell bodies or nuclei for the upper motor neuron system—located within the brain; responsible for initiating voluntary movement
• Axons from these cell bodies—form tracts (rubrospinal, corticospinal, vestibulospinal, reticulospinal) that descend from the brain to synapse on interneurons in the spinal cord
• Interneuronal axons—then synapse on large alpha motor neurons in the ventral gray matter of the spinal cord • Large alpha motor neurons—are cell bodies of origin for the lower motor neuron system, which is responsible for spinal reflexes • Collections of lower motor neurons in the cervical and lumbar intumescences—give rise to axons that form the ventral nerve roots, the spinal nerves, and (ultimately) the peripheral nerves that innervate limb muscles • Evaluation of limb reflexes—determines which system (upper or lower motor neuron) is involved
• Upper motor neurons and their axons—have inhibitory influence on the large alpha motor neurons of the lower motor neuron system; maintain normal muscle tone and normal spinal reflexes; if upper motor neuron system is injured, spinal reflexes are no longer inhibited or controlled and reflexes become exaggerated or hyperreflexic • Large alpha motor neurons or their processes (peripheral nerves)—also help to maintain normal muscle tone and normal spinal reflexes; if lower motor neuron system is injured, spinal reflexes cannot be elicited (areflexic) or are

reduced (hyporeflexic) and muscle wasting is usually severe within 5–7 days of injury

SYSTEMS AFFECTED
Nervous

SIGNALMENT
Any species

SIGNS
General Comments
Limb weakness—acute or gradual onset

Historical Findings
• Owner may describe the patient as being "down," unable to move, walk, or get up
• Many focal compressive spinal cord diseases begin with ataxia and progress to weakness and finally to paralysis.

Physical Examination Findings
• Usually normal, unless the disease process is systemic • Patient usually alert • If in pain, patient may resent handling and manipulation during the examination.
• Aortic emboli (ischemic neuromyopathy)—patient may be paraplegic and areflexic or hyporeflexic on examination; femoral pulses absent; limbs often cold; nail beds often blue

Neurologic Examination Findings
• Confirm that the problem is weakness or paralysis. • Localize problem to either lower or upper motor neuron system. • If limbs are paralyzed—likely bladder is also paralyzed, negating voluntary urination • Tetraparesis with exaggerated spinal reflexes in all limbs—lesion is most likely located at C1-C5 spinal cord segments or in the brain • Tetraparesis with normal or depressed front limb spinal reflexes and exaggerated pelvic limb spinal reflexes—lesion is most likely located at C6-T2 spinal cord segments • Tetraparesis with depressed spinal reflexes and muscle tone in all limbs—lesion is most likely diffuse muscle or peripheral nerve problem, or located at both the cervical (C6-T2 spinal cord segments) and lumbar spinal cord intumescences (L4-S2 spinal cord segments)
• Normal front limbs but paraparesis/paraplegia with exaggerated pelvic limb spinal reflexes—lesion is most likely located at T3-L3 spinal cord segments • Normal front limbs but paraparesis/ paraplegia with depressed to absent pelvic limb spinal reflexes—lesion is most likely located at L4 spinal cord segment and caudally • Normal front limb and pelvic limb motor activity but flaccid tail/anus and urinary and/or fecal incontinence—lesion is most likely located at S2 spinal cord segment and caudally • Normal front limbs but paraparesis/paraplegia and depressed patellar reflexes–lesion is most likely located at spinal cord segments L4–6, which are located in vertebral bodies L3–4. • Normal front limbs but paraparesis/paraplegia, exaggerated patellar reflexes, and weak flexor and sciatic reflexes—if only the spinal cord is affected (no root involvement), lesion is likely located

at spinal cord segments L6-S2, which are located in vertebral bodies L4-L6

CAUSES
Generalized Quadriplegia
• Lower motor neuron—acute onset: coonhound paralysis, botulism, tick paralysis, fulminating form of myasthenia gravis, or protozoal myoneuritis; more gradual onset: polyneuropathies and polymyopathies from toxicity, infection, inflammation, endocrinopathy, metabolic disease, or congenital/inherited disease • Upper motor neuron—cervical spinal cord or multifocal cord diseases: disk herniation; diskospondylitis; fibrocartilaginous embolism; trauma; neoplasia; myelitis of many causes; malformations of the spine or spinal cord

Paraplegia
• Upper motor neuron—disk herniation; diskospondylitis; fibrocartilaginous embolism; neoplasia; trauma; congenital malformations of spine or spinal cord; degenerative myelopathy • Lower motor neuron—fibrocartilaginous embolism; disk herniation; lumbosacral instability; diskospondylitis; trauma; neoplasia; spina bifida

Generalized Quadriplegia with Cranial Nerve Deficits, Seizures, or Stupor
Upper motor neuron—diseases of the brain stem: encephalitis; neoplasia; trauma; vascular accidents; congenital or inherited disorders

RISK FACTORS
• Breeds at risk for degenerative disk disease—dachshunds, poodles, cocker spaniels, and beagles • Hunting dogs—at risk for coonhound paralysis • Roaming animals—at risk for spinal cord trauma
• Breeds at risk for atlantoaxial luxation—toy and small breeds • Breeds at risk for lumbosacral instability—large breeds; working breeds; German shepherds • Breeds at risk for cervical vertebral malformation/stenosis/instability syndrome (wobbler syndrome)—large breeds; Doberman pinschers; Great Danes

 DIAGNOSIS

DIFFERENTIAL DIAGNOSIS
• Weak or paralyzed pelvic limbs—make sure femoral pulses are present and normal; aortic or femoral artery emboli may lead to lower motor neuron paraparesis or paraplegia
• Spinal reflexes—localize weakness to the cervical, thoracolumbar, or lower lumbar cord segments • Acute onset—be careful when moving the patient because of the possibility of trauma

CBC/BIOCHEMISTRY/URINALYSIS
Usually normal, unless inflammatory diseases involved

OTHER LABORATORY TESTS
• Urinary tract inflammation—bacterial culture of urine may be positive in diskospondylitis cases
• Diskospondylitis—diagnose by spinal radiography (intervertebral disk space lysis); perform a *Brucella* titer; consider blood and urine bacterial cultures
• Exercise-induced weakness—determine acetylcholine receptor antibody titers (test for myasthenia gravis); check serum creatine kinase concentration (polymyositis or polymyopathy), RBC count (anemia or polycythemia), and blood glucose concentration (hypoglycemia); check for cardiac arrhythmia and hypoxia via ECG and thoracic radiography; perform muscle biopsy
• Lower motor neuron weakness or muscle pain, muscle atrophy, or hypertrophy—determine creatine kinase concentration to help diagnose polymyositis; perform muscle and nerve biopsy; evaluate *Neospora caninum* and *Toxoplasma gondii* serum titers
• Suspected myelitis or meningitis—dog: perform titers for *N. caninum*, *T. gondii*, Rocky Mountain spotted fever, *Ehrlichia* spp., and canine distemper virus; cat: perform serum titers for *T. gondii* and *Cryptococcus neoformans* and evaluate spinal fluid for sign of feline infectious peritonitis virus and *C. neoformans*

IMAGING
• Spinal radiography—lesion localized to the spinal cord; may reveal disk herniation, diskospondylitis, bony tumor, congenital vertebral malformation, and fracture or luxation • Myelography—required if survey radiography is not diagnostic and when considering surgery • CT or MRI—if lesion can be precisely localized or if more information is required after myelography localizes the lesion; will likely replace myelography for imaging the spine once the technology becomes more accessible
• Diskospondylitis—may collect aspirate of the intervertebral space using fluoroscopy; perform cytology and culture to isolate the infectious agent

DIAGNOSTIC PROCEDURES
• CSF analysis—do before myelography to detect myelitis and meningitis; if high protein or cell numbers are found, a culture is warranted; save some fluid for infectious disease titer analysis • Needle electromyography and motor nerve conduction velocity—may help with diagnosis of generalized lower motor neuron signs; better characterize the lesion and help determine the prognosis in some cases
• Muscle and nerve biopsy—generalized lower motor neuron weakness

TREATMENT
• Inpatient—with severe weakness or paralysis until bladder function can be ascertained
• Hand feeding—with diffuse lower motor neuron signs, swallowing can be affected; until it is certain that the patient can swallow properly • Feeding from an elevated platform—recommended for animals with megaesophagus until it resolves
• Activity—restrict until spinal trauma and disk herniation can be ruled out • Physical therapy—important for paralyzed patients; tone muscles and keep joints flexible
• Bedding—move paralyzed patients away from soiled bedding; check and clean frequently to prevent urine scalding and superficial pyoderma; use padded bedding or a waterbed to help prevent decubital ulcer formation • Turning—turn quadriplegic patients from side to side four to eight times daily; prevent hypostatic lung congestion and decubital ulcer formation • Surgery—for disk herniation, fracture, and some neoplasias and congenital conditions; often the quickest and most effective method of improving the neurologic status

MEDICATIONS
DRUG(S) OF CHOICE
• Methylprednisolone sodium succinate—30 mg/kg IV followed by 15 mg/kg 2 and 6 hr later; may be beneficial for suspected trauma, disk herniation, or fibrocartilaginous embolism; acute upper motor neuron signs
• Pyridostigmine bromide—0.5–3.0 mg/kg PO q8–12h; for suspected myasthenia gravis; administer while waiting for titer results
• Acute generalized lower motor neuron signs—check for ticks; dip with appropriate insecticides, if necessary

CONTRAINDICATIONS
Corticosteroids—do not use with diskospondylitis or fungal or protozoal myelitis/meningitis; do not use with myasthenia gravis associated with aspiration pneumonia

PRECAUTIONS
Corticosteroids—associated with gastrointestinal ulceration and hemorrhage, delayed wound healing, and heightened susceptibility to infection

ALTERNATIVE DRUG(S)
• Dexamethasone—0.5–1 mg/kg q24–48h
• Prednisolone—1–2 mg/kg q12–24h

FOLLOW-UP
PATIENT MONITORING
• Neurologic examinations—daily to monitor status • Bladder—evacuate (via manual expression or catheterization) three to four times a day to prevent overdistention and subsequent bladder atony; once bladder function has returned, patient can be managed at home

POSSIBLE COMPLICATIONS
• Urinary tract infection, bladder atony, urine scalding and pyoderma, constipation, decubital ulcer formation • Aspiration pneumonia—with generalized lower motor neuron disease or in any quadriplegic patient
• Myelomalacia—with severe spinal cord trauma or disk herniations • Respiratory compromise or paralysis—with myelomalacia or generalized lower motor neuron disease

MISCELLANEOUS
ASSOCIATED CONDITIONS
N/A

AGE-RELATED FACTORS
N/A

ZOONOTIC POTENTIAL
N/A

PREGNANCY
Contraindicated in paralyzed patients

ABBREVIATIONS
• CSF = cerebrospinal fluid
• CT = computed tomography
• ECG = electrocardiogram
• MRI = magnetic resonance imaging
• RBC = red blood cell

Suggested Reading

Davies C, Shell L. Neurological problems. In: Common small animal medical diagnoses: an algorithmic approach. Philadelphia: Saunders, 2002:36–59.

de Lahunta A. Veterinary neuroanatomy and clinical neurology. 2nd ed. Philadelphia: Saunders, 1983.

Oliver JE, Lorenz MD, Kornegay JN. Tetraparesis, hemiparesis, and ataxia. In: Handbook of veterinary neurology. 3rd ed. Philadelphia: Saunders. 1997:173–215.

Wheeler SJ, Sharp NJH. Diagnosis and differential diagnosis. In: Small animal spinal disorders. London: Mosby-Wolfe, 1994: 31–56.

Withrow SJ. Localization and diagnosis of spinal cord lesions in small animals. Part 1. Compend Contin Educ Pract Vet 1980;2: 464–474.

Author Linda G. Shell
Consulting Editor Joane M. Parent

PARANEOPLASTIC SYNDROMES

 BASICS

DEFINITION
A clinical anomaly resulting from the noninvasive actions of a tumor. Usually results from the abnormal secretion of a hormone or hormone-like product (hormone type or amount) that causes an inappropriate clinical response.

PATHOPHYSIOLOGY
Depends entirely on how the target of the hormone product responds to inappropriate stimulation

SYSTEMS AFFECTED
Varied, depending on the response of the hormone target

GENETICS
No basis

INCIDENCE/PREVALENCE
• No good data, but most are considered rare.
• Hypercalcemia is reported in up to 20% of dogs with lymphosarcoma.
• Approximately 75% of humans with cancer have some paraneoplastic disorder during the course of their illness.

GEOGRAPHIC DISTRIBUTION
None recognized

SIGNALMENT
Any dog or cat with a histologically malignant (most common) or benign cancer (rare)

SIGNS
Vary with syndrome and organ systems affected

CAUSES
Inappropriate hormone or hormone-like peptide secretion by a tumor

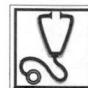 **DIAGNOSIS**

DIFFERENTIAL DIAGNOSIS
Varies with syndrome; see table.

CBC/BIOCHEMISTRY/URINALYSIS
Helpful in identifying and monitoring several of the reported syndromes

 TREATMENT

• Depends on the underlying tumor and the clinical manifestations of the paraneoplastic syndrome • The usual principle is to treat the underlying neoplasm rather than to try to control the clinical signs of the paraneoplastic syndrome. • Sometimes, trying to manage clinical signs is appropriate for palliation if control of the primary tumor is impossible.

 MEDICATIONS

DRUG(S)
Depends on underlying tumor type

 FOLLOW-UP

PATIENT MONITORING
As for underlying tumor type

 MISCELLANEOUS

Suggested Reading
Morrison WB. Paraneoplastic syndromes and the tumors that cause them. In: Morrison WB, ed. Cancer in dogs and cats: medical and surgical management. 2nd ed. Jackson Hole, WY: Teton NewMedia, 2002: 731–744.
Author Wallace B. Morrison
Consulting Editor Wallace B. Morrison

Paraneoplastic Syndromes and Tumors that Cause Them

Syndrome	Primary tumor association (dog)	Primary tumor association (cat)	Primary mechanism
Alopecia	Adrenal carcinoma	Pancreatic carcinoma	Dogs: due to an excess of cortisol production; most often associated with hyperadrenocorticism. Cats: mechanism unknown. See Adenocarcinoma, Pancreas, and Hyperadrenocorticism (Cushing's Disease)
Cachexia	Many	Many	Severe metabolic derangements likely caused by cytokines and hormones (e.g., tumor necrosis factor, interferons, interleukins, insulin, growth hormone; may result from alterations in lipid, protein, and carbohydrate metabolism that create a net energy loss in spite of adequate caloric intake; anaerobic metabolic pathways of cancer cells may play a role in some cases, other causes of cachexia in cancer patients include bowel obstruction, inappetence, malabsorption, maldigestion, and external nutrient loss in effusion, urine, or exudates See Weight Loss and Cachexia
Cutaneous flushing syndrome	Pheochromocytoma; mast cell tumor	Not reported	Inappropriate release of vasoactive substances, such as histamine, causes paroxysmal flushing of the skin
Disseminated intravascular coagulation	Hemangiosarcoma; carcinoma; others	Myeloproliferative disease inflammatory	See Disseminated Intravascular Coagulation
Diencephalic syndrome	Astrocytoma	Not reported	Tumor is present in the diencephalon region of the brain; excess of growth hormone results in dramatic weight loss (without acromegaly) despite adequate caloric intake; other hypothalamic signs (e.g., adipsia, inability to maintain body temperature) may be observed
Eosinophilia	Fibrosarcoma; mammary carcinoma	Transitional cell carcinoma of urinary bladder; mast cell tumor; lymphosarcoma	May be due to stimulation of eosinophil precursors by products such as interleukin-2, -3, and -5 and granulocyte-macrophage colony-stimulating factor

PARANEOPLASTIC SYNDROMES

Fever	Many	Many	Involves resetting the hypothalamic "set point" by cytokines (e.g., interleukin-1, tumor necrosis factor, others that cause the local synthesis of prostaglandin [PGE$_2$] within the hypothalamus) that coordinate the autonomic, endocrine, and behavioral components of the febrile response See Fever
Gastroduodenal ulceration	Non–islet cell pancreatic neoplasia; mast cell tumor	Mast cell tumor	Inappropriate gastrin secretion (non–islet cell tumor) or excess histamine secretion (mast cell)
Immune complex disorders	Lymphocytic leukemia; primary erythrocytosis	Lymphosarcoma	Secondary to antigen-antibody–immune complex activation; glomerulonephritis is most recognized problem
Hypercalcemia	Lymphosarcoma; anal sac apocrine gland carcinoma; multiple myeloma; others	Lymphosarcoma; multiple myeloma; others	Dogs with lymphosarcoma and apocrine gland carcinoma: involves excess parathyroid hormone–related protein (PTHrP) Cats: mechanism unexplored See Hypercalcemia
Hypertrophic osteopathy	Metastatic and primary tumors of the lung	Metastatic and primary tumors of the lung	Characterized by rapid periosteal new bone growth in a nodular or smooth linear pattern on radiographs; precise mechanism is unknown, but partly involves the neural afferent stimulation and increased blood flow to the extremities; afferent impulses traveling in the vagus and intercostal nerves from the lesion to the CNS may initiate this syndrome
Hyperviscosity syndrome	Immunoglobulin-secreting tumor (e.g., multiple myeloma, lymphosarcoma)	Immunoglobulin-secreting tumor	Follows the accumulation of large immunoglobulin proteins or polymerized small immunoglobulin proteins in the blood that result in decreased blood flow from increased viscosity See Multiple Myeloma, Lymphosarcoma, and Paraproteinemia
Hypoglycemia	Insulinoma; benign and malignant smooth muscle tumors; large mesenchymal tumors	Insulinoma	Usually involves excessive glucose utilization or the excess production of insulin or insulin-like factors See Insulinoma
Myasthenia gravis	Thymoma; others	Mediastinal mass	Exact mechanism is unknown See Myasthenia Gravis
Myelofibrosis	Non–islet cell pancreatic tumors; lymphosarcoma; myelodysplastic syndromes	Myelodysplastic syndromes; feline leukemia virus infection	See Myelodysplastic Syndromes
Neutrophilic leukocytosis	Fibrosarcoma; others	Carcinoma	Production of a granulocyte-monocyte stimulating peptide is likely cause
Nodular dermatofibrosis	Renal cystadenocarcinoma in German shepherds	Not reported	Unknown, but involves proliferation of fibroblasts
Peripheral nerve syndromes	Various	Not reported	Unknown, but usually subclinical and secondary to changes in myelination
Polycythemia	Renal sarcoma and carcinoma; others	Not reported	Inappropriate secretion of erythropoietin or erythropoietin-like peptides See Polycythemia and Polycythemia Vera
Thrombocytopathy	Immunoglobulin-secreting tumors	Immunoglobulin-secreting tumors	Immunoglobulin molecules inhibit normal platelet aggregation See Thrombocytopathies
Thrombocytopenia	Hemangiosarcoma	Lymphosarcoma	Thrombocytopenia, primary immune mediated or secondary to myelophthisis See Thrombocytopenia
Thrombocytosis	Myeloproliferative disorders	Myeloproliferative disorders	Overproduction of cytokines that stimulate thrombopoietin production (e.g., interleukin-1,-3, -6, -11 See Thrombocytosis
Superficial necrolytic dermatitis (metabolic epidermal necrosis, hepatocutaneous syndrome, necrolytic migratory erythema)	Hepatic neoplasia; pancreatic neoplasia	Pancreatic neoplasia	Many names used to describe similar clinical entities; usually observed in patients with hepatic disease and less commonly with glucagon-secreting pancreatic tumors; sometimes referred to as glucagonoma syndrome; exact mechanism is unclear but may be due to the catabolic effects of glucagons on keratinocyte metabolism, abnormal zinc metabolism, or aberrant fatty acid metabolism; may see associated glucose intolerance or diabetes mellitus

PARAPHIMOSIS AND PHIMOSIS

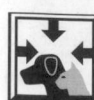

BASICS

OVERVIEW
• Phimosis—inability to protrude the penis beyond the preputial orifice
• Paraphimosis—penis protrudes from the preputial orifice and cannot be returned to its normal position
• Priapism—prolonged extrusion of an erect penis not associated with sexual arousal; can result from excessive parasympathetic stimulation or decreased venous outflow from the corpus cavernosum penis; relatively rare condition in dogs and cats

SIGNALMENT
• Dogs and cats
• German shepherds and golden retrievers—observed congenital preputial stenosis, possibly hereditary
• Siamese cats—one report noted 6 of 7 cases of priapism were in Siamese cats.

SIGNS
• Phimosis—may be undetected until patient is unsuccessful in attempts to copulate; severe defects in the neonate interfere with urination; may cause pooling of urine in preputial cavity, which may cause balanoposthitis, leading to septicemia
• Paraphimosis—short duration: only sign may be licking of an exteriorized penis; after some hours of exposure: may see ischemic necrosis and urethral obstruction; edema and swelling may make differentiation from priapism difficult

CAUSES & RISK FACTORS
• Phimosis—caused by an abnormally small preputial orifice; may be congenital or acquired (e.g., caused by injury or disease); may be associated with a persistent penile or preputial frenulum, a thin band of connective tissue joining the penis and prepuce along the ventral glans
• Paraphimosis—usually associated with erection and/or copulation; hair surrounding the preputial orifice is trapped against the surface of the penis, especially the bulbus glandis, preventing retraction; moderately stenotic preputial orifice may contribute; injuries; os penis fractures; neurological disease (encephalomyelitis, intervertebral disk disease); balanoposthitis; penile swelling (neoplasia, strangulation with foreign body)
• Priapism—cause often unknown; trauma during mating; chronic distemper encephalomyelitis; penile thromboembolism; amphetamine use

DIAGNOSIS

DIFFERENTIAL DIAGNOSIS
Paraphimosis—exposure of the glans penis caused by abnormality of the retractor penis muscles or preputial muscles, large preputial opening, short prepuce, or priapism

CBC/BIOCHEMISTRY/URINALYSIS
• Usually normal
• Phimosis in neonates—may note severe balanoposthitis and evidence of septicemia (e.g., leukocytosis, neutrophilia progressing to neutropenia, positive urine cultures)

OTHER LABORATORY TESTS
N/A

IMAGING
N/A

DIAGNOSTIC PROCEDURES
N/A

TREATMENT

Phimosis
• Surgical enlargement of the preputial orifice
• Persistent penile frenulum (dogs)—remove the band of tissue holding the glans penis to the parietal lamina of prepuce

Paraphimosis
• Requires immediate treatment—after 24 hr, tissue damage and urethral obstruction may necessitate penile amputation; goal is to replace the penis in a normal position
• Indwelling urinary catheter—if urethral patency is in question
• Remove foreign objects
• Lubricate the penis
• Apply compresses of hypertonic glucose solutions
• Surgically enlarge the preputial orifice, if necessary
• Castration is not effective; paraphimosis is not a testosterone-dependent disease

Priapism
• Identifying the underlying cause is often not possible before ischemia of the penis occurs; penile amputation and perineal urethrostomy usually required due to irreparable ischemic necrosis of the penis; castration is not effective

• Penile amputation and perineal urethrostomy—indicated for cats with difficulty urinating
• Abdominal compression bandage and indwelling urinary catheter—maintain the penis within the prepuce; may also reduce localized edema

MEDICATIONS

DRUG(S)
Antibiotic ointments—maintain treatment; prevent adhesions between the penis and prepuce

CONTRAINDICATIONS/POSSIBLE INTERACTIONS
N/A

FOLLOW-UP

EXPECTED COURSE AND PROGNOSIS
• Phimosis—fair to good if identified prior to development of septicemia
• Paraphimosis and priapism—guarded to poor for return to breeding activity; fair to good for life with early successful medical management or penile amputation with perineal urethrostomy

MISCELLANEOUS

Suggested Reading
Burke TJ. Small animal reproduction and infertility. Philadelphia: Lea & Febiger, 1986.
Feldman EC, Nelson RW. Canine and feline endocrinology and reproduction. Philadelphia: Saunders, 1987:692–693.
Gunn-Moore DA, Brown PJ, Holt PE, Gruffydd-Jones T. Priapism in seven cats. J Sm Anim Pract 1995;36:262–266.
Johnston SD, Root Kustritz MV, Olson PNS. Disorders of the canine penis and prepuce. In: Canine and feline theriogenology. Philadelphia: Saunders, 2001:356–367.
Johnston SD, Root Kustritz MV, Olson PNS. Disorders of the feline penis and prepuce. In: Canine and feline theriogenology. Philadelphia: Saunders, 2001:539–543.
Authors Carlos R. F. Pinto and Rolf E. Larsen
Consulting Editor Sara K. Lyle

BASICS

OVERVIEW
• The presence in the blood of an abnormal protein (paraprotein or M component) produced by a single clone of cells. The paraprotein may be composed of whole immunoglobulin molecules, subunits, light chains, or heavy chains. This disorder is commonly seen with plasma cell neoplasms, such as multiple myeloma, or other lymphoproliferative diseases, such as CLL or lymphoma. • Primary signs are related to the underlying neoplasm and could be related to bony invasion or bone marrow infiltration. • Markedly elevated serum paraprotein levels can produce signs of HVS.

SYSTEMS AFFECTED
• Musculoskeletal—bone lysis by the neoplastic cells can cause lameness and pathologic fractures • Nervous—bony lysis of the vertebrae can cause neurologic signs; disorientation, seizures, cranial nerve deficits, or vestibular signs may be associated with HVS • Hemic/lymph/immune—myelophthisis may cause anemia, leukopenia, or thrombocytopenia: hemostasis may be compromised by paraprotein interference with platelet and coagulation factor function; decreased normal immunoglobulin levels increase susceptibility to infection • Ophthalmic—HVS can cause retinal detachment or retinal hemorrhage • Cardiovascular—HVS can cause tachycardia or a gallop rhythm • Renal/urologic—renal failure is possible secondary to tumor infiltration, HVS causing renal hypoxia, proteinuria, hypercalcemia of malignancy, or infection

SIGNALMENT
• Dogs—middle aged to older • Cats (rare)—older • No sex predilection

SIGNS
• Lethargy and weakness • Lameness • Epistaxis or gingival bleeding • Petechiae or ecchymoses • Blindness or retinal hemorrhage • Polyuria and polydipsia • Seizures or dementia

CAUSES & RISK FACTORS
• Factors contributing to multiple myeloma—genetic predisposition, viral infections, chronic immune stimulation, and exposure to carcinogens have all been suggested • Dogs living in industrial areas or exposed to chemicals such as paints or solvents appear to be at higher risk for lymphoma. • Feline leukemia virus causes lymphosarcoma in cats.

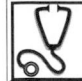 DIAGNOSIS

DIFFERENTIAL DIAGNOSIS
• Other causes of monoclonal gammopathy—ehrlichiosis, leishmaniasis, chronic inflammatory processes (e.g., pyoderma), amyloidosis, plasmacytic gastroenteritis, and FIP • Other causes of polyclonal gammopathy—systemic mycoses, hemoparasitic infections, FIP, chronic autoimmune disease, and neoplasms (lymphoma, mast cell tumor) • Bleeding—in most cases, due to paraproteinemia and thrombocytopenia; other possibilities: paraneoplastic autoimmune immune-mediated thrombocytopenia/pathia and vasculitis • HVS—see Hyperviscosity Syndrome

CBC/BIOCHEMISTRY/URINALYSIS
• Anemia/leukopenia/thrombocytopenia—secondary to myelophthisis or autoimmune mechanisms; marked lymphocytosis associated with CLL or lymphoma within the bone marrow • Total protein and globulin—elevated • Albumin—may be low • Calcium—may be high secondary to malignancy, renal failure, or bony lysis • Urea and creatinine—may be elevated secondary to primary renal azotemia • Proteinuria—caused by light chains (i.e., Bence Jones protein); not detected on routine test; immunoassay or electrophoresis on the urine sample is much more likely to detect Bence Jones protein

OTHER LABORATORY TESTS
• Protein electrophoresis—to identify a monoclonal spike • Immunoelectrophoresis—helps to define the type of gammopathy (i.e., IgG, IgA, or IgM) • Viscosimetry—may help define HVS • Serology for *Ehrlichia* or FCoV

IMAGING
• Radiology of affected bones—to identify a potential site to aspirate or biopsy • Skeletal survey or bone scan—to define extent of lytic lesions • Thoracic and abdominal radiography or abdominal ultrasonography—for evidence of enlarged lymph nodes or organomegaly suggestive of lymphoma

OTHER DIAGNOSTIC PROCEDURES
• Bone marrow aspiration/biopsy—plasma cells > 5% consistent with multiple myeloma; myelophthisis associated with other lymphoproliferative diseases • Bone biopsy of lytic lesion—rarely required to diagnose multiple myeloma • Lymph node aspiration—to identify neoplastic population of lymphocytes with lymphoma; to identify amastigotes of *Leishmania* or morulae of *Ehrlichia* • Organ cytology or histopathology—for neoplastic populations of cells, infectious agents (e.g., immunofluorescence for FCoV

in macrophages), or amyloid; note: coagulopathies may prevent invasive diagnostics

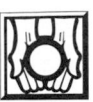 TREATMENT
• Supportive care depending on the manifestation of disease and the organ systems affected • HVS—see Hyperviscosity Syndrome • Chemotherapy for neoplastic processes, such as multiple myeloma, CLL, or lymphoma

 MEDICATIONS

DRUG(S)
• Antibiotics for infections secondary to immunocompromise • See specific diseases for specific drugs.

 FOLLOW-UP
• See specific diseases • Electrophoresis may be monitored as an indication of response to therapy.

 MISCELLANEOUS

ASSOCIATED CONDITIONS
Immunologic incompetence

AGE-RELATED FACTORS
None

SYNONYMS
• Monoclonal gammopathy • M protein

SEE ALSO
• Hyperviscosity Syndrome
• Lymphosarcoma—Cats
• Lymphosarcoma—Dogs
• Multiple Myeloma

ABBREVIATIONS
• CLL = chronic lymphocytic leukemia
• FCoV = feline coronavirus
• FIP = feline infectious peritonitis
• HVS = hyperviscosity syndrome

Suggested Reading

Hohenhaus AE. Syndromes of hyperglobulinemia: diagnosis and therapy. In: Bonagura JD, Kirk RW, eds. Kirk's current veterinary therapy XII. Philadelphia: Saunders, 1995:523–530.

Vail DM. Plasma cell neoplasms. In: Withrow SJ, MacEwen EG, eds. Small animal clinical oncology. Philadelphia: Saunders, 2001: 626–638.

Author Julie Armstrong
Consulting Editor Stephen Kruth

PATELLAR LUXATION

 BASICS

DEFINITION
Medial or lateral displacement of the patella from its normal anatomic position in the femoral trochlea

PATHOPHYSIOLOGY
• May be mild to severe; different degrees of clinical and pathologic changes; classified into grades I–IV
• Common musculoskeletal changes—tibial rotation on its long axis; bowing of the distal and proximal tibia; shallow to absent femoral trochlea; dysplasia of the femoral and tibial epiphysis; displacement of the quadriceps muscle group

SYSTEMS AFFECTED
Musculoskeletal

GENETICS
• Recessive, polygenic, and multifocal inheritances proposed
• Hereditary factor in Devon rex cats

INCIDENCE/PREVALENCE
• One of the most common stifle joint abnormalities in dogs
• Medial—> 75% of cases
• Bilateral involvement—50% of cases
• Uncommon in cats, but may be more common than suspected because most affected cats are not lame

GEOGRAPHIC DISTRIBUTION
N/A

SIGNALMENT
Species
• Predominantly dogs
• Rarely cats

Breed Predilections
• Most common in toy and miniature dog breeds
• Dogs—miniature and toy poodles; Yorkshire terriers; Pomeranians; Pekingese; Chihuahuas; Boston terriers

Mean Age and Range
Clinical signs—may develop soon after birth; generally after 4 months of age

Predominant Sex
Risk for females 1.5 times that for males

SIGNS
General Comments
Depend on grade (severity), amount of degenerative arthritis, chronicity of disease, and occurrence of other stifle joint abnormalities (e.g., cruciate ligament rupture)

Historical Findings
• Persistent abnormal hindlimb carriage and function in neonates and puppies
• Occasional skipping or intermittent hindlimb lameness—worsens in young to mature dogs
• Sudden signs of lameness—owing to minor trauma or worsening DJD in mature animals

Physical Examination Findings
• Grade I—patella can be manually luxated; patella reduces when pressure is released.
• Grade II—patella can be manually luxated or can spontaneously luxate with flexion of the stifle joint; patella remains luxated until it is manually reduced or the patient extends the joint and derotates the tibia in the opposite direction of luxation.
• Grades I and II—patient intermittently carries the affected limb with the stifle joint flexed.
• Grade III—patella remains luxated most of the time but can be manually reduced with the stifle joint in extension; flexion and extension of the stifle joint result in reluxation of the patella.
• Grade IV—patella is permanently luxated and cannot be manually repositioned; may be up to 90° of rotation of the proximal tibial plateau; shallow or missing femoral trochlea; displacement of quadriceps muscle group in the direction of luxation
• Grades III and IV—crouching, bowlegged (genu varum) or knock-kneed (genu valgum) stance for medial or lateral luxations, respectively; most of the body weight is transferred to the front limbs.
• Pain—may be elicited with chondromalacia of the patella or femoral trochlea

CAUSES
• Congenital
• Traumatic

RISK FACTORS
• Coxa vara—decreased femoral neck–femoral shaft axis; associated with medial luxation
• Coxa valga—increased femoral neck–femoral shaft axis; associated with lateral luxation
• Excessive anteversion—forward inclination of the femoral head and neck

 DIAGNOSIS

DIFFERENTIAL DIAGNOSIS
• Cranial cruciate ligament rupture—distinguished by palpation of cranial drawer motion; concurrent in 15%–20% of cases
• Avulsion fracture of the tibial tubercle—causes laxity of the quadriceps mechanism; results in patellar instability
• Rupture of the patellar tendon—causes proximal displacement of the patella and instability
• Malunion and malalignment of fractures of the femur or tibia—may result in displacement of the quadriceps muscle group
• Craniodorsal hip luxation—often concurrent with grade I luxation owing to laxity of the quadriceps muscle group; laxity spontaneously resolves after reduction of the hip luxation.

CBC/BIOCHEMISTRY/URINALYSIS
N/A

OTHER LABORATORY TESTS
N/A

IMAGING
• Craniocaudal and mediolateral radiographs of the stifle joint—indicated for all grade III and IV luxations; include the joint above (hip) and below (hock) to detect bowing and/or torsion of the femur and tibia.
• Skyline radiographs of the femoral trochlea—help determine its shape (shallow, flattened, or convex)

DIAGNOSTIC PROCEDURES
Arthrocentesis and synovial fluid analysis—slightly increase in mononuclear cells (generally < 2000 cells/mL)

PATHOLOGIC FINDINGS
• Gross—cartilage wear lesions of the patella and femoral trochlea; osteophytes at the joint capsule–bone interface; joint capsule redundancy on the side opposite of luxation; fibrosis and contracture on the side of luxation
• Microscopic—cartilage fibrillation and loss of glycosaminoglycan content; synovitis

TREATMENT

APPROPRIATE HEALTH CARE
• Outpatient—all grade I and some grade II luxations
• Inpatient (surgery)—most grade II and all grade III and IV luxations

NURSING CARE
• Cryotherapy (ice packing)—initiated immediately after surgery; 15–20 min every 8 hr for 3–5 days
• Range-of-motion exercises of the stifle joint—as soon as tolerated

ACTIVITY
Normal to restricted, depending on severity

DIET
Weight control—important for decreasing the load and, therefore, stress on the stifle joint

CLIENT EDUCATION
• Discuss the heritability of the condition.
• Warn client of the possibility of DJD development.
• Inform client of the increased risk of cranial cruciate ligament disease.
• Warn client that the condition could worsen over time (e.g., from grade I to grade II).

SURGICAL CONSIDERATIONS
• Bone deformity (e.g., shallow trochlea or tibial tubercle deviation)—requires surgical bone reconstruction; assumed in all grade II or higher luxations
• Trochleoplasty—arthroplastic procedure; deepen trochlear sulcus
• Trochlear sulcoplasty—curettage technique; remove hyaline cartilage and cancellous bone to deepen the sulcus; fibrocartilage eventually resurfaces the trochlea.
• Recession sulcoplasty—taco shell technique; remove a V-shaped wedge; preserves the hyaline cartilage; after the trochlea is deepened, the osteochondral bone wedge is replaced; creates a new sulcus composed of hyaline cartilage; preferred technique for most patients
• Trochlear chondroplasty—cartilage flap technique; useful only in young patients (< 6 months); create a distally based cartilage flap; remove subchondral bone beneath it; replace flap to line the new sulcus; preserves hyaline cartilage to cover the bottom of the sulcus; fibrocartilage covers the sides.
• Transposition of the tibial tubercle—realign the longitudinal axis of the quadriceps

mechanism so that it is centered over the femoral trochlea; osteotomize the tibia tubercle, transpose it opposite the direction of luxation, and stabilize it with pins and a tension band wire.
• Imbrication of the joint capsule and supporting soft tissues on the side opposite the luxation—helps pull the patella over
• Desmotomy or releasing incision—made on the side toward which the patella is luxated
• Patellar and tibial antirotational suture ligaments—reinforce stretched supporting soft tissue structures
• Corrective osteotomy—realigns the longitudinal axis of the hindlimb; generally indicated in only grade III and IV luxations

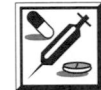

MEDICATIONS

DRUG(S) OF CHOICE
NSAIDs—minimize pain; decrease inflammation; may try buffered or enteric-coated aspirin (10–25 mg/kg PO q8–12h), carprofen (2.2 mg/kg PO q12h), etodolac (10–15 mg/kg PO once daily), phenylbutazone (3–7 mg/kg PO q8h, total dose < 800 mg/day), meclofenamic acid (0.5 mg/kg PO q12h), or piroxicam (0.3 mg/kg PO q24h for 3 days, then q48h), or deracoxib (3–4 mg/kg PO q24h for 7 days for postoperative pain) (1–2 mg/kg PO q24h for long-term treatment over 7 days)

CONTRAINDICATIONS
Avoid corticosteroids because of potential side effects and articular cartilage damage associated with long-term use.

PRECAUTIONS
NSAIDs—gastrointestinal irritation may preclude their use.

POSSIBLE INTERACTIONS
N/A

ALTERNATIVE DRUG(S)
Chondroprotective drugs (e.g., polysulfated glycosaminoglycans, glucosamine, and chondroitin sulfate)—may help limit cartilage damage and degeneration

FOLLOW-UP

PATIENT MONITORING
• Post-trochleoplasty—encourage early, active use of the limb.
• Limit exercise for 4 weeks; prevent jumping.

• Onset of an acute non–weight-bearing lameness—may indicate cranial cruciate ligament disease
• Yearly examinations—to assess progression

PREVENTION/AVOIDANCE
• Discourage breeding of affected animals.
• Do not repeat dam–sire breedings that result in affected offspring.

POSSIBLE COMPLICATIONS
Recurrence after surgical stabilization—reported to be as high as 48%; usually of a lower grade than the original luxation

EXPECTED COURSE AND PROGNOSIS
• With surgical treatment—> 90% of patients are free from lameness and clinical dysfunction.
• DJD—radiographic evidence in almost all affected stifle joints

MISCELLANEOUS

ASSOCIATED CONDITIONS
Cranial cruciate ligament disease

AGE-RELATED FACTORS
N/A

ZOONOTIC POTENTIAL
N/A

PREGNANCY
N/A

SEE ALSO
Arthritis (Osteoarthritis)

ABBREVIATIONS
DJD = degenerative joint disease
NSAIDs = nonsteroidal antiinflammatory drugs

Suggested Reading
Arnoczky S, Tarvin G. Surgical repair of patella luxations and fractures. In: Bojrab MJ, ed. Current techniques in small animal surgery. 4th ed. Philadelphia: Lea & Febiger, 1998:1237–1244.
Brinker WO, Piermattei DL, Flo GL. Patellar luxations. In: Brinker WO, Piermattei DL, Flo GL, eds. Handbook of small animal orthopedics and fracture repair. 3rd ed. Philadelphia, Saunders, 1997:516–534.
Slocum B, Slocum TD. Patella luxation. In: Bojrab MJ, ed. Current techniques in small animal surgery. 4th ed. Philadelphia: Lea & Febiger, 1998:1222–1236.
Willauer C, Vasseur P. Clinical results of surgical correction of medial luxation of the patella in dogs. Vet Surg 1987;16:31–36.
Author Peter D. Schwarz
Consulting Editor Peter K. Shires

PATENT DUCTUS ARTERIOSUS

 BASICS

DEFINITION
Persistent patency of the fetal ductus arteriosus connecting the descending aorta to the pulmonary artery

PATHOPHYSIOLOGY
Flow across a PDA is typically from the aorta to pulmonary artery (left to right). The hemodynamic consequences depend on the magnitude of the shunt, the pulmonary vascular resistance, and intercurrent heart defects. Small shunt volumes are well tolerated; moderate-to-large shunt volumes cause left-sided CHF from volume overload. Much less frequently, a large-diameter PDA causes pulmonary vascular injury, high pulmonary vascular resistance, pulmonary hypertension, and reversal of the shunt (Eisenmenger's physiology or "reversed" PDA), with bidirectional shunting across the PDA. Patients affected with right-to-left shunting suffer from arterial desaturation and hypoxia-triggered polycythemia.

SYSTEMS AFFECTED
• Cardiovascular—volume overload (left-to-right shunt) or pulmonary vascular disease and polycythemia (right-to-left shunt) • Respiratory—if pulmonary edema develops • Hemic/Lymph/Immune—if polycythemia develops

GENETICS
Genetically transmitted (polygenic model) defect in many canine breeds, including the miniature poodle, collie, Maltese, Shetland sheepdog, German shepherd, cocker spaniel, Pomeranian, and Labrador retriever

INCIDENCE/PREVALENCE
Second most common congenital heart defect in dogs; prevalence estimated to be 6.5–8 cases per 1000 live births. Very uncommon malformation in cats

SIGNALMENT
Species Dogs and cats

Breed Predilections See genetics

Mean Age and Range
• Vast majority identified during the initial vaccination sequence • Onset of signs related to CHF—weeks to many years

Predominant Sex
Dogs—females predisposed

SIGNS
General Comments
• Onset of reversed PDA—quite sudden in dogs (usually before 4 months of age); can develop more gradually in cats • No significant documentation that shunt reversal begins after 6 months of age, but signs related to reversed shunting may be overlooked; onset of related problems has been reported in dogs older than 5 years of age.

Historical Findings
• Respiratory distress, coughing, exercise intolerance • Stunted growth • Right-to-left shunting PDA—exertional rear limb weakness and complications of polycythemia and hyperviscosity (seizures or sudden death related to arrhythmias or right to left embolus) • Signs usually precipitated by exercise

Physical Examination Findings
• Typically, continuous, machinery-type murmur loudest over pulmonary artery at the left craniodorsal cardiac base; localized in some dogs; murmur may be loud over the manubrium sterni in small dogs; often a concurrent systolic murmur of mitral regurgitation at the left apex. The murmur in cats or in puppies < 6 weeks of age may not be obviously continuous, but more resemble a long systolic and early diastolic murmur. • Loud murmurs—associated with a palpable precordial thrill • Arterial pulses—hyperkinetic ("waterhammer") • Caudoventral displacement of the ventricular apex • Tachypnea, respiratory distress, and inspiratory crackles—may indicate left-sided CHF • Rapid, irregular cardiac rhythm with variable-intensity arterial pulses if atrial fibrillation develops • In right-to-left shunting ("reversed") PDA findings differ—no continuous murmur, normal arterial pulses, and a prominent right ventricular impulse; may be a systolic ejection murmur and a tympanic, or split, second heart sound; may be a prominent jugular pulse • Classic feature of right-to-left shunting PDA is differential cyanosis: pink cranial, but cyanotic caudal, mucous membranes; in severe secondary polycythemia, the cranial mucous membranes may also be cyanotic.

CAUSES
Genetically predisposed in most cases

RISK FACTORS
Genetic predisposition in dogs; risk factors in cats are unknown.

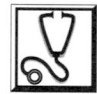 DIAGNOSIS

DIFFERENTIAL DIAGNOSIS
• Principal auscultatory differentials are congenital aortic stenosis with aortic insufficiency (to-and-fro systolic/diastolic murmur) and ventricular septal defect with aortic valve prolapse into the defect (causing both systolic and diastolic murmurs). • Very rare causes of continuous murmurs—arteriovenous fistula of the lung or related to thyroid neoplasia, aorticopulmonary communication, rupture of the aorta into the right atrium or right ventricle, and coronary artery fistula
• Simplified by Doppler echocardiography

CBC/BIOCHEMISTRY/URINALYSIS
Usually normal unless right-to-left shunting; then may be variable degrees of polycythemia (PCV 58–80%)

OTHER BLOOD TESTS
Reversed PDA—low femoral arterial pO_2; comparable to a pO_2 obtained by careful puncture of the carotid or brachial artery using a 25-gauge needle. Pulse oximetry of the cranial membranes compared to the rectum may document the disparity in hemoglobin saturations.

IMAGING
Thoracic Radiographic Findings
• Lateral projection—variable degrees of left heart enlargement; typically pulmonary over-circulation; frequently the lobar pulmonary veins are larger than the attendant arteries, related to high left atrial pressure or incipient heart failure • Dorsoventral view (preferable to accentuate the aorta) demonstrates cardiac elongation (left ventricular enlargement), left auricular enlargement, and dilation of the descending aorta (called a "ductus bump"); the main pulmonary artery is dilated. • Left-sided CHF—evident as distended pulmonary veins, increased interstitial/alveolar densities • Reversed PDA—heart usually normal sized, but the contour of the right cardiac border is more prominent on the DV view, and the pulmonary circulation appears normal to reduced; the main pulmonary artery and proximal lobar branches are dilated; a ductus bump generally is seen on the DV view.

Echocardiographic Findings
• Left atrium, left ventricle, and main pulmonary artery are dilated; right ventricle is normal, except in cats in which it is more likely to be hypertrophied to varying degrees; the ductal ampulla and the distal ductus can generally be imaged from the left cranial hemithorax. • Left ventricular systolic function (shortening fraction) is normal to reduced; may be markedly decreased in larger dogs with long-standing PDA • Doppler studies demonstrate continuous flow into the main pulmonary artery (from the ductus); often concurrent pulmonary insufficiency, related to dilation of the pulmonary artery and mitral regurgitation caused by left-sided cardiac dilatation; transmitral flow velocity and transaortic flow velocity are high because of increased volume and left atrial pressure; aortic velocities can be augmented substantially (up to 2.5–3.0 m/sec), mimicking findings of mild subvalvular aortic stenosis. • Right-to-left shunting PDA—small left heart chambers, right atrial dilation, right ventricular hypertrophy, and dilation of the main and branch pulmonary arteries; contrast echocardiography is useful to confirm the diagnosis; inject saline in the cephalic vein while imaging the abdominal aorta.

Angiographic Findings
• Echocardiography has completely supplanted angiography for the diagnosis. • Angiographic demarcation is useful during interventional procedures such as coil occlusion of the ductus; injection of contrast material into the descend-

ing aorta demonstrates whether the ductus is tapered or short and wide, information crucial to catheter-occlusion techniques.

DIAGNOSTIC PROCEDURES

Electrocardiography
• ECG—rarely needed for diagnosis of PDA; used to diagnose auscultable arrhythmias
• Atrial fibrillation—observed infrequently, related to marked dilatation of the left atrium
• Typical abnormalities include widened P waves (atrial enlargement) and increased-amplitude QRS complexes in the left caudal leads (II, aVF, III) and left precordial leads.

PATHOLOGIC FINDINGS
• Necropsy findings in left-to-right shunting PDA include pulmonary edema, cardiomegaly (left sided), and dilation of the aorta and pulmonary artery. • Right-to-left shunting PDA—right ventricular hypertrophy, dilation of the pulmonary artery, and prominent bronchial arteries; ductal diameter is invariably very wide, generally approaching that of the descending aorta. Pulmonary arterioles are thick; there may be necrotizing arteritis.

 TREATMENT

APPROPRIATE HEALTH CARE
• Manage pulmonary edema with furosemide and, if necessary, oxygen and cage rest; following stabilization, occlude the PDA promptly. • Can schedule stable animals for elective surgery; but do not delay procedure; asymptomatic dogs as young as 7–8 weeks of age show no higher operative mortality than older dogs. • Dogs with polycythemia caused by right-to-left shunting PDA—periodic phlebotomy to maintain the PCV < 65% (typically 62–65%).

DIET
Normal; but restricted sodium intake if CHF.

CLIENT EDUCATION
• Surgery—do not delay; mortality is higher and left ventricular function impaired if clinical signs develop. Following successful surgery and a 2-week convalescence, the dog can be treated normally.

SURGICAL CONSIDERATIONS
• Surgery can generally proceed within 24–48 h of medical stabilization. • Standard therapy involves ductal ligation via left thoracotomy; surgical and perioperative mortality should be < 8% for all cases. • Catheter-delivered occlusion devices, including thrombogenic Gianturco coils that can occlude the ductus in some animals • Never correct right-to-left PDA surgically; the right ventricle will not be able to eject against the pulmonary vascular resistance without the "pop-off" of the PDA.

 MEDICATIONS

DRUG(S) OF CHOICE
• Treat pulmonary edema with furosemide (2–4 mg/kg q6–12h PO, SQ, IM, or IV as required); can be discontinued when the PDA is closed • When surgery is not an option—prescribe furosemide, enalapril (0.5 mg/kg q12–24h PO), and digoxin (0.005 mg/kg q12h PO) to control CHF. • To control severe, life-threatening CHF—can use direct vasodilators such as hydralazine (1–2 mg/kg q12h PO) or sodium nitroprusside (1–5 μg/kg/min)

CONTRAINDICATIONS
• In left-to-right PDA—drugs that increase systemic vascular resistance and arterial blood pressure, except as needed for anesthesia and surgery • In right-to-left PDA—drugs that lead to systemic arterial vasodilation and reduce systemic arterial blood pressure

PRECAUTIONS
• Measure digoxin levels. • Monitor arterial blood pressure, renal function, and serum electrolytes to identify problems related to diuretic and vasodilator therapies.

ALTERNATIVE DRUG(S)
• Prostaglandin inhibitors (e.g., indomethacin) do *not* close PDAs effectively in dogs.
• Consider hydroxyurea to treat severe polycythemia unresponsive to phlebotomy; consult a specialist regarding use. Some dogs experience side-effects of hydroxyurea requiring discontinuation of treatment. The drug is not always effective.

 FOLLOW-UP

PATIENT MONITORING
• Pain management is appropriate and also shortens the recovery time. Consider a fentanyl patch, placed 8–12 hours before anesthetic induction. Instill local anesthetic in the surgical wound prior to closure. Post-operatively administer opiates to control pain for at least 24–48 hr. • Postoperative—vital signs and dyspnea related to pneumothorax indicated postoperatively; provide analgesics for 24–48 hr. • Cardiac auscultation postoperatively and at suture removal; if sounds are normal, no further follow-up or diagnostic studies required. • Persistent, continuous murmur indicates either incomplete closure of the ductus, recannulization (rule out infection), or a concurrent cardiac defect. Systolic murmurs variably heard postoperatively should abate by time of suture removal. Reinvestigate unexpected murmurs by Doppler echocardiography. When only partial ligation at surgery, consider referral to a cardiologist for coil occlusion. • Sudden illness, fever, or acute respiratory signs postoperatively—consider

bacterial infection of the ligation site and recannulization of the ductus with hematogenous pneumonia; aggressive antibiotic therapy needed; consult surgical specialist or cardiologist

PREVENTION/AVOIDANCE
Do not breed affected animals.

POSSIBLE COMPLICATIONS
• Left-sided CHF • Cardiac arrhythmias
• Recannulization of the ductus
• Perioperative death (from torn ductus), bleeding, or infection • Pulmonary vascular disease with pulmonary hypertension, reversed shunting, exercise intolerance, and polycythemia • Pulmonary or systemic embolization from a dislodged coil; hemolysis from coil-induced RBC fragmentation

EXPECTED COURSE AND PROGNOSIS
• Infrequently dogs remain asymptomatic for life. Unless the defect is closed, approximately 50–60% of dogs die from CHF within 1 year of diagnosis. PDA in a dog > 3 years should be evaluated on a case-by-case basis with appropriate consultation as needed. • Surgery performed prior to onset of moderate-to-severe CHF—excellent; approximately 5–8% surgical/perioperative mortality • Moderate-to-severe CHF is related to either left ventricular myocardial failure or atrial fibrillation—guarded; referral to a specialist advised • Dogs with right-to-left shunting PDA can live for several years but often die suddenly; infrequently, dogs live beyond 5 years of age (especially cocker spaniels). • Cats—varies from rapidly progressive left-sided CHF to gradual development of pulmonary vascular disease; even right-sided CHF can develop in cats with PDA and pulmonary vascular disease.

 MISCELLANEOUS

ASSOCIATED CONDITIONS
Typically an isolated defect, but may occur in conjunction with other congenital heart lesions that are more likely in larger breeds.

PREGNANCY
Carries greater risk for CHF in pregnant bitches (and affected dogs should not be bred); offspring carry greater risk for large PDA or reversed shunting due to pulmonary vascular disease.

ABBREVIATIONS
• CHF = congestive heart failure • PCV = packed cell volume • PDA = patent ductus arteriosus

Suggested Reading
Bonagura JD, Lehmkuhl LB. Congenital heart disease. In: Fox PR, Sisson D, Moise NS. Textbook of canine and feline cardiology. Philadelphia: Saunders, 1999:471–535.
Author John D. Bonagura
Consulting Editors Tilley and Smith

PECTUS EXCAVATUM

 BASICS

OVERVIEW
• Deformity of the sternum and costal cartilages that results in a dorsal to ventral narrowing of the chest, primarily in the caudal aspect
• May note secondary abnormalities of respiratory and cardiovascular function from restriction of ventilation and cardiac compression
• Most cases are congenital.
• Concurrent cardiac defects common
• Speculated that upper respiratory obstruction at a young age may cause abnormal respiratory gradients and subsequent pectus excavatum
• Some patients demonstrate swimmer syndrome—neonatal dogs lack the ability to posture properly and remain in sternal recumbency, which may lead to invagination of the sternum.

SIGNALMENT
• Dogs and cats
• Brachycephalic breeds predisposed
• Most common age—4 weeks to 3 months

SIGNS
• Dyspnea
• Exercise intolerance
• Weight loss
• Hyperpnea
• Recurrent pulmonary infections
• Cough
• Vomiting
• Cyanosis
• Poor appetite
• Episodes of mild upper respiratory disease
• Thoracic defect—easily palpated or seen
• Respiratory problems—common; increased inspiratory effort; inspiratory stridor; moist rales (with infection)
• Cardiac murmurs associated with concurrent cardiac defects or compression of the heart common
• Heart sounds—often muffled, especially over the right hemithorax
• No correlation between severity of signs and the severity of anatomic or physiologic abnormalities
• Swimmer syndrome—possible; limbs not adducted properly; ambulation impaired

CAUSES & RISK FACTORS
• Genetic predisposition—may exist
• Puppies raised on surfaces causing poor footing may be predisposed to swimmer syndrome.
• Dogs predisposed to respiratory obstructive processes have a higher risk than others.

 DIAGNOSIS

DIFFERENTIAL DIAGNOSIS
• Numerous causes of dyspnea, cyanosis, hyperpnea, and cough
• Physical examination and radiographic evaluation—rule out the most common differentials.
• Tracheal malformations or collapse
• Cardiac disease
• Electric cord bite
• Hemothorax
• Pyothorax
• Pneumonia
• Allergic bronchitis
• Stenotic nares
• Elongated soft palate

CBC/BIOCHEMISTRY/URINALYSIS
N/A

OTHER LABORATORY TESTS
N/A

IMAGING
• Radiographs—confirm the diagnosis; readily reveal deformities that cause decreased thoracic volume; cardiac malposition common (heart shifted to the left of midline and sometimes cranially); may note cardiac

enlargement (may be artifact of malpositioning); may note evidence of concurrent disease in the lung fields; heart shadow shift to the left may expose the right hilus and encourage a diagnosis of pulmonary disease.
• Echocardiography—fully evaluate cardiac status; eliminate primary cardiac disease; detect possible concurrent cardiac defects.

DIAGNOSTIC PROCEDURES
N/A

TREATMENT
• Surgery—only available modality
• Decision to repair deformities—made on the basis of clinical signs
• Mild disease (only a flat chest)—patient may become normal without surgical intervention; try manual medial compression of the thorax by the owners or with a splint.
• Moderate or severe disease—surgical candidate; frontosagittal and vertebral indexes provide objective criteria for determining severity.
• Technique may be dictated by the age; young patient with a compliant sternum and ribs may do well with external coaptation; old patient with a less compliant thorax may need partial sternotomy.

• Surgery benefits patients with concurrent respiratory distress; benefits unknown with no respiratory distress but with moderate or severe deformity
• Asymptomatic patient may develop respiratory distress; patients with clinical signs of disease may show progression.
• Puppies with swimmer syndrome—place on surfaces with excellent footing; careful toggling of front and rear legs may improve adduction.
• Brachycephalic breeds with concurrent upper airway problems—may benefit from surgery directed at these problems

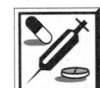

MEDICATIONS

DRUG(S)
Treat underlying or secondary medical conditions.

CONTRAINDICATIONS/POSSIBLE INTERACTIONS
Anesthesia—patients require constant monitoring; respiratory support should be available.

FOLLOW-UP
• Examinations—dictated by clinical signs or when surgical intervention has been precluded
• No specific actions for avoiding disease; genetic factors may sometimes be involved.
• Progression of respiratory signs—may develop in asymptomatic or mildly symptomatic patients
• Prognosis—guarded for all patients; depends on properly timed and expertly administered intervention

MISCELLANEOUS

ASSOCIATED CONDITIONS
• Cardiac defects
• Swimmer syndrome

Suggested Reading
Boudrieau RJ, Fossum TW, Hartsfield SM, et al. Pectus excavatum in dogs and cats. Compend Contin Educ Pract Vet 1990; 12:341–355.
Author Justin H. Straus
Consulting Editor Lynelle R. Johnson

PEDIATRIC BEHAVIOR PROBLEMS—CATS

 BASICS

DEFINITION

Undesirable behaviors exhibited by kittens between birth and puberty. Behaviors in this age range are particularly vulnerable to environmental influence, both physical and social. Behaviors acquired during this period may be difficult to ameliorate. Preventive measures, in the form of client education, are extremely important. For discussion of litter box problems, see Housesoiling—Cats.

PATHOPHYSIOLOGY

Most pediatric behavior problems are normal, species-typical behaviors. Pathophysiological substrates have not been identified for abnormal behaviors owing to lack of early experience, such as neophobia, defensive behaviors, and uninhibited play aggression.

SYSTEM AFFECTED

Behavioral

GENETICS

Possible paternal influences for fearfulness in kittens.

INCIDENCE/PREVALENCE

Unknown

GEOGRAPHIC DISTRIBUTION

Unknown

SIGNALMENT

Species: Cats

Breed Predilections: None

Mean Age and Range: Precise data unknown

Predominant Sex: None

SIGNS

General Comments

• Defensive behaviors include hiding, fleeing, and aggression. • Play is composed of components of other behavioral sequences, often predatory and intraspecific fighting. Play can be solitary, with objects, or social. Social play is often accompanied by signals that indicate the activity is play and not a "serious" encounter. The bites are inhibited and claws not fully extended. Play is modulated to accommodate the partner. If one partner escalates the intensity, the other usually follows suit. If play gets too rough, one partner may signal that the activity is too rough, e.g., vocalize, quit, or become defensively aggressive and inflict injury. Play directed towards people or other animals in the house may be unwelcome, either due to frequency or intensity.

Historical Findings

Fear and Defensive Behaviors Due to Lack of Early Experience
• No exposure to people between 3–7 weeks of age • Behaviors associated with fear, e.g., dilated pupils, piloerection, defensive postures, hissing, hiding, fleeing, aggression • Has always been afraid of people

Fear and Defensive Behaviors Related to Early Trauma
Normal until experienced traumatic event, e.g., abuse, attack by another animal

Fear and Defensive Behaviors Related to Correction Techniques
Normal until "corrected" by person, e.g., spanked, electric shock, hit on the nose, yelled at, or chased

Aggressive Play Directed Towards People
• Unsolicited attacks by kitten directed towards people • Inhibited bites, may indent the skin, and light scratches with claws. If skin soft or fragile, the wounds may break the skin. • If a person runs away, puts feet up, or tries to brush kitten away, the intensity of the play may increase. • No vocalizations • Generally starts as a kitten but may continue into adulthood. • Usually single kitten household • Often ritualized, occurring in same locations and same time of day. • Ambushes are common. • Often directed to specific persons.

Aggressive Play Directed Towards Other Cats in the Household
• Unsolicited attacks by kitten directed towards other cat • Other cat either runs and hides or responds by hissing, threatening, or seriously attacking kitten. • Other cat is usually over 10 years old.

Uninhibited Aggressive Play Directed Towards People
• Signs similar to normal aggressive play except more intense • Bites are not as inhibited and usually break the skin.

Normal Play Directed Towards Objects in the Household
• Bursts of solitary play that include intense running across household furnishings
• Shredding objects or propelling self along back underneath furniture • Knocks over objects and removes them from horizontal surfaces

Physical Examination Findings

Fear and Defensive Behaviors Due to Lack of Early Experience
• Extremely aroused and generally aggressive
• Behaviors associated with extreme fear

Other Listed Pediatric Problems
• Normal physical

CAUSES

Fear and Defensive Behaviors Due to Lack of Early Experience

Lack of exposure to people when between 3 and 7 weeks of age

Fear and Defensive Behaviors Related to Early Trauma

• Abuse • Attack by other animal • Sensitization to a stimulus due to exposure to extremely high intensity of the stimulus

Fear and Defensive Behaviors Related to Correction Techniques

Hitting, spanking, chasing, and yelling by people

Aggressive Play Directed Towards People or Other Cats in the Household

Normal species-typical behavior

Uninhibited Aggressive Play Directed Towards People

• Orphan-reared with no littermates or other cats to play with • Rough play encouraged by people • Teasing kitten

Normal Play Directed Towards Objects in the Household

Normal species-typical behavior

RISK FACTORS

Aggressive Play Directed Towards People or Other Cats in the Household

• The only young cat in the household
• The longer the delay before sufficient and appropriate exposure to people, the poorer the prognosis.

Uninhibited Aggressive Play Directed Towards People

• The longer the delay between 3 weeks of age and when an orphan-reared kitten experiences play with other kittens and/or cats, the more likely uninhibited aggressive play will occur.
• Adolescent or juvenile male human in household

Normal Play Directed Towards Objects in the Household

• Lack of environmental stimuli • No appropriate toys available • Little or no interactive play with people or other animals • Only kitten or pet in household

 DIAGNOSIS

DIFFERENTIAL DIAGNOSIS

Fearful and Defensive Behaviors

• Differentiate based on history or by testing with different stimuli. • Central nervous system diseases, e.g., infectious, toxic or neoplastic

Play Behaviors

• Often presented as "psychomotor epilepsy" by owners or referring professional

CBC/BIOCHEMISTRY/URINALYSIS

Extremely frightened kittens may have elevated corticosteroids, ACTH, and glucose levels.

OTHER LABORATORY TESTS N/A

IMAGING N/A

DIAGNOSTIC PROCEDURES N/A

 TREATMENT

APPROPRIATE HEALTH CARE

Outpatient

ACTIVITY

Many pediatric behavior problems can be alleviated or reduced by enriching the kitten's environment, e.g., provide movable toys, engage in interactive play, allow the kitten access to windows, don't shut in small, barren rooms.

DIET

Unknown

CLIENT EDUCATION

Fear and Defensive Behaviors Due to Lack of Early Experience

• Gradual exposure to people without forcing any interactions • In general, the kitten should be housed where it is comfortable, can remove itself from view but be continuously/very frequently aware of people. • Counterconditioning is also required. Initially, food can be put in or near the hiding area. Gradually the food is placed further from the hiding area and closer to where a person is stationary. No attempt should be made to grab the kitten. Eventually, several variables can be manipulated, depending on the intensity of the fear of the kitten. The food can be left progressively further from the hiding place while people engage in their normal activities. The food may eventually be placed on a person's lap. Toys on strings can be used to entice the kitten to play. Eventually the kitten may accept stroking, then holding. • Important principles to remember are to let the kitten make the advances—not the person—and avoid scaring the kitten. Frightened kittens can bite and scratch.

Fear and Defensive Behaviors Related to Early Trauma

• Identify the stimuli that elicit the fearful and/or defensive behaviors. • Employ behavior modification techniques similar to above. See section on behavior modification.

Fear and Defensive Behaviors Related to Correction Techniques

• Identify and cease inappropriate punitive behaviors of people. • Identify the stimuli that elicit the fearful and/or defensive behaviors. • Employ behavior modification techniques similar to above. See section on behavior modification.

Aggressive Play Directed Towards People

• The most effective treatment is to acquire an additional kitten of the same size and temperament. The kittens will play with each other, and attacks directed towards people should diminish. • Identify the circumstances in which the attacks occur and redirect the play to another object (e.g., string, ball). • Do not encourage escalation of play with evasive actions or mild aversive techniques. • Can use a startling stimulus as a punisher. Such a stimulus will not work unless it is paired with the act of attacking and used every time the kitten attacks and, in addition, the kitten will become afraid of the person. Possible startling stimuli are water, foghorns, compressed air, and citronella spray. • Do not hit, kick, or snap kitten on nose with fingers. Such actions frequently elicit an immediate serious aggressive response from kitten and/or induce residual fear and fear-induced aggression towards that person thereafter. • Interactive play with kitten using toys or objects that move • Frequent trimming of tips of claws helps reduce damage.

Aggressive Play Directed Towards Other Cats in the Household

• Acquire an additional kitten of the same size and temperament of the problem kitten. • If ac-

quiring another kitten is not an option, the problem kitten and older cat must have restricted access to each other. • Startling, punitive techniques would aversively affect the older cat.

Uninhibited Aggressive Play Directed Towards People

• Except for acquiring additional kitten, treatments would be similar to those used for normal aggressive play. The problem kitten might injure a second kitten. • Declawing is an option.

Normal Play Directed Towards Objects in the Household

• Put valuable, breakable, or dangerous objects away. • Provide appropriate toys for kitten. • Interactive play with kitten using toys or objects that move • Prohibit access to items. • "Booby-traps" or self-activated punishers might be used to keep kitten away from a few select objects or areas. Excessive use of such items might result in generalized anxiety. • Provide scratching posts. • Frequent trimming of tips of claws. Trimming kittens' nails is often most easily accomplished if the kitten is released for a few minutes between each nail nip. • Softclaws or beads applied to claws • Declawing is an option. Although there is some controversy about the humaneness of this procedure, several studies indicate that declawing is not psychologically harmful to cats.

MEDICATIONS

DRUG(S) None

CONTRAINDICATIONS N/A

PRECAUTIONS N/A

POSSIBLE INTERACTIONS N/A

FOLLOW-UP

PATIENT MONITORING

• Two, 12 and 26 weeks after the initial consultation, re-check by phone or during subsequent visits. • Be sure clients are not inappropriately applying aversive techniques. Such procedures may induce fear and aggression in the kitten.

PREVENTION/AVOIDANCE

• Kitten behavior problems can be prevented. • Between 3 and 7 weeks of age, kittens should experience positive interactions with people. • Clients with children in the household should specifically be advised to prohibit roughhouse play with kittens. • Provide education in the form of verbal advice, pamphlets, videos, books, or lists thereof at routine office visits or special kitten appointments.

POSSIBLE COMPLICATIONS

Clients apply punitive techniques that result in fear, anxiety, and defensive aggression in the kitten.

EXPECTED COURSE AND PROGNOSIS

Fear and Defensive Behaviors Due to Lack of Early Experience or Related to Early Trauma

• It may take months, or even years, to acclimate the kitten to people; kittens will vary in the degree to which they acclimate; some kittens may never be comfortable around people. • If clients report no improvement, it may be that they are inadvertently reinforcing escape and defense behaviors by advancing towards the kitten. • The longer the interval between 3 weeks of age and lack of exposure to people, the poorer the prognosis. • The more intense the early trauma, the poorer the prognosis.

Fear and Defensive Behaviors Related to Correction Techniques

• Should resolve within weeks if clients follow advice • The more frequent the correction, the poorer the prognosis

Normal Play Behaviors Directed Towards People, Other Cats, and Household Objects

Appropriately followed treatment protocols should result in quick reduction or resolution of problem. If not resolving, follow-up appointment is needed.

Uninhibited Aggressive Play Directed Towards People

Guarded prognosis

MISCELLANEOUS

AGE-RELATED FACTORS

Fear and Defensive Behaviors Due to Lack of Early Experience

After birth, there appears to be a sensitive period, 3–7 weeks, during which a kitten must be exposed to prevent fearful and defensive responses to people.

Play-Related Behavior Problems

Should decline as the cat matures

ZOONOTIC POTENTIAL

Aggressive behaviors can inflict serious harm to people.

Suggested Reading

Borchelt PL, Voith VL. Aggressive behavior in cats. In: Voith VL, Borchelt PL, eds. Readings in companion animal behavior. Trenton, NJ: Veterinary Learning Systems, 1996:208–216.

Hunthausen W, Seksel K. Preventative behavioural medicine. In: Horwitz DF, Mills D, and Heath S, eds. BSAVA manual of canine and feline behavioural medicine. Gloucester, BSAVA, 2002:49–60.

Voith VL (videotape). An Introduction to Animal Behavior Problems. Animal Care Training Programs. Denton, TX. 1996.

Author Victoria L. Voith

Consulting Editor Debra F. Horwitz

PEDIATRIC BEHAVIOR PROBLEMS—DOGS

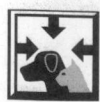

BASICS

DEFINITION
For the most part, these problems include behaviors that are normal and common to most puppies but not acceptable to the family. They require some degree of modification and shaping to become acceptable. Training problems include destructive chewing, playbiting, jumping on people, and getting on counters or furniture.

PATHOPHYSIOLOGY
None

SYSTEMS AFFECTED
Behavioral

GENETICS
Activity levels and behaviors of young pups likely to be similar to those of their parents.

INCIDENCE/PREVALENCE
Common to most puppies

GEOGRAPHIC DISTRIBUTION
May be more frequent in urban areas where opportunities to exercise are less available

SIGNALMENT

Species
Dogs

Breed Predilection
Working breeds selected for high energy levels

Mean Age and Range
Four to nine months of age, but may persist until late in the second year

Predominant Sex
Somewhat increased frequency and intensity in male dogs

SIGNS

Destructive Chewing
The pet chews and damages family members' furniture, possessions, etc. This initially occurs in the presence of family members but may be more secretive once the pet has been caught and punished several times.

Playbiting
The pet bites hands, legs, and/or clothing. Bites are usually inhibited but can cause injuries owing to sharp deciduous teeth. Growling and barking may be present but usually has a tone with a higher pitch than that associated with more serious types of aggression such as fear or possessive aggression. Play attacks are usually triggered by some movement by a family member but can be very spontaneous without apparent provocation or stimulus.

Jumping on People
The pet jumps up against and places paws against family members and/or visitors. This typically occurs during greetings but may occur when the pet wants attention or something the person is holding.

Getting On Counters/Furniture
The pet gets on furniture to access objects to chew or the family's food. The pet jumps on furniture during play, to get attention, or to rest.

CAUSES

General
Inadequate owner control, supervision, training, exercise, and/or mental stimulation can be underlying causes of these problems.

Destructive Chewing
• Poor nutrition, inadequate amounts of food, insufficient or uninteresting toys.
• Mice or other small mammals in the walls or flooring
• Food spilled on carpeting or furniture
• Escape behavior

Playbiting
Rough play, teasing, and encouraging the pet to bite hands and feet

Jumping on People
Long confinement periods, especially in a very small enclosure. Excited greetings by family members and visitors.

Getting on Counters/Furniture
• Insufficient or uninteresting toys
• Tempting objects or food left on furniture
• No comfortable surface on the floor on which to rest

DIAGNOSIS

DIFFERENTIAL DIAGNOSIS

Destructive Chewing
Separation anxiety may occur in young dogs but is more common in adults. The pet typically exhibits significant signs of predeparture anxiety and very excited greetings. The destructive behavior occurs virtually every time the puppy loses access to a family member(s) and is usually directed toward exit ways or personal possessions of the family.

Playbiting
• Fear aggression—Aggressive behavior is accompanied by signs of fear and/or submission. The behavior occurs when the pet is in a situation it perceives as threatening. Growling may have a higher pitch and be accompanied by yipes.
• Possessive aggression—The behavior occurs in specific situations where there is competition for a resource. The pet typically stiffens and hovers over the guarded object. Growling has a deep pitch. Piloerection may occur, as might lunging and snapping.
• Viral encephalitis, toxicosis—Biting is usually accompanied by other signs of illness.

Jumping on People
None

Getting on Counters/Furniture
None

CBC/BIOCHEMISTRY/URINALYSIS
N/A

OTHER LABORATORY TESTS
N/A

IMAGING
N/A

DIAGNOSTIC PROCEDURES
N/A

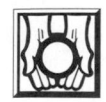

TREATMENT

APPROPRIATE HEALTH CARE
Outpatient

ACTIVITY
• Provide as much vigorous exercise as possible that is within acceptable health parameters for the individual.
• *Fetch/Drop It* is an excellent game for providing exercise and reminding the pet that the owner has control of resources. It will also help family members retrieve objects from the pet that he shouldn't have.

DIET
Feed enough food at optimum times to keep the pet satiated in order to decrease its motivation to get on counters, get into trash, or chew on inanimate objects.

CLIENT EDUCATION

General
• Discuss important tenets of the use of rewards and punishment, including timing, consistency, and intensity. Impress upon the owner that harsh or physical punishment should be avoided. Family members must be counseled to never strike the pet, thump its nose, shake it by the scruff, roll it on its back, or squeeze the lips against its teeth in an attempt to stop mouthing or biting. These approaches may increase the severity of the problem, ruin the bond with the pet and lead to more serious problems, such as fear and aggression. On the other hand, family members should constantly look for and reward acceptable behaviors.
• Teach the owner to teach the pet to sit on command by using food-lure training.
• Teach the owner how to properly use confinement and train the pet to accept it.

Destructive Chewing
• Provide interesting toys.
• Experiment with different types of toys to find types the pet prefers.
• Offer toys in which small amounts of food can be wedged or hidden to make them more attractive.
• Reward acceptable chewing with praise and by tossing treats when the pet chews its toys.
• Keep forbidden objects out of reach.

• Close doors and use baby gates to restrict access to objects.
• Spray objects that need to be protected with safe, aversive-tasting substances.
• Use a motion-activated alarm to keep the pet away from objects that need to be protected.
• Interrupt any unacceptable chewing with a sharp "No," the noise of a shake can, the "hiss" from a can of compressed air, or an air horn. Any of these interruptive methods should be used with some attention to the pet's temperament. They should be avoided or tempered in intensity so that a fear response is not elicited from the pet.
• Close supervision or safe confinement may be necessary for up to two years of age.

Playbiting
• Provide plenty of exercise to reduce reactivity and impulsivity.
• Have toys available at all times to toss and distract the pet. Use food-laced toys to divert the pet's attention and keep it occupied.
• Use a leash and head halter as needed for more control.
• Place the pet in time-out when it is out of control and the family cannot devote the time needed to shape the behavior or wear the pet out with exercise.
• Avoid games that encourage playbiting hands or feet.
• The puppy should be enrolled in puppy classes as early as possible (eight to ten weeks of age).
• Take control of the pet by controlling resources and making it sit before receiving toys, food, play, and attention.
• Ignore any pushy social behavior by the puppy, such as whining, barking, or pawing for attention.
• Saying "Ouch" very loudly and walking away from the pet should immediately interrupt any hard bites during play.
• Physical corrections should be avoided and could cause fear, anxiety, and aggression.

Jumping on People
• Avoid play and games during which the pet jumps up on people.
• Teach the pet to sit on command.
• Every time the pup approaches for attention or to greet someone, quickly place a small treat or toy in front of its mouth and ask it to sit.
• If the pet jumps up, the behavior can be interrupted with a sharp noise (see Destructive Chewing, above).
• It is extremely important that all family members be very consistent in responding to this problem and shaping the pet's behavior.

Getting on Counters/Furniture
• Keep food and interesting objects off counters and furniture during the early training period.

• Constantly supervise or place the pet in a safe confinement area.
• Provide interesting toys for mental stimulation and to keep the pet focused on objects on the floor.
• Use motion-activated alarms or air canisters to teach the pet to stay off furniture and counters when unsupervised.
• Keep the pet well fed so it is not hungry and therefore less likely to look for food on tables and counters.
• Provide a doggie bed on the floor.

MEDICATIONS

DRUG(S) OF CHOICE
• Drugs are generally not indicated.
• On rare occasions a small amount of a phenothiazine (e.g., acepromazine) or an antihistamine (e.g., diphenhydramine) might be considered for sedation during the early training period when friends visit and the pet is not yet under control.

CONTRAINDICATIONS
None

PRECAUTIONS
N/A

POSSIBLE INTERACTIONS
N/A

ALTERNATIVE DRUG(S)
None

FOLLOW-UP

PATIENT MONITORING
• Follow-up appointments must be determined on a case-by-case consideration.
• Phone follow-ups at approximately ten days, thirty days, and three months following the initial visit are usually helpful.
• A trained support staff member can play an important roll in helping with client follow-up.

PREVENTION/AVOIDANCE
• An adequate amount of supervision and confinement
• Begin food-lure-reward obedience training in the home at seven to eight weeks of age. Enroll in a puppy class at eight to ten weeks of age.
• Large amounts of physical exercise and mental stimulation
• Provide information about normal young pet behavior and needs (especially mental and physical stimulation) during various growth phases so the family knows what to expect.
• Suggest safe and interesting toys.

POSSIBLE COMPLICATIONS
• Damaged household objects and clothing
• The family's food eaten by the pet
• Intestinal foreign bodies/obstructions
• Minor skin injuries from playbites
• A guest is knocked down and injured.
• A weakened bond with the pet

EXPECTED COURSE AND PROGNOSIS
Prognosis is generally good. The frequency and intensity of the behaviors will decrease with age. Jumping up on people and playbiting can usually be quickly controlled if the family is consistent with training. The tendency to occasionally chew on the family's possessions or explore counters for food and other objects may last until 12 to 24 months of age, when the pet becomes behaviorally mature and less active.

MISCELLANEOUS

ASSOCIATED CONDITIONS
None

AGE-RELATED FACTORS
None

ZOONOTIC POTENTIAL
N/A

Suggested Reading and Videos

Ackerman L, Landsberg G, Hunthausen W, eds. Dog behavior and training: veterinary advice for owners. Neptune, NJ: TFH Publications, 1996.

American Animal Hospital Association behavior pamphlets. (Playbiting, Destructive Puppy Behavior, Leadership and Control, and more). American Animal Hospital Association, 12575 W. Bayaud Ave., Lakewood, CO 80228, 1-800-252-2242, 1998.

Dunbar I. Sirius Puppy Training (video). James and Kenneth Publishers, 2140 Shattuck Ave #2406, Berkeley, CA 94704, 510-658-8588.

Hunthausen W, Seksel K. Preventative behavioural medicine. In: Horwitz DF, Mills D, and Heath S, eds. BSAVA manual of canine and feline behavioural medicine. Gloucester, England: BSAVA, 2002:49–60.

Landsberg GL, Hunthausen WL, Ackerman L. Handbook of behaviour problems of the dog and cat. 2nd ed. Philadelphia: Saunders, 2003.

Scidmore K, McConnell PB. Puppy primer, published by Dog's Best Friend, Ltd., P.O. Box 447, Black Earth, WI 53515, 608-767-2435, 1996.

Author Wayne Hunthausen
Consulting Editor Debra F. Horwitz

PELGER-HUËT ANOMALY

 BASICS

OVERVIEW
• An inherited disorder characterized by leukocyte nuclear hyposegmentation in the presence of a mature coarse chromatin pattern
• Limited breeding studies suggest autosomal dominant transmission of the anomaly in dogs and cats; however, autosomal dominant transmission with incomplete penetrance occurs in Australian shepherds.
• Heterozygous anomaly—usual phenotype; neutrophils resemble bands and metamyelocytes; not associated with immunodeficiency, predisposition to infection, or abnormalities of leukocyte function
• Homozygous anomaly—usually lethal in utero; survivors may have leukocytes with round to oval nuclei on stained blood smear.
• Skeletal abnormalities—homozygous anomaly and chondrodysplasia reported in one stillborn kitten; heterozygous anomaly and skeletal anomalies (chondrodysplasia and brachygnathia) reported in Samoyeds; not linked conclusively to Pelger-Huët anomaly in either species

SIGNALMENT
Several breeds of dogs (e.g., American foxhounds, Australian shepherds, basenjis) and domestic shorthair cats

SIGNS

Historical Findings
Parents or siblings may be affected.

Physical Examination Findings
No abnormalities

CAUSES & RISK FACTORS
Genetic defect with probable autosomal dominant transmission (or proven autosomal dominant trait with incomplete penetrance in Australian shepherd dogs)

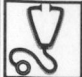 **DIAGNOSIS**

DIFFERENTIAL DIAGNOSIS
• Severe inflammation or bacterial infection often associated with toxic change of neutrophils
• FeLV or FIV infection in cats with altered cellular maturation
• Drug-induced alterations in cellular morphology, especially encountered with use of sulfa drugs
• Preleukemic maturation disturbances

CBC/BIOCHEMISTRY/URINALYSIS
• Serendipitous finding during WBC differential count
• On stained blood smear, nuclear hyposegmentation of neutrophils (persistent left shift without toxic changes), eosinophils, basophils, and monocytes

OTHER LABORATORY TESTS
None

IMAGING
None

OTHER DIAGNOSTIC PROCEDURES
• Bone marrow biopsy—stained smear reveals nuclear hyposegmentation of leukocytes and nuclear hypolobulation of megakaryocytes; blast cell count within reference intervals
• Hereditary nature of disease revealed by examination of blood smears from parents and siblings; if relatives are unavailable for study, demonstrated by prospective test mating

 TREATMENT

None needed, because no associated clinical disease

 MEDICATIONS

DRUG(S)
None

CONTRAINDICATIONS/POSSIBLE INTERACTIONS
None

 FOLLOW-UP

PATIENT MONITORING
None

PREVENTION/AVOIDANCE
• Inform owner to avoid unnecessary laboratory testing or inappropriate drug administration in future.
• Provide genetic counseling to eliminate trait from breeding animals.
• Breed affected heterozygotes and select normal offspring for future matings to preserve desirable genetic lines.

POSSIBLE COMPLICATIONS
• When heterozygotes are bred, litter size may be small because homozygous phenotype is usually a lethal trait.
• Association with chondrodysplasia or other skeletal abnormalities not yet confirmed

EXPECTED COURSE AND PROGNOSIS
• Heterozygous anomaly—normal life span
• Homozygous anomaly—usually lethal (fetal resorption)

 MISCELLANEOUS

ASSOCIATED CONDITIONS
Fetal resorption (homozygous embryos)

PREGNANCY
Fetal resorption (homozygous embryos)

ABBREVIATIONS
• FeLV = feline leukemia virus
• FIV = feline immunodeficiency virus

Suggested Reading
Latimer KS, Campagnoli RP, Danilenko DM. Pelger-Huët anomaly in Australian shepherds, 87 cases (1991–1997). Comp Haematol Int 2000;10:9–13.
Author Kenneth S. Latimer
Contributing Editor Stephen A. Kruth

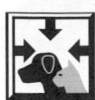

BASICS

OVERVIEW
Describes a condition in which the neck of the bladder is located extremely caudally in the pelvic canal and the urethra is shortened or displaced; most often associated with incontinence in young intact female dogs, but some dogs with pelvic bladder do not exhibit urinary incontinence

SIGNALMENT
• Dogs and rarely cats; the difference in prevalence between species is presumably because the cat has a longer urethra than a dog of similar size.
• May occur in dogs of both sexes, either intact or neutered, but primarily affects young intact female dogs (< 1 year of age); usually detected in male dogs after neutering

SIGNS
• Incontinence is usually intermittent, and there are voluntary urinations.
• Involuntary dribbling of urine from the vulva or prepuce
• Urinary "soiling" of the perineum, tail, or caudal thighs; urine spots or pools of urine where the dog has been lying down or sleeping
• May be asymptomatic

CAUSES & RISK FACTORS
Incontinence that accompanies a pelvic bladder is attributed to two components of the disorder: (1) the extreme caudal displacement of the bladder into the pelvic canal, limiting bladder distension, and (2) the abnormal position of the urethra in these animals. The urethra takes on a variety of appearances, from short and dilated to S-shaped.

DIAGNOSIS

DIFFERENTIAL DIAGNOSIS
• Causes of intermittent or continuous incontinence—ectopic ureter, urethral incompetence, hormonal incontinence, urge incontinence, urinary tract infection, neurologic conditions, detrusor instability
• The level of incontinence caused by a pelvic bladder often exceeds that seen with urethral incompetence or hormone-responsive incontinence.

CBC/BIOCHEMISTRY/URINALYSIS
• Hematologic and biochemical analysis may be indicated in patients with polyuric disorders.
• Urinalysis may reveal evidence of urinary tract infection (e.g., pyuria, hematuria, and bacteriuria) or polyuria (e.g., low urine specific gravity).

• Urine culture may be indicated if urinalysis is suggestive of urinary tract infection.

OTHER LABORATORY TESTS
N/A

IMAGING
• Abdominal radiographs may reveal a caudally displaced bladder; interpret cautiously if the bladder is not distended.
• Use contrast radiography in juvenile animals exhibiting urinary incontinence.
• Excretory urography also may allow visualization of the kidneys, ureteral terminations, urinary bladder, and urethra.
• Retrograde vaginourethrography allows visualization of the vaginal vault, urethra, and urinary bladder.
• Double-contrast cystourethrography may be required for full visualization of the urinary bladder and urethra.
• After maximum dilation with infusion of carbon dioxide or contrast medium, most of the bladder remains within the pelvic canal.
• There may be a short, widened urethra or a urethra with a prominently convoluted appearance.
• Ultrasonography of the kidneys and urinary bladder can be used to identify uroliths, masses, hydronephrosis or hydroureter, and evidence of pyelonephritis.

DIAGNOSTIC PROCEDURES
• Neurologic examination—a cursory assessment of caudal spinal and peripheral nerve function is provided by examination of anal tone, tail tone, perineal sensation, and bulbospongiosus reflexes; results are normal.
• Urodynamic procedures—consider cystometrography and urethral pressure profilometry to evaluate urinary bladder and urethral function more objectively. Detrusor function is usually normal; however, higher threshold pressures may be generated at lower volumes. The functional urethral length is shortened, and intraurethral pressure is frequently decreased.
• Cystoscopy may be beneficial in ruling out other anatomical abnormalities (e.g., ectopic ureter).

TREATMENT
• Usually outpatient
• Identify urinary tract infection and treat appropriately.
• Surgical procedures such as seromuscular flap, colposuspension, cystourethropexy, and Teflon or collagen implants have been described for the treatment of patients refractory to medical management. Treat patients refractory to medical management with a combination of α-adrenergic agonists and diethylstilbestrol before attempting surgical correction.

MEDICATIONS

DRUG(S)
• α-Adrenergic agonists (e.g., phenylpropanolamine, phenylephrine, pseudoephedrine) and/or estrogen (diethylstilbestrol) therapy
• Imipramine—a tricyclic antidepressant with α-agonist actions—provides an alternative method of treatment, but often needs to be administered in combination with phenylpropanolamine.

CONTRAINDICATIONS/POSSIBLE INTERACTIONS
Adrenergic agonists are contraindicated in animals with cardiac disease, renal disease, and hypertensive disorders.

FOLLOW-UP

PATIENT MONITORING
• Periodically, for urinary tract infection
• Patients receiving α-adrenergic agonists—check for adverse effects of the drug, including tachycardia, anxiety, and hypertension.
• After seeing a therapeutic effect, slowly reduce the dosage and frequency of administration of medications to the minimum required.

POSSIBLE COMPLICATIONS
• Recurrent and ascending urinary tract infection
• Urine scald and perineal and ventral dermatitis
• Refractory and unmanageable incontinence

MISCELLANEOUS

ASSOCIATED CONDITIONS
• Urethral incompetence/urethral dysplasia
• Urinary tract infection

Suggested Reading
Lane IF, Lappin MR. Urinary incontinence and congenital urogenital anomalies in small animals. In: Kirk RW, Bonagura JD, eds. Current veterinary therapy XII. Philadelphia: Saunders, 1995:1022–1026.
Mahaffey MB, Barsanti JA, et al. Pelvic bladder in dogs without urinary incontinence. J Am Vet Med Assoc 1984;184(12):1477.
Rawlings C, Barsanti JA, Mahaffey MB, Bement S. Evaluation of colposuspension for treatment of incontinence in spayed female dogs. J Am Vet Med Assoc 2001;219:770–775.
Author Mary Anna Labato
Consulting Editors Larry G. Adams and Carl A. Osborne

PEMPHIGUS

BASICS

OVERVIEW
• A group of autoimmune dermatoses characterized by varying degrees of ulceration, crusting, and pustule and vesicle formation • Affects the skin and sometimes mucous membranes

PATHOPHYSIOLOGY
• Tissue-bound autoantibody directed at interepidermal cell antigen is deposited within the intercellular spaces, causing epidermal cell separation and cell rounding (acantholysis). • Severity of ulceration and disease—related to depth of autoantibody deposition within the skin • Types—foliaceus, vulgaris, erythematosus, and vegetans • Foliaceus—autoantibody deposition in the superficial layers of the epidermis • Vulgaris—lesions more severe; mediated by autoantibody deposition just above the basement membrane zone; results in deeper ulcer formation

SYSTEMS AFFECTED
Skin/Exocrine—autoantibody is tissue-bound

GENETICS
N/A

INCIDENCE/PREVALENCE
• Uncommon group of diseases • Foliaceus—most common type • Erythematosus—relatively common; may be a more benign variant of pemphigus foliaceus or may be a crossover syndrome of pemphigus and lupus erythematosus • Vulgaris—second most common type; the most severe form • Vegetans—rarest type; possibly a relatively benign variant of pemphigus vulgaris

GEOGRAPHIC DISTRIBUTION
N/A

SIGNALMENT
Species
• Foliaceus, erythematosus, and vulgaris—dogs and cats • Vegetans—dogs only

Breed Predilections
• Foliaceus—akitas, bearded collies, chow chows, dachshunds, Doberman pinschers, Finnish spitzes, Newfoundlands, and schipperkes • Erythematosus—collies, German shepherds, and Shetland sheepdogs

Mean Age and Range
Usually middle-aged to old animals

Predominant Sex
None

SIGNS
Foliaceus
• Scales, crust, pustules, epidermal collarettes, erosions, erythema, alopecia, and footpad hyperkeratosis with fissuring • Occasional vesicles are transient. • Common involvement—head, ears, and footpads; often becomes generalized • Mucosal and mucocutaneous lesions uncommon • Cats—nipple and nailbed involvement common • Sometimes lymphadenopathy, edema, depression, fever, and lameness (if footpads involved); however, patients are often in good health. • Variable pain and pruritus • Secondary bacterial infection possible

Erythematosus
• As for pemphigus foliaceus • Lesions usually confined to head, face, and footpads • Mucocutaneous depigmentation more common than with other forms

Vulgaris
• Ulcerative lesions, erosions, epidermal collarettes, blisters, and crusts • More severe than pemphigus foliaceus and erythematosus • Affects mucous membranes, mucocutaneous junctions, and skin; may become generalized • Oral ulceration frequent • Axillae and groin areas often involved • Positive Nikolsky sign (new or extended erosive lesion created when lateral pressure is applied to the skin near an existing lesion) • Variable pruritus and pain • Anorexia, depression, and fever • Secondary bacterial infections common

Vegetans
• Pustule groups become eruptive papillomatous lesions and vegetative masses that ooze. • Oral involvement has not been noted. • No systemic illness

CAUSES
Unknown

RISK FACTORS
Unknown

DIAGNOSIS

DIFFERENTIAL DIAGNOSIS
Foliaceus
• Bacterial folliculitis • Dermatophytosis • Demodicosis • Candidiasis • Keratinization disorders • Lupus erythematosus • Pemphigus erythematosus • Subcorneal pustular dermatosis • Drug eruption • Zinc-responsive dermatitis • Dermatomyositis • Tyrosinemia • Mycosis fungoides • Lymphoreticular malignancies • Metabolic epidermal necrosis • Sterile eosinophilic pustulosis • Linear IgA dermatosis

Erythematosus
• Pemphigus foliaceus • Systemic lupus erythematosus • Discoid lupus erythematosus • Nasal pyoderma • Demodicosis • Dermatophytosis • Epidermolysis bullosa simplex • Uveodermatologic syndrome

Vulgaris
• Bullous pemphigoid • Systemic lupus erythematosus • Toxic epidermal necrolysis • Drug eruption • Mycosis fungoides • Lymphoreticular neoplasia • Ulcerative stomatitis causes • Erythema multiforme

Vegetans
• Pemphigus vulgaris • Bacterial folliculitis • Pemphigus foliaceus • Lichenoid dermatoses • Cutaneous neoplasia

CBC/BIOCHEMISTRY/URINALYSIS
• Abnormalities uncommon • Leukocytosis and hyperglobulinemia sometimes noted

OTHER LABORATORY TESTS
• Antinuclear antibody—may be weakly positive in pemphigus erythematosus only

IMAGING
N/A

DIAGNOSTIC PROCEDURES
• Cytology of aspirates or impression smears of pustules or crusts—acantholytic cells and neutrophils • Bacteriologic culture—identify secondary bacterial infections

PATHOLOGIC FINDINGS
• Biopsies of lesional or perilesional skin—acantholysis and intraepidermal clefting; microabscess or pustule formation; surface acantholytic keratinocytes • Location of epidermal lesions—varies with disease; pemphigus foliaceous and erythematosus have subcorneal or intragranular clefting and acantholysis; pemphigus vulgaris and vegetans have suprabasilar clefting. • Immunopathology of biopsied skin via immunofluorescent antibody assays or immunohistochemical testing—may demonstrate positive staining in the intercellular spaces in 50%–90% of cases; results can be affected by concurrent or previous corticosteroid (or other immunosuppressive drug) administration; indirect immunofluorescence usually negative; pemphigus erythematosus may demonstrate staining of basement membranes and intercellular spaces.

TREATMENT

APPROPRIATE HEALTH CARE
• Initial inpatient supportive therapy for severely affected patients • Outpatient treatment with initial frequent hospital visits (every 1–3 weeks); taper to every 1–3 months when remission is achieved and the patient is on a maintenance medical regimen.

NURSING CARE
Severely affected patients may need antibiotics and soaks.

ACTIVITY
N/A

DIET
Low-fat—to avoid pancreatitis predisposed by corticosteroids and (possibly) azathioprine therapy

CLIENT EDUCATION
Advise client that the patient should avoid the sun, because UV light may exacerbate lesions.

SURGICAL CONSIDERATIONS
N/A

MEDICATIONS

DRUG(S)

Pemphigus Vulgaris and Foliaceus
Corticosteroids
• Prednisone or prednisolone—1.1–2.2 mg/kg/day PO divided q12h to initiate control
• Minimum maintenance—0.5 mg/kg PO q48h
• Taper dosage at 2–4-week intervals by 5–10 mg per week.

Cytotoxic Agents
• More than half of patients require the addition of other immunomodulating drugs.
• Generally work synergistically with prednisone, allowing reduction in dose and side effects of the corticosteroid
• Azathioprine—2.2 mg/kg PO q24h, then q48h (dogs); infrequently used in cats, owing to potential for marked bone marrow suppression; feline dose 1 mg/kg q24–48h
• Chlorambucil—0.2 mg /kg daily; best choice for cats
• Cyclophosphamide—50 mg/m² PO BSA q48h (dogs)
• Cyclosporine—15–27 mg/kg daily PO; limited application
• Dapsone—1 mg/kg PO q8h; then as needed (dogs); limited application

Chrysotherapy
• Often used in conjunction with prednisone
• Aurothioglucose—administer a test dose of 1 mg IM (animals < 25 kg) or 5 mg IM (animals > 25 kg) 1st week; 2 mg IM (animals < 25 kg) or 10 mg IM (animals > 25 kg) 2nd week; then 1 mg/kg IM weekly until a clinical response is noted (generally a lag phase of 6–8 weeks); then 1 mg/kg IM every 2–4 weeks for maintenance
• Auranofin—0.1–0.2 mg/kg PO q12–24h

Pemphigus Erythematosus and Vegetans
• Oral prednisone or prednisolone—1.1 mg/kg PO q24h; then q48h; then to the lowest maintenance dose possible; may be stopped when in remission
• Topical steroids may be sufficient in mild cases.

CONTRAINDICATIONS
N/A

PRECAUTIONS
• Corticosteroids—polyuria, polydipsia, polyphagia, temperament changes, diabetes mellitus, pancreatitis, and hepatotoxicity
• Azathioprine—pancreatitis
• Cytotoxic drugs—leukopenia, thrombocytopenia, nephrotoxicity, and hepatotoxicity
• Chrysotherapy—leukopenia, thrombocytopenia, nephrotoxicity, dermatitis, stomatitis, and allergic reactions
• Cyclophosphamide—hemorrhagic cystitis
• Immunosuppression—can predispose animal to *Demodex,* cutaneous and systemic bacterial and fungal infection

POSSIBLE INTERACTIONS
N/A

ALTERNATIVE DRUG(S)

Alternative Corticosteroids
• Use instead of prednisone if undesirable side effects or poor response occur
• Methylprednisolone—0.8–1.5 mg/kg PO q12h; for patients that tolerate prednisone poorly
• Triamcinolone—0.2–0.3 mg/kg PO q12h; then 0.05–0.1 mg/kg q48–72h
• Glucocorticoid pulse therapy—11 mg/kg IV methylprednisolone sodium succinate for 3 consecutive days to induce remission; limited application

Topical Steroids
• Hydrocortisone cream
• More potent topical corticosteroids—0.1% betamethasone valerate, fluocinolone acetonide, or 0.1% triamcinonide; q12h; then q24–48h

Miscellaneous
Tetracycline and niacinamide—500 mg PO q8h (dogs > 10 kg); half doses for dogs < 10 kg; limited application

FOLLOW-UP

PATIENT MONITORING
• Monitor response to therapy. • Monitor for medication side effects—routine hematology and serum biochemistry, especially patients on high doses of corticosteroids, cytotoxic drugs, or chrysotherapy; check every 1–3 weeks, then every 1–3 months when in remission.

PREVENTION/AVOIDANCE
N/A

POSSIBLE COMPLICATIONS
N/A

EXPECTED COURSE AND PROGNOSIS

Pemphigus Vulgaris and Foliaceus
• Therapy with corticosteroids and cytotoxic drugs needed • Patients may require medication for life. • Monitoring necessary • Side effects of medications may affect quality of life. • May be fatal if untreated (especially pemphigus vulgaris) • Secondary infections cause morbidity and possible mortality (especially pemphigus vulgaris).

Pemphigus Erythematosus and Vegetans
• Relatively benign and self-limiting
• Oral corticosteroids may eventually be tapered to low maintenance doses; may be stopped in some patients
• Dermatosis develops if untreated; systemic symptoms rare
• Prognosis fair

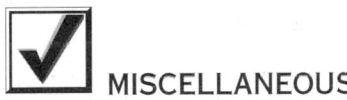

MISCELLANEOUS

ASSOCIATED CONDITIONS
N/A

AGE-RELATED FACTORS
N/A

ZOONOTIC POTENTIAL
None

PREGNANCY
Avoid steroids and cytotoxic drugs during pregnancy.

SYNONYMS
None

Suggested Reading

Ackerman LJ. Immune-mediated skin diseases. In: Morgan RV, ed. Handbook of small animal practice. 3rd ed. Philadelphia: Saunders, 1997:941–943.

Angarano DW. Autoimmune dermatosis. In: Nesbitt GH, ed. Contemporary issues in small animal practice: dermatology. New York: Churchill Livingstone, 1987:79–94.

Rosenkrantz WS. Pemphigus foliaceous. In: Griffin CE, Knochka KW, MacDonald JM, et al., eds. Current veterinary dermatology. St. Louis: Mosby, 1993:141–148.

Author Margaret S. Swartout
Consulting Editor Karen Helton Rhodes

PERIANAL FISTULA

 BASICS

OVERVIEW
Chronic inflammatory condition characterized by multiple, painful, progressive, ulcerating sinuses or, much less frequently, true fistulous tracts involving the perianal region

SIGNALMENT
• Dogs
• German shepherd dogs primarily; Irish setters
• Middle-aged dogs with mean age of 5–7 years; range, 7 months to 14 years
• No gender predisposition, but incidence higher in sexually intact dogs

SIGNS
• Vary with the severity and extent of involvement
• Dyschezia
• Tenesmus
• Hematochezia
• Constipation
• Diarrhea
• Malodorous mucopurulent anal discharge
• Ulceration of the perianal skin with sinus tract formation
• Licking and self-mutilation
• Reluctance to sit; posturing difficulties; and personality changes
• Pain on manipulation of tail and examination of perianal area
• Fecal incontinence
• Anorexia
• Weight loss

CAUSES & RISK FACTORS
• Cause not clearly defined, but immune-mediated disease and anatomic factors have been implicated, particularly in German shepherds
• An association with colitis in German shepherd dogs has also been proposed.
• A genetic predisposition, based on breed incidence, has been proposed but not proven.
• Low tail carriage and a broad tail base—speculated risk factors predisposing the dog to inflammation and infection because of poor ventilation, accumulation of feces, moisture, and secretions; only a small percentage of dogs with this conformation become affected
• High density of apocrine sweat glands in the cutaneous zone of the anal canal of German shepherd dogs

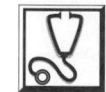 DIAGNOSIS

DIFFERENTIAL DIAGNOSIS
• Other inflammatory processes—e.g., anusitis, hydradenitis suppurativa
• Chronic anal sac abscess
• Perianal adenoma or adenocarcinoma with ulceration and drainage
• Rectal fistula

CBC/BIOCHEMISTRY/URINALYSIS
• Usually normal
• Patients with inflammation may have an inflammatory leukogram.

OTHER LABORATORY TESTS
N/A

IMAGING
N/A

DIAGNOSTIC PROCEDURES
• Presumptive diagnosis—based on clinical signs and results of physical examination
• Definitive diagnosis—made by biopsy of the affected area
• Colonoscopy with biopsy—may reveal associated colitis

 TREATMENT

APPROPRIATE HEALTH CARE
Outpatient medical therapy recommended initially in all cases

NURSING CARE
• Postoperative warm packing of the affected area—but many of these dogs are apprehensive about manipulations of the perianal area
• Daily hydrotherapy and/or antiseptic lavage—if wounds are left open to heal by second intention

DIET
• Dietary modification—fiber-enhanced or hypoallergenic diet for associated colitis or proctitis
• Stool softeners—with pain or tenesmus

SURGICAL CONSIDERATIONS
• Surgical treatment—indicated when there is incomplete response or recurrence
• No technique is uniformly successful—selection of a specific surgical technique is based on severity of the lesions, acceptability of likely complications and side-effects, and surgeon preference
• Surgical options—surgical debridement (deroofing) with fulguration by chemical cautery or electrocautery; surgical resection followed by primary closure or second intention healing; radical excision of the rectal ring with modified rectal pull-through; laser resection followed by primary closure
• Primary objective of surgery—complete removal or destruction of diseased tissue while preserving normal tissue and function
• Anal sacculectomy—perform with any of these surgical techniques

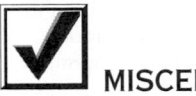
• Multiple procedures—may be necessary for complete resolution
• Tail amputation—has been recommended to change the local environment and to make the area more accessible for topical therapy; not routinely performed

 MEDICATIONS

DRUG(S) OF CHOICE

Cyclosporine
• Low dose—2–3 mg/kg PO q24h (100–200 ng/mL trough levels)
• High dose—5–7 mg/kg PO q24h (400–600 ng/mL trough levels)
• If low dose regimen is chosen and there is no response or incomplete response, use high dose.
• To achieve trough levels of 400–600 ng/mL—cyclosporine 2.5–3.5 mg/kg PO q24h and ketoconazole 5–10 mg/kg PO; ketoconazole inhibits metabolism of cyclosporine, allowing higher blood levels for a given dose
• Continue treatment at least 4 weeks after complete resolution of fistula.
• Consider surgery with incomplete resolution or recurrence.

ALTERNATIVE DRUG(S)
• Azathioprine—has been used to decrease the severity of lesions prior to surgery; unlikely to result in complete resolution by itself
• Corticosteroids (2 mg/kg PO q12h) and a hypoallergenic diet for 6 weeks—may yield partial or complete resolution (about 33% of cases); most dogs do not improve; corticosteroid side effects are common
• Antibiotics and analgesics—may be indicated in some cases

CONTRAINDICATIONS/POSSIBLE INTERACTIONS
• Consult package insert for a complete list of possible interactions and adverse effects.
• Immunosuppressive agents increase the risk of infection.
• Cyclosporine—use with caution in patients with renal or hepatic disease; levels may increase with administration of calcium channel blockers and metoclopramide; levels can decrease with administration of trimethoprim sulfate, omeprazole, and terbinafine
• Ketoconazole—use with caution in patients with hepatic disease and thrombocytopenia; antacids, anticholinergics, and H_2 blockers inhibit absorption
• Azathioprine—may cause bone marrow suppression

 FOLLOW-UP

PATIENT MONITORING
• Assess cyclosporine trough levels at 5–7 days, then every 3–4 weeks.
• Reexamine to assess healing, signs of recurrence, and associated complications.

POSSIBLE COMPLICATIONS
• Recurrence
• Failure to heal
• Dehiscence of surgical site
• Tenesmus
• Fecal incontinence
• Anal stricture
• Flatulence
• The incidence of postoperative complications is directly related to the severity of the disease and the surgical technique performed
• Iatrogenic Cushing's disease from corticosteroids

EXPECTED COURSE AND PROGNOSIS
• Guarded for complete resolution except in mildly affected patients
• Clients often become frustrated with the difficulty of attaining definitive resolution.

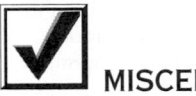 **MISCELLANEOUS**

ASSOCIATED CONDITIONS
• Colitis
• Constipation and/or obstipation may develop.

PREGNANCY
Use caution with medication and surgery

SEE ALSO
• Colitis and Proctitis
• Constipation and Obstipation
• Dyschezia and Hematochezia

Suggested Reading

Harkin KR, Walshaw R, Mullaney TP. Association of perianal fistula and colitis in the German shepherd dog: response to high-dose prednisone and dietary therapy. J Am Anim Hosp Assoc 1996;32:515–520.

Hedlund CS. Surgery of the perineum, rectum, and anus. In: Fossum TW, ed. Small animal surgery. 2nd ed. St. Louis: Mosby, 2002:414–449.

Patricelli AJ, Hardie RJ, McAnulty JF. Cyclosporine and ketoconazole for the treatment of perianal fistulas in dogs. J Am Vet Med Assoc 2002;220:1009–1016.

Author Eric R. Pope
Section Editor Albert E. Jergens

PERICARDIAL EFFUSION

 BASICS

DEFINITION
Abnormally high volume of fluid within the pericardial sac; cardiac tamponade is the clinical result of hemodynamic compromise.

PATHOPHYSIOLOGY
Accumulation of effusion exceeds elastic, or stretching, capabilities of the pericardial sac; further accumulation leads to high intrapericardial pressure. Cardiac tamponade occurs when intrapericardial pressure exceeds cardiac diastolic filling pressure. The right atrium and right ventricle normally have the lowest cardiac filling pressure and are predominantly affected. The resultant reduction in cardiac filling (preload reduction) diminishes forward blood flow, resulting in low cardiac output. In animals with chronic pericardial disease, low cardiac output activates compensatory mechanisms that lead to fluid accumulation. Congestive signs are typically manifested as right-sided CHF. Animals with acutely developing effusions typically exhibit signs of weakness or collapse.

SYSTEMS AFFECTED
• Cardiovascular—signs of low cardiac output and CHF • Hepatobiliary—chronic passive congestion with mildly to moderately high liver enzymes • Renal/Urologic—prerenal azotemia • Respiratory—tachypnea or pleural effusion

GENETICS
N/A

INCIDENCE/PREVALENCE
N/A

GEOGRAPHIC DISTRIBUTION
N/A

SIGNALMENT

Species
Dogs; uncommon in cats

Breed Predilection
Golden retrievers and German shepherds sare predisposed to right atrial hemangiosarcoma and idiopathic effusion.

Mean Age and Range
Middle-aged to old dogs are predisposed.

Predominant Sex
Male dogs are predisposed to idiopathic effusion.

SIGNS

General Comments
Chronic pericardial effusion often causes ascites without a cardiac murmur.

Historical Findings
• Lethargy • Anorexia • Weakness • Exercise intolerance • Abdominal distension • Syncope or collapse

Physical Examination Findings
Acute pericardial effusion
• Pallor • Slow capillary refill time • Weak arterial pulses • Weakness, syncope, collapse • Tachypnea • Tachycardia
Chronic pericardial effusion
• Jugular vein distension • Ascites • Muffled heart sounds • Weak arterial pulses • Pulsus paradoxus • Pallor • Slow capillary refill time • Weakness • Tachypnea • Tachycardia

CAUSES
• Neoplasia—hemangiosarcoma, heart-base tumor (chemodectoma), thyroid carcinoma, mesothelioma, metastatic neoplasia, and lymphoma (cats) • Idiopathic—benign or hemorrhagic • Coagulopathy—intoxication with vitamin K antagonist rodenticide, thrombocytopenia, other coagulopathies • Infection—feline infectious peritonitis, coccidioidomycosis, bacterial pericarditis • Congenital disorders—peritoneopericardial hernia • Left atrial tear or cardiac trauma • CHF • Foreign body • Constrictive pericarditis with fibrosis

RISK FACTORS
N/A

 DIAGNOSIS

DIFFERENTIAL DIAGNOSIS
• CHF secondary to other causes (e.g., chronic valvular disease and cardiomyopathy), hepatic failure, abdominal neoplasm with hemorrhage, protein-losing nephropathy or enteropathy • Usually a cardiac murmur or gallop in animals with heart failure is caused by cardiomyopathy or valvular disease. • Other causes of ascites (e.g., hepatic failure, hypoproteinemia, intraabdominal neoplasia, and hemorrhage caused by coagulopathy)—characteristically result in remarkable abnormalities on CBC and biochemistry profile, with a lack of jugular venous distention. Examination of the jugular vein can be extremely helpful in differentiating these conditions from heart failure.

CBC/BIOCHEMISTRY/URINALYSIS
• CBC—usually normal; anemia possible in animals with hemangiosarcoma, lymphoma, or coagulopathy; red cell morphology may be abnormal (e.g., nucleated red blood cells, schistocytes, and acanthocytes); may be thrombocytopenia in animals with hemangiosarcoma
• Biochemistry profile—often normal; may be mild to moderately high liver enzymes (in animals with chronic passive hepatic congestion), mild azotemia (typically prerenal), and mild electrolyte abnormalities (e.g., hyponatremia, hypochloremia, and hyperkalemia)
• Urinalysis—usually normal with normal renal concentrating ability unless a diuretic has been administered

OTHER LABORATORY TESTS
• Clotting times (e.g., activated partial thromboplastin time and one-stage prothrombin time)—prolonged in animals with vitamin K antagonist rodenticide intoxication
• Feline infectious peritonitis titers may be high in cats.
• Cats with lymphoma may be positive for feline leukemia virus.

IMAGING

Thoracic Radiographic Findings
• Mild-to-severe cardiac enlargement; cardiac silhouette often globoid and often very sharp edges on the dorsoventral view because of lack of cardiac motion artifact
• Mild-to-moderate pleural effusion in some patients
• Ascites in many patients
• Large caudal vena cava in some patients

Echocardiography
• Superior diagnostic test to confirm diagnosis
• Echo-free space clearly identified between the pericardium and the epicardial surface of the heart
• Often demonstrates the cause of pericardial effusion in patients with neoplasia (e.g., right atrial hemangiosarcoma and heart base tumor around aorta) or peritoneopericardial hernia

DIAGNOSTIC PROCEDURES

Electrocardiographic Findings
• Sinus tachycardia in many patients; occasionally ventricular or supraventricular arrhythmias
• Low-voltage QRS complexes (< 1 mV in leads I, II, III, aVR, aVL, and aVF) in dogs.
• ST segment elevation in some patients
• Electrical alternans, a regular (1-to-1 or 2-to-1) variation in QRS-T wave height or morphology, results from the heart swinging back and forth within the pericardial sac in some patients.

 TREATMENT

APPROPRIATE HEALTH CARE
Cardiac tamponade requires immediate pericardiocentesis; if uncomfortable with performing pericardiocentesis, referral to individuals with competence in this technique is strongly advised. Repeated pericardiocentesis may be needed; surgery may be indicated in selected dogs. Pericardiocentesis is rarely required in the cat.

PERICARDIOCENTESIS
• Place the patient in sternal recumbency. Clip haircoat on the right thorax between the 3rd and 8th intercostal spaces from above the costochondral junction ventrally to the sternum. The right side of the thorax is

preferred over the left because of less likelihood of coronary artery laceration. Simultaneous ECG monitoring is advised to detect arrhythmias due to contact between the needle or catheter and the myocardium. Echocardiography is useful to identify the best intercostal space, but if not available, perform pericardiocentesis at the 5th intercostal space just below the costochondral junction. After aseptic skin preparation and local anesthetic block with lidocaine, advance a long (~2 cm), large (~18 gauge) catheter into the pericardial sac; may obtain a small amount of clear pleural fluid before advancement of the catheter into the pericardial sac. In dogs, pericardial effusion is usually hemorrhagic, but some patients have a serous or serosanguineous effusion. Remove as much effusion as possible. If arrhythmias develop, reposition the needle or catheter.
• Unless the patient has active hemorrhage into the pericardial sac, the effusion obtained by pericardiocentesis should not clot and should have a packed cell volume that differs from that of peripheral blood. The supernatant of the effusion is often xanthochromic.

NURSING CARE
Unless the patient has marked dehydration, fluids are generally not required or recommended for chronic pericardial effusion. Mild volume expansion may be useful in selected animals with acute pericardial effusion due to intrapericardial hemorrhage—0.45 NaCl with 2.5% dextrose is preferred by some. Administer oxygen to dogs with tachypnea or signs of hemodynamic instability.

SURGICAL CONSIDERATIONS
• Pericardectomy may be useful in the treatment of chemodectoma or heart-base tumor.
• If idiopathic—may respond to pericardiocentesis; pericardectomy is indicated if it recurs.
• Surgery and chemotherapy are generally ineffective in the treatment of right atrial hemangiosarcoma.
• Thoracoscopy allows for pericardectomy with reduced risk and reduced postoperative pain.

MEDICATIONS

DRUG(S) OF CHOICE
• Drugs should not be used in place of pericardiocentesis.
• Diuretics—may help reduce ascites but can lead to progressive azotemia and renal dysfunction and worsen the patient's

weakness; can use diuretics such as furosemide or spironolactone if client refuses pericardiocentesis, but in low dosage, with caution; generally not advised
• Vitamin K—indicated for patients with rodenticide anticoagulant intoxication
• Appropriate antibiotics—indicated for infection by susceptible organism causing infectious pericarditis
• Chemotherapy—may be useful to treat effusion caused by lymphosarcoma; usually ineffective in the treatment of atrial hemangiosarcoma and heart-base tumor

CONTRAINDICATIONS
Digitalis, vasodilators, and angiotensin-converting enzyme inhibitors—reported to be relatively or absolutely contraindicated

PRECAUTIONS
Diuretic administration often leads to weakness and prerenal azotemia.

POSSIBLE INTERACTIONS
N/A

ALTERNATIVE DRUG(S)
• Systemic or intrapericardial chemotherapy may be attempted to treat right atrial hemangiosarcoma; generally ineffective
• Corticosteroids by systemic or intrapericardial administration—may be useful in selected patients with idiopathic pericardial effusion
• Azathioprine at a dosage of 1 mg/kg PO q24h for 3 months—can be considered for recurrent idiopathic pericardial effusion; not commonly used and, like steroids, has not been evaluated in prospective trials to confirm efficacy in idiopathic pericardial effusion

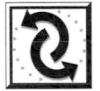

FOLLOW-UP

PATIENT MONITORING
• ECG—advised during first 24 hours because pericardiocentesis often leads to ventricular arrhythmias
• Pericardial effusion may recur at any stage; examination and echocardiography at 10–14 days and every 2–4 months recommended to detect idiopathic pericardial effusion

POSSIBLE COMPLICATIONS
• Hypotension or shock
• Pneumothorax, arrhythmias, and myocardial injury secondary to pericardiocentesis

EXPECTED COURSE AND PROGNOSIS
• Right atrial hemangiosarcoma—poor; tumor is highly malignant, usually not resectable at the time of diagnosis, and minimally responsive to chemotherapy; pericardectomy may result in exsanguination.

• Chemodectoma—fair; slow-growing tumor, late to metastasize; pericardectomy often resolves clinical signs; survival of up to 3 years has been reported following pericardectomy.
• Prognosis is good with idiopathic pericardial effusion; approximately 50% of cases resolve after 1 or 2 pericardiocenteses; pericardectomy is generally curative (~85% success) in persistent cases.

MISCELLANEOUS

ASSOCIATED CONDITIONS
Hemangiosarcoma of the spleen

AGE-RELATED FACTORS
• Idiopathic pericardial effusion may be more common in middle-aged to elderly dogs.
• Hemangiosarcoma and heart-base tumors are more common in elderly dogs.

ZOONOTIC POTENTIAL
Coccidioidomycosis

SYNONYMS
• Cardiac tamponade
• Pericardial tamponade
• Pericarditis

SEE ALSO
• Anticoagulant Rodenticide Toxicity
• Atrial Tear
• Chemodectoma
• Coccidioidomycosis
• Feline Infectious Peritonitis
• Hemangiosarcoma, Heart
• Myocardial Tumors
• Pericarditis

ABBREVIATIONS
CHF = congestive heart failure

Suggested Reading
Miller MW, Sisson DD. Pericardial disorders. In: Ettinger SJ, Feldman F.C, eds. Textbook of veterinary internal medicine. 5th ed. Philadelphia: Saunders, 2000:923–936.
Sisson D, Thomas WP. Pericardial disease and cardiac tumors. In: Fox PR, Sisson D, Moise NS, eds. Textbook of canine and feline cardiology. 2nd ed. Philadelphia: Saunders, 1999:679–702.
Smith FWK Jr, Rush JE. Diagnosis and treatment of pericardial effusion. In: Bonagura JD, ed. Kirk's current veterinary therapy XIII. Philadelphia: Saunders, 1999:772–777.
Author John E. Rush
Consulting Editors Larry P. Tilley and Francis W. K. Smith, Jr.

PERICARDITIS

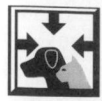

BASICS

OVERVIEW
• Inflammatory condition of the parietal (pericardial sac) and/or visceral (epicardium) pericardium; clinical syndromes caused by pericardial effusion, constrictive pericarditis, inflammatory extension to surrounding tissues (pleural, myocardium), or the underlying cause of the pericarditis • In dogs—most commonly seen as idiopathic hemorrhagic pericarditis, a mild inflammatory condition that can lead to life-threatening pericardial effusion and tamponade

SIGNALMENT
• Dogs and rarely cats • Idiopathic hemorrhagic pericarditis more common in young to middle-aged, medium to large-breed dogs (e.g., great Pyrenees, Great Dane, Saint Bernard, golden retriever); males predisposed • Others depend on the underlying disease.

SIGNS
• Cats—rarely seen on examination.
• Dogs—signs usually caused by low cardiac output and right heart failure secondary to cardiac tamponade (i.e., anorexia, weakness, collapse, ascites, dyspnea, diminished pulse strength, tachycardia, muffled heart sounds, jugular distension or pulsation); similar to those often seen in animals with constrictive pericarditis and pericardial effusion, which may coexist (constrictive-effusive pericarditis).

CAUSES & RISK FACTORS
• Idiopathic hemorrhagic pericarditis—unknown • Dogs—blunt or penetrating trauma and bacterial or fungal infection (e.g., tuberculosis, coccidioidomycosis, actinomycosis, nocardiosis, and infection with *Pasteurella* spp) • Cats—trauma or infection (e.g., FIP, *Staphylococcus aureus*, *Escherichia coli*, *Streptococcus*, *Actinomyces*, *Cryptococcus*, and possibly *Toxoplasma*.)

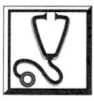

DIAGNOSIS

DIFFERENTIAL DIAGNOSIS
• Other causes of pericardial effusion (e.g., neoplasia, left atrial rupture, right-sided CHF, peritoneal-pericardial diaphragmatic hernia, and pericardial cysts) • Other causes of right-sided congestive heart failure (e.g., cardiomyopathy, myocarditis, tricuspid or pulmonary valve disease, congenital heart disease, and severe left-sided congestive heart failure) • Other causes of abdominal effusion (e.g., neoplastic effusion, hemorrhage, and hypoproteinemia) • Other causes of weakened arterial pulses or collapse (e.g., cardiomyopathy, shock, hypoadrenocorticism, arrhythmias, saddle thrombus, and aortic stenosis) • May be concealed by multisystemic signs relating to the underlying disease

CBC/BIOCHEMISTRY/URINALYSIS
Leukocytosis in some animals with a systemic inflammatory condition, but not dogs with idiopathic hemorrhagic pericarditis

IMAGING

Thoracic Radiography
• May suggest pericardial effusion (rounded cardiac silhouette), particularly when chronic effusion allows slow but marked expansion of the pericardium; absence of this finding does not rule out pericardial effusion or pericarditis • May see radiodense foreign objects • Intrapericardial injection of gas after pericardiocentesis (pneumopericardiography) may reveal space-occupying lesions; neoplastic lesions may be difficult to distinguish from granulomas or cysts.

Echocardiography
• Two-dimensional echocardiography is preferred for evaluation of effusion, cardiac tamponade, and neoplasia; diagnosis by direct visualization. • Doppler echocardiography may suggest constrictive physiology with demonstration of substantial respiratory-associated variation in pulmonary venous flow or mitral inflow. Fixed pericardial volume results in marked interdependence of the two ventricular volumes.

Cardiac Catheterization
Constrictive pericardial physiology is difficult to diagnose but may be recognized by simultaneous pressure measurements from the right and left ventricles showing pressure equalization of the two sides at an elevated end-diastolic pressure. Atrial tracings show a rapid drop in pressure in early diastole followed by an early rise to plateau at an elevated end-diastolic pressure.

DIAGNOSTIC PROCEDURES

Electrocardiographic Findings
May see small QRS complexes, electrical alternans, S-T segment elevation, and arrhythmias

Fluid Analysis
Cytologic examination of pericardial effusion—usually not helpful because it cannot differentiate the most common causes, neoplastic and idiopathic; can potentially reveal an etiologic agent and rule out a suppurative process; cytologic evaluation of effusion or pericardial biopsy provides the definitive diagnosis of pericarditis.

Other Procedures
• If an infectious agent is suspected, aerobic and anaerobic cultures of the effusion are indicated. • Histopathologic examination of the pericardium

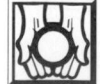

TREATMENT
• Pericardiocentesis and partial pericardectomy for severe effusion. Right

heart failure may cause or result from pericardial effusion; medical treatment of heart failure is appropriate in the former. Effusion due to idiopathic pericarditis in dogs may subside after one or more pericardiocenteses. For pericardial effusion, thoracic exploration with partial pericardectomy prevents effusions from limiting cardiac function and allows surgical débridement, retrieval of specimens for histopathologic examination, removal of foreign objects, and evaluation for neoplastic or granulomatous disease. Thorascopic pericardectomy may provide similar therapeutic benefit but more limited diagnostic evaluation • Constrictive pericarditis with extensive involvement of the epicardium may require epicardial stripping to relieve the constriction and relieve adhesions between the epicardium and pericardium; this is a difficult procedure with high mortality.

MEDICATIONS

DRUG(S)
• Treat infectious disease with chemotherapeutic agents determined through culture and sensitivity testing. • Steroid administration in dogs with idiopathic hemorrhagic pericarditis has been recommended, but efficacy is unknown; this is also true of azathioprine recommended at 1.0 mg/kg q24h for 3 months.

CONTRAINDICATIONS/POSSIBLE INTERACTIONS
• Fluid therapy exacerbates right heart failure • Diuretics and preload reducers—relatively contraindicated in animals with cardiac tamponade • Steroids may exacerbate an infection.

FOLLOW-UP
Pericardial effusion may recur if the pericardium is intact. Occasionally, clinically important pleural effusion may occur after pericardectomy; echocardiography or thoracic radiography is recommended.

MISCELLANEOUS

Suggested Reading
Miller MW, Sisson DD. Pericardial disorders. In: Ettinger SJ, Feldman EC, eds. Textbook of veterinary internal medicine. 5th ed. Philadelphia: Saunders, 2000:923–936.
Author Donald J. Brown
Consulting Editors Larry P. Tilley and Francis W. K. Smith, Jr.

BASICS

OVERVIEW
• Results from a defect in the musculature of the pelvic diaphragm
• Allows herniation of retroperitoneal fat or pelvic viscera through the pelvic diaphragm
• Organ systems potentially involved—GI, musculoskeletal, urologic, reproductive

SIGNALMENT
• Much more common in dogs than cats
• Almost exclusively (95%) male dogs
• Usually older than 5 years of age
• Boston terriers, collies, boxers, Pekingese, and mongrels overrepresented

SIGNS

Historical Findings
• Tenesmus
• Stranguria/dysuria if prostate or bladder entrapment
• Painful defecation
• Flatulence
• Fecal or urinary incontinence (rare)

Physical Examination Findings
• Fluctuant perineal swelling—unilateral or bilateral
• Defect in pelvic diaphragm palpable per rectum

CAUSES & RISK FACTORS
• Unknown
• Suggested causes include congenital pelvic muscle weakness, gonadal hormone imbalance, prostatic disease, chronic constipation/tenesmus, concurrent rectal disease (diverticulum, sacculation, deviation)

DIAGNOSIS

DIFFERENTIAL DIAGNOSIS
• Perianal or perineal neoplasia is usually a firm irregular swelling.
• Anal sac disease (abscess, cellulitis) is usually painful and localized to the anal sacs.

CBC/BIOCHEMISTRY/URINALYSIS
• No consistent changes
• Complete laboratory analysis recommended to look for concurrent diseases in older patients.
• May be azotemic if urinary obstruction is due to bladder entrapment

OTHER LABORATORY TESTS
N/A

IMAGING
• Plain radiographs document extent of rectal/colonic dilatation.
• GI contrast radiography differentiates rectal deviation from rectal sacculation or diverticulum.
• Contrast cystography demonstrates bladder entrapment.
• Ultrasonography (abdominal, perineal) may demonstrate prostatic, bladder, and/or GI entrapment.

DIAGNOSTIC PROCEDURES
N/A

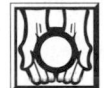
TREATMENT
• Inpatient surgical management; not an emergency unless bladder or GI entrapment with obstruction
• Surgery indicated to reduce hernia and repair muscular defect
• Internal obturator flap herniorrhaphy technique has the lowest recurrence rate.
• May use semitendinosus muscle flap to repair large ventral hernias, especially when other surgeries have failed
• Can perform colopexy/cystopexy in conjunction with, or independent of, herniorrhaphy to prevent herniation of rectum and urinary bladder, respectively
• Concurrent castration is recommended.
• High-fiber diet may help obtain a soft, formed stool; if colonic fecal overdistension occurs with bulk-fiber diets, a low-residue diet is indicated.
• Warn owners that underlying cause may not be corrected by surgery.

MEDICATIONS

DRUG(S)
• Use stool softeners as needed to maintain a soft, formed stool, and thus reduce straining.
• Perioperative prophylactic antibiotics are justified; choose one with broad-spectrum activity against gram-negative organisms.

CONTRAINDICATIONS/POSSIBLE INTERACTIONS
N/A

FOLLOW-UP

PREVENTION/AVOIDANCE
Early neutering of male dogs reduces risk.

POSSIBLE COMPLICATIONS
Immediate postsurgical complications include infection, fecal incontinence, sciatic nerve entrapment, and rectal prolapse.

EXPECTED COURSE AND PROGNOSIS
Overall recurrence rate 10–50% following repair

MISCELLANEOUS

ASSOCIATED CONDITIONS
• Megacolon
• Prostatic disease
• Dyschezia
• Tenesmus

ABBREVIATION
GI = gastrointestinal

Suggested Reading
Anderson MA, Constantinescu GM, Mann FA. Perineal hernia repair in the dog. In: Bojrab MJ, ed., Current techniques in small animal surgery. 4th ed. Philadelphia: Lippincott Williams & Wilkins, 1998: 555–564.

Author Bradford C. Dixon
Consulting Editor Albert E. Jergens

PERIODONTAL DISEASE

 BASICS

DEFINITION
Inflammation of some or all of the tooth's support structures (gingiva, cementum, periodontal ligament, and alveolar bone); compared with gingivitis (inflammation of the marginal gingiva), periodontitis indicates some degree of periodontal attachment tissue loss.

PATHOPHYSIOLOGY
• An intact epithelial barrier and high rate of epithelial turnover and surface desquamation prevent bacteria from gaining direct access to tissue.
• Some bacterial products may diffuse through the junctional epithelium to reach the underlying gingival connective tissue; normal host defense mechanisms limit the penetration of these products and their damaging effects.
• Fluctuations in the host–parasite equilibrium may result in cycles of either diminished or increased intensity of the inflammatory response; it may be possible to think of periodontitis as the outcome of an imperfectly balanced host–parasite interaction.
• Caused by bacteria located in the gingival crevice; initially a pellicle forms on the enamel surface of a clean tooth; the pellicle is composed of proteins and glycoproteins deposited from saliva and gingival crevicular fluid; the pellicle attracts aerobic Gram-positive bacteria (mostly actinomycetes and streptococci); more bacteria soon adhere, forming plaque; within days the plaque thickens, becomes mineralized and transforms into calculus, which is rough and irritating to the gingiva; the underlying bacteria run out of oxygen and anaerobic motile rods and spirochetes begin to populate the subgingival area; more plaque builds on top of the calculus; endotoxins released by anaerobic bacteria cause tissue destruction and bone-loss periodontitis.

SYSTEMS AFFECTED
Microscopic hepatic, renal, and CNS lesions are found in some animals.

SIGNALMENT
Dogs and cats 6 months and older may be affected.

SIGNS

Physical Examination Findings
• Grade 1 inflammation—confined to tissues of the marginal gingiva
• Grade 2 inflammation—edema; gingival bleeding on probing (up to 25% attachment loss)
• Grade 3—as above; pustular discharge; slight-to-moderate bone loss (25–50% attachment loss)
• Grade 4—as above; mobility; severe bone loss (> 50% attachment loss)

CAUSES
• Gingivitis—dogs; *Streptococcus* and *Actinomyces* spp.
• Periodontitis—dogs; pigmented and nonpigmented bacteroides (*Porphyromonas gingivalis*, *Prevotella* spp., *Bacteroides* spp.), *Fusobacterium* spp.
• Cats—*Peptostreptococcus, Actinomyces,* and *Porphyromonas* spp.
• Soft diet promotes periodontal disease through accumulation of plaque

RISK FACTORS
• Toy breeds with crowded teeth
• Dogs that groom themselves—causes hair to be imbedded in the gingival sulcus
• Other debilitating illnesses
• Poor nutritional state

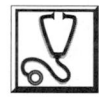 DIAGNOSIS

DIFFERENTIAL DIAGNOSIS
• Pemphigus
• Lupus
• Oral neoplasia
• Stomatitis

CBC/BIOCHEMISTRY/URINALYSIS
N/A

OTHER LABORATORY TESTS

IMAGING
• Radiography—important diagnostic tool; as much as 60% of disease is hidden below the gum line.

• No radiographic changes in grades 1 and 2 disease (gingivitis)
• Early radiographic signs of grade 3 disease include loss of density and sharpness of the crestal bone; as periodontal disease progresses, loss of lamina dura mineralization apically and furcation involvement in multirooted teeth
• Severe periodontal disease appears radiographically as loss of bone support around one or more roots; bone loss may be horizontal (a decrease in bone height around one or more teeth), vertical (infrabony defect), or oblique (a combination of both).

DIAGNOSTIC PROCEDURES
• Periodontal probing—"probing depth": distance between free gingival margin and apical extent of pocket; probing depths > 2 mm in the dog and 1 mm in the cat are abnormal
• "Attachment loss" measures between CEJ and apical extent of pocket; normally the gingival sulcus is located at the CEJ; any attachment loss is abnormal.

 TREATMENT

• The ultimate goal of periodontal therapy is to control plaque; a willing patient and a client who can provide home care are important considerations in creating a therapy plan.
• Grade 1 or 2—professional cleaning, hand scaling, polishing, irrigation, application of fluoride
• Grade 3—pocket depths: 3–6 mm in dogs, 2–4 mm in cats; above plus closed-root planing and subgingival curettage
• After thoroughly cleaning moderate pocket, placement of a local antibiotic gel (Doxirobe, Atrix Laboratories, Fort Collins, CO) can help rejuvenate periodontal tissues and may reduce pocket depth.
• Grade 4—pocket depth > 6 mm in dogs, 4 mm in cat; surgery needed to either expose the root for treatment (open-flap curettage) or extract
• If 2–3 mm of healthy, attached gingiva is present—apically reposition flap to decrease pocket depth in areas of alveolar bone loss; if not enough healthy gingiva remains to apically reposition flap; rotated flap (from

adjacent gingiva), free gingival flap, or extraction
• Bone replacement procedures—with two-, three-, four-walled infrabony pockets
• Guided tissue regeneration—use tissue barriers to separate gingival tissue and root surface.
• Periodontal splinting—can be used especially in the incisor areas to help stabilize mobile teeth; criteria for splinting include normal periodontal support on both sides of the tooth (teeth) to be stabilized, strict home care, and a cooperative patient who will not chew on hard objects and destroy the splint.

MEDICATIONS

DRUG(S) OF CHOICE
Clindamycin is approved for dental infections; may be used for a week before periodontal treatment, 20 min before anesthesia, postoperatively for 7–10 days, and/or, in a pulse therapy fashion, given the first 5 days of each month.

Home Care
• Fluoride—stannous fluoride preparations (Omni Gel and Gel Kam) help control periodontal disease by reducing plaque deposition on the surface of enamel and also decrease dental pain; use 0.4% strength in patients with stage 3 and 4 periodontal disease, especially those with exposed root surfaces.
• Chlorhexidine—the most effective product to inhibit plaque formation in humans; bacteriostatic and bactericidal against bacteria, fungi, and some viruses; once absorbed it continues to be effective for up to 24 hr; in humans, to be maximally effective, it is swished in the mouth for 1 min twice daily; the contact time of application is important for binding to the tooth and gingival sulcus; 1-min oral rinsing is difficult to accomplish in animals; chlorhexidine can be applied with a gauze sponge or cotton-tipped applicators, as a spray, or with finger brushes.
• CHX Guard solution (VRx Products, Harbor City, CA) contains chlorhexidine

gluconate 0.12% plus zinc gluconate, which promotes healing of ulcerated tissue; CHX gel chlorhexidine gluconate 0.12%; the gel allows greater binding time and has a pleasant taste.
• DentiVet toothpaste (Virbac, Fort Worth, TX) contains chlorhexidine gluconate, zinc, and sodium hexamethylphosphate; Hexarinse contains 0.12% chlorhexidine, cetylpyridinium, chloride, and zinc.
• Novaldent—chlorhexidine acetate 0.1%
• Lactoperoxidase system enhanced enzyme products—have antibacterial properties that decrease plaque (CET, CET Forte toothpastes, CET Chews, CET Spray-VRx Product).
• Diet-hard biscuit foods are preferable to soft sticky foods.
• T/D tartar control diet (Hills)—specifically indicated to control tartar in dogs and cats
• Amount and type of home care products dispensed depends on dental periodontal pathology.
Stage 1 and 2—daily brushing with dentifrice
Stage 3, established periodontal disease—daily brushing with fluoride-containing toothpaste plus twice-weekly application of stannous fluoride gel and pulse therapy antibiotics
Stage 4, advanced periodontal disease—zinc ascorbate gel (Maxi-Guard-Addison Biologics Inc) 3–4 times daily to help regenerate cellular collagen, plus 0.2% chlorhexidine spray twice daily; or CHX-Guard (VRx Products), a combination of chlorhexidine gluconate and zinc, and pulse therapy antibiotics; after 2 weeks, can substitute stannous fluoride gel twice weekly for the chlorhexidine spray

CONTRAINDICATIONS
N/A

PRECAUTIONS
N/A

POSSIBLE INTERACTIONS
Do not use chlorhexidine and fluoride products concurrently; binding both products may inactivate them; better to wait 30 min to 1 hr between use of a dentifrice containing fluoride and a chlorhexidine rinse or gel

ALTERNATIVE DRUG(S)
• Tetracycline
• Clavamox
• Flagyl

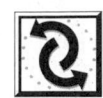

FOLLOW-UP

PATIENT MONITORING
The degree of periodontal pathology dictates recall interval; some patients are checked weekly, while others can be evaluated every 3–6 months.

POSSIBLE COMPLICATIONS
N/A

MISCELLANEOUS

ASSOCIATED CONDITIONS
N/A

AGE-RELATED FACTORS
N/A

ZOONOTIC POTENTIAL
N/A

PREGNANCY
N/A

SYNONYMS
N/A

SEE ALSO
N/A

ABBREVIATION
CEJ = cementoenamel junction

Suggested Reading
Harvey CE. Periodontal disease in dogs. Vet Clin North Am 1998;28:1111–1128.
Wiggs RB, Lobprise HB. Veterinary dentistry: principles and practice. Philadelphia: Lippincott Raven, 1997.
Author Jan Bellows
Consulting Editor Heidi B. Lobprise

PERIPHERAL EDEMA

 BASICS

DEFINITION
Edema is focal or diffuse excessive accumulation of tissue fluid within the interstitium; often at gravitative surfaces, whether localized or generalized

PATHOPHYSIOLOGY
- High capillary hydrostatic pressure
- Increased capillary permeability
- Lymphatic drainage abnormality
- Low plasma colloid osmotic pressure

SYSTEMS AFFECTED
- Skin/Exocrine • Musculoskeletal

GENETICS
- Dominantly inherited primary lymphedema has been described in poodles.
- Lethal congenital edema has been documented in bull dogs.

INCIDENCE/PREVALENCE
Variable

GEOGRAPHIC DISTRIBUTION
N/A

SIGNALMENT

Species
Dogs and cats

Breed Predilection
Primary or congenital lymphedema has been reported in bull dogs, poodles, Old English sheep dogs, and Labradors.

Mean Age and Range
None

Predominant Sex
None

SIGNS

Historical Findings
- Allergic or other immune, cardiac, hepatic, or other organic disease • Trauma • Exposure to toxic (venomous) or infectious agents such as ticks or other arachnids

Physical Examination Findings
- Unexplained weight gain may be noted initially; otherwise early detection is unlikely.
- Noninflammatory subcutaneous edema is often first recognized at the dependent thorax or abdomen or distal limbs.
- Inflammatory edema may be noted in nondependent foci of the interstitium.

CAUSES

Localized or Single-Limb Edema
- High capillary hydrostatic pressure • Venous or arterial obstruction, e.g., thrombosis or postcaval syndrome • Arteriovenous fistula
- Increased capillary permeability • Focal or multifocal immune, infectious, or toxic (chemical or biologic) insults (e.g., snake bite or bee sting) • Trauma • Burns • Lymphatic obstruction • Sterile (juvenile pyoderma) or infectious lymphangitis • Primary or metastatic neoplastic invasion of lymphatic tissue • Congenital aplasia or dysgenesis of the lymphatic system

Regional or Generalized Edema
- High capillary hydrostatic pressure
- Congestive heart failure (CHF) • Cardiac tamponade • Cranial or caudal vena caval thrombosis • Renal failure and hypernatremia (salt retention) • Paralysis or prolonged recumbency with subsequent failure of the venous pump • Tourniquet effect of a bandage • Increased capillary permeability
- Systemic immune, infectious, or toxic insults (e.g., sepsis or vasculitis) • Lymphatic abnormalities • Acquired regional traumatic, immune, infectious, or neoplastic process
- Congenital aplasia or other lymphatic dysgenesis • Low plasma colloid osmotic pressure • Protein-losing disease (e.g., nephrotic syndrome or intestinal lymphangiectasia) • Failure to produce protein (e.g., cirrhosis) • Exudative protein loss (e.g., severe burn)

RISK FACTORS
Variable

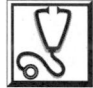 **DIAGNOSIS**

DIFFERENTIAL DIAGNOSIS
- Peripheral edema secondary to myxedema or inflammation is typically nonpitting.
- Bilateral forelimb edema with jugular venous distention implies cranial vena caval syndrome.
- Bilateral rear limb edema with or without ascites implies either hypoalbuminemia or caudal vena caval obstruction.
- Fore and/or rear limb edema with jugular venous distension, hydrothorax, and/or ascites implies cardiac disease.
- Focal edema with bruit and fremitus implies an arteriovenous fistula.
- Focal edema with erythema may be secondary to an insect or other bite.
- Multifocal or diffuse edema with petechiation and/or ecchymosis may be associated with a coagulopathy or vasculitis.

CBC/BIOCHEMISTRY/URINALYSIS
- Leukocytosis suggests inflammatory or infectious disease.
- Thrombocytopenia may be secondary to vasculitis (e.g., Rocky Mountain spotted fever [RMSF]), systemic lupus erythematosus (SLE), or a coagulopathy (e.g., disseminated intravascular coagulation [DIC]).
- Panhypoproteinemia is consistent with gastrointestinal disease, but diarrhea is not an obligatory clinical sign.
- Panhypoproteinemia and hypocholesterolemia are seen with intestinal lymphangiectasia.
- Hypoalbuminemia may occur with hepatic failure.
- Hypoalbuminemia with proteinuria suggests glomerular disease.
- Hypoalbuminemia with proteinuria and hypercholesterolemia in an edematous patient defines nephrotic syndrome.

OTHER LABORATORY TESTS
- Antithrombin (AT) III assay indicated in conditions with albumin loss
- Further delineate thrombocytopenia with a bone marrow biopsy, antinuclear antibody (ANA), *Ehrlichia* and RMSF titers, and a coagulation profile.
- Panhypoproteinemia may dictate a need for intestinal biopsy.
- Hypoalbuminemia may warrant liver function testing (e.g., bile acid test, hepatic biopsy)
- Confirm proteinuria with a urine protein: creatinine ratio.
- Bacterial and fungal cultures of blind fistulae may prove useful.
- Fungal or other titers of infectious disease may be warranted.
- Pleural or peritoneal fluid analysis is suggested if effusion is present.
- Low resting thyroid hormone (T_4) should be elaborated with a thyrotropin-releasing hormone (TRH) stimulation test, free T_4 by equilibrium dialysis, or thyroid-stimulating hormone (TSH) concentration.

IMAGING
- Suspected heart disease necessitates thoracic radiographs and echocardiogram.
- Angiography (e.g., venacavagram) may help define a vascular obstruction.
- Diagnostic ultrasound may help to delineate a vascular occlusion.
- Thermography and perfusion scans (e.g., scintigraphy) are esoteric but have been used to diagnose occlusive vascular disease.

DIAGNOSTIC PROCEDURES
- Fine-needle aspiration of an affected area for cytology and culture may be helpful.
- Biopsy and deep culture may help define an underlying cause for edema.

PATHOLOGIC FINDINGS
Depend on cause of the edema

 TREATMENT

APPROPRIATE HEALTH CARE
Depend on the cause of the edema

NURSING CARE
- Application of warm compresses is recommended for patients with edema secondary to infection.

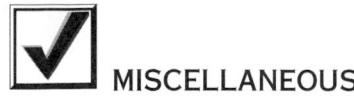

• Good nursing care required to prevent decubital ulceration in recumbent patients

ACTIVITY
Depends on cause of edema—e.g., exercise restriction is recommended in patients with congestive heart failure

DIET
Depends on the cause of edema—e.g., patients with protein-losing nephropathy require a restricted protein diet

CLIENT EDUCATION
Depends on the cause of edema

SURGICAL CONSIDERATIONS
• Surgery such as lymphangioplasty, thrombectomy, or lymphaticovenous shunt may be palliative.
• Amputation of the edematous limb is sometimes indicated.
• Arteriovenous fistulae may be treated by various surgical methods.

 MEDICATIONS

DRUG(S)
• Anaphylaxis—epinephrine (1 mg/mL) at 0.01 mL/kg IM or SC to a maximum of 0.02–0.05 mL; prednisone sodium succinate, 10–30 mg/kg IV; antihistamines are of equivocal benefit once anaphylaxis ensues.
• Lymphedema—benzopyrone use yields variable results in veterinary medicine; rutin, 50 mg/kg PO q8h, has been mixed with food for cats with chylothorax.
• Cardiogenic edema—combinations of positive or negative inotropes, vasodilators, and diuretics commonly used in patients with CHF
• Immune-mediated edema requires immunosuppressive therapy (e.g., prednisone and cyclophosphamide)
• Vasculitis and edema secondary to rickettsial disease typically respond to tetracycline (22 mg/kg PO q8h) or doxycycline (5 mg/kg PO q12h).
• Edema in association with other infectious agents requires antifungal therapy or antibiotic therapy (ideally dictated by culture and sensitivity).
• Myxedema secondary to hypothyroidism should respond gradually to T_4 supplementation.
• Edema associated with toxic insults may be slowed with antidotes (e.g., antivenom).
• Anticoagulant therapy (e.g., heparin and warfarin) may benefit patients with DIC or AT III depletion, respectively.
• Vascular volume expanders such as hydroxy-

ethyl starch or plasma often benefit patients with low plasma oncotic pressure; very-low-dose furosemide in a constant-rate infusion of 0.1 mg/kg/h has been effective in conjunction with a volume expander

CONTRAINDICATIONS
• Diuretics generally aggravate edema of non-cardiogenic origin.
• Steroids may worsen edema secondary to infectious disease.
• Epinephrine—generally contraindicated in shock except in anaphylaxis
• Propranolol (β-blocker)—contraindicated in patients predisposed to bronchospasm

PRECAUTIONS
• Avoid IM injections in patients with thrombocytopenia.
• Taper patients on long-term steroid therapy so that endogenous steroid production resumes.
• Use epinephrine cautiously in patients predisposed to ventricular fibrillation.
• Use enalapril cautiously in patients with renal disease.
• Long-term antibiotic therapy may facilitate a superinfection by a fungus (e.g., Candida) or resistant bacteria.
• Monitor anticoagulants closely to avoid fatal hemorrhage.

 FOLLOW-UP

PATIENT MONITORING
• Repeat complete blood counts, chemistries, and urine protein:creatinine ratios for blood dyscrasias and serum and urine protein concentrations, respectively • Weekly assessment of prothrombin or partial thromboplastin time for patients on warfarin or heparin, respectively • Serial biopsies of affected tissue such as kidney in glomerulonephritis may help to prognosticate. • Repeat cultures or acute and convalescing titers for patients suffering from an infectious disease • Periodic T_4 assay for patients receiving thyroid supplementation

PREVENTION/AVOIDANCE
Depends on the cause of the edema

POSSIBLE COMPLICATIONS
• Decubital ulceration • Fatal hemorrhage
• Fatal thrombosis • Refractory cardiac, gastrointestinal, hepatic, or renal failure
• Malnutrition • Cerebral edema and herniation • Resistant infection and sepsis

EXPECTED COURSE AND PROGNOSIS
Depends on cause of the edema

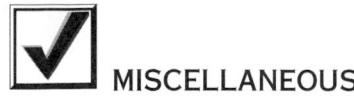 MISCELLANEOUS

ASSOCIATED CONDITIONS
Pericardial, pleural, or peritoneal effusion

AGE-RELATED FACTORS
Vascular anomalies or primary lymphedema are generally documented in juvenile patients (e.g., anasarca).

ZOONOTIC POTENTIAL
• Recent tick exposure is a common element in pets and their owners who may suffer simultaneously from rickettsial disease.
• Certain protozoal (Leishmania), fungal (Sporothrix), and bacterial (Brucella) organisms may transfer to people via direct contact.

PREGNANCY
Brucellosis has been associated with vulvar edema, necrotizing vasculitis, and embryonic death or fetal abortion.

SYNONYMS
Anasarca

SEE ALSO
• Ascites • Chylothorax • Cirrhosis and Fibrosis of the Liver • Hyperlipidemia
• Hypoalbuminemia • Lymphedema
• Proteinuria • Thrombocytopenia
• Vasculitis, Cutaneous • Vasculitis, Systemic

ABBREVIATIONS
• AT III = antithrombin III
• RMSF = Rocky Mountain spotted fever
• T_4 = thyroid hormone
• TRH = thyrotropin-releasing hormone
• TSH = thyroid-stimulating hormone

Suggested Reading

Bright JM. Peripheral edema. In: Ettinger SJ, Feldman EC, eds. Textbook of veterinary internal medicine. 4th ed. Philadelphia: Saunders, 1995:100–103.

Fossum TW, King LA, Miller MW, et al. Lymphedema. Clinical signs, diagnosis and treatment. J Vet Intern Med 1992;6:312–319.

Fossum TW, Miller MW. Lymphedema. Etiopathogenesis. J Vet Intern Med 1992;6:283–293.

Suter FP, Fox PR. Peripheral vascular disease. In: Ettinger SJ, Feldman EC, eds. Textbook of veterinary internal medicine. 4th ed. Philadelphia: Saunders, 1995.

Author Marc Elie

Consulting Editors Larry P. Tilley and Francis W. K. Smith, Jr.

PERIPHERAL NEUROPATHIES (POLYNEUROPATHIES)

BASICS

DEFINITION
Diseases that affect many peripheral motor, sensory, autonomic, and/or cranial nerves, in any combination

PATHOPHYSIOLOGY
• Inherited or acquired • Primary pathologic process—destruction or degeneration of the ventral horn cells (neuronopathy), primary demyelination, or axonal degeneration (with secondary demyelination)

SYSTEMS AFFECTED
• Nervous—primarily peripheral nervous system; possible involvement of the cranial nerves • Other organ systems—many may be involved in the primary disease process.

GENETICS
• Most inherited as autosomal recessive disorders • Spinal muscular atrophy in Brittany spaniels—autosomal dominant disorder

INCIDENCE/PREVALENCE
• Inherited—rare • Peripheral nerve involvement in metabolic and neoplastic diseases—incidence unknown • Inflammatory—uncommon; coonhound paralysis most frequently encountered (somewhat seasonal prevalence: highest in fall and early winter)

GEOGRAPHIC DISTRIBUTION
• Coonhound paralysis—confined to North and Central America and parts of South America • Distal denervating disease—most common in dogs in the UK; not reported elsewhere • Other polyneuropathies—no evidence of a geographic distribution

SIGNALMENT

Species
Dogs and cats

Breed Predilections
INHERITED
Spinal Muscular Atrophy
• Brittany spaniels, Swedish Lapland dogs, English pointers, German shepherds, rottweilers • Progressive neuronopathy—cairn terriers
Axonopathies
• Giant axonal neuropathy—German shepherds • Progressive axonopathy—boxers • Primary hyperoxaluria—domestic shorthair cats • Laryngeal paralysis–polyneuropathy complex—Dalmatians and rottweilers • Distal polyneuropathy—Birman cats • Distal sensorimotor polyneuropathy—rottweilers
Demyelination
Hypertrophic neuropathy—Tibetan mastiffs
Lysosomal Storage Diseases
• Globoid cell leukodystrophy—West Highland whites, cairn terriers, domestic shorthair kittens • a-L-fucosidosis—springer spaniels • G_{M1} gangliosidosis type II—Siamese and mixed-breed cats • Sphingomyelinosis—Siamese cats • Ceroid

lipofuscinosis—English setters, Chihuahuas, Siamese cats • Sensory neuropathy—long-haired dachshunds, English pointers, border collies
ACQUIRED
• Coonhound paralysis—because of their use, coonhounds have a higher incidence than other breeds. • Clinical diabetic polyneuropathy—more common in cats than dogs • Insulinomas—German shepherds, boxers, Irish setters, standard poodles, and collies

Mean Age and Range
INHERITED
• Usually begin at < 6 months of age • Feline hyperchylomicronemia—usually > 8 months • Feline hyperoxaluria—5–9 months • Rottweiler distal polyneuropathy—> 1 year • Giant axonal neuropathy in German shepherds—14–16 months • Intermediate and chronic forms of spinal muscular atrophy in heterozygote Brittany spaniels—6–12 months
ACQUIRED
• Secondary to neoplasia and insulinoma-associated hypoglycemia—tend to occur in middle-aged and old animals • *Neospora* polyradiculoneuritis—most commonly seen in dogs < 6 months of age; highest incidence 2–4 months

Predominant Sex
N/A

SIGNS

Historical Findings
INHERITED
• Most—slow, progressive; generalized weakness, muscle tremors, muscle atrophy, often with a plantigrade/palmigrade stance and gait • Sensory neuropathies—may see self-mutilation or ataxia • Lysosomal storage diseases—evidence of slowly progressive CNS involvement common; head tremors, ataxia, dysmetria, seizures, blindness, dementia, and depression • Giant axonal neuropathy of German shepherds—rapidly progressive generalized weakness (< 3 weeks)
ACQUIRED
• Rapid or slow progression • Rapidly progressive course—an initial stiff, stilted gait, leading to progressive generalized paresis or paralysis (coonhound paralysis, distal denervating disease) • Slowly progressive course—generalized weakness and muscle atrophy; in the distal polyneuropathies (diabetic cat), a plantigrade stance • Dysautonomia—primarily an acute onset (< 48 hr) of depression, anorexia, constipation, third eyelid protrusion, vomiting, and urinary incontinence • Metabolic—owner reports the non-neurologic clinical signs associated with the initiating defect. • Paraneoplastic—primary tumor may be clinically silent at the time of presentation.

Physical Examination Findings
• Motor and sensorimotor—tetraparesis to tetraplegia, hyporeflexia to areflexia, hypotonia to atonia, and muscle atrophy classic; muscle tremors common • Sensory—proprioceptive

deficits; hypothenia to anesthesia, without muscle atrophy or hyporeflexia (except in boxers) • Hypothyroidism—associated with generalized polyneuropathy, laryngeal paralysis, megaesophagus, facial nerve paralysis, and peripheral vestibular disease • Lysosomal storage diseases—hepatosplenomegaly common • Paraneoplastic—may be evidence of neoplasia • Dysautonomia—dry rhinarium, xerostomia, low tear production, bradycardia, and anal areflexia • Primary feline hyperchylomicronemia—lipid granulomata, which can be palpated under the skin and in the abdomen, common • Primary hyperoxaluria (cats)—enlarged, painful kidneys on abdominal palpation • Cranial nerve abnormalities (including dysphonia and aphonia)—variable

CAUSES

Acquired
• Immune—primary or secondary; may be seen with SLE or other immune diseases (e.g., polymyositis, glomerulonephritis, polyarthritis, and pemphigus) • Metabolic—diabetes mellitus (cats), hypothyroidism, and insulinoma; may be associated with (adeno) carcinomas, malignant melanoma, mast cell tumor, osteosarcoma, multiple myeloma, or lymphosarcoma • Infectious—*Neospora caninum;* FeLV • Cancer drugs—vincristine; vinblastine; cisplatin; colchicine • Toxic—thallium; organophosphates; carbon tetrachloride; lindane • Idiopathic

RISK FACTORS
Development of associated specific diseases (metabolic, immune, neoplastic) or exposure to associated specific drugs/toxins or causal factors (raccoon saliva)

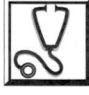

DIAGNOSIS

DIFFERENTIAL DIAGNOSIS
• Acute—botulism; tick paralysis; acute disseminated or multifocal myelopathies • Chronic—polymyopathy; chronic disseminated or multifocal myelopathies

CBC/BIOCHEMISTRY/URINALYSIS
• Standard laboratory tests—do not reflect occurrence of polyneuropathy; often indicate possible underlying metabolic or neoplastic disease • High serum creatine kinase—indicates an accompanying myopathy

OTHER LABORATORY TESTS
• None with respect to the actual polyneuropathy • ANA, lupus erythematosus preparation, and Coombs test—assist in the diagnosis of immune disease • Low TSH stimulation test, low T_4, low free T_4, and high endogenous TSH—hypothyroidism • Amended insulin:glucose ratio—> 30 supports the diagnosis of an insulinoma • Serology—assists in the diagnosis of *N. caninum* and FeLV infection • Low specific leukocyte lysosomal enzymes—indicate specific storage diseases • High plasma epinephrine and norepinephrine levels—

dysautonomia • High serum cholesterol, triglycerides, and very low density lipoprotein—hyperchylomicronemia • Hyperoxaluria and L-glyceric aciduria—seen in primary hyperoxaluria (cats) • Monoclonal gammopathy—multiple myeloma

IMAGING
• Thoracic and abdominal radiographs—important in the diagnosis of megaesophagus; demonstrate ileus, bladder atony, constipation, and delayed gastric emptying in dysautonomia • Radiography and ultrasound—help the search for a neoplastic cause

DIAGNOSTIC PROCEDURES
• Electrophysiology (EMG, motor and sensory nerve conduction and action potential amplitudes, and late wave studies)—cornerstone for diagnosis • Lumbar CSF analysis—valuable in diagnosing nerve root involvement • Muscle biopsy—confirms evidence of denervation (myofiber angular atrophy type I and II) • Peripheral nerve biopsy—further delineates disease process

PATHOLOGIC FINDINGS
• Degree of axonal degeneration, demyelination, and/or neuronal cell body degeneration depends on the specific condition. • Anatomic distribution of the lesion along the peripheral nerves (proximal, distal or widespread) depends on the specific condition.

TREATMENT

APPROPRIATE HEALTH CARE
• Usually outpatient • Inpatient—observe acute polyradiculoneuropathies closely for respiratory failure in the early progressive phase of disease.

NURSING CARE
• Dysautonomia—may require intensive IV fluid therapy and/or parenteral feeding • Physiotherapy—an excellent ancillary treatment

ACTIVITY
No restrictions, if ambulatory

DIET
• Generally no special management, unless megaesophagus or dysphagia occurs • Hyperchylomicronemia—low-fat diet alone can resolve the polyneuropathy within 2–3 months. • Paralysis—make sure the patient can reach food and water. • Regurgitation and/or vomiting (e.g., in dysautonomia)—temporarily halt oral intake. • Diabetes mellitus—important to carefully monitor food intake

CLIENT EDUCATION
• Inform client that treatment of the primary cause may not lead to reversal of the peripheral nerve signs, and, in some cases, deterioration will continue. • Inform client that many polyneuropathies are idiopathic, despite extensive diagnostic workup.

SURGICAL CONSIDERATIONS
Paraneoplastic—treat the primary tumor via surgery, chemotherapy, or radiation.

MEDICATIONS

DRUG(S) OF CHOICE
• Inherited—most are untreatable. • Acquired—principal goal is usually to treat the primary cause, if identified, with the hope that the secondary polyneuropathy will improve or resolve after appropriate therapy; not always successful • Chronic progressive or relapsing—most likely of immune origin; may improve with long-term immunosuppressive corticosteroid therapy (prednisone at 1–2 mg/kg PO q12h), azathioprine (2.2 mg/kg PO q24h), or cyclophosphamide (50 mg/m² q48h); response of individual patient variable • SLE-related—treat as for chronic progressive or relapsing polyneuropathy. • Neoplasia—immunosuppressive corticosteroid therapy may improve the polyneuropathy without specific action against the primary tumor. • *Neospora*-associated polyradiculoneuritis—best treated with clindamycin (5.5 mg/kg PO q12h); efficacy is questionable. • Dysautonomia—treat symptomatically with IV fluid therapy, artificial tears, metoclopramide (0.2–0.4 mg/kg PO q8h), bethanechol (cats: 0.5–2.5 mg SC q12h or 2.5–10 mg PO q6–8h; dogs: 0.5–15 mg SC q12h or 2.5–30 mg PO q6–8h), and physostigmine eye drops.

CONTRAINDICATIONS
Corticosteroid therapy—contraindicated in *Neospora*-associated polyradiculoneuritis and coonhound paralysis

PRECAUTIONS
N/A

POSSIBLE INTERACTIONS
N/A

ALTERNATIVE DRUG(S)
N/A

FOLLOW-UP

PATIENT MONITORING
Repeat neurologic examinations.

PREVENTION/AVOIDANCE
• Avoid breeding patients with inherited or *Neospora*-associated (placental transfer of the organism from the bitch) diseases. • Avoid contact with raccoons for dogs with a previous history of coonhound paralysis.

POSSIBLE COMPLICATIONS
• Inherited—continued neurologic deterioration, eventually leading to inability to successfully ambulate • Acute or chronic progressive—severe muscle atrophy and resultant pressure sores; urinary tract infection; muscle fibrosis and contracture; aspiration pneumonia

EXPECTED COURSE AND PROGNOSIS
• Purely demyelinating conditions have a more rapid course of improvement than those involving axonal degeneration (the majority), which can take months for partial or complete recovery, if at all. • Inherited—most have a poor to hopeless prognosis for any recovery of peripheral nerve function (except hyperchylomicronemia in cats). • Acute polyradiculoneuritis (coonhound paralysis)—good long-term prognosis; may take weeks to months to recover ambulation • Metabolic—fair to good prognosis with successful treatment of the primary metabolic abnormality; insulinomas have a high recurrence rate. • Other acquired—most show continued deterioration despite treatment; guarded to poor prognosis; sometimes progression is slow and insidious over many months or years.

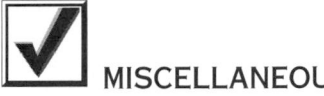

MISCELLANEOUS

ASSOCIATED CONDITIONS
N/A

AGE-RELATED FACTORS
N/A

ZOONOTIC POTENTIAL
N/A

PREGNANCY
• Metabolic—some have a significant affect on pregnant patients • High-dose corticosteroids and other immunosuppressive agents—contraindicated during pregnancy

SYNONYMS
N/A

SEE ALSO
See Causes

ABBREVIATIONS
• ANA = antinuclear antibody • CSF = cerebrospinal fluid • EMG = electromyography • FeLV = feline leukemia virus • SLE = systemic lupus erythematosus • TSH = thyroid-stimulating hormone

Suggested Reading

Cuddon PA. Feline neuromuscular diseases. Feline Pract 1994;22:7–13.

Cummings JF. Canine inflammatory polyneuropathies. In: Kirk RW, Bonagura JD, eds. Current veterinary therapy XI. Small animal practice. Philadelphia: Saunders, 1992:1034–1037.

Summers BA, Cummings JF, de Lahunta A. Diseases of the peripheral nervous system. In: Veterinary neuropathology. St. Louis: Mosby, 1994:424–501.

Towell TL, Shell LC. Endocrinopathies that affect peripheral nerves of cats and dogs. Compend Contin Educ Pract Vet 1994; 16:157–161.

Author Paul A. Cuddon

Consulting Editor Joane M. Parent

PERIRENAL PSEUDOCYSTS

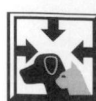

BASICS

OVERVIEW

Capsulogenic renal cyst, capsular cyst, pararenal pseudocyst, capsular hydronephrosis, perirenal cyst, and *perirenal pseudocyst* are terms used to describe renomegaly caused by accumulation of fluid between the kidney and its surrounding capsule. One or both kidneys are affected.

SIGNALMENT

• Primarily old male cats (>8 years)
• When detected in young cats, the disease is usually unilateral.
• Rare in dogs; the difference in prevalence between species may be related to the prominent network of subcapsular veins that characterize feline kidneys.

SIGNS

• Maybe none
• Nonpainful, large abdomen common
• Signs of concomitant renal failure in some animals

CAUSES & RISK FACTORS

• Cause of perirenal accumulation of fluid—not completely understood; a dynamic, not a static, process
• Cytologic and biochemical evaluation of pseudocyst fluid may aid understanding of pathophysiologic mechanisms.
• Transudate-type fluid may accumulate because of high capillary hydrostatic pressure or lymphatic obstruction. Some cats have histopathologic evidence of renal fibrosis, but it is not known whether progressive renal parenchymal contraction occludes lymphatics and blood vessels, promoting transudation of fluid.
• Perirenal accumulation of transudate can also result from ruptured renal cysts.
• Accumulation of perirenal urine may indicate disruption of the renal pelvis or proximal ureter.
• Accumulation of blood in pseudocysts can result from external trauma, surgery, neoplastic erosion of blood vessels, rupture of aneurysms, coagulopathies, or paracentesis.

DIAGNOSIS

DIFFERENTIAL DIAGNOSIS

• Causes of renomegaly include renal neoplasia, hydronephrosis, polycystic kidney disease (common), feline infectious peritonitis, and mycotic or bacterial nephritis (less common).
• Ascites and enlargement of other abdominal organs can cause nonpainful distension.

CBC/BIOCHEMISTRY/URINALYSIS

• Results unremarkable unless animal has renal insufficiency
• Azotemia and inappropriately low urinary specific gravity (<1.035) indicate concomitant renal failure.

OTHER LABORATORY TESTS

N/A

IMAGING

• Renomegaly is commonly detected by survey radiography.
• Excretory urography and ultrasonography delineate normal or small kidneys beneath an abnormally wide fluid-filled intracapsular space.

DIAGNOSTIC PROCEDURES

Examination of aspirate of intracapsular material may reveal a modified transudate (acellular, low-protein fluid), hemorrhage, or urine (fluid creatinine concentration several times higher than serum creatinine concentration).

TREATMENT

• Perirenal pseudocysts are not immediately life-threatening.
• Some animals need no treatment.
• Many patients require further diagnostic evaluation and treatment for concomitant renal failure.
• Capsulectomy or pseudocyst fenestration is generally associated with amelioration of abdominal distention and abdominal organ displacement. However, progression of renal disease usually remains unabated.
• Surgical omentalization of pseudocyst has also been utilized in the management of abdominal distention.

• Long-term response unknown
• Avoid nephrectomy, to preserve maximal renal function.
• Decompress by paracentesis with a needle and syringe for temporary relief.
• Pseudocysts usually refill in 1–2 weeks; paracentesis can then be repeated.

MEDICATIONS

DRUG(S)

Consider appropriate antimicrobic (i.e., lipid soluble antibiotic chosen on the basis of antimicrobial susceptibility) if the pseudocyst becomes infected.

CONTRAINDICATIONS/POSSIBLE INTERACTIONS

N/A

FOLLOW-UP

• Monitor patients periodically (every 2–6 months) for development of renal failure.
• Short-term prognosis—appears favorable with or without pseudocyst decompression in patients with no evidence of renal dysfunction
• Long-term prognosis—not known because it is not known whether perirenal pseudocysts are associated with underlying lesions in the renal parenchyma that may be progressive.
• Survival is related to the degree and progression of renal dysfunction.

MISCELLANEOUS

Suggested Reading

Beck JA, Bellenger CR, Lamb WA, et al. Perirenal pseudocysts in 26 cats. Aust Vet J 2000;78:166–171.
Lulich JP, Osborne CA, Polzin DJ. Cystic diseases of the kidney. In: Osborne CA, Finco DR, eds. Canine and feline nephrology and urology. Philadelphia: Williams & Wilkins, 1995:460–483.

Authors Jody P. Lulich and Carl A. Osborne
Consulting Editors Larry G. Adams and Carl A. Osborne

PERITONEOPERICARDIAL DIAPHRAGMATIC HERNIA

BASICS

OVERVIEW
- Embryologic malformation of the ventral midline allowing communication between the pericardial and peritoneal cavities
- May be associated with other congenital malformations including congenital malformations, sternal deformities (especially in cats), cranial abdominal hernia, and ventricular septal defects
- Signs may be due to large amounts of abdominal viscera compressing the heart or lungs and incarceration of abdominal organs (e.g., liver and small bowel).

SIGNALMENT
- Dogs and cats
- Age when clinical signs first occur varies; more than one-third of patients are 4 years of age or older.
- Weimaraners and Persians may be predisposed.
- No evidence that lesions are hereditary, but have been reported in littermates

SIGNS

General Comments
Depend on the nature and amount of abdominal contents that herniate

Historical Findings
- Vomiting
- Diarrhea
- Weight loss
- Abdominal pain
- Coughing
- Dyspnea

Physical Examination Findings
- Muffled heart sounds
- Displaced or attenuated apical cardiac impulse
- Palpable sternal deformity or cranial abdominal hernia
- Cardiac tamponade and signs of right-sided congestive heart failure (rare)

CAUSES & RISK FACTORS
- Embryologic malformation
- Prenatal injury of the septum transversum and pleuroperitoneal folds

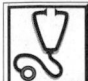

DIAGNOSIS

DIFFERENTIAL DIAGNOSIS
- Never an acquired traumatic defect because no natural direct communication exists between the peritoneal and pericardial cavities after birth
- Pericardial effusion

CBC/BIOCHEMISTRY/URINALYSIS
No associated hematologic or biochemical alterations

OTHER LABORATORY TESTS
N/A

Imaging
- Radiographic findings depend on size of defect and amount of herniated abdominal contents; caudal heart border and diaphragm may overlap; thoracic radiographs may show an "empty" abdomen and possible multiple radiographic densities
- Positive and negative contrast peritoneography have been used to evaluate the diaphragm. Injection of 1–2 mL per kilogram body weight of water-soluble positive-contrast into the peritoneal cavity followed by right and left lateral, sternal, and dorsal recumbent radiographs allows complete evaluation of the diaphragm. Identification of contrast within the pleural space confirms the diagnosis of diaphragmatic rupture. Air, carbon dioxide, or nitrous oxide may also be used.
- Barium series may demonstrate bowel loops crossing the diaphragm and within the pericardial sac.
- Nonselective angiography outlines the cardiac chambers within the large cardiac silhouette.
- Echocardiography gives a definitive diagnosis.

Diagnostic Procedures
ECG may show small complexes if abdominal contents have herniated or if marked effusion is present.

TREATMENT
Surgical closure of the hernia after returning viable organs to their normal location is usually curative. In asymptomatic adult patients with small hernias, treatment may not be indicated.

MEDICATIONS

DRUG(S)
- Myocardial contractility is unaffected in most patients; drugs for improving cardiac output are not indicated.
- Can give symptomatic treatment based on nature and amount of abdominal contents that are herniated

CONTRAINDICATIONS/POSSIBLE INTERACTIONS
Drugs that reduce ventricular afterload (e.g., arteriolar vasodilators) or preload (e.g., venous dilators and diuretics) are not useful and can cause reduction of ventricular filling, hypotension, and low cardiac output.

FOLLOW-UP
Prognosis after surgery is excellent in animals with no other significant congenital anomalies or complicating factors.

MISCELLANEOUS

Suggested Reading
Kienle RD. Pericardial disease and cardiac neoplasia. In: Kittleson MD. Kienle RD, eds. Small animal cardiovascular medicine. St. Louis: Mosby, 1999:413.
Neiger R. Peritoneopericardial diaphragmatic hernia in cats. Compend Contin Educ 1996:461–479.

Author Larry P. Tilley
Consulting Editors Larry P. Tilley and Francis W. K. Smith, Jr.

PERITONITIS

 BASICS

DEFINITION
An inflammatory process involving the serous membrane of the abdominal cavity

PATHOPHYSIOLOGY
• Insult to the peritoneal cavity, whether localized or generalized, leads to an inflammatory process characterized by vasodilation, cellular infiltration, stimulation of pain fibers, and development of adhesions.
• Extent and severity depend on type of insult.

SYSTEMS AFFECTED
• Gastrointestinal
• Cardiovascular
• Renal/Urologic
• Hemic/Lymphatic/Immune

GENETICS
N/A

INCIDENCE/PREVALENCE
N/A

GEOGRAPHIC DISTRIBUTION
N/A

SIGNALMENT
Species
Dogs and cats

Breed Predilections
None

Mean Age and Range
None

Predominant Sex
None

SIGNS
• Abdominal pain—localized or generalized; patient usually resents palpation
• A "praying" position—for relief; similar to that sometimes seen with pancreatitis
• Vomiting common
• Hypotension and shock—may develop rapidly
• Tachycardia—often noted; a variety of arrhythmias may be detected.
• Fever—not consistent; when noted with other signs of peritonitis suggests bacterial contamination of the abdominal cavity

CAUSES
Primary Peritonitis
• Uncommon
• Results from direct infection through hematogenous spread of the causative agent (e.g., FIP)

Secondary Peritonitis
• Predominant form
• Results from disruption of the abdominal cavity or hollow viscus
• Septic or chemical contamination—from dehiscence of surgical sites, penetrating abdominal wounds, blunt abdominal trauma, severe pancreatitis, pyometra, liver, or prostatic abscesses; also rupture of the gallbladder, urinary bladder, or bile duct

RISK FACTORS
• Trauma
• Gastrointestinal surgery
• Undetected abscess of liver, pancreas, prostate, uterine stump

 DIAGNOSIS

DIFFERENTIAL DIAGNOSIS
Other causes of abdominal pain or distention, sepsis, and shock

CBC/BIOCHEMISTRY/URINALYSIS
• Neutrophilic leukocytosis most common finding; may be a left shift; degenerative left shift or development of neutropenia may portend a worsening prognosis.
• Hemoconcentration common
• Hypoproteinemia—owing to exudation of albumin
• Hypokalemia
• Azotemia
• Metabolic acidosis
• Hypoglycemia—may indicate sepsis

OTHER LABORATORY TESTS
N/A

IMAGING
Ultrasound
May identify free fluid within the abdomen; abscesses of the pancreas, liver, or prostate; and rupture of the gallbladder

Radiography
• Findings inconsistent and depend on cause
• Loss of abdominal detail (ground-glass appearance suggests fluid in the abdominal cavity)—do not confuse with dehydration or lack of intra-abdominal fat
• Standing lateral view—may see free fluid line
• Left lateral recumbent view with a horizontal beam—may see free gas within the abdominal cavity
• Generalized ileus associated with free abdominal gas and a visible fluid line—may support the diagnosis; consider other causes of ileus
• Contrast procedures—usually not warranted; may complicate management if contrast material enters the abdominal cavity; avoid barium if gastrointestinal perforation is suspected.

DIAGNOSTIC PROCEDURES
• Abdominocentesis and diagnostic peritoneal lavage—safe and reliable
• Paracentesis—empty urinary bladder; aseptically prepare centesis site; use a 22-gauge needle or Teflon catheter to penetrate the abdominal cavity; sometimes a few drops of abdominal fluid may be recovered; if not successful, use a 3-mL syringe to apply gentle negative pressure; tap all four quadrants (i.e., four separate needle punctures).
• Diagnostic Peritoneal Lavage—if abdominal fluid not recovered by paracentesis; empty urinary bladder; aseptically prepare site; gravity infuse 20 mL/kg warm sterile saline into the abdominal cavity; may gently roll patient from side to side to increase recovery of the lavage fluid; no need to recover entire amount of infused fluid
• Cytology—collect samples into EDTA tubes; note color and clarity of the fluid and presence of fibrin before submitting to the laboratory.
• Culture and sensitivity—collect samples into sterile clot tubes.
• Suspected chemical peritonitis—analyze abdominal fluid for BUN and creatinine (to detect urine leakage), amylase (for pancreatitis), alkaline phosphatase (for intestinal trauma), and bilirubin (for bile leakage).
• Suspected FIP—may submit abdominal fluid for protein electrophoresis and globulin determination.

PATHOLOGIC FINDINGS
N/A

TREATMENT

APPROPRIATE HEALTH CARE

Inpatient—intensive monitoring; supportive care

NURSING CARE

Intravenous Fluid Therapy

• Critical for correction of hemodynamic disturbances and electrolyte and acid–base abnormalities
• Balanced electrolyte solution—lactated Ringer's solution or Normosol-R usually acceptable
• Potassium and glucose—may need to supplement
• Replacement rate—may initially be as high as 45 mL/kg/hr (cats) and 90 mL/kg/hr (dogs); adjust rate frequently as patient status changes; if supplemented with potassium, the rate should not exceed 0.5 mEq/kg/hr of potassium.

ACTIVITY

Usually limited as a result of hospitalization and confinement

DIET

• Dictated by cause, when identified, and any concurrent conditions (e.g., heart disease)
• Feeding tube, if necessary, may be placed for nutritional support (e.g., esophagostomy, gastrostomy, enterostomy).
• Adequate nutrition—essential to optimize outcome

CLIENT EDUCATION

• Advise client of the high rate of morbidity and, in some cases, mortality.
• Inform client that extensive monitoring and intensive care may be costly.

SURGICAL CONSIDERATIONS

• Decision to treat medically or surgically—dictated by cause (if known), patient's response to initial treatment, and owner's financial constraints
• Mild cases that seem to respond to medical therapy—surgery may not be required.
• Known bacterial contamination or suspected chemical peritonitis—surgical intervention necessary
• Inform clients who decline surgery of the possible consequences; even with surgical attention, many animals will succumb.
• Exploratory laparotomy—prepare skin in anticipation of a large surgical field; if source of infection can be identified, remove or

correct it; collect fluid sample for gram staining; use monofilament absorbable or nonabsorbable suture within the abdomen (avoid multifilament nonabsorbable suture and catgut); before closing, thoroughly lavage the abdomen with 200–300 ml/kg sterile saline solution, warmed to body temperature.
• Leaving the abdomen open or closed—determined by degree of contamination, ability to remove all debris, severity of the illness, and anticipation of septic complications; closed: use a routine closure; open: partially close and apply a sterile laparotomy pad and secure bandaging; consult a detailed surgical text for management of open peritoneal drainage.

 MEDICATIONS

DRUG(S) OF CHOICE

• Antimicrobials—broad-spectrum (against gram-positive and gram-negative, aerobic, and anaerobic organisms); when possible, based on culture and sensitivity
• Results of culture and sensitivity pending—try a combination of an aminoglycoside (e.g., amikacin, gentamicin) and a cephalosporin (e.g., cefazolin) or a penicillin (e.g., ampicillin)
• Ampicillin sodium—22 mg/kg IV q8h
• Gentamicin—2–3 mg/kg IV q8h
• Pain control—consider if indicated.

CONTRAINDICATIONS

Glucocorticoids and NSAIDs—use is controversial

PRECAUTIONS

• Aminoglycosides—use with caution if renal function is impaired.
• Adequate hydration—essential to enhance safety of these drugs

POSSIBLE INTERACTIONS

N/A

ALTERNATIVE DRUG(S)

Fluoroquinolone—enrofloxacin or orbifloxacin; substitute for an aminoglycoside, especially with impaired renal function

 FOLLOW-UP

PATIENT MONITORING

• Fluid balance, electrolyte balance, acid–base status—monitor closely
• Frequency of monitoring—varies with patient's condition and response to treatment

• CBC, chemistry profile, urinalysis—every 1–2 days during periods of intensive monitoring, even in patients who are responding

PREVENTION/AVOIDANCE

Prevention—difficult except when specific risk factors are identified (e.g., pyometra)

POSSIBLE COMPLICATIONS

• If underlying cause is not identified and managed, patient is at risk for complications.
• Open peritoneal drainage—herniation of abdominal contents
• Adhesions

EXPECTED COURSE AND PROGNOSIS

• Prognosis—depends on rapid identification and successful management of the underlying cause and appropriate follow-up care
• Septic peritonitis—open peritoneal drainage may improve survival.

 MISCELLANEOUS

ASSOCIATED CONDITIONS

N/A

AGE-RELATED FACTORS

N/A

ZOONOTIC POTENTIAL

N/A

PREGNANCY

N/A

SEE ALSO

Sepsis and Bacteremia

ABBREVIATIONS

• BUN = blood urea nitrogen
• EDTA = ethylene diamine tetraacetic acid
• FIP = feline infectious peritonitis

Suggested Reading

Greenfield CL, Walshaw R. Open peritoneal drainage for treatment of contaminated peritoneal cavity and septic peritonitis in dogs and cats: 24 cases (1980–1986). J Am Vet Med Assoc 1987;191:100–105.
Seim HB. Management of peritonitis. In: Bonagura JD, ed., Current veterinary therapy XII. Philadelphia: Saunders, 1995:764–770.
Author Sharon Fooshee Grace
Consulting Editor Stephen C. Barr

PETECHIA/ECCHYMOSIS/BRUISING

BASICS

DEFINITION
Pinpoint (petechia) or larger (ecchymosis) hemorrhage in the skin or mucous membranes secondary to abnormal primary hemostasis (platelet or vessel-wall mediated); may appear spontaneously or following minimal trauma

PATHOPHYSIOLOGY
• Thrombocytopenia and/or defective platelet function (i.e., thrombocytopathia) cause impaired primary hemostasis (failure of platelet plug formation).
• Main mechanisms of thrombocytopenia—increased destruction, e.g., immune mediated; decreased production, e.g., myelophthisis or chemotherapy-induced myelosuppression; increased consumption, e.g., disseminated intravascular coagulation (DIC); and sequestration, e.g., splenic torsion or neoplasia
• Main mechanisms of congenital thrombocytopathia—deficient or abnormal von Willebrand factor (most common); defects in platelet membrane glycoproteins, e.g., Glanzmann's thrombasthenia in otter hounds and Great Pyrenees (rare); defects in platelet storage granules, e.g., storage pool disease in Persian cats or American cocker spaniels (rare); defects in signal transduction, e.g., in basset hounds or spitzs (rare). Note: a combination of the latter two mechanisms is seen in collies.
• Main mechanisms of acquired platelet dysfunction are drug (NSAID)- or uremia-induced inhibition of prostaglandin metabolism. Other causes are paraproteinemia, liver disease, immune-mediated causes, and possibly anemia.
• Vascular hemostatic defects—generally caused by increased capillary permeability, e.g., RMSF or FIP-associated vasculitis, or altered dermal vascular support, e.g., hyperadrenocorticism or Ehlers-Danlos syndrome

SYSTEMS AFFECTED
• Hemic/Lymph/Immune
• Skin/Exocrine—petechia/ecchymosis/bruising
• Respiratory—epistaxis
• Renal/Urologic—hematuria
• Gastrointestinal—melena/hematochezia
• Ophthalmic—scleral/retinal hemorrhage, secondary glaucoma and uveitis
• Neurologic—variable depending on location of bleeding

SIGNALMENT
• Doberman pinschers and Scottish terriers are overrepresented for von Willebrand deficiency. Many other breeds have von Willebrand's disease.
• See specific thrombopathias for breed-associated disorders.
• An inherited thrombocytopenia with giant platelets is seen in King Charles cavalier spaniels.
• Immune-mediated thrombocytopenia is suggested to have a genetic predisposition because of the high prevalence in cocker spaniels, toy poodles, and Old English sheepdogs. Middle-aged female dogs also are at increased risk.
• Cats—less common than dogs

SIGNS
N/A

CAUSES

Thrombocytopenia
• Immune mediated—idiopathic, drug induced, paraneoplastic, and infection induced (e.g., viral, rickettsial, bacterial, or fungal)
• Infectious, e.g., ehrlichiosis, RMSF, leptospirosis, FIP, FeLV, or cytauxzoonosis
• Bone marrow suppression, e.g., estrogen toxicity or chemotherapy
• Bone marrow infiltration—myeloproliferative or lymphoproliferative diseases, e.g., multiple myeloma or lymphoma
• Sequestration in liver and/or spleen secondary to vascular neoplasia, or torsions.
• Consumption, e.g., DIC or recent extensive mucosal and serosal hemorrhage, such as with rodenticide poisoning

Thrombocytopathy
Congenital or acquired disorders affecting platelet adhesion, aggregation; see Pathophysiology

Vascular Disease
Vasculitis secondary to infection such as RMSF or FIP; also with immune-mediated vasculitis; see specific disease(s)

Coagulation Factor Deficiency
Clinical signs are not usually associated with petechia or ecchymosis. Most commonly seen is hemorrhage into body cavities as well as hemarthosis and hematomas.

RISK FACTORS
• The occurrence of any of the diseases mentioned or breed predispositions. Severe von Willebrand's disease is seen in German shorthaired pointers, Shetland sheepdogs, Scottish terriers and Chesapeake Bay retrievers.
• History of NSAID use
• Recent vaccination has been suggested as a risk factor for immune-mediated thrombocytopenia.

DIAGNOSIS

DIFFERENTIAL DIAGNOSIS
• Usually are not mistaken for anything else. Some inflammatory skin lesions may look like petechia. A glass slide can be placed over the site of hemorrhage and pressure applied to blanch the skin. If it is hemorrhage, it will not disappear; if the lesion is secondary to inflammation, the skin will blanch.

CBC/BIOCHEMISTRY/URINALYSIS
• Platelets are low, either by direct count or by estimation on a well-made blood smear. One platelet per high power field (hpf) represents approximately 15×10^9/L. An average of 10–30 platelets per hpf corresponds to a normal platelet count. If the platelet count is greater than 100×10^9/L, consider other causes of primary hemostasis abnormalities.
• RBC fragmentation is associated with DIC or microangiopathies.
• *Ehrlichia morulae* or other hemoparasites may be seen on a peripheral blood smear.
• Patients with myeloproliferative or lymphoproliferative disease, myelofibrosis, or a history of chemotherapy or administration of drugs such as estrogens may be concurrently leukemic or have other cytopenias.
• Biochemical analysis—identify renal or liver disease as well as hyperglobulinemia.
• Urinalysis—identify hematuria. Proteinuria—may suggest concurrent immune-mediated disease, such as glomerulonephritis, and increase the suspicion of systemic lupus erythematosus

OTHER LABORATORY TESTS
• Coagulation studies (APTT, PT, FDP, D-dimer, antithrombin III concentration) help diagnose DIC. Platelet counts less than 10×10^9/L will interfere with ACT assay.
• Von Willebrand factor antigen assay—necessary to confirm von Willebrand's disease
• Platelet function tests—may be necessary to rule out platelet function disorders
• Serum and urine protein electrophoresis (looking for Bence-Jones proteins)—indicated if hyperglobulinemia noted
• Protein:creatinine ratio—if proteinuria noted on urine analysis. An elevated ratio may be suggestive of concurrent glomerulonephritis.
• FeLV/FIV testing—underlying cause of thrombocytopenia
• Antinuclear antibody titer—helps to diagnose systemic lupus erythematosus if there is evidence of other immune-mediated disease
• ACTH stimulation test or LDDST may be indicated if hyperadrenocorticism is suspected
• Serology—aid to diagnose ehrlichiosis or RMSF

• PCR—for underlying infections such as *Ehrlichia platys* or *Haemobartonella felis*

IMAGING
• Three-view thoracic radiography—look for evidence of metastasis or primary neoplasia. Identify enlarged lymph nodes or signs suggestive of underlying infectious disease.
• Abdominal radiography to assess spleen and liver size. Identify enlarged sublumbar lymph nodes or an abdominal mass consistent with hemangiosarcoma.
• Abdominal ultrasonography to identify underlying architectural abnormalities in various organs, which suggest underlying neoplasia, infection, or inflammation. Evaluate mesenteric lymph nodes for signs of neoplasia, infection, or inflammation.

DIAGNOSTIC PROCEDURES
• Buccal mucosal bleeding time (BMBT) is indicated if the platelets are above 100 × 10^9/L; prolonged BMBT suggests a thrombopathia. Thrombocytopenic patients also have a prolonged BMBT. Normal range is less than 4 minutes in dogs and less than 2 minutes in cats.
• Most invasive procedures are contraindicated in patients with bleeding disorders, except bone marrow aspiration and core biopsy. These procedures are indicated if there are cytopenias, hypergammaglobulinemia, or evidence of leukemia.
• Invasive diagnostic procedures may be performed with less risk if platelet concentrate can be administered during the procedure to decrease the risk of hemorrhage.

TREATMENT
• Usually as an inpatient until a definitive diagnosis has been made
• Minimize activity to reduce the risk of even minor trauma.
• Discontinue any medications that may alter platelet function, e.g., aspirin and other NSAIDs.
• Discontinue medication that is associated with immune-mediated thrombocytopenia, such as methimazole in cats.
• Maintain fluid volume with a balanced electrolyte solution.
• Avoid subcutaneous and intramuscular injections as well as venipuncture from the jugular vein.
• Blood or platelet transfusions may be necessary and life saving before a definitive diagnosis is been made. Ensure blood samples are collected prior to transfusion for

diagnostic testing such as coagulation tests, serology, or PCR.
• No specific treatment is available for congenital thrombopathias, other than DDAVP, which can be used for type I von Willebrand's disease to help control bleeding. It can also be given to blood donors prior to blood collection if the recipient needs surgery. See von Willebrand's Disease for additional details. Acquired thrombopathias need to have the underlying disease corrected. Hyperadrenocorticism can be treated—see specific chapter. There is no treatment for Ehlers-Danlos syndrome. The underlying disease needs to be treated when treating vasculitis. See specific chapters.

MEDICATIONS

DRUG(S)
Depends on the underlying diagnosis

CONTRAINDICATIONS
Avoid subcutaneous and intramuscular injectable medications whenever possible.

PRECAUTIONS
Avoid NSAIDs and other drugs that inhibit hemostasis, other than heparin in DIC.

POSSIBLE INTERACTIONS
N/A

FOLLOW-UP
Daily platelet count for patients with thrombocytopenia until an adequate response is seen. See specific diseases for details.

POSSIBLE COMPLICATIONS
• Death or morbidity caused by hemorrhage into brain, gut, or other organs
• Shock caused by hemorrhagic hypovolemia

MISCELLANEOUS

ASSOCIATED CONDITIONS
N/A

AGE-RELATED FACTORS
None

ZOONOTIC POTENTIAL
None

SYNONYMS
• Hemorrhagic diatheses
• Bleeding

SEE ALSO
• Disseminated Intravascular Coagulation
• Hyperadrenocorticism
• Myeloproliferative Disorders
• Thrombocytopathies
• Thrombocytopenia, Immune-mediated and Non–Immune-mediated
• von Willebrand's Disease

ABBREVIATIONS
• ACT = activated clotting time
• ACTH = adrenocorticotrophic hormone
• APTT = activated partial thromboplastin time
• DDAVP = deamino-8-D-arginine vasopressin
• DIC = disseminated intravascular coagulation
• FDP = fibrinogen degradation products
• FeLV = feline leukemia virus
• FIP = feline infectious peritonitis
• FIV = feline immunodeficiency virus
• LDDST = low-dose dexamethasone suppression test
• NSAID = nonsteroidal antiinflammatory drug
• PCR = polymerase chain reaction
• PT = prothrombin time
• RMSF = Rocky Mountain spotted fever

Suggested Reading

Brooks M, Catalfamo JL. Platelet dysfunction. In: Bonagura JD, Kirk RW, eds. Kirk's current veterinary therapy XIII. Small animal practice. Philadelphia: Saunders, 2000:442–447.

Callan MB. Petechiae and ecchymoses. In: Ettinger SJ, ed. Textbook of veterinary internal medicine. Philadelphia: Saunders, 2000:218–222.

Grindem CB. Infectious and immune-mediated thrombocytopenia. In: Bonagura JD, Kirk RW, eds. Kirk's current veterinary therapy XIII. Small animal practice. Philadelphia: Saunders, 2000:438–442.

Ruiz de Gopegui R, Feldman BF. Platelets and von Willebrand's disease. In: Ettinger SJ, ed. Textbook of veterinary internal medicine. Philadelphia: Saunders, 2000: 1817–1828.

Russell KE, Grindem CB. Secondary thrombocytopenia. In: Feldman BF, Zinki JG, Jain NC, eds. Schalm's veterinary hematology. Philadelphia: Lippincott Williams & Wilkins, 2000:469–477.

Author Julie Armstrong
Consulting Editor Stephen Kruth

PETROLEUM HYDROCARBON TOXICOSES

 BASICS

DEFINITION

• The term "petroleum hydrocarbons" refers to a diverse collection of products that have been purified from the extremely complex hydrocarbon mixture that is crude oil.
• Although crude oil intoxication is an important problem in wildlife and large animals, small animal poisoning most commonly results from exposure to refined commercial products. These include such disparate mixtures as fuels, solvents, lubricants, and waxes. Further complicating the clinician's task is the fact that petroleum-based solvents are often used as "inert" carriers for other potential toxicants (e.g., pesticides, paints, medications). • In theory, each of the hundreds of compounds that make up even a relatively simple commercial product like gasoline has its own physical, chemical, and toxicologic characteristics, all of which must be considered in the clinical management of poisoning. In practice, however, most petroleum products can be "lumped" into a few relatively broad categories on the basis of volatility, viscosity, and chemical additives. Mixtures with high boiling points (low volatility), such as asphalt, mineral oil, and waxes, are relatively nontoxic. Products with relatively low boiling points, such as benzene or turpentine, tend to be more readily aspirated and more likely to cause chemical pneumonitis. In general, products that are more volatile also tend to be more lipophilic and thus more readily absorbed systemically. Products with high aromatic content, such as benzene, are also more predisposed to systemic toxicity.
• Certain nonpetroleum-origin hydrocarbons, such as turpentine and linseed oil, are similar enough to be considered with petroleum-based products of similar molecular weight.
• Storage in inappropriate containers and failure to clean up spills are common causes of exposure in pets. Cats may ingest significant amounts of gasoline or other hydrocarbons by grooming themselves after topical contamination. Pets are often poisoned by folk remedies involving gasoline, kerosene, and other products as tonics or vermifuges. Gasoline and other solvents are used in an attempt to remove sticky material from an animal's coat.

PATHOPHYSIOLOGY

• In general, the most acutely life-threatening effects of hydrocarbon ingestion result from aspiration-induced pneumonitis. • Viscosity and surface tension are strong determinants of pneumotoxic potential. Low viscosity permits hydrocarbons to penetrate further into smaller airways. Low surface tension increases their tendency to "wet" pulmonary surfaces. For example, aspiration of as little as 0.1 mL of a low-viscosity hydrocarbon (e.g., hexane) may produce severe pneumonitis, whereas a high-viscosity product (e.g., motor oil) may not even penetrate past the major airways. • Topical exposure to hydrocarbon-based solvents (e.g., petroleum distillates, turpentine) may result in irritation and even necrosis of skin and cornea. • Systemic toxicity is a possibility after oral or topical exposure. Although there are no quantitative data readily applicable to small animals, systemic toxicity has been reported in human beings following topical exposure or inhalation and should be considered when evaluating pets that have received a heavy topical exposure. This is especially important in small animals (e.g., puppies, kittens, rodents), which have a relatively high body surface area–to-mass ratio. Systemic uptake and thus toxicity are also enhanced by factors such as a long hair coat, which traps the product against the skin.

SYSTEMS AFFECTED

• Respiratory • Gastrointestinal • Nervous • Skin

INCIDENCE/PREVALENCE

The incidence of this problem is low compared with that of common infectious diseases, but a single-veterinarian small animal practice may expect to see 1 to 10 cases per year.

SIGNS

General Comments

• Pneumonitis is the most serious complication associated with ingesting volatile petroleum hydrocarbons (e.g., gasoline). Signs referable to the respiratory system usually occur within a few minutes to 1–2 hr postingestion. The central nervous and gastrointestinal systems may also be affected, but death, if it occurs, usually results from respiratory failure. • If aspiration occurs simultaneously with ingestion, there will be choking, coughing, gagging, and varying degrees of dyspnea. Direct damage of airway components and bronchospasm may result in hypoxia. Cyanosis may also develop immediately as alveolar oxygen is displaced by hydrocarbon vapor.

Historical Findings

• Signs of hydrocarbon poisoning are seldom sufficiently characteristic to permit diagnosis without at least a strong index of suspicion from the history. A history of (possible) exposure is essential to the diagnosis of hydrocarbon intoxication. • Respiratory involvement, when present, is usually progressive over the first 24–48 hr, then gradually resolves 3–10 days following exposure. Animals that remain asymptomatic for 6–12 hr after ingestion are unlikely to develop respiratory illness. • Human patients report a burning sensation in the mouth and pharynx immediately after ingestion of gasoline. Animals appear to experience the same symptoms after ingesting hydrocarbons, in addition to slobbering, champing the jaws, shaking the head, and pawing at the muzzle.

Physical Examination

• Astute observers may note a hydrocarbon odor on the animal's breath or coat. • Fever usually occurs in 3–4 hr following aspiration, but may occur in less than an hour or as much as 24 hr. • The irritant properties of petroleum products may result in vomiting, colic, and diarrhea after oral exposure. The severity and indeed the presence of such signs are a function of the dose and the individual hydrocarbon. Heavy aliphatic hydrocarbons (e.g., mineral oil) may produce mild diarrhea but little else. Lighter hydrocarbons (e.g., gasoline) are more likely to produce colic and vomiting. • The *systemic* signs of acute hydrocarbon intoxication are principally those of central nervous system derangement. Intoxicated animals exhibit vertigo, ataxia, and mental confusion. Hydrocarbons produce depression and narcosis in most cases, but tremors and convulsions have also been reported in a few. If the dose is very high, the animal may become comatose and die prior to exhibiting signs of pneumonitis, although this is very rare. • The heartbeat may be irregular as a result of myocardial sensitization to endogenous catecholamines, or there may be a complete collapse if the animal is stressed. Myocardial sensitization may persist for as much as 24–48 hr after apparent recovery from the neurologic effects of intoxication.

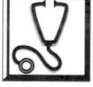 **DIAGNOSIS**

DIFFERENTIAL DIAGNOSIS

• A number of infectious diseases, toxins, and/or injuries may result in respiratory signs similar to hydrocarbon aspiration. However, only very acute processes (e.g., trauma, chylothorax) exhibit a similar rapidity of onset. • The diverse spectrum of neurologic effects sometimes seen in hydrocarbon intoxication may be confused with those of acute ethylene glycol or drug intoxication.

CBC/BIOCHEMISTRY/URINALYSIS

• Urine will be negative for ethylene glycol; serum osmolality will be normal. • Although a CBC may indicate stress, it is usually normal early in the course of the condition.

OTHER LABORATORY TESTS

• A simple spot test involves mixing vomitus or gastric contents vigorously with warm water. If gasoline or other petroleum distillates are present, they will float to the surface. Care must be taken to distinguish between petroleum products and dietary lipids. The former usually have a characteristic odor. • Most petroleum products lighter than kerosene, if isolated and absorbed onto a paper towel, evaporate relatively quickly and have a characteristic odor. • Chemical analysis of ingesta or postmortem tissues is useful forensically but is not practical for clinical evaluation of the acute case. If chemical analysis is to be conducted, take samples as quickly as practical and freeze in airtight containers to prevent loss due to volatilization.

IMAGING
• Radiographic abnormalities may lead or lag the onset of clinical signs slightly, but are readily observed within a few hours of ingestion in all cases that develop pneumonitis. • Radiographic findings are typical of aspiration pneumonia and consist of fine, perihilar densities and extensive infiltrates in ventral portions of the lungs. These are worst at 3–4 days, then gradually improve. Not all animals with radiographic signs of hydrocarbon aspiration develop respiratory signs, and radiographic changes usually persist past the resolution of clinical signs.

PATHOLOGIC FINDINGS
• If aspiration has occurred, the principal lesions will be in the respiratory tract. Pulmonary lesions are bilateral and typically involve caudoventral portions of the lung. The earliest lesions include hyperemia, edema, and hemorrhage into the airways. Foreign matter may be grossly visible in the smaller airways. Later, there is bronchospasm, emphysema, and atelectasis. Pneumatoceles, pneumothorax, and subcutaneous emphysema result from airway collapse. There may be ulcerations in the mucosa of the trachea and larger airways. • Bacterial pneumonia occasionally supervenes and may result in abscesses. • Systemic toxicity very occasionally results in hepatic, myocardial, and/or renal tubular necrosis if the animal survives > 24 hr.

TREATMENT

APPROPRIATE HEALTH CARE
• In all cases of uncomplicated (i.e., not contaminated with some other, more toxic substance) petroleum hydrocarbon ingestion, the primary goal is to minimize the risk of aspiration. • If the amount ingested was small, and especially if the hydrocarbon ingested was known to be one of the less volatile, more viscous products (e.g., motor oil, grease), cage rest and observation may be all that is required. • If the volume ingested was substantial and the product involved is one known to cause systemic toxicity (e.g., benzene), activated charcoal or gastric lavage is indicated within the first 4–6 hr

postexposure. • If the product contains other, highly toxic substances (e.g., pesticide), gastric decontamination may be indicated, despite the risk of aspiration. If lavage is to be attempted, it is essential that precautions be taken to prevent possible aspiration of stomach contents. Emetics are contraindicated except as a very last resort to clear some other highly toxic constituent (e.g., pesticide) from the gastrointestinal tract.
• Respiratory effects should be treated symptomatically. Supplemental oxygen, continuous positive airway pressure, and mechanical ventilation should be used as needed. However, because pneumomediastinum, pneumatoceles, and pneumothorax are common complications of hydrocarbon pneumonitis, positive pressure systems must be used with caution. Also, since the lungs are the major route of elimination for many hydrocarbons, closed or semi-closed systems should be purged frequently. • Topical exposure may be treated by gently bathing with warm water and a mild detergent shampoo. If the hair coat is especially heavy or matted, it may be necessary to clip the contaminated areas to prevent systemic absorption and minimize skin damage.
• Symptomatic treatment of petroleum burns may involve topical antibacterials or other agents as necessary. • Very viscous hydrocarbons (e.g., tar, waxes) may also be removed with mild detergents. Because they are not readily absorbed, they pose only a cosmetic and skin irritation problem and are not as critical to remove. Lipophilic materials (e.g., butter, lard, mechanics hand cleaner) may also be useful, but the use of solvents is not recommended.

NURSING CARE
Cage rest is indicated, both for its beneficial effects on the healing process and to minimize the effects of excitement-induced catecholamines on a potentially sensitized myocardium.

CLIENT EDUCATION
Despite decades of public service messages about the dangers of household chemicals, many pet owners persist in improperly storing and using petroleum products. Presentation of an exposed animal, whether actually intoxicated or not, gives the clinician a golden opportunity to reinforce the necessity of keeping all such products out of the reach of pets and children.

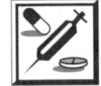

MEDICATIONS

DRUG(S)
• In the past, oral mineral or vegetable oil was recommended to increase the viscosity of petroleum hydrocarbons and thus decrease the risk of aspiration. Oils also produce a

mild catharsis, decreasing the period during which the petroleum product might be absorbed. However, retrospective studies in children suggest that such treatment actually increases the likelihood of aspiration pneumonia, and the use of such oils is no longer recommended. • The routine use of antibiotics is of questionable value. Hydrocarbon pneumonitis is largely nonbacterial in origin. In one experimental study in which dogs were given an intratracheal dose of kerosene, parenteral ampicillin and dexamethasone did not reduce the respiratory rate or radiographic, gross, or microscopic pulmonary lesions. However, given the potentially severe consequences of bacterial complications and the relatively nil downside to antibiotic use, it may be prudent to use some form of antimicrobial prophylaxis if vomiting has occurred.
• Corticosteroids have been associated with increased numbers of positive lung cultures in retrospective studies and are thus contraindicated. • Bronchospasm may be treated with β_2-agonists in case the myocardium has been unduly sensitized.

PRECAUTIONS
Induce emesis only as a last resort and only in cases where there is a high degree of certainty that leaving the foreign material in the gut poses a greater hazard than aspiration.

FOLLOW-UP

PATIENT MONITORING
Monitor patients for 3–4 days to ensure that ingested hydrocarbons have cleared the gastrointestinal tract and no pulmonary sequelae have occurred.

EXPECTED COURSE AND PROGNOSIS
Although the diversity of this class of products precludes any absolute prediction, most hydrocarbon exposures respond well to conservative, supportive therapy.

MISCELLANEOUS

Suggested Reading
Raisbeck MF. Petroleum hydrocarbons. In: Peterson ME, Talcott PA, eds. Small animal toxicology. Philadelphia: Saunders, 2001:666–676.
Reese E, Kimbrough RD. Acute toxicity of gasoline and some additives. Environ Health Perspect 1993;101:115–131.
Seymour FK, Henry JA. Assessment and management of acute poisoning by petroleum products. Hum Exp Toxicol 2001;20:551–562.
Author Merl F. Raisbeck
Consulting Editor Gary Osweiler

PHEOCHROMOCYTOMA

 BASICS

DEFINITION
• Tumor of the adrenergic portion of the sympathetic nervous system • Tumors arise from chromaffin cells of the adrenal medulla and rarely from extraadrenal chromaffin cells (paragangliomas).

PATHOPHYSIOLOGY
• Most commonly involve the adrenal medulla; the vast majority are unilateral • Can vary in size from small nodules 0.5 cm in diameter to large, space-occupying intraabdominal masses; the larger the tumor the more frequently there are related clinical signs. • Approximately 50% are classified as malignant because of either local tissue invasion or distant metastasis. • Distant metastasis is most commonly observed in the liver, lungs, spleen, kidney, brain, pancreas, bone, and vertebral canal; metastasis to regional lymph nodes is also frequent • Pheochromocytomas produce clinical signs by direct invasion of adjacent structures (kidney, aorta, or caudal vena cava) and by production of epinephrine, norepinephrine, and less commonly dopamine. • The predominant clinical signs result from a1-mediated vasoconstriction and b1-mediated cardiac chronotropic and inotropic effects that cause systemic hypertension or tachyarrhythmias.

SYSTEMS AFFECTED
• Cardiovascular • Respiratory • Behavior • Neuromuscular • Renal/Urologic • Gastrointestinal • Ophthalmic

INCIDENCE/PREVALENCE
Uncommon disease in dogs; rare in cats

SIGNALMENT

Species
Dogs and cats

Breed Predilections
None

Mean Age and Range
• Median age is 11 years; range is 1–16 years of age • The great majority of affected dogs are ≥ 7 years old.

SIGNS

General Comments
Difficult to diagnose antemortem; 48–85% of reported pheochromocytomas have been identified unexpectedly during necropsy examination or exploratory surgery

Historical Findings
• Clinical signs are often episodic or acute. • Common presenting signs are (in decreasing order of frequency) generalized weakness, collapse, anorexia, lethargy/depression, vomiting, tachypnea, and polyuria/polydipsia. • Less common presenting complaints are diarrhea, weight loss, rear limb edema, abdominal distension, epistaxis, acute blindness, pacing, and seizures.

Physical Examination Findings
• Related to excessive catecholamine release or tumor invasion of adjacent structures; abnormalities not always present • Respiratory—tachypnea is one of the most common; dyspnea or abnormal lung sounds are less commonly observed • Cardiovascular—tachycardia or cardiac arrhythmias are very common; epistaxis is occasionally noted; some patients present in cardiovascular shock • Neuromuscular—weakness, loss of muscle mass, shaking, muscle tremors, head tilt, and rarely strabismus, nystagmus, and/or seizures • Ocular—blindness, retinal detachment, retinal hemorrhage, and tortuous retinal vessels may occur in dogs with prolonged or severe hypertension

CAUSES
Pheochromocytomas are chromaffin cell tumors.

 DIAGNOSIS

DIFFERENTIAL DIAGNOSIS
• Primary differentials include causes of systemic hypertension such as renal disease, hyperadrenocorticism, hyperthyroidism, primary hyperaldosteronism, and essential hypertension. • Hyperadrenocorticism can closely mimic, and may occur simultaneously with, pheochromocytomas.

CBC/BIOCHEMISTRY/URINALYSIS
• Decreased plasma volume may result in an increased PCV; also some evidence indicates that catecholamines may cause increased kidney erythropoietin release. • Any anemia is usually mild and nonregenerative and is thought to be secondary to chronic disease or chronic low-grade hemorrhage. • A mature neutrophilic leukocytosis is the most common leukogram abnormality. • The most common serum biochemistry abnormality is elevated liver enzymes; no apparent correlation exists between elevated liver enzymes and hepatic metastasis. • Hypercholesterolemia is frequently noted. • Proteinuria, seen in up to 50% of patients, results from hypertensive glomerulonephropathy.

OTHER LABORATORY TESTS
• In humans, a diagnosis of pheochromocytoma is confirmed by demonstrating elevated levels of serum or urine catecholamines and their metabolites. • In veterinary medicine, these tests are rarely done because of their technical difficulty, expense, and unavailability and the lack of documented normal reference values. • Quantification of urinary catecholamines and their metabolites from a 24-hr urine collection is the preferred method of confirming a diagnosis of pheochromocytoma in humans. • Test sensitivity is greatly enhanced by assays for urinary catecholamines (dopamine, epinephrine, and norepinephrine) and their metabolites (metanephrine, normetanephrine, and vanillylmandelic acid). • Urine must be acidified (pH , 3.0) and kept cold during collection and transport to the laboratory.

Phentolamine Suppression Test
• Phentolamine is an intravenous α-receptor antagonist that lowers blood pressure by inhibiting catecholamine-mediated vasoconstriction; test can only be performed if patient is hypertensive • After obtaining a baseline blood pressure, administer 0.5–1.5 mg of phentolamine as an IV bolus; measure blood pressure every 30 sec for 3 min, then every minute for 7 min. • If the patient's blood pressure decreases by at least 35 mm Hg systolic or 25 mm Hg diastolic and the decrease lasts for a minimum of 5 min, the result is considered positive; in humans, the test has been associated with a large number of false positives. This test has not been evaluated in dogs with pheochromocytomas.

Clonidine Suppression Test
• Clonidine is an α-adrenergic agonist that acts to decrease centrally mediated release of catecholamines. • Clonidine should not suppress catecholamine secretion from pheochromocytomas. • Results of this suppression test are affected by individual circulating catecholamine levels • This test has not been performed in dogs.

IMAGING

Abdominal Radiography
• A cranial abdominal mass has been detected in up to 56% of patients; ~7% of pheochromocytomas have had radiographically detectable calcification. • Tumor extension into the adjacent kidney or liver lobule may cause abnormalities in their radiographic contours.

Thoracic Radiography
• Common thoracic abnormalities are generalized cardiomegaly, right or left ventricular enlargement, and pulmonary edema or congestion; thoracic radiographs are also indicated to evaluate for metastatic disease. • Pulmonary metastasis has been detected radiographically in approximately 11% of evaluated patients; in one study, 50% of pulmonary metastatic lesions were not detected on radiographs.

Abdominal Ultrasonography
• An abdominal mass was identified in 50–83% of patients evaluated with ultrasound; the origin of the mass frequently cannot be identified. • Pheochromocytomas are usually unilateral; the contralateral adrenal gland usually is normal in size, shape, and echo texture. • Ultrasonography is relatively sensitive for identifying tumor invasion of the caudal vena cava and other adjacent structures and for detecting intraabdominal metastasis; however, in one study, tumor invasion of adjacent tissues was missed in 75% of affected animals examined.

OTHER IMAGING MODALITIES
• Computed tomography (CT scan) and magnetic resonance imaging (MRI) are very sensitive imaging methods for detection of adrenal masses and intraabdominal metastasis. • Metaiodobenzylguanidine scan is a new imaging technique used to detect pheochromocytomas in humans with a high index of clinical suspicion but with a negative CT scan.

DIAGNOSTIC PROCEDURES

Arterial Blood Pressure

Identification of systemic hypertension (systolic blood pressure > 160 mm Hg, diastolic > 100 mm Hg) is highly variable in canine patients with pheochromocytoma; therefore, normal blood pressure does not rule out a diagnosis of pheochromocytoma.

Electrocardiography (ECG)

Sinus tachycardia is the most common ECG abnormality; ventricular premature contractions are less commonly observed.

Adrenal Testing

Hyperadrenocorticism is one of the primary differential diagnoses for patients with clinical signs consistent with a pheochromocytoma. In addition, hyperadrenocorticism reportedly occurs concurrently in up to 20% of canine patients with pheochromocytomas.

PATHOLOGIC FINDINGS

• Grossly, pheochromocytomas are dark-red to tan, and multinodular. • They arise from the adrenal medulla; the surrounding adrenal cortex is compressed into a thin surrounding shell of tissue. • Histologically, pheochromocytomas are composed of round to cuboidal cells with granular eosinophilic cytoplasm.• Immunohistochemical staining of tumor tissues with chromogranin A or synaptophysin will allow differentiation of pheochromocytomas.

 TREATMENT

APPROPRIATE HEALTH CARE

• Surgical removal of the tumor is the only treatment modality that may be curative. • Surgical exploration and biopsy are usually required for a definitive diagnosis. • Medical therapy is most commonly used to stabilize patients prior to surgery or in patients with nonresectable or metastatic tumors; medical therapy is only palliative and can be conducted on an outpatient basis. • Patients that are presented in a hypertensive crisis represent a diagnostic and therapeutic challenge; these patients require intensive emergency and critical care.

CLIENT EDUCATION

Survival times of > 1–3 years are possible following successful surgical tumor removal, even in dogs with tumor invasion of adjacent tissues or blood vessels; however, perioperative mortality rates of close to 50% have been reported.

SURGICAL CONSIDERATIONS

Preoperative Care

• Severe hypertension and cardiac arrhythmias are life-threatening complications that commonly develop during anesthetic induction and tumor removal in patients with pheochromocytomas. • Marked hypotension commonly develops following tumor removal. • Phenoxybenzamine, a noncompetitive adrenergic α antagonist, is given for 2–3 weeks prior to surgery; the initial dosage is 0.25 mg/kg q12h; the dosage can be incrementally increased until the patient's clinical signs and blood pressure

are controlled; the maximum dosage is 1.5 mg/kg q12h in canines and 0.5 mg/kg q12h in cats.

Complications and Patient Monitoring

• Common complications—hypertension, severe tachycardia, other cardiac arrhythmias, and hypovolemia/hypotension • Closely monitor the ECG, central venous pressure (CVP) and blood pressure. • Hypotension and hypovolemia may develop following tumor removal or secondary to uncontrolled hemorrhage; hypotension is best treated by volume expansion with IV fluid therapy; adequacy of fluid therapy is based on normalization of blood pressure and maintaining the patient's CVP between 5 and 10 mm H_2O.

Anesthesia

• The anesthetic protocol should include agents that do not directly or indirectly cause the release of catecholamines or sensitize tissues to their effects. • Appropriate drugs are diazepam, oxymorphone, midazolam, and acepromazine (low dosage) or combinations of the above. • Atropine or glycopyrrolate should not be a routine part of the preinduction protocol because they can predispose the patient to life-threatening tachycardia. • Anesthetic induction should be as stress-free as possible; emergency drugs (phentolamine, sodium nitroprusside, propranolol, esmolol, and lidocaine) should be readily available, and the appropriate dosages and/or infusion rates predetermined. • Anesthesia is induced with a narcotic agent or propofol; propofol should be used cautiously because it occasionally causes histamine release that can induce tumor catecholamine secretion. • Maintain anesthesia with isoflurane, since it causes less sensitization of the myocardium to catecholamines than does halothane.

Surgery

• The surgeon should be prepared to do an adrenalectomy, nephrectomy, and thrombectomy even if the preoperative evaluation showed no evidence of tumor invasion of adjacent organs or vessels. • Arterial blood pressure typically increases dramatically when the tumor is manipulated and falls acutely following tumor removal.

 MEDICATIONS

DRUG(S) OF CHOICE

• Hypertension can be treated with phentolamine (0.02–0.1 mg/kg IV to effect) or sodium nitroprusside (0.5–15 µg/kg/min constant-rate IV infusion); sodium nitroprusside is a direct-acting vasodilator with an immediate onset and a short duration of activity. • Cardiac arrhythmias and severe tachycardia—common problems; usually respond to β-blocking agents such as propranolol (0.03–0.1 mg/kg IV to effect) or esmolol (0.5 mg/kg slow IV bolus followed by 0.05–0.2 mg/kg/min IV infusion)

CONTRAINDICATIONS

• Metoclopramide can cause tumor catecholamine secretion and thus initiate a hyper-

tensive crisis. • Anesthetic agents—morphine, meperidine, xylazine, and ketamine

PRECAUTIONS

See Anesthetic Considerations.

ALTERNATIVE DRUG(S)

α-Methyltyrosine has been used to reduce catecholamine secretion and ameliorate clinical signs in humans with inoperable or metastatic disease; it inhibits tyrosine hydroxylase, the rate-limiting enzyme in catecholamine synthesis; this drug has not been used in dogs or cats.

 FOLLOW-UP

PATIENT MONITORING

• Blood pressure and CVP—closely in the immediate postoperative period (24–72 h) • Blood pressure and ECG—at least monthly in patients being treated long-term for ongoing hypertension and/or cardiac arrhythmias

POSSIBLE COMPLICATIONS

Postoperative—intraabdominal hemorrhage, hypotension, peritonitis, sepsis, or unresolved hypertension

EXPECTED COURSE AND PROGNOSIS

• Survival times > 3 years have been reported in dogs following tumor removal. • Prognosis in general is guarded and is commonly adversely affected by concurrent diseases.

 MISCELLANEOUS

ASSOCIATED CONDITIONS

• Most dogs with pheochromocytomas have concurrent organ dysfunction, neoplasms, or other diseases. • Hyperadrenocorticism has been observed in up to 20% of dogs with pheochromocytomas.

SEE ALSO

• Hyperadrenocorticism (Cushing's Disease)
• Hypertension, Systemic

Suggested Readings

Barthez PB, Marks SL, Woo J, et al. Pheochromocytoma in dogs: 61 cases (1984–1995). J Vet Intern Med 1997;11:272–278.

Gilson SD, Withrow SJ, Orton EC. Surgical treatment of pheochromocytoma: technique, complications, and results in six dogs. Vet Surg 1994;23:195–200.

Locke-Bohannon LG, Mauldin GA. Canine pheochromocytoma: diagnosis and management. Compendium 2001;23:807–815.

Rosentein DA. Diagnostic imaging in canine pheochromocytoma. Vet Radiol Ultrasound 2000;41:499–506.

Author Nicole Bennett, John W. Tyler
Consulting Editor Deborah S. Greco

PHOSPHOFRUCTOKINASE DEFICIENCY

BASICS

OVERVIEW
• Phosphofructokinase is the most important rate-controlling enzyme in glycolysis and RBCs; intensely exercising skeletal muscles depend heavily on anaerobic glycolysis for energy.
• Affected dogs have compensated hemolytic anemia and mild myopathy caused by markedly reduced total phosphofructokinase activity in both tissues.
• Anemia develops because of insufficient generation of ATP to maintain normal RBC shape, ionic composition, and deformability and because RBCs from affected dogs are alkaline fragile and lyse when blood pH is slightly high.

SIGNALMENT
• English springer spaniels and American cocker spaniels
• Transmitted as an autosomal recessive trait
• Affected homozygous animals generally not recognized as abnormal before 1 year of age

SIGNS
• Some animals exhibit mild clinical signs that go unrecognized for years; others regularly exhibit episodes of severe illness.
• Depression or weakness concomitant with episodes of red to brown pigmenturia; hemoglobinuria less likely to be recognized in female dogs, because of the sex difference in urination pattern
• Mild lethargy with slight fever during mild hemolytic episodes
• Marked lethargy, weakness, pale or icteric mucous membranes, mild hepatosplenomegaly, muscle wasting, and fever as high as 41°C (106°F) possible during severe hemolytic crises
• Intravascular hemolysis can be caused by hyperventilation-induced alkalemia associated with exercise or excitement.
• Signs of muscle dysfunction—usually limited to exercise intolerance and slightly diminished muscle mass, but muscle cramping and severe progressive myopathy can occur
• Heterozygous carrier animals appear clinically normal.

CAUSES & RISK FACTORS
Deficiency of the muscle-type subunit of phosphofructokinase—markedly reduced total activity in RBCs and skeletal muscle

DIAGNOSIS

DIFFERENTIAL DIAGNOSIS
• Other causes of hemolytic anemia—immune-mediated hemolytic anemia, haemobartonellosis, babesiosis, Heinz body hemolytic anemia, microangiopathic hemolytic anemia, and pyruvate kinase deficiency
• Affected dogs—negative Coombs test, no parasites or Heinz bodies in stained blood films, seronegative for *Babesia* spp., and no evidence of DIC or heartworm disease
• Differentiated from pyruvate kinase deficiency by specific enzyme assays or DNA test

CBC/BIOCHEMISTRY/URINALYSIS
• Persistent compensated hemolytic anemia
• MCV usually 80–90 fL
• Reticulocyte counts generally 10–30%
• PCV values generally 30–40%; during hemolytic crises may decrease to ≤ 15%
• Bilirubinuria—often markedly high in male dogs
• Hemoglobinuria in association with episodes of intravascular hemolysis
• Serum—slightly high potassium, magnesium, calcium, urea, AST, total protein, and globulin; slightly to moderately high LDH,

ALP, iron, and bilirubin; markedly high bilirubin in association with a hemolytic crisis; markedly high urea and creatinine if renal failure develops secondary to hemoglobin nephrosis or shock

OTHER LABORATORY TESTS

• Measure RBC phosphofructokinase activity—easily identify affected animals older than 3 months; heterozygous carrier dogs have approximately one-half normal activity.

• Perform DNA test by PCR technology—clearly differentiate normal and carrier animals of any age.

IMAGING
N/A

DIAGNOSTIC PROCEDURES
N/A

 ### TREATMENT

• Bone marrow transplantation is the only cure.

• In patients with severe intravascular hemolysis, IV fluid therapy minimizes the chance of acute renal failure.

• Blood transfusions usually not needed, but should be given if anemia becomes life-threatening

 ### MEDICATIONS

DRUG(S)
For fever that often accompanies intravascular hemolysis and potentiates hemolytic crisis—aspirin (10 mg/kg PO q12h) or dipyrone (0.055 mL of 50% solution/kg SC q8h).

CONTRAINDICATIONS/POSSIBLE INTERACTIONS
None

 ### FOLLOW-UP

• Infrequently, affected dogs may die during a hemolytic crisis because of anemia or renal failure.

• Affected animals can have a normal life span if properly managed.

• Owners should avoid placing affected dogs in stressful situations or subjecting them to strenuous exercise, excitement, or high environmental temperatures.

 ### MISCELLANEOUS

ABBREVIATIONS
• ALP = alkaline phosphatase
• AST = aspartate aminotransferase
• DIC = disseminated intravascular coagulation
• LDH = lactate dehydrogenase
• MCV = mean cell volume
• PCR = polymerase chain reaction
• PCV = packed cell volume

Suggested Reading

Giger U. Erythrocyte phosphofructokinase and pyruvate kinase deficiencies. In: Feldman BF, Zinkl JG, Jain NC, eds. Schalm's veterinary hematology, 5th ed. Philadelphia: Lippincott Williams & Wilkins, 2000;1020–1025.

Harvey JW. Congenital erythrocyte enzyme deficiencies. Vet Clin North Am Small Anim Pract 1996;26:1003–1011.

Author John W. Harvey
Consulting Editor Stephen A. Kruth

PHYSALOPTEROSIS

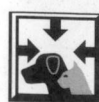

BASICS

OVERVIEW
• Stomach worm, *Physaloptera* spp., of dogs, cats
• Gastritis caused by small number of parasites, even single-worm infections
• No extraintestinal involvement
• Infective larvae carried by coprophagous grubs, beetles, and other bugs

SIGNALMENT
Dogs and cats; any age or sex

SIGNS
• Vomiting
• Small 2.5- to 5-cm worms with cuticular collars and spiral tails seen in vomitus

CAUSES & RISK FACTORS
Physaloptera, spirurid worms, transmitted as infective larvae in coprophagous beetles, bugs, or transport hosts such as birds, rodents, and frogs

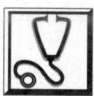

DIAGNOSIS

DIFFERENTIAL DIAGNOSIS
• Other spirurid infections (e.g., *Spirocerca,* the esophageal worm) produce similar eggs and may cause projectile vomiting.
• Viral, bacterial infections
• Foreign objects in the stomach
• Noxious substances accidentally ingested
• The trichostrongylid *Ollulanus* can cause chronic vomiting (colony and feral cats)—no eggs in feces; larvae, adults in vomitus

CBC/BIOCHEMISTRY/URINALYSIS
Usually normal

OTHER LABORATORY TESTS
N/A

IMAGING
Abdominal radiography, including contrast studies, to eliminate other causes of vomiting

DIAGNOSTIC PROCEDURES
• Fecal examination for ovoid-to-ellipsoidal eggs 30–40 × 20 μm, thick-shelled, larvated
• Endoscopy—adult worms seen with gastroscopy; worm retrieval and identification

TREATMENT
Outpatient treatment

MEDICATIONS
With no migration beyond the stomach wall, use adulticide anthelmintics with release in stomach.

DRUG(S)
• Fenbendazole 50 mg/kg PO q24h for 5 days
• Dichlorvos packets/tabs as single dose or biweekly
• Anthelmintic use is extra-label
• Pyrantel pamoate 5 mg/kg twice at 3-week interval or 20 mg/kg once; repeat if signs persist.
• Medication to reduce gastritis—histamine H_2-antagonists (e.g., famotidine 0.5 mg/kg PO q24h); sucralfate 0.25–1 g PO q8–12h in the dog; 0.25 g PO q8–12h in the cat

CONTRAINDICATIONS/POSSIBLE INTERACTIONS
• Do not give organophosphates to heartworm-positive dogs or cats.
• Do not give dichlorvos concurrently with other organophosphates such as insecticides.

FOLLOW-UP
Fecal examination after 2 weeks to determine drug effect.

MISCELLANEOUS

Suggested Reading

Bowman DD, Lynn RC, Eberhard ML. Georgi's parasitology for veterinarians, 8th ed. St. Louis: Saunders (Elsevier Science), 2003:213–214,1999.
Bowman DD, Hendrix CM, Lindsay DS, Barr SC. Feline clinical parasitology. Ames: Iowa State University Press, 2002:262–265, 299–304.
Campbell KL, Graham JC. *Physaloptera* infection in dogs and cats. Comp Cont Vet Practice 21:299–314,1999.

Acknowledgment

The author and editors acknowledge the prior contributions of Dr. Robert M. Corwin, who authored this topic in the previous edition.
Author Julie Ann Jarvinen
Consulting Editor Albert E. Jergens

BASICS

OVERVIEW
• *Yersinia pestis*—gram-negative, bipolar staining rod; an Enterobacteriaceae; reservoir includes wild rodents (sylvatic), ground squirrels, prairie dogs, rabbits, bobcats, coyotes • Occurs worldwide
• U.S.—reported cases from New Mexico, Arizona, California, Colorado, Idaho, Nevada, Oregon, Texas, Utah, Washington, Wyoming, and Hawaii • Common from May to October • Infected vectors (fleas) transmit the bacterium in bite. • Bacteria—rapidly migrate from skin lymphatics to regional lymph nodes; survive phagocytosis (because of capsule protection) and multiply in lymph nodes; phagocytic cells rupture and organism is resistant to further phagocytosis.
• Infection—fever and painful lymphadenopathy (bubo); intense local inflammation results in bubonic plague; intermittent bacteremia; lymph nodes may rupture; may become septicemic with or without lymph node involvement • Cats—highly susceptible to infection; severe fatal disease • Dogs—naturally resistant to infection

SIGNALMENT
Cats and rarely dogs

SIGNS
• Dogs—may exhibit mild febrile signs and depression • Cats—are unique among carnivores in exhibiting bubonic, pneumonic, and septicemic forms of plague.
Bubonic (Cats)
• Most common form • Incubation period—2–7 days after flea bite or after eating infected rodent • Duration of illness variable
• Buboes—head and neck; marked lymphadenopathy (hemorrhagic, necrotic, edematous); if patient survives long enough, lymph nodes abscess, rupture, and drain through fistula tracts to skin. • Fever—39.5–40.5°C (103–105°F) • Depression
• Vomiting/diarrhea • Dehydration
• Enlarged tonsils • Anorexia • Ocular discharge • Weight loss • Ataxia • Coma
• Oral ulcers
Septicemic (Cats)
• Rare • Septicemia without lymphadenopathy or abscess formation
• Other signs same as for bubonic

CAUSES & RISK FACTORS
• Hunter (outdoor) cats—greater risk of contacting wild rodent populations and rodent fleas • Travel to endemic areas—western United States and Hawaii
• Environment—homes or pet with heavy flea infestation; homes with large nearby rodent population (e.g., garbage food source or wood pile)

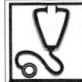 DIAGNOSIS

DIFFERENTIAL DIAGNOSIS
Fight wound abscess—*Pasteurella multocida; Staphylococcus aureus*

CBC/BIOCHEMISTRY/URINALYSIS
• Leukocytosis with left shift and marked toxic changes • Thrombocytopenia—with DIC • High liver enzyme activity and hyperbilirubinemia

OTHER LABORATORY TESTS
• Serology—Communicable Disease Center and/or state health department; cats and dogs develop high passive hemagglutinating titers to fraction 1A (capsule antigen) 8–12 days postinfection; may see fourfold rise in titer between acute and convalescent serum samples; high titers persist > 1 year in surviving animals • Prolonged clotting times—with DIC

IMAGING N/A

DIAGNOSTIC PROCEDURES
• Culture isolation—by reference laboratory; definitive (large numbers of gram-negative coccobacilli with bipolar staining); samples from antemortem clinical material (abscess, lymph node, peripheral blood) before treatment is given or from postmortem tissue (lymph node, abscess, liver, spleen)
• Fluorescent antibody test—quick presumptive method for identifying infected animals; samples same as for culture

PATHOLOGIC FINDINGS
• Acutely ill cats—few lesions; enlarged lymph nodes (buboes) on head and neck; enlarged liver and spleen • Lymph nodes—destruction of normal architecture; hemorrhagic necrosis; extracellular bacteria

 TREATMENT

• Inpatient
• High mortality if not treated early
• Treat aggressively with intravenous fluids to counteract septicemia.
• Treat DIC, if indicated.
• Treat patient for fleas.

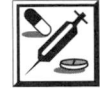 MEDICATIONS

DRUG(S)
• Treat all suspect cases empirically until laboratory confirmation is obtained.

• Systemic antimicrobials—use in all patients except those with lung involvement (such patients should be euthanized because of high zoonotic potential).
• Tetracyclines—oxytetracyclines, tetracycline, chlortetracycline; 25 mg/kg PO q8h for 10 days; parenteral, 7.5 mg/kg q12h
• Doxycycline—effectiveness not established but probably effective
• Chloramphenicol—30–50 mg/kg PO q8h
• Gentamicin, trimethoprim-sulfamethoxazole, and kanamycin—use if the other listed drugs cannot be used.

CONTRAINDICATIONS/POSSIBLE INTERACTIONS N/A

 FOLLOW-UP

PATIENT MONITORING
DIC—common later in infection, if disease not treated early

PREVENTION/AVOIDANCE
• Limit travel with pet to avoid endemic areas. • Endemic areas—keep pet on a leash to limit/control exposure to wild rodents and their fleas; periodically spray or dust pet and home for flea control. • Neuter cats—limit hunting behavior and wild rodent exposure.
• Rodents—eliminate animals and their habitats near houses and outbuildings (e.g., wood piles, garbage piles); store food in rodent-proof containers.

EXPECTED COURSE AND PROGNOSIS
• Prognosis—poor if not treated early
• Pneumonic plague has greatest risk of death

 MISCELLANEOUS

ZOONOTIC POTENTIAL
• High; do not mistake for bite abscesses or tularemia • Risk of exposure via bites of fleas or contact with infected tissue in blood

ABBREVIATION
DIC = disseminated intravascular coagulation

Suggested Reading
Rollag OJ, Skeels MR, Nims LJ, et al. Feline plague in New Mexico: report of five cases. J Am Vet Med Assoc 1981;179:1381–1383.
Author Patrick L. McDonough
Consulting Editor Stephen C. Barr

PLASMA CELL GINGIVITIS AND PHARYNGITIS

BASICS

OVERVIEW
An uninhibited, excessive immune inflammatory response affecting the oral cavity in cats

SIGNALMENT
• Cat
• Purebred breeds predisposed—Abyssinian, Persian, Himalayan, Burmese, Siamese, and Somali

SIGNS
• Ptyalism
• Halitosis
• Dysphasia
• Anorexia—prefers soft food
• Weight loss
• Scruffy haircoat
• Erythematous, ulcerative, proliferative lesions affecting the gingiva, glossopalatine arches, tongue, lips, buccal mucosa, and/or hard palate
• Gingival inflammation completely surrounds the tooth, compared with gingivitis, which usually only occurs on the buccal and labial surfaces.
• May extend to the glossopharyngeal arches as well as the palate

CAUSES & RISK FACTORS
• Cause unknown; bacterial, viral, and immunologic etiologies suspected
• Significant findings of feline coronavirus in one study
• Immunosuppression from FeLV or FIV can also lead to nonresponsive infections; most affected cats are negative for FeLV and FIV.

DIAGNOSIS

DIFFERENTIAL DIAGNOSIS
• Periodontal disease
• Oral malignancy
• Eosinophilic granuloma complex

CBC/BIOCHEMISTRY/URINALYSIS
• Polyclonal gammopathy secondary to antibody production following bacterial invasion into periodontal tissues
• Leukocytosis and eosinophilia may be present.

OTHER LABORATORY TESTS
N/A

IMAGING
Intraoral radiographs to evaluate periodontal disease and feline oral odontoclastic resorptions

DIAGNOSTIC PROCEDURES
Biopsy (especially unilateral lesions) to rule out neoplasia—primarily squamous cell carcinoma

TREATMENT

• First-line therapy involves teeth cleaning above and below the gingiva as well as strict home care and treatment (extraction) for teeth affected with grades 3 and 4 periodontal disease and/or feline odontoclastic resorptive lesions.
• Currently, the only treatment that consistently delivers 60–80% (depending on the study) cure without the use of follow-up medications is extraction of all teeth distal to the canines.
• To aid the extractions; flap all quadrants and use a high-speed bur with water spray to remove a trough of bone where the roots were, thus removing most of the keratinized gingiva, periodontal ligament, and periradicular alveolar bone; before suturing, "smooth down" the alveolar socket to remove sharp edges.
• If patients do not respond to extraction of the teeth distal to the canines, remove all teeth; when extracting the teeth, pay meticulous attention to removing all tooth substance; take intraoral radiographs before and after surgery; postoperative application of fluocinonide 0.05% (Lidex Gel) to the gingival margin helps in the healing process.
• Refractory cases with extensive proliferative lesion in the caudal oral cavity and pharynx warrant a more guarded prognosis.

MEDICATIONS

DRUG(S)
• Medication and other therapies have been used with limited long-term success; lack of permanent response to conventional oral hygiene, antibiotics, antiinflammatory drugs, and immunosuppressives is typical.

• Antibiotics—clindamycin (5 mg/kg q12h), metronidazole, amoxicillin, ampicillin, enrofloxacin, tetracycline
• Corticosteroids—prednisone (2 mg/kg initially daily, followed by every other day); methylprednisolone acetate 2 mg/kg q7–30 days) may also help control inflammation.
• Gold Salts Solganol (Shering)—1 mg/kg IM every week until improvement (up to 4 months), then every 14–35 days
• Chlorambucil—2 mg/m² orally every other day or 20 mg/m² every other week
• Bovine Lactoferrin (40 mg/kg) applied to the oral mucous membranes
• CO_2 laser to remove the inflamed tissue
• Megestrol acetate 1 mg/kg
• Levamisole
• Cyclophosphamide
• Cyclosporine

CONTRAINDICATIONS/POSSIBLE INTERACTIONS
N/A

FOLLOW-UP
N/A

MISCELLANEOUS

ABBREVIATIONS
FeLV = feline leukemia virus
FIV = feline immunodeficiency virus

Suggested Reading
Harvey CE, Emily PP. Small animal dentistry. St. Louis: CV Mosby, 1993.
Wiggs RB, Lobrise HB. Veterinary dentistry: principles and practice. Philadelphia: Lippincott-Raven, 1997.
Author Jan Bellows
Consulting Editor Heidi B. Lobprise

PLASMACYTOMA, MUCOCUTANEOUS

BASICS

OVERVIEW
• Tumor of plasma cell origin
• Rapid development
• May be a subtype of extramedullary plasmacytoma that is a primary tumor of soft tissue origin or may be metastasis of primary osseous multiple myeloma

SIGNALMENT
• Dogs and rarely cats
• Most common in mixed-breed dogs and cocker spaniels
• Age at diagnosis (dogs)—mean, 9.7 years; median, 10.5 years
• Both sexes affected equally

SIGNS
• Usually raised or ulcerated solid nodule, 0.25–6.0 cm in diameter
• Tumor of the lips—typically small
• Usually solitary
• Rarely polypoid
• Common locations—mouth, feet, trunk, and ears
• Occasionally occurs with multiple myeloma or lymphosarcoma, developing together or at different times
• Systemic signs rare

CAUSES & RISK FACTORS
Unknown

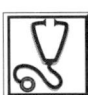

DIAGNOSIS

DIFFERENTIAL DIAGNOSIS
• Other round cell tumors—lymphosarcoma; mast cell tumor; histiocytoma; transmissible venereal tumor
• Poorly differentiated carcinoma
• Amelanotic melanoma
• Biopsy—distinguishes from other tumors

CBC/BIOCHEMISTRY/URINALYSIS
Usually normal, unless patient has multiple myeloma or lymphosarcoma

OTHER LABORATORY TESTS
N/A

IMAGING
No evidence of metastasis or bony lysis will be seen.

DIAGNOSTIC PROCEDURES
• Cytologic examination of fine-needle aspirate—reveals moderate to marked cellularity; round to polyhedral individual tumor cells with discrete margins and prominent anisocytosis and anisokaryosis; round to oval nuclei with fine to coarse chromatin and no visible nucleoli; cytoplasm stains lightly basophilic.
• Histologic—usually well circumscribed and easily identifiable

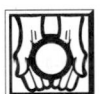

TREATMENT
• Occasionally invasive—aggressive surgical excision recommended
• Radiotherapy—successful in some patients

MEDICATIONS

DRUG(S)
Chemotherapy not recommended

CONTRAINDICATIONS/POSSIBLE INTERACTIONS
N/A

FOLLOW-UP

PATIENT MONITORING
Usually none, unless accompanied by multiple myeloma or lymphosarcoma

EXPECTED COURSE AND PROGNOSIS
Excellent in most patients

MISCELLANEOUS

ASSOCIATED CONDITIONS
• Multiple myeloma
• Lymphosarcoma (lymphoma)—dogs
• Cats—may note systemic amyloidosis

SEE ALSO
• Amyloidosis
• Lymphosarcoma—dogs
• Multiple Myeloma

Suggested Reading
Rakich PM, Latimer KS, Weiss R, Steffens WL. Mucocutaneous plasmacytomas in dogs. 75 cases (1980–1987). J Am Vet Med Assoc 1989;194:803–810.
Author Wallace B. Morrison
Consulting Editor Wallace B. Morrison

PLEURAL EFFUSION

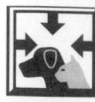 BASICS

DEFINITION
Abnormal accumulation of fluid within the pleural cavity

PATHOPHYSIOLOGY
• More than normal production or less than normal resorption of fluid • Alterations in hydrostatic and oncotic pressures or vascular permeability and lymphatic function may contribute to fluid accumulation.

SYSTEMS AFFECTED
• Respiratory • Cardiovascular

GENETICS
N/A

INCIDENCE/PREVALENCE
N/A

GEOGRAPHIC DISTRIBUTION
N/A

SIGNALMENT
Species
Dogs and cats

Breed Predilection
Varies with underlying cause

Mean Age and Range
Varies with underlying cause

Predominant Sex
Varies with underlying cause

SIGNS
General Comments
Depend on the fluid volume, rapidity of fluid accumulation, and the underlying cause

Historical Findings
• Dyspnea • Tachypnea • Orthopnea
• Open-mouth breathing • Cyanosis
• Exercise intolerance • Lethargy
• Inappetence • Cough

Physical Examination Findings
• Dyspnea—respirations often shallow and rapid • Muffled or inaudible heart and lung sounds ventrally • Preservation of breath sounds dorsally • Dullness ventrally on thoracic percussion

CAUSES
High Hydrostatic Pressure
• CHF • Overhydration • Intrathoracic neoplasia

Low Oncotic Pressure
Hypoalbuminemia—occurs in protein-losing enteropathy, protein-losing nephropathy, and liver disease

Vascular or Lymphatic Abnormality
• Infectious—bacterial, viral, or fungal
• Neoplasia (e.g., mediastinal lymphosarcoma, thymoma, mesothelioma, primary lung tumor, and metastatic disease) • Chylothorax (e.g., from lymphangiectasia, CHF, cranial vena caval obstruction, neoplasia, fungal infections, heartworms, diaphragmatic hernia, lung lobe torsion, trauma) • Diaphragmatic hernia • Hemothorax (e.g., from trauma, neoplasia, coagulopathy) • Lung lobe torsion • Pulmonary thromboembolism • Pancreatitis

RISK FACTORS
N/A

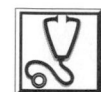 DIAGNOSIS

DIFFERENTIAL DIAGNOSIS
• Historical or physical evidence of external trauma—consider hemothorax or diaphragmatic hernia.
• Fever suggests an inflammatory, infectious, or neoplastic cause.
• Murmurs, gallops, or arrhythmias combined with jugular venous distension or pulsation suggest an underlying cardiac cause.
• Concurrent ascites suggests FIP, CHF (mainly dogs), severe hypoalbuminemia, diaphragmatic hernia, disseminated neoplasia, or pancreatitis.
• In cats, decreased compressibility of the cranial thorax suggests a cranial mediastinal mass.
• Concurrent ocular changes (e.g., chorioretinitis and uveitis) suggest FIP or fungal disease.

CBC/BIOCHEMISTRY/URINALYSIS
• Hemogram results may be abnormal in patients with pyothorax, FIP, neoplasia, or lung lobe torsion.
• Severe hypoalbuminemia (generally < 1 g/dL to cause effusion) suggests protein-losing enteropathy, protein-losing nephropathy, or liver disease.
• Hyperglobulinemia (polyclonal) suggests FIP.

OTHER LABORATORY TESTS
• Fluid analysis should include physical characteristics (i.e., color, clarity, odor, clots), pH, glucose, total protein, total nucleated cell count, and cytologic examination; Table 1 provides characteristics of various pleural fluid types and their disease associations.
• In cats the LDH concentration in transudates is < 200 IU/L and in exudates it is > 200 IU/L.
• Pleural fluid pH < 6.9 suggests pyothorax in cats.
• Glucose concentration in pleural fluid usually parallels levels in serum. In cats, pyothorax and malignancy lower pleural fluid glucose concentration relative to serum glucose concentration; thus pleural fluid with a normal pH and low glucose concentration suggests malignancy in cats.
• Serologic tests for feline leukemia virus (if patient has mediastinal lymphosarcoma), feline immunodeficiency virus (if patient has pyothorax), and coronavirus (if FIP is suspected) are available.
• Cardiac disease suspected—consider a heartworm test in dogs and cats and a thyroid evaluation in cats.
• Infection suspected—do aerobic and anaerobic bacterial culture and sensitivity tests and consider special stains (e.g., gram and acid-fast stains) of the fluid.
• FIP suspected—consider protein electrophoresis of the fluid; γ-globulin level > 32% of total protein strongly suggests a diagnosis of FIP.
• Chyle suspected—do an ether clearance test or Sudan stain of the pleural fluid, and triglyceride and cholesterol evaluations of the fluid and serum.

IMAGING
Radiographic Findings
• Used to confirm pleural effusion; should not be performed until after thoracocentesis in dyspneic patients with evidence of pleural effusion on physical examination
• Evidence of pleural effusion includes separation of lung borders away from the thoracic wall and sternum by fluid density in the pleural space, fluid-filled interlobar fissure lines, loss or blurring of the cardiac and diaphragmatic borders, blunting of the lung margins at the costophrenic angles (ventrodorsal view), and widening of the mediastinum (ventrodorsal view).
• Rounding of the caudal lung lobe borders (lateral view)—most common in patients with fibrosing pleuritis caused by chylothorax, pyothorax, or FIP
• Unilateral effusion—most common in patients with chylothorax and pyothorax; hemothorax, pulmonary neoplasia, diaphragmatic hernias, and lung lobe torsion
• Evaluate post-thoracocentesis radiographs carefully for cardiomegaly, intrapulmonary lesions, mediastinal masses, diaphragmatic hernia, lung lobe torsion, and evidence of trauma (e.g., rib fractures).
• Can diagnose a diaphragmatic hernia with positive-contrast peritoneography
• Can evaluate the thoracic duct by positive contrast lymphangiography

Echocardiographic Findings
• Ultrasonographic evaluation of the thorax is recommended whenever cardiac disease, a diaphragmatic hernia, or cranial mediastinal mass is suspected.
• Echocardiography is easiest to perform before thoracocentesis, provided the patient is stable.

DIAGNOSTIC PROCEDURES
• Thoracocentesis—allows characterization of the fluid type and determination of potential underlying cause
• Exploratory thoracotomy or thoracoscopy—to obtain biopsy specimens of lung, lymph nodes, or pleura, if indicated

TREATMENT

• First, thoracocentesis to relieve respiratory distress; if the patient is stable after thoracocentesis, outpatient treatment may be possible for some diseases. Most patients are hospitalized because they require intensive management such as indwelling chest tubes (e.g., patients with pyothorax) or thoracic surgery.
• Preventing fluid reaccumulation requires treatment based on a definitive diagnosis.
• Surgery is indicated for management of some neoplasias, diaphragmatic hernia repair, lymphangiectasia (i.e., thoracic duct ligation), foreign body removal, and lung lobe torsion (lung lobectomy).
• Pleuroperitoneal shunts may relieve clinical signs in animals with intractable pleural effusion.

MEDICATIONS

DRUG(S) OF CHOICE
• Treatment varies with specific disease.
• Diuretics generally reserved for patients with diseases causing fluid retention and volume overload (e.g., CHF)

CONTRAINDICATIONS
N/A

PRECAUTIONS
• Avoid drugs that depress respirations or decrease blood pressure.

• Inappropriate use of diuretics predisposes the patient to dehydration and electrolyte disturbances without eliminating the effusion.

POSSIBLE INTERACTIONS
N/A

ALTERNATIVE DRUG(S)
N/A

FOLLOW-UP

PATIENT MONITORING
Radiographic evaluation is key to assessment of treatment in most patients.

PREVENTION/AVOIDANCE
N/A

POSSIBLE COMPLICATIONS
• Death due to respiratory compromise
• Reexpansion pulmonary edema may develop after pleural effusion is manually removed.

EXPECTED COURSE AND PROGNOSIS
Vary with underlying cause, but usually guarded to poor

MISCELLANEOUS

ASSOCIATED CONDITIONS
N/A

AGE-RELATED FACTORS
N/A

ZOONOTIC POTENTIAL
N/A

PREGNANCY
N/A

SYNONYMS
• Hydrothorax = transudates and modified transudates • Pyothorax = empyema, septic pleuritis

SEE ALSO
See Causes.

ABBREVIATIONS
• CHF = congestive heart failure • FIP = feline infectious peritonitis • LDH = lactate dehydrogenase

Suggested Reading
Padrid P. Pulmonary diagnostics. In: August JR, ed. Consultations in feline internal medicine 3. Philadelphia: Saunders, 1997:292–302.
Sherding RG, Birchard SJ. Pleural effusion. In: Birchard SJ, Sherding RG, eds. Saunders manual of small animal practice, 2nd ed. Philadelphia: Saunders, 2000:670– 680.
Smeak DD, Birchard SJ, McLoughlin MA, et al. Treatment of chronic pleural effusion with pleuroperitoneal shunts in dogs: 14 cases (1985–1999). J Am Vet Med Assoc. 2001;219(11):1590–1597.
Author Francis W. K. Smith, Jr.
Consulting Editor Larry P. Tilley and Francis W. K. Smith, Jr.

Table 1.

	Transudate	Modified Transudate	Nonseptic Exudate	Septic Exudate	Chyle	Hemorrhage
Characterization of Pleural Fluid						
Color	Colorless to pale yellow	Yellow or pink	Yellow or pink	Yellow to red-brown	Milky white	Red
Turbidity	Clear	Clear to cloudy	Clear to cloudy; fibrin	Cloudy to opaque; fibrin	Opaque	Opaque
Protein (g/dl)	<1.5	2.5–5.0	3.0–8.0	3.0–7.0	2.5–6.0	>3.0
Nucleated cells/μl	<1,000	1,000–7,000 (LSA up to 100,000)	5,000–20,000 (LSA up to 100,000)	5,000–300,000	1,000–20,000	Similar to peripheral blood
Cytology	Mostly mesothelial cells	Mostly macrophages and mesothelial cells; few nondegenerate PMNs; neoplastic cells in some cases	Mostly nondegenerate PMNs and macrophages; neoplastic cells in some cases	Mostly degenerate PMNs; also macrophages; bacteria	Small lymphocytes, PMNs, and macrophages	Mostly RBCs; macrophages with erythrophagocytosis
Disease associations	Hypoalbuminemia (protein-losing nephropathy, protein-losing enteropathy, or liver disease); early CHF	CHF; neoplasia; diaphragmatic hernia; pancreatitis	FIP; neoplasia; diaphragmatic hernia; lung lobe torsion	Pyothorax	Lymphangiectasia, CHF, cranial vena cava obstruction, neoplasia, fungal, dirofilariasias, diaphragmatic hernia, lung lobe torsion, trauma	Trauma, coagulopathy, neoplasia, lung lobe torsion

Modified from Sherding RG. Diseases of the pleural cavity, In: Sherding RG, ed. The cat: diseases and clinical management. 2nd ed. New York: Churchill Livingstone, 1994; 1061.

LSA = lymphoma • CHF = congestive heart failure • FIP = feline infectious peritonitis • RBC = red blood cells • PMN = polymorphonuclear cells

PNEUMOCYTOSIS

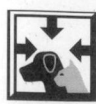

BASICS

OVERVIEW
• *Pneumocystis carinii*—saprophyte of the mammalian respiratory tract whose life cycle is completed in the alveolar spaces; classified as an atypical fungal organism, based on analysis of nucleic acids • Infections—dogs, clinical; cats, subclinical; usually confined to the respiratory tract; a reported case of disseminated disease in the dog • Transmission of infection—to susceptible animal within a species; strain differences may account for the lack of interspecies transmission

SIGNALMENT
• Dogs • No clinical infection reported in cats • Dachshunds < 12 months of age—majority of reported cases; suspected as having a congenital immunodeficiency • Clinical disease reported in a Shetland sheepdog, Cavalier King Charles spaniels, a beagle, and a Yorkshire terrier • Animals with predilection for impaired immunity (e.g., the very young or old) seem to carry an increased risk for overgrowth of the organism • No sex predilection

SIGNS
• Respiratory difficulty progressing over 1–4 weeks • Exercise intolerance—often a primary complaint • Coughing • Gradual weight loss • Vomiting and diarrhea—occasionally noted • Cachexia • Slight fever • Dyspnea • Tachycardia • Increased lung sounds on thoracic auscultation • Cyanosis—with severe infections • Previous history of recurrent infections

CAUSE & RISK FACTORS
• *P. carinii* • Humans—increased risk with immunodeficiency (e.g., HIV), stress, immunosuppressive therapy, and concurrent pulmonary infection • Dogs—factors that affect human risk may play a role • Affected Dachshunds appear to have T and B cell abnormalities (i.e., combined variable immunodeficiency)

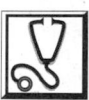

DIAGNOSIS

DIFFERENTIAL DIAGNOSIS
• Infectious tracheobronchitis • Bacterial bronchopneumonia—e.g., secondary to ciliary dyskinesis • Viral, *Toxoplasma*, *Mycoplasma*, parasitic, or mycotic pneumonitis • Pulmonary infiltration with eosinophils • Disseminated neoplasia • Noncardiogenic pulmonary edema • Congestive heart failure

CBC/BIOCHEMISTRY/URINALYSIS
• Changes usually nonspecific • Leukocytosis with neutrophilia and a left shift • Eosinophilia and monocytosis • Erythrocytosis—secondary to chronic hypoxia

OTHER LABORATORY TESTS
• Arterial blood gases—hypoxemia; hypocapnia; increase in blood pH; and increased alveolar-arterial oxygen tension difference • Serologic tests—not reliable for diagnosis because of possible underlying immunodeficiency • Immunoglobulin fraction quantification—hypogamma-globulinemia: IgA, IgG, and IgM deficiencies

IMAGING

Thoracic Radiography
• Changes not specific for *P. carinii* • Diffuse mild interstitial pattern with peribronchial opacification • More advanced cases have greater opacification with alveolar pattern and effacement of borders. • Middle lung lobes more severely affected than the cranioventral lung lobes • Cardiac changes minimal, but cor pulmonale may develop as a result of increased pulmonary vascular resistance resulting in tracheal elevation, right-sided heart enlargement, and pulmonary artery enlargement

DIAGNOSTIC PROCEDURES
• Definitive diagnosis made by direct visualization of *P. carinii* in respiratory fluids or biopsy specimens • Transtracheal aspiration and bronchoalveolar lavage—shown to be reliable methods for obtaining diagnostic samples • Direct lung fine-needle aspiration and lung biopsy—most reliable diagnostic procedures; carry the greatest risk for complications • Impression smears—may be made before tissue fixation • Immunohis-tochemical kits available—positive result is specific and highly diagnostic; may be used on cytologic, formalin-fixed, and paraffin-embedded material; note: host species–specific antigenic variation has been demonstrated and may cause false-negative results

PATHOLOGIC FINDINGS
• Lungs—firm, consolidated, and pale brown or gray; fluid not expressed from cut surfaces; do not collapse when the chest cavity is opened; small amounts of pleural fluid may be noted • Right heart—may find some degree of enlargement • Alveolar spaces—may be filled with amorphous, foamy, eosinophilic material with a honeycombed appearance; macrophages; few neutrophils; septa may be thickened and fibrosed; trophozoites and cyst stages may be identified • Generalized lymphoid tissue atrophy reported

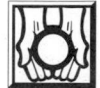

TREATMENT
• Inpatient—oxygen administration for hypoxemic patients; decrease exposure of immunocompromised patients to other pathogens • Nebulization with chemo-therapeutic agents may provide some benefit. • Cage rest or restricted exercise • Intravenous fluid as deemed necessary • Coupage and physical therapy

MEDICATIONS

DRUG(S)
• Trimethoprim-sulfonamide—15 mg/kg PO q6h for 3 weeks; first-choice drug • Pentamidine isethionate—4 mg/kg IM q24h for 2 weeks • Carbutamide—50 mg/kg IM q12h for 3 weeks • Drug combinations—dapsone and pyrimethamine; trimethoprim and atovaquone

CONTRAINDICATIONS/POSSIBLE INTERACTIONS
Pentamidine isethionate—impaired renal function; hepatic dysfunction; hypoglycemia; hypotension; hypocalcemia; urticaria; hematologic disorders; localized pain at injection site

FOLLOW-UP

PATIENT MONITORING
• Serial blood gases, pulse oximetry, and thoracic radiography—provide valuable prognostic information; monitor response to therapy • Pentamidine isethionate—check BUN and glucose daily; discontinue or decrease dosage if azotemia or other complications are noted • Monitor for resolution of cough and dyspnea • Clinical course variable • Early treatment of less severely affected patients associated with improved outcomes

MISCELLANEOUS

ZOONOTIC POTENTIAL
Little to none

ABBREVIATION
BUN = blood urea nitrogen

Suggested Reading

Kirberger RM, Lobetti RG. Radiographic aspects of *Pneumocystis carinii* pneumonia in the miniature dachshund. Vet Radiol Ultrasound 1998;39:313–317.

Lobetti R. Common variable immunodeficiency in miniature dachshunds affected with *Pneumocystis carinii* pneumonia. J Vet Diagn Invest 2000;12:39–45.

Lobetti RG, Leisewitz AL, Spancer JA. *Pneumocystis carinii* in the miniature dachshund: case report and literature review. J Small Anim Pract 1996;37:280–285.

Author Tania N. Davey
Consulting Editor Stephen C. Barr

BASICS

OVERVIEW
• Inflammation of the lungs caused by inhaled material (e.g., oral ingesta, regurgitated material, and vomitus) and subsequent pulmonary dysfunction; develops when laryngeal reflexes function improperly or are overwhelmed; thus a consequence of an underlying problem • Pulmonary dysfunction—caused by a combination of factors; (1) obstruction—large particles obstruct large airways, causing acute respiratory distress (extremely rare); particulates cause direct obstruction of small airways and indirect obstruction from bronchospasm and the production of mucus and exudate; (2) aspiration of gastric acid—results in marked damage to the respiratory epithelium and surfactant; may cause bronchospasm and occasionally ARDS; (3) bacterial pneumonia—common component in regurgitated material, food, or pharyngeal flora; may initiate an immediate infection or a secondary infection occurring later in the course of disease

SIGNALMENT
Dogs more commonly affected than cats

SIGNS
• May be peracute, acute, or chronic • Cough • Respiratory distress • Tachypnea • Fever • Cyanosis • Exercise intolerance • Nasal discharge • Depending on underlying cause: • Regurgitation • Vomiting • Dysphagia • Altered consciousness—depression, post-ictus, dementia, sedation, and anesthesia • Stertor or stridor

CAUSES & RISK FACTORS
• Pharyngeal abnormalities—local paralysis (e.g., idiopathic, focal myasthenia gravis, and traumatic nerve damage); generalized neuromuscular disease; cricopharyngeal motor dysfunction; anatomic malformations; postoperative laryngoplasty • Esophageal abnormalities • Megaesophagus • Reflux esophagitis • Esophageal obstruction—mass, foreign body, stricture • Bronchoesophageal fistula • Altered consciousness • Sedation • Anesthesia—during or recovery from • Postictus • Forebrain disease • Severe metabolic disturbance • Iatrogenic cause • Force feeding • Tube feeding—improper technique; misplacement of tube • Mineral oil administration

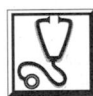

DIAGNOSIS

DIFFERENTIAL DIAGNOSIS
• Bacterial pneumonia—component of cases; may develop for reasons other than the overt aspiration of foreign material • Lung lobe abscess—consolidated appearance radiographically; may be a sequela to aspiration pneumonia, bacterial pneumonia, or foreign body

CBC/BIOCHEMISTRY/URINALYSIS
• Neutrophilic leukocytosis with a left shift • WBC count—may be normal • Nonregenerative anemia associated with chronic inflammatory disease

OTHER LABORATORY TESTS
• Arterial blood gas analysis—hypoxemia expected; $PaCO_2$ generally low but may be high with large airway obstruction or systemic neuromuscular disease • Other tests—pursue underlying cause; antiacetylcholine antibodies for suspected myasthenia gravis; ANA, thyroid function, or adrenal function for suspected polyneuropathy

IMAGING
• Thoracic radiography—bronchoalveolar pattern most severe in the gravity-dependent lung lobes (e.g., right middle and cranial and left middle); may take up to 24 hr for pattern to develop after acute aspiration; scrutinize for evidence of esophageal or mediastinal disease. • Contrast swallowing study—ideally with fluoroscopy; provides evidence of swallowing or esophageal dysfunction that may predispose the patient to aspiration

DIAGNOSTIC PROCEDURES
• Tracheal wash—collect material for bacterial culture and sensitivity testing; collect before administering antibiotics; infection often caused by multiple organisms with unpredictable susceptibility • Bronchoscopy—for suspected large airway obstruction based on breathing pattern, auscultation, or radiographic findings; collect airway samples • Appropriate tests to investigate underlying causes

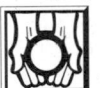

TREATMENT
• Oxygen—respiratory distress; if distress persists, provide ventilatory support. • Intravenous fluids—indicated for shock or dehydration, or if oral intake is withheld; avoid overhydration, which may exacerbate secondary edema. • Oral intake—withhold until primary problem identified and managed, particularly in acutely affected, unstable patients • Cage rest—for respiratory distress • Do not allow patient to remain laterally recumbent on one side for more than 2 hr. • Once stable, mild exercise may assist in generating a productive cough and facilitating airway clearance. • Saline nebulization and coupage—recommended for consolidation or if resolution is proceeding slowly • Airway suction—indicated only if aspiration is observed (e.g., during recovery from anesthesia) • Lavage—contraindicated; forces material deeper into lungs; any gastric acid neutralized in seconds

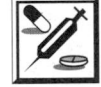

MEDICATIONS

DRUG(S)
• Antibiotic therapy—ideally, withhold until an airway specimen is collected for cytology and C/S; if signs of sepsis or severe compromise, ampicillin with sulbactam plus a fluoroquinolone IV or ampicillin with sulbactam plus an aminoglycoside IV; otherwise, ampicillin with sulbactam IV or amoxicillin with clavulanate PO; adjust antibiotic selection based on results of airway cytology, C/S, and clinical response; continue for 10 days after resolution of clinical and radiographic signs. • Bronchodilators (e.g., theophylline and terbutaline)—may cause dramatic improvement in some cases, but have the potential to worsen V:Q mismatch; most often helpful in cats and in dogs with either acute aspiration or auscultable wheezes. • Short-acting corticosteroids—may be administered once to combat inflammation with peracute life-threatening aspiration

CONTRAINDICATIONS/POSSIBLE INTERACTIONS
• Diuretics—generally contraindicated; drying of airways reduces mucociliary clearance • Corticosteroids—generally contraindicated; predispose patient to infection • Fluoroquinolone antibiotics and chloramphenicol—may prolong clearance of theophylline-derivative bronchodilators, resulting in signs of toxicity

FOLLOW-UP

PATIENT MONITORING
• Radiographs, arterial blood gas analysis, and clinical signs—monitor response to treatment. • Radiographs—evaluate every 3–7 days initially to determine appropriateness of treatment; then every 1–2 weeks • If signs do not resolve or suddenly worsen—possible recurrence of aspiration or a secondary infection; repeat diagnostic evaluation, including examination of tracheal wash fluid.

PREVENTION/AVOIDANCE
The underlying cause must be identified and managed.

POSSIBLE COMPLICATIONS
• Secondary infection common • ARDS—may develop, particularly after aspiration of gastric acid • Abscessation or foreign body granuloma rare

EXPECTED COURSE AND PROGNOSIS
• Prognosis—depends on severity of signs when patient is examined and the ability to correct the underlying problem • Acute, severe aspiration—can be fatal • Recurrence—likely if underlying cause is not or cannot be addressed

MISCELLANEOUS

SEE ALSO
• Acute Respiratory Distress Syndrome • Megaesophagus • Pneumonia, Bacterial

ABBREVIATIONS
• ANA = antinuclear antibody • ARDS = acute respiratory distress syndrome • C/S = culture and sensitivity • V:Q = ventilation:perfusion

Suggested Reading
Hawkins EC. Aspiration pneumonia. In: Bonagura JD, Kirk RW, eds. Current veterinary therapy XII. Philadelphia: Saunders, 1995:915–919.
Marik PE. Aspiration pneumonitis and aspiration pneumonia. N Engl J Med 2001;344:665–671.

Author Eleanor C. Hawkins
Consulting Editor Lynelle R. Johnson

PNEUMONIA, BACTERIAL

BASICS

DEFINITION
The fully developed inflammatory response to virulent bacteria in lung parenchyma characterized by exudation of cells and fluid into conducting airways and alveolar spaces

PATHOPHYSIOLOGY
• Bacteria—enter the lower respiratory tract primarily by the inhalation or aspiration routes; enter less commonly by the hematogenous route; infections incite an overt inflammatory reaction.
• Tracheobronchial tree and lungs—normally not continuously sterile • Oropharyngeal bacteria—frequently aspirated; may be present for an unknown interval in the normal tracheobronchial tree and lung; have the potential to cause or complicate respiratory infection; cloud interpretation of airway and lung cultures • Respiratory infection—development depends on the complex interplay of many factors: size, inoculation site, number of organisms and their virulence, and resistance of the host • Viral infections—alter bacterial colonization patterns; increase bacterial adherence to respiratory epithelium; reduce mucociliary clearance and phagocytosis; thus may allow resident bacteria to invade the lower respiratory tract • Exudative phase—inflammatory hyperemia; serous exudation of high-protein fluid into interstitial and alveolar spaces • Leukocytic emigration phase—leukocytes infiltrate the airways and alveoli; consolidation, ischemia, tissue necrosis, and atelectasis owing to bronchial occlusion, obstructive bronchiolitis, and impaired collateral ventilation • Mortality—associated with severe hypoxemia (low arterial oxygen concentration) and sepsis

SYSTEMS AFFECTED
Respiratory—primary or secondary infection

GEOGRAPHIC DISTRIBUTION
Widespread

SIGNALMENT

Species
More common in dogs than in cats

Breed Predilection
Dogs—sporting breeds, hounds, working breeds, and mixed breeds > 12 kg

Mean Age and Range
Dogs—range, 1 month to 15 years; many cases in dogs < 1 year old

Predominant Sex
Dogs—60% males

SIGNS

Historical Findings
• Cough • Fever • Labored breathing • Exercise intolerance • Anorexia and weight loss • Lethargy • Nasal discharge

Physical Examination Findings
• Cough • Fever • Difficult or rapid breathing • Abnormal breath sounds on auscultation—increased intensity or bronchial breath sounds, crackles, and wheezes • Weight loss • Serous or muco-purulent nasal discharge • Lethargy • Dehydration

CAUSES

Dogs
• *Bordetella bronchiseptica* and *Streptococcus zooepidemicus*—primary bacterial pathogens • Isolates—most thought to be opportunistic invaders; usually one or two bacterial pathogens, but may see three or more; gram-negative species and *Mycoplasma* spp. predominate in single and mixed infections. • *B. bronchiseptica, Escherichia coli, Klebsiella pneumoniae, Pasteurella multocida, Staphylococcus* spp., *Streptococcus* spp., *Mycoplasma* spp., and *Pseudomonas aeruginosa*—most common isolates • Anaerobic bacteria—found in pulmonary abscesses and aspiration pneumonia

Cats
• Bacterial pathogens—poorly documented; *B. bronchiseptica* and *Pasteurella* spp. most frequently reported • Carrier state—may exist; periods of shedding *B. bronchiseptica* after stress; infected queens may not shed organism prepartum but begin shedding postpartum, serving as a source of infection for kittens.

RISK FACTORS
• Pre-existing viral, mycoplasmal, parasitic, or fungal respiratory infection • Regurgitation, dysphagia, or vomiting • Reduced level of consciousness—stupor, coma, and anesthesia • Thoracic trauma or surgery • Bronchial foreign body • Bronchiectasis • Immunosuppressive therapy—chemotherapy and glucocorticoids • Severe metabolic disorders—uremia, diabetes mellitus, hyperadrenocorticism, and hypoadrenocorticism • Functional or anatomic defects—tracheal hypoplasia, cleft palate, primary ciliary dyskinesia, megaesophagus, laryngeal paralysis • Sepsis • Intravenous catheter placement • Protein–calorie malnutrition • Immunodeficiency • Age—very young more susceptible to fatal infections • Phagocyte dysfunction—FeLV and diabetes mellitus • Complement deficiency—rare • Selective IgA deficiency • Combined T cell and B cell dysfunction—rare

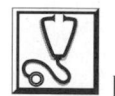

DIAGNOSIS

DIFFERENTIAL DIAGNOSIS
• Viral pneumonia—canine distemper virus and canine adenovirus • Rickettsial pneumonia—ehrlichiosis and Rocky Mountain spotted fever • Protozoal pneumonia—toxoplasmosis • Parasitic pneumonia—capillariasis, paragonimiasis, and dirofilariasis • Fungal pneumonia—histoplasmosis, blastomycosis, coccidioidomycosis, and cryptococcosis • Eosinophilic pneumonia • Bacterial or fungal rhinitis • Chronic sinusitis • Pharyngitis • Tonsillitis • Infectious tracheobronchitis • Pulmonary abscess • Pleural infection—pyothorax • Bronchial foreign body

CBC/BIOCHEMISTRY/URINALYSIS
Inflammatory leukogram—neutrophilic leukocytosis with or without a left shift; absence does not rule out the diagnosis.

OTHER LABORATORY TESTS
• Arterial blood gas analysis—values correlate well with the degree of physiologic disruption; sensitive monitor of progress during treatment; $PaO_2 < 80$ torr on room air = mild or moderate hypoxemia; $PaO_2 < 60$ torr on room air = severe hypoxemia • Blood culture—may help identify causal agent

IMAGING

Thoracic Radiography
Alveolar pattern characterized by increased pulmonary densities (margins indistinct; air bronchograms or lobar consolidation); patchy or lobar alveolar pattern with a cranial ventral lung lobe distribution

DIAGNOSTIC PROCEDURES
• Microbiologic (aerobic and anaerobic bacteria culture) and cytologic examinations for definitive diagnosis • Samples—transtracheal washing, bronchoscopy, bronchoalveolar lavage (with or without bronchoscope), or fine-needle lung aspiration • Septic inflammation with degenerate neutrophils predominating • Recent antibiotic administration—nonseptic inflammation likely • Bacteria—visible microscopically in < 50% of affected dogs; always culture specimens, even if no bacteria are seen on cytologic examination.

PATHOLOGIC FINDINGS

Gross
• Irregular consolidation in cranioventral regions • Consolidated lung—varies from dark red to gray-pink to more gray, depending on age of patient and nature of the process • Palpable firmness of the tissue—single most important gross criterion

Histopathologic
• Nidus of inflammation—bronchiolar-alveolar junction
• Early—bronchioles and adjacent alveoli filled with neutrophils and an admixture of cell debris, fibrin, and macrophages; necrotic to hyperplastic epithelium
• Later—neutrophilic, fibrinous, hemorrhagic, or necrotizing inflammation, depending on virulence of bacteria and host response

TREATMENT

APPROPRIATE HEALTH CARE
Inpatient—recommended with multisystemic signs (e.g., anorexia, high fever, weight loss, and lethargy)

NURSING CARE
• Maintain normal systemic hydration—important to aid mucociliary clearance and secretion mobilization; use a balanced multielectrolyte solution.
• Nebulization with saline aerosol—results in more rapid resolution if used with physiotherapy and antibacterials
• Physiotherapy—mild forced exercise, chest wall coupage, tracheal manipulation to stimulate mild cough, and postural drainage; may enhance clearance of secretions; always do immediately after nebulization; avoid allowing the patient to lie in one position for a prolonged time.
• Oxygen therapy—for respiratory distress

ACTIVITY
Restrict during treatment (inpatient or outpatient), except as part of physiotherapy after aerosolization.

DIET
• Ensure normal intake with food high in protein and energy density.
• Enteral or parenteral nutritional support—indicated in severely ill patients

CLIENT EDUCATION
Warn client that high morbidity and mortality are associated with severe hypoxemia and sepsis.

SURGICAL CONSIDERATIONS
Surgery (lung lobectomy)—may be indicated with pulmonary abscessation or bronchopulmonary foreign body with secondary pneumonia; may be indicated if patient is unresponsive to conventional treatment and disease is limited to one or two lobes

MEDICATIONS

DRUG(S) OF CHOICE
Antimicrobials
• Antimicrobials are best selected based on results of culture and susceptibility testing from tracheal wash or other pulmonary specimens.
• Reasonable initial antimicrobial choices pending culture results include amoxicillin–clavulanic acid, cephalexin, chloramphenicol, or trimethoprim-sulfonamide.
• Gram-positive cocci—ampicillin, ampicillin-sulbactam; amoxicillin; amoxicillin–clavulanic acid; azithromycin; chloramphenicol, erythromycin; gentamicin; trimethoprim-sulfonamide; first-generation cephalosporins
• Gram-negative rods—amikacin; chloramphenicol; gentamicin; trimethoprim-sulfonamide; enrofloxacin; marbofloxacin; carboxypenicillins
• *Bordetella*—tetracyclines; amikacin; chloramphenicol; gentamicin; enrofloxacin; kanamycin; azithromycin
• *Mycoplasma*—doxycycline, enrofloxacin, marbofloxacin, chloramphenicol
• Anaerobes—amoxicillin–clavulanic acid; chloramphenicol; metronidazole; clindamycin
• Continue treatment for at least 10 days beyond clinical resolution; usually a total of 3 weeks or longer

CONTRAINDICATIONS
Anticholinergics and antihistamines—may thicken secretions and inhibit mucokinesis and exudate removal from airways

PRECAUTIONS
Antitussives—use with caution and only for short intervals to control intractable cough; potent, centrally acting agents may inhibit mucokinesis and exudate removal from airways.

POSSIBLE INTERACTIONS N/A

ALTERNATIVE DRUG(S)
Expectorants—recommended by some clinicians; no objective evidence that they increase mucokinesis or mobilization of secretions

FOLLOW-UP

PATIENT MONITORING
• Arterial blood gases—most sensitive monitor of progress • Auscultate patient thoroughly several times daily. • Thoracic radiographs—improve more slowly than the clinical appearance

PREVENTION/AVOIDANCE
• Vaccination—against upper respiratory viruses; against *B. bronchiseptica* if a dog is boarded or exposed to large numbers of other animals • Catteries—environmental strategies to lower population density and improve hygiene help control outbreaks of bordetellosis.

POSSIBLE COMPLICATIONS
Young dogs infected with *B. bronchiseptica* may develop chronic bronchitis.

EXPECTED COURSE AND PROGNOSIS
• Prognosis—good with aggressive antibacterial and supportive therapy; more guarded in young animals, patients with immunodeficiency, and patients that are debilitated or have severe underlying disease
• Prolonged infection—potential for chronic bronchitis or bronchiectasis in any patient

MISCELLANEOUS

ASSOCIATED CONDITIONS
• Frequently develops secondary to underlying metabolic diseases—hyperadrenocorticism; diabetes mellitus; uremia • Frequently develops secondary to underlying functional or anatomic abnormalities—cleft palate; tracheal hypoplasia; primary ciliary dyskinesia; laryngeal paralysis; megaesophagus
• Bronchiectasis—both predisposing factor and potential complication

AGE-RELATED FACTORS
• Young puppies and kittens—may have a poorer prognosis; puppies often develop long-term complications (e.g., chronic bronchitis).
• Underlying functional and anatomic problems and immunodeficiencies—suspect in young patients.

ZOONOTIC POTENTIAL N/A

PREGNANCY
Bitches or queens infected with *B. bronchiseptica*—may transmit infection to neonates

SEE ALSO
• Bordetellosis—Cats • Pneumonia, Aspiration • Tracheobronchitis, Infectious—Dogs

ABBREVIATION
FeLV = feline leukemia virus

Suggested Reading
Angus JC, Jang SS, Hirsh DC. Microbiological study of transtracheal aspirates from dogs with suspected lower respiratory tract disease: 264 cases (1989–1995). J Am Vet Med Assoc 1997;210:55–58.
Ford RB. Bacterial pneumonia. In: Bonagura JD, ed. Current veterinary therapy XIII. Philadelphia: Saunders, 2000:812–815.
Hawkins EC. Tracheal wash and bronchoalveolar lavage in the management of respiratory disease. In: Kirk RW, Bonagura JD, eds. Current veterinary therapy XI. Philadelphia: Saunders, 1992:795–800.
Jameson PH, King LA, Lappin MR, et al. Comparison of clinical signs, diagnostic findings, organisms isolated, and clinical outcome in dogs with bacterial pneumonia: 93 cases (1986–1991). J Am Vet Med Assoc 1995;206:206–209.
Johnson LR. Respiratory therapeutics. In: August JR, ed. Consultations in feline internal medicine 4. Philadelphia: Saunders, 2001:283–290.
Author Philip Roudebush
Consulting Editor Lynelle R. Johnson

PNEUMONIA, EOSINOPHILIC

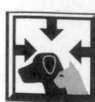

BASICS

DEFINITION
The fully developed inflammatory response to antigens in lung parenchyma characterized by exudation of cells and fluid into lung interstitium, conducting airways, and alveolar spaces

PATHOPHYSIOLOGY
• Immunologic basis—supporting evidence generally accepted; mechanisms involved not yet clarified
• Evolution of disease—likely determined by characteristics of antigens, the host response, and the regulation of that response
• Three disease patterns—eosinophilic pneumonitis, allergic bronchitis, and pulmonary eosinophilic granulomatosis
• Antigens enter the lower respiratory tract by inhalation or hematogenous routes.
• Chronic exposure to antigens—elicits a humoral and cellular immune response
• Allergic or hypersensitivity pulmonary disorders—associated with an abnormal humoral antibody response and a cell-mediated immunoregulatory defect
• Immunoglobulin classes involved—IgE, IgG, and others
• High numbers of activated macrophages and T-lymphocytes and depressed suppressor T-cell activity—alter cell-mediated immunity
• Inflammatory infiltration—of lung interstitium and alveolar spaces
• Severely affected patients develop marked granulomatous disease.
• Occult heartworm disease with pneumonitis—microfilaria become entrapped in the pulmonary circulation.
• Allergic bronchial disease—response to infection or colonization of the airways with a fungal organism, usually *Aspergillus* spp.
• Mortality—associated with severe hypoxemia (e.g., low arterial oxygen concentration) and (rarely) severe hemoptysis

SYSTEMS AFFECTED
• Respiratory
• Cardiovascular—may see cor pulmonale

GENETICS
N/A

INCIDENCE/PREVALENCE
N/A

GEOGRAPHIC DISTRIBUTION
Widespread

SIGNALMENT
Species
Dogs

Breed Predilection
Siberian husky

Mean Age and Range
All ages

Predominant Sex
None

SIGNS
General Comments
Extremely variable, depending on the severity

Historical Findings
• Cough—unresponsive to antibacterial therapy
• Fever
• Labored breathing
• Exercise intolerance
• Anorexia
• Lethargy
• Weight loss
• Nasal discharge

Physical Examination Findings
• Harsh, moist cough
• Fever
• Dyspnea
• Abnormal breath sounds on auscultation—increased-intensity breath sounds; crackles; wheezes; decreased sound can occur
• Weight loss
• Peripheral lymphadenopathy—rare
• Mucopurulent nasal discharge

CAUSES
• Aeroallergens—spores or hyphae from fungi and actinomycetes; pollen; insect antigens
• Parasitic antigens—heartworm microfilaria, respiratory parasites

RISK FACTORS
• Living in a heartworm-endemic area without receiving preventive medication
• Dusty or moldy environment

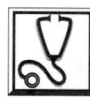

DIAGNOSIS

DIFFERENTIAL DIAGNOSIS
• Parasitic pneumonia—capillariasis; paragonimiasis; dirofilariasis
• Fungal pneumonia—histoplasmosis; blastomycosis; coccidioidomycosis; cryptococcosis
• For eosinophilic pneumonitis—bacterial pneumonia; viral pneumonia (e.g., canine distemper virus and canine adenovirus); rickettsial pneumonia (e.g., ehrlichiosis and Rocky Mountain spotted fever); protozoal pneumonia (e.g., toxoplasmosis); congestive heart failure
• For allergic bronchitis—infectious tracheobronchitis; chronic bronchitis
• For pulmonary eosinophilic granulomatosis—neoplasia (including lymphomatoid granulomatosis); pulmonary abscess; bronchial foreign body

CBC/BIOCHEMISTRY/URINALYSIS
• Inflammatory leukogram—neutrophilic leukocytosis with or without a left shift, eosinophilia, basophilia, or monocytosis
• Hyperglobulinemia—suggests occult dirofilariasis

OTHER LABORATORY TESTS
Arterial Blood Gas Analysis
• Values correlate well with the degree of physiologic disruption; sensitive monitor of patient's progress during treatment
• Hypoxemia—mild or moderate, $PaO_2 < 80$ torr on room air; severe, $PaO_2 < 60$ torr on room air

Other
• Heartworm microfilaria and antigen tests—positive results suggest dirofilariasis or eosinophilic pneumonitis associated with microfilaria trapped in the lung.
• Protein electrophoresis—β-globulin spike (hyperbetaglobulinemia) often found with occult dirofilariasis

IMAGING
• Radiographic findings depend on extent and severity of disease.
• Thoracic radiographs—help document the severity of pulmonary artery disease; reveal interstitial pneumonitis in dogs with dirofilariasis
• Eosinophilic pneumonitis—linear or miliary interstitial pattern that resembles changes seen with early pulmonary edema or fungal pneumonia; alveolar pattern characterized by increased pulmonary densities with indistinct margins in severely affected patients; tortuous, large pulmonary arteries and right-sided cardiomegaly in patients with dirofilariasis
• Allergic or eosinophilic bronchitis—bronchial pattern with bronchi extending into the periphery of the lung (tram/railroad track and donut signs)
• Eosinophilic granuloma—multiple nodular lesions of variable sizes in different lung lobes; patchy, focal alveolar densities; tracheobronchial lymphadenopathy

DIAGNOSTIC PROCEDURES
• Cytologic examination of aspirates, washings, or brushings—definitive diagnosis: eosinophilic inflammation predominates; may note other types of inflammatory cells; carefully examine specimens for antigenic sources (e.g., parasites, fungi, or neoplasia).

- Transtracheal washing
- Bronchoscopy; yellow-green mucus, polypoid mucosal proliferation, partial airway collapse
- Bronchoalveolar lavage—with or without bronchoscope
- Fine-needle lung aspiration and examination
- Intradermal skin testing—rarely may identify allergens
- Fecal examinations—routine flotation, direct smear, sediment examination, and Baermann technique; when negative, respiratory parasitic infection less likely

PATHOLOGIC FINDINGS
- Gross—diffuse, patchy, or nodular firm lesions; usually pale or mottled
- Histopathologic—eosinophilic, lymphocytic, and macrophagic infiltration of alveolar walls and alveolar spaces; as the disease progresses, interstitial infiltrative process becomes fibrotic with obliteration of alveolar spaces, and granulomas may be dispersed within the interstitial fibrosis.

 TREATMENT

APPROPRIATE HEALTH CARE
Inpatient—recommended with multisystemic signs (e.g., anorexia, weight loss, or lethargy)

NURSING CARE
- Dehydration—hinders mucociliary clearance and secretion mobilization; maintain normal systemic hydration with a balanced multielectrolyte solution.
- Supplemental oxygen—for respiratory distress

ACTIVITY
Restricted during treatment (inpatient or outpatient)

DIET
Ensure normal intake.

CLIENT EDUCATION
Warn client that morbidity and mortality are associated with severe hypoxemia.

SURGICAL CONSIDERATIONS
May remove lung lobes with large granulomas

 MEDICATIONS

DRUG(S) OF CHOICE
- Corticosteroids—prednisolone or prednisone at 2–4 mg/kg/day until clinical signs begin to resolve; then taper slowly.
- Heartworm adulticidal therapy—for heartworm-positive patient; initiate after the patient has been stabilized with corticosteroids and rest.

- Itraconazole or ketoconazole—may be used with confirmed allergic bronchopulmonary fungal infection, which is a rare condition; use antifungal drugs only if the fungal infection is confirmed by cytologic examination or culture.

CONTRAINDICATIONS
N/A

PRECAUTIONS
N/A

POSSIBLE INTERACTIONS
N/A

ALTERNATIVE DRUG(S)
- Other immunosuppressive drugs (e.g., cyclosporine, cyclophosphamide, azathioprine, and mercaptopurine)—may use when corticosteroids are contraindicated or have been ineffective
- Bronchodilators—may be helpful, particularly if wheezes are auscultated or labored respiratory effort is observed; see Asthma, Bronchitis—Cats, and/or Bronchitis, Chronic (COPD)

 FOLLOW-UP

PATIENT MONITORING
- Arterial blood gases—most sensitive monitor of progress
- Auscultate patient thoroughly several times daily.
- Thoracic radiographs—improve more slowly than the clinical appearance

PREVENTION/AVOIDANCE
- Routine heartworm-prevention medication
- Change patient's environment if an aeroallergen is suspected.

POSSIBLE COMPLICATIONS
Pulmonary thromboembolism—patients treated with adulticide for dirofilariasis

EXPECTED COURSE AND PROGNOSIS
- If primary allergen is identified and eliminated—prognosis good for mild cases
- If allergen is not identified—prognosis for control good; many patients require long-term treatment with steroids.
- Heartworm infection—prognosis depends on severity of pulmonary hypertension, cor pulmonale, and thromboembolism.
- Eosinophilic granulomatosis—prognosis guarded; often disease is progressive.

 MISCELLANEOUS

ASSOCIATED CONDITIONS
- Dirofilariasis
- Bronchopulmonary fungal infection

AGE-RELATED FACTORS
N/A

ZOONOTIC POTENTIAL
N/A

PREGNANCY
Corticosteroids and other immunosuppressive drugs are contraindicated in pregnant animals.

SYNONYMS
- Allergic bronchitis
- Eosinophilic bronchitis or bronchopneumopathy
- Bronchitic pulmonary eosinophilia
- Allergic bronchopulmonary aspergillosis
- Allergic alveolitis
- Eosinophilic pneumonitis
- Eosinophilic pneumonia
- Hypersensitivity pneumonitis
- Eosinophilic pulmonary granulomatosis
- Extrinsic allergic alveolitis
- Occult heartworm pneumonia
- Parasitic pulmonary eosinophilia
- Pulmonary infiltrates with eosinophilia (PIE)

SEE ALSO
- Cough
- Dyspnea, Tachypnea, and Panting
- Heartworm Disease—Dogs
- Lymphomatoid Granulomatosis
- Respiratory Parasites

Suggested Reading

Calvert CA, Rawlings CA. Pulmonary manifestations of heartworm disease. Vet Clin North Am Small Anim Pract 1985;15:991–1009.

Calvert CA. Eosinophilic pulmonary granulomatosis. In: Kirk RW, Bonagura JD, eds. Current veterinary therapy XI. Philadelphia: Saunders, 1992:813–816.

Clercx, Peeters D, Snaps F, et al. Eosinophilic bronchopneumopathy in dogs. J Vet Intern Med 2000;14:282–291.

Corcoran BM, Thoday KL, Henfrey JI, et al. Pulmonary infiltration with eosinophils in 14 dogs. J Small Anim Pract 1991;32:494–502.

Hawkins EC. Tracheal wash and bronchoalveolar lavage in the management of respiratory disease. In: Kirk RW, Bonagura JD, eds. Current veterinary therapy XI. Philadelphia: Saunders, 1992:795–800.

Kuehn NF, Roudebush P. Allergic lung disease. In: Allen DG, ed. Small animal medicine. Philadelphia: Lippincott, 1991: 423–432.

Author Philip Roudebush
Consulting Editor Lynelle R. Johnson

PNEUMONIA, FUNGAL

BASICS

DEFINITION
Inflammation of the pulmonary interstitial, lymphatic, and peribronchial tissues caused by deep mycotic infection

PATHOPHYSIOLOGY
• Mycelial fungal elements—inhaled from contaminated soil; organisms then colonize the lungs • Dimorphic fungi—grow in the yeast phase at body temperature • Systemic dissemination of yeast common in dogs and cats • Clinical signs determined by organ systems affected • Pulmonary interstitial involvement—may cause hypoxia • Airway involvement—may cause cough • Cell-mediated immunity—important response to fungal infection; leads to pyogranulomatous inflammation

SYSTEMS AFFECTED
• Depend on the specific fungal disease (see also chapters dealing with specific fungi) • Blastomycosis—about 85% of dogs and cats have respiratory involvement; diffuse interstitial or bronchial pneumonia most common; solitary mass lesions seen; tracheobronchial lymphadenopathy may contribute to cough; nasal infection occasionally detected • Histoplasmosis—diffuse interstitial pneumonia common, especially in cats; tachypnea or dyspnea seen in only 50% of cats and < 50% of dogs; perihilar or mediastinal lymphadenopathy often contributes to cough. • Coccidioidomycosis—diffuse interstitial or bronchial pneumonia common in dogs but less common in cats; perihilar or mediastinal lymphadenopathy common • Cryptococcosis—nasal involvement most common in cats; lungs usually subclinically affected by small multifocal granulomas in dogs • Systemic aspergillosis—pneumonia noted only in systemically affected patients and usually involves *Aspergillus terreus; A. fumigatus* more common with rhinitis

GENETICS
Breed susceptibilities may be related to defects in cell-mediated immunity.

INCIDENCE/PREVALENCE
Depends on geographic distribution

GEOGRAPHIC DISTRIBUTION
• Blastomycosis—endemic in U.S. Southeast and Midwest along the Mississippi, Ohio, Missouri, and Tennessee rivers and southern Great Lakes; also in southern Midatlantic states • Histoplasmosis—similar to but more widely distributed than *Blastomycosis;* pockets of disease in Texas, Oklahoma, and California • Coccidioidomycosis—U.S. Southwest from Texas to California • Cryptococcosis and aspergillosis—sporadically throughout the U.S.

SIGNALMENT

Species
Dogs and less commonly in cats

Breed Predilection
• Systemic mycosis—large-breed dogs kept outdoors or used for hunting or field trials; Doberman pinschers and rottweilers may be predisposed to more severe disseminated disease. • Cryptococcosis—cocker spaniels may be overrepresented. • Systemic aspergillosis—German shepherds may be overrepresented.

Mean Age And Range
• Young animals (< 4 years) predisposed • Any age may be affected.

Predominant Sex
Males affected 2–4 times more often than females

SIGNS

General Comments
• Depend primarily on the organ systems involved • Multisystemic illness apparent

Historical Findings
• Chronic weight loss and inappetence • Fever • Oculonasal discharge • Coughing—may be prominent; seen inconsistently even with marked pulmonary disease • Dyspnea or exercise intolerance common • Labored breathing—more common in cats; sign of severe disease in both dogs and cats • Acute blindness or blepharospasm—if eyes are affected • Cutaneous nodules—uncommon until draining tracts appear • Lameness—common if the feet are affected or if osteomyelitis develops

Physical Examination Findings
• Depression and emaciation—may note in chronically affected patients • Fever—about 50% of patients • Harsh, loud breath sound—common on auscultation • Crackles—may be prominent, especially in cats • Cough—may be induced on tracheal palpation • Dyspnea—at rest with severe disease • Blastomycosis—multiple cutaneous and subcutaneous nodules with draining tracts; uveitis; granulomatous retinal detachment common • Coccidioidomycosis (dogs)—severe pain caused by osteomyelitis common • Histoplasmosis (dogs)—emaciation and diarrhea (often bloody) prominent

CAUSES
• *Blastomyces dermatitidis*—lungs primary route of infection • *Histoplasma capsulatum*—lungs and possibly gastrointestinal tract primary routes of infection

• *Coccidioides immitis*—lungs primary route of infection • *Cryptococcus neoformans*—nasal cavity primary route of infection with direct extension into the eyes or CNS • *Aspergillus* spp.—nasal cavity and lungs primary routes of infection

RISK FACTORS
• Blastomycosis, histoplasmosis, and cryptococcosis—environmental exposure to soils rich in organic matter; exposure to bird droppings or other fecal matter may predispose patient to blastomycosis and cryptococcosis • Coccidioidomycosis—environmental exposure to sandy, alkaline soil after periods of rainfall; outdoor activities (hunting and field trials); immunosuppression (especially poor cell-mediated immunity) may contribute to systemic spread of fungal infection; test cats for FeLV and FIV. • Prednisone—may markedly worsen the disease • Antineoplastic chemotherapy • Lymphoreticular neoplasia

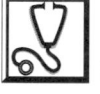

DIAGNOSIS

DIFFERENTIAL DIAGNOSIS
• Parasitic pneumonia • Bacterial pneumonia • Chronic bronchial disease • Metastatic neoplasia • Lymphoreticular and histiocytic neoplasia • Eosinophilic lung disease • Lymphomatoid granulomatosis • Idiopathic pyogranulomatous disease • FIP or other vasculitic disease • Pulmonary edema

CBC/BIOCHEMISTRY/URINALYSIS
• Depend on the systems affected • Moderate leukocytosis with or without a left shift • Lymphopenia common • Leukopenia—may note with histoplasmosis • Thrombocytopenia and nonregenerative anemia common • Hyperglobulinemia and hypoalbuminemia common • Hypercalcemia—occasionally • Liver enzymes—more likely to be high with histoplasmosis • Urinalysis usually normal • Proteinuria—may detect • Organisms—may see in urine (rarely) if the kidneys or lower urinary tract are affected

OTHER LABORATORY TESTS
• Serologic testing—yields both false-positive and false-negative results; high incidence of seropositivity may represent previous or subclinical infection in endemic areas.

• Latex agglutination test—for capsular antigen; highly reliable for cryptococcosis
• Cytologic or histologic identification of the organism—definitive diagnosis
• Culture—not usually necessary; may be difficult

IMAGING
• Thoracic radiography—diffuse nodular interstitial and peribronchial infiltrates; nodular densities may coalesce to granulomatous masses with indistinct edges; tracheobronchial lymphadenopathy common; large focal granulomas more likely in cats than in dogs
• Appendicular or axial skeleton radiography—osteolysis with periosteal proliferation; soft tissue swelling
• Abdominal ultrasonography—may reveal granulomas or large lymph nodes
• Ocular ultrasonography—may reveal a retrobulbar mass

DIAGNOSTIC PROCEDURES
• Impression smear or aspirate of a skin nodule—most likely to yield organisms
• Fine-needle aspirate of the lung—more likely to be diagnostic than transtracheal aspirate or bronchoalveolar lavage specimen
• Lymph node aspirate or biopsy
• CSF tap—with cryptococcosis
• Examination of bone marrow or splenic aspirate—with histoplasmosis
• Biopsy—may be needed

PATHOLOGIC FINDINGS
• Pyogranulomatous inflammation
• Organisms—usually seen with blastomycosis, histoplasmosis, and cryptococcosis; sometimes difficult to find coccidioidomycosis

 TREATMENT

APPROPRIATE HEALTH CARE
• Outpatient—if patient is still eating
• Inpatient evaluation and treatment—dehydration, anorexia, and severe hypoxia

NURSING CARE
Administration of fluids, potassium, oxygen, and antibiotics as needed

ACTIVITY
Restricted

DIET
• Feed high-protein, calorically dense food.
• Histoplasmosis accompanied by marked gastrointestinal involvement—highly digestible food

CLIENT EDUCATION
• Inform client that < 70% of dogs and a smaller percentage of cats are likely to respond to treatment.

• Warn client that treatment is expensive and will probably be necessary for at least 2 months
• Advise client to clean areas in the environment with high organic matter or feces

SURGICAL CONSIDERATIONS
None

 MEDICATIONS

DRUG(S) OF CHOICE
• Itraconazole—5–10 mg/kg PO daily; most often used first; must be given with food
• Amphotericin B—0.5 mg/kg (dogs) or 0.25 mg/kg (cats) IV 3 times a week to a total dose of 8 mg/kg if used alone or 4 mg/kg if used with an azole drug (e.g., itraconazole); administer in 200–500 mL of D_5W; best used with itraconazole or ketoconazole for severely affected patients
• Amphotericin B—alternative; 0.5–0.8 mg/kg 2–3 times per week; to reduce nephrotoxicity, may give subcutaneously diluted in 0.45% saline/2.5% dextrose solution (400 mL for cats, 500 mL for dogs < 20 kg, 1000 mL for dogs > 20 kg)
• Fluconazole—10 mg/kg PO q12h; drug of choice for cryptococcosis and patients with CNS or urinary tract involvement

CONTRAINDICATIONS
Corticosteroids

PRECAUTIONS
• Azole drugs—do not use with severe liver disease.
• Amphotericin B—do not use in azotemic or dehydrated patients; stop use if BUN > 50 mg/dL or creatinine > 3.0 mg/dL.
• Itraconazole and the other azole drugs—anorexia; increase in liver enzymes; cutaneous vasculitis

POSSIBLE INTERACTIONS
• Antacids and anticonvulsants—may lower the blood concentration of itraconazole

ALTERNATIVE DRUG(S)
• Ketoconazole—10–30 mg/kg; may be effective; longer treatment is necessary; relapse common
• Lipid-complexed amphotericin B—1–2 mg/kg IV q48h for 12 treatments; nephrotoxicity low; diuresis not required

 FOLLOW-UP

PATIENT MONITORING
• Liver enzymes—evaluated monthly while patient is on itraconazole, fluconazole, or ketoconazole • BUN and creatinine—measure before each dose of amphotericin B.
• Thoracic radiographs—re-evaluate before discontinuing treatment.

PREVENTION/AVOIDANCE
Monitor for signs of recurrence

POSSIBLE COMPLICATIONS
• Blindness is usually permanent.
• Renal failure from amphotericin B

EXPECTED COURSE AND PROGNOSIS
• Blastomycosis—requires a minimum of 2 months of treatment; 60%–70% of dogs are cured by itraconazole; those not cured usually relapse.
• Others—continued until 1 month past remission
• Systemic aspergillosis—prognosis not as good as for other causes
• Relapse—may occur up to 1 year after treatment

 MISCELLANEOUS

ASSOCIATED CONDITIONS
None

AGE-RELATED FACTORS
Young animals predisposed

ZOONOTIC POTENTIAL
Infections in people—primarily from a common environmental source; no direct transmission from animals to humans, except by penetrating wounds contaminated by the organism

PREGNANCY
• Fungal abortion possible
• Azole antifungals—teratogenic; do not use in pregnant animals.

SEE ALSO
• Aspergillosis • Blastomycosis
• Coccidioidomycosis • Cryptococcosis
• Histoplasmosis

ABBREVIATIONS
• CSF = cerebrospinal fluid
• FeLV = feline leukemia virus
• FIP = feline infectious peritonitis
• FIV = feline immunodeficiency virus

Suggested Reading

Greene CE, ed. Infectious diseases of the dog and cat. 2nd ed. Philadelphia: Saunders, 1998.
Taboada J. Systemic mycoses. In: Morgan RV, ed. Handbook of small animal practice. 3rd ed. Philadelphia: Saunders, 1997: 1113–1126.
Taboada J. Systemic mycoses. In: Ettinger SJ, Feldman EC, eds. Textbook of veterinary internal medicine. 5th ed. Philadelphia: Saunders, 2000:453–477.
Wolf AM. Antifungal agents. In: August JR, ed. Consultations in feline internal medicine 2. Philadelphia: Saunders, 1994.

Author Joseph Taboada
Consulting Editor Lynelle R. Johnson

PNEUMONIA, INTERSTITIAL

BASICS

DEFINITION
A form of pneumonia in which the inflammatory process occurs in alveolar walls and alveolar interstitium

PATHOPHYSIOLOGY
Results from either aerogenous injury to the alveolar epithelium (type I or II pneumocytes) or hematogenous injury to the alveolar capillaries. Alveolar wall damage often occurs secondary to inflammation and antigen-antibody complex deposition. Progression from acute to chronic interstitial pneumonia may occur, leading to alveolar fibrosis +/− interstitial mononuclear cell accumulation and persistent type II pneumocyte hyperplasia.

SYSTEMS AFFECTED
• Respiratory • Cardiovascular (cor pulmonale may develop)

GEOGRAPHIC DISTRIBUTION
Angiostrongylus vasorum is found in Europe, Asia, and Africa (rare in United States)

SIGNALMENT
• Canine distemper virus is most common in dogs 3–6 months of age. Greyhounds, Siberian huskies, Weimaraners, Samoyeds, and Alaskan malamutes are over-represented and severely affected. • Endogenous lipid pneumonia (EnLP) most commonly affects older cats of either sex. • Feline immunodeficiency virus (FIV) is most frequently seen in middle-aged to older male cats. • Pulmonary interstitial fibrosis is most commonly recognized in the middle- to old-age West Highland white terrier +/− white Cairn terriers. A Staffordshire bull terrier has also been reported. An acute fibrosing alveolitis has been reported in one West Highland white terrier and one Scottish terrier. One 7 year-old, domestic shorthaired cat with the desquamative interstitial pneumonitis (DIP) form of interstitial fibrosis has been reported. • *Pneumocystis carinii*—Miniature dachshunds < 1 year of age at risk. Also described in two Cavalier King Charles spaniels and a sheltie. • Toxoplasmosis most commonly affects middle-aged male cats.

SIGNS
Dependent on severity of disease • Tachypnea, coughing, dyspnea, orthopnea, cyanosis, open-mouth breathing, exercise intolerance, abnormal breath sounds on auscultation (commonly end-inspiratory and early expiratory crackles), +/− hemoptysis • Mild fever and oculonasal discharge are often present with canine adenovirus-2 infection. • Gastrointestinal signs, fever, oculonasal discharge, hyperkeratosis of the footpads, and neurologic deficits or myoclonus may be seen with canine distemper virus infection. • Fever, anorexia, upper respiratory tract inflammation or infection, lymphadenopathy, weight loss, stomatitis, and/or neurologic abnormalities may be seen in cats with FIV. • Animals with paraquat toxicity

often display vomiting, oliguria, diarrhea, and oropharyngeal ulcers (+/− hyperexcitability and neurologic signs in the early phase).
• Retinitis, uveitis, neurologic signs, and/or gastrointestinal signs with toxoplasmosis.

CAUSES AND RISK FACTORS

Congenital
Bronchiolitis obliterans–organizing pneumonia (BOOP) has been described secondary to primary ciliary dyskinesia in one dog; bronchial dysgenesis may lead to EnLP in the cat.

Metabolic
Uremic pneumonopathy, BOOP may occur in conjunction with uremic pneumonopathy, hepatic disease, or pancreatitis in cats.

Neoplastic
Neoplasia may lead to bronchiectasis or BOOP.

Idiopathic
Pulmonary interstitial fibrosis and DIP, some cases of EnLP, BOOP, primary pulmonary alveolar proteinosis (PAP)

Inflammatory
EnLP is most commonly seen in cats with bronchitis and bronchiectasis or necrotizing bronchiolitis; pulmonary interstitial fibrosis most likely occurs secondary to immune stimulation and/or immune complex deposition.

Infectious
• Dogs—canine distemper virus, canine adenovirus-2, *Pneumocystis carinii*, *Angiostrongylus vasorum*, *Toxoplasma*. BOOP is often secondary to pulmonary infections in humans and has been produced experimentally by infecting dogs with adenovirus or *Mycoplasma*.
• Cats—toxoplasmosis, FIV

Toxic
Inhalation of dusts, gases, or vapors, thiacetarsemide. BOOP is often secondary to inhaled toxins in humans, exogenous lipid pneumonia has been reported following the administration and aspiration of petroleum-based products to cats, secondary PAP, paraquat toxicity (respiratory embarrassment typically occurs 3 days post-exposure).

Vascular
Disseminated intravascular coagulation, microembolism, circulating larval migrans, pulmonary arterial thrombosis may precipitate EnLP in cats.

DIAGNOSIS

DIFFERENTIAL DIAGNOSIS
• Airway disease • Bronchopneumonia • Heartworm disease • Embolic pneumonia • Granulomatous pneumonia • Neoplasia • Cardiac disease

CBC/BIOCHEMISTRY/URINALYSIS
• May see neutrophilia, eosinophilia, lymphocytosis, hyperglobulinemia; polycythemia may be present if the animal is hypoxemic.
• Immune-mediated thrombocytopenia has been reported with *Angiostrongylus vasorum*.

• Neutropenia or high liver enzymes and bilirubin possible with *Toxoplasma* • High liver enzymes and bilirubin (dogs only) possible with hepatotoxicity due to thiacetarsemide therapy and occasionally with paraquat toxicity. • Severe azotemia and isosthenuria with uremic pneumonopathy; renal failure may occur secondary to paraquat toxicity.

OTHER LABORATORY TESTS
• Arterial blood gas measurement and calculation of alveolar-arterial (A–a) gradient to assess degree of respiratory impairment; $PaO_2 < 80$ mmHg indicates mild-moderate hypoxemia, $PaO_2 < 60$ mmHg indicates severe hypoxemia, A–a gradient > 15 indicates venous admixture.
• Serologic and other tests for infectious causes.
• Fecal examination for *Toxoplasma* and *Angiostrongylus vasorum* (preferably a Baermann technique) • Toxicologic analysis of the urine or serum to diagnose paraquat toxicity in live animals.

IMAGING

Thoracic Radiographic Findings
• A focal or diffuse, mild to severe interstitial to bronchial to alveolar pattern might be present (+/− hyperinflation or incomplete thoracic expansion). Dilated bronchi may be seen with bronchiectasis or BOOP. • Right heart enlargement and hepatosplenomegaly may be present secondary to pulmonary hypertension (+/− retraction of peripheral lung edges and/or flattening of the diaphragm). • Pleural effusion is occasionally seen in many of the interstitial pneumonias.

Computed Tomography or Magnetic Resonance Imaging
Variable findings that are not well described in the veterinary literature are possible. CT or MRI may help guide surgeon in obtaining a diagnostic biopsy. Dilated bronchi are common with bronchiectasis and BOOP.

OTHER DIAGNOSTIC PROCEDURES
• Electrocardiography—arrhythmias may occur with severe hypoxia or systemic disease. Enlarged S waves in lead II suggestive of right ventricular hypertrophy if pulmonary hypertension present • Pulmonary function tests.
• Open lung biopsy is the most definitive diagnostic test. • Endotracheal or transtracheal wash, bronchoscopy with bronchoalveolar lavage, and/or fine needle aspirate of lungs might be useful (e.g., may visualize trophozoite or cysts of *Pneumocystis carinii* or *Toxoplasma* or see L1 larvae with *Angiostrongylus vasorum*); cultures frequently reveal the presence of secondary bacterial infections. With pulmonary alveolar proteinosis, an opaque white material is retrieved following washing of the airways and cytology shows a dense granular substance with abundant lipid and stains PAS-positive. • Echocardiogram may reveal evidence of pulmonary hypertension.
• An elevation in pulmonary artery pressure might be present if measured using a pulmonary artery catheter.

PATHOLOGIC FINDINGS

• *Angiostrongylus vasorum*—thrombosing arteritis and fibrotic peribronchitis may be seen, in addition to parasites present within the arterioles of the lung parenchyma. • See specific chapters for other infectious causes. • BOOP—Polypoid plugs of loose, fibrous tissue fill the bronchioles and alveoli, foamy macrophages are often present within the alveoli, and variable inflammatory infiltrate with type II pneumocyte reactivity and hyperplasia of the small airway smooth muscle is common. Interstitial fibrosis may be present. • Idiopathic pulmonary fibrosis—lungs may grossly appear as a "honeycomb lung" in advanced stages. Alveolar septal fibrosis and alveolar epithelialization with type II pneumocyte hyperplasia +/− septal and intra-alveolar hemosiderophages and islands of squamous metaplasia. • Lipid pneumonias—macroscopic lesions may include subpleural, parenchymal, or perivascular white, firm nodules. Accumulation of lipid-laden macrophages in the alveoli is seen histologically. A mixed pattern of inflammation is common, as well as cholesterol clefts and multinucleated giant cells. • Paraquat toxicity—the lungs are heavy, edematous, and hemorrhagic. Emphysematous bullae and pneumomediastinum commonly present. Histologic changes following ingestion or inhalation include necrosis of type I pneumocytes, edema, hemorrhage, and type II pneumocyte proliferation. If the animal survives, the lungs become pale and develop severe interstitial and intra-alveolar fibrosis. Evidence of hepatic, renal, cardiac, and adrenal gland injury is commonly present as well. • PAP—Alveolar spaces are distended with a PAS staining eosinophilic proteinaceous material. Intra-alveolar cholesterol clefts and mucus-laden macrophages with mild mixed-inflammatory infiltrates are common. • Uremic pneumonopathy—pulmonary edema and calcification of smooth muscle and/or alveolar walls are seen in this condition.

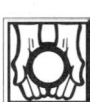

TREATMENT

• Inpatient care and monitoring for animals with evidence of respiratory distress. Oxygen therapy via cage, intranasal, mask, or flow-by.
• Exercise restriction for animals with increased respiratory effort
• Minimize exposure to house dust, vapors, chemical fumes, or tobacco smoke.
• Weight loss is indicated if obese.
• Humidification of the inspired air with a nebulizer or vaporizer may help to liquefy secretions.
• Use a harness rather than a restraint collar.

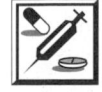

MEDICATIONS

DRUG(S)

• Inhaled corticosteroids (e.g., fluticasone q12h) or bronchodilators (e.g., terbutaline q12h) using an Optichamber spacer and appropriate size mask might be beneficial in animals that require these therapies (see below).
• Antitussives may be helpful in noninfectious diseases: butorphanol tartrate (0.5 mg/kg PO q 6–12h, 0.05–0.1 mg/kg if given SC, IM, or IV); codeine phosphate (0.5–2.0 mg/kg PO q12h in dogs and 0.25–4.0 mg/kg PO q12h in cats [caution is recommended in this species]), or dextromethorphan (0.05–0.1 mg/kg up to 5 mg q6–12h).
• Bronchodilators might be helpful: sustained release theophylline (20 mg/kg PO q12h in the dog or q24h in the cat) clenbuterol hydrochloride (1–5 μg/kg PO q12h in dogs and 1 μg/kg PO q12h in cats), terbutaline sulfate (0.01 mg/kg SC, IM, or IV q8–12h, dog or cat), 0.03 mg/kg PO q8–12h in the dog or 0.312–0.625 mg total dose PO q8–12h in the cat
• *Angiostrongylus vasorum*—levamisole, 7.5 mg/kg PO q24h for two days followed by 10 mg/kg PO q24h for two days +/− aspirin or corticosteroids concurrently. Alternative therapies include fenbendazole, mebendazole, and ivermectin.
• BOOP—corticosteroids have been used with clinical success in one case report (prednisone, 2.2 mg/kg PO q24h).
• Idiopathic pulmonary fibrosis—Antiinflammatory steroid therapy with prednisolone (0.5–1.0 mg/kg PO q24–48h, most helpful in animals with a predominant lymphocytic inflammation) and bronchodilators +/− antitussives or antibiotics if indicated.
• Paraquat toxicity–vomition and activated charcoal therapy is indicated if recent ingestion is known. Supportive care, diuresis using furosemide (most effective in the first 3 days following ingestion to enhance excretion), oxygen therapy as needed, +/− immunosuppressive dexamethasone, cyclophosphamide, nicotinamide, superoxide dismutase, and vitamin Λ.
• PAP—therapeutic bronchoalveolar lavage
• Antimicrobial therapy should be used as indicated by results of culture and sensitivities.

PRECAUTIONS

Immunosuppressive therapy can exacerbate secondary infections.

FOLLOW-UP

PATIENT MONITORING

• Have owners observe clinical response to therapy. • Repeat physical examination/chest auscultation, chest radiographs, lab test, and arterial blood gas analysis as indicated.

PREVENTION/AVOIDANCE

• Avoid proximity to toxic fumes or paraquat (not legally sold in the US). • Vaccinate and deworm animals as recommended.

POSSIBLE COMPLICATIONS

Secondary pulmonary infections are common with most forms of interstitial pneumonia.

EXPECTED COURSE AND PROGNOSIS

• Guarded with *Pneumocystis carinii*, Toxo-plasma, *Angiostrongylus vasorum*, canine adenovirus-2, canine distemper virus, and EnLP
• Poor long-term prognosis with idiopathic pulmonary fibrosis (mean survival time from the beginning of clinical signs ≅ 17 months) • Poor prognosis with clinical FIV and uremic pneumonopathy • Paraquat toxicity is commonly fatal in dogs, although there is up to a 75% recovery rate in man.

MISCELLANEOUS

ASSOCIATED CONDITIONS

• Canine adenovirus-2 is sometimes associated with infectious tracheobronchitis and may coexist with canine distemper virus infection.
• Secondary infectious pneumonias are common sequelae to interstitial pneumonia.

AGE-RELATED FACTORS

Young, free-roaming animals are more likely to succumb to infectious diseases.

ZOONOTIC POTENTIAL

Toxoplasmosis, if animal is shedding oocysts

PREGNANCY

Transplacental infection with *Toxoplasma* and canine distemper virus is possible.

SEE ALSO

• Bronchiectasis • Canine Distemper • Feline Immunodeficiency Virus Infection (FIV)
• Infectious Canine Tracheobronchitis (Kennel Cough) • Pneumocystosis • Toxoplasmosis

ABBREVIATIONS

• BOOP = bronchiolitis obliterans with organizing pneumonia • DIP = desquamative interstitial pneumonitis • EnLP = endogenous lipid pneumonia • PAP = pulmonary alveolar proteinosis • PAS = periodic acid–Schiff

Suggested Reading

Corcoran BM, Cobb M, Martin WS, et al. Chronic pulmonary disease in West Highland white terriers. Vet Rec 1999; 144:611–616.

Jones DJ, Norris CR, Samii VF, Griffey SM. Endogenous lipid pneumonia in cats: 24 cases (1985–1998). J Am Vet Med Assoc 2000;216:1437–1440.

Phillips S, Barr S, Dykes N, et al. Bronchiolitis obliterans with organizing pneumonia in a dog. J Vet Intern Med 2000;14:204–207.

Silverstein D, Greene C, Gregory C, et al. Pulmonary alveolar proteinosis in a dog. J Vet Intern Med 2000;14(5):546–551.

Author Deborah C. Silverstein
Consulting Editor Lynelle R. Johnson

PNEUMOTHORAX

 BASICS

DEFINITION

• Air accumulation in the pleural space; it is categorized as traumatic or spontaneous. Spontaneous—a closed pneumothorax occurring in the absence of trauma; spontaneous pneumothorax is primary if it occurs in the absence of underlying pulmonary pathology, but secondary if associated pulmonary disease is evident.
• Closed pneumothorax—no defects in the thoracic wall • Open pneumothorax—defect in the thoracic wall such that the pleural space communicates with the atmosphere
• Tension pneumothorax—pleural pressure in a closed pneumothorax exceeds atmospheric pressure, causing further restriction of lung expansion; typically due to a pleural or pulmonary flap-like defect that allows leakage of air into the pleural space, then closes because of increased pleural pressure

PATHOPHYSIOLOGY

• The pleural space is normally a potential space between the visceral and parietal pleura. It contains a thin layer of fluid that contributes to the "tethering" of the lungs to the thoracic wall. Pleural pressure is normally sub-atmospheric. Air accumulation in the pleural space breaks the surface tension seal of the pleural fluid, and the lungs can collapse away from the thoracic wall. • Closed pneumothorax—air leakage is from the pulmonary parenchyma or a large airway. On inspiration, pleural pressure drops, pulling more air into the pleural space, which is then trapped there. This leads to progressive compression of the lung by the pleural space. The pleural pressure rises in proportion to the amount of air accumulated in the pleural space. When the pleural pressure is higher than atmospheric pressure, it is called a tension pneumothorax and can lead to total collapse of the lung. • Open pneumothorax—may or may not have associated pulmonary pathology; the pleural pressure equals atmospheric pressure, leading to lung collapse. • Hypoxemia develops secondary to pulmonary parenchymal collapse. Tidal volume is reduced and leads to hypoventilation with hypercapnia. • High intrathoracic pressures can reduce venous return to the heart, further compromising the cardiovascular system. • Cats and dogs with pneumothorax usually have bilateral disease; if the mediastinum is intact, it can present as a unilateral problem.

SYSTEMS AFFECTED

• Respiratory • Cardiovascular

GENETICS

N/A

INCIDENCE/PREVALENCE

Traumatic pneumothorax occurs in >40% of cases with chest trauma and in 11–18% of dogs and cats presented for vehicular trauma.

GEOGRAPHIC DISTRIBUTION

N/A

SIGNALMENT

Species

Dogs and cats

Breed Predilection

Spontaneous pneumothorax—more common in large, deep-chested dogs

Median Age and Range

N/A

Predominant Sex

N/A

SIGNS

Historical Findings

• Traumatic—recent trauma. Recent anesthesia and intubation raises possibility of tracheal trauma. Recent thoracocentesis performed or recent jugular venipuncture—possible iatrogenic cause
• Spontaneous—may have previous history of pulmonary disease; usually acute, but can have a slowly progressive onset

Physical Examination Findings

• Tachypnea • Dyspnea • Orthopnea
• Shallow, rapid abdominal breathing common • Tachycardia • Reduced lung sounds dorsally—can be difficult to appreciate in very dyspneic animals.
Traumatic Pneumothorax
Additional signs include the following:
• Other signs of trauma, including shock
• May or may not have evidence of thoracic trauma • Open pneumothorax—obvious thoracic wall trauma present • Pale mucous membranes; overt cyanosis in severe cases
• Subcutaneous emphysema in some cases with pneumomediastinum and/or tracheal trauma

CAUSES

• Blunt trauma • Penetrating thoracic injuries
• Penetrating cervical injuries • Post-thoracocentesis • Post-thoracotomy
• Esophageal perforation • Endotracheal tube–associated tracheal trauma • Migrating pulmonary foreign body • Pulmonary neoplasia • Pulmonary abscess • Pneumonia
• Mycotic pulmonary granuloma • Parasitic pulmonary disease (*Paragonimus*)
• Congenital pulmonary cyst • Pulmonary bullae • Pulmonary blebs • Diffuse emphysema

RISK FACTORS

• Trauma • Thoracocentesis • Thoracotomy
• Overinflation of endotracheal cuff
• Migrating plant awns • Pulmonary pathology

 DIAGNOSIS

DIFFERENTIAL DIAGNOSIS

• Pleural effusion • Diaphragmatic hernia
• Pulmonary contusions

CBC/BIOCHEMISTRY/URINALYSIS

Neutrophilia with a left shift if pulmonary infection or inflammatory disease

OTHER LABORATORY TESTS

Arterial blood gases—hypoxemia, hypocapnia, or hypercapnia may occur.

IMAGING

Thoracic Radiography

• Delay until patient is stable; may not be able to get more than one view if patient becomes distressed • Air in pleural space visible, pulmonary vascular pattern does not extend to the chest wall—horizontal beam radiograph with animal in lateral recumbency is the most sensitive view. • Often pneumomediastinum • Pulmonary pathology may be obscured by lung lobe collapse; may need to repeat radiographs following thoracocentesis • Traumatic pneumothorax—evaluate for other traumatic injury such as contusions, rib fractures, diaphragmatic hernia, hemothorax, foreign bodies (bullets, arrowhead). • Spontaneous pneumothorax—evaluate for any sign of parenchymal pathology.

Thoracic Computed Tomography

Investigation of spontaneous pneumothorax if unable to define pulmonary pathology on plain radiographs

DIAGNOSTIC PROCEDURES

• Thoracocentesis—confirms diagnosis; remove maximal amount of air from pleural space. • Bronchoscopy—if evidence of tracheal or large airway trauma

PATHOLOGIC FINDINGS

• Will vary depending on underlying disease
• Gross evaluation—may be able to visualize pulmonary blebs, pulmonary or airway tears, pulmonary parenchymal disease or pulmonary masses • Histopathology—blebs are most commonly found at the apex and are contained entirely within the pleura; bullae are lined by pleura, fibrous pulmonary tissue, and emphysematous lung.

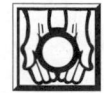 **TREATMENT**

APPROPRIATE HEALTH CARE

• Inpatient care until air accumulation has stopped or has stabilized at a level that is not life-threatening
• All dyspneic animals should have thoracocentesis and a maximal amount of air removed. ALWAYS provide oxygen therapy

until patient's ability to oxygenate is established.
• Analgesia with an opioid-type drug if significant injuries following trauma—use low end of the dose range of a μ-agonist. It gives the best analgesia and can be reversed if required.
• Thoracocentesis can be performed with an intravenous catheter attached to an extension set and stopcock or via a butterfly needle. No need to perform thoracocentesis on non-dyspneic animals. If large open chest wound—cover as cleanly as possible; will require surgical closure once animal is stable
• Tube thoracostomy—used if unable to stabilize with thoracocentesis or if have to do repeat thoracocentesis for continued pneumothorax; chest tube placement (under local or general anesthesia)—skin entrance site aseptically prepared in dorsal caudal quadrant of lateral thorax; skin incision similar in size to the tube is made over rib space 11–12 or 12–13; skin is then pulled cranially by an assistant so that the incision now lies over rib spaces 7–8 or 8–9. Chest tube is then placed, aiming cranioventrally; skin can be released and a subcutaneous tunnel is formed; thoracic radiographs should be performed after chest tube placement.
• If pneumothorax is rapidly accumulating—continuous chest tube suction via one-, two- or three-bottle drainage system with an underwater seal. If pneumothorax is not severe or is resolving—intermittent tube aspiration via a stopcock
• Heimlich valves—unidirectional valves used to prevent introduction of air into chest tubes. These are very easily occluded with small amounts of fluid secretions. Not recommended for any length of time or in very small patients.
• In emergency situation of life-threatening tension pneumothorax—consider emergency thoracotomy to convert problem to an open pneumothorax; animal can then be intubated and positive pressure–ventilated until stabilized
• Open traumatic pneumothorax—surgery as soon as patient is stable
• Closed traumatic pneumothorax—rarely requires surgical intervention
• Spontaneous pneumothorax—exploratory thoracotomy often performed via median sternotomy if location of lesion is unknown

NURSING CARE
• Oxygen therapy via cage, nasal cannula, E-collar covered in plastic wrap, mask, or flow-by. Humidify oxygen source if giving oxygen therapy for more than a few hours.
• Intravenous fluids required in most cases of trauma, but may not be indicated in cases of spontaneous pneumothorax
• Chest tube maintenance—ensure all connections are air-tight (cable ties are

excellent for securing connections); ensure that tube is attached to animal at two points to reduce chance of inadvertent tube removal. Clean tube site and change dressing once daily. Do not allow animal to chew at chest tube.

ACTIVITY
Strict rest for at least a week following resolution of pneumothorax in an effort to minimize the chance of recurrence

DIET
N/A

CLIENT EDUCATION
• Traumatic pneumothorax—discuss possibility of a chest tube and several days' hospitalization; some animals may require surgery.
• Spontaneous pneumothorax—discuss possibility of underlying pulmonary disease that may make resolution challenging and recurrence possible. Warn owner that even with thoracotomy, the source of the pneumothorax may not be found.

SURGICAL CONSIDERATIONS
• Do not use positive-pressure ventilation for closed pneumothorax. Place chest tube prior to ventilation or await thoracotomy prior to ventilation.
• Thoracoscopy—may allow visualization of local lesion; allows instillation of substances for pleurodesis.
• Thoracotomy—if lesion is not evident, can fill thorax with saline and look for bubbles as sign of a leak. Partial or full lung lobectomy for localized lesions. Traumatic lacerations may be sutured. In some cases the location of the leak may not be evident at surgery.
• Pleurodesis with mechanical abrasion of the pleura or instillation of an inflammatory substance, such as talc, into the pleural space

 MEDICATIONS

DRUG(S) N/A

CONTRAINDICATIONS N/A

PRECAUTIONS N/A

POSSIBLE INTERACTIONS N/A

 FOLLOW-UP

PATIENT MONITORING
• Respiratory rate—increased rate suggests reoccurrence of pneumothorax. • Serial thoracic radiographs in an attempt to quantitate accumulation of air • Pulse oximetry if breathing room air can help determine oxygenation status • Arterial blood gases give the best evaluation of oxygenation status.

• Central venous (jugular) blood gases can be used to evaluate ventilation status via P_{VCO_2}.
• Rate of air production from chest tube, on continuous drainage with a 3-bottle suction system—need to count bubbles; if intermittent aspiration, can quantitate with syringe

PREVENTION/AVOIDANCE
Keep pets confined—less likely to be injured.

POSSIBLE COMPLICATIONS
• Death from hypoxemia and cardiovascular compromise • Re-expansion pulmonary edema following thoracocentesis • Incorrect placement of chest tube—lung lobe laceration, cardiac puncture, diaphragmatic laceration, liver trauma • Pleural infection from thoracocentesis or chest drain

EXPECTED COURSE AND PROGNOSIS
• Traumatic pneumothorax—if thoracic trauma is not severe, the prognosis is good with thoracocentesis +/– chest drain placement. With severe thoracic trauma, patient can deteriorate despite all efforts to stabilize it. • Spontaneous pneumothorax—prognosis depends on underlying cause. If there is a single, focal lesion that can be surgically resected, the prognosis is good. If unable to locate lesion or diffuse pulmonary disease is present—prognosis is poor; without surgery, majority will recur; with surgery, the recurrence rate is decreased and the time interval before recurrence is increased.

 MISCELLANEOUS

ASSOCIATED CONDITIONS N/A

AGE-RELATED FACTORS N/A

ZOONOTIC POTENTIAL N/A

PREGNANCY N/A

SYNONYMS
Punctured lung

SEE ALSO
Dyspnea, Tachypnea, and Panting

Suggested Reading
Holstinger RH, Ellison GW. Spontaneous pneumothorax. Compend Contin Educ Pract Vet 1995;17:197–210.
Krahwinkel DJ, Barton W. et al. Factors associated with survival in dogs and cats with pneumothorax. J Vet Emerg Crit Care 1999;9(1):7–12.
Orron EC: Pleura and pleural space. In: Slatter DH ed. Textbook of Small Animal Surgery. Philadelphia: Saunders, 1985;547–565.
Sahn SA, Heffner JE. Spontaneous pneumothorax. N Engl J Med 2000;342(12):868–874.
Author Kate Hopper
Consulting Editor Lynelle R. Johnson

PODODERMATITIS

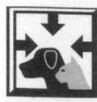 BASICS

DEFINITION

An inflammatory, multifaceted complex of diseases that involves the feet of dogs and, less commonly, cats

PATHOPHYSIOLOGY

• Depends on the underlying cause
• Causes include infectious, allergic, auto-immune, endocrine/metabolic, neoplastic, and environmental diseases
• Psychogenic dermatoses rarely involved

SYSTEMS AFFECTED

Skin/Exocrine—primary or secondary infection (bacterial, fungal, or parasitic); neoplasia; target organ for underlying autoimmune, endocrine, or other systemic disease; paronychia (ungual folds, claw folds)

GENETICS

N/A

INCIDENCE/PREVALENCE

• Dogs—common
• Cats—uncommon

SIGNALMENT

Species

Dogs and cats

Breed Predilections

• Short-coated breeds (dogs)—most commonly affected; English bulldogs, great Danes, basset hounds, mastiffs, bull terriers, boxers, dachshunds, Dalmatians, German short-haired pointers, and weimaraners
• Long-coated breeds (dogs)—German shepherds, Labrador retrievers, golden retrievers, Irish setters, and Pekingese
• Cats—none

Mean Age and Range

Any age

Predominant Sex

• Dogs—male • Cats—none

SIGNS

General Comments

The history and physical findings vary considerably depending on the underlying cause.

Historical Findings

• History—extremely important; determine environment and general husbandry (e.g., indoor vs. outdoor, working dog vs. pet, unsanitary conditions, other pets affected, trauma, contact irritants, hookworms)
• Seasonality—suggests atopic dermatitis, allergic contact dermatitis, or irritant contact dermatitis
• Lesions elsewhere on the body—may aid in diagnosis of cause
• Response to previous therapy—antibiotics, antifungals, and corticosteroids
• Diet, travel history, and other medical problems—important in investigation

Physical Examination Findings

Infectious (Dogs)
• Tissues—may be erythematous and edematous, nodules, inflammatory plaques (fungal "kerions"), ulcers, fistulae, hemorrhagic bullae, or serosanguineous or seropurulent discharge • Feet—may be grossly swollen, may have pitting edema of the metacarpal and metatarsal areas
• Skin—may be alopecic and moist owing to constant licking; patient may have some degree of pain, pruritus, and paronychia
• Regional lymph nodes may be enlarged.

Infectious (Cats)
• Painful paronychia, involving one or more claws • Higher incidence of nodular, often ulcerated lesions, compared to dog
• Footpads and periungual areas—commonly involved
• Interdigital spaces—seldom affected
• Scaly and crusted lesions—occasionally seen

Allergic (Dogs)
• Feet—erythematous and alopecic, secondary to pruritus; dorsal surface usually more severely affected
• Salivary staining may be evident.
• Allergic contact dermatitis—uncommon cause; dermatitis of the ventral interdigital surfaces is usually worse, although the whole paw may be involved.

Allergic (Cats)
Single or multiple, exudative or ulcerated, eosinophilic, pruritic plaques of the digits, periungual, and interdigital spaces

Immune-mediated (Dogs)
• Crusts and ulcerations—most common lesions; occasionally vesicles or bullae are seen
• All four feet may be affected, especially the nailbeds and footpads. • Hyperkeratotic and erosive dermatitis of the footpads—common finding in pemphigus foliaceus

Immune-mediated (Cats)
• Lesions—generally involve the footpad, including hyperkeratosis and ulceration
• Lameness and paronychia—may occur

Endocrine/Metabolic (Dogs)
• Lesions—usually consistent with secondary infectious pododermatitis
• Hepatocutaneous syndrome—rare condition; signs of skin disease precede the onset of signs of internal disease; lesions include hyperkeratosis and ulceration of the footpads.

Endocrine/Metabolic (Cats)
Whitish nodules resembling candle wax; may be caused by cutaneous xanthomatosis; seen with diabetes mellitus

Neoplastic
• Dogs—lesions usually nodules, possible ulceration or pruritus; usually only one foot is involved; multiple foot involvement with nailbed squamous cell carcinoma reported
• Cats—tumors appear as nodules; variably ulcerated and painful; localized destruction variable, depends on the tumor type

Environmental (Dogs and Cats)
• Depends on underlying cause
• Lesions—involve one digit or foot (foreign body, trauma) or multiple digits (irritant contact dermatitis, thallium toxicity, housed on rough surface or in moist environment)
• Chronic interdigital inflammation, ulceration, pyogranulomatous abscesses, draining tracts, or swelling, with or without pruritus

Miscellaneous
• Hyperkeratosis of the footpads (dogs)—associated with several diseases (e.g., zinc-responsive dermatosis, generic dog food dermatosis, and idiopathic digital hyperkeratosis)
• Nodules without draining tracts (dogs)—associated with sterile pyogranulomas in several breeds and nodular dermatofibrosis of the German shepherds and golden retrievers
• Hypomelanosis of the footpads (cats)—associated with vitiligo • Hypermelanosis of the footpads (cats)—associated with lentigo simplex • Polydactylism and syndactylism (cats)—common in certain families

CAUSES

Infectious (Dogs)

• Bacterial—*Staphylococcus intermedius, Pseudomonas* spp., *Proteus* spp., *Mycobacterium* spp., *Nocardia* spp., or *Actinomyces* spp.
• Fungal—dermatophytes, intermediate mycoses (sporotrichosis, mycetoma), or deep mycoses (blastomycosis, cryptococcosis)
• Parasitic—*Demodex canis, Pelodera strongyloides,* and hookworms
• Protozoal—leishmaniasis

Infectious (Cats)

• Bacterial—same as dog, plus *Pasteurella* spp.
• Fungal—same as dog, excluding blastomycosis • Parasitic—*Neotrombicula autumnalis, Notoedres cati,* or *Demodex* spp.
• Protozoal—*Anatrichosoma cutaneum*

Allergic

• Dogs—atopy; food hypersensitivity; allergic contact dermatitis
• Cats—atopy; rare for flea allergy dermatitis, adverse food reaction (food hypersensitivity), or contact dermatitis to involve paws

Immune-mediated

• Dogs—pemphigus foliaceus; systemic lupus erythematosus; erythema multiforme; toxic epidermal necrolysis; vasculitis; cold agglutinin disease; pemphigus vulgaris; bullous pemphigoid; epidermolysis bullosa acquisita
• Cats—pemphigus foliaceus; systemic lupus erythematosus; erythema multiforme; toxic epidermal necrolysis; vasculitis; cold agglutinin disease; plasma cell pododermatitis

Endocrine/Metabolic

• Dogs—hypothyroidism; hyperadrenocorticism; hepatocutaneous syndrome (necrolytic migratory erythema)

- Cats—hypothyroidism; hyperadrenocorticism; cutaneous xanthomatosis (secondary to diabetes mellitus); endocrine pododermatitis rare

Neoplastic
- Higher incidence in cats than in dogs
- Dogs—squamous cell carcinomas; melanomas; mast cell tumors; keratoacanthomas; inverted papillomas; eccrine adenocarcinomas
- Cats—papillomas; spinocellular epithelioma; trichoepithelioma; fibrosarcoma; malignant fibrous histiocytoma; metastatic primary adenocarcinoma of the lung; other metastatic carcinomas

Environmental
- Dogs—irritant contact dermatitis; trauma; concrete and gravel dog runs; excessive exercise; clipper burn; foreign bodies (grass awns, bristle-like hairs of short-coated dogs); thallium toxicity
- Cats—irritant contact dermatitis; foreign bodies; thallium toxicity

Miscellaneous
- Dogs—sterile interdigital granulomas; see Physical Examination Findings
- Cats—see Physical Examination Findings

RISK FACTORS
- Lifestyle and general husbandry conditions—influence development
- Excess exercise, abrasive or moist housing, poor grooming, and/or lack of preventive medical practice may predispose an animal or exacerbate condition

DIAGNOSIS

DIFFERENTIAL DIAGNOSIS
See Signs and Causes

CBC/BIOCHEMISTRY/URINALYSIS
- Depend on the underlying cause
- Rarely used in the initial workup

OTHER LABORATORY TESTS
Endocrine tests, serology, or immune studies—rarely used in the initial workup; indications depend on results of initial workup.

IMAGING
- Radiographs and ultrasound—rarely used in the initial workup
- Neoplastic—depending on the underlying cause, may be necessary to confirm system disease or stage tumors

DIAGNOSTIC PROCEDURES
- Skin scrapings, fungal culture, and a stained smear of any exudate or pustule contents
- Biopsy—histopathology, bacterial and fungal culture, and potentially for immunopathology
- Food elimination diet • Intradermal skin testing • Endocrine tests

- Dogs—biopsies indicated if skin scrapings are negative and lesions (nodules, draining tracts) are seen
- Cats—biopsies may be indicated in all cases, because pedal dermatosis is relatively rare.

PATHOLOGIC FINDINGS
Vary depending on the underlying cause

TREATMENT

APPROPRIATE HEALTH CARE
Outpaient, unless surgery is indicated

NURSING CARE
Foot soaks, hot packing, and/or bandaging may be necessary, depending on cause.

ACTIVITY
Depends on severity of the lesions and the underlying cause

DIET
Hypoallergenic diet—determine food hypersensitivity

CLIENT EDUCATION
- Depends on underlying cause and severity of condition • Discuss husbandry, lifestyle, and preventive medical practices.
- For allergic, immune-mediated, or endocrine causes, client must understand that condition will be managed, not cured

SURGICAL CONSIDERATIONS
- Melanomas and squamous cell carcinomas—very poor prognosis; early diagnosis necessitates removal of the digit, digits, or paw
- Infectious—may benefit from surgical débridement of devitalized tissue before medical therapy

MEDICATIONS

DRUG(S) OF CHOICE
- Long-term antibiotics, antifungals, anti-inflammatory, or immunosuppressive levels of corticosteroids, chemotherapeutic agents, hormone-replacement therapy, or zinc supplementation
- Depend on the underlying cause and secondary infections

CONTRAINDICATIONS
N/A

PRECAUTIONS
Depend on the treatment protocol selected for the underlying cause; see specific drugs and their precautions

POSSIBLE INTERACTIONS
Depend on the underlying cause and treatment protocol selected

ALTERNATIVE DRUG(S)
N/A

FOLLOW-UP

PATIENT MONITORING
Depends on the underlying cause and treatment protocol selected

PREVENTION/AVOIDANCE
- Environmental cause—good husbandry and preventive medical practices should avoid recurrence.
- Allergic cause—important to avoid the allergen (inhalant or food), if possible

POSSIBLE COMPLICATIONS
Depend on the underlying cause and treatment protocol selected

EXPECTED COURSE AND PROGNOSIS
- Success of therapy depends on finding the underlying cause; often the cause is unknown; even when the cause is known, management can be frustrating owing to relapses or lack of affordable therapeutics.
- Often the disease can only be managed and not cured.
- Surgical intervention is sometimes the only option.

MISCELLANEOUS

ASSOCIATED CONDITIONS
N/A

AGE-RELATED FACTORS
Depend on the underlying cause

ZOONOTIC POTENTIAL
Not usually; depends on the underlying cause

PREGNANCY
Avoid systemically administered corticosteroids, antifungals, chemotherapeutic agents, azathioprine, and certain antimicrobials (e.g., enrofloxacin) in pregnant animals.

SYNONYMS
N/A

SEE ALSO
See Causes

Suggested Reading
Foil CS. Disorders of the feet and claws. Paper presented at the 11th Kal Kan Symposium.
Guaguere E, Hubert B, Delabre C. Feline pyodermatoses. Vet Dermatol 1992;3:1–12.
White SD. Pododermatitis. Vet Dermatol 1989;1:1–18.
Author K. Marcia Murphy
Consulting Editor Karen Helton Rhodes

POISONING (INTOXICATION)

 BASICS

DEFINITION
• Acutely ill patients are often diagnosed as poisoned when no other diagnosis is obvious.
• Direct efforts toward stabilizing the patient.
• Make the diagnosis after determining pre-existing conditions and initially controlling clinical signs.
• Goals of treatment—providing emergency intervention; preventing further exposure; preventing further absorption; applying specific antidotes; hastening elimination; providing supportive measures; offering client education
• Suspected intoxication—suspected toxic materials and specimens may be valuable from a medicolegal aspect; maintain a proper chain of physical evidence; keep good medical records.
• Valuable time can be saved by applying the appropriate treatment for a suspected or known intoxicant.

Initial Instructions to Client
• May be beneficial to subsequent treatment
• Transport patient to a veterinarian as soon as possible.
• Delayed transport—keep patient warm; avoid any other stress.
• Warn onlookers about the condition of the patient.
• May need to muzzle the patient
• Transport uncontaminated vomitus and suspected toxic materials and their containers to the hospital.
• Use clean plastic containers or glass jars for the specimens.

 DIAGNOSIS

DIFFERENTIAL DIAGNOSIS
• Definitive diagnosis—difficult; animals come in contact with a vast array of toxicants; see Appendix IV: Clinical Toxicosis—Systems Affected and Clinical Effects
• Resources for emergencies—National Poison Control Center; state diagnostic laboratories; local poison control centers; great value for cases of suspected intoxication, especially when labels or containers are available
• When suspected compound and clinical signs do not concur—treat the signs; disregard the label
• Confirmation of diagnosis—by chemical analysis (may occur after the fact); accurate diagnosis and detailed records may help with future patients affected by the same intoxicant and are invaluable in medicolegal proceedings.

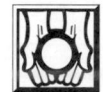 TREATMENT

SUPPORTIVE
• Control of body temperature
• Maintenance of respiratory and cardiovascular function
• Control of acid–base balance
• Alleviation of pain
• Control of CNS disorders—see specific topics

EMERGENCY
• Establishment of a patent airway
• Artificial respiration
• Cardiac massage—external or internal
• Application of defibrillation techniques
• After stabilization—may proceed with more specific therapeutic measures

PREVENT ABSORPTION
• Major treatment factor
• First remove patient from the affected environment.
• Available measures—washing; judicious use of emetics; gastric lavage techniques; use of adsorbents and cathartics

Washing Skin
• External toxicants
• Wash patient's skin to remove the noxious agent.
• **CAUTION:** avoid contamination of the people handling the patient.

Emetics
• Of little value beyond 4 hr after ingestion; most material will have passed to the duodenum.
• Do not induce in unconscious or severely depressed patients or after ingestion of strong acids, alkalis, petroleum distillates, tranquilizers, or other antiemetics.
• Apomorphine—most effective and most reliable for use in dogs and cats; availability at any given time unknown; small animals, 0.04 mg/kg IV or 0.08 mg/kg IM, SC; control adverse clinical signs caused by apomorphine with an appropriate intravenous narcotic antagonist (e.g., naloxone at 0.04 mg/kg).
• Ipecac—little efficacy; never use when activated charcoal is part of the therapeutic regimen.
• Xylazine—intravenous administration; used with some success in dogs and cats

Activated Charcoal
• Does not detoxify but prevents absorption if properly used
• Highly absorptive of many toxicants—organophosphate insecticides; other insecticides; rodenticides; mercuric chloride; strychnine; other alkaloids (e.g., morphine and atropine); barbiturates; ethylene glycol

POISONING (INTOXICATION)

- Ineffective against cyanide
- Administered in combination with emetics—increases efficacy of toxicant elimination by emesis
- Use a bathtub or some other easily cleansed area when administering activated charcoal to small animals.
- Dosage—1–5 g/kg body weight in a concentration of 1 g charcoal/5–10 mL water three to four times a day for 2–3 days
- Some charcoal should remain in the stomach and be followed by a cathartic to prevent desorption of the toxicant.
- Cathartic—sodium sulfate; administered 30 min after administration of the charcoal

Gastric Lavage

- An effective means of emptying the stomach
- Stomach tube size—use the largest possible; a good rule: use the same size as the cuffed endotracheal tube (1 mm = 3 Fr).
- Volume of water or lavage solution for each washing—5–10 mL/kg body weight
- Infusion and aspiration cycle—repeated 10–15 times
- Activated charcoal in the solution enhances the effectiveness.
- Precautions—(1) use low pressure to prevent forcing the toxicant into the duodenum; (2) reduce the infused volume in obviously weakened stomachs (e.g., in a patient that has ingested a caustic or corrosive toxicant); (3) do not force the stomach tube through either the esophagus or the stomach wall.

Oils

- Mineral or vegetable oil—of value for lipid-soluble toxicants
- Mineral oil (liquid petrolatum)—inert; less likely to be absorbed
- Use with a cathartic.
- Sodium sulfate—1 g/kg PO; more efficient agent for evacuation of the bowel than is magnesium sulfate; preferred with activated charcoal and mineral oil

Enemas

- Colonic lavage or high enema—may hasten the elimination of toxicants from the gastrointestinal tract
- Warm water with Castile soap—excellent solution
- Commercially available preparations are available that act as osmotic agents.
- Take care to avoid the induction of dehydration and electrolyte imbalances with overzealous treatment.
- Avoid hexachlorophene soaps in cats.

ENHANCE ELIMINATION

- Absorbed toxicants—generally excreted by the kidneys; may be excreted by other routes (e.g., bile, feces, lungs, and other body secretions)
- Renal excretion—may be manipulated in many animals
- Urinary excretion—may be enhanced by the use of diuretics or by altering the pH of the urine

Diuretics

- To enhance urinary excretion of toxicants—requires maintenance of adequate renal function
- Minimum urine flow cannot be established—must use peritoneal dialysis
- Agents of choice—mannitol (1.0–2.0 g/kg IV q6h) and furosemide (5 mg/kg q6–8h)

Manipulating Urine pH

- Classic pharmacologic technique
- Acidic compounds remain ionized in alkaline urine; alkaline compounds remain ionized in acidic urine
- Long-term urinary acidification—ammonium chloride (200 mg/kg PO daily in divided doses) and ethylenediamine dihydrochloride (1–2 tablets q8h for the average-sized dog)
- Physiologic saline—good, rapid, urinary acidifying agent

- Sodium bicarbonate—5 mEq/kg/hr; may be used as an alkalinizing agent

Peritoneal Dialysis

- Indicated for oliguria or anuria
- Indicated for simple removal of absorbed toxicants in patient with normal renal function
- pH of the solution—may be altered to maintain the ionized state of the offending compound

MEDICATIONS

Specific antidotes or procedures are available for the more common toxicants; see specific topic

FOLLOW-UP

Specific monitoring depends on the toxicant and the patient's signs and laboratory abnormalities.

MISCELLANEOUS

ABBREVIATION
CNS = central nervous system

Suggested Reading
Bailey EM, Garland T. Toxicologic emergencies. In: Murtaugh RJ, Kaplan PM, eds., Veterinary emergency and critical care medicine. St. Louis: Mosby Year Book, 1992:427–452.

Authors E. Murl Bailey and Tam Garland
Consulting Editor Gary D. Osweiler

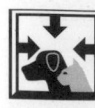

BASICS

DEFINITION
• Nonsuppurative meningoencephalomyelitis of unknown cause
• Associations with Borna disease virus suspected but not proven
• Neurons in the thoracic spinal cord appear preferentially affected.
• Lesions are also seen in the cervical and lumbar spinal cord, brainstem, and cerebrum.
• Axonal degeneration and demyelination in ventral and lateral funiculi of spinal cord occur secondary to neuronal necrosis.

SIGNALMENT
• Domestic shorthair cats and a few purebreds
• Age range—2 months to 6.5 years

• Females more commonly affected than males

SIGNS
• Vary with location of CNS lesion
• Chronic, progressive incoordination of hind or all four limbs
• Seizures in a few patients

CAUSES & RISK FACTORS
Viral cause suspected but not proven

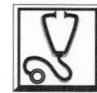

DIAGNOSIS

DIFFERENTIAL DIAGNOSIS
• FIP
• Toxoplasmosis
• Fungal infection
• Bacterial infection

CBC/BIOCHEMISTRY/URINALYSIS
• Laboratory changes not well characterized
• Nonspecific changes (e.g., leukopenia and nonregenerative anemia) rare

OTHER LABORATORY TESTS
N/A

IMAGING
N/A

DIAGNOSTIC PROCEDURES
• Mononuclear pleocytosis with mild to moderately high CSF protein (few data)
• Serum or CSF antibody titers—not thoroughly evaluated

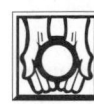

TREATMENT

Not attempted in any of the reported cases

MEDICATIONS

DRUG(S)
• No drug therapy used in reported cases.
• Because lesions are nonsuppurative, steroid therapy may palliate clinical signs, at least temporarily.

CONTRAINDICATIONS/POSSIBLE INTERACTIONS
N/A

FOLLOW-UP
N/A

MISCELLANEOUS

ABBREVIATIONS
• CNS = central nervous system
• CSF = cerebrospinal fluid
• FIP = feline infectious peritonitis

Suggested Reading
Berg A-L. Borna disease in cats. In: Bonagura JD, ed. Kirk's current veterinary therapy XIII. Small animal practice. Philadelphia: Saunders, 2000:976–978.
Lundgren AL. Feline non-suppurative meningoencephalomyelitis. A clinical and pathological study. J Comp Pathol 1992; 107:411–425.
Vandevelde M, Braund KG. Polioencephalomyelitis in cats. Vet Pathol 1979; 16:420–427.
Author Karen Dyer Inzana
Consulting Editor Joane M. Parent

POLYARTHRITIS, EROSIVE, IMMUNE-MEDIATED

BASICS

DEFINITION
An immune-mediated inflammatory disease of joints that results in erosion of articular cartilage

PATHOPHYSIOLOGY
• Pathogenesis—inciting cause unknown as extrapolated from human rheumatoid arthritis research; likely perpetuated by cell-mediated immunity; predominance of CD4+ helper T lymphocytes and immune complex depositions found in synovium of affected joints; leukocytes, leukocyte enzymes, cell-mediated immunity, immune complexes, and autoallergic reactions are directed against cartilage components; leads to an inflammatory response and complement activation
• Destructive enzymes—released from inflammatory cells, synoviocytes, and chondrocytes; damage the articular cartilage, leading to erosive changes
• IEP—associated with an abnormal antigenic response to host immunoglobulin, similar to human rheumatoid arthritis
• EPG and FCPP—offending antigens unknown

SYSTEMS AFFECTED
Musculoskeletal—diarthrodial joints

GENETICS
Not known to be hereditary

INCIDENCE/PREVALENCE
Rare

GEOGRAPHIC DISTRIBUTION
N/A

SIGNALMENT
Species
• Dogs—IEP; EPG
• Cats—FCPP

Breed Predilections
• Small or toy breeds (dogs)—more susceptible to IEP
• Greyhounds—only breed known to be susceptible to EPG

Mean Age and Range
• IEP (dogs)—young to middle-aged (8 months to 8 years)
• EPG—young greyhounds (3–30 months) more susceptible
• FCPP (cats)—onset at 1.5–4.5 years of age

Predominant Sex
FCPP—reported to affect only male cats

SIGNS
General Comments
Nonerosive and erosive forms of immune-mediated inflammatory disease initially appear similar

Historical Findings
• Dogs and cats—initial symmetric stiffness, especially after rest, or intermittent shifting leg lameness and swelling of affected joints
• Cats—may note a more insidious onset; may note shifting leg lameness
• Joint swelling—may be evident, especially in the carpi and tarsi
• Usually no history of trauma
• May also note vomiting, diarrhea, anorexia, pyrexia, depression, and lymphadenopathy
• Often cyclic—may appear to respond to antibiotic therapy, but may be undergoing spontaneous remission

Physical Examination Findings
• Stiffness of gait, lameness, decreased range of motion, crepitus, and joint swelling and pain in one or more joints
• Joint instability, subluxation, and luxation—depend on duration of disease
• Lameness—mild weight-bearing to more severe non–weight-bearing
• Diarthrodial joints—all may be affected; IEP and FCPP usually affect the carpi, tarsi, and phalangeal joints; EPG usually affects the carpi, proximal interphalangeal joints, tarsi, elbow, stifle, and hip.

CAUSES
• Unknown
• Immunologic mechanism likely
• *Mycoplasma spumans* (EPG)—cultured from one affected greyhound; not isolated in other patients
• FeLV and FeSFV—linked to cats with FCPP

RISK FACTORS
N/A

DIAGNOSIS

DIFFERENTIAL DIAGNOSIS
• Idiopathic polyarthritis
• Infectious arthritis
• Systemic lupus erythematosus
• Reactive polyarthritis
• Neoplasia
• Osteoarthritis—primary or secondary

CBC/BIOCHEMISTRY/URINALYSIS
• Usually normal
• Hemogram—may note leukocytosis, neutrophilia, and hyperfibrinogenemia

OTHER LABORATORY TESTS
• Rheumatoid factor—positive in only about 25% of IEP patients
• Coombs' test and antinuclear antibody titer—normal
• Serum titers for *Borrelia*, *Ehrlichia*, and *Rickettsia*—should be normal
• Serologic evidence of FeSFV—found in all FCPP patients
• Serologic evidence of FeLV exposure—found in 50% or fewer of FCPP patients

IMAGING
Radiography
• Earliest finding is periarticular soft tissue swelling
• Severe disease—joint capsular distention; osteophytosis; soft tissue thickening; narrowed joint spaces; subchondral sclerosis; decreased trabecular bone density; bony ankylosis in severely affected joints
• Cyst-like lucencies—occasionally seen in subchondral bone
• Chronic disease—subluxation, luxation, and obvious joint deformity

DIAGNOSTIC PROCEDURES
• Arthrocentesis and synovial fluid analysis—essential for diagnosis
• Synovial fluid—typically cloudy with normal viscosity; large number of nondegenerate neutrophils (10,000–100,000 cells/mL); submit for bacterial culture and sensitivity
• Biopsy of synovial tissue—helps make the diagnosis, rules out other arthritides and neoplasia

PATHOLOGIC FINDINGS
• Erosion of articular cartilage—particularly near the periphery at synovial attachments
• Eburnation and sclerosis of subchondral bone with full-thickness cartilage loss—chronic disease
• Synovial membrane—grossly thickened; may see villous projections
• Granulation tissue (pannus)—may invade the margins of articular cartilage, and arise from the marrow cavity to destroy cartilage at central regions of the joint
• Enthesiophytes—at joint capsular attachments and adjacent to the joint
• Histopathology of the synovial membrane—typically reveals villous synovial hyperplasia, hypertrophy, and lymphoplasmacytic inflammatory infiltrate
• Synovial fluid—cloudy; increased volume

TREATMENT

APPROPRIATE HEALTH CARE
Usually outpatient

NURSING CARE
• Physical therapy—range-of-motion exercises, massage, and swimming; may be indicated for severe disease
• Bandages and/or splints—to prevent further breakdown of the joint; may be indicated for severe disease with greatly compromised ambulation

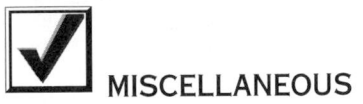

ACTIVITY
Limited to minimize aggravation of clinical signs

DIET
Weight reduction—to decrease stress placed on affected joints

CLIENT EDUCATION
Warn clients of the poor prognosis for cure and complete resolution.

SURGICAL CONSIDERATIONS
• Healing rates—may be long and protracted; range of recovery levels
• Surgery—generally not recommended as a good treatment option
• Arthroplasty—total hip replacement, femoral head ostectomy; may consider
• Arthrodesis—in selective cases of joint pain and joint instability; carpus; generally yields the best results and is a good salvage option; shoulder, elbow, stifle or hock: less predictable results

MEDICATIONS

DRUG(S) OF CHOICE

IEP
• NSAIDs (dogs)—unrewarding
• Prednisone—1.5–2.0 mg/kg PO q12h for 10–14 days as initial therapy; slowly taper over several weeks to 1.0 mg/kg PO q48h if synovial fluid cell counts return to < 4000 cells/mL and mononuclear cells predominate; add cytotoxic drugs if clinical signs persist or synovial fluid analysis is abnormal
• Combination of glucocorticoids and cytotoxic drugs—recommended for synergistic effect; may try cyclophosphamide, azathioprine, 6-mercaptopurine, methotrexate, or leflunomide
• Cyclophosphamide—patient < 10 kg: 2.5 mg/kg; patient 10–50 kg: 2.0 mg/kg; patient > 50 kg: 1.75 mg/kg; agent given orally q24h for 4 consecutive days of each week; can give concurrently with prednisone, the dose of prednisone may be decreased by half.
• Azathioprine or 6-mercaptopurine—2.0 mg/kg PO q24h for 14–21 days, then give q48h; give prednisone as for cyclophosphamide, but on alternating days
• Leflunomide—dog dose 4 mg/kg PO q24h; dosage may be adjusted after several days to maintain trough level of 20 μg/mL.
• Remission—usually induced by combination chemotherapy within 2–16 weeks; determined by resolution of clinical signs and confirmation of a normal synovial fluid analysis
• Discontinue cytotoxic drugs 1–3 months after remission is achieved.
• Maintaining remission—alternate-day glucocorticoid therapy (prednisone 1.0 mg/kg PO) is generally successful; if clinical signs or synovial effusion recurs, may require long-term cytotoxic drug therapy; if clinical signs do not recur in 2–3 months, may stop the glucocorticoid; if clinical signs recur after glucocorticoid is stopped, reinstitute treatment
• Aurothiomalate (chrysotherapy)—1 mg/kg IM weekly; successfully alleviates symptoms

EPG
• Treatment is unrewarding.
• Antibiotics, NSAIDs, glucocorticoids, cytotoxic drugs, and polysulfated glycosaminoglycan (Adequan)—fail to induce remission

FCPP
• Treatment may help slow progression.
• Prednisone (2 mg/kg q12h) and cyclophosphamide (2.5 mg/kg q24h)—typically used as described for IEP

CONTRAINDICATIONS
• Cytotoxic drugs—do not use with chronic infections or bone marrow suppression (cats with FCPP)
• Chrysotherapy—do not use with renal disease owing to nephrotoxicity

PRECAUTIONS
• Glucocorticoids—long-term use may lead to Cushing's disease
• Cytotoxic drugs—frequently induce bone marrow suppression; monitor CBC: if leukocyte count < 6000 cells/mL and platelet count < 125,000 cells/mL, discontinue for 1 week, then reinstitute at three-quarters dose when counts return to normal
• Thiopurines generally cause bone marrow suppression at 2–6 weeks; cyclophosphamide, at several months.
• Cyclophosphamide—limit to < 4 months; sterile hemorrhagic cystitis may develop; immediately discontinue if symptoms occur
• Leflunomide requires a plasma trough level for monitoring; is intestinally necrotizing to dogs at higher dosages.

POSSIBLE INTERACTIONS
None known

ALTERNATIVE DRUG(S)
See Drugs of Choice

FOLLOW-UP

PATIENT MONITORING
• Treatment is often frustrating and requires frequent reevaluation.
• Clinical deterioration—requires a change in drug selection or dosage, or surgical intervention
• Important to try to induce remission; allowing the disease to smolder uncontrolled will increase risk of secondary degenerative joint disease

PREVENTION/AVOIDANCE
N/A

POSSIBLE COMPLICATIONS
N/A

EXPECTED COURSE AND PROGNOSIS
• Progression likely
• Long-term prognosis poor
• Cure is not expected; remission is the goal.

MISCELLANEOUS

ASSOCIATED CONDITIONS
N/A

AGE-RELATED FACTORS
N/A

ZOONOTIC POTENTIAL
N/A

PREGNANCY
N/A

SEE ALSO
Polyarthritis, Nonerosive, Immune-Mediated

ABBREVIATIONS
• EPG = erosive polyarthritis of greyhounds
• FCPP = feline chronic progressive polyarthritis
• FeLV = feline leukemia virus
• FeSFV = feline syncytium-forming virus
• IEP = idiopathic erosive polyarthritis

Suggested Reading
Beale BS. Arthropathies. In: Bloomberg MS, Taylor RT, Dee J, eds. Canine sports medicine and surgery. Philadelphia: Saunders, 1998:517–532.
Goring RL, Beale BS. Immune mediated arthritides. In: Bojrab MJ, ed. Disease mechanisms in small animal surgery. Philadelphia: Lea & Febiger, 1993:742–750.
Pedersen NC, Morgan JP, Vasseur PB. Joint diseases of dogs and cats. In: Ettinger SJ, Feldman EC, eds. Textbook of veterinary internal medicine—diseases of the dog and cat. 5th ed. Philadelphia: Saunders, 2000:1862–1886.
Ralphs SC, Beale BS, Whitney WO, Liska W. Idiopathic erosive polyarthritis in six dogs (description of the disease and treatment with bilateral pancarpal arthrodesis). J Vet Comp Orthop Traumatol 2000; 13:191–196.
Ralphs SC, Beale BS. Canine idiopathic erosive polyarthritis. Compendium 2000; 22:671–677, 703.
Authors Brian Beale and Deanna Worley
Consulting Editor Peter Shires

POLYARTHRITIS, NONEROSIVE, IMMUNE-MEDIATED

BASICS

DEFINITION
An immune-mediated inflammatory disease of joints that does not cause erosive change; includes idiopathic polyarthritis, SLE, polyarthritis associated with chronic disease (chronic infectious, neoplastic, or enteropathic disease), polyarthritis-polymyositis syndrome, polymyositis syndrome, polyarthritis-meningitis syndrome, polyarthritis nodosa, familial renal amyloidosis in Chinese shar-pei dogs, lymphocytic-plasmacytic synovitis, juvenile-onset polyarthritis of Akitas, and the proliferative form of FCPP

PATHOPHYSIOLOGY
• Pathogenesis—involves a type III hypersensitivity reaction; immune complexes deposited within the synovial membrane; inflammatory response and complement activation ensue, leading to clinical signs of arthritis
• SLE—nuclear material from various cells becomes antigenic, leading to formation of autoantibodies (antinuclear antibody)

SYSTEMS AFFECTED
Musculoskeletal—diarthrodial joints

GENETICS
Not known to be hereditary

INCIDENCE/PREVALENCE
• Idiopathic—most common in dogs
• Other forms uncommon

GEOGRAPHIC DISTRIBUTION
N/A

SIGNALMENT

Species
Dogs and cats

Breed Predilections
• Idiopathic—large- (more common) and small-breed dogs; uncommon in cats; German shepherds, Doberman pinschers, retrievers, spaniels, pointers, toy poodles, Lhasa apsos, Yorkshire terriers, and Chihuahuas overrepresented
• SLE—tendency to affect large-breed dogs; collies, German shepherds, poodles, terriers, beagles, and Shetland sheepdogs
• Secondary to administration of sulfa drugs—increased sensitivity in Doberman pinschers
• Polyarthritis-meningitis syndrome—reported in weimaraners, German shorthaired pointers, boxers, Bernese mountain dogs, beagles, rottweilers, and Japanese Akitas
• Amyloidosis and synovitis—prominent features of a syndrome affecting young shar-pei dogs
• Juvenile onset—polyarthritis reported in Akitas
• Lymphocytic-plasmacytic synovitis in German shepherds and other large breed dogs

Mean Age and Range
Dogs—young to middle-aged

Predominant Sex
FCPP—male cats only

SIGNS

General Comments
Nonerosive and erosive forms of immune-mediated inflammatory disease initially appear similar

Historical Findings
• Dogs and cats—acute onset; single- or multiple-limb lameness
• Lameness—may shift from leg to leg
• Usually no history of trauma
• May also note vomiting, diarrhea, anorexia, pyrexia, polyuria, or polydypsia
• May also note signs associated with systemic disease or infections (pyometra, prostatitis, or diskospondylitis), or neoplastic disease
• Often cyclic—may appear to respond to antibiotic therapy, but may be undergoing spontaneous remission
• Disease may develop when patient is being treated with (sulfur-containing) antibiotics.

Physical Examination Findings
• Stiffness of gait, lameness, decreased range of motion, crepitus, and joint swelling and pain in one or more joints
• Lameness—mild weight-bearing to more severe non–weight-bearing
• Diarthrodial joints—all may be affected; usually stifle, elbow, carpus, and tarsus

CAUSES
• Unknown for most
• Immunologic mechanism likely
• Chronic—associated with antigenic stimulation along with concurrent meningitis, gastrointestinal disease, neoplasia, urinary tract infection, periodontitis, bacterial endocarditis, heartworm disease, pyometra, chronic otitis media or externa, fungal infections, and chronic *Actinomyces* or *Salmonella* infections
• May occur secondary to a hypersensitivity reaction involving the deposition of drug-antibody complexes in the blood vessels of the synovium; suspected antibiotics include sulfas, cephalosporins, lincomycin, erythromycin, and penicillins.
• FeLV and FeSFV—linked to FCPP

RISK FACTORS
N/A

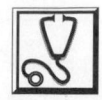

DIAGNOSIS

DIFFERENTIAL DIAGNOSIS
• Early erosive polyarthritides
• Infectious arthritis
• Joint trauma
• Polymyositis

CBC/BIOCHEMISTRY/URINALYSIS
• Usually normal
• Hemogram—may show leukocytosis, neutrophilia, and hyperfibrinogenemia
• Hematologic abnormalities (e.g., thrombocytopenia and hemolytic anemia)—seen in only 10%–20% of patients with SLE

OTHER LABORATORY TESTS
• Positive lupus erythematosus preparation or positive antinuclear antibody test—dogs with SLE
• Serum titers (*Borrelia*, *Ehrlichia*, and *Rickettsia*)—should be normal
• Serologic evidence of FeSFV—found in all FCPP patients
• Serologic evidence of FeLV exposure—found in 50% or fewer of cats with FCPP

IMAGING
• Primary radiographic change—joint capsular distention
• May see enthesiophytosis in prolonged or recurrent disease

DIAGNOSTIC PROCEDURES
• Arthrocentesis and synovial fluid analysis—essential for diagnosis
• Synovial fluid—typically appears cloudy with normal viscosity; large increase in nondegenerate neutrophils (20,000–200,000 cells/mL); submit for bacterial culture and sensitivity
• Synovial biopsy—may help diagnosis

PATHOLOGIC FINDINGS
• Joint capsule—may be thickened; synovial effusion
• Synovial hypertrophy and hyperplasia—associated with a mononuclear cell infiltrate
• Neutrophils—seen in the synovial tissues owing to chemotaxis

POLYARTHRITIS, NONEROSIVE, IMMUNE-MEDIATED

TREATMENT

APPROPRIATE HEALTH CARE
Usually outpatient

NURSING CARE
• Physical therapy—range-of-motion exercises and swimming; may be indicated for severe disease
• Bandages and/or splints—to prevent further breakdown of the joint; may be indicated for severe disease with compromised ambulation

ACTIVITY
Limited to minimize aggravation of clinical signs

DIET
Weight reduction—to decrease stress placed on affected joints

CLIENT EDUCATION
Warn client of poor prognosis for cure and complete resolution.

SURGICAL CONSIDERATIONS
N/A

MEDICATIONS

DRUG(S) OF CHOICE
• Typical therapy—initial trial of glucocorticoids; if poor response, then combination chemotherapy (glucocorticoids and cytotoxic drugs)
• Eliminate underlying causes if possible—chronic disease; offending antibiotic.
• Complete remission—usually achieved in 2–16 weeks; determined by resolution of clinical signs and confirmation of normal synovial fluid analysis
• Recurrence rate—30%–50% once therapy is discontinued
• Prednisone—1.5–2.0 mg/kg PO q12h for 10–14 days as initial treatment; synovial fluid cell counts < 4000 cells/mL and mononuclear cells predominate: slowly taper over several weeks to 1.0 mg/kg PO q48h; clinical signs persist or abnormal synovial fluid analysis: add cytotoxic agents; no clinical signs after 2–3 months of alternate-day therapy: discontinue
• Combination of glucocorticoids and cytotoxic drug—recommend for synergistic effect; may try cyclophosphamide or a thiopurine (azathioprine or 6-mercaptopurine)

• Cyclophosphamide—patient < 10 kg: 2.5 mg/kg; patient 10–50 kg: 2.0 mg/kg; patient > 50 kg: 1.75 mg/kg; agent given PO q24h for 4 consecutive days of each week; given concurrently with prednisone (as described above; some clinicians reduce the total steroid dose by half)
• Azathioprine or 6-mercaptopurine—2.0 mg/kg PO q24h for 14–21 days, then q48h; given concurrently with prednisone as for cyclophosphamide, but on alternating days
• Leflunomide—may be used synergistically with azathioprine, prednisone, and cyclophosphamide (4.0 mg/kg q24h for dogs). After several days, adjust dose to plasma trough levels of 20 μg/mL
• Discontinue cytotoxic drugs 1–3 months after remission is achieved.
• Maintaining remission—alternate-day glucocorticoid therapy (prednisone, 1.0 mg/kg PO) is generally successful; clinical signs or synovial neutrophilia recur: long-term cytotoxic drug therapy may be necessary; clinical signs do not recur after 2–3 months: may stop the glucocorticoid; clinical signs recur after glucocorticoid is stopped: continue treatment

FCPP
• Treatment may slow progression
• Prednisone (2 mg/kg q12h) and cyclophosphamide (2.5 mg/kg)—typically as described above

CONTRAINDICATIONS
• Do not use cytotoxic drugs with chronic infections or bone marrow suppression (cats with FCPP)
• Avoid using glucocorticoids with NSAIDs such as aspirin, carprofen, etodolac, and deracoxib as gastric ulceration may result

PRECAUTIONS
• Glucocorticoids—long-term use may lead to iatrogenic Cushing's disease
• Cytotoxic drugs—frequently induce bone marrow suppression; monitor CBC weekly (see Polyarthritis, Erosive, Immune-Mediated)
• Leflunomide may cause intestinal necrosis with overdosing.

POSSIBLE INTERACTIONS
None known

ALTERNATIVE DRUG(S)
See Drugs of Choice.

FOLLOW-UP

PATIENT MONITORING
Clinical deterioration—indicates a change in drug selection or dosage

PREVENTION/AVOIDANCE
N/A

POSSIBLE COMPLICATIONS
N/A

EXPECTED COURSE AND PROGNOSIS
• Recurrence—seen intermittently
• SLE and FCPP—progression common; guarded prognosis
• Other forms—good prognosis

MISCELLANEOUS

ASSOCIATED CONDITIONS
N/A

AGE-RELATED FACTORS
N/A

ZOONOTIC POTENTIAL
N/A

PREGNANCY
N/A

ABBREVIATIONS
• FCPP = feline chronic progressive polyarthritis
• FeLV = feline leukemia virus
• FeSFV = feline syncytium-forming virus
• SLE = systemic lupus erythematosus
• NSAID = nonsteroidal antiinflammatory drug

Suggested Reading
Beale BS. Arthropathies. In: Bloomberg MS, Taylor RT, Dee J, eds. Canine sports medicine and surgery. Philadelphia: Saunders, 1998:517–532.
Goring RL, Beale BS. Immune mediated arthritides. In: Bojrab MJ, ed. Disease mechanisms in small animal surgery. Philadelphia: Lea & Febiger, 1993:742–750.
Pedersen NC. Joint diseases of dogs and cats. In: Ettinger SJ, ed. Textbook of veterinary internal medicine. 5th ed. Philadelphia: Saunders, 2000:1862–1886.
Authors Brian S. Beale and Scott P. Hammel
Consulting Editor Peter Shires

POLYCYSTIC KIDNEY DISEASE

 BASICS

OVERVIEW
Disorder in which large portions of normally differentiated renal parenchyma are displaced by multiple cysts; renal cysts develop in pre-existing nephrons and collecting ducts; both kidneys are invariably involved, probably because the disease is inherited.

SIGNALMENT
• Persian and other long-haired cats are affected more commonly than other breeds.
• Dog breeds affected include cairn terriers and beagles.

SIGNS
• Cysts often remain undetected until they become large and numerous enough to contribute to renal failure or abdominal enlargement; thus patients typically are clinically normal during initial stages of cyst formation and growth.
• May detect bosselated (lumpy) kidneys by abdominal palpation
• Most renal cysts are not painful when palpated, but acute secondary infection of cysts may be associated with rapid distension of the renal capsule and pain.

CAUSES & RISK FACTORS
• Autosomal-dominant inheritance in Persian cats

• The stimuli for renal cyst formation remains obscure; genetic, endogenous, and environmental factors appear to influence the process.
• Endogenous compounds hypothesized to stimulate cellular hyperplasia and contribute to cyst development include parathyroid hormone, vasopressin, cAMP, and endotoxins of enteric microbes.
• Cystogenic chemicals include diphenylthiazole, nordihydroguaiarectic acid, diphenylamine, trichlorophenoxyacetic acid, and long-acting corticosteroids.

 DIAGNOSIS

DIFFERENTIAL DIAGNOSIS
• Other multicystic diseases of the kidneys
• Glomerulocystic disease of collie
• Renal cystadenocarcinoma associated with nodular fibrosis in German shepherd dogs
• Renal cysts associated with chronic renal failure or renal dysplasia
• Noncystic causes of renomegaly
• Renal neoplasia
• Hydronephrosis
• Perirenal pseudocysts
• Feline infectious peritonitis
• Mycotic or bacterial nephritis

CBC/BIOCHEMISTRY/URINALYSIS
• Results usually unremarkable unless patient has renal insufficiency
• Hematuria is rare.

OTHER LABORATORY TESTS
• Cyst fluid can be clear, cloudy, or hemorrhagic, and the fluid from different cysts in the same kidney can differ.
• Bacterial culture of cyst fluid helps in diagnosing concomitant infection.
• Hypertension is uncommon without renal failure.

IMAGING
Radiography
Survey radiography and intravenous urography are insensitive methods of confirming cystic disease.

Ultrasonography
• Reveals anechoic cavitating lesions characterized by sharply marginated smooth walls and distal enhancement, which are diagnostic
• Cysts detected in cats as young as 7 weeks; screening cats younger than 6 months is associated with higher false negative rate.
• Reveals hypoechoic cystic cavities in some patients with cysts infected with bacteria
• Used to detect cysts in other organs (e.g., liver), which helps to differentiate polycystic kidney disease from acquired multicystic disorders of the kidneys

DIAGNOSTIC PROCEDURES
Evaluation of fine-needle aspirates of the kidney may allow differentiation of cystic disease from other diseases that cause renomegaly.

TREATMENT

• Usually not immediately life-threatening, but bacterial nephritis and cyst involvement warrants immediate measures to prevent sepsis and mortality
• Spontaneous resolution of cysts is not documented in dogs or cats; with time, most cysts increase in size and number, often compressing adjacent normally functioning renal parenchyma.
• Elimination of renal cysts and associated renal parenchymal lesions is not yet feasible; treatment is often limited to minimizing the pathophysiologic consequences of renal cyst formation (i.e., renal failure, renal infection, hematuria, and pain).
• Can use percutaneous aspiration of fluid from large renal cysts to minimize pain and compression of adjacent normal renal parenchyma. This procedure is impractical for kidneys with hundreds of cysts. Periodic aspiration of fluid (weekly to biweekly) is needed to maintain reduced cyst volume.
• Some patients may require treatment for concomitant renal failure.
• Avoid nephrectomy but may consider if infected cysts are associated with sepsis
• Disease eradication by selective breeding of unaffected

MEDICATIONS

DRUG(S)

• Bacterial infection of cysts has been observed in cats. Unless infection is accompanied by pyelonephritis, bacteria may not be observed in urine. Consider parenchymal infection when renal cysts are associated with renal pain and fever, even in absence of bacteriuria.
• Treatment of infected cysts requires special consideration. The acidic nature of cyst fluid and its containment by an epithelial barrier might inhibit establishment of bactericidal concentrations of commonly used acidic antibiotics (e.g., cephalosporins and penicillins) within cystic lumens. Alkaline, lipid-soluble antibiotics (e.g., trimethoprim-sulfonamide combinations, enrofloxacin, chloramphenicol, tetracycline, and clindamycin), which penetrate epithelial barriers and become ionized and trapped in cyst lumens, have been recommended for humans with infected cysts and should be considered for veterinary patients.

FOLLOW-UP

• Monitor patients every 2–6 months for associated disease (e.g., renal failure, renal infection, and pain).
• In the absence of sepsis, the short-term prognosis appears to be favorable without treatment.
• The long-term prognosis for patients with polycystic kidney disease often depends on the severity and progression of renal failure.

MISCELLANEOUS

Suggested Reading

Biller DS, DiBartola SP, Eaton KA, et al. Inheritance of polycystic kidney disease in Persian cats. Hered 1996;87:1–5.
Lulich JP, Osborne CA, Polzin DJ. Cystic diseases of the kidney. In: Osborne CA, Finco DR, eds. Canine and feline nephrology and urology. Baltimore: Williams & Wilkins, 1995:460–470.

Authors Jody P. Lulich and Carl A. Osborne
Consulting Editors Larry G. Adams and Carl A. Osborne

POLYCYTHEMIA

 BASICS

DEFINITION
Higher than reference range values for PCV, hemoglobin concentration, and RBC count because of a relative or absolute increase in the number of circulating RBCs

PATHOPHYSIOLOGY
• Number of circulating RBCs affected by changes in plasma volume, rate of RBC destruction or loss, splenic contraction, erythropoetin (EPO) secretion, and rate of bone marrow production
• Erythropoiesis also affected by hormones from the adrenal cortex, thyroid gland, ovary, testis, and anterior pituitary gland; normal PCV maintained by an endocrine loop

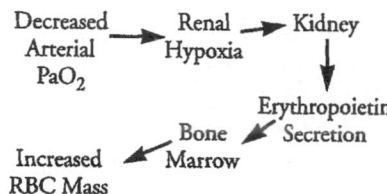

• Classified as relative, transient, or absolute
• Relative—develops when a decrease in plasma volume, usually caused by dehydration, produces a relative increase in circulating RBCs
• Transient—caused by splenic contraction, which injects concentrated RBCs into the circulation; because splenic contraction is a momentary response to epinephrine, this type is usually not a major diagnostic consideration.
• Absolute—characterized by an absolute increase in the circulating RBC mass as a result of an increase in bone marrow production; either primary or secondary to an increase in the production of EPO
• Primary absolute (polycythemia rubra vera)—a myeloproliferative disorder characterized by the uncontrolled but orderly production of excessive numbers of mature RBCs
• Secondary absolute—caused by a physiologically appropriate release of EPO resulting from chronic hypoxemia or by an inappropriate and excessive production of EPO or an EPO-like substance in an animal with normal SaO_2

SYSTEMS AFFECTED
• Cardiovascular, Respiratory, Nervous, Renal/Urologic—hyperviscosity and poor perfusion and oxygenation of tissues, which are related directly to the high PCV, especially values > 60%
• Animals with absolute polycythemia have expanded blood volume, whereas those with relative polycythemia (dehydration) have decreased volume; both types can compromise tissue perfusion and oxygenation.

SIGNALMENT
• Reference values for PCV, hemoglobin, and RBC count vary with geographic location and breed.
• Animals at altitudes > 6000 ft have higher values than those at sea level.
• Brachycephalic breeds have higher PCV values than do normocephalic breeds.
• Large, excitable breeds are prone to splenic contraction.
• Greyhounds typically have high PCV; normal range is 50–65%.

SIGNS

General Comments
Vary with the degree of polycythemia

Historical Findings
• Transient—excitement or vigorous exercise
• Absolute—lethargy, anorexia, epistaxis, seizures, or stunted growth

Physical Examination Findings
• Relative—dehydration caused by vomiting, diarrhea, or lack of water intake and oliguria
• Absolute—lethargy, low exercise tolerance, behavioral change, brick red or cyanotic mucous membranes, sneezing, bilateral epistaxis, large size and tortuosity of retinal and sublingual vessels, and cardiopulmonary impairment
• Primary absolute—variable degrees of splenomegaly, hepatomegaly, thrombosis, and hemorrhage; occasional seizure
• Secondary absolute caused by tissue hypoxia—clinical signs of hypoxemia caused by chronic pulmonary disease, cardiac disease or anomaly with right to left shunting, or hemoglobinopathy
• Secondary absolute caused by inappropriate EPO secretion—signs associated with neoplasia, space-occupying renal lesion, or endocrine disorder

CAUSES
• Relative (common)—vomiting, diarrhea, diminished water intake, diuresis, hyperventilation, renal disease, and shift of plasma water to interstitium or gastrointestinal lumen
• Transient—excitement, anxiety, seizures, and restraint
• Primary absolute—rare myeloproliferative disorder
• Secondary absolute caused by tissue hypoxia—chronic pulmonary disease, cardiac disease or anomaly with right to left shunting, high altitude, brachycephalic breed conformation, methemoglobinemia, and impairment of renal blood supply
• Secondary absolute caused by inappropriate EPO secretion (rare)—renal cyst or tumor, hydronephrosis, hyperadrenocorticism, hyperthyroidism, pheochromocytoma, nasal fibrosarcoma, hepatic neoplasia, and hyperandrogenism

RISK FACTORS
None

 DIAGNOSIS

DIFFERENTIAL DIAGNOSIS
• Moderately high PCV and total plasma protein with concurrent dehydration—suggest relative polycythemia
• Secondary absolute—caused by diseases that produce chronic hypoxemia or by space-occupying lesions of the kidney, endocrine disorders, and neoplasms that produce EPO or an EPO-like substance independent of hypoxia
• Polycythemia vera—diagnosed by elimination of other causes

LABORATORY FINDINGS

Drugs That May Alter Laboratory Results
Dilutional effect of fluid therapy on PCV and total plasma protein

Disorders That May Alter Laboratory Results
Concurrent anemia, hypoproteinemia, or dehydration can affect interpretation of PCV and total plasma protein values.

Valid if Run in Human Laboratory?
Yes.

CBC/BIOCHEMISTRY/URINALYSIS

Assessment begins with CBC and total plasma protein measurement; additional tests selected as indicated; noted in following table (Inc = Increase, Dec = Decrease):

Mechanism	Relative Dehydration	Absolute Primary Myeloproliferative	Absolute Secondary Hypoxemia	Absolute Secondary Excess EPO
PCV	Inc	Marked Inc > 60%	Marked Inc > 60%	Marked Inc > 60%
TPP	Inc	N	N	N
SaO$_2$		N > 90%	Dec << 90%	N > 90%
EPO		N/Dec	Inc	Inc
Bone marrow		------- Erythroid Hyperplasia -------		
Other	Prerenal Azotemia	Inc WBC Inc Platelets		

OTHER LABORATORY TESTS

• SaO$_2$ and EPO determinations—diagnose absolute polycythemia
• Hormone assays—assessment of endocrine dysfunction; EPO samples can be sent to a human testing laboratory; control sample from a normal animal (not a blood donor) should also be submitted
• Extensive overlap in EPO values exists between normal and affected animals; in some animals with secondary absolute polycythemia, low or normal EPO values have been reported.

IMAGING

Radiography and ultrasonography to detect cardiopulmonary disease and space-occupying lesions of the kidneys

DIAGNOSTIC PROCEDURES

Pulse oximetry to determine oxygen saturation of the blood

TREATMENT

• Relative—rehydration with IV fluids appropriate for the primary cause; assessment of renal function, gastrointestinal system, acid–base status, and electrolyte balance important to the selection of the fluid
• Absolute—phlebotomy recommended (20 mL/kg over one to several days) to reduce the RBC mass to a PCV of 55%; blood volume should be replaced concurrently with isotonic fluids to prevent hypotension, cardiovascular collapse, and thrombosis
• Secondary caused by inappropriate EPO production—phlebotomy and removal of the EPO source
• Secondary caused by hypoxemia—the high PCV is an appropriate compensatory response; thus phlebotomy may be dangerous; if indicated, remove blood at a slower rate (5 mL/kg); a higher PCV (60–65%) may be necessary to sustain life until the cause of hypoxemia can be corrected
• Polycythemia vera—phlebotomy (20 mL/kg) and hydroxyurea; frequency of bleeding and dosage adjusted to maintain a PCV of 55% in dogs and 45% in cats

MEDICATIONS

DRUG(S) OF CHOICE
Polycythemia vera—hydroxyurea (30–50 mg/kg PO q24h, dogs; 30 mg/kg q24h, cats)

CONTRAINDICATIONS
Phlebotomy may be contraindicated in patients with hypoxemia.

PRECAUTIONS
Removal of blood at a rapid rate can cause hypotension and cardiovascular collapse.

POSSIBLE INTERACTIONS
None

ALTERNATIVE DRUG(S)
Polycythemia vera—chlorambucil (0.2 mg/kg PO q24h, dogs and cats) or busulfan (2.0–4.0 mg/m² PO q24h, dogs)

FOLLOW-UP

PATIENT MONITORING
• PCV, total plasma protein, urine output, and body weight 2–3 times daily in severely dehydrated animals until normal hydration is maintained
• Patients being treated for polycythemia vera by chemotherapy—monitor weekly for changes in PCV, neutrophil count, and platelets during the initial treatment; then monthly for adjustment of chemotherapy and periodic phlebotomy

POSSIBLE COMPLICATIONS
• Hyperviscosity in patients with absolute polycythemia, especially polycythemia vera, may lead to thrombosis, infarction, or hemorrhage.
• Chemotherapy may cause bone marrow suppression.

MISCELLANEOUS

ASSOCIATED CONDITIONS
None

AGE-RELATED FACTORS
None

ZOONOTIC POTENTIAL
None

PREGNANCY
N/A

SYNONYM
Erythrocytosis

SEE ALSO
• Hyperviscosity Syndrome
• Polycythemia Vera

ABBREVIATIONS
• EPO = erythropoietin
• PCV = packed cell volume
• RBC = red blood cell
• SaO$_2$ = arterial oxygen saturation
• TPP = total plasma protein
• WBC = white blood cell

Suggested Reading
Cook SM, Lothrop CD. Serum erythropoietin concentrations measured by radioimmunoassay in normal, polycythemic, and anemic dogs and cats. J Vet Intern Med 1994;8:18–25.
Hasler AH, Giger U. Serum erythropoietin values in polycythemic cats. J Am Anim Hosp Assoc 1996;12:294–301.
Moore KW, Stepien RL. Hydroxyurea for treatment of polycythemia secondary to right-to-left shunting patent arteriosus in 4 dogs. J Vet Intern Med 2001;15:418–421.
Author Peter S. MacWilliams
Consulting Editor Stephen A. Kruth

POLYCYTHEMIA VERA

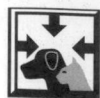

BASICS

OVERVIEW
Myeloproliferative disorder that results in high blood viscosity secondary to an increased RBC mass

SIGNALMENT
• Dogs and cats
• Primarily old animals

SIGNS
• Gradual in onset; runs a chronic course
• Depression
• Anorexia
• Weakness
• Polydipsia and polyuria
• Erythema of skin and mucous membranes
• Dilated and tortuous retinal blood vessels
• Splenomegaly and hepatomegaly uncommon

CAUSES & RISK FACTORS
Unknown

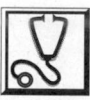

DIAGNOSIS

DIFFERENTIAL DIAGNOSIS
• Severe dehydration
• Renal neoplasia
• Chronic pyelonephritis
• Hyperadrenocorticism
• Androgen stimulation
• Pulmonary disease
• Cardiac disease with right-to-left shunts

CBC/BIOCHEMISTRY/URINALYSIS
• High PCV
• Absolute increase in RBC mass
• Prerenal azotemia possible
• Leukocytosis in 50% of dogs

OTHER LABORATORY TESTS
• PaO$_2$—normal
• Serum erythropoietin concentration—low to zero
• Cytologic examination of bone marrow and core biopsy

IMAGING
• Radiography—assess kidneys and cardiopulmonary system
• Abdominal ultrasonography—assess kidneys and adrenal glands
• Echocardiography—evaluate for right-to-left cardiac shunts
• Intravenous pyelogram—assess kidneys
• Imaging studies—normal in affected animals

DIAGNOSTIC PROCEDURES
• Bone marrow biopsy
• Electrocardiography—assess heart disease

TREATMENT
• Phlebotomy and concurrent replacement with intravenous isotonic fluids—quick relief of signs during clinical crisis
• Hydroxyurea—inhibit intracellular DNA synthesis and retard bone marrow proliferation.

MEDICATIONS

DRUG(S)
Hydroxyurea—40–50 mg/kg divided twice daily; titrate to response and toxicity (dogs and cats).

CONTRAINDICATIONS/POSSIBLE INTERACTIONS
Hydroxyurea—potentially myelosuppressive; frequent blood monitoring advised

FOLLOW-UP
Periodic reexaminations—CBC and platelet count to monitor toxic effects of hydroxyurea on bone marrow

MISCELLANEOUS

SEE ALSO
Polycythemia

ABBREVIATION
PCV = packed cell volume
RBC = red blood cell

Suggested Reading
Hamilton TA. The leukemias. In: Morrison WB, ed. Cancer in dogs and cats: medical and surgical management. Baltimore: Williams & Wilkins, 1998:721–729.
Morrison WB. Polycythemia. In: Ettinger SJ, Feldman EC, eds., Textbook of veterinary internal medicine. 4th ed. Philadelphia: Saunders, 1995;197–199.

Author Wallace B. Morrison
Consulting Editor Wallace B. Morrison

BASICS

OVERVIEW
Increased food intake

PATHOPHYSIOLOGY
• Failure to assimilate or loss of nutrients (e.g., maldigestion/malabsorption syndromes such as exocrine pancreatic insufficiency) • Inability to use nutrients (e.g., diabetes mellitus, poor-quality diets, gastrointestinal parasites) • Hypoglycemia (e.g., insulinoma, insulin overdose) • Increased metabolic rate or demand (e.g., hyperthyroidism, cold environments, pregnancy, lactation) • Psychologic or learned behaviors (e.g., palatable diets, competition, drugs such as anticonvulsants or glucocorticoids)

SYSTEMS AFFECTED
• Musculoskeletal—overweight patients are susceptible to arthritis and other orthopedic problems. • Integument—obese animals, especially cats, are susceptible to dermatitis. • Respiratory—obesity exacerbates dyspnea in patients with respiratory disease. • Cardiovascular—obesity can worsen clinical cardiac disease.

SIGNALMENT
Dogs and cats

SIGNS
Historical Findings
• Eating more frequently and/or a greater quantity than normal • Weight loss may occur with certain disease states (e.g., exocrine pancreatic insufficiency, diabetes mellitus, hyperthyroidism). • PU/PD occurs in some patients (diabetes mellitus, hyperthyroidism, hyperadrenocorticism).

Physical Examination Findings
Patients may have excessive body fat, but those with an underlying medical problem (e.g., exocrine pancreatic insufficiency, diabetes mellitus, hyperthyroidism) may be thin.

CAUSES & RISK FACTORS
Physiologic
• Pregnancy • Lactation • Growth • Response to a cold environment • Increased exercise

Pathologic
• Diabetes mellitus • Hyperthyroidism—cats • Hyperadrenocorticism—dogs • Exocrine pancreatic insufficiency • Gastrointestinal parasites • Insulinoma • Insulin overdose • Lymphangiectasia • Growth hormone—secreting pituitary tumor • Megaesophagus • Lymphocytic plasmacytic enteritis—cats; uncommon • Neoplasms of the brain—rare • Gastrointestinal neoplasms—rare

Iatrogenic
• Corticosteroids • Progestins • Benzodiazepines • Anticonvulsants • Palatable food/overfeeding • Poor diets • Competition for food

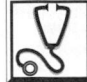 DIAGNOSIS

DIFFERENTIAL DIAGNOSIS
PU/PD (excessive trips to food/water area)—differentiate by observation

CBC/BIOCHEMISTRY/URINALYSIS
• Neutrophilia, monocytosis, lymphopenia, and eosinopenia with hyperadrenocorticism, and in patients receiving corticosteroids • Hyperglycemia with diabetes mellitus, growth hormone–secreting pituitary tumors (cats, insulin-resistant diabetes mellitus) and hyperadrenocorticism (mild) • Hypercholesterolemia with recent food intake, hyperadrenocorticism, and diabetes mellitus, and in patients receiving corticosteroids • High ALP and ALT activity with hyperadrenocorticism (dogs), hyperthyroidism (cats), and diabetes mellitus, and in patients receiving corticosteroids • Hypoproteinemia with protein-losing enteropathies (e.g., lymphangiectasia, inflammatory bowel disease) • Hypoglycemia in patients with insulinoma or insulin overdose • Low urine specific gravity with diabetes mellitus, hyperthyroidism, and hyperadrenocorticism, and in patients receiving corticosteroids • Glucosuria, possibly ketonuria, with diabetes mellitus

OTHER LABORATORY TESTS
• Fecal examination to rule out gastrointestinal parasites • Serum trypsin-like immunoreactivity to diagnose exocrine pancreatic insufficiency • Total serum T_4 to rule out hyperthyroidism (cats); T_3 suppression testing if hyperthyroidism is suspected but serum total T_4 is normal. • Low-dose dexamethasone suppression or ACTH stimulation test to diagnose hyperadrenocorticism; plasma ACTH level or high-dose dexamethasone suppression testing to differentiate pituitary-dependent hyperadrenocorticism from adrenal tumor if hyperadrenocorticism is confirmed with the low-dose dexamethasone suppression test or ACTH stimulation test • Serum insulin levels in hypoglycemic patients to rule out insulinoma

IMAGING
• Abdominal radiology may demonstrate hepatomegaly associated with hyperadrenocorticism, diabetes mellitus, and corticosteroid administration. • Abdominal ultrasonography may demonstrate an adrenal mass or bilateral adrenomegaly (hyperadrenocorticism), hepatomegaly (hyperadrenocorticism, diabetes mellitus, and corticosteroid administration), bowel wall thickening or bowel wall layering disruption (inflammatory bowel disease, lymphoma, lymphangiectasia), and pancreatic masses (insulinoma).

DIAGNOSTIC PROCEDURES
Endoscopy with biopsy of the upper gastrointestinal tract to rule out gastrointestinal diseases

 TREATMENT

• Usually outpatient medical management • Polyphagia without weight gain or with weight loss is more likely due to a medical problem; evaluate the animal prior to food restriction or manipulation. • Once pathologic causes of polyphagia have been excluded, limit the amount of food available, feed a reduced-calorie diet, or increase exercise if obesity or weight gain is present. • The average animal's daily caloric need can be estimated by the formula $30 \times$ weight (kg) + 70. • Chew toys can be used as a substitute for food.

 MEDICATIONS

DRUG(S)
• See specific disease chapters for detailed therapy • Drug-induced—attempt to taper or discontinue drug. • If a compulsive eating disorder is suspected, drugs such as clomipramine or amitriptyline (1–3 mg/kg PO q12h) may be used.

CONTRAINDICATIONS/POSSIBLE INTERACTIONS N/A

 FOLLOW-UP

PATIENT MONITORING
Monitor body weight in patients with nonpathologic causes of polyphagia.

POSSIBLE COMPLICATIONS
• Obesity in nonpathologic polyphagia • Weight loss/emaciation in pathologic causes of polyphagia • Worsening of respiratory or cardiovascular disease processes in obese patient

 MISCELLANEOUS

ASSOCIATED CONDITIONS
Obesity

PREGNANCY
A normal physiologic response to pregnancy

SYNONYMS
• Hyperphagia • Eating disorder

SEE ALSO
Obesity

Suggested Reading
Monroe WE. Anorexia and polyphagia. In: Ettinger SJ, Feldman EC, eds. Textbook of veterinary internal medicine. Philadelphia: Saunders, 1995:18–21.

Author Katherine A. Houpt
Consulting Editor Debra F. Horwitz

POLYPOID CYSTITIS

BASICS

OVERVIEW
Polypoid cystitis is a chronic inflammatory condition of the urinary bladder characterized by villous or polypoid protrusions from the mucosa. Polypoid projections are diffusely located over the bladder surface and can cause mucosal ulceration, which results in intermittent hematuria. The gross appearance of polyps cannot be distinguished from that of bladder neoplasms such as transitional cell carcinoma (TCC). Polypoid cystitis in dogs is due to chronic irritation of the mucosa from either infection or inflammation, and has been reported secondary to urinary catheterization in humans. Signs are related to the mucosal irritation and include pollakiuria, dysuria, and hematuria.

SIGNALMENT
• Dogs
• No reported cases in cats
• The populations at risk are dogs with chronic urinary tract infections (UTI) or urolithiasis.

SIGNS
• May be initially asymptomatic
• Hematuria is the most common sign.
• Pollakiuria and dysuria may also be present and are due to physical irritation of the polyps.
• Urethral obstruction could occur if enough polyps are located in the trigone area of the bladder.
• Ureteral obstruction may occur if polyps surround the ureteral orifice.

CAUSES & RISK FACTORS
• Causes for polypoid cystitis in dogs have not been well documented but may be associated with UTI or urolithiasis.
• Chronic infection and inflammation secondary to indwelling urinary catheters have been related to cases of polypoid cystitis in humans.

DIAGNOSIS

DIFFERENTIAL DIAGNOSIS
• Polypoid cystitis should be considered in cases of hematuria, pollakiuria, dysuria, and recurrent UTI.
• Bladder neoplasms (such as TCC), UTI, and urolithiasis are the major differential diagnoses.

CBC/BIOCHEMISTRY/URINALYSIS
• Serum biochemistry should be normal in most cases of polypoid cystitis unless concurrent pyelonephritis is present, causing azotemia.
• Urinalysis will reveal hematuria, pyuria, and transitional epithelial cells.

OTHER LABORATORY TESTS
• Urine should be cultured by sterile catheterization or at the time of cystoscopy, but not by cystocentesis until TCC has been ruled out. This will prevent potential abdominal spread of TCC.
• At cystoscopy or cystotomy, polyps should be submitted for both histopathology and culture (including aerobic and anaerobic bacteria and *Mycoplasma* spp.).

IMAGING
• Plain radiographs may show a normal bladder or may reveal concurrent urolithiasis.
• Double-contrast cystography or positive contrast cystography may reveal irregular polyploid masses in the bladder lumen and/or a thickened bladder wall. The most common location of involvement is the cranioventral bladder wall. Single large polyps with a narrow or broad base occur rarely.
• Urinary tract ultrasound may show polypoid/mass-like lesions along the mucosal surface of the bladder, especially in the cranioventral aspect.

DIAGNOSTIC PROCEDURES
Cystoscopy or cystotomy is essential for obtaining a histopathologic diagnosis of polypoid cystitis. Cystotomy or cystoscopy will show erythematous, polypoid lesions over the bladder surface that cannot be visually differentiated from TCC. Cystoscopic biopsies should be obtained by removal of polyps by biopsy forceps at the base of the polyp as close to the bladder wall as possible. Full-thickness biopsies may be required to definitively exclude TCC.

PATHOLOGIC FINDINGS
• Gross changes in the bladder reveal single or multiple small masses ranging from 1 to 10 mm in size. The masses may be nodular or pedunculated on a stalk.
• Histopathologic changes reveal polypoid projection of hyperplastic epithelium that covers a core of proliferative connective tissue with edema, congestion, and inflammation.

TREATMENT

• Remove the polyps either by cystoscopy or cystotomy. Polyps can be individually removed or cauterized at cystoscopy or cystotomy.
• Partial cystectomy may be required to remove the affected area of the bladder.
• Treatment of the underlying cause for the chronic inflammation may prevent further recurrence of the polyps.
• Effective treatment of concurrent UTI is essential.

MEDICATIONS

DRUG(S)

Select an antibiotic based on culture of urine and polyp tissue. The patient should receive antibiotic therapy for a minimum of four to six weeks.

CONTRAINDICATIONS/POSSIBLE INTERACTIONS

N/A

FOLLOW-UP

PATIENT MONITORING

• A urine culture should be performed 7 to 10 days after antimicrobial therapy is initiated, to confirm urine sterility. Follow-up urinalysis and urine cultures should also be performed by cystocentesis 7 days after antimicrobial therapy has ceased and one month post therapy.
• Ultrasonographic reevaluation of the urinary tract is recommended at 1, 3, and 6 months.

PREVENTION/AVOIDANCE

Control of predisposing factors such as UTI and urolithiasis.

POSSIBLE COMPLICATIONS

• Chronic UTIs
• Possibility of pyelonephritis
• Complete obstruction of ureters or urethra

EXPECTED COURSE AND PROGNOSIS

• The expected course is favorable and the prognosis good for these cases if the underlying cause is treated.
• Rarely patients with polypoid cystitis have developed TCC several years after initial diagnosis. It is unknown if some of these cases could be early carcinoma in situ.

MISCELLANEOUS

ASSOCIATED CONDITIONS

• Urinary tract infection, which can also predispose to pyelonephritis
• Urolithiasis

AGE-RELATED FACTORS

No age-related factors have been reported.

SEE ALSO

• Hematuria
• Transitional Cell Carcinoma, Renal Bladder, Urethra
• Urinary Tract Infections
• Urinary Tract Obstruction
• Urolithiasis

ABBREVIATIONS

• TCC = transitional cell carcinoma
• UTI = urinary tract infection

Suggested Reading

Cooper JE, Brearley MJ. Urothelial abnormalities in the dog. Vet Rec 1986;118:513–514.
Johnstone SD, Osborne CA, Stevens JB. Canine polyploid cystitis. J Am Vet Med Assoc 1975;166:1155–1160.

Authors Kate E. Hill and Larry G. Adams
Consulting Editors Larry G. Adams and Carl A. Osborne

POLYURIA AND POLYDIPSIA

 BASICS

DEFINITION
• Polyuria—greater than normal urine production (dogs, > 45 mL/kg/day; cats, > 40 mL/kg/day) • Polydipsia—greater than normal water consumption (dogs, > 90 mL/kg/day; cats, > 45 mL/kg/day)

PATHOPHYSIOLOGY
• Urine production and water consumption (thirst) are controlled by interactions between the kidneys, pituitary gland, and hypothalamus. Volume receptors within the cardiac atria and aortic arch also influence thirst and urine production. Polyuria may occur when the quantity of functional antidiuretic hormone (ADH) synthesized in the hypothalamus or released from the posterior pituitary is limited or when the kidneys fail to respond normally to ADH. Polydipsia occurs when the thirst center in the anterior hypothalamus is stimulated. • In most patients, polydipsia occurs as a compensatory response to polyuria to maintain hydration. The patient's plasma becomes relatively hypertonic and activates thirst mechanisms. Occasionally, polydipsia is the primary process and polyuria is the compensatory response. Then, the patient's plasma becomes relatively hypotonic because of excessive water intake, and ADH secretion is reduced, resulting in polyuria.

SYSTEMS AFFECTED
• Renal/urologic—kidneys • Endocrine-metabolic—pituitary gland and hypothalamus • Cardiovascular—alterations in "effective" circulating volume

SIGNALMENT
• Dogs and cats • Congenital (e.g., central diabetes insipidus, nephrogenic diabetes insipidus, portal-vascular anomalies, and certain renal diseases), hypoadrenocorticism, and some causes of primary polydipsia predominantly affect young dogs. • Renal failure, hyperadrenocorticism, hyperthyroidism, and neoplastic disorders affecting the pituitary and hypothalamus predominantly affect middle-aged and older dogs and cats.

SIGNS
N/A

CAUSES
• Primary polyuria due to impaired renal response to ADH—renal failure, hyperadrenocorticism (dogs), hyperthyroidism (cats), pyelonephritis, leptospirosis, hypoadrenocorticism, pyometra, hepatic failure, hypercalcemia, hypokalemia, renal medullary solute washout, dietary protein restriction, drugs, congenital nephrogenic diabetes insipidus • Primary polyuria caused by osmotic diuresis—diabetes mellitus, primary renal glucosuria, postobstructive diuresis, some diuretics (e.g., mannitol and furosemide), ingestion or administration of large quantities of solute (e.g., sodium chloride or glucose), and hypersomatotropism • Primary polyuria due to ADH deficiency—idiopathic, traumatic, neoplastic, or congenital-origin central diabetes insipidus; some drugs (e.g., alcohol and phenytoin) • Primary polydipsia—behavioral problem, pyrexia, pain, or organic disease of the anterior hypothalamic thirst center of neoplastic, traumatic, or inflammatory origin

RISK FACTORS
• Renal disease or liver disease • Selected endocrine and electrolyte disorders • Administration of diuretics, corticosteroids, and anticonvulsants • Low-protein diets designed for dissolution of struvite uroliths in dogs • Young, hyperactive, large-breed dogs appear to be at higher than normal risk for primary polydipsia.

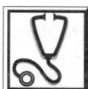 DIAGNOSIS

DIFFERENTIAL DIAGNOSIS

Differentiating Similar Signs
• Differentiate polyuria from an abnormal increase in the frequency of urination (pollakiuria). Pollakiuria is often associated with dysuria, stranguria, or hematuria. Patients with polyuria void large quantities of urine; patients with pollakiuria typically void small quantities of urine. Confirm polyuria/polydipsia by measuring 24-hr water intake or urine output (a 3- to 5-day collection period is used to increase reliability). • Alternatively, measuring urinary specific gravity may provide evidence of adequate urine-concentrating ability (dogs, 1.030; cats, 1.035), which rules out polyuria/polydipsia.

Differentiating Causes
• Renal failure, hyperadrenocorticism, and diabetes mellitus are common causes of polyuria/polydipsia in dogs. Renal failure, hyperthyroidism, and diabetes mellitus are common causes of polyuria/polydipsia in cats. Rule out these conditions before seeking less common disorders. • If associated with progressive weight loss—consider renal failure, diabetes mellitus, hyperthyroidism, hepatic failure, pyometra, pyelonephritis, and malignancy-induced hypercalcemia • If associated with polyphagia—consider diabetes mellitus, hyperthyroidism, and hyperadrenocorticism • If associated with bilateral alopecia and other cutaneous problems—consider hyperadrenocorticism and other endocrinologic disorders • If associated with uremic breath and uremic stomatitis—consider renal failure • If associated with vomiting—consider renal failure, hypoadrenocorticism, pyelonephritis, hepatic failure, hypercalcemia, hypokalemia, hyperthyroidism, and diabetes mellitus; occasionally, vomiting occurs after rapid consumption of a large quantity of water • If associated with recent estrus (within the previous 2 months) in a middle aged intact female—consider pyometra • If associated with abdominal distention—consider hepatic failure, hyperadrenocorticism, pyometra, and nephrotic syndrome • If associated with lymphadenopathy or anal sac mass—consider hypercalcemia of malignancy • If associated with palpable thyroid nodule—consider hyperthyroidism • If associated with hypertensive retinopathy—consider renal failure, hyperthyroidism, diabetes mellitus, and hyperadrenocorticism • If associated with behavioral or neurologic disorder—consider hepatic failure, primary polydipsia, or central diabetes insipidus • If associated with marked polydipsia, in which patients almost continuously seek and consume water from any source—consider primary polydipsia, central diabetes insipidus, and congenital nephrogenic diabetes insipidus

CBC/BIOCHEMISTRY/URINALYSIS
• Serum sodium concentration may help differentiate primary polyuria from primary polydipsia. Measuring serum osmolality is preferred; calculated serum osmolality is not an acceptable substitute. • Relative hypernatremia or high serum osmolarity suggests primary polyuria (values typically trend to or exceed the high end of the normal range). • Hyponatremia or low serum osmolarity suggests primary polydipsia (values typically trend to or decline below the normal range), except in animals with hypoadrenocorticism, which have hyponatremia and primary polyuria.
• Azotemia is consistent with renal causes for polyuria/polydipsia but may also indicate dehydration resulting from inadequate compensatory polydipsia. • Unexpectedly low BUN concentrations suggest hepatic failure.
• High hepatic enzyme activities are consistent with hyperadrenocorticism (especially when the value for ALP exceeds that for ALT), hyperthyroidism, hepatic failure, pyometra, and diabetes mellitus. Administration of some drugs that promote polyuria/polydipsia (e.g., anticonvulsants and corticosteroids) elevates hepatic enzyme activities. • Persistent hyperglycemia is consistent with diabetes mellitus. • Hyperkalemia, particularly if associated with hyponatremia, suggests possible hypoadrenocorticism or therapy with potassium-sparing diuretics. • Hypercalcemia and hypokalemia can cause, or occur in association with, other diseases that cause polyuria/polydipsia (e.g., chronic renal failure may be associated with both; hypoadrenocorticism may be associated with hypercalcemia).
• Hypercalcemia induces polyuria only when it results from increased ionized calcium concentration. • Hypoalbuminemia supports renal or hepatic causes of polyuria/polydipsia.
• Neutrophilia is consistent with pyelonephritis, pyometra, hyper-

adrenocorticism, and corticosteroid administration. • Urinary specific gravity values between 1.001 and 1.003 particularly suggest primary polydipsia, central diabetes insipidus, or congenital nephrogenic diabetes insipidus. • Glucosuria supports a diagnosis of diabetes mellitus or renal glucosuria; pyuria, white blood cell casts, and/or bacteriuria should prompt consideration of pyelonephritis.

OTHER LABORATORY TESTS

• ACTH stimulation or dexamethasone suppression tests to rule out hyperadreno-corticism in middle-aged to older dogs in which initial findings do not explain polyuria/polydipsia.
• Serum thyroxine concentration to rule out hyperthyroidism in middle-aged and old cats
• Urine culture—chronic pyelonephritis cannot be conclusively ruled out by absence of pyuria or bacteriuria.
• Cytologic examination of lymph node aspirate may provide evidence of lymphosarcoma, which induces polyuria by hypercalcemic nephrotoxicity or direct infiltration of renal tissues.

IMAGING

Abdominal survey radiography and ultrasonography may provide additional evidence of renal (e.g., primary renal diseases and urinary obstruction), hepatic (e.g., microhepatica, portal vascular anomalies, and hepatic infiltrate), adrenal (e.g., adrenal mass or bilateral adrenal hypertrophy suggesting hyperadrenocorticism), or uterine (e.g., pyometra) disorders that can contribute to polyuria/polydipsia.

DIAGNOSTIC PROCEDURES

Modified Water Deprivation with ADH Response Testing (see Appendix)

• Differentiates central diabetes insipidus from primary polydipsia and nephrogenic diabetes insipidus. Rule out other causes for polyuria/polydipsia before performing this test.
• Most useful for patients with marked polyuria/polydipsia and hyposthenuria
• Water deprivation testing is contraindicated in dehydrated and azotemic patients, but ADH response testing may be performed safely in these patients.
• Patients that concentrate urine adequately in response to water deprivation are presumed to have primary polydipsia.
• Patients that fail to concentrate urine adequately in response to properly designed water deprivation tests but further concentrate their urine in response to administration of exogenous ADH have central diabetes insipidus.
• Patients that fail to concentrate urine adequately in response to water deprivation and also fail to further concentrate urine in response to administration of exogenous ADH have nephrogenic diabetes insipidus.

TREATMENT

• Serious medical consequence for the patient is rare if patient has free access to water and is willing and able to drink. Until the mechanism of polyuria is understood, discourage owners from limiting access to water. Direct treatment at the underlying cause.
• Provide polyuric patients with free access to water unless they are vomiting. If polyuric patients are vomiting, give replacement maintenance fluids parenterally. Also provide fluids parenterally when other conditions limit oral intake or dehydration persists despite polydipsia.
• Base fluid selection on knowledge of the underlying cause for fluid loss. In most patients, lactated Ringer's solution is an acceptable replacement fluid.
• When dehydration has resulted from withholding water, or when urine is hyposthenuric, providing oral water or parenteral administration of dextrose 5% in water may be preferred to lactated Ringer's solution.
• Primary polydipsia—treat by gradually limiting water intake to a normal daily volume. It may be necessary to reduce water intake over days to weeks to avoid such undesirable behavior as increased barking, urine consumption, or other patterns of bizarre behavior. Monitor the patient closely to avoid iatrogenic dehydration. Salt (1 g/30 kg q12h) or sodium bicarbonate (0.6 g/30 kg q12h) may be given orally to help reestablish the renal medullary solute gradient. Consider behavior modification if water restriction alone is unsuccessful.

MEDICATIONS

DRUG(S) OF CHOICE
Vary with underlying cause

CONTRAINDICATIONS
Do not administer ADH (or any of its synthetic analogs, such as DDAVP) to patients with primary polydipsia because of the risk of inducing water intoxication.

PRECAUTIONS
Until renal and hepatic failure have been excluded as potential causes for polyuria/polydipsia, use caution in administering any drug eliminated via these pathways.

POSSIBLE INTERACTIONS
N/A

ALTERNATIVE DRUG(S)
N/A

FOLLOW-UP

PATIENT MONITORING
• Hydration status by clinical assessment of hydration and serial evaluation of body weight
• Fluid intake and urine output—provide a useful baseline for assessing adequacy of hydration therapy

POSSIBLE COMPLICATIONS
Dehydration

MISCELLANEOUS

ASSOCIATED CONDITIONS
• Bacterial urinary tract infection—patients appear to be at particular risk of developing urinary tract infection as a consequence of urinary catheterization • Urinary incontinence may develop in dogs with concurrent urethral sphincter dysfunction, presumably because of increased bladder-filling associated with polyuria.

AGE-RELATED FACTORS
N/A

ZOONOTIC POTENTIAL
N/A

PREGNANCY
N/A

SYNONYMS
N/A

SEE ALSO
• Congenital and Developmental Renal Disorders • Diabetes Insipidus • Diabetes Mellitus • Fanconi Syndrome • Hepatic Failure, Acute • Hyperadrenocorticism • Hypercalcemia • Hyperthyroidism • Hypoadrenocorticism • Hypokalemia • Portovascular Anomalies • Pyelonephritis • Pyometra • Renal Failure, Acute and Chronic • Urinary Tract Obstruction

ABBREVIATIONS
• ADH = antidiuretic hormone
• ALP = alkaline phosphatase
• ALT = alanine aminotransferase
• BUN = blood urea nitrogen
• DDAVP = trademark for preparation of vasopressin

Suggested Reading
Feldman EC, Nelson RW. Canine and feline endocrinology and reproduction. Philadelphia: Saunders, 1996:2–37.
Meric SM. Polyuria and polydipsia. In: Ettinger SJ, Feldman EC, eds. Textbook of veterinary internal medicine. Philadelphia: Saunders, 2000:85–89.
Author David J. Polzin
Consulting Editors Larry G. Adams and Carl A. Osborne

PORTOSYSTEMIC SHUNTING, ACQUIRED

BASIC

OVERVIEW
Acquired portosystemic shunts (APSS) develop subsequent to portal hypertension

SIGNALMENT
• Most common—dogs with chronic liver disease; also occurs in dogs with juvenile fibrosing liver disease, noncirrhotic portal hypertension; dogs with PSVA unable to accommodate surgical ligation • Cats—with end stage of fibrosing form of polycystic liver disease or severe cholangiohepatitis syndrome; with portal venous atresia or hypoplasia; unable to accommodate surgical ligation of PSVA • Dogs and cats—subsequent to chronic (> 6 weeks) extrahepatic bile duct obstruction • Certain disorders—have age or breed incidence (See Juvenile Fibrosing Liver Disease; Cirrhosis and Fibrosis of the Liver; Hepatitis, Chronic Active); polycystic disease in cats more common in Persians and Himalayans

SIGNS
• Clinical signs represent sequelae of impaired hepatic function and portosystemic shunting; depend on chronicity of underlying disorder • Episodic hepatic encephalopathy—predominates; may include neurobehavioral abnormalities, blindness, polyuria and polydipsia, anorexia, lethargy, vomiting, and neurologic signs that localize to the cerebrum or brain stem or suggest a transverse myelopathy; signs often improve with fluid therapy (with dextrose and potassium), broad-spectrum antibiotics, lactulose, and dietary protein restriction (see Hepatic Encephalopathy) • Ascites—common; waxes and wanes • Hypertensive splanchnic vasculopathy—associated with gastroduodenal ulceration; may progress to perforation and septic peritonitis, life-endangering blood loss due to coexistent coagulopathy, or severe hepatic encephalopathy because of potent encephalogenic effect of enteric blood; causes anorexia, vomiting, diarrhea, and abdominal pain • Urogenital—obstructive uropathy due to ammonium biurate urolithiasis: hematuria; pollakiuria; dysuria

CAUSES & RISK FACTORS
• Multiple tortuous vessels—represent circulatory engagement of normally present but unused vascular channels bridging between the splanchnic and systemic circulatory beds • Lack of valves in the portal vein—allows blood to follow "a path of least resistance" • Portal hypertension—resulting from many disease processes: importantly, diffuse hepatic fibrosis with or without cirrhosis; chronic unresolved extrahepatic bile duct occlusion (> 6 weeks); other causes,

including portal venous thromboembolism, idiopathic portal hypertension, and hepatic sinusoidal outflow obstruction (zone 3, hepatic venous, vena caval involvement); less commonly, disorders impairing perfusion of the splanchnic segment of portal vein (thromboembolism, stricture, strangulation) and, rarely, hypoplasia of portal vein (lack of development internal or external to the liver as a congenital malformation) and congenital or acquired hepatic AV fistula(e) (that arterialize the portal circulation); see Hypertension, Portal • May lead to episodic development of hepatic encephalopathy associated with ingestion of high-protein food, enteric hemorrhage (bleeding tendencies), azotemia, alkalemia, electrolyte disturbances, blood transfusions or hemolysis, infections, and administration of certain drugs • Hyperammonemia and impaired transformation of uric acid to water-soluble allantoin results in ammonium urate urolithiasis.

DIAGNOSIS

DIFFERENTIAL DIAGNOSIS
• CNS signs—infectious disorders (e.g., FIP, canine distemper, toxoplasmosis, FeLV- or FIV-related infections); toxicities (e.g., lead, mushrooms, recreational drugs); hydrocephalus; idiopathic epilepsy; metabolic disorders (e.g., severe hypoglycemia, hypokalemia or hyperkalemia, hypocalcemia) • Gastrointestinal signs—bowel obstruction; dietary indiscretion; foreign body ingestion; inflammatory bowel disease • Urinary tract signs—bacterial urinary tract infection; urolithiasis • Polyuria and polydipsia—disorders of urine concentration (e.g., diabetes insipidus, abnormal adrenal function, hypercalcemia, primary polydipsia, congenital or acquired renal disease) • Causes of abdominal effusion—cardiopulmonary disorders causing right-sided heart failure; pericardial disease; primary inflammatory hepatopathies; infiltrative hepatic disease (e.g., neoplasia, amyloid); nonhepatic abdominal disorders associated with effusions (e.g., splenic torsion, visceral neoplasia, carcinomatosis); or peritonitis: chemical (e.g., bile, urine, chyle) or septic

CBC/BIOCHEMISTRY/URINALYSIS
• CBC—microcytosis reflects portosystemic shunting; mild nonregenerative anemia common; poikilocytosis (cats); target cells (dogs)
• Biochemistry—low BUN, low to normal creatinine, glucose, albumin, and cholesterol are common; liver enzyme activity variable (ALP usually high in young patients [bone isoenzyme]); bilirubin may be high; changes depend on underlying cause • Urinalysis—

variable urine concentration; ammonium urate crystalluria, hematuria, pyuria, and proteinuria due to mechanical inflammation/infection secondary to urolithiasis

OTHER LABORATORY TESTS
• TSBA—sensitive indicators; normal to modestly high fasting and markedly high postprandial values (postprandial TSBA usually > 100 μmol/L) suggest a "shunting pattern" • Blood ammonia values—sensitive indicators for hepatic encephalopathy; however, less reliable than TSBA because of analytic/methodologic issues (samples cannot be frozen or mailed for analyses; analytic reactions unstable) • Ammonia tolerance testing—most reliable method of demonstrating hyperammonemia; **Caution:** may promote iatrogenic hepatic encephalopathy • Coagulation tests—increased PT, APTT, and PIVKA reflect severity of liver dysfunction, synthetic failure, DIC, and vitamin K adequacy; PIVKA useful in deciding on need for supplemental vitamin K therapy • Abdominal effusion—usually a pure or modified transudate; high serum albumin:effusion albumin ratio (> 1.1), consistent with portal hypertension

IMAGING

Abdominal Radiography
• Liver size depends on underlying cause; microhepatica: common in dogs with chronic liver disease or variant of PSVA causing ascites; variable in cats • Abdominal effusion • Ammonium urate calculi—radiolucent unless combined with radiodense minerals

Radiographic Portovenography
Demonstrates multiple APSS; usually detected by ultrasonography; not a recommended procedure as associated with morbid side effects

Abdominal Ultrasonography
• Liver size depends on underlying cause • Discloses altered parenchymal and biliary tract echogenicity • Portosystemic collaterals—well defined by color-flow Doppler interrogation confirming hepatofugal portal flow; tortuous acquired shunts typically adjacent to kidneys or spleen • Abdominal effusion • Uroliths may be observed in renal pelvis or urinary bladder • Intrahepatic AV fistula—pulsating vascular structure within enlarged liver lobe, along with abdominal effusion and APSS; see Arteriovenous Malformation of Liver • Color-flow Doppler may detect portal thrombi

Colorectal Scintigraphy
• Sensitive and noninvasive test • Confirms presence of portosystemic shunting; cannot differentiate PSVA from APSS • Administer technetium-99m pertechnetate rectally; gamma camera imaging determines rate of isotope appearance in liver versus heart; calculate shunt fraction from time/activity plots ($\leq$ 15% is normal)

DIAGNOSTIC PROCEDURES

Fine-needle Aspiration Cytology

• Hepatic aspiration—22-gauge needle aspirates cannot differentiate disorders causing portosystemic shunting • Liver biopsy—open surgical wedge biopsy or laparoscopic sampling (cup biopsy forceps); obtaining tissue from several liver lobes is advised; inadequate tissue sampling to confirm a definitive diagnosis may occur with core needle biopsy technique

PATHOLOGIC FINDINGS

• Gross—small, irregularly contoured liver with chronic liver disease (cirrhosis, fibrosis) • Normal to large size in early venous outflow obstruction (Budd-Chiari, venoocclusive disease); normal size if portal venous thrombi present; small liver if congenital portal atresia present • Large liver lobe (remainder of liver normal to small size) with hepatic AV fistula • Normal to small—idiopathic portal hypertension or noncirrhotic portal hypertension

 TREATMENT

APPROPRIATE HEALTH CARE

Inpatient—severe signs of hepatic encephalopathy; for supportive care

NURSING CARE

• See Hepatic Encephalopathy

DIET

• Nutritional support—essential to maintain body condition and optimal management of hepatic encephalopathy; balanced, restricted-protein diet important; protein allocation titrated to patient response in combination with treatments ameliorating hepatic encephalopathy; use commercial diet formulated for liver disease or moderate renal insufficiency; dogs: dairy and soy protein best sources; cats: pure carnivores must have meat-derived protein; titrated protein with 0.5 g/kg allocation additions, adjustments every 5–7 days; use cottage cheese or calcium caseinate in dogs • Optimize dietary protein tolerance—see Hepatic Encephalopathy. • Parenteral nutrition—see Hepatic Encephalopathy

CLIENT EDUCATION

• Depends on underlying cause • Warn client about signs of hepatic encephalopathy and potential for ammonium biurate obstructive uropathy in males; male dogs may require permanent prescrotal urethrostomy. • Educate client on how to use diuretics on an as-needed basis to mobilize abdominal effusion. • Educate client on how to adjust oral medications and enemas on an as-needed basis to ameliorate hepatic encephalopathy

 MEDICATIONS

DRUG(S)

• Enteric hemorrhage—associated with hypertensive splanchnic vasculopathy (ulcerations in gastroduodenal region) and coagulopathy; no evidence that prophylactic use of acid blockers or gastroprotectants reduces risk; treat symptomatic animal with H_2blocker (famotidine preferred) and sucralfate; may require critical care for blood component and DDAVP therapy (see Coagulopathy of Liver Disease) • Abdominal effusion—sequentially measure body weight and girth; enforce exercise restriction (improves renal perfusion and sodium and water elimination), dietary sodium restriction, diuretics (combined use of furosemide and spironolactone); furosemide (0.5–2 mg/kg PO q12–24h) and spironolactone (0.5–2 mg/kg PO q12h, use a single doubled dose for loading one time): dose titrations based on response every 4 days using 25%–50% dose increases; therapeutic abdominocentesis used when ascites resistant to conservative measures or compromises food intake, ventilation, or sleep: requires aseptic technique, concurrent polyionic fluid and colloid administration optimize safety.

PRECAUTIONS

• Remain aware of altered drug metabolism related to reduced first-pass extraction (portosystemic shunting), altered hepatic metabolism/biotransformation, and reduced protein binding (if hypoalbuminemic). • Remain vigilant for diuretic-induced dehydration and electrolyte dysregulation.

POSSIBLE INTERACTIONS

• Avoid metoclopramide if using spironolactone (blocks effect); avoid nonsteroidal antiinflammatory drugs as these may inhibit furosemide-induced diuresis and potentiate renal injury.

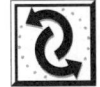 FOLLOW-UP

PATIENT MONITORING

• Reevaluate patient's at-home behavior as a reflection of hepatic encephalopathy. • Monitor clinical signs, appetite, body condition and weight, abdominal girth, CBC, serum biochemistry, and urine (ammonium biurate crystalluria); TSBA not useful for sequential evaluation as these are consistently high in patients with APSS and patients treated with ursodeoxycholic acid (drug measured in the assay). • Adjust medical management to reduce episodic hepatic encephalopathy, ammonium urate crystalluria and potential for urolith formation, and

occurrence of abdominal effusion. • Inspect patient carefully for evidence of clinical bleeding; determine need for intermittent chronic vitamin K administration by parenteral route (PIVKA test).

PREVENTION/AVOIDANCE

• Early treatment of acquired liver disease and expedient correction of EHBDO to minimize hepatic fibrosis and remodeling • Careful consideration of the propriety of complete ligation of PSVA either by surgical or ameroid band techniques

POSSIBLE COMPLICATIONS

• Treat underlying disorder • Enteric hemorrhage due to hypertensive vasculopathy; may require acute intensive care to manage hypovolemia, coagulopathy, and ensuing hepatic encephalopathy and surgical resection of involved gut segment • Dehydration, contraction alkalosis, azotemia—complications of diuretics • Death—from liver failure, complications of hepatic encephalopathy, hepatic coma, lethal enteric hemorrhage, or sepsis

EXPECTED COURSE AND PROGNOSIS

• Varies with the underlying cause • Management of chronic liver disease or hepatic fibrosis using a polypharmacy approach seemingly extends life. • Animals with noncirrhotic portal hypertension and juvenile hepatic fibrosis may live > 8 years if managed successfully during initial symptomatic interval and if definitive diagnosis is ascertained.

 MISCELLANEOUS

ASSOCIATED CONDITIONS

• Ammonium urate urolithiasis • Ascites • Coagulopathy • Hepatic Encephalopathy • Enteric bleeding/ulceration • Obstructive uropathy

SYNONYMS

Portovascular anastomosis

SEE ALSO

• Ascites • Cirrhosis and Fibrosis of the Liver • Coagulopathy of Liver Disease • Hepatic Encephalopathy • Hepatitis, Chronic Active • Juvenile Fibrosing Liver Disease • Portosystemic Vascular Anomaly, Congenital

ABBREVIATIONS

• APSS = acquired portosystemic shunt • APTT = activated partial thromboplastin time • AV = arteriovenous • EHBDO = extrahepatic bile duct obstruction • PIVKA = proteins invoked by vitamin K absence or antagonism • PSVA = portosystemic vascular anomaly • PT = prothrombin time • TSBA = total serum bile acids

Author Sharon A. Center
Consulting Editor Sharon A. Center

PORTOSYSTEMIC VASCULAR ANOMALY, CONGENITAL

 BASICS

DEFINITION
• Congenital PSVA—venous malformations bridging the portal and systemic circulations that permit portal blood to circumvent the liver (hepatofugal circulation); may be intra-hepatic or extrahepatic; most are single vessels; patients may also have portal venous hypoplasia external to or within the liver
• APSS—develop subsequent to portal hypertension; see Portosystemic Shunting, Acquired

PATHOPHYSIOLOGY
• Hepatofugal circulation—eliminates hepatocellular cleansing of portal blood that contains toxins derived from the gut; deprives liver of gut-derived hepatotrophic substances, resulting in microhepatica • Usually episodic hepatic encephalopathy associated with ingestion of high-protein food, gastrointestinal bleeding, dehydration, azotemia, alkalosis, electrolyte disturbances, blood transfusion, hemolysis, infections, catabolism, and administration of certain drugs • Hyperammonemia and impaired transformation of uric acid to water-soluble allantoin: ammonium urate crystalluria or calculi

SYSTEMS AFFECTED
• Nervous—episodic hepatic encephalopathy
• Gastrointestinal—intermittent inappetence; vomiting; diarrhea; pica; ptyalism (cats)
• Urogenital—large kidneys (especially in dogs); ammonium urate urolithiasis; 50% of males dogs cryptorchid

GENETICS
• Kindreds affected—Yorkshire terriers, cairn terriers, Maltese, miniature schnauzers, Irish wolfhounds; Old English sheepdogs
• Suspected polygenic trait

INCIDENCE/PREVALENCE
Relatively uncommon

GEOGRAPHIC DISTRIBUTION
Reported in North America, Japan, Europe

SIGNALMENT

Species
Dogs and cats

Breed Predilections
• Higher risk—purebred dogs; mixed-breed cats • Especially common in Yorkshire terriers, Maltese dogs • Extrahepatic PSVA—small-breed dogs; cats • Intrahepatic PSVA—large-breed dogs

Mean Age and Range
Usually in young animals; 4 weeks to 12 years

Predominant Sex N/A

SIGNS

Historical Findings
• Episodic hepatic encephalopathy—predominates; episodes transiently improve with fluid therapy, broad-spectrum antibiotics, and lactulose • Cats initially thought to have upper respiratory infection based on display of ptyalism • Signs initiate with weaning of puppy or kitten to commercial food • Stunted growth common • CNS signs—weakness; pacing; ataxia; disorientation; head pressing; blindness; behavioral changes: aggression (cats), vocalization, hallucinations; seizures; coma • Gastrointestinal signs—inappetence; vomiting; diarrhea; pica • Urinary signs—polyuria and polydipsia; ammonium urate crystalluria: pollakiuria, dysuria; hematuria; urethral (rarely ureteral) urolith obstruction

Physical Examination Findings
Normal appearance; stunted stature; microhepatica; hepatic encephalopathy; golden- or copper-colored irises in non–blue-eyed and non-Persian cats; ascites and edema (rare)

CAUSES
• Congenital malformations • APSS in animals with congenital PSVA—develop subsequent to congenital or surgically induced portal hypertension; rare portal atresia in dogs, more common in cats

RISK FACTORS
PSVA—purebred dogs, especially terrier-type breeds; particular kindreds may be affected

 DIAGNOSIS

DIFFERENTIAL DIAGNOSES
• CNS signs—infectious disorders (e.g., FIP, canine distemper, toxoplasmosis, FeLV- or FIV-related infections); toxicities (e.g., lead, mushrooms, recreational drugs); hydrocephalus; idiopathic epilepsy; metabolic disorders (e.g., severe hypoglycemia, hypokalemia or hyperkalemia, hypocalcemia)
• Gastrointestinal signs—bowel obstruction; dietary indiscretion; foreign body ingestion; inflammatory bowel disease • Urinary tract signs—bacterial urinary tract infection; urolithiasis • Polyuria and polydipsia—disorders of urine concentration (e.g., diabetes insipidus, abnormal adrenal function, hypercalcemia, primary polydipsia)
• Primary liver disease—distinguished via diagnostic imaging and liver biopsy
• Abnormal liver function suggesting PSVA but lacking macroscopic shunt—hepatoportal MVD • APSS—many differentials; see Portosystemic Shunting, Acquired

CBC/BIOCHEMISTRY/URINALYSIS
• CBC—microcytosis; mild nonregenerative anemia; poikilocytosis (cats); target cells (dogs) • Biochemistry—low BUN, creatinine, glucose, and cholesterol common; liver enzyme activity variable (ALP usually high in young patients [bone isoenzyme]); bilirubin normal, hypoalbuminemia inconsistent and mild • Urinalysis—dilute urine; ammonium urate crystalluria, hematuria, pyuria, and proteinuria due to mechanical inflammation and infection secondary to metabolic calculi

OTHER LABORATORY TESTS
• TSBA—sensitive indicators; random fasting values may be within normal reference range; 2-hr postprandial values markedly high (usually > 100 μmol/L) • Blood ammonia values—sensitive indicators for hepatic encephalopathy and shunting but less reliable than TSBA in practice because of analytic/methodologic issues (samples for ammonia assay cannot be frozen or mailed for analysis) • Ammonia tolerance testing—most reliable method of demonstrating hyperammonemia; **Caution:** may cause clinical signs of hepatic encephalopathy
• Coagulation tests—dogs: increased APTT and PIVKA usually not associated with bleeding • Abdominal effusion—postsurgical complication; cytologic/physicochemical analysis usually a pure or modified transudate

IMAGING

Abdominal Radiography
• Microhepatica—common in dogs, variable in cats • Renomegaly (PSVA) • Abdominal effusion (APSS) only after surgical ligation in dogs; in some cats with portal atresia before surgery • Ammonium urate urolithiasis—radiolucent unless combined with radiodense mineral shell

Radiographic Portovenography
• Gold standard for confirming PSVA—contrast study outlining portal venous flow via contrast injection into a mesenteric vein, splenic vein, or splenic pulp, or venous phase of cranial mesenteric angiogram or mesenteric phase of jugular systemic contrast injection
• Verifies shunt location—intrahepatic versus extrahepatic; extrahepatic if caudal extent of shunt is caudal to thoracic vertebra 13; intrahepatic if caudal extent of shunt cranial to thoracic vertebra 13

Abdominal Ultrasonography
• Subjective microhepatica; hypovascularity; and observation of shunting vessel • Color-flow Doppler—assists in shunt localization; interrogate vena cava cranial to phrenicoabdominal vein and vena cava junction (turbulence here supports extrahepatic PSVA) • Intrahepatic shunts—easily imaged • Renomegaly • Urolithiasis common (cystic, renal pelvis, rarely ureteral)

Colorectal Scintigraphy
• Sensitive noninvasive test—confirms shunting • Cannot differentiate PSVA and APSS or intra- and extrahepatic PSVA
• Administer technetium-99m pertechnetate rectally; image with gamma camera to determine rate of isotopic appearance in liver versus heart; calculate shunt fraction from time activity plots; shunt fraction ≤ 15% is normal; PSVA shunt fractions usually > 60%

PORTOSYSTEMIC VASCULAR ANOMALY, CONGENITAL

DIAGNOSTIC PROCEDURES
• Fine-needle aspiration cytology—cannot differentiate PSVA • Liver biopsy—open surgical wedge biopsy or laparoscopic sampling (cup biopsy forceps), obtaining tissue from several liver lobes, provides the best diagnostic sampling; inadequate tissue samples common with needle biopsy procedures for confirming PSVA; avoid sampling caudate lobe: fewest lesions

PATHOLOGIC FINDINGS
• Gross—small, smooth-surfaced liver; actual PSVA may be difficult to verify at autopsy; young animals with extrahepatic portal atresia may have multiple APSS; diagnosis of intrahepatic atresia or hypoplasia controversial • Microscopic—small non-perfused portal venules; increased zone 1 and 3 lymphatics; multiple cross-sections of portal arterioles; scattered lipogranulomas containing hemosiderin (variable); lobular atrophy; in some dogs, marked zone 3 vacuolation with apparent lipid and nonsuppurative inflammation impinging on hepatic venule may suggest high surgical risk and/or poor response

TREATMENT

APPROPRIATE HEALTH CARE
Inpatient—severe signs of hepatic encephalopathy; for supportive care and initiation of medical management prior to liver biopsy and surgical ligation

NURSING CARE
Hepatic Encephalopathy
See topic on Hepatic Encephalopathy for patient management.

DIET
• Nutritional support—essential to maintain body condition and optimize hepatic encephalopathy management
• Balanced, protein-restricted diet—recommended; thereafter, protein allocation titrated to response in combination with treatments ameliorating hepatic enceph-alopathy; as tolerated, add 0.5 g/kg protein (use cottage cheese or calcium caseinate in dogs) adjustments observed over 5- to 7-day intervals

CLIENT EDUCATION
• Surgical ligation—expect improvement but may not be curative • Clinical signs—may persist, requiring chronic nutritional and medical management • Surgical/anesthetic risks—10%–29% mortality; depends on surgeon experience and critical care

SURGICAL CONSIDERATIONS
• Surgical PSVA ligation—optimal goal of total ligation; often only partial ligation achieved (surgical decision based on influence of temporary shunt occlusion on portal pressure and splanchnic circulation); surgical assessment of extent of ligation proven inaccurate • Ameroid constrictor—reduces immediate surgical risks of ligation; **Caution:** may later result in APSS in some patients
• Hepatic encephalopathy—should mitigate with medical management before surgery
• Intrahepatic PSVA—most difficult to ligate
• Portography advised for all patients—to verify location of PSVA and ensure correct vessel(s) identified and ligated • Postoperative complications—portal venous thrombi; severe portal hypertension; mesenteric ischemia; endotoxemia; seizures; sepsis; acute pancreatitis; hemorrhage • Intraoperative hypothermia—especially in very small patients; complicates recovery • Emergency surgery—rarely required for ligature removal
• Abdominal effusion—common after shunt ligation; alone, does not indicate pathologic portal hypertension leading to APSS; watch closely for signs of mesenteric ischemia (bloody diarrhea, abdominal pain, failure to recover from surgery/anesthesia, unexplained tachycardia, hyper- or hypothermia); monitor effusion via girth circumference measurements and body weight • Synthetic colloids increase bleeding risks. • ICU monitoring—recommended postoperatively for 72–96 hr

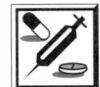

MEDICATIONS

DRUG(S)
See Hepatic Encephalopathy

PRECAUTIONS
Remain aware of altered drug metabolism related to reduced first-pass extraction (portosystemic shunting), altered hepatic metabolism/biotransformation, and reduced protein binding (with hypoalbuminemia)

FOLLOW-UP

PATIENT MONITORING
• Reevaluate—patient's at-home behavior; body condition, girth circumference, (immediately postoperative) and weight; CBC (resolution of microcytosis), biochemistry, and urinalysis (resolution of features under Diagnosis) • TSBA (small-breed dogs)—do not substantiate surgical success; common coexistent MVD

POSSIBLE COMPLICATIONS
See Surgical Considerations

PREVENTION/AVOIDANCE
If multiple portosystemic shunts are identified—do not recommend surgical ligation; likely another underlying liver disease causing portal hypertension; rarely portal atresia/hypoplasia

EXPECTED COURSE AND PROGNOSIS
• Cannot predict individual response
• Dogs—ligation improves signs in 70%–80% • Cats—substantial subset develops APSS • Postsurgery—continue management of hepatic encephalopathy until reevaluation of clinical condition
• Some patients—indefinite treatment of hepatic encephalopathy • Partial ligation—may proceed to full shunt attenuation (scar, stricture, clot formation at site of ligation)
• Ameroid constrictor—may proceed to full ligation within only a few days (twisting after placement); may cause APSS
• Increased risk for poor outcome in certain small dogs (see Pathologic Findings) and cats

MISCELLANEOUS

ASSOCIATED CONDITIONS
• Ammonium urate urolithiasis • Copper-colored iris (cats) • Cryptorchidism (dogs)
• Hepatic encephalopathy

AGE-RELATED FACTORS
PSVA—surgical outcome may be good in young and old patients, especially those with minimal signs of hepatic encephalopathy

PREGNANCY
Affected bitches can carry litters to term.

SYNONYMS
• Portacaval shunt • Portovascular anastomosis

SEE ALSO
• Hepatic Encephalopathy • Juvenile Fibrosing Liver Disease • Portosystemic Shunting, Acquired

ABBREVIATIONS
• APSS = acquired portosystemic shunt
• APTT = activated partial thromboplastin time • MVD = microvascular dysplasia
• PIVKA = proteins invoked by vitamin K absence or antagonism • PSVA = portosystemic vascular anomaly • TSBA = total serum bile acids

Suggested Reading
Center SA. Hepatic vascular diseases. In: Guilford WG, Center SA, Strombeck DR, et al., eds. Strombeck's small animal gastroenterology. 3rd ed. Philadelphia: Saunders, 1996:802–846.
Wolschrijn DF, Mahapokai W, Rothuizen J, et al: Gauged attenuation of congenital portosystemic shunts: results in 160 dogs and 15 cats. Vet Q 2000;22:94–98.
Authors Susan E. Johnson & Sharon Center
Consulting Editor Sharon A. Center

POXVIRUS INFECTION—CATS

BASICS

OVERVIEW
• Member of the genus *Orthopoxvirus,* family Poxviridae
• Enveloped DNA virus, resistant to drying (viable for years) but readily inactivated by most disinfectants
• Geographically limited to Eurasia
• Relatively common

SIGNALMENT
• Cats—domestic and exotic
• No age, sex, or breed predisposition

SIGNS
• Skin lesions—multiple, circular; dominant feature; usually develop on head, neck, or forelimbs
• Primary lesions—crusted papules, plaques, nodules, crateriform ulcers, or areas of cellulitis or abscesses
• Secondary lesions—erythematous nodules that ulcerate and crust; often widespread; develop after 1–3 weeks
• Pruritus variable
• Systemic—20% of cases; anorexia; lethargy; pyrexia; vomiting; diarrhea; oculonasal discharge; conjunctivitis; pneumonia

CAUSES & RISK FACTORS
• Reservoir host—wild rodents
• Infection thought to be acquired during hunting; most common in young adults and active hunters, often from rural environment
• Lesions—often develop at the site of a bite wound (presumably inflicted by the prey animal carrying the virus)
• Most cases occur in autumn, when small wild mammals are at maximum population and most active.
• Severe cutaneous and systemic signs with poor prognosis are frequently associated with immunosuppression (iatrogenic or co-infection with FeLV or FIV).
• Cat-to-cat transmission—rare; causes only subclinical infection

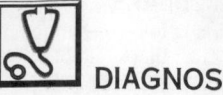

DIAGNOSIS

DIFFERENTIAL DIAGNOSIS
• Bacterial and fungal infections
• Eosinophilic granuloma complex
• Neoplasia—particularly mast cell tumor; lymphosarcoma
• Miliary dermatitis

CBC/BIOCHEMISTRY/URINALYSIS
Noncontributory

OTHER LABORATORY TESTS
Serologic testing—demonstrate rising titers; hemagglutination inhibition, virus neutralizing, complement fixation, or ELISA; titers may remain high for months or years.

IMAGING
N/A

DIAGNOSTIC PROCEDURES
• Virus isolation from scab material—definitive diagnosis; 90% positive

• Electron microscopy of extracts of scab, biopsy, or exudate—rapid presumptive diagnosis; 70% positive
• Skin biopsy—characteristic histologic changes of epidermal hyperplasia and hypertrophy; multilocular vesicle and ulceration; large eosinophilic intracytoplasmic inclusion bodies
• Polymerase chain reaction

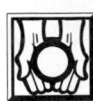 **TREATMENT**

• No specific treatment
• Supportive (antibiotics, fluids) when necessary
• Elizabethan collar—to prevent self-induced damage

 MEDICATIONS

DRUG(S)
Antibiotics—prevent secondary infections

CONTRAINDICATIONS/POSSIBLE INTERACTIONS
Immunosuppressive agents (e.g., gluco-corticoids and megestrol acetate)—absolutely contraindicated because they can induce fatal systemic disease

 FOLLOW-UP

PREVENTION/AVOIDANCE
• Natural reservoir host is possibly small rodents; cats infected incidentally
• Vaccines—none available; vaccinia virus may be considered for valuable zoo collections, but its effects in nondomestic cats have not been investigated

EXPECTED COURSE AND PROGNOSIS
• Most cats recover spontaneously in 1–2 months.
• Healing may be delayed by secondary bacterial skin infection.
• Prognosis is poor with severe respiratory or pulmonary involvement.

 **MISCELLANEOUS**

ZOONOTIC POTENTIAL
• Rare human pox virus infections have been linked to contact with infected cats with skin lesions; use basic hygiene precautions (disposable gloves) when handling infected cats.
• May cause painful skin lesion and severe systemic illness, particularly in the very young or elderly, people with a pre-existing skin condition, and the immunodeficient.

ABBREVIATIONS
• ELISA = enzyme-linked immunosorbent assay
• FeLV = feline leukemia virus
• FIV = feline immunodeficiency virus

Suggested Reading
Gaskell RM, Bennett M. Feline poxvirus infection. In: Chandler EA, Gaskell CJ, Gaskell RM, eds. Feline medicine and therapeutics. Oxford, UK: Blackwell Scientific, 1994:515–520.
Author J. Paul Woods
Consulting Editor Stephen C. Barr

PRIMARY CILIARY DYSKINESIA

BASICS

OVERVIEW
• Congenital disorder caused by ciliary dys-function
• Cilia—complex structures lining various organs, including the upper and lower respiratory tracts, auditory tubes, ventricles of the brain, spinal canal, oviducts, and efferent ducts of the testes; sperm flagellum is a modified cilium.
• Ciliary beating—normally coordinated by an intricate mechanochemical interaction of numerous proteins contained within each cilium; characteristically uncoordinated (dyskinetic) or absent in affected dogs; cilia often, but not invariably, have structural lesions.
• Clinical signs predominate in ciliated organs—lack of mucociliary clearance in the respiratory tract (recurrent bacterial rhino-sinusitis, bronchopneumonia) and auditory canal (secretory otitis media); chronic inflammation and obstruction of the airways (bronchiectasis); male infertility (live but immotile or hypomotile spermatozoa; may also see unexplained oligospermia and azoospermia)
• Hydrocephalus and situs inversus—common but variable features; genesis of these lesions not determined
• Diagnosis—confirmed by demonstrating the absence of tracheal mucociliary clearance and the presence of a specific ultrastructural lesion in respiratory cilia or sperm flagella; established in patients without ultrastructural ciliary lesions by in vitro analysis of ciliary function
• Dogs with chronic respiratory tract disease and situs inversus (e.g., Kartagener syndrome)—in all probability have primary ciliary dyskinesia and do not warrant an extensive workup

SIGNALMENT
• Genetic disease—probable autosomal recessive mode of inheritance
• Signs typically develop at an early age (days to 5 weeks); dogs have remained asymptomatic for prolonged periods (6 months to 10 years).
• Reported only in purebred dogs—Bichon Frises, border collies, bull mastiffs, Chihuahuas, shar peis, chow chows, Dalmatians, Doberman pinschers, English cocker spaniels, English pointers, English setters, English springer spaniels, golden retrievers, Gordon setters, long-haired dachshunds, miniature poodles, Old English sheepdogs, Newfoundlands, and rottweilers

• Kartagener syndrome—unpublished observations in a Norwegian elkhound, a West Highland white terrier, and a domestic shorthair cat

SIGNS

Historical Findings
• Young purebred dog
• Chronic sneezing and coughing—may produce copious amounts of mucoid to mucopurulent material
• Despite dramatic response to antibiotics, patients have continuous serous to mucoid nasal discharge and relapse after treatment is stopped.
• Family history—large litters tend to have > 1 affected animal; progeny from prior matings of the dam and sire may have been affected.
• Fertility—females fertile; males characteristically not

Physical Examination Findings
• Bilateral, mucopurulent nasal discharge
• Moist, productive cough that can be elicited by exercise or tracheal palpation
• Tachypnea, dyspnea, and cyanosis—may be seen
• Diffuse increase in lung sounds of variable intensity—typically auscultated; sounds from the ventral thorax diminish with more advanced lung disease (consolidation).
• Heart sounds—may be inaudible with severe bronchopneumonia; loudest on the right side of thorax with situs inversus totalis (Kartagener syndrome)
• Hydrocephalus—common; but clinical signs (e.g., dome-shaped calvarium and CNS dysfunction) rarely observed

CAUSES & RISK FACTORS
• Genetic disease
• Inbreeding

DIAGNOSIS

DIFFERENTIAL DIAGNOSIS
• Congenital (e.g., neutrophil dysfunction and immunoglobulin deficiency) or acquired disease (e.g., canine distemper) that develops in young dogs and produces chronic rhino-sinusitis and bronchopneumonia
• Recurrent aspiration pneumonia
• Chronic bacterial pneumonia—caused by resident organisms, inadequate antimicrobial therapy, foreign body, abscess, or other persistent nidus of infection
• Bronchoesophageal fistula

CBC/BIOCHEMISTRY/URINALYSIS
• Mature neutrophilic leukocytosis and normal or high numbers of lymphocytes—common

• Lymphocyte numbers—help distinguish from canine distemper viral infection, which typically produces marked lymphopenia
• With severe bronchopneumonia—may see left shift and toxic change in the blood neutrophils
• Old dogs—may note hyperglobulinemia
• With chronic hypoxemia—may see polycythemia

OTHER LABORATORY TESTS
• Blood gas analysis—may reveal hypoxemia and normocapnia or hypocapnia
• Transtracheal lavage—typically recovers a mucoid to mucopurulent material characterized cytologically as a purulent exudate; one or more bacterial species commonly cultured
• *Mycoplasma* spp. and *Pasteurella multocida*— most common isolates; *Mycoplasma* too small to see in a cytologic specimen and requires special culture medium to recover

IMAGING

Radiography
• Changes consistent with broncho-pneumonia and sometimes bronchiectasis
• Mirror image reversal of viscera (situs inversus) involving the thorax or abdomen or both body cavities—common
• Thickened or sclerotic tympanic bullae (secretory otitis media) and radiopaque rhinoliths—may note in old patients

Mucociliary Scintigraphy
• Tracheal mucus clearance—determined with radiopharmaceuticals (^{99m}Tc-macroaggregated albumin) and γ camera imaging; no clearance observed in affected patients
• Mucociliary clearance—determine before ultrastructural analysis of cilia (avoids unnecessary use of electron microscopy); normal results exclude the diagnosis.

Magnetic Resonance Imaging
Moderate to severe dilation of the lateral cerebral ventricles—found in many patients

DIAGNOSTIC PROCEDURES

Electron Microscopy
• Ultrastructural lesions in the cilia—most patients; identify by pinch biopsy of the nasal or bronchial mucosa; dynein arm deficiency, abnormal microtubular patterns, lack of central pair of microtubules, and random orientation reported.
• Diagnostic significance—specific lesion must be found in a high percentage of cilia; same defect must be found in cilia from multiple locations (e.g., nasal and bronchial cilia and sperm flagella) and from affected litter mates.
• Acquired ultrastructural lesions—common in humans (and presumably dogs) with

chronic respiratory tract infection; vary; typically involve < 20% of cilia; evaluation of cilia from cells cultured in vitro can be used to distinguish primary versus acquired ultrastructural lesions.
• Dogs with primary ciliary dyskinesia but no ultrastructural ciliary lesions have been described.

Other
• In vitro analysis of ciliary beat frequency and synchrony—confirms diagnosis in patients with no ultrastructural lesions
• Electrocardiogram—inversion of lead I and transposition of leads II and III in patients with thoracic situs inversus or isolated dextrocardia

PATHOLOGIC FINDINGS

Upper Respiratory Tract
• Chronic bacterial rhinitis—characterized by a mucoid to mucopurulent exudate overlaying an inflamed mucosa
• Histologic—mucosa infiltrated with plasma cells and neutrophils and has mucous gland hyperplasia; may note hypoplastic nasal turbinates, atresia of the frontal sinuses, frontal sinusitis, nasal polyps, and rhinoliths

Lower Respiratory Tract
• Lesions—vary with severity of bronchopneumonia and chronicity of disease
• Mucoid to mucopurulent material—observed throughout the airways
• Gross lung lesions—atelectasis, bronchiectasis, and subpleural emphysema; most pronounced in the ventral aspect of the cranial and middle lung lobes and in the cranioventral portion of the caudal lung lobes
• Histologic—bronchitis, bronchiolitis, and bronchiectasis

Miscellaneous
• Severe dilatation of the lateral cerebral ventricles—may be noted
• Situs inversus of thoracic viscera or abdominal viscera or both (situs inversus totalis) may occur.
• Impaction of one or both middle ears with a sterile gelatinous material (secretory otitis media) may be seen.

 TREATMENT
• Airway secretions—cleared by the shear force produced by expiration and coughing
• Routine exercise—may enhance mucus clearance by increasing respiration and inducing coughing
• Daily positioning of patient in dorsal recumbency—may promote postural drainage of mucus from dependent airways; may facilitate expectoration

• Supplemental oxygen therapy—may be needed during acute episodes of life-threatening bronchopneumonia

 MEDICATIONS

DRUG(S)
• Antibiotics—for respiratory infections; selected on the basis of bacterial culture and sensitivity testing; duration varies with the severity of infection; continuous therapy often rendered ineffective by colonization with resistant bacteria

CONTRAINDICATIONS/POSSIBLE INTERACTIONS
• Radiographic contrast medium used for bronchography—patient cannot clear it; may eventually elicit a pyogranulomatous inflammatory reaction

Anesthesia
• Patients have impaired gas exchange and, therefore, have increased risk of complications.
• Goal—minimize respiratory depression and recovery time
• Preanesthetic medication with narcotics—contraindicated
• Anticholinergics—increase dead air space by bronchodilatation; give only at induction.
• Nitrous oxide—do not use if obstructed bullae are noted in the lungs.
• Assisted or controlled ventilation—adjust ventilator to provide a long expiratory phase to prevent air trapping.
• Suction endotracheal tube and trachea intermittently during prolonged periods of anesthesia.
• Patients positioned on their backs are at greater risk for complications; because of small airway obstruction, atelectasis, and pulmonary fibrosis in the dependent portions of the lung, a severe ventilation–perfusion mismatch may develop.
• Postanesthesia—keep patient in sternal recumbency until it is fully recovered.

 FOLLOW-UP

POSSIBLE COMPLICATIONS
• High ambient temperature—may produce hyperthermia and potential heat stroke because of reduced capacity for evaporative heat loss through the lungs
• Subpleural cysts—bronchiectatic cysts, interstitial cysts, and emphysematous bullae; may develop from prolonged air entrapment; may rupture, producing pneumothorax

• Chronic hypoxemia in association with a small pulmonary vascular bed—may precipitate pulmonary artery hypertension, cor pulmonale, and right-sided heart failure
• Persistent bacterial infections in the airways—may result in systemic reactive amyloidosis

EXPECTED COURSE AND PROGNOSIS
• The clinical course of disease and longevity of patients—highly variable
• Appropriate antibiotic treatment and pulmonary physical therapy—may result in prolonged survival; reactive systemic amyloidosis and cor pulmonale are potential sequelae of chronic bacterial infection of the airways.
• Patients < 1 year old—may develop chronic rhinosinusitis or bronchopneumonia with periodic exacerbations that can be life-threatening
• Patients > 1 year old—clinical disease varies considerably; despite persistent lack of mucociliary clearance, may become virtually asymptomatic for respiratory disease; may continue to have mucoid to mucopurulent nasal discharge, sneezing, and coughing but with less frequent acute exacerbations of bronchopneumonia
• Symptomatic patients who survive several years develop progressive pulmonary disease characterized by ventral consolidation of the lungs and bronchiectasis.
• Appropriate treatment may result in a normal life span; patients may, however, die during the acute episodes of bronchopneumonia.

 MISCELLANEOUS

SEE ALSO
Pneumonia, Bacterial

Suggested Reading
Clercx C, Peeters D, Beths T, et al. Use of ciliogenesis in the diagnosis of primary ciliary dyskinesia in a dog. J Am Vet Med Assoc 2000;217:1681–1685.
Daniel GB, Edwards DF, Harvey RC, Kabalka GW. Communicating hydrocephalus in dogs with congenital ciliary dysfunction. Dev Neurosci 1995;17:230–235.
Edwards DF, Patton CS, Kennedy JR. Primary ciliary dyskinesia in the dog. Probl Vet Med 1992;4:291–319.
Author David F. Edwards
Consulting Editor Lynelle R. Johnson

PROLAPSED GLAND OF THE THIRD EYELID (CHERRY EYE)

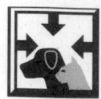 BASICS

OVERVIEW
• Gland of the third eyelid—normally anchored by a fibrous attachment to the periorbita beneath the third eyelid
• Weak attachment—several breeds of dogs and cats; predisposes animals to unilateral or bilateral prolapse

SIGNALMENT
• Dogs and cats
• Dogs—usually in young dogs (aged 6 months to 2 years); common breeds: cocker spaniels, bulldogs, beagles, bloodhounds, lhasa apsos, shih tzus, other brachycephalic breeds
• Cats—rare; occurs in Burmese and Persians

SIGNS
• Oval, hyperemic mass protruding from behind the leading edge of the third eyelid
• May be unilateral or bilateral
• May see accompanying epiphora, hyperemic conjunctiva, or blepharospasm
• Additional swelling and hyperemia caused by environmental irritation and desiccation of the exposed gland

CAUSES & RISK FACTORS
• Congenital weakness of the attachment of the gland of the third eyelid
• Inheritance unknown

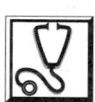 DIAGNOSIS

DIFFERENTIAL DIAGNOSIS
• Scrolled or everted cartilage of the third eyelid—seen in Wiemaraners, Great Danes, German short-haired pointers, and other breeds in which the T-shaped cartilage of the third eyelid is rolled away from the surface of the eye instead of conforming to the surface of the cornea
• Neoplasia of the third eyelid—usually seen in old animals; may see squamous cell carcinoma, lymphosarcoma, or fibrosarcoma; may be origin of adenoma or adenocarcinoma; small incisional biopsy is indicated in old patients (> 7–9 years) to differentiate
• Orbital fat prolapse—may dissect anteriorly between the conjunctiva and globe; occasionally occurs in the medial canthus and simulates a prolapsed gland of the third eyelid

CBC/BIOCHEMISTRY/URINALYSIS
N/A

OTHER LABORATORY TESTS
N/A

IMAGING
N/A

DIAGNOSTIC PROCEDURES
N/A

 TREATMENT

• Surgical replacement of the gland—see Suggested Reading
• Excision of the gland—avoid; gland produces up to 50% of the aqueous tear film; puts patient at substantial risk for developing KCS at it ages
• Elizabethan collar—recommended to prevent self-trauma

 MEDICATIONS

DRUG(S)
Topical antiinflammatory medications—may be used before and after surgery to lessen swelling

CONTRAINDICATIONS/POSSIBLE INTERACTIONS
N/A

 FOLLOW-UP

• Recurrence—5%–20%, depending on the surgical procedure; re-replacement of the gland is encouraged.
• If unilateral, warn client that the other gland may develop a prolapse and that no preventive procedure or medication exists.

 MISCELLANEOUS

SYNONYM
Cherry eye

ABBREVIATION
KCS = keratoconjunctivitis sicca

Suggested Reading
Stanley RG, Kaswan RL. Modification of the orbital rim anchorage method for surgical replacement of the gland of the third eyelid in dogs. J Am Vet Med Assoc 1994; 205:1412–1414.
Author Brian C. Gilger
Consulting Editor Paul E. Miller

BASICS

OVERVIEW
• Forward displacement of the globe, with the eyelids trapped posterior to the eyeball
• Frequently associated with head trauma and usually occurs peracutely
• Potentially vision threatening
• May cause bradycardia secondary to traction on the retrobulbar muscles and the associated oculocardiac reflex (regulated through the trigeminal and vagus nerves)

SIGNALMENT
• More common in the brachycephalic breeds due to the prominence of the eyes, relatively shallow orbits, and large palpebral fissures
• May occur in any species or breed if the traumatic force is severe enough

SIGNS

General Comments
Globe positioned anterior to the eyelids

Possible Accompanying Signs
• Abnormalities in pupil size—dilated or constricted
• Corneal ulceration and/or desiccation
• Intraocular inflammation
• Fractures of the bony orbit or other parts of the skull
• Subconjunctival or intraocular hemorrhage
• Rupture of the globe
• Brain trauma
• Trauma to the contralateral eye
• Shock
• Other signs associated with trauma

Associated Signs After Repositioning
• Dorsolateral strabismus—due to rupture of the inferior oblique and medial rectus muscles
• Blindness
• Dilated pupil
• Decreased tear production
• Corneal desiccation
• Decreased corneal sensitivity

CAUSES & RISK FACTORS
• Trauma—primary cause; relatively minor force in brachiocephalic breeds; usually severe force in dolichocephalic and mesocephalic breeds
• Retrobulbar tumor or severe cellulitis or other infection—rare

DIAGNOSIS

DIFFERENTIAL DIAGNOSIS
• Buphthalmia—enlargement of the globe; rarely acute; eyelids still positioned correctly, but may not be able to close completely over the globe
• Exophthalmia—forward displacement of the globe; but eyelids positioned correctly; may be acute; rarely peracute; eye cannot be retropulsed due to a mass-effect (e.g., neoplasia, retrobulbar polymyositis, infection, or cellulitis) in the retrobulbar tissues.

CBC/BIOCHEMISTRY/URINALYSIS
Normal, unless secondary to trauma

OTHER LABORATORY TESTS
N/A

IMAGING
Skull radiographs—may show fractures due to trauma

DIAGNOSTIC PROCEDURES
N/A

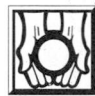

TREATMENT
• Keep the cornea lubricated.
• Assess the patient overall before performing surgery on the globe.
• Treat primary condition, as necessary.
• Treat shock and head trauma, if necessary.

Repositioning the Globe
• Perform as soon as possible once the patient is stable.
• Performed under sedation and local anesthesia or, if the patient is stable, under general anesthesia
• Fluorescein—stain the cornea prior to repositioning
• Preplace two or three temporary tarsorrhaphy mattress sutures through the eyelids, exiting at the lid margins, crossing across to the other lid, entering at the lid margin, and reversing the procedure.
• Lateral canthotomy—may ease tension on the eyelids and allow easier suture placement
• While protecting the globe (a lubricated scalpel blade handle can serve this function), tie the preplaced sutures and reposition the globe; suture the lateral canthotomy closed.
• If the optic nerve is definitely severed, or the globe is ruptured, infected, or desiccated; enucleation may be a better choice than repositioning.

MEDICATIONS

DRUG(S)
• Systemic and topical broad-spectrum antibiotics—until sutures are removed
• Systemic corticosteroids—usually used at least initially; may be continued on a chronic basis with marked periorbital and retrobulbar swelling
• Topical corticosteroids—may be used with associated intraocular inflammation (uveitis) or hyphema, as long as no corneal or conjunctival ulcers exist
• Topical atropine—for intraocular inflammation or hyphema; relieve ciliary spasm and lower the risk of synechiae

CONTRAINDICATIONS/POSSIBLE INTERACTIONS
• Topical corticosteroids—do not use with ulcerations.
• Systemic corticosteroids—do not use with retrobulbar infection.

FOLLOW-UP

PATIENT MONITORING
• Suture removal—usually done sequentially, rather than all at once, starting 10–14 days after repositioning. Integrity of the globe, vision, and cornea—reassessed 10–14 days after surgery

POSSIBLE COMPLICATIONS
• Most patients retain a dorsolateral strabismus, which may improve with time. • Schirmer tear tests—perform after suture removal; may note decreased tear production • Neurotrophic keratitis with chronic ulceration secondary to corneal denervation

EXPECTED COURSE AND PROGNOSIS
• Most affected eyes can be salvaged; majority caused by trauma will be blind (more common in the dolichocephalic than in the brachycephalic breeds). • Normal retinal vessels and optic nerve, normal IOP, and a short time from occurrence to repair—relatively favorable prognosis for maintaining vision • Positive menace response or direct or consensual pupillary light reflex originating from the injured eye—good prognosis for maintaining vision • Pupil size at the time of the injury—not necessarily an accurate prognostic indicator; mydriasis may be the result of trauma to the optic nerve (if permanent, results in blindness) or damage to the oculomotor nerve (does not affect vision) • Miosis—does not necessarily indicate a good prognosis for vision; most likely cause is uveitis (if severe enough, pupillary constriction occurs even with retinal or optic nerve damage)

MISCELLANEOUS

SEE ALSO
Orbital Diseases (Exophthalmos, Enophthalmos, Strabismus)

ABBREVIATION
• IOP = intraocular pressure

Suggested Reading
Slatter D. Fundamentals of veterinary ophthalmology. 2nd ed. Philadelphia: Saunders, 1990.
Author Stephanie L. Smedes
Consulting Editor Paul E. Miller

PROSTATIC CYSTS

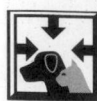

BASICS

OVERVIEW
• Prostatic cysts in the dog include diffuse epithelial cystic change from androgen-dependent benign prostatic hypertrophy (BPH), retention cysts within the prostatic parenchyma that are cavitating, fluid-filled lesions with a distinct capsule, and para-prostatic cysts that are cavitating, fluid-filled lesions with a distinct capsule located outside of the prostatic parenchyma. Prostatic cysts range in diameter from a few mm to more than 20 cm.
• Paraprostatic cysts usually arise craniolateral to the prostate, displacing the bladder cranially and ventrally, or caudal to the prostate in the pelvis, as possible dilated embryonal remnants of the wolffian ducts.
• Pathogenesis is unknown, but the occurrence of retention cysts in dogs with estrogen-secreting Sertoli cell tumors causes speculation that these cysts are dilations of prostatic acini secondary to estrogen-induced squamous metaplasia.

SIGNALMENT
• Male intact dogs
• Age range 2–12 years, mean age 8.0 years
• Large dogs are more commonly affected than small dogs.

SIGNS
• Asymptomatic
• Lethargy and anorexia
• Abdominal distention
• Tenesmus if the cyst compresses the rectum
• Dysuria if the cyst compresses the urethra
• Sanguineous urethral discharge in the presence of BPH

CAUSES & RISK FACTORS
• Benign prostatic hypertrophy
• Androgenic hormones
• Estrogenic hormones

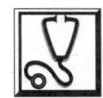

DIAGNOSIS

DIFFERENTIAL DIAGNOSIS
• BPH—distinguished by ultrasound
• Prostatic abscess—distinguished by ultrasound and semen culture
• Distended urinary bladder—distinguished by cystocentesis, imaging
• Caudal abdominal mass of undetermined origin—distinguished by imaging

CBC/BIOCHEMISTRY/URINALYSIS
No abnormalities

OTHER LABORATORY TESTS
• Examination of prostatic fluid collected by ejaculation or prostatic massage confirms absence of infection.
• Culture and cytology of cyst fluid collected by ultrasound-guided fine-needle aspiration or by aspiration at surgical exploration reveal sterile clear or sanguineous fluid consistent with prostatic fluid.

IMAGING
Retrograde contrast urethrocystography followed by prostatic ultrasonography confirms presence, location, echo-texture, and size of prostatic cysts, and differentiates retention cysts from paraprostatic cysts.

DIAGNOSTIC PROCEDURES
Collection of prostatic fluid by ejaculation followed by prostatic imaging is recommended prior to fine-needle aspiration of cystic fluid in order to rule out presence of bacterial infection.

PATHOLOGIC FINDINGS
Epithelial cysts within the prostatic parenchyma occur with parenchymal hypertrophy and hyperplasia; squamous metaplasia of the ducts and alveoli may be present. Retention cysts and paraprostatic cysts are lined by a single layer of prostatic epithelium or fibrous connective tissue and contain clear to sanguineous fluid with fibrin.

 TREATMENT
• Intraprostatic cysts (epithelial, retention) respond to prostatic involution, which may be induced by castration or by the 5 alpha-reductase inhibitor finasteride.
• Large retention cysts and paraprostatic cysts should be surgically resected partially or completely, depending on adherence to surrounding structures, or marsupialized and drained for 1–2 months.
• Simple drainage of the cyst(s) is not recommended, as persistence of the capsule usually results in recurrence.

 MEDICATIONS

DRUG(S)
Prostatic parenchyma and diffuse epithelial cysts involute following treatment with the 5 alpha-reductase inhibitor finasteride (0.1–1.0 mg/kg) given orally once daily for 2 to 4 months. Finasteride prevents conversion of testosterone to dihydrotestosterone, causing prostatic involution without adversely affecting libido or spermatogenesis. BPH recurs following cessation of finasteride therapy. Paraprostatic cysts do not respond to finasteride treatment.

CONTRAINDICATIONS/POSSIBLE INTERACTIONS
N/A

 FOLLOW-UP
• Imaging assessment of cyst size at 4-week intervals following treatment
• Standard postoperative monitoring of marsupialized stoma, if any

 MISCELLANEOUS

ABBREVIATION
BPH = benign prostatic hypertrophy

Suggested Reading
Rawlings CA, Mahaffey MB, Barsanti JA, et al. Use of partial prostatectomy for treatment of prostatic abscesses and cysts in dogs. J Am Vet Med Assoc 1997;211: 868–871.
Stowater JL, Lamb CR. Ultrasonographic features of paraprostatic cysts in nine dogs. Vet Rad 1989;30:232–239.
White RAS, Herrtage ME, Dennis R. The diagnosis and management of paraprostatic and prostatic retention cysts in the dog. J Small Anim Pract 1987;28:551–574.
Author Shirley D. Johnston
Consulting Editors Larry G. Adams & Carl A. Osborne

PROSTATITIS AND PROSTATIC ABSCESS

 BASICS

DEFINITION

Acute Prostatitis

Infection of the canine prostate with bacteria, mycoplasmas, and/or fungi with systemic signs of fever, anorexia, lethargy, pain, and inflammatory exudate in prostatic fluid. Presence of abscessation is variable, occurring in 15 of 25 dogs with prostatitis in one study. Abscesses occasionally rupture into the peritoneal cavity, causing sepsis, shock, and rarely death.

Chronic Prostatitis

Subclinical (recent or long-term) infection of the canine prostate in the absence of prostatic abscessation and polysystemic signs. Affected animals are asymptomatic except for presence of inflammatory exudate in the prostatic fluid, which causes infertility. Chronic prostatitis may occur after or independently of acute prostatitis.

PATHOPHYSIOLOGY

• Predisposing pathology is gross and/or microscopic benign prostatic hypertrophy (BPH), which occurs under the influence of dihydrotestosterone (DHT) in more than 80% of intact male dogs over five years of age.
• BPH is characterized by large, irregularly-shaped, well-vascularized prostatic alveoli and branching infoldings of epithelium with microcysts containing sanguineous prostatic fluid; if infected, these can become abscesses.
• Infection of the hypertrophied canine prostate develops most commonly from ascent of normal urethral flora—rarely from blood-borne bacteria and/or from penetrating wounds introducing bacteria or fungi to the scrotum (see Causes). The prostate of the intact male dog constantly secretes prostatic fluid, which is deposited into the prostatic urethra and then flows both into the urinary bladder and out the tip of the penile urethra. With prostatitis, prostatic fluid containing blood, inflammatory exudate, and bacteria or fungi is deposited into the urinary bladder and discharged intermittently from the tip of the penis.

SYSTEMS AFFECTED

• Gastrointestinal—tenesmus if the enlarged prostate compresses the rectum
• Hemic/Lymphatic/Immune—Mature or immature neutrophilia in acute prostatitis
• Polysystemic—septic shock if prostatic abscesses rupture, tachycardia, poor tissue perfusion, elevated temperature, and focal or generalized peritonitis • Renal/Urologic—dysuria if the enlarged prostate compresses the urethra; deposition of prostatic fluid with inflammatory exudate into the urinary bladder • Reproductive—pain at copulation and reduction in libido; infertility from infected prostatic fluid in the ejaculate

GENETICS

No known genetic basis

INCIDENCE/PREVALENCE

High in intact male dogs over five years of age. Infection is reported in 40% of dogs with prostatic disease.

SIGNALMENT

Species

Dogs

Breed Predilection

All breeds and mixed breeds

Mean Age and Range

Middle-aged; mean age range, 7 to 11 years

Predominant Sex

Intact male dogs

SIGNS

Acute Prostatitis

• Lethargy/depression • Anorexia • Tenesmus • Dysuria • Pyrexia • Pain at prostatic or caudal abdominal palpation • Sanguineous urethral discharge • Stiff hind limb gait • Septic shock (rare)

Chronic Prostatitis

• Asymptomatic • Tenesmus • Dysuria • Sanguineous urethral discharge

CAUSES

• Infection of the hypertrophied prostate with ascending urethral flora, including *Escherichia coli*, *Staphylococcus* spp., *Streptococcus* spp., *Proteus mirabilis*, *Klebsiella* spp., *Enterobacter* spp., *Hemophilus* spp., *Pseudomonas* spp., *Pasteurella* spp., anaerobic bacteria, and *Mycoplasma* (most common) • Infection of the hypertrophied prostate with systemic bacterial infection, including *Brucella canis* • Systemic or local puncture wound infection with *Blastomyces dermatitidis*

RISK FACTORS

• Increasing age • Presence of functional testes in affected dogs • BPH • Historical androgen or estrogen administration • Impaired host defense mechanisms (immunosuppression, catheterization of the urethra)

 DIAGNOSIS

DIFFERENTIAL DIAGNOSIS

• BPH without infection, distinguished by semen culture • Prostatic cysts, distinguished by ultrasound and semen culture • Prostatic neoplasia, distinguished by ultrasound and tissue biopsy • Abdominal mass or abscess, distinguished by abdominal imaging

CBC/BIOCHEMISTRY/URINALYSIS

• CBC abnormalities in acute prostatitis and abscessation include immature neutrophilia and toxic neutrophils; immature neutropenia may occur with sepsis. Seventy-five percent of dogs with prostatic abscesses exhibit neutrophilia. Most dogs with chronic

prostatitis have a normal CBC. • Serum chemistry abnormalities are variable with acute prostatitis. In one study, 35% of dogs with prostatic abscesses had chemistry abnormalities, of which elevated serum alkaline phosphatase was the most common. Most dogs with chronic prostatitis have normal serum chemistries. • Urinalysis abnormalities include presence of blood, purulent exudate, and causative microbes; these arise not from primary urinary tract infection but from deposition of infected prostatic fluid into the urinary bladder.

OTHER LABORATORY TESTS

• Gross examination, cytology and culture of whole semen or the prostatic fluid (third) fraction of semen or fluid collected at prostatic massage yields inflammatory exudate with aerobic bacteria, anaerobic bacteria, *Mycoplasma*, or fungi. Normal prostatic fluid should contain less than 10,000 colony-forming bacterial units per mL, and less than five leukocytes per high power field following fluid centrifugation. • Although infection with *Brucella canis* is uncommon, because of the zoonotic potential of this infection, *B. canis* serology is recommended in all dogs with suspected prostatitis, with follow-up culture of semen for *B. canis* if serology is positive.

IMAGING

Survey radiography of the caudal abdomen, retrograde cystourethrography, and prostatic ultrasonography are indicated in order to evaluate prostatic size, echo-texture, and presence of cavitating prostatic lesions, if any. The prostate is enlarged if its greatest cranio-caudal diameter measured on a line parallel to the line connecting the sacral promontory to the anterior aspect of the pubis on a lateral radiograph exceeds 70% of the length of the distance between the sacral promontory and the anterior aspect of the pubis.

DIAGNOSTIC PROCEDURES

• Collection and evaluation of prostatic fluid in seminal plasma and collection of prostatic fluid by prostatic massage in dogs reluctant to ejaculate. • Ultrasound-directed percutaneous fine-needle aspirate of the prostate or of cavitating lesions of the prostate is not recommended unless the dog has been treated with specific antibiotics for 24 hours prior to the procedure in order to avoid creation of sepsis along the needle track.

PATHOLOGIC FINDINGS

• Gross pathology of the infected prostate includes enlargement, variable loss of symmetry and the dorsal median raphe, and variable presence of fluid-filled abscesses within or on the surface of the gland. Enlargement may be focal, multifocal, or diffuse. • Bacterial or fungal infection causes suppurative (bacterial) or granulomatous (fungal) inflammation of the gland.

Inflammatory lesions may be focal, multifocal, or diffuse. Abscesses contain accumulations of purulent fluid exudate. • Biopsy of the infected prostate is not recommended, because diagnostic imaging and examination of prostatic fluid are diagnostic, and because biopsy may result in spread of infection to adjacent tissues.

 TREATMENT

APPROPRIATE HEALTH CARE

• Acute prostatitis, prostatic abscess, and rupture of prostatic abscesses into the peritoneal cavity are potentially life-threatening emergencies that can lead to septic shock and death. Affected patients should be hospitalized and diagnostic samples (blood, urine, semen, imaging) collected immediately. • Dogs with chronic prostatitis may be seen as outpatients for diagnostic procedures and started on specific therapy when laboratory results are available.

NURSING CARE

• Dogs with acute prostatitis or prostatic abscess should have an intravenous line placed and antimicrobial therapy initiated. • The patient should be assessed for likelihood of abscess rupture and peritonitis, which warrants intravenous fluid therapy for septic shock.

ACTIVITY

Breeding should be avoided until bacteria have been cleared from the prostatic fluid.

CLIENT EDUCATION

• Castration should be recommended for dogs with acute prostatitis and/or prostatic abscess, as castration induces permanent prostatic involution. • If maintenance of breeding potential is necessary, long-term or intermittent treatment with finasteride is recommended to induce prostatic involution; routine rechecks at 2–3 month intervals for semen culture, semen cytology, and prostatic imaging are recommended. BPH recurs over time in intact male dogs after treatment with finasteride is discontinued, and BPH increases risk of recurrence of prostatitis.

SURGICAL CONSIDERATIONS

• Surgical management of prostatic abscesses should be deferred until after initiation of antimicrobial therapy and prostatic involution; involution is associated with resolution of abscesses, often making surgery unnecessary. • Castration is recommended for induction of prostatic involution in non-breeding dogs with prostatitis; castration should be deferred until after identification and treatment (for at least one week) of the causative bacterial/fungal agent; alternatively, medical involution of the prostate may be induced with finasteride. • Placement of Penrose drains, marsupialization, partial prostatectomy, and

use of an ultrasonic surgical aspirator have been advocated for treatment of prostatic abscesses in dogs; however, these procedures have been associated with a high percentage of short- and long-term adverse sequelae, including abscess recurrence.

 MEDICATIONS

DRUG(S)

Eradicating Infection

• Choice of antimicrobial agent is based on culture and sensitivity findings in the prostatic fluid, antibiotic lipid solubility (which enhances its ability to diffuse into prostatic tissue in therapeutic concentrations), and assessment of acute or chronic status of the infection. • Antibiotics known to diffuse into normal prostatic tissue in therapeutic concentrations include chloramphenicol, erythromycin, fluoroquinolones, and trimethoprim, the antibiotics of choice in chronic prostatitis; in acute prostatitis, the blood-prostate barrier is disrupted, and almost any antibiotic will penetrate the prostatic parenchyma in therapeutic concentrations. • Emergency antibiotic treatment of choice in dogs with acute prostatitis and/or abscess, administered after collection of prostatic fluid for culture, is amoxicillin/clavulanate (25 mg/kg PO q8h) with enrofloxacin (5 mg/kg PO q12h).

Inducing Prostatic Involution

• Treatment of choice for inducing permanent prostatic involution is castration. • Alternatively, the 5 α-reductase inhibitor finasteride (0.1–1.0 mg/kg PO q24h) for 2 to 4 months induces involution of the prostatic parenchyma and diffuse epithelial cysts and abscesses. • Finasteride prevents conversion of testosterone to DHT, thereby causing prostatic involution without adversely affecting libido or spermatogenesis. • BPH recurs following cessation of finasteride therapy.

CONTRAINDICATIONS

Estrogens and androgens cause squamous metaplasia of the prostate and BPH, respectively.

PRECAUTIONS

Long-term therapy with trimethoprim may lead to keratoconjunctivitis sicca and/or hypothyroidism.

 FOLLOW-UP

PATIENT MONITORING

• Repeated evaluation of semen culture, cytology, and prostatic imaging • Intervals between reevaluations vary with severity of signs, presence of an abscess, selection of

castration or finasteride therapy for prostatic involution, and use of the dog in a breeding program; these range from 1- to 8-week intervals, with recheck recommended prior to breeding. • Continue patient monitoring until the dog has been castrated.

PREVENTION/AVOIDANCE

Castration is recommended to induce prostatic involution, resolution of BPH, and prevention of recurrence.

POSSIBLE COMPLICATIONS

• Recurrence of infection if prostatic involution is not induced • Surgical drainage of abscesses is associated with many complications, including urinary incontinence, recurrent abscessation, hypoproteinemia, scrotal edema, anemia, sepsis, and shock.

EXPECTED COURSE AND PROGNOSIS

• Prognosis is good to excellent except in the case of rupture of prostatic abscesses into the peritoneal cavity, with resulting peritonitis. • Castration prevents recurrence and improves prognosis. • Surgical management of prostatic abscesses is associated with complications and a poorer prognosis than medical/surgical induction of prostatic involution.

 MISCELLANEOUS

ASSOCIATED CONDITIONS

When prostatic fluid is infected, it deposits blood, inflammatory exudate, and microbial organisms into the urinary bladder which, if detected in a urine sample collected by cystocentesis, may be misinterpreted as primary urinary tract infection.

AGE-RELATED FACTORS

Incidence of BPH increases with age, especially after 5 years of age.

ZOONOTIC POTENTIAL

Rare. *Brucella canis* and *Blastomyces dermatitidis* have been isolated from the urine of dogs with prostatic infection, but human infection from these sources has not been reported.

SEE ALSO

• Benign Prostatic Hyperplasia • Dysuria and Pollakiuria • Hematuria • Peritonitis • Prostatic Cysts • Shock, Septic

ABBREVIATIONS

• BPH = benign prostatic hypertrophy • DHT = dihydrotestosterone

Suggested Reading

Johnston SD, Kamolpatana K, Root-Kustritz MV, Johnston GR. Prostatic disorders in the dog. Animal Reprod Sci 2000;60–61: 405–415.

Author Shirley D. Johnston

Consulting Editors Larry G. Adams and Carl A. Osborne

PROSTATOMEGALY

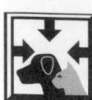 BASICS

DEFINITION
Abnormally large prostate gland determined by rectal or abdominal palpation or by abdominal radiography or prostatic ultrasonography; enlargement can be symmetrical or asymmetrical, painful or nonpainful. Normal prostate size varies with age, body size, castration status, and breed, so determination of enlargement is subjective.

PATHOPHYSIOLOGY
Enlargement can result from epithelial cell hyperplasia or hypertrophy (e.g., benign prostatic hyperplasia), neoplasia of prostatic epithelium or stroma, cystic change within the prostatic parenchyma, or inflammatory cell infiltration (e.g., acute and chronic bacterial prostatitis and prostatic abscess).

SYSTEMS AFFECTED
• Renal/Urologic
• Reproductive

SIGNALMENT
• Dogs
• Typically noted in middle-aged to older males

SIGNS
• Maybe none
• Straining to defecate
• Ribbonlike stools
• Dysuria
• Urethral outflow obstruction

CAUSES
• Benign prostatic hyperplasia
• Squamous metaplasia
• Adenocarcinoma
• Transitional cell carcinoma
• Sarcoma
• Metastatic neoplasia
• Acute bacterial prostatitis
• Prostatic abscess
• Chronic bacterial prostatitis
• Prostatic cyst

RISK FACTORS
• Castration lowers the risk of benign prostatic hyperplasia and bacterial prostatitis.
• Risk of adenocarcinoma may be increased in neutered dog.

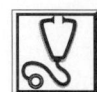 DIAGNOSIS

DIFFERENTIAL DIAGNOSIS
• Benign prostatic hyperplasia—typically causes nonpainful symmetrical enlargement of the prostate gland; not found in neutered dogs
• Primary or metastatic neoplasia—typically causes painful, nonsymmetrical enlargement of the prostate gland; weight loss, impaired appetite, rear limb weakness observed in some patients; suspect neoplasia in neutered dogs.
• Acute bacterial prostatitis—typically results in slight-to-moderate symmetric or nonsymmetrical enlargement of the prostate gland with prostatic pain; fever, impaired appetite, rear limb weakness, and painful abdomen observed in some patients.
• Chronic bacterial prostatitis—signs similar to those seen in animals with acute prostatitis or those related to recurrent lower urinary tract infection (e.g., dysuria and hematuria); systemic signs less common than in acute bacterial prostatitis; bacterial prostatitis uncommon in neutered dogs
• Prostatic abscess—may result in signs similar to those in patients with acute or chronic prostatitis; abscess rupture causes fever and caudal abdominal pain.
• Prostatic cysts—may cause a palpable caudal abdominal mass, straining to urinate, or straining to defecate; patient may also be asymptomatic.

CBC/BIOCHEMISTRY/URINALYSIS
• CBC normal in patients with benign prostatic hyperplasia
• Leukocytosis in patients with acute and chronic (occasionally) bacterial prostatitis, prostatic abscess, and prostatic neoplasia (occasionally)
• High bilirubin and alkaline phosphatase (ALP) in some patients with prostatic abscess
• Urinalysis—normal or hematuria in patients with benign prostatic hyperplasia
• Pyuria, hematuria, proteinuria, and bacteriuria in patients with bacterial prostatitis
• Pyuria, hematuria, proteinuria, and, occasionally, neoplastic cells in dogs with prostatic neoplasia

OTHER LABORATORY TESTS
Serum prostatic esterase concentration is high in dogs with benign prostatic hyperplasia.

IMAGING
Radiographic Findings
• Prostatomegaly
• Prostatic mineralization more likely in dogs with prostatic neoplasia

Ultrasonographic Findings
• Abscess or cyst—hypoechoic or anechoic lesions with distal enhancement
• Acute bacterial prostatitis—uniform prostatic echogenicity
• Benign prostatic hyperplasia—uniform prostatic echogenicity; small fluid-filled cysts in some patients
• Chronic bacterial prostatitis—focal or diffuse hyperechogenicity
• Prostatic neoplasia—focal to multifocal areas of coalescing echogenicity and acoustic shadowing (if mineralization)

DIAGNOSTIC PROCEDURES
• Examination of prostatic fluid obtained by ejaculation or prostatic massage may reveal changes similar to those seen on urinalysis.

- Bacterial culture of prostatic fluid typically reveals >100,000 bacteria/mL in dogs with bacterial prostatitis.
- Transrectal aspiration biopsy (specimen obtained by a Franzen needle guide) or urethral catheter biopsy reveals neoplastic cells in some dogs with prostatic carcinoma.
- Needle biopsy with ultrasound guidance provides visualization of the area to be sampled and increases the likelihood of obtaining a diagnostic sample; take care to avoid rupturing a prostatic abscess.

 TREATMENT

- Varies with the cause of prostatomegaly
- Surgical castration—indicated in symptomatic dogs with benign prostatic hyperplasia and after acute infection resolves in dogs with bacterial prostatitis
- Surgical drainage—indicated in dogs with prostatic abscess or large prostatic cysts
- External beam radiotherapy may provide palliation in patients with prostatic carcinoma.

 MEDICATIONS

DRUG(S) OF CHOICE

Benign Prostatic Hyperplasia
If castration is not acceptable, the following drugs may produce a temporary response:
- Finasteride (0.1–0.5 mg/kg/day for up to 4 months)
- Megestrol acetate (0.11 mg/kg PO daily for 3 weeks)
- Medroxyprogestcronc (3 mg/kg SC)

Bacterial Prostatitis
Chose antibiotics on the basis of antibacterial sensitivity testing of the isolated organism and ability of the antibiotic to diffuse into prostatic fluid in therapeutic concentrations; good choices for latter include trimethoprim/sulfa, chloramphenicol, and enrofloxacin.

Prostatic Carcinoma
Chemotherapy has not been proved beneficial; can consider combination therapy with cyclophosphamide and doxorubicin.

CONTRAINDICATIONS
N/A

PRECAUTIONS
Long-term administration of megestrol acetate or medroxyprogesterone can cause diabetes mellitus.

POSSIBLE INTERACTIONS
N/A

ALTERNATIVE DRUG(S)
N/A

 FOLLOW-UP

PATIENT MONITORING
- Abdominal radiographs or prostatic ultrasonography to assess efficacy of treatment in benign prostatic hyperplasia, prostatic carcinoma, or bacterial prostatitis
- Urine and prostatic fluid culture to access efficacy of treatment in patients with bacterial prostatitis

POSSIBLE COMPLICATIONS
- Urethral obstruction
- Rectal obstruction

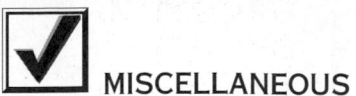 **MISCELLANEOUS**

ASSOCIATED CONDITIONS
N/A

AGE-RELATED FACTORS
Prostatic carcinoma typically diagnosed in 8- to 10-year-old dogs

ZOONOTIC POTENTIAL
N/A

PREGNANCY
N/A

SYNONYMS
N/A

SEE ALSO
- Adenocarcinoma, Prostate
- Benign Prostatic Hyperplasia
- Prostatic Cysts
- Prostatitis and Prostatic Abscess

ABBREVIATION
ALP = alkaline phosphatase

Suggested Reading
Barsanti JA, Finco DR. Canine prostatic diseases. In: Ettinger SJ, ed. Textbook of veterinary internal medicine. Philadelphia: Saunders, 1989:1662–1685.
Kay ND. Diseases of the prostate gland. In: Birchard SJ, Sherding RD, eds. Saunders manual of small animal practice. Philadelphia: Saunders, 1994:865–871.
Authors Jeffrey S. Klausner and Margaret V. Root-Kustritz
Consulting Editors Larry G. Adams and Carl A. Osborne

PROTEIN-LOSING ENTEROPATHY

 BASICS

DEFINITION
• A group of diseases characterized by excessive loss of serum proteins into the gastrointestinal lumen
• Diseases associated with PLE include primary gastrointestinal disease and systemic disorders such as lymphatic disease or congestive heart failure.

PATHOPHYSIOLOGY
• Under physiologic conditions two-thirds of normal protein loss in dogs occurs through the small intestine.
• Plasma proteins that leak into the gastrointestinal lumen are rapidly digested into constituent amino acids that can be reabsorbed and utilized for the synthesis of new proteins.
• This normal loss of plasma proteins can be accelerated by gastrointestinal mucosal disease or by decreased lymphatic drainage from the intestines.
• Gastrointestinal loss of plasma proteins is associated with loss of both albumin and globulin.
• In response to increased gastrointestinal protein loss, the liver increases the synthesis of albumin. However, the liver cannot increase albumin synthesis to more than twice the normal output.
• When protein loss exceeds protein synthesis, hypoproteinemia results.
• Severe hypoproteinemia causes decreased plasma oncotic pressure, which may be associated with hemodynamic changes and may lead to effusion into body cavities or peripheral edema.

SYSTEMS AFFECTED
• Gastrointestinal—primary gastrointestinal disease that may be associated with diarrhea, vomiting, or other clinical signs of GI disease
• Lymphatic—lymphangiectasia
• Hemodynamic—ascites or pleural effusion due to decreased oncotic pressure leading to abdominal discomfort or even dyspnea
• Respiratory—dyspnea due to pleural effusion
• Skin—subcutaneous edema

GENETICS
The hereditary nature of PLE or specific causes of PLE has not been studied but a genetic predisposition in breeds with increased prevalence of the disease is likely.

INCIDENCE/PREVALENCE
True incidence and prevalence of PLE are unknown. Many dogs with subacute or acute gastroenteritis have transient PLE.

GEOGRAPHIC DISTRIBUTION
N/A

SIGNALMENT

Species
Dogs and cats

Breed Predilection
Breeds of dogs with an increased prevalence of protein-losing enteropathy include the soft-coated Wheaten terrier, basenji, Yorkshire terrier, and Norwegian Lundehund.

Mean Age and Range
Any age

Predominant Sex
None

SIGNS

General Comments
Clinical signs are variable.

Historical findings
• Diarrhea (chronic, continuous or intermittent, watery to semisolid), weight loss, and lethargy are most frequently reported. However, a significant number of dogs with PLE have normal stools.
• Vomiting is reported uncommonly.

Physical Examination Findings
• Ascites, dependent edema, and dyspnea from pleural effusion may be detected with marked hypoproteinemia.
• Abdominal palpation may reveal thickened bowel loops.

CAUSES

Disorders of Lymphatics
• Intestinal lymphangiectasia
• Gastrointestinal lymphosarcoma
• Granuloma of the small bowel or mesentery
• Congestive heart failure leading to lymphatic hypertension

Diseases Associated with Increased Mucosal Permeability or Mucosal Ulceration
• Viral gastroenteritis—parvovirus and others
• Bacterial gastroenteritis—small intestinal bacterial overgrowth (SIBO), salmonellosis, and others
• Fungal gastroenteritis—histoplasmosis and others
• Parasitic enteritis—hookworms, whipworms, and others
• Inflammatory bowel disease—lymphocytic, lymphocytic-plasmacytic, eosinophilic gastroenteritis
• Adverse food reactions—food allergy, food intolerance, and others
• Mechanical enteropathies—chronic intussusception, chronic foreign body, and others
• Intestinal neoplasia—lymphosarcoma, carcinoma
• Gastric or intestinal ulcers

RISK FACTORS
• Gastrointestinal disease
• Lymphatic disorders
• Heart disease

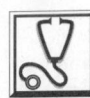 DIAGNOSIS

DIFFERENTIAL DIAGNOSIS
• Hypoalbuminemia due to PLE must be differentiated from other causes of hypoalbuminemia.
• Hypoalbuminemia due to hepatic failure is most often associated with a normal or even increased serum globulin concentration. Hepatic enzymes may be elevated, serum BUN and cholesterol may be decreased, serum pre- and postprandial bile acid concentrations may be increased.
• Hypoalbuminemia due to protein losing nephropathy (PLN, mild in patients with fever or hyperadrenocorticism, moderate to severe in patients with glomerulonephritis, severe in patients with amyloidosis) is commonly associated with a normal or even increased serum globulin concentration—ruled out by a normal urine protein/creatinine ratio.
• Hypoalbuminemia due to severe blood loss is associated with hypoglobulinemia—blood loss can be excluded by measurement of PCV and a thorough physical examination; in some cases a test for fecal occult blood may be necessary
• Inadequate protein intake (i.e., starvation) is a rare cause of hypoalbuminemia
• Hypoalbuminemia due to PLE is often associated with hypoglobulinemia—confirmation by an increased fecal α_1-proteinase inhibitor concentration (must be assessed in naturally-passed and freshly-frozen fecal samples from 3 consecutive days).

CBC/BIOCHEMISTRY/URINALYSIS
• Hypoalbuminemia and frequently hypoglobulinemia (panhypoproteinemia)
• Hypocalcemia—secondary to hypoalbuminemia
• Hypocholesterolemia can be seen.
• Lymphopenia may be seen with lymphangiectasia.

OTHER LABORATORY TESTS
• Increased fecal α_1-proteinase inhibitor concentration
• Once PLE has been identified as the cause of the hypoalbuminemia, specific tests may be useful to determine the specific cause of PLE—multiple fecal examinations (smears and flotations) to rule out intestinal

parasitism as a cause of PLE; serum cobalamin and folate concentrations to diagnose SIBO or cobalamin deficiency; plasma turbidity test to detect abnormal fat absorption.
• Others as needed

IMAGING
• Thoracic radiographs may show evidence of cardiac or fungal disease.
• Abdominal radiographs may show evidence of a mechanical enteropathy or other causes of PLE.
• Abdominal ultrasound also may show evidence of a mechanical enteropathy or other causes of PLE.
• Cardiac ultrasound may show evidence of cardiac disease.

DIAGNOSTIC PROCEDURES
• Feeding trial—to rule out adverse reactions to food
• Rectal mucosal scraping—to rule out histoplasmosis
• Endoscopy allows mucosal visualization and biopsy (however, a diagnosis of lymphangiectasia requires full-thickness biopsies).
• Abdominal exploratory laparotomy may show dilated intestinal lymphatics and allows for full-thickness biopsies of intestines and lymph nodes.
• Can use radioactive label to document protein loss through the gastrointestinal tract; the gold standard is ^{51}Cr-labeled albumin; other radioactive labels used successfully include ^{51}Cr-labeled EDTA and ^{111}In-labeled transferrin—all of these tests are, however, impractical in most clinical settings

PATHOLOGIC FINDINGS

PLE
PLE is not associated with any specific gross or histopathologic lesions. Instead, lesions identified are those of the specific cause of PLE.

Intestinal Lymphangiectasia
• Gross pathology—visualization of dilated lymphatics in the mesentery and on the serosal surface of intestines; may see yellow-white nodules and foamy granular deposits adjacent to lymphatics.
• Histopathology—a ballooning distortion of villi caused by markedly dilated lacteals; the villi can be edematous, and some have a blunted appearance; mucosal edema is usually present, and diffuse or multifocal accumulations of lymphocytes and plasma cells can be identified in the lamina propria.
• Other causes of PLE may also lead to specific gross or histopathologic changes. See chapters covering those conditions.

 TREATMENT

NURSING CARE
• In cases of severe hypoalbuminemia and complications due to the hypoalbuminemia plasma transfusions, hetastarch, or dextran should be considered in order to increase plasma oncotic pressure when clinical signs from edema or effusion are severe.
• Abdominocentesis in cases with compromise from severe abdominal effusion

ACTIVITY
Normal

DIET
Modified depending on the underlying cause of PLE

CLIENT EDUCATION
Prepare clients for long-term therapy; spontaneous cures are rare.

SURGICAL CONSIDERATIONS
• Hypoalbuminemia increases postoperative morbidity because of slow wound healing
• Some causes of PLE (e.g., intussusception, chronic foreign body, and some intestinal neoplasias) require surgical intervention.

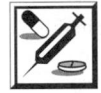 MEDICATIONS

DRUG(S) OF CHOICE
There is no pharmacologic therapy for PLE itself. Instead the underlying cause of PLE must be addressed. See Treatment for these conditions.

CONTRAINDICATIONS
N/A

PRECAUTIONS
N/A

POSSIBLE INTERACTIONS
N/A

ALTERNATIVE DRUG(S)
Diuretics such as furosemide have been used by some to control edema and pleural effusion. However, they do not work well because of decreased plasma oncotic pressure and may be associated with side effects.

 FOLLOW-UP

PATIENT MONITORING
Check body weight, serum albumin concentration, and evidence of recurrent clinical signs (pleural effusion, ascites, and/or edema). Frequency is dependent on the severity of the condition.

PREVENTION/AVOIDANCE
N/A

POSSIBLE COMPLICATIONS
• Respiratory difficulty from pleural effusion
• Severe protein-calorie malnutrition
• Intractable diarrhea

EXPECTED COURSE AND PROGNOSIS
• Prognosis is guarded
• Primary disease cannot be treated in many cases.

 MISCELLANEOUS

ASSOCIATED CONDITIONS
Soft-coated Wheaten terriers may have protein-losing nephropathy (PLN) in conjunction with PLE.

AGE-RELATED FACTORS
N/A

ZOONOTIC POTENTIAL
Histoplasmosis, hookworms, and coccidia have zoonotic potential to humans.

PREGNANCY
N/A

SYNONYMS
N/A

ABBREVIATIONS
• PLE = protein-losing enteropathy
• PLN = protein-losing nephropathy
• SIBO = small intestinal bacterial overgrowth

Suggested Reading

Berry CR, Guilford WG, Koblik PD, et al. Scintigraphic evaluation of four dogs with protein-losing enteropathy using ^{111}Indium-labeled transferrin. Vet Radiol Ultrasound 1997;38:221–225.

Fossum TW. Protein-losing enteropathy. Semin Vet Med Surg (Small Anim) 1989; 4:219–225.

Hall EJ, Batt RM. Enhanced intestinal permeability to ^{51}Cr-labeled EDTA in dogs with small intestinal disease. J Am Vet Med Assoc 1990;196:91–95.

Tams TR, Twedt DC. Canine protein-losing gastroenteropathy syndrome. Compend Contin Educ Pract Vet 1981;3:105–114.

Williams DA. Malabsorption, small intestinal bacterial overgrowth, and protein-losing enteropathy. In: Strombeck DR, Guilford WG, Center SA, et al. eds. Small animal gastroenterology. Philadelphia: Saunders, 1996;367–380.

Author Jörg M. Steiner
Consulting Editor Albert E. Jergens

PROTEINURIA

 BASICS

DEFINITION
• Proteinuria is a subjective increase in urinary protein detected by dipstick analysis, or objectively, a urinary protein:creatinine ratio > 0.5–1 or a 24-hour urine protein content > 20 mg/kg.
• Microalbuminuria is the presence of low, yet abnormal, concentrations of albumin in the urine (1–30 mg/dl) that are below the limit of detection of standard urine dipsticks.

PATHOPHYSIOLOGY
• Greater than normal delivery of low-molecular-weight plasma proteins to the glomerulus • Excessive leakage of larger-molecular-weight proteins (e.g., albumin) across the glomerular basement membrane secondary to altered permselectivity of the glomerulus • Reduced tubular reabsorptive capacity for proteins, or exudation of blood or serum into the lower urinary tract

SYSTEMS AFFECTED
• Renal/Urologic—longstanding glomerular proteinuria causes tubular damage with subsequent isosthenuria and renal failure.
• Cardiovascular—systemic hypertension is common in patients with glomerular disease; severe glomerular proteinuria can lead to edema and a hypercoagulable state; hypercoagulation is brought about by several mechanisms, including hyperfibrinogenemia, platelet abnormalities, and loss of antithrombin III; the pathogenesis of edema is also complex, with both primary renal sodium retention and decreased plasma oncotic pressure being involved.

INCIDENCE/PREVALENCE
In a study of urinalysis data from 500 dogs at a large referral hospital, the prevalence of proteinuria was approximately 19%.

SIGNALMENT
• Dogs and cats (less common)
• Glomerular proteinuria may be the initial manifestation of the familial renal diseases seen in soft-coated wheaten terriers, bull terriers, English cocker spaniels, Samoyeds, beagles, Bernese mountain dogs, and Chinese shar peis.

SIGNS
• Vary with underlying cause and severity of proteinuria
• None directly attributed to proteinuria

CAUSES
Preglomerular Proteinuria
• Functional proteinuria—strenuous exercise, fever, hypothermia, seizures, or venous congestion; poorly documented as a cause of proteinuria in dogs and cats
• Overload proteinuria—tubular resorptive capacity exceeded by large amounts of low-molecular-weight plasma proteins in the glomerular filtrate (e.g., excessive hemolysis or rhabdomyolysis, neoplastic production of paraproteins or Bence-Jones proteins)

Glomerular Proteinuria
• Glomerulonephritis (e.g., mesangial proliferative, membranoproliferative, proliferative), glomerulonephropathy (e.g., membranous nephropathy), minimal change disease, hereditary nephritis, amyloidosis, focal segmental glomerulosclerosis, glomerulosclerosis • In general, amyloidosis results in the heaviest proteinuria, although dogs with other glomerular diseases (e.g., membranous nephropathy) can also have very heavy proteinuria.

Postglomerular Proteinuria
• Tubular dysfunction resulting in failure of tubular protein reabsorption can cause mild-to-moderate postglomerular proteinuria.
• Hemorrhage or inflammation of the urogenital tract

RISK FACTORS
• Chronic inflammatory (e.g., infectious and immune-mediated) and neoplastic diseases can lead to development of glomerulo-nephritis or, less commonly, amyloidosis. Examples include dirofilariasis, ehrlichiosis, borreliosis, chronic bacterial infections (e.g., endocarditis, pyoderma), pyometra, FIV, mast cell tumor, lymphosarcoma, hyperadreno-corticism, and systemic lupus erythematosus.
• Systemic hypertension • Chronic hyper-lipidemia (e.g., miniature schnauzer)
• Hematuria and pyuria • Multiple myelomas can produce paraproteins resulting in Bence-Jones proteinuria.

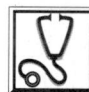 DIAGNOSIS

DIFFERENTIAL DIAGNOSIS
• Need to differentiate preglomerular, glomerular, and postglomerular causes
• Patients with glomerular proteinuria are frequently asymptomatic or have signs attributable to an underlying disease process; many have vague signs of weight loss and lethargy; some have signs of uremia, hypertension, edema, cavitary effusion, and/or thromboembolism.
• Patients with lower urinary tract disorders and postglomerular proteinuria may have dysuria, pollakiuria, inappropriate urination, and/or hematuria.

CBC/BIOCHEMISTRY/URINALYSIS
• The urine dipstick and sulfosalicylic acid (SSA) tests allow qualitative and semiquantitative assessment of urine protein content, respectively. These screening tests are quick and inexpensive; however, results of both are affected by urine concentration and must be interpreted in light of urinary specific gravity. • Low urinary protein (trace or 1+) may be normal in a concentrated urine sample. These methods may not detect high amounts of protein in samples of dilute urine. • Contamination with quaternary ammonium compounds causes false-positive urine dipstick colorimetric (tetrabromphenol blue) test results. • Results of the SSA turbidimetric test (Bumintest Tabs) are falsely increased by radiographic contrast media, penicillins, sulfisoxazole, or the urine preservative thymol. • False-positive urine dipstick test results occur when urine is highly alkaline (pH > 8–9) or when the dipstick is immersed in the urine for a prolonged period of time. • SSA test results are falsely decreased by very alkaline urine and increased by uncentrifuged urine.
• If proteinuria is detected by these methods, the urine sediment should be evaluated for hematuria, pyuria, or bacteriuria. Hematuria alone does not increase urine albumin content above the negligible range (i.e., > 1mg/dl) until there is a visible color change in the urine or until RBCs are too numerous to count using standard urinalysis methods. Data for the urine protein:creatinine ratio in urine samples with only microscopic hematuria are similar. In one study of the effects of inflammation on urine protein determination, 67% of dogs with varying degrees of pyuria had negligible urine albumin concentrations (< 1 mg/dl) and 81% had normal urine protein:creatinine ratios (< 0.4). • Repeat the urinary protein screening test in dogs and cats with proteinuria that initially have a normal urinary sediment examination or have been treated for urinary tract inflammation or hemorrhage. If proteinuria is transient and the urine sediment is normal, consider functional proteinuria or false-positive test results. • Glomerular proteinuria should be suspected in any animal that has concurrent proteinuria and hypoalbuminemia, although not all animals with glomerular disease are hypoalbuminemic. As disease progresses, other cliniopathologic changes consistent with renal failure may develop.

OTHER LABORATORY TESTS
• Urinary protein should be quantified by urinary protein:creatinine ratio or 24-hour urinary protein determination in dogs and cats that have hypoalbuminemia and/or repeatedly positive urine dipstick or SSA tests in the absence of lower urinary tract hemorrhage or inflammation.
• Suspect glomerular disease if the urinary protein:creatinine ratio or 24-hour urine protein content is abnormal, concurrent hypoalbuminemia is detected, little evidence supports primary tubular disease, and/or a large amount of albuminuria has been detected by electrophoresis. In such dogs, make aggressive attempts to identify an underlying disease (e.g., neoplasia,

ehrlichiosis, dirofilariasis, systemic lupus erythematosus, hyperadrenocorticism, chronic bacterial infection).
• Microalbuminuria can be detected in dogs using a point of care immunoassay or quantitation by ELISA. Microalbuminuria has been shown to be an early predictor of proteinuria, as traditionally defined, in 3 canine models of glomerular disease. If microalbuminuria is detected via one of these tests, the test should be repeated in 2–4 weeks. If repeatedly positive, the dog may be at risk for development of glomerular disease and should be thoroughly evaluated for an underlying cause.

IMAGING
Ultrasound and radiographs may identify an underlying infectious, inflammatory, or neoplastic disease process. Ultrasound may provide information about structural changes suggesting primary renal disease (e.g., loss of corticomedullary distinction, hyperecho-genicity, and irregular surface margin) or evidence in support of lower urinary tract disease (e.g., postglomerular proteinuria).

DIAGNOSTIC PROCEDURES
Renal biopsy is needed to specifically diagnose the glomerular disease when an underlying disease cannot be identified or proteinuria has persisted for several months following treatment of the underlying disease. Samples should be processed for light, electron, and immunofluorescence microscopy.

PATHOLOGIC FINDINGS
There are no pathologic findings specific for proteinuria.

 TREATMENT

APPROPRIATE HEALTH CARE
Most dogs and cats with proteinuria can be managed as outpatients. Inpatient care may be required during select diagnostic evaluation (e.g., renal biopsy) or when there are complications associated with renal failure in animals with glomerular proteinuria.

NURSING CARE
Physical therapy and exercise may limit formation or assist in the mobilization of edema in patients with glomerular proteinuria and hypoalbuminemia. For these patients, cage confinement should be avoided.

ACTIVITY
Maintain normal activity if proteinuria is the only laboratory abnormality.

DIET
If glomerular disease is suspected, feed a diet moderately reduced in protein.

CLIENT EDUCATION N/A

SURGICAL CONSIDERATIONS N/A

 MEDICATIONS

DRUG(S) OF CHOICE
An angiotensin-converting enzyme inhibitor should be given to dogs, and possibly cats, with glomerular proteinuria. See chapters describing Azotemia and Uremia; Nephrotic syndrome; Glomerulonephritis; Amyloidosis.

CONTRAINDICATIONS N/A

PRECAUTIONS
Drugs that are highly bound to albumin may have an altered effect if proteinuria is severe enough to cause hypoalbuminemia. Lower dosages of warfarin may be required for effective anticoagulation. In the presence of hypoalbuminemia or chronic renal failure, higher doses of furosemide may be required to mobilize edema effectively; however, this should be done cautiously. See chapter on Hypoalbuminemia.

POSSIBLE INTERACTIONS N/A

ALTERNATIVE DRUG(S)
See chapters describing Azotemia and Uremia; Nephrotic Syndrome; Glomerulonephritis; and Amyloidosis.

 FOLLOW-UP

PATIENT MONITORING
• The urinary protein:creatinine ratio should be used to assess progression of glomerular disease and response to treatment. Urine albumin content can also be used in those dogs that have microalbuminuria but may or may not have proteinuria as traditionally defined. • The urinary protein:creatinine ratio or urine albumin content should be assessed for months after resolution of any treatable underlying disease. • Monitor serum creatinine concurrently; in some patients, reduced proteinuria or reduced albuminuria may actually reflect deteriorating renal function. • Assess disease progression and subsequent therapeutic changes on the basis of trends noted in repeat urinary protein:creatinine ratio or urine albumin content rather than on one or two data points.

PREVENTION/AVOIDANCE
• All adult dogs and cats should have annual urinalyses, which should include determination of urine protein and/or albumin. If proteinuria or albuminuria is detected, the tests should be repeated in 2–4 weeks. Dogs or cats with persistent proteinuria or microalbuminuria of glomerular origin should be evaluated more thoroughly for underlying causes of glomerular injury. Potential underlying causes

should be eliminated or managed. If proteinuria or albuminuria persists and all potential underlying causes have been managed appropriately or underlying causes were not identified, the dog or cat should be evaluated for protein-losing nephropathy via renal biopsy and managed appropriately. See Glomerulonephritis; Amyloidosis.

POSSIBLE COMPLICATIONS
• Edema • Thromboembolism • Systemic hypertension • Poor wound healing

EXPECTED COURSE AND PROGNOSIS
• Vary with the cause of proteinuria
• Postglomerular proteinuria due to hemorrhage or inflammation and preglomerular proteinuria will resolve following resolution of the inciting cause.
• Most diseases associated with failure of tubular protein reabsorption will be progressive. • Glomerular diseases are, in general, progressive, although spontaneous remissions have been reported. Animals with persistent glomerular proteinuria may develop renal tubular damage resulting in renal failure and eventual uremia and death. The rate of progression is highly variable. Some dogs die shortly after the initial detection of proteinuria, while others remain alive for years.

 MISCELLANEOUS

ASSOCIATED CONDITIONS
Heavy proteinuria can be associated with hypoalbuminemia, hypoglobulinemia (rare), hypercholesterolemia, low antithrombin III, thrombocytosis, and hyperfibrinogenemia.

PREGNANCY
Some drugs used in the treatment of diseases associated with proteinuria may be contraindicated in pregnancy.

SEE ALSO
• Amyloidosis • Azotemia and Uremia
• Glomerulonephritis • Hematuria
• Hypoalbuminemia • Nephrotic Syndrome
• Pyuria

ABBREVIATIONS
• FIV = feline immunodeficiency virus
• SSA = sulfosalicylic acid

Suggested Reading
Hurley K, Vaden SL. Proteinuria in dogs and cats—a diagnostic approach. In: Bonagura JD, ed. Kirk's current veterinary therapy XII. Philadelphia; Saunders, 1995:937–940.
Vaden SL, Pressler BM, Lappin MR, et al. Urinary tract inflammation has a variable effect on urine albumin concentrations. J Vet Intern Med: 2002;16:378.
Author Shelly L. Vaden
Consulting Editors Larry G. Adams and Carl A. Osborne

PROTOTHECOSIS

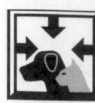

BASICS

OVERVIEW
• *Prototheca wickerhamii* and *P. zopfii*—single-celled achlorophyllous blue-green algae (Chlorophyta) that can cause disease in warm-blooded animals
• Humans and cats—usually localized infection of the skin or gastrointestinal tract
• Dogs—usually widely disseminated disease

SIGNALMENT
• Dogs and cats—uncommon
• Dogs—medium-large, middle-aged females most frequently affected

SIGNS

Historical Findings
Dogs
• Intermittent and chronic bloody diarrhea
• Chronic weight loss
• Blindness
• Neurologic disease
• Cutaneous lesions
Cats
Chronic cutaneous or mucous membrane ulceration with few systemic signs

Physical Examination Findings
Dogs
• Depend on organ system involvement
• Most often disseminated
• Hemorrhagic colitis
• Severe weight loss
• Debilitation
• Blindness with posterior segment disease and/or retinal granulomas and/or detached retinas not infrequent
• CNS—depression, ataxia, vestibular signs, and paresis may be seen.
• Ragged ulcers and crusts found on the extremities and mucosal surfaces—a few cases with cutaneous infection
Cats
Large cutaneous nodules on the limbs or face

CAUSES & RISK FACTORS
• Dogs—usually *P. zopfii;* one reported case of *P. wickerhamii* infection
• Cats—usually *P. wickerhamii*
• Basis for the pathogenicity of Prototheca unknown
• Organism—ecological niche is raw and treated sewage; survive as contaminants of water, soil, and food; occasionally isolated from fresh fecal samples from healthy individuals
• Dogs and humans—depressed cell-mediated immunity may predispose to gastrointestinal and disseminated infections with *P. zopfii.*
• Cats—no known predisposing factors

DIAGNOSIS

DIFFERENTIAL DIAGNOSIS
• Systemic—systemic mycoses
• Cutaneous—systemic and subcutaneous mycoses; mycobacterioses

CBC/BIOCHEMISTRY/URINALYSIS
• Dogs—often normal; depends on organ system affected; organism occasionally seen in urine sediment
• Cats—almost always normal

OTHER LABORATORY TESTS
CSF tap—may find pleocytosis with mononuclear cells; increased protein; organisms

IMAGING
N/A

DIAGNOSTIC PROCEDURES

Cytology
• Most common definitively diagnostic test; use Wright-Giemsa stain

• Rectal or colonic mucosa, anterior chamber aspirations, CSF taps, cutaneous aspirations
• Organisms—unicellular, nonpigmented, oval; 1.5–16 μm in diameter; cell walls often appear folded; diagnostic characteristic is endospore formation with internal septation in two planes.

Histopathology

Biopsy specimens—identification of organisms may be diagnostic; special stains (GMS or PAS) or IFA stains used at the CDC

Culture

• Grow on Sabouraud dextrose agar at 25–37°C (77–97°F) in 2 to 7 days; or on blood agar.
• Specific identification accomplished by IFA at the CDC.

PATHOLOGIC FINDINGS

Dogs

• Small granulomatous foci   may be found in many organs, especially kidneys
• Colonic muscularis and myocardium
• Nodular thickening of the gastrointestinal mucosa with ulceration
• Granulomas—poorly organized; mixed with other inflammatory cells
• Organisms—contained within macrophages and multinucleate giant cells; may be masses in the colon and kidney with minimal inflammatory response; may be masses in all layers and subjacent fascia and muscle of cutaneous lesions (ulceration frequent)

Cats

Cutaneous masses—localized; extend deep into subcutaneous tissues; consist of granulomatous inflammation and mixed cell inflammation; made up primarily by organisms

TREATMENT

• Dogs—depends on organ system(s) involved
• Cats—excision of localized cutaneous masses is primary therapeutic modality.

MEDICATIONS

DRUG(S)

• Amphotericin B—use for localized disease after surgical excision; 0.25–0.5 mg/kg IV 3 times weekly or until a total dose of 8 mg/kg; or lipid formulation; concurrent administration of tetracyclines may provide synergistic effect; lipid formulations may be more efficacious and less toxic for cutaneous disease; reported effective for ocular disease
• Ketoconazole, fluconazole, and itraconazole—may use in conjunction with amphotericin B, as consolidation treatment, or as sole agents for less life-threatening disease
• Alternative treatments—clotrimazole (locally for *P. wickerhamii*); potassium iodide

CONTRAINDICATIONS/POSSIBLE INTERACTIONS

N/A

FOLLOW-UP

EXPECTED COURSE AND PROGNOSIS

• Difficult to eradicate with drug therapy
• No well-defined therapeutic protocol
• Dogs—prognosis guarded to grave
• Cats—prognosis fair to good for cutaneous disease if lesions can be completely excised

MISCELLANEOUS

ZOONOTIC POTENTIAL

None recorded

ABBREVIATIONS

• CSF = cerebrospinal fluid
• GMS = Gomori methenamine silver
• IFA = immunofluorescent antibody test
• PAS = periodic acid–Schiff

Suggested Reading

Greene CE. Protothecosis. In: Greene CE, ed. Infectious diseases of the dog and cat. Philadelphia: Saunders, 1998:430–435.
Author Carol S. Foil
Consulting Editor Stephen C. Barr

PRURITUS

 BASICS

DEFINITION
The sensation that provokes the desire to scratch, rub, chew, or lick; an indicator of inflamed skin

PATHOPHYSIOLOGY
• A specific end organ has not been found.
• The sensation of itch is conducted by A δ fibers and C fibers of the peripheral nervous system to the dorsal root of the spinal cord.
• The axons, some of which cross over, ascend via the lateral spinothalamic tract and synapse in the caudal thalamus and then to the sensory cortex.
• Other factors can modify the perception of pruritus at this level.

SYSTEMS AFFECTED
Skin/Exocrine—in severe cases, the mental state of the animal may also be affected.

SIGNALMENT
Highly variable; depends on the underlying cause

SIGNS
• The act of scratching, licking, biting, or chewing
• For some animals, evidence of self-trauma and cutaneous inflammation is necessary to make the diagnosis if the history is incomplete.
• Cats—can be secretive lickers; alopecia without inflammation may be the only sign

CAUSES
• Parasitic—fleas, scabies, *Demodex, Otodectes, Notoedres, Cheyletiella,* trombicula, lice, *Pelodera,* endoparasite migration
• Allergic—parasite, atopy, food, contact, drug, bacterial hypersensitivity
• Bacterial/fungal—*Malassezia* pachydermatis
• Miscellaneous—primary and secondary seborrhea, calcinosis cutis, cutaneous neoplasia, immune-mediated dermatosis; psychogenic diseases and endocrine dermatosis variable

RISK FACTORS
N/A

 DIAGNOSIS

DIFFERENTIAL DIAGNOSIS
• Alopecia—in most cases, a clear history of pruritus is noted; without pruritus, may accompany endocrine diseases; some animals may excessively lick themselves without the owner's knowledge; demodicosis, dermatophytosis, bacterial pyoderma, seborrhea, some cutaneous neoplasms, and unusual diseases (e.g., leishmaniasis) may cause alopecia with varying degrees of inflammation and pruritus.
• History—often the most important guide to necessary tests; severe condition, which constantly keeps the patient and owner awake, suggests scabies, flea allergy/infestation, food allergy, or cutaneous yeast infection; all but the latter typically have an acute onset
• Uncomplicated atopy—initially very steroid responsive; originally seasonal; often progresses to nonseasonal, pruritic disease with a predilection for the face, feet, ears, forelimbs, axilla, and rump; flea- and food-allergic animals are predisposed to atopy and may show similar signs

CBC/BIOCHEMISTRY/URINALYSIS
N/A

OTHER LABORATORY TESTS
N/A

IMAGING
N/A

DIAGNOSTIC PROCEDURES
• Skin scrapes, epidermal cytology, and dermatophyte cultures (with microscopic identification)—identify primary or co-existing diseases caused by parasites or other microorganisms
• Wood's lamp—do not use as the sole means of diagnosing or excluding dermatophytosis, owing to false negatives and misinterpretations of fluorescence.

Allergy Testing
• Two methods—skin testing (intradermal skin testing) and blood testing; skin testing is the historical standard and the preferred method; some veterinary dermatologists use both tests

• Skin testing—identifies individual allergens; takes into account the important allergy-associated immunoglobulins (IgGd and systemic as well as localized IgE)
• Blood testing—commercial tests for allergies measure only serum IgE, not IgGd; disadvantage, some tests determine groups or mixes of allergens
• Allergy extract—correlate positive reactions with the history; then formulate the immunotherapy solution; contains a mixture of specific allergens, based on the history, test results, and the veterinarian's (or the laboratory's) clinical experience; concentration may vary with the type of test done and may affect the success rate

Skin Biopsy
• Useful when associated lesions are unusual and an immune-mediated disease is expected or the history and physical findings do not correlate
• Results should be interpreted by a trained veterinary dermatopathologist.

Trial Courses
Canine Scabies
• Can be difficult to diagnose
• Skin scrapes often negative
• Trial course (lime sulfur, ivermectin) often necessary to rule out
• Ivermectin—use caution; associated with idiosyncratic reactions and death
Food Allergy
• Blood and skin tests—not recommended for diagnosis
• Hypoallergenic dietary trial most appropriate test
• Trial—must include only novel food; use a diet that has been confirmed as hypoallergenic through clinical trials; avoid meat-flavored treats and medicines (heartworm preventives); continue trial until patient improves or for 8–10 weeks; if improvement is noted, reintroduce original diet and monitor for itching for 7–14 days; return of itching may occur within hours; reintroduction of original diet confirms food allergy

TREATMENT

• More than one disease may be contributing to the itching; if treatment for an identified condition does not result in improvement, consider other causes.
• Use of a mechanical restraint (e.g., Elizabethan collar) can help but is seldom feasible in the long term.

MEDICATIONS

DRUG(S) OF CHOICE

Topical Therapy
• Helpful for mild cases
• Localized—sprays, lotions, and creams
• Generalized—shampoos
• Colloidal oatmeal—available in all forms; may be very beneficial; duration of effect usually < 2 days
• Antihistamines—beneficial effect not demonstrated
• Anesthetics—very short duration of effect
• Antibacterial shampoo—controls bacterial infections; some (e.g., benzoyl peroxide or iodine) may exacerbate the condition
• Lime sulfur—may be antipruritic; has antiparasitic, antibacterial, and antifungal properties; disadvantages are bad odor and staining
• Steroids—most useful topical medication; excessive use causes localized and systemic side effects; hydrocortisone mildest and most common; stronger drugs (e.g., betamethasone) more effective, more expensive, and cause more side effects; some contain ingredients (e.g., alcohol) that increase irritation
• Low-dose triamcinolone spray @ 0.015 concentration as a body spray (Genesis from Allerderm/Virbac)
• Sometimes the application of any substance, including water (especially warm water), can worsen itching sensation; cool water is often soothing.

Systemic Therapy
• Three pathways lead to inflammation and itching.
• Steroids—block all three pathways; undesirable side effects; consider drugs that block individual pathways
• Antihistamines—hydroxyzine, diphenhydramine, and chlorpheniramine; block only one pathway

• ω-3 and ω-6 fatty acids—available as powder, liquid, and capsules; help block individual pathways that lead to inflammation; 6–8 weeks until maximum effect is observed; prevent rather than stop inflammation; help control dry or flaky skin
• Psychogenics—can help control itching; amitriptyline (Elavil; a human antidepressant) has rather potent antihistaminic actions in dogs, with side effects similar to antihistamines; doxepin is similar; fluoxetine (Prozac) used with variable success in treating canine lick granuloma (acral lick dermatitis); diazepam (Valium) has been beneficial; reports of acute hepatotoxicity in cats
• The use of nonsteroid drugs is less convenient but diminishes the potential for serious side effects; if not totally effective in controlling clinical signs, they often help reduce the amount of steroids necessary to decrease itching.
• Cyclosporine (Neoral) 5mg/kg/day

CONTRAINDICATIONS
• Sometimes the application of anything topically, including water and products containing alcohol, iodine, and benzoyl peroxide, can exacerbate itching; cool water may be soothing.
• Steroids—avoid with infectious causes

PRECAUTIONS

Steroids
• Most well-known drugs used to control itching
• Significant long-term and not always obvious side effects
• Used wisely, usually safe
• Avoid long-term daily administration of oral corticosteroids (including prednisone or methylprednisolone).
• Avoid long-term daily or alternate-day administration of triamcinolone (Vetalog).
• Short-term use seldom causes serious problems.
• Avoid with a history of pancreatitis, diabetes mellitus, calcinosis cutis, demodicosis, dermatophytosis, and other infectious diseases.

POSSIBLE INTERACTIONS
N/A

ALTERNATIVE DRUG(S)
Immunosuppressive drugs (e.g., azathioprine)—use in extremely rare cases; because of potential profound side effects, reserve for cases in which euthanasia is being considered or when all other treatments have failed.

FOLLOW-UP

PATIENT MONITORING
• Multiple causes (e.g., flea allergy, inhalant allergy, and pyoderma) common; eradication or control of one cause may not be enough to reduce the condition.
• Food- and airborne/inhalant-allergic animals may do well during winter on a hypoallergenic diet; clinical signs may return in the warmer months in association with inhalant allergies.
• Monitor patients receiving chronic steroids every 3–6 months for signs of iatrogenic Cushing disease.

POSSIBLE COMPLICATIONS
• Client frustration due to the chronic nature of pruritus
• Skin scrapes and other tests may be initially negative or normal but may later become diagnostic.
• Complications common with chronic steroid use

MISCELLANEOUS

ASSOCIATED CONDITIONS
N/A

AGE-RELATED FACTORS
N/A

ZOONOTIC POTENTIAL
Some causes (e.g., sarcoptic mange)

PREGNANCY
N/A

SEE ALSO
See Causes

Suggested Reading
Bevier DE. Long-term management of atopic disease in the dog. Vet Clin North Am Small Anim Pract 1995;25:1487–1505.
Authors W. Dunbar Gram and Nicola Williamson
Consulting Editor Karen Helton Rhodes

PSEUDORABIES VIRUS INFECTION

BASICS

OVERVIEW
• Uncommon but highly fatal disease of dogs and cats, usually occurring in animals that have contact with swine
• Characterized by sudden death, often without characteristic signs or with signs that include hypersalivation, intense pruritus, and neurologic changes

SIGNALMENT
• Domestic and exotic dogs and cats
• Other domestic animals—swine, cattle, sheep, and goats
• Primarily farm dogs and cats, with no breed or age predilection

SIGNS
• Sudden death
• Hypersalivation
• Rapid and labored breathing
• Fever
• Vomiting
• Neurologic—depression and lethargy, ataxia, convulsions, reluctance to move, recumbency, intense pruritus and self-mutilation, coma, and death

CAUSES & RISK FACTORS
• Pseudorabies virus (herpesvirus suid)—an α-herpesvirus
• Contact with swine
• Eating contaminated, uncooked meat or offal from swine
• Ingestion of infected rats

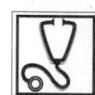

DIAGNOSIS

DIFFERENTIAL DIAGNOSIS
• Rabies—in the furious form, affected dog or cat will attack anything that moves; no pruritus or sudden death; immunofluorescent antibody test of brain positive
• Canine distemper—no hypersalivation, sudden death, or personality change; respiratory and gastrointestinal signs common
• Poisoning (organophosphate, lead, strychnine, inorganic arsenic)—no pruritus or personality change; history of exposure to toxin; signs consistent with toxicity

CBC/BIOCHEMISTRY/URINALYSIS
No characteristic changes

OTHER LABORATORY TESTS
Serologic assays—reveal pseudorabies virus antibodies if an animal recovers

IMAGING
N/A

DIAGNOSTIC PROCEDURES
• Immunofluorescent antibody test—brain tissue
• Viral isolation—affected tissues
• Animal (rabbit) inoculation

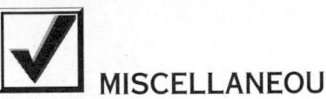

PATHOLOGIC FINDINGS
• Severe skin lesions—caused by self-mutilation from intense pruritus
• Histopathologic examination—glial and ganglion cells of neurologic tissues reveal Cowdry type A intranuclear inclusion bodies
• Nonsuppurative meningoencephalitis in the medulla oblongata

 TREATMENT

• Dogs and cats—no known effective treatment
• General supportive therapy and prevention of self-injury indicated

 MEDICATIONS

DRUG(S)
• None specific
• Antiherpetic antivirals—not evaluated for dogs and cats

• Rapid course makes successful use of antiviral drugs unlikely.

CONTRAINDICATIONS/POSSIBLE INTERACTIONS
None

 FOLLOW-UP

PREVENTION/AVOIDANCE
• Avoid contact with infected swine, the reservoir host.
• Avoid ingestion of contaminated pork.
• Avoid ingestion of infected rats.
• Cat-to-cat and dog-to-dog transmission usually does not occur.

EXPECTED COURSE AND PROGNOSIS
• Classic (cats)—60% of cases; lasts 24–36 hr; almost invariably fatal
• Atypical (cats)—40% of cases; lasts > 36 hr; almost invariably fatal

MISCELLANEOUS

ZOONOTIC POTENTIAL
Mild potential for human infection; take precautions when treating infected animals and handling infected tissues and fluids.

Suggested Reading
Gustafson DP. Pseudorabies (Aujeszky's disease, mad itch, infectious bulbar paralysis). In: Holzworth J, ed. Diseases of the cat. Philadelphia: Saunders, 1987:242–246.
Author Fred W. Scott
Consulting Editor Stephen C. Barr

PTYALISM

 BASICS

DEFINITION
- Excessive production of saliva
- Pseudoptyalism is the excessive release of saliva that has accumulated in the oral cavity.

PATHOPHYSIOLOGY
- Saliva is constantly produced and secreted into the oral cavity from the salivary glands (parotid, sublingual, mandibular, zygomatic, buccal).
- Normal saliva production may appear excessive in patients with an anatomic abnormality that allows saliva to dribble out of the mouth or with a condition that affects swallowing.
- Salivation increases because of excitation of the salivary nuclei in the brain stem.
- Stimuli that lead to this are taste and tactile sensations involving the mouth and tongue.
- Higher centers in the CNS can also excite or inhibit the salivary nuclei.
- Lesions involving either the CNS or the oral cavity can cause excessive salivation.
- Diseases that affect the pharynx, esophagus, and stomach can also stimulate excessive production of saliva.

SYSTEMS AFFECTED
N/A

SIGNALMENT
- Dogs and cats
- Young animals are more likely to have ptyalism caused by a congenital problem such as portosystemic shunt and from ingestion of a toxin, caustic agent, or foreign body.
- Yorkshire terrier, Maltese terrier, Australian cattle dog, miniature schnauzer, and Irish wolfhound breeds have a relatively higher incidence of congenital portosystemic shunt.
- Megaesophagus is hereditary in wire-haired fox terriers and miniature schnauzers; familial predispositions have been reported in the German shepherd, Newfoundland, Great Dane, Irish setter, Chinese shar-pei, greyhound, and retriever breeds, as well as in Siamese cats.
- Congenital hiatal hernia has been recognized in the Chinese shar-pei.
- Giant breeds, such as St. Bernard and mastiff, are known for excessive drooling.

SIGNS

Historical Findings
- Anorexia—seen most often in patients with oral lesions, gastrointestinal disease, and systemic disease
- Eating behavior changes—patients with oral disease or cranial nerve dysfunction may refuse to eat hard food, not chew with the affected side (patients with unilateral lesions), hold the head in an unusual position while eating, or drop prehended food
- Other behavioral changes—irritability, aggressiveness, and reclusiveness are common, especially in patients with a painful condition

- Dysphagia—may be seen if inability to swallow
- Regurgitation—in patients with esophageal disease
- Vomiting—secondary to gastrointestinal or systemic disease
- Pawing at the face or muzzle—patients with oral discomfort or pain
- Neurologic signs—patients that have been exposed to causative drugs or toxins and those with hepatic encephalopathy following consumption of a meal high in protein

Physical Examination Findings
- Periodontal disease—inflammation may cause ptyalism
- Stomatitis—ulceration and inflammation of many different causes is associated with ptyalism
- Mass in the oral cavity
- Lesions of the tongue—inflammation, ulceration, mass, and foreign body
- Lesions of the oropharynx—inflammation, ulceration, and mass, especially involving the soft palate and glossopalatine arch
- Blood in the saliva—suggests bleeding from the oral cavity, pharynx, or esophagus
- Halitosis—usually caused by oral cavity disease, but also by esophageal and gastric disease
- Facial pain—caused by oral cavity or pharyngeal disease
- Dysphagia—caused by oral cavity, pharyngeal, or neuromuscular disease or abnormally large retropharyngeal lymph nodes
- Cranial nerve deficits—trigeminal nerve (CN V) lesions can cause drooling due to inability to close the mouth; facial nerve palsy (CN VII) can cause drooling from the affected side; glossopharyngeal (CN IX), vagus (CN X), and hypoglossal (CN XII) nerve lesions can cause a loss of the gag reflex or inability to swallow
- Salivary gland problem—inflamed, necrotic, or painful salivary glands can cause ptyalism (rare)
- Cheilitis or acne—persistent drooling can lead to dermatologic lesions

CAUSES

Conformational Disorder of the Lips
Particularly in giant-breed dogs

Oral and Pharyngeal Diseases
- Foreign body (e.g., linear foreign body, such as a sewing needle)
- Neoplasm
- Abscess
- Gingivitis or stomatitis—secondary to periodontal disease, FeLV infection in cats, viral upper respiratory infection, immune-mediated disease (e.g., lymphoplasmacytic stomatitis, pemphigus vulgaris), uremia, ingestion of a caustic agent, poisonous plant, or burns (e.g., those from biting on an electrical cord)
- Neurologic or functional disorder of the pharynx

Salivary Gland Diseases
- Foreign body
- Neoplasm
- Sialoadenitis
- Hyperplasia
- Infarction
- Sialocele (ranula)

Esophageal or Gastrointestinal Disorders
- Esophageal foreign body
- Esophageal neoplasm
- Esophagitis—secondary to ingestion of a caustic agent or poisonous plant
- Gastroesophageal reflux
- Hiatal hernia
- Megaesophagus
- Gastric distension/volvulus
- Gastric ulcer

Metabolic Disorders
- Hepatoencephalopathy (especially in cats)—caused by congenital or acquired portosystemic shunt or hepatic failure
- Hyperthermia
- Uremia

Neurologic Disorders
- Rabies
- Pseudorabies in dogs
- Botulism
- Tetanus
- Dysautonomia
- Disorders that cause dysphagia
- Disorders that cause facial nerve palsy or a dropped jaw
- Disorders that cause seizures—during a seizure, ptyalism may occur because of autonomic discharge or reduced swallowing of saliva and may be exacerbated by chomping of the jaws
- Nausea associated with vestibular disease

Drugs and Toxins
- Those that are caustic (e.g., household cleaning products and some common house plants)
- Those with a disagreeable taste (especially in cats)—many antibiotics and anthelmintics
- Those that induce hypersalivation, including organophosphate compounds, cholinergic drugs, insecticides containing boric acid, pyrethrin and pyrethroid insecticides, ivermectin (dogs), fluids containing benzoic acid derivatives (cats), clozapine (a tricyclic dibenzodiazepine), caffeine, and illicit drugs such as amphetamines, cocaine, and opiates
- Animal venom (e.g., black widow spiders, Gila monsters, and North American scorpions)
- Toad and newt secretions
- Plant consumption or prehension (e.g., poinsettia, *Dieffenbachia*) may cause increased salivation

RISK FACTORS
N/A

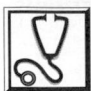

DIAGNOSIS

DIFFERENTIAL DIAGNOSIS
• Differentiating causes of ptyalism and pseudoptyalism requires a thorough history, including vaccination status, current medications, possible toxin exposure, and duration of ptyalism.
• May be able to distinguish salivation associated with nausea (signs of depression, lip smacking, and retching) from dysphagia by observing the patient
• Complete physical examination (with special attention to the oral cavity and neck) and neurologic examination are critical; wear examination gloves when rabies exposure is possible.

CBC/BIOCHEMISTRY/URINALYSIS
• CBC—often normal; leukocytosis in patients with immune-mediated or infectious disease
• Stress leukogram—common in animals that have ingested a caustic agent or organophosphate
• FeLV-infected cats may have leukopenia and nonregenerative anemia.
• Possible microcytosis with portosystemic shunts
• Biochemical analysis—usually normal except in patients with renal disease (azotemia, hyperphosphatemia, decreased urine specific gravity) and hepatoencephalopathy (possibly elevated hepatic enzyme activities, decreased BUN, decreased albumin and decreased glucose)
• Marked ptyalism can result in hypokalemia and acidosis from the loss of potassium and bicarbonate-rich saliva.

OTHER LABORATORY TESTS
• Serologic FeLV and FIV testing in cats with oral lesions
• Fasting and postprandial bile acids when hepatoencephalopathy is suspected
• Serum cholinesterase concentration to detect organophosphate toxicosis
• Postmortem fluorescent antibody testing of the brain if rabies is suspected

IMAGING
• Survey radiography of the oral cavity, neck, and thorax when foreign body or neoplasm is suspected
• Ultrasonographic evaluation, portal venography, or portal scintigraphy may help diagnose a portosystemic shunt
• Fluoroscopic evaluation of swallowing may be useful in dysphagic patients.

DIAGNOSTIC PROCEDURES
• Biopsy and histopathology of mucocutaneous lesions—possibly including immunofluorescence testing when immune-mediated disease (e.g., pemphigus vulgaris) is suspected
• Cytologic examination of oral lesions or fine-needle aspiration of oral mass and regional lymph nodes.
• Biopsy and histopathology of oral lesion, salivary gland, or mass
• Consider esophagoscopy or gastroscopy if lesions distal to the oral cavity are suspected.

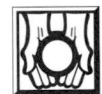

TREATMENT
• Treat the underlying cause (refer to sections pertaining to specific conditions)
• Symptomatic treatment to reduce the flow of saliva—generally unnecessary, may be of little value to the patient, and may mask other signs of the underlying cause and so delay diagnosis; only recommended when hypersalivation is prolonged and severe and, if possible, after the underlying condition has been diagnosed
• Nutritional supplementation (esophagostomy, gastrostomy tubes, etc.) may be needed in patients with ptyalism and anorexia secondary to severe oral, gastrointestinal, or metabolic causes.

MEDICATIONS

DRUG(S) OF CHOICE
• Atropine (0.05 mg/kg SC q8h)—can give symptomatically to reduce the flow of saliva
• Petroleum jelly—can apply to areas of the face constantly wet from saliva, to help prevent moist dermatitis
• Astringent solutions applied for 10 min q8–12h—can be used to treat areas of moist dermatitis
• Crystalloid fluids—give IV or SC to treat dehydration caused by prolonged or severe ptyalism

CONTRAINDICATIONS
N/A

PRECAUTIONS
N/A

POSSIBLE INTERACTIONS
N/A

ALTERNATIVE DRUG(S)
N/A

FOLLOW-UP

PATIENT MONITORING
• Depends on the underlying cause (see Causes)
• Continually monitor hydration, serum electrolytes, and nutritional status, especially in dysphagic or anorexic animals.

POSSIBLE COMPLICATIONS
• Dehydration
• Hypokalemia
• Acidosis
• Moist dermatitis

MISCELLANEOUS

ASSOCIATED CONDITIONS
N/A

AGE-RELATED FACTORS
N/A

ZOONOTIC POTENTIAL
Rabies

PREGNANCY
N/A

SYNONYMS
• Hypersalivation
• Drooling
• Sialorrhea

SEE ALSO
• Gastroesophageal Reflux
• Gingivitis
• Hepatic Encephalopathy
• Megaesophagus
• Stomatitis

ABBREVIATIONS
• BUN = blood urea nitrogen
• CN = cranial nerve
• CNS = central nervous system
• FeLV = feline leukemia virus
• FIV = feline immunodeficiency virus

Suggested Reading

DeBowes LJ. Ptyalism. In: Ettinger SJ, ed., Veterinary internal medicine. 5th ed. Philadelphia: Saunders, 2000;107–110.
Spangler WL, Cubertson MR. Salivary gland disease in dogs and cats: 245 cases (1985–1988). J Am Vet Med Assoc 1991;198:465–469.

Acknowledgment

The author acknowledges the prior contributions of Dr. N. C. Myers III, who authored this topic in a previous edition.
Author John Crandell
Consulting Editor Albert E. Jergens

PUG ENCEPHALITIS (MENINGOENCEPHALITIS)

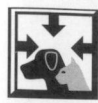

BASICS

OVERVIEW
• One of the breed-restricted encephalitides defined by highly characteristic morphologic features
• Similar to the described necrotizing encephalitis of Maltese dogs
• Differs from necrotizing encephalitis of Yorkshire terriers by clinical and pathologic features
• Sporadic disease; known for many years; occurs worldwide
• A genetic basis is probable.
• Affects the CNS

SIGNALMENT
• Pug dogs; also described in a Pekingese dog
• Age range—6 months to 7 years

SIGNS
• Generalized seizures—most common; may be the only sign at onset
• Typical for cortical involvement—circling, blindness, visual hemifield loss
• Cervical rigidity sometimes seen

CAUSES & RISK FACTORS
• Unknown
• An infectious agent might be suspected.

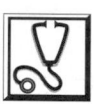

DIAGNOSIS

DIFFERENTIAL DIAGNOSIS
Neoplasia and other inflammatory or infectious diseases

CBC/BIOCHEMISTRY/URINALYSIS
Usually normal

OTHER LABORATORY TESTS
N/A

IMAGING
CT and MRI (brain)—nonspecific changes; may help support the clinical diagnosis considering breed and age

DIAGNOSTIC PROCEDURES
• CSF analysis—pleocytosis (200–550 leukocytes/mm³) with mononuclear cells; lymphocytes predominating cell population; mild protein elevation
• Brain biopsy—should help confirm or support the diagnosis in vivo

PATHOLOGIC FINDINGS
• Extensive necrosis and nonsuppurative inflammation of the cerebral gray and white matter
• Inflammatory changes are severe.

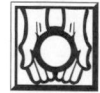

TREATMENT
• Inpatient or outpatient
• No specific treatment known
• Supportive only—prevent seizures

MEDICATIONS

DRUG(S)
• None specific
• Seizures—phenobarbital (2–8 mg/kg PO q12h); monitor serum concentrations.
• Inflammatory response—corticosteroids; prednisolone or prednisone (1–2 mg/kg PO q24h for the first 1–2 weeks; then taper dosage slowly)

CONTRAINDICATIONS/POSSIBLE INTERACTIONS
N/A

FOLLOW-UP

PATIENT MONITORING
• Monitor serum concentration of phenobarbital.
• Perform regular clinical and neurologic examinations.

PREVENTION/AVOIDANCE
N/A

POSSIBLE COMPLICATIONS
N/A

EXPECTED COURSE AND PROGNOSIS
• May be acute
• Status epilepticus may develop.
• Often chronic for months or even years, but neurologic signs are progressive.
• Prognosis—guarded

MISCELLANEOUS

ASSOCIATED CONDITIONS
In one patient, myocardial necrosis was seen in addition to the encephalitic lesions.

PREGNANCY
• Report of three patients in Japan with a history of pregnancy before onset of clinical signs
• Other more extended studies report patients of both sexes.

SEE ALSO
• Necrotizing Encephalitis in Yorkshire Terriers
• Necrotizing Meningoencephalitis of Maltese Dogs
• Seizures (Convulsions, Status Epilepticus)—Dogs

ABBREVIATIONS
• CNS = central nervous system
• CSF = cerebrospinal fluid
• CT = computed tomography
• MRI= magnetic resonance imaging

Suggested Reading

Beltran WA, Ollivet FF. Homonymous hemianopia in a pug dog with necrotising meningoencephalitis. J Small Anim Pract 2000; 41:161–164.

Cantile C, Chianini F. Arispici M, Fatzer R. Necrotizing meningoencephalitis associated with cortical hippocampal hamartia in a Pekingese dog. Vet Pathol 2001; 38:119–120.

Cordy DR, Holliday TA. A necrotizing meningoencephalitis of pug dogs. Vet Pathol 1989;26:191–194.

Author Andrea Tipold
Consulting Editor Joane M. Parent

PULMONARY CONTUSIONS

BASICS

OVERVIEW
• Hemorrhage in the lung parenchyma caused by tearing and crushing during direct trauma to the thorax • Relatively small volumes of blood in the lungs may markedly compromise lung function by causing ventilation–perfusion mismatch. • In patients in shock with capillary damage, the hemorrhage may later be accompanied by pulmonary edema after fluid resuscitation.

SIGNALMENT
• Dogs and cats • No specific breed, age, or sex predilection

SIGNS
• Historical findings consistent with blunt trauma • Tachypnea • Abnormal respiratory effort • Postural adaptations to respiratory distress • Cyanotic or pale mucous membranes • Auscultation of harsh bronchovesicular sounds or crackles • Expectoration of blood or blood-tinged fluid

CAUSES & RISK FACTORS
• Blunt trauma • Motor vehicle accidents • Falls from a height • Abuse—beating • Coagulopathy • von Willebrand factor deficiency

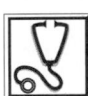

DIAGNOSIS

DIFFERENTIAL DIAGNOSIS
• Hemothorax—may cause dull lung sounds; may see pleural effusion on thoracic radiographs • Pneumothorax—may cause dull lung sounds; may see pleural air on thoracic radiographs • Diaphragmatic hernia—distinguished radiographically • Coagulopathy—may cause pulmonary hemorrhage; distinguished by coagulation testing and platelet count • Acute onset of pulmonary hemorrhage—may be a feature of some neoplasms (e.g., hemangiosarcoma); occasionally accompanies pulmonary infarction associated with bacterial endocarditis and heartworm disease

CBC/BIOCHEMISTRY/URINALYSIS
• CBC—may reveal anemia or mature neutrophilia • Serum biochemistry profile—may demonstrate hypoproteinemia, indicating blood loss; may reveal damage to other organ systems • Urinalysis—usually normal

IMAGING
Thoracic radiographs—usually reveal patchy areas of alveolar pattern, focal or asymmetrical; always perform in trauma patients after stabilization to rule out hemothorax, pneumothorax, and diaphragmatic hernia.

DIAGNOSTIC PROCEDURES
• Examination of transtracheal wash—may demonstrate excessive numbers of erythrocytes and macrophages; culture to monitor for development of a superimposed bacterial infection. • Pulse oximetry or arterial blood gas analysis—may confirm hypoxemia

TREATMENT
• Usually inpatient for stabilization • Support respiratory function, stabilize cardiovascular function, and resuscitate if necessary. • Assess and treat injuries to other organ systems. • Restrict activity, minimize stress, and observe carefully for deterioration of respiratory function during the first 24 hours after trauma. • Respiratory support—oxygen supplementation for hypoxemia; intubation and positive-pressure ventilation in severely affected patients; nebulization of saline to facilitate clearance of respiratory secretions; coupage and physical therapy to facilitate clearance of respiratory secretions if no rib fractures • Shock—fluids may be required to support cardiovascular function; if possible, be conservative with fluid administration because it may lead to deterioration of pulmonary function by creating and exacerbating pulmonary edema; to minimize edema development, consider synthetic colloids in animals with hypoproteinemia. • Blood or plasma transfusion—consider if hemorrhage has resulted in anemia or with a coagulopathy. • Nutritional support—if needed to maintain body condition and immune status

MEDICATIONS

DRUG(S)
Low-dose diuretics—furosemide (0.5–2 mg/kg IV, IM); used only when hemorrhage is accompanied by edema, and respiratory distress is severe

CONTRAINDICATIONS/POSSIBLE INTERACTIONS
Diuretics—no value in the early stages and may, in fact, be harmful; cause diuresis and decrease intravascular volume, which is contraindicated for shock; however, after fluid resuscitation, some pulmonary edema may accompany hemorrhage, and the edema and respiratory distress may be responsive to diuretic therapy.

FOLLOW-UP

PATIENT MONITORING
• Monitor respiratory rate and effort, mucous membrane color, heart rate and pulse quality, and lung sounds • Measure PCV and total solids and perform pulse oximetry and arterial blood gas analysis for 24 hours. • Monitor ECG frequently to detect ventricular arrhythmias. • Radiographs—repeated in 48 hours to ensure that the contusions are resolving.

PREVENTION AND AVOIDANCE
Rely on appropriate restriction of the animal to prevent exposure to trauma.

POSSIBLE COMPLICATIONS
• Bacterial pneumonia—owing to systemic immunosuppression, reduced pulmonary defenses, and aspiration of gastrointestinal tract contents • Development of a moist productive cough and failure to improve within 48 hours—suspect pneumonia. • Patients with severe shock may develop ARDS (less common).

EXPECTED COURSE AND PROGNOSIS
• Usually deterioration of respiratory function occurs during the initial 12–24 hours after trauma, and then gradually improves. • Marked clinical improvement in respiratory status generally occurs within 48 hours, with a more gradual resolution of radiographic lesions. • If patient fails to improve after 48 hours, evaluate for complications or concurrent disease.

MISCELLANEOUS

ASSOCIATED CONDITIONS
• Fractured ribs • Flail chest • Ruptured trachea, bronchi, or esophagus • Cardiac arrhythmias—ventricular • Other possible complications of trauma

ABBREVIATIONS
• ARDS = acute respiratory distress syndrome • PCV = packed cell volume

Suggested Reading
Campbell VL, King LG. Pulmonary function, ventilator management and outcome of dogs with thoracic trauma and pulmonary contusions: 10 cases (1994–1998). J Am Vet Med Assoc 2000;217:1505–1509.

Hackner SG. The emergency management of traumatic pulmonary contusions. Compend Contin Educ Pract Vet 1995;17:677–686.

Powell LL, Rozanski EA, Tidwell AS, Rush JE. A retrospective analysis of pulmonary contusion secondary to motor vehicular accidents in 143 dogs: 1994–1997. J Vet Emerg Crit Care 1999;9:127–136.
Author Lesley G. King
Consulting Editor Lynelle R. Johnson

PULMONARY EDEMA

 BASICS

DEFINITION
An accumulation of extravascular fluid in the pulmonary interstitial and alveolar spaces

PATHOPHYSIOLOGY
In normal lungs, fluid exudes from the pulmonary capillaries into the interstitial space and returns to the circulation via the pulmonary lymphatic vessels, a dynamic process that depends upon capillary and interstitial hydrostatic and oncotic pressures and capillary and alveolar epithelial permeability. When increased hydrostatic pressure occurs, there is damage to the capillary/alveolar membrane and edema results. When fluid formation exceeds fluid removal by the lymphatic vessels, pulmonary edema results. When edema becomes clinically important, pulmonary gas exchange is impaired, and clinical signs develop.

SYSTEMS AFFECTED
- Respiratory
- Cardiovascular
- CNS

GENETICS
N/A

INCIDENCE/PREVALENCE
N/A

GEOGRAPHIC DISTRIBUTION
N/A

SIGNALMENT
Species
Dogs and cats

Breed Predilection
None

Mean Age and Range
- Immature and mature animals with cardiac disease
- Animals of any age affected by noncardiac causes

Predominant Sex
N/A

SIGNS
General Comments
Clinical signs depend upon the cause and severity of edema and the rapidity of onset.

Historical Findings
- Tachypnea
- Dyspnea
- Dry cough (uncommon in cats)
- Open-mouth breathing (common in cats)

Physical Examination Findings
- May be no auscultable abnormalities
- Crackles at end inspiration
- Crackles and wheezes during inspiration and expiration
- Pink-tinged, frothy secretions from nares and mouth (end-stage)
- Cardiac murmurs, gallops, and arrhythmias (patients with cardiogenic pulmonary edema)

CAUSES
High Capillary Hydrostatic Pressure
- Cardiogenic—cardiomyopathy (i.e., dilated, hypertrophic, intermediate, and restrictive), mitral valvular endocardiosis, ruptured chordae tendineae, thyrotoxicosis, endocarditis, aortic valve disease, patent ductus arteriosus, ventricular septal defect, and arrhythmias
- Noncardiogenic—overzealous intravenous fluid administration, anemia

Low Capillary Oncotic Pressure
- Hypoproteinemia
- Overzealous IV fluid administration

High Capillary or Alveolar Epithelial Permeability (ARDS)
- Pneumonia
- Toxins (e.g., smoke, gastric contents, and snake venom)
- Heatstroke, disseminated intravascular coagulation
- Near-drowning
- Circulating endotoxins, shock

High Negative Intrathoracic or Interstitial Pressure
- Upper airway obstruction
- Reexpansion of atelectatic lung

Unknown Mechanisms
Neurogenic (e.g., seizures, head trauma, and electrocution)

RISK FACTORS
Heart disease

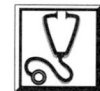 DIAGNOSIS

DIFFERENTIAL DIAGNOSIS
- Must differentiate from other causes of coughing or dyspnea such as upper airway obstruction, tracheitis, bronchitis, pneumonia, heartworm disease, collapsing trachea, respiratory foreign body, and neoplasia; thoracic radiographs and hematologic testing help exclude these.
- Many patients with cardiogenic pulmonary edema have other signs of heart disease (e.g., murmur, arrhythmias, and tachycardia).

- The character of the cough (i.e., dry versus moist) and dyspnea (i.e., expiratory versus inspiratory) may better define the cause of the clinical signs.

CBC/BIOCHEMISTRY/URINALYSIS
- Help evaluate noncardiogenic causes of pulmonary edema
- Generally normal in patients with cardiogenic edema; may see stress leukogram, prerenal azotemia, and high liver enzymes because of passive congestion or poor forward cardiac output

OTHER LABORATORY TESTS
Arterial blood gas analysis documents hypoxemia, but does not correlate well with the severity of pulmonary edema.

IMAGING
Thoracic Radiographic Findings
- Signs of pulmonary edema vary with the severity and cause of the edema.
- An interstitial or alveolar lung pattern is characteristic of pulmonary edema.
- Cardiogenic pulmonary edema—often associated with cardiomegaly (most often left atrium or auricular appendage) and pulmonary venous enlargement; early edema in dogs is often situated in the hilar region; becomes diffuse in patients with advanced heart failure; usually symmetrical, but may start out in the right caudal lung lobe; usually patchy and diffuse in cats
- Neurogenic pulmonary edema—often situated in the caudal dorsal lung field

Echocardiography
May confirm cardiac disease but cannot identify pulmonary edema

DIAGNOSTIC PROCEDURES
- Pulmonary capillary wedge pressure, an indicator of left atrial pressure, can be measured with a Swan-Ganz catheter temporarily "wedged" in the pulmonary artery; usually high pressure (> 20–25 mm Hg) in patients with cardiogenic pulmonary edema
- When used correctly, pulse oximetry correlates well with arterial oxygen saturation of hemoglobin. An SpO_2 of 90%–100% correlates to a $PaO_2 > 60$ mmHg.
- Central venous pressure not always high in animals with left heart failure

PATHOLOGIC FINDINGS
- Fluid accumulates in the pulmonary interstitium and alveoli; lungs usually normal color but often heavy and "wet"
- Lungs may not collapse completely when the thorax is opened.
- May see white or pink-tinged froth in the trachea and small airways

TREATMENT

APPROPRIATE HEALTH CARE
• Whether to treat the patient as an inpatient or outpatient depends on the degree of respiratory compromise and the underlying cause of the edema.
• If respiratory distress—minimal handling and supplemental oxygen (6–10 L/min, oxygen concentrations initially of 50%–100%) are indicated; postpone diagnostic tests until the patient's condition is more stable; intubate and ventilate if necessary.

NURSING CARE
• Oxygen therapy as needed
• Fluid therapy in animals with pulmonary edema is challenging. Hypovolemic patients in heart failure are hard to manage with parenteral fluid therapy. Small volumes of isotonic saline solutions may be most appropriate for volume replacement if plasma cannot be used. Once circulating volumes are restored, low sodium (0.45% NaCl in 2.5% dextrose) or sodium-free (D5W) fluids can maintain hydration without further increasing total body sodium. Monitor patients closely for worsening edema by auscultation and thoracic radiography. Central venous or pulmonary capillary wedge pressures—may use to assist with fluid management; neither should be relied upon exclusively

ACTIVITY
Cage rest or exercise restriction is recommended until the edema resolves.

DIET
Restrict sodium (< 13 mg/kg/day; < 90 mg/100 g of dry food) in patients with cardiogenic edema.

CLIENT EDUCATION
Cardiogenic pulmonary edema signals advanced heart disease; long-term prognosis is guarded to poor. Many patients respond well to initial medical management, but the owner must monitor closely for the earliest signs of dyspnea, tachypnea, or coughing (dogs) that might signal recurrence.

SURGICAL CONSIDERATIONS
Resolve pulmonary edema prior to anesthesia.

 MEDICATIONS

DRUG(S) OF CHOICE

To Reduce Edema
• Diuretics (e.g., furosemide, hydrochloro-thiazide, and spironolactone)
• Vasodilators (e.g., nitroglycerin, nitroprusside, hydralazine, and enalapril)

To Improve Oxygen Delivery to Alveoli (May Be Useful)
Bronchodilators (e.g., aminophylline, theophylline, terbutaline)

To Reduce Anxiety (Use Only If Necessary)
• Morphine (dogs only)
• Acepromazine
• Diazepam

To Increase Capillary Oncotic Pressure (Noncardiogenic Pulmonary Edema)
• Plasma
• Intravenous colloids (e.g., dextran and hetastarch)

To Treat Increased Capillary Permeability (Noncardiogenic Pulmonary Edema)
• Treat the underlying cause.
• Consider corticosteroids.

CONTRAINDICATIONS
• Unless specifically indicated, drugs with negative inotropic actions are contraindicated in animals with cardiogenic pulmonary edema.
• Morphine in patients with neurogenic pulmonary edema

PRECAUTIONS
Reduced cardiac output, hypotension, and prerenal azotemia may occur with overzealous use of a diuretic or vasodilator.

POSSIBLE INTERACTIONS
N/A

ALTERNATIVE DRUG(S)
Addition of a thiazide diuretic or spironolactone to furosemide may benefit patients with refractory cardiogenic pulmonary edema.

 FOLLOW-UP

PATIENT MONITORING
Thoracic radiographs to assess treatment

PREVENTION/AVOIDANCE
N/A

POSSIBLE COMPLICATIONS
Cardiogenic Pulmonary Edema
• Often recurs, since the inciting cause is rarely eliminated
• Response to treatment is a good indicator of short-term prognosis.

EXPECTED COURSE AND PROGNOSIS
• Long-term—guarded with cardiogenic edema because underlying disease generally cannot be cured; exception: some forms of congenital heart disease
• Noncardiogenic edema—quite variable; depends on the underlying cause; prognosis often good if underlying cause can be corrected

 MISCELLANEOUS

ASSOCIATED CONDITIONS
N/A

AGE-RELATED FACTORS
N/A

ZOONOTIC POTENTIAL
N/A

PREGNANCY
N/A

SYNONYMS
Pulmonary congestion

SEE ALSO
• Congestive Heart Failure, Left-Sided
• Cough
• Dyspnea
• Pulmonary Edema, Noncardiogenic

ABBREVIATIONS
• ARDS = adult respiratory distress syndrome
• CNS = central nervous system
• D5W = 5% dextrose in water
• SpO$_2$ = arterial hemoglobin saturation estimated by pulse oximetry

Suggested reading
Cooke K, Snyder P. Fluid therapy in the cardiac patient. Vet Clin North Am 1998;28(3)663–676.
Harpster N. Pulmonary edema. In: Kirk RW, ed. Current veterinary therapy X. Philadelphia: Saunders, 1989:385–392.
Ware W, Bonagura JB. Pulmonary edema. In: Fox PR, Sisson D, Moise NS. eds. Textbook of canine and feline cardiology. Philadelphia: Saunders, 1999:251–264.
Author Patti S. Snyder
Consulting Editors Larry P. Tilley and Francis W. K. Smith, Jr.

PULMONARY EDEMA, NONCARDIOGENIC

 BASICS

DEFINITION
The accumulation of edema fluid in the pulmonary interstitium and alveoli, in the absence of heart disease

PATHOPHYSIOLOGY
• Common cause of all forms—increased pulmonary vascular permeability, which is associated with leakage of fluid into the interstitium and alveoli; if severe, may be followed by an inflammatory response and accumulation of neutrophils and macrophages in the interstitium and alveoli
• Several mechanisms may contribute to changes in pulmonary vascular permeability.
• Systemic release of catecholamines—may lead to systemic vasoconstriction, temporarily shunting blood into the pulmonary circulation and leading to transient pulmonary circulatory overload and endothelial damage; probably occurs in patients with neurogenic edema, electric cord bites, and upper airway obstruction
• Increased negativity of intrathoracic pressure induced by inspiratory attempts against an airway obstruction
• Pulmonary manifestation of a generalized inflammatory response—systemic inflammatory response syndrome; develops in patients with sepsis or pancreatitis
• For all forms, the inciting insult may trigger a cascade inflammatory response that often worsens over 24-hours following after the initial episode.
• Severity of clinical manifestation—varies, ranging from mild to severe; the most seriously affected patients may progress from normal to death in as little as a couple of hours after the incident.

SYSTEMS AFFECTED
• Respiratory
• Hemic/Lymphatic/Immune—if severe and causing respiratory failure, may be associated with DIC
• Cardiovascular—hypotension, tachycardia, and shock
• Renal/Urologic—acute renal failure

GENETICS
Unknown

INCIDENCE/PREVALENCE
Uncommon

GEOGRAPHIC DISTRIBUTION
N/A

SIGNALMENT

Species
Mainly dogs, occasionally cats

Breed Predilection
None specific; brachycephalic dogs are more prone to airway obstruction.

Mean Age and Range
• Higher incidence in puppies < 1 year old
• Young—associated with strangulation, head trauma, and electric cord bites
• Old—associated with laryngeal obstruction and neoplasia

Predominant Sex
None

SIGNS

General Comments
Vary, depending on underlying cause and severity

Historical Findings
• Predisposing cause—airway obstruction; electric cord bite; seizures; head trauma
• Acute onset of dyspnea

Physical Examination Findings
• Mild to severe dyspnea
• Increased respiratory rate and effort; open-mouthed breathing
• Postural adaptations to respiratory distress (severe)
• Unwillingness to lie down
• Pale or cyanotic mucous membranes (severe)
• Harsh sounds (early, mild) or generalized crackles (late, severe) on auscultation
• Expectoration of pink froth or bubbles; in severely affected intubated patient, may note large volumes of bloody fluid flowing out through the endotracheal tube
• Normal cardiac auscultation; may note arrhythmias; tachycardia common

CAUSES
• Upper airway obstruction—laryngeal paralysis; choke-chain injury; mass; abscess
• Electric cord bite
• Acute neurologic disease—head trauma; prolonged seizures
• Smoke inhalation
• Systemic inflammatory response syndrome— sepsis; endotoxemia; pancreatitis
• Anaphylaxis (cats)

RISK FACTORS
• Hypoproteinemia
• Crystalloid fluid resuscitation

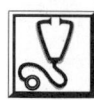 DIAGNOSIS

DIFFERENTIAL DIAGNOSIS
• Cardiogenic pulmonary edema
• Pulmonary infection—bacterial, viral, or fungal pneumonia
• Pulmonary neoplasia
• Pulmonary hemorrhage
• Pulmonary thromboembolism

CBC/BIOCHEMISTRY/URINALYSIS
• Leukocytosis but possibly leukopenia and thrombocytopenia—owing to neutrophil sequestration in the lung and platelet consumption
• Biochemistries—usually normal; may note hypoalbuminemia owing to pulmonary protein loss; mild hyperglycemia reported
• Urinalysis—usually normal

OTHER LABORATORY TESTS
• Arterial blood gas analysis—usually demonstrates mild to severe hypoxemia and hypocapnia; results are not specific but indicate the severity of pulmonary dysfunction.
• Coagulation testing (severely affected patients)—may reveal mild to moderate prolongation of PT and PTT because of consumption and DIC

IMAGING
• Thoracic radiographs—vital; may simply reveal prominent interstitial pattern with mild or early disease; may note alveolar infiltrates with moderate or severe disease; alveolar infiltrates in the dorsocaudal lung fields common; alveolar infiltrates may be seen in other lung fields, are sometimes asymmetrical and demonstrate predominant right-sided involvement.
• Echocardiography—rule out cardiogenic pulmonary edema.

DIAGNOSTIC PROCEDURES
• Pulse oximetry—noninvasive, continuous monitoring of arterial hemoglobin saturation; provides information about the severity and progression of pulmonary dysfunction
• Pulmonary artery wedge pressure—confirms noncardiogenic origin; not commonly performed

PATHOLOGIC FINDINGS
• Lungs—may be heavy, red, or congested; may fail to collapse; may exhibit a wet cut surface; may note foam in the major airways
• Histopathologic—depend on severity of the insult; early, mild: may note eosinophilic amorphous material filling the alveoli or may be near normal because fluid removed in processing; severe: alveolar hyaline membranes, alveolitis, and interstitial inflammatory infiltrates with neutrophils and macrophages evident and accompanied by atelectasis, vascular congestion, and hemorrhage; may be found within hours of a severe insult

PULMONARY EDEMA, NONCARDIOGENIC

TREATMENT

APPROPRIATE HEALTH CARE
• Inpatient vs. outpatient—depends on the severity of clinical manifestation of respiratory dysfunction; depends on the underlying cause of disease (e.g., dogs with upper airway obstruction or severe seizures may require hospitalization)
• Make every effort to resolve and treat the underlying cause (e.g., relieve airway obstruction or treat seizures).
• Mild to moderate—patients generally improve on their own within 24–48 hours with complete resolution; offer support of pulmonary and cardiovascular function while the lung repairs.
• Severe—difficult to treat; may require PPV because of respiratory failure; many patients die despite extensive supportive care.

NURSING CARE
• Minimize stress in dyspneic animals.
• Oxygen therapy—vital in moderate to severe disease; administer via a mask or hood, nasal catheter, or oxygen cage; inspired oxygen concentration depends on the severity of disease; most patients do well on 40%–50% oxygen, but severe disease may require 80%–100% to sustain life
• Severe—may require PPV and PEEP
• Fluid therapy with a balanced electrolyte—give as replacement solution with dehydration or shock; use caution with fluids if animal is dyspnic.
• Plasma or synthetic colloids—consider with hypoproteinemia; improve oncotic pressure, minimizing movement of fluid into the lungs

ACTIVITY
Dogs with moderate to severe hypoxia and respiratory distress—rest and minimal stress vital for minimizing oxygen requirements

DIET
N/A

CLIENT EDUCATION
• Warn client that the condition may worsen before improving.
• Inform client that severe disease which progresses rapidly to fulminant pulmonary edema and respiratory failure is associated with a very poor prognosis.

SURGICAL CONSIDERATIONS
Relevant only for treating the underlying cause

MEDICATIONS

DRUG(S) OF CHOICE
• Damaged endothelium in the pulmonary vasculature—no specific treatment available
• Inflammatory response—generated by a variety of mediators and cascades; cannot be blocked by one specific anti-inflammatory drug that leads to resolution of the edema
• Diuretics—often ineffective; edema is caused by changes in permeability, not high hydrostatic pressure; may use furosemide cautiously in boluses of 0.5–2 mg/kg IV, IM or at 0.1–1 mg/kg/hr IV in a continuous infusion
• Corticosteroids—minimize swelling with upper airway obstruction; generally ineffective for pulmonary inflammatory response; may predispose patients to infectious complications (e.g., bacterial pneumonia); if used, recommend an antiinflammatory dosage (e.g., dexamethasone sodium phosphate at 0.05–0.1 mg/kg IV)

CONTRAINDICATIONS
N/A

PRECAUTIONS
Diuretics (e.g., furosemide)—excessive use may cause dehydration and a marked decrease in intravascular volume with minimal resolution of edema; low intravascular volume may exacerbate cardiovascular collapse or shock.

POSSIBLE INTERACTIONS
N/A

ALTERNATIVE DRUG(S)
N/A

FOLLOW-UP

PATIENT MONITORING
• Observe respiratory rate and pattern and auscultate frequently (every 2–4 hours) for the first 24–48 hours, depending on severity of disease.
• If dyspnea, assess pulmonary function by pulse oximetry or arterial blood gas analysis (initially every 2–4 hours).
• Perform PCV and total solids and evaluate mucous membranes, pulse quality, heart rate, and urine output every 2–4 hours to assess cardiovascular status and possible progression to shock.

PREVENTION/AVOIDANCE
• Avoid contact with electric wire.
• Correct airway obstruction.
• Treat seizures and high intracranial pressure.

POSSIBLE COMPLICATIONS
Usually none if patient recovers from the acute crisis

EXPECTED COURSE AND PROGNOSIS
• Mild to moderate—uneventful resolution of signs in 24–72 hours; no specific treatment required except for oxygen and careful fluid supplementation
• Overall survival rates—80%–100%
• Long-term prognosis—excellent for recovered patients

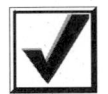

MISCELLANEOUS

ASSOCIATED CONDITIONS
Acute respiratory distress syndrome

AGE-RELATED FACTORS
N/A

ZOONOTIC POTENTIAL
N/A

PREGNANCY
N/A

SYNONYMS
• Shock lung
• Traumatic wet lung
• Acute alveolar failure
• Capillary leak syndrome
• Progressive respiratory distress
• Congestive atelectasis
• Hemorrhagic lung syndrome

SEE ALSO
Acute respiratory distress syndrome (ARDS)

ABBREVIATIONS
• DIC = disseminated intravascular coagulation
• PCV = packed cell volume
• PEEP = positive end-expiratory pressure
• PPV = positive-pressure ventilation
• PT = prothrombin time
• PTT = partial thromboplastin time

Suggested Reading
Drobatz KJ, Concannon K. Noncardiogenic pulmonary edema. Compend Contin Educ Pract Vet 1994;16:333–346.
Drobatz KJ, Saunders HM, Pugh C, Hendricks JC. Noncardiogenic pulmonary edema 26 cases (1987–1993). J Am Vet Med Assoc 1995;206:1732–1736.
Kerr LY. Pulmonary edema secondary to upper airway obstruction in the dog: a review of nine cases. J Am Anim Hosp Assoc 1989;25:207–212.
Kolata RJ, Burrows CF. The clinical features of injury by chewing electrical cords in dogs and cats. J Am Anim Hosp Assoc 1981;17:219–222.
Author Lesley G. King
Consulting Editor Lynelle R. Johnson

PULMONARY FIBROSIS

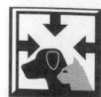 **BASICS**

OVERVIEW
• Fibrosis +/− varying degrees of inflammation of the lung interstitium
• Affects pulmonary mechanics, alters ventilation–perfusion ratios, and leads to chronic tachypnea
• Characterized by sequential acute lung injury that results in a progressive accumulation of fixed fibrosis with architectural distortion
• The initiating causes—unknown; in humans, > 100 known agents can incite alveolar inflammation.
• Also known as cryptogenic alveolitis or usual interstitial pneumonia

SIGNALMENT
• Dogs and cats
• West Highland white terriers and other terriers predisposed
• Affected animals usually middle-aged to old

SIGNS

Historical Findings
• Open-mouth breathing
• Exercise intolerance
• Cough (nonproductive)

Physical Examination Findings
• Dyspnea
• Increased respiratory rate and effort
• Cyanosis
• Auscultation—reveals bilateral end-inspiratory and early expiratory crackles

CAUSES & RISK FACTORS
• Usually idiopathic
• Viral infections—canine distemper; adenovirus; parainfluenza
• Toxins or drugs—paraquat; kerosene; nitrofurantoin
• Oxygen toxicosis
• Acute pancreatitis
• Environmental insults

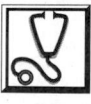 **DIAGNOSIS**

DIFFERENTIAL DIAGNOSIS
• Generalized cardiogenic pulmonary edema—accompanied by left-sided heart enlargement and pulmonary venous distention; response to diuretic expected
• Fungal pneumonia and metastatic neoplasia—associated with an interstitial pattern; usually diagnosed by results of cytologic examination and culture of transtracheal wash or bronchoalveolar lavage

specimen and by identification of organisms or neoplastic cells from other affected organs
• Obesity, end expiration, and poor film quality—cause increase in lung density

CBC/BIOCHEMISTRY/URINALYSIS
Polycythemia caused by chronic hypoxemia

OTHER LABORATORY TESTS
N/A

IMAGING
• Radiography—bilateral, diffuse increase in interstitial pattern; right-sided cardiomegaly may be caused by chronic lung disease
• Echocardiography—may document right heart enlargement
• Doppler echocardiography—may demonstrate pulmonary hypertension
• High-resolution CT—patchy peripheral reticular abnormalities with intralobular linear opacities, irregular septal thickening, subpleural dilation of distal air spaces, and traction brachiectasis reported in people

DIAGNOSTIC PROCEDURES
• Arterial blood gas measurements—hypoxemia and high alveolar–arterial oxygen difference
• Cytologic examination of bronchoalveolar lavage specimen—nontoxic neutrophil count exceeding 20% of cells in dogs with alveolitis or fibrosis
• Bacterial, *Mycoplasma,* and fungal cultures—no growth
• Open lung biopsy—proliferative interstitial pneumonia

PATHOLOGIC FINDINGS
• Proliferation of atypical and multinucleated alveolar epithelial cells
• Thickening of interalveolar septa
• Intra-alveolar hemorrhage and edema
• Intracapillary and intra-alveolar fibrin deposits
• Macrophages and alveolar epithelial cells in alveolar lumina
• Masson trichrome staining—reveals increase in interalveolar septal collagen

 TREATMENT
• Inpatient if oxygen is needed
• Goals—supportive therapy; control signs and enhance quality of life; manifestations of disorder do not occur until pulmonary gas exchange is severely compromised.
• Obesity—may impair diaphragmatic function; may cause early, small airway closure; may impede ventilation; weight loss lessens signs of respiratory impairment.
• Eliminate exposure to dusts or fumes.

 MEDICATIONS

DRUG(S)
• Antiinflammatory dosage of prednisone—1 mg/kg PO q12h for 2 weeks; then taper over the next month; recommended if no underlying infection; most beneficial early in the course of disease
• Concurrent use of azathioprine, antifibrotic agents, or immune modulators—may offer additional benefit
• Bronchodilators—may diminish signs
• Administer oxygen during acute exacerbation.

CONTRAINDICATIONS/POSSIBLE INTERACTIONS
• Steroids—may predispose patient to overt infection; not advised unless bacterial and fungal cultures are negative
• Nonselective β-blockers—may cause bronchoconstriction
• Diuretics—decrease pulmonary clearance mechanisms owing to airway dehydration; may predispose patient to infection

 FOLLOW-UP
• Monitor with serial arterial blood gas measurements and cytologic examination of bronchoalveolar lavage specimens.
• Progressive condition with a guarded prognosis
• Pulmonary hypertension and right heart failure—may develop with any severe, chronic lung disease
• Bullous emphysema and spontaneous pneumothorax—may develop as a result of severe alveolar damage

 MISCELLANEOUS

SEE ALSO
Pneumonia, interstitial

Suggested Reading
Bonagura JD, Hamlin RL, Gaber CE. Chronic respiratory disease in the dog. In: Kirk RW, ed. Current veterinary therapy X. Philadelphia: Saunders, 1989:361–368.
Gross TD, Humminghake GW. Idiopathic pulmonary fibrosis. N Engl J Med 2001;345:517–525.
Lobetti RG, Mulner R, Lane E. Chronic idiopathic pulmonary fibrosis in five dogs. J Am Anim Hosp Assoc 2001;37:119–127.
Author Rosemary A. Henik
Consulting Editor Lynelle R. Johnson

BASICS

OVERVIEW
• Both calcification and ossification; may be generalized or localized
• Discrete—if individual mineral deposits can be identified
• Diffuse—preclude identification of individual deposits
• Calcification—dystrophic or metastatic; dystrophic occurs secondary to tissue degeneration or inflammation; metastatic: occurs secondary to metabolic disease; may be normal (e.g., the pleura in old dogs or premature calcification of the tracheal and bronchial cartilages in chondrodystrophic breeds); often a sign of inactivity of a lesion, thus most focal calcifications are functionally unimportant.
• Ossification—also called heterotopic bone formation; calcification of a bony matrix; pulmonary ossification in the form of small, multiple nodules (osteomas) common in normal dogs
• Generalized pulmonary mineralizations of unknown cause—reported in dogs and cats under descriptive terms: pulmonary alveolar microlithiasis or pumice stone lung, bronchiolar microlithiasis, idiopathic pulmonary calcification or ossification

SIGNALMENT
Older dogs and cats

SIGNS
Historical Findings
• None if focal pulmonary mineralization is incidental finding
• Exercise intolerance
• Cough

Physical Examination Findings
• Dyspnea
• High respiratory rate and abnormal effort
• Cyanosis
• Abnormal breath sounds

CAUSES & RISK FACTORS
• Often idiopathic
• Metastatic calcification—secondary to metabolic disease that induces high serum calcium concentration and/or bone resorption (e.g., hyperadrenocorticism, primary or secondary hyperparathyroidism, hypervitaminosis D, and renal failure)
• Hyperadrenocorticism—may cause dystrophic mineralization owing to the gluconeogenic and catabolic effects of high cortisol levels on proteins; calcium binds to the organic matrix of the abnormal proteins.
• Alveolar and bronchial microlith—may be secondary to exudative or granulomatous lung disease

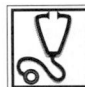 DIAGNOSIS

DIFFERENTIAL DIAGNOSIS
• Dystrophic calcification secondary to chronic pulmonary inflammatory disease
• Atypical pulmonary neoplasia
• Histoplasmosis or tuberculosis granuloma—usually with hilar lymph node calcification
• Alveolar microlithiasis
• Barium sulfate aspiration
• Interstitial pulmonary edema—will respond to diuretic; differentiated by bone scintigraphy

CBC/BIOCHEMISTRY/URINALYSIS
• Hypercalcemia—with hyperparathyroidism, neoplasia, or hypervitaminosis D
• Polycythemia—with chronic hypoxemia
• Stress leukogram, low urine specific gravity, and high ALP—may see in dogs with hyperadrenocorticism

OTHER LABORATORY TESTS
Arterial blood gas measurements—may note hypoxemia

IMAGING
Thoracic radiographs—generalized or localized, discrete or diffuse abnormalities, ranging from an unstructured interstitial pattern to mineralized nodules within the pulmonary parenchyma; may see pleural effusion

DIAGNOSTIC PROCEDURES
• Cytologic examination of transtracheal wash or bronchoalveolar lavage specimen—reveals inflammatory cells with underlying inflammation or infection; microliths appear as nonstaining crystalline concretions.
• Bacterial and fungal cultures—results depend on underlying cause.
• Delayed bone phase scintigraphy (^{99m}Tc-methylene diphosphonate)—generalized pulmonary uptake if sufficient osteoid is being produced
• Lung biopsy—firm, noncompressible, and variably resistant to blunt dissection because of mineralizations

 TREATMENT

None indicated if localized form found in asymptomatic patient

 MEDICATIONS

DRUG(S)
• Bronchodilators—relief of dyspnea and respiratory muscle fatigue
• Antimicrobial or antifungal—with positive bacterial or fungal culture
• Treat underlying metabolic disease—mitotane for hyperadrenocorticism; chemotherapy for neoplasia

CONTRAINDICATIONS/POSSIBLE INTERACTIONS
Fluid loading—may exacerbate dyspnea and right heart failure

 FOLLOW-UP

POSSIBLE COMPLICATIONS
Pleural effusion, chronic obstructive bronchitis, or emphysematous bullae—may develop owing to severe chronic pulmonary disease

 MISCELLANEOUS

ABBREVIATION
ALP = alkaline phosphatase

Suggested Reading
Suter PF, Lord PF. Thoracic radiography: a text atlas of thoracic diseases of the dog and cat. Wettswil, Switzerland: 1984.
Author Rosemary A. Henik
Consulting Editor Lynelle R. Johnson

PULMONARY THROMBOEMBOLISM

 **BASICS**

DEFINITION
Develops when a thrombus lodges in the pulmonary arterial tree and occludes blood flow to the lung served by that artery

PATHOPHYSIOLOGY
• Pulmonary thromboemboli associated with heartworm disease occur in situ in the pulmonary vessels; in most other instances, the origin of the thrombus is unclear.
• Potential sites of origin include the right atrium, vena cava, jugular veins, and femoral or mesenteric veins; these venous thrombi are carried in the bloodstream to the lungs, where they lodge in the pulmonary circulation.
• Abnormal blood flow (stasis), vascular endothelial damage, and altered coagulability (hypercoagulable state) are believed to predispose to thrombus formation.
• In most patients, pulmonary thrombo-embolism is a complicating feature of another primary disease process.

SYSTEMS AFFECTED
• Respiratory—diminished pulmonary blood flow leads to arterial hypoxemia and dyspnea.
• Cardiovascular—pulmonary hypertension may result, leading to right ventricular enlargement, right ventricular failure, and reduced cardiac output.

GENETICS
N/A

INCIDENCE/PREVALENCE
• Not known—likelihood of pulmonary thromboembolism increases in animals with abnormal coagulation or severe systemic disease.
• Uncommon diagnosis in dogs and cats

GEOGRAPHIC DISTRIBUTION
N/A

SIGNALMENT
Species
Dogs and cats
Breed Predilection
No predisposition; disease may be more common in medium- and large-breed dogs
Mean Age and Range
More frequently seen in mature and old dogs
Predominant Sex
N/A

SIGNS
Historical Findings
• Often reflect the primary disease
• Occasionally the reason for initial examination; in such a patient, peracute dyspnea, anorexia, collapse, cough or hemoptysis, weakness, and inability to sleep or get comfortable may be historical complaints.

Physical Examination Findings
• Tachypnea and dyspnea in most animals
• Tachycardia, weak arterial pulses, jugular vein distension, pale or cyanotic mucous membranes, delayed capillary refill time, and split second heart sound in some animals

CAUSES
• Heartworm disease
• Neoplasia
• Hyperadrenocorticism (Cushing's disease)
• Protein-losing nephropathy (renal loss of antithrombin III) or enteropathy
• Cardiac disease
• Immune-mediated hemolytic anemia
• Pancreatitis
• Orthopedic trauma or surgery
• Sepsis
• Disseminated intravascular coagulopathy
• Liver disease

RISK FACTORS
• Coagulopathy, especially any hypercoagulable state
• Diseases listed under "Causes" are associated.
• Estrogen administration and airplane travel may be causative.

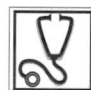 **DIAGNOSIS**

DIFFERENTIAL DIAGNOSIS
• Other diseases that cause clinically important dyspnea and hypoxemia without profound radiographic findings include upper airway obstruction, laryngeal paralysis, and diffuse airway disease processes (e.g., toxin inhalation and interstitial pneumonia).
• Upper airway obstruction often manifests as inspiratory dyspnea; lung sounds often loudest over the trachea or larynx
• Should be a leading diagnostic consideration in a patient with acute onset of dyspnea and a disease known to be associated with pulmonary thromboembolism

CBC/BIOCHEMISTRY/URINALYSIS
• Results often reflect the underlying disease.
• Leukocytosis may develop.

OTHER LABORATORY TESTS
• Arterial blood gases often show arterial hypoxemia (PaO_2 often < 65 mm Hg) and low $PaCO_2$ with respiratory alkalosis.
• Metabolic and respiratory acidosis may develop in severely affected patients.
• Coagulation profile may show high fibrin degradation products, high fibrinogen, or alterations in one-stage PT and activated PTT.

IMAGING
Thoracic Radiographic Findings
Normal or pulmonary artery enlargement or pruning, cardiomegaly, interstitial and alveolar lung patterns, small-volume pleural effusion, or areas of regional hyperlucency

Echocardiographic Findings
Right ventricular enlargement, an enlarged pulmonary artery segment, or diminished size of the left ventricular cavity in some patients; infrequently a thrombus is imaged in the right heart or the pulmonary artery.

Angiographic Findings and Radionuclide Studies
• Usually required for definitive diagnosis
• Right-sided cardiac catheterization with pulmonary angiography may permit identification of an intravascular thrombus or regions of reduced pulmonary blood flow.
• Nonselective angiography has a low level of diagnostic success, especially in medium- and large-breed dogs.
• Combined ventilation and perfusion scans with radioisotopes permit identification of well-ventilated lung regions that do not receive blood flow; when thoracic radiographs are nearly normal, a perfusion scan alone may suffice.

DIAGNOSTIC PROCEDURES
Electrocardiography
• Acute cor pulmonale—right axis deviation, P pulmonale, ST segment deviation, large T waves
• Arrhythmias

PATHOLOGIC FINDINGS
• Thrombi in the major branches of the pulmonary arteries
• Some patients exhibit multiple smaller thrombi in small vessels of the pulmonary arteries, eventually leading to marked respiratory dysfunction and death.

TREATMENT

APPROPRIATE HEALTH CARE
Always treat patients suspected of having pulmonary thromboembolism as inpatients until hypoxemia is resolved.

NURSING CARE
• Administer IV fluids cautiously unless preexisting volume depletion exists; they may contribute to the development of right-sided congestive heart failure.
• Administer oxygen if dyspnea exists and/or $PaO_2 < 65$ mm Hg.

ACTIVITY
Restrict to prevent worsening hypoxemia or syncope.

DIET
N/A

CLIENT EDUCATION
• Alert client that disease is often fatal; further episodes are likely unless an underlying cause is identified and corrected; sudden death is not unusual.
• Treatment with anticoagulant medications can lead to bleeding; frequent reevaluation of clotting times (e.g., PT and PTT) is needed for successful management; anticoagulant administration may be required for several months even after resolution of the causative disease.

SURGICAL CONSIDERATIONS
Requires cardiopulmonary bypass and is not available at most institutions; even if available, extrapolation from human literature suggests probable high surgical mortality.

MEDICATIONS

DRUG(S) OF CHOICE
• Always identify and treat the underlying disease; if this is unlikely to be successful, aggressive efforts to treat pulmonary thromboembolism will probably be in vain.
• Heparin may help prevent further thrombi from developing; low dosages are probably inadequate for management; a dosage of 200–300 units/kg SC q8h is indicated.
• Thrombolytic drug administration (e.g., streptokinase and tissue plasminogen activator) may also be useful in

hemodynamically unstable cases; these drugs are expensive and carry a higher risk of bleeding complications.
• Warfarin—usually indicated for long-term treatment (0.1 mg/kg q24h), with dosage adjustments to maintain a PT 1.5–2 times the baseline value

CONTRAINDICATIONS
N/A

PRECAUTIONS
Warfarin—interacts with many other drugs; degree of anticoagulation may change after giving these drugs; dose titration may be difficult in patients with diseases that result in coagulopathy. Review the mechanism of action and pharmacology of the antithrombotic drugs before use.

POSSIBLE INTERACTIONS
N/A

ALTERNATIVE DRUG(S)
N/A

FOLLOW-UP

PATIENT MONITORING
• Serial arterial blood gases—may help determine improvement in respiratory function
• Check PT every 3 days initially for adjusting warfarin dosage to achieve a PT 1.5–2 times the baseline value. International normalization ratios are recommended to minimize the effects of test kit variability on PT results. Check weekly after an effective dosage is achieved (typically no sooner than 2 weeks).

PREVENTION/AVOIDANCE
• Activity or physical therapy may improve venous blood flow and prevent development of venous thrombi in immobile patients with severe systemic disease.
• Aspirin may have some preventive role but is inadequate as treatment.
• Heparin may be administered to animals predisposed to the development of pulmonary thromboembolism (200 units/kg IV initially and 75 units/kg SC q4–8h).

POSSIBLE COMPLICATIONS
Clinically important bleeding complications may arise in patients treated with anticoagulant drugs. Bleeding may occur from any organ system. Anticipate active

bleeding or anemia necessitating blood or plasma transfusion and have blood products readily available.

EXPECTED COURSE AND PROGNOSIS
Generally guarded to poor; depends on resolution of the precipitating cause. For irreversible diseases (e.g., some neoplasias and advanced protein-losing nephropathy), prognosis is poor long-term; it is somewhat better for patients with thromboembolism due to trauma or sepsis.

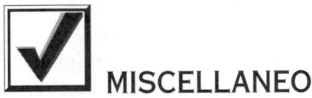

MISCELLANEOUS

ASSOCIATED CONDITIONS
See Causes and Risk Factors.

AGE-RELATED FACTORS
N/A

ZOONOTIC POTENTIAL
N/A

PREGNANCY
N/A

SYNONYMS
Pulmonary embolism, PTE

SEE ALSO
• Disseminated Intravascular Coagulation
• Heartworm Disease
• Hyperadrenocorticism (Cushing's Disease)
• Immune-mediated Hemolytic Anemia
• Nephrotic Syndrome
• Sepsis and Bacteremia

ABBREVIATIONS
• PT = prothrombin time
• PTT = partial thromboplastin time

Suggested Reading

Hawkins EC. Pulmonary parenchymal diseases. In: Ettinger SJ, Feldman EC, eds. Textbook of veterinary internal medicine. 5th ed. Philadelphia: Saunders, 2000:1061–1091.
LaRue MJ, Murtaugh RJ. Pulmonary thromboembolism in dogs: 47 cases (1986–1987). J Am Vet Med Assoc 1990;197:1368–1372.
Norris CR, Griffey SM, Samii VF. Pulmonary thromboembolism in cats: 29 cases (1987–1997). J Am Vet Med Assoc 1999;215:1650–1654.

Author John E. Rush
Consulting Editors Larry P. Tilley and Francis W. K. Smith, Jr.

PULMONIC STENOSIS

 BASICS

DEFINITION
Congenital narrowing of the right ventricular outflow tract, obstructing the passage of flow from the right ventricle to the pulmonary artery; usually valvular, but may be subvalvular or supravalvular

PATHOPHYSIOLOGY
The stenosis causes a pressure overload of the right ventricle, resulting in concentric hypertrophy. The right ventricle develops high systolic pressures to overcome the stenosis, whose magnitude correlates with the severity of the stenosis. The difference between the high right ventricular pressure and the normal pulmonary artery pressure (i.e., the pressure gradient) is often used to describe the severity of the stenosis. Hypertrophy of the right ventricle increases the risk of ischemia and arrhythmias, and the geometric changes in right ventricular shape may result in secondary tricuspid insufficiency. With exercise, the right ventricle may be unable to increase stroke volume adequately. Tricuspid insufficiency with or without myocardial failure of the right ventricle may lead to high right atrial pressures, and R-CHF. A concurrent atrial septal defect or patent foramen ovale may cause right-to-left shunting, especially with exercise, which may result in cyanosis on exertion. Mild pulmonic stenosis usually produces no significant hemodynamic effects apart from an ejection murmur.

SYSTEMS AFFECTED
• Cardiovascular—R-CHF, arrhythmias
• Hepatobiliary—hepatomegaly with R-CHF
• Nervous—cerebral hypoperfusion during exercise

GENETICS
Inherited defect in beagles; polygenic mode of transmission suggested

INCIDENCE/PREVALENCE
• Most surveys show PS to be the third most common congenital cardiac defect in dogs, comprised 21% of congenital heart defects in one study
• Uncommon in cats, especially as an isolated defect; comprised 3% of congenital heart defects in one study

GEOGRAPHIC DISTRIBUTION
N/A

SIGNALMENT

Species
Dogs and cats

Breed Predilection
English bulldog, Scottish terrier, wirehaired fox terrier, miniature schnauzer, West Highland white terrier, Chihuahua, Samoyed, mastiff, cocker spaniel, beagle, boxer

Mean Age and Range
Present from birth and may be detected as a murmur in puppies; if murmur is not detected, affected animals may not be identified until clinical signs develop later in life.

Predominant Sex
A predilection for males in English bulldogs and possibly other breeds.

SIGNS

General Comments
• Mild stenosis—usually no clinical signs
• Severely affected patients—may develop CHF, exertional syncope, or sudden death

Historical Findings
• Abdominal distension
• Dyspnea
• Exertional syncope, exercise intolerance or sudden death
• Asymptomatic

Physical Examination Findings
• Systolic murmur loudest over the left heart base; may radiate widely
• Murmur—midsystolic or holosystolic, and crescendo–decrescendo
• Louder murmurs with a precordial thrill—generally associated with more severe stenosis
• Arrhythmias may occur; the heart rate may be high in CHF.
• Other signs of CHF include ascites, jugular venous distension, and tachypnea.

CAUSES
Congenital

RISK FACTORS
N/A

 DIAGNOSIS

DIFFERENTIAL DIAGNOSIS

Similar Murmurs May Be Found With:
• Aortic stenosis
• Ventricular or atrial septal defects with marked left-to-right shunting
• Tetralogy of Fallot

R-CHF Associated with a Murmur May Be Seen With:
• Acquired valvular disease (endocardiosis)
• Dilated cardiomyopathy

CBC/BIOCHEMISTRY/URINALYSIS
Generally unremarkable

OTHER LABORATORY TESTS
N/A

IMAGING

Radiographic Findings
• Thoracic radiographs usually show right-sided cardiac enlargement, with a poststenotic pulmonary artery bulge visible on the dorso-ventral view at 1–2 o'clock.
• The caudal vena cava may be wide, and ascites may be present with or without pleural effusion in congestive failure.

Echocardiographic Findings
• Right ventricular hypertrophy, with flattening of the interventricular septum and a "figure-of-eight" appearance on short axis views in severe cases
• Can usually image the site of the stenosis, but may be more difficult when the valve is hypoplastic; dysplastic pulmonic valves appear as thickened echodense leaflets; fused leaflets have abnormal motion with systolic doming; discrete subvalvular or supravalvular stenoses may appear as a localized hyperechoic narrowing.
• Localized hypertrophy may be seen in the right ventricular infundibular region.
• May see poststenotic dilation of the pulmonary artery

Doppler Echocardiography
• Can use spectral Doppler to measure the elevated pulmonary artery flow velocity to calculate the pressure gradient across the stenosis. Pressure gradients under 50 mm Hg generally represent mild stenosis; those over 100 mm Hg indicate severe stenosis.
• Color-flow Doppler may reveal tricuspid regurgitation.

Angiography
• Selective cardiac angiography can help identify the precise morphologic abnormalities prior to surgery; may image dysplastic valves and hypertrophy of the infundibulum and supravalvular crest more clearly
• Useful in identifying pulmonic stenosis caused by an anomalous coronary artery encircling the right ventricular outflow tract, which may affect the choice of therapy; recommended for English bulldogs because this anomaly is reported frequently

DIAGNOSTIC PROCEDURES

Electrocardiography
• QRS complex waveform changes include deep S waves in leads I, II, III, and aVF and right axis deviation.
• Atrial fibrillation may occur with severe right atrial enlargement.

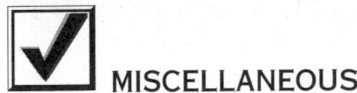
Cardiac Catheterization
Pressure measurement by this technique is rarely necessary for diagnosis; pressure gradients can be assessed noninvasively with Doppler echocardiography.

PATHOLOGIC FINDINGS
• Various forms exist; most result in right ventricular hypertrophy and poststenotic dilation of the pulmonary artery; infundibular hypertrophy may occur proximal to the obstruction.
• Hypoplastic pulmonic valve, with thickened leaflets ("dysplastic pulmonic valve")
• Normal pulmonic valve annulus with fused commissures
• Anomalous coronary arteries
• Discrete supravalvular or subvalvular stenosis, with possible concurrent tricuspid dysplasia
• Fibromuscular bands dividing the right ventricular inflow and outflow tracts ("double-chambered right ventricle")

TREATMENT

APPROPRIATE HEALTH CARE
Most managed as outpatients; initial hospitalization of those with severe CHF may be better.

Nursing Care
Rarely, pleural effusions may need draining; ascites is usually treated medically.

Activity
Exercise should be restricted in cases with syncope or congestive failure, and severe exertion should be avoided in asymptomatic cases with severe stenosis.

Diet
Low-salt diets may benefit those with refractory ascites.

Client Education
• Mildly affected animals may lead normal lives.
• Severely affected patients may benefit from interventions such as balloon catheter dilation or surgery; prognosis is guarded once congestive signs develop.
• Do not breed affected animals.

Surgical Considerations
• Balloon catheter dilation—relatively safe procedure that involves passing a catheter across the stenosis and inflating a balloon to dilate the obstruction; in many cases, the pressure gradient is significantly reduced, especially when the lesion is caused by fused commissures; less successful with dysplastic or hypoplastic valves and contraindicated with anomalous coronary arteries
• Alternative surgical techniques include valvulotomy or patch-graft procedures; mortality rates tend to be higher than with balloon valvuloplasty.

MEDICATIONS

DRUG(S) OF CHOICE
If signs of CHF, treat ascites with furosemide (2–4 mg/kg PO q8–12h); in refractory failure, it may be worth adding spironolactone (1–2 mg/kg PO q12h); treat atrial fibrillation with digoxin (0.22 mg/m² PO q12h).

CONTRAINDICATIONS
Vasodilators (e.g., hydralazine) may cause hypotension without relieving the stenosis and are best avoided.

PRECAUTIONS
Avoid overuse of diuretics; administer intravenous fluids (when required) cautiously to avoid exacerbating congestive signs. ACE inhibitors may be helpful with congestive signs, but may cause hypotension. Low doses should be used and blood pressure monitored.

POSSIBLE INTERACTIONS
N/A

ALTERNATIVE DRUG(S)
N/A

FOLLOW-UP

PATIENT MONITORING
Use serial echocardiograms to follow the pressure gradient and cardiac chamber size.

PREVENTION/AVOIDANCE
Do not breed affected animals.

POSSIBLE COMPLICATIONS
• R-CHF
• Arrhythmias
• Exercise intolerance
• Exertional syncope
• Sudden death

EXPECTED COURSE AND PROGNOSIS
• Mildly affected animals may remain asymptomatic with a normal life span.
• Severely affected animals have a guarded prognosis because they may develop CHF or sudden death; clinical signs are generally more common in animals over 1 year of age.

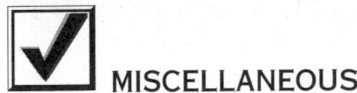
MISCELLANEOUS

ASSOCIATED CONDITIONS
• Ventricular septal defects, atrial septal defects, and patent foramen ovale
• English bulldogs described with a single right coronary artery from which an anomalous left main coronary artery arises and then encircles and constricts the base of the pulmonic valve

AGE-RELATED FACTORS
Defect and murmur are present from birth.

ZOONOTIC POTENTIAL
None

PREGNANCY
Do not breed affected animals.

SYNONYMS
Pulmonary stenosis

SEE ALSO
• Congestive Heart Failure, Right-sided
• Murmurs, Heart

ABBREVIATIONS
• ACE = angiotensin-converting enzyme
• PS = pulmonic stenosis
• R-CHF = right-sided congestive heart failure

Suggested Reading
Buchanan JW. Pathogenesis of single right coronary artery and pulmonic stenosis in English Bulldogs. J Vet Intern Med 2001;15:101–104.
Bussadori C, DeMadron E, Santilli RA, Borgarelli M. Balloon valvuloplasty in 30 dogs with pulmonic stenosis: effect of valve morphology and annular size on initial and 1-year outcome. J Vet Intern Med 2001;15:553–558.
Fingland RB, Bonagura JD, Myer CW. Pulmonic stenosis in the dog: 29 cases (1975–1984). J Am Vet Med Assoc 1986;189:218–226.
Martin MWS, Godman M, Luis Fuentes V, et al. Assessment of balloon pulmonary valvuloplasty in six dogs. J Small Anim Pract 1992;33:443–449.
Orton EC, Bruecker KA, McCracken TO. An open patch-graft technique for correction of pulmonic stenosis in the dog. Vet Surg 1990;19:148–154.
Sisson DD, Thomas WP, Bonagura JD. Congenital heart disease. In: Ettinger SJ, Feldman EC, eds. Textbook of veterinary internal medicine. Philadelphia: Saunders, 2000;737–787.

Author Virginia Luis Fuentes
Consulting Editors Larry P. Tilley and Francis W. K. Smith, Jr.

PUPPY STRANGLES (JUVENILE CELLULITIS)

BASICS

OVERVIEW
• An uncommon granulomatous and pustular disorder of puppies
• Rarely seen in adult dogs
• The face, pinnae, and submandibular lymph nodes are the most common sites.
• Immunopathogenesis unknown

SIGNALMENT
• Dogs
• Age range—usually between 3 weeks and 4 months
• Predisposed breeds—golden retrievers, dachshunds, and Gordon setters

SIGNS
• Acutely swollen face (eyelids, lips, and muzzle)
• Submandibular lymphadenopathy
• A marked pustular and exudative dermatitis, which frequently fistulates, develops within 24–48 hr.
• Purulent otitis externa
• Lesions often become crusted.
• Affected skin is usually painful.
• Lethargy—50% of cases
• Anorexia, pyrexia, and a sterile suppurative arthritis—25% of cases
• A sterile pyogranulomatous panniculitis (rare) over the trunk, preputial, or perianal area; lesions may appear as fluctuant subcutaneous nodules that fistulate.

CAUSES & RISK FACTORS
• Cause and pathogenesis unknown
• An immune dysfunction with a heritable cause is suspected.

DIAGNOSIS

DIFFERENTIAL DIAGNOSIS
• Staphylococcal dermatitis
• Demodicosis
• Drug eruption
• Deep fungal infection

CBC/BIOCHEMISTRY/URINALYSIS
No specific changes noted

OTHER LABORATORY TESTS
• Cytology—pyogranulomatous inflammation with no microorganisms; nondegenerate neutrophils
• Culture—sterile

IMAGING
N/A

PUPPY STRANGLES (JUVENILE CELLULITIS)

DIAGNOSTIC PROCEDURES
- Skin biopsy
- Multiple discrete or confluent granulomas and pyogranulomas—clusters of large epithelioid macrophages and neutrophils
- Sebaceous glands and apocrine glands may be obliterated.
- Suppurative changes in the dermis—predominate in later stages
- Panniculitis

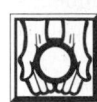 TREATMENT
- Early and aggressive therapy, because scarring may be severe
- Topical therapy—may be soothing and palliative; adjunct to corticosteroids

 MEDICATIONS

DRUG(S)
- Corticosteroids—high doses required; prednisone (2.2 mg/kg divided twice daily for at least 2 weeks)
- Do not taper too rapidly.
- Chemotherapeutics—rare resistant cases
- Adult dogs with panniculitis may require longer therapy.
- Antibiotics—if there is evidence of secondary bacterial infection; as an adjunct therapy with immunosuppressive doses of steroids

CONTRAINDICATIONS/POSSIBLE INTERACTIONS
None

 FOLLOW-UP
- Most cases do not recur.
- Scarring may be a problem, especially around the eyes.

 MISCELLANEOUS

Suggested Reading
Scott DW, Miller WH, Griffin CE. eds. Muller & Kirk's small animal dermatology. Philadelphia: Saunders, 1995:938–941.
Author Karen Helton Rhodes
Consulting Editor Karen Helton Rhodes

PYELONEPHRITIS

 BASICS

DEFINITION
A microbial colonization of the upper urinary tract including the renal pelvis, collecting diverticula, renal parenchyma, and ureters; because it is not usually limited to the renal pelvis and parenchyma, a more descriptive term is *upper urinary tract infection;* this chapter is limited to bacterial pyelonephritis.

PATHOPHYSIOLOGY
• Infection of any portion of the urinary tract usually requires some impairment of normal host defenses against urinary tract infection (see chapter on lower urinary tract infection); normal defenses against ascending urinary tract infection include mucosal defense barriers, ureteral peristalsis, ureterovesical flap valves, and an extensive renal blood supply. Pyelonephritis usually occurs by ascension of microbes causing lower urinary tract infection. In dogs and cats, hematogenous seeding of the kidneys does not usually cause pyelonephritis. Regardless of the route of infection, an upper urinary tract infection is frequently accompanied by lower urinary tract infection.
• Can develop secondarily to infection of metabolic nephroliths; upper urinary tract infection with urease-producing bacteria can predispose to formation of struvite nephroliths.
• Obstruction of an infected kidney or ureter can cause septicemia (so-called urosepsis).

SYSTEMS AFFECTED
• Renal/Urologic
• Can cause urosepsis, thus affecting any body system

GENETICS
N/A

INCIDENCE/PREVALENCE
• Unknown
• Probably occurs much more commonly than is recognized clinically, because many animals with pyelonephritis are asymptomatic or have signs limited to lower urinary tract infection.

GEOGRAPHIC DISTRIBUTION
N/A

SIGNALMENT
Species
Dogs affected more commonly than cats
Breed Predilection
N/A
Mean Age and Range
Mean age of affected dogs and cats unknown; dogs of any age can be affected. Cats over 10 years of age are more likely to develop urinary tract infection than cats less than 10 years of age.

Predominant Sex
Unknown; dogs—urinary tract infection affects more females than males; cats—urinary tract infection is uncommon and occurs with similar frequency in males and females

SIGNS
General Comments
Many patients are asymptomatic or have signs of lower urinary tract infection only.
Historical Findings
• None
• Polyuria/polydipsia (PU/PD)
• Abdominal or lumbar pain
• Signs associated with lower urinary tract infection—e.g., dysuria, pollakiuria, stranguria, hematuria, and malodorous or discolored urine
Physical Examination Findings
• None
• Pain upon palpation of kidneys
• Fever

CAUSES
Usually, ascending urinary tract infection caused by aerobic bacteria; most common isolates are *Escherichia coli* and *Staphylococcus* spp.; other bacteria, including *Proteus, Streptococcus, Klebsiella, Enterobacter,* and *Pseudomonas* spp., which frequently infect the lower urinary tract, may ascend into the upper urinary tract. Anaerobic bacteria, ureaplasma, and fungi rarely infect the upper urinary tract.

RISK FACTORS
• Ectopic ureters, vesicoureteral reflux, congenital renal dysplasia, and lower urinary tract infection; conditions that predispose to urinary tract infection—e.g., diabetes mellitus, hyperadrenocorticism, exogenous steroid administration, renal failure, urethral catheterization, urine retention, uroliths, urinary tract neoplasia, perineal urethrostomy
• In cats with experimentally induced lower urinary tract disease, indwelling urinary catheters combined with administration of exogenous steroids frequently resulted in pyelonephritis.

 DIAGNOSIS

DIFFERENTIAL DIAGNOSIS
• Clinical diagnosis of pyelonephritis is usually presumptive, based on results from CBC, biochemical analysis, urinalysis, urine culture, and diagnostic imaging; definitive diagnosis is not usually required for planning treatment.
• Since many dogs and cats lack specific symptoms attributable to pyelonephritis, any patient with urinary tract infection could potentially have pyelonephritis; the best methods for differentiating between upper

and lower urinary tract infection are ultrasonography or excretory urography.
• Consider the possibility of pyelonephritis, since patients are frequently asymptomatic; consider as a differential diagnosis for dogs or cats with fever of unknown origin, PU/PD, chronic renal failure, or lumbar/abdominal pain.

CBC/BIOCHEMISTRY/URINALYSIS
• CBC—results often normal with chronic pyelonephritis; leukocytosis and neutrophilia with a left shift detected in some patients
• Biochemistry—usually normal unless chronic pyelonephritis leads to chronic renal failure (azotemia with an inappropriate urinary specific gravity)
• Urinalysis reveals hematuria, pyuria, proteinuria, bacteriuria, and leukocyte casts in some animals. Leukocyte casts are diagnostic for renal inflammation and usually result from pyelonephritis. Observe dilute urine specific gravity in patients with nephrogenic diabetes insipidus, which may occur secondary to pyelonephritis. Absence of abnormalities does not rule out pyelonephritis.

OTHER LABORATORY TESTS
• Quantitative urine culture to confirm urinary tract infection; see chapter on lower urinary tract infection for interpretation.
• Dogs with chronic pyelonephritis may have a negative urine culture and require multiple urine cultures to confirm urinary tract infection.

IMAGING
• Ultrasonography or excretory urography are the best methods for presumptively differentiating between upper and lower urinary tract infection. Experimentally, ultrasonography is more useful than excretory urography for identification of mild-to-moderate acute pyelonephritis.
• Ultrasonographic findings supporting pyelonephritis include dilation of the renal pelvis and proximal ureter and a hyperechoic mucosal margin line within the renal pelvis and/or proximal ureter.
• Excretory urography may reveal dilation and blunting of the renal pelvis with lack of filling of the collecting diverticula, dilation of the proximal ureter, and decreased opacity of the nephrogram phase and of the contrast media in the collecting system.
• In patients with acute pyelonephritis, the kidneys may be large; in patients with chronic pyelonephritis, the kidneys may be small, with an irregular surface contour.
• Concomitant nephroliths detected in some patients by survey radiography, ultrasonography, or excretory urography

DIAGNOSTIC PROCEDURES
• Definitive diagnosis requires urine cultures obtained from the renal pelvis or parenchyma,

or histopathology from a renal biopsy. Pyelocentesis can be performed percutaneously using ultrasound guidance or during exploratory surgery; can obtain specimen for culture from the renal pelvis (or from nephroliths) during nephrotomy
• To confirm the diagnosis, the biopsy specimen must include the renal cortex and medulla; thus renal biopsy should be performed by open surgery and only if necessary.
• May have a patchy distribution and can be missed by needle biopsy.

PATHOLOGIC FINDINGS
• Kidneys affected by chronic pyelonephritis have areas of infarction and scarring on the capsular surface in some animals. The renal pelvis and collecting diverticula may be dilated and distorted from chronic infection and inflammation. Purulent exudate is occasionally noted in the renal pelvis.
• Histologic findings include papillitis, pyelitis, interstitial nephritis, and leukocyte casts in tubular lumens.

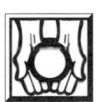 TREATMENT

APPROPRIATE HEALTH CARE
Outpatient unless animal has septicemia or renal failure

NURSING CARE
N/A

ACTIVITY
Unlimited

DIET
Modification recommended in animals with concomitant chronic renal failure or nephrolithiasis

CLIENT EDUCATION
• Recurrent pyelonephritis may be asymptomatic. Unresolved chronic pyelonephritis may lead to chronic renal failure; diagnostic follow-up is important to document resolution of pyelonephritis.
• In patients with nephroliths, resolution is unlikely unless the nephroliths are removed.

SURGICAL CONSIDERATIONS
• Complete obstruction of the upper urinary tract of a patient with pyelonephritis may result in urosepsis and should be corrected by surgery (or lithotripsy for nephroliths).
• Infected nephroliths—surgically remove, medically dissolve (struvite), or fragment by extracorporeal shock wave lithotripsy; use periprocedural antibiotics to reduce the risk of urosepsis when manipulating infected nephroliths
• Unilateral nephrectomy is usually not effective for elimination of suspected unilateral pyelonephritis.

 MEDICATIONS

DRUG(S) OF CHOICE
• Base antibiotic selection on urine culture and sensitivity testing.
• Antibiotics should be bactericidal, achieve good serum and urine concentrations, and not be nephrotoxic.
• High serum and urinary antibiotic concentrations do not necessarily ensure high tissue concentrations in the renal medulla; thus chronic pyelonephritis may be difficult to eradicate.
• Give orally administered antibiotics at full therapeutic dosages for 4–6 weeks.
• Do not use drugs that achieve good concentrations in urine but poor concentrations in serum (e.g., nitrofurantoin).

CONTRAINDICATIONS
Do not use aminoglycosides unless no other alternatives exist on the basis of urine culture and sensitivity testing.

PRECAUTIONS
Trimethoprim/sulfa combinations can cause side effects (keratoconjunctivitis sicca, blood dyscrasias, polyarthritis) when administered for more than 4 weeks.

POSSIBLE INTERACTIONS
N/A

ALTERNATIVE DRUG(S)
N/A

 FOLLOW-UP

PATIENT MONITORING
Do urine cultures and urinalysis during antibiotic administration (~ 5–7 days into treatment) and 1 and 4 weeks after antibiotics are finished.

PREVENTION/AVOIDANCE
Eliminate factors predisposing to urinary tract infection; correct ectopic ureters.

POSSIBLE COMPLICATIONS
Renal failure, recurrent pyelonephritis, struvite nephrolithiasis, septicemia, septic shock, metastatic infection (e.g., endocarditis, polyarthritis)

EXPECTED COURSE AND PROGNOSIS
• Patients with pyelonephritis—fair to good, with a return to normal health unless the patient also has nephrolithiasis, chronic renal failure, or some other underlying cause for urinary tract infection (e.g., obstruction or neoplasia)
• Established infection of the renal medulla may be difficult to resolve because of poor tissue penetration of antibiotics. • Patients with chronic renal failure caused by

pyelonephritis—prognosis determined by the severity and rate of progression of the chronic renal failure
• Recurrent pyelonephritis is likely if infected nephroliths are not removed.

 MISCELLANEOUS

ASSOCIATED CONDITIONS
Hyperadrenocorticism, exogenous glucocorticoid administration, chronic renal failure, hyperthyroidism (cats), and diabetes mellitus are associated with lower urinary tract infection, which can ascend into the ureters and kidneys.

AGE-RELATED FACTORS
N/A

ZOONOTIC POTENTIAL
N/A

PREGNANCY
Use antibiotics that are safe for the pregnant bitch or queen.

SYNONYMS
Upper urinary tract infection, pyelitis

SEE ALSO
• Lower Urinary Tract Infection
• Nephrolithiasis
• Renal Failure, Chronic
• Urinary Tract Obstruction
• Urolithiasis, Struvite—Canine
• Urolithiasis, Struvite—Feline

ABBREVIATIONS
PU/PD = polyuria and polydipsia

Suggested Reading
Senior DF. Management of difficult urinary tract infections. In: Bonagura JD, ed. Current Veterinary Therapy, XIII. Philadelphia: Saunders, 2000:883–886.
Lees GE, Forrester SD. Update: bacterial urinary tract infections. In: Kirk RW, Bonagura JD, eds. Current Veterinary Therapy XI. Philadelphia: Saunders, 1992:909–914.
Lulich JP, Osborne CA. Fungal urinary tract infections. In: Kirk RW, Bonagura JD, eds. Current veterinary therapy XI. Philadelphia: Saunders, 1992:914–919.
Lulich JP, Osborne CA. Bacterial infections of the urinary tract. In: Ettinger SJ, Feldman EC, eds. Textbook of veterinary internal medicine. 4th ed. Philadelphia: Saunders, 1995:1775–1788.
Neuwirth L, Mahaffey M, Crowell W, et al. Comparison of excretory urography and ultrasonography for detection of experimentally induced pyelonephritis in dogs. Am J Vet Res 1993;54:660–669.
Author Larry G. Adams
Consulting Editors Larry G. Adams and Carl A. Osborne

PYODERMA

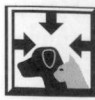 **BASICS**

DEFINITION
Bacterial infection of the skin

PATHOPHYSIOLOGY
Skin infections occur when the surface integrity of the skin has been broken, the skin has become macerated by chronic exposure to moisture, normal bacterial flora have been altered, circulation has been impaired, or immunocompetency has been compromised.

SYSTEMS AFFECTED
Skin/Exocrine

GENETICS
N/A

INCIDENCE/PREVALENCE
• Dogs—very common
• Cats—uncommon

GEOGRAPHIC DISTRIBUTION
N/A

SIGNALMENT
Species
Dogs and cats

Breed Predilections
• Breeds with short coats, skin folds, or pressure calluses
• German shepherds develop a severe, deep pyoderma that may only partially respond to antibiotics and frequently relapses.

Mean Age and Range
Age of onset usually related to underlying cause

Predominant Sex
N/A

SIGNS
General Comments
• Superficial—usually involves the trunk; extent of lesions may be obscured by the hair coat.
• Deep—often affects the chin, bridge of the nose, pressure points, and feet; may be generalized

Historical Findings
• Acute or gradual onset
• Variable pruritus—underlying cause may be pruritic or the staphylococcal infection itself may be pruritic

Physical Examination Findings
• Papules
• Pustules
• Hemorrhagic bullae
• Crusts
• Epidermal collarettes
• Circular erythematous or hyperpigmented spots
• Target lesions
• Alopecia, moth-eaten hair coat
• Scaling
• Lichenification
• Abscess
• Furunculosis, cellulitis

CAUSES
• *Staphylococcus intermedius*—most frequent
• *Pasteurella multocida*—an important pathogen in cats
• Deep—may be complicated by gram-negative organisms (e.g., *E. coli*, *Proteus* spp., *Pseudomonas* spp.)
• Rarely caused by higher bacteria (e.g., *Actinomyces*, *Nocardia*, *Mycobacteria*, *Actinobacillus*)

RISK FACTORS
• Allergy—flea; atopy; food; contact
• Parasites—especially *Demodex*
• Fungal infection—dermatophyte
• Endocrine disease—hypothyroidism; hyperadrenocorticism; sex hormone imbalance
• Immune incompetency—glucocorticoids; young animals
• Seborrhea—acne; schnauzer comedo syndrome
• Conformation—short coat; skin folds
• Trauma—pressure points; grooming; scratching; rooting behavior; irritants
• Foreign body—foxtail; grass awn

DIAGNOSIS

DIFFERENTIAL DIAGNOSIS
• Allergy—pruritus usually precedes the rash; pruritus will not resolve with resolution of the pyoderma.
• Endocrine problem causing a relapsing pyoderma—consider if pruritus resolves with resolution of the pyoderma; reports of poly-dipsia, polyuria, pendulous abdomen, leth-argy, weight gain, and/or signs of feminization
• Flea allergy or atopy—may be seasonal
• Pustular disease—superficial staphylococcal

pyoderma; dermatophytosis; demodicosis; pemphigus foliaceus; and subcorneal pustular dermatosis
• Furunculosis—deep staphylococcal pyoderma; higher bacterial infection; demodicosis; dermatophytosis; opportunistic fungal infections; deep fungal infections; panniculitis; and zinc-responsive dermatosis
• Superficial pyoderma in short-coated breeds is often misdiagnosed as urticaria, because of the acute onset of pruritic papules misdiagnosed as hives.

CBC/BIOCHEMISTRY/URINALYSIS
• Superficial—normal or may reflect the underlying cause (e.g., anemia due to hypothyroidism; stress leukogram and high serum alkaline phosphatase due to Cushing disease; eosinophilia due to parasitism)
• Generalized, deep—may show leukocytosis with a left shift and hyperglobulinemia; also changes related to the underlying cause

OTHER LABORATORY TESTS
N/A

IMAGING
N/A

DIAGNOSTIC PROCEDURES
• Skin scrapings, dermatophyte culture, intradermal allergy testing, hypoallergenic food trial, endocrine tests—identify the underlying cause
• Skin biopsy
• Direct smear from intact pustule—neutrophils engulfing bacteria
• Cytology—differentiate pemphigus foliaceus (acantholytic keratinocytes) and deep fungal infections (blastomycosis, cryptococcosis) from pyodermas; tissue grains may identify filamentous organisms characteristic of higher bacteria.

Culture
• Usually positive for *S. intermedius*
• Other gram-negative organisms besides staphylococci and higher bacteria may be cultured from deep pyodermas.
• Contents of an intact pustule—most reliable results
• Punch biopsy obtained by sterile technique—if no pustules are noted; more likely to get false-negative results
• Freshly expressed exudate from a draining tract or beneath a crust—may yield the pathogen or a contaminant; least reliable method

PATHOLOGIC FINDINGS
- Subcorneal pustules
- Intraepidermal neutrophilic microabscesses
- Perifolliculitis
- Folliculitis
- Furunculosis
- Nodular to diffuse dermatitis
- Panniculitis
- Inflammatory reaction—suppurative or pyogranulomatous
- Tissue grains within pyogranulomas—observed most often with *Staphylococcus, Actinomyces, Actinobacillus,* and *Nocardia*
- Special stains—identify gram-negative bacteria or acid-fast organisms

TREATMENT

APPROPRIATE HEALTH CARE
Usually outpatient, except for severe, generalized deep pyodermas

NURSING CARE
- Severe, generalized, deep—may require IV fluids, parenteral antibiotics, or daily whirlpool baths
- Benzoyl peroxide or chlorhexidine shampoos—remove surface debris
- Whirlpool baths—deep pyodermas; remove crusted exudate; encourage drainage

ACTIVITY
No restriction

DIET
- Hypoallergenic if secondary to food allergy; otherwise a high-quality, well-balanced dog food
- Avoid high-protein, poor-quality "bargain" diets and excessive supplementation.

CLIENT EDUCATION
N/A

SURGICAL CONSIDERATIONS
Fold pyodermas require surgical correction to prevent recurrence.

MEDICATIONS

DRUG(S) OF CHOICE
- *S. intermedius* isolates—usually susceptible to cephalosporins, cloxacillin, oxacillin, methicillin, amoxicillin-clavulanate, erythro-mycin, and chloramphenicol; somewhat less responsive to lincomycin and trimethoprim-sulfonamide; frequently resistant to amoxicillin, ampicillin, penicillin, tetracycline, and sulfonamides
- Amoxicillin-clavulanate—most isolates of *Staphylococcus* and *P. multocida* susceptible; generally effective for skin infections in cats
- Superficial—initially may be treated empirically with one of the antibiotics listed above.
- Recurrent, resistant, or deep—base antibiotic therapy on culture and sensitivity testing
- Multiple organisms with different antibiotic sensitivities—choose antibiotic on basis of staphylococcal susceptibility.

CONTRAINDICATIONS
Steroids—will encourage resistance and recurrence even when used concurrently with antibiotics

PRECAUTIONS
- Erythromycin, lincomycin, and oxacillin—vomiting; administer with small amount of food
- Gentamicin and kanamycin—renal toxicity usually precludes their prolonged systemic use.
- Trimethoprim-sulfa—associated with keratoconjunctivitis sicca, fever, hepatotoxicity, polyarthritis, and hematologic abnormalities
- Chloramphenicol—use with caution in cats; may cause mild, reversible anemia in dogs

POSSIBLE INTERACTIONS
Trimethoprim-sulfa—may lead to low thyroid test results

ALTERNATIVE DRUG(S)
Staphage lysate, staphoid AB, or autogenous bacterins—may improve antibiotic efficacy and decrease recurrence in a small percentage of cases

FOLLOW-UP

PATIENT MONITORING
Administer antibiotics for a minimum of 2 weeks beyond clinical cure; this is usually about 1 month for superficial pyodermas, and 2–3+ months for deep pyodermas.

PREVENTION/AVOIDANCE
- Routine bathing with benzoyl peroxide or chlorhexidine shampoos—may help prevent recurrences
- Some cases that continue to relapse may be managed with subminimal inhibitory concentrations of antibiotics (long-term/low-dose).
- Padded bedding—may ease pressure point pyodermas
- Topical benzoyl peroxide gel or mupirocin ointment may be helpful adjunct therapies

POSSIBLE COMPLICATIONS
Bacteremia and septicemia

EXPECTED COURSE AND PROGNOSIS
Likely to be recurrent or nonresponsive if underlying cause is not identified and effectively managed

MISCELLANEOUS

ASSOCIATED CONDITIONS
N/A

AGE-RELATED FACTORS
- Impetigo—affects young dogs before puberty; associated with poor husbandry; often requires only topical therapy
- Superficial pustular dermatitis—occurs in kittens; associated with overzealous "mouthing" by the queen
- Pyoderma secondary to atopy—usually begins at 1–3 years of age
- Pyoderma secondary to endocrine disorders—usually begins in middle adulthood

ZOONOTIC POTENTIAL
- Cutaneus tuberculosis—rare
- Feline leprosy—unknown

PREGNANCY
N/A

SEE ALSO
- Acne—Cats
- Acne—Dogs
- Interdigital Dermatitis
- Perianal Fistula
- Pododermatitis

Suggested Reading

Muller GH, Kirk RW, Scott DW. Small animal dermatology. 4th ed. Philadelphia: Saunders, 1989.

Authors Ellen C. Codner and Karen Helton Rhodes

Consulting Editor Karen Helton Rhodes

PYOMETRA AND CYSTIC ENDOMETRIAL HYPERPLASIA

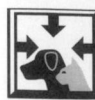 **BASICS**

DEFINITION
• Cystic endometrial hyperplasia—hormonally mediated, progressive pathologic change in the uterine lining
• Pyometra—secondary to cystic endometrial hyperplasia; develops when bacterial invasion of the abnormal endometrium leads to intraluminal accumulation of purulent exudate

PATHOPHYSIOLOGY
• Normal cycling bitches—2-month diestrus, with ovarian secretion of progesterone after every estrus
• Repeated exposure of the endometrium to high concentrations of estrogen followed by high concentrations of progesterone without pregnancy—leads to cystic endometrial hyperplasia
• Bacteria—secretions provide excellent media for growth; ascend from the vagina through the partially open cervix during proestrus and estrus; normal vaginal flora; *Escherichia coli* most common isolate

SYSTEMS AFFECTED
• Reproductive
• Renal/Urologic
• Hemic/Lymphatic/Immune
• Hepatobiliary

GENETICS
No predisposition known

INCIDENCE/PREVALENCE
Incidence—accurate assessment cannot be made because most dogs and cats in the U.S. undergo elective ovariohysterectomy

GEOGRAPHIC DISTRIBUTION
N/A

SIGNALMENT

Species
Dogs and cats

Breed Predilection
N/A

Mean Age and Range
• Usually > 6 years old
• Young animals—especially if treated with exogenous estrogen or progestogen
• Dogs—usually diagnosed 1–12 weeks after estrus
• Cats—onset relative to estrus more variable
• Pyometra of the uterine stump in spayed animals—may develop any time after ovariohysterectomy

Predominant Sex
Female only

SIGNS

Historical Findings
Closed cervix—signs of systemic illness, progressing to signs of septicemia and shock

Physical Examination Findings
• Uterus—palpably large; careful palpation may allow determination of size; overly aggressive palpation may induce rupture; with open cervix, may not be palpably large
• Vaginal discharge—depends on cervical patency; sanguinous to mucopurulent
• Depression and lethargy
• Anorexia
• Polyuria and polydipsia
• Vomiting
• Abdominal distension

CAUSES
• Dogs—the unique, repeated exposure of the endometrium to estrogen followed by exposure to progesterone
• Cats—may be the result of estrogen at estrus followed by a progestational phase, caused by induction of ovulation by coitus or other (as yet undefined) stimuli

RISK FACTORS
• Old, nulliparous females may be predisposed.
• Pharmacologic use of estrogen (mismate) shots during midestrus to early diestrus
• No correlation with pseudopregnancy in dogs

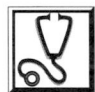 **DIAGNOSIS**

DIFFERENTIAL DIAGNOSIS
• Pregnancy
• Other causes of polyuria and polydipsia—diabetes mellitus; hyperadrenocorticism; primary renal disease
• Severe vaginal disease

CBC/BIOCHEMISTRY/URINALYSIS
• Neutrophilia—immature; more severe with closed cervix
• Mild, normocytic, normochromic anemia
• Hyperglobulinemia and hyperproteinemia
• Azotemia
• ALT and ALP—high with septicemia or severe dehydration
• Electrolyte disturbances—depend on clinical course
• Urinalysis—sample collected by catheterization of the urinary bladder (least traumatic and most diagnostically accurate)

OTHER LABORATORY TESTS
• Cytologic examination of vaginal discharge—regenerative polymorphonuclear cells and bacteria; may be indistinguishable from the purulent discharge associated with vaginal disease (e.g., vaginitis, vaginal mass, foreign object, and vaginal anatomic anomaly)
• Bacterial culture and sensitivity test of vaginal discharge—not helpful in confirming diagnosis (bacteria cultured are usually normal vaginal flora); useful in determining appropriate antibiotic use
• Serologic testing for *Brucella canis*—rapid slide agglutination test used as a screen; sensitive but not specific. If positive, recheck by an agar gel immunodiffusion test (Cornell University Diagnostic Laboratory, 607-253-3900) or bacterial culture of whole blood, lymph node aspirate, or vaginal discharge.

IMAGING

Radiography
• Detect a large uterus.
• Rule out pregnancy—45 days after ovulation; 43–54 days after breeding.
• Pyometra—uterus may appear as a distended, tubular structure in the caudal ventral abdomen.

Ultrasonography
• Assess size of uterus and extent of cystic endometrial hyperplasia; nature of uterine contents
• Rule out pregnancy—20–24 days after ovulation.
• Normal uterine wall—not visible as a distinct entity
• Pyometra or cystic endometrial hyperplasia—associated with a thickened uterine wall and intraluminal fluid
• Pyometra—may occur with pregnancy in dogs (rare)

DIAGNOSTIC PROCEDURES
Vaginoscopy—indicated only in dogs with purulent vulvar discharge and no apparent uterine enlargement; allows determination of site of origin of the vaginal discharge; not possible in cats

PATHOLOGIC FINDINGS
• Endometrium (dogs and cats)—described as cobblestone (either condition)
• Cystic endometrial surface—covered by malodorous, mucopurulent exudate; thickened because of increased endometrial gland size and cystic gland distension

 TREATMENT

APPROPRIATE HEALTH CARE
• Inpatient
• Pyometra—life-threatening condition if the cervix is closed

PYOMETRA AND CYSTIC ENDOMETRIAL HYPERPLASIA

NURSING CARE
Supportive care—immediate intravenous fluid administration and antibiotics

ACTIVITY
N/A

DIET
N/A

CLIENT EDUCATION
• Inform client that ovariohysterectomy is the preferred treatment.
• Recommend medical treatment only for valuable breeding animals that are not azotemic and have an open cervix; warn client that nonprogestational, estrus-suppressing drugs must be given for life.
• Warn client that medical treatment of closed-cervix pyometra can be associated with uterine rupture and peritonitis (see Contraindications).
• Inform client that medical treatment probably does not cure underlying cystic endometrial hyperplasia in patients with either open- or closed-cervix pyometra but may enable some affected bitches to reproduce.

SURGICAL CONSIDERATIONS
• Pyometra (open and closed cervix)—ovariohysterectomy preferred treatment; chronic progressive disease
• Closed-cervix pyometra—use caution during ovariohysterectomy; enlarged uterus may be friable.
• Uterine rupture or leakage of purulent material from the uterine stump—repeated lavage of the peritoneal cavity with sterile saline

MEDICATIONS

DRUG(S) OF CHOICE

Antibiotics
• Empirical, pending results of bacterial culture and sensitivity test
• All patients with pyometra
• Common choices—ampicillin (20 mg/kg PO q8h); enrofloxacin (Baytril; 2.5 mg/kg PO q12h)

PGF$_{2\alpha}$
• Recommended dosages for only the native compound; dosages for analogues not well defined
• Cats—0.1–0.5 mg/kg SC q12–24h for 2–5 days until the size of the uterus nears normal
• Dogs—0.05–0.25 mg/kg SC q12–24h for 2–7 days until the uterus nears normal size as determined by palpation, radiography, or ultrasound
• In luteal phase (serum progesterone > 2 ng/mL)—may use 0.05–0.25 mg/kg SC q12h for 4 days

• Once-daily dosing—causes smooth muscle contractions and subsequent uterine evacuation
• Twice-daily dosing—causes luteolysis and a subsequent decrease in serum progesterone concentration
• Re-evaluate patient 2–4 weeks after discontinuation; if the uterus has increased in size or the patient still has marked vaginal discharge, the protocol can be repeated.
• Ovariohysterectomy—performed in patients refractory to prostaglandin, i.e., uterus still enlarged or vaginal discharge still present after two courses of medical treatment

CONTRAINDICATIONS
• PGF$_{2\alpha}$ with closed-cervix pyometra—strong myometrial contractions may cause uterine rupture or force purulent exudate through the oviducts, causing secondary peritonitis.
• PGF$_{2\alpha}$ in a valuable breeding animal—always rule out pregnancy before administering.

PRECAUTIONS
• PGF$_{2\alpha}$—not approved for use in dogs and cats
• Side effects of PGF$_{2\alpha}$—referable to contraction of smooth muscle; include hypersalivation; emesis; defecation; intense grooming of the flanks and vulva (cats); appear within minutes of injection; subside within 30–60 min; severity diminishes throughout the treatment regimen; may be diminished by diluting the drug with an equal volume of sterile saline before subcutaneous injection and by walking dogs for 20–30 min after injection

POSSIBLE INTERACTIONS
N/A

ALTERNATIVE DRUG(S)
• Drugs that enhance the immune response (e.g., estrogens) or induce myometrial contractility (e.g., oxytocin and ergot alkaloids)—unreliable
• Antibiotics—not efficacious as sole treatment unless the uterus is of normal size and the serum progesterone is < 2 ng/mL

FOLLOW-UP

PATIENT MONITORING
• Discharge from the hospital when the uterus is of near normal size and clinical signs have lessened in severity or disappeared; re-evaluate in 2–4 weeks.
• Antibiotics—administration continued for 3–4 weeks
• Vaginal discharge—may persist for up to 4 weeks
• Serial CBC—WBC count rises precipitously after ovariohysterectomy, because bone

marrow continues to release polymorpho-nuclear neutrophils into the bloodstream, from which they can no longer enter the uterus.

PREVENTION/AVOIDANCE
• Next proestrus—obtain a specimen of the anterior vagina for bacterial culture using a guarded culture swab.
• Treat bitch with an appropriate antibiotic for 3 weeks.
• Breed during that estrus—the gravid uterus may be less susceptible to re-infection; bitch with underlying cystic endometrial hyperplasia has limited breeding life (best to get the desired number of pups as soon as possible); bitch not more likely to clear the disease spontaneously if allowed to cycle without being bred

POSSIBLE COMPLICATIONS
Bitch may enter estrus sooner after treatment than anticipated if medical treatment induced premature luteolysis.

EXPECTED COURSE AND PROGNOSIS
Dogs—underlying cystic endometrial hyperplasia still exists; predisposed to recurrence; breed patient to desired stud dogs in a timely manner; recommend ovariohysterectomy as soon as breeding life is over; use of subfertile stud dogs not recommended

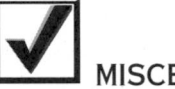 MISCELLANEOUS

ASSOCIATED CONDITIONS
Pyometra of the uterine stump in spayed animals—may develop any time after ovariohysterectomy; may be associated with an ovarian remnant

AGE-RELATED FACTORS
N/A

ZOONOTIC POTENTIAL
N/A

PREGNANCY
PGF$_{2\alpha}$—always rule out pregnancy before administration to valuable breeding animals; effective pregnancy-terminating agent

ABBREVIATIONS
• ALP = alkaline phosphatase
• ALT = alanine aminotransferase
• PGF$_{2\alpha}$ = prostaglandin F$_{2\alpha}$

Suggested Reading
Hardy RM, Osborne CA. Canine pyometra: pathophysiology, diagnosis and treatment of uterine and extrauterine lesions. J Am Anim Hosp Assoc 1974;10:245–268.
Author Margaret V. Root Kustritz
Consulting Editor Sara K. Lyle

PYOTHORAX

 BASICS

DEFINITION
Accumulation of pus within the pleural cavity, usually associated with infection

PATHOPHYSIOLOGY
• Infectious—generally arises from transpulmonary, transesophageal, or transthoracic inoculation of bacteria into the pleural space, with subsequent suppurative pleuritis
• Dogs—commonly associated causes: inhaled grass awn or other foreign object and penetrating wound to the thorax
• Cats—most common cause: penetrating bite wound
• Secondary to systemic infection or pneumonia—uncommon

SYSTEMS AFFECTED
• Respiratory
• Hemic/Lymphatic/Immune
• Renal/Urologic—protein-losing glomerulopathy

GENETICS
N/A

INCIDENCE/PREVALENCE
N/A

GEOGRAPHIC DISTRIBUTION
N/A

SIGNALMENT

Species
Dogs and cats

Breed Predilection
• Dogs—hunting and sporting breeds
• Cats—domestic shorthair

Mean Age and Range
Dogs and cats—median ~4 years

Predominant Sex
• Dogs—none
• Cats—males, because of tendency to fight

SIGNS

General Comments
• Often insidious in nature, with few clinical signs until late in the course of disease
• Respiratory compromise—often not severe until the disease is advanced

Historical Findings
• Diminished activity
• Collapse after exercising and slow recovery
• Weight loss and partial anorexia
• Temporary improvement with antibiotic therapy
• Confirm history of fights or puncture wounds

Physical Examination Findings
• Tachypnea—usually apparent; may be mild and not associated with dyspnea
• Cachexia—often observed
• Cough—may be observed

• Pyrexia—usually low-grade, may be observed
• Thoracic auscultation—may reveal muffled heart sounds, diminished lung sounds ventrally, and amplified lung sounds dorsally
• Cats—may show few clinical signs before onset of apparently acute respiratory distress, collapse, and septic shock
• Injury to the thoracic wall—may not be apparent or may be healed at the time of examination
• Perform thorough palpation and inspection of the thorax for evidence of scarring or fibrosis.

CAUSES
• Infectious—dogs: *Actinomyces* spp., *Nocardia* spp., *Bacteroides* spp., *Corynebacterium, Escherichia coli,* fungal agents, and *Streptococcus* spp.; cats: oral commensals (e.g., *Pasteurella multocida* and *Bacteroides* spp.) most common; frequency of isolation of these organisms may vary geographically; obligate anaerobes common, especially in cats
• Neoplastic—rarely with intrathoracic tumors secondary to tumor necrosis

RISK FACTORS
• Dogs—hunting, field trials, and other strenuous outdoor sporting activities
• Cats—outdoor lifestyle and fighting

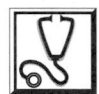 **DIAGNOSIS**

DIFFERENTIAL DIAGNOSIS
Other pleural effusions—chylothorax and hemothorax; nonseptic exudates (FIP or neoplasia); transudative effusions; differentiated via cytologic examination

CBC/BIOCHEMISTRY/URINALYSIS
• Marked neutrophilic leukocytosis with a (usually regenerative) left shift, monocytosis, and anemia of chronic disease
• Regenerative anemia—may be seen with substantial hemorrhage into the pleural cavity
• Biochemistry—often normal
• Possible hyperglobulinemia—due to inflammation
• Hypoalbuminemia—from renal loss
• Mildly high ALP
• Prerenal azotemia—may note if the patient is dehydrated
• Organ-specific changes—if other organs are secondarily infected (e.g., pyelonephritis and hepatitis)
• Proteinuria—possible with glomerulopathy

OTHER LABORATORY TESTS
• Serologic test for fungus may be positive.
• Cats—may be FeLV- or FIV-positive

IMAGING
• Radiography—unilateral or bilateral pleural effusion with pleural fissure lines; abscesses within the pulmonary parenchyma possible

• Ultrasonography—pleural effusion; may show marked amount of fibrinous deposition in the pleural space

DIAGNOSTIC PROCEDURES

Thoracocentesis
• Cytologic evaluation—often necessary to confirm the diagnosis, because many effusions appear grossly hemorrhagic
• Gram stains—may facilitate early identification of pathogenic organisms
• Sulfa granules (small accumulations of purulent debris) in the exudate—characteristic of infection by filamentous organisms (e.g., *Actinomyces* and *Nocardia*)
• Organisms are often seen on cytologic examination, often within neutrophils.
• Degenerative neutrophils abundant
• The effusion is often malodorous/putrid, especially in cats.

Microbiology
• Culture all fluid samples aerobically and anaerobically.
• Many of the filamentous, microaerophilic, and anaerobic organisms are slow-growing, so cultures should be maintained for 2–4 weeks.
• Sulfa granules—maceration may enhance culturing; contain higher concentrations of bacteria
• Fungal organisms—culture depends on history and geographic location.
• Urine samples—culture with suspected pyelonephritis.

PATHOLOGIC FINDINGS
• Fibrinous and suppurative pleuritis, with or without pulmonary abscessation
• Glomerulonephritis

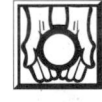 **TREATMENT**

APPROPRIATE HEALTH CARE
• Inpatient—often for several weeks
• Treat like any abscess; drainage is critical, without which resolution is highly unlikely.

NURSING CARE
• Continuous evacuation via tube thoracostomy with low-pressure suction through a perforated tube; use a large-bore tube to minimize occlusion; continue until net drainage is < 2–3 mL/kg/day and intracellular bacteria are no longer visible on gram stain; drainage may be slightly higher with red rubber tubes, because they are more irritating.
• Cats—usually require general anesthesia for tube placement
• Dogs with severe respiratory compromise—may substitute local anesthesia and regional analgesia for general anesthesia
• Periodic thoracic radiography—to ensure that bilateral tube placement is not necessary, tube placement is adequate, and there is no pocketing or loculation of exudate; determine

any primary pulmonary pathologic change that may not have been apparent on initial examination.

• Thoracic lavage—every 6–8 hours with warm, sterile saline; may help break down consolidated debris

• Coupage (rapid thoracic percussion)—may help remove consolidated debris

• Repeat bacterial culture if the patient fails to improve.

ACTIVITY

• Inpatient—encourage the patient to exercise lightly (10 min every 6–8 hours); promotes ventilatory efforts and helps break down pleural adhesions

• After discharge, gradually increase exercise over 2–4 months.

DIET

• High-calorie food

• Protein replacement is usually unnecessary.

CLIENT EDUCATION

Warn client that the duration of treatment (inpatient and outpatient) is long and expensive.

SURGICAL CONSIDERATIONS

• Surgery—associated with higher mortality; contraindicated unless the patient has pulmonary abscessation, pleural fibrosis, lung-lobe torsion, or extensive loculation of the pus that limits effective thoracic drainage

• Identified foreign body via thoracic imaging (radiography, ultrasound, CT, or MRI)—thoracotomy and retrieval indicated; grass awns are rarely found, even during surgery; attempted surgical retrieval is not recommended unless foreign body is visualized via imaging.

• Surgery may be indicated if pus is restricted to the mediastinum.

MEDICATIONS

DRUG(S) OF CHOICE

Antimicrobials

• Ultimately, choice determined by in vitro results of sensitivity testing

• Suspected specific pathogen—may initiate treatment before culture results are available; choose on the basis of common antibiotic sensitivities of particular organisms; *Actinomyces* spp. and *Bacteroides* (non-*fragilis*) spp. often susceptible to amoxicillin; *Nocardia* spp. often susceptible to potentiated sulfonamides; obligate anaerobic bacteria (including *B. fragilis*) susceptible to amoxicillin–clavulanic acid, chloramphenicol, and usually metronidazole; *Pasteurella* spp. often susceptible to potentiated penicillins

• Ampicillin or amoxicillin with a β-lactamase inhibitor—good initial choice for most patients; ampicillin and sulbactam (20

mg/kg IV q8h) followed by amoxicillin–clavulanic acid (25 mg/kg PO q8h) when medications can be given orally

• Trimethoprim-sulfa, aminoglycosides, and quinolones—generally ineffective

• Multiple antibiotics occasionally necessary

• Dosages are generally high (e.g., amoxicillin, 40 mg/kg PO q8h) to allow adequate distribution into the pleural cavity; may need to continue drug for several months and occasionally indefinitely

Analgesics

• Generally not required

• With severe discomfort—may use intrapleural anesthesia (e.g., bupivacaine mixed with the lavage fluid)

CONTRAINDICATIONS

Glucocorticoids and immunosuppressive agents—avoid with infectious pyothorax

PRECAUTIONS

Potentiated sulfas—may be associated with keratoconjunctivitis sicca, polyarthropathy, hypothyroidism, thrombocytopenia, and anemia, especially with prolonged use

POSSIBLE INTERACTIONS

N/A

ALTERNATIVE DRUG(S)

No specific suspected organism and culture and sensitivity results pending—use amoxicillin owing to its high efficacy against anaerobic bacteria and low probability of complications or toxicity; may consider clindamycin

FOLLOW-UP

PATIENT MONITORING

• Measure net thoracic fluid production—determine when thoracic drains may be removed.

• Evaluate thoracic radiographs—ensure adequate evacuation of fluid.

• Antibiotics—continue for 1 month after the patient is clinically normal, the hemogram is normal, and there is no radiographic evidence of fluid reaccumulation; average duration of therapy is 3–4 months but may continue for 6–12 months or longer.

• Assess CBC and radiographs monthly—residual radiographic changes may be permanent, but fluid should be absent.

PREVENTION AND AVOIDANCE

Avoid activity that predisposes the animal to the disease (often not practical).

POSSIBLE COMPLICATIONS

• Incorrect insertion of the drainage tube—may prevent adequate drainage or produce pneumothorax; too proximal a placement may put pressure on the brachial arteries and

veins, resulting in unilateral limb edema or lameness; lung laceration during placement

• Persistent, recurrent pyothorax—compartmentalization of pus; premature discontinuation of treatment

• Chronic fibrosing pleuritis and poor performance upon apparent recovery—may be treated surgically on occasion

• Persistent mediastinitis

EXPECTED COURSE AND PROGNOSIS

• With aggressive management—prognosis fair to excellent

• With repeated intermittent antibiotic therapy only or with inadequate drainage—prognosis poor

• Return to performance—depends on chronicity of disease and level of management

MISCELLANEOUS

ASSOCIATED CONDITIONS

• Retroperitoneal abscessation and diskospondylitis caused by migration of a foreign body through the diaphragm into the retroperitoneal space—occasionally seen • Glomerulonephropathy

AGE-RELATED FACTORS

N/A

ZOONOTIC POTENTIAL

Fungal infection during in vitro isolation

PREGNANCY

N/A

SYNONYMS

• Empyema • Suppurative pleuritis
• Pleurisy

SEE ALSO

• Chylothorax • Dyspnea, Tachypnea, and Panting • Pleural Effusion

ABBREVIATIONS

• ALP = alkaline phosphatase • FeLV = feline leukemia virus • FIP = feline infectious peritonitis • FIV = feline immunodeficiency virus

Suggested Reading

Edwards DF. Actinomycosis and nocardiosis. In: Greene CE, ed. Infectious diseases of the dog and cat. 2nd ed. Philadelphia: Saunders, 1998:303–313.

Greene CE. Pleural infections. In: Greene CE, ed. Infectious diseases of the dog and cat. 2nd ed. Philadelphia: Saunders, 1998:592–594.

Walker AL, Jang SS, Hirsh D.C. Bacteria associated with pyothorax of dogs and cats: 98 cases (1989–1998). J Am Vet Med Assoc 2000;216:359–363.

Author Mark Rishniw

Consulting Editor Lynelle R. Johnson

PYRETHRIN AND PYRETHROID TOXICITY

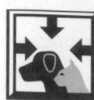

BASICS

OVERVIEW
• Insecticides • Pyrethrins—natural; derived from *Chrysanthemum cinerariaefolium* and related plant species • Pyrethroids—synthetic; include allethrin, cypermethrin, deltamethrin, fenvalerate, fluvalinate, permethrin, phenothrin, and tetramethrin • Affect the nervous system—reversibly prolong sodium conductance in nerve axons, resulting in repetitive nerve discharges; enhanced effect in hypothermic mammals and cold-blooded animals

SIGNALMENT
Adverse reactions occur more frequently in cats; small dogs; and young, old, sick, or debilitated animals. Reactions may occur when cats interact closely with permethrin spot-on treated dogs.

SIGNS
• Result from immune-mediated allergic hypersensitivity and anaphylactic reactions, genetic-based idiosyncratic reactions, and neurotoxic reactions; may be challenging to differentiate among these • Mild—hypersalivation; paw flicking; ear twitching; mild depression; vomiting; diarrhea • Moderate to serious—protracted vomiting and diarrhea; marked depression; ataxia; muscle tremors (must be differentiated from paw flicking and ear twitching) • Extreme dermal or oral overdose—may produce seizures or death • Cats—especially sensitive to concentrated permethrin-containing products labeled for use on dogs; may develop muscle tremors, ataxia, seizures, hyperthermia, and death within hours • Allergic reactions—urticaria; hyperemia; pruritus; anaphylaxis; shock; respiratory distress; (rarely) death • Idiosyncratic reactions—not allergic; resemble toxic reactions at much lower doses • Death—thoroughly investigate to rule out predisposing underlying conditions

CAUSES & RISK FACTORS
• Cats—more sensitive; less-efficient metabolic pathways, extensive grooming habits, and long haircoats that can retain large quantities of topically applied product • Patients with subnormal body temperatures after bathing, anesthesia, or sedation—predisposed to clinical signs

DIAGNOSIS

DIFFERENTIAL DIAGNOSIS
• Exposure history (amount and frequency of product usage), type and severity of clinical signs, and onset and duration of clinical signs—must be consistent before a tentative diagnosis can be made • Organophosphorous compounds, carbamate, or D-limonene toxicosis • Strychnine, metaldehyde, tremorgenic mycotoxins, methylxanthines, amphetamines, alcohol intoxication from isopropyl alcohol–based sprays • With sudden death—flea bite anemia, cardiomyopathy, or hyperthyroidism • Anaphylactic and idiosyncratic reactions

OTHER LABORATORY TESTS
• Pyrethrins—analytical tests for detection in tissues or fluids not generally available • Pyrethroids—some types can be detected in tissues to confirm exposure. • Cholinesterase activity—not reduced; may rule out exposure to organophosphate or carbamate insecticides

TREATMENT
• Adverse reactions (salivation, paw flicking, and ear twitching)—often mild and self-limiting
• Patient saturated with spray products—dry with a warmed towel; brush
• Continued mild signs—bathe at home with a mild hand dishwashing detergent.
• Progression to tremors and ataxia—hospitalize
• Seriously affected patient—fluid support with balanced electrolyte solution recommended
• Maintenance of a normal body temperature—critical
• Bath upon stabilization with liquid hand-dishwashing detergent and warm water is critical.

MEDICATIONS

DRUG(S)
• Tremors or seizures—especially for cats exposed to permethrin; methocarbamol (Robaxin-V injectable at 55–220 mg/kg IV not to exceed 330 mg/kg/day; administer one-half dose slowly IV, wait until the patient begins to relax, continue administration to effect; do not exceed 2 mL/min injection rate, and start with lower dose initially)
• Diazepam at low dosages has been used to control minor hyperesthesia. Seizure control has been achieved with pentobarbital and inhalant anesthetics. Methocarbimol remains the agent of choice
• Activated charcoal (2.0 g/kg PO) is rarely beneficial or recommended. Most formulations are rapidly absorbed liquids containing water, various alcohols, or hydrocarbon solvents.

• Emetics—rarely warranted; most formulations are rapidly absorbed liquids containing water, various alcohols, or hydrocarbon solvents; do not use with hydrocarbon solvent exposure (potential for aspiration); if indicated, if the patient is asymptomatic, and if it is within 1–2 hr of ingestion: induced with 3% hydrogen peroxide (2.2 mL/kg, maximum 45 mL) after feeding

CONTRAINDICATIONS/POSSIBLE INTERACTIONS
• Atropine sulfate—not antidotal; avoid; may cause tachycardia, CNS stimulation, disorientation, drowsiness, respiratory depression, and even seizures
• Judiciously avoid hypothermia.

FOLLOW-UP

PREVENTION/AVOIDANCE
• Proper application of flea-control products— greatly reduces incidence of adverse reactions; correct dose of most sprays: 1–2 pumps of a typical trigger sprayer per pound body weight • Reduction of salivation by sensitive cats (sprays)—spray onto a grooming brush; evenly brush through haircoat. • Liquids—term *dip* common; never submerge animal; pour on body; sponge to cover dry areas. • Premise products—do not apply topically unless labeled for such use; after treating house or yard, do not allow animal in the area until product has dried and environment has been ventilated. • Do not apply dog-only products on cats. • Do not use permethrin spot-on products on dogs in households with cats

EXPECTED COURSE AND PROGNOSIS
• Hypersalivation—may recur for several days after use of flea-control product when patient (especially cat) grooms itself
• Most clinical signs (mild to severe) resolve within 24–72 hr.

MISCELLANEOUS

SEE ALSO
• Organophosphate and Carbamate Toxicity
• Poisoning (Intoxication)

Suggested Reading
Hansen SR, Villar D, Buck WB, et al. Pyrethrins and pyrethroids in dogs and cats. Compend Contin Educ Pract Vet 1994;16:707–713.
Authors Steven R. Hansen and Elizabeth A. Curry-Galvin
Consulting Editor Gary D. Osweiler

BASICS

OVERVIEW
• RBCs require energy in the form of ATP for maintenance of shape, deformability, active membrane transport, and limited synthetic activities; mature RBCs lack mitochondria and depend on anaerobic glycolysis for ATP generation.
• PK catalyzes an important rate-controlling, ATP-generating step in glycolysis; consequently, energy metabolism is markedly impaired in PK-deficient RBCs, resulting in shortened RBC life-span and anemia; bone marrow attempts to compensate by erythroid hyperplasia, with marked reticulocytosis in peripheral blood.

SIGNALMENT
• Autosomal recessive trait recognized in basenjis, beagles, West Highland white terriers, Cairn terriers, miniature poodles, dachshunds, Chihuahuas, pugs, American Eskimo dogs, and Abyssinian, Somali, and domestic shorthair cats
• Affected homozygous animals generally not recognized as abnormal until several months of age or until adulthood

SIGNS
• Exercise intolerance
• Pale mucous membranes
• Tachycardia
• Systolic heart murmurs
• Often splenomegaly or hepatomegaly
• Icterus rarely seen
• Affected dogs may be slightly smaller than normal for their breed and age and may exhibit weakness and muscle wasting.
• Heterozygous carriers asymptomatic

CAUSES & RISK FACTORS
• RBCs from normal adult dogs exhibit only one PK isozyme (the R-type).
• Breed-specific defects in the *PKLR* gene result in erythrocyte PK deficiency in dogs.
• A common molecular defect has been described in cats.

DIAGNOSIS

DIFFERENTIAL DIAGNOSIS
• Other causes of hemolytic anemia—immune-mediated hemolytic anemia, haemobartonellosis, babesiosis, Heinz body hemolytic anemia, microangiopathic hemolytic anemia, and phosphofructokinase deficiency
• Affected dogs—negative Coombs test, no parasites or Heinz bodies in stained blood films, seronegative for *Babesia* spp., and no evidence of DIC or heartworm disease
• In contrast to phosphofructokinase, affected dogs do not exhibit episodes of intravascular hemolysis and hemoglobinuria; these deficiencies are differentiated by specific enzyme assays or DNA tests.

CBC/BIOCHEMISTRY/URINALYSIS
• Macrocytic hypochromic anemia, with PCV values of 16%–28% and uncorrected reticulocyte counts of 15%–50%
• Normal or slightly high leukocyte counts with mature neutrophilia
• Normal to slightly high platelet count
• Moderate to marked polychromasia, anisocytosis, and numerous nucleated RBCs on stained blood films
• Poikilocytosis in some animals, especially in splenectomized dogs
• Possible abnormal clinical chemistry findings, such as hyperferremia, mild hyperbilirubinemia, and slightly high ALT and ALP activities; dogs with liver failure may have hypoalbuminemia
• Normal urinalysis, except for bilirubinuria in dogs

OTHER LABORATORY TESTS
• Total RBC PK activity—low value diagnostic in cats and some dogs; many affected dogs have normal or high activities because of the expression of an M_2 isozyme that does not normally occur in mature RBCs; approximately 50% of normal in heterozygous animals
• Additional assays (e.g., enzyme heat stability test, measurement of RBC glycolytic intermediates, electrophoresis of isozymes, and enzyme immunoprecipitation)—to reach a diagnosis in dogs whose total enzyme activity is not low
• DNA diagnostic tests—for screening basenji and West Highland white terriers

IMAGING
N/A

DIAGNOSTIC PROCEDURES
N/A

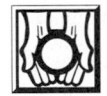

TREATMENT
Affected animals can only be cured by bone marrow transplantation.

MEDICATIONS

DRUG(S)
Although not adequately evaluated, long-term treatment with iron-chelating drugs, such as deferoxamine mesylate, might prolong the life expectancy of affected animals.

CONTRAINDICATIONS/POSSIBLE INTERACTIONS
None

FOLLOW-UP
• Hepatic iron overload—develops in affected dogs; can result in cirrhosis
• Myelofibrosis and osteosclerosis—develop in affected dogs with age; thus most die by 4 years of age as a result of bone marrow or liver failure
• Severe anemia with minimal reticulocytosis or abnormal liver function tests and ascites secondary to hypoalbuminemia indicate the terminal stage of the disease in dogs.
• The long-term consequences of this deficiency in cats have not been reported.

MISCELLANEOUS

ABBREVIATIONS
• ALP = alkaline phosphatase
• ALT = alanine aminotransferase
• DIC = disseminated intravascular coagulation
• PCV = packed cell volume
• PK = pyruvate kinase

Suggested Reading

Giger U. Erythrocyte phosphofructokinase and pyruvate kinase deficiencies. In: Feldman BF, Zinkl JG, Jain NC, eds. Schalm's veterinary hematology, 5th ed. Philadelphia: Lippincott Williams & Wilkins, 2000;7020–1025.
Harvey JW. Congenital erythrocyte enzyme deficiencies. Vet Clin North Am Small Anim Pract 1996;26:1003–1011.
Author John W. Harvey
Consulting Editor Stephen Kruth

PYTHIOSIS

BASICS

DEFINITION
An infectious disease affecting primarily the skin or GI tract of dogs and cats. It is caused by the aquatic pathogen *Pythium insidiosum*, an organism classified in the class Oomycetes.

PATHOPHYSIOLOGY
• The infective form of *P. insidiosum* is thought to be the motile biflagellate zoospore, which is released into warm water environments and is chemotactically attracted to damaged tissue and animal hair. Animals are likely infected when they enter or ingest water that contains infective zoospores. • *P. insidiosum* is considered a pathogenic rather than opportunistic organism because immune suppression is not a prerequisite for infection. • In the GI tract, *P. insidiosum* infection causes chronic pyogranulomatous disease manifested by severe segmental transmural thickening of one or more areas of the stomach or intestine. • In the skin, pythiosis typically results in the development of nonhealing wounds and invasive masses that contain ulcerated nodules and draining tracts.

SYSTEMS AFFECTED
• GI and cutaneous forms of disease are encountered with equal frequency in the dog. In cats, which are infrequently infected, the cutaneous form is more common. With the exception of occasional dissemination to regional lymph nodes, pythiosis usually affects only one body system in each patient. • GI pythiosis most often affects the gastric outflow region, proximal small intestine, ileocolic junction, or colon. Rarely, the esophagus may be affected. • In dogs with GI disease, *P. insidiosum*–induced local thromboembolic events or vascular invasion may lead to bowel wall ischemia and GI perforation or hemoabdomen. • Dogs with cutaneous pythiosis most often are presented for solitary or multiple cutaneous or subcutaneous lesions involving the extremities, tailhead, ventral neck, perineum, or medial thigh. • In cats, cutaneous lesions or subcutaneous masses involving retrobulbar, periorbital, or nasopharyngeal regions, the tailhead, or the footpads have been observed. • Multisystemic involvement is rare.

GENETICS
Although large-breed dogs are most often affected, no genetic predisposition has been documented.

INCIDENCE/PREVALENCE
• Dependent on geographic distribution
• Affected animals are presented for signs of disease usually in the fall or early winter months.

GEOGRAPHIC DISTRIBUTION
• Disease caused by *P. insidiosum* occurs primarily in tropical and subtropical areas of the world. • In the United States, pythiosis occurs most often in states bordering the Gulf of Mexico; however, it has also been documented in Oklahoma, Arkansas, Missouri, Kentucky, Tennessee, North and South Carolina, Virginia, southern Indiana, and New Jersey. • Outside the United States, pythiosis has been reported in Australia, Brazil, Burma, Colombia, Costa Rica, Indonesia, Japan, New Guinea, and Thailand.

SIGNALMENT

Species
Dogs and, less commonly, cats

Breed Predilection
• Large-breed dogs, especially those used in hunting or field trial work near water
• Labrador retrievers are overrepresented.
• German shepherds may be predisposed to cutaneous pythiosis.

Mean Age and Range
Animals less than 3 years old are most likely to be infected.

Predominant Sex
Males are affected more often than females, possibly because of increased exposure.

SIGNS

General Comments
Affected dogs are not usually severely ill until late in the course of disease.

Historical Findings
• Chronic weight loss and intermittent vomiting are the most common signs.
• Diarrhea may be evident if the colon or a large segment of the small intestine is affected.
• Regurgitation is noted with rare esophageal disease. • Cutaneous disease is characterized by nodules that ulcerate and drain.

Physical Examination Findings
GI Pythiosis
• Emaciation is common. • An abdominal mass is often palpable. • Despite severe weight loss, affected dogs are usually bright and alert. • Fever is occasionally noted. • Systemic signs and abdominal pain may occur with intestinal obstruction, infarction, or perforation.
Cutaneous Pythiosis
• Cutaneous or subcutaneous lesions appear as nonhealing wounds; boggy, edematous regions; or poorly defined nodules that become ulcerated. Multiple tracts draining a serosanguinous or purulent exudate often are present.

CAUSES
P. insidiosum

RISK FACTORS
• Environmental exposure to swampy areas, bayous, ponds, or lakes containing infective zoospores
• Outdoor activities such as hunting

DIAGNOSIS

DIFFERENTIAL DIAGNOSIS

GI Pythiosis
• Intestinal obstruction caused by a foreign body or chronic intussusception • Histoplasmosis • Gastric or intestinal lymphosarcoma • Gastric carcinoma • Other GI neoplasia • Inflammatory bowel disease
• Basidiobolomycosis, prototfecosis • Histiocytic or idiopathic colitis

Cutaneous Pythiosis
• Lagenidiosis (caused by oomycotic pathogens in the genus *Lagenidium*) • Zygomycosis (infections caused by *Basidiobolus* or *Conidiobolus* spp.) • Other mycotic skin diseases, such as cryptococcosis, coccidioidomycosis, sporotrichosis, eumycotic mycetoma, and phaeohyphomycosis
• Nodular bacterial skin diseases, such as actinomycosis, mycobacteriosis, botryomycosis, and brucellosis • Protothecosis or nodular leishmaniasis • Noninfectious pyogranulomatous diseases, such as foreign-body reaction, idiopathic nodular panniculitis, sebaceous nodular adenitis, and canine cutaneous sterile pyogranuloma/ granuloma syndrome • Cutaneous neoplasia
• Systemic vasculitis and cutaneous embolic disease

CBC/BIOCHEMISTRY/URINALYSIS
• Laboratory findings are nonspecific.
• Eosinophilia, leukocytosis, and anemia of chronic disease may occur. • Hyperglobulinemia and/or hypoalbuminemia may be noted in chronically affected dogs. • Hypokalemia, hyponatremia, hypochloridemia, and metabolic alkalosis may be noted in dogs with gastric outflow obstruction. • Hypercalcemia was reported in a single affected dog.
• Urinalysis usually normal

OTHER LABORATORY TESTS
Serology—a sensitive and specific ELISA test is available through the Pythium Laboratory at Louisiana State University

IMAGING
• Abdominal radiography may reveal an obstructive pattern, bowel wall thickening, or abdominal mass. • Abdominal ultrasonography may reveal segmental transmural thickening of the stomach, proximal small intestine, or ileocolic junction. Granulomas or enlarged lymph nodes may be evident in the mesentery.

DIAGNOSTIC PROCEDURES
• Biopsy of gastrointestinal or skin lesions will demonstrate histologic changes that are suggestive of, but not definitive for, pythiosis.

• Definitive diagnosis is based on culture; tissue samples should be submitted to an experienced laboratory via overnight shipping at room temperature. • An immunohisto-chemical stain can be used to identify *P. insidiosum* hyphae in histologic sections. • A nested PCR assay can be used for the definitive identification of cultured isolates or organisms in tissue samples.

PATHOLOGIC FINDINGS
• Histologically, GI and skin lesions are characterized by pyogranulomatous and eosinophilic inflammation associated with broad (4–6 micron), irregularly branching, infrequently septate hyphae with thick, nonparallel walls. • Predominance of eosinophils within the inflammatory reaction helps to differentiate pythiosis and zygomycosis from other mycotic infections. • Hyphal organisms are usually not visible on hematoxylin and eosin stained sections, but are readily visualized with a silver stain. • Dogs with GI lesions typically have severe segmental thickening of portions of stomach and/or bowel, often with obstruction of the intestinal lumen. • Mesenteric lymph-adenopathy is often noted, but the presence of *P. insidiosum* hyphae within lymph nodes is uncommon. • Histologically, GI pythiosis is characterized by mucosal ulceration, lymphoplasmacytic and eosinophilic inflammation in the lamina propria, and granulomatous inflammation within the submucosa and muscularis.

TREATMENT

APPROPRIATE HEALTH CARE
The treatment of choice is aggressive surgical excision of all infected tissue. Unfortunately, many animals are not presented to the veterinarian until late in the disease, when complete resection is not possible.

NURSING CARE
Supportive care should include fluids, potassium, nutritional support, and antibiotics as needed.

ACTIVITY
Limit activity

DIET
Feed a highly digestible, calorie-dense diet.

CLIENT EDUCATION
• Treatment is expensive. • Prognosis is guarded to poor unless a complete resection is feasible.

SURGICAL CONSIDERATIONS
• Attempt wide surgical excision to obtain 5- to 6-cm margins even if medical therapy is contemplated. • Amputation is recommended

for treatment of extremity lesions. • Enlarged mesenteric lymph nodes should be biopsied but often do not contain infective hyphae, thus do not have to be removed. • Dogs often improve after obstructive lesions are resected, even if significant disease is still grossly evident. • Postoperative medical therapy with itraconazole and terbinafine (see below) for 2–3 months is recommended to decrease the chance of recurrence. • Reevaluation of ELISA serology 2–3 months after surgery is an excellent prognostic indicator.

MEDICATIONS

DRUG(S) OF CHOICE
• Itraconazole (10 mg/kg PO daily) combined with terbinafine (5–10 mg/kg PO daily) appears to be most effective. Although controlled studies have not been performed, the efficacy of this combination is probably 20%–25% in dogs with nonresectable or partially resectable lesions. • Medical therapy should be continued for a minimum of 4–6 months. • Give itraconazole with food.

CONTRAINDICATIONS
Although corticosteroids may cause a temporary improvement in clinical signs, their use is contraindicated.

PRECAUTIONS
• Azole drugs should not be used in animals with severe liver disease. • Anorexia, high liver enzymes, and cutaneous vasculitis are the most common adverse affects of itraconazole.

POSSIBLE INTERACTIONS
Antacids and anticonvulsants may decrease blood levels of itraconazole.

ALTERNATIVE DRUG(S)
• ABLC has shown efficacy in a limited number of dogs with GI pythiosis. Its use is recommended when the patient cannot tolerate oral medications. • Dose of ABLC is 2–3 mg/kg (dog) or 0.5–1 mg/kg (cat) IV 3×/week for 9–12 treatments (total dose of 24–30 mg in the dog). The drug should be diluted in 5% dextrose to a concentration of 1 mg/mL and given IV over 45–90 minutes. • ABLC should not be used in animals that are azotemic or hypokalemic. • Side effects, such as chills, trembling, fever, anorexia, and vomiting, may be noted during ABLC infusion.

FOLLOW-UP

PATIENT MONITORING
• ELISA serology can be used to monitor response to therapy; serology should be

checked 2–3 months after surgery, or every 3 months during medical therapy. • Abdominal ultrasonography is useful in reevaluating intestinal lesions. • Medical management may reduce nonresectable lesions to the point that they become resectable. • Liver enzymes should be evaluated monthly while patient is on itraconazole. • Serum BUN, creatinine, and potassium should be evaluated before each dose of ABLC is administered.

PREVENTION/AVOIDANCE
Monitor for signs of recurrence.

POSSIBLE COMPLICATIONS
Acute abdomen and death from GI thrombosis and perforation

EXPECTED COURSE AND PROGNOSIS
• Prognosis is guarded to poor unless a complete resection is possible. • Less than 25% of affected animals are cured with medical therapy alone.

MISCELLANEOUS

ASSOCIATED CONDITIONS
None

AGE-RELATED FACTORS
Young animals are predisposed.

ZOONOTIC POTENTIAL
Infections in people are very rare and are from a common environmental source. There is no evidence of direct transmission from animals to humans.

PREGNANCY
Azole antifungals are teratogenic and should not be used in pregnant animals.

SYNONYMS
Phycomycosis, Swamp Cancer

ABBREVIATIONS
ABLC = amphotericin B lipid complex
ELISA = enzyme-linked immunosorbent assay
PCR = polymerase chain reaction

Suggested Reading

Grooters AM, Gee MK. Development of a nested PCR assay for the detection and identification of *Pythium insidiosum*. J Vet Intern Med 2002;16:147–152.

Grooters AM, Leise BS, Lopez MK, et al. Development and evaluation of an enzyme-linked immunosorbent assay for the serodiagnosis of pythiosis in dogs. J Vet Intern Med 2002;16:142–146.

Thomas RC, Lewis DT. Pythiosis in dogs and cats. Compend Contin Ed Pract Vet 1998;20:63–74.

Authors Amy Grooters and Joseph Taboada
Consulting Editor Albert E. Jergens

PYURIA

 BASICS

DEFINITION
• WBCs (i.e., neutrophils, eosinophils, mono-cytes, lymphocytes, or plasma cells) in urine
• More than five WBCs per high-power field is generally considered abnormal, but the number of WBCs found in urinary sediment depends on method of collection, sample volume and concentration, degree of cellular destruction after collection, and laboratory technique.

PATHOPHYSIOLOGY
• Large numbers of WBCs in voided urine samples indicate active inflammation some-where along the urogenital tract.
• Can be associated with any pathologic process (infectious or noninfectious) that causes cellular injury or death; tissue damage evokes exudative inflammation characterized by evidence of leukocytic extravasation (pyuria) and increased vascular permeability (hematuria and proteinuria).

SYSTEMS AFFECTED
• Renal/Urologic—urethra, urinary bladder, ureters, and kidneys • Genital—prepuce, prostate, vagina, and uterus

SIGNALMENT
Dogs and cats

SIGNS

General Comments
Inflammation can cause clinical signs localized to the site(s) of injury or may be accompanied by systemic manifestations. Historical and physical examination findings depend on the underlying cause, organ(s) affected, degree of organ dysfunction, and magnitude of systemic inflammatory responses. Nonobstructive lesions confined to the urinary bladder, urethra, vagina, or prepuce rarely cause systemic signs of inflammation. Systemic signs may accompany generalized inflammatory lesions of the kidneys, prostate, or uterus.

Physical Examination Findings
Local Effects of Inflammation
• Erythema of mucosal surfaces—e.g., redness of vaginal or preputial mucosa
• Tissue swelling—e.g., renomegaly, prostatomegaly, mural thickening of urinary bladder or urethra
• Exudation of leukocytes and protein-rich fluid—e.g., pyuria, purulent urethral or vagi-nal discharge, pyometra, or prostatic abscess
• Pain—e.g., adverse response to palpation, dysuria, pollakiuria, stranguria
• Loss of function—e.g., polyuria, dysuria, pollakiuria, urinary incontinence
Systemic Effects of Inflammation
• Fever • Depression • Anorexia
• Dehydration

CAUSES

Kidney
• Pyelonephritis—e.g., bacterial, fungal, parasitic, or mycoplasmal • Nephrolith(s)
• Neoplasia • Trauma • Immune-mediated

Ureter
• Ureteritis—e.g., bacterial
• Ureterolith(s) • Neoplasia

Urinary Bladder
• Cystitis—e.g., bacterial, mycoplasmal, fungal, or parasitic • Urocystolith(s)
• Neoplasia • Trauma • Overdistension—urethral obstruction • Pharmacologic—cyclophosphamide

Urethra
• Urethritis—e.g., bacterial, fungal, or mycoplasmal
• Urethrolith(s)
• Neoplasia
• Trauma
• Foreign body

Prostate
• Prostatitis/abscess—e.g., bacterial or fungal
• Neoplasia

Penis/Prepuce
• Balanoposthitis
• Neoplasia
• Foreign body

Uterus
Pyometra/metritis—e.g., bacterial

Vagina
• Vaginitis—bacterial, mycoplasmal, viral, or fungal
• Neoplasia
• Foreign body
• Trauma

RISK FACTORS
• Any disease process, diagnostic procedure, or therapy that alters normal host urinary tract defenses and predisposes to infection
• Any disease process, dietary factor, or therapy that predisposes to formation of metabolic uroliths

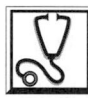 **DIAGNOSIS**

DIFFERENTIAL DIAGNOSIS

Voided Specimens
• Rule out vaginitis—signs include vaginal discharge, erythema of vaginal mucosa, licking of vulva, and attracting male dogs.
• Rule out pyometra, metritis—signs include vaginal discharge, large uterus, pyrexia, depression, anorexia, polyuria, polydipsia, and a recent history of estrus, parturition, or progestin administration.
• Rule out balanoposthitis—signs include preputial discharge, erythema of preputial or penile mucosa, and licking of prepuce.

• Rule out prostatitis, prostatic abscess, or prostatic neoplasia—signs include urethral discharge, prostatomegaly, pyrexia, depression, dysuria, tenesmus, caudal abdominal pain, and stiff gait.
• Rule out urethritis, urethroliths, urethral neoplasms—signs include dysuria, pollakiuria, stranguria, and/or palpable uroliths or mass lesions in the urethra.
• Rule out inflammatory disorders of urinary bladder and kidneys.

Specimens Collected by Cystocentesis
• Rule out urethral obstruction—signs include stranguria, anuria, and a large overdistended urinary bladder.
• Rule out prostatic and urethral disorders (see previous text); purulent prostatic or urethral exudates can reflux into the urinary bladder.
• Rule out cystitis, urocystoliths, and urinary bladder neoplasia—signs may include dysuria, pollakiuria, stranguria, and/or palpable uroliths or mass lesions in the urinary bladder.
• Rule out pyelonephritis—signs may include pyrexia, depression, anorexia, polyuria, polydipsia, renal pain, and renomegaly.
• Rule out posttraumatic pyuria—signs may include history of trauma, including iatrogenic

LABORATORY FINDINGS

Drugs That May Alter Laboratory Results
• WBCs lyse rapidly in hypotonic or alkaline urine. Administration of alkalinizing agents (e.g., sodium bicarbonate, potassium citrate, chlorothiazide, or acetazolamide) or agents that produce hypotonic urine (e.g., diuretics and glucocorticoids) may falsely decrease urine WBC numbers.
• Nitrofurantoin, cephalosporins, and gentamicin can cause false-positive leukocyte esterase reactions with reagent strip (dipstick) methods.
• Urinary WBC concentrations can be low in patients with inflammatory disorders who have been given steroidal or nonsteroidal antiinflammatory drugs.

Disorders That May Alter Laboratory Results
• Disorders associated with diminished WBC function or absolute neutropenia can artificially lower WBC values.
• Disorders associated with production of hypotonic urine or alkaline urine artificially lower WBC values.

Miscellaneous Factors That May Alter Laboratory Results
• False-negative leukocyte esterase reaction in dogs when urine is tested by the reagent strip (dipstick) method
• False-positive and false-negative leukocyte esterase reaction in cats when urine is tested by the reagent strip (dipstick) method

Valid If Run in Human Laboratory?
Valid if urinary sediment is examined microscopically; invalid if only leukocyte esterase reagent strip (dipstick) method is used.

CBC/BIOCHEMISTRY/URINALYSIS
• Pyuria in specimens collected by voiding, manual compression, or catheterization indicates an inflammatory lesion involving at least the urinary or genital tracts.
• Pyuria in specimens collected by cystocentesis localizes the site of inflammation to at least the urinary tract, but does not exclude the urethra and genital tract. Reflux of prostatic exudates into the urinary bladder may result in pyuria in patients with prostatic disease.
• Pyuria associated with WBC casts is unequivocal evidence of renal parenchymal inflammation.
• Generalized renal injury may be associated with concomitant leukocytosis, isosthenuria, and azotemia.
• Pyuria associated with bacteria, fungi, or parasite ova in sufficient numbers to be seen by microscopic sediment examination indicates that the inflammatory lesion was caused or complicated by urinary tract infection.
• Pyuria associated with neoplastic cells indicates neoplasia. Diagnosis of urinary tract neoplasia by cytologic examination of urine may be complicated by epithelial cell hyperplasia and atypia caused by urinary tract inflammation or the physiochemical properties of urine (pH and tonicity).

OTHER LABORATORY TESTS
• Perform quantitative urine culture on all patients with pyuria; it provides the most definitive means of identifying and characterizing bacterial urinary tract infection.
• Negative urine culture results suggest a noninfectious cause of inflammation (e.g., uroliths, neoplasia) or inflammation associated with urinary tract infection caused by fastidious organisms (e.g., mycoplasmas and viruses).
• Cytologic evaluation of urinary sediment, prostatic fluid, urethral or vaginal discharges, or biopsy specimens obtained by catheter or needle aspiration may help evaluate patients with localized urinary or genital tract disease. Cytologic examination may establish a definitive diagnosis of urinary tract neoplasia, but negative cytologic findings do not rule out neoplasia.

IMAGING
Survey abdominal radiography, contrast urethrocystography and cystography, urinary tract ultrasonography, and excretory urography are important means of identifying and localizing underlying causes.

DIAGNOSTIC PROCEDURES
• Urethrocystoscopy—indicated in patients with persistent lesions of the lower urinary tract for which a definitive diagnosis has not been established by other, less invasive, means
• Light microscopic evaluation of tissue specimens—indicated in patients with lesions of the urinary or genital tracts for which a definitive diagnosis has not been established by other, less invasive, means; tissue specimens may be obtained by catheter biopsy, cystoscopy and forceps biopsy, or exploratory laparotomy; aspiration and punch biopsy techniques may be used to evaluate the prostate gland.

TREATMENT
• Treatment varies, depending on the underlying cause and specific organs involved.
• Pyuria associated with systemic signs of illness (i.e., pyrexia, depression, anorexia, vomiting, dehydration, leukocytosis, polyuria, and polydipsia) or urinary obstruction warrants aggressive diagnostic evaluation and initiation of specific, supportive, and/or symptomatic treatment.

MEDICATIONS
DRUG(S)
Depend on underlying cause

CONTRAINDICATIONS
• Avoid glucocorticoids or other immunosuppressive agents in patients suspected of having urinary or genital tract infection.
• Avoid potentially nephrotoxic drugs (e.g., gentamicin) in febrile, dehydrated, or azotemic patients and those suspected of having pyelonephritis, septicemia, or preexisting renal disease.

PRECAUTIONS N/A

POSSIBLE INTERACTIONS N/A

FOLLOW-UP
PATIENT MONITORING
Response to treatment by serial urinalyses, including examination of urine sediment; collect specimens from most patients by cystocentesis to avoid contamination by preputial or vaginal exudates; perform transurethral catheterization if the expected benefits outweigh the risk of iatrogenic bacterial urinary tract infection.

POSSIBLE COMPLICATIONS
• Infectious and noninfectious inflammatory disorders of the urinary tract can cause primary renal failure, urinary obstruction, uremia, septicemia, and death.
• Pyuria is a potential risk factor for formation of matrix or matrix-crystalline urethral plugs and subsequent urethral obstruction in male cats.

MISCELLANEOUS
ASSOCIATED CONDITIONS
• Hematuria
• Proteinuria
• Bacteriuria

AGE-RELATED FACTORS N/A

ZOONOTIC POTENTIAL N/A

PREGNANCY N/A

SYNONYMS
Leukocyturia

SEE ALSO
• Dysuria and Pollakiuria
• Hematuria
• Lower Urinary Tract Infection
• Proteinuria
• Pyelonephritis

ABBREVIATION
WBC = white blood cell

Suggested Reading

Ling GV. Bacterial infections of the urinary tract. In: Ettinger SJ, Feldman EC, eds. Textbook of veterinary internal medicine. 5th ed. Philadelphia: Saunders, 2000:1678–1686.
Lulich JP, Osborne CA, Bartges JW, et al. Canine lower urinary tract disorders. In: Ettinger SJ, Feldman EC, eds. Textbook of veterinary internal medicine. 5th ed. Philadelphia: Saunders, 2000:1747–1781.
Osborne CA, Kruger JM, Lulich JP, et al. Feline lower urinary tract diseases. In: Ettinger SJ, Feldman EC, eds. Textbook of veterinary internal medicine. 5th ed. Philadelphia: Saunders, 2000:1710–1747.
Osborne CA, Stevens JB, Lulich JP, et al. A clinician's analysis of urinalysis. In: Osborne CA, Finco DR, eds. Canine and feline nephrology and urology. 2nd ed. Baltimore: Williams & Wilkins, 1995:136–205.

Authors John M. Kruger, Carl A. Osborne, and Cheryl L. Swenson
Consulting Editors Larry G. Adams and Carl A. Osborne

Q FEVER

BASICS

OVERVIEW
• Caused by the zoonotic rickettsia *Coxiella burnetii*
• Infection—most commonly by inhalation or ingestion of organisms while feeding on infected body fluids (urine, feces, milk, or parturient discharges), tissues (especially placenta), or carcasses of infected animal reservoir hosts (cattle, sheep, goats); can occur after tick exposure (many species of ticks implicated)
• Lungs—thought to be main portal of entry to systemic circulation
• Organism replicates in vascular endothelium; causes widespread vasculitis; severity depends on the pathogenicity of the strain of organism; vasculitis results in necrosis and hemorrhage in lungs, liver, and CNS
• An extended latent period exists after recovery until chronic immune-complex phenomena develop; organism reactivated out of the latent state during parturition, resulting in large numbers entering the placenta, parturient fluids, urine, feces, and milk
• Endemic worldwide

SIGNALMENT
Cats and dogs

SIGNS

Historical Findings
• Fever
• Lethargy
• Depression
• Anorexia
• Abortion—especially cats
• Ataxia and seizures—especially dogs

Physical Examination Findings
• Usually asymptomatic
• Multifocal neurologic signs—dogs

CAUSES & RISK FACTORS
• *C. burnetii*
• Exposure to infected animals (especially following parturition) and ticks

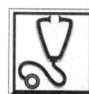

DIAGNOSIS

DIFFERENTIAL DIAGNOSIS
• Cats—other causes of abortion: infections (viral rhinotracheitis, panleukopenia, FeLV, toxoplasmosis, bacteria including coliforms, *Streptococci, Staphylococci, Salmonellae*); fetal defects; maternal problems (nutrition, genital tract abnormalities); environmental stress; endocrine disorders (hypoluteidism)
• Dogs—other causes of encephalitis

CBC/BIOCHEMISTRY/URINALYSIS
Nonspecific

OTHER LABORATORY TESTS

Serology
• Collect 2–3 mL of serum and refrigerate, for organism identification.
• Collect tissue sample (e.g., placenta) and refrigerate, for animal inoculation.
• Tests available from the New Mexico Department of Agriculture, Veterinary Diagnostic Services, 700 Camino de Salud NE, Albuquerque, NM 87106

IMAGING
N/A

DIAGNOSTIC PROCEDURES
N/A

TREATMENT
• Alert client of possible zoonotic risk.
• Inpatient—avoids zoonotic risk to client
• Wear gloves and masks when treating an infected animal or when attending an aborting cat.

MEDICATIONS

DRUG(S)
• Tetracycline—22 mg/kg PO q8h for 2 weeks
• Doxycycline—20 mg/kg PO q12h for 1 week
• Enrofloxacin—10 mg/kg PO q12h for 1 week; should be effective but no clinical reports; effective in vitro

CONTRAINDICATIONS/POSSIBLE INTERACTIONS
N/A

FOLLOW-UP

• Difficult to determine success of therapy because many animals spontaneously improve

• Even asymptomatic cases should be aggressively treated because of the zoonotic potential.
• Utility of predicting success of therapy based on serologic improvement unknown

MISCELLANEOUS

ZOONOTIC POTENTIAL
• Major zoonotic potential
• By the time a diagnosis is made in a cat or dog, human exposure and infection have occurred.
• Instruct owners and people in contact with the pet to seek medical advice immediately.
• Humans contract the disease by inhalation of infected aerosols (e.g., after parturition); children commonly infected from ingestion of raw milk but are usually asymptomatic

• Previous urban outbreaks have been related to exposure to infected cats.
• Incubation period from time of contact until the first signs of illness—5–32 days
• Person-to-person transmission possible

ABBREVIATIONS
• CNS = central nervous system
• FeLV = feline leukemia virus

Suggested Reading
Greene CE, Breitschwerdt EB. Rocky mountain spotted fever, Q fever, and typhus. In: Greene CE, ed. Infectious diseases of the dog and cat. 2nd ed. Philadelphia: Saunders, 1998:155–165.
Author Stephen C. Barr
Consulting Editor Stephen C. Barr

RABIES

BASICS

DEFINITION
A severe, invariably fatal, viral polioencephalitis of warm-blooded animals, including humans

PATHOPHYSIOLOGY
Virus—enters body through a wound (usually from a bite of rabid animal) or via mucous membranes; replicates in myocytes; spreads to the neuromuscular junction and neurotendinal spindles; travels to the CNS via intraaxonal fluid within peripheral nerves; spreads throughout the CNS; finally spreads centrifugally within peripheral, sensory, and motor neurons

SYSTEMS AFFECTED
• Nervous—clinical encephalitis, either paralytic or furious
• Salivary glands—contain large quantities of infectious virus particles that are shed in saliva

GENETICS
None

INCIDENCE/PREVALENCE
• Incidence of disease within infected animals, high (approaches 100%)
• Prevalence—overall low; can be significant in enzootic areas; especially high in underdeveloped countries where vaccination of dogs and cats is not routinely carried out

GEOGRAPHIC DISTRIBUTION
• Worldwide
• Exceptions—British Isles, Australia, New Zealand, Hawaii, Japan, and parts of Scandinavia
• Species adapted strains—specific geographic distributions within endemic countries

SIGNALMENT

Species
• All warm-blooded animals, including dogs, cats, and humans
• U.S.—four strains endemic within fox, raccoon, skunk, and bat populations; all four strains can be transmitted to dogs and cats.

Breed Predilections
None

Mean Age and Range
None, but adult animals that come in contact with wildlife at most risk

Predominant Sex
None

SIGNS

General Comments
• Quite variable; atypical presentation is the rule rather than the exception.
• Three progressive stages of disease—prodromal; furious; and paralytic

Historical Findings
• Change in attitude—solitude; apprehension, nervousness, anxiety; unusual shyness or aggressiveness
• Erratic behavior—biting or snapping; licking or chewing at sight of wound; biting at cage; wandering and roaming; excitability; irritability; viciousness
• Disorientation
• Muscular—incoordination; seizures; paralysis
• Change in tone of bark
• Excess salivation or frothing

Physical Examination Findings
• All or some of the historical findings
• Mandibular and laryngeal paralysis, with dropped jaw
• Inability to swallow
• Hypersalivation
• Fever

CAUSES
Rabies virus—a single-stranded RNA virus; genus *Lyssavirus;* family Rhabdoviridae

RISK FACTORS
• Exposure to wildlife, especially skunks, raccoons, bats, and foxes
• Lack of adequate vaccination against rabies
• Bite or scratch wounds from unvaccinated dogs, cats, or wildlife
• Exposure to aerosols in bat caves
• Immunocompromised animal—use of modified live virus rabies vaccine

DIAGNOSIS

DIFFERENTIAL DIAGNOSIS
• Must seriously consider rabies for any dog or cat showing unusual mood or behavior changes or exhibiting any unaccountable neurologic signs; CAUTION: handle with considerable care to prevent possible transmission of the virus to individuals caring for or treating the animal.
• Any neurologic disease—brain tumor; viral encephalitis
• Head wound—identify lesions from wound
• Laryngeal paralysis
• Choking
• Pseudorabies virus infection

CBC/BIOCHEMISTRY/URINALYSIS
No characteristic hematologic or biochemical changes

OTHER LABORATORY TESTS
N/A

IMAGING
N/A

DIAGNOSTIC PROCEDURES
• CSF—minimal increased protein and leukocyte counts may be seen.
• DFA test of nervous tissue—rapid and sensitive test; collect brain, head, or entire body of a small animal that has died or has been euthanized; chill sample immediately; submit to a state-approved laboratory for rabies diagnosis; CAUTION: use extreme care when collecting, handling, and shipping these specimens.
• DFA test of dermal tissue—skin biopsy of the sensory vibrissae of the maxillary area, including deeper subcutaneous hair follicles

PATHOLOGIC FINDINGS
• Gross changes—generally absent, despite dramatic neurologic disease
• Histopathologic changes—acute to chronic polioencephalitis; gradual increase in the severity of the nonsuppurative inflammatory process in the CNS as disease progresses; large neurons within the brain may contain the classic intracytoplasmic inclusions (Negri bodies).

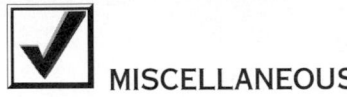

RABIES

TREATMENT

APPROPRIATE HEALTH CARE
Strictly inpatient

NURSING CARE
Administer with extreme caution.

ACTIVITY
• Confine to secured quarantine area with clearly posted signs indicating suspected rabies.
• Runs or cages should be locked; only designated people should have access.
• Feed and water without opening the cage or run door.

DIET
Soft, moist food; most patients will not eat.

CLIENT EDUCATION
• Thoroughly inform client of the seriousness of rabies to the animal and the zoonotic potential.
• Ask client about any human exposure (e.g., contact, bite) and strongly urge client to see a physician immediately.
• Local public health official must be notified.

SURGICAL CONSIDERATIONS
• Generally none
• Skin biopsy—may help establish antemortem diagnosis; must be confirmed by identification from CNS tissue

MEDICATIONS

DRUG(S) OF CHOICE
• No treatment
• Once the diagnosis is certain, euthanasia is indicated.

CONTRAINDICATIONS
None

PRECAUTIONS
N/A

POSSIBLE INTERACTIONS
N/A

ALTERNATIVE DRUG(S)
N/A

FOLLOW-UP

PATIENT MONITORING
• All suspected rabies patients should be securely isolated and monitored for any development of mood change, attitude change, or clinical signs that might suggest the diagnosis.
• An apparently healthy dog or cat that bites or scratches a person should be monitored for a period of 10 days; if no signs of illness occur in the animal within 10 days, the person has had no exposure to the virus; dogs and cats do not shed the virus for more than 3 days before development of clinical disease.
• An unvaccinated dog or cat that is bitten or exposed to a known rabid animal must be quarantined for up to 6 months or according to local or state regulations.

PREVENTION/AVOIDANCE
• Vaccines (dogs and cats)—vaccinate according to standard recommendations and state and local requirements; all dogs and cats with any potential exposure to wildlife or other dogs; vaccinate after 12 weeks of age; then 12 months later; then every 3 years using a vaccine approved for 3 years; use only inactivated vaccines for cats.
• Rabies-free countries—entering dogs and cats are quarantined for long periods, usually 6 months.
• Disinfection—any contaminated area, cage, food dish, or instrument must be thoroughly disinfected; use a 1:32 dilution (4 ounces per gallon) of household bleach to quickly inactivate the virus.

POSSIBLE COMPLICATIONS
From paralysis or attitude changes

EXPECTED COURSE AND PROGNOSIS
• Prognosis—grave; almost invariably fatal
• All dogs and cats with clinical infection will succumb within 7–10 days of onset of clinical signs.

MISCELLANEOUS

ASSOCIATED CONDITIONS
None

AGE-RELATED FACTORS
None

ZOONOTIC POTENTIAL
• Extreme
• Humans must avoid being bitten by a rabid animal or an asymptomatic animal that is incubating the disease.
• Rabies cases must be strictly quarantined and confined to prevent exposure to humans and other animals.
• Local and state regulations must be adhered to carefully and completely.

PREGNANCY
Infection during pregnancy will be fatal to dam.

SYNONYMS
Rage

ABBREVIATIONS
• CNS = central nervous system
• CSF = cerebrospinal fluid
• DFA = direct immunofluorescent antibody

Suggested Reading
Barr MC, Olsen CW, Scott FW. Feline viral diseases. In: Ettinger SJ, Feldman EC, eds. Veterinary internal medicine. Philadelphia: Saunders; 1995:409–439.
Eng TR, Fishbein DB. National Study Group on rabies. Epidemiologic factors, clinical findings, and vaccination status of rabies in cats and dogs in the United States in 1988. J Am Vet Med Assoc 1990;197:201–209.
Greene CE, Dreesen DW. Rabies. In: Greene CE, ed. Infectious diseases of the dog and cat. 2nd ed. Philadelphia: Saunders, 1998:114–126.
Jenkins SR, Auslander M, Conti L, et al. Compendium of animal rabies prevention and control, 2002. J Am Vet Med Assoc 2002;221:44–48.
Krebs JW, Strine TW, Smith JS, et al. Rabies surveillance in the United States during 1993. J Am Vet Med Assoc 1994;205: 1695–1709.
Author Fred W. Scott
Consulting Editor Stephen C. Barr

RECTAL AND ANAL PROLAPSE

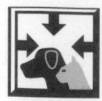

BASICS

OVERVIEW
• Eversion of one or more layers of the rectum through the anus
• An anal prolapse (incomplete prolapse) is a protrusion of anorectal mucosa through the external anal orifice.
• A rectal prolapse (complete prolapse) is a double-layer invagination of the full thickness of the rectal tube through the anal orifice.

SIGNALMENT
• Dogs and cats (especially Manx)
• Any age, sex, or breed
• High prevalence for young, parasitized dogs or cats with diarrhea

SIGNS
• Persistent tenesmus
• Incomplete prolapse—protrusion of a portion of the circumference of the rectal mucosa that typically appears worse immediately after defecation and then subsides
• Complete prolapse appears as a tubular hyperemic mass protruding from the anus.
• Chronic prolapses may be dark blue or black in color or the mucosa may be ulcerated.

CAUSES & RISK FACTORS
• Gastrointestinal disorders that cause diarrhea and tenesmus, such as parasitism, colitis/enteritis, constipation/obstipation, rectal foreign body, rectal deviation and diverticulum, proctitis, and rectal or anal tumors
• Urogenital disorders, such as cystitis, urolithiasis, prostatitis, prostatic hypertrophy, and dystocia
• Tenesmus following perineal, rectal, or urogenital surgery (e.g., perineal herniorrhaphy)

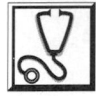

DIAGNOSIS

DIFFERENTIAL DIAGNOSIS
• Prolapsed intussusception—rule out by passing a blunt probe between the mass and the anus (the probe should not penetrate more than 1–2 cm before contacting the fornix; if the probe easily passes 5–6 cm, then suspect prolapsed intussusception) or by abdominal ultrasonography (look for increased intestinal layering)
• Neoplasia—rule out by palpation, fine needle aspiration and cytology, and/or biopsy and histopathology

CBC/BIOCHEMISTRY/URINALYSIS
• Usually normal
• Inflammatory or stress leukogram may be present.

OTHER LABORATORY TESTS
Fecal examination may confirm parasitism.

IMAGING
• Abdominal radiography and ultrasonography—usually normal
• Abdominal radiography—may demonstrate foreign body, prostatomegaly, cystic calculi, or colonic fecal distention
• Abdominal ultrasonography—may demonstrate prostatomegaly, cystic calculi, bladder wall thickening, or intussusception

DIAGNOSTIC PROCEDURES
• Rectal examination to palpate for perineal hernia
• Colonoscopy may help evaluate recurrent prolapse for an underlying cause.

PATHOLOGIC FINDINGS
Assess viability of the prolapsed tissue by surface appearance and tissue temperature—vital tissue appears swollen and hyperemic, and red blood exudes from the cut surface; devitalized tissue appears dark purple or black, and dark cyanotic blood exudes from the cut surface; ulcerations may be present.

TREATMENT
• Must identify and treat underlying cause
• Conservative medical management—gently replace prolapsed tissue through the anus with the use of lubricants and gentle massage; osmotic agents may help if severe swelling exists
• Use of an epidural may facilitate treatment and relieve discomfort.
• Place a pursestring suture to aid retention and prevent acute recurrence; place the suture loose enough to allow room for defecation.
• Decrease straining with stool softeners.
• Colopexy recommended for recurrent viable prolapses
• When prolapse is devitalized, rectal resection and anastomosis are necessary.

MEDICATIONS

DRUG(S) OF CHOICE
• Appropriate anesthetic/analgesics as needed
• Consider epidural to facilitate surgery and reduce postoperative straining.
• Appropriate perioperative antibiotics are recommended (e.g., cefoxitin sodium [30 mg/kg IV]) for resection anastomosis.

• Topical agents to aid in reduction—50% dextrose solution and KY Jelly
• Stool softeners—docusate sodium (dogs, 50–200 mg PO q8–12h; cats, 50 mg PO q12–24h) or lactulose (10 g/15 mL of solution, 1 mL/4.5 kg q8–12h to effect); continue for 2–3 weeks after removal of the pursestring suture
• Feed a low-residue diet until pursestring suture is removed.

CONTRAINDICATIONS/POSSIBLE INTERACTIONS
N/A

FOLLOW-UP

PATIENT MONITORING
• Pursestring suture removal in 5–7 days
• Examine for rectal stricture if straining persists following anastomosis.

POSSIBLE COMPLICATIONS
• Recurrence—especially if underlying cause is not eliminated
• Postoperative—may include anastomosis dehiscence within 5–7 days postoperatively or rectal stricture
• Fecal incontinence after resection (sensory incontinence resulting from removal of receptors in rectal wall)

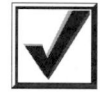

MISCELLANEOUS

ASSOCIATED CONDITIONS
Intestinal parasitism

SEE ALSO
• Colitis and Proctitis
• Dyschezia and Hematochezia
• Intussusception

Suggested Reading
DeNovo RC, Bright RM: Rectoanal disease. In: Ettinger SJ, Feldman EC, eds. Textbook of veterinary internal medicine. Philadelphia: Saunders, 2000:1257–1270.
Hedlund CS: Surgery of the perineum, rectum, and anus. In: Fossum TW, ed. Small animal surgery. 2nd ed. St. Louis: Mosby, 2002:414–449.

Acknowledgment
The author and editors acknowledge the prior contributions of Dr. Michelle J. Waschak, who authored this topic in the previous edition.
Author Eric R. Pope
Section Editor Albert E. Jergens

BASICS

OVERVIEW
• Diminution in the size of the rectal or anal lumen either from cicatricial contracture or scarring as a result of wound healing or chronic inflammation or from proliferative neoplastic disease • Gastrointestinal function is compromised because of outflow obstruction. • No genetic basis reported

SIGNALMENT
• Dogs and cats • No age, breed, or gender predilection reported

SIGNS
• Vary with severity of the lesion • Dyschezia • Tenesmus • Constipation • Hematochezia • Mucoid feces • Large-bowel diarrhea • Secondary megacolon can develop.

CAUSES & RISK FACTORS
• Inflammatory—rectoanal abscess, anal sacculitis, perianal fistulas, proctitis, foreign body, fungal infection (e.g., histoplasmosis, pythiosis) • Traumatic—lacerations • Neoplastic—rectal adenocarcinoma, leiomyoma, rectal polyps • Iatrogenic—rectal anastomosis, rectal mass excision, rectal biopsy • Congenital—atresia ani

DIAGNOSIS

DIFFERENTIAL DIAGNOSIS
• Space-occupying processes that lead to diminished rectal capacity (extraluminal rectal compression [e.g., prostatic disease, pelvic fractures], intraluminal rectal obstruction [e.g., pseudocoprostasis, foreign body]) and functional constriction (rectal muscle spasms) • Differentiate by rectal palpation and imaging.

CBC/BIOCHEMISTRY/URINALYSIS
• Usually normal • Patients with inflammation or infection may have an inflammatory leukogram.

OTHER LABORATORY TESTS
N/A

IMAGING
• Survey abdominal radiography and contrast studies (e.g., barium, air, or double-contrast enema and barium gastrointestinal series) may reveal consistent narrowing of the rectal luminal diameter. • Contrast radiography requires adequate patient preparation (warm water enemas ± polyethylene glycol 30–50 mL/kg PO 12 and 6 h prior to procedure) followed by instillation of 10 mL of barium/kg through a balloon catheter. • A combination of air and barium allows the best visualization of the colonic mucosa and aids in determining the extent of the lesion;

lesions in close proximity to the anus may be difficult to delineate. • Abdominal ultrasonography may reveal thickening and altered architecture if infiltrative rectocolonic disease is present (e.g., pythiosis, neoplasia).

DIAGNOSTIC PROCEDURES
• Digital rectal palpation to characterize and determine the extent and location of the stricture • Proctoscopy/colonoscopy may be useful to visualize a stricture, determine the extent of the lesion, and procure a biopsy specimen. • Colonic scrapings may aid in cytological diagnosis of fungal (histoplasmosis) and neoplastic diseases. • Biopsy and evaluate the lesion histopathologically to classify the disease process and establish a prognosis.

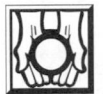

TREATMENT
• Resolve the underlying cause before specifically treating the stricture when possible. • Direct medical treatment at either palliation by use of stool softeners and enemas or the elimination of infective agents or inflammatory conditions. • Give fluid therapy to optimize hydration prior to administering an enema to constipated or obstipated patients. • Anesthesia may be necessary for enema administration. • Surgical treatment ranges from balloon dilation or bougienage for benign superficial strictures to partial or complete resection for more extensive lesions (see Suggested Reading for greater detail). • Radiotherapy and/or chemotherapy may benefit the treatment of some neoplasms.

MEDICATIONS

DRUG(S)
• Stool softeners—docusate sodium (dogs, 50–200 mg PO q8–12h; cats, 50 mg PO q12–24h); lactulose (10 g/15 mL of solution, 1 mL/4.5 kg q8–12h to effect) • Corticosteroids—can use prednisone to treat noninfectious inflammatory conditions (0.5–1 mg/kg PO q24h or divided q12h) and after balloon dilation or bougienage to prevent stricture recurrence • Chemotherapy may be indicated for various neoplasms. • Antifungal therapy if fungal infection present • Appropriate perioperative antimicrobial therapy has been advocated in conjunction with balloon dilation or surgical therapy; choose one with a broad spectrum of activity against anaerobes and coliforms (e.g., cefoxitin sodium [30 mg/kg IV]).

CONTRAINDICATIONS/POSSIBLE INTERACTIONS
• Corticosteroids when infection is possible

• Corticosteroids may adversely affect healing after surgical correction of the stricture.

FOLLOW-UP

PATIENT MONITORING
• Resolution or recurrence of clinical signs • Patients with neoplastic lesions—recurrence and metastatic disease

POSSIBLE COMPLICATIONS
• Medical treatment—can include inefficacy, diarrhea, and adverse effects of medications • Balloon dilation can result in deep rectal tears, hemorrhage, or possibly full-thickness perforation. • Surgical treatment—fecal incontinence, secondary stricture formation, and wound dehiscence

EXPECTED COURSE AND PROGNOSIS
• Varies with the severity of the stricture • Patients with benign strictures that are readily managed medically or with balloon dilation or bougienage may have a good long-term outcome. • Surgical resection has more guarded prognosis because of the frequency of complications. • Most patients with recognizable clinical signs have a guarded to poor prognosis for complete resolution.

MISCELLANEOUS

AGE-RELATED FACTORS
Atresia ani is seen within weeks of birth.

SEE ALSO
• Colitis and Proctitis • Constipation and Obstipation • Dyschezia and Hematochezia • Histoplasmosis • Perianal Fistula • Pythiosis • Rectoanal Polyps

Suggested Reading

Biery DN. The large bowel. In: Thrall DE, ed. Textbook of veterinary diagnostic radiology. Philadelphia: Saunders, 1986:513–514.

DeNovo RC, Bright RM: Rectoanal disease. In: Ettinger SJ, Feldman EC, eds. Textbook of veterinary internal medicine. Philadelphia: Saunders, 2000:1257–1270.

Matthiesen D, Marretta SM. Diseases of the rectum and anus. In: Slatter D, ed. Textbook of small animal surgery. 2nd ed. Philadelphia: Saunders, 1993:627–644.

Niebauer GW. Rectoanal disease. In: Bojrab MJ, ed. Disease mechanisms in small animal surgery. 2nd ed. Philadelphia: Lea & Febiger, 1993:271–284.

Acknowledgment

The author and editors acknowledge the contributions of Dr. James L. Cook and Dr. Michelle J. Waschak, who authored this topic in the previous edition.

Author Eric R. Pope
Section Editor Albert E. Jergens

RECTOANAL POLYPS

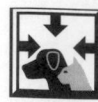

BASICS

OVERVIEW
Most rectoanal polyps are benign growths located in the distal rectum. Histopathologic evaluation typically reveals adenomas, but lesions may undergo malignant transformation.

SIGNALMENT
- Dogs and, rarely, cats
- Middle-aged to old
- No breed or sex predilection

SIGNS
- Hematochezia
- Mucus-covered feces
- Tenesmus
- Dyschezia
- Soft, well-vascularized, friable, and often ulcerated mass(es) may be seen or palpated rectally.
- Usually single but multiple polyps can occur
- May be pedunculated or broad-based sessile masses

CAUSES & RISK FACTORS
Unknown

DIAGNOSIS

DIFFERENTIAL DIAGNOSIS
- Carcinoma *in situ* and adenocarcinoma
- Other neoplasias—leiomyoma, lymphoma, papilloma
- Proctitis
- Pythiosis
- Incomplete rectal prolapse

CBC/BIOCHEMISTRY/URINALYSIS
Usually normal

OTHER LABORATORY TESTS
N/A

IMAGING
N/A

DIAGNOSTIC PROCEDURES
- Rectal palpation
- Direct visualization through anus
- Colonoscopy—recommended to evaluate the entire rectum and colon for additional polyps

- Cytologic examination of polyp aspirate or scraping may help the initial diagnosis.
- Histopathologic examination of excised tissue is required for definitive diagnosis and to assess completeness of the excision.

PATHOLOGIC FINDINGS
- Adenomatous polyp
- Adenomatous hyperplasia
- Carcinoma *in situ*

TREATMENT
- Surgical excision is the treatment of choice.
- Most polyps can be exteriorized directly through the anus and removed with submucosal resection.
- Close the mucosal defect with absorbable sutures, avoiding compromise of the lumen diameter.
- Lesions that cannot be exteriorized may be removable transanally by electrosurgery with endoscopic guidance or can be directly exposed through a dorsal rectal approach.

MEDICATIONS

DRUG(S)
• Appropriate perioperative antibiotics are recommended (e.g., cefoxitin sodium [30 mg/kg IV]).
• Stool softeners may help decrease tenesmus—docusate sodium (dogs, 50–200 mg PO q8–12h; cats, 50 mg PO q12–24h) or docusate calcium (dogs, 50–100 mg PO q12–24h; cats, 50 mg PO q12–24h)
• Alternative stool softener—lactulose (1 mL/4.5 kg PO q8h to effect)

CONTRAINDICATIONS/POSSIBLE INTERACTIONS
N/A

FOLLOW-UP

PATIENT MONITORING
• Examine the excision site 14 days after surgery and again at 3 and 6 months to ensure absence of recurrence or stricture.
• Twice yearly examination thereafter to assess for recurrence

POSSIBLE COMPLICATIONS
• Recurrence
• Rectal stricture (rare)

EXPECTED COURSE AND PROGNOSIS
• Dogs with focal single adenomas have a good prognosis with a low rate of recurrence.
• Dogs with multiple and/or diffuse lesions (involvement of < 50% of circumference of rectal wall) have much higher rates of recurrence.

MISCELLANEOUS

SEE ALSO
• Adenocarcinoma, Anal Sac/Perianal/Rectal
• Dyschezia and Hematochezia
• Rectal Prolapse

Suggested Reading
DeNovo RC, Bright RM. Rectoanal disease. In: Ettinger SJ, Feldman EC, eds. Textbook of veterinary internal medicine. Philadelphia: Saunders, 2000:1257–1270.
Hedlund CS. Surgery of the perineum, rectum, and anus. In: Fossum TW, ed. Small animal surgery. 2nd ed. St. Louis: Mosby, 2002:414–449.
Niebauer GW. Rectoanal disease. In: Bojrab MJ, ed. Disease mechanisms in small animal surgery. 2nd ed. Philadelphia: Lea & Febiger, 1993:271–284.
Valerius KD, Powers BE, McPherron MA, et al. Adenomatous polyps and carcinoma *in situ* of the canine colon and rectum: 34 cases (1982–1994). J Am Anim Hosp Assoc 1997;33:156–160.

Acknowledgment
The author and editors acknowledge the prior contribution of Dr. Michelle J. Waschak, who authored this topic in the previous edition.

Author Eric R. Pope
Section Editor Albert E. Jergens

RED EYE

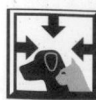 **BASICS**

DEFINITION
Hyperemia of the eyelids or ocular vasculature, or hemorrhage within the eye

PATHOPHYSIOLOGY
• Active dilation of ocular vessels—in response to extraocular or intraocular inflammation or passive congestion
• Hemorrhage from existing or newly formed blood vessels

SYSTEMS AFFECTED
Ophthalmic—eye and/or ocular adnexa

SIGNALMENT
Dogs and cats

SIGNS

Historical Findings
Depend on cause

Physical Examination Findings
• Depend on cause
• May affect one or both eyes
• Result of systemic disease—abnormalities in other organ systems common

CAUSES
• Virtually every case fits into one or more of the following categories.
• Blepharitis
• Conjunctivitis
• Keratitis
• Episcleritis or scleritis
• Anterior uveitis
• Glaucoma
• Hyphema
• Orbital disease—usually the orbital abnormality is more prominent.

RISK FACTORS
• Systemic infectious or inflammatory diseases
• Immunocompromise

• Coagulopathies
• Systemic hypertension
• Topical ophthalmic medications—aminoglycosides; pilocarpine; epinephrine
• Neoplasia
• Trauma

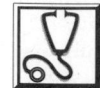 **DIAGNOSIS**

DIFFERENTIAL DIAGNOSIS
More than one cause may occur simultaneously.

Similar Signs
• Rule out normal variations.
• Palpebral conjunctiva—normally redder than bulbar conjunctiva
• One or two large episcleral vessels—may be normal if the eye is otherwise quiet
• Transient mild hyperemia—with excitement, exercise, and straining
• Horner's syndrome—may cause mild conjunctival vascular dilation; differentiated by other signs and pharmacologic testing

Causes
• Superficial (conjunctival) vessels—originate near the fornix; move with the conjunctiva; branch repeatedly; blanch quickly with topical 2.5% phenylephrine or 1:100,000 epinephrine; suggest ocular surface disorders (e.g., conjunctivitis, superficial keratitis, blepharitis)
• Deep (episcleral) vessels—originate near the limbus; branch infrequently; do not move with the conjunctiva; blanch slowly or incompletely with topical sympathomimetics; suggest episcleritis or intraocular disease (e.g., anterior uveitis or glaucoma)
• Discharge—mucopurulent to purulent: typical of ocular surface disorders and blepharitis; serous or none: typical of intraocular disorders

• Swollen or inflamed eyelids—indicate blepharitis
• Corneal opacification, neovascularization, or fluorescein stain retention—suggests keratitis
• Aqueous flare or cell (increased protein or cells in the anterior chamber)—confirms diagnosis of anterior uveitis
• Pupil—miotic: common with anterior uveitis; dilated: common with glaucoma; normal: with blepharitis and conjunctivitis
• Abnormally shaped or colored irides—suggests anterior uveitis
• Luxated or cataractous lenses—suggests glaucoma or anterior uveitis
• IOP—high: diagnostic for glaucoma; low: suggests anterior uveitis
• Loss of vision—suggests glaucoma, anterior uveitis, or severe keratitis
• Glaucoma and anterior uveitis—may complicate hyphema

CBC/BIOCHEMISTRY/URINALYSIS
• Typically normal, except with anterior uveitis, glaucoma, or hyphema secondary to systemic disease
• See Anterior Uveitis—Dogs; Anterior Uveitis—Cats; Hyphema

OTHER LABORATORY TESTS
Depend on cause

IMAGING
• Chest radiographs—consider with anterior uveitis or if intraocular neoplasia is a possibility.
• Abdominal radiography or ultrasonography—may help rule out infectious or neoplastic causes
• Ocular ultrasonography—if the ocular media are opaque; may define the extent and nature of intraocular disease or identify an intraocular tumor

DIAGNOSTIC PROCEDURES
Tonometry—must perform in every patient with an unexplained red eye

Ocular Surface Disorders
• Aerobic bacterial culture and sensitivity profile—with a purulent discharge, chronic disease, or if the response to treatment is poor
• Schirmer tear test
• Cytologic examination of affected tissue—lid; conjunctiva; cornea
• Cats—consider PCR or IFA test on corneal or conjunctival scrapings for feline herpesvirus and *Chlamydia;* collect sample before fluorescein staining to avoid false-positive results on IFA
• Fluorescein stain
• Conjunctival biopsies—with chronic conjunctivitis or with a mass lesion
• See specific disease—conjunctivitis; blepharitis; keratitis

Intraocular Disorders
• Fluorescein stain
• See specific disease—uveitis; hyphema; glaucoma

TREATMENT
• Usually outpatient
• Elizabethan collar—considered to prevent self-trauma
• Avoid dirty environments or those that may lead to ocular trauma, especially if topical corticosteroids are used.
• Because there is a narrow margin for error, consider referral if you cannot attribute the condition to one of the listed causes, if you cannot rule out glaucoma on the initial visit, or if the diagnosis is so uncertain that administration of a topical antibiotic alone or a topical corticosteroid alone would be questionable.
• Few causes are fatal; however, a workup may be indicated (especially with anterior uveitis and hyphema) to rule out potentially fatal systemic diseases.
• Deep corneal ulcers and glaucoma—may be best treated surgically

MEDICATIONS

DRUG(S) OF CHOICE
• Depends on specific cause
• Generally, control ocular pain, inflammation, infection, and IOP
• Aspirin—10–15 mg/kg PO q8–12h; may control mild ocular inflammation and pain pending test results
• Flunixin meglumine—0.5 mg/kg IV one time; may be used in dogs with severe ocular inflammation pending test results

CONTRAINDICATIONS
• Topical corticosteroids—contraindicated if the cornea retains fluorescein stain
• Systemic corticosteroids—avoid until infectious systemic causes have been ruled out

PRECAUTIONS
• Topical aminoglycosides—may be irritating; may impede reepithelization if used frequently or at high concentrations
• Topical solutions—may be preferable to ointments if corneal perforation is possible
• Atropine—may exacerbate KCS and glaucoma
• NSAIDs—use with caution in hyphema

POSSIBLE INTERACTIONS
N/A

ALTERNATIVE DRUG(S)
N/A

FOLLOW-UP

PATIENT MONITORING
• Depends on cause
• Repeat ophthalmic examinations—as required to ensure that IOP, ocular pain, and inflammation are well controlled

• The greater the risk of loss of vision, the more closely the patient needs to be followed; may require daily or more frequent examination

POSSIBLE COMPLICATIONS
• Death
• Loss of the eye or permanent vision loss
• Chronic ocular inflammation and pain

MISCELLANEOUS

ASSOCIATED CONDITIONS
Numerous systemic diseases

AGE-RELATED FACTORS
N/A

ZOONOTIC POTENTIAL
See Anterior Uveitis—Dogs; Anterior Uveitis—Cats

PREGNANCY
Systemic corticosteroids may complicate pregnancy.

SEE ALSO
See Causes

ABBREVIATIONS
IFA = immunofluorescent antibody
IOP = intraocular pressure
KCS = keratoconjunctivitis sicca
PCR = polymerase chain reaction

Suggested Reading
Gelatt KN, ed. Veterinary ophthalmology. 3rd ed. Philadelphia: Lippincott Williams & Wilkins, 1999.
Slatter DS. Fundamentals of veterinary ophthalmology. 3rd ed. Philadelphia: WB Saunders Co., 2001.
Author Paul E. Miller
Consulting Editor Paul E. Miller

REGURGITATION

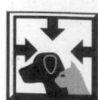 BASICS

DEFINITION
Passive, retrograde movement of esophageal contents into the pharyngeal or oral cavity

PATHOPHYSIOLOGY
Regurgitation results from a loss of normal esophageal contractions. In the normal esophagus, the presence of a food bolus in the proximal esophagus stimulates afferent sensory neurons. Signals are transferred centrally, via the vagus and glossopharyngeal nerves; to the nucleus solitarius. Motor impulses travel back via the vagus nerve to stimulate striated muscle (canine) and striated and smooth muscle (feline) to cause esophageal contraction. Lesions anywhere along this pathway may lead to regurgitation.

SYSTEMS AFFECTED
• Gastrointestinal—dysphagia, weight loss
• Respiratory—aspiration pneumonia
• Musculoskeletal—weakness, weight loss
• Nervous—polyphagia

GENETICS
Regurgitation due to megaesophagus can be inherited in wire-haired fox terriers (autosomal recessive) and miniature schnauzers (autosomal dominant or 60% penetrance autosomal recessive).

INCIDENCE/PREVALENCE
N/A

GEOGRAPHIC DISTRIBUTION
N/A

SIGNALMENT

Species
Dogs (more commonly) and cats

Breed Predilections
• Wire-haired fox terriers, miniature schnauzers. Other predisposed breeds include Great Danes, German shepherds, Irish setters, Labrador retrievers, Newfoundlands, shar peis.
• Siamese and Siamese-related cats

Mean Age and Range
• Congenital cases present soon after birth or at weaning from liquid to solid foods.
• Acquired cases may be seen at any age, depending on the etiology.

Predominant Sex
No gender predilection has been identified.

SIGNS

General Comments
• Owners often report vomiting; veterinarian must differentiate vomiting from regurgitation.
• Regurgitation—passive; little to no abdominal effort; no prodromal phase; regurgitated material has increased amounts of thick mucus.
• Vomiting—active process; prodromal phase; vomited material has increased bile staining
• The shape of the expelled material, presence of undigested food, and length of time from ingestion to regurgitation or vomiting are less helpful to differentiate.

Historical Findings
• Vomiting (per owner)
• Dysphagia
• Coughing
• Ravenous appetite
• Weight loss
• Other signs, depending upon underlying etiology

Physical Examination Findings
• Cervical swelling may be noted.
• Ptyalism
• Halitosis
• Increased respiratory noises
• Nasal discharge (and fever, if concurrent pneumonia)
• Cachexia
• Weakness

CAUSES

Congenital Pharyngeal
• Cleft or short palate
• Cricopharyngeal achalasia
• Myasthenia gravis

Congenital Esophageal
• Persistent right aortic arch
• Megaesophagus
• Glycogen storage disease
• Diverticulum

Acquired Pharyngeal
• Foreign bodies
• Neoplasia
• Rabies
• Toxicity (botulism)
• Myopathy/neuropathy

Acquired Esophageal
• Megaesophagus
• Myasthenia gravis
• Idiopathic
• Gastric dilatation/volvulus
• Gastroesophageal reflux
• Stricture
• Neoplasia
• Endocrine disease
• Hiatal hernia
• Gastroesophageal intussusception
• Periesophageal masses
• Dysautonomia
• Myopathy/neuropathy
• Foreign bodies
• Granulomatous disease
• Toxicity (lead)

RISK FACTORS
Risk for foreign body and toxin ingestion

 DIAGNOSIS

DIFFERENTIAL DIAGNOSIS
Differentiate vomiting from regurgitation.

CBC/BIOCHEMISTRY/URINALYSIS
• No pathognomonic changes for regurgitation
• Inflammatory leukogram if aspiration pneumonia
• Most helpful for evaluation of underlying etiology: e.g., erythrocyte changes with lead toxicity, elevated CK with myopathy, hyperkalemia and hyponatremia with hypoadrenocorticism, hypercholesterolemia with hypothyroidism.

OTHER LABORATORY TESTS
These elucidate etiologies of acquired conditions causing regurgitation and include ACTH stimulation test (hypoadrenocorticism); thyroid serology (hypothyroidism); acetylcholine receptor antibody level (myasthenia gravis); blood lead levels (toxicity).

IMAGING
• Thoracic and cervical radiography—evidence of a gas-, fluid-, or ingesta-filled esophagus with megaesophagus; may also show aspiration pneumonia, foreign bodies, hiatal hernia.
• Contrast studies—both liquid barium and barium-coated food for obstructive disorders **Caution:** Esophagram may increase risk for aspiration with megaesophagus.
• Fluoroscopy—for pharyngeal dysfunction and esophageal motility disorders
• Other imaging studies include scintigraphy and manometry for motility and ultrasound for pharyngeal or cervical masses.

DIAGNOSTIC PROCEDURES
• Esophagoscopy can be useful for esophagitis, strictures, neoplasia, and foreign bodies.
• Electromyography (EMG) and nerve/muscle biopsies for neuropathy or myopathy
• Transtracheal wash if aspiration pneumonia

PATHOLOGIC FINDINGS
Gross and histologic findings depend upon underlying etiology and presence of complicating factors.

TREATMENT

APPROPRIATE HEALTH CARE
• Therapy for underlying etiology should be instituted.
• Most important aspects are meeting nutritional requirements and treating or preventing aspiration pneumonia

NURSING CARE
• Aspiration pneumonia may require oxygen therapy, nebulization/coupage, fluid therapy with balanced electrolyte solution.
• These animals may be recumbent and require soft bedding and should be maintained in sternal recumbency or turned to alternate down side every 4 hr.

ACTIVITY
Depending on etiology, restricted activity is not necessary.

DIET
• Experimentation with different food consistencies is essential. Liquid gruel, small meatballs, blenderized slurries may be used.
• Some cases benefit from gastrostomy feedings.
• Both food and water should be elevated, and the animal should be maintained in an upright position 10–15 minutes after eating or drinking.

CLIENT EDUCATION
• Most cases of megaesophagus require lifelong therapy, even if an underlying etiology is found. Client dedication is important for long-term management.
• Most animals will succumb to aspiration pneumonia.

SURGICAL CONSIDERATIONS
• Surgical intervention is indicated for vascular ring anomalies, cricopharyngeal myotomy, and other congenital lesions.
• Balloon dilation is indicated for cases of esophageal stricture.

MEDICATIONS

DRUG(S) OF CHOICE
• Antibiotics for aspiration pneumonia (broad spectrum or based on culture and sensitivity from tracheal wash)
• Specific therapy for underlying etiology if indicated
• Prokinetics—metoclopramide (0.2–0.4 mg/kg SC or PO q 6–12h) increases lower esophageal sphincter tone, increases gastric motility, and may increase esophageal motility. Cisapride (0.5 mg/kg PO q 8–12h) is more effective for esophageal reflux than metoclopramide; however it has no effect on esophageal motility. Other motility agents (e.g., nizatidine) have not been evaluated for esophageal motility.
• H_2 blockers for esophagitis—ranitidine (1–2 mg/kg PO, IV q12h), cimetidine (4–10 mg/kg PO, SC, IM, IV q6h), famotidine (0.5–1 mg/kg PO, SC, IM, IV q12–24h)

CONTRAINDICATIONS
N/A

PRECAUTIONS
Absorption of orally administered drugs may be compromised. Injectable forms should be used when applicable.

POSSIBLE INTERACTIONS
N/A

ALTERNATIVE DRUG(S)
N/A

FOLLOW-UP

PATIENT MONITORING
• Animals with aspiration pneumonia should have thoracic radiographs and complete blood counts checked until resolution, or if recurrence is suspected.

• Animals should be monitored and weighed to ensure adequate caloric intake.

PREVENTION/AVOIDANCE
N/A

POSSIBLE COMPLICATIONS
• Aspiration pneumonia
• Others depending on presence of other diseases (e.g., hypothyroidism)

EXPECTED COURSE AND PROGNOSIS
• Older animals with idiopathic megaesophagus have a poor prognosis.
• Aspiration pneumonia is the typical cause of death or euthanasia.

MISCELLANEOUS

ASSOCIATED CONDITIONS
Aspiration pneumonia

AGE-RELATED FACTORS
Young animals may regain some esophageal function with appropriate therapy.

ZOONOTIC POTENTIAL
None

PREGNANCY
N/A

SEE ALSO
• Dysautonomia (Key-Gaskell Syndrome)
• Dysphagia
• Esophagitis
• Megaesophagus
• Myasthenia Gravis
• Pneumonia, Bacterial

Suggested Reading
Guilford G. Approach to clinical problems in gastroenterology. In: Strombeck's small animal gastroenterology, 3rd Ed. Philadelphia: Saunders, 1996:50–58.
Guilford G, Strombeck D. Diseases of swallowing. In: Strombeck's small animal gastroenterology, 3rd Ed. Philadelphia: Saunders, 1996:211–235.
Author Jo Ann Morrison
Consulting Editor Albert E. Jergens

RENAL FAILURE, ACUTE

 **BASICS**

DEFINITION
Acute renal failure (ARF) is a syndrome characterized by sudden onset of filtration failure by the kidneys; accumulation of uremic toxins; dysregulation of fluid, electrolyte, and acid–base balance; and appearance of the clinical signs of uremia. It is potentially reversible if diagnosed quickly and treated aggressively. Although postrenal azotemia fulfills these criteria, the following discussion refers generally to intrinsic acute renal failure.

PATHOPHYSIOLOGY
Initiated by ischemia, nephrotoxins, systemic inflammatory disease, or intrinsic renal disease; renal excretory failure is perpetuated by multiple factors including (1) reduced glomerular surface area and permeability, (2) low renal blood flow, (3) intratubular obstruction by tubular debris, (4) cellular and interstitial edema, and (5) "backleak" of filtrate across damaged tubular epithelia; resolution occurs by renal regeneration and repair

SYSTEMS AFFECTED
• Renal • GI • Nervous • Respiratory
• Musculoskeletal • Hemic/Lymph/Immune

INCIDENCE/PREVALENCE
• Prevalence is substantially lower than that of chronic renal failure (CRF). • Prevalence may increase in the fall and winter with greater exposure of animals to antifreeze containing ethylene glycol, and wet environments supporting leptospirosis.

SIGNALMENT

Species
Dogs and cats

Breed Predilections
None

Mean Age and Range
• Six to eight years peak incidence in dogs
• Older animals at greater risk

SIGNS

Historical Findings
Sudden onset of anorexia, listlessness, vomiting (± blood), diarrhea (± blood), halitosis, ataxia, seizures, known toxin exposure, recent medical or surgical conditions, and oliguria/anuria or polyuria

Physical Examination Findings
Normal body condition and haircoat (no evidence of chronicity), depression, dehydration (sometimes overhydration), variable scleral injection, oral ulceration, glossitis, necrosis of the tongue, uremic breath, hypothermia, fever, tachypnea, bradycardia, nonpalpable urinary bladder, and large, painful, firm, kidneys

CAUSES

Hemodynamic/Hypoperfusion
Shock, malignant hypertension, heart failure, thromboembolism (e.g., disseminated intravascular coagulation, vasculitis, and transfusion reaction), heatstroke, excessive vasoconstriction (e.g., administration of nonsteroidal anti-inflammatory drug [NSAID]), excessive vasodilation (e.g., administration of angiotensin-converting enzyme inhibitor or antihypertensive drug), and prolonged anesthesia

Nephrotoxic
Administration of antimicrobials (e.g., aminoglycoside, sulfonamide, and cephalosporin), amphotericin B, chemotherapeutic agent (e.g., cisplatin and doxorubicin), thiacetarsamide, NSAIDs, radiographic contrast agents, ethylene glycol, heavy metals (e.g., lead, mercury, arsenic, and thallium), insect or snake venom, heme pigment, calcium, grape or raisin ingestion (dogs), and lily ingestion (cats).

Intrinsic and Systemic Disease
Leptospirosis, immune-mediated glomerulonephritis and arteritis, pancreatitis, septicemia, DIC, hepatic failure, heat stroke, transfusion reaction, bacterial endocarditis, pyelonephritis, cortical necrosis, and lymphosarcoma. Unilateral or bilateral ureteral obstruction with calcium oxalate uroliths is common cause of ARF in cats.

RISK FACTORS
• Endogenous—preexisting renal disease, dehydration, hypovolemia, hypotension, advanced age, concurrent disease, hyponatremia, hypokalemia, hypocalcemia, and acidosis • Exogenous—drugs (e.g., furosemide, NSAIDs, prolonged anesthesia, aminoglycoside), diet (e.g., low sodium, calculogenic, acidifying), prolonged surgery, trauma, multiple organ disease, and high environmental temperature

 DIAGNOSIS

DIFFERENTIAL DIAGNOSIS
• Prerenal azotemia—oliguria, concentrated urine specific gravity (dogs, ≥ 1.030; cats, ≥ 1.035), correctable with fluid repletion
• Postrenal azotemia—anuria, dysuria, stranguria, large bladder, urethral obstruction, and uroperitoneum • CRF—polyuria, polydipsia, chronic history of illness, loss of body condition, and anemia • Prerenal on CRF—clinical and laboratory features of CRF but partially correctable with fluid repletion • Prerenal on ARF—acute-onset uremia, partially correctable with fluid repletion • Hypoadrenocorticism—hyponatremia, hyperkalemia, and "flat" ACTH stimulation test • Pancreatitis—markedly high serum lipase, cranial abdominal pain, high trypsin–like immunoreactivity, hyperbilirubinemia, and high liver enzyme activity
• Hepatorenal syndrome—clinical and laboratory evidence of hepatic failure

CBC/BIOCHEMISTRY/URINALYSIS
• Normal or high PCV, variable leukocytosis, and lymphopenia • Progressive (moderate to severe) increases in BUN, creatinine, and phosphate; variably high potassium and glucose; and variably low bicarbonate and calcium
• Inability to concentrate urine (≥ 1.020), mild-to-moderate proteinuria, glucosuria; variably high number of casts, WBCs, RBCs, and tubular epithelial cells; variable bacteriuria and crystalluria (calcium oxalate)

OTHER LABORATORY TESTS
• Enzymuria—high urinary α-glutamyl transpeptidase, N-acetyl-β-D-glucosaminidase predicts early nephrotoxic tubular damage in some patients • Metabolic acidosis common; mixed disorders may occur
• Leptospirosis titer—≥ 1:800 or rising if patient infected • Ethylene glycol concentration—positive if patient poisoned; increased serum osmolality or osmolar gap

IMAGING
• Routine and contrast radiography—kidneys are normal to large, with smooth contours, bilaterally or asymmetric ("big kidney-little kidney" syndrome) with ureteral obstruction—seek small radiodensities in the retroperitoneum. Percutaneous nephropyeleography (ureteral obstruction)
• Ultrasonography—hyperechoic kidneys suggest ethylene glycol toxicity. Pelvic and/or ureteral dilation or calcific densities suggest outflow obstruction.

DIAGNOSTIC PROCEDURES
• Catheterize to monitor urine output—helps establish the diagnosis and formulates treatment and prognosis: anuria, ≤ 0.1 mL/kg/h; oliguria, ≤ 0.25 mL/kg/h; nonoliguria, ≥ 2 mL/kg/h • Fine-needle aspiration—may establish lymphosarcoma as cause of enlarged kidneys. • Percutaneous renal biopsy—helps establish the cause, severity, and potential reversibility of injury; later in the course of disease (4-6 weeks) it may help predict ongoing renal repair and permanence of renal damage.

PATHOLOGIC FINDINGS
Nephrosis or nephritis, calcium oxalate crystals, interstitial edema, and lack of interstitial fibrosis; the subacute stage is characterized by attenuated epithelium, interstitial fibrosis and mineralization, cellular infiltration, and variable tubular regeneration

TREATMENT

APPROPRIATE HEALTH CARE
Inpatient management; eliminate inciting insults; discontinue nephrotoxic drugs; establish and maintain hemodynamic stability; ameliorate life-threatening fluid imbalances, biochemical abnormalities, and uremic toxicities; induce emesis; institute gastric lavage and administer activated charcoal, cathartics,

and specific antidotes to patients with acute poisoning; early hemodialysis can eliminate dialyzable toxins.

NURSING CARE
• Hypovolemia—correct estimated fluid deficits with normal (0.9%) saline or balanced polyionic solution within 2–4 hr; replace blood losses by whole blood transfusion; once the patient is hydrated, ongoing fluid requirements are provided by 5% dextrose for insensible requirements (approximately 20–25 mL/kg/ day) and balanced electrolyte solution equal to urinary and other losses (i.e., vomiting and diarrhea); avoid overhydration.
• Hypervolemia—stop fluid administration and eliminate excess fluid by diuretic administration or dialysis.

DIET
• Restrict oral intake until vomiting subsides. For most patients, endogenous fat and protein stores supply requisite calories during early phases of dietary restriction; thereafter moderately protein-restricted diets or enteral feeding solutions are used to control azotemia and supply caloric requirements. • Parenteral nutrition (vomiting animals)—provide caloric requirements by 30–50% dextrose and 20% emulsified lipid solution; protein requirements (dogs, 3–4 g/100 kcal; cats, 5–6 g/100 kcal) provided by 8.5% amino acid mixture via central venous catheter • Enteral feeding (anorectic, nonvomiting animals)—caloric and protein requirements supplied by blended commercial prescription renal diet or commercial formulated liquid diet; enteral feedings can be force-fed or given by naso-esophageal, pharyngostomy, gastrostomy, or enterostomy tube.

CLIENT EDUCATION
Inform of the poor prognosis for complete recovery, potential for morbid complications of treatment (e.g., fluid overload, sepsis, and multiple organ failure), expense of prolonged hospitalization, alternatives to conventional medical management (i.e., peritoneal dialysis, hemodialysis, and renal transplantation), and zoonotic potential of leptospirosis.

SURGICAL CONSIDERATIONS
• Ureterotomy or ureteral transplantation may be required for acute ureteral obstruction.
• Renal transplantation may provide long-term survival for patients (particularly cats) with fulminating ARF.

MEDICATIONS

DRUG(S) OF CHOICE

Inadequate Urine Production
• Ensure patient is fluid-volume-replete; provide additional isonatric fluid to achieve mild (3–5%) volume expansion; failure to induce

diuresis by fluid replacement indicates severe parenchymal damage or underestimation of fluid deficit; if fluid-replete, administer diuretics and/or dopamine. • Hypertonic mannitol (10–20%)—0.5–1.0 g/kg IV over 15–30 min; if effective, continue as intermittent IV bolus q4–6h or 1.0–2.0 mg/kg/min IV continuous-rate infusion (CRI); if ineffective, discontinue • Furosemide (alternative or subsequent to mannitol)—2–6 mg/kg IV; if effective, continue q8h; if ineffective, discontinue or combine with dopamine • Dopamine—1–5 μg/kg/min IV in 5% dextrose as CRI; synergistic with furosemide; if effective, continue as CRI; if ineffective, combine with furosemide or discontinue • If these treatments fail to induce diuresis within 4–6 hr, consider dialysis.

Acid–Base Disorders
Administer bicarbonate if serum bicarbonate ≤ 15 mEq/L; bicarbonate replacement: mEq − bicarbonate deficit × body weight (kg) × 0.3; give half IV over 30 min and the remainder over 2–4 hr; then reassess

Hyperkalemia
See Hyperkalemia

Vomiting
• NPO until vomiting subsides • Reduce gastric acid production—famotidine (0.5–1.0 mg/kg IM, IV q12–24h) or ranitidine (2 mg/kg IV q8–12h) or omeprazole (0.7–2.0 mg/kg PO q24h [dogs]) • Mucosal protectant—sucralfate (0.5–1.0 g PO q6–8h) • Antiemetics—metoclopramide (0.2–0.5 mg/kg SC, IV, or IM q6–8h; 0.01–0.02 mg/kg/h CRI)

CONTRAINDICATIONS
Avoid nephrotoxic agents and overhydration.

PRECAUTIONS
Modify dosages of all drugs that require renal metabolism or elimination.

POSSIBLE INTERACTIONS
Metoclopramide may impair the effects of dopamine.

ALTERNATIVE DRUG(S)
Control of vomiting—chlorpromazine (0.2–0.5 mg/kg IM q6–12h), prochlorperazine (0.1–0.2 mg/kg IM q6–8h), acepromazine (0.005–0.05 mg/kg IM, SC q8–12h), or trimethobenzamide (3.0 mg/kg IM q6–8h) can be used to treat vomiting but may be associated with CNS depression, vasodilatation, and hypotension.

Peritoneal or Hemodialysis
• Dialysis can stabilize the patient until renal function is restored, corrective procedures or surgeries are implemented, renal transplantation; without dialysis, most oliguric patients die before renal repair can occur • Specific indications include severe oliguria or anuria, life-threatening fluid overload, life-threatening electrolyte or acid–base disturbance, BUN ≥

100 mg/dL, serum creatinine ≥ 10 mg/dL, clinical course refractory to conservative treatment for more than 24 hr, perioperative stabilization, and poisoning with a dialyzable toxin.

FOLLOW-UP

PATIENT MONITORING
Fluid, electrolyte, and acid–base balances; body weight; urine output; and clinical status; daily

PREVENTION/AVOIDANCE
Anticipate the potential for ARF in patients that are hemodynamically unstable, receiving nephrotoxic drugs, have multiple organ failure, or are undergoing prolonged anesthesia and surgery; maintenance of hydration, mild saline volume expansion, and administration of mannitol may be preventive.

POSSIBLE COMPLICATIONS
Seizures, coma, cardiac arrhythmias, congestive heart failure, pulmonary edema, uremic pneumonitis, GI bleeding, hypovolemic shock, sepsis, cardiopulmonary arrest, and death

EXPECTED COURSE AND PROGNOSIS
• Infectious etiologies have a better prognosis for recovery than toxic causes. • Nonoliguric ARF—milder than oliguric; recovery may occur over 2–6 weeks, but the prognosis remains guarded to unfavorable • Oliguric ARF—predicts extensive renal injury, is difficult to manage, and has a poor prognosis for recovery; recovery signaled by a sudden (and often excessive) increase in urine production and a sluggish and incomplete return of renal function over 4–12 weeks; dialysis extends the potential for renal regeneration and repair • Anuric ARF—generally fatal; dialysis required for renal repair; recovery of renal function is usually incomplete • Oligoanuric ARF with multiple organ failure—generally fatal, usually requires dialysis

MISCELLANEOUS

ZOONOTIC POTENTIAL
Leptospirosis has infectious and zoonotic potential; avoid contact with infective urine.

PREGNANCY
A rare complication of pregnancy in animals; promoted by acute metritis, pyometra, and postpartum sepsis or hemorrhage

SYNONYMS
Acute tubular necrosis, acute uremia, lower nephron nephrosis, vasomotor nephropathy
Author Larry D. Cowgill
Consulting Editors Larry G. Adams and Carl A. Osborne

RENAL FAILURE, CHRONIC

 BASICS

DEFINITION

Azotemia and urine specific gravity < 1.030 in dogs and < 1.035 in cats; results from primary renal disease that has persisted for months to years; characterized by irreversible renal dysfunction that tends to deteriorate progressively over months to years.

PATHOPHYSIOLOGY

More than approximately 75% reduction in functional renal mass results in impaired urine-concentrating ability (leading to polyuria and polydipsia [PU/PD]) and retention of nitrogenous waste products of protein catabolism (leading to azotemia). Severe chronic renal failure (CRF) results in uremia. Decreased erythropoietin and calcitriol production by the kidneys results in hypoproliferative anemia and renal secondary hyperparathyroidism, respectively.

SYSTEMS AFFECTED

• Renal/Urologic—impaired renal function leading to PU/PD and signs of uremia
• Nervous, Gastrointestinal, Musculoskeletal, and other body systems—secondarily affected by uremia • Hemic/Lymph/Immune—anemia

GENETICS

Inherited in the following breeds (mode of inheritance, known or suspected, indicated in parentheses):
• Abyssinian cats (autosomal dominant with incomplete penetrance) • Persian cats (autosomal dominant) • Bull terrier (autosomal dominant) • Cairn terrier (autosomal recessive) • German shepherd (autosomal dominant) • Samoyed (X-linked dominant)
• English cocker spaniel (autosomal recessive)

INCIDENCE/PREVALENCE

• Reportedly 9 cases per 1000 dogs examined and 16 cases per 1000 cats examined • Prevalence increases with age—in animals >15 years of age, reportedly 57 cases per 1000 dogs examined and 153 cases per 1000 cats examined

GEOGRAPHIC DISTRIBUTION

N/A

SIGNALMENT

Species
Dogs and cats

Breed Predilection
All breeds of dogs and cats are affected. Familial renal disease resulting in CRF has been reported in the basenji, beagle, bull terrier, Cairn terrier, chow chow, Doberman pinscher, English cocker spaniel, German shepherd, golden retriever, Lhasa apso, miniature schnauzer, Norwegian elkhound, rottweiler, Samoyed, Chinese shar pei, shih tzu, soft-coated wheaten terrier, and standard poodle, and in Abyssinian cats.

Mean Age and Range
Mean age at diagnosis is approximately 7 years in dogs and 9 years in cats. Animals of any age can be affected, but prevalence increases with increasing age.

Predominant Sex
None

SIGNS

General Comments
Clinical signs are related to the severity of renal dysfunction and the presence or absence of complications such as hypertension. Cats with mild CRF may be asymptomatic. An animal with stable CRF may decompensate, resulting in a uremic crisis.

Historical Findings
• PU/PD (less frequent in cats than dogs)
• Anorexia • Lethargy • Vomiting • Weight loss • Nocturia • Constipation • Diarrhea
• Acute blindness—because of hypertension
• Seizures or coma—late • Cats may also have ptyalism and muscle weakness with cervical ventroflexion (because of hypokalemic myopathy).

Physical Examination Findings
• Small, irregular kidneys (or enlarged kidneys secondary to polycystic kidney disease or lymphoma) • Dehydration • Cachexia • Mucous membrane pallor • Oral ulceration • Uremic breath odor • Constipation • Hypertensive retinopathy • Renal osteodystrophy

CAUSES
• Most are idiopathic, and the disease is termed *chronic generalized nephropathy.* • Include familial and congenital renal disease, nephrotoxins, hypercalcemia, hypokalemic nephropathy, glomerulonephritis, amyloidosis, pyelonephritis, polycystic kidney disease, nephroliths, chronic urinary obstruction, drugs, lymphoma, leptospirosis (following acute renal failure), FIP (cats), and, possibly, diabetes mellitus

RISK FACTORS
Aging, hypercalcemia, hypokalemia (cats), hypertension, urinary tract infection, diabetes mellitus

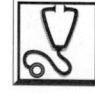 **DIAGNOSIS**

DIFFERENTIAL DIAGNOSIS
• See chapter on polyuria/polydipsia for differential diagnosis.
• Azotemia—includes causes of prerenal and postrenal azotemia, acute renal failure, and hypoadrenocorticism
• Prerenal azotemia—characterized by azotemia with urine specific gravity > 1.030 in dogs and > 1.035 in cats
• Postrenal azotemia—characterized by azotemia with obstruction or rupture of the excretory system
• Acute renal failure—differentiated by normal renal size, cylindruria, lack of indications of chronicity (e.g., nonregenerative anemia and renal secondary hyperparathyroidism), and recent nephrotoxin exposure or hypotensive episode
• Hypoadrenocorticism—characterized by hyponatremia, hyperkalemia with decreased cortisol response to ACTH stimulation

CBC/BIOCHEMISTRY/URINALYSIS
• Nonregenerative anemia
• Azotemia (high BUN and creatinine), hyperphosphatemia, acidosis (low total CO_2), hyperamylasemia, hyperlipasemia, hypokalemia or hyperkalemia, and hypercalcemia or hypocalcemia
• Urine specific gravity < 1.030 in dogs and < 1.035 in cats; mild proteinuria

OTHER LABORATORY TESTS
• Urinary protein:creatinine ratio to determine magnitude of proteinuria.
• Microalbuminuria assay to screen for early evidence of glomerular injury

IMAGING
• Abdominal radiographs may demonstrate small kidneys (or large kidneys secondary to polycystic kidney disease or lymphoma).
• Ultrasound demonstrates small kidneys and hyperechoic renal parenchyma with less apparent distinction between the cortex and medulla in some animals. Animals with lymphoma often have renomegaly with hypoechoic renal parenchyma. See also Congenital/Developmental Renal Disorders, Pyelonephritis, Nephrolithiasis, Hydronephrosis, and Polycystic Kidneys.

DIAGNOSTIC PROCEDURES
• Direct or indirect blood pressure determinations indicated to detect hypertension
• Renal biopsy helpful in selected patients to document underlying cause—especially in patients with glomerular disease, familial renal disease, lymphoma, and FIP—but renal biopsy not indicated in most dogs and cats

PATHOLOGIC FINDINGS
• Gross findings—small kidneys with a lumpy or granular surface; renal capsule frequently adheres to the renal parenchyma.
• Histopathologic findings—frequently nonspecific; chronic generalized nephropathy or end-stage kidneys; findings are specific for diseases causing CRF in some patients.

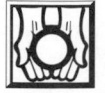 **TREATMENT**

APPROPRIATE HEALTH CARE
Patients with compensated CRF may be managed as outpatients; patients in uremic crisis should be managed as inpatients.

NURSING CARE
• Patients in uremic crisis—correct fluid and electrolyte deficits with intravenous fluid

therapy (e.g., lactated Ringer's solution); correct dehydration over 2–6 hours to prevent additional renal injury from ischemia
• Subcutaneous fluid therapy (daily or every other day) may benefit patients with moderate-to-severe CRF.

ACTIVITY
Unrestricted

DIET
• Reduced dietary protein, phosphorus, and sodium with adequate buffering capacity (alkalinizing diet); supplemental n-3 fatty acids may be beneficial.
• Recommendations for animals with mild-to-moderate renal failure are controversial; some authors suggest that protein restriction is not required until the patient has moderate-to-severe renal failure.
• Free access to fresh water at all times

CLIENT EDUCATION
• Tends to progress to terminal CRF over months to years
• Heritability of familial renal diseases

SURGICAL CONSIDERATIONS
• Avoid hypotension during anesthesia, to prevent additional renal injury.
• Renal transplantation has been successfully performed in dogs and cats with advanced disease.

MEDICATIONS

DRUG(S) OF CHOICE

Uremic Crisis
• Cimetidine (dogs, 10 mg/kg IV initial dose followed by 5 mg/kg IV q8–12h; cats, 2.5–5 mg/kg IV q8–12h) to minimize nausea and vomiting
• Potassium chloride in IV fluids or potassium gluconate PO (2–6 mEq/cat/day) as needed to correct hypokalemia

Compensated CRF
• Famotidine (dogs, 0.5–1 mg/kg PO q24h; cats, 5 mg/cat PO q48h) to minimize nausea
• Potassium gluconate (2–6 mEq/cat/day PO) as needed for hypokalemia
• Intestinal phosphate binders (e.g., aluminum carbonate, 30–100 mg/kg/day PO with meals) as needed to correct hyperphosphatemia (see Renal Secondary Hyperparathyroidism)
• Calcitriol (see Hyperparathyroidism, Renal Secondary)
• Erythropoietin (see Anemia of Chronic Renal Disease)
• Angiotensin-converting enzyme (ACE) inhibitors (e.g., enalapril or benazepril, 0.5 mg/kg PO q24h) or amlodipine (dogs, 0.1 mg/kg PO q24h; cats, 0.18 mg/kg or 0.625–1.25 mg/cat PO q24h) as needed for hypertension. Amlodipine is more effective than ACE inhibitors in cats with CRF-induced hypertension. If refractory to

monotherapy, consider combination of amlodipine and ACE inhibitor with frequent monitoring of blood pressure.
• Oxazepam (2.5 mg/cat PO) as needed to increase appetite

CONTRAINDICATIONS
Avoid nephrotoxic drugs (aminoglycosides, cisplatin, amphotericin B) and corticosteroids

PRECAUTIONS
• Reduce dosage or prolong dosing interval of drugs eliminated by the kidneys, including cimetidine, enalapril, ranitidine, and metoclopramide.
• Use ACE inhibitors with caution; monitor patient for worsening of azotemia or proteinuria.
• Use caution with NSAIDs.

POSSIBLE INTERACTIONS
Cimetidine or trimethoprim may cause artifactual increases in the serum creatinine concentration by reducing tubular secretion in dogs with CRF.

ALTERNATIVE DRUG(S)
• Metoclopramide (0.2–0.4 mg PO or SC q6–8h) can be used in addition to H_2-receptor antagonists to treat uremic vomiting.
• Ranitidine (0.5–2 mg/kg PO or IV q12h) or cimetidine (5 mg/kg q8–12h for dogs; 2.5–5 mg/kg q8–12h for cats) may be used instead of famotidine for uremic gastritis.
• Hemodialysis and renal transplantation are available at selected referral hospitals.

FOLLOW-UP

PATIENT MONITORING
Dogs and cats with CRF should be monitored at regular intervals, depending on therapy and severity of disease; initially weekly for patients receiving calcitriol or erythropoietin; reevaluate patients with mild-to-moderate CRF every 1–3 months.

PREVENTION/AVOIDANCE
Do not breed animals with familial renal disease.

POSSIBLE COMPLICATIONS
Systemic hypertension, uremic stomatitis, gastroenteritis, anemia, secondary urinary tract infection

EXPECTED COURSE AND PROGNOSIS
• Short-term—depends on severity • Long-term—guarded to poor because CRF tends to be progressive over months to years

MISCELLANEOUS

ASSOCIATED CONDITIONS
• Hyperthyroidism in cats • Urinary tract infection • Systemic hypertension

AGE-RELATED FACTORS
Increased incidence in older animals; normal renal function decreases with aging.

ZOONOTIC POTENTIAL
None

PREGNANCY
Patients with mild CRF may maintain pregnancy; those with moderate-to-severe disease may be infertile or have spontaneous abortions; breeding of female patients not recommended

SYNONYMS
• Kidney failure • Chronic renal disease

SEE ALSO
• Anemia of Chronic Renal Disease
• Azotemia and Uremia
• Congenital/Developmental Renal Disorders
• Hydronephrosis • Hyperparathyroidism, Renal Secondary • Hypertension, Systemic
• Nephrolithiasis • Polycystic Kidneys
• Polyuria/Polydipsia • Proteinuria
• Pyelonephritis • Renal Failure, Acute
• Urinary Tract Obstruction

ABBREVIATIONS
• ACE = angiotensin converting enzyme
• CRF = chronic renal failure • FIP = feline infectious peritonitis • NSAID = nonsteroidal antiinflammatory drug • PU/PD = polyuria/polydipsia

Suggested Reading
DiBartola SP. Familial renal disease in dogs and cats. In: Ettinger SJ, Feldman EC, eds. Textbook of veterinary internal medicine. 4th ed. Philadelphia: Saunders, 1995:1796–1801.
Finco DR, Brown SA, Barsanti JA, et al. Recent developments in the management of progressive renal failure. In: Bonagura JD, ed. Kirk's Current veterinary therapy XIII. Philadelphia: Saunders, 2000:861–864.
Gregory CR. Renal transplantation in cats. Compend Contin Educ Pract Vet 1993;15:1325–1339.
Polzin DJ, Osborne CA, Adams LG, Lulich JP. Medical management of feline chronic renal failure. In: Kirk RW, Bonagura JD, eds. Current veterinary therapy XI. Philadelphia: Saunders, 1992:848–853.
Polzin DJ, Osborne CA, Bartges JW, et al. Chronic renal failure. In: Ettinger SJ, Feldman EC, eds. Textbook of veterinary internal medicine. 4th ed. Philadelphia: Saunders, 1995:1734–1760.

Author Larry G. Adams
Consulting Editors Larry G. Adams and Carl A. Osborne

RENAL TUBULAR ACIDOSIS

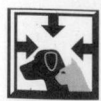

BASICS

OVERVIEW
A rare syndrome that refers to the development of metabolic acidosis because of either reduced bicarbonate reabsorption from the proximal renal tubule (proximal or type 2 renal tubular acidosis) or reduced hydrogen ion secretion in the distal tubule (distal or type 1 renal tubular acidosis); proximal renal tubular acidosis has not been documented as an isolated entity in dogs but has been observed as part of Fanconi syndrome; the following discussion is limited to distal renal tubular acidosis.

SIGNALMENT
• Reported in 5 dogs and 3 cats
• No apparent breed or sex predilection
• Age range at time of diagnosis, 1–8 years

SIGNS
• Anorexia and lethargy—most common
• Others depend on the presence or absence of associated diseases (e.g., pyelonephritis).
• Panting
• Weakness—related to hypokalemia
• Polyuria
• Polydipsia
• Vomiting
• Weight loss
• Hematuria
• Dysuria—related to urolithiasis
• Fever

CAUSES & RISK FACTORS
• Associated with distal renal tubular acidosis in human beings; may be primary (i.e., inherited), or secondary to other inherited diseases (e.g., Ehlers-Danlos syndrome), toxins and drugs (e.g., amphotericin B), altered calcium metabolism causing nephrocalcinosis (e.g., hypervitaminosis D), autoimmune and hypergammaglobulinemic disorders (e.g., multiple myeloma, systemic lupus erythematosus) and tubulointerstitial nephropathies
• In cats, distal renal tubular acidosis has been associated with pyelonephritis (two cases) and hepatic lipidosis (one case).
• In dogs, all clinical reports of distal renal tubular acidosis appeared to be idiopathic; struvite urolithiasis (one case) occurred secondary to distal renal tubular acidosis; distal renal tubular acidosis has also been caused by experimentally induced renal ischemia.

DIAGNOSIS

DIFFERENTIAL DIAGNOSIS
Consider other diseases that may cause a normal anion gap metabolic acidosis (e.g., diarrhea).

CBC/BIOCHEMISTRY/URINALYSIS
• Vary depending on associated diseases
• Hypokalemia (because of increased renal excretion) in some animals; may be severe enough to cause muscle weakness
• Alkaline urine—pH > 6.0, assuming urinary tract infection is absent

OTHER LABORATORY TESTS
Blood gas analysis and evaluation of serum electrolytes reveal normal anion gap metabolic acidosis.

IMAGING
May detect uroliths radiographically

DIAGNOSTIC PROCEDURES

The key diagnostic feature is normal anion gap metabolic acidosis accompanied by an inappropriately alkaline urine pH (> 6.0). In some patients in which no nonrenal cause for a normal anion gap metabolic acidosis can be found and the urine pH is 6.0 (or very close to it), an acid load may be required to demonstrate distal renal tubular acidosis—administer ammonium chloride (200 mg/kg PO, dogs); drain the bladder hourly; urinary pH (measured by a pH meter) should decrease to < 6.0 (often < 5.5) within 3–6 h; avoid this test if there is severe acidosis.

TREATMENT

• Individualize depending on the nature and severity of associated conditions.
• Typically, less bicarbonate is needed to resolve metabolic acidosis associated with distal renal tubular acidosis than is needed to resolve acidosis associated with proximal renal tubular acidosis.

• Hypokalemia may resolve with bicarbonate administration alone, or potassium supplementation may be required.

MEDICATIONS

DRUG(S)
• Sodium bicarbonate—10–50 mg/kg q8–12h PO
• Potassium supplementation—potassium gluconate; cats: 2–8 mEq/day divided q12h PO; dogs (depending on body size): 2–44 mEq/day divided q12h PO, if required

CONTRAINDICATIONS/POSSIBLE INTERACTIONS
N/A

FOLLOW-UP

• Serial blood gas analyses every 3–5 days until acid–base status has normalized
• Monitor serum electrolytes, particularly potassium, as needed.

• Long-term prognosis depends on the nature and severity of associated conditions; may be reasonably good in patients without other diseases and that respond well to bicarbonate therapy, but little information exists on the long-term course of this disease

MISCELLANEOUS

SEE ALSO
• Acidosis, Metabolic
• Hypokalemia

Suggested Reading

Bartges JW. Disorders of renal tubules. In: Ettinger SJ, Feldman EC, eds. Textbook of veterinary intenal medicine. 5th ed. Philadelphia:Saunders, 2000:1704–1710.

Author Darcy H. Shaw
Contributing Editors Larry G. Adams and Carl A. Osborne

RENOMEGALY

 BASICS

DEFINITION
One or both kidneys are abnormally large as detected by abdominal palpation or radiography.

PATHOPHYSIOLOGY
The kidneys may become abnormally large because of abnormal cellular infiltration (e.g., inflammation, infection, and neoplasia), urinary tract obstruction, acute tubular necrosis, or development of renal cysts or pseudocysts.

SYSTEMS AFFECTED
• Renal/Urologic
• Gastrointestinal—inappetence, vomiting, diarrhea, or melena due to gastrointestinal irritation or ulceration in patients with uremia
• Endocrine/Metabolic—metabolic acidosis due to decreased elimination of acid by kidneys and inability to reclaim bicarbonate
• Hemic/Lymph/Immune—anemia due to blood loss or decreased red blood cell survival in patients with uremia; increased susceptibility to infections due to immune dysfunction in patients with uremia
• Nervous—depression and lethargy associated with effect of uremic toxins on central nervous system
• Respiratory—tachypnea or respiratory distress due to uremic pneumonitis or compensatory response for metabolic acidosis

SIGNALMENT
Dogs and cats

SIGNS

Historical Findings
• Lethargy
• Loss of appetite
• Weight loss
• Vomiting
• Diarrhea
• Polyuria and polydipsia
• Discolored urine
• Abdominal enlargement

• Lameness (rarely) because of hypertrophic osteopathy associated with renal neoplasia

Physical Examination Findings
• Abnormally large abdomen
• Abdominal mass
• Abdominal pain
• One or both kidneys palpably large
• Dehydration
• Pale mucous membranes
• Oral ulcers
• Foul-smelling breath

CAUSES

Neoplasia
• Lymphoma—most often occurs in cats and causes bilateral renomegaly; some patients have unilateral renomegaly.
• Renal carcinoma—most common renal tumor of dogs; often causes unilateral renomegaly; very malignant and rapidly metastatic to distant sites such as lungs
• Nephroblastoma—also called Wilms' tumor; a congenital renal tumor that affects young dogs, although it may not be diagnosed until the patient is much older; biologic behavior varies; usually unilateral
• Sarcomas—usually cause unilateral renomegaly and behave malignantly
• Cystadenocarcinoma—bilateral renal tumor that occurs in German shepherd dogs; often associated with skin lesions (i.e., nodular dermatofibrosis)

Inflammation/Infection
• Leptospirosis—may cause bilateral renomegaly and acute renal failure in dogs
• Feline infectious peritonitis—causes bilateral renomegaly in cats; some cats have unilateral renomegaly
• Renal abscess—localized abscess within renal parenchyma usually causes unilateral renomegaly in dogs and cats.

Developmental/Acquired Disorders
• Hydronephrosis—can cause unilateral or bilateral renomegaly in dogs and cats; develops secondarily to ureteral obstruction (e.g., urolithiasis, ureteral strictures, and neoplasia at trigone of urinary bladder) and ectopic ureters

• Polycystic kidney disease—causes bilateral renomegaly in cats and often leads to chronic renal failure; may be more common in Persians and domestic longhair cats
• Hematoma—occurs secondarily to trauma; infrequent cause of renomegaly in dogs and cats
• Compensatory hypertrophy—causes unilateral renomegaly and occurs secondarily to abnormality of the other kidney (e.g., renal hypoplasia, renal dysplasia, or nephrectomy)
• Ethylene glycol toxicosis—can cause bilateral renomegaly secondary to renal tubular swelling and renal infiltration by calcium oxalate crystals

RISK FACTORS
• Feline leukemia virus infection predisposes cats to development of renal lymphoma.
• Exposure to infectious diseases such as leptospirosis and feline infectious peritonitis increases risk of developing renomegaly associated with these disorders.

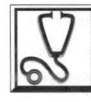 **DIAGNOSIS**

DIFFERENTIAL DIAGNOSIS
• Must distinguish from other abdominal masses
• Confirmation may require diagnostic imaging procedures or exploratory celiotomy.

CBC/BIOCHEMISTRY/URINALYSIS
• Leukocytosis in patients with infectious, inflammatory, and neoplastic causes of renomegaly
• Nonregenerative anemia secondary to chronic renal failure or inflammatory disorders in some
• Polycythemia and extreme leukocytosis accompany some renal neoplasms (rare).
• Hyperglobulinemia in some patients with infectious or inflammatory disorders (e.g., feline infectious peritonitis)
• Azotemia, hyperphosphatemia, and low urine specific gravity (dogs, <1.030; cats, <1.035) in patients with renal failure

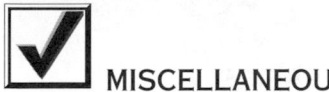
- Hematuria and proteinuria in some patients with renal neoplasia
- Neoplastic cells rarely observed in urine of patients with renal neoplasia

OTHER LABORATORY TESTS
- Test cats for feline leukemia virus infection.
- Do serum protein electrophoresis to distinguish between polyclonal and monoclonal hyperglobulinemia in patients with hyperglobulinemia.
- Do paired titers for *Leptospira* spp. 3–4 weeks apart in dogs with suspected leptospirosis.

IMAGING

Radiographic Findings
- Survey abdominal radiographs indicated to confirm renomegaly
- Kidneys on the ventrodorsal view are >3 or 3.5 times the length of the second lumbar vertebra in cats or dogs, respectively.
- Can use excretory urography to confirm presence of renomegaly, hydronephrosis, and space-occupying masses of the kidneys
- Thoracic radiography indicated to detect metastases in patients with renal neoplasia.

Ultrasonographic Findings
- Helpful to confirm diagnosis and identify potential causes such as polycystic kidney disease, perirenal pseudocysts, hydronephrosis, neoplastic mass, abscess, and subcapsular hematoma
- Dogs with leptospirosis may have increased cortical echogenicity, perinephric effusion, or a medullary band of increased echogenicity.

DIAGNOSTIC PROCEDURES
- Examination of fine-needle aspirate can confirm presence of renal cyst, abscess, and neoplasia (especially lymphoma).
- If no definitive diagnosis is made by cytologic evaluation of renal aspirates, renal biopsy may be indicated.

TREATMENT
- Diagnose and treat underlying cause if possible.
- Usually treat as an outpatient unless patient is dehydrated or has decompensated renal failure.
- If the patient is healthy otherwise, feed normal diet and allow normal exercise.
- If the patient cannot maintain hydration, administer lactated Ringer's solution or a maintenance fluid either intravenously or subcutaneously.
- If the patient has dehydration or continuing fluid losses such as vomiting or diarrhea, administer fluids intravenously to correct hydration deficits, maintain daily fluid requirements, and replace ongoing losses.

MEDICATIONS

DRUG(S) OF CHOICE
Vary with the cause

CONTRAINDICATIONS
Avoid nephrotoxic drugs.

PRECAUTIONS
N/A

POSSIBLE INTERACTIONS
N/A

ALTERNATIVE DRUG(S)
N/A

FOLLOW-UP

PATIENT MONITORING
Perform physical examination and weigh patient to assess hydration status.

POSSIBLE COMPLICATIONS
- Renal failure, depending on underlying cause of renomegaly
- Paraneoplastic syndromes caused by production of hormone-like substances by renal neoplasms

MISCELLANEOUS

ASSOCIATED CONDITIONS
N/A

AGE-RELATED FACTORS
N/A

ZOONOTIC POTENTIAL
Leptospirosis can be spread by contact with infected urine.

PREGNANCY
N/A

SYNONYMS
None

SEE ALSO
- Ethylene Glycol Poisoning
- Feline Infectious Peritonitis
- Hydronephrosis
- Leptospirosis
- Lymphosarcoma—Feline
- Polycystic Kidneys
- Renal Carcinoma

Suggested Reading

Cuypers MD, Grooters AM, Williams J, et al. Renomegaly in dogs and cats. Part I. Differential diagnosis. Compend Contin Educ Pract Vet 1997;19:1019–1033.

Forrest LJ, O'Brien RT, Tremelling MS, et al. Sonographic findings in 20 dogs with leptospirosis. Vet Radiol Ultrasound 1993;39:337–340.

Klein MK, Cockerell GL, Harris CK, et al. Canine primary renal neoplasms: A retrospective review of 54 cases. J Am Anim Hosp Assoc 1988;24:443–452.

Lulich JP, Osborne CA, Walter PA, et al. Feline idiopathic polycystic kidney disease. Compend Contin Educ Pract Vet 1988;10:1030–1041.

Mooney SC, Hayes AA, Matus RE, et al. Renal lymphoma in cats: 28 cases (1977–1984). J Am Vet Med Assoc 1987;191:1473–1477.

Osborne C, Stevens J, Perman V. Kidney biopsy. Vet Clin North Am (Small Anim Pract) 1974;4:351–365.

Author S. Dru Forrester

Consulting Editors Larry G. Adams and Carl A. Osborne

REOVIRUS INFECTIONS

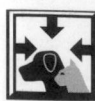

BASICS

OVERVIEW
• Respiratory enteric orphan virus (reovirus)—genus in the family Reovirus; nonenveloped, double-stranded RNA virus; isolated from respiratory and enteric tracts; not associated with any known disease (hence *orphan*)
• Ubiquitous in geographic distribution and host range, virtually every species of mammal, including humans
• Virus—infects mature epithelial cells on luminal tips of the intestinal villi; causes cellular destruction, resulting in villous atrophy (similar to rotavirus and coronavirus)
• Loss of absorptive capability and loss of brush border enzymes (e.g., disaccharidases) leads to osmotic diarrhea.

SIGNALMENT
Dogs and cats

SIGNS

Dogs
• Conjunctivitis
• Rhinitis
• Tracheobronchitis—minor role
• Pneumonia
• Diarrhea
• Encephalitis—rare

Cats
• Generally mild disease
• Respiratory illness
• Conjunctivitis
• Gingivitis
• Ataxia
• Diarrhea

CAUSES & RISK FACTORS
• Predominantly excreted from respiratory and digestive tract; acquired by inhalation and oral ingestion
• Infection is common; specific disease has not been reproduced.

• Other viral pathogens—infections observed repeatedly; speculated that reovirus may have an immunosuppressive effect that aggravates such infections

DIAGNOSIS

DIFFERENTIAL DIAGNOSIS
• Canine viral enteritis—canine parvovirus; canine coronavirus; canine astrovirus; canine calicivirus; canine herpesvirus; canine distemper virus; canine rotavirus
• Canine infectious tracheobronchitis—canine parainfluenza; *Bordetella bronchiseptica;* mycoplasmas; canine adenovirus types 1 and 2; canine herpesvirus; canine distemper virus
• Feline upper respiratory disease—feline rhinotracheitis virus; feline calicivirus; *Chlamydia;* mycoplasma; bacterial infection

CBC/BIOCHEMISTRY/URINALYSIS
Noncontributory

OTHER LABORATORY TESTS
• Virus isolation—cytopathic effect slow to develop
• Histopathology—large intracytoplasmic inclusion bodies

IMAGING
N/A

DIAGNOSTIC PROCEDURES
N/A

 TREATMENT
• Doubtful that reovirus is an important pathogen
• No vaccines developed
• Other control measures ignored

 MEDICATIONS

DRUG(S)
N/A

CONTRAINDICATIONS/POSSIBLE INTERACTIONS
N/A

 FOLLOW-UP
N/A

 MISCELLANEOUS

ZOONOTIC POTENTIAL
• Infection can spread among individuals of the same or different species.

• The role (if any) that animals serve as a reservoir for virus or as a possible source of human infection unknown
• Humans—by early childhood, the vast majority demonstrate serologic evidence of past reovirus infection; difficult to link to disease; majority of infections must be asymptomatic or blend imperceptibly with minor respiratory and gastrointestinal illness of infancy and early childhood

Suggested Reading
Pedersen NC. Feline infectious diseases. American Veterinary Publications, Inc., 1988:69–70.
Thein P, Scheid R. Mammalian reoviral infections. In: Steele JH, ed. CRC handbook series in zoonoses. Vol. 2: Viral zoonoses. Boca Raton, FL: CRC, 1981: 191–216.
Author J. Paul Woods
Consulting Editor Stephen C. Barr

RESPIRATORY PARASITES

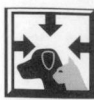 BASICS

DEFINITION
Helminths and arthropods that reside in the respiratory tract or pulmonary vessels of dogs and cats

PATHOPHYSIOLOGY
Infestation with parasites causes irritant allergic rhinitis, bronchitis, pneumonitis, or arteritis, depending on the location of the organism within the respiratory system.

SYSTEMS AFFECTED
• Respiratory
• Cardiovascular
• Hepatic—with hepatopulmonary migration of some parasites

GENETICS
N/A

INCIDENCE/PREVALENCE
Depends on parasite

GEOGRAPHIC DISTRIBUTION
• *Pneumonyssoides caninum*—worldwide
• *Oslerus (Filaroides) osleri*—worldwide
• *Filaroides hirthi*—North America
• *Filaroides milksi*—North America; Europe
• *Aelurostrongylus abstrusus*—worldwide
• *Capillaria aerophila*—North America
• *Crenosoma vulpis*—worldwide
• *Paragonimus kellicotti*—North America
• *Eucoleus boehmi*—North America

SIGNALMENT
Species
Dogs and cats

Breed Predilections
None

Mean Age and Range
N/A

Predominant Sex
N/A

SIGNS
General Comments
• Three basic categories—upper respiratory, lower respiratory, and vascular; based on location and lifestyle of parasite
• Often insidious and chronic, with few clinical signs
• Respiratory compromise often not severe

Historical Findings
• Upper respiratory—sneezing; nasal discharge (serous, sanguinous); reverse sneezing; nasal irritation or rubbing
• Lower respiratory—chronic coughing non-responsive to empirical treatment

Physical Examination Findings
• Upper respiratory—similar to historical findings; variable
• Lower respiratory—elicitable cough; occasionally harsh lung sounds; often cause coughing in cats

CAUSES
• Upper respiratory—*Pneumonyssus caninum* (nasal mites); *Eucoleus boehmi*; *Crenosoma vulpis*
• Lower respiratory—dogs and cats: *Capillaria aerophila* (rare in cats), *Paragonimus kellicotti* (lung fluke); dogs: *Filaroides osleri* (*Oslerus osleri*), *Filaroides hirthi*, *Filaroides milksi*, *Crenosoma vulpis*; cats: *Aelurostrongylus abstrusus*

RISK FACTORS
• Depends on the specific parasite—some have intermediate or paratenic hosts that must be ingested by the definitive host, putting scavenging animals at higher risk
• *Crenosoma vulpis*—snails
• *Paragonimus kellicotti*—snails; crabs; shellfish
• *Aelurostrongylus abstrusus*—snails and slugs; transport hosts: rodents, frogs, lizards, birds
• Multianimal households with unhygienic living conditions—allows fecal–oral or direct-contact transmission

 DIAGNOSIS

DIFFERENTIAL DIAGNOSIS
• Upper respiratory—other causes of epistaxis, rhinitis, or sinusitis (see specific topics)
• Lower respiratory—allergic bronchitis (nonparasitic); chronic bronchitis; infectious tracheobronchitis; allergic pneumonitis; bronchopneumonia; granulomatous pneumonia; pulmonary granulomatosis; hepatopulmonary migration of enteric helminths

CBC/BIOCHEMISTRY/URINALYSIS
• CBC—variable; may note eosinophilia, basophilia (especially with heartworm disease), neutrophilia, and monocytosis
• Biochemistry—often normal; high liver enzyme activity with some parasites during early stages as a result of hepatic migration if burden is substantial
• Urinalysis—normal; may see proteinuria with heartworm disease

OTHER LABORATORY TESTS
N/A

IMAGING
• Thoracic radiography—often unrewarding; generalized interstitial pattern; granulomatous masses (especially right caudal lobe) with *Paragonimus*; pneumothorax if rupture of a cyst containing *Paragonimus*

DIAGNOSTIC PROCEDURES
Sputum examination—may reveal eggs or larvae (L-1)

Fecal Examination
• Lung flukes, *Capillaria*, and *Eucoleus*—may shed eggs into the feces
• Other lungworm eggs—usually hatch within the respiratory system; necessary to extract larva from feces via the Baermann method
• Multiple examinations often necessary; negative results do not rule out infection.

Rhinoscopy/Bronchoscopy
• Upper respiratory—examination via retrograde pharyngoscopy or rhinoscopy with antegrade flushing of anesthetic gas; often allows visualization of nasal mites; retrograde nasal lavage and cytologic examination of fluid may be helpful.
• Lower respiratory—may see tracheal and bronchial parasites and parasitic nodules; occasionally may be removed for definitive identification; bronchoalveolar lavage may allow extraction of larvae or worms from alveoli.
• May attempt anthelmintic response therapeutic trial

PATHOLOGIC FINDINGS
• Upper respiratory—may find nasal mites or worms in sinuses and nasal cavity
• Lower respiratory—may see pulmonary nodules throughout the parenchyma or within bronchi

TREATMENT

APPROPRIATE HEALTH CARE
Outpatient—upper and lower respiratory parasites; may need repeated examinations to monitor response

ACTIVITY
No restrictions unless severe pulmonary dysfunction occurs with upper or lower respiratory parasites

DIET
No special restrictions

CLIENT EDUCATION
• Explain that treatment response and duration depend on the type of parasite.
• Warn client of the risk of recurrence in dogs that maintain lifestyles conducive to transmission of the parasites (e.g., hunting, sporting dogs, and multidog households).

SURGICAL CONSIDERATIONS
N/A

MEDICATIONS

DRUG(S) OF CHOICE
• Anthelmintics—few studies confirm efficacy; most data anecdotal
• *Pneumonyssoides caninum*—ivermectin at 200–400 μg/kg SC, PO for 2 treatments 2 weeks apart; **NOTE:** not registered for use in dogs at this dosage; dosage contraindicated in collies, collie breeds, and Australian shepherds because of high incidence of toxicity; try pyrethrin/pyrethroid inhalation (e.g., Shelltox Ministrips) instead; milbemycin oxime at 0.5–1.0 mg/kg PO weekly for 3 weeks
• *Aelurostrongylus abstrusus*—fenbendazole at 50 mg/kg PO q24h for 4 days, repeat after 10 days; ivermectin at 200 μg/kg SC q24h for 3 days or PO for 5 days; **NOTE:** ivermectin not registered for use in cats at this dosage
• Other upper and lower respiratory parasites—fenbendazole at 50–100 mg/kg PO q24h for 7–14 days or longer with evidence of persistent infestation; variable success with ivermectin at 200 μg/kg every week for 2–4 treatments

• *Crenosoma vulpis*—reported to be susceptible to diethylcarbamazine (dosage unknown), fenbendazole at 50 mg/kg PO q24h for 7 days
• *Paragonimus kellicotti*—praziquantel at 25 mg/kg PO, SC for 3 days; fenbendazole at 50–100 mg/kg PO q24h for 10–14 days
• Antiinflammatory agents—generally not required; may reduce efficacy of anthelmintic

CONTRAINDICATIONS
Ivermectin—not registered for use in dogs or cats other than for heartworm prophylaxis; contraindicated at dosages > 50 μg/kg in breeds with known increased sensitivity (collies, collie breeds, and Australian shepherds)

PRECAUTIONS
Ivermectin—use caution when considering treatment with ivermectin; after administration at 200 μg/kg, observe for adverse side effects for 4–6 hr.

POSSIBLE INTERACTIONS
N/A

ALTERNATIVE DRUG(S)
N/A

FOLLOW-UP

PATIENT MONITORING
• Serial fecal Baermann larval extractions or examination for eggs—some anthelmintics may suppress egg or larval production in some species.
• Repeating bronchoscopic examination—may help assess efficacy of treatment for lower respiratory parasites
• Resolution of clinical signs—suggests response to treatment; does not indicate complete clearance of parasites
• Peripheral eosinophilia, if noted initially, may subside with treatment

PREVENTION AND AVOIDANCE
• Avoid activity that predisposes to infestations (often not practical).
• Avoid contact with wildlife reservoirs (especially wild canides).
• Consider prophylactic treatment for heartworm.

POSSIBLE COMPLICATIONS
• Chronic pulmonary damage—possible with persistent and heavy lower respiratory parasite burdens

• Infestations rarely fatal
• Nasal mites have been associated with gastric dilation and volvulus

EXPECTED COURSE AND PROGNOSIS
• With aggressive management—prognosis usually fair to excellent; variable
• Return to performance—depends on chronicity of disease and level of chronic pulmonary damage by lower respiratory parasites
• Recurrence possible

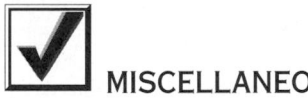

MISCELLANEOUS

ASSOCIATED CONDITIONS
N/A

AGE-RELATED FACTORS
N/A

ZOONOTIC POTENTIAL
N/A

PREGNANCY
N/A

SYNONYMS
• Lungworm infestation—*Aelurostrongylus, Capillaria, Crenosoma, Filaroides, Paragonimus*
• Nasal mite infestation—*Pneumonyssus caninum*

SEE ALSO
• Heartworm Disease—Cats
• Heartworm Disease—Dogs
• Pneumonia, Eosinophilic

Suggested Reading
Foreyt WJ. Veterinary parasitology reference manual. Pulman: Washington State University, Board of Regents, 1989.
Marks SL, Moore MP, Rishniw M. *Pneumonyssus caninum:* the canine nasal mite. Compend Contin Educ Pract Vet 1994;16:577–582.
Shaw DH, Conboy GA, Hogan PM, et al. Eosinophilic bronchitis caused by *Crenosoma vulpis* infection in dogs. Can Vet J 1996;37:361–363.
Soulsby EJL. Helminths, arthropods and protozoa of domesticated animals. 7th ed. Philadelphia: Lea & Febiger, 1982.
Urquhart GM, Armour J, Duncan JL, et al. Veterinary parasitology. UK: Longman Scientific, 1987. London, UK: Blackwell Science, 1996.
Author Mark Rishniw
Consulting Editor Lynelle R. Johnson

RETAINED PLACENTA

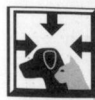 BASICS

OVERVIEW
• Dogs—placenta retained beyond the immediate postpartum period; placentas usually passed within 15 minutes of birth of a puppy; may develop acute metritis secondary to retained placenta
• Cats—may retain placentas for days without signs of illness
• Extremely uncommon

SIGNALMENT
• Dogs—most common in toy dog breeds
• Cats—rare

SIGNS

Historical Findings
• Recent parturition
• Continued vulvar discharge of lochia
• Owner may note number of placentas passed; not always reliable

Physical Examination Findings
• Green lochia vulvar discharge
• Palpation of firm mass in uterus—not always possible

CAUSES & RISK FACTORS
• Toy breed
• Large litter size
• Dystocia

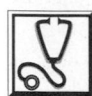 DIAGNOSIS

DIFFERENTIAL DIAGNOSIS
• Postpartum metritis—physical examination and vaginal cytologic examination show no signs of infection with uncomplicated condition; may develop concurrently
• Retained fetus—differentiated by radiography or ultrasonography

CBC/BIOCHEMISTRY/URINALYSIS
Usually normal when uncomplicated

OTHER LABORATORY TESTS
Vaginal cytologic examination—parabasal epithelial cells; may note erythrocytes; biliverdin clumps

IMAGING
Ultrasonography—echogenic but nonfetal mass within the uterus

DIAGNOSTIC PROCEDURES
Celiotomy or hysterotomy—may be required for diagnosis

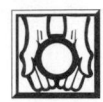 TREATMENT

• Outpatient for healthy bitch or queen
• Instruct owner to monitor temperature and observe for signs of systemic illness.
• Ovariohysterectomy—curative; recommend if future breeding is not a consideration
• Surgical removal—indicated if medical treatment is unsuccessful and the bitch develops metritis

MEDICATIONS

DRUG(S)
• Oxytocin—known or suspected condition in otherwise healthy cats and dogs; dogs, 0.5 U/kg IM up to 20 U; cats, 0.5–3.0 U IM)
• May precede oxytocin treatment with calcium gluconate (10%); dogs, 3–10 ml IV, given slowly
• Metritis—treat accordingly (see Metritis)

CONTRAINDICATIONS/POSSIBLE INTERACTIONS
Do not give progestational drugs

 FOLLOW-UP

• Monitor temperature and physical condition
• Acute metritis (dogs)—may develop if the placenta is not passed; fair to good prognosis for recovery with treatment
• Prognosis for future reproduction—good without metritis; fair to poor with metritis

 MISCELLANEOUS

SEE ALSO
Metritis

Suggested Reading
Feldman EC, Nelson RW. Canine and feline endocrinology and reproduction, 2nd ed. Philadelphia: Saunders, 1996:586–675.
Author Joni L. Freshman
Consulting Editor Sara K. Lyle

RETINAL DEGENERATION

BASICS

DEFINITION
• Degeneration of the retina from any cause, inherited or acquired • Inherited—generalized PRA; a group of progressive retinal diseases; may be subdivided into photoreceptor dysplasias (begin before the retina fully develops, < 12 weeks) and photoreceptor degenerations (begin after the retina matures)

PATHOPHYSIOLOGY
• A number of genetic defects in photoreceptor metabolism have been identified. • May be secondary to retinal pigment epithelial or choroidal disease (central PRA, ornithine deficiency, and the mucopolysaccharidoses) • Also may be idiopathic, secondary to diffuse or focal inflammation and scarring (e.g., chorioretinitis), nutritional deficiency, or previous retinal detachment

SYSTEMS AFFECTED
Ophthalmic

GENETICS

Dogs
• PRA—autosomal recessive in most breeds, especially collies, Irish setters, miniature poodles, cocker spaniels, and Labrador retrievers • Central PRA—autosomal dominant with incomplete penetrance in Labrador retrievers • Inheritance in many breeds not determined • Neuronal ceroid lipofuscinosis—autosomal recessive (proven or presumed) in most breeds studied • Hemeralopia—autosomal recessive cone dysplasia in Alaskan malamutes; undetermined inheritance in miniature poodles

Cats
• Rod–cone dysplasia (Abyssinians)—autosomal dominant: clinical signs at 4 months; autosomal recessive: may be blind by 2 years • Also may have later onset of 2 years, vision problems by 4 years • Isolated reports of both dominant and reces-sive inheritance in young Persians and domestic shorthair cats • Gyrate atrophy—autosomal recessive; ornithine aminotransferase deficiency

INCIDENCE/PREVALENCE
• Hereditary—prevalence greater in dogs than in cats • Taurine deficiency—uncommon now that cat foods are appropriately supplemented

GEOGRAPHIC DISTRIBUTION
Central PRA—more common in dogs from Europe than from the United States

SIGNALMENT

Species
Dogs and cats

Breed Predilections
Hereditary—Dogs (many breeds) • Retinal dysplasia—Bedlington terrier, Sealyham terrier, English springer spaniel, cocker spaniel, and others. • Early-onset

PRA—Irish setters; collies; Norwegian elkhounds; miniature schnauzers; Belgian shepherds • Late-onset PRA—miniature and toy poodles; American and English cocker spaniels; Labrador retrievers; Tibetan terriers; miniature longhair dachshunds; akitas; Samoyeds • Central PRA—Labradors; golden retrievers; border collies; collies; Shetland sheepdogs; Briards; others • Neuronal ceroid lipofuscinosis—English setters; Dalmatians; Tibetan terriers; collies • SARD—Brittany spaniels; miniature schnauzer; dachshunds Hereditary—Cats • Abyssinians • Siamese • Persians • Domestic shorthairs

Mean Age and Range
• Early PRA and dystrophies—3–4 months to 2 years • Late PRA—clinical signs > 4–6 years • SARD—middle-aged to old

Predominant Sex
• PRA—none, except possibly X-linked recessive condition in Siberian huskies • SARD—70% are female

SIGNS

Historical Findings
• PRA (dog)—a gradually progressing nyctalopia (night blindness) that ultimately affects vision in bright light; may note dilated pupils or brighter tapetal reflex at night; may appear to be acutely blind (when patient finally becomes totally blind or is moved to unfamiliar surroundings) • Hemeralopia—rare; cones degenerate; day vision lost • Central PRA (dogs)—rare in the US; central vision lost; may never become completely blind; may have difficulty locating stationary objects in bright light (especially hunting breeds) • SARD—vision lost in 1–4 weeks; polyuria, polydipsia, and polyphagia common

Physical Examination Findings
• If severe—direct and consensual pupillary light reflexes impaired or nearly abolished • Tapetal hyperreflectivity and nontapetal depigmentation or mottled hyperpigmentation; eventually, retinal blood vessel attenuation and optic nerve atrophy • PRA (dogs)—cataracts common • SARD (dogs)—obesity; hepatomegaly; may note slow or absent pupillary light reflexes • Taurine-deficient retinopathy (cats)—begins as a spot in area centralis; then horizontal band forms superior to the optic nerve; finally, diffuse degeneration and hyperreflectivity • Postinflammatory retinal scars—focal or multifocal lesions manifest as areas of tapetal hyperreflectivity or altered pigmentation • Retinal dysplasia may be associated with Samoyeds and Laborador Retrievers. • Retinal dysplasia may also be associated with multiple other ocular anomalies in Akitas, Doberman pinschers.

CAUSES

Degenerative
• PRA—genetic; affects both eyes symmetrically • Chronic or uncontrolled glaucoma—

retinal and optic nerve atrophy • Secondary to scarring from previous multifocal or diffuse retinal detachment or inflammation

Anomalous
• Rod–cone photoreceptor dysplasias—genetically inherited; affect both eyes • Other dysplasias—may be multifocal and non-blinding (e.g., in English springer spaniels and Labrador retrievers)

Metabolic
• Mucopolysaccharidosis—mixed-breed dogs; Siamese and domestic shorthair cats • Ornithine aminotransferase deficiency—a mitochondrial enzyme; progressive and total gyrate atrophy of the choroid and retina

Neoplastic
• Neoplastic cell infiltrate • Scars from previous retinal detachment if treated

Nutritional
• Severe deficiency of vitamin E or A (dogs and cats)—experimentally may cause partial or complete degeneration • Taurine deficiency (cats)—causes retinal degeneration and dilated cardiomyopathy

Infectious/Immune
See Retinal Detachment; Chorioretinitis

Idiopathic
• SARD—dogs; • See Retinal Detachment; Chorioretinitis

Toxic
• Idiosyncratic reaction to griseofulvin or enrofloxacin (cats). • Concurrent administration of ketamine hydrochloride and methylnitrosourea induces diffuse degeneration (cats).

RISK FACTORS
• Ocular disease—cataracts; posterior segment inflammation; chorioretinitis; retinal detachment; glaucoma • Taurine-deficient diet—dog food fed to cats • Heredity • Cats—enrofloxacin dose should not exceed 5 mg/kg/day. Toxicity noted at lower doses

DIAGNOSIS

DIFFERENTIAL DIAGNOSIS
• See Blind Quiet Eye • Acute vision loss—pupillary light reflex slow or absent: SARD, optic neuritis, retinal detachment, unrecognized PRA, or glaucoma; pupillary light reflex normal: rapidly developing diabetic cataracts or visual cortex disease • Slowly progressive visual loss—PRA; cataracts; severe corneal disease (e.g., pigmentation, scarring, or edema); chronic retinitis; chorioretinitis; vitreal inflammation (e.g., posterior uveitis); differentiated by ophthalmic examination

CBC/BIOCHEMISTRY/URINALYSIS
• Usually normal, unless secondary to a systemic disease • SARD (dogs)—results may be consistent with hyperadrenocorticism, which patient may have

OTHER LABORATORY TESTS
• ACTH-stimulation and dexamethasone-suppression tests—with SARD; • Taurine concentration (cats)—diffuse degeneration, especially with dilated cardiomyopathy
• Serum and urine (may collect on dry filter paper) ornithine concentrations (cats)—elevated with ornithine aminotransferase deficiency

Genetic Testing
• Genetic testing on blood samples—OptiGen® LLC provides genetic testing on blood samples for several varieties of genetically inherited eye diseases and some other metabolic diseases. New tests for a variety of breeds are steadily being developed. Details on tests available, samples needed, and how to interpret test results may be found at *www.Optigen.com* or contact Optigen at Cornell Business & Technology Park, 767 Warren Road, Suite 300, Ithaca, New York 14850. Telephone: 607-257-0301.
• Test results often allow identification of affected, nonaffected, and probable carriers with good confidence. Results can help direct breedings to avoid getting affected dogs.

IMAGING
• Thoracic radiographs and cardiac ultrasound (cats)—may be indicated with suspected taurine-deficient condition • Abdominal radiographs and ultrasound (dogs)—may be indicated with SARD • CT or MRI—occasionally used to rule out causes of central blindness (e.g., optic nerve damage, cortical blindness, and SARD with pituitary adenoma)

DIAGNOSTIC PROCEDURES
• Complete ophthalmic examination
• Electroretinography confirms blindness not apparent on ophthalmoscopy; minimal or no response with severe condition (SARD, late PRA); normal with optic neuritis and CNS blindness

PATHOLOGIC FINDINGS
• Thin retina • Edges of focal retinal scars—sharply delineated; course of blood vessels not altered • Hyperpigmented areas—associated with postinflammatory scars or central PRA
• Histologic characteristics of end-stage degenerations—marked photoreceptor atrophy; generalized reduction in retinal cell destiny • Lipopigment accumulated in the neuroepithelium—central PRA

 TREATMENT

DIET
Cats—food should contain 500–750 ppm taurine.

CLIENT EDUCATION
• Patient visually impaired—inform client that the condition is irreversible but nonpainful. • Advise client that blind dogs should be watched or kept on a leash if they are outside, not in fenced yards, or in an area with a pool. • Suggest playing with toys that make sounds. • Inform client that dogs can memorize their environment and that unless the family moves or rearranges the furniture, most blind animals function well. • Suggest applying perfume to legs of furniture to help the patient memorize the environment and identify the location of objects. • Warn client that some old blind animals with other problems such as hearing loss or senility may not adapt well to blindness. • Warn client that some blind animals experience behavioral changes such as increased aggression or reduced activity. • Assure clients that animals with only one blind eye can function normally. • Blind cats may adapt better than dogs but should probably be kept indoors.

SURGICAL CONSIDERATIONS
Not indicated in patients with blind, nonpainful *eyes*

 MEDICATIONS

DRUG(S)
• None currently effective • Pyridoxine supplementation (cats)—for ornithine aminotransferase deficiency; may increase activity of the enzyme; has not clinically arrested or reversed degeneration • Adequate dietary taurine—may halt the progression of the taurine-deficient retinopathy

CONTRAINDICATIONS
N/A

PRECAUTIONS
Cataract surgery—do not perform in patients with retinal degeneration; electroretinography is useful for avoiding unnecessary surgery.

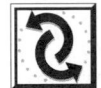 **FOLLOW-UP**

PATIENT MONITORING
• Serial fundic examinations—at 3–6-month intervals; confirm progressive degeneration if the diagnosis is in doubt; will note obvious signs of degeneration over weeks in the retinas of dogs with SARD • Developing and progressing cataracts—with PRA; watch for painful complications (e.g., glaucoma and uveitis).

PREVENTION/AVOIDANCE
• Do not breed animals suspected of having inherited PRA. • Do not breed known carriers (e.g., offspring of an affected animal).

POSSIBLE COMPLICATIONS
• Cataracts • Glaucoma • Uveitis • Ocular trauma as a result of visual impairment—corneal trauma with ulceration or perforation • Obesity—secondary to reduced activity

EXPECTED COURSE AND PROGNOSIS
• Inherited PRA—progresses to complete blindness; progression often slow enough for patient to adapt to visual loss; nonpainful
• Degeneration from previous inflammation or trauma—usually does not progress unless a systemic disease causes persistent (e.g., uveodermatologic syndrome) or recurrent ocular inflammation (e.g., blastomycosis and toxoplasmosis) • SARD—irreversible blindness • Transient taurine deficiency (cats)—degeneration may halt at any stage (e.g., a horizontal hyperreflective band over the optic nerve).

 **MISCELLANEOUS**

ASSOCIATED CONDITIONS
SARD—adrenal or pituitary hyperadrenocorticism

AGE-RELATED FACTORS
N/A

ZOONOTIC POTENTIAL
N/A

PREGNANCY
N/A

SYNONYMS
• PRA—progressive rod–cone degeneration; retinal atrophy, retinal dystrophy; dysplasia
• Taurine-deficient retinopathy—previously called feline central retinal degeneration

SEE ALSO
• Blind Quiet Eye • Chorioretinitis • Retinal Detachment

ABBREVIATIONS
• ACTH = adrenocorticotropic hormone
• CNS = central nervous system • CT = computed tomography • MRI = magnetic resonance imaging • PRA = progressive retinal atrophy • PRD = photoreceptor dysplasia, retinal dystrophy • SARD = sudden acquired retinal degeneration

Suggested Reading
Gelatt KN, van der Woerlt A, Ketring KL, et al. Enrofloxacin-associated retinal degeneration in cats. Vet Ophthalmol 2001;4(2):99–106.
Narfström K, Ekesten B. Diseases of the canine ocular fundus. In: Gelatt KN, ed. Veterinary ophthalmology. 3rd ed. Philadelphia: Lippincott Williams & Wilkins, 1999;869–933.
Author Patricia J. Smith
Consulting Editor Paul E. Miller

RETINAL DETACHMENT

 BASICS

DEFINITION
Any separation of the neural retina from the RPE at the outer segment–neuroepithelium interface

PATHOPHYSIOLOGY
• Subretinal space—potential space between the RPE and neural retina in which fluid or exudates accumulate • Characterized by its etiopathogenesis—one or a combination of rhegmatogenous (retinal tear), subretinal exudation, or traction
Rhegmatogenous
• A tear that may be related to age, cataracts, or retinal degeneration • Allows vitreous to move into the subretinal space and results in detachment • Probably the predominant type that occurs in association with cataracts and after cataract surgery • Usually requires some vitreous abnormality (e.g., liquefaction)
Exudative
• Fluid accumulates in the subretinal space because of breakdown of the blood–retinal barrier. • Fluid—may be serous, hemorrhagic, or exudative (e.g., granulomatous in patients with blastomycosis chorioretinitis) • Hematogenous pathogenetic factors—common • Vasculitis, hypertension, and hyperviscosity—may cause serous detachment with or without hemorrhage

Traction
• Traction on the retina—usually by fibrous or fibrovascular tissue; raises the retina from the underlying RPE • Occurs after trauma or inflammation

SYSTEMS AFFECTED
• Ophthalmic—retina • Nervous—vision may be severely compromised or permanently lost. • May be manifestation of a systemic disease

GENETICS
• Depends on cause—dogs with hereditary cataracts or lens luxations may develop rhegmatogenous detachment. Some breeds (Shih tzu, poodle) may have a problem of retinal tear and detachment from primary vitreous.

INCIDENCE/PREVALENCE
• Exudative—most common in dogs and cats • Rhegmatogenous—more common in dogs than in cats because of the greater prevalence of cataracts and cataract surgery

SIGNALMENT
Species
Dogs and cats
Breed Predilections
• Depends on cause • Terrier breeds—predisposed to primary lens luxation, which may contribute to retinal tear and detachment with or without surgery • Breeds that develop cataracts • Shih tzus—appear to be predis-

posed to spontaneous rhegmatogenous detachments owing to abnormal vitreous (significant vitreous liquefaction)

Mean Age and Range
• Depends on cause • More common in old patients—cataracts and systemic diseases (e.g., hypertension, neoplasia, and immune-mediated disease) are often age-related

Predominant Sex
N/A

SIGNS
• Blindness or reduced vision • Dilated pupil with slow or no pupillary light reflex • Blood vessels or a membrane is usually observed easily through the pupil just behind the lens. • Vitreous abnormalities—liquefaction, hemorrhage, or syneresis (liquefaction); common • Interruption or alteration of the course of blood vessels owing to retinal elevation • With clear subretinal fluid—vessels may cast shadows on the tapetum or RPE • Depend on any underlying systemic diseases • See Chorioretinitis for signs of inflammation.

CAUSES
• Bilateral—suggests a systemic problem • Toxic—idiosyncratic reactions to drugs (e.g., trimethoprim-sulfa in dogs, griseofulvin in cats)
Degenerative
• End-stage progressive retinal atrophy (degeneration)—may lead to retinal hole formation and detachment • Chronic glaucoma with globe stretching and retinal thinning
Anomalous
• Optic nerve colobomas—Collie eye anomaly • Multiple ocular anomalies—Akitas or any breed • Severe retinal dysplasia—oculoskeletal dysplasia in Labrador retrievers, Samoyeds, English springer spaniels, and Bedlington terriers • RPE dysplasia—Australian shepherds • Congential ocular defect—any young animal; congenital or juvenile retinal detachment
Metabolic
• Systemic hypertension • Hypothyroidism • Hyperviscosity • Polycythemia • Hypoxia with hemorrhagic complications • Dogs—renal failure or pheochromocytoma with systemic hypertension, hypothyroidism, hypercholesterolemia, and hyperproteinemia (e.g., with multiple myeloma) • Bilateral (cats)—probably most often caused by systemic hypertension either as a primary condition or secondary to renal failure or hyperthyroidism
Neoplastic
• Any primary or metastatic neoplasm • Commonly associated with multiple myeloma, lymphosarcoma, granulomatous meningoencephalitis, and intraocular masses—ciliary body adenocarcinoma or melanoma
Infectious
• Infectious retinitis or chorioretinitis—may cause focal or diffuse detachment • Infection may extend from or to the

CNS—see Chorioretinitis.
Immune-mediated/Inflammatory
• Immune complex disease—may cause vasculitis or inflammation that may result in exudative detachment • Dogs—SLE; uveodermatologic syndrome • Cats—periarteritis nodosa; SLE
Idiopathic
• If all other causes are ruled out, including retinal tears • Idiopathic steroid-responsive detachment—reported in giant-breed dogs, but may occur in any breed
Trauma
• Bilateral—probably never occurs • Penetrating injury or foreign body that causes retinal tears or intraocular hemorrhage—may cause partial or complete detachment • Severe blunt trauma with inflammation or hemorrhage • Surgical trauma—may contribute to retinal tearing

RISK FACTORS
• Systemic hypertension • Old age • Hypermature cataracts • Luxated lenses • Extracapsular or intracapsular lens extraction

 DIAGNOSIS

DIFFERENTIAL DIAGNOSIS
• Ophthalmic examination—usually sufficient for diagnosis • Blindness or impaired vision—optic neuritis; glaucoma; cataracts; progressive retinal atrophy; SARDS; CNS disease • Dilated pupil with slow or absent pupillary light reflexes—glaucoma; oculomotor nerve lesion; optic neuritis; progressive retinal atrophy; SARDS • Membrane or vessels associated with or behind lens—persistent tunica vasculosa lentis; persistent pupillary membranes; fibrovascular membrane secondary to intraocular neoplasia or inflammation

CBC/BIOCHEMISTRY/URINALYSIS
• Typically normal if the problem is confined to the eye • Abnormalities consistent with an associated systemic disease process

OTHER LABORATORY TESTS
• Depend on suspected systemic problem • Protein electrophoresis • Documentation of Bence-Jones protein in urine • Coagulation profile • Bacterial culture of ocular or body fluids • Thyroid hormone measurement • Serologic testing for infectious diseases—see Chorioretinitis.

IMAGING
• Thoracic radiograph—search for lymphadenopathy, metastatic disease, or infiltrates consistent with infectious agents. • Radiographs of the spine—may reveal bony changes consistent with multiple myeloma • Ocular ultrasound—identify retinal detach-

ments, intraocular masses, and sometimes lens luxations; especially helpful if the ocular media is not clear • Cardiac ultrasound (cats)—may be indicated with hypertensive retinopathy

DIAGNOSTIC PROCEDURES

• Single or repeated blood pressure measurement—may reveal hypertension; mean arterial pressure in dogs and cats usually < 160 mm Hg • CSF tap—indicated with signs of CNS disease or optic neuritis • Vitreocentesis or subretinal fluid aspirate—may be performed if other diagnostic tests failed to yield a cause and an infectious agent or neoplasia is suspected; may aggravate the inflammation or induce hemorrhage, which may lessen the chance of the retina reattaching and restoring vision

PATHOLOGIC FINDINGS

• Retina separated from the RPE and underlying choroid
• May note masses or subretinal exudate
• Chronic—results in retinal atrophy and a tombstone appearance to the RPE

TREATMENT

APPROPRIATE HEALTH CARE

• Depends on the physical condition of the patient
• Usually outpatient
• Acute blindness—vision may be restored if the underlying cause is rapidly identified and treated; make every attempt to determine the cause.
• Degeneration occurs rapidly—provide therapy, whether surgical or medical, as soon as possible after diagnosis.
• Rhegmatogenous—an ophthalmologist may be able to provide surgical treatment.

NURSING CARE

As appropriate for any associated systemic disease; see Retinal Degeneration.

ACTIVITY

• Restrict until reattachment has occurred.
• Supervise irreversibly blind patients.

DIET

N/A

CLIENT EDUCATION

• Explain that retinal detachment (especially if bilateral) may be a sign of systemic disease, so diagnostic testing is important.
• Inform client that retinal detachment associated with lens luxation or cataract surgery has a bilateral potential, so both eyes should be observed closely.
• Inform client that retinal detachments may be reversible with return of vision if the underlying cause is treated and the detachment is caught early.
• Advise client that blind pets, especially cats,

can adapt remarkably well and live a good quality life (see Retinal Degeneration).

SURGICAL CONSIDERATIONS

• Rhegmatogenous—may be surgically repaired; refer patient to an ophthalmologist.
• Laser retinopexy—may reverse detachments associated with optic disk colobomas with Collie eye anomaly; may stabilize partial/small detachments

MEDICATIONS

DRUG(S) OF CHOICE

• Depend on underlying systemic causes, which should be identified and treated appropriately
• Systemic prednisone—2 mg/kg divided q12h for 3–10 days, then taper; if systemic mycosis is ruled out and the detachment is believed to be immune-mediated; may facilitate retinal reattachment; for immune-mediated disease, taper medications very slowly over months.
• Antiinflammatory doses of prednisone—0.5 mg/kg, then taper; may be useful for exudative detachments of an infectious nature as long as the underlying disease is being definitively treated
• Antihypertensive agents—amlodipine 0.25 mg/kg PO q24h in dogs and cats, others such as propranolol can be used if amlodipine fails to control hypertension. Higher doses of amlodipine can be tolerated in certain individuals.

CONTRAINDICATIONS

Systemic corticosteroids—do not use unless systemic mycosis is ruled out or is being definitively treated.

PRECAUTIONS

N/A

POSSIBLE INTERACTIONS

N/A

ALTERNATIVE DRUG(S)

• Chemotherapeutic agents—suggested for treatment of neoplastic conditions (e.g., lymphosarcoma or multiple myeloma)
• Azathioprine (dogs)—2 mg/kg preoperatively q24h initially, then 0.5–1 mg/kg q48h; to control inflammation; may be required in addition to steroids for uveodermatologic syndrome or idiopathic immune-mediated detachment; avoid in cats.

FOLLOW-UP

PATIENT MONITORING

• Depends on underlying cause and type of medical treatment • Azathioprine—obtain an initial CBC, then every 1–2 weeks for the first 1–3 months; monitor every 1–2 months

for bone marrow suppression (if noted, reduce the dose or discontinue). • Monitor blood pressure in hypertensive cases

PREVENTION/AVOIDANCE

N/A

POSSIBLE COMPLICATIONS

• Permanent blindness • Cataracts • Glaucoma • Chronic ocular pain • Death if secondary to a systemic disease process

EXPECTED COURSE AND PROGNOSIS

• Prognosis for vision with complete detachment—guarded • Blindness—may develop in days to weeks even if reattachment occurs (earlier with exudative than with serous detachments) • Vision may return if the underlying cause is removed and reattachment occurs. • Focal or multifocal chorioretinitis—does not markedly impair vision; will leave scars • Systemic disease or neoplasia with ocular manifestations—may influence the prognosis for life

MISCELLANEOUS

ASSOCIATED CONDITIONS

• Exudative—systemic disease • Cataracts • Trauma • Traction and/or rhegmatogenous—vitreal hemorrhage or inflammation

AGE-RELATED FACTORS

N/A

PREGNANCY

N/A

SEE ALSO

• Blind Quiet Eye • Chorioretinitis • Retinal Degeneration

ABBREVIATIONS

• CSF = cerebrospinal fluid • CNS = central nervous system • RPE = retinal pigment epithelium • SARD = sudden acquired retinal degeneration • SLE = systemic lupus erythematosus

Suggested Reading

Gelatt KN, ed. Veterinary ophthalmology. 3rd ed. Philadelphia: Lippincott Williams & Wilkins, 1999.

Mathor S, Syme H, Brown CA, et al. Effects of the calcium channel blocker amlodipine in cats with surgically induced hypertensive renal insufficiency. AJVR 2002;63(6): 833–839.

Millichamp NJ, Dziezyc J. Small animal ophthalmology. Vet Clin North Am Small Anim Pract 1990;20:564.

Author Patricia J. Smith
Consulting Editor Paul E. Miller

RETINAL HEMORRHAGE

 BASICS

DEFINITION
• Focal or generalized areas of bleeding into part or all layers of the retina
• May be acute or chronic

PATHOPHYSIOLOGY
• Depends on cause
• May result from a variety of causes
• Trauma-induced retinal detachments—may tear retinal blood vessels
• Often involved in congenital malformations, concurrent vascular abnormalities, and neo-vascularization syndromes
• May note a retinopathy in conjunction with diabetes mellitus—includes the formation of vascular microaneurysms with accompanying hemorrhage or exudation
• Intoxications, systemic clotting, neoplastic disorders, systemic fungal disease—may cause focal or more widespread hemorrhage
• Systemic hypertension and immune-mediated diseases (e.g., those causing anemia)—may cause local hemorrhage in conjunction with vascular abnormalities and/or complete or partial retinal detachments

SYSTEMS AFFECTED
Ophthalmic

SIGNALMENT
• Any breed, age, or sex
• Cause may have a genetic basis and be highly breed and age specific—young collies with collie eye anomaly; Labrador retrievers with congenital vitreoretinal dysplasia
• Hereditary breed-specific congenital defects that might cause detachment or severe retinal dysplasia—collies and shelties with collie eye anomaly; Labradors, Sealyhams, Bedlington terriers, and springer spaniels with retinal dysplasia

SIGNS
Historical findings
• Often none
• Vision loss
• Bumping into objects

Physical Examination Findings
• Depend on underlying cause
• Evidence of bleeding elsewhere—petechia; ecchymoses; melena; hematuria
• Leukocoria (whitish appearing pupil) with or without reddish coloration behind the lens
• Absent of menace response
• Abnormal pupillary responses

CAUSES
Congenital
• Retinal detachment secondary to congenital malformation
• Vitreoretinal dysplasia

Acquired
• Trauma
• Systemic hypertension (especially old cats)—renal disease; cardiac disease; hyperthyroidism; hyperadrenocorticism; idiopathic
• Intoxication—dicumarol; paracetamol; sulfonamide; Estradurin
• Systemic mycosis—cryptococcosis
• Neoplasia—lymphosarcoma
• Plasma cell myeloma
• Hematologic disorders—blood-clotting disorder (von Willebrand disease); severe anemia; thrombocytopenia; monoclonal gammopathy and hyperviscosity syndrome
• Diabetic retinopathy
• Retinal detachment

RISK FACTORS
• Systemic hypertension
• Hematologic

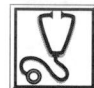 DIAGNOSIS

DIFFERENTIAL DIAGNOSIS
Signs
• Reddish coloration of the pupil—may indicate vitreal hemorrhage; impossible to rule out concurrent retinal hemorrhage
• Generalized or local blurring or lack of fundus detail—usually no reddish coloration without vitreal or retinal hemorrhage

Causes (Vitreal Hemorrhage)
• Young dogs—may be associated with abnormal persistence of the hyaloid vascular system (e.g., hereditary PHTVL/PHPV and some forms of multiple developmental ocular anomalies)
• Neoplasia
• Lens luxation
• Uveitis
• Glaucoma
• Severe inflammatory changes in the vitreous—associated with ocular infections due to penetrating injuries, foreign bodies, and spread from local or systemic diseases (e.g., systemic mycosis)

CBC/BIOCHEMISTRY/URINALYSIS
• Usually normal unless secondary to a systemic disease

• Hyperglycemia and/or glucosuria—may note with diabetic retinopathy
• High BUN or serum creatinine and proteinuria—common in cats with retinal detachment and hemorrhage secondary to systemic hypertension

OTHER LABORATORY TESTS
Complete workup—suspected systemic disease; includes thyroid and adrenal endocrine tests, serologic tests for infectious agents, and immune studies

IMAGING
Ocular ultrasound—may demonstrate retinal detachment

DIAGNOSTIC PROCEDURES
• Ophthalmic examination with a penlight—usually permits diagnosis of complete retinal detachment with partial retinal hemorrhage; detached neuroretina may often be visualized through the pupil as a whitish veil of tissue.
• Indirect ophthalmoscopy—diagnosis of funduscopic and vitreal changes; may evaluate depth of the hemorrhage by its shape and color; preretinal (between the external limiting membrane and the vitreous body): often shaped as a boat keel and light red; intraretinal: more rounded and darker
• Vitreous paracentesis and cytologic examination—aid in the diagnosis for suspected neoplasia
• Blood pressure measurement—indicated in all patients with severe retinal and vitreal hemorrhage

 TREATMENT

• Usually initially treated as inpatients—sometimes in intensive care for maximal follow-up
• Intoxications—often require specific treatment
• Consider referral for a more detailed ophthalmic examination, including ultrasound, before attempting empirical therapy.
• Retinal detachment—cage rest until the retina is reattached
• Discuss euthanasia for severe bilateral hemorrhage in young pups with congenital abnormalities (of the breeds listed under Signalment)
• Advise client that unilaterally affected dogs can function as pets but should not be used for breeding, a fact not always obvious to the owner.
• Surgery—for some forms of retinal detachment; refer patient to an ophthalmologist.

MEDICATIONS

DRUG(S) OF CHOICE
• Depend on underlying cause
• Systemic corticosteroids—workup is declined and infectious disease is unlikely; prednisolone (1–2 mg/kg/day for 7–14 days, then taper; long-term treatment up to 4–6 weeks); especially for retinal detachment as a sequela to trauma
• Chloramphenicol or other systemic broad-spectrum antibiotic—suspected infectious disease; may be administered concurrently with corticosteroids
• Primary systemic hypertension—treat as required; often combined with corticosteroid treatment (as above), diuretics (e.g., furosemide, 3–4 mg/kg/day for 5–7 days), and calcium channel blockers
• Oral azathioprine—1–2 mg/kg/day up to a week, then taper; for immune-mediated retinal detachments; combine with systemic corticosteroids; perform a CBC, platelet count, and liver enzyme analysis every 2 weeks for the first 2 months, then periodically.
• Itraconazole—for cryptococcosis or other deep fungal infection; see Cryptococcosis or appropriate systemic mycosis

CONTRAINDICATIONS
• Systemic corticosteroids and other immuno-suppressive drugs—do not use in manifest infectious processes in the posterior segment of the eye
• Systemic NSAIDs—contraindicated with bleeding disorders, impaired renal function, or preexisting hypersensitivities; predispose patient to gastrointestinal ulceration

PRECAUTIONS
NSAIDs—flunixin meglumine and aspirin commonly used but may exacerbate bleeding; either may be administered to control intraocular inflammation in dogs. Use with caution in cats (see Contraindications).

POSSIBLE INTERACTIONS
N/A

ALTERNATIVE DRUG(S)
• Flunixin meglumine—0.5 mg/kg IV; single dose; may be used in dogs if infectious causes have not been ruled out
• Oral azathioprine—may be used in immune-mediated fundus disease; see Drug(s) of Choice

FOLLOW-UP

PATIENT MONITORING
• Repeated monitoring—required to ensure that condition subsides and retinal morphology normalizes
• Preretinal hemorrhages—usually absorbed within a few weeks to several months if localized
• Larger or repeated hemorrhages—may be followed by fibroblastic processes; may lead to the formation of fibrous preretinal membranes and vitreoretinal adhesions, which may cause vitreoretinal traction and retinal detachment
• Intraretinal hemorrhage—resorbed within several weeks to months; may produce retinal scarring

POSSIBLE COMPLICATIONS
• Blindness
• Impaired vision
• Chronic uveitis
• Glaucoma

MISCELLANEOUS

ASSOCIATED CONDITIONS
• Trauma—may often note concurrent lesions in other parts of the eye or body
• Hypertension—cardiac, renal disease, hyperthyroidism, or hyperadrenocorticism—common; may cause systemic medical problems that must be monitored
• Intoxication—often a generalized bleeding disorder affecting other organs
• *Cryptococcus* infection—often causes concurrent leptomeningitis and pneumonitis

• Lymphosarcoma—may affect several parts of the body; fatal disease
• Hematologic disorders—cause systemic disease; symptoms depend on pathophysiology; anemia and recurrent bleeding common
• Secondary cataracts—may develop within weeks after the onset of diabetes mellitus in dogs

AGE-RELATED FACTORS
• May occur at any age
• May be a sequela to congenital diseases (usually have a hereditary background) or to developmental disease processes (see Causes)

ZOONOTIC POTENTIAL
N/A

PREGNANCY
Corticosteroids and immunosuppressive drugs may cause complications.

SEE ALSO
• Chorioretinitis
• Hypertension, Systemic
• Hyphema
• Retinal Detachment

ABBREVIATIONS
NSAID = nonsteroidal antiinflammatory drug
PHPV = persistent hyperplastic primary vitreous
PHTVL = persistent hyperplastic tunica vasculosa lentis

Suggested Reading
Narfström K, Eksten B. Diseases of the canine ocular fundus. In: Gelatt KN ed., Veterinary ophthalmology. 3rd ed. Philadelphia: Lippincott Williams & Wilkins: 1999:869–933.
Peiffer RL, Petersen-Jones SM. Small animal ophthalmology. A problem-oriented approach. London: Saunders, 1997.
Petersen-Jones SM, Crispin SM. Manual of small animal ophthalmology. Gloucestershire, UK: British Small Animal Veterinary Association, 1993.

Author Kristina Narfström
Consulting Editor Paul E. Miller

RHABDOMYOMA

BASICS

OVERVIEW
- An extremely rare, benign, striated muscle tumor that occurs only half as frequently as its malignant counterpart
- Cardiac—usual site; probably congenital; exhibits no potential for malignant transformation
- Extracardiac—very rare; reported in the tongue and larynx in dogs and pinna in cats

SIGNALMENT
- Dogs and cats
- Extracardiac—affects mostly middle-aged animals
- No sex or breed predilections identified

SIGNS
- Cardiac—none; rarely, signs of right-sided congestive heart failure
- Extracardiac—localized swelling

CAUSES & RISK FACTORS
Unknown

DIAGNOSIS

DIFFERENTIAL DIAGNOSIS

Cardiac Location
- Rhabdomyosarcoma
- Lymphosarcoma
- Hemangioma or hemangiosarcoma
- Fibroma or fibrosarcoma
- Chondroma
- Myxoma
- Myxofibroma
- Mesothelioma
- Neurofibroma
- Teratoma
- Lipofibroma
- Lymphangioendothelioma
- Mixed spindle cell sarcoma

Skeletal Muscle Location
- Rhabdomyosarcoma
- Lipoma or liposarcoma
- Mast cell tumor
- Fibrosarcoma
- Nonneoplastic, inflammatory disease

Lingual Location
- Squamous cell carcinoma
- Granular cell myoblastoma
- Rhabdomyosarcoma
- Malignant melanoma
- Mast cell tumor
- Fibrosarcoma

Laryngeal Location
- Oncocytoma
- Rhabdomyosarcoma
- Extramedullary plasmacytoma
- Osteosarcoma
- Chondrosarcoma
- Fibrosarcoma
- Mast cell tumor
- Squamous cell carcinoma

CBC/BIOCHEMISTRY/URINALYSIS
Normal

OTHER LABORATORY TESTS
N/A

IMAGING
- Radiography—generally reveals soft tissue density; not helpful with extracardiac forms
- Echocardiography (cardiac)—may reveal a pedunculated mass or an infiltrative mass, most often affecting the cardiac ventricles; the interventricular septum appears to be the most common site

DIAGNOSTIC PROCEDURES
- ECG—arrhythmias may be noted
- Biopsy
- Cytologic examination of an aspirate—occasionally suggests a mesenchymal neoplasm; usually does not afford a definitive diagnosis

PATHOLOGIC FINDINGS
- Useful immunohistochemical markers—vimentin, actin, desmin, and myoglobin; differentiate striated muscle neoplasms from other spindle cell neoplasms
- Embryonic disease—actin is considered the most reliable marker because embryonic rhabdomyoblasts stain positive for actin before staining positive for desmin
- May be difficult to differentiate from other eosinophilic granular cell neoplasms; oncocytoma of larynx
- Transmission election microscopy may also be helpful for differentiating these tumors.

TREATMENT
- Cardiac—none
- Extracardiac—surgical excision
- Partial glossectomy involving 40%–60% of the tongue is well tolerated by dogs.
- Unlike other laryngeal tumors, rhabdomyomas are minimally invasive and can be successfully removed with preservation of function.

MEDICATIONS

DRUG(S)
N/A

CONTRAINDICATIONS/POSSIBLE INTERACTIONS
N/A

FOLLOW-UP
- Evaluate monthly for the first 3 months; then at 3–6-month intervals for another year.
- Cardiac—cardiac decompensation progressing to congestive heart failure may develop.

MISCELLANEOUS

SEE ALSO
- Rhabdomyosarcoma
- Rhabdomyosarcoma, Urinary Bladder

Suggested Reading
Mansfield CS, Callanan JJ, McAllister H. Intra-atrial rhabdomyoma causing chyloperi-cardium and right-sided congestive heart failure in a dog. Vet Rec 2000;147:264–267.
O'Hara AJ, McConnell M, Wyatt K, et al. Laryngeal rhabdomyoma in a dog. Aust Vet J 2001;79:817–821.

Acknowledgment
The author and editors acknowledge the prior contributions of Dr. James P. Thompson, who authored this topic in the previous edition.

Author Anthony J. Mutsaers
Consulting Editor Wallace B. Morrison

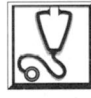 BASICS

OVERVIEW
• A malignant tumor derived from striated muscle (adult variety) or embryonic, pluripotent mesenchymal cells (juvenile variety)
• Most common striated muscle tumor in animals, but represents < 1% of spontaneous neoplasms
• Typically shows diffuse and infiltrative growth characteristics
• Reported in laryngeal, lingual, and cardiac locations
• Aggressive and widespread metastasis can occur to lungs, liver, spleen, kidneys, and adrenal glands.
• Has been reported as an injection site–related sarcoma in cats.

SIGNALMENT
• Dogs and cats
• Adult variety—middle-age to old animals
• Juvenile variety—young dogs
• No sex or breed predilection

SIGNS
• Large, diffuse, soft tissue mass generally of skeletal muscle
• May metastasize within the primary muscle (multiple nodules)
• Signs of right-sided congestive heart failure may occur with the cardiac form.

CAUSES & RISK FACTORS
Unknown

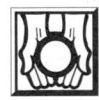 DIAGNOSIS

DIFFERENTIAL DIAGNOSIS
Skeletal Muscle Location
• Fibrosarcoma
• Mast cell neoplasia
• Rhabdomyoma
• Lipoma, infiltrative lipoma, or liposarcoma
Laryngeal Location
• Squamous cell carcinoma
• Adenocarcinoma
• Undifferentiated carcinoma
• Osteosarcoma
• Chondrosarcoma
• Fibrosarcoma

• Myxochondroma
• Leiomyoma
• Oncocytoma
• Melanoma
Lingual Location
• Squamous cell carcinoma
• Granular cell myoblastoma
• Rhabdomyoma
• Fibrosarcoma
• Mast cell tumor
• Lymphoma
• Malignant melanoma
• Hemangioma/hemangiosarcoma
Cardiac Location
• Hemangiosarcoma
• Chemodectoma
• Rhabdomyoma
• Ectopic thyroid tumor
• Ectopic parathyroid tumor
• Lymphoma
• Metastatic neoplasia

CBC/BIOCHEMISTRY/URINALYSIS
• Usually normal
• May cause hypoglycemia

OTHER LABORATORY TESTS
N/A

IMAGING
Dense, soft tissue mass

DIAGNOSTIC PROCEDURES
Cytologic examination—reveals a malignant mesenchymal neoplasm; usually does not provide a definitive diagnosis (requires histopathologic examination)

PATHOLOGIC FINDINGS
• Two varieties based on histomorphologic features
• Adult—large, pleomorphic, elongated tumor cells that may have cross-striation and eosinophilic cytoplasm
• Juvenile—embryonal and alveolar features
• Transmission electron microscopy—may be required for definitive diagnosis
• Immunohistologic examination—may be required for definitive diagnosis; useful markers: actin, desmin, and myoglobin

 TREATMENT
• Surgical excision—difficult because of invasiveness
• Partial glossectomy involving 40%–60% of the tongue is well tolerated by dogs.

• Total laryngectomy with permanent tracheostomy may be required for laryngeal tumors.
• Amputation of an affected limb—consider
• Radiotherapy—may be helpful for localized, low grade/well differentiated tumors

 MEDICATIONS

DRUG(S)
• Chemotherapy—may provide palliation; no specific regimens evaluated
• Discussion of plans with a veterinary oncologist is recommended if considering chemotherapy for this tumor.

CONTRAINDICATIONS/POSSIBLE INTERACTIONS
Chemotherapy—may be myelosuppressive and cause gastrointestinal toxicity; very important to monitor carefully; do not use without prior experience.

 FOLLOW-UP
Physical examination, thoracic radiography, and abdominal ultrasound—monthly for 3 months; then every 3–6 months

✔ MISCELLANEOUS

SEE ALSO
• Rhabdomyoma
• Rhabdomyosarcoma, Urinary Bladder

Suggested Reading
Lascelles BDX, McInnes E, Dobson JM, et al. Rhabdomyosarcoma of the tongue in a dog. J Small Anim Pract 1998;39:587–591.
Perez J, Perez-Rivero A, Montoya A, et al. Right-sided heart failure in a dog with primary cardiac rhabdomyosarcoma. J Am Anim Hosp Assoc 1998;34:208–211.

Acknowledgment
The author and editors acknowledge the prior contributions of Dr. James P. Thompson, who authored this topic in the previous edition.
Author Anthony J. Mutsaers
Consulting Editor Wallace B. Morrison

RHABDOMYOSARCOMA, URINARY BLADDER

 **BASICS**

OVERVIEW
• A malignant tumor derived from pluri-potent or striated myoblastic cells of mesenchymal origin that surround the developing Müllerian or Wolffian ducts
• May also be reported as "botryoid" rhabdomyosarcomas due to their grapelike appearance
• Metastasis—extension to visceral organs and lymph nodes occurs; prevalence not clearly defined
• Constitutes < 1% of all bladder tumors

SIGNALMENT
• Most occur in female, large-breed dogs < 18 months of age
• St. Bernard—may be overrepresented
• Cats—very rare

SIGNS
• Predominantly consistent with lower urinary tract disease
• Hematuria
• Stranguria
• Pollakiuria
• Urine retention possible

CAUSES & RISK FACTORS
Unknown

 DIAGNOSIS

DIFFERENTIAL DIAGNOSIS
• Bacterial cystitis
• Urocystolithiasis
• Transitional cell carcinoma
• Squamous cell carcinoma
• Fibroma or fibrosarcoma
• Lymphoma
• Bladder polyps
• Granulomatous urethritis

CBC/BIOCHEMISTRY/URINALYSIS
• Blood tests usually normal
• Urinalysis—usually reveals hematuria
• Cytologic examination of urine sediment—may find cellular pleomorphism and cross-striations consistent with rhabdomyosarcoma

OTHER LABORATORY TESTS
• Commercially available urinary bladder tumor antigen tests will not be helpful as they were designed for transitional cell carcinoma. Also false positive results are seen with hematuria.

IMAGING
• Bladder ultrasonography or double-contrast cystourethrography
• Intravenous pyelography—evaluate any trigonal mass; assess the ureters and renal pelves

DIAGNOSTIC PROCEDURES
Diagnosis confirmed from histopathologic specimens obtained from exploratory surgery or possibly cystoscopy

PATHOLOGIC FINDINGS
• Useful immunohistochemical markers—vimentin, actin, desmin, and myoglobin; differentiate striated muscle neoplasms from other spindle cell neoplasms
• Ultrastructural information from transmission electron microscopy may also be useful.

RHABDOMYOSARCOMA, URINARY BLADDER

TREATMENT

• Surgical excision recommended, but difficult because of invasiveness
• Surgical resection—may be enhanced by bladder submucosal saline injection to aid in establishing a dissection plane

MEDICATIONS

DRUG(S)

• Adjuvant chemotherapy—recommended; assist in control or elimination of residual neoplastic disease after surgical resection.
• Results with chemotherapy in controlled trials have not been reported.
• A 21-day cycle—used successfully in one dog; doxorubicin (30 mg/m² IV on day 0) and cyclophosphamide (75 mg/m² PO on days 3, 4, 5, and 6); administer a total of four cycles; tumor cell growth indicates clear evidence of chemotherapy resistance.

CONTRAINDICATIONS/POSSIBLE INTERACTIONS

Chemotherapy may be toxic; seek advice before initiating treatment if you are unfamiliar with cytotoxic drugs.

FOLLOW-UP

• Evaluate every 21 days during chemotherapy and every 3–6 months thereafter; include a physical examination, CBC, serum biochemistry profile, and urinalysis.
• Thoracic radiography and abdominal ultrasonography—every 3–6 months during the first year after surgery

MISCELLANEOUS

ASSOCIATED CONDITIONS

• Hypertrophic osteopathy—occasionally
• Concurrent bacterial cystitis common; choose antibiotics on the basis of bacterial culture and sensitivity testing

SYNONYMS

• Botryoid rhabdomyosarcoma (i.e., grapelike appearance)
• Embryonal rhabdomyosarcoma

SEE ALSO

• Rhabdomyoma
• Rhabdomyosarcoma

Suggested Reading

Kuwamura M, Yoshida M, Yamate J, et al. Urinary bladder rhabdomyosarcoma (sarcoma botryoides) in a young Newfoundland dog. J Vet Med Sci 1998;60:619–621.
Senior DF, Lawrence DT, Gunson C, et al. Successful treatment of botryoid rhabdomyosarcoma in the bladder of a dog. J Am Anim Hosp Assoc 1993;29:386–390.

Acknowledgment

The author and editors acknowledge the prior contributions of Dr. James P. Thompson, who authored this topic in the previous edition.
Author Anthony J. Mutsaers
Consulting Editor Wallace B. Morrison

RHINITIS AND SINUSITIS

BASICS

DEFINITION
• Rhinitis—inflammation of the nasal epithelium • Sinusitis—inflammation and irritation of the paranasal sinuses. Includes the frontal sinus and maxillary recess in dogs, frontal and sphenopalatine sinuses in cats • The nasal cavity communicates directly with the paranasal sinuses; thus rhinitis and sinusitis often occur together (rhinosinusitis).

PATHOPHYSIOLOGY
Inflammation and irritation stimulate serous glandular secretion in the nasal mucosa. With chronicity, opportunistic bacterial infections develop in the compromised nasal mucosa causing the discharge to become mucoid or mucopurulent. Erosion into the richly vascularized nasal mucosa leads to hemorrhage and epistaxis. Chronic erosive processes (neoplasia, fungi, chronic bacterial inflammation) can cause bony lysis.

SYSTEMS AFFECTED
• Respiratory—usually confined to nasal turbinates and nasolacrimal ducts. Nasal discharge may occasionally be seen with lower airway disease. • Nervous—fungal and neoplastic disease can invade the brain via destruction of the cribriform plate. • Ocular—epiphora with inflammation of the nasolacrimal ducts. Conjunctivitis, keratitis, and/or corneal ulcerations with viral rhinitis. Chorioretinitis with canine distemper or *Cryptococcus*. • Oral Cavity—Calicivirus, FeLV, FIV are associated with stomatitis, glossitis, faucitis. Tooth root abscess or oronasal fistula

INCIDENCE/PREVALENCE
• Primary bacterial rhinosinusitis rare in both dogs and cats • Idiopathic and chronic rhinosinusitis is common in cats. • Dog—in 42 dogs, neoplasia was the most common cause of nasal signs followed by inflammatory rhinitis.

SIGNALMENT

Species
Dogs and cats

Breed Predilection
• Brachycephalic cats more prone to chronic rhinitis • Dolichocephalic dogs more prone to *Aspergillus* infection and nasal tumors

Mean Age and Range
• Cats—acute viral rhinosinusitis more common in young kittens (6–12 weeks) or unvaccinated cats. Inflammatory polyps more common in young cats. • Congenital diseases (cleft palate) more common in young animals. • Neoplasia and dental disease is more common in older animals. • Foreign bodies more common in young dogs.

Predominant Sex
No sex predilection

SIGNS

Historical Findings
• Sneezing, nasal discharge, epistaxis • Discharge usually is serous initially and becomes mucoid, mucopurulent, serosanguinous, or hemorrhagic. • Unilateral discharge suggests foreign body, tooth root abscess, neoplasia, or fungal infection. • Bilateral discharge more common with viral or bacterial rhinosinusitis, inflammatory rhinitis, pharyngeal disease, or congenital abnormalities • Facial deformity—usually with fungal or neoplastic disease • Reverse sneezing more common in dogs, inappetence more common in cats

Physical Examination Findings
• Decreased nasal air flow, bilateral or unilateral • Evaluate oral cavity for tooth root abscess, oronasal fistula, or ulcers • Increase in tracheal sensitivity or cough possible • Look for epiphora, conjunctivitis, Horner's syndrome (middle ear disease) • Fundic examination—chorioretinitis with viral or fungal rhinitis

CAUSES

Dogs
Primary inciting causes
• Fungal disease—*Aspergillus fumigatus, Penicillium* spp, *Rhinosporidium seeberi, Blastomycoses dermatitidis, Cryptococcus neoformans* are rare causes. • Tooth root abscess • Foreign body • Congenital abnormalities such as cleft palate or primary ciliary dyskinesia • Parasitic causes—nasal mites (*Pneumonyssoides caninum*), *Capillaria aerophagia* • Intranasal neoplasia—adenocarcinoma most common (31.5%). Other tumors include chondrosarcomas, osteosarcomas, or lymphoma. • Immune-mediated rhinitis—allergic rhinitis rare, lymphoplasmacytic rhinitis more common. • Other infectious diseases include canine distemper or *Bordetella bronchiseptica*. • Local trauma may cause bone or turbinate deformity and predispose to chronic rhinitis.
Secondary causes
• Lower airway disease may cause signs of rhinitis. • Epistaxis can be related to hypertension, thrombocytopenia, thrombocytopathia, or rarely other coagulopathies.

Cats
Primary inciting causes
• Viral infections—herpesvirus-1 and calicivirus = 90% of acute infections and/or chlamydial rhinosinusitis (<5%). *Bordetella bronchiseptica* can be a primary pathogen in cats but its significance in cats is unknown. FIV/FeLV infections or co-infections commonly present with chronic rhinitis. • Fungal disease—*Cryptococcus neoformans* most common, also consider *Aspergillus* and *Penicillium* (rare in cats). • Neoplasia—adenocarcinoma and lymphoma most common • Nasopharyngeal polyps in young cats. Cats can develop nasopharyngeal webbing/stenosis secondary to chronic infection or trauma. • Allergic rhinitis rare • Foreign bodies • Parasitic infection • Congenital abnormalities include cleft palate

Secondary causes
• Epistaxis due to coagulopathy or hypertension less common in cats • Cats with vomition can aspirate into the nasopharynx.

RISK FACTORS
• Dolichocephalic breeds—fungal disease • Brachycephalic cats—rhinosinusitis

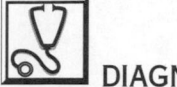

DIAGNOSIS

DIFFERENTIAL DIAGNOSIS
Rule out secondary causes of rhinitis including coagulopathy, hypertension, lower airway disease, chronic vomition.

CBC/BIOCHEMISTRY/URINALYSIS
• Hemogram is nonspecific—may show leukocytosis, neutrophilia, eosinophilia with infectious agents. Leukopenia may be seen with specific infectious agents such as FeLV, FIV, canine distemper. Regenerative anemia with severe blood loss from coagulopathy. Non-regenerative anemia with chronic disease or neoplasia. Thrombocytopenia seen with coagulopathies or severe blood loss. Thrombocytosis seen commonly with systemic inflammation • Serum biochemistry and urinalysis typically normal.

OTHER LABORATORY TESTS
• FeLV and FIV serologic tests • Latex agglutination test for cryptococcal capsular antigen. • Aspergillus titers—false positives and negatives possible • Coagulation profile if epistaxis present

IMAGING
• Radiography—chest radiographs if lower airway disease, neoplasia, or fungal disease suspected. • Dental radiographs highly sensitive for detecting periodontal disease. • Skull radiographs are useful but do not differentiate among inflammatory rhinitis, fungal infection, and neoplastic disease. Bony lysis can be seen with fungal or neoplastic disease. Loss of turbinate structures can be seen with fungal, neoplastic, or chronic inflammatory disease.
• Nasopharyngeal polyps occasionally seen within the nasopharynx. The open-mouth ventrodorsal or intra-oral ventrodorsal views provide superior evaluation of the nasal cavity without superimposition of the mandible.
• CT/MRI—CT thought to be superior to plain radiography in evaluating the extent of the disease and for assessing the integrity of the cribriform plate. Also useful in evaluating presence of disease in palate, nasopharyngeal meatus, maxillary sinus, periorbital tissues, and cribriform plate. Infectious rhinitis and neoplasia cannot be differentiated on the degree of contrast enhancement used during CT.

DIAGNOSTIC PROCEDURES

Cytology
Nasal swab or flush is generally non-diagnostic. On occasion *Cryptococcus, Aspergillus,* or neoplastic cells observed

Culture
• Bacterial culture not very useful owing to broad spectrum of naturally occurring bacteria in nasal cavity. Most animals with rhinitis have secondary bacterial infection. • Fungal culture can be unrewarding, since 40% of normal dogs had positive culture for Aspergillus or Penicillium, and fungal infection can occur secondary to underlying neoplasia. Fungal culture of a visualized lesion on endoscopy can aid diagnosis.

Biopsy
Techniques include flushing, core biopsy, pinch biopsies, and surgical biopsies. A pinch biopsy should be considered before a surgical biopsy as it is less invasive. Excessive hemorrhage can be controlled with topical epinephrine at 1:100,000.

Endoscopy
• An otoscope evaluates only the rostral nares. A rigid endoscope can be guided to the ethmoid turbinates, although iatrogenic hemorrhage is a common sequelae. A flexible bronchoscope provides good visualization, and can be used to visualize the caudal choanae by retroflexing into the caudal nasopharynx. • Guided biopsy is possible with rigid and flexible endoscopy, although difficult in cats owing to size limitation.

Surgery
Exploratory rhinotomy most invasive diagnostic tool, can be most useful for difficult biopsies, foreign body removal, or mass removal.

PATHOLOGIC FINDINGS
Chronic inflammation causes turbinate resorption, mucosal ulceration and necrosis with a resultant increase in space within the nasal cavity. Neoplasia and fungus also cause destruction but replace it with proliferative tissue. White-yellow plaques common with fungal infections.

TREATMENT

APPROPRIATE HEALTH CARE
Depends on underlying cause

NURSING CARE
Humidification can aid in moistening and mobilizing nasal secretions. Saline intranasal infusion helpful if tolerated. Clean the nares.

ACTIVITY
No change unless in respiratory distress

DIET
Soft or warmed food for cats with a decreased appetite

CLIENT EDUCATION
Signs of chronic rhinitis in cats can be variably controlled but are rarely eliminated.

SURGICAL CONSIDERATIONS
• Rhinotomy is reserved for obtaining a biopsy or foreign body/mass removal. In most instances it does not carry an advantage over endoscopy.

• Surgical debulking of nasal tumors only shown to increase survival time if combined with radiation therapy
• Useful for polyp removal

MEDICATIONS

DRUG(S)

Antibiotics
• May help with secondary bacterial rhinitis, however will not resolve the underlying primary problem. Selection of antibiotic is mainly empirical (common isolates include *Staphylococcus, Streptococcus, Neisseria, Bacillus, E. coli*, and *Pasturella multocida*); culture not useful owing to presence of normal nasal flora • Tetracyclines—helpful with chlamydial rhinitis. May need long-term doxycycline therapy for 6–8 weeks (5 mg/kg PO q12h). • Chloramphenicol is also effective against Chlamydia (dogs: 50 mg/kg PO q12h, cats: 12.5–20 mg/kg PO q12h).

Antifungals
See Cryptococcosis and Aspergillosis chapters for detailed treatment discussion

Human alpha-interferon
Anecdotal at this point—30 IU PO q24h

L-lysine
Experimentally decreases FHV replication in cell culture and may be useful in chronic herpesvirus infection—250–500 mg PO q24h for life.

Anti-inflammatory agents
Piroxicam, a non-steroidal anti-inflammatory, is being used empirically for palliation of nasal tumors, either as sole agent or in conjunction with chemotherapy (0.3 mg/kg PO q24h, then taper to q48h). When chemotherapeutics combined with radiation therapy in dogs, survival time extended to 8–20 months.

Steroids
Use with presumptive allergic rhinitis—prednisolone at 1 mg/kg divided PO q12h.

Antihistamines
Efficacy is debated—clemastine 1.34 mg PO q12h for cats and small dogs, 2.68 mg PO q12h for medium to large breed dogs or hydroxyzine 2.2 mg/kg PO q8–12h.

Anti-Parasitics
Ivermectin 300 mcg/kg PO once weekly for 3–4 treatments or milbemycin oxime 1.0 mg/kg PO once weekly for 3 weeks for treatment of nasal mites.

CONTRAINDICATIONS
Avoid chronic steroid use with chronic viral rhinitis owing to danger of immunosuppression.

PRECAUTIONS
• Piroxicam can cause GI ulceration.
• Tetracyclines may stain teeth of young animals.

POSSIBLE INTERACTIONS
Use of piroxicam and corticosteroids together is contraindicated.

FOLLOW-UP

PATIENT MONITORING
Clinical assessment and monitoring for relapse

PREVENTION/AVOIDANCE
• Vaccinations in kittens can lessen severity and duration of infection with calicivirus or herpesvirus. • Consider removing chronically affected cats from catteries.

POSSIBLE COMPLICATIONS
• Extension of fungal or neoplastic invasion into brain. • Seizures and other neurologic signs are possible if topical antifungal therapy is used when the cribriform plate is not intact.

EXPECTED COURSE AND PROGNOSIS
• Dependent on etiology and extent of disease
• Acute viral/bacterial rhinitis—carries good prognosis, chronic rhinitis is frustrating to the owners and veterinarians. • Fungal—fair to guarded prognosis depending on invasiveness
• Neoplastic—3–5 months with no treatment. Life expectancy can be extended up to 20–23 months with radiation therapy.

MISCELLANEOUS

ZOONOTIC POTENTIAL
Cryptococcus, Aspergillus, Penicillium are thought to be transmissible to humans via shared environment. No documentation to support transmission directly from dogs or cats

PREGNANCY
Ketoconazole, itraconazole, flucytosine are teratogenic.

SEE ALSO
• Aspergillosis • Cryptococcosis • Epistaxis
• Nasal and Nasopharyngeal Polyps • Nasal Discharge (Sneezing, Reverse Sneezing)
• Respiratory Parasites • Stertor and Stridor

ABBREVIATIONS
• FeLV = feline leukemia virus • FHV = feline herpesvirus • FIV = feline immunodeficiency virus

Suggested Reading
Gartrell CL, O'Handley PA, and Perry RL. Canine nasal disease—part I. Compend Contin Educ 1995;17(3):323–326.
Gartrell CL, O'Handley PA, and Perry RL. Canine nasal disease—part II. Compend Contin Educ 1995;17(4):539–547.
Russo M, Lamb CR, Jakovljevic S. Distinguishing rhinitis and nasal neoplasia by radiography. Vet Radiol Ultrasound 2000;41(2):118–124.
Tasker S, Knottenbelt CM, Munro EA. Aetiology and diagnosis of persistent nasal disease in the dog: a retrospective study of 42 cases. J Small Anim Pract 1999;40(10):473–478.
Author Carrie J. Miller
Consulting Editor Lynelle R. Johnson

RHINOSPORIDIOSIS

 BASICS

OVERVIEW
• A rare chronic fungal infection of the mucous membranes of dogs; generally forms a cauliflower-like mass that often protrudes from the nostril; reported in one cat
• Respiratory system affected
• Worldwide distribution
• Endemic areas—Argentina, Sri Lanka, and India
• U.S.—most infections have been reported in the southern states.

SIGNALMENT
• Reported in 13 dogs, 7 of which were males
• No apparent breed predilection
• Reported in one cat

SIGNS
• Anterior nasal cavity—most common site
• Sneezing, epistaxis, and stertorous breathing—most prominent

• Mass—often seen protruding from the nostril; usually single and polypoid; may be lobulated or sessile; surface may have white or yellowish superficial flecks, which are fungal sporangia.
• Humans—reported sites: vagina, penis, conjunctival sac, and ears

CAUSES & RISK FACTORS
• *Rhinosporidium seeberi*
• Suspected that stagnant fresh water and arid environment increase likelihood of occurrence

 DIAGNOSIS

DIFFERENTIAL DIAGNOSIS
• Nasal neoplasia
• Nasal inflammatory polyp

CBC/BIOCHEMISTRY/URINALYSIS
Usually normal

OTHER LABORATORY TESTS
None

IMAGING
Radiographs of nasal cavity—generally normal; mass located in the anterior nasal cavity and does not invade turbinates

DIAGNOSTIC PROCEDURES
Impression smears—reveal organisms from nasal mass; use new methylene blue stain or periodic acid–Schiff stain.

PATHOLOGIC FINDINGS
Histopathology
• Examination of mass—papillomatous hyperplasia; ulceration of the epithelium; fibrovascular stroma
• Identification of the organism is diagnostic.
• An intense inflammatory reaction will be seen if organisms are released into the surrounding tissues.

TREATMENT

• Good nursing care important; anorexia and dehydration not typically reported
• Cage confinement or other means of exercise restriction—helpful if epistaxis occurs
• Surgical excision of the mass—treatment of choice; approach through the external nares or rhinotomy; failure to remove the entire mass will likely result in regrowth.

MEDICATIONS

DRUG(S)

• Ketoconazole has been used with limited success.
• Dapsone—used to treat humans; report of use in one dog (1.1 mg/kg PO q8–12h) with favorable response but no cure; however, it has severe side effects.

CONTRAINDICATIONS/POSSIBLE INTERACTIONS

Dapsone (dogs)—hepatotoxicity; anemia; neutropenia; thrombocytopenia; gastrointestinal signs; skin reactions

FOLLOW-UP

If surgical approach was through the external nasal orifice, monitor patient closely for regrowth; difficult to remove the entire mass

MISCELLANEOUS

ZOONOTIC POTENTIAL

• No known risk of direct transmission to humans by handling of infected dogs
• Organism is infectious to humans.

Suggested Reading

Breitschwerdt EB, Castellano MC. Rhinosporidiosis. In: Greene CE, ed. Infectious diseases of the dog and cat. Philadelphia: Saunders, 1998:402–404.
Caniatti M, Roccabianca P, Scanziani E, et al. Nasal rhinosporidiosis in dogs: four cases from Europe and a review of the literature. Vet Rec 1998;142:334–338.
Wallin LL, Coleman GD, Froeling J, Parker GA. Rhinosporidiosis in a domestic cat. Med Mycol 2001;39:139–141.

Author Gary D. Norsworthy
Consulting Editor Stephen C. Barr

RIGHT BUNDLE BRANCH BLOCK

BASICS

DEFINITION
Conduction delay or block in the right bundle branch resulting in late activation of the right ventricle; the block can be complete or incomplete. (Figures 1 and 2)

ECG Features
• A right axis deviation and wide QRS ($\geq$ 0.08 sec in dogs; $\geq$ 0.06 in cats) in most patients
• Large, wide S waves in leads I, II, III, and aVF

PATHOPHYSIOLOGY
• The right bundle branch is anatomically vulnerable to injury because it is a thin strand of tissue and has a long undivided course.
• No hemodynamic compromise

SYSTEMS AFFECTED
Cardiovascular

GENETICS
N/A

INCIDENCE/PREVALENCE
• Dogs—most frequent form of intraventricular conduction defect
• Cats—not as frequent as left anterior fascicular block

GEOGRAPHIC DISTRIBUTION
N/A

SIGNALMENT
Species
Dogs and cats

Breed Predilections
In beagles, incomplete right bundle branch block can result from a genetically determined localized variation in right ventricular wall thickness.

Predominant Sex
N/A

SIGNS
Historical Findings
• Usually an incidental ECG finding—does not cause hemodynamic abnormalities
• Observed signs are usually associated with the underlying condition.

Physical Examination Findings
• Splitting of heart sounds because of asynchronous activation of ventricles in some patients
• Does not cause signs of hemodynamic compromise

CAUSES
• Occasionally seen in normal and healthy dogs and cats
• Congenital heart disease
• Chronic valvular fibrosis
• After surgical correction of a cardiac defect
• Trauma caused by cardiac needle puncture to obtain blood sample
• Trauma from other causes
• Chronic infection with *Trypanosoma cruzi* (Chagas' disease)
• Neoplasia
• Heartworm disease
• Acute thromboembolism
• Cardiomyopathy
• Hyperkalemia (most commonly in cats with urethral obstruction)

RISK FACTORS
N/A

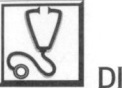

DIAGNOSIS

DIFFERENTIAL DIAGNOSIS
• Right ventricular enlargement—absence of right ventricular enlargement on thoracic radiographs or echocardiogram supports a diagnosis of right bundle branch block.
• Can also be confused with ventricular ectopic beats (especially if the block is intermittent), but consistent PR intervals and no pulse deficits with right bundle branch block

CBC/BIOCHEMISTRY/URINALYSIS
• None specific
• Serum potassium may be extremely high in cats with urethral obstruction.

OTHER LABORATORY TESTS
• Occult heartworm test may be positive in dogs or cats.
• Chagas' indirect fluorescent antibody test, direct hemagglutination, and complement fixation test may be positive in dogs.

IMAGING
• Echocardiogram may show structural heart disease; absence of right heart enlargement supports the diagnosis.
• Thoracic and abdominal radiographs may show masses or pulmonary metastatic lesions; traumatic injuries could cause localized or diffuse pulmonary densities.

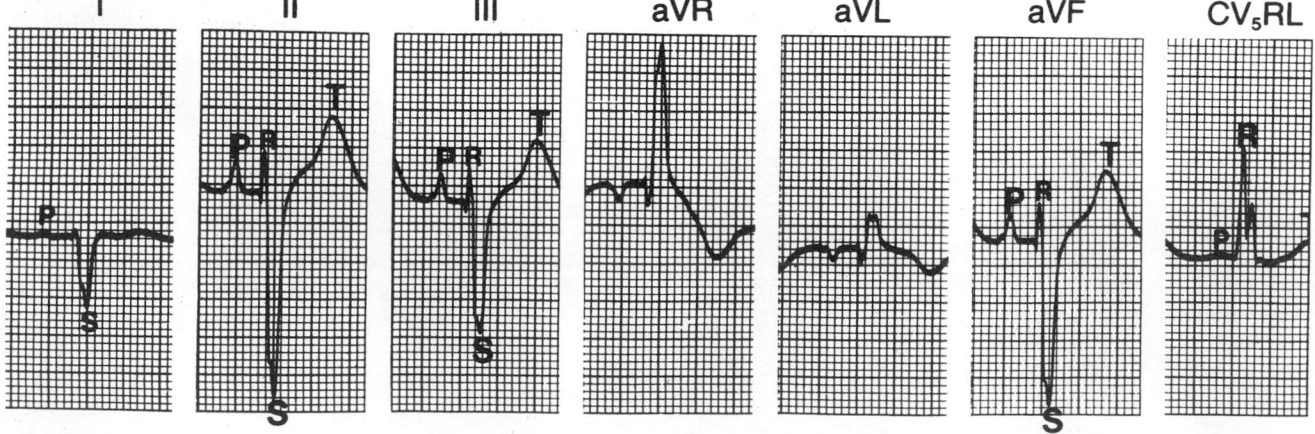

Figure 1.

Right bundle branch block in a dog. The electrocardiographic features include QRS duration of 0.08 sec; positive QRS complex in aVR, aVL, and CV5RL (M shaped); and large wide S waves in leads I, II, III, and aVF. There is a right axis deviation (approximately −110°) (50 mm/sec, 1 cm = 1 mV). (From: Tilley LP. Essentials of canine and feline electrocardiography. 3rd ed. Baltimore: Lippincott Williams & Wilkins, 1992, with permission.)

DIAGNOSTIC PROCEDURES
• Electrocardiography
• Echocardiography

PATHOLOGIC FINDINGS
Possible lesions or scarring on endocardial surface in the path of the bundle branches; applying Lugol's iodine to the endocardial surface within 2 hr postmortem gives clear visualization of the conduction system.

 TREATMENT

APPROPRIATE HEALTH CARE
Direct treatment toward the underlying cause.

NURSING CARE
N/A

ACTIVITY
Unrestricted

DIET
No modifications unless required to manage underlying condition

CLIENT EDUCATION
• Does not cause hemodynamic abnormalities itself
• The lesion causing the block could progress, leading to more serious arrhythmias or complete heart block.

SURGICAL CONSIDERATIONS
N/A

 MEDICATIONS

DRUG(S) OF CHOICE
Not required unless needed to manage underlying condition

CONTRAINDICATIONS
N/A

PRECAUTIONS
N/A

POSSIBLE INTERACTIONS
N/A

ALTERNATIVE DRUG(S)
N/A

 FOLLOW-UP

PATIENT MONITORING
Serial ECG may show resolution of the lesion or progression to complete heart block.

PREVENTION/AVOIDANCE
N/A

POSSIBLE COMPLICATIONS
• The causative lesion could progress, leading to a more serious arrhythmia or complete heart block.
• First- or second-degree AV block may indicate involvement of the left bundle branch.

EXPECTED COURSE AND PROGNOSIS
No hemodynamic compromise

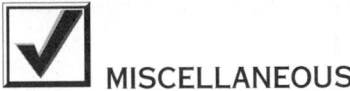 **MISCELLANEOUS**

ASSOCIATED CONDITIONS
N/A

AGE-RELATED FACTORS
N/A

ZOONOTIC POTENTIAL
N/A

PREGNANCY
N/A

SYNONYMS
None

SEE ALSO
• Atrioventricular Block, Complete
• Atrioventricular Block, First-degree
• Atrioventricular Block, Second-degree
• Left Anterior Fascicular Block
• Left Bundle Branch Block

ABBREVIATION
• AV = atrioventricular

Suggested Reading
Tilley LP. Essentials of canine and feline electrocardiography. 3rd ed. Baltimore: Williams & Wilkins, 1992.
Authors Larry P. Tilley and Naomi L. Burtnick
Consulting Editors Larry P. Tilley and Francis W. K. Smith, Jr.

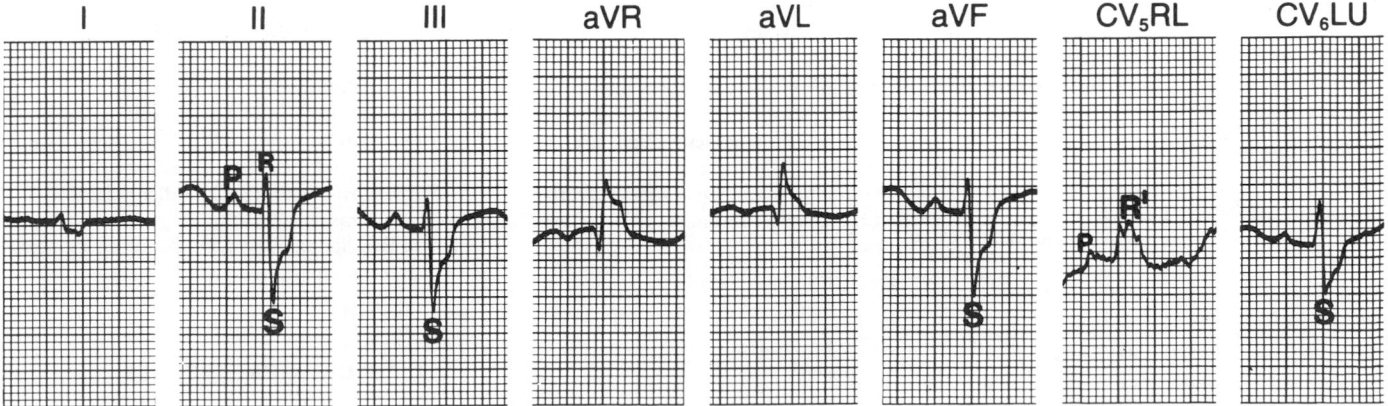

Figure 2.

Right bundle branch block in a cat with the dilated form of cardiomyopathy. The QRS duration is 0.08 sec (4 boxes). Large and wide S waves are present in leads I, II, III, aVF, and CV₆LU. The QRS in CV₅RL has a wide R wave (M-shaped). There is a marked axis deviation (approximately −90°). (From: Tilley LP: Essentials of canine and feline electrocardiography, 3rd ed. Baltimore: Lippincott Williams & Wilkins, 1992, with permission.)

ROCKY MOUNTAIN SPOTTED FEVER

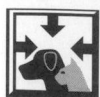

BASICS

DEFINITION
• A tick-borne rickettsial disease, caused by *Rickettsia rickettsii*, that affects dogs and is considered the most important rickettsial disease in humans
• Antibodies to *R. akari* (causative agent of rickettsialpox in humans) have been found in dogs from New York, NY. Unknown if causes disease in dogs.
• Other as yet undefined rickettsial organisms may also cause clinical signs in dogs.

PATHOPHYSIOLOGY
• Vector—American dog tick (*Dermacentor variabilis*), found east of the Great Plains; wood tick (*D. andersoni*), found from the Cascades to the Rocky Mountains
• Transmission—via the saliva of the vector or blood transfusion; tick must be attached for 5–20 hr to infect host (humans, dogs, and cats) or reservoir host (rodents and dogs).
• Incubation period—2 days to 2 weeks
• Infection—organism invades and multiplies in vascular endothelium; causes microvascular hemorrhage, platelet aggregation (thrombocytopenia), vasoconstriction, increased vascular permeability, increased plasma loss into the interstitial space (organ swelling), hypotension, and eventually DIC and shock; leads to widespread vasculitis in organs with endarterial circulation (cause of clinical signs)

SYSTEMS AFFECTED
• Multisystemic involvement
• Hemic/Lymphatic/Immune—bleeding tendency from thrombocytopenia, vasculitis, lymphadenopathy, splenomegaly
• Musculoskeletal—joint pain
• Ophthalmic—conjunctivitis, scleral injection
• Nervous—stupor, seizures, vestibular deficits, coma, cervical pain
• Respiratory—dyspnea, cough
• Skin/Exocrine—edema of extremities, face
• Cardiovascular—vasculitis, hypotension, shock

GENETICS
N/A

INCIDENCE/PREVALENCE
• Tick season—late March to the end of September
• Prevalence—overall infections in ticks < 2%; varies by geographic locality

GEOGRAPHIC DISTRIBUTION
• North and South America
• U.S.—no accurate data for dogs; similar distribution as for humans: eastern seaboard states (especially the Carolinas), Mississippi River valley, and south-central states; serosurvey of shelter dogs from Rhode Island: 21%

SIGNALMENT
Species
Dogs

Breed Predilections
• Purebred dogs seem more prone to developing clinical illness than do mixed-breed dogs.
• German shepherds—more common

Mean Age and Range
Any age

Predominant Sex
None

SIGNS
Historical Findings
• Fever—within 2–3 days of tick attachment
• Lethargy
• Depression
• Anorexia
• Swelling (edema)—lips, scrotum, prepuce, ears, extremities
• Stiff gait—especially with scrotal or prepucial swelling
• Spontaneous bleeding—sneezing, epistaxis
• Respiratory distress
• Neurologic—ataxia, head tilt
• Ocular pain

Physical Examination Findings
• Both clinical and subclinical illness occur.
• Clinical—variable in severity; lasts 2–4 weeks untreated
• Ticks may still be present in acute cases.
• Pyrexia
• Cutaneous lesions—edema of face, limbs, prepuce, scrotum
• Extremities—necrosis
• Conjunctivitis
• Scleral injection
• Respiratory—dyspnea, exercise intolerance resulting from pneumonitis, increased bronchovesicular sounds
• Generalized lymphadenopathy
• Neurologic—vestibular dysfunction, altered mental status, seizures
• Myalgia/arthralgia
• Petechia
• Ecchymoses—ocular, oral, genital regions; 20% of patients
• Hemorrhagic diathesis—epistaxis, melena, hematuria; in severe cases
• Cardiac arrhythmias—sudden death
• DIC and death from shock—in severe acute cases

CAUSES
R. rickettsii

RISK FACTORS
• Exposure to ticks
• Co-infection with other pathogens (tick borne)

DIAGNOSIS

DIFFERENTIAL DIAGNOSIS
• Canine ehrlichiosis—*Ehrlichia canis;* not seasonal; can be clinically indistinguishable from Rocky Mountain spotted fever (especially acute cases); differentiate with serologic testing; both respond to same treatment.
• Immune-mediated thrombocytopenia—not usually associated with fever or lymphadenopathy; differentiate with serologic testing; may treat for both until results are known
• Systemic lupus erythematosus—antinuclear antibody titer usually negative with Rocky Mountain spotted fever; serologic testing diagnostic
• Brucellosis—scrotal edema; serologic testing diagnostic

CBC/BIOCHEMISTRY/URINALYSIS
CBC
• Thrombocytopenia (~40% of cases)—partly due to antiplatelet antibody
• Megathrombocytosis mild anemia (normochromic, normocytic), mild leukopenia (early in infection), leukocytosis (and monocytosis)—as disease becomes more chronic

Biochemistry
• Usually nonspecific
• Mild increases in ALT, ALP, BUN, creatinine, and total bilirubin (rare)
• Hypercholesterolemia—consistently found; cause unknown
• Hypoalbuminemia—from vascular endothelial damage
• Azotemia, hyponatremia, hypochloremia, and metabolic acidosis have all been reported.

Urinalysis
• Proteinuria—with or without azotemia; from glomerular/tubular damage
• Hematuria—coagulation defects

OTHER LABORATORY TESTS
• Serum titers—take 2–3 weeks to rise; may be negative in very acute cases
• Paired titers—perform 3 weeks apart; four-fold increase between acute and convalescent titers; avoid misdiagnosis because of considerable cross-reactivity with other rickettsial organisms
• High titers can be detected for up to 1 year after treatment.

IMAGING
N/A

DIAGNOSTIC PROCEDURES
• Direct immunofluorescence—skin biopsies obtained by local anesthesia and punch biopsies from affected lesions; detect rickettsial antigens as early as 3–4 days postinfection
• CSF—often normal; may show an increase in protein and nucleated cells

PATHOLOGIC FINDINGS
• Widespread petechia, splenomegaly, and generalized hemorrhagic lymphadenopathy
• Necrotizing vasculitis with perivascular cell infiltration (mononuclear and neutrophilic)
• Vascular lesions—most prominent in the skin, kidneys, myocardium, meninges, retina, pancreas, gastrointestinal tract, and urinary bladder • Hepatic and focal myocardial necrosis, nodular gliosis in the brain, and interstitial pneumonia common
• Special stains—to identify organisms

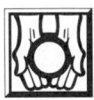

TREATMENT

APPROPRIATE HEALTH CARE
Inpatient until stable and showing response to treatment

NURSING CARE
• Dehydration—balanced electrolyte solution; use cautiously because of increased vascular permeability and expanded extracellular fluid volume (exacerbating cerebral and pulmonary edema)
• Anemia—blood transfusion
• Hemorrhage from thrombocytopenia—platelet-rich plasma or a blood transfusion

ACTIVITY
Restricted

DIET N/A

CLIENT EDUCATION
• Prognosis—good in acute cases with appropriate and prompt therapy • Response occurs within hours of treatment. • If treatment is not instituted until CNS signs occur or later in the disease process, mortality is high; patient with CNS signs may die within hours.

SURGICAL CONSIDERATIONS
If surgery is required for other reasons, blood transfusion may be needed to correct anemia and/or thrombocytopenia.

MEDICATIONS

DRUG(S) OF CHOICE
• Doxycycline—synthetic derivative of tetracycline, 10 mg/kg PO q12h for 10 days; or IV for 5 days if patient is vomiting
• Prednisone—concurrent use; anti-inflammatory or immunosuppressive dose; given early in course of disease does not seem to be detrimental to the clinical recovery

CONTRAINDICATIONS
• Tetracyclines (or derivatives)—do not use in patients < 6 months because of permanent yellowing of the teeth.
• Renal insufficiency—do not use tetracycline; doxycycline may be given (also excreted via the gastrointestinal tract).

• Enrofloxacin—avoid in young dogs because articular cartilage damage can occur (preceded by lameness); gastrointestinal upset (vomiting, anorexia)

PRECAUTIONS
Chloramphenicol
• Avoid if serologic confirmation will be conducted after treatment has started; reduces titers to a greater extent than will tetracyclines
• Warn client of public health risks; directly interferes with heme and bone marrow synthesis
• Avoid use in dogs with thrombocytopenia, pancytopenia, or anemia.

POSSIBLE INTERACTIONS
None

ALTERNATIVE DRUG(S)
• Tetracyclines, chloramphenicol, and enrofloxacin—equally efficacious if used early
• Oxytetracycline and tetracycline—22 mg/kg PO q8h for 14 days; effective and less expensive
• Chloramphenicol—puppies < 6 months of age; 20 mg/kg PO q8h for 14 days; recommended to avoid yellow discoloration of erupting teeth
• Enrofloxacin—3 mg/kg PO q8h for 7 days

FOLLOW-UP

PATIENT MONITORING
Monitor platelet count every 3 days until normal.

PREVENTION/AVOIDANCE
• Control tick infestation on dogs—use dips or sprays containing dichlorvos, chlorfenvinphos, dioxathion, propoxur, or carbaryl
• Flea and tick collars—may reduce reinfestation; reliability is unproven.
• Avoid tick-infested areas.
• Environment—tick eradication impossible; organism maintained in rodents and other reservoir hosts
• Removing ticks by hand—use gloves (see Zoonotic Potential); ensure mouth parts are removed, because a foreign body reaction is likely to result if they are left in place.

COMPLICATIONS N/A

EXPECTED COURSE AND PROGNOSIS
• Early antibiotic treatment—reduces fever and albumin extravasation and improves patient's attitude within 24–48 hr
• Platelet counts—repeat every 3 days after initiating treatment until within normal range; should return to normal within 2–4 days after initiating treatment
• Serologic titers—lower in treated than in untreated dogs; titers remain positive during convalescence.
• Naturally infected dogs never seem to become reinfected.

• Acute cases—excellent prognosis with appropriate treatment
• With CNS disease—poor prognosis

MISCELLANEOUS

ASSOCIATED CONDITIONS
None

AGE-RELATED FACTORS
None

ZOONOTIC POTENTIAL
• Incidence (humans)—dropping in the U.S.; mid-1992–mid-1993: 300 cases; earlier incidence: up to 1000 cases/year
• Mainly young adults and children infected
• Source of infection (humans)—from ticks that are transferred from dogs; not from dogs directly; when removing infected ticks from dogs
• Major clinical signs (humans)—mimic those in dogs; mainly fever and headache; neurologic signs occur later; skin rash appreciated in only 50% of patients
• Treatment with tetracyclines results in a rapid recovery.

PREGNANCY N/A

ABBREVIATIONS
• ALP = alkaline phosphatase
• ALT = alanine aminotransferase
• CSF = cerebrospinal fluid
• DIC = disseminated intravascular coagulation

Suggested Reading
Breitschwerdt EB, Davidson MG, Aucoin DP, et al. Efficacy of chloramphenicol, enrofloxacin, and tetracycline for treatment of experimental Rocky Mountain spotted fever in dogs. Antimicrob Agents Chemother 1991;35:2375–2381.
Breitschwerdt EB, Davidson MG, Hegarty BC, et al. Prednisolone at anti-inflammatory or immunosuppressive dosages in conjunction with doxycycline does not potentiate the severity of *Rickettsia rickettsii* infection in dogs. Antimicrob Agents Chemother 1997;41:141–147.
Gasser AM, Birkenheuer AJ, Breitschwerdt EB. Canine Rocky Mountain spotted fever: a retrospective study of 30 cases. J Am Anim Hosp Assoc 2001;37:41–48.
Greene CE, Breitschwerdt EB. Rocky Mountain spotted fever, Q fever, and typhus. In: Greene CE, ed. Infectious diseases of the dog and cat. 2nd ed. Philadelphia: Saunders, 1998;155–165.
Author Stephen C. Barr
Consulting Editor Stephen C. Barr

ROTAVIRUS INFECTIONS

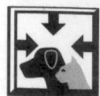 **BASICS**

OVERVIEW
• Nonenveloped, double-stranded RNA virus; *rota* (Latin; "wheel") for shape of the capsid; genus within the family Reoviridae; relatively resistant to environmental destruction (acid and lipid solvents); unique double capsid protects virus from inactivation in the upper gastrointestinal tract
• Wide host range, identified in almost every species investigated
• Most significant cause of severe gastro-enteritis in young children (< 2 years) and animals throughout the world
• Transmission—fecal–oral contamination
• Infection—affects mature epithelial cells on luminal tips of the intestinal villi; causes swelling, degeneration, and desquamation; denuded villi contract; results in villous atrophy with loss of absorptive capability and loss of brush border enzymes (e.g., disaccharidases); leads to osmotic diarrhea

SIGNALMENT
• Dogs and cats
• Pups < 12 weeks old and more often < 2 weeks old—diarrhea
• Kittens and young cats (<6 months of age)—more susceptible to infection

SIGNS
• Dogs—most infections subclinical or limited to relatively mild, nonspecific watery to mucoid diarrhea, anorexia, and lethargy; rare fatalities reported
• Cats—primarily subclinical or mild diarrhea; with co-infections or in stressed conditions, more severe clinical disease may occur.

CAUSES & RISK FACTORS
• Rotavirus
• Young animals with immature immune systems at increased risk

 DIAGNOSIS

DIFFERENTIAL DIAGNOSIS
• Canine viral enteritis—canine parvovirus; canine coronavirus; canine astrovirus; canine calicivirus; canine herpesvirus; canine distemper virus; canine reovirus
• Feline viral enteritis—feline parvovirus (feline panleukopenia virus); FeLV; feline coronavirus; feline astrovirus; feline calicivirus
• Other causes of enteritis—bacteria (e.g., *Salmonella, Campylobacter, Clostridium*); fungi; protozoa; parasites; foreign bodies; intussusception; allergies; toxicants

CBC/BIOCHEMISTRY/URINALYSIS
Noncontributory

OTHER LABORATORY TESTS
• Serology—not recommended; most animals (e.g., 85% of dogs) carry antibodies owing to previous exposure or from passive antibody immunization transfer from the bitch or queen; must demonstrate fourfold difference in acute and convalescent serum samples
• Direct electron microscopy—detects virus in feces; rapid; lack of sensitivity
• Immunoelectron microscopy—more sensitive and specific than direct electron microscopy; not commonly available
• ELISA—detect common group rotavirus antigen in feces; Rotazyme (Abbott Laboratories, North Chicago, IL)
• Virus isolation
• Polymerase chain reaction

IMAGING
N/A

DIAGNOSTIC PROCEDURES
Histology—swollen small intestinal villi; mild infiltration by macrophages and neutrophils; virus detected by fluorescent antibody test

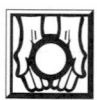 **TREATMENT**

• Symptomatic for diarrhea—fluids, electrolytes, and dietary restriction

• Antibiotic therapy not indicated
• Principal protection—probably antibodies in milk of immune bitch or queen

 MEDICATIONS

DRUG(S)
N/A

CONTRAINDICATIONS/POSSIBLE INTERACTIONS
N/A

 **FOLLOW-UP**

N/A

 MISCELLANEOUS

ZOONOTIC POTENTIAL
• Rotaviruses are not host-specific; thus, affected puppy or kitten may pose a potential human health hazard, particularly for infants.
• Exercise care when handling fecal material from pets with diarrhea.
• Humans—diarrhea; infants in developed countries: high morbidity and low mortality (attributed to fluid therapy); infants and young children in developing countries: leading cause of life-threatening diarrhea

ABBREVIATIONS
• ELISA = enzyme-linked immunosorbent assay
• FeLV = feline leukemia virus

Suggested Reading
Hoskins JD. Canine viral enteritis. In: Greene CE, ed. Infectious diseases of the dog and cat. 2nd ed. Philadelphia: Saunders, 1998:40–49.
Pedersen NC. Feline rotavirus. In: Appel M, ed. Virus infections of carnivores. New York: Elsevier Science, 1987:259–260.
Author J. Paul Woods
Consulting Editor Stephen C. Barr

ROUNDWORMS (ASCARIASIS)

BASICS

OVERVIEW
• Ascariasis of dogs, especially pups, is caused by *Toxocara canis,* and, of cats, by *Toxocara cati;* both host species are infected by *Toxascaris leonina.*
• These are relatively large, robust worms up to 10–12 cm long, so distension of the small intestine often leads to colic, interference with gut motility, and inability to use food.
• Because of transplacental transmission to fetuses, pups may be born with a developing worm burden.
• Over first month of life, infected neonatal pups may rapidly debilitate with abdominal pain, prior to appearance of eggs in stool.
• Kittens may be similarly affected by transcolostral transmission.
• Older pups and kittens may become infected by ingesting infective eggs disseminated on premises by dams with postgestational infections.
• *Toxascaris* may be transmitted by eggs or by predation of transport hosts (rodents) infected with dormant infective larvae.

SIGNALMENT
Dogs and cats; clinically especially important in pups and kittens

SIGNS

Historical Findings
• Abdominal distension
• Colic
• Cachexia
• Poor nursing or appetite
• Scant feces
• Coughing—due to larval migration
• Whole litter may be affected

Physical Examination Findings
• Weakness, loss of condition, cachexia
• Abdominal distension—often with distended intestines palpable

CAUSES & RISK FACTORS
• *Toxocara* infection
• Infected bitch or queen
• Food or environment contaminated with feces
• Concurrent enteric infections

DIAGNOSIS

DIFFERENTIAL DIAGNOSIS
• Hookworm infection
• *Strongyloides* infection

CBC/BIOCHEMISTRY/URINALYSIS
Usually normal

OTHER LABORATORY TESTS
N/A

IMAGING
N/A

DIAGNOSTIC PROCEDURES
• Fecal egg examination of pups, kittens > 3 weeks of age
• *Toxocara* egg—spherical, with pitted outer shell membrane, single dark cell (zygote filling interior), 80–85 μm *(T. canis),* ~ 75 μm *(T. cati)*
• *Toxascaris* egg—ovoid, with smooth exterior shell membrane, 1- or 2-cell, not filling interior, light cytoplasm, 80 × 70 μm
• Necropsy findings of siblings that have died of similar signs

TREATMENT
• Acute severe cases—inpatients; supplement with intravenous fluids
• Educate client to possibility of sudden death or chronic debilitation.
• Treat bitch or queen with adulticide/ larvicide anthelmintic (fenbendazole) to decrease likelihood of subsequent litter and mature maternal infections.

MEDICATIONS

DRUG(S)

Adulticide/Larvicide Anthelmintics
• Fenbendazole 50 mg/kg PO q24h for 3 days
• Milbemycin oxime tabs monthly

Adulticide Anthelmintics
• Dichlorvos twice monthly
• Pyrantel + praziquantel tablets for cats; febantel + praziquantel + pyrantel pamoate tablets for dogs
• Ivermectin + pyrantel pamoate monthly
• Pyrantel pamoate 5 mg/kg PO in dogs; 10–20 mg/kg in cats (extra-label) monthly
• Selamectin 6 mg/kg topically once in cats for *T. cati*; extra-label in dogs.

CONTRAINDICATIONS/POSSIBLE INTERACTIONS
• Organophosphates in heartworm-positive patients
• Do not give dichlorvos concurrently with other organophosphates such as insecticides.

FOLLOW-UP
Monitor fecal egg counts posttreatment.

MISCELLANEOUS

AGE-RELATED FACTORS
Greater clinical concern in neonates

ZOONOTIC POTENTIAL
Visceral larva migrans may follow ingestion of infective eggs.

SYNONYMS
Ascariasis

Suggested Reading
Bowman DD, Lynn RC, Eberhard ML. Georgi's parasitology for veterinarians, 8th ed. St. Louis: Saunders (Elsevier Science), 2003:206–211.
Bowman DD, Hendrix CM, Lindsay DS, Barr SC. Feline clinical parasitology. Ames: Iowa State University Press, 2002:273–287.

Acknowledgment
The author and editors acknowledge the prior contributions of Dr. Robert M. Corwin, who authored this topic in the previous edition.
Author Julie Ann Jarvinen
Consulting Editor Albert E. Jergens

SALIVARY MUCOCELE

BASICS

OVERVIEW
• Salivary mucoceles are non–epithelial-lined cavities filled with saliva that has leaked from a damaged salivary gland or duct and are surrounded by granulation tissue that forms secondary to inflammation caused by the free saliva. • There are four major pairs of salivary glands: parotid, mandibular, sublingual, zygomatic. Smaller buccal salivary glands are located in the soft palate, lips, tongue, and cheeks. • Types of mucoceles are listed in Table 1. The most common type occurs with rupture of the sublingual duct.

SYSTEMS AFFECTED
Gastrointestinal

SIGNALMENT
• Three times more frequent in dogs than in cats • All breeds are susceptible. Commonly affected breeds include miniature poodles (pharyngeal mucoceles), German shepherds, dachshunds, and Australian silky terriers. • Slight predisposition of males compared to females • No age predisposition

SIGNS
Cervical Mucocele
• Soft, fluctuant, minimal or non-painful gradually developing cervical mass • Pain is usually manifested only during the acute-manifestation phase of the mucocele.
Ranula
• Sublingual, soft, frog-like swelling (L. rana, frog) • Often blood-tinged saliva secondary to self-trauma while eating
Zygomatic Mucocele
• Periorbital facial swelling • Exophthalmos • Divergent strabismus • Periocular pain • Pressure-related neuropathy of the optic nerve
Pharyngeal Mucocele
• Abnormal tongue movement • Respiratory distress • Dysphagia

CAUSES & RISK FACTORS
Cause is rarely identified. Suspected causes: • Blunt trauma to the head and neck (choke chains) • Bite wound • Penetrating foreign body • Ear canal surgery • Sialoliths

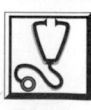

DIAGNOSIS
• Diagnosis is based on history, visual examination, and paracentesis of the mass. • Determine the site of origin with help of oral examination, palpation, sialography, or exploration of the mucocele.

DIFFERENTIAL DIAGNOSIS
• Sialoadenitis (second most common salivary disease, usually involving the mandibular gland, often concurrent with sialoceles) • Sialoadenosis • Salivary neoplasia (rare; mandibular gland most commonly involved; benign neoplasms exclusively found in cats) • Sialoliths (calcium phosphate or carbonate) • Cervical abscess • Salivary gland infarction (95% occur in mandibular gland) • Foreign body • Hematoma • Cystic or neoplastic lymph nodes • Tonsil cysts • Thyroglossal cysts (rare, congenital) • Cystic Rathke's pouch and branchial cysts (rare congenital)

CBC/BIOCHEMISTRY/URINALYSIS
Laboratory abnormalities are rarely seen.

OTHER LABORATORY TESTS N/A
IMAGING
• Rarely needed • Plain cervical radiographs only to identify sialoliths, foreign bodies, or neoplasia • Skull radiographs sometimes helpful to differentiate neoplastic disease from zygomatic mucocele, if cytologic evaluation is indeterminate • Sialography (injection of iodinated, water-soluble contrast agent into the salivary duct) is reserved for patients with trauma, previous surgeries, or fistulous draining tracts.

DIAGNOSTIC PROCEDURES
Aseptic Paracentesis
• Differentiates mucoceles from neoplasia, abscesses, and sialadenitis • Aspirated fluid is viscous, yellowish, clear, or blood-tinged with a low cell count. Inflamed sialoceles are characterized by low-grade chronic plasmacytic-lymphocytic inflammation. • Cytologic evaluation (Wright's stain) reveals diffuse or irregular clumps of pink to violet staining mucin, large phagocytic cells with small, round nuclei and foamy cytoplasm, intermixed salivary gland epithelial cells, and nondegenerate neutrophils in small numbers. • Stain with a mucus-specific stain (e.g., periodic acid–Schiff) for definitive diagnosis.

TREATMENT
• Patients with acute respiratory distress (pharyngeal mucoceles) might need to be intubated or have a temporary tracheostomy performed.

• Complete surgical excision of the involved gland-duct complex and drainage of the mucocele is the treatment of choice. Prolonged drainage can be achieved with marsupialization of ranulas and pharyngeal mucoceles and with placement of Penrose drains in cervical mucoceles.

MEDICATIONS

DRUG(S)
Antibiotics based on bacteriologic evaluation, if concurrent abscess or sialadenitis.

CONTRAINDICATIONS
Non-surgical treatment of salivary mucoceles with repeated drainage or injection of cauterizing or anti-inflammatory agents is not curative, and will complicate subsequent surgery by causing abscessation or fibrosis.

FOLLOW-UP

PATIENT MONITORING
• Daily bandage changes with Penrose drain placement. • Penrose drains are usually removed 24 to 72 hours following surgery. • Drain site should heal by second intention and contraction following marsupialization.

POSSIBLE COMPLICATIONS
Uncommon:
• Seroma formation • Infection • Mucocele recurrence

EXPECTED COURSE AND PROGNOSIS
• Excellent prognosis with complete surgical excision • Previous infection or injection complicates successful surgical excision.

MISCELLANEOUS

ASSOCIATED CONDITIONS
Sialoadenitis

SYNONYMS
• Sialocele • Salivary cyst • Honey cyst

Suggested Reading
Hedlund CS. Salivary mucoceles. In: Fossum TW, ed., Small animal surgery. 2nd ed. St. Louis: Mosby, 2002:302–307.
Author Susanne K. Lauer
Consulting Editor Albert E. Jergens

Table 1

Types of Mucoceles		
Salivary Mucocele Type	Location	Gland/Duct Involved
Cervical mucocele	Intermandibular space, jaw angle, upper cervical region	Sublingual
Ranula	Sublingual tissues	Mandibular or sublingual
Pharyngeal mucocele	Pharyngeal wall	Sublingual
Zygomatic mucocele	Ventral to the globe	Zygomatic
Parotid mucocele	Angle of the jaw, ventral to ear	Parotid
Complex mucoceles	Depending on gland/duct involvement (see above)	Two or more glands/ducts

SALMON POISONING DISEASE

BASICS

OVERVIEW
• Infection with the rickettsial organism *Neorickettsia helminthoeca*
• Organism—invades small intestinal epithelium and associated lymphoid tissue; systemic infection eventually develops.
• Occurs in the northern Pacific rim of the U.S.

SIGNALMENT
• Dogs of all ages
• No sex or breed predisposition

SIGNS
• Diarrhea
• Vomiting
• Lymphadenopathy
• Nasal and ocular discharge
• Fever

CAUSES & RISK FACTORS
• Ingestion of raw fish containing the trematode vector or *Neorickettsia helminthoeca* organisms
• Eating raw fish in an endemic area is a risk factor.

DIAGNOSIS

DIFFERENTIAL DIAGNOSIS
• Poisoning
• Canine parvovirus type 2
• Ehrlichiosis
• Canine distemper

CBC/BIOCHEMISTRY/URINALYSIS
No specific findings

OTHER LABORATORY TESTS
N/A

IMAGING
N/A

DIAGNOSTIC PROCEDURES
• Giemsa stain—aspirate of enlarged lymph node; reveals intracytoplasmic rickettsial bodies
• Fecal examination—reveal operculated eggs of the trematode *Nanophyetus salmincola*

PATHOLOGIC FINDINGS
• Changes in lymphoid tissue—enlarged, yellowish, prominent white foci
• Intestinal contents—frequently contain free blood

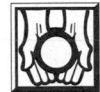

TREATMENT
• Inpatient—acutely ill patients
• Treat as for canine ehrlichiosis.
• Supportive therapy—fluids with electrolytes; basic measures to control diarrhea

MEDICATIONS

DRUG(S)
• Oxytetracycline—7.5–10 mg/kg IV q12h for 14 days; 20 mg/kg PO q12h
• Tetracycline—15–20 mg/kg PO q8h for 14 days
• Chloramphenicol—40–50 mg/kg PO q8h for 14 days
• Praziquantel—20–30 mg/kg SC or PO q24h for 3 days to kill flukes

FOLLOW-UP

PATIENT MONITORING
Monitor hydration, electrolytes, acid–base balance, and body temperature.

PREVENTION /AVOIDANCE
• Prevent animals from eating raw fish.
• Inform client of necessity to act quickly and consider other dogs that may have eaten the same raw fish.

EXPECTED COURSE AND PROGNOSIS
• Animals likely to succumb within 5–10 days of infection unless treated
• With early diagnosis and treatment—prognosis good
• Untreated—often fatal

MISCELLANEOUS

ASSOCIATED CONDITIONS
• Elokomin fluke fever agent—similar rickettsia; causes a more mild form of the disease
• Infection with *Nanophyetus salmincola* does not itself cause severe clinical disease.

ZOONOTIC POTENTIAL
No reported risk to humans

Suggested Reading
Gorham JR, Foreyt WJ. Salmon poisoning disease. In: Greene CE, ed. Infectious diseases of the dog and cat. 2nd ed. Philadelphia: Saunders, 1998:135–139.
Author Johnny D. Hoskins
Consulting Editor Stephen C. Barr

SALMONELLOSIS

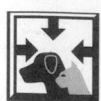

BASICS

DEFINITION
A bacterial disease that causes enteritis, septicemia, and abortions and is caused by many different serotypes of *Salmonella*

PATHOPHYSIOLOGY
• *Salmonella*—a gram-negative bacterium; colonizes the small intestine (ileum); adheres to and invades the enterocytes; eventually enters and multiplies in the lamina propria and local mesenteric lymph nodes; cytotoxin (cell death) and enterotoxin (increases cAMP) are produced; inflammation occurs; and prostaglandin synthesis ensues; results in secretory diarrhea and mucosal sloughing • Uncomplicated gastroenteritis—organisms are stopped at the mesenteric lymph node stage; patient has only diarrhea, vomiting, and dehydration • Bacteremia and septicemia following gastroenteritis—more serious disease; focal extraintestinal infections (abortion, joint disease) or endotoxemia may result; may lead to organ infarction, generalized thrombosis, DIC, and death • Some patients recover from the septicemic form but suffer prolonged recovery as a result of their debilitated state.

SYSTEMS AFFECTED
• Gastrointestinal—enterocolitis; inflammation, mucosal sloughing, secretory diarrhea • Systemic disease (e.g., bacteremia, focal infections, septicemia)—multiorgan infarction, thrombosis, abscesses, meningitis, osteomyelitis, abortion

GENETICS
Genetic susceptibility not well known

INCIDENCE/PREVALENCE
• True incidence unknown • Most infections subclinical • Dogs—clinical disease most often seen in the young and pregnant; fecal/rectal swab survey of clinically normal domestic pets, boarding kennels, and veterinary hospitals shows incidences of 30%, 16.7%, and 21.5%, respectively. Common in racing greyhounds and racing sled dogs • Cats—have a high natural resistance; stressed hospitalized animals at high risk; fecal survey of normal cats and cats from a research colony shows incidences of 18% and 10.6%, respectively; Shelter cats more likely to have *Salmonella* in feces; pandemics of salmonellosis in migrating songbirds (usually *typhimurium*) in spring create epidemics in bird-hunting cats.

GEOGRAPHIC DISTRIBUTION
Worldwide

SIGNALMENT
Species
Dogs and cats

Breed Predilections
None

Mean Age and Range
• Dogs—clinical disease manifests in neonatal/immature puppies and in pregnant bitches; most adult carrier dogs clinically normal • Cats—adults highly resistant

Predominant Sex
N/A

SIGNS
General Comments
Disease severity—subclinical (carrier state: *Salmonella* shed in stool) to mild, moderate, and severe clinical cases in neonatal and stressed adult dogs and cats; subclinical infection more common than clinical disease (rare)

Historical Findings
• Diarrhea • Vomiting • Fever • Malaise • Anorexia • Vaginal discharge/abortion—dogs • Chronic febrile illness—persistent fever, anorexia, malaise without diarrhea

Physical Examination Findings
• Asymptomatic carrier states—no clinical signs • Gastroenteritis—anorexia; malaise/lethargy; depression fever (39–40°C; 102–104°F); diarrhea with mucus and/or blood; progressive dehydration; abdominal pain; tenesmus; pale mucous membranes; mesenteric lymphadenopathy; weight loss • Gastroenteritis with bacteremia and septicemia, septic shock, or endotoxemia—pale mucous membranes; weakness; cardiovascular collapse; tachycardia; tachypnea • Focal extraintestinal infections—conjunctivitis; uterus/abortion; cellulitis; pyothorax • Cats—may exhibit syndrome of a chronic febrile illness (without gastrointestinal signs); persistent fever; prolonged illness with vague, nonspecific clinical signs; and left shift on leukogram • Recovering patients—may exhibit chronic intermittent diarrhea for 3–4 weeks; may shed *Salmonella* in stool for 6 weeks or longer

CAUSES
• Any one of more than 2000 serotypes of salmonellae • Two or more simultaneous serotypes in a host animal not uncommon

RISK FACTORS
Disease Agent
Salmonella serotype—virulence factors, infectious dose, and route of exposure • Host factors that increase susceptibility • Age—neonatal/young dogs and cats; immature immune system • Overall health status—debilitated young animals or adults: other concurrent disease, parasitism; young animals: immature gastrointestinal tract, poorly developed normal microbial flora • Disrupted gastrointestinal bacteria flora (adult cats)—antimicrobial treatment; subsequent exposure to salmonellae during hospitalization

Environmental Factors
• Coprophagia spreads infection. • Dehydrated (dry) pet food—known to harbor salmonellae; semimoist foods (e.g., kibble and dog biscuits) usually not as risky • Pig ear dog

treats contaminated by *Salmonella* • Horse meat fed to exotic felids • Grooming habits—may result in *Salmonella*-contaminated hair coat, which contaminates cage or run environment, feed and water dishes • Dense population—research colony, boarded animals, shelter/pound animals; overcrowded housing; unsanitary conditions; exposure to other infected (or carrier) animals—buildup of *Salmonella* in the environment; more efficient fecal–oral cycling; high opportunity for fecal exposure; stress factors

Hunting/Stray Animals
• Scavenging for food—exposure to garbage, contaminated food/water, dead animals • Exposure to other infected (or carrier) animals • Exposure to infected raw meat

Hospitalized Animals
Nosocomial exposure (plus stress) or activation (by stress) of preexisting asymptomatic (carrier) *Salmonella* infection, especially in animals treated with antimicrobial drugs

Vaccinated Cats
Death in kittens (likely to be infected by *Salmonella* subclinically) post-vaccination, with high titers of modified line panleukopenia vaccine

DIAGNOSIS

DIFFERENTIAL DIAGNOSIS
• Acute gastroenteritis—vomiting, diarrhea, infectious enteritis; differentiate by serology and/or culture • Viral gastroenteritis—feline panleukopenia, FeLV, FIV, feline enteric coronavirus, canine enteric coronavirus, canine parvovirus, rotavirus, canine distemper • Bacterial gastroenteritis—*E. coli, Campylobacter jejuni, Yersinia enterocolitica* • Bacterial overgrowth syndrome—*Clostridium difficile, Clostridium perfringens* • Parasites—helminths (hookworms, ascarids, whipworms, strongyloides); protozoa (*Giardia, Coccidia, Cryptosporidia*); Rickettsiae; salmon poisoning • Acute gastritis—erosions or ulcers • Dietary-induced distress—overeating, abrupt changes, starvation, thirst, allergy or food intolerance, indiscretions (foreign material, garbage) • Drug or toxin-induced distress • Extraintestinal disorders/metabolic disease

CBC/BIOCHEMISTRY/URINALYSIS
• CBC—variable; depends on stage of illness • Neutropenia initially • Left shift with toxic neutrophils • Nonregenerative anemia • Lymphopenia • Thrombocytopenia • Hypoalbuminemia • Electrolyte imbalances

OTHER LABORATORY TESTS N/A

IMAGING N/A

DIAGNOSTIC PROCEDURES
• Fecal/rectal culture—positive; special media needed

• Fecal leukocytes—positive
• Blood cultures—positive in patients with bacteremia
• Joint fluid—may be culture-positive
• Subclinical carrier states—chronic; intermittent fecal culture positive (> 6 weeks)
• **NOTE:** use of antimicrobials in a patient before sampling may produce false-negative cultures.

PATHOLOGIC FINDINGS
• Gross lesions—only in severely affected patients
• Cultures of ileum, mesenteric lymph node, liver/spleen, and bone marrow—positive

TREATMENT

APPROPRIATE HEALTH CARE
• Outpatient—uncomplicated gastroenteritis (without bacteremia) and carrier states
• Inpatient—with bacteremia/septicemia and for gastroenteritis in neonatal/immature animals that are rapidly debilitated by diarrhea

NURSING CARE
• Varies according to severity of illness—assess percentages of dehydration, body weight, ongoing fluid loss, shock, PCV/total protein, electrolytes, acid–base status

Uncomplicated Gastroenteritis
• Supportive care—fluid and electrolyte replacement
• Parenteral, balanced, polyionic isotonic solution (lactated Ringer's)
• Oral fluids—hypertonic glucose solutions; for secretory diarrhea
• Plasma transfusions—if serum albumin < 2 g/dL

Neonates, Aged, and Debilitated Animals
• Plasma transfusions
• Supportive care—as outlined above

ACTIVITY
• Isolate inpatients—all patients in acute stages may shed large numbers of salmonellae in the stool.
• Restrict activity with cage rest, monitor, and provide warmth—acutely ill, bacteremic/septicemic, and chronically ill animals.

DIET
Restrict food 24–48 hr; gradually introduce a highly digestible, low-fat diet.

CLIENT EDUCATION
Instruct client to wash hands frequently and to restrict access to patient in acute stages of the disease; large numbers of salmonellae may be shed in the stool.

SURGICAL CONSIDERATIONS N/A

MEDICATIONS

DRUG(S) OF CHOICE

Asymptomatic Carrier State
• Antimicrobials—contraindicated
• Quinolone drugs—demonstrated clearing of carrier states in humans; more controlled trials in animals needed

Uncomplicated Gastroenteritis
• Antimicrobials not indicated
• Locally acting intestinal adsorbents and protectants

Neonates, Aged, and Debilitated Animals
• Glucocorticoids—shown to reduce mortality in endotoxic shock • Antimicrobial therapy—indicated; culture and susceptibility testing/MIC necessary to assess drug-resistance problems • Trimethoprim-sulfa—15 mg/kg PO or SC q12h • Enrofloxacin—5 mg/kg PO or IM q12h • Norfloxacin—22 mg/kg PO q12h • Chloramphenicol—dogs: 50 mg/kg PO, IV, IM, or SC q8h; cats: 50 mg/kg total PO, IV, IM, or SC q12h

CONTRAINDICATIONS
None

PRECAUTIONS
• Chloramphenicol and trimethoprim-sulfa—use cautiously in neonatal and pregnant patients. • Fluoroquinolones—avoid use in pregnant, neonatal, or growing animals (medium-sized dogs < 8 months of age; large or giant breeds < 12–18 months of age) because of cartilage lesions.

POSSIBLE INTERACTIONS N/A

ALTERNATIVE DRUG(S) N/A

FOLLOW-UP

PATIENT MONITORING
• Fecal culture—repeat monthly for few months to assess development of carrier state
• Other animals—monitor for secondary spread of infection • Advise client to contact veterinarian if patient shows signs of recurring disease.

PREVENTION/AVOIDANCE
• Keep animals healthy—proper nutrition; no raw meat; vaccinate for other infectious diseases; clean and disinfect cages, runs, and food and water dishes frequently; store food and feeding utensils properly • Reduce over-crowding—pounds, shelters, kennels, catteries, and research colonies • New arrivals—isolate and screen; monitor for sickness before mixing with other animals. • Experimental live attenuated vaccine shows promise, especially for racing dogs. • Important to protect animals being treated with antimicrobial drugs from

exposure to a salmonella-contaminated environment (e.g., an animal hospital)

POSSIBLE COMPLICATIONS
• Spread of infection not uncommon within household to other animals or humans
• Development of chronic infection with diarrhea • Recurrence of disease with stress

EXPECTED COURSE AND PROGNOSIS
• Uncomplicated gastroenteritis—prognosis excellent; frequently self-limited; patients recover with good nursing care. • Recovered animals may shed *Salmonella* intermittently for months or longer as a recovered carrier.
• Neonatal, aged, stressed animals—can develop septicemia and systemic disease; can be severe and debilitating; may lead to death if untreated

MISCELLANEOUS

ASSOCIATED CONDITIONS N/A

AGE-RELATED FACTORS
Clinical disease is frequently seen in neonatal and aged animals.

ZOONOTIC POTENTIAL
• High potential, especially in children, elderly, immunosuppressed, and antimicrobial drug users • Multi-drug resistant *Salmonella* isolated from kittens with enteritis • Acutely ill animals shed large numbers of salmonellae in stool.
• Grooming habits allow rapid contamination of animal's fur and environment. • Isolation is needed.

PREGNANCY
• May complicate disease • Abortion—may be a sequela to infection • Antimicrobial therapy—take into account the effect on the fetus.

SYNONYMS
Songbird fever

ABBREVIATIONS
• DIC = disseminated intravascular coagulation • FeLV = feline leukemia virus • FIV = feline immunodeficiency virus • MIC = minimal inhibitory concentration • PCV = packed cell volume

Suggested Reading
Dow SW, Jones RL, Henik RA, Husted PW. Clinical features of salmonellosis in cats: six cases (1981–1986). J Am Vet Med Assoc 1989;194:1464–1466.
Greene CE. Salmonellosis. In: Greene CE, ed. Infectious diseases of the dog and cat. Philadelphia: Saunders, 1998:235–240
Morse EV, Duncan MA. Canine salmonellosis: prevalence, epizootiology, signs, and public health significance. J Am Vet Med Assoc 1975;167:817–820.
Author Patrick L. McDonough
Consulting Editor Stephen C. Barr

SARCOPTIC MANGE

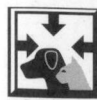

BASICS

OVERVIEW
A nonseasonal, intensely pruritic, highly contagious parasitic skin disease of dogs caused by *Sarcoptes scabiei* var. canis mites. The mites burrow through the stratum corneum and cause intense pruritus by mechanical irritation and production of irritating secretions and allergenic substances that produce a hypersensitivity reaction in sensitized dogs.

SIGNALMENT
• Affects dogs of all ages and breeds • In multiple-dog households, more than one dog usually shows symptoms.

SIGNS
• Nonseasonal, intense pruritus • Ear pinnae are usually affected with a mild to severe alopecic crusting dermatitis; ear canals are often not affected. • Alopecia and erythema with a papular rash develop on the elbows, hocks, ventral abdomen, and chest; severely affected dogs have generalized alopecic crusting papular rash and are intensely pruritic. • Some dogs have minimal skin lesions (erythema) with only mild pruritus. • Treatment with antihistamines or anti-inflammatory doses of steroids typically does not reduce the pruritus.

CAUSES & RISK FACTORS
• Exposure to infected dogs 2–6 weeks before the development of symptoms • Close contact with other dogs, especially by way of animal shelters, boarding kennels, groomers, and veterinarians' offices

DIAGNOSIS

DIFFERENTIAL DIAGNOSIS
• Atopy, food allergy, and scabies—can look exactly alike
• Folliculitis (pyoderma, demodicosis, dermatophytosis)
• *Malassezia* dermatitis
• *Cheyletiella*
• Trombiculosis (chiggers)
• Contact dermatitis
• *Pelodera* dermatitis

OTHER LABORATORY TESTS
ELISA—technique to identify *Sarcoptes*-infested dogs; has shown good results (sensitivity = 84.2%, specificity = 89.5%), and is available at the University of Georgia.

DIAGNOSTIC PROCEDURES
• Response to scabicidal treatment—most common method for diagnosing scabies; any dog with clinical signs suggestive of sarcoptic mange should be treated for scabies. • Positive

pinnal-pedal reflex—rubbing the ear margin between the thumb and forefinger should induce the dog to scratch with its hind leg; occurs in 80% of cases (sensitivity = 81.8%, specificity = 93.8%) • Skin scrapings—positive in only 20% of scabies cases; mites and ova are extremely difficult to find; false-negative results are common. • Fecal flotation–occasionally reveals mites or ova; adult mites are 200–400 μm in size and have short unjointed stalks extending from the distal portion of the leg

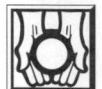

TREATMENT
• Any dog with nonseasonal pruritus should be treated with a scabicide (even if skin scraping results are negative) to definitively rule out sarcoptic mange. When scabicidal dips are used, the entire dog must be treated. • Treatment failures are often linked to the owner's reluctance to apply dip to the dog's face and ears. • All in-contact dogs should be treated, even those with no clinical signs, because they may be asymptomatic carriers. • Because of the hypersensitivity reaction to the scabies mites, it can take as long as 4–6 weeks for the pruritus and clinical signs to resolve. • *Sarcoptes* mites usually perish quickly in the environment; however, the mites have been reported to survive for up to 3 weeks. Therefore, thorough cleaning and treatment of the dog's environment are recommended.

MEDICATIONS

DRUG(S) OF CHOICE
• Selamectin (Revolution; Pfizer, New York, NY)—labeled for treatment of scabies when applied every 30 days; application every 2–4 weeks for at least three treatments may be more effective • Ivermectin—effective; 0.2–0.4 mg/kg SC or PO every 1–2 weeks for three to four treatments (for at least 1 month); do not use in herding breeds or heartworm-positive dogs • Milbemycin (Interceptor; Novartis AH, Greensboro, NC)—may be effective when used at 0.75 mg/kg PO q24h or 2 mg/kg PO every week for 3 weeks • Alternative ivermectins that may be effective—doramectin 0.2–0.6 mg/kg SC or IM every week for three to six treatments • Amitraz dip (250 ppm)—may be effective when used every week for a minimum of three treatments; treatment failures may occur unless the entire body is covered, including the face and ears
• Alternative dips—2%–3% solution of lime sulfur (LymDyp; DVM Pharmaceuticals, Miami, FL); mercaptomethyl phthalimide dip (phosmet); applied weekly and continue

for a minimum of 6 weeks, making sure that the entire body is covered, including the face and ears • Topical antiseborrheic therapy in conjunction with scabicidal therapy—helps speed clinical resolution of the scaling, crusting lesions • Systemic antibiotics—may be needed for 21 days or longer to resolve any secondary pyodermas

CONTRAINDICATIONS/POSSIBLE INTERACTIONS
Do not use ivermectin in collies, Shetland sheepdogs, old English sheepdogs, Australian shepherds, and their cross-breeds—increased risk of ivermectin toxicity in herding-type breeds

FOLLOW-UP
• Response to therapy may require 4–6 weeks. • Topical scabicidal treatments are more prone to failure because of incomplete application of the treatment solution. • Reinfection may occur if contact with infected animals continues.

MISCELLANEOUS

POSSIBLE COMPLICATIONS
Approximately 30% of dogs with *Sarcoptes* infections will also react to house dust mite antigens on intradermal skin testing, suggesting that house dust mite allergy may be a possible sequeala to scabies infection.

ZOONOTIC POTENTIAL
Sarcoptic mange is zoonotic. People who come in close contact with an affected dog may develop a pruritic, papular rash on their arms, chest, or abdomen. Human lesions are usually transient and should resolve spontaneously after the affected dog(s) have been treated. If the lesions on people persist, advice from a human dermatologist should be sought.

ABBREVIATION
ELISA = enzyme-linked immunosorbent assay

Suggested Reading
De Jaham C, Henry CJ. Treatment of canine sarcoptic mange using milbemycin oxime. Can Vet J 1995;36:42–43.
Lower KS, Medleau L, Hnilica KA. Evaluation of an enzyme-linked immunosorbent assay (ELISA) for the serological diagnosis of sarcoptic mange in dogs. Vet Dermatol 2001;12:315–320.
Scott DW, Miller WH, Griffin CE. Muller & Kirk's small animal dermatology. 6th ed. Philadelphia: Saunders, 2001:476–483.
Author Keith A. Hnilica
Consulting Editor Linda Medleau

BASICS

OVERVIEW
• Thoracic limb extension associated with hind limb paralysis after acute and usually severe spinal cord lesion cranial to L2 and caudal to the cervical intumescence
• Posture—caused by the release of the border cells, interneurons located in the lumbar spinal cord (mainly L2–4) and normally inhibiting the extensor motor neurons of the cervical intumescence

SIGNALMENT
• Any dog suffering from a severe thoraco-lumbar spinal cord injury

SIGNS
• Forelimbs—rigidly extended; normal gait and postural reactions (because the lesion is caudal to the cervical intumescence)
• Hindlimbs—depend on the severity and location of the lesion; usually upper motor neuron in type, but may be lower motor neuron

CAUSES & RISK FACTORS
Road accident and intervertebral disk disease—most common

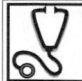 DIAGNOSIS

DIFFERENTIAL DIAGNOSIS
• Decerebrate rigidity—observed with brain stem disease in which all four limbs are rigid and upper motor neuron dysfunction occurs in all limbs; patient is unconscious.
• Decerebellate rigidity—observed with cerebellar disease in which the forelimbs are rigid but the hind limbs are flexed; consciousness may be normal but is usually altered
• Cervical spinal cord injury—may have extensor hypertonia in the forelimbs; upper motor neuron and proprioceptive deficits of all limbs are also seen

CBC/BIOCHEMISTRY/URINALYSIS
N/A

OTHER LABORATORY TESTS
N/A

IMAGING
Radiology (myelography, CT, MRI)—demonstrate the thoracolumbar spinal lesion

DIAGNOSTIC PROCEDURES
N/A

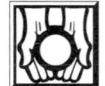 TREATMENT

• Directed toward the underlying thoraco-lumbar lesion
• No specific treatment available
• Condition resolves if adequate spinal cord function is restored.

 MEDICATIONS

DRUG(S)
As indicated for underlying spinal cord disease

CONTRAINDICATIONS/POSSIBLE INTERACTIONS
N/A

 FOLLOW-UP

• Posture may persist for days to weeks; not an indication of a hopeless prognosis
• With rapid and aggressive treatment, the patient may recover, especially if there is pain perception caudal to the lesion.

 MISCELLANEOUS

Suggested Reading
de Lahunta A. Veterinary neuroanatomy and clinical neurology. 2nd ed. Philadelphia: Saunders, 1983:185.
Author Mary O. Smith
Consulting Editor Joane M. Parent

SCHISTOSOMIASIS—DOGS

 BASICS

OVERVIEW
• *Heterobilharzia americanum*—schistosomatid parasite of raccoons
• Eggs passed in the feces of raccoons hatch to release miracidia that penetrate snail hosts. After a period of development and asexual multiplication, the snails release cercariae that infect the next host (can be dogs) by skin penetration. After penetrating the skin, the larvae undergo a migration to the lung, and then make their way to the mesenteric veins where separate males and females form pairs. Eggs laid by female worms are carried to the intestinal wall where they erode their way through to the lumen to be passed in the feces. Other eggs are carried to the liver or other organs by the bloodstream where they lodge and cause granulomatous disease.
• Dogs infected when in contact with water containing cercariae
• Restricted to southeastern US. Dog cases reported from Texas, Florida, Louisiana, and North Carolina

SIGNALMENT
• Dogs, typically adult, that have access to swampy areas or bayou

SIGNS
• Diarrhea (sometimes hemorrhagic) most common presenting sign
• Mild anemia, weight loss, hyperproteinemia, vomiting, and hypercalcemia

CAUSES & RISK FACTORS
Swimming in areas contaminated with cercariae from miracidia

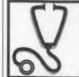 DIAGNOSIS

DIFFERENTIAL DIAGNOSIS
• Coccidiosis
• Bacterial diarrhea
• Viral enteritis

CBC/BIOCHEMISTRY/URINALYSIS
• Mild anemia and eosinophilia
• Proteinuria

OTHER LABORATORY TESTS
ELISA—performed by private laboratory, College of Veterinary Medicine, North Carolina State University

IMAGING
• Contrast radiographs and ultrasound may reveal thickened bowel walls.

DIAGNOSTIC PROCEDURES
Eggs with miracidia can be identified in feces, but feces must be kept in saline—not water—or miracidia will spontaneously hatch, making diagnosis impossible.
• Identify eggs using fecal flotation using sugar solution of specific gravity of 1.3, or fecal sedimentation. Routine fecal flotation will not detect these heavy eggs.
• Several of the past cases have been diagnosed after laparotomy.

 TREATMENT

Inpatient care for the first few days of treatment would probably be warranted, as the response to worm kill may require supportive care.

 MEDICATIONS

DRUG(S)
• Praziquantel (50 mg/kg, PO, once)
• Fenbendazole (50 mg/kg, PO, q24h for 10 days).

 FOLLOW-UP

Check feces after 1 to 2 months to ensure that it does not contain eggs.

 MISCELLANEOUS

In Japan and other countries with endemic *Schistosoma japonicum,* dogs can be infected with this human and zoonotic species.

ABBREVIATION
ELISA = enzyme-linked immunosorbent assay

ZOONOTIC POTENTIAL
Stages in the dog pose no threat to staff or owners. People entering the same waterways could develop lesions.

Suggested Reading
Flowers JR, et al. *Heterobilharzia americana* infection in a dog. J Am Vet Med Assoc 2002;220:193–196.
Author Dwight D. Bowman
Consulting Editor Stephen C. Barr

BASICS

OVERVIEW
• Tumors of nerve sheath origin, arising from Schwann cells
• Peripheral nerve sheath tumor—proposed term to include schwannomas, neuro-fibromas, and neurofibrosarcomas, because all arise from the same cell

SIGNALMENT
• Dogs and rarely cats
• Dogs—mean age, 8.7 years
• No breed predilection
• Slight male predisposition (1.4:1)

SIGNS
• Chronic, progressive forelimb lameness and muscle atrophy—most common
• Hind limbs—may be primarily affected; less common
• Peripheral neuropathy (self-mutilation)—occasionally
• Palpable mass—> 50% of patients
• Horner's syndrome—with cervical involvement

CAUSES & RISK FACTORS
None identified

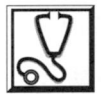

DIAGNOSIS

DIFFERENTIAL DIAGNOSIS
• Orthopedic disease
• Other neurologic disease—intervertebral disk disease
• Other neoplasia—lymphoma

CBC/BIOCHEMISTRY/URINALYSIS
Usually normal

OTHER LABORATORY TESTS
CSF analysis—usually unrewarding

IMAGING
• Plain radiography—rarely helpful
• Myelography—may be helpful with dorsal or ventral nerve root involvement
• CT or, ideally, MRI—provides the most information regarding extent and location of disease

DIAGNOSTIC PROCEDURES
Electromyography—consistently reveals abnormal, spontaneous electrical activity in muscles of the affected limb

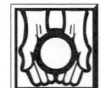

TREATMENT
• Surgical excision—treatment of choice
• Distal mass—limb may still be functional after excision.
• Amputation—usually required
• Laminectomy—necessary with nerve root involvement
• Local recurrence after surgery common
• Radiotherapy—deserves further evaluation

MEDICATIONS

DRUG(S)
• Chemotherapy—no successful management described
• Corticosteroids—may help reduce peri-tumoral edema; may temporarily relieve clinical signs

CONTRAINDICATIONS/POSSIBLE INTERACTIONS
N/A

FOLLOW-UP

EXPECTED COURSE AND PROGNOSIS
• Recurrence after surgical excision—common; up to 72% of cases
• The more distal the tumor, the better the possibility of a surgical cure.
• Median disease-free interval with brachial or lumbosacral plexus involvement—7.5 months
• Median disease-free interval with dorsal or ventral nerve root involvement—1 month
• Metastasize—(rarely) to regional lymph nodes or lungs

MISCELLANEOUS

ABBREVIATION
CSF = cerebrospinal fluid

Suggested Reading
Brehm DM, Vite CH, Steinberg HS, et al. A retrospective evaluation of 51 cases of peripheral nerve sheath tumors in the dog. J Am Anim Hosp Assoc 1995;31:349–359.
LeCouteur RA. Tumors of the nervous system. In: Withrow SJ, MacEwen EG, eds. Small animal clinical oncology. Philadelphia: Saunders, 2001:500–531.
Morrison WB. Cancer affecting the nervous system. In: Morrison WB, ed. Cancer in dogs and cats: medical and surgical management. Baltimore: Williams & Wilkins, 1998:655–665.

Author Ruthanne Chun
Consulting Editor Wallace B. Morrison

SEBACEOUS ADENITIS

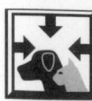 BASICS

OVERVIEW
• An inflammatory disease process directed against the cutaneous adnexal structures (sebaceous glands)
• May be genetically inherited, immune-mediated, or metabolic
• Initial defect—a keratinization disorder or an abnormality in lipid metabolism (accumulation of toxic intermediate metabolites)

SIGNALMENT
• Young adult to middle-aged dogs
• Two forms—one in long-coated and one in short-coated breeds
• Predisposed—standard poodles, akitas, Samoyeds, and vizslas

SIGNS

Long-coated Breeds
• Symmetrical, partial alopecia
• Dull brittle hair
• Tightly adherent silver-white scale
• Follicular casts around hair shaft
• Small tufts of matted hair
• Lesions—often first observed along dorsal midline and dorsum of the head
• Severe—secondary bacterial folliculitis, pruritus, and malodor
• Akitas—often relatively severely affected

Short-coated Breeds
• Alopecia—moth-eaten, circular, or diffuse
• Mild scaling
• Affects the trunk, head, and ears
• Secondary bacterial folliculitis rare

CAUSES & RISK FACTORS
Mode of inheritance is being studied

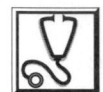 DIAGNOSIS

DIFFERENTIAL DIAGNOSIS
• Primary seborrhea—keratinization disorder
• Bacterial folliculitis
• Demodicosis
• Dermatophytosis
• Endocrine skin disease

CBC/BIOCHEMISTRY/URINALYSIS
N/A

OTHER LABORATORY TESTS
N/A

IMAGING
N/A

DIAGNOSTIC PROCEDURES
• Skin scrapings—normal
• Dermatophyte culture—negative
• Endocrine function tests—normal
• Skin biopsies

PATHOLOGIC FINDINGS
• Nodular granulomatous to pyogranulomatous inflammatory reaction at the level of the sebaceous glands
• Orthokeratotic hyperkeratosis and follicular cast formation; more prominent in long-coated breeds
• Advanced—complete loss of sebaceous glands; periadnexal fibrosis

• Destruction of entire hair follicle and adnexal unit rare

TREATMENT

• Clinical signs may wax and wane irrespective of treatment.
• Controlled studies have not been done to document efficacy of any therapy.
• Results extremely variable; response may depend on severity of disease at the time of diagnosis.
• Akita—breed most refractory to treatment

MEDICATIONS

DRUG(S)
• Propylene glycol and water—50–75% mixture; spray every 24 hr to affected areas

• Baby oil—soak affected areas for 1 hr; follow with multiple shampoos to remove oil and scales
• Derm Cap (1 extra-strength) and evening primrose oil (500 mg)—q12h PO; possible side effects include vomiting, diarrhea, and flatulence.
• Isotretinoin (Accutane)—1 mg/kg q12h PO; reduce to 1 mg/kg q24h after 1 month and to 1 mg/kg q48h after 2 months; continue as needed for maintenance.
• Cyclosporine (Sandimmune)—5 mg/kg q12h PO; side effects include vomiting, diarrhea, gingival hyperplasia, hirsutism, papillomatous skin lesions, increased incidence of infections, nephrotoxicity, and hepatotoxicity.
• Bactericidal antibiotics and Sulf-Oxydex shampoo—for secondary bacterial folliculitis

CONTRAINDICATIONS/POSSIBLE INTERACTIONS
N/A

FOLLOW-UP

Urge owners to register affected dogs so that mode of inheritance can be determined.

MISCELLANEOUS

Suggested Reading

Rosser EJ. Sebaceous adenitis. In: Griffin CE, Kwochka KW, MacDonald JM, eds. Current veterinary dermatology. St. Louis: Mosby, 1993:211–214.

Authors Ellen C. Codner and Karen Helton Rhodes

Consulting Editor Karen Helton Rhodes

SEIZURES (CONVULSIONS, STATUS EPILEPTICUS)—CATS

 BASICS

DEFINITION
• Clinical manifestation of excessive discharge of hyperexcitable cerebrocortical neurons • Clinical signs vary depending on the area of the brain involved in the seizure discharge generation and propagation.

PATHOPHYSIOLOGY
• Intracranial and extracranial causes of seizures—result in focal or diffuse hyper-excitability of cerebrocortical neurons • High-frequency and sustained seizure activity may recruit other parts of the brain into the epileptic discharge and cause neuronal damage, leading to more frequent and refractory seizures (in both acute and chronic seizure disorders).

SYSTEMS AFFECTED
Nervous

GENETICS
Inherited (primary or genetic or idiopathic) epilepsy is rare in cats.

INCIDENCE/PREVALENCE
Seizure disorders are much less frequent in cats than in dogs.

SIGNALMENT
Cats of any age, breed, or sex

SIGNS

General Comments
• Sudden onset; short duration (usually < 2 min); abrupt termination; often followed by postictal disturbances (e.g., mental confusion, apparent blindness) • May occur as isolated events, cluster seizures (> two within 24 hr), or status epilepticus (one sustained or serial seizures lasting > 30 min) • Primary generalized—diffuse onset within both cerebral hemispheres; manifest with unconsciousness and bilateral, symmetric motor activity involving the whole body (e.g., tonic-clonic or convulsive seizures) • Partial—focal onset in one cerebral hemisphere; limited spreading within one or both cerebral hemispheres; may be preceded by an aura (behavioral changes within the few seconds or minutes of the ictus onset) or followed by localized (unilateral) postictal deficits (e.g., motor, menace, proprioceptive), even if seizure appears generalized from the onset (partial seizure with rapid secondary generalization) • Simple partial—no consciousness alteration; unilateral, often localized motor signs (e.g., facial twitching); contralateral to the seizure focus • Complex partial—most common; consciousness alterations; unilateral or bilateral (symmetric or asymmetric) motor signs; bizarre behavioral activity common

Historical Findings
• Seizure history (e.g., age at first seizure; type, initial and subsequent frequency)—may reveal important clues about the underlying cause (e.g., partial seizures are always caused by structural brain lesions)

Physical Examination Findings
• Physical or fundic abnormalities—may be related to the seizures, indicating multisystemic disease (e.g., infectious, metabolic, neoplastic) • Unilateral or bilateral but asymmetric deficits in the menace response, nasal septum sensation, hopping and proprioceptive positioning—structural brain lesion in the contralateral forebrain; common but often subtle, and must be looked for carefully • Bilateral symmetric deficits—may be caused by diffuse brain dysfunction owing to intracranial or extracranial diseases or to postictal disturbances • Multifocal neurologic deficits—multifocal CNS involvement; usually caused by infectious or noninfectious encephalomyelitides

CAUSES

Extracranial
• Metabolic—severe hypoglycemia and hypocalcemia; advanced hepatic encephalopathy and renal failure • Toxicities—many intoxications in their advanced stages • Hypoxic—polycythemia; cardiovascular diseases

Intracranial
• Functional (idiopathic and genetic) epilepsy—poorly documented • Structural brain lesions—most common; active lesions: meningoencephalitis of unknown but suspected viral or perhaps immune-mediated origin, feline ischemic encephalopathy (seizures may be the only sign in the atypical form), and brain tumors (e.g., meningiomas) common; infectious encephalitides (e.g., FIP, toxoplasmosis, bacterial and fungal infections, cuterebral myiasis) less frequent; static lesions, such as in postencephalitic, postanoxic, ischemic (e.g., birth-related, polycythemia-related cerebrovascular accidents, feline ischemic encephalopathy) and post-traumatic epilepsy possibly frequent

RISK FACTORS
Any brain lesion involving the forebrain

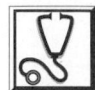 **DIAGNOSIS**

DIFFERENTIAL DIAGNOSIS

Similar Signs
• Syncope—sudden loss of consciousness and muscle tone resulting in flaccid recumbency and followed by complete recovery within seconds; differentiated by history and physical examination (e.g., episodes induced by stress or exercise, cardiovascular abnormalities such as heart murmur and arrhythmias) • Sleep disorders—violent movements occurring exclusively during sleep; patient may be aroused by external stimulations and exhibit a normal waking behavior (no postictal disturbances)

Causes
• Extracranial—rare; cause an acute onset of multiple or continuous generalized convulsive seizures and no focal neurologic deficits • Metabolic and hypoxic disorders—other historical, clinical, and laboratory signs • Thiamine deficiency—rare; probably does not cause real seizures but bilateral vestibular signs • Toxins—a progression from shaking to trembling and finally to sustained status epilepticus until treatment or death • Structural brain lesions—look for carefully; partial seizures, including aura or localized postictal deficits; neurologic deficits of forebrain origin; active lesions: acute onset of high-frequency seizures (status epilepticus, cluster seizures or > one seizure within the first 4–6 weeks) with no signs of extracranial causes; progressive or regressive course; static lesions: low to moderate initial frequency; no or slow subsequent increase in frequency

CBC/BIOCHEMISTRY/URINALYSIS
• Usually normal unless multisystemic disease (e.g., metabolic, infectious) exists • Polycythemia—PCV usually > 60%

OTHER LABORATORY TESTS
• Serology testing—FeLV, FIV, FIP, and *Toxoplasma gondii*; usually noncontributory without concurrent systemic signs; FIP and *Toxoplasma* do not reliably identify active infection; FeLV and FIV rarely cause primary clinical CNS disease • Bile acid testing—indicated only with classic signs of hepatic encephalopathy (i.e., episodic depression, dementia, and hypersalivation that develop and resolve over hours)

IMAGING
• Skull radiography—usually unrewarding; may reveal calcified meningiomas or associated calvarial hyperostosis • CT or MRI (brain)—MRI most useful in identifying and defining structural brain lesions

DIAGNOSTIC PROCEDURES
CSF analysis—detects active brain diseases; findings often nonspecific

 TREATMENT

APPROPRIATE HEALTH CARE
• Known cause—treat, if possible • Prompt and aggressive antiepileptic drug therapy—> one single seizure every 6–8 weeks; cluster seizures; status epilepticus (convulsive or nonconvulsive) • Goal—< one single seizure every 6–8 weeks • Severe ongoing cluster seizures or status epilepticus—emergency

inpatient; aggressive parenteral antiepileptic drug therapy

CLIENT EDUCATION

• Emphasize the importance of the diagnostic work-up (but do not delay initiation of symptomatic antiepileptic drug therapy if indicated). • Discuss the treatment goal, potential drug side effects and toxicity, and the need for close medical follow-up.
• Instruct the client to keep a seizure calendar.
• Discuss the importance of consulting the clinic before modifying treatment and the risk of abrupt medication withdrawal. • Outline an emergency plan in the eventuality of cluster seizures or status epilepticus.

SURGICAL CONSIDERATIONS

Brain tumor excision—complete or debulking; combined or not with radiation and/or chemotherapy; convexity meningiomas bear a good prognosis following surgical excision (do not recur, or do so over a 1- to 3-year period)

MEDICATIONS

DRUG(S) OF CHOICE

Chronically Recurrent Seizures

• Phenobarbital—2–2.5 mg/kg PO q12h; when seizures occur at < 3–7 day intervals, initiate therapy with one loading dose (15–20 mg/kg slow IV; marked sedation will dissipate within a few hours) • Diazepam—second choice; 0.5–1.0 mg/kg PO divided q8–12h

Severe Cluster Seizures and Status Epilepticus

• If no ongoing seizures at presentation—initiate phenobarbital therapy with one loading dose (15–20 mg/kg slow IV); continue with oral maintenance dosage 12 hr later; if > one seizure reoccurs, administer parenteral diazepam (IV bolus and infusion) • Ongoing seizures—diazepam 0.5–1.0 mg/kg IV bolus (administer in rectum only if IV access is impossible); may repeat if gross seizure activity has not stopped within 3–5 min; immediately start a 0.25–0.5 mg/kg/hr infusion in maintenance fluids in an in-line burette; prepare only 1–2 hr of infusion at a time to limit the adsorption of diazepam into the plastic; use a fluid pump; only if continuous infusion cannot be administered, give repeated 0.5 mg/kg IV boluses (three to four at 30-min interval, starting 30 min after the initial 1 mg/kg bolus) • Persistent seizures—give another diazepam IV bolus, and increase the infusion rate to 0.5–1.0 mg/kg/hr and/or add phenobarbital (5–10 mg/kg IV bolus and add 2–3 mg/cat/hr to the diazepam infusion); dilute the phenobarbital solution for dosage accuracy • When seizures have been controlled for at least 6 hr, slowly decrease the infusion rate by 25% q4–6h. • Phenobarbital—initiate or continue orally as soon as patient can safely

swallow • Severe seizures refractory to IV diazepam and phenobarbital treatment protocol—may proceed to anesthesia with IV propofol or pentobarbital; intubate and oxygenate if necessary; ensure adequate anesthetic care and monitoring; do not confound dysphoric anesthetic recovery with seizure recurrence • Dexamethasone—0.25 mg/kg q12–24h for 1–3 days; may give when extremely severe seizures (prolonged or frequent, convulsive or nonconvulsive) have occurred; may be contraindicated in patients with infectious diseases; interferes with CSF analysis

CONTRAINDICATIONS

• Thiamine, glucose, and calcium—do not administer unless a deficiency is documented
• Acepromazine, ketamine, xylazine, tricyclic antidepressants (e.g., amitriptyline), bronchodilators (e.g., aminophylline, terbutaline, theophylline), and estrogens—do not administer to any patient with documented or potential seizures; lower seizure threshold

ALTERNATIVE DRUG(S)

Potassium bromide—20–30 mg/kg/day in one or two daily doses; may be used as a third-line maintenance drug; one initial loading dose (300–400 mg/kg divided into three or four subdoses administered with food at 3- to 4-hr intervals) may be given if < 3–4 weeks between seizures

FOLLOW-UP

PATIENT MONITORING

• CBC, biochemistry, and urinalysis—evaluate before initiation of maintenance oral antiepileptic drug therapy; then monitor along with antiepileptic drug concentration every 6–12 months • Serum drug concentration—measure at steady state, 10–14 days (phenobarbital) or 5–7 days (diazepam) after maintenance treatment initiation, and after any dosage modification; adjust dosage to reach the optimal concentration of 100–130 μmol/L (23–30 μg/L) for phenobarbital or 200–500 ng/L for total benzodiazepines; calculate new dosage = actual dosage ÷ actual serum drug concentration × optimal drug concentration to be reached • If the patient remains seizure free for > 6–12 months, attempt to wean from antiepileptic drug over a few months; if seizures recur more often than one single seizure every 6–8 weeks, resume treatment.
• Adequate seizure control not obtained despite optimal serum concentration of phenobarbital or diazepam—add diazepam to phenobarbital or vice versa; if seizures are still not well controlled, add potassium bromide: measure serum bromide concentration 2 weeks after treatment initiation (should be 50% of the maximum a given dosage will produce at steady state 2 months after treatment onset); adjust dosage (calculate) to

reach an optimal concentration of 15–20 mmol/L at steady state; feed a regular diet to insure stable chloride intake (increases bromide elimination); consult a veterinary neurologist for fourth-line drugs.

POSSIBLE COMPLICATIONS

• Hypersensitivity to phenobarbital—thrombocytopenia, neutropenia, pruritus, and swelling of the feet (noted in a few patients); repeat the CBC within a few weeks of treatment initiation; may need to discontinue (substitute diazepam)
• Diazepam—acute hepatic necrosis: monitor liver enzymes 5–7 days after treatment initiation; discontinue drug if elevated (substitute potassium bromide) • Potassium bromide—feline asthma, potentially severe and life threatening (fatalities reported); contraindicated in patients with actual or historical asthma; discontinue treatment if asthma develops (substitute another drug); use with caution and regular monitoring.

EXPECTED COURSE AND PROGNOSIS

• Depend on the underlying cause and response to treatment • Rational and aggressive diagnostic and therapeutic procedures lead to a good outcome in most patients (well-controlled epilepsy or absence of seizures), including many with severe and initially refractory seizures.

MISCELLANEOUS

AGE-RELATED FACTORS

Kittens may have a higher metabolic rate as compared with adults and require a higher phenobarbital dosage to reach an optimal serum concentration; may need to decrease dosage when maturity is reached (measure serum concentration at 10–12 months of age and adjust dosage, if necessary)

ABBREVIATIONS

• CNS = central nervous system • CSF = cerebrospinal fluid • CT = computed tomography • FeLV = feline leukemia virus
• FIP = feline infectious peritonitis • FIV = feline immunodeficiency virus • MRI = magnetic resonance imaging • PCV = packed cell volume

Suggested Reading

Parent JM, Quesnel AD. Seizures in cats. Vet Clin North Am Small Anim Pract 1996; 26:811–825.

Quesnel AD, Parent JM, McDonell W. Clinical management and outcome of cats with seizure disorders: 30 cases (1991–1993). J Am Vet Med Assoc 1997;210:72–77.

Quesnel AD, Parent JM, McDonell W, et al. Diagnostic evaluation of cats with seizure disorders: 30 cases (1990–1993). J Am Vet Med Assoc 1997;210:65–71.

Author Andrée D. Quesnel
Consulting Editor Joane M. Parent

SEIZURES (CONVULSIONS, STATUS EPILEPTICUS)—DOGS

 BASICS

DEFINITION

• The manifestation of abnormal neuronal hyperactivity involving the cerebral cortical neurons • Clinical appearance depends on the extent and location of the neuronal hyper-activity; frequently convulsive • Status epilepticus—results from continuous seizure activity lasting at least 30 min or from seizures repeated at brief intervals for 30 min or more, without complete recovery between seizures; may be convulsive, which is a life-threatening medical emergency • Epilepsy—recurrence of seizures from primary brain origin; primary: no gross or microscopic structural abnormalities; secondary: seizures are the result of a structural cerebral disease; cryptogenic: seizure pattern strongly suggests a secondary cause (e.g., partial seizure) but the diagnostic work up fails to reveal a cause

PATHOPHYSIOLOGY

• Originate from the thalamocortex; result in a paroxysmal disorganization of one or several brain functions; part or entire brain may be involved • Type largely determined by extent of brain involvement • Basic disorder—most commonly localized in the brain, but metabolic abnormalities may lead to encephalopathies and seizure activity • As more seizures occur, the tendency for neuronal damage and the propensity for developing more seizures or status epilepticus increase.

SYSTEMS AFFECTED

Nervous

SIGNALMENT

Dogs of any breed, age, or sex

SIGNS

General Comments

• Seizures—transient altered mentation, salivation, urination, and defecation during the ictal phase; aimless pacing, blindness, polydipsia, or polyphagia during the postictal phase; recumbency usually the result of involuntary tonic–clonic muscle activity; period of disorientation, confusion, and apparent blindness follows; most occur while patient is resting • Generalized or partial • Generalized—patient is unconscious; convulsions (tonic–clonic motor seizures) predominate; nonconvulsive (absence seizures) rare • Partial—patient is conscious; localized onset; indicate focal cerebral disease; may generalize; complex: alteration of consciousness; simple: normal mental status • Complex partial—often symmetrical; motor activity often predominates on one side (the side opposite to the cerebral lesion).

Historical Findings

• Obtain a description of the entire event. • Determine if the patient knows a seizure is coming (aura). • Aura—beginning of a seizure; indicates a partial onset even if the seizure rapidly generalizes • Patient may be known epileptic • Inquire about the presence of behavioral changes in the few days/weeks preceding seizure/status onset. This suggests structural disease.

Physical Examination Findings

• First 30 minutes of status—salivation, hyperthermia, tachycardia, arrhythmia increased blood pressure • Late stage status epilepticus—difficulty breathing, weak pulse, low blood pressure, poor capillary refill

CAUSES

Extracranial

• Metabolic—hypoglycemia; hypocalcemia; acute renal failure; hepatic encephalopathy • Toxins (e.g., metaldehyde in slug bait)

Intracranial

• Degenerative—storage diseases; anoxia; vas-cular accident; senile changes • Anomalous—hydrocephalus; other congenital malforma-tions • Neoplasia—primary (gliomas, menin-gioma); secondary (metastatic) • Inflam-matory or infectious—viral (e.g., canine distemper); fungal; protozoal (*Neospora, Toxoplasma*); rickettsial (ehrlichiosis, Rocky Mountain spotted fever); bacterial • Idio-pathic or immune-mediated—granulomatous meningoencephalomyelitis; eosinophilic meningoencephalomyelitis; pug encephalitis; necrotizing meningoencephalitis of Maltese dogs; necrotizing encephalitis of Yorkshire terriers • Traumatic—acute • Epilepsy—primary (idiopathic or genetic); secondary (postencephalitic or post-traumatic glial scar)

 DIAGNOSIS

DIFFERENTIAL DIAGNOSIS

Similar Signs

• Convulsive status is rapidly recognized based on history or observation of a dog that is in lateral recumbency, unresponsive, head/neck possibly in dorsiflexion, tonic/clonic movements of limbs, excessive salivation, and has been seizing for over 30 minutes. • Syncope—sudden loss of consciousness and muscle tone; results in recumbency and flaccidity; may be difficult to differentiate from absence seizure (nonconvulsive generalized seizure) without EEG and ECG recordings; sudden onset; rapid and complete recovery • Narcolepsy—excessive daytime sleepiness; periods of unconsciousness are frequent daily; elicited by excitement such as eating and playing • Obsessive–compulsive behaviors or stereotypies—complex and goal-directed behaviors; abnormal behavior can be stopped, early in the course of the disorder.

Causes

• Extracranial—generalized seizures; no lateralizing neurologic deficits; no aura at the onset • Seizurogenic toxins—progression from shaking to trembling to status epilepticus; seizures continue until treatment or death. • Active brain diseases—likely with an acute onset of multiple seizures in the absence of extracranial causes (more than two seizures within the first week), occurrence of partial seizures, and/or presence of neurologic deficits interictally including behavioral changes • Idiopathic or primary epilepsy—differentiated by age and breed; progressive onset of generalized seizures; and a normal CBC, biochemical profile, urinalysis, and neurologic examination

CBC/BIOCHEMISTRY/URINALYSIS

• Infectious CNS diseases—blood test results may reflect multisystemic involvement. • Metabolic acidosis—common • Hyper-glycemia—in the early stages • Hypogly-cemia—in the advanced stages (especially in the small breeds) • Creatine kinase—mild to markedly high; with or without myoglobu-linuria; result of muscle necrosis • Hepatic and renal dysfunction • DIC in advanced stage of status epilepticus

OTHER LABORATORY TESTS

• Suspected hepatic encephalopathy—bile acid testing; seizures are rare; accompanied interictally by abnormal behavior such as unawareness, dementia, and aimless pacing • Hypoglycemia—fasting blood glucose and an amended insulin:glucose ratio; dogs > 5 years old with an onset of occasional seizures • Viral, fungal, rickettsial, and protozoal diseases—serology indicated if systemic signs are noted and laboratory abnormalities suggest such a disease.

IMAGING

• MRI scan (brain)—most useful imaging modality; defines location, extent, and nature of structural abnormalities

DIAGNOSTIC PROCEDURES

• CSF analysis—indicated whenever an intracranial structural cause is suspected; titers may be useful for diagnosing some infectious diseases when combined with serum titers. • Surface EEG—usually unrewarding for detecting epileptic waves if animal still clinically convulsing due to muscle artifacts; • EEG monitoring—once clinical seizure activity has stopped, to evaluate for presence of epileptic waves

 TREATMENT

• Outpatient—isolated seizures • Inpatient—cluster seizures (> 3 seizures/24 hr); status epilepticus; treat rapidly and aggressively. • Treat early: the more seizures occur, the more drugs required for control and the more time needed for recovery.

SEIZURES (CONVULSIONS, STATUS EPILEPTICUS)—DOG

NURSING AND SUPPORTIVE CARE
• Constantly supervise the hospitalized patient. • Cool down if hyperthermic • Install IV line for drug and fluid administration • Use 0.9% sodium chloride over 5% glucose to avoid drug precipitation. • Draw blood for emergency measurement of blood gases, glucose, calcium, and antiepileptic drug levels if patient already treated

CLIENT EDUCATION
• Inform client that antiepileptic treatment in such cases is only symptomatic and may not help until the primary cause is addressed.

MEDICATIONS

DRUG(S) OF CHOICE

Convulsive Cluster Seizures or Status Epilepticus

Diazepam
• Administer as a 0.5–1.0 mg/kg IV bolus; repeat 5 min later if gross motor activity has not subsided; follow immediately with 0.5–1.0 mg/kg/hr as a constant-rate infusion added to the maintenance fluids in an in-line burette (prepare only 1–2 hr of infusion at a time to avoid adsorption to the plastic line).
• Rectal—should not replace intravenous administration in an emergency situation; use only in the rare instance when an IV access cannot be obtained; may diminish or stop the gross motor seizure activity to allow IV catheter placement

Phenobarbital
• Add if seizures persist after second diazepam bolus or during CRI; administer at a constant rate of infusion if the patient is already being treated with the drug or as a loading dose if the patient is new to the drug • Loading dose (total mg) = (desired serum level mg/L) × (body weight kg) × (0.8 L/kg); optimal therapeutic range = 100–120 µmol/L (23–28 mg/L): Administer one-quarter of the loading dose every 15 min until the desired effect is reached. • If the patient is already on the drug, obtain a serum level before administering the IV bolus. • Can also administer as a 2–5 mg/kg IV bolus; follow with 2–6 mg/dog/hr as a constant-rate infusion added to the diazepam infusion;
• Once seizures have been controlled for 4–6 hr, gradually wean the patient off the infusion over as many hours. • Start or resume oral maintenance antiepileptic treatment using phenobarbital and/or potassium bromide as soon as the patient can swallow.

Other
• If seizures continue, propofol is administered at 2–8 mg/kg as a slow IV bolus. It can be followed with a CRI 0.1–0.6 mg/kg/minute. • Potassium bromide—no place in the treatment of convulsive status epilepticus; takes too long to reach

therapeutic serum levels • Dexamethasone— 0.25 mg/kg 1–3 times a day for 1–3 days; reduce cerebral edema • Corticosteroids—use for acute treatment of cerebral edema secondary to severe inflammatory CNS disease, even if infectious

Complex Partial Status
• Frequently difficult to control; unknown if recurrence worsens the underlying epilepsy; thus usually not treated aggressively • If treatment is applied, treat as for convulsive cluster seizures or status epilepticus.
• Diazepam and phenobarbital—both have been proven effective experimentally
• Potassium bromide—in humans, more effective against generalized seizures

CONTRAINDICATIONS
• Acepromazine, aminophylline, and xylazine—do not use in patients with historical, ongoing, or potential seizure disorders; lower seizure threshold
• Steroids—avoid if considering a CSF analysis; alter CSF parameters

PRECAUTIONS
• Phenobarbital—highly protein bound and metabolized by the liver; with hypoalbuminemia or liver disease, lower dose and monitor levels closely; do not abruptly discontinue (may precipitate seizure activity); for status epilepticus, add cautiously to diazepam because the drugs potentiate each other, and cardiac and respiratory depression may ensue.
• Steroids—contraindicated in infectious diseases, but one dose of dexamethasone (0.25 mg/kg) may help decrease brain edema when impending brain herniation or life-threatening brain edema is suspected.

POSSIBLE INTERACTIONS
• Cimetidine and chloramphenicol—interfere with the metabolism of phenobarbital • Each time a drug is added to phenobarbital or to other chronic antiepileptic treatment, refer to pharmacology texts for possible interactions.

ALTERNATIVE DRUG(S)
Pentobarbital—anesthetize patients in status epilepticus that fail to respond to intravenous diazepam and phenobarbital; antiepileptic activity of propofol is superior to pentobarbital; if possible, monitor anesthetized patient with surface EEG to evaluate treatment response.

FOLLOW-UP

PATIENT MONITORING
• Inpatients should be under constant supervision and monitored for seizure activity. • Note that eyelid or lip twitching in a heavily sedated patient is a sign of ongoing seizure activity. • Patient may need 7–10 days before returning to normal after status

epilepticus; vision returns last. • Epilepsy secondary to treated primary disease (e.g., *Ehrlichia canis*)—slowly and gradually (over months) wean patient off the antiepileptic drug after 6 months without seizures; if seizures recur, reinstate the drug.

POSSIBLE COMPLICATIONS
• Phenobarbital—hepatotoxicity after chronic treatment with serum drug levels in the middle to upper therapeutic range; acute neutropenia (rare) in the first few weeks of use requires permanent withdrawal from the drug • Seizures may continue despite adequate antiepileptic drug serum levels; refractoriness to diazepam may develop rapidly. • Status epilepticus, leading to death
• Permanent neurologic deficits (e.g., blindness, abnormal behavior, cerebellar signs) may follow severe status epilepticus regardless of the cause.

MISCELLANEOUS

ASSOCIATED CONDITIONS

Status Epilepticus
• Hyperthermia • Acid–base and electrolyte imbalances • Anoxia • Pulmonary edema
• Arrhythmias • Aspiration pneumonia
• Cardiovascular collapse • Death

AGE-RELATED FACTORS
• Primary and idiopathic epilepsy—6 months to 5 years of age; more severe and often refractory when onset is at < 2 years of age
• Phenobarbital—higher dose needed in puppies (< 5 months) to reach the therapeutic range; minimum initial dose of 5 mg/kg q12h is advised; measure serum levels every 5 days until optimal levels are reached.

SEE ALSO
• Epilepsy, Idiopathic, Genetic, Primary
• Narcolepsy and Cataplexy • Stupor and Coma • Syncope

ABBREVIATIONS
• CNS = central nervous system • CRI = constant rate infusion • CSF = cerebrospinal fluid • DIC = disseminated intravascular coagulation • ECG = electrocardiogram
• EEG = electroencephalogram • MRI = magnetic resonance imaging

Suggested Reading
Bateman SW, Parent JM. A retrospective study of dogs presented for status epilepticus or cluster seizures: 156 cases (1990–1995). J Am Vet Med Assoc 219:1024, 2000.
Parent J, Poma R. Single seizure, cluster seizures, and status epilepticus. In: WE Wingfield and MR Raffe, eds. The veterinary ICU Book. Jackson, WY: Teton New-Media, 2002:871–879.
Author Joane M. Parent
Consulting Editor Joane M. Parent

SEMINOMA

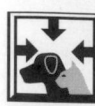

BASICS

OVERVIEW
• Benign, unilateral, solitary tumor of the testis
• Usually < 2 cm in diameter; often difficult to palpate
• Exists in 1 in 9 dogs > 4 years; 71% not detected by physical examination
• One-third found in a cryptorchid testis; extrascrotal tumors more common in the right testis

SIGNALMENT
• Usually old male dogs
• Mean age, 10 years
• No breed predisposition
• Cats—extremely rare; one reported case of malignant tumor with metastasis

SIGNS
• Usually none
• Palpable testicular mass in 29% of cases
• Rarely associated with feminization from estrogen excess (see Sertoli Cell Tumor)

CAUSES & RISK FACTORS
Cryptorchidism

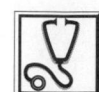

DIAGNOSIS

DIFFERENTIAL DIAGNOSIS
• Sertoli cell tumor
• Interstitial cell tumor

CBC/BIOCHEMISTRY/URINALYSIS
Usually normal unless evidence of male feminization syndrome

OTHER LABORATORY TESTS
N/A

IMAGING
Ultrasound—tumors < 3 cm in diameter usually hypoechoic; > 5 cm in diameter usually mixed echo pattern

DIAGNOSTIC PROCEDURES
• Castration
• Histopathologic examination

TREATMENT
• Castration
• Radiotherapy—reported effective in patients with regional metastasis

 MEDICATIONS

DRUG(S)
N/A

CONTRAINDICATIONS/POSSIBLE INTERACTIONS
N/A

 FOLLOW-UP

PREVENTION/AVOIDANCE
N/A

POSSIBLE COMPLICATIONS
None likely

EXPECTED COURSE AND PROGNOSIS
• After castration—recovery usually complete; prognosis excellent
• Usually benign; occasional metastasis to regional lymph nodes, visceral organs, lungs, and other sites

 MISCELLANEOUS

ASSOCIATED CONDITIONS
• Prostate disease
• Perianal adenoma
• Perineal hernia

Suggested Reading

McDonald RK, Walker M, Legendre AM, et al. Radiotherapy of metastatic seminoma in the dog. J Vet Intern Med 1988;2:103–107.

Morrison WB. Cancers of the reproductive tract. In: Morrison WB, ed. Cancer in dogs and cats: medical and surgical management. Baltimore: Williams & Wilkins, 1998: 581–590.

Author Wallace B. Morrison
Consulting Editor Wallace B. Morrison

SEPARATION ANXIETY SYNDROME

BASICS

DEFINITION
A distress response dogs may experience when separated from the person or persons to whom they are most attached, usually their owner(s). This distress may result in problem behaviors in the absence or perceived absence of the owner, including episodes of destruction, vocalization, and elimination. Separation anxiety is a subset of separation-related problems that may have different underlying motivations including fear, anxiety, overattachment to owners, and lack of appropriate stimulation or interactions.

PATHOPHYSIOLOGY
Unknown

SYSTEMS AFFECTED
• Behavioral—escape attempts, howling, whining, depression • Cardiovascular—tachycardia • Endocrine/Metabolic—increased cortisol levels, stress-induced hyperglycemia • Gastrointestinal—inappetence, gastrointestinal upset • Musculoskeletal—self-induced trauma resulting from escape attempts • Nervous—adrenergic/noradrenergic overstimulation • Respiratory—tachypnea • Skin/Exocrine—acral lick dermatitis

GENETICS
None known

INCIDENCE/PREVALENCE
Speculated that 7–28% of companion dogs experience some degree of separation anxiety syndrome

SIGNALMENT

Species
Primarily dogs; possible in cats

Breed Predilection
N/A

Mean Age and Range
Any age, most commonly in dogs > 6 months; may increase in prevalence in dogs > 8 yrs

Predominant Sex
None recorded

SIGNS

General Comments
Destruction, vocalization, and elimination in the absence of the owner alone are not diagnostic for separation anxiety.

Historical Findings
• Destruction, vocalization (whining, howling, barking) and indoor elimination are most commonly reported. Destruction often targets windows and doors and/or owner possessions. • Other signs include behavioral depression, anorexia, drooling, hiding, shaking, panting, pacing, attempts to prevent owner departure, and self-trauma from lick lesions. An occasional case presents with diarrhea while the owner is gone. • Owners may indicate signs of strong pet-owner attachment, usually excessive attention-seeking behaviors and following behaviors. Excited and prolonged greeting behavior upon owner return regardless of the length of the absence is frequently reported. • In cats, elimination problems in the owner's absence may be linked to separation-related anxiety. • Separation distress behavior(s) occurs regardless of the length of owner absence and tend to occur within 30 minutes of owner departure. • Specific triggers may be identified, such as getting keys, putting on outer garments, or packing the car. • May occur on every departure and absence or only with atypical departures such as after-work, evening, or weekend departures; the reverse pattern may also be seen.

Physical Examination Findings
• Usually normal • Injuries possible in escape attempts or while engaging in destructive activities • Skin lesions from excessive licking • Rare cases of dehydration from drooling or diarrhea due to stress

CAUSES
Specific causes are unknown. Speculated causal factors include: • Improper socialization to owner departure and absence • Lack of appropriate pet-owner interactions • Prolonged contact with humans without learning to be alone • Traumatic episodes during owner absence • Cognitive decline

RISK FACTORS
• Suspected but not proven risk factors include adoption from humane shelters, periods of extended time with preferred person such as during vacation or illness, boarding, lack of detachment when young. • Geriatric animals seem to be overrepresented. • Possible correlation between separation anxiety and noise phobias such as thunderstorm phobias

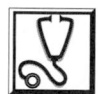

DIAGNOSIS

DIFFERENTIAL DIAGNOSIS
• Vocalization due to outdoor influences, territorial displays, or fears • Destructive behaviors—occur both when the owner is present and absent (e.g., territorial destructive displays at windows and doors; destruction due to fear-producing stimuli such as noises and thunderstorms) • Housesoiling due to inadequate housetraining, illness, endocrine dysfunction, cognitive decline • Licking due to primary dermatologic conditions • Fear-based conditions that mimic separation anxiety behaviors • Barrier frustration—dogs unable to be confined in crates or behind barriers but who are fine if not confined • Cognitive dysfunction syndrome

CBC/BIOCHEMISTRY/URINALYSIS
Abnormalities, if present, suggest alternate diagnosis or concurrent medical disease.

OTHER LABORATORY TESTS
As indicated by history

IMAGING
As indicated by history

DIAGNOSTIC PROCEDURES
• Questionnaires targeting cognitive decline are advisable for geriatric dogs. • Skin biopsies if a primary dermatologic condition is suspected • CSF tap to identify infectious or inflammatory conditions • Endoscopy with biopsies if gastrointestinal signs are persistent

PATHOLOGIC FINDINGS
None specific to this condition

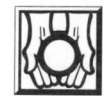

TREATMENT

ACTIVITY
Regular, scheduled daily exercise and playtime are beneficial.

DIET
No dietary changes are necessary unless diarrhea is also present.

CLIENT EDUCATION

General Comments
Owners need realistic expectations of the time course of treatment and the need for behavior modification in order to have successful resolution of the problem. Problem behavior may take weeks or months to resolve depending on severity and duration of the problem. Treatment components include:

Changing the Predictive Value of Pre-Departure Cues
• Habituation exercises • Presentation of pre-departure cues (picking up keys, walking to the door) without leaving • Repeated 2–4 times daily until the dog does not respond to cues with anxious behaviors (panting, pacing, following, or increased vigilance) • Goal is to disassociate the cues with departures and diminish the anxious response.

Counterconditioning (Response Substitution)
• Teaching the dog to sit/stay near the typical exit door • Gradually increase the distance between the dog and owner toward the door. • Owner slowly progresses toward the door, increasing the time away on each trial. • Eventually elements of departure, such as opening and closing the door, are added. • Finally, the owner steps outside the door and returns.

Classical Counterconditioning
• Leaving the dog a delectable food treat or food-stuffed toy on departure • Associating departure with something pleasant

Changing Departure and Return Routine
• Ignore the pet for 15–30 minutes prior to departure and upon return. • On return attend to the dog only when it is calm and quiet; may, however, allow the dog outside to eliminate

Independence Training
• Teaching the dog to be more independent of the owner(s) • All attention is at owner initiation—owner begins and ends attention ses-sions. • No attention on pet demand • Must be earned by the pet by performing a task such as "sit" • Decreasing following behavior while the owner is home • Teaching the dog to stay in another location away from the owner

Graduated Planned Departures and Absences
• Begun after dog is habituated to pre-departure cues • Use short absences to teach the dog how to be left home alone. • Departures must be short enough not to elicit a separation distress response. • Goal—animal learns consistency of owner return and to experience departure and absence without anxiety. • Departures must be just like real departures (owner must do all components of departure including leaving in the car if that is how they usually depart). Owner will leave a safety cue (radio or television on, ring a bell) on planned departures only (must not be used on departures where length of absence is not controlled, such as work departures). Initial departures must be very short, 1–5 minutes. • Length of absence is slowly increased at 3–5 minute intervals if no signs of distress were evident at the shorter interval. • Increase in interval must be variable; intersperse short (1–3 minute) with longer (5–20 minute) departures. • If destruction, elimination, or vocalization occur, departure was too long. • If departures and absences are continued even though distress behaviors are present, the dog will get worse. • Audio tapes for vocalization can help monitor progress. • Once the pet can be left for 2–3 hours on a planned departure, it often can be left all day. • Cue is slowly phased out over time or can be used indefinitely.

Arrangements for the Pet During Retraining and Owner Absence
• Allow no more destructive activity if possible. • Mixing up or eliminating triggering departure cues may help diminish the anxious responses. • Doggy daycare arrangements or pet sitters • Gradual conditioning to a crate; • Crates are not recommended unless the dog is already crate-trained and comfortable being left in a crate

SURGICAL CONSIDERATIONS
If the animal is on medication, care should be exercised prior to administering anesthesia.

MEDICATIONS

DRUG(S) OF CHOICE
Clomipramine Hydrochloride
• Tricyclic antidepressant—drug of first choice and only drug approved for use in the treat-ment of separation anxiety in dogs • Approved for dogs older than 6 months of age • Dosage: 2–4 mg/kg total daily dose (canine). May be administered as one dose or divided and given twice daily. Must be given daily, not on an "as needed" basis, as it may take 2–4 weeks before behavioral effect is evident • Side effects—vomiting, diarrhea, and lethargy

CONTRAINDICATIONS
• Clomipramine should not be used in con-junction with monoamine oxidase inhibitors (MAOIs) such as amitraz and selegiline, nor within 14 days before or after an MAOI. • Use with caution in patients showing cardiac con-duction disturbances. • Caution advised using in conjunction with CNS active drugs inclu-ding general anesthesia, neuroleptic, anti-cholinergic, and sympathomimetic drugs. • Practitioners are urged to read package insert for contraindications.

PRECAUTIONS
• Improperly applied behavioral modification may make dogs more anxious rather then less anxious. • Crating can result in serious physical damage to the pet if it attempts to escape and should only be recommended cautiously for those animals that are already crate-trained.

POSSIBLE INTERACTIONS
Serotonin syndrome with MAOI and SSRI in combination with clomipramine

ALTERNATIVE DRUG(S)
• Tricyclic antidepressants (TCA) such as amitriptyline (dog: 1–2 mg/kg q12h) • Selective serotonin reuptake inhibitors (SSRIs) such as fluoxetine (dog: 0.5–1 mg/kg q24h) • Benzodiazepines such as alprazolam (dog: 0.01–0.1 mg/kg q8–12h) • DAP (dog-appeasing pheromone). Synthetic analogue of the natural appeasing pheromones of the nursing bitch which calm puppies; used to calm dogs in fearful, stressful, and anxiety situations such as separation anxiety and noise phobias; available as a plug-in diffuser

FOLLOW-UP

PATIENT MONITORING
Good client follow-up is necessary to monitor both the behavioral treatment plan and medication if prescribed. Weekly follow-up is best in the early stages to access efficacy of the treatment plan and owner compliance with instructions. Once the dog has become more independent, habituated to pre-departure cues, and calmer on departures and returns, graduated planned departures may be implemented.

PREVENTION/AVOIDANCE
Teaching animals how to be left home alone, making animals independent

POSSIBLE COMPLICATIONS
Injuries during escape attempts and ongoing destruction and elimination disrupt the human-animal bond and result in pet relinquishment.

EXPECTED COURSE AND PROGNOSIS
Separation anxiety often responds well to behavioral modification with or without medication. Some severe cases can be very resistant to treatment. Other concurrent behavioral disorders may make resolution more difficult. Drug therapy alone is rarely curative for most behavioral disorders. Realistically, drug therapy can be expected to decrease the anxiety associated with owner departure but the dog still must be taught how to be left alone during owner absences.

MISCELLANEOUS

ASSOCIATED CONDITIONS
Other anxiety conditions including noise phobias, generalized anxiety, fears, and compulsive disorders.

AGE-RELATED FACTORS
Common behavior problem in senior dogs

PREGNANCY
No drugs approved for use in pregnant animals

SYNONYMS
• Separation anxiety • Hyperattachment

SEE ALSO
• Cognitive Dysfunction Syndrome
• Excessive Vocalization

ABBREVIATIONS
• MAOI = monoamine oxidase inhibitor
• SSRI = selective serotonin reuptake inhibitor
• TCA = tricyclic antidepressant

Suggested Reading
Horwitz DF. Separation-related problems in dogs. In: Horwitz DF, Mills D, and Heath S, eds. BSAVA Manual of canine and feline behavioural medicine. Gloucester, UK: BSAVA, 2002.

King JN, Simpson, BS, Overall KL, et al. Treatment of separation anxiety in dogs with clomipramine: results from a prospec-tive, randomised, double-blind, placebo-controlled, parallel-group multicenter clini-cal trial. Appl Anim Behav Sci 2000; 67:255–275.

Takeuchi Y, Houpt KA, Scarlett JM. Evalua-tion of treatments for separation anxiety in dogs. J Am Vet Med Assoc 2000; 217:342–345.

Author Debra F. Horwitz
Consulting Editor Debra F. Horwitz

SEPSIS AND BACTEREMIA

BASICS

DEFINITION
• Bacteremia—defined as the presence of bacterial organisms in the bloodstream
• Sepsis—systemic response to bacterial infection (e.g., fever, hypotension)
• Terms are not synonymous, although often used interchangeably

PATHOPHYSIOLOGY
• Shedding of bacterial organisms into the bloodstream—may occur transiently, intermittently, or continually
• The most critical host response for elimination of bacteremia—provided by mononuclear phagocyte system of the spleen and liver; activation leads to release of numerous cellular mediators (cytokines), some of which are beneficial and others detrimental; may lead to death of the host
• Neutrophils—relatively more important for defense against extravascular infection
• Bacteremia—transient, subclinical event or may escalate to overt sepsis when the immune system is overwhelmed; generally of more pathologic significance when the bloodstream is invaded from venous or lymphatic drainage sites

SYSTEMS AFFECTED

Cardiovascular
• With peracute development of septicemia—increased or decreased cardiac output, decreased systemic vascular resistance, and increased vascular permeability; ultimately, refractory hypotension develops, leading to multiorgan failure and death.
• Endocarditis—may develop; presence of bacteremia alone is not sufficient for induction; multiple factors involving both the host and the bacterial organism must be favorable for bacterial adherence to heart valves.

Hemic/Lymphatic/Immune
• Coagulation disorders and thromboembolism
• Kidney and myocardium especially prone to septic embolization
• With chronic bacteremia—antigenic stimulation of the immune system may lead to immune-complex deposition.

Other
• Respiratory
• Gastrointestinal
• Hepatobiliary

SIGNALMENT
• Dogs and cats
• No age, sex, or breed predispositions reported.
• Large-breed male dogs—predisposed to bacterial endocarditis and discospondylitis

SIGNS

General Comments
• Development may be acute or may occur in a vague or episodic fashion.
• Variable and may involve multiple organ systems
• May be confused with those of immune-mediated disease
• Clinical—more severe when gram-negative organisms are involved
• Dogs that develop overt sepsis—the earliest signs are usually referable to the gastrointestinal tract
• Cats—respiratory system more commonly involved

Physical Examination Findings
• Intermittent or persistent fever
• Lameness
• Depression
• Tachycardia
• Heart murmur
• Weakness

CAUSES
• Dogs—gram-negative organisms (especially *E. coli*) most common; gram-positive cocci and obligate anaerobes also important; polymicrobial infection reported in about 20% of dogs with positive blood cultures
• Cats—bloodstream pathogens usually gram-negative bacteria from the Enterobacteriaceae family or obligate anaerobes; *Salmonella* most common gram-negative organism cultured
• *Pseudomonas aeruginosa*—uncommon isolate from animal blood cultures

RISK FACTORS
• Peracute—pyometra and disruption of the gastrointestinal tract most often associated
• More protracted onset—infections of the skin, upper urinary tract, oral cavity, and prostate
• Hyperadrenocorticism, diabetes mellitus, liver or renal failure, splenectomy, malignancy, and burns—predisposing factors
• Immunodeficient state—chemotherapy, FIV, splenectomy; particular risk
• Glucocorticoids—considered an important risk factor for bacteremia; allows greater multiplication of bacteria in extravascular tissues
• Intravenous catheter—provides rapid venous access for bacteria
• Indwelling urinary catheters—may be a predisposing factor

DIAGNOSIS

DIFFERENTIAL DIAGNOSIS
• Consider other causes of fever, heart murmur, joint or back pain, or hypotension.
• Clinical signs of more chronic bacteremia may be confused with immune-mediated disease.

CBC/BIOCHEMISTRY/URINALYSIS
• Neutrophilic leukocytosis with a left shift and an associated monocytosis—most common hematologic abnormalities
• Neutropenia—may develop
• Hypoalbuminemia and a high ALP (up to two times upper limit of normal)—up to 50% of affected dogs
• Hypoglycemia—about 25% of affected dogs

OTHER LABORATORY TESTS
• With suspected catheter-induced sepsis—submit catheter tip for culture.
• Urine culture—may be useful; positive culture does not determine if urinary tract is primary or secondary source of infection.

IMAGING
May identify source of bacteremia (e.g., pyometra) or secondarily infected organs (e.g., discospondylitis)

DIAGNOSTIC PROCEDURES

Blood Culture
• Indications—any patient that develops fever (or hypothermia), leukocytosis (especially with a left shift), neutropenia, shifting leg lameness, recent onset or changing heart murmur, or any sign of sepsis that cannot be explained
• Essential for confirming suspected bacteremia and for optimizing management of the patient; one study of critically ill animals reported approximately 75% of cats and 50% of dogs had positive blood cultures.
• Clinical findings—not reliable for discriminating between particular types of bacteria
Guidelines
• Current antimicrobial therapy—does not preclude collection of blood cultures; advise laboratory that patient is receiving antibiotics; steps can be taken to inactivate certain medications.
• Anaerobic cultures—special bottles may not be necessary.
• Sets (pairs) of samples—inform laboratory that for each submitted pair of bottles, one is for aerobic culture and the other for anaerobic.

- Collect at least two (and preferably three) sets of samples—improves chance of obtaining a positive culture and facilitates interpretation of results
- Volume—the greater the volume of collected blood, the better the chances of obtaining positive cultures; often only a few organisms present per milliliter of blood; 10 mL of blood per culture recommended; may not be possible for cats and small dogs; have an assortment of culture bottles available (including 25, 50, and 100 mL); small bottles useful for small patients for maintaining appropriate blood-to-culture broth ratio
- Timing—for most patients, sufficient to take three cultures over a 24-hr period; for critically ill patients, take three cultures over a 2-hr period.

Collection
- Bottles—warm to room temperature; apply alcohol or iodine to the rubber stopper.
- Patient—clip hair; thoroughly disinfect skin before venipuncture, to avoid contamination; wipe with 70% alcohol, then apply an iodine-based disinfectant; allow a minimum of 1 min of contact time with the skin.
- Withdrawing blood—wearing a sterile glove, palpate the vein; draw blood into a sterile syringe; evacuate all air from the syringe; attach a new needle before inoculating blood into the bottles.
- Samples—maintain culture bottles at room temperature for transport to the laboratory.

Media
- Commercial multipurpose nutrient broth media—recommended
- A medium that supports growth of both aerobes and anaerobes—ideal
- Often the laboratory that processes the culture will supply culture bottles.

Interpretation of Results
- Single positive culture—not possible to distinguish true bacteremia from sample contamination
- Two or more positive cultures identified as the same organism desired
- Coagulase-negative staphylococci, α-hemolytic streptococci, and *Acinetobacter*—probably contamination
- *Enterobacteriaceae, Bacteroidaceae, Pseudomonas aeruginosa, Staphylococcus aureus, Staphylococcus intermedius*, β-hemolytic streptococci, and yeasts—nearly always clinically significant bacteremia
- Negative results from two or three successive cultures—generally eliminates bacteremia owing to common pathogens; some less common bacteria may take several weeks to grow.

TREATMENT

- Success—requires early identification of the problem and aggressive intervention; careful monitoring essential, because the status of patient may change rapidly
- Hypotension—intravenous fluids; isotonic fluids (e.g., lactated Ringer) at a rate up to 90 mL/kg/hr in dogs and 55 mL/kg/hr in cats; use caution when hypoalbuminemia or increased vascular permeability is a concern
- Volume expanders (e.g., hydroxyethyl starch)—may help maintain oncotic pressure
- With hypoglycemia—may add dextrose to intravenous fluids
- Electrolytes and acid–base balance—correct abnormalities.
- Abscesses—locate and drain
- External sources of infection—give appropriate attention to wound care and bandage changes.
- Internal sources of infection (e.g., pyometra or disruption of the bowel)—surgical intervention essential
- Nutritional support—provide by assisted feeding or placement of a feeding tube.

MEDICATIONS

DRUG(S) OF CHOICE
- Antibiotics—usually selected before culture and sensitivity results available; empiric therapy acceptable while waiting for results; do not delay treatment.
- Antimicrobials—give intravenously; direct therapy to cover all possible bacterial organisms (gram-positive and negative; aerobic and anaerobic)
- If patient not in shock—a good choice is a first-generation cephalosporin; dogs and cats: administer cefazolin at 40 mg/kg IV as a loading dose; then 20–30 mg/kg IV q6–8h (dogs and cats).
- Aminoglycosides—add to protocol if more aggressive therapy is warranted; administer gentamicin at 2–4 mg/kg IV q8h (dogs and cats).

CONTRAINDICATIONS
Glucocorticoids and NSAIDs—value in treating septic shock; do not improve survival unless given within the first few hours of the onset; may complicate the clinical picture in potentially ischemic organs (e.g., gastrointestinal tract and kidneys)

PRECAUTIONS
Aminoglycosides—use with caution with renal impairment.

POSSIBLE INTERACTIONS
None

ALTERNATIVE DRUG(S)
None

FOLLOW-UP

PATIENT MONITORING
- Aminoglycoside therapy—monitor renal function.
- Blood pressure and ECG—monitor, if indicated.

POSSIBLE COMPLICATIONS
Gram-negative septicemia—high rate of mortality; death owing to hypotension, electrolyte and acid–base disturbances, and endotoxemic shock

MISCELLANEOUS

ASSOCIATED CONDITIONS
- Suspected discospondylitis (dogs)—may need to screen for *Brucella canis*
- See Risk Factors for possible underlying diseases

AGE-RELATED FACTORS
N/A

ZOONOTIC POTENTIAL
N/A

PREGNANCY
N/A

SYNONYMS
- Septic shock
- Septicemia

SEE ALSO
- Abscessation
- Anaerobic Infection
- Endocarditis, Infective
- Shock, Septic

ABBREVIATIONS
- ALP = alkaline phosphatase
- FIV = feline immunodeficiency virus

Suggested Reading
Dow SW, Jones RL. Bacteremia: pathogenesis and diagnosis. Compend Contin Educ Pract Vet 1989;11:432–444.
Morresey PR. Synthesis of proinflammatory mediators in endotoxemia. Compend Contin Educ 2001;23:829–836.
Purvis D, Kirby R. Systemic inflammatory response syndrome: septic shock. Vet Clin North Am Small Anim Pract 1994; 24:1225–1247.
Author Sharon Fooshee Grace
Consulting Editor Stephen C. Barr

SERTOLI CELL TUMOR

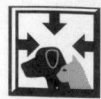

BASICS

OVERVIEW
• Common testicular tumor in dogs
• Between 10% and 14% are malignant and metastasize to regional lymph nodes and other abdominal and thoracic organs.

SIGNALMENT
• Old male dogs
• Cats—extremely rare; two reported cases of malignant tumor with metastasis

SIGNS
• Unilaterally large testicle with atrophy of the unaffected testicle
• Feminization syndrome—gynecomastia; galactorrhea; atrophy of penis; pendulous prepuce; attraction to other male dogs; standing in the female position to urinate
• Squamous metaplasia of the prostate and prostatomegaly—occasionally
• Dermatologic changes—nonpruritic alopecia; thinning of the haircoat; hyperpigmentation
• Abdominal mass—if patient is cryptorchid
• Inguinal location possible

CAUSES & RISK FACTORS
Cryptorchid testicles are 13–13.6 times more likely to develop neoplasia than are scrotally located testicles.

DIAGNOSIS

DIFFERENTIAL DIAGNOSIS
• Interstitial cell tumor
• Seminoma
• Hyperadrenocorticism
• Hypothyroidism
• More likely to have an abdominal location than other testicular tumors; high testicular temperature in the abdominal location may destroy spermatogenic cells and leave Sertoli cells unregulated.

CBC/BIOCHEMISTRY/URINALYSIS
Nonregenerative anemia, leukopenia, and thrombocytopenia associated with hyperestrogenism

OTHER LABORATORY TESTS
• Serum estradiol concentration high in most patients
• Serum progesterone concentration high in most patients

IMAGING
Variable echotexture on ultrasound

DIAGNOSTIC PROCEDURES
Castration and histopathologic examination of appropriate tissue

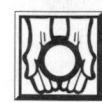

TREATMENT
Castration

MEDICATIONS

DRUG(S)
N/A

CONTRAINDICATIONS/POSSIBLE INTERACTIONS
N/A

FOLLOW-UP

PATIENT MONITORING
N/A

PREVENTION/AVOIDANCE
N/A

POSSIBLE COMPLICATIONS
None unless associated with surgery or estrogen excess

EXPECTED COURSE AND PROGNOSIS
• Good in most patients
• Guarded if severe cytopenias develop because of hyperestrogenism

MISCELLANEOUS

ASSOCIATED CONDITIONS
• 25–29% of dogs with Sertoli cell tumor develop male feminization syndrome.
• About 70% of intra-abdominal testicular tumors in dogs are associated with male feminization syndrome.
• Hyperestrogenism can cause hematopoietic failure.

Suggested Reading
Metzger FL, Hattel AL, White DG. Hematuria, hyperestrogenemia, and hyperprogesteronemia due to a sertoli-cell tumor in a bilaterally cryptorchid dog. Canine Pract 1993;18:32–35.
Morrison WB. Cancers of the reproductive tract. In: Morrison WB, ed. Cancer in dogs and cats: medical and surgical management. Baltimore: Williams & Wilkins 1998: 581–590.

Author Wallace B. Morrison
Consulting Editor Wallace B. Morrison

SEX HORMONE–RESPONSIVE DERMATOSES

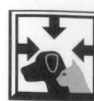

BASICS

DEFINITION
Uncommon alopecias and dermatoses suspected to result from an imbalance of sex hormones; often defined on the basis of stimulatory response to sex hormone therapy

SIGNALMENT
See Causes

SIGNS
• Alopecia—localized alopecia more common than generalized; initially involves the perineum, ventrum, thighs, and cervical areas; later involves the caudodorsal back and flank; flank alopecia may be the first or only sign in some patients with hyperestrogenism and may be seasonal in some spayed females
• Fur—may be soft or dry and brittle
• Nipples, mammary glands, vulva, prepuce, testicles, ovaries, and prostate—often abnormal
• Secondary seborrhea, pruritus, pyoderma, comedones, ceruminous otitis externa, and hyperpigmentation—variable
• Tail gland hyperplasia and perianal gland hyperplasia with macular melanosis—dogs with testicular tumors
• Urinary incontinence—estrogen- and testosterone-responsive conditions

CAUSES & RISK FACTORS

Estrogen-responsive—Females (Ovarian Imbalance II)
• Possible deficiency or imbalance of estrogen; serum estradiol concentrations may be normal
• Inadequate production of adrenal sex hormones
• Cutaneous defect in the sex hormone receptor/metabolism system
• Rare in dogs
• Extremely rare in cats
• Predisposed breeds—dachshunds and boxers
• Primarily seen in young adults
• May occur after ovariohysterectomy in noncycling, intact females
• Occasionally seen during pseudopregnancy
• Variant—cyclical flank alopecia and hyperpigmentation; noted in Airedales, boxers, and English bulldogs; may worsen in winter

Hyperestrogenism—Females (Ovarian Imbalance I)
• Estrogen excess or imbalance owing to cystic ovaries, ovarian tumors (rare), or exogenous estrogen overdose
• Abnormal peripheral conversion of sex hormones
• Ectopic production of sex hormones
• Animals with normal serum estrogen concentrations may have increased numbers of estrogen receptors in the skin.
• Rare in dogs
• Extremely rare in cats

• English bulldogs may be predisposed to cystic ovaries.
• Generally, middle-aged and old intact female dogs

Hyperestrogenism—Male Dogs with Testicular Tumors
• Estrogen excess (or rarely hyperprogesteronism) due to Sertoli cell tumor (most common), seminoma, or interstitial cell tumor (rarely)
• Cryptorchidism predisposes animals to the formation of testicular tumors.
• Intact males; usually middle-aged or older
• Predisposed breeds—boxers, Shetland sheepdogs, Weimaraners, German shepherds, Cairn terriers, Pekingese, and collies
• Associated with male pseudohermaphrodism in miniature schnauzers

Hyperandrogenism Associated with Testicular Tumors
Androgen-producing testicular tumors (especially interstitial cell tumors) in intact male dogs

Idiopathic Male Feminizing Syndrome
• Undetermined
• Serum sex hormone concentrations normal
• Blockage of androgen receptors in the skin may prevent attachment of testosterone.
• Intact, middle-aged male dogs

Testosterone-responsive—Males
• Rare
• Old castrated male dogs
• Afghan hounds overrepresented
• Extremely rare in cats
• Suspected hypoandrogenism or a possible defect in the skin sex hormone–receptor system

Castration-responsive
• Intact males with normal testicles
• Estradiol, testosterone, and progesterone—variably high, low, or normal
• Onset 1–4 years or older
• Predisposed breeds—chow chows, Samoyeds, keeshonds, Pomeranians, huskies, malamutes, and miniature poodles

Adrenal Sex Hormone Imbalance (Adrenal Hyperplasia–like Syndrome)
• Adrenal enzyme (21-hydroxylase) deficiency resulting in excessive adrenal androgen or progesterone secretion
• Males and females, intact or neutered
• Onset 1–5 years of age
• Pomeranians predisposed

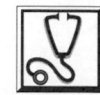

DIAGNOSIS

DIFFERENTIAL DIAGNOSIS
• Hypothyroidism and hyperadrenocorticism—critical to rule out first; these diseases generally cause truncal alopecia first;

REMEMBER: sex hormones can change the affinity of binding proteins, so that the baseline total T_4 can be normal or above normal in dogs with hyperandrogenemia or hypoestrogenemia.
• Growth hormone–responsive/adrenal hyperplasia dermatosis
• Follicular dysplasia
• Dachshunds—pattern baldness
• Keratinization disorders
• Allergic skin disease

CBC/BIOCHEMISTRY/URINALYSIS
• Usually unremarkable
• Bone marrow hypoplasia or aplasia is noted occasionally in states of estrogen excess, owing to testicular tumors in male and hyperestrogenism in female dogs.

OTHER LABORATORY TESTS
• Serum estrogen/estradiol concentrations—sometimes high (30%–40% of patients) with hyperestrogenism of female dogs, hyperestrogenism in male dogs with testicular tumors, and castration-responsive dermatosis; rarely helpful in estrogen-responsive dermatosis, because serum estradiol 17β concentrations in spayed females are similar to intact females
• Serum testosterone and progesterone—sometimes elevated in animals with castration-responsive dermatosis; occasionally elevated with hyperestrogenism (ovarian imbalance) in female dogs
• Serum sex hormone concentrations—often normal, treat according to the suspected diagnosis based on clinical signs; by ruling out other disorders, and by noting the response to therapy.

Combined ACTH Stimulation and Adrenal Reproductive Hormone Test
• Obtain plasma and serum before injection; administer ACTH (cosyntropin 0.5 IU/kg IV or ACTH gel 0.22 USP U/kg IM); obtain plasma and serum 1 hr later (and a 2-hr sample if ACTH gel is used)
• Partial deficiency of 21-hydroxylase enzyme results in accumulation of steroid precursors (e.g., progesterone, 17-hydroxyprogesterone, androstenedione, and DHEAS), resulting in dermatosis of Pomeranians and other breeds; clinically similar to growth hormone–responsive dermatosis

GnRH (Cystorelin) Response Test
• Demonstrates response of gonads to stimulation
• Especially useful when basal hormones are normal
• Determine baseline serum estradiol, testosterone, and progesterone before injection; administer GnRH (0.22 mg/kg IV); obtain serum samples 1–2 hr later; determine levels of the three sex hormones; values vary with lab.

IMAGING
Radiography, ultrasonography, and laparoscopy—detect cystic ovaries, ovarian tumors, testicular tumors (scrotal and abdominal), sublumbar lymphadenopathy, and possible thoracic metastases of malignant tumors

DIAGNOSTIC PROCEDURES
• Preputial cytology—may demonstrate cornification of cells (similar to bitch in estrus) in patients with advanced testicular feminizing tumors
• Skin biopsy

PATHOLOGIC FINDINGS
• General endocrinopathy findings (see above)—all syndromes, except hyperandrogenism due to testicular tumors
• Perivascular dermatitis—may be seen in pruritic animals (male feminizing syndrome, hyperestrogenism of female dogs)
• Sebaceous glands—relatively spared in estrogen-responsive dermatosis of female dogs and in testosterone-responsive dermatosis of male dogs
• Hair follicles—hypereosinophilic tricholemmal keratinization ("flame follicles") may be seen with castration-responsive dermatosis

 TREATMENT
• Cryptorchid animals—do not breed (prevention and avoidance of problems); neuter when young
• Exploratory laparotomy—diagnosis and treatment (e.g., ovariohysterectomy and castration) for ovarian cysts and tumors and abdominal testicular tumors
• Castration—castration-responsive dermatosis and scrotal testicular tumors
• Discontinue excessive exogenous estrogen administration

 MEDICATIONS

DRUG(S)

Estrogen-Responsive Dermatosis
• Spayed females—DES at 0.02 mg/kg (maximum, 1 mg) PO q24h for 14–21 days; stop for 1 week; repeat cycle until hair regrowth; then give 2–3 times weekly to maintain hair coat; discontinue during estrus and resume maintenance when estrus subsides; if no response, try methyltestosterone (see below) or milbolerone (at 30 μg [dogs < 11 kg] or 50 μg [dogs 11–23 kg]) until hair regrowth and then taper to maintenance
• Intact females—DES (5 mg PO q24h) until bloody discharge; if no response after 7 days,

double the dose; give until proestrus day 2 (maximum, 14 days total) until sanguineous vaginal discharge and vulvar edema are noted; then for 2 days more; then LH (5 mg IM) on day 5 of proestrus; then FSH on days 9 and 11 of proestrus
• Alternative treatment—FSH (0.75 mg/kg IM daily) until signs of estrus appear

Testosterone-responsive (Males)/Some Estrogen-responsive (Female Dogs)
• Methyltestosterone—0.5–1.0 mg/kg (maximum, 30 mg) PO q48h until response; may take 1–3 months; after hair regrowth is complete, 2–3 times/week for maintenance;
• Respositol testosterone (2 mg/kg [maximum, 30 mg] IM every 1–4 months) as needed to maintain normal hair coat

Hyperestrogenism—Female Dogs
• Consider o,p'-DDD (Lysodren) or L-deprenyl.
• Alternative treatments—GnRH or hCG
• Tamoxifen—may be useful

Other Conditions
• Castration-responsive alopecia—may respond to hCG (50 IU/kg IM twice weekly for 6 weeks) or testosterone (see above) if castration is not possible
• Adrenal 21-hydroxylase enzyme deficiency—o,p'-DDD (Lysodren) if adrenal sex hormones are high; beginning dose 15–25 mg/kg PO q24h for 7 days; maintenance doses (15–25 mg/kg PO every 5–14 days) titrated to maintain post-ACTH-stimulation cortisol within the baseline range

General Treatment
• Topical antiseborrheic therapy—conditions with associated keratinization defects and comedones
• Antibiotics—associated pyodermas
• Prednisone—for pruritus if infections and bone marrow suppression have been ruled out; 0.5 mg/kg PO q12h for 5–7 days; then 0.5 mg q24h for 5–7 days; then 0.5 mg/kg q48h for 7 days

CONTRAINDICATIONS
N/A

POSSIBLE INTERACTIONS
N/A

 FOLLOW-UP

PATIENT MONITORING
• DES supplementation—CBC for bone marrow hypoplasia or aplasia every 2 weeks for the first month; then every 3–6 months
• Testosterone supplementation—serum biochemistry with an emphasis on liver enzymes every 3–4 weeks for the first 3 months; every 4–6 months

• o,p'-DDD—electrolytes with ACTH-stimulation testing every 3 months

POSSIBLE COMPLICATIONS
• Estrogen—bone marrow hypoplasia (uncommon); aplasia (uncommon); signs of estrus (rare)
• methyltestosterone—cholangiohepatitis (rare); behavior changes (uncommon); seborrhea oleosa
• o,p'-DDD—potential toxicities (e.g., vomiting, diarrhea, collapse, and iatrogenic hypoadrenocorticism)
• Tamoxifen—vulvar swelling; discontinue until signs of estrus are gone

EXPECTED COURSE AND PROGNOSIS
• Estrogen-responsive—regrowth of hair may take about 3 months and may be transient
• Female hyperestrogenism—improvement should occur within 3–6 months after ovariohysterectomy
• Estrogen- and androgen-secreting tumors—resolution of signs noted within 3–6 months of castration; bone marrow aplasia associated with hyperestrogenism usually does not respond to castration, and the prognosis for recovery is grave; relapse after a positive response to castration may indicate metastasis, and if confirmed, the prognosis is poor
• Castration-responsive—response noted 2–4 months after castration
• Testosterone therapy—may result in hair regrowth in 4–12 weeks
• Adrenal sex hormone imbalance—response seen 4–12 weeks after adrenal hyperplasia therapy with o,p'-DDD

 MISCELLANEOUS

ABBREVIATIONS
• ACTH = adrenocorticotropic hormone
• DES = diethylstilbestrol
• DHEAS = dehydroepiandrosterone sulfate
• FSH = follicle-stimulating hormone
• GnRH = gonadotropin-releasing hormone
• hCG = human chorionic gonadotropin
• LH = luteinizing hormone
• o,p'-DDD = 1,1-(o,p'-dichlorodiphenyl)-2,2-dichloroethane

Suggested Reading
Schmeitzel LP. Sex hormone-related and growth hormone-related alopecias. Vet Clin North Am Small Anim Pract 1990; 20:1579–1601.
Author Margaret S. Swartout
Consulting Editor Karen Helton Rhodes

SEXUAL DEVELOPMENT DISORDERS

 BASICS

DEFINITION
• Errors in the establishment of chromosomal, gonadal, or phenotypic sex that cause abnormal sexual differentiation
• Variety of patterns from ambiguous genitalia to apparently normal genitalia with sterility

PATHOPHYSIOLOGY
Normal sexual differentiation—establishment of chromosomal sex at fertilization (either XX or XY), development of gonadal sex, and development of phenotypic sex

Disorders of Chromosomal Sex
• Defects in the number or structure of the sex chromosomes—chromosomal nondisjunction during meiosis leads to trisomy, monosomy; mitotic nondisjunction of a single zygote leads to mosaicism; fusion of zygotes leads to chimerism
• XXY (Klinefelter) syndrome—79, XXY (dog); 39, XXY (cat); hypoplastic testes; phenotypic male (normal to hypoplastic genitalia); sterile; some tortoiseshell male cats
• XO (Turner) syndrome—77, XO (dog); 37, XO (cat); dysgenetic ovaries; phenotypic female; infantile genitalia; sterile
• XXX syndrome—79, XXX; ovaries without follicles; female phenotype; high FSH and LH; dogs
• True hermaphrodite chimera—XX/XY or XX/XXY; ovarian and testicular tissue; phenotypic sex depends on amount of testicular tissue; dogs and cats
• XX/XY chimera with testes and XY/XY chimera with testes—vary from phenotypic female with abnormal genitalia to male with possible fertility; dogs and cats (some tortoiseshell males)

Disorders of Gonadal Sex
• Gonadal differentiation—normally determined by the sex chromosome constitution; Sry (located on the Y chromosome) encodes a protein that initiates testis differentiation; other genes likely involved in testis differentiation (Sox9)
• Sex reversed—affected individuals have gonads that do not agree with chromosomal sex; only Sry-negative XX sex reversal has been reported in the dog; has not been described in cats • XX sex reversed, XX true hermaphrodite—ovaries and testes (or ovotestis); phenotypic female or partially masculinized female phenotype; varies from normal to abnormal vulva, normal-sized to large clitoris, uterus, oviducts, epididymis, and vas deferens; rarely fertile; dogs only
• XX sex reversed, XX males—testes (usually cryptorchid); epididymis, vas deferens, prostate; bicornuate uterus, but oviducts absent; hypoplastic penis and prepuce; hypospadias common; dogs only

Disorders of Phenotypic Sex
• Phenotypic sex differentiation (tubular reproductive tract and external genitalia)—depends on gonadal sex; basic embryonic plan is female; male phenotype results only if testes capable of secreting müllerian inhibiting substance and testosterone are present; chromosomal and gonadal sex agree; internal or external genitalia ambiguous
• Female pseudohermaphrodite—XX; ovaries; masculinized genitalia (mild clitoral enlargement to nearly normal male genitalia); oviducts, uterus, cranial vagina; prostate variably present; caused by sex steroid administration during pregnancy; dogs only
• Persistent müllerian duct syndrome (male pseudohermaphrodite)—XY; testes (unilateral or bilateral cryptorchid); all wolffian and müllerian duct derivatives present; penis, prepuce, and scrotum usually normal; dogs and cats • Hypospadias (defect in androgen-dependent masculinization)—XY; abnormal location of urinary orifice (from glans penis to perineum); external genitalia unambiguous; testes (can be cryptorchid); dogs • Testicular feminization (defect in androgen-dependent masculinization)—XY; testes (often abdominal); no wolffian or müllerian duct derivatives; vulva externally; cats

SYSTEMS AFFECTED
• Reproductive—anomalies of the gonads, tubular tract, and external genitalia
• Renal/Urologic—occasionally affected (e.g., incontinence, hematuria, and cystitis)
• Skin/Exocrine—perivulvar dermatitis (hypoplastic vulva); perineal or peripreputial dermatitis (hypospadias); hyperpigmentation (testicular neoplasia)

GENETICS
• Chromosomal sex abnormalities—usually caused by random events during gamete formation or early embryonic development
• Gonadal sex abnormalities—XX sex reversal in American cocker spaniels inherited as an autosomal recessive trait; XX sex reversal in beagles, German shorthaired pointers inheritance consistent with autosomal recessive trait; XX sex reversal considered familial in English cocker spaniels, Chinese pugs, Kerry blue terriers, Norwegian elkhound, Weimaraners
• Phenotypic sex abnormalities—PMDS in miniature schnauzers inherited as an autosomal recessive trait with expression limited to XY individuals; hypospadias considered inherited in Boston terriers; testicular feminization (cats only) probably X-linked

INCIDENCE/PREVALENCE
• Generally rare • In affected breeds—may be common within families or even within the breed as a whole

GEOGRAPHIC DISTRIBUTION
N/A

SIGNALMENT
Species
Dogs and cats

Breed Predilections
Dogs—American cocker spaniels; beagles; German shorthaired pointers; English cocker spaniels; Chinese pugs; Kerry blue terriers; Norwegian elkhound; Weimaraners; basset hounds; miniature schnauzers; Boston terriers

Mean Age and Range
• Disorders congenital; defects present at birth • Affected individuals with normal external genitalia may not be identified until breeding age or at routine gonadectomy.

Predominant Sex
Found in both phenotypic females and phenotypic males

SIGNS
General Comments
• Depend on the type of disorder
• Listed here are the possible findings for any of the conditions; not all occur with each specific disorder.

Historical Findings
• Failure to cycle • Infertility and sterility (male or female) • Vulva, clitoris, prepuce, or penis—abnormal size, shape, or location
• Urine stream—abnormal location
• Affected phenotypic males attractive to other males • Urinary incontinence
• Vulvar discharge

Physical Examination Findings
• Vulva normal or hypoplastic • Clitoris normal or enlarged; os clitoris • Perivulvar dermatitis and vulvar discharge • Testes scrotal, unilateral, or bilateral cryptorchid
• Penis and prepuce normal or hypoplastic
• Urethral meatus normal or abnormal location • Dermatologic signs of hyperestrogenism in males • Abdominal mass

CAUSES
• Congenital—heritable or nonheritable
• Exogenous steroid hormone administration during gestation

RISK FACTORS
Androgen or progestogen administration during pregnancy (canine female pseudohermaphrodite)

 DIAGNOSIS

DIFFERENTIAL DIAGNOSIS
Individuals with Unambiguous Genitalia
• Infertility (female)—male infertility; mistimed breeding; subclinical cystic endometrial hyperplasia; hypothyroidism
• Failure to cycle (female)—silent heat; hypothyroidism; hypercorticism; previous gonadectomy • Infertility (male)—female infertility; mistimed breeding; exogenous drug use affecting fertility; orchitis or

SEXUAL DEVELOPMENT DISORDERS

epididymitis; testicular degeneration or hypoplasia; prostatitis

CBC/BIOCHEMISTRY/URINALYSIS
• Usually normal • Urinalysis—may reveal evidence of cystitis with anatomic abnormalities that affect the location of the urethral meatus

OTHER LABORATORY TESTS
• Sex steroid hormones (progesterone, testosterone, and estradiol)—generally below the normal range; may be normal with some mild disorders (patient not sterile)
• Karyotyping—required to define chromosomal sex • Polymerase chain reaction test for Sry—XX sex reversal (not commercially available) • Androgen-binding studies on genital fibroblasts—testicular feminization (not commercially available)

IMAGING
• Routine radiography and ultrasonography—may be of diagnostic value for suspected abdominal mass (e.g., testicular neoplasia with PMDS, testicular feminization, or XX sex reversal); males with signs referable to pyometra (uterus present with female pseudohermaphrodite or PMDS)
• Contrast studies of the lower urogenital tract—may be useful in diagnosing female pseudohermaphrodites

DIAGNOSTIC PROCEDURES N/A

PATHOLOGIC FINDINGS

Gross
• All patients—a precise description of the external genitalia: particular attention given to the size and location of the vulva or prepuce; presence and appearance of the clitoris, penis, scrotum, prostate, caudal vagina, or os clitoris; position of the urinary orifice (necessary to term the phallic structure as penis or clitoris)
• Most patients with no identified chromosomal abnormalities—exploratory laparotomy to determine the location and morphology of the gonads and internal genitalia

Histopathologic
• Examination of all tissues removed—paramount for defining the type of disorder
• Gonads—vary from nearly normal architecture to dysgenetic or a combination of ovary and testis (ovotestis)
• Essential to describe the components of the müllerian and/or wolffian duct system, if found

TREATMENT

APPROPRIATE HEALTH CARE
• Usually outpatient
• Inpatient—exploratory laparotomy

NURSING CARE
Phenotypic females with perivulvar dermatitis secondary to a hypoplastic vulva and phenotypic males with hypospadias—local therapy for improvement of dermatologic sequelae, as necessary; see Dermatoses, Erosive or Ulcerative

ACTIVITY N/A

DIET N/A

CLIENT EDUCATION
• Advise client to allow sterilization of affected individuals.
• Advise client to remove carriers of heritable disorders from the breeding program.

SURGICAL CONSIDERATIONS
• Gonadectomy and hysterectomy (if a uterus is found)—recommended
• Amputation of an enlarged clitoris—recommended when the mucosal surface is repeatedly traumatized
• Reconstructive surgery of the prepuce and malformed penis—dogs; may be necessary with XX male syndrome or hypospadias

MEDICATIONS

DRUG(S) N/A

CONTRAINDICATIONS
Avoid androgen or progestogen use during pregnancy.

PRECAUTIONS N/A

POSSIBLE INTERACTIONS N/A

FOLLOW-UP

PREVENTION/AVOIDANCE
• Sterilize individuals with heritable disorders.
• Remove carriers of heritable disorders from the breeding program

POSSIBLE COMPLICATIONS
• Infertility • Sterility • Urinary tract problems—incontinence; cystitis • Testicular neoplasia • Pyometra

EXPECTED COURSE AND PROGNOSIS
N/A

MISCELLANEOUS

ASSOCIATED CONDITIONS N/A

AGE-RELATED FACTORS
Patients not diagnosed at an early age—pyometra (e.g., PMDS; female pseudohermaphrodite); testicular neoplasia (e.g., PMDS; testicular feminization; XX sex reversal)

PREGNANCY N/A

SYNONYMS
• Hermaphrodites • Pseudohermaphrodites
• Intersexes • Klinefelter syndrome
• Turner syndrome

SEE ALSO
Cryptorchidism

ABBREVIATIONS
• FSH = follicle-stimulating hormone
• LH = luteinizing hormone
• PMDS = persistent müllerian duct syndrome

Suggested Reading
Johnston SD, Root Kustritz MV, Olson PN. Disorders of the canine ovary. In: Johnston SD, Root Kustritz MV, Olson PN. Canine and feline theriogenology. Philadelphia: Saunders, 2001:193–205.

Johnston SD, Root Kustritz MV, Olson PN. Disorders of the feline ovaries. In: Johnston SD, Root Kustritz MV, Olson PN. Canine and feline theriogenology. Philadelphia: Saunders, 2001:453–462.

Meyers-Wallen VN. Inherited abnormalities of sexual development in dogs and cats. In: Concannon PW, England G, Verstegen J, eds. Recent advances in small animal reproduction. Ithaca, NY: International Veterinary Information Service (www.ivis.org), 2001; document no. A1217.0901.

Meyers-Wallen VN. CVT update: inherited disorders of the reproductive tract in dogs and cats. In: Kirk, RW, Bonagura JD, eds. Current veterinary therapy XIII. Philadelphia: Saunders, 2000:904–909.

Meyers-Wallen VN, Schlafer D, Barr I, Lovell-Badg R, Heyzner A. Sry-Negative XX sex reversal in purebred dogs. Molec Reprod Dev 1999;53:266–273.

Authors Sara K. Lyle and Vicki N. Meyers-Wallen

Consulting Editor Sara K. Lyle

SHAKER SYNDROME (GENERALIZED TREMOR SYNDROME)

BASICS

OVERVIEW
Whole body tremor

SIGNALMENT
• Dogs
• Most often in young to middle-aged dogs
• Dogs with white hair coats (e.g., Maltese and West Highland white terriers)—historically have been overrepresented; but disease found in dogs with other coat colors especially miniature pinschers
• Both sexes affected

SIGNS
• Diffuse body tremoring
• Initially, can be confused with signs of apprehension or hypothermia

CAUSES & RISK FACTORS
Most often associated with mild inflammatory CNS disease

DIAGNOSIS

DIFFERENTIAL DIAGNOSIS
Other causes of weakness, apprehension, hypothermia, and seizure

CBC/BIOCHEMISTRY/URINALYSIS
Usually normal

OTHER LABORATORY TESTS
N/A

IMAGING
N/A

OTHER DIAGNOSTIC PROCEDURES
CSF analysis—mild (< 20 WBC × 10/L) monocytic or lymphocytic pleocytosis with normal protein content in most patients; can be normal

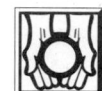

TREATMENT
Inpatient or outpatient

MEDICATIONS

DRUG(S)
• Corticosteroids—reduce the inflammatory response; prednisolone or prednisone (1–2 mg/kg divided q12h) for the first 1–2 weeks
• Depending on clinical response, taper dosage slowly (usually over 4–6 months); assess periodically for clinical deterioration; if dosage is reduced too rapidly, clinical signs may recur, necessitating reinduction of initial dosage
• Many patients do not require further treatment.

CONTRAINDICATIONS/POSSIBLE INTERACTIONS
Corticosteroids—may be contraindicated with infectious encephalitis

SHAKER SYNDROME (GENERALIZED TREMOR SYNDROME)

 FOLLOW-UP

PATIENT MONITORING
Weekly evaluations for approximately 1 month; then monthly until corticosteroids are discontinued

PREVENTION/AVOIDANCE
N/A

POSSIBLE COMPLICATIONS
N/A

EXPECTED COURSE AND PROGNOSIS
• Clinical signs usually subside in 3–7 days from onset of steroid treatment.

• In some patients, recurrence necessitates reinstitution of corticosteroids.
• A small percentage of patients require every-other-day, low-dose corticosteroids, indefinitely, to maintain remission.

 MISCELLANEOUS

SYNONYMS
• Idiopathic Cerebellitis
• Shaker Syndrome

SEE ALSO
Tremors

ABBREVIATION
CNS = central nervous system
CSF = cerebrospinal fluid
WBC = white blood cell

Suggested Reading

Bagley RS, Kornegay JN, Wheeler SJ, et al. Generalized tremors in Maltese: clinical findings in seven cases. J Am Anim Hosp Assoc 1993;29:141–145.
Wagner SO, Podell M, Fenner WR. Generalized tremors in dogs: 24 cases (1984–1995). J Vet Med Assoc 1997;211:731–735
Author Rodney S. Bagley
Consulting Editor Joane M. Parent

SHOCK, CARDIOGENIC

 BASICS

DEFINITION
Results from profound impairment of cardiac function, leading to a decrease in stroke volume and cardiac output, venous congestion, and peripheral vasoconstriction
• Cardiac dysfunction may be caused by hypertrophic or dilated cardiomyopathies, pericardial tamponade, outflow obstructions, thrombosis, severe endocardiosis, heartworm disease, or severe arrhythmias.
• Cardiac "pump" failure may also be secondary to systemic diseases causing myocardial dysfunction such as sepsis.
• Results in hypotension and compromised tissue perfusion, with reduced tissue oxygen delivery

PATHOPHYSIOLOGY
• Most causative conditions are associated with markedly depressed left or right ventricular function, but conditions that cause cardiac compression, leading to inadequate ventricular filling, such as pericardial effusion, or conditions causing severe ventricular inflow or outflow obstruction, may also play a role.
• Associated with greatly diminished stroke volume and cardiac output
• Severe hypotension causes tissue hypoperfusion.
• Compensatory neuroendocrine responses cause peripheral vasoconstriction, which further impairs tissue perfusion. Tissue hypoperfusion causes organ ischemia and energy depletion, leading to abnormal organ function, which exacerbates the shock state. Secondary organs affected include the brain, heart, lung, liver, and kidneys.
• Patients display signs of low output failure. As shock progresses, CHF may develop.
• Rises in left atrial pressure and pulmonary venous pressure may lead to pulmonary edema.

SYSTEMS AFFECTED
• Cardiovascular—primary cardiac dysfunction is causative; cardiac dysfunction (i.e., reduced myocardial contractility) may occur secondary to sepsis; low cardiac output affects coronary blood flow, resulting in myocardial hypoperfusion that exacerbates myocardial dysfunction; cardiac arrhythmias may develop, further compromising myocardial function.
• Respiratory—as cardiac dysfunction progresses, increases in left atrial pressure result in pulmonary venous congestion and development of pulmonary edema; pulmonary gas exchange is affected and hypoxemia results.
• Renal Urologic—systemic hypotension and renal hypoperfusion may result in oliguria, ischemic tubular damage, and development of acute renal failure.
• Hepatobiliary—hepatic congestion may result from right-sided CHF (R-CHF) in cases of right ventricular dysfunction. Hepatic hypoperfusion may lead to increased hepatocellular enzyme concentration.
• Musculoskeletal—low cardiac output and muscle hypoperfusion lead to skeletal muscle weakness.
• Nervous—central nervous system depression occurs in response to organ hypoperfusion.

SIGNALMENT
• Dogs and cats
• Any breed, age, or sex

SIGNS

Historical Findings
• Cardiac decompensation may be associated with a history of previously compensated heart disease and cardiac drug administration.
• A suspicion of previously undiagnosed cardiac disease may result from a history of coughing, exercise intolerance, weakness or syncope.

Physical Examination Findings
• Pale mucous membranes
• Prolonged capillary refill time
• Weak femoral pulse
• Muscle weakness
• Mental dullness
• Possible cardiac arrhythmias
• Cool extremities and hypothermia
• Variable heart rate and respiratory rate
• Harsh lung sounds and crackles
• Cough

CAUSES

Primary Cardiac Disease
• Dilated cardiomyopathy—large-breed dogs, or cats with taurine deficiency
• Hypertrophic or intermediate cardiomyopathy in young male cats
• Severe mitral insufficiency or other end-stage valvular disease in dogs
• Tachy- or bradyarrhythmias
• Pericardial tamponade or constriction

Secondary Cardiac Dysfunction
• Sepsis may result in reduced cardiac contractility.
• Hyperkalemia
• Pulmonary thromboembolism
• Tension pneumothorax

RISK FACTORS
Concurrent illness causing hypoxemia, acidosis, electrolyte imbalances, or the release of cytokines that may affect myocardial function

 DIAGNOSIS

DIFFERENTIAL DIAGNOSIS

Differentiating Similar Signs
Differentiate cardiogenic shock associated with circulatory collapse from compensated cardiac failure; cardiogenic shock is associated with significant reduction in cardiac output, hypotension, tissue hypoperfusion, and evidence of multiorgan dysfunction as evidenced by oliguria, muscle weakness, and mental depression.

Differentiating Causes
• Severe mitral insufficiency—detect by auscultation of a left-sided systolic murmur and the presence of bounding femoral pulses.
• Pericardial effusion—muffled heart sounds, tachycardia, and weak femoral pulses (possibly pulsus paradoxus)
• Dilated cardiomyopathy—weak apex beat and weak femoral pulses
• Cardiac arrhythmias—auscultation and asynchrony of femoral pulses

CBC/BIOCHEMISTRY/URINALYSIS
Usually normal; hyponatremia, high hepatocellular enzyme concentrations, and mild hypoalbuminemia in some patients

OTHER LABORATORY TESTS
Blood gas analysis or pulse oximetry may reveal hypoxemia or metabolic acidosis.

IMAGING

Radiographic Findings
Thoracic radiography may reveal cardiomegaly (cardiomyopathy, pericardial effusion) or evidence of pulmonary edema (CHF).

Echocardiography
May document cardiomyopathy, valvular disease, depressed myocardial contractility, or pericardial tamponade

DIAGNOSTIC PROCEDURES
• Blood pressure measurement may document hypotension.
• Electrocardiography may aid in the detection of arrhythmias.

TREATMENT
• Treat as inpatient; the degree of cardiac dysfunction necessitates intensive medical treatment.
• Pericardiocentesis is essential for patients displaying pericardial tamponade.
• Provide minimal fluid therapy until cardiac function is improved, with the use of positive inotropes or vasodilators or by decompression of a pericardial effusion, as CHF may be exacerbated.
• Oxygen supplementation is important; it can be administered by oxygen cage, mask, or nasal cannula.
• Inform owner of the danger of imminent cardiac arrest in all patients.

MEDICATIONS

DRUG(S) OF CHOICE
• Provide positive inotropic cardiac support to patients with reduced myocardial contractility—digoxin (0.005 mg/kg hourly for up to 4 doses) or dobutamine (5–20 µg/kg/min), given intravenously (dogs)
• Cats with hypertrophic cardiomyopathy may benefit from the use of a calcium channel blocker or a β-blocker.

• Dogs with ventricular arrhythmias may require antiarrhythmic therapy with lidocaine hydrochloride (2 mg/kg loading dose followed by 50 µg/kg/min), given intravenously. Ventricular tachycardia is rare in cats; if lidocaine is needed in a cat, use 1/10 the dose recommended for dogs and administer it slowly while monitoring for signs of neurotoxicity.
• Diuretic therapy may be required for patients in CHF.
• Vasodilator therapy (enalapril, 0.25–0.5 mg/ kg PO, or sodium nitroprusside, 5–10 µg/kg/ min IV) may improve cardiac output by reducing afterload; monitor blood pressure closely.

CONTRAINDICATIONS
• Avoid diuretic therapy in patients with pericardial effusion.
• Avoid calcium channel and β-blockers in patients with reduced myocardial contractility.

PRECAUTIONS
• Vasodilator therapy without positive inotropic support may further compromise tissue perfusion in patients with myocardial dysfunction.
• Monitoring blood pressure and indicators of perfusion (mental status, urine production, body temperature, muscle strength, capillary refill time) may be helpful.
• Use infusion pumps for constant rate infusions of sodium nitroprusside or dobutamine.

POSSIBLE INTERACTIONS
N/A

ALTERNATIVE DRUG(S)
Dopamine may be used as an alternative to dobutamine at a dose of 5–10 µg/kg/min (dogs).

FOLLOW-UP

PATIENT MONITORING
• Heart rate, pulse intensity, mucous membrane color, respiratory rate, lung sounds, urine output, mentation, and rectal temperature during treatment with inotropic drugs or fluids; cardiovascular monitoring by ECG, measurement of central venous pressure, and blood pressure is useful; blood pressure must

be monitored if sodium nitroprusside therapy is used.
• Blood gas analysis and pulse oximetry to follow tissue oxygenation and acid-base balance
• PCV, serum total protein, serum electrolytes, hepatocellular enzymes, blood urea nitrogen, and serum creatinine

POSSIBLE COMPLICATIONS
• Cardiac arrhythmias
• Acid-base disturbances
• Pulmonary edema
• Renal dysfunction
• Syncope
• Hepatic dysfunction
• Cardiac arrest

MISCELLANEOUS

ASSOCIATED CONDITIONS
N/A

AGE-RELATED FACTORS
N/A

ZOONOTIC POTENTIAL
N/A

PREGNANCY
N/A

SYNONYMS
N/A

SEE ALSO
• Atrioventricular Valve Endocardiosis
• Congestive Heart Failure, Left-sided
• Congestive Heart Failure, Right-sided
• Dilated Cardiomyopathy—Dogs
• Hypertrophic Cardiomyopathy—Cats
• Pericardial Effusion

ABBREVIATION
CHF = congestive heart failure

Suggested Reading
Shoemaker WC. Diagnosis and treatment of shock syndromes. In: Shoemaker WC, et al., eds. Textbook of critical care. Philadelphia: Saunders, 1995:85–101.
Author Nishi Dhupa
Consulting Editors Larry P. Tilley and Francis W. K. Smith, Jr.

SHOCK, HYPOVOLEMIC

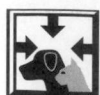

BASICS

DEFINITION
Hypovolemia occurs when blood volume is diminished by whole blood loss or extra-cellular fluid losses. If initial blood loss is severe or compensatory mechanisms fail, adequate coronary and cerebral perfusion cannot be achieved, and hypovolemic shock exists.

PATHOPHYSIOLOGY
Caused by significant whole blood loss or extracellular fluid losses (third-space accumu-lations, vomiting, diarrhea, burns) leading to hypovolemic shock; normal compensatory mechanisms include splenic and venous constriction to shunt blood from venous capacitance vessels to the central arterial circulation, peripheral arteriolar vasoconstric-tion to help maintain diastolic blood pressure, and increased heart rate to increase cardiac output. The aim is to support coronary and cerebral perfusion, which occurs at the expense of visceral and other peripheral organ perfu-sion; the resultant compromise of oxygen and nutrient delivery to the tissues is characteristic. Therapeutic steps that restore blood volume via exogenous administration of fluids can reestab-lish visceral organ perfusion. If excessive hypo-perfusion and hypotension persist, peripheral tissue ischemia leads to multiorgan failure. In the presence of hypoxia and accumulation of noxious metabolic products, peripheral arter-ioles lose their ability to remain constricted; as they dilate, blood begins to pool in tissue capillary beds. At this stage, the animal has moved from early, compensatory, vasoconstric-tive shock to the decompensatory, vasodilative, irreversible stage of hypovolemic shock. Essen-tial blood volume becomes sequestered, venous return and cardiac output are compromised, and organs fail.

SYSTEMS AFFECTED
• Cardiovascular—compensatory responses to all forms of early shock involve increased heart rate, contractility, and peripheral vasoconstriction, all effects that result from sympathetic activation and serve to maintain blood pressure. Sympathetic activation of the heart increases oxygen demands in the face of reduced oxygen delivery. Arrhythmias may result and can intensify shock by further decreasing cardiac output. Prolonged shock decreases cardiac function because of poor coronary perfusion and hypoxia.
• Respiratory—hyperventilation may occur in an attempt to compensate for the progressive metabolic acidosis that develops; as shock progresses, respiratory failure may result from respiratory muscle fatigue secondary to ischemia.
• Renal/Urologic—renal function is compro-mised because of splanchnic vasoconstriction and reduced renal blood flow and glomerular filtration. Progressive renal ischemia leads to oliguria, azotemia, and acute renal failure.
• Gastrointestinal—compromise of gastroin-testinal mucosal blood flow during compen-sation for hypovolemia leads to ischemic mucosal necrosis, hemorrhage, mucosal sloughing, and potential for bacterial translocation; intense pancreatic vasoconstric-tion may cause release of vasoactive and cardiodepressant polypeptides.
• Hepatobiliary—hepatic ischemia results in release of hepatocellular enzymes; hepatic reticuloendothelial system dysfunction leads to reduced bacterial clearance and predisposes to bacteremia and endotoxemia.

SIGNALMENT
N/A

SIGNS

Historical Findings
May be associated with a history of trauma and blood loss, burn injury, severe vomiting and diarrhea, or bleeding associated with surgery

Physical Examination Findings
Early or compensatory shock:
• Tachycardia
• Normal or high arterial blood pressure
• Bounding peripheral pulses
• Hyperemic mucous membranes
• Rapid capillary refill time
• Tachypnea
• Pale mucous membranes, if associated with blood loss; evidence of bleeding or traumatic injuries, if trauma-related
Late or decompensatory shock:
• Tachycardia or bradycardia
• Poor peripheral pulses
• Pale mucous membranes
• Prolonged capillary refill time
• Cool extremities
• Hypothermia
• Mental depression or stupor
• Oliguria
• Tachypnea
• Extreme weakness

CAUSES
• Traumatic blood loss into body cavities or lungs, into fracture sites, or from wounds
• Severe gastrointestinal bleeding associated with corticosteroids or nonsteroidal anti-inflammatory drug therapy, neoplasia, or thrombocytopenia
• Severe epistaxis secondary to intranasal infection, neoplasia, or thrombocytopenia
• Intrathoracic or intraabdominal hemorrhage secondary to coagulation disorders or antico-agulant rodenticide toxicity
• Fluid loss from extensive burn injury, severe vomiting, or diarrhea

RISK FACTORS
• Exposure to possible trauma or burn injury
• Exposure to anticoagulant rodenticides
• Concurrent illness causing thrombocyto-penia or coagulopathy
• Exposure to potentially hazardous situations such as roadways

DIAGNOSIS

DIFFERENTIAL DIAGNOSIS
Must differentiate hypovolemic shock asso-ciated with circulatory collapse from compen-sated hypovolemia or dehydration—circulatory collapse is associated with tachycardia or bradycardia, reduced cardiac output, hypotension, reduced tissue perfusion and evidence of multiorgan dysfunction such as skeletal muscle weakness, mental depression, and oliguria.

CBC/BIOCHEMISTRY/URINALYSIS
• Anemia and hypoproteinemia in animals with blood loss
• Hemoconcentration and electrolyte disturbances in patients with fluid loss caused by gastrointestinal disease or burns
• Hypoproteinemia associated with protein loss in gastrointestinal disease or burns
• Urinalysis may support a diagnosis of hypovolemia and a renal water conservation response (high urine specific gravity).
• If renal ischemia progresses, may be evidence of renal failure (casts in urine)

OTHER LABORATORY TESTS
Blood gas analysis may reveal hypoxemia and acid–base disturbances.

IMAGING
Thoracic radiography may reveal microcardia and pulmonary vascular underperfusion associated with severe hypovolemia.

DIAGNOSTIC PROCEDURES
• Blood pressure measurement may document hypotension.
• Electrocardiography may reveal cardiac arrhythmias
• Central venous pressure monitoring allows objective monitoring of hypovolemia and guides fluid therapy.
• Coagulation profile may document coagulopathy or thrombocytopenia with body cavity or mucosal blood loss.
• Endoscopy or abdominal ultrasonography may help locate a source of blood loss in the gastrointestinal tract.

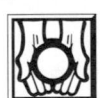

TREATMENT
• Inpatient because of circulatory collapse
• Vigorous fluid therapy to increase effective circulatory volume
• Use balanced electrolyte solutions at initial rate of up to 90 mL/kg for dogs and 40 mL/kg for cats.
• May use colloidal solutions such as whole blood, hydroxyethyl starch (Hetastarch), or dextrans in combination with crystalloid solutions to retain fluid within the vascular space.

• Colloids—20 mL/kg will allow concurrent reduction of crystalloid fluid dosage to 1/4–1/2 the usual shock dosage; indicated for severe hypovolemia; also may use in severe protein loss (e.g., burn patients). A 7.5% solution of hypertonic saline may also be used (5 mL/kg IV bolus) for rapid volume resuscitation.
• Oxygen supplementation—essential; can be administered by oxygen cage, mask, or nasal cannula

MEDICATIONS
DRUG(S) OF CHOICE
Refractory hypovolemic shock—may use positive inotropic therapy (dobutamine, 5–10 µg/kg/min) or vasopressor therapy (dopamine 5–20 µg/kg/min) to raise systemic blood pressure

CONTRAINDICATIONS
N/A

PRECAUTIONS
N/A

POSSIBLE INTERACTIONS
N/A

ALTERNATIVE DRUG(S)
May use vasopressor agents (e.g., phenylephrine or norepinephrine) instead of dopamine

FOLLOW-UP
PATIENT MONITORING
• The aim of aggressive therapy is to obtain a positive trend and reverse the hypovolemic shock state.
• Physical parameters such as heart rate, pulse intensity, mucous membrane color, respiratory rate, urine output, mentation, and rectal temperature
• Cardiovascular—ECG, central venous pressure, and blood pressure recommended; can use blood gas analysis and pulse oximetry to follow tissue oxygenation and acid–base balance

• Should measure PCV, serum total protein, serum electrolytes, hepatocellular enzymes, blood urea nitrogen, and serum creatinine

POSSIBLE COMPLICATIONS
• Electrolyte and acid–base disturbances
• Severe anemia and hypoproteinemia
• Cardiac arrhythmias
• Renal dysfunction
• Hepatic dysfunction
• Gastrointestinal ischemia and hemorrhage and bacterial translocation
• Cardiac arrest

MISCELLANEOUS
ASSOCIATED CONDITIONS
N/A

AGE-RELATED FACTORS
N/A

PREGNANCY
N/A

SYNONYMS
N/A

SEE ALSO
• Anemia, Regenerative
• Hypoalbuminemia
• Hypoxemia

Suggested Reading
Mandell DC, King LG. Fluid therapy in shock. Vet Clin North Am Small Anim Pract. 1998;28(3):623–644.
Shoemaker WC. Diagnosis and treatment of shock syndromes. In: Shoemaker WC, et al., eds. Textbook of critical care. Philadelphia: Saunders, 1995:85–101.
Author: Nishi Dhupa
Consulting Editors: Larry P. Tilley and Francis W. K. Smith, Jr.

SHOCK, SEPTIC

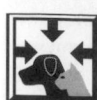

BASICS

DEFINITION
Develops as a complication of overwhelming systemic infection. Sepsis is defined as a systemic inflammatory response to infection. Occurs in severe sepsis and is associated with hypoperfusion or hypotension that may or may not respond to fluids or pharmacologic cardiovascular support to maintain arterial pressure.

PATHOPHYSIOLOGY
Results from cardiovascular and/or vasomotor failure caused by circulating endotoxin and inflammatory mediator release. Gram-positive or gram-negative, aerobic or anaerobic, systemic bacterial infection is the most common underlying cause. The primary event is hypovolemia caused by pyrexia, dehydration, and vascular fluid leakage (because of increased microvascular permeability). Differential vasoconstriction and vasodilation of microvascular beds causes pooling of blood and differential tissue perfusion. Vasculitis and thromboembolic events further compromise tissue perfusion. The ultimate result is tissue hypoxemia and metabolic acidosis, leading to multiple organ failure. In gram-negative bacterial sepsis, endotoxin (a lipopolysaccharide component of the outer bacterial membrane) plays a key role in the activation of the complement and fibrinolytic pathways. Endotoxin also stimulates macrophages to release cytokines, including tumor necrosis factor and interleukin-1, which in turn amplify the systemic response to endotoxin by stimulating neutrophils, endothelial cells, and platelets, and the release of other cellular mediators that are ultimately responsible for the cardiorespiratory and systemic manifestations of septic shock. Gram-positive bacteria produce other bacterial products capable of activating the same mediator responses.

SYSTEMS AFFECTED
• Cardiovascular—cardiac dysfunction (i.e., reduced myocardial contractility) may occur secondary to sepsis due to ischemia and circulating myocardial depressant factors. Differential vasoconstriction and vasodilation occur in capillary beds because of a loss of local vascular autoregulation, in response to ischemia and locally vasoactive metabolites and inflammatory mediators. Vascular endothelial damage results in permeability changes,

fluid leakage, and DIC. Increased blood viscosity impairs microcirculatory flow and leads to aggregation of red blood cells and platelets in low-flow vessels. Peripheral circulatory failure is typical of septic shock and leads to tissue hypoxemia.
• Respiratory—pulmonary edema and pulmonary thromboembolism may be associated with sepsis. Pulmonary edema may be caused by myocardial failure or may be noncardiogenic in origin (i.e., related to vascular leakage of fluids). Noncardiogenic edema may progress to ARDS following development of widespread lung injury. Pulmonary changes may cause potentially severe hypoxemia.
• Renal/Urologic—the kidney initially compensates for reduced blood flow by increasing efferent arteriolar tone, which helps maintain glomerular filtration rate. As circulatory compromise progresses, the protective mechanisms fail, causing a diminished glomerular filtration rate and abnormalities of intrarenal blood flow. Renal ischemia lead to oliguria and acute renal failure.
• Gastrointestinal—severe vasoconstriction and ischemia can lead to necrosis of gastric and intestinal mucosa, in turn leading to erosions, mucosal sloughing, and hemorrhage. Bowel injury results in absorption of bacteria and toxins, which predisposes to bacteremia and endotoxemia.
• Hepatobiliary—hepatic ischemia causes high hepatocellular enzyme concentrations, hyperbilirubinemia, and possible coagulation factor deficiency. Reticuloendothelial system dysfunction reduces bacterial clearance.

SIGNALMENT
Dogs and cats of any breed, age, and sex

SIGNS

Historical Findings
• Possible history of known infection such as urinary tract infection or prostatitis
• Previous surgery possible
• Immunosuppressive conditions, such as diabetes mellitus, hyperadrenocorticism, or chemotherapy regimens, possible

Physical Examination Findings
Early or compensatory shock:
- Tachycardia
- Normal or high arterial blood pressure
- Bounding peripheral pulses
- Hyperemic mucous membranes
- Rapid capillary refill time
- Pyrexia
- Tachypnea
Late or decompensatory shock:
- Tachycardia or bradycardia
- Poor peripheral pulses

- Pale mucous membranes
- Prolonged capillary refill time
- Cool extremities
- Hypothermia
- Mental depression or stupor
- Oliguria
- Dyspnea
- Petechiation
- Peripheral edema
- Dyspnea and tachypnea
- Gastrointestinal bleeding
- Extreme weakness

CAUSES
• Gastrointestinal mucosal compromise from hypovolemia or ischemia, resulting in bacterial translocation and endotoxemia
• Urinary tract infection (e.g., pyelonephritis)
• Prostatitis and prostatic abscessation
• Gastrointestinal rupture
• Septic peritonitis
• Pneumonia
• Bacterial endocarditis
• Bite wounds

RISK FACTORS
• Concurrent condition causing immunocompromise and predisposing to sepsis; examples include diabetes mellitus, hyperadrenocorticism, high-dosage steroids, or chemotherapy
• Old or young age

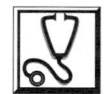

DIAGNOSIS

DIFFERENTIAL DIAGNOSIS
Clinical features include fever, inflammatory response, and circulatory collapse. Septic shock associated with circulatory collapse must be differentiated from systemic infection with adequate compensatory cardiovascular response. Circulatory collapse is associated with tachycardia or bradycardia, reduced cardiac output, hypotension, reduced tissue perfusion, and evidence of multiorgan dysfunction such as mental depression, oliguria, and DIC.

CBC/BIOCHEMISTRY/URINALYSIS
• Leukocytosis with a left shift and possible toxic changes in cells; overwhelming septic shock may be associated with marked leukopenia.
• Hemoconcentration, or anemia and hypoproteinemia in patients with blood loss.
• Hypoalbuminemia secondary to vascular permeability changes and fluid leakage
• High hepatocellular enzyme concentrations and bilirubinemia

- Azotemia (e.g., high BUN, high creatinine)
- Thrombocytopenia
- Urinalysis may show evidence of urinary tract infection (bacteria, whole cells, blood) or acute renal failure (casts).

OTHER LABORATORY TESTS
- Coagulation profile may show prolongation of the activated partial thromboplastin and prothrombin times, increased fibrin degradation products and thrombocytopenia; all consistent with DIC
- Blood gas analysis may reveal hypoxemia and acid–base disturbances.

IMAGING
- Thoracic radiography may reveal evidence of pneumonia, pyothorax, pulmonary edema, or pulmonary thromboembolism.
- Echocardiography may document depressed myocardial contractility, vegetative valvular lesions secondary to bacterial endocarditis, or right ventricular overload secondary to pulmonary hypertension (due to ARDS or pulmonary thromboembolism).
- Abdominal ultrasonography may help detect underlying abdominal disease such as pyelonephritis, abscessation, and peritonitis.

DIAGNOSTIC PROCEDURES
- Electrocardiography may document arrhythmias associated with myocardial depression, ischemia, and acidosis.
- Blood pressure measurement may document hypotension.
- Aerobic and anaerobic blood cultures may identify an infectious source of sepsis.

 TREATMENT
- Inpatient because of circulatory collapse
- Surgically excise any source of sepsis (e.g., an abscess); aggressive treatment and life support may be required. Vigorous fluid therapy is needed to increase effective circulating volume. Use balanced electrolyte solutions at initial rate of up to 90 mL/kg/h for dogs and 40 mL/kg/h for cats. Colloidal solutions such as hydroxyethyl starch (Hetastarch) or dextrans may be used in combination with crystalloid solutions to retain fluid within the vascular space. Synthetic colloids (20 mL/kg) allow reducing the concurrent crystalloid fluid dosage to 1/4–1/2 the usual dosage for shock. A 7.5% solution of hypertonic saline may be used (5 mL/kg IV bolus) for rapid volume resuscitation.
- Oxygen supplementation—as important as fluid replacement; administer by oxygen cage, mask, or nasal cannula.

 MEDICATIONS

DRUG(S) OF CHOICE
- Refractory septic shock—systemic blood pressure may be raised through the use of positive inotropic agents or vasopressors. Dobutamine (5–20 μg/kg/min) can be used as a positive inotrope in myocardial depression. Dopamine (5–20 μg/kg/min) can be used for vasopressor support. Supply both drugs as constant-rate infusions.
- Broad-spectrum antibiotics administered intravenously are essential; while awaiting results of blood, urine, or tissue cultures, initiate treatment with one of the following combinations: ampicillin or cephalexin and gentamicin or enrofloxacin; metronidazole can be used with either of these combinations.
- Sodium bicarbonate may be given intravenously to a patient with severe metabolic acidosis. Calculate the bicarbonate dose with the equation 0.3 mEq × body weight (kg) × base deficit. Give 1/2 the dose slowly IV over a 20-min period and the rest in crystalloid fluids over 4 hours. If unable to calculate the plasma bicarbonate, administer 0.5–1 mEq/kg as directed above.

CONTRAINDICATIONS
N/A

PRECAUTIONS
When using dopamine or dobutamine, watch for development of tachyarrhythmias; high doses of dopamine may also cause excessive peripheral vasoconstriction.

POSSIBLE INTERACTIONS
Sodium bicarbonate and dopamine or dobutamine cannot be administered in the same intravenous line.

ALTERNATIVE DRUG(S)
Vasopressor agents (e.g., phenylephrine or norepinephrine) may be used instead of dopamine.

 FOLLOW-UP

PATIENT MONITORING
- Heart rate, pulse intensity, mucous membrane color, respiratory rate, lung sounds, urine output, mentation; and rectal temperature during aggressive treatment with fluids or inotropic drugs

- ECG and measurement of central venous pressure and blood pressure are useful; use blood gas analysis and pulse oximetry to follow tissue oxygenation and acid–base balance.
- PCV, serum total protein, serum electrolytes, hepatocellular enzymes, blood urea nitrogen, and serum creatinine

POSSIBLE COMPLICATIONS
- Electrolyte and acid–base disturbances
- Cardiac arrhythmias
- Pulmonary edema or ARDS
- Pulmonary thromboembolism
- DIC
- Renal dysfunction
- Hepatic dysfunction
- Gastrointestinal ischemia and bacterial translocation
- Cerebral edema and seizures
- Pancreatitis
- Vasculitis and peripheral edema
- Cardiac arrest

 MISCELLANEOUS

ASSOCIATED CONDITIONS
N/A

AGE-RELATED FACTORS
N/A

PREGNANCY
N/A

SYNONYMS
N/A

SEE ALSO
- Bacteremia and Septicemia
- Disseminated Intravascular Coagulation
- Hypoxemia

ABBREVIATIONS
- ARDS = acute respiratory distress syndrome
- DIC = disseminated intravascular coagulation

Suggested Reading
Betshel SO, Gurn V, Miller CW, et al. Canine toxic shock syndrome: An emerging disease? Adv Exp Med Biol 1997;418:189–192.
Shoemaker WC. Diagnosis and treatment of shock syndromes. In: Shoemaker WC, et al., eds. Textbook of critical care. Philadelphia: Saunders, 1995:85–101.
Author Nishi Dhupa
Consulting Editors Larry P. Tilley and Francis W. K. Smith, Jr.

SHOULDER, LIGAMENT, AND TENDON CONDITIONS

BASICS

DEFINITION
• Make up the majority of causes for lameness in the canine shoulder joint, excluding osteochondritis dissecans lesions

PATHOPHYSIOLOGY

Bicipital Tenosynovitis
• Strain injury to the tendon of the biceps brachii • Mechanism of injury—direct trauma; indirect trauma (more common) • Pathologic changes—from partial disruption of the tendon to chronic inflammatory changes, including dystrophic calcification
• Proliferation of the fibrous connective tissue and adhesions between the tendon and the sheath—limit motion; cause pain

Fibrotic Contracture of the Infraspinatus Muscle
• Primary muscle–tendon disorder—not a neuropathy • Fibrous tissue—replaces normal muscle–tendon unit architecture • Loss of elasticity • Functional shortening of the muscle and tendon • Degeneration and atrophy of affected muscle • Partial muscle disruption—likely caused by direct or indirect trauma

Other
• Rupture of the biceps brachii tendon of origin—strain injury or disruption of the tendinous fibers at or near the junction with the supraglenoid tubercle of the scapula
• Mineralization of the supraspinatus tendon—degenerative condition; granular grayish white calcium deposited between the fibers of the tendon; unknown cause; probably the result of overuse and indirect trauma
• Avulsion or fracture of the supraspinatus tendon—overuse injury; variable amount of bone is avulsed from the greater tubercle of the proximal humerus

SYSTEMS AFFECTED
Musculoskeletal

INCIDENCE/PREVALENCE
Common cause of forelimb lameness

SIGNALMENT

Species
Dogs

Breed Predilections
Medium- to large-breed dogs

Mean Age and Range
• Skeletally mature dogs ≥ 1 year of age
• Usually 3–7 years of age

SIGNS

General Comments
• Depend on the severity and chronicity of the disease • Atrophy of the spinati muscles—consistent finding for all conditions

Historical Findings
• Bicipital tenosynovitis—onset usually insidious; often of several months' duration; may be a traumatic incident as the inciting cause; subtle, intermittent lameness that worsens with exercise • Rupture of the biceps brachii tendon of origin—similar to bicipital tenosynovitis; may have acute onset due to a known traumatic event; usually subtle, chronic lameness that worsens with exercise
• Mineralization of the supraspinatus tendon—onset usually insidious; chronic lameness that worsens with activity
• Avulsion/fracture of the supraspinatus tendon—similar to mineralization of supraspinatus tendon • Fibrotic contracture of the infraspinatus muscle—usually sudden onset during a period of outdoor exercise (e.g., hunting); shoulder lameness and tenderness gradually disappears within 2 weeks; condition results in chronic, persistent lameness 3–4 weeks later, which is not particularly painful

Physical Examination Findings
• Bicipital tenosynovitis—short and limited swing phase of gait owing to pain on extension and flexion of the shoulder; pain inconsistently demonstrated on manipulation of shoulder; pain most evident by applying deep digital pressure over the tendon in the intertubercular groove region while simultaneously flexing the shoulder and extending the elbow • Rupture of the biceps brachii tendon—similar • Mineralization of the supraspinatus tendon—similar; manipulations often do not produce pain; may palpate firm swelling over the greater tubercle
• Avulsion or fracture of the supraspinatus tendon—similar to mineralization of the supraspinatus tendon • Fibrotic contracture of the infraspinatus muscle—usually not painful on manipulation; internal rotation (pronation) of the shoulder joint—patient incapable; when forced, caudal aspect of the scapula elevates off the trunk and becomes more prominent, when patient is standing—elbow adducted; paw abducted and outwardly rotated; when patient is walking—lower limb swings in a lateral arc (circumduction) as the paw is advanced during the stride; marked atrophy of the infraspinatus muscle on palpation

CAUSES
• Indirect or direct trauma—likely • Strain injury (indirect trauma)—most common

RISK FACTORS
• Overexertion • Poor conditioning before performing athletic activities • Obesity

DIAGNOSIS

DIFFERENTIAL DIAGNOSIS
• Luxation or subluxation of the shoulder joint—often a history of trauma with an acute onset of lameness; often severe lameness with marked pain on manipulation of the shoulder joint • Osteosarcoma of the proximal humerus—progressive lameness with varying degrees of pain on manipulation of the shoulder; may note swelling and tenderness of the proximal humerus • Brachial plexus nerve sheath tumor—slow, insidious, progressive lameness over a period of months; marked atrophy of the spinati muscles with chronic disease; may feel a firm mass deep in the axillary region that is painful to digital pressure

IMAGING

Radiology
• Required for differentiation • Craniocaudal and mediolateral views necessary for all patients
Bicipital Tenosynovitis
• Generally normal
• Mediolateral view (chronic disease)—reveals bony reaction on the supraglenoid tubercle, dystrophic calcification of the bicipital tendon, sclerosis of the floor of the intertubercular groove, and osteophytes in the intertubercular groove • Hyperflexed CP-CD or CD-CP view (tangential) of the intertubercular groove—important for identifying the location of calcification; CP-CD view taken with patient in sternal recumbency (radiographic cassette placed on top of the forearm) with the elbow hyperflexed; CD-CP view taken with patient in dorsal recumbency with the shoulder joint hyperflexed and the limb rotated externally approximately 30°; position the radiographic tube directly over the scapulohumeral joint
Rupture of the Biceps Brachii Tendon of Origin
• Normal • Chronic disease—may see bony, irregular reaction on the supraglenoid tubercle
Mineralization of the Supraspinatus Tendon
• Mediolateral view—generally reveals calcification • Occurs cranial and immediately medial to the greater tubercle of the proximal humerus • Superimposition on the greater tubercle of the humerus—requires high-quality images • Tangential or skyline view of the intertubercular region of the proximal humerus—as for bicipital tenosynovitis; eliminates superimposition; allows distinction from calcification of the biceps brachii tendon • Density(ies)—smooth or irregular; multiple lesions common • Often bilateral radiographically but rarely produces bilateral lameness
Avulsion/Fracture of the Supraspinatus Tendon
• Similar to mineralization of the supraspinatus tendon • Bone fragment—origin may be seen as a defect in the greater tubercle of the humerus; generally not as radiographically dense as that identified with mineralization of the supraspinatus tendon
Fibrotic Contracture of the Infraspinatus Muscle
Radiographically normal
Ultrasonography
• May help identify bicipital tenosynovitis and rupture of the biceps brachii tendon of origin
Contrast Arthrography
• Helps identify bicipital tenosynovitis • Useful for determining the location of calcific densities near the intertubercular groove • Incomplete filling of the tendon sheath—may indicate proliferative inflammatory synovitis and adhesions between the tendon sheath and intertubercular groove

DIAGNOSTIC PROCEDURES
• Joint tap and analysis of synovial fluid—identify intraarticular disease; fluid should be straw colored with normal to decreased vis-

cosity; cytologic evaluation: < 10,000 nucleated cells/µl (> 90% are mononuclear cells) • Arthroscopic exploration of the shoulder joint—diagnose bicipital tenosynovitis and rupture of the biceps brachii tendon of origin; confirm lack of intraarticular disease

PATHOLOGIC FINDINGS

• Bicipital tenosynovitis—grossly, mineralization of the biceps tendon; osteophytosis of the intertubercular groove; proliferative synovitis; and fibrous adhesions between the biceps tendon and its synovial sheath; histologically, synovial proliferation, edema, fibrosis, dystrophic mineralization, and lymphocytic-plasmacytic infiltration of the tendon and synovium • Rupture of the biceps brachii tendon of origin—grossly, partial to complete rupture of the biceps tendon at its insertion on the supraglenoid tubercle, proliferative synovitis, and fibrous adhesions between the biceps tendon and its synovial sheath; histologically, synovial proliferation, edema, fibrosis, and occasional dystrophic mineralization • Mineralization of the supraspinatus tendon—grossly, tendon often looks normal, but longitudinal incision reveals numerous pockets of mineralized debris within the fibers; histologically, chondromucinous stromal degeneration of the tendon with multiple foci of dystrophic mineralization • Avulsion or fracture of the supraspinatus tendon—grossly, tendon often looks normal, but longitudinal incision reveals bone fragment(s) surrounded by a fibrous tissue capsule; usually see a corresponding bony defect in the greater tubercle • Fibrotic contracture of the infraspinatus muscle—grossly, atrophied, fibrotic, and contracted muscle, normal tendon, and (commonly) adhesions to the underlying joint capsule; histologically, degeneration, atrophy, and fibroplasia within the damaged muscle

TREATMENT

APPROPRIATE HEALTH CARE

• Outpatient—early diagnosis • Inpatient—chronic, severe disease requires surgical intervention. • Bicipital tenosynovitis—50%–75% success with medical treatment; requires surgery with evidence of chronic changes and failure of medical management • Rupture of the biceps brachii tendon of origin generally requires surgery • Mineralization of the supraspinatus tendon—may be an incidental finding; requires surgery after excluding other causes of lameness and medical treatment • Avulsion or fracture of the supraspinatus tendon—often requires surgery because of persistent bone fragment irritation of the tendon • Fibrotic contracture of the infraspinatus muscle—requires surgery

NURSING CARE

• Cryotherapy (ice packing)—immediately postsurgery; helps reduce inflammation and swelling at the surgery site; performed 15–20 min every 8 hr for 3–5 days • Regional massage

and range-of-motion exercises—improve flexibility; decrease muscle atrophy

ACTIVITY

• Medical treatment—requires strict confinement for 4–6 weeks; activity; premature return to normal likely exacerbates signs and induces a chronic state. • Postsurgery—depends on procedure performed

DIET

Weight control—decrease the load applied to the painful joint

SURGICAL CONSIDERATIONS

• Bicipital tenosynovitis—recommended with poor response to medical treatment and chronic disease; goal: eliminate movement of the biceps tendon within the inflamed synovial sheath by performing a tenodesis of the bicipital tendon; remove the tendon from its origin on the scapular supraglenoid tubercle and reattach it to the proximal lateral aspect of the humerus. • Rupture of the biceps brachii tendon of origin—tenodesis is the treatment of choice; reattach tendon to the proximal lateral aspect of the humerus using either a screw and spiked washer or passing the tendon through a bone tunnel and suturing it to the supraspinatus tendon. • Mineralization of the supraspinatus tendon—longitudinally incise the tendon; remove the calcium deposits. • Avulsion or fracture of the supraspinatus tendon—remove the bone fragment(s) • Fibrotic contracture of the infraspinatus muscle—tenotomy and excision of part of the tendon of insertion; often feel a distinct pop after excision of the last adhesion, which allows complete range of motion of the shoulder joint.

MEDICATIONS

DRUG(S) OF CHOICE

Bicipital Tenosynovitis

• Intraarticular injection of a corticosteroid—initial treatment of choice • Systemic treatment (NSAIDs or steroids)—not as effective • Do not inject into a septic joint; perform complete synovial fluid analysis if any doubt. • Prednisolone acetate—20–40 mg, depending on size • Lameness markedly improved but not eliminated—give a second injection in 3–6 weeks • Incomplete resolution—recommend surgery

NSAIDs and Analgesics

• May be used for symptomatic treatment • May try buffered or enteric-coated aspirin (10–25 mg/kg PO q8–12h), carprofen (2.2 mg/kg PO q12h), etodolac (10–15 mg/kg PO q24h), phenylbutazone (3–7 mg/kg PO q8h, total dose < 800 mg/day), meclofenamic acid (0.5 mg/kg PO q12h), piroxicam (0.3 mg/kg PO q24h for 3 days, then q48h), or deracoxib (3–4 mg/kg PO q24h for 7 days for postoperative pain) (1–2 mg/kg PO q24h for long-term treatment over 7 days)

CONTRAINDICATIONS

• Avoid corticosteroids because of the potential side effects and articular cartilage damage

associated with long-term use. • Direct injection of a corticosteroid into the biceps tendon—may promote further tendon disruption and eventual rupture

PRECAUTIONS

NSAIDs—gastrointestinal irritation may preclude use.

ALTERNATIVE DRUG(S)

Chondroprotective drugs (e.g., polysulfated glycosaminoglycans, glucosamine, and chondroitin sulfate)—may help limit associated cartilage damage and degeneration

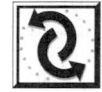

FOLLOW-UP

PATIENT MONITORING

• Most patients require a minimum of 1–2 months of rehabilitation after treatment.

EXPECTED COURSE AND PROGNOSIS

• Medically managed bicipital tenosynovitis—often successful after one or two treatments (50%–75% of cases) with no chronic changes • Surgically treated bicipital tenosynovitis—good to excellent results (90% of cases); recovery to full function may take 2–8 months • Surgically treated tenodesis of the bicipital brachii tendon—good to excellent prognosis; > 85% of patients show improved return to function. • Surgically treated mineralization of the supraspinatus tendon—good to excellent prognosis; recurrence possible but uncommon • Surgically treated avulsion or fracture of the supraspinatus tendon—good to excellent prognosis; recurrence possible but uncommon • Surgically treated fibrotic contracture of the infraspinatus muscle—good to excellent prognosis; patients uniformly return to normal limb function

MISCELLANEOUS

ABBREVIATIONS

CD = craniodorsal
CP = cranioposterior
NSAID = nonsteroidal antiinflammatory drug

Suggested Reading

Flo GL, Middleton D. Mineralization of the supraspinatus tendons in dogs. J Am Vet Med Assoc 1990:197:95–97.

Rivers B, Wallace L, Johnston GR. Biceps tenosynovitis in the dog: radiographic and sonographic findings. Vet Comp Orthop Trauma 1992;5:51–57.

Stobie D, Wallace LJ, Lipowitz AJ, et al. Chronic bicipital tenosynovitis in dogs: 29 cases (1985–1992). J Am Vet Med Assoc 1995;207:201–207.

Author Peter D. Schwarz
Consulting Editor Peter K. Shires

SICK SINUS SYNDROME

BASICS

DEFINITION

A disorder of impulse formation within, and conduction out of, the sinus node; it also affects subsidiary pacemakers and the specialized conduction system of the atria, AV node, His bundle, and bundle branches.

ECG Features

• Arrhythmias noted with SSS include any or all of the following: inappropriate sinus bradycardia, sinus arrest, sinoatrial exit block, slow ectopic atrial rhythm, or alternating periods of sinus bradyarrhythmias and SVT
• Paroxysms of SVT may alternate with prolonged periods of sinus node inertia and often AV nodal inertia as well, producing tachycardia–bradycardia syndrome, a variant of SSS (Figure 1)
• P waves and QRS complexes are usually normal.
• P waves may be abnormal or absent with slow atrial ectopic rhythm or junctional escape rhythm.

PATHOPHYSIOLOGY

• ECG manifestations may preceed development of clinical signs.
• Clinical signs usually result from the failure of subsidiary pacemakers to generate escape rhythms when sinus node dysfunction occurs.
• The common clinical manifestations reflect transient decreases in organ perfusion, particularly reduced cerebral perfusion.
• Rarely, congestive heart failure develops

SYSTEMS AFFECTED

• Cardiovascular
• Nervous, musculoskeletal, and renal systems may be secondarily affected because of hypoperfusion.

GENETICS

May be heritable in miniature schnauzers

INCIDENCE/PREVALENCE

N/A

SIGNALMENT

Species

Dogs

Breed Predilections

• Miniature schnauzers (may be heritable)
• Noted commonly in cocker spaniels, dachshunds, and West Highland white terriers

Mean Age and Range

Most dogs > 6 years old

Predominant Sex

Female

SIGNS

Historical Findings

• Clinical signs vary from asymptomatic to weakness, syncope, collapse, and/or seizures.
• Sudden death is infrequent.

Physical Examination Findings

• Heart rate may be abnormally rapid or abnormally slow.
• Pauses may be noted.
• Some patients appear normal.

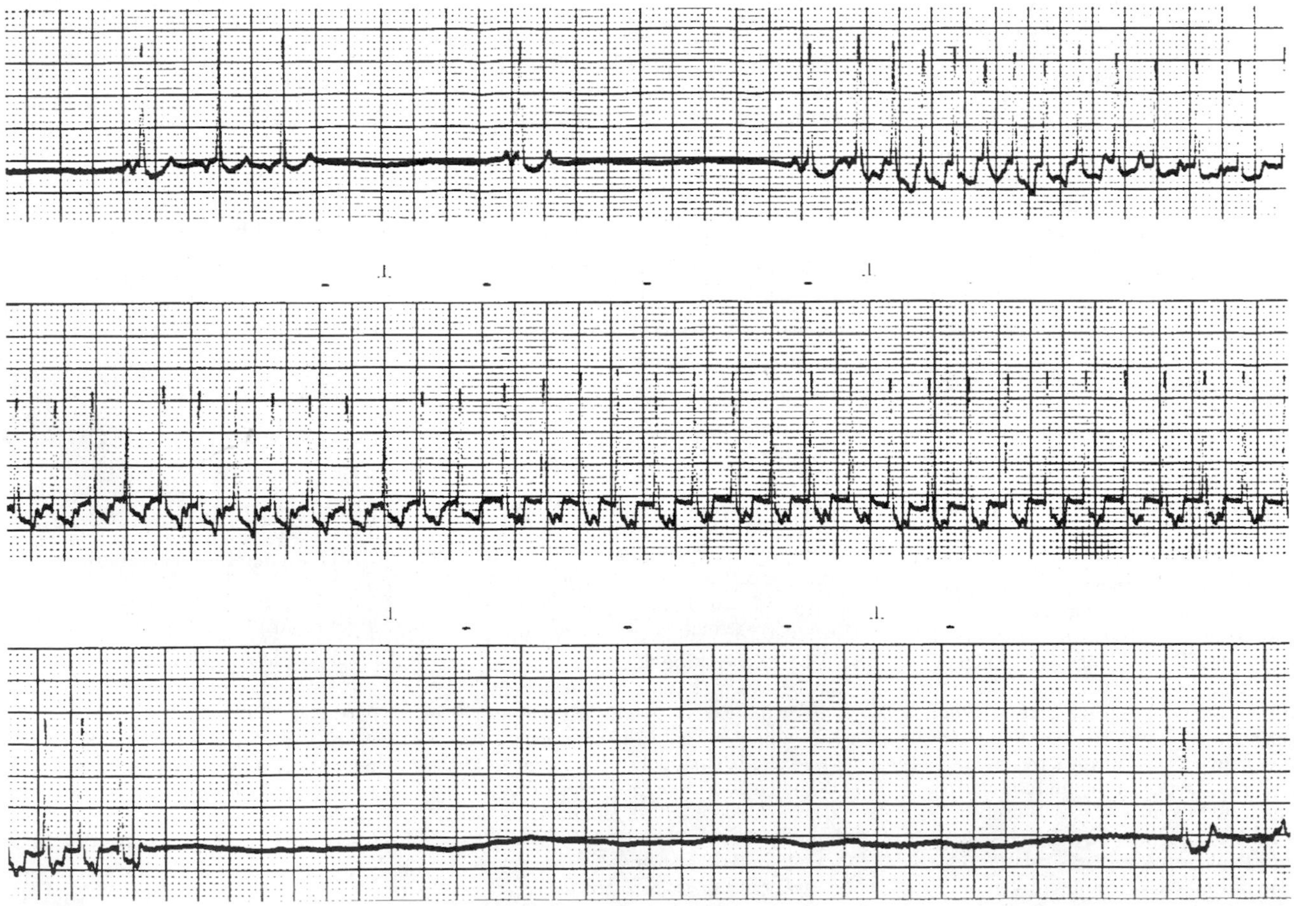

Figure 1.

A continuous lead II ECG rhythm strip recorded from a dog with bradycardia-tachycardia syndrome, a variant of sick sinus syndrome. The dog's rhythm is initially a relatively slow ectopic atrial rhythm (negative P waves; heart rate 150 beats/minute) followed by brief asystole. The third pause is followed by supraventricular tachycardia with a rate of approximately 300 beats/minute. The tachycardia terminates abruptly and is followed by 6.7 seconds of asystole (paper speed = 25 mm/s).

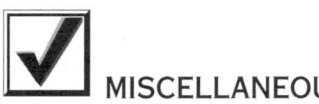

SICK SINUS SYNDROME

CAUSES
- Idiopathic
- Familial in miniature schnauzers
- Metastatic disease
- Ischemic disease

RISK FACTORS
N/A

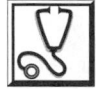

DIAGNOSIS

DIFFERENTIAL DIAGNOSIS
- Healthy dogs may exhibit sinus bradycardia (rate as low as 30 beats/min) and sinus pauses (as long as 3 sec) normally during sleep.
- Bradycardia and sinus arrest due to normal or enhanced vagal tone
- Drug-induced (digitalis, β-adrenergic antagonists, α_2-adrenergic agonists, calcium channel antagonists, cimetidine, opioids)
- Seizures or syncope due to noncardiac disease
- Atrial standstill secondary to hyperkalemia or atrial disease
- Weakness due to neurologic, musculoskeletal, or metabolic diseases

CBC/BIOCHEMISTRY/URINALYSIS
Normal

OTHER LABORATORY TESTS
N/A

IMAGING
N/A

DIAGNOSTIC PROCEDURES
- Atropine response testing—indicated in dogs with sinus bradycardia, sinus arrest, and sinoatrial exit block. Administer atropine (0.04 mg/kg IM), and evaluate the ECG 20–30 min later. A normal (positive) response is > 50% increase in heart rate with abolishment of pauses; dogs with SSS generally have no response or an incomplete response to atropine.
- Electrophysiologic testing of sinus node recovery time and sinoatrial conduction time
- 24-hr ambulatory ECG (Holter) or event monitoring to correlate clinical signs with arrhythmia

PATHOLOGIC FINDINGS
Vary with cause

TREATMENT

APPROPRIATE HEALTH CARE
- Hospitalization rarely necessary except for electrophysiologic testing or pacemaker implantation
- Do not treat asymptomatic animals.

ACTIVITY
Avoid vigorous exercise and stressful situations.

DIET
Modifications unnecessary

CLIENT EDUCATION
Owner should be aware that medical management is often ineffective.

SURGICAL CONSIDERATIONS
- Permanent pacemaker necessary for dogs failing to respond to medical treatment and those exhibiting unacceptable medication side effects
- Permanent pacemaker usually required for dogs with bradycardia-tachycardia syndrome

MEDICATIONS

DRUG(S)
- Do not treat asymptomatic animals.
- Symptomatic dogs are grouped into those showing primarily bradycardia, sinus arrest, and/or sinoatrial exit block and those with supraventricular tachycardia followed by sinus arrest.
- Atropine-responsive symptomatic dogs with bradycardia or sinus arrest—anticholinergic agents (propantheline: small dogs 3.75–7.5 mg PO q8–12h, medium dogs 15 mg PO q8h, large dogs 30 mg PO q8h; hyoscyamine: 0.003–0.006 mg/kg q8h)
- Dogs with bradycardia and sinus arrest—may try theophylline (Theo-Dur, 20 mg/kg PO q12h), terbutaline (0.2 mg/kg PO q8–12h), or hydralazine (1.0–2.0 mg/kg PO q8–12h) if anticholinergic drugs are ineffective
- Dogs with bradycardia-tachycardia whose clinical signs are due to tachycardia or tachycardia-induced sinus arrest—can give digoxin (0.005 mg/kg PO q12h) or atenolol (0.5–1.0 mg/kg PO q12–24h) in attempt to suppress the SVT (monitor closely for exacerbation of bradycardia)

CONTRAINDICATIONS
Avoid drugs that may worsen sinus node dysfunction (e.g., β-adrenergic antagonists, calcium channel blocking agents, phenothiazines, class I and III antiarrhythmic agents, opioids, cimetidine, α_2-adrenergic agonists).

PRECAUTIONS
- Attempts to manage bradycardia-tachycardia syndrome medically without prior pacemaker implantation carry significant risk because drugs used to control SVT may worsen the bradyarrhythmias, and vice versa.
- Adverse effects of anticholinergic medication (constipation, difficulty voiding, keratoconjunctivitis sicca, emesis) occur commonly.

FOLLOW-UP

PATIENT MONITORING
- ECG in asymptomatic patients—to detect progression of disease
- ECG in patients treated medically or with pacemaker implantation

POSSIBLE COMPLICATIONS
Rarely, reduced cerebral or renal perfusion results in chronic renal dysfunction or CNS damage.

EXPECTED COURSE AND PROGNOSIS
- Good, following pacemaker implantation in animals without congestive heart failure
- Medical management—often ineffective; initial beneficial effects often not sustained

MISCELLANEOUS

AGE-RELATED FACTORS
N/A

SYNONYMS
- Bradycardia-tachycardia syndrome
- Tachycardia-bradycardia syndrome

SEE ALSO
- Sinus Arrest or Sinoatrial Block
- Supraventricular Tachycardia
- Sinus Bradycardia

ABBREVIATIONS
- AV = atrioventricular
- ECG = electrocardiogram
- SSS = sick sinus syndrome
- SVT = supraventricular tachycardia

Suggested Reading

Belic N, Talano JV. Current concepts in sick sinus syndrome: I. Anatomy, physiology, and pharmacologic causes. Arch Intern Med 1985;145:521–523.

Belic N, Talano JV. Current concepts in sick sinus syndrome: II. ECG manifestation and diagnostic and therapeutic approaches. Arch Intern Med 1985;145:722–726.

Reiffel JA. Normal sinus rhythm and its variants. In: Podrid PJ, Kowey PR, eds. Cardiac arrhythmia—mechanisms, diagnosis, and management. Baltimore: Williams & Wilkins, 1995:752–767.

Tilley LP. Essentials of canine and feline electrocardiography. 3rd ed. Baltimore: Williams & Wilkins, 1992.

Saito D, Matsubara K, Yamanari H, et al. Effects of oral theophylline on sick sinus syndrome. J Am Coll Cardiol 1993; 21:1119–1204.

Author Janice McIntosh Bright

Consulting Editors Larry P. Tilley and Francis W. K. Smith, Jr.

SINUS ARREST AND SINOATRIAL BLOCK

 BASICS

DEFINITION
• Sinus arrest—a disorder of impulse formation caused by slowing or cessation of spontaneous sinus nodal automaticity; failure of the SA node to initiate an impulse at the expected time. P-P interval does not equal a multiple of basic P-P interval.
• Sinoatrial block—a disorder of impulse conduction; an impulse formed within the sinus node fails to depolarize the atria or does so with delay; most commonly the basic rhythmicity of the sinus node is not disturbed and the duration of the pause is a multiple of the basic P-P interval. Classified into first-, second-, and third-degree SA block (similar to degrees of AV block). Difficult to diagnose first- and third-degree SA block from ECG. Second-degree SA block most common: Mobitz type I (Wenckebach) SA block—P-P interval progressively shortens prior to a pause; duration of pause is less than two P-P cycles; Mobitz type II SA block—duration of pause occurring after a sinus beat is exact multiple (two, three, or four times normal) of basic P-P interval.

ECG Features
• A normal P wave exists for each QRS complex with a pause equal to or greater than twice the normal P-P interval; rhythm is regularly irregular or irregular with pauses (Figure 1).
• Junctional or ventricular escape beats—if pauses significantly prolonged. Subsidiary pacemaker takes over rhythm with escape beats normally from AV; junctional tissue or Purkinje fibers.
• Surface ECG cannot differentiate sinus arrest from block in the dog because of normal R-R interval variation (sinus arrhythmia).

PATHOPHYSIOLOGY
• Sympathetic and parasympathetic influences can alter spontaneous sinus node depolariza-tion; vagal stimulation of acetylcholine, which binds to SA nodal receptor sites, can slow automaticity of the sinus node by reducing the slope of phase 4 depolarization; sympathetic stimulation releases norepineph-rine that binds to β_1 receptors on the SA node, enhancing spontaneous SA nodal discharge rate.
• Postdrive inhibition phenomenon occurs when sinus arrest follows a run of ectopic beats. The sinus node requires a warming-up period until its usual rate of automaticity is reestablished.
• Intrinsic disease of the sinus node may affect the balance between the parasympa-thetic and sympathetic efferent traffic to the SA node and its spontaneous discharge rate.
• Duration of sinus arrest may be long and possibly irreversible when the sinus node is suppressed by an ectopic tachycardia, particularly with severe underlying heart disease. Persistent sinus arrest not due to any drug often indicates SSS.

SYSTEMS AFFECTED
Cardiovascular—clinical signs of weakness or syncope may appear if sinus arrest or block causes sufficiently long periods (generally 5 seconds or longer) of ventricular asystole with no escape beats initiated by latent pacemakers.

GENETICS
• Seen in purebred pugs with hereditary stenosis of the bundle of His
• Seen in female miniature schnauzers predisposed to SSS
• Congenitally deaf Dalmatian coach hounds often have abnormal SA node and multiple atrial arteries.

INCIDENCE/PREVALENCE
• Normal incidental finding in brachycephalic breeds of dogs in which inspiration causes a reflex increase in vagal tone
• Common in dog breeds predisposed to SSS
• Uncommon in cats

GEOGRAPHIC DISTRIBUTION
N/A

SIGNALMENT
Species
Dogs and cats

Breed Predilections
• Brachycephalic breeds
• Breeds predisposed to SSS (e.g., miniature schnauzers, dachshunds, cocker spaniels, pugs, and West Highland white terriers)

Mean Age and Range
If associated with SSS, generally older animal

Predominant Sex
In association with SSS, older females

SIGNS
General Comments
Generally no clinical significance by itself if terminated by sinus node depolarization again or latent pacemakers promptly escape to prevent ventricular asystole

Historical Findings
• Usually none
• Signs of low cardiac output (e.g., weakness and syncope) may occur with failure of the SA node to fire on time if no lower pacemaker focus takes over the rhythm.
• Sudden death is possible with prolonged periods of ventricular asystole.

Physical Examination Findings
• May be normal
• Heart sounds following a pause may be louder than usual because the ventricles had longer to fill and eject a larger amount of blood.
• Extremely slow heart rate if arrest or block is prolonged or frequent
• With significant pathologic cardiac disease—may be findings consistent with poor cardiac output (e.g. prolonged perfusion time, pale mucous membranes, weak femoral pulses)

CAUSES
Physiologic
• Vagal stimulation secondary to coughing, pharyngeal irritation
• Ocular or carotid sinus pressure
• Surgical manipulation

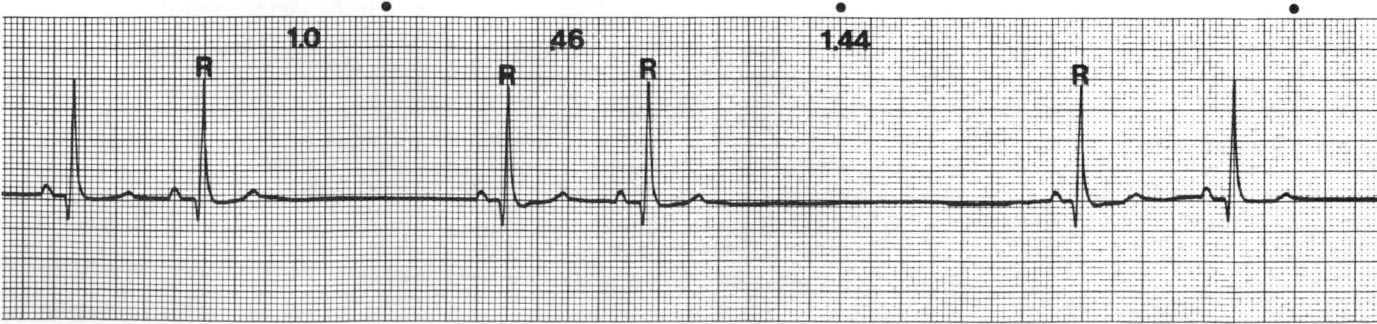

Figure 1.

Intermittent sinus arrest in a brachycephalic breed with an upper respiratory disorder and episodes of fainting. The pauses (1 and 1.44 sec) are greater than twice the nor-mal R-R interval (0.46). (From: Tilley LP: Essentials of canine and feline electrocardiography. 3rd ed. Baltimore: Williams & Wilkins, 1992, with permission.)

SINUS ARREST AND SINOTRIAL BLOCK

Pathologic
- Degenerative heart disease (fibrosis)
- Dilatory heart disease
- Acute myocarditis
- Neoplastic heart disease
- SSS
- Irritation of vagus nerve secondary to thoracic or cervical neoplasia
- Electrolyte imbalance
- Drug toxicity (e.g., digoxin)

RISK FACTORS
- Certain drugs, including digitalis, quinidine, propranolol, xylazine, acepromazine
- Respiratory tract disease
- Vagal maneuvers

DIAGNOSIS

DIFFERENTIAL DIAGNOSIS
- Marked sinus arrhythmia and sinus bradycardia
- Not always possible to differentiate sinus arrest from SA block without direct recordings of sinus node discharge; pauses that are precise multiples of the dominant beat interval suggest sinus block

CBC/BIOCHEMISTRY/URINALYSIS
Serum electrolyte abnormalities in some animals, especially hyperkalemia (serum K^+ > 5.7 mEq/L)

OTHER LABORATORY TESTS
N/A

IMAGING
- Thoracic radiographs if neoplastic or cardiac disease suspected
- Cardiac ultrasound if structural or neoplastic heart disease suspected

DIAGNOSTIC PROCEDURES
- Provocative atropine response test to assess sinus node function. Administer 0.04 mg/kg atropine IM; evaluate ECG lead II rhythm strip 30 min later for response. Resolution of the arrhythmia with atropine administration suggests high vagal tone as the underlying cause.
- Ambulatory monitoring may reveal prolonged periods of failure of impulses from the SA node if signs of weakness or syncope present.
- In people, a period of sinus arrest following right carotid massage that lasts longer than 3 sec suggests inappropriate sinus responsiveness.
- Electrophysiologic studies of sinus node
- Serum digoxin concentration, if applicable; assay 6–8 hr post pill; therapeutic serum concentrations are typically 0.8–1.5 ng/mL.

PATHOLOGIC FINDINGS
Histologic study of the SA node may reveal necrosis, fibrosis, and/or degenerative changes in the sinus node.

TREATMENT

APPROPRIATE HEALTH CARE
Asymptomatic sinus arrest or block does not require therapy. If clinical signs, therapeutic approach depends on cause, underlying cardiac status, and severity of symptoms. Any indicated treatment may be outpatient unless pacemaker implantation is necessary, which necessitates hospital management.

NURSING CARE
Correct any electrolyte abnormalities that may be contributing.

ACTIVITY
Unrestricted unless signs of weakness, syncope, or CHF develop

DIET
N/A

CLIENT EDUCATION
An artificial pacemaker may be necessary when patient is symptomatic and non-responsive to medical management

SURGICAL CONSIDERATIONS
Implantation of an artificial demand pacemaker in animals with clinical signs nonresponsive to therapy

MEDICATIONS

DRUG(S) OF CHOICE
- If patient is symptomatic, consider atropine (0.02 mg/kg IV, 0.04 mg/kg IM), glycopyrrolate (0.005–0.01 mg/kg IV, IM), or isoproterenol (10 μg/kg IM, SC q6h or dilute 1 mg in 500 mL of 5% dextrose or Ringer's solution, and infuse IV 0.5–1 mL/min [1–2 μg/min] or to effect)
- If responsive to injectable anticholinergic drugs (e.g., atropine)—can prescribe oral propantheline bromide (0.25–0.5 mg/kg q8–12h) or hyocyamine (0.003–0.006 mg/kg q8h) for at-home management; bronchodilator therapy with aminophylline, theophylline, albuterol, or terbutaline can also be considered for oral therapy

CONTRAINDICATIONS
If patient is symptomatic secondary to prolonged pauses, discontinue any drugs that may be causative (e.g., digitalis, β-blockers, calcium channel blockers)

PRECAUTIONS
Avoid drugs that depress SA node function.

POSSIBLE INTERACTIONS
N/A

ALTERNATIVE DRUG(S)
If medical therapy does not resolve signs, consider a ventricular demand artificial pacemaker.

FOLLOW-UP

PATIENT MONITORING
When indicated, periodic serial ECG evaluation to assess therapeutic efficacy and possible progression to a more serious dysrhythmia

PREVENTION/AVOIDANCE
N/A

POSSIBLE COMPLICATIONS
If associated with primary cardiac disease, CHF may develop and necessitate appropriate therapies.

EXPECTED COURSE AND PROGNOSIS
If cause is SSS, symptomatic patient may respond well to medical intervention; if poorly responsive, permanent pacemaker implantation would improve prognosis markedly

MISCELLANEOUS

ASSOCIATED CONDITIONS
- Sick sinus syndrome • Sinus arrhythmia
- Sinus bradycardia

AGE-RELATED FACTORS
N/A

ZOONOTIC POTENTIAL
N/A

PREGNANCY
N/A

SYNONYMS
- Sinus block • Sinus pause

SEE ALSO
- Sick Sinus Syndrome • Sinus Arrhythmia
- Sinus Bradycardia

ABBREVIATIONS
- AV = atrioventricular • CHF = congestive heart failure • ECG = electrocardiogram
- SA = sinoatrial • SSS = sick sinus syndrome

Suggested Reading
Chung EK. Manual of cardiac arrhythmias. 1st ed. New York: Yorke Medical Books, 1986.

Kittleson MD, Kienle RD. Small animal cardiovascular medicine. St. Louis: Mosby, 1998.

Tilley LP, Goodwin J, eds. Manual of canine and feline cardiology. 3rd ed. Philadelphia: Saunders, 2000.

Tilley LP, ed. Essentials of canine and feline electrocardiography. 3rd ed. Baltimore: Williams & Wilkins, 1992.

Author Deborah J. Hadlock
Consulting Editors Larry P. Tilley and Francis W. K. Smith, Jr.

SINUS ARRHYTHMIA

 BASICS

DEFINITION
• Normal sinus impulse formation characterized by a phasic variation in sinus cycle length. An irregular R-R interval is present that has more than 10% variation in sinus cycle length (or variability of 0.12 seconds [dog], 0.10 seconds [cat], or more exists between successive P waves).
• Two basic forms exist—respiratory sinus arrhythmia: P-P interval cyclically shortens during inspiration due primarily to reflex inhibition of vagal tone and lengthens during expiration; nonrespiratory sinus arrhythmia: phasic variation in P-P interval unrelated to the respiratory cycle

ECG Features
Other than the irregular rhythm, all other criteria for sinus rhythm are present.
• Normal heart rate
• Positive P wave in leads, I, II, III, and aVF, unless a wandering pacemaker is present, where the P waves may be positive, diphasic, or negative temporarily
• A P wave is present for every QRS complex.
• A QRS complex is present for every P wave.
• PR interval is relatively constant

PATHOPHYSIOLOGY
• Sinus node discharge rate depends on the two opposing influences of the autonomic nervous system. Vagal stimulation decreases spontaneous sinus nodal discharge rate and predominates over sympathetic stimulation. During inspiration, feedback from the respiratory and cardiac centers in the medulla produces cardiac acceleration by decreasing vagal restraint on the sinus node; the opposite occurs during exhalation. The genesis of sinus arrhythmia (SA) also depends on reflexes involving stretch receptors in the lung, pressure-volume sensory receptors in the heart (Bainbridge, baroreceptor), blood vessels, and chemical factors of the blood.

SYSTEMS AFFECTED
Cardiovascular—generally no hemodynamic consequence, but marked SA may produce a long enough sinus pause to produce syncope if not accompanied by an escape rhythm

GENETICS
N/A

INCIDENCE/PREVALENCE
Most frequent form of arrhythmia in the dog

SIGNALMENT

Species
• Common and normal in dogs
• Uncommon, usually abnormal in cats

Breed Predilections
• Brachycephalic breeds predisposed
• Dogs—bulldogs, Lhasa apsos, Pekingese, pugs, shar-peis, shih tzus, boxers
• Cats—Persians, Himalayans

Mean Age and Range
N/A

Predominant Sex
N/A

SIGNS

General Comments
Uncommon, but weakness may develop if pauses between beats are excessively long; syncope can occur when a marked sinus arrhythmia and sinus bradycardia develop

Historical Findings
• Respiratory SA—none
• Nonrespiratory SA—may be findings related to underlying disease

Physical Examination Findings
• May be normal
• Irregular rhythm on auscultation
• May be findings related to specific disease accentuating vagal tone (e.g., stertor and stridor in a patient with brachycephalic airway syndrome)

CAUSES
• Normal cyclic change in vagal tone associated with respiration in the dog; heart rate increases with inspiration and decreases with expiration
• Underlying conditions that increase vagal tone—high intracranial pressure, gastrointestinal disease, respiratory disease, cerebral disorders, digitalis toxicity
• Carotid sinus massage or ocular pressure (vagal maneuver) may accentuate

RISK FACTORS
• Brachycephalic conformation
• Digoxin therapy
• Any disease that increases vagal tone

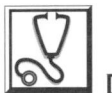 DIAGNOSIS

DIFFERENTIAL DIAGNOSIS
• Auscultation of SA is often confusing; ECG helps differentiate normal SA from true pathologic arrhythmia.
• Wandering sinus pacemaker frequently associated and a variant of sinus arrhythmia. Site of impulse formation shifts within the sinoatrial node or to an atrial focus or AV node, changing the configuration of the P wave.
• Important to differentiate normal SA from pathologic arrhythmias including atrial premature complexes, SSS, slow atrial fibrillation, and AV dissociation

CBC/BIOCHEMISTRY/URINALYSIS
N/A

OTHER LABORATORY TESTS
Cats with chronic respiratory disease may be positive for feline leukemia or feline immunodeficiency virus.

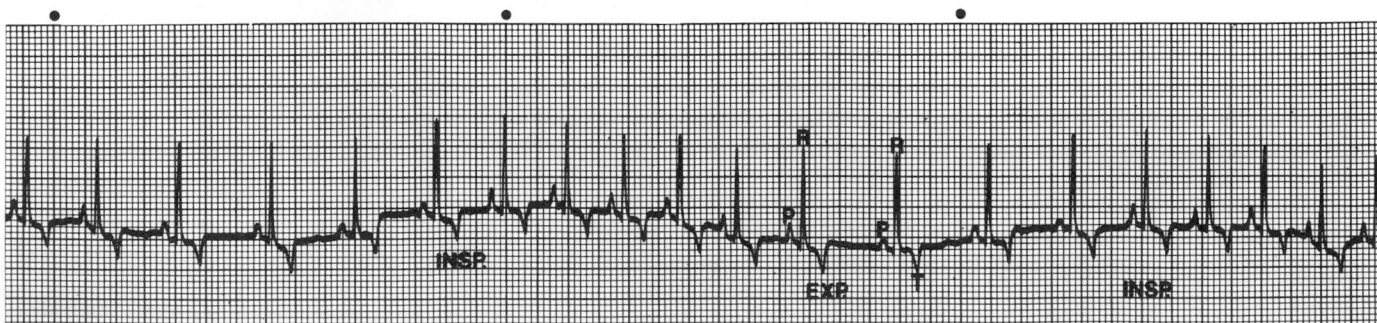

Figure 1.

Respiratory sinus arrhythmia with an average rate of 120/min (paper speed, 25 mm/sec; 6 complexes between one set of time lines × 20). The rate increases during inspiration (*INSP*) and decreases during expiration (*EXP*). The fluctuation of the baseline correlates with the movement of the electrodes by the thoracic cavity. Variation in P wave amplitude is due to a wandering sinus pacemaker, which often accompanies sinus arrhythmia. (From: Tilley LP: Essentials of canine and feline electrocardiography. 3rd ed. Baltimore: Williams & Wilkins, 1992, with permission.)

IMAGING
Radiographs of head and neck to assess for abnormal anatomic conformation that might predispose to airway problems

DIAGNOSTIC PROCEDURES
• Pharyngoscopy/laryngoscopy if upper airway disease suspected
• Atropine challenge test (administer atropine 0.04 mg/kg IM followed by ECG in 30 min) if associated with sinus bradycardia and primary dysfunction of sinus node is suspected

PATHOLOGIC FINDINGS
See specific disease

TREATMENT

APPROPRIATE HEALTH CARE
Generally, specific treatment required only when associated with symptomatic sinus bradycardia; if not related to respiration, underlying cause is treated. If patient is suffering respiratory distress, appropriate inpatient management indicated until patient is stable

NURSING CARE
None unless associated with underlying disease (see also below)

ACTIVITY
Not restricted unless associated with specific disease; (e.g., brachycephalic animals may need to limit exercise, especially in high ambient temperatures)

DIET
Caloric restriction for obese animals with airway compromise

CLIENT EDUCATION
None unless associated with specific disease

SURGICAL CONSIDERATIONS
None unless associated with specific disease

MEDICATIONS

DRUG(S) OF CHOICE
• Generally no therapy indicated; this is a normal rhythm.
• Infectious respiratory diseases require appropriate antibiotic therapy.
• If associated with symptomatic sinus bradycardia or sinus arrest or block, anticholinergics may be indicated—atropine (0.04 mg/kg IM, SC) or glycopyrrolate (0.01 mg/kg IM, SC)

CONTRAINDICATIONS
Stop administering digoxin if toxicity is a problem.

PRECAUTIONS
Avoid atropine in patients with respiratory disease; it dehydrates respiratory secretions.

POSSIBLE INTERACTIONS
N/A

ALTERNATIVE DRUG(S)
N/A

FOLLOW-UP

PATIENT MONITORING
Only if associated with specific disease

PREVENTION/AVOIDANCE
N/A

POSSIBLE COMPLICATIONS
N/A

EXPECTED COURSE AND PROGNOSIS
N/A

MISCELLANEOUS

ASSOCIATED CONDITIONS
• SSS
• Brachycephalic airway syndrome
• Asthma
• Chronic obstructive pulmonary disease

AGE-RELATED FACTORS
Generally more pronounced in young adult

ZOONOTIC POTENTIAL
N/A

PREGNANCY
Increased incidence of arrhythmias

SYNONYMS
• Respiratory SA = phasic SA
• Nonrespiratory SA = nonphasic SA; sinus irregularity
• Ventriculophasic SA—form of nonphasic SA in which atrial cycles containing ventricular complexes are shorter than those in which they are absent (ex: advanced AV block)

SEE ALSO
• Brachycephalic Airway Syndrome
• Sick Sinus Syndrome
• Sinus Arrest and Block

ABBREVIATIONS
• AV = atrioventricular
• ECG = electrocardiogram
• SA = sinus arrhythmia
• SSS = sick sinus syndrome

Suggested Reading

Braunwald E, ed. Heart disease. 5th ed. Philadelphia: Saunders, 1997.
Chung EK. Manual of cardiac arrhythmias. 1st ed. New York: Yorke Medical Books, 1986.
Tilley LP, ed. Essentials of canine and feline electrocardiography. 3rd ed. Baltimore: Williams & Wilkins, 1992.
Tilley LP, Goodwin J. eds. Manual of canine and feline cardiology. 3rd ed. Philadelphia: Saunders, 2000.
Author Deborah J. Hadlock
Consulting Editors Larry P. Tilley and Francis W. K. Smith, Jr.

SINUS BRADYCARDIA

 BASICS

DEFINITION
Sinus rhythm in which impulses arise from the sinoatrial node at slower-than-normal rate

ECG Features
• Dogs—sinus rate < 70 bpm (< 60 bpm in giant breeds) • Cats—sinus rate < 120 bpm at home or < 150 bpm at the clinic • Rhythm regular, often with a slight variation in R-R interval; may be irregular if bradycardia due to high vagal tone; often coexists with sinus arrhythmia • Normal P wave for each QRS complex • P-R interval constant

PATHOPHYSIOLOGY
• May represent normal physiologic response to athletic training; may result from enhanced cardiac parasympathetic tone or decreased sympathetic tone as well as from intrinsic changes in the sinus node; changes in sinoatrial nodal discharge frequency are usually produced by the cardiac autonomic nerves • May represent pathophysiologic response due to high vagal tone, change in blood pH, PCO_2, PO_2, or serum electrolyte derangements

SYSTEMS AFFECTED
Cardiovascular—most instances benign arrhythmia and may be beneficial by producing a longer period of diastole and increased ventricular filling time; can be associated with syncope if due to abnormal reflex (neurocardiogenic) or intrinsic disease of sinus node

GENETICS
Female miniature schnauzers predisposed to SSS, which may cause bradycardia

INCIDENCE/PREVALENCE
Common in the dog, less common in cats

SIGNALMENT

Species
Dogs and cats

Breed Predilections
Bradycardia associated with SSS: miniature schnauzers, cocker spaniels, dachshunds, pugs, and West Highland white terriers

Mean Age and Range
• Decreased prevalence with advancing age unless associated with intrinsic disease of SA node • SSS typically seen in geriatric patients

Predominant Sex
With SSS, older females

SIGNS

General Comments
Importance depends on cause. • May be insignificant or serious, depending upon signs and underlying cause

Historical Findings
• May be none • Lethargy • Exercise intolerance • Syncope • Episodic ataxia • Seizures

Physical Examination Findings
• Pulse rate slow • Hypothermia may be present.

CAUSES

Physiologic
• Athletic conditioning • Hypothermia • Intubation • Sleep

Pathophysiologic
High vagal tone associated with gastrointestinal, respiratory, neurologic, and pharyngeal diseases

Pathologic
• High intracranial pressure • Hyperkalemia • Hypercalcemia • Hypocalcemia • Hypermagnesemia • Hypoxemia • Hypothyroidism • May precede cardiac arrest • SSS • Feline dilated cardiomyopathy • Sinoatrial block • Neurocardiogenic • Vasovagal • Carotid sinus hyperactivity • Situational (micturition, defecation, cough, swallowing)

Pharmacologic
• General anesthesia • Phenothiazines • β-Blockers • Digitalis • Calcium channel blockers • Xylazine

RISK FACTORS
• Any situation or disease that may increase parasympathetic tone • Oversedation • Hypoventilation under anesthesia

 DIAGNOSIS

DIFFERENTIAL DIAGNOSIS
• Persistent and marked SB should raise possibility of SSS • Clinical signs may mimic cerebral dysfunction.

CBC/BIOCHEMISTRY/URINALYSIS
• Hyperkalemia, hypercalcemia, hypocalcemia, or hypermagnesemia possible • CBC and serum chemistry profile may reveal changes associated with metabolic disease such as renal failure.

OTHER LABORATORY TESTS
• Serum T_4 and T_3, free T_4 (FT_4), and TSH assay if hypothyroidism suspected • Measure serum digoxin concentration, if applicable, 6–8 hr after last dose; normal therapeutic serum concentration should be 0.8–1.5 ng/mL.

IMAGING
Survey radiographs and ultrasound may reveal evidence of cardiac, renal, or other organ abnormalities.

DIAGNOSTIC PROCEDURES
• Provocative atropine response test to assess sinus node function—administer atropine 0.04 mg/kg IM; follow-up ECG 30 min post–atropine administration; lower doses of atropine have increased tendency to cause initial accentuation of sinus bradycardia and first- or second-degree AV block because of centrally mediated increase in vagal tone. • 24-hr Holter monitoring or ECG event recorder useful if transient bradyarrhythmia is suspected cause for clinical signs

PATHOLOGIC FINDINGS
Depends on primary disease, if any

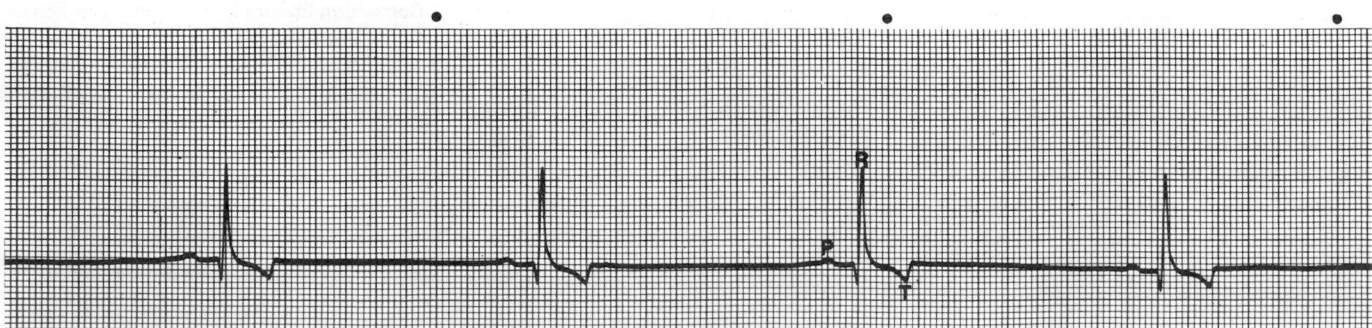

Figure 1.

Sinus bradycardia at a rate of 75 beats/min in a cat during anesthetic complications during surgery. (From: Tilley LP: Essentials of canine and feline electrocardiography, 3rd ed. Baltimore: Williams & Wilkins, 1992, w/permission.)

TREATMENT

APPROPRIATE HEALTH CARE

• Many animals exhibit no clinical signs and require no treatment. In dogs without structural heart disease, heart rates as low as 40–50 bpm generally provide normal cardiac output at rest. • Therapeutic approaches—vary markedly; depend on the mechanism for SB, the ventricular rate, and severity of clinical signs • Inpatient or outpatient management—depends on underlying cause and clinical status of patient

NURSING CARE

• Provide general supportive therapy including intravenous fluid therapy for hypothermic and hypovolemic patients.
• Discontinue any causative drug.
• Correct any serious electrolyte imbalance with appropriate fluid therapy.

ACTIVITY

No restrictions unless patient has symptomatic SB related to structural heart disease; then exercise restriction recommended until medical and/or surgical intervention

DIET

Special considerations may be indicated if cause is associated with electrolyte imbalance secondary to renal disease

CLIENT EDUCATION

• Discuss importance of complying with daily medical management when treating underlying disease. • Advise that persistent symptomatic bradycardia may necessitate permanent pacemaker implantation for reliable long-term management.

SURGICAL CONSIDERATIONS

• If progressive bradycardia occurs during anesthesia and is attributed to hypoventilation, immediately discontinue inhalation anesthetics and provide adequate ventilation; atropine is generally ineffective in this situation. • If surgical manipulation triggering vagal reflexes (eye, vagus nerve, larynx) is anticipated, pretreatment with atropine (0.04 mg/kg IM, SC) or glycopyrrolate (0.005–0.01 mg/kg IM, SC) may prevent bradycardia. • Severe bradycardia may precipitate cardiopulmonary arrest; identify the causative agent or condition for effective management.

MEDICATIONS

DRUG(S) OF CHOICE

• If patient is hypothyroid, supplement with L-thyroxine

• For severe hypocalcemia (< 6 mg/dL) administer 10% calcium gluconate (0.5–1.5 mL/kg IV) slowly over 15–30 min; monitor with ECG.
• For symptomatic drug-induced bradycardias, disorders causing excessive vagal tone, and initial management of bradycardia associated with SSS, administer atropine (0.02 mg/kg IV) or glycopyrrolate (0.005–0.01 mg/kg IV); anticholinergic therapy may be continued short-term using atropine (0.04 mg/kg IM, SC q6–8h) or glycopyrrolate (0.01 mg/kg IM, SC q6–8h).
• Consider propantheline bromide (0.25–0.5 mg/kg PO q8–12h) or hyoscyamine (0.003–0.006 mg/kg PO q8h), theophylline (Theo-Dur 10–20 mg/kg PO q12h, dogs; 25 mg/kg PO q24h, cats), and/or terbutaline (0.2 mg/kg PO q8h, dogs; 0.625 mg/cat PO, cats) to manage symptomatic bradycardia associated with SA node disease.
• For temporary management of symptomatic persistent bradycardia until pacing can be accomplished, consider continuous IV infusion of isoproterenol (1–2 µg/min or to effect) or dobutamine (2.5–20 µg/kg/min IV infusion, dogs; 1–5 µg/kg/min IV infusion, cats).

CONTRAINDICATIONS

Parasympatholytic agents contraindicated for acidotic, hypercarbic patients under anesthesia (hypoventilation); bradycardia in this setting may protect the myocardium by decreasing oxygen consumption.

PRECAUTIONS

• Close ECG monitoring recommended when administering calcium solutions for treatment of hypocalcemia; if QT interval shortening or bradycardia, stop administration temporarily.
• In patients with heart disease, a lower initial dose of L-thyroxine is advised to allow adaptation to higher metabolic rate.
• Administer atropine selectively; rapid IV administration may predispose to ventricular arrhythmias by altering autonomic balance.

POSSIBLE INTERACTIONS N/A

ALTERNATIVE DRUG(S)

• Bradycardia associated with structural heart disease is most reliably treated by permanent pacemaker implantation.
• Glycopyrrolate may have longer vagal blocking effect and cause less frequent ventricular ectopic beats than atropine.

FOLLOW-UP

PATIENT MONITORING

• Assess postpill serum T_4 4–6 hr after dose, 30 and 60 days after starting treatment.
• Addison's disease—assess electrolytes every 3–4 months after patient is stable.

• ECG check of pacemaker function and pacing rate is recommended during each follow-up examination.

PREVENTION/AVOIDANCE

• Maintain normal PAO_2 under anesthesia with proper ventilation; monitor with pulse oximetry or blood gases. • Avoid hypothermia intraoperatively.

POSSIBLE COMPLICATIONS

Malfunctioning pacemaker

EXPECTED COURSE AND PROGNOSIS

• Signs, if present, should resolve with correction of causative metabolic or endocrine problem • Treatment of symptomatic SB with a permanent pacemaker generally offers a good prognosis.

MISCELLANEOUS

ASSOCIATED CONDITIONS

• SSS • Heart block • Sinus arrhythmia

AGE-RELATED FACTORS N/A

ZOONOTIC POTENTIAL N/A

PREGNANCY

Postparturient hypocalcemia usually develops 1–4 weeks postpartum, but can occur at term, prepartum, or late lactation.

SYNONYMS N/A

SEE ALSO

• Digoxin Toxicity • Eclampsia
• Hypercalcemia • Hyperkalemia
• Hypermagnesemia • Hypocalcemia
• Hypothermia • Hypothyroidism
• Organophosphate and Carbamate Toxicity
• Sick Sinus Syndrome

ABBREVIATIONS

• ECG = electrocardiogram
• SA = sinoatrial
• SB = sinus bradycardia
• SSS = sick sinus syndrome
• T_4 = thyroxine
• T_3 = triiodothyronine
• TSH = thyroid stimulating hormone

Suggested Reading
Miller MS, Tilley LP, Smith FWK, Fox PR. Electrocardiography. In: Fox PR, Sisson D, Moise NS, eds. Textbook of canine and feline cardiology. Philadelphia: Saunders, 1999:67–106.
Smith FWK, Hadlock DJ. Electrocardiography. In: Miller MS, Tilley LP, eds. Manual of canine and feline cardiology. 2nd ed. Philadelphia: Saunders, 1995:47–74.
Tilley LP, ed. Essentials of canine and feline electrocardiography. 3rd ed. Baltimore: Williams & Wilkins, 1992.
Author Deborah J. Hadlock
Consulting Editors Larry P. Tilley and Francis W. K. Smith, Jr.

SINUS TACHYCARDIA

 BASICS

DEFINITION
Disturbance of sinus impulse formation; acceleration of the sinoatrial node beyond its normal discharge rate. (Figure 1)

ECG Features
• Dogs—HR > 160 bpm (toy breeds HR > 180 bpm; giant breeds HR > 140 bpm; puppies HR > 220 bpm) • Cats—HR > 240 bpm • ECG shows a regular rhythm with possible slight variation in R-R interval • Normal P wave (may be peaked) for each QRS complex with constant P-R interval • P waves may be partially or completely fused with preceding T waves. • Generally has a gradual onset and termination

PATHOPHYSIOLOGY
• Accelerated phase 4 diastolic depolarization of sinus nodal cells generally responsible for ST • Enhanced adrenergic effect or cholinergic inhibition results in high rate of sinus impulse formation; changes in heart rate usually involve a reciprocal action of the parasympathetic and sympathetic divisions of the autonomic nervous system.

SYSTEMS AFFECTED
Cardiovascular—cardiac output = heart rate × stroke volume. Changes in heart rate affect preload, afterload, and contractility, which determine stroke volume; severe tachycardia can compromise cardiac output. Rapid rates shorten diastolic filling time, and particularly in diseased hearts, the increased heart rate can fail to compensate for decreased stroke volume, resulting in decreased cardiac output and coronary blood flow. Chronic tachycardias can cause cardiac dilation.

GENETICS
N/A

INCIDENCE/PREVALENCE
• Most common benign arrhythmia in the dog and cat • Most common rhythm disturbance in the postoperative patient

GEOGRAPHIC DISTRIBUTION
N/A

SIGNALMENT
Species
Dogs and cats
Breed Predilections
N/A
Mean Age and Range
N/A
Predominant Sex
N/A

SIGNS
General Comments
Often no clinical signs because condition is a natural response to a variety of physiologic or pathophysiologic stresses

Historical Findings
Clinical signs, if present, most often referable to something other than the arrhythmia, occurring as a result of some other disease process. If associated with primary cardiac disease, weakness, exercise intolerance, or syncope may be reported

Physical Examination Findings
• High HR • May otherwise be normal if not associated with a pathologic condition • Pale mucous membranes if associated with anemia or CHF • Fever may be present. • Signs of CHF (e.g., dyspnea, cough, cyanosis, ascites) when ST is associated with primary cardiac disease

CAUSES
Physiologic
• Exercise • Pain • Restraint • Excitement
Pathologic
• Fever • CHF • Hyperthyroidism • Shock • Anemia • Infection • Hypoxia • Pulmonary thromboembolism • Hypotension • Hypovolemia • Functional pheochromocytoma
Pharmacologic
• Atropine
• Epinephrine
• Ketamine
• Quinidine
• Xanthine bronchodilators
• β-Agonists
• Light anesthesia

RISK FACTORS
• Thyroid medications
• Primary cardiac diseases
• Inflammation
• Pregnancy

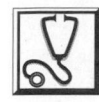 DIAGNOSIS

DIFFERENTIAL DIAGNOSIS
Must differentiate from atrial tachycardia, atrial flutter with 2:1 AV block, and AV junctional tachycardia; as sinus rate increases, the P wave appears closer to the T wave of the previous beat, and at very rapid rates, it becomes difficult to distinguish this condition from other pathologic SVT.

CBC/BIOCHEMISTRY/URINALYSIS
• Low PCV if patient is anemic
• Leukocytosis with left shift if inflammation or infection is causative

OTHER LABORATORY TESTS
• High serum T_4 or free T_4 concentration (cats) if secondary to hyperthyroidism
• T_3 suppression test or TRH response test if T_4 values are normal and hyperthyroidism is suspected
• 24-hr urine sample collection for catecholamine assay and their metabolites in diagnosis of pheochromocytoma; provocative testing to induce hypertension with histamine and glucagon or hypotension with phentolamine may be useful but is not practical.

IMAGING
• Thoracic radiographs to evaluate for evidence of primary cardiac disease
• Echocardiogram to evaluate for any structural cardiac disease
• Thyroid scan to evaluate for hyperthyroidism
• Abdominal ultrasound and angiography to evaluate for adrenal mass

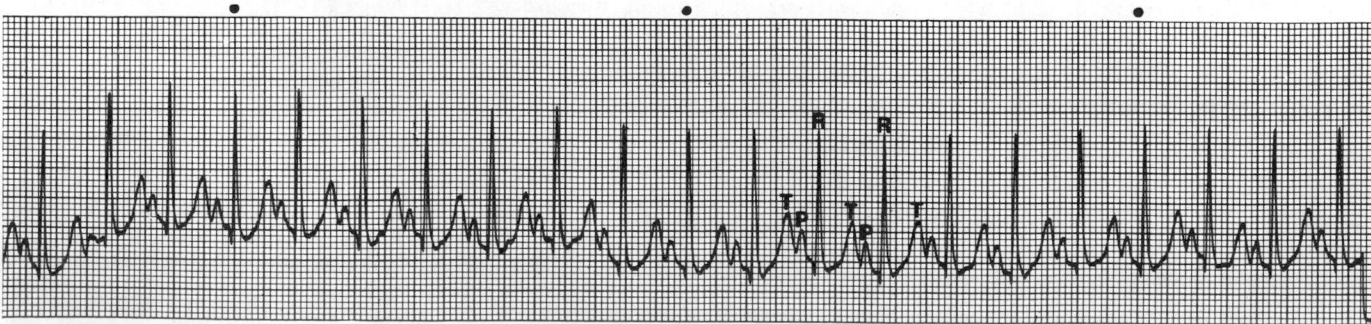

Figure 1.

Sinus tachycardia at a rate of 272/min in a dog in shock. The rhythm is sinus because the P waves are normal, the P-R relationship is normal, and the rhythm is regular. (From: Tilley LP: Essentials of canine and feline electrocardiography. 3rd ed. Baltimore: Williams & Wilkins, 1992, with permission.)

• CT and MRI very sensitive for detecting adrenal masses

DIAGNOSTIC PROCEDURES
• Consider nonpharmacologic vagal maneuver to differentiate from other supraventricular tachyarrhythmias; carotid sinus or ocular pressure may terminate ectopic SVT. With ST, vagal maneuvers produce gradual, transient slowing of the HR if any. Less commonly, varying degrees of AV block (usually first-degree or Wenckebach) may occur transiently. ECG monitoring is recommended during these vagal maneuvers.
• A precordial thump may be used to differentiate ST from other SVT. ST will not be affected, whereas the SVT may stop for at least one or two beats.
• Serial arterial blood pressure measurement may document hypertension in patients with hyperthyroidism, pheochromocytoma, or renal disease.

PATHOLOGIC FINDINGS
• None if associated with physiologic or pharmacologic cause
• Pathologic findings depend on the primary disease process.

 TREATMENT

APPROPRIATE HEALTH CARE
• Identify and correct underlying cause whenever possible
• Whether inpatient or outpatient depends on clinical status of patient and primary disease, if any (e.g., if CHF, treat as outpatient unless animal is dyspneic or severely hypotensive).

NURSING CARE
Depends on whether associated with a specific disease

ACTIVITY
Exercise restriction recommended if symptomatic cardiac disease

DIET
Sodium restriction generally advised in hypertension and CHF

CLIENT EDUCATION
Discuss importance of managing any primary disease appropriately, with medical or surgical intervention.

SURGICAL CONSIDERATIONS
• Thyroidectomy recommended for hyperthyroidism (cats)
• Tumor removal is the definitive treatment for patients with pheochromocytoma.

 MEDICATIONS

DRUG(S) OF CHOICE
• Establish underlying cause and treat appropriately; specific antiarrhythmic therapy is generally limited to patients in CHF or those with secondary cardiac disease due to hyperthyroidism or hypertension
• Dogs—if CHF is the cause, administer digoxin along with a diuretic and angiotensin-converting enzyme (ACE) inhibitor. If ST persists despite digoxin, consider adding a β-blocker (e.g., atenolol 0.25–1.0 mg/kg PO q12–24h) or calcium channel blocker (e.g., diltiazem at 0.5–1.5 mg/kg PO q8h) after congestion is con-trolled.
• Cats—if ST is associated with hyperthyroidism without CHF, a β-blocker (e.g., atenolol 6.25–12.5 mg/cat PO q24h) may lower the HR. Consider digoxin (0.0312 mg PO q24h, average-size cat, tablet preferred) if chronic hyperthyroidism with CHF or for treatment of primary dilated cardiomyopathy. If ST associated with hypertrophic cardiomyopathy, administer diltiazem (1.75–2.4 mg/kg PO q8h) or use sustained-release form of diltiazem (XR or CD 10 mg/kg PO q24h).

CONTRAINDICATIONS
Avoid drugs such as atropine or catecholamines (epinephrine) that may further increase the HR.

PRECAUTIONS
β-Blockers and calcium channel antagonists can worsen signs of congestion and lower cardiac output in patients with systolic dysfunction.

POSSIBLE INTERACTIONS
See manufacturer's insert for specific drug.

ALTERNATIVE DRUG(S)
• If associated with pericardial effusion, avoid drug therapy and perform pericardiocentesis.
• If associated with a certain drug (e.g., hydralazine, bronchodilators), discontinue the medication or adjust the dose.

 FOLLOW-UP

PATIENT MONITORING
Depends on specific disease—for CHF, serial ECG, thoracic radiographs, BUN, creatinine, and serum electrolytes; for hyperthyroidism, serial serum T_4, CBC, and biochemistry

PREVENTION AVOIDANCE
Minimize stress, exercise, and dietary sodium, if heart disease.

POSSIBLE COMPLICATIONS
• Weakness or syncope if associated with low cardiac output • Development of CHF if persistent ST associated with heart disease

EXPECTED COURSE AND PROGNOSIS
• Arrhythmia usually resolves with correction of the underlying cause. • Poor despite treatment if arrhythmia is associated with CHF • Favorable for remission of ST when hyperthyroidism is controlled medically, surgically, or by radioactive iodine

 MISCELLANEOUS

ASSOCIATED CONDITIONS
N/A

AGE-RELATED FACTORS
N/A

ZOONOTIC POTENTIAL
N/A

PREGNANCY
• Increase in cardiac output in late pregnancy (third trimester) largely due to an accelerated HR • Pregnancy of multiple fetuses in humans associated with an even higher HR; increased susceptibility to arrhythmias, including ST

SYNONYMS
N/A

SEE ALSO
• Atrial Fibrillation and Flutter • Congestive Heart Failure, Left-sided • Congestive Heart Failure, Right-sided • Hyperthyroidism • Pheochromocytoma • Supraventricular Tachycardia

ABBREVIATIONS
• AV = atrioventricular • BUN = blood urea nitrogen • CHF = congestive heart failure • CT = computed tomography • ECG = electrocardiogram • HR = heart rate • MRI = magnetic resonance imaging • ST = sinus tachycardia • SVT = supraventricular tachycardia • T_4 = thyroxine • T_3 = triiodothyronine • TRH = thyrotropin-releasing hormone

Suggested Reading
Braunwald E, ed. Heart disease. 5th ed. Philadelphia: Saunders, 1997.
Kittleson MD, Kienle RD. Small animal cardiovascular medicine. St. Louis: Mosby, 1998.
Miller MS, Tilley LP, Smith FWK, Fox PR. Electrocardiography. In: Fox PR, Sisson D, Moise NS, eds. Textbook of canine and feline cardiology. Philadelphia: Saunders, 1999:67–106.
Smith FWK, Hadlock DJ. Electrocardiography. In: Miller MS, Tilley LP, eds. Manual of canine and feline cardiology, 2nd ed. Philadelphia: Saunders, 1995:47–74.
Author Deborah J. Hadlock
Consulting Editors Larry P. Tilley and Francis W. K. Smith, Jr

SJÖGREN-LIKE SYNDROME

BASICS

OVERVIEW
• A systemic autoimmune disease characterized by keratoconjunctivitis sicca, xerostomia, and lymphoplasmacytic adenitis
• Underlying mechanism unknown; however, autoantibodies directed against glandular tissues have been identified.
• Associated with other autoimmune or immune-mediated diseases, such as rheumatoid arthritis and pemphigus

SIGNALMENT
• Higher incidence in several canine breeds—English bulldogs, West Highland white terriers, and miniature schnauzers
• Chronic disease of adult dogs
• Cats unaffected

SIGNS

Historical Findings
• Adult onset
• Conjunctivitis and keratitis
• Keratitis sicca most prominent clinical feature

Physical Examination Findings
• Blepharospasm
• Conjunctival hyperemia
• Corneal lesions (opacity to ulceration)
• Gingivitis
• Stomatitis

CAUSES & RISK FACTORS
• Possible genetic predisposition in breeds with high incidence
• Develops concurrently with other immune-mediated and autoimmune diseases

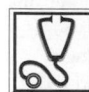

DIAGNOSIS

DIFFERENTIAL DIAGNOSIS
• Other causes of keratoconjunctivitis sicca—canine distemper, trauma, and drug toxicities
• Keratoconjunctivitis sicca associated with other immune-mediated diseases—atopy, lymphocytic thyroiditis, polymyositis, systemic lupus erythematosus, rheumatoid arthritis, and pemphigoid diseases

CBC/BIOCHEMISTRY/URINALYSIS
Normal

OTHER LABORATORY TESTS
• Hypergammaglobulinemia revealed by serum protein electrophoresis
• Positive antinuclear antibody test
• Positive lupus erythematosus cell test
• Positive rheumatoid factor test
• Positive indirect fluorescent antibody test for autoantibodies

IMAGING
N/A

DIAGNOSTIC PROCEDURES
Schirmer tear test (0–5 mm/min)

PATHOLOGIC FINDINGS
• Histopathologic changes in salivary glands—lymphoplasmacytic adenitis
• Conjunctival biopsy—reveals conjunctivitis

TREATMENT
• Directed at controlling keratoconjunctivitis sicca
• Any concurrent disease must be medically managed
• May include administration of anti-inflammatory or immunosuppressive drugs
• Surgical management of keratoconjunctivitis sicca indicated in animals that fail to respond to medical treatment

MEDICATIONS
DRUG(S)
• Topical tear preparations
• Appropriate topical antibiotics for secondary bacterial infection
• Immunosuppressive or anti-inflammatory drugs
• For more aggressive medical treatment and surgical intervention, see Keratoconjunctivitis Sicca.

CONTRAINDICATIONS/POSSIBLE INTERACTIONS
Use of topical steroids in patients with acute keratoconjunctivitis sicca may cause corneal ulceration and is, therefore, not recommended.

FOLLOW-UP
• Re-examine patients weekly until keratoconjunctivitis sicca controlled
• Additional monitoring may be indicated to manage underlying or concurrent disease.
• Immunosuppressive drugs—monitor patients every other week for possible side effects.
• Prognosis variable and depends on existence of concurrent disease

MISCELLANEOUS
SEE ALSO
Keratoconjunctivitis Sicca

Suggested Reading
Quimby FW, Schwartz RS, Poskitt T, et al. A disorder of dogs resembling Sjögren's syndrome. Clin Immunol Immunopathol 1979;12:471–476.
Author Paul W. Snyder
Consulting Editor Stephen A. Kruth

SMALL INTESTINAL BACTERIAL OVERGROWTH

BASICS

DEFINITION
• A clinical syndrome caused by an increase in number or shift in species of microorganisms that make up the small intestinal microflora. • Usually multiple species are present; the species may change with time. • Small intestinal bacterial overgrowth (SIBO) in dogs has previously been defined as $>10^4$ anaerobic and/or $>10^5$ total bacterial colony–forming units (cfu)/mL of fasting duodenal juice; these criteria are now controversial in dogs. • Currently, there is no consensus on the definition and diagnostic criteria for SIBO. Bacterial counts reported in clinically healthy dogs range from 0 to $>10^9$ cfu/mL for aerobic bacteria and from 0 to $>10^8$ cfu/mL for anaerobic bacteria in clinically healthy dogs. • SIBO differs from colonization of the alimentary tract by known pathogenic bacteria with virulence factors (e.g., *Salmonella* spp., *Campylobacter jejuni*, etc.) or overgrowth of toxigenic *Clostridium perfringens* in the colon.

PATHOPHYSIOLOGY
• Bacteria are constantly ingested with food and/or saliva. • Most are destroyed by gastric acid or antibacterial factors in the small intestine. • Bacteria that survive are eliminated from the small intestine by normal intestinal motility. • The ileocolic valve is a physiological barrier between the highly populated colon and less populated small intestine. • When these natural defenses fail and excessive bacteria persist in the upper small intestine, they may cause pathology even though they are not obligate pathogens. • Reported pathophysiologic mechanisms include deconjugation of bile acids (may lead to fat malabsorption); dehydroxylation of fatty acids (may lead to diarrhea); destruction of brush border enzymes, damage of carrier proteins, and competition for nutrients (e.g., cobalamin) may lead to malabsorption of carbohydrates and malnutrition. SIBO can lead to sufficient mucosal damage to cause protein-losing enteropathy. • Anaerobic bacteria (e.g., *Bacteroides* spp. and *Clostridium* spp.) have been considered to more likely cause pathology than many aerobic bacteria. • It has also been hypothesized that an abnormal host response (e.g., loss of tolerance) to a normal intestinal microflora may lead to SIBO.

SYSTEMS AFFECTED
• Gastrointestinal—normal absorptive function is disrupted, resulting in weight loss with or without diarrhea or vomiting. • Hepatobiliary—the portal vein carries bacterial toxins and other substances from the small intestine into the liver (may or may not be significant).

GENETICS
• No genetic basis has been established. • Some breeds (German shepherds, shar peis) appear to be at increased risk. • Decreased IgA concentrations have been associated with SIBO. • A genetic susceptibility for a dysregulation in cell mediated immune response to a normal luminal microflora is suspected to occur in human beings—similar mechanisms may lead to enteropathies in dogs (not proven).

INCIDENCE/PREVALENCE
Unknown

GEOGRAPHIC DISTRIBUTION N/A

SIGNALMENT

Species
• Dogs • Cats—unknown; clinically healthy cats can have $>10^8$ cfu/mL in duodenal juice.

Breed Predilections
Subjectively, German shepherds and shar peis have an increased incidence.

Mean Age and Range
• Unknown • Identified in dogs <1 year of age and >8 years of age

Predominant Sex
N/A

SIGNS

General Comments
Can cause signs of small intestinal disease

Historical Findings
• Weight loss possible despite a reasonable appetite—principal sign • Chronic diarrhea—common • Vomiting and borborygmus—occasional/variable • Clinical signs of underlying disease in secondary SIBO may be present • May wax and wane or be continuous

Physical Examination Findings
• Weight loss and poor body condition • May have evidence of diarrhea. • Intestinal thickening is unexpected unless other infiltrative intestinal disease is also present. • Signs typical of infection (e.g., fever, depression) are unexpected.

CAUSES

Idiopathic or Primary SIBO

Secondary SIBO (more common)
• Altered small intestinal anatomy—inherited or acquired (e.g., congenital blind loop, partial obstructions, neoplasia, foreign body, intussusception, stricture, adhesion, and diverticulum) • Decreased intestinal motility (e.g., hypothyroidism, autonomic neuropathies) • Exocrine pancreatic insufficiency (EPI)—approximately 70% of dogs with EPI have concurrent SIBO. • Hypochlorhydria or achlorhydria—spontaneous or iatrogenic (e.g., H_2-blocker) • Immunodeficiency, decreased mucosal defense, and preexisting intestinal disease

RISK FACTORS
• IgA deficiency—suspected • Intestinal disease (e.g., inflammatory bowel disease [IBD], adverse food reactions, parasite infestation) that affects local defense mechanisms

DIAGNOSIS

DIFFERENTIAL DIAGNOSIS
• Maldigestion—EPI • Malabsorption • Intestinal parasites (especially *Giardia*)

CBC/BIOCHEMISTRY/URINALYSIS
• Usually normal • Hypoalbuminemia—rare; when present, it suggests particularly severe intestinal disease and warrants an aggressive diagnostic and therapeutic approach

OTHER LABORATORY TESTS

Serum Cobalamin and Folate
• Serum folate may be increased (folate-producing bacteria) and cobalamin may be decreased (many bacterial species compete for cobalamin). • High specificity, low sensitivity—if both altered then highly suggestive. Some dogs with symptomatic SIBO have normal serum cobalamin and folate concentrations.

Breath Hydrogen Analysis
• Mammalian cells cannot synthesize hydrogen but bacteria can. Thus an early peak in hydrogen in the expiratory air reflects microbial activity in the small intestine. • Not routinely available • Some false-negative and false-positive results occur.

Unconjugated Serum Bile Acids (SUBA)
• The increased bacterial flora leads to deconjugation of bile acids in the small intestine. • Under investigation; appears to have low sensitivity and specificity.

IMAGING
N/A—may reveal findings indicative of an underlying cause, such as an intestinal mass or partial obstruction.

DIAGNOSTIC PROCEDURES

Qualitative and Quantitative Bacterial Culture
• Aerobic and anaerobic bacteria from fasted, upper intestinal fluid has been considered the "gold standard." • Invasive—requires endoscopy or laparoscopy. • Recent work would suggest that the criterion of $>10^4$ anaerobic and/or $>10^5$ total bacterial cfu/mL of intestinal fluid may be too low, leading to false-positive results. • No standardized protocols are established for sampling, handling, and culturing of duodenal juice leading to high variability in bacterial counts.

Therapeutic Trials
• Treat for SIBO and observe the results. • Simple and inexpensive • Main difficulty—interpreting the results; more than one disease

(e.g., IBD plus SIBO, dietary intolerance plus SIBO) may be present, and lack of clinical response to antibiotics might lead to incorrect conclusion that SIBO is absent; incorrect antibiotic selection might also cause failure of clinical response.

PATHOLOGIC FINDINGS
• No evidence seen at surgery or endoscopy
• Histopathology and cytology of small intestinal mucosa—typically unremarkable

TREATMENT

APPROPRIATE HEALTH CARE
• Outpatient medical management
• Results/improvement may take a few days to several weeks.

NURSING CARE
• Usually none
• Supportive care for emaciated or hypoalbuminemic patients is rarely needed.

ACTIVITY
Unrestricted

DIET
• Highly digestible, restricted in fat
• Antigen-restricted diets recommended if a concurrent adverse food reaction is suspected
• Diet containing fructo-oligosaccharides is the only diet that has been shown to be beneficial in some patients

CLIENT EDUCATION
• Some patients show clinical improvement in days—the diarrhea stops.
• Some patients require weeks of therapy before demonstrating improvement—treat for at least 2–3 weeks before concluding that therapy is ineffective.
• Any concurrent or predisposing diseases (e.g., IBD, EPI, dietary intolerance/allergy, alimentary tract neoplasia, partial obstruction) must also be treated.
• Continual or repeated treatment is often required; rarely permanent resolution with one course of therapy.

SURGICAL CONSIDERATIONS
Indicated for some primary causes of SIBO (i.e., partial obstruction, diverticulum, or intestinal mass).

MEDICATIONS

DRUG(S) OF CHOICE
• Broad-spectrum, orally administered antibiotics effective against both aerobic and anaerobic bacteria are preferred.
• Tylosin (15 mg/kg PO q12h)—primary choice in the US; usually a powder (designed to be used in poultry); administered in the

food; can be used long-term; very safe and inexpensive; for small dogs the drug should be reformulated; in larger dogs the dose can be approximated by administering the drug in food.
• Oxytetracycline (20 mg/kg PO q8h) is secreted in bile and undergoes enterohepatic circulation—limited availability in the US; do not administer with food (calcium in the diet chelates oxytetracycline and renders it ineffective).
• Metronidazole (10–20 mg/kg PO q8h)—used to treat SIBO because of its activity against anaerobic bacteria; may also have immunomodulatory effects; possibly useful in treating IBD.
• Dogs with SIBO may be cobalamin deficient, and parenteral supplementation of vitamin B_{12} is indicated (dogs 5–15 kg: 500 µg vitamin B_{12}; dogs > 15 kg: up to 1000 µg vitamin B_{12}; dose regimen is typically one dose weekly for six weeks, one dose every two weeks for six weeks, one dose a month later; serum cobalamin and folate concentrations should be reevaluated a month after the last dose.

CONTRAINDICATIONS N/A

PRECAUTIONS
• Must use oxytetracycline carefully in patients with significant hepatic disease.
• Avoid oxytetracyclines in very young patients.
• Renal disease can occur with high doses of oxytetracyclines.
• Oxytetracycline may cause fever, abdominal pain, hair loss, and depression in cats.

POSSIBLE INTERACTIONS N/A

ALTERNATIVE DRUG(S)
Dogs with EPI plus SIBO—concurrent therapy for SIBO is indicated only if enzyme replacement alone does not resolve the diarrhea and/or lead to weight gain.

FOLLOW-UP

PATIENT MONITORING
• Body weight and (in hypoproteinemic patients) serum albumin concentration—most important parameters; improvement suggests effective therapy.
• Diarrhea should also resolve.
• If diarrhea persists despite improved body weight and/or increased serum albumin concentration, investigation for concurrent intestinal disease is indicated.

PREVENTION/AVOIDANCE N/A

POSSIBLE COMPLICATIONS
Although unproven, SIBO may predispose to IBD in some dogs.

EXPECTED COURSE AND PROGNOSIS
Primary SIBO without complicating factors (e.g., IBD, lymphoma)—prognosis with appropriate antimicrobial therapy is usually good.

MISCELLANEOUS

ASSOCIATED CONDITIONS
• SIBO has been suspected as a cause of IBD in some patients. • Consider the possibility of concurrent EPI.

AGE-RELATED FACTORS N/A

ZOONOTIC POTENTIAL N/A

PREGNANCY
Avoid oxytetracycline and metronidazole, especially during early pregnancy.

SYNONYMS N/A

SEE ALSO
• Diarrhea, Chronic—Cats • Diarrhea, Chronic—Dogs • Exocrine Pancreatic Insufficiency • Giardiasis • Inflammatory Bowel Disease • Lymphosarcoma—Cats • Lymphosarcoma—Dogs

ABBREVIATIONS
• cfu = colony-forming units
• EPI = exocrine pancreatic insufficiency
• IBD = inflammatory bowel disease
• SIBO = small intestinal bacterial overgrowth

Suggested Reading

German AJ, Day MJ, Ruaux CG, Steiner JM, Williams DA. Comparison of direct and indirect tests for small intestinal bacterial overgrowth and antibiotic-responsive diarrhea in dogs. J Vet Intern Med 2003; 17(1):33–43.

Johnston KL. Small intestinal bacterial overgrowth. Vet Clin North Am Small Anim Pract 1999;29(2):523–550.

Rutgers HC, Batt RM, Elwood CM, Lamport A. Small intestinal bacterial overgrowth in dogs with chronic intestinal disease. J Am Vet Med Assoc 1995;206(2):187–193.

Willard MD, Simpson RB, Fossum TW, et al. Characterization of naturally developing small intestinal bacterial overgrowth in 16 German shepherd dogs. J Am Vet Med Assoc 1994;204(8):1201–1206.

Acknowledgment

The authors and editors acknowledge the prior contributions of Dr. Michael D. Willard, who authored this topic in the previous edition.
Authors Jan S. Suchodolski and Jörg M. Steiner
Consulting Editor Albert E. Jergens

SMOKE INHALATION

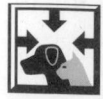

BASICS

OVERVIEW
- Injury occurs as a result of direct heat damage to the upper airway and nasal mucosa; inhalation of carbon monoxide, which decreases tissue oxygen delivery by preferentially binding to hemoglobin; inhalation of other toxins (e.g., oxidants and aldehydes) that directly irritate the airway, and inhalation of particulate matter that adheres to the airways and alveoli.
- Extent of damage depends on the degree and duration of exposure and the material that was burning.
- Dogs and cats may have serious lung injury with little cutaneous or oral evidence of burning.
- Lung reaction—initially bronchoconstriction, airway edema, and mucus production; then an inflammatory response, necrotizing tracheobronchitis, and pulmonary fluid accumulation owing to increased capillary permeability
- Superimposed bacterial infections—common cause of morbidity late in the disease; most patients show progression of lung dysfunction in the initial 2–3 days after exposure.

SIGNALMENT
Dogs and cats

SIGNS
- Historical findings consistent with exposure
- Patient may have a smoky odor.
- Tachypnea and increased depth of respiration
- Inspiratory effort that suggests upper airway obstruction by edema
- Postural adaptations to respiratory distress
- Mucous membranes may be cherry red (owing to carbon monoxyhemoglobin) pale, or cyanotic.
- Auscultation of wheezes, harsh bronchovesicular sounds, or crackles
- Cough

CAUSES & RISK FACTORS
Exposure to smoke, usually because of being trapped in a burning building

DIAGNOSIS

DIFFERENTIAL DIAGNOSIS
N/A

CBC/BIOCHEMISTRY/URINALYSIS
- Neutropenia—poor prognostic sign; indicates neutrophil sequestration in the lungs
- Thrombocytopenia—may suggest platelet sequestration or consumption
- Serum chemistry profile—may reveal hypoxic damage to other organ systems (e.g., kidneys or liver)
- Urinalysis—usually normal

OTHER LABORATORY TESTS
N/A

IMAGING
Thoracic radiographs—always take to establish a baseline; findings vary from normal to a bronchointerstitial or alveolar pattern; cranioventral alveolar infiltrates suggest aspiration pneumonia.

DIAGNOSTIC PROCEDURES
- Cytologic examination and culture of a transtracheal wash specimen—perform for suspected superimposed bacterial tracheobronchitis or pneumonia; results usually reveal an acute suppurative reaction with excessive mucus, neutrophils, and alveolar macrophages; bacteria may be seen, but the absence of obvious bacteria does not rule out a bacterial infection.
- Pulse oximetry or arterial blood gas analysis—may confirm hypoxemia; of less value for determining tissue oxygen delivery when carbon monoxyhemoglobin occurs
- Bronchoscopy—may demonstrate the severity of airway damage; bronchoalveolar lavage allows collection of appropriate samples for cytologic examination or culture.

TREATMENT
- Initial management—stabilization of respiratory function; establishment of a patent airway; severe upper airway edema or obstruction may require intubation or tracheostomy.
- Oxygen—administer immediately after rescue from the fire to displace carbon monoxide from hemoglobin; use the highest available concentration for at least 2–4 hours (longer in more severely affected patients) deliver by mask, hood, cage, or nasal line; after elimination of carbon monoxyhemoglobin, continue supplementation at 40%–60% as needed.
- Fluid administration—may be required with shock to support cardiovascular function but should be conservative, if possible, to minimize pulmonary edema; use synthetic colloids (e.g., hetastarch) with hypoproteinemia; high requirements with extensive dermal burns (usually considerable loss of fluid and protein from the skin surface)
- Blood or plasma transfusions—may be necessary
- Nebulization of saline—facilitates clearance of respiratory secretions
- Coupage and physical therapy—facilitate clearance of respiratory secretions
- Nutritional support—if needed to maintain body condition and immune status

MEDICATIONS

DRUG(S)
- Suspected bacterial infection—consider broad-spectrum antibiotics after appropriate specimens for bacterial culture have been obtained.

- Severe edema—may try diuretics (e.g., furosemide at 0.5–2 mg/kg IV, IM), but usually of little benefit; single early dose of corticosteroids may decrease airway edema.

CONTRAINDICATIONS/POSSIBLE INTERACTIONS
- Diuretics—may decrease the intravascular volume without a major beneficial effect on airway function or pulmonary edema
- Corticosteroids—use only if absolutely necessary; may predispose the patient to bacterial infection

FOLLOW-UP

PATIENT MONITORING
- Carefully monitor respiratory rate and effort, mucous membrane color, heart rate and pulse quality, auscultation of the lungs, and PCV and total solids for 24–72 hours.
- Repeat radiographs in 48 hours—ensure condition is resolving; monitor for bacterial pneumonia.
- Pulse oximetry and arterial blood gas analysis—as needed to monitor the degree of hypoxemia and response to treatment

POSSIBLE COMPLICATIONS
- Bacterial tracheobronchitis or pneumonia—owing to systemic immunosuppression and reduced pulmonary defenses, including poor mucociliary clearance
- Moist productive cough, fever, and failure to improve within 48 hours—provokes suspicion of pneumonia
- Profound, generalized pulmonary inflammatory response or severe systemic inflammatory response syndrome—may develop ARDS
- Severely affected patients may develop neurologic sequelae including seizures or cerebral edema

EXPECTED COURSE AND PROGNOSIS
- Most patients deteriorate during the initial 24–48 hours after smoke exposure and then gradually improve, unless they develop bacterial pneumonia or ARDS.
- Severe burns or organ injury—associated with a poor prognosis

MISCELLANEOUS

ABBREVIATION
ARDS = acute respiratory response syndrome

Suggested Reading
Drobatz KJ, Walker L, Hendricks JC. Smoke exposure in cats: 22 cases (1986–1997). J Am Vet Med Assoc 1999;215:1312–1316.
Drobatz KJ, Walker LM, Hendricks JC. Smoke exposure in dogs: 27 cases (1988–1997). J Am Vet Med Assoc 1999;1306–1311.
Author Lesley G. King
Consulting Editor Lynelle R. Johnson

BASICS

OVERVIEW

Coral Snakes
• Two clinically important subspecies in North America—*Micrurus fulvius fulvius,* eastern coral snake (North Carolina to the north; southern Florida to the south; West of the Mississippi River) and *M. fulvius tenere,* Texas coral snake (west of Mississippi; in Arkansas, Louisiana, and Texas)
• Family Elapidae—fixed front fangs
• Color pattern—bands fully encircling the body; red, yellow, and black; distinguished from the harmless tricolored king snake by the arrangement of the bands: if yellow (caution) and red (danger) color bands touch, then stay clear; relatively small head; black snout; round pupils

Bites
• Relatively uncommon—snake's reclusive behavior and nocturnal habits
• Often occur on the lip
• Onset of clinical signs may be delayed several hours (up to 18 hr) after envenomation.
• Victims develop bulbar paralysis.
• Primary cause of death—respiratory collapse

SIGNALMENT
Dogs and cats

SIGNS
• Bulbar paralysis—affecting cranial motor nerves, respiratory tract, and skeletal muscles; acute flaccid quadriplegia
• Salivation—caused by dysphagia
• Dyspnea
• Dysphonia
• Hyporeflexive spinal reflexes

CAUSES & RISK FACTORS
Size of the snake

DIAGNOSIS

DIFFERENTIAL DIAGNOSIS
• Myasthenia gravis
• Botulism
• Polyradiculoneuritis
• Tick bite paralysis

CBC/BIOCHEMISTRY/URINALYSIS
• Hemolysis
• RBC burring
• May note high creatine kinase
• Hemoglobinuria

OTHER LABORATORY TESTS
N/A

IMAGING
N/A

DIAGNOSTIC PROCEDURES
N/A

TREATMENT
• Inpatient—hospitalized for a minimum of 48 hr
• Specific antivenin available (*M. fulvius*)—equine origin (Wyeth); cross-reactivity for both subspecies
• First aid—generally avoid; most effective measure is rapid transport to a veterinary facility for antivenin administration;
• **CAUTION:** do not wait for onset of clinical signs.
• Antivenin unavailable—provide ventilatory support for several days in a critical care facility.

MEDICATIONS

DRUG(S)
• *M. fulvius* antivenin (Wyeth)—indicated if the history includes recent coral snake interaction; evidence of puncture wounds; clinical signs consistent with coral snake envenomation; administer 1–2 vials; additional vials may be necessary (technique same as for pit viper antivenin)
• Broad-spectrum antibiotic for 7–10 days

CONTRAINDICATIONS/POSSIBLE INTERACTIONS
• Corticosteroids—not indicated
• Observe the same precautions outlined for pit viper antivenin administration (see Snake Venom Toxicity—Pit Vipers)

FOLLOW-UP
• Marked clinical signs may last 1–1.5 weeks.
• Full recovery may take months as receptors regenerate.

MISCELLANEOUS

Suggested Reading
Peterson M, Meerdink G. Venomous bites and stings. In: Kirk RW, ed., Current veterinary therapy X. Philadelphia: Saunders, 1989:177–186.
Author Michael E. Peterson
Consulting Editor Gary D. Osweiler

SNAKE VENOM TOXICOSIS—PIT VIPERS

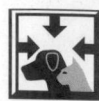

BASICS

OVERVIEW
• Pit vipers—*Crotalus* spp. (rattlesnakes), *Sistrurus* spp. (pigmy rattlesnakes and massassauga), and *Agkistrodon* spp. (copperheads and cottonmouth water moccasins); retractable fangs; heat-seeking pit between the nostril and eye; triangle-shaped head
• Range—throughout the continental U.S.
• Toxicity—considered hematoxic; several species have subpopulations with lethal neurotoxic components (e.g., Mojave rattlesnake); general ranking of severity: (1) rattlesnakes, (2) moccasins, (3) copperheads
• Venom—enzymes: hyaluronidase and phospholipase A (cause local tissue injury) and others that interfere with the coagulation cascade (cause major coagulation defects); nonenzymatic polypeptides: affect the cardiovascular and respiratory systems
• Bite—85% of victims have altered laboratory values and clinically important swelling; severe hypotension from pooling of blood within the splanchnic (dogs) or pulmonary (cats) vessels; fluid loss from the vascular compartment secondary to severe peripheral edema

SIGNALMENT
Dogs and cats

SIGNS

General Comments
May be delayed for 8 hr after envenomation

Historical Findings
• Outdoors, rural setting
• Owner saw bite or heard snake

Physical Examination Findings
• Puncture wounds on head and forelimbs in most animals
• Local tissue swelling and pain surrounding bite site
• Bruising, with possible necrosis and sloughing of bite site tissue
• Ecchymosis and petechiation of tissues and mucous membranes
• Hypotension and shock
• Tachycardia
• Shallow respiration
• Depression and lethargy
• Nausea and excessive salivation

CAUSES & RISK FACTORS

Snake-associated
• Toxic peptide fraction:enzyme fraction ratio—higher in spring; lower in fall; high in very young snakes
• Amount of venom production since last bite
• Aggressiveness and motivation of snake

Victim-associated
• Bite site—bites to tongue and torso are of major concern.
• Size of victim
• Elapsed time between bite and initiation of treatment
• Activity level of victim after the bite—activity increases absorption of venom.

DIAGNOSIS

DIFFERENTIAL DIAGNOSIS
• Angioedema secondary to insect envenomation
• Blunt trauma
• Penetrating wound
• Animal bite
• Penetration of foreign body
• Draining abscess

CBC/BIOCHEMISTRY/URINALYSIS
• Hemoconcentration
• Burring of RBCs within first 24 hr
• Thrombocytopenia
• Hypokalemia
• High creatine kinase
• Hematuria or myoglobinuria

OTHER LABORATORY TESTS
Clotting tests—may note prolonged ACT, PT, and PTT; may note high FDP

IMAGING
N/A

DIAGNOSTIC PROCEDURES
ECG—may detect ventricular arrhythmia, especially in severely depressed patients

TREATMENT
• Tissue reaction around the bite site—not a reliable indicator of systemic toxicity
• Bite location—may affect uptake of venom; bites to tongue and torso are of major concern.
• First aid measures—calming patient; transporting quickly to a veterinary facility
• Intravenous fluids—correct hypotension

MEDICATIONS

DRUG(S)
• Antivenin (Crotalidae polyvalent, equine origin)—1 vial mixed with 200 mL crystalloid fluids administered slowly IV with careful monitoring of the inner pinna for onset of hyperemia (indicator of possible allergic reaction)
• Allergic reaction—stop antivenin; give diphenhydramine; after 5 min, restart antivenin infusion at a slower rate

CONTRAINDICATIONS/POSSIBLE INTERACTIONS
• CAUTION: In animals receiving β-blockers, the onset of anaphylaxis may be masked, therefore, the condition may be more advanced once recognized and more difficult to treat effectively.
• Corticosteroids—of no value
• DMSO—enhances uptake and spread of venom
• Heparin—do not use.

FOLLOW-UP
• Repeated laboratory analysis—6 hr after admission to hospital
• Clinical signs—may last 1–1.5 weeks

MISCELLANEOUS

ABBREVIATIONS
• ACT = activated clotting time
• DMSO = dimethyl sulfoxide
• ECG = electrocardiogram
• FDP = fibrin degradation products
• PT = prothrombin time
• PTT = partial thromboplastin time

Suggested Reading
Peterson M, Meerdink G. Venomous bites and stings. In: Kirk RW, Bonagura D, eds. Current veterinary therapy X. Philadelphia: Saunders, 1989:177–186.

Author Michael E. Peterson
Consulting Editor Gary D. Osweiler

SPERMATOCELE/SPERM GRANULOMA

BASICS

OVERVIEW
• Spermatocele—a cystic distension of the efferent ductules or epididymis containing spermatozoa, usually associated with loss of patency of the duct
• Sperm granuloma—the granulomatous inflammatory reaction that develops when spermatozoa escape from the efferent ductules or epididymal duct into the surrounding tissue; clinically important when bilateral obstruction of the duct system leads to azoospermia

SIGNALMENT
Dogs and cats

SIGNS
• Suspected in azoospermic dog with normal-sized testes
• Rarely associated with pain or visible or palpable lesions

CAUSES & RISK FACTORS
• Trauma causing a break in the epididymal duct—releases sperm antigens into the surrounding tissue
• Adenomyosis—invasion of the epithelial lining cells of the epididymis into the muscular layers; may be a factor; associated with excess estrogenic stimulation
• Epithelial hyperplasia of the epididymis—may be a precursor of adenomyosis; not often seen in dogs < 2.5 years old; noted to some degree in 75% of dogs > 7.75 years old; risk increases with age.
• Complication of vasectomy—especially when surgical technique was not meticulous
• Congenital anomaly

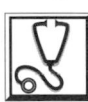

DIAGNOSIS

DIFFERENTIAL DIAGNOSIS
• Azoospermia (dogs)—testicular degeneration; hypoplasia; retrograde ejaculation; incomplete ejaculation

• Scrotal signs (e.g., pain and palpable lesions; dogs)—epididymitis; orchitis; scrotal dermatitis

CBC/BIOCHEMISTRY/URINALYSIS
• Urinalysis (cystocentesis) after ejaculation—rule out retrograde ejaculation
• CBC and biochemistry profile—usually normal

OTHER LABORATORY TESTS
• Assay for canine FSH—high concentration associated with degeneration and hypoplasia; normal concentration in azoospermic dogs with normal-sized testicles associated with bilateral blockage of the epididymis or retrograde ejaculation
• Alkaline phosphatase concentration of seminal plasma—azoospermic samples with AP < 5000 U/L consistent with bilateral epididymal blockage or incomplete ejaculation; see Infertility, Male—Dogs

IMAGING
N/A

DIAGNOSTIC PROCEDURES
Surgical testicular biopsy—allows identification of epididymis; spermatoceles appear as yellow cysts within the epididymis

PATHOLOGIC FINDINGS
Histologic examination of testicular specimen—complete spermatogenesis in an azoospermic dog indicates blockage

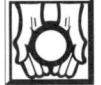

TREATMENT
• Azoospermic dogs—rarely spontaneously recover
• Bilateral blockage of the epididymis—probably not treatable except by micro-surgical anastomosis of the ductus deferens to the cystic structure or patent segment of the epididymis; few attempts have been made to perform this procedure in dogs

MEDICATIONS

DRUG(S)
None recognized as effective in unblocking the duct system.

FOLLOW-UP

EXPECTED COURSE AND PROGNOSIS
• Unilateral sperm granuloma—fair to guarded for fertility; breeding management will improve fertility; see Breeding, Timing
• Bilateral sperm granuloma—poor prognosis for fertility

MISCELLANEOUS

SEE ALSO
• Breeding, Timing
• Infertility, Male—Dogs

ABBREVIATION
FSH = follicle-stimulating hormone

Suggested Reading
Althouse GC, Evans LE, Hopkins SM. Episodic scrotal mutilation with concurrent bilateral sperm granuloma in a dog. J Am Vet Med Assoc 1993;202:776–778.
Mayenco Aguirre AM, Garcia Fernandez P, Sanchez Muela M. Sperm granuloma in the dog: complication of vasectomy. J Sm Anim Pract 1996;37:392–393.
McEntee K. Reproductive pathology of domestic animals. New York: Academic Press, 1990:309–332.
Authors Carlos R. F. Pinto and Rolf E. Larsen
Consulting Editor Sara K. Lyle

SPERMATOZOAL ABNORMALITIES

BASICS

OVERVIEW
• Teratozoospermia—presence of significant amounts of spermatozoal abnormalities; teratozoospermia is considered present if spermatozoal abnormalities are ≥ 40% in the ejaculate. • Optimal fertility is expected in dogs with at least 80% morphologically normal spermatozoa. • High percentage of spermatozoal abnormalities may cause infertility; expect a decrease in fertility in dogs with ≥ 40% of spermatozoal abnormalities in their ejaculate. • Some fertile cats inherently have ≥ 40% spermatozoal abnormalities. • Spermatozoal abnormalities are sometimes classified into primary and secondary defects; primary defects occur during spermatogenesis, and secondary defects occur during transport and storage within the epididymis.

SIGNALMENT
• Dogs and cats of any age; older dogs and cats most likely to have other age-related diseases or conditions affecting overall sperm quality. • No breed predilection for dogs or cats; Irish wolfhounds reported to have significantly lower semen quality than dogs of other breeds • English springer spaniels affected with fucosidosis • Dogs affected with primary ciliary dyskinesia—reported in many breeds; see Primary Ciliary Dyskinesia.

SIGNS
• Infertility after appropriately timed mating to several reproductively proven bitches • Spermatozoal abnormalities found during routine breeding soundness evaluation

CAUSES AND RISK FACTORS
Congenital
• Dogs with fucosidosis—lysosomal storage disease caused by a deficiency of the enzyme α-L-fucosidase; spermatogenesis (acrosomal defects) and sperm maturation (retention of proximal droplets) are impaired; English springer spaniels—autosomal recessive inheritance pattern • Primary ciliary dyskinesia—ultrastructural abnormality of cilia causing absent or abnormal motility of ciliated cells; affected animals are infertile; reported in many breeds; probably autosomal recessive inheritance • Idiopathic—dogs, cats with inherent poor sperm morphology • Testicular hypoplasia—tortoiseshell or calico tom cat

Acquired
• Conditions disrupting normal testicular thermoregulation—trauma; hematocele; hydrocele; orchitis; epididymitis; prolonged fever secondary to systemic infections; obesity (increased scrotal fat); animal not adapted to high environmental temperatures; exercise-induced heat exhaustion • Infections of the reproductive tract—prostatitis; brucellosis; orchitis; epididymitis • Drugs—anabolic steroids; androgens; estrogens; progestogens; corticosteroids; chemotherapeutic agents; ketoconazole; amphotericin B; cimetidine • Testicular neoplasia • Prolonged sexual abstinence • Overuse • Testicular degeneration

DIAGNOSIS

DIFFERENTIAL DIAGNOSIS
Excessive numbers of kinked or coiled tails may be iatrogenic artifacts caused by the stain; re-examine the sample under phase contrast microscopy after dilution with formalin phosphate—buffered saline solution.

OTHER LABORATORY TESTS
• Hormonal profile—concentrations of gonadotropin and steroid hormones in plasma or serum should be determined to rule out endocrinopathies. • Azoospermic ejaculates (absence of sperm cells)—should be examined for the presence of alkaline phosphatase to confirm azoospermia; complete ejaculates have >5,000 U/L of alkaline phosphatase. • Any dog being referred to a veterinarian because of infertility should be tested for brucellosis.

IMAGING
Ultrasonography—useful to diagnose conditions that may affect sperm morphology such as testicular tumors, orchitis, hydrocele, hematocele, spermatocele

DIAGNOSTIC PROCEDURES
• Light microscopic evaluation of dry-mount slide—eosin-nigrosin stain (Society for Theriogenology stain; Lane Manufacturing, Denver, CO) or modified Giemsa stain (Diff-Quik; Baxter Healthcare, Deerfield, IL) are used to stain spermatozoa; recommended to prepare slides on a heated slide warmer; faster drying decreases the incidence of artifacts such as kinked tails or coiled tails; a minimum of 100 (preferably 200) sperm cells are counted under 1000× magnification • Phase contrast microscopic evaluation of wet-mount slide—samples diluted with formalin phosphate-buffered saline solution; verify whether a high percentage of kinked or coiled tails seen on a stained slide is staining artifact. • Electron microscopy—determine spermatozoon ultrastructure to further evaluate sperm morphology

PATHOLOGIC FINDINGS
• Biopsy—incisional biopsy or testicular fine-needle aspirate to determine status of spermatogenesis • Absence of spermatids or spermatocytes—impaired spermatogenesis • Neoplasia • Inflammation—peritubular lymphocytic accumulation • Degenerative changes • Hypoplasia

TREATMENT
• There is no a specific treatment for spermatozoal abnormalities; if applicable, the underlying disease or condition should be treated accordingly. • Antibiotics and anti-inflammatory agents for infectious diseases • Unilateral orchiectomy for unilateral testicular tumors or severe orchitis • Sexual rest for edema or hematocele associated with trauma • Frequent semen collection may temporarily improve sperm quality in dogs or cats with idiopathic teratozoospermia. • Remove the dog or cat from environments that cause extreme heat stress. • Alter exercise program to reduce heat stress.

MEDICATIONS

DRUG(S) None

CONTRAINDICATIONS
• Exogenous hormones—anabolic steroids; estrogens; testosterone; progestogens • Glucocorticoids • Chemotherapeutic agents • Ketoconazole; amphotericin B • Cimetidine

FOLLOW-UP

PATIENT MONITORING
• If an underlying cause is identified and treated, a sperm evaluation should be performed at 30 and 60 days after the condition is resolved. • In cases due to reversible causes, a complete improvement in sperm morphology does not occur before 60 days (approximate length of a complete spermatogenic cycle).

PREVENTION/AVOIDANCE
• Climate-controlled environment for animals not adapted to high environmental temperatures • Avoid heat exhaustion during exercise or grooming.

MISCELLANEOUS

SEE ALSO
• Epididymitis/Orchitis • Infertility, Male—Dogs • Primary Ciliary Dyskinesia

Suggested Reading
Johnston SD, Kustritz MVR, Olson PNS. Clinical approach to infertility in the male dog. In: Canine and feline theriogenology. Philadelphia: Saunders, 2001:370–387.

Author Carlos R. F. Pinto
Consulting Editor Sara K. Lyle

SPIDER VENOM TOXICOSIS—BLACK WIDOW

BASICS

OVERVIEW
- Black widow spider—*Latrodectus* spp.; females toxic; 2–2.5 cm in length; shiny black; red or orange hourglass mark on the ventral abdomen; immature female brown with red to orange stripes that change into the hourglass shape as she darkens to black and ages
- Bites—may be dry (no venom injected)
- Range—genus found in every state except Alaska; often found around buildings and human habitation
- Venom—contains α-latrotoxin, a potent neurotoxin; opens cation-selective channels at the presynaptic nerve terminal; causes massive release of acetylcholine and norepinephrine, which causes sustained muscular spasms

SIGNALMENT
Dogs and cats

SIGNS

Historical Findings
- Usually sudden onset
- May be delayed several days with mild envenomation

Physical Examination Findings
Dogs
- Progressive muscle fasciculations
- Severe pain
- Cramping of large muscle masses
- Abdominal rigidity without tenderness
- Marked restlessness, writhing, and contorted spasms
- Hypertension and tachycardia anticipated
- May note bronchorrhea, hypersalivation, hyperesthesia, lymph node tenderness, regional numbness, facial swelling (*Latrodectus* facies)
- Rhabdomyolysis possible
Cats
- Early, marked paralysis
- Severe pain—manifested by howling and loud vocalizations

- Excessive salivation and restlessness
- Vomiting—not unusual to vomit up the spider
- Diarrhea
- Muscle tremors and cramping
- Ataxia and inability to stand—becomes adynamic and atonic
- Respiratory collapse
- Death without antivenin

CAUSES & RISK FACTORS
- Very young or old age—increased risk
- Systemic hypertension—increased risk

DIAGNOSIS

DIFFERENTIAL DIAGNOSIS
- Back pain from disk disease
- Acute abdomen

CBC/BIOCHEMISTRY/URINALYSIS
- Leukocytosis
- High creatine kinase—with severe muscle spasms
- Albuminuria

OTHER LABORATORY TESTS
Normal stool hemoccult test

IMAGING
Normal abdominal radiographs

DIAGNOSTIC PROCEDURES
N/A

TREATMENT
- Inpatient—supportive care
- Monitor respiratory status.

MEDICATIONS

DRUG(S)
- Antivenin (Lyovac (*Latrodectus*), equine origin)—1 vial mixed with 100 mL crystalloid solution IV given slowly with monitoring of the inner ear pinna for evidence of hyperemia (indicator of allergic response); dose usually sufficient for response within 30 min; with proper use, reactions are rare
- Allergic reaction—stop antivenin; diphenhydramine; after 5–10 min, restart antivenin at a slower rate
- Muscle spasms and severe pain are controlled by careful intravenous administration of narcotics or benzodiazepines at lowest effective dosage to avoid respiratory depression; methocarbamol (Robaxin) relieves muscle spasms but has no effect on hypertension or respiratory depression.
- Intractable hypertension—sodium nitroprusside

CONTRAINDICATIONS/POSSIBLE INTERACTIONS
Intravenous fluids with hypertension

FOLLOW-UP
- Weekly monitoring of the wound site until healed
- Prognosis—uncertain for days; cats, usually fatal without antivenin
- Weakness, fatigue, and insomnia—may persist for months

MISCELLANEOUS

Suggested Reading
Peterson ME, Meerdink G. Venomous bites and stings. In: Kirk RW, Bonagura D, eds. Current veterinary therapy X. Philadelphia: Saunders, 1989:177–186.
Author Michael E. Peterson
Consulting Editor Gary D. Osweiler

SPIDER VENOM TOXICOSIS—BROWN RECLUSE FAMILY

 BASICS

OVERVIEW
• Brown recluse family—*Loxosceles* spp.; 8–15 mm in body size; legs 2–3 cm long; violin-shaped pattern on cephalothorax with the neck of the fiddle extending caudally; active at night
• Distribution—found throughout the southern U.S. and up the Mississippi River valley to southern Wisconsin
• Bites—usually occur when spider becomes trapped in bedding; induce necrotic arachnidism, an indolent dermatonecrotic lesion mediated by the venom enzyme sphingomyelinase D, direct hemolysis of erythrocytes, platelet aggregation, renal failure, coagulopathy, and death

SIGNALMENT
Dogs and cats

SIGNS
• Local pain and stinging (may last 6–8 hr); followed by pruritus and soreness
• Classic target lesion—ischemic area with a dark central eschar on an uneven erythematous background; after 2–5 weeks, central eschar may slough, leaving a deep, nonhealing ulcer that usually spares muscle tissue.
• Less common—hemolytic anemia with hemoglobinuria in the first 24 hr
• Other possible systemic manifestations within the first 2–3 days after envenomation—fever; chills; rash; weakness; leukocytosis; nausea; arthralgia

CAUSES & RISK FACTORS
N/A

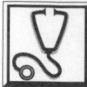 **DIAGNOSIS**

DIFFERENTIAL DIAGNOSIS
• Bacterial or mycobacterial infection
• Decubitus ulcer
• Third-degree burn
• Hemolytic anemia
• Jaundice
• Thrombocytopenia
• Ehrlichiosis
• RBC parasitism

CBC/BIOCHEMISTRY/URINALYSIS
• Anemia
• Leukocytosis
• Thrombocytopenia
• Hemoglobinuria

OTHER LABORATORY TESTS
Coagulation profile—may reveal prolonged clotting times

IMAGING
N/A

DIAGNOSTIC PROCEDURES
N/A

 TREATMENT
• Routine wound care—may need aggressive supportive care
• Supportive care—fluid therapy; presumptive treatment of bacterial superinfection; (rarely) blood transfusion
• Mild, local envenomation—usually responds to cool compresses
• Necrotic lesions—may need débridement after erythema has subsided
• Severe envenomation—may require skin grafting after the lesion reaches full maturity

 MEDICATIONS

DRUG(S)
• Antibiotics—prevent secondary infection

CONTRAINDICATIONS/ POSSIBLE INTERACTIONS
• Do not use heat—exacerbates condition
• Early surgical excision may cause larger defect than supportive care alone.
• Hyperbaric oxygen, dapsone, electric shock, and steroids have been proposed for treatments, but subsequently have been demonstrated to be ineffective.

 FOLLOW-UP
Monitor wound site weekly until healed.

 MISCELLANEOUS

ABBREVIATION
G6PD = glucose-6-phosphate dehydrogenase

Suggested Reading
Peterson ME, Meerdink G. Bites and stings of venomous animals. In: Kirk RW, ed. Current veterinary therapy X. Philadelphia: Saunders, 1989:177–186.
Author Michael E. Peterson
Consulting Editor Gary D. Osweiler

SPINAL DYSRAPHISM (HYDROSYRINGOMYELIA, MYELODYSPLASIA)

 BASICS

OVERVIEW
• Abnormal spinal cord development along the median plane leading to a variety of structural anomalies (e.g., hydromyelia, duplicated or absent central canal, syringomyelia, and aberrations in the dorsal median septum and ventral medial fissure)
• Thoracic and lumbar spinal segments most commonly affected
• The term *dysraphism* suggests an abnormality in closure of the neural tube; the term *myelodysplasia* may be preferable

SIGNALMENT
Nonprogressive
• Dogs and cats
• Weimaraners—hereditary
• Has been reported in English bulldogs, Samoyeds, Dalmatians, English setters, golden retrievers, Rottweilers
• No sex predilection
• Apparent by 3–6 weeks of age
Progressive
• Adult Cavalier King Charles Spaniels described with syringohydromyelia resulting from occipital bone malformation (Chiari I malformation)
• Adult Pomeranian described with cervical syringomyelia and hydrocephalus
• Adult fox terrier with progressive paresis in the left pelvic limb

SIGNS
• Vary in severity
• Weimaraners—simultaneous flexion and extension of pelvic limbs (bunny hopping); proprioceptive deficits, base wide stance, and crouched pelvic limb posture
• Cavalier King Charles spaniels—progressive forelimb weakness, paraparesis; paroxysmal involuntary flank or shoulder scratching; apparent neck, thoracic limb, or ear pain

CAUSES & RISK FACTORS
• Genetic—weimaraners; homozygous condition lethal; heterozygotes clinically affected
• In utero spinal cord damage caused by infection, trauma, and vascular compromise may cause syringomyelia (cavitation of the spinal cord).
• Idiopathic in isolated patients

• Hydrosyringomyelia may be acquired as result of infection, trauma, or neoplasia.

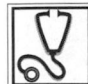 DIAGNOSIS

DIFFERENTIAL DIAGNOSIS
• Clinically differentiated from common spinal cord diseases because it is present at birth and nonprogressive
• Intervertebral disc disease, myelitis, and neoplasia must be differentiated from progressive causes of syringohydromyelia.

CBC/BIOCHEMISTRY/URINALYSIS
Usually normal

OTHER LABORATORY TESTS
N/A

IMAGING
• Survey and contrast spinal radiography—associated vertebral column anomalies and spinal cord compression in some patients
• Without sophisticated imaging techniques, an antemortem diagnosis may be impossible to make in dogs other than weimaraners.
• MRI is most definitive and useful imaging modality for syringohydromyelia, occipital bone malformations, hydrocephalus, and cerebellar herniation (Chiari malformation).
• CT can reveal hydrocephalus and syringohydromyelia.

OTHER DIAGNOSTIC PROCEDURES
N/A

TREATMENT
• Mildly affected animals—may be acceptable pets
• Severely affected animals may benefit from a canine cart; consider euthanasia.
• Surgical considerations—foramen magnum remodeling (with occipital malformation) or laminectomy, ± drainage of syrinx (with syringomyelia) may arrest progression or improve course of progressive neurologic signs.

 MEDICATIONS

DRUG(S)
• If urinary tract infection—treat with antibiotics based on culture and sensitivity of urine.
• Hydrosyringomyelia—corticosteroids: may improve signs by decreasing CSF production and edema formation; carbonic anhydrase inhibitors (acetozolamide 3.5–7.5 mg/kg/q8–12hrs; methazolamide 5 mg/kg q8–12h) may alleviate signs by reducing CSF production.

CONTRAINDICATIONS/POSSIBLE INTERACTIONS
N/A

 FOLLOW-UP

• Secondary urinary tract infection—seen in severely affected animals; owing to disorders of micturition
• Avoid decubitus ulcers and urine and fecal scalds by properly caring for recumbent patients.

 MISCELLANEOUS

ASSOCIATED CONDITIONS
Congenital vertebral arch (e.g., spina bifida) and vertebral body-disk malformation (e.g., hemivertebra and block vertebra)—alone often do not cause clinical signs

ABBREVIATIONS
CSF = cerebrospinal fluid
CT = computed tomography
MRI = magnetic resonance imaging

Suggested Reading
Bailey CS, Morgan JP. Congenital malformations. In: Moore MP, ed. Diseases of the spine. Vet Clin North Am Small Anim Pract 1992;22:985–1015.
Rusbridge C, MacSweeny JE, Davies JV, et al. Syringohydromyelia in Cavalier King Charles spaniels. J Am Anim Hosp Assoc 2000 Jan–Feb; 36(1):34–41.
Summers BA, Cummings JH, de Lahunta A. Veterinary pathology. St. Louis: Mosby, 1995.
Author Richard J. Joseph
Consulting Editor Joane M. Parent

SPLENIC TORSION

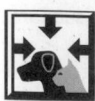

BASICS

OVERVIEW
• May occur as a separate entity or in association with gastric dilatation-volvulus syndrome
• Acute or chronic
• Pathophysiology—unknown
• Systems affected—Hemic/Lymphatic/ Immune and Cardiovascular
• Isolated splenic torsion uncommon

SIGNALMENT
• More common in large-breed, deep-chested dogs, such as German shepherds and Great Danes
• No sex predilection

SIGNS

Historical Findings
• Acute—cardiovascular collapse and abdominal pain
• Chronic—intermittent anorexia, vomiting, weight loss, and possibly hemoglobinuria

Physical Examination Findings
• Pale mucous membranes, tachycardia, and other signs of hypoperfusion
• Palpable abdominal mass

CAUSES & RISK FACTORS
• Large breed and deep chest (dogs)
• Prior stretching of gastrosplenic, phrenico-splenic, and splenocolic ligaments
• Historical gastric dilatation
• Excessive exercise, rolling, and retching may contribute

DIAGNOSIS

DIFFERENTIAL DIAGNOSIS
• Other splenic disease (e.g., neoplasia and immune-mediated disease)
• Acute gastrointestinal disease with abdominal pain
• Other causes of intravascular hemolysis

CBC/BIOCHEMISTRY/URINALYSIS
• Anemia
• Thrombocytopenia
• Leukocytosis
• High liver enzyme values
• Hemoglobulinuria

OTHER LABORATORY TESTS
Coagulation test—DIC (prolonged prothrombin time, partial thromboplastin time, and fibrin split products) because of accelerated consumption

IMAGING

Abdominal Radiography
• Cranial or midabdominal mass may be seen.
• Spleen may be abnormally located.

Abdominal Ultrasound
• Splenic congestion
• Dilated splenic veins
• Splenic infarction

DIAGNOSTIC PROCEDURES
ECG—may show ventricular arrhythmias

PATHOLOGIC FINDINGS
Splenic congestion and infarction

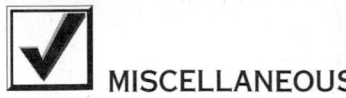

 TREATMENT

- Surgical emergency
- After adequate cardiovascular stabilization, a splenectomy should be performed without untwisting the splenic pedicle.
- A permanent gastropexy should also be performed because of the association with gastric dilatation-volvulus syndrome.
- A splenic specimen should be submitted for histopathologic examination.
- Fluid support and cardiovascular monitoring indicated after splenectomy

 MEDICATIONS

DRUG(S)

- No specific drugs required
- Postoperative pain relief advised
- Heparin (75 IU/kg SC q8h) or plasma transfusion may be considered if DIC documented

CONTRAINDICATIONS/POSSIBLE INTERACTIONS

None

 FOLLOW-UP

Surgical correction considered curative

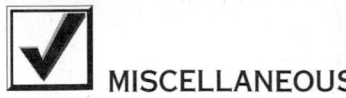 **MISCELLANEOUS**

ABBREVIATION

- DIC = disseminated intravascular coagulation

Suggested Reading

Neath PJ, Brookman DJ, Saunders HM. Retrospective analysis of 19 cases of isolated torsion of the splenic pedicle in dogs. J Small Anim Pract 1997;38:337–392.

Author Elizabeth A. Rozanski

Consulting Editor Stephen A. Kruth

SPLENOMEGALY

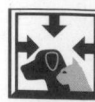 BASICS

DEFINITION
Enlargement of the spleen; characterized as either diffuse or nodular

PATHOPHYSIOLOGY
• Spleen functions—removal of senescent and abnormal erythrocytes; filtration and phagocytosis of antigenic particles; production of lymphocytes and plasma cells; reservoir for erythrocytes and platelets; hematopoiesis, as required • Many disorders affect the function of the spleen and clinical signs influenced by altered splenic function.

Diffuse
Four General Pathologic Mechanisms
• Inflammation (splenitis)—associated with infectious agents; classified according to cell type (e.g., suppurative, necrotizing, eosinophilic, lymphoplasmacytic, and granulomatous-pyogranulomatous)
• Lymphoreticular hyperplasia—hyperplasia of mononuclear phagocytes and lymphoid elements (in response to antigens); accelerated erythrocyte destruction • Congestion—associated with impaired venous drainage
• Infiltration—involves cellular invasion of the spleen or deposition of abnormal substances

Nodular
Associated with neoplastic (tumor) or non-neoplastic disorders (hemorrhage, infection, or inflammation)

SYSTEMS AFFECTED
N/A

SIGNALMENT
• Dogs and cats • Splenic torsion—over-represented in large, deep-chested breeds (e.g., German shepherds, Great Danes)
• Hemangiosarcoma—middle-aged animals; large breeds; more common in males than in females; predilection in German shepherds, golden retrievers, and Labrador retrievers
• Prominent spleen—may be normal in certain breeds (German shepherds, Scottish terriers)

SIGNS

General Comments
• May reflect the underlying disease rather than primary disease of the spleen • Splenic enlargement—often nonspecific

Historical Findings
• Hemoabdomen secondary to splenic hematoma or hemangiosarcoma (dogs)—weakness, collapse • Lymphosarcoma, mast cell tumor, FIP, and lymphoplasmacytic enteritis (cats)—diarrhea; vomiting; anorexia
• Vague abdominal pain and mild to modest distention • Lethargy with splenic torsion

Physical Examination Findings
• Enlarged spleen on abdominal palpation; nonpalpable spleen does not preclude enlargement • Dogs—smooth or irregular surface • Cats—usually diffuse; uniform enlargement • Splenic hemorrhage—may note pallor and tachycardia • Massive enlargement and/or splenic rupture—may note abdominal distention • Coagulopathy owing to primary splenic or underlying disease—may result in petechia and ecchymosis • Infiltrative or inflammatory disease—implied by hepatomegaly, thickened intestines, and/or enlarged mesenteric lymph nodes • Lymphosarcoma—suggested by concurrent peripheral lymphadenopathy
• Cardiac arrhythmias—may be sign of clinically significant cardiac abnormalities affecting the spleen; ventricular arrhythmias are associated with splenic hemangiosarcoma

CAUSES

Dogs
Inflammation (Splenitis)
• Suppurative—penetrating abdominal wound; migrating foreign body; endocarditis; sepsis; infection secondary to splenic torsion
• Necrotizing—usually secondary to torsion or neoplasia; anaerobes; *Salmonella*; acute infectious canine hepatitis
• Eosinophilic—eosinophilic gastroenteritis
• Lymphoplasmacytic—subacute or chronic infectious disorder; infectious canine hepatitis; ehrlichiosis; pyometra; *Brucella*; *Leishmania*
• Granulomatous—histoplasmosis; *Leishmania*
• Pyogranulomatous—blastomycosis; *Mycobacterium*; sporotrichosis
Hyperplasia
• Infection—bacterial endocarditis; diskospondylitis; *Brucella*
• Immune-mediated disease—SLE; hemolytic disease; thrombocytopenia
Congestion
Tranquilizers; barbiturates; portal hypertension; right-sided heart failure; splenic torsion
Infiltration
• Neoplasia—lymphosarcoma; acute and chronic leukemia; malignant histiocytosis; multiple myeloma; systemic mastocytosis
• Extramedullary hematopoiesis—immune-mediated hemolytic anemia or thrombocytopenia; chronic anemia; infectious disease; malignancy; SLE
• Amyloidosis

Cats
Inflammation
• Lymphoplasmacytic—lymphoplasmacytic enteritis; *Haemobartonella*; pyometra
• Pyogranulomatous—FIP, *Mycobacterium*
• Eosinophilic—hypereosinophilic syndrome
• Granulomatous—histoplasmosis; mycobacteriosis

• Suppurative—penetrating wound or migrating foreign body; septicemia; salmonellosis; toxoplasmosis
• Necrotizing—salmonellosis
Hyperplasia
• Haemobartonellosis
• Chronic hemolysis • SLE • Immune stimulation
Congestion
• Portal hypertension • Congestive heart failure
Infiltration
• Neoplastic—mast cell tumor (most common); lymphosarcoma; myeloproliferative disease; lymphoproliferative disease; malignant histiocytosis; multiple myeloma
• Non-neoplastic—amyloidosis, extramedullary hematopoiesis

RISK FACTORS
Cats—FeLV, FIP

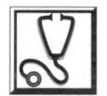 DIAGNOSIS

DIFFERENTIAL DIAGNOSIS
Other cranial organomegaly or masses

CBC/BIOCHEMISTRY/URINALYSIS

Dogs
• Regenerative anemia secondary to splenic bleeding or hemolytic disease
• Spherocytes—hemolysis, microangiopathic shearing
• Leukocytosis with a left shift—may indicate infectious or inflammatory conditions, marked regenerative stimulation, or extramedullary hematopoiesis
• Thrombocytopenia—from increased consumption (DIC) secondary to hemangiosarcoma, increased destruction or sequestration, or decreased production
• Hypercalcemia may be associated with neoplasia, especially lymphosarcoma.
• Hyperglobulinemia may be associated with neoplasia or ehrlichial infections.
• Hemoglobinemia and hyperbilirubinemia—may occur with microangiopathic anemia, splenic torsion, hemangiosarcoma, and immune-mediated anemia with spleen as site of extravascular RBC removal

Cats
• Direct RBC examination for hemoparasites
• Regenerative anemia and splenomegaly—may indicate haemobartonellosis
• Macrocytosis and nonregenerative anemia—suggest retroviral infection or myeloproliferative disease
• Eosinophilia—suggests hypereosinophilic syndrome, systemic mastocytosis, or lymphosarcoma
• Circulating blast cells—indicate myeloproliferative or lymphoproliferative disorder

- Nucleated RBCs—may accompany extramedullary hematopoiesis
- Thrombocytopenia—from increased consumption (DIC), increased destruction, decreased production, or sequestration

OTHER LABORATORY TESTS
- FeLV and FIV testing
- Buffy coat smears—circulating mast cells (may occur with inflammatory disease and neoplasia); blast cells
- Coagulation panel—DIC commonly seen with hemangiosarcoma (includes prolonged clotting times, hypofibrinogenemia, and increased FDPs; D-dimers too sensitive for clinical application in differential diagnoses)

IMAGING
Abdominal Radiography
- Confirms or detects splenomegaly
- May provide evidence for the underlying cause—concurrent hepatomegaly may indicate infiltrative disease or right-sided heart disease; splenic torsion may occur secondary to gastric dilation or volvulus
- Effusion—may indicate hemorrhage from splenic rupture (hemangiosarcoma, hematoma) or portal hypertension influencing circulation to the spleen

Thoracic Radiography
- Three views (right and left lateral and dorsal-ventral views)—screen for metastasis and underlying disease

Abdominal Ultrasonography
- Distinguishes between diffuse and nodular patterns of disease
- Diffuse enlargement with normal parenchyma—may be noted with congestion or cellular infiltration
- Reduced echogenicity—may be seen with splenic torsion, splenic vein thrombosis, lymphosarcoma, or leukemia
- Nodular abnormalities easily identified
- Complex, mixed echogenic pattern—hemangiosarcoma
- Hematomas—variable echogenicity; may have internal septation and encapsulation and pass through a stage where they resemble target lesions suggesting neoplasia
- Can identify concurrent abdominal diseases affecting liver, kidneys, intestines, and lymph nodes
- Cannot differentiate between benign and malignant splenic disorders

Echocardiography
Evaluation of the right atrium—indicated when hemangiosarcoma is suspected (based on ultrasonographic appearance and hematologic findings): mass supports diagnosis of hemangiosarcoma

DIAGNOSTIC PROCEDURES
Fine-Needle Aspiration
- Procedure—place patient in right lateral or dorsal recumbency; use a 23- or 25-gauge, 2.5–3.75 cm (1–1.5 in.) needle; diffuse: may aspirate without ultrasonography; nodular: requires ultrasound guidance to sample lesions
- Specimens—evaluate cytologically for infectious agents (most commonly found in macrophages); identify the predominant inflammatory cell type
- Neoplastic infiltrates—classified as epithelial, mesenchymal, or discrete (round cell)

Bone Marrow Aspiration
- Indicated with cytopenias before splenectomy (spleen may be the main hematopoietic source)
- May yield a diagnosis of infectious disease (e.g., ehrlichiosis, mycosis) or hematopoietic neoplasia

 TREATMENT
- Depends on underlying cause; supportive nursing care as needed
- Important to determine if splenomegaly is appropriate for systemic conditions
- Treatment and prognosis after splenectomy—based on histopathologic results

SURGICAL CONSIDERATIONS
Splenectomy
- With anemia or leukopenia—rule out bone marrow aplasia before surgery; spleen may be the source of hematopoietic precursors
- Indicated for splenic torsion, splenic rupture, splenic masses considered likely to be hemangiosarcomas, and mast cell infiltration (cats)
- Exploratory celiotomy—permits direct evaluation of all abdominal organs

 MEDICATIONS
DRUG(S)
Depend on underlying disease
CONTRAINDICATIONS
N/A
PRECAUTIONS
N/A
POSSIBLE INTERACTIONS
N/A

 FOLLOW-UP
PATIENT MONITORING
Ventricular arrhythmias (dogs)—associated with splenic mass lesions; may occur before,

during, and up to 3 days after surgery for splenectomy; evaluate (auscultation and electrocardiogram) surgical candidates before anesthesia; continuous cardiac monitoring during surgery and postoperatively

POSSIBLE COMPLICATIONS
- Asplenic patient—increased risk of infection
- Postoperative sepsis—uncommon complication • Antibiotics—indicated in asplenic patients receiving immunosuppressive therapy, if any sign of infection is noted

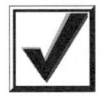 MISCELLANEOUS
ASSOCIATED CONDITIONS
N/A
AGE-RELATED FACTORS
N/A
ZOONOTIC POTENTIAL
A variety of infectious diseases may involve the spleen
PREGNANCY
N/A
SEE ALSO
See Causes
ABBREVIATIONS
- DIC = disseminated intravascular coagulation
- FDPs = fibrin degradation products
- FeLV = feline leukemia virus
- FIP = feline infectious peritonitis
- SLE = systemic lupus erythematosus

Suggested Reading
Hammer AS, Couto CG. Disorders of the lymph nodes and spleen. In: Scherding RG, ed. The cat: diseases and clinical management. 2nd ed. New York: Churchill Livingstone, 1994:671–689.
Neer MT. Clinical approach to splenomegaly in dogs and cats. Compendium 1996;18:35–48.
Spangler WL, Culbertson MR. Prevalence and type of splenic diseases in cats: 455 cases (1985–1991). J Am Vet Med Assoc 1992;201:773–776.
Spangler WL, Culbertson MR. Prevalence and type of splenic diseases in dogs: 1480 cases (1985–1989). J Am Vet Med Assoc 1992;200:829–834.
Spangler WL, Kass PH. Pathologic factors affecting postsplenectomy survival in dogs. J Vet Intern Med 1997;11:166–171.
Authors Angelyn M. Cornetta and Cheryl E. Balkman
Consulting Editor Sharon A. Center

SPONDYLOSIS DEFORMANS

BASICS

OVERVIEW
• Degenerative, noninflammatory condition of the vertebral column characterized by the production of osteophytes along the ventral, lateral, and dorsolateral aspects of the vertebral endplates
• Most common location—dogs: thoraco-lumbar spine in the area of the anticlinal vertebra and the upper lumbar vertebrae; cats: thoracic vertebrae reported in 68% of asymptomatic domestic cats

SIGNALMENT
• Dogs and cats
• Dogs—commonly seen in large breeds, especially German shepherds; also boxers, Airedale terriers, and cocker spaniels
• Occurrence increases with age; 50% of dogs by 6 years and 75% by 9 years; may be evident in young dogs with an inherited predisposition
• Females affected more than males

SIGNS

General Comments
• Patients are typically asymptomatic; lesions of minor clinical importance
• Pain may follow fracture of bony spurs or bridges.

Historical Findings
• Stiffness
• Restricted motion
• Pain

Physical Examination Findings
Neurologic deficits referable to the spinal cord or nerve root compression unusual

CAUSES & RISK FACTORS
• Repeated microtrauma
• Major trauma
• Inherited predisposition

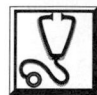

DIAGNOSIS

DIFFERENTIAL DIAGNOSIS
• Diskospondylitis—differentiated by radiographic evidence of end-plate lysis
• Spinal osteoarthritis—degeneration of the articular facet joints

CBC/BIOCHEMISTRY/URINALYSIS
Normal

OTHER LABORATORY TESTS
N/A

IMAGING
Spinal radiography—initially shows osteophytes as triangular projections several millimeters from the edge of the vertebral body; with progression, they appear to bridge the intervertebral space; true ankylosis rare

DIAGNOSTIC PROCEDURES
Myelography and CT or MRI—for unusual cases; demonstrate an atypical dorsal osteophyte compressing the spinal cord or nerve roots or encroaching on critical soft tissue structures

TREATMENT
• Inform owner that the condition is usually an asymptomatic, incidental finding and is probably not responsible for the clinical signs.
• Back pain or neurologic deficits—perform a neurodiagnostic evaluation of the spine in consideration of surgical intervention.
• Spondylosis—treat as outpatient with strict rest and analgesic administration or possibly acupuncture.
• Obesity—recommend a weight-reduction program.

MEDICATIONS

DRUG(S)
Use only when the patient is exhibiting signs.

NSAIDs
• Preferred to steroids in dogs unless the patient has neurologic deficits, because of fewer side effects
• Administer after feeding and in combination with an antacid (cimetidine at 6–10 mg/kg PO q8h or ranitidine at 1–2 mg/kg PO q12h) or a gastrointestinal protector (misoprostol at 3–5 µg/kg PO q6–8h) to reduce the possibility of gastrointestinal ulceration
• Carprofen (Rimadyl)—2.2 mg/kg PO q12h in dogs
• Etodolac (Etogesic)—5–15 mg/kg once a day in dogs
• Deracoxib (Deramaxx)—1–2 mg/kg once a day in dogs

• Aspirin—dogs: buffered, enteric-coated aspirin (e.g., Ascriptin or Ecotrin) at 10–20 mg/kg q8–12h); adult cats: a baby aspirin or one-quarter of a 325-mg aspirin tablet every 3 days
• Other NSAIDs should be used cautiously, because they are more likely to cause gastrointestinal ulceration.
• Acetaminophen (Tylenol)—5 mg/kg PO q12h PO in dogs only; non-NSAID analgesic

Corticosteroids
• Prednisone—0.5–1.0 mg/kg divided q12h; taper to alternate days or less, if possible
• Use only in patients with neurologic deficits
• Acupuncture—Dry needle or electroacupuncture at a weekly or biweekly treatment interval and tapered to as needed basis can be very effective in relief of pain; useful in animals that don't tolerate medication or when clients "prefer a natural alternative"

CONTRAINDICATIONS/POSSIBLE INTERACTIONS
• Acetaminophen (Tylenol)—do not use in cats.
• Avoid prolonged administration of NSAIDs or combinations of NSAIDs and steroids because of risk of gastrointestinal ulceration.

FOLLOW-UP
• Gradually return the animal to normal activity after signs have subsided for several weeks.
• Relapse can occur with strenuous activity.

MISCELLANEOUS

ABBREVIATIONS
• CT = computed tomography
• MRI = magnetic resonance imaging

Suggested Reading
Morgan JP, Hansson K, Miyabayashi T. Spondylosis deformans in the female beagle dog. A radiographic study. J Small Anim Pract 1989;30[8]:457–460.
Romatowski J. Spondylosis deformans in the dog. Compend Contin Educ Pract Vet 1986;8:531–536.
Author Richard J. Joseph
Consulting Editor Joane M. Parent

BASICS

OVERVIEW
• A zoonotic fungal disease that may affect the integument or lymphatics or be generalized
• Caused by the virtually ubiquitous dimorphic fungus *Sporothrix schenckii,* which typically infects via direct inoculation; direct inoculation not a requirement

SIGNALMENT
• Cats, dogs, and humans
• Dogs—more commonly seen in hunting dogs because of the increased likelihood of puncture wounds associated with thorns or splinters
• Cats—intact male cats that roam outdoors and fight because of the increased likelihood of puncture wounds and acquiring the disease from their opponents

SIGNS
Historical Findings
• Previous trauma or puncture wound in the affected area—variable finding
• Poor response to previous antibacterial therapy

Physical Examination Findings
• Cutaneous form—dog: associated with numerous nodules, which may drain or crust, typically affecting the head or trunk; cat: lesions often initially appear as wounds or abscesses, mimicking wounds associated with fighting, found on the head, lumbar region, or distal limbs
• Cutaneolymphatic form—usually an extension of the cutaneous form; spreads via the lymphatics, resulting in new nodules and draining tracts or crusts; lymphadenopathy common
• Disseminated form—associated with the systemic signs of malaise and fever; consider the potential of an underlying immunosuppressive disease as a contributing factor

CAUSES & RISK FACTORS
• Animals exposed to soil rich in decaying organic debris appear to be predisposed.
• Puncture wounds associated with foreign bodies provide an increased opportunity for infection in dogs; cat scratches provide a similar opportunity in roaming cats.
• Immunosuppressive disease—risk factor for the disseminated form

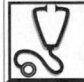 DIAGNOSIS

DIFFERENTIAL DIAGNOSIS
• Various bacterial and fungal diseases—consider when symptoms include a nodular granulomatous disease and draining tracts
• Neoplastic conditions
• Parasitic infections (*Demodex* or *Pelodera*)

CBC/BIOCHEMISTRY/URINALYSIS
N/A

OTHER LABORATORY TESTS
N/A

IMAGING
N/A

DIAGNOSTIC PROCEDURES
• **REMEMBER:** this is a zoonotic disease and proper precautions should be taken to prevent infection; absence of a break in the skin does not protect against the disease • Cytology of the exudate and staining—cats: often the only test necessary to confirm infection; cigar- to round-shaped yeast may be found intracellularly or free in the exudate; dogs: special fungal stains (PAS or GMS) may aid in the diagnosis; a negative finding does not rule out the disease • Cultures of the deeply affected tissue—often require surgery to obtain an adequate sample; alert the laboratory that sporotrichosis is a differential diagnosis; secondary bacterial infections common

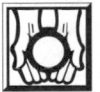 TREATMENT

• Remember the zoonotic potential when treating patients.
• Sometimes outpatient treatment may be considered.

 MEDICATIONS

DRUG(S)
SSKI
• Treatment of choice—dogs: 40 mg/kg PO q8h with food; cats: 20 mg/kg PO q12h with food
• Continue for 30 days after resolution of the clinical lesions.
• Dogs—if signs of iodism are noted (dry hair coat, excessive scales, nasal or ocular discharge, vomiting, depression, or collapse), discontinue for 1 week; mild symptoms, reinitiate at the same dose; severe or recurrent symptoms, consider other drugs
• Cats—signs of iodism (depression, vomiting, anorexia, twitching, hypothermia, and

cardiovascular collapse) are more common; if noted, discontinue; use other drugs

Ketoconazole and Itraconazole
• Show encouraging results for fungal diseases in cats and dogs
• Dogs—ketoconazole: 15 mg/kg PO q12h, preferably with an acidic meal (e.g., tomato juice), until 1 month after clinical resolution; resolution should occur within approximately 3 months; side effects relatively mild, anorexia most common; acute hepatopathy, pruritus, alopecia, and lightening of the hair color reported
• Cats—ketoconazole: 5–10 mg/kg PO q12–24h, or itraconazole 10 mg/kg/day preferably with an acidic meal until 1 month after clinical resolution; side effects include gastrointestinal disturbances, depression, fever, jaundice, and neurologic signs; may be necessary to alternate drugs

CONTRAINDICATIONS/POSSIBLE INTERACTIONS
N/A

 FOLLOW-UP

PATIENT MONITORING
Reevaluate every 2 to 4 weeks for clinical signs and side effects associated with treatment.

PREVENTION/AVOIDANCE
Although difficult, try to determine the source of the original infection to prevent repeat infections.

EXPECTED COURSE AND PROGNOSIS
Unresponsive to therapy—not unexpected; consider alternative treatment or combined treatment regimens (SSKI and ketoconazole); itraconazole relatively untested but promising

 MISCELLANEOUS

ZOONOTIC POTENTIAL
Zoonotic; proper precautions and client education are of paramount importance.

ABBREVIATIONS
GMS = Gomori's methamine silver (stain)
PAS = periodic acid–Schiff (stain)
SSKI = supersaturated potassium iodide

Suggested Reading
Scott DW, Miller WH, Griffin CE. Muller and Kirk's small animal dermatology. 5th ed. Philadelphia: Saunders, 1995.
Author Dunbar Gram
Consulting Editor Karen Helton Rhodes

SQUAMOUS CELL CARCINOMA, DIGIT

BASICS

OVERVIEW
• Malignant tumor arising from the sub-ungual epithelium
• Cats—metastasis to one or multiple digits from other cutaneous sites reported
• Dogs—most common digital tumor

SIGNALMENT
• Dogs and rarely cats
• Large breeds and black dogs—predisposed; particularly standard poodles and Labrador retrievers
• Median age, 10 years; may occur in dogs as young as 4 years old

SIGNS
• Swelling of digit—reason for examination
• May note ulceration
• Multiple digits—rarely in dogs; may be seen in cats as part of a metastatic process
• Lymph node and lung metastasis—reported; uncommon at the time of examination (13%)

CAUSES & RISK FACTORS
• Cause—unknown
• Risk factors—hereditary; black skin pigmentation

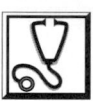

DIAGNOSIS

DIFFERENTIAL DIAGNOSIS
• Nail bed infection
• Other tumors—melanoma; soft tissue sarcomas; mast cell tumor

CBC/BIOCHEMISTRY/URINALYSIS
N/A

OTHER LABORATORY TESTS
N/A

IMAGING
• Thoracic radiographs—important to rule out metastatic disease; results typically normal at the time of diagnosis
• Radiographs of the affected foot—reveal lysis of the third phalanx of the affected digit in 75% of patients

DIAGNOSTIC PROCEDURES
• Wedge biopsy of abnormal tissue—required to confirm diagnosis
• Lymph node biopsy—may be indicated

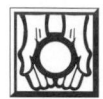

TREATMENT
• Amputation of the affected digit at the level of the metacarpal (or metatarsal) phalangeal joint—treatment of choice
• Complete surgical excision of the primary lesion and no evidence of metastasis—no additional treatment required

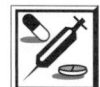

MEDICATIONS

DRUG(S)
• Multiple affected digits owing to metastasis (cats)—surgery not an option because digits from multiple limbs are generally affected; pain control with piroxicam (0.3 mg/kg q24–28h) may offer temporary relief; benefit of chemotherapy unknown

CONTRAINDICATIONS/POSSIBLE INTERACTIONS
None

FOLLOW-UP
• Survival time following complete surgical excision is dependent on location of the tumor or the digit—squamous cell carcinoma originating from subungual epithelium: 95% 1-year and 74% 2-year survival; squamous cell carcinoma originating in other parts of digit: 60% 1-year and 44% 2-year survival
• Benefit of chemotherapy has not been established.
• Recurrence is not anticipated with complete resection.

MISCELLANEOUS

Suggested Reading

Marino DJ, Matthiesen DT, Stefanacci JD, Moroff SD. Evaluation of dogs with digit masses: 117 cases (1981–1991). J Am Vet Med Assoc 1995;207:726–728.
O'Brien MG, Berg J, Engler SJ. Treatment by digital amputation of subungual squamous cell carcinoma in dogs: 21 cases (1987–1988). J Am Vet Med Assoc 1992; 201:759–761.

Author Robyn Elmslie
Consulting Editor Wallace B. Morrison

BASICS

OVERVIEW
• Malignant tumor arising from the squamous epithelium of the skin of the pinnae
• Occasionally involves the ear canal
• Most are very invasive but very slow to metastasize.
• Most common in animals that have had high exposure to sunlight

SIGNALMENT
• Cats and rarely dogs
• Common in cats with white or light-colored fur and skin
• Mean age at time of diagnosis—12 years (range, 7–24 years)

SIGNS
• Lesions develop slowly over months to years.
• Precancerous stage—characterized by crusty eczematous lesions of the edge of the pinnae that flare up and regress repeatedly
• Proliferation and ulceration of the ear signal the true cancerous phase; ear becomes extensively disfigured if left untreated.
• Metastatic disease uncommon

CAUSES & RISK FACTORS
• Prolonged sunlight exposure—important cause
• White fur and light skin pigmentation—risk factors

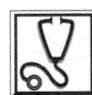

DIAGNOSIS

DIFFERENTIAL DIAGNOSIS
• Classic clinical findings—help differentiate from other neoplastic conditions

• Lesions on the pinnae caused by vasculitis or cryoglobulinemia—may resemble squamous cell carcinoma

CBC/BIOCHEMISTRY/URINALYSIS
N/A

OTHER LABORATORY TESTS
N/A

IMAGING
Thoracic radiographs—may help definitively rule out the rare pulmonary metastasis

DIAGNOSTIC PROCEDURES
• Biopsy of pinna—confirm diagnosis.
• Cytologic—evaluate lymph nodes; may help definitively rule out metastasis.

PATHOLOGIC FINDINGS
Distinguished microscopically by characteristic groups of epithelial cells and keratinizing cells forming keratin pearls

TREATMENT
• Aggressive surgical excision—required; must amputate the pinnae below the demarcation of unhealthy tissue
• Histologic evaluation of the surgical margins—essential to assess completeness of surgical excision
• Photodynamic therapy—alternative to amputation; results less predictable; more than one treatment often required
• Cryosurgery—successful for small lesions
• Hyperthermia—reported to be beneficial

MEDICATIONS

DRUG(S)
• Etretinate—0.75–1 mg/kg q24h; used successfully to prevent progression of precancerous lesions

• Vitamin E—400–600 IU PO q12h; may be beneficial to prevent or delay progression of precancerous lesions
• Bleomycin—10–20 IU/m^2 SC once per week; has been used systemically to treat advanced disease
• Chemotherapy—benefit not yet established

CONTRAINDICATIONS/POSSIBLE INTERACTIONS
None

FOLLOW-UP
• Limit sun exposure—may prevent development of new lesions
• Sunscreen and tattooing—useful for preventing development of new lesions
• Early treatment of crusting lesions on the ears by cryosurgery or surgical excision is recommended.
• Prognosis—good if complete surgical excision is achieved

MISCELLANEOUS

Suggested Reading

Dorn CR, Taylor D. Sunlight exposure and the risk of developing cutaneous and oral squamous cell carcinoma in white cats. J Natl Cancer Inst 1971;46:1073–1078.
London CA, Dubilzeig RR, et al. Evaluation of dogs and cats with tumors of the ear canal: 145 cases (1978–1992). J Am Vet Med Assoc 1996;208:1413–1418.

Author Robyn Elmslie
Consulting Editor Wallace B. Morrison

SQUAMOUS CELL CARCINOMA, GINGIVA

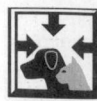

BASICS

OVERVIEW
- Progressive, rapid (weeks), local invasion of neoplastic epithelial cells within the oral cavity in dogs and cats
- The most common oral malignancy in cats and second most common in dogs
- Highly invasive to the bone with a nonencapsulated, raised, irregular, ulcerated, or necrotic surface
- Metastasis—rare in cats; spread to lymph nodes more common than to the lungs; in dogs, metastasis is site dependent. Rostral oral lesions have a low metastatic rate. Caudal oral or tonsillar lesions have an increased metastatic rate.
- Cause of death—secondary to local recurrence, dysphagia, and subsequent cachexia

SIGNALMENT
- Dogs and cats
- Mean age (dogs and cats)—10.5 years (range, 3–15 years)
- More common in medium- and large-breed dogs

SIGNS

Historical Findings
- Excessive salivation
- Dysphagia
- Halitosis
- Bloody oral discharge
- Weight loss

Physical Examination Findings
- Loose teeth
- Facial deformity
- Cervical lymphadenomegaly—occasionally
- Rostral mandible—most common site

CAUSES & RISK FACTORS
None identified

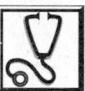

DIAGNOSIS

DIFFERENTIAL DIAGNOSIS
- Other oral malignancy
- Epulis
- Abscess
- Benign polyp
- Tonsillar lymphoma

CBC/BIOCHEMISTRY/URINALYSIS
Usually normal

OTHER LABORATORY TESTS
Cytologic evaluation—obtain impression smear from an incisional biopsy specimen (wedge); may yield diagnosis. Cytology of enlarged regional lymph nodes should be done to evaluate for metastatic disease.

IMAGING
- Skull radiography—evaluate bone involvement deep to the mass.
- Thoracic radiography—detect pulmonary metastasis (uncommon).

DIAGNOSTIC PROCEDURES
Large, deep tissue biopsy (down to bone)—required to sufficiently differentiate from other oral malignancies

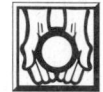

TREATMENT

SURGERY
- Radical surgical excision—required (e.g., hemimandibulectomy); usually well tolerated by patient; survival improves when excisional margins are free of neoplastic cells; margins of at least 2 cm necessary
- Cryosurgery—indicated for small lesions minimally adherent to the bone

RADIATION
- Considerable long-term control if inoperable; most plans attempt 40–60 Gy over 3–6 weeks; combined with low-dose cisplatin chemotherapy improves overall survival; combined with hyperthermia does not improve overall survival; complications common in cats (mucositis, anorexia, and dehydration requiring aggressive supportive care)
- Lingual squamous cell carcinoma surgery or radiation therapy results in 50% having a 1-year survival time.
- Soft foods—may be recommended to prevent tumor ulceration or after radical oral excision
- Photodynamic therapy—17 months of local control in dogs

MEDICATIONS

DRUG(S)
- Cisplatin (dogs)—60–70 mg/m^2 IV once every 3–4 weeks for four treatments; provides marked palliation of clinical signs; response depends on severity of the localized or metastatic lesion; nephrotoxic must use with saline diuresis (18.3 mL/kg/hr IV over 6 hr; give cisplatin after 4 hr)

- Butorphanol—0.4 mg/kg IM; before and after cisplatin; reduces emesis
- Local control (palliation) by intralesionally administered cisplatin has been reported.
- Piroxicam (dogs)—0.3 mg/kg PO daily; may be useful to induce partial remission in some patients. May cause ulcerative gastritis

CONTRAINDICATIONS/POSSIBLE INTERACTIONS
- Cisplatin—never use in cats.
- Chemotherapy may be toxic; seek advice if unfamiliar with cytotoxic drugs.

FOLLOW-UP

- Survival after excision (dogs)—1 year, 25%–45%; 2-year, 20%–35%
- Median survival after excision (dogs)—7–11 months; survival improves when excisional margins are free of neoplastic cells.
- Survivals after excision and radiotherapy (dogs)—mean, 7 months; median 8 months; range, 0–27 months
- Survival after excision (cats)—mean, 2.5 months; median, 14 months; range, 0–36 months
- Median survival after excision and radiotherapy (cats)—14 months; range, 1–36 months
- Cause of death—related to local recurrence and secondary anorexia and cachexia
- Overall prognosis—poor in cats because most tumors are locally invasive and diagnosed late in the course of disease

MISCELLANEOUS

Suggested Reading
Hutson CA, Willauer CC, Walder EJ, et al. Treatment of mandibular squamous cell carcinoma in cats by use of mandibulectomy and radiotherapy: seven cases (1987–1989). J Am Vet Med Assoc 1992;201:777–781.

Oakes MG, Lewis DD, Hedlund CS, et al. Canine oral neoplasia. Compend Contin Educ Pract Vet 1993;15:15–31.

Authors Kevin A. Hahn and Kimberly P. Freeman

Consulting Editor Wallace B. Morrison

BASICS

OVERVIEW
• Rare primary tumor of bronchial epithelial origin with squamous metaplasia (epidermoid carcinoma)
• Commonly develops in the right caudal lung lobe in dogs and the left caudal lung lobe in cats
• High metastatic potential, especially if regional lymph nodes are positive

SIGNALMENT
• Dogs and cats
• Mean age—dogs, 11 years; cats, 12 years
• No breed predilection

SIGNS

Historical Findings
• Sometimes none
• Harsh, nonproductive cough
• Dyspnea
• Lethargy or exercise intolerance
• Cachexia and weight loss
• Lameness—resulting from bone metastasis

Physical Examination Findings
• Tachypnea
• Wheeze
• Hemoptysis
• Hypertrophic osteopathy
• Neuromyopathy and paraplegia
• Digital lesions (metastasis) in cats

CAUSES & RISK FACTORS
Approximately 74% of patients come from an urban environment.

DIAGNOSIS

DIFFERENTIAL DIAGNOSIS
• Bronchogenic cysts
• Bullae and blebs
• Abscesses
• Paragonimus
• Eosinophilic lung disease
• Other primary lung neoplasm
• Metastatic pulmonary neoplasm
• Aspiration pneumonia

CBC/BIOCHEMISTRY/URINALYSIS
• Neutrophilic leukocytosis
• Hypercalcemia rare

OTHER LABORATORY TESTS
Cytology—examination of tissue obtained by endoscopic bronchial brushing or fine-needle aspiration; may provide tentative diagnosis

IMAGING
• Survey thoracic radiographs—solitary mass arising from a single focus most common appearance
• Right caudal lung lobes in dogs and the left caudal lung lobe in cats common
• Margins—well circumscribed; sharp demarcation from other surrounding normal parenchyma
• Arises from larger bronchi
• Trachea or mainstem bronchi—displaced or compressed
• Partial or complete airway obstruction and peripheral atelectasis

DIAGNOSTIC PROCEDURES
Tissue biopsy—definitive diagnosis

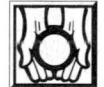

TREATMENT
• Surgery—wide and complete resection of affected lung lobe; best opportunity for long-term control; examine tracheobronchial lymph nodes; manually palpate all remaining lung lobes; biopsy of lymph nodes advised, even if they appear normal; removal is best, but frequently difficult and thus not often done
• Chemotherapy—best to start when there is residual disease that can be measured on radiographs or ultrasound; may administer before or after surgery; best to have some tumor present so it is possible to evaluate response

MEDICATIONS

DRUG(S)
• Cisplatin—60 mg/m^2 IV every 3 or 4 weeks for four treatments; nephrotoxic, so must use with saline diuresis (18.3 mL/kg/hr IV over 6 hr; give cisplatin after 4 hr

• Butorphanol—0.4 mg/kg IM before and after cisplatin; reduces emesis
• Doxorubicin—dogs > 10 kg: 30 mg/m^2 IV once every 2 weeks for five treatments; dogs < 10 kg and cats: 1 mg/kg; has provided marked palliation

CONTRAINDICATIONS/POSSIBLE INTERACTIONS
• Cisplatin—never use in cats.
• Chemotherapy may be toxic; seek advice before treatment if you are unfamiliar with cytotoxic drugs.

FOLLOW-UP
• Survival if left untreated or with evidence of metastatic disease—usually < 3 months
• Median survival with complete excision of primary tumor and tracheobronchial lymph nodes negative for neoplastic cells (dogs and cats)—> 300 days
• Median survival with incomplete surgical excision of primary tumor or tracheo-bronchial lymph nodes positive for neoplastic cells (dogs and cats)—< 75 days
• Pleural effusion—poor prognosis

MISCELLANEOUS

Suggested Reading

Frazier DL, Hahn KA. Cancer chemotherapeutics. In: Hahn KA, Richardson RC, eds., Cancer chemotherapy, a veterinary handbook. Baltimore: Williams & Wilkins, 1995:77–150.

Hahn KA, Anderson TA. Tumors of the respiratory tract. In: Bonagura JD, ed. Kirk's current veterinary therapy XIII. Philadelphia: Saunders, 1998:500–505.

Authors Kevin A. Hahn and Avenelle Turner
Consulting Editor Wallace B. Morrison

SQUAMOUS CELL CARCINOMA, NASAL AND PARANASAL SINUSES

BASICS

OVERVIEW
• Progressive local invasion of neoplastic keratinizing and nonkeratinizing squamous epithelium arising from within the nasal and paranasal sinuses
• Keratinizing—tend to arise from the nasal area
• Nonkeratinizing—tend to arise from the frontal sinus region
• Transitional (intermediate) in a nonkeratinizing form—classified as undifferentiated
• Slowly progressive (months)
• Commonly bilateral
• Approximately 35% of patients have extension to the brain and seizures; usually nonkeratinizing tumors
• Prevalence (nasal neoplasia)—0.3%–8% of all tumors in dogs and cats
• Keratinizing and nonkeratinizing—28.5% of all nasal neoplasia in dogs
• Only adenocarcinomas occur more frequently.

SIGNALMENT
• More common in dogs than in cats
• Dogs—median age, 9.5 years (range, 3–16 years); male predilection for keratinizing form (3.4:1)

SIGNS

Historical Findings
• Intermittent and progressive unilateral to bilateral epistaxis and/or mucopurulent discharge—median duration, 3 months
• Epiphora
• Sneezing
• Halitosis
• Anorexia
• Seizures secondary to cranial invasion

Physical Examination Findings
• Nasal discharge
• Facial deformity or exophthalmia
• Pain on nasal or paranasal sinus examination
• Obstruction of nasal airflow (unilateral or bilateral)

CAUSES & RISK FACTORS
Unknown

DIAGNOSIS

DIFFERENTIAL DIAGNOSIS
• Bacterial sinusitis—uncommon
• Viral infection—cats
• Cryptococcosis—cats
• Aspergillosis; other fungal infection
• Foreign body
• Trauma
• Tooth root abscess
• Oronasal fistula
• Coagulopathy
• Hypertension
• Parasites

CBC/BIOCHEMISTRY/URINALYSIS
Usually normal

OTHER LABORATORY TESTS
Cytologic and bacterial examination—rarely helpful

IMAGING
• Skull radiographs—reveal typical pattern of asymmetrical destruction of caudal turbinates; superimposition of a soft tissue mass; may see fluid density in the frontal sinuses secondary to outflow obstruction
• Thoracic radiographs—detect pulmonary metastasis (uncommon)
• CT or MRI—best method for observing integrity of cribriform plate or orbital invasion

DIAGNOSTIC PROCEDURES
• Deep tissue biopsy—necessary for definitive diagnosis
• Bacterial culture—often positive
• Rhinoscopy—reveals soft, friable, fleshy mass; tumor often obscured by exudate; avoid progressing caudally into the cribriform plate
• Cytology of regional lymp nodes—detect metastatic disease

TREATMENT
• Surgery alone—not curative
• Turbinectomy—may be performed before external (teletherapy) or internal (brachytherapy) irradiation
• Inpatient radiotherapy—36–60 Gy; with or without surgery; best clinical control in dogs

MEDICATIONS

DRUG(S)
• Cisplatin (dogs only)—60–70 mg/m², IV once every 3 weeks for four treatments; may be a good option; nephrotoxic, so must use with saline diuresis (18.3 mL/kg/hr IV over 6 hr; give cisplatin after 4 hr)
• Butorphanol—0.4 mg/kg IM; before and after cisplatin will reduce emesis

CONTRAINDICATIONS/POSSIBLE INTERACTIONS
• Cisplatin—never use in cats
• Chemotherapy may be toxic; seek advice before initiating treatment if you are unfamiliar with cytotoxic drugs.

FOLLOW-UP

PATIENT MONITORING
Skull radiography, CT, and MRI—when signs recur

POSSIBLE COMPLICATIONS
• Rhinitis—after turbinectomy and radiotherapy; usually subsides in 1–2 months
• Secondary fungal rhinitis—occasionally after turbinectomy

EXPECTED COURSE AND PROGNOSIS
• Median survival if left untreated—3–5 months
• Survival with radiotherapy—1 year, 38%–57% (dogs and cats); 2 years, 30%–48% (dogs); median 8–25 months (dogs); median, 1–36 months (cats)
• Median survival after cisplatin (dogs)—22 weeks; may provide marked palliation of clinical signs
• Local recurrence with extension to the brain—common; brain involvement is a poor prognostic sign.
• Nasal squamous cell carcinoma in the dog may carry poorer prognosis than other nasal tumors: one report median survival time with radiotherapy 6.1 months

MISCELLANEOUS

Suggested Reading

Adams WM, Withrow SJ, Walshaw R, et al. Radiotherapy of malignant nasal tumors in 67 dogs. J Am Vet Med Assoc 1987; 191:311–315.

Patnaik AK. Canine sinonasal neoplasms: clinicopathological study of 285 cases. J Am Anim Hosp Assoc 1989;25:103–114.

Rogers KS, Walker MA, Helman RG. Squamous cell carcinoma of the canine nasal cavity and frontal sinus: eight cases. J Am Anim Hosp Assoc 1996;32:103–110.

Theon AP, Peaston AE, Madewell BR, et al. Irradiation of nonlymphoproliferative neoplasms of the nasal cavity and paranasal sinuses in 16 cats. J Am Vet Med Assoc 1994;204:78–83.

Authors Kevin A. Hahn and Janet K. Carreras
Consulting Editor Wallace B. Morrison

SQUAMOUS CELL CARCINOMA, NASAL PLANUM

BASICS

OVERVIEW
• Malignant tumor of squamous epithelial cells of the nasal planum
• Locally invasive and rarely metastasizes

SIGNALMENT
• Common in cats; rare in dogs
• Mean age—cats, 8.5–12.1 years; dogs, 9–10 years
• No reported sex or breed predilection
• More likely to develop in animals with a lightly pigmented nose

SIGNS
• Slow progression
• May begin as superficial crusting and scabbing, progress to carcinoma in situ, and develop into superficial and then invasive erosive carcinoma
• Dogs—sneezing; epistaxis; swelling of planum

CAUSES & RISK FACTORS
• Exposure to ultraviolet light
• Absence of protective pigment

DIAGNOSIS

DIFFERENTIAL DIAGNOSIS
Biopsy—differentiate from immune-mediated disease, eosinophilic granuloma complex, and other neoplasms

CBC/BIOCHEMISTRY/URINALYSIS
Usually normal

OTHER LABORATORY TESTS
N/A

IMAGING
• Thoracic radiographs—evaluate for metastasis (rare)
• CT or MRI—defines posterior extent of tumor to guide resection

DIAGNOSTIC PROCEDURES
Cytologic—fine-needle aspirate of large lymph nodes; detect metastasis

PATHOLOGIC FINDINGS
• Lesions—may vary in appearance depending on stage of disease; typically ulcerative not proliferative
• Histopathologic—characterized by irregular masses or cords of epidermal cells that proliferate downward into the dermis
• Keratin formation, horn pearls, desmosomes, mitotic figures, and cellular atypia—frequent

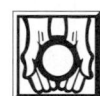

TREATMENT

• Superficial—surgery, cryosurgery, intralesional carboplatin, irradiation, or photodynamic therapy
• Etretinate—synthetic retinoid; may be useful for early precancerous lesions
• Invasive—requires radical surgical excision and adjunctive radiotherapy
• Immediate postoperative nutritional support may be required, especially for cats.

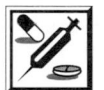

MEDICATIONS

DRUG(S)
Chemotherapy—not yet evaluated

CONTRAINDICATIONS/POSSIBLE INTERACTIONS
N/A

FOLLOW-UP

PATIENT MONITORING
• Physical examination and thoracic radiography—1, 3, 6, 9, 12, 18, and 24 months after treatment
• Biopsy—any suspicious lesion

PREVENTION/AVOIDANCE
• Limit sun exposure, especially between 10:00 A.M. and 2:00 P.M.
• Yearly tattoos on nonpigmented areas may be helpful.
• Sunscreens ineffective

POSSIBLE COMPLICATIONS
N/A

EXPECTED COURSE AND PROGNOSIS
• Survival with radiotherapy alone (cats)—mean, 17.7 months; 1 year, 61.5% with 81.8% recurrence
• Median survival with surgery (nosectomy) alone (cats)—over 22 months
• Recurrence with radiotherapy alone (8 dogs)—100%; mean time to recurrence, 2.9 months
• Dogs—surgery alone may be curative if the lesions are superficial.
• Prognosis—good for small, noninvasive tumors; guarded for invasive tumors

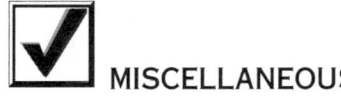

MISCELLANEOUS

ASSOCIATED CONDITION
Secondary bacterial infection

ABBREVIATIONS
• CT = computed tomography
• MRI = magnetic resonance imaging

Suggested Reading
Thomas RC, Fox LE. Tumors of the skin and subcutis. In: Morrison WB, ed. Cancer in dogs and cats: medical and surgical management. Philadelphia: Lippincott Williams & Wilkins, 1998:489–510.
Author Joanne C. Graham
Consulting Editor Wallace B. Morrison

SQUAMOUS CELL CARCINOMA, SKIN

BASICS

DEFINITION
• Malignant tumor of squamous epithelium
• Bowen's disease (cats)—multicentric squamous cell carcinoma in situ

PATHOPHYSIOLOGY
Metastasis—to any site; more commonly to regional lymph nodes and lungs

SYSTEMS AFFECTED
Skin/Exocrine—skin and metastatic sites

GENETICS
Unknown

INCIDENCE/PREVALENCE
Represents 9%–25% of all skin tumors in cats and 4%–18% in dogs

GEOGRAPHIC DISTRIBUTION
More prevalent in sunny climates and high altitudes (high ultraviolet light exposure)

SIGNALMENT
Species
Dogs and cats

Breed Predilection
• Cats—none reported; patients often have light or unpigmented skin.
• Dogs—Scottish terriers, Pekingese, boxers, poodles, Norwegian elkhounds, Dalmatians, beagles, whippets, and white English bull terriers may be predisposed; large breeds with black skin and haircoats may be predisposed to multiple squamous cell carcinoma involving the digits.

Mean Age and Range
• Dogs—9 years
• Cats—9–12.4 years

Predominant Sex
None

SIGNS
Historical Findings
• Crusts, ulcer, or mass that may have been present for months and unresponsive to conservative treatment

• Bowen's disease (cats)—skin becomes pigmented; ulcer forms in the center; followed by a painful scabby lesion that may expand peripherally
• Lips, nose, and pinna involvement—may start out as a shallow crusting lesion that progresses to a deep ulcer
• Facial skin involvement (cats)
• Nail bed involvement (dogs)

Physical Examination Findings
• Proliferative or erosive skin lesions
• Most common sites—cats: nasal planum, eyelids, lips, and pinna; dogs: toes, scrotum, nose, legs, and anus
• Flank and abdomen involvement
• Bowen's disease (cats)—may note 2 to > 30 lesions on the head, digits, neck, thorax, shoulders, and ventral abdomen; hair in the lesion epilates easily; crusts cling to the epilated hair shaft.

CAUSES
• Unknown
• Exposure to ultraviolet irradiation

RISK FACTORS
• Prolonged exposure to ultraviolet light
• Light or nonpigmented skin
• Previous thermal injury—burn scar

DIAGNOSIS

DIFFERENTIAL DIAGNOSIS
• Often misdiagnosed as draining abscesses or infected wounds on the basis of gross appearance
• Digit involvement—sometimes confused with nail bed infection and osteomyelitis
• Biopsy and histopathology—distinguish from eosinophilic granuloma complex, immune-mediated disease, mast cell tumor, and cutaneous lymphosarcoma

CBC/BIOCHEMISTRY/URINALYSIS
Usually normal

OTHER LABORATORY TESTS
None

IMAGING
• Thoracic radiography—detects lung metastasis
• Abdominal radiography—evaluates and monitors sublumbar lymph nodes, if clinically relevant
• Radiography of extremities—with digital tumor; determines extent of underlying bone involvement

DIAGNOSTIC PROCEDURES
• Cytologic examination—fine-needle aspirate; evaluate large lymph nodes for metastasis
• Biopsy—needed to confirm diagnosis

PATHOLOGIC FINDINGS
Gross
• Ulcerative tumors—most common; may appear shallow and crusted and progress to deep craters
• Proliferative tumors—may have a cauliflower-like appearance; may ulcerate and bleed easily
• Bowen's disease—painful ulcers that scab over and expand peripherally to reach more than 4 cm in diameter

Histopathologic
• Cords or irregular masses of epidermal cells infiltrating into the dermis and subcutis
• Large numbers of horn (keratin) pearls in well-differentiated tumors
• Desmosomes and mitotic figures common
• Bowen's disease—dysplastic, highly ordered keratinocytes proliferate, replacing normal epidermis, but do not penetrate the basement membrane into the surrounding dermis.

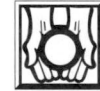

TREATMENT

APPROPRIATE HEALTH CARE
• Invasive tumors—inpatient; require aggressive surgical excision or radiotherapy
• Superficial tumors—surgery, cryosurgery, photodynamic therapy, or irradiation
• Topical synthetic retinoids—may be useful for early superficial lesions

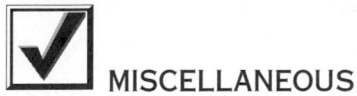
SQUAMOUS CELL CARCINOMA, SKIN

NURSING CARE
Interventional parenteral nutrition (feeding tube)—with nasal planum resection

ACTIVITY
• Dictated by the location of the tumor and the type of treatment
• Generally limit until sutures are removed, if surgery has been done

DIET
Normal

CLIENT EDUCATION
• Inform client about the benefit of early diagnosis and treatment.
• Discuss risk factors associated with the development of the tumor (ultraviolet light exposure).

SURGICAL CONSIDERATIONS
• Wide surgical excision—treatment of choice; skin flaps and body wall reconstruction sometimes required
• Digit involvement—amputation
• Pinna involvement—may require partial or total resection
• Invasive tumors of the nares—removal of the nasal planum recommended
• Radiotherapy—recommended for inoperable tumors or as adjunct to surgery

MEDICATIONS

DRUG(S) OF CHOICE
• Adjunctive chemotherapy—recommended with incomplete surgical excision, non-resectable mass, and metastasis
• Cisplatin (dogs), carboplatin, and mitoxantrone—reported to induce partial and complete remission; generally of short duration; small number of patients
• Intralesional sustained-release chemotherapeutic gel implants (dogs)—contain either 5-fluorouracil or cisplatin; effective

CONTRAINDICATIONS
• Cisplatin—do not use in cats, causes severe hydrothorax, pulmonary edema, and death; do not use in dogs with concurrent renal disease, potentially nephrotoxic
• 5-Fluorouracil—contraindicated in cats

PRECAUTIONS
Chemotherapeutics—follow published guidelines and protocols for safe use; be familiar with potential side effects.

POSSIBLE INTERACTIONS
None

ALTERNATIVE DRUG(S)
Topical synthetic retinoids—may be useful for early superficial lesions

FOLLOW-UP

PATIENT MONITORING
• Physical examination and radiography—1, 3, 6, 9, 12, 18, and 24 months after treatment or if the owner thinks the tumor is recurring
• Thoracic radiography at each recheck examination. Abdominal radiography or ultrasound if the lesion is on the caudal portion of the patient

PREVENTION/AVOIDANCE
• Limit sun exposure, especially between the hours of 10:00 A.M. and 2:00 P.M.
• Yearly tattoos on nonpigmented areas may be helpful.
• Sunscreens—usually licked off by the patient; may help in some areas (e.g., pinna)

POSSIBLE COMPLICATIONS
N/A

EXPECTED COURSE AND PROGNOSIS
Prognosis—good with superficial lesions that receive appropriate treatment; guarded with invasive lesions and those involving the nail bed or digit

☑ MISCELLANEOUS

ASSOCIATED CONDITIONS
N/A

AGE RELATED FACTORS
N/A

ZOONOTIC POTENTIAL
N/A

PREGNANCY
N/A

SEE ALSO
Squamous Cell Carcinoma, Nasal Planum

ABBREVIATIONS
N/A

Suggested Reading
Himsel CA, Richardson RC, Craig JA. Cisplatin chemotherapy for metastatic squamous cell carcinoma in two dogs. J Am Vet Med Assoc 1986;189:1575–1578.

Marks S. Clinical evaluation of etretinate (Tegison) for the treatment of preneoplastic and early neoplastic cutaneous squamous cell carcinoma in dogs. Vet Can Soc Newslett 1990;14:4–5.

O'Brien MG, Berg J, Engler SJ. Treatment by digital amputation of subungual squamous cell carcinoma in dogs: 21 cases (1987–1988). J Am Vet Med Assoc 1992; 201:759–761.

Ruslander D, Kaser-Hotz B, Sardinas JC. Cutaneous squamous cell carcinoma in cats. Compendium Contin Educ Small Anim 1997;19:1119–1129.

Thomas RC, Fox LE. Tumors of the skin and subcutis. In: Morrison WB, ed. Cancer in dogs and cats: medical and surgical management. Baltimore: Williams & Wilkins, 1998:489–510.
Author Joanne C. Graham
Consulting Editor Wallace B. Morrison

SQUAMOUS CELL CARCINOMA, TONGUE

 BASICS

OVERVIEW

• Rare tumor that occurs more commonly in cats than in dogs
• Cats—most commonly located on the ventrolateral surface of the body of the tongue at the level of the reflection of the frenulum
• Dogs—most commonly located on the dorsum of the tongue
• Usually grows rapidly
• Highly metastatic by way of lymphatic vessels to regional lymph nodes and lungs (37%–43% at examination)

SIGNALMENT

• Most dogs and cats middle-aged or old (> 7 years)
• No breed or sex predilection in dogs

SIGNS

Historical Findings

• Excessive salivation ulceration
• Halitosis
• Dysphagia
• Bloody oral discharge
• Weight loss

Physical Examination Findings

• Tongue mass—may be small, white, cauliflower-like, nodular lesions with a broad base on examination
• Loose teeth
• Facial deformity
• Cervical lymphadenomegaly—occasionally

CAUSES & RISK FACTORS

None identified

 DIAGNOSIS

DIFFERENTIAL DIAGNOSIS

• Other lingual malignancy
• Abscess
• Benign polyp

CBC/BIOCHEMISTRY/URINALYSIS

Usually normal

OTHER LABORATORY TESTS

Cytologic—impression smear obtained from an incisional biopsy specimen (wedge); may yield diagnosis

IMAGING

• Skull radiography—rarely demonstrates bone involvement deep to the mass
• Thoracic radiographs—required to evaluate lungs for metastasis

DIAGNOSTIC PROCEDURES

• Extensive physical examination of the cervical region—detect lymphadenomegaly (mandibular and retropharyngeal nodes)
• Deep tissue biopsy—necessary for definitive diagnosis

 TREATMENT

• Surgical—most are inoperable; aggressive excision may be warranted; function of the tongue after recuperation is usually acceptable.
• Postsurgical care (e.g., gastrotomy tube) by owner often required
• Partial glossectomy—may be performed on the rostral half (mobile tongue) or longitudinal half of the tongue (40%–60% removed); more than 50% of patients have incomplete surgical margins.
• Other surgical methods (e.g., electrocautery and cryosurgery) do not offer any additional advantage to conventional excision.
• Cervical lymphadenectomy—rarely curative; perform only for diagnosis or before adjuvant therapy.
• Response to radiotherapy—poor (< 7 weeks)

 MEDICATIONS

DRUG(S)

• Chemotherapy—no effective agents available for local or systemic control

CONTRAINDICATIONS/POSSIBLE INTERACTIONS

Chemotherapy may be toxic; seek advice before initiating treatment if you are unfamiliar with cytotoxic drugs.

 FOLLOW-UP

• Prognosis—grave, owing to extensive local disease and high rate of metastasis
• Few patients survive > 6 months after diagnosis
• Survival after surgical excision—1 year, < 25%
• Survival with incomplete resection and mitoxantrone chemotherapy (1 dog)—27 months
• Survival with incomplete resection and localized radiotherapy combined with cisplatin chemotherapy (1 dog)—6 weeks
• Cause of death—secondary to local recurrence, dysphagia, and subsequent cachexia

 MISCELLANEOUS

Suggested Reading

Carpenter LG, Withrow SJ, Powers BE, et al. Squamous cell carcinoma of the tongue in 10 dogs. J Am Anim Hosp Assoc 1993; 29:17–24.

Evans SM, Shofer F. Canine oral nontonsillar squamous cell carcinoma: prognostic factors for recurrence and survival following orthovoltage radiation therapy. Vet Radiol 1988; 29:133–137.

Schmidt BR, Glickman NW, DeNicola DB, et al. Evaluation of piroxicam for the treatment of oral squamous cell carcinoma in dogs. J Am Vet Med Assoc 2001;218: 1783–1786.

Authors Kevin A. Hahn and Avenelle Turner
Consulting Editor Wallace B. Morrison

SQUAMOUS CELL CARCINOMA, TONSIL

BASICS

OVERVIEW
- Rapid and progressive local invasion by cords of neoplastic squamous epithelium arising from the tonsillar fossa into tonsillar lymphoid tissue
- Local extension common
- Quick to metastasize to lymph nodes (> 98%), lungs (> 63%), and other distant organs (>20%)
- Composes 20%–25% of all oral tumors and 50% of all intraoral tumors in dogs and cats
- Commonly unilateral, affecting the right more than the left tonsil

SIGNALMENT
- Middle-aged or old (range, 2.5–17 years) dogs and cats
- No known breed or sex predilection

SIGNS

Historical Findings
- Excessive salivation
- Halitosis
- Dysphagia
- Bloody oral discharge
- Weight loss

Physical Examination Findings
- Abnormally large tonsil (oral mass)
- Cervical lymphadenomegaly possible

CAUSES & RISK FACTORS
- Exact cause unknown
- Ten times more common in animals living in an urban environment than in those living in a rural environment

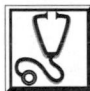

DIAGNOSIS

DIFFERENTIAL DIAGNOSIS
- Lymphoma (generally associated with lymphadenomegaly)
- Abscess
- Salivary gland tumor
- Metastatic neoplasm (melanoma)
- Mast cell tumor
- Tonsillitis

CBC/BIOCHEMISTRY/URINALYSIS
Usually normal

OTHER LABORATORY TESTS
Cytologic—impression smear obtained from an incisional biopsy specimen (wedge); may yield diagnosis

IMAGING
- Skull radiography—rarely demonstrates bone involvement deep to the mass
- Thoracic radiography—detect lung metastasis; 10%–20% positive for metastasis at presentation
- Cervical radiography—evaluate retropharyngeal lymph nodes

DIAGNOSTIC PROCEDURES
- Thorough physical examination of the cervical region—detect abnormally large, regional lymph nodes (e.g., mandibular and retropharyngeal)
- Large, deep tissue biopsy—required to sufficiently differentiate from other oral malignancies

TREATMENT
- Surgery—most are inoperable; aggressive excision may be warranted in patients with airway obstruction; tonsillectomy, when done, should be bilateral.
- Postoperative care (e.g., gastrotomy tube) by owner is often required.
- Other surgical methods (e.g., electrocautery and cryosurgery)—no advantage over conventional excision
- Cervical lymphadenectomy—rarely curative; perform only for diagnosis or before adjuvant therapy.
- Regional radiotherapy—partial responses observed (24–63 Gy) and palliation of signs (3–9 months)

MEDICATIONS

DRUG(S)
Chemotherapy—no effective agents available for local or systemic control; anecdotal reports of cisplatin or bleomycin having been used with limited success

CONTRAINDICATIONS/POSSIBLE INTERACTIONS
Chemotherapy may be toxic; seek advice before initiating treatment if you are unfamiliar with cytotoxic drugs.

FOLLOW-UP
- Prognosis—grave owing to extensive local disease and high rate of metastasis; few patients survive > 6 months after diagnosis
- Local recurrence common with regional extension to tongue, pharynx, and lymph nodes
- Median survival after localized radiotherapy (dogs)—110 days
- Median survival after systemic chemotherapy (dogs)—60–130 days
- Median survival after localized radiotherapy combined with systemic chemotherapy (e.g., doxorubicin and cisplatin; dogs)—270 days
- Survival after surgical excision (dogs)— 1 year, < 10%
- Metastasis—common on examination; leading cause of death regardless of treatment

MISCELLANEOUS

Suggested Reading

Brooks MB, Matus RE, Leifer CE, et al. Chemotherapy versus chemotherapy plus radiotherapy in the treatment of tonsillar squamous cell carcinoma in the dog. J Vet Intern Med 1988;2:206–211.

Buhles WC, Theilen GH. Preliminary evaluation of bleomycin in feline and canine squamous cell carcinoma. Am J Vet Res 1973; 34:289–291.

Postorino-Reeves NC, Turrel JM, Withrow SJ. Oral squamous cell carcinoma in the cat. J Am Anim Hosp Assoc 1993;29:438–441.

Authors Kevin A. Hahn and Avenelle I. Turner
Consulting Editor Wallace B. Morrison

STAPHYLOCOCCAL INFECTIONS

 BASICS

OVERVIEW

• *Staphylococcus*—gram-positive, facultatively anaerobic, spherical bacteria; *staphyle* (Greek; "bunch of grapes") from characteristic microscopic arrangement in clusters; produces a variety of infections characterized by pus formation involving all tissues of the body; can produce toxins (superantigens) that exert profound systemic signs (fever, hypotension, shock, multiorgan failure, death)
• Ubiquitous; live free in environment and as commensal parasites of skin and upper respiratory tract
• Pathogenic and nonpathogenic strains; wide spectrum of virulence, host range, and site specificities; not strictly host or site specific
• Pathogenic strains—possess extracellular toxins and enzymes (e.g., coagulase, staphylokinase, hemolysin, epidermolysins); staphylocoagulase in more pathogenic strains (e.g., *S. aureus, S. intermedius*)

SIGNALMENT

• Dogs and cats
• Very young—susceptible because of incomplete, developing immunity
• Old, debilitated—susceptible because of impaired host defenses
• Immunocompromised—more susceptible

SIGNS

• Fever
• Anorexia
• Pain
• Can affect every organ system
• Abscesses and infections of the skin, eyes, ears, respiratory system, genitourinary tract, skeleton, and joints—common
• Dogs—pyoderma; otitis externa; cystitis; prostatitis; pneumonia; abscesses; osteomyelitis; discospondylitis; arthritis; mastitis; bacteremia; endocarditis; wound infections; toxic shock syndrome
• Cats—abscesses; oral infections; otitis externa; conjunctivitis; metritis; cholangiohepatitis; cystitis; bacteremia

CAUSES & RISK FACTORS

• Opportunistic pathogens
• Disease—from disturbance of the natural host–parasite equilibrium when local and general defense mechanisms are significantly lowered (e.g., chronic debilitating diseases)
• Secondary infection—allergies (atopy, food, fleas); endocrinopathies (hypothyroidism, hyperadrenocorticism); parasites (demodicosis); seborrhea
• Burns or wounds—complications
• Transmission—airborne organisms; carriers; and direct contact (droplet nuclei)

 DIAGNOSIS

DIFFERENTIAL DIAGNOSIS

• Dermatitis—allergies, seborrhea, immune-mediated
• Other infectious causes—viruses, bacteria, fungi, *Rickettsia*, protozoa
• Neoplasia
• Immune-mediated diseases

CBC/BIOCHEMISTRY/URINALYSIS

• Normal or high WBCs
• Biochemistry—may suggest underlying cause (e.g., hypothyroidism, hyperadrenocorticism)
• Urinalysis—pyuria (with or without bacteriuria) with cystitis

OTHER LABORATORY TESTS

• Direct microscopy
• Gram stain
• Cytology—neutrophils and cocci singly or in pairs, short chains, or irregular clusters
• Culture—avoid superficial contamination; collect samples by aspiration, wash, or biopsy; do not overinterpret a positive isolation; organisms can be isolated from normal animals.
• Organisms survive up to 48 hr in clinical specimens when kept cool (4°C; 40°F), particularly on swabs containing a holding medium
• Antibiotic susceptibility testing

IMAGING

Radiology—osteolytic and osteoproliferative lesions with osteomyelitis; interstitial or alveolar pulmonary pattern with pneumonia; radiodense uroliths (struvite)

DIAGNOSTIC PROCEDURES

CSF—if meningitis or discospondylitis suspected

PATHOLOGIC FINDINGS

Characteristic abscess lesion—necrotic tissue, fibrin, and a large number of neutrophils

 TREATMENT

• Properly handle and dispose of contaminated objects.
• Organism resistant to many environmental insults and common disinfectants
• Topical antibacterial cleaning of wounds and pyoderma—may be beneficial

 MEDICATIONS

DRUG(S)

• Antibiotic resistance—great propensity owing to production of β-lactamase, which inactivates penicillins; may carry plasmids (segments of genetic material that may carry genes for antimicrobial resistance) that can be transferred to other strains of staphylococci or species of bacteria
• History of previous antimicrobial therapy for staphylococcal infection—culture and antibiotic susceptibility testing indicated
• Nonpenicillinase-producing strains—penicillin G at 10,000–20,000 U/kg IM, SC q12–24h or penicillin V at 8–30 mg/kg PO q8h
• Penicillinase-producing strains—use penicillinase-resistant drugs
• First-generation cephalosporins—rarely resistant; cephalexin at 22 mg/kg PO q8h; cefadroxil at 22 mg/kg PO q8–12h
• β-lactamase-resistant synthetic penicillins—rarely resistant; oxacillin at 22–40 mg/kg PO q8h; dicloxacillin at 10–25 mg/kg PO q8h; and clavulanic acid-potentiated amoxicillin at 12.5–25 mg/kg PO q8–12h
• Gentamicin—rarely resistant; 2–4 mg/kg IV, IM, SC q8h
• Enrofloxacin—rarely resistant; 2.5–5 mg/kg PO, IM q12h
• Trimethoprim-potentiated sulfonamides—infrequently resistant; 30 mg/kg IV, PO q12h
• Chloramphenicol—infrequently resistant; 40–50 mg/kg IV, IM, SC, PO q8–12h
• Penicillin allergy—try cephalosporin, clindamycin, or vancomycin
• Methicillin-resistant (express mecA gene) *Staphylococcus* occasionally isolated from dogs

CONTRAINDICATIONS/POSSIBLE INTERACTIONS

Avoid immunosuppressive drugs.

 FOLLOW-UP

N/A

 MISCELLANEOUS

ZOONOTIC POTENTIAL

• Possible
• Most people and pets carry their own pathogenic staphylococcal flora; disease not caused by mere exposure

ABBREVIATION

CSF = cerebrospinal fluid

Suggested Reading

Cox HU. Staphylococcal infections. In: Greene CE, ed. Infectious diseases of the dog and cat. Philadelphia: Saunders, 1998: 214–217.
Author J. Paul Woods
Consulting Editor Stephen C. Barr

BASICS

OVERVIEW
• Steatitis is inflammation of fatty tissue.
• Nutrition is involved in the pathology of the condition. Ingestion of large amounts of dietary unsaturated fats without sufficient antioxidant activity may result in peroxidation with subsequent fat necrosis and steatitis. Steatitis can also occur secondary to infection, inflammatory disorder, vasculopathy, neoplasia, and immune-mediated disease. Some cases are idiopathic.
• Rare disease, becoming less prevalent with addition of antioxidants to standard pet food

SIGNALMENT
Species
• Predominantly cats
• Reported in dogs with concurrent diseases (e.g., pancreatic carcinoma)

Breed Predilection
None

Mean Age and Range
• Young to middle-aged cats (4 months–7 years)
• Older dogs

Predominant Sex
None

SIGNS
• Decreased appetite
• Lethargy
• Reluctance to move, jump, play
• Pain with handling or with abdominal palpation
• Fever
• Lumpy subcutaneous tissue (fat)

CAUSES & RISK FACTORS
• Vitamin E deficiency
• Decreased antioxidant capacity with subsequent free-radical peroxidation of lipids
• Oily fish–based diet (red tuna, whitefish, sardines, mackerel); rarely, liver-based diet
• Homemade diet with large fish base
• Large amounts of dietary unsaturated fatty acids
• Obesity

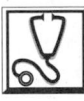

DIAGNOSIS

DIFFERENTIAL DIAGNOSIS
• Nutritional osteodystrophy
• Peritonitis (any cause)
• Subcutaneous abscess, infection
• Spinal meningitis, hyperesthesia (any cause)
• Feline infectious peritonitis (FIP)
• Myositis (any cause)
• Pancreatic disease

CBC/BIOCHEMISTRY/URINALYSIS
• Severe neutrophilic leukocytosis +/− a left shift
• Mild normocytic, normochromic anemia
• Occasional eosinophilia
• Nonspecific changes due to inflammation/fever (mildly elevated liver enzyme activity, creatine kinase elevation, azotemia)
• Blood test results indicative of concurrent disorder

OTHER LABORATORY TESTS
N/A

IMAGING
• Mottled subcutaneous, inguinal, or falciform fat
• Loss of contrast in abdominal cavity

DIAGNOSTIC PROCEDURES
Biopsy

PATHOLOGIC FINDINGS
• Lumpy, granular subcutaneous fat
• Normal to yellowish to orange coloration of body fat
• Fat edema, mineralization, necrosis, with inflammatory infiltrate
• Predominantly neutrophils, mixed inflammation including lymphocytes, plasma cells, and macrophages
• Lobular and septal pyogranulomatous panniculitis
• Intracellular/extracellular ceroid pigment (inert product of unsaturated fatty acid peroxidation)

TREATMENT

NURSING CARE
• Attention to patient comfort level
• Steps to encourage appetite
• Treatment of concurrent disorders

ACTIVITY
Limited owing to discomfort

DIET
• Remove fish products from diet
• Feed nutritionally complete, balanced, commercially prepared cat food
• May require enteral feeding (e.g., PEG-tube, esophagostomy feeding tube)

CLIENT EDUCATION
• Importance of balanced diet
• Any alterations in feline diet must be made gradually

MEDICATIONS

DRUG(S)
• Vitamin E (α-tocopherol acetate), 10–25 IU PO q12h
• Corticosteroids at an anti-inflammatory dose
• S-adenosylmethionine (SAMe) as an antioxidant at 18 mg/kg/day PO

CONTRAINDICATIONS/POSSIBLE INTERACTIONS
Corticosteroids contraindicated with active infection

FOLLOW-UP

PATIENT MONITORING
May require weeks to months for resolution

PREVENTION/AVOIDANCE
Feed a balanced commercial cat food diet.

POSSIBLE COMPLICATIONS
• Anorexia
• Hepatic lipidosis

EXPECTED COURSE AND PROGNOSIS
• Protracted recovery
• Good prognosis once ingestion of proper diet is established

MISCELLANEOUS

ASSOCIATED CONDITIONS
• Pancreatic carcinoma
• Chylous ascites
• Peritonitis

SYNONYMS
• Pansteatitis
• "Yellow fat disease"
• Panniculitis

SEE ALSO
• Adenocarcinoma, pancreas
• Peritonitis

ABBREVIATION
PEG tube = percutaneous endoscopically-placed gastrostomy tube

Suggested Reading
Hoskins JD. Nutrition and Nutritional Problems. In: Hoskins JD, ed. Veterinary pediatrics. 3rd ed. Philadelphia: Saunders, 2001; 487–488.
Author Craig B. Webb
Consulting Editor Deborah S. Greco

STEROID-RESPONSIVE MENINGITIS-ARTERITIS—DOGS

 BASICS

OVERVIEW
• May be acute or protracted
• Lesions—most impressive in CNS, affecting the meninges and the meningeal arteries; also vascular changes in the heart, liver, kidney, and gastrointestinal system
• Genetic factors—may play a role; suspected in beagle colonies
• Worldwide occurrence

SIGNALMENT
• Dogs
• Beagles, Bernese mountain dogs, toller retrievers, and boxers predisposed; every breed can be affected.
• Affects mostly young adult dogs of both sexes; age range 5–18 months

SIGNS
• Classical (acute)—hyperesthesia; cervical rigidity; stiff gait; fever of up to 42°C (107.6°F)
• Protracted—further neurologic deficits, usually reflecting a spinal cord or multifocal lesion

CAUSES & RISK FACTORS
• Cause unknown
• Pathologic and laboratory data and marked response to steroids—suggest an immune-mediated disease related to a dysregulation of IgA production
• Epidemiologic observations—altered immune response may be triggered by an environmental factor, possibly of infectious nature

 DIAGNOSIS

DIFFERENTIAL DIAGNOSIS
• Acute—bacterial meningitis; tumors of the meninges (histiocytosis, meningioma, lymphosarcoma)
• Protracted—bacterial meningitis; tumors of the meninges (histiocytosis, meningioma, lymphosarcoma); viral encephalitides; granulomatous meningoencephalitis; protozoal infections

CBC/BIOCHEMISTRY/URINALYSIS
• Acute—leukocytosis with neutrophilia and left shift; high erythrocyte sedimentation rate
• Protracted—CBC noncontributory

OTHER LABORATORY TESTS
• IgA levels (serum and CSF)—usually high; strongly supports the diagnosis, especially with protracted disease

IMAGING
Myelography, MRI, or CT—exclude tumors

DIAGNOSTIC PROCEDURES

CSF Analysis
• Acute—mild to clear elevation of protein; pleocytosis with several hundreds to thousands of leukocytes, predominantly polymorphonuclear cells
• Protracted—normal or slightly high protein; mild to moderate pleocytosis with mixed cell population or with a predominance of mononuclear cells

PATHOLOGIC FINDINGS

Acute
• Marked meningitis with invasion of macrophages, plasma cells, lymphocytes, and varying numbers of polymorphonuclear cells, mostly in the meninges of the cervical region
• Lesions of the meningeal arteries—more degenerative with perivascular inflammation

Protracted
• Marked fibrous thickening and focal mineralization of the leptomeninges
• Arterial walls—many are thickened with considerable stenosis owing to cellular proliferation of the intima and fibrosis.

 TREATMENT

• Inpatient—at onset, fluid therapy and ice packs useful for high body temperature
• Outpatient—after initial treatment, owners may dispense medication.
• Regular controls—must be initiated; inform owner about side effects of long-term steroid treatment.
• Activity—do not alter (prevention of muscle atrophy).

STEROID-RESPONSIVE MENINGITIS-ARTERITIS—DOGS

 MEDICATIONS

DRUG(S)
• Initial signs and pleocytosis of the CSF mild—NSAIDs; carefully monitor the patient.
• First relapse or symptoms become worse with massive pleocytosis in the CSF—start long-term treatment (6 months) with prednisolone (4 mg/kg PO q24h for 1–2 days; then taper slowly); re-examine patient (including a CSF collection and blood profile) every 4–6 weeks after the initiation of therapy
• Neurologic examination and CSF become normal—reduce steroid dose
• Persistent pleocytosis—continue same steroid dosage
• Treatment may be stopped after about 6 months.
• Immunosuppressive drugs (purine analogs)—azathioprine (1.5 mg/kg PO q48h) if patient does not respond well to prednisolone alone; used in combination
• Consider protecting patient against ulceration in the gastrointestinal tract.

CONTRAINDICATIONS/POSSIBLE INTERACTIONS
• Corticosteroids—high-dose treatment can lead to serious complications; nonlife threatening side effects (polyuria, polydipsia, polyphagia and weight gain); not tolerated in about 5% of dogs

 FOLLOW-UP

PATIENT MONITORING
Clinical control examinations—every 4–6 weeks; include blood examination and CSF collection; until steroids discontinued

PREVENTION/AVOIDANCE
Strictly control treatment schedule to prevent frequent relapses.

POSSIBLE COMPLICATIONS
• Hypoxic lesions of the spinal cord or the brain—protracted disease; may result in gait abnormalities and seizures
• Side effects of immunosuppressive treatment—bacterial infections; bleeding in the gastrointestinal tract; pancreatitis

EXPECTED COURSE AND PROGNOSIS
• Acute—prognosis relatively good in young dogs and with early aggressive therapy
• Protracted cases with frequent relapses—prognosis guarded; controlled studies note about 60% of dogs are cured after immunosuppressive treatment

 MISCELLANEOUS

ASSOCIATED CONDITIONS
Polyarthritis

AGE-RELATED FACTORS
Old animals do not tolerate long-term steroid treatment well; but condition is rare in dogs > 5 years of age.

PREGNANCY
Avoid pregnancy during treatment.

SEE ALSO
• Juvenile Polyarteritis (Beagle Pain Syndrome)

SYNONYMS
• Aseptic meningitis
• Canine juvenile polyarteritis syndrome
• Corticosteroid-responsive meningomyelitis

ABBREVIATIONS
• CNS = central nervous system
• CSF = cerebrospinal fluid
• CT = computed tomography
• NSAID = nonsteroidal antiinflammatory drug

Suggested Reading
Cizinauskas S, Jaggy A, Tipold A. Long-term treatment of dogs with steroid-responsive meningitis-arteritis: clinical, laboratory and therapeutic results. J Small Anim Pract 2000;41:295–301.
Author Andrea Tipold
Consulting Editor Joane M. Parent

STERTOR AND STRIDOR

BASICS

DEFINITION
• Abnormally loud sounds that result from air passing through a narrowed nasopharynx, pharynx, larynx, or trachea and meeting resistance because of partial obstruction of these regions
• Discontinuous sounds heard without a stethoscope
• **Stertor**—low-pitched snoring sound that usually arises from the vibration of flaccid tissue or fluid; usually arises from pharyngeal airway obstruction
• **Stridor**—higher-pitched sounds that result when relatively rigid tissues are vibrated by the passage of air; result of nasal or laryngeal partial or complete obstruction or cervical tracheal collapse

PATHOPHYSIOLOGY
• Airway obstruction causes turbulence as air passes through a narrowed passage; with worsening obstruction or increasing air velocity, the amplitude of the sound increases as the tissue, secretion, or foreign body composing the obstruction is vibrated.
• Obstruction sufficient to increase the work of breathing causes increased respiratory muscle effort, and the turbulence is exacerbated; inflammation and edema of the tissues in the region of the obstruction may develop, further reducing the airway lumen and further increasing the work of breathing, creating a vicious circle.

SYSTEM AFFECTED
Respiratory

SIGNALMENT

Species
Dogs and cats

Breed Predilections
• Common in brachycephalic breeds
• Inherited laryngeal paralysis—identified in Bouvier des Flandres, Siberian husky, bulldogs, and Dalmatians
• Acquired laryngeal paralysis—over-represented in certain giant breeds (e.g., St. Bernards and Newfoundlands) and large breeds (e.g., Irish setters, Labradors, and golden retrievers)

Mean Age and Range
• Affected brachycephalic dogs and dogs with inherited laryngeal paralysis are typically younger than 1 year of age when owners detect a problem.
• Acquired laryngeal paralysis typically occurs in older dogs.
• Cats—diagnosed less commonly than are dogs; no obvious age pattern

Predominant Sex
• No sex predilection for any cause, although inherited laryngeal paralysis, has a 3:1 male predominance

SIGNS
• Change or loss of voice
• Partial obstruction—produces an increase in airway sounds before producing an obvious change in respiratory pattern or gas exchange
• Owners may indicate that the sound has existed for as long as several years.
• Breath sounds audible from a distance without a stethoscope—suspect narrowing of upper airway.
• Nature of the sound—ranges from abnormally loud to obvious fluttering to high-pitched squeaking, depending on the degree of airway narrowing
• May note increased respiratory effort and paradoxical respiratory movements (chest wall collapses inward during inspiration and springs outward during expiration) when the effort is extreme; are often accompanied by obvious postural changes (e.g., abducted forelimbs, extended head and neck, and open-mouth breathing)

CAUSES
• Brachycephalic airway syndrome (stenotic nares, elongated soft palate, laryngeal edema, collapsed larynx, everted or edematous laryngeal saccules)
• Nasopharyngeal stenosis
• Laryngeal paralysis—inherited or acquired
• Laryngeal neoplasia—benign or malignant
• Granulomatous laryngitis
• Tracheal collapse
• Tracheal stenosis
• Tracheal neoplasia
• Tracheal foreign bodies
• Nasopharyngeal polyps
• Acromegaly
• Neuromuscular dysfunction (e.g., myasthenia gravis, brain stem disease, polyneuropathy, polymyopathy, hypothyroidism)
• Anesthesia or sedation—only if predisposing anatomy exists
• Cystic Rathke cleft
• Cleft soft palate
• Aplasia of soft palate
• Redundant pharyngeal mucosal fold
• Soft palate mass
• Nasopharyngeal mass
• Edema or inflammation of the palate, pharynx, and larynx (including everted mucosal lining of the laryngeal ventricles)—secondary to coughing, vomiting or regurgitation, turbulent airflow, upper respiratory infection, and hemorrhage
• Secretions (e.g., pus, mucus, and blood) in the airway lumen—acutely after surgery; a normal conscious animal would cough out or swallow them
• Foreign bodies in the airway lumen

RISK FACTORS
• High ambient temperature
• Fever
• High metabolic rate—as occurs with hyperthyroidism or sepsis
• Exercise
• Anxiety or excitement
• Any respiratory or cardiovascular disease that increases ventilation
• Turbulence caused by the increased airflow may lead to swelling and worsen the airway obstruction
• Eating or drinking

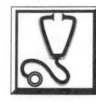

DIAGNOSIS

DIFFERENTIAL DIAGNOSIS
• Must differentiate sounds of pharyngeal, laryngeal, and tracheal narrowing from sounds arising elsewhere in the respiratory system
• The entire area from cricopharynx to trachea is auscultated for areas of high-pitched sounds caused by narrowing.
• Nasal and tracheal narrowing and severe or extensive narrowing of the bronchi—may cause increased respiratory sounds
• If the sound persists when the patient opens its mouth, a nasal cause can virtually be ruled out.
• If the sound occurs only during expiration, it is likely that intrathoracic airway narrowing is the cause.
• If the abnormal sounds are loudest during inspiration, they are from extrathoracic disease.
• If the owner describes a change in voice, the larynx is the likely abnormal site.
• Without helpful indicators, systematically auscultate over the nose, pharynx, larynx, and trachea to identify the point of maximal intensity of any abnormal sound and to identify the phase of respiration when it is most obvious.
• Important to identify the anatomic location from which the abnormal sound arises and to seek exacerbating causes (see Risk Factors; e.g., a chronic airway obstruction may become manifest when the patient is exposed to extremely high ambient temperatures)

CBC/BIOCHEMISTRY/URINALYSIS
N/A

OTHER LABORATORY TESTS
N/A

IMAGING
• Lateral radiographs of the head and neck—may help identify abnormal soft tissues of the airway (e.g., elongated soft palate or a nasal polyp); limited use for identifying laryngeal paralysis, although experienced radiographers can identify abnormally dilated or swollen laryngeal saccules; cartilaginous destruction is

suggestive of neoplasia or granulomatous laryngitis; may allow further evaluation of external masses compressing the upper airway
• Radiography and fluoroscopy—important for assessing the cardiorespiratory system; rule out other or additional causes of respiratory difficulty; such conditions may add to an underlying upper airway obstruction, causing a subclinical condition to become symptomatic.

DIAGNOSTIC PROCEDURES

Pharyngoscopy and Laryngoscopy
• Definitive diagnostic tests for direct visualization of pharyngeal or laryngeal changes
• Require heavy sedation that preserves laryngeal function
• Remember that the patient's ability to use muscles to open the airway is compromised by anesthesia; veterinarian and clients must determine if they are prepared to carry out surgical remedies if indicated
• If correctable conditions are not identified and corrected—patient's recovery from anesthesia may be complicated by severe airway obstruction; must be prepared to perform a tracheostomy if airway is obstructed and a definitive surgical remedy cannot be pursued immediately
• Assess timing and degree of movement of the vocal folds during light anesthesia—evaluate laryngeal paralysis.
• Normal palate—thin; just barely overlaps the tips of the epiglottis; easily displaced dorsally using the blade of the laryngoscope
• Overlong soft palate—thick; usually inflamed; may lie as much as 1 cm or more past the tip of the epiglottis
• Patient should be as stable as possible before undergoing general anesthesia, but do not unduly delay procedure; appropriate surgical treatment is usually the only means of reducing the airway obstruction

TREATMENT
• Keep patient cool, quiet, and calm—anxiety, exertion, and pain lead to increased ventilation, potentially worsening the obstruction.
• Hypoxia and hypoventilation occur with prolonged severe obstruction; supplemental oxygen not always critical for sustaining patients with partial airway collapse
• Closely monitor effects of sedatives; sedatives may relax the upper airway muscles and worsen the obstruction; be prepared with emergency means for securing the airway if complete obstruction occurs. Diazepam preferred

• Extreme airway obstruction—attempt an emergency intubation; if obstruction prevents intubation, emergency tracheostomy or passage of a tracheal catheter to administer oxygen may be the only available means for sustaining life; a tracheal catheter can only briefly sustain oxygenation while a more permanent solution is sought.
• Utilization of small balloon catheters may be useful in dislodging foreign bodies.
• Surgery—biopsy (histopathology), management (tracheostomy while awaiting pathology reports or resolving inflam-mation/infection), or resolution (excision, correction of defect, removal of foreign bodies)

MEDICATIONS

DRUG(S)
• Medical approaches—appropriate only if the underlying cause is infection, edema, inflammation, or hemorrhage; anatomic or neurologic causes are not amenable to symptomatic medical treatment.
• Steroids—may be indicated if edema or inflammation is thought to be an important contributor; effect with intravenous administration should be apparent in approximately 1 hr

CONTRAINDICATIONS
N/A

PRECAUTIONS
Sedatives and anesthetics

POSSIBLE INTERACTIONS
N/A

ALTERNATIVE DRUG(S)
N/A

FOLLOW-UP

PATIENT MONITORING
Respiratory rate and effort need to be closely monitored. When owner chooses to take an apparently stable patient home, or if continual observation is not feasible, inform client that complete obstruction could occur

PREVENTION/AVOIDANCE
Advise client to avoid exercise, high ambient temperatures, and extreme excitement.

POSSIBLE COMPLICATIONS
• Serious complications may occur without therapy to relieve the obstruction; these include airway edema, pulmonary edema

(may progress to life-threatening acute lung injury), and hypoventilation; may require tracheostomy and/or artificial ventilation.
• Take particular care when inducing general anesthesia or when using sedatives in any patient with upper airway obstruction.
• Inform client that the patient can make the transition from being a noisy breather to having an obstructed airway in a few minutes or even seconds.

EXPECTED COURSE AND PROGNOSIS
• Varies with underlying cause
• Even with surgical treatment, some degree of obstruction may remain for 7–10 days due to swelling.

MISCELLANEOUS

ASSOCIATED CONDITIONS
N/A

AGE-RELATED FACTORS
N/A

ZOONOTIC POTENTIAL
N/A

PREGNANCY
N/A

SYNONYM
Snoring

SEE ALSO
• Acromegaly—Cats
• Brachycephalic Airway Syndrome
• Hypothyroidism
• Laryngeal Disease
• Myasthenia Gravis
• Nasal and Nasopharyngeal Polyps
• Tracheal Collapse

Suggested Reading
Hendricks JC. Brachycephalic airway syn-drome. Update on respiratory disease. Vet Clin North Am Small Anim Pract 1989; 19:1167–1188.
Hendricks JC. Respiratory condition in criti-cal patients. Vet Clin North Am Small Anim Pract 1989;19:1167–1188.
Nelson AW. Upper respiratory system. In: Slatter D, ed. Textbook of small animal surgery. 2nd ed. Philadelphia: Saunders, 1993:733–776.

Acknowledgment
The author and editors acknowledge the prior contributions of Dr. Joan C. Hendricks, who authored this topic in the previous edition.

Author James C. Prueter
Consulting Editor Lynelle R. Johnson

STOMATITIS

BASICS

DEFINITION
An inflammation of the soft tissues of the oral cavity, which may be caused by many different stimuli of local or systemic origin.

PATHOPHYSIOLOGY
Inflammation and other changes may develop in the normal oral mucosa because of the tremendous amount of vasculature in the area and its proximity to the external environment.

SYSTEMS AFFECTED
• Gastrointestinal—prehension and mastication
• Behavioral—varying degrees of interest in food may result; patients may approach food and attempt to masticate with varying degrees of difficulty.
• Ophthalmic—periorbital swelling, exophthalmos, protrusion of nictitating membrane, resistance to retropulsion of the globe, orbital cellulitis, conjunctivitis, and other ophthalmic manifestations of posterior maxillary disease because of its proximity to the orbital structures
• Skin/Exocrine—may be inflammation of the skin around the lips because of ptyalism; other conditions may affect the skin around the oral cavity because of its proximity to lesions affecting the cheek or lips

SIGNALMENT
• Dog and cat
• Ulcerative stomatitis in Maltese—higher incidence in males
• Juvenile-onset periodontitis in young cats

• Oral eosinophilic granuloma—most commonly in Siberian husky (may be hereditary)
• Gingival hyperplasia in large breeds
• Rapidly progressive periodontitis seen mostly in young adult animals such as the greyhound and the shih tzu
• Lymphocytic plasmocytic stomatitis in cats
• Localized juvenile periodontitis in the maxillary or mandibular incisor region—especially common in miniature schnauzer

SIGNS
• Halitosis
• Pain
• Ulcerated lesions
• Ptyalism
• Edema
• Extensive plaque and calculus

CAUSES

Anatomic
• Periodontal disease due to overcrowding of teeth
• Lip frenulum attachment
• Tight-lip syndrome in shar-pei

Metabolic
• Uremia and high ammonia levels in saliva
• Vasculitis and xerostomia seen with diabetes mellitus
• Macroglossia and puffy lips as seen with hypoparathyroidism

Immune-Mediated
• Pemphigus foliaceous
• Pemphigus vulgaris
• Bullous pemphigoid
• Systemic lupus erythematosus and discoid lupus erythematosus in the dog
• Acute hypersensitivity to drugs

Infectious
• Opportunistic oral flora secondary to oral lesions

• Mycotic stomatitis
• Systemic infections
• Leptospirosis: petechia
• Feline leprosy (mycobacterium): raised plaques
• Calicivirus or herpesvirus infections—cat
• Canine distemper
• Viral papillomatosis—dogs

Trauma
• Irritation from calculus
• Foreign objects—gum-chewers syndrome
• Electrical cord shock
• Chemical burns
• Lacerations
• Snake bite
• Blows
• Trauma of the palate from base-narrow mandibular canine teeth

Toxic
• Certain plants
• Chemotherapy
• Radiotherapy
• Chemical irritants

RISK FACTORS
N/A

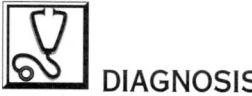

DIAGNOSIS

DIFFERENTIAL DIAGNOSIS
• Oral ulcers
• Chronic ulcerative periodontal stomatitis (CUPS)
• Idiopathic osteomyelitis

CBC/BIOCHEMISTRY/URINALYSIS
Useful to detect systemic disease

OTHER LABORATORY TESTS
• Immunologic testing
• Mycotic cultures

- Virus isolation
- Toxicologic studies
- Serum protein electrophoresis
- Endocrine tests

IMAGING

Radiography to identify osseous or dental abnormalities

DIAGNOSTIC PROCEDURES

Biopsy

TREATMENT

- Correct nutritional or hydration deficiencies as needed, on an inpatient or outpatient basis
- Can place feeding tube if necessary
- Dental disease or periodontal disease present should be treated
- Sometimes most or all teeth must be extracted to resolve stomatitis.

MEDICATIONS

DRUG(S) OF CHOICE

Antimicrobials
- Broad-spectrum antibiotics
- Amoxicillin-clavulanate
- Clindamycin
- Metronidazole—10 mg/kg q12h PO or 40–50 mg/kg as a loading dose on the first day, followed by 20–25 mg/kg q8h for 7 days or less
- Doxycycline—5 mg/kg PO loading dose, 2.5 mg/kg PO 12 h later, and 2.5 mg/kg PO once daily thereafter
- Chlorhexidine solution or gel (CHX, VRx Products, Harbor City, CA)—plaque retardant

- Maxi-Guard (Addison Biological Laboratory, Fayette, MO) zinc-organic acid solutions and gels to promote tissue healing and retard plaque accumulation

Antiinflammatory Drugs
- Prednisolone or prednisone
- For eosinophilic ulcer: 2–4.4 mg/kg PO once a day; for chronic cases use 0.5–1.0 mg/kg PO every other day.
- For adjunctive therapy of feline plasma cell gingivitis–pharyngitis; may improve inflammation and appetite

CONTRAINDICATIONS
- Hypersensitivity to medication
- Glucocorticoid use with systemic mycotic infections

PRECAUTIONS
N/A

POSSIBLE INTERACTIONS
N/A

ALTERNATIVE DRUG(S)
N/A

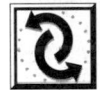

FOLLOW-UP

PATIENT MONITORING
- Laboratory tests when systemic disease is involved
- Oral rinses and brushing the teeth with oral medications may be helpful, especially with periodontal disease.

POSSIBLE COMPLICATIONS
Bacteremia from periodontal disease can cause renal, cardiac, hepatic, and pulmonary disease.

MISCELLANEOUS

ASSOCIATED CONDITIONS
Periodontal disease is probably the leading cause of other oral disorders.

AGE-RELATED FACTORS
Periodontal disease associated with calculus is seen most often in old dogs and cats and in susceptible breeds.

ZOONOTIC POTENTIAL
- Dental prophylaxis procedures have caused human infections.
- Safety glasses and a mask are recommended when performing such procedures.

PREGNANCY
N/A

SYNONYMS
- Trench mouth
- St. Vincent's stomatitis, an ulceromembranous stomatitis due to *Fusobacterium* spp. and spirochetes

SEE ALSO
N/A

ABBREVIATIONS
N/A

Suggested Reading
Harvey CE, Emily PP. Oral lesions of soft tissues and bone: differential diagnosis. In: Harvey CE, Emily PP, eds. Small animal dentistry. St. Louis: CV Mosby, 1993:42–88.
Wiggs RB, Lobprise HB. Veterinary dentistry. Philadelphia: Lippincott-Raven. 1997:104–139.
Author Larry Baker
Consulting Editor Heidi B. Lobprise

STREPTOCOCCAL INFECTIONS

BASICS

OVERVIEW
• *Streptococcus*—gram-positive, nonmotile, spherical bacteria; grow in pairs or chains; commensal organisms; normal flora of the upper respiratory tract, oropharynx, lower genital tract, and skin; under appropriate conditions, capable of infecting all areas of body; primary infections involve respiratory, circulatory, integumentary, urogenital, or central nervous systems; frequent secondary invader of body tissues
• Classified by ability to hemolyze RBCs and produce zone on blood agar plates around bacterial colony—α-hemolytic (green zone of partial hemolysis); β-hemolytic (clear zone of hemolysis); γ-hemolytic (no change; non-hemolytic); β-hemolytic usually more pathogenic than α-hemolytic, which is more pathogenic than nonhemolytic strains
• Hemolytic strains further subdivided by antigenic differences in cell wall carbohydrates—Lancefield serogroups A–H and K–T (e.g., group G *S. canis*); some groups more likely to be associated with disease, depending on species (e.g., group G associated with cats and dogs; group A associated with humans)
• Produce exotoxins—streptolysins (hemolysins), streptokinases, deoxyribonucleases, and hyaluronidases

SIGNALMENT
• Dogs and cats
• Very young—more prone to infection because of incomplete, developing immunity; particularly kittens born to primiparous queen

SIGNS
• Vary with site of infection and host immunocompetence
• Weakness
• Coughing
• Dyspnea
• Fever
• Hematemesis
• Hematuria
• Lymphadenopathy
• Dogs—septicemia; endometritis; vaginitis; mastitis; fading puppies; abortion; urinary tract infection; pyelonephritis; pneumonia; necrotizing fasciitis; streptococcal shock syndrome
• Cats—septicemia; peritonitis; cervical lymphadenitis; pharyngitis; tonsillitis; fading kitten

CAUSES & RISK FACTORS
• Age, exposure, and immune response—important for determining disease
• Virulence—depends on cellular products, surface components, and related substances
• Opportunistic—wounds, trauma, surgical procedures, viral infections, or immuno-suppressive conditions
• FeLV, FIP, immunodeficiency, respiratory viral infections, feline lower urinary tract disease—predisposing conditions
• Maternal antibodies generally protect puppies and kittens against clinical disease.
• Carrier state occurs

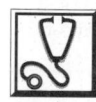

DIAGNOSIS

DIFFERENTIAL DIAGNOSIS
Other infectious causes—viruses, bacteria, fungi, *Rickettsia*, protozoa

CBC/BIOCHEMISTRY/URINALYSIS
• Normal or high WBCs with neutrophilic inflammatory response with a left shift or degenerative left shift
• Cocci—may be found in circulating neutrophils in overwhelming sepsis
• Biochemistry—may suggest predisposing conditions
• Urinalysis—pyuria (with or without bacteruria) with cystitis

OTHER LABORATORY TESTS
• Direct microscopy
• Gram stain—of exudates; reveals chains of and single gram-positive cocci
• Culture—affected tissues; exudate or needle aspirates; confirms diagnosis
• Antibiotic susceptibility testing

IMAGING
Radiographs—interstitial or alveolar pulmonary pattern with pneumonia; radiodense uroliths (struvite)

DIAGNOSTIC PROCEDURES
N/A

PATHOLOGIC FINDINGS
• Acute inflammation—gross or microscopic abscesses
• Septicemia—postmortem reveals omphalophlebitis, peritonitis, hepatitis, pneumonia, and myocarditis.

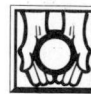

TREATMENT
• Good nursing care
• Rehydrate.
• Drain and flush abscess.
• Debride necrotic tissue.

MEDICATIONS

DRUG(S)
• Penicillin—first choice; penicillin G at 10,000–20,000 U/kg IM, SC q12–24h or penicillin V at 8–30 mg/kg PO q8h
• Ampicillin—20–30 mg/kg IV, IM, SC, PO q8h; alone or in combination with gentamicin at 2–4 mg/kg IV, IM, SC q8h; for group B
• Prophylactic treatment—all kittens born to primiparous queens indicated for neonatal infections

CONTRAINDICATIONS/POSSIBLE INTERACTIONS
Avoid immunosuppressive drugs

FOLLOW-UP

PREVENTION/AVOIDANCE
• Avoid overcrowding and poor environmental sanitation
• Prevention in newborns—dipping navel and umbilical cord in 2% tincture of iodine
• Prevention in colonies—avoid overcrowding; maintain clean feeders; segregate infected animals.

MISCELLANEOUS

ZOONOTIC POTENTIAL
• Dogs and cats may show no clinical signs with group A streptococci but may serve as a reservoir for human infection.
• Streptococci isolated from people are usually of human not animal origin.

ABBREVIATIONS
• FeLV = feline leukemia virus
• FIP = feline infectious peritonitis

Suggested Reading
Greene CE, Prescott JF. Streptococcal and other gram-positive bacterial infections. In: Greene CE, ed. Infectious diseases of the dog and cat. Philadelphia: Saunders, 1998: 205–214.
Author J. Paul Woods
Consulting Editor Stephen C. Barr

STRONGYLOIDIASIS

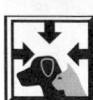 **BASICS**

OVERVIEW
• Neonatal infection of paramucosa of small intestine by *Strongyloides stercoralis* (*canis*)
• Transcolostral transmission to neonates, skin penetration by infective larvae, or ingestion of infective larvae; may persist by autoinfection
• Relatively host-specific; possibly transmission to humans
• Cats: natural *S. stercoralis* infection not reported; *S. tumefaciens* causes parasite containing adenomatous mass in colon.

SIGNALMENT
• Dogs and cats
• Neonatal diarrhea of pups and kittens with transcolostral transmission

SIGNS

Historical Findings
• Neonatal diarrhea or constipation
• Dermatitis

Physical Examination Findings
• Debilitated pups or kittens
• Dermatitis

CAUSES & RISK FACTORS
• Transcolostral transmission
• Possibility of autoinfection
• Skin penetration by infective larvae

 DIAGNOSIS

DIFFERENTIAL DIAGNOSIS
• *Toxocara* infections
• Viral infections

CBC/BIOCHEMISTRY/URINALYSIS
Usually normal

OTHER LABORATORY TESTS
N/A

IMAGING
N/A

DIAGNOSTIC PROCEDURES
• Fecal examination for small (~ 50 μm long), larvated eggs
• Concentrate and examine fluid from fresh or cultured feces for filariform larvae.

 TREATMENT

Usually outpatient unless intravenous fluid supplementation needed for dehydration

 MEDICATIONS

DRUG(S)
Adulticide/larvicide recommended for neonatal infection of small intestine with possible respiratory migration by infective larvae
• Fenbendazole 50 mg/kg PO q24h PO for 5 days
• Anthelmintic use extra-label
• Ivermectin 0.2 mg/kg SC as single dose; repeat treatment may be needed
• Thiabendazole 100–150 mg/kg PO 3 days repeated weekly until feces negative for larvae

CONTRAINDICATIONS/POSSIBLE INTERACTIONS
Difficulty with administration of efficacious anthelmintic

 FOLLOW-UP

• Fecal examination for *Strongyloides* larvae or eggs posttreatment
• Repeat exam monthly for 6 mo post treatment.

 MISCELLANEOUS

ZOONOTIC POTENTIAL
Humans may experience dermatitis and severe abdominal discomfort.

Suggested Reading
Bowman DD, Lynn RC, Eberhard ML. Georgi's parasitology for veterinarians, 8th ed. St. Louis: Saunders (Elsevier Science), 2003:197–201, 290–291, 305.
Bowman DD, Hendrix CM, Lindsay DS, Barr SC. Feline clinical parasitology. Ames: Iowa State University Press, 2002:235–241.

Acknowledgment
The author and editors acknowledge the prior contributions of Dr. Robert M. Corwin, who authored this topic in the previous edition.
Author Julie Ann Jarvinen
Consulting Editor Albert E. Jergens

STRYCHNINE POISONING

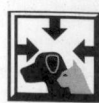

BASICS

OVERVIEW
• Strychnine—potent convulsant; alkaloid toxin; derived from the seeds of *Strychnos nux-vomica* and *S. ignatii;* used to kill rats, moles, gophers, and predators
• Rapid absorption
• Onset of clinical signs—10 min to 2 hr
• Effects—reversibly blocks the binding of the inhibitory neurotransmitter glycine; results in an unchecked reflex stimulation; eliminated as hepatic metabolites and as the parent compound in the urine
• Cause of death—apnea and hypoxia due to rigidity of the respiration muscles
• Baits—containing > 0.5% strychnine limited to use by certified applicators; containing < 0.5% strychnine available to the general public

SIGNALMENT
Dogs and cats

SIGNS
• Violent tetanic seizures—may be initiated by physical, visible, or auditory stimuli
• Extensor rigidity
• Muscle stiffness
• Opisthotonus
• Tachycardia
• Hyperthermia
• Apnea
• Vomiting—rare

CAUSES & RISK FACTORS
• Malicious poisoning—fairly common
• Direct exposure to baits—more common in dogs than other species
• Relay toxicosis by the ingestion of poisoned rodents and birds has occurred.
• LD_{50}—dogs, > 0.2 mg/kg; cats, 0.5 mg/kg

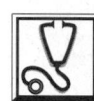

DIAGNOSIS

DIFFERENTIAL DIAGNOSES
• Other toxicants—lead; nicotine; amphetamines; metaldehyde; chocolate; zinc phosphide; tremorogenic mycotoxins; antidepressants; 4-aminopyridine; cocaine; pyrethrins or pyrethroids; 1080 (fluoroacetate); caffeine; LSD; organochlorine insecticides
• Systemic diseases—uremia; hepatic failure; neoplasia; hypoglycemia; encephalitides; heat stroke; trauma; ischemia; tetanus

CBC/BIOCHEMISTRY/URINALYSIS
• High creatine kinase and lactate dehydrogenase
• Myoglobinuria

OTHER LABORATORY TESTS
• Analysis of stomach content, liver, kidney, or urine—reveal strychnine; if death is too rapid, kidney and urine are negative
• Blood gases—reveal acidosis

IMAGING
N/A

DIAGNOSTIC PROCEDURES
• **CAUTION:** do not induce a seizure with a stimulus; it is *not* diagnostic and may be lethal.
• Blood pressure—may reveal systemic hypertension

PATHOLOGIC FINDINGS
• Associated with trauma from the seizure activity
• Baits—often found in the stomach contents; may be color-coded red or green

 TREATMENT

GENERAL LIFE SUPPORT
• Inpatient—may require treatment for as long as 48 hr
• Primary goals—prevent asphyxia; control seizures; may require complete anesthesia and artificial respiration
• Keep patient in a quiet, dimly lit room.
• Cool water baths—for hyperthermia

DECONTAMINATION
• Lessens duration and severity of signs
• Gastric or enterogastric lavage—lessens absorption
• Fluid diuresis—enhances elimination; normal saline with 5% mannitol (7 mg/kg/hr)

• Emesis—do not induce unless it is within minutes of the ingestion and the patient is asymptomatic

 MEDICATIONS

DRUG(S)
• Decontamination—activated charcoal (2 g/kg); cathartic (sorbitol at 2.1 g/kg or magnesium sulfate at 0.5 g/kg)
• Seizure control—diazepam (may not be effective); pentobarbital (to effect); glycerol guaiacolate (110 mg/kg IV, repeated as needed); methocarbamol (150 mg/kg IV, repeated at 90 mg/kg as needed); inhalation anesthesia
• Urinary acidification—ammonium chloride (150 mg/kg); enhances elimination

CONTRAINDICATIONS/POSSIBLE INTERACTIONS
• Do not acidify with ammonium chloride if the patient is acidotic.

• Do not use ketamine.
• Do not use morphine.

 FOLLOW-UP

• Monitor for secondary renal damage from myoglobinuria and possible tubular cast development.
• Prognosis—guarded until seizures are controlled; good after seizures are controlled

 MISCELLANEOUS

SEE ALSO
Poisoning (Intoxication)

Suggested Reading
Osweiler GD. Strychnine poisoning. In: Kirk RW, ed. Current veterinary therapy VIII. Philadelphia: Saunders, 1983:98–100.
Author Jeffery O. Hall
Consulting Editor Gary D. Osweiler

STUPOR AND COMA

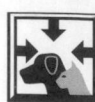

BASICS

DEFINITION
• Stupor—unconscious but arousable with noxious stimuli • Coma—unconscious and not arousable with noxious stimuli

PATHOPHYSIOLOGY
ARAS—network of neurons situated in the core of the brain stem; functions as the arousal system for the cerebral cortex; any severe pathologic change (either anatomic or metabolic) that causes interruption can lead to depression, stupor, or coma.

SYSTEMS AFFECTED
• Nervous • Cardiovascular • Respiratory • Ophthalmic

SIGNALMENT
• Dogs and cats • No breed, age, or sex predilection

SIGNS

Historical Findings
• The possibility of trauma or unsupervised roaming • Past medical problems of significance—diabetes mellitus and insulin therapy; hypoglycemia; cardiovascular problems; hypoxic episodes; renal failure; liver failure; neoplasia • Record a description of the patient's environment—possible heatstroke; hypothermia; drowning; exposure to drugs, narcotics, and toxins (e.g., ethylene glycol, lead, anticoagulants), including owner's medications • Onset may be acute or slowly progressive, depending on underlying cause.

Physical Examination Findings
• Look for evidence of external or internal trauma. • Examine for severe hypothermia or hyperthermia. • Evidence of hypoxia or cyanosis, ecchymosis or petechiation, or cardiac or respiratory insufficiency—warrants investigation for metabolic causes • Carefully palpate for evidence of neoplasia. • Retinal hemorrhages or distended vessels—hypertension • Papilledema—cerebral edema • Retinal detachment—infectious, neoplastic, or hypertensive causes • Chorioretinitis—infectious causes (distemper, FeLV-related diseases, toxoplasmosis, cryptococcosis, or FIP) • Sustained bradycardia (with normal serum potassium)—midbrain, pontine, or medullary lesion

Neurologic Examination Findings
• Determine level of consciousness and whether patient is arousable.
• Pupillary light reflexes—small responsive pupils: cerebral or diencephalic lesion; dilated unresponsive pupils (unilateral or bilateral) or fixed in midposition: midbrain or severe medullary lesions
• Oculocephalic reflex (when cervical manipulation is possible)—loss of physiologic vestibular nystagmus: brain stem involvement

• Respiratory patterns—Cheyne-Stokes respiration: severe, diffuse cerebral or diencephalic lesion; hyperventilation: midbrain lesion; ataxic or apneustic breathing: pons or medulla lesion
• Cranial nerves—no deficits with lesion of cerebrum-diencephalon; deficits of cranial nerve III: midbrain lesion; deficits of cranial nerves V–XII: pons and medulla lesions
• Postural changes—decerebrate rigidity: midbrain lesion

CAUSES
• Drugs—narcotics; depressants; ivermectin
• Anatomic—hydrocephalus
• Metabolic—severe hypoglycemia; hyperglycemia; hyperosmolar syndromes; hypernatremia; hyponatremia; hepatic encephalopathy; hypoxemia; hypercarbia; hypothermia; hyperthermia; hypotension; coagulopathies; renal failure; lysosomal storage disease
• Nutritional—hypoglycemia; thiamine deficiency
• Neoplastic (primary)—meningioma; astrocytoma; gliomas; choroid plexus papilloma; pituitary adenoma; others
• Metastatic—hemangiosarcoma; lymphosarcoma; mammary carcinoma; others
• Inflammatory noninfectious—granulomatous meningoencephalomyelitis
• Infectious—bacterial; viral (distemper, FIP); parasitic (aberrant larva migrans); protozoal (neosporosis, toxoplasmosis); fungal (cryptococcosis, blastomycosis, histoplasmosis, coccidioidomycosis, actinomycosis); rickettsial
• Idiopathic—epilepsy (poststatus epilepticus)
• Immune-mediated—vasculitis and thrombocytopenia leading to hemorrhage
• Traumatic
• Toxins—ethylene glycol; lead; rodenticide anticoagulants; others
• Vascular—hemorrhage (bleeding disorders, hypertension); infarction (feline ischemic encephalopathy, microfilaria, or migrating adult heartworm)

RISK FACTORS
• Diabetes mellitus—insulin therapy
• Insulinomas
• Severe heat or cold exposure without protection
• Free-roaming animals—trauma
• Young and unvaccinated animals

DIAGNOSIS

DIFFERENTIAL DIAGNOSIS

Similar Signs
• Other altered states of consciousness—narcolepsy (intermittent episodes of deep sleep with spontaneous recovery); syncope (temporary loss of consciousness with spontaneous recovery); collapse and severe

depression (patient is conscious with depressed mentation and motor activity)

Causes
• Acute onset—most commonly caused by toxins, drugs, trauma, or vascular accidents
• Slow progression of neurologic signs without systemic abnormalities—suggests primary neurologic disorders of inflammatory, neoplastic, or anatomic causes
• Bilateral diffuse cortical signs—metabolic diseases, toxins, systemic infection, drugs, and nutritional causes
• Brain stem signs—trauma, inflammation, neoplasia, vascular accidents, or commonly from progression of cerebral disease causing tentorial herniation

CBC/BIOCHEMISTRY/URINALYSIS

CBC
• Lead toxicity—may show nucleated red blood cells or basophilic stippling
• Severe infection—inflammatory hemogram
• Severe anemia—suggests hypoxemia

Biochemistry
May see hypoglycemia, hyperglycemia, hypernatremia, azotemia, hyperosmolarity, and other metabolic derangements

Urinalysis
• Diabetes mellitus—glycosuria
• End-stage renal disease—isosthenuria
• Immune-mediated disease or severe infection—proteinuria
• Hepatic encephalopathy—ammonium biurate crystals
• Ethylene glycol toxicity—calcium oxalate or hippurate crystals

OTHER LABORATORY TESTS
• Serum ethylene glycol test and measure osmolar gap—acute onset
• Serum ammonia concentrations and preprandial and postprandial bile acids—high levels indicate hepatic encephalopathy.
• Serum and CSF titers—suspected infectious disease (e.g. distemper, FIP, rickettsial diseases, cryptococcosis, blastomycosis, histoplasmosis, *Neospora caninum*, toxoplasmosis)
• Arterial blood gases—evidence of hypoxemia; severe pH changes; hypercarbia
• Coagulogram—including PT, PTT, fibrinogen, FDP, platelet count, antithrombin III, and buccal bleeding time; suspected intracranial bleeding or thrombosis
• Serologic testing—FeLV, FIV, and heartworm disease

IMAGING
• Survey radiographs (chest and abdomen)—evidence of organ compromise, infiltration, or neoplasia
• Skull radiographs—fractures in trauma cases
• MRI—best modality for detecting acute hemorrhage within the cranial vault or brain
• CT (skull)—method of choice for detecting depressed fractures or penetrating foreign bodies

DIAGNOSTIC PROCEDURES
• CSF analysis—include immunoglobulin concentrations and titers for infectious diseases; perform when there is no evidence of trauma, increased ICP, coagulopathies, or metabolic disease.
• BAER—determine brainstem function
• ECG—determine cardiac dysfunction; abnormalities may contribute to stupor or coma or may be caused by brain disease.

TREATMENT
• Hydration—maintained with a balanced electrolyte crystalloid solution
• The head should be level with the body or elevated to a 20° angle; the head should never be lower than the body to avoid increase in ICP.
• Avoid triggering a cough or sneeze reflex during intubation or oxygen supplementation by nasal cannula; may severely elevate ICP; lidocaine (dogs: 0.75 mg/kg IV) given before intubation can blunt the gag and cough reflex.
• PaCO$_2$—maintain between 35 and 45 mm Hg; hyperventilating may reduce cerebral blood flow and ICP; PaO$_2$ must be above 50 mm Hg to maintain cerebral blood flow autoregulation; use peripheral veins, leaving the jugular vein blood flow unobstructed; shifting blood volume into the jugular veins is an important compensatory mechanism during high ICP.
• Prevent thrashing, seizures, or any other form of uncontrolled motor activity; may elevate ICP; diazepam infusion (0.5–1 mg/kg/hr) may be required for seizures.
• Meticulous nursing care to prevent secondary complications of recumbency—eye lubrication; aseptic technique with catheters; turning to avoid hypostatic lung congestion; hygiene
• Surgical decompression and exploration—seriously consider if neurologic signs worsen, including cerebral dysfunction that is progressing to midbrain signs with a history of trauma or bleeding (tentorial herniation), high ICP not responsive to medical therapy (if monitoring instrumentation available), depressed skull fracture fragments, and penetrating foreign body.
• Nutrition—maintain during the unconscious period; adjust nutritional requirements to compensate for metabolic demands.
• Motility modifier cisapride (0.5 mg/kg bid–tid) may be necessary

MEDICATIONS

DRUG(S) OF CHOICE

Poor Perfusion
• Use a minimal amount of crystalloids, because they contribute to brain edema; a combination of large molecular weight colloids (e.g., hetastarch) with crystalloids allows small fluid volume resuscitation.
• Do not use colloids if there is intracranial hemorrhage.
• Maintain systolic arterial blood pressure > 90 mm Hg with crystalloids and/or colloids; avoid hypertension.

High ICP
• Hyperventilation or diuretic therapy
• Furosemide—0.75 mg/kg IV; lowers CSF production and ICP
• Mannitol—0.1–0.5 g/kg IV bolus q2h for 3–4 doses in dogs and 2–3 doses in cats; improves brain blood flow and lowers ICP; given after furosemide

Underlying Disease
• Glucocorticosteroids—inflammatory and space-occupying intracranial abnormalities
• Lactulose enemas and fluid support—hepatic encephalopathy
• Fluid diuresis—renal failure
• Rehydration and insulin—diabetes mellitus with hyperosmolality; lower glucose slowly.
• Glucose supplementation—hypoglycemia
• Support the intravascular volume; cool—hyperthermia.
• Support the intravascular volume; warm—hypothermia.
• Gastric lavage and instillation of activated charcoal with a cathartic—suspected toxic ingestion
• Specific toxins may require specific therapeutics (e.g., ethylene glycol treated with ethanol and peritoneal dialysis).
• Antibiotics—use agents that cross the blood–brain barrier for suspected bacterial infections (e.g., trimethoprim-sulfa, chloramphenicol, and metronidazole); use broad-spectrum agents if the blood–brain barrier is interrupted (e.g., first-generation cephalosporins).
• Adjust crystalloid fluid selection to correct electrolyte disorders.

CONTRAINDICATIONS
• Do not allow the head to lie below plane of body.
• Colloids—do not use when there is intracranial hemorrhage

PRECAUTIONS
• Avoid hypertension.
• Avoid intravascular volume overload.

• Mannitol and hypertonic saline—may worsen neurologic status when there is intracranial hemorrhage
• Hyperventilating—maintain PaCO$_2$ > 25 mm Hg; do not perform for extended time periods (> 48 hr)

POSSIBLE INTERACTIONS
N/A

ALTERNATIVE DRUG(S)
N/A

FOLLOW-UP

PATIENT MONITORING
• Repeat neurologic examinations—detect deterioration of function that warrants aggressive therapeutic intervention • Blood pressure—keep fluid therapy adequate for perfusion while avoiding hypertension • Blood gases—assess need for oxygen supplementation or ventilation; monitor PCO$_2$ when hyperventilating • Blood glucose—ensure an adequate blood level to maintain brain functions while avoiding hyperosmolality
• ECG—detect arrhythmias that may affect perfusion, oxygenation, and cerebral blood flow • ICP—detect marked elevations; track success of therapeutics • Electrolytes—detect hypernatremia and hypokalemia.

POSSIBLE COMPLICATIONS
N/A

MISCELLANEOUS

SEE ALSO
Brain Injury (Head Trauma and Hypoxia)

ABBREVIATIONS
• ARAS = ascending reticular activating system • BAER = brainstem auditory-evoked response • CSF = cerebrospinal fluid
• ECG = electrocardiogram • FDP = fibrin degradation product • FeLV = feline leukemia virus • FIP = feline infectious peritonitis • FIV = feline immunodeficiency virus • ICP = intracranial pressure
• PT = prothrombin time • PTT = partial thromboplastin time

Suggested Reading
Bagley RS. Pathophysiologic sequelae of intracranial disease. Vet Clin North Am Small Anim Pract 1996;26:711–733.
Chrisman CL. Coma and altered states of consciousness. In: Problems in small animal neurology. Philadelphia: Lea & Febiger, 1991:219–233.

Author Rebecca Kirby
Consulting Editor Joane M. Parent

SUBINVOLUTION OF PLACENTAL SITES

BASICS

OVERVIEW
• Failure or delay of normal postpartum uterine involution
• Failure of eosinophilic masses of collagen at placental sites to slough at 3–4 weeks postpartum
• Failure of fetal trophoblastic cells to regress normally; instead, they invade the maternal myometrium
• Cause—unknown; hormonal or uterine basis not suspected

SIGNALMENT
• Dogs only
• Bitches < 3 years
• Seen with first litter
• No breed predilections

SIGNS

Historical Findings
• Patient presented 6–12 weeks postpartum
• Serosanguineous vulvar discharge beyond 6 weeks postpartum
• No systemic signs

Physical Examination Findings
• Serosanguineous vulvar discharge
• Firm, spherical structures within uterus on abdominal palpation

CAUSES & RISK FACTORS
• Unknown
• Hormonal—unlikely, because only some of the placental sites may be involved
• Uterine disease—unlikely, because of high first litter prevalence

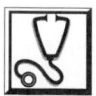

DIAGNOSIS

DIFFERENTIAL DIAGNOSIS
• Metritis—differentiated by vaginal cytology and physical examination
• Vaginitis—differentiated by vaginal cytology
• Vaginal neoplasia—differentiated by vaginal cytology and vaginal endoscopy
• Uterine neoplasia—differentiated by ultrasonography or exploratory laparotomy
• Cystitis—differentiated by vaginal cytology and urinalysis

• Coagulopathy—differentiated by clotting times
• Trauma
• Endogenous estrogen stimulation—bitch with an extremely shortened interestrous interval
• Exogenous estrogen stimulation

CBC/BIOCHEMISTRY/URINALYSIS
Usually normal

OTHER LABORATORY TESTS
Serology for *Brucella canis* negative

IMAGING
Uterine ultrasonography—focal uterine wall thickening; echogenic fluid in the lumen

DIAGNOSTIC PROCEDURES
• Vaginal cytologic examination—key for diagnosis; reveals erythrocytes and parabasal epithelial cells; may note pathognomonic trophoblastic cells
• Guarded anterior vaginal culture—if vaginal cytologic examination or hemogram supports a diagnosis of secondary metritis

PATHOLOGIC FINDINGS
• Gross—sites characterized by a thickened, hemorrhagic area that may be nodular
• Histopathologic—definitive diagnosis; eosinophilic collagen masses with trophoblasts extending into the myometrium

TREATMENT
• Usually outpatient
• Spontaneous remission—occurs before or at next cycle
• Medical—for rare development of anemia, metritis, or peritonitis
• Severely affected patients—may require blood transfusion (rare)
• Warn owner of the rare possibility of excessive hemorrhage; instruct owner to monitor mucous membrane color.
• Ovariohysterectomy—curative; treatment of choice if future breeding not desired
• Surgical curettage of subinvoluted sites—may also be performed

MEDICATIONS

DRUG(S)
Generally not successful

CONTRAINDICATIONS/POSSIBLE INTERACTIONS
• Ecbolics—may cause uterine rupture
• Progestational drugs—increase the risk of metritis, which may mimic pyometra

FOLLOW-UP

PATIENT MONITORING
• Mucous membrane color and amount of discharge
• Packed cell volume—if anemia is a concern
• Changes in discharge color or odor and vaginal cytologic examination and culture—diagnose secondary infection

POSSIBLE COMPLICATIONS
Infection, blood-loss anemia, or uterine rupture—rare

EXPECTED COURSE AND PROGNOSIS
• Spontaneous resolution—the norm
• Recurrence—not expected
• Prognosis for future reproduction—excellent with spontaneous resolution

MISCELLANEOUS

Suggested Reading
Johnston SD. Subinvolution of placental sites. In: Kirk RW, ed. Current veterinary therapy IX. Philadelphia: Saunders, 1986: 1231–1233.
Johnston SD, Root Kustritz MV, Olson PNS. Periparturient disorders in the bitch. In: Johnston SD, Root Kustritz MV, Olson PNS, eds. Canine and feline theriogenology. Philadelphia: Saunders, 2001:129–145.
Wheeler SL. Subinvolution of placental sites in the bitch. In: Morrow DA, ed. Current therapy in theriogenology 2. Philadelphia: Saunders, 1986:513–515.

Author Joni L. Freshman
Consulting Editor Sara K. Lyle

SUPERFICIAL NECROLYTIC DERMATITIS

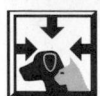

BASICS

OVERVIEW
• A rare canine disorder
• Usually a cutaneous marker for advanced hepatic disease or concurrent hepatic disease and diabetes mellitus
• Rarely associated with a glucagon-secreting pancreatic tumor
• Lesions—pathogenesis unclear; result of keratinocyte degeneration and necrosis; hyperglucagonemia, hypoaminoacidemia, zinc and essential fatty acid deficiencies believed to play a direct or indirect role

SYSTEMS AFFECTED
• Skin/Exocrine—eroded, erythematous, and crusting lesions around the mouth and eyes and on the legs, feet, and genitalia
• Hepatobiliary—hepatic cirrhosis or vacuolar hepatopathy with parenchymal collapse and nodular hyperplasia
• Endocrine/Metabolic—glucagon-secreting pancreatic tumor

SIGNALMENT
• Dogs
• No breed predilection
• Often old dogs
• Males more likely affected

SIGNS
• Skin lesions—usually precede clinical evidence of internal disease by weeks or months; usually the presenting complaint; consist of erythema, crusts, and erosions or ulcerations affecting the muzzle, mucocutaneous areas of the face, distal limbs, feet, and external genitalia
• Footpads—usually hyperkeratotic and affected with fissures and ulcerations; pain associated with walking
• Secondary bacterial and/or fungal infections—often associated with footpad lesions

CAUSES & RISK FACTORS
• Specific cause unknown
• Keratinocyte degeneration and necrosis—probably result from cellular starvation or other nutritional imbalance
• Nutritional imbalance—probably hypoaminoacidemia or deficiencies in essential fatty acids and zinc; due to metabolic abnormalities caused by high serum glucagon levels, liver dysfunction, or a combination
• No risk factors have been identified.

DIAGNOSIS

DIFFERENTIAL DIAGNOSIS
• Pemphigus foliaceus
• Systemic lupus erythematosus
• Zinc-responsive dermatosis
• Toxic epidermal necrolysis
• Drug eruption
• Distal extremity erythema and footpad hyperkeratosis—unique; strongly suggest the diagnosis

CBC/BIOCHEMISTRY/URINALYS
• Anemia—may be noted; usually normocytic, normochromic, and nonregenerative
• RBC abnormalities—polychromasia; anisocytosis; poikilocytosis; and target cells
• ALP, ALT, and AST—high activity
• Total bilirubin and bile acid levels—high
• BSP retention
• Biochemistry abnormalities are not seen in dogs with glucagon-secreting tumors.
• Most patients develop borderline or frank hyperglycemia.

OTHER LABORATORY TESTS
• Elevated plasma glucagon levels—consistently present with glucagon-secreting tumors; variably observed with chronic hepatic disorders
• Hypoaminoacidemia common
• High insulin levels may be noted.

IMAGING
Abdominal radiography and ultrasonography—usually unremarkable with glucagon-secreting pancreatic tumors; abnormalities compatible with hepatic cirrhosis or vacuolar hepatopathy and nodular hyperplasia seen with advanced liver disease

DIAGNOSTIC PROCEDURES
Skin biopsies—important diagnostic tool; sample early lesions because chronic lesions rarely show the unique epidermal edema

PATHOLOGIC FINDINGS
• Skin biopsies—diffuse parakeratotic hyperkeratosis with high-level intracellular and intercellular epidermal edema are unique; irregular epidermal hyperplasia and mild superficial perivascular dermatitis
• Chronic lesions—marked parakeratotic hyperkeratosis and epidermal hyperplasia; also noted with zinc deficiency

TREATMENT
• Usually as outpatients
• Patients with signs of liver failure may need to be hospitalized for supportive care.
• Surgical excision of glucagon-secreting tumors—can be curative if diagnosis is made before metastasis; unfortunately, this is rarely the case.
• Most cases are associated with chronic irreversible liver disease.
• Inform clients that this disorder indicates concurrent severe internal disease with a poor prognosis.
• Hydrotherapy and shampoos—help remove crusts; lessen pruritus and pain.

MEDICATIONS

DRUG(S)
• Specific treatment—attempt to correct the underlying disease; not usually accomplished
• Nonspecific symptomatic therapy—antibiotics and antifungal drugs for secondary skin infections
• Glucocorticoids—improve skin lesions; may induce a diabetic crisis because patients are either prediabetic or overtly diabetic at diagnosis; may induce ascites if patient has chronic severe liver disease; prednisone or prednisolone: usual initial dosage of 0.5–1.0 mg/kg daily; maintain at lowest possible alternate-day dosage
• Zinc sulfate or gluconate—10 mg/kg daily; results unrewarding
• Essential fatty acids—not beneficial
• Amino acid hyperalimentation

CONTRAINDICATIONS/POSSIBLE INTERACTIONS
N/A

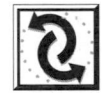

FOLLOW-UP

POSSIBLE COMPLICATIONS
• Liver failure • Secondary bacterial and/or fungal skin infections

EXPECTED COURSE AND PROGNOSIS
Prognosis poor; survival time reported as 5 months after development of skin lesions

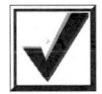

MISCELLANEOUS

ASSOCIATED CONDITIONS
Diabetes mellitus—usually nonketoacidotic

SYNONYMS
• Hepatocutaneous syndrome
• Necrolytic migratory erythema
• Metabolic epidermal necrosis
• Canine diabetic dermatosis

ABBREVIATIONS
• ALP = alkaline phosphatase
• ALT = alanine aminotransferase
• AST = aspartate aminotransferase
• BSP = sulfobromophthalein

Suggested Reading
Scott DW, Miller WH, Griffin GE. Endocrine and metabolic diseases. In: Muller & Kirk's small animal dermatology. 5th ed. Philadelphia: Saunders, 1995:706–710.
Author Sheila M. F. Torres
Consulting Editor Karen Helton Rhodes

SUPRAVENTRICULAR TACHYCARDIA

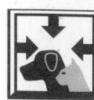 BASICS

DEFINITION
Repetitive supraventricular premature depolarizations that usually originate from a site other than the sinus node, such as the atrial myocardium or atrioventricular junctional tissue

ECG Features
• Heart rate—rapid, 150–350 bpm in dogs
• Rhythm usually very regular (R-R interval is constant) and may be sustained, but there can be frequent or infrequent short runs of supraventricular tachycardia (SVT), so-called paroxysmal SVT. Rarely, the rhythm during the tachycardia will be irregular, suggesting abnormal automaticity as the etiology.
• Usually the QRS complexes are typical of normal sinus complexes, narrow and upright in lead II. In some cases a coexisting bundle branch block or aberrant ventricular conduction makes it difficult, if not impossible, to differentiate an SVT from a ventricular tachycardia by examining the ECG.
• P waves can be positive or negative in lead II and typically differ in configuration from the sinus P waves. P waves may be buried in the previous T wave and therefore not visualized.
• Atrioventricular conduction is usually normal (1:1), but various levels of functional second-degree AV block may occur at higher atrial rates (2:1, 3:1, 4:1, etc).

PATHOPHYSIOLOGY
• May result from a reentrant mechanism or from abnormal automaticity in an ectopic focus. Reentrant SVT produces a very regular rhythm; SVT due to an automatic focus in atrial myocardium can be irregular.
• Most cases in dogs respond to drugs that specifically alter conduction and refractoriness in the AV junctional tissue, suggesting AV junctional reentry as the mechanism.
• Recent electrophysiologic studies revealed that some SVT in dogs is related to a congenital accessory pathway between the atria and ventricles that allows the electrical impulses to travel freely between the atria and ventricles without traversing the AV node and without conduction delay; in these patients, the SVT is caused by reentry through the accessory pathway and the AV node.

SYSTEMS AFFECTED
Cardiovascular
Rarely CHF develops secondary to progressive myocardial failure associated with a chronically high heart rate.

Neuromuscular
Syncope or generalized episodic weakness due to reduced cardiac output and oxygen delivery

GENETICS
Labrador retrievers suspected on the basis of clinical data to have a genetic predisposition to congenital accessory pathway

SIGNALMENT
Species
Dogs and less commonly cats

Breed Predilections
Labrador retrievers are overrepresented in the literature.

SIGNS
General Comments
• Clinical signs may relate to the underlying cause.
• Dogs with slow SVT or infrequent paroxysmal SVT exhibit no clinical signs.
• Dogs with fast SVT (heart rate usually > 300 bpm) generally exhibit weakness or collapse.

Historical Findings
• Owners are generally unaware of the arrhythmia.
• Coughing or breathing abnormalities in dogs with CHF
• Possible episodes of weakness or collapse

Physical Examination Findings
• Rapid, usually regular heart rhythm
• May have evidence of poor peripheral perfusion—pale mucous membranes, a prolonged capillary refill time, and weak pulses
• May have no signs other than the rapid heart rate
• Findings may reflect an underlying cardiac condition (e.g., heart murmur).

CAUSES
• Chronic valvular disease
• Cardiomyopathy
• Congenital heart disease
• Cardiac neoplasia
• Systemic disorders
• Ventricular preexcitation
• Electrolyte imbalances
• Digoxin toxicity
• Idiopathic

RISK FACTORS
• Heart disease • Genetics in Labrador retrievers

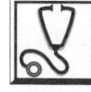 DIAGNOSIS

DIFFERENTIAL DIAGNOSIS
• Sinus tachycardia
• Atrial flutter
• Atrial fibrillation
• Ventricular tachycardia (SVT with right bundle branch block or aberrant conduction can look like ventricular tachycardia; resolution of arrhythmia after lidocaine administration usually confirms ventricular tachycardia)

IMAGING
• Echocardiography (including Doppler studies) may help characterize the type and severity of underlying cardiac disorders.
• When viewed on an echocardiogram during bursts of SVT, the left ventricle has a normal end-systolic diameter and a small end-diastolic diameter, resulting in a decreased shortening fraction because of inadequate filling.
• Usually left or right atrial enlargement in dogs with SVT secondary to other cardiac disorders

DIAGNOSTIC PROCEDURES
• Long-term ambulatory (Holter) recording of the ECG may detect paroxysmal SVT in cases of unexplained syncope; Holter monitors may also help characterize the rate and frequency of sustained SVT and are useful in evaluating therapy.
• Sustained SVT must be distinguished from sinus tachycardia because the two arrhythmias have different implications and treatment. A precordial thump may help differentiate sinus tachycardia from SVT when the heart rate is in the 150–250 bpm range; it will usually stop an SVT for at least 1 or 2 beats, while a sinus tachycardia will not slow. A vagal maneuver (e.g., ocular pressure or carotid sinus massage) may break an SVT abruptly but only gradually slows sinus tachycardia.

PATHOLOGIC FINDINGS
N/A

 TREATMENT

APPROPRIATE HEALTH CARE
• Asymptomatic patients can be managed on an outpatient basis; patients with a sustained SVT or signs of heart failure should be hospitalized until stable.
• SVT is a medical emergency in dogs that exhibit weakness and collapse; non-pharmacologic interventions that may break an SVT include vagal maneuvers, precordial thump, and electrical cardioversion
• Vagal maneuvers are often unsuccessful but may be used initially because of their ease of administration and noninvasive nature.
• Delivering a precordial thump can successfully (> 90% of the time) terminate an SVT in dogs, but this maneuver may break the rhythm for only a brief period. At other times the rhythm remains converted. To perform a precordial thump, the dog is placed on its right side and the left apex beat is located. This region is then "thumped" with a fist while recording the ECG. Electrical cardioversion or intracardiac electrophysiologic pacing methods may be considered in extreme cases.

NURSING CARE
Treat CHF and correct any underlying electrolyte or acid–base disturbances.

ACTIVITY
Restrict until arrhythmia has been controlled

DIET
Mild to moderate sodium restriction if in CHF

CLIENT EDUCATION
Owners should observe patients closely for signs of low cardiac output such as weakness and collapse.

SURGICAL CONSIDERATIONS
Consider transvenous catheter ablation for patients with accessory pathways.

MEDICATIONS

DRUG(S) OF CHOICE

Emergency Therapy
Administer one of the following drugs:
- Calcium channel blockers—verapamil (0.05 mg/kg boluses IV over 3–5 min up to 3 times) or diltiazem (0.05–0.25 mg/kg IV over 5–15 min)
- β-Adrenergic blockers—propranolol (0.02 mg/kg slow IV boluses up to a total dose of 0.1 mg/kg) or esmolol (0.25–0.5 mg/kg slow IV bolus administration followed by a constant-rate infusion of 50–200 μg/kg/min); moderate-to-severe myocardial failure is a relative contraindication to the administration of these drugs at these doses.

Long-term Therapy
- Digoxin—administer at either a maintenance oral dose or double the maintenance dose for the first day to produce a therapeutic serum concentration more rapidly; contraindicated in patients with accessory pathways

- β-Adrenergic blocker—(propranolol 0.3–1 mg/kg PO q8h or atenolol 0.2–1 mg/kg PO q12–24h) can be administered as long as the patient does not have underlying moderate-to-severe myocardial failure
- Diltiazem is the calcium channel blocker of choice for long-term control of SVT. The dosage required to control SVT has not been reported in the dog. Diltiazem is used more frequently to control the ventricular rate in patients with atrial fibrillation at a dosage of 0.5–1.5 mg/kg PO q8h. In our clinic, we generally start in this dosage range but almost always need to increase the dose to 2.0–3.0 mg/kg PO q8h to effect control of SVT.
- Class I antiarrhythmic agents such as quinidine and procainamide can be tried when the aforementioned drugs are ineffective or when the SVT is thought to be due to an automatic, rather than a reentrant, rhythm. SVT caused by an automatic atrial focus may produce an irregular rhythm and may be refractory to conventional drug therapy. When the SVT is due to an accessory pathway, these drugs are more effective.

CONTRAINDICATIONS
Avoid use of calcium channel blockers in combination with β-blockers; clinically significant bradyarrhythmias can develop.

PRECAUTIONS
Calcium channel blockers and β-adrenergic blockers have negative inotropic properties and should be used cautiously in dogs with documented myocardial failure.

POSSIBLE INTERACTIONS
N/A

ALTERNATIVE DRUG(S)
Emergency treatment—intravenous adenosine (1–12 mg IV rapidly). Adenosine is very expensive and short-lived; intravenous verapamil (0.5 mg/kg slow bolus) can be repeated twice.

FOLLOW-UP

PATIENT MONITORING
Serial ECG or Holter monitoring

POSSIBLE COMPLICATIONS
Syncope and CHF

EXPECTED COURSE AND PROGNOSIS
Most is controlled effectively with medication.

MISCELLANEOUS

ASSOCIATED CONDITIONS
Accessory pathways in some patients

AGE-RELATED FACTORS
In young dogs without evidence of structural heart disease, suspect a reentrant tachycardia involving an accessory pathway.

SYNONYMS
Atrial tachycardia, junctional tachycardia

SEE ALSO
Atrial Fibrillation and Atrial Flutter

ABBREVIATIONS
- CHF = congestive heart failure
- SVT = supraventricular tachycardia

Suggested Reading
Atkins CE, Wright KN. Supraventricular tachycardia associated with accessory pathways in dogs. In: Bonagura JD, ed. Current veterinary therapy XII. Philadelphia: WB Saunders, 1995:807–810.

Wright KN. Assessment and treatment of supraventricular tachyarrhythmias. In: Bonagura JD, ed. Kirk's current veterinary therapy XIII. Philadelphia: WB Saunders. 1999:726–730.

Author Richard D. Kienle

Consulting Editors Larry P. Tilley and Francis W. K. Smith, Jr.

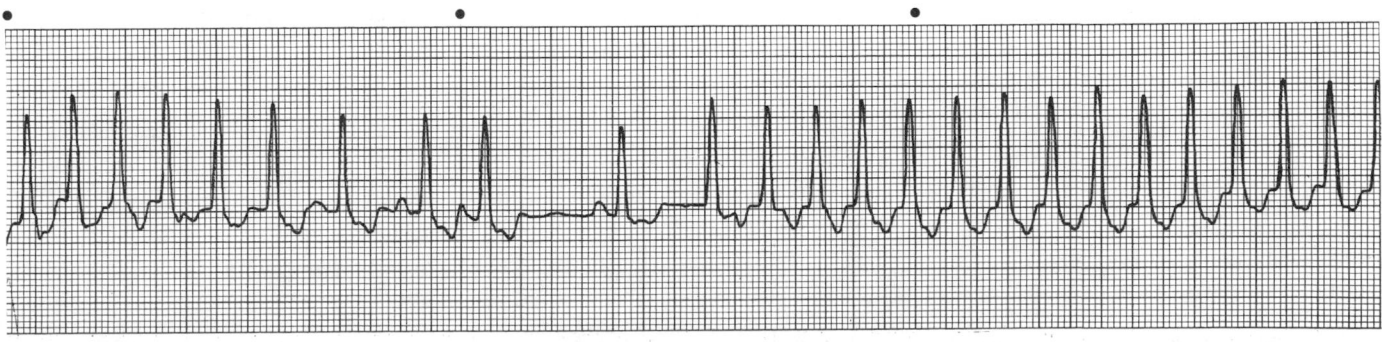

Figure 1.

Sinus with an atrial premature complex and paroxysmal supraventricular tachycardia. Abrupt initiation and termination of the tachycardia help distinguish it from sinus tachycardia (lead II, 50 mm/sec, 1 cm = 1 mV). (From: Tilley LP: Essentials of canine and feline electrocardiography. 3rd ed. Baltimore: Williams & Wilkins, 1992, with permission.)

SYNCOPE

BASICS

DEFINITION
Temporary loss of consciousness and vascular tone associated with loss of postural tone, with spontaneous recovery

PATHOPHYSIOLOGY
Inadequate cerebral perfusion and delivery of oxygen and metabolic substrates leads to loss of consciousness and motor tone; impaired cerebral perfusion can result from changes in vasomotor tone, cerebral disease, and low cardiac output caused by structural heart disease or arrhythmias.

SYSTEMS AFFECTED
• Nervous
• Cardiovascular

SIGNALMENT

Species
Dogs and cats

Breed Predilection
• Sick sinus syndrome—cocker spaniel, miniature schnauzer, pug, dachshund
• Ventricular arrhythmias—boxer

Mean Age and Range
More common in old animals

Predominant Sex
N/A

SIGNS
N/A

CAUSES

Cardiac Causes
• Bradyarrhythmias—sinus bradycardia, sinus arrest, second-degree atrioventricular (AV) block, complete AV block, atrial standstill
• Tachyarrhythmias—ventricular tachycardia, supraventricular tachycardia, atrial fibrillation
• Low cardiac output (nonarrhythmic)—cardiomyopathy, AV valve endocardiosis, subaortic stenosis, pulmonic stenosis, heartworm disease, pulmonary embolism, cardiac tumor, cardiac tamponade

Neurologic and Vasomotor Instability
• Vasovagal syncope—emotional stress and excitement may cause heightened sympathetic stimulation, leading to transient tachycardia and hypertension, which is followed by a compensatory rise in vagal tone, leading to excessive vasodilation without a compensatory rise in heart rate and cardiac output; bradycardia often occurs.
• Situational syncope refers to syncope associated with coughing, defecation, urination, and swallowing.
• Carotid sinus hyperactivity may cause hypotension and bradycardia—often the cause of syncope when one pulls on a dog's collar

Miscellaneous Causes
• Drugs that affect blood pressure and regulation of autonomic tone

• Hypoglycemia, hypocalcemia, and hyponatremia (rare)
• Hyperviscosity syndromes (e.g., polycythemia and paraproteinemia) cause sludging of blood and impaired cerebral perfusion (rare).

RISK FACTORS
• Heart disease
• Sick sinus syndrome
• Drug therapy—vasodilators (e.g., calcium channel blockers, ACE inhibitors, hydralazine, and nitrates), phenothiazines (e.g., acepromazine), antiarrhythmics, and diuretics

DIAGNOSIS

DIFFERENTIAL DIAGNOSIS

Differential Signs
• Must differentiate from other altered states of consciousness, including seizures and narcolepsy (a sleep disorder)
• Seizures are often associated with a prodromal and postictal period; syncope occurs without warning, and animal usually has rapid, spontaneous recovery. Unlike syncope, seizure activity is usually associated with tonic clonic muscle activity rather than flaccidity.
• Like syncope, narcolepsy occurs suddenly, results in muscle flaccidity, and resolves spontaneously. Unlike syncope, narcolepsy can last for minutes and can be terminated by loud noises or harsh external stimuli.
• Must differentiate from other causes of collapse such as musculoskeletal disease and neuromuscular disease (e.g., myasthenia gravis), which are not associated with loss of consciousness

Differential Causes
• Syncope with excitement or stress suggests vasovagal syncope.
• Syncope with coughing, urination, or defecation suggests situational syncope.
• Syncope with exercise suggests low-output states associated with arrhythmias or structural heart disease.
• A murmur supports heart disease but does not confirm cardiac cause for syncope.

CBC/BIOCHEMISTRY/URINALYSIS
• Usually normal
• Hypoglycemia or electrolyte disturbance in some animals

OTHER LABORATORY TESTS
• If animal is hypoglycemic, measure insulin concentration on same sample. Calculate an amended insulin:glucose ratio to rule out insulinoma. • If animal is hyponatremic or hyperkalemic, consider an ACTH stimulation test. • If low cardiac output is suspected, rule out occult heartworm disease.

IMAGING

Echocardiography
May detect structural heart disease that could lower cardiac output

DIAGNOSTIC PROCEDURES
• Have owner monitor heart rate during any syncopal episode.
• Electroencephalogram, computed tomography of the head, cerebrospinal fluid (CSF) tap if CNS origin suspected

Electrocardiographic Findings
• Post-exercise ECG may reveal intermittent arrhythmia.
• Holter monitoring (24-hour ECG recording) or use of an ECG event (loop) recorder—useful for evaluating arrhythmic causes
• Carotid sinus massage with ECG and blood pressure monitoring useful in evaluating carotid sensitivity

TREATMENT

APPROPRIATE HEALTH CARE
• Avoid or discontinue medications likely to precipitate syncope. • Treat as outpatient unless important heart disease is evident.

NURSING CARE
N/A

ACTIVITY
See Client Education.

DIET
N/A

CLIENT EDUCATION
• Minimize stimuli that precipitate episodes.
• Low cardiac output—minimize activity.
• Vasovagal—minimize excitement and stress.
• Cough—remove collar.

SURGICAL CONSIDERATIONS
N/A

MEDICATIONS

DRUG(S) OF CHOICE

Bradyarrhythmias
• Correct metabolic causes.
• Anticholinergics (e.g., atropine, propantheline bromide) • Sympathomimetics (e.g., isoproterenol, bronchodilators) • Pacemaker implantation in some patients

Tachyarrhythmias
• Atrial arrhythmias—administer digoxin, β-blocker, or diltiazem.
• Ventricular arrhythmias—administer lidocaine, procainamide, mexiletine, sotalol, or β-blockers.

Low Cardiac Output
Institute treatment to improve cardiac output, which varies according to specific cardiac disease.

Vasovagal
• Theophylline or aminophylline—sometimes helpful; mechanism of action in this setting is unclear

• β-Blockers (e.g., atenolol, propranolol, and metoprolol) may indirectly prevent vagal stimulation by blocking the initial sympathetic response.
• Anticholinergics (e.g., propantheline bromide and hyoscyamine) may blunt the vagal response.

CONTRAINDICATIONS
N/A

PRECAUTIONS
Drugs that lower blood pressure

POSSIBLE INTERACTIONS
N/A

ALTERNATIVE DRUG(S)
N/A

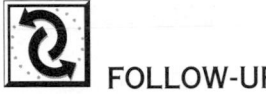 **FOLLOW-UP**

PATIENT MONITORING
ECG or Holter monitoring to assess efficacy of antiarrhythmic therapy

PREVENTION/AVOIDANCE
See Client Education.

POSSIBLE COMPLICATIONS
• Death
• Trauma when collapse occurs

EXPECTED COURSE AND PROGNOSIS
Most noncardiac causes are not life-threatening; cardiac causes may be treated, but syncope in patients with cardiac disease may suggest higher mortality risk.

 MISCELLANEOUS

ASSOCIATED CONDITIONS
N/A

AGE-RELATED FACTORS
N/A

ZOONOTIC POTENTIAL
N/A

PREGNANCY
N/A

SYNONYMS
Fainting

SEE ALSO
• Myasthenia Gravis
• Narcolepsy and Cataplexy
• Seizures (Convulsions, Status Epilepticus)—Cats
• Seizures (Convulsions, Status Epilepticus)—Dogs

Suggested Reading
Kapoor WN. Syncope and hypotension. In: Braunwald E, ed. Heart disease: a textbook of cardiovascular medicine. 5th ed. Philadelphia: Saunders, 1997:863–876.
Rush JE. Syncope and episodic weakness. In: Fox PR, Sisson D, Moise NS, eds. Textbook of canine and feline cardiology. Philadelphia: Saunders, 1999:446–455.
Author Francis W. K. Smith, Jr.
Consulting Editors Larry P. Tilley and Francis W. K. Smith, Jr.

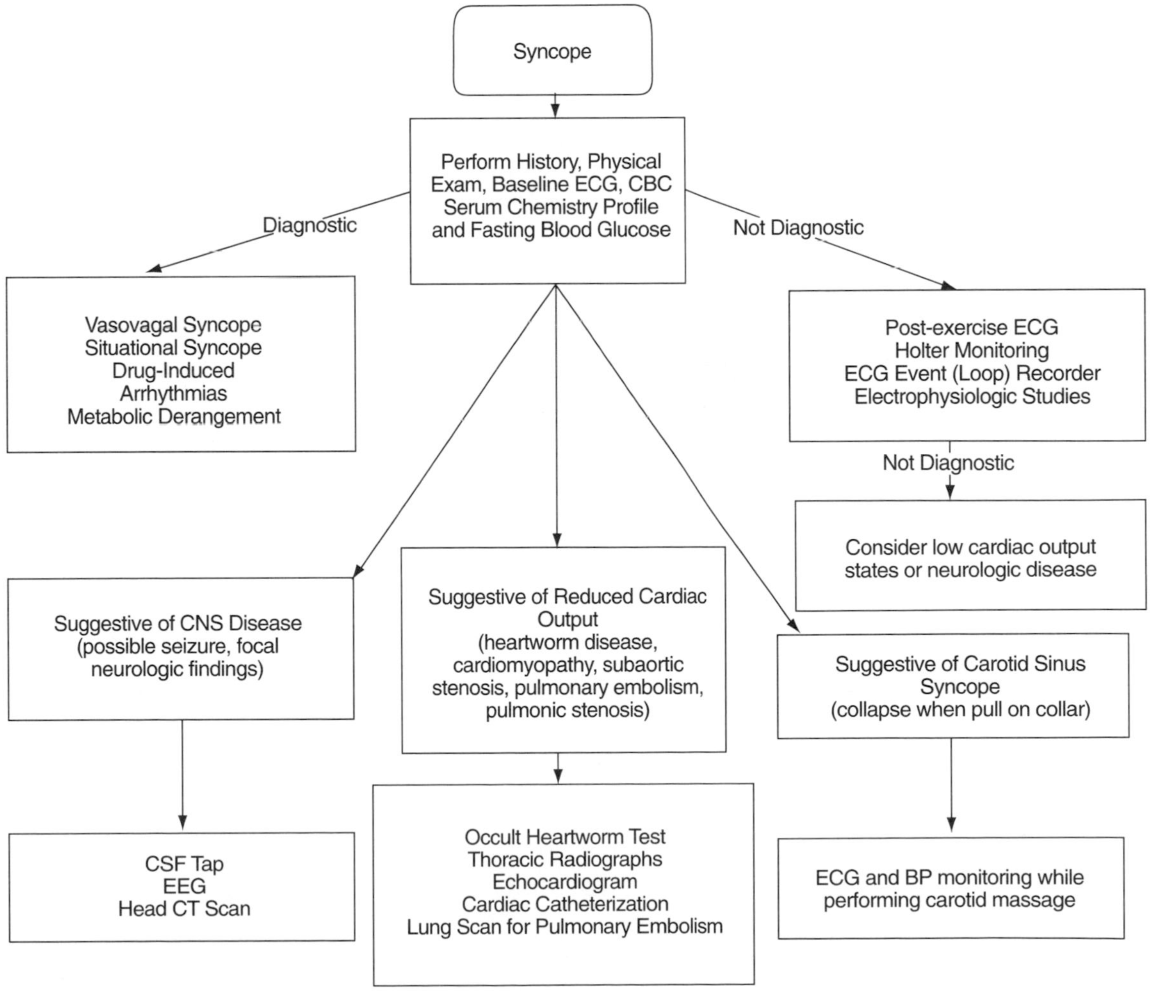

Syncope

↓

Perform History, Physical Exam, Baseline ECG, CBC Serum Chemistry Profile and Fasting Blood Glucose

Diagnostic ← → Not Diagnostic

Diagnostic:
Vasovagal Syncope
Situational Syncope
Drug-Induced
Arrhythmias
Metabolic Derangement

Suggestive of CNS Disease (possible seizure, focal neurologic findings)
↓
CSF Tap
EEG
Head CT Scan

Suggestive of Reduced Cardiac Output (heartworm disease, cardiomyopathy, subaortic stenosis, pulmonary embolism, pulmonic stenosis)
↓
Occult Heartworm Test
Thoracic Radiographs
Echocardiogram
Cardiac Catheterization
Lung Scan for Pulmonary Embolism

Not Diagnostic:
Post-exercise ECG
Holter Monitoring
ECG Event (Loop) Recorder
Electrophysiologic Studies
↓
Not Diagnostic
↓
Consider low cardiac output states or neurologic disease

Suggestive of Carotid Sinus Syncope (collapse when pull on collar)
↓
ECG and BP monitoring while performing carotid massage

SYNOVIAL SARCOMA

BASICS

OVERVIEW
• Malignant neoplasm believed to arise from primitive mesenchymal precursor cells outside the synovial membrane of joints and bursa; precursor cells have the ability to differentiate into epithelial or fibroblastic cells; thus tumor may have components of both epithelial and mesenchymal neoplasia.
• Highly locally invasive; potential to metastasize in > 40% of cases
• Most common sites—appendicular skeleton, specifically elbow, stifle, and scapulohumeral regions

SIGNALMENT
• Dogs—large-breed dogs of either sex; median age, 9 years
• Cats—rarely reported

SIGNS
• Slowly progressive lameness
• Palpable mass
• Weight loss
• Anorexia

CAUSES & RISK FACTORS
Unknown

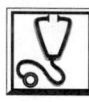

DIAGNOSIS

DIFFERENTIAL DIAGNOSIS
• Other primary neoplasia—chondrosarcoma; fibrosarcoma; osteosarcoma
• Metastatic neoplasia—prostatic carcinoma
• Other primary bone diseases—osteoarthritis; osteomyelitis

CBC/BIOCHEMISTRY/URINALYSIS
No consistent abnormalities

OTHER LABORATORY TESTS
N/A

IMAGING
• Radiographs of the primary lesion—show both bone and joint involvement; increased soft tissue opacity in and around the involved joints common; may note periosteal reaction
• Thoracic radiographs—screen for metastatic disease

DIAGNOSTIC PROCEDURES
• Biopsy—definitive diagnosis; ideally, obtain both soft tissue and bony components for histologic evaluation.
• Regional lymph nodes—palpate; obtain fine-needle aspirates, if possible.

TREATMENT
Radical surgical excision (amputation)—treatment of choice

MEDICATIONS

DRUG(S)
• Chemotherapy—definitive regimen not described; isolated case reports of response to doxorubicin and cyclophosphamide;
• Higher tumor grades are more likely to metastasize; these cases should be treated with adjuvant chemotherapy.
• Pain management—NSAIDs, as necessary

CONTRAINDICATIONS/POSSIBLE INTERACTIONS
N/A

FOLLOW-UP

PATIENT MONITORING
Monitor for local recurrence and pulmonary metastatic disease—every 2–3 months for the first year; every 6 months thereafter

EXPECTED COURSE AND PROGNOSIS
• Clinical course—may be protracted over months to years
• Localized disease—prognosis excellent; median survival > 48 months
• Median survival with amputation alone—17 months
• Metastatic disease, specific histologic criteria (e.g., high mitotic rate, high percent tumor necrosis, and high nuclear pleomorphism), and positive immunocytochemical staining for cytokeratin—prognosis poor; median survival, < 4 months

MISCELLANEOUS

PREGNANCY
Do not breed animals who are undergoing chemotherapy.

ABBREVIATION
NSAID = nonsteroidal antiinflammatory drug

Suggested Reading
MacEwen EG, Powers BE, Macy D, Withrow SJ. Soft tissue sarcomas. In: Withrow SJ, MacEwen EG, eds. Small animal clinical oncology. Philadelphia: Saunders, 2001: 283–304.
Vail DM, Powers BE, Getzy DM, et al. Evaluation of prognostic factors for dogs with synovial sarcoma: 36 cases (1986–1991). J Am Vet Med Assoc 1994;205:1300–1307.

Author Ruthanne Chun
Consulting Editor Wallace B. Morrison

BASICS

OVERVIEW
• Adult tapeworm infections of small intestine with *Taenia* spp., esp. *T. pisiformis* of dogs and *T. taeniaeformis* of cats, *Dipylidium caninum*, *Echinococcus* spp., and *Mesocestoides* of dogs and cats
• Taeniids are transmitted by predation of rabbits or rodents; *Dipylidium caninum* is flea-vectored; flea maggots ingest tapeworm eggs from cat or dog feces, and adult fleas transmit infection when ingested by dogs or cats. Others transmitted by preying on birds, reptiles, or small mammals
• No apparent harm done to host by intestinal adults, but can result in mild perianal pruritus
• *Mesocestoides* larvae (tetrathyridia) can infect peritoneal cavity and cause potentially fatal ascites, anorexia, and leucocytosis.

SIGNALMENT
Dogs and cats

SIGNS
• Chains of segments or single segments in feces (except *Echinococcus*)
• Dragging or rubbing anus on ground because of perianal pruritus with *Dipylidium*
• Segments pasted to perianal skin

CAUSES & RISK FACTORS
• Taeniid infections—eating viscera of birds, reptiles, rabbits, rodents
• *Dipylidium* infections—fleas in environment

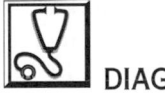

DIAGNOSIS

DIFFERENTIAL DIAGNOSIS
Anal sac impaction

CBC/BIOCHEMISTRY/URINALYSIS
Normal

OTHER LABORATORY TESTS
N/A

IMAGING
N/A

DIAGNOSTIC PROCEDURES
• Squash segments in water or saline between two glass slides; examine for eggs
• *Dipylidium*—Scotch tape pressed to perianal skin for egg packets; single egg ~50 μm diameter; pale yellow, hexacanth embryo
• *Taenia*—eggs spherical, brown, ~30–35 μm; hexacanth embryo (6 apparent hooks on embryo); indistinguishable from *Echinococcus* eggs
• *Mesocestoides*—eggs oval, thin shell; hexacanth embryo; abdominocentesis to detect larvae in peritoneal fluid by microscopy or PCR

TREATMENT
• For intestinal infection—outpatient
• Discuss need for flea control to prevent recurrence of *Dipylidium*.
• For larval peritoneal *Mesocestoides* infection in patient; remove ascites fluid and lavage peritoneum to remove larvae.

MEDICATIONS

DRUG(S)
• Fenbendazole effective at 50 mg/kg PO q24h for 3 days for *Taenia* in dogs; for peritoneal larval *Mesocestoides* infection: 50–100 mg/kg PO q24 h for 4–8 weeks (extra-label)
• Praziquantel 5–7.5 mg/kg PO, SC, or IM; praziquantel/pyrantel pamoate for cats; praziquantel/pyrantel pamoate/febantel for dogs; for *Taenia*, *Echinococcus*, *Mesocestoides* (extra-label) and *Dipylidium*
• Epsiprantel 5.5 mg/kg PO for dogs, 2.8 mg/kg PO cats, for *Taenia*, *Dipylidium*
• Flea control necessary for control of *Dipylidium*

CONTRAINDICATIONS/POSSIBLE INTERACTIONS
Do not use praziquantel or epsiprantel for puppies or kittens < 4 weeks old.

FOLLOW-UP
Fecal examination for tapeworm segments

MISCELLANEOUS

ZOONOTIC POTENTIAL
• Children may be at risk for *Dipylidium* infections by ingestion of flea vector.
• Ingestion of *Echinococcus* eggs causes hydated disease.

SYNONYM
Cestodiasis

ABBREVIATION
PCR = polymerase chain reaction

Suggested Reading
Bowman DD, Lynn RC, Eberhard ML. Georgi's parasitology for veterinarians, 8th ed. St. Louis: Saunders (Elsevier Science), 2003:138–146, 148–153.

Acknowledgment
The author and editors acknowledge the prior contributions of Dr. Robert M. Corwin, who authored this topic in the previous edition.
Author Julie Ann Jarvinen
Consulting Editor Albert E. Jergens

TAURINE DEFICIENCY

 BASICS

OVERVIEW
• Taurine is an essential amino acid in the diet of cats; they must conjugate bile acids with taurine and cannot synthesize enough to cope with this obligatory loss, so diets deficient in taurine cause taurine deficiency in cats. All cat food manufacturers add taurine to their feline diets. Taurine is not an essential amino acid in dogs and so most canine diets do not contain added taurine.
• Taurine is found throughout the body, with highest concentrations in excitable tissues (e.g., myocardium, central nervous system, and retina), where its exact function remains a mystery. It probably helps maintain osmolar gradients and may help regulate calcium movement. Taurine is actively concentrated in myocardial cells by a membrane pump that is under the influence of catecholamines.
• Taurine deficiency results in retinal degeneration and myocardial failure (i.e., decreased myocardial contractility), a condition commonly termed dilated cardiomyopathy (DCM), which has been identified in domestic cats, foxes, and some dogs. In each, the myocardial failure was usually fully or partially reversible with dietary taurine supplementation.

SIGNALMENT
• Cats—DCM due to taurine deficiency is rare because taurine is added to most cat foods.
• Dogs—American cocker spaniels with DCM are almost uniformly taurine-deficient; most golden retrievers with DCM are probably taurine-deficient. Some dogs with DCM that are members of breeds that do not commonly get DCM or mixed breed dogs with DCM have a low plasma taurine concentration.

SIGNS
See Cardiomyopathy, Dilated (Cats and Dogs)

CAUSES & RISK FACTORS
• Cats fed home-cooked diets (e.g., vegetarian or boiled-meat diets) are at risk; rarely a cat with DCM that is on a commercial diet will have a low plasma taurine concentration.
• Dogs—breed predisposition and cystinuria are risk factors.

 DIAGNOSIS

DIFFERENTIAL DIAGNOSIS
Idiopathic dilated cardiomyopathy or myocardial failure due to another cause; see Cardiomyopathy, Dilated (Cats and Dogs)

CBC/BIOCHEMISTRY/URINALYSIS
• No characteristic abnormalities
• Cystinuria in some dogs

OTHER LABORATORY TESTS
• Obtain a heparinized blood sample, place it on ice, and centrifuge within 30 min. Do not allow clotting, because platelets are rich in taurine. Avoid hemolysis. A plasma taurine concentration below 50–60 nmoles/mL is too low in dogs and cats. Heparinized whole blood can also be analyzed; a whole-blood concentration below 200 nmoles/mL is too low.
• Prolonged fasting in cats can produce a low plasma taurine concentration; the whole-blood concentration stays within the normal range longer.

IMAGING
Myocardial failure is diagnosed by identifying an increase in end-systolic diameter, usually with a compensatory smaller increase in end-diastolic diameter and a reduced shortening fraction on an echocardiogram.

DIAGNOSTIC PROCEDURES
Examine any taurine-deficient patient for central retinal degeneration.

 TREATMENT

• Use conventional heart failure therapy until taurine supplementation has caused significant echocardiographic and clinical improvement; drug therapy can usually be discontinued after 3–6 months of taurine supplementation in both dogs and cats that respond to supplementation.
• Most cats in heart failure do better if they are sent home, as long as the owner can provide good nursing care.

 MEDICATIONS

DRUG(S)
• Supplement taurine (cats: 250 mg PO q12h; dogs: 250–1000 mg PO q12h), usually for life

• Taurine supplements—can obtain from health food stores without a prescription; they are relatively inexpensive.
• Carnitine supplementation (1 g PO q12h) is also recommended for American cocker spaniels.

CONTRAINDICATIONS/POSSIBLE INTERACTIONS
No known adverse effects of taurine supplementation; excess taurine is eliminated in the urine.

 FOLLOW-UP

Routine examinations for a patient with heart failure; repeat echocardiogram in 3–6 months to document improvement. If no improvement, can discontinue taurine supplementation

 MISCELLANEOUS

ABBREVIATION
DCM = dilated cardiomyopathy

Suggested Reading
Kittleson MD, Keene B, Pion PD, Loyer CG, and the MUST Study Investigators. Results of the Multicenter Spaniel Trial (MUST): taurine- and carnitine-responsive dilated cardiomyopathy in American cocker spaniels with decreased plasma taurine concentration. J Vet Intern Med 1997; 11(4):204–211.
Kramer GA, Kittleson MD, Fox PR, et al. Plasma taurine concentrations in normal dogs and in dogs with heart disease. J Vet Intern Med 1995;9:253–258.
Pion PD, Kittleson MD, Rogers QR, Morris JG. Myocardial failure in cats associated with low plasma taurine: a reversible cardiomyopathy. Science 1987;237:764–768.
Sanderson SL, Osborne CA, Lulich JP, et al. Evaluation of urine carnitine and taurine excretion in 5 cystinuric dogs with carnitine and taurine deficiency. J Vet Intern Med 2000;15:94–100.
Author Mark D. Kittleson
Consulting Editors Larry P. Tilley and Francis W. K. Smith, Jr.

TEMPOROMANDIBULAR JOINT—DISLOCATION/LUXATION/INTERMITTENT

BASICS

OVERVIEW
Disorders of the TMJ lead to an alteration of the normal function of the masticatory system as the mobility and function of the joint are compromised. Genetic, traumatic, degenerative, or idiopathic causes may result in pain, occlusal dysfunction, joint laxity, chronic arthritis, or open-mouth locking.

SIGNALMENT
• No breed, sex, or age predisposition in most TMJ disorders • Open-mouth mandibular locking—basset hounds; Irish setters • There may be a genetic predisposition in certain breeds (e.g., basset hounds) to develop TMJ disorders

SIGNS
General
• Difficulty opening mouth • Difficulty closing mouth • Laxity or excessive lateral movement of the mandible • Pain when masticating, yawning, and/or vocalizing

Specific
• TMJ luxation/subluxation—history of trauma or mouth locked open; radiographic evidence of luxation • Open-mouth mandibular locking—coronoid process of the mandible "slips" lateral to the ventral surface of the zygomatic arch and is locked in that position; large bulge palpated on affected side of face • Traumatic injury—evidence of trauma; mouth dropped open; mobility of mandible (may have multiple fractures); radiographs indicate fracture
• Osteoarthritis/chronic post-traumatic changes—crepitation and pain when eating or if mandible is forced to move; radiographs may show osseous reaction indicative of arthritic changes

CAUSES & RISK FACTORS
• Patients at a higher risk to experience injuries—young; free roaming
• Trauma may cause fractures or a luxation resulting in immediate problems, as well as future degenerative problems • Mandibular neurapraxia—carrying heavy objects by mouth • MMM—adult; large breed (e.g., German shepherds)

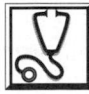

DIAGNOSIS

DIFFERENTIAL DIAGNOSIS
• Craniomandibular osteopathy • Primary or secondary hyperparathyroidism • Mandibular neurapraxia—stretching of the nerve branches (motor) of the masticatory muscles;

usually caused by carrying heavy objects in the mouth; mandible hangs open but can be easily closed manually • MMM—auto-immune disease of type 2M myofibers of masticatory muscles supplied by trigeminal nerve with necrosis, phagocytosis, and fibrosis; trismus progresses to total inability to open jaws

CBC/BIOCHEMISTRY/URINALYSIS
Findings are expected to be within normal limits

OTHER LABORATORY TESTS
• Serum autoantibodies to type 2M myosin—to rule out MMM • Muscle biopsy—to rule out MMM • Cytology of fluid aspirated from TMJ—may be beneficial in diagnosis of a polyarthropathy in which the articular surfaces of the joint are inflamed

IMAGING
• Skull radiography—essential to perform proper radiographic technique in order to visualize the TMJs • MRI—gold standard for imaging the TMJ

DIAGNOSTIC PROCEDURES
• Usually none • MRI may aid in visualizing a radiographic lesion in the TMJ

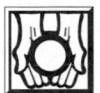

TREATMENT

• Definitive treatment is aimed at eliminating or altering the etiologic factor responsible for the disorder, as well as correcting the problem.
• TMJ luxation—traumatic: luxation often occurs in a rostral direction; place a "dowel" (pencil) across the mouth between the carnassial teeth; gently close the rostral portion of the mouth with a gentle "push" to reduce the luxation (push caudally for a rostral luxation); chronic luxation may not reduce and may require surgery
• Open-mouth mandibular locking—immediate attention; sedate animal, open the mouth further, and apply gentle pressure on the bulging coronoid process to allow it to slip back under the zygomatic arch; surgical management: excise ventral portion of the zygomatic arch and/or a dorsal portion of the coronoid process to relieve future lockings
• Injury or fracture at TMJ—depends on extent of damage; fixation is difficult; condylectomy sometimes necessary
• Chronic osteoarthritis or ankylosis—if severe, condylectomy may be needed
• "Dropped jaw" (trigeminal neurapraxy)—conservative treatment: rest, anti-inflammatory drugs
• MMM—immunosuppressant medications; possible forcible, gradual opening of mouth

MEDICATIONS

DRUG(S) OF CHOICE
• Analgesics—for painful disorders
• Antiinflammatory drugs—for post-operative pain and chronic inflammation
• Muscle relaxants—help prevent increased muscle activity due to chronic pain response

FOLLOW-UP

PATIENT MONITORING
Each case should be carefully followed because of the progressive changes that may occur in the TMJ, especially after traumatic injury.

PREVENTION/AVOIDANCE
Avoid situations that allow for trauma (pets running loose).

POSSIBLE COMPLICATIONS
In many cases after surgical treatment involving TMJ disorders, arthritis may develop later.

EXPECTED COURSE AND PROGNOSIS
Depend on the disorder afflicting the TMJ and the degree to which it is affected

MISCELLANEOUS

PREGNANCY
Condition is typically unaffected by pregnancy. However, if medical treatment is considered, agents such as corticosteroids should not be used in pregnant patients.

SEE ALSO
Maxillary and Mandibular Fractures

ABBREVIATIONS
• MMM = masticatory muscle myositis
• MRI = magnetic resonance imaging
• TMJ = temporomandibular joint

Suggested Reading
Harvey CE, Emily PP. Small animal dentistry. Philadelphia: Mosby-Year Book, 1993: 85–88.
Okeson JP. Management of temporo-mandibular disorders and occlusion. St. Louis: Mosby-Year Book, 1998.
Wiggs RB, Lobprise HB. Clinical oral pathology. In: Wiggs RB, Lobprise HB. Veterinary dentistry: principles and practice. Philadelphia: Lippincott-Raven, 1997:127–130.
Authors Heidi B. Lobprise and Bonnie C. Bloom
Consulting Editor Heidi B. Lobprise

TESTICULAR DEGENERATION AND HYPOPLASIA

 BASICS

OVERVIEW

- Degeneration—histologic changes in the testes after puberty; may be differentiated from hypoplasia by the increased thickness of the basement membrane in the degenerated testis
- Hypoplasia—a variety of histologic lesions thought to be congenital (although often not obvious until after puberty) or heritable

SIGNALMENT

- Dogs and cats
- Dogs—any age or breed; hypoplasia, generally young; degeneration, generally old
- Tortoiseshell cats—may be fertile; usually linked with sex chromosome abnormalities (see Sexual Development Disorders)

SIGNS

- Infertility
- Oligospermia (low numbers of spermatozoa in the ejaculate) or azoospermia (no spermatozoa in the ejaculate)
- Hypoplasia (dogs)—rarely any physical signs other than small testes
- Degeneration (dogs)—any previous scrotal or testicular lesion can be related

CAUSES & RISK FACTORS

Degeneration
- Heat
- Irradiation
- Metals—lead salts; cadmium; organic mercurial compounds
- Nitrogen-containing and halogenated compounds
- Other toxins
- Orchitis
- Steroid hormones—estrogen secreted by a Sertoli cell tumor
- Other hormonal abnormalities—hypothyroidism; hypocortisolism; hyperadrenocorticism
- Increasing age—6.3% of beagles maintained to 7.75 years had incomplete spermatogenesis
- Arterial sclerosis
- Some chemotherapeutic agents—cimetidine; ketoconazole; nitrofurans
- Any previous scrotal or testicular lesion may be related

Hypoplasia
- Klinefelter (XXY) syndrome
- Hypogonadotropic hypogonadism—may be acquired from traumatic or neoplastic lesion of the pituitary
- XX sex reversal—female pseudohermaphroditism

 DIAGNOSIS

DIFFERENTIAL DIAGNOSIS

- Degeneration—old, azoospermic or severely oligospermic previously fertile dogs with small testes
- Hypoplasia—young, azoospermic, never-fertile dogs with small testes
- Spermatocele
- Sperm granuloma
- Orchitis
- Neoplasia
- Ejaculatory failure—retrograde ejaculation; incomplete ejaculation

CBC/BIOCHEMISTRY/URINALYSIS
N/A

OTHER LABORATORY TESTS

- Canine FSH assay—differentiate from blockage (spermatocele); high concentration indicates incomplete spermatogenesis associated with hypoplasia or degeneration
- Alkaline phosphatase concentration of seminal plasma—rule out incomplete ejaculation; samples with AP < 5000 U/L consistent with complete ejaculation

IMAGING
Ultrasonography—testicular size; homogenicity of the parenchyma

DIAGNOSTIC PROCEDURES

- Semen evaluation—primary diagnostic procedure; dog: always obtained by use of an artificial vagina or collection cone; cat: obtained by electroejaculation, when available; collect two ejaculates on separate days; establish azoospermia or oligospermia
- Testicular biopsy (for azoospermia)—fine-needle: identify long spermatids and spermatozoa; Tru-Cut (tissue plug) or open incision: most complete histopathologic diagnosis; fix tissue for sectioning in Bouin or Zenker fixative
- Karyotype—identify extra X chromosome or other numerical or structural chromosome anomaly

PATHOLOGIC FINDINGS

- Normal spermatogenesis—indicates blockage in azoospermic dogs
- Basement membrane thickness—differentiates hypoplasia from degeneration

 TREATMENT

- Degeneration linked to pituitary, adrenal gland, thyroid gland, or other metabolic disruption—goal is to correct the underlying cause.

- No specific diagnosis—may try gonadotropic hormones; rare anecdotal success

 MEDICATIONS

DRUG(S)

- hCG—500 IU SC 2 times a week
- GnRH—1 µg/kg SC with or with hCG (1600 IU IM)

CONTRAINDICATIONS/POSSIBLE INTERACTIONS
N/A

 **FOLLOW-UP**

PATIENT MONITORING
Suspected testicular degeneration (dogs)—a repeat semen analysis performed at least 60 days after correcting any identified underlying cause is needed before reversibility can be assessed.

EXPECTED COURSE AND PROGNOSIS

- Hypoplasia (dogs)—prognosis for fertility poor
- Degeneration (dogs)—prognosis for fertility depends on the cause, site, and extent of injury; usually guarded to poor

 MISCELLANEOUS

SEE ALSO
- Infertility, Male—Dogs
- Sexual Development Disorders
- Spermatocele/Sperm Granuloma

ABBREVIATIONS
- FSH = follicle-stimulating hormone
- hCG = human chorionic gonadotropin

Suggested Reading

Axner E, Strom B, Linde-Forsberg C, et al. Reproductive disorders in 10 domestic male cats. J Sm Anim Pract 1996;37:394–401.

Johnston SD, Root Kustritz MV, Olson PNS. Disorders of the canine penis and prepuce. In: Canine and feline theriogenology. Philadelphia: Saunders, 2001:356–367.

McEntee K. Reproductive pathology of domestic animals. San Diego: Academic Press, 1990:262–263.

Authors Carlos R.F. Pinto and Rolf E. Larsen
Consulting Editor Sara K. Lyle

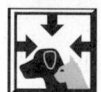

BASICS

OVERVIEW
• *Clostridium tetani*—an obligate, anaerobic, spore-forming, gram-positive rod found in soil and as part of the normal bacterial flora of the intestinal tract of mammals with a predilection for contaminated, necrotic, anaerobic wounds (puncture, surgery, lacerations, burns, frostbite, open fractures, abrasions)
• Germinating spores—in wounds produce potent exotoxin tetanospasmin (tetanus toxin); resistant to disinfectants and to the effects of environmental exposure
• Found worldwide, especially in the tropics

SIGNALMENT
• Dogs—occasionally
• Cats—rarely (especially localized tetanus)

SIGNS
Historical Findings
• Appear a few days to few months after spores enter wound (fracture, surgery, and puncture) • Wound—often necrotic; but may have healed over

Physical Examination Findings
Localized
• Mild rigidity of muscles or leg nearest the site of spore inoculation (wound)
• Stiffness of (hind) limbs; stilted gait; mild weakness and incoordination
• Can resolve spontaneously—reflects partial immunity to tetanospasmin
• Can be prodromal to generalized disease—when enough toxin gains access to CNS
Progressive/Generalized
• Tail—stretches out; progressive tetany of muscles to point of sawhorse appearance
• Convulsions (clonic)—limbs; whole body (opisthotonus); pain during contractions
• Difficulty breathing—dyspnea • Difficulty opening jaws—lockjaw, trismus • Difficulty eating—dysphagia • Eyes—lids retract (visus sardonicus); third eyelid prolapses when head is touched; eyeballs recede into orbit (enophthalmos) • Wrinkled forehead • Erect ears • Grinning appearance—commissure of lips retracted • Salivation • Fever, painful urination (dysuria) and constipation—may be seen • Tetanic muscle spasms—from stimulation (sudden movement, sound, touch) • Death—during spasm of laryngeal and respiratory muscles (fatal acute asphyxia); when respiratory muscles are sufficiently paralyzed

CAUSES & RISK FACTORS
• Unattended wounds (e.g., punctures, surgical, compound bone fractures)—portal of entry for spores • Outdoor pets—greater opportunity for acquiring wounds

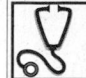

DIAGNOSIS

DIFFERENTIAL DIAGNOSIS
Intoxications mimicking tetanus—lead and strychnine poisoning

CBC/BIOCHEMISTRY/URINALYSIS
• Initial leukopenia; switch to moderate leukocytosis; then gradual return to normal range • AST and CPK—some increase; result of muscle damage during later stages of disease • Urinalysis—essentially normal; high myoglobin from muscles damaged by constant excitation

OTHER LABORATORY TESTS
• Serology—antitetanus antibody often undetectable in serum • Culture—wounds and serum; usually unrewarding to culture for *C. tetani* or to detect toxin (by mouse neutralization); CSF and blood cultures for bacterial pathogens of meningitis

TREATMENT

• Inpatient—good supportive and constant nursing care important; prolonged period (3–4 weeks) • Feeding—patients often have difficulty in prehending food unless helped; pay particular attention to what consistency of food the patient easily ingests; placement of a gastrotomy tube may be necessary; force feeding or feeding with a stomach tube may exacerbate tetanic state, so not advised • Hydration—maintain with oral water; if inadequate, give a balanced intravenous fluid • Keep patient in darkened, quiet area; do not disturb • Keep patient on soft bedding; prevent decubital ulcers • Airway and ventilation—assess; may be necessary to perform endotracheal intubation; trachcostomy may be necessary later
• Urinary and fecal retention—may occur as a result of hypertonic anal and urethral sphincters; urinary catheterization and enemas (to relieve constipation) may be necessary

MEDICATIONS

DRUG(S)
Sedation
• To control reflex spasms and convulsions
• Phenothiazines—drugs of choice; chlorpromazine; with or without barbiturates (e.g., phenobarbital) • Heart rate—may drop when phenothiazines are used in combination; if < 60 beats/min, reverse the bradycardia with glycopyrrolate • Diazepam—alternative to phenobarbital
Tetanus
• First test for hypersensitivity reaction.
• Human tetanus immunoglobulin—administer 500–3000 U IM at multiple sites, especially proximal to wound; or use equine tetanus antitoxin (10,000 U IV) • Administer adsorbed tetanus toxoid intramuscularly.

Antibiotics
• Have no effect against toxin already bound to nerves • Penicillin—administer systemically and locally into the wound; 20,000 IU/kg q12h for 5 days; use crystalline penicillin on the first day and procaine penicillin thereafter

CONTRAINDICATIONS/POSSIBLE INTERACTIONS
• Avoid glucocorticoids and atropine.
• Avoid narcotics—depress respiratory center

FOLLOW-UP

PATIENT MONITORING
• Prevent decubital ulcers and peripheral nerve palsies—cautiously move stabilized patient • Monitor blood pressure and ECG.
• Bronchopneumonia possible • Constipation possible

PREVENTION/AVOIDANCE
• Vaccinate—tetanus toxoid • Prevent skin wound trauma—clear runs and yards of wire, glass, etc. • Wound management—early and thorough irrigation with hydrogen peroxide; debridement, draining, especially in known tetanus-prone wounds • Penicillin—administer for minimum of 3 days for all deep contaminated wounds

EXPECTED COURSE AND PROGNOSIS
• Prognosis—depends on number of factors; the more toxin bound to nerves, the poorer the prognosis; improve by removing source of additional toxin (debriding and cleaning wound). • Course of recovery—slow; requires rehabilitation to regain full use of limbs; most recover in 1 week; some have a course of 3–4 weeks; unattended disease usually fatal
• Hiatal hernia possible with gastroesophageal reflux and regurgitation

MISCELLANEOUS

ZOONOTIC POTENTIAL
None, but tetanus spores ubiquitous in environment

ABBREVIATIONS
• AST = aspartate aminotransferase
• CNS = central nervous system
• CPK = creatine phosphokinase
• CSF = cerebrospinal fluid

Suggested Reading
Greene CE. Tetanus. In: Greene CE, ed. Infectious diseases of the dog and cat. Philadelphia: Saunders, 1998:267–273.
Author Patrick L. McDonough
Consulting Editor Stephen C. Barr

TETRALOGY OF FALLOT

BASICS

OVERVIEW
• A congenital cardiac malformation that consists of a VSD, pulmonic stenosis, an overriding aorta, and right ventricular hypertrophy (Figure 1). The VSD is usually large, with an area that equals or exceeds that of the open aortic valve. The essential developmental abnormality is probably a cranial deviation of a component of the infundibular septum; the other defects are secondary. Some reserve the term for malformations that strictly fulfill the above criteria; others apply it more liberally to include patients that have a VSD and right ventricular outflow tract obstruction.
• Hemodynamics are determined primarily by the size of the VSD and the severity of right ventricular outflow tract obstruction. A large VSD allows equilibration of left and right ventricular pressures, with shunt direction determined by the relationship between peripheral vascular resistance and the resistance to right ventricular ejection. Severe right ventricular outflow tract obstruction results in a right-to-left shunt with cyanosis and compensatory erythrocytosis as prominent clinical features.
• An uncommon congenital defect, but the most common congenital cardiac

malformation that causes cyanosis in dogs and cats

SIGNALMENT
• Dogs and cats—uncommon in both
• English bulldogs and keeshonds predisposed

SIGNS

Historical Findings
• Weakness
• Syncope
• Shortness of breath

Physical Examination Findings
• A systolic ejection murmur at the left heart base, caused by right ventricular outflow tract obstruction in most patients; some with hyperviscosity and severe pulmonary stenosis do not have murmurs.
• Cyanosis—in most patients; degree of cyanosis depends on the direction and volume of shunt. If right ventricular outflow tract obstruction is mild, the direction of the shunt may be left to right; in this case, cyanosis is absent and the pathophysiology is that of an isolated VSD.
• Arterial pulses usually normal
• Congestive heart failure occurs rarely, possibly because the right ventricle can unload into the left.

CAUSES & RISK FACTORS
Congenital; monogenic inheritance of a continuum of conotruncal defects that

includes tetralogy of Fallot has been shown in keeshonds. Genetic factors probably contribute to development of naturally occurring disorder.

DIAGNOSIS

DIFFERENTIAL DIAGNOSIS
• Pulmonic stenosis, aortic stenosis, ventricular septal defect, and atrial septal defect can all cause left basilar ejection murmurs.
• Patients with severe pulmonic stenosis and a right-to-left atrial level shunt may have similar findings on physical examination.
• Other anatomic right-to-left shunts (PDA or VSD with pulmonary hypertension) do not typically cause murmurs; differential cyanosis (mucous membranes in head are pink and those in caudal portions of body are cyanotic) are observed if a PDA shunts right to left.

CBC/BIOCHEMISTRY/URINALYSIS
• Compensatory erythrocytosis if the shunt is right to left
• Other clinicopathologic findings usually normal

OTHER LABORATORY TESTS
N/A

IMAGING

Thoracic Radiographic Findings
• Variable degree of right ventricular enlargement
• Ascending aorta may be prominent.
• Pulmonary vessels are small.

Echocardiographic Findings
• Right ventricular hypertrophy
• Large VSD visualized directly
• Straddling of the VSD by the aorta
• Narrow infundibulum and/or abnormal pulmonic valve
• Doppler evidence of pulmonic stenosis
• Contrast echocardiography delineates a right-to-left shunt.

Angiocardiography
• Reveals VSD, right ventricular hypertrophy, pulmonic stenosis, and direction of shunt
• Nonselective angiography may confirm the diagnosis in small animals.

DIAGNOSTIC PROCEDURES

Electrocardiographic Findings
• Right ventricular hypertrophy pattern in most dogs and cats
• Various intraventricular conduction disturbances observed in cats

Oximetry
Used to confirm peripheral desaturation of hemoglobin

TREATMENT
• Most can be treated as outpatients.
• Exercise restriction recommended
• Definitive surgical correction requires cardiopulmonary bypass.
• Palliative surgical procedures that enhance pulmonary blood flow have been performed.
• Treat erythrocytosis by periodic phlebotomy to maintain a PCV of 62–68%.

MEDICATIONS

DRUGS
Nonselective β-adrenergic antagonists such as propranolol may be palliative; they act as negative inotropes and prevent the physiologic drop in peripheral vascular resistance that occurs during exercise. These hemodynamic effects serve to limit right-to-left shunting. Propranolol may also favorably affect the oxyhemoglobin dissociation curve.

CONTRAINDICATIONS/POSSIBLE INTERACTIONS
Vasodilators contraindicated

FOLLOW-UP
• Monitor PCV every 1–3 months.
• Breeding affected animals is not advised.
• Bacterial endocarditis, neurologic complications associated with erythrocytosis, arrhythmias, and sudden death are potential sequelae.
• Prognosis is poor; most patients with clinical signs live less than 1 year, although survivals > 3 years have been documented.

MISCELLANEOUS

ABBREVIATIONS
• PDA = patent ductus arteriosus
• VSD = ventricular septal defect

Suggested Reading
Kittleson MD. Tetralogy of Fallot. In Kittleson MD, Kienle RD, eds. Small animal cardiovascular medicine. St. Louis: Mosby, 1998:240–247.

Author Jonathan A. Abbott
Consulting Editors Larry P. Tilley and Francis W. K. Smith, Jr.

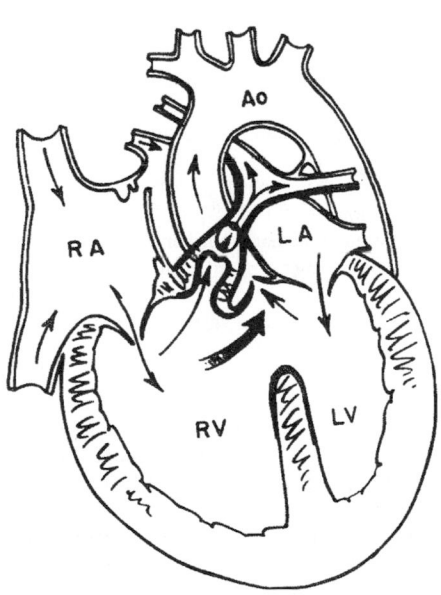

Figure 1.

Classic tetralogy of Fallot. RA = right atrium, LA = left atrium, RV = right ventricle, LV = left ventricle, AO = aorta. (From Roberts W. Adult congenital heart disease. Philadelphia: F.A. Davis Co., 1987, with permission.)

THIRD EYELID PROTRUSION

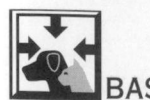

BASICS

DEFINITION
Abnormal protrusion (elevation) of the third eyelid

PATHOPHYSIOLOGY
• Dogs—movement of the third eyelid is passive.
• Cats—partial sympathetic nervous control of the third eyelid
• Results from a space-occupying mass in the orbit pushing the third eyelid forward, enophthalmia, sympathetic denervation of the eye, or a painful eye

SYSTEMS AFFECTED
• Ophthalmic—third eyelid(s); orbit; eyeball
• Nervous—autonomic nervous system

SIGNALMENT
See Causes.

SIGNS
• May have none
• May be associated with primary condition—exophthalmus; enophthalmus; blepharospasm; Horner's syndrome
• Unilateral or bilateral—depending on cause

CAUSES

Unilateral
Blepharospasm
• Painful ocular condition—corneal ulcer; glaucoma; uveitis; or ocular foreign body
• May cause the globe to be retracted and secondary third eyelid elevation
Space-occupying Orbital Mass
• Often an abscess or neoplasm
• May displace the third eyelid anteriorly
• Usually causes exophthalmus
• Abscess—generally seen in young patients; usually acute onset; painful on palpation
• Neoplasm—usually seen in old patients; gradual onset; frequently not painful (see Orbital Diseases)
Enophthalmus
• Globe—recedes into the orbit, causing third eyelid to appear elevated
• Unilateral—may be caused by trauma, orbital fat atrophy, and inflammation; may be secondary to orbital neoplasia in cats (see Orbital Diseases)
Microphthalmus or Phthisis Bulbi
• Small globes—cause the third eyelid to appear elevated

• Microphthalmus—congenital; may be idiopathic; inherited in specific breeds (collie eye anomaly); may result from toxin ingestion (griseofulvin in pregnant cats)
• Phthisis bulbi—occurs with severe damage to the globe (severe uveitis, glaucoma, or trauma); ciliary body fails to produce aqueous humor; diminished; small, fibrotic globe from chronic inflammation
Other
• Horner's syndrome—clinical signs develop after sympathetic denervation; elevated third eyelid; enophthalmus; ptosis (drooping upper eyelid); miosis (see Horner's Syndrome)
• Neoplasia of the third eyelid—adenocarcinoma of the gland of the third eyelid and squamous cell carcinoma of eyelid most common
• Cherry eye—see Prolapsed Gland of the Third Eyelid (Cherry Eye)
• Everted or scrolled cartilage of the third eyelid—seen in Wiemaraners, Great Danes, German short-haired pointers, and other breeds; the T-shaped cartilage of the third eyelid is rolled away from the surface of the eye instead of conforming to the corneal surface.
• Symblepharon—postinflammatory adhesions between the third eyelid and cornea or conjunctiva

Bilateral
Exophthalmus
• Space-occupying lesions of both orbits
• Usually caused by inflammatory lesions (e.g., eosinophilic myositis and extraocular muscle polymyositis)
Conformational
• Breed-specific—Doberman pinschers and pointers
• Deep orbits and prominent third eyelids
• Not pathologic
• No treatment needed
Plasmoma
• Immune-mediated thickening and hyperemia of the leading edge of the third eyelid
• Seen almost exclusively in German shepherds
• May be associated with chronic superficial keratitis (pannus)
Other
• Blepharospasm
• Enophthalmus—caused by dehydration, bilateral orbital fat atrophy secondary to severe cachexia, and chronic masticatory muscle myositis
• Haw syndrome (cats)—idiopathic bilateral elevation of the third eyelids; all other aspects of the ophthalmic examination are normal; usually resolves in 3–4 weeks without treatment

• Dysautonomia (Key-Gaskell syndrome)—bilateral elevated third eyelids; dilated nonresponsive pupils; KCS; dry mucosal surfaces; anorexia; lethargy; regurgitation; megaesophagus; bradycardia; megacolon; distended bladder (see Dysautonomia)
• Tranquilizers—many (e.g., acepromazine) cause bilateral third eyelid elevation
• Fatigue—may cause transient third eyelid elevation, especially in dogs prone to ectropion

RISK FACTORS
Depend on cause

DIAGNOSIS

DIFFERENTIAL DIAGNOSIS
• Most common causes of acute onset of unilateral condition—ocular pain (e.g., corneal ulcer and uveitis); orbital inflammation (e.g., orbital abscess and cellulitis)
• Middle-aged or old patient with unilateral, nonpainful condition—third eyelid or orbital neoplasm likely
• All patients—must rule out a small eye (microphthalmus or phthisis bulbi) and Horner's syndrome
• Likely causes of bilateral condition—systemic illness (e.g., dehydration, cachexia, and dysautonomia); associated with conformational abnormalities
• Prolapsed gland of the third eyelid—medial aspect of the third eyelid swollen; the third eyelid itself usually normal

CBC/BIOCHEMISTRY/URINALYSIS
• Leukocytosis and a left shift—with orbital inflammatory processes
• Blood work—generally unrewarding in differentiating causes

OTHER LABORATORY TESTS
Dysautonomia—confirmed by measuring urine and plasma catecholamine concentrations and pharmacologic testing of the autonomic nervous system

IMAGING
• Thoracic radiography—all patients with Horner's syndrome to rule out intrathoracic cause of sympathetic denervation; patients with suspected neoplasia to evaluate for metastatic disease
• Orbital ultrasound—recommended to help localize suspected orbital mass and define its nature (e.g., solid or cystic)

• CT or MRI—further define suspected or known orbital mass
• Skull radiographs—rarely show signs of orbital disease unless the lesion is very large and destructive

DIAGNOSTIC PROCEDURES
• Thorough ophthalmic examination
• Slit-lamp biomicroscope or some other source of magnification—recommended to help localize any potential ocular abnormality
• All patients with unilateral condition—examine both surfaces of the third eyelid and the conjunctival cul-de-sac carefully for a foreign body or symblepharon.
• Pharmacologic testing—localize lesion(s) with Horner syndrome (see Horner's Syndrome)
• Exploratory surgery and biopsy—may be only means to make a definitive diagnosis for a suspected orbital or third eyelid mass

Cytology
• For suspected mass lesions—orbital mass or mass of the third eyelid; fine-needle aspirate; may help make the diagnosis
• Unguided fine-needle aspiration—attempt only if the mass is anterior to the equator of the eye.
• Ultrasonography-guided fine-needle aspiration—for masses posterior to the eye; help avoid delicate retrobulbar structures
• Third eyelid scrapings (German shepherds with suspected plasmoma)—reveal plasma cells and lymphocytes

 TREATMENT
• Depends on cause
• Painful condition—remove the cause of the irritation (e.g., foreign body); treat the primary ocular condition
• Orbital cellulitis and abscess—generally respond well to systemically administered antibiotics
• Orbital neoplasms—usually require wide surgical excision via an orbital exenteration; may require adjunct therapeutic modalities (e.g., radiotherapy or chemotherapy) if excision is incomplete
• Microphthalmic eyes—usually none required; remove the globes if painful or subject to recurrent conjunctivitis
• Pathologic globes—enucleate to prevent formation of intraocular sarcomas (cats)

• Horner's syndrome—treat cause, if known (~ 50% of dogs and cats); otherwise will usually resolve without treatment in 4–12 weeks
• Surgical removal of the entire third eyelid—indicated for third eyelid neoplasia; may require adjunct therapeutic modalities (e.g., radiotherapy or chemotherapy) if the surgical margins are not free of neoplasm
• Radiotherapy around the eye—may result in severe keratitis, dry eye, and cataracts; discuss enucleation with the client before initiating treatment.
• Orbital exenteration—may be warranted if the mass extends into the orbit
• Plasmomas—usually controlled with topically applied medications; not cured; inform client that some form of treatment will likely be needed for the life of the patient; topical corticosteroids (0.1% dexamethasone or 1% prednisolone acetate; q6h initially, reduced to q24h when the lesion appears resolved); topical 1% cyclosporine (q12h) also effective
• Haw syndrome—usually resolves in 3–4 weeks without treatment
• Dysautonomia—see Dysautonomia.

 **MEDICATIONS**

DRUG(S) OF CHOICE
See Treatment.

CONTRAINDICATIONS
Topical corticosteroids—never use with a corneal ulcer

PRECAUTIONS
N/A

POSSIBLE INTERACTIONS
N/A

ALTERNATIVE DRUG(S)
N/A

 FOLLOW-UP

PATIENT MONITORING
Malignant neoplasm—take thoracic radiographs every 3–6 months to monitor for metastatic disease.

POSSIBLE COMPLICATIONS
Neoplasm—extension to or infection of adjacent orbital structures (e.g., eye, orbit,

orbital sinuses, and cranial cavity) possible; metastasis to distant sites (usually thorax or liver) possible (approximately 90% are malignant)
• Vision loss—from the lesion itself; from the elevation; from treatment (e.g., radiotherapy and exenteration)

 **MISCELLANEOUS**

ASSOCIATED CONDITIONS
N/A

AGE-RELATED FACTORS
• Middle-aged to old patients—at risk for neoplastic diseases of the third eyelid and orbit
• Young patients—at risk for congenital abnormalities; affected by inflammatory conditions of the third eyelid more frequently than are old animals

ZOONOTIC POTENTIAL
N/A

PREGNANCY
N/A

SYNONYMS
• Elevated third eyelid
• Haw syndrome (cats)

SEE ALSO
• Ectropion
• Entropion
• Horner's Syndrome
• Orbital Diseases (Exophthalmus, Enophthalmus, Strabismus)
• Prolapsed Gland of the Third Eyelid (Cherry Eye)

ABBREVIATION
KCS = keratoconjunctivitis sicca

Suggested Reading
Sharp NH, Nash AS, Griffiths IR. Feline dysautonomia (the Key-Gaskell syndrome): a clinical and pathological study of forty cases. J Small Anim Pract 1985; 25:599–615.
Ward DA. Diseases and surgery of the canine nictitating membrane. In: Gelatt KN, ed. Veterinary Ophthalmology, 3rd ed. Philadelphia: Lippincott Williams & Wilkins, 1999; 609–618.
Author Brian C. Gilger
Consulting Editor Paul E. Miller

THROMBOCYTOPATHIES

BASICS

OVERVIEW
• Acquired or hereditary defects that can affect any of the main functions of the platelets, including activation, adhesion, and aggregation
• Affected animals typically have normal platelet counts but have spontaneous or excessive bleeding; mucosal bleeding is the most common sign.

SIGNALMENT
• Hereditary platelet function defects diagnosed at all ages, but may first appear in young animals when excessive bleeding occurs with loss of deciduous teeth
• Acquired defects—any breed of dog or cat
• Von Willebrand disease—many breeds of dogs and rarely cats (see von Willebrand Disease)
• Basset hound hereditary thrombopathia—widespread in this breed
• Spitz thrombopathia—Spitz
• Type I Glanzmann thromboasthenia—otter hounds (thromboasthenic thrombopathia) and Great Pyrenees
• Platelet function defect—gray collies with cyclic hematopoiesis
• Chediak-Higashi syndrome—Persian cats (rare in other breeds)
• Delta-storage pool disease—American cocker spaniels
• Other platelet function defects—boxers, mixed breeds

SIGNS
• Spontaneous bleeding in some animals, often associated with mucosal surfaces
• Epistaxis
• Auricular hematomas in basset hounds with hereditary thrombopathia
• Prolonged bleeding in some animals during diagnostic or surgical procedures

CAUSES & RISK FACTORS

Acquired–Drugs
• Anesthetic and sedative agents, except barbiturates and isoflurane
• Antibiotics, especially penicillins. Fluoroquinolones and cefazolin have minimal effects.
• Antihistamines—H_1 and H_2 blockers. Famotidine has less effect than cimetidine or ranitidine.
• NSAIDs (e.g., aspirin) inhibit platelet function by preventing the formation of thromboxane A_2, a potent platelet agonist. This effect is less pronounced to absent with more selective cyclooxygenase-2 antagonists (e.g., meloxicam, deracoxib).
• Secondary to systemic disease—uremia, pancreatitis, liver disease, immune-mediated thrombocytopenia (rarely significant) and neoplastic disorders (both hematopoietic and nonhematopoietic neoplasms)

Hereditary
• Von Willebrand disease—a deficiency of von Willebrand's factor, which is critical for platelet adhesion
• Basset hound hereditary thrombopathia and Spitz thrombopathy—platelet aggregation defects
• Aggregation defect caused by lack of the fibrinogen receptor—otter hounds and great Pyrenees with type I Glanzmann thromboasthenia, a deficiency of the platelet glycoproteins necessary for fibrinogen binding
• Aggregation defect caused by lack of normal constituents in the platelet dense granules—gray collies with cyclic hematopoiesis and Chediak-Higashi syndrome
• Deficiency in delta-storage pool of ADP—American cocker spaniels.
• Suspected secretion/signal transduction disorder described in a Boxer and mixed-breed dog

DIAGNOSIS

DIFFERENTIAL DIAGNOSIS
Other acquired or hereditary bleeding disorders characterized by bleeding that is more severe than the bleeding seen in most animals with acquired or hereditary platelet function defects

CBC/BIOCHEMISTRY/URINALYSIS
• Anemia, if bleeding is severe; regenerative or nonregenerative
• Platelet counts typically normal in dogs with thrombocytopathies, but low counts seen in some otter hounds
• Giant platelets in some otter hounds
• Large pink cytoplasmic granules in granulocytes with or without granules in monocytes in cats with Chediak-Higashi syndrome
• Biochemical profile—no specific changes

OTHER LABORATORY TESTS
• Von Willebrand disease assay—in animals suspected of having this disease
• Platelet function testing—in select laboratories to document and characterize hereditary platelet function defects
• Coagulation tests (PT and APTT)—to eliminate DIC or a vitamin K antagonist from the differential diagnosis; APTT may be prolonged in some animals with von Willebrand disease

DIAGNOSTIC PROCEDURES
• Mucosal bleeding time–platelet function defects; normal buccal mucosal bleeding time measured using a spring-loaded lancet that makes an incision 6 mm long by 1 mm deep (Simplate, bioMérieux, Inc, Durham NC) is less than 4–5 min in dogs, and less than 2–3 min in cats

TREATMENT

• Many affected animals have spontaneous bleeding that is not life threatening.
• Before surgery, identify animals with platelet function defects by buccal mucosal bleeding time to allow preparation to prevent excessive bleeding during the procedure.
• Platelet transfusion—20 mL/kg (minimum 10 mL/kg) fresh whole blood, platelet-rich plasma or fresh frozen plasma (contains platelet particles) or 1 unit/10 kg (minimum 1 unit/30 kg) platelet concentrate or cryoprecipitate. Also appropriate (except for platelet concentrate) for von Willebrand disease. Transfuse prophylactically or if critical hemorrhage is noted.
• Whole blood or packed red cell transfusion to correct anemia—bleeding due to thrombocytopathia is worse in the presence of anemia
• Consider using topical hemostatic agents.
• In animals with acquired platelet function disorders, treat the underlying disease process or withdraw the offending agent.
• Minimize IM and SC injections. Apply extended pressure after IV injections, IV catheterization, and invasive procedures.
• Avoid overexuberant fluid therapy.
• Restrict activity during a bleeding episode.
• Avoid hard foods (gingival bleeding).

MEDICATIONS

DRUG(S)
• Desmopressin acetate [DDAVP] (1 μg/kg SC or IV diluted in 20 mL saline

administered over 10 min) to dogs with von Willebrand disease during a bleeding episode (if effective, effect lasts 2–3 hours).
• Desmopressin is beneficial in many thrombocytopathies in humans, so consider using in dogs.
• Give desmopressin to donor 30 min before collection of blood for transfusion to dogs with von Willebrand disease or thrombocytopathia.
• Lithium carbonate (10 mg/kg PO q12h) enhances platelet function in normal dogs, but there is limited clinical experience with the drug.

CONTRAINDICATIONS/POSSIBLE INTERACTION
• NSAIDs that interfere with platelet function. Opioids are preferred for analgesia. If NSAID use required, use more selective cyclooxygenase-2 inhibitors (e.g., meloxicam, deracoxib)
• Antibiotics that interfere with platelet function–clinically most relevant with all penicillins
• Anticoagulants

FOLLOW-UP

• Take special precautions when performing surgical procedures on these animals.
• Make owner aware that animals with hereditary platelet function defects may have recurring bleeding episodes, but fatal bleeds are uncommon.
• If a hereditary defect is identified, do not use the animal for breeding.

MISCELLANEOUS

SEE ALSO
Von Willebrand Disease, Thrombocytopenia

ABBREVIATIONS
• ADP = adenosine diphosphate
• APTT = activated partial thromboplastin time
• DDAVP = 1 deamino-8-D-arginine vasopressin
• DIC = disseminated intravascular coagulation
• NSAID = nonsteroidal antiinflammatory drug
• PT = prothrombin time

Suggested Reading
Callan MB. Treatment of primary hemostatic disorders. Proceedings of the 19th Annual Veterinary Medical Forum of the American College of Veterinary Internal Medicine, 2001:517–519.
de Gopegui RR, Feldman BF. Platelets and von Willebrand's disease. In: Ettinger SL, Feldman EC, eds. Textbook of veterinary internal medicine. 5th ed. Philadelphia: Saunders, 2000:1817–1828.

Acknowledgment
The author and editors acknowledge the prior contribution of Dr. William J. Reagan, who authored this topic in the previous edition.
Author Anthony C.G. Abrams-Ogg
Consulting Editor Stephen A. Kruth

THROMBOCYTOPENIA

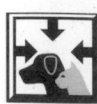

BASICS

DEFINITION
• Platelet count below the lower limit of reference range • Reference range varies with method of platelet counting; Animal Health Laboratory (Guelph, Ontario) reference range using Advia 120 hematology system (Bayer HealthCare, Monheim, Germany): 117,000–418,000/μL (dogs), 93,000–514,000/μL (cats): the lower limit in cats is probably due to platelet clumping • Mild thrombocytopenia: 80,000/μL—lower limit of reference range; moderate thrombocytopenia: 20,000–80,000/μL; severe thrombocytopenia: < 20,000/μL

PATHOPHYSIOLOGY
• Platelets are produced by megakaryocytes in the bone marrow and released into the bloodstream, where they circulate for up to 7 days. • In the normal state, the platelet count remains stable because production of platelets is equivalent to removal of platelets from the circulation and there is a splenic reserve. • Thrombocytopenia is caused by decreased production and increased sequestration, use, destruction, or loss of platelets. • Thrombocytopenia may result in spontaneous or excessive hemorrhage.

SYSTEMS AFFECTED
• Hemorrhage may occur into any organ system. • Clinical hemorrhage—most commonly recognized in the skin/exocrine and gastrointestinal systems, followed by the renal/urologic and respiratory systems; less commonly recognized in the ophthalmic, nervous, and reproductive systems

INCIDENCE/PREVALENCE
Hemorrhage due to thrombocytopenia is uncommon (dogs) or rare (cats) in general practice.

GEOGRAPHIC DISTRIBUTION
Varies with infectious agents and use of cytotoxic therapy

SIGNALMENT

Species
• Dogs and cats • Primary IMT rare in cats

Breed Predilections
• Primary IMT—more common in cocker spaniels, poodles, and Old English sheepdogs • Hereditary asymptomatic thrombocytopenia with macroplatelets—described in Cavalier King Charles spaniels • Hereditary asymptomatic mild thrombocytopenia—described in greyhounds

Mean Age And Range
• Any age • Primary IMT—more common in middle-aged dogs

Predominant Sex
• Primary IMT—more common in female dogs

SIGNS

General Comments
• Increased surgical hemorrhage may occur at platelet counts < 80,000/μL. • Microscopic

spontaneous hemorrhage may occur at platelet counts < 50,000/μL. • There is mild, moderate, and severe risk of spontaneous clinical hemorrhage at platelet counts of < 20,000/μL, < 10,000/μL, and < 5000/μL, respectively. • These figures are guidelines only because of variation in methods of platelet counting and imprecision of low platelet counts. • Concurrent platelet function defect, von Willebrand's disease, vasculitis, coagulopathy, or sepsis increases risk of hemorrhage. • Dogs with IMT have a lower risk of hemorrhage for a given platelet count. • Cats have a lower risk of hemorrhage than do dogs.

Historical Findings
• Spontaneous or excessive mucous membrane, cutaneous, gastrointestinal, nasal, and urinary bleeding • Lethargy and collapse • Dyspnea and coughing

Physical Examination Findings
• Petechiae and ecchymoses in skin and mucous membranes • Persistent bleeding from wounds and venipuncture sites • Melena, hematochezia, hematemesis • Hematuria • Ocular hemorrhages • Splenomegaly, hepatomegaly • Pale mucous membranes • Weakness • Dyspnea, hemoptysis • Heart murmur • Fever • Neurologic signs • Excessive bleeding in estrus

CAUSES
• Decreased production—hereditary; neoplasia in bone marrow • Sertoli cell tumor; infectious agents • immune-mediated; drugs • irradiation. Thrombocytopenia varies from mild to severe, and may be an isolated hematologic abnormality or a feature of generalized bone marrow failure. • Increased sequestration—splenomegaly. Severe thrombocytopenia is uncommon • Increased use—DIC • local thrombosis; vasculitis. Severe thrombocytopenia is uncommon. • Increased destruction • primary IMT or IMT secondary to neoplasia; infectious agents; aseptic inflammation; drugs. Most common cause of severe thrombocytopenia in dogs • Increased loss—hemorrhage due to vitamin K antagonist poisoning may result in mild to moderate thrombocytopenia; hemorrhage due to major trauma may result in mild to severe thrombocytopenia after volume resuscitation with crystalloids, colloids, or platelet-poor blood products

RISK FACTORS
• Infectious agents and diseases associated with thrombocytopenia—FeLV; FIV; distemper; parvoviruses; *Ehrlichia canis; Ehrlichia platys;* Rocky Mountain spotted fever; leptospirosis; bacterial sepsis; *Cytauxzoon felis;* histoplasmosis; and heartworm • Potentially any neoplasm—neoplasms most commonly identified include hemangiosarcoma, lymphoma, and acute leukemias • Cytotoxic therapy—predictable myelosuppression; lomustine causes a cumulative thrombocytopenia • Potentially any drug—drugs with known risk for causing unpredictable myelosuppression or IMT include estrogen, gold compounds, phenylbutazone, phenobarbital (dogs) chloramphenicol, griseofulvin, propylthiouracil, and methimazole (cats); drugs with reported idiosyncratic reactions causing myelosuppression include cepha-

losporins and albendazole (dogs, cats), sulfonamides, angiotensin-converting enzyme inhibitors (dogs), and ribavirin • Vaccination within 1 month—for IMT

DIAGNOSIS

DIFFERENTIAL DIAGNOSIS
• Measurement error due to platelet clumping—most likely to occur with traumatic venipuncture and in cats • Clerical error • Local hemorrhage—rule out trauma, gastrointestinal ulceration, and primary intranasal, urinary and reproductive tract, and ophthalmic disorders • von Willebrand's disease—petechiae, ecchymoses, and ocular hemorrhages unusual • Coagulopathy—petechiae, gastrointestinal hemorrhage, and epistaxis unusual; subcutaneous swellings, swollen joints, hemothorax, and hemoabdomen may be present

CBC/BIOCHEMISTRY/URINALYSIS
• Disregard platelet count from a QBC analyzer if there is an error message; confirm thrombocytopenia reported by an automated hematology analyzer by microscopic examination of a blood smear; examine feather edge for platelet clumps; estimate platelet count from red cell monolayer where about 50% of cells are touching; each platelet-per-oil immersion field represents 15,000–25,000/μL; if there are > 2 platelets per oil field, spontaneous bleeding is unlikely; if there are > 4 platelets per oil field, there is minimal risk of excessive bleeding • Concurrent nonregenerative anemia and neutropenia—thrombocytopenia probably due to decreased production • Shift platelets—there is some platelet production occurring (quantification standards similar to reticulocytosis not established) • Regenerative anemia—rule out hemorrhage, or IMHA concurrent with IMT (supported by spherocytosis with or without agglutination) • Neutrophilia and left shift—rule out bacterial/fungal sepsis, nonseptic inflammation, and nonspecific stimulation of granulopoiesis • Eosinophilia—rule out heartworm disease. • Schistocytes—rule out DIC. • Morulae in blood cells—rule out *Ehrlichia* spp. • Proteinuria—rule out concurrent glomerulonephritis (SLE).

OTHER LABORATORY TESTS
• von Willebrand's factor antigen—rule out von Willebrand's disease. • PT, APTT, ACT—normal PT rules out vitamin K antagonism; positive results increase likelihood of DIC • Fibrinogen degradation products—positive result increases likelihood of DIC • FeLV and FIV tests—rule out retroviral infection. • Serum titers—rule out ehrlichial infections, Rocky Mountain spotted fever, and leptospirosis • Bacterial/fungal cultures of abnormal organs, blood, and urine—rule out bacterial or fungal sepsis • Heartworm antigen test—rules out dirofilariasis • Antiplatelet antibody and antimegakaryocyte antibody tests—negative results help rule out IMT, but tests are not widely available • Coombs test—positive result increases likelihood of concurrent IMHA

• Antinuclear antibody test—positive result increases likelihood of SLE.

IMAGING
Radiography and ultrasonography to identify splenomegaly, hepatomegaly, internal neoplasms, foci of infection, and internal bleeding

DIAGNOSTIC PROCEDURES
Bone marrow biopsy—to rule out reduced platelet production: neoplasia in bone marrow, histoplasmosis, maturation arrest, marrow aplasia, myelofibrosis, and marrow necrosis; no specific finding that rules in or out immune-mediated megakaryocytic hypoplasia

TREATMENT

APPROPRIATE HEALTH CARE
• Platelet transfusion—20 mL/kg (minimum 10 mL/kg) fresh whole blood, platelet-rich plasma, or fresh frozen plasma (contains platelet particles), or 1 unit/10 kg (minimum 1 unit/30 kg) platelet concentrate or cryoprecipitate; transfuse if critical hemorrhage is noted or prophylactically if platelet count < 5000–10,000/µL; most useful when thrombocytopenia is due to reduced production or loss, less useful in splenomegaly and DIC, and least useful in IMT • Whole blood or packed red cell transfusion to correct anemia—bleeding due to thrombocytopenia is worse in the presence of anemia • Do not drain hematomas unless causing a problem (e.g., tracheal compression)

NURSING CARE
• Minimize IM and SC injections. Apply extended pressure after IV injections, IV catheterization, and invasive procedures. Avoid jugular venipuncture. Bone marrow biopsy is safe.
• Avoid overexuberant fluid therapy.

CLIENT EDUCATION
If underlying cause of severe thrombocytopenia cannot be identified and treated, treatment will fail because of limited ability to provide extensive platelet transfusions.

SURGICAL CONSIDERATIONS
• Surgery may be required to eliminate neoplasm, septic focus, or splenic torsion. • May need extensive perioperative and intraoperative transfusions • Consider using topical hemostatic agents.

MEDICATIONS

DRUG(S) OF CHOICE
• DIC—heparin (70–100 U/kg IV over 30 min or SC q8h); see Disseminated Intravascular Coagulation • IMT—prednisone (2 mg/kg PO q12–24h for at least two weeks, then tapered) with or without other immunosuppressive agents; see Thrombocytopenia, Primary Immune-mediated • Rickettsial diseases—doxycycline, tetracycline, or oxytetracycline; see Ehrlichiosis and Rocky Mountain Spotted Fever

• Bacterial infections—cefazolin (30 mg/kg IV q8h) and enrofloxacin (5 mg/kg IV over 20 min or IM q12–24h) • Lymphoma and leukemia—anticancer chemotherapy • Central nervous system hemorrhage—dexamethasone (0.25 mg/kg IV or PO q8–24h) • Hyphema—topical prednisolone acetate 1% or dexamethasone sodium phosphate 0.1% q6–8h, and topical atropine 1% q8–12h

CONTRAINDICATIONS
• NSAIDS that interfere with platelet function—opioids are preferred for analgesia; if NSAID use required, use more selective cyclooxygenase-2 inhibitors (e.g., meloxicam, deracoxib) • Other drugs that interfere with platelet function—clinically relevant in severe thrombocytopenia with all penicillins; see Thrombocytopathies

PRECAUTIONS
• Heparin may aggravate hemorrhage due to thrombocytopenia. • Corticosteroid therapy may exacerbate infection and promote gastrointestinal ulceration. • Enrofloxacin not approved for IV use; visual disturbances occur rarely in cats

ALTERNATIVE DRUG(S)
• Recombinant human interleukin-11 (Neumega; Wyeth, Collegeville, PA)—50 µg/kg SC q24h for a maximum of 2 weeks; most useful to stimulate platelet production when thrombocytopenia is caused by cytotoxic therapy; neutralizing antibody formation occurs after 2 weeks; expensive • Lithium carbonate—10 mg/kg PO q12h; stimulates platelet production but limited clinical experience; inexpensive • Aminocaproic acid—plasmin inhibitor; limited clinical experience; contraindicated in DIC; dose reported for degenerative myelopathy in dogs: about 12.5–15 mg/kg PO q8h; human dosage about 10 times that for dogs

FOLLOW-UP

PATIENT MONITORING
• Amount of bleeding—control of clinical hemorrhage is most important parameter to monitor to judge effectiveness of treatment • Platelet counts—daily until patient is stable, then weekly until platelets return to normal range Serial coagulation profiles—if DIC suspected

POSSIBLE COMPLICATIONS
Excessive bleeding, which can be fatal

EXPECTED COURSE AND PROGNOSIS
Vary with cause of thrombocytopenia

MISCELLANEOUS

ASSOCIATED CONDITIONS
• If thrombocytopenia is from reduced production, there may be concurrent anemia from erythroid hypoplasia and neutropenia. • IMT may be an isolated abnormality or associated with

other immune-mediated disorders (e.g., IMHA, hypothyroidism, SLE).

AGE-RELATED FACTORS
Varies with cause—e.g., FeLV in younger cats, IMT in middle-aged dogs, neoplasia in older dogs

ZOONOTIC POTENTIAL
Thrombocytopenia may be due to a zoonotic infection (e.g., leptospirosis).

PREGNANCY
• Corticosteroid therapy may cause fetal loss.
• Treatment of animals with rickettsial diseases with tetracycline or doxycycline can cause fetal abnormalities. • Because conditions causing thrombocytopenia are likely to result in fetal loss, placing emphasis on therapy for the dam despite effects on the fetuses should be considered.

SEE ALSO
• Anemia, Immune-mediated • Sepsis and Bacteremia • Cytauxzoonosis • Disseminated Intravascular Coagulation • Canine Distemper • Ehrlichiosis • Feline Immunodeficiency Virus Infection (FIV) • Feline Leukemia Virus Infection (FeLV) • Heartworm Disease—Cats; Heartworm Disease—Dogs • Histoplasmosis • Leptospirosis • Lupus Erythematosus, Systemic (SLE) • Neutropenia • Pancytopenia • Petechiae, Ecchymoses, Bruising • Rocky Mountain Spotted Fever • Splenomegaly • Thrombocytopathies • Thrombocytopenia, Primary Immune-mediated • Vasculitis Systemic

ABBREVIATIONS
• ACT = activated clotting time • APTT = activated partial thromboplastin time • DIC = disseminated intravascular coagulation • FeLV = feline leukemia virus • FIV = feline immunodeficiency virus • IMHA = immune-mediated hemolytic anemia • IMT = immune-mediated thrombocytopenia • NSAID = nonsteroidal antiinflammatory drug • PT = prothrombin time • QBC = quantitative buffy coat • SLE = systemic lupus erythematosus

Suggested Reading
Abrams-Ogg ACG. Management of hemorrhage due to thrombocytopenia. Proceedings of the 20th Annual ACVIM Forum. Lakewood, CO: American College of Veterinary Internal Medicine, 2002:577–579.
Grinden CB, Breischwerdt EB, Corbett WT, Jans HE. Epidemiologic survey of thrombocytopenia in dogs: a report of 987 cases. Vet Clin Pathol 1991;20:38–43.
Jordan HL, Grindem CB, Breitschwerdt EB. Thrombocytopenia in cats: a retrospective study of 41 cases. J Vet Intern Med 1993; 7:261–265.

Acknowledgment
The author and editors acknowledge the prior contributions of Dr. William J. Reagan, who authored this topic in the previous edition.

Author Anthony C.G. Abrams-Ogg
Consulting Editor Stephen A. Kruth

THROMBOCYTOPENIA, PRIMARY IMMUNE-MEDIATED

BASICS

DEFINITION
Immune-mediated destruction of platelets with no identifiable cause

PATHOPHYSIOLOGY
Autoantibodies (primarily IgG) bound to the platelet surface result in premature platelet destruction by macrophages.

SYSTEMS AFFECTED
• Skin/Exocrine • Gastrointestinal • Respiratory • Ophthalmic • Renal/Urologic

GENETICS
• Predisposition is suggested by high disease prevalence in several breeds. • Mode of inheritance is complex and poorly understood.

INCIDENCE/PREVALENCE
• Common in dogs: 5% of hospital admissions in one study; reported incidence is 3 to 18%. • Rare in cats

GEOGRAPHIC DISTRIBUTION
• No regional differences • Regional variations in the prevalence of infectious causes of thrombocytopenia influence the likelihood that a patient with thrombocytopenia has primary IMT.

SIGNALMENT

Species
• Common in dogs • Rare in cats

Breed Predilection
• Cocker spaniels, poodles, and Old English sheepdogs • Any breed, including crossbreeds, can be affected.

Mean Age and Range
• Most common in middle-aged dogs • Reported age range is 8 months to 17 years.

Predominant Sex
Females, spayed or intact, are affected twice as frequently as males.

SIGNS

Historical Findings
• Anorexia, lethargy, weakness • Epistaxis, hematochezia, mucosal hemorrhages

Physical Examination Findings
• Lethargy and weakness • Mucosal and cutaneous petechiae and ecchymoses • Hyphema • Retinal hemorrhages • Melena • Hematemesis • Epistaxis • Mucous membrane pallor • Central nervous system or intraocular hemorrhage can lead to neurologic signs or blindness, respectively. • Fever, hepatosplenomegaly, and lymphadenomegaly are unusual in dogs with primary IMT.

CAUSES
• Unknown • In dogs, may occur with SLE and secondary to drug administration (potentially any drug, but especially potentiated sulfonamide antibiotics), neoplasia (especially lymphoma), dirofilariasis, and ehrlichiosis • In cats, may occur secondary to FeLV or FIV infection

RISK FACTORS
May be preceded by vaccination or a stressful event

DIAGNOSIS

DIFFERENTIAL DIAGNOSIS
• Diagnosis is made by excluding other causes of thrombocytopenia; the extent to which other causes of thrombocytopenia can or need to be definitively excluded varies; in many cases, history, physical examination, and results of screening blood tests (see CBC/Biochemistry/Urinalysis) are sufficient to establish a working diagnosis. • Response to treatment can be used for diagnostic confirmation. • DIC—to rule out, perform a coagulation profile • Hemorrhage (especially due to anticoagulant rodenticide toxicity) may cause mild to moderate thrombocytopenia but will not cause petechial hemorrhages; coagulation testing can investigate anticoagulant rodenticide toxicity.
• Secondary IMT—investigate history of drug exposure, heartworm status, *Ehrlichia* titers, and evidence of lymphadenopathy or hepatosplenomegaly; response to doxycycline treatment can be used to investigate ehrlichiosis. • Other signs of SLE (e.g., mucocutaneous ulceration, polyarthritis, polymyositis, protein-losing nephropathy) should prompt ANA and LE tests. • Vasculitis (ehrlichiosis, Rocky Mountain spotted fever, leptospirosis, sepsis, babesiosis, bartonellosis, systemic mycoses)—fever and evidence of renal and/or liver disease on chemistry profile are more consistent with ehrlichiosis, Rocky Mountain spotted fever, leptospirosis, sepsis, babesiosis, bartonellosis, or systemic mycosis; titers and response to doxycycline can be used to investigate rickettsial disease; titers and response to ampicillin can be used to investigate leptospirosis; clinical signs, blood and urine cultures, and response to broad-spectrum antibiotics can be used to investigate bacterial sepsis; serology and PCR testing can be used to investigate babesiosis; serology can be used to investigate bartonellosis; thoracic radiographs, serology, and cytology can be used to investigate systemic mycoses. • Hemangiosarcoma—abdominal palpation (splenomegaly), ultrasonography, coagulation profile • Snake envenomation—history • Splenomegaly causes only mild thrombocytopenia (not < 100,000/ μL); diagnose by abdominal palpation, radiographs, and ultrasonography. • Bone marrow disease can cause thrombocytopenia of variable severity; neutropenia or nonregenerative anemia in a patient with thrombocytopenia should prompt consideration of bone marrow aspiration or core biopsy. • Estrogen toxicity—history, palpate testes, preputial cytology, bone marrow aspirates • Greyhounds, Shiba Inus, and Cavalier King Charles spaniels have lower platelet counts than other breeds.
• Pseudothrombocytopenia can be caused by platelet clumping, presence of many large platelets (especially in Cavalier King Charles spaniels), or inappropriate automated hematology analyzer settings; thrombocytopenia should always be verified by blood smear evaluation. • The most common causes of thrombocytopenia in cats are infectious diseases (FeLV, FIV, toxoplasmosis, rickettsial disease), neoplasia (especially lymphoproliferative and myeloproliferative disease), and thromboembolism secondary to underlying cardiac disease; test for FeLV, FIV, and *Haemobartonella*; *Ehrlichia risticii* titers, because infection in cats may lead to thrombocytopenia; doxycycline treatment trial for *Haemobartonellosis* and ehrlichiosis; bone marrow aspiration or core biopsy if bone marrow disease is suspected from the CBC

CBC/BIOCHEMISTRY/URINALYSIS
• Peripheral blood smear evaluation enables rapid in-house assessment of platelet numbers, although a CBC is necessary to quantify its severity. • Dogs with primary IMT usually have marked thrombocytopenia (platelets < 50,000/ μL). • High mean platelet volume or presence of large platelets on blood smear evaluation indicates that bone marrow production of platelets is increased. • Low mean platelet volume (microthrombocytosis) suggests IMT. • Some patients will have neutrophilia. • Neutropenia suggests bone marrow disease or sepsis. • Anemia may occur from hemorrhage or concurrent immune-mediated hemolytic anemia and will be regenerative if there has been sufficient time (5–7 days) for the bone marrow to respond. • Many fragmented red blood cells (schistocytes or schizocytes) support DIC, hemangiosarcoma, or heartworm disease as the cause. • Autoagglutination or numerous spherocytes support a diagnosis of immune-mediated hemolytic anemia; thrombocytopenia in these patients is likely to be due to either IMT or DIC • Biochemical profile is usually normal, although liver enzymes are often mildly to moderately high in dogs with concurrent AIHA. • Hematuria may be present.

OTHER LABORATORY TESTS
• The utility of tests for antiplatelet autoantibodies in dogs with thrombocytopenia is uncertain. • The platelet factor 3 test is not specific for IMT. • Megakaryocyte immunofluorescence is not highly sensitive, and its specificity is uncertain. • Increased platelet-bound IgG is a highly sensitive but nonspecific test. • Coagulation profiles can be done to investigate DIC and anticoagulant rodenticide toxicity. • Antinuclear antibody and lupus erythematosus tests are indicated in patients with clinical signs and laboratory abnormalities that support SLE. • Serology for ehrlichiosis, Rocky Mountain spotted fever, dirofilariasis, and leptospirosis may be indicated.

IMAGING
Radiographs and ultrasound can be obtained to investigate other causes of thrombocytopenia, such as hemangiosarcoma, lymphoma, hemorrhage, and systemic mycosis.

THROMBOCYTOPENIA, PRIMARY IMMUNE-MEDIATED

DIAGNOSTIC PROCEDURES

• Bone marrow evaluation is not routinely necessary. • Indications for bone marrow aspiration or core biopsy include neutropenia, presence of blast cells on blood smear evaluation, nonregenerative anemia, history of exposure to exogenous estrogens, or thrombocytopenia that is refractory to immunosuppressive therapy. • Response to immunosuppressive treatment can be used for diagnostic confirmation of primary IMT. • A doxycycline treatment trial can be used in patients suspected of having rickettsial infections. • Doxycyclines and corticosteroids can be administered concurrently to treat both IMT and rickettsial infections

TREATMENT

APPROPRIATE HEALTH CARE

Treat as outpatient unless hemorrhaging is severe or other diagnostic procedures are required.

NURSING CARE

• Hypovolemia or anemia can be managed by administration of crystalloid or colloid solutions, packed red blood cells, or whole blood. • Platelet transfusions are rarely necessary, and multiple units of platelets must be administered to have any appreciable effect on platelet numbers.

CLIENT EDUCATION

• Strict rest is important to minimize hemorrhage. • Animals with severe hemorrhage, seizures, or changes in mental status should be brought to the hospital for monitoring. • Unnecessary medications and NSAIDs should be avoided.

SURGICAL CONSIDERATIONS

• Splenectomy is an option for dogs refractory to other treatments. • Increased risk of bleeding in dogs with < 30,000 platelets/µL.

MEDICATIONS

DRUG(S)

• Corticosteroids—prednisone or prednisolone at an induction dose of 1–3 mg/kg q12h or dexamethasone at an induction dose of 0.1–0.6 mg/kg q24h • Vincristine 0.02 mg/kg IV can repeat weekly if needed. • Other immunosuppressive medications are often combined with corticosteroids for initial treatment of primary IMT in dogs; whether this improves treatment success is uncertain. • The majority of dogs with IMT will attain a platelet count > 50,000–100,000/ µL within 7 days of commencing treatment. • Failure of patients to respond to initial treatment should prompt reconsideration of the diagnosis. • Treatment options for dogs refractory to initial treatment include increasing the dose of

corticosteroid or using an alternate corticosteroid; cyclophosphamide (200 mg/kg PO or IV weekly), azathioprine (2 mg/kg PO q24h induction dose), danazol (5 mg/kg PO q12h), cyclosporine (Neoral [Novartis, East Hanover, NJ] 2.5–5 mg/kg PO q12h; monitor blood level), human immunoglobulin concentrate (0.5–1.5 g/kg IV over 2–4 hr), or splenectomy. • Once the platelet count normalizes, taper immunosuppressive medications to cessation over 4–6 months • Sucralfate and antacids can be administered if gastric ulceration is suspected. • Cats usually respond well to immunosuppressive doses of prednisone or prednisolone (1–3 mg/kg PO q12h).

CONTRAINDICATIONS

NSAIDs

PRECAUTIONS

• Any unnecessary medications should be discontinued, because they may induce secondary IMT. • High-dose corticosteroids may cause gastrointestinal ulceration; dexamethasone may be more ulcerogenic than is prednisone. • Long-term treatment with corticosteroids can result in iatrogenic hyperadrenocorticism. • Excessive immunosuppression can predispose to infections by opportunistic pathogens. • Cytotoxic medications can cause bone marrow suppression. • Dose tapering too rapidly after remission may predispose to recurrence.

POSSIBLE INTERACTIONS

Combination therapy causes increasing immunosuppression, which can predispose to opportunistic infections.

FOLLOW-UP

PATIENT MONITORING

• Platelet count daily to every few days until platelet numbers exceed 50,000/µL, then weekly until platelet numbers normalize (in some patients the platelet count may never return to normal range) • Platelet counts should be performed weekly or every 2 weeks during the period of drug dose tapering. • Animals with severe hemorrhage, seizures, or changes in mental status should be brought to the hospital for monitoring.

PREVENTION/AVOIDANCE

• Whether MLV vaccination will induce recurrence is uncertain; unnecessary vaccinations should be avoided. • Minimize stress that may initiate recurrence. • If medications are suspected to have caused secondary IMT, they should never again be administered to the patient.

POSSIBLE COMPLICATIONS

• Death from hemorrhagic shock or central nervous system hemorrhage • Gastrointestinal ulceration

EXPECTED COURSE AND PROGNOSIS

• Most dogs with primary IMT will have platelet count increases to < 50,000–100,000/µL within 7–10 days of starting corticosteroid treatment, either alone or in conjunction with other immunosuppressive medications. • Approximately 50% of dogs with primary IMT will experience only one episode of disease. • Approximately 50% of dogs will experience recurrence. • The mortality rate for dogs is ~ 30%.

MISCELLANEOUS

ASSOCIATED CONDITIONS

Approximately 20% of dogs with primary IMT also have AIHA.

PREGNANCY

Use of immunosuppressive drugs may cause fetal damage or abortion.

SYNONYMS

• Idiopathic thrombocytopenic purpura (ITP)
• Autoimmune thrombocytopenia
• Autoimmune thrombocytopenic purpura (ATP)

SEE ALSO

• Anemia, Immune-mediated • Disseminated Intravascular Coagulation (DIC) • Ehrlichiosis • Thrombocytopenia

ABBREVIATIONS

• AIHA = autoimmune hemolytic anemia • ANA = antinuclear antibody • DIC = disseminated intravascular coagulation • FeLV = feline leukemia virus • FIV = feline immunodeficiency virus • IMT = immune-mediated thrombocytopenia • LE = lupus erythematosus • MLV = modified live virus • NSAID = nonsteroidal antiinflammatory drug • PCR = polymerase chain reaction • SLE = systemic lupus erythematosus

Suggested Reading

Breitschwerdt EB. Infectious thrombocytopenia in dogs. Compend Contin Educ Pract Vet 1988;10:1177–1190.

Jordan HL, Grindem CB, Breitschwerdt EB. Thrombocytopenia in cats: a retrospective study of 41 cases. J Vet Intern Med 1993; 7:261–265.

Lewis DC. Management of refractory immune thrombocytopenia. ACVIM Proc 1997;15:94–96.

Lewis DC, Meyers KM. Canine idiopathic thrombocytopenic purpura. J Vet Intern Med 1996;10:207–218.

Rozanski EA, Callan MB, Hughes D, et al. Comparison of platelet count recovery with use of vincristine and prednisone or prednisone alone for treatment of severe immune-mediated thrombocytopenia in dogs. J Am Vet Med Assoc 2002;220:477–481.

Author David C. Lewis

Consulting Editor Stephen A. Kruth

THROMBOCYTOSIS

 BASICS

DEFINITION
• Platelet count above the upper limit of reference range
• Reference range varies with method of platelet counting. Animal Health Laboratory, Guelph, Ontario, reference range using Advia 120 Hematology System—117,000–418,000/µL (dogs); 93,000–514,000/µL (cats).
• Severe thrombocytosis is defined as a platelet count above 1,000,000/µL.

PATHOPHYSIOLOGY
• Can be caused by overproduction of platelets, decreased clearance of platelets, and decreased sequestration of platelets.
• Overproduction occurs secondary to neoplastic proliferation and/or to bone marrow stimulation by thrombopoietin and factors such as IL-1, IL-3, IL-6, and IL-11.
• For most associated diseases, the exact mechanisms are not well documented.

SYSTEMS AFFECTED
• Usually does not cause systemic abnormalities
• Thrombosis not commonly observed. Although animals with severe thrombocytosis are considered at higher risk, in humans there is no direct correlation with platelet count and thrombosis.
• The risk of thrombosis is increased with concurrent altered blood flow, endothelial cell damage, and increased coagulation factor function.
• Thrombosis can cause organ dysfunction. Systems most likely to be clinically affected by thrombosis are cardiovascular, gastrointestinal, hemic/lymphatic/immune (spleen), nervous, renal/urologic, and respiratory.
• Bleeding not commonly observed; if the patient has a concurrent platelet function defect, bleeding can occur. This is most likely in essential thrombocythemia and megakaryocytic leukemia. Mucosal bleeding is most common—see Thrombocytopenia and Thrombocytopathies.

GENETICS
N/A

INCIDENCE/PREVALENCE
• Mild to moderate thrombocytosis is common in dogs and cats.
• Severe thrombocytosis is uncommon.

SIGNALMENT
Species
• Dogs and cats. Excitement-induced thrombocytosis more common in cats
Breed Predilections
• None

Mean Age and Range
• Any age, but many disorders that cause thrombocytosis occur more frequently in older animals (e.g., neoplasia and hyperadrenocorticism). Excitement-induced thrombocytosis more common in young animals

Predominant Sex
• None

SIGNS
General Comments
• Usually none directly attributable to the thrombocytosis
• Clinical signs are those of the underlying disease, thrombosis, or bleeding.

CAUSES
Primary Thrombocytosis–Neoplastic Proliferation in Bone Marrow
• Essential thrombocythemia (platelet leukemia)
• Megakaryoblastic leukemia (platelet count may be elevated, normal, or low)
• Myelofibrosis

Secondary (Reactive) Thrombocytosis—Bone Marrow Stimulation
• Iron deficiency
• Regenerative anemia–acute hemorrhage and hemolysis
• Endocrine disorders—diabetes mellitus, hyperadrenocorticism, hypothyroidism
• Neoplasia
• Septic and nonseptic inflammation—infections, gingivitis, enteritis, colitis, pancreatitis, hepatitis, glomerulonephritis, polyarthritis
• Rebound thrombocytosis in patients recovering from immune-mediated thrombocytopenia
• Drugs—corticosteroids, antibiotics, vincristine, vinblastine, rebound thrombocytosis in patients recovering from thrombocytopenia caused by anticancer chemotherapy

Secondary (Reactive) Thrombocytosis–reduced splenic clearance
• Excitement, exercise, stress (splenic contraction)
• Fractures or soft tissue trauma (splenic contraction)
• Postsplenectomy

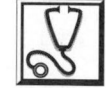 **DIAGNOSIS**

DIFFERENTIAL DIAGNOSIS
• Mass—consider thrombocytosis associated with neoplasia
• Diarrhea and vomiting—consider associated inflammatory conditions of the gastrointestinal tract.
• Polydipsia and polyuria—consider associated hyperadrenocorticism, diabetes mellitus, glomerulonephritis.
• Weight gain, bilateral alopecia, and dry hair coat—consider associated hypothyroidism.
• Gastrointestinal or integumentary chronic blood loss—consider associated iron deficiency.
• Polyarthritis, dermatitis, polymyositis, and glomerulonephritis—consider SLE.
• Splenectomy—consider reduced sequestration of platelets.
• Drug therapy (e.g., corticosteroids, antibiotics, vincristine, and other antineoplastic drugs)—consider drug-induced thrombocytosis.
• Bone fracture or soft tissue trauma—consider thrombocytosis associated with trauma.
• Excited patients during venipuncture—consider excitement-induced splenic contraction.
• Essential thrombocytosis diagnosed by ruling out other causes of thrombocytosis

CBC/BIOCHEMISTRY/URINALYSIS
• Mild normocytic normochromic nonregenerative anemia—consider hypothyroidism or neoplasia
• Microcytic hypochromic anemia—consider iron deficiency
• Regenerative anemia with spherocytosis with or without agglutination—consider immune-mediated hemolytic anemia.
• Inflammatory leukogram—consider secondary thrombocytosis associated with an inflammatory response
• Concurrent neutrophilia and lymphocytosis—consider excitement-induced thrombocytosis
• High hepatocellular and cholestatic liver enzymes with or without high bilirubin—consider hepatic disease
• High lipase and amylase—consider pancreatitis
• Stress leukogram, fasting hyperglycemia, high liver enzyme activity, including alkaline phosphatase—consider hyperadrenocorticism
• Fasting hyperglycemia and glucosuria—consider diabetes mellitus
• Regenerative anemia without spherocytosis or agglutination—consider acute hemorrhage
• Severe nonregenerative anemia with or without dacryocytes and with or without neutropenia—consider myelofibrosis
• Blast cells or bone marrow precursor cells in the circulation—consider myeloproliferative disorders, including megakaryoblastic leukemia and basophilic leukemia
• Moderate to severe thrombocytosis, macro-platelets, hypogranulation or hypergranulation with or without basophilia—consider the myeloproliferative disorder essential thrombocythemia; diagnosis made by ruling out all other causes of thrombocytosis.

• Concurrent hyperkalemia—consider release of intracellular potassium of platelets during clotting

OTHER LABORATORY TESTS
• Serum T_4 concentration with or without TSH and free T_4 concentration—hypothyroidism
• ACTH stimulation or low-dose dexamethasone-suppression test—hyperadrenocorticism
• Serum iron, ferritin, and total iron-binding capacity—iron deficiency
• FeLV and FIV tests in cats with myeloproliferative disorders

IMAGING
To detect internal organomegaly, neoplasm, inflammatory disease, and traumatic injury.

DIAGNOSTIC PROCEDURES
• Examination of bone marrow aspirate and core biopsy—myeloproliferative disorder, iron deficiency, and myelofibrosis
• Endoscopy—gastrointestinal disease
• Biopsy of any internal or external mass

PATHOLOGIC FINDINGS
Gastrointestinal ulceration, organomegaly, histologic changes in endocrine organs, internal neoplasm, histologic changes in bone marrow as on biopsy, site of inflammation, traumatic injury

 TREATMENT

APPROPRIATE HEALTH CARE
• Usually no specific treatment is required unless there is bleeding due to concurrent thrombocytopathia—see Thrombocytopathies.
• Treat underlying disease, and platelet count will return to normal.
• Excitement-induced thrombocytosis is usually transient.
• Consider plateletpheresis for severe thrombocytosis, especially if there are other risk factors for thrombosis.

NURSING CARE
Usually no specific treatment is required unless there is bleeding due to thrombocytopathia–see Thrombocytopathies.

ACTIVITY
Strenuous exercise should be avoided in animals at risk for thrombosis.

DIET
Avoid hard foods with thrombocytopathia (gingival bleeding).

CLIENT EDUCATION
Thrombocytosis does not usually require specific treatment.

SURGICAL CONSIDERATIONS
None specific for thrombocytosis. Surgery may be required to eliminate gastrointestinal ulcer, neoplasm, or focus of inflammation, and to correct traumatic injuries.

 MEDICATIONS

DRUG(S) OF CHOICE
• No treatment in most cases
• Consider aspirin (0.5 mg/kg PO q12h, dog; 25 mg/kg PO twice a week, cat) if severe thrombocytosis, especially if there are other risk factors for thrombosis.
• Radiophosphorus or hydroxyurea for essential thrombocythemia

CONTRAINDICATIONS
If platelet function is abnormal, do not use NSAIDs or other drugs that interfere with platelet function. See Thrombocytopenia and Thrombocytopathies.

PRECAUTIONS
Corticosteroids may increase the risk of thrombosis.

POSSIBLE INTERACTIONS
Aspirin may increase the risk of gastrointestinal ulceration in dogs treated with corticosteroids—minimal risk at low antithrombotic doses.

ALTERNATIVE DRUG(S)
• Anagrelide is a platelet count–lowering drug used to treat essential thrombocythemia in humans.
• Ticlopidine, clopidogrel, abciximab, eptifibatide, and tirofiban are antithrombotic drugs used to impair platelet function in humans.

 **FOLLOW-UP**

PATIENT MONITORING
• CBC as needed to monitor the underlying disease process and platelet count
• Thrombocytosis will resolve once the primary disease is controlled.

PREVENTION/AVOIDANCE
See appropriate sections on underlying conditions.

POSSIBLE COMPLICATIONS
• Thrombosis
• Spontaneous or excessive bleeding if platelet function defect

EXPECTED COURSE AND PROGNOSIS
• Secondary thrombocytosis—prognosis for thrombocytosis is excellent; prognosis overall varies with underlying disease.

• Essential thrombocythemia—most treated cases have responded to therapy and survived over 1 year.
• Megakaryocytic leukemia—poor prognosis

 MISCELLANEOUS

ASSOCIATED CONDITIONS
• Pseudohyperkalemia, caused by release of potassium from platelets during clotting in vitro, most often associated with moderate to severe thrombocytosis
• Plasma potassium should be normal.
• Polycythemia vera and other myeloid leukemias

AGE-RELATED FACTORS
Excitement-induced thrombocytosis more common in cats, especially kittens, than in dogs

SYNONYM
• Thrombocythemia–strictly, "thrombocythemia" refers to primary clonal increases in platelet counts, whereas "thrombocytosis" refers to secondary causes

SEE ALSO
• Anemia, Iron Deficiency
• Hyperadrenocorticism (Cushing's Disease)
• Hypothyroidism
• Myelofibrosis
• Thrombocytopathies
• Thrombocytopenia

ABBREVIATIONS
• ACTH = adrenocorticotropic hormone
• FeLV = feline leukemia virus
• FIV = feline immunodeficiency virus
• IL = interleukin
• NSAID = nonsteroidal antiinflammatory drug
• SLE = systemic lupus erythematosus
• TSH = thyroid-stimulating hormone

Suggested Reading

de Gopegui RR, Feldman BF. Platelets and von Willebrand's disease. In: Ettinger SL, Feldman EC, eds. Textbook of veterinary internal medicine. 5th ed. Philadelphia: Saunders, 2000:1817–1828.

Hammer AS. Thrombocytosis in dogs and cats: a retrospective study. Comp Haematol Int 1991;1:181–186.

Mandell CP. Essential thrombocythemia and reactive thrombocytosis. In: Feldman BF, Zinkl JG, Jain NC, eds. Schalm's veterinary hematology. 5th ed. Philadelphia: Lippincott Williams & Wilkins, 2000:501–508.

Acknowledgment

The author and editors acknowledge the prior contributions of Dr. William J. Reagan, who authored this topic in the previous edition.

Author Anthony C.G. Abrams-Ogg
Consulting Editor Stephen A. Kruth

THUNDERSTORM PHOBIAS

BASICS

OVERVIEW
Thunderstorm phobia is a disorder in which there is persistent and exaggerated fear of storms, or the stimuli associated with storms. Pathophysiology involves physiologic, emotional, and behavioral components

SYSTEMS AFFECTED
• Behavioral—avoidance or escape attempts • Cardiovascular—tachycardia • Endocrine/metabolic—increased cortisol levels, stress-induced hyperglycemia • Gastrointestinal—inappetence, gastrointestinal upset • Musculoskeletal—self-induced trauma resulting from escape attempts • Nervous—adrenergic/noradrenergic overstimulation • Respiratory—tachypnea • Skin/exocrine—acral lick dermatitis

SIGNALMENT
• Occurs in both dogs and cats, but dogs are more often presented for treatment. • Affected dogs show even distributions of sex and neuter status. • Any breed can be affected. In one study, thunderstorm phobias were most prevalent among herding breeds. • A genetic predisposition is suspected. • Dogs may begin exhibiting signs as puppies, but may not be presented for treatment until adulthood.

SIGNS

Historical Findings
• One or more of the following occurs during storms: panting, pacing, trembling, remaining near the owner, hiding, salivating, destructiveness, excessive vocalization, self-inflicted trauma, and inappropriate elimination. • Stimuli that elicit fear include rain, lightning, thunder, strong winds, and possibly changes in barometric pressure and static electricity.

Physical Examination Findings
Unremarkable, except for self-inflicted injuries

CAUSES AND RISK FACTORS
Exact cause is unknown, but may include combinations of the following: • Lack of exposure to storms early in development • Unintentional reinforcement of fear response by owner • Highly aversive experience, such as exposure to a violent storm • Genetic predisposition for emotional reactivity

DIAGNOSIS

DIFFERENTIAL DIAGNOSIS
• Conditions causing similar behavioral responses include separation anxiety, barrier frustration, and noise phobias. • Medical conditions causing similar signs include metabolic, cardiac, neurological, dermatologic, and GI disorders, or any condition that causes pain or discomfort.

CBC/BIOCHEMISTRY/URINALYSIS
Results should be within normal ranges.

OTHER LABORATORY TESTS
Tests for thyroid or adrenal disease may be indicated.

IMAGING
• Radiographs to help identify sources of pain • CT scan or MRI to detect certain cerebral abnormalities

DIAGNOSTIC PROCEDURES
• Electrocardiogram to detect cardiac conduction abnormalities • Skin biopsies if a primary dermatological condition is suspected • CSF tap to identify infectious or inflammatory conditions • GI endoscopy with biopsies if GI signs are persistent

TREATMENT

Environment
Avoid crate confinement if risk of injury.

Behavior Modification
• Neither punish nor attempt to comfort the animal during storms. • Desensitization and counterconditioning are often used in combination. • Desensitization involves exposure to the recorded stimulus at a volume that does not elicit fear. The volume is gradually increased only if the animal remains calm. • Counterconditioning involves teaching a response (sit, relax) that is incompatible with the fear response. • Audio recordings of storms are commercially available. Other than storm sounds, it is difficult to reproduce the natural stimuli that occur during thunderstorms. • Improper use of these exercises can worsen the condition. • Exercises will be ineffective in animals that do not react to recorded thunderstorm sounds.

MEDICATIONS

DRUG(S) OF CHOICE
• Use of medications is considered extra-label. • Azapirones, tricyclic antidepressants (TCAs), and selective serotonin reuptake inhibitors (SSRIs) require 2–4 weeks for effect and must be given daily during storm season to control anxiety. They can be used in combination with fast-acting benzodiazepines.

Benzodiazepines
• Drugs of choice • Use for acute, short-term control of anxiety • Diazepam—Dog: 0.5–1 mg/kg PO PRN; Cat: 1–3 mg/cat PO q12h • Alprazolam—Dog: 0.02 mg/kg PO q4–12h; Cat: 0.125–0.25 mg/cat PO q12h

Azapirones
Buspirone—Dog: 1 mg/kg PO q8–12h; Cat: 2.5–7.5 mg/cat PO q12h

Tricyclic Antidepressants (TCAs)
• Amitriptyline—Dog: 1–3 mg/kg PO q12h; Cat: 0.5–2 mg/kg PO q24h • Clomipramine—Dog: 2 mg/kg PO q12h; Cat: 2.5–5.0 mg/cat PO q24h • Side effects: sedation, anticholinergic effects, and cardiac conduction disturbances if predisposed

Selective Serotonin Reuptake Inhibitors
• Fluoxetine: Dog: 1–1.5 mg/kg PO q24h; Cat: 0.5–1 mg/kg PO q24h • Side effects: inappetence and irritability

Phenothiazine Tranquilizers
• Acepromazine—Dog: 0.1–1 mg/kg PO q6–8h • Poor anti-anxiety properties • Use *only* when chemical restraint is necessary to prevent injury

CONTRAINDICATIONS/POSSIBLE INTERACTIONS
• Use benzodiazepines with caution in cats and aggressive dogs—disinhibition of aggression possible. • Avoid using TCAs and phenothiazines in breeding males, patients with seizure disorders, cardiac disease, diabetes mellitus, glaucoma, or thyroid disease. • Decrease dose or avoid use of these medications in geriatric patients and patients with impaired hepatic or renal function. • TCAs, SSRIs, and phenothiazines should never be combined with monoamine oxidase inhibitors (Anipryl, mitoban). • TCAs and phenothiazines should not be used in combination with antihistamines, anticholinergic agents, thyroid supplements, and other antidepressants.

FOLLOW-UP

PATIENT MONITORING
With medication use, CBC and biochemistry profiles should be monitored periodically.

PREVENTION/AVOIDANCE
• Puppies and kittens should be exposed to a variety of stimuli under benign conditions. • Ignore mild signs of anxiety during storms to avoid reinforcing these behaviors.

POSSIBLE COMPLICATIONS
Severe injuries and property damage.

EXPECTED COURSE AND PROGNOSIS
Prognosis depends on severity, duration, and the ability to prevent injuries. The condition is likely to progress if left untreated.

MISCELLANEOUS

PREGNANCY
Medications have not been evaluated in pregnant animals.

ABBREVIATIONS
• GI = gastrointestinal • SSRI = selective serotonin reuptake inhibitor • TCA = tricyclic antidepressant

Suggested Reading
Voith VL, Borchelt PL. Fears and phobias in companion animals. In: Voith VL, Borchelt PL, eds. Readings in companion animal behavior. Trenton, NJ: Veterinary Learning Systems, 1996:140–151.
Author Lynne M. Seibert
Consulting Editor Debra F. Horwitz

THYMOMA

BASICS

OVERVIEW
• Originates from thymic epithelium
• Infiltrated with mature lymphocytes

SIGNALMENT
• Rare in dogs and cats
• Most common in medium- and large-breed dogs
• Dogs—mean age, 9 years
• Cats—mean age, 10 years

SIGNS
• Coughing
• Tachypnea
• Dyspnea
• Swelling of the head, neck, or forelimbs—cranial caval syndrome
• Muscle weakness and megaesophagus—caused by myasthenia gravis

CAUSE & RISK AFACTORS
N/A

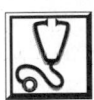

DIAGNOSIS

DIFFERENTIAL DIAGNOSIS
• Lymphoma
• Branchial cyst
• Ectopic thyroid carcinoma
• Chemodectoma
• Mesothelioma

CBC/BIOCHEMISTRY/URINALYSIS
Lymphocytosis—occasionally

OTHER LABORATORY TESTS
N/A

IMAGING
Thoracic radiographs—may reveal a cranial mediastinal mass, pleural effusion, and megaesophagus

DIAGNOSTIC PROCEDURES
• Cytologic—shows mature lymphocytes and epithelial cells
• Evaluate for myasthenia gravis—patients with signs of muscle weakness, dysphagia, or regurgitation

TREATMENT
• Inpatient
• Surgical excision—treatment of choice; tends to be highly invasive and difficult to resect in dogs and less invasive and easier to remove in cats; use an intercostal approach for small masses and a sternotomy for large masses.
• Radiotherapy—potentially beneficial by reducing the lymphoid component of the mass; median survival time 248 days in dogs and 720 days in cats

MEDICATIONS

DRUG(S)
• Chemotherapy—little information available
• Prednisone (20 mg/m^2 q48h) and cyclophosphamide (50–100 mg/m^2 q48h)—used in a very limited number of patients, two of which had a partial remission
• Myasthenia gravis—treat with prednisone and anticholinesterase drugs until the tumor can be removed.

CONTRAINDICATIONS/POSSIBLE INTERACTIONS
Immunosuppressive drugs—do not use to treat myasthenia gravis with aspiration pneumonia.

FOLLOW-UP
• Thoracic radiography—every 3 months; monitor for recurrence
• Cure—possible if tumor is surgically resectable
• Prognosis—poor with nonresectable tumor

MISCELLANEOUS

ASSOCIATED CONDITIONS
Concurrent nonthymic tumors, polymyositis, and other autoimmune diseases—20%–40% of patients

SEE ALSO
Myasthenia Gravis

Suggested Reading

Atwater SW, Powers BE, Park RD, et al. Thymoma in dogs: 23 cases (1980–1991). J Am Vet Med Assoc 1994;205:1007–1013.

Morrison WB. Nonpulmonary intrathoracic cancer. In: Morrison WB, ed. Cancer in dogs and cats: medical and surgical management. Jackson, Wyoming: Teton NewMedia, 2002:513–526.

Author Terrance A. Hamilton
Consulting Editor Wallace B. Morrison

TICK PARALYSIS

 BASICS

DEFINITION
Flaccid, lower motor neuron paralysis caused by salivary neurotoxins from certain species of female ticks

PATHOPHYSIOLOGY
• Tick—injects salivary neurotoxins that probably interfere with the depolarization/ acetylcholine release mechanism in the presynaptic nerve terminal, leading to reduction in the release of acetylcholine
• *Ixodes holocyclus* tick infestation—neurotoxin depends strongly on temperature; one adult tick is sufficient to cause neurologic signs, but a large larval or nymphal *Ixodes* tick infestation can also induce signs.
• Signs—occur 6–9 days after initial tick attachment
• Not all infested animals develop tick paralysis; not all adult female ticks produce the toxin.

SYSTEMS AFFECTED
• Nervous—peripheral nervous system and the neuromuscular junction most affected by the neurotoxin; cranial nerves can become involved, including the vagal, facial, and trigeminal nerves; sympathetic system also affected
• Respiratory—may see paralysis of the intercostal muscles and diaphragm; caudal brain stem respiratory center may be affected

GENETICS
No genetic basis

INCIDENCE/PREVALENCE
• North America and Australia—somewhat seasonal (more prevalent in the summer months); in the warmer areas (southern U.S.; northern Australia) may become a year-round problem
• Overall incidence—low in the U.S.; higher in Australia

GEOGRAPHIC DISTRIBUTION
• U.S.—*Dermacentor variabilis*: wide distribution over the eastern two-thirds of the country and in California and Oregon; *D. andersoni*: from the Cascades to the Rocky Mountains; *Amblyomma americanum*: from Texas and Missouri to the Atlantic Coast; *A. maculatum*: high temperature and humidity of the Atlantic and Gulf of Mexico seaboards

• Australia—limited to the coastal areas of the east; especially associated with areas of bush and scrub

SIGNALMENT

Species
• Australia—dogs and cats
• U.S.—dogs; cats appear to be resistant

Breed Predilections
None

Mean Age and Range
Any age

Predominant Sex
N/A

SIGNS

Historical Findings
• Patient walked in a wooded area approximately 1 week before onset of signs.
• Onset—gradual; starts with unsteadiness and weakness in the pelvic limbs

Neurologic Examination Findings
Non-Ixodes Tick
• Once neurologic signs appear, there is rapid ascending lower motor neuron paresis to paralysis.
• Patient becomes recumbent in 1–3 days, with hyporeflexia to areflexia and hypotonia to atonia.
• Pain sensation preserved
• Cranial nerve dysfunction—not a prominent feature; may note facial weakness and reduced jaw tone; sometimes dysphonia and dysphagia early in the course
• Respiratory paralysis—uncommon in the U.S.; may occur in severely affected patients
• Urination and defecation usually normal
Ixodes Tick
• Neurologic signs—much more severe and rapidly progressive; ascending motor weakness can progress to paralysis within a few hours
• Sialosis, megaesophagus, and vomiting or regurgitation characteristic
• Sympathetic nervous system—mydriatic and poorly responsive pupils; hypertension; tachyarrhythmias; high pulmonary capillary hydrostatic pressure; pulmonary edema
• Caudal medullary respiratory center— additive to the peripheral pulmonary changes, causing progressive fall in respiratory rate without a change in tidal volume, resulting in hypoxia, hypercapnia, and respiratory acidosis

• Respiratory muscle paralysis—much more prevalent; dogs and cats progress to dyspnea, cyanosis, and respiratory paralysis within 1–2 days if not treated

CAUSES

United States
• *D. variabilis*—common wood tick
• *D. andersoni*—Rocky Mountain wood tick
• *A. americanum*—lone star tick
• *A. maculatum*—Gulf Coast tick

Australia
I. holocyclus—secretes a far more potent neurotoxin than that of the North American species

RISK FACTORS
• Environments that harbor ticks

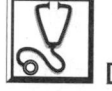 **DIAGNOSIS**

DIFFERENTIAL DIAGNOSIS
• Botulism
• Acute polyneuropathy
• Coonhound paralysis
• Acute polyradiculoneuritis
• Distal denervating disease
• Generalized (diffuse) or multifocal myelopathy

CBC/BIOCHEMISTRY/URINALYSIS
Normal

OTHER LABORATORY TESTS
Arterial blood gases—severely affected patients; low PaO_2, high $PaCO_2$, and low pH

IMAGING
Thoracic radiography (*Ixodes* tick)— megaesophagus

DIAGNOSTIC PROCEDURES
• Thoroughly search for a tick—head, neck, body and limbs, ear canals, mouth, rectum, vagina, prepuce, and in between the digits and foot pads; immediately remove tick.
• Electrodiagnostics (electromyogram)— normal insertion activity and an absence of spontaneous myofiber activity (no fibrillations and positive sharp waves); lack of motor unit action potentials; motor nerve stimulation is followed by either a dramatic decrease in amplitude or a complete absence of compound muscle action potentials.

PATHOLOGIC FINDINGS
N/A

TREATMENT

APPROPRIATE HEALTH CARE
Inpatient—any neurologic dysfunction suggesting tick paralysis; hospitalize until either a tick is found and removed or appropriate treatment to kill a hidden tick is performed.

NURSING CARE
• Inpatient supportive care—essential until patient begins to show signs of recovery
• Oxygen cage—hypoventilation and hypoxia
• Artificial ventilation—respiratory failure
• Intravenous fluid therapy—generally not required unless recovery is prolonged

ACTIVITY
• Keep patient in a quiet environment.
• *Ixodes* tick paralysis—keep patient in a cool, air-conditioned area; toxin is temperature-sensitive; avoid activity to prevent increase in body temperature.

DIET
• Withhold food and water if patient has dysphagia or vomiting/regurgitation.

CLIENT EDUCATION
• Non-*Ixodes* tick—inform client that good nursing care is essential, although the patient's recovery is rapid after removal of ticks.
• *Ixodes* tick—warn client that signs often continue to worsen despite tick removal; thus more aggressive treatment to neutralize the toxin must be undertaken

SURGICAL CONSIDERATIONS
N/A

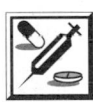 MEDICATIONS

DRUG(S) OF CHOICE
• U.S.—if the tick cannot be found, dip the patient in an insecticidal bath; often the only treatment needed
• Australia—must neutralize circulating toxin via hyperimmune serum (0.5–1 mg/kg IV),

depending on severity of clinical signs; if severe, phenoxybenzamine, an α-adrenergic antagonist (1 mg/kg IV diluted in saline and given slowly over 20 min), appears to be beneficial in relieving the sympathetic effects; acepromazine (0.5–1 mg/kg IV) can be used as an alternative (it has α-adrenergic blocking effects).

CONTRAINDICATIONS
• Drugs that interfere with neuromuscular transmission are contraindicated (e.g., tetracyclines, aminoglycosides, and procaine penicillin).
• *Ixodes* tick—atropine contraindicated in the advanced stages of disease or with marked bradycardia

PRECAUTIONS
Ixodes tick—administer intravenous fluids at a very slow rate to avoid further complications of pulmonary congestion

POSSIBLE INTERACTIONS
N/A

ALTERNATIVE DRUG(S)
N/A

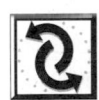 FOLLOW-UP

PATIENT MONITORING
• Non-*Ixodes* tick—reassess neurologic status after tick removal at least daily—should see rapid improvement in muscle strength in animals
• *Ixodes* tick—monitor neurologic status and respiratory and cardiovascular functions continuously and intensively even after tick removal, because of the residual effect of neurotoxin.

PREVENTION/AVOIDANCE
• Vigilantly check for ticks after exposure (at least every 2–3 days); signs do not occur for 4–6 days after tick attachment.
• Weekly insecticidal baths or the use of insecticide-impregnated collars help.
• Short-term acquired immunity develops after exposure to *Ixodes* neurotoxin.

POSSIBLE COMPLICATIONS
No long-term complications if the patient survives the acute effects of the toxin

EXPECTED COURSE AND PROGNOSIS
• Non-*Ixodes* tick—prognosis good to excellent if ticks are removed; recovery occurs in 1–3 days.
• *Ixodes* tick—prognosis often guarded; recovery prolonged; death in 1–2 days without treatment

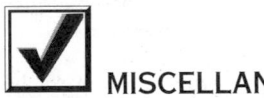 MISCELLANEOUS

ASSOCIATED CONDITIONS
N/A

AGE-RELATED FACTORS
N/A

ZOONOTIC POTENTIAL
Although humans can acquire the disease by being bitten by the same ticks (especially in Australia), tick paralysis is not transmitted to humans from affected pets.

PREGNANCY
Unknown

SEE ALSO
• Coonhound Paralysis (Idiopathic Polyradiculoneuritis)
• Peripheral Neuropathies (Polyneuropathies)

Suggested Reading
Braund KG. Clinical syndromes in veterinary neurology. 2nd ed. St. Louis: Mosby, 1994.
Ilkiw JE. Tick paralysis in Australia. In: Kirk RW, ed. Current veterinary therapy VIII. Small animal practice. Philadelphia: Saunders, 1983:691–693.
Malik R, Farrow BRH. Tick paralysis in North America and Australia. Vet Clin North Am 1991;21:157–171.
Author Paul A. Cuddon
Consulting Editor Joane M. Parent

TICKS AND TICK CONTROL

BASICS

DEFINITION
• Dogs and cats may be parasitized by hard ticks of the family Ixodidae.
• Ectoparasites that feed only on the blood of their hosts; arthropods; closely related to scorpions, spiders, and mites
• Transmitted microbial pathogens—protozoa, helminths, fungi, bacteria, rickettsiae, and viruses
• May cause toxicosis, hypersensitivity, paralysis, and blood-loss anemia

PATHOPHYSIOLOGY
• Hard ticks—four life stages: egg, larva, nymph, and adult; larvae and nymphs must feed to repletion before detaching and molting; as adult female ixodid ticks engorge, they may increase their weight by more than 100-fold; after detachment, females may lay thousands of eggs.
• Blood-loss anemia—from heavy infestations
• Damage to the integument—tick mouth parts cut through the host's skin; bites are generally painless; local irritation and infection may occur.
• Salivary secretion of neurotoxins—may lead to systemic signs (tick paralysis); local action may cause impaired hemostasis and immune suppression.
• Pathogens—acquired when ticks feed on infected reservoir hosts (often rodents and small feral mammals); sometimes transovarial transmission occurs and infected eggs hatch and produce infected larvae; greatest potential for systemic disease occurs when infections acquired in early life stages are transmitted to new hosts when the next stage feeds; may affect virtually any organ system
• Transmission of pathogens and toxins—often requires periods of attachment from hours to days; the essentially painless bite allows adequate feeding times.

SYSTEMS AFFECTED
• Skin/Exocrine—irritation secondary to bite
• Hemic/Lymphatic/Immune—blood-loss anemia
• Nervous—neurotoxin-induced paralysis

Genetics
N/A

INCIDENCE/PREVALENCE
N/A

GEOGRAPHIC DISTRIBUTION
• Strong geographic specificities exist for some tick species; thus geographic prevalence of associated diseases
• *Ixodes scapularis*—Lyme disease; midwest, northeast, and parts of the southeast

• *Ixodes pacificus*—western coastal states
• *Rhipicephalus sanguineus*—found throughout the continental U.S.; but canine ehrlichiosis and babesiosis most common in the southeast

SIGNALMENT

Species
• Dogs and cats
• Cats are thought to be quite efficient at removing ticks, but tick attachment and subsequent tick-vectored diseases are routinely diagnosed.

Breed Predilections
None

Mean Age and Range
None

Predominant Sex
None

SIGNS
• Attached ticks or tick feeding cavities from which ticks have detached may be seen on the skin.
• Associated tick-borne diseases (borreliosis, ehrlichiosis, babesiosis, Rocky Mountain spotted fever, and others)—vary with the organ system(s) affected
• Irritation caused by ticks and subsequent self-trauma—may lead to pyotraumatic dermatitis ("hot spots") in dogs

CAUSES
• Direct contact with questing ticks
• Ticks—attracted to hosts by motion, variation in light patterns, warmth, presence of carbon dioxide, and host-associated odors

RISK FACTORS
• Large hunting breeds (dogs)—considered to be at high risk, because they are likely to come in contact with environments harboring questing ticks
• Domestic animals—can be in close contact with ticks owing to encroachment of ticks into suburban environments and expansion of suburban environment into surrounding forests, prairies, and coast line areas

DIAGNOSIS

• Ticks—examine the skin for attached ticks or tick feeding cavities
• Tick-borne diseases—evaluate epidemiologic considerations for each disease, history of tick parasitism, and complete clinical examination

DIFFERENTIAL DIAGNOSIS
N/A

CBC/BIOCHEMISTRY/URINALYSIS
N/A

OTHER LABORATORY TESTS
N/A

IMAGING
N/A

DIAGNOSTIC PROCEDURES
N/A

PATHOLOGIC FINDINGS
N/A

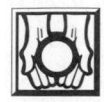

TREATMENT

APPROPRIATE HEALTH CARE
• Outpatient after removal of ticks
• Removal—do as soon as possible to limit time available for neurotoxin or pathogen transmission; grasp ticks close to the skin with fine-pointed tweezers and gently pull free; species with short, strong mouth parts (e.g., *Dermacentor*) usually pull free with host skin attached; species with long, fragile mouth parts (e.g., *Ixodes*) often leave fragments of mouth parts embedded in the feeding cavity.

NURSING CARE
Wash feeding cavity with soap and water; generally sufficient to prevent local inflammation or secondary infection

ACTIVITY
N/A

DIET
N/A

CLIENT EDUCATION
Inform client that application of hot matches, Vaseline, or other materials not only fails to cause tick detachment but allows for longer periods of attachment and feeding.

SURGICAL CONSIDERATIONS
N/A

MEDICATIONS

DRUG(S) OF CHOICE
See Prevention/Avoidance

CONTRAINDICATIONS
N/A

PRECAUTIONS
N/A

POSSIBLE INTERACTIONS
N/A

ALTERNATIVE DRUG(S)
N/A

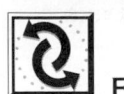

FOLLOW-UP

PATIENT MONITORING
N/A

PREVENTION/AVOIDANCE
• Avoid environments that harbor ticks; may be difficult except for pets kept strictly indoors
• Tick control—essential to realize that this does not always equal control of tick-borne diseases; often the goal is the perceived absence of ticks on the host animal.
• Pets—owners report complete tick control even though there may be some period of attachment and tick feeding or live ticks may spend some time crawling on the animal after they have been exposed to lethal levels of an acaricide; immature ticks of some species (*R. sanguineus* and *I. scapularis*) may be undetected because of their minute size.
• Tick-borne pathogens—may be transmitted very rapidly (viruses) or may require several hours (*Rickettsia rickettsii*) or days (*Borrelia burgdorferi*)

Insecticides and Acaricides
• In the U.S., the EPA licenses agents as effective against various species of pests.
• Control—inferred as providing control of diseases carried by that species; although this may be correct in some or all cases, veterinarians should be sophisticated enough to require demonstration of efficacy in prevention of disease transmission before accepting a disease-control claim at face value
• A recent study has demonstrated that an amitraz-impregnated collar (Preventic Plus, Virbac/Allerderm) could interrupt the transmission of *Borrelia burgdorferi* from infected ticks to dogs treated with the collar; challenging because ticks are widely dispersed in the environment, spend a relatively short time on their hosts, posses great reproductive capacities, and have long lifetimes
• Acaricidal collars (Preventic) and spot treatments (Frontline and K9 Advantix)—have gained wide use; ease of application is as important as efficacy; direct marketing to pet owners of veterinarian-dispensed products has been a major factor in shifting tick control away from OTC formulations
• Bathing, spraying, or powdering with appropriate organophosphate- or pyrethrin-containing products has become far less common with the advent of new convenient and effective products.

POSSIBLE COMPLICATIONS
Tick-borne diseases or tick paralysis

EXPECTED COURSE AND PROGNOSIS
N/A

MISCELLANEOUS

ASSOCIATED CONDITIONS
• Canine babesiosis—vectored by *R. sanguineus;* caused by protozoan parasite *Babesia canis;* infects canine RBCs, leading to sludging in capillaries and destruction in the spleen
• Rocky Mountain spotted fever—vectored by *Dermacentor variabilis;* caused by *R. rickettsii;* invades vascular endothelial tissues, leading to necrotizing vasculitis
• Canine ehrlichiosis—vectored by *R. sanguineus;* caused by *Ehrlichia canis;* infects mononuclear cells and platelets
• Granulocytic ehrlichiosis—emerging disease; caused by *E. equi;* infects granulocytes, leading to nonspecific signs and fever
• Lyme disease—vectored by *I. scapularis* and *I. pacificus;* caused by *Borrelia burgdorferi;* dogs may develop fevers associated with arthritis or syndromes leading to complete heart block, protein-losing nephropathy, and neurologic abnormalities.
• Canine hepatozoonosis—caused by protozoal organism *Hepatozoon canis* after the dog ingests an infected *R. sanguineus* or *A. maculatum;* cysts and pyogranulomas in the muscles and other tissues associated with myositis and renal failure, often leading to death in chronic cases
• Tick paralysis—caused by a neurotoxin; affects acetylcholine synthesis and/or liberation at the neuromuscular junction of the host animal; signs (typified by ascending flaccid paralysis often initially affecting the pelvic limbs) develop 5–9 days after tick attachment.

Vaccines
• Currently for "prevention" of only Lyme disease; two types for dogs: whole-cell, killed bacterin (since 1990) and Osp A (since 1996)
• Safety and efficacy—peer-reviewed published data for dogs naturally exposed to *B. burgdorferi* available only for bacterin; 1969 dogs received a total of 4033 doses of bacterin during a 20-month period; 4498 control dogs were not vaccinated; immunization was found to be safe regardless of previous history of Lyme disease or exposure to *B. burgdorferi;* 38 (1.9%) of vaccinated dogs had minor reactions that resolved without complications immediately or within 72 hr after vaccination; cumulative incidence of Lyme disease was 1.0% in vaccinated dogs and 4.7% in control dogs; 40% of vaccinated dogs had serologic evidence of infection with *B. burgdorferi*

before vaccination but the incidence of Lyme disease was only 2%; incidence of Lyme disease in infected control dogs was 4.8%; thus vaccination of infected dogs was associated with about a 50% decrease in the incidence of Lyme disease. Continued clinical experience with the whole-cell bacterin has reinforced published safety and efficacy data. A new peer-reviewed study of bacterin published in 2002 demonstrated a preventable fraction of 92.2%.

AGE-RELATED FACTORS
N/A

ZOONOTIC POTENTIAL
• Ticks may parasitize many different species of mammals, birds, and reptiles at different stages in their developmental cycles; infections acquired in early life stages may be transmitted when ticks feed again in the next stage.
• Humans, if parasitized, may be exposed to babesiosis, Rocky Mountain spotted fever, ehrlichiosis, borreliosis, or tick paralysis.

PREGNANCY
N/A

SYNONYMS
Acariasis

SEE ALSO
• Babesiosis
• Ehrlichiosis
• Hepatozoonosis
• Lyme Disease (Borreliosis)
• Rocky Mountain Spotted Fever
• Tick Bite Paralysis

Suggested Reading

Elfassy OJ, Goodman FW, Levy SA, et al. Efficacy of an amitraz-impregnated collar in preventing transmission of *Borrelia burgdorferi* by adult *Ixodes scapularis* to dogs. J Am Vet Med Assoc 2001;219:185–189.

Hoskins JD, ed. Tick-transmitted disease, Vet Clin North Am 1991:21.

Levy SA, Barthold SW, Dombach DM, et al. Canine borreliosis. Compend Cont Ed 1993;15:833–848.

Levy, S.A., Use of a C6 ELISA tests to evaluate the efficacy of a whole-cell bacterin for the prevention of naturally transmitted canine *Borrelia burgdorferi* infection. J Vet Ther 2002;3(4):420–424.

Sonenshine DE. Biology of ticks. Vol. 2. New York: Oxford University Press, 1993.

Author Steven A. Levy
Consulting Editor Karen Helton Rhodes

TOAD VENOM TOXICOSIS

BASICS

OVERVIEW
• Two species of primary concern—Colorado River toad (*Bufo alvarius*) and marine toad (*B. marinus*); marine toad more toxic; both can be fatal.
• Toads—most active during periods of high humidity (the monsoon season of late summer in the desert Southwest for Colorado River toads); most encounters occur during the evening, night, or early morning.
• Toxin—produced from the parotid glands; defensive; rapidly absorbed across the victim's mucous membranes; contains several major components: indole alkyl amines (similar to the street drug LSD), cardiac glycosides, and noncardiac sterols

SIGNALMENT
Primarily dogs; rarely, ferrets and cats

SIGNS
General Comments
Rapid onset

Historical Findings
• Crying and pawing at the mouth
• Ataxia or stiff gaited
• Seizures

Physical Examination Findings
• Profuse hypersalivation
• Hyperexcitability with vocalization
• Brick red buccal mucous membranes
• Hyperthermia
• Collapse
• Marked cardiac ventricular arrhythmia—less common with Colorado River toad intoxication
• Cyanosis
• Dyspnea

CAUSES & RISK FACTORS
• Living in proximity to toads
• Moist, warm, outside environment
• Outdoor animal

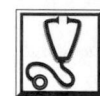

DIAGNOSIS

DIFFERENTIAL DIAGNOSIS
Caustics or other oral irritants

CBC/BIOCHEMISTRY/URINALYSIS
May note hyperkalemia

OTHER LABORATORY TESTS
N/A

IMAGING
N/A

DIAGNOSTIC PROCEDURES
Electrocardiogram—may reveal ventricular arrhythmias

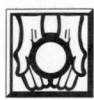

TREATMENT

• Marine toad intoxication—medical emergency; death common
• Decontamination—flush mouth with copious quantities of water for 5–10 min
• Hyperthermia (> 40.6°C; 105°F)—provide a cool bath; remove patient from bath once temperature reaches 39.4°C (103°F).
• Rapid evaluation of cardiac activity necessary

MEDICATIONS

DRUG(S)
• Atropine—0.04 mg/kg IM, SC; reduces the amount of salivation; helps prevent aspiration; use with bradycardia, heart block, or other sinoatrial node alterations as a result of the digitalis-like effect of the toxin
• Atropine—not recommended if severe trachycardia present
• Propranolol (Inderal)—2 mg/kg IV (see Contraindications); rapid administration may be required to combat tachyarrhythmias; may be repeated in 20 min; may need continuous intravenous infusion (0.02–0.2 mg/kg) for persistent arrhythmias
• Anesthesia with pentobarbital (dogs)—increases tolerance to intoxication

• In severe cases, treatment with digoxin-specific Fab fragments may be indicated.

CONTRAINDICATIONS/POSSIBLE INTERACTIONS
• Cardiac disease or bronchial asthma—patient may not tolerate the generally recommended high dose of propranolol; try propranolol at 0.5 mg/kg as a slow IV bolus; monitor cardiac rhythm and stop injection when it normalizes.
• Anesthetics (e.g., pentobarbital)—may depress function of an already compromised myocardium; use with caution.

FOLLOW-UP
• Continuous electrocardiographic monitoring—recommended until the patient is fully recovered

• Colorado River toad intoxication—patients usually normal within 30 min of onset of treatment; death relatively uncommon if treated; do not underestimate the risk of secondary heatstroke.
• Marine toad intoxication—medical emergency; death common

MISCELLANEOUS

Suggested Reading
Palumbo NE, Perri SF. Toad poisoning. In: Kirk RW, ed. Current veterinary therapy VIII. Philadelphia: Saunders, 1983: 160–162.
Author Michael E. Peterson
Consulting Editor Gary D. Osweiler

TOOTH FRACTURE

BASICS

DEFINITION
• Traumatic tooth injuries may involve fracture of enamel, dentin, and cement or damage to the periodontium.
• May involve the crown and root of the affected tooth
• Classified as uncomplicated if they do not involve pulpal exposure and complicated if the pulp is exposed by the fracture line

PATHOPHYSIOLOGY
• Untreated pulpal exposure invariably leads to pulpitis and eventually pulpal necrosis and periapical pathology.
• Pulpitis and pulpal necrosis may also occur with uncomplicated fractures, particularly if the fracture line is close to the pulp chamber, which exposes a large number of wide-diameter dentinal tubules and allows communication between the pulp and the external environment.

SYSTEMS AFFECTED
Oral cavity initially, but a focus of infection in the oral cavity may cause systemic complications

GENETICS
N/A

INCIDENCE/PREVALENCE
N/A

GEOGRAPHIC DISTRIBUTION
N/A

SIGNALMENT

Species
Dogs and cats

Breed Predilections
None

Mean Age and Range
Any age

Predominant Sex
None

SIGNS

Crown Fractures
• Clinical loss of tooth crown substance; may affect enamel only, or enamel and dentin; fracture line may be transverse or oblique

• Uncomplicated fractures with the fracture line close to the pulp chamber—pale pink pulp is visible through the dentin; gentle exploring will not allow the explorer into the pulp cavity
• In complicated crown fractures, the pulp chamber is open and readily accessed with an explorer.
• The fresh complicated fracture is associated with hemorrhage from the pulp.
• Older fractures may exhibit a necrotic pulp; clinically the pulp chamber is filled with dark necrotic material, and the tooth is often discolored.

Root Fractures
• May occur at any point along the root surface; often in combination with fracture of the crown, but may occur in isolation
• Fracture line may be transverse or oblique; segments may remain aligned or be displaced.
• Clinical signs indicating a possible root fracture include pain on closure of the mouth or during open mouth breathing.
• Abnormal horizontal or vertical mobility of a periodontally sound tooth may raise suspicion of a root fracture.

CAUSES & RISK FACTORS
Generally the result of a traumatic incident (e.g., road traffic accident, blunt blow to the face, chewing on hard objects)

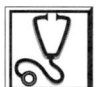

DIAGNOSIS

DIFFERENTIAL DIAGNOSIS
• Crown fracture—none
• Root fracture—luxation; definitive diagnosis of root fractures is by radiography

CBC/BIOCHEMISTRY/URINALYSIS
N/A

OTHER LABORATORY TESTS
N/A

IMAGING
• Radiographs are mandatory.
• Intraoral radiographic technique and dental intraoral film are required.
• Radiographs reveal the full extent of the lesion and allow treatment planning.

• Radiographs are required for adequate performance of endodontic procedures and monitoring treatment outcome.

DIAGNOSTIC PROCEDURES
• Transillumination to help determine tooth vitality: shine a brightlight through the tooth (otoscope light); a vital tooth should transilluminate well

PATHOLOGIC FINDINGS
Untreated pulpal exposure invariably leads to pulpitis and eventual pulpal necrosis and periapical pathology.

TREATMENT

Uncomplicated Crown Fractures
Remove sharp edges with a bur and seal the exposed dentin tubules with a suitable liner or restorative material.

Complicated Crown Fractures
All require endodontic therapy if the tooth is to be maintained; extraction is preferable to no treatment at all.

Mature Tooth
• Recent fracture in the mature tooth with the pulp still vital—two options exist, partial pulpectomy and direct pulp capping (vital pulpotomy) followed by restoration or conventional root canal therapy and restoration
• For partial pulpectomy and direct pulp capping to succeed, the procedure should be carried out within hours of the injury.
• Tell the client at the beginning that the procedure may not be the final treatment—the tooth may require standard root canal treatment later if the pulp becomes necrotic.
• When the pulp is already chronically inflamed or necrotic, standard root canal therapy and restoration are the treatments of choice if the tooth is periodontally sound.

Immature Tooth
• A vital pulp is required for continued root development; as long as the pulp is vital the treatment of choice is partial pulpectomy and direct pulp capping, followed by restoration.
• If the pulp is necrotic, no further root development will occur; necrotic immature teeth need endodontic treatment to be

maintained; remove the necrotic tissue and pack the root canal with calcium hydroxide paste; some apexogenesis (physiologic event, continued root development) and apexification (closure of the apex, induced by treatment) can be stimulated if this procedure is performed; change the calcium hydroxide every 6 months until the apex is closed when a standard root canal is performed.

• Immature teeth may be present in the mature animal if trauma to the developing teeth caused pulp necrosis; treat such teeth as you would any immature teeth.

Root Fractures

• Treatment of crown and root fractures depends on how far below the gingival margin the fracture line extends.

• If the fracture line does not involve the pulp and does not extend more than 4–5 mm below the gingival margin, restorative dentistry can be performed; if the fracture extends more than 5 mm below the gingival margin and involves the pulp, the tooth should usually be extracted.

• The fracture level determines the choice of treatment for horizontal root fractures; a fracture in the apical region carries a better prognosis than one close to the gingival margin.

• A horizontal fracture of the coronal part of the root usually mandates tooth extraction; the main exception is the lower canine, since jaw stability and strength depend on the canine roots. If the root is periodontally sound it must receive endodontic treatment after removal of the coronal portion;

• Horizontal midroot and apical fractures will heal if the tooth is immobilized; horizontal root fractures can heal by means of a dentinocemental callus, a fibrous union, or an osteofibrous union.

• If the pulp of the coronal fragment becomes necrotic the fracture will not heal; endodontic treatment of the coronal segment is indicated; the apical segment may be left in situ if there is no radiographic evidence of periapical pathology; if radiographic evidence of periapical pathology exists, remove the apical segment.

MEDICATIONS

DRUG(S) OF CHOICE

A broad-spectrum bacteriocidal antibiotic drug for 5 to 7 days may be indicated, e.g., when longstanding infection is present.

CONTRAINDICATIONS/POSSIBLE INTERACTIONS

None

PRECAUTIONS

None

POSSIBLE INTERACTIONS

None

ALTERNATIVE DRUG(S)

None

FOLLOW-UP

PATIENT MONITORING

• Check a partial pulpectomy and direct pulp-capping procedure with postoperative radiographs after 6 and 12 months, or at intervals determined by clinical signs, to detect pulp death and consequent periapical changes indicating the need for root canal treatment.

• Check the outcome of conventional root canal therapy radiographically 6–12 months postoperatively; evidence of periapical pathology at this time indicates the need for further endodontic therapy or extraction of the tooth; further endodontic therapy consists of redoing the root canal therapy, often in conjunction with surgical endodontics.

• Check root fractures radiographically 6–12 months postoperatively.

• Check uncomplicated fractures postoperatively with radiographs at 4–6 months to assess periapical status.

PREVENTION/AVOIDANCE

• Avoid situations in which teeth are likely to be damaged; keep animal from chewing on hard objects such as rocks.

• To avoid complications, institute treatment within hours of injury.

POSSIBLE COMPLICATIONS

• Untreated pulpal exposure invariably leads to pulpitis and eventual pulpal necrosis and periapical pathology.

• Arrested development of immature teeth

EXPECTED COURSE AND PROGNOSIS

Vary with vitality of the pulp, location of the fracture, and whether the tooth is mature or immature; see Treatment section for detailed discussion

MISCELLANEOUS

ASSOCIATED CONDITIONS

None

AGE-RELATED FACTORS

Treatment of mature and immature teeth differs; see Treatment section.

ZOONOTIC POTENTIAL

None

PREGNANCY

N/A

SYNONYMS

None

SEE ALSO

N/A

ABBREVIATIONS

None

Suggested Reading

Gorrel C, Penman S, Emily P. Handbook of small animal oral emergencies. New York: Pergamon Press, 1993.

Gorrel C, Robinson J. Endodontic therapy. In: Crossley DA, Penman S, eds. Manual of small animal dentistry. Gloucester, UK: British Small Animal Veterinary Association. 1995

Author Cecilia Gorrel

Consulting Editor Heidi B. Lobprise

TOOTH LUXATION OR AVULSION

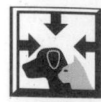

BASICS

OVERVIEW
• Luxation of a tooth can be either vertical (i.e., an intrusion or extrusion) or lateral.
• An intrusion occurs when the tooth is pushed apically into the alveolar bone.
• An extrusion occurs when the tooth is dislocated vertically partially out of the alveolus.
• Lateral luxation—the affected tooth is tipped in either a labial or a palatal/lingual direction; can occur when trauma pushes the crown in one direction and the root in the opposite direction; always associated with a fracture of the lingual or labial alveolar bone plate that allows the tooth to luxate rather than fracture
• An avulsed tooth has been totally luxated from its alveolus.

SIGNALMENT
Dog and cats

SIGNS
• Intrusion—tooth appears shorter than normal; no tooth mobility detected
• Extrusion—tooth appears longer than normal and is mobile both vertically and horizontally
• Lateral luxation—tooth crown is displaced in either a labial or palatal/lingual direction
• Avulsion—intact tooth is totally displaced from its alveolus

CAUSES & RISK FACTORS
• Luxation/avulsion—usually results from a traumatic incident (e.g., road traffic accident or dog fight)
• The trauma causes injury to the periodontium, thus allowing abnormal tooth mobility and malpositioning.
• The upper canine tooth is the most commonly luxated/avulsed tooth.
• Advanced periodontitis will predispose

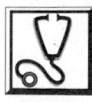

DIAGNOSIS

DIFFERENTIAL DIAGNOSIS
• Luxation—root fracture where the coronal segment is displaced
• Avulsion—tooth lost due to severe periodontitis

CBC/BIOCHEMISTRY/URINALYSIS
Noncontributory

OTHER LABORATORY TESTS
N/A

IMAGING

General
• Radiographs are mandatory.
• Intraoral radiographic technique and dental X-ray film are required.

Radiographic Findings
• Intrusion—narrowing of the periodontal ligament space in the apical region
• Extrusion—widening of the periodontal ligament, especially in the apical section
• Lateral luxation—widening and narrowing of the periodontal ligament space and fracture of the alveolar bone plate
• Avulsion—empty but intact alveolus

TREATMENT
• Replace and fix the tooth in its normal position; bond with acrylic splints and fine ligature wire—an effective method of achieving stabilization and occlusal alignment.
• Handle the avulsed tooth only by its crown and rinse gently with sterile saline solution; if severely contaminated, the tooth root can be gently cleaned with sterile gauze swabs moistened with saline.
• Be gentle; tooth handling should be kept to a minimum; it is essential not to remove the periodontal ligament from the root; a viable periodontal ligament is necessary for healing.
• Replace the tooth in its bony socket; there is usually no need to remove the blood clot from the alveolus; the tooth is just firmly placed in its bony socket and fixed in that position.
• Contraindications for repositioning a luxated or avulsed tooth are deciduous teeth, severe periodontitis, caries or resorptive lesion.
• The two most important factors determining the result of treatment are the length of time the avulsed tooth has been out of its bony socket and the medium in which the tooth has been stored during this period.
• The sooner an avulsed tooth is reimplanted the better the prognosis; optimal results are achieved if the tooth is reimplanted within 30 min of avulsion; do not let the avulsed tooth dry prior to reimplantation; the best medium for storing an avulsed tooth is saline; if not available, use milk.
• Advise clients to place the tooth in either saline or milk and bring the affected animal in for treatment as quickly as possible.
• The appliance for fixation is usually left in place for 4–6 weeks; maintain oral hygiene during this period; a water pick or curved-tip syringe is used to flush debris from between the splint, teeth, and soft tissue; rinsing the oral cavity with chlorhexidine solution is also useful.
• The appliances are removed with pliers or high-speed drill; at this stage the tooth should be stable or very slightly mobile; take radiographs; if the tooth is still loose, reimplantation has failed and it should be extracted.

MEDICATIONS

DRUG(S)
• Use of a broad-spectrum bacteriocidal antibiotic is recommended; if oral hygiene is maintained, only a short course is necessary.
• If no oral hygiene measures are possible, antibiotics may be indicated throughout the period of fixation.
• Daily rinsing with 0.12% chlorhexidine gluconate solution will diminish the need for prolonged administration of antibiotics.

CONTRAINDICATIONS/POSSIBLE INTERACTIONS
N/A

FOLLOW-UP
• An avulsed tooth invariably develops pulpal necrosis; the tooth must receive endodontic therapy to prevent development of periapical pathology.
• Best to perform endodontic therapy when the appliance is removed
• External root resorption and ankylosis commonly follow reimplantation.
• Luxated teeth often suffer pulp necrosis; check at regular intervals.
• Signs of pulp pathology (e.g., tooth discoloration or radiographic evidence of periapical pathology) are indications for endodontic treatment.

MISCELLANEOUS

Suggested Reading
Gorrel C, Penman S, Emily P. Handbook of small animal oral emergencies. New York: Pergamon Press, 1993.
Gorrel C, Robinson J. Endodontic therapy. In: Crossley DA, Penman S, eds. Manual of small animal dentistry. British Small Animal Veterinary Association 1995:168–181.
Author Cecilia Gorrel
Consulting Editor Heidi B. Lobprise

TOOTH ROOT ABSCESS (APICAL ABSCESS)

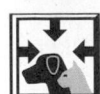

BASICS

OVERVIEW
• An abscess is a localized collection of pus in a cavity formed by the disintegration of tissues. • Can divide into "acute" and chronic phases on the basis of severity of pain and presence or absence of systemic signs and symptoms • Accumulation of inflammatory cells at the apex of a nonvital tooth—periapical abscess • Acute exacerbation of a chronic periapical abscess is called a *phoenix abscess.* • An abscess spreads along the pathway of least resistance from the tooth apex, resulting in osteomyelitis and, if perforated through the cortex, a cellulitis that can burst through the skin to create a cutaneous sinus. • Systemic spread of bacteria (bacteremia and pyemia) can affect other organ systems.

SIGNALMENT
Species
• Dogs and cats • Can occur in deciduous and permanent dentition • Usually occurs in active animals that bite or chew a lot • Can involve any teeth; canines and carnassial teeth are most commonly affected.

SIGNS
• Tooth is visibly broken—90% of cases • Tooth may appear discolored. • Tooth is not sensitive to cold or hot liquids or foods—**Note:** acute tooth fracture with pulp exposure would be sensitive. • Facial swelling • Cutaneous sinus exuding pus • Facial sensitivity may be slight. • Increased accumulation of plaque and calculus on the affected side of the mouth • Animal does not want to chew, especially on the affected side • Tooth may be asymptomatic for a long time but will be affected sooner or later. • Tooth may be clinically asymptomatic, yet nonapparent problems, such as bacteremia, may be occurring. • Tooth may be sensitive to percussion. • A deep "vertical" periodontal pocket may extend to the apex of the affected tooth. • Putrid smell • Tooth may be loose and painful on palpation. • May have facial lymphadenitis • Sinusitis—maxillary sinus is most commonly affected.

CAUSES & RISK FACTORS
• Any pulpal trauma • Direct blow causing fracture of the crown of severe pulpitis and pulpal necrosis • Defense (fighting)—the canines are most commonly affected • Chewing hard objects (e.g., bones, hooves, rocks, wood, especially with knots)—carnassials are most commonly affected) • Malocclusive trauma • "Tugging" rags with puppies • Previous surgical repair to an area around the dentition—bone plating for fracture repair • Bacteria—the pulp can be affected by bacteria from dental caries, exposed dentinal tubules • Septicemia—documented in humans but not yet proven in animals • Thermal heat resulting in pulpal necrosis—electrical cord burns • Immature patients (< 18 months) • Small animals on long-term corticosteroids • Diabetes or Cushing's disease

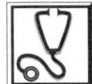

DIAGNOSIS

DIFFERENTIAL DIAGNOSIS
• Feline odontoclastic resorptive lesions—radiographs show no apical lucency or abscessation. • Squamous cell carcinoma and fibrosarcoma—rapidly growing and invasive; displace and increase mobility of the teeth. • Cementomas—radiographically show enlarged apical roots with a thin radiolucent zone continuous with the periodontal ligament • Ameloblastoma—displaces and increases mobility to the teeth; slowly enlarges • Cysts—radiographs usually show a very large lytic area; can mimic apical abscesses, and apical abscesses, can become cystic (radicular cysts, apical periodontal granulomas); conventional endodontic treatment is unsuccessful; primordial cyst occurs at the site of a congenitally missing tooth and radiographically has a round oval radiolucency with a thin radiopaque border. • Dentigerous cyst—occurs from the follicular cyst of an impacted or embedded tooth (usually the first premolars in dogs); radiographs show a tooth within the cyst.

CBC/BIOCHEMISTRY/URINALYSIS
CBC may show a leucocytosis and/or a mild regenerative anemia.

IMAGING
• Key diagnostic aid—demonstrates thickening of the apical periodontal ligament; ill-defined radiolucency; shows bone loss at the apex as the lesion becomes chronic • As the lesion progresses, radiographic lesions consistent with osteomyelitis and cellulitis occur. • If fistulization has occurred, can place a gutta percha cone into the sinus and take a radiograph to identify the affected tooth • Transillumination with a strong fiberoptic light can help the clinician by distinguishing between a vital and necrotic pulp.

DIAGNOSTIC PROCEDURES
• Surgical removal of the abscess site (surgical endodontics) or extraction • Endodontic treatment evaluation in 6 months to a year

PATHOLOGIC FINDINGS
• Apical area has a central area of liquefaction necrosis containing disintegrating neutrophils and cellular debris, surrounded by macrophages, lymphocytes, and plasma cells; can see bacteria • Chronic changes as above, but tracts lead away from the central lesion and can be lined with epithelium; may be osteomyelitis and cellulitis lesions or the outer portion of granulation tissue becomes fibrotic and a capsule develops (radicular cyst and/or a periapical periodontal granuloma)

TREATMENT
• Drainage and elimination of the focus of infection • Extraction of the tooth involved, with curettage of the apical infected area • Endodontic treatment of the involved tooth • Surgical endodontic treatment of the involved tooth if the apical lesion is large • Chronic conditions require surgical removal of the granulation tissue and curettage of the tract. • After treatment, cold packs on the area will help reduce inflammation. • Complete rest for a few days • Give nothing hard to chew for a few days.

MEDICATIONS

DRUG(S)
• Antibiotics preoperatively to prevent systemic spread of infection • Broad-spectrum antibiotic postoperatively for 7–10 days • Analgesics preoperatively, intraoperatively, and postoperatively for 3–4 days • If a surgical endodontic treatment or an extraction was performed, a protective collar may be required.

CONTRAINDICATIONS/POSSIBLE INTERACTIONS
N/A

FOLLOW-UP
• Recheck 10 days postoperatively. • General examination of the area; percussion to test for sensitivity, healing of the extraction or surgical endodontic site, and integrity of the endodontic access fillings • Recheck in 6 months to a year; repeat radiographs to see if the lesion has resolved (in endodontic treatment). • Avoid traumatic injuries (e.g., letting the dog chase cars). • Eliminate bones, hooves, and other chewable hard objects. • Stop throwing rocks or wood for the dog to retrieve. • Decrease fighting. • Curtail bite work—avoid handler sleeves that have tears or hole in them • Check the mouth regularly for broken or discolored teeth.

MISCELLANEOUS

Suggested Reading
Neville BW, Damm DD, Allen CM, Bouguot JE. Oral & maxillofacial pathology. Philadelphia: Saunders, 1995:96–121.
Author James M. G. Anthony
Consulting Editor Heidi B. Lobprise

TOXOPLASMOSIS

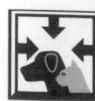

BASICS

DEFINITION
Toxoplasma gondii—an obligate intracellular coccidian protozoan parasite that infects nearly all mammals; Felidae the definitive hosts; all other warm-blooded animals are intermediate hosts.

PATHOPHYSIOLOGY
• Severity and manifestation—depend on location and degree of tissue injury caused by tissue cysts • Infection—acquired by ingestion of tissue cysts or oocysts; organisms spread to extraintestinal organs via blood or lymph; results in focal necrosis to many organs (heart, eye, CNS) • Acute disseminated infection rarely fatal • Chronic disease—tissue cysts form; low-grade disease; usually not clinically apparent unless immunosuppression or concomitant illness allows organism to proliferate, causing an acute inflammatory response • Clinical disease—often associated with other infections that cause severe immunosuppression (e.g., canine distemper, FIP, and FeLV).

SYSTEMS AFFECTED
• Multisystemic—usually the same in cats and dogs • Ophthalmic—approximately 80% of affected cats have evidence of intraocular inflammation, most commonly uveitis.

GENETICS N/A

INCIDENCE/PREVALENCE
• Approximately 30% of cats and up to 50% of people serologically positive for *T. gondii* • Most animals asymptomatic

GEOGRAPHIC DISTRIBUTION
Worldwide

SIGNALMENT
Species
Cats more commonly symptomatic than dogs
Breed Predilections
None
Mean Age and Range
In one study, mean age 4 years; range 2 weeks to 16 years
Predominant Sex
Male cats—more common

SIGNS
General Comments
• Determined mainly by site and extent of organ damage • Acute—at the time of initial infection • Chronic—reactivation of encysted infection; caused by immunosuppression
Historical Findings
• Nonspecific signs of lethargy, depression, and anorexia
• Weight loss
• Fever
• Ocular discharge, photophobia, miotic pupils (cats)

• Respiratory distress
• Neurologic—ataxia; seizures; tremors; paresis/paralysis; cranial nerve deficits
• Digestive tract—vomiting; diarrhea; abdominal pain; jaundice
• Stillborn kittens

Physical Examination Findings
Cats
• Most severe in transplacentally infected kittens, which may be stillborn or die before weaning
• Surviving kittens—anorexia; lethargy; high fever unresponsive to antibiotics; reflect necrosis/inflammation of lungs (dyspnea, increased respiratory noises), liver (icterus, abdominal enlargement from ascites), and CNS (encephalopathic)
• Respiratory and gastrointestinal (postnatal)—most common; anorexia; lethargy; high fever unresponsive to antibiotics; dyspnea; weight loss; icterus; vomiting; diarrhea; abdominal effusion
• Neurologic (postnatal)—seen in < 10% of patients; blindness; stupor; incoordination; circling; torticollis; anisocoria; seizures
• Ocular signs (postnatal)—common; uveitis (aqueous flare, hyphema, mydriasis); iritis; detached retina; iridocyclitis; keratic precipitates
• Rapid course—acutely affected patient with CNS and/or respiratory involvement
• Slow course—patients with reactivation of chronic infection

Dogs
• Young—usually generalized infection; fever; weight loss; anorexia; tonsillitis; dyspnea; diarrhea; vomiting
• Old—tend to localized infections; mainly associated with neural and muscular systems
• Neurologic—quite variable; usually reflect diffuse neurologic inflammation; seizures; tremors; ataxia; paresis; paralysis; muscle weakness; and tetraparesis
• Ocular—rare; similar to those found in cats
• Cardiac involvement—occurs; usually not clinically apparent

CAUSES
T. gondii

RISK FACTORS
Immunosuppression—may predispose to infection or reactivation: FeLV, FIV, FIP, haemobartonellosis, canine distemper, and glucocorticoid or antitumor chemotherapy or post–renal transplant.

DIAGNOSIS

DIFFERENTIAL DIAGNOSIS
Cats
• Intraocular disease (anterior uveitis)—FIP; FeLV; FIV; immune-mediated; trauma; lens-induced; corneal ulceration with reflex uveitis

• Dyspnea (respiratory signs)—asthma; cardiogenic; pneumonia (bacterial, fungal, parasitic); neoplasia; heartworm disease; pleural disease (effusions); diaphragmatic hernia; chest wall injury • Neurologic (causes of meningoencephalitis)—viral (FIP, rabies, pseudorabies); fungal (cryptococcosis, blastomycosis, histoplasmosis); parasitic (cuterebriasis, coenurosis, aberrant heartworm migration); bacterial; idiopathic disease (feline polioencephalomyelitis)
Dogs
• Often associated with other immuno-suppressive diseases—e.g., signs of distemper may be seen. • Neurologic—usually in very young dogs; differentiate from *Neospora caninum* (both produce CNS and neuromuscular disease) • Consider other conditions causing multifocal signs—infectious or inflammatory toxicity; metabolic disease

CBC/BIOCHEMISTRY/URINALYSIS
CBC (Cats)
• Most show mild normocytic normochromic anemia.
• Leukopenia—approximately 50% of patients with severe disease; mainly owing to lymphopenia
• Neutropenia—alone or in addition to lymphopenia and a degenerative left shift
• Leukocytosis—may occur during recovery

Biochemistry
• ALT and AST—marked increase in most patients
• Hypoalbuminemia
• Cats—icterus seen in approximately 25% of patients; mildly low serum calcium concentrations often seen with pancreatitis; amylase levels unreliable

Urinalysis (Cats)
• Mild proteinuria—small proportion of patients
• Bilirubinuria—especially with icterus

OTHER LABORATORY TESTS
Serology
• IgM, IgG, and antigen serum titers—most definitive information from one sample; determine type of infection (active, recent, chronic) with a follow-up sample taken 3 weeks later; titers available from Veterinary Diagnostic Laboratory, College of Veterinary Medicine, Colorado State University, Fort Collins, CO 80523
• IgM—single serologic titer of choice for diagnosis of active infection; elevated 2 weeks postinfection (usually coincides with onset of clinical signs); persists for a maximum of 3 months; then falls; prolonged titer: reactivation or delay in antibody class shift to IgG (result of immunosuppression from FeLV or FIV infection or steroid therapy)

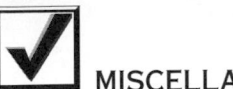

• IgG—titers rise 2–4 weeks postinfection; persist > 1 year; single high titer not diagnostic for active infection; fourfold increase over a 3-week period suggests active infection
• Antigen—positive 1–4 weeks postinfection; because it remains positive during active or chronically persistent infections, does not add much to antibody titer results

IMAGING
Radiographs—may see mixed pattern of patchy alveolar and interstitial pulmonary infiltrates, pleural and abdominal effusions, and hepatomegaly

DIAGNOSTIC PROCEDURES
• CSF—high leukocyte count (both mononuclear cells and neutrophils) and protein in encephalopathic patients
• Cytology—organism rarely detected in body fluids during acute infection (CSF, pleural or peritoneal effusions); broncho-alveolar lavage effective in identifying organisms in affected cats with signs of pulmonary involvement
• Fecal—evaluation with Sheather sugar solution may be diagnostic; fecal oocyst shedding rarely occurs during clinical disease; oocysts may be detected on routine examination in asymptomatic cats but are morphologically indistinguishable from *Hammondia* spp. and *Besnoitia;* distinguish organisms via mouse inoculation

PATHOLOGIC FINDINGS
• Necrotic foci—up to 1 cm; most often in liver, pancreas, mesenteric lymph nodes, and lungs; necrosis of brain (1-cm areas of discoloration)
• Ulcers and granulomas—may be seen in stomach and small intestine

 TREATMENT

APPROPRIATE HEALTH CARE
• Usually outpatient
• Inpatient—severe disease; patient cannot maintain adequate nutrition or hydration.
• Confine—patients with neurologic signs

NURSING CARE
Dehydration—intravenous fluids

CLIENT EDUCATION
• Cats—prognosis guarded in patients needing therapy; response to therapy inconsistent • Neonates and severely immunocompromised animals—prognosis worse

SURGICAL CONSIDERATIONS
N/A

 MEDICATIONS

DRUG(S) OF CHOICE
• Clindamycin—25–50 mg/kg PO or IM daily, divided into two doses, for at least 2 weeks after clinical signs clear
• 1% prednisone drops—every 8 hours for 2 weeks for uveitis; use concurrently

PRECAUTIONS
Clindamycin—anorexia, vomiting, and diarrhea (dose dependent)

ALTERNATIVE DRUG(S)
• Sulfadiazine (30 mg/kg PO q12h) in combination with pyrimethamine (0.5 mg/kg PO q12h) for 2 weeks; can cause depression, anemia, leukopenia, and thrombocytopenia, especially in cats.
• Folinic acid (5 mg/day) or brewer's yeast (100 mg/kg/day)—correct bone marrow suppression caused by sulfadiazine/pyrimethamine therapy

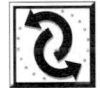 FOLLOW-UP

PATIENT MONITORING
Clindamycin
• Examine 2 days after initiation treatment—clinical signs (fever, hyperesthesia, anorexia, uveitis) should begin to resolve; uveitis should resolve completely within 1 week. • Examine 2 weeks after initiation of treatment—assess neuromuscular deficits; should partially resolve (some deficits permanent owing to CNS or peripheral neuromuscular damage)
• Examine 2 weeks after owner-reported resolution of signs—assess discontinuing treatment; some neuromuscular deficits permanent

PREVENTION/AVOIDANCE
Cats
• Diet—prevent ingestion of raw meat, bones, viscera, or unpasteurized milk (especially goat's milk); or mechanical vectors (flies, cockroaches); feed only well-cooked meat. • Behavior—prevent free roaming to hunt prey (birds, rodents) or to enter buildings where food-producing animals are housed.

POSSIBLE COMPLICATIONS N/A

EXPECTED COURSE AND PROGNOSIS
• Prognosis—guarded; varied response to drug treatment • Acute—prompt and aggressive therapy often successful • Residual deficits (especially neurologic) cannot be predicted until after a course of therapy.
• Ocular disease—usually responds to appropriate therapy • Severe muscular or neurologic disease—usually chronic debility

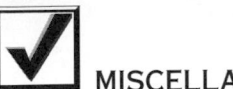 MISCELLANEOUS

ASSOCIATED CONDITIONS
• Young dogs—distemper • Cats—FeLV, FIP, and FIV; FIV infection does not affect clinical outcome or the ability of the animal to mount a protective immune response to subsequent reinfection. Renal transplant

AGE-RELATED FACTORS
Disease worse in neonates

ZOONOTIC POTENTIAL
• Considerable • Cats—healthy animal with a positive antibody titer poses little danger to humans; animal with no antibody titer at more risk of becoming infected, shedding oocysts in the feces, and constituting a risk to humans • Avoid contact with oocysts or tissue cysts—do not feed raw meat; wash hands and surfaces (cutting boards) after preparing raw meat; boil drinking water if source is unreliable; keep sandboxes covered to prevent cats from defecating in them; wear gloves when gardening; wash hands and vegetables before eating to avoid contact with oocyst soil contamination; empty cat litter boxes daily (oocysts need at least 24 hr to become infective); disinfect litter boxes with boiling water; control stray cat population to avoid oocyst contamination of environment.
• Pregnant women—avoid all contact with a cat that is excreting oocysts in feces; avoid contact with soil and cat litter; do not handle or eat raw meat (to kill organism, cook to 66°C; 150°F).

PREGNANCY
• Parasitemia during pregnancy—spread of organism to fetus; probably does not happen unless first-time infection of dam occurs during pregnancy (as with humans)
• Placental transmission rare

ABBREVIATIONS
• ALT = alanine aminotransferase
• AST = aspartate aminotransferase
• FeLV = feline leukemia virus
• FIP = feline infectious peritonitis
• FIV = feline immunodeficiency virus

Suggested Reading
Dubey JP. Toxoplasmosis. J Am Vet Med Assoc 1994;205:1593–1598.
Dubey JP, Lappin MR. Toxoplasmosis and neosporosis. In: Greene CE, ed. Infectious diseases of the dog and cat. Philadelphia: Saunders, 1998:493–509.
Author Stephen C. Barr
Consulting Editor Stephen C. Barr

TRACHEAL COLLAPSE

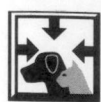 **BASICS**

DEFINITION
• Dynamic reduction in the luminal diameter of the large conducting airway with respiration • May involve the cervical trachea, the intrathoracic trachea, or both segments • Compression of the trachea or bronchi as a result of hilar lymphadenopathy or external mass lesions—not considered part of this condition

PATHOPHYSIOLOGY
• Hypocellular tracheal cartilage identified in some patients • Lack of chondroitin sulfate and/or decreased glycoproteins within the cartilage matrix results in a reduction in bound water and loss of turgidity in the cartilage. • Abnormalities in the cartilage structure may represent defects in chondrogenesis associated with primary genetic influences, nutritional deficiencies, or possibly degenerative changes caused by long-standing airway disease. • Collapse—weak cartilage allows flattening of the tracheal ring structure; trachea collapses in a dorsoventral direction when pressures change within the airway lumen. • Increased tension on the trachealis dorsalis muscle or neurogenic atrophy of the muscle causes stretching of the dorsal tracheal membrane with protrusion into the airway lumen. • Coughing—mechanical trauma to the tracheal mucosa from collapse of the dorsal tracheal membrane exacerbates airway edema and inflammation and may lead to pseudomembrane formation. • Abnormal pressure gradients develop along the trachea during inspiration, which lead to increased inspiratory effort and dynamic collapse of the airway. • Chronic increase in respiratory effort may lead to secondary abnormalities in laryngeal structure and function. • Upper airway obstruction worsens clinical signs. • High intrapleural pressure during expiration leads to collapse of the intrathoracic trachea. • Small airway disease heightens airway pressure gradient and potentiates collapse; may be perpetuated by chronic cough and airway inflammation, leading to more widespread pulmonary dysfunction

SYSTEMS AFFECTED
• Respiratory—lower respiratory tract infection or inflammation owing to poor clearance of secretions and bacteria
• Cardiovascular—pulmonary hypertension
• Nervous—may be involved when syncope develops from hypoxia or a vasovagal reflex associated with cough

GENETICS
Unknown

INCIDENCE/PREVALENCE
Common clinical entity

GEOGRAPHIC DISTRIBUTION
Worldwide

SIGNALMENT

Species
Primarily dogs, rarely cats

Breed Predilection
• Miniature poodles, Yorkshire terriers, Chihuahuas, Pomeranians, and other small and toy breeds • Occasionally seen in young, large-breed dogs

Mean Age and Range
• Middle-aged to elderly—onset of signs at 4–14 years of age
• Severely affected animals < 1 year of age

Predominant Sex
None

SIGNS

Historical Findings
• Usually worsened by excitement, heat, humidity, exercise, or obesity
• Dry honking cough • May have chronic history of intermittent coughing or difficulty breathing • Retching—often observed; occurs from an attempt to clear respiratory secretions from the larynx • Tachypnea, exercise intolerance, and/or respiratory distress—common • Cyanosis or syncope—may see in severely affected individuals

Physical Examination Findings
• Increased tracheal sensitivity—virtually always seen • Dyspnea—inspiratory dyspnea with cervical collapse; expiratory with intrathoracic collapse • Wheezing or musical tracheal sounds when ausculting over a region of narrowed trachea • An end-expiratory snap—may be heard when large segments of the intrathoracic airway collapse during forceful expiration • Wheezes or crackles—indicate concurrent small airway disease
• Mitral insufficiency murmurs—often found concurrently in small-breed dogs
• Normal to low heart rate and/or marked sinus arrhythmia—common in dogs with tracheal collapse, unless marked respiratory distress occurs • Loud second heart sound—suggests pulmonary hypertension
• Hepatomegaly—cause unknown

CAUSES
• Congenital, nutritional, or familial defects of chondrogenesis
• Chronic small airway disease

RISK FACTORS
• Obesity
• Pulmonary infection or inflammation
• Upper airway obstruction

 DIAGNOSIS

DIFFERENTIAL DIAGNOSIS
• Infectious tracheobronchitis
• Tracheal or laryngeal obstruction or foreign body
• Chronic bronchitis
• Pneumonia—viral, bacterial, fungal, parasitic, eosinophilic
• Bronchiectasis

CBC/BIOCHEMISTRY/URINALYSIS
CBC—may show an inflammatory leukogram secondary to chronic stress or pneumonia

OTHER LABORATORY TESTS
N/A

IMAGING

Thoracic Radiography
• Collapse identified in 60% of affected patients
• Inspiratory radiographs—show cervical collapse
• Expiratory radiographs—show intrathoracic tracheal collapse; may also note collapse of the mainstem bronchus and ballooning of the cervical trachea
• Bronchitis, pneumonia, or bronchiectasis—may be identified
• Right-sided heart enlargement—may be seen secondary to chronic pulmonary disease and cor pulmonale

Fluoroscopy
Dynamic collapse of the cervical or intrathoracic trachea and/or dorsal tracheal membrane—may be more easily identified after induction of cough

DIAGNOSTIC PROCEDURES

Tracheal Wash
Use oral intubation (rather than the transtracheal approach) with a small endotracheal tube and a sterile catheter when obtaining samples for cytologic examination and bacterial culture and sensitivity.

Bronchoscopy
• Grade severity of collapse; identify small airway disease.
• Grade I—slight protrusion of the dorsal tracheal membrane into the airway lumen; diameter reduced by < 25%
• Grade II—reduction of the tracheal lumen by 50%
• Grade III—reduction of the tracheal lumen by 75%; trachealis muscle brushing the tracheal mucosa

- Grade IV—tracheal rings flattened; < 10% of the tracheal lumen can be seen; may note a double lumen trachea when the trachealis muscle contacts the ventral surface of the trachea and the rings have bowed dorsally
- Submit airway samples for cytologic examination and bacterial culture and sensitivity testing; specific cultures for *Mycoplasma* are recommended.

Cytology
- Unremarkable in uncomplicated airway collapse
- Sepsis and suppuration along with marked bacterial growth of a pathogen—suggests pulmonary infection
- Neutrophils without intracellular bacteria or marked bacterial growth—indicates airway inflammation

PATHOLOGIC FINDINGS
- Trachealis muscle—greatly elongated
- Cartilage rings—flattened
- May note tracheal inflammation or pseudomembrane formation
- Hypocellularity of the cartilage with low glycoproteins and chondroitin sulfate—may be noted via histopathologic examination or electron microscopy
- May see changes associated with chronic obstructive pulmonary disease

 TREATMENT

APPROPRIATE HEALTH CARE
- Outpatient—stable patients
- Inpatient—oxygen therapy and heavy sedation for severe dyspnea

NURSING CARE
Oxygen therapy and heavy sedation—severely dyspneic patients

ACTIVITY
- Severely limited until patient is stable
- During management of disease—gentle exercise recommended to encourage weight loss

DIET
- Most affected dogs improve after losing weight.
- Institute weight-loss program with a high-fiber reducing diet.
- Feed 60% of total daily requirement of calories; use a slow weight-loss program

CLIENT EDUCATION
- Warn client that obesity, overexcitement, and humid conditions may precipitate a crisis.
- Advise client to use a harness instead of a collar.

SURGICAL CONSIDERATIONS
- Upper airway obstructive disorder (e.g., laryngeal paralysis, everted laryngeal saccule)—may improve after corrective surgery
- Placement of C-shaped stents in selected patients (primarily with cervical collapse) by a skilled surgeon—shown to improve quality of life and reduce clinical signs when adequate stabilization of the airway can be achieved and when chronic pulmonary changes do not limit resolution of disease
- Consider likelihood of complications after surgery (e.g., persistent cough, dyspnea, or laryngeal paralysis); some patients may require a permanent tracheostomy.
- Intraluminal stents helpful in selected cases

 MEDICATIONS

DRUG(S) OF CHOICE
- Sedation and cough suppression—butorphanol (0.05 mg/kg SC); addition of acepromazine (0.025 mg/kg SC) may enhance sedative effects and further reduce the cough reflex; narcotic cough suppressants (butorphanol at 0.5–1.0 mg/kg PO q4–8h or hydrocodone at 0.22 mg/kg PO q4–8h) effective for chronic treatment
- Dilation of small airways and lowering pressure gradients with lower airway disease—sustained-release theophylline (10–20 mg/kg q12h), or terbutaline (1.25–5.0 mg/dog q8–12h); bronchodilators have no effect on tracheal diameter.
- Reduction of tracheal inflammation—prednisone (0.5–1.0 mg/kg PO q12h; taper to q48h) for 5–7 days may help.

CONTRAINDICATIONS
None

PRECAUTIONS
Avoid long-term steroid use because of the propensity for weight gain and diseases associated with immunosuppression.

POSSIBLE INTERACTIONS
Theophylline metabolism—increased by concurrent treatment with ketoconazole or phenobarbital, which results in inadequate plasma concentration; decreased by fluoroquinolones (e.g., enrofloxacin), erythromycin, cimetidine, steroids, β-blockers, mexiletine, and thiabendazole, which results in toxic plasma concentration and gastrointestinal upset, nervousness, or tachycardia; adjust dosages when concurrent use is necessary.

ALTERNATIVE DRUG(S)
Robitussin DM—may provide palliation

 FOLLOW-UP

PATIENT MONITORING
- Body weight • Exercise tolerance • Pattern of respiration • Incidence of cough

PREVENTION/AVOIDANCE
- Avoid obesity in breeds commonly afflicted.
- Avoid heat and humidity. • Use harnesses.

POSSIBLE COMPLICATIONS
Intractable dyspnea leading to respiratory failure or euthanasia

EXPECTED COURSE AND PROGNOSIS
- Combinations of medications along with weight control may reduce clinical signs.
- Surgery—may benefit some patients, primarily those with cervical collapse
- Patient will cough throughout life.
- Prognosis—based on bronchoscopic evidence of airway obstruction

 MISCELLANEOUS

ASSOCIATED CONDITIONS
- Chronic bronchitis • Laryngeal paralysis
- Everted laryngeal saccules • Pulmonary hypertension • Breeds of dogs that develop tracheal collapse also commonly have mitral insufficiency.

AGE-RELATED FACTORS
N/A

PREGNANCY
N/A

SEE ALSO
Bronchitis, Chronic (COPD)

Suggested Reading

Buback JL, Boothe HW, Hobson HP. Surgical treatment of tracheal collapse in dogs: 90 cases (1983–1993). J Am Vet Med Assoc 1996;308:380–384.

Johnson LR, McKiernan BC. Diagnosis and medical management of tracheal collapse. Sem Vet Med Surg 1995;10:101–108.

McKiernan BC. Current uses and hazards of bronchodilator therapy. In Kirk RW, Bonagura JD, eds. Current veterinary therapy XI. Philadelphia: Saunders, 1992: 660–668.

White RAS, Williams JM. Tracheal collapse. Is there really a role for surgery? A survey of 100 cases. J Small Anim Pract 1994; 35:191–196.

Author Lynelle R. Johnson
Consulting Editor Lynelle R. Johnson

TRACHEAL PERFORATION

BASICS

OVERVIEW
Tracheal perforation is a loss of the integrity of the tracheal wall, allowing leakage of air into surrounding tissues, creating subcutaneous emphysema, pneumomediastinum, and potentially pneumopericardium, pneumothorax, and pneumoretroperitoneum. It can be caused by penetrating trauma, intraluminal trauma (iatrogenic), or blunt cervical or thoracic trauma. Severity can range from small perforation to complete tracheal avulsion. In patients with complete avulsion, the mediastinal tissues can form a pseudomembrane, maintaining airway patency.

SYSTEMS AFFECTED
• Respiratory—due to compromise of the airway and possible development of pneumothorax
• Skin—subcutaneous emphysema, initially cervical but can progress to entire body
• Cardiovascular—pneumothorax and tension pneumothorax (especially if positive pressure ventilation is used) can cause decreased venous return and decreased cardiac output.
• Others (Nervous, Musculoskeletal)—depending on severity of hypoxia

SIGNALMENT
Dogs and cats—no breed, age, or sex predilection

SIGNS
• Onset of clinical signs can be immediate or up to one week after perforation.
• Subcutaneous emphysema and respiratory distress are the most common signs.
• Other signs include anorexia, lethargy, gagging, coughing, inspiratory stridor, and shock.

CAUSES AND RISK FACTORS
• Penetrating cervical wounds such as bite wounds or missiles (e.g., gunshots, arrows)
• Iatrogenic perforation due to transtracheal wash or inadvertently during jugular venipuncture
• Anesthesia and intubation with failure to deflate the cuff or stabilize the endotracheal tube before repositioning the patient, or from overinflation of the endotracheal cuff, causing a tracheal tear; overinflation of cuff is proven to cause tracheal rupture, and causes a linear tear in trachealis muscle in the region of the thoracic inlet or intrathoracic trachea; seen most often with anesthesia for dental procedures and endotracheal washes—overinflation of cuff may be more common with these procedures.
• Blunt trauma (motor vehicle accident or falling from height) can cause intrathoracic tracheal avulsion.

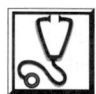

DIAGNOSIS

DIFFERENTIAL DIAGNOSIS
• Anesthesia—barotrauma resulting in alveolar rupture from closed pop-off valve or positive-pressure ventilation to high airway pressures.
• Penetrating wounds—perforation of the esophagus or severe cervical bite wounds can cause subcutaneous emphysema and airway compression.
• Post–blunt trauma—pulmonary contusions, pneumothorax, rib fractures.
• Other differentials include: intrathoracic tracheal compression by mediastinal mass, anticoagulant rodenticide–induced hemorrhage, spontaneous pneumothorax, pleural effusion, and bronchoesophageal fistula.

CBC/BIOCHEMISTRY/URINALYSIS
Usually normal

OTHER LABORATORY TESTS
Arterial blood gas analysis may show hypoxia, hypercarbia, and respiratory acidosis if ventilation is severely impaired.

IMAGING
• Lateral cervical and thoracic radiographs are essential for diagnosing tracheal perforation. Subcutaneous emphysema, pneumomediastinum, pneumopericardium, and finally pneumothorax can be seen.
• In cases of tracheal avulsion, the site of disruption may be visible.
• Abdominal radiographs may show a pneumoretroperitoneum.

DIAGNOSTIC PROCEDURES
• Pulse oximetry may show low oxygen saturation.
• Tracheoscopy can be used to confirm tracheal perforation or avulsion and characterize the severity, although false negative examinations can occur.

TREATMENT
• Hospitalization is indicated.
• Oxygen supplementation should be provided.
• Minimal handling to reduce stress
• Medical management is usually appropriate for iatrogenic perforation; most will heal spontaneously with supportive therapy.

• If pneumothorax develops, thoracocentesis and even thoracostomy tubes may be indicated.
• If patient does not stabilize or decompensates, surgical exploration is indicated.
• Tracheal rupture secondary to blunt trauma or penetrating wounds usually requires surgical therapy.
• During anesthesia in patients with tracheal avulsion, only the proximal segment should be intubated initially, using an undersized endotracheal tube, and positive-pressure ventilation should be avoided to prevent disruption of the pseudomembrane.
• Cervical tracheal perforation is approached via ventral midline. Damaged areas of the trachea should be debrided and repaired with 3-0 to 5-0 monofilament absorbable suture.
• Tracheal resection and anastomosis is indicated in cases of severe tracheal damage or tracheal avulsion. Proximal and distal tracheal segments are aligned with pre-placed sutures of 3-0 to 5-0 monofilament absorbable sutures.
• Intrathoracic tracheal avulsion is usually approached via a right lateral 3rd or 4th intercostal thoracotomy. The distal tracheal segment is located and intubated with a sterile endotracheal tube for maintenance of an airway and anesthesia once the pseudomembrane has been opened. After pre-placement of sutures, an endotracheal tube should then be guided caudally from the proximal segment into the distal segment by the surgeon.

 MEDICATIONS

DRUG(S)
Broad-spectrum antibiotic therapy is indicated if perforation is due to bite wounds until culture and sensitivity results are obtained.

CONTRAINDICATIONS/POSSIBLE INTERACTIONS
• Sedation should be used with caution—may decrease respiratory drive and precipitate crisis
• Corticosteroids are not indicated unless there is a large degree of upper airway swelling.

 FOLLOW-UP

PATIENT MONITORING
• Monitor respiratory rate and effort, mucous membrane color, capillary refill time, pulse quality, heart rate, and perform auscultation frequently, especially when patient first presents and also after surgical intervention.
• Pulse oximetry and/or arterial blood gases may be useful.
• Thoracic radiographs can monitor degree of pneumomediastinum and pneumothorax present, and help detect development of tracheal stenosis.

PREVENTION/AVOIDANCE
• Use of 3-ml syringe for cuff inflation for cats and small dogs to prevent overinflation of cuff
• Disconnect endotracheal tube from anesthetic circuit when repositioning patient.
• Prevent stylet from extending beyond end of endotracheal tube when used during intubation.

POSSIBLE COMPLICATIONS
• Tracheal stricture and stenosis at site of perforation or repair
• Dehiscence of tracheal anastomosis site
• Sepsis (rare)

• Death, particularly at induction of anesthesia in cases with complete tracheal avulsion

EXPECTED COURSE AND PROGNOSIS
• Majority of cases will respond well to appropriate therapy.
• Complete tracheal avulsion has a more guarded prognosis owing to the difficulties that may be encountered during stabilization and anesthesia, and without surgery has an extremely poor prognosis due to stricture formation 2–3 weeks post trauma and risk of sudden death.
• If tracheal rupture extends to the carina, death may occur intraoperatively due to difficulty maintaining an airway during repair.

 MISCELLANEOUS

ASSOCIATED CONDITIONS
When tracheal perforation is caused by blunt trauma, pulmonary contusions, pneumothorax, rib fractures, and hemothorax may result.

PREGNANCY
Hypoxia caused by airway embarrassment may result in fetal distress and death.

Suggested Reading
Hardie EM, Spodnick GJ, Gilson SD, et al. Tracheal rupture in cats: 16 cases (1983–1998). J Am Vet Med Assoc 1999; 214:508–512.
Authors Lori S. Waddell and David A. Puerto
Consulting Editor Lynelle R. Johnson

TRANSITIONAL CELL CARCINOMA: RENAL, BLADDER URETHRA

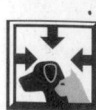

BASICS

DEFINITION
Malignancy arising from the transitional epithelium of the kidney, ureters, urinary bladder, urethra, prostate, or vagina

PATHOPHYSIOLOGY
Flea-control products (organophosphates and carbamate) and cyclophosphamide—possible causal agents

SYSTEMS AFFECTED
Renal/Urologic
• Kidneys—less commonly affected than other renal sites; may be primary site
• Urinary bladder (may include ureters)—trigone most commonly affected site in dogs; local invasion of the distal ureter also common; may lead to postrenal azotemia; apex more often affected than is the trigone in cats
• Urethra—second most common site in dogs; may find urethral obstruction and postrenal azotemia
Other
• Reproductive—vagina less commonly affected but may be primary site; prostate may be involved by local invasion or may be primary site
• Metastatic sites—regional lymph nodes and lungs most common; may also spread to bones
• Paraneoplastic organ involvement—hypertrophic osteopathy has been reported secondary to transitional cell carcinoma of the urinary bladder

GENETICS
Possible genetic basis in Scottish terriers

INCIDENCE/PREVALENCE
• Dogs—< 1% of all reported malignancies
• Rare in cats

GEOGRAPHIC DISTRIBUTION
N/A

SIGNALMENT
Middle-aged to old, spayed, female small-breed dogs most commonly reported

Species
Dogs and cats

Breed Predilections
• Dogs—Scottish terriers, west Highland white terriers, Shetland sheepdogs, American Eskimo dogs, and dachshunds; may occur in any breed
• Cats—none

Mean Age and Range
• Dogs—8 years; range, 1–15+ years
• Cats—7 years; range, 3–16 years

Predominant Sex
Female

SIGNS

General Comments
Similar to those of bacterial urinary tract infection; for patients showing temporary or no response to appropriate antibiotics, consider transitional cell carcinoma; may temporarily respond to antibiotic therapy

Historical Findings
• Recurrent stranguria, pollakiuria, hematuria, dysuria, urinary incontinence, or any combination

Physical Examination Findings
• Often normal
• Mass—occasionally palpable in the caudal abdomen and urinary bladder region
• Urethral or vaginal—may be palpable on rectal examination
• Enlarged intrapelvic or sublumbar lymph nodes—rarely palpable

CAUSES
• Dogs—see Risk Factors
• Cats—unknown

RISK FACTORS
Dogs—obesity, environmental carcinogens, chronic exposure to flea-control products, and long-term or a large bolus dose of cyclophosphamide

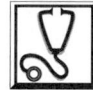

DIAGNOSIS

DIFFERENTIAL DIAGNOSIS
• Urinary tract infection
• Urolithiasis
• Vaginitis
• Prostatitis
• Other primary neoplasia or metastatic neoplasia

CBC/BIOCHEMISTRY/URINALYSIS
• Usually normal
• Biochemistry—may show signs of renal and/or postrenal azotemia with ureteral or urethral obstruction
• Urinalysis—often reveals epithelial cells with multiple criteria of malignancy; interpret cytologic examination with caution if the sample is inflammatory, because epithelial cells may exhibit criteria of malignancy in the presence of inflammation.
• Avoid cystocentesis because seeding of tumor cells along needle tract is possible.

OTHER LABORATORY TESTS
Urine culture and sensitivity testing—indicated because concurrent urinary tract infection is common

IMAGING
• Thoracic radiography—metastatic patterns: multiple well-defined interstitial nodules, interstitial pattern more pronounced than normal, and alveolar infiltrates; up to 37% of dogs have metastatic disease at the time of examination.
• Abdominal radiography—probably will not reveal specific urinary bladder disease unless the mass is mineralized (rare); may reveal sublumbar lymphadenomegaly
• Double-contrast cystography—dogs: lesion(s) usually at trigone of the urinary bladder; cats lesion(s) usually at the apex of the urinary bladder
• Intravenous pyelography, voiding urethrogram, or vaginogram—sometimes indicated
• Ultrasonography—helps identify location and extent of disease; excellent for monitoring response to treatment

DIAGNOSTIC PROCEDURES
• Biopsy—gold standard for definitive diagnosis
• Exploratory laparotomy—reasonable method for obtaining specimens of the primary tumor and regional lymph nodes
• Cystoscopy—less invasive way to view lesions and retrieve specimens
• Ultrasound-guided biopsy—not recommended, because seeding of the biopsy tract with viable tumor cells is likely

PATHOLOGIC FINDINGS
• Irregular to diffuse thickening of the urinary bladder mucosa
• Metastasis possible

TRANSITIONAL CELL CARCINOMA, RENAL, BLADDER, URETHRA

 TREATMENT

APPROPRIATE HEALTH CARE
• Outpatient—stable patients
• Radiotherapy (intraoperative and fractionated)—reported to result in longer survival times and better local control than chemotherapy; potential side effects: urinary bladder stricture and fibrosis with urinary incontinence

NURSING CARE
N/A

ACTIVITY
Normal

DIET
Normal, unless concurrent renal failure

CLIENT EDUCATION
• Warn client that the long-term prognosis is poor but palliation is often attainable.
• Inform client that the tumor is not usually surgically resectable in dogs.

SURGICAL CONSIDERATIONS
• Highly exfoliative and highly transplantable tumor; multiple reports of surgically induced seeding; replace all surgical instruments and gloves after contact with the tumor.
• Surgery may result in a cure if the mass is surgically resectable.
• Wide surgical margins necessary; up to 50% of the urinary bladder may be resected with minimal loss of function.
• Tube cystostomy placement—may greatly prolong survival times by bypassing urethral obstruction

 MEDICATIONS

DRUG(S) OF CHOICE
• Piroxicam (Feldene)—0.3 mg/kg PO q24h with food; reported to have activity in up to 20% of cases
• Cisplatin—50–70 mg/m² IV every 3 weeks; conventional agent; reported activity not > 20%

• Mitoxantrone—5.5 mg/m² IV every 3 weeks
• Other agents (doxorubicin, or doxorubicin/cyclophosphamide combination) may have activity.
• Piroxicam (0.3 mg/kg PO q24h) and mitoxantrone (5 mg/m² IV q21d for 4 doses); reported to have activity in ≤ 40% of cases.

CONTRAINDICATIONS
• Piroxicam—do not use with known gastrointestinal erosions or ulcers; do not use with renal insufficiency; not evaluated in cats
• Cisplatin—do not use in cats; do not use with renal insufficiency

PRECAUTIONS
• Cisplatin or piroxicam (dogs)—monitor for renal insufficiency; patients may have renal damage caused by hydroureter, hydronephrosis, or pyelonephritis
• Seek advice before initiating treatment if you are unfamiliar with cytotoxic drugs.

POSSIBLE INTERACTIONS
• Cisplatin and piroxicam—do not use concurrently because of the risk of cumulative nephrotoxicity
• Cisplatin—do not use concurrently with other nephrotoxic drugs

ALTERNATIVE DRUG(S)
Antibiotics—administered as necessary

 FOLLOW-UP

PATIENT MONITORING
• Contrast cystography or ultrasonography—every 6–8 weeks; assess response to treatment
• Thoracic radiography—every 2–3 months; detect metastatic disease

PREVENTION/AVOIDANCE
N/A

POSSIBLE COMPLICATIONS
• Urethral or ureteral obstruction and renal failure
• Metastatic disease to regional lymph nodes, lungs, or bone
• Recurrent urinary tract infection

• Urinary incontinence
• Myelosuppression or gastrointestinal toxicity secondary to chemotherapy
• Gastrointestinal ulceration secondary to piroxicam therapy

EXPECTED COURSE AND PROGNOSIS
• Long-term prognosis grave
• Progressive disease probable
• Median survival—no treatment, 4–6 months; with treatment, 6–12 months

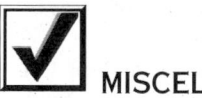 MISCELLANEOUS

ASSOCIATED CONDITIONS
• Recurrent urinary tract infection
• Paraneoplastic hypertrophic osteopathy

AGE-RELATED FACTORS
N/A

ZOONOTIC POTENTIAL
N/A

PREGNANCY
N/A

SEE ALSO
N/A

ABBREVIATIONS
N/A

Suggested Reading
Chun R, Knapp DW, Widmer WR, et al. Cisplatin treatment of transitional cell carcinoma of the urinary bladder in dogs: 18 cases (1983–1993). J Am Vet Med Assoc 1996;209:1588–1591.
Knapp DW. Tumors of the urinary system. In: Withrow ST, MacEwen EG, eds. Small animal clinical oncology. Philadelphia: Saunders, 2001:490–499.
Morrison WB. Cancers of the urinary tract. In: Morrison WB, ed. Cancer in dogs and cats: medical and surgical management. Baltimore: Williams & Wilkins, 1998:569–579.
Author Ruthanne Chun
Consulting Editor Wallace B. Morrison

TRANSMISSIBLE VENEREAL TUMOR

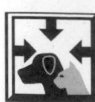

BASICS

OVERVIEW
• Sexually transmitted, naturally occurring tumor
• Appears to be more common in temperate areas and large cities

SIGNALMENT
Usually young, intact dogs of either sex

SIGNS
• Red, friable, lobulated mass on the mucosa of the vagina or penis
• Oral or nasal mucosa may also be affected.
• Blood dripping from the prepuce or vagina
• Excessive licking of the genital area
• Tumor protrusion

CAUSES & RISK FACTORS
• Direct transplantation of tumor cells onto abraded mucosa, either by coitus or oral transmission
• Intact, free-roaming dogs—at greater than average risk

DIAGNOSIS

DIFFERENTIAL DIAGNOSIS
• Other neoplasms—squamous cell carcinoma; cutaneous lymphoma
• Vaginal hyperplasia

CBC/BIOCHEMISTRY/URINALYSIS
• Usually normal
• Free-catch urine—hematuria and abnormal cells may be noted.

OTHER LABORATORY TESTS
N/A

IMAGING
• Thoracic radiographs—part of a thorough staging procedure; although rarely metastatic
• Abdominal radiography or ultrasonography—may be useful in staging

DIAGNOSTIC PROCEDURES
• Careful palpation of regional lymph nodes
• Examination of impression smears or aspirate of the tumor—reveals homogenous sheets of round to oval cells with prominent nucleoli, scant cytoplasm, and multiple clear cytoplasmic vacuoles
• Biopsy—provides definitive diagnosis

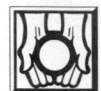

TREATMENT

• May spontaneously regress; treatment recommended because spontaneous remission is not reliable
• Surgical excision of small tumors—often followed by recurrence
• Radiotherapy alone—may be curative
• Medical treatment with vincristine—usually curative

MEDICATIONS

DRUG(S)
• Vincristine sulfate—0.5–0.7 mg/m² IV once weekly for 2 weeks beyond complete resolution of gross disease
• Partial or no remission—try doxorubicin (30 mg/m² IV every 3 weeks)

CONTRAINDICATIONS/POSSIBLE INTERACTIONS
• Myelosuppression secondary to vincristine or doxorubicin administration
• Doxorubicin—may be cardiotoxic; use with caution once a cumulative dose of 150 mg/m² is reached.
• Vincristine and doxorubicin—tissue sloughing if administered perivascularly; always administer through a patent IV catheter.
• Seek advice before initiating treatment if you are unfamiliar with cytotoxic drugs.

FOLLOW-UP

PATIENT MONITORING
CBC and platelet count—before each chemotherapy treatment

PREVENTION/AVOIDANCE
• Spay or neuter
• Prevent animals from roaming free.

POSSIBLE COMPLICATIONS
• Tumor recurrence after incomplete surgical excision or reexposure
• Metastatic disease uncommon

EXPECTED COURSE AND PROGNOSIS
Usually an excellent response to treatment (primarily chemotherapy or radiotherapy) and an excellent prognosis

MISCELLANEOUS

PREGNANCY
• Do not treat pregnant animals with chemotherapy.
• Animals may be infected with transmissible venereal tumor during coitus.

Suggested Reading
MacEwen EG. Transmissible venereal tumor. In: Withrow SJ, MacEwen EG, eds. Philadelphia: Saunders, 2001:651–656.
Morrison WB. Cancers of the reproductive tract. In: Morrison WB, ed. Cancer in dogs and cats: medical and surgical management. Baltimore: Williams & Wilkins, 1998: 581–590.
Rogers KS, Walker MA, Dillon HB. Transmissible venereal tumor: a retrospective study of 29 cases. J Am Anim Hosp Assoc 1998;34:463–470.
Author Ruthanne Chun
Consulting Editor Wallace B. Morrison

BASICS

OVERVIEW
• Traumatic myocarditis is the term applied to the syndrome of arrhythmias that sometimes complicates blunt trauma; it is a misnomer, because myocardial lesions (if present) are more likely to take the form of necrosis than inflammation.
• Direct cardiac injury is not required for development of posttraumatic arrhythmia; extracardiac conditions are likely to have equal or greater etiologic importance.
• Ventricular tachyarrhythmias occur in most affected patients; supraventricular arrhythmias and bradyarrhythmias are uncommon. Ventricular rhythms that complicate blunt trauma are often relatively slow and detected only during pauses in the sinus rhythm; they are most appropriately referred to as AIVRs. The QRS complexes are wide and bizarre; the rate is > 100 bpm but generally < 160 bpm. Usually, these rhythms are electrically and hemodynamically benign.
• Dangerous ventricular tachycardias can also complicate blunt trauma and can also evolve from seemingly benign AIVRs, compromising perfusion and placing the patient at risk for sudden death.

SIGNALMENT
Dogs; rarely cats

SIGNS

Historical Findings
• Trauma, most often from road accidents
• Arrhythmias often noticed within 48 hours of trauma

Physical Examination Findings
• Arrhythmias may be inapparent if the rate of an AIVR closely matches the sinus rate.
• Rapid, irregular rhythms in some patients
• Signs of poor peripheral perfusion (e.g., weakness, pale mucous membranes, and weak femoral pulses) in patients with rapid, poorly tolerated ventricular rhythms

CAUSES & RISK FACTORS
• Blunt trauma
• Hypoxia
• Autonomic imbalance
• Electrolyte derangements
• Acid–base disturbances

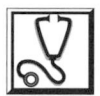

DIAGNOSIS

DIFFERENTIAL DIAGNOSIS
AIVRs should be differentiated from ventricular tachycardia.

• AIVRs—usually initiated by late diastolic ventricular (escape) complexes or fusion complexes; heart rate is generally 100–160 bpm.
• Ventricular tachycardia—usually initiated by a ventricular premature complex; heart rates exceed 160 bpm.

CBC/BIOCHEMISTRY/URINALYSIS
• Creatine kinase, liver enzymes, and lactic dehydrogenase often high because of organ trauma
• Electrolyte derangements (particularly hypokalemia and hypomagnesemia) predispose to ventricular arrhythmia

OTHER LABORATORY TESTS
N/A

IMAGING

Thoracic Radiographic Findings
Evidence of trauma, including pneumothorax, rib fractures, and pulmonary contusion in some patients

DIAGNOSTIC PROCEDURES

Electrocardiographic Findings
Ventricular arrhythmias, as previously discussed

TREATMENT
• Treat extracardiac conditions, including pain, electrolyte derangements, and hypoxia, which can predispose to ventricular arrhythmia.
• Thoracic radiographs for all patients with blunt trauma; identify and remedy disorders such as pneumothorax.
• The need for antiarrhythmic therapy is predicated on clinical signs and the electrocardiographic character of the arrhythmia; pharmacologic suppression of AIVR is usually unnecessary.
• Fluid therapy for shock

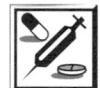

MEDICATIONS

DRUG(S)
• First treat rapid ventricular rhythms or those associated with hemodynamic compromise with lidocaine (2 mg/kg boluses IV); a total of 8 mg/kg can be administered over 10–12 min. Start a lidocaine infusion (25–75 (µg/kg/min) once the rhythm is stabilized with lidocaine boluses

• If lidocaine administration fails to convert to sinus rhythm, try procainamide, β-blockers such as esmolol or propranolol, or even class III agents such as bretylium.
• Consider DC conversion while animal is under anesthesia or heavy sedation, to treat rapid, hemodynamically unstable ventricular rhythms that do not respond to drug therapy.
• Antiarrhythmic agents are not necessarily benign; they can worsen existing arrhythmias and provide a substrate for development of new arrhythmias (proarrhythmia); weigh the relative risk or benefit carefully at every step.

CONTRAINDICATIONS/POSSIBLE INTERACTIONS
N/A

FOLLOW-UP
• ECG monitoring of animals with arrhythmias is recommended; generally, the arrhythmias that complicate blunt trauma are self-limiting and resolve within 48–72 hours.
• If antiarrhythmic therapy deemed necessary, it can often be discontinued after 2–5 days.
• Although dangerous arrhythmias occasionally complicate blunt trauma, the prognosis usually depends on the severity of extracardiac injury.

MISCELLANEOUS

SEE ALSO
• Shock, Cardiogenic
• Idioventricular Rhythm
• Ventricular Tachycardia

ABBREVIATIONS
• AIVR = accelerated idioventricular rhythm
• DC = direct current

Suggested Reading
Abbott JA. Traumatic myocarditis. In: Bonagura JD, ed. Kirk's Current veterinary therapy XII. Philadelphia: Saunders, 1995: 846–830.

Author Jonathan A. Abbott
Consulting Editors Larry P. Tilley and Francis W. K. Smith, Jr.

TREMORS

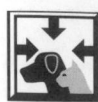 **BASICS**

DEFINITION
Rhythmic, oscillatory, involuntary movement of all or part of the body

PATHOPHYSIOLOGY
• Abnormal movement caused by the alternate or synchronous contraction of reciprocally innervated, antagonistic muscles
• Synchronous contraction—force or duration of contraction is slightly different in the opposing muscles, resulting in biphasic, to-and-fro movement.

SYSTEMS AFFECTED
• Nervous
• Musculoskeletal—muscle weakness or pain

SIGNALMENT
• Dogs and cats
• Age depends on cause.

Dogs
• Generalized tremor syndrome—usually young to middle-aged
• Variety of hair coat colors, including white
• Hypomyelination—6–8 weeks old; chow chows, springer spaniels, Samoyeds, Weimaraners, and Dalmatians
• Idiopathic transient head tremor—Doberman pinschers, English bulldogs, and Labrador retrievers

SIGNS
• Localized or generalized
• Localized—most often involves the head or the pelvic limbs

CAUSES

Head
• Cerebellar abnormalities—degenerative; congenital; inflammatory; immune-mediated; toxic causes
• Idiopathic—Doberman pinschers and English bulldogs overrepresented
• Genetic
• Inflammatory—encephalitides
• Trauma
• Drug administration—doxorubicin; diphenhydramine; metoclopramide

Pelvic Limb Tremor
• May be a sign of weakness or pain in the lumbosacral area
• Metabolic—renal failure; hypoparathyroidism; hypoglycemia
• Compressive lesions of the spine or nerve roots—lumbosacral stenosis; cauda equina syndrome; spinal cord tumor; diskospondylitis
• Peripheral neuropathy; neuromuscular junction abnormality; myopathy
• Poor perfusion to pelvic muscles—right-to-left shunting patent ductus arteriosus; other cardiopulmonary diseases
• Unknown—pelvic limbs in older dogs (senile tremor)

Generalized Tremor
• Hypomyelination
• Intoxications—organophosphates; hexachlorophene; bromethalin
• Degenerative neurologic disease—storage disease; spongiform encephalopathy
• Idiopathic generalized tremor syndrome—white shaker dog syndrome

RISK FACTORS
• Any encephalitis or degenerative neurologic disease—storage disease and spongiform encephalopathy
• Treatment with doxorubicin, diphenhydramine, or metoclopramide

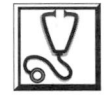 **DIAGNOSIS**

DIFFERENTIAL DIAGNOSIS

Similar Signs
• Shaking, shuddering, myotonia, and myoclonus—tremor usually more consistent, rhythmic, to-and-fro movements of similar amplitude that persist throughout the waking state and stop during sleep
• Weakness—tremor associated with weakness usually occurs when the muscles are forced to work (e.g., during standing, walking, and running).
• Tetany—usually a more consistent extension of the limbs and facial muscles without an extension–flexion cycle of movement

• Seizures—short duration; may be associated with autonomic disturbances (e.g., urination, defecation, and salivation) and alterations of consciousness
• Reflex myoclonus—Labrador retrievers and Dalmatians; characterized by prolonged episodes of extensor rigidity with tactile or auditory stimulus and voluntary exercise

Localized to the Head
Diseases of the lumbosacral spinal cord and associated peripheral nerves; musculoskeletal diseases
• Localized to the pelvic limbs
• Assess for additional neurologic deficits suggesting cerebellar disease; often a clinical sign of cerebellar disease; intention tremor that worsens when the patient attempts to move the head in a goal-oriented manner; may also involve the whole body; ataxia and dysmetria help determine the neuroanatomic diagnosis.
• Idiopathic condition—breed-specific (e.g., Doberman pinschers, English bulldogs); patient usually young at onset; sporadic; occurs at a frequency of 2–4 Hz; up-and-down (yes) or side-to-side (no) direction; anatomic origin unknown; small percentage of dogs have encephalitis.

Generalized
• Young dog (6–8 weeks)—congenital myelination abnormality; check breed incidences
• Young adult dog—assess history for toxin exposure; consider generalized tremor syndrome, especially with a white hair coat.

CBC/BIOCHEMISTRY/URINALYSIS
• Usually normal with an associated primary brain disease
• Localized to the head or pelvic limbs—assess for occult metabolic disease; may find hypoglycemia, hypocalcemia, and abnormal renal function
• Some myopathies are characterized by high creatine kinase.

OTHER LABORATORY TESTS
N/A

IMAGING
• Localized to the pelvic limbs—radiography, myelography, epidurography, CT, and MRI; reveal lumbosacral, spinal, or vertebral abnormalities
• Generalized or localized to the head—CT and MRI of the brain and radiography of the spine usually normal
• Maltese dogs with generalized tremor syndrome—CT; reveals hydrocephalus; importance of this finding uncertain
• Hypomyelination—MRI; may reveal evidence of lack of myelin

DIAGNOSTIC PROCEDURES
• CSF analysis—usually helpful in establishing diagnosis of generalized tremor syndrome and other causes of encephalitis
• Suspected lumbosacral syndrome—survey radiography; CSF analysis; electromyography of limb muscles; myelography; CT; and MRI; look for evidence of a lumbar spinal compressive lesion.
• Suspected primary brain disease—CSF analysis (assess underlying brain inflammation); CT or MRI (assess intracranial structures); BAER (assess central auditory pathways and overall brainstem function)

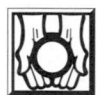 TREATMENT
• Treat the underlying primary disease.
• Outpatient, unless surgical treatment is indicated (lumbosacral disease that requires decompression and stabilization)
• Avoid excitement and exercise—may worsen many tremors
• Generalized tremor of primary brain origin—patient may lose weight; monitor weight and modify oral intake accordingly
• Most of the causes in adult dogs are treatable.
• Degenerative neurologic diseases (e.g., storage disease and spongiform encephalopathy)—no treatment available
• Hypomyelination—generally not treatable; some breeds improve with maturity (e.g., chow chows)

• Idiopathic head tremor—no effective treatment available; benign tremor that occurs sporadically; has few health consequences
• Drug-induced—consider an alternate drug.
• Suspected intoxication—remove patient from further exposure; consult with a poison control center for possible antidote.

 MEDICATIONS

DRUG(S) OF CHOICE
• Usually do not respond to muscle relaxants or anticonvulsants (e.g., phenobarbital or diazepam)
• Corticosteroids—immunosuppression; for generalized tremor syndrome
• Antibiotics—for diskospondylitis; choose on the basis of culture and sensitivity of the lesion, blood, or urine.
• Cerebellar diseases—depends on the diagnosis

CONTRAINDICATIONS
Sympathomimetic drugs—may worsen condition

PRECAUTIONS
N/A

POSSIBLE INTERACTIONS
N/A

ALTERNATIVE DRUG(S)
N/A

 FOLLOW-UP

PATIENT MONITORING
• Monitor the primary disease.
• Corticosteroids for generalized tremor syndrome—monitor weekly initially to assess response to treatment.

POSSIBLE COMPLICATIONS
N/A

☑ MISCELLANEOUS

ASSOCIATED CONDITIONS
N/A

AGE-RELATED FACTORS
N/A

ZOONOTIC POTENTIAL
N/A

PREGNANCY
N/A

SYNONYMS
• Shaking
• Shuddering

SEE ALSO
• Cerebellar Degeneration
• Hypomyelination
• See also Causes

ABBREVIATIONS
• BAER = brainstem auditory-evoked response
• CSF = cerebrospinal fluid
• CT = computed tomography
• MRI = magnetic resonance imaging

Suggesting Reading
Bagley RS. Tremor syndromes in dogs: diagnosis and treatment. J Small Anim Pract 1992;33:485–490.
Cuddon PA. Tremor syndromes. Prog Vet Neurol 1990;1:285–299.
De Lahunta A. Veterinary neuroanatomy and clinical neurology. 2nd ed. Philadelphia: Saunders, 1983.
Farrow BH. Generalized tremor syndrome. In: Kirk RW, ed. Current veterinary therapy IX. Philadelphia: Saunders, 1986:880–881.
Kornegay JN, Thomson CE. Trembling and shaking. In: Ettinger SJ, ed. Textbook of veterinary internal medicine: diseases of the dog and cat. 3rd ed. Philadelphia: Saunders, 1989:54–56.
Wagner SO, Podell M, Fenner WR. Generalized tremors in dogs: 24 cases (1984–1995). J Am Vet Med Assoc 1997;211:731–735.
Author Rodney S. Bagley
Consulting Editor Joane M. Parent

TRIGEMINAL NEURITIS

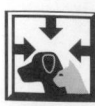 BASICS

OVERVIEW
• Acute onset of inability to close the jaw owing to bilateral dysfunction of the mandibular branch of the trigeminal nerves
• Nerve injury—from bilateral nonsuppurative neuritis, demyelination, and (occasionally) fiber degeneration of all branches of trigeminal nerve and ganglion

SIGNALMENT
• Primarily adult dogs
• Rare in cats

SIGNS
• Acute onset of a dropped jaw
• Inability to close the mouth
• Drooling
• Difficulty in prehending food
• Messy eating
• No apparent deficits in sensory perception
• Swallowing intact

CAUSES & RISK FACTORS
• Unknown
• Possibly immune-mediated

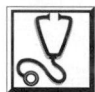 DIAGNOSIS

DIFFERENTIAL DIAGNOSIS
• Musculoskeletal disorders of the temporomandibular joints and jaw—differentiated by history of trauma and pain and physical examination findings
• Rabies—always initially consider until there is sufficient evidence to rule it out.
• Neoplasia—both mandibular nerves secondary to myelomonocytic leukemia, lymphosarcoma, and neurofibrosarcoma reported; usually does not have an acute onset
• Masticatory muscle myositis—trismus; jaw is difficult to open.

CBC/BIOCHEMISTRY/URINALYSIS
Usually normal

OTHER LABORATORY TESTS
N/A

IMAGING
N/A

DIAGNOSTIC PROCEDURES
• No specific test
• Skull radiography, examination of bone marrow aspirate, and muscle biopsy—rule out the differentials

 TREATMENT

• Outpatient if owner is able to help the patient eat and drink
• Patient cannot prehend and move food and water to the throat; requires help when eating and drinking
• Patient is able to lap and swallow food offered by a large syringe placed in the corner of mouth with the head slightly elevated.
• Fluids—administer subcutaneously; may be necessary to maintain hydration
• Pharyngostomy or gastrostomy tubes—rarely necessary to maintain adequate food intake

 MEDICATIONS

DRUG(S)
Corticosteroids—no indication that they help recovery

CONTRAINDICATIONS/POSSIBLE INTERACTIONS
Steroids—use with caution; dehydration may develop from steroid-induced polyuria and polydipsia in a patient that relies on its owner for water intake

 FOLLOW-UP

• Self-limiting disorder
• Full recovery in 2–4 weeks
• Occasional masticatory muscle atrophy but without trismus

 MISCELLANEOUS

Suggested Reading
Mayhew PD, Bush WW, Glass EN. Trigeminal neuropathy in dogs: a retrospective study of 29 cases (1991–2000). J Am Anim Hosp Assoc 2002;38:262–270.
Author T. Mark Neer
Consulting Editor Joane M. Parent

BASICS

OVERVIEW
• *Francisella tularensis*—small gram-negative coccobacillus; type A, more virulent, found in rabbits and ticks; type B, waterborne, found in rodents and ticks; in North America principally found in wild lagomorphs (cottontail, jack, snowshoe) and rodents (moles, squirrels, muskrats, beavers); facultative intracellular parasite; survives and grows in liver-producing granulomas and/or abscesses • Peak occurrence—late spring; June–August; December
• Northern Hemisphere—absent from United Kingdom, Africa, South America, Australia; in U.S. most cases found in Missouri, Alaska, Oklahoma, South Dakota, Tennessee, Kansas, Colorado, Illinois, Utah, and Maine.
• Infection—ingestion of tissue or body fluids of an infected mammal or contaminated water; bitten by blood-sucking arthropod (tick), flies, mites, midges, fleas, or mosquitos; few bacteria needed to infect cats through skin, airways, or conjunctiva; larger number required to infect through the gastrointestinal tract • Skin contact—organism multiplies locally (papule) 3–5 days after contact; ulcerates 2–4 days later; spreads via lymphatics to regional LN and bloodstream; results in septicemia (lung, liver, spleen, LN, bone marrow) • Ingestion—may involve lymphadenopathy of cervical and mesenteric LN followed by septicemic spread; distribution of lesions to face, oral cavity, tonsils, intestines, and LN • Acute disease—2–7 days after contact with organism

SIGNALMENT
• Cats—occasionally • Dogs—rarely

SIGNS
• Sudden onset of anorexia, lethargy, fever (40–41°C; 104–106°F) • Enlarged palpable submandibular and cervical LN • Tender abdomen, palpable mesenteric LN, hepatomegaly—depending on stage of disease
• Multifocal white patches or ulcers along glossopalatine arches and tongue • Icterus

CAUSES & RISK FACTORS
• Organism—all *Francisella* biogroups may infect cats but may differ in virulence; some cats may have mild infection
• Hunter or outdoor cats in endemic areas
• Infected wildlife in the area of hunting activity
• Exposure to infected blood-sucking parasites

DIAGNOSIS

DIFFERENTIAL DIAGNOSIS
• Any acute disease state manifested by acute lymphadenopathy, malaise, oral ulceration,

and fatal outcome—consider tularemia
• Bubonic plague (*Yersinia pestis*)—western U.S.
• Pseudotuberculosis (*Yersinia pseudotuberculosis*)—usually vomiting and diarrhea

CBC/BIOCHEMISTRY/URINALYSIS
• Initially severe panleukopenia; then leukocytosis with left shift, toxic neutrophils, thrombocytopenia
• Hyperbilirubinemia
• Hyponatremia
• Hypoglycemia
• Alanine aminotransferase—elevated
• Bilirubinuria
• Hematuria

OTHER LABORATORY TESTS
Serology with tube agglutination or ELISA—possible; difficult to perform, except in reference laboratory

IMAGING N/A

DIAGNOSTIC PROCEDURES
• Direct smear—lesion or biopsy; difficult to see organism on Gram staining
• Cultural isolation—by reference laboratory; blood, pleural fluid, LN aspirate onto cysteine- or cystine-containing media; not recoverable on routine laboratory media; **CAUTION:** use extreme care when working with infected specimens or isolates
• Direct fluorescent antibody testing—clinical materials or tissues; rapid assay of infection status

PATHOLOGIC FINDINGS
• Multifocal white patches or ulcers along glossopalatine arches and tongue
• Oral, tonsillar ulceration
• Lymphadenopathy of cervical, retropharyngeal, or submandibular LN with abscessation
• Diffuse intestinal lesions
• Mesenteric lymphadenopathy, hepatosplenomegaly, and icterus

TREATMENT
• Inpatient with good nursing care
• Early treatment important to prevent high mortality
• Treat for ectoparasites.

MEDICATIONS

DRUG(S)
• Treat all cases empirically until laboratory confirmation obtained

Cats
• Little information available on the efficacy of antimicrobials because of high mortality if patient not treated early • Early treatment

with amoxicillin (20 mg/kg PO q8h for 5–7 days or 20 mg/kg IM or SC q12h for 5 days) in combination with gentamicin (4.4 mg/kg IM or SC q12h once and then q24h thereafter until a clinical response or until 7 days) has been successful.
• Fluoroquinolones are showing promise as a potential new treatment drug (ciprofloxacin).

CONTRAINDICATIONS/POSSIBLE INTERACTIONS N/A

FOLLOW-UP

PATIENT MONITORING
Monitor for DIC—may occur late in the infection

PREVENTION/AVOIDANCE
• Travel with pet—avoid endemic areas
• Endemic areas—confine animals to control exposure to and ingestion of wildlife and their ectoparasites (ticks); ecoparasite control by periodic spraying or dusting of animal and pastures • Neuter cats—limit hunting behavior and wildlife exposure • Take precautions to limit contamination of food and water with carcasses of infected wildlife.

EXPECTED COURSE AND PROGNOSIS
Prognosis poor if not treated early; prognosis poor if mesenteric LN palpable

MISCELLANEOUS

ZOONOTIC POTENTIAL
• High • All personnel in contact with patient or body fluids must use face mask, gloves, and gowns to avoid infection. • Isolate patients
• In emerging disease areas, cat ownership is a disease risk for humans • Bites pose a risk for humans. • Do not mistake for bite abscess in cats or plague.

SYNONYMS
• Rabbit fever • Deerfly fever • Market men's disease

ABBREVIATIONS
• DIC = disseminated intravascular coagulation • ELISA = enzyme-linked immunosorbent assay • LN = lymph node(s)

Suggested Reading
Rohrbach BW. Tularemia. J Am Vet Med Assoc 1988;193:428–432.
Author Patrick L. McDonough
Consulting Editor Stephen C. Barr

TYZZER DISEASE

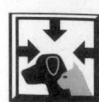

BASICS

OVERVIEW
• *Clostridium piliformis* (formerly *Bacillus piliformis*)—gram-negative bacterium; 0.5 × 10–40 μm in size; an obligate intracellular pathogen
• Infection—organism thought to initially proliferate in intestinal epithelial cells; spreads to the liver via the hepatic portal vein; hepatic colonization associated with multifocal periportal hepatic necrosis

SIGNALMENT
• Dogs and cats
• Any age; young at higher risk
• Rodents—clinically affected

SIGNS
• Rapid onset of lethargy, depression, anorexia, abdominal discomfort, hepatomegaly, and abdominal distention; followed by hypothermia
• Death—within 24–48 hr
• Fecal matter—diarrhea infrequent; small amounts of pasty feces more common

CAUSES & RISK FACTORS
• *C. piliformis*
• Contact with rodents—may be a risk factor
• Neonates and immunocompromised animals (e.g., distemper, FeLV, feline panleukopenia, familial hyperlipo-proteinemia)—seem to be at greatest risk

DIAGNOSIS

DIFFERENTIAL DIAGNOSIS
• Diagnosis usually made at necropsy—rapid and highly fatal disease diagnosis
• Distinguished from other causes of sudden death and acute hepatitis

CBC/BIOCHEMISTRY/URINAYSIS
• ALT—marked elevations in blood samples taken shortly before death

OTHER LABORATORY TESTS
• Serology—identify latent infections in rodent colonies; could be used to investigate illness in dogs and cats
• Isolation of organism—requires inoculation of mice, embryonating eggs, or cell culture

IMAGING
N/A

DIAGNOSTIC PROCEDURES
N/A

PATHOLOGIC FINDINGS

Gross
• Multifocal whitish gray to hemorrhagic foci throughout the liver; may also occur in other viscera
• Focal myocarditis, thickening and congestion of the intestine, mesenteric lymphadenopathy—reported

Histologic
• Multifocal hepatic necrosis
• Necrotic ileitis or colitis
• Intracellular filamentous organisms—usually numerous; difficult to visualize with H&E; require silver stains (e.g., modified Steiner or Warthin-Starry)

 TREATMENT
• None effective

 MEDICATIONS

DRUG(S)
None

CONTRAINDICATIONS/POSSIBLE INTERACTIONS
None

 FOLLOW-UP

PREVENTION/AVOIDANCE
• Avoid predisposing factors—may limit disease

 MISCELLANEOUS

ABBREVIATIONS
• ALT = alanine aminotransferase
• FeLV = feline leukemia virus
• H&E = hematoxylin and eosin

Suggested Reading
Jones BR, Green CE. Tyzzer's disease. In: Greene CE, ed. Infectious diseases of the dog and cat. Philadelphia: Saunders, 1998:242–243.
Author Kenneth W. Simpson
Consulting Editor Stephen C. Barr

UNRULY BEHAVIORS: JUMPING, DIGGING, CHASING, STEALING

BASICS

DEFINITION
• Jumping—standing on rear legs with front legs on a person or object or leaping in the air with or without landing against the person
• Digging—using paws to scrape a surface as though attempting to excavate the substrate
• Chasing—pursuing a moving person, animal, or object
• Stealing—the taking of an item not intended to be utilized by the dog

PATHOPHYSIOLOGY
• All are within the range of normal dog behaviors. • Insufficient activity may contribute to all. • Jumping up as part of excessive greeting can be associated with separation anxiety. • Digging can be associated with an obsessive-compulsive disorder (OCD) or be associated with a seizure disorder.

SYSTEMS AFFECTED
• Behavioral • Nervous

GENETICS
N/A

INCIDENCE/PREVALENCE
Unknown

GEOGRAPHIC DISTRIBUTION
N/A

SIGNALMENT

Species
Dogs

Breed Predilection
• Herding and hunting breeds may be more likely to chase. • Hunting breeds (including the terrier breeds) may be more likely to dig.

Mean Age and Range
More common in younger dogs, but occur at any age

Predominant Sex
N/A

SIGNS

Historical Findings
• Jumping up on people occurs more commonly in association with arrivals or departures or greeting at other times; it is also associated with exploring the contents of countertops or tables. • Digging often occurs in areas along a fence line or areas of recent gardening, at rodent holes, and on interior flooring with or without owner presence.
• Items displaced or food items missing from surfaces are common complaints in stealing.

Physical Examination Findings
• Usually unremarkable • Nails worn down
• Pain on abdominal palpation may suggest an organic disease. • Neurologic examination may suggest an organic disease.

CAUSES
• Jumping up is a normal greeting and play behavior. Excitement, encouragement of the behavior by others, or inadvertent rewarding of the behavior perpetuates it. Separation anxiety may result in excessive jumping on owners when returning home or leaving.
• Digging is a normal behavior. Presence of rodents, anxiety, regulation of body temperature, under-stimulation or lack of adequate exercise, food caching or retrieval, escape from confinement, pain (particularly abdominal), obsessive-compulsive disorder, and neurologic disease can all be causes of digging. • Stealing is a normal acquisitive behavior. It can be caused by a dog trying to get an owner's attention or by the desire for a food item. • Chasing is a normal behavior. Causes include herding, hunting, play, and defense.

RISK FACTORS
• Inadequate exercise
• Under-stimulation
• Stealing food—special or weight-reduction diets
• Chasing—lack of exposure to fast moving stimuli at a young age, common in herding breeds

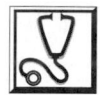

DIAGNOSIS

DIFFERENTIAL DIAGNOSIS

Digging
• Separation anxiety—escapes or attempts escape from confined areas in the owner's absence. Presence of other signs consistent with separation anxiety, including vocalization, urination, defecation, other destruction, or salivation, in the owner's absence. • Other anxiety or phobia (thunderstorm or other stimulus such as plane) • Pain, particularly abdominal—splinting of abdomen, other gastrointestinal signs, urinary tract signs, with dog appearing to have difficulty getting comfortable • OCD (such as light chasing and digging for the light)—behavior usually occupies a large percentage of the dog's time, interferes with normal functioning, and can be difficult to interrupt. • Neurologic disease—presence of other neurologic abnormalities such as seizures

CBC/BIOCHEMISTRY/URINALYSIS
• Usually unremarkable • May be abnormalities consistent with system affected

OTHER LABORATORY TESTS
As indicated to rule out source of pain or neurologic disease (bile acids, CSF analysis)

IMAGING
Radiographs, ultrasound, MRI, or CT scan as indicated by physical exam findings

DIAGNOSTIC PROCEDURES
CSF tap to rule out neurologic disorder

PATHOLOGIC FINDINGS
N/A

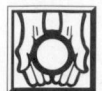

TREATMENT

APPROPRIATE HEALTH CARE
Outpatient management

NURSING CARE
None

ACTIVITY
Increase the dog's daily exercise.

DIET
N/A

CLIENT EDUCATION

Jumping
• During training, prevention of the undesired jumping-up behavior is essential.
• A head collar and leash greatly facilitate training. • Visitors can be greeted outside or inside with the dog on a leash and head collar, or the dog's access to the situation can be restricted by placing it in another room until the visitor is seated. • Teach "sit" and "stay" as an alternative method to greet people. • When the dog is calm and tractable, practice sitting for a food reward in different areas of the house. • Sessions should be short—3–5 minutes with 8–12 repetitions per session. • Food should be highly palatable and small (1/4″ square or larger, depending on the size and weight of the dog). • Add the word "stay" when the duration of sitting is a few seconds; take a step away, return to the dog and give the food reward. Build up the time away from the dog to 3–5 minutes. • Repeat exercises near the door and with the addition of leaving and returning. • Next ask the dog to sit for a food reward when returning from work or other absences of a few hours' duration. • Familiar visitors can enter, ask the dog to sit, and give a food reward. • Alternatively, the owner can reward the dog for remaining seated as people enter.
• Eventually the food rewards can be reduced to intermittent use. • Dogs that like to retrieve and are too excited to remain seated may do better if a ball is tossed as a visitor enters. This is more beneficial if a dog has been taught to sit prior to an item's being tossed again. • The owner should avoid increasing the dog's excitement by walking calmly to the door and speaking in a quiet voice. • People should avoid rewarding the jumping with attention such as pushing the dog off. Do not acknowledge or interact with the dog; hold arms against the body, and turn body away from the dog. Some dogs will stop jumping and ignore the person. • Stepping on the dog's toes or squeezing the paws and

UNRULY BEHAVIORS: JUMPING, DIGGING, CHASING, STEALING

activities like these are cruel and can lead to aggression.

Digging

• Digging associated with temperature regulation occurs in hot or cold weather to help cool a dog or conserve heat for a dog. Adequate heated or cooled shelter should minimize this problem. • Digging associated with rodents can occur inside or out. This behavior is likely to persist until the rodents are removed. • Digging associated with separation anxiety, escaping a phobic stimulus, or OCD should resolve with treatment of those conditions. Dogs with separation anxiety should not be left alone in the yard for extended periods of time. • For digging in the owner's presence or not associated with any of the above, the owner should increase the dog's exercise and activity. Aerobic exercise should occur before leaving the dog unsupervised in the yard. The provision of interactive toys like automatic tennis ball throwers may be helpful. • If the digging persists, create an area where it is acceptable for the dog to dig. A children's sandbox can be used for this purpose or an area can be marked off with wood and filled with sand or topsoil. Initially bury toys or food items with the dog observing, so the dog is directed to and rewarded for digging in the specific area. • Supervision is necessary to redirect the dog to another activity as it starts to dig. Aversive stimuli (loud noise, water spray) can be used to interrupt the digging but may not affect the digging when the owner is absent. Remote activated aversive stimuli (a motion detector on a garden hose), stones, or putting water in the dug area might prevent digging in that specific area but may not affect digging in other areas.

Chasing

• A head collar can be extremely helpful in controlling the dog in the presence of the chase stimulus. Herding breeds exhibit a phenotypic behavior that may respond better to control and management than to treatment. • Dogs that chase will need to be desensitized (gradually exposed to) and counter-conditioned (taught a different response) to the stimulus. • The owner should practice the same sit-and-stay exercises as described above, with the addition of a "look" command using a treat brought up to the owner's eye. This will help get the dog's attention and focus it back on the owner when it sees the moving stimulus. • Sessions should be 3–5 minutes, with numerous repetitions per session. Initially work with the dog inside without distractions, having it sit, stay, and look. • Next work in a quiet yard with the dog on a leash, have the dog sit, stay, step away, return, look, and give the food

reward. When the dog is successful, the process can be repeated in a more distracting part of the yard. If the dog is too distracted, the owner should work with the dog at times of day when there are fewer distractions (i.e., passers-by, traffic). • The owner should first work with the dog without the chase stimulus present. If the owner is able to keep the dog's attention, the owner should then stage the chase stimulus (like a bike or person jogging) to pass by at a great distance while working with the dog. The owner might need to increase the speed of the repetitions and rewards. • Each day, if the dog is able to ignore the chase stimulus, the owner should move a few inches closer to it. If the dog is unable to ignore the chase stimulus, the distance should be increased. When the dog is able to ignore the chase stimulus in the yard, the owner can incorporate the same exercise on a walk. When the owner sees the chase stimulus, he or she should ask the dog to sit, stay, and look, and then reward the dog.

Stealing

• The dog's attempts to initiate play and chase may result in stealing. • Adequate attention, exercise, and toys before the owner becomes preoccupied (e.g., making dinner, working, watching TV) will help to decrease this motivation for stealing. • Owners should not engage in chasing the dog. They should ignore the dog and walk away, get a treat, and call the dog to them. While the dog is in the process of dropping the item, the owner can say "drop," "good dog," and give the dog the treat. The dog is being rewarded for relinquishing the item. • The owner may want to give a second treat so there is no "race" for the dropped item. The item should be placed out of view and not shown to the dog. • If the dog retreats under furniture, the owner should not pursue it. If the dog feels threatened or cornered, it may defend itself aggressively. • For food stealing, food needs to be placed out of the dog's reach, since acquiring food is highly rewarding. • Products that can interrupt and are mildly aversive can help correct the stealing behavior. Motion detectors can be helpful in deterring stealing behavior. Traditional ones sound an alarm when motion is detected. A new one for pets is a motion-activated compressed air sprayer. If the dog steals food because it is on a diet, low-calorie foods like raw or cooked vegetables can be added to the dog's food so it is less hungry.

SURGICAL CONSIDERATIONS

None

MEDICATIONS

DRUG(S) OF CHOICE
None

CONTRAINDICATIONS
N/A

PRECAUTIONS
N/A

POSSIBLE INTERACTIONS
N/A

ALTERNATIVE DRUG(S)
N/A

FOLLOW-UP

PATIENT MONITORING
Every 2–3 weeks initially

PREVENTION/AVOIDANCE
Close supervision, exercise, and exposing the dog to different stimuli as a young puppy can help to prevent some of the unruly behaviors.

POSSIBLE COMPLICATIONS
Injury as a result of escaping a fence, chasing a stimulus, or ingesting an inappropriate item

EXPECTED COURSE AND PROGNOSIS
Generally good response to treatment for jumping, digging, and stealing if the owner is consistent. Chasing behaviors may be more difficult and resistant to treatment.

MISCELLANEOUS

AGE-RELATED FACTORS
Younger dogs need more activity than many owners anticipate.

SEE ALSO
• Compulsive Disorders—Dogs
• Fears, Phobias, and Anxieties—Dogs
• Separation Anxiety Syndrome

ABBREVIATIONS
• CSF = cerebrospinal fluid
• CT = computed tomography
• MRI = magnetic resonance imaging
• OCD = obsessive-compulsive disorder

Suggested Reading
Landsberg G, Hunthausen W, Ackerman L. Unruly behaviors. In: Handbook of behaviour problems of the dog and cat. Oxford, UK: Butterworth-Heinemann, 1997:65–78.

Author Marsha R. Reich
Consulting Editor Debra F. Horwitz

BASICS

OVERVIEW
Occurrence of a urolith (calculus) within a ureter; most ureteroliths originate in the renal pelves and so commonly occur in association with nephroliths. Many uroliths that enter the ureter continue to the bladder without impedance, but uroliths may cause partial or complete obstruction of the ureter, resulting in dilation of the proximal ureter and renal pelves and subsequent destruction of renal parenchyma.

SIGNALMENT
• Dogs and cats • Breed, age, and sex predispositions vary with type of nephrolith. • See Nephrolithiasis.

SIGNS
• May be initially asymptomatic • Pain (ureteral colic) during passage of ureteroliths or following acute ureteral obstruction • Renomegaly if ureteral obstruction leads to hydronephrosis • Unilateral ureteral obstruction results in azotemia and uremic clinical signs only when the function of the contralateral kidney is compromised. • Signs referable to a lower urinary tract infection and septicemia may be present concurrently. • Ureteral rupture may occur, resulting in urine accumulation in the retroperitoneal space.

CAUSES & RISK FACTORS
• For a list of causes, see chapters on each urolith type. • Prior treatment of nephroliths by extracorporeal shock wave lithotripsy (ESWL), medical dissolution, or surgery to remove nephroliths may be additional risk factors.

DIAGNOSIS

DIFFERENTIAL DIAGNOSIS
• Consider in all cases of renal failure, unilateral or bilateral renomegaly, abdominal pain, or fluid accumulation in the retroperitoneal space • Radiopacities on abdominal radiographs that may be confused with ureteroliths include particulate fecal material in the colon, mammary gland nipples, peritoneoliths, calcified lymph nodes, and mineralization of the renal pelvis. • Radiolucent ureteroliths may be difficult to differentiate from ureteral blood clots. Other causes of ureteral obstruction include intraluminal tumors, ureteroceles, ureteral strictures (following surgery or trauma), and extraluminal compression. Hydroureter and hydronephrosis may occur because of ureteral ectopia, pyelonephritis, and obstruction of the ureteral opening at the trigone, most commonly due to transitional cell carcinoma of the bladder.

CBC/BIOCHEMISTRY/URINALYSIS
These tests evaluate renal function and screen for concurrent disease before the treatment of ureterolithiasis. They do not directly contribute to the diagnosis of ureterolithiasis. Urinalysis, serum calcium concentration, and fractional excretion of electrolytes may permit estimation of urolith composition pending results of definitive analysis.

OTHER LABORATORY TESTS
• Submit all retrieved ureteroliths for quantitative analysis to determine appropriate preventive strategies. • Patients (other than dalmatians and bulldogs) with urate stones should be evaluated for portosystemic shunts.

IMAGING
• Radiopaque ureteroliths may be visualized with survey radiographs. If obstruction and hydronephrosis have occurred, renomegaly may be apparent. If ureteral rupture occurs, contrast in the retroperitoneal space may be lost. • Small uroliths may not be visualized on radiographs even if they are radiopaque. • When ureteroliths are suspected, but cannot be documented, an intravenous urogram may help to identify the obstruction and will also distinguish ureteral rupture from retroperitoneal hemorrhage. In many instances the damaged tubules do not concentrate dye adequately, resulting in poor delineation of the ureter; in these cases contrast injection by nephropyelocentesis may be useful. • Ultrasound is valuable for detecting hydronephrosis or hydroureter • Changes suggesting pyelonephritis may also be observed by ultrasound. The dilated proximal ureter may be traced to the ureterolith and thus allow direct observation of it. • Ureteroliths in the middle or distal ureter are less frequently observed sonographically.

DIAGNOSTIC PROCEDURES
• Nuclear scintigraphy has been advocated to determine each kidney's contribution to the total GFR, but since GFR measurements cannot be used to predict the functional recovery possible following the relief of obstruction, nuclear scintigraphy alone should not determine whether or not to preserve or surgically remove a kidney. • Voiding urohydropropulsion may be performed to retrieve ureteroliths that have spontaneously passed into the bladder.

PATHOLOGIC FINDINGS
• Gross changes in the kidney—progressive dilation of the pelves and calyces; in advanced cases, the kidney may be transformed into a thin-walled sac with only a thin shell of atrophic cortical parenchyma; ureteral dilation proximal to the site of obstruction is typical. • Microscopic changes—begin with dilation of the tubules, which then atrophy, separate, and are replaced by diffuse cortical fibrosis; the glomeruli are relatively well preserved in the residual cortical tissue.

TREATMENT
• Remove ureteroliths that are causing obstruction (i.e., causing hydronephrosis or hydroureer) or which have not moved on sequential radiographs. • Ureteroliths in dogs have been successfully treated with ESWL. • Surgical techniques recommended for removal of ureteroliths vary, depending on the site of obstruction, the presence or absence of infection, and the degree of function of the associated kidney. Ureteroneocystotomy may be performed for ureteroliths in the middle and distal ureter: the ureter proximal to the obstruction is excised and reimplanted into the bladder. Ureteroliths in the proximal ureter are removed by ureterotomy. Concurrent placement of a nephrostomy catheter is recommended. Performance of a ureterotomy or ureteroneocystotomy requires experience in microsurgical techniques, particularly in cats. When the contralateral kidney functions normally or when severe hydronephrosis or pyelonephritis is present in the affected kidney, ureteronephrectomy may be appropriate.

MEDICATIONS

DRUG(S)
• Medical dissolution is largely ineffective. • Therapy aimed at prevention of recurrent disease is imperative following relief of obstruction.

CONTRAINDICATIONS/POSSIBLE INTERACTIONS
• Medical therapy designed to promote the dissolution or prevent the recurrence of uroliths is not totally benign. Some patients will not tolerate the high salt concentration, protein restriction, acidification, or related management procedures that may be required. Take particular care in patients with high metabolic demands, such as growth or lactation, and in animals with congestive heart failure or renal failure. • Attempts to prevent one type of urolith may promote formation of a second type.

FOLLOW-UP

PATIENT MONITORING
Following successful removal of ureteroliths, recheck every 3–6 months for recurrence of uroliths and to ensure owner compliance with preventive measures; urinalysis, radiographs (or ultrasound) and a urine culture are usually appropriate.

PREVENTION/AVOIDANCE
• Elimination of factors predisposing to the development of urolithiasis • Specific therapy depends on the mineral composition of the urolith. Refer to chapters on individual urolith types for appropriate preventive measures.

POSSIBLE COMPLICATIONS
Hydronephrosis, renal failure, recurrent urinary tract infection, pyelonephritis, sepsis, ureteral rupture

EXPECTED COURSE AND PROGNOSIS
Highly variable; if unilateral disease is present and recurrence is prevented, the prognosis is good.

MISCELLANEOUS

ASSOCIATED CONDITIONS
Commonly associated with uroliths elsewhere in the urinary tract, especially nephroliths

AGE-RELATED FACTORS
Geriatric dogs that are poor surgical candidates may be treated with ESWL.

PREGNANCY A contraindication to ESWL

SEE ALSO
• Hydronephrosis • Nephrolithiasis • Pyelonephritis • Renal Failure, Chronic • Urinary Tract Obstruction • Urolithiasis

ABBREVIATIONS
• ESWL = extracorporeal shock wave lithotripsy
• GFR = glomerular filtration rate

Suggested Reading
Kyles AE, Stone EA, Gookin J, et al. Diagnosis and surgical management of obstructive ureteral calculi in cats: 11 cases (1993–1996). J Am Vet Med Assoc 1998;213:1150–1156.
Authors Harriet M. Syme and Larry G. Adams
Consulting Editors Larry G. Adams and Carl A. Osborne

BASICS

OVERVIEW
• Occurs when the mucosal lining of the distal portion of the urethra prolapses through the external urethral orifice • Exact pathophysiology unknown; see Causes and Risk Factors • Systems affected include urinary, reproductive (bleeding may sometimes only occur during penile erection), and hemic/lymph/immune (blood loss can be severe enough to cause anemia, especially in smaller breeds of dogs).
• Prolapsed urethras often appear as a congested, pea-shaped mass protruding from the distal end of the penis. They often are associated with varying degrees of hemorrhage. Excessive licking may result in further traumatic damage to the exposed urethral mucosa.

SIGNALMENT
• Dogs • Most common in English bulldogs and Boston terriers • Mean age, 18 months; range, 4 months to 5 years
• Reported in male dogs only

SIGNS

Historical Findings
• Intermittent or persistent bleeding from the urethra independent of urination
• Intermittent or persistent licking of the penis
• Depending on the underlying cause, dysuria and pollakiuria caused by concomitant disorders may also be present.

Physical Examination Findings
• Red to purple, pea-sized, doughnut-shaped mass protruding from the distal end of the penis • Pale mucous membranes if bleeding is severe • Uroliths may be palpable in the urinary bladder or urethra.

CAUSES & RISK FACTORS
• May result from sexual excitement and/or unrelated disorders (e.g., infections, uroliths) of the lower urinary tract • Increased intraabdominal pressure secondary to dysuria associated with urocystoliths may be a predisposing factor.
• Other proposed causes include abnormal development of the urethra with superimposed increased intraabdominal pressure as a consequence of brachycephalic airway syndrome, dysuria, or sexual activity. This increased intraabdominal pressure could impair venous return of blood through the pudendal veins, predisposing susceptible dogs to engorgement of the corpus spongiosum surrounding the distal urethra. • Breed predisposition (bulldogs and Boston terriers) • Abnormal urethral anatomy associated with increased intraabdominal pressure secondary to upper airway obstructive syndrome, any cause of persistent dysuria, and/or sexual excitement may be risk factors. Increased intraabdominal pressure could impair venous return of blood through the pudendal veins, predisposing susceptible dogs to engorgement of the corpus spongiosum surrounding the distal urethra.

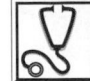 DIAGNOSIS

DIFFERENTIAL DIAGNOSIS
• Prostatic disease • Persistent penile frenulum
• Fractures of the os penis • Testicular disease
• Urethritis • Urethroliths • Coagulopathy
• Urethral neoplasia

CBC/BIOCHEMISTRY/URINALYSIS
• CBC—may reveal regenerative anemia
• Serum biochemistries—usually normal
• May not detect significant hematuria in urine collected by cystocentesis, but a voided urine sample may reveal hematuria.

OTHER LABORATORY TESTS
Coagulation profile may rule out coagulopathy.

IMAGING
• Survey abdominal radiographs—useful to rule out radiodense uroliths and to evaluate the prostate gland • Double-contrast cystography and positive-contrast urethrography—useful to rule out radiolucent uroliths, other urethral disorders, and prostatic disease • Abdominal ultrasonography—useful to evaluate the prostate and urinary bladder further

DIAGNOSTIC PROCEDURES
• Ejaculation—useful to evaluate urethra during penile erection; some urethral prolapses are present only during penile erection. • Evaluation of ejaculates may also facilitate evaluation of prostatic fluid for evidence of prostatic disease.

 TREATMENT

• May not be required if prolapsed urethra is asymptomatic or only associated with episodic bleeding • If prolapsed urethra is present only during penile erection, consider castration prior to attempting surgical removal of prolapsed tissue; diethylstilbestrol given for 3–6 weeks after surgery may reduce frequency of erections.
• Consider surgery for patients with excessive bleeding, pain, or extensive ulceration and/or necrosis of the prolapsed tissue. Also consider surgery if troublesome relapses are associated with medical management. • Satisfactory results have been obtained by manual reduction of the prolapse followed by urethropexy.
• If surgery is necessary, Elizabethan collars or similar restraint devices may be needed to prevent licking-induced trauma to the surgical site.
• Regardless of treatment chosen, advise the owner that recurrence is possible. • Because brachycephalic breeds are at risk for this problem, use caution in choosing an anesthetic regimen; monitor brachycephalic breeds carefully during anesthesia to ensure maintenance of adequate oxygenation.

 MEDICATIONS

DRUG(S)
• Bacterial urethritis warrants use of appropriate antibiotics.
• May need to consider using diethylstilbestrol for 3–6 weeks after surgery to reduce frequency of erections

CONTRAINDICATIONS/POSSIBLE INTERACTIONS
Because of the possibility of bone marrow suppression, consider risk:benefit ratios before giving estrogens, especially if patients are already anemic.

 FOLLOW-UP

PATIENT MONITORING
At least 7–10 days following surgery, for evidence of severe hemorrhage or recurrence of urethral prolapse

PREVENTION/AVOIDANCE
If urethral prolapse is associated with penile erection, advise owners to prevent contact with female dogs or other situations likely to cause penile erection.

POSSIBLE COMPLICATIONS
Advise owners that postsurgical recurrence of prolapse may occur, especially if no underlying cause has been detected and eliminated or controlled.

EXPECTED COURSE AND PROGNOSIS
• Urethral prolapse may persist without significant sequelae. Therefore, some dogs may not require therapy.
• Other dogs may not have any further problems after castration and/or surgical correction of a prolapsed urethra.
• If the underlying cause(s) persists, postsurgical recurrence is common.

 MISCELLANEOUS

ASSOCIATED CONDITIONS
• Concurrent urethritis is common.
• Concurrent urolithiasis may be a predisposing cause. • May be present during, or worsened by, penile erection

Suggested Reading
Kirsch JA, Hauptman JG, Walshaw R. A urethropexy technique for surgical treatment of urethral prolapse in the male dog. J Am Anim Hosp Assoc 2002;38:381–384.
Osborne CA, Sanderson SL. Medical management of urethral prolapse in male dogs. In: Bonagura JD, Kirk RW, eds. Current veterinary therapy XII. Philadelphia: Saunders, 1995:1027–1029.
Authors Sherry L. Sanderson and Carl A. Osborne
Consulting Editors Larry G. Adams and Carl A. Osborne

URINARY RETENTION, FUNCTIONAL

BASICS

DEFINITION
Incomplete voiding not associated with urinary obstruction

PATHOPHYSIOLOGY
Usually a disorder of the voiding phase of micturition; incomplete voiding results from hypocontractility of the urinary bladder (detrusor atony) or from inappropriately excessive outlet resistance (functional urinary obstruction).

SYSTEMS AFFECTED
• Renal/Urologic
• Endocrine/Metabolic
• Nervous

SIGNALMENT
More common in male than in female dogs and cats; see Causes.

SIGNS
• Palpably distended resting urinary bladder; after attempts by the animal to void, palpable distension may persist or inappropriate residual urine can be measured (normal < 0.5 mL/kg).
• Affected animals may demonstrate ineffective, frequent, or no attempts to void.
• Urine stream may be weak, attenuated, or interrupted.
• Abdominal distension, abdominal pain, or signs of postrenal azotemia may predominate in rare cases or with urinary tract rupture.
• May be an occult finding in patients with recurrent urinary tract infection
• Overflow urinary incontinence may occur

CAUSES

Hypocontractility of the Urinary Bladder Detrusor Muscle (Detrusor Atony)
• Most commonly develops as a sequel to acute or chronic urinary bladder overdistension; many patients have a history of neurologic dysfunction or previous urinary obstruction.
• Neurogenic causes include lesions of the pelvic nerves, sacral spinal cord, and suprasacral spinal cord.
• Lesions of the sacral spinal cord (e.g., congenital malformations, cauda equina compression, lumbosacral disk disease, and vertebral fractures/dislocations) can result in a flaccid, overdistended urinary bladder with weak outlet resistance.
• Lesions of the suprasacral spinal cord (e.g., intervertebral disk protrusion, spinal fractures, and compressive neoplasms) can result in a distended, firm urinary bladder that is difficult to express.
• Electrolyte disturbances, including hyperkalemia, hypokalemia, hypocalcemia,

and hypercalcemia, and other metabolic disturbances associated with generalized muscle weakness can also affect detrusor muscle contractility.
• Detrusor atony with urine retention is a feature of dysautonomia, a disturbance of autonomic ganglia primarily encountered in cats in Great Britain; the disorder has also been described in dogs in certain geographic regions of the United States.
• Some dogs with hyperadrenocorticism have polyuria, urinary bladder distention and mild urine retention.

Functional Urinary Obstruction
• Occurs when excessive or inappropriate outlet resistance prevents complete voiding during urinary bladder contraction
• In patients with suprasacral spinal lesions or midbrain disorders, urethral outlet resistance becomes uninhibited and remains inappropriately excessive or fails to coordinate with voiding contractions (detrusor-urethral dyssynergia). The condition has been associated with sacral lesions, local neuropathy, and idiopathic causes.
• Excessive urethral resistance, usually attributed to smooth or striated muscular components of the urethra (urethrospasm), may be seen after urethral obstruction or urethral or pelvic surgery, urethral inflammation, or prostatic disease.

RISK FACTORS
• Feline lower urinary tract disease
• Urethral obstruction
• Pelvic or urethral surgery
• Anticholinergic medications

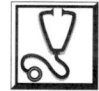

DIAGNOSIS

DIFFERENTIAL DIAGNOSIS
• When no voiding is observed, must be differentiated from oliguria, anuria, and urinary tract rupture
• Must be differentiated from physical and mechanical obstruction; clinical signs of urinary obstruction include pollakiuria, stranguria, and hematuria; patients with mechanical obstruction may void a few drops of urine after long periods of straining.
• Neurologic findings in dogs with supraspinal lesions affecting micturition include paralysis or paresis of pelvic ± thoracic limbs, hyperreflexia of affected limbs, and cervical, thoracolumbar, and lumbar pain. The urinary bladder is usually distended, firm, and difficult to express. In patients with chronic or partial lesions, reflexive voiding may return, characterized by incomplete, involuntary detrusor contractions with outlet spasticity.

• Neurologic findings in dogs with sacral lesions affecting micturition include pelvic limb paresis with hyporeflexia, depressed anal and tail tone, perineal sensory loss, and depressed bulbospongiosus reflexes. Lumbosacral pain may be the only sign in some dogs. The urinary bladder is typically distended, flaccid, and fairly easy to express.
• A urine stream that can be initiated but is abruptly tapered or halted is typical of idiopathic detrusor-urethral dyssynergia. Manual palpation may confirm detrusor contractions, which persist after flow terminates, and may suggest a high residual volume of urine.
• In patients recovering from urinary obstruction, inability to void may result from reobstruction, excessive (functional) urethral resistance, or detrusor atony caused by over-distension. If the urinary bladder can be expressed with gentle manual compression of the urinary bladder, detrusor atony is likely. If resistance to manual expression is encountered and urethral obstruction can be ruled out by examination or catheterization, functional obstruction is likely.
• Clinical signs accompanying urine retention in patients with dysautonomia may include mydriasis, prolapsed third eyelids, regurgitation or vomiting, and diarrhea or constipation.

CBC/BIOCHEMISTRY/URINALYSIS
• Results of hemogram and serum biochemical profile may rule in or rule out metabolic causes of muscle weakness; also used to detect severity of postrenal azotemia
• Urinalysis and urine sediment examination may reveal evidence of urinary tract infection or inflammation.

OTHER LABORATORY TESTS
N/A

IMAGING
• Contrast cystourethrography or vagino-urethrography—use to rule out obstructive lesions.
• Myelography, epidurography or computed tomography—use to localize neurologic lesions.

DIAGNOSTIC PROCEDURES
• Neurologic examination—a brief assessment of caudal spinal and peripheral nerve function is provided by examination of anal tone, tail tone, perineal sensation, and bulbospongiosus reflexes.
• Urethral catheterization—may be required to rule out urethral obstruction; catheters should pass easily in animals with no mechanical obstruction and in those with extramural urethral compression (e.g., that caused by a smooth bladder neck mass, a large prostate gland, or a caudal abdominal mass).

• Testing for dysautonomia includes a number of tests of autonomic responses.
• Urodynamic procedures—may use to confirm detrusor atony or functional urethral obstruction or to document detrusor-urethral dyssynergia; detrusor areflexia may be documented by cystometrographic studies; inappropriate urethral resistance or urethral spasm occasionally is documented by resting urethral profilometry; combined cystometry and urethral pressure measurements or uroflow studies are necessary to document dyssynergia.

 TREATMENT

• Usually managed as inpatients until adequate voiding function returns
• Address primary disorders such as electrolyte disturbances and neurologic lesions and correct if possible.
• Manage azotemia, electrolyte imbalances, and acid–base disturbances associated with acute urine retention appropriately.
• Identify urinary tract infection and treat appropriately.
• May consider surgical options for salvaging urethral patency in some patients; perineal urethrostomy may be required in male cats with unmanageable distal urethral resistance.
• Keep the urinary bladder small by intermittent or indwelling catheterization or frequent manual compression; intermittent or indwelling urinary catheterization may be required temporarily to ensure urine flow.

 MEDICATIONS

DRUG(S) OF CHOICE

Detrusor Atony
• Bethanechol (5–25 mg/dog PO q8h; 1.25–5.0 mg/cat q8h)—a cholinergic, parasympathomimetic agent; may increase detrusor contractile input in partially denervated or acutely overdistended urinary bladders
• Metoclopramide—a dopamine antagonist with prokinetic activity in the gastrointestinal tract; may stimulate detrusor contraction as well
• Cisapride—a smooth muscle prokinetic agent; thought to enhance acetylcholine release; may promote bladder emptying; availability limited to veterinary compounding pharmacies

Functional Urethral Obstruction
• Prazosin, 1 mg/15 kg [dogs] or 0.25–0.5 mg/cat PO q12–24h, or phenoxybenzamine,

approximately 0.25 mg/kg PO q12h—α-adrenergic antagonists reduce smooth muscle contraction in the urethra; more effective in dogs than in cats
• Diazepam—a short-acting, central skeletal muscle relaxant; relaxes striated muscle of the external urethral sphincter
• Acepromazine—a phenothiazine tranquilizer; has general muscle relaxant and α-blocking effects on urethral tone; may be effective in cats with excessive urethral resistance
• Dantrolene—another striated muscle relaxant; acts via calcium antagonist properties; appears to be effective in reducing distal urethral resistance in cats
• Baclofen—a spinal reflex inhibitor; acts as a skeletal muscle relaxant; clinical use in small animals has been limited.

CONTRAINDICATIONS

• Baclofen in cats
• Acepromazine, phenoxybenzamine, and prazosin have vasodilatory effects—avoid in volume-depleted or azotemic patients as well as those with cardiac disease.
• Acepromazine and diazepam can cause sedation; avoid in lethargic patients.

PRECAUTIONS

• Ensure an adequate outlet for urine flow before administering bethanechol. Phenoxybenzamine or prazosin is administered concurrently, since bethanechol can increase muscular contraction of the urinary bladder neck and proximal urethra.
• Prazosin may cause potent "first-dose" hypotension; initial dosage should be one half of total dosage.
• Acute hepatopathy—described as a rare complication of oral administration of diazepam in cats

POSSIBLE INTERACTIONS

Concurrent administration of cisapride may enhance the sedative effect of diazepam.

ALTERNATIVE DRUG(S)

N/A

 FOLLOW-UP

PATIENT MONITORING

• As treatment progresses, assess residual urine volume by urinary bladder palpation or by periodic urinary catheterization.
• In most patients, can slowly withdraw medications after primary causes are corrected and adequate voiding function has been sustained for several days
• Perform periodic urinalysis in patients with chronic urine retention to detect urinary tract infection.

• Advise clients that complete voiding function may not return and that pets should be monitored for signs of complete obstruction or uremia.

POSSIBLE COMPLICATIONS

• Lower urinary tract and ascending infection
• Permanent detrusor muscle injury and atony; urinary bladder or urethral rupture
• Postrenal azotemia

 MISCELLANEOUS

ASSOCIATED CONDITIONS

• Urinary tract infection
• Azotemia

AGE-RELATED FACTORS

N/A

ZOONOTIC POTENTIAL

N/A

PREGNANCY

Bethanechol is contraindicated.

SYNONYMS

• Dysfunctional voiding
• Neuropathic bladder
• Reflex dyssynergia, detrusor-urethral dyssynergia
• Urethrospasm

SEE ALSO

• Azotemia and Uremia
• Dysuria and Pollakiuria
• Feline Idiopathic Lower Urinary Tract Disease
• Intervertebral Disk Disease, Thoracolumbar
• Lumbosacral Stenosis
• Prostatitis and Prostatic Abscess
• Urinary Tract Obstruction

Suggested Reading

Barsanti JA. Urinary incontinence. In: Lorenz MD, Cornelius LM, eds. Small animal medical diagnosis. 2nd ed. Philadelphia: Lippincott, 1993:345–356.
Fisher JR, Lane IF, Cribb AE. Medical management of voiding dysfunction. Vet Med 2003;98:67–73.
Lane IF. Diagnosis and management of urinary retention. Vet Clin North Am Small Anim Pract 2000;30:25–57.
Lees GE. Management of voiding disability following relief of urethral obstruction. In: August J, ed. Consultations in feline internal medicine. 2nd ed. Philadelphia: Saunders, 1994:365–372.

Author India F. Lane
Consulting Editors Larry G. Adams and Carl A. Osborne

URINARY TRACT OBSTRUCTION

 BASICS

DEFINITION
Restricted flow of urine from the kidneys through the urinary tract to the external urethral orifice

PATHOPHYSIOLOGY
• Excess resistance to urine flow through the urinary tract develops because of lesions affecting the excretory pathway, which cause increased pressure in the urinary space proximal to the obstruction and may cause abnormal distension of this space with urine. Ensuing pathophysiologic consequences depend on the site, degree, and duration of obstruction. Complete obstruction produces a pathophysiologic state equivalent to oliguric acute renal failure.
• Perforation of the excretory pathway with extravasation of urine is functionally equivalent.

SYSTEMS AFFECTED
• Renal/Urologic
• Gastrointestinal, Cardiovascular, Nervous, and Respiratory systems as uremia develops

SIGNALMENT
• Dogs and cats
• More common in males than females

SIGNS

Historical Findings
• Pollakiuria (common)
• Stranguria
• Reduced velocity or caliber of the urine stream or no urine flow during voiding
• Gross hematuria
• Signs of uremia that develop when urinary tract obstruction is complete (or nearly complete): lethargy, dull attitude, reduced appetite, and vomiting

Physical Examination Findings
• Excessive (i.e., overly large or turgid) or inappropriate (i.e., remains after voiding efforts), palpable distension of the urinary bladder
• Uroliths are often palpable in the urethras of obstructed male dogs.
• Occasionally, palpable renomegaly is discovered in an animal with chronic partial ureteral obstruction, especially when the lesion is unilateral.
• Signs of severe uremia—dehydration, weakness, hypothermia, bradycardia with moderate hyperkalemia, high rate of shallow respirations, stupor or coma, seizures occurring terminally, tachycardia resulting from ventricular dysrhythmias induced by severe hyperkalemia
• Signs of perforation of the excretory pathway—leakage of urine into the peritoneal cavity causes abdominal pain and distension; leakage of urine into periurethral spaces causes pain and swelling in intrapelvic or perineal tissues, depending on the site of the urethral injury; fever

CAUSES

Intraluminal Causes
• Solid or semisolid structures including uroliths, urethral plugs in cats, blood clots, and sloughed tissue fragments
• Most common site—the urethra
• Urolithiasis—most common cause in male dogs
• Urethral plugs—most common cause in male cats

Intramural Causes
• Neoplasia of the bladder neck or urethra—common cause in dogs
• Pyogranulomatous inflammatory lesions in the urethra—seen occasionally in dogs
• Fibrosis at a site of prior injury or inflammation can cause stricture or stenosis, which may impede urine flow or may be a site where intraluminal debris becomes lodged.
• Prostatic disorders in male dogs
• Edema, hemorrhage, or spasm of muscular components can occur at sites of intraluminal (e.g., urethral) obstruction and contribute to persistent or recurrent obstruction to urinary flow after removal of the intraluminal material. Tissue changes might develop because of injury inflicted by the obstructing material, by the manipulations used to remove the obstructing material, or both.
• Ruptures, lacerations, and punctures—usually caused by traumatic incidents

Miscellaneous Causes
• Displacement of the urinary bladder into a perineal hernia
• Neurogenic (see Urinary Retention, Functional)

RISK FACTORS
• Urolithiasis, particularly in males
• Feline lower urinary tract disease, particularly in males
• Prostatic disease in male dogs

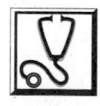 DIAGNOSIS

DIFFERENTIAL DIAGNOSIS
• Repeated unproductive squatting in the litter box by a cat that has a urethral obstruction can be misinterpreted as constipation.
• Animals whose efforts to urinate are not observed by their owners can be examined because of signs referable to uremia without a history of possible obstruction.
• Evaluation of any patient with azotemia should include consideration of possible postrenal causes (e.g., urinary obstruction).

See chapter on Azotemia and Uremia for differential diagnosis of this problem.
• Patients with a ruptured urinary bladder can exhibit clinical signs (e.g., anorexia, vomiting, diarrhea, depression, lethargy, weakness, and collapse) and laboratory test results (azotemia, hyperkalemia and hyponatremia) similar to those commonly seen in patients with hypoadrenocorticism (Addison's disease).
• Once existence of urinary obstruction is recognized, diagnostic efforts focus on detecting the presence and evaluating the magnitude of abnormalities secondary to obstruction, and identifying the location, cause, and completeness of the impediment(s) to urine flow.

CBC/BIOCHEMISTRY/URINALYSIS
• Results of a hemogram are usually normal, but a stress leukogram may be seen.
• Biochemistry analysis reveals azotemia, hyperphosphatemia, metabolic acidosis, hyperkalemia, and decreased ionized calcium proportional to the duration of complete obstruction.
• Hematuria and proteinuria are common; crystalluria supports a diagnosis of urolithiasis, and atypical epithelial cells may be seen in patients with neoplasia.

OTHER LABORATORY TESTS
Uroliths passed or retrieved should be sent for crystallographic analysis to determine their composition.

IMAGING

Abdominal Radiography
• Uroliths—often demonstrated by survey radiography; some are difficult or impossible to see because of their size, composition, or location.
• Positive-contrast urethrography is the most sensitive method of detecting intraluminal and intramural lesions of the urethra; double-contrast cystography is the most sensitive method of detecting lesions of the bladder lumen and wall.
• Upper urinary tract (i.e., ureter or renal pelvis) obstruction can be detected by excretory urography if enough renal function is preserved on the affected side(s) so that radiographic contrast media is excreted and sufficiently concentrated to be seen proximal to the obstruction.

Abdominal Ultrasonography
Ultrasonography is highly sensitive for detecting lesions of the bladder and proximal urethra (including the prostate gland in male dogs) and upper urinary tract (i.e., ureter or renal pelvis) obstruction.

DIAGNOSTIC PROCEDURES
• Electrocardiography may detect abnormalities secondary to hyperkalemia, including tall T waves, prolonged PR interval, bradycardia, and atrial standstill.

URINARY TRACT OBSTRUCTION

• Urinary catheterization has diagnostic and therapeutic value. As the catheter is inserted, the location and nature of obstructing material may be determined. Some or all of the obstructing material (e.g., small uroliths and feline urethral plugs) may be induced to pass out of the urethra distally for identification and analysis. Retrograde irrigation of the urethral lumen may propel intraluminal debris toward the bladder. Although intramural lesions sometimes are detected during catheterization, catheter insertion can be normal. Animals that cannot urinate despite generating adequate intravesicular pressure (i.e., excessive outlet resistance) and have urethras that can be readily catheterized and irrigated either have intramural lesions or functional urinary retention.

• Cytologic evaluation of specimens obtained from the urinary tract with the assistance of catheters may be diagnostic, particularly for carcinoma of the urethra or bladder and some prostatic diseases. Prostatic massage or physical manipulation of the catheter tip positioned near the suspected lesion is used to produce cell-rich specimens that are retrieved through the catheter by aspiration or washing with saline in an attached syringe.

• Cystoscopy can be helpful, particularly in female dogs with intramural lesions of the bladder neck or urethra.

TREATMENT

APPROPRIATE HEALTH CARE

• Complete obstruction is a medical emergency that can be life-threatening; treatment should usually be started immediately.

• Partial obstruction—not necessarily an emergency, but these patients may be at risk for developing complete obstruction; may cause irreversible urinary tract damage if not treated promptly

• Treat as an inpatient until the patient's ability to urinate has been restored.

• Surgery is sometimes required.

• Long-term management and prognosis depend on the cause of the obstruction.

• Treatment has three major components: combating the metabolic derangements associated with postrenal uremia (e.g., dehydration, hypothermia, acidosis, hyperkalemia, and azotemia); restoring and maintaining a patent pathway for urine outflow; and implementing specific treatment for the underlying cause of urine retention.

• Urinary diversion by tube cystostomy is useful in selected cases.

NURSING CARE

Give fluid therapy to patients with dehydration or azotemia. Give fluids intravenously if systemic derangements are moderately severe or worse. Lactated Ringer's solution is the fluid of choice, except for patients with severe hyperkalemia (i.e., >8.0 mEq/L and/or ECG changes), in which the fluid of choice is 0.45% saline and 2.5% dextrose solution with addition of sodium bicarbonate (1–2 mEq/kg slow bolus). Normal saline with added dextrose (2.5% IV) is an alternative fluid choice for patients with dehydration and hyperkalemia. Combat cardiotoxic effects of hyperkalemia that are immediately life-threatening by giving calcium gluconate (2–10 mL 10% solution IV slowly to effect). As soon as hyperkalemia and its effects have abated, use lactated Ringer's solution.

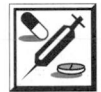

MEDICATIONS

DRUG(S)

Procedures for relief of obstruction often require, or are facilitated by, giving sedatives or anesthetics. When substantial systemic derangements exist, start fluid administration and other supportive measures first. Careful decompression of the bladder by cystocentesis may be performed before anesthesia and catheterization. Calculate the dosage of sedative or anesthetic drug using the low end of the recommended range or give only to effect. Isoflurane is the anesthetic of choice; however, certainly a variety of other anesthetics or sedatives can give satisfactory results.

CONTRAINDICATIONS

Avoid intramuscular ketamine in patients with complete obstruction, because it is excreted through the kidneys. If the obstruction cannot be eliminated, prolonged sedation may result.

PRECAUTIONS

Avoid drugs that reduce blood pressure or induce cardiac dysrhythmia until dehydration and hyperkalemia are resolved.

FOLLOW-UP

PATIENT MONITORING

• Assess urine production and hydration status frequently, and adjust fluid administration rate accordingly.

• Verify ability to urinate adequately or use urinary catheterization to combat urine retention.

• Indwelling catheterization with closed drainage is appropriate if catheter insertion requires chemical restraint or is unduly traumatic, but frequent brief catheterization is a better choice if catheter can readily be inserted repeatedly (i.e., as in some male dogs).

• When the ECG indicates life-threatening changes, use continuous monitoring initially to guide treatment and evaluate response.

POSSIBLE COMPLICATIONS

• Death

• Injury to the excretory pathway while trying to relieve obstruction

• Hypokalemia during postobstruction diuresis

• Recurrence of obstruction

MISCELLANEOUS

ASSOCIATED CONDITIONS

• Bradycardia secondary to hyperkalemia

• Azotemia, hyperphosphatemia, and metabolic acidosis

AGE-RELATED FACTORS

In old dogs, the underlying cause of obstruction (e.g., tumor and prostate disease) often is difficult to treat effectively.

PREGNANCY

N/A

SYNONYM

Urethral obstruction

SEE ALSO

• Azotemia and Uremia

• Feline Idiopathic Lower Urinary Tract Disease

• Hydronephrosis

• Hyperkalemia

• Urinary Retention, Functional

Suggested Reading

Labato MA. Urologic emergencies. In: Murtaugh RJ, Kaplan PM, eds. Veterinary emergency and critical care medicine. St. Louis: Mosby-Year Book, 1992:295–320.

Lane IF. Urinary obstruction and functional urine retention. In: Ettinger SJ, Feldman EC, eds. Textbook of veterinary internal medicine. 5th ed. Philadelphia: Saunders, 2000:93–96.

Osborne CA, Kruger JM, Lulich JP, et al. Feline lower urinary tract diseases. In: Ettinger SJ, Feldman EC, eds. Textbook of veterinary internal medicine. 5th ed. Philadelphia: Saunders, 2000:1733–1739.

Stone EA, Barsanti JA. Urologic surgery of the dog and cat. Philadelphia: Lea & Febiger, 1992.

Waldrow DR. Urine diversion by tube cystostomy. In: Bonagura JD, ed. Kirk's current veterinary therapy XIII. 13th ed. Philadelphia: Saunders, 2000:870–871.

Author George E. Lees

Consulting Editors Larry G. Adams and Carl A. Osborne

UROLITHIASIS, CALCIUM OXALATE

 BASICS

DEFINITION
Formation of calcium oxalate uroliths within the urinary tract and associated clinical conditions

PATHOPHYSIOLOGY
Presence of hypercalciuria, hyperoxaluria, hypocitraturia, and defective crystal growth inhibitors

Hypercalciuria
In dogs, normocalcemic hypercalciuria is thought to result from either intestinal hyper-absorption of calcium (so-called absorptive hypercalciuria) or reduced renal tubular reabsorption of calcium (so-called renal-leak hypercalciuria). Hypercalcemic hypercalciuria results from excessive glomerular filtration of mobilized calcium, which overwhelms normal renal tubular reabsorptive mechanisms (called resorptive hypercalciuria, since excessive bone resorption is associated with high serum calcium concentrations).

Hyperoxaluria
In humans, hyperoxaluria is associated with inherited abnormalities of excessive oxalate synthesis (i.e., primary hyperoxaluria), excess consumption of foods containing high quantities of oxalate or oxalate precursors, pyridoxine deficiency, and disorders associated with fat malabsorption.

Hypocitraturia
Urine citrate inhibits calcium oxalate urolith formation. By complexing with calcium ions to form the relatively soluble salt calcium citrate, citrate reduces the quantity of calcium available to bind with oxalate. In normal dogs, acidosis is associated with low urinary citrate excretion, whereas alkalosis promotes urinary citrate excretion.

Defective Crystal Growth Inhibitors
In addition to urinary concentration of calculogenic minerals, large-molecular-weight proteins in urine, such as nephrocalcin, have a profound ability to enhance solubility of calcium oxalate. Preliminary studies of urine obtained from dogs with calcium oxalate uroliths revealed that nephrocalcin had fewer carboxyglutamic acid residues than nephrocalcin isolated from normal dog urine.

Feeding Diets Promoting Urine Acidification
Epidemiologic studies report this is a consistent risk factor in cats. In several species, acid urine is associated with hypercalciuria (bone mobilization, increased calcium filtration, decreased renal tubular reabsorption) and hypocitraturia (increased renal tubular reabsorption).

SYSTEMS AFFECTED
Renal/urologic

INCIDENCE/PREVALENCE
In dogs, calcium oxalate accounts for approximately 30–35% of the uroliths removed from the lower urinary tract and 40% of those removed from the upper urinary tract. In cats, calcium oxalate accounts for approximately 50–55% of the uroliths removed from the lower urinary tract and 50% of those retrieved from the upper urinary tract.

GEOGRAPHIC DISTRIBUTION
Ubiquitous

SIGNALMENT

Species
Dogs and cats

Breed Predilections
• Dogs—reported in many breeds. Six breeds represent 60% of cases: miniature schnauzer, Lhasa apso, Yorkshire terrier, bichon frise, Shih Tzu, and miniature poodle.
• Cats—Himalayan, Scottish fold, Persian, ragdoll, and Burmese are at greater risk.

Mean Age and Ranges
• Dogs—8.5 ± 3 years; 60%, 6–11 years
• Cats—97% > 2 years; 53%, 7–15 years

Predominant Sex
Mostly male dogs (73%) and male cats (55%)

SIGNS

General Comments
• None in some animals
• Depend on location, size, and number of uroliths.
• Animals with nephroliths are typically asymptomatic but may have persistent hematuria.
• Ureteral obstruction associated with contralateral microrenale, ipsilateral hydronephrosis, and acute uremia occur frequently in cats.

Historical Findings
• Typical signs of urocystoliths or urethroliths include pollakiuria, dysuria, and hematuria.
• Nephroureteroliths common in cats with renal failure

Physical Examination Findings
• Detection of urocystoliths by abdominal or urethral palpation; failure to palpate uroliths does not exclude them from consideration.
• A thickened and contracted bladder wall palpable in some patients, especially in cats
• Large urinary bladder if patient has complete urethral obstruction (more common in cats)
• Urocystoliths with irregular contours uncommonly cause complete urethral obstruction.

CAUSES
See Pathophysiology

RISK FACTORS
• Calcium supplements independent of meals
• Excessive dietary protein and vitamin D promote hypercalciuria.
• Additional dietary oxalate (e.g., chocolate and peanuts) and ascorbic acid promote hyperoxaluria.
• Exogenous or endogenous exposure to a high concentration of glucocorticoids, diets that promote formation of acidic urine, and furosemide promote hypercalciuria.
• Pyridoxine (vitamin B_6)-deficient diets (e.g., homemade) promote hyperoxaluria.
• Consumption of dry diets is associated with a higher risk for calcium oxalate urolith formation than consumption of canned diets.

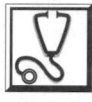 DIAGNOSIS

DIFFERENTIAL DIAGNOSIS
• Other common causes of hematuria, dysuria, and pollakiuria, with or without urethral obstruction, include urinary tract infection and urinary tract neoplasia.
• Other common radiodense uroliths include those composed of magnesium ammonium phosphate, calcium phosphate, and silica (dogs)

CBC/BIOCHEMISTRY/URINALYSIS
• Results usually unremarkable
• Urinary sediment evaluation may reveal calcium oxalate crystals, but absence of crystalluria does not exclude uroliths as a possibility.
• Hypercalcemia or azotemia (rare in dogs, more common in cats)

OTHER LABORATORY TESTS
Quantitative mineral analysis of uroliths retrieved during voiding, by voiding uro-hydropropulsion, by aspiration into a urinary catheter, or by cystoscopy or cystotomy

IMAGING
Calcium oxalate uroliths are radiodense and easily detected by survey radiography; intravenous urography, pyelography, or ultrasonography is required to verify ureteral obstruction.

DIAGNOSTIC PROCEDURES
N/A

PATHOLOGIC FINDINGS
N/A

 TREATMENT

APPROPRIATE HEALTH CARE
• Retrograde urohydropropulsion to flush urethral stones back into the urinary bladder or voiding urohydropropulsion to eliminate small bladder stones can be performed on an

outpatient basis. Voiding urohydropropulsion is contraindicated in patients with urethral obstruction.

• Shock wave lithotripsy and surgery require short periods of hospitalization.

NURSING CARE
N/A

ACTIVITY
Reduce during the period of tissue repair after surgery

DIET
• No reports of dissolution of calcium oxalate uroliths with special diets
• Hypercalcemia in cats without evidence of hyperparathyroidism or malignancy is sometimes minimized by use of Prescription Diet Feline w/d (Hill's).

CLIENT EDUCATION
• Urolith removal does not alter the factors responsible for their formation; eliminating risk factors is necessary to minimize recurrence.
• Approximately 60% of dogs with a normal serum calcium concentration reform uroliths within 3 years.
• Patients with hypercalcemia typically reform uroliths at a faster rate.

SURGICAL CONSIDERATIONS
• Consider surgical removal of uroliths from patients with obstruction or dysuria if they cannot be removed by nonsurgical methods (e.g., voiding urohydropropulsion) or if clinical signs cannot be alleviated by flushing uroliths back into the urinary bladder.
• Shock wave lithotripsy is an alternative to surgery for removal of nephroliths and ureteroliths.
• Consider parathyroidectomy for patients with primary hyperparathyroidism and hypercalcemia.

MEDICATIONS

DRUG(S) OF CHOICE
No available drugs effectively dissolve calcium oxalate uroliths.

CONTRAINDICATIONS
None

PRECAUTIONS
Steroids and furosemide promote calciuria.

POSSIBLE INTERACTIONS
N/A

ALTERNATIVE DRUG(S)
N/A

FOLLOW-UP

PATIENT MONITORING
• Postsurgical radiographs are essential to verify complete urolith removal.
• To prevent repeat surgery, evaluate abdominal radiography every 3–5 months to detect urolith recurrence early. Small uroliths are easily removed by voiding urohydropropulsion or catheter retrieval.

PREVENTION/AVOIDANCE
• If patient is hypercalcemic, correct underlying cause. Consider Prescription Diet w/d for cats with idiopathic hypercalciuria; administer potassium citrate to minimize aciduria.
• If patient is normocalcemic, consider diet with reduced oxalate and protein that does not promote formation of acidic urine (Prescription Diet Canine u/d, Prescription Diet Feline c/d-oxl, Prescription Diet Feline k/d, or Prescription Diet Feline w/d, Hills Pet Products). Ideally, the diet should contain additional water (canned diets) and citrate, and have adequate phosphorus and magnesium. Avoid supplementation with vitamins C and D.
• Reevaluate patient 2–4 weeks after initiation of diet therapy to verify appropriate urine dilution (specific gravity < 1.020 for dogs and < 1.030 for cats), appropriate urine pH ($\geq$6.5), and amelioration of crystalluria. Do not use inappropriately collected or stored urine samples (e.g., urine collected by owners, refrigerated, or contaminated with debris) to monitor therapeutic efficacy. To promote less-concentrated urine consider canned formulations of food or add water to all types of food. If urine is acidic, consider additional potassium citrate (75 mg/kg PO q12h); adjust dosage to achieve a pH between 6.5 and 7.5. Vitamin B$_6$ (2–4 mg/kg PO q24–48h) may help minimize oxalate excretion, especially for animals fed homemade or pyridoxine-deficient diets.

POSSIBLE COMPLICATIONS
• Urocystoliths can pass into and obstruct the urethra in male dogs and cats, especially if the patient is dysuric; managed by retrograde urohydropropulsion
• Dogs that do not consume their daily requirement of the urolith prevention diet can develop various degrees of protein calorie malnutrition.
• Diet-associated hyperlipidemia develops in some patients. Miniature schnauzers with hereditary hyperlipidemia and predisposition to pancreatitis can develop pancreatitis when consuming the prevention diet, in which case Prescription Diet Canine w/d (Hills) can be

used as an alternative. This diet should be supplemented with potassium citrate as needed to maintain a urine pH between 6.5 and 7.5.

EXPECTED COURSE AND PROGNOSIS
• Approximately 60% of dogs with normal serum calcium concentration reform uroliths in 3 years. Treatment to minimize recurrence is helpful. Patients with hypercalcemia typically reform uroliths at a faster rate.
• Comparable data are not available for cats.

MISCELLANEOUS

ASSOCIATED CONDITIONS
Any condition predisposing to hypercalciuria (e.g., hyperadrenocorticism, acidemia, hypervitaminosis D, and hyperparathyroidism) or hyperoxaluria (e.g., vitamin B$_6$ deficiency, hereditary hyperoxaluria, and ingestion of chocolate and peanuts)

AGE-RELATED FACTORS
Rare in young animals

ZOONOTIC POTENTIAL
None

PREGNANCY
Diets used to prevent calcium oxalate uroliths are not appropriate.

SYNONYMS
Oxalate urolithiasis

SEE ALSO
Crystalluria

ABBREVIATIONS
N/A

Suggested Reading

Lulich JP, Osborne CA. Voiding urohydropropulsion: a nonsurgical technique for removal of urocystoliths. In: Bonagura JD, Kirk RW, eds. Current veterinary therapy XII. Philadelphia: Saunders, 1995; 1003–1006.

Lulich JP, Osborne CA, Felice L. Calcium oxalate urolithiasis: cause, detection and control. In: August JR, ed. Consultations in feline internal medicine. Philadelphia: Saunders, 1994;343–349.

Lulich JP, Osborne C, Thumchai R, et al. Management of canine calcium oxalate urolith recurrence. Compend Contin Educ Pract Vet. 1998;20:178–189.

McClain HM, Barsanti JA, Bartges JW. Hypercalcemia and calcium oxalate urolithiasis in cats: a report of five cases. J Am Anim Hosp Assoc 1999;35:297–301.

Authors Jody P. Lulich and Carl A. Osborne
Consulting Editors Larry G. Adams and Carl A. Osborne

UROLITHIASIS, CALCIUM PHOSPHATE

 BASICS

OVERVIEW
- Formation of calcium phosphate uroliths within the urinary tract and the associated clinical condition
- Calcium phosphate uroliths represent 1–2 % of uroliths from dogs and cats submitted to laboratories for analysis
- Calcium phosphate uroliths—commonly called apatite uroliths
- Hydroxyapatite and carbonate apatite are the most common forms; brushite (calcium hydrogen phosphate dihydrate) and whitiockite (tricalcium phosphate) are less common.
- A greater percentage of calcium phosphate uroliths are found in the kidneys than in the urinary bladder.

SIGNALMENT
- Dogs and cats
- Rarely detected in animals less than 1 year old
- No other distinguishing trends for breed, age, and gender in dogs or cats

SIGNS
- Depend on location, size, and number of uroliths
- None in some patients
- Typically, pollakiuria, dysuria, hematuria, and urethral obstruction
- Animals with nephroureteroliths—typically asymptomatic but may have persistent hematuria or signs referable to concomitant renal failure (primarily cats)

CAUSES & RISK FACTORS
- Calcium phosphate—commonly a minor component of struvite and calcium oxalate uroliths
- Pure calcium phosphate uroliths—usually associated with metabolic disorders such as primary hyperparathyroidism, renal tubular acidosis, and excessive dietary calcium and phosphorus
- Nephroliths, urocystoliths, and urethroliths composed of blood clots mineralized with calcium phosphate suggest dystrophic mineralization of tissue, in contrast to metastatic mineralization reflecting abnormal calcium and phosphorus metabolism.
- Other risk factors include concentrated urine, vitamin D supplements, hypercalciuria, mineral supplements, and alkaline urine (hydroxyapatite and carbonate apatite).

 DIAGNOSIS

DIFFERENTIAL DIAGNOSIS
- Other common causes of hematuria, dysuria, and pollakiuria, with or without urethral obstruction, include urinary tract infection and urinary tract neoplasia.
- Magnesium ammonium phosphate, calcium oxalate, cystine, and silica are other radiodense uroliths.
- Metastatic or dystrophic mineralization of urinary tract parenchyma may resemble uroliths.

CBC/BIOCHEMISTRY/URINALYSIS
- Usually unremarkable
- Hypercalcemia or azotemia rarely detected; postrenal azotemia in some animals with complete obstruction
- Urinary sediment analysis reveals amorphous crystals in some patients; brushite (calcium hydrogen phosphate dihydrate) forms are elongated, rectangular, lath-shaped crystals.

OTHER LABORATORY TESTS
- Quantitative analysis of retrieved uroliths necessary to confirm their mineral composition
- Serum concentrations of parathyroid hormone, parathyroid hormone–related peptide, and hydroxycholecalciferol may help establish underlying causes.

IMAGING
- Uroliths are radiodense, often detected by survey radiography
- Calcium phosphate uroliths may be detected by ultrasonography.

OTHER DIAGNOSTIC PROCEDURES
Calcium phosphate uroliths in the urethra and bladder may be detected by cystoscopy.

 TREATMENT

- Medical dissolution of calcium phosphate uroliths remains a goal for the future.
- Consider surgery for removal of clinically active uroliths
- Nonsurgical methods of removing uroliths from the lower urinary tract include voiding urohydropropulsion, aspiration into a urinary catheter, and lithotripsy.
- Correction of hyperparathyroidism or other causes of hypercalcemia should minimize further urolith formation.

 MEDICATIONS

DRUG(S)
No effective medications available for dissolving calcium phosphate uroliths

CONTRAINDICATIONS/POSSIBLE INTERACTIONS
N/A

 FOLLOW-UP

PATIENT MONITORING
- Radiography after surgery to verify complete urolith removal—essential
- Abdominal radiography or ultrasonography every 3–4 months to enhance early detection of urolith recurrence and prevent the need for repeat surgery
- Small uroliths are easily removed by voiding urohydropropulsion or catheter retrieval.

PREVENTION/AVOIDANCE
- A diet formulated to prevent formation of calcium oxalate uroliths may help prevent recurrence.
- Prescription Diet Canine U/D (Hill's Pet Nutrition) is formulated to reduce calcium excretion, is phosphorus-restricted, and reduces formation of concentrated urine.
- Because of the high moisture content of canned foods and their tendency to promote dilute urine, canned diets are more effective than dry diets in preventing recurrence.
- Avoid excessive acidification or alkalinization of urine.

 MISCELLANEOUS

SYNONYMS
Apatite uroliths

Suggested Reading

Kruger JM, Osborne CA, Lulich JP. Canine calcium oxalate uroliths: etiopathogenesis, diagnosis, management. Vet Clin North Am Small Anim Pract 1999;29:141–159.

Lulich JP, Osborne CA, Bartges JW, et al. Canine lower urinary tract disorders. In: Ettinger S, Feldman EC, eds. Textbook of veterinary internal medicine. Philadelphia: Saunders, 2000;1747–1781.

Authors Jody P. Lulich and Carl A. Osborne
Consulting Editors Larry G. Adams and Carl A. Osborne

BASICS

OVERVIEW
• Formation of polycrystalline concretions (i.e., uroliths, calculi, or stones) composed of organic cystine in the urinary tract • Occurs in dogs and cats with cystinuria, an inborn error of metabolism characterized by abnormal transport of cystine and other amino acids (including ornithine, lysine, and arginine) by the renal tubules • Cystine—normally present in low concentrations in plasma; is freely filtered at the glomerulus, and most is actively reabsorbed in the proximal tubules; much less is reabsorbed from the glomerular filtrate by cystinuric dogs than by normal dogs, and some may even have net cystine secretion.
• Cystine—relatively insoluble in acid urine; becomes more soluble in alkaline urine
• Unless protein intake is severely restricted, cystinuric dogs have no detectable abnormalities associated with amino acid loss, with the exception of formation of cystine uroliths. Excessive loss of arginine in urine predisposes cats to hyperammonemic encephalopathy. Some cystinuric dogs may have carnitinuria. The exact mechanism of cystine urolith formation is unknown. Because not all cystinuric dogs form uroliths, cystinuria is a predisposing, rather than a primary, cause of cystine urolith formation. • The precise mode of inheritance of canine cystinuria is unknown. In past years, this genetic disorder considered gender-linked in all affected breeds. However, cystinuria in Newfoundlands was recently reported to have a simple autosomal recessive pattern of transmission. In Newfoundlands, parents of cystinuric dogs are either cystinuric or carriers, although littermates may be cystinuric, cystinuric carriers, or normal.

SIGNALMENT
• Dogs and cats • Canine cystinuria primarily affects adult (mean age at diagnosis, 5 years; range, 3 months to 14 years) males but may also affect females. It occurs in many breeds, especially dachshund, English bulldog, Newfoundland, Staffordshire bull terrier, and Welsh corgi dogs. Cystine uroliths may be detected in Newfoundlands less than 1 year old. • Feline cystinuria primarily affects adult (mean age at diagnosis, 3.5 years; range, 4 months to 12 years) males and females; most commonly recognized in the domestic shorthair and Siamese breeds

SIGNS
• Depend on location, size, and number of uroliths; affected animals may be asymptomatic • Typical signs of urocystoliths include pollakiuria, dysuria, and hematuria. • Typical signs of urethroliths include pollakiuria, dysuria, and sometimes voiding of small smooth uroliths. Complete outflow obstruction may result in postrenal uremia. • Nephroliths are typically asymptomatic but may be associated

with manifestations of hydronephrosis and renal insufficiency.

CAUSES & RISK FACTORS
Cystinuria is a risk factor.

Breed Predisposition
• In young and middle-aged dogs with previous history of cystine urolithiasis—recurrence within 6–12 months following surgery unless prophylactic therapy is given • Urolith formation—enhanced by acidic urine, highly concentrated urine, incomplete and infrequent micturition

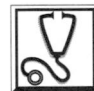

DIAGNOSIS

DIFFERENTIAL DIAGNOSIS
• Uroliths mimic other causes of pollakiuria, dysuria, hematuria, and/or outflow obstruction. • Differentiate from other types of uroliths, especially ammonium urate in English bulldogs, by urinalysis, radiography, and quantitative analysis of voided or retrieved uroliths.

CBC/BIOCHEMISTRY/URINALYSIS
• Cystine crystals are six-sided and are insoluble in acetic acid. • Positive urine cyanide-nitroprusside test

OTHER LABORATORY TESTS
• Urinary amino acid profiles—reveal abnormal quantities of cystine and, in some dogs and cats, lysine, arginine, ornithine, and other amino acids • Quantitative mineral analysis of uroliths, and other amino acids retrieved during voiding, by voiding urohydropropulsion, or by aspiration into a urinary catheter

IMAGING
• Radiography—the radiodensity of cystine uroliths compared with soft tissue is similar to that of struvite and silica, less than that of calcium oxalate and calcium phosphate, and greater than that of ammonium urate; when large enough, cystine uroliths can be detected by survey radiography. • Ultrasonography—can detect cystine uroliths, but does not provide information about the radiodensity or their shape

DIAGNOSTIC PROCEDURES
Urethrocystoscopy may detect cystine urethroliths and urocystoliths.

TREATMENT
• Medical dissolution of uroliths by a combination of N-(2-mercaptopropionyl)-glycine (2-MPG) and dietary therapy; Hill's Prescription Diet Canine u/d reduces urinary excretion of cystine, promotes formation of alkaline urine, and reduces urine concentration; it is used in conjunction with 2-MPG for urolith dissolution and is often effective alone in preventing recurrence of cystine uroliths.
• Remove small urocystoliths by voiding urohydropropulsion or surgery.

MEDICATIONS

DRUG(S)

Urine Alkalinizers
• Consider for patients that have acidic urine despite dietary therapy and control of urease-positive urinary tract infections. • Data derived from studies in cystinuric humans suggest that dietary sodium may enhance cystinuria; thus potassium citrate may be preferable to sodium bicarbonate as a urine alkalinizer. Give enough potassium citrate (40–75 mg/kg q12h) to maintain a urine pH of 7.5.

Thiol-containing Drugs
• 2-MPG decreases the urine concentration of cystine by combining with cysteine to form cysteine-2-MPG, which is more soluble than cystine. • 2-MPG (Thiola-Mission Pharmacal) may be given at a dosage of 15–20 mg/kg q12h to dissolve canine cystine uroliths in conjunction with dietary therapy. In our hospital, mean dissolution time was 78 days (range, 11–211 days). • 2-MPG may be given at a lower dosage (5–10 mg/kg PO q12h) to prevent recurrent canine cystine uroliths, if dietary therapy is not optimal. • Drug-induced adverse events associated with 2-MGP are uncommon in dogs; they include reversible Coombs-positive spherocytic anemia, thrombocytopenia, glomerular proteinuria, myopathy, aggressiveness, and increased hepatic enzyme activity. • The efficacy and safety of 2-MPG has not been evaluated in cystinuric cats.

FOLLOW-UP
• Prevention of recurrence with dietary management or 2-MPG • Monitor urolith dissolution at 30-day intervals by urinalysis and survey or contrast radiography or ultrasonography. • Although cystine uroliths tend to recur, recurrence does not happen in all cystinuric dogs and cats. • In some older dogs, the rate of recurrence declines as a consequence of a reduction in the magnitude of cystinuria.

MISCELLANEOUS

ABBREVIATION
2-MPG = N-(2-mercaptopropionyl)-glycine

Suggested Reading
Osborne CA, Sanderson SL, Lulich JP, et al. Canine cystine urolithiasis. Vet Clin North Am 1999;29:193–211.
Authors Carl A. Osborne, Jody P. Lulich, and Lisa Ulrich
Consulting Editors Larry G. Adams and Carl A. Osborne

UROLITHIASIS, STRUVITE—CATS

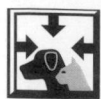 **BASICS**

DEFINITION
Struvite uroliths and struvite urethral plugs have physical and etiopathogenic differences; thus, these terms should not be used as synonyms. Struvite uroliths are polycrystalline concretions composed primarily of magnesium ammonium phosphate and small quantities of matrix. Struvite feline urethral plugs commonly are composed of large quantities of matrix mixed with magnesium ammonium phosphate. Some urethral plugs are composed primarily of organic matrix, sloughed tissue, blood, and/or inflammatory reactants.

PATHOPHYSIOLOGY
• See Urolithiasis, Struvite—Dogs.
• The most commonly encountered form of naturally occurring feline urethral plugs contains relatively large quantities of matrix in addition to minerals, especially struvite. Risk factors associated with formation of MAP crystals contained in urethral plugs are similar to those associated with formation of struvite uroliths. Prevention or control of these risk factors should minimize the recurrence of the struvite component of urethral plugs. Specific causes and composition of urethral plug matrix have not yet been classified. One hypothesis is that plug matrix follows urinary tract infections, especially by viruses.

SYSTEMS AFFECTED
Renal/Urologic—upper and lower urinary tract

INCIDENCE/PREVALENCE
• The prevalence of feline struvite uroliths has been declining during the past decade in association with special diets designed to dissolve and prevent this type of stone.
• Currently, struvite makes up less than 40% of uroliths in the feline lower urinary tract. Of these, 95% are sterile.
• Struvite has been detected in approximately 8% of feline nephroliths.
• Struvite remains the most common (80%) mineral in matrix-crystalline urethral plugs.

SIGNALMENT
Species
Cats (see Urolithiasis, Struvite—Dogs)

Breed Predilection
None

Mean Age and Range
• Mean age at time of diagnosis is 7 years (range, < 1 to 22 years).
• Sterile struvite uroliths do not affect immature cats; infection-induced struvite may occur in immature cats.

Predominant Sex
• Struvite uroliths are more common in females (55%) than in males (45%).
• Struvite urethral plugs primarily affect males.

SIGNS
General Comments
• Affected cats may be asymptomatic.
• Depend on location, size, and number of uroliths

Historical Findings
• Typical signs of urocystoliths include pollakiuria, dysuria, and hematuria.
• Typical signs of urethroliths include pollakiuria, dysuria, and sometimes voiding of small, smooth uroliths; signs of postrenal uremia (e.g., anorexia and vomiting) are found in some cats with outflow obstruction.
• Manifestations of renal insufficiency (polyuria and polydipsia) are found in some cats with nephroliths.
• Signs typical of outflow obstruction (e.g., dysuria, large painful urinary bladder, and signs of postrenal uremia) are found in cats with struvite urethral plugs.

Physical Examination Findings
• A thickened, firm, contracted bladder wall is found in some cats with urocystoliths.
• Detection of urocystoliths by palpation is unreliable.
• Urethral plugs or uroliths may be detected by examination of the distal penis and penile urethra.
• Outflow obstruction results in an enlarged urinary bladder and signs of postrenal uremia.

CAUSES
See Pathophysiology.

RISK FACTORS
• For formation of sterile struvite uroliths—include mineral composition, energy content, and moisture content of diets; urine-alkalinizing metabolites in diets; quantity of diet consumed; ad libitum versus meal-feeding schedules; formation of concentrated urine; and retention of urine
• Elimination or control may result in dissolution of sterile struvite uroliths and prevention of their recurrence.
• Probable for infection-induced struvite urolithiasis—include urinary tract infection with urease-producing microbial pathogens, abnormalities in local host defenses that allow bacterial urinary tract infections (including perineal urethrostomies), and the quantity of urea (the substrate of urease) excreted in urine
• The normal small diameter of the distal urethra of male cats predisposes them to obstruction with plugs and uroliths.

 DIAGNOSIS

DIFFERENTIAL DIAGNOSIS
• Uroliths mimic other causes of pollakiuria, dysuria, hematuria, and/or outflow obstruction.
• Differentiate struvite uroliths and urethral plugs from other types of uroliths by signalment, urinalysis, urine culture, radiography, ultrasonography, cystoscopy, and quantitative analysis of voided or retrieved uroliths or plugs.

CBC/BIOCHEMISTRY/URINALYSIS
• Complete outflow obstruction may cause postrenal azotemia (e.g., high BUN, creatinine, and phosphorus).
• Magnesium ammonium phosphate crystals typically appear as colorless, orthorhombic (having three unequal axes intersecting at right angles), coffin-like prisms. They often have three to eight sides.

OTHER LABORATORY TESTS
• Pretreatment quantitative bacterial urine cultures (preferably with specimen obtained by cystocentesis) yield bacterial urinary tract infections in only 1–3% of affected patients.
• Quantitative mineral analysis is the accepted standard of practice for uroliths and urethral plugs retrieved during voiding, by voiding urohydropropulsion, by aspiration into a urinary catheter, or by cystoscopy.
• Bacterial culture of inner portions of infection-induced struvite uroliths may be of value.

IMAGING
Radiography
• Struvite uroliths—radiodense; may be detected by survey radiography; some struvite urethral plugs may be detected by survey radiography.
• The size and number of uroliths are not a reliable index of probable efficacy of dissolution therapy.
• Contrast urethrocystography helps identify the site(s) of urethral obstruction and urethral strictures.

Ultrasonography
• Detects location, size, and number of uroliths, but does not indicate degree of radiodensity or shape of uroliths
• Determines precise location, size, and number of uroliths

DIAGNOSTIC PROCEDURES
Cystoscopy reveals location, number, size, and shape of urethroliths and urocystoliths.

PATHOLOGIC FINDINGS
Urethral plugs may contain red blood cells, white cells, transitional epithelial cells, bacteria, and/or viruses in addition to matrix and minerals.

TREATMENT

APPROPRIATE HEALTH CARE
• Retrograde urohydropropulsion to eliminate urethral stones, lavage to remove urethral plugs, voiding urohydropropulsion to eliminate bladder and urethral stones, and/or surgery require short periods of hospitalization.
• Medical dissolution of struvite uroliths is an outpatient strategy.

NURSING CARE
N/A

ACTIVITY
If dietary management is used, monitor outdoor activity.

DIET
• Sterile and infection-induced struvite urocystoliths and nephroliths may be dissolved by feeding a calculolytic diet (Prescription Diet Feline s/d; Hill's Pet Nutrition).
• Continue diet therapy for 1 month after survey radiographic evidence of urolith dissolution.
• Struvite crystalluria may be minimized by feeding magnesium-restricted urine-acidifying diets.
• Canned (moist) foods help to reduce urine concentration of calculogenic metabolites and promote increased frequency of normal voiding.

CLIENT EDUCATION
• If dietary management is used, limit access to other foods and treats.
• Short-term (weeks to months) treatment with a calculolytic diet (Hill's Feline s/d) ± antibiotics as needed is effective in dissolving struvite uroliths. Avoid feeding calculolytic diets to immature cats.
• Owners of cats with infection-induced struvite urocystoliths must comply with dosage schedule for antibiotic therapy.

SURGICAL CONSIDERATIONS
• Ureteroliths cannot be dissolved. Consider surgery for persistent ureteroliths associated with morbidity.
• Urethroliths cannot be medically dissolved. Consider voiding urohydropropulsion to remove urethroliths or urethral plugs. Alternatively, move urethroliths into the bladder by retrograde urohydropropulsion.
• Immovable urethroliths, recurrent urethral plugs, or strictures of the distal urethra may require perineal urethrostomy.
• Nephroliths causing outflow obstruction, or associated with nonfunctioning kidneys cannot be dissolved medically.
• Consider surgical correction if uroliths are obstructing urine outflow, and/or if correctable abnormalities predisposing to recurrent

urinary tract infection are identified by radiography or other means.
• Uroliths and urethral plugs should be localized before considering surgical correction.
• Radiographs should be obtained immediately following surgery to verify that all uroliths were removed.

MEDICATIONS

DRUG(S)
Dietary dissolution of infection-induced urocystoliths or nephroliths requires oral administration of appropriate antibiotics, chosen on the basis of bacterial culture and antimicrobial susceptibility tests. Give antibiotics at therapeutic dosages until the urinary tract infection is eradicated and no radiographic evidence of uroliths exists.

CONTRAINDICATIONS
Do not give urine acidifiers to azotemic patients or immature cats.

PRECAUTIONS
Azotemic patients are at increased risk for adverse drug events.

FOLLOW-UP

PATIENT MONITORING
Check rate of urolith dissolution at monthly intervals by urinalysis, urine culture, survey or contrast radiography, or ultrasonography.

PREVENTION/AVOIDANCE
• Recurrent sterile struvite uroliths may be prevented by using acidifying, magnesium-restricted diets or urine acidifiers. Do not administer urine acidifiers with acidifying diets.
• Monitor patients whose urine has been acidified for calcium oxalate crystalluria. Change management protocol if persistent calcium oxalate crystalluria develops.
• In patients at risk for both struvite and calcium oxalate crystalluria, focus on preventing calcium oxalate uroliths. Struvite uroliths can be medically dissolved; recurrent calcium oxalate uroliths cannot be dissolved.
• Infection-induced struvite urolithiasis can be prevented by eradicating and controlling urinary tract infections. Use of magnesium-restricted, acidifying diets is an ancillary method of prevention.

POSSIBLE COMPLICATIONS
• Urocystoliths may pass into and obstruct the urethra of male cats, especially if the patient is persistently dysuric. Urethral obstruction may be managed by retrograde urohydropropulsion.

• Dysuria may be minimized by treatment of bacterial urinary tract infection, and by administration of an anticholinergic drug (e.g., propantheline bromide, 7.5 mg PO q3days).
• An indwelling transurethral catheter increases the risk for iatrogenic bacterial urinary tract infection and/or urethral stricture.

EXPECTED COURSE AND PROGNOSIS
In our hospital, the mean time for dissolution of feline sterile urocystoliths was 1 month (range, 2 weeks to 5 months). The mean time for dissolution of infection-induced struvite urocystoliths was 10 weeks (range, 9–12 weeks).

MISCELLANEOUS

ASSOCIATED CONDITIONS
Any disease that predisposes to bacterial urinary tract infection

AGE-RELATED FACTORS
Infection-induced struvite is the most common urolith in immature cats. Sterile struvite is rare in immature cats.

SYNONYMS
FUS • Feline urologic disease • Feline lower urinary tract disease

SEE ALSO
• Lower Urinary Tract Infection
• Nephrolithiasis
• Urolithiasis, Struvite—Dogs

ABBREVIATION
MAP = magnesium ammonium phosphate

Suggested Reading
Osborne CA, Lulich JP, Kruger JM, et al. Feline urethral plugs: etiology and pathophysiology. Vet Clin North Am 1996; 26:233–254

Osborne CA, Lulich JP, Thumchai R, et al. Feline urolithiasis: etiology and pathophysiology. Vet Clin North Am 1996; 26:217–232.

Osborne CA, Lulich JP, Thumchai R, et al. Diagnosis, medical treatment, and prognosis of feline urolithiasis. Vet Clin North Am 1996;26:589–628.

Osborne CA, Kruger JM, Lulich JP, et al. Feline lower urinary tract diseases. In: Ettinger SJ, Feldman EC, eds. Textbook of veterinary internal medicine. 5th ed. Philadelphia: Saunders, 1999; 1710–1747

Authors Carl A. Osborne, John M. Kruger, and Jody P. Lulich
Consulting Editors Larry G. Adams and Carl A. Osborne

UROLITHIASIS, STRUVITE—DOGS

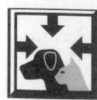

BASICS

DEFINITION
Formation of polycrystalline concretions (i.e., uroliths, calculi, or stones) composed of MAP, or struvite, in the urinary tract.

PATHOPHYSIOLOGY

Infection-induced Struvite
• Urine must be supersaturated with MAP for struvite uroliths to form. MAP supersaturation of urine may be associated with several factors, including urinary tract infections with urease-producing microbes, alkaline urine, genetic predisposition, and diet. • If animals are affected by urinary tract infections caused by urease-producing microbes (especially species of *Staphylococcus, Proteus,* and *Ureaplasma*) and their urine contains sufficient urea, the result is a unique combination of concomitant elevations in the concentrations of ammonium (NH_4^+), phosphate (PO_4^{3-}), and carbonate (CO_3^{2-}) in an alkaline environment. These conditions favor formation of uroliths containing struvite ($MgNH_4PO_4 \cdot 6H_2O$), calcium apatite [$Ca_{10}(PO_4)6(OH_2)_2$], and carbonate apatite [$Ca_{10}(PO_4)6CO_3$]. • Consumption of dietary protein in excess of the daily requirement for anabolism results in formation of urea from catabolism of amino acids. Hyperammonuria, hypercarbonaturia, and alkaluria mediated by microbial urease depend on the quantity of urea (the substrate of urease) in urine.
• Abnormal urinary excretion of minerals as a result of enhanced glomerular filtration rate, reduced tubular reabsorption, or enhanced tubular secretion is not required for initiation and growth of infection-induced struvite uroliths; however, metabolic and anatomic abnormalities may indirectly induce struvite uroliths by predisposing to urinary tract infections.

Sterile Struvite
• Dietary or metabolic factors may be involved in the genesis of sterile struvite uroliths in these species. • Microbial urease is not involved in formation of sterile struvite uroliths.

SYSTEMS AFFECTED
Renal/Urologic

GENETICS
• The high incidence of struvite uroliths in some breeds of dogs such as miniature schnauzers suggests a familial tendency. We hypothesize that susceptible miniature schnauzers inherit some abnormality of local host defenses of the urinary tract that increases their susceptibility to urinary tract infection. • Sterile struvite uroliths were found in a family of English cocker spaniels.

INCIDENCE/PREVALENCE
Struvite uroliths account for approximately 50% of stones affecting the canine lower urinary tract and 33% of stones affecting the upper urinary tract.

GEOGRAPHIC DISTRIBUTION
Ubiquitous

SIGNALMENT

Species
Dogs (see Urolithiasis, Struvite—Cats)

Breed Predilection
• Miniature schnauzer, shih tzu, bichon frise, miniature poodle, cocker spaniel, and Lhasa apso • Any breed may be affected.

Mean Age and Range
• Mean age, 6 years (range, <1 to >19 years) • Most uroliths in immature dogs are infection-induced struvite.

Predominant Sex
More common in females (85%) than males (15%), which may be related to the greater propensity of females to develop bacterial UTI

SIGNS

General Comments
• None in some dogs • Signs depend on location, size, and number of uroliths

Historical Findings
• Typical signs of urocystoliths include pollakiuria, dysuria, and hematuria; sometimes small, smooth uroliths are voided. • Typical signs of urethroliths include pollakiuria and dysuria; sometimes small, smooth uroliths are voided. • Nephroliths may be associated with manifestations of renal insufficiency. Obstruction to urine outflow with bacterial urinary tract infection may result in generalized pyelonephritis and septicemia.

Physical Examination Findings
• Uroliths may be palpated in the urinary bladder and urethra. • Obstruction of the urethra may cause enlargement of the urinary bladder. • Obstruction of a ureter may cause enlargement of the associated kidney.
• Complete urine outflow obstruction combined with bacterial infection may cause ascending urinary tract infection, signs of renal failure, and signs of septicemia.

CAUSES
• Urinary tract disorders that predispose to infections with urease-producing bacteria, fungal pathogens, or ureaplasma in patients whose urine contains a large quantity of urea
• Specific causes of sterile struvite uroliths are unknown.

RISK FACTORS
• Exogenous or endogenous exposure to high concentrations of glucocorticoids predispose to bacterial urinary tract infection.
• Abnormal retention of urine • Alkaline urine decreases the solubility of struvite.

DIAGNOSIS

DIFFERENTIAL DIAGNOSIS
• Uroliths mimic other causes of pollakiuria, dysuria, hematuria, and/or outflow obstruction. • Differentiate from other types of uroliths by signalment, urinalysis, urine culture, radiography, and quantitative analysis of voided or retrieved uroliths.

CBC/BIOCHEMISTRY/URINALYSIS
• Complete outflow obstruction can cause postrenal azotemia (e.g., high BUN, creatinine, and phosphorus). • Magnesium ammonium phosphate crystals typically appear as colorless, orthorhombic (having three unequal axes intersecting at right angles), coffinlike prisms. They may have three to six or more sides and often have oblique ends.

OTHER LABORATORY TESTS
• Quantitative bacterial culture of urine, preferably collected by cystocentesis
• Bacterial culture of inner portions of infection-induced struvite uroliths
• Quantitative mineral analysis of uroliths retrieved during voiding, by voiding urohydropropulsion, by aspiration into a urinary catheter, or by cystoscopy

IMAGING
• Struvite uroliths are radiodense and may be detected by survey radiography.
• Ultrasonography—can detect uroliths, but provides no information about their density or shape • Determine precise location, size, and number of uroliths; the size and number are not a reliable index of probable efficacy of dissolution therapy

TREATMENT

APPROPRIATE HEALTH CARE
• Retrograde urohydropropulsion to eliminate urethral stones, voiding urohydropropulsion to eliminate bladder and urethral stones, shock-wave lithotripsy, and/or surgery require short periods of hospitalization. • Medical dissolution of struvite uroliths is an outpatient strategy.

NURSING CARE
N/A

ACTIVITY
If dietary management is used, monitor outdoor activity.

DIET
• Infection-induced and sterile struvite urocystoliths and nephroliths may be dissolved by feeding a calculolytic diet (Prescription Diet Canine s/d; Hill's Pet Nutrition). • Continue calculolytic diet

therapy for 1 month beyond survey radiographic evidence of urolith dissolution. • Avoid use of the protein-restricted diet in patients with protein-calorie malnutrition. The calculolytic diet is designed for short-term (weeks to months) dissolution therapy, rather than long-term (months to years) prophylactic therapy. If used, monitor the patient for evidence of protein malnutrition. Avoid prolonged feeding of the calculolytic diet to immature dogs.

CLIENT EDUCATION
• If dietary management is used, limit access to other foods and treats. • Short-term treatment with a calculolytic diet and administration of antibiotics has been effective in dissolving struvite uroliths. • Comply with dosage schedule for antibiotic therapy

SURGICAL CONSIDERATIONS
• Ureteroliths cannot be dissolved; consider surgery or shock-wave lithotripsy for persistent ureteroliths associated with morbidity. • Urethroliths cannot be medically dissolved; consider voiding urohydropropulsion if the urethroliths are likely to pass through the entire length of the urethra. Alternatively, move urethroliths into the bladder by retrograde urohydropropulsion. • Immovable urethroliths may require urethrotomy or urethrostomy. • Nephroliths causing outflow obstruction or associated with nonfunctioning kidneys cannot be dissolved medically. • Consider surgical correction if uroliths are obstructing urine outflow and/or if correctable abnormalities predisposing to recurrent urinary tract infection are identified by radiography or other means.

MEDICATIONS

DRUG(S)
• Dietary dissolution of infection-induced urocystoliths or nephroliths requires oral administration of appropriate antibiotics, chosen on the basis of quantitative bacterial culture and antimicrobial susceptibility tests. Give antibiotics at therapeutic dosages until there is no radiographic evidence of uroliths and there is laboratory confirmation of eradication of urinary tract infection. • Patients with infection-induced struvite urocystoliths associated with persistent bacterial infection with urease-producing bacteria and refractory to dietary and antibiotic dissolution may be given AHA (Lithostat, Mission Pharmacal, 12.5 mg/kg PO q12 h). AHA is a urease inhibitor that blocks hydrolysis of urea to ammonia.

CONTRAINDICATIONS
AHA is teratogenic and should not be given to pregnant dogs.

PRECAUTIONS
• Diet-induced polyuria will reduce the concentration of antimicrobial drugs in urine; consider this fact when calculating antimicrobic dosages. • Prolonged administration of AHA at higher doses induces abnormalities in bilirubin metabolism in some dogs. • Higher doses of AHA may induce a reversible hemolytic anemia.

FOLLOW-UP

PATIENT MONITORING
Rate of urolith dissolution at monthly intervals by urinalysis, urine culture, ultrasonography, and/or survey or contrast radiography

PREVENTION/AVOIDANCE
• Infection-induced struvite urolithiasis may be prevented by eradicating and controlling infections by urease-producing bacteria. • Recurrent sterile struvite uroliths may be prevented by use of acidifying, magnesium-restricted diets (Prescription Diet Canine c/d, Hill's) or urine acidifiers. • Monitor patients whose urine has been acidified for calcium oxalate crystalluria. Change management protocol if persistent calcium oxalate crystalluria develops. • In patients at risk for both struvite and calcium oxalate crystalluria, focus on prevention of calcium oxalate uroliths—struvite uroliths can be medically dissolved if they recur; recurrent calcium oxalate uroliths cannot be dissolved.

POSSIBLE COMPLICATIONS
• Benefits and risks are associated with feeding struvitolytic diets. Not all patients qualify for dietary medical management, including those with (1) abnormal fluid accumulation, (2) azotemic primary renal failure, and (3) predispositions to pancreatitis (especially miniature schnauzers with hyperlipidemia). • Urocystoliths may pass into and obstruct the urethra of male dogs, especially if the patient is persistently dysuric. Urethral obstruction may be managed by retrograde urohydropropulsion. • Dysuria may be minimized by antimicrobic treatment of bacterial urinary tract infections and oral administration of anticholinergic drugs (e.g., propantheline). • Dogs that do not consume their daily requirement of the calculolytic diet may develop varying degrees of protein calorie malnutrition. This can be prevented by proper calculation of the daily dietary requirement and adjustment in the quantity of diet fed on the basis of serial physical examination. • Diet-associated polyuria will result in voiding increased urine volume. This may be associated with varying degrees of urinary incontinence in neutered female dogs with a predisposition to estrogen-responsive incontinence.

EXPECTED COURSE AND PROGNOSIS
• In our hospital, the mean time for dissolution of infection-induced urocystoliths was approximately 3 months (range, 2 weeks to 7 months). The mean time for dissolution of infection-induced struvite nephroliths was 6 months (range, 2–10 months). The mean time for dissolution of sterile struvite urocystoliths was 6 weeks (range, 4–12 weeks). • Compliance with dietary recommendations is suggested by a reduced concentration of urea in serum (10 mg/dL), and a low urine specific gravity (1.004–1.014). • If uroliths increase in size during dietary management or do not begin to decrease in size after approximately 4–8 weeks of appropriate medical management, alternative methods should be considered. Difficulty in inducing complete dissolution of uroliths by creating urine undersaturated with struvite should prompt consideration that (1) the wrong mineral component was identified, (2) the nucleus of the uroliths has a different mineral composition than other portions of the urolith, and (3) the owner is not complying with medical recommendations.

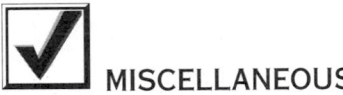

MISCELLANEOUS

ASSOCIATED CONDITIONS
Any disease that predisposes to bacterial urinary tract infection

AGE-RELATED FACTORS
Infection-induced struvite is the most common form of urolith in immature dogs.

PREGNANCY
• AHA is teratogenic. • The calculolytic diet is not designed to sustain pregnancy.

SYNONYMS
Phosphate calculi • Infection stones • Urease stones • Triple-phosphate stones

ABBREVIATIONS
• AHA = acetohydroxamic acid • MAP = magnesium ammonium phosphate • UTI = urinary tract infection

Suggested Reading

Osborne CA, Lulich JP, Bartges JW, et al. Canine and feline urolithiasis: relationship of etiopathogenesis to treatment and prevention. In: Osborne CA, Finco DR, eds. Canine and feline nephrology and urology. Baltimore: Williams & Wilkins, 1995:798–888.

Osborne CA, Lulich JP, Polzin DJ, et al. Medical dissolution and prevention of canine struvite urolithiasis: twenty years of experience. Vet Clin North Am 1999;29:73–111.

Authors Carl A. Osborne, Jody P. Lulich, and David J. Polzin

Consulting Editors Larry G. Adams and Carl A. Osborne

UROLITHIASIS, URATE

BASICS

DEFINITION
Uroliths composed of uric acid, sodium urate, or ammonium urate

PATHOPHYSIOLOGY
• Impaired conversion of uric acid to allantoin causes high concentration of uric acid in serum and urine.

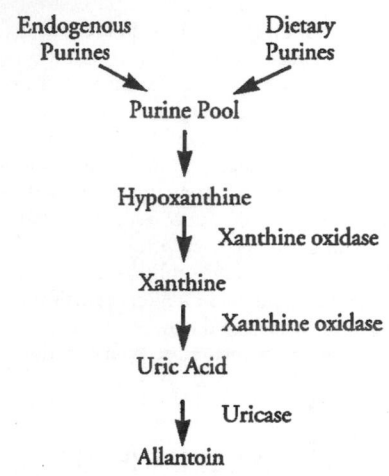

• Patients with portosystemic shunt may develop ammonium urate uroliths because of impaired metabolism of uric acid and ammonia.

SYSTEMS AFFECTED
Renal/urologic

GENETICS
Dalmatians have a breed predisposition to forming urate urolithiasis; the genetics of this condition are unknown.

INCIDENCE/PREVALENCE
Approximately 5–8% of uroliths retrieved from dogs and cats

SIGNALMENT
Species
Dogs and cats

Breed Predilections
Dalmatian, English bulldog, and breeds at risk for portosystemic shunt (e.g., Yorkshire terrier)

Mean Age and Range
• Mean age in patients without portosystemic shunt is 3.5 years (range, 0.5 to > 10 years)
• Mean age in patients with portosystemic shunt is < 1 year (range, 0.1 to > 10 years).

Predominant Sex
• More common in male dogs without portosystemic shunt • No sex predilection in dogs with portosystemic shunt or cats

SIGNS
Historical Findings
• Hematuria • Dysuria • Possible hepatic encephalopathy in patients with portosystemic shunt

Physical Examination Findings
• Urethral obstruction • No signs in some patients

CAUSES
Rule out portosystemic shunt

RISK FACTORS
• High purine intake (glandular meat)
• Persistent aciduria in a predisposed animal

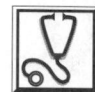

DIAGNOSIS

DIFFERENTIAL DIAGNOSIS
Other causes of lower or upper urinary tract disease

CBC/BIOCHEMISTRY/URINALYSIS
• Aciduria • Urate crystalluria • Azotemia in patients with urinary outflow obstruction • Low BUN in patients with portosystemic shunt.

OTHER LABORATORY TESTS
Liver function tests such as bile acids have abnormal results in patients with portosystemic shunt.

IMAGING
• Urate uroliths may be radiolucent; may need intravenous pyelogram (IVP) to detect nephroliths or double contrast cystography to detect urocystoliths • Microhepatica in patients with portosystemic shunt • Ultrasonography may reveal small uroliths and portosystemic shunts.

DIAGNOSTIC PROCEDURES
Liver biopsy; bile acids, ammonia

PATHOLOGIC FINDINGS
In patients with portosystemic shunt, liver biopsy may reveal hepatic atrophy and/or dysplasia.

TREATMENT

APPROPRIATE HEALTH CARE
Urethral or ureteral obstruction may require inpatient treatment. Urate uroliths can be dissolved on outpatient basis.

NURSING CARE
Fluid therapy to correct dehydration

ACTIVITY
Usually not restricted, except after surgery

DIET
For dissolution and prevention, a low-purine, urine-alkalinizing diet

CLIENT EDUCATION
Recurrence of uroliths is possible.

SURGICAL CONSIDERATIONS
• Cystotomy, urethrotomy, or nephrotomy to remove uroliths • Portosystemic shunt ligation

MEDICATIONS

DRUG(S)
Allopurinol (15 mg/kg PO q12h), a xanthine oxidase inhibitor, for dissolution (see algorithm 1)

CONTRAINDICATIONS
Glucocorticoids and other immunosuppressive drugs may promote hyperuricosuria.

PRECAUTIONS
Allopurinol is contraindicated in animals with renal failure and is not effective in animals with portosystemic shunts.

POSSIBLE INTERACTIONS
Skin eruption with use of allopurinol and ampicillin

FOLLOW-UP

PATIENT MONITORING
See algorithm 2

PREVENTION/AVOIDANCE
Low-purine, urine-alkalinizing diet

POSSIBLE COMPLICATIONS
• Urethral obstruction • Uroliths likely to recur if no preventive measures

EXPECTED COURSE AND PROGNOSIS
• Medical dissolution takes an average of 4 weeks. • Medical dissolution usually not successful with portosystemic shunt

MISCELLANEOUS

ASSOCIATED CONDITIONS
Portosystemic shunt

AGE-RELATED FACTORS
N/A

PREGNANCY
Low-protein diet is not recommended for pregnant or lactating animal.

SEE ALSO
• Portosystemic Shunting, Acquired • Portosystemic Vascular Anomaly, Congenital • Urolithiasis, Xanthine

ABBREVIATION
IVP = intravenous pyelogram

Suggested Reading
Bartges JW, Osborne CA, Felice LJ. Canine xanthine uroliths: risk factor management. In: Kirk RW, Bonagura JD, eds. Current

veterinary therapy XI. Philadelphia: WB
Saunders, 1992:900–905.
Bartges JS, Osborne CA, Lulich JP, et al. Ca-
nine urate urolithiasis: Etiopathogenesis, di-
agnosis, and management. Vet Clin North
Am Small Anim Pract 1996;26:589–628.

Lulich JP, Osborne CA, Bartges JW, et al. Ca-
nine lower urinary tract disorders. In:
Ettinger SJ, Feldman EC, ed. Textbook of
veterinary internal medicine. 5th ed.
Philadelphia: Saunders, 2000:1747–1781.
Osborne CA, Lulich JP, Thumchai R, et al.

Diagnosis, medical treatment, and progno-
sis of feline urolithiasis. Vet Clin North Am
Small Anim Pract 1996;26:161–192.
Author Joseph W. Bartges
Consulting Editors Larry G. Adams and Carl
A. Osborne

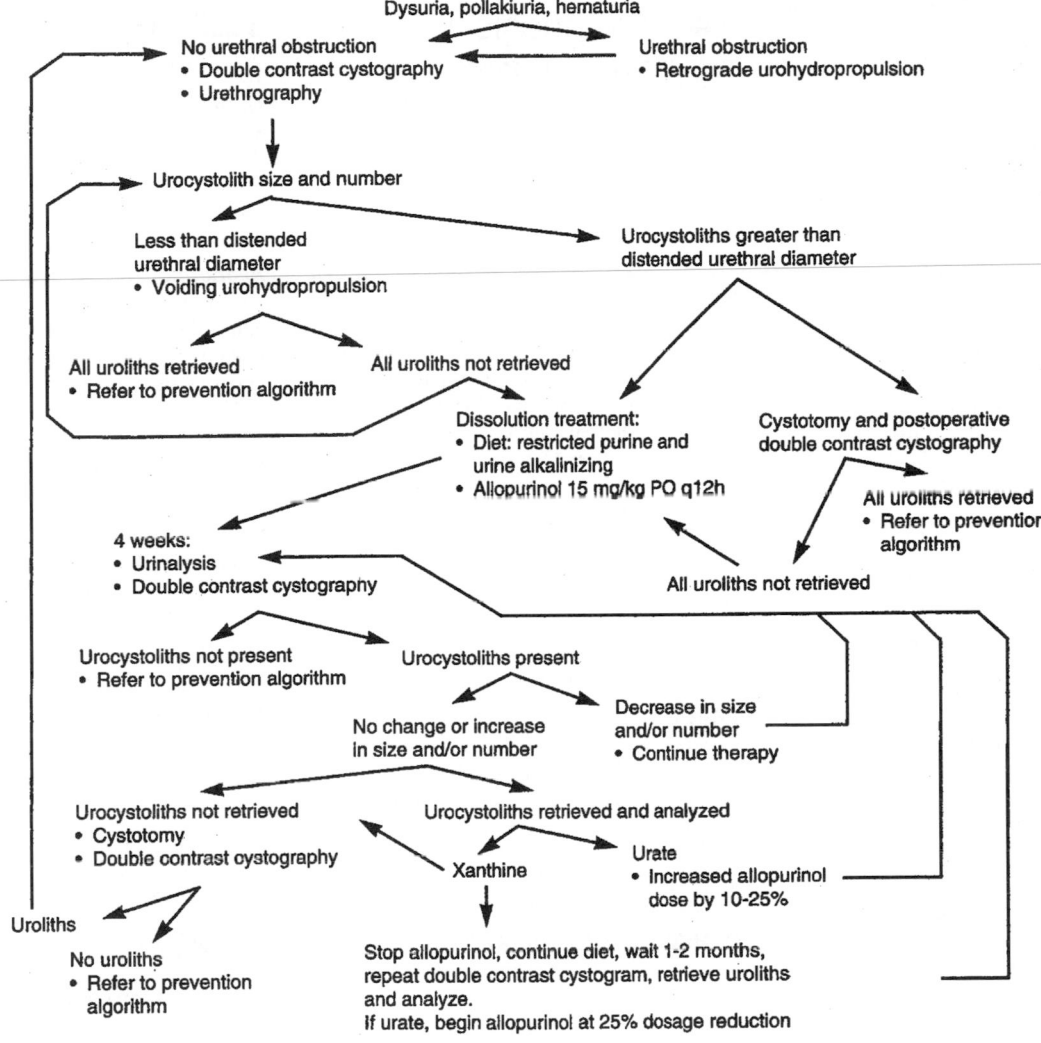

Figure 1.

Algorithm for Treatment of Urate Urocystolithiasis

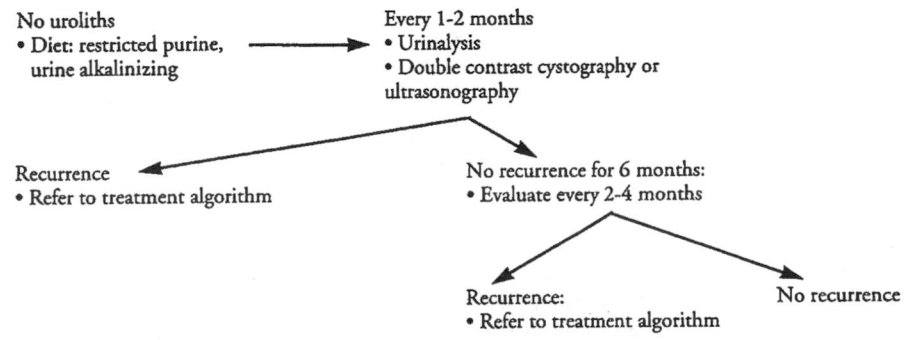

Figure 2.

Algorithm for Prevention of Urate Urocystolithiasis

UROLITHIASIS, XANTHINE

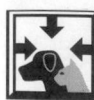

BASICS

OVERVIEW
• Xanthine, a degradation product of purine metabolism, is converted to uric acid by the enzyme xanthine oxidase. Naturally occurring (enzyme deficiency) or drug-induced (allopurinol) impairment of xanthine oxidase ultimately results in hyperxanthinemia and xanthinuria. • In naturally occurring xanthinuria, a familial or congenital defect in xanthine oxidase activity is likely. A breed predisposition has not been identified in cats (number = 64). In Cavalier King Charles spaniels, an autosomal recessive mode of inheritance has been postulated to occur.
• In dogs, acquired xanthinuria is a common complication of treatment of urate urolithiasis or leishmaniasis with allopurinol. Consumption of high purine diets increases the risk of xanthinuria in patients treated with allopurinol. • Because xanthine is the least soluble of the purines excreted in urine, xanthinuria may be associated with formation of xanthine uroliths.

SIGNALMENT
• Dogs and cats. Naturally occurring xanthinuria is more commonly observed in cats than in dogs. • In dogs, allopurinol-induced xanthinuria may affect any breed, age, or gender. Naturally occurring xanthinuria, hypoxanthinuria, and xanthine uroliths have been observed in young Cavalier King Charles spaniels. • In cats, xanthine uroliths primarily affect adult males and females (mean age at diagnosis = 2.9 years; range = 4 months to 12 years). They have been most commonly recognized in the domestic shorthair and domestic longhair breeds.

SIGNS
• Signs are dependent on location, size, and number of uroliths. Affected animals may be asymptomatic. • Typical signs of urocystoliths include pollakiuria, dysuria, and hematuria.
• Typical signs of urethroliths include pollaki-uria, dysuria, and sometimes voiding of small, smooth, yellow uroliths. Complete outflow obstruction may result in post-renal uremia.
• Nephroliths are typically asymptomatic, but may be associated with manifestations of hydronephrosis and renal insufficiency.

CAUSES AND RISK FACTORS
• Xanthinuria is a risk factor for xanthine urolithiasis. • Canine breed predisposition may include Cavalier King Charles spaniels.
• In young and middle-aged cats with previous history of xanthine urolithiasis, uroliths often recur within 3 to 12 months following removal unless prophylactic therapy has been initiated. • Urolith formation is enhanced by acid urine pH, highly

concentrated urine, incomplete and infrequent micturition. • In animals given excessive allopurinol, xanthinuria is enhanced by failure to appropriately restrict dietary purine precursors.

DIAGNOSIS

DIFFERENTIAL DIAGNOSIS
• Uroliths mimic other causes of pollakiuria, dysuria, hematuria, and/or outflow obstruction.
• Differentiate from other types of uroliths, especially ammonium urate, by urinalysis, radiography, and quantitative analysis of voided or retrieved uroliths.

CBC/BIOCHEMISTRY/URINALYSIS
• Xanthine crystals in urine sediment cannot be distinguished from many forms of ammonium urate or amorphous urates by light microscopy. All these crystals are usually brown or yellow-brown and may form spherules of varying size.

OTHER LABORATORY TESTS
• Infrared spectroscopy is required to differentiate xanthine uroliths from uroliths composed of ammonium urate, sodium urate, and uric acid.
• High-pressure liquid chromatography of urine to detect xanthine, hypoxanthine, and other purine metabolites

IMAGING
• Radiography—The radiodensity of pure xanthine uroliths is similar to that of soft tissue and therefore cannot be reliably detected by survey radiography.
• Ultrasonography, double-contrast cystography, and intravenous urography aid in detecting uroliths and their location.

OTHER DIAGNOSTIC PROCEDURES
• Xanthine urethroliths and urocystoliths may be detected by urethrocystoscopy.
• Small uroliths for analysis may be retrieved by aspiration via a transurethral catheter or voiding urohydropulsion.

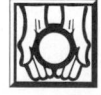

TREATMENT
• Medical protocols that consistently promote dissolution of xanthine uroliths have not been developed.
• Removal of small urocystoliths by voiding urohydropulsion
• Surgery remains the most reliable method to remove larger active uroliths from the lower urinary tract.
• Minimize further growth of existing uroliths by reducing dietary risk factors.
• Pending further studies, in cats with naturally occurring xanthine uroliths, consider canned renal-failure diets in an

attempt to increase urine volume, to minimize purine precursors, and to minimize formation of acid urine.
• Perineal urethrostomies may minimize recurrent urethral obstruction in male cats.

MEDICATIONS

DRUGS

Urine Alkalinizers
• Consider in patients that have acid urine despite dietary therapy.
• A sufficient quantity of potassium citrate or sodium bicarbonate should be given to sustain a urine pH of 7.0 to 7.5.

Allopurinol
• When treating urate urolithiasis in dogs, adjust dosage of allopurinol in context of magnitude of concentration of urine uric acid and quantity of dietary purines (see Urolithiasis, Urate).
• In dogs, allopurinol-induced uroliths may dissolve by discontinuing allopurinol therapy but continuing the low purine diet.

CONTRAINDICATIONS/POSSIBLE INTERACTIONS
Do not give allopurinol to cats or dogs with naturally occurring xanthine uroliths.

FOLLOW-UP
• Monitor urolith dissolution at 30-day intervals by urinalysis and contrast radiography or ultrasonography.
• Although naturally occurring xanthine uroliths tend to be recurrent, recurrence does not occur in all xanthinuric cats and dogs.

MISCELLANEOUS

ASSOCIATED CONDITIONS
• Urate urolithiasis
• Nephrolithiasis

SEE ALSO
• Crystalluria
• Urolithiasis, Urate

Suggested Reading
Bartges JW, Osborne CA, Felice LJ: Canine xanthine uroliths: risk factor management. In: Kirk RW, Bonagura JD, eds. Current veterinary therapy XI. Philadelphia: Saunders, 1992:900–905.
Osborne CA, Lulich JP, Bartges JW et al: Drug-induced urolithiasis. Vet Clin N Amer 29:251–266, 1999.

Authors Carl A. Osborne and Joseph W. Bartges
Consulting Editors Larry G. Adams and Carl A. Osborne

BASICS

OVERVIEW
Failure of the uterine muscles to expel fetuses

Primary
• Uterine muscles do not contract normally at parturition
• Large-breed dog with an abnormally small litter—uterine contractions may not be induced.
• Overstretching of the myometrium by large litters—uterine contractions may not be induced.

Secondary
• Pup not delivered within 2 hours
• May develop during a prolonged parturition or after dystocia with subsequent uterine muscle failure (see Dystocia)

SIGNALMENT
• Dogs
• Noted in some small breeds
• Seen in nervous, obese, older, and under-exercised females
• Possibly with small litters in all breeds

SIGNS
• Primary—lack of onset of parturition at the end of gestation; patient is bright and alert; may detect cervical dilation on vaginoscopy; may see small green-tinged vaginal discharge
• Secondary—patient usually has prolonged dystocia; may note one or two normal deliveries, after which labor ceases, even though there are more fetuses in the uterus

CAUSES & RISK FACTORS
• Primary—result of muscles that do not respond to hormonal stimuli; receptors that failed to develop; or hormones that are lacking, not released, or imbalanced; obesity and lack of exercise main causal factors
• Secondary—obstruction in the reproductive tract; absolute or relative fetal oversize; fetal deficiency of adrenocorticoid hormone; faulty fetal presentation, position, and posture
• Progesterone administration—mimics condition

DIAGNOSIS

DIFFERENTIAL DIAGNOSIS
• Primary—pseudopregnancy
• Secondary—obstructive dystocia

CBC/BIOCHEMISTRY/URINALYSIS
• Primary—normal; may be useful if cesarean section is indicated
• Secondary—may note low serum calcium and blood glucose

OTHER LABORATORY TESTS
Presumptive diagnosis—labor has not started after > 24 hours since the prepartum drop in rectal temperature, or serum progesterone < 2 ng/mL for 36 hours.

IMAGING
• Radiography—number and disposition of the fetus(es)
• Ultrasonography—fetal stress and viability

DIAGNOSTIC PROCEDURES
N/A

TREATMENT
• True primary inertia—may not respond to medical treatment; immediate cesarean section indicated if ultrasonography documents fetal stress (heart rate < 150 or > 250 bpm)
• Medical treatment—contraindicated with obstructive dystocia and uterine rupture (rare)

MEDICATIONS

DRUG(S)

Oxytocin
• Small doses induce effective uterine contractions.
• Total dose—small breeds, 1–2 IU SC, IM; medium breeds, 3–4 IU SC, IM; large breeds, 5–6 IU SC, IM; may be repeated in 45 min
• No progress after two to three injections—surgery indicated
• May try adding 5–10 IU to 1 L 5% dextrose; administer intravenously at a maintenance dosage rate; if no effective contractions within 10–15 min, surgery indicated; if contractions are induced, wait 1–1.5 hours before performing surgery.

Other
• Calcium—2–10 mL slow IV bolus of 10% calcium gluconate; stop immediately if cardiac arrhythmias are detected.
• Glucose—10–20% dextrose in a slow intravenous infusion

CONTRAINDICATIONS/POSSIBLE INTERACTIONS
• Obstructive dystocia or uterine rupture (rare)
• Overtreatment with oxytocin—induces nonproductive tetanic contractions
• Prostaglandins—may induce contractions; have not worked in author's experience

FOLLOW-UP

PATIENT MONITORING
• Successful medical treatment—make sure all placentae have passed.
• Evaluate dam for endocrine and reproductive tract disease, which may have been a predisposing factor.

PREVENTION/AVOIDANCE
Proper feeding and adequate exercise—prevent obesity during pregnancy.

POSSIBLE COMPLICATIONS
Death of pups—too much time elapses from time when labor should have started until treatment is initiated.

EXPECTED COURSE AND PROGNOSIS
• Primary—may recur at subsequent parturition dates
• Puppy survival—prognosis good if treatment is instituted on the date of expected parturition

MISCELLANEOUS

AGE-RELATED FACTORS
Relatively old bitches more prone

SEE ALSO
Dystocia

Suggested Reading
Davidson A. Periparturient problems in the bitch. In: Proceedings of the Annual Meeting of the Society for Theriogenology, Montreal, September 17–20. Nashville: Society for Theriogenology, 1997:231–235.
Feldman EC, Nelson RW. Canine female reproduction. In: Feldman EC, Nelson RW. Canine and feline endocrinology. Philadelphia: Saunders, 1987:399–480.
Linde-Forsberg C, Eneroth A. Parturition. In: Simpson GM, England GCW, Harvey M, eds. Manual of small animal reproduction and neonatology. Cheltenham, UK: British Small Animal Veterinary Medical Association, 1998:127–142.

Author Klaas Post
Consulting Editor Sara K. Lyle

UTERINE TUMORS

 BASICS

OVERVIEW
• Rare tumors, arising from the uterine smooth muscle and epithelial tissues
• Compose 0.3%–0.4% of tumors in dogs and 0.2%–1.5% in cats
• Dogs—usually benign; leiomyomas, 85%–90%; leiomyosarcoma, 10%; other types (e.g., carcinoma, fibroma, fibrosarcoma, lipoma) rare
• Cats—usually malignant (adenocarcinoma); include leiomyoma, leiomyosarcoma, fibrosarcoma, fibroma, and lipoma
• Metastasis—may occur with malignant forms

SIGNALMENT
• Dogs and cats
• No breed predilection reported
• Middle-aged to old animals usually affected

SIGNS
• Dogs—often clinically silent and discovered incidentally; vaginal discharge; pyometra; abdominal organ compression or secondary metastatic signs
• Cats—vaginal discharge; abnormal estrous cycles; polyuria; polydipsia; vomiting; abdominal distention; signs related to metastatic disease

CAUSES & RISK FACTORS
Intact sexual status

 DIAGNOSIS

DIFFERENTIAL DIAGNOSIS
• Pyometra
• Other midcaudal abdominal masses

CBC/BIOCHEMISTRY/URINALYSIS
No specific abnormalities

OTHER LABORATORY TESTS
N/A

IMAGING
• Abdominal radiographs—may detect a midcaudal abdominal mass
• Thoracic radiographs—recommended; assess for metastasis
• Ultrasonography—may reveal uterine mass

DIAGNOSTIC PROCEDURES
• Cytologic evaluation—with abdominal effusion
• Histopathologic examination—necessary for definitive diagnosis

 TREATMENT

Ovariohysterectomy—treatment of choice

 MEDICATIONS

DRUG(S)
Doxorubicin, cisplatin, and carboplatin—rational choices for palliation of malignant or metastatic disease

CONTRAINDICATIONS/POSSIBLE INTERACTIONS
• Doxorubicin—carefully monitor patients with underlying cardiac disease; consider pretreatment and serial echocardiograms and ECG
• Cisplatin—do not use in dogs with pre-existing renal disease; do not use without appropriate and concurrent diuresis; do not use in cats (fatal).
• Chemotherapy may be toxic; seek advice if unfamiliar with these agents.

 FOLLOW-UP

PATIENT MONITORING
• Malignant—consider thoracic and abdominal radiographs every 3 months.
• CBC, biochemical profile, and urinalysis (if using cisplatin)—perform before each chemotherapy treatment.

EXPECTED COURSE AND PROGNOSIS
Prognosis—excellent (cure) if benign; guarded if malignant; after chemotherapy, unknown

 MISCELLANEOUS

ASSOCIATED CONDITIONS
Renal cystadenocarcinoma and nodular dermatofibrosis—reported in German shepherds with uterine leiomyoma

ABBREVIATION
ECG = electrocardiogram

Suggested Reading
Klein MK. Tumors of the female reproductive system. In: Withrow SJ, MacEwen EG, eds. Small animal clinical oncology. 2nd ed. Philadelphia: Saunders, 1996:347–355.
Morrison WB. Cancers of the reproductive tract. In: Morrison WB, ed. Cancer in dogs and cats: medical and surgical management. Baltimore: Williams & Wilkins, 1998: 581–590.
Author Renee Al-Sarraf
Consulting Editor Wallace B. Morrison

BASICS

OVERVIEW
• The most common intraocular tumor in cats
• Usually arise from the anterior iridal surface with extension to the ciliary body and choroid
• Tend to be flat and diffuse, not nodular (unlike intraocular melanomas in dogs)
• Initially has a benign clinical and histologic appearance
• Unique feature—may develop metastatic disease up to several years later
• Metastatic rate may be up to 63%.

SIGNALMENT
• No sex or breed predisposition
• Average age of affected cats is 9.5 years, though can affect any age adult cat

SIGNS

Historical Findings
• Iris color change
• Secondary glaucoma leading to mydriasis or buphthalmia, resulting in blindness

Physical Examination Findings
• Iris surface—thickened, irregular, usually pigmented, though can be nonpigmented
• Lesions—focal to diffuse; usually flat; slowly progressive; may involve one or both eyes
• Advanced disease—often see pigmented tumor cells in the aqueous; homogeneously thickened iris
• May note drainage angle infiltration, which may result in secondary glaucoma

CAUSES & RISK FACTORS
N/A

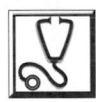

DIAGNOSIS

DIFFERENTIAL DIAGNOSIS
• Freckles on the surface of the iris that do not appear to change over time—may be benign pigmented lesions; more likely variants of iris melanoma
• Heterochromia irides—congenital, nonprogressive alteration in iridal pigmentation
• Most closely resembles iridal color change that results from chronic anterior uveitis
• Limbal melanomas—benign behavior; tend to be focal, superiorly located, flat to slightly raised limbal masses that do not invade the uveal tract unless they are very large

CBC/BIOCHEMISTRY/URINALYSIS
Normal

OTHER LABORATORY TESTS
N/A

IMAGING
• Thoracic radiographs and abdominal ultrasonography—help determine extent of metastatic disease
• Recommended presurgically and every 6 months after the diagnosis

DIAGNOSTIC PROCEDURES
• Complete ophthalmic examination, including tonometry and gonioscopy
• Fine-needle aspiration of the iridal surface ("vacuuming")—diagnostic value questionable; not beneficial for staging
• Iridal biopsy—may be performed, not beneficial for staging the disease
• Melanoma cells in the iridocorneal angle and ciliary venous plexus suggest that metastatic cells have spread through the body, but metastases may not be evident until a few years later
• Anterior segment fluorescein angiography may become a useful clinical diagnostic technique in the future

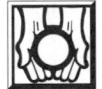

TREATMENT
• Enucleation—in early to moderate cases, some ophthalmologists prefer a conservative approach consisting of periodic examinations and serial photography to monitor the growth progress of the lesion(s)
• Cats with iridal thickening and iridocorneal angle involvement, with and without glaucoma, had similar survival times when compared with unaffected age-matched control cats.
• Advanced lesions consisting of infiltrative iris involvement including the posterior epithelium and ciliary body had decreased survival times presumably as a result of metastatic disease.
• When enucleating, use a gentle technique; in humans enucleation has been associated with metastasis if not done.
• Laser (diode) photoablation—has been used to treat freckle-like lesions with apparent success; no controlled or long-term follow-up studies

MEDICATIONS

DRUG(S)
N/A

CONTRAINDICATIONS/POSSIBLE INTERACTIONS
N/A

FOLLOW-UP

PATIENT MONITORING
• IOP—quarterly monitoring if surgical options are declined; mild elevation may be treated with oral or topical carbonic anhydrase inhibitors (e.g., methazolamide at approximately 6 mg PO q12–24h); secondary glaucoma is best controlled by enucleation.
• Common metastasis sites—liver, lungs, regional lymph nodes; monitor periodically.

EXPECTED COURSE AND PROGNOSIS
• One long-term study shows that patients with early iris melanoma have no increased risk of life-threatening metastasis compared to controls, but patients with advanced lesions had dramatically shortened survival times.
• Lesions—focal, multifocal to diffuse; usually flat; pigmentation over months to years (i.e., variable); may involve one or both eyes
• Advanced disease—often see pigmented tumor cells in the aqueous; homogeneously thickened iris causing abnormal pupil shape and change in pupil mobility
• Prognosis—guarded, even with enucleation; metastasis may not become apparent for several years or diagnosed on necropsy.

MISCELLANEOUS

SYNONYMS
• Iris melanoma
• Diffuse iris melanoma

ABBREVIATION
IOP = intraocular pressure

Suggested Reading
Dubielzig RR. Ocular neoplasia in small animals. Vet Clin North Am Small Anim Pract 1990;20:837–848.
Glaze MB, Gelatt KN. Feline ophthalmology. In: Veterinary ophthalmology. Philadelphia: Lippincott Williams & Wilkins, 1999: 1026–1027.
Kalishman JB, Chappell RJ, Flood LA, Dubielzig RR, et al. A matched observational study of survival in cats with enucleation due to diffuse iris melanoma. Vet Ophthalmol 1998;1:25–29.
Author Carmen Colitz
Consulting Editor Paul E. Miller

UVEAL MELANOMA—DOGS

BASICS

OVERVIEW
- Melanomas of the anterior uvea (e.g., iris and ciliary body) and posterior uvea (choroid)
- Most common primary intraocular neoplasm in dogs
- Usually benign and unilateral; often destructive to the eye
- Most often affect the anterior uvea
- Anterior uveal—4% rate of vascular metastasis to lungs and viscera
- Choroidal—rarely metastasize

SIGNALMENT
- No breed or sex predilection
- Anterior uveal—average age 8–10 years
- Choroidal melanoma—average age 6.5 years
- Range—2 months to 17 years

SIGNS

Anterior Uveal
- Pigmented scleral or corneal mass
- Pigmented mass visible in the anterior chamber or posterior to the pupillary margin
- Irregular pupil
- Uveitis
- Glaucoma
- Hyphema
- No vision loss—unless mass obstructs the pupil or glaucoma has developed

Choroidal
- Often missed because of tumor location
- Posterior segment mass on funduscopy

CAUSES & RISK FACTORS
- Idiopathic
- Potential transformation of flat, pigmented iris freckles into melanomas
- Young Labrador retrievers—presumed autosomal recessive inheritance

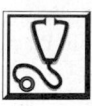

DIAGNOSIS

DIFFERENTIAL DIAGNOSIS
- Nonneoplastic uveal proliferations—iris freckles are not raised
- Diffuse iris hyperpigmentation secondary to chronic uveitis
- Uveal cysts—transilluminate and may move freely within the eye, unlike melanomas
- Granulomatous masses

- Ocular perforation with uveal prolapse
- Other ocular neoplastic conditions
- Outward scrolling of pupillary margin owing to uveitis (ectropion uvea)

CBC/BIOCHEMISTRY/URINALYSIS
Usually normal

OTHER LABORATORY TESTS
N/A

IMAGING
Ultrasonography—may help determine the extent of the mass

DIAGNOSTIC PROCEDURES
- Slit-lamp biomicroscopy—determine size and location of mass
- Transillumination of mass
- Tonometry
- Indirect ophthalmoscopy—with or without concomitant scleral indentation
- Gonioscopy—evaluate drainage angle for tumor extension
- Ocular ultrasonography—if cornea opaque and cannot visualize deeper ocular structures

PATHOLOGIC FINDINGS
- Usually restricted to the enucleated globe; biopsy not practical
- Two cell types usually seen—plump cells filled with melanin; spindle cells
- Benign appearance and low mitotic index (< 2 mitotic figures per high power field) common
- Mitotic index—most reliable criterion for malignancy; ≥ 4 for clinically malignant tumors
- When submitting eyes for histologic evaluation, request bleached tissue sections and mitotic index.
- Best if veterinary ocular pathologist evaluates globe

TREATMENT
- Usually benign, may opt to monitor every 3–6 months
- Young Labrador retrieves—aggressive growth, need surgery
- Counsel the client about enucleation; the procedure often causes the client emotional distress.
- Emphasize that the condition is unilateral, sparing the fellow eye, and that one-eyed animals function very well.

- Indications for enucleation—size of the mass increases rapidly; eye cannot be salvaged; mass spreads diffusely within the eye; visual function significantly impaired; extraocular invasion; secondary complications (e.g., glaucoma, signs of pain, and hemorrhage)
- Enucleation technique—use gentle surgical technique to prevent showering of tumor cells into the vascular circulation; avoid tension on optic chiasm, as could blind fellow eye; exenterate the entire orbital contents, if extrascleral extension is noted.
- Other surgical treatments—infrequently used; sector iridectomy and iridocyclectomy of discrete small masses
- Laser treatment of small iris tumors—promising, recently developed procedure

MEDICATIONS

DRUG(S)
N/A

CONTRAINDICATIONS/POSSIBLE INTERACTIONS
N/A

FOLLOW-UP
- Postoperative thoracic and abdominal radiography or ultrasonography—at 6 and 12 months if the mitotic index is high or the patient has extrascleral, vascular, or optic nerve extension
- Evaluate the enucleation site for tumor recurrence.

MISCELLANEOUS

Suggested Reading
Cook CS, Wilkie DA. Treatment of presumed iris melanoma in dogs by diode laser photocoagulation: 23 cases. Vet Ophthalmol 1999;2:217–225.
Wilcock BP, Peiffer RL. Morphology and behavior of primary ocular melanomas in 91 dogs. Vet Pathol 1986;23:418–424.
Author Terri L. McCalla
Consulting Editor Paul E. Miller

UVEODERMATOLOGIC SYNDROME (VKH)

BASICS

OVERVIEW
• Rare syndrome similar to Vogt-Koyanagi-Harada syndrome in humans
• Considered to be an autoimmune disorder resulting in concurrent granulomatous uveitis and depigmenting dermatitis and rare meningoencephalitis

SIGNALMENT
• Reported in dogs, especially akitas, Samoyeds, and Siberian huskies
• No apparent age or sex predilections

SIGNS
• Sudden-onset uveitis—may be painful and progress to blindness; concurrent or subsequent leukoderma of the nose, lips, and eyelids
• Footpads, scrotum, anus, and hard palate may also become depigmented.
• Ulcerations may develop.
• Meningoencephalitis—reported (rare)

CAUSES & RISK FACTORS
• Thought to be an autoimmune disease; antiretinal antibodies have been found in affected dogs.
• Exposure to sunlight—exacerbates symptoms

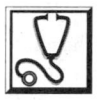

DIAGNOSIS

DIFFERENTIAL DIAGNOSIS
• Immune-mediated skin diseases—pemphigus complex, systemic lupus erythematosus, and discoid lupus erythematosus, pemphigoid
• Neoplasia and numerous other inflammatory and infectious skin diseases that can cause depigmentation
• Skin biopsies, negative ANA titers, and a normal retinal examination—help differentiate these diseases

CBC/BIOCHEMISTRY/URINALYSIS
Usually normal

OTHER LABORATORY TESTS
N/A

IMAGING
N/A

DIAGNOSTIC PROCEDURES
• Biopsy and dermatopathology—best interpreted by a veterinarian experienced in detecting the sometimes subtle differences in pathologic patterns; early lesions have a lichenoid interface pattern with large histiocytes and pronounced pigmentary incontinence; hydropic degeneration of the epidermal basal cell rare
• Evaluate the retina.

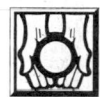

TREATMENT
• Aggressive and rapid initiation of immunosuppressive therapy is recommended to prevent formation of posterior synechiae and secondary glaucoma, cataracts, or blindness.
• Retinal examinations—most important means of monitoring progress; improvement in dermatologic lesions may not reflect the retinal pathology.
• Enucleation—sometimes recommended because of pain

MEDICATIONS

DRUG(S)
• Corticosteroids—initial high doses of prednisone (1.1–2.2 mg/kg PO q12–24h) and azathioprine (1.5–2.5 mg/kg PO q24h) recommended; taper dosages and frequencies to every other day for chronic use; some patients may improve with the initial use of prednisone alone, but the potential sequelae of delayed aggressive therapy warrant the additional use of azathioprine.

• Topical or subconjunctival steroids and cycloplegics—may be indicated with anterior uveitis

CONTRAINDICATIONS/POSSIBLE INTERACTIONS
Prednisone and azathioprine—anemia, leukopenia, thrombocytopenia, high serum alkaline phosphatase levels, vomiting, and pancreatitis; conduct biweekly serum chemistries and CBCs, including platelet counts, initially; decrease after the condition has stabilized and the dose and frequency have been tapered

FOLLOW-UP
• Weekly or biweekly examinations including retinal evaluations—recommended initially for monitoring side effects associated with therapeutics; retinal examinations are important because improvement in dermatologic lesions may not indicate improvement in the retinal lesions.
• Azathioprine may be discontinued after a few months of therapy; prednisone may be necessary indefinitely.
• Iatrogenic hyperadrenocorticism—often a result of the steroid therapy

MISCELLANEOUS

ABBREVIATION
ANA = antinuclear antibody

Suggested Reading
Scott DW, Miller WH, Griffen CE. Small animal dermatology. 5th ed. Philadelphia: Saunders, 1995.
Author Dunbar Gram
Consulting Editor Karen Helton Rhodes

VACCINE-ASSOCIATED SARCOMA

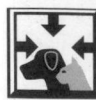 **BASICS**

DEFINITION
A sarcoma developing at the site of injection of a vaccine. Vaccines most commonly implicated in sarcoma formation are those used for rabies and feline leukemia virus. Other types of injectable vaccine and nonvaccine products have rarely been associated with sarcoma development in cats.

PATHOPHYSIOLOGY
• Unknown, but believed that local inflammation is an antecedent event.
• Dysregulation of the cell cycle regulating gene p53 is involved in most tumors.
• These tumors also overexpress PDGF, which may cause the transformation of normal fibroblasts to sarcoma.
• FeLV and FIV are not involved in the pathogenesis of these tumors.
• Initial reports focused on vaccine adjuvants containing aluminum as a potential etiologic agent.
• The role of aluminum is unclear because not all adjuvants used in vaccines associated with sarcoma formation contain aluminum.

SYSTEMS AFFECTED
• Primarily the subcutaneous tissues, skin, and associated muscle.
• These tumors frequently metastasize.

INCIDENCE/PREVALENCE
Estimated prevalence is between 1 and 10 cases per 10,000 cats following rabies and leukemia virus vaccination.

SIGNALMENT
All cats susceptible

SIGNS
• Lesions occur at site of vaccination. They often resemble postvaccine-site granulomas.
• These tumors are highly invasive and rapidly growing.
• Metastasis rates are reported to be 22.5–24%.
• Metastasis to the lungs is most common, but occurs frequently to regional lymph nodes and the skin.
• Advanced lesions are large, fixed, and occasionally ulcerated.

CAUSES
Vaccination with FeLV or rabies vaccine is the overwhelming cause.

RISK FACTORS
• Risk increases with frequency and number of vaccinations given.
• Risk of sarcoma formation following a single injectable vaccination in the cervical/interscapular region is 50% higher than for cats not receiving a vaccination.
• Risk of cats given two vaccinations at this site is 127% higher, and the risk with three or four vaccines is 175% higher than for cats not receiving vaccinations in the cervical/interscapular region.

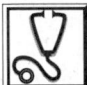 **DIAGNOSIS**

• Record location, shape, and size of all masses occurring at injection sites.
• Assume lesions are malignant until proven otherwise.
• Masses at vaccination sites persisting for longer than 3 months, larger than 2 cm diameter, or increasing in size 1 month after injection should be biopsied.

• Distinguishing a vaccine-sarcoma from a granuloma is vital.
• Tissue biopsy by incision or cutting needle is advised.
• Fine-needle aspiration biopsy is unreliable.
• Always plan biopsy so that subsequent surgery can completely remove the lesion and the biopsy site.
• Advanced lesions should also be biopsied prior to definitive treatment.

DIFFERENTIAL DIAGNOSIS
Granuloma or other neoplasia

CBC/BIOCHEMISTRY/URINALYSIS
Usually unaffected

OTHER LABORATORY TESTS
FeLV and FIV testing should be done. Neither virus plays a role in the pathogenesis of these tumors.

IMAGING
• Three view radiographs of thorax and two of the abdomen should be made to assess for metastasis.
• CT images should be done whenever possible. CT generally demonstrates more invasion into normal tissues surrounding the grossly visible tumor than can be determined by physical examination and facilitates treatment planning.

DIAGNOSTIC PROCEDURES
Incisional or needle biopsy done so that any later surgery attempting cure includes the biopsy tract.

PATHOLOGIC FINDINGS
Fibrosarcoma is the most common vaccine-associated sarcoma type.

VACCINE-ASSOCIATED SARCOMA

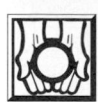

TREATMENT

- Effective treatment is difficult.
- Contrast CT scan prior to aggressive surgery done by a board-certified surgeon results in substantially longer time to first recurrence than surgery done by practitioner.
- Radiation therapy before or after definitive surgery will substantially enhance survival.
- Chemotherapy with doxorubicin may not enhance survival.

CLIENT EDUCATION

Do not overvaccinate. Use informed-consent forms, and discuss risks of vaccination with owners.

SURGICAL CONSIDERATIONS

- Aggressive surgery is vital to increase time to recurrence and overall survival.
- CT scans prior to surgery will help plan the surgery and radiation therapy.
- Surgical drains should be avoided because they help disseminate cancer cells to new locations.

MEDICATIONS

N/A. Most effective treatment is with aggressive surgery and radiation therapy.

FOLLOW-UP

Recheck at appropriate intervals.

PREVENTION/AVOIDANCE

- Assess the risks of exposure to diseases, and compare them to the risks of vaccine-associated sarcoma formation.
- Do not over-vaccinate.
- Vaccinate for rabies, panleukopenia, herpes-1, and caliciviruses no more frequently than every 3 years.
- Vaccination for FeLV is advised only for cats older than 16 weeks that are not restricted to a closed indoor environment that is free of FeLV.
- Avoid other vaccines unless there is a documented risk of exposure.

POSSIBLE COMPLICATIONS

Recurrence and/or new lesions are likely.

EXPECTED COURSE AND PROGNOSIS

- Referral to a board-certified surgeon is highly recommended.
- Median time to first recurrence reported to be 66 days following surgery by referring DVM versus 274 days if surgery performed by a board-certified surgeon.
- Median time to first recurrence following radical excision reported to be 325 days versus 79 days following local excision.
- Several studies report radiation therapy before or after aggressive surgery will further lengthen time to first recurrence and survival.
- Consult an oncologist for latest recommendations.

MISCELLANEOUS

ZOONOTIC POTENTIAL

None

SYNONYMS

Vaccine-caused sarcoma

SEE ALSO

Fibrosarcoma

ABBREVIATIONS

- FeLV = feline leukemia virus
- FIV = feline immunodeficiency virus
- PDGF = platelet-derived growth factor

Suggested Reading

Cronin K, Page RL, Spodnick G, et al. Radiation therapy and surgery for fibrosarcoma in 33 cats. Vet Radiol Ultrasound 1998; 39:51–56.

Hershey AE, Soremno KU, Hendrick MJ, et al. Prognosis for presumed feline vaccine-associated sarcoma after excision: 61 cases (1986–1996). J Am Vet Med Assoc 2000; 216:58–61.

Kass PH, Barnes WG, Spangler WL, et al. Epidemiologic evidence for a causal relationship between vaccination and fibrosarcoma tumorigenesis in cats. J Am Vet Med Assoc 1993;203:396–405.

Morrison WB. Vaccine-associated sarcoma. In: Morrison WB, ed. Cancer in dogs and cats: medical and surgical management. Jackson, WY: Teton New Media, 2002: 461–468.

Richards J, Rodan I, Elston T, et al. 2000 Report of the American Association of Feline Practitioners and the Academy of Feline Medicine Advisory Panel on Feline Vaccines. AAFP, 2000.

Author Wallace B. Morrison
Consulting Editor Wallace B. Morrison

VACUOLAR HEPATOPATHY

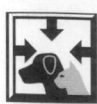

BASIC

DEFINITION
• Vacuolar glycogen hepatopathy—reversible vacuolar change in hepatocytes in dogs, associated with glucocorticoid treatment, hyperadrenocorticism (iatrogenic or spontaneous), chronic illnesses in other organs, and sex hormone abnormalities due to adrenal hyperplasia; usually typified by high ALP and GGT activity without signs of hepatic insufficiency • Similar but remarkably severe histologic changes in hepatocutaneous disease • Vacuolar hepatopathy with discrete lipid inclusions—associated with idiopathic hyperlipidemia; with combined lipid and glycogen in diabetes mellitus

PATHOPHYSIOLOGY
• Glucocorticoids—cause reversible glycogen accumulation in hepatocytes within 2–3 days of administration; injectable and respiratory forms usually induce more severe changes than do oral, topical, ocular, cutaneous, or aural applications (unless long term) • Cell swelling—leads to parenchymal enlargement and hepatomegaly • Response (dogs)—marked individual variation related to type, route, dosage, duration of treatment, and especially individual sensitivity; may develop even with low-dose, short-term oral medication • May develop with systemic diseases not related to glucocorticoid exposure or adrenal hyperplasia/neoplasia • Associated with significant non-hepatobiliary health problems that involve inflammation—suggests a relationship with stress (endogenous glucocorticoid release) or acute phase reactants

SYSTEMS AFFECTED
• Hepatobiliary—usually minimal impairment of hepatic function • Systemic effects of adrenocortical hormones or a primary systemic disease

INCIDENCE/PREVALENCE
• Dogs—common; glycogen vacuolation occurs in up to 33% of patients undergoing liver biopsy; many patients identified through laboratory and ultrasound imaging (see below) • Cats—extremely rare; vacuolation usually due to triglyceride accumulation

SIGNALMENT

Species
Dogs; rarely cats

Breed Predilections
Breeds predisposed to hyperadrenocorticism (e.g., miniature poodles, dachshunds, boxers, Boston terriers), Scottish terriers (sex hormone adrenal hyperplasia, hyperlipidemia), and others with hyperlipidemia (miniature schnauzers)

Mean Age and Range
• Middle-aged to old dogs—when caused by spontaneous hyperadrenocorticism (> 75% older than 9 years); when associated with chronic inflammation or neoplasia • Dogs of any age—iatrogenic disease subsequent to glucocorticoid administration • Young dogs—idiopathic hyperlipidemia

Predominant Sex N/A

SIGNS

General Comments
• Often related to multisystemic effects of glucocorticoids or other systemic illness causing stress • Rarely, signs of hepatic disease or failure; hepatic failure may predominate in dogs with hepatocutaneous vacuolar hepatopathy (see Diabetic Hepatopathy)

Historical Findings
• Glucocorticoid excess—polyuria and polydipsia; polyphagia; endocrine alopecia; abdominal distention; muscle weakness; panting; lethargy • Adrenal overproduction of sex hormones—endocrine alopecia with hyperpigmentation, polyuria and polydipsia, in some but not all • Other causes—depend on the affected system

Physical Examination Findings
• Hepatomegaly • Relate to glucocorticoid excess or underlying disease; depend on severity and duration

CAUSES
• Glucocorticoid administration • Hyperadrenocorticism • Adrenal hyperplasia—overproduction of multiple steroid hormones • Systemic diseases associated with an acute-phase response or stress—e.g., severe dental disease, inflammatory bowel disease, chronic pancreatitis, systemic neoplasia (especially lymphoma), chronic infections (urinary tract, skin), hypothyroidism, inborn errors of lipid metabolism (lipid or glycogen accumulation)

RISK FACTORS
• Pharmacologic doses of glucocorticoids
• Breeds at risk for hyperadrenocorticism
• Breeds at risk for hyperlipidemia—miniature schnauzers, Shetland sheepdogs, beagles

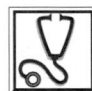

DIAGNOSIS

DIFFERENTIAL DIAGNOSES
• Most other diffuse hepatopathies (especially those causing hepatomegaly and high serum hepatic enzyme activities)—passive congestion; neoplasia (primary or metastatic to the liver); inflammatory disease; anticonvulsant hepatopathy; hepatocellular swelling associated with diabetes mellitus (lipid vacuolation); hepatic distention due to amyloid (rare) • Distinguishing features of vacuolar hepatopathy—most cases have more severe increases in serum ALP and GGT activities relative to ALT and AST; normal serum bilirubin concentration; normal to mild abnormalities in hepatic function tests (TSBA concentrations); heterogeneous or homogeneous hyperechoic liver on ultrasonography (may see nodules suggestive of "Swiss cheese" pattern); characteristic cytologic features on hepatic fine-needle aspiration and biopsy • If laboratory and clinical signs are compatible with the disorder and another underlying cause is not evident or the patient is symptomatic for adrenal disease: assess the pituitary adrenal axis, adrenal steroid hormones, and adrenal ultrasound image

CBC/BIOCHEMISTRY/URINALYSIS

CBC
• Depends on underlying disease • Nonregenerative anemia—chronic inflammation or hypothyroidism • Relative polycythemia—hyperadrenocorticism • Stress leukogram—hyperadrenocorticism; glucocorticoid treatment; stress (chronic disease) • Thrombocytosis—neoplasia; hyperadrenocorticism; splenic disease

Biochemistry
• ALP and GGT markedly high activities; ALP glucocorticoid isoenzyme consistent but does not differentiate this disorder as most other liver disorders also show this isoenzyme pattern; ALT and AST activities variable (low or very high) • Serum albumin and total bilirubin—usually normal; high bilirubin unusual and indicates another hepatobiliary or hemolytic process • Hypercholesterolemia—hyperadrenocorticism or adrenal hyperplasia; some inborn errors of lipid metabolism; hypothyroidism; pancreatitis; nephrotic syndrome

OTHER LABORATORY TESTS
• TSBA—sensitive indicators of hepatic function; random fasting values and 2-hr postprandial values often normal, but may be modestly increased (rarely > 75–100 μM/L) • Ammonia tolerance test—usually normal • ALP glucocorticoid isoenzyme—high in adrenal gland–associated vacuolar change and other diffuse hepatopathies; rules out but does not confirm adrenal gland abnormalities (most other liver disorders also show increases in this isoenzyme) • Pituitary adrenal axis—evaluate with ACTH-response test (include sex hormone profile if cortisol response inconsistent with hyperadrenocorticism); LDDST • Dexamethasone suppression test—LDDST and HDDST; may help differentiate adrenal versus primary pituitary disorder; endogenous ACTH—may help differentiate adrenal versus primary pituitary disorder; Urine cortisol:creatinine ratio—helps rule out hyperadrenocorticism; less reliable than ACTH-stimulation or LDDST as spurious high values may develop in stressed patients or in patients with non-adrenal illness; values more reliable if urine collected at home in nonstressful environment • Thyroid testing—rules out hypothyroidism • Triglyceride determinations—quantify extent of hyperlipidemia • PLI—may indicate chronic "smoldering" pancreatic or bowel inflammation

IMAGING
• Abdominal radiography—reveals hepatomegaly and possibly other underlying conditions • Thoracic radiography—may reveal lymphadenopathy, metastatic disease, cardiac or pulmonary disorders; when hyperadrenocorticism not likely • Abdominal ultrasonog-

raphy—reveals hepatomegaly and diffuse hyperechoic hepatic parenchyma or multifocal mottling; multifocal lesions may suggest nodules (Swiss cheese pattern); may disclose underlying primary visceral disease (e.g., mesenteric lymphadenopathy) and adrenal size (adrenal glands may be large with hyperadrenocorticism or chronic stress)

DIAGNOSTIC PROCEDURES
• Hepatic fine-needle aspiration cytology—22- or 25-gauge, 2.5–3.75 cm (1–1.5 in.) needle; may aspirate diffusely enlarged liver without ultrasound guidance; aspirate representative regions using ultrasound with multifocal echogenic pattern and sampling tissue with different echogenicity • Hepatic biopsy—verifies vacuolar change; excludes primary hepatic disease if other systemic diagnoses have not been made; methods: ultrasound-guided needle, laparoscopy (recommended), or laparotomy (if visceral inspections and biopsies are indicated) • Cytologic features—vacuolar distention of hepatocytes causing a "rarification" or granular and fragile appearance of the hepatocyte cytosol; bile canalicular casts may be observed; pure vacuolar change is not associated with inflammatory infiltrates; may have associated extramedullary hematopoiesis that may be misinterpreted as inflammation • Tissue culture and sensitivity testing—if suppurative inflammation suspected on aspiration cytology or biopsy; aerobic and anaerobic bacteria, fungal, as appropriate • Coagulation assessments—PT, APTT, ACT, fibrinogen, PIVKA, and mucosal bleeding time; usually normal; lack of dependable association of test findings with bleeding and low predictive capabilities of tests for iatrogenic hemorrhage recognized

PATHOLOGIC FINDINGS
• Gross—variable; normal liver; mild to moderate hepatomegaly; mild surface irregularity to marked nodularity; loss of normal lobular pattern • Microscopic—abnormalities usually pathognomonic; marked vacuolization and ballooning of hepatocytes in a zone 2 (between portal triads and hepatic venule) or 3 (adjacent to hepatic venule) or diffuse distribution; mild hepatic degeneration/necrosis; small focal aggregates of neutrophils associated with extramedullary hematopoiesis; with severe diffuse vacuolation, stromal collapse and formation of nodules surrounded by a thin reticulin rim and marked nodule formation may be seen

TREATMENT

APPROPRIATE HEALTH CARE
Outpatient—common for underlying disease

ACTIVITY Normal

DIET
• Hyperlipidemia or pancreatitis—fat restriction • Obesity—cautious energy restriction; treat primary disease

SURGICAL CONSIDERATIONS
• Depend on underlying conditions
• Adrenocortical masses may be resected
• Hypophyseal masses—resection only by experienced surgeons; if surgical experience limited, pituitary mass lesions better treated with radiation

MEDICATIONS

DRUG(S) OF CHOICE
• Depend on underlying disease • Pituitary-dependent hyperadrenocorticism or adrenal hyperplasia syndrome (abnormal sex hormones)—usually treated medically once diagnosis confirmed; op'-DDD, ketoconazole, or trilostane (latter two medications impair enzymes necessary for adrenal steroid synthesis); L-deprenyl usually ineffective • Management of causal inflammatory conditions that may require immunosuppressive or anti-inflammatory medications—use very low dosage of glucocorticoids combined with other medications (see Alternative Drugs); better choice is to avoid glucocorticoids and use alternative medications (e.g., azathioprine, mycophenolate, cyclosporine) • Neoplasia—tumor resection and/or chemotherapy and radiation • Dental disease—antibiotic therapy; appropriate dental procedures • Pyelonephritis, chronic dermatitis, or other infectious disorders—long-term antimicrobial treatment based on microbial culture and sensitivity tests • Hypothyroidism—supplemental thyroxine

CONTRAINDICATIONS
• Avoid hepatotoxic drugs • Beware of drug interactions if using ketoconzaole (impairs metabolism of certain other drugs)

PRECAUTIONS
Glucocorticoids—use caution when using these drugs in all patients; use an alternate-day protocol if possible with prednisone or prednisolone to reduce severity of induced vacuolar hepatopathy and influence on pituitary-adrenal axis (may not be advisable depending on underlying disease); use with special caution in dogs with hyperlipidemia, as there is great risk for worsening hyperlipidemia causing clinical signs (e.g., pancreatitis) and hepatocellular vacuolation

ALTERNATIVE DRUG(S)
Metronidazole, azathioprine, chlorambucil, cyclophosphamide, mycophenolate, or cyclosporine—may be considered for patients with immune-mediated disorders managed with glucocorticoids

FOLLOW-UP

PATIENT MONITORING
• Hepatomegaly—abdominal palpation; imaging with radiography or ultrasonography
• Normalizing enzymes—biochemistry
• Adrenal function—ACTH-stimulation test

to assess treatment efficacy • Neoplasia—repeat physical exam and imaging studies • Control of infection—repeat cultures • Hyperlipidemia—assess plasma lipemia, triglycerides, and cholesterol

PREVENTION/AVOIDANCE
• Limit administration of glucocorticoids to confirmed conditions requiring anti-inflammatory or immunosuppressive therapy • Use alternate-day therapy (if possible) with prednisone titrated to lowest effective dose

POSSIBLE COMPLICATIONS
Numerous—related to multisystemic effects of glucocorticoids and associated conditions

EXPECTED COURSE AND PROGNOSIS
• Most patients do not develop a symptomatic disorder, even with chronic glucocorticoid therapy. • Some patients develop very high serum enzyme activities and a symptomatic disorder persisting for weeks, even after short-term glucocorticoid therapy. • Laboratory and hepatic morphologic abnormalities are completely reversible before hepatic nodule formation by stromal dropout

MISCELLANEOUS

ASSOCIATED CONDITIONS
• Pulmonary thromboembolism and neuropathy due to hyperadrenocorticism • Pancreatitis due to hyperlipidemia

PREGNANCY
Reproductive failure with glucocorticoid excess—testicular atrophy; abnormal estrus

SYNONYMS
• Glucocorticoid hepatopathy • Steroid hepatopathy • Corticosteroid hepatopathy • Vacuolar change

SEE ALSO
• Diabetic Hepatopathy
• Hyperadrenocorticism (Cushing's Disease)
• Hyperlipidemia

ABBREVIATIONS
• ACT = activated clotting time • ACTH = adrenocorticotropic hormone • APTT = activated partial thromboplastin time • HDDST = high-dose dexamethasone suppression test • LDDST = low-dose dexamethasone suppression test • PIVKA = proteins invoked by vitamin K absence or antagonism • PLI = pancreatic lipase immunoreactivity • PT = prothrombin time • TSBA = total serum bile acids

Suggested Reading
Center SA. Hepatic lipidosis, glucocorticoid hepatopathy, vacuolar hepatopathy, storage disorders, amyloidosis and iron toxicity. In: Guilford WG, Center SA, Strombeck DR, et al., eds. Strombeck's small animal gastroenterology. 3rd ed. Philadelphia: Saunders, 1996:766–801.

Authors Keith P. Richter and Sharon Center
Consulting Editor Sharon A. Center

VAGINAL DISCHARGE

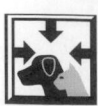 **BASICS**

DEFINITION
Any substance emanating from the vulvar labia

PATHOPHYSIOLOGY
May originate from several distinct sources, depending in part on the age and reproductive status of the patient; from urinary tract, uterus, vagina, vestibule, clitoris, or perivulvar skin; may be normal or abnormal

SYSTEMS AFFECTED
• Reproductive
• Renal/Urologic
• Skin/Exocrine

GENETICS
N/A

INCIDENCE/PREVALENCE
• Unknown
• Since there are many causes of vaginal discharge (several of which are normal processes), it would be considered a common reason for seeking veterinary attention.

GEOGRAPHIC DISTRIBUTION
N/A

SIGNALMENT
• Prepubertal bitches—anomalies and prepubertal vaginitis more common
• Estrual and postpartum bitches—normal discharges common
• Postestrual, pregnant, and postpartum bitches—may be more serious

SIGNS

Historical Findings
• Discharge from the vulva
• Spotting
• Scooting
• Attracting males
• Parturition—with postpartum discharge
• Estrus during the preceding 2 months—with pyometra

Physical Examination Findings
• Blood
• Lochia
• Pus
• Urine
• Feces

CAUSES

Serosanguinous
• Normal during proestrus and sometimes into estrus
• Urinary tract infection
• Foreign body
• Vaginal neoplasia—transmissible venereal tumor; leiomyoma
• Vaginal trauma
• Fetal death
• Vaginal hematoma
• Ovarian neoplasia

Lochia and Postpartum
• Normal postpartum discharge—for 6–8 weeks
• Subinvolution of placental sites—discharge lasting longer than 8 weeks
• Retained placentas
• Metritis

Purulent Exudate
• Normal in early diestrus (slight)
• Prepubertal vaginitis
• Primary vaginitis
• Secondary vaginitis—from anomaly, foreign body, urinary tract infection, clitoral hypertrophy, vaginal neoplasia, and fetal death
• Pyometra
• Embryonic and fetal death
• Postpartum metritis
• Perivulvar dermatitis
• Zinc toxicity—reported

Other
• Urine or feces—with congenital anomaly
• Acquired perivulvar dermatitis can also be mistaken for vaginal discharge
• Urine from ectopic ureters or incontinence from hypoestrogenism
• Normal mucus discharge during pregnancy

RISK FACTORS
• Exogenous androgens—may cause clitoral hypertrophy
• Prophylactic antibiotics—may alter the normal vaginal flora
• Exogenous estrogens given during late estrus and diestrus—predispose patient to pyometra

 DIAGNOSIS

DIFFERENTIAL DIAGNOSES
• History and signalment—establish risk of anomaly and hormonal influences (e.g., estrus, diestrus, pregnancy, and parturition)
• Source and type of the discharge—must be identified by appropriate diagnostics

CBC/BIOCHEMISTRY/URINALYSIS
• Leukocytosis with a left shift—with pyometra or metritis
• High BUN and creatinine—with pyometra
• Isosthenuria—with polyuria and polydipsia associated with pyometra
• Urinary tract infection—may be noted
• Otherwise, unremarkable

OTHER LABORATORY TESTS
• Serum progesterone concentration—determine if the bitch is in diestrus and more likely to have pyometra
• Rapid slide agglutination test—helps rule out *Brucella canis*

IMAGING
• Radiography—detects a large uterus in patients with metritis or pyometra and later stages of fetal death; cannot differentiate early pregnancy from pyometra
• Contrast radiography of the vagina—helps rule out vaginal neoplasia, urethrovaginal stricture, and rectovaginal stricture
• Ultrasonography—determines pregnancy as early as the 14th day of diestrus; heartbeats seen as early as the 20th day of diestrus; fetal heartbeats and movement rule out fetal death; fetal distress considered if fetal heart rate < 200 bpm

VAGINAL DISCHARGE

DIAGNOSTIC PROCEDURES
• Vaginal bacterial culture—via guarded culturette; perform before doing any other vaginal procedure.
• Vaginal cytologic examination—determines if the discharge is purulent, blood, or feces; extent of cornification determines the estrogen influence and helps establish whether the bitch is in proestrus or estrus.
• Vaginoscopy—reveals anomalies and bands; may need an endoscope to see the anterior vagina; cervix not usually seen by endoscopy (except possibly in large dogs); differentiates fluid emanating from the uterus from vaginal and vestibular discharges
• Digital examination of the vagina—helps identify vaginal anomalies (e.g., bands, strictures, and persistent hymen) and tumors
• Cystocentesis and bacterial culture—helps rule out urinary tract infection
• Biopsy of vaginal mass—rules out neoplasia

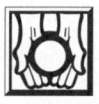

TREATMENT
• Outpatient, unless metritis or pyometra noted (ovariohysterectomy may be indicated)
• Medical treatment for pyometra—performed in a hospital and with great care
• Remove or treat any inciting cause—foreign body; neoplasia; anomaly; urinary tract infection; exogenous androgens or estrogens.
• Prepubertal vaginitis—usually resolves spontaneously after the first estrus
• Supportive fluids—for pyometra if the patient is not extremely ill; for metritis if the patient is ill
• Subinvolution of placental sites—rarely requires treatment

MEDICATIONS

DRUG(S) OF CHOICE
• Pyometra—prostaglandin and systemic antibiotics if the patient is not extremely ill (see Pyometra and Cystic Endometrial Hyperplasia)
• Prepubertal vaginitis—diethylstilbestrol to induce estrus may help; long-term effects not documented; 5 mg PO q24h for up to 7 days; day 1 of bleeding is day 1 of the induced cycle; continue treatment for an additional 2 days.
• Primary vaginitis—systemic antibiotics; vaginal douches
• Metritis—systemic antibiotics if the patient is ill
• Transmissible venereal tumor—vincristine

CONTRAINDICATIONS
Many antibiotics are contraindicated during pregnancy.

PRECAUTIONS
• Estrogens—increase the risk of pyometra if given during diestrus
• Prostaglandins—cause transient vomiting, diarrhea, and possibly hypotension

POSSIBLE INTERACTIONS
Estrogen during diestrus—associated with increased risk of pyometra

ALTERNATIVE DRUG(S)
N/A

FOLLOW-UP

PATIENT MONITORING
Ultrasonography or radiography—determine uterine size and contents with pyometra or metritis

POSSIBLE COMPLICATIONS
Toxic shock—with severe pyometra or metritis

MISCELLANEOUS

ASSOCIATED CONDITIONS
N/A

AGE-RELATED FACTORS
• Puppies—prepubertal vaginitis; anomalies; ectopic ureters
• Old animals—pyometra

ZOONOTIC POTENTIAL
B. canis—common with postpartum lochia caused by abortion or stillbirth; rare with vaginitis

PREGNANCY
Many antibiotics are contraindicated during pregnancy.

SEE ALSO
See Causes.

Suggested Reading
Bouchard G. Estrus induction in the bitch using DES. Proceedings of the Annual Meeting of the Society of Theriogenology, Kansas City, 1994:176–184.
Johnson CA. Diagnosis and treatment of chronic vaginitis in the bitch. Vet Clin North Am Small Anim Pract 1991;21:523–531.
Johnston SD, Root-Kustritz MV, Olson PN. Periparturient disorders in the bitch. In: Canine and feline theriogenology. Philadelphia: Saunders, 2001:225–242.
Memon MA, Mickelson WD. Clinical management of bitches with vaginal discharge during pregnancy. Semin Vet Med Surg Small Anim 1994;9:38–40.
Romagnoli SE, Johnston SD. Vulvar discharge. In: Allen DG, ed. Small animal medicine. Philadelphia: Lippincott, 1991:763–779.
Wykes PM, Soderberg SF. Disorders of the canine vagina. In: Morgan RV, ed. Handbook of small animal practice. 2nd ed. New York: Churchill Livingstone, 1992:661–666.
Author Bruce E. Eilts
Consulting Editor Sara K. Lyle

VAGINAL HYPERPLASIA AND PROLAPSE

BASICS

OVERVIEW
• Protrusion of spherical or donut-shaped mass from vulva during proestrus or estrus
• Type I—slight eversion of the vaginal floor but no protrusion through the vulva
• Type II—vaginal tissue prolapses through the vulvar opening (tongue-shaped mass)
• Type III—donut-shaped eversion of the entire vaginal wall, including the urethral orifice, which can be seen ventrally on the prolapsed tissue
• Exaggerated response of vaginal mucosa to estrogen
• Despite the name, the change seen histopathologically is consistent with edema rather than hyperplasia or hypertrophy
• Severe prolapse—may affect the urethra and prevent normal urination

SIGNALMENT
• Young (< 3 years of age), large-breed bitches
• Predisposed breeds—large and brachycephalic breeds (boxers, mastiffs, English bulldogs, St. Bernards); Labrador and Chesapeake Bay retrievers; German shepherds; springer spaniels; Walker hounds; Airedale terriers
• Hereditary component probable

SIGNS

Historical Findings
• Onset of proestrus or estrus
• Although rare, can be seen during diestrus or at parturition
• Licking of vulvar area
• Failure to allow copulation
• Dysuria
• Previous occurrence

Physical Examination Findings
• Protrusion of round, tongue-shaped, or donut-shaped tissue mass from the vulva
• Vaginal examination—locate lumen and urethral orifice; types I and II: lumen is dorsal to the prolapse; type III: lumen is central to the prolapse; urethral orifice is ventral to the prolapse with all three types
• Tissue may be dry or necrotic

CAUSES & RISK FACTORS
• Estrogen stimulation
• Genetic predisposition

DIAGNOSIS

DIFFERENTIAL DIAGNOSIS
• Vaginal polyp—differentiated by vaginal examination
• Vaginal neoplasia—transmissible venereal tumor and leiomyoma; differentiated by signalment, stage of cycle, and vaginal examination

CBC/BIOCHEMISTRY/URINALYSIS
N/A

OTHER LABORATORY TESTS
N/A

IMAGING
N/A

DIAGNOSTIC PROCEDURES
Biospsy (old bitch)—differentiate from neoplasia

TREATMENT
• Outpatient; unless urethral obstruction
• Breeding—possible by artificial insemination

VAGINAL HYPERPLASIA AND PROLAPSE

• Prolapsed tissue—keep clean and lubricated with sterile water-soluble lubricant
• Elizabethan collar and clean indoor environment—minimize tissue trauma
• Instruct client to monitor patient's ability to urinate
• Regression—usually begins in late estrus; should be resolved during early diestrus
• Recurrence rate—66–100% at next estrous cycle
• Ovariohysterectomy—prevents recurrence; may hasten resolution
• Severe condition—requires surgical reduction or resection; if possible, perform when the mass is beginning to regress; 25% recurrence at next cycle after surgery

 MEDICATIONS

DRUG(S)
GnRH (2.2 μg/kg IM) or hCG (1000 IU IM)—if breeding not planned that cycle; may hasten ovulation and resolution; not effective if given after ovulation

CONTRAINDICATIONS/POSSIBLE INTERACTIONS
Avoid progestational drugs, because they can induce pyometra

 FOLLOW-UP

PATIENT MONITORING
Monitor health of prolapsed tissue and the ability to urinate

PREVENTION/AVOIDANCE
Ovariohysterectomy—recommended owing to genetic component and likelihood of recurrence

POSSIBLE COMPLICATIONS
Type III—may affect urethra and prevent normal urination

EXPECTED COURSE AND PROGNOSIS
• Medical treatment—prognosis for recovery good, except with urethral involvement
• Surgical intervention for type III—prognosis good

 MISCELLANEOUS

ABBREVIATIONS
• GnRH = gonadotropin-releasing hormone
• hCG = human chorionic gonadotropin

Suggested Reading

Johnston SD. Vaginal prolapse. In: Kirk RW, ed. Current veterinary therapy X. Philadelphia: Saunders, 1989:1302–1305.
Johnston SD, Root Kustritz MV, Olson PNS. Disorders of the canine vagina, vestibule, and vulva. In: Johnston SD, Root Kustritz MV, Olson PNS, eds. Canine and feline theriogenology. Philadelphia: Saunders, 2001:225–242.
Post K, Van Haaften BV, Okkens AC. Vaginal hyperplasia in the bitch: literature review and commentary. Can Vet J 1991;32:35–37.
Wykes PM. Disease of the vagina and vulva in the bitch. In: Morrow DA, ed. Current therapy in theriogenology 2. Philadelphia: Saunders, 1986:476–481.
Author Joni L. Freshman
Consulting Editor Sara K. Lyle

VAGINAL MALFORMATIONS AND ACQUIRED LESIONS

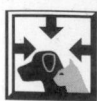 BASICS

DEFINITION
• Altered anatomic architecture owing to congenital anomalies (imperforate hymen, dorsoventral septum, hymenal constriction, and cysts) and acquired conditions (vaginal hyperplasia, foreign bodies, strictures, adhesions, and neoplasia)

PATHOPHYSIOLOGY

Congenital
• Normal embryological development—the paired paramesonephric (müllerian) ducts fuse to form the uterine body, cervix, and vagina; urogenital sinus forms the vestibule, urethra, and urinary bladder; hymen (composed of the epithelial linings of the paramesonephric ducts and urogenital sinus and an interposed layer of mesoderm) normally disappears by birth
• Errors during embryonic development—imperforate hymens; dorsoventral septa hymenal constrictions (including vestibulo-vaginal stenoses); cysts

Acquired
• Vaginal scarring—response to trauma or inflammation; with mature scarring, may note adhesions or strictures, which narrow the diameter of the vagina
• Vaginal hyperplasia (dogs)—result of an exaggerated response of the vaginal mucosa to estrogen; effect produced is edema rather than hyperplasia or hypertrophy
• Neoplastic processes—extraluminal leiomyoma most common; usually old patients; no effect of ovarian status on occurrence

SYSTEMS AFFECTED
• Reproductive—principal effect: interference with natural mating and whelping; frequent concurrent problem: vaginitis
• Renal/Urologic—ascending urinary tract infections not uncommon; may note urinary incontinence in conjunction with congenital malformations of the hymenal area (inter-relationship not understood)
• Skin/Exocrine—usually see perivulvar dermatitis secondary to vaginitis or urinary incontinence

GENETICS
Congenital—heritable component may be suspected; no direct evidence

INCIDENCE/PREVALENCE
• Incidence (congenital)—unknown; conditions may be asymptomatic, especially if the female is never used for breeding
• Prevalence (vaginal septa)—in one study, reported as 0.03% of all cases seen

SIGNALMENT

Species
Dogs and cats

Breed Predilections
• Congenital—none identified
• Vaginal hyperplasia—large breeds more prone

Mean Age and Range
• Congenital lesion (e.g., imperforate hymen, stenosis, septa)—young (< 2 years of age) intact or spayed females
• Vaginal hyperplasia—young (< 2 years of age) intact females
• Acquired lesion (adhesions and strictures)—postpubertal females of any age
• Neoplasia—mean age, 10 years; ovarian status has no effect

SIGNS

Historical Findings
• Vaginal discharge
• Excessive licking of vulva
• Frequent or inappropriate urination
• Stranguria or dyschezia
• Urinary incontinence
• Attractive to males
• Refuses mating
• Mass at vulvar labia

Physical Examination Findings
• Usually normal
• Evidence of vaginal discharge or perivulvar dermatitis common
• Hypoplastic vulva occasionally seen

CAUSES
• Congenital
• Inflammatory
• Hormonal
• Traumatic
• Neoplastic

RISK FACTORS
N/A

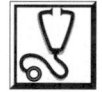 DIAGNOSIS

DIFFERENTIAL DIAGNOSIS
• Vaginitis—concurrent with many malformations; differentiated by vaginoscopy and positive contrast vaginography
• Urinary tract infection—differentiated by vaginal cytology and concurrent urinalysis on a sample collected by cystocentesis
• Pyometra—differentiated by CBC, biochemistry profiles, and abdominal ultrasonography

CBC/BIOCHEMISTRY/URINALYSIS
• CBC and biochemistry—usually normal
• Urinalysis—may show evidence of a secondary ascending urinary tract infection

OTHER LABORATORY TESTS
N/A

IMAGING

Positive-contrast Vaginography
• Defines vaginal vault to the cervix, urethra, cranial vestibule, and urinary bladder
• Defines the cervical canal and uterine lumen in intact patient in estrus
• Identifies strictures, septa, persistent hymens, masses, rectovaginal fistulas, urethrovaginal fistulas, vaginal rupture, and diverticula
• Patients should fast for 24 hours; give enema 2 hours before the procedure.
• Place patient under sedation or general anesthesia.
• Pass a balloon-tipped Foley catheter in the vestibule; inflate balloon; infuse aqueous iodinated contrast media (1 mL/kg); avoid overdistention and underdistention.
• Urinary incontinence—may require excretory urography to rule out ectopic ureters or an intrapelvically positioned bladder neck

Abdominal Ultrasonography
• Much of the vagina is not accessible owing to the bony pelvis
• Cranial vaginal masses—may occasionally be imaged
• Aid visualization by infusing saline into the vagina before examination.

DIAGNOSTIC PROCEDURES
• Order in which procedures are performed is important; they are listed here in the recommended order.
• Vaginal culture—identify secondary infections; guarded culturette recommended to avoid contamination from the vestibule and caudal vagina (see Vaginal Discharge; Vaginitis)
• Vaginal cytology—identify stage of the estrous cycle; reveal inflammatory or neoplastic cells (see Breeding, Timing)
• Digital examination of the vestibule and caudal vagina—measure the diameter; identify caudal strictures or masses; note the size and conformation of the vulva; patient standing with abdomen supported; sedation or anesthesia may be required.
• Vaginoscopy—identify strictures, adhesions, septa, diverticula, masses, and foreign bodies; may use a variety of specula; a long (16–20 cm), hollow, rigid type (e.g., infant proctoscope) with either a fiberoptic or halogen light source recommended; match the speculum's diameter to size of the patient; postcervical fold normal (obscures visualization of the external os of the cervix)
• Imaging—when results of previous procedures suggest an anatomic abnormality; vaginography and/or ultrasonography

PATHOLOGIC FINDINGS

Congenital
• Imperforate hymen—thin fenestrated membrane, dorsoventral band(s), or a thick membrane at the vestibulovaginal junction; simplest, most common defect; remainder of the genital tract normal
• Dorsoventral septum—oriented dorsoventrally in the vagina, cranial to the vestibulovaginal junction; may note a double

VAGINAL MALFORMATIONS AND ACQUIRED LESIONS

cervix (most common variant); double vagina, or divided uterine fundus (rare)
• Hymenal constriction, vaginal hypoplasia, or vaginal aplasia—moderate to severe constriction at the vestibulovaginal junction (also called vestibulovaginal stenosis); vagina, cervix, uterus, vulva may be absent or hypoplastic

Acquired
• Strictures and adhesions—may be identified anywhere in the vagina or vestibule; result of prior trauma and/or inflammation; persistent vaginitis, refusal to mate, dystocia, or problems with micturition common
• Vaginal hyperplasia and prolapse
• Vaginal neoplasia—usually leiomyoma; usually extraluminal in the wall of the vestibule; leiomyosarcomas, transmissible venereal tumors, lipomas, mast cell tumors, epidermoid carcinomas, squamous cell carcinomas, fibromas, fibrosarcomas, and invasive urinary tract carcinomas reported
• Foreign bodies—plant material, sticks, and swabs; occasionally found

TREATMENT

APPROPRIATE HEALTH CARE
• Usually outpatient, until nature of the defect is ascertained
• Inpatient—for positive contrast vaginography

NURSING CARE
Manual dilation—digitally or with a smooth rigid object; may attempt in patients that have an imperforate hymen or mild vestibulovaginal stenosis; may be performed in a sedated patient gradually over a course of several treatments; may be performed in an anesthetized patient at one time to maximal dilation; variable success; typically leads to reduction, but not complete resolution, of clinical signs

ACTIVITY
N/A

DIET
N/A

CLIENT EDUCATION
N/A

SURGICAL CONSIDERATIONS
• Resection, transection, excision—many minor congenital (e.g., imperforate hymen, small dorsoventral septa) and acquired lesions (small strictures or adhesions in the caudal portion of the vagina or masses)
• Episiotomy—usually required for adequate surgical access
• T-shaped vaginoplasty—described for vestibulovaginal stenoses; resection appears to provide superior results

• Transendoscopic laser ablation—one report for correcting a dorsoventral septum in an English bulldog that subsequently bred and delivered four pups vaginally
• Ovariohysterectomy—patient has no breeding value; exhibits signs only during estrus
• Vaginal ablation (vaginectomy cranial to the external urethral orifice) and ovariohysterectomy—patient has no breeding value; concurrent severe, refractory vaginitis at all stages of the estrous cycle

MEDICATIONS

DRUG(S) OF CHOICE
• Concurrent vaginitis—common; usually resolves with correction of the anatomic defect; for severe condition, hasten resolution with appropriate local and antibiotic therapy (see Vaginitis)
• Stenotic lesions—corticosteroids (prednisone: 1 mg/kg PO q24h) used in conjunction with manual dilation in an attempt to prevent recurrence; high recurrence rates with or without steroids

CONTRAINDICATIONS
N/A

PRECAUTIONS
N/A

POSSIBLE INTERACTIONS
N/A

ALTERNATIVE DRUG(S)
N/A

FOLLOW-UP

PATIENT MONITORING
N/A

PREVENTION/AVOIDANCE
Congenital lesions—possibly inherited, but not confirmed; for a familial line with a high number of affected individuals, recommend sterilization of affected individuals and their parents

POSSIBLE COMPLICATIONS
• Dystocia, urinary tract infections, incontinence, and vaginitis—with vaginal malformations; with patients that fail to respond to treatment
• Strictures and adhesions—may be postoperative complications of surgical procedures aimed at correcting abnormalities

EXPECTED COURSE AND PROGNOSIS
• Depend on the severity of the lesion and the degree of inflammation after treatment
• Prognosis after treatment for imperforate hymens, short dorsoventral bands, or caudal

strictures or adhesions—fair to good for improvement of clinical signs; fair to guarded for complete resolution of signs and normal fertility
• Prognosis for hymenal constrictions, vaginal hypoplasia or severe cranial strictures or adhesions—guarded to poor for complete resolution of signs and normal fertility; with concurrent severe vaginitis, the best recommendation is vaginal ablation

MISCELLANEOUS

ASSOCIATED CONDITIONS
• Urinary tract infections
• Vaginitis
• Urinary incontinence

AGE-RELATED FACTORS
• Congenital—more likely in young bitches of any ovarian status
• Vaginal hyperplasia—more likely in young intact bitches
• Neoplasia of the vagina or vestibule—more likely in old bitches of any ovarian status

ZOONOTIC POTENTIAL
N/A

PREGNANCY
• Some patients may be bred by artificial insemination; the possibility for a vaginal delivery is unlikely
• Warn owner that an elective cesarean section would probably be required

SEE ALSO
• Transmissible Venereal Tumor
• Vaginal Discharge
• Vaginal Hyperplasia and Prolapse
• Vaginitis

Suggested Reading
Johnston SD, Root Kustritz MV, Olson PNS. Disorders of the canine vagina, vestibule, and vulva. In: Canine and feline theriogenology. Philadelphia: Saunders, 2001:225–242.
Johnston SD, Root Kustritz MV, Olson PNS. Disorders of the feline vagina, vestibule, and vulva. In: Canine and feline theriogenology. Philadelphia: Saunders, 2001:472–473.
Kyles AE, Vaden S, Hardie EM, Stone EA. Vestibulovaginal stenosis in dogs: 18 cases (1987–1995). J Am Vet Med Assoc 1996; 209:1889–1893.
Root MV, Johnston SD, Johnston GR. Vaginal septa in dogs: 15 cases (1983–1992). J Am Vet Med Assoc 1995;206:56–58.
Wykes PM, Soderberg SF. Disorders of the canine vagina. In: Morgan RV, ed., Handbook of small animal practice. 2nd ed. New York: Churchill Livingstone, 1992:661–666.
Author Sara K. Lyle
Consulting Editor Sara K. Lyle

VAGINAL TUMORS

BASICS

OVERVIEW
• Second most common reproductive tumor, composing 2.4%–3.0% of all tumors in dogs
• Dogs—86% benign smooth muscle tumors (e.g., leiomyoma, fibroleiomyoma, and fibroma); lipoma, transmissible venereal tumor, mast cell tumor, squamous cell carcinoma, leiomyosarcoma, hemangiosarcoma, osteosarcoma, or extension of primary urinary tract carcinomas also reported
• Cats—extremely rare; usually of smooth muscle origin
• Hormonal influence—speculated to be involved in the etiopathogenesis

SIGNALMENT
• Dogs—mean age, 10.2–11.2 years
• Cats—no data available

SIGNS
Dogs
• Extraluminal—slow-growing perineal mass; vulvar discharge; dysuria; pollakiuria; vulvar licking; dystocia
• Intraluminal—mass protruding from the vulva (often at estrus); vulvar discharge; stranguria; dysuria; tenesmus
Cats
• Firm mass
• Constipation

CAUSES & RISK FACTORS
• Intact sexual status
• Nulliparous bitches more commonly affected

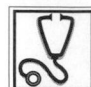

DIAGNOSIS

DIFFERENTIAL DIAGNOSIS
• Vaginal prolapse
• Urethral neoplasia
• Uterine prolapse
• Clitoral hypertrophy
• Vaginal polyp • Vaginal abscess
• Vaginal hematoma

CBC/BIOCHEMISTRY/URINALYSIS
No consistent abnormalities

OTHER LABORATORY TESTS
N/A

IMAGING
• Abdominal radiography—may detect cranial extension of a mass
• Ultrasonography, vaginography, and urethrocystography—may help delineate mass

DIAGNOSTIC PROCEDURES
• Vaginoscopy with cytologic examination of an aspirate—may help determine cell type
• Histopathologic examination—often necessary for definitive diagnosis

PATHOLOGIC FINDINGS
• Intraluminal—vestibular wall; protruding into the vulva; may occur singularly or as multiple masses
• Extraluminal—vestibular roof; causing a bulging of the perineum

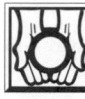

TREATMENT
• Surgical excision and concurrent ovariohysterectomy—treatment of choice
• Postoperative radiotherapy—may be of benefit for sarcoma
• Laser surgery with radiotherapy—reported anecdotally

MEDICATIONS

DRUG(S)
• Postoperative therapy—no standard established
• Doxorubicin, cisplatin, or carboplatin—rational choice to palliate malignant or metastatic disease

CONTRAINDICATIONS/POSSIBLE INTERACTIONS
• Doxorubicin—carefully monitor with underlying cardiac disease; consider pretreatment and serial echocardiograms and ECG
• Cisplatin—do not use in cats (fatal); do not use in dogs with renal disease; always use appropriate and concurrent diuresis.
• Chemotherapy may be toxic; seek advice if you are unfamiliar with chemotherapeutic drugs.

 FOLLOW-UP

PATIENT MONITORING
• Thoracic and abdominal radiographs—consider every 3 months if tumor is malignant.
• CBC (doxorubicin, cisplatin, carboplatin), biochemical profile (cisplatin), urinalysis (cisplatin)—perform before each chemotherapy treatment

EXPECTED OUTCOME AND PROGNOSIS
• Prognosis—good with complete excision; guarded if incomplete excision; poor with metastatic disease; poor with carcinoma or squamous cell tumor
• Recurrence—15% (leiomyoma) without concurrent ovariohysterectomy

 MISCELLANEOUS

• Dogs—may be an incidental finding at necropsy
• Cats—reported concurrent cystic ovaries and mammary gland adenocarcinoma

ABBREVIATION
ECG = electrocardiogram

Suggested Reading
Manithaiudom K, Johnston SD. Clinical approach to vaginal/vestibular masses in the bitch. Vet Clin North Am Small Anim Pract 1991;21:509–521.
Morrison WB. Cancers of the reproductive tract. In: Morrison WB, ed. Cancer in dogs and cats: medical and surgical management. Baltimore, Williams & Wilkins, 1998: 581–590.
Author Renee Al-Sarraf
Consulting Editor Wallace B. Morrison

VAGINITIS

BASICS

DEFINITION
Inflammation of the vagina or vestibule

PATHOPHYSIOLOGY
• Primary bacterial or viral—not common
• Generally involves a predisposing factor—anomaly; chemical irritation; neoplasia; vaginal trauma; foreign body
• Other sources of discharge—uterus; clitoris; perivulvar skin; urinary tract

SYSTEMS AFFECTED
Reproductive

GENETICS
N/A

INCIDENCE/PREVALENCE
• Not common
• Reported as 7 in 1000 cases in a 5-year period

GEOGRAPHIC DISTRIBUTION
N/A

SIGNALMENT

Species
Primarily dogs

Breed Predilection
None

Mean Age and Range
• Anomalies and prepubertal vaginitis—suspect in prepubertal bitches.
• May occur at any age, in any breed, or with any ovarian status

Predominant Sex
N/A

SIGNS

Historical Findings
• Discharge from the vulva
• Pollakiuria
• Vaginal licking
• Spotting
• Scooting
• Attracting males

Physical Examination Findings
• Discharge from the vagina
• Possibly, inflamed vulva and vagina

CAUSES
• Prepubertal vagina
• Foreign bodies
• Urinary tract infections
• Vaginal trauma
• Urine or feces contamination in patients with congenital anomaly
• May be incited by acquired problems
• Urine contamination in patients with ectopic ureters
• Incontinence owing to hypoestrogenism
• Vaginal neoplasia—transmissible venereal tumor; leiomyoma
• Bacterial—*Pasteurella; Streptococcus; E. coli; Pseudomonas; Mycoplasma; Chlamydia; Brucella canis*
• Viral—herpes
• Vaginal hematoma
• Vaginal abscess
• Exogenous androgens
• Vestibulovaginal stricture
• Zinc toxicity reported

RISK FACTORS
• Clitoral hypertrophy caused by exogenous androgens
• Alteration of normal vaginal bacterial flora owing to administration of prophylactic antibiotics that allow overgrowth of pathogenic species
• Anomalies in prepubertal bitches

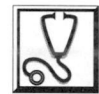

DIAGNOSIS

DIFFERENTIAL DIAGNOSES
• History and signalment—establish risk of anomaly; possibility of prepubertal vaginitis
• Normal serosanguinous discharge—during proestrus; sometimes continues into estrus
• Slight purulent exudate—may be normal in early diestrus; usually see neutrophils on cytologic examination
• Normal postpartum discharge—for up to 6–8 weeks; odorless, dark brown or bloody discharge; substantial amounts are normal for up to 4 weeks
• Subinvolution of the placental sites—when discharge lasts longer than 6–8 weeks postpartum
• Urinary tract infection
• Foreign body
• Pyometra
• Metritis
• Retained placentas
• Clitoral hypertrophy
• Embryonic or fetal death
• Urine or feces contamination owing to congenital anomaly or acquired condition
• Perivulvar dermatitis—may appear as vaginal discharge
• Urine contamination with ectopic ureter
• Incontinence owing to hypoestrogenism
• Normal mucus discharge during pregnancy
• Vaginal neoplasia—transmissible venereal tumor; leiomyoma
• Vaginal trauma
• Vaginal hematoma
• Vaginal abscess
• Ovarian neoplasia
• Zinc toxicity

CBC/BIOCHEMISTRY/URINALYSIS
• Routine laboratory tests usually within normal limits
• Voided urine samples—may note inflammatory cells

OTHER LABORATORY TESTS
• Serum progesterone concentration—determines if patient is in diestrus; slight diestrual discharge may be normal; high concentration increases possibility of pyometra or pregnancy
• Rapid slide agglutination test—helps rule out *Brucella canis*

IMAGING
• Contrast radiography of the vagina—rules out vaginal neoplasia; foreign body; vestibulovaginal, urethrovaginal, and rectovaginal stricture
• Ultrasonography—aids in identifying some intraluminal vaginal masses; distend the vagina with saline to greatly enhance visualization.

DIAGNOSTIC PROCEDURES

Vaginal Culture
• Guarded culturette
• Perform before any other vaginal procedure.
• Only 5% of normal bitches that were cultured repeatedly had negative cultures.
• Most common vaginal isolates from normal and infertile bitches—*Pasteurella; Streptococcus*
• Less common isolates—*E. coli; Staphylococcus*
• Most common mixed culture—*Pasteurella, Streptococcus,* and *E. coli*
• Most common pure culture—*Pasteurella*
• More organisms usually grow during estrus than at other stages of the estrus cycle, but the types do not change.

Vaginal Cytologic Examination
• Determine if the discharge is pus, blood, or feces
• Septic inflammation—seen in older patients
• Extent of cornification—determines the estrogen influence; helps establish if the patient is in proestrus or estrus and if the discharge is normal

Vaginoscopy
• Detects an anomaly, band, mass, foreign body, hematoma, abscess, or inflamed vagina or vestibule

- Endoscope—may be needed to see anterior vagina
- Cannot normally see cervix by endoscopy, except possibly in large dogs
- Determines the most cranial origin of the discharge—differentiates uterine from vaginal and vestibular sources

Other
- Digital examination of the vagina—identify vaginal anomalies such as bands, strictures, or persistent hymen; palpate tumors.
- Biopsy of vaginal masses—rule out neoplasia.

PATHOLOGIC FINDINGS
N/A

TREATMENT

APPROPRIATE HEALTH CARE
- Usually treated as outpatients
- Inpatient—surgical management of anatomic anomalies, foreign bodies, or neoplasia

NURSING CARE
N/A

ACTIVITY
Not altered

DIET
Not altered

CLIENT EDUCATION
- Inform client that prepubertal vaginitis normally resolves after the first estrus and that antibiotic therapy is not needed.
- Inform client that vaginitis in adults is often associated with a correctable predisposing factor.
- Discuss ovariohysterectomy and isolation of patients infected with *B. canis.*
- Inform client that exogenous androgens and estrogens must be removed.

SURGICAL CONSIDERATIONS
- Remove or treat any inciting causes—foreign body; neoplasia; anomaly.
- Vaginectomy—has been used in refractory patients

MEDICATIONS

DRUG(S) OF CHOICE

Primary Vaginitis
- Appropriate systemic antibiotics—normally eradicate susceptible bacteria within 24 hours

- Vaginal douches—0.05% chlorhexidine or 0.5% povidone-iodine, twice daily until the discharge resolves; reported to be beneficial

Prepubertal Vaginitis
- Estrus induction—may be helpful; long-term effects not documented
- DES—5 mg PO q24h for up to 7 days; count day 1 of bleeding as day 1 of induced cycle; continue treatment for an additional 2 days; may help persistent condition in patients that were spayed before puberty

CONTRAINDICATIONS
Many antibiotics are contraindicated during pregnancy.

PRECAUTIONS
Estrogens given during diestrus increase the chance of pyometra.

POSSIBLE INTERACTIONS
- Exogenous estrogen administered during diestrus
- Exogenous androgen

ALTERNATIVE DRUG(S)
Prepubertal—estrus induction with DES may help refractory cases; long-term effects not documented

FOLLOW-UP

PATIENT MONITORING
- Prepubertal patients—re-examine after the first estrus or physical maturity.
- Mature patients with no predisposing factors—re-examine after a 14-day course of antibiotics.
- If condition persists—reevaluate for an underlying or another cause; perform another vaginal bacterial culture and sensitivity test.

PREVENTION/AVOIDANCE
Because some cases become refractory after the patient is spayed, there may be some rationale for delaying ovariohysterectomy until after the first estrus in prepubertal patients with a chronic condition.

POSSIBLE COMPLICATIONS N/A

EXPECTED COURSE AND PROGNOSIS
- Prepubertal—normally resolves after the first estrus

- Adults—usually resolves if the causative factor is removed; antibiotic therapy and vaginal douches may hasten recovery of uncomplicated chronic cases to within 2 weeks.

MISCELLANEOUS

ASSOCIATED CONDITIONS
N/A

AGE-RELATED FACTORS
Puppies—prepubertal vaginitis, anomalies, and ectopic ureters

ZOONOTIC POTENTIAL
B. canis—rare in patients with vaginitis, but should be considered

PREGNANCY
Many antibiotics are contraindicated during pregnancy.

SYNONYMS
N/A

SEE ALSO
See Causes.

ABBREVIATION
DES = diethylstilbestrol

Suggested Reading
Bjurström L, Linde-Forsberg C. Long-term study of aerobic bacteria of the genital tract in breeding bitches. Am J Vet Res 1992; 53:665–669.
Holt PE, Sayle, B. Congenital vestibulovaginal stenosis in the bitch. J Small Anim Pract 1988;22:67–75.
Johnson CA. Diagnosis and treatment of chronic vaginitis in the bitch. Vet Clin North Am Small Anim Pract 1991;21:523–531.
Strom B, Linde-Forsberg C. Effects of ampicillin and trimethoprim-sulfamethoxazole on the vaginal bactrial-flora of bitches. Am J Vet Res 1993;54:891–896.
van Duijkeren E. Significance of the vaginal bacterial flora in the bitch: a review. Vet Rec 1992;131:367–369.
Wykes PM, Soderberg SF. Disorders of the canine vagina. In: Morgan RV, ed. Handbook of small animal practice. 2nd ed. New York: Churchill Livingstone, 1992:661–666.

Author Bruce E. Eilts
Consulting Editor Sara K. Lyle

VASCULAR RING ANOMALIES

 **BASICS**

OVERVIEW

Right Aortic Arch
• Entrapment of the esophagus by a persistent right fourth aortic arch (dextropositioned aorta) on the right and dorsally, the base of the heart and pulmonary artery ventrally, and ductus or ligamentum arteriosum on the left and dorsally
• Causes megaesophagus cranial to the obstruction at the base of the heart

Double Aortic Arch
• Entrapment of the esophagus by a functional aortic arch on the right, an atretic aortic arch on the left, the base of the heart and pulmonary artery ventrally, and ductus or ligamentum arteriosum on the left and dorsally
• Causes megaesophagus cranial to the obstruction at the base of the heart; also causes some tracheal compression

SIGNALMENT
• Dogs and cats
• Seen most commonly in German shepherds, Irish setters, and Boston terriers

SIGNS
• Regurgitation of undigested solid food in animals < 6 months old
• Malnourishment in many animals
• Time between eating and regurgitation varies
• Signs of aspiration pneumonia (e.g., cough, tachypnea or dyspnea) in some animals

CAUSES & RISK FACTORS
N/A

 DIAGNOSIS

DIFFERENTIAL DIAGNOSIS
• Congenital megaesophagus
• Stricture, diverticulum, or esophageal foreign body
• Esophageal motility disorder in shar-peis

CBC/BIOCHEMISTRY/URINALYSIS
• Results usually normal
• High WBC in some animals with aspiration pneumonia

OTHER LABORATORY TESTS
N/A

IMAGING
• Thoracic radiography—shows food-filled cranial esophagus or signs of aspiration pneumonia in some animals
• Contrast esophagography—confirms megaesophagus extending to the heart base
• Fluoroscopy—may be used to differentiate esophageal motility disorders
• Angiography—may be needed to differentiate between specific vascular ring anomalies

OTHER DIAGNOSTIC PROCEDURES
Esophagoscopy can be used to differentiate esophageal motility disorders.

 TREATMENT
• Surgical correction of the vascular entrapment is indicated.
• Medical management of concurrent aspiration pneumonia may be necessary.
• Feeding procedures for megaesophagus may also be necessary for a prolonged period.
• Supportive care with oxygen may be needed in animal with aspiration pneumonia.

 MEDICATIONS

DRUG(S)
Broad-spectrum antibiotics, such as enrofloxacin (2.5 mg/kg q12h) and amoxicillin (10–15 mg/kg q12h) should be instituted in animals with aspiration pneumonia.

CONTRAINDICATIONS/POSSIBLE INTERACTIONS
N/A

 **FOLLOW-UP**

EXPECTED COURSE AND PROGNOSIS
• Prognosis for resolution of the problem, even after surgery, is guarded to poor.
• Complications of malnourishment and aspiration pneumonia are common and severe.
• Esophageal function is often permanently compromised.

Suggested Reading
Bonagura JD, Lehmkuhl LB. Congenital heart disease. In: Fox PR, Sisson D, Moise NS, eds. Textbook of canine and feline cardiology. 2nd ed. Philadelphia: Saunders, 1999:471–535.
Goodwin J. Double aortic arch. In: Tilly LP, Smith FWK, eds. The 5-minute veterinary consult. 2nd ed. Philadelphia: Lippincott Williams & Wilkins, 2000:636.

Author Carroll Loyer
Consulting Editors Larry P. Tilley and Francis W. K. Smith, Jr.

BASICS

OVERVIEW
- An inflammation of blood vessels with a neutrophilic (leukocytoclastic/nonleukocytoclastic), lymphocytic, rarely eosinophilic, granulomatous, or mixed cell type
- Pathomechanisms—type III (immune complex) and type I (immediate) reactions

SIGNALMENT
- Any age, breed, or sex may be affected.
- Dachshunds and rottweilers may be predisposed.
- Varies depending on cause

SIGNS
- Palpable purpura
- Hemorrhagic bullae
- Necrosis and "punched out" ulcers
- Affects the extremities (paws, pinnae, lips, tail, and oral mucosa) and may be painful
- Anorexia, depression, pyrexia, pitting edema of the extremities, polyarthropathy, and myopathy—depend on the underlying cause

CAUSES & RISK FACTORS
- Idiopathic
- Drug-induced
- Vaccine-induced (especially rabies vaccine)
- Food hypersensitivities
- Tick-borne diseases—Rocky Mountain spotted fever, ehrlichiosis, Lyme's disease
- Autoimmune
- Neoplasia

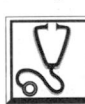

DIAGNOSIS

DIFFERENTIAL DIAGNOSIS
- See Causes & Risk Factors
- Ear margin seborrhea, chemical and thermal burns, toxic epidermal necrolysis, erythema multiforme, and sepsis

CBC/BIOCHEMISTRY/URINALYSIS
Usually normal

OTHER LABORATORY TESTS
- Sepsis, disseminated intravascular coagulation, systemic lupus erythematosus, Rocky Mountain spotted fever, and rheumatoid arthritis—abnormalities may be noted
- Consider serologic testing for parasitic and infectious disease in high-risk areas.
- Consider immunodiagnostics—ANA titer, Coombs test and cold agglutinin tests

IMAGING
N/A

DIAGNOSTIC PROCEDURES
- Skin scrapings—possible demodicosis (with secondary sepsis)
- Biopsy of early lesion—submit to a dermatopathologist; findings depend on the underlying cause, but usually include neutrophilic (leukocytoclastic/nonleukocytoclastic), lymphocytic, eosinophilic, or granulomatous, mixed cells in and around the vessels; vascular necrosis and fibrin thrombi may be prominent; perivascular hemorrhage and edema may occur
- Vasculitis—perform representative cultures (blood, urine, skin, etc.) if CBC, chemistry screen, or urinalysis reveal systemic disease.

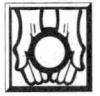

TREATMENT
- Underlying disease—first priority in clinical management
- No systemic abnormalities—treat as outpatient with no alterations in food or water intake
- Systemic disease—inpatient care must be recommended
- Inform owner that the prognosis is guarded until a cause is found; prognosis is based on the cause.

MEDICATIONS

DRUG(S)
- First line of therapy while awaiting histopathology results, if no drug reaction is suspected—antibiotics
- Immune-mediated disease with concurrent vasculitis—prednisone (2–4 mg/kg q24h)
- No known underlying cause or prednisolone alone does not work—try dapsone (1 mg/kg q8h) or sulfasalazine (20–40 mg/kg q8h).
- Pentoxifylline 15 mg/kg PO TID. Trental® thought to have fewer side effect than generics
- Alkylating agents including chlorambucil and azathioprine have been added to regimens to decrease the need for corticosteroids.

CONTRAINDICATIONS/POSSIBLE INTERACTIONS
- Dapsone and sulfasalazine—not recommended with pre-existing renal disease, hepatic disease, or blood dyscrasias

- Sulfasalazine—not recommended with pre-existing or borderline keratoconjunctivitis sicca; use with caution in cats; may displace highly protein-bound drugs (e.g., methotrexate, warfarin, phenylbutazone, thiazide diuretics, salicylates, probenecid, and phenytoin); bioavailability decreased by antacids; may decrease bioavailability of folic acid or digoxin; blood levels may be decreased if concurrently administering ferrous sulfate or other iron salts
- Pentoxifylline—may increase prothrombin times; may decrease blood pressure

FOLLOW-UP
- Patients receiving prednisolone or dapsone—initially monitor every 2 weeks with a CBC, chemistry screen, and urinalysis; if a specific underlying disease is found, then monitor appropriately.
- If no underlying disease is found, vasculitis may be difficult to treat and the prognosis is guarded.
- Immunosuppressive therapies should always be reduced to the lowest possible therapeutic dose.

MISCELLANEOUS

PREGNANCY
- Corticosteroids and dapsone—do not use in pregnant animals
- Sulfasalazine—use during pregnancy only when absolutely necessary

ABBREVIATION
- ANA = antinuclear antibody

Suggested Reading

Greek JS. New therapeutics in dermatology. Vet Med 1996.

Marsella R, Nicklin CF, Munson JW, Roberts SM. Pharmacokinetics of pentoxifylline in dogs after oral and intravenous administration. Am J Vet Res 2000;61(6):631–637.

Mueller GH, Kirk RW, Scott DW, eds. Small animal dermatology. 4th ed. Philadelphia: Saunders, 1989.

Nichols PR, Morris DO, Beale KM. A retrospective study of canine and feline cutaneous vasculitis. Vet Derm 2001;12(5):255–264.

Authors Karen A. Kuhl and Jean S. Greek
Consulting Editor Karen Helton Rhodes

VASCULITIS, SYSTEMIC

BASICS

OVERVIEW
• Blood vessel inflammation caused by endothelial injury or extension of adjacent inflammation or infection • Endothelial damage by infectious agent, parasite infestation, endotoxin, or immune complex deposition initiates local inflammation, neutrophil accumulation, and complement activation. Neutrophils release lysosomal enzymes, leading to necrosis of vessel wall, thrombosis, and hemorrhage. In humans and dogs with polyarteritis nodosa, intimal proliferation and vessel wall degeneration and necrosis predominate and lead to hemorrhage, thrombosis, and necrosis of involved vessels and adjacent tissues in most patients. • Nondermal vasculitis (e.g., renal, hepatic, and serosal surfaces of body cavities) may be the mechanism leading to development of clinically apparent signs of systemic disease (e.g., polyarthritis and proteinuria) without causing obvious external lesions.

SIGNALMENT
Dogs and cats

SIGNS

Historical Findings
• Provocative drug (e.g., penicillin, sulfonamides, streptomycin, and hydralazine) given to sensitized animal • Exposure to ticks • Poor dirofilariasis prophylaxis in endemic area

Physical Examination Findings
• Swelling • Ulceration • Necrosis of affected skin, especially mucous membranes, mucocutaneous junctions, pinnae edges, and footpads • Systemic signs reflecting organ involvement (e.g., hepatic, renal, and CNS) • Systemic signs of illness (e.g., lethargy, lymphadenopathy, pyrexia, vague signs of pain, and weight loss) • Cutaneous lesions of polyarteritis nodosa (subcutaneous nodules—less common in dogs than in people) • Signs associated with underlying infectious or immune-related disease (e.g., thrombocytopenia and polyarthropathy)

CAUSES & RISK FACTORS

Infectious
• Parasitic (i.e., heart and pulmonary arteries)—*Dirofilaria immitis, Angiostrongylus vasorum*
• Viral—e.g., feline infectious peritonitis and canine coronavirus infection
• Rickettsial—e.g., Rocky Mountain spotted fever and ehrlichiosis
• Bacterial—sepsis

Immune-related
• Systemic lupus erythematosus • Rheumatoid arthritis–like arthropathy • Lupus-like drug reaction • Type III hypersensitivities (e.g., to food, sulfonamides, and penicillin) • Polyarteritis nodosa • Neoplasia • Uremia

DIAGNOSIS

DIFFERENTIAL DIAGNOSIS
• Cutaneous signs developing after administration of medication implicate drug reaction (usually not immediate, may develop after days or weeks).
• Vasculitis associated with polyarthropathy and pyrexia implicates immune or infectious cause.
• Cold hemagglutinin disease suggested by distribution of cyanotic or necrotic lesions (nose, ears, toes, tail tip, prepuce) and history of exposure to cold

CBC/BIOCHEMISTRY/URINALYSIS
Results depend on underlying disease

OTHER LABORATORY TESTS
• Serologic tests may aid diagnosis of tick-related (i.e., rickettsial) disease
• ANA titer positive in patient with SLE, may also be positive in patients with other systemic illnesses
• Occult heartworm test positive in patient with dirofilariasis
• *Angiostrongylus* infestation diagnosed by fecal examination and cytologic examination of tracheal wash

IMAGING
Radiographs help diagnose dirofilariasis and *Angiostrongylus* infection.

DIAGNOSTIC PROCEDURES
• Skin biopsy specimen from edge of developing lesion may be diagnostic for vasculitis but may not reveal cause.
• Immunofluorescence test of skin biopsy specimen may rule out pemphigus and pemphigoid diseases.
• If allergic response is suspected, resolution of signs upon discontinuation of suspect medication or food supports diagnosis.

 TREATMENT
• Usually resolution of underlying condition and supportive care
• If untreatable or unknown underlying condition—glucocorticoid, immunosuppressive (e.g., cyclophosphamide, azathioprine), and other drugs (e.g., dapsone and sulfasalazine) are occasionally effective, but clinical trials of efficacy have not been reported in animals.

 MEDICATIONS

DRUG(S)
• Infectious or immune-related—treat underlying disease (see specific condition); supportive care

• Lupus-like drug reactions—discontinue drug; supportive care
• Type III hypersensitivity—discontinue drug; supportive care
• Polyarteritis nodosa—glucocorticoids and cyclophosphamide (unknown value)
• "Idiopathic" vasculitis—if other causes have been ruled out, administer dapsone (1 mg/kg PO q8h for 14 days, then 1 mg/kg PO q12h for 14 days, then 1 mg/kg PO q24h; may eventually be decreased to q48h to maintain remission); alternative—sulfasalazine (45 mg/kg PO q8h). Neither drug's effectiveness is well documented. Pentoxifylline has been used in limited numbers of cases at doses of 400 mg q 24 to 48 hr. Immunosuppressive doses of corticosteroids may be helpful in idiopathic cases.

CONTRAINDICATIONS/POSSIBLE INTERACTIONS
• Do not administer sulfasalazine to patients sensitive to sulfonamides.
• Pentoxifylline is a methylxanthine derivative and may reduce blood pressure.

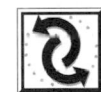 **FOLLOW-UP**
• Patients undergoing treatment with dapsone—monitor CBC and liver enzymes for side effects (e.g., hemolytic anemia, methemoglobinemia, and hepatopathy)

• Patients undergoing treatment with sulfasalazine—monitor for keratoconjunctivitis sicca, blood dyscrasias, and hepatopathy

 MISCELLANEOUS

SEE ALSO
• Leukocytoclastic vasculitis
• Lupus erythematosus, systemic
• Pemphigus
• Vasculitis, cutaneous

ABBREVIATIONS
• ANA = antinuclear antibody
• CNS = central nervous system
• SLE = systemic lupus erythematosus

Suggested Reading
Greek JS. New therapeutics in dermatology. Vet Med Nov 1996;91:90.
Suter PF, Fox PR. Peripheral vascular disease. In: Ettinger SJ, Feldman EC, eds. Textbook of veterinary internal medicine. 4th ed. Philadelphia: Saunders, 1995:1068–1083.
Author Jean S. Greek
Consulting Editors Larry P. Tilley and Francis W. K. Smith, Jr.

VENTRICULAR FIBRILLATION

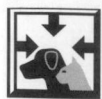 **BASICS**

DEFINITION
Ventricular rhythm associated with loss of organized ventricular activity resulting in cardiac muscle fibrillation

ECG Features
• Rapid, chaotic, irregular rhythm with bizarre waves or oscillations (Figures 1 and 2)
• No P waves
• No QRS complexes
• Oscillations may be large (coarse fibrillation) or small (fine fibrillation)

PATHOPHYSIOLOGY
Loss of organized ventricular activity results in acute and profound drop in cardiac output, usually followed by death.

SYSTEMS AFFECTED
• Cardiovascular
• All organ systems affected by loss of perfusion

GENETICS
N/A

INCIDENCE/PREVALENCE
Unknown

GEOGRAPHIC DISTRIBUTION
None

SIGNALMENT

Species
Dogs and cats

Breed Predilection
None

Mean Age and Range
Unknown, but probably more common in old animals

SIGNS

Historical Findings
• Severe systemic illness or cardiac disease in many patients
• Previous cardiac arrhythmias in some patients

Physical Examination Findings
• Cardiac arrest
• Collapse
• Death

CAUSES
• Anoxia
• Aortic stenosis
• Autonomic imbalances, especially high sympathetic tone or administration of catecholamines
• Cardiac surgery
• Drug reactions—e.g., anesthetic agents, especially halothane and ultrashort-acting barbiturates, digoxin
• Electrical shock
• Electrolyte and acid–base imbalances
• Hypothermia
• Myocardial injury
• Myocarditis
• Shock

RISK FACTORS
Any severe systemic illness or heart disease

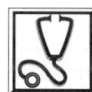 **DIAGNOSIS**

DIFFERENTIAL DIAGNOSIS
Rule out ECG artifact. Reapply ECG clips and ensure good skin contact and adequate alcohol applied to leads.

CBC/BIOCHEMISTRY/URINALYSIS
Abnormalities generally relate to the underlying metabolic problem that causes ventricular fibrillation

OTHER LABORATORY TESTS
N/A

IMAGING
N/A

DIAGNOSTIC PROCEDURES
N/A

PATHOLOGIC FINDINGS
N/A

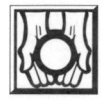 **TREATMENT**

APPROPRIATE HEALTH CARE
• Rapidly fatal rhythm requiring immediate, aggressive treatment
• Patient will probably die without electrical cardioversion.

Direct Current Defibrillation
• External countershock—50–100 watt-sec (small patients); 100–360 watt-sec (large patients)
• Internal countershock—10–25 watt-sec (small patients); 25–100 watt-sec (large patients)
• Repeat twice if first attempts fail.
• Start at the low end and increase power with each shock.
• If no access to electrical defibrillator, administer a precordial thump. Apply a sharp blow

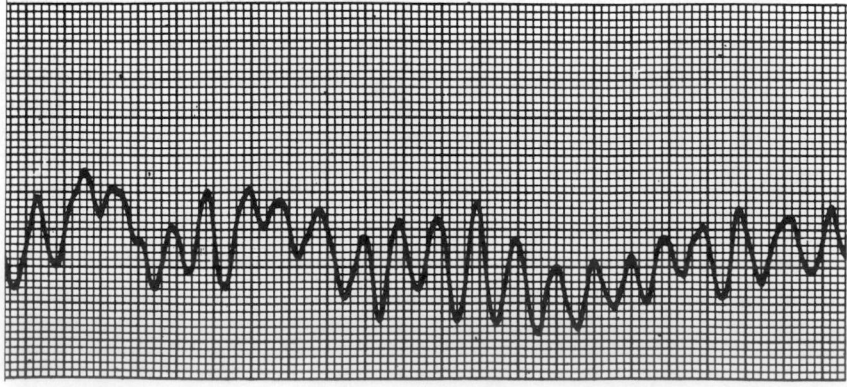

Figure 1.

Coarse ventricular fibrillation. (From: Tilley LP: Essentials of canine and feline electrocardiography. 3rd ed. Baltimore: Williams & Wilkins, 1992, with permission.)

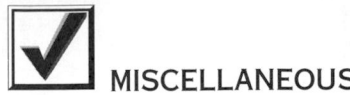

with your open fist to the chest wall over the heart. Rarely successful, but you have nothing to lose.

NURSING CARE
Treat any problems such as hypothermia, hyperkalemia, and acid–base disorders.

ACTIVITY
N/A

DIET
N/A

CLIENT EDUCATION
If the patient is converted back to a sinus rhythm, warn the owner that the patient is at high risk for recurrence of the arrhythmia in the immediate postresuscitation period.

SURGICAL CONSIDERATIONS
N/A

MEDICATIONS

DRUG(S) OF CHOICE
• Institute CPCR.
• Epinephrine (0.2 mg/kg IV, IT, IL; double the dose and dilute with equal volume of saline for IT administration)—may change fine fibrillation to coarse fibrillation and increase the chances of electrical cardioversion
• Once animal is successfully converted, administer lidocaine to lower the risk of refibrillation or development of ventricular tachycardia.

CONTRAINDICATIONS
None

PRECAUTIONS
Lidocaine raises the fibrillation threshold, but makes defibrillation more difficult.

POSSIBLE INTERACTIONS
Bretylium is recommended in humans to treat recurrent ventricular fibrillation, but in dogs and cats this drug may precipitate ventricular arrhythmias, including ventricular fibrillation.

ALTERNATIVE DRUG(S)
Chemical conversion can be attempted if no access to electrical defibrillator. Administer 1.0 mEq potassium/kg and 6.0 mg acetyl-choline/kg IC; rarely successful

FOLLOW-UP

PATIENT MONITORING
• CBC, urinalysis, biochemistry profile, arterial blood gases, and acid–base status
• If primary cardiac disease is suspected—echocardiogram and thoracic radiographs
• Monitor ECG closely and frequently.

PREVENTION/AVOIDANCE
Careful monitoring of critically ill patients to prevent and correct acid–base disturbances, hypotension, and hypoxemia

POSSIBLE COMPLICATIONS
• Death
• DIC and multiorgan failure

EXPECTED COURSE AND PROGNOSIS
Most patients die because of either the arrhythmia or the underlying disease.

✓ MISCELLANEOUS

ASSOCIATED CONDITIONS
None

AGE-RELATED FACTORS
None

ZOONOTIC POTENTIAL
None

PREGNANCY
N/A

SYNONYMS
None

SEE ALSO
Cardiopulmonary Arrest

ABBREVIATIONS
• CPCR = cardiopulmonary cerebral resuscitation
• DIC = disseminated intravascular coagulation
• IC = intracardiac
• IL = intralingual
• IT = intratracheal

Suggested Reading
Crowe DT, Fox PR, Devey JJ, Spreng D. Cardiopulmonary and cerebral resuscitation. In: Fox PR, Sisson D, Moise NS, eds. Textbook of canine and feline cardiology. 2nd ed. Philadelphia: Saunders, 1999: 427–454.
Tilley LP. Essentials of canine and feline electrocardiography. 3rd ed. Baltimore: Williams & Wilkins, 1992.
Author Francis W. K. Smith, Jr.
Consulting Editors Larry P. Tilley and Francis W. K. Smith, Jr.

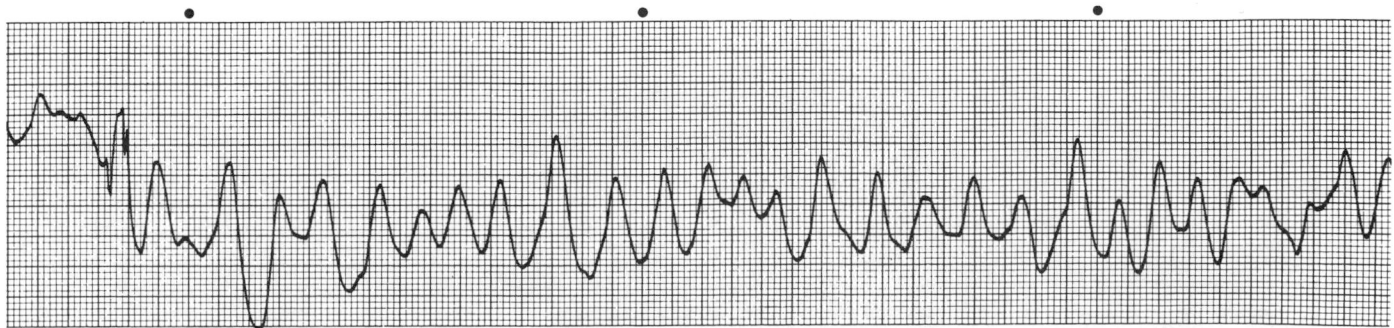

Figure 2.

Ventricular flutter-fibrillation in a cat with severe myocardial damage from an 11-story fall. The complexes are very wide, bizarre, tall, and rapid. (From: Tilley LP: Essentials of canine and feline electrocardiography. 3rd ed. Baltimore: Williams & Wilkins, 1992, with permission.)

VENTRICULAR PREMATURE COMPLEXES

 **BASICS**

DEFINITION
Single cardiac impulse initiated within the ventricles instead of the sinus node

ECG Features
• QRS complexes typically wide and bizarre (Figures 1 and 2)
• P waves dissociated from the QRS complexes

PATHOPHYSIOLOGY
Mechanisms include increased automaticity, reentry, and delayed afterdepolarizations.

SYSTEMS AFFECTED
Cardiovascular—secondary effects on other systems because of poor perfusion

GENETICS
N/A

INCIDENCE/PREVALENCE
Unknown

GEOGRAPHIC DISTRIBUTION
N/A

SIGNALMENT

Species
Dog and cat

Breed Predisposition
• Common in large-breed dogs with cardio-myopathy, especially boxers and Doberman pinschers
• Inherited ventricular arrythmia in German shepherds
• Common in cats with cardiomyopathy; occasionally seen in cats with hyperthyroidism

Mean Age and Range
Seen in all age groups

SIGNS

Historical Findings
• Weakness
• Exercise intolerance
• Syncope
• Sudden death
• Often asymptomatic

Physical Examination Findings
• Irregular rhythm associated with pulse deficits; may auscult splitting of the first or second heart sound
• May be normal if arrhythmia is intermittent and absent during examination
• May observe signs of CHF (e.g., cough, dyspnea) or murmur, depending on the cause of arrhythmia

CAUSES
• Cardiomyopathy
• Congenital defects (especially subaortic stenosis)
• Chronic valve disease
• Gastric dilitation and volvulus
• Traumatic myocarditis (dogs)
• Digitalis toxicity
• Hyperthyroidism (cats)
• Cardiac neoplasia
• Myocarditis
• Pancreatitis

RISK FACTORS
• Hypokalemia
• Hypomagnesemia
• Acid–base disturbances
• Hypoxia

 DIAGNOSIS

DIFFERENTIAL DIAGNOSIS
• Supraventricular premature beats with bundle branch block
• Look for P waves associated with the wide QRS complexes; an atrial premature complex with aberrant conduction has an associated P wave.
• An atrial premature complex is usually followed by a noncompensatory pause.
• A ventricular premature complex is usually followed by a compensatory pause (Fig. 1).

CBC/BIOCHEMISTRY/URINALYSIS
• Hypokalemia and hypomagnesemia predispose animals to ventricular arrhythmias and blunt the response to class 1 antiarrhythmic drugs (e.g., lidocaine, procainamide, mexiletine, and quinidine).
• High amylase and lipase if condition is secondary to pancreatitis

OTHER LABORATORY TESTS
High T_4 (cats) if condition is secondary to hyperthyroidism

IMAGING
Echocardiography may reveal structural heart disease.

DIAGNOSTIC PROCEDURES
Long-term ambulatory (Holter) recording of the ECG to detect transient ventricular arrhythmias in patients with unexplained syncope or weakness

PATHOLOGIC FINDINGS
Vary with underlying cause

 TREATMENT

APPROPRIATE HEALTH CARE
Generally outpatient basis

NURSING CARE
Varies with underlying cause

ACTIVITY
Restrict if the arrhythmia is accompanied by clinical signs or evidence of structural heart disease.

DIET
N/A

CLIENT EDUCATION
Alert owner to potential for the arrhythmia worsening and syncope or sudden death.

SURGICAL CONSIDERATIONS
• Continuous ECG monitoring recommended while anesthetized
• Premedicating the patient with acepromazine (0.02–0.05 mg/kg) raises the threshold for ventricular fibrillation.
• Mask inductions not recommended; sympathetic release during mask induction can aggravate arrhythmia.

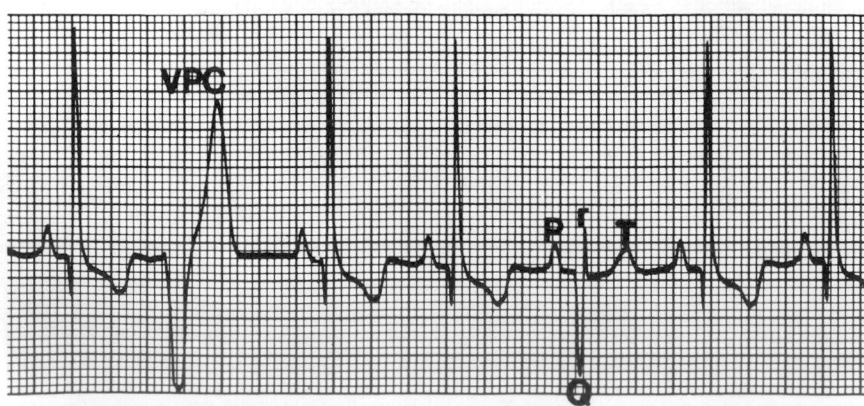

Figure 1.

VPC and a fusion complex (fifth complex) in a dog with myocarditis from a pancreatitis. A fusion complex is the simultaneous activation of the ventricle by impulses coming from the SA node and the ventricular ectopic foci. The QRS complex is intermediate in form. (From: Tilley LP: Essentials of canine and feline electrocardiography. 3rd ed. Baltimore: Williams & Wilkins, 1992, with permission.)

MEDICATIONS

DRUG(S) OF CHOICE

General Comments
• Correct any hypokalemia or hypomagnesemia.
• Drug therapy in the absence of clinical signs—controversial; studies in humans with asymptomatic VPCs and myocardial infarctions demonstrated a high incidence of sudden death when treatment is initiated with class 1 antiarrhythmic agents; no similar studies in veterinary patients
• The author generally does not prescribe antiarrhythmic drugs unless there is evidence of clinical signs of low cardiac output (e.g. episodic weakness or syncope) or the belief that the patient is at high risk of sudden death, based on presence of R on T phenomenon or breed association with VPCs and sudden death (e.g., boxers and Doberman pinschers).
• If antiarrhythmic therapy is initiated in an attempt to lower the risk of sudden death, the author usually chooses a β-blocker; no studies have been done to confirm efficacy of β-blockers for prevention of sudden death in dogs or cats.

Dogs
• Patient not in CHF or hypotensive—initiate therapy with a β-blocker such as propranolol (0.2–1 mg/kg PO q8h), atenolol (0.2–1 mg/kg q12h), or metoprolol (0.2–1 mg/kg PO q8–12h).
• Patient in CHF or hypotensive—initiate therapy with a class I antiarrhythmic agent such as procainamide (8–20 mg/kg PO q6–8h) or mexiletine (5–8 mg/kg PO q8h).
• Combine a class I antiarrhythmic drug with a β-blocker if important arrhythmia persists.

Cats
Atenolol (6.25 mg PO q12h)

CONTRAINDICATIONS
Avoid atropine, catecholamines (e.g., epinephrine and dopamine) until arrhythmia is controlled.

PRECAUTIONS
• Use β-blockers cautiously in animals with CHF; they initially depress myocardial contractility.
• Use digoxin cautiously; it can potentially aggravate ventricular arrhythmias.
• Drugs that prolong the action potential (e.g., sotalol) may worsen arrythmia in German shepherds with inherited ventricular arrhythmia.

POSSIBLE INTERACTIONS
Quinidine and amiodarone raise serum digoxin levels.

ALTERNATIVE DRUG(S)
• Consider sotalol (1–3.5 mg/kg PO q12h) or amiodarone (5–10 mg/kg PO q12h) for refractory arrhythmias in dogs (generally reserved for ventricular tachycardia).
• Consider sotalol (10–20 mg/cat PO q12h) or procainamide (3–8 mg/kg PO q6–8h) for cats that do not tolerate β-blockers.

FOLLOW-UP

PATIENT MONITORING
• Holter monitoring preferred for monitoring severity of the arrhythmia and efficacy of antiarrhythmic therapy; the goal of antiarrhythmic therapy is to reduce the frequency of ventricular ectopy by > 75%.
• Serial ECGs are not as useful as Holter monitoring—VPCs and paroxysmal ventricular tachycardia can occur sporadically through the day.
• Serum digoxin levels in patients receiving that medication

PREVENTION/AVOIDANCE
Correct predisposing factors such as hypokalemia, hypomagnesemia, myocardial hypoxia, and digoxin toxicity.

POSSIBLE COMPLICATIONS
Syncope, sudden death

EXPECTED COURSE AND PROGNOSIS
• If cause is metabolic—condition may resolve with good prognosis.

• If condition is associated with cardiac disease—prognosis is guarded; VPCs may increase the risk of sudden death.

MISCELLANEOUS

ASSOCIATED CONDITIONS
N/A

AGE-RELATED FACTORS
N/A

ZOONOTIC POTENTIAL
N/A

PREGNANCY
N/A

SYNONYMS
N/A

SEE ALSO
• Digoxin Toxicity
• Myocarditis
• Trypanosomiasis (Chagas' Disease)
• Ventricular Tachycardia

ABBREVIATIONS
• bpm = beats per minute
• CHF = congestive heart failure
• VPC = ventricular premature complex

Suggested Reading
Calvert CA. Diagnosis and management of ventricular arrhythmias in Doberman pinschers with cardiomyopathy. In: Bonagura JD, ed. Kirk's current veterinary therapy XII. Philadelphia: Saunders, 1995:799–806.
Knight DH. Reason must supersede dogma in the management of ventricular arrhythmias. In: Bonagura JD, ed. Kirk's current veterinary therapy XIII. Philadelphia: Saunders, 2000:730–733.
Tilley LP. Essentials of canine and feline electrocardiography. 3rd ed. Baltimore: Williams & Wilkins, 1992.
Author Francis W. K. Smith, Jr.
Consulting Editors Larry P. Tilley and Francis W. K. Smith, Jr.

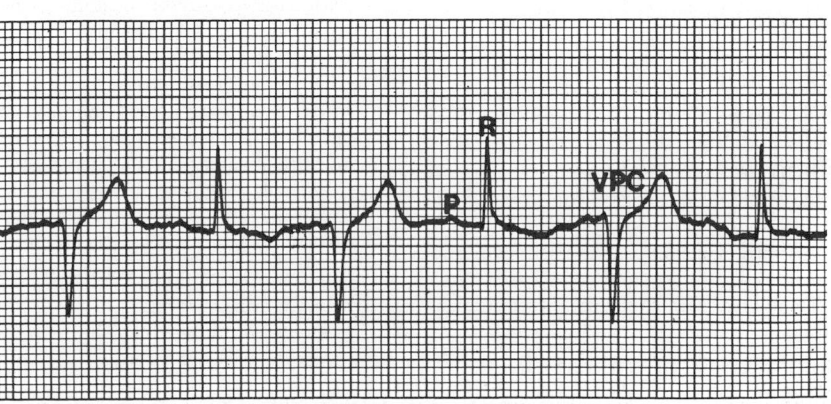

Figure 2.
Ventricular bigeminy. Every other complex is a VPC from the same focus. Each is coupled (interval the same between it and the adjacent sinus complex) to the preceding normal complex. (From: Tilley LP: Essentials of canine and feline electrocardiography. 3rd ed. Baltimore: Williams & Wilkins, 1992, with permission.)

VENTRICULAR SEPTAL DEFECT

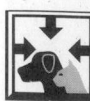

BASICS

DEFINITION
An anomalous communication between the two ventricles (Figure 1). The defect may be in the inlet, outlet, muscular, or membranous septum. Most VSDs in small animals are perimembranous and subcristal, meaning that the defect is subaortic with a right ventricular orifice that is beneath the septal leaflet of the tricuspid valve.

PATHOPHYSIOLOGY
• A VSD results in a pulmonary systemic shunt—direction and volume of the shunt are determined by the size of the defect, the relationship of the pulmonary and systemic vascular resistances, and the presence of other anomalies
• Most VSDs in dogs and cats are small and therefore restrictive (i.e., the difference between left and right ventricular pressures is maintained). Moderate-sized VSDs have an area > 40% of the area of the open aortic valve; they are only partially restrictive and result in various degrees of right ventricular hypertension. Large VSDs—area as large or larger than the open aortic valve; they are nonrestrictive, and right ventricular pressure is necessarily systemic. Only moderate and large defects impose a pressure load upon the right ventricle.
• In a patient with normal resistance to right ventricular ejection, the direction of the shunt is left to right, which increases pulmonary venous return and imposes a volume load on the left atrium and ventricle. With large shunts, left ventricular congestive failure can develop.
• Generally, the left ventricle unloads into the pulmonary arterial system during systole; unless the defect is of moderate size or large, the right ventricle is spared.

SYSTEMS AFFECTED
• Respiratory—if pulmonary edema develops
• Cardiovascular—theoretically, a large shunt could result in pulmonary vascular disease, pulmonary hypertension, and shunt reversal (i.e., Eisenmenger's syndrome). This is uncommon in small animals; if shunt reversal, usually early in life

GENETICS
Breed predispositions recognized; no genetic transmission established

INCIDENCE/PREVALENCE
One of the most common congenital cardiac malformations in cats, comprising 15% of cases with congenital cardiac defects in one study. Less common in dogs, occurring in 10% of cases with congenital cardiac defects in one study

GEOGRAPHIC DISTRIBUTION
N/A

SIGNALMENT

Species
Dogs and cats

Breed Predilections
English bulldog, English springer spaniel, basset hound, Akita, West Highland white terrier, Lakeland terrier

Mean Age and Range
Most defects detected during routine examination of puppies and kittens

Predominant Sex
N/A

SIGNS

Historical Findings
• Usually asymptomatic
• Clinical signs of left ventricular failure include dyspnea, exercise intolerance, syncope, and cough.

Physical Examination Findings
• Systolic murmur with a restrictive VSD. Murmur—typically loud, band-shaped, and heard best over the right hemithorax; may be a softer, midsystolic murmur of functional pulmonic stenosis heard over the left heart base; a diastolic decrescendo murmur results if the VSD undermines anatomic support of the aortic valve, causing aortic regurgitation. Patients with right-to-left shunts generally have no murmurs.
• Split second heart sound in some patients
• Femoral pulses usually normal
• Mucous membranes—pink, unless pulmonary hypertension causes a right-to-left shunt and arterial hypoxemia
• Tachycardia, dyspnea, and crackles may be evident if left ventricular failure occurs.

CAUSES
Congenital; may have a genetic basis

RISK FACTORS
N/A

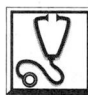

DIAGNOSIS

DIFFERENTIAL DIAGNOSIS
• Other congenital cardiac malformations that cause systolic murmurs include atrioventricular valve dysplasia, aortic or pulmonary stenosis, and complex malformations such as tetralogy of Fallot.
• The "to-and-fro" murmur that results when aortic valve regurgitation complicates a VSD must be distinguished from the continuous murmur of patent ductus arteriosus.
• Generally, diagnosis of congenital cardiac malformations requires echocardiographic evaluation including Doppler studies.

CBC/BIOCHEMISTRY/URINALYSIS
• Results usually normal
• Uncommon right-to-left shunting results in compensatory erythrocytosis.

• Patients with severe CHF may have prerenal azotemia.

OTHER LABORATORY TESTS
N/A

IMAGING

Thoracic Radiography
• Radiographic appearance is determined by the size and direction of the shunt. Thoracic radiographs may be normal if the VSD is small. Larger defects cause various degrees of left or even generalized cardiac enlargement. Pulmonary hyperperfusion with prominence of the main pulmonary artery segment may be apparent. CHF is manifest as pulmonary edema.
• Patients with right-to-left shunts have right-sided cardiomegaly; the pulmonary arteries are large proximally but distally attenuated, and the pulmonary veins are small because of reduced pulmonary perfusion.

Echocardiography
• Two-dimensional echocardiographic study may demonstrate left atrial enlargement with left ventricular dilation and hypertrophy. Systolic myocardial function is usually preserved. Right ventricular hypertrophy is apparent only if the defect is moderate-sized or large or if the VSD is one aspect of a complex malformation. Careful study usually demonstrates the defect. Evaluate echocardiographic images critically; the artifact of "septal drop-out" is very common.
• The diagnosis is confirmed by Doppler interrogation of the interventricular septum. If the defect is restrictive, spectral Doppler reveals a discrete, high-velocity systolic jet. The shunt may be seen directly by color-flow Doppler.
• Contrast echocardiography may help in the diagnosis of a right-to-left VSD.

Cardiac Catheterization
Selective cardiac catheterization allows visualization of the defect by contrast angiocardiography and calculation of the shunt fraction (QP/QS) and pulmonary vascular resistance.

OTHER DIAGNOSTIC PROCEDURES

Electrocardiographic Findings
• Evidence of left atrial enlargement, left ventricular hypertrophy, or even right ventricular hypertrophy in some animals
• Right ventricular enlargement pattern in most animals if the shunt is right-to-left because of pulmonary hypertension or pulmonic stenosis

PATHOLOGIC FINDINGS
Size of the defect determines the degree of chamber enlargement and hypertrophy; pulmonary edema and possibly ascites are seen in patients with CHF.

VENTRICULAR SEPTAL DEFECT

TREATMENT

APPROPRIATE HEALTH CARE
Clinical signs are related to CHF; most patients can be treated as outpatients.

NURSING CARE
N/A

ACTIVITY
Restrict if animal has CHF; need not restrict asymptomatic patients with small defects

DIET
Moderate sodium restriction recommended for patients with CHF

CLIENT EDUCATION
Definitive surgical correction is not widely available; if CHF develops, it is terminal, even with palliative care.

SURGICAL CONSIDERATIONS
Consider definitive surgical repair of the defect during cardiopulmonary bypass for moderate and large defects in which the QP/QS exceeds 2.5. Cardiopulmonary bypass is presently performed at a small number of veterinary centers. Consider pulmonary artery banding as a palliative procedure for patients with moderate or large shunts and CHF.

MEDICATIONS

DRUG(S) OF CHOICE
Furosemide, enalapril, and digoxin—recommended for animals with CHF (see Congestive Heart Failure, Left-Sided)

CONTRAINDICATIONS
Vasodilators—contraindicated or used only with great caution in patients with complex malformations that include stenotic lesions.

PRECAUTIONS
ACE inhibitors and digoxin must be used cautiously if patient has renal dysfunction.

POSSIBLE INTERACTIONS
N/A

ALTERNATIVE DRUG(S)
N/A

FOLLOW-UP

PATIENT MONITORING
Periodic echocardiographic or radiographic evaluation suggested for patients without clinical signs

PREVENTION/AVOIDANCE
Breeding affected animals is not recommended.

POSSIBLE COMPLICATIONS
• Left ventricular congestive failure
• Bacterial endocarditis
• Pulmonary hypertension
• Arrhythmias

EXPECTED COURSE AND PROGNOSIS
• Patients with small shunts may have a normal life span; isolated, restrictive VSDs usually do not cause clinical signs.
• Concurrent anomalies such as pulmonic stenosis or aortic insufficiency worsen the prognosis.
• Patients with overt CHF may live 6–18 months with medical treatment.
• The development of pulmonary hypertension and shunt reversal is uncommon.

MISCELLANEOUS

ASSOCIATED CONDITIONS
• VSD may be one component of complex malformations such as tetralogy of Fallot.

• Aortic valve insufficiency resulting from a poorly supported aortic valve complicates the condition in some patients.
• In cats, VSD may be associated with an atrial septal defect and atrioventricular valve abnormalities as part of a complete atrioventricular septal defect (endocardial cushion defect.)

AGE-RELATED FACTORS
The murmur of VSD becomes apparent shortly after birth, when pulmonary vascular resistance drops.

ZOONOTIC POTENTIAL
N/A

PREGNANCY
High risk in patients with large defects; breeding affected animals is not recommended.

SYNONYMS
Interventricular septal defect

SEE ALSO
• CHF, Left-Sided
• Tetralogy of Fallot

ABBREVIATIONS
• ACE = angiotensin-converting enzyme
• CHF = congestive heart failure
• VSD = ventricular septal defect

Suggested Reading
Bonagura JD, Lehmkuhl LB. Congenital heart disease. In: Fox PR, Sisson D, Moise NS, eds., Textbook of canine and feline cardiology. Philadelphia: Saunders, 1999: 471–535.
Kittleson MD. Septal defects. In: Small animal cardiovascular medicine. St. Louis: Mosby, 1998:231–239.
Author Jonathan A. Abbott
Consulting Editors Larry P. Tilley and Francis W. K. Smith, Jr.

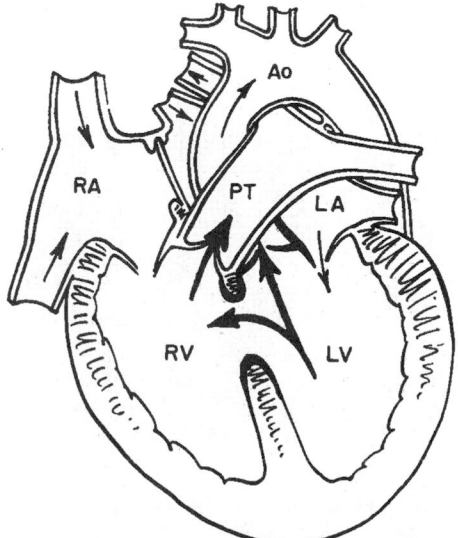

Figure 1.

Ventricular Septal Defect. The defect is an unobstructed communication. Right ventricular hypertrophy and pulmonary hypertension are associated. Left-to-right shunting is shown. RA = right atrium, LA = left atrium, RV = right ventricle, LV = left ventricle, AO = aorta, PT = pulmonary trunk. (From Roberts W. Adult Congenital Heart Disease. Philadelphia: FA Davis, 1987, with permission.)

VENTRICULAR STANDSTILL (ASYSTOLE)

 BASICS

DEFINITION
Absence of ventricular complexes on the ECG or absence of ventricular activity (electrical–mechanical dissociation)

ECG Features
Ventricular asystole can result from severe sinoatrial block or arrest or by third-degree AV block (Figure 1) without a junctional or ventricular escape rhythm; ECG features include:
• P waves present if patient has complete AV block
• P waves absent during asystole if patient has severe sinoatrial block or arrest
• No QRS complexes
• Electrical-mechanical dissociation—a recorded ECG cardiac rhythm (P–QRS–T) and no effective cardiac output or palpable femoral pulse

PATHOPHYSIOLOGY
Ventricular asystole represents cardiac arrest; if the ventricular rhythm is not restored in 3–4 min, irreversible brain injury can occur

SYSTEMS AFFECTED
• Cardiovascular
• All organ systems affected by loss of perfusion

GENETICS
N/A

INCIDENCE/PREVALENCE
Unknown

GEOGRAPHIC DISTRIBUTION
None

SIGNALMENT

Species
Dogs and cats

Breed Predilection
None

Mean Age and Range
Unknown

SIGNS

Historical Findings
• Severe systemic illness or cardiac disease in many patients
• Other cardiac arrhythmias in some
• Syncope

Physical Examination Findings
• No ventricular pulse can be palpated.
• Cardiac arrest
• Collapse
• Death

CAUSES
• Complete AV block with absence of ventricular or junctional escape rhythm
• Severe sinus arrest or block
• Hyperkalemia (Figure 2)

RISK FACTORS
• Any severe systemic illness (e.g., severe acidosis and hyperkalemia) or heart disease
• Hypoadrenocorticism causing hyperkalemia
• Urinary tract rupture of obstruction, resulting in hyperkalemia

 DIAGNOSIS

DIFFERENTIAL DIAGNOSIS
Rule out ECG artifact; reapply ECG clips and make sure skin contact is good and adequate alcohol is applied to leads.

CBC/BIOCHEMISTRY/URINALYSIS
Severe hyperkalemia possible cause

OTHER LABORATORY TESTS
N/A

IMAGING
N/A

DIAGNOSTIC PROCEDURES
Systemic blood pressure—readable pressure absent

PATHOLOGIC FINDINGS
N/A

 TREATMENT

APPROPRIATE HEALTH CARE
• Asystole is a frequently fatal rhythm requiring immediate aggressive treatment.
• Artificial pacing with a transvenous pacemaker may succeed if myocardium is mechanically responsive.
• DC electrical conversion is not effective unless the rhythm can first be converted to ventricular fibrillation with medications.

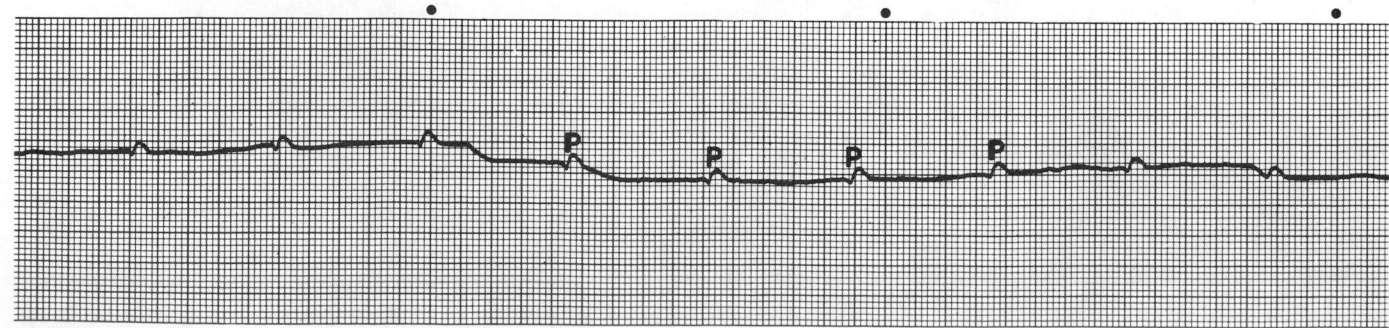

Figure 1.

Ventricular asystole in a dog with severe complete AV block. Only P waves (atrial activity) are present; there is no ventricular activity. (Lead II, 50 mm/sec, 1 cm = 1 mV) (From: Tilley LP: Essentials of canine and feline electrocardiography. 3rd ed. Baltimore: Williams & Wilkins, 1992, with permission.)

VENTRICULAR STANDSTILL (ASYSTOLE)

NURSING CARE
Treat any treatable problems such as hypothermia, hyperkalemia, and acid–base disorders.

ACTIVITY
N/A

DIET
N/A

CLIENT EDUCATION
None

SURGICAL CONSIDERATIONS
None

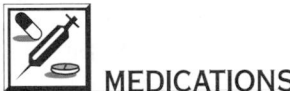

MEDICATIONS

DRUG(S) OF CHOICE
• Institute cardiopulmonary resuscitation.
• Epinephrine—0.2 mg/kg IV, IT, or IL (double the dose for IT administration and deliver with equal volume of saline)
• Atropine—0.05 mg/kg IV, IT, or IL (double the dose for IT administration and deliver with equal volume of saline)
• Sodium bicarbonate—1 mEq/kg IV for each 10 min of cardiac arrest
• Dexamethasone and dopamine may be helpful in patients with electrical-mechanical dissociation

CONTRAINDICATIONS
Drugs that depress sinus node or AV node conduction in patients with sinus arrest or heart block (e.g., β-blockers, calcium channel blockers, digoxin)

PRECAUTIONS
None

POSSIBLE INTERACTIONS
None

ALTERNATIVE DRUG(S)
Calcium gluconate—patients with ventricular standstill and hyperkalemia

FOLLOW-UP

PATIENT MONITORING
• If animal is resuscitated—evaluate CBC, biochemical analysis, and urinalysis.
• If animal survives and primary cardiac disease is suspected—an echocardiogram and thoracic radiographs
• ECG—closely and frequently

PREVENTION/AVOIDANCE
Careful monitoring of critically ill patients to prevent and correct acid–base disturbances, hypotension, and hypoxemia

POSSIBLE COMPLICATIONS
• Death
• DIC and multiorgan failure

EXPECTED COURSE AND PROGNOSIS
Patients that arrest frequently have recurrent arrest.

MISCELLANEOUS

ASSOCIATED CONDITIONS
None

AGE-RELATED FACTORS
None

ZOONOTIC POTENTIAL
None

PREGNANCY
None

SYNONYMS
Ventricular asystole

SEE ALSO
• Atrioventricular Block, Complete (Third Degree)
• Cardiopulmonary Arrest
• Sinus Arrest and Sinoatrial Block

ABBREVIATIONS
• AV = antrioventricular
• DC = direct current
• DIC = disseminated intravascular coagulation
• IL = intralingual
• IT = intratracheal

Suggested Reading
Tilley LP. Essentials of canine and feline electrocardiography. 3rd ed. Baltimore: Williams & Wilkins, 1992.
Author Francis W. K. Smith, Jr.
Consulting Editors Larry P. Tilley and Francis W. K. Smith, Jr.

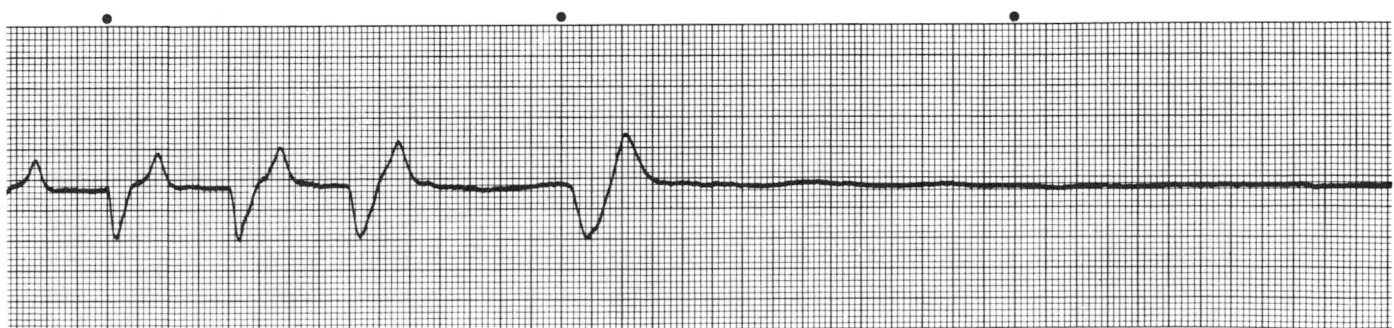

Figure 2.

Ventricular asystole in a cat with severe hyperkalemia (11 mEq/L) from urethral obstruction. No P waves or QRS complexes are seen after four wide and bizarre QRS complexes (atrial standstill with delayed ventricular conduction). (Lead II, 50 mm/sec, 1 cm = 1 mV) (From: Tilley LP: Essentials of canine and feline electrocardiography. 3rd ed. Baltimore: Williams & Wilkins, 1992, with permission.)

VENTRICULAR TACHYCARDIA

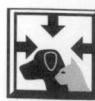

BASICS

DEFINITION

ECG Features
- Three or more ventricular premature contractions in a row
- May be intermittent (paroxysmal) or sustained; heart rate > 150 bpm with a regular rhythm
- QRS complexes—typically wide and bizarre
- If P waves—dissociated from the QRS complexes (Figure 1)

PATHOPHYSIOLOGY
Potentially life-threatening arrhythmia, usually signifying myocardial disease or metabolic derangement; mechanisms include increased automaticity, reentry, and delayed afterdepolarizations.

SYSTEMS AFFECTED
Cardiovascular system, with secondary effects on other systems because of poor perfusion

GENETICS
- Ventricular arrhythmias and sudden cardiac death hereditary in German shepherds, but mode of inheritance not determined
- Arrhythmogenic boxer cardiomyopathy— probably inherited

INCIDENCE/PREVALENCE
Common arrhythmia in dogs; uncommon in cats

GEOGRAPHIC DISTRIBUTION
None

SIGNALMENT

Species
Dogs and cats

Breed Predilection
- German shepherds with sudden cardiac death
- Commonly seen in large-breed dogs with cardiomyopathy, especially boxers and Doberman pinschers

Mean Age and Range
- All age groups
- German shepherds with sudden cardiac death—usually present at 4–6 months of age
- Boxers with arrhythmogenic cardiomyopathy—usually present at 4–6 years of age
- Doberman pinschers with occult cardiomyopathy typically develop ventricular arrhythmias beginning at 3–6 years of age, but can occur much earlier; frequency and severity of the arrhythmia usually increases over time.

SIGNS

Historical Findings
- Weakness
- Exercise intolerance
- Syncope
- Sudden death
- May be asymptomatic

Physical Examination Findings
- Paroxysmal or sustained tachycardia
- May be normal if arrhythmia is paroxysmal and absent during examination
- Signs of congestive heart failure (CHF) or murmur may be present, depending on cause of arrhythmia

CAUSES
- Cardiomyopathy
- Congenital defects (especially subaortic stenosis)
- Chronic valve disease
- Gastric dilation and volvulus
- Traumatic myocarditis (dogs)
- Digitalis toxicity
- Hyperthyroidism (cats)
- Cardiac neoplasia
- Myocarditis
- Pancreatitis

RISK FACTORS
- Hypokalemia
- Hypomagnesemia
- Acid–base disturbances
- Hypoxemia

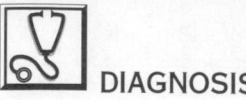

DIAGNOSIS

DIFFERENTIAL DIAGNOSIS
Supraventricular tachycardia with bundle branch block. If P waves can be identified, look for association between P waves and QRS complexes. If there is a consistent P-R interval, then the rhythm is supraventricular with bundle branch block. If no association between P waves and QRS complexes, the rhythm is probably ventricular tachycardia. If P waves cannot be identified, use response to lidocaine to differentiate. Termination of arrhythmia after administration of lidocaine supports ventricular tachycardia.

CBC/BIOCHEMISTRY/URINALYSIS
- Hypokalemia and hypomagnesemia predispose animal to ventricular tachycardia and blunt response to class 1 antiarrhythmic drugs (e.g., lidocaine, procainamide, mexiletine, and quinidine).
- High amylase and lipase if arrhythmia is secondary to pancreatitis

OTHER LABORATORY TESTS
High T_4 (cats) if arrhythmia is secondary to hyperthyroidism

IMAGING
Echocardiography may reveal structural heart disease.

DIAGNOSTIC PROCEDURES
Long-term ambulatory (Holter) recording of the ECG—for detection of transient ventricular arrhythmias in patients with unexplained syncope or weakness

PATHOLOGIC FINDINGS
Vary with underlying cause

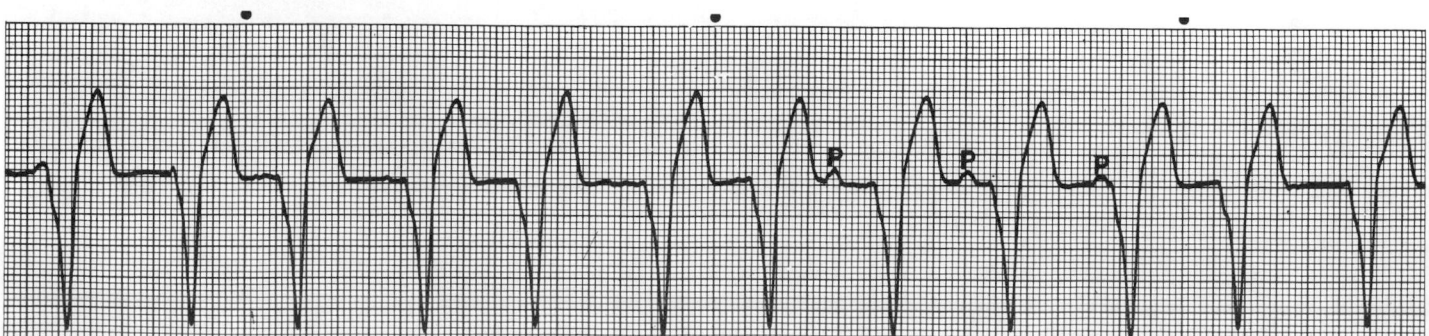

Figure 1.

Ventricular tachycardia. The wide and bizarre QRS complexes occur at a rate of 160 beats/min, with no relationship to the P waves. There are more QRS complexes than P waves. Ventricular tachycardia should be treated as soon as possible. Acid-base and electrolyte abnormalities should always be corrected. (From: Tilley LP: Essentials of canine and feline electrocardiography. 3rd ed. Baltimore: Williams & Wilkins, 1992, with permission.)

TREATMENT

APPROPRIATE HEALTH CARE
Treat as inpatient until arrhythmia is controlled and patient is hemodynamically stable.

NURSING CARE
Varies with underlying cause

ACTIVITY
Restrict

DIET
N/A

CLIENT EDUCATION
Alert the owner to the potential for sudden death.

SURGICAL CONSIDERATIONS
• Continuous ECG monitoring while animal is anesthetized
• Control arrhythmia prior to inducing general anesthesia.
• Premedication with acepromazine (0.02–0.05 mg/kg) raises the threshold for ventricular fibrillation.
• Mask inductions not recommended in patients with ventricular arrhythmias; sympathetic release during mask induction can aggravate the arrhythmia.

MEDICATIONS

DRUG(S) OF CHOICE
Correct any hypokalemia or hypomagnesemia.

Dogs
• Administer lidocaine slowly in 2 mg/kg IV boluses (up to 8 mg/kg total) to convert to sinus rhythm; follow with lidocaine infusion, 25–75 µg/kg/min.
• If lidocaine fails—administer procainamide slowly in 2 mg/kg IV boluses (up to 20 mg/kg total) to convert to sinus rhythm; follow with procainamide infusion at 20–50 µg/kg/min or 8–20 mg/kg IM q6h.
• If lidocaine and procainamide both fail to convert the rhythm, administer magnesium sulfate diluted in normal saline or D₅W at 25–30 mg/kg IV over 5–10 min. If the arrhythmia improves, administer the same dosage in intravenous fluids over the next 4–8 hours.
• If the patient does not respond to lidocaine, procainamide, or magnesium, administer slow IV boluses of esmolol (a short-acting β-blocker) at 0.05–0.1 mg/kg q5min to a cumulative dose of 0.5 mg/kg, or as a 50–200 µg/kg/min constant rate infusion.

• When the patient is stable, give mexiletine (5–8 mg/kg PO q8h), sotalol (1–3.5 mg/kg PO q12h), or procainamide (8–20 mg/kg PO q6–8h).
• Combine previous drugs (except sotalol) with a β-blocker (e.g., propranolol or atenolol) if arrhythmia persists.
• In boxers, sotalol or a combination of mexiletine and atenolol (0.3–0.6 mg/kg q12h) is the most effective therapy.

Cats
• Use lidocaine cautiously and only for sustained ventricular tachycardia; neurotoxicity is common in cats. Use one-tenth of the dosage used for dogs.
• Atenolol (6.25–12.5 mg PO q12h) is preferred in cats.

CONTRAINDICATIONS
• Avoid atropine, catecholamines (e.g., epinephrine, dopamine), and digoxin until arrhythmia is controlled.

PRECAUTIONS
• Use β-blockers cautiously in animals with CHF.
• Sotalol and other drugs that prolong the action potential duration may worsen arrhythmia in the inherited ventricular arrhythmia of German shepherds.

POSSIBLE INTERACTIONS
Quinidine and amiodarone raise digoxin levels.

ALTERNATIVE DRUG(S)
• Consider amiodarone (5–10 mg/kg PO q12h) for refractory arrhythmias in dogs.
• Consider sotalol (10–20 mg/cat q12h) or procainamide (3–8 mg/kg PO, q6–8h) for refractory arrhythmias in cats.

FOLLOW-UP

PATIENT MONITORING
• Holter monitoring is preferred for monitoring severity of the arrhythmia and efficacy of antiarrhythmic therapy; the goal of antiarrhythmic therapy is to reduce the frequency of ventricular ectopy by > 75%.
• Serial ECGs and telemetry can be used—not as useful as Holter monitoring because ventricular premature complexes and paroxysmal ventricular tachycardia can occur sporadically through the day
• Serum digoxin levels in patients receiving that medication

PREVENTION/AVOIDANCE
Correct predisposing factors such as hypokalemia, hypomagnesemia, myocardial hypoxia, and digoxin toxicity.

POSSIBLE COMPLICATIONS
• Syncope
• Sudden death

EXPECTED COURSE AND PROGNOSIS
• If cause is metabolic—condition may resolve with a good prognosis.
• If condition is associated with cardiac disease—prognosis guarded; ventricular tachycardia may increase the risk of sudden death.
• Approximately 50% of German shepherds with ventricular tachycardia and inherited sudden death syndrome die acutely within the first year of life.

MISCELLANEOUS

ASSOCIATED CONDITIONS
N/A

AGE-RELATED FACTORS
N/A

ZOONOTIC POTENTIAL
None

PREGNANCY
N /A

SYNONYMS
None

SEE ALSO
• Digoxin Toxicity
• Myocarditis
• Trypanosomiasis (Chagas' Disease)
• Ventricular Premature Complexes

ABBREVIATIONS
• bpm = beats per minute
• CHF = congestive heart failure

Suggested Reading
Meurs KM, Spier AW, Wright NA, et al. Comparison of the effects of four antiarrhythmic treatments for familial ventricular arrhythmias in boxers. J Am Vet Med Assoc 2002;221[4]:52–527.
Moise NS, Gilmour RF Jr. Inherited sudden cardiac death in German shepherds. In: Kirk RW, Bonagura JD, eds. Current veterinary therapy XI. Philadelphia: Saunders, 1992:749–751.
Tilley LP. Essentials of canine and feline electrocardiography. 3rd ed. Baltimore: Williams & Wilkins, 1992.
Author Francis W. K. Smith, Jr.
Consulting Editors Larry P. Tilley and Francis W. K. Smith, Jr.

VESICOURACHAL DIVERTICULA

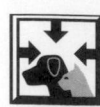 BASICS

OVERVIEW
• A common congenital anomaly of the urinary bladder that occurs when the portion of the urachus (i.e., a fetal conduit that allows passage of urine from the bladder to the placenta) located at the bladder vertex fails to close; the result is a blind diverticulum of variable size that protrudes from the bladder vertex.
• Other characteristics include congenital microscopic diverticula (microscopic lumens that may persist at the bladder vertex).
• Acquired macroscopic diverticula develop after the onset of concurrent but unrelated acquired lower urinary tract diseases; presumably, urethral obstruction or detrusor hyperactivity induced by inflammation causes high intraluminal pressure and subsequent enlargement of microscopic diverticula.
• Congenital macroscopic diverticula, most likely caused by impaired urine outflow, develop before or soon after birth and persist indefinitely.

SIGNALMENT
• Dogs and cats
• Frequently encountered in cats with acquired lower urinary tract diseases; twice as common in male cats as in female cats
• No breed or age predisposition

SIGNS
• Depend on concomitant disorders predisposing to formation of macroscopic vesicourachal diverticula
• Hematuria, dysuria, pollakiuria, or signs of urethral obstruction in some patients with concurrent acquired lower urinary tract diseases

CAUSES & RISK FACTORS
• Persistent congenital microscopic diverticula—cause unknown
• Congenital microscopic diverticula—risk factors for acquired macroscopic diverticula
• Diseases associated with increased bladder intraluminal pressure (e.g., bacterial urinary tract infection, uroliths, urethral plugs, and idiopathic disease) —risk factors for acquired macroscopic diverticula

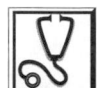 DIAGNOSIS

DIFFERENTIAL DIAGNOSIS
• Persistent (or patent) urachus—characterized by inappropriate loss of urine through the umbilicus
• Persistent urachal ligaments are nonpatent fibrous remnants of the urachus, connecting the bladder vertex to the umbilicus.
• Urachal cysts are focal accumulations of fluid in isolated segments of a persistent urachus. They may be aseptic or septic.

CBC/BIOCHEMISTRY/URINALYSIS
• Abnormal findings related to the underlying disorder that causes vesicourachal diverticula, unless complicated by concurrent acquired lower urinary tract diseases
• Abnormal findings related to secondary urinary tract infection

OTHER LABORATORY TESTS
N/A

IMAGING
• Congenital and acquired macroscopic diverticula—best identified by positive-contrast urethrocystography
• Radiographs obtained with the bladder completely, then partially distended with contrast medium, may facilitate detection of small diverticula.

DIAGNOSTIC PROCEDURES
N/A

PATHOLOGIC FINDINGS
• Extramural macroscopic diverticula appear as convex or conical luminal projections from the bladder vertex.
• Intramural microscopic diverticula appear as transitional epithelium-lined lumens persisting at the bladder vertex from the level of the submucosa to subserosa.

TREATMENT

• Many macroscopic diverticula in cats (and probably dogs) are acquired and self-limiting if the underlying disease is eliminated.
• Direct treatment efforts toward eliminating underlying cause(s) of lower urinary tract disease.
• Consider diverticulectomy if a macroscopic diverticulum persists in a patient with persistent or recurrent bacterial urinary tract infection despite appropriate antimicrobial therapy.

 MEDICATIONS

DRUG(S)
N/A

CONTRAINDICATIONS/POSSIBLE INTERACTIONS
N/A

 FOLLOW-UP

PATIENT MONITORING
If bacterial urinary tract infection persists or recurs despite proper antimicrobial therapy, the status of the diverticulum should be reevaluated by contrast radiography.

PREVENTION/AVOIDANCE
Avoid diagnostic procedures or treatments that alter normal host urinary tract defenses and predispose to urinary tract infection.

POSSIBLE COMPLICATIONS
Persistent congenital macroscopic diverticula are risk factors for recurrent bacterial urinary tract infection.

EXPECTED COURSE AND PROGNOSIS
• Congenital microscopic diverticula are usually clinically silent unless complicated by concurrent lower urinary tract disease.
• Acquired macroscopic diverticula typically heal in 2–3 weeks after amelioration of clinical signs of lower urinary tract disease.
• Diverticulectomy and appropriate antimicrobial therapy usually resolve recurrent urinary tract infection in patients with persistent congenital macroscopic diverticula.

 MISCELLANEOUS

ASSOCIATED CONDITIONS
• Persistent congenital macroscopic diverticula are potential risk factors for recurrent bacterial urinary tract infections.
• Acquired macroscopic diverticula are typically encountered in patients with concurrent lower urinary tract diseases.

SEE ALSO
• Feline Lower Urinary Tract Disease
• Lower Urinary Tract Infection

Suggested Reading
Osborne CA, Johnston GR, Kruger JM, et al. Etiopathogenesis and biological behavior of feline vesicourachal diverticula. Vet Clin North Am 1987;17:697.
Authors John M. Kruger and Carl A. Osborne
Consulting Editors Larry G. Adams and Carl A. Osborne

VESTIBULAR DISEASE, GERIATRIC—DOGS

BASICS

DEFINITION
Acute nonprogressive disturbance of the peripheral vestibular system in old dogs

PATHOPHYSIOLOGY
• Unknown
• Suspected abnormal flow of the endolymphatic fluid in the semicircular canals of the inner ear secondary to disturbance in production, circulation, or absorption of the fluid
• Possible intoxication of the vestibular receptors or inflammation of the vestibular portion of the vestibulocochlear nerve (cranial nerve VIII)
• Often incorrectly referred to as a stroke (disease is neither central in location nor suspected to be vascular or ischemic in origin)

SYSTEMS AFFECTED
Nervous—peripheral vestibular system

GENETICS
N/A

INCIDENCE/PREVALENCE
• Common, sporadic, acquired disease of old dogs

GEOGRAPHIC DISTRIBUTION
N/A

SIGNALMENT

Species
Dogs

Breed Predilections
• None reported
• Seems to occur more frequently in medium-to-large breeds

Mean Age and Range
Geriatric; patients usually > 8 years old

Predominant Sex
N/A

SIGNS

General Comments
• Signs of peripheral vestibular dysfunction
• Severe disease—do not incorrectly attribute the signs (especially the gait) to a CNS location.

Historical Findings
• Sudden onset of imbalance, disorientation, reluctance to stand, and (usually) head tilt and irregular eye movements
• May be preceded or accompanied by nausea and vomiting

Physical Examination Findings
• Head tilt—mild to marked; directed toward the side of the lesion; occasionally bilateral disease with erratic side-to-side movements with or without mild tilt in the direction of the more severely affected side
• Abnormal nystagmus (resting or positional)—in early stages common; either horizontal or rotatory with the fast phase always in a direction opposite to the head tilt; with bilateral disease, may have depressed or absent physiologic eye movements (i.e., abnormal conjugate eye movements)
• Mild to marked disorientation and vestibular ataxia with a tendency to lean or fall in the direction of the head tilt
• Strength and proprioception normal; with severe disease, patient may be reluctant to stand, making assessment of gait difficult; with bilateral disease, may have base-wide stance.

CAUSES
Unknown

RISK FACTORS
N/A

DIAGNOSIS

DIFFERENTIAL DIAGNOSIS
• Primarily distinguished by the acute onset and rapid improvement without specific treatment
• Otitis media and interna—may have concurrent ipsilateral facial nerve (cranial nerve VII) paresis or paralysis, deafness, or Horner syndrome; otitis externa with ruptured tympanic membrane supports diagnosis of otitis media and interna.
• Ototoxic drugs—eliminated by history
• Trauma—may cause similar acute changes; differentiated by history, results of physical examination, and other neurologic deficits
• Hypothyroid neuropathy—not as acute in onset; associated with clinical signs of hypothyroidism and possible cranial nerve VII deficit

CBC/BIOCHEMISTRY/URINALYSIS
• Generally normal
• Hemoconcentration secondary to dehydration
• Unrelated concurrent disorders (e.g., renal and hepatic disease) associated with geriatric state may cause other laboratory abnormalities.

OTHER LABORATORY TESTS
N/A

IMAGING
• Usually none
• Radiographs of bullae or preferably CT or MRI may be required to rule out otitis media and interna

DIAGNOSTIC PROCEDURES
BAER—to assess cochlear portion of cranial nerve VIII; may help to evaluate for otitis media and interna; since only the vestibular portion of cranial nerve VIII should be affected with geriatric vestibular disease. Deafness may be present as an unrelated aging change.

PATHOLOGIC FINDINGS
None reported

TREATMENT

APPROPRIATE HEALTH CARE
• Usually outpatient
• Severe disease—patients that cannot ambulate or require intravenous fluid support should be hospitalized during the initial stages.

NURSING CARE
• Treatment supportive, including rehydration and intravenous fluids if required
• Keep recumbent patients warm and dry using soft, absorbent bedding

VESTIBULAR DISEASE, GERIATRIC—DOGS

• Severe disease—physical therapy, including passive manipulation of limbs and moving body to alternate sides, may be required initially

ACTIVITY
Restrict activity as required by the degree of disorientation and vestibular ataxia.

DIET
• No modification usually required
• Nausea, vomiting, and severe disorientation—initially withhold oral intake.

CLIENT EDUCATION
Reassure client that although the initial signs can be alarming and incapacitating, the prognosis for rapid improvement and recovery is excellent.

SURGICAL CONSIDERATIONS
N/A

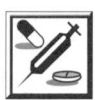 MEDICATIONS

DRUG(S) OF CHOICE
• Sedatives—for severe disorientation and ataxia; diazepam (2–10 mg/dog PO q8h)
• Antiemetic drugs or drugs against motion sickness—may be beneficial; dimenhydrinate (4–8 mg/kg PO, IM, IV q8h)
• Glucocorticoids—do not alter the course of the disease; not recommended, especially in old patients whose fluid intake may be low
• Antibiotics—advised when otitis media and interna cannot be ruled out; trimethoprim-sulfa (15 mg/kg PO q12h or 30 mg/kg PO q12–24h); first-generation cephalosporin (e.g., cephalexin 10–30 mg/kg PO q6–12h); amoxicillin/clavulanic acid (12.5–25 mg/kg PO q12h)

CONTRAINDICATIONS
N/A

PRECAUTIONS
N/A

POSSIBLE INTERACTIONS
N/A

ALTERNATIVE DRUG(S)
N/A

 FOLLOW-UP

PATIENT MONITORING
• Neurologic examination of outpatient—repeat 2–3 days later to confirm stabilization and initial improvement.
• Discharge inpatient when able to ambulate and resume eating and drinking.

PREVENTION/AVOIDANCE
N/A

POSSIBLE COMPLICATIONS
Fluid and electrolyte imbalances and decompensation of renal insufficiency (if exists)—may follow vomiting and/or insufficient fluid and food intake

EXPECTED COURSE AND PROGNOSIS
• Improvement of clinical signs within approximately 72 hr with resolution of vomiting and improvement of nystagmus and vestibular ataxia
• Head tilt and ataxia—significant improvement usually occurs over 7–10 days; if no improvement other causes of peripheral vestibular disease should be explored; mild head tilt may persist.
• Most should be explored patients return to normal within 2–3 weeks.
• Recurrence—rare; brief return of signs may occur with stress (e.g., anesthesia); repeat episodes of geriatric vestibular disease can occur on the same or opposite side but are uncommon

 MISCELLANEOUS

ASSOCIATED CONDITIONS
N/A

AGE-RELATED FACTORS
Only geriatric dogs affected

ZOONOTIC POTENTIAL
N/A

PREGNANCY
N/A

SYNONYMS
• Canine idiopathic vestibular disease
• Old dog vestibular syndrome

SEE ALSO
• Head Tilt (Vestibular Disease)
• Otitis Media and Interna

ABBREVIATIONS
• BAER = brain stem auditory-evoked response
• CNS = central nervous system
• CT = computed tomography
• MRI = magnetic resonance imaging

Suggested Reading

de Lahunta A. Veterinary neuroanatomy and clinical neurology. 2nd ed. Philadelphia: Saunders, 1983.
Oliver JE, Lorenz MD, Kornegay JN. Handbook of veterinary neurology, 3rd ed. Philadelphia: Saunders, 1997:222–223.
Parent JM, Cochrane SM. Head tilt. In: Allen DG, ed. Small animal medicine. Philadelphia: Lippincott, 1991:753–759.
Author Susan M. Cochrane
Consulting Editor Joane M. Parent

VESTIBULAR DISEASE, IDIOPATHIC—CATS

 BASICS

DEFINITION
Acute nonprogressive disturbance of the peripheral vestibular system of cats

PATHOPHYSIOLOGY
• Unknown
• Suspected abnormal flow of the endo-lymphatic fluid in the semicircular canals of the inner ear, secondary to a disturbance in the production, circulation, or absorption of the fluid
• Possible intoxication of the vestibular receptors or inflammation of the vestibular portion of the vestibulocochlear nerve (cranial nerve VIII)

SYSTEMS AFFECTED
Nervous—peripheral vestibular system

Genetics
N/A

Incidence/Prevalence
• Sporadic acquired disease
• None reported

Geographic Distribution
N/A

SIGNALMENT

Species
Cats

Breed Predilections
N/A

Mean Age and Range
Any age; rarely observed in cats < 1 year old

Predominant Sex
N/A

SIGNS

General Comments
Limited to signs associated with peripheral vestibular disturbance

Historical Findings
Sudden onset of severe disorientation, falling and rolling, leaning, vocalizing, and crouched posture with tendency to panic when picked up

Physical Examination Findings
• Head tilt—always toward the side of the lesion; occasionally bilateral disease with wide, side-to-side excursion of the head, and possibly mild tilt toward the most severely affected side
• Resting nystagmus—usually horizontal, but may be rotatory with the fast phase always in direction opposite to the head tilt; with bilateral disease, the abnormal nystagmus is mild or not present, and physiologic nystagmus or conjugate eye movements are diminished to absent
• Vestibular ataxia with tendency to roll and fall toward the side of the head tilt
• Preservation of strength and normal proprioception; with bilateral disease, patient may be reluctant to ambulate, preferring to stay in a crouched posture or having wide abduction of the limbs

CAUSES
• Unknown
• Previous upper respiratory tract infection—suspected in some patients; relationship not confirmed; in limited necropsy data no evidence of inflammation

RISK FACTORS
• Reports of an increase in cases in the summer and early fall, possibly after outbreaks of upper respiratory disease; but not been proven; disease can occur throughout the year

 DIAGNOSIS

DIFFERENTIAL DIAGNOSIS
• Diagnosis made on the basis of peripheral vestibular signs that improve rapidly without specific treatment
• Otitis media and interna (bacterial and parasitic)—may have concurrent ipsilateral facial nerve (cranial nerve VII) paresis or paralysis, Horner's syndrome, deafness, ruptured tympanic membrane, otitis externa, and radiographic changes in tympanic bulla; signs usually not as acute or severe at onset and not self-limiting
• Nasopharyngeal polyp(s)—may cause unilateral or bilateral peripheral vestibular signs; concurrent tympanic bulla involvement characteristic; signs usually not as acute and severe at onset and not self-limiting
• Blue-tailed lizard ingestion—southeastern U.S.; thought to produce a similar acute, unilateral, peripheral vestibular syndrome; vomiting, salivation, irritability, and trembling also noted; most patients recover without specific treatment.
• Aminoglycoside toxicity, especially strepto-mycin—may cause acute unilateral or bilateral peripheral vestibular syndrome or hearing loss; differentiated by history of drug use

CBC/BIOCHEMISTRY/URINALYSIS
Normal

OTHER LABORATORY TESTS
None required

IMAGING
• None usually necessary
• Radiographs of tympanic bullae preferably. CT or MRI—occasionally required to evaluate for otitis media and interna

DIAGNOSTIC PROCEDURES
• BAER—may help rule out other causes (e.g., otitis media and interna; nasopharyngeal polyps); with idiopathic vestibular disease hearing should not be affected since disease limited to the vestibular apparatus

PATHOLOGIC FINDINGS
None reported

VESTIBULAR DISEASE, IDIOPATHIC—CATS

TREATMENT

APPROPRIATE HEALTH CARE
- Usually outpatient
- Inpatient—severely affected patient may require a short period of hospitalization for supportive care

NURSING CARE
- Treatment supportive only
- Severe disease—may require initial intravenous or subcutaneous fluids; maintain patient in quiet, well-padded cage initially.

ACTIVITY
Restricted according to the degree of disorientation and ataxia

DIET
- No specific changes or restrictions required
- Patient may be initially reluctant to eat and drink, possibly because of the disorientation or nausea.

CLIENT EDUCATION
Reassure client that, despite initial alarming and incapacitating signs, the prognosis for rapid and complete recovery is excellent.

SURGICAL CONSIDERATIONS
N/A

MEDICATIONS

DRUG(S) OF CHOICE
- Sedatives—for severe disorientation and rolling; diazepam (1–5 mg/cat PO q8–12h) and acepromazine (0.05–0.10 mg/kg IM, SC, IV; to a maximum of 1 mg)
- Antiemetic drugs and drugs against motion sickness—usually ineffective
- Glucocorticoids—do not alter the course of the disease; not recommended

- Antibiotics—have been recommended in the acute phase if otitis media and interna cannot be ruled out; trimethoprim-sulfa (30 mg/kg PO q12–24h); a first-generation cephalosporin (e.g., cephalexin (10–30 mg/kg PO q6–12h); amoxicillin/clavulanic acid (62.5 mg/cat PO q12h)

CONTRAINDICATIONS
N/A

PRECAUTIONS
N/A

POSSIBLE INTERACTIONS
N/A

ALTERNATIVE DRUG(S)
N/A

FOLLOW-UP

PATIENT MONITORING
- Neurologic examination of outpatient—repeat in approximately 72 hr to confirm stabilization and initial improvement.
- Discharge inpatient when it is able to ambulate and resume eating and drinking.

PREVENTION/AVOIDANCE
N/A

POSSIBLE COMPLICATIONS
- Uncommon
- Dehydration and electrolyte imbalance (rare)

EXPECTED COURSE AND PROGNOSIS
- Marked improvement especially in the resting nystagmus within 72 hr, with progressive improvement of the gait and head tilt
- Patients usually normal within 2–3 weeks
- Head tilt—final sign to resolve; mild residual tilt may remain.
- If signs do not improve rapidly, other causes of vestibular disease should be pursued.

- Rarely recurs; mild head tilt and ataxia may temporarily return with stress (e.g., general anesthesia)

MISCELLANEOUS

ASSOCIATED CONDITIONS
N/A

AGE-RELATED FACTORS
N/A

ZOONOTIC POTENTIAL
N/A

PREGNANCY
N/A

SYNONYMS
- Feline vestibular syndrome
- Idiopathic vestibular neuropathy

SEE ALSO
- Head Tilt
- Otitis Media and Interna

ABBREVIATIONS
BAER = brain stem auditory-evoked response
CT = computed tomography
MRI = magnetic resonance imaging

Suggested Reading
de Lahunta A. Veterinary neuroanatomy and clinical neurology. Philadelphia: Saunders, 1983.
Oliver JE, Lorenz MD. Handbook of veterinary neurologic diagnosis. Philadelphia: WB Saunders, 1993.
Parent JM, Cochrane SM. Head tilt. In: Allen DG, ed. Small animal medicine. Philadelphia: Lippincott, 1991:753–759.
Author Susan M. Cochrane
Consulting Editor Joane M. Parent

VITAMIN A TOXICITY

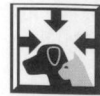

BASICS

OVERVIEW
• Skeletal disease that occurs after excessive intake of vitamin A
• High concentrations of vitamin A—inhibits intramembranous and endochondral ossification, resulting in dystrophic calcification of the skeleton

SIGNALMENT
• Cats aged 2–9 years
• No breed or sex predilections recognized

SIGNS

Historical Findings
• Daily diet high in liver or vitamin A supplementation (e.g., liver or cod liver oil) for > 14 weeks

• Lethargy
• Anorexia
• Weight loss

Physical Examination Findings
• Resentment of handling
• Marsupial-like sitting position with the forelimbs raised
• Weight-bearing lameness—most notable in the forelimbs, as osseous proliferation impinges on spinal nerves
• Cutaneous hypersensitivity or hyposensitivity over the cervical and forelimb regions
• Cervical, joint, and/or spinal stiffness
• Unkempt hair coat from inability to groom
• Constipation

CAUSES & RISK FACTORS
• Diet that includes large amounts of raw liver (usually beef or sheep)
• Excessive intake of vitamin A supplement—cod liver oil can contain > 1000 IU/mL of vitamin A.

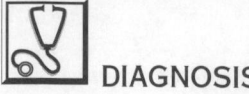

DIAGNOSIS

DIFFERENTIAL DIAGNOSIS
• Osteomyelitis
• Multiple cartilaginous exostoses
• Neoplasia

CBC/BIOCHEMISTRY/URINALYSIS
• Neutrophilic leukocytosis with stress leukogram
• Stress-induced hyperglycemia

OTHER LABORATORY TESTS
N/A

IMAGING
Radiography—new bone formation involving the cervical vertebrae (often extending from C1 to T2), the sternum, and the costal cartilages; new periosteal bone formation on metaphyses or surrounding joints; bony arthrodesis of joints

DIAGNOSTIC PROCEDURES
N/A

TREATMENT

• Stop feeding patient raw liver or supplementing with vitamin A.
• Use a balanced commercial cat food.

MEDICATIONS

DRUG(S)
Analgesics intended for cats—as required

CONTRAINDICATIONS/POSSIBLE INTERACTIONS
Avoid NSAIDs, except for aspirin (cats)

FOLLOW-UP

• Mature cats—reversal of most signs, except those related to bony arthrodesis
• Young cats—permanent retardation of long-bone growth; appositional bone formation returns to normal
• Skeletal improvement—detected by radiographic and clinical changes
• Plasma concentrations of vitamin A—decrease to normal within a few weeks after dietary change; may note high vitamin A content of the liver for years

MISCELLANEOUS

SEE ALSO
Poisoning (Intoxication)

ABBREVIATION
NSAID = nonsteroidal antiinflammatory drug

Suggested Reading
Fry PD. Hypervitaminosis A in the cat. Vet Intern 1989;1:16–31.
Goldman AL. Hypervitaminosis A in a cat. J Am Vet Med Assoc 1992;200:1970–1972.
Seawright AA, English PB. Hypervitaminosis A and deforming cervical spondylosis of the cat. J Compend Pathol 1967;77:29–39.
Author Johnny D. Hoskins
Consulting Editor Gary D. Osweiler

VITAMIN D TOXICITY

 BASICS

DEFINITION

A hypercalcemic disorder resulting from ingestion of vitamin D rodenticide preparations, excessive dietary supplementation, ingestion of congeners of vitamin D metabolites used for treatment of psoriasis, or diets high in vitamin D

PATHOPHYSIOLOGY

• Cholecalciferol is metabolized to 25-hydroxycholecalciferol in the liver. 25-Hydroxycholecalciferol is metabolized to several metabolites in the kidney, including calcitriol, the most potent metabolite in terms of enhancing calcium absorption from the gut and calcium resorption from bones under physiologic conditions. • 25-Hydroxy-cholecalciferol is the predominant circulating and active metabolite in cholecalciferol toxicity. • Calcipotriol (Dovonex), a congener of calcitriol, does not require activation; has immediate but limited action because it has a short half-life of 100 minutes • 25-Hydroxy-cholecalciferol calcitriol, and calcipotriol increase absorption of calcium from the gut, stimulate bone resorption, and enhance calcium absorption in renal distal tubules, resulting in hypercalcemia (serum calcium > 12.5 mg/dL). • Serum phosphorus is also increased. • The outcome is metastatic and dystropic mineralization of soft tissues.

SYSTEMS AFFECTED

• Musculoskeletal—demineralization; muscle tremors • Renal/urologic—calcification and renal failure • Gastrointestinal—anorexia; mineralization; emesis; hematemesis; constipation • Cardiovascular—mineralization, arrhythmias • Nervous—seizures • Respiratory—mineralization; dyspnea

INCIDENCE/PREVALENCE

• Cholecalciferol rodenticide toxicosis—most common cause of vitamin D poisoning in dogs and cats • Calcipotriol (Dovonex) antipsoriasis medication—leading cause of vitamin D congener toxicity in dogs • Overall incidence of vitamin D toxicity is not known

SIGNALMENT

Species

• Dogs and cats • Other species

Mean Age and Range

All ages affected; younger dogs (< 6 months) and cats are the most sensitive

SIGNS

General Comments

• Calcipotriol—signs develop within 6–12 hr postingestion • Cholecalciferol rodenticides—signs develop within 12–36 hr postingestion

Historical Findings

• Vomiting • CNS depression • Weakness • Anorexia • Polydipsia • Polyuria • Diarrhea • Melena • Hematemesis • Loss in body weight • Constipation • Seizures • Muscle tremors

Physical Examination Findings

• Renal pain on palpation • Gastrointestinal hemorrhage • Abdominal pain • Hyper-salivation • Oropharyngeal erosive lesions • Bradycardia; ventricular premature contractions • Dyspnea

CAUSES

• Ingestion of cholecalciferol rodenticides or congeners of calcitriol (e.g., calcipotriol [Dovonex]), excessive dietary supplementation with vitamin D, or diets high in vitamin D • Cholecalciferol rodenticides (0.075%)—include Quintox, Rampage, Ortho Rat-B-Gone, and Ortho Mouse-B-Gone; a single toxic dose is 2–3 mg/kg body weight in dogs; single lethal dose is 13 mg (520,000 IU)/kg body weight • Ingesting 1.8–3.6 μg/kg body weight of calcipotriol is toxic to dogs. • In dogs, daily ingestion of vitamin D 2000–4000 IU/kg for 1–2 weeks may cause chronic toxicosis. The National Research Council's recommended daily requirement for growing dogs is 0.55 μg (22 IU)/kg body weight. • Chronic intake of 50–100 μg cholecalciferol/kg body weight was toxic to dogs in 2–3 weeks; 15 mg vitamin D2 weekly was toxic to puppies in 2 months.

RISK FACTORS

• Pre-existing renal, cardiac, or CNS diseases • Neoplasia • Primary hyperparathyroidism • Hypoadrenocorticism • Granulomatous diseases (e.g., blastomycosis) • Juvenile hypercalcemia

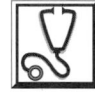 DIAGNOSIS

DIFFERENTIAL DIAGNOSIS

• Other hypercalcemic disorders, including lymphosarcoma and other malignancies, hypoadrenocorticism, chronic renal failure, primary hyperparathyroidism, and granulomatous lesions in soft tissues. Vitamin D and congener toxicosis can be differentiated from these diseases because it suppresses iPTH. In other conditions, iPTH is either normal or increased. • Anticoagulant rodenticide toxicity—due to hematemesis and melena

CBC/BIOCHEMISTRY/URINALYSIS

• Calcium—hypercalcemia (total serum calcium > 12.5 mg/dL, ionized calcium > 6.6 mg/dL). Hypercalcemia is immediate (2–3 hr) and transient (will decline to normal within 24 hr postingestion) in case of

calcipotriol ingestion. In case of chole-calciferol rodenticide toxicity, hypercalcemia is evident 12 hr postingestion and persists for weeks if not treated. • Hyperphosphatemia (> 8 mg/dL) • Hypokalemia • Azotemia • Hyposthenuria, proteinuria, and glucosuria • Metabolic acidosis • Calcipotriol—other abnormalities noted include hypoalbu-minemia, increased ALP, ALT and AST activity, thrombocytopenia, prolonged APTT, and increased fibrinogen concentration

OTHER LABORATORY TESTS

• Currently there are no confirmatory tests for calcipotriol intoxication. Serum 25-hydroxy vitamin D and calcitriol are normal. • The calcium-to-phosphorus ratio in renal cortex of deceased dogs is in the range of 0.4–0.9 for all vitamin D–related intoxications. • Renal cortical 25-hydroxy vitamin D concentration > 80 nmol/L supports a diagnosis of cholecalciferol toxicosis. • Biliary 25-hydroxy vitamin D concentration > 100 nmol/L supports a diagnosis of cholecalciferol toxicosis. • Serum 25-hydroxy vitamin D concentration is increased at least 10 times normal (normal ranges: dogs, 85–285 nmol/L; cats, 65–170 nmol/L) in cholecalciferol toxicosis. • Serum 1,25 dihydroxy vitamin D is only transiently increased and is of limited diagnostic value.

IMAGING

• Ultrasonography—renal, gastric wall, lung hyperechogenicity

DIAGNOSTIC PROCEDURES

• ECG—may show bradycardia, sinus tachycardia, and ventricular premature complexes • Endoscopy—may reveal erosive/hemorrhagic gastric mucosa. Tubular Necrosis

PATHOLOGIC FINDINGS

• Diffuse mineralization of gastric wall and intestines; hemorrhage in gastric mucosa; mineralization of the soft palate, salivary glands, or other soft tissues • Necrosis and mineralization of myocardium and large blood vessels • Mineralization of glomerular mesangium and capsule, and renal tubular basement membranes • Tubular necrosis

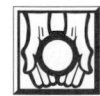 TREATMENT

APPROPRIATE HEALTH CARE

• Calcipotriol—emergency treatment is recommended; disease is characterized by acute transient hypercalcemia with massive soft tissue mineralization; prognosis is guarded, and hospitalization is required for patients presented 24 hr postingestion • Cholecalciferol—once clinical signs show (usually 24–36 hr postingestion), gastric decontamination is not worthwhile as absorption is already complete • All cases of vitamin D toxicosis require hospitalization for at least 48 hr postingestion for close observation.

Emetics
• A "must-do" in case of calcipotriol ingestion. Because of the peracute nature of this condition, the earliest clinical signs will show within a few hours of ingestion.
• Recommended if pet is seen ingesting a cholecalciferol rodenticide product before clinical signs show • Syrup of ipecac (dogs, 1–2 mL/kg; cats, 3.3 mL/kg) or hydrogen peroxide (5–25 mL/5 kg) orally. If vomiting has not occurred within 15–20 min, repeat dose once. • Apomorphine (0.25 mg subconjunctivally)

NURSING CARE
• Correct dehydration and electrolyte imbalances (hypokalemia). • Enhance calciuresis with fluid therapy—strongly recommended for all patients • Peritoneal dialysis with a calcium-free dialysate—for severe azotemia and hypercalcemia • Blood transfusion—if anemia is severe • Antibiotic therapy—to prevent secondary bacterial infection because of broken defense barrier in gut • Parenteral alimentation—recommended to rest the gut and to overcome anorexia

DIET
Offer low-calcium, low-phosphorus diets

CLIENT EDUCATION
• Caution client to keep all rodenticide products in places that are inaccessible to pets. • Caution client to secure all medications where pets cannot reach them. • Warn client that vitamin D toxicity is a severe and costly disease to treat because prolonged therapy and hospitalization are usually required.

MEDICATIONS

DRUG(S) OF CHOICE
• Biphosphonates (e.g., pamidronate disodium)—to treat hypercalcemia • Salmon calcitonin—to treat hypercalcemia

Decontamination of Gastrointestinal Tract
• Within 6 hr of vitamin D ingestion
• Emetic and activated charcoal plus saline or osmotic cathartics • Dogs—apomorphine 0.02–0.04 mg/kg IV, IM, SC, or subconjunctivally • Cats—xylazine 0.4–0.5 mg/kg IV • Activated charcoal powder (1–4 g/kg) combined with a saline cathartic (magnesium or sodium sulfate, 250 mg/kg)—orally or by gastric tube

Hypercalcemia Reduction
• Pamidronate disodium (Aredia; Ciba-Geigy, Tarrytown, NY)—1.3–2.0 mg/kg in 0.9% sodium chloride by slow IV infusion over 2–4 hr; repeat once 3–4 days later; do not combine with salmon calcitonin as this has no added benefit • Salmon calcitonin—4–6 IU IM or SC every 2–3 weeks; because of limited efficacy and because patients may become refractory, combine calcitonin therapy with corticosteroids or increase dose up to 10–20 IU/kg • Prednisolone—dogs and cats: 2–6 mg/kg IM q12h • Furosemide—dogs: 2–6 mg/kg; cats: 1–4 mg/kg SC, IV, or IM q8–12h

Seizure Control
Diazepam—0.5 mg/kg IV, repeat as necessary

Control of Ventricular Premature Contractions
Lidocaine—50 μg/kg/min

Gastrointestinal Protection
• Sucralfate—1-g slurry PO q6h
• Famotidine—15 mg IV q12h

Antiemetics
Metoclopramide—6 mg SC q8h

PRECAUTIONS
• Supratherapeutic doses of pamidronate disodium—may worsen renal failure
• Salmon calcitonin—associated with side effects: anorexia, anaphylaxis, and emesis
• Xylazine—may aggravate respiratory depression and result in vagal-mediated slowing of the heart rate; yohimbine (0.1 mg/kg IV) is the antidote to xylazine
• Prolonged prednisolone therapy—may result in adrenocortical suppression; taper doses gradually over a 2–4 week treatment period

FOLLOW-UP

PATIENT MONITORING
• Following pamidronate therapy—serum calcium and BUN; measure 24, 48, and 72 hr following exposure; if hypercalcemia is present, fluid diuresis is recommended; if hypercalcemia is still present, repeat pamidronate infusion 72 or 96 hr after the first infusion, then monitor serum calcium and BUN q48h • Following calcitonin therapy—serum calcium and BUN; monitor q24h and continue adjusting dose until calcium returns to normal (24–48 hr for calcipotriol, or 2–4 weeks for cholecalciferol)
• Calcipotriol causes short-term hypercalcemia (24–48 hr) with massive soft tissue mineralization; requires long-term aggressive fluid and supportive therapy; cholecalciferol-induced hypercalcemia is persistent, requiring long-term management plus supportive care

PREVENTION/AVOIDANCE
• Keep rodenticides and medications out of reach of pets. • Avoid diets that are high in vitamin D.

POSSIBLE COMPLICATIONS
• Chronic renal failure—inability to concentrate urine • Secondary bacterial infection—due to injury in the gut
• Subclinical renal, cardiovascular, and gastrointestinal injury—due to mineralization

EXPECTED COURSE AND PROGNOSIS
• Calcipotriol—guarded prognosis unless aggressive therapy is given immediately because of peracute nature of condition and associated massive soft tissue mineralization
• Cholecalciferol—depends on severity and duration of hypercalcemia; if high unresponsive hypercalcemia is present or if severe mineralization occurs before therapy is initiated, prognosis is poor • Usual course—2–4 weeks

MISCELLANEOUS

AGE-RELATED FACTORS
Distinguish from normal juvenile hypercalcemia

PREGNANCY
Teratogenic effects—calcipotriol and vitamin D have antiproliferative effects and potential for teratogenesis

SYNONYMS
• Cholecalciferol toxicosis • Calcipotriol toxicosis • Vitamin D congener toxicosis
• Dovonex toxicosis

ABBREVIATIONS
• ALP = alanine phosphatase • ALT = alanine aminotransferase • APTT = activated partial thromboplastin time • AST = aspartate aminotransferase • BUN = blood urea nitrogen • CNS = central nervous system • ECG = electrocardiography
• iPTH = intact parathyroid hormone

Suggested Reading
Drazner FH. Hypercalcemia in the dog and cat. J Vet Med Assoc 1981;178:1252–1256.
Fan TM, Simpson KW, Center SA, Yeager A. Calcipotriol toxicity in a dog. J Small Anim Pract 1998;39:581–586.
Rumbeiha WK, Braselton WE, Nachreiner R, et al. The post-mortem diagnosis of cholecalciferol toxicosis: a novel approach and differentiation from ethylene glycol toxicosis. J Vet Diagn Invest 2000;12:426–432.
Rumbeiha WK, Fitzgerald SD, Kruger JM, et al. Use of pamidronate disodium to reduce cholecalciferol-induced toxicosis in dogs. Am J Vet Res 2000;61:9–13.
Author Wilson K. Rumbeiha
Consulting Editor Gary D. Osweiler

VOMITING, ACUTE

BASICS

DEFINITION
• Forceful, reflex expulsion of gastric contents from the oral cavity
• Acute vomiting is defined as vomiting of short duration (< 7 days) and variable frequency.

PATHOPHYSIOLOGY
• A complex set of reflex activities under central neurologic control involving the coordination of GI, abdominal, and respiratory musculature
• Often preceded by prodromal signs of nausea that can include depression, shivering, hiding or seeking comfort, hypersalivation, lip licking, frequent swallowing, and retching
• Occurs when the VC in the medulla is stimulated by afferent activity from several sources
• Stimulation can occur from stretch receptors, chemoreceptors, and osmoreceptors located throughout the GI tract, hepatobiliary system, genitourinary system, peritoneum, and pancreas.
• The CTZ, when stimulated by a variety of drugs and toxins, can also stimulate the VC.
• Higher centers can lead to psychogenic vomiting, and input from the vestibular apparatus (e.g., motion sickness, vestibular disease) can stimulate the VC.

SYSTEMS AFFECTED
• Cardiovascular—hypovolemia, causing tachycardia, pale mucous membranes, and weak pulses; hypokalemia can cause arrhythmias
• GI—reflux esophagitis
• Metabolic—electrolyte and acid–base abnormalities (e.g., hypokalemia, hyponatremia, hypochloremia, metabolic alkalosis), prerenal azotemia, and dehydration
• Respiratory—aspiration pneumonia, rhinitis from ingesta refluxed into the nasopharynx
• Nervous—depression

SIGNALMENT
No age, breed, or sex predisposition

SIGNS

Historical Findings
• Variable vomiting of food and/or fluid (either clear, bile-, or blood-stained)
• Ingestion of foreign material
• Variable lethargy and appetite loss; may see diarrhea and/or melena

Physical Examination Findings
• May include dehydration, (e.g., dry mucous membranes, reduced skin turgor, pale mucous

membranes, tachycardia, weak pulses), fluid-filled bowel loops, excessive gut sounds, abdominal pain (localized [e.g., foreign body, pancreatitis, pyelonephritis, hepatic disease] vs. diffuse [e.g., peritonitis, severe enteritis]), or abdominal mass (e.g., foreign body, intussusceptum, torsed viscus)
• May note diarrhea or melena on rectal examination
• May see fever with infectious and inflammatory causes

CAUSES
• Adverse food reactions—indiscretions (eating rapidly, ingestion of foreign material); intolerances (e.g., sudden diet change, allergies)
• Drugs—antibiotics, antiinflammatories (corticosteroid and NSAIDs), chemotherapeutics, digitalis, narcotics, xylazine, thiacetarsamide
• GI inflammation—infectious enteritis: viruses (parvo, distemper, corona), bacteria (salmonella, Campylobacter); hemorrhagic gastroenteritis
• Gastroduodenal ulcers
• GI obstruction—foreign bodies, intussusception, neoplasia, volvulus, ileus, constipation
• Systemic disease—uremia, hepatic failure, sepsis, acidosis, electrolyte imbalance (hypokalemia, hypocalcemia, hypercalcemia)
• Abdominal disorders—pancreatitis, peritonitis, pyometra
• Endocrine disease—hypoadrenocorticism, diabetic ketoacidosis
• Neurologic disease—vestibular disturbances, meningitis, encephalitis, CNS trauma
• Parasitism—*Tricuspis* (dogs), ascarids, *Giardia, Physaloptera* (dogs), *Ollulanus tricuspis* (cats), salmon poisoning (dogs)
• Toxins—lead, ethylene glycol, zinc, mycotoxins, household plants
• Miscellaneous—anaphylaxis, heat stroke, motion sickness, pain, fear

RISK FACTORS
N/A

DIAGNOSIS

DIFFERENTIAL DIAGNOSIS

Differentiating Similar Signs
• Vomiting usually includes hypersalivation, retching, and forceful contractions of the abdominal muscles and diaphragm.
• Must always be differentiated from regurgitation, which is the effortless expulsion of fluid or food from the esophagus or pharyngeal

cavity, and dysphagia (difficulty in swallowing), which is observed during eating or drinking
• Animals that are vomiting may have disorders that additionally cause regurgitation, and frequent vomiting can lead to reflux esophagitis and regurgitation.

Differentiating Causes
• Classify patients as serious or nonserious cases.
• If no signs of serious vomiting (e.g., dehydration, lethargy, fever, anorexia, or abdominal pain), can assess with a thorough history and physical examination alone
• When indications of serious vomiting exist, when frequency intensifies, or when signs do not resolve over 2–3 days, obtain a minimum database (including CBC, biochemical analysis, urinalysis, and survey abdominal radiographs) in an attempt to find the primary cause.

CBC/BIOCHEMISTRY/URINALYSIS
• In nonsevere vomiting the hemogram, biochemical profile, and urinalysis are typically normal.
• Anemia with pan-hypoproteinemia with severe gastric ulceration and bleeding
• Dehydration—may see hemoconcentration (high PCV and total protein)
• May see a stress leukogram
• Infectious or inflammatory causes—may see an inflammatory leukogram
• Differentiate prerenal azotemia from renal causes by urine specific gravity.
• Acute hepatopathies—may see elevated liver enzymes and serum bilirubin or hypoglycemia
• Pancreatitis—may see elevated lipase, amylase, and liver enzymes and hypocalcemia
• Hyponatremia, hyperkalemia, and azotemia suggest hypoadrenocorticism.
• Hyperglycemia with glucosuria and ketonuria indicates ketoacidotic diabetic mellitus.

OTHER LABORATORY TESTS
Additional blood tests for specific diseases when indicated (e.g., blood lead level, ethylene glycol assay, ACTH stimulation testing for hypoadrenocorticism, and cPLI or TLI testing for pancreatitis).

IMAGING
• Survey abdominal radiographs are often normal, but radiodense foreign bodies, segmental ileus, or gastric distension indicating volvulus or outflow obstruction may be observed; serosal detail may be lost ("ground glass" appearance) with pancreatitis or peritonitis; a mass effect or haziness in the right cranial quadrant or persistent gas in the descending duodenum may indicate pancreatitis.

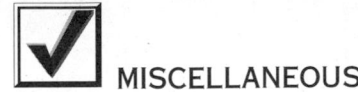
• Can use contrast radiography to evaluate for radiolucent foreign bodies, obstruction, intussusception, or volvulus
• Can use abdominal ultrasonography to visualize a focally dilated bowel loop indicating an obstruction or a multilamellar abdominal mass indicating an intussusception or to confirm an enlarged hypoechoic pancreas typical of pancreatitis

DIAGNOSTIC PROCEDURES
Endoscopy may be useful to assess for gastroduodenal ulceration and gastric and proximal duodenal foreign bodies.

TREATMENT
• The most frequent cause of acute vomiting is dietary indiscretion.
• Patients with nonserious vomiting are treated on an outpatient basis, resting the GI tract by keeping the animal NPO for 12–24 hr.
• If vomiting resolves, initially offer small amounts of water or ice cubes and if vomiting does not recur, follow with an easily digestible, low-fat, single-protein and single-carbohydrate source diet such as non-fat cottage cheese or skinless white chicken and rice at a 1:3 ratio.
• Recovery from nonserious vomiting is usually rapid and spontaneous.
• If vomiting does not recur, wean the patient back onto the normal diet over 4–5 days.
• Patients with serious vomiting should be hospitalized and treated initially NPO with intravenous crystalloid fluids while further diagnostics are performed.

MEDICATIONS
• NPO followed by a bland diet usually will control nonserious vomiting.
• Antiemetics can be used for frequent vomiting.

DRUG(S) OF CHOICE
• May use antiemetics in patients with severe vomiting causing electrolyte and/or acid–base disturbances or reflux esophagitis
• Several antiemetics are available for both dogs and cats—phenothiazine derivatives that act at the CTZ and VC include chlorproma-

zine (0.5–4 mg/kg SC q8h) and metoclopramide, a dopamine antagonist and motility modifier that acts at the CTZ and on local receptors in the gut (0.2–0.5 mg/kg PO or SC q6–8h, or 1–2 mg/kg/day as a CRI); H_1-receptor antagonists acting on the CTZ can be used in motion sickness (e.g., diphenhydramine 2–4 mg/kg PO, IM q6–8h)
• Patients with ulceration—can use H_2-receptor antagonists such as ranitidine (1–2 mg/kg PO, SC, IV q12h) and/or the gastric mucosal protectant sucralfate (250 mg/cat PO q8–12h, 250–1000 mg/dog PO q8–12h)
• Fever or mucosal injury (hematemesis, melena)—antibiotics may be indicated (e.g.. ampicillin, cephalothin)

CONTRAINDICATIONS
• Use phenothiazines with caution in dehydrated patients because of possible hypotension from their α-receptor antagonist effect; they also lower the seizure threshold and should be avoided in epileptics.
• Do not use anticholinergics; they can cause gastric atony and intestinal ileus, which could exacerbate vomiting.
• Do not use metoclopramide in patients with GI obstruction, because of its prokinetic effect.

PRECAUTIONS
Use antiemetics carefully; they may suppress vomiting and mask progressive disease or hamper an important means of monitoring response to primary therapy.

POSSIBLE INTERACTIONS
Anticholinergics negate the effect of metoclopramide.

ALTERNATIVE DRUG(S)
N/A

FOLLOW-UP

PATIENT MONITORING
• If frequency of vomiting increases or serious problems occur, hospitalize animals for treatment and obtain appropriate data.
• If vomiting persists beyond 7 days despite conservative therapy, pursue appropriate testing for chronic vomiting.

POSSIBLE COMPLICATIONS
N/A

MISCELLANEOUS

ASSOCIATED CONDITIONS
See Systems Affected

AGE-RELATED FACTORS
Young animals are more likely to ingest foreign objects and acquire viral, bacterial, and parasitic disease.

ZOONOTIC POTENTIAL
N/A

PREGNANCY
Misoprostol, a synthetic prostaglandin used most often in treatment or prevention of gastric ulceration, is contraindicated in pregnant animals.

SYNONYMS
N/A

SEE ALSO
• Diarrhea, Acute
• Gastroduodenal Ulcer Disease

ABBREVIATIONS
ACTH = adrenocorticotropic hormone
cPLI = canine pancreatic lipase immunoreactivity
CRI = continuous-rate infusion
CTZ = chemoreceptor trigger zone
GI = gastrointestinal
PCV = packed cell volume
TLI = trypsin-like immunoreactivity
VC = vomiting center

Suggested Reading

Guilford WG, Strombeck DR. Acute gastritis. In: Guilford WG, et al., eds. Small animal gastroenterology. Philadelphia: Saunders, 1996:261–274.
Hall JA. Diseases of the stomach. In: Ettinger SJ, Feldman EC, eds. Textbook of veterinary internal medicine. Philadelphia: Saunders, 2000:1154–1181.
Twedt DC. Vomiting. In: Ettinger SJ, Feldman EC, eds. Textbook of veterinary internal medicine. Philadelphia: Saunders, 2000:117–120.
Author John Hart Jr.
Consulting Editors Albert E. Jergens

VOMITING, CHRONIC

BASICS

DEFINITION
Chronic vomiting is defined as either intermittent episodes of vomiting that have not responded to symptomatic treatment or persistent vomiting of long duration with variable frequency.

PATHOPHYSIOLOGY
Vomiting occurs when the vomiting center, located within the medulla oblongata, is activated by humoral or neural stimulation of various peripheral receptors sensitive to chemicals, inflammation, and changes in osmolality.

SYSTEMS AFFECTED
• Endocrine/Metabolic—dehydration, electrolyte and acid–base imbalances, prerenal azotemia • Cardiovascular—hypovolemia or electrolyte and acid–base imbalances can cause arrhythmias • Gastrointestinal—gastroesophageal reflux, esophagitis, and subsequent esophageal stricture • Respiratory system—aspiration pneumonia • Neurologic system—altered mentation

SIGNALMENT
• Dogs and cats • Young animals are more likely to ingest foreign bodies; linear foreign bodies are more common in cats. • Confirmed or suspected breed predispositions—Lhasa apso, shih tzu, and other brachycephalic breeds are prone to pyloric stenosis; basenjis, German shepherds, and shar-peis are prone to inflammatory bowel diseases; rottweilers are prone to gastric eosinophilic granuloma; Airedale terriers are prone to pancreatic carcinoma; beagles, Bedlington terriers, cocker spaniels, Doberman pinschers, Labrador retrievers, Skye terriers, and standard poodles are prone to chronic hepatitis

SIGNS

Historical Findings
• Vomiting, regurgitation, or both, of food, clear or bile-stained fluid, hematemesis, decreased appetite or anorexia, pica, melena, polydipsia, and abdominal distension are typical of gastric disease. • Diarrhea and weight loss are more characteristic of intestinal disease. • Signs such as weakness, polyuria, or jaundice relate to other underlying metabolic diseases.

Physical Examination Findings
• May see poor haircoat, weight loss, abdominal distention, abdominal pain, palpably thickened bowel loops, or abdominal masses • Dry, pale, mucous membranes occur if the patient is dehydrated or anemic. • Increased gut sounds occasionally auscultated • Rectal examination may detect diarrhea, hematochezia, or melena.

CAUSES

Esophageal Disease
• Hiatal hernia • Gastroesophageal reflux
• Distal esophagitis

Infectious Disease
• *Helicobacter*-related gastritis • Histoplasmosis • Pythiosis • Small intestinal bacterial overgrowth (SIBO) • Disseminated aspergillosis • Gastric parasites—*Physaloptera* spp. • Intestinal parasitism

Metabolic Diseases
• Renal disease • Hepatic disease • Biliary disease • Hypoadrenocorticism • Chronic pancreatitis • Ketoacidotic diabetes mellitus • Metabolic acidosis • Electrolyte abnormalities—hypokalemia, hyperkalemia, hyponatremia, hypercalcemia can alter motility

Inflammatory Bowel Disease (IBD)
• Lymphocytic, plasmacytic, eosinophilic, or granulomatous • Gastritis, enteritis, or colitis

Obstructive GI Disease
• Foreign body • Congenital pyloric stenosis • Chronic pyloric hypertrophic gastropathy • Intussusception

Neoplastic Disease
• Gastric polyps • GI lymphosarcoma, adenocarcinoma, fibrosarcoma • Pancreatic adenocarcinoma • Pancreatic gastrin-secreting tumor (gastrinoma) • Systemic mastocytosis

Neurologic
• Cerebral edema • CNS tumors • Encephalitis/meningoencephalitis • Vestibulitis

Motility Disorders
• Chronic enterogastric reflux • Diabetic gastroparesis • Postgastric dilatation • Post-surgical—gastric, pyloric, duodenal • Electrolyte imbalances

Miscellaneous
• Drug-induced (e.g., NSAIDs, glucocorticoids, antibiotics, antifungals) • Food intolerance/allergy • Toxicity

Additional Causes in Cats
• Parasitic—dirofilariasis, *Ollulanus tricuspis,* giardiasis • Inflammatory—cholecystitis, cholangiohepatitis • Metabolic—hyperthyroidism • Functional—obstipation

RISK FACTORS
Breed-associated disease (see Signalment)

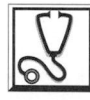

DIAGNOSIS

DIFFERENTIAL DIAGNOSIS
• Initially, vomiting must be differentiated from dysphagia and regurgitation. • Dysphagia—characterized by difficulty with prehension and initiation of swallowing; indicates abnormality in the oral cavity, pharynx, or proximal esophagus • Regurgitation is a passive retrograde movement into the oronasal cavity of fluid and undigested food that has not yet reached the stomach. • Regurgitation—occurs without retching (forceful abdominal contractions); localizes disease to the esophagus • Vomiting is often preceded by restlessness, nausea, salivation, and repeated swallowing. • Retching and expulsion of partially digested food and clear or bile-stained liquid, sometimes with digested blood that resembles coffee-grounds—typical observations of vomiting patients • Vomiting patients may also regurgitate because of secondary esophagitis. • Vomiting—the hallmark of gastric disease; however, many intestinal and nongastrointestinal diseases cause vomiting • Diarrhea, abnormal stool, or significant weight loss is more suggestive of intestinal disease. • Changes in activity or mentation, or signs such as polyuria, weakness, or jaundice indicate that vomiting is secondary to metabolic abnormalities caused by renal, adrenal, or hepatic disease. • If vomiting persists for 5–7 days or if vomiting occurs intermittently several days per week, it is classified as chronic vomiting. • A thorough diagnostic workup is indicated.

CBC/BIOCHEMISTRY/URINALYSIS
• CBCs are usually normal with primary gastric disease. • Chronic GI bleeding can cause a nonregenerative anemia, often with characteristics of iron deficiency (microcytosis, hypochromasia, thrombocytosis). • Acute GI bleeding can cause either regenerative or nonregenerative anemia, depending on severity and duration. • Nonregenerative anemia occurs secondary to chronic metabolic or chronic inflammatory diseases. • Inflammatory bowel diseases, chronic pancreatitis, cholangiohepatitis, and cholecystitis may cause neutrophilic leukocytosis and monocytosis. • Eosinophilia can occur from eosinophilic gastroenteritis, adrenocortical insufficiency, and GI nematodes. • Dehydration increases the packed cell volume and total protein. • Biochemistry—diagnostic and therapeutic information; normal results rule out metabolic disease as a cause of chronic vomiting. • Electrolyte and acid–base imbalances usually do not indicate the cause of vomiting but do reflect severity of losses and can help to localize disease. • Include total CO_2 in the biochemical assessment of any chronically vomiting patient. • Hypochloremic metabolic alkalosis, often with hypokalemia, indicates substantial loss of gastric content, most consistent with gastric outflow obstruction; vomiting from acute pancreatitis or renal failure can cause similar changes. • Hyperkalemia in the vomiting patient indicates hypoadrenocorticism or oliguric or anuric renal failure; occasionally, enteritis caused by trichuriasis or bacterial infection (salmonellosis) mimics hypoadrenocorticism. • Metabolic acidosis is common in dehydrated patients and those with renal failure, diabetic ketoacidosis, and severe gastroenteritis with diarrhea. • Increased liver enzyme activity, hypoalbuminemia, hyperbilirubinemia, hypoglycemia, or low urea nitrogen concentration indicates liver disease. • Increased blood and urine glucose concentration, with or without ketonemia or ketonuria, is diagnostic for diabetes mellitus. • Hyperglobulinemia may indicate chronic inflammation or infection. • Hypoalbuminemia and lymphopenia occur secondary to a protein-losing enteropathy

caused by infiltrative intestinal diseases such as lymphocytic plasmacytic gastroenteritis, neoplasia, histoplasmosis, or primary intestinal lymphangiectasia. • Hypocholesterolemia may also be seen with lymphangiectasia. • Urinalysis is used to rule out such nongastrointestinal causes of chronic vomiting as renal failure or diabetic ketoacidosis. • Acid urine in the hypokalemic, hypochloremic, alkalotic patient indicates substantial loss of gastric content as would occur with gastric outflow obstruction.

OTHER LABORATORY TESTS
• ACTH stimulation test is used to confirm hypoadrenocorticism. • Amylase, lipase, and trypsin-like immunoreactivity help confirm pancreatitis. • Bile acid concentration is used to help confirm hepatobiliary disease.

IMAGING
• Survey radiographs of the abdomen help identify foreign bodies, GI distension with fluid or gas, and displacement, malposition, and shape or size changes of abdominal organs. • Survey thoracic radiographs are used to evaluate for pulmonary metastatic or infectious disease. • Abdominal contrast radiographs help identify foreign bodies, GI wall masses or infiltrative disease, mucosal ulceration, delayed gastric emptying, and motility disorders. • Abdominal ultrasonography is done to seek parenchymal abnormalities of the liver, kidneys, pancreas, and GI tract to identify an underlying cause of chronic vomiting. • CT and MRI further evaluate for parenchymal abnormalities of abdominal organs.

DIAGNOSTIC PROCEDURES
• Gastroduodenoscopy—allows direct inspection of the gastric and intestinal lumen to identify gross mucosal lesions and foreign bodies and provides a method of biopsy to evaluate for microscopic disease
• Laparoscopy or exploratory laparotomy is used for more extensive diagnostic and therapeutic procedures.

TREATMENT
• Specific treatment, elimination of underlying causes, and supportive therapy • If vomiting persists, stop oral intake of food and water for several days. • Use fluid therapy to replace deficits and to provide for maintenance and ongoing losses. • If acid–base status is unknown or if hypochloremic metabolic alkalosis is present, use 0.9% normal saline. • If metabolic acidosis is present, use lactated Ringer's solution. • Supplement potassium if hypokalemia is present; 20 mEq of KCl/L of fluid can be safely added for replacement and maintenance. • Debilitated patients and those in poor nutritional condition may need parenteral or enteral nutrition. • Dietary therapy for patients with suspected food allergy or with IBD should use a diet containing a single-source protein novel to the patient, given for a minimum of 4–6

weeks. • Give blood transfusion to severely anemic patients with evidence of active GI bleeding. • Use surgical treatment if uncontrolled hemorrhage, obstruction, or perforation is seen.

MEDICATIONS
DRUG(S)
• Use anti-ulcer medications for patients with evidence of upper GI bleeding (e.g., hematemesis or melena). • Antisecretory drugs such as H_2-receptor blockers (e.g., cimetidine, ranitidine, famotidine, nizatidine) or proton-pump inhibitors such as omeprazole (more potent than H_2-receptor blockers and permit once-daily dosing)—ranitidine 2 mg/kg PO, IV q12h; omeprazole 0.7 mg/kg PO q24h
• Protectants such as sucralfate (0.5–1 g/dog PO q8–12h; 0.25 g/cat PO q 8–12h) to accelerate gastric mucosal healing
• Antibiotics—indicated for treatment of *Helicobacter*-associated gastritis, as an adjunct to corticosteroids in the treatment of IBD, and to treat SIBO syndrome • Suggested treatment of *Helicobacter*-associated gastritis—amoxicillin 22 mg/kg PO q8h plus omeprazole 0.7 mg/kg PO q24h; metronidazole 10 mg/kg PO q8h can be added if response is inadequate; azithromycin 5 mg/kg PO q12h is an effective alternative to amoxicillin • Metronidazole—effective in some cases of mild IBD and is used in combination with corticosteroids to treat IBD
• SIBO syndrome—tetracycline, metronidazole, amoxicillin, and tylosin in addition to correcting the underlying cause
• Use corticosteroids in conjunction with dietary changes and sometimes antibiotics to treat biopsy-confirmed IBD (e.g., lymphocytic-plasmacytic, eosinophilic, granulomatous)
• Azathioprine or cyclophosphamide—can use as alternatives in patients that do not respond to corticosteroids or in conjunction with corticosteroids to decrease the dosage of corticosteroids required to control symptoms • Can use the prokinetic drugs metoclopramide or erythromycin to treat delayed gastric emptying not associated with obstructive disease
• Pyrantel pamoate is effective for *Physaloptera*; fenbendazole is effective for *Ollulanus*.
• Animals with chronic GI bleeding that develop microcytic hypochromic anemia may require iron supplementation. • Treatment for neoplasia depends on tumor type and location; most require surgical resection, some with adjunctive chemotherapy. • GI lymphosarcoma is usually treated with chemotherapy.
• Paraneoplastic hypersecretion of gastric acid, as occurs with mastocytosis and gastrin-secreting pancreatic tumors, is best treated with potent antisecretory drugs such as omeprazole to diminish gastritis, gastric ulcer, and chronic vomiting. • Reserve antiemetics for patients with persistent vomiting unresponsive to treatment of the underlying disease.

• Phenothiazines (e.g., chlorpromazine, phenylethylpirazine) block at both the CTZ and vomiting center; limit use to 48–72 hours—chlorpromazine 0.5 mg/kg SC, IM q6–8h • Prokinetic drugs (e.g., metoclopramide)—metoclopramide also blocks the CTZ; can use both indefinitely to treat motility disorders; metoclopramide 0.2–0.5 mg/kg IV, IM, PO q6–8h • Vomiting caused by chemotherapy is best treated with ondansetron 0.5–1 mg/kg IV, PO given 30 min before chemotherapy.

CONTRAINDICATIONS
Do not give α-adrenergic blockers such as chlorpromazine to dehydrated patients; they can cause hypotension.

PRECAUTIONS
• Use antiemetics with caution; they can mask an underlying problem. • Metoclopramide can cause depression, restlessness, agitation, and other behavioral changes, particularly in cats. • Corticosteroids are immunosuppressive and are a risk factor for development of GI ulceration; use caution when treating IBD with corticosteroids at high dosages or for long periods. • Azathioprine is myelotoxic; do a CBC for neutropenia and thrombocytopenia every 2 weeks for the first 2 months of treatment and monthly thereafter. • Do not use anticholinergics as antiemetics; they can cause gastric atony and gastric retention, which can exacerbate vomiting. • Metoclopramide and cisapride are contraindicated in patients with GI obstruction.

POSSIBLE INTERACTIONS
Cimetidine and ranitidine interfere with hepatic metabolism of theophylline, phenytoin, and warfarin, and should not be used concurrently with these drugs.

MISCELLANEOUS
ZOONOTIC POTENTIAL
Helicobacter heilmanii and *H. felis* may have zoonotic potential; they have been isolated from humans with chronic gastritis, most of whom have had close contact with dogs or cats.

ABBREVIATION
CTZ = chemoreceptor trigger zone.

Suggested Reading
Guilford WG, Center SA, Williams DA, Meyer DJ. Chronic gastric diseases. In: Strombeck's small animal gastroenterology. 3rd ed. Philadelphia: Saunders, 1996: 275–302.
Willard M. Diseases of the stomach. In: Ettinger SJ, Feldman ED, eds. Textbook of veterinary internal medicine. 5th ed. Philadelphia: Saunders, 2000:1154–1181.
Authors Robert C. DeNovo and Christine C. Jenkins
Consulting Editor Albert E. Jergens

VON WILLEBRAND DISEASE

 BASICS

DEFINITION
• A complex inherited defect of hemostasis related to defects in synthesis or function of vWF
• The most common inherited bleeding disorder in dogs

PATHOPHYSIOLOGY
• vWF—a large, multimeric glycoprotein consisting of identical subunits that are synthesized mostly by endothelial cells; circulates in the plasma as a macromolecular complex with factor VIII; is required for platelet adhesion to collagen and for stabilizing and preventing rapid clearance of factor VIII from the circulation
• Various defects in the vWF gene may cause deficient synthesis of vWF or production of dysfunctional vWF; these defects may cause platelet function defects and delayed coagulation of blood.

SYSTEMS AFFECTED
Hemic/Lymph/Immune—bleeding diathesis with hemorrhages in a variety of organs but especially at surgical sites and mucosal surfaces

GENETICS
• An autosomal trait; the pattern in most dogs fits a model in which each normal allele affects production of about 50% of normal vWF levels.
• Described as autosomal recessive disease in Scottish terriers and Chesapeake Bay retrievers

INCIDENCE/PREVALENCE
Prevalence of a low concentration of vWF—extremely variable in different breeds; reported estimates of 68%–73% in Doberman pinschers, 18%–28% in Shetland sheepdogs, and 16%–30% in Scottish terriers

GEOGRAPHIC DISTRIBUTION
None

SIGNALMENT

Species
• Dogs
• Rare in cats

Breed Predilections
• Described in at least 60 breeds of dogs
• Breeds with a known high prevalence—Airedale terriers, Basset hounds, dachshunds, Doberman pinschers, German shepherds, golden retrievers, keeshonds, Manchester terriers, miniature schnauzers, Pembroke Welsh corgis, rottweilers, Shetland sheepdogs, Scottish terriers, and standard poodles

Mean Age and Range
Present from birth

Predominant Sex
Males and females affected

SIGNS

General Comments
Can be subclinical or manifested as a bleeding diathesis, most commonly as a consequence of surgery or some form of injury.

Historical Findings
• Previous abnormal bleeding associated with teething or disproportionate hemorrhage associated with minor injury
• Many dogs survive ear cropping or tail docking without serious bleeding.

Physical Examination Findings
• Gastrointestinal bleeding
• Hematuria
• Bleeding around gums at teething
• Epistaxis
• Vaginal or penile bleeding
• Petechiae are uncommon, despite the platelet function defect.

CAUSES
• Divided into three classifications
• Type I—quantitative defect with low vWF concentration; most common pattern; clinical severity varies; typical of Doberman pinschers, Airedales, and the one-third of shelties with detectable vWF
• Type II—qualitative defect with selective depletion of high molecular weight multimers; described in German shorthaired and wire-haired pointers
• Type III—severe form of type I with virtually undetectable vWF; typical of the defect in Scottish terriers, Chesapeake Bay retrievers, Dutch Kooiker dogs, and about two-thirds of affected Shetland sheepdogs

RISK FACTORS
Hypothyroidism may exacerbate the bleeding tendency in affected animals.

 DIAGNOSIS

DIFFERENTIAL DIAGNOSIS
• Classic hemophilia—defective synthesis of factor VIII is usually associated with much lower factor VIII activity and with a more severe bleeding tendency, including spontaneous hemorrhages in body cavities, deep muscle masses, and joints.
• Other inherited or acquired hemostatic defects

CBC/BIOCHEMISTRY/URINALYSIS
• Anemia proportional to the degree of blood loss
• Neutrophilia and mild left shift secondary to hemorrhage
• Mild reticulocytosis
• Normal platelet count

OTHER LABORATORY TESTS
• PT—normal
• APTT—normal in most dogs, even those with severe deficiency of vWF
• vWF assay—the test of choice for diagnosis; normal range reported as > 70% of normal reference pools of dogs; ELISA method may be used: < 7% indicates either a homozygous defect or severe (penetrant) heterozygous animal, 7%–50% usually indicates heterozygous animal (either asymptomatic carrier or bleeder), < 30% may indicate a hemorrhagic tendency

IMAGING
N/A

DIAGNOSTIC PROCEDURES
Buccal mucosal bleeding time—the most useful test for predicting bleeding problems in dogs suspected of being affected; use of a gauze strip tied around the maxilla to cause venous engorgement in the folded-back upper lip increases the sensitivity of the test; normal bleeding time for this method is 1.7–4.2 min (mean, 2.6 min); bleeding time does not identify all animals at risk for abnormal bleeding after surgery.

PATHOLOGIC FINDINGS
Hemorrhage is the only associated abnormality, which can occur at any site but most commonly occurs at sites of injury and mucosal surfaces.

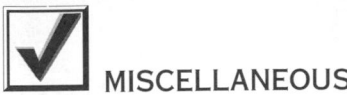

TREATMENT

APPROPRIATE HEALTH CARE
Inpatient monitoring if bleeding

NURSING CARE
After surgery, affected dogs should be monitored for abnormal bleeding for at least 48 hr before release from the hospital.

ACTIVITY
Usually it is not necessary to limit the activity of affected dogs, because of the low frequency of spontaneous hemorrhages.

DIET
N/A

CLIENT EDUCATION
• Genetic testing is available for some affected breeds (www.vetgen.com).
• Explain pattern of inheritance to owners along with the options for screening related animals for the defect; carriers generally have an intermediate concentration of vWF but some have vWF levels in the normal range.
• Animals that have had bleeding episodes—inform owners about early signs that indicate bleeding and options for early treatment with fresh frozen plasma or cryoprecipitate

SURGICAL CONSIDERATIONS
Steps should be taken to minimize the risk of bleeding problems in patients undergoing elective surgery.

MEDICATIONS

DRUG(S) OF CHOICE
• Cryoprecipitate—a concentrated form of vWF and factor VIII; if available, the treatment of choice
• Fresh plasma or fresh-frozen plasma in patients without anemia and fresh whole blood in patients with anemia—practical, effective treatment; transfusion with plasma at 10 mL/kg twice daily is generally effective for controlling bleeding in affected dogs; favorable responses are seen at a lower dosage in some dogs.
• In contrast to classic hemophilia, control of the bleeding is usually achieved with one or two transfusions.

CONTRAINDICATIONS
Drugs such as aspirin, and other nonsteroidal anti-inflammatory agents, which are known to inhibit platelet function, should be avoided.

PRECAUTIONS
N/A

POSSIBLE INTERACTIONS
N/A

ALTERNATIVE DRUG(S)
• Evidence exists that thyroid supplementation decreases the bleeding tendency and may increase the vWF concentration in hypothyroid dogs.
• Desmopressin acetate (1 μg/kg SC) has been shown to increase the vWF concentration and shorten the bleeding time in some affected dogs and may be helpful in reducing the risk of bleeding associated with surgery; this should not be viewed as an equal alternative to plasma transfusion, which is the most effective method of treating bleeding episodes. Desmopressin also is useful in increasing vWF concentration in dogs used as blood donors.

FOLLOW-UP

PATIENT MONITORING
Observe closely for hemorrhage associated with trauma or surgical procedures.

PREVENTION/AVOIDANCE
• Inherited disorder; perform genetic screening prior to breeding.
• Pretreatment with DDAVP may help prevent excessive bleeding during surgery.

POSSIBLE COMPLICATIONS
Hemorrhage

EXPECTED COURSE AND PROGNOSIS
• May be subclinical or manifested as a bleeding diathesis, most commonly as a consequence of surgery, toenail clipping, or some form of injury
• Course and prognosis vary with the concentration of vWF.

MISCELLANEOUS

ASSOCIATED CONDITIONS
None

AGE-RELATED FACTORS
Bleeding tendency may decline with age.

ZOONOTIC POTENTIAL
None

PREGNANCY
Risk of bleeding at parturition

SYNONYMS
None

ABBREVIATIONS
• APTT = activated partial thromboplastin time
• DDAVP = 1 deamino-8-D-arginine vasopressin
• ELISA = enzyme-linked immunosorbent assay
• PT = prothrombin time
• vWF = von Willebrand factor

Suggested Reading

Brooks M, Dodds WJ, Raymond SL. Epidemiologic features of von Willebrand's disease in Doberman pinschers, Scottish terriers, and Shetland sheepdogs: 260 cases (1984–1988). J Am Vet Med Assoc 1992; 200:1123–1127.

Gopegui RR, Feldman BF. Platelets and von Willebrand's disease. In: Ettinger SJ, Feldman EC, eds. Textbook of veterinary internal medicine. 5th ed. Philadelphia: Saunders, 2000:1824–1825.

Johnson GS. Canine von Willebrand's disease. In: Feldman BF, ed. Hemostasis. Vet Clin North Am Small Anm 1988; 18:195–229.

Raymond SL, Jones DW, Brooks MB, Dodds WJ. Clinical and laboratory features of a severe form of von Willebrand disease in Shetland sheepdogs. J Am Vet Med Assoc 1990;197:1342–1346.

Stokol T, Parry BW. Canine von Willebrand disease; a review. Aust Vet Pract 1993; 23:94–103.

Author Gary J. Kociba
Consulting Editor Stephen A. Kruth

WEIGHT LOSS AND CACHEXIA

 BASICS

DEFINITION
• Weight loss is considered clinically important when it exceeds 10% of the normal body weight and is not associated with fluid loss.
• Cachexia is defined as a general physical wasting and malnutrition characterized by weight loss, muscle wasting, anorexia, and general debilitation that is associated with a chronic disease.

PATHOPHYSIOLOGY
• Weight loss can result from many different pathophysiologic mechanisms that share a common feature—energy requirement exceeding energy intake
• Insufficient caloric intake can be caused by (1) a high energy demand (e.g., that characteristic of a hypermetabolic state); (2) inadequate energy intake, including insufficient quantity or quality of food, or inadequate nutrient assimilation (e.g., with anorexia, dysphagia, regurgitation, or malabsorption–maldigestion disorders); (3) excessive loss of nutrients or fluid, which can occur in patients with gastrointestinal losses, glucosuria, proteinuria, or extensive skin lesions (burns, excoriations, etc.)

SYSTEMS AFFECTED
All body systems may be affected by weight loss depending on the underlying disease and severity of illness.

SIGNALMENT
Dogs and cats

SIGNS

Historical Findings
• Clinical signs of particular diagnostic value in patients with weight loss are whether the appetite is normal, increased, decreased, or absent, and the presence or absence of fever.
• Historical information is extremely important and should evaluate the type and quantity of diet being offered, the patient's daily activity, environment, pregnancy, appetite, signs of gastrointestinal disease (e.g., vomiting, diarrhea, stool color/consistency, dysphagia, regurgitation)

Physical Examination Findings
Evaluation should be aimed at detecting any abnormality that may be associated with an underlying disease (see Causes).

CAUSES

Dietary Causes
• Insufficient quantity
• Poor quality
• Inedible food—decreased palatability
• Spoiled diets
• Diets that have lost nutrients because of prolonged storage

Anorexia

Pseudoanorexia
• Inability to smell, prehend, or chew food
• Dysphagia
• Regurgitation
• Vomiting

Malabsorptive Disorders
• Infiltrative and inflammatory bowel disease
• Lymphangiectasia
• Severe intestinal parasitism

Maldigestive Disorders
• Exocrine pancreatic insufficiency

Metabolic Disorders
• Organ failure—cardiac failure, hepatic failure, and renal failure
• Hypoadrenocorticism
• Hyperthyroidism (especially cats)
• Cancer cachexia

Excessive Nutrient Loss
• Protein-losing enteropathy
• Protein-losing nephropathy
• Diabetes mellitus
• Extensive skin lesions (e.g., burns)

Neuromuscular Disease
• Lower motor neuron disease
• CNS disease—usually associated with anorexia or pseudoanorexia

Excessive Use of Calories
• Increased physical activity
• Prolonged or extreme cold environment
• Hyperthyroidism
• Pregnancy or lactation
• Increased catabolism—fever, infection, inflammation, cancer

RISK FACTORS
See Causes above.

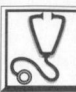 **DIAGNOSIS**

• First confirm weight loss by comparing the current weight to previous weights.
• If previous weights are not available, subjectively assess the patient for cachexia, emaciation, dehydration, or other clues that would confirm the owner's complaint of weight loss.
• After weight loss is confirmed, seek the underlying cause.

DIFFERENTIAL DIAGNOSIS
• First categorize the weight loss as occurring with a normal, increased, or decreased appetite.
• The list of likely differential diagnoses for a patient with weight loss despite a normal or increased appetite can be significantly different than for patients with decreased appetite or anorexia.
• Determine what the patient's appetite was at the onset of weight loss; any condition can lead to anorexia if it persists long enough for the patient to become debilitated.
• The patient's age may provide a clue as to the underlying cause (e.g., portosystemic shunt in a young dog and hyperthyroidism in an older cat).
• Also seek causes of pseudoanorexia (e.g., loss of sense of smell, dysphagia, and disorders of the oral cavity, head and neck).
• Fever suggests that the underlying cause may be infectious or inflammatory (e.g., immune-mediated disease, pancreatitis, or neoplasia).
• Absence of fever is more consistent with metabolic causes of weight loss such as cardiac, renal, or hepatic failure.

CBC/BIOCHEMISTRY/URINALYSIS
Help identify infectious, inflammatory, and metabolic diseases

OTHER LABORATORY TESTS
• Determined by the clinician's list of most likely differential diagnoses on the basis of the specific findings of the history and physical examination, and initial database
• Perform serologic feline leukemia virus (FeLV) and feline immunodeficiency virus (FIV) tests in any cat with weight loss of unknown cause.
• Measure serum T_4 concentration in any cat > 5 years old with weight loss of unknown cause, especially (but not restricted to) cats with a normal or increased appetite.

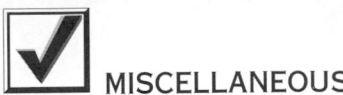

• Examine serial fecal flotations and direct smears to exclude intestinal parasitism.
• Specific organ function tests are necessary if indicated by historical, physical examination, and initial database findings.
• Examples include a serum TLI for exocrine pancreatic insufficiency, an ACTH stimulation test for hypoadrenocorticism, pre- and postprandial serum bile acids for hepatobiliary disease, and a urine protein:creatinine ratio if protein-losing nephropathy is suspected.
• Fecal digestive studies and assays of fecal α_1-protease inhibitor activity may help identify protein-losing enteropathies.

IMAGING
• The most useful diagnostic imaging techniques vary, depending on other clinical findings and suspected underlying causes.
• Thoracic radiography may be particularly helpful in diagnosing thoracic disease, including cardiac failure, pulmonary disease, and metastatic neoplasia.
• Abdominal radiography or ultrasonography may be useful.

DIAGNOSTIC PROCEDURES
• Vary depending on initial diagnostic findings and the suspected underlying cause of weight loss
• If gastrointestinal disease is suspected, examine multiple biopsy specimens taken from the indicated portions of the gastrointestinal tract by endoscopy or exploratory laparotomy.
• If indications for exploratory laparotomy exist—obtain multiple biopsy specimens from the suspected organ or organs as well as from other routinely biopsied abdominal organs such as liver, multiple sites along the gastrointestinal tract, ± pancreas, ± mesenteric lymph nodes.

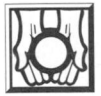

TREATMENT
• The most important treatment principle is to treat the underlying cause of the weight loss.
• Must provide sufficient caloric nutrition in the form of adequate amounts of an appropriate, high-quality diet fed in the form or manner that best allows patient utilization; this requires calculating the patient's caloric needs

and may require assisted enteral feeding with nasogastric, pharyngostomy, esophagostomy, gastrostomy, or jejunostomy tubes
• If enteral feeding is considered inappropriate, parenteral feeding may become necessary.
• Determine caloric requirements from formulas for basal (resting) energy requirement (BER) multiplied by an illness/infection/injury factor to yield a maintenance energy requirement (MER]:

$$BER = 70 \times (\text{patient's weight in kg})^{0.75}$$

or approximately 30 (patient's weight in kg) + 70 for animals weighing over 2 kg and less than 45 kg. Illness factors tend to range from 1.0 to 1.5, depending on the severity and nature of the underlying disorder.

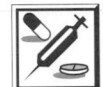

MEDICATIONS

DRUG(S) OF CHOICE
• Depend on the underlying cause of the weight loss; see specific topic for each condition, including anorexia.
• See other sections regarding specific disorders or problems.

CONTRAINDICATIONS
N/A

PRECAUTIONS
N/A

POSSIBLE INTERACTIONS
N/A

ALTERNATIVE DRUG(S)
N/A

FOLLOW-UP

PATIENT MONITORING
The necessity for frequent patient monitoring and the methods required depend on the underlying cause of the weight loss; however, the patient should be weighed regularly and frequently.

POSSIBLE COMPLICATIONS
See Causes.

MISCELLANEOUS

ASSOCIATED CONDITIONS
See Causes.

AGE-RELATED FACTORS
N/A

ZOONOTIC POTENTIAL
N/A

PREGNANCY
Pregnancy and lactation can be associated with weight loss due to increased calorie expenditure.

SYNONYMS
N/A

SEE ALSO
See Causes (refer to specific sections).

ABBREVIATIONS
ACTH = Adrinocorticotropic hormone
BER = basal (resting) energy requirement
CNS = central nervous system
MER = maintenance energy requirement
TLI = trypsin-like immunoreactivity

Suggested Reading
Carnevale JM, et al. Nutritional assessment: guidelines to selecting patients for nutritional support. Comp Cont Ed 1991; 13:255–261.
Greco DS. Changes in body weight. In: Ettinger SJ, ed. Veterinary internal medicine. 5th ed. Philadelphia: Saunders, 2000: 72–74.
Hill RC. A rapid method of estimating maintenance energy requirement from body surface area in inactive dogs and in cats. J Am Vet Med Assoc 1993;202:1814–1816.
Willard M: Clinical manifestations of gastrointestinal disorders. In: Nelson RW, Couto CG, eds. Essentials of small animal internal medicine. St. Louis: Mosby Year Book, 1992:274–275.

Acknowledgment
The author and editors acknowledge the prior contributions of Drs. Daniel Harrington and Nathaniel C. Myers III, who authored this topic in the previous edition.
Author John Crandell
Consulting Editor Albert E. Jergens

WHIPWORMS (TRICHURIASIS)

 BASICS

OVERVIEW

• *Trichuris vulpis,* the whipworm, in the cecum of dogs *(T. felis* in cats) may cause bloody diarrhea and large-bowel inflammation. Feline trichuriasis rare in US.
• Infection is usually not patent with eggs in feces until 3 months; may be clinical before patency (90 days)
• Infective eggs ingested to establish cecal infection
• No extraintestinal migration
• Eggs persist in environment for months to years.

SIGNALMENT

Dogs of any age

SIGNS

Historical Findings

Intermittent large-bowel diarrhea—often mucus and fresh blood (hematochezia) in feces

Physical Examination Findings

Acute to chronic debilitation

CAUSES & RISK FACTORS

• Ingestion of infective trichurid eggs from contaminated environment
• Eggs persist in environment (i.e., in soil) for months to years.

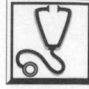 DIAGNOSIS

DIFFERENTIAL DIAGNOSIS

• Bacterial (spirochaetal) infections of cecum
• Hookworm infection
• Capillarid infections (eggs similar in appearance but smaller)

CBC/BIOCHEMISTRY/URINALYSIS

Normal

OTHER LABORATORY TESTS

N/A

IMAGING

N/A

DIAGNOSTIC PROCEDURES

Fecal flotation; trichurid eggs ovoid with prominent bipolar plugs, brown color, single cell (zygote) within egg shell membranes; 90 × 45 μm

TREATMENT

Outpatient

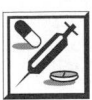

MEDICATIONS

DRUG(S)

• Fenbendazole 50 mg/kg PO q24h for 3–5 days; repeat monthly three times.
• Febantel/praziquantel/pyrantel pamoate
• Dichlorvos given twice, 3–4 weeks apart
• Milbemycin oxime monthly

CONTRAINDICATIONS/POSSIBLE INTERACTIONS

• Organophosphates in heartworm-positive dogs
• Do not give dichlorvos concurrently with other organophosphates such as insecticides.

FOLLOW-UP

Fecal examination for trichurid eggs 3–4 weeks following treatment

MISCELLANEOUS

SYNONYMS

Trichuriasis

Suggested Reading

Bowman DD, Lynn RC, Eberhard ML. Georgi's parasitology for veterinarians. 8th ed. St, Louis: Saunders (Elsevier Science), 2003:228–229.

Bowman DD, Hendrix CM, Lindsay DS, Barr SC. Feline clinical parasitology. Ames: Iowa State University Press, 2002:348–350.

Acknowledgment

The author and editors acknowledge the prior contributions of Dr. Robert M. Corwin, who authored this topic in the previous edition.

Author Julie Ann Jarvinen
Consulting Editor Albert E. Jergens

WOBBLER SYNDROME (CERVICAL VERTEBRAL INSTABILITY)

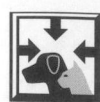

BASICS

DEFINITION
• Encompasses compressive spinal cord lesions affecting the cervical spine (primarily caudal) in large- and giant-breed dogs; may be disk related or vertebral related
• Disk related—mature dogs; arising from type II disk herniation with accompanying vertebral ligamentous hypertrophy, presumably caused by joint instability; C5–6 and C6–7 primarily involved; C3–4 and C4–5 may be involved.
• Vertebral-related—young dogs; arising from developmental abnormalities causing malformation and malarticulation of the vertebral column; all cervical joints may be affected.

PATHOPHYSIOLOGY
Compression of the cervical spinal cord

SYSTEMS AFFECTED
Nervous

GENETICS
No inheritance specifically identified, but many factors may be under genetic control

INCIDENCE/PREVALENCE
Reported in numerous breeds of large dogs

GEOGRAPHIC DISTRIBUTION
N/A

SIGNALMENT
Species
Dogs

Breed Predilections
• Disk related—Doberman pinschers; seen in small breeds as well (e.g., chihuahua)
• Vertebral related—Great Danes

Mean Age and Range
• Disk related—mature, > 2 years old; most patients > 5 years
• Vertebral related—young, generally < 2 years old

Predominant Sex
N/A

SIGNS

General Comments
Highly variable, depending on the degree of compression and duration of lesion

Historical Findings
• Acute or chronic onset
• Progressive or nonprogressive nature

Physical Examination Findings
• Variable neck pain
• Difficulty rising to a standing posture
• Variable muscle atrophy, especially in forelimbs
• Worn toenails
• Ataxia—involves all four limbs but to a lesser degree in the forelimbs; normal, decreased, or absent postural reactions in all limbs; lower or upper motor neuron signs in forelimbs and upper motor neuron signs in hind limbs
• Pain perception usually intact

CAUSES
• Disk-related—disk degeneration or vertebral instability
• Vertebral-related—nutritionally related malformation or malarticulation

RISK FACTORS
• Disk-related—none specifically identified
• Vertebral related—large, rapidly growing dogs

DIAGNOSIS

DIFFERENTIAL DIAGNOSIS
• Disk-related—trauma, diskospondylitis, primary disk disease, neoplasia, and inflammatory spinal cord diseases; differentiated by breed incidence, results of CSF analysis, and radiographic studies
• Vertebral-related—same as for disk related; juvenile orthopedic diseases

CBC/BIOCHEMISTRY/URINALYSIS
Usually normal

OTHER LABORATORY TESTS
N/A

IMAGING

Survey Cervical Radiography
• Disk-related—may be normal or show narrowing of the disk space suggesting disk herniation
• Vertebral-related—may show abnormal articular facet shape or density, subluxation, malformed vertebral bodies, stenosis of the vertebral canal, and misshapen dorsal spinal processes

Myelography
• Disk-related—soft tissue compression of the spinal cord by the dorsal annulus of the disk, dorsal longitudinal ligament, and dorsal ligamentum flavum
• Vertebral-related—compression of the spinal cord due to proliferation of the articular facets, remodeling of vertebral bodies, and other bony causes of stenosis of the spinal canal

MRI
Clearly defines spinal cord, ligaments, intervertebral disks, nerve roots, spinal nerves; it is preferred diagnostic imaging method.

DIAGNOSTIC PROCEDURES
CSF analysis—may be normal or show high protein owing to compressive degeneration of the spinal cord

PATHOLOGIC FINDINGS
• White and gray matter necrosis at the level of compression
• Wallerian-type degeneration of white matter above and below area of compression

TREATMENT

APPROPRIATE HEALTH CARE
Inpatient—requires surgery

NURSING CARE
• Nonambulatory—keep patient on soft bedding (synthetic fleece) to avoid bed sores.
• Bladder catheterization—avoids manual expression and urine scalding
• Passive and active manipulation of the limbs to avoid reduced range of motion

WOBBLER SYNDROME (CERVICAL VERTEBRAL INSTABILITY)

ACTIVITY
Limit to avoid exacerbation of the condition

DIET
Vertebral related disease—discontinue excessive use of dietary supplements; control food intake.

CLIENT EDUCATION
• Depending on the chronicity of the disease, inform client that neurologic deficits may remain.
• Inform client that the goal of treatment is to stop the progression.
• Advise client that physiotherapy is usually required to maximize return of function.

SURGICAL CONSIDERATIONS

Decompression
• Ventral spondylectomy—best suited for solitary lesions compressing from the floor of the spinal canal
• Multiple sites can be operated ventrally if care is taken to keep the "slots" as small as possible and not connect adjacent "slots," leaving at least 1/3 of the vertebral body of the middle vertebra intact
• Dorsal laminectomy—best for multiple sites of involvement or when compression is mainly from the roof of the spinal canal; disk-related and developmental diseases

Other
• Fenestration—prevents additional sites of involvement; disk-related disease
• Stabilization/fusion—controversial for disk-related caudal cervical compression; advocates: primary lesion is unstable, which should be stabilized; opponents: stabilization without decompression does nothing for the compressive lesion and may actually precipitate additional damage at the disk spaces on either side of the fused space.

 MEDICATIONS

DRUG(S) OF CHOICE
Glucocorticosteroids—in combination with surgery, the most advantageous therapeutic approach; without surgery, useful only in mildly affected patients

CONTRAINDICATIONS
N/A

PRECAUTIONS
Observe for signs of gastroenteritis and cystitis.

POSSIBLE INTERACTIONS
N/A

ALTERNATIVE DRUG(S)
N/A

 FOLLOW-UP

PATIENT MONITORING
• Repeat neurologic examinations—as necessary to evaluate response to treatment

PREVENTION/AVOIDANCE
• Limit running and jumping.
• Avoid collar; use body harness instead.

POSSIBLE COMPLICATIONS
Disk related—adjacent sites may become involved

EXPECTED COURSE AND PROGNOSIS
• Acute—immediate aggressive treatment necessary for best outcome
• Chronic progressive—the earlier surgery is performed, the better the outcome; paralyzed patients often cannot be helped

 MISCELLANEOUS

ASSOCIATED CONDITIONS
N/A

AGE-RELATED FACTORS
• Disk-related—old dogs
• Developmental related—young dogs

ZOONOTIC POTENTIAL
N/A

PREGNANCY
Use of glurocorticosteroids is contra-indicated.

SYNONYMS
• Disk related—spondylolisthesis; vertebral subluxation; caudal cervical spondylopathy; cervical spondylopathy
• Vertebral related—vertebral stenosis; cervical vertebral stenotic myelopathy; cervical spondylopathy

SEE ALSO
• Intervertebral Disk Disease, Cervical
• Osteochondrosis

ABBREVIATION
MRI = magnetic resonance imaging

Suggested Reading
Lipsitz D, Levitski RE, Chauvet AE, et al. Magnetic resonance imaging features of cervical stenotic myelopathy in 21 dogs. Vet Radiol Ultrasound 2001;42:20–27.
Oliver JE, Lorenz MD, Kornegay JN. Handbook of veterinary neurology. 3rd ed. Philadelphia: Saunders, 1997.
Rusbridge C, Wheeler SJ, Torrington AM, et al. Comparison of two surgical techniques for the management of cervical spondylomyelopathy in Dobermans. J Small Anim Pract 1998;39:425–431.
Sharp NJH, Cofone M, Robertson ID, et al. Computed tomography in the evaluation of caudal cervical spondylomyelopathy of the Doberman pinscher. Vet Radiol Ultrasound 1995;36:100–108.
Summers BA, Cummings JF, de Lahunta. Veterinary neuropathology. St. Louis: Mosby, 1995:198–199.

Author Patricia J. Luttgen
Consulting Editor Joane M. Parent

WOLFF-PARKINSON-WHITE SYNDROME

BASICS

DEFINITION
• Ventricular preexcitation occurs when impulses originating in the sinoatrial node or atrium activate a portion of the ventricles prematurely through an accessory pathway without going through the AV node; the remainder of the ventricles is activated normally through the usual conduction system. • WPW syndrome consists of ventricular preexcitation with episodes of paroxysmal supraventricular tachycardia. (Figures 1 and 2)

ECG Features of Ventricular Preexcitation
• Normal heart rate and rhythm • Normal P waves • Short P-R interval (dogs, < 0.06 sec; cats, < 0.05 sec) • Widened QRS (small dogs, > 0.05 sec; large dogs, > 0.06 sec; cats, > 0.04 sec), often with slurring or notching of the upstroke of the R wave (delta wave)

ECG Features of Ventricular Preexcitation with WPW Syndrome
• Extremely rapid heart rate (dogs, often > 300 bpm; cats, approaching 400–500 bpm) • P waves may be difficult to recognize. • QRS complexes may be normal, wide with delta wave, or very wide and bizarre, depending on the circuit. • Conduction is usually 1:1 (i.e., one P wave for every QRS complex).

PATHOPHYSIOLOGY
• Can be associated with congenital or acquired cardiac defects in dogs or cats • May be associated with hypertrophic cardiomyopathy in cats • Hemodynamic compromise during episodes of supraventricular tachycardia with WPW syndrome

SYSTEMS AFFECTED
Cardiovascular

GENETICS N/A

INCIDENCE/PREVALENCE
Unknown

SIGNALMENT
Species
Dogs and cats
Breed Predilections
N/A
Mean Age and Range
N/A
Predominant Sex
N/A

SIGNS
Historical Findings
• None in patients with ventricular preexcitation • Syncope in patients with WPW syndrome
Physical Examination Findings
• None in animals with ventricular preexcitation • Rapid heart rate in animals with WPW syndrome

CAUSES
Congenital Heart Disease
• Congenital defect limited to the conduction system • Atrial septal defect in dogs or cats • Tricuspid valvular dysplasia in dogs
Acquired Heart Disease
Hypertrophic cardiomyopathy in cats

RISK FACTORS N/A

DIAGNOSIS

DIFFERENTIAL DIAGNOSIS
• Ventricular preexcitation—differentiate from other causes of short P-R intervals (e.g., fever, hyperthyroidism, and anemia); these conditions do not cause delta waves. • Narrow complex WPW syndrome—differentiate from other supraventricular arrhythmias (e.g., atrial tachycardia, atrial flutter, and atrial fibrillation); WPW syndrome is most easily recognized after conversion to normal heart rate and rhythm. • Alternating WPW syndrome should not be confused with ventricular bigeminy. • Wide complex WPW syndrome must be differentiated from ventricular tachycardia. • Short PR interval may be correlated with a normal QRS complex if the anomalous pathway bypasses the AV node and connects to the bundle of His (i.e., Lown-Ganong-Levine syndrome).

CBC/BIOCHEMISTRY/URINALYSIS
Normal

OTHER LABORATORY TESTS
Normal

IMAGING
Echocardiography may show structural heart disease.

CV₆LU

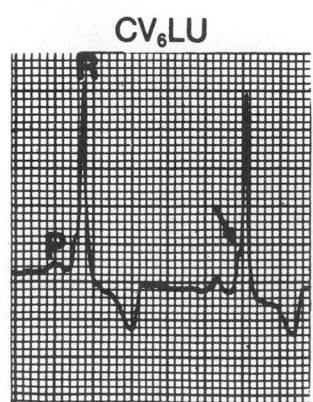
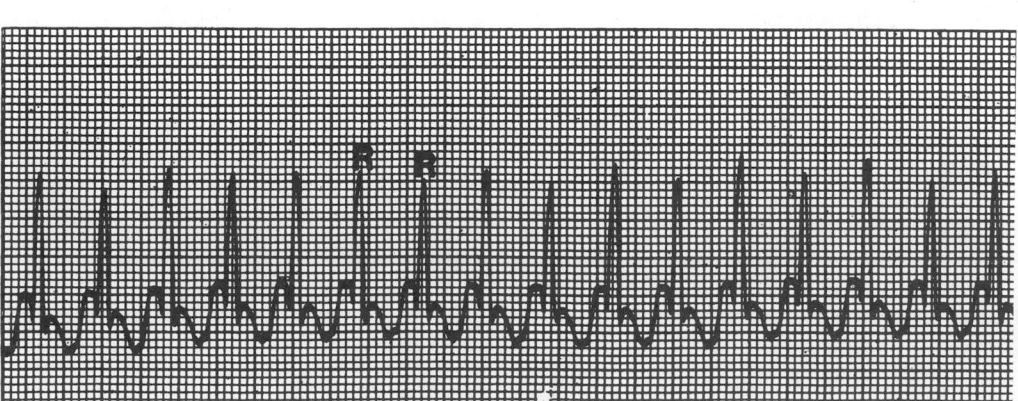

Figure 1.

Wolff-Parkinson-White syndrome (canine). Ventricular preexcitation represented by the short P-R interval, wide QRS complex, and delta wave (arrow) in CV6LU. Paroxysms of supraventricular tachycardia are represented in the long lead II rhythm strip. (From: Tilley LP: Essentials of canine and feline electrocardiography. 3rd ed. Baltimore: Lippincott Williams & Wilkins, 1992, with permission.)

WOLFF-PARKINSON-WHITE SYNDROME

DIAGNOSTIC PROCEDURES
Electrocardiography

PATHOLOGIC FINDINGS
• Pathologic findings vary with underlying cause.
• Possibility of no organic heart lesions

 TREATMENT

APPROPRIATE HEALTH CARE
• Ventricular preexcitation without tachycardia—no treatment needed
• WPW syndrome requires conversion by ocular or carotid sinus pressure, direct current shock (the most effective treatment), or drugs.

ACTIVITY
May need to be limited with WPW until supraventricular tachycardias are controlled

CLIENT EDUCATION
WPW—explain the need to identify and treat the underlying cause in addition to therapy for supraventricular tachycardia.

SURGICAL CONSIDERATIONS
Catheter ablation with radiofrequency current—a relatively recent technique that allows accessory pathways to be destroyed or ablated by a transvenous catheter positioned at the site of the pathway; can be preferred alternative to lifelong therapy with drugs

 MEDICATIONS

DRUG(S) OF CHOICE
• A variety of drugs are used in humans; opinions differ on agents of choice.
• Lidocaine IV bolus (2 mg/kg) followed by IV drip (25–75 µg/kg/min CRI—dogs only)

• Procainamide (8–20 mg/kg q8h—dogs only)
• Propranolol (cats, 2.5–5 mg PO q8–12h; dogs, 0.2–1.0 mg/kg PO q8h) or atenolol (cats, 6.2–12.5 mg PO q24h; dogs, 0.25–1.0 mg/kg PO q12h)
• Diltiazem may be effective (cats, 1–2.5 mg/kg PO q8h; dogs, 0.5–1.5 mg/kg PO q8h)

CONTRAINDICATIONS
• Digitalis, verapamil, and propranolol may be contraindicated—by slowing conduction through the AV node, these drugs may favor conduction through the anomalous pathways.
• Cats—propranolol and atenolol are the drugs of choice.

PRECAUTIONS
N/A

POSSIBLE INTERACTIONS
N/A

ALTERNATIVE DRUG(S)
N/A

 FOLLOW-UP

PATIENT MONITORING
Serial ECG

PREVENTION/AVOIDANCE
N/A

POSSIBLE COMPLICATIONS
None expected

EXPECTED COURSE AND PROGNOSIS
Depends on severity of the underlying cause; most WPW patients respond to therapy for supraventricular tachycardia—favorable prognosis

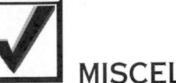 MISCELLANEOUS

ASSOCIATED CONDITIONS N/A

AGE-RELATED FACTORS N/A

ZOONOTIC POTENTIAL N/A

PREGNANCY N/A

SYNONYMS
None

ABBREVIATIONS
• AV = atrioventricular • bpm = beats per minute • WPW = Wolff-Parkinson-White

Suggested Readings
Al-Khatib SM, Pritchett ELC. Clinical features of Wolff-Parkinson-White syndrome. Am Heart J 1999;138:403–413.
Hill BL, Tilley LP. Ventricular preexcitation in seven dogs and nine cats. J Am Vet Med Assoc 1985;187:1026–1031.
Tilley LP. Essentials of canine and feline electrocardiography. 3rd ed. Baltimore: Williams & Wilkins, 1992.
Wright KN. Assessment and treatment of supraventricular tachyarrhythmias. In: Bonagura JD, ed. Kirk's current veterinary therapy XIII. Philadelphia: Saunders, 2000:726–729.
Authors Larry P. Tilley and Naomi L. Burtnick
Consulting Editors Larry P. Tilley and Francis W. K. Smith, Jr.

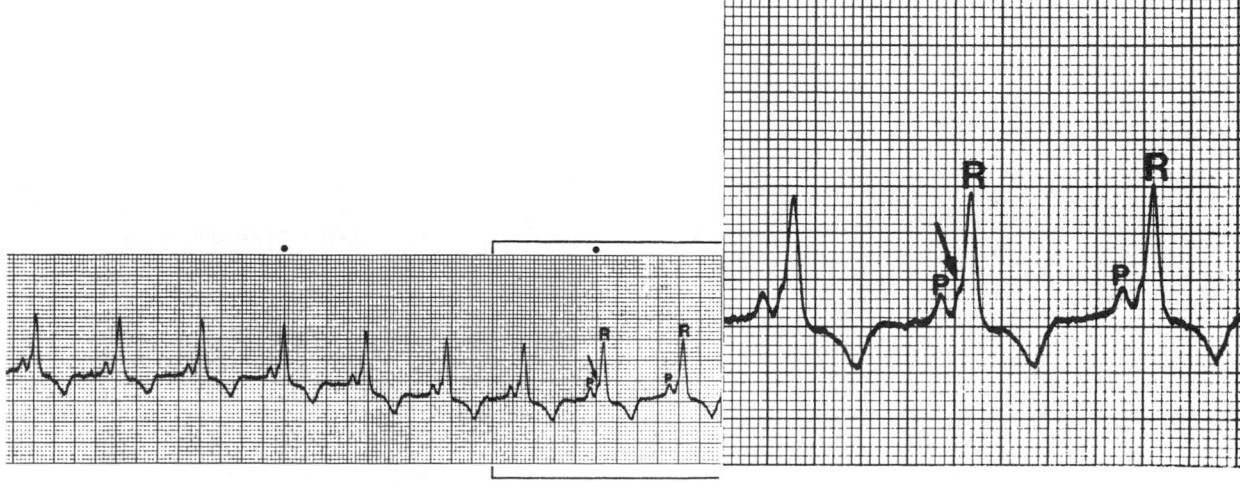

Figure 2.

Ventricular preexcitation in a cat with episodes of fainting. The P waves are normal, the P-R interval is short, and the QRS complex is wide; delta waves (arrow) are present. (From: Tilley LP: Essentials of canine and feline electrocardiography. 3rd ed. Baltimore: Lippincott Williams & Wilkins, 1992, with permission.)

ZINC TOXICITY

 ## BASICS

OVERVIEW
• Toxicity from the ingestion of zinc-containing objects
• Causes severe intravascular hemolysis and gastrointestinal irritation; may cause multiple organ failure (e.g., renal, hepatic, pancreatic, and cardiac), DIC, and cardiopulmonary arrest

SIGNALMENT
Most frequently reported in dogs

SIGNS
• Pale mucous membranes
• Hemoglobinuria
• Hemoglobinemia
• Anorexia
• Vomiting
• Diarrhea
• Icterus

CAUSES & RISK FACTORS
Ingestion of zinc-containing objects: nuts from transport cages and plumbing parts; staples; galvanized metal (nails); pieces from board games; zippers; miscellaneous toys; jewelry; American pennies minted after 1982; Canadian pennies minted after 1996; zinc-containing skin preparations rare (zinc oxide sunblock, Desitin, calamine lotion)

 ## DIAGNOSIS

DIFFERENTIAL DIAGNOSIS
• Immune-mediated hemolytic anemia
• Babesia
• Onion and garlic toxicosis
• Mothball toxicosis (naphthalene)
• Caval syndrome

CBC/BIOCHEMISTRY/URINALYSIS
• Severe intravascular hemolytic anemia
• High nucleated RBC counts
• Basophilic stippling
• Target cells
• Polychromasia
• Hemoglobinuria
• High BUN, creatinine, ALP, ALT, high amylase and lipase—may indicate multiple organ failure

OTHER LABORATORY TESTS
• Serum zinc levels often exceed 5 ppm (approximate normal range: 0.70–2.0 ppm for dogs and cats).
• Blood must be collected in non–zinc contaminated blood tubes.
• Coagulation panel—may indicate DIC (prolonged PT and PTT, hypofibrino-genemia, thrombocytopenia, and high FDP)

IMAGING
• Abdominal imaging—*may* reveal metallic object in the gastrointestinal tract
• Often the zinc object has passed (via vomit or feces) by the time the patient is admitted.

DIAGNOSTIC PROCEDURES
ECG—may reveal arrhythmias and ST-segment abnormalities

 ## TREATMENT
• Rapid removal of the zinc object by endoscopy or laparotomy—imperative
• Maintain hydration—acute renal failure is a serious sequela
• Severe intravascular hemolysis—may require blood transfusion
• Inform client about the hazards of ingesting zinc-containing objects (especially American pennies minted after 1982)

 ## MEDICATIONS

DRUG(S)
• Heparin—150 U/kg SC q6h; for DIC
• H$_2$-receptor blockers—cimetidine, ranitidine; may help reduce stomach acidity and the rate of release of zinc
• CaEDTA—100 mg/kg diluted in 5% dextrose SC, divided into four doses per day (treatment as for lead poisoning)
• Penicillamine—110 mg/kg/day PO divided 6–8h for 5–14 days (treatment as for lead poisoning)

CONTRAINDICATIONS/POSSIBLE INTERACTIONS
Avoid aminoglycoside antibiotics and other potential nephrotoxins—risk of acute renal failure

 ## FOLLOW-UP

PATIENT MONITORING
• ECG—monitor for evidence of arrhythmias and ST-segment alterations.
• Coagulation profile, PCV, RBC, amylase, lipase, BUN, creatinine, ALP, and ALT—monitor for the first 72 hr after zinc removal
• Monitor serum zinc levels.

EXPECTED COURSE AND PROGNOSIS
• Multiple organ failure, DIC, pancreatic disease, cardiopulmonary arrest—potential outcomes
• Rapid removal of the source of zinc—may provide progressive improvement over 48–72 hr; complete recovery possible

 ## MISCELLANEOUS

SEE ALSO
Poisoning (Intoxication)

ABBREVIATIONS
• ALP = alkaline phosphatase
• ALT = alanine aminotransferase
• BUN = blood urea nitrogen
• DIC = disseminated intravascular coagulation
• FDP = fibrin degradation products
• PCV = packed cell volume
• PT = prothrombin time
• PTT = partial thromboplastin time
• RBC = red blood cells

Suggested Reading
Ogden L. Zinc toxicosis. In: Kirk RW, Bonagura JD, eds. Current veterinary therapy XI. Philadelphia: Saunders, 1992: 197–200.
Talcott PA. Zinc poisoning. In: Peterson ME, Talcott PA, eds. Small animal toxicology. Philadelphia: Saunders, 2001:756–761.

Acknowledgment
The author and editors acknowledge the prior contributions of Dr. Kathryn M. Meurs, who authored this topic in the previous edition.
Author Patricia A. Talcott
Consulting Editor Gary D. Osweiler

APPENDIX I

NORMAL REFERENCE RANGES FOR LABORATORY TESTS

Table I-A.

Normal Hematologic Values			
Test	Units	Dogs	Cats
WBC	$10 \times 3/mm^3$	6.0–17.0	5.5–19.5
RBC	$10 \times 6/mm^3$	5.5–8.5	6.0–10
Hemoglobin	g/dL	12.0–18.0	9.5–15
Hematocrit	%	37.0–55.0	29–45
Mean corpuscular volume	fL	60.0–77.0	41.0–54
Mean corpuscular hemoglobin	pg	19.5–26	13.3–17.5
Mean corpuscular hemoglobin concentration	%	32.0–36.0	31–36
Platelet count (automated)	$10 \times 3/mm^3$	200–500	150–600
Platelet count (manual)	$10 \times 3/mm^3$	164–510	230–680
Neutrophils	%	60–77	35–75
	Absolute	3000–11,500	2500–12,500
Bands	%	0–3	0–3
	Absolute	0–510	0–585
Lymphocytes	%	12–30	20–55
	Absolute	1000–4800	1500–7000
Monocytes	%	3–10	1–4
	Absolute	180–1350	0–850
Eosinophils	%	2–10	2–12
	Absolute	1000–1250	0–1500
Basophils	%	0–1	0–1
	Absolute	0–100	0–100
Reticulocyte count	%	0.5–1.5	0.0–1.0
Corrected	%	0.0–1.0	0.0–1.0
Absolute	$/mm^3$	0–80,000	0–50,000

From Abbott Cell Dyne 3500; IDEXX Veterinary Services.
It is important to realize that normal values vary among individual laboratories.

Table I-B.

Normal Biochemical Values

Test	Units	Dogs	Cats
Blood urea nitrogen (BUN)	mg/dL	7–27	15–34
Creatinine	mg/dL	0.4–1.8	0.8–2.3
Cholesterol	mg/dL	112–328	82–218
Glucose	mg/dL	60–125	70–150
Alkaline phosphatase (ALP)	IU/L	10–150	0–62
Alanine aminotransferase (ALT)	IU/L	5–60	28–76
Aspartate aminotransferase (AST)	IU/L	5–55	5–55
Total protein	g/dL	5.1–7.8	5.9–8.5
Albumin	g/dL	2.6–4.3	2.4–4.1
Globulin	g/dL	2.3–4.5	3.4–5.2
Albumin-globulin ratio		0.75–1.9	0.6–1.5
Sodium	mEq/L	141–156	147–156
Potassium	mEq/L	4.0–5.6	3.9–5.3
Sodium-potassium ratio		27–40	> 27.0
Chloride	mEq/L	105–115	111–125
Total CO_2	mEq/L	17–24	13–25
Anion gap	mEq/L	12–24	13–27
Calcium	mg/dL	7.5–11.3	7.5–10.8
Phosphorus	mg/dL	2.1–6.3	3.0–7.0
Total bilirubin	mg/dL	0–0.4	0.0–0.4
Direct bilirubin	mg/dL	0.0–0.1	0.0–0.1
Indirect bilirubin	mg/dL	0–0.3	0.0–0.3
Lactate dehydrogenase (LDH)	IU/L	50–380	46–350
Creatine kinase (CK or CPK)	IU/L	10–200	64–440
Gamma glutamyl transferase (GGT)	IU/L	0–10	1–7
Uric acid	mg/dL	0–2	0–1
Amylase	IU/L	500–1500	500–1500
Lipase	U/L	100–500	10–195
Magnesium	mEq/L	1.8–2.4	1.8–2.4
Trigiycendes	mg/dL	20–150	20–90
Bile acids:			
Fasting	μmol/L	0.0–5.0	0.0–5.0
Postprandial	μmol/L	< 25	< 15
Random	μmol/L	< 25	< 15
Total iron	μg/dL	33–147	33–134
Unsaturated iron binding capacity	μg/dL	127–340	105–205
Total iron binding capacity	μg/dL	282–386	169–325

From Hitachi Chemistry Analyzer model 747 IDEXX Veterinary Services.
It is important to realize that normal values vary among individual laboratories.

Table I-C.

Conversion Table for Hematologic Units

	Example values		Conversion factors	
Analyte	Traditional	SI*	Traditional to SI	SI to Traditional
Hemoglobin	15.0 g/dL	150 g/L	10	0.1
HCT or PCV	45%	0.45 L/L	0.01	100
Erythrocytes	$6.0 \times 10^6/mm^3$	$6.0 \times 10^{12}/L$	10^6	10^{-6}
MCV	$75 \mu^3$	75 fL	No change	No change
MCH	$25 \mu\mu g$	25 pg	No change	No change
MCHC	33 g/dL	330 g/L	10	0.1
WBC	$15.0 \times 10^3/mm^3$	$15.0 \times 10^9/L$	10^6	10^{-6}
Platelets	$250 \times 10^3/mm^3$	$250 \times 10^9/L$	10^6	10^{-6}

*Système International d'Unités
Modified from Appendices. In: Bonagura JD, ed. Kirk's current veterinary therapy XIII. Philadelphia: WB Saunders, 2000:1209 (with permission).

Table I-D.

Conversion Table for Clinical Biochemical Units

Analyte	Traditional unit (with examples)	Conversion factor	SI unit (with examples)
Alanine aminotransferase	0–40 U/L	1.00	0–40 U/L
Albumin	2.8–4.0 g/dL	10.0	28–40 g/L
Alkaline phosphatase	30–150 U/L	1.00	30–150 U/L
Ammonia	10–80 μg/dL	0.5871	5.9–47.0 μmol/L
Amylase	200–800 U/L	1.00	200–800 U/L
Aspartate aminotransferase	0–40 U/L	1.00	0–40 U/L
Bile acids (total)	0.3–2.3 μg/mL	2.45	0.74–5.64 μmol/L
Bilirubin	0.1–0.2 mg/dL	17.10	2–4 μmol/L
Calcium	8.8–10.3 mg/dL	0.2495	2.20–2.58 mmol/L
Carbon dioxide	22–28 mEq/L	1.00	22–28 mmol/L
Chloride	95–100 mEq/L	1.00	95–100 mmol/L
Cholesterol	100–265 mg/dL	0.0258	2.58–5.85 mmol/L
Copper	70–140 μg/dL	0.1574	11.0–22.0 μmol/L
Cortisol	2–10 μg/dL	27.59	55–280 nmol/L
Creatine kinase	0–130 U/L	1.00	0–130 U/L
Creatinine	0.6–1.2 mg/dL	88.40	50–110 μmol/L
Fibrinogen	200–400 mg/dL	0.01	2.0–4.0 g/L
Folic acid	3.5–11.0 μg/L	2.265	7.93–24.92 nmol/L
Glucose	70–110 mg/dL	0.05551	3.9–6.1 mmol/L
Iron	80–180 μg/dL	0.1791	14–32 μmol/L
Lactate	5–20 mg/dL	0.1110	0.5–2.0 mmol/L
Lead	150 μg/dL	0.04826	7.2 μmol/L
Lipase, Sigma-Tietz (37° C)	≤ 1 ST U/dL	280	≤ 280 U/L
Lipase, Cherry-Crandall (30° C)	0–160 U/L	1.00	0–160 U/L
Lipids (total)	400–850 mg/dL	0.01	4.0–8.5 g/L
Magnesium	1.8–3.0 mg/dL	0.4114	0.80–1.20 mmol/L
Mercury	≤ 1.0 μg/dL	49.85	≤ 50 nmol/L
Osmolality	280–300 mOsm/kg	1.00	280–300 mmol/kg
Phosphorus	2.5–5.0 mg/dL	0.3229	0.80–1.6 mmol/L
Potassium	3.5–5.0 mEq/L	1.0	3.5–5.0 mmol/L
Protein (total)	5–8 g/dL	10.0	50–80 g/L
Sodium	135–147 mEq/L	1.00	135–147 mmol/L
Testosterone	4.0–8.0 mg/mL	3.467	14.0–28.0 nmol/L
Thyroxine	1–4 μg/dL	12.87	13–51 nmol/L
Triglyceride	10–500 mg/dL	0.0113	0.11–5.65 mmol/L
Urea nitrogen	10–20 mg/dL	0.3570	3.6–7.1 nmol/L
Uric acid	3.6–7.7 mg/dL	59.44	214–458 μmol/L
Urobilinogen	0–4.0 mg/dL	16.9	0.0–6.8 μmol/L
Vitamin A	90 μg/dL	0.03491	3.1 μmol/L
Vitamin B_{12}	300–700 ng/L	0.738	221–516 pmol/L
Vitamin E	5.0–20.0 mg/L	2.32	11.6–46.4 μmol/L
D-xylose	30–40 mg/dL	0.06666	2.0–2.71 mmol/L
Zinc	75–120 μg/dL	0.1530	11.5–18.5 μmol/L

From Appendices. In: Bonagura JD, ed. Kirk's current veterinary therapy XIII. Philadelphia: WB Saunders, 2000:1214 (with permission).

APPENDIX II

Table II-A.

ENDOCRINE TESTING

Endocrine Function Testing Protocols

ADRENAL GLAND DISORDERS

ACTH STIMULATION TEST

Dogs

Administer 20 IU ACTH gel IM or 0.25 mg synthetic ACTH IV or IM (Cortrosyn, Organon Pharmaceuticals, West Orange, NJ).
ACTH Gel
Serum samples should be obtained before and 2 hours after injection of ACTH for cortisol assay.
Synthetic ACTH
Serum samples should be obtained before and 1 hour after injection of ACTH for cortisol assay.

Cats

Administer 0.125 mg synthetic ACTH IV. Serum samples should be obtained before and 1 hour after injection of ACTH for cortisol assay.

Interpretation

Screening for Cushing's Disease
An exaggerated response to ACTH is consistent with Cushing's disease. High normal cut-off values differ slightly between laboratories.
Screening for Hypoadrenocorticism
Pre- and postcortisol determinations < 1 μg/dL (30 nmol/L) are consistent with hypoadrenocorticism.
Monitoring Mitotane or Ketoconazole Therapy for Cushing's Disease
Pre- and postcortisol determinations should be within the normal basal cortisol range.

LOW-DOSE DEXAMETHASONE SUPPRESSION TEST (LDDST)

Dogs

Administer 0.015 mg/kg dexamethasone (Azium) IV or IM. Obtain serum samples before and 4 and 8 hours after injection of dexamethasone for cortisol assay.

Cats

Administer 0.1 mg/kg dexamethasone (Azium, Schering-Plough, Union, NJ) IV or IM. Obtain serum sample before and 4 and 8 hours after injection of dexamethasone for cortisol assay.

Interpretation

Three Basic Patterns
Lack of Suppression
All cortisol values remain above 1 μg/dL (30 nmol/L). This pattern is consistent with Cushing's disease.
Suppression
Cortisol values fall below 1 μg/dL (30 nmol/L) at 4 and 8 hours. This pattern suggests that the animal does not have Cushing's disease.
Escape from Suppression
Cortisol value falls below 1 μg/dL (30 nmol/L) at 4 hours and rises above 1 μg/dL at 8 hours. This pattern is consistent with pituitary-dependent Cushing's disease.

HIGH-DOSE DEXAMETHASONE SUPPRESSION TEST (HDDST)

Administer 1 mg/kg dexamethasone (Azium) IV or IM. Obtain serum samples before and 4 and 8 hours after injection of dexamethasone for cortisol assay.

Interpretation

Any cortisol determination that falls below 1.5 μg/dL (45 nmol/L) at any point during the 8-hour testing period is considered suppression. Suppression after a high dose of dexamethasone is consistent with pituitary-dependent Cushing's disease. Lack of suppression (all cortisol values remain above 1.5 μg/dL) is diagnostic of a pituitary or adrenal tumor.

THYROID GLAND DISORDERS

TSH STIMULATION TEST

Administer 0.5 U/kg TSH (maximum dose 5 U) IV. Obtain serum samples before and 6 hours after injection of TSH for T_4 determination.

Interpretation

Post-TSH T_4 levels < 3 μg/dL (35 nmol/L) are consistent with hypothyroidism.

TRH STIMULATION TEST

Administer 0.1 mg/kg TRH IV. Obtain serum samples before and 4 hours after TRH injection for T_4 determination.

Interpretation

An increase in T_4 concentration $< 50\%$ after TRH administration is consistent with hypothyroidism.

T_3 SUPPRESSION TEST

Obtain a blood sample for determination of T_4 and T_3. The serum is removed and kept refrigerated or frozen. Administer T_3 (Cytomel, SmithKline Beecham, Philadelphia, PA) PO at a dosage of 25 μg/cat q8h for 2 days. On the morning of the third day, administer 25 μg of T_3, and 2–4 hours later obtain a second blood sample for T_3 and T_4 determinations. The basal (day 1) and postoral T_3 serum samples should be submitted to the laboratory together to avoid interassay variation.

Interpretation

Serum T_4 concentration after administration of T_3 > 1.5 μg/dL (20 nmol/L) is consistent with hyperthyroidism.

GASTRINOMA

SECRETIN STIMULATION TEST

Administer 2 units of secretin/kg IV. Take blood samples before administration of secretin and then 2, 5, 10, 15, and 30 minutes later. Assay the samples for gastrin.

Interpretation

Dogs with gastrinomas have a rise in gastrin levels after the injection of secretin. In three reported cases, two dogs had a rise in gastrin levels 2 times baseline 5 minutes after secretin injection, and one dog had a rise in gastrin levels 1.4 times baseline 5 minutes after secretin injection. Normal dogs have a decline in gastrin levels after administration of secretin.

CALCIUM CHALLENGE TEST

Administer 2 mg/kg of calcium gluconate IV over a 1-minute period or administer 5 mg/kg of calcium gluconate as an IV infusion over several hours.

Obtain a blood sample before calcium administration and then 15, 30, 60, 90, and 120 minutes after calcium administration. Assay the samples for gastrin.

Interpretation

Two reported patients with gastrinoma had a doubling of the gastrin level 60 minutes after the calcium infusion.

SEX HORMONE DISORDERS

GN-RH STIMULATION TEST

Administer 0.5–1.0 μg of Gn-RH/kg IM. Obtain blood samples before Gn-RH administration and 1 hour later. Assay blood samples for testosterone.

Interpretation

Normal dogs have baseline testosterone levels between 0.5–5 ng/mL, and after administration of Gn-RH the testosterone levels rise above 5 ng/mL. Animals with hypoandrogenism have lower values.

HCG STIMULATION TEST

Administer 44 IU of hCG/kg IM. Obtain blood samples before hCG administration and 4 hours later. Assay blood samples for testosterone.

Interpretation

Normal dogs have baseline testosterone levels between 0.5–5 ng/mL, and after administration of hCG, the testosterone levels rise above 5 ng/mL. Animals with hypoandrogenism have lower values.

DIABETES INSIPIDUS

MODIFIED WATER DEPRIVATION TEST

Rule out other causes of polyuria and polydipsia (especially hyperadrenocorticism). Begin water restriction 3 days before abrupt water deprivation.

Day 1	130–165 mL/kg/day
Day 2	100–125 mL/kg/day
Day 3	65–70 mL/kg/day (normal maintenance requirement)

The morning of the fourth day, discontinue food and water. Start the test. Weigh the patient and empty the bladder. Weigh at 1–2 hour intervals. Monitor carefully for dehydration and depression. When 5% of body weight is lost or azotemia develops, empty the bladder and check urine specific gravity. Consider plasma vasopressin determination at this point.

Interpretation

If the urine specific gravity is > 1.025 (dogs) or > 1.030 (cats), stop the test. The patient does not have diabetes insipidus. If the urine specific gravity is not > 1.025 (dogs) or > 1.030 (cats), administer 0.55 U/kg aqueous vasopressin IM (maximum dose 5 U). Empty the bladder and check urine specific gravity at 30, 60, and 120 minutes postadministration. If urine specific gravity increases $< 10\%$, nephrogenic diabetes insipidus is indicated; if it increases 10%–50%, partial central diabetes insipidus is indicated; if it increases 50%–800%, complete central diabetes insipidus is indicated.

Table II-B.

Tests of the Endocrine System*

Hormone	Unit	Dogs	Cats
Adrenocorticotropic hormone, basal (ACTH, plasma)	pmol/L	2–15	1–20
Aldosterone[†] (plasma)			
Basal	pmol/L	14–957	194–388
Post-ACTH	pmol/L	197–2103	277–721
Cortisol (serum or plasma, urine)			
Basal	nmol/L	25–125	15–150
Post-ACTH	nmol/L	200–550	130–450
Post–low-dose dexamethasone (0.01 or 0.015 mg/kg)	nmol/L	≤ 40	≤ 40
Post–high-dose dexamethasone (0.1 or 1.0 mg/kg)[‡]	nmol/L	≤ 40	≤ 40
Urinary cortisol-creatinine ratio	$\times 10^{-6}$	8–24,[†] 10[§]	—
Insulin, basal (serum)	pmol/L	35–200	35–200
Intact parathormone[†] (serum)	pmol/L	2–13	0–4
Progesterone (serum or plasma, female)	mmol/L	≤ 3.0 in anestrus, proestrus	≤ 3.0 in anestrus, proestrus
		50–220 in diestrus, pregnancy	50–220 in diestrus, pregnancy
Testosterone (serum or plasma, male)	nmol/L	1–20	1–20
Thyroxine (T_4, serum)			
Basal	nmol/L	12–50	10–50
Post–thyroxine-stimulating hormone (TSH)	nmol/L	> 45	> 45
Triiodothyronine (T_3) suppression[‖]	nmol/L	—	≤ 20
Triiodothyronine, basal (T_3, serum)	nmol/L	0.7–2.3	0.5–2.0

*Prepared with the assistance of ME Peterson, The Animal Medical Center, New York, NY. Unless indicated otherwise, values in this table are adapted from Kemppainen RJ, Zerbe CA. Common endocrine diagnostic tests: normal values and interpretations. In: Kirk RW, ed. Current veterinary therapy X. Philadelphia: WB Saunders, 1989:961–968. Hormone determinations are variable between laboratories. The laboratory performing the analysis should provide reference values. Before submitting samples for hormone determinations, consult the laboratory for sample specifications, use of anticoagulants, and sample preservation. General sampling conditions are discussed in Reimers TJ. Guidelines for collection, storage, and transport of samples for hormone assay. In: Kirk RW, ed. Current veterinary therapy X. Philadelphia: WB Saunders, 1989:968–973. Factors that affect serum thyroid and adrenocortical hormone concentrations in dogs are discussed in Reimers TJ, Lawler DF, Sutaria PM, et al. Effects of age, sex, and body size on serum concentrations of thyroid and adrenocortical hormones in dogs. Am J Vet Res 1990;51:454.

†Provided by RF Nachreiner, Animal Health Diagnostic Laboratory, Endocrine Diagnostic Section, Michigan State University.

‡This test is used after adrenocortical hyperfunction has been confirmed. It is used to differentiate adrenal tumor (where no suppression is seen) from pituitary-dependent cases (where suppression occurs but is variable).

§From Stolp R, Rijnberk A, Meiher JC, Croughs RJM. Urinary corticoids in the diagnosis of canine hyperadrenocorticism. Res Vet Sci 1983;34:141. Rijnberk A, van Wees A, Mol JA. Assessment of two tests for the diagnosis of canine hyperadrenocorticism. Vet Rec 1988;122:178–180.

‖From Peterson ME, Ferguson DC. Thyroid diseases. In: Ettinger SJ, ed. Textbook of veterinary internal medicine. Diseases of the dog and cat. 3rd ed. Philadelphia: WB Saunders, 1989:1632–1675.

From Appendices. In: Bonagura J, ed. Kirk's current veterinary therapy XIII. Philadelphia: WB Saunders, 2000:1223 (with permission).

Table II-C.

Conversion Table for Hormone Assay Units

Hormone	Unit Traditional	Unit SI	Conversion factors Traditional to SI	Conversion factors SI to Traditional
Aldosterone	ng/dL	pmol/L	27.7	0.036
Corticotropin (ACTH)	pg/mL	pmol/L	0.22	4.51
Cortisol	μg/dL	mmol/L	27.59	0.36
β-endorphin	pg/mL	pmol/L	0.289	3.43
Epinephrine	pg/mL	pmol/L	5.46	0.183
Estrogen (estradiol)	pg/mL	pmol/L	3.67	0.273
Gastrin	pg/mL	ng/L	1.00	1.00
Glucagon	pg/mL	ng/L	1.00	1.00
Growth hormone (GH)	ng/mL	μg/L	1.00	1.00
Insulin	μU/mL	pmol/L	7.18	0.139
α-melanocyte–stimulating hormone (α-MSH)	pg/mL	pmol/L	0.001	1.00
Norepinephrine	pg/mL	nmol/L	0.006	169
Pancreatic polypeptide (PP)	mg/dL	mmol/L	0.239	4.18
Progesterone	ng/mL	mmol/L	3.18	0.315
Prolactin	ng/mL	μg/L	1.00	1.00
Renin	ng/mL/hr	ng/L/sec	0.278	3.60
Somatostatin	pg/mL	pmol/L	0.611	1.64
Testosterone	ng/mL	nmol/L	3.47	0.288
Thyroxine (T_4)	μg/dL	nmol/L	12.87	0.078
Triiodothyronine (T_3)	ng/dL	nmol/L	0.0154	64.9
Vasoactive intestinal polypeptide (VIP)	pg/mL	pmol/L	0.301	3.33

Contributed by ME Peterson, The Animal Medical Center, New York, NY.
From Appendices. In: Bonagura JD, ed. Kirk's current veterinary therapy XIII. Philadelphia: WB Saunders, 2000:1223 (with permission).

APPENDIX III

APPROXIMATE NORMAL RANGES FOR COMMON MEASUREMENTS IN DOGS AND CATS

	Dog	Cat
Heart rate (bpm)	60–180	140–220
Capillary refill time	< 2 sec	< 2 sec
Body temperature	99.5–102.5° F	100.5–102.5° F
	37.5–39.2° C	38.1–39.2° C
Mean arterial pressure (mm Hg)	90–120	100–150
Blood volume (mL/kg)	75–90	47–66
Cardiac output		
(mL/kg/min)	100–200	167 ± 39
(L/M^2/min)	4.72 ± 1.09	
Systemic resistance		
(mm Hg/mL/kg/min)	0.64 ± 0.16	
(dynes/sec/cm)	2162 ± 458	
Mean pulmonary arterial pressure (mm Hg)	14 ± 3	
Central venous pressure (cm H_2O)	3 ± 4	
Pulmonary artery occlusion pressure (mm Hg)	5 ± 2	
Urine output	1–2 mL/kg/hr	1–2 mL/kg/hr
Breathing rate (breaths/min)	10–30	24–42
Minute ventilation (mL/kg/min)	170–350	200–350
Oxygen delivery		
(mL/kg/min)	29 ± 8	
(mL/M^2/min)	815 ± 234	
Oxygen consumption		
(mL/kg/min)	4–11	3–8
(mL/M^2/min)	198 ± 53	
Arterial Po_2 (mm Hg)	85–105	100–115
Arterial So_2	> 95	> 95
Arterial Pco_2 (mm Hg)	30–44	28–35
Arterial pH	7.36–7.46	7.34–7.43
Bicarbonate (mEq/L)	20–25	17–21
Base deficit (mEq/L)	0 to −4	−1 to −8
Total plasma proteins (g/dL)	6.0–8.0	6.8–8.3
Albumin (g/dL)	2.5–3.5	1.9–3.9
Packed cell volume (%)	37–55	29–48
Hemoglobin (g/dL)	12–18	9–15.1
Sodium (mEq/L)	145–154	151–158
Potassium (mEq/L)	4.1–5.3	3.6–4.9
Chloride (mEq/L)	105–116	113–121
Total CO_2 (mEq/L)	16–26	15–21

Modified from Aldrich J, Haskins SC. Monitoring the critically ill patient. In: Current veterinary therapy XII. Philadelphia: WB Saunders, 1995;98–105 (with permission).

APPENDIX IV

NORMAL VALUES FOR THE CANINE AND FELINE ELECTROCARDIOGRAM

RATE

	Dog	60 to 140 beats/min for giant breeds
		70 to 160 beats/min for adult dogs
		Up to 180 beats/min for toy breeds
		Up to 220 beats/min for puppies
	Cat	Range: 120 to 240 beats/min
		Mean: 197 beats/min

RHYTHM

	Dog	Normal sinus rhythm
		Sinus arrhythmia
		Wandering sinoatrial pacemaker
	Cat	Normal sinus rhythm
		Sinus tachycardia (physiologic reaction to excitement)

MEASUREMENTS (lead II, 50 mm/sec, 1 cm = 1 mV)

Dog	P wave	Width: maximum, 0.04 second; 0.05 second in giant breeds
		Height: maximum, 0.4 mV
	P-R interval	Width: 0.06 to 0.13 second
	QRS complex	Width: maximum, 0.05 second in small breeds
		maximum, 0.06 second in large breeds
		Height of R wave*: maximum, 3.0 mV in large breeds
		maximum, 2.5 mV in small breeds
	S-T segment	No depression: not more than 0.2 mV
		No elevation: not more than 0.15 mV
	T wave	Can be positive, negative, or biphasic
		Not greater than one-fourth amplitude of R wave
		Amplitude range ± 0.05–1.0 mV in any lead
	Q-T interval	Width: 0.15 to 0.25 second at normal heart rate; varies with heart rate (faster rates have shorter Q-T intervals and vice versa)
Cat	P wave	Width: maximum, 0.04 second
		Height: maximum, 0.2 mV
	P-R interval	Width: 0.05 to 0.09 second
	QRS complex	Width: maximum, 0.04 second
		Height of R wave: maximum, 0.9 mV
	S-T segment	No depression or elevation
	T wave	Can be positive, negative, or biphasic—most often positive
		Maximum amplitude: 0.3 mV
	Q-T interval	Width: 0.12 to 0.18 second at normal heart rate (range 0.07 to 0.20 second); varies with heart rate (faster rates have shorter Q-T intervals and vice versa)

MEAN ELECTRICAL AXIS (frontal plane)

	Dog	+40 to +100 degrees
	Cat	0 to +160 degrees (not valid in many cats)

PRECORDIAL CHEST LEADS (values of special importance)

	Dog	CV_5RL (rV_2): T wave positive, R wave not greater than 3.0 mV
		CV_6LL (V_2): S wave not greater than 0.8 mV, R wave not greater than 3.0 mV*
		CV_6LU (V_4): S wave not greater than 0.7 mV, R wave not greater than 3.0 mV*
		V_{10}: negative QRS complex, T wave negative except in Chihuahuas
	Cat	CV_6LL (V_2): R wave not greater than 1.0 mV
		CV_6LU (V_4): R wave not greater than 1.0 mV
		V_{10}: T wave negative, R/Q not greater than 1.0 mV

*Not valid for thin, deep-chested dogs under 2 years of age.
Source: Tilley, LP. Essentials of canine and feline electrocardiography, interpretation and treatment. 3rd edition. Baltimore: Williams & Wilkins, 1992 (with permission).

CLINICAL TOXICOSIS—SYSTEMS AFFECTED AND CLINICAL EFFECTS

Neurologic Toxicants

Excitation or stimulation of nervous system
  Amphetamine
  Aminopyridine
  Caffeine
  Cyanide
  Ergot (*Claviceps* spp.)
  Fluoroacetate
  Lead
  Metaldehyde
  Moonseed (*Menispermum canadense*)
  Mycotoxins
  Nicotine
  Organochlorine insecticides
  Organophosphate insecticides
  Phenols and chlorophenols
  Strychnine
  Theobromine
  Theophylline
  Water hemlock (*Cicuta* spp.)
Depression, coma
  Alcohols
  Antihistamines
  Barbiturates
  Carbon monoxide
  Hydrocarbons, aliphatic
  Hydrocarbons, aromatic
  Hydrocarbons, halogenated
  Lead
  Mercury
  Morphine derivatives
  Salicylates
  Snake venoms
Loss of motor control
  Botulinum
  Buckeye (*Aesculus* spp.)
  Carbon disulfide
  Curare
  Ergot
  Ethylene glycol
  Hexachlorophene
  Lead
  Nicotine
  Organophosphates
  Triaryl phosphates
Autonomic stimulation
  Atropine
  Carbamate insecticides
  Fly mushroom (*Amanita muscaria*)
  Organophosphate insecticides
Behavioral changes
  Belladonna alkaloids
  Ergot
  Lead
  Lysergic acid diethylamide (LSD)
  Marijuana
  Morning glory
  Nutmeg
  Opium derivatives
  Organochlorine insecticides
  Periwinkle
  Peyote

Gastrointestinal Toxicants

Stomatitis, pharyngitis
  Acids and alkalis
  Aldehydes
  Chromium salts
  Fertilizer
  Mercuric salts
  Detergents
  Petroleum distillates
  Phenol
Salivation
  Amanita muscaria
  Ammonia
  Cresol
  Metaldehyde
  Nicotine
  Organophosphates
  Thallium
Dry mouth
  Amphetamine
  Antihistamine
  Atropine
  Belladonna
  Opiates
Gastroenteritis
  Amanita spp.
  Antimony
  Arsenic
  Barium
  Bismuth
  Cantharidin
  Copper salts
  Croton oil
  Detergents, soaps, sanitizers
  Digitalis toxins
  Iron
  Lead
  Mercury
  Mushrooms
  Phenoxy herbicides
  Phosphorus
  Plants (see Appendix VII)
  Staphylococcus toxins
  Thallium
  Zinc phosphide

Hepatotoxins

Acetaminophen
Aflatoxin
Amanita phalloides
Blue-green algae
Coal tar derivatives
Copper
Halogenated hydrocarbons
Iron
Petroleum distillates
Phosphorus

Nephrotoxins

Inadvertent nephrotoxins
  Aldehydes
  Amanita mushrooms

Arsenic
Bismuth
Cadmium
Cresols
Dichromate
Ethylene glycol
Halogenated hydrocarbons
Mercury
Ochratoxins
Oxalates
Petroleum distillates
Phenols
Thallium
Turpentine
Volatile oils (e.g., pennyroyal oil or oil of juniper)
Nephrotoxic drugs
  Acetaminophen
  Amphotericin B
  Bacitracin
  Gentamicin
  Kanamycin
  Neomycin
  Polymyxin B
  Sulfonamides
  Vancomycin

Blood Toxicants

Methemoglobin
  Acetaminophen
  Aniline derivatives
  Chlorate
  Copper
  Methylene blue
  Nitrite
  Nitrobenzene
Hemolysis
  Acetaminophen*
  Aniline
  Arsine
  Chlorates
  Copper
  Methylene blue*
  Nitrobenzene
  Onions
  Snake venoms
  Turpentine
  Red maple leaves
Aplastic anemia, leukopenia, thrombo-cytopenia
  Arsenicals
  Aspirin
  Benzene
  Chloramphenicol
  Cytostatic agents
  Estrogens
  Phenylbutazone
  Toluene
  Trichlorethylene
Coagulopathy
  Aflatoxin
  Aspirin
  Coumarin rodenticides

*Especially in cats

CLINICAL TOXICOSIS—SYSTEMS AFFECTED AND CLINICAL EFFECTS (CONT'D)

Phosphorus
Sulfonamides

Cardiovascular Toxicants

Tachycardia and arrhythmias
  Adrenaline
  Aminophylline
  Amphetamine
  Aminoglycoside antibiotics
  Atropine
  Caffeine
  Cyanide
  Dinitrophenol
  Fluorocarbons
  Nicotine
  Thallium
Bradycardia
  Barium
  Cardiac glycosides
  Digitalis
  Morphine
  Opiates
  Oleander
  Red squill
Myocardial damage
  Amanita phalloides
  Barium
  Carbon monoxide
  Oleander
  Phosphorus
  Thallium

Vascular necrosis
  Ergot
  Lead
  Mercury
  Selenium

Respiratory Toxicants

Air pollutants (nitrogen dioxide, sulfur dioxide)
Allergens
Ammonia
Alphanaphthyl thiourea rodenticide
Chlorine
Gasoline, kerosene
Organophosphate insecticides
Ozone
Paraquat herbicide
Thallium

Ocular Toxicants

Mydriasis
  Amanita mushrooms
  Atropine
  Belladonna
  Methanol
Miosis
  Heroin
  Morphine
  Nicotine
  Organophosphates
Optic neuropathy
  Arsenicals
  Lead

Mercury
Methanol
Thallium
Vitamin A

General Signs

Fever
  Atropine
  Carbon monoxide
  Dinitrophenol
  Lead
  Metaldehyde
  Organochlorine insecticides
Hypothermia
  Alcohol
  Arsenic
  Barbiturates
  Heroin
  Morphine
  Oxalates
  Phenols
Cyanosis
  Carbon dioxide
  Hydrogen sulfide
  Nitrite
  Paraquat
Pink skin color
  Arsenic
  Carbon monoxide
  Cyanide
  Mercury
  Thallium

From Osweiler G. A brief guide to clinical toxicosis in small animals. In: Kirk RW, ed. Current veterinary therapy IX. Philadelphia: WB Saunders, 1986:132–135 (with permission).

APPENDIX VI

TOXIC AGENTS AND THEIR SYSTEMIC ANTIDOTES—DOSAGE AND METHOD OF TREATMENT

Toxic agent	Systemic antidote	Dosage and method of treatment
Acetaminophen	N-acetylcysteine (Mucomyst, Apothecon)	150 mg/kg loading dose PO or IV, then 50 mg/kg q4h for 17–20 additional doses
Amphetamines	Chlorpromazine	1 mg/kg IM or IV; administer only half the dosage if barbiturates have been given; blocks excitation
Arsenic, mercury, and other heavy metals except cadmium, lead, silver, selenium, and thallium	Dimercaprol (BAL, Hynson, Wescott & Dunning)	10% solution in oil; give small animals 2.5–5.0 mg/kg IM q6h for 2 days then q12h for the next 10 days or until recovery. (Note: With severe acute poisoning, 5 mg/kg should be given only on the first day.)
	D-Penicillamine (Cuprimine, Merck)	Developed for chronic mercury poisoning; now seems most promising drug; no reports on dosage in animals; give 3–4 mg/kg q6h
Atropine, belladonna alkaloids	Physostigmine salicylate	0.1–0.6 mg/kg (do not use neostigmine)
Barbiturates	Doxapram	2% solution; give small animals 3–5 mg/kg IV only (0.14–0.25 mL/kg); repeat as necessary. (Note: The above is reliable only when depression is mild; in animals with deeper levels of depression, ventilatory support [and oxygen] is preferable.)
Bromides	Chlorides (sodium or ammonium salts)	0.5–1.0 g PO daily for several days; hasten excretion
Carbon monoxide	Oxygen	Pure oxygen at normal or high pressure; artificial respiration; blood transfusion
Cholecalciferol	Calcitonin (Calcimar, Rhône-Poulenc Rorer)	4 IU/kg SC or IM q8–12h
Cholinergic agents	Atropine sulfate	0.02–0.04 mg/kg, as needed
Cholinesterase inhibitors	Atropine sulfate	0.2 mg/kg, repeated as needed for atropinization; treat cyanosis (if present) first; blocks only muscarinic effects: atropine in oil may be injected for prolonged effect. Avoid atropine intoxication!
Cholinergic agents and cholinesterase inhibitors (organophosphates, some carbamates; but not carbaryl, morphine, succinylcholine, or carbam piloxime)	Pralidoxime chloride (2-PAM)	5% solution; 20–50 mg/kg IM or by slow IV (0.2–1.0 mg/kg) injection (maximum dose is 500 mg/min), repeat as needed; 2-PAM alleviates nicotinic effect and regenerates cholinesterase; phenothiazine tranquilizers are contraindicated
Copper	D-Penicillamine (Cuprimine)	See Arsenic
Coumarin-derivative anticoagulants	Vitamin K₁ (AquaMEPHYTON, 5-mg capsules or 1% emulsion, Merck)	Give 3–5 mg/kg SC or PO per day with canned food; treat 7 days for warfarin-type, treat 21–30 days for second-generation anticoagulant rodenticides; oral therapy more effacious than parenteral
	Fresh whole blood, fresh plasma, or fresh frozen plasma	Blood transfusion, 10–25 mL/kg, as required
Curare	Neostigmine methylsulfate	Solution: 1:5000 or 1:2000 (1 mL = 0.2 or 0.5 mg/mL): dosage is 0.005 mg/5 kg SC; follow with IV injection of atropine (0.04 mg/kg)
	Edrophonium chloride (Tensilon, Roche)	1% solution: give 0.05–1.0 mg/kg IV
	Ventilatory support	
Cyanide	Methemoglobin (sodium nitrite is used to form methemoglobin)	1% solution of sodium nitrite; dosage is 16 mg/kg IV (1.6 mL/kg)
	Sodium thiosulfate	Follow with 20% solution of sodium thiosulfate at dosage of 30–40 mg/kg (0.15–0.2 mL/kg) IV; if treatment is repeated, use only sodium thiosulfate. (Note: Both of the above may be given simultaneously as follows: 0.5 mL/kg of combination consisting of 10 g sodium nitrite, 15 g sodium thiosulfate distilled water q.s. to 250 mL; dosage may be repeated once; if further treatment is required, give only 20% solution thiosulfate at 0.2 mL/kg.)
Digitalis glycosides, oleander, and Bufo toads	Potassium chloride	Dogs: 0.5–2.0 g PO in divided doses or, in serious cases, a diluted solution given IV by slow drip (ECG monitoring is essential)
	Diphenylhydantoin	25 mg/min IV until ventricular arrhythmias are controlled
	Propranolol (β-blocker)	0.5–1.0 mg/kg IV or IM as needed to control cardiac arrhythmias (ECG monitoring is essential)
	Atropine sulfate	0.02–0.04 mg/kg as needed for cholinergic and arrhythmia control
Fluoride	Calcium borogluconate	3–10 mL of 5%–10% solution
Fluoroacetate (compound 1080)	Glyceryl monoacetate (monoacetin, Sigma)	0.1–0.5 mg/kg IM hourly for several hours (total 2–4 mg/kg), or diluted (0.5–1.0% solution IV; danger of hemolysis); monoacetin is available only from chemical supply houses
	Acetamide	Animal may be protected if acetamide is given before or simultaneously with compound 1080 (experimental)
	Pentobarbital	May protect against lethal dose (experimental). (Note: All treatments are generally unrewarding.)
Hallucinogens (LSD, phencyclidine hydrochloride [PCP])	Diazepam (Valium, Roche)	As needed—avoid respiratory depression (2–5 mg/kg)
Heparin	Protamine sulfate	1% solution; give 1.0–1.5 mg by slow IV injection to antagonize each 1 mg of heparin; reduce dose as time increases between heparin injection and start of treatment (after 30 minutes, give only 0.5 mg)

TOXIC AGENTS AND THEIR SYSTEMIC ANTIDOTES—DOSAGE AND METHOD OF TREATMENT (CONT'D)

Toxic agent	Systemic antidote	Dosage and method of treatment
Iron salts	Deferoxamine mesylate (Desferal, Ciba)	Dosage for animals not yet established; dosage for humans is 5 g of 5% solution PO, then 20 mg/kg IM q4–6h; in case of shock, dosage is 40 mg/kg by IV drip over 4-hour period; may be repeated in 6 hours, then 15 mg/kg by drip q8h
Lead	Calcium disodium edetate (CaEDTA)	Maximum safe dosage is 75 mg/kg per 24 hours (only for severe case); EDTA is available in 20% solution; for IV drip, dilute in 5% glucose to 0.5%; for IM, add procaine to 20% solution to give 0.5% concentration of procaine
	EDTA and BAL	BAL is given as 10% solution in oil (a) In severe cases (CNS involvement with > 100 μg lead per 100 g whole blood), give 4 mg/kg BAL only as initial dose; follow after 4 hours and q4h for 3–4 days with BAL and EDTA (12.5 mg/kg) at separate IM sites; skip 2 or 3 days and then treat again for 3–4 days; (b) In subacute cases with < 100 μg lead per 100 g whole blood, give only 50 mg EDTA/kg per 24 hours for 3–5 days;
	Penicillamine (Cuprimine)	May use after either treatment (a) or (b) with 100 mg/kg per day PO for 1–4 weeks
	Thiamine hydrochloride	Experimental to treat CNS signs; 5 mg/kg IV q12h for 1–2 weeks; give slowly and watch for untoward reactions
Metaldehyde	Diazepam (Valium)	2–5 mg/kg IV to control tremors
	Triflupromazine	0.2–2.0 mg/kg IV
	Pentobarbital	To effect
Methanol	Ethanol	Give 1.1 g/kg (4.4 mL/kg) of 25% solution IV; then give 0.5 g/kg (2.0 mL/kg) q4h for 4 days; to prevent or correct acidosis, use sodium bicarbonate 0.4 g/kg IV; activated charcoal, 5 g/kg PO if within 4 hours of ingestion
Methemoglobinemia-producing agents (nitrites, chlorates)	Methylene blue (not recommended for cats)	1% solution (maximum concentration); give by slow IV injection, 8.8 mg/kg (0.9 mL/kg), and repeat if necessary; to prevent fall in blood pressure in cases of nitrite poisoning, use a sympathomimetic drug (ephedrine or epinephrine)
Morphine and related drugs	Naloxone hydrochloride (Narcan, Endo)	0.1 mg/kg IV; do not repeat if respiration is not satisfactory
	Levallorphan tartrate (Lorfan, Roche)	Give IV 0.1–0.5 mL of solution containing 1 mg/mL. (Note: Use either of the antidotes only in acute poisoning. Ventilatory support may be indicated. Activated charcoal is also indicated.)
Oxalates	Calcium	10% solution of calcium gluconate IV; give 3–20 mL (to control hypocalcemia)
Phenothiazine	Methamphetamine hydrochloride (Desoxyn, Abbott)	0.1–0.2 mg/kg; treatment for hypovolemic shock may be required
	Diphenhydramine hydrochloride	For CNS depression, 2–5 mg/kg IV to treat extrapyramidal signs
Phytotoxins and botulin	Antitoxins not available commercially (attempt to obtain through Centers for Disease Control)	As indicated for specific antitoxins; examples of phytotoxins: ricin, abrin, robin, crotin
Plants		Treat signs as necessary (see Appendix VII)
Red squill	Atropine sulfate, propranolol, potassium chloride	As for digitalis and oleander
Snake bite		
Rattlesnake, copperhead, water moccasin	Antivenin (Crotalidae) Polyvalent (Wyeth), Trivalent Crotalidae (Fort Dodge)	Caution: equine origin; administer 1–2 vials IV, slowly, diluted in 250–500 mL of saline or lactated Ringer's solution; also administer antihistamines; corticosteroids are contraindicated
Coral snake	Coral Snake (Wyeth)	Caution: equine origin; may be used as with pit viper antivenin
Spider bite		
Black widow	Antivenin (Merck)	Caution: equine origin; administer IV undiluted
	Dantrolene sodium (Dantrium, Norwich-Eaton)	For neurologic signs, 1 mg/kg IV, followed by 1 mg/kg PO q4h
Brown recluse	Dapsone	1 mg/kg q12h for 10 days
Strontium	Calcium salts	Usual dose of calcium borogluconate
	Ammonium chloride	0.2–0.5 g PO 3–4 times daily
Strychnine and brucine	Pentobarbital	Give IV to effect; higher dose is usually required than that required for anesthesia; place animal in warm, quiet room
	Amobarbital	Give slow IV to effect; duration of sedation is usually 4–6 hours
	Methocarbamol (Robaxin, AH Robins)	10% solution; average first dosage is 149 mg/kg IV (range, 40–300 mg); repeat half dosage as needed
	Glyceryl guaiacolate	110 mg/kg IV, 5% solution; repeat as necessary
	Diazepam (Valium)	2–5 mg/kg; controls convulsions
Thallium	Diphenylthiocarbazone	Dogs: 70 mg/kg PO q8h for 6 days; hastens elimination but is partially toxic
	Prussian blue	0.2 mg/kg PO in 3 divided doses daily
	Potassium chloride	Give simultaneously with thiocarbazone or Prussian blue, 2–6 g PO daily in divided doses

IM = intramuscularly; IV = intravenously; PO = orally; SC = subcutaneously; q = every; h = hour; q.s. = sufficient quantity; ECG = electrocardiogram; CNS = central nervous system.
From Bailey EM Jr, Garland T. Toxicologic emergencies. In: Murtaugh RJ, Kaplan PM, eds. Veterinary emergency and critical care medicine. St. Louis: Mosby, 1992:443–446.

TOXIC PLANTS AND THEIR CLINICAL SIGNS—ANTIDOTES AND TREATMENT

Plant and characteristics	Clinical signs	Antidotes and treatment
Angel's trumpet (*Datura* spp.) Garden annual with white trumpet-shaped flowers Whole plant toxic; toxicity highest in seeds	Thirst, GI atony, disturbed vision, delirium, hallucinations	Parasympathomimetic drugs
Autumn crocus (*Colchicum autumnale*) Houseplant Whole plant toxic; toxicity highest in bulbs	Burning sensation in throat and mouth, thirst, nausea, diarrhea	Fluids; analgesics and atropine to alleviate colic and diarrhea
Azalea (*Rhododendron* spp.) Garden, landscape plant Leaves and flowers are toxic Honey made from flower nectar is toxic	Burning sensation in mouth, salivation, emesis, diarrhea, muscular weakness, dimness of vision, bradycardia, arrhythmia, hypotension EMERGENCY CONDITION	Do not use emetics. Use activated charcoal. Fluid replacement and respiratory support are required. Treat heart block with isoproterenol.
Belladonna lily (*Amaryllis* spp.) Garden, potted plant Bulbs are most toxic	Nausea, diarrhea, hypotension, depression, liver damage	Gastric lavage, charcoal, fluids, and supportive treatment
Bittersweet (*Celastrus* spp.) Weed, vine with red berries Immature fruits are toxic	Gastric irritation, fever, diarrhea	Fluids
Bleeding heart (*Dicentra* spp.) Garden, woods, potted plant Roots more toxic than leaves	Vomiting, diarrhea, convulsions or paralysis	Fluids and seizure control
Castor bean (*Ricinus communis*) Garden annual, grows to 2 m Seeds are 1 cm, dark and light mottled, and highly toxic	Latent period; colic, emesis, diarrhea, thirst	Emesis, charcoal, fluids, and electrolytes
Chinaberry tree (*Melia azedarach*) Ornamental tree in temperate to subtropical areas Fruit and bark are most toxic	Faintness, ataxia, mental confusion, intense gastritis, emesis, diarrhea	Fluid and electrolyte replacement
Christmas rose (*Helleborus niger*) Houseplant Entire plant is toxic	Pain in mouth and abdomen, nausea, emesis, colic, diarrhea, arrhythmia, hypotension	Gastric lavage or emesis; activated charcoal or saline cathartics to decontaminate the GI tract
Daphne (*Daphne mezereum*) Landscape shrub Entire plant is toxic	Vesication and edema of the lips and oral cavity, salivation, thirst, abdominal pain, emesis, hemorrhagic diarrhea	Fluid and electrolyte replacement
Delphinium or larkspur (*Delphinium* spp.) Outdoor garden, mountains; tall with blue flowers Seeds more toxic than leaves	Trembling, ataxia, weakness, salivation	GI detoxification; physostigmine to treat muscarinic signs
English holly (*Ilex* spp.) Landscape plant Fruit is toxic	Nausea, vomiting, diarrhea	Fluid and electrolyte replacement
English ivy (*Hedera helix*) Houseplant Fruit and leaves are toxic	Salivation, thirst, emesis, gastroenteritis, diarrhea, dermatitis	Corticosteroids to treat dermal response; treat other signs symptomatically
Foxglove (*Digitalis purpurea*) Outdoor gardens Entire plant is toxic (especially leaves)	Nausea, emesis, abdominal pain, diarrhea, bradycardia, arrhythmia with prolonged P-R interval and hypokalemia	GI decontamination with activated charcoal or saline cathartics. Treat hypokalemia and give lidocaine for ventricular arrhythmia.
Golden chain (*Laburnum anagyroides*) Landscape tree with long chains of yellow flowers Entire plant is toxic	Emesis, depression, weakness, incoordination, mydriasis, tachycardia	GI decontamination with lavage or emesis followed by activated charcoal
Horse chestnut or buckeye (*Aesculus* spp.) Landscape or forest tree; palmate leaves Nuts and twigs most toxic	Gastroenteritis, diarrhea, dehydration, electrolyte imbalance	Fluid and electrolyte replacement, demulcents, and therapy for gastroenteritis
Iris or flag (*Iris* spp.) Perennial garden flower Rootstock most toxic	Colic, nausea, vomiting, diarrhea	Fluid and electrolyte replacement

TOXIC PLANTS AND THEIR CLINICAL SIGNS—ANTIDOTES AND TREATMENT (CONTINUED)

Plant and characteristics	Clinical signs	Antidotes and treatment
Irish potato (*Solanum tuberosum*) Vegetable garden Vines, green skin, and sprouts are toxic	Colic, diarrhea, salivation, ataxia, weakness, bradycardia, hypotension. Signs may vary from atropine-like to cholinesterase inhibition. Use antidotes accordingly and with caution.	GI decontamination. If atropine-like signs predominate, use physostigmine. If salivation and diarrhea are present, use atropine cautiously.
Jack-in-the-pulpit (*Arisaema triphyllum*) Woods and gardens of temperate zones Entire plant is toxic	Glossitis, pharyngitis, oral inflammation, edema, salivation	Irrigate mouth with water. Cool liquids or demulcents held in mouth may relieve signs.
Lantana (*Lantana camara*) Garden and wild in mild temperate to tropical areas; bright orange and yellow flowers Foliage and immature berries are toxic	Weakness, lethargy, vomiting, diarrhea, mydriasis, bradypnea. Advanced signs are cholestasis, bilirubinemia, and photosensitization.	GI decontamination, fluids, and respiratory support. Protect from sunlight and treat for hepatic insufficiency.
Lily, including Easter lily, tiger lily (*Lilium* spp.), daylily (*Hemerocallis* spp.)	Depression, oliguria, renal failure in cats as a result of toxic tubular necrosis	Prompt GI decontamination and supportive therapy for renal failure. Toxin presently is unknown.
Lily-of-the-valley (*Convallaria majalis*) Garden ornamental Seeds and flowers more toxic than leaves	Colic, vomiting, diarrhea, bradycardia, arrhythmia	Decontaminate GI tract with lavage and charcoal. Avoid emetics. Lidocaine to treat ventricular arrhythmias; treat as for other digitalis glycoside overdose, including correction of hyperkalemia.
Lupine (*Lupinus* spp.) Garden ornamental Seeds more toxic than leaves	Salivation, ataxia, seizures, dyspnea	GI decontamination, control of seizures
Mistletoe (*Phoradendron* spp.) Parasitic shrub on other trees Access to pets in homes at holiday time Leaves, stems, and berries are moderately toxic	Emesis, colic, diarrhea, mydriasis, hypovolemia	Fluid and electrolyte replacement; demulcents for gastroenteritis
Monkshood (*Aconitum* spp.) Perennial garden ornamental Entire plant is toxic	Glossitis, pharyngitis, salivation, nausea, emesis, impaired vision, bradycardia	GI decontamination, fluid and electrolyte replacement. Manage similar to digitalis glycoside overdose, with caution about potassium administration.
Moonseed (*Menispermum canadense*) Woody vine of forests Fruit is most toxic	Convulsions	Maintain airway and support respiration as needed. Control seizures with least medication possible (e.g., diazepam).
Morning glory (*Ipomoea purpurea* and *Ipomoea tricolor*) Garden annual, potted plant Seeds most toxic Occasionally used as hallucinogen	Nausea, mydriasis, hallucinations, decreased reflexes, diarrhea, hypotension	Activated charcoal; dark, quiet surroundings; tranquilization with diazepam
Mountain laurel (*Kalmia* spp.) Native of eastern and southeastern woods, mountains Leaves and flowers are toxic Honey from nectar also toxic	Oral irritation, salivation, emesis, diarrhea, weakness, impaired vision, bradycardia, hypotension, AV block	Emetics are contraindicated. Use activated charcoal, fluid replacement, and respiratory support as needed. Isoproterenol to treat AV block as needed.
Narcissus, daffodil, jonquil (*Narcissus* spp.) Garden ornamental bulb Bulb is most toxic	Nausea, emesis, hypotension, diarrhea	Gastric lavage, charcoal, fluid replacement, supportive treatment for gastroenteritis
Nettle (*Urtica dioica*) Garden weed Hairs on leaves contain toxin that enters skin on contact	Oral irritation and pain, salivation, swelling and edema of nose and periocular areas or other areas of skin contact	Antihistamines and atropine may control appropriate signs. Local or systemic anti-inflammatory supportive therapy to treat affected contact areas.
Oleander (*Nerium oleander*) Landscape shrub 1–3 m tall Whole plant is extremely toxic	Nausea, early signs of vomiting, colic, diarrhea; bradycardia and arrythmia with hyperkalemia develop soon after; EMERGENCY CONDITION	Gastric lavage or induced emesis; activated charcoal or saline cathartics. Treat as for digitalis glycoside overdose, including correction of hyperkalemia. Lidocaine or other appropriate drugs for arrhythmia.
Philodendron (*Monstera* and *Philodendron* spp.) Houseplant Leaves are slightly to moderately toxic	Painful irritation, edema of lips, mouth, tongue, and throat; reported nephrotoxic to cats	Cool liquids or demulcents held in mouth may aid relief

TOXIC PLANTS AND THEIR CLINICAL SIGNS—ANTIDOTES AND TREATMENT (CONTINUED)

Plant and characteristics	Clinical signs	Antidotes and treatment
Poinsettia (*Euphorbia pulcherrima*) Garden or potted plant, especially at Christmas holidays Sap of stem and leaves is mildly to moderately irritant or toxic	Irritation of mouth; may cause vomiting, diarrhea, and dermatitis	Demulcents and fluids to prevent dehydration
Rhubarb (*Rheum rhaponticum*) Garden plant Raw or canned Leaves are high in oxalates	Vomiting, diarrhea, and occasionally icterus. Renal failure develops from oxalate nephrosis.	Early GI decontamination is important. Demulcents and fluid replacement. Treat possible oxalate nephrosis.
Rosary pea or precatory bean (*Abrus precatorius*) Native of Caribbean islands Seeds (when broken or chewed) are highly toxic Illegal to import into United States	Nausea, vomiting, diarrhea, weakness, tachycardia, possible renal failure, coma, death	Emesis or lavage followed with charcoal, demulcents, fluids, and electrolytes. Vitamin C may improve survival.
Thorn apple or jimsonweed (*Datura stramonium*) Annual weed, some species are ornamental (*Datura metel*) Entire plant is toxic, but seeds are most toxic and available Relatively common drug abuse plant used as hallucinogen	Thirst, disturbances of vision, delirium, mydriasis, GI atony. Signs similar to atropine overdose.	Parasympathomimetic drug (e.g., physostigmine)
Tobacco (*Nicotiana tabacum*) Garden plant, weed, cigarettes Whole plant is toxic	Rapid onset of salivation, nausea, emesis, tremors, incoordination, and ataxia, followed by collapse and respiratory failure; EMERGENCY CONDITION	Assist ventilation and vascular support first to save the animal. After respiratory support, decontaminate the GI tract with lavage and activated charcoal.
Wisteria (*Wisteria* spp.) Woody vine or shrub with blue to white legume flowers Entire plant is toxic	Nausea, abdominal pain, prolonged vomiting	Antiemetics and fluid replacement therapy
Yellow jessamine (*Gelsemium sempervirens*) Mild temperate to subtropical climates Yellow trumpet-shaped flowers grow on evergreen vines	Abdominal pain, bradypnea, paresis, seizures, hypothermia	Symptomatic and supportive therapy of respiration and cardiovascular function. GI decontamination and fluid replacement therapy.
Yew (*Taxus cuspidata* and *Taxus baccata*) Evergreen landscape shrub with two-ranked flat needle Whole plant (except ripe fruit) is toxic	Acute onset or sudden death. Affected animals show trembling, muscle weakness, dyspnea, collapse, arrhythmia, and heart block.	Symptomatic and supportive therapy of respiration and cardiovascular function. GI decontamination and fluid replacement therapy.

Contributed by Gary Osweiler, College of Veterinary Medicine, Iowa State University, Ames, IA.

PAIN MANAGEMENT

Table VIII-A

Recommended Parenteral Opioid Dosages and Indications

Opioid	Dose/Route/Duration	Indications	Comments
Butorphanol	Dog: 0.2–0.4 mg/kg IM, IV, or SC Cat: 0.2–0.4 mg/kg; IM, IV, or SC Duration: 1–3 hr	Mild to moderate pain	Mild or no sedation; mild ventilatory depression
Buprenorphine	Dog: 0.005–0.02 mg/kg IM, IV, or SC Cat: 0.005–0.015 mg/kg IM, IV, or SC Duration: 3–8 hr	Mild to moderate pain	Prolonged sleep times; may be difficult to antagonize
Morphine	Dog: 0.2–1.0 mg/kg IM or SC; 0.05–0.4 mg/kg IV Cat: 0.05–0.2 mg/kg IM or SC Duration: 3–6 hr	Moderate to severe pain	Sedation; respiratory depression; bradycardia; nausea; hypothermia; dysphoria in cats without pain or with large dosage; rapid IV injection may cause histamine release.
Hydromorphone	Dog: 0.05–0.2 mg/kg IM, IV, or SC Cat: 0.05–0.2 mg/kg IM, IV, or SC Duration: 3–6 hr	Moderate to severe pain	Similar side effects as those observed with morphine, but less vomiting
Fentanyl	Dog: 0.002–0.01 mg/kg IV or IM Cat: 0.001–0.005 mg/kg IV or IM Duration: 0.5–2 hr	Mild to moderate pain; CRI necessary for long-term analgesia	Sedation; respiratory depression; bradycardia; nausea; inadequate duration of analgesia from single IV bolus or IM injection

CRI = constant rate infusion.

Table VIII-B

Recommended Dispensable Opioid Dosages and Indications

Opioid	Dose/Route/Duration	Indications	Comments
Codeine	Dog: 1.0–2.0 mg/kg PO Cat: 0.1–1.0 mg/kg PO **(see Comments)** Duration: 4–8 hr	Mild to moderate pain	Minimal side effects; when dosed with acetaminophen, avoid in dogs with liver disease or Heinz body anemia; **do not use in combination with acetaminophen in cats**
Butorphanol	Dog: 0.5–1.0 mg/kg PO Cat: 0.5–1.0 mg/kg PO Duration: 2–4 hr	Mild to moderate pain	Mild or no sedation; mild ventilatory depression

Table VIII-C

Recommended Parenteral NSAID Dosages and Indications

NSAID	Dosage/Route/Duration	Indications	Comments
Carprofen (injectable)	Dog: 2–4 mg/kg IV, SC q24hr Cat: 1.0 mg/kg SC only once	Mild to moderate pain	Primarily used perioperatively before switching to oral formulation; GI irritation and altered renal function
Meloxicam (injectable)	Dog: 0.2 mg/kg initially IM, IV, or SC; 0.1 mg/kg thereafter SC Cat: 0.1–0.2 mg/kg initially IM, IV, or SC; 0.05–0.1 mg/kg thereafter SC Duration: 24 hr	Mild to moderate pain	Can be mixed with food; GI irritation and altered renal function
Ketoprofen (injectable)	Dog: 1.0–2.0 mg/kg initially IM, IV, or SC; 0.5–1.0 mg/kg thereafter SC Cat: 1.0–2.0 mg/kg initially IM, IV, or SC; 0.5–1.0 mg/kg thereafter SC Duration: 24 hr	Mild to moderate pain; approved in Canada for dogs and cats and in the U.S. for horses	GI irritation and altered renal function. Dosing should not exceed 5 days for dogs and 3 days for cats

GI = gastrointestinal; NSAID = nonsteroidal anti-inflammatory drug.

PAIN MANAGEMENT

Table VIII-D

Recommended Dispensable NSAID Dosages and Indications			
NSAID	Dosage/Route/Duration	Indications	Comments
Carprofen (tablets and chewables)	Dog: 1.0–2.0 mg/kg PO q24hr Cat: 1.0 mg/kg PO (1 dose only) Duration: 12–24 hr	Mild to moderate pain; approved in the U.S. for dogs	Toxicity associated with chronic use in cats; minimal toxicity in dogs with chronic use, but may cause GI irritation and altered renal function in some patients
Deracoxib (chewable tablets)	Dog (postoperative pain: 3.0–4.0 mg/kg PO q24hr as needed for 7 days) Dog (osteoarthritis): 1–2 mg/kg PO q24hr for long-term treatment over 7 days Duration: 24 hr	Pain and inflammation associated with osteoarthritis. Post-operative pain and inflammation associated with orthopedic surgery in dogs with osteoarthritis. Post-operative ≥1.8 kg; approved in the U.S.	GI irritation and altered renal function
Tepoxalin (oral lyopnilisate)	Dog: 10–20 mg/kg PO initially; 10 mg/kg thereafter Cat: not used Duration: 24 hr	Mild to moderate pain and inflammation; approved for dogs in the U.S.; perioperative administration not recommended	GI irritation and altered renal function. Dual inhibitor of the 5-LO and COX enzymes; 7-day washout recommended when switching from another NSAID
Etodolac (tablets)	Dog: 10–15 mg/kg PO Cat: not used Duration: 24 hr	Mild to moderate pain; approved for dogs in the U.S.	Hypoproteinemia; GI irritation and altered renal function
Aspirin (tablets)	Dog: 10–25 mg/kg PO Cat: 10–15 mg/kg PO Duration: 8–12 hr for dogs, 24–72 hr for cats	Mild to moderate pain and inflammation	GI irritation and altered renal function; more likely at higher doses
Meloxicam (oral liquid suspension)	Dog: 0.2 mg/kg initially PO; 0.1 mg/kg thereafter PO Cat: 0.1–0.2 mg/kg initially PO; 0.05–0.1 mg/kg thereafter PO Duration: 24 hr	Mild to moderate pain; approved for dogs in Canada	GI irritation; can be mixed with food. Cats should not be given meloxicam for > 5 days.
Ketoprofen (tablets)	Dog: 1.0–2.0 mg/kg initially PO; 0.5–1.0 mg/kg thereafter PO Cat: 1.0–2.0 mg/kg initially PO; 0.5–1.0 mg/kg thereafter PO Duration: 24 hr	Mild to moderate pain; approved in Canada for dogs and cats and in the U.S. for horses	GI irritation and altered renal functions Limit administration to 5 days for both dogs and cats
Acetaminophen (tablets and oral liquid suspension)	Dog: 10–15 mg/kg PO Cat: contraindicated Duration (in dogs): 8–12 hr	Mild to moderate pain; low anti-inflammatory action	**Toxic to cats**; often given in combination with codeine to dogs (see oral analgesic preparations)

GI = gastrointestinal; NSAID = nonsteroidal antiinflammatory drug.

Table VIII-E

Dosages and Indications for Selected Drugs Used to Treat Neuropathic Pain			
Drug	Dosage/Route	Duration (PO)	Comments
Ketamine (NMDA antagonist)	Dog: 0.1–1.0 mg/kg IM, SC, or PO Cat: 0.1–1.0 mg/kg IM or SC	4–6 hr 4–6 hr	Low doses potentiate postoperative analgesics. Do not use with intracranial hypertension.
Amitriptyline (tricyclic antidepressant)	Dog: 1.0 mg/kg PO Cat: 2.5–10.0 mg/kg PO	12–24 hr 24 hr	Used to potentiate or prolong analgesia
Gabapentin (anticonvulsant)	Dog: 1.0–15.0 mg/kg PO Cats: 1.0–15.0 mg/kg PO	24 hr 24 hr	Usually associated with few side effects Has shown good results in human and animal studies

To select and administer an adjuvant analgesic properly, the veterinarian should be aware of the drug's clinical pharmacology. The following information about the drug is necessary: (1) approved indication, (2) unapproved indication (e.g., as an analgesic) widely accepted in veterinary medical practice, (3) common side effects and potentially serious adverse effects, (4) pharmacokinetic features, and (5) specific dosing guidelines for pain.

NMDA = N-methyl-D-aspartate

APPENDIX IX

5-MINUTE CONSULT DRUG FORMULARY

Drug Name (Trade or Other Names)	Pharmacology and Indications	Adverse Effects and Precautions	Dosing Information and Comments	Formulations	Dosage
Acemannan (Acemannan immuno-stimulant)	Immunostimulant. A polysaccharide acetyl-ated mannan extract from aloe. Proposed to stimulate T-cell activity in animals. It has been used to treat tumors in dogs and cats. It may stimulate tumor necrosis factor (TNF) and other cytokine release.	No reported side effects	After reconstitution, shake well to dissolve. Use within 4 hours after preparation. Beneficial effect is controversial. There has been a lack of demonstrated effect on lymphocyte blasto-genic response in cats.	10 mg vials reconstitu-ted to 1 mg/mL	Intraperitoneal (1 mg/kg) and intralesional injection (2 mg) every week for 6 treatments
Acepromazine (PromAce and many generic brands)	Phenothiazine tranquili-zer. Inhibits action of dopamine as neuro-transmitter. Used for sedation and preanes-thetic purposes.	Phenothiazines can cause sedation as a common side effect. May lower seizure threshold and cause α-adrenergic blockade. Produces extrapyramidal side effects in some individuals.	Usually used as pre-anesthetic in combina-tion with other drugs. When used as pre-anesthetic, dose is ordinarily 0.02–0.2 mg/kg IM, SC, IV.	5, 10, 25 mg tablet and 10 mg/mL injection	Dog: .5–2.2 mg/kg PO q6–8h, or 0.02–0.1 mg/kg IV, IM, SC. Do not exceed 3 mg total dose in dogs Cat: 1.13–2.25 mg/kg PO q6–8h, or 0.02–0.1 mg/kg IM, SC, IV.
Acetaminophen (Tylenol and many generic brands)	Analgesic agent. Exact mechanism of action is not known. *Not* a pros-taglandin synthesis inhibitor.	Well tolerated in dogs at doses listed. High doses have caused liver toxicity. Do *not* administer to cats.	Many OTC formulations available. Acetamino-phen with codeine may have greater analgesic efficacy in some animals.	120, 160, 325, 500 mg tablets	Dog: 15 mg/kg q8h PO. Cat: not recommended.
Acetaminophen with codeine (Tylenol with codeine and many generic brands)	Same as above, except the opiate codeine is added to enhance analgesia	See Codeine and Acetaminophen.	See Codeine and Acetaminophen.	Oral solution and tablets. Many forms, for example: 300 mg acetaminophen plus either 15, 30, or 60 mg codeine.	Follow dosing recommenda-tions for codeine.
Acetylcysteine (Mucomyst)	Decreases viscosity of secretions. Used as mucolytic agent in eyes and in bronchial nebu-lizing solutions. However, as a donator of sulfhy-dral group, used as antidote for intoxications (e.g., acetaminophen toxicosis in cats).	May cause sensitiza-tion with prolonged topical administration. May react with certain materials in nebulizing equipment.	Available as agent for decreasing viscosity of respiratory secretions, but most common use is as a treatment for intoxications	20% solution	Antidote: 140 mg/kg (loading dose), then 70 mg/kg q4h IV or PO for 5 doses Eye: 2% solution topically q2h
Acetylsalicylic acid	See Aspirin.				
ACTH	See Corticotropin.				
Activated charcoal	See Charcoal, activated.				
Adequan	See Polysulfated glyco-saminoglycan (PSGAG).				
Albendazole (Valbazen)	Benzimidazole antipara-sitic drug. Inhibits glucose uptake in parasites.	At approved doses, there is a wide margin of safety. Adverse effects can include anorexia, lethargy, and bone marrow toxicity. At high doses, has been asso-ciated with bone marrow toxicity (J Am Vet Med Assoc 213:44–46, 1998). Adverse effects are possible when administered for longer than 5 days.	Used primarily as anti-helmintic, but also has demonstrated efficacy for giardiasis	113.6 mg/mL suspen-sion and 300 mg/mL paste	25–50 mg/kg q12h PO × 3 days For giardia, use 25 mg/kg q12h × 2 days.

Drug Name (Trade or Other Names)	Pharmacology and Indications	Adverse Effects and Precautions	Dosing Information and Comments	Formulations	Dosage
Albuterol (Proventil, Ventolin)	β_2-adrenergic agonist. Bronchodilator. Stimulates β_2 receptors to relax bronchial smooth muscle. May also inhibit release of inflammatory mediators, especially from mast cells.	Causes excessive β-adrenergic stimulation at high doses (tachycardia, tremors). Arrhythmias occur at toxic doses. Avoid use in pregnant animals.	Doses are primarily derived from extrapolation of human dose. Well-controlled efficacy studies in veterinary medicine are not available. Onset of action is 15–30 min; duration of action may be as long as 8 hr.	2, 4, 5 mg tablets; 2 mg/5 mL syrup	20–50 mcg/kg q6–8h; or up to maximum of 100 mcg/kg q6h.
Allopurinol (Lopurin, Zyloprim)	Decreases production of uric acid by inhibiting enzymes responsible for uric acid	May cause skin reactions (hypersensitivity)	Used in people primarily for treating gout. In animals, used to decrease formation of uric acid uroliths.	100, 300 mg tablets	10 mg/kg q8h, then reduce to 10 mg/kg q24h, PO. For leishmaniasis, use 10 mg/kg q12h PO for at least 4 months.
Alumunium carbonate gel (Basaljel)	Antacid (neutralizes stomach acid), and phosphate binder in intestine	Generally safe. May interact with other drugs administered orally.	Antacid doses are designed to neutralize stomach acid, but duration of acid suppression is short.	Capsules (equivalent to 500 mg aluminum hydroxide)	10–30 mg/kg PO q8h (with meals)
Aluminium hydroxide gel (Amphojel)	Antacid (neutralizes stomach acid), and phosphate binder in intestine	Generally safe. May interact with other drugs administered orally.	Antacid doses are designed to neutralize stomach acid, but duration of acid suppression is short.	64 mg/mL oral suspension; 600 mg tablet	10–30 mg/kg PO q8h (with meals)
Amikacin (Amiglyde-V [veterinary] and Amikin [human])	Aminoglycoside antibacterial drug (inhibits protein synthesis). Mechanism is similar to other aminoglycosides (see Gentamicin sulfate), but may be more active than gentamicin.	May cause nephrotoxicosis with high doses or prolonged therapy. May also cause ototoxicity and vestibulotoxicity. (See Gentamicin sulfate.)	Once-daily doses are designed to maximize peak minimum inhibitory concentration (MIC) ratio. Consider therapeutic drug monitoring for chronic therapy. (See also Gentamicin sulfate.)	50, 250 mg/mL injection	Dog and cat: 6.5 mg/kg q8h IV, IM, SC; or Dog; 15–30 mg/kg q24h IV, IM, SC; Cat: 10–14 mg/kg q24h IV, IM, SC
Aminopentamide (Centrine)	Antidiarrheal drug. Anticholinergic (blocks acetylcholine at parasympathetic synapse).	Use cautiously in animals with GI stasis or when anticholinergic drugs are contraindicated (e.g., glaucoma).	Dosing guidelines based on manufacturer's recommendation	0.2 mg tablets; 0.5 mg/mL injection	Dog: 0.01–0.03 mg/kg q8–12h IM, SC, PO. Cat: 0.1 mg/cat q8–12h IM, SC, PO.
Aminophylline (many [generic])	Bronchodilator. Aminophylline is a salt of theophylline, formulated to enhance oral absorption without gastric side effects. It is converted to theophylline after ingestion.	Causes excitement and possible cardiac side effects with high concentrations. (See Theophylline.)	See also Theophylline. Therapeutic drug monitoring is recommended for chronic therapy.	100, 200 mg tablet; 25 mg/mL injection	Dog: 10 mg/kg q8h PO, IM, IV. Cat: 6.6 mg/kg q12h PO.
6-Aminosalicylic acid	See Mesalamine, Olsalazine.				
Amiodarone (Cordarone)	Class III antiarrhythmic agent with potassium-blocking properties; indicated for severe refractory atrial and ventricular arrhythmias	Most common effect in dogs is decreased appetite. Prolonged QT interval is a concern. Other adverse effects include: bradycardia, chronic heart failure (CHF), hypotension, atrioventricular (AV) block, thyroid dysfunction, pulmonary fibrosis, and hepatotoxicity. Acute cardiac toxicity has been observed in dogs.	Use as last resort for recurrent hemodynamically unstable ventricular tachycardia; takes weeks to achieve therapeutic levels. Typically, loading doses are administered, followed by maintenance dose. Safe doses for injection have not been established.	200 mg tablets; 50 mg/mL injection	Dog: Dose range is 10–20 mg/kg PO q12h; typically start with 25 mg/kg q12h PO x 4 days, followed by 25 mg/kg q24h PO thereafter. Cat: no safe dose established.

Drug Name (Trade or Other Names)	Pharmacology and Indications	Adverse Effects and Precautions	Dosing Information and Comments	Formulations	Dosage
Amitraz (Mitaban)	Antiparasitic drug for ectoparasites. Used for treatment of mites, including *Demodex*. Inhibits monoamine oxidase in mites.	Causes sedation in dogs (α_2-agonist), which may be reversed by yohimbine or atipamezole. When high doses are used, other side effects reported include pruritus, polyuria and polydipsia (PU/PD), bradycardia, hypothermia, hyperglycemia, and (rarely) seizures.	Manufacturer's dose should be used initially. But, for refractory cases, this dose has been exceeded to produce increased efficacy. Doses that have been used include: 0.025, 0.05, and 0.1% concentration applied 2× week and 0.125% solution applied to 1/2 body every day for 4 weeks to 5 months.	10.6 mL concentrated dip (19.9%)	10.6 mL per 7.5 L water (0.025% solution). Apply 3–6 topical treatments q14d. For refractory cases, this dose has been exceeded to produce increased efficacy. Doses that have been used include: 0.025, 0.05, and 0.1% concentration applied 2× week and 0.125% solution applied to 1/2 body every day for 4 weeks to 5 months.
Amitriptyline hydrochloride (Elavil)	Tricyclic antidepressant drug. Action is via inhibition of uptake of serotonin and other transmitters at presynaptic nerve terminals. Used in animals to treat variety of behavioral disorders, such as anxiety. Used in cats for chronic idiopathic cystitis.	Multiple side effects are associated with tricyclic antidepressants, such as antimuscarinic effects (dry mouth, rapid heart rate) and antihistamine effects (sedation). High doses can produce life-threatening cardiotoxicity. In cats, reduced grooming, weight gain, and sedation are possible.	Doses are primarily based on empiricism. There are no controlled efficacy trials available for animals. There is evidence for success treating idiopathic cystitis in cats. (J Am Vet Med Assoc. 213:1282–1286, 1998.)	10, 25, 50, 75, 100, 150 mg tablets; 10 mg/mL injection	Dog: 1–2 mg/kg PO q12–24h. Cat: 5–10 mg per cat/day PO; cystitis: 2 mg/kg/day (2.5–7.5 mg/cat/day).
Amlodipine besylate (Norvasc)	Calcium channel–blocking drug of the dihydropyridine class. Decreases calcium influx in cardiac and vascular smooth muscle. Its greatest effect is as a vasodilator. In cats and dogs, it is used to treat hypertension.	Can cause hypotension and bradycardia. Use cautiously with other vasodilators.	In cats, efficacy has been established at 0.625 mg/cat once daily. If cats are large size (> 4.5 kg) or refractory, increase to higher dose (J Vet Int Med 12:157–162, 1998).	2.5, 5, and 10 mg tablets	Dog: 2.5 mg/dog, or 0.1 mg/kg once daily PO Cat: 0.625 mg/cat initially, PO once daily, and increase if needed to 1.25 mg/cat (average is 0.18 mg/kg)
Ammonium chloride (generic)	Urine acidifier	Do not use in patients with systemic acidemia. May be unpalatable when added to some animals' food.	Doses are designed to maximize urine acidifying effect.	Available as crystals	Dog: 100 mg/kg q12h PO Cat: 800 mg/cat (approximately 1/3 to 1/4 tsp) mixed with food daily
Amoxicillin (Amoxi-Tabs, Biomox, and other brands. [Omnipen, Principen, Totacillin are human forms])	β-lactam antibiotic. Inhibits bacterial cell wall synthesis. Generally broad-spectrum activity. Used for a variety of infections in all species.	Usually well tolerated. Allergic reactions are possible. Diarrhea is common with oral doses.	Dose recommendations vary depending on the susceptibility of bacteria and location of infection. Generally, more frequent or higher doses needed for gram-negative infections.	50, 100, 150, 200, 400 mg tablets. 250 and 500 mg capsules (human forms).	6.6–20 mg/kg q8–12h PO
Amoxicillin trihydrate (Amoxi-Tabs, Amoxi-Drops, Amoxil, and others)	β-lactam antibiotic. Inhibits bacterial cell wall synthesis. Generally broad-spectrum activity, but resistance is common.	Use cautiously in animals allergic to penicillin-like drugs.	Dose requirements vary depending on susceptibility of bacteria.	50, 100, 200, 400 mg tablets. 50 mg/mL oral suspension.	6–20 mg/kg q8–12h PO
Amoxicillin + clavulanate potassium (Clavamox)	β-lactam antibiotic + β-lactamase inhibitor (clavulanate/clavulanic acid)	Same as for amoxicillin	Same as for amoxicillin	62.5, 125, 250, 375 mg tablets and 62.5 mg/mL suspension	Dog: 12.5–25 mg/kg q12h PO Cat: 62.5 mg/cat q12h PO. Consider administering these doses q8h for gram-negative infections.

Drug Name (Trade or Other Names)	Pharmacology and Indications	Adverse Effects and Precautions	Dosing Information and Comments	Formulations	Dosage
Amphotericin B (Fungizone)	Antifungal drug. Fungicidal for systemic fungi, by damaging fungal membranes.	Produces a dose-related nephrotoxicosis. Also produces fever, phlebitis, and tremors.	Administer IV via slow infusion diluted in fluids, and monitor renal function closely. When preparing IV solution, do not mix with electrolyte solutions (use D-5-W, for example); administer NaCl fluid loading before therapy. (One study administered this drug subcutaneously: Aust Vet J 73:124, 1996.)	50-mg injectable vial	0.5 mg/kg IV (slow infusion) q48h to a cumulative dose of 4–8 mg/kg
Amphotericin B, liposomal formulation (ABLC, Abelcet)	Same indications as for conventional amphotericin B. Liposomal formulations may be used at higher doses, and safety margin is increased. Expense is much higher than for conventional formulations.	Renal toxicity is the most dose-limiting effect.	Higher doses can be used compared to conventional formulation of amphotericin B. Dilute in 5% dextrose in water to 1 mg/mL, and administer IV over 1–2 hours.	100 mg/20 mL in lipid formulation	Dog: 2–3 mg/kg IV 3 times/week for 9–12 treatments to a cumulative dose of 24–27 mg/kg Cat: 1 mg/kg IV 3 times/week for 12 treatments
Ampicillin (Omnipen, Principen, others [human forms])	β-lactam antibiotic. Inhibits bacterial cell wall synthesis.	Use cautiously in animals allergic to penicillin-like drugs.	Dose requirements vary depending on susceptibility of bacteria. Absorbed approximately 50% less, compared with amoxicillin, when administered orally. Generally, more frequent or higher doses needed for gram-negative infections.	250, 500 mg capsules; 125, 250, 500 mg vials of ampicillin sodium. Ampicillin trihydrate: 10 and 25 g vials for injection.	Ampicillin sodium: 10–20 mg/kg q6–8h IV, IM, SC or 20–40 mg/kg q8h PO. Ampicillin trihydrate: Dog: 10–50 mg/kg q12–24h IM, SC. Cat: 10–20 mg/kg q12–24h IM, SC. Dogs and cats: doses as high as 100 mg/kg have been used for some resistant infections, such as those caused by enterococci.
Ampicillin + sulbactam (Unasyn)	Ampicillin plus a β-lactamase inhibitor (sulbactam). Sulbactam has similar activity as clavulanate.	Same as for ampicillin	Same as for amoxicillin + clavulanate	2:1 combination for injection. 1.5 and 3 g vials.	10–20 mg/kg IV, IM q8h
Ampicillin trihydrate (Polyflex)	β-lactam antibiotic. Inhibits bacterial cell wall synthesis.	Use cautiously in animals allergic to penicillin-like drugs.	Absorption is slow and may not be sufficient for acute serious infection.	10, 25 mg vials for injection	Dog: 10–50 mg/kg q12–24h IM, SC Cat: 10–20 mg/kg q12–24h IM, SC
Amprolium (Amprol, Corid)	Antiprotozoal drug. Antagonizes thiamine in parasites. Used for treatment of coccidiosis, especially in puppies.	Toxicity observed only at high doses (CNS signs due to thiamine deficiency).	Usually administered as feed additive to livestock. For dogs, 30 mL of 9.6% amprolium has been added to 3.8 L of drinking water for control of coccidiosis.	9.6% (9.6 g/100 mL) oral solution; soluble powder	1.25 g of 20% amprolium powder to daily feed, or 30 mL of 9.6% amprolium solution to 3.8 L of drinking water for 7 days
Antacid drugs	See Aluminum hydroxide, Magnesium hydroxide, Calcium carbonate.				
Apomorphine hydrochloride (generic)	Emetic drug. Causes emesis via dopamine release or direct effects on chemoreceptor trigger zone	Produces emesis before serious adverse effects occur. Use cautiously in cats that may be sensitive to opiates.	Consult local poison center or pharmacist for availability.	6 mg tablets	0.02–0.04 mg/kg IV IM, 0.1 mg/kg SC, or instill 0.25 mg in conjunctiva of eye (dissolve 6 mg tablet in 1–2 mL of saline)
Ascorbic acid (Vitamin C)	Vitamin. Used as acidifier.	Toxicity only at very high doses	Primarily used as nutritional supplement, but high doses have been used for treatment of certain diseases.	Various forms, including 250 mg/ml sodium ascorbate	100–500 mg/animal/day (diet supplement), or 100 mg/animal q8h (urine acidification)

Drug Name (Trade or Other Names)	Pharmacology and Indications	Adverse Effects and Precautions	Dosing Information and Comments	Formulations	Dosage
L-Asparaginase (Elspar)	Anticancer agent. Purified enzyme from *E. coli*. Used in lymphoma protocols. Depletes cancer cells of asparagine and interferes with protein synthesis.	Hypersensitivity, allergic reactions	Usually used in combination with other drugs in cancer chemotherapy protocols	10,000 U per vial for injection	Dog: 400 U/kg IM weekly or 10,000 U/m² weekly × 3 weeks Cat: 400 U/kg SC weekly
Aspirin (many generic and brand names [Bufferin, Ascriptin])	Nonsteroidal anti-inflammatory drug (NSAID). Anti-inflammatory action is generally considered to be caused by inhibition of prostaglandins. Used as analgesic, anti-inflammatory, and anti-platelet drug.	Narrow therapeutic index. High doses frequently cause vomiting. Other GI effects can include ulceration and bleeding. Cats susceptible to salicylate intoxication because of slow clearance. Use cautiously in patients with coagulopathies because of platelet inhibition.	Analgesic and anti-inflammatory doses have primarily been derived from empiricism. Antiplatelet doses are lower because of prolonged effect of aspirin on platelets. When administering aspirin, giving buffered forms or administering with food may decrease stomach irritation. Enteric-coated formulations are not recommended for dogs and cats.	81, 325 mg tablets	Mild analgesia: (dog) 10 mg/kg q12h. Anti-inflammatory: dog: 20–25 mg/kg q12h; cat: 10–20 mg/kg q48h. Antiplatelet: dog: 5–10 mg/kg q24–48h; cat: 80 mg q48h.
Atenolol (Tenormin)	β-adrenergic blocker. Relatively selective for β₁-receptor. Used primarily as an antiarrhythmic or for other cardiovascular conditions to slow sinus rate.	Bradycardia and heart block are possible. May produce bronchospasm in sensitive patients.	Dosing precautions are similar to other β-blocking drugs. Atenolol is reported to be less affected by changes in hepatic metabolism than other β-blockers. Dose in animals based on Am J Vet Res 57: 1050–1053, 1996.	25, 50, 100 mg tablets; 25 mg/mL oral suspension; and 0.5 mg/mL ampules for injection	Dog: 6.25–12.5 mg/dog q12h (or 0.25–1.0 mg/kg q12–24h) Cat: 6.25–12.5 mg/cat q12h (approx. 3 mg/kg)
Atipamezole (Antisedan)	α₂-antagonist. Used to reverse α₂-agonists, such as medetomidine and xylazine.	Safe. Can cause some initial excitement in some animals shortly after reversal.	When used to reverse medetomidine, inject same volume as used for medetomidine.	5 mg/mL injection	Inject same volume as used for medetomidine.
Atracurium (Tracrium)	Neuromuscular blocking agent (nondepolarizing). Competes with acetylcholine at neuromuscular end plate. Used primarily during anesthesia or other conditions in which it is necessary to inhibit muscle contractions.	Produces respiratory depression and paralysis. Neuromuscular blocking drugs have no effect on analgesia.	Administer only in situations in which careful control of respiration is possible. Doses may need to be individualized for optimum effect. Do not mix with alkalinizing solutions or lactated Ringer's solution.	10 mg/mL injection	0.2 mg/kg IV initally, then 0.15 mg/kg every 30 min (or IV infusion at 3–8 mcg/kg/min)
Atropine (many generic brands)	Anticholinergic agent (blocks acetylcholine effect at muscarinic receptor), parasympatholytic. Used primarily as adjunct to anesthesia or other procedures to increase heart rate and decrease respiratory and gastrointestinal secretion. Also used as antidote for organophosphate intoxication.	Potent anticholinergic agent. Do not use in patients with glaucoma, intestinal ileus, gastroparesis, or tachycardia. Side effects of therapy include xerostomia, ileus, constipation, tachycardia, urine retention.	Used ordinarily as adjunct with anesthesia or other procedures. Do not mix with alkaline solutions.	400, 500, 540 mcg/mL injection; 15 mg/mL injection	0.02–0.04 mg/kg q6–8h IV, IM, SC; 0.2–0.5 mg/kg (as needed) for organophosphate and carbamate toxicosis.

Drug Name (Trade or Other Names)	Pharmacology and Indications	Adverse Effects and Precautions	Dosing Information and Comments	Formulations	Dosage
Auranofin (triethylphosphine gold) (Ridaura)	Used for gold therapy (chrysotherapy). Mechanism of action is unknown, but may relate to immunosuppressive effect on lymphocytes. Used primarily for immune-mediated diseases.	Adverse effects include dermatitis, nephrotoxicity, and blood dyscrasias.	Use of this drug has not been evaluated in veterinary medicine. No controlled clinical trials are available to determine efficacy in animals. It has been suggested that this product (oral) is not as effective as injectable products, such as aurothioglucose.	3 mg capsules	0.1–0.2 mg/kg q12h PO
Aurothioglucose (Solganol)	Used for gold therapy (chrysotherapy). Mechanism of action is unknown, but may relate to immunosuppressive effect on lymphocytes. Used primarily for immune-mediated diseases (such as dermatologic disease).	Adverse effects include dermatitis, nephrotoxicity, and blood dyscrasias.	Use of this drug has not been evaluated in veterinary medicine. No controlled clinical trials are available to determine efficacy in animals. This drug is often used in combination with other immunosuppressive drugs, such as corticosteroids.	50 mg/mL injection	Dogs <10 kg: 1 mg IM first week, 2 mg IM second week, 1 mg/kg/week maintenance Dogs >10 kg: 5 mg IM first week, 10 mg IM second week, 1 mg/kg/week maintenance Cat: 0.5–1 mg/cat every 7 days IM
Azathioprine (Imuran)	Thiopurine immunosuppressive drug. Acts to inhibit T cell lymphocyte function. This drug is metabolized to 6-mercaptopurine, which may account for immunosuppressive effects. Used to treat various immune-mediated disease.	Bone marrow suppression is most serious concern. Cats particularly are susceptible. There has been some association with development of pancreatitis when administered with corticosteroids.	Usually used in combination with other immunosuppressive drugs (such as corticosteroids) to treat immune-mediated disease. Some evidence suggests that it is contraindicated in cats because of bone marrow effects. Doses of 2.2 mg/kg in cats have produced toxicity.	50 mg tablets; 10 mg/mL for injection	Dog: 2 mg/kg q24h PO initially then 0.5–1 mg/kg q48h Cat (use cautiously): 0.3 mg/kg q24h PO initially, then q48h, with careful monitoring
Azithromycin (Zithromax)	Azalide antibiotic. Similar mechanism of action as macrolides (erythromycin), which is to inhibit bacteria protein synthesis via inhibition of ribosome. Spectrum is primarily gram-positive.	Has not been in common use in veterinary medicine to establish adverse effects. Vomiting is likely with high doses. Diarrhea may occur in some patients.	Azithromycin may be better tolerated than erythromycin. Primary difference from other antibiotics is the high intracellular concentrations achieved.	250 mg capsules, 250 and 600 mg tablets, 100 or 200 mg/5 mL oral suspension, and 500 mg vials for injection	Dog: 10 mg/kg PO once every 5 days, or 3.3 mg/kg q24h for three days Cat: 5 mg/kg PO q48h
AZT (Azidothymidine)	See Zidovudine.				
Bactrim (sulfamethoxazole + trimethoprim) (See Trimethoprim-sulfonamide combinations.					
BAL (British antilewisite)	See Dimercaprol.				
Benazepril (Lotensin)	Angiotensin-converting enzyme (ACE) inhibitor. See Captopril and Enalapril for details. Used for hypertension and heart failure.	Similar to those for captopril and enalapril	Dose is based on approved use in dogs in Europe and Canada. Monitor renal function and electrolytes 3–7 days after initiating therapy and periodically thereafter.	5,10, 20, 40 mg tablets	Dog: 0.25–0.5 mg/kg q24h PO Cat (systemic hypertension and renal disease): 0.5–1 mg/kg q24h PO

Drug Name (Trade or Other Names)	Pharmacology and Indications	Adverse Effects and Precautions	Dosing Information and Comments	Formulations	Dosage
Betamethasone (Celestone)	Potent, long-acting corticosteroid. Anti-inflammatory and immunosuppressive effects are approximately 30× more than cortisol. Anti-inflammatory effects are complex, but primarily via inhibition of inflammatory cells and suppression of expression of inflammatory mediators. Use is for treatment of inflammatory and immune-mediated disease.	Side effects from corticosteroids are many and include polyphagia, PU/PD, and hypothalamic-pituitary-adrenal (HPA) axis suppression. Adverse effects include GI ulceration, hepatopathy, diabetes, hyperlipidemia, decreased thyroid hormone, decreased protein synthesis and wound healing, and immunosuppression.	Dosing schedules are based on desired effect. Anti-inflammatory effects are seen at doses of 0.1–0.2 mg/kg, immunosuppressive effects at 0.2–0.5 mg/kg.	600 mcg (0.6 mg) tablets; 3 mg/mL sodium phosphate injection	Anti-inflammatory effects: 0.1–0.2 mg/kg q12–24h PO Immunosuppressive effects: 0.2–0.5 mg/kg q12–24h PO
Bethanechol chloride	Muscarinic, cholinergic agonist. Parasympathomimetic. Stimulates gastric and intestinal motility, but primarily used to increase contraction of urinary bladder.	High doses of cholinergic agonists will increase motility of GI tract and cause abdominal discomfort and diarrhea. Can cause circulatory depression in sensitive animals.	Administer injection SC only, not IV. Doses are derived from extrapolation of human doses or via empiricism. There are no well-controlled efficacy studies available for veterinary species.	No longer commercially available. However, available through compounding pharmacies	Dog: 5–15 mg/dog q8h PO Cat: 1.25–5 mg/cat q8h PO
Bisacodyl (Dulcolax)	Laxative/cathartic. Acts via local stimulation of GI motility, most likely by irritation of bowel. Used primarily as laxative or for procedures in which bowel evacuation is necessary.	Avoid use in patients with renal disease. Avoid overuse.	Available as OTC tablet. Doses are derived from extrapolation of human doses or via empiricism. There are no well-controlled efficacy studies available for veterinary species. Onset of action is approx. 1 hr.	5 mg tablets	5 mg/animal q8–24h PO
Bismuth subsalicylate (Pepto-Bismol)	Antidiarrhea agent and GI protectant. Precise mechanism of action is unknown, but anti-prostaglandin action of salicylate component may be beneficial for enteritis. Bismuth component is efficacious for treating infections caused by spirochete bacteria (Helicobacter gastritis).	Adverse effects are uncommon; however, salicylate component is absorbed systemically, and overuse should be avoided in animals that cannot tolerate salicylates (such as cats and animals allergic to aspirin). Owners should be warned that bismuth will discolor stools.	Available as OTC product. Doses are derived from extrapolation of human doses or via empiricism. There are no well-controlled efficacy studies available for veterinary species.	Oral suspension: 262 mg/15 mL, or 525 mg/mL in extra strength formulation; 262 mg tablets	1–3 mL/kg/day (in divided doses) PO
Bismuth subcarbonate	Same as for bismuth subsalicylate				0.3–3.0 g q4h PO
Bleomycin (Blenoxane)	Anticancer, antibiotic agent. Used for treatment of various sarcomas and carcinomas. Exact mechanism of action is unknown, but may bind to DNA and prevent synthesis.	Causes local reaction at site of injection. Causes pulmonary toxicity in people as well as fever and chills, but side effects are not well documented in veterinary species.	Injectable solution usually used in combination with other anticancer agents. Consult anticancer protocols for details regarding use.	15 U vials for injection	Dog: 10 U/m² IV or SC for 3 days, then 10 U/m² weekly (maximum cumulative dose 200 U/m²)
Bromide	See Potassium bromide.				
Bunamidine hydrochloride (Scolaban)	Used as anticestodal agent. Primarily to treat tapeworm infections in dogs and cats. Mechanism of action is to damage integrity of protective integument on parasite.	Vomiting and diarrhea have occurred after use. Avoid use in young animals.	Do not break tablets. Administer tablets on empty stomach. Do not feed for 3 hr after administration.	400 mg tablets	20–50 mg/kg once PO

Drug Name (Trade or Other Names)	Pharmacology and Indications	Adverse Effects and Precautions	Dosing Information and Comments	Formulations	Dosage
Bupivacaine hydrochloride (Marcaine, and generics)	Local anesthetic. Inhibits nerve conduction via sodium channel blockade. Longer-acting and more potent than lidocaine or other local anesthetics.	Adverse effects rare with local infiltration. High doses absorbed systemically can cause nervous system signs (tremors and convulsions). After epidural administration, respiratory paralysis is possible with high doses.	Used for local infiltration or infusion into epidural space. One may admix 0.1 mEq sodium bicarbonate per 10 mL solution to increase pH, decrease pain from injection, and increase onset. Use immediately after mixing with bicarbonate.	2.5 and 5 mg/mL solution injection	1 mL of 0.5% solution per 10 cm for an epidural
Buprenorphine hydrochloride (Buprenex ([Vetergesic in the UK])	Opioid analgesic. Partial μ-receptor agonist, κ-receptor antagonist. 25–50 × more potent than morphine. Buprenorphine may cause less respiratory depression than other opiates.	Adverse effects are similar to other opiate agonists, except there may be less respiratory depression. Dependency from chronic use may be less than with pure agonists.	Used for analgesia, often in combination with other analgesics or in conjunction with general anesthesia. Longer acting than morphine. Only partially reversed by naloxone	0.3 mg/mL solution	Dog: 0.006–0.02 mg/kg IV, IM, SC q4–8h Cat: 0.005–0.01 mg/kg IV, IM, q4–8h
Buspirone (BuSpar)	Antianxiety agent. Acts to block release of serotonin by binding to presynaptic receptors. In veterinary medicine, has been primarily used for treatment of urine spraying in cats.	Some cats show increased aggression; some cats show increased affection to owners.	Some efficacy trials suggest effectiveness for treating urine spraying in cats. There may be a lower relapse rate compared to other drugs.	5, 10 mg tablets	Dog: 2.5–10 mg/dog q12–24h PO or 1–2 mg/kg q12h PO Cat: 2.5–5 mg/cat q24h PO (may be increased to 5–7.5 mg per cat twice daily for some cats)
Busulfan (Myleran)	Anticancer agent. Bifunctional alkylating agent and acts to disrupt DNA of tumor cells. Used primarily for lymphoreticular neoplasia.	Leukopenia is most severe side effect.	Usually used in combination with other anticancer agents. Consult specific protocol for details.	2 mg tablets	3–4 mg/m² q24h PO
Butorphanol tartrate (Torbutrol, Torbugesic)	Opioid analgesic. κ-receptor agonist and weak μ-receptor antagonist. Butorphanol is used for perioperative analgesia, chronic pain, and as an antitussive agent.	Adverse effects are similar to other opioid analgesic drugs. Sedation is common at analgesic doses. Respiratory depression can occur with high doses. Dysphoric effects have been observed with these agonist/antagonist drugs.	Often used in combination with anesthetic agents or in conjunction with other analgesic drugs.	1, 5, 10 mg tablets; 0.5 or 10 mg/mL injection	Dog: (antitussive) 0.055 mg/kg q6–12h SC or 0.55 mg/kg PO; (preanesthetic) 0.2–0.4 mg/kg IV, IM, SC (with acepromazine); (analgesic) 0.2–0.4 mg/kg q2–4h Cat (analgesic): 0.2–0.8 mg/kg q2–6h, IV, SC or 1.5 mg/kg PO q4–8h
Calcitriol (Rocaltrol, Calcijex)	Used to treat calcium deficiency and diseases such as hypocalcemia associated with hypoparathyroidism. Not indicated as vitamin D supplement. Action is to increase calcium absorption in intestine. Also used to lower parathormone levels in patients with renal secondary hyperthyroidism	Overdose can result in hypercalcemia.	Doses should be adjusted in each patient according to response and monitoring of calcium plasma concentration . (hypoparathyroidism) or parathormone levels (renal secondary hyperparathyroidism	Available as injection (Calcijex) and capsules (Rocaltrol); 0.25, 0.5 mcg capsules, 1 or 2 mcg/mL injection	Dog: for hypoparathyroidism: 0.25–0.5 mcg/dog/day; for renal secondary hyperparathyroidism: 2.5–3.5 ng/kg PO q24h Cat: for hypoparathyroidism: 0.25 mcg/cat q48h (or 0.01–0.04 mg/kg/day); for renal secondary hyperparathyroidism: 2.5–3.5 ng/kg PO q24h
Calcium carbonate (many brands available: Titralac, Tums, generic)	Used as oral calcium supplement for hypocalcemia. Used as antacid to treat gastric hyperacidity and GI ulcers. Neutralizes stomach acid. Also used as intestinal phosphate binder for hyperphosphatemia.	Few side effects. Increased calcium concentrations are possible. Drug interactions: Avoid use with oral fluoroquinolones (e.g., ciprofloxacin, enrofloxacin) as it may decrease their absorption.	Doses are primarily derived from extrapolation of human doses. When used as calcium supplement, doses should be adjusted according to serum calcium concentrations.	Many tablets or oral suspension, e.g., 650 mg tablets (contain 260 mg calcium ion)	5–10 mL of oral solution q4–6h PO; for phosphate binder: 60–100 mg/kg/day in divided doses PO
Calcium chloride (generic)	Calcium supplement. Used in acute situations to supplement as electrolyte replacement or as a cardiotonic.	Overdose with calcium is possible. Do not administer IV solution SC or IM because it may cause tissue necrosis.	Injection is (27.2 mg of calcium ion [1.36 mEq]) per mL. Usually used in emergency situations. Intracardiac administration has been performed, but avoid injections into the myocardium.	10% (100 mg/mL) solution	0.1–0.3 mL/kg IV (slowly)

Drug Name (Trade or Other Names)	Pharmacology and Indications	Adverse Effects and Precautions	Dosing Information and Comments	Formulations	Dosage
Calcium citrate (Citracal [OTC])	Calcium supplement. Used in treatment of hypocalcemia, such as with hypoparathyroidism.	Hypercalcemia possible with oversupplementation	Doses should be adjusted according to serum calcium concentration.	950 mg tablets (contain 200 mg calcium ion)	Dog: 20 mg/kg/day PO (with meals) Cat: 10–30 mg/kg q8h PO (with meals)
Calcium disodium EDTA	See Edetate calcium disodium.				
Calcium gluconate (Kalcinate, and generic)	Calcium supplement. Used in treatment of hypocalcemia, such as with hypoparathyroidism. Used in electrolyte deficiency.	Hypercalcemia possible with oversupplementation	Injection is 97 mg (9.5 mg of calcium ion [0.47 mEq]) per mL. 500 mg tablets contain 45 mg of calcium ion. Avoid administration of IV solution IM or SC because it will cause tissue necrosis.	10% (100 mg/mL) injection	0.5–1.5 mL/kg IV (slowly)
Calcium lactate (generic)	Generally same comments as for other calcium supplements		Calcium lactate contains 130 mg of calcium ion per gram.	OTC tablets	Dog: 0.5–2.0 g/dog/day PO (in divided doses) Cat: 0.2–0.5 g/cat/day PO (in divided doses)
Captopril (Capoten)	ACE inhibitor. Inhibits conversion of angiotensin I to angiotensin II. May have other vasodilating properties. Generally used to treat hypertension and congestive heart failure.	Hypotension possible with excessive doses. May cause azotemia in some patients, especially when administered with potent diuretics (furosemide). Drug interactions: Use cautiously with diuretics, potassium supplements. NSAIDs may diminish antihypertensive effect.	Monitor patients carefully to avoid hypotension. With all ACE inhibitors, monitor electrolytes and renal function 3–7 days after initiating therapy and periodically thereafter. Use of captopril has been replaced by enalapril in many patients.	25 mg tablet	Dogs: 0.5–2 mg/kg q8–12h PO Cats: 3.12–6.25 mg/cat q8h PO
Carbenicillin (Geopen, Pyopen)	β-lactam antibiotic. Inhibits bacterial cell wall synthesis. Active against Pseudomonas and other gram-negative bacteria.	Use cautiously in patients sensitive to penicillins (e.g., allergy).	Carbenicillin injection often is administered with an aminoglycoside. Do not mix with aminoglycosides prior to administration, or inactivation will result.	1, 2, 5, 10, and 30 g vials for injection	40–50 mg/kg, and up to 100 mg/kg q6–8h IV, IM, SC
Carbenicillin indanyl sodium (Geocillin)	Same as for carbenicillin. Primary use is for treating infections of lower urinary tract.	Same as for carbenicillin	Oral formulation of carbenicillin, but attains concentrations that are only sufficient for treating urinary tract infections. Do not use for systemic infections.	500 mg tablets	10 mg/kg q8h PO
Carbimazole (neo-mercazole)	Antithyroid drug similar to methimazole but with perhaps fewer side effects.	See Methimazole.	Used in Europe. Clinical experience in U.S. is limited.	Available in Europe	Cat: 5 mg/cat q8h PO (induction), followed by 5 mg/cat q12h PO
Carboplatin (Paraplatin)	Anticancer agent. Used for treating various carcinomas. Interrupts replication of DNA in tumor cells by cross-linking. Used for squamous cell carcinoma and other carcinomas, melanoma, osteosarcomas, and other sarcomas. Action is similar to cisplatin (see Cisplatin for further details).	Dose-limiting toxicosis is myelosuppression. May cause anemia, leukopenia, or thrombocytopenia. Carboplatin may induce renal toxicity. Compared to cisplatin, carboplatin is less emetogenic and less nephrotoxic. In cats, causes a dose-limiting neutropenia and thrombocytopenia (nadir at day 17).	Available for reconstitution for injection. Do not use with administration sets containing aluminum, because of incompatibility. Usually administered in specific anticancer protocols.	50 and 150 mg vial for injection	Dog: 300 mg/m² every q3–4 weeks IV Cat: 200–250 mg/m² every 4 weeks IV

Drug Name (Trade or Other Names)	Pharmacology and Indications	Adverse Effects and Precautions	Dosing Information and Comments	Formulations	Dosage
Carprofen (Rimadyl; Zenecarp in the UK)	NSAID. Used for treatment of pain and inflammation, particularly pain and inflammation associated with osteoarthritis. Shown to be safe and effective for perioperative use for surgical pain either by injection or PO. Carprofen's action may be via cyclooxygenase inhibition but is relatively COX-1 sparing. Other mechanisms also may explain its efficacy.	Most common adverse effects in clinical patients have been GI (vomiting, nausea, diarrhea). Other adverse effects are more rare and include idiosyncratic hepatotoxicosis. If they occur, signs of hepatotoxicosis appear 2–3 weeks after beginning therapy. Perioperative use has not adversely affected renal function or bleeding times. Avoid use with other NSAIDs or with corticosteroids.	Doses are based on manufacturer's field trials and U.S. registration data. Clinical trials conducted with canine patients with osteoarthritis and surgical patients. There is not sufficient safety information available to recommend carprofen for use in cats. Injectable carprofen administered for surgery may be given 2 hours prior to the procedure.	25, 75, 100 mg tablets (regular and chewable); 50 mg/mL injectable solution	Dog: 4.4 mg/kg/day PO, administered either once a day or divided into 2.2 mg/kg q12h; 4.4 mg/kg/day SC, administered once daily or 2.2 mg/kg q12h. To control postoperative pain, administer prior to surgery. Cat: not recommended
Carvedilol (Coreg)	Nonselective β-blocker with α-blocking and antioxidant properties; indicated for systemic hypertension and upregulation of β-receptors in animals with myocardial failure	Bradycardia, CHF due to initial myocardial depression. Adverse effects from nonselective β-blockade are possible, including weakness and bronchospasm.	Typical starting dose is 0.2 mg/kg q12h, then gradually titrate the dose upward to 0.4 mg/kg. If signs of heart failure worsen at higher doses, lower to the previously well-tolerated dose.	3.125, 6.25, 12.5, 25 mg tablets	Dog: 0.2–0.4 mg/kg q12h PO Cat: no dose established
Cascara sagrada (many brands [e.g., Nature's Remedy])	Stimulant cathartic. Action is believed to be by local stimulation of bowel motility. Used as laxative to treat constipation or evacuate bowel for procedures.	Overuse can cause electrolyte losses.	Available in various OTC products.	100 and 325 mg tablets	Dog: 1–5 mg/kg/day PO Cat: 1–2 mg/cat/day
Castor oil (generic)	Stimulant cathartic. Action is believed to be by local stimulation of bowel motility. Used as laxative to treat constipation or evacuate bowel for procedures.	Overuse can cause electrolyte losses. Castor oil has been known to stimulate premature labor in pregnancy.	Available as OTC product	Oral liquid (100%)	Dog: 8–30 mL/day PO Cat: 4–10 mL/day PO
Cefaclor (Ceclor)	Cephalosporin antibiotic. Action is similar to other β-lactam antibiotics, which is to inhibit synthesis of bacterial cell wall, leading to cell death. Cephalosporins are divided into 1st, 2nd, or 3rd generation, depending on spectrum of activity. Consult package insert or specific reference for spectrum of activity of individual cephalosporin. Cefaclor is a 2nd-generation cephalosporin.	All cephalosporins are generally safe; however, sensitivity can occur in individuals (allergy). Rare bleeding disorders have been known to occur with some cephalosporins.	Used primarily when resistance has been demonstrated to 1st-generation cephalosporins	250, 500 capsules and 25 mg/mL oral suspension	15 mg/kg q8h PO
Cefadroxil (Cefa-Tabs, Cefa-Drops)	See Cefaclor. Cefadroxil is a 1st-generation cephalosporin.	See Cefaclor. Cefadroxil has been known to cause vomiting after oral administration in dogs.	Spectrum of cefadroxil is similar to other 1st-generation cephalosporins. For susceptibility test, use cephalothin as test drug.	50 mg/mL oral suspension; 50, 100, 200, 1000 mg tablet	Dog: 22 mg/kg q12h, up to 30 mg/kg q12h PO Cat: 22 mg/kg q24h PO
Cefazolin sodium (Ancef, Kefzol, and generic)	See Cefadroxil. Cefazolin is a 1st-generation cephalosporin.	See Cefaclor. For cefazolin, use cephalothin to test susceptibility.	Commonly used 1st-generation cephalosporin as injectable drug for prophylaxis for surgery as well as for acute therapy for serious infections.	50 and 100 mg/50 mL for injection	20–35 mg/kg q8h IV, IM. For perisurgical use: 22 mg/kg q2h during surgery.

Drug Name (Trade or Other Names)	Pharmacology and Indications	Adverse Effects and Precautions	Dosing Information and Comments	Formulations	Dosage
Cefdinir (Omnicef)	Oral 3rd-generation cephalosporin. Activity includes staphylococci and many gram-negative bacilli. Other characteristics are similar to those of other drugs in this class.	Similar to those of other oral cephalosporins.	Use in veterinary medicine has not been reported. Use and doses are extrapolated from human medicine.	300 mg capsules, 25 mg/mL oral suspension	Dose not established. Human dose is 7 mg/kg q12h PO.
Cefixime (Suprax)	See Cefaclor. Cefixime is a 3rd-generation cephalosporin.	See Cefaclor.	Although not approved for veterinary use, pharmacokinetic studies in dogs have provided recommended dosages.	20 mg/mL oral suspension and 200 and 400 mg tablets	10 mg/kg q12h PO; for cystitis: 5 mg/kg q12–24h PO
Cefotaxime sodium (Claforan)	See Cefaclor. Cefotaxime is a 3rd-generation cephalosporin. Cefotaxime is used when resistance is encountered to other antibiotics or when infection is in central nervous system.	See Cefaclor.	3rd-generation cephalosporin used when resistance encountered to 1st- and 2nd-generation cephalosporins.	500 mg; 1, 2, and 10 g vials for injection	Dog: 50 mg/kg IV, IM, SC q12h Cat: 20–80 mg/kg q6h IV, IM
Cefotetan disodium (Cefotan)	See Cefaclor. Cefotetan is 2nd-generation cephalosporin.	See Cefaclor.	2nd-generation cephalosporin similar to cefoxitin, but may have longer half-life in dogs.	1, 2, and 10 g vials for injection	30 mg/kg q8h IV, SC
Cefoxitin sodium (Mefoxin)	See Cefaclor. Cefoxitin is a 2nd-generation cephalosporin. May have increased activity against anaerobic bacteria.	See Cefaclor.	2nd-generation cephalosporin, which is often used when activity against anaerobic bacteria is desired.	1, 2, and 10 g vials for injection	30 mg/kg q6–8h IV
Cefpodoxime proxetil (Vantin)	Oral 3rd generation cephalosporin. Activity includes gram-negative bacilli resistant to first generation cephalosporins. Activity also includes staphylococcus.	No adverse effects reported for animals, but be aware of possibility of reactions seen with other oral cephalosporins (e.g., vomiting, diarrhea, allergy).	Use for infections (e.g., UTI) resistant to other oral drugs.	100, 200 mg tablets; 10 or 20 mg/mL oral suspension	10 mg/kg q8h PO for systemic infections; 10 mg/kg q12h PO for urinary tract infections
Ceftazidime (Fortaz, Ceptaz, Tazicef)	3rd-generation cephalosporin. Ceftazidime has more activity than other cephalosporins against Pseudomonas aeruginosa.	See Cefaclor.	3rd-generation cephalosporin. May be reconstituted with 1% lidocaine for IM injection.	Vials (0.5, 1, 2, 6 g) reconstituted to 280 mg/mL	Dog and cat: 30 mg/kg q6h IV, IM Dog: 30 mg/kg q4–6h SC
Ceftiofur (Naxcel [ceftiofur sodium]; Excenel [ceftiofur HCl]).	See Cefaclor. Ceftiofur is a unique cephalosporin that does not fit into a distinct class; however, its spectrum resembles many of the 3rd-generation cephalosporins.	See Cefaclor. Ceftiofur is primarily used only for urinary tract infections.	Available as powder for reconstitution prior to injection. After reconstitution, stable for 7 days when refrigerated or 12 hrs at room temperature, or frozen for 8 weeks. Excenel is not approved for use in dogs.	50 mg/mL injection	2.2–4.4 mg/kg SC q24h (for urinary tract infections)
Cephalexin (Keflex and generic forms)	See Cefaclor. Cephalexin is a 1st-generation cephalosporin.	See Cefaclor. For cephalexin, use cephalothin to test susceptibility.	Although not approved for veterinary use, trials in dogs with pyoderma show similar efficacy.	250, 500 mg capsules; 250, 500 mg tablets; 100 mg/mL or 125, 250 mg/5 mL oral suspension	10–30 mg/kg q6–12h PO; for pyoderma, 22–35 mg/kg q12h PO
Cephalothin sodium (Keflin)	See Cefaclor.	See Cefaclor.	1st-generation cephalosporin. Used as test drug for susceptibility tests of other 1st-generation cephalosporins.	1 and 2 g vials for injection	10–30 mg/kg q4–8h IV, IM
Cephapirin (Cefadyl)	See Cefaclor. Cephapirin is a 1st-generation cephalosporin.	See Cefaclor.		500 mg, 1, 2, 4 g vials for injection	10–30 mg/kg q4–8h IV, IM
Cephradine (Velosef)	See Cefaclor. Cephradine is a 1st-generation cephalosporin.	See Cefaclor.		250, 500 mg capsules, and 250, 500 mg, 1 and 2 g vials for injection	10–25 mg/kg q6–8h PO

Drug Name (Trade or Other Names)	Pharmacology and Indications	Adverse Effects and Precautions	Dosing Information and Comments	Formulations	Dosage
Charcoal, activated (Acta-Char, Charco-dote, Toxiban, generic)	Adsorbent. Used primarily to adsorb drugs and toxins in intestine to prevent their absorption	Not absorbed systemically. Safe for administration	Available in variety of forms; usually used as treatment of poisoning. Many commercial preparations contain sorbitol, which acts as flavoring agent and promotes intestinal catharsis.	Oral suspension	1–4 g/kg PO (granules); 6–12 mL/kg (suspension)
Chlorambucil (Leukeran)	Cytotoxic agent. Acts in similar manner as cyclophosphamide as alkylating agent. Used for treatment of various tumors and immuno-suppressive therapy.	Myelosuppression is possible. Cystitis does not occur with chloram-bucil as with cyclophos-phamide.	Consult anticancer drug protocol for specific regimens.	2 mg tablets	Dog: 2–6 mg/m² q24h initially, then q48h PO Cat: 0.1–0.2 mg/kg q24h initially, Then q48h PO
Chloramphenicol and chloramphenicol palmitate (Chloromyce-tin, generic forms)	Antibacterial drug. Mechanism of action is via inhibition of protein synthesis via binding to ribosome. Broad spectrum of activity. Florfenicol acts via similar mechanism and has been substituted in some animals. (See Florfenicol.)	Bone marrow suppression is possible with high doses or prolonged treatment (especially in cats). Avoid use in pregnant or neonatal animals. Drug interactions with other drugs (e.g., barbiturates) possible because chloramphenicol will inhibit hepatic microsomal enzymes.	Chloramphenicol use based on susceptibility data. Chloramphenicol palmitate requires active enzymes and should not be administered to fasted (or anorectic) animals. Note: Some forms of chloramphenicol are no longer available in the U.S.	30 mg/mL oral suspension (palmitate), 250 mg capsules, and 100, 250, and 500 mg tablets	Dog: 40–50 mg/kg q8h PO Cat: 12.5–20 mg/kg q12h PO
Chloramphenicol sodium succinate (Chloromycetin, generic)	Injection form of choramphenicol. Converted by liver to parent drug.	Same as for chloram-phenicol.	Injectable solution converted to chloramphenicol by hepatic metabolism	100 mg/mL injection	Dog: 40–50 mg/kg q6–8h IV, IM Cat: 12.5–20 mg/cat q12h IV, IM
Chlorothiazide (Diuril)	Thiazide diuretic. Inhibits sodium reabsorption in distal renal tubules. Used as diuretic and antihyper-tensive. Since it decreases renal excretion of calcium, it also has been used to treat calcium-containing uroliths.	Do not use in patient with elevated calcium. May cause electrolyte imbalance, such as hypokalemia	Not as effective as high-ceiling diuretics (such as furosemide).	250 and 500 mg tablets, 50 mg/mL oral suspension, and injection	20–40 mg/kg q12h PO or IV
Chlorpheniramine maleate (Chlor-Trimeton, Phenetron, and others)	Antihistamine (H₁-blocker). Blocks action of histamine on receptors. Also may have direct anti-inflammatory action. Used most often to prevent allergic reactions. Used for pruritus therapy in dogs and cats.	Sedation is most common side effect. Anti-muscarinic effects (atropine-like effects) also are common.	Chlorpheniramine is included as ingredient in many OTC cough/cold and allergy medications.	4, 8 mg tablets	Dog: 4–8 mg/dog q12h PO (up to a maximum of 0.5 mg/kg q12h) Cat: 2 mg/cat q12h PO
Chlorpromazine (Thorazine)	Phenothiazine tranquilizer/antiemetic. Inhibits action of dopamine as neuro-transmitter. Most often used as central anti-emetic. Also used for sedation and preanesthetic purposes.	Causes sedation. May lower seizure threshold and causes α-adrenergic blockade. Produces extrapyramidal side effects in some individuals.	Used for vomiting caused by toxins, drugs, or GI disease. Higher doses than listed in dose section have been used with cancer chemotherapy (2 mg/kg q3h SC).	25 mg/mL injection solution	Dog: 0.5 mg/kg q6–8h IM, SC Cat: 0.2–0.4 mg/kg q6–8h IM, SC
Chlortetracycline (generic)	Tetracycline antibacterial drug. Inhibits bacterial protein synthesis by interfering with peptide elongation by ribosome. Bacteriostatic agent with broad spectrum of activity.	Avoid use in young animals; may bind to bone and developing teeth. High doses have caused renal injury.	Broad-spectrum antibiotic. Used for routine infections and intracellular pathogens	Powdered feed additive	25 mg/kg q6–8h PO
Chorionic gonadotropin	See Gonadotropin, chorionic				

Drug Name (Trade or Other Names)	Pharmacology and Indications	Adverse Effects and Precautions	Dosing Information and Comments	Formulations	Dosage
Cimetidine (Tagamet [OTC and prescription])	Histamine-2 antagonist (H$_2$-blocker). Blocks histamine stimulation of gastric parietal cells to decrease gastric acid secretion. Used to treat ulcers and gastritis.	Adverse effects usually seen only with decreased renal clearance. In people, CNS signs may occur with high doses. *Drug interactions:* May increase concentrations of other drugs used concurrently (e.g., theophylline) because of inhibition of hepatic enzymes.	Precise doses needed to treat ulcers have not been established. Doses are derived from gastric secretory studies.	100, 200, 300, 400, 800 mg tablets; 60 mg/mL oral solution; 6 mg/mL injection	10 mg/kg q6–8h IV, IM, PO (in renal failure, administer 2.5–5 mg/kg q12h IV, PO)
Ciprofloxacin (Cipro)	Fluoroquinolone antibacterial. Acts to inhibit DNA gyrase and inhibit cell DNA and RNA synthesis. Bactericidal. Broad antimicrobial activity	Avoid use in dogs 4 weeks to 7 months of age. High concentrations may cause CNS toxicity, especially in animals with renal failure. Use cautiously in epileptic patients. Causes occasional vomiting. IV solution should be given slowly (over 30 min).	Doses are based on plasma concentrations needed to achieve sufficient plasma concentration above MIC. Efficacy studies have not been performed in dogs or cats. Ciprofloxacin is not absorbed orally as well as enrofloxacin.	250, 500, 750 mg tablets; 2 mg/mL injection	10–20 mg/kg q24h PO, IV
Cisapride	Prokinetic agent. Stimulates gastric and intestinal motility by either acetylcholine action, activity on serotonin receptors, or direct effect on smooth muscle. Used for gastric reflux, gastroparesis, ileus, constipation.	Contraindicated in patients with GI obstruction	Doses are based on extrapolation from human doses, experimental studies, and anecdotal evidence. Efficacy studies have have not been performed in dogs or cats.	No longer commercially available. However, available through compounding pharmacies	Dog: 0.1–0.5 mg/kg q8–12h PO (as high as 0.5–1.0 mg/kg) Cat: 2.5–5 mg/cat q8–12h PO (as high as 1 mg/kg q8h)
Cisplatin (Platinol)	Anticancer agent. Used for treating various solid tumors, including osteosarcoma. Action is believed to be similar to bifunctional alkylating agents and interrupts replication of DNA in tumor cells.	Nephrotoxicity is the most limiting factor to cisplatin therapy. In cats, causes a dose-related, species-specific, primary pulmonary toxicosis. Vomiting may occur in dogs with administration. Transient thrombocytopenia may occur in dogs.	To avoid toxicity, fluid loading before administration using sodium chloride should be performed. Antiemetic agents are often administered before therapy to decrease vomiting.	1 mg/mL injection	Dog: 60–70 mg/m^2 every 3–4 weeks IV (administer fluid for diuresis with therapy) Cat: Do not administer to cats
Clarithromycin (Biaxin)	Macrolide antibiotic with bacteriostatic activity. Spectrum includes primarily gram-positive bacteria. Resistance is expected for most gram-negative bacteria. Efficacy is not established for animals. Most common use in people is for treatment of *Helicobacter* gastritis, and respiratory infections.	Well tolerated in animals. Most common side side effects are vomiting, nausea, and diarrhea.	Doses are not established for animals due to lack of clinical trials. Dose recommendations are extrapolated from human or empirical use.	250, 500 mg tablets; 25 and 50 mg/mL oral suspension	7.5 mg/kg q12h PO
Clavamox	See Amoxicillin/ clavulanate potassium.				
Clavulanic acid	See Amoxicillin/ clavulanate potassium.				
Clemastine (Tavist, Contac 12 Hour Allergy, and generic)	Antihistamine (H$_1$-blocker). Blocks action of histamine on tissues. Used primarily for treatment of allergy. Some evidence suggests that clemastine is more effective than other antihistamines for pruritus in dogs.	Sedation is most common side effect.	Used for short-term treatment of pruritus in dogs. May be more efficacious when combined with other anti-inflammatory drugs. Tavist syrup contains 5.5% alcohol.	1.34 mg tablets (OTC), 2.64 mg tablets (Rx), and 0.134 mg/mL syrup	Dog: 0.05–0.1 mg/kg q12h PO

Drug Name (Trade or Other Names)	Pharmacology and Indications	Adverse Effects and Precautions	Dosing Information and Comments	Formulations	Dosage
Clindamycin (Antirobe [veterinary], Cleocin [human])	Antibacterial drug of the lincosamide class (similar in action to macrolides). Inhibits bacterial protein synthesis via inhibition of bacterial ribosome. Primarily bacteriostatic, with spectrum of activity primarily against gram-positive bacteria and anaerobes.	Generally well tolerated in dogs and cats. Oral liquid product may be unpalatable to cats. Lincomycin and clindamycin may alter bacterial population in intestine and cause diarrhea; for this reason, do not administer to rodents or rabbits.	Most doses are based on manufacturer's drug approval data and efficacy trials. See dosing column for specific guidelines for different infections.	Oral liquid 25 mg/mL; 25, 75, and 150 mg capsules, and 150 mg/mL injection (Cleocin)	Dog: 11–33 mg/kg q12h PO; for periodontal and soft tissue infection, 5.5–33 mg/kg q12h PO Cat: 11–33 mg/kg q24h PO; for skin and anaerobic infections, 11 mg/kg q12h PO; for toxoplasmosis, 12.5–25 mg/kg PO q12h.
Clofazimine (Lamprene)	Antimicrobial agent used to treat feline leprosy. Slow bactericidal effect on *Mycobacterium leprae*.	Adverse effects have not been reported in cats. In people, the most serious adverse effects are GI.	Doses based on empiricism or extrapolation of human studies	50 and 100 mg capsules	Cat: 1 mg/kg up to a maximum of 4 mg/kg/day PO
Clomipramine (Clomicalm [veterinary]; Anafranil [human])	Tricyclic antidepressant (TCA) drug. Used in people to treat anxiety and depression. Used in animals to treat variety of behavioral disorders, including obsessive-compulsive disorders and separation anxiety. Action is via inhibition of uptake of serotonin at presynaptic nerve terminals.	Reported adverse effects include sedation, reduced appetite. Other side effects associated with TCAs are antimuscarinic effects (dry mouth, rapid heart rate) and antihistamine effects (sedation). Overdoses can produce life-threatening cardiotoxicity.	When adjusting doses, one may initiate therapy with low dose and increase gradually. There may be a 2–4 week delay after initiation of therapy before beneficial effects are seen. (J Am Vet Med Assoc 213:1760–1766, 1998).	5, 20, 80 mg tablets (veterinary); 10, 25, 50 mg tablets (human)	Dog: 1–3 mg/kg/day q12h PO Cat: 1–5 mg per cat q12–24h PO
Clonazepam (Klonopin)	Benzodiazepine. Action is to enhance inhibitory effects of γ-aminobutyric acid (GABA) in CNS. Used for antiseizure action, sedation, and treatment of some behavioral disorders.	Side effects include sedation and polyphagia. Some animals may experience paradoxical excitement.	Doses are based primarily on reports from human medicine, empiricism, or experimental studies. No clinical efficacy studies have been performed in dogs or cats.	0.5, 1, and 2 mg tablets	0.5 mg/kg q8–12h PO
Clorazepate dipotassium (Tranxene)	Benzodiazepine. Action is to enhance inhibitory effects of GABA in CNS. Used for antiseizure action, sedation, and treatment of some behavioral disorders.	Side effects include sedation and polyphagia. Some animals may experience paradoxical excitement.	Doses are based primarily on reports from human medicine, empiricism, or experimental studies. No clinical efficacy studies have been performed in dogs or cats. Clorazepate tablets degrade quickly in presence of light, heat, or moisture. Keep in original packaging or in tightly sealed container.	3.75, 7.5, 11.25, 15, and 22.5 mg tablets	2 mg/kg q12h PO
Cloxacillin sodium (Cloxapen, Orbenin, Tegopen)	β-lactam antibiotic. Inhibits bacterial cell wall synthesis. Spectrum is limited to gram-positive bacteria, especially staphylococci.	Use cautiously in animals allergic to penicillin-like drugs.	Doses based on empiricism or extrapolation from human studies. No clinical efficacy studies available for dogs or cats. Oral absorption is poor; if possible, administer on empty stomach.	250, 500 mg capsules, 25 mg/mL oral solution	20–40 mg/kg q8h PO
Codeine (generic)	Opiate agonist. Mechanism is similar to morphine, except with approximately 1/10 potency of morphine. (see Morphine for other details.)	See Morphine.	Available as codeine phosphate and codeine sulfate oral tablets. Doses listed for analgesia are considered initial doses; individual patients may need higher doses, depending on degree of tolerance or pain threshold.	15, 30, 60 mg tablets, 5 mg/mL syrup, 3 mg/mL oral solution	Dog: (analgesia) 0.5–1 mg/kg q4–6h PO (antitussive) 0.1–0.3 mg/kg q4–6h PO Cat: (analgesia) 0.5 mg/kg q6h PO (antitussive) 0.1 mg/kg q6h PO

Drug Name (Trade or Other Names)	Pharmacology and Indications	Adverse Effects and Precautions	Dosing Information and Comments	Formulations	Dosage
Colchicine (generic)	Anti-inflammatory agent. Used primarily to treat gout. In animals, used to decrease fibrosis and development of hepatic failure (possibly by inhibiting formation of collagen).	Do not administer to pregnant animals. Adverse effects are not well documented in animals. Colchicine may cause dermatitis in people.	Doses based on empiricism. There are no well controlled efficacy studies in veterinary species.	500, 600 mcg tablets and 500 mcg/mL ampule injection	0.01–0.03 mg/kg q24h PO
Colony-stimulating factor (Amgen)	Stimulates granulocyte development in bone marrow. Used primarily to regenerate blood cells to recover from cancer chemotherapy or other therapy.		Doses based on limited experimental information performed in dogs. (J Am Vet Med Assoc 200:1957, 1992.)		2.5 mcg/kg q12h SC
Corticotropin (ACTH) (Acthar)	Used for diagnostic purposes to evaluate adrenal gland function. Stimulates normal synthesis of cortisol from adrenal gland.	Adverse effects unlikely when used as single injection for diagnostic purposes.	Doses established by measuring normal adrenal response in animals. See also Cosyntropin.	80 U/mL gel	Response test: Collect pre-ACTH sample and inject 2.2 IU/kg IM. Collect post-ACTH sample at 2 hr in dogs and at 1 and 2 hr in cats.
Cosyntropin (Cortrosyn)	Cosyntropin is a synthetic form of corticotropin (ACTH) used for diagnostic purposes only. In humans, it is preferred over corticotropin because it is less allergenic.	Same as for corticotropin	Same as for corticotropin. Use for diagnostic purposes only; not intended for treatment of hypoadrenocorticism.	250 mcg per vial	ACTH response test: collect pre-ACTH sample and inject 5 mcg/kg IV (dog) or 125 mcg (0.125 mg) IV (cat) and collect post sample at 30 and 60 min. Maximum dosage for dog should be 250 mcg.
Cyanocobalamin (Vitamin B$_{12}$) (many)	Vitamin B analogue	Adverse effects rare except in high over-doses.	Same as for other vitamin B preparations	100 mcg/mL injection	Dog: 100–200 mcg/day PO, SC Cat: 50–100 mcg/day PO, SC
Cyclophosphamide (Cytoxan, Neosar)	Cytotoxic agent. Bifunctional alkylating agent. Disrupts base-pairing and inhibits DNA and RNA synthesis. Cytotoxic for tumor cells and other rapidly dividing cells. Used primarily as adjunct for cancer chemotherapy and as immunosuppressive therapy	Bone marrow suppression is most common adverse effect. Can produce severe neutropenia (that usually is reversible). Vomiting and diarrhea may occur in some patients. Dogs are susceptible to bladder toxicity (sterile hemorrhagic cystitis). May cause hair loss when used in some chemotherapeutic protocols	Cyclophosphamide is usually administered with other drugs (other cancer drugs in cancer protocols or corticosteroids) when used for immunosuppressive therapy. Consult specific anticancer protocols for specific regimens.	25 mg/mL injection; 25, 50 mg tablet.	Anticancer: 50 mg/m^2 once daily 4 days/week PO, or 150–300 mg/m^2 IV, and repeat in 21 days Immunosuppressive therapy: 50 mg/m^2 (approx. 2.2 mg/kg) q48h PO, or 2.2 mg/kg once daily for 4 days/week Cat: 6.25–12.5 mg/cat once daily 4 days/week
Cyclosporine (Neoral, Sandimmune, Optimmune [ophthalmic]. Other name for cyclosporine is cyclosporin A)	Immunosuppressive drug. Suppresses induction of T cell lymphocytes.	Can cause vomiting, diarrhea, anorexia. Nephrotoxicity may occur. In comparison to other immunosuppressive drugs, does not cause myelosuppression. Drug interactions: Cimetidine, erythromycin, or ketoconazole may increase cyclosporine concentrations when used concurrently.	Adjust dose via monitoring if possible. Suggested trough blood concentration range (whole blood assay) is 300–400 ng/mL. Neoral oral products are absorbed more predictably than Sandimmune. Neoral may produce 50% higher blood concentrations in some patients. Oral solution can be diluted to make it more palatable. Topical cyclosporine has been used successfully as treatment for keratoconjunctivitis sicca.	Neoral: 25 and 100 mg microemulsion capsules; 100 mg/mL oral solution (for microemulsion) Sandimmune: 100 mg/mL oral solution; 25, 100 mg capsules Optimmune: 0.2% ointment	Dog: 3–7 mg/kg/day PO. Dose for atopic dermatitis may be changed to 5 mg/kg q48h in some patients. Cat: 3–5 mg/kg/day PO
Cyproheptadine hydrochloride (Periactin)	Phenothiazine with antihistamine and anti-serotonin properties. Used as appetite stimulant (probably by altering serotonin activity in appetite center)	May cause increased appetite and weight gain	Clinical studies have not been performed in veterinary medicine. Use is based primarily on empiricism and extrapolation from human results. Syrup contains 5% alcohol.	4 mg tablet; 2 mg/5 mL syrup	Antihistamine: 0.5–1.1 mg/kg q8–12h PO Appetite stimulant: 2 mg/cat PO Feline asthma: 1–2 mg/cat q12h PO

Drug Name (Trade or Other Names)	Pharmacology and Indications	Adverse Effects and Precautions	Dosing Information and Comments	Formulations	Dosage
Cytarabine (cytosine arabinoside) (Cytosar)	Anticancer agent. Exact mechanism is not known. Probably inhibits DNA synthesis. Used for lymphoma and leukemia protocols.	Bone marrow suppression. Causes vomiting and nausea	Consult anticancer protocols for precise dosing regimens.	100 mg vial	Dog (lymphoma): 100 mg/m^2 once daily, or 50 mg/m^2 twice daily for 4 days IV, SC Cat: 100 mg/m^2 once daily for 2 days
Dacarbazine (DTIC)	Anticancer agent. Monofunctional alkylating agent. Used for melanoma.	Leukopenia, nausea, vomiting, diarrhea. Do not use in cats.	Consult anticancer protocol for specific regimens.	200 mg vial for injection	Dog: 200 mg/m^2 for 5 days every 3 weeks IV; or 800–1000 mg/m^2 every 3 weeks IV
Dalteparin sodium (Fragmin)	Low molecular weight heparin (LMWH); anticoagulant; indicated for prevention of thromboembolism in at-risk patients. It has been used in cats with left atrial enlargement secondary to cardiomyopathy or prior embolism. Anti-Xa: anti-IIa ratio: 2.7	Better tolerated than unfractionated (conventional) heparin. Bleeding may be a problem.	No need to monitor clotting times as with conventional (unfractionated) heparin when dalteparin is used at recommended dosages	16 mg (2500 U)/0.2 mL; 32 mg (5000 U)/0.2 mL prefilled syringes for injection; 64 mg (10,000) U/mL multidose vials for injection	Dog: 70 U/kg q24h SC. Cat: 100 U/kg q24h SC (can increase to q12h) for high-risk patients. Lower doses of 50 U/kg q24 SC can be used in low-risk patients.
Danazol (Danocrine)	Gonadotropin inhibitor. Suppresses luteinizing hormone (LH) and follicle-stimulating hormone (FSH) (and estrogen synthesis. In humans, used for endometriosis. May reduce destruction of platelets or RBC in immune-mediated disease.	May cause signs similar to other androgenic drugs. Adverse effects have not been reported in animals. Gonadotropin inhibitor.	When used to treat autoimmune disease, usually used in conjunction with other drugs (e.g., corticosteroids).	50, 100, 200 mg capsules	5–10 mg/kg q12h PO
Dantrolene sodium (Dantrium)	Muscle relaxant. Inhibits calcium leakage from sarcoplasmic reticulum. In addition to muscle relaxation, it has been used for malignant hyperthermia. Also has been used to relax urethral muscle in cats.	Muscle relaxants can cause weakness in some animals.	Doses have been primarily extrapolated from experimental studies or extrapolation of human studies. No clinical trials available in veterinary medicine. Studies in which dantrolene relaxed urethra in cats used 1 mg/kg IV.	100 mg capsule and 0.33 mg/mL injection	For prevention of malignant hyperthermia: 2–3 mg/kg IV For muscle relaxation: dog: 1–5 mg/kg q8h PO; cat: 0.5–2 mg/kg q12h PO
Dapsone (generic)	Antimicrobial drug used primarily for treatment of mycobacterium. May have some immunosuppressive properties or inhibit function of inflammatory cells. Used primarily for dermatologic diseases in dogs and cats.	Hepatitis and blood dyscrasias may occur. Toxic dermatologic reactions have been seen in people. *Drug interactions:* Do not administer with trimethoprim (may increase blood concentrations).	Doses are derived from extrapolation of human doses or empiricism. No well-controlled clinical studies have been performed in veterinary medicine.	25 and 100 mg tablets	1.1 mg/kg q8–12h PO
Deferoxamine mesylate (Desferal)	Chelating agent with strong affinity for trivalent cations. Used to treat acute iron toxicosis. Indicated in cases of severe poisoning. Deferoxamine also has been used to chelate aluminum and facilitate removal.	Adverse effects have not been reported in animals. Allergic reactions and hearing problems have occurred in people.	100 mg of deferoxamine binds 8.5 mg of ferric iron. Monitor serum iron concentrations to determine severity of intoxication and success of therapy. Contact local poison control center for guidance. Successful therapy is indicated by monitoring urine color (orange-rose color change to urine indicates chelated iron is being eliminated).	500 mg vial for injection	10 mg/kg IV, IM q2h for 2 doses, then 10 mg/kg q8h for 24 hr
Deprenyl (L-deprenyl)	See Selegiline.				

Drug Name (Trade or Other Names)	Pharmacology and Indications	Adverse Effects and Precautions	Dosing Information and Comments	Formulations	Dosage
Deracoxib (Deramaxx)	NSAID of the coxib class; high COX-1:COX-2 in vitro inhibitory ratio. Indicated for the control of postoperative pain and inflammation associated with orthopedic surgery and pain and inflammation associated with osteoarthritis.	Most common adverse effect from clinical trials has been GI (vomiting and diarrhea). In safety studies at doses above 25 kg/mg, reduced body weight, melena, and vomiting occurred.	Recommended doses are for dogs weighing > 1.8 kg (4 lb). Safety has not been established for dogs under 4 months of age, dogs used for breeding, pregnant or lactating dogs, or for cats.	25, 100 mg tablets; chewable tablets	Dog (postoperative pain): 3.0–4.0 mg/kg q24h PO as needed for 7 days Dog (osteoarthritis): 1–2 mg/kg PO q24h for long-term treatment over 7 days Cat: safe dose not established
DES	See Diethylistilbestrol.				
Desmopressin acetate (DDAVP)	Synthetic peptide similar to antidiuretic hormone (ADH). Used as replacement therapy for patients with diabetes insipidus. Desmopressin also has been used for treatment of patients with mild to moderate von Willebrand's disease prior to surgery or other procedure that may cause bleeding.	No side effects reported. In people, it rarely has caused thrombotic events.	Desmopressin is used only for central diabetes insipidus. Duration of effect is variable (8–20 hr). It is ineffective for treatment of nephrogenic diabetes insipidus or polyuria from other causes. Intranasal product has been administered as eye drops in dogs. Onset of effect is within 1 hr. (J Am Vet Med Assoc 205:170, 1994; J Am Vet Med Assoc 209:1884, 1996). Oral tablets are available for humans.	4 and 15 mcg/mL injection and desmopressin acetate nasal solution 100 mcg/mL (0.01%) metered spray. Tablets 0.1 and 0.2 mg.	Diabetes insipidus: 2–4 drops (2 mcg) q12–24h intranasally or in eye. 0.05–0.1 mg q12h PO as needed von Willebrand's disease treatment: 1 mcg/kg (0.01 mL/kg) SC, IV, diluted in 20 mL of saline administered over 10 min
Desoxycorticosterone pivalate (Percorten-V, DOCP, or DOCA pivalate)	Mineralocorticoid. Used for adrenocortico-insufficiency (hypoadrenocorticism). No glucocorticoid activity.	Excessive mineralocorticoid effects with high doses.	Initial dose based on studies performed in clinical patients. Individual doses may be based on monitoring electrolytes in patients. Actual interval between doses may range from 14–35 days. (J Vet Intern Med 11: 43–49, 1997.)	Injection	1.5–2.2 mg/kg every 25 days IM
Detomidine (Dormosedan)	α_2-adrenergic agonist. More potent and more specific than xylazine. Used primarily for anesthesia and analgesia.	Potent α_2-agonist. Produces sedation and ataxia. Cardiac depression, heart block, and hypotension possible with high doses.	Doses not established for small animals; used primarily for horses	10 mg/mL injection	Doses not established for small animals
Dexamethasone (Dexamethasone solution and dexamethasone sodium phosphate) (Azium solution in polyethylene glycol. Sodium phosphate forms include: Decaject SP, Dexavet, and Dexasone. Tablets include Decadron and generic)	Corticosteroid. Dexamethasone has approximately 30× potency of cortisol. Multiple anti-inflammatory effects (see Betamethasone).	Multiple side effects. (See Betamethasone.)	Doses based on severity of underlying disease (see Betamethasone). Dexamethasone is used for testing hyperadrenocorticism. Low-dose dexamethasone suppression test: dogs 0.01 mg/kg IV, cats 0.1 mg/kg IV, and collect sample at 0, 4, and 8 hours. For high-dose dexamethasone suppression test: dogs 0.1 mg/kg, cats 1.0 mg/kg.	Azium solution, 2 mg/mL. Sodium phosphate forms are 3.33 mg/mL. 0.25, 0.5, 0.75, 1, 1.5, 2, 4, 6 mg tablets.	Anti-inflammatory: 0.07–0.15 mg/kg q12–24h IV, IM, PO For shock, spinal injury: 2.2–4.4 mg/kg IV (of sodium phosphate form)
Dextran (Dextran 70, Gentran 70)	Synthetic colloid used for volume expansion. High molecular weight fluid replacement. Primarily used for acute hypovolemia and shock	Only limited use in veterinary medicine, and adverse effects have not been reported. In people, coagulopathies are possible because of decreased platelet function. Anaphylactic shock also has occurred.	Used primarily in critical care situations. Delivered via constant rate infusion slowly. Monitor patient's cardiopulmonary status carefully during administration.	Injectable solution 250, 500, 1000 mL	10–20 mL/kg IV to effect

Drug Name (Trade or Other Names)	Pharmacology and Indications	Adverse Effects and Precautions	Dosing Information and Comments	Formulations	Dosage
Dextromethorphan (Benylin and others)	Centrally acting anti-tussive drug. Shares similar chemical structure as opiates, but does not affect opiate receptors. Appears to directly affect cough receptor.	Adverse effects not reported in veterinary medicine. High over-dose may cause sedation.	Many OTC preparations that may contain other ingredients (e.g., anti-histamines, decongestants, and acetaminophen)	Available in syrup, capsule, and tablet. Many OTC products	0.5–2 mg/kg q6–8h PO
Dextrose solution 5% (D-5-W)	Sugar added to fluid solutions. Isotonic	High doses produce pulmonary edema.	Commonly used fluid solution administered via constant rate infusion. *Not* a maintenance solution	Fluid solution for IV administration	40–50 mL/kg q24h IV
Diazepam (Valium and generic)	Benzodiazepine. Central-acting CNS depressant. Mechanism of action appears to be via potentiation of GABA-receptor mediated effects in CNS. Used for sedation, anesthetic adjunct, anticonvulsant, and behavioral disorders. Diazepam metabolized to desmethyldiazepam (nordiazepam) and oxazepam.	Sedation is most common side effect. May cause paradoxical excitement in dogs. Causes polyphagia. In cats, idiopathic fatal hepatic necrosis has been reported.	Clearance in dogs is many times faster than in people (half-life in dogs less than 1 hr) requires frequent administration. For treatment of status epilepticus, may be administered IV or rectally. Avoid administration IM.	2, 5 mg tablets; 5 mg/mL solution for injection	Preanesthetic: 0.5 mg/kg IV Status epilepticus: 0.5 mg/kg IV, 1 mg/kg rectal; repeat if necessary Appetite stimulant (cat): 0.2 mg/kg IV For behavior treatment in cats: 1–4 mg per cat q12–24 hr PO
Dichlorphenamide (Daranide)	Carbonic anhydrase inhibitor. Diuretic. Acts to inhibit enzyme that forms hydrogen and bicarbonate ions. Reduces plasma bicarbonate concentration, producing systemic metabolic acidosis and alkaline diuresis. Primarily used to treat glaucoma.	Sulfonamide derivative. Use cautiously in animals sensitive to sulfonamides. Hypokalemia may occur in some patients. Severe metabolic acidosis is rare.	Dichlorphenamide is not used as diuretic, but is most commonly employed to treat glaucoma. May be combined with other antiglaucoma agents	50 mg tablets	3–5 mg/kg q8–12h PO
Dichlorvos (Task)	Antiparasitic drug, used primarily to treat hookworms, roundworms, whipworms. Kills parasites by anticholinesterase action.	Do not use in heartworm-positive patients. Overdoses can cause organophosphate intoxication. (Treat with 2-PAM, atropine).	Doses based on manufacturer's recommendations	10, 25 mg tablets	Dog: 26.4–33 mg/kg PO Cat: 11 mg/kg PO
Dicloxacillin sodium (Dynapen)	β-lactam, antibiotic. Inhibits bacterial cell wall synthesis. Spectrum is limited to gram-positive bacteria, especially staphylococci.	Use cautiously in animals allergic to penicillin-like drugs.	No clinical efficacy studies available for dogs or cats. In dogs, oral absorption is very low and may not be suitable for therapy (J Vet Pharmacol Ther 21:414–417, 1998). Administer, if possible, on empty stomach.	125, 250, 500 mg capsules, 12.5 mg/mL oral suspension	11–55 mg/kg q8h PO
Diethylcarbamazine (DEC) (Caricide, Filaribits)	Heartworm preventative. For action, see Piperazine.	Safe in all species. Reactions can occur in animals with positive microfilaria.	Doses based on manufacturer's recommendations. Specific protocols for heartworm administration may be based on region of country.	50, 60, 180, 200, 400 mg chewable tablets	Heartworm prophylaxis: 6.6 mg/kg q24h PO
Diethylstilbestrol (DES)	Synthetic estrogen compound. Used for estrogen replacement in animals. DES is most commonly used to treat estrogen-responsive incontinence in dogs. Also has been used to induce abortion in dogs	Side effects may occur that are caused by excess estrogen. Estrogen therapy may increase risk of pyometra and estrogen-sensitive tumors.	Doses listed are for treating urinary incontinence and vary depending on response. Titrate dose to individual patients. Although used to induce abortion, it was *not* efficacious in one study that administered 75 mcg/kg.	1, 5 mg tablets; 50 mg/mL injection (no longer manufactured in U.S., but available from compounding pharmacist)	Dog: 0.1–1.0 mg/dog q24h PO Cat: 0.05–0.1 mg/cat q24h PO

Drug Name (Trade or Other Names)	Pharmacology and Indications	Adverse Effects and Precautions	Dosing Information and Comments	Formulations	Dosage
Difloxacin hydrochloride (Dicural)	Fluoroquinolone antibacterial drug. Acts via inhibition of DNA gyrase in bacteria to inhibit DNA and RNA synthesis. Bactericidal with broad spectrum of activity. Used for variety of infections, including skin infections, wound infections, and pneumonia	Adverse effects include seizures in epileptic animals, arthropathy in young animals, vomiting at high doses. *Drug interactions:* May increase concentrations of theophylline if used concurrently. Coadministration with di- and trivalent cations (e.g., sucralfate) may decrease absorption. Ocular safety not established in cats	Dose range can be used to adjust dose, depending on severity of infection and susceptibility of bacteria. Bacteria with low MIC can be treated with low dose; susceptible bacteria with higher MIC should be treated with higher dose. Difloxacin is primarily eliminated in feces rather than urine (urine is < 5% of clearance). Sarafloxacin is an active desmethyl metabolite.	11.4, 45.4, and 136 mg tablets	Dog: 5–10 mg/kg q24h PO (see dosing information guidelines)
Digitoxin (Crystodigin [no longer available from some distributors])	Cardiac ionotropic agent. Increases cardiac contractility and decreases heart rate. Mechanism is via inactivation of cardiac muscle sodium-potassium ATPase. Beneficial effects for heart failure may occur via neuroendocrine effects (alters sensitivity of baroreceptors).	Digitalis glycosides have narrow therapeutic index. May cause variety of arrhythmias in patients (e.g., heart block, ventricular tachycardia). Causes vomiting, anorexia, diarrhea. Adverse effects are potentiated by hypokalemia, reduced by hyperkalemia.	Used in heart failure for ionotropic effect and to decrease heart rate. Used in supraventricular arrhythmias to decrease ventricular response to atrial stimulation. May be used with other cardiac drugs. Monitor concentrations in patients to determine optimum therapy.	0.05, 0.1 mg tablets	0.02–0.03 mg/kg q8h PO
Digoxin (Lanoxin, Cardoxin)	Cardiac ionotropic agent. Increases cardiac contractility and decreases heart rate. Mechanism is via inactivation of cardiac muscle sodium-potassium ATPase. Beneficial effects for heart failure may occur via neuroendocrine effects (alters sensitivity of baroreceptors). Used in heart failure for ionotropic effect and to decrease heart rate. Used in supraventricular arrhythmias to decrease ventricular response to atrial stimulation.	Digitalis glycosides have narrow therapeutic index. May cause variety of arrhythmias in patients (e.g., heart block, ventricular tachycardia). Causes vomiting, anorexia, diarrhea. Adverse effects potentiated by hypokalemia, reduced by hyperkalemia. Some breeds of dogs (Doberman pinschers) and cats are more sensitive to adverse effects.	Monitor patients carefully. Optimum plasma concentration is 1–2 ng/mL. Adverse effects common at concentration above 3.5 ng/mL. When dosing, calculate dose on lean body weight. Doses should be 10% less for elixir because of increased absorption.	0.0625, 0.125, 0.25 mg tablets; 0.05 mg/mL elixir	Dog: < 20 kg body weight: 0.01 mg/kg q12h; > 20 kg use 0.22 mg/m² q12h PO (subtract 10% for elixir) Dog (rapid digitalization): 0.0055–0.011 mg/kg q1h IV to effect Cat: 0.08–0.01 mg/kg q48h PO (approximately 1/4 of a 0.125 mg tablet/cat)
Dihydrotachysterol (DHT, vitamin D) (Hytakerol)	Vitamin D analogue. Used for treatment of hypocalcemia, especially hypoparathyroidism associated with thyroidectomy. Vitamin D promotes absorption and utilization of calcium.	Overdose may cause hypercalcemia. Avoid use in pregnant animals because it may cause fetal abnormalities. Use cautiously with high doses of calcium-containing preparations.	Available as oral solution, tablets, and capsules. Doses for individual patients should be adjusted by monitoring serum calcium concentrations.	0.125 mg tablets; 0.5 mg/mL oral liquid	0.01 mg/kg/day PO; for acute treatment, administer 0.02 mg/kg initially, then 0.01–0.02 mg/kg q24–48h PO thereafter
Diltiazem (Cardizem, Dilacor)	Calcium channel–blocking drug. Blocks calcium entry into cells via blockade of slow channel. Produces vasodilation, negative chronotropic effects. Used for supraventricular arrhythmias in dogs; hypertrophic cardiomyopathy in cats	Hypotension, cardiac depression, bradycardia, AV block. May cause anorexia in some patients	Consider higher dose of 5 mg/kg in dogs. Experimental work showed that when doses of 2.5 and 5 mg/kg were compared in dogs, only the higher dose of 5 mg/kg produced effective results (J Vet Int Med 7(6):358–367, 2001)	30, 60, 90, 120 mg tablets. 5 mg/mL injection. Extended release capsules are 60, 90, 120, 180, 240, 300 mg.	Dog: 0.5–1.5 mg/kg q8h PO, 0.25 mg/kg over 2 min IV (repeat if necessary) Cat: 1.75–2.4 mg/kg q8h PO For Dilacor XR or Cardizem CD, dose is 10 mg/kg once daily PO. Dilacor capsules contain 60-mg tablets for dosing cats.

Drug Name (Trade or Other Names)	Pharmacology and Indications	Adverse Effects and Precautions	Dosing Information and Comments	Formulations	Dosage
Dimenhydrinate (Dramamine, [Gravol in Canada])	Antihistamine drug. Converted to active diphenhydramine. (See Chlorpheniramine.)	See Chlorpheniramine.	See Chlorpheniramine. There have been no clinical studies on the use of dimenhydrinate. It is primarily used empirically for treatment of vomiting.	50 mg tablets and 50 mg/mL injection	Dog: 4–8 mg/kg q8h PO, IM, IV Cat: 12.5 mg/cat q8h IV, IM, PO
Dimercaprol (BAL) (BAL in Oil)	Chelating agent. Used to treat lead, gold, arsenic toxicity.	Adverse effects not reported in veterinary medicine. In people, sterile absesses occur at injection site. High doses have caused seizures, drowsiness, and vomiting.	Use as soon as possible after intoxicant exposure. Alkalinization of urine will increase toxin removal. For lead intoxication, may be used with edetate calcium.	Injection	4 mg/kg q4h IM
Dinoprost tromethamine	See Prostaglandin F$_{2\alpha}$				
Dioctyl calcium sulfosuccinate	See Docusate calcium.				
Dioctyl sodium sulfosuccinate	See Docusate sodium.				
Diphenhydramine hydrochloride (Benadryl)	Antihistamine (see Chlorpheniramine)	See Chlorpheniramine.	Antihistamine used primarily for allergic disease in animals.	Available OTC; 2.5 mg/mL elixir; 25, 50 mg capsules and tablets; 50 mg/mL injection	Dog: 25–50 mg/dog q8h IV, IM, PO Cat: 2–4 mg/kg q6–8h PO or 1 mg/kg IM, IV.
Diphenoxylate (Lomotil)	Opiate agonist. Stimulates smooth muscle segmentation in intestine, as well as electrolyte absorption. Used for acute treatment of nonspecific diarrhea.	Adverse effects have not been reported in veterinary medicine. Diphenoxylate is poorly absorbed systemically and produces few systemic side effects. Excessive use can cause constipation.	Doses are based primarily on empiricism or extrapolation of human dose. Clinical studies have not been performed in animals. Contains atropine, but dose is not high enough for significant systemic effects.	2.5 mg tablets	Dog: 0.1–0.2 mg/kg q8–12h PO Cat: 0.05–0.1 mg/kg q12h PO
Diphenylhydantoin	See Phenytoin.				
Diphosphonate disodium etidronate	See Etidronate disodium.				
Dipyridamole (Persantine)	Platelet inhibitor. Mechanism of action is attributed to increased levels of cyclic adenosine monophosphate (cAMP) in platelet, which decreases platelet activation. Indicated to prevent thromboembolism	Adverse effects have not been reported in animals.	Used primarily in people to prevent thromboembolism. Use in animals has not been reported. When used in people, it is combined with other antithrombotic agents (e.g., warfarin).	25, 50, 75 mg tablets; 5 mg/mL injection	4–10 mg/kg q24h PO
Dipyrone	Antipyretic. No longer available commercially. (Previous use in animals was at 28 mg/kg q8h IV, IM, SC.)				
Disopyramide (Norpace [Rythmodan in Canada])	Antiarrhythmic agent of Class I. Depresses myocardial electrophysiologic conduction rate	Adverse effects have not been reported in animals. High doses may cause cardiac arrhythmias.	Not commonly used in veterinary medicine. Other antiarrhythmic drugs are preferred.	100, 150 mg capsules (10 mg/mL injection in Canada only)	Dog: 6–15 mg/kg q8h PO
Dithiazanine iodide (generic)	Microfilaricidal drug for dogs. Also effective for hookworms, roundworms, and whipworms	Adverse effects are rare. Causes vomiting in some dogs. Causes discoloration of feces	Before ivermectin and similar drugs, this was the only microfilaricidal agent for dogs. Not commonly used and may not be commercially available anymore	10, 50, 100, 200 mg tablets	Dog: (heartworm) 6.6–11 mg/kg q24h PO for 7–10 days (other parasites) 22 mg/kg PO

Drug Name (Trade or Other Names)	Pharmacology and Indications	Adverse Effects and Precautions	Dosing Information and Comments	Formulations	Dosage
Dobutamine hydrochloride (Dobutrex)	Adrenergic agonist. Action is primarily to stimulate myocardium via action on cardiac β_1-receptors. Increases heart contraction without increase in heart rate. Some action may occur via α-receptors. Primarily used for acute treatment of heart failure	May cause tachycardia and ventricular arrhythmias at high doses or in sensitive individuals.	Dobutamine has a very rapid elimination half-life (minutes) and therefore must be administered via carefully monitored constant rate infusion. When mixing, avoid alkalinizing solutions. Usually dilute in 5% dextrose solution (e.g., 250 mg in 1 L 5% dextrose).	250 mg/20 mL vial for injection (12.5 mg/mL)	Dog: 5–20 mcg/kg/min IV infusion Cat: 0.5–2 mcg/kg/min IV infusion
Docusate calcium (Surfak, Doxidan)	Stool softener (surfactant). Acts to decrease surface tension to allow more water to accumulate in the stool	No adverse effects reported in animals. In people, high doses have caused abdominal discomfort.	Doses are based on extrapolations from humans or empiricism. No clinical studies reported for animals. Docusate calcium products may contain stimulant cathartic phenolphthalein, which should be used cautiously in cats.	60 mg tablets (and many others)	Dog: 50–100 mg/dog q12–24h PO Cat: 50 mg/cat q12–24h PO
Docusate sodium (Colace, Doxan, Doss; many OTC brands)	See Docusate calcium.	See Docusate calcium.	See Docusate calcium.	50, 100 mg capsules; 10 mg/mL liquid	Dog: 50–200 mg/dog q8–12h PO Cat: 50 mg/cat q12–24h PO
Domperidone (Motilium)	Motility modifier (similar to metoclopramide)	See Metoclopramide.	Not available in U.S., only in Canada	Not available in U.S.	2–5 mg/animal PO, q8–12h has been used
Dopamine hydrochloride (Intropin)	Adrenergic agonist. Action is primarily to stimulate myocardium via action on cardiac β_1-receptors. There is some suggestion that dopamine increases renal perfusion via action on renal dopaminergic receptors; however, clinical evidence for beneficial effect is lacking.	May cause tachycardia and ventricular arrhythmias at high doses or in sensitive individuals	Dopamine has a very rapid elimination half-life (minutes) and therefore must be administered via carefully monitored constant rate infusion. When mixing, avoid alkalinizing solutions. Administer in 5% dextrose solution or lactated Ringer's solution. Mix 200–400 mg in 250 to 500 mL of fluid.	40, 80, or 160 mg/mL	2–10 mcg/kg/min IV infusion
Doxapram hydrochloride (Dopram)	Respiratory stimulant via action on carotid chemoreceptors and subsequent stimulation of respiratory center. Used to treat respiratory depression or to stimulate respiration post anesthesia. May also increase cardiac output.	Adverse effects not reported in animals. Cardiovascular effects and convulsions have occurred with high doses in people. Contraindicated in newborn humans because it contains benzyl alcohol as vehicle	Used for short-term treatment only. No longer available from manufacturer.	20 mg/mL injection	5–10 mg/kg IV; neonate: 1–5 mg SC, sublingual, or via umbilical vein
Doxorubicin (Adriamycin)	Anticancer agent. Acts to intercalate between bases on DNA, disrupting DNA and RNA synthesis in tumor cell. Doxorubicin also may affect tumor cell membranes. Used for treatment of various neoplasias, including lymphoma	Most common acute effects are anorexia, vomiting, and diarrhea. Dose-related toxicity also includes bone marrow suppression, hair loss (in certain breeds), and cardiotoxicity. Cardiotoxicity limits the total dose administered (usually not to exceed 200 mg/m^2).	Regimen listed may differ for various tumors. Consult specific anticancer protocol for guidelines. Dose must be infused IV (over 20–30 min). Animals may require antiemetic and antihistamine (diphenhydramine) prior to therapy. Monitor ECG during therapy. Dose according to body weight may be more effective for small dogs.	2 mg/mL injection	Dog: 30 mg/m^2 IV every 21 days, or: > 20 kg, use 30 mg/m^2 and < 20 kg, use 1 mg/kg. Cat: 1 mg/kg IV every 3 weeks

Drug Name (Trade or Other Names)	Pharmacology and Indications	Adverse Effects and Precautions	Dosing Information and Comments	Formulations	Dosage
Doxycycline (Vibramycin and generic forms)	Tetracycline antibiotic. Mechanism of action of tetracyclines is to bind to 30S ribosomal subunit and inhibit protein synthesis. Usually bacteriostatic. Broad spectrum of activity including bacteria, some protozoa, *Rickettsia, Ehrlichia*	Severe adverse reactions not reported with doxycycline. Tetracyclines in general may cause renal tubular necrosis at high doses. Tetracyclines can affect bone and teeth formation in young animals. *Drug interactions:* Tetracyclines bind to calcium-containing compounds, which decreases oral absorption.	Many pharmacokinetic and experimental studies have been conducted in small animals, but no clinical studies. Ordinarily considered the drug of choice for *Rickettsia* and *Ehrlichia* infections in dogs. Doxycycline IV infusion is stable for only 12 hr at room temperature and 72 hr if refrigerated.	10 mg/mL oral suspension; 100 mg tablets; 100 mg injection vial	3–5 mg/kg q12h PO IV or 10 mg/kg q24h PO For *Rickettsia* in dogs: 5 mg/kg q12h
Edetate calcium disodium (CaNa$_2$ EDTA, Calcium Disodium Versenate)	Chelating agent. Indicated for treatment of acute and chronic lead poisoning. Sometimes used in combination with dimercaprol	No adverse effects reported in animals. In people, allergic reactions (release of histamine) occur after IV administration	May be used with dimercaprol. Equally effective when administered IV or IM, but IM injection may be painful. Ensure adequate urine flow before the first dose.	20 mg/mL injection	25 mg/kg q6h SC, IM, IV for 2–5 days
Edrophonium (Tensilon and others)	Cholinesterase inhibitor. Causes cholinergic effects by inhibiting metabolism of acetylcholine. Very short acting and ordinarily is only used for diagnostic purposes (e.g., for myasthenia gravis). Also has been used to reverse neuromuscular blockade of nondepolarizing agents (pancuronium)	Short acting, so side effects are minimal. Excessive muscarinic/cholinergic effects may occur with high doses (counteract with atropine).	Usually used only for determination of diagnosis of myasthenia gravis in patients. Too short acting to be used for therapy.	10 mg/mL injection	Dog: 0.11–0.22 mg/kg IV Cat: 2.5 mg/cat IV
Enalapril maleate (Enacard, Vasotec)	ACE inhibitor (see Captopril for details). Used for vasodilation and treatment of heart failure. Primarily used in dogs, but may benefit some cats in heart failure.	(See Captopril.) May cause azotemia in some patients; carefully monitor patients receiving high doses of diuretics. *Drug interactions:* Use cautiously with other hypotensive drugs and diuretics. NSAIDs may decrease vasodilating effects.	Doses are based on clinical trials conducted in dogs by manufacturer. For dogs, start with once-daily administration and increase to q12h if needed. Other drugs used for treatment of heart failure may be used concurrently. With all ACE inhibitors, monitor electrolytes and renal function 3–7 days after initiating therapy and periodically thereafter.	2.5, 5, 10, 20 mg tablets	Dog: 0.5 mg/kg q12–24h PO Cat: 0.25–0.5 mg/kg q12–24h PO, or 1.0–1.25 mg/cat/day
Enflurane (Ethrane)	Inhalent anesthetic	Adverse effects (not related to anesthesia) not reported in animals	Titrate dose for each individual with anesthetic monitoring.	Available as solution for inhalation	Induction: 2%–3%; Maintenance: 1.5%–3%
Enilconazole (Imaverol, Clinafarm EC)	Azole antifungal agent for topical use only. Like other azoles, inhibits membrane synthesis (ergosterol) in fungus. Highly effective for dermatophytes	Administered topically. Adverse effects have not been reported.	Imaverol is available only in Canada as 10% emulsion. In the U.S., Clinafarm EC is available for use in poultry units as 13.8% solution. Dilute solution to at least 50:1, and apply topically every 3–4 days for 2–3 weeks. Enilconazole also has been instilled as 1:1 dilution into nasal sinus for nasal aspergillosis.	10% or 13.8% emulsion	Nasal aspergillosis: 10 mg/kg q12h instilled into nasal sinus for 14 days (10% solution diluted 50/50 with water) Dermatophytes: dilute 10% solution to 0.2%, and wash lesion with solution 4 times at 3–4 day intervals.

Drug Name (Trade or Other Names)	Pharmacology and Indications	Adverse Effects and Precautions	Dosing Information and Comments	Formulations	Dosage
Enoxaparin (Lovenox)	LMWH; anticoagulant; indicated for prevention of thromboembolism in at-risk patients. It has been used in cats with left atrial enlargement secondary to cardiomy-opathy or prior to embolism. Anti-Xa: anti-IIa ratio: 3.8	Bleeding may be a problem.	No need to monitor clotting times as with conventional (unfractio-nated) heparin when enoxaparin is used at recommended dosages. Better tolerated than unfractionated (conventional) heparin.	30 mg/0.3 mL, 40 mg/ 0.4 mL, 60 mg/0.6 mL, 80 mg/0.8 mL, and 100 mg/1 mL prefilled syringes for injection	1 mg/kg q12–24h SC
Enrofloxacin (Baytril)	Fluoroquinolone anti-bacterial drug. Acts via inhibition of DNA gyrase in bacteria to inhibit DNA and RNA synthesis. Bactericidal. Broad spectrum of activity	Adverse effects include seizures in epileptic animals, arthropathy in dogs 4–28 weeks of age, vomiting in dogs and cats at high doses. Blindness in cats has been reported. *Drug interactions:* May increase concentrations of theophylline if used concurrently. Coadmin-istration with di- and trivalent cations (e.g., sucralfate) may decrease absorption.	In dogs, low dose of 5 mg/kg/ day is used for sensitive organisms with MIC of 0.12 mcg/mL or less, or urinary tract infection; dose of 5–10 mg/kg/day is used for organisms with MIC of 0.12–0.5 mcg/mL; dose of 10–20 mg/kg/day is used for organisms with MIC of 0.5–1.0 mcg/mL. Solution is not approved for IV use but has been administered via this route safely if given slowly.	68 and 22.7 mg tablets. Taste Tabs are 22.7, 68, and 136 mg. 22.7 mg/mL injection. Otic formulation containing enrofloxacin/silver sulfadiazine.	Dog: 5–20 mg/kg/ q24h PO, IV, IM (see dosing information guidelines) Cat: 5 mg/kg q24h PO, IM Do not administer to cats at doses higher than 5 mg/kg and do not administer to cats IV.
Ephedrine (many, generic)	Adrenergic agonist. Agonist on α- and β₁-adrenergic receptors but not β₂-receptors. Used as vasopressor, e.g., administered during anesthesia. CNS stimu-lant. Also has been used to treat urinary inconti-nence because of action on bladder sphincter muscle	Adverse effects related to excessive adrenergic activity (e.g., peripheral vasoconstriction and tachycardia)	Used primarily in acute situations to increase blood pressure and urinary incontinence in dogs	25, 50 mg/mL injection	Urinary Incontinence: 4 mg/kg, or 12.5–50 mg/dog q8–12h PO (2–4 mg/kg for cats) Vasopressor: 0.75 mg/kg IM, SC, repeat as needed
Epinephrine hydrochloride (Adrenalin Chloride and generic forms)	Adrenergic agonist. Nonselectively stimu-lates α- and β₂-adrener-gic receptors. Used primarily for emergency situations to treat cardiopulmonary arrest and anaphylactic shock	Overdose will cause excessive vasocon-striction and hyper-tension. High doses can cause ventricular arrhythmias. When high doses are used for cardiopulmonary arrest, an electrical defibrillator should be available.	Doses are based on experimental studies, primarily in dogs. Clinical studies are not available. IV doses are ordinarily used, but endotracheal admini-stration is acceptable when IV access is not available. Intraosseous route also has been used, and doses are equivalent to IV. When endotracheal route is used, the dose is higher and duration of effect may be longer than with IV administration. There appears to be no advantage to intra-cardiac injection compared to IV administration.	1 mg/mL (1:1000) injection solution	Cardiac arrest: 10–20 mcg/kg IV *or* 200 mcg/kg endotra-cheal (may be diluted in saline before administration) Anaphylactic shock: 2.5–5 mcg/kg IV *or* 50 mcg/kg endotracheal (may be diluted in saline)
Epsiprantel (Cestex)	Anticestodal agent (similar to praziquantel)	See Praziquantel.	See Praziquantel	Coated tablet	Dog: 5.5 mg/kg PO Cat: 2.75 mg/kg PO
Ergocalciferol (vitamin D₂) (Calciferol, Drisdol)	Vitamin D analogue. Used for vitamin D deficiency and as treat-ment of hypocalcemia, especially that associ-ated with hypothyroid-ism. Vitamin D pro-motes absorption and utilization of calcium.	Overdose may cause hypercalcemia. Avoid use in pregnant ani-mals because it may cause fetal abnormal-ities. Use cautiously with high doses of calcium-containing preparations.	Should not be used for renal hypoparathyroid-ism because of inability to convert to active compound. Available as oral solution, tablets, capsules, and injection. Doses for individual patients should be adjusted by monitoring serum calcium concen-trations.	400 U tablets (OTC); 50,000 U tablets (1.25 mg); 500,000 U/mL (12.5 mg/mL) injection	500–2000 U/kg/day PO

Drug Name (Trade or Other Names)	Pharmacology and Indications	Adverse Effects and Precautions	Dosing Information and Comments	Formulations	Dosage
Ertapenem (Invanz)	Carbapenem antibiotic of the β-lactam group. Like meropenem and imipenem, highly active against a broad spectrum of bacteria, including those resistant to other drugs. Ertapenem is not as active against *Pseudomonas* as meropenem or imipenem. High protein binding in people allows for infrequent dosing.	Well tolerated in animals. CNS toxicity may be possible with high doses. Allergy to β-lactam antibiotics is possible.	Dosing information is extrapolated from human medicine or limited empirical use in veterinary medicine. As with other carbapenems, use only when organisms are resistant to other drugs.	1 g vial for injection	15 mg/kg q12h IV or SC
Erythromycin (many brands and generic)	Macrolide antibiotic. Inhibits bacteria by binding to 50S ribosome and inhibiting protein synthesis. Spectrum of activity limited primarily to gram-positive aerobic bacteria. Used for skin and respiratory infections.	Most common side effect is vomiting (probably caused by cholinergic-like effect or motilin-induced motility). May cause diarrhea in some animals. Do not administer PO to rodents or rabbits.	There are several forms of erythromycin, including the ethylsuccinate and estolate esters, and stearate salt for oral administration. There is no convincing data to suggest that one form is absorbed better than another, and one dose is included for all. Only erythromycin gluceptate and lactate are to be administered IV. Motilin-like effect on GI motility occurs at low dose.	250 mg capsules or tablets	10–20 mg/kg q8–12h PO; prokinetic effects at 0.5–1.0 mg/kg q8–12h PO
Erythropoietin (r-HuEPO) (Epogen, epoetin alfa [r-HuEPO])	Human recombinant erythropoietin. Hematopoietic growth factor that stimulates erythropoiesis. Used to treat nonregenerative anemia (Compend Contin Educ 14: 25–34, 1992; J Am Vet Med Assoc 212:521–528, 1998).	Since this product is a human recombinant product, it may induce local and systemic allergic reactions in animals. Injection site pain and headache have occurred in people. Seizures also have occurred. Delayed anemia may occur because of cross-reacting antibodies against animal erythropoietin (reversible when drug is withdrawn).	Use has been based on clinical reports in dogs and cats. The only form currently available is a human recombinant product.	2000 units/mL injection	Doses range from 35 or 50 U/kg 3 times/week to 400 U/kg/week SC (adjust dose to hematocrit of 30%–34%).
Esmolol hydrochloride (Brevibloc)	β-blocker. Selective for β₁-receptor. The difference between esmolol and other β-blockers is the short duration of action. Indicated for short-term control of heart rate and arrhythmias	Same as other precautions for β-blockers (see Propranolol.)	Indicated for short-term IV therapy only. Doses are based primarily on empiricism or extrapolation of human dose. No clinical studies have been reported in animals.	10 mg/mL injection	500 mcg/kg IV, which may be given as 0.05–0.1 mg/kg slowly every 5 min or 50–200 mcg/kg/min infusion
Estradiol cypionate (ECP, Depo-Estradiol Cypionate, generic)	Semisynthetic estrogen compound. Used primarily to induce abortion in animals	High risk of endometrial hyperplasia and pyometra. High doses can produce leukopenia, thrombocytopenia, and fatal aplastic anemia.	Ordinarily, 22 mcg/kg is administered once IM during days 3–5 of estrus or within 3 days of mating. However, in one study, a dose of 44 mcg/kg was more efficacious than 22 mcg/kg when given during estrus or diestrus.	2 mg/mL injection	Dog: 22–44 mcg/kg IM (total dose not to exceed 1.0 mg) Cat: 250 mcg/cat IM between 40 hrs and 5 days of mating
Etidronate disodium (Didronel)	Bisphosphonate drug. Used to treat osteoporosis and hypercalcemia. Decreases bone turnover, inhibits osteoclast activity, retards bone resorption, and decreases rate of osteoporosis	Adverse effects not reported for animals. In people, GI problems are common.	At high doses, may inhibit mineralization of bone. In people, alendronate has replaced etidronate because of side effects.	200, 400 mg tablets; 50 mg/mL injection	Dog: 5 mg/kg q24h PO Cat: 10 mg/kg q24h PO

Drug Name (Trade or Other Names)	Pharmacology and Indications	Adverse Effects and Precautions	Dosing Information and Comments	Formulations	Dosage
Etodolac (EtoGesic, veterinary; Lodine, human)	An NSAID of the pyranocarboxylic acid group. Inhibits inflammatory prostaglandins.	NSAIDs may cause GI ulceration. Other adverse effects caused by NSAIDs include decreased platelet function and renal injury. In clinical trials with etodolac, some dogs at recommended doses showed weight loss, loose stools, or diarrhea. At high doses, etodolac caused GI ulceration in dogs.	Studies in dogs showed etodolac to be more efficacious than placebo for treatment of arthritis.	150 and 300 mg tablets	Dog: 10–15 mg/kg q24h PO Cat: Dose not established
Famotidine (Pepsid)	Histamine H_2-receptor antagonist. (See Cimetidine for details.)	See Cimetidine.	See Cimetidine. Clinical studies for famotidine have not been performed, therefore optimal dose for ulcer prevention and healing is not known.	10 mg tablet; 10 mg/mL injection	0.1–0.2 mg/kg q12h PO, IV, SC, IM
Felbamate (Felbatol)	Anticonvulsant. Usually used when dogs are refractory to other anticonvulsants. Mechanism may be via antagonism at the N-methyl-D-aspartate (NMDA) receptor and block effects of excitatory amino acids.	Not documented with use in dogs. In people, the most severe reactions have been hepatotoxicity and aplastic anemia. It may increase phenobarbital concentrations.	Dosing has been empirical. See dosage section. Starting doses are 200–400 mg/dog and increased to maximum of 600 mg for small dogs and 1200 mg for large dogs q8h.	120 mg/mL oral liquid; 400 and 600 mg tablets	Dog: Start with 15–20 mg/kg q8h PO. Or 200 mg/dog q8h for small dogs and 400 mg/dog q8h for larger dogs. Increase dose gradually by 200 mg increments until seizure control. Maximum dose for small dogs is 600 mg/dog q8h and for large dogs is 1200 mg/dog q8h
Fenbendazole (Panacur, Safe-Guard)	Benzimidazole antiparasite drugs. (See Albendazole). Effective for treatment of Giardia (Am J Vet Res 59: 61–63, 1998).	Good safety margin, but vomiting and diarrhea have been reported. No known contraindications.	Dose recommendations based on clinical studies by manufacturer. Granules may be mixed with food. In studies for treatment of Giardia, it was safer than other treatments.	Panacur granules 22.2% (222 mg/g); 100 mg/mL oral suspension	50 mg/kg/day × 3 days PO
Fentanyl citrate (Sublimaze, generic)	Synthetic opiate analgesic. Approximately 80–100 times more potent than morphine. (See Morphine for more details.)	Adverse effects similar to morphine.	Doses are based on empiricism and experimental studies. No clinical studies have been reported. In addition to fentanyl injection, transdermal fentanyl is available (see below).	250 mg/5 mL injection	0.02–0.04 mg/kg IV q2h IM SC or 0.01 mg/kg IV, IM, SC (with acetylpromazine or diazepam); for analgesia: 0.01 mg/kg q2h IV, IM, SC
Fentanyl, transdermal (Duragesic)	Same as for fentanyl. Transdermal fentanyl incorporates fentanyl into adhesive patches applied to skin of dogs and cats. Studies have determined that patches release sustained levels of fentanyl for 72–108 hours in dogs and cats. One 100 mcg/hr patch is equivalent to 10 mg/kg of morphine q4h IM.	Adverse effects have not been reported. However, if adverse effects are observed (e.g., respiratory depression, excess sedation, excitement in cats), remove patch and, if necessary, administer naloxone.	Patches available in sizes of 25, 50, 75, and 100 mcg/hr. Patch size is related to release rate of fentanyl. Studies have determined that 25 mcg/hr patches are appropriate for cats; 50 mcg/hr patches are appropriate for dogs 10–20 kg. Follow manufacturer's recommendations carefully when applying patches.	25, 50, 75, and 100 mcg/hr patch	Dog: 10–20 kg, 50 mcg/hr patch every 72 hr Cat: 25 mcg patch every 118 hr
Ferrous sulfate (many OTC brands)	Iron supplement	High doses cause stomach ulceration.	Recommendations based on dose needed to increase hematocrit	Many	Dog: 100–300 mg/dog q24h PO Cat: 50–100 mg/cat q24h PO
Finasteride (Proscar)	Inhibits conversion of testosterone to dihydrotestosterone (DHT). Since DHT stimulates prostate growth, this drug has been used for benign prostatic hypertrophy.	No adverse effects reported in dogs. Contraindicated in pregnancy	Doses based on study in dogs (J Am Vet Med Assoc 59:762–764, 1998)	5 mg tablets	Dog: 0.1 mg/kg PO q24h (or 5 mg tablet q24h in 10–50 kg dogs)

Drug Name (Trade or Other Names)	Pharmacology and Indications	Adverse Effects and Precautions	Dosing Information and Comments	Formulations	Dosage
Florfenicol (Nuflor)	Chloramphenicol derivative with same mechanism of action as chloramphenicol (inhibition of protein synthesis) and broad antibacterial spectrum. It has been used in situations in which chloramphenicol is not available.	Use in dogs and cats has been limited, therefore adverse effects have not been reported. Chloramphenicol has been linked to dose-dependent bone marrow depression, and similar reactions may be possible with florfenicol. However, there does not appear to be a risk of aplastic anemia, as for chloramphenicol.	Dose form is only approved for use in cattle, and these doses have not been thoroughly evaluated in small animals. Doses listed are derived from pharmacokinetic studies. Sustained effect in cattle from IM and SC administration does not appear to be long lasting in dogs. Injectable formulation for cattle has been administered, if necessary, orally to small animals.	300 mg/mL injectable solution	Dog: 20 mg/kg q6h PO, IM, q6h Cat: 22 mg/kg q8h IM, PO
Fluconazole (Diflucan)	Azole antifungal drug. Similar mechanism as other azole antifungal agents. Inhibits ergosterol synthesis in fungal cell membrane. Fungistatic. Efficacious against dermatophytes and variety of systemic fungi	Adverse effects have not been reported from fluconazole administration. Compared to ketoconazole, has less effect on endocrine function. However, increased liver enzyme plasma concentrations and hepatopathy are possible. Compared to other oral azole antifungals, fluconazole is absorbed more predictably and completely, even on an empty stomach.	Doses for fluconazole are primarily based on studies performed in cats for treatment of cryptococcosis. Efficacy for other infections has not been reported. The primary difference between fluconazole and other azoles is that fluconazole attains higher concentrations in the CNS.	50, 100, 150 or 200 mg tablets; 10 or 40 mg/mL oral suspension; 2 mg/mL IV injection	Dog: 10–12 mg/kg q24h, PO Cat: 50 mg/cat q12h–24h
Flucytosine (Ancobon)	Antifungal drug. Used in combination with other antifungal drugs for treatment of cryptococcosis. Action is to penetrate fungal cells and is converted to fluorouracil, which acts as antimetabolite.	Adverse effects have not been reported in animals.	Flucytosine is used primarily to treat cryptococcosis in animals. Efficacy is based on flucytosine's ability to attain high concentrations in cerebrospinal fluid (CSF). Flucytosine may be synergistic with amphotericin B.	250 mg capsule; 75 mg/mL oral suspension	25–50 mg/kg q6–8h PO (up to a maxiumum dose of 100 mg/kg q12h PO)
Fludrocortisone Acetate (Florinef)	Mineralocorticoid. Used as replacement therapy in animals with adrenal atrophy/adrenocortical insufficiency. Has high potency of mineralocorticoid activity compared to glucocorticoid activity	Adverse effects are primarily related to glucocorticoid effects with high doses. Long-term treatment for hypoadrenocorticism may result in glucocorticoid side effects.	Dose should be adjusted by monitoring patient response (i.e., monitoring electrolyte concentrations). In some patients, it is administered with a glucocorticoid and sodium supplementation.	100 mcg (0.1 mg) tablets	Dog: 0.2–0.8 mg per dog or 0.02 mg/kg q24h PO (15–30 mcg/kg) Cat: 0. 1–0.2 mg per cat q24h PO
Flumazenil (Romazicon)	Benzodiazepine receptor antagonist. Used as reversal agent after benzodiazepine administration in people (not commonly used in veterinary medicine)	No adverse effects reported in animals	Used primarily to block effects of benzodiazepine drugs. May be used to treat toxicity caused by high doses of benzodiazepines (e.g., diazepam). Although used experimentally for hepatic encephalopathy, it is not recommended for this use.	100 mcg/mL (0.1 mg/mL) injection	0.2 mg (total dose) as needed IV
Flumethasone (Flucort)	Potent glucocorticoid anti-inflammatory drug. Potency is approximately 15× that of cortisol. See Dexamethasone for additional details.	See Dexamethasone.	See Dexamethasone. Doses are based on severity of underlying disease (see dose table).	0.5 mg/mL injection	Anti-inflammatory uses: 0.15–0.3 mg/kg q12–24h IV, IM, SC

Drug Name (Trade or Other Names)	Pharmacology and Indications	Adverse Effects and Precautions	Dosing Information and Comments	Formulations	Dosage
Flunixin meglumine (Banamine)	NSAID. Acts to inhibit cyclooxygenase (COX) enzyme, which synthesizes prostaglandins. Other anti-inflammatory effects may occur (such as effects on leukocytes), but have not been well characterized. Used primarily for short-term treatment of moderate pain and inflammation	Most severe adverse effects related to GI system. Causes gastritis, GI ulceration with high doses or prolonged use. Renal ischemia has also been documented. Therapy in dogs should be limited to 4 consecutive days. Avoid use in pregnant animals near term. *Drug interactions:* Ulcerogenic effects are potentiated when administered with corticosteroids.	Not approved for small animals, but has been shown in experimental studies to be an effective prostaglandin synthesis inhibitor. Approved for use in small animals in Europe	250 mg packet granules; 10, 50 mg/mL injection	1.1 mg/kg once IV, IM, SC or 1.1 mg/kg/day 3 day/week PO Ophthalmic: 0.5 mg/kg once IV
5-Fluorouracil (Fluorouracil)	Anticancer agent. Antimetabolite. Action is via inhibition with nucleic acid synthesis.	Causes mild leukopenia, thrombocytopenia. CNS toxicity. Do not use in cats.	Used in anticancer protocols. Consult anticancer treatment protocol for precise dosage and regimen.	50 mg/mL vial	Dog: 150 mg/m² once/week IV Cat: do not use.
Fluoxetine (Prozac)	Antidepressant drug. Used to treat behavioral disorders, such as obsessive-compulsive disorders and dominance aggression. Mechanism of action appears to be via selective inhibition of serotonin reuptake and down-regulation of 5-HT1 receptors.	Fewer adverse effects (especially antihistamine, antimuscarinic effects) compared to other antidepressant drugs. Serious adverse effects have not been reported in animals, but decreased appetite may be common. In cats, nervousness and increased anxiousness have been observed.	Use of fluoxetine in animals is largely experimental. Doses have been derived empirically and use is based primarily on anecdotal experience. Because of long half-life, accumulation in plasma may take several days to weeks.	10 and 20 mg capsules; 4 mg/mL oral solution	Dog: 0.5 mg/kg/day initially PO, then increase to 1 mg/kg/day PO (average dose is 10–20 mg/dog) Cat: 0.5–4 mg/cat q24h PO
Follicle-stimulating hormone (FSH)	See Urofollitropin.				
Fomepizole (4-methylpyrazole, Antizol-Vet)	Antidote for ethylene glycol (antifreeze) intoxication. Inhibits dehydrogenase enzyme that converts ethylene glycol to toxic metabolite. Should be used early for maximum success	Methylpyrazole was safe and effective in dogs in clinical trials, if used within 8 hours of poisoning.	Used for emergency management of ethylene glycol intoxication. Experimental studies have demonstrated effectiveness in dogs, but in cats, ethanol is more effective. (J Am Vet Med Assoc 209: 1880, 1996.) Admix 0.9% sodium chloride before administration.	5% solution in a 1.5 mL vial	20 mg/kg initially IV, then 15 mg/kg at 12 and 24 hr intervals, then 5 mg at 36 hrs
Furazolidone (Furoxone)	Oral antiprotozoal drug with activity against *Giardia*. May have some activity against bacteria in intestine. Not used for systemic therapy	Adverse effects not reported in animals. In people, mild anemia, hypersensitivity, and disturbance of intestinal flora have been reported.	Clinical studies have not been reported for animals. Doses and recommendations are based on extrapolation from humans. Other drugs, such as fenbendazole, may be preferred for *Giardia*.	100 mg tablets	4 mg/kg q12h for 7–10 days PO
Furosemide (Lasix, generic)	Loop diuretic. Inhibits sodium and water transport in ascending loop of Henle, which produces diuresis. Also may have vasodilating properties, increasing renal perfusion, and decreasing preload	Adverse effects primarily related to diuretic effect (loss of fluid and electrolytes). Administer conservatively in animals receiving ACE inhibitors to decrease risk of azotemia.	Recommendations are based on extensive clinical use of furosemide in animals.	12.5, 20, 50 mg tablets; 10 mg/mL oral solution; 50 mg/mL injection	Dog: 2–6 mg/kg q8–12h (or as needed) IV, IM, SC, PO Cat: 1–4 mg/kg q8–24h IV, IM, SC, PO
Gemfibrozil (Lopid)	Cholesterol-lowering agent	Adverse effects have not been reported in animals.	Used primarily in people to treat hyperlipidemia. Clinical studies have not been performed in animals.	300 mg capsules; 600 mg tablets	7.5 mg/kg q12h PO

Drug Name (Trade or Other Names)	Pharmacology and Indications	Adverse Effects and Precautions	Dosing Information and Comments	Formulations	Dosage
Gentamicin sulfate (Gentocin)	Aminoglycoside antibiotic. Action is to inhibit bacteria protein synthesis via binding to 30S ribosome. Bactericidal. Broad spectrum of activity except streptococci and anaerobic bacteria	Nephrotoxicity is the most dose-limiting toxicity. Ensure that patients have adequate fluid and electrolyte balance during therapy. Ototoxicity, vestibulotoxicity also are possible. *Drug interactions:* When used with anesthetic agents, neuromuscular blockade is possible. Do not mix in vial or syringe with other antibiotics.	Dosing regimens are based on sensitivity of organisms. Some studies have suggested that once-daily therapy (combining multiple doses into a single daily dose) is as efficacious as multiple treatments. Activity against some bacteria (e.g., *Pseudomonas*) is enhanced when combined with a β-lactam antibiotic. Nephrotoxicity is increased with persistently high trough concentrations.	50 and 100 mg/mL solution for injection	Dog: 2–4 mg/kg q8h, or 9–14 mg/kg q24h IV, IM, SC Cat: 3 mg/kg q8h, or 5–8 mg/kg q24h IV, IM, SC
Glibenclamide	British name for glyburide				
Glipizide (Glucotrol)	Sulfonylurea oral hypoglycemic agent. Used as oral treatment in the management of diabetes mellitus, particularly in cats. Response rate is approximately 40%. This drug acts to increase secretion of insulin from pancreas, probably by interacting with sulfonylurea receptors on β cells. These drugs also may increase sensitivity of existing insulin receptors.	It may cause dose-related vomiting, anorexia, increased bilirubin, and elevated liver enzymes in some cats. Causes hypoglycemia, but less so than insulin. In people, increased cardiac mortality is possible. *Drug interactions:* Many drug interactions have been reported in people. It is not known if these occur in animals. Use cautiously with β-blockers, antifungal drugs, anticoagulants, fluoroquinolones, sulfonamides, and others (consult package insert).	Oral hypoglycemic agents are successful in people only for non–insulin-dependent diabetes. There has been only limited use in animals. Similar drugs include acetohexamide, chlorpropamide, glyburide, gliclazide, and tolazamide. Since response to oral hypoglycemic agents in cats is unpredictable, it is recommended to use a trial first of at least 4 weeks. If the cat responds, the drug can be continued; otherwise, insulin may be indicated. Feed cats a high-fiber diet when using oral hypoglycemic agents. Efficacy in cats is unpredictable.	5, 10 mg tablets	Cat: 2.5 mg/cat q12h PO, up to 5 mg/cat q12h PO if lower dose is not sufficient to affect glucose
Glucosamine and Chondroitin sulfate (Cosequin)	Cosequin is brand name for combination of glucosamine HCl and chondroitin sulfate. According to manufacturer, these compounds stimulate synthesis of synovial fluid and inhibit degradation and improve healing of articular cartilage. Used primarily for degenerative joint disease.	Adverse effects have not been reported, although hypersensitivity is possible.	Doses are based primarily on empiricism and manufacturer's recommendations. No published trials of efficacy are available.	Regular (RS) and double strength (DS) capsules.	Dog: 1–2 RS capsules per day (2–4 capsules of DS for large dogs) Cat: 1 RS capsule daily
Glyburide (DiaBeta, Micronase, Glynase)	Sulfonylurea hypoglycemic agent. See Glipizide.	See Glipizide.	See Glipizide.	1.25, 2.5, 5 mg tablets	Cat: 0.2 mg/kg daily PO
Glycerin (generic)	Used to treat acute glaucoma	No adverse effects reported		Oral solution	1–2 mL/kg, up to q8h PO
Glycopyrrolate (Robinul-V)	Anticholinergic drug (for mechanism, see Atropine.) Glycopyrrolate may have less effect on CNS compared to atropine because of lower CSF levels. May have longer duration of action than atropine.	Adverse effects attributed to antimuscarinic (anticholinergic) effects. (see Atropine.)	Glycopyrrolate is often used in combination with other agents, particularly anesthetic drugs.	0.2 mg/mL injection	0.005–0.01 mg/kg IV, IM, SC

Drug Name (Trade or Other Names)	Pharmacology and Indications	Adverse Effects and Precautions	Dosing Information and Comments	Formulations	Dosage
Gold sodium thiomalate (Myochrysine)	Gold therapy (for mechanism, see Aurothioglucose).	See Aurothioglucose.	Clinical studies have not been performed in animals. Efficacy and safety of this product are not available for animals. Aurothioglucose generally is used more often than Myochrysine.	Injection	1–5 mg IM on first week, then 2–10 mg IM on second week, then 1 mg/kg once/week IM maintenance
Gold therapy	See Aurothioglucose, Gold sodium thiomalate, or Auranofin.				
GoLYTELY	Oral solution for producing catharsis	See Polyethylene glycol electrolyte solution.			
Gonadorelin (GnRH, LHRH) (Factrel)	Stimulates synthesis and release of luteinizing hormone (LH) and, to a lesser degree, follicle-stimulating hormone (FSH). Used to induce luteinization.	Adverse effects have not been reported in animals.	Gonadotropin has been used to manage various reproductive disorders. Consult specific reference on reproductive problems in animals to guide therapy.	50 mcg/mL injection	Dog: 50–100 mcg/dog q24–48h IM Cat: 25 mcg/cat once IM
Gonadotropin, chorionic (HCG) (Profasi, Pregnyl, generic, A.P.L.)	Action of HCG is identical to that of leutinizing hormone (LH). Used to induce luteinization in animals.	Adverse effects have not been reported in animals.	Consult specific reference on reproductive problems in animals to guide therapy.	Injection sizes of 5000, 10,000, and 20,000 U H vials	Dog: 22 U/kg q24–48h IM, or 44 U once IM Cat: 250 U/cat once IM
Gonadotropin-releasing hormone	See Gonadorelin.				
Granisetron (Kytril)	Antiemetic drug that acts by inhibiting serotonin (5-HT) receptors. Used primarily for antiemetic during chemotherapy	None reported in dogs or cats.	Doses extrapolated from human uses.	1 mg tablets and 1 mg/mL injection	0.01 mg/kg IV (in people, dose is 1 mg/person PO)
Griseofulvin (microsize) (Fulvicin U/F)	Antifungal drug. Incorporates into skin layers and inhibits mitosis of fungi. Antifungal activity is limited to dermatophytes.	Adverse effects in animals include teratogenicity in cats; anemia and leukopenia in cats; anorexia, depression, vomiting, and diarrhea. Do not administer to pregnant cats.	A wide range of doses has been reported. Doses listed here represent the current consensus. Griseofulvin should be administered with food to enhance absorption.	125, 250, 500 mg tablets; 25 mg/mL oral suspension; 125 mg/mL oral syrup	50 mg/kg q24h PO (up to a maximum dose of 110–132 mg/kg/day in divided treatments)
Griseofulvin (ultra-microsize) (Fulvicin P/G, Gris-PEG)	Same as above	Same as above	Same as above. Ultra-microsize is absorbed to a greater extent, and doses should be less than microsize.	100, 125, 165, 250, 330 mg tablets	30 mg/kg/day in divided treatments PO
Growth hormone (hGH, somatrem, somatropin) (Protropin, Humatrope, Nutropin)	Growth hormone, also known as human growth hormone. Used to treat growth hormone deficiencies	Growth hormone is diabetogenic in all animals. Excess growth hormone causes acromegaly.	There is only limited clinical experience in animals. Dose form must be reconstituted with sterile diluent before use. Prepared solution is stable for 14 days, if refrigerated.	5 and 10 mg per vial	0.1 U/kg 3 times/week for 4–6 weeks, SC IM (usual human pediatric dose is 0.18–0.3 mg/kg/week)
Halothane (Fluothane)	Inhalent anesthetic. Exact mechanism of action is unknown.	Adverse effects related to anesthetic effects (e.g., cardiovascular and respiratory depression). Hepatotoxicosis has been reported in people.	Use of inhalent anesthetics requires careful monitoring. Dose is determined by depth of anesthesia.	250 mL bottle	Induction: 3%; Maintenance: 0.5%–1.5%
Hemoglobin glutamer (Oxyglobin)	Hemoglobin glutamer (bovine) used as oxygen-carrying fluid in dogs with varying causes of anemia	Transient hemoglobinuria. Adverse pulmonary effects can occur from rapid administration. Adverse effects have been skin discoloration, cardiovascular effects, vomiting, diarrhea, and anorexia.	Administer using aseptic technique. Do not administer with other fluids or drugs in the same IV line. Do not mix with other medications. 90% of dose is eliminated in 5–7 days.	13 g/dL polymerized hemoglobin of bovine origin in 125 mL single-dose bags	Dog: One-time dose of 10–30 mL/kg IV at rate up to 10 mL/kg/hr

Drug Name (Trade or Other Names)	Pharmacology and Indications	Adverse Effects and Precautions	Dosing Information and Comments	Formulations	Dosage
Heparin sodium (Liquaemin ([US]; Hepalean [Canada])	Anticoagulant. Potentiates anticoagulant effects of antithrombin III. Used primarily for prevention of thrombosis	Adverse effects caused by excessive inhibition of coagulation: bleeding	Dose adjustments should be performed by monitoring clotting times. For example, dose is adjusted to maintain activated partial thromboplastin time (APTT) to 1.5 to 2× normal.	1000 and 10,000 U/mL injection	100–200 U/kg IV loading dose, then 100–300 U/kg q6–8h SC. Low-dose prophylaxis (dog and cat): 70 units/kg q8–12h SC
Hetastarch	See Hydroxyethyl starch (HES).				
Hycodan	See Hydrocodone bitartrate.				
Hydralazine (Apresoline)	Vasodilator. Antihypertensive. Used to dilate arterioles and decrease afterload. Primarily used for treatment of CHF and other cardiovascular disorders characterized by high peripheral vascular resistance.	Adverse effects attributed to excess vasodilation. Monitor patients for hypotension. May dangerously decrease cardiac output. Allergic reactions (lupus-like syndrome) have been reported in people and are related to acetylator status, but have not been reported in animals.	Use in heart failure may accompany other drugs, such as digoxin and diuretics. It is advised to monitor patient for hypotension to adjust dosage.	10 mg tablets; 20 mg/mL injection	Dog: 0.5 mg/kg (initial dose), titrate to 0.5–2 mg/kg q12h PO Cat: 2.5 mg/cat q12–24h PO
Hydrochlorothiazide (HydroDIURIL, generic)	Thiazide diuretic. Inhibits sodium reabsorption in distal renal tubules. Used as diuretic and antihypertensive. Since it decreases renal excretion of calcium, it also has been used to treat calcium-containing uroliths.	Do not use in patient with elevated calcium. May cause electrolyte imbalance, such as hypokalemia	Not as potent as loop diuretics (such as furosemide). Clinical efficacy has not been established in veterinary patients.	10, 100 mg/mL oral solution and 25, 50, and 100 mg tablets	2–4 mg/kg q12h PO
Hydrocodone bitartrate (Hycodan)	Opiate agonist. Used primarily for antitussive action (see Codeine). Hycodan contains homatropine, but other combinations may contain guaifenesin or acetaminophen.	Oral opiate. See Codeine.	Hydrocodone is combined with atropine in the product Hycodan. Atropine can decrease respiratory secretions, but probably does not have significant clinical effects at doses in this preparation (1.5 mg homatropine per 5 mg tablet).	5 mg tablets and 1 mg/mL syrup	Dog: 0.22 mg/kg q4–8h PO Cat: no dose available
Hydrocortisone (Cortef and generic)	Glucocorticoid anti-inflammatory drug. Hydrocortisone has weaker anti-inflammatory effects and greater mineralocorticoid effects compared with prednisolone or dexamethasone (see Dexamethasone for other details). Also used for replacement therapy	Adverse effects are attributed to excessive glucocorticoid effects (see Betamethasone).	Dose requirements are related to severity of disease.	5, 10, 20 mg tablets	Replacement therapy: 1–2 mg/kg q12h PO Anti-inflammatory: 2.5–5 mg/kg q12h PO
Hydrocortisone sodium succinate (Solu-Cortef)	Same as hydrocortisone, except that this is a rapid-acting, injectable product	Same as for hydrocortisone	Same as for hydrocortisone. Prepare vials according to manufacturer.	Various size vials for injection	Shock: 50–150 mg/kg IV q8h for two days Anti-inflammatory: 5 mg/kg q12h IV
Hydroxyethyl starch (HES, hetastarch)	Synthetic colloid volume expander (used in same manner as dextran). Used primarily to treat acute hypovolemia and shock	Only limited use in veterinary medicine; therefore, adverse effects have not been reported. May cause allergic reactions. Coagulopathies are rare at usual doses.	Used in critical care situations. Infused via constant rate infusion. HES appears to be more effective and to produce fewer side effects than dextran. Infuse slowly.	Injection	10–20 mL/kg IV to effect

Drug Name (Trade or Other Names)	Pharmacology and Indications	Adverse Effects and Precautions	Dosing Information and Comments	Formulations	Dosage
Hydroxyurea (Hydrea)	Antineoplastic agent. Used in combination with other anticancer modalities for treatment of certain tumors. Has been used to treat polycythemia vera	Only limited use in veterinary medicine. No adverse effects have been reported. In people, hydroxyurea causes leukopenia, anemia, thrombocytopenia.	Limited use in veterinary medicine	500 mg capsules	Dog: 50 mg/kg PO q24h, 3 days/week Cat: 25 mg/kg PO q24h, 3 days/week
Hydroxyzine (Atarax)	Antihistamine of the piperazine class. Used primarily to treat pruritus in animals	Side effects of therapy are related primarily to antihistamine effects. Sedation occurs in some animals.	Clinical studies have shown hydroxyzine to be somewhat effective for treatment of pruritus in dogs.	10, 25, 50 mg tablets; 2 mg/mL oral solution	Dog: 1–2 mg/kg q6–8h IM, PO Cat: safe dose not established
Ibuprofen (Motrin, Advil, Nuprin)	NSAID (see Flunixin meglumine)	Safe doses have not been established for dogs and cats. Vomiting and severe GI ulceration and hemorrhage have been reported in dogs.	Avoid use, especially in dogs.	200, 400, 600, 800 mg tablets	Safe dose not established
Imipenem (Primaxin)	β-lactam antibiotic with broad-spectrum activity. Action is similar to other β-lactam (see Amoxicillin). Imipenem is the most active of all β-lactams. Used primarily for serious, multiple-resistant infections	Allergic reactions may occur with β-lactam antibiotics. With rapid infusion or in patients with renal insufficiency, neurotoxicity may occur (seizures). Vomiting and nausea are possible. IM or SC injections may cause pain in dogs.	Doses and efficacy studies have not been determined in animals. Recommendations are based on studies performed in humans and extrapolation from humans. Reserve the use of this drug for only resistant, refractory infections. Observe manufacturer's instructions carefully for proper administration. For IV administration, add to IV fluids. For IM administration, add 2 mL lidocaine (1%); suspension is stable for only 1 hour.	250 or 500 mg vials for injection	Dog: 5 mg/kg IV, IM, or SC q4h Cat: Dose not established, but often used at same dose as dogs
Imipramine (Tofranil)	Tricyclic antidepressant drug (TCA). Used in people to treat anxiety and depression. Used in animals to treat variety of behavioral disorders, including obsessive-compulsive disorders. Action is via inhibition of uptake of serotonin at presynaptic nerve terminals.	Multiple side effects are associated with TCAs, such as antimuscarinic effects (dry mouth, rapid heart rate) and antihistamine effects (sedation). Overdoses can produce life-threatening cardiotoxicity.	Doses are primarily based on empiricism. There are no controlled efficacy trials available for animals. There may be a 2–4 week delay after initiation of therapy before beneficial effects are seen.	10, 25, 50 mg tablets	2–4 mg/kg q12–24h PO
Indomethacin (Indocin)	NSAID (see Flunixin meglumine)	Causes severe GI ulceration and hemorrhage in dogs. Do not use.	Do not use in dogs.		Safe dose has not been established.
Insulin, regular crystalline	Insulin has multiple effects associated with utilization of glucose. Used to treat diabetes mellitus in dogs and cats	Adverse effects primarily related to overdoses (hypoglycemia)	Doses should be carefully adjusted in each patient, depending on response. Monitor plasma/serum glucose concentrations. For cats with ketoacidosis, alternative dosing regimen has used 0.2 U/kg IM initially, then 0.1 U/kg IM every hour until glucose level < 300, then 0.25–0.4 U/kg SC q6h.	100 U/mL injection	Ketoacidosis: animals < 3 kg, 1 U/animal initially, then 1 U/animal q1h; animals 3–10 kg, 2 U/animal initially, then 1 U/animal q1h; animals > 10 kg, 0.25 U/kg initially, then 0.1 U/kg q1h IM (for cats, see dosing information section)
Insulin, NPH isophane	Same as above	Same as above	Same as above	100 U/mL injection	Dog < 15 kg; 1 U/kg q24h SC (to effect); dog > 25 kg: 0.5 U/kg q24h SC (to effect) Cat: NPH not recommended for cats

Drug Name (Trade or Other Names)	Pharmacology and Indications	Adverse Effects and Precautions	Dosing Information and Comments	Formulations	Dosage
Interferon (interferon-α, HuIFN-α) (Roferon)	Human interferon. Used to stimulate the immune system in patients.	Adverse effects have not been reported in animals.	Doses and indications for animals have primarily been based on extrapolation of human recommendations or limited experimental studies. (J Am Vet Med Assoc 199:1477, 1991.) To prepare, add 3 million U to 1 L sterile saline and divide into aliquots and freeze. Thaw as needed for 30 U/mL solution.	3 million U/vial	Cat: 15–30 U per cat SC or IM q24h for 7 days and repeated every other week
Iodide	See Potassium iodide.				
Ipecac syrup (Ipecac)	Emetic drug. For emergency treatment of poisoning. Active ingredient is thought to be emetine.	No adverse effects with acute therapy for poisoning. Chronic administration can lead to myocardial toxicity.	Available as non-prescription drug. Onset of vomiting may require 20–30 min.	Oral solution; 30 mL bottle	Dog: 3–6 mL per dog PO Cat: 2–6 mL per cat PO
Ipodate	Cholecystographic agent. Used as treatment for hyperthyroidism in cats. Used as alternative to methimizole, radiation therapy, or surgery.	No adverse effects reported	Use of ipodate has been experimental, and precise doses have not been evaluated. In one study, 2/3 of treated cats responded.	Formulated into 50 mg capsules. (These may have to be formulated for cats.)	Cat: 15 mg/kg q12h PO. Most common dose has been 50 mg/cat q12h.
Iron	See Ferrous sulfate.				
Isoflurane (AErrane)	Inhalent anesthetic. See Halothane.	See Halothane.	See Halothane.	100 mL bottle	Induction: 5% Maintenance: 1.5%–2.5%
Isoproterenol (Isuprel)	Adrenergic agonist. Stimulates both β_1- and β_2-adrenergic receptors. Used to stimulate heart (inotropic and chronotropic). Also used to relax bronchial smooth muscle for acute treatment of bronchoconstriction.	Adverse effects are related to excessive adrenergic stimulation and are seen primarily as tachycardia and tachyarrhythmias.	Short half-life. Must be infused via constant rate infusion or repeated if administered IM or SC. Recommended for short-term use only.	Ampules for injection, 0.2 mg/mL	10 mcg/kg q6h IM, SC; or dilute 1 mg in 500 mL of 5% dextrose or Ringer's solution and infuse IV 0.5–1 mL/min (1–2 mcg/min), or to effect
Isosorbide dinitrate (Isordil, Isorbid, Sorbitrate)	Nitrate vasodilator. Causes vasodilation via generation of nitric oxide. Relaxes vascular smooth muscle, especially venous. Reduces preload in patients with CHF. In people, it is primarily used to treat angina.	Adverse effects are primarily related to overdoses that produce excess vasodilation and hypotension. Tolerance may develop with repeated doses.	Generally, doses are titrated to individual, depending on response.	2.5, 5, 10, 20, 30, 40 mg tablets; 40 mg capsules	2.5–5 mg/animal q12h PO (or 0.22–1.1 mg/kg q12h PO)
Isosorbide mononitrate (Monoket)	Same comments as for isosorbide dinitrate, except that this is a biologically active form of isosorbide dinitrate. Compared to isosorbide dinitrate, it does not undergo first-pass metabolism and is completely absorbed orally.	Same as for isosorbide dinitrate and nitroglycerin	Generally absorbed better than isosorbide dinitrate	10, 20 mg tablets	5 mg/dog two doses per day 7 hours apart PO
Isotretinoin (Accutane)	Keratinization stabilizing drug. Isotretinoin reduces sebaceous gland size and inhibits sebaceous gland activity, and decreases sebum secretion. In people, it is primarily used to treat acne. In animals, it has been used to treat sebaceous adenitis.	Absolutely contraindicated in pregnant animals. Adverse effects not reported for animals, although experimental studies have demonstrated that it can cause focal calcification (such as in myocardium and vessels)	Use in veterinary medicine is confined to limited clinical experience and extrapolation from human reports.	10, 20, 40 mg capsules	1–3 mg/kg/day (up to a maximum recommended dose of 3–4 mg/kg/day PO)

Drug Name (Trade or Other Name)	Pharmacology and Indications	Adverse Effects and Precautions	Dosing Information and Comments	Formulations	Dosage
Itraconazole (Sporanox)	Azole (triazole) antifungal drug. See Ketoconazole for mechanism of action. Active against dermatophytes and systemic fungi, such as *Blastomyces*, *Histoplasma*, and *Coccidioides*	Itraconazole is better tolerated than ketoconazole. However, vomiting and hepatotoxicosis are possible, especially at high doses. In one study, hepatotoxicosis was more likely at high doses. 10%–15% of dogs will develop high liver enzyme levels. High doses in cats caused vomiting and anorexia.	Doses are based on studies in animals in which itraconazole has been used to treat blastomycosis in dogs. In cats, lower doses have been effective for dermatophytes (see dosage section). Other uses or doses are based on empiricism or extrapolation from human literature.	100 mg capsules and 10 mg/mL oral liquid	Dog: 2.5 mg/kg q12h, or 5 mg/kg q24h PO For *Malassezia* dermatitis: 5 mg/kg q24h PO for 2 days, repeated each week for 3 weeks. Cat: 5 mg/kg q12h PO. For dermatophyte infection in cats: 1.5–3.0 mg/kg (up to 5 mg/kg) q24h PO for 15 days
Ivermectin (Heartgard, Ivomec, Eqvalan liquid)	Antiparasitic drug. Neurotoxic to parasites by potentiating effects of inhibitory neurotransmitter GABA.	Toxicity may occur at high doses, and in breeds in which ivermectin crosses blood–brain barrier. Sensitive breeds include collies, Australian shepherds, shelties, and Old English sheepdogs. Toxicity is neurotoxic, and signs include depression, ataxia, difficulty with vision, coma, and death. Ivermectin appears to be safe for pregnant animals. Do not administer to animals under 6 weeks of age. Animals with high microfilaremia may show adverse reactions to high doses.	Doses vary, depending on use. Heartworm prevention is lowest dose, other parasites require higher doses. Heartgard is only form approved for small animals; for other indications, large animal injectable products are often administered PO, IM, or SC to small animals. For demodectic therapy, it is advised to start with 100 mcg/kg/day and increase dose by 100 mcg/kg/day to 600 mcg/kg/day (Compendium 20:459–469, 1998).	1% (10 mg/mL) injectable solution; 10 mg/mL oral solution; 18.7 mg/mL oral paste; 68, 136, and 272 mcg tablets	Heartworm preventative: 6 mcg/kg every 30 days PO in dogs and 24 mcg/kg every 30 days PO in cats Microfilaricide: 50 mcg/kg PO 2 wks after adulticide therapy. Ectoparasite therapy (dogs and cats): 200–300 mcg/kg IM, SC, PO. Endoparasites (dogs and cats): 200–400 mcg/kg weekly SC, PO. *Demodex* therapy: start with 100 mcg/kg/day and increase dose by 100 mcg/kg/day to 600 mcg/kg/day for 60–120 days PO (Compendium 20:459–469, 1998).
Kanamycin (Kantrim)	Aminoglycoside antibiotic. See Gentamicin, Amikacin for details.	Shares same properties with other aminoglycosides (see Amikacin, Gentamicin)	See Gentamicin.	200, 500 mg/mL injection	10 mg/kg q12h or 20 mg/kg q24h IV IM, SC
Kaolin + pectin Kaopectate)	Antidiarrheal compound. Kaolin may act as adsorbent for endotoxins, and pectin may protect intestinal mucosa.	Side effects are uncommon.	Efficacy has not been established for treatment of diarrhea in animals.	Oral suspension, 12 oz	1–2 mL/kg q2–6h PO
Ketamine (Ketalar, Ketavet, Vetalar)	Anesthetic agent. NMDA receptor antagonist. Exact mechanism of action is not known, but appears to act as dissociative agent. Ketamine has little analgesic activity. Rapidly metabolized and eliminated in most animals.	Causes pain with IM injection. Tremors, spasticity, and convulsive seizures have been reported. Increases cardiac output compared to other anesthetic agents. Do not use in animals with head injury because it may elevate CSF pressure.	Often used in combination with other anesthetics and anesthetic adjuncts, such as xylazine, acepromazine, or diazepam. IV doses generally less than IM doses.	100 mg/mL injection solution	Dog: 5.5–22 mg/kg IV, IM (recommend adjunctive sedative or tranquilizer treatment). Cat: 2–25 mg/kg IV, IM (recommend adjunctive sedative or tranquilizer treatment). Dog and cat: Dose for constant rate infusion: 0.5 mg/kg IV followed by 10 mcg/kg/min. May be used in combination with other analgesics
Ketoconazole (Nizoral)	Azole (imidazole) antifungal drug. Similar mechanism of action as other azole antifungal agents. Inhibits ergosterol synthesis in fungal cell membrane. Fungistatic. Efficacious against dermatophytes and variety of systemic fungi, such as *Histoplasma*, *Blastomyces*, and *Coccidioides*.	Adverse effects in animals include dose-related vomiting, diarrhea, and hepatic injury. Enzyme elevations are common. Do not administer to pregnant animals. Ketoconazole causes endocrine abnormalities, most specifically, inhibition of cortisol synthesis. *Drug interactions:* Ketoconazole will inhibit metabolism of other drugs (anticonvulsants, cyclosporine, cisapride).	Oral absorption depends on acidity in stomach. Do not administer with antisecretory drugs or antacids. Because of endocrine effects, ketoconazole has been used for short-term treatment of hyperadrenocorticism.	200 mg tablets; 100 mg/mL oral suspension (only available in Canada)	Dog: 10–15 mg/kg q8–12h PO. For *Malassezia canis* infection: 5 mg/kg q24h PO. For hyperadrenocorticism: 15 mg/kg q12h PO. Cat: 5–10 mg/kg q8–12h PO.

Drug Name (Trade or Other Names)	Pharmacology and Indications	Adverse Effects and Precautions	Dosing Information and Comments	Formulations	Dosage
Ketoprofen (Orudis KT [human OTC tablet]; Ketofen [veterinary injection])	NSAID (See Flunixin meglumine)	All NSAIDs share similar adverse effect of GI toxicity (see Flunixin meglumine). Ketoprofen has been administered for 5 consecutive days in dogs, without serious adverse effects. Most common side effect is vomiting. GI ulceration is possible in some animals.	Although not approved in the U.S., ketoprofen is approved for small animals in other countries. Doses listed are based on approved use in those countries. It is available as OTC drug for humans in the U.S.	12.5 mg tablet (OTC); 25, 50, 75 mg Rx human form; 100 mg/mL injection for horses	1 mg/kg q24h PO for up to 5 days. Initial dose can be given via injection at up to 2 mg/kg SC, IM, IV.
Ketorolac tromethamine (Toradol)	NSAID. Used for short-term relief of pain and inflammation. Acts by inhibiting cyclooxygenase enzyme (COX). Use of ketorolac has been evaluated clinically in dogs but not cats.	NSAIDs may cause GI ulceration. Ketorolac may cause gastrointestinal lesions if administered more frequently than q8h. Do not administer more than 2 doses.	Available as 10 mg tablet and injection for IV or IM use. Clinical studies in dogs have shown safety and efficacy. Dosing q12h is recommended to avoid GI problems.	10 mg tablets; 15 and 30 mg/mL injection, in 10% alcohol	Dog: 0.5 mg/kg q8–12h PO, IM, IV Cat: safe dose not established
Lactated Ringer's solution (many)	Fluid solution for replacement. IV administration.	Administer IV fluids only in carefully monitored patients.	Fluid requirements vary depending on animal's needs (replacement vs maintenance). Consult fluid therapy reference for optimum rate. Rate listed here is for maintenance and shock.	250, 500, 1000 mL bags	Maintenance: 40–50 mL/kg/day IV. For shock therapy—dog: 90 mL/kg IV; cat: 60–70 mL/kg IV.
Lactulose (Chronulac, generic)	Laxative. Produces laxative effect by osmotic effect in colon. Lactulose also has been used for treatment of hyperammonemia (hepatic encephalopathy) because it decreases blood ammonia concentrations via lowering pH of colon, thus ammonia in colon is not as readily absorbed.	Excessive use may cause fluid and electrolyte loss.	In veterinary medicine, clinical studies to establish efficacy are not available. In addition to doses cited, 20–30 mL/kg of 30% solution retention enema has been used in cats.	10 g/15 mL	Constipation: 1 mL/4.5 kg q8h (to effect) PO. Hepatic encephalopathy—dog: 0.5 mL/kg q8h PO; cat: 2.5–5 mL/cat q8h PO.
L-Dopa	See Levodopa.				
Leucovorin (folinic acid) (Wellcovorin and generic)	Leucovorin is a reduced form of folic acid, which is converted to active folic acid derivatives for purine and thymidine synthesis. It is used as antidote for folic acid antagonists.	Allergic reactions have been reported in people.	Used primarily as rescue for overdoses of folic acid antagonists (methotrexate). Clinical studies have not been reported in veterinary medicine. It is not established whether leucovorin will prevent toxicity from trimethoprim–sulfonamide administration.	5, 10, 15, 25 mg tablets; 3 or 5 mg/mL injection	With methotrexate administration: 3 mg/m² IV IM PO. As antidote for pyrimethamine toxicosis: 1 mg/kg q24h PO.
Levamisole (Levasole, Tramisol, Ergamisol)	Antiparasitic drug of the imidazothiazole class. Mechanism of action due to neuromuscular toxicity to parasites. Levamisole has been used for endoparasites in dogs and as microfilaricide. In people, levamisole is used as immunostimulant to aid in treatment of colorectal carcinoma and malignant melanoma.	May produce cholinergic toxicity. May cause vomiting in some dogs.	In heartworm-positive dogs, it may sterilize female adult heartworms. Levamisole has also been used as an immunostimulant; however, clinical reports of its efficacy are not available.	0.184 g bolus; 11.7 g per 13 g packet; 50 mg tablet (Ergamisol)	Dog: hookworms, 5–8 mg/kg once PO (up to 10 mg/kg PO for 2 days); microfilaricide, 10 mg/kg q24h PO for 6–10 days; immunostimulant, 0.5–2 mg/kg 3 times/week PO. Cat: endoparasites, 4.4 mg/kg once PO; lungworms, 20–40 mg/kg q48h for 5 treatments PO

Drug Name (Trade or Other Names)	Pharmacology and Indications	Adverse Effects and Precautions	Dosing Information and Comments	Formulations	Dosage
Levodopa (L-dopa) (Larodopa)	Converted to dopamine after crossing blood–brain barrier. Stimulates CNS dopamine receptors. In people, used for treating Parkinson's disease. In animals, has been used for treating hepatic encephalopathy.	Adverse effects in animals have not been reported. In people, dizziness, mental changes, difficult urination, and hypotension are among the reported adverse effects.	Clinical studies have not been reported in veterinary medicine. Titrate dose for each patient.	100, 250, 500 mg tablets or capsules	Hepatic encephalopathy: 6.8 mg/kg initially, then 1.4 mg/kg q6h PO
Levothyroxine sodium (Soloxine, Thyro-Tabs, Synthroid)	Replacement therapy for treating patients with hypothyroidism. Levothyroxine is T_4, which is converted in most patients to the active T_3.	High doses may produce thyrotoxicosis, which is uncommon (compared to people). *Drug interactions:* Patients receiving corticosteroids may have decreased ability to convert T_4 to T_3.	Thyroid supplementation should be guided by testing to confirm diagnosis and post-medication monitoring to adjust dose.	0.1–0.8 mg tablets (in 0.1 mg increments)	Dog: 18–22 mcg/kg q12h PO (adjust dose via monitoring) Cat: 10–20 mcg/kg/day PO (adjust dose via monitoring)
Lidocaine (Xylocaine and generic brands)	Local anesthetic. (See Bupivacaine for mechanism of action.) Lidocaine is also used commonly for acute treatment of cardiac arrhythmias. Class I antiarrhythmic. Decreases phase 0 depolarization without affecting conduction. Not useful for supraventricular arrhythmias.	High doses cause CNS effects (tremors, twitches, and seizures). Lidocaine can produce cardiac arrhythmias, but has greater effect on abnormal cardiac tissue than normal tissue. Cats are more susceptible to adverse effects, and lower doses should be used.	When used for local infiltration, many formulations contain epinephrine to prolong activity at injection site. Avoid epinephrine in patients with cardiac arrhythmias. Note that human formulations may contain epinephrine, but no veterinary formulations contain epinephrine. To increase pH, increase onset of action, and decrease pain from injection, one may add 1 mEq sodium bicarbonate to 10 mL lidocaine (use immediately after mixing).	5, 10, 15, 20 mg/mL injection	Dog (antiarrhythmic): 2–4 mg/kg IV (to a maximum dose of 8 mg/kg over 10-min period); 25–75 mcg/kg/min IV infusion; 6 mg/kg q1.5h IM. Cat (antiarrhythmic): 0.25–0.75 mg/kg IV slowly, or 10–40 mcg/kg/min infusion. For epidural (dog and cat): 4.4 mg/kg of 2% solution.
Lincomycin (Lincocin)	Lincosamide antibiotic, similar in mechanism to clindamycin and erythromycin. Spectrum includes primarily gram-positive bacteria. Used for pyoderma and other soft tissue infections.	Adverse effects uncommon. Lincomycin has caused vomiting and diarrhea in animals. Do *not* administer orally to rodents and rabbits.	Action of lincomycin and clindamycin are similar enough that clindamycin can be substituted for lincomycin.	100, 200, 500 mg tablets	15–25 mg/kg q12h PO. For pyoderma, doses as low as 10 mg/kg q12h have been used.
Liothyronine (Cytomel)	Thyroid supplement. Liothyronine is equivalent to T_3.	Adverse effects have not been reported (see Levothyroxine sodium).	See Levothyroxine sodium. Doses of liothyronine should be adjusted on the basis of monitoring T_3 concentrations in patients.	60 mcg tablets	4.4 mcg/kg q8h PO. For T_3 suppression test in cats: collect presample for T_4 and T_3, administer 25 mcg q8h for 7 doses, then collect postsamples for T_3 and T_4 after last dose.
Lisinopril (Prinivil, Zestril)	ACE inhibitor. See Captopril for details. Used for treatment of CHF and hypertension.	See Captopril for details. Lisinopril has not been used extensively in animals to document adverse effects. Lisinopril appears to be better tolerated than captopril.	Clinical studies using lisinopril in animals have not been reported. See comments for Captopril and Enalapril maleate. With all ACE inhibitors, monitor electrolytes and renal function 3–7 days after initiating therapy and periodically thereafter.	2.5, 5, 10, 20, 40 mg tablets	Dog: 0.5 mg/kg q24h PO Cat: no dose established
Lithium carbonate (Lithotabs)	Stimulates granulopoiesis and elevates neutrophil pool in animals. In people, it is used for treatment of depression. CNS effect is related to decreased concentrations of neurotransmitters.	Adverse effects have not been reported in animals. In people, cardiovascular problems, drowsiness, and diarrhea are among the adverse effects.	Use in animals is not common. It has been used experimentally to increase neutrophils following cancer therapy.	150, 300, 600 mg capsules; 300 mg tablets; 300 mg/5 mL syrup	Dog: 10 mg/kg q12h PO Cat: not recommended
Lomotil	See Diphenoxylate.				

Drug Name (Trade or Other Names)	Pharmacology and Indications	Adverse Effects and Precautions	Dosing Information and Comments	Formulations	Dosage
Lomustine (CCNU) (CeeNU)	Anticancer drug—alkylating agent in the nitrosourea class. Chemotherapeutic agent. Highly lipid-soluble and crosses blood–brain barrier. Used for lymphoma and brain tumors	Myelosuppression, hepatotoxicosis, vomiting	Administering on empty stomach decreases nausea. Monitor hemogram for evidence of myelosuppression.	10, 40, 100 mg capsules	Dog: Moderate and early myelosuppression was reported at doses of 90 mg/m² PO given every 3 weeks. Cat: 30–60 mg/m² PO every 3 weeks or 10 mg PO every 3 weeks
Loperamide (Imodium and generic)	Opiate agonist. Stimulates smooth muscle segmentation in intestine, as well as electrolyte absorption. Used for acute treatment of nonspecific diarrhea	Loperamide does not produce systemic opiate adverse effects because it is a substrate for P-glycoprotein (P-gp). Therefore, its systemic effects are low and it does not cross the blood-brain barrier. However, some breeds (e.g., collies, Australian shepherds, and collie-mixed breeds) may be susceptible to adverse effects because of a deletion of the P-gp. Also, drugs that inhibit P-gp, such as quinidine, cyclosporine, ketoconazole, and calcium-channel blockers, could produce a drug interaction. In any animal, excessive use can cause constipation.	Doses are based primarily on empiricism or extrapolation of human dose. Clinical studies have not been performed in animals.	2 mg tablet; 0.2 mg/mL oral liquid	Dog: 0.1 mg/kg q8–12h PO Cat: 0.08–0.16 mg/kg q12h PO
Lufenuron (Program)	Antiparasitic. Used for controlling fleas in animals. Inhibits development in hatching fleas. May be used for dermatophytes in dogs and cats, although efficacy has been questioned by some experts	Adverse effects have not been reported. Appears to be relatively safe during pregnancy and in young animals	Lufenuron may control flea development with administration once every 30 days in animals.	45, 90, 135, 204.9, 409.8 mg tablets; 135, and 270 mg suspension per unit pack	Dog: 10 mg/kg PO every 30 days Cat: 30 mg/kg PO every 30 days Cat injection: 10 mg/kg SC every 6 mos Antifungal dose—Dogs: 80 mg/kg Cats: 100 mg/kg. In endemic areas (e.g., catteries) treat cats once a month
Lufenuron + milbemycin oxime (Sentinel tablets and Flavor Tabs)	Combination of two antiparasitic drugs. See Lufenuron or Milbemycin oxime. Used to protect against fleas, heartworms, roundworms, hookworms, and whipworms	See Lufenuron or Milbemycin oxime.	See Lufenuron or Milbemycin oxime.	Milbemycin oxime/ lufenuron ratio is as follows: 2.3/46 mg tablets;5.75/115, 11.5/230, and 23/460 mg Flavor Tabs.	Dog: Administer one tablet, every 30 days. Each tablet formulated for size of dog. Cat: This product is not registered for cats
Luteinizing hormone	See Gonadorelin.				
L-Lysine	Amino acid for treatment of herpes infections. Oral supplementation for cats with feline herpesvirus-1 (FHV-1) infection is associated with reduced viral shedding.	Well tolerated in cats	Doses listed will reduce viral shedding.	Supplied as a powder that can be mixed with food	Cat: 400 mg PO/day
Magnesium citrate (Citroma, Citro-Nesia [Citro-Mag in Canada])	Saline cathartic. Acts to draw water into small intestine via osmotic effect. Fluid accumulation produces distention, which promotes bowel evacuation. Used for constipation and bowel evacuation prior to certain procedures	Adverse effects have not been reported in animals. However, fluid and electrolyte loss can occur with overuse. Magnesium accumulation may occur in patients with renal impairment. Drug interactions: Magnesium-containing cathartics decrease oral absorption of ciprofloxacin and other fluoroquinolones.	Commonly used to evacuate bowel prior to surgery or diagnostic procedures. Onset of action is rapid.	Oral solution	2–4 mL/kg/day PO

Drug Name (Trade or Other Names)	Pharmacology and Indications	Adverse Effects and Precautions	Dosing Information and Comments	Formulations	Dosage
Magnesium hydroxide (milk of magnesia)	Same as for magnesium citrate. Magnesium hydroxide also is used as oral antacid to neutralize stomach acid.	Same as for magnesium citrate.	See Magnesium citrate.	Oral liquid	Antacid: 5–10 mL/kg q4–6h PO. Cathartic (dog): 15–50 mL/kg PO. Cathartic (cat): 2–6 mL/cat q24h PO.
Magnesium sulfate (Epsom salts)	Same as for magnesium citrate.	See Magnesium citrate.	See Magnesium citrate.	Crystals. Many generic preparations	Dog: 8–25 g/dog q24h PO Cat: 2–5 g/cat q24h PO
Mannitol (Osmitrol)	Hyperosmotic diuretic. Increases plasma osmolality, which draws fluid from tissues to plasma. Antiglaucoma agent. Used for treatment of edema and reducing intraocular pressure. Mannitol also has been used to promote urinary excretion of certain toxins.	Causes fluid and electrolyte imbalance. Do not use in dehydrated patients. Use cautiously when intracranial bleeding is suspected because it may increase bleeding. Administration that is too rapid may expand the extracellular volume excessively.	Use only in patients in which fluid and electrolyte balance can be monitored. Once solutions are prepared, discard unused portions.	5%–25% solution for injection	Diuretic: 1 g/kg of 5%–25% solution IV to maintain urine flow. Glaucoma or CNS edema: 0.25–2 g/kg of 15%–25% solution over 30–60 min IV (repeat in 6 hr, if necessary).
Marbofloxacin (Zeniquin)	Fluoroquinolone antimicrobial. Same mechanism as enrofloxacin and ciprofloxacin. Spectrum includes staphylococci, gram-negative bacilli, and some Pseudomonas.	Same precautions as enrofloxacin. May cause some nausea and vomiting at high doses. Avoid use in young animals. Safe for cats (ocular safety) at recommended dose.	Same dosing guidelines as for other fluoroquinolones. Higher doses are needed for organisms with higher MIC values. Safety data not available for cats. Doses published for European use may be lower than those U.S. approved for dogs.	25, 50, 100, and 200 mg tablets	2.75–5.55 mg/kg q24h PO
MCT oil (medium chain triglyceride oil [many sources])	Medium chain triglycerides. Used to treat hepatic encephalopathy	Adverse effects not reported in veterinary medicine. May cause diarrhea in some patients.	Results of clinical trials using MCT oil have not been reported. Many enteral feeding formulas contain MCT oil (many polymeric formulations).	Oral liquid	1–2 mL/kg q24h in food
Meclizine (Antivert, generic)	Antiemetic and antihistamine. Used for treatment of motion sickness. Action may be caused by central anticholinergic actions. Also may suppress chemoreceptor trigger zone (CRTZ)	Adverse effects have not been reported in animals. Anticholinergic (atropine-like) effects may cause side effects.	Results of clinical studies in animals have not been reported. Use in animals is based on experience in people or anecdotal experiences in animals.	12.5, 25, 50 mg tablets	Dog: 25 mg q24h PO (for motion sickness, administer 1 hr prior to traveling) Cat: 12.5 mg q24h PO
Meclofenamate sodium (Arquel, Meclofen)	NSAID. Used for treatment of arthritis and other inflammatory disorders. (See Flunixin meglumine.)	Adverse effects have not been reported in animals, but adverse effects common to other NSAIDs are possible. (See Flunixin meglumine.)	Results of clinical studies in animals have not been reported. Use in animals is based on experience in people or anecdotal experiences in animals. Administer with food.	50, 100 mg capsules	Dog: 1 mg/kg q24h for up to 5 days PO
Medetomidine (Domitor)	α_2-adrenergic agonist (see Xylazine). Used primarily as sedative, anesthetic adjunct, and analgesia.	α_2-agonists decrease sympathetic output. Cardiovascular depression may occur. Medetomidine will cause an initial bradycardia and hypertension.	May be used for sedation, analgesia, and minor surgical procedures. Should be reversed with equal volume of atipamezole	1.0 mg/mL injection	750 mcg/m^2 IV or 1000 mcg/m^2 IM
Medium chain triglycerides	See MCT oil.				
Medroxyprogesterone acetate (Depo-Provera [injection]; Provera [tablets])	Progestin hormone. Derivative of acetoxyprogesterone. In animals, used as progesterone hormone treatment to control estrus cycle. Also used for management of some behavioral and dermatologic disorders (such as urine spraying in cats and alopecia)	Adverse effects include polyphagia, polydipsia, adrenal suppression (cats), increased risk of diabetes, pyometra, diarrhea, and increased risk of neoplasia.	Clinical studies in animals have studied primarily the reproductive use and effects on behavioral use. Medroxyprogesterone acetate may have fewer side effects than megestrol acetate.	150, 400 mg/mL suspension injection; 2.5, 5, 10 mg tablets	1.1–2.2 mg/kg q7d IM. For behavioral use, 10–20 mg/kg is injected SC. For prostatic disease in dogs, use 3–5 mg/kg IM, SC.

Drug Name (Trade or Other Names)	Pharmacology and Indications	Adverse Effects and Precautions	Dosing Information and Comments	Formulations	Dosage
Megestrol acetate (Ovaban)	See Medroxyprogesterone.	See Medroxyprogesterone.	See Medroxyprogesterone.	5 mg tablets	Dog—proestrus: 2 mg/kg q24h PO for 8 days; anestrus: 0.5 mg/kg q24h PO for 30 days; behavior: 2–4 mg/kg q24h for 8 days (reduce dose for maintenance). Cat—dermatologic therapy or urine spraying: 2.5–5 mg/cat q24h PO for one week, then reduce to 5 mg once or twice/week; suppress estrus: 5 mg/cat/day for 3 days, then 2.5–5 mg once/week for 10 weeks.
Melarsomine (Immiticide)	Organic arsenical compound used for heartworm therapy. Heartworm adulticide. Arsenicals alter glucose uptake and metabolism in heartworms.	Adverse effects: pulmonary thromboembolism (7–20 days after therapy), anorexia (13% incidence), injection site reaction (myositis) (32% incidence), lethargy or depression (15% incidence). Causes elevations of hepatic enzymes. High doses ($3\times$) can cause pulmonary inflammation and death. If high doses are administered, dimercaprol (3 mg/kg IM) may be used as antidote.	Dose regimens are based on severity of heartworm disease. Consult current reference to determine class of disease (class I–IV). Class I and II are least severe. Class IV is most severe, and should not be treated with adulticide before surgery. Avoid human exposure. (Wash hands after handling, or wear gloves.) Do not freeze solutions after they are prepared.	25 mg/mL injection. After reconstitution, retains potency for 24 hrs.	Dog: Administer via deep IM injection. Class I and II dogs: 2.5 mg/kg q24h for two consecutive days. Class III dogs: 2.5 mg/kg once, then in 1 mo, two additional doses 24 hrs apart
Meloxicam (Mobic [human drug], Metacam [veterinary drug]	NSAID of the oxicam class. Melox-icam is relatively COX-1–sparing and has high COX-1: COX-2 ratio. It has been used in dogs and cats for pain and osteoarthritis.	Adverse effects are GI and include vomiting, diarrhea, and ulceration.	In studies performed in dogs, higher doses (up to 0.5 mg/kg) were more effective than lower doses but were associated with a higher incidence of GI adverse effects (Am J Vet Res 58:626, 1997). Meloxicam has been used in dogs and cats in Europe. Oral suspension is in a palatable flavor, 0.1 mg per drop (15 drops = 1 mL), which may be added to pet's food.	7.5 mg tablets (human); 0.5% injection, 1.5 mg/mL (veterinary); injection form is not available in the U.S.	Dog: 0.2 mg/kg initial loading dose, then 0.1 mg/kg q24h PO Cat: single antipyretic dose, 0.3 mg/kg; long-term dose, 0.1 mg/kg q48–72h PO
Melphalan (Alkeran)	Anticancer agent. Alkylating agent, similar in action to cyclophosphamide	Adverse effects related to its action as an anticancer agent. Causes myelosuppression.	Used to treat multiple myeloma and certain carcinomas.	2 mg tablets	1.5 mg/m^2 (or 0.1–0.2 mg/kg) q24h PO for 7–10 days (repeat every 3 weeks)
Meperidine (Demerol)	Synthetic opioid agonist with activity primarily at the μ-opiate receptor. Similar in action to morphine, except with approximately 1/7 of the potency. 75 mg meperidine IM or 300 mg PO has similar potency as 10 mg morphine.	Side effects similar to other opiates. See Morphine.	Although comparative clinical studies have not been conducted in animals, meperidine is considered an effective analgesic in dogs and cats, but with short duration.	50, 100 mg tablets; 10 mg/mL syrup; 25, 50, 75, 100 mg/mL injection	Dog: 5–10 mg/kg IV, IM as often as q2–3h (or as needed) Cat: 3–5 mg/kg IV, IM q2–4h (or as needed)
Mepivacaine (Carbocaine-V)	Local anesthetic of the amide class (see Bupivacaine). Medium potency and duration of action, compared to bupivacaine. Compared to lidocaine, longer-acting, but equal potency	See Bupivacaine. Mepivacaine may cause less irritation to tissues than lidocaine.	See Bupivacaine. For epidural use, do not exceed 8 mg/kg total dose. Duration of epidural is 2.5–3 hrs.	2% (20 mg/mL) injection	Variable dose for local infiltration. For epidural, 0.5 mL of 2% solution every 30 sec until reflexes are absent

Drug Name (Trade or Other Names)	Pharmacology and Indications	Adverse Effects and Precautions	Dosing Information and Comments	Formulations	Dosage
6-Mercaptopurine (Purinethol)	Anticancer agent. Antimetabolite agent that inhibits synthesis of purines in cancer cells.	Many side effects are possible that are common to anticancer therapy (many of which are unavoidable), including bone marrow suppression and anemia.	Used for various forms of cancer, including leukemia and lymphoma. Consult specific anticancer protocol for specific regimen.	50 mg tablets	50 mg/m^2 q24h PO
Meropenem (Merrem IV)	Broad-spectrum carbapenem antibiotic; indicated primarily for resistant infections caused by bacteria resistant to other drugs. Bactericidal. More active than imipenem and ertapenem.	Risks similar to those of other β-lactam antibiotics. Meropenem does not cause seizures as frequently as imipenem. SC injections may cause slight hair loss at injection site.	Dosage guidelines have been extrapolated from pharmacokinetic studies in animals and not tested for efficacy in animals. Meropenem is more soluble than imipenem and can be injected via bolus rather than administered in fluid solutions.	500 mg/20 mL or 1g/30 mL vial for injection	8 mg/kg q12h SC up to 12 mg/kg q8h SC (for *Pseudomonas*); IV dose, 12 mg/kg q8h
Mesalamine (Asacol, Mesasal, Pentasa)	5-Aminosalicylic acid. Used as treatment for colitis. Action is not precisely known, but suppresses inflammation in colon. Component of sulfasalazine.	See Sulfasalazine. Mesalamine alone has not been associated with side effects in animals.	Mesalamine use has not been reported in animals from clinical trials; however, it has been used as a substitute for sulfasalazine in animals that cannot tolerate sulfonamides.	400 mg tablets; 250 mg capsules	Veterinary dose has not been established. The usual human dose is 400–500 mg q6–8h (also see Sulfasalazine, Olsalazine).
Metamucil	Bulk-forming laxative containing psyllium. See Psyllium for details.				
Metaproterenol (Alupent, Metaprel)	β-adrenergic agonist. β$_2$-specific. Used primarily for bronchodilation. See Albuterol for further details.	Adverse effects related to excessive β-adrenergic stimulation. See Albuterol.	Results of clinical studies in animals have not been reported. Use in animals (and doses) is based on experience in people or anecdotal experience in animals. β$_2$-agonists also have been used in people to delay labor (inhibit uterine contractions).	10, 20 mg tablets; 5 mg/mL syrup; and inhalers	0.325–0.65 mg/kg q4–6h PO
Methazolamide (Neptazane)	Carbonic anhydrase inhibitor. Produces less diuresis than others (see Dichlorphenamide and Acetazolamide).	Use cautiously in patients sensitive to sulfonamides. (See Acetazolamide, Dichlorphenamide.)	Used to treat glaucoma in patients. May be used with other glaucoma agents. (See Acetazolamide, Dichlorphenamide.)	25, 50 mg tablets	2–3 mg/kg q8h PO
Methanamine hippurate (Hiprex, Urex)	Urinary antiseptic. Converted to formaldehyde in acidic urine to produce antibacterial/antifungal effect. Active against a wide range of bacteria. Resistance does not develop. Less effective against Proteus, which produces an alkaline urine pH. Not effective for systemic infections	Although formaldehyde formation in bladder may be irritating, in people, high doses were required (>8 gm/day). In animals, no adverse effects have been reported.	Results of clinical studies in animals have not been reported. Use in animals is based on experience in people, or anecdotal experience in animals. Urine must be acidic fo methenamine to convert to formaldehyde (monitor pH periodically). pH below 5.5 is optimal. Supplement with ascorbic acid or ammonium chloride to lower pH.	1 gm tablets.	Dog: 500 mg/dog q12h PO Cat: 250 mg/cat q12h PO
Methenamine mandelate (Mandelamine and generic)	Urinary antiseptic. (See Methenamine hippurate.)	See Methenamine hippurate.	See Methenamine hippurate.	1 g tablets; granules for oral solution; 50 and 100 mg/mL oral suspension	10–20 mg/kg q8–12h PO

Drug Name (Trade or Other Names)	Pharmacology and Indications	Adverse Effects and Precautions	Dosing Information and Comments	Formulations	Dosage
Methimazole (Tapazole)	Antithyroid drug. Used for treating hyperthyroidism, primarily in cats. Action is to serve as substrate for thyroid peroxidase and decrease incorporation of iodide into tyrosine molecules.	In people, it has caused agranulocytosis and leukopenia. In cats, lupus-like reactions are possible, such as vasculitis and bone marrow changes. Well tolerated in dogs.	Use in cats is based on experimental studies in hyperthyroid cats. Methimazole has, for the most part, replaced propylthiouracil for use in cats. Adjust maintenance dose by monitoring T_4 levels. Twice daily dosing in cats shown to be more effective than once daily dosing	5 and 10 mg tablets	Cat: 2.5 mg per cat q12h PO × 7–14 days, then 5–10 mg per cat PO q12h, and monitor T_4 concentrations
DL-Methionine	See Racemethionine.				
Methocarbamol (Robaxin-V)	Skeletal muscle relaxant. Depresses polysynaptic reflexes. Used for treatment of skeletal muscle spasms.	Causes some depression and sedation of the CNS.	Results of clinical studies in animals have not been reported. Use in animals (and doses) is based on experience in people or anecdotal experience in animals.	500, 750 mg tablets; 100 mg/mL injection	44 mg/kg q8h PO on the first day, then 22–44 mg/kg q8h PO
Methohexital (Brevital)	Barbiturate anesthetic. See Thiopental sodium for details. Methohexital is about 2–3 × more potent than pentothal, but with shorter duration.	See Thiopental sodium.	See Thiopental sodium.	0.5, 2.5, and 5 g vials for injection	3–6 mg/kg IV (give slowly to effect)
Methotrexate (MTX, Mexate, Folex, Rheumatrex, and generic)	Anticancer agent. Used for various carcinomas, leukemia, and lymphomas. Action is via antimetabolite action. Analogue of folic acid that binds dihydrofolate reductase. Inhibits DNA, RNA, and protein synthesis. In people, methotrexate is also commonly used for autoimmune diseases, such as rheumatoid arthritis.	Anticancer drugs cause predictable (and sometimes unavoidable) side effects that include bone marrow suppression, leukopenia, and immunosuppression. Hepatotoxicity has been reported in people from methotrexate therapy. *Drug interactions:* Concurrent use with NSAIDs may cause severe methotrexate toxicity. Do not administer with pyrimethamine, trimethoprim, or sulfonamides.	Use in animals has been based on experimental studies. There is only limited clinical information available. Consult specific anticancer protocols for precise dosage and regimen.	2.5 mg tablets; 2.5 or 25 mg/mL injection	2.5–5 mg/m² q48h PO (dose depends on specific protocol). Dog: 0.3–0.5 mg/kg once/week IV. Cat: 0.8 mg/kg IV every 2–3 weeks
Methoxamine (Vasoxyl)	Adrenergic agonist. Sympathomimetic. α_1-adrenergic agonist. Specific for α_1-receptors	Adverse effects related to excessive stimulation of α_1-receptor (prolonged peripheral vasoconstriction). Reflex bradycardia may occur.	Used primarily in critical care patients or during anesthesia to increase peripheral resistance and increase blood pressure. Short onset and duration of action	20 mg/mL injection	200–250 mcg/kg IM, or 40–80 mcg/kg IV
Methoxyflurane (Metofane)	Inhalant anesthetic. See Halothane.	See Halothane. Methoxyflurane has been reported to cause hepatic injury in animals. *Drug Interactions:* Labeling recommendations in some countries state that flunixin should not be administered to animals receiving methoxyflurane anesthesia.	See Halothane.	4 oz bottle for inhalation	Induction: 3% Maintenance: 0.5%–1.5%
Methylene blue 0.1% (generic, also called new methylene blue)	Antidote for intoxication. Used to treat methemoglobinemia. Methylene blue acts as reducing agent to reduce methemoglobin to hemoglobin.	Methylene blue can cause Heinz body anemia in cats, but is safe when used at therapeutic doses listed here.	Comparison of effects for intoxication has only been performed in experimental studies. One study demonstrated that acetylcysteine produced the best response; methylene blue also was helpful in some cats. (Am J Vet Res 56:1529, 1995.)	1% solution (10 mg/mL)	1.5 mg/kg IV, slowly, once

Drug Name (Trade or Other Names)	Pharmacology and Indications	Adverse Effects and Precautions	Dosing Information and Comments	Formulations	Dosage
Methylprednisolone (Medrol)	Glucocorticoid anti-inflammatory drug. (See Betamethasone, Prednisolone.) Compared to prednisolone, methylprednisolone is 1.25 × more potent.	Same as for other glucocorticoids (see Betamethasone.) Manufacturer suggests that methylprednisolone causes less PU/PD than prednisolone.	Use of methylprednisolone is similar to that of other corticosteroids. Dose adjustment should be made to account for difference in potency. (See dose section.)	1, 2, 4, 8, 18, 32 mg tablets	0.22–0.44 mg/kg q12–24h PO. Compared to prednisolone, methylprednisolone is 1.25 × more potent.
Methylprednisolone acetate (Depo-Medrol)	Depot form of methylprednisolone. Slowly absorbed from IM injection site, producing glucocorticoid effects for 3–4 weeks in some animals. Used for intralesional therapy, intra-articular therapy, and inflammatory conditions	Many adverse effects are possible from use of corticosteroids (see Betamethasone).	Use of methylprednisolone acetate should be evaluated carefully because one injection will cause glucocorticoid effects that persist for several days to weeks.	20 or 40 mg/mL suspension for injection	Dog: 1 mg/kg (or 20–40 mg/dog) IM every 1–3 weeks Cat: 10–20 mg/cat IM every 1–3 weeks
Methylprednisolone sodium succinate (Solu-Medrol)	Same as methylprednisolone, except that this is a water-soluble formulation intended for acute therapy when high IV doses are needed for rapid effect. Used for treatment of shock and CNS trauma.	Adverse effects are not expected from single administration; however, with repeated use, other side effects are possible (see Betamethasone).	Results of clinical studies in animals have not been reported. Use in animals (and doses) is based on experience in people or anecdotal experience in animals.	1 and 2 g and 125 and 500 mg vials for injection	For emergency use: 30 mg/kg IV and repeat at 15 mg/kg in 2–6 hr, IV. For replacement or anti-inflammatory therapy, see Prednisolone.
Methyltestosterone (Android, generic)	Anabolic androgenic agent. Used for anabolic actions or testosterone hormone replacement therapy (androgenic deficiency). Testosterone has been used to stimulate erythropoiesis.	Adverse effects caused by excessive androgenic action of testosterone. Prostatic hyperplasia is possible in male dogs. Masculinization can occur in female dogs. Hepatopathy is more common with oral methylated testerone formulations.	See also Testosterone cypionate, Testosterone propionate. Use of testosterone androgens has not been evaluated in clinical studies in veterinary medicine. Use is based primarily on experimental evidence or experiences in people.	10, 25 mg tablets	Dog: 5–25 mg/dog q24–48h PO Cat: 2.5–5 mg/cat q24–48h PO
Metoclopramide (Reglan, Maxolon)	Prokinetic drug. Centrally acting antiemetic. Stimulates motility of upper GI tract. Action is to inhibit dopamine receptors and enhance action of acetylcholine in GI tract. Used primarily for gastroparesis and treatment of vomiting. It is not effective for dogs with gastric dilation.	Adverse effects are primarily related to blockade of central dopaminergic receptors. Adverse effects similar to what is reported for phenothiazines (e.g., acepromazine) have been reported, in addition to behavioral changes. Do not use in epileptic patients or with diseases caused by GI obstruction.	Results of clinical studies in animals have not been reported. Use in animals (and doses) is based on experience in people or anecdotal experience in animals. Most use is for general antiemetic purposes, but doses as high as 2 mg/kg have been used to prevent vomiting during cancer chemotherapy.	10, 5 mg tablet; 1 mg/mL oral solution; 5 mg/mL injection	0.2–0.5 mg/kg q6–8h IV, IM, PO (or continuous IV infusion, of 0.1–0.2 mg/kg/hr)
Metoprolol tartrate (Lopressor)	Adrenergic-blocking agent. β_1-adrenergic blocker. Similar properties to propranolol, except that metoprolol is specific for β_1-receptor. Used to control tachyarrhymias and slow heart rate.	Adverse effects are primarily caused by excessive cardiovascular depression (decreased inotropic effects). May cause heart block. Use cautiously in animals prone to bronchoconstriction.	Results of clinical studies in animals have not been reported. Use in animals (and doses) is based on experience in people or anecdotal experience in animals.	50, 100 mg tablets; 1 mg/mL injection	Dog: 5–50 mg/dog (0.5–1.0 mg/kg) q8h PO Cat: 2–15 mg/cat q8h PO

Drug Name (Trade or Other Names)	Pharmacology and Indications	Adverse Effects and Precautions	Dosing Information and Comments	Formulations	Dosage
Metronidazole (Flagyl and generic)	Antibacterial and anti-protozoal drug. Disrupts DNA in organism via reaction with intracellular metabolite. Action is specific for anaerobic bacteria. Resistance is rare. Active against some protozoa, including *Giardia;* however, other drugs, such as fenbendazole, have been used for *Giardia*.	Most severe adverse effect is caused by toxicity to CNS. High doses have caused lethargy, CNS depression, ataxia, vomiting, and weakness. Metronidazole may be mutagenic. Fetal abnormalities have not been demonstrated in animals with recommended doses, but use cautiously during pregnancy. Cats may find broken tablets unpalatable.	Metronidazole is one of the most commonly used drugs for anaerobic infections. Although it is effective for giardiasis, other drugs used for giardiasis include albendazole, fenbendazole, and quinacrine. CNS toxicity is dose-related. Maximum dose that should be administered is 50–65 mg/kg/day in any species. Although tablets have been broken or crushed for oral administration to cats, they find these unpalatable.	250, 500 mg tablet; 50 mg/mL suspension; 5 mg/mL injection	For anaerobes—dog: 15 mg/kg q12h, or 12 mg/kg q8h PO; cat: 10–25 mg/kg q24h PO. For *Giardia*—dog: 12–15 mg/kg q12h for 8 days PO; cat: 17 mg/kg (1/3 tablet per cat) q24h for 8 days.
Mexiletine (Mexitil)	Antiarrhythmic drug. Used for ventricular arrhythmias. Mechanism of action is to block fast sodium channel. Class IB antiarrhythmic agent.	May produce arrhythmias. Use cautiously in animals with liver disease.	Results of clinical studies in animals have not been reported. Use in animals (and doses) is based on experience in people or anecdotal experience in animals.	150, 200, 250 mg capsules	Dog: 5–8 mg/kg q8–12h PO (use cautiously)
Mibolerone (Cheque Drops)	Androgenic steroid. Used to suppress estrus.	Do not use in Bedlington terriers. Do not use with perianal adenoma or carcinoma. Many bitches show clitoral enlargement or discharge from treatment. Do not use in cats.	Treatment ordinarily is initiated 30 days prior to onset of estrus. It is not recommended to be used for more than 2 years.	55 mcg/mL oral solution	Dog: (2.6–5 mcg/kg/day PO) 0.45–11.3 kg, 30 mcg; 11.8–22.7 kg, 60 mcg; 23–45.3 kg, 120 mcg; >45.8 kg, 180 mcg. Cat: safe dose not established.
Midazolam (Versed)	Benzodiazepine. Action is similar to other benzodiazepines (see Diazepam). Used as anesthetic adjunct.	Use very cautiously IV, especially with opiates. IV midazolam has caused serious cardiorespiratory depression.	Routine clinical use is not common. Clinical trials have not been reported. Compared to other benzodiazepines, midazolam can be administered IM.	5 mg/mL injection	Dog: 0.1–0.25 mg/kg IV IM or 0.1–0.3 mg/kg/hr IV infusion Cat: (sedation) 0.05 mg/kg IV (induction) 0.3–0.6 mg/kg IV; combined with 3 mg/kg ketamine
Milbemycin oxime (Interceptor, Interceptor Flavor Tabs, and SafeHeart)	Antiparasitic drug. Action is similar to ivermectin. Acts as GABA agonist in nervous system of parasite. Used as heartworm preventative, miticide, and microfilaricide. Used to control infections of hookworm, roundworms, and whipworms. At high doses, it has been used to treat *Demodex* infections in dogs.	In susceptible dogs (collie breeds), milbemycin may cross the blood–brain barrier and produce CNS toxicosis (depression, lethargy, coma). At doses used for heartworm prevention, this effect is less likely.	Doses vary, depending on parasite treated. Consult dose column. Treatment of *Demodex* requires high dose administered daily (J Am Vet Med Assoc 207:1581, 1995). See also Lufenuron + milbemycin oxime.	2.3, 5.75, 11.5, and 23 mg tablet	Dog—microfilaricide: 0.5 mg/kg; *Demodex:* 2 mg/kg q24h PO for 60–120 days; heartworm prevention and control of endoparasites: 0.5 mg/kg every 30 days PO. Cat: for heartworm and endoparasite control, 2.0 mg/kg every 30 days PO.
Mineral oil (generic)	Lubricant laxative. Increases water content of stool. Used to increase passage of feces for treatment of impaction and constipation.	Adverse effects have not been reported. Chronic use may decrease absorption of fat-soluble vitamins.	Use is empirical. No clinical results reported.	Oral liquid	Dog: 10–50 mL/dog q12h PO Cat: 10–25 mL/cat q12h PO
Minocycline (Minocin)	Tetracycline antibiotic. Similar to doxycycline in pharmacokinetics. (See Doxycycline.)	See other tetracycline (Doxycycline). Adverse effects have not been reported for minocycline. Oral absorption is not affected by calcium products as with other tetracyclines.	Minocycline has received little attention for clinical use in North America. Clinical use has not been reported, but properties are similar to doxycycline.	50, 100 mg tablets; 10 mg/mL oral suspension	5–12.5 mg/kg q12h PO

Drug Name (Trade or Other Names)	Pharmacology and Indications	Adverse Effects and Precautions	Dosing Information and Comments	Formulations	Dosage
Misoprostol (Cytotec)	Prostaglandin E$_2$ analogue. Prostaglandins provide a cytoprotective role in the GI mucosa. Misoprostol is used to prevent gastritis and ulcers associated with NSAID therapy.	Adverse effects are caused by effects of prostaglandins. Most common side effects are GI discomfort, vomiting, and diarrhea. Do *not* administer to pregnant animals; may cause abortion.	Doses and recommendations are based on clinical trials in which misoprostol was administered to prevent GI mucosal injury caused by aspirin.	0.1 mg (100 mcg), 0.2 mg (200 mcg) tablets	Dog: 2–5 mcg/kg q6–8h PO Cat: dose not established
Mithramycin	Older name for plicamycin				
Mitotane (*o,p*′-DDD) (Lysodren)	Adrenocortical cytotoxic agent. Causes suppression of adrenal cortex. Used to treat adrenal tumors and pituitary-dependent-hyperadrenocorticism (PDH).	Adverse effects, especially during induction period, include lethargy, anorexia, ataxia, depression, vomiting. Corticosteroid supplementation (e.g., hydrocortisone or prednisolone) may be administered to minimize side effects.	Dose and frequency often are based on patient response. Adverse effects are common during initial therapy. Administration with food increases oral absorption. Maintenance dose should be adjusted on the basis of periodic cortisol measurements and ACTH stimulation tests. (See also Vet Rec 122:486, 1988.) Cats usually have not responded to mitotane treatment.	500 mg tablets	Dog—for PDH: 50 mg/kg/day (in divided doses) PO for 5–10 days, then 50–70 mg/kg/week PO; for adrenal tumor: 50–75 mg/kg/day for 10 days, then 75–100 mg/kg/week PO
Mitoxantrone (Novantrone)	Anticancer antibiotic. Similar to doxorubicin in action (see Doxorubicin). Used for leukemia, lymphoma, and carcinomas.	As with all anticancer agents, certain adverse effects are predictable, unavoidable, and related to drug's action. Mitoxantrone produces myelosuppression, vomiting, anorexia, and GI upset, but may be less cardiotoxic than doxorubicin.	Proper use of mitoxantrone usually follows a specific anticancer protocol. Consult specific protocol for dosing regimen.	2 mg/mL injection	Dog: 6 mg/m² IV every 21 days Cat: 6.5 mg/m² IV every 21 days
Morphine sulfate (generic)	Opioid agonist, analgesic. Prototype for other opioid agonists. Action of morphine is to bind to μ- and κ-opiate receptors on nerves and inhibit release of neurotransmitters involved with transmission of pain stimuli (such as substance P). Morphine also may inhibit release of some inflammatory mediators. Central sedative and euphoric effects related to μ-receptor effects in brain.	Like all opiates, side effects from morphine are predictable and unavoidable. Side effects from morphine administration include sedation, constipation, and bradycardia. Respiratory depression occurs with high doses. Tolerance and dependence occur with chronic administration. Cats are more sensitive to excitement than other species.	Effects from morphine administration are dose dependent. Low doses (0.1–0.25 mg/kg) produce mild analgesia. Higher doses (up to 1 mg/kg) produce greater analgesic effects and sedation. Usually morphine is administered IM, IV, or SC, but delayed-release tablets have been used in dogs experimentally, but dose is higher (1–3 mg/kg q12h). Epidural administration has been used for surgical procedures.	1 and 15 mg/mL injection; 30, 60 mg delayed-release tablets	Dog: 0.1–1 mg/kg IV, IM, SC (dose is escalated as needed for pain relief) q4–6h. Oral dose: 1 mg/kg PO q4–6h Epidural: 0.1 mg/kg Cat: 0.1 mg/kg IM SC q3–6h (or as needed)
Moxidectin (canine form: ProHeart; equine oral gel: Quest; cattle pour-on: Cydectin)	Antiparasitic drug. Neurotoxic to parasites by potentiating effects of inhibitory neurotransmitter GABA. Used for endo- and ecto-parasites, as well as heartworm prevention.	Toxicity may occur at high doses and in species in which ivermectin crosses blood–brain barrier (collie-breeds). Toxicity is neurotoxic, and signs include depression, ataxia, difficulty with vision, coma, and death.	Similar use as ivermectin. Extreme caution is recommended if equine formulation is considered for use in small animals. Toxic overdoses are likely because the equine formulation is highly concentrated.	30, 68, 136 mcg tablets for dogs; 20 mg/mL equine oral gel; and 5 mg/mL cattle pour-on	Dog—heartworm prevention: 3 mcg/kg q30d PO; endoparasites: 25–300 mcg/kg *Demodex:* 500 mcg/kg/day for 21–22 weeks
Moxifloxacin (Avelox)	Fluoroquinolone antibiotic of the new (4th) generation. Similar to other fluoroquinolones, except with greater activity against gram positive and anaerobic bacteria.	Similar to those of other fluoroquinolones. Because of the increased spectrum of action on anaerobic bacteria, greater GI disturbance is expected from oral dose.	Doses and recommendations based primarily on limited clinical experience and extrapolation from human studies	400 mg tablet	10 mg/kg q24h PO

Drug Name (Trade or Other Names)	Pharmacology and Indications	Adverse Effects and Precautions	Dosing Information and Comments	Formulations	Dosage
Myochrysine	See Gold sodium thiomalate				
Naloxone (Narcan)	Opiate antagonist. Used to reverse effects from opiate agonists (such as morphine). Naloxone may be used to reverse sedation, anesthesia, and adverse effects caused from opiates.	Adverse effects are not reported. Tachycardia and hypertension have been reported in people.	Administration may have to be individualized based on response in each patient. Naloxone's duration of action is short in animals (60 min) and may have to be repeated.	20 or 400 mcg/mL injection	0.01–0.04 mg/kg IV, IM, SC, as needed, to reverse opiate
Naltrexone (Trexan)	Opiate antagonist. Similar to naloxone, except that it is longer acting and administered orally. Used in people for treatment of opiate dependence. In animals, it has been used for treatment of some obsessive-compulsive behavioral disorders.	Adverse effects have not been reported in animals.	Treatment for obsessive-compulsive disorders in animals has been reported with naltrexone. Relapse rates may be high.	50 mg tablets	Dog: For behavior problems: 2.2 mg/kg q12h PO
Nandrolone decanoate (Deca-Durabolin)	Anabolic steroid. Derivative of testosterone. Anabolic agents are designed to maximize anabolic effects while minimizing androgenic action (see also Methyltestosterone). Anabolic agents have been used for reversing catabolic conditions, increasing weight gain, increasing muscling in animals, and stimulating erythropoiesis.	Adverse effects from anabolic steroids can be attributed to the pharmacologic action of these steroids. Increased masculine effects are common. Increased incidence of some tumors has been reported in people. 17α-methylated oral anabolic steroids (oxymetholone, stanozolol, and oxandrolone) are associated with hepatic toxicity.	Results of clinical studies in animals have not been reported. Use in animals (and doses) is based on experience in people or anecdotal experience in animals.	50, 100, 200 mg/mL injection	Dog: 1–1.5 mg/kg/week IM Cat: 1 mg/kg/week IM
Naproxen (Naprosyn, Naxen, Aleve [naproxen sodium])	NSAID. Action is similar to other NSAIDs (see Flunixin meglumine).	Naproxen is a potent NSAID. Adverse effects attributed to GI toxicity are common to all NSAIDs (see Flunixin meglumine). Naproxen has produced serious ulceration in dogs because elimination in dogs is many-fold slower than in people or horses.	Results of clinical studies in animals have not been reported. Use in animals (and doses) is based on pharmacokinetic studies in experimental animals. Use caution when using the OTC formulation designed for people because the tablet size is much larger than safe dose for dogs. 220 mg naproxen sodium is equivalent to 200 mg naproxen.	220 mg tablet (OTC); 25 mg/mL oral suspension; 250, 375, 500 mg tablets (Rx)	Dog: 5 mg initially, then 2 mg/kg q48h PO
Neomycin (Biosol)	Aminoglycoside antibiotic. For mechanism, and other effects, see Gentamicin, Amikacin. Neomycin differs from other aminoglycosides because it is only administered topically or orally. Systemic absorption is minimal from oral absorption.	Although oral absorption is so small that systemic adverse effects are unlikely, some oral absorption has been demonstrated in young animals (calves). Alterations in intestinal bacterial flora from therapy may cause diarrhea.	Neomycin is primarily used for oral treatment of diarrhea. Efficacy for this indication (especially for nonspecific diarrhea) is questionable. Used also for treatment of hepatic encephalopathy	500 mg bolus; 200 mg/mL oral liquid	10–20 mg/kg q6–12h PO
Neostigmine bromide and neostigmine methylsulfate (Prostigmin; Stiglyn)	Anticholinesterase drug. Cholinesterase inhibitor. Inhibits breakdown of acetylcholine at synapse. Antimyasthenic drug. Used primarily for treatment of myasthenia gravis or as an antidote for neuromuscular blockade caused neuromuscular blocking drugs.	Adverse effects are related to drug's pharmacologic effects: excessive cholinergic stimulation (muscarinic effects), which include diarrhea, salivation, respiratory problems, vomiting, CNS effects, muscle twitching, or used to treat overdose.	Compared to other drugs in this class (e.g., pyridostigmine) produces more severe muscarinic effects. Neostigmine has been used for diagnostic purposes also (see Edrophonium). When injected for diagnosis or treatment of myasthenia, it is recommended to use atropine to counteract side effects	15 mg tablet (neostigmine bromide); 0.25, 0.5 mg/mL injection (neostigmine methylsulfate)	2 mg/kg/day PO (in divided doses, to effect). Injection—antimyasthenic: 10 mcg/kg IM, SC, as needed; antidote for neuromuscular block: 40 mcg/kg IM or SC; diagnostic aid for myasthenia gravis: 40 mcg/kg IM or 20 mcg/kg IV

Drug Name (Trade or Other Names)	Pharmacology and Indications	Adverse Effects and Precautions	Dosing Information and Comments	Formulations	Dosage
Nifedipine (Adalat, Procardia)	Calcium channel–blocking drug of the dihydropyridine class. Action is similar to other calcium channel–blocking drugs, except nifedipine is more specific for vascular smooth muscle than cardiac tissue. Used for smooth muscle relaxation, vasodilation.	Adverse effects have not been reported in veterinary medicine. Most common side effect is hypotension.	Use of nifedipine is limited in veterinary medicine. Other calcium channel blockers, such as diltiazem, are used to control heart rhythm.	10, 20 mg capsules	Animal dose not established. In people, the dose is 10 mg/person three times a day and increased in 10 mg increments to effect.
Nitrates	See Nitroglycerin ointment, Isosorbide dinitrate.				
Nitrofurantoin (Macrodantin, Furalan, Furatoin, Furadantin, and generic)	Antibacterial drug. Urinary antiseptic. Action is via reactive metabolites that damage DNA. Therapeutic concentrations are reached only in the urine. Not to be used for systemic infections.	Adverse effects include nausea, vomiting, and diarrhea. Turns urine color rust-yellow brown. Do not administer during pregnancy.	Two dosing forms exist. Microcrystalline is rapidly and completely absorbed. Macrocrystalline (Macrodantin) is more slowly absorbed and causes less GI irritation. Urine should be at acidic pH for maximum effect. Administer with food to increase absorption.	Macrodantin and generic: 25, 50, 100 mg capsules; Furalan, Furatoin, and generic: 50, 100 mg tablets; Furadantin: 5 mg/mL oral suspension	10 mg/kg/day divided into four daily treatments, then 1 mg/kg at night PO
Nitroglycerin ointment (Nitrol, Nitro-Bid, Nitrostat)	Nitrate. Nitrovasodilator. Relaxes vascular smooth muscle (especially venous) via generation of nitric oxide. Used primarily in heart failure to reduce preload or decrease pulmonary hypertension. In people, used to treat angina pectoris.	Adverse effects from nitrates are related to their pharmacologic action. Most significant adverse effect is hypotension. Methemoglobinemia can occur with accumulation of nitrites, but is a rare problem.	Tolerance can develop with repeated, chronic use. Use should be intermittent for optimum effect. Nitroglycerin has high presystemic metabolism, and oral availability is poor. When using ointment, 1 inch of ointment is approximately 15 mg.	0.5, 0.8, 1, 5, 10 mg/mL injection; 2% ointment; transdermal systems (0.2 mg/hr patch)	Dog: 4–12 mg (up to 15 mg) topically q12h Cat: 2–4 mg topically q12h (or 1/4 inch of ointment per cat)
Nitroprusside (Nitropress)	Nitrate vasodilator. See Nitroglycerin ointment. Nitroprusside is used only as an IV infusion, and patients should be monitored carefully during administration.	Severe hypotension is possible during therapy. Monitor patients carefully during administration. Cyanide is generated via metabolism during nitroprusside treatment, especially at high infusion rates. Cyanide toxicity is possible with nitroprusside therapy. Sodium thiosulfate has been used in people to prevent cyanide toxicity. Methemoglobinemia is possible, and if necessary, treated with methylene blue.	Nitroprusside is administered via IV infusion. IV solution should be delivered in 5% dextrose solution (e.g., add 50 mg to 250 mL of 5% dextrose). Protect from light. Discard solution if color change is observed. Titrate dose carefully in each patient.	50 mg vial for injection	1–5 mcg/kg/min up to a maximum of 10 mcg/kg/min IV infusion
Nizatidine (Axid)	Histamine H_2 blocking drug. See Cimetidine. Same as cimetidine, except up to 10× more potent.	See Cimetidine and Ranitidine. Side effects from nizatidine have not been reported in animals.	Results of clinical studies in animals have not been reported. Use in animals (and doses) is based on experience in people or anecdotal experience in animals. Nizatidine and ranitidine have been shown to stimulate gastric emptying and colonic motility via anticholinesterase activity.	150, 300 mg capsules	Dog: 2.5–5 mg/kg q24h PO
Norfloxacin (Noroxin)	Fluoroquinolone antibacterial drug. Same action as ciprofloxacin, except spectrum of activity is not as broad as with enrofloxacin or ciprofloxacin.	Adverse effects have not been reported in animals. Some effects are expected to be similar to cipro/enrofloxacin administration.	Use in animals (and doses) is based on pharmacokinetic studies in experimental animals, experience in people, or anecdotal experience in animals.	400 mg tablets	22 mg/kg q12h PO

Drug Name (Trade or Other Names)	Pharmacology and Indications	Adverse Effects and Precautions	Dosing Information and Comments	Formulations	Dosage
Olsalazine (Dipentum)	Anti-inflammatory drug for treating colitis. Two molecules of amino-salicylic acid joined by an azobond. (See Mesalamine).	See Mesalamine.	See Mesalamine. Olsalazine is used in patients that cannot tolerate sulfasalazine.	500 mg tablets	Dose not established, but 5–10 mg/kg q8h PO has been used. (The usual human dose is 500 mg twice daily.)
Omeprazole (Prilosec [formerly Losec]; equine formulation [a paste]: GastroGard)	Proton pump inhibitor. Omeprazole inhibits gastric acid secretion by inhibiting the K^+/H^+ pump. Omeprazole is more potent and longer acting than most available antisecretory drugs. Used for treatment and prevention of GI ulcers.	Side effects have not been reported in animals. However, in people, there is concern about hypergastrinemia with chronic use. *Drug interactions:* Do not administer with drugs that depend on stomach acid for absorption (e.g., ketoconazole).	Due to omeprazole's potency and accumulation in gastric cells, infrequent administration is possible. Lansoprazole is a newer drug of this class, but has not been used in animals.	20 mg capsules and equine paste	Dog: 20 mg/dog q24h PO (or 0.7 mg/kg q24h). Cat: not recommended
Ondansetron (Zofran)	Antiemetic drug. Ondansetron's action is to inhibit action of serotonin (blocks 5-HT$_3$ receptors). Used primarily to inhibit vomiting associated with chemotherapy.	Adverse effects have not been reported in animals. Some effects may be indistinguishable from concurrent cancer drugs.	Ondansetron has been used infrequently in veterinary medicine due to its expense. Granisetron is a similar drug not yet evaluated in veterinary medicine.	4, 8 mg tablets; 2 mg/mL injection	0.5 to 1.0 mg/kg IV or PO 30 min prior to administration of cancer drugs. To control vomiting due to other causes, doses as low as 0.1–0.2 mg/kg IV q6–12h may be considered.
o,p'-DDD	See Mitotane				
Orbifloxacin (Orbax)	Fluoroquinolone antimicrobial. Same mechanism as enrofloxacin and ciprofloxacin. Spectrum includes staphylococci, gram-negative bacilli, and some *Pseudomonas*.	Same precautions as enrofloxacin. May cause some nausea and vomiting at high doses. Avoid use in young animals. Blindness in cats has not been reported with doses ≤ 15 mg/kg/day.	Dose range is wide to account for susceptibility of bacteria. Most susceptible bacteria should be treated with low dose. More resistant bacteria, such as *Pseudomonas*, should be treated with high dose.	5.7, 22.7, and 68 mg tablets	2.5 to 7.5 mg/kg q24h PO
Ormetoprim + sulfadimethoxine	Trimethoprim-like drug used in combination with sulfadimethoxine. (See Primor.)				
Oxacillin (Prostaphlin and generic)	β-lactam antibiotic. Inhibits bacterial cell wall synthesis. Spectrum is limited to gram-positive bacteria, especially staphylococci.	Use cautiously in animals allergic to penicillin-like drugs.	Doses based on empiricism or extrapolation from human studies. No clinical efficacy studies available for dogs or cats. Administer on empty stomach, if possible.	250, 500 mg capsules; 50 mg/mL oral solution	22–40 mg/kg q8h PO
Oxazepam (Serax)	Benzodiazepine. Central-acting CNS depressant. Mechanism of action appears to be via potentiation of GABA–receptor mediated effects in CNS. Used for sedation and to stimulate appetite.	Sedation is most common side effect. Causes polyphagia. In cats, fatal hepatic necrosis has been reported from diazepam.	Doses based on empiricism. There have been no clinical trials in veterinary medicine.	15 mg tablets	Cat: appetite stimulant, 2.5 mg/cat PO
Oxtriphylline (Choledyl-SA)	Choline theophyllinate. Methylxanthine bronchodilator, similar in mechanism to theophylline.	See Theophylline.	Adverse effects similar to theophylline (see Theophylline). Some formulations (Theocon) contain oxtriphylline and guaifenesin. When administering slow-release tablet, do not crush tablet.	400, 600 mg tablets (oral solutions and syrup available in Canada, but not U.S.)	Dog: 47 mg/kg (equivalent to 30 mg/kg theophylline) q12h PO
Oxybutynin chloride (Ditropan)	Anticholinergic agent. Inhibits smooth muscle spasms via blocking action of acetylcholine. Used primarily to increase bladder capacity and to decrease spasms of urinary tract.	Adverse effects are related to anticholinergic effects (see Atropine), but are less frequent compared to other anticholinergic drugs. Administer physostigmine for overdose.	Results of clinical studies in animals have not been reported. Use in animals (and doses) is based on experience in people or anecdotal experience in animals.	5 mg tablets	Dog: 5 mg/dog q6–8h PO

Drug Name (Trade or Other Names)	Pharmacology and Indications	Adverse Effects and Precautions	Dosing Information and Comments	Formulations	Dosage
Oxymetholone (Anadrol)	Anabolic steroid. See Nandrolone decanoate (there are no differences in efficacy among the anabolic steroids.)	See Nandrolone decanoate.	See Nandrolone decanoate.	50 mg tablets	1–5 mg/kg q24h PO
Oxymorphone (Numorphan)	Opioid agonist. Action is similar to morphine, except that oxymorphone is more lipophilic than morphine and 10–15× more potent than morphine.	See Morphine.	See Morphine. There is some evidence that oxymorphone may have fewer cardiovascular effects compared to morphine. Since oxymorphone is more lipophilic, it is readily absorbed from epidural injection.	1.5 and 1 mg/mL injection	Analgesia: 0.1–0.2 mg/kg IV, SC, IM (as needed), redose with 0.05–0.1 mg/kg q1–2h; preanesthetic: 0.025–0.05 mg/kg IM or SC; Sedation: 0.05–0.02 mg/kg (with or without acepromazine) IM, SC
Oxytetracycline (Terramycin)	Tetracycine antibiotic. (See Tetracycline.) Same mechanism and spectrum as tetracycline. Oxytetracycline may be absorbed to higher extent.	Generally safe. Use cautiously in young animals. See precautions for tetracycline.	Oral dose forms are from large-animal use. Use of injectable long-acting forms has not been studied in small animals.	250 mg tablets; 100, 200 mg/mL injection	7.5–10 mg/kg IV q12h; 20 mg/kg q12h PO
Oxytocin (Pitocin, Syntocinon [nasal solution], and generic)	Stimulates uterine muscle contraction via action on specific oxytoxin receptors. Used to induce or maintain normal labor and delivery in pregnant animals. Does not increase milk production but will stimulate contraction leading to milk ejection.	Adverse effects are uncommon if used carefully. Fetal stress and progression of normal labor should be monitored closely.	Used to induce labor. In people, oxytocin is administered via injection, constant IV infusion, and intranasal solution. Repeat up to 3× every 30–60 min. (maximum dose is 3 units/cat).	10, 20 U/mL injection; 40 U/mL nasal solution	Dog: 5–20 U/dog IM or SC (repeat every 30 min for primary inertia) Cat: 2.5–3 U/cat IM or IV
2-PAM	See Pralidoxime chloride.				
Pamidronate (Aredia)	Bisphosphonate drug; they slow the formation and dissolution of hydroxyapatite crystals. Is used in animals to decrease calcium in conditions that cause hypercalcemia, such as cancer and vitamin D toxicosis.	No serious adverse effects have been identified; however, use in animals has been uncommon.	Bisphosphonates may be effective in animals for treatment of hypercalcemia of cancer and vitamin D toxicosis.	Available as 30, 60, and 90 mg vials for injection	Dog: 2 mg/kg IV, SC. Treatment of cholecalciferol toxicosis: 1.3–2 mg/kg × two treatments after toxin exposure. For IV infusion, dilute in fluid solution and administer over several hours (dilute 30 mg pamidronate in 250 mL of fluids).
Pancreatic enzyme	See Pancrelipase.				
Pancrelipase (Viokase)	Pancreatic enzyme. Used to treat pancreatic exocrine insufficiency. Provides lipase, amylase, and protease.	Adverse effects not reported.	Mix with food when administering, approximately 20 minutes prior to feeding.	16,800 U of lipase, 70,000 U of protease, and 70,000 U of amylase per 0.7 g. Also capsules and tablets.	Dog: Mix 2 tsp powder with food per 20 kg body weight, or 1–3 tsp/0.45 kg of food Cat: 1/2 tsp per cat with food
Pancuronium bromide (Pavulon)	Nondepolarizing neuromuscular blocker (see Atracurium)	See Atracurium.	See Atracurium.	1, 2 mg/mL injection	0.1 mg/kg IV, or start with 0.01 mg/kg and add 0.01 mg/kg doses every 30 min
Pantoprazole sodium (Protonix, Protonix IV)	Ulcer treatment. Proton pump inhibitor; indicated for treatment of gastroduodenal ulcer disease and gastroesophageal reflux. Pantoprazole is the first proton pump inhibitor for IV use. Antisecretory effects persist for > 24 hrs.	Side effects have not been reported in animals. However, in humans, there is concern about hypergastrinemia with chronic use.	Give IV dose over 15 minutes, and do not mix with other drugs that may interfere with stability.	40 mg delayed-release tablets; 0.4 mg/mL vials for IV injection	0.5 mg/kg q24h IV for 7–10 days for acute treatment of GI ulcer. For gastrin-secreting tumors, 1 mg/kg q12h IV
Paregoric (corrective Mixture)	Paregoric (opium tincture) is an outdated product used to treat diarrhea. Paregoric contains 2 mg of morphine in every 5 mL of paregoric.	See opiates (e.g., Morphine).	Use of paregoric has been replaced by more specific products, such as loperamide or diphenoxylate.	2 mg morphine per 5 mL of paregoric	0.05–0.06 mg/kg q12h PO

Drug Name (Trade or Other Names)	Pharmacology and Indications	Adverse Effects and Precautions	Dosing Information and Comments	Formulations	Dosage
Paroxetine (Paxil)	Selective serotonin re-uptake inhibitor (SSRI) much like fluoxetine (Prozac) in action. Used for obsessive-compulsive disorders, aggression, and other behavioral problems.	Some effects similar to fluoxetine, but in some animals, paroxetine is better tolerated.	Dosing recommendations are empirical.	10, 20, 30, 40 mg tablets	Dog: 0.5–1 mg/kg q24h PO Cat: 1/8 to 1/4 of a 10 mg tablet q24h PO
Penicillamine (Cuprimine, Depen)	Chelating agent for lead, copper, iron, and mercury. Used primarily in animals for treatment of copper toxicity and hepatitis associated with accumulation of copper. It also has been used to treat cystine calculi. Penicillamine has been used in people to treat rheumatoid arthritis.	Do not use in pregnant animals. In people, allergic reactions have been reported, as well as agranulocytosis and anemia.	Administer on an empty stomach (2 hrs before meals).	125, 250 mg capsules and 250 mg tablets	10–15 mg/kg q12h PO
Penicillin G benzathine (Benza-Pen and other names)	All benzathine penicillin G is combined with procaine penicillin G in commercial formulation.	Same as for other penicillins (see Amoxicillin)	Benzathine is not recommended for therapy because concentrations are too low to be therapeutic.	150,000 U/mL combined with 150,000 U/mL of procaine penicillin G	24,000 U/kg q48h IM
Penicillin G potassium; Penicillin G sodium (many brands)	β-lactam antibiotic. Action is similar to other penicillins (see Amoxicillin). Spectrum of penicillin G is limited to gram-positive bacteria and anaerobes.	Same as for other penicillins (see Amoxicillin)	See other penicillins (Amoxicillin).	5–20 million U vials	20,000–40,000 U/kg q6–8h IV or IM
Penicillin G procaine (generic)	Same as other forms of penicillin G, except procaine penicillin is absorbed slowly, producing concentrations for 12–24 hrs after injection.	Same as for other penicillins (see Amoxicillin)	Same as for other penicillins (amoxicillin). Avoid SC injection with procaine penicillin G.	300,000 U/mL suspension	20,000–40,000 U/kg q12–24h IM
Penicillin V (Pen-Vee)	Oral penicillin. Otherwise, same as other penicillins. Not highly absorbed, and narrow spectrum in comparison with other penicillin derivatives.	Same as for other penicillins (see Amoxicillin)	Same as for other penicillins (amoxicillin). Penicillin V should be administered on an empty stomach for maximum absorption (250 mg = 400,000 U).	250, 500 mg tablets	10 mg/kg q8h PO
Pentazocine (Talwin-V)	Synthetic opiate analgesic. Action is as agonist-antagonist (similar to buprenorphine or butorphanol).	Adverse effects similar to other opiates (see Butorphanol tartrate or Morphine)	See other opiates.	30 mg/mL injection	Dog: 1.65–3.3 mg/kg q4h IM Cat: 2.2–3.3 mg/kg q4h IV, IM, SC
Pentobarbital (Nembutal and generic)	Short-acting barbiturate anesthetic. Action is via nonselective CNS depression. Pentobarbital usually is used as IV anesthetic. Used to control severe seizures in animals. Duration of action may be 3–4 hrs.	Adverse effects are related to anesthetic action (see Thiopental sodium). Cardiac and respiratory depression is common.	Pentobarbital has narrow therapeutic index. When administering IV, inject first half of dose initially, then remainder of calculated dose gradually, until anesthetic effect is achieved.	50 mg/mL	25–30 mg/kg IV
Pentoxifylline (Trental)	Methylxanthine. Pentoxifylline is used primarily as a rheological agent in people (increases blood flow through narrow vessels). It may have anti-inflammatory action via inhibition of cytokine synthesis. Used in dogs for some dermatoses (dermatomyositis) and vasculitis.	May cause similar signs as other methylxanthines (see Theophylline). Nausea and vomiting have been reported in people. When broken tablet is administered to cats, the taste is unpleasant.	Results of clinical studies in animals have not been reported. Use in animals (and doses) is based on experience in people or anecdotal experience in animals.	400 mg tablets	Dog—dermatologic use: 10 mg/kg q12h PO. For other uses: 10 mg/kg q8–12h PO, or 400 mg/dog for most animals. Cat: 1/4 of a 400 mg tablet (100 mg) q8–12h PO

Drug Name (Trade or Other Names)	Pharmacology and Indications	Adverse Effects and Precautions	Dosing Information and Comments	Formulations	Dosage
Pepto-Bismol	See Bismuth subsalicylate.				
Phenobarbital (Luminal and generic)	Long-acting barbiturate. See other barbiturates (Thiopental sodium). Phenobarbital's major use is as an anticonvulsant, in which it potentiates inhibitory actions of GABA.	Adverse effects are dose-related. Phenobarbital causes polyphagia, sedation, ataxia, and lethargy. Some tolerance develops to side effects after initial therapy. Hepatotoxicity has been reported in some dogs receiving high doses.	Phenobarbital doses should be carefully adjusted via monitoring serum/plasma concentrations. Optimum range for therapeutic effect is 15–40 mcg/mL.	15, 30, 60, 100 mg tablets; 30, 60, 65, and 130 mg/mL injection; 4 mg/mL oral elixir solution	Dog: 2–8 mg/kg q12h PO Cat: 2–4 mg/kg q12h PO Status epilepticus: administer in increments of 10–20 mg/kg IV (to effect)
Phenoxybenzamine (Dibenzyline)	α_1-adrenergic antagonist. Binds α_1-receptor on smooth muscle, causing relaxation. Potent vasodilator. Used primarily to treat peripheral vasoconstriction. In some animals, has been used to relax urethral smooth muscle.	Causes prolonged hypotension in animals. Use carefully in animals with cardiovascular compromise.	Results of clinical studies in animals have not been reported. Use in animals (and doses) is based on experience in people or limited experimental experience in animals.	10 mg capsules	Dog: 0.25 mg/kg q8–12h PO, or 0.5 mg/kg q24h. Cat: 2.5 mg/cat q8–12h, or 0.5 mg/kg q12h PO. (In cats, doses as high as 0.5 mg/kg IV have been used to relax urethral smooth muscle.)
Phentolamine mesylate (Regitine, [Rogitine in Canada])	Nonselective α-adrenergic blocker. Vasodilator. Blocks stimulation of α-receptors on vascular smooth muscle. Primarily used to treat hypertension.	May cause excess hypotension with high doses or in animals that are dehydrated. May cause tachycardia.	Results of clinical studies in animals have not been reported. Use in animals (and doses) is based on experience in people or anecdotal experience in animals. Titrate dose for each patient to produce desired vasodilation.	5 mg vials for injection	0.02–0.1 mg/kg IV
Phenylbutazone (Butazolidin and generic)	NSAID. See Flunixin meglumine. Phenylbutazone is used primarily for arthritis and various forms of musculoskeletal pain and inflammation.	Phenylbutazone is generally well-tolerated in dogs, but there is no data for cats. Adverse effects possible are GI toxicity (see Flunixin meglumine). Do not administer injectable formulation IM. Phenylbutazone causes bone marrow depression in people, which also is possible in dogs.	Doses are based primarily on manufacturer's recommendations and clinical experience. There have been no comparative trials demonstrating efficacy of one NSAID over another. Not approved in U.S. for cats, but has been used in cats in Europe.	100, 200, 400 mg and 1g tablets; 200 mg/mL injection	Dog: 15–22 mg/kg q8–12h (44 mg/kg/day) PO or IV (800 mg/dog maximum) Cat: 6–8 mg/kg q12h IV or PO
Phenylephrine (Neo-Synephrine)	Specific adrenergic agonist; specific for α_1-receptor; same as methoxamine.	Same as for methoxamine	Same as for methoxamine. Phenylephrine also is used commonly as topical vasoconstrictor (as in nasal decongestants).	10 mg/mL injection; 1% nasal solution	0.01 mg/kg every 15 min IV; 0.1 mg/kg every 15 min IM or SC
Phenylpropanolamine (PPA) (Dexatrim, Propagest, Proin PPA, Propalin syrup)	Adrenergic agonist. Used as decongestant, mild bronchodilator, and to increase tone of urinary sphincter. (See Ephedrine, Pseudoephedrine).	Adverse effects are attributed to excess stimulation of adrenergic (α and β) receptors. See Ephedrine. Side effects: tachycardia, cardiac effects, CNS excitement, restlessness, and appetite suppression.	Phenylpropanolamine is available in variety of dose forms, usually used for treatment of cough/colds in people. Many preparations contain other ingredients.	15, 25, 30, 50 mg tablets; 25, 50, 75 mg liver-flavored tablet and 25 mg/mL vanilla-flavored oral solution	Dog: 1.5–2 mg/kg q12h PO
Phenytoin (Dilantin)	Anticonvulsant. Depresses nerve conduction via blockade of sodium channels. Also classified as class I antiarrhythmic. Commonly used as anticonvulsant in people, but not effective in dogs and not used in cats.	Adverse effects: sedation, gingival hyperplasia, skin reactions, CNS toxicity. Do not administer to pregnant animals.	Because of short half-life and poor efficacy in dogs and questionable safety in cats, other anticonvulsants are used as first choice before phenytoin.	30, 125 mg/mL oral suspension; 30, 100 mg capsules; 50 mg/mL injection	Dog: (Antiepileptic) 20–35 mg/kg q8h. (Antiarrhythmic) 30 mg/kg q8h PO or 10 mg/kg IV over 5 min

Drug Name (Trade or Other Names)	Pharmacology and Indications	Adverse Effects and Precautions	Dosing Information and Comments	Formulations	Dosage
Physostigmine (Antilirium)	Cholinesterase inhibitor. Antidote for anticholinergic intoxication, especially intoxication that exhibits CNS signs. Major difference between physostigmine and neostigmine or pyridostigmine is that physostigmine crosses blood–brain barrier and the others do not.	Adverse effects attributed to excessive cholinergic effects (treat overdoses with atropine)	Physostigmine is indicated primarily only for treatment of intoxication. For routine systemic use of anticholinesterase drug, neostigmine and pyridostigmine have fewer side effects. When used, frequency of dose may be increased, based on observation of effects.	1 mg/mL injection	0.02 mg/kg q12h IV
Phytonadione	See Vitamin K$_1$.				
Phytomenadione	See Vitamin K$_1$.				
Pimobendan (Vetmedin)	Phosphodiesterase 3 inhibitor and a calcium sensitizer that acts as an inotropic vasodilator. Currently licensed in Europe for treating CHF due to dilated cardiomyopathy and valvular insufficiency.	Potentially arrhythmogenic. Use cautiously in dogs with atrial fibrillation.	Currently not available in the U.S. but is undergoing experimental studies	2.5 and 5 mg capsules	Dog: 4–8 kg (body weight), 1.25 mg q12h; 8–20 kg, 2.5 mg q12h; 20–40 kg, 5 mg q12h; 40–60 kg, 10 mg q12h; > 60 kg, 15 mg q12h Cat: dose not established
Piperacillin (Pipracil)	β-lactam antibiotic of the acylureido-penicillin class. Similar to other penicillins, except with high activity against *Pseudomonas aeruginosa*. Also good activity against streptococci.	Same precautions as for other injectable penicillins (e.g., ampicillin)	Reconstituted solution should be used within 24 hours (or 7 days if refrigerated). Piperacillin is combined with tazobactam (β-lactamase inhibitor) in Zosyn.	2, 3, 4, 40 g vials for injection	40 mg/kg IV or IM q6h
Piperazine (many)	Antiparasitic compound. Produces neuromuscular blockade in parasite through inhibition of neurotransmitter, which causes paralysis of worms. Used primarily for treatment of helminth (ascarid) infections.	Remarkably safe in all species	Used to treat all species for roundworms	860 mg powder; 140 mg capsules; 170, 340, and 800 mg/mL oral solution	44–66 mg/kg PO, administered once
Piroxicam (Feldene and generic)	NSAID of the oxicam class. Clinical effects are similar to other NSAIDs (see Aspirin, Flunixin meglumine). Piroxicam has been used for treatment of transitional cell carcinoma in dogs.	Elimination of piroxicam is slow; use cautiously in dogs. Adverse effects are primarily GI toxicity (ulcers); see Flunixin meglumine.	Piroxicam is primarily used to treat arthritis and other musculoskeletal conditions, but there are reports of its activity for treating certain tumors (e.g., transitional cell carcinoma of bladder).	10 mg capsules	Dog: 0.3 mg/kg q48h PO Cat: dose not established, but doses similar to those used in dogs have been given
Pitressin (ADH)	See Vasopressin and Desmopressin acetate.				
Plicamycin (old name is mithramycin) (Mithracin)	Anticancer agent. Action is to combine with DNA in presence of divalent cations and inhibit DNA and RNA synthesis. Lowers serum calcium. May have direct action on osteoclasts to decrease serum calcium. Used for carcinomas and treatment of hypercalcemia.	Adverse effects have not been reported in animals. In people, hypocalcemia and GI toxicity have been reported. May cause bleeding problems. *Drug interactions:* Do not use with drugs that may increase the risk of bleeding (e.g., NSAIDs, heparin, or anticoagulants).	Results of clinical studies in animals have not been reported. Use in animals (and doses) is based on experience in people or anecdotal experience in animals.	2.5 mg injection	Antihypercalcemic (dogs or cats): 25 mcg/kg q24h IV (slow infusion) over 4 hrs; antineoplastic (dogs): 25–30 mcg/kg q24h IV (slow infusion) for 8–10 days

Drug Name (Trade or Other Names)	Pharmacology and Indications	Adverse Effects and Precautions	Dosing Information and Comments	Formulations	Dosage
Polyethylene glycol electrolyte solution (GoLYTELY)	Saline cathartic. (See Magnesium citrate.) Nonabsorbable compounds that increase water secretion into bowel via osmotic effect. Used for bowel evacuation prior to surgical or diagnostic procedure.	Water and electrolyte loss with high doses or prolonged use. (See also Magnesium citrate.)	Used primarily to evacuate bowel as preparation for procedures	Oral solution	25 mL/kg, repeat in 2–4 hr PO
Polysulfated glycosaminoglycan (PSGAG) (Adequan Canine)	Large molecular weight compounds similar to normal constituents of healthy joints. Chondroprotective. Inhibits enzymes that may degrade articular cartilage. Used primarily to treat or prevent degenerative joint disease.	Adverse effects are rare. Allergic reactions are possible. PSGAG has heparin-like effects and may potentiate bleeding problems in some animals.	Doses are derived from empirical evidence, experimental studies, and clinical studies in dogs. (see Compend Contin Educ 16:501, 1994; or J Am Vet Med Assoc 204:1245, 1994). Although effective for acute arthritis, may not be as effective for chronic arthropathy.	100 mg/mL injection in 5 mL vial (for horses, vials are 250 mg/mL)	4.4 mg/kg IM, twice weekly for up to 4 weeks
Potassium bromide (KBr)	Anticonvulsant. Anticonvulsant action is to stabilize neuronal cell membranes. Bromide ordinarily is used in patients refractory to phenobarbital.	Adverse effects are related to high levels of bromide. Signs of toxicosis are CNS depression, weakness, ataxia. Consider using sodium bromide in patients with hypoadrenocorticism.	Bromide usually is administered in combination with phenobarbital. Monitor serum bromide concentrations to adjust dose. Effective plasma concentrations should be 1–2 mg/mL, but if used alone (without phenobarbital), higher concentrations of 2–4 mg/mL may be needed. Diets high in chloride will cause shorter half-life and need for higher dose. Sodium bromide can be substituted for potassium bromide. Note that 30 mg/kg potassium bromide is equal to 20 mg/kg of elemental bromide.	Usually prepared as oral solution. (No commercial formulation, but can be formulated by a pharmacist)	Standard starting dose: 30–40 mg/kg q24h PO. If administered without phenobarbital, higher doses of up to 40–50 mg/kg by monitoring plasma concentrations. Rapid IV loading dose: 800 mg/kg (sodium bromide) given over 8 hours slowly IV. Rapid oral loading dose: 400–600 mg/kg PO divided over 3–4 days. Slow (60 day) oral loading dose: 60 mg/kg/day (30 mg/kg q12h) for 60 days, then monitor blood level. If in therapeutic range, switch to maintenance dose of 20–30 mg/kg/day.
Potassium chloride (generic)	Potassium supplement. Used for treatment of hypokalemia. Usually added to fluid solutions.	Toxicity from high potassium concentrations can be dangerous. Hyperkalemia can lead to cardiovascular toxicity (bradycardia and arrest) and muscular weakness. Oral potassium supplements can cause nausea and stomach irritation.	1 g of potassium chloride provides 13.41 mEq of potassium. When potassium is supplemented in fluids, do not administer at a rate faster than 0.5 mEq/kg/hr.	Various concentrations for injection (usually 2 mEq/mL). Oral suspension and oral solution.	0.5 mEq potassium/kg/day, or supplement 10–40 mEq/500 mL of fluids, depending on serum potassium
Potassium citrate (generic, Urocit-K)	Alkalinizes urine and may increase urine citric acid. Used for calcium oxalate urolithiasis. Also used for renal tubular acidosis.	Same as potassium chloride.	1 g of potassium citrate provides 9.26 mEq of potassium.	5 mEq tablet. Some forms are in combination with potassium chloride.	2.2 mEq/100 kCal of energy q24h PO; or 40–75 mg/kg q12h PO
Potassium gluconate (Kaon, Tumil-K, generic)	Same as for potassium chloride. Used for renal tubular acidosis.	Same as for potassium chloride	1 g of potassium gluconate provides 4.27 mEq of potassium.	2 mEq tablets; 500 mg tablets; Kaon elixir is 20 mg/15 mL elixir.	Dog: 0.5 mEq/kg q12–24h PO Cat: 2–8 mEq/day divided twice daily, PO
Potassium phosphate	Phosphorus supplement. Used for severe hypophosphatemia associated with diabetic ketoacidosis.				0.03–0.12 mmol/kg/hour IV
Pralidoxime chloride (2-PAM) (Protopam)	Used for treatment of organophosphate toxicosis	Adverse effects have not been reported.	When treating intoxication, consult poison control center for precise guidelines.	50 mg/mL injection	20 mg/kg q8–12h; initial dose IV slow, or IM

Drug Name (Trade or Other Names)	Pharmacology and Indications	Adverse Effects and Precautions	Dosing Information and Comments	Formulations	Dosage
Praziquantel (Droncit)	Antiparasitic drug. Action on parasites related to neuromuscular toxicity and paralysis via altered permeability to calcium. Used primarily to treat infections caused by tapeworms.	Vomiting occurs at high doses. Anorexia and transient diarrhea have been reported. Safe in pregnant animals.	Dose recommendations based on label dose supplied by manufacturer.	23, 34 mg tablet; 56.8 mg/mL injection	Dog (oral dose)—<6.8 kg: 7.5 mg/kg PO, once; >6.8 kg: 5 mg/kg PO, once. Dog (injection)—≤2.3 kg: 7.5 mg/kg IM or SC, once; 2.7–4.5 kg: 6.3 mg/kg IM or SC, once; ≤5 kg: 5 mg/kg IM or SC, once. Cat (oral dosage)—<1.8 kg: 6.3 mg/kg PO, once; >1.8 kg: 5 mg/kg PO, once. For *Paragonimus* infection use 25 mg/kg q8h PO for 2–3 days. Cat (injection)—5 mg/kgIM or SC.
Prazocin (Minipress)	α_1-adrenergic blocker. Relaxes smooth muscle, especially of vasculature. Prazocin is used as vasodilator and to relax smooth muscle (occasionally urethral muscle).	High doses cause vasodilation and hypotension.	Titrate dose to needs of individual patient. Results of clinical studies in animals have not been reported. Use in animals (and doses) is based on experience in people or anecdotal experience in animals.	1, 2, 5 mg capsules	0.5–2 mg/animal (1 mg/15 kg) q8–12h PO
Prednisolone (Delta-Cortef and many others)	Glucocorticoid anti-inflammatory drug. Potency is approximately 4× cortisol. (See Betamethasone for details.)	All glucocorticoids produce expected (and sometimes unavoidable) side effects. See Betamethasone for partial list of side effects.	Doses for prednisolone are based on severity of underlying condition. Doses listed are for dogs. Cats often require 2× the dog dose.	5 and 20 mg tablets	Dog (cats often require 2× dog dose)—anti-inflammatory: 0.5–1 mg/kg q12–24h IV, IM, PO initially, then taper to q48h; immunosuppressive: 2.2–6.6 mg/kg/day IV, IM, PO initially, then taper to 2–4 mg/kg q48h; replacement therapy: 0.2–0.3 mg/kg/day PO; shock, spinal trauma: see Prednisolone sodium succinate
Prednisolone sodium succinate (Solu-Delta-Cortef)	Same as for prednisolone, except that this is a water-soluble formulation intended for acute therapy when high IV doses are needed for rapid effect. Used for treatment of shock and CNS trauma	Adverse effects are not expected from single administration; however, with repeated use, other side effects are possible (see Betamethasone).	See Prednisolone.	100, 200 mg vials for injection (10 and 50 mg/mL)	Shock: 15–30 mg/kg IV (repeat in 4–6 hr) CNS trauma: 15–30 mg/kg IV, taper to 1–2 mg/kg q12h
Prednisone (Deltasone and generic; Meticorten for injection)	Same as for prednisolone, except that, after administration, prednisone is converted to prednisolone	Same as for prednisolone	Same as for prednisolone. There are no known contraindications in which prednisolone is preferred over prednisone.	1, 2.5, 5, 10, 20, 25, and 50 mg tablets; 1 mg/mL syrup (Liquid Pred in 5% alcohol) and 1 mg/mL oral solution (in 5% alcohol)	Same as for prednisolone.
Primidone (Mylepsin, Neurosyn [Mysoline in Canada])	Anticonvulsant. Primidone is converted to phenylethylmalonamide and phenobarbital, both of which have anticonvulsant activity, but most of activity (85%) is probably due to phenobarbital. See Phenobarbital for more details.	Adverse effects are same as for phenobarbital. Primidone has been associated with idiosyncratic hepatotoxicity in dogs. Although some labels caution its use in cats, one study in experimental cats determined that it is safe if used at recommended doses.	See Phenobarbital. When monitoring therapy with primidone, phenobarbital plasma concentrations should be measured to estimate anticonvulsant effect.	50 and 250 mg tablets	8–10 mg/kg q8–12h as initial dose PO, then adjust via monitoring to 10–15 mg/kg q8h.
Primor (ormetoprim + sulfadimethoxine) (Primor)	Antibacterial drug. Ormetoprim inhibits bacterial dihydrofolate reductase, sulfonamide competes with *p*-aminobenzoic acid (PABA) for synthesis of nucleic acids. Bactericidal/bacteriostatic. Broad antibacterial spectrum and active against some coccidia.	Several adverse effects have been reported from sulfonamides (See Trimethoprim/sulfonamides). No adverse effects reported from ormetoprim.	Doses listed are based on manufacturer's recommendations. Controlled trials have demonstrated efficacy for treatment of pyoderma on once-daily schedule.	Combination tablet (ormetoprim + sulfadimethoxine)	27 mg/kg on first day, followed by 13.5 mg/kg q24h PO

Drug Name (Trade or Other Names)	Pharmacology and Indications	Adverse Effects and Precautions	Dosing Information and Comments	Formulations	Dosage
Procainamide (Pronestyl, Procanbid, generic)	Antiarrhythmic drug. Class I antiarrhythmic used primarily for treatment of ventricular arrhythmias. Action is to inhibit sodium influx into cardiac cell via sodium channel blockade.	Adverse effects include cardiac arrhythmias, cardiac depression, tachycardia, and hypotension. In people, procainamide produces hypersensitivity effects (lupus-like reactions), but these have not been reported in animals. *Drug interactions:* Cimetidine may increase plasma concentrations.	Since dogs do not produce active metabolite (*N*-acetyl-procainamide), dose may be higher to control some arrhythmias compared to dose for people. Monitor plasma concentrations during chronic therapy (effective plasma concentration in experimental dogs is 20 mcg/mL). In animals, there is no evidence that slow-release oral formulations produce longer duration of sustained blood concentrations.	250, 375, 500 mg tablet or capsule; 100, 500 mg/mL injection	Dog: 10–30 mg/kg q6h PO (q8h for continuous release [CR]) to a maximum dose of 40 mg/kg; 8–20 mg/kg IV, IM; 25–50 mcg/kg/min IV infusion. Cat: 3–8 mg/kg IM, PO q6–8h
Prochlorperazine + isopropamide (Darbazine)	Combination product. Chlorpromazine is a central-acting dopamine antagonist (antiemetic); isopropamide is an anticholinergic drug (atropine-like effects). Used primarily to control vomiting in animals.	Side effects are attributed to each component. Prochlorperazine produces phenothiazine-like effects (see Acepromazine). Isopropamide produces antimuscarinic effects (see Atropine). Use of antimuscarinic drugs is contraindicated in animals with gastroparesis and should be used cautiously in animals with diarrhea.	Doses are based on manufacturer's recommendations	No. 1, 2, and 3 capsules	Dog and cat: 0.14–0.2 mL/kg q12h SC Dog 2–7 kg: 1–#1 capsule q12h PO Dog 7–14 kg: 1–#2 capsule q12h PO Dog > 14 kg: 1–#3 capsule q12h PO
Progesterone, repositol	See Medroxyprogesterone acetate.				
Promethazine (Phenergan)	Phenothiazine with strong antihistamine effects. Used for treatment of allergy and as antiemetic (motion sickness).	Adverse effects include sedation and antimuscarinic (atropine-like) effects. Both phenothiazine effects (see Acepromazine) and anticholinergic (see Atropine) effects are possible in some patients.	Results of clinical studies in animals have not been reported. Use in animals (and doses) is based on experience in people or anecdotal experience in animals.	6.25 and 25 mg/5 mL syrup; 12.5, 25, 50 mg tablets; 25, 50 mg/mL injection	0.2–0.4 mg/kg q6–8h IV, IM, PO (up to a maximum dose of 1 mg/kg)
Propantheline bromide (Pro-Banthine)	Anticholinergic (antimuscarinic) drug. Blocks acetylcholine receptor to produce parasympatholytic effects (atropine-like effects). (See Atropine.) Used to decrease smooth muscle contraction and secretion of GI tract. Used to treat vagal-mediated cardiovascular effects.	Side effects are attributed to excess anticholinergic (antimuscarinic) effects (see Atropine). Treat overdoses with physostigmine.	Propantheline has not been evaluated in clinical trials in animals, but propantheline is often the drug of choice for oral therapy in cases in which an anticholinergic effect is desired.	7.5, 15 mg tablet	0.25–0.5 mg/kg q8–12h PO
Propiopromazine (Tranvet, Largon)	Phenothiazine sedative. Also has antiemetic, antihistaminic actions.	See other phenothiazines (Acepromazine).	Results of clinical studies in animals have not been reported. Use in animals (and doses) is based on experience in people or anecdotal experience in animals.	20 mg/mL injection	1.1–4.4 mg/kg q12–24h

Drug Name (Trade or Other Names)	Pharmacology and Indications	Adverse Effects and Precautions	Dosing Information and Comments	Formulations	Dosage
Propofol (Rapinovet [veterinary]; Diprivan [human])	Anesthetic. Used for induction or producing short-term general anesthesia. Mechanism of action is not well-defined, but may be barbiturate-like. Propofol may be used as induction agent, followed by inhalation with halothane or isoflurane.	Apnea and respiratory depression is most common adverse effects. Adverse effects attributed to general anesthetic properties.	Propofol is primarily used for general anesthesia, or adjunct for general anesthesia. Propofol's advantage over other agents is smooth, rapid recovery. Use strict aseptic technique for administration. Propofol may be diluted in 5% dextrose, lactated Ringer's solution, or 0.9% saline, but not to less than 2 mg/mL concentration.	1% (10 mg/mL) injection in 20 mL ampules	6.6 mg/kg IV slowly over 60 sec. Constant rate IV infusions have been used at 2 mg/kg/hr
Propranolol (Inderal)	β-adrenergic blocker. Nonselective for β_1- and β_2-adrenergic receptors. Class II antiarrhythmic. Used primarily to decrease heart rate, cardiac conduction, tachyarrhythmias, and blood pressure.	Adverse effects related to β_1-blocking effects on heart. Causes cardiac depression, decreases cardiac output. β_2-blocking effects can cause bronchoconstriction. Decreases insulin secretion.	Usually, dose is titrated according to patient's response. Start with low dose and increase gradually to desired effect. Clearance relies on hepatic blood flow; use cautiously in animals with impaired hepatic perfusion.	10, 20, 40, 60, 80, and 90 mg tablets; 1 mg/mL injection; 4 and 8 mg/mL oral solution	Dog: 20–60 mcg/kg over 5–10 min IV; 0.2–1 mg/kg PO q8h (titrate dose to effect) Cat: 0.4–1.2 mg/kg (2.5–5 mg/cat) PO q8h
Propylthiouracil (PTU) (generic, Propyl-Thyracil)	Antithyroid drug. See Methimazole. Compared to methimizole, PTU inhibits conversion of T_4 to T_3.	Adverse effects in cats include hemolytic anemia, thrombocytopenia, and other signs of immune-mediated disease. (J Am Vet Med Assoc 184:806, 1984.)	Use of PTU in most cats has been replaced with methimazole.	50 and 100 mg tablets	11 mg/kg q12h PO
Prostaglandin $F_{2\alpha}$ (dinoprost) (Lutalyse)	Prostaglandin induces leutolysis. Has been used to treat open pyometra in animals. Use for inducing abortion has been questioned.	Side effects include vomiting, diarrhea, and abdominal discomfort.	Use in treating pyometra should be monitored carefully.	5 mg/mL solution for injection	Pyometra (dog): 0.1–0.2 mg/kg, once daily for 5 days SC; (cat): 0.1–0.25 mg/kg, once daily for 5 days SC. Abortion (dog): 0.025–0.05 mg (25–50 mcg/kg) q12h IM; (cat): 0.5–1 mg/kg IM for 2 injections.
Pseudoephedrine (Sudafed, and many others [some formulations have other ingredients])	Adrenergic agonist. Similar to ephedrine, phenylpropanolamine in action. Used to increase peripheral resistance, as a decongestant, and in animals to treat urinary incontinence.	Side effects attributed to adrenergic effects (excitement, rapid heart rate, arrhythmias) (see Ephedrine, Phenylpropanolamine)	Although clinical trials have not been conducted for comparison, it is believed that pseudoephedrin's action and efficacy is similar to ephedrine and phenylpropanolamine.	30, 60 mg tablets; 120 mg capsules; 6 mg/mL syrup	Dog: 0.2–0.4 mg/kg (or 15–60 mg/dog) q8–12h PO
Psyllium (Metamucil and others)	Bulk-forming laxative. Use for treatment of constipation and bowel evacuation. Action is to absorb water and expand to provide increased bulk and moisture content to the stool, which encourages normal peristalsis and bowel motility.	Adverse effects have not been reported in animals. Intestinal impaction can occur with overuse, or in patients with inadequate fluid intake.	Results of clinical studies in animals have not been reported. Use in animals (and doses) is based on experience in people or anecdotal experience in animals.	Available as powder	1 tsp/5–10 kg (added to each meal)
Pyrantel pamoate (Nemex, Strongid)	Antiparasitic drug. Acts to block ganglionic neurotransmission via cholinergic action.	No adverse effects reported	Dose recommendations based on manufacturer's recommendations	180 mg/mL paste; 50 mg/mL suspension	Dog: 5 mg/kg once PO and repeat in 7–10 days Cat: 20 mg/kg once PO
Pyridostigmine bromide (Mestinon, Regonol)	Anticholinesterase. Same as for neostigmine, except that pyridostigmine has longer duration of action.	Same as for neostigmine, except that adverse effects may persist longer. *Drug interactions:* Since this product contains bromide, use cautiously in patients already receiving bromide (e.g., potassium bromide for epilepsy).	Same as for neostigmine	12 mg/mL oral syrup; 60 mg tablets; 5 mg/mL injection	Antimyasthenic: 0.02–0.04 mg/kg q2h IV, or 0.5–3 mg/kg q8–12h PO Antidote for muscle blockade: 0.15–0.3 mg/kg IM, IV

Drug Name (Trade or Other Names)	Pharmacology and Indications	Adverse Effects and Precautions	Dosing Information and Comments	Formulations	Dosage
Pyridoxine	Vitamin B$_6$				
Pyrimethamine (Daraprim)	Antibacterial, antiprotozoal drug. Blocks dihydrofolate reductase enzyme, which inhibits synthesis of reduced folate and nucleic acids. Activity of pyrimethamine is more specific against protozoa than bacteria.	When administered with trimethoprim-sulfonamide combinations, anemia has been observed. Folic or folinic acid has been supplemented to prevent anemia, but benefit of this treatment is unclear.	Used either alone or in combination with sulfonamides	25 mg tablets	Dog: 1 mg/kg q24h PO for 14–21 days (5 days for *Neosporum caninum*) Cat: 0.5–1 mg/kg q24h PO for 14–28 days
Quibron	See Theophylline.				
Quinacrine (Atabrine [no longer available in U.S.])	Outdated antimalarial drug. Used occasionally for treatment of protozoa (*Giardia*). Inhibits nucleic acid synthesis in parasite.	Side effects are common. Vomiting occurs after oral administration.	Doses listed are for treatment of *Giardia*.	100 mg tablets	Dog: 6.6 mg/kg q12h PO for 5 days Cat: 11 mg/kg q24h PO for 5 days
Quinidine gluconate (Quinaglute, Duraquin)	Antiarrhythmic drug. Class I antiarrhythmic. Action is to inhibit sodium influx via blockade of sodium channels. Used to treat ventricular arrhythmias and occasionally atrial fibrillation.	Side effects with quinidine are more common than procainamide and include nausea and vomiting. Adverse effects: hypotension, tachycardia (due to antivagal effect). *Drug interactions:* Co-administration with digoxin may increase digoxin concentrations.	Quinidine is not used as commonly as other Class I antiarrhythmic drugs. Doses calculated according to amount of quinidine base in each product. 324 mg quinidine gluconate = 202 mg quinidine base.	324 mg tablets; 80 mg/mL injection	Dog: 6–20 mg/kg q6h IM; 6–20 mg/kg q6–8h PO (of base)
Quinidine polygalacturonate (Cardioquin)	Same as for quinidine gluconate	Same as for quinidine gluconate	Doses calculated according to amount of quinidine base in each product	275 mg tablets	Dog: 6–20 mg/kg q6h PO (of base) (275 mg quinidine polygalacturonate = 167 mg quinidine base)
Quinidine sulfate (Cin-Quin, Quinora)	Same as for quinidine gluconate	Same as for quinidine gluconate	Doses calculated according to amount of quinidine base in each product. 300 mg quinidine sulfate = 250 mg quinidine base.	100, 200, 300 mg tablets; 200, 300 mg capsules; 200 mg/mL injection	Dog: 6–20 mg/kg q6–8h PO (of base); 5–10 mg/kg IV
Racemethionine (DL-methionine) (Uroeze, Methio-Form, and generic. Human forms include Pedameth, Uracid, and generic.)	Urinary acidifer. Lowers urinary pH. Also has been used to protect against acetaminophen overdose in people by restoring hepatic concentrations of glutathione. In people, it also is used to treat dermatitis caused by urinary incontinence (reduces urine ammonia).	Adverse effects have not been reported. Do not use in patients with metabolic acidosis or hepatic function impairment. Do not use in young cats.	Used for urinary acidification. Use for acetaminophen toxicity has been replaced by acetylcysteine.	500 mg tablets, powders added to animal's food; 75 mg/5 mL pediatric oral solution; 200 mg capsules	Dog: 150–300 mg/kg q24h PO Cat: 1–1.5 g/cat PO (added to food each day)
Ranitidine (Zantac)	Histamine H$_2$-antagonist. See Cimetidine for details. Same as cimetidine except 4–10× more potent and longer acting.	See Cimetidine. Ranitidine may have fewer effects on endocrine function and drug interactions, compared to cimetidine.	See Cimetidine. Pharmacokinetic information in dogs suggests that ranitidine may be administered less often than cimetidine to achieve continuous suppression of stomach acid secretion. Ranitidine may stimulate stomach emptying and colon motility via anticholinesterase action.	75, 150, 300 mg tablets; 150, 300 mg capsules; 25 mg/mL injection	Dog: 2 mg/kg q8h IV, PO Cat: 2.5 mg/kg q12h IV; 3.5 mg/kg q12h PO.
Retinoids	See Isotretinoin and Vitamin A				
Retinol	See Vitamin A.				
Riboflavin (vitamin B$_2$)	See Vitamin B$_2$.				

Drug Name (Trade or Other Names)	Pharmacology and Indications	Adverse Effects and Precautions	Dosing Information and Comments	Formulations	Dosage
Rifampin (Rifadin)	Antibacterial. Action is to inhibit bacterial RNA synthesis. Spectrum of action includes staphylococci and mycobacteria. Other susceptible bacteria include streptococci. Used in people primarily for treatment of tuberculosis	Adverse effects not reported in animals, but in people, hypersensitivity and flulike symptoms are reported. *Drug interactions:* Multiple drug interactions are possible. Induces cytochrome P-450 enzymes. Drugs affected include barbiturates, chloramphenicol, and corticosteroids.	Results of clinical studies in animals have not been reported. Use in animals (and doses) is based on experience in people or anecdotal experience in animals. Rifampin is highly lipid soluble and has been used to treat intracellular infections. Administer on an empty stomach.	150, 300 mg capsules; injection solution: 600 mg Rifadin IV	5 mg/kg q12–24h PO
Ringer's solution, lactated (generic)	IV solution for replacement	Monitor pulmonary pressure when infusing high doses.	When administering IV fluid solution, monitor rate and electrolyte concentrations carefully.	250, 500, 1000 mL bags for infusion	40–50 mg/kg/day IV, SC, IP
Salicylate	See Aspirin.				
Selamectin (Revolution)	Topical parasiticide and heartworm prevention	Transient localized alopecia with or without inflammation at or near the site of application was observed in approximately 1% of 691 treated cats. Other signs observed rarely included GI signs, anorexia, lethargy, salivation, tachypnea, and muscle tremors.	Recommended for use in dogs 6 weeks of age or older and in cats 8 weeks of age or older	Available in six separate dose strengths	The recommended minimum dose is 6 mg/kg topically; see insert.
Selegiline (deprenyl) (Anipryl [also known as deprenyl and L-deprenyl]; human dose form is Eldepryl)	Action is to inhibit specific monoamine oxidase (MAO type B). Specifically, it appears to inhibit degradation of dopamine in CNS. In people, it is primarily used to treat Parkinson's disease and other neurodegenerative diseases (in combination with levodopa). In dogs, it is approved to control clinical signs of pituitary-dependent hyperadrenocorticism (Cushing's disease) and to treat cognitive dysfunction in geriatric dogs.	Adverse effects have not been reported in dogs. However, amphetamine-like signs can be produced in experimental animals. At high doses in dogs, hyperactivity has been observed (doses > 3 mg/kg).	In the multicenter trial performed by Deprenyl Animal Health, Inc. selegiline controlled the clinical signs of >70% of dogs with hyperadrenocorticism. However, other investigators have reported efficacy rates as low as 20%	2, 5, 10, 15, and 30 mg tablets	Dog: Begin with 1 mg/kg q24h PO. If there is no response within 2 months, increase dose to maximum of 2 mg/kg q24h PO. Cat: dose not established.
Senna (Senokot)	Laxative. Acts via local stimulation or via contact with intestinal mucosa	Adverse effects not reported for animals	Doses and indications are not well established for veterinary medicine. Use is strictly through anecdotal experience.	Granules in concentrate, or syrup	Dog (syrup): 5–10 ml/dog q24h; (granules): 1/2–1 tsp/dog q24h PO Cat (syrup): 5 mL/cat q24h; (granules) 1/2 teaspoon per cat q24h (with food)
Septra (sulfamethoxazole + trimethoprim)	See Trimethoprim + sulfadiazine.				
Sevoflurane	Inhalant anesthetic				Induction: 8% Maintenance: 3% – 6% to effect
Sodium bicarbonate (NaHCO₃) (generic, baking soda, Soda Mint)	Alkalizing agent. Antacid. Used to treat systemic acidosis or to alkalize urine. Increases plasma and urinary concentrations of bicarbonate	Adverse effects attributed to alkalizing activity. *Drug interactions:* When administered orally, interaction may occur to decrease absorption of other drugs (partial list includes anticholinergic drugs, ketoconazole, fluoroquinolones, tetracyclines).	When used for systemic acidosis, doses should be adjusted on basis of blood gas measurements or assessment of acidosis. Doses vary depending on underlying condition (see dosage section). Note: 8.5% solution = 1 mEq/mL of NaHCO₃.	325, 520, 650 mg tablets; injection of various strengths (4.2% to 8.4%), and 1 mEq/mL	Acidosis: 0.5–1 mEq/kg IV. Renal failure: 10 mg/kg q8–12h PO. Alkalization of urine: 50 mg/kg q8–12h PO (1 tsp is approximately 2 g).

Drug Name (Trade or Other Names)	Pharmacology and Indications	Adverse Effects and Precautions	Dosing Information and Comments	Formulations	Dosage
Sodium chloride 0.9% (generic)	Sodium chloride is used for IV infusion as replacement fluid.	Not a balanced electrolyte solution. Long-term infusion may cause electrolyte imbalace.	Rate of infusion varies depending on patient needs.	500, 1000 mL infusion	40–50 mL/kg/day IV, SC, IP
Sodium chloride 7.5% (generic)	Concentrated sodium chloride used for acute treatment of hypovolemia	Not a balanced electrolyte solution. Long-term infusion may cause electrolyte imbalace.	Hypertonic saline is used for short-term infusion for rapid replacement of vascular volume.	Infusion	2–8 mL/kg IV
Sodium iodide 20% (Iodopen, generic)	Used to treat iodine deficiency	Overuse causes iodism (burning of mouth, gastric irritation, skin lesions).		100 mcg elemental iodide (118 mcg sodium iodide) per mL injection	20–40 mg/kg q8–12h PO
Sodium thiomalate	See Gold sodium thiomalate.				
Somatrem, somatropin	See Growth hormone.				
Sotalol (Betapace)	Nonspecific β- (β₁ and β₂) adrenergic blocker (class II antiarrhythmic). Action is similar to propranolol (1/3 potency); however, its beneficial effect may be caused more by the other antiarrhythmic effects. In addition to being a class II antiarrhythmic drug, sotalol may have some class III (potassium channel–blocking) activity.	Adverse effects have not been reported for animals but are expected to be similar to propranolol. Like many antiarrhythmics, it may have some proarrhythmic activity. Negative inotropic effects may cause concern in some animals with poor contractility.	There is little reported use in veterinary medicine, but in some animals, it has been a beneficial antiarrhythmic, e.g., animals with cardiomyopathy. In people, it may be a more effective maintenance agent than other drugs for controlling arrhythmias.	80, 160, 240 mg	1–2 mg/kg q12h PO
Spironolactone (Aldactone)	Potassium-sparing diuretic. Action is to interfere with sodium reabsorption in distal renal tubule. Spironolactone competitively inhibits the action of aldosterone. Used for treating high blood pressure, and congestion caused by heart failure.	Can produce hyperkalemia in some patients. Do not use in dehydrated patients. *Drug interactions:* NSAIDs may interfere with action. Avoid supplements that are high in potassium.	Spironolactone usually is used with diuretic agent when used for CHF. Recent studies in humans show benefits in cardiac remodelling and patient survival. Spironolactone will cause slight false increase in plasma digoxin concentrations measured by some assays.	25, 50, 100 mg tablets	2–4 mg/kg q24h PO (or 1–2 mg/kg q12h PO)
Stanozolol (Winstrol-V)	Anabolic steroid. Stanozolol has been used to decrease negative nitrogen balance in animals with chronic renal failure. There are no documented differences in efficacy among the anabolic steroids. (See Nandrolone decanoate.)	See Nandrolone decanoate.	See Nandrolone decanoate.	50 mg/mL injection; 2 mg tablets	Dog: 2 mg/dog (or range of 1–4 mg/dog) q12h PO; 25–50 mg/dog/week IM Cat: 1 mg/cat q12h PO; 25 mg/cat/week IM
Succimer (Chemet)	Used in treatment of lead toxicosis. Chelates lead and other heavy metals, such as mercury and arsenic.	No known adverse effects	Doses based on studies in dogs (J Am Vet Med Assoc 208:371, 1996.)	100 mg capsules	Dog: 10 mg/kg q8h PO for 5 days,then 10 mg/kg q12h PO for 2 more weeks Cat: 10 mg/kg q8h PO for 2 weeks
Sucralfate (Carafate, [Sulcrate in Canada])	Gastric mucosa protectant. Antiulcer agent. Action of sucralfate is to bind to ulcerated tissue in GI tract to aid healing of ulcers. There is some evidence that sucralfate may act as a cytoprotectant (via prostaglandin synthesis). Used to treat or prevent ulcers.	Adverse effects have not been reported. Not absorbed systemically. *Drug interactions:* Sucralfate may decrease absorption of other orally administered drugs (e.g., fluoroquinolones and tetracyclines) via chelation with aluminum.	Dosing recommendations are based largely on empiricism. There have not been clinical trials of efficacy in animals. Sucralfate may be administered concurrently with histamine type-2 inhibitors (e.g., cimetidine).	1 g tablets; 200 mg/mL oral suspension	Dog: 0.5–1 g q8–12h PO Cat: 0.25 g q8–12h PO

Drug Name (Trade or Other Names)	Pharmacology and Indications	Adverse Effects and Precautions	Dosing Information and Comments	Formulations	Dosage
Sufentanil citrate (Sufenta)	Opiod agonist. Action of fentanyl derivatives is via μ-receptor. See Fentanyl citrate, Morphine. Sufentanil is 5–7× more potent than fentanyl. 13–20 mcg of sufentanil produces analgesia equal to 10 mg of morphine.	Adverse effects similar to other opiates (see Morphine)	When used for anesthesia, often animals are premedicated with acepromazine or benzodiazepine.	50 mcg/mL injection	2 mcg/kg IV, up to a maximum dose of 5 mcg/kg
Sulfadiazine (generic, combined with trimethoprim in Tribrissen)	Sulfonamides compete with PABA for enzyme that synthesizes dihydrofolic acid in bacteria. Synergistic with trimethoprim. Broad spectrum of activity, including some protozoa. Bacteriostatic.	Adverse effects associated with sulfonamides include allergic reactions, type II and III hypersensitivity, hypothyroidism (with prolonged therapy), keratoconjunctivitis sicca, and skin reactions.	Usually, sulfonamides are combined with trimethoprim or ormetoprim in 5:1 ratio. There is no clinical evidence that one sulfonamide is more or less toxic or efficacious than another.	500 mg tablets	100 mg/kg IV, PO (loading dose), followed by 50 mg/kg q12h IV, PO (see also Trimethoprim + sulfadiazine).
Sulfadimethoxine (Albon, Bactrovet, and generic)	See Sulfadiazine.	See Sulfadiazine.	See Sulfadiazine. Sulfadimethoxine is combined with ormetoprim in Primor.	125, 250, 500 mg tablets; 400 mg/mL injection; 50 mg/mL suspension	55 mg/kg PO (loading dose), followed by 27.5 mg/kg q12h PO
Sulfamethazine (many brands [e.g., Sulmet])	See Sulfadiazine.	See Sulfadiazine.	See Sulfadiazine.	30 g bolus	100 mg/kg PO (loading dose), followed by 50 mg/kg q12h PO
Sulfamethoxazole (Gantanol)	See Sulfadiazine.	See Sulfadiazine.	See Sulfadiazine.	500 mg tablets	100 mg/kg PO (loading dose), followed by 50 mg/kg q12h PO
Sulfasalazine (sulfapyridine + mesalamine) (Azulfidine [Salazopyrin in Canada])	Sulfonamide + anti-inflammatory drug. Used for treatment of colitis. Sulfonamide has little effect, salicylic acid (mesalamine) has anti-inflammatory effects (see Mesalamine).	Adverse effects are all attributed to sulfonamide component. (See Sulfadiazine.) Keratoconjunctivitis sicca has been reported.	Usually used for treatment of idiopathic colitis, often in combination with dietary therapy.	500 mg tablets	Dog: 10–30 mg/kg q8–12h PO (see also Mesalamine, Olsalazine) Cat: 20 mg/kg q12h PO
Sulfisoxazole (Gantrisin)	See Sulfadiazine. Sulfisoxizole is primarily used only for treating urinary tract infections.	See Sulfadiazine.	See Sulfadiazine.	500 mg tablets; 500 mg/5 mL syrup	50 mg/kg q8h PO (urinary tract infections)
Tamoxifen (Nolvadex)	Nonsteroid estrogen receptor blocker. Also has weak estrogenic effects. Tamoxifen may also increase release of gonadotropin-releasing hormone (Gn-RH). Used as adjunctive treatment for certain tumors	Adverse effects have not been thoroughly documented in animals. However, in people, tamoxifen causing increased tumor pain has been reported. Do not use in pregnant animals. *Drug interactions:* Reacts with antiulcer drugs	Consult specific anti-cancer protocols for doses and regimens.	10 mg tablets (tamoxifen citrate)	Veterinary dose not established. Human dose is 10 mg q12h PO.
Taurine (generic)	Nutritional supplement for cats. Used in prevention and treatment of ocular and cardiac disease (cardiomyopathy) caused by taurine deficiency	Adverse effects have not been reported.	Routine supplementation with taurine may not be necessary in cats that are receiving a balanced diet.	Available in powder	Dog: 500 mg q12h PO Cat: 250 mg/cat q12h PO
Telazol	See Tiletamine + zolazepam.				
Tepoxalin oral lyophilisate (Zubrin)	Analgesic drug and NSAID. Used to treat pain and inflammation in dogs, particularly osteoarthritis. Tepoxalin has lipoxygenase-inhibiting effects (decreases leukotrienes), and the active metabolite has cyclooxygenase-inhibiting effects (decreases prostaglandins), which is longer acting.	Most common adverse effects from the clinical trials have been GI-related (nausea, vomiting, diarrhea)	When switching animals from another NSAID or corticosteroid to tepoxalin, allow 7-day washout. Long-term safely of tepoxalin has not been established in cats; therefore, avoid use in cats.	50, 100, and 200 mg tablets (Zydis freeze-dried tablet)	Dog: 10–20 mg/kg PO initially, 10 mg/kg q24h PO thereafter Cat: safe dose not established

Drug Name (Trade or Other Names)	Pharmacology and Indications	Adverse Effects and Precautions	Dosing Information and Comments	Formulations	Dosage
Terbutaline (Brethine, Bricanyl)	β-adrenergic agonist. β₂-specific. Used primarily for bronchodilation. See Albuterol for further details.	Adverse effects related to excessive β-adrenergic stimulation. See Albuterol for list of adverse effects.	Used primarily for bronchodilation. May be administered orally, IM, or SC. Terbutaline (and other β₂-agonists) have also been used in people to delay labor (dose in people is 2.5 mg q6h PO).	2.5, 5 mg tablets; 1 mg/mL injection (equivalent to 0.82 mg/mL)	Dog: 1.25–5 mg/dog q8h PO or 3–5 mcg/kg SC Cat: 0.1–0.2 mg/kg q12h SC or 0.625 mg/cat (1/4 of 2.5 mg tablet) q12h PO
Testosterone cypionate ester (Andro-Cyp, Andronate, Depo-Testosterone, and other forms)	Testosterone ester. Similar effects as methyltestosterone. Testosterone esters are administered IM to avoid first-pass effects. Esters in oil are absorbed more slowly from IM injection. Esters are then hydrolyzed to free testosterone.	See Methyltestosterone.	See Methyltestosterone.	100, 200 mg/mL injection	1–2 mg/kg every 2–4 weeks IM (see also Methyltestosterone)
Testosterone propionate ester (Testex, [Malogen in Canada])	Testosterone ester for injection. Similar effects as methyltestosterone. Testosterone esters are administered IM to avoid first-pass effects. Esters in oil are absorbed more slowly from IM injection. Esters are then hydrolyzed to free testosterone.	See Methyltestosterone.	See Methyltestosterone.	100 mg/mL injection	0.5–1 mg/kg 2–3 times/week IM
Tetracycline (Panmycin)	Tetracycline antibiotic. Mechanism of action of tetracyclines is to bind to 30S ribosomal subunit and inhibit protein synthesis. Usually bacteriostatic. Broad spectrum of activity, including bacteria, some protozoa, *Rickettsia*, *Ehrlichia*.	Tetracyclines in general may cause renal tubular necrosis at high doses. Tetracyclines can affect bone and teeth formation in young animals. Tetracyclines have been implicated in drug fever in cats. Hepatotoxicity may occur at high doses in susceptible individuals. *Drug interactions:* Tetracyclines bind to calcium-containing compounds, which decreases oral absorption.	Pharmacokinetic and experimental studies have been conducted in small animals, but no clinical studies. Do not use outdated solutions.	250, 500 mg capsules; 100 mg/mL suspension	15–20 mg/kg q8h PO; or 4.4–11 mg/kg q8h IV, IM
Thenium closylate (Canopar)	Antiparasitic drug. Used to treat hookworms (*Ancylostoma* and *Uncinaria*).	Tablet is bitter if coating is broken. May cause occasional vomiting after oral administration.	Doses listed are based on recommendations from manufacturer.	500 mg tablets	Dogs >4.5 kg: 500 mg PO once, repeat in 2–3 weeks; 2.5–4.5 kg: 250 mg q12h for 1 day, repeat in 2–3 weeks
Theophylline (many brands and generic)	Methylxanthine bronchodilator. Mechanism of action is unknown, but may be related to increased cAMP or antagonism of adenosine. There appears to be anti-inflammatory action as well as bronchodilating action.	Adverse effects: nausea, vomiting, diarrhea. With high doses, tachycardia, excitement, tremors, and seizures are possible. Cardiovascular and CNS adverse effects appear to be less frequent in dogs than in people.	Plasma concentrations of theophylline should be monitored in patients receiving chronic therapy to maintain plasma concentrations between 10 and 20 mcg/mL. Doses for slow-release tablets are unique for each product (see Theophylline, sustained-release and Aminophylline).	100, 125, 200, 250, 300 mg tablets; 27 mg/5 mL oral solution or elixir; injection in 5% dextrose	Dog: 9 mg/kg q6–8h PO Cat: 4 mg/kg q8–12h PO (see also Aminophylline)

Drug Name (Trade or Other Names)	Pharmacology and Indications	Adverse Effects and Precautions	Dosing Information and Comments	Formulations	Dosage
Theophylline sustained-release capsules and tablets (Inwood Laboratories)	Same as for theophylline. Sustained-release preparations are used to decrease frequency of administration.	Same as for theophylline	Same as for theophylline. Doses listed in this section apply only to theopylline extended release products manufactured by Inwood Laboratories. Other manufacturers formulation may not have the same release.	200 and 300 mg tablets 125 and 200 mg capsules	Dog: 10 mg/kg q12h PO Cat: Dose not established
Thiabendazole (Omnizole, Equizole)	Benzimidazole anthelmintic. (See Fenbendazole, Albendazole).	Adverse effects uncommon	Ordinarily administered to horses and cattle. Experience in small animals is limited.	2 or 4 g per oz (30 mL) suspension or liquid	Dog: 50 mg/kg q24h for 3 days, repeat in 1 month; for respiratory parasites, 30–70 mg/kg q12h PO Cat: for *Strongyloides*, 125 mg/kg q24h for 3 days
Thiamine (vitamin B$_1$) (Bewon and others)	Vitamin B$_1$ used for treatment of vitamin deficiency	Adverse effects are rare because water-soluble vitamins are easily excreted. Riboflavin may discolor the urine.	Vitamin B supplements are administered often in combination.	250 mcg/5 mL elixir; tablets of various size from 5 mg to 500 mg; 100 and 500 mg/mL injection	Dog: 10–100 mg/dog q24h PO Cat: 5–30 mg/cat q24h PO (up to a maximum dose of 50 mg/cat q24h)
Thiamylal sodium (Surital, Bio-Tal)	No longer available in U.S. Use has been replaced by thiopental.				
Thioguanine (6-TG) (generic)	Anticancer agent. Antimetabolite of purine analog type. Inhibits DNA synthesis in cancer cells.	Adverse effects, as with any anticancer drugs, are expected (see 6-Mercaptopurine). Immunosuppression and leukopenia are common.	Thioguanine is often combined with other agents for treatment of cancer. Consult specific reference on cancer therapy for guidance.	40 mg tablets	Dog: 40 mg/m^2 q24h PO Cat: 25 mg/m^2 PO q24h × 1–5 days, then repeat every 30 days
Thiomalate sodium	See Gold sodium thiomalate.				
Thiopental sodium (Pentothal)	Ultra-short-acting barbiturate. Used primarily for induction of anesthesia or for short duration of anesthesia (10–15 min procedures). Anesthesia is produced by CNS depression, without analgesia. Anesthesia is terminated by redistribution in the body.	Adverse effects are related to the anesthetic effects of the drug. Severe adverse effects are caused by respiratory and cardiovascular depression. Overdoses are caused by rapid or repeated injections. Avoid extravasation outside of vein.	Therapeutic index is low. Use only in patients in which it is possible to monitor cardiovascular and respiratory functions. Often administered with other anesthetic adjuncts.	Various size vials from 250 mg to 10 g (mix to desired concentration)	Dog: 10–25 mg/kg IV (to effect) Cat: 5–10 mg/kg IV (to effect)
Thiotepa (generic)	Anticancer agent. Alkylating agent of the nitrogen mustard type (similar to cyclophosphamide). Used for various tumors, especially malignant effusions.	Adverse effects are similar to other anticancer agents and alkylating drugs (many of which are unavoidable). Bone marrow suppression is the most common effect.	One should consult specific cancer chemotherapy protocol for guidance on administration. Thiotepa usually is administered directly into body cavities.	15 mg injection (usually in solution of 10 mg/mL)	0.2–0.5 mg/m^2 weekly, or daily for 5–10 days IM, intracavitary, or intratumor
Thyroid hormone	See Levothyroxine sodium and Liothyronine.				
Thyroid-releasing hormone (TRH)	Used to detect hyperthyroidism when T$_4$ is not elevated		Used for diagnostic purposes	Injection	Collect baseline T$_4$, followed by 0.1 mg/kg IV. Collect post-TRH T$_4$ sample at 4 hrs.
Thyrotropin, thyroid-stimulating hormone (TSH) (Thytropar)	Thyroid-stimulating hormone is used for diagnostic testing. Stimulates normal secretion of thyroid hormone.	Adverse reactions rare. In people, allergic reactions have occurred.	To prepare solution, add 2 mL NaCl to 10 U vial. Reconstituted solutions retain potency for 2 weeks at 2°–8°C. Consult testing laboratory for specific guidelines for thyroid testing.	10 U vial	Dog: Collect baseline sample, followed by 0.1 U/kg UIV (maximum dose is 5 U); collect post-TSH sample at 6 hrs.

Drug Name (Trade or Other Names)	Pharmacology and Indications	Adverse Effects and Precautions	Dosing Information and Comments	Formulations	Dosage
Ticarcillin (Ticar, Ticillin)	β-lactam antibiotic. Action similar to ampicillin/amoxicillin. Spectrum similar to carbenicillin. Ticarcillin is primarily used for gram-negative infections, especially those caused by *Pseudomonas*.	Adverse effects are uncommon. However, allergic reactions are possible. High doses can produce seizures and decreased platelet function. *Drug interactions*: Do not combine in same syringe or in vial with aminoglycosides.	Ticarcillin is synergistic and often combined with aminoglycosides (e.g., amikacin, gentamicin). 1% lidocaine may be used for reconstitution to decrease pain from IM injection.	6 g/50 mL vial; vials containing 1, 3, 6, 20, and 30 g	33–50 mg/kg q4–6h IV, IM
Ticarcillin + clavulanate (Timentin)	Same as ticarcillin, except clavulanic acid has been added to inhibit bacterial β-lactamase and increase spectrum. Clavulanate does not increase activity against *Pseudomonas*, however.	Same as for ticarcillin	Same as for ticarcillin	3 g per vial for injection	Dose according to rate for ticarcillin
Tiletamine + zolazepam (Telazol, Zoletil)	Anesthetic. Combination of tiletamine (dissociative anesthetic agent similar in action to ketamine) and zolazepam (benzodiazepine similar in action to diazepam). Produces short duration (30 min) of anesthesia.	Wide margin of safety. Side effects include excessive salivation (may be antagonized with atropine), erratic recovery, and muscle twitching.	Administer by deep IM injection. (Consult manufacturer's package insert for dosing information for dogs and cats.)	50 mg of each component per mL	Dog (minor procedures): 6.6–10 mg/kg IM (short-term anesthesia) 10–13 mg/kg IM Cat (minor procedures): 10–12 mg/kg IM (surgery) 14–16 mg/kg IM
Tobramycin (Nebcin)	Aminoglycoside antibacterial drug. Similar mechanism of action and spectrum as amikacin, gentamicin.	Adverse effects similar to those of amikacin, gentamicin.	Dosing requirements vary depending on bacterial susceptibility. See dose schedules for gentamicin and amikacin.	40 mg/mL injection	Dog: 2–4 mg/kg q8h IV, IM, SC or 9–14 mg/kg q24h IV, IM, SC Cat: 3 mg/kg q8h IV, IM, SC or 5–8 mg/kg q24h, IV, IM, SC
Tocanide (Tonocard)	Antiarrhythmic drug. Considered an oral analogue of lidocaine. Class I antiarrhythmic.	In dogs, anorexia and GI toxicity have been reported. Arrhythmias, vomiting, ataxia also are possible. (In one study, 35% of dogs showed GI effects.)	Limited experience in animals. However, clinical studies demonstrate efficacy. Therapeutic concentrations are 6–10 mcg/mL.	400, 600 mg tablets	Dog: 15–20 mg/kg q8h PO Cat: no dose established
Trandolapril (Mavik)	ACE inhibitor. Similar in mechanism to captopril and enalapril. Used for management of CHF. Converted to active trandolaprilat after administration.	Same adverse effects as for other ACE inhibitors	Not used extensively in veterinary patients	1, 2, 4 mg tablets	Not established for dogs. Dose in people is 1 mg/person/day to start, then increase to 2–4 mg/day.
Triamcinolone (Vetalog, Triamtabs, Aristocort, generic)	Glucocorticoid anti-inflammatory drug. See Betamethasone for details. Triamcinolone has potency that is approximately equal to methylprednisolone (about 5× cortisol and 1.25× prednisolone), although some dermatologists suggest that potency is higher.	Adverse effects are similar to other corticosteroids (see Betamethasone).	See Prednisolone. Note that cats may require higher doses than dogs (sometimes 2×).	Veterinary (Vetalog) 0.5 and 1.5 mg tablets. Human form: 1, 2, 4, 8, 16 mg tablets; 10 mg/mL injection.	Anti-inflammatory: 0.5–1 mg/kg q12–24h PO, then taper dose to 0.5–1 mg/kg q48h PO. (However, manufacturer recommends doses of 0.11 to 0.22 mg/kg/day.)
Triamcinolone acetonide (Vetalog)	Same as for triamcinolone, except that injectable suspension is slowly absorbed from IM or intralesional injection site. Used for intralesional therapy of tumors and similar purposes as methyl-prednisolone acetate.	See Methylprednisolone acetate. When used for ocular injections, there is some concern that granulomas may occur at injection site.	See Prednisolone.	2 or 6 mg/mL suspension injection; 0.5 and 1.5 mg tablets	0.1–0.2 mg/kg IM, SC, repeat in 7–10 days. Intralesional: 1.2–1.8 mg, or 1 mg for every cm diameter of tumor every 2 weeks

Drug Name (Trade or Other Names)	Pharmacology and Indications	Adverse Effects and Precautions	Dosing Information and Comments	Formulations	Dosage
Triamterene (Dyrenium)	Potassium-sparing diuretic. Similar action as spironolactone, except that spirono-lactone has competitive inhibiting effect of al-dosterone; triamterene does not.	See Spironolactone.	Little clinical experi-ence available for triamterene. There is no convincing evidence that triamterene is more effective than spironolactone.	50, 100 mg capsules	1–2 mg/kg q12h PO
Tribrissen	See Trimethoprim + sulfadiazine.				
Trientine hydrochloride (Syprine)	Chelating agent. Used to chelate copper when penicillamine cannot be tolerated in a patient.	Adverse effects have not been reported in animals.	Used only in patients that cannot tolerate penicillamine. Gener-ally induces less cupruresis than penicillamine.	250 mg capsules	10–15 mg/kg q12h PO
Trifluoperazine (Stelazine)	Phenothiazine. Used for treatment of anxiety, to produce sedation, antiemetic. Action is believed to be via an-tagonism of dopamine (similar to aceproma-zine); antiemetic action may be via antimus-carinic action.	Adverse effects not reported in animals, but are expected to be similar to other phenothiazines. See Acepromazine, Prochlorperazine + isopropamide.	Results of clinical stud-ies in animals have not been reported. Use in animals (and doses) is based on experience in people or anecdotal experience in animals.	10 mg/mL oral solution; 1, 2, 5, 10 mg tablets; 2 mg/mL injection	0.03 mg/kg IM q12h
Triflupromazine (Vesprin)	Phenothiazine. Similar action as other pheno-thiazines, except tri-flupromazine may have stronger antimuscarinic activity than other phenothiazines. Used for antiemetic action.	Adverse effects have not been reported in animals. Adverse effects possible include anticholinergic effects.	Same as for other phenothiazines.	10, 20 mg/mL injection	0.1–0.3 mg/kg IM, PO q8–12h
Triiodothyronine	See Liothyronine.				
Trilostane (Vetoryl)	Used for treatment of hypercortisolemia (Cushing's syndrome) in dogs. 3-β-hydroxysteroid dehydrogenase inhibitor, in dogs, for treatment of pituitary-dependent hyperadrenocorticism (PDH).	In one study, adverse effects consisted of 1 dog with transient lethargy and 1 dog with anorexia. Otherwise, it has been well tolerated. One should check elec-trolyte levels in treated patients because trilostane decreases aldosterone.	Trilostane is an effica-cious and safe medica-tion for treatment of dogs with PDH. It is reg-istered in Europe for treatment of PDH but is not commercially avail-able at this time in the U.S. It has been im-ported by veterinarians after obtaining permis-sion from the Food and Drug Administration. Dose should be adjusted in individual patients based on cor-tisol measurements.	60 mg capsules	Dog: median dose is 6.1 mg/kg/day but range is 3.9–9.2 mg/kg/day PO, which is adjusted based on cortisol measurements. General dose is 30 mg q24h PO for dogs that weigh <5 kg and 60 mg q24h PO for dogs that weigh ≥ 5 kg.
Trimeprazine tartrate (Temaril [Panectyl in Canada])	Phenothiazine with antihistamine activity (similar to prometha-zine). Used for treating allergies and motion sickness.	Adverse effects similar to those of prometh-azine.	There is evidence that trimeprazine is more effective when com-bined with prednisone for treatment of pruritus. Combination product is Temaril-P.	2.5 mg/5 mL syrup; 2.5 mg tablet	0.5 mg/kg q12h PO
Trimethobenzamide (Tigan, and others)	Antiemetic. Mechanism of action is not under-stood.	Adverse effects not reported in animals.	Efficacy as antiemetic not reported in animals.	100 mg/mL injection; 100, 250 mg capsules	Dog: 3 mg/kg q8h IM PO Cat: not recommended
Trimethoprim + sulfadiazine (Tribrissen, Tucoprim, and others)	Combines the anti-bacterial drug action of trimethoprim and a sulfonamide. Together, the combination is synergistic, with a broad spectrum of activity.	Adverse effects primar-ily caused by sulfona-mide component. (See Sulfadiazine.)	Dosage recommenda-tions vary. There is evidence that 30 mg/kg/day is efficacious for pyoderma; for other infections, 30 mg/kg twice daily has been recommended.	30, 120, 240, 480, 960 mg tablet (all formula-tions have ratio of 5:1 sulfa:trimethoprim)	15 mg/kg q12h PO, or 30 mg/kg q12–24h PO (for *Toxoplasma*: 30 mg/kg q12h PO)

Drug Name (Trade or Other Names)	Pharmacology and Indications	Adverse Effects and Precautions	Dosing Information and Comments	Formulations	Dosage
Trimethoprim + sulfamethoxazole (Bactrim, Septra, and generic forms)	Combines the antibacterial drug action of trimethoprim and a sulfonamide. Together, the combination is synergistic, with a broad spectrum of activity.	Adverse effects primarily caused by sulfonamide component. (See Sulfadiazine.)	Dosage recommendations vary. There is evidence that 30 mg/kg/day is efficacious for pyoderma; for other infections, 30 mg/kg twice daily has been recommended.	480, 960 mg tablet; 240 mg/5 mL oral suspension (all formulations have ratio of 5:1 sulfa:trimethoprim)	15 mg/kg q12h PO, or 30 mg/kg q12–24h PO
Tripelennamine (Pelamine, PBZ)	Histamine (H_1) blocker. Similar in action as other antihistamines (see Chlorpheniramine maleate). Used to treat allergic disease	Adverse effects similar to other antihistamines. See Chlorpheniramine maleate. Members of this class (ethanolamines) have greater antimuscarinic effects than other antihistamines.	There are no clinical reports of use in veterinary medicine. No evidence that it is more efficacious than other drugs in this class.	25, 50 mg tablets; 20 mg/mL injection	1 mg/kg q12h PO
TSH (thyroid-stimulating hormone)	See Thyrotropin.				
Tylosin (Tylocine, Tylan, Tylosin tartrate)	Macrolide antibiotic. (See Erythromycin for mechanisms of action and spectrum of activity.)	May cause diarrhea in some animals. Do not administer orally to rodents or rabbits.	Tylosin is rarely used in small animals. Powdered formulation (tylosin tartrate) has been administered on food for control of signs of colitis in dogs. Tablets are approved in Canada for treatment of colitis.	Available as soluble powder 2.2 g tylosin per tsp (tablets for dogs in Canada)	Dog and cat: 7–15 mg/kg q12–24h PO Dog (for colitis): 10–20 mg/kg q8h with food; if there is a response, increase the interval to q12–24h
Urofollitropin (FSH) (Metrodin)	Stimulates ovulation. Contains FSH. In people, it is used in combination with HCG to stimulate ovulation and induce pregnancy.	Side effects have not been reported in animals. In people, thromboembolism or severe ovarian hyperstimulation syndrome has been reported.	Results of clinical studies in animals have not been reported. Use in animals is based on experience in people.	75 U per vial for injection	Doses not established
Ursodiol (ursodeoxycholate) (Actigall)	Hydrophilic bile acid. Anticholelithic. Used for treatment of liver diseases. Increases bile flow. In dogs, may alter pool of circulating bile acids, displacing the more hydrophobic bile acids. In people, it is used to prevent or treat gallstones.	Adverse effects not reported in animals. May cause diarrhea.	Results of clinical studies in animals have not been reported. Use in animals (and doses) is based on experience in people or anecdotal experience in animals. Administer with meals.	300 mg capsules	10–15 mg/kg q24h PO
Valproic acid (Depakene [valproic acid]; Depakote [divalproex] [Epival is Canadian brand])	Anticonvulsant. Used, usually in combination with phenobarbital, to treat refractory epilepsy in animals. Action is not known, but it may increase GABA concentrations in the CNS.	Adverse effects have not been reported in animals, but hepatic failure has been reported in people. Sedation may be seen in some animals. Do not use in pregnant animals. Drug interactions: May cause bleeding if used with drugs that inhibit platelets.	Valproic acid is listed here with divalproex. Divalproex is composed of both valproic acid and sodium valproate. Equivalent oral doses of divalproex sodium and valproic acid deliver equivalent quantities of valproate ion.	125, 250, 500 mg tablets (Depakote); 250 mg capsules; 50 mg/mL syrup (Depakene)	Dog: 60–200 mg/kg q8h PO; or 25–105 mg/kg q24h PO when administered with phenobarbital

Drug Name (Trade or Other Names)	Pharmacology and Indications	Adverse Effects and Precautions	Dosing Information and Comments	Formulations	Dosage
Vancomycin (Vancocin, Vancoled)	Antibacterial drug. Mechanism of action is to inhibit cell wall and cause bacterial cell lysis (via mechanism different from that of β-lactams). Spectrum includes staphylococci, streptococci, and enterococci (but not gram-negative bacteria). Used primarily for treatment of resistant staphylococci and enterococci.	Adverse effects have not been reported in animals. Administer IV; causes severe pain and tissue injury if administered IM or SC. Do not administer rapidly; use slow infusion, if possible (e.g., over 30 min). Adverse effects in people include renal injury (more common with older products that contained impurities) and histamine release.	Vancomycin use is not common in animals, but is valuable for treatment of enterococci or staphylococci that are resistant to other antibiotics. Doses are derived from pharmacokinetic studies in dogs. Monitoring of trough plasma concentrations is recommended to ensure proper dose. Maintain trough concentration above 5 mcg/mL. Infusion solution can be prepared in 0.9% saline or 5% dextrose, but not alkalinizing solutions.	Vials for injection (0.5 to 10 g)	Dog: 15 mg/kg q6–8h IV infusion Cat: 12–15 mg/kg q8h IV infusion
Vasopressin (ADH) (Pitressin)	Antidiuretic hormone. Vasopressin is used for treatment of polyuria caused by central diabetes insipidus. Not effective for polyuria caused by renal disease.	Adverse effects have not been reported. Allergic reactions have been reported in people. Increase in blood pressure has been reported in people.	Doses are adjusted on the basis of monitoring of water intake and urine output. See also Desmopressin acetate.	20 U/mL (aqueous)	10 U IV, IM
Verapamil (Calan, Isoptin)	Calcium channel blocking drug of the nondihydropyridine group. Blocks calcium entry into cells via blockade of slow channel. Produces vasodilation, negative chronotropic effects.	Hypotension, cardiac depression, bradycardia, AV block. May cause anorexia in some patients.	Diltiazem preferred over verapamil in patients with heart failure because of less cardiac suppression. Oral formulation not absorbed sufficiently (of the active stereoisomer) for adequate effects.	40, 80, 120 mg tablet; 2.5 mg/mL injection	Dog: 0.05 mg/kg every 10–30 min IV (maximum cumulative dose is 0.15 mg/kg); oral dose is not established
Vinblastine (Velban)	Similar to vincristine. Sometimes used as an alternative to vincristine. Do not use to increase platelet numbers (may actually cause thrombocytopenia).	Does not produce neuropathy as vincristine does, but there may be a higher incidence of myelosuppression. Causes tissue necrosis if injected outside vein.	Vinblastine is used in cancer chemotherapy protocols for various tumors. Consult specific chemotherapy protocol for regimens.	1 mg/mL injection	2 mg/m^2 IV (slow infusion) once/week
Vincristine (Oncovin, Vincasar, generic)	Anticancer agent. Vincristine causes arrest of cancer cell division by binding to microtubules and inhibiting mitosis. Used in combination chemotherapy protocols. Vincristine also increases numbers of functional circulating platelets and is used for thrombocytopenia.	Generally well tolerated. Less myelosuppressive than other anticancer drugs. Neuropathy has been reported but is rare. Constipation can occur. Very irritating to tissues. Avoid extravasation outside vein during administration.	Vincristine is used in cancer chemotherapy protocols for various tumors. Consult specific chemotherapy protocol for regimens.	1 mg/mL injection	Antitumor: 0.5–0.7 mg/m^2 IV (or 0.025–0.05 mg/kg) once/week For thrombocytopenia: 0.02 mg/kg IV once/week
Viokase	See Pancrelipase.				
Vitamin A (retinoids) (Aquasol A)	Vitamin A supplement. See also Isotretinoin for analogues used for other conditions.	Excessive doses can cause bone or joint pain, dermatitis.	Dosing of vitamin is expressed as U or retinol equivalents (RE), or mcg of retinol. 1 RE = 1 mcg of retinol. 1 RE of vitamin A = 3.33 U of retinol.	Oral solution: 5000 U (1500 RE)/0.1 mL; 10,000, 25,000 and 50,000 U tablets	625–800 U/kg q24h PO (see dosing information section)
Vitamin B$_1$	See Thiamine.				
Vitamin B$_2$ (riboflavin)	Vitamin B$_2$ supplement	Adverse effects are rare because water-soluble vitamins are easily excreted. Riboflavin may discolor the urine.	Not necessary to supplement in animals with well-balanced diets	Various size tablets in increments from 10–250 mg	Dog: 10–20 mg/day PO Cat: 5–10 mg/day PO

Drug Name (Trade or Other Names)	Pharmacology and Indications	Adverse Effects and Precautions	Dosing Information and Comments	Formulations	Dosage
Vitamin B₁₂ (cyanocobalamin)	Vitamin B₁₂ supplement. Vitamin B₁₂ has been used to treat some forms of anemia.	Adverse effects are rare because water-soluble vitamins are easily excreted.	Not necessary to supplement in animals with well-balanced diets	Various size tablets in increments from 25–1000 mcg, and injection	Dog: 100–200 mcg/day PO, SC Cat: 50–100 mcg/day PO, SC
Vitamin C (ascorbic acid) (see Ascorbic acid)	Used to treat vitamin C deficiency and occasionally used as urine acidifier. Insufficient data to show that ascorbic acid is effective for preventing cancer or cardiovascular disease.	Adverse effects have not been reported in animals. High doses may increase risk of oxalate stones in bladder.	Not necessary to supplement in animals with well-balanced diets	Tablets of various sizes, and injection	100–500 mg/day
Vitamin D	See Dihydrotachysterol or Ergocalciferol.				
Vitamin E (alpha tocopherol) (Aquasol E and generic)	Vitamin considered as antioxidant. Used as supplement and as treatment of some immune-mediated dermatoses.	Side effects have not been reported.	Vitamin E has been proposed as treatment for a wide range of human illnesses, but evidence for efficacy in animals is lacking.	Wide variety of capsules, tablets, oral solution available (e.g., 1000 U/capsule)	100–400 U q12h PO (or 400–600 U q12h PO for immune-mediated skin disease)
Vitamin K₁ (phytonadione, phytomenadione) (AquaMEPHYTON [injection], Mephyton [tablets]; Veta-K1 [capsules])	Vitamin K₁ used to treat coagulopathies caused by anticoagulant toxicosis (warfarin or other rodenticides). (Anticoagulants deplete vitamin K in the body, which is essential for synthesis of clotting factors.)	Side effects have not been reported.	Consult poison control center for specific protocol if specific rodenticide is identified. Use vitamin K₁ for acute therapy because it is more highly bioavailable. Administer with food to enhance absorption. Phytonadione and phytomenadione are synthetic lipid-soluble forms of vitamin K₁. Menadiol is vitamin K₄, which is converted in the body to vitamin K₃ (menadione).	2 or 10 mg/mL injection; Mephyton is 5 mg tablet; Veta-K1 is 25 mg capsule.	Short-acting rodenticides: 1 mg/kg/day IV, IM, SC, PO for 10–14 days Long-acting rodenticides: 2.5–5 mg/kg/day IV, IM, SC, PO for 3–4 weeks.
Warfarin (Coumadin, generic)	Anticoagulant. Depletes vitamin K, which is responsible for generation of clotting factors. Used to treat hypercoagulable disease, prevent thromboembolism.	Adverse effects are attributable to decreased clotting. Drug interactions: Other drugs may potentiate warfarin's action (including aspirin, chloramphenicol, phenylbutazone, ketoconazole, cimetidine)	Warfarin response is individualistic. For optimum therapy, adjust dose by monitoring clotting time. For example, in some patients, dose is adjusted to maintain prothrombin time at 1.5–2 × to 2–2.5 × normal (or INR of 2–3). Consult specific reference for guidance (Current Veterinary Therapy XII, page 868).	1, 2, 2.5, 4, 5, 7.5, 10 mg tablets	Dog: 0.1–0.2 mg/kg q24h PO Cat (thromboembolism): Start with 0.5 mg/cat q24h PO and adjust dose based on clotting time assessment.
Xylaxine (Rompun, and generic)	α₂-adrenergic agonist. Used primarily for anesthesia and analgesia.	Produces sedation and ataxia. Cardiac depression, heart block, and hypotension are possible with high doses. Produces emesis after IV injection, especially in cats.	Often used in combination with other drugs, e.g., ketamine	20 and 100 mg/mL injection	Dog: 1.1 mg/kg IV; 2.2 mg/kg IM Cat: 1.1 mg/kg IM (emetic [cats only] dose is 0.4–0.5 mg/kg IV)
Yohimbine (Yobine)	α₂-adrenergic antagonist. Used primarily to reverse actions of xylazine or detomidine.	High doses can cause tremors and seizures.	Reverses signs of sedation and anesthesia caused by α₂-agonists	2 mg/mL injection	0.11 mg/kg IV, or 0.25–0.5 mg/kg SC, IM

Drug Name (Trade or Other Names)	Pharmacology and Indications	Adverse Effects and Precautions	Dosing Information and Comments	Formulations	Dosage
Zidovudine (AZT) (Retrovir)	Antiviral drug. In people, used to treat AIDS. In animals, has been experimentally used for treatment of feline leukemia virus (FeLV) and feline immunodeficiency virus (FIV) viral infection in cats. AZT acts to inhibit the viral enzyme, reverse transcriptase, which prevents conversion of viral RNA into DNA.	Anemia and leukopenia are adverse effects. Monitor the packed cell volume in treated cats, and perform a complete blood count periodically.	At this time, experience with using AZT for treating viral disease in animals is largely experimental or anecdotal. Consult a more-detailed reference for guidance (Feline Pract 23:16, 1995). It may have helped some cats with FIV and may prevent persistent FeLV.	10 mg/mL syrup; 10 mg/mL injection	Cat: 15 mg/kg q12h PO to 20 mg/kg q8h PO (doses as high as 30 mg/kg/day also have been used)
Zolazepam	See Tiletamine + zolazepam.				
Zonisamide (Zonegran)	Anticonvulsant drug. Used to treat epilepsy in dogs when other drugs have not been effective. Used usually with other drugs. Mechanism of action is uncertain: may affect GABA or block calcium and sodium channels.	Structure resembles sulfonamides; therefore, one should be cognizant of sulfonamide-like reactions in dogs (e.g. keratoconjunctivitis sicca).	Doses are based on limited studies in animals. Zonisamide has been used only in selected patients that have been refractory to other anticonvulsants.	100 mg capsule in a two-piece capsule	Dog: 5–10 mg/kg q12h PO.

Key to Table Abbreviations:

ACE	angiotensin converting enzyme
CHF	congestive heart failure
CNS	central nervous system
COX	cyclooxygenase
CSF	cerebrospinal fluid
g	gram
GABA	gamma amino butyric acid
GI	gastrointestinal
IM	Intramuscular
INR	International normalization ratio
IV	Intravenous
mcg	micrograms
mg	milligram
MIC	minimum inhibitory concentration
mL	milliliter
NSAID	nonsteroidal antiinflammatory drug
OTC	Over the counter (without prescription)
PO	per os (oral)
PU/PD	polyuria and polydipsia
q	every, as in q8h = every 8 hours
Rx	Prescription only
SC	Subcutaneous
U	Units

DISCLAIMER FOR DOSE TABLES:
Note: Doses listed are for dogs *and* cats, unless otherwise listed. Many of the doses listed are extra-label, or are human drugs not approved for animals administered in an extra-label manner. Doses listed are based on best available information at the time of table editing. The author cannot ensure efficacy or absolute safety of drugs used according to recommendations in this table. Adverse effects may be possible from drugs listed in this table of which authors were not aware at the time of table preparation. Veterinarians using this table are encouraged to consult current literature, product labels and inserts, and the manufacturer's disclosure information for additional information on adverse effects, interactions, and efficacy that were not identified at the time these tables were prepared.

APPENDIX X

CONVERSION TABLES

Table X-A.

kg	m²		kg	m²
0.5	0.06		26.0	0.88
1.0	0.10		27.0	0.90
2.0	0.15		28.0	0.92
3.0	0.20		29.0	0.94
4.0	0.25		30.0	0.96
5.0	0.29		31.0	0.99
6.0	0.33		32.0	1.01
7.0	0.36		33.0	1.03
8.0	0.40		34.0	1.05
9.0	0.43		35.0	1.07
10.0	0.46		36.0	1.09
11.0	0.49		37.0	1.11
12.0	0.52		38.0	1.13
13.0	0.55		39.0	1.15
14.0	0.58		40.0	1.17
15.0	0.60		41.0	1.19
16.0	0.63		42.0	1.21
17.0	0.66		43.0	1.23
18.0	0.69		44.0	1.25
19.0	0.71		45.0	1.26
20.0	0.74		46.0	1.28
21.0	0.76		47.0	1.30
22.0	0.78		48.0	1.32
23.0	0.81		49.0	1.34
24.0	0.83		50.0	1.36
25.0	0.85			

Conversion Table of Weight to Body Surface Area (In Square Meters) for Dogs

Although the above chart was compiled for dogs, it can also be used for cats. More precise values are represented in the formula BSA in $m^2 = (K \times W^{2/3}) \times 10^{-4}$; where m^2 = square meters, BSA = body surface area, W = weight in g, and K = constant of 10.1 in dogs and 10.0 in cats.

Table X-B.

Approximate Equivalents for Degrees Fahrenheit and Celsius*			
°F	°C	°F	°C
0	−17.8	98	36.7
32	0	99	37.2
85	29.4	100	37.8
86	30.0	101	38.3
87	30.6	102	38.9
88	31.1	103	39.4
89	31.7	104	40.0
90	32.2	105	40.6
91	32.7	106	41.1
92	33.3	107	41.7
93	33.9	108	42.2
94	34.4	109	42.8
95	35.0	110	43.3
96	35.5	212	100.0
97	36.1		

*Temperature conversion: °Celsius to °Fahrenheit, (°C)(9/5) + 32°; °Fahrenheit to °Celsius, (°F − 32°)(5/9).

Table X-C.

Weight-Unit Conversion Factors		
Units Given	*Units Wanted*	*For Conversion, Multiply by*
lb	g	453.6
lb	kg	0.4536
oz	g	28.35
kg	lb	2.2046
kg	mg	1,000,000.
kg	g	1000.
g	mg	1000.
g	μg	1,000,000.
mg	μg	1000.
mg/g	mg/lb	453.6
mg/kg	mg/lb	0.4536
μg/kg	μg/lb	0.4536
Mcal	kcal	1000.
kcal/kg	kcal/lb	0.4536
kcal/lb	kcal/kg	2.2046
ppm	μg/g	1.
ppm	mg/kg	1.
ppm	mg/lb	0.4536
mg/kg	%	0.0001
ppm	%	0.0001
mg/g	%	0.1
g/kg	%	0.1

APPENDIX XI

HOTLINES EVERY VETERINARIAN SHOULD KNOW

ANIMAL BLOOD BANK HOTLINE—800-243-5759
A 24-hour hotline that focuses on transfusion medicine (particularly blood component therapy), recommending dosages and infusion rates, at no cost to caller

ANIMAL POISON HOTLINE—888-232-8870
A 24-hour hotline staffed by veterinary professionals, toxicologists, and pharmacologists for pet owners and veterinarians. Fee $35 per incident, payable by credit card; veterinarians can set up an account. No charge for follow-up calls. Sponsored by the North Shore Animal League of America in New York City and PROSAR International Animal Poison Center.

ASPCA NATIONAL ANIMAL POISON CONTROL CENTER (ALLIED AGENCY OF THE UNIVERSITY OF ILLINOIS COLLEGE OF VETERINARY MEDICINE)—888-426-4435
Fee $45 per case; credit cards only; no extra charge for follow-up calls. **900-680-0000**—Fee $45 per case. The charge is billed directly to caller's phone. Follow-up calls can be made for no additional charge by dialing **888-426-4435**. There is no charge when the call involves a product covered by the Animal Product Safety Service.

DEA TOLL-FREE NUMBER FOR OFFICE OF DIVERSION CONTROL, REGISTRATION SECTION—800-882-9539

EASTERN VETERINARY BLOOD BANK—800-949-EVBB (800-949-3822)
A 24-hour, commercial blood bank that focuses on transfusion medicine; gives recommendations and referrals to distribution centers when it cannot ship the requested product; for complicated cases, offers a paid consultation service

FDA/CVM: DRUGS, DEVICES, ANIMAL FEEDS—888-FDA-VETS (888-332-8387)
Calls to report suspected adverse drug experiences will be forwarded to the CVM's Division of Epidemiology and Surveillance; voice-mail messages can be left during nonbusiness hours.

FDA/CVM SHORTAGE COORDINATOR—301-827-6641
Calls to report shortages of medically necessary veterinary drugs

HEMOPET—714-891-2022
A national, full-service, nonprofit blood bank and educational network for animals, in Garden Grove, CA, accessible 24 hours.

IMPAIRED VETERINARIANS INFORMATION LINE—800-321-1473
Information on and referrals for assistance with chemical impairment; sponsored by the AVMA.

MIDWEST ANIMAL BLOOD SERVICES—517-851-8244
A 24-hour, commercial, all-species blood bank providing blood components, blood typing services, and transfusion medicine consultation (special emphasis on red blood cell typing and transplantation matching)

NATIONAL PESTICIDE INFORMATION CENTER—800-858-7378; *email, npic@ace.orst.edu*
Service sponsored by the EPA and Oregon State University provides information about pesticide products and poisonings, toxicology, environmental chemistry, and other pesticide-related issues

PET LOSS SUPPORT HOTLINES (GRIEF COUNSELING)
530-752-4200 or 800-565-1526—Staffed by University of California–Davis veterinary students
630-325-1600—Staffed by Chicago VMA veterinarians and staff
607-253-3932—Staffed by Cornell University veterinary students
352-392-4700; then dial 1 and 4080—Staffed by University of Florida veterinary students
217-244-2273(CARE) or 877-394-2273(CARE)—Staffed by University of Illinois veterinary students
888-ISU-PLSH (888-478-7574)—Staffed by Iowa State University veterinary students and community volunteers
517-432-2696—Staffed by Michigan State University veterinary students
614-292-1823, *e-mail, petloss@osu.edu*—Staffed by The Ohio State University veterinary students
508-839-7966—Staffed by Tufts University veterinary students
540-231-8038—Staffed by Virginia-Maryland Regional College of Veterinary Medicine students
509-335-5704—Staffed by Washington State University veterinary students

USDA VOICE RESPONSE SERVICE—800-545-8732
Up-to-date interstate shipping regulations, emergency notices, and animal care regulations for shipping pets on airlines

USP VETERINARY PRACTITIONERS' REPORTING PROGRAM—800-4-USP-PRN (800-487-7776)
Veterinarians may report any type of problem (adverse reactions, quality concerns, medication errors, etc.) encountered with the use of medical products in animals. Information is shared with manufacturers, regulatory agencies, and the AVMA. Call to make a report or request reporting forms. Reports can also be submitted electronically at *http://www.usp.org*. Reporting forms are available 24 hours a day through our on-demand faxback system. Call our toll-free number, press 1, then enter #9401.

Compiled by the Publications Division, American Veterinary Medical Association (AVMA). Phone numbers current as of January 1, 2003. Modified from J Am Vet Med Assoc 2003;222:590 (with permission).

INDEX

Text in **boldface** denotes chapter discussions.